Bailey & Love's SHORT PRACTICE of SURGERY

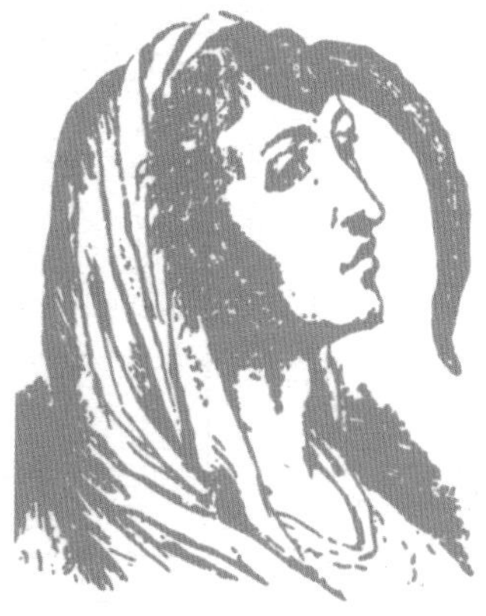

Sebaceous horn
(The owner, the widow Dimanche, sold water-cress in Paris)

A favourite illustration of Hamilton Bailey and McNeill Love, and well known to readers of earlier editions of Short Practice.

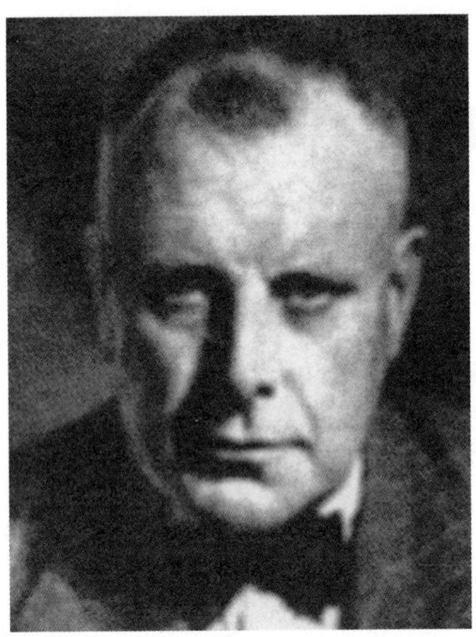

Henry Hamilton Bailey 1894–1961

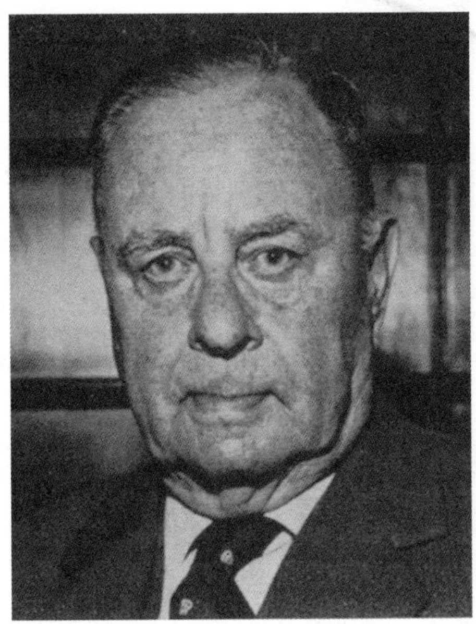

Robert J. McNeill Love 1891–1974

Skilled surgeons, inspirational teachers, dedicated authors

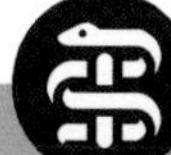

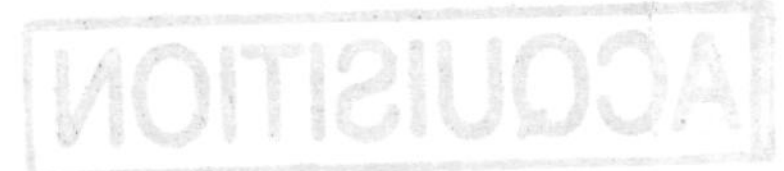

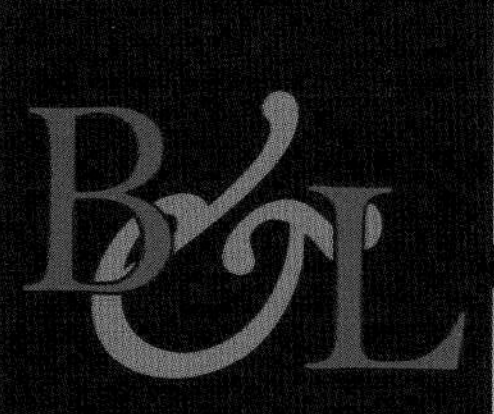

Bailey & Love's

SHORT PRACTICE of SURGERY

27th EDITION

Edited by

PROFESSOR SIR NORMAN WILLIAMS
MS FRCS FMedSci FRCP FRCP(Ed) FRCA FDS(Hon) FACS(Hon) FRCS(I)(Hon) FRCS(Ed)(Hon)
Senior Clinical Advisor to the Secretary of State for Health; Past President, The Royal College of Surgeons of England 2011–2014; Emeritus Professor of Surgery, Barts and The London School of Medicine and Dentistry, Queen Mary University of London, London, UK

PROFESSOR P. RONAN O'CONNELL
MD FRCS(I) FRCPS(Glas) FRCS(Ed)
Head of Section of Surgery and Surgical Specialties, University College Dublin, St Vincent's University Hospital, Dublin, Ireland

PROFESSOR ANDREW W. MCCASKIE
MMus MD FRCS FRCS (T&O)
Professor of Orthopaedic Surgery and Head of Department of Surgery, University of Cambridge; Honorary Consultant, Addenbrooke's Hospital, Cambridge University Hospitals NHS Foundation Trust, Cambridge, UK

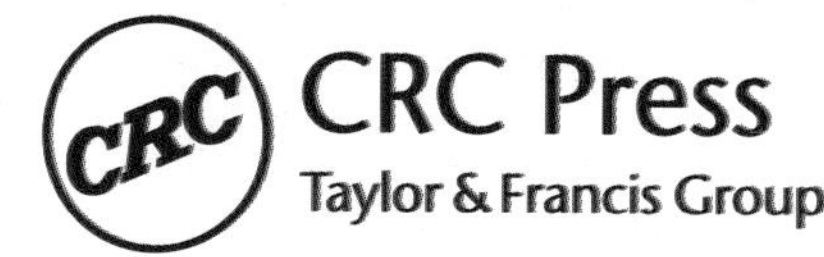

CRC Press
Taylor & Francis Group

First published in Great Britain in 1932

This 27th edition published in 2018 by
CRC Press
Taylor & Francis Group
6000 Broken Sound Parkway NW, Suite 300
Boca Raton, FL 33487-2742

Printed and bound in India by Replika Press Pvt. Ltd.

Printed on acid-free paper

International Standard Book Number-13: 978-1-4987-9650-7 (Pack – Paperback and eBook)
International Standard Book Number-13: 978-1-138-03166-1 (Pack – Hardback and eBook)
International Standard Book Number-13: 978-1-138-03164-7 (International Student Edition; restricted territorial availability)

Library of Congress Cataloging-in-Publication Data

Names: Williams, Norman S., 1947- editor. | O'Connell, P. Ronan, editor. | McCaskie, A. W., editor.
Title: Bailey & Love's short practice of surgery / [edited by] Norman Williams, P. Ronan O'Connell, Andrew McCaskie.
Other titles: Bailey and Love's short practice of surgery | Short practice of surgery.
Description: 27th edition. | Boca Raton, FL : CRC Press, 2017.
Identifiers: LCCN 2017015906 (print) | LCCN 2017018725 (ebook) | ISBN 9781315111087 (General eBook) | ISBN 9781351617994 (Adobe eBook) | ISBN 9781351617987 (ePub eBook) | ISBN 9781351617970 (Mobipocket eBook) | ISBN 9781138031661 (hardback : alk. paper) | ISBN 9781498796507 (pbk. : alk. paper) | ISBN 9781138031647 (international edition pbk. : alk. paper).
Subjects: | MESH: Surgical Procedures, Operative | Perioperative Care.
Classification: LCC RD31 (ebook) | LCC RD31 (print) | NLM WO 500 | DDC 617--dc23
LC record available at https://lccn.loc.gov/2017015906

Visit the Taylor & Francis Web site at
http://www.taylorandfrancis.com

and the CRC Press Web site at
http://www.crcpress.com

Contents

Preface viii
Contributors x
Acknowledgements xvii
Sayings of the great xx

PART 1: BASIC PRINCIPLES

1 Metabolic response to injury 2
The late Kenneth Fearon

2 Shock and blood transfusion 12
Karim Brohi

3 Wounds, healing and tissue repair 24
Michael John Earley

4 Tissue engineering and regeneration 33
Andrew W. McCaskie & John Andrew Bradley

5 Surgical infection 42
Peter Lamont

6 Tropical infections and infestations 57
Pradip K. Datta, Pawanindra Lal & Sanjay De Bakshi

7 Basic surgical skills and anastomoses 84
Mark G. Coleman

8 Principles of laparoscopic and robotic surgery 105
Hutan Ashrafian, Sanjay Purkayastha & Ara Darzi

9 Principles of paediatric surgery 119
Anthony Lander

10 Principles of oncology 139
Robert J.C. Steele & Alastair Munro

11 Surgical audit and research 161
Jonothan J. Earnshaw & Birgit Whitman

12 Surgical ethics and law 170
Robert Wheeler

13 Human factors, patient safety and quality improvement 176
Frank B.V. Keane & Ken Mealy

PART 2: INVESTIGATION AND DIAGNOSIS

14 Diagnostic imaging 190
Matthew Matson, Muaaze Ahmad & Niall Power

15 Gastrointestinal endoscopy 216
James O. Lindsay & Philip Woodland

16 Tissue and molecular diagnosis 234
Roger M. Feakins

PART 3: PERIOPERATIVE CARE

17 Preoperative care including the high-risk surgical patient 254
Medha Vanarase-Pandit, Pierre Foex & Anand Sardesai

18 Anaesthesia and pain relief 269
Vivek Mehta & Serene Hsi-Lin Chang

19 Nutrition and fluid therapy 278
John MacFie

20 Postoperative care 290
Anand Sardesai & Fay Gilder

21 Day case surgery 301
Douglas McWhinnie & Ian Jackson

PART 4: TRAUMA

22 Introduction to trauma 310
Peter Giannoudis & Bob Handley

23 Early assessment and management of severe trauma 322
Chris Moran & Dan Deakin

24 Traumatic brain injury 328
Harry J.C.J. Bulstrode & Antonio Belli

25 Neck and spine — 338
John Crawford & Douglas Hay

26 Maxillofacial trauma — 355
David A. Koppel

27 Torso trauma — 364
Ken Boffard & Elias Degiannis

28 Extremity trauma — 381
Lee Van Rensburg

29 Disaster surgery — 409
Mamoon Rashid

30 Conflict surgery — 424
Jon Clasper & Phill Pearce

PART 5: ELECTIVE ORTHOPAEDICS

31 History taking and clinical examination in musculoskeletal disease — 436
Stephen M. McDonnell & Hemant G. Pandit

32 Sports medicine and sports injuries — 463
Gina Allen

33 The spine — 471
Brian J.C. Freeman & Chris Lavy

34 Upper limb — 488
David Limb & Sam Vollans

35 Hip and knee — 511
Vikas Khanduja & Wasim Sardar Khan

36 Foot and ankle — 524
Bob Sharp

37 Musculoskeletal tumours — 534
Paul Cool & Craig Gerrand

38 Infection of the bones and joints — 549
Martin A. McNally & Philippa C. Matthews

39 Paediatric orthopaedics — 561
Deborah M. Eastwood

PART 6: SKIN AND SUBCUTANEOUS TISSUE

40 Skin and subcutaneous tissue — 592
Adam R. Greenbaum & Christopher L.H. Chan

41 Burns — 617
Michael P.H. Tyler & Sudip J. Ghosh

42 Plastic and reconstructive surgery — 633
Tim Goodacre

PART 7: HEAD AND NECK

43 Cranial neurosurgery — 652
Harry J.C.J. Bulstrode & William P. Gray

44 The eye and orbit — 672
Keith R. Martin

45 Cleft lip and palate: developmental abnormalities of the face, mouth and jaws — 686
David A. Koppel

46 The ear, nose and sinuses — 703
Iain J. Nixon, Iain Hathorn & Alex Bennett

47 Pharynx, larynx and neck — 725
Terry M. Jones

48 Oral cavity malignancy — 760
Andrew G. Schache

49 Disorders of the salivary glands — 776
Mark McGurk & Leandros-Vassilios F. Vassiliou

PART 8: BREAST AND ENDOCRINE

50 The thyroid gland — 800
Iain J. Nixon & Richard M. Adamson

51 The parathyroid glands — 823
Ruth S. Prichard

52 The adrenal glands and other abdominal endocrine disorders — 838
Tom W.J. Lennard

53 The breast — 860
Richard C. Sainsbury

PART 9: CARDIOTHORACIC

54 Cardiac surgery — 884
Jonathan R. Anderson & Mustafa Zakkar

55 The thorax — 914
Carol Tan & Ian Hunt

PART 10: VASCULAR

56 Arterial disorders — 942
Rob Sayers & Robert S.M. Davies

57 Venous disorders — 969
Ian C. Chetter & Dan Carradice

58 Lymphatic disorders — 995
Gneneswar Atturu, David A. Russell & Shervanthi Homer-Vanniasinkam

PART 11: ABDOMINAL

59 History and examination of the abdomen 1016
P. Ronan O'Connell

60 Abdominal wall, hernia and umbilicus 1022
Bruce Tulloh & Stephen J. Nixon

61 The peritoneum, omentum, mesentery and retroperitoneal space 1047
Charles H. Knowles

62 The oesophagus 1067
Derek Alderson

63 Stomach and duodenum 1106
Tim Underwood & John N. Primrose

64 Bariatric and metabolic surgery 1144
Richard Welbourn & Dimitri Pournaras

65 The liver 1153
Robert P. Jones & Graeme J. Poston

66 The spleen 1176
O. James Garden

67 The gallbladder and bile ducts 1188
Kevin C.P. Conlon

68 The pancreas 1212
Satyajit Bhattacharya

69 The small intestine 1240
Gordon Lawrence Carlson & Mattias Soop

70 The large intestine 1258
Gordon Lawrence Carlson & Jonathan Epstein

71 Intestinal obstruction 1280
Jim Hill

72 The vermiform appendix 1299
Jürgen Mulsow

73 The rectum 1318
David Jayne & Hiba Fatayer

74 The anus and anal canal 1339
Karen Nugent

PART 12: GENITOURINARY

75 Urinary symptoms and investigations 1374
J. Kilian Mellon

76 Kidneys and ureters 1398
J. Kilian Mellon

77 The urinary bladder 1423
Freddie C. Hamdy

78 The prostate and seminal vesicles 1456
David E. Neal & Greg Shaw

79 Urethra and penis 1477
Ian Eardley

80 Testis and scrotum 1497
Ian Eardley

81 Gynaecology 1513
Monica Mittal, Prasanna Raj Supramaniam & Christian Becker

PART 13: TRANSPLANTATION

82 Transplantation 1532
John Andrew Bradley

APPENDICES

Appendix 1:
Common instruments used in general surgery 1560
Pradip K. Datta

Appendix 2:
Fundamental principles in the operating theatre and the importance of global health 1563
Alan Norrish & Chris Lavy

Index 1567

Preface to 27th Edition

When Hamilton Bailey and McNeil Love published the first edition of their venerated textbook in 1932 the surgical world was a very different place to that of today. There were no antibiotics, no joint replacement, no open heart surgery, no transplantation and many other procedures that we now take for granted had simply not been invented. Medicine as a whole and surgery in particular never stands still. Surgeons continually strive to innovate so that they can tackle conditions and diseases previously thought to be beyond reach. They do this against a background of new discoveries in both the physical and biological sciences. Such breakthroughs make some surgical procedures redundant but others stimulate new approaches. This is seen in all specialties and consequently it is important for textbooks not only to keep pace with new developments but also to ensure that a balanced view is taken of their place in the therapeutic armamentarium. In developing the 27th edition of this much-loved textbook, we have striven to keep this in the forefront of our minds and those of our contributors. Nevertheless, in addition to considering the place of innovation, it is important not to 'throw the baby out with the bathwater'. We have therefore ensured that the basic tenets of surgical practice that have stood the test of time remain where appropriate.

Since the last edition great strides have been made in certain areas and we have ensured that these have been embedded in the book. For instance, in colorectal surgery a tipping point has been reached whereby more elective surgery is performed laparoscopically than by open technique. Similarly, in vascular surgery there has been an explosion in the use of interventional radiology to treat conditions that were previously the sole province of the surgeon. Stenting of aortic aneurysms (EVAR), for instance, is rapidly replacing elective open operations and, in many instances, is being used for treating leaking aneurysms, with a concomitant marked reduction in mortality. Damage control surgery is an increasingly important part of trauma management, in both civilian and conflict settings. Such developments also highlight the important role of the multidisciplinary team and the realisation that modern surgical care can no longer be provided in isolation. This concept is reiterated throughout the book and is also why the importance of human factors is emphasised in the chapter on patient safety, which is a relatively new science of how humans behave physically and psychologically in relation to particular environments. There is no more intense environment than an operating theatre, so how a surgical team interacts is crucial to the outcome for a patient undergoing a surgical procedure. This also applies, of course, outside the operating theatre because multidisciplinary working is now paramount to the delivery of safe and effective patient care. There is no doubt that in recent years regulation of medical practice has become tighter. Whereas in certain jurisdictions some may feel that this has become stifling, there is no doubt that regulation is here to stay. Needless to say, we should all be aware of our responsibilities to patients, both morally and ethically, and, although most need no reminding, the law is continually changing as test cases are brought before the courts. Hence, we draw the attention of the reader to the revamped chapter on ethics and the law, the tenets of which we must all abide by.

Throughout the text, we have also endeavoured to point out where we and our authors think the specialty is moving. Exciting developments are on the horizon. For instance, genome sequencing will have a marked effect on how we practise in certain specialties, none more so than oncology. Robotics is likely to improve many more surgical procedures and tissue engineering will become more commonplace. In order to accommodate these advances, it has been necessary to streamline some of the more established chapters, otherwise the book would become unwieldy. As a consequence, we have ensured that the 'Further reading' list at the end of each chapter has been brought up to date, allowing readers to delve further if they so wish.

We are very conscious that the book is popular throughout the world and consequently we have ensured that those diseases that are prevalent outside Europe and North America are included. Where relevant we have involved experts who are used to dealing with such maladies. The chapter on tropical infections and infestations is such an example.

We have also endeavoured in this edition to be more consistent in its layout, ensuring that we use a similar format for tables, graphs and diagrams. Nevertheless, we have been sure to keep the biographical details of individual scientists and practitioners, which have been beloved of all readers throughout the generations. Similarly, we have retained the section on surgical instruments. Although some are now very much of historical interest, they are part of our heritage and students and indeed established practitioners will, we hope, find these vignettes fascinating. We have been told that the Summary boxes are very much appreciated by both undergraduate and postgraduate students revising, sometimes in haste, before exams and hence our authors have ensured that these are up to date.

A book as comprehensive as this could never have been completed without the dedication and professionalism of our contributors. They have invariably answered our demands with alacrity and accuracy, appreciating the responsibility that goes with informing the readership of such a respected and established textbook. We are extremely grateful for all their efforts because we are conscious that a textbook such as this can never rest on its laurels. If it is to remain in the higher echelons of surgical tomes it must have the very best contributors and we believe that we have brought together such a cadre in the present edition. This in no way diminishes the contributions of the authors from the previous edition who are no longer involved. They, for a variety of reasons including retirement, have passed on the baton. We are grateful to them for magnanimously stepping down and making way for 'new blood' and none more so than our previous co-editor Professor Christopher Bulstrode. Chris helped revamp the 23rd, 24th, 25th and 26th Editions and these would never have been as successful without his dedicated efforts. Chris's place in the editorial team has been taken by Andrew McCaskie who has streamlined the trauma and orthopaedic sections as well as overseeing other chapters.

Readers of *Bailey & Love* have always been an integral part of the development of the book over the years and the present editorial group relish your feedback, which we know from experience will be forthcoming. Such input is vital if the book is to continue to reach the very high standards expected from each new edition. This has been a labour of love for all of us involved in this edition and we do hope it fulfils your needs, no matter whether you are an undergraduate student exploring the exciting world of surgical practice for the first time, a postgraduate trainee studying for exams or an established consultant who wishes to refresh his or her memory.

We wish you all well in your careers no matter which specialty you choose to practise in and we very much hope that the 27th and indeed subsequent editions of *Bailey & Love* accompany you on your travels through this most rewarding of professions.

Norman S. Williams
P. Ronan O'Connell
Andrew W. McCaskie

Contributors

Richard M. Adamson MBBS FRCS(ORL-HNS)
Consultant Ear, Nose and Throat Surgeon
University of Edinburgh ENT Department
Edinburgh, UK

Muaaze Ahmad MBChB FRCR
Consultant Radiologist
Barts Health NHS Trust
London, UK

Derek Alderson MD
President, Royal College of Surgeons of England
Emeritus Professor of Surgery
University of Birmingham
Honorary Consultant Surgeon
University Hospitals NHS Trust
Queen Elizabeth Hospital
Birmingham, UK

Gina Allen BM DCH MRCP MRCGP FRCR MFSEM MScSEM DipESSR
Musculoskeletal Radiologist and Sports Physician
Oxford University and St Lukes Radiology Oxford Ltd
Oxford, UK

Jonathan R. Anderson FRCS(C-Th) FFST(Ed)
Consultant Cardiothoracic Surgeon
Hammersmith Hospital
London, UK

Hutan Ashrafian BSc(Hons) MBBS PhD MBA MRCS
Department of Surgery and Cancer and Institute of Global Health Innovation
Imperial College London
Bariatric and Metabolic Surgical Unit
Chelsea and Westminster Hospital
London, UK

Gnaneswar Atturu MS ChM FRCS
Locum Consultant Vascular and Trauma Surgeon
Leeds Vascular Institute
Leeds General Infirmary
Leeds, UK

Sanjay De Bakshi MS(Cal) FRCS(Eng) FRCS(Ed)
Head of Department of Surgery
Calcutta Medical Research Institute
Kolkata, India

Christian Becker MD
Associate Professor
Consultant Gynaecologist and Subspecialist in Reproductive Medicine
Nuffield Department of Obstetrics and Gynaecology
University of Oxford
John Radcliffe Hospital
Oxford, UK

Antonio Belli MD FRCS FRCS(SN)
Professor of Trauma Neurosurgery
Director of the NIHR Surgical Reconstruction and Microbiology Research Centre
University of Birmingham
Birmingham, UK

Alex Bennett MBBS DLO FRCS(ORL-HNS) MEd DIC
Consultant Ear, Nose and Throat Surgeon
University of Edinburgh ENT Department
Edinburgh, UK

Satyajit Bhattacharya MS MPhil FRCS
Consultant Hepato-Pancreato-Biliary Surgeon
The Royal London Hospital
London, UK

Ken Boffard BSc(Hons) MB BCh FRCS FRCS(Ed) FRCPS(Glas) FCS(SA) FACS(Hon)
Professor Emeritus
Department of Surgery
University of the Witwatersrand
Trauma Director and Academic Head
Netcare Milpark Academic Trauma Centre
Johannesburg, South Africa

John Andrew Bradley PhD, FRCS
Emeritus Professor of Surgery
Cambridge University
Cambridge, UK

Karim Brohi FRCS FRCA
Professor of Trauma Sciences
Barts and the London School of Medicine and Dentistry
Queen Mary, University of London
London, UK

Harry J.C.J. Bulstrode PhD
Clinical Lecturer in Neurosurgery
University of Cambridge
Cambridge, UK

Gordon Lawrence Carlson BSc(Hons) MBChB(Hons) MD FRCS FRCS(Gen) FRCS(Ed)
Consultant Surgeon and Honorary Professor of Surgery
University of Manchester
Salford Royal Hospital NHS Foundation Trust
Salford, UK

Dan Carradice MBChB MD(Hons) FRCS PGC Med US(Dist) PGD(Health Econ)
Senior Lecturer
Hull York Medical School
Consultant Vascular and Endovascular Surgeon
Hull and East Yorkshire Hospitals NHS Trust
Hull and York, UK

Christopher L.H. Chan BSc(Hons) PhD FRCS(Eng) FRCS(Gen Surg)
Consultant Colorectal Surgeon
Barts Health NHS Trust
London, UK

Serene Hsi-Lin Chang MBBS MD FRCA
Consultant Anaesthetist
Ng Teng Fong General Hospital
Singapore
Honorary Fellow, Pain and Anaesthesia Research Centre
St Bartholomew's Hospital and Biomedical Engineering Research Group
City University
London, UK

Ian C. Chetter MBChB MD FRCS PGC Med US(Dist) PGD Clin Ed
Chair of Surgery
Hull York Medical School
Consultant Vascular Surgeon
Hull and East Yorkshire Hospitals NHS Trust
Hull and York, UK

Jon Clasper CBE DPhil DM FRCSEd(Orth) Col L/RAMC
Emeritus Professor and Consultant Orthopaedic Surgeon
Military Clinical Director DMG (SE)
Visiting Professor in Bioengineering
Imperial College London
Clinical Lead
The Royal British Legion Centre for Blast Injury Studies
London, UK

Mark G. Coleman, MBChB MD(Hons) FRCS FRCPS(Glas) FFST(RCSEd)
Consultant Surgeon
Derriford Hospital, Plymouth
Senior Lecturer (Associate Professor)
Plymouth University Peninsula School of Medicine and Dentistry
Plymouth, UK

Kevin C.P. Conlon MA MCh MBA FRCS(I) FACS FRCS(Ed) FRCPS(Glas) FTCD
Professor of Surgery
Trinity College Dublin
Consultant HPB Surgeon
St. Vincent's University Hospital
Dublin, Ireland

Paul Cool MD MMedSc(Res) DipStat FRCS(Ed) FRCS(Orth)
Consultant Orthopaedic and Oncological Surgeon
Robert Jones and Agnes Hunt Orthopaedic Hospital NHS Foundation Trust
Oswestry, UK

John Crawford BSc MBBS FRCS FRCS(Orth)
Consultant Orthopaedic Spinal Surgeon
Department of Neurosurgery
Cambridge University Hospital NHS Foundation Trust
Cambridge, UK

Professor the Lord Darzi of Denham OM KBE PC FRS FMedSci
Professor of Surgery
Imperial College London
St Mary's Hospital Campus
London, UK

Pradip K. Datta MBE MS FRCS(Ed) FRCS(Eng) FRCS(I) FRCS(Glas)
Honorary Consultant Surgeon
Caithness General Hospital
Wick, UK

Robert S.M. Davies MBChB MMedSci(Med Ed) MD FRCS
Consultant Vascular Surgeon and Honorary Senior Lecturer
University Hospitals of Leicester
Leicester, UK

Dan Deakin FRCS(T&O)
Consultant Orthopaedic Trauma Surgeon
Nottingham University Hospital
Nottingham, UK

Elias Degiannis MD PhD FRCS(Glasg) FCS(SA) FACS
Professor Emeritus, Department of Surgery
University of the Witwatersrand Medical School
Netcare Milpark Academic Trauma Center and Leratong Hospital
Johannesburg, South Africa

Ian Eardley MA MChir FRCS(Urol) FEBU
Consultant Urologist
Leeds Teaching Hospital Trust
Leeds, UK

Michael John Earley MB MCh FRCS(I) FRCS(Plast)
Consultant Plastic Surgeon and Associate Clinical Professor
The Children's University Hospital
Temple Street and Mater Misericordiae University Hospital
Dublin, Ireland

Jonathan J. Earnshaw DM FRCS
Consultant Vascular Surgeon
Cheltenham General Hospital
Cheltenham, UK

Deborah M. Eastwood MB FRCS
Consultant Paediatric Orthopaedic Surgeon
Great Ormond St Hospital for Children and the Royal National Orthopaedic Hospital
London, UK

Jonathan Epstein MA MD FRCS
Consultant Surgeon
Salford Royal NHS Foundation Trust
Salford, UK

Hiba Fatayer MBBS MSc MRCS
Specialist Registrar in General Surgery
Leeds Teaching Hospitals NHS Trust
Leeds, UK

Roger M. Feakins MB BCh BAO BA MD FRCPI FRCPath
Consultant Histopathologist and Professor of Gastrointestinal Pathology
Department of Histopathology
Barts Health NHS Trust
London, UK

The late Professor Kenneth Fearon, MD, FRCPS(Glas) FRCS(Ed) FRCS
Professor of Surgical Oncology and Honorary Consultant, Colorectal Surgeon, Clinical Surgery
School of Clinical Science
University of Edinburgh
Royal Infirmary
Edinburgh, UK

Pierre Foex DPhil FRCA FMedSci
Emeritus Nuffield Professor of Anaesthetics
Nuffield Division of Anaesthetics
John Radcliffe Hospital
Oxford, UK

Brian J.C. Freeman MB BCh BAO DM(Nott) FRCS(T&O) FRACS(Ortho) FAOrthA
Professor of Spinal Surgery
University of Adelaide
Head of Spinal Services
Royal Adelaide Hospital
Adelaide
Senior Visiting Specialist
Women's and Children's Hospital
Clinical Director
Centre for Orthopaedic and Trauma Research
Adelaide, Australia

O. James Garden CBE BSc MBChB MD FRCS(Ed) FRCP(Ed) FRSE FRCS(Can)(Hons) FRACS(Hons) FACS(Hons) FRCS(Hons) FCSHK(Hons) FRCS(I)(Hons)
Regius Professor of Clinical Surgery
University of Edinburgh
Royal Infirmary
Edinburgh, UK

Craig Gerrand MD FRCS(Ed)(T&O)
Consultant Orthopaedic Surgeon
North of England Bone and Soft Tissue Tumour Service
Newcastle upon Tyne Hospitals NHS Foundation Trust
Newcastle upon Tyne, UK

Sudip J. Ghosh MBBS MS FRCS(Plast)
Consultant Plastic Reconstructive and Burns Surgeon
Stoke Mandeville Hospital
Aylesbury, UK

Peter Giannoudis MD FACS FRCS
Professor of Trauma and Orthopaedic Surgery
School of Medicine
University of Leeds
Leeds, UK

Fay Gilder MBBS FRCA
Consultant Anaesthetist
Cambridge University Hospitals NHS Foundation Trust
Cambridge, UK

Tim Goodacre MBBS BSc FRCS
Consultant Plastic Surgeon
Oxford University Hospitals NHS Foundation Trust
Oxford, UK

William P. Gray MB MD FRCS(I) FRCS(SN)
Professor of Neurosurgery
Director Wales BRAIN Unit
Neuroscience and Mental Health Research Institute
School of Medicine
Cardiff University
Cardiff, UK

Adam R. Greenbaum MBBS MBA PhD FRCS(Plast) FEBOPRAS FACS
Consultant Plastic and Reconstructive Surgeon
Auckland and the Waikato
New Zealand

Freddie C. Hamdy MD MA FRCS FRCS(Ed)(Urol) FMedSci
Nuffield Professor of Surgery and Professor of Urology
University of Oxford
Director, Division of Surgery and Oncology
Oxford University Hospitals NHS Foundation Trust
Oxford, UK

Bob Handley MBChB FRCS
Consultant Trauma and Orthopaedic Surgeon
John Radcliffe Hospital
Oxford, UK

Iain Hathorn BSc MBChB DOHNS PGCME FRCSEd(ORL-HNS)
Consultant Ear, Nose and Throat Surgeon
University of Edinburgh ENT Department
Edinburgh, UK

Douglas Hay MBBS FRCS(Orth)
Consultant Orthopaedic Spinal Surgeon
Department of Neurosurgery
Cambridge University Hospital NHS Foundation Trust
Cambridge, UK

Jim Hill MDChB ChM FRCS
Clinical Professor of Colorectal Surgery
Manchester Royal Infirmary and Manchester Academic Health Science Centre
Manchester, UK

Shervanthi Homer-Vanniasinkam BSc MD FRCS(Ed) FRCS
Consultant Vascular Surgeon
Leeds Vascular Institute
Leeds General Infirmary
Leeds, UK

Ian Hunt FRCS(CTh)
Consultant Thoracic Surgeon
Department of Thoracic Surgery
St George's Hospital
London, UK

Ian Jackson MBChB FRCA
Chief Clinical Information Officer
York Teaching Hospital NHS Foundation Trust
York, UK

David Jayne BSc MBChB MD FRCS
Professor of Surgery
University of Leeds and Leeds Teaching Hospitals NHS Trust
Leeds, UK

Terry M. Jones BSc FRCSEd FRCS(ORL-HNS) MD SFHEA FASE(RCS)
Professor of Head and Neck Surgery
Institute of Translational Medicine
University of Liverpool
Liverpool, UK

Robert P. Jones BSc MBChB PhD MRCS
Lecturer in Surgery
Institute of Translational Medicine
University of Liverpool
Liverpool, UK

Frank B.V. Keane MD FRCS FRCS(I) FRCPS(Glas)(Hons) FRCP(Ed)(Hons) FRCPI(Hons)
Joint Lead, National Clinical Programme in Surgery
Royal College of Surgeons in Ireland
Former Consultant Colorectal Surgeon
Adelaide and Meath Hospital
Dublin, Ireland

Wasim Sardar Khan MBChB MSc PhD MRCS FRCS(Tr&Orth)
University Lecturer and Honorary Consultant Trauma and Orthopaedic Surgeon
Addenbrooke's Hospital
Cambridge University Hospitals NHS Foundation Trust
Cambridge, UK

Vikas Khanduja MA(Cantab) MSc FRCS FRCS(Tr&Orth)
Consultant Orthopaedic Surgeon
Research Lead – Elective Clinical Trials
Addenbrooke's Hospital
Cambridge University Hospitals NHS Foundation Trust
Cambridge, UK

Charles H. Knowles BChir PhD FRCS
Professor of Surgery and Honorary Consultant Colorectal Surgeon
Barts Health NHS Trust
The Blizard Institute
Barts and the London School of Medicine and Dentistry
Queen Mary, University of London
London, UK

David A. Koppel MB BS BDS FDS FRCS
Consultant Craniofacial/Oral and Maxillofacial Surgeon
Regional Maxillofacial Unit
Queen Elizabeth University Hospital, Royal Hospital for Children
Glasgow, UK

Pawanindra Lal MS DNB MNAMS FIMSA FCLS FRCS(Ed) FRCS(Glas) FRCS(Eng) FACS
Director Professor of Surgery
Maulana Azad Medical College (University of Delhi) and Associated Lok Nayak Hospital
New Delhi, India

Peter Lamont MD FRCS FEBVS
Consultant Vascular Surgeon
Bristol, Bath and Weston Vascular Network
Bristol, UK

Anthony Lander PhD FRCS(Paed) DCH
Consultant Paediatric Surgeon
Birmingham Children's Hospital
Birmingham, UK

Chris Lavy OBE MD MCh FRCS(Eng)
Professor of Orthopaedic and Tropical Surgery
University of Oxford
Honorary Consultant Spine Surgeon
Oxford University Hospitals
Oxford, UK

Tom W.J. Lennard MBBS MD FRCS
Professor of Surgery and Associate Dean
Newcastle University
Newcastle upon Tyne, UK

David Limb BSc FRCSEd(Orth)
Consultant Orthopaedic Surgeon
Leeds Teaching Hospitals Trust
Leeds, UK

James O. Lindsay PhD FRCP
Consultant Gastroenterologist
Barts Health NHS Trust
The Royal London Hospital
Reader in Inflammatory Bowel Disease
Queen Mary University of London
London, UK

Andrew W. McCaskie MMus MD FRCS FRCS(T&O)
Professor of Orthopaedic Surgery and Head of Department of Surgery
University of Cambridge
Honorary Consultant
Addenbrooke's Hospital
Cambridge University Hospitals NHS Foundation Trust
Cambridge, UK

Stephen M. McDonnell MBBS BSc MD FRCS(T&O)
University Lecturer and Consultant Orthopaedic Surgeon
Addenbrooke's Hospital
Cambridge University Hospitals NHS Foundation Trust
Cambridge, UK

John MacFie MD FRCS(Eng) FRCS(Ed) FRCS(Glas) FRCP(Ed)
Professor of Surgery and Consultant Surgeon
University of Hull, York NHS Trust at Scarborough Hospital
Scarborough, UK

Mark McGurk MD BDS FRCS FDSRCS DLO
Professor of Oral and Maxillofacial Surgery
University College London Hospital
London, UK

Martin A. McNally MB BCH MD(Res) FRCS(Ed) FRCS(Orth)
Consultant in Limb Reconstruction
Nuffield Orthopaedic Centre
Oxford University Hospitals
Honorary Senior Clinical Lecturer in Orthopaedic Surgery
University of Oxford
Oxford, UK

Douglas McWhinnie MD(Hons) FRCS
Professor of Clinical Education and Consultant General and Vascular Surgeon
University of Buckingham
Milton Keynes University Hospital NHS Foundation Trust
Milton Keynes, UK

Keith R. Martin MA BM BCh DM MRCP FRCOphth
Professor of Ophthalmology
University of Cambridge
Cambridge, UK

Matthew Matson MRCP FRCR
Divisional Director of Imaging
Barts Health NHS Trust
London, UK

Philippa C. Matthews BMBS MRCP DTM&H DPhil(Oxon) FRCPath
Wellcome Trust Clinical Research Fellow
Nuffield Department of Medicine
University of Oxford
Honorary Consultant in Infectious Diseases and Microbiology
Oxford University Hospitals NHS Foundation Trust
Oxford, UK

Ken Mealy MD FRCS(I) FRCS(Ed)
Joint Lead, National Clinical Programme in Surgery
Royal College of Surgeons in Ireland
Consultant General Surgeon
Wexford General Hospital
Wexford, Ireland

Vivek Mehta MBBS MD FRCA FFPMRCA
Consultant in Pain Medicine and Neuromodulation
Director, Pain and Anaesthesia Research Centre
St Bartholomew's and Royal London Hospital
Barts Health NHS Trust
London, UK

J. Kilian Mellon MD FRCS(Urol)
Consultant Urological Surgeon
Leicester General Hospital
Leicester, UK

Monica Mittal Intercalated BSc MBBS MRCOG
Subspecialist Trainee in Reproductive Medicine and Surgery
Specialist Registrar in Obstetrics and Gynaecology
Oxford University Hospitals NHS Foundation Trust
Oxford, UK

Chris Moran MD FRCS(Ed)
National Clinical Director for Trauma
NHS-England
Professor of Orthopaedic Trauma Surgery
Nottingham University Hospital
Nottingham, UK

Jürgen Mulsow MD FRCS(I)
Consultant General and Colorectal Surgeon
Department of Colorectal Surgery and National Centre for Peritoneal Malignancy
Mater Misericordiae University Hospital
Dublin, Ireland

Alastair Munro BSc FRCR FRCP(E) FRCS(Ed)
Honorary Professor
School of Medicine
University of St Andrews
St Andrews, UK

David E. Neal CBE FMedSci FRCS
Senior Visiting Fellow and Professor Emeritus of Surgical Oncology
University of Cambridge
Cambridge, UK

Iain J. Nixon MB ChB FRCS(ORL-HNS) PhD
Consultant Ear, Nose and Throat Surgeon
University of Edinburgh
Edinburgh, UK

Stephen J. Nixon FRCS(Ed) FRCP(Ed)
Consultant Surgeon
Royal Infirmary of Edinburgh
Edinburgh, UK

Alan Norrish BSc(Hons) MB BChir LLM PhD FRCS(Orth)
Associate Lecturer
School of Clinical Medicine
University of Cambridge
Consultant Orthopaedic Surgeon
Cambridge University Hospitals NHS Foundation Trust
Cambridge, UK

Karen Nugent MA MS MEd FRCS
Consultant Colorectal Surgeon
University of Southampton
Southampton, UK

P. Ronan O'Connell MD FRCS(I) FRCPS(Glas) FRCS(Edin)
Professor, Head of Section of Surgery and Surgical Specialties
University College Dublin
St Vincent's University Hospital
Dublin, Ireland

Hemant G. Pandit DPhil FRCS(T&O)
Professor of Orthopaedic Surgery and Honorary Consultant
Director of Research and Innovation
University of Leeds
Leeds
Professor of Orthopaedic Surgery
University of Oxford
Oxford, UK

Phill Pearce MA MBBS MRCS RAF
Registrar in General Surgery
Royal British Legion Centre for Blast Injury Studies
Imperial College London
London
Academic Department of Military Surgery and Trauma
Royal Centre for Defence Medicine
Frimley Park, UK

Graeme J. Poston MS DSc FRCS(Eng) FRCS(Ed)
Professor of Surgery
Northwestern Hepatobiliary Unit
Aintree University Hospital
Liverpool, UK

Dimitri Pournaras PhD FRCS
Registrar in Upper Gastrointestinal and General Surgery
Addenbrooke's Hospital
Cambridge University Hospitals NHS Foundation Trust
Cambridge, UK

Niall Power MD MRCP(I) FRCR
Consultant Radiologist
Royal Free Hospital
London, UK

Ruth S. Prichard MD FRCS(I)
Consultant Endocrine and Breast Surgeon
St Vincent's University Hospital
Dublin, Ireland

John N. Primrose FMedSci
Professor of Surgery
University of Southampton
Southampton General Hospital
Southampton, UK

Sanjay Purkayastha BSc MBBS MD FRCS(Gen Surg)
Consultant Surgeon
General, Laparoscopic, Bariatric and Upper GI Surgery
St Mary's Hospital
Imperial College Healthcare NHS Trust
Senior Lecturer in Bariatric Surgery
Imperial College
London, UK

Mamoon Rashid FRCS FCPS(Pak)
Professor of Plastic and Reconstructive Surgery
Shifa College of Medicine
Consultant Plastic Surgeon and Programme Director
Shifa International Hospital
Islamabad, Pakistan

Lee Van Rensburg MBBCh FRCS(Tr&Orth)
Consultant Orthopaedic Surgeon
Addenbrooke's Hospital
Cambridge University Hospitals NHS Foundation Trust
Cambridge, UK

David A. Russell MB ChB MD FRCS(Gen Surg)
Consultant Vascular Surgeon
Leeds Vascular Institute
Leeds General Infirmary
Leeds, UK

Richard C. Sainsbury MBBS MD FRCS
Honorary Reader in Surgery
University College London
Consultant Surgeon
London Breast Clinic
London, UK

Anand Sardesai MB BS MD FRCA
Consultant Anaesthetist
Addenbrooke's Hospital
Cambridge University Hospitals NHS Foundation Trust
Cambridge, UK

Rob Sayers MD FRCS
Honorary Professor of Vascular Surgery
Leicester Royal Infirmary
Leeds, UK

Andrew G. Schache PhD FDSRCS FRCS(OMFS)
Clinical Senior Lecturer in Head and Neck Surgery
University of Liverpool
Honorary Consultant in Oral and Maxillofacial – Head and Neck Surgery
Aintree University Hospitals NHS Foundation Trust
Liverpool, UK

Bob Sharp BM BCh MA FRCS FRCS(Tr&Orth)
Consultant Orthopaedic Surgeon
Oxford University Hospitals
The Nuffield Orthopaedic Centre
Oxford, UK

Greg Shaw MD FRCS(Urol)
Consultant Urologist
University College London Hospitals NHS Foundation Trust
Honorary Senior Lecturer
University College and Queen Mary College
London, UK

Mattias Soop MD PhD
Consultant Surgeon and Honorary Reader in Surgery
The University of Manchester
Manchester Academic Health Science Centre
Salford Royal NHS Foundation Trust
Salford, UK

Robert J.C. Steele MB ChB MD FRCS(Ed) FRSE
Head of Academic Surgery and Head of Cancer Division
Medical Research Institute, Division of Cancer
Ninewells Hospital and Medical School
Dundee, UK

Prasanna Raj Supramaniam MBChB MSc MRCOG
Specialist Registrar in Obstetrics and Gynaecology
Oxford University Hospitals NHS Foundation Trust
Oxford, UK

Carol Tan FRCS(C-Th)
Consultant Thoracic Surgeon
Department of Thoracic Surgery
St George's Hospital
London, UK

Bruce Tulloh MB MS(Melb) FRACS FRCS(Ed)
Consultant General Surgeon
Department of Surgery
Royal Infirmary of Edinburgh
Edinburgh, UK

Michael P.H. Tyler MB CHM FRCS(Plast)
Consultant Plastic Reconstructive and Burns Surgeon
Stoke Mandeville Hospital
Aylesbury, UK

Tim Underwood PhD FRCS
Professor of GI Surgery
University of Southampton
Southampton, UK

Medha Vanarase-Pandit MD FRCA Cert Med Ed
Consultant Anaesthetist
Leeds Teaching Hospitals NHS Trust
Leeds, UK

Leandros-Vassilios F. Vassiliou DDS MD MSc FRCS
Department of Head and Neck
Guy's Hospital
London, UK

Sam Vollans FRCS(Ed)(Orth)
Consultant Orthopaedic Surgeon
Leeds Teaching Hospitals Trust
Leeds, UK

Richard Welbourn MD FRCS
Consultant Upper Gastrointestinal and Bariatric Surgeon
Honorary Reader in Bariatric Surgery
University of Bristol
Musgrove Park Hospital
Taunton, UK

Robert Wheeler MS LLB(Hons) LLM FRCS
Consultant Neonatal and Paediatric Surgeon
Director, Department of Clinical Law
University Hospital of Southampton
Southampton, UK

Birgit Whitman PhD
Head of Research Governance
University of Bristol
Bristol, UK

Philip Woodland MBBS PhD MRCP
Consultant Gastroenterologist
Barts Health NHS Trust
The Royal London Hospital
Honorary Senior Lecturer in Upper GI Medicine
Queen Mary, University of London
London, UK

Mustafa Zakkar PhD FRCS(C-Th)
NIHR Clinical Lecturer in Cardiothoracic Surgery
University of Bristol and Bristol Heart Institute
Bristol, UK

Acknowledgements

In this day and age, it is impossible to produce a book like Bailey and Love without the contribution of numerous talented individuals. Although it is impractical to mention all those who have played a part in producing the 27th Edition, it would be remiss not to express our gratitude to the following key players.

Henry Spilberg initiated the new edition as commissioning editor under the supervision of Jo Koster and was very much involved in the early planning. His role was subsequently taken over by Miranda Bromage following his departure for pastures green. Miranda's diligence and experience has been invaluable and we are enormously indebted to her wise counsel. Cherry Allen, as Editorial Assistant has been key in liaising with the editors and the contributors, ensuring manuscripts have been received on time and has been responsible for ensuring the smooth handover of the text to the production team. The latter has been headed by Paul Bennett who has provided an extremely professional service. His and his team's attention to detail has been very much valued and we hope is reflected in a first class product.

Chapter 5, *Surgical infection*, contains some material from '*Surgical infection*' by David J. Leaper. The material has been revised and updated by the current author.

Chapter 7, *Basic surgical skills and anastomoses*, contains some material from '*Basic surgical skills and anastomoses*' by David J. Leaper and William E.G. Thomas. The material has been revised and updated by the current author.

Chapter 9, *Principles of paediatric surgery*, contains some material from '*Principles of paediatric surgery*' by Mark Stringer. The material has been revised and updated by the current author.

Chapter 12, *Surgical ethics and law*, contains some material from '*Surgical ethics*' by Len Doyal. The material has been revised and updated by the current author.

Chapter 14, *Diagnostic imaging*, contains some material from '*Diagnostic imaging*' by the current authors and Gina Allen, which has been revised and updated for this edition.

Chapter 17, *Preoperative care including the high-risk surgical patient*, contains some material from '*Pre operative preparation*' by current authors Medha Vanarase-Pandit and Pierre Foex, and Kevin Tremper, Lisa Leonard and Sarah Barton, and '*Perioperative management of the high-risk patient*' by Mridula Rai, Kevin D. Johnston, Rupert M. Pearse and Richard M. Langford. The material has been revised and updated by the current authors.

Chapter 18, *Anaesthesia and pain relief*, contains some material from '*Anaesthesia and pain relief*' by current author Vivek Mehta, and Richard Langford and Jagannath Halder. The material has been revised and updated by the current authors.

Chapter 20, *Postoperative care*, contains some material from '*Postoperative care*' by Jay Kini, current author Anand Sardesai, and Alistair Pace and Nicholas C.M. Armitage. The material has been revised and updated by the current authors.

Chapter 23, *Early assessment and management of trauma*, contains some material from '*Early assessment and management of trauma*' by Dinesh Nathwani and Joseph Windley. The material has been revised and updated by the current authors.

Chapter 24, *Traumatic brain injury*, contains some material from '*Head injury*' by Richard Stacey and John Leach. The material has been revised and updated by the current authors.

Chapter 25, *Neck and spine*, contains some material from '*Neck and spine*' by Ashley Poynton. The material has been revised and updated by the current authors.

Chapter 26, *Maxillofacial trauma*, contains some material from '*Maxillofacial trauma*' by Charles Perkins. The material has been revised and updated by the current author.

Chapter 28, *Extremity trauma*, contains some material from '*Extremity trauma*' by Parminder Singh. The material has been revised and updated by the current author.

Chapter 31, *History taking and clinical examination in musculoskeletal disease*, contains some material from '*History taking and clinical examination in musculoskeletal disease*' by

Parminder Singh and current author Hemant G. Pandit. The material has been revised and updated by the current authors.

Chapter 32, *Sports medicine and sports injuries*, contains some material from '*Sports medicine and sports injuries*' by D.L. Back and Jay Smith. The material has been revised and updated by the current authors.

Chapter 33, *The spine*, contains some material from '*The spine*' by the current authors and Gavin Bowden, which has been revised and updated for this edition.

Chapter 34, *Upper limb*, contains some material from '*Upper limb – pathology, assessment and management*' by Vinay Takwale, Irfan Khan and Srinath Kamineni. The material has been revised and updated by the current authors.

Chapter 35, *Hip and knee*, contains some material from '*Hip and knee*' by Hermant G. Pandit, Andrew Bernett, current author Vikas Khanduja and Richard N. Villar. The material has been revised and updated by the current authors.

Chapter 36, *Foot and ankle*, contains some material from '*Foot and ankle*' by Mark Davies, Matthew C. Solan and Vikas Khanduja. The material has been revised and updated by the current author.

Chapter 38, *Infection of the bones and joints*, contains some material from '*Infection of the bones and joints*' by the current authors and Philip Bejon, which has been revised and updated for this edition.

Chapter 39, *Paediatric orthopaedics*, contains some material from '*Paediatric orthopaedics*' by the current author and Joanna Hicks, which has been revised and updated for this edition.

Chapter 43, *Cranial neurosurgery*, contains some material from '*Elective Neurosurgery*' by John Leach and Richard Kerr. The material has been revised and updated by the current authors.

Chapter 44, *The eye and orbit*, contains some material from '*The eye and orbit*' by Colm O'Brien, Hugo Henderson and Jonathan Jagger. The material has been revised and updated by the current author.

Chapter 45, *Cleft lip and palate: developmental abnormalities of the face, mouth and jaws*, contains some material from '*Cleft lip and palate: developmental abnormalities of the face, mouth and jaws*' by William P. Smith. The material has been revised and updated by the current author.

Chapter 46, *The ear, nose and sinuses*, contains some material from '*The nose and sinuses*' by Robert W. Ruckley and current author Iain J. Nixon, and '*The ear*' by Grant Bates. The material has been revised and updated by the current authors.

Chapter 47, *Pharynx, larynx and neck*, contains some material from '*Pharynx, larynx and neck*' by Rishi Sharma, Martin Birchall, Jonathan D. Jagger and Hugo W.A. Henderson. The material has been revised and updated by the current author.

Chapter 48, *Oral cavity malignancy*, contains some material from '*Oropharyngeal cancer*' by William P. Smith. The material has been revised and updated by the current author.

Chapter 49, *Disorders of the salivary glands*, contains some material from '*Disorders of the salivary glands*', by William P. Smith. The material has been revised and updated by the current authors.

Chapter 50, *The thyroid glands*, contains some material from '*The thyroid and parathyroid glands*' by Zygmunt H. Krukowski. The material has been revised and updated by the current author.

Chapter 51, *The parathyroid glands*, contains some material from '*The thyroid and parathyroid glands*' by Zygmunt H. Krukowski. The material has been revised and updated by the current author.

Chapter 52, *The adrenal glands and other abdominal endocrine disorders*, contains some material from '*Adrenal glands and other endocrine disorders*' by Matthias Rothmund. The material has been revised and updated by the current author.

Chapter 54, *Cardiac surgery*, contains some material from '*Cardiac surgery*' by current author Jonathan Anderson and Ian Hunt. The material has been revised and updated by the current authors.

Chapter 55, *The thorax*, contains some material from '*The thorax*' by Tom Treasure. The material has been revised and updated by the current authors.

Chapter 56, *Arterial disorders*, contains some material from '*Arterial disorders*' by John A. Murie. The material has been revised and updated by the current author.

Chapter 57, *Venous disorders*, contains some material from '*Venous disorders*' by Peter McCollum, current author Ian Chetter and Kevin Burnand. The material has been revised and updated by the current authors.

Chapter 58, *Lymphatic disorders*, contains some material from '*Lymphatic disorders*' by current author Shervanthi Homer-Vanniasinkam and Andrew Bradbury. The material has been revised and updated by the current authors.

Chapter 59, *History and examination of the abdomen*, contains some material from *'History and examination of the abdomen'*, by Mohan de Silva, V. Sitaram and Simon Paterson-Brown. The material has been revised and updated by the current author.

Chapter 60, *Abdominal wall, hernia and umbilicus*, contains some material from *'Hernias, umbilicus and abdominal wall'* by Andrew N. Kingsnorth, Giorgi Giorgobiani and David H. Bennett. The material has been revised and updated by the current authors.

Chapter 61, *The peritoneum, omentum, mesentery and retroperitoneal space*, contains some material from *'The peritoneum, omentum, mesentery and retroperitoneal space'* by Jerry Thompson. The material has been revised and updated by the current author.

Chapter 64, *Bariatric and metabolic surgery*, contains some material from *'Bariatric surgery'* by John Baxter. The material has been revised and updated by the current author.

Chapter 65, *The liver*, contains some material from *'The liver'* by Rahul S. Koti, Sanjeev Kanoria and Brian R. Davidson. The material has been revised and updated by the current authors.

Chapter 69, *The small intestine*, contains some material from *'The small and large intestines'* by current author Gordon Carlson, Jonathan Epstein, Neil J. McC. Mortensen and Shazad Ashraf. The material has been revised and updated by the current authors.

Chapter 70, *The large intestine*, contains some material from *'The small and large intestines'* by Neil J. McC. Mortensen and Shazad Ashraf. The material has been revised and updated by the current authors.

Chapter 71, *Intestinal obstruction*, contains some material from *'Intestinal obstruction'* by Marc Christopher Winslet. The material has been revised and updated by the current author.

Chapter 72, *The vermiform appendix*, contains some material from *'The vermiform appendix'* by P. Ronan O'Connell. The material has been revised and updated by the current author.

Chapter 73, *The rectum*, contains some material from *'The rectum'* by Sue Clark. The material has been revised and updated by the current author.

Chapter 74, *The anus and anal canal*, contains some material from *'The anus and anal canal'* by the current author and Peter Lunniss, which has been revised and updated for this edition.

Chapter 76, *The kidneys and ureters*, contains some material from *'The kidneys and ureters'* by Christopher G. Fowler. The material has been revised and updated by the current author.

Chapter 77, *The urinary bladder*, contains some material from *'The urinary bladder'* by David E. Neal. The material has been revised and updated by the current author.

Chapter 79, *Urethra and penis*, contains some material from *'Urethra and penis'* by Christopher G. Fowler. The material has been revised and updated by the current author.

Chapter 80, *Testis and scrotum*, contains some material from *'Testis and scrotum'* by Christopher G. Fowler. The material has been revised and updated by the current author.

Chapter 81, *Gynaecology*, contains some material from *'Gynaecology'* by Stephen Kennedy and Enda McVeigh. The material has been revised and updated by the current author.

We acknowledge advice, beyond their chapter contribution, from Anand Sardesai in relation to anaesthetics, and Lee Van Rensburg, in relation to trauma.

Sayings of the great

Both Hamilton Bailey and McNeill Love, when medical students, served as clerks to Sir Robert Hutchinson, 1871–1960, who was Consulting Physician to the London Hospital and President of the Royal College of Physicians. They never tired of quoting his 'medical litany', which is appropriate for all clinicians and, perhaps especially, for those who are surgically minded.

> From inability to leave well alone;
> From too much zeal for what is new and contempt for what is old;
> From putting knowledge before wisdom, science before art, cleverness before common sense;
> From treating patients as cases; and
> From making the cure of a disease more grievous than its endurance,
> Good Lord, deliver us.

To which may be added:

> The patient is the centre of the medical universe around which all our works revolve and towards which all our efforts trend.
>
> J.B. Murphy, 1857–1916, Professor of Surgery, Northwestern University, Chicago, IL, USA

> To study the phenomenon of disease without books is to sail an uncharted sea, while to study books without patients is not to go to sea at all.
>
> Sir William Osler, 1849–1919, Professor of Medicine, Oxford, UK

> A knowledge of healthy and diseased actions is not less necessary to be understood than the principles of other sciences. By and acquaintance with principles we learn the cause of disease. Without this knowledge a man cannot be a surgeon. … The last part of surgery, namely operations, is a reflection on the healing art; it is a tacit acknowledgement of the insufficiency of surgery. It is like an armed savage who attempts to get that by force which a civilised man would by stratagem.
>
> John Hunter, 1728–1793, Surgeon, St George's Hospital, London, UK

Investigating Nature you will do well to bear ever in mind that in every question there is the truth, whatever our notions may be. This seems perhaps a very simple consideration; yet it is strange how often it seems to be disregarded. If we had nothing but pecuniary rewards and worldly honours to look to, our profession would not be one to be desired. But in its practice you will find it to be attended with peculiar privileges; second to none in intense interest and pure pleasures. It is our proud office to tend the fleshy tabernacle of the immortal spirit, and our path, if rightly followed, will be guided by unfettered truth and love unfeigned. In the pursuit of this noble and holy calling I wish you all God-speed.

Promoter's address, Graduation in Medicine, University of Edinburgh, August, 1876, by Lord Lister, the Founder of Modern Surgery

Surgery has undergone many great transformations during the past fifty years, and many are to be thanked for their contributions – yet when we think of how many remain to be made, it should rather stimulate our inventiveness than fuel our vanity.

Sir Percival Pott, 1714–88, Surgeon, St Bartholomew's Hospital, London, UK

If you cannot make a diagnosis at least make a decision!
Sir Harry Platt, 1897–1986,
Professor of Orthopaedics, Manchester, and President of the Royal College of Surgeons England, London, UK

If the surgeon cuts a vessel and knows the name of that vessel, the situation is serious; if the anaesthetist knows the name of that vessel, the situation is irretrievable.

Maldwyn Morgan 1938–
Anaesthetist, Hammersmith Hospital, London, UK

PART 1

Basic principles

1 Metabolic response to injury 2
2 Shock and blood transfusion 12
3 Wounds, healing and tissue repair 24
4 Tissue engineering and regeneration 33
5 Surgical infection 42
6 Tropical infections and infestations 57
7 Basic surgical skills and anastomoses 84
8 Principles of laparoscopic and robotic surgery 105
9 Principles of paediatric surgery 119
10 Principles of oncology 139
11 Surgical audit and research 161
12 Surgical ethics and law 170
13 Human factors, patient safety and quality improvement 176

Chapter 1

Metabolic response to injury

Learning objectives

To understand:

- Classical concepts of homeostasis
- Mediators of the metabolic response to injury
- Physiological and biochemical changes that occur during injury and recovery
- Changes in body composition that accompany surgical injury
- Avoidable factors that compound the metabolic response to injury
- Concepts behind optimal perioperative care

BASIC CONCEPTS IN HOMEOSTASIS

In the eighteenth and nineteenth centuries, a series of eminent scientists laid the foundations of our understanding of homeostasis and the response to injury. The classical concepts of homeostasis and the response to injury are:

- 'The stability of the "milieu intérieur" is the primary condition for freedom and independence of existence' (Claude Bernard); i.e. body systems act to maintain internal constancy.
- 'Homeostasis: the coordinated physiological process which maintains most of the steady states of the organism' (Walter Cannon); i.e. complex homeostatic responses involving the brain, nerves, heart, lungs, kidneys and spleen work to maintain body constancy.
- 'There is a circumstance attending accidental injury which does not belong to the disease, namely that the injury done, has in all cases a tendency to produce both the deposition and means of cure' (John Hunter); i.e. responses to injury are, in general, beneficial to the host and allow healing/survival.

In essence, the concept evolved that the constancy of the 'milieu intérieur' allowed for the independence of organisms, that complex homeostatic responses sought to maintain this constancy, and that within this range of responses were the elements of healing and repair. These ideas pertained to normal physiology and mild/moderate injury. In the modern era, such concepts do not account for disease evolution following major injury/sepsis or the injured patient who would have died but for artificial organ support. Such patients exemplify less of the classical homeostatic control system (signal detector–processor–effector regulated by a negative feedback loop) and more of the 'open loop' system, whereby only with medical/surgical resolution of the primary abnormality is a return to classical homeostasis possible.

As a consequence of modern understanding of the metabolic response to injury, elective surgical practice seeks to reduce the need for a homeostatic response by minimising the primary insult (minimal access surgery and 'stress-free' perioperative care). In emergency surgery, where the presence of tissue trauma/sepsis/hypovolaemia often compounds the primary problem, there is a requirement to augment artificially homeostatic responses (resuscitation) and to close the 'open' loop by intervening to resolve the primary insult (e.g. surgical treatment of major abdominal sepsis) and provide organ support (critical care) while the patient comes back to a situation in which homeostasis can achieve a return to normality.

Summary box 1.1

Basic concepts

- Homeostasis is the foundation of normal physiology
- 'Stress-free' perioperative care helps to preserve homeostasis following elective surgery
- Resuscitation, surgical intervention and critical care can return the severely injured patient to a situation in which homeostasis becomes possible once again

Claude Bernard, 1813–1878, Professor of Physiology, The College de France, Paris, France.
Walter Bradford Cannon, 1871–1945, Professor of Physiology, Harvard University Medical School, Boston, MA, USA.
John Hunter, 1728–1793, surgeon, St George's Hospital, London, UK. He is regarded as 'The Father of Scientific Surgery'. To further his knowledge of venereal disease he inoculated himself with syphilis in 1767.

This chapter aims to review the mediators of the stress response, the physiological and biochemical pathway changes associated with surgical injury and the changes in body composition that occur following surgical injury. Emphasis is laid on why knowledge of these events is important to understand the rationale for modern 'stress-free' perioperative and critical care.

THE GRADED NATURE OF THE INJURY RESPONSE

It is important to recognise that the response to injury is graded: the more severe the injury, the greater the response (**Figure 1.1**). This concept not only applies to physiological/metabolic changes but also to immunological changes/sequelae. Thus, following elective surgery of intermediate severity, there may be a transient and modest rise in temperature, heart rate, respiratory rate, energy expenditure and peripheral white cell count. Following major trauma/sepsis, these changes are accentuated, resulting in a systemic inflammatory response syndrome (SIRS), hypermetabolism, marked catabolism, shock and even multiple organ dysfunction (MODS). It is important to recognise that genetic variability plays a key role in determining the intensity of the inflammatory response. Moreover, in certain circumstances, the severity of injury does not lead to a simple dose-dependent metabolic response, but rather leads to quantitatively different responses.

Not only is the metabolic response graded, but it also evolves with time. In particular, the immunological sequelae of major injury evolve from a proinflammatory state driven primarily by the innate immune system (macrophages, neutrophils, dendritic cells) into a compensatory anti-inflammatory response syndrome (CARS) characterised by suppressed immunity and diminished resistance to infection. In patients who develop infective complications, the latter will drive ongoing systemic inflammation, the acute phase response and continued catabolism.

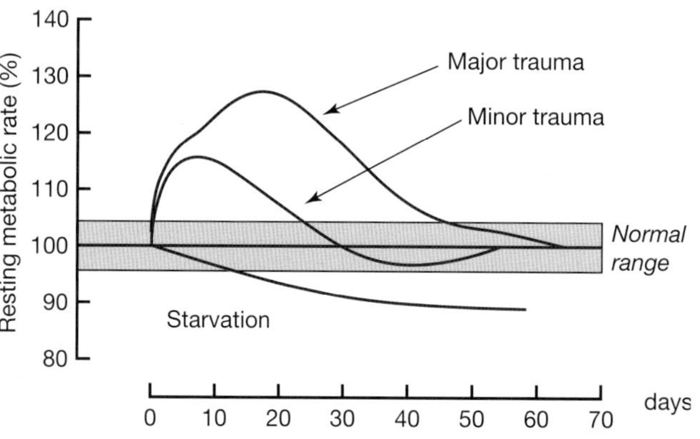

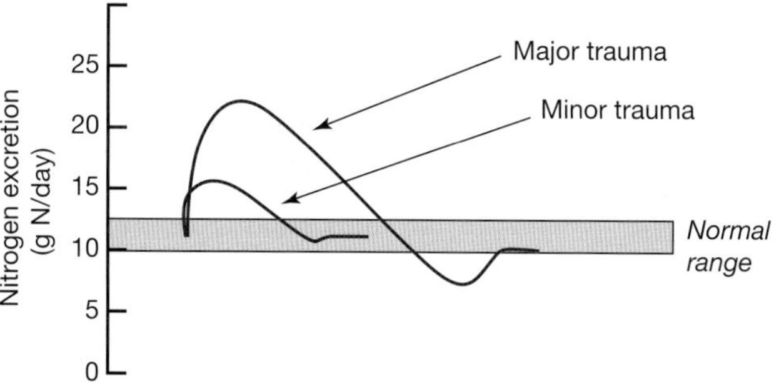

Figure 1.1 Hypermetabolism and increased nitrogen excretion are closely related to the magnitude of the initial injury and show a graded response.

MEDIATORS OF THE METABOLIC RESPONSE TO INJURY

The classical neuroendocrine pathways of the stress response consist of afferent nociceptive neurones, the spinal cord, thalamus, hypothalamus and pituitary (**Figure 1.2**). Corticotrophin-releasing factor (CRF) released from the hypothalamus increases adrenocorticotrophic hormone (ACTH) release from the anterior pituitary. ACTH then acts on the adrenals to increase the secretion of cortisol. Hypothalamic activation of the sympathetic nervous system causes release of adrenaline and also stimulates release of glucagon. Intravenous infusion of a cocktail of these 'counter-regulatory' hormones (glucagon, glucocorticoids and catecholamines) reproduces many aspects of the metabolic response to injury. There are, however, many other players, including alterations in insulin release and sensitivity, hypersecretion of prolactin and growth hormone (GH) in the presence of low circulatory insulin-like growth factor-1 (IGF-1) and inactivation of peripheral thyroid hormones and gonadal function. Of note, GH has direct lipolytic, insulin-antagonising and proinflammatory properties.

Summary box 1.2

Neuroendocrine response to injury/critical illness

The neuroendocrine response to severe injury/critical illness is biphasic:

- **Acute phase** characterised by an actively secreting pituitary and elevated counter-regulatory hormones (cortisol, glucagon, adrenaline). Changes are thought to be beneficial for short-term survival
- **Chronic phase** associated with hypothalamic suppression and low serum levels of the respective target organ hormones. Changes contribute to chronic wasting

The innate immune system (principally macrophages) interacts in a complex manner with the adaptive immune system (T cells, B cells) in co-generating the metabolic response to injury (**Figure 1.2**). Proinflammatory cytokines including interleukin-1 (IL-1), tumour necrosis factor alpha (TNFα), IL-6 and IL-8 are produced within the first 24 hours and act directly on the hypothalamus to cause pyrexia. Such cytokines also augment the hypothalamic stress response and act directly on skeletal muscle to induce proteolysis while inducing acute phase protein production in the liver. Proinflammatory cytokines also play a complex role in the development of peripheral insulin resistance. Other important proinflammatory mediators include nitric oxide ([NO]

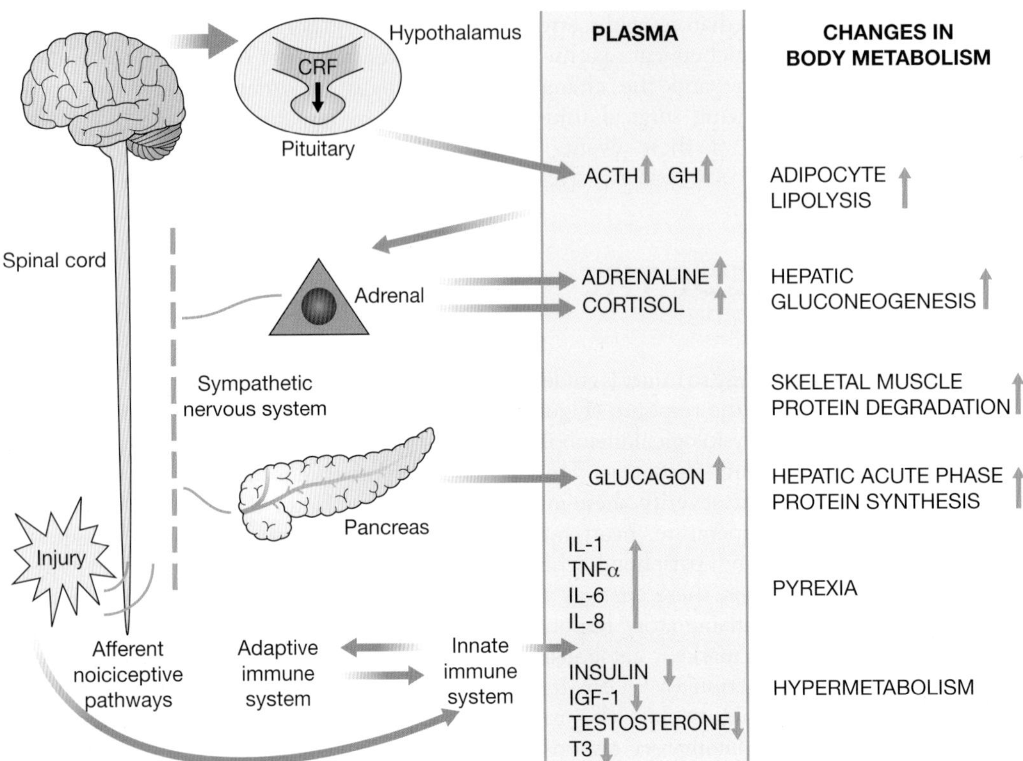

Figure 1.2 The integrated response to surgical injury (first 24–48 hours): there is a complex interplay between the neuroendocrine stress response and the proinflammatory cytokine response of the innate immune system.

via inducible nitric oxide synthetase [iNOS]) and a variety of prostanoids (via cyclooxygenase-2 [Cox-2]). Changes in organ function (e.g. renal hypoperfusion/impairment) may be induced by excessive vasoconstriction via endogenous factors such as endothelin-1.

Within hours of the upregulation of proinflammatory cytokines, endogenous cytokine antagonists enter the circulation (e.g. interleukin-1 receptor antagonist [IL-1Ra] and TNF-soluble receptors [TNF-sR-55 and 75]) and act to control the proinflammatory response. A complex further series of adaptive changes includes the development of a Th2-type counterinflammatory response (regulated by IL-4, -5, -9 and -13 and transforming growth factor beta [TGFβ]) which, if accentuated and prolonged in critical illness, is characterised as the CARS and results in immunosuppression and an increased susceptibility to opportunistic (nosocomial) infection. Within inflamed tissue the duration and magnitude of acute inflammation as well as the return to homeostasis are influenced by a group of local mediators known as specialised proresolving mediators (SPM) that include essential fatty acid-derived lipoxins, resolvins, protectins and maresins. These endogenous resolution agonists orchestrate the uptake and clearance of apoptotic polymorphonuclear neutrophils and microbial particles, reduce proinflammatory cytokines and lipid mediators as well as enhancing the removal of cellular debris in the inflammatory milieu. Thus, both at the systemic level (endogenous cytokine antagonists – see above) and at the local tissue level, the body attempts to limit/resolve inflammation driven dyshomeostasis.

Summary box 1.3

Systemic inflammatory response syndrome following major injury

- Is driven initially by proinflammatory cytokines (e.g. IL-1, IL-6 and TNFα)
- Is followed rapidly by increased plasma levels of cytokine antagonists and soluble receptors (e.g. IL-1Ra, TNF-sR)
- If prolonged or excessive may evolve into a counterinflammatory response syndrome

There are many complex interactions among the neuroendocrine, cytokine and metabolic axes. For example, although cortisol is immunosuppressive at high levels, it acts synergistically with IL-6 to promote the hepatic acute phase response. ACTH release is enhanced by proinflammatory cytokines and the noradrenergic system. The resulting rise in cortisol levels may form a weak feedback loop attempting to limit the proinflammatory stress response. Finally, hyperglycaemia may aggravate the inflammatory response via substrate overflow in the mitochondria, causing the formation of excess oxygen free radicals and also altering gene expression to enhance cytokine production.

At the molecular level, the changes that accompany systemic inflammation are extremely complex. In a recent study using network-based analysis of changes in mRNA expression in leukocytes following exposure to endotoxin, there were changes in the expression of more than 3700 genes with over half showing decreased expression and the remainder increased expression. The cell surface receptors, signalling mechanisms and transcription factors that initiate these events are also complex, but an early and important player involves the nuclear factor kappa B (NFκB)/*relA* family of transcription factors. A simplified model of current understanding of events within skeletal muscle is shown in Figure 1.3.

THE METABOLIC STRESS RESPONSE TO SURGERY AND TRAUMA: THE 'EBB AND FLOW' MODEL

In the natural world, if an animal is injured, it displays a characteristic response, which includes immobility, anorexia and catabolism.

Summary box 1.4

Physiological response to injury

The natural response to injury includes:

- Immobility/rest
- Anorexia
- Catabolism

The changes are designed to aid survival of moderate injury in the absence of medical intervention.

In 1930, Sir David Cuthbertson divided the metabolic response to injury in humans into 'ebb' and 'flow' phases (Figure 1.4). The ebb phase begins at the time of injury and lasts for approximately 24–48 hours. It may be attenuated by proper resuscitation, but not completely abolished. The ebb phase is characterised by hypovolaemia, decreased basal metabolic rate, reduced cardiac output, hypothermia and lactic acidosis. The predominant hormones regulating the ebb phase are catecholamines, cortisol and aldosterone (following activation of the renin–angiotensin system). The magnitude of this neuroendocrine response depends on the degree of blood loss and the stimulation of somatic afferent nerves at the site of injury. The main physiological role of the ebb phase is to conserve both circulating volume and energy stores for recovery and repair.

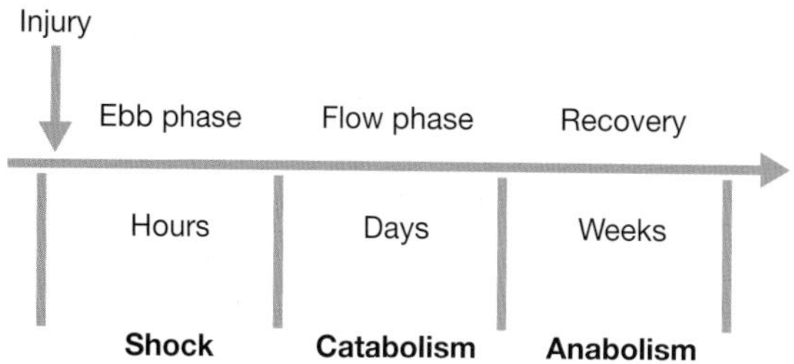

Figure 1.4 Phases of the physiological response to injury (after Cuthbertson 1930).

Following resuscitation, the ebb phase evolves into a hypermetabolic flow phase, which corresponds to SIRS. This phase involves the mobilisation of body energy stores for recovery and repair, and the subsequent replacement of lost or damaged tissue. It is characterised by tissue oedema (from vasodilatation and increased capillary leakage), increased basal metabolic rate (hypermetabolism), increased cardiac output, raised body temperature, leukocytosis, increased oxygen consumption and increased gluconeogenesis. The flow phase may be subdivided into an initial catabolic phase, lasting approximately 3–10 days, followed by an anabolic phase, which may last for weeks if extensive recovery and repair are required following serious injury. During the catabolic phase, the increased production of counter-regulatory hormones (including catecholamines, cortisol, insulin and glucagon) and inflammatory cytokines

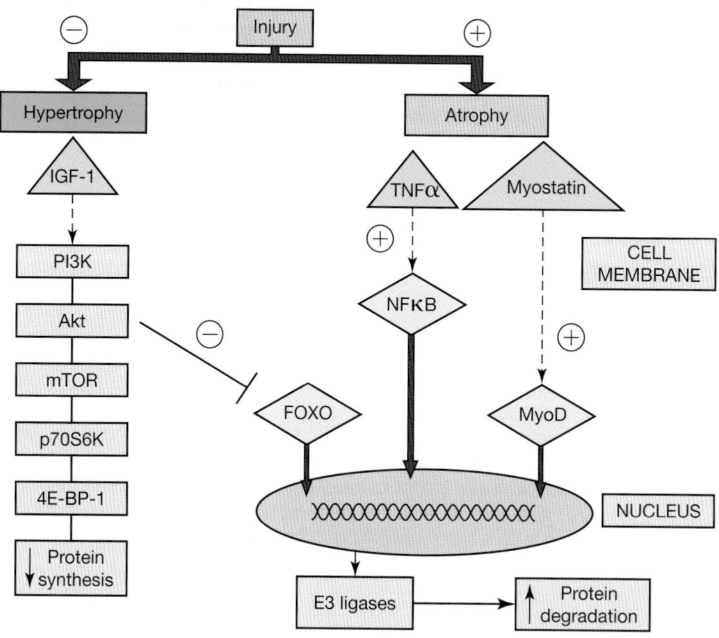

Figure 1.3 The major catabolic and anabolic signalling pathways involved in skeletal muscle homeostasis. FOXO, forkhead box sub-group O; mTOR, mammalian target of rapamycin; MyoD, myogenic differentiation factor D; NFκB, nuclear factor kappa B; PI3K, phosphatidylinositol 3-kinase; p70S6K, p70S6 kinase; TNFα, tumour necrosis factor alpha; 4E-BP-1, eukaryotic initiation translation factor 4E binding protein 1.

Sir David Paton Cuthbertson, 1900–1989, biochemist, Director of the Rowett Research Institute, Glasgow, UK.

(e.g. IL-1, IL-6 and TNFα) results in significant fat and protein mobilisation, leading to significant weight loss and increased urinary nitrogen excretion. The increased production of insulin at this time is associated with significant insulin resistance and, therefore, injured patients often exhibit poor glycaemic control. The combination of pronounced or prolonged catabolism in association with insulin resistance places patients within this phase at increased risk of complications. Obviously, the development of complications will further aggravate the neuroendocrine and inflammatory stress responses, thus creating a vicious catabolic cycle.

Summary box 1.5

Purpose of neuroendocrine changes following injury

The constellation of neuroendocrine changes following injury acts to:

- Provide essential substrates for survival
- Postpone anabolism
- Optimise host defence

These changes may be helpful in the short term, but may be harmful in the long term, especially to the severely injured patient who would otherwise not have survived without medical intervention.

KEY CATABOLIC ELEMENTS OF THE FLOW PHASE OF THE METABOLIC STRESS RESPONSE

There are several key elements of the flow phase that largely determine the extent of catabolism and thus govern the metabolic and nutritional care of the surgical patient. It must be remembered that, during the response to injury, not all tissues are catabolic. Indeed, the essence of this coordinated response is to allow the body to reprioritise limited resources away from peripheral tissues (muscle, adipose tissue, skin) and towards key viscera (liver, immune system) and the wound (**Figure 1.5**).

Hypermetabolism

The majority of trauma patients (except possibly those with extensive burns) demonstrate energy expenditures approximately 15–25% above predicted healthy resting values. The predominant cause appears to be a complex interaction between the central control of metabolic rate and peripheral energy utilisation. In particular, central thermodysregulation (caused by the proinflammatory cytokine cascade), increased sympathetic activity, abnormalities in wound circulation (ischaemic areas produce lactate, which must be metabolised by the adenosine triphosphate [ATP]-consuming hepatic Cori cycle; hyperaemic areas cause an increase in cardiac output), increased protein turnover and nutritional support may all increase patient energy expenditure. Theoretically, patient energy expenditure could rise even higher than observed levels following surgery or trauma, but several features of standard intensive care (including bed rest, paralysis, ventilation and external temperature regulation) counteract the hypermetabolic driving forces of the stress response. Furthermore, the skeletal muscle wasting experienced by patients with prolonged catabolism actually limits the volume of metabolically active tissue (see below).

Summary box 1.6

Hypermetabolism

Hypermetabolism following injury:

- Is mainly caused by an acceleration of energy-dependent metabolic cycles
- Is limited in modern practice on account of elements of routine critical care

Alterations in skeletal muscle protein metabolism

Muscle protein is continually synthesised and broken down with a turnover rate in humans of 1–2% per day, and with a greater amplitude of changes in protein synthesis (± twofold) than breakdown (± 0.25-fold) during the diurnal cycle. Under normal circumstances, synthesis equals breakdown and muscle bulk remains constant. Physiological stimuli that promote net muscle protein accretion include feeding (especially extracellular amino acid concentration) and exercise. Paradoxically, during exercise, skeletal muscle

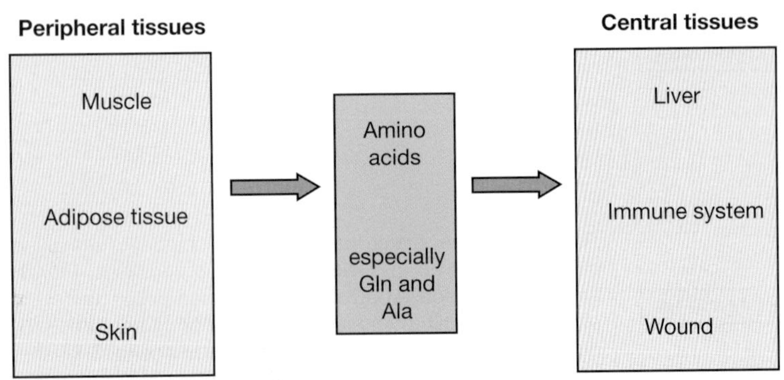

Figure 1.5 During the metabolic response to injury, the body reprioritises protein metabolism away from peripheral tissues and towards key central tissues such as the liver, immune system and wounds. One of the main reasons why the reutilisation of amino acids derived from muscle proteolysis leads to net catabolism is that the increased glutamine and alanine efflux from muscle is derived, in part, from the irreversible degradation of branched chain amino acids. Ala, alanine; Gln, glutamine.

Carl Ferdinand Cori, 1896–1984, Professor of Pharmacology, and later of Biochemistry, Washington University Medical School, St Louis, MI, USA and his wife Gerty Theresa Cori, 1896–1957, who was also Professor of Biochemistry at the Washington University Medical School. In 1947 the Coris were awarded a share of the Nobel Prize for Physiology or Medicine 'for their discovery of how glycogen is catalytically converted'.

protein synthesis is depressed, but it increases again during rest and feeding.

During the catabolic phase of the stress response, muscle wasting occurs as a result of an increase in muscle protein degradation (via enzymatic pathways), coupled with a decrease in muscle protein synthesis. The major site of protein loss is peripheral skeletal muscle, although nitrogen losses also occur in the respiratory muscles (predisposing the patient to hypoventilation and chest infections) and in the gut (reducing gut motility). Cardiac muscle appears to be mostly spared. Under extreme conditions of catabolism (e.g. major sepsis), urinary nitrogen losses can reach 14–20 g/day; this is equivalent to the loss of 500 g of skeletal muscle per day. It is remarkable that muscle catabolism cannot be inhibited fully by providing artificial nutritional support as long as the stress response continues. Indeed, in critical care, it is now recognised that 'hyperalimentation' represents a metabolic stress in itself, and that nutritional support should be at a modest level to attenuate rather than replace energy and protein losses.

The predominant mechanism involved in the wasting of skeletal muscle is the ATP-dependent ubiquitin–proteasome pathway (**Figure 1.6**), although the lysosomal cathepsins and the calcium–calpain pathway play facilitatory and accessory roles.

Clinically, a patient with skeletal muscle wasting will experience asthenia, increased fatigue, reduced functional ability, decreased quality of life and an increased risk of morbidity and mortality. In critically ill patients, muscle weakness may be further worsened by the development of critical illness myopathy, a multifactorial condition that is associated with impaired excitation–contraction coupling at the level of the sarcolemma and the sarcoplasmic reticulum membrane.

Summary box 1.7

Skeletal muscle wasting

- Provides amino acids for the metabolic support of central organs/tissues
- Is mediated at a molecular level mainly by activation of the ubiquitin–proteasome pathway
- Can result in immobility and contribute to hypostatic pneumonia and death if prolonged and excessive

Alterations in hepatic protein metabolism: the acute phase protein response

The liver and skeletal muscle together account for >50% of daily body protein turnover. Skeletal muscle has a large mass but a low turnover rate (1–2% per day), whereas the liver has a relatively small mass (1.5 kg) but a much higher protein turnover rate (10–20% per day). Hepatic protein synthesis is divided roughly 50:50 between renewal of structural proteins and synthesis of export proteins. Albumin is the major export protein produced by the liver and is renewed at the rate of about 10% per day. The transcapillary escape rate (TER) of albumin is about ten times the rate of synthesis, and short-term changes in albumin concentration are most probably due to increased vascular permeability. Albumin TER may be increased three-fold following major injury/sepsis.

In response to inflammatory conditions, including surgery, trauma, sepsis, cancer or autoimmune conditions, circulating peripheral blood mononuclear cells secrete a range of proinflammatory cytokines, including IL-1, IL-6 and TNFα.

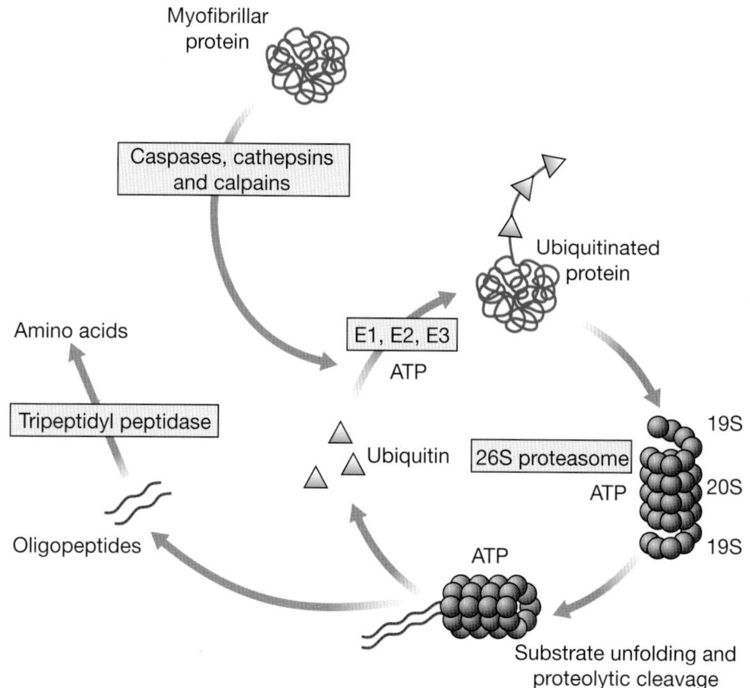

Figure 1.6 The intercellular effector mechanisms involved in degrading myofibrillar protein into free amino acids. The ubiquitin–proteasome pathway is a complex multistep process, which requires adenosine triphosphate and results in the tagging of specific proteins with ubiquitin for degradation of proteasome. E1, ubiquitin-activating enzyme; E2, ubiquitin-conjugating enzyme; E3, ubiquitin ligase.

These cytokines, in particular IL-6, promote the hepatic synthesis of positive acute phase proteins, e.g. fibrinogen and C-reactive protein (CRP). The acute phase protein response (APPR) represents a 'double-edged sword' for surgical patients as it provides proteins important for recovery and repair, but only at the expense of valuable lean tissue and energy reserves.

In contrast to the positive acute phase reactants, the plasma concentrations of other liver export proteins (the negative acute phase reactants) fall acutely following injury, e.g. albumin. However, rather than representing a reduced hepatic synthesis rate, the fall in plasma concentration of negative acute phase reactants is thought principally to reflect increased transcapillary escape, secondary to an increase in microvascular permeability (see above). Thus, increased hepatic synthesis of positive acute phase reactants is not compensated for by reduced synthesis of negative reactants.

Summary box 1.8

Hepatic acute phase response

The hepatic acute phase response represents a reprioritisation of body protein metabolism towards the liver and is characterised by:

- **Positive** reactants (e.g. CRP): plasma concentration ↑
- **Negative** reactants (e.g. albumin): plasma concentration ↓

Insulin resistance

Following surgery or trauma, postoperative hyperglycaemia develops as a result of increased glucose production combined with decreased glucose uptake in peripheral tissues. Decreased glucose uptake is a result of insulin resistance which is transiently induced within the stressed patient. Suggested mechanisms for this phenomenon include the action of proinflammatory cytokines and the decreased responsiveness of insulin-regulated glucose transporter proteins. The degree of insulin resistance is proportional to the magnitude of the injurious process. Following routine upper abdominal surgery, insulin resistance may persist for approximately 2 weeks.

Postoperative patients with insulin resistance behave in a similar manner to individuals with type II diabetes mellitus. The mainstay of management of insulin resistance is intravenous insulin infusion. Insulin infusions may be used in either an intensive approach (i.e. sliding scales are manipulated to normalise the blood glucose level) or a conservative approach (i.e. insulin is administered when the blood glucose level exceeds a defined limit and discontinued when the level falls). While some studies of postoperatively ventilated patients in the intensive care unit (ICU) have suggested that maintenance of normal glucose levels using intensive insulin therapy can significantly reduce both morbidity and mortality, others have not. The risks of adverse events following significant hypoglycaemia as a consequence of intensive insulin therapy have led most ICUs to adopt a more conventional approach to glycaemic control. It should be noted that diabetic patients whose glycaemic control has been poor prior to their critical illness pose a particular challenge.

CHANGES IN BODY COMPOSITION FOLLOWING INJURY

The average 70-kg male can be considered to consist of fat (13 kg) and fat-free mass (or lean body mass: 57 kg). In such an individual, the lean tissue is composed primarily of protein (12 kg), water (42 kg) and minerals (3 kg) (**Figure 1.7**). The protein mass can be considered as two basic compartments, skeletal muscle (4 kg) and non-skeletal muscle (8 kg), which includes the visceral protein mass. The water mass (42 litres) is divided into intracellular (28 litres) and extracellular (14 litres) spaces. Most of the mineral mass is contained in the bony skeleton.

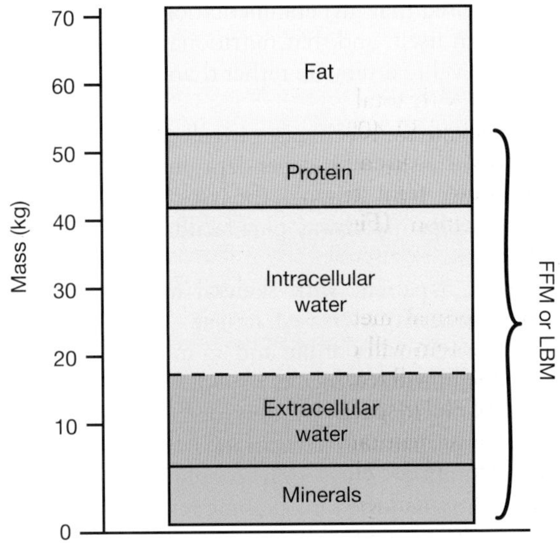

Figure 1.7 The chemical body composition of a normal 70-kg male. FFM, fat-free mass; LBM, lean body mass.

The main labile energy reserve in the body is fat, and the main labile protein reserve is skeletal muscle. While fat mass can be reduced without major detriment to function, loss of protein mass results not only in skeletal muscle wasting, but also in depletion of visceral protein status. Within lean issue, each 1 g of nitrogen is contained within 6.25 g of protein, which is contained in approximately 36 g of wet weight tissue. Thus, the loss of 1 g of nitrogen in urine is equivalent to the breakdown of 36 g of wet weight lean tissue. Protein turnover in the whole body is of the order of 150–200 g per day. A normal human ingests about 70–100 g protein per day, which is metabolised and excreted in urine as ammonia and urea (i.e. approximately 14 g N/day). During total starvation, urinary loss of nitrogen is rapidly attenuated by a series of adaptive changes. Loss of body weight follows a similar course (**Figure 1.8**), thus accounting for the survival of hunger strikers for a period of 50–60 days. Following major injury, and particularly in the presence of ongoing septic complications, this adaptive change fails to occur, and there is a state of 'autocannibalism', resulting in continuing urinary nitrogen losses of 10–20 g N/day (equivalent to 500 g of wet weight lean tissue

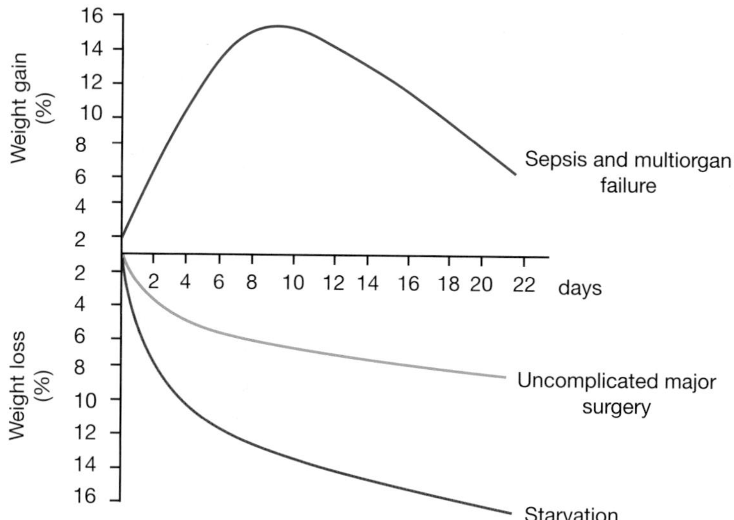

Figure 1.8 Changes in body weight that occur in serious sepsis, after uncomplicated surgery and in total starvation.

per day). As with total starvation, once loss of body protein mass has reached 30–40% of the total, survival is unlikely.

Critically ill patients admitted to the ICU with severe sepsis or major blunt trauma undergo massive changes in body composition (**Figure 1.8**). Body weight increases immediately on resuscitation with an expansion of extracellular water by 6–10 litres within 24 hours. Thereafter, even with optimal metabolic care and nutritional support, total body protein will diminish by 15% in the next 10 days, and body weight will reach negative balance as the expansion of the extracellular space resolves. In marked contrast, it is now possible to maintain body weight and nitrogen equilibrium following major elective surgery. This can be achieved by blocking the neuroendocrine stress response with epidural analgesia/other related techniques and providing early oral/enteral feeding. Moreover, the early fluid retention phase can be avoided by careful intraoperative management of fluid balance, with avoidance of excessive administration of intravenous saline.

Summary box 1.9

Changes in body composition following major surgery/critical illness

- Catabolism leads to a **decrease** in fat mass and skeletal muscle mass
- Body weight may paradoxically **increase** because of expansion of extracellular fluid space

AVOIDABLE FACTORS THAT COMPOUND THE RESPONSE TO INJURY

As noted previously, the main features of the metabolic response are initiated by the immune system, cardiovascular system, sympathetic nervous system, ascending reticular formation and limbic system. However, the metabolic stress response may be further exacerbated by anaesthesia, dehydration, starvation (including preoperative fasting), sepsis, acute medical illness or even severe psychological stress (**Figure 1.9**). Attempts to limit or control these factors can be beneficial to the patient.

Summary box 1.10

Avoidable factors that compound the response to injury

- Continuing haemorrhage
- Hypothermia
- Tissue oedema
- Tissue underperfusion
- Starvation
- Immobility

Volume loss

During simple haemorrhage, pressor receptors in the carotid artery and aortic arch, and volume receptors in the wall of the left atrium, initiate afferent nerve input to the central nervous system (CNS), resulting in the release of both aldosterone and antidiuretic hormone (ADH). Pain can also stimulate ADH release. ADH acts directly on the kidney to cause fluid retention. Decreased pulse pressure stimulates the juxtaglomerular apparatus in the kidney and directly activates the renin–angiotensin system, which in turn increases aldosterone release.

Aldosterone causes the renal tubule to reabsorb sodium (and consequently also conserve water). ACTH release also augments the aldosterone response. The net effects of ADH and aldosterone result in the natural oliguria observed after surgery and conservation of sodium and water in the extracellular space. The tendency towards water and salt retention is exacerbated by resuscitation with saline-rich fluids. Salt and water retention can result in not only peripheral oedema, but also visceral oedema (e.g. in the stomach). Such visceral oedema has been associated with reduced gastric emptying, delayed resumption of food intake and prolonged hospital

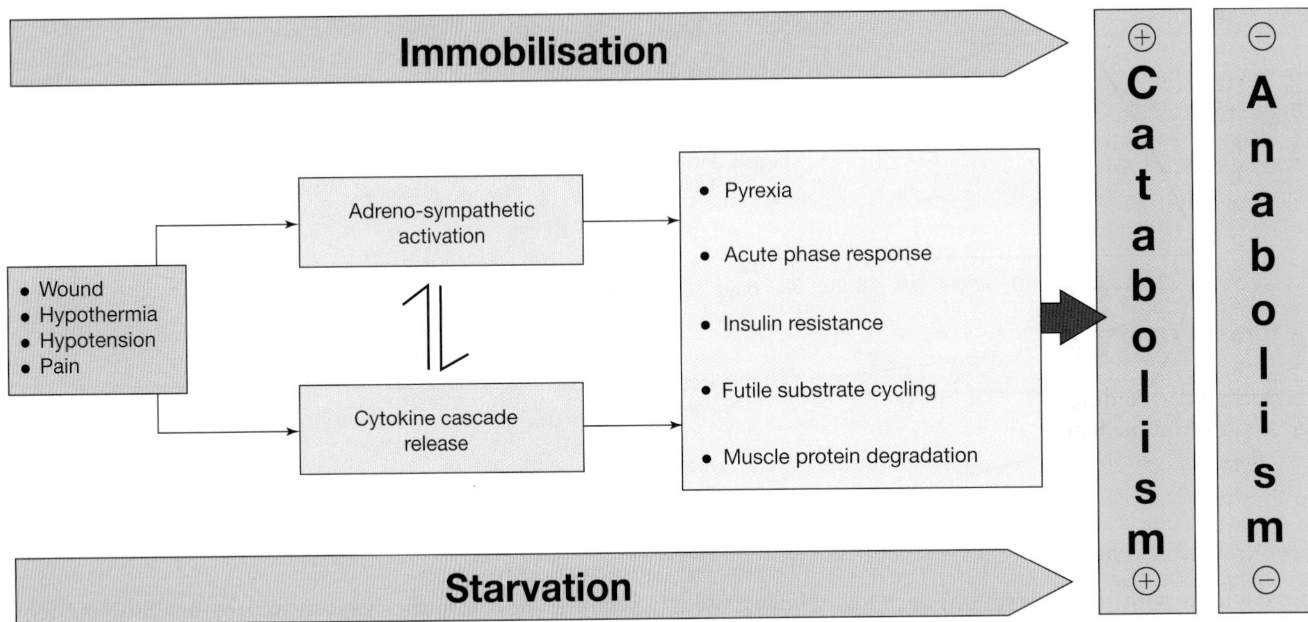

Figure 1.9 Factors that exacerbate the metabolic response to surgical injury include hypothermia, uncontrolled pain, starvation, immobilisation, sepsis and medical complications.

stay. Careful limitation of intraoperative administration of balanced crystalloids so that there is no net weight gain following elective surgery has been proven to reduce postoperative complications and length of stay.

Hypothermia

Hypothermia results in increased elaboration of adrenal steroids and catecholamines. When compared with normothermic controls, even mild hypothermia results in a two- to three-fold increase in postoperative cardiac arrhythmias and increased catabolism. Randomised trials have shown that maintaining normothermia by an upper body forced-air heating cover reduces wound infections, cardiac complications and bleeding and transfusion requirements.

Tissue oedema

During systemic inflammation, fluid, plasma proteins, leukocytes, macrophages and electrolytes leave the vascular space and accumulate in the tissues. This can diminish the alveolar diffusion of oxygen and may lead to reduced renal function. Increased capillary leak is mediated by a wide variety of mediators including cytokines, prostanoids, bradykinin and nitric oxide. Vasodilatation implies that intravascular volume decreases, which induces shock if inadequate resuscitation is not undertaken. Meanwhile, intracellular volume decreases, and this provides part of the volume necessary to replenish intravascular and extravascular extracellular volume.

Systemic inflammation and tissue underperfusion

The vascular endothelium controls vasomotor tone and microvascular flow, and regulates trafficking of nutrients and biologically active molecules. When endothelial activation is excessive, compromised microcirculation and subsequent cellular hypoxia contribute to the risk of organ failure. Maintaining normoglycaemia with insulin infusion during critical illness has been proposed to protect the endothelium, probably, in part, via inhibition of excessive iNOS-induced NO release.

Starvation

During starvation, the body is faced with an obligate need to generate glucose to sustain cerebral energy metabolism (100 g of glucose per day). This is achieved in the first 24 hours by mobilising glycogen stores and thereafter by hepatic gluconeogenesis from amino acids, glycerol and lactate. The energy metabolism of other tissues is sustained by mobilising fat from adipose tissue. Such fat mobilisation is mainly dependent on a fall in circulating insulin levels. Eventually, accelerated loss of lean tissue (the main source of amino acids for hepatic gluconeogenesis) is reduced as a result of the liver converting free fatty acids into ketone bodies, which can serve as a substitute for glucose for cerebral energy metabolism. Provision of 2 litres of intravenous 4% dextrose/0.18% sodium chloride as maintenance intravenous fluids for surgical patients who are fasted provides 80 g of glucose per day and has a significant protein-sparing effect. Avoiding unnecessary fasting in the first instance and early oral/enteral/parenteral nutrition form the platform for avoiding loss of body mass as a result of the varying degrees of starvation observed in surgical patients. Modern guidelines on fasting prior to anaesthesia allow intake of clear fluids up to 2 hours before surgery. Administration of a carbohydrate drink at this time reduces perioperative anxiety and thirst and decreases postoperative insulin resistance.

Immobility

Immobility has long been recognised as a potent stimulus for inducing muscle wasting. Inactivity impairs the normal meal-derived amino acid stimulation of protein synthesis in skeletal muscle. Avoidance of unnecessary bed rest and active early mobilisation are essential measures to avoid muscle wasting as a consequence of immobility.

CONCEPTS BEHIND ENHANCED RECOVERY AFTER SURGERY

Current understanding of the metabolic response to surgical injury and the mediators involved has led to a reappraisal of traditional perioperative care. There is now a strong scientific rationale for avoiding unmodulated exposure to stress, prolonged fasting and excessive administration of intravenous (saline) fluids (**Figure 1.10**). The widespread adoption of minimal access (laparoscopic) surgery is a key change in surgical practice that can reduce the magnitude of surgical injury and enhance the rate of patients' return to homeostasis and recovery. It is also important to realise that modulating the stress/inflammatory response at the time of surgery may have long-term sequelae over periods of months or longer. For example, β-blockers and statins have been shown to improve long-term survival after major surgery. It has been suggested that these effects may be due to suppression of innate immunity at the time of surgery. Equally, in 'open' surgery the use of epidural analgesia to reduce pain, block the cortisol stress response and attenuate postoperative insulin resistance may, via effects on the body's protein economy, favourably affect many of the patient-centred outcomes that are important to postoperative recovery. Due to the reduction in wound size and tissue trauma, it should be noted that epidural analgesia is no longer recommended for laparoscopic surgery. Patient controlled analgesia is usually sufficient. Adjuncts such as 'one shot' spinal diamorphine and/or a 6–12-hour infusion of intravenous lidocaine have been suggested to be opiate sparing, to improve gut function and enhance overall recovery.

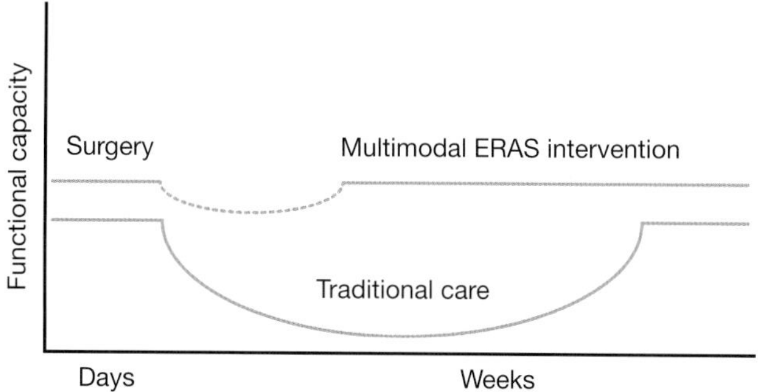

Figure 1.10 Enhanced recovery after surgery (ERAS) programmes can be modulated by multimodal enhanced recovery programmes (optimal nutritional and metabolic care to minimise the stress response).

Summary box 1.11

A proactive approach to prevent unnecessary aspects of the surgical stress response

- Minimal access techniques
- Blockade of afferent painful stimuli (e.g. epidural analgesia, spinal analgesia, wound catheters)
- Minimal periods of starvation
- Early mobilisation

FURTHER READING

Bessey PQ, Watters JM, Aoki TT, Wilmore DW. Combined hormonal infusion simulates the metabolic response to injury. *Ann Surg* 1984; **200**: 264–81.

Cuthbertson DP. The disturbance of metabolism produced by bone and non-bony injury, with notes on certain abnormal conditions of bone. *Biochem J* 1930; **24**: 1244.

Fearon KCH, Ljungqvist O, von Meyenfeldt M *et al*. Enhanced recovery after surgery: a consensus review of clinical care for patients undergoing colonic resection. *Clin Nutr* 2005; **24**: 466–77.

Finfer S, Chittock DR, Su SY *et al*., NICE-SUGAR Study Investigators. Intensive versus conventional glucose control in critically ill patients. *N Engl J Med* 2009; **360**: 1283–97.

Finfer S, Chittock DR, Su SY *et al*., NICE-SUGAR Study Investigators. Intensive versus conventional glucose control in critically ill patients with traumatic brain injury: long term follow-up in a subgroup of patients from the NICE-SUGAR study. *Intensive Care Med* 2015; **41**: 1037–47.

Ljungqvist O. Insulin resistance and outcomes in surgery. *J Clin Endocrinol Metab* 2010; **95**: 4217–19.

Lobo DN, Bostock KA, Neal KR *et al*. Effect of salt and water balance on recovery of gastrointestinal function after elective colonic resection: a randomised controlled trial. *Lancet* 2002; **359**: 1812–18.

Moore FO. *Metabolic care of the surgical patient*. Philadelphia, PA: WB Saunders Company, 1959.

Scott MJ, Baldini G, Fearon KC *et al*. Enhanced Recovery After Surgery (ERAS) for gastrointestinal surgery, part 1: pathophysiological considerations. *Acta Anaesthesiol Scand* 2015; **59**: 1212–31.

Van den Berghe G, Wonters P, Weckers F *et al*. Intensive insulin therapy in the critically ill patient. *N Engl J Med* 2001; **345**: 1359–67.

Vanhorebeek O, Langounche L, Van den Berghe G. Endocrine aspects of acute and prolonged critical illness. *Nat Clin Pract Endocrinol Metab* 2006; **2**: 20–31.

Wilmore DW. From Cuthbertson to fast-track surgery: 70 years of progress in reducing stress in surgical patients. *Ann Surg* 2002; **236**: 643–8.

Chapter 2

Shock and blood transfusion

Learning objectives

To understand:

- The pathophysiology of shock and ischaemia–reperfusion injury
- The different patterns of shock and the principles and priorities of resuscitation
- Appropriate monitoring and end points of resuscitation
- Use of blood and blood products, the benefits and risks of blood transfusion

INTRODUCTION

Shock is the most common and therefore the most important cause of death of surgical patients. Death may occur rapidly due to a profound state of shock, or be delayed due to the consequences of organ ischaemia and reperfusion injury. It is important therefore that every surgeon understands the pathophysiology, diagnosis and priorities in management of shock and haemorrhage.

SHOCK

Shock is a systemic state of low tissue perfusion that is inadequate for normal cellular respiration. With insufficient delivery of oxygen and glucose, cells switch from aerobic to anaerobic metabolism. If perfusion is not restored in a timely fashion, cell death ensues.

Pathophysiology

Cellular

As perfusion to the tissues is reduced, cells are deprived of oxygen and must switch from aerobic to anaerobic metabolism. The product of anaerobic respiration is not carbon dioxide but lactic acid. When enough tissue is underperfused, the accumulation of lactic acid in the blood produces a systemic metabolic acidosis.

As glucose within cells is exhausted, anaerobic respiration ceases and there is failure of sodium/potassium pumps in the cell membrane and intracellular organelles. Intracellular lysosomes release autodigestive enzymes and cell lysis ensues. Intracellular contents, including potassium, are released into the blood stream.

Microvascular

As tissue ischaemia progresses, changes in the local milieu result in activation of the immune and coagulation systems. Hypoxia and acidosis activate complement and prime neutrophils, resulting in the generation of oxygen free radicals and cytokine release. These mechanisms lead to injury of the capillary endothelial cells. These, in turn, further activate the immune and coagulation systems. Damaged endothelium loses its integrity and becomes 'leaky'. Spaces between endothelial cells allow fluid to leak out and tissue oedema ensues, exacerbating cellular hypoxia.

Systemic

CARDIOVASCULAR

As preload and afterload decrease, there is a compensatory baroreceptor response resulting in increased sympathetic activity and release of catecholamines into the circulation. This results in tachycardia and systemic vasoconstriction (except in sepsis – see below).

RESPIRATORY

The metabolic acidosis and increased sympathetic response result in an increased respiratory rate and minute ventilation to increase the excretion of carbon dioxide (and so produce a compensatory respiratory alkalosis).

RENAL

Decreased perfusion pressure in the kidney leads to reduced filtration at the glomerulus and a decreased urine output. The renin–angiotensin–aldosterone axis is stimulated, resulting in further vasoconstriction and increased sodium and water reabsorption by the kidney.

ENDOCRINE

As well as activation of the adrenal and renin–angiotensin systems, vasopressin (antidiuretic hormone) is released from the hypothalamus in response to decreased preload and results in vasoconstriction and resorption of water in the renal collecting system. Cortisol is also released from the adrenal cortex, contributing to the sodium and water resorption and sensitising cells to catecholamines.

Ischaemia-reperfusion syndrome

During the period of systemic hypoperfusion, cellular and organ damage progresses due to the direct effects of tissue hypoxia and local activation of inflammation. Further injury occurs once normal circulation is restored to these tissues. The acid and potassium load that has built up can lead to direct myocardial depression, vascular dilatation and further hypotension. The cellular and humoral elements activated by the hypoxia (complement, neutrophils, microvascular thrombi) are flushed back into the circulation where they cause further endothelial injury to organs such as the lungs and the kidneys. This leads to acute lung injury, acute renal injury, multiple organ failure and death. Reperfusion injury can currently only be attenuated by reducing the extent and duration of tissue hypoperfusion.

Classification of shock

There are numerous ways to classify shock, but the most common and most clinically applicable is one based on the initiating mechanism.

All states are characterised by systemic tissue hypoperfusion, and different states may coexist within the same patient.

Summary box 2.1

Classification of shock

- Hypovolaemic shock
- Cardiogenic shock
- Obstructive shock
- Distributive shock
- Endocrine shock

Hypovolaemic shock

Hypovolaemic shock is due to a reduced circulating volume. Hypovolaemia may be due to haemorrhagic or non-haemorrhagic causes. Non-haemorrhagic causes include poor fluid intake (dehydration), excessive fluid loss due to vomiting, diarrhoea, urinary loss (e.g. diabetes), evaporation, or 'third-spacing' where fluid is lost into the gastrointestinal tract and interstitial spaces, as for example in bowel obstruction or pancreatitis.

Hypovolaemia is probably the most common form of shock, and to some degree is a component of all other forms of shock. Absolute or relative hypovolaemia must be excluded or treated in the management of the shocked state, regardless of cause.

Cardiogenic shock

Cardiogenic shock is due to primary failure of the heart to pump blood to the tissues. Causes of cardiogenic shock include myocardial infarction, cardiac dysrhythmias, valvular heart disease, blunt myocardial injury and cardiomyopathy. Cardiac insufficiency may also be due to myocardial depression caused by endogenous factors (e.g. bacterial and humoral agents released in sepsis) or exogenous factors, such as pharmaceutical agents or drug abuse. Evidence of venous hypertension with pulmonary or systemic oedema may coexist with the classical signs of shock.

Obstructive shock

In obstructive shock there is a reduction in preload due to mechanical obstruction of cardiac filling. Common causes of obstructive shock include cardiac tamponade, tension pneumothorax, massive pulmonary embolus or air embolus. In each case, there is reduced filling of the left and/or right sides of the heart leading to reduced preload and a fall in cardiac output.

Distributive shock

Distributive shock describes the pattern of cardiovascular responses characterising a variety of conditions, including septic shock, anaphylaxis and spinal cord injury. Inadequate organ perfusion is accompanied by vascular dilatation with hypotension, low systemic vascular resistance, inadequate afterload and a resulting abnormally high cardiac output.

In anaphylaxis, vasodilatation is due to histamine release, while in high spinal cord injury there is failure of sympathetic outflow and adequate vascular tone (neurogenic shock). The cause in sepsis is less clear but is related to the release of bacterial products (endotoxin) and the activation of cellular and humoral components of the immune system. There is maldistribution of blood flow at a microvascular level with arteriovenous shunting and dysfunction of cellular utilization of oxygen.

In the later phases of septic shock there is hypovolaemia from fluid loss into interstitial spaces and there may be concomitant myocardial depression, complicating the clinical picture (*Table 2.1*).

Endocrine shock

Endocrine shock may present as a combination of hypovolaemic, cardiogenic or distributive shock. Causes of endocrine shock include hypo- and hyperthyroidism and adrenal insufficiency. Hypothyroidism causes a shock state similar to that of neurogenic shock due to disordered vascular and cardiac responsiveness to circulating catecholamines. Cardiac output falls due to low inotropy and bradycardia. There may also be an associated cardiomyopathy. Thyrotoxicosis may cause a high-output cardiac failure.

Adrenal insufficiency leads to shock due to hypovolaemia and a poor response to circulating and exogenous catecholamines. Adrenal insufficiency may be due to pre-existing Addison's disease or be a relative insufficiency due to a pathological disease state, such as systemic sepsis.

Thomas Addison, 1799–1860, physician, Guy's Hospital, London, UK, described the effects of disease of the suprarenal capsules in 1849.

TABLE 2.1 Cardiovascular and metabolic characteristics of shock.

	Hypovolaemia	Cardiogenic	Obstructive	Distributive
Cardiac output Vascular resistance	Low High	Low High	Low High	High Low
Venous pressure	Low	High	High	Low
Mixed venous saturation Base deficit	Low High	Low High	Low High	High High

Severity of shock

Compensated shock

As shock progresses, the body's cardiovascular and endocrine compensatory responses reduce flow to non-essential organs to preserve preload and flow to the lungs and brain. In compensated shock, there is adequate compensation to maintain central blood volume and preserve flow to the kidneys, lungs and brain. Apart from a tachycardia and cool peripheries (vasoconstriction, circulating catecholamines), there may be no other clinical signs of hypovolaemia.

However, this cardiovascular state is only maintained by reducing perfusion to the skin, muscle and gastrointestinal tract. There is a systemic metabolic acidosis and activation of humoral and cellular elements within the underperfused organs. Although clinically occult, this state will lead to multiple organ failure and death if prolonged, due to the ischaemia–reperfusion effect described above under **Ischaemia–reperfusion syndrome**. Patients with occult hypoperfusion (metabolic acidosis despite normal urine output and cardiorespiratory vital signs) for more than 12 hours have a significantly higher mortality, infection rate and incidence of multiple organ failure (see below, **Multiple organ failure**).

Decompensation

Further loss of circulating volume overloads the body's compensatory mechanisms and there is progressive renal, respiratory and cardiovascular decompensation. In general, loss of around 15% of the circulating blood volume is within normal compensatory mechanisms. Blood pressure is usually well maintained and only falls after 30–40% of circulating volume has been lost.

Mild shock

Initially there is tachycardia, tachypnoea, a mild reduction in urine output and the patient may exhibit mild anxiety. Blood pressure is maintained although there is a decrease in pulse pressure. The peripheries are cool and sweaty with prolonged capillary refill times (except in septic distributive shock).

Moderate shock

As shock progresses, renal compensatory mechanisms fail, renal perfusion falls and urine output dips below 0.5 mL/kg per hour. There is further tachycardia, and now the blood pressure starts to fall. Patients become drowsy and mildly confused.

Severe shock

In severe shock, there is profound tachycardia and hypotension. Urine output falls to zero and patients are unconscious with laboured respiration.

Pitfalls

The classic cardiovascular responses described (*Table 2.2*) are not seen in every patient. It is important to recognise the limitations of the clinical examination and to recognise patients who are in shock despite the absence of classic signs.

CAPILLARY REFILL

Most patients in hypovolaemic shock will have cool, pale peripheries, with prolonged capillary refill times. However, the actual capillary refill time varies so much in adults that it is not a specific marker of whether a patient is shocked, and patients with short capillary refill times may be in the early stages of shock. In distributive (septic) shock, the peripheries will be warm and capillary refill will be brisk, despite profound shock.

TACHYCARDIA

Tachycardia may not always accompany shock. Patients who are on beta-blockers or who have implanted pacemakers are unable to mount a tachycardia. A pulse rate of 80 in a fit young adult who normally has a pulse rate of 50 is very abnormal. Furthermore, in some young patients with penetrating trauma, where there is haemorrhage but little tissue damage, there may be a paradoxical bradycardia rather than tachycardia accompanying the shocked state.

TABLE 2.2 Clinical features of shock.

	Compensated	Mild	Moderate	Severe
Lactic acidosis	+	++	++	+++
Urine output	Normal	Normal	Reduced	Anuric
Conscious level	Normal	Mild anxiety	Drowsy	Comatose
Respiratory rate	Normal	Increased	Increased	Laboured
Pulse rate	Mild increase	Increased	Increased	Increased
Blood pressure	Normal	Normal	Mild hypotension	Severe hypotension

BLOOD PRESSURE

It is important to recognise that hypotension is one of the last signs of shock. Children and fit young adults are able to maintain blood pressure until the final stages of shock by dramatic increases in stroke volume and peripheral vasoconstriction. These patients can be in profound shock with a normal blood pressure.

Elderly patients who are normally hypertensive may present with a 'normal' blood pressure for the general population but be hypovolaemic and hypotensive relative to their usual blood pressure. Beta-blockers or other medications may prevent a tachycardic response. The diagnosis of shock may be difficult unless one is alert to these pitfalls.

Consequences

Unresuscitatable shock

Patients who are in profound shock for a prolonged period of time become 'unresuscitatable'. Cell death follows from cellular ischaemia and the ability of the body to compensate is lost. There is myocardial depression and loss of responsiveness to fluid or inotropic therapy. Peripherally there is loss of the ability to maintain systemic vascular resistance and further hypotension ensues. The peripheries no longer respond appropriately to vasopressor agents. Death is the inevitable result.

This stage of shock is the combined result of the severity of the insult and delayed, inadequate or inappropriate resuscitation in the earlier stages of shock. Conversely, when patients present in this late stage, and have minimal responses to maximal therapy, it is important that the futility of treatment is recognised and valuable resources are not wasted.

Multiple organ failure

As techniques of resuscitation have improved, more and more patients are surviving shock. Where intervention is timely and the period of shock is limited, patients may make a rapid, uncomplicated recovery. However the result of prolonged systemic ischaemia and reperfusion injury is end-organ damage and multiple organ failure.

Multiple organ failure is defined as two or more failed organ systems. There is no specific treatment for multiple organ failure. Management is supporting of organ systems, with ventilation, cardiovascular support and haemofiltration/dialysis until there is recovery of organ function. Multiple organ failure currently carries a mortality of 60%; thus, prevention is vital by early aggressive identification and reversal of shock.

Summary box 2.2

Effects of organ failure

- Lung: Acute respiratory distress syndrome
- Kidney: Acute renal insufficiency
- Clotting: Coagulopathy
- Cardiac: Cardiovascular failure

RESUSCITATION

Immediate resuscitation manoeuvres for patients presenting in shock are to ensure a patent airway and adequate oxygenation and ventilation. Once 'airway' and 'breathing' are assessed and controlled, attention is directed to cardiovascular resuscitation.

Conduct of resuscitation

Resuscitation should not be delayed in order to definitively diagnose the source of the shocked state. However, the timing and nature of resuscitation will depend on the type of shock and the timing and severity of the insult. Rapid clinical examination will provide adequate clues to make an appropriate first determination, even if a source of bleeding or sepsis is not immediately identifiable. If there is initial doubt about the cause of shock, it is safer to assume the cause is hypovolaemia and begin with fluid resuscitation, and then assess the response.

In patients who are actively bleeding (major trauma, aortic aneurysm rupture, gastrointestinal haemorrhage), it is counterproductive to institute high-volume fluid therapy without controlling the site of haemorrhage. Increasing blood pressure merely increases bleeding from the site while fluid therapy cools the patient and dilutes available coagulation factors. Thus operative haemorrhage control should not be delayed and resuscitation should proceed in parallel with surgery.

Conversely, a patient with bowel obstruction and hypovolaemic shock must be adequately resuscitated before undergoing surgery otherwise the additional surgical injury and hypovolaemia induced during the procedure will exacerbate the inflammatory activation and increase the incidence and severity of end-organ insult.

Fluid therapy

In all cases of shock, regardless of classification, hypovolaemia and inadequate preload must be addressed before other therapy is instituted. Administration of inotropic or chronotropic agents to an empty heart will rapidly and permanently deplete the myocardium of oxygen stores and dramatically reduce diastolic filling and therefore coronary perfusion. Patients will enter the unresuscitatable stage of shock as the myocardium becomes progressively more ischaemic and unresponsive to resuscitative attempts.

First-line therapy, therefore, is intravenous access and administration of intravenous fluids. Access should be through short, wide-bore catheters that allow rapid infusion of fluids as necessary. Long, narrow lines, such as central venous catheters, have too high a resistance to allow rapid infusion and are more appropriate for monitoring than fluid replacement therapy.

Type of fluids

There is continuing debate over which resuscitation fluid is best for the management of shock. There is no ideal resuscitation fluid, and it is more important to understand how and when to administer it. In most studies of shock resuscitation there is no overt difference in response or outcome between crystalloid solutions (normal saline, Hartmann's solution, Ringer's lactate) or colloids (albumin or commercially available products). Furthermore, there is less volume benefit to the administration of colloids than had previously been thought, with only 1.3 times more crystalloid than colloid administered in blinded trials. On balance, there is little evidence to support the administration of colloids, which are more expensive and have worse side-effect profiles.

Most importantly, the oxygen carrying capacity of crystalloids and colloids is zero. If blood is being lost, the ideal replacement fluid is blood, although crystalloid therapy may be required while awaiting blood products.

Hypotonic solutions (dextrose etc.) are poor volume expanders and should not be used in the treatment of shock unless the deficit is free water loss (e.g. diabetes insipidus) or patients are sodium overloaded (e.g. cirrhosis).

Dynamic fluid response

The shock status can be determined dynamically by the cardiovascular response to the rapid administration of a fluid bolus. In total, 250–500 mL of fluid is rapidly given (over 5–10 minutes) and the cardiovascular responses in terms of heart rate, blood pressure and central venous pressure are observed. Patients can be divided into 'responders', 'transient responders' and 'non-responders'.

Responders have an improvement in their cardiovascular status that is sustained. These patients are not actively losing fluid but require filling to a normal volume status.

Transient responders have an improvement, but this then reverts to the previous state over the next 10–20 minutes. These patients have moderate ongoing fluid losses (either overt haemorrhage or further fluid shifts reducing intravascular volume).

Non-responders are severely volume depleted and are likely to have major ongoing loss of intravascular volume, usually through persistent uncontrolled haemorrhage.

Vasopressor and inotropic support

Vasopressor or inotropic therapy is not indicated as first-line therapy in hypovolaemia. As discussed above, administration of these agents in the absence of adequate preload rapidly leads to decreased coronary perfusion and depletion of myocardial oxygen reserves.

Vasopressor agents (phenylephrine, noradrenaline) are indicated in distributive shock states (sepsis, neurogenic shock) where there is peripheral vasodilatation, and a low systemic vascular resistance, leading to hypotension despite a high cardiac output. Where the vasodilatation is resistant to catecholamines (e.g. absolute or relative steroid deficiency) vasopressin may be used as an alternative vasopressor.

In cardiogenic shock, or where myocardial depression has complicated a shock state (e.g. severe septic shock with low cardiac output), inotropic therapy may be required to increase cardiac output and therefore oxygen delivery. The inodilator dobutamine is the agent of choice.

Monitoring

The **minimum** standard for monitoring of the patient in shock is continuous heart rate and oxygen saturation monitoring, frequent non-invasive blood pressure monitoring and hourly urine output measurements. Most patients will need more aggressive invasive monitoring, including central venous pressure and invasive blood pressure monitoring.

Summary box 2.3

Monitoring for patients in shock

Minimum
- ECG
- Pulse oximetry
- Blood pressure
- Urine output

Additional modalities
- Central venous pressure
- Invasive blood pressure
- Cardiac output
- Base deficit and serum lactate

Cardiovascular

Cardiovascular monitoring at minimum should include continuous heart rate (ECG), oxygen saturation and pulse waveform and non-invasive blood pressure. Patients whose state of shock is not rapidly corrected with a small amount of fluid should have central venous pressure monitoring and continuous blood pressure monitoring through an arterial line.

CENTRAL VENOUS PRESSURE

There is no 'normal' central venous pressure (CVP) for a shocked patient, and reliance cannot be placed on an individual pressure measurement to assess volume status. Some patients may require a CVP of 5 cmH_2O, whereas some may require a CVP of 15 cmH_2O or higher. Further, ventricular compliance can change from minute to minute in the shocked state, and CVP is a poor reflection of end diastolic volume (preload).

CVP measurements should be assessed dynamically as response to a fluid challenge (see above). A fluid bolus (250–500 mL) is infused rapidly over 5–10 minutes.

The normal CVP response is a rise of 2–5 cmH_2O which gradually drifts back to the original level over 10–20 minutes. Patients with no change in their CVP are empty and require further fluid resuscitation. Patients with a large, sustained rise in CVP have high preload and an element of cardiac insufficiency or volume overload.

Alexis Frank Hartmann, 1898–1964, paediatrician, St Louis, MO, USA, described the solution; should not be confused with the name of Henri Albert Charles Antoine Hartmann, French surgeon, who described the operation that goes by his name.
Sidney Ringer, 1835–1910, Professor of Clinical Medicine, University College Hospital, London, UK.

CARDIAC OUTPUT

Cardiac output monitoring allows assessment of not only the cardiac output but also the systemic vascular resistance and, depending on the technique used, end diastolic volume (preload) and blood volume. Use of invasive cardiac monitoring with pulmonary artery catheters is becoming less frequent as new non-invasive monitoring techniques, such as Doppler ultrasound, pulse waveform analysis and indicator dilution methods, provide similar information without many of the drawbacks of more invasive techniques.

Measurement of cardiac output, systemic vascular resistance and preload can help distinguish the types of shock present (hypovolaemia, distributive, cardiogenic), especially when they coexist. The information provided guides fluid and vasopressor therapy by providing real-time monitoring of the cardiovascular response.

Measurement of cardiac output is desirable in patients who do not respond as expected to first-line therapy, or who have evidence of cardiogenic shock or myocardial dysfunction. Early consideration should be given to instituting cardiac output monitoring for patients who require vasopressor or inotropic support.

Systemic and organ perfusion

Ultimately, the goal of treatment is to restore cellular and organ perfusion. Ideally, therefore, monitoring of organ perfusion should guide the management of shock. The best measure of organ perfusion and the best monitor of the adequacy of shock therapy remains the urine output. However, this is an hourly measure and does not give a minute-to-minute view of the shocked state. The level of consciousness is an important marker of cerebral perfusion, but brain perfusion is maintained until the very late stages of shock, and hence is a poor marker of adequacy of resuscitation (*Table 2.3*).

Currently, the only clinical indicators of perfusion of the gastrointestinal tract and muscular beds are the global measures of lactic acidosis (lactate and base deficit) and the mixed venous oxygen saturation.

BASE DEFICIT AND LACTATE

Lactic acid is generated by cells undergoing anaerobic respiration. The degree of lactic acidosis, as measured by serum lactate level and/or the base deficit, is sensitive for both diagnosis of shock and monitoring the response to therapy. Patients with a base deficit over 6 mmol/L have a much higher morbidity and mortality than those with no metabolic acidosis. Furthermore, the length of time in shock with an increased base deficit is important, even if all other vital signs have returned to normal (see occult hypoperfusion below under **End points of resuscitation**).

These parameters are measured from arterial blood gas analyses, and therefore the frequency of measurements is limited and they do not provide minute-to-minute data on systemic perfusion or the response to therapy. Nevertheless, the base deficit and/or lactate should be measured routinely in these patients until they have returned to normal levels.

MIXED VENOUS OXYGEN SATURATION

The percentage saturation of oxygen returning to the heart from the body is a measure of the oxygen delivery and extraction by the tissues. Accurate measurement is via analysis of blood drawn from a long central line placed in the right atrium. Estimations can be made from blood drawn from lines in the superior vena cava, but these values will be slightly higher than those of a mixed venous sample (as there is relatively more oxygen extraction from the lower half of the body). Normal mixed venous oxygen saturation levels are 50–70%. Levels below 50% indicate inadequate oxygen delivery and increased oxygen extraction by the cells. This is consistent with hypovolaemic or cardiogenic shock.

High mixed venous saturations (>70%) are seen in sepsis and some other forms of distributive shock. In sepsis, there is disordered utilisation of oxygen at the cellular level, and arteriovenous shunting of blood at the microvascular level. Therefore, less oxygen is presented to the cells, and those cells cannot utilise what little oxygen is presented. Thus, venous blood has a higher oxygen concentration than normal.

TABLE 2.3 Monitors for organ/systemic perfusion.

	Clinical	Investigational
Systemic perfusion		Base deficit
		Lactate
		Mixed venous oxygen saturation
Organ perfusion		
Muscle	–	Near-infrared spectroscopy
		Tissue oxygen electrode
Gut	–	Sublingual capnometry
		Gut mucosal pH
		Laser Doppler flowmetry
Kidney	Urine output	–
Brain	Conscious level	Tissue oxygen electrode
		Near-infrared spectroscopy

Christian Johann Doppler, 1803–1853, Professor of Experimental Physics, Vienna, Austria, enunciated the Doppler principle in 1842.

Patients who are septic should therefore have mixed venous oxygen saturations above 70%; below this level, they are not only in septic shock but also in hypovolaemic or cardiogenic shock. Although the S_vO_2 level is in the 'normal' range, it is low for the septic state, and inadequate oxygen is being supplied to cells that cannot utilise oxygen appropriately. This must be corrected rapidly. Hypovolaemia should be corrected with fluid therapy, and low cardiac output due to myocardial depression or failure should be treated with inotropes (dobutamine), to achieve a mixed venous saturation greater than 70% (normal for the septic state).

New methods for monitoring regional tissue perfusion and oxygenation are becoming available, the most promising of which are muscle tissue oxygen probes, near-infrared spectroscopy and sublingual capnometry. While these techniques provide information regarding perfusion of specific tissue beds, it is as yet unclear whether there are significant advantages over existing measurements of global hypoperfusion (base deficit, lactate).

End points of resuscitation

It is much easier to know when to start resuscitation than when to stop. Traditionally, patients have been resuscitated until they have a normal pulse, blood pressure and urine output. However, these parameters are monitoring organ systems whose blood flow is preserved until the late stages of shock. A patient therefore may be resuscitated to restore central perfusion to the brain, lungs and kidneys and yet continue to underperfuse the gut and muscle beds. Thus, activation of inflammation and coagulation may be ongoing and lead to reperfusion injury when these organs are finally perfused, and ultimately multiple organ failure.

This state of normal vital signs and continued underperfusion is termed 'occult hypoperfusion'. With current monitoring techniques, it is manifested only by a persistent lactic acidosis and low mixed venous oxygen saturation. The time spent by patients in this hypoperfused state has a dramatic effect on outcome. Patients with occult hypoperfusion for more than 12 hours have two to three times the mortality of patients with a limited duration of shock.

Resuscitation algorithms directed at correcting global perfusion end points (base deficit, lactate, mixed venous oxygen saturation) rather than traditional end points have been shown to improve mortality and morbidity in high-risk surgical patients. However, it is clear that, despite aggressive regimes, some patients cannot be resuscitated to normal parameters within 12 hours by fluid resuscitation alone. More research is underway to identify the pathophysiology behind this and investigate new therapeutic options.

HAEMORRHAGE

Haemorrhage must be recognised and managed aggressively to reduce the severity and duration of shock and avoid death and/or multiple organ failure. Haemorrhage is treated by arresting the bleeding – not by fluid resuscitation or blood transfusion. Although necessary as supportive measures to maintain organ perfusion, attempting to resuscitate patients who have ongoing haemorrhage will lead to physiological exhaustion (coagulopathy, acidosis and hypothermia) and subsequently death.

Pathophysiology

Haemorrhage leads to a state of hypovolaemic shock. The combination of tissue trauma and hypovolaemic shock leads to the development of an endogenous coagulopathy called acute traumatic coagulopathy (ATC). Up to 25% of trauma patients develop ATC within minutes of injury and it is associated with a four-fold increase in mortality. It is likely that ATC exists whenever there is the combination of shock and tissue trauma (e.g. major surgery). ATC is a component of trauma-induced coagulopathy (TIC), which is ultimately multifactorial (**Figure 2.1**).

Ongoing bleeding with fluid and red blood cell resuscitation leads to a dilution of coagulation factors which worsens the coagulopathy. In addition, the acidosis induced by the hypoperfused state leads to decreased function of the coagulation proteases, resulting in coagulopathy and further haemorrhage. The reduced tissue perfusion includes reduced blood supply to muscle beds. Underperfused muscle is unable to generate heat and hypothermia ensues. Coagulation functions poorly at low temperatures and there is further haemorrhage, further hypoperfusion and worsening acidosis and hypothermia. These three factors result in a downward spiral leading to physiological exhaustion and death (**Figure 2.1**).

Medical therapy has a tendency to worsen this effect. Intravenous blood and fluids are cold and exacerbate hypothermia. Further heat is lost by opening body cavities during surgery. Surgery usually leads to further bleeding and many crystalloid fluids are themselves acidic (e.g. normal saline has a pH of 6.7). Every effort must therefore be made to rapidly identify and stop haemorrhage, and to avoid (preferably) or limit physiological exhaustion from coagulopathy, acidosis and hypothermia.

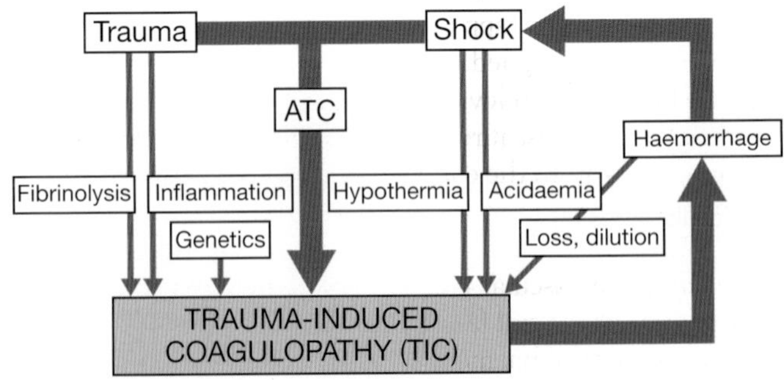

Figure 2.1 Trauma-induced coagulopathy.

Definitions

Revealed and concealed haemorrhage

Haemorrhage may be revealed or concealed. Revealed haemorrhage is obvious external haemorrhage, such as exsanguination from an open arterial wound or from massive haematemesis from a duodenal ulcer.

Concealed haemorrhage is contained within the body cavity and must be suspected, actively investigated and controlled. In trauma, haemorrhage may be concealed within the chest, abdomen, pelvis, retroperitoneum or in the limbs with contained vascular injury or associated with long-bone fractures. Examples of non-traumatic concealed haemorrhage include occult gastrointestinal bleeding or ruptured aortic aneurysm.

Primary, reactionary and secondary haemorrhage

Primary haemorrhage is haemorrhage occurring immediately due to an injury (or surgery). Reactionary haemorrhage is delayed haemorrhage (within 24 hours) and is usually due to dislodgement of a clot by resuscitation, normalisation of blood pressure and vasodilatation. Reactionary haemorrhage may also be due to technical failure, such as slippage of a ligature.

Secondary haemorrhage is due to sloughing of the wall of a vessel. It usually occurs 7–14 days after injury and is precipitated by factors such as infection, pressure necrosis (such as from a drain) or malignancy.

Surgical and non-surgical haemorrhage

Surgical haemorrhage is due to a direct injury and is amenable to surgical control (or other techniques such as angioembolisation). Non-surgical haemorrhage is the general ooze from all raw surfaces due to coagulopathy and cannot be stopped by surgical means (except packing). Treatment requires correction of the coagulation abnormalities.

Degree and classification

The adult human has approximately 5 litres of blood (70 mL/kg children and adults, 80 mL/kg neonates). Estimation of the amount of blood that has been lost is difficult, inaccurate and usually underestimates the actual value.

External haemorrhage is obvious, but it may be difficult to estimate the actual volume lost. In the operating room, blood collected in suction apparatus can be measured and swabs soaked in blood weighed.

The haemoglobin level is a poor indicator of the degree of haemorrhage because it represents a concentration and not an absolute amount. In the early stages of rapid haemorrhage, the haemoglobin concentration is unchanged (as whole blood is lost). Later, as fluid shifts from the intracellular and interstitial spaces into the vascular compartment, the haemoglobin and haematocrit levels will fall.

The amount of haemorrhage can be classified into classes 1–4 based on the estimated blood loss required to produce certain physiological compensatory changes (*Table 2.4*). Although conceptually useful, there is variation across ages (the young compensate well, the old very poorly), variation among individuals (e.g. athletes versus the obese) and variation due to confounding factors (e.g. concomitant medications, pain).

TABLE 2.4 Traditional classification of haemorrhagic shock.

	Class			
	1	2	3	4
Blood volume lost as percentage of total	<15%	15–30%	30–40%	>40%

Treatment should therefore be based upon the degree of hypovolaemic shock according to vital signs, preload assessment, base deficit and, most importantly, the dynamic response to fluid therapy. Patients who are 'non-responders' or 'transient responders' are still bleeding and must have the site of haemorrhage identified and controlled.

Management

Identify haemorrhage

External haemorrhage may be obvious, but the diagnosis of concealed haemorrhage may be more difficult. Any shock should be assumed to be hypovolaemic until proven otherwise and, similarly, hypovolaemia should be assumed to be due to haemorrhage until this has been excluded.

Immediate resuscitative manoeuvres

Direct pressure should be placed over the site of external haemorrhage. Airway and breathing should be assessed and controlled as necessary. Large-bore intravenous access should be instituted and blood drawn for cross-matching (see **Cross-matching** below). Emergency blood should be requested if the degree of shock and ongoing haemorrhage warrants this.

Identify the site of haemorrhage

Once haemorrhage has been considered, the site of haemorrhage must be rapidly identified. Note this is not to identify the exact location definitively, but rather to define the next step in haemorrhage control (operation, angioembolisation, endoscopic control).

Clues may be in the history (previous episodes, known aneurysm, non-steroidal therapy for gastrointestinal [GI] bleeding) or examination (nature of blood – fresh, melaena; abdominal tenderness, etc.). For shocked trauma patients, the external signs of injury may suggest internal haemorrhage, but haemorrhage into a body cavity (thorax, abdomen) must be excluded with rapid investigations (chest and pelvis x-ray, abdominal ultrasound or diagnostic peritoneal aspiration).

Investigations for blood loss must be appropriate to the patient's physiological condition. Rapid bedside tests are more appropriate for profound shock and exsanguinating haemorrhage than investigations such as computed tomography (CT) which take time. Patients who are not actively bleeding can have a more methodical, definitive work-up.

Haemorrhage control

The bleeding, shocked patient must be moved rapidly to a place of haemorrhage control. This will usually be in the operating room but may be the angiography or endoscopy suite. These patients require surgical and anaesthetic support and full monitoring and equipment must be available.

Haemorrhage control must be achieved rapidly to prevent the patient entering the triad of coagulopathy–acidosis–hypothermia and physiological exhaustion. There should be no unnecessary investigations or procedures prior to haemorrhage control to minimise the duration and severity of shock. This includes prolonged attempts to volume resuscitate the patient prior to surgery, which will result in further hypothermia and clotting factor dilution until the bleeding is stopped. Attention should be paid to correction of coagulopathy with blood component therapy to aid surgical haemorrhage control.

Surgical intervention may need to be limited to the minimum necessary to stop bleeding and control sepsis. More definitive repairs can be delayed until the patient is haemodynamically stable and physiologically capable of sustaining the procedure. This concept of tailoring the operation to match the patient's physiology and staged procedures to prevent physiological exhaustion is called 'damage control surgery' – a term borrowed from the military which ensures continued functioning of a damaged ship above conducting complete repairs which would prevent rapid return to battle.

Once haemorrhage is controlled, patients should be aggressively resuscitated, warmed and coagulopathy corrected. Attention should be paid to fluid responsiveness and the end points of resuscitation to ensure that patients are fully resuscitated and to reduce the incidence and severity of organ failure.

Summary box 2.4

Damage control surgery

- Arrest haemorrhage
- Control sepsis
- Protect from further injury
- Nothing else

Damage control resuscitation

These concepts have been combined into a new paradigm for the management of trauma patients with active haemorrhage called damage control resuscitation (DCR). The four central strategies of DCR are:

1 Anticipate and treat acute traumatic coagulopathy.
2 Permissive hypotension until haemorrhage control.
3 Limit crystalloid and colloid infusion to avoid dilutional coagulopathy.
4 Damage control surgery to control haemorrhage and preserve physiology.

Damage control resuscitation strategies have been shown to reduce mortality and morbidity in patients with exsanguinating trauma and may be applicable in other forms of acute haemorrhage.

TRANSFUSION

The transfusion of blood and blood products has become commonplace since the first successful transfusion in 1818. Although the incidence of severe transfusion reactions and infections is now very low, in recent years it has become apparent that there is an immunological price to be paid from the transfusion of heterologous blood, leading to increased morbidity and decreased survival in certain population groups (trauma, malignancy). Supplies are also limited, and therefore the use of blood and blood products must always be judicious and justifiable for clinical need (*Table 2.5*).

TABLE 2.5 History of blood transfusion.

1492	Pope Innocent VIII suffers a stroke and receives a blood transfusion from three 10-year-old boys (paid a ducat each). All three boys died, as did the pope later that year
1665	Richard Lower in Oxford conducts the first successful canine transfusions
1667	Jean-Baptiste Denis reports successful sheep–human transfusions
1678	Animal–human transfusions are banned in France because of the poor results
1818	James Blundell performs the first successful documented human transfusion in a woman suffering post-partum haemorrhage. She received blood from her husband and survived
1901	Karl Landsteiner discovers the ABO system
1914	The Belgian physician Albert Hustin performed the first non-direct transfusion, using sodium citrate as an anticoagulant
1926	The British Red Cross instituted the first blood transfusion service in the world
1939	The Rhesus system was identified and recognised as the major cause of transfusion reactions

Blood and blood products

Blood is collected from donors who have been previously screened before donating, to exclude any donor whose blood may have the potential to harm the patient, or to prevent possible harm that donating a unit of blood may have on the donor. In the UK, up to 450 mL of blood is drawn, a maximum of three times each year. Each unit is tested for evidence of hepatitis B, hepatitis C, HIV-1, HIV-2 and syphilis. Donations are leukodepleted as a precaution against variant Creutzfeldt–Jakob disease (this may also reduce the immunogenicity of the transfusion). The ABO and rhesus D blood groups are determined, as well as the presence of irregular red cell antibodies. The blood is then processed into subcomponents.

Whole blood

Whole blood is now rarely available in civilian practice because it has been seen as an inefficient use of the limited resource. However, whole blood transfusion has significant advantages over packed cells as it is coagulation factor rich and, if fresh, more metabolically active than stored blood.

Hans Gerhard Creutzfeldt, 1885–1946, neurologist, Kiel, Germany.
Alfons Maria Jakob, 1884–1931, neurologist, Hamburg, Germany.
Karl Landsteiner, 1868–1943, Professor of Pathological Anatomy, University of Vienna, Austria. In 1909 he classified the human blood groups into A, B, AB and O. For this he was awarded the Nobel Prize for Physiology or Medicine in 1930.

Packed red cells

Packed red blood cells are spun-down and concentrated packs of red blood cells. Each unit is approximately 330 mL and has a haematocrit of 50–70%. Packed cells are stored in a SAG-M solution (saline–adenine–glucose–mannitol) to increase shelf life to 5 weeks at 2–6°C. (Older storage regimes included storage in CPD: citrate–phosphate–dextrose solutions, which have a shelf life of 2–3 weeks.)

Fresh-frozen plasma

Fresh-frozen plasma (FFP) is rich in coagulation factors and is removed from fresh blood and stored at −40 to −50°C with a 2-year shelf life. It is the first-line therapy in the treatment of coagulopathic haemorrhage (see below under **Management of coagulopathy**). Rhesus D-positive FFP may be given to a rhesus D-negative woman although it is possible for seroconversion to occur with large volumes owing to the presence of red cell fragments, and Rh-D immunisation should be considered.

Cryoprecipitate

Cryoprecipitate is a supernatant precipitate of FFP and is rich in factor VIII and fibrinogen. It is stored at −30°C with a 2-year shelf life. It is given in low fibrinogen states or factor VIII deficiency.

Platelets

Platelets are supplied as a pooled platelet concentrate and contain about 250×10^9/L. Platelets are stored on a special agitator at 20–24°C and have a shelf life of only 5 days. Platelet transfusions are given to patients with thrombocytopenia or with platelet dysfunction who are bleeding or undergoing surgery.

Patients are increasingly presenting on antiplatelet therapy such as aspirin or clopidogrel for reduction of cardiovascular risk. Aspirin therapy rarely poses a problem but control of haemorrhage on the more potent platelet inhibitors can be extremely difficult. Patients on clopidogrel who are actively bleeding and undergoing major surgery may require almost continuous infusion of platelets during the course of the procedure. Arginine vasopressin or its analogues (DDAVP) have also been used in this patient group, although with limited success.

Prothrombin complex concentrates

Prothrombin complex concentrates (PCC) are highly purified concentrates prepared from pooled plasma. They contain factors II, IX and X. Factor VII may be included or produced separately. It is indicated for the emergency reversal of anticoagulant (warfarin) therapy in uncontrolled haemorrhage.

Autologous blood

It is possible for patients undergoing elective surgery to predonate their own blood up to 3 weeks before surgery for retransfusion during the operation. Similarly, during surgery blood can be collected in a cell-saver which washes and collects red blood cells which can then be returned to the patient.

Indications for blood transfusion

Blood transfusions should be avoided if possible, and many previous uses of blood and blood products are now no longer considered appropriate. The indications for blood transfusion are as follows:

- Acute blood loss, to replace circulating volume and maintain oxygen delivery;
- Perioperative anaemia, to ensure adequate oxygen delivery during the perioperative phase;
- Symptomatic chronic anaemia, without haemorrhage or impending surgery.

Transfusion trigger

Historically, patients were transfused to achieve a haemoglobin >10 g/dL. This has now been shown not only to be unnecessary but also to be associated with an increased morbidity and mortality compared with lower target values. A haemoglobin level of 6 g/dL is acceptable in patients who are not actively bleeding, not about to undergo major surgery and are not symptomatic. There is some controversy as to the optimal haemoglobin level in some patient groups, such as those with cardiovascular disease, sepsis and traumatic brain injury. Although, conceptually, a higher haemoglobin level improves oxygen delivery, there is little clinical evidence at this stage to support higher levels in these groups (*Table 2.6*).

TABLE 2.6 Perioperative red blood cell transfusion criteria.

Haemoglobin level (g/dL)	Indications
<6	Probably will benefit from transfusion
6–8	Transfusion unlikely to be of benefit in the absence of bleeding or impending surgery
>8	No indication for transfusion in the absence of other risk factors

Blood groups and cross-matching

Human red cells have on their cell surface many different antigens. Two groups of antigens are of major importance in surgical practice – the ABO and rhesus systems.

ABO system

These proteins are strongly antigenic and are associated with naturally occurring antibodies in the serum. The system consists of three allelic genes – A, B and O – which control synthesis of enzymes that add carbohydrate residues to cell surface glycoproteins. A and B genes add specific residues while the O gene is an amorph and does not transform the glycoprotein. The system allows for six possible genotypes although there are only four phenotypes. Naturally occurring antibodies are found in the serum of those lacking the corresponding antigen (*Table 2.7*).

Blood group O is the universal donor type as it contains no antigens to provoke a reaction. Conversely, group AB individuals are 'universal recipients' and can receive any ABO blood type because they have no circulating antibodies.

TABLE 2.7 ABO blood group system.

Phenotype	Genotype	Antigens	Antibodies	Frequency (%)
O	OO	O	Anti-A, anti-B	46
A	AA or AO	A	Anti-B	42
B	BB or BO	B	Anti-A	9
AB	AB	AB	None	3

Rhesus system

The rhesus D (Rh(D)) antigen is strongly antigenic and is present in approximately 85% of the population in the UK. Antibodies to the D antigen are not naturally present in the serum of the remaining 15% of individuals, but their formation may be stimulated by the transfusion of Rh-positive red cells, or acquired during delivery of a Rh(D)-positive baby.

Acquired antibodies are capable, during pregnancy, of crossing the placenta and, if present in a Rh(D)-negative mother, may cause severe haemolytic anaemia and even death (hydrops fetalis) in a Rh(D)-positive fetus *in utero*. The other minor blood group antigens may be associated with naturally occurring antibodies, or may stimulate the formation of antibodies on relatively rare occasions.

Transfusion reactions

If antibodies present in the recipient's serum are incompatible with the donor's cells, a transfusion reaction will result. This usually takes the form of an acute haemolytic reaction. Severe immune-related transfusion reactions due to ABO incompatibility result in potentially fatal complement-mediated intravascular haemolysis and multiple organ failure. Transfusion reactions from other antigen systems are usually milder and self-limiting.

Febrile transfusion reactions are non-haemolytic and are usually caused by a graft-versus-host response from leukocytes in transfused components. Such reactions are associated with fever, chills or rigors. The blood transfusion should be stopped immediately. This form of transfusion reaction is rare with leukodepleted blood.

Cross-matching

To prevent transfusion reactions, all transfusions are preceded by ABO and rhesus typing of both donor and recipient blood to ensure compatibility. The recipient's serum is then mixed with the donor's cells to confirm ABO compatibility and to test for rhesus and any other blood group antigen–antibody reaction.

Full cross-matching of blood may take up to 45 minutes in most laboratories. In more urgent situations, 'type specific' blood is provided which is only ABO/rhesus matched and can be issued within 10–15 minutes. Where blood must be given emergently, group O (universal donor) blood is given (O– to females, O+ to males).

When blood transfusion is prescribed and blood is administered, it is essential that the correct patient receives the correct transfusion. Two healthcare personnel should check the patient details against the prescription and the label of the donor blood. In addition, the donor blood serial number should also be checked against the issue slip for that patient. Provided these principles are strictly adhered to the number of severe and fatal ABO incompatibility reactions can be minimised.

Complications of blood transfusion

Complications from blood transfusion can be categorised as those arising from a single transfusion and those related to massive transfusion.

Complications from a single transfusion

Complications from a single transfusion include:

- incompatibility haemolytic transfusion reaction;
- febrile transfusion reaction;
- allergic reaction;
- infection:
  - bacterial infection (usually due to faulty storage);
  - hepatitis;
  - HIV;
  - malaria;
- air embolism;
- thrombophlebitis;
- transfusion-related acute lung injury (usually from FFP).

Complications from massive transfusion

Complications from massive transfusion include:

- coagulopathy;
- hypocalcaemia;
- hyperkalaemia;
- hypokalaemia;
- hypothermia.

In addition, patients who receive repeated transfusions over long periods of time (e.g. patients with thalassaemia) may develop iron overload. (Each transfused unit of red blood cells contains approximately 250 mg of elemental iron.)

Management of coagulopathy

Correction of coagulopathy is not necessary if there is no active bleeding and haemorrhage is not anticipated (not due for surgery). However, coagulopathy following or during massive transfusion should be anticipated and managed aggressively. Prevention of dilutional coagulopathy is central to the damage control resuscitation of patients who are actively bleeding.

This is the prime reason for delivering balanced transfusion regimes matching red blood cell packs with plasma and platelets. Based on moderate evidence, when red cells are transfused for active haemorrhage, it is best to match each red cell unit with one unit of FFP and one of platelets (1:1:1). This will reduce the incidence and severity of subsequent dilutional coagulopathy. Crystalloids and colloids should be avoided for the same reason.

The balanced transfusion approach cannot, however, correct coagulopathy. Therefore, coagulation should be monitored routinely, either with point-of-care testing (thromboelastometry) or with laboratory tests (fibrinogen, clotting times). Underlying coagulopathies should be treated in addition to the administration of 1:1:1 balanced transfusions.

There are pharmacological adjuncts to blood component therapy. The antifibrinolytic tranexamic acid is the most commonly administered. It is usually administered empirically to bleeding patients because effective point-of-care tests of fibrinolysis are not yet routinely available. There is little evidence to support the use of other coagulation factor concentrates at this time.

Blood substitutes

Blood substitutes are an attractive alternative to the costly process of donating, checking, storing and administering blood, especially given the immunogenic and potential infectious complications associated with transfusion.

There are several oxygen-carrying blood substitutes under investigation in experimental animal or early clinical trials. Blood substitutes are either biomimetic or abiotic. Biomimetic substitutes mimic the standard oxygen-carrying capacity of the blood and are haemoglobin based. Abiotic substitutes are synthetic oxygen carriers and are currently primarily perfluorocarbon based.

Haemoglobin is seen as the obvious candidate for developing an effective blood substitute. Various engineered molecules are under clinical trials, and are based on human, bovine or recombinant technologies. Second-generation perfluorocarbon emulsions are also showing potential in clinical trials.

FURTHER READING

Duchesne JC, McSwain NE Jr, Cotton BA *et al.* Damage control resuscitation: the new face of damage control. *J Trauma* 2010; **69**: 976–90.

Glen J, Constanti M, Brohi K; Guideline Development Group. Assessment and initial management of major trauma: summary of NICE guidance. *BMJ* 2016; **353**: i3051.

Harris T, Thomas GO, Brohi K. Early fluid resuscitation in severe trauma. *BMJ* 2012; **345**: e5752.

Nguyen HB, Jaehne AK, Jayaprakash N *et al.* Early goal-directed therapy in severe sepsis and septic shock: insights and comparisons to ProCESS, ProMISe, and ARISE. *Crit Care* 2016; **20**(1): 160.

Pearse RM, Ackland GL. Perioperative fluid therapy. *BMJ* 2012; **344**: e2865.

Rossaint R, Bouillon B, Cerny V *et al.* The European guideline on management of major bleeding and coagulopathy following trauma: fourth edition. *Crit Care* 2016; **20**: 100.

Sihler KC, Nathans AB. Management of severe sepsis in the surgical patient. *Surg Clin N Am* 2006; **86**: 1457–81.

Chapter 3

Wounds, healing and tissue repair

Learning objectives

To understand:

- Normal healing and how it can be adversely affected
- How to manage wounds of different types, of different structures and at different sites
- Aspects of disordered healing that lead to chronic wounds
- The variety of scars and their treatment
- How to differentiate between acute and chronic wounds

INTRODUCTION

Wound healing is a mechanism whereby the body attempts to restore the integrity of the injured part. This falls far short of tissue regeneration by pluripotent cells, seen in some amphibians, and is often detrimental, as seen in the problems created by scarring, such as adhesions, keloids, contractures and cirrhosis of the liver. Several factors may influence healing. However, a clean incised wound in a healthy person where there is no skin loss will follow a set pattern as outlined below.

Summary box 3.1

Factors influencing healing of a wound

- Site of the wound
- Structures involved
- Mechanism of wounding
  - Incision
  - Crush
  - Crush avulsion
- Contamination (foreign bodies/bacteria)[a]
- Loss of tissue
- Other local factors
  - Vascular insufficiency (arterial or venous)
  - Previous radiation
  - Pressure
- Systemic factors
  - Malnutrition or vitamin and mineral deficiencies
  - Disease (e.g. diabetes mellitus)
  - Medications (e.g. steroids)
  - Immune deficiencies (e.g. chemotherapy, acquired immunodeficiency syndrome [AIDS])
  - Smoking

[a] In explosions, the contamination may consist of tissue such as bone from another individual.

NORMAL WOUND HEALING

This is variously described as taking place in three or four phases, the most commonly agreed being:

1 the inflammatory phase;
2 the proliferative phase;
3 the remodelling phase (maturing phase).

Occasionally, a haemostatic phase is referred to as occurring before the inflammatory phase, or a destructive phase following inflammation consisting of the cellular cleansing of the wound by macrophages (**Figure 3.1**).

The inflammatory phase begins immediately after wounding and lasts 2–3 days. Bleeding is followed by vasoconstriction and thrombus formation to limit blood loss. Platelets stick to the damaged endothelial lining of vessels, releasing adenosine diphosphate (ADP), which causes thrombocytic aggregates to fill the wound. When bleeding stops, the platelets then release several cytokines from their alpha granules. These are platelet-derived growth factor (PDGF), platelet factor IV and transforming growth factor beta (TGFβ). These attract inflammatory cells such as polymorphonuclear leukocytes (PMN) and macrophages. Platelets and the local injured tissue release vasoactive amines, such as histamine, serotonin and prostaglandins, which increase vascular permeability, thereby aiding infiltration of these inflammatory cells. Macrophages remove devitalised tissue and microorganisms while regulating fibroblast activity in the proliferative phase of healing. The initial framework for structural support of cells is provided by fibrin produced by fibrinogen. A more historical (Latin) description of this phase is described in four words: *rubor* (redness), *tumor* (swelling), *calor* (heat) and *dolor* (pain).

The proliferative phase lasts from the third day to the third week, consisting mainly of fibroblast activity with the production of collagen and ground substance (glycosaminogly-

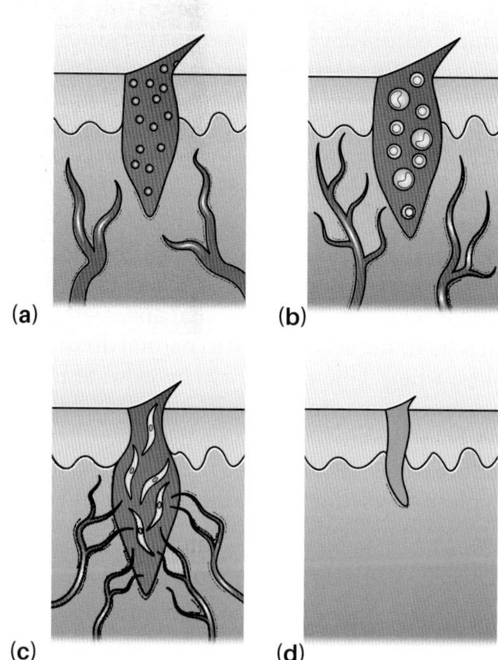

Figure 3.1 The phases of healing. (**a**) Early inflammatory phase with platelet-enriched blood clot and dilated vessels. (**b**) Late inflammatory phase with increased vascularity and increase in polymorphonuclear leukocytes and lymphocytes (round cells). (**c**) Proliferative phase with capillary buds and fibroblasts. (**d**) Mature contracted scar.

cans and proteoglycans), the growth of new blood vessels as capillary loops (angioneogenesis) and the re-epithelialisation of the wound surface. Fibroblasts require vitamin C to produce collagen. The wound tissue formed in the early part of this phase is called granulation tissue. In the latter part of this phase, there is an increase in the tensile strength of the wound due to increased collagen, which is at first deposited in a random fashion and consists of type III collagen. This proliferative phase with its increase of collagen deposition is associated with wound contraction, which can considerably reduce the surface area of a wound over the first 3 weeks of healing.

The remodelling phase is characterised by maturation of collagen (type I replacing type III until a ratio of 4:1 is achieved). There is a realignment of collagen fibres along the lines of tension, decreased wound vascularity, and wound contraction due to fibroblast and myofibroblast activity. This maturation of collagen leads to increased tensile strength in the wound which is maximal at the 12th week post injury and represents approximately 80% of the uninjured skin strength.

NORMAL HEALING IN SPECIFIC TISSUES

Bone

The phases are as above, but periosteal and endosteal proliferation leads to the formation of callus, which is immature bone consisting of osteoid (mineralised by hydroxyapatite and laid down by osteoblasts). In the remodelling phase, cortical structure and the medullary cavity are restored. If fracture ends are accurately opposed and rigidly fixed, callus formation is minimal and primary healing occurs. If a gap exists, then secondary healing may lead to delayed union, non-union or malunion.

Nerve

Distal to the wound, Wallerian degeneration occurs. Proximally, the nerve suffers traumatic degeneration as far as the last node of Ranvier. The regenerating nerve fibres are attracted to their receptors by neurotrophism, which is mediated by growth factors, hormones and other extracellular matrix trophins. Nerve regeneration is characterised by profuse growth of new nerve fibres which sprout from the cut proximal end. Overgrowth of these, coupled with poor approximation, may lead to neuroma formation.

Tendon

Although repair follows the normal pattern of wound healing, there are two main mechanisms whereby nutrients, cells and new vessels reach the severed tendon. These are intrinsic, which consists of vincular blood flow and synovial diffusion, and extrinsic, which depends on the formation of fibrous adhesions between the tendon and the tendon sheath. The random nature of the initial collagen produced means that the tendon lacks tensile strength for the first 3–6 weeks. Active mobilisation prevents adhesions limiting range of motion, but the tendon must be protected by splintage in order to avoid rupture of the repair.

ABNORMAL HEALING

Some of the adverse influences on wound healing are listed in *Summary box 3.1*. Delayed healing may result in loss of function or poor cosmetic outcome. The aim of treatment is to achieve healing by primary intention and so reduce the inflammatory and proliferative responses.

Summary box 3.2

Classification of wound closure and healing

- Primary intention
  - Wound edges opposed
  - Normal healing
  - Minimal scar
- Secondary intention
  - Wound left open
  - Heals by granulation, contraction and epithelialisation
  - Increased inflammation and proliferation
  - Poor scar
- Tertiary intention (also called delayed primary intention)
  - Wound initially left open
  - Edges later opposed when healing conditions favourable

Augustus Volney Waller, 1816–1870, general practitioner of Kensington, London, UK (1842–1851), subsequently worked as a physiologist in Bonn, Germany; Paris, France; Birmingham, UK; and Geneva, Switzerland.
Louis Antoine Ranvier, 1835–1922, physician and histologist who was a professor in the College of France, Paris, France, described these nodes in 1878.

Healing by primary intention is also known as healing by first intention. This occurs when there is apposition of the wound edges and minimal surrounding tissue trauma that causes least inflammation and leaves the best scar. Delayed primary intention healing occurs when the wound edges are not opposed immediately, which may be necessary in contaminated or untidy wounds. The inflammatory and proliferative phases of healing are well established when delayed closure of the wound is carried out. This is also called healing by tertiary intention in some texts and will result in a less satisfactory scar than would result after healing by primary intention. Secondary healing or healing by secondary intention occurs in wounds that are left open and allowed to heal by granulation, contraction and epithelialisation.

TYPES OF WOUNDS – TIDY VERSUS UNTIDY

The site injured, the structures involved in the injury and the mechanism of injury (e.g. incision or explosion) all influence healing and recovery of function. This has led to the management of wounds based upon their classification into tidy and untidy (*Table 3.1* and **Figure 3.2**).

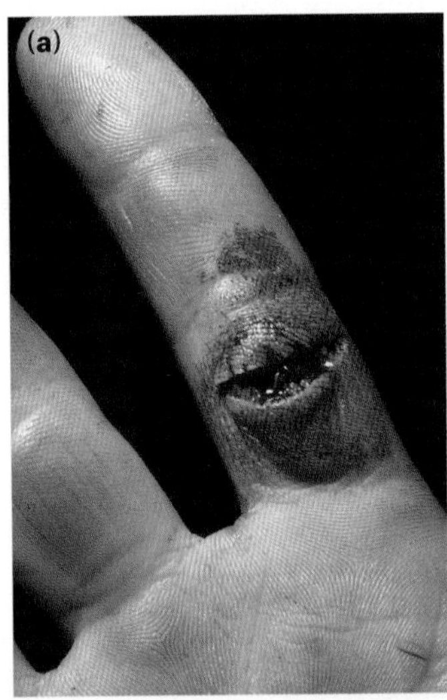

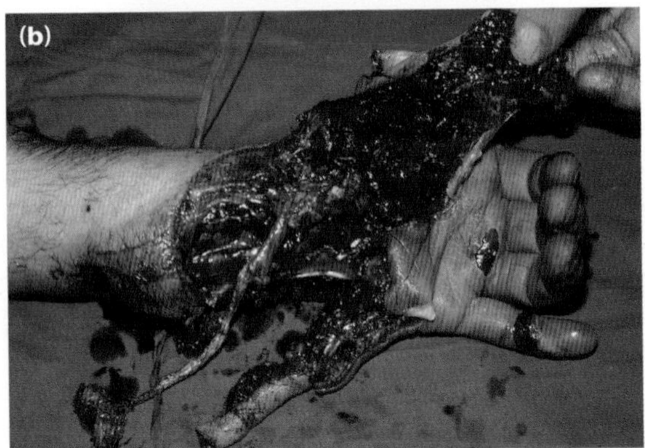

Figure 3.2 **(a)** Tidy incised wound on the finger. **(b)** Untidy avulsed wound on the hand.

The surgeon's aim is to convert untidy to tidy by removing all contaminated and devitalised tissue.

Primary repair of all structures (e.g. bone, tendon, vessel and nerve) may be possible in a tidy wound, but a contaminated wound with dead tissue requires debridement on one or several occasions before definitive repair can be carried out (the concept of 'second look' surgery). This is especially true in injuries caused by explosions, bullets or other missiles, where the external wound itself may appear much smaller than the wider extent of the injured tissues deep to the surface. Multiple debridements are often required after crushing injuries in road traffic accidents or in natural disasters such as earthquakes, where fallen masonry causes widespread muscle damage and compartment syndromes (see Compartment syndromes below). Any explosion where there are multiple victims at the same site or where there has been a suicide-related explosion will carry the risk of tissue and viral contamination. Appropriate tests for hepatitis viruses and human immunodeficiency virus (HIV) are required.

TABLE 3.1 Tidy versus untidy wounds.

Tidy	Untidy
Incised	Crushed or avulsed
Clean	Contaminated
Healthy tissues	Devitalised tissues
Seldom tissue loss	Often tissue loss

MANAGING THE ACUTE WOUND

The surgeon must remember to examine the whole patient according to acute trauma life support (ATLS) principles. A stab wound in the back can be missed just as easily in the reality of the accident and emergency room as in a fictitious detective novel. The wound itself should be examined, taking into consideration the site and the possible structures damaged (**Figure 3.3**). It is essential to assess movement and sensation while

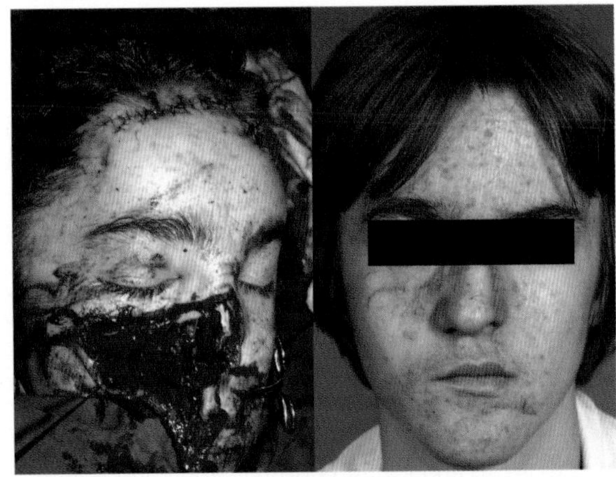

Figure 3.3 Facial trauma – apparent tissue loss but none found after careful matching.

The term **'debridement'** was introduced by the great French surgeon in Napoleon's army, Dominique Jean Larrey (1766–1842). He used it to describe the removal of bullets, bits of cloth, loose bits of bone and soft tissue.

watching for pain and listening to the patient. Tetanus cover should be noted and appropriate treatment carried out.

A bleeding wound should be elevated and a pressure pad applied. Clamps should not be put on vessels blindly because nerve damage is likely and vascular anastomosis is rendered impossible.

In order to facilitate examination, adequate analgesia and/or anaesthesia (local, regional or general) are required. General anaesthesia is often needed in children. With limb injuries, particularly those of the hand, a tourniquet should be used in order to facilitate visualisation of all structures. Due care should be taken with tourniquet application, avoiding uneven pressure and noting the duration of tourniquet time.

After assessment, a thorough debridement is essential. Abrasions, 'road rash' (following a fall from a motorbike) and explosions all cause dirt tattooing and require the use of a scrubbing brush or even excision under magnification. A wound should be explored and debrided to the limit of blood staining. Devitalised tissue must be excised until bleeding occurs, with the obvious exceptions of nerves, vessels and tendons. These may survive with adequate revascularisation subsequently or after being covered with viable tissue such as that brought in by skin or muscle flaps.

The use of copious saline irrigation or pulsed jet lavage (where the instrumentation is available) can be less destructive than knife or scissors when debriding. However, it has been suggested that pulsed jet lavage can implant dirt into a deeper plane and care should be taken to avoid this complication. Muscle viability is judged by the colour, bleeding pattern and contractility. In a tidy wound, repair of all damaged structures may be attempted. Repair of nerves under magnification (loupes or microscope) using 8/0 or 10/0 monofilament nylon is usual. Vessels such as the radial or ulnar artery may be repaired using similar techniques. Tendon repairs, particularly those in the hand, benefit from early active mobilisation because this minimises adhesions between the tendon and the tendon sheath (see above under **Tendon** for extrinsic tendon healing mechanism).

Skin cover by flap or graft may be required as skin closure should always be without tension and should allow for the oedema typically associated with injury and the inflammatory phase of healing. A flap brings in a new blood supply and can be used to cover tendon, nerve, bone and other structures that would not provide a suitable vascular base for a skin graft. A skin graft has no inherent blood supply and is dependent on the recipient site for nutrition.

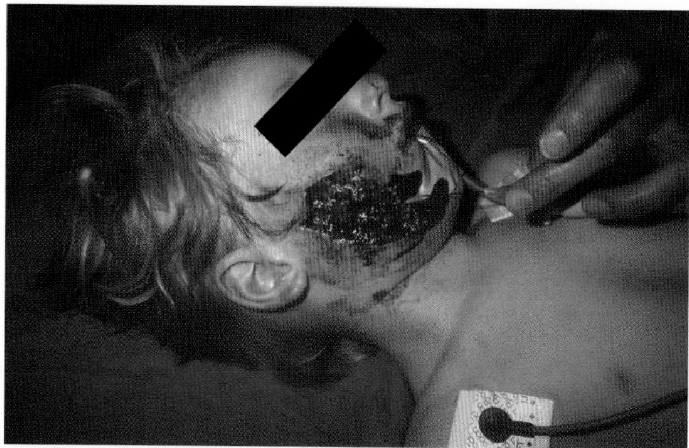

Figure 3.4 Dog bite in a child.

Summary box 3.3

Managing the acute wound

- Cleansing
- Exploration and diagnosis
- Debridement
- Repair of structures
- Replacement of lost tissues where indicated
- Skin cover if required
- Skin closure without tension
- All of the above with careful tissue handling and meticulous technique

SOME SPECIFIC WOUNDS

Bites

Most bites involve either puncture wounds or avulsions. Bites from small animals are common in children (**Figure 3.4**) and require cleansing and treatment according to the principles outlined in *Summary box 3.3*, usually under general anaesthetic.

Injuries to the ear, tip of nose and lower lip are most usually seen in victims of human bites. A boxing-type injury of the metacarpophalangeal joint may result from a perforating contact with the teeth of a victim. Anaerobic and aerobic organism prophylaxis is required as bite wounds typically have high virulent bacterial counts.

Puncture wounds

Wounds caused by sharp objects should be explored to the limit of tissue blood staining. Needle-stick injuries should be treated according to the well-published protocols because of hepatitis and HIV risks. X-ray examination should be carried out in order to rule out retained foreign bodies in the depth of the wound.

Haematoma

If large, painful or causing neural deficit, a haematoma may require release by incision or aspiration. In the gluteal or thigh region, there may be an associated disruption of fat in the form of a fat fracture, which results in an unsightly groove but intact skin. An untreated haematoma may also calcify and therefore require surgical exploration if symptomatic.

Degloving

Degloving occurs when the skin and subcutaneous fat are stripped by avulsion from the underlying fascia, leaving neurovascular structures, tendon or bone exposed. A degloving injury may be open or closed. An obvious example of an open degloving is a ring avulsion injury with loss of finger

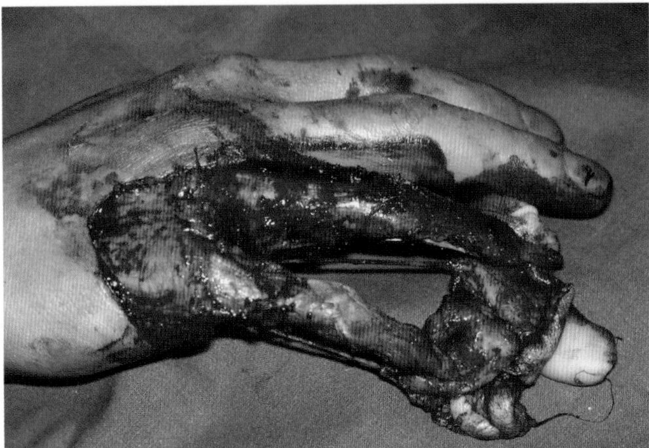

Figure 3.5 Degloving hand injury.

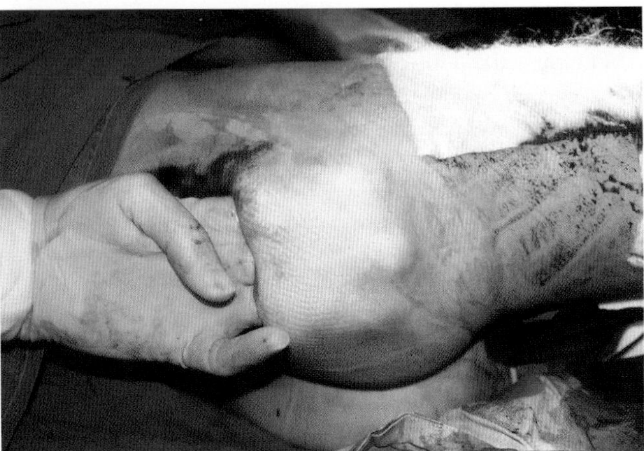

Figure 3.6 Degloving buttock injury.

skin (Figure 3.5). A closed degloving may be a rollover injury, typically caused by a motor vehicle over a limb. Such an injury will extend far further than expected, and much of the limb skin may be non-viable (Figure 3.6). Examination under anaesthetic is required with a radical excision of all non-bleeding skin, as judged by bleeding dermis. Fluoroscein can be administered intravenously while the patient is anaesthetised. Under ultraviolet light, viable (perfused) skin will show up as a fluorescent yellowish green colour, and the non-viable skin for excision is clearly mapped out. However, the main objection to this method is that of possible anaphylactic shock due to fluoroscein sensitivity. Most surgeons therefore rely upon serial excision until punctate dermal bleeding is obvious. Split-skin grafts can be harvested from the degloved non-viable skin and meshed (Figure 3.7) to cover the raw areas resulting from debridement.

Compartment syndromes

Compartment syndromes typically occur in closed lower limb injuries. They are characterised by severe pain, pain on passive movement of the affected compartment muscles, distal sensory disturbance and, finally, by the absence of pulses distally (a late sign). They can occur with an open injury if the wound does not extend into the affected compartment.

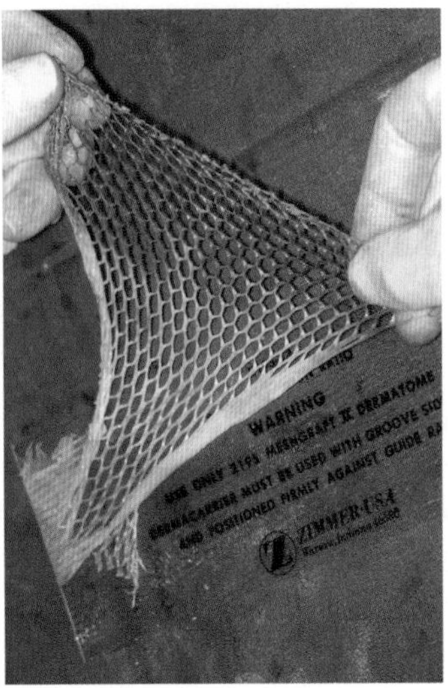

Figure 3.7 Meshed split-skin graft.

Compartment pressures can be measured using a pressure monitor and a catheter placed in the muscle compartment. If pressures are constantly greater than 30 mmHg or if the above clinical signs are present, then fasciotomy should be performed. Fasciotomy involves incising the deep muscle fascia and is best carried out via longitudinal incisions of skin, fat and fascia (Figure 3.8). The muscle will then be seen bulging out through the fasciotomy opening. The lower limb can be decompressed via two incisions, each being lateral to the subcutaneous border of the tibia. This gives access to the two posterior compartments and to the peroneal and anterior compartments of the leg. In crush injuries that present several days after the event, a late fasciotomy can be dangerous because dead muscle produces myoglobin which, if suddenly released into the blood stream, causes myoglobinuria with glomerular blockage and renal failure. In the late treatment of lower limb injuries, therefore, it may be safer to amputate the limb once viable and non-viable tissues have been demarcated.

High-pressure injection injuries

The use of high-pressure devices in cleaning, degreasing and painting can cause extensive closed injuries through

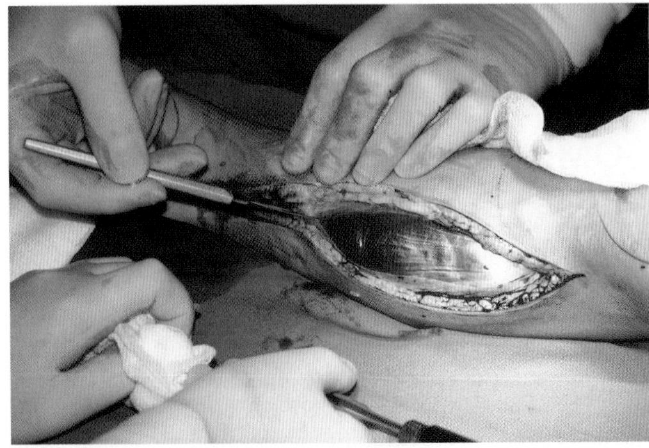

Figure 3.8 Fasciotomy of the lower leg.

small entry wounds. The liquid injected spreads along fascial planes, a common site being from finger to forearm. The tissue damage is dependent upon the toxicity of the substance and the injection pressure. Treatment is surgical, with wide exposure, removal of the toxic substance and thorough debridement. Preoperative x-rays may be helpful where air or lead-based paints can be seen. It should be noted that amputation rates following high-pressure injection injuries are reported as being over 45%. Delayed or conservative treatment is therefore inappropriate.

CHRONIC WOUNDS

A chronic wound may be defined as one that fails to heal in the expected time for a wound of that type, which is usually less than 3 weeks. Delays in healing can occur at any phase but most often occur in the inflammatory phase.

Leg ulcers

In resource-rich countries, the most common chronic wounds are leg ulcers. An ulcer can be defined as a break in the epithelial continuity. A prolonged inflammatory phase leads to overgrowth of granulation tissue, and attempts to heal by scarring leave a fibrotic margin. Necrotic tissue, often at the ulcer centre, is called slough. The more common aetiologies are listed in *Summary box 3.4*.

A chronic ulcer, unresponsive to dressings and simple treatments, should be biopsied to rule out neoplastic change, a squamous cell carcinoma known as a Marjolin's ulcer being the most common. Effective treatment of any leg ulcer depends on treating the underlying cause, and diagnosis is therefore vital. Arterial and venous circulation should be assessed, as should sensation throughout the lower limb. Surgical treatment is only indicated if non-operative treatment has failed or if the patient suffers from intractable pain. Meshed skin grafts (**Figure 3.7**) are more successful than sheet grafts and have the advantage of allowing mobilisation, as any tissue exudate can escape through the mesh. It should be stressed that the recurrence rate is high in venous ulceration, and patient compliance with a regime of hygiene, elevation and elastic compression is essential.

Summary box 3.4

Aetiology of leg ulcers

- Venous disease leading to local venous hypertension (e.g. varicose veins)
- Arterial disease, either large vessel (atherosclerosis) or small vessel (diabetes)
- Arteritis associated with autoimmune disease (rheumatoid arthritis, lupus, etc.)
- Trauma – could be self-inflicted
- Chronic infection – tuberculosis/syphilis
- Neoplastic – squamous or basal cell carcinoma, sarcoma

Pressure sores

These can be defined as tissue necrosis with ulceration due to prolonged pressure. Less preferable terms are bed sores, pressure ulcers and decubitus ulcers. They should be regarded as preventable but occur in approximately 5% of all hospitalised patients (range 3–12% in published literature). There is a higher incidence in paraplegic patients, in the elderly and in the severely ill patient. The most common sites are listed in *Summary box 3.5*.

A staging system for description of pressure sores devised by the American National Pressure Ulcer Advisory Panel is shown in *Table 3.2*.

Summary box 3.5

Pressure sore frequency in descending order

- Ischium
- Greater trochanter
- Sacrum
- Heel
- Malleolus (lateral then medial)
- Occiput

TABLE 3.2 Staging of pressure sores.

Stage	Description
1	Non-blanchable erythema without a breach in the epidermis
2	Partial-thickness skin loss involving the epidermis and dermis
3	Full-thickness skin loss extending into the subcutaneous tissue but not through underlying fascia
4	Full-thickness skin loss through fascia with extensive tissue destruction, maybe involving muscle, bone, tendon or joint

If external pressure exceeds the capillary occlusive pressure (over 30 mmHg), blood flow to the skin ceases, leading to tissue anoxia, necrosis and ulceration (**Figure 3.9**). Prevention

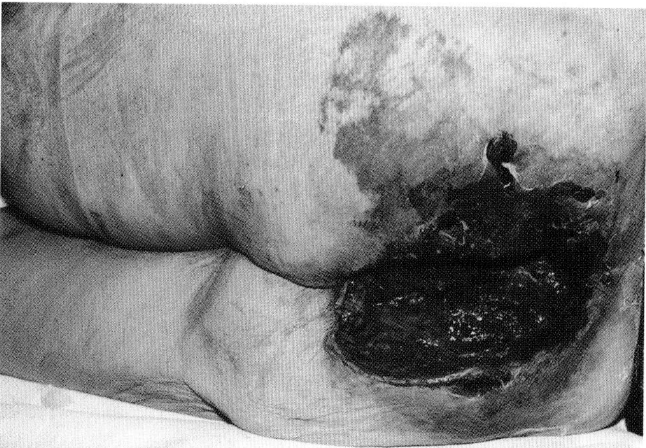

Figure 3.9 Pressure ulcer.

Jean-Nicholas Marjolin, 1780–1850, surgeon, Paris, France, described the development of carcinomatous ulcers in scars in 1828.

is obviously the best treatment, with good skin care, special pressure dispersion cushions or foams, the use of low air loss and air-fluidised beds and urinary or faecal diversion in selected cases. Pressure sore awareness is vital, and the bed-bound patient should be turned at least every 2 hours, with the wheelchair-bound patient being taught to lift themselves off their seat for 10 seconds every 10 minutes. It should be stressed that the most important treatment is to treat the cause of the pressure sore and that surgical treatment is a last resort often doomed to failure if the cause persists.

Surgical management of pressure sores follows the same principles involved in acute wound treatment (*Summary box 3.4*). The patient must be well motivated, clinically stable with good nutrition and adhere to the preventative measures advised postoperatively. Preoperative management of the pressure sore involves adequate debridement, and the use of vacuum-assisted closure (VAC) may help to provide a suitable wound for surgical closure (see below). The aim is to fill the dead space and to provide durable sensate skin. Large skin flaps that include muscle are best and, occasionally, an intact sensory innervated area can be included (e.g. extensor fascia lata flap with lateral cutaneous nerve of the thigh). If possible, use a flap that can be advanced further if there is recurrence and that does not interfere with the planning of neighbouring flaps that may be used in the future.

Vacuum-assisted closure

This is now more correctly known as negative pressure wound closure. Applying intermittent negative pressure of approximately −125 mmHg appears to hasten debridement and the formation of granulation tissue in chronic wounds and ulcers. A foam dressing is cut to size to fit the wound. A perforated wound drain is placed over the foam, and the wound is sealed with a transparent adhesive film. A vacuum is then applied to the drain (**Figure 3.10**). Negative pressure may act by decreasing oedema, by removing interstitial fluid and by increasing blood flow. As a result, bacterial counts decrease and cell proliferation increases, thereby creating a suitable bed for graft or flap cover.

NECROTISING SOFT-TISSUE INFECTIONS

These are rare but often fatal. They are most commonly polymicrobial infections with Gram-positive aerobes (*Staphylococcus aureus*, *S. pyogenes*), Gram-negative anaerobes (*Escherichia coli*, *Pseudomonas*, *Clostridium*, *Bacteroides*) and beta-haemolytic *Streptococcus*. There is usually a history of trauma or surgery with wound contamination. Sometimes, the patient's own defence mechanisms may be deficient. These infections are characterised by sudden presentation and rapid progression. The fact that deeper tissues are involved often leads to a late or missed diagnosis (**Figure 3.11**). Clinical signs are shown in *Summary box 3.6*.

There are two main types of necrotising infections: clostridial (gas gangrene) and non-clostridial (streptococcal gangrene and necrotising fasciitis). The variant of necrotising fasciitis with toxic shock syndrome results from *Streptococcus pyogenes* and is often called the 'flesh-eating bug' in this situation. Treatment consists of appropriate antibiotics with wide surgical excision. Tissue biopsies are essential for histological

Summary box 3.6

Signs and symptoms of necrotising infections

- Unusual pain
- Oedema beyond area of erythema
- Crepitus
- Skin blistering
- Fever (often absent)
- Greyish drainage ('dishwater pus')
- Pink/orange skin staining
- Focal skin gangrene (late sign)
- Shock, coagulopathy and multiorgan failure

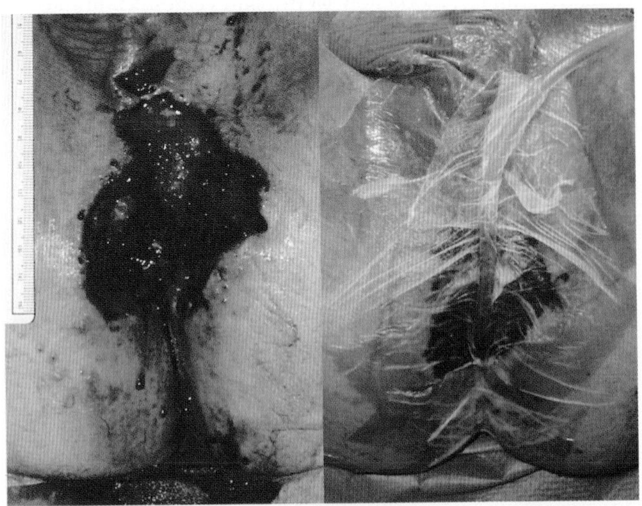

Figure 3.10 Vacuum-assisted closure dressing of a large wound.

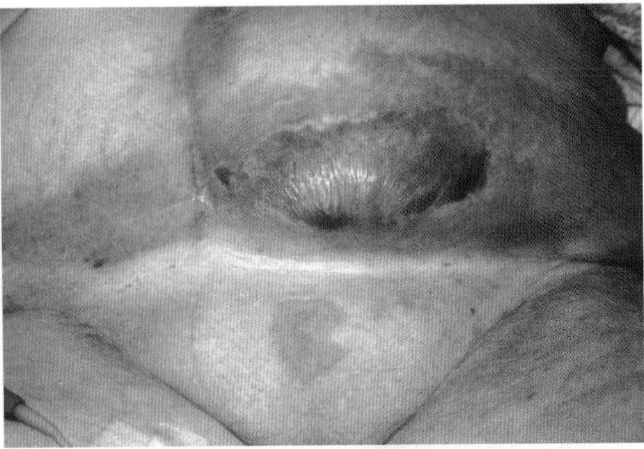

Figure 3.11 Necrotising fasciitis of the anterior abdominal wall.

Hans Christian Joachim Gram, 1853–1938, Professor of Pharmacology (1891–1900) and of Medicine (1900–1923), Copenhagen, Denmark, described this method of staining bacteria in 1884.

diagnosis and culture to obtain appropriate antibiotic sensitivity information. The raw areas resulting from excision often require skin grafting. Treatment is surgical excision, with tissue biopsies being sent for culture and diagnosis. Wide raw areas requiring skin grafting often result.

SCARS

The maturation phase of wound healing has been discussed above and represents the formation of what is described as a scar. The immature scar becomes mature over a period lasting a year or more, but it is at first pink, hard, raised and often itchy. The disorganised collagen fibres become aligned along stress lines with their strength being in their weave rather than in their amount (this has been compared with steel wool being slowly woven into a cable). As the collagen matures and becomes denser, the scar becomes almost acellular as the fibroblasts and blood vessels reduce. The external appearance of the scar becomes paler, while the scar becomes softer, flattens and its itchiness diminishes. Most of these changes occur over the first three months but a scar will continue to mature for one to two years. Tensile strength will continue to increase but would not be expected to exceed 60–80% that of normal skin.

Scars are often described as being atrophic, hypertrophic and keloid. An atrophic scar is pale, flat and stretched in appearance, often appearing on the back and in areas of tension. It is easily traumatised as the epidermis and dermis are thinned. Excision and resuturing may only rarely improve such a scar.

A hypertrophic scar is defined as excessive scar tissue that does not extend beyond the boundary of the original incision or wound. It results from a prolonged inflammatory phase of wound healing and from unfavourable scar siting (i.e. across the lines of skin tension). In the face, these are known as the lines of facial expression.

A keloid scar is defined as excessive scar tissue that extends beyond the boundaries of the original incision or wound (**Figure 3.12**). Its aetiology is unknown, but it is associated with elevated levels of growth factor, deeply pigmented skin, an inherited tendency and certain areas of the body (e.g. a triangle whose points are the xiphisternum and each shoulder tip).

The histology of both hypertrophic and keloid scars shows excess collagen with hypervascularity, but this is more marked in keloids where there is more type III collagen.

The treatment of both hypertrophic and keloid scars is difficult and is summarised in *Summary box 3.7*.

Hypertrophic scars improve spontaneously with time, whereas keloid scars do not.

Summary box 3.7

Treatment of hypertrophic and keloid scars

- Pressure – local moulds or elasticated garments
- Silicone gel sheeting (mechanism unknown)
- Intralesional steroid injection (triamcinolone)
- Excision and steroid injections[a]
- Excision and postoperative radiation (external beam or brachytherapy)[a]
- Intralesional excision (keloids only)
- Laser – to reduce redness (which may resolve in any event)
- Vitamin E or palm oil massage (unproven)

[a]All excisions are associated with high rates of recurrence.

AVOIDABLE SCARRING

If an acute wound has been managed correctly (see *Summary box 3.3*), most of the problems described above should not occur. However, the surgeon should always stress to the patient that there will be a scar of some description after wounding, be it planned or accidental. A dirt-ingrained (tattooed) scar is usually preventable by proper initial scrubbing and cleansing of the wound (**Figure 3.13**). Late treatment may require excision of the scar or pigment destruction by laser.

Mismatched or misaligned scars result from a failure to recognise normal landmarks, such as the lip vermilion/white roll interface, eyelid and nostril free margins and hair lines such as

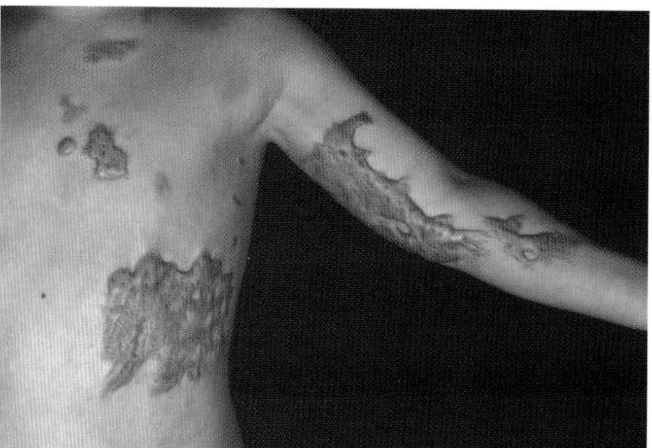

Figure 3.12 Multiple keloid scars.

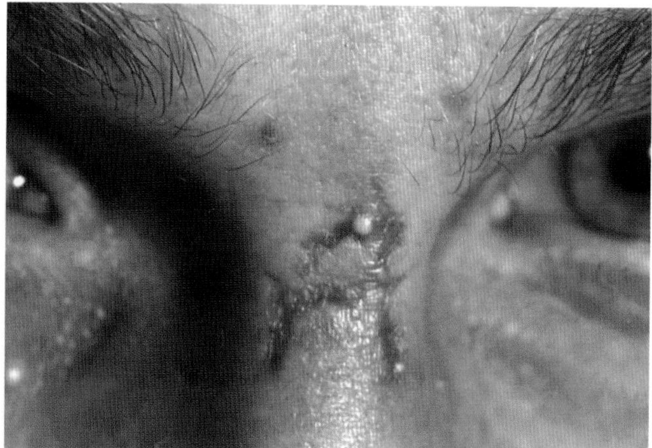

Figure 3.13 Dirt-ingrained scar.

Laser is an acronym for Light Amplification by Stimulated Emission of Radiation. A laser is an intense beam of monochromatic light.

those relating to eyebrows and moustache. Treatment consists of excision and resuturing.

Poorly contoured scars can be stepped, grooved or pincushioned. Most are caused by poor alignment of deep structures such as muscle or fat, but trapdoor or pincushioned scars are often unavoidable unless the almost circumferential wound can be excised initially. Late treatment consists of scar excision and correct alignment of deeper structures or, as in the case of a trapdoor scar, an excision of the scar margins and repair using W or Z-plasty techniques.

Suture marks may be minimised by using monofilament sutures that are removed early (3–5 days). Sutures inserted under tension will leave marks. Wounds can be strengthened post suture removal by the use of sticky strips. Fine sutures (6/0 or smaller) placed close to the wound margins tend to leave less scarring. Subcuticular suturing avoids suture marks either side of the wound or incision.

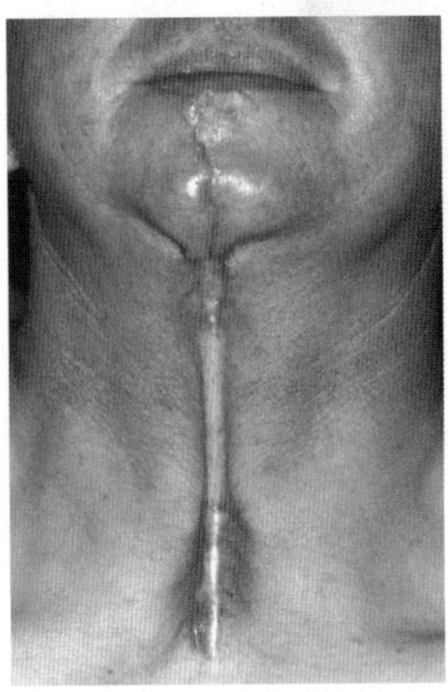

Figure 3.15 Post-traumatic (chainsaw) midline neck contracture.

CONTRACTURES

Where scars cross joints or flexion creases, a tight web may form restricting the range of movement at the joint. This may be referred to as a contracture and can cause hyperextension or hyperflexion deformity (**Figure 3.14**). In the neck, it may interfere with head extension (**Figure 3.15**). Treatment may be simple involving, multiple Z-plasties (**Figure 3.16**), or more complex, requiring the inset of grafts or flaps. Splintage and intensive physiotherapy are often required postoperatively.

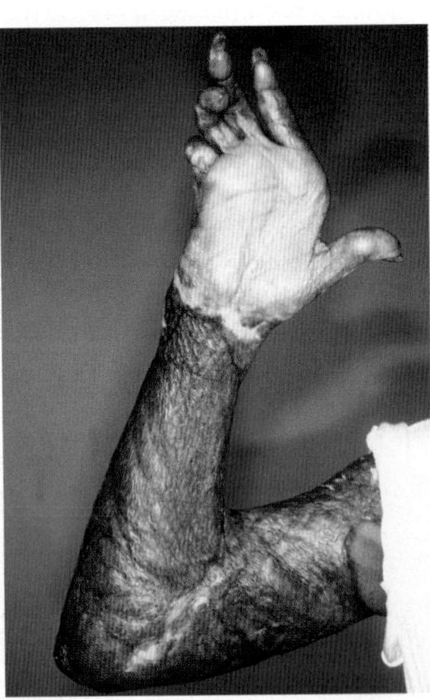

Figure 3.14 Burn contractures showing hyperextended fingers and hyperflexed elbow.

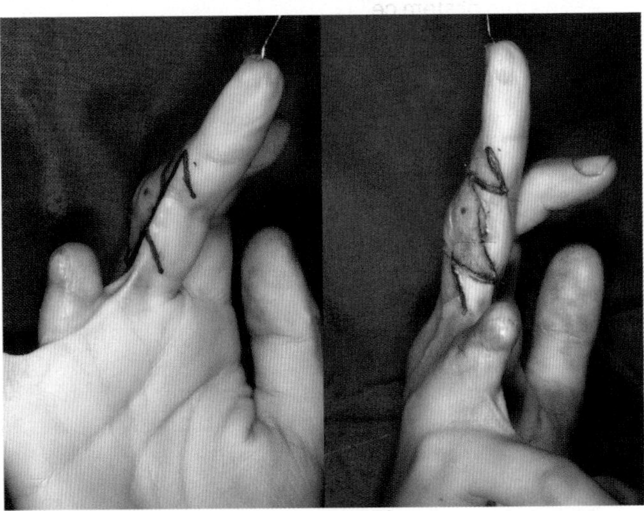

Figure 3.16 Multiple Z-plasty release of finger contracture.

FURTHER READING

Brown DL, Borschel GH. *Michigan manual of plastic surgery*. Baltimore, MD: Lippincott, Williams & Wilkins, 2004.

Georgiade GS, Riefkokl R, Levin LS. *Georgiade plastic, maxillofacial and reconstructive surgery*, 3rd edn. Baltimore, MD: Williams & Wilkins, 1997.

McGregor AD, McGregor, IA. *Fundamental techniques of plastic surgery*, 10th edn. Edinburgh: Churchill Livingstone, 2000.

Richards AM, MacLeod T, Dafydd H. *Key notes on plastic surgery*. Oxford: Wiley-Blackwell, 2012.

Thomas S. *An introduction to the use of vacuum assisted closure*. World Wide Wounds, 2001; available from: www.worldwidewounds.com.

Westaby S. *Wound care*. London: William Heinemann Medical Books Ltd, 1985.

Chapter 4

Tissue engineering and regeneration

Learning objectives

To understand:

- The potential opportunities afforded by tissue engineering and regenerative medicine
- The nature of stem cells, including somatic and adult stem cells, embryonic stem cells, fetal stem cells and induced pluripotent stem cells
- The role and range of scaffolds for tissue engineering
- The different approaches for seeding scaffolds and bioreactor technology
- The main safety issues and current limitations to clinical application

INTRODUCTION

Tissue engineering and regenerative medicine are relatively new but rapidly expanding multidisciplinary fields of clinical medicine, which have the potential to revolutionise the treatment of a wide range of human diseases. The ability of tissues to undergo spontaneous repair and regeneration is highly variable but in many cases very limited. Bone, for example, is one of the few tissues able to undergo effective regeneration, so long as the defective tissue is not too extensive. Adjacent cartilage, on the other hand, in common with most tissues, has little or no propensity for spontaneous regeneration, in terms of quality and quantity, following injury or arthritic disease. The limited ability of tissues to repair themselves has driven the desire to develop cell therapy and tissue engineering approaches to repair or replace diseased and damaged tissues. In most cases this involves the implantation of cells and tissues that have been expanded *in vitro* (outside the body), either as a cell therapy or with cells seeded into natural or synthetically based tissue scaffolds. However, cells (with or without expansion) and cellularised or cell-free scaffolds may also be implanted into areas of tissue injury with the aim of promoting *in vivo* (inside the body) regeneration and repair of tissues. This chapter provides a brief overview of tissue engineering and regenerative therapy, highlighting the opportunities, challenges and likely future directions.

OPPORTUNITIES

The potential impact of tissue engineering and regenerative therapies is so far-reaching that practising surgeons should be aware of the opportunities afforded to improve radically the management of patients. Stem cell therapy has the potential to provide treatment for a wide range of diseases, including spinal cord injury and neurodegenerative conditions, cardiovascular disease, degenerative retinal conditions, type I diabetes and diseases of the musculoskeletal system. The field of tissue engineering is of particular relevance to surgeons because many of the potential future clinical applications are for conditions where surgeons are closely involved in assessment and treatment (*Table 4.1*). Selected examples include

TABLE 4.1 Examples of tissues created by tissue engineering and conditions they may be used to treat.

Tissue	Conditions treated
Skin	Burns and skin defects after excision or trauma
Cardiac muscle	Heart failure
Heart valves	Congenital and acquired valvular heart disease
Cartilage	Degenerative and traumatic joint disorders
Trachea and bronchus	Congenital and acquired stenosis and resection for malignancy
Bladder	Congenital bladder malformation, and cystectomy
Anal/bladder sphincter	Incontinence
Pancreatic islets	Insulin-dependent diabetes
Large blood vessels	Atheromatous, aneurysmal and traumatic arterial disease
Oesophagus	Benign stenosis, and resection for malignancy
Small intestine	Intestinal failure after surgical resection for Crohn's disease, cancer or ischaemia

repair or replacement of injured or diseased cartilage, skin, pancreatic islets, bladder, intestine, heart tissue, arteries, larynx and bronchus. A longer-term goal in tissue engineering is the replacement of diseased whole organs such as the liver and kidney, although the technical challenges here are enormous.

Surgeons are integral to many of the multidisciplinary research teams currently undertaking translational research in the field and will play a vital role in the future delivery and assessment of many of the treatments based on tissue engineering and regenerative therapy. In addition to its direct therapeutic application, tissue engineering also has the potential to provide *in vitro* tissues that can be used to model human disease and to test therapeutic drugs for efficacy and toxicity. It is important to emphasise, however, that while the potential benefit of cell therapy and tissue engineering is undeniable, there are many technical, regulatory and safety issues to be addressed for it to have wide clinical impact.

Summary box 4.1

Tissue engineering and regenerative therapies have potential to provide:

- Treatment for a wide range of diseases
- Clinical applications in surgical assessment and treatment
- Models to test therapeutic efficacy and toxicity

THE KEY AREAS OF UNDERPINNING SCIENCE

Advances in both the biological and physical sciences underpin the fields of tissue engineering and regenerative therapy (**Figure 4.1**). In the biological sciences, new discoveries in stem cell biology have been key, particularly an understanding of the different types of stem cell, and how these can be derived and directed *in vitro* to differentiate into specialised cell types. In material sciences, major advances in the manufacture of scaffolds, on which to seed cells or to encourage specific interaction with host cells, have been key. In particular, design goals relate to scaffolds that possess both the physical and the biological characteristics that allow cells to create tissues, and potentially even organs, for therapeutic purposes. Key also have been engineering advances in the development of the many different types of bioreactors that provide an appropriate physical environment for growing engineered tissues *in vitro*, outside the body in the laboratory.

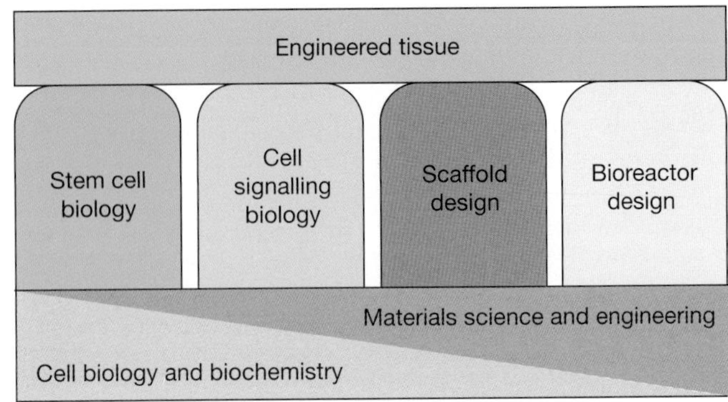

Figure 4.1 Underpinning science in tissue engineering and cell therapy.

There is considerable commercial interest in tissue engineering and regenerative therapy and this is contributing to the rapid pace of development in these areas. Notwithstanding the potential offered by these therapies, it should be emphasised that the whole field is still at a relatively early stage of development. While there are examples where tissue engineering and regenerative therapies have already been introduced into clinical practice (e.g. for repair of damaged cartilage), most potential regenerative therapies have not yet entered routine surgical practice, as there are considerable barriers to be overcome before this translational step can be achieved.

SOURCE OF CELLS FOR TISSUE ENGINEERING

Both fully differentiated cells (somatic cells) and stem cells are being used for tissue engineering and regenerative therapy, but most of the focus is on the use of stem cells, particularly somatic stem cells (SSCs) such as mesenchymal stem cells, and induced pluripotent stem cells (iPSCs). The major features of the different cell types are listed in *Table 4.2*.

Somatic cells

Fully differentiated specialised cells (somatic cells) obtained from normal tissues have been used for tissue engineering and

TABLE 4.2 Cells used in tissue engineering and regenerative therapy.

Cell type	Somatic cells	SSCs	hESCs	Fetal cells	iPSCs
Ease of availability	Limited	Good	Moderate	Moderate	Good
Expansion *in vitro*	Limited	Good	Excellent	Good	Excellent
Pluripotency	No	Limited	Excellent	Limited	Excellent
Ethical concerns	No	No	Yes	Yes	Yes*
Risk of malignancy	None	Low	Moderate	Moderate	Moderate
Autologous	Yes	Yes	No	No	Yes
Likely future use	Limited	High	Limited	Limited	High

hESCs, human embryonic stem cells; iPSCs, induced pluripotent stem cells; SSCs, somatic stem cells. *Note iPSCs avoid some of the ethical issues associated with hESCs.

regenerative therapy with some degree of success. For example, skin has been engineered using cultured epithelial cells grown *in vitro* and used to treat patients with burn injuries. Chondrocytes have been isolated, expanded *in vitro*, and implanted into areas of deficient cartilage in a procedure called autologous chondrocyte implantation. Bladder wall has also been engineered using a combination of smooth muscle cells and uroepithelial cells expanded *in vitro* and grown on a scaffold before reimplantation. Such tissues can be grown using cells obtained from the intended recipient by tissue biopsy (autologous cells) or using cells obtained from deceased unrelated donors (allogeneic cells). The major advantage of the former source is that after implantation they are not rejected by the recipient's immune system and hence there is no requirement for immunosuppression (see Chapter 82 for a description of immunosuppressive agents and their side effects).

For other indications, the use of fully differentiated specialised cells is not practical in most situations because such cells are not readily available in sufficient numbers and they have only limited proliferative ability *in vitro*, which means their numbers cannot be readily expanded to sufficient levels. To overcome these limitations, the major focus in the field of cell therapy has been on the use of stem cells.

Stem cells

Stem cells are undifferentiated or non-specialised cells that are able, through cell division, to renew themselves indefinitely. Crucially, they are also able, when provided with the appropriate stimuli, to differentiate into one or more of the different types of specialised cell found in tissues and organs. Because of their unique ability to undergo self-renewal when cultured *in vitro* and to be directed to differentiate into specialised cell types, they have enormous potential for use as cell-based therapies. There are several different types of stem cell with different characteristics, all of which have potential uses in regenerative medicine.

Stem cells can be classified according to whether they are derived from the early embryo (embryonic stem cells), tissues from the fetus (fetal stem cells), later in development (adult or somatic stem cells) or whether they are derived by reprogramming adult specialised cells to become pluripotent stem cells (iPSCs).

Adult tissue resident or somatic stem cells (SSCs)

Stem cells resident in the different tissues and organs are responsible for providing replacements for specialised cells that have reached the end of their functional lifespan either through natural attrition or because of damage and disease. In certain tissues and organs, notably the bone marrow and gut, stem cells regularly divide and differentiate into specialised cells to replace senescent or damaged cells in the blood and the gastrointestinal mucosa, respectively. Stem cells in other organs, such as the heart or central nervous system, are less able to effect repair or replacement. SSCs have the capacity to differentiate into a limited number of specialised cell types (i.e. they are multipotent). Among the best characterised types of SSCs are haematopoeitic stem cells, mesenchymal stem or stromal cells (MSCs), endothelial progenitor cells and neural stem cells. While haematopoeitic stem cells are widely used for treatment of haematological malignancies, the somatic stem cell type that has been most widely used for tissue engineering and regenerative therapy is the MSC.

Mesenchymal stem and stromal cells

MSCs are multipotent stromal cells that can be sourced from a variety of tissues, including bone marrow, adipose tissue and umbilical cord. Morphologically they resemble fibroblasts. They are adherent to plastic, express certain cell surface markers (CD105, CD73 and CD90), and do not express the cell surface markers associated with haematopoietic stem cells (such as CD34 and CD45). MSCs were initially shown to have the ability to be directed to differentiate into a variety of specialised cell types of the mesodermal lineages, including osteoblasts, chondrocytes, adipocytes, tenocytes and myocytes (**Figure 4.2**). Recent studies suggest that they may also be directed into cells of the ectoderm and endoderm lineages.

Of further clinical importance, MSCs have potent trophic and anti-inflammatory properties, attributable to their ability to produce growth factors (including vascular endothelial growth factor (VEGF), insulin-like growth factor (IGF), hepatocyte growth factor (HGF)), and prostaglandin E2. MSCs for therapeutic use can be isolated from bone marrow (iliac crest aspiration) or from subcutaneous fat (liposuction) which is less invasive and gives a high yield of MSCs. In both cases, MSCs are isolated *in vitro* on the basis of their adherence to plastic. They can then be used either immediately, or after expansion of their numbers by *in vitro* culture. Alternatively, MSCs can be differentiated into the desired lineage *in vitro* by addition of suitable growth factors and chemicals.

The relative ease of cell acquisition has meant that autologous MSCs have been used clinically in a variety of settings such as treatment of burns and to repair defects in cartilage. More clinical evidence is required in terms of efficacy and mechanism of action, as it is not entirely clear whether a given clinical effect resulting from MSC administration is attributable to their ability to contribute directly to tissue regeneration, or due to immunomodulatory and paracrine effects resulting from their ability to release trophic mediators that promote tissue repair by recipient cells (**Figure 4.2**).

Embryonic stem cells (ESCs)

In the embryo, stem cells are able to give rise to all of the different cell types of the body (i.e. they are totipotent). ESCs are obtained from the inner cell mass of the early human blastocyst (days 4–5 after fertilisation) using embryos that have been created through *in vitro* fertilisation for treatment of infertility, and are surplus to those needed for reimplantation. The technique for isolating and growing hESCs in culture was developed by James Thompson at the University of Wisconsin, Madison, USA in 1998.

ESCs have much greater proliferative ability than MSCs and, as already noted, can differentiate into all types of specialised cells, unlike MSCs. However, their use has major

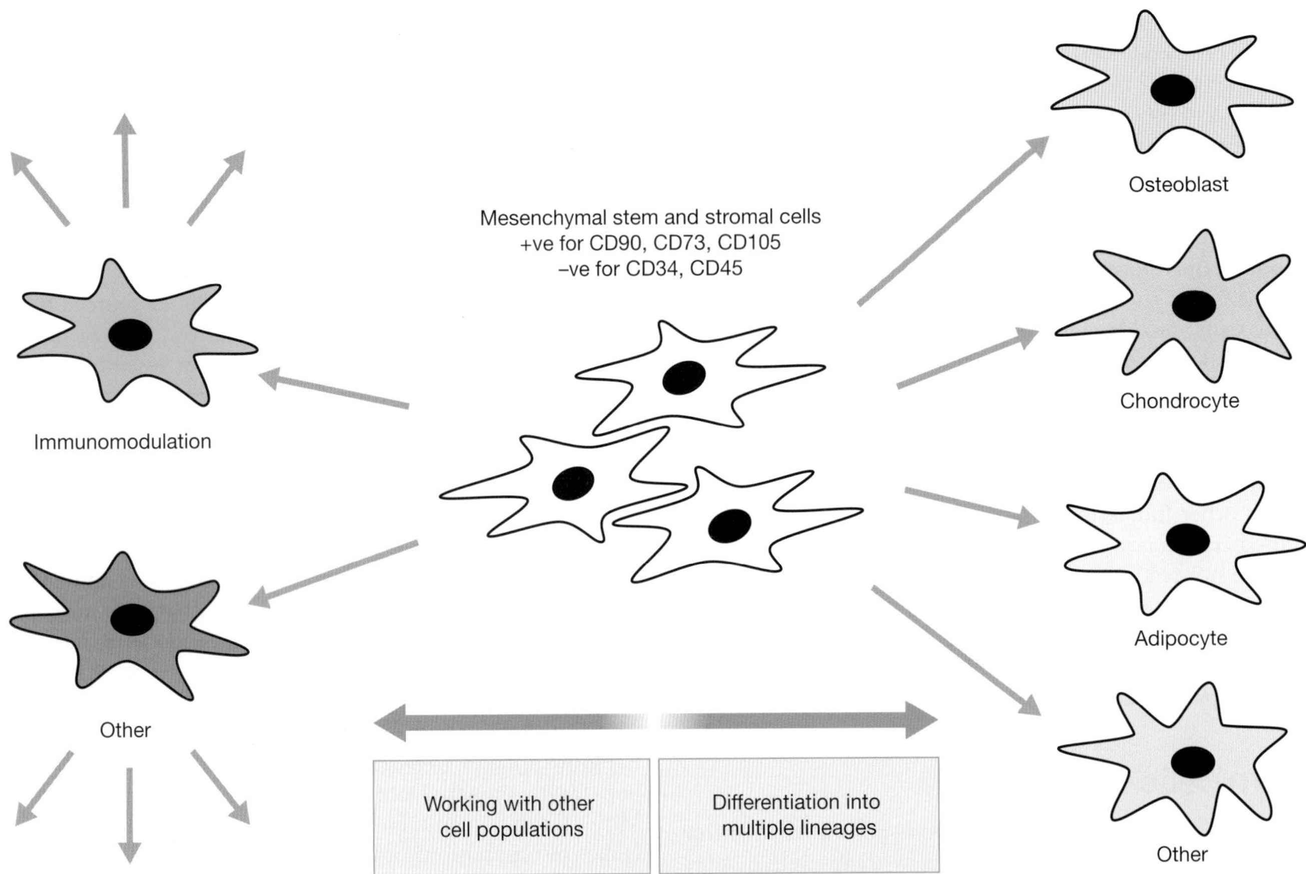

Figure 4.2 Proposed characteristics of mesenchymal stem and stromal cells relevant to tissue engineering and regenerative medicine.

limitations, one of which is ethical. The surplus embryos used for derivation of ESCs would otherwise be discarded, but because they need to be destroyed to obtain ESCs the approach has raised major ethical and political debate. The dominant view in many countries, including the UK, is that the potential therapeutic benefits of ESCs justify their use but there are very strict guidelines for their derivation, and to date their clinical use has been very limited. Cells from ESCs would be allogeneic and therefore be at risk of immunological rejection. It would, in principle, be possible to produce ESCs that were autologous for an intended recipient by the process of somatic cell nuclear transfer, i.e. transferring the nucleus from a somatic cell of the intended recipient into an oocyte that has had its nucleus removed. The transferred somatic cell nucleus, containing the human leukocyte antigen (HLA) genes and all of the other genetic information from the donor, is turned into a pluripotent stem cell that can be used as cell therapy for the donor of the nucleus.

Fetal stem cells

Stem cells can also be obtained from the blood, bone marrow and other tissues of aborted fetuses (fetal stem cells). These proliferate *in vitro* as efficiently as ESCs and are pluripotent. They have been used as cell therapy in a variety of clinical settings, including Parkinson's disease, diabetes and spinal cord injury. In some studies they showed early promise but the magnitude of any clinical benefits is controversial. The use of fetal stem cells also poses ethical challenges, although perhaps not to the extent seen with ESCs.

Induced pluripotent stem cells (iPSCs)

The discovery in 2006 by Shinya Yamanaka, building on the earlier work of John Gurdon, that certain types of specialised adult cells could be reprogrammed using genetic manipulation to become embryonic-like iPSCs was a major breakthrough. Using retroviral or lentiviral transfection to introduce a combination of transcription factors (OCT3/4, SOX2, and either Kruppel-like factor and C-MYC (together designated the OSKM reprogramming factors) or NANOG and LIN28), it was shown that specialised somatic cells can be reprogrammed to become stem cells. Moreover, iPSCs proliferate *in vitro* as efficiently as ESCs and are pluripotent, thereby circumventing concerns about the use of human embryos. Importantly, the development of iPSCs also means that, at least in principle, an intended recipient of stem cell therapy can themselves provide a source of stem cells (e.g. from a skin biopsy or blood sample) that can then be directed to differentiate into the desired specialised cell type for therapy; because such cells would be autologous they would not provoke an immunological rejection response (**Figure 4.3**). Alternatively, iPSCs could be obtained from a number of volunteer donors selected on the basis of their

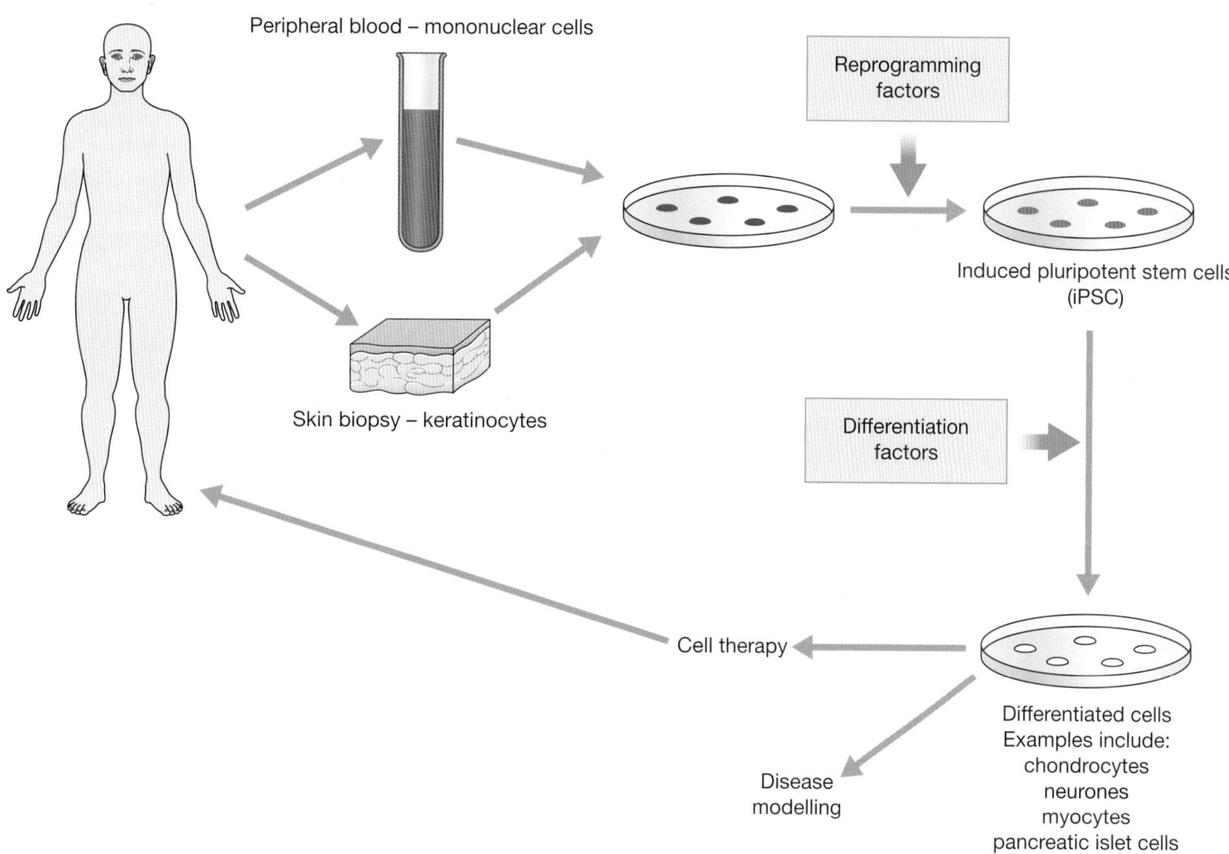

Figure 4.3 Schematic diagram showing the principles of iPSC therapy. Mononuclear cells from peripheral blood or keratinocytes from a skin biopsy are cultured *in vitro* and then reprogrammed to become iPSC by addition of reprogramming factors. The iPSC are then expanded, and selected differentiation factors added to promote differentiation of iPSCs into the desired specialised cell type for use as therapy.

HLA type and stored to create a national or international tissue bank of iPSCs. Lines of iPSCs could then be chosen from the bank to provide a fully or partially matched cell transplant for recipients, eliminating or reducing the need for immunosuppression to prevent immunological rejection.

One of the problems of reprogramming somatic cells to become iPSCs using retroviruses is that genomic integration of the virus may lead to activation of oncogenic genes, causing tumorigenesis. To reduce this risk, non-retroviral vectors have been used (such as adenovirus and Sandai virus vectors, that do not insert their own genes into the host cell genome), or plasmids, episomal vectors and synthetic RNA. There has also been much recent progress in identifying combinations of small molecules, growth factors and chemicals that mimic the effect of viral transfection with transcription factors and obviate the need for viral vectors altogether. The production process from sourcing cells (e.g. skin fibroblasts or peripheral blood mononuclear cells) to obtaining an adequate number of validated iPSCs may take several weeks.

In vitro differentiation of stem cells to specialised tissue cells

There is an enormous research effort aimed at better understanding the factors responsible for cell fate decisions, and establishing effective and reproducible protocols that can be used to differentiate stem cells *in vitro* into the desired type of specialised cell. Typically such protocols use culture in chemically defined media containing cocktails of small molecules that stimulate or inhibit key signalling pathways, along with cytokines, growth factors and chemicals. Many protocols include the addition of critical amounts of Activin, bone-morphogenetic protein-4 (BMP4) and fibroblast growth factor-2 (FGF2) at specific time points during culture, but protocols vary widely. For example, exposure of iPSCs to a combination of retinoic acid and BMP4 promotes differentiation along the ectoderm and then the keratinocyte lineage. Alternatively, culture of iPSCs on a Matrigel® scaffold in defined media supplemented with ascorbic acid and exposed sequentially to a glycogen synthase kinase (GSK) inhibitor followed by an inhibitor of Wnt signalling promotes the development of immature cardiomyocytes.

It is becoming increasingly clear that exposure to certain biomaterials and the physical attributes of a scaffold, including its surface characteristics, also promote stem cell differentiation along a particular lineage. Mechanical stress also influences cell fate decisions.

Protocols for differentiation often promote stem cells to differentiate in steps through intermediate stages that mirror normal *in vivo* development. In other words, sequential exposure to different factors is used first to differentiate ESCs or iPSCs into either endoderm, mesoderm or ectoderm lineages, followed by further differentiation into the specific lineage desired. After stem cells have been subjected to *in vitro* differentiation, it is essential that the purity of the differentiated cells and the absence of undifferentiated stem cells are confirmed, to reduce the risk of tumour transmission. The cells must also be fully phenotyped and their function confirmed before they are used for therapeutic purposes.

SCAFFOLDS FOR TISSUE ENGINEERING

The complex anatomical arrangement of the different cell types in tissues and organs is absolutely integral to their normal function, and the importance of structural integrity is evident in many diseases where deranged tissue structure and tissue remodelling is associated with a failure in function. Stem cells and their progeny are able, when cultured under conventional tissue culture conditions, to form cell sheets or small three-dimensional collections of cells (organoids), but they are not able under such conditions spontaneously to assume the complex anatomical relationships seen in normal tissues. To do so they need to be provided with an appropriate scaffold that gives physical support and shape to the engineered tissue, mimicking extracellular matrix. This allows cells to attach, and delivers the cell signals necessary to guide the cell growth, migration and differentiation to form a functional tissue. Tissue engineering typically utilises rigid or semi-rigid scaffolds (usually three-dimensional) that are porous (**Figure 4.4**) and act as templates on which to seed donor cells and guide them to restore a functional tissue or organ that can then be implanted in the recipient. Scaffolds may be derived from intact human tissue (natural scaffolds) or from engineered implantable biomaterials (artificial scaffolds). The general requirements that a scaffold must provide are listed in *Table 4.3*, and the choice of scaffolds that best fulfils the requirements for tissue engineering will depend on the nature of the tissue to be engineered.

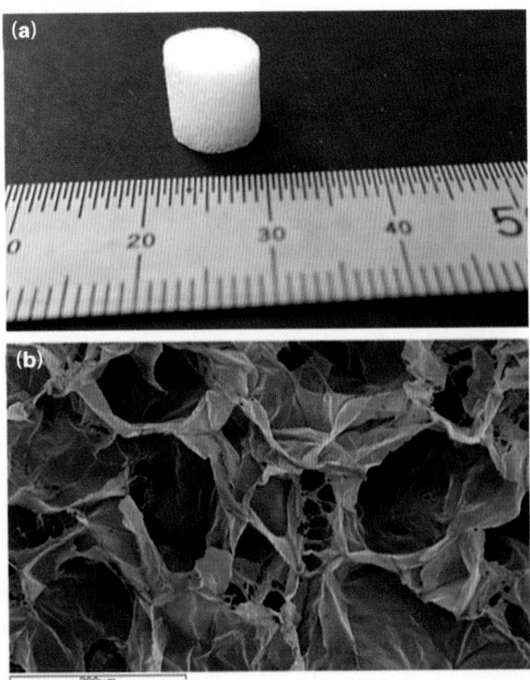

Figure 4.4 An example of a porous scaffold in research development, manufactured using collagen. (**a**) Macroscopic view of collagen scaffold. (**b**) Overview of a scanning electron microscopy (SEM) image that shows the structure of collagen scaffold (courtesy of Prof S Best and Prof R Cameron, University of Cambridge).

TABLE 4.3 Requirements of a scaffold used in tissue engineering.
Provide structural support for cells
Allow cells to attach, migrate and proliferate
Enable oxygen, nutrients and regulatory factors access to all cells
Deliver signals to promote cell migration and proliferation
Biocompatible, non-immunogenic and ideally biodegradable

Summary box 4.2

Regenerative scaffolds can:

- Provide physical support and shape to the engineered tissue
- Guide cell growth, migration and differentiation
- Be natural or artificial

Natural scaffolds

Natural scaffolds may be obtained by treatment of human (or other animal) tissues or organs to remove the resident cell types, leaving behind the extracellular matrix that preserves the intricate architecture of the tissue or organ, onto which to seed new cells. Natural scaffolds not only act as a physical scaffold that allows the natural architecture of the tissue to be preserved, but they may also provide key cell signals that guide the growth and differentiation of the cells used to repopulate the scaffold. Typically, natural scaffolds are obtained either by immersing tissues in detergent or perfusing them with detergent via the arterial tree. This effectively destroys most or all of the cellular elements of the tissue or organ but leaves the collagen-rich extracellular matrix largely intact. Variable protocols have been used successfully to achieve decellurisation, and the optimal approach probably varies according to the type of tissue or organ being used to create the scaffold. The use of natural scaffolds may be particularly suited to certain applications where deceased donor tissue is relatively easy to source, for example to engineer lengths of trachea. The use of natural scaffolds to engineer whole organs such as the kidney or liver has the advantage that the extremely intricate three-dimensional structure of the organ is preserved and this would be extremely challenging to achieve using engineered biocompatible materials. Moreover, decellularised organ scaffolds provide an opportunity to repopulate the scaffold with autologous cells derived from the potential recipient to create an organ that is not susceptible to immunological rejection, thereby avoiding the need for immunosuppressive drugs and their attendant side effects. However, a significant disadvantage of using decellularised scaffolds to engineer whole organs is the need to use a whole human organ for each organ to be engineered; the availability of such organs is likely to be limited.

Summary box 4.3

Natural scaffolds:

- Can be prepared by removal of the resident cell types from tissue, for example with detergent
- Consist of tissue extracellular matrix, which can preserve intricate anatomical structures

Artificial scaffolds

The materials used to create artificial scaffolds are highly variable, and new materials are being developed continually. Different scaffold characteristics are required for engineering different types of tissue but all scaffolds need to be biocompatible and in most settings they should be biodegradable and bioreabsorbable. Scaffolds encompass both natural and synthetic materials. Natural materials used include various polysaccharides, collagen, fibrin, gelatin and cellulose, while synthetic materials include various synthetic polymers such as polylactide (PLA) and polyglycolide (PGA), and graphene. Bioactive ceramics such as calcium phosphates (e.g. hydroxyapatite) and bioactive glasses have been widely used for skeletal repair. Synthetic biodegradable polymers are commonly used and have the advantage that they can be produced under standard conditions that ensure reproducible physical characteristics. Scaffolds can also be fabricated using a blend of natural and synthetic components to optimise their performance.

Most artificial scaffolds are fabricated with a porous three-dimensional structure, and a wide variety of designs are in use. The application of computational design and three-dimensional printing technology has revolutionised the development of artificial scaffolds. Hydrogel scaffolds composed of cross-linked hydrophilic polymers are also increasingly used in tissue engineering because of their favourable physical and chemical characteristics. They are able to absorb very large amounts of aqueous fluid while maintaining their three-dimensional shape and structural integrity. They are fabricated from naturally occurring (e.g. collagen and fibrin) or artificial (egg PLA) cross-linked polymers and can be impregnated with growth factors to promote cellularisation.

Electrospinning technology is being utilised increasingly to produce scaffolds composed of fibres with a diameter at the nanoscale level. The fibres can be spun using blends of different synthetic polymers or blends of synthetic and natural polymers, depending on the desired characteristics of the scaffold. Scaffolds based on microspheres have also been utilised. Recent developments in materials science have led to the creation of increasingly complex and innovative artificial scaffolds for tissue engineering, including composite materials (e.g. combining ceramics with polymers to gain the advantages of each), and the production of so called 'smart scaffolds' having biomimetic properties that provide biophysical cues or cellular signals to instruct and guide cell behaviour.

Historically, a limitation of traditional artificial scaffolds is that they do not incorporate a vasculature that can be used in the potential recipient to restore the vascular integrity of the transplanted tissue or organ. However, recent innovations that allow a vascular network to be created by three-dimensional printing suggest that this limitation may be overcome. Such technology also allows the design and production of scaffolds that have the structural properties (e.g. pore size and diffusion characteristics) needed to provide the necessary cues for cell differentiation and migration. Artificial scaffolds can be engineered to incorporate molecules that aid retention of particular cell growth factors, including angiogenic growth factors such as vascular endothelial growth factor (VEGF), to provide a local environment conducive to the growth of a functional tissue construct.

Summary box 4.4

Artificial scaffolds include:

- Natural materials, synthetic polymers, bioactive ceramics and glasses
- New or 'smart' materials that have biomimetic properties

Approaches to cell seeding of scaffolds and bioreactors

Cellularisation of scaffolds can be achieved *in vitro* (outside the body) by a variety of methods and the most appropriate seeding system may to some extent depend on the type of tissue being engineered (*Table 4.4*). This is a rapidly developing area and it is only possible here to outline the principles of different approaches to cell seeding. The aim is to achieve a rapid seeding of viable cells with high seeding efficiency and uniform and effective penetration of cells into the scaffold. Some systems incorporate mechanisms to deliver mechanical stress or electrical stimulation to promote cellularisation.

The most simple but possibly least effective method is static cell seeding, where a concentrated cell suspension is placed in direct contact with the scaffold. The seeding efficiency and penetration of cells into the scaffold are generally low, although scaffolds can be coated with various agents to increase the efficiency of cell attachment.

Dynamic cell seeding techniques include a range of systems in which either the scaffold is rotated in the medium containing the cells or both the scaffold and cell suspension are rotated together. Rotation in some systems occurs at

TABLE 4.4 Approaches for seeding cells into scaffolds.
Static cell seeding
Dynamic cell seeding
Magnetic cell seeding
Pressure and vacuum seeding
Photopolymerised hydrogels
Bioreactor perfusion systems

a sufficiently high speed to generate centrifugal forces. Dynamic seeding techniques increase seeding efficiency, shorten the duration of the culture period needed and may help penetration of cells into the scaffold.

Magnetic cell seeding makes use of magnetic forces to direct cells into the scaffold. Essentially, the cells are first labelled, either by using supramagnetic microbeads coated with a ligand that specifically binds to molecules on the cell surface or by culturing them with cationic liposomes that contain supramagnetic ferrous particles. Magnets are then used to attract the cells into the scaffold. This enables rapid seeding of the scaffold but a potential concern is that the magnetic particles used may have adverse effects.

Photopolymerised hydrogel scaffolds offer a completely different approach to cell seeding. Essentially, the cells are suspended in an aqueous monomer solution and ultraviolet light is used to promote polymerisation of the hydrogel scaffold. Alternatively, to increase cell adherence to the surface of polymerised hydrogel scaffolds, an arginine–glycine–aspartic acid adhesion peptide can be incorporated.

Another approach to cell seeding uses differential pressure or vacuum seeding systems to force cells into the pores of the scaffold. Again this reduces the time needed to seed cells but the pressures used may potentially reduce cell viability.

Finally, one of the more complex approaches to cell seeding is to use scaffold perfusion systems. These may take the form of bioreactor perfusion systems for tissue engineering, or whole organ perfusion systems in the case of decellularised organ scaffolds.

CHALLENGES TO ENGINEERING TISSUE *IN VITRO*

There are many technical challenges to successful engineering of tissues *in vitro*. Delivery of adequate oxygen and nutrients uniformly to three-dimensional tissue constructs is problematic, as is ensuring that the varying nutritional and growth requirements of different cell types grown simultaneously are met.

The difficulties of tissue engineering vary considerably according to the nature of the tissue or organ being engineered. Flat tissues such as skin, cornea and cartilage present fewer problems than complex tubular structures such as trachea, bronchus and blood vessels. Hollow organs, such as bladder and gut, present a much greater challenge, and complex solid organs such as the liver and kidney present the greatest challenge of all. Obtaining adequate numbers of differentiated cells, maintaining their viability and ensuring that they maintain their function and do not revert to undesirable cell types are all important challenges.

IMPLANTATION OF ENGINEERED TISSUE

Irrespective of the nature of the engineered scaffold and the cell types used to populate it, after it is implanted it will only effect successful repair if it becomes fully integrated into adjacent normal tissue and can be remodelled appropriately in the recipient. An important consideration that is often not addressed sufficiently is that many tissues in the body, notably tissues in the musculoskeletal system and the cardiovascular system, are subject to considerable mechanical stress. Engineered tissues are not subjected to relevant mechanical stresses during their fabrication *in vitro* and their behaviour in response to mechanical loading after implantation is a major determinant of their ability to perform successfully. The development of innovative high-resolution three-dimensional imaging techniques to evaluate engineered tissue before and after implantation is key to refining the design of engineered tissues and assessing their functional integration after implantation.

SAFETY CONCERNS

The major safety concerns of cell-based therapy and tissue engineering are listed in *Table 4.5*. One of the most serious concerns is that of tumour formation and malignant transformation. The risk of tumour formation varies according to the cell type used, the genetic modification strategy used to transform the stem cells, the site of transplantation and whether the cells are autologous or allogeneic. The direct risk of tumour formation by the transplanted cells relates specifically to ESCs and iPSCs and there appears to be little risk with SSCs. The ability of stem cells to form teratomas is one of the hallmarks of pluripotency, and the risk of this happening following stem cell therapy may be reduced by ensuring that only cells that have been fully differentiated *in vitro* and not those that are still pluripotent are used for therapy. The risk of malignancy may also be reduced by the choice of *in vitro* strategy used to differentiate stem cells prior to use: use of viral vectors that do not integrate into the genome or of non-viral approaches to differentiation reduces the risk of malignant transformation. There is also interest in developing techniques for directly reprogramming somatic cells to adopt the function of a different cell type without having to make them first revert back to the pluripotent state – so-called transdifferentiation.

Another major concern is that of transmitting infection. It is essential that if allogeneic stem cells are used they are screened to exclude infection and that cells and engineered tissues are prepared according to Good Manufacturing Practice (GMP) guidelines to avoid bacterial infection during in vitro culture prior to use. As already noted, if allogeneic stem cells are used for tissue engineering and regenerative therapy they may be susceptible to graft rejection, and immunosuppressive therapy may be necessary.

TABLE 4.5 Risks of cell-based therapy.
Tumour formation
Genetic and epigenetic abnormalities
Transmission of infection
Poor viability and loss of function
Differentiation to undesired cell-types
Rejection (allogeneic cells)
Side effects of immunosuppression (allogeneic cells)

FUTURE DIRECTIONS

Tissue engineering and regenerative strategies hold out great hope for effectively repairing or replacing tissues in a wide number of human diseases. The field is moving rapidly, underpinned by new developments in stem cells and scaffold design. The use of mesenchymal stem and stromal cell based therapies and iPSC based therapies is likely to dominate, in conjunction with improved bioactive scaffold designs that can be reproducibly manufactured and seeded, sometimes with multiple cell types, by sophisticated bioreactors that incorporate dynamic culture systems.

It is likely that patient stratification will further refine therapy options. The ability to phenotype, to genotype and to profile patients at a molecular level will allow more detailed characterisation of patient subgroups and staging of disease. This would refine the surgical approach to many diseases, including regenerative procedures.

Over the next decade it is likely that major advances will be made in the clinical translation of tissue engineering and regenerative therapies across a broad range of applications. Numerous clinical studies are currently being undertaken, many with promising early results, and the number of studies is set to rise considerably. However, caution is required and there are many examples where engineered tissues have failed to live up to their early promise. The pace of development is so rapid that regulatory authorities will have difficulty keeping up.

It is important that the clinical use of tissue engineering is subject to rigorous evaluation, and that novel developments are only used in the context of appropriate clinical trials where the potential benefits and limitations are fully examined before they are introduced into routine clinical practice. The field is becoming increasingly commercialised and the cost and practicality of regenerative therapies, especially personalised autologous therapies, will need to be addressed.

FURTHER READING

Fisher S. *Handbook of regenerative medicine and tissue engineering*. New York: Hayle Medical, 2015.

Giannoudis P, Jones E, Yang X, McGonagle D. *Mesenchymal stem cells and skeletal regeneration*. Cambridge: Academic Press, 2013.

Van Blitterswijk C, Jan De Boer J. *Tissue engineering*, 2nd edn. Amsterdam: Elsevier, 2015.

Warburton D. *Stem cells, tissue engineering and regenerative medicine*. Singapore: World Scientific, 2014.

Chapter 5

Surgical infection

Learning objectives

To understand:
- The characteristics of the common surgical pathogens and their sensitivities
- The factors that determine whether a wound will become infected
- The classification of sources of infection and their severity
- The clinical presentation of surgical infections
- The indications for and choice of prophylactic antibiotics
- The spectrum of commonly used antibiotics in surgery and the principles of therapy

To learn:
- Koch's postulates
- The management of abscesses

To appreciate:
- The importance of aseptic and antiseptic techniques and delayed primary or secondary closure in contaminated wounds

To be aware of:
- The causes of reduced resistance to infection (host response)

To know:
- The definitions of infection, particularly at surgical sites
- What basic precautions to take to avoid surgically relevant hospital acquired infections

HISTORY OF SURGICAL INFECTION

Surgical infection, particularly surgical site infection (SSI), has always been a major complication of surgery and trauma and has been documented for 4000–5000 years. The Egyptians had some concepts about infection, as they were able to prevent putrefaction using their skills in mummification. Their medical papyruses also describe the use of salves and antiseptics to prevent SSIs. This 'prophylaxis' had also been known earlier by the Assyrians, although less well documented. It was described again independently by the Greeks. The Hippocratic teachings described the use of antimicrobials, such as wine and vinegar, which were widely used to irrigate open, infected wounds before delayed primary or secondary wound closure. A belief common to all these civilisations, and indeed even later to the Romans, was that, whenever pus was localised in an infected wound, it needed to be drained.

Galen recognised that this localisation of infection (suppuration) in wounds inflicted in the gladiatorial arena often heralded recovery, particularly after drainage (*pus bonum et laudabile*). Sadly, this dictum of laudable pus was misunderstood by many later healers, who thought that it was the production of pus that was desirable. Until well into the Middle Ages, some practitioners promoted suppuration in wounds by the application of noxious substances, including faeces, in the misguided belief that healing could not occur without pus formation. Theodoric of Cervia, Ambroise Paré and Guy de Chauliac observed that clean wounds, closed primarily, could heal without infection or suppuration.

An understanding of the causes of infection came in the nineteenth century. Microbes had been seen under the

Hippocrates was a Greek Physician, and by common consent 'The Father of Medicine'. He was born on the Greek island of Cos off Turkey about 460 BC and probably died in 375 BC.

Galen, 130–200, Roman physician, commenced practice as Surgeon to the Gladiators at Pergamum (now Bregama in Turkey) and later became personal physician to the Emperor Marcus Aurelius and to two of his successors. He was a prolific writer on many subjects, amongst them anatomy, medicine, pathology and philosophy. His work affected medical thinking for 15 centuries after his death. (Gladiator is Latin for 'swordsman'.)

Theodoric of Cervia. Theodoric, 1210–1298, Bishop of Cervia, published a book on surgery ca. 1267.

Ambroise Paré, 1510–1590, French military surgeon, also worked at the Hotel Dieu, Paris, France.

Guy de Chauliac, ?1298–1368, physician and chaplain to Pope Clement VI at Avignon, France and the author of *Chirurgia Magna*, which was published about 1363.

microscope, but Koch laid down the first definition of infective disease (Koch's postulates). Koch's postulates do not cover every eventuality though. Organisms of low virulence may not cause disease in normal hosts but may be responsible for disease in immunocompromised hosts. Some hosts may develop subclinical disease and yet still be a carrier of the organism capable of infecting others. Also, not every organism that causes disease can be grown in culture, the commonly quoted one being *Mycobacterium leprae* which causes leprosy.

Summary box 5.1

Koch's postulates proving whether a given organism is the cause of a given disease

- It must be found in every case
- It should be possible to isolate it from the host and grow it in culture
- It should reproduce the disease when injected into another healthy host
- It should be recovered from an experimentally infected host

The Austrian obstetrician Ignac Semmelweis showed that puerperal sepsis could be reduced from over 10% to under 2% by the simple act of hand washing between cases, particularly between postmortem examinations and the delivery suite. He was ignored by his contemporaries and died at the age of 47 in an insane asylum before the value of his work was accepted two decades later with the recognition that infections were caused by microbes.

Louis Pasteur recognised through his germ theory that microorganisms were responsible for infecting humans and causing disease. Joseph Lister applied this knowledge to the reduction of colonising organisms in compound fractures by using antiseptics. The principles of antiseptic surgery were soon enhanced with aseptic surgery at the turn of the twentieth century. As well as killing the bacteria on the skin before surgical incision (antiseptic technique), the conditions under which the operation was performed were kept free of bacteria (aseptic technique). This technique is still employed in modern operating theatres.

The concept of a 'magic bullet' (*Zauberkugel*) that could kill microbes but not their host became a reality with the discovery of sulphonamide chemotherapy in the mid-twentieth century. The discovery of the antibiotic penicillin is attributed to Alexander Fleming in 1928, but it was not isolated for clinical use until 1941, by Florey and Chain. The first patient to receive penicillin was Police Constable Alexander in Oxford. He scratched his mouth while pruning roses and developed abscesses of the face and eyes leading to a severe staphylococcal bacteraemia. He responded to treatment and made a partial recovery before the limited batch of penicillin ran out, following which he relapsed and died. Since then there has been a proliferation of antibiotics with broad-spectrum activity and antibiotics today remain the mainstay of antimicrobial therapy.

Many staphylococci today have become resistant to penicillin. Often bacteria develop resistance through the acquisition of β-lactamases, which break up the β-lactam ring present in the molecular structure of many antibiotics. The acquisition of extended spectrum β-lactamases (ESBLs) is an increasing concern in some gram-negative organisms that cause urinary tract infections because it is difficult to find an antibiotic effective against them. In addition, there is increasing concern about the rising resistance of many other bacteria to antibiotics, in particular the emergence of methicillin-resistant *Staphylococcus aureus* (MRSA) and glycopeptide-resistant enterococci (GRE), which are also relevant in general surgical practice.

The introduction of antibiotics for prophylaxis and for treatment, together with advances in anaesthesia and critical care medicine, has made possible surgery that would not previously have been considered. Faecal peritonitis is no longer inevitably fatal, and incisions made in the presence of such contamination can heal primarily without infection in over 90% of patients with appropriate antibiotic therapy. Despite this, it is common practice in many countries to delay wound closure in patients in whom the wound is known to be contaminated or dirty. Waiting for the wound to granulate and then performing a delayed primary or secondary closure may be considered a better option in such cases.

Summary box 5.2

Advances in the control of infection in surgery

- Aseptic operating theatre techniques have enhanced the use of antiseptics
- Antibiotics have reduced postoperative infection rates after elective and emergency surgery
- Delayed primary, or secondary, closure remains useful in heavily contaminated wounds

Surgical site infection in patients who have contaminated wounds, who are immunosuppressed or who are undergoing prosthetic surgery is now the exception rather than the rule since the introduction of prophylactic antibiotics. The evidence for this is of the highest level. The use of prophylactic

---

Robert Koch, 1843–1910, Professor of Hygiene and Bacteriology, Berlin, Germany, stated his 'Postulates' in 1882.

Ignac Semmelweis, 1818–1865, Professor of Obstetrics, Budapest, Hungary.

Louis Pasteur, 1822–1895, French chemist, bacteriologist and immunologist, Professor of Chemistry at the Sorbonne, Paris, France.

Joseph Lister (Lord Lister), 1827–1912, Professor of Surgery, Glasgow, Scotland (1860–1869), Edinburgh, Scotland (1869–1877) and King's College Hospital, London (1877–1892).

Sir Alexander Fleming, 1881–1955, Professor of Bacteriology, St Mary's Hospital, London, England, discovered *Penicillium notatum* in 1928.

Howard Walter Florey (Lord Florey of Adelaide), 1898–1968, Professor of Pathology, the University of Oxford, Oxford, England.

Sir Ernst Boris Chain, Professor of Biochemistry, Imperial College, London, England. Fleming, Florey and Chain shared the 1945 Nobel Prize for Physiology or Medicine for their work on penicillin.

Hans Christian Joachim Gram, 1853–1938, Professor of Pharmacology (1891–1900) and of Medicine (1900–1923), Copenhagen, Denmark, described this method of staining bacteria in 1884.

antibiotics in clean, non-prosthetic surgery is of less value as infection rates are low and the indiscriminate use of antibiotics simply encourages the emergence of resistant strains of bacteria.

MICROBIOLOGY OF SURGICAL INFECTION

Common bacteria causing surgical infection

Streptococci

Streptococci form chains and are Gram positive on staining (**Figure 5.1**). The most important is the β-haemolytic *Streptococcus*, which resides in the pharynx of 5–10% of the population. In the Lancefield A–G carbohydrate antigens classification, it is the group A *Streptococcus*, also called *Streptococcus pyogenes*, that is the most pathogenic. It has the ability to spread, causing cellulitis, and to cause tissue destruction through the release of enzymes such as streptolysin, streptokinase and streptodornase.

Streptococcus faecalis is an enterococcus in Lancefield group D. It is often found in synergy with other organisms, as are the γ-haemolytic *Streptococcus* and *Peptostreptococcus*, which is an anaerobe.

Both *Streptococcus pyogenes* and *Streptococcus faecalis* may be involved in wound infection after large bowel surgery, but the α-haemolytic *Streptococcus viridans* is not associated with wound infections.

All the streptococci remain sensitive to penicillin and erythromycin. The cephalosporins are a suitable alternative in patients who are allergic to penicillin.

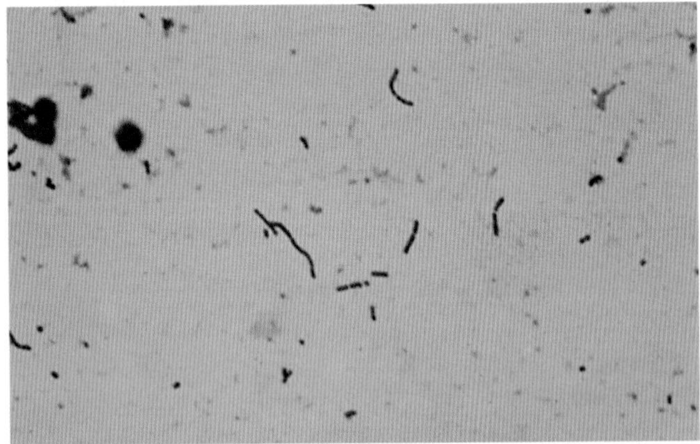

Figure 5.1 Streptococci.

Staphylococci

Staphylococci form clumps and are Gram positive (**Figure 5.2**). *Staphylococcus aureus* is the most important pathogen in this group and is found in the nasopharynx of up to 15% of the population. It can cause suppuration in wounds and around implanted prostheses. Some strains are resistant to many common antibiotics (especially methicillin resistant *Staphylococcus aureus*, MRSA) and so are difficult to treat. MRSA can be found in the nose of asymptomatic carriers amongst both patients and hospital workers, a potential source of infection after surgery. In parts of northern Europe, the prevalence of MRSA infections has been kept at very low levels using 'search and destroy' methods, which use screening techniques to look for MRSA in patients before they come in to hospital for elective surgery so that any carriers can be treated before their admission for surgery. Local policies on the management of MRSA depend on the prevalence of MRSA, the type of hospital, the clinical specialty and the availability of facilities. Widespread swabbing, ward closures, isolation of patients and disinfection of wards by deep cleaning all have to be carefully considered.

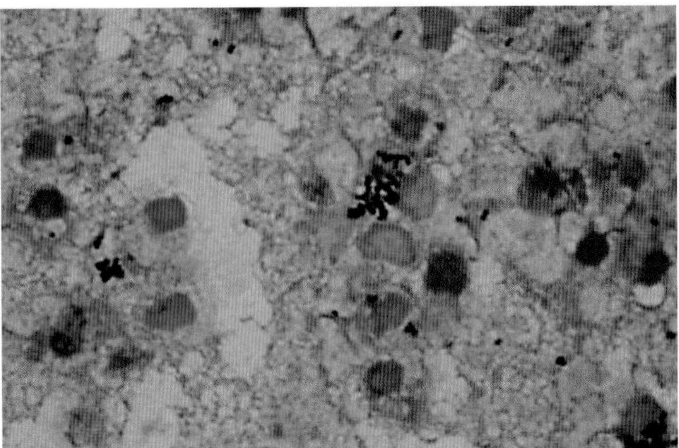

Figure 5.2 Staphylococcal pus.

Staphylococcal infections are usually suppurative and localised. Most hospital *Staphylococcus aureus* strains are now β-lactamase producers and so are resistant to penicillin, but many strains remain sensitive to flucloxacillin, vancomycin, aminoglycosides and some cephalosporins. There are several novel and innovative antibiotics becoming available that have high activity against resistant strains. Some have the advantage of good oral activity (linezolid), some have a wide spectrum (teicoplanin), some have good activity in bacteraemia (daptomycin) but all are relatively expensive, and some have side effects involving marrow, hepatic and renal toxicity. Their use is justified but needs to be controlled by tight local policies and guidelines that involve clinical microbiologists.

Staphylococcus epidermidis (previously *Staphylococcus albus*), also known as coagulase-negative staphylococcus, was regarded as a non-pathogenic commensal organism commonly found on the skin, but is now recognised as a major threat in vascular and orthopaedic prosthetic surgery and in indwelling vascular cannulas/catheters. The bacteria form biofilms which adhere to prosthetic surfaces and limit the effectiveness of antibiotics.

Clostridia

Clostridial organisms are gram-positive, obligate anaerobes, which produce resistant spores (**Figure 5.3**). *Clostridium perfringens* is the cause of gas gangrene, and *C. tetani* causes tetanus after implantation into tissues or a wound.

Clostridium difficile is the cause of pseudomembranous colitis, where destruction of the normal colonic bacterial flora by

Rebecca Graighill Lancefield, 1895–1981, American bacteriologist, classified streptococci in 1933.

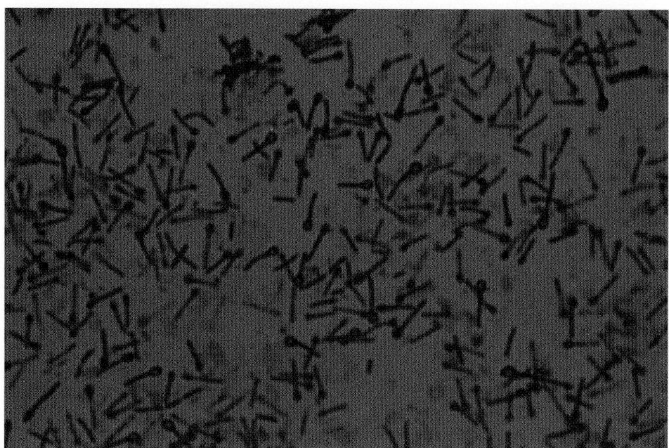
Figure 5.3 *Clostridium tetani* (drumstick spores).

antibiotic therapy allows an overgrowth of the normal gut commensal C. *diff* to pathological levels. Any antibiotic may cause this phenomenon, although the quinolones such as ciprofloxacin seem to be the highest risk, especially in elderly or immunocompromised patients. In its most severe form, the colitis may lead to perforation and the need for emergency colectomy with an associated high mortality. Treatment involves resuscitation and antibiotic therapy with metronidazole or vancomycin. The fibrinous exudate is typical and differentiates the colitis from other inflammatory diseases; laboratory recognition of the toxin is an early accurate diagnostic test.

Aerobic gram-negative bacilli

These bacilli are normal inhabitants of the large bowel. *Escherichia coli* and *Klebsiella* spp. are lactose fermenting; *Proteus* is non-lactose fermenting. Most organisms in this group act in synergy with *Bacteroides* to cause SSIs after bowel operations (in particular, appendicitis, diverticulitis and peritonitis). *Escherichia coli* is a major cause of urinary tract infection, although most aerobic gram-negative bacilli can be involved, particularly in relation to urinary catheterisation. There is increasing concern about the development of extended spectrum β-lactamases (ESBLs) in many of this group of bacteria, which confer resistance to many antibiotics, particularly cephalosporins.

Pseudomonas spp. tend to colonise burns and tracheostomy wounds, as well as the urinary tract. Once *Pseudomonas* has colonised wards and intensive care units, it may be difficult to eradicate. Surveillance of cross-infection is important in outbreaks. Hospital strains become resistant to β-lactamase as resistance can be transferred by plasmids. Wound infections need antibiotic therapy only when there is progressive or spreading infection with systemic signs. The aminoglycosides and the quinolones are effective, but some cephalosporins and penicillin may not be. Many of the carbapenems (e.g. meropenem) are useful in severe infections.

Bacteroides

Bacteroides are non-spore-bearing, strict anaerobes that colonise the large bowel, vagina and oropharynx. *Bacteroides fragilis* is the principal organism that acts in synergy with aerobic gram-negative bacilli to cause SSIs, including intra-abdominal abscesses after colorectal or gynaecological surgery. They are sensitive to the imidazoles (e.g. metronidazole) and some cephalosporins (e.g. cefotaxime).

Sources of infection

The infection of a wound can be defined as the invasion of organisms into tissues following a breakdown of local and systemic host defences, leading to either cellulitis, lymphangitis, abscess formation or bacteraemia. The infection of most surgical wounds is referred to as superficial surgical site infection (SSSI). The other categories include deep SSI (infection in the deeper musculofascial layers) and organ space infection (such as an abdominal abscess after an anastomotic leak).

Pathogens resist host defences by releasing toxins, which favour their spread, and this is enhanced in anaerobic or frankly necrotic wound tissue. *Clostridium perfringens*, which is responsible for gas gangrene, releases proteases such as hyaluronidase, lecithinase and haemolysin, which allow it to spread through the tissues. Resistance to antibiotics can be acquired by previously sensitive bacteria by transfer through plasmids.

The human body harbours approximately 10^{14} organisms. They can be released into tissues before, during or after surgery, contamination being most severe when a hollow viscus perforates (e.g. faecal peritonitis following a diverticular perforation). Any infection that follows surgery may be termed endogenous or exogenous, depending on the source of the bacterial contamination. Endogenous organisms are present on or in the patient at the time of surgery, whereas exogenous organisms come from outside the patient. In modern hospital practice, endogenous organisms colonising the patient are by far the most common source of infection.

Summary box 5.3

Classification of sources of infection

- Endogenous: present in or on the host e.g. SSSI following contamination of the wound from a perforated appendix
- Exogenous: acquired from a source outside the body such as the operating theatre (inadequate air filtration, poor antisepsis) or the ward (e.g. poor hand-washing compliance). The cause of hospital acquired infection (HAI)

Microorganisms are normally prevented from causing infection in tissues by intact epithelial surfaces, most notably the skin. These surfaces are broken down by trauma or surgery. In addition to these mechanical barriers, there are other protective mechanisms, which can be divided into:

- **chemical**: low gastric pH;
- **humoral**: antibodies, complement and opsonins;
- **cellular**: phagocytic cells, macrophages, polymorphonuclear cells and killer lymphocytes.

Theodor Albrecht Edwin Klebs, 1834–1913, Professor of Bacteriology successively at Prague, Czechoslovakia, Zurich, Switzerland and The Rush Medical College, Chicago, IL, USA.

All of these natural mechanisms may be compromised by surgical intervention and treatment.

The chance of developing an SSI after surgery is also determined by the pathogenicity of the organisms present and by the size of the bacterial inoculum. The more virulent the organism or the larger the extent of bacterial contamination, the more likely is wound infection to occur. Host factors are also important, so a less virulent organism or a lower level of wound contamination may still result in a wound infection if the host response is impaired (see *Summary box* 5.5). Devitalised tissue, excessive dead space or haematoma, all the results of poor surgical technique, increase the chances of infection. The same applies to foreign materials of any kind, including sutures and drains. If there is a silk suture in tissue, the critical number of organisms needed to start an infection is reduced logarithmically. Silk should not be used to close skin as it causes suture abscesses for this reason. These principles are important to an understanding of how best to prevent infection in surgical practice.

Summary box 5.4

Factors that determine whether a wound will become infected

- Host response
- Virulence and inoculum of infective agent
- Vascularity and health of tissue being invaded (including local ischaemia as well as systemic shock)
- Presence of dead or foreign tissue
- Presence of antibiotics during the 'decisive period'

The decisive period

There is up to a 4-hour interval before bacterial growth becomes established enough to cause an infection after a breach in the tissues, whether caused by trauma or surgery. This interval is called the 'decisive period' and strategies aimed at preventing infection from taking a hold become ineffective after this time period. It is therefore logical that prophylactic antibiotics should be given to cover this period and that they could be decisive in preventing an infection from developing, before bacterial growth takes a hold. The tissue levels of antibiotics during the period when bacterial contamination is likely to occur should be above the minimum inhibitory concentration (MIC_{90}) for the expected pathogens.

Reduced resistance to infection

Reduced resistance to infection has several causes, particularly those that impair the inflammatory response. Host response is weakened by malnutrition, which can be recognised clinically, and most easily, as recent rapid weight loss that can be present even in the presence of obesity. Metabolic diseases such as diabetes mellitus, uraemia and jaundice, disseminated malignancy and acquired immmune deficiency syndrome (AIDS) are other contributors to infection and a poor healing response, as are iatrogenic causes including the immunosuppression caused by radiotherapy, chemotherapy or steroids (**Figures 5.4 and 5.5**).

Summary box 5.5

Risk factors for increased risk of wound infection

- Malnutrition (obesity, weight loss)
- Metabolic disease (diabetes, uraemia, jaundice)
- Immunosuppression (cancer, AIDS, steroids, chemotherapy and radiotherapy)
- Colonisation and translocation in the gastrointestinal tract
- Poor perfusion (systemic shock or local ischaemia)
- Foreign body material
- Poor surgical technique (dead space, haematoma)

When enteral feeding is suspended during the perioperative period, and particularly with underlying disease such as cancer, immunosuppression, shock or sepsis, bacteria (particularly aerobic gram-negative bacilli) tend to colonise the normally sterile upper gastrointestinal tract. They may then translocate to the mesenteric nodes and cause the release of endotoxins (lipopolysaccharide in bacterial cell walls), which

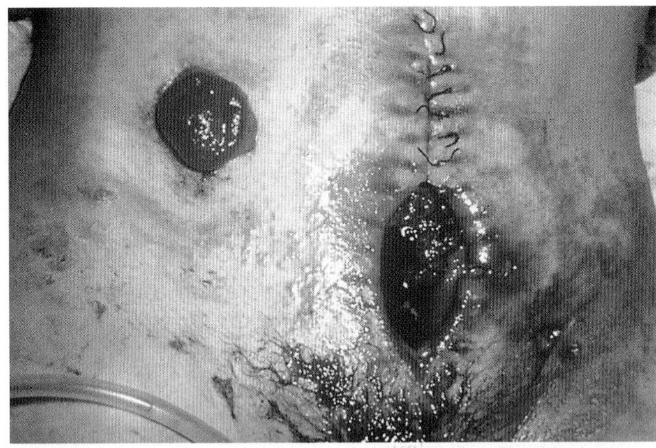

Figure 5.4 Major wound infection and delayed healing presenting as a faecal fistula in a patient with Crohn's disease on steroid treatment.

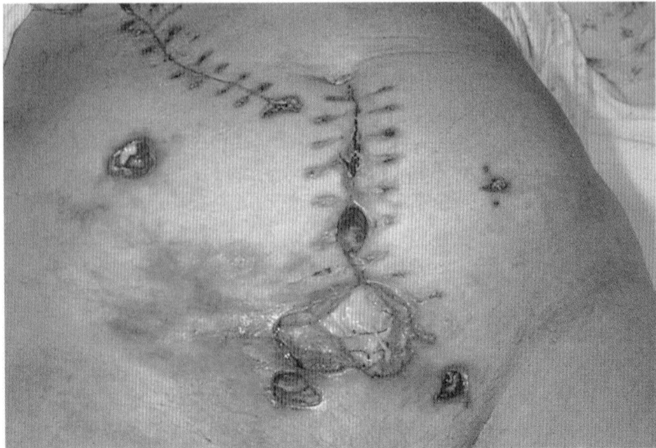

Figure 5.5 Delayed healing relating to infection in a patient on high-dose steroids.

can be one cause of a harmful systemic inflammatory response through the excessive release of proinflammatory cytokines and activation of macrophages (**Figure 5.6**). In the circumstances of reduced host resistance to infection, microorganisms that are not normally pathogenic may start to behave as pathogens. This is known as opportunistic infection. Opportunistic infection with fungi is an example, particularly when prolonged and changing antibiotic regimes have been used.

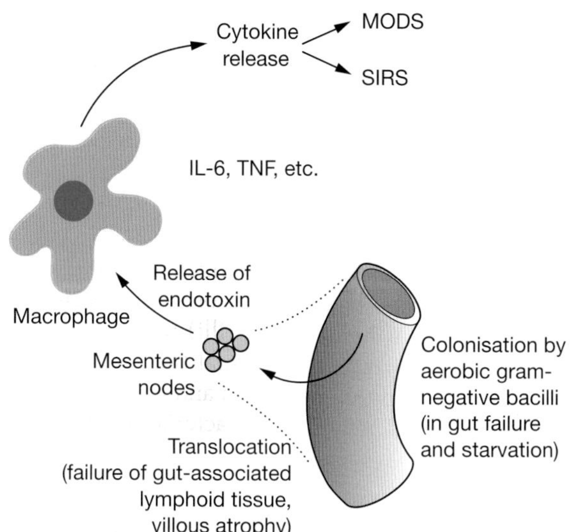

Figure 5.6 Gut failure, colonisation and translocation related to the development of systemic inflammatory response syndrome (SIRS) and multiple organ dysfunction syndrome (MODS). IL, interleukin; TNF, tumour necrosis factor.

PRESENTATION OF SURGICAL INFECTION

Major and minor surgical site infection (SSI)

Infection acquired from the environment or the staff following surgery or admission to hospital is termed hospital acquired infection (HAI). There are four main groups: respiratory infections (including ventilator-associated pneumonia), urinary tract infections (mostly related to urinary catheters), bacteraemia (mostly related to indwelling vascular catheters) and SSIs.

A major SSI is defined as a wound that either discharges significant quantities of pus spontaneously or needs a secondary procedure to drain it (**Figure 5.7**). The patient may have systemic signs such as tachycardia, pyrexia and a raised white cell count.

Summary box 5.6

Major wound infections
- Significant quantity of pus
- Delayed return home
- Patients are systemically ill

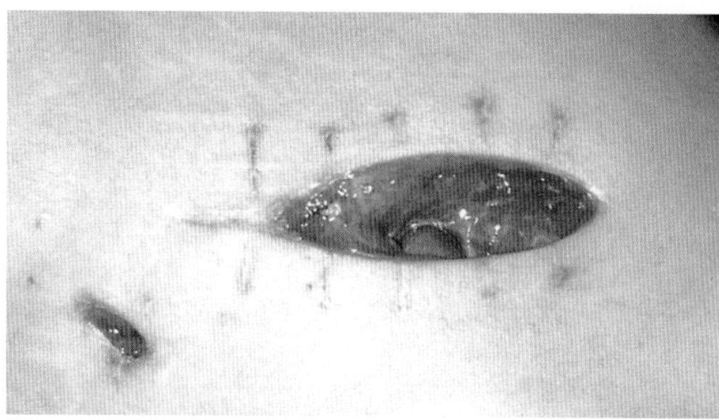

Figure 5.7 Major wound infection with superficial skin dehiscence.

Minor wound infections may discharge pus or infected serous fluid but are not associated with excessive discomfort, systemic signs or delay in return home (**Figure 5.8**). The differentiation between major and minor and the definition of SSI is important in audits and clinical trials of antibiotic prophylaxis. There are scoring systems for the severity of wound infection, which are particularly useful in surveillance and research. Examples are the Southampton (*Table 5.1*) and ASEPSIS systems (*Table 5.2*).

Accurate surveillance can only be achieved using trained, unbiased and blinded assessors. Most include surveillance for a 30-day postoperative period. The US Centers for Disease Control (CDC) definition insists on a 30-day follow-up period for non-prosthetic surgery and 1 year after implanted hip and knee surgery.

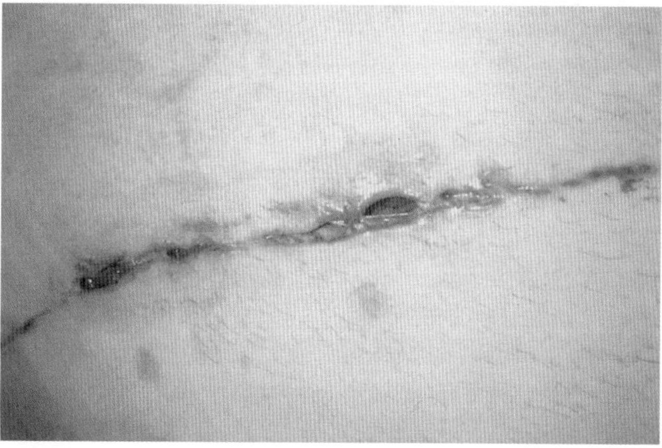

Figure 5.8 Minor wound infection that settled spontaneously without antibiotics.

Localised infection

ABSCESS

An abscess presents all the clinical features of acute inflammation originally described by Celsus: *calor* (heat), *rubor* (redness), *dolor* (pain) and *tumor* (swelling). To these can be added *functio laesa* (loss of function: if it hurts, the infected part is not used). Abscesses usually follow a puncture wound of some kind, which may have been forgotten, as well as surgery, but can be metastatic in all tissues following bacteraemia.

Aulus Aurelius Cornelius Celsus, 25 BC–50 AD, Roman surgeon and the author of *De Re Medico Libri Octo*.

TABLE 5.1 Southampton wound grading system.

Grade	Appearance
0	Normal healing
I	Normal healing with mild bruising or erythema
Ia	Some bruising
Ib	Considerable bruising
Ic	Mild erythema
II	Erythema plus other signs of inflammation
IIa	At one point
IIb	Around sutures
IIc	Along wound
IId	Around wound
III	Clear or haemoserous discharge
IIIa	At one point only (≤2 cm)
IIIb	Along wound (>2 cm)
IIIc	Large volume
IIId	Prolonged (>3 days)
Major complication	
IV	Pus
IVa	At one point only (≤2 cm)
IVb	Along wound (>2 cm)
V	Deep or severe wound infection with or without tissue breakdown; haematoma requiring aspiration

TABLE 5.2 The ASEPSIS wound score.

Criterion	Points
Additional treatment	0
Antibiotics for wound infection	10
Drainage of pus under local anaesthesia	5
Debridement of wound under general anaesthesia	10
Serous discharge[a]	Daily 0–5
Erythema[a]	Daily 0–5
Purulent exudate[a]	Daily 0–10
Separation of deep tissues[a]	Daily 0–10
Isolation of bacteria from wound	10
Stay as inpatient prolonged over 14 days as result of wound infection	5

[a] Scored for 5 of the first 7 days only, the remainder being scored if present in the first 2 months.

Pyogenic organisms, predominantly *Staphylococcus aureus*, cause tissue necrosis and suppuration. Pus is composed of dead and dying white blood cells, predominantly neutrophils, that have succumbed to bacterial toxins. An abscess is surrounded by an acute inflammatory response composed of a fibrinous exudate, oedema and the cells of acute inflammation. Granulation tissue (macrophages, fibroblasts and new blood vessel proliferation) forms later around the suppurative process and leads to collagen deposition. If it is not drained or resorbed completely, a chronic abscess may result. If it is partly sterilised with antibiotics, an antibioma may form.

Abscesses contain hyperosmolar material that draws in fluid. This increases the pressure and causes pain. If they spread, they usually track along planes of least resistance and point towards the skin. Wound abscesses may discharge spontaneously by tracking to a surface, but may need drainage through a surgical incision. Most abscesses relating to surgical wounds take 7–10 days to form after surgery. As many as 75% of SSIs present after the patient has left hospital and may thus be overlooked by the surgical team.

Abscess cavities need cleaning out after incision and drainage and are traditionally encouraged to heal by secondary intention. When the cavity is left open to drain freely, there is no need for antibiotic therapy as well. Antibiotics should be used if the abscess cavity is closed after drainage, but the cavity should not be closed if there is any risk of retained loculi or foreign material. Thus a perianal abscess can be incised and drained, the walls curretted and the skin closed with good results using appropriate antibiotic therapy, but a pilonidal abscess has a higher recurrence risk after such treatment because a nidus of hair may remain in the subcutaneous tissue adjacent to the abscess. Some small breast abscesses can be managed by simple needle aspiration of the pus and antibiotic therapy.

Summary box 5.7

Abscesses

- Abscesses need drainage
- Modern imaging techniques may allow guided needle aspiration
- Antibiotics are indicated if the abscess cavity is not left open to drain freely
- An open abscess cavity heals by secondary intention

Persistent chronic abscesses may lead to sinus or fistula formation. In a chronic abscess, lymphocytes and plasma cells are seen. There is tissue sequestration and later calcification may occur. Certain organisms are associated with chronicity, and sinus and fistula formation. Common ones are *Mycobacterium* and *Actinomyces*. They should not be forgotten when these complications occur and persist.

Perianastomotic contamination may be the cause of an abscess but, in the abdomen, abscesses are more usually the result of anastomotic leakage. An abscess in a deep cavity such as the pleura or peritoneum may be difficult to diagnose or locate even when there is strong clinical suspicion that it is present (**Figure 5.9**). Plain or contrast radiographs may not be helpful, but ultrasonography, computed tomography (CT), magnetic resonance imaging (MRI) and isotope labelled white cell scans are all useful and may allow guided aspiration without the need for surgical intervention.

CELLULITIS AND LYMPHANGITIS

Cellulitis is a non-suppurative, invasive infection of tissues, which is usually related to the point of injury.There is poor localisation in addition to the cardinal signs of spreading inflammation. Such infections presenting in surgical practice

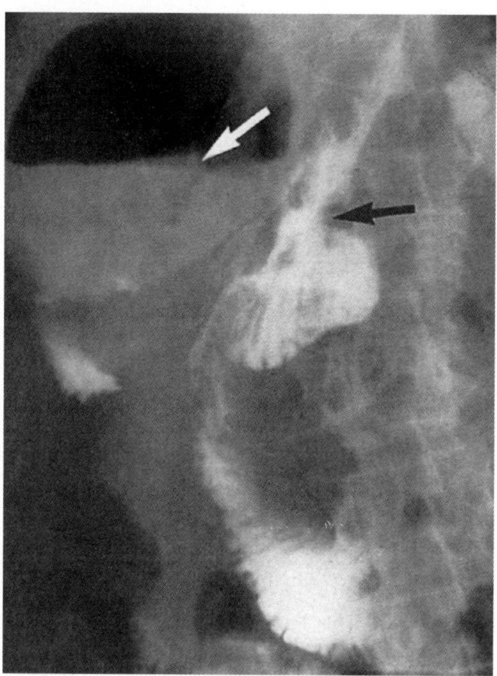

Figure 5.9 Plain radiograph showing a subphrenic abscess with a gas/fluid level (white arrow). Gastrografin is seen leaking from the oesophagojejunal anastomosis (after gastrectomy) towards the abscess (black arrow).

are typically caused by organisms such as β-haemolytic streptococci (**Figure 5.10**), staphylococci (**Figure 5.11**) and *C. perfringens*. Tissue destruction, gangrene and ulceration may follow, which are caused by release of proteases.

Systemic signs (the old-fashioned term is toxaemia) are common, with chills, fever and rigors. These events follow the release of toxins into the circulation, which stimulate a cytokine-mediated systemic inflammatory response even though blood cultures may be negative.

Lymphangitis is part of a similar process and presents as painful red streaks in affected lymphatics draining the source of infection. Lymphangitis is often accompanied by painful lymph node groups in the related drainage area.

Summary box 5.8

Cellulitis and lymphangitis

- Non-suppurative, poorly localised
- Commonly caused by streptococci, staphylococci or clostridia
- Blood cultures are often negative

Specific local wound infections

GAS GANGRENE

Gas gangrene is caused by *C. perfringens*. These gram-positive, anaerobic, spore-bearing bacilli are widely found in nature, particularly in soil and faeces. This infection is particularly relevant to military and trauma surgery. Patients who are immunocompromised, diabetic or have malignant disease are at greater risk, particularly if they have wounds containing necrotic or foreign material, resulting in anaerobic conditions. Military wounds provide an ideal environment as the kinetic energy of high-velocity missiles or shrapnel causes extensive tissue damage. The cavitation which follows passage of a missile through the tissues causes a 'sucking' entry wound, leaving clothing and environmental soiling in the wound in addition to devascularised tissue. Gas gangrene wound infections are associated with severe local wound pain and crepitus (gas in the tissues, which may also be visible on plain radiographs). The wound produces a thin, brown, sweet-smelling exudate, in which Gram staining will reveal bacteria. Oedema and spreading gangrene follow the release of collagenase, hyaluronidase, other proteases and alpha toxin. Early systemic complications with circulatory collapse and organ failure follow if prompt action is not taken.

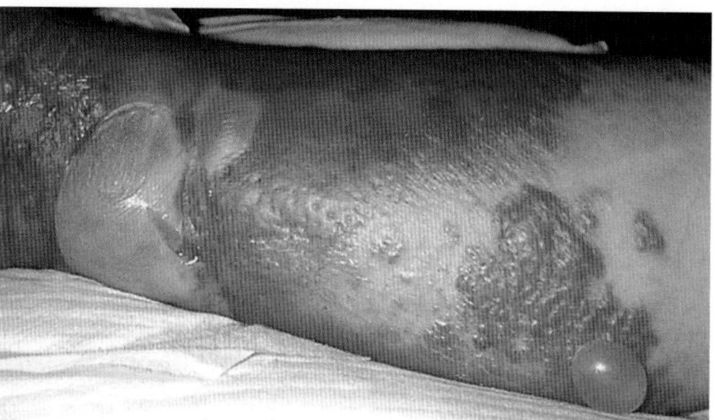

Figure 5.10 Streptococcal cellulitis of the leg following a minor puncture wound.

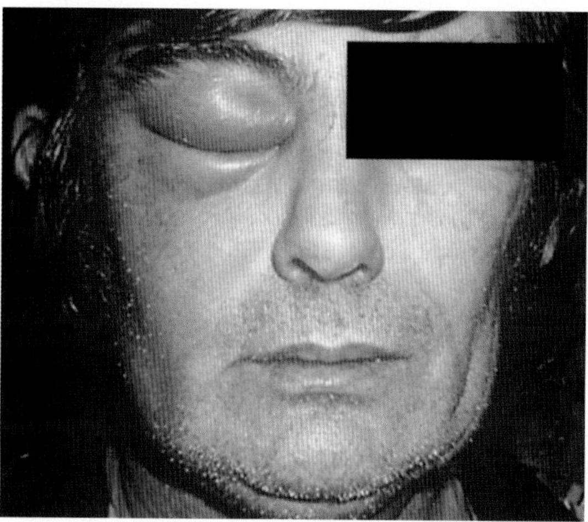

Figure 5.11 Staphylococcal cellulitis of the face and orbit following severe infection of an epidermoid cyst of the scalp.

Summary box 5.9

Gas gangrene

- Caused by *Clostridium perfringens*
- Gas and smell are characteristic
- Immunocompromised patients are most at risk
- Antibiotic prophylaxis is essential when performing amputations to remove dead tissue

Antibiotic prophylaxis should always be considered in patients at risk, especially when amputations are performed for peripheral vascular disease with open necrotic ulceration. Once gas gangrene infection is established, large doses of intravenous penicillin and aggressive debridement of affected tissues are required.

CLOSTRIDIUM TETANI

This is another anaerobic, terminal spore-bearing, gram-positive bacterium, which can cause tetanus following implantation into tissues or a wound (which may have been trivial or unrecognised and forgotten). The spores are widespread in soil and manure, and so the infection is more common in traumatic civilian or military wounds. The signs and symptoms of tetanus are mediated by the release of the exotoxin tetanospasmin, which affects myoneural junctions and the motor neurones of the anterior horn of the spinal cord. A short prodromal period, which has a poor prognosis, leads to spasms in the distribution of the short motor nerves of the face followed by the development of severe generalised motor spasms including opsithotonus, respiratory arrest and death. A longer prodromal period of 4–5 weeks is associated with a milder form of the disease. The entry wound may show a localised small area of cellulitis. Exudate or aspirate may give a sample that can be stained to show the presence of gram-positive rods. Prophylaxis with tetanus toxoid is the best preventative treatment but, in an established infection, minor debridement of the wound may need to be performed and antibiotic treatment with benzylpenicillin provided in addition. Relaxants may also be required, and the patient will require ventilation in severe forms, which are associated with a high mortality. The administration of antitoxin using human immunoglobulin ought to be considered for both at-risk wounds and established infection.

The toxoid is a formalin-attenuated vaccine and should be given in three separate doses to give protection for a 5-year period, after which a single 5-yearly booster confers immunity. It should be given to all patients with open traumatic wounds who are not immunised. At-risk wounds are those when there is late presentation, when there is devitalisation of tissue or when there is wound soiling. For these wounds, a booster of toxoid should be given or, if the patient is not immunised at all, a three-dose course is given together with prophylactic benzylpenicillin, but the use of antitoxin is controversial because of the risk of toxicity and allergy.

SYNERGISTIC SPREADING GANGRENE (SYNONYM: SUBDERMAL GANGRENE, NECROTISING FASCIITIS)

This condition is not caused by clostridia. A mixed pattern of organisms is responsible: coliforms, staphylococci, *Bacteroides* spp., anaerobic streptococci and peptostreptococci have all been implicated, acting in synergy. Often, aerobic bacteria destroy the living tissue, allowing anaerobic bacteria to thrive. Abdominal wall infections are known as Meleney's synergistic gangrene and scrotal infections as Fournier's gangrene (Figure 5.12). Patients are almost always immunocompromised, with conditions such as diabetes mellitus. The wound initiating the infection may have been minor, but severely contaminated wounds are more likely to be the cause. Severe wound pain, signs of spreading inflammation with crepitus and smell are all signs of the infection spreading. Untreated, it will lead to widespread local gangrene and systemic multisystem organ failure. The subdermal spread of gangrene is always much more extensive than appears from initial examination. Broad-spectrum antibiotic therapy must be combined with aggressive circulatory support. Locally, there should be wide excision of necrotic tissue and laying open of affected areas. The debridement may need to be extensive, and patients who survive may need large areas of skin grafting.

Systemic infection

Bacteraemia

Bacteraemia is unusual following superficial SSIs, which tend to drain through the wound, but common after deep space SSIs such as follow an intestinal anastomotic breakdown. It is usually transient and can follow procedures undertaken through infected tissues (particularly instrumentation in infected bile or urine). It may also occur through bacterial infection of indwelling intravenous cannulae, which should be replaced regularly in order to avoid colonisation. Bacteraemia is important when a prosthesis has been implanted, as infection of the prosthesis can occur through haematogenous spread. Aerobic gram-negative bacilli are often responsible, but *Staphylococcus aureus* and fungi may be involved, particularly after the use of broad-spectrum antibiotics.

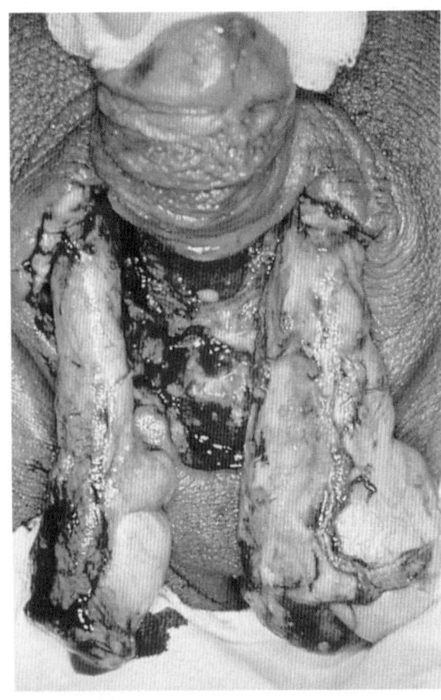

Figure 5.12 A classic presentation of Fournier's gangrene of the scrotum with 'shameful exposure of the testes' following excision of the gangrenous skin.

Frank Lamont Meleney, 1889–1963, Professor of Clinical Surgery, Columbia University, New York, NY, USA.

Jean Alfred Fournier, 1832–1915, syphilologist, the founder of the Venereal and Dermatological Clinic, Hôpital St. Louis, Paris, France.

Summary box 5.10

Bacteraemia

- Common after anastomotic breakdown
- Dangerous if the patient has a prosthesis, which can become infected
- May be associated with systemic organ failure

Systemic inflammatory response syndrome (SIRS)

SIRS is a systemic manifestation of sepsis (see *Table 5.3*), although the syndrome may also be caused by multiple trauma, burns or pancreatitis without infection. Serious infection, such as secondary peritonitis, may lead to SIRS through the release of lipopolysaccharide endotoxin from the walls of dying gram-negative bacilli (mainly *Escherichia coli*) or other bacteria or fungi. This and other toxins stimulate the release of cytokines from macrophages (see **Figure 5.6**). SIRS should not be confused with bacteraemia although the two may coexist.

Septic manifestations and multiple organ dysfunction syndrome (MODS) in SIRS are mediated by the release of proinflammatory cytokines such as interleukin-1 (IL-1) and tumour necrosis factor alpha (TNFα). These cytokines normally stimulate neutrohil adhesion to endothelial surfaces adjacent to the source of infection and cause them to migrate through the blood vessel wall by chemotaxis, where they can attack the bacterial invasion. A respiratory burst occurs within such activated neutrophils, releasing lysosomal enzymes, oxidants and free radicals which are involved in killing the invading bacteria, but which may also damage adjacent cells. Coagulation, complement and fibrinolytic pathways are also stimulated as part of the normal inflammatory response. This response is usually beneficial to the host and is an important aspect of normal tissue repair and wound healing. In the presence of severe sepsis or bacteraemia, this response may become harmful to the host if it occurs in excess, when it is known as the systemic inflammatory response syndrome or SIRS. There are high circulating levels of cytokines and activated neutrophils which stimulate fever, tachycardia and tachypnoea. The activated neutrophils adhere to vascular endothelium in key organs remote from the source of infection and damage it, leading to increased vascular permeability, which in turn leads to cellular damage within the organs, which become dysfunctional and give rise to the clinical picture of multiple organ dysfunction syndrome or MODS. In its most severe form, MODS may progress into multiple system organ failure (MSOF). Respiratory, cardiac, intestinal, renal and liver failure ensue in combination with circulatory failure and shock. In this state, the body's resistance to infection is reduced and a vicious cycle develops where the more organs that fail, the more likely it becomes that death will follow despite all that a modern intensive care unit can do for organ support.

TABLE 5.3 Definitions of systemic inflammatory response syndrome (SIRS) and sepsis.

SIRS is ***Two of:*** hyperthermia (>38°C) or hypothermia (<36°C) tachycardia (>90/min, no β-blockers) or tachypnoea (>20/min) white cell count >12 × 10^9/litre or <4 × 10^9/litre
Sepsis is SIRS with a documented infection
Severe sepsis or sepsis syndrome is sepsis with evidence of failure of one or more organs: respiratory (acute respiratory distress syndrome), cardiovascular (septic shock follows compromise of cardiac function and fall in peripheral vascular resistance), renal (usually acute tubular necrosis), hepatic, blood coagulation systems or central nervous system

Summary box 5.11

Definitions of infected states

- SSI is an infected wound or deep organ space
- SIRS is the body's systemic response to severe infection
- MODS is the effect that SIRS produces systemically
- MSOF is the end stage of uncontrolled MODS

Viral infections relevant to surgery

Hepatitis

Both hepatitis B and hepatitis C carry risks in surgery as they are blood-borne pathogens that can be transmitted both from the surgeon to the patient and *vice versa*. The usual mode of transmission is blood to blood contact through a needle-stick injury or a cut. Many cases of hepatitis B are asymptomatic and a surgeon may carry the virus without being aware of it. As there is an effective vaccine against hepatitis B, surgeons should know their immune status to hepatitis B and be vaccinated against it. Hepatitis C infection often becomes chronic with the risk of significant liver damage, but is potentially curable with interferon-alpha and ribavirin treatment, so surgeons who are exposed to an infection risk should seek medical advice and antibody measurement. Transmission of hepatitis C from surgeon to patient is extremely rare.

HIV

The type I human immunodeficiency virus (HIV) is one of the viruses of surgical importance because it can be transmitted by body fluids, particularly blood. It is a retrovirus that has become increasingly prevalent through sexual transmission (both homo- and heterosexual), intravenous drug addiction and in infected blood products used to treat haemophiliacs in particular. The risk in surgery is mostly through needle-stick injury during operations.

After exposure, the virus binds to CD4 receptors with a subsequent loss of CD4+ cells, T helper cells and other cells

Theodor Escherich, 1857–1911, Professor of Paediatrics, Vienna, Austria, discovered the *Bacterium coli commune* in 1886.

involved in cell-mediated immunity, antibody production and delayed hypersensitivity. Macrophages and gut-associated lymphoid tissue (GALT) are also affected. The risk of opportunistic infections (such as *Pneumocystis carinii* pneumonia, tuberculosis and cytomegalovirus) and neoplasms (such as Kaposi's sarcoma and lymphoma) is thereby increased.

In the early weeks after HIV infection, there may be a flu-like illness and, during the phase of seroconversion, patients present the greatest risk of HIV transmission. It is during these early phases that drug treatment, highly active antiretroviral therapy (HAART), is most effective through the ability of these drugs to inhibit reverse transcriptase and protease synthesis, which are the principal mechanisms through which HIV can progress. These drugs suppress the virus but do not clear it completely from the body, and treated patients can still transmit the virus to others. Within 2 years, untreated HIV can progress to acquired immune deficiency syndrome (AIDS) in 25–35% of patients.

Involvement of surgeons with HIV or hepatitis patients (universal precautions)

Patients may present to surgeons for operative treatment if they have a surgical disease and they are known to be infected or 'at risk', or because they need surgical intervention related to their illness for vascular access or a biopsy when they are known to have hepatitis, HIV infection or AIDS. Particular care should be taken when there is a risk of splashing/aerosol formation, particularly with power tools. Universal precautions have been drawn up by the CDC in the United States and largely adopted by the National Health Service (NHS) in the UK (in summary):

- use of a full face mask ideally, or protective spectacles;
- use of fully waterproof, disposable gowns and drapes, particularly during seroconversion;
- boots to be worn, not clogs, to avoid injury from dropped sharps;
- double gloving needed (a larger size on the inside is more comfortable);
- allow only essential personnel in theatre;
- avoid unnecessary movement in theatre;
- respect is required for sharps, with passage in a kidney dish;
- a slow meticulous operative technique is needed with minimised bleeding.

AFTER CONTAMINATION

Needle-stick injuries are commonest on the non-dominant index finger during operative surgery. Hollow needle injury carries the greatest risk of viral transmission. The injured part should be washed under running water and the incident reported. Local policies dictate whether post-exposure antiretroviral treatment should be given. Occupational health advice is required after high-risk exposure, together with the need for hepatitis/HIV testing and the option for continuation in an operative specialty.

PREVENTION OF SURGICAL INFECTION

Preoperative preparation

A short preoperative hospital stay lowers the risk of acquiring MRSA, multiply resistant coagulase-negative staphylococci (MRCNS) and other antibiotic-resistant organisms from the hospital environment. Medical and nursing staff should always wash their hands after any patient contact. Alcoholic hand gels can act as a substitute for hand washing, but do not destroy the spores of *Clostridium difficile*, which may cause pseudomembranous colitis, especially in immunocompromised patients or those whose gut flora is suppressed by antibiotic therapy. Although the need for clean hospitals, emphasised by the media, is logical, the 'clean your hands campaign' is beginning to result in falls in the incidence of HAIs. Staff with open, infected skin lesions should not enter the operating theatres. Ideally, neither should affected patients, especially if they are having a prosthesis implanted. Antiseptic baths (usually chlorhexidine) are popular in Europe, but there is no hard evidence for their value in reducing wound infections. Preoperative skin shaving should be undertaken in the operating theatre immediately before surgery as the SSI rate after clean wound surgery may be doubled if shaving is performed the night before, because minor skin injury enhances superficial bacterial colonisation. Cream depilation is messy and hair clipping is best, with the lowest rate of infection.

Scrubbing and skin preparation

When washing the hands prior to surgery, dilute alcohol-based antiseptic hand soaps such as chlorhexidine or povidone–iodine should be used for hand washing, and the scrub should include the nails.

One application of a more concentrated alcohol-based antiseptic is adequate for skin preparation of the operative site. This leads to a >95% reduction in bacterial count but caution should be taken not to leave a pool of alcohol-based fluid on the skin which could ignite with diathermy and burn the patient.

Theatre technique and discipline also contribute to low infection rates. Numbers of staff in the theatre and movement in and out of theatre should be kept to a minimum. Careful and regular surveillance is needed to ensure the quality of instrument sterilisation, aseptic technique and theatre ventilation. Laminar flow systems direct clean, filtered air over the operating field, with any air potentially contaminated as it passes over the incision then directed away from the patient. Operator skill in gentle manipulation and dissection of tissues is much more difficult to audit, but dead spaces and haematomas should be avoided. There is no evidence that drains, incision drapes or wound guards help to reduce wound infection. There is a high level of evidence that both the perioperative avoidance of hypothermia and the use of supplemental oxygen during recovery significantly reduce the rate of SSIs.

Moritz Kaposi, 1837–1902, Professor of Dermatology, Vienna, Austria, described pigmented sarcoma of the skin in 1872.

Prophylactic antibiotics

Prophylactic antibiotics are used when there is a risk of wound contamination with bacteria during surgery. The theoretical degree of contamination, proposed by the National Research Council (USA) over 40 years ago, relates well to infection rates (*Table 5.4*). The value of antibiotic prophylaxis is low in non-prosthetic clean surgery, with most trials showing no clear benefit because infection rates without antibiotics are so low. The exception to this is where a prosthetic implant is used, as the results of infection are so catastrophic that even a small risk of infection is unacceptable.There is undisputed evidence that prophylactic antibiotics are effective in reducing the risk of infection in clean-contaminated and contaminated operations. When wounds are heavily contaminated or when an incision is made into an abscess, a 5-day course of therapeutic antibiotics may be justified on the assumption that the wound is inevitably infected and so treatment is needed rather than prophylaxis.

If antibiotics are given to prevent infection after surgery or instrumentation, they should be used before bacterial growth becomes established (i.e. within the decisive period). Ideally, maximal blood and tissue levels should be present at the time at which the first incision is made and before contamination occurs. Tissue levels of the antibiotic should remain high throughout the operation and antibiotics with a short tissue half life should be avoided. Intravenous administration at induction of anaesthesia is therefore optimal, as unexpected delays in the timing of surgery may occur before then and antibiotic tissue levels may fall off before the surgery starts. In long operations or when there is excessive blood loss, or when unexpected contamination occurs, antibiotics may be repeated at 4-hourly intervals during the surgery, because tissue antibiotic levels often fall faster than serum levels. There is no evidence that further doses of antibiotics after surgery are of any value in prophylaxis against infection and the practice can only encourage the development of antibiotic resistance. The choice of an antibiotic depends on the expected spectrum of organisms likely to be encountered, which will depend on the site and type of surgery and whether or not the patient has any antibiotic allergies. Hospitals in the UK now have standardised antibiotic prophylaxis policies which take account of the above factors and are only deviated from with microbiological advice.

Patients with known valvular disease of the heart (or with any implanted vascular or orthopaedic prosthesis) should have prophylactic antibiotics during dental, urological or open viscus surgery, to prevent bacterial colonisation of the valve or prosthesis during the transient bacteraemia which can occur during such surgery.

TABLE 5.4 SSI rates relating to wound contamination with and without using antibiotic prophylaxis.

Type of surgery	Infection rate with prophylaxis (%)	Infection rate without prophylaxis (%)
Clean (no viscus opened)	1–2	1–2
Clean-contaminated (viscus opened, minimal spillage)	3	6–9
Contaminated (open viscus with spillage or inflammatory disease)	6	13–20
Dirty (pus or perforation, or incision through an abscess)	7	40

Summary box 5.12

Antibiotic prophylaxis

- Not required in clean surgery unless a prosthesis is implanted
- Use antibiotics that are effective against expected pathogens within local hospital guidelines
- Plan for single-shot intravenous administration at induction of anaesthesia
- Repeat only during long operations or if there is excessive blood loss
- Patients with heart valve disease or a prosthesis should be protected from bacteraemia caused by dental work, urethral instrumentation or visceral surgery

Postoperative wound infections

The majority of wound infections arise from endogenous sources within the patient, but exogenous SSI may also occur from bacteria present in the ward or staff and so can be related to poor hospital standards. Strict attention to ward cleanliness, gloving before touching patient wounds and hand washing between all patient contacts are important preventive measures. An outbreak of wound infections on the ward with bacteria having the same antibiotic sensitivity profile implies an exogenous source of infection, which needs to be investigated by swabbing all staff and work surfaces. It may need temporary ward closure and a deep clean to eradicate the infection source.

Now that patients are discharged more quickly after surgery and many procedures are performed as day cases, many SSIs are missed by the surgical team unless they undertake a prolonged and carefully audited follow-up with primary care doctors. Suppurative wound infections take 7–10 days to develop, and even cellulitis around wounds caused by invasive organisms (such as β-haemolytic *Streptococcus*) takes 3–4 days to develop. Major surgical infections with systemic signs (**Figure 5.13**), evidence of spreading infection, cellulitis or bacteraemia need treatment with appropriate antibiotics. The choice may need to be empirical initially but is best based on culture and sensitivities of isolates harvested at surgery or from culture of wound fluids or wound swabs. Although the identification of organisms in surgical infections is necessary for audit and wound surveillance purposes, it is usually 2–3 days before sensitivities are known (**Figures 5.14 and 5.15**). It is illogical to withhold antibiotics until results are available but, if clinical response is poor by the time sensitivities are known, then antibiotics can be changed. Such changes are unusual if the empirical choice of antibiotics is sensible; change of antibiotics promotes resistance and risks complications, such as *C. difficile* enteritis.

If an infected wound is under tension, or there is clear evidence of suppuration, sutures or clips need to be removed, with curettage if necessary, to allow pus to drain adequately. In severely contaminated wounds, such as an incision made

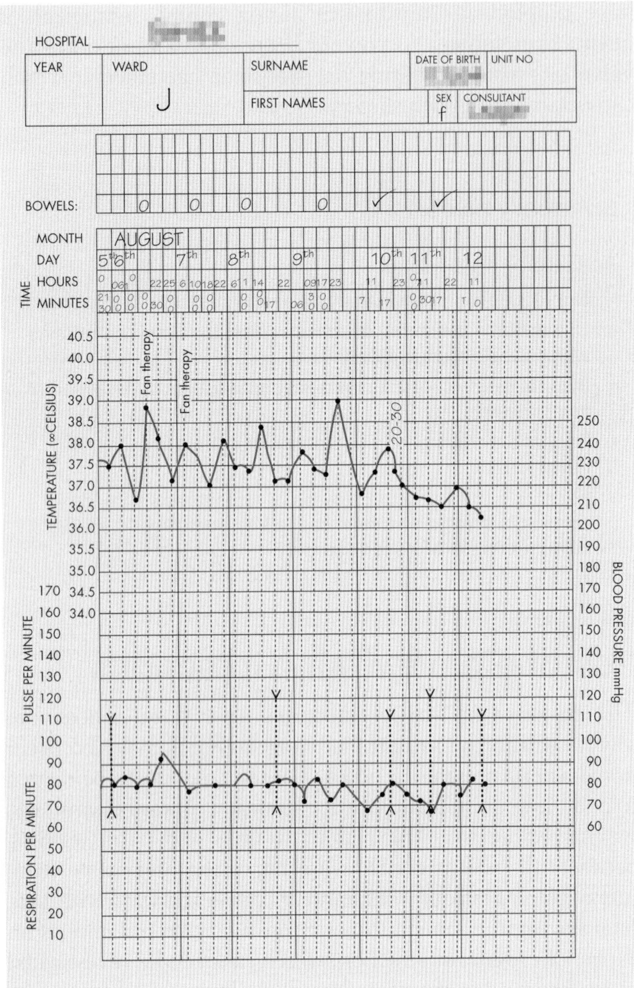

Figure 5.13 Classic swinging pyrexia related to a perianastomotic wound abscess that settled spontaneously on antibiotic therapy.

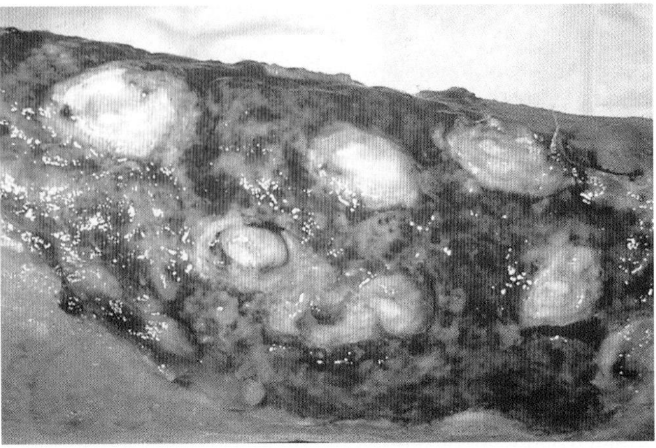

Figure 5.14 Mixed streptococcal infection of a skin graft with very poor 'take'.

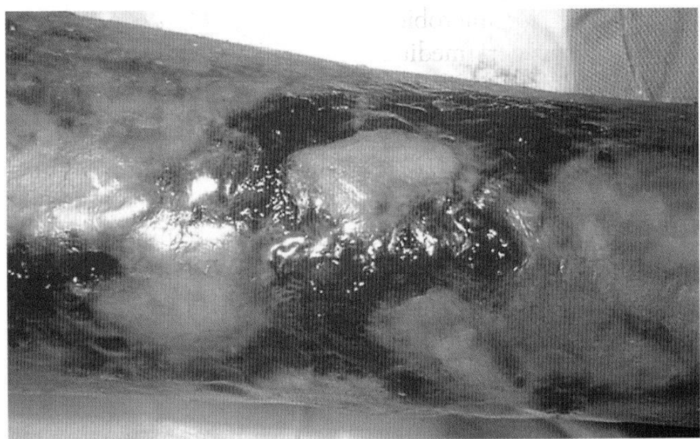

Figure 5.15 After 5–6 days of antibiotics, the infection shown in Figure 5.14 is under control, and the skin grafts are clearly viable.

for drainage of an abscess, it is logical to leave the skin open. Delayed primary or secondary closure can be undertaken when the wound is clean and granulating (**Figures 5.16 and 5.17**). Some heavily infected wounds may be left to heal by secondary intention, with no attempt at closure, particularly where there is a loss of skin cover and healthy granulation tissue develops (**Figure 5.18**). While the end result may be excessive scarring, that can always be revised with plastic surgery under clean surgical conditions at a later stage. Leaving wounds open after a 'dirty' operation, such as laparotomy for faecal peritonitis, is not practised as widely in the UK as in the USA or mainland Europe.

Summary box 5.13

Surgical incisions through infected or contaminated tissues

- When possible, tissue or pus for culture should be taken before antibiotic cover is started
- The choice of antibiotics is empirical until sensitivities are available
- Heavily contaminated wounds are best managed by delayed primary or secondary closure

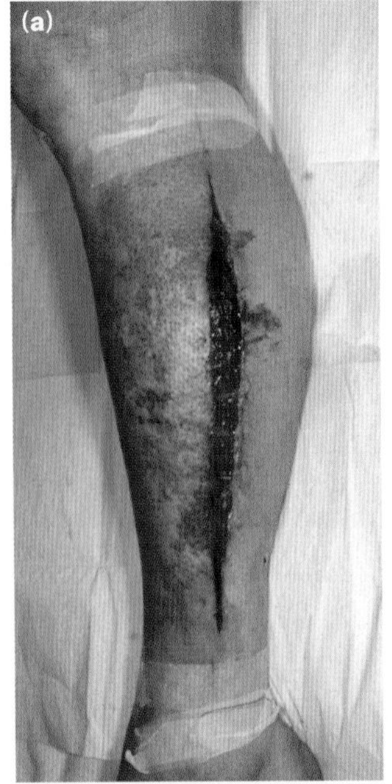

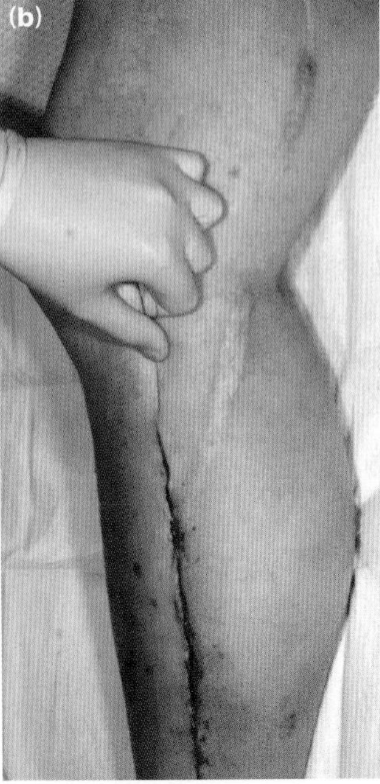

Figure 5.16 (**a, b**) Delayed primary closure of fasciotomy wound after 3–5 days.

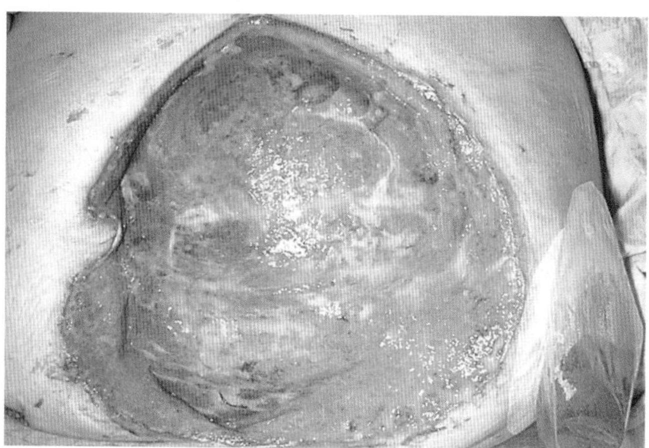

Figure 5.17 Skin layers left open to granulate after laparotomy for faecal peritonitis, ready for skin grafting.

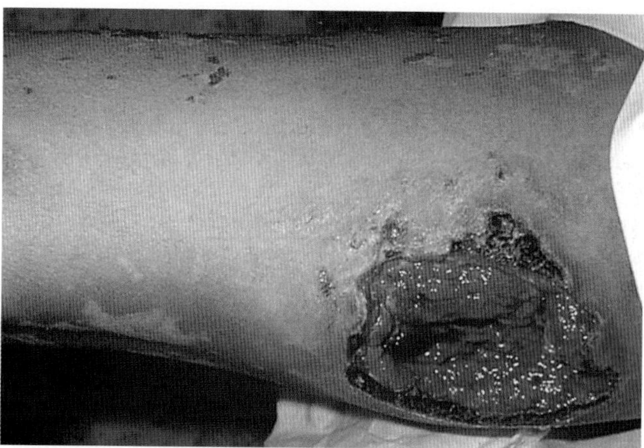

Figure 5.18 Infected animal bite/wound of the upper thigh, treated by open therapy following virulent staphylococcal infection.

When taking pus from infected wounds, specimens should be sent fresh for microbiological culture. Swabs should be placed in transport medium, but the larger the volume of pus sent, the more likely is the accurate identification of the organism involved. Providing the microbiologist with as much information as possible and discussing the results with them gives the best chance of the most appropriate antibiotic treatment. If bacteraemia is suspected, but results are negative, then repeat specimens for blood culture may need to be taken. A rapid report on infective material can be based on an immediate Gram stain.

Topical antiseptics should only be used on heavily contaminated wounds for a short period to clear infection as they inhibit epithelial ingrowth and so impair wound healing.

ANTIMICROBIAL TREATMENT OF SURGICAL INFECTION

Principles

Antimicrobials may be used to prevent or treat established surgical infection.

> **Summary box 5.14**
>
> **Principles for the use of antibiotic therapy**
> - Antibiotics do not replace surgical drainage of infection
> - Only spreading infections or signs of systemic infection justify the use of antibiotics
> - Whenever possible, the organism and sensitivity should be determined

The use of antibiotics for the treatment of established surgical infection ideally requires recognition and determination of the sensitivities of the causative organisms. Antibiotic therapy should not be held back if it is indicated, the choice being empirical and later modified depending on microbiological findings. Once antibiotics have been administered, it may not be possible to grow bacteria from the wound and so the opportunity to ascertain the most appropriate antibiotic sensitivities is lost if a patient's condition does not improve on empirical antibiotic therapy. Antibiotics alone are rarely sufficient to treat SSIs, which may also need open drainage and debridement.

There are two approaches to antibiotic treatment:

- A **narrow-spectrum antibiotic** may be used to treat a known sensitive infection; for example, MRSA (which may be isolated from pus) is usually sensitive to vancomycin or teicoplanin, but not flucloxacillin.
- **Combinations of broad-spectrum antibiotics** can be used when the organism is not known or when it is suspected that several bacteria, acting in synergy, may be responsible for the infection. For example, during and following emergency surgery requiring the opening of perforated or ischaemic bowel, any of the gut organisms may be responsible for subsequent peritoneal or bacteraemic infection. In this case, a broad spectrum antibiotic such as teicoplenin or meropenem effective against a wide range of aerobic bacteria is combined with metronidazole, effective against anaerobic bacteria. Alternatively, triple therapy is used with amoxacillin, gentamicin and metronidazole. The use of such broad-spectrum antibiotic strategies should be guided by specialist microbiological advice. If clincal response is poor after 3–4 days, there should be a re-evaluation with a review of charts and further investigations requested to exclude the development or persistence of infection such as a collection of pus.

Antibiotics used in treatment and prophylaxis of surgical infection

Antimicrobials may be produced by living organisms (antibiotics) or by synthetic methods. Some are bactericidal, e.g. penicillins and aminoglycosides, and others are bacteriostatic, e.g. tetracycline and erythromycin. In general, penicillins act upon the bacterial cell wall and are most effective against bacteria that are multiplying and synthesising new cell wall materials. The aminoglycosides act at the ribosomal level, preventing or distorting the production of proteins required to maintain the integrity of the enzymes in the bacterial cell. Hospital and Formulary guidelines should be consulted for doses and monitoring of antibiotic therapy.

Penicillin

Benzylpenicillin has proved most effective against gram-positive pathogens, including most streptococci, the clostridia and some of the staphylococci that do not produce β-lactamase. It is still effective against *Actinomyces*, which is a rare cause of chronic wound infection. It may be used specifically to treat spreading streptococcal infections. Penicillin is valuable even if other antibiotics are required as part of multiple therapy for a mixed infection. Some serious infections, e.g. gas gangrene, require high-dose intravenous benzylpenicillin.

Flucloxacillin

Flucloxacillin is resistant to β-lactamases and is therefore of use in treating infections with penicillinase-producing staphylococci which are resistant to benzylpenicillin, but it has poor activity against other pathogens. It has good tissue penetration and therefore is useful in treating soft tissue infections and osteomyelitis.

Ampicillin, amoxicillin and co-amoxiclav

Ampicillin and amoxicillin are β-lactam penicillins and can be taken orally or may be given parenterally. Both are effective against Enterobacteriaceae, *Enterococcus faecalis* and the majority of group D streptococci, but not species of *Klebsiella* or *Pseudomonas*. Clavulanic acid has no antibacterial activity itself, but it does inactivate β-lactamases, so can be used in conjunction with amoxicillin. The combination is known as co-amoxiclav and is useful against β-lactamase producing bacteria that are resistant to amoxicillin on its own. These include resistant strains of *Staphylococcus aureus*, *E. coli*, *Haemophilus influenzae*, *Bacteroides* and *Klebsiella*.

Piperacillin and ticarcillin

These are ureidopenicillins with a broad spectrum of activity against a broad range of gram-positive, gram-negative and anaerobic bacteria. Both are used in combination with β-lactamase inhibitors (tazobactam with piperacillin and clavulanic acid with ticarcillin). They are not active against MRSA but are used in the treatment of septicaemia, hospital-acquired pneumonia and complex urinary tract infections, where they are active against *Pseudomonas* and *Proteus* spp. and have a synergistic effect when used with aminoglycosides such as gentamicin.

Cephalosporins

There are several β-lactamase-susceptible cephalosporins that are of value in surgical practice: cefuroxime, cefotaxime and ceftazidime are widely used. The first two are most effective in intra-abdominal skin and soft-tissue infections, being active against *Staphylococcus aureus* and most Enterobacteriaceae. As a group, the enterococci (*Streptococcus faecalis*) are not sensitive to the cephalosporins. Ceftazidime, although active against the gram-negative organisms and *Staphylococcus aureus*, is also effective against *Pseudomonas aeruginosa*. These cephalosporins may be combined with an aminoglycoside, such as gentamicin, and an imidazole, such as metronidazole, if anaerobic cover is needed.

Aminoglycosides

Gentamicin and tobramycin have similar activity and are effective against gram-negative Enterobacteriaceae. Gentamicin is effective against many strains of *Pseudomonas*, although resistance has been recognised. All aminoglycosides are inactive against anaerobes and streptococci. Serum levels immediately before and 1 hour after intramuscular injection must be taken 48 hours after the start of therapy, and dosage should be modified to satisfy peak and trough levels. Ototoxicity and nephrotoxicity may follow sustained high toxic levels and therefore single, large doses may be safer. Use needs to be discussed with the microbiologist and local policies should be observed.

Vancomycin and teicoplanin

These glycopeptide antibiotics are most active against gram-positive aerobic and anaerobic bacteria and have proved to be effective against MRSA, so are often used as prophylactic antibiotics when there is a high risk of MRSA. They are ototoxic and nephrotoxic, so serum levels should be monitored. They are effective against *C. difficile* in cases of pseudomembranous colitis.

Carbapenems

Meropenem, ertapenem and imipenem are members of the carbapenems. They are stable to β-lactamase, have useful broad-spectrum anaerobic as well as gram-positive activity and are effective for the treatment of resistant organisms, such as ESBL-resistant urinary tract infections or serious mixed-spectrum abdominal infections (peritonitis).

Metronidazole

Metronidazole is the most widely used member of the imidazole group and is active against all anaerobic bacteria. It is particularly safe and may be administered orally, rectally or intravenously. Infections caused by anaerobic cocci and strains of *Bacteroides* and *Clostridia* can be treated, or prevented, by its use. Metronidazole is useful for the prophylaxis and treatment of anaerobic infections after abdominal, colorectal and pelvic surgery and in the treatment of *C. difficile* pseudomembranous colitis.

Ciprofloxacin

Quinolones, such as ciprofloxacin, have a broad spectrum of activity against both gram-positive and gram-negative bacteria but are particularly useful against *Pseudomonas* infections. Many UK hospitals have restricted their use as a preventive measure against the development of *C. difficile* enterocolitis.

FURTHER READING

Fraise AP, Bradley C. *Ayliffe's control of healthcare associated infection: a practical handbook*. London: Hodder Arnold, 2009.

Fry DE. *Surgical infections*. London: JP Medical Ltd, 2013.

Sawyer RG, Hedrick TL. *Surgical infections, an issue of surgical clinics*. New York: Elsevier – Health Sciences Division, 2014.

Thomas WEG, Reed MWR, Wyatt MG. *Oxford textbook of fundamentals of surgery*. Oxford: Oxford University Press, 2016.

Torok E, Moran E, Cooke F. *Oxford handbook of infectious diseases and microbiology*, 2nd edn. Oxford: Oxford University Press, 2016.

Chapter 6

Tropical infections and infestations

Learning objectives

To be able to list:

- The common surgical infections and infestations that occur in the tropics

To appreciate:

- That many patients do not seek medical help until late in the course of the disease because of socioeconomic reasons

To be able to describe:

- The emergency presentations of the various conditions, as patients may not seek treatment until they are very ill

To be able to:

- Diagnose and treat these conditions, particularly as emergencies. The ease of global travel has connected areas where tropical infections are common to areas where they are not. Patients with such an infection who are recently returned from the tropics will mostly present as emergencies

To realise:

- That the ideal management involves a multidisciplinary approach between the surgeon, physician, radiologist, pathologist and microbiologist. In case of doubt, in a difficult situation, there should be no hesitation in seeking help from a specialist centre.

INTRODUCTION

Most surgical conditions in the tropics (regions of the Earth surrounding the equator) are associated with parasitic infestations and infections related to poor hygeinic conditions. With the ease of international travel, diseases that are common in the tropics may present in areas of the world where they are not commonly seen, especially as emergencies.

This chapter deals with the conditions that a surgeon might occasionally see when working in an area where such diseases are uncommon. Typically the patient would be a visitor from a tropical climate or a local resident who has visited the tropics either on holiday or to work. The life cycles of the parasites will not be described. For academic interest readers may refer to the 24th edition of this book should they wish to learn details of the parasitology. The principles of surgical treatment are dealt with in the appropriate sections although, for operative details, referral to a relevant textbook is advised.

AMOEBIASIS

Introduction

Amoebiasis is caused by *Entamoeba histolytica*. The disease is common in the Indian subcontinent, Africa and parts of Central and South America, where almost half the population is infected. The majority remain asymptomatic carriers. The mode of infection is via the faeco-oral route, and the disease occurs as a result of substandard hygiene and sanitation; therefore, the population from the poorer socioeconomic strata are more vulnerable. Amoebic liver abscess, the commonest extraintestinal manifestation, occurs in less than 10% of the infected population and, in endemic areas, is much more common than pyogenic abscess. Patients who are immunocompromised and alcoholics are more susceptible to infection.

Pathogenesis

The organism enters the gut through food or water contaminated with the cyst. In the small bowel, the cysts hatch, and a large number of trophozoites are released and carried to the colon where flask-shaped ulcers form in the submucosa. The trophozoites multiply, ultimately forming cysts, which enter the portal circulation or are passed in the faeces as an infective form that infects other humans as a result of insanitary conditions.

Having entered the portal circulation, the trophozoites are filtered and trapped in the interlobular veins of the liver. They multiply in the portal triads, causing focal infarction of hepatocytes and liquefactive necrosis as a result of proteolytic enzymes produced by the trophozoites. The areas of necrosis eventually coalesce to form the abscess cavity. The term 'amoebic hepatitis' is used to describe the microscopic picture in the absence of macroscopic abscess, a differentiation only in theory because the medical treatment is the same.

The right lobe is involved in 80% of cases, the left in 10% and the remainder are multiple. One possible explanation for the more common involvement of the right lobe of the liver is that blood from the superior mesenteric vein runs on a straighter course through the portal vein into the larger lobe. The abscesses are most common high in the diaphragmatic surface of the right lobe. This may cause pulmonary symptoms and chest complications. The abscess cavity contains chocolate-coloured, odourless, 'anchovy sauce'-like fluid that is a mixture of necrotic liver tissue and blood. There may be secondary infection of the abscess which causes the pus to smell. While pus in the abscess is sterile unless secondarily infected, trophozoites may be found in the abscess wall in a minority of cases. Untreated abscesses are likely to rupture.

Chronic infection of the large bowel may result in a granulomatous lesion along the large bowel, most commonly seen in the caecum, called an amoeboma.

Summary box 6.1

Amoebiasis - pathology

- *Entamoeba histolytica* is the most common pathogenic amoeba in humans
- The vast majority of carriers are asymptomatic
- Insanitary conditions and poor personal hygiene encourage transmission of the infection
- In the small intestine, the parasite hatches into trophozoites, which invade the submucosa to produce flask-shaped ulcers
- In the portal circulation, the parasite causes liquefactive necrosis in the liver, producing an abscess, the commonest extraintestinal manifestation
- The majority of abscesses occur in the right lobe of the liver
- A mass in the course of the large bowel may indicate an amoeboma

Clinical features

The typical patient with amoebic liver abscess is a young adult male with a history of insidious onset of non-specific symptoms, such as abdominal pain, anorexia, fever, night sweats, malaise, cough and weight loss. These symptoms gradually progress to more specific symptoms of pain in the right upper abdomen and right shoulder tip, hiccoughs and a non-productive cough. A past history of bloody diarrhoea or travel to an endemic area raises the index of suspicion.

Examination reveals a patient who is toxic and anaemic. The patient will have upper abdominal rigidity, tender hepatomegaly, tender and bulging intercostal spaces, overlying skin oedema, a pleural effusion and basal pneumonitis – the last feature is usually a late manifestation. Occasionally, a tinge of jaundice or ascites may be present. Rarely, the patient may present as an emergency due to the effects of rupture of an abscess into the peritoneal, pleural or pericardial cavity.

Amoeboma

This is a chronic granuloma arising in the large bowel, most commonly seen in the caecum. It is prone to occur in longstanding amoebic infection that has been treated intermittently with drugs without completion of a full course, a situation that arises from indiscriminate self-medication, particularly in resource-poor countries. Hence this is more often seen in such countries.

This can easily be mistaken for a carcinoma. An amoeboma should be suspected when a patient from an endemic area with generalised ill health and pyrexia has a mass in the right iliac fossa with a history of blood-stained mucoid diarrhoea. Such a patient is highly unlikely to have a carcinoma because altered bowel habit is not a feature of right-sided colonic carcinoma. While iron deficiency anaemia is a classical elective presentation of a caecal carcinoma, the same is present in an amoeboma because of chronic malnutrition.

Investigations

The haematological and biochemical investigations reflect the presence of a chronic infective process: anaemia, leukocytosis, raised inflammatory markers – erythrocyte sedimentation rate (ESR) and C-reactive protein (CRP) – hypoalbuminaemia and deranged liver function tests, particularly elevated alkaline phosphatase.

Serological tests are more specific, with the majority of patients showing antibodies in serum. These can be detected by tests for complement fixation, indirect haemagglutination (IHA), indirect immunofluorescence and enzyme-linked immunosorbent assay (ELISA). These tests are extremely useful in detecting acute infection in non-endemic areas. IHA has a very high sensitivity in acute amoebic liver abscess in non-endemic regions and remains elevated for some time. The persistence of antibodies in a large majority of the population in endemic areas precludes its use as a diagnostic investigation in those locations. In these cases, tests, such as counter-immunoelectrophoresis, are more useful for detecting acute infection.

While flexible sigmoidoscopy is routine in any patient with blood-stained altered bowel habit, an outpatient rigid sigmoidoscopy using a disposable instrument may be a prudent first choice if amoebic infection is suspected in the presence of bloody mucoid diarrhoea. Most amoebic ulcers occur in the rectosigmoid and are therefore within reach of the sigmoidoscope; shallow skip lesions and 'flask-shaped' or 'collar-stud' undermined ulcers may be seen, and can be biopsied or scrapings can be taken along with mucus for immediate microscopic examination. The presence of trophozoites distinguishes the condition from ulcerative colitis.

Imaging techniques

On ultrasound, an abscess cavity in the liver is seen as a hypoechoic or anechoic lesion with ill-defined borders; internal echoes suggest necrotic material or debris **(Figure 6.1)**.

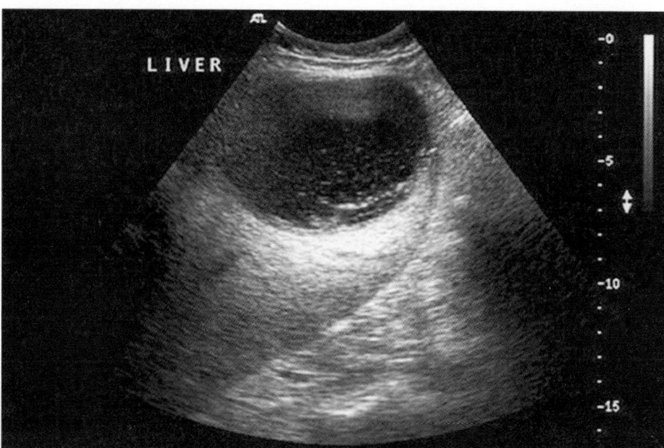

Figure 6.1 Ultrasound of the liver showing a large amoebic liver abscess with necrotic tissue in the right lobe.

The investigation is very accurate and is used for aspiration, both diagnostic and therapeutic. Where there is doubt about the diagnosis, a computed tomography (CT) scan may be helpful (**Figure 6.2**).

Diagnostic aspiration is of limited value except for establishing the typical colour of the aspirate, which is sterile and odourless unless it is secondarily infected.

A CT scan may show a raised right hemidiaphragm, a pleural effusion and evidence of pneumonitis (**Figure 6.3**).

An 'apple-core' deformity on barium enema would arouse suspicion of a carcinoma. A colonoscopy with biopsy is mandatory because the radiological and macroscopic appearance may be indistinguishable from a carcinoma. In doubtful cases, vigorous medical treatment is given, and the patient undergoes colonoscopy again in 3–4 weeks, as these masses are known to regress completely on a full course of drug therapy. If symptoms persist even partially following full medical treatment in a patient who has recently returned from an endemic area, a colonic carcinoma must be excluded forthwith. This is because a dormant colonic carcinoma may become apparent as a result of infestation with amoebic dysentery causing 'traveller's diarrhoea'. However, it must be borne in mind that an amoeboma and a carcinoma can coexist.

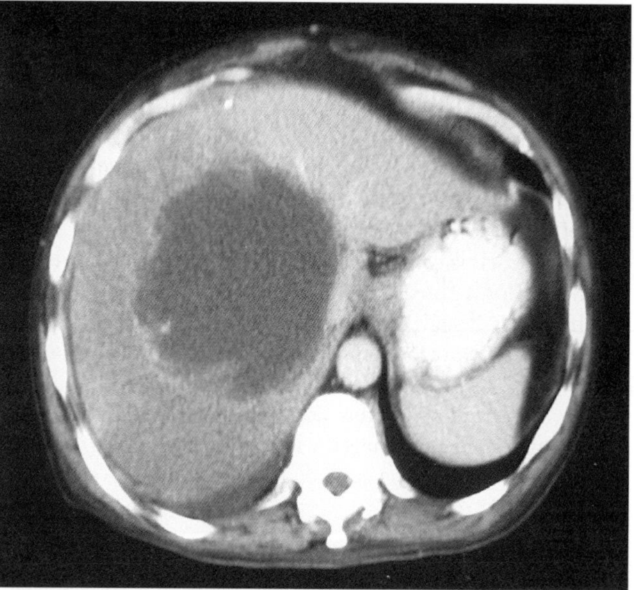

Figure 6.2 Computed tomographic scan showing an amoebic liver abscess in the right lobe.

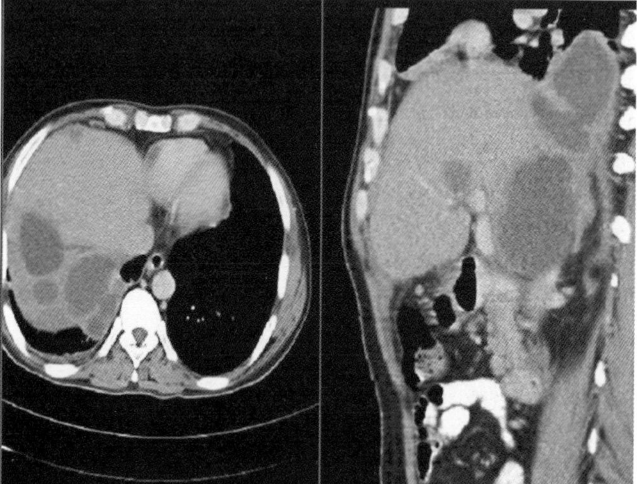

Figure 6.3 Computed tomographic scans showing multiple amoebic liver abscesses with extension into the chest.

Summary box 6.2

Diagnostic pointers for infection with *Entamoeba histolytica*

- Bloody mucoid diarrhoea in a patient from an endemic area or following a recent visit to such a country
- Upper abdominal pain, fever, cough, malaise
- In chronic cases, a mass in the right iliac fossa may be an amoeboma but caecal cancer must be excluded by colonoscopy and biopsy
- Sigmoidoscopy shows typical ulcers – biopsy and scrapes may be diagnostic
- Serological tests are highly sensitive and specific outside endemic areas
- Ultrasound and CT scans are the imaging methods of choice

Treatment

Medical treatment is very effective and should be the first choice in the elective situation, with surgery being reserved for complications. Metronidazole and tinidazole are the effective drugs. After treatment with metronidazole and tinidazole, diloxanide furoate, which is not effective against hepatic infestation, is used for 10 days to destroy any intestinal amoebae.

Aspiration is carried out when imminent rupture of an abscess is expected. Aspiration also helps the penetration of metronidazole, and so reduces the morbidity when carried out with drug treatment in a patient with a large abscess. If there is evidence of secondary infection, appropriate drug treatment is added. The threshold for aspirating an abscess in the left lobe should be lower because of its proximity to the pericardium.

Surgical treatment should be reserved for the complications of rupture into the pleural (usually the right side), peritoneal or pericardial cavities. Resuscitation, drainage and appropriate lavage with vigorous medical treatment are the key principles. In the large bowel, severe haemorrhage and toxic megacolon are rare complications. In these patients, the general principles of a surgical emergency apply, the principles of management being the same as for any toxic megacolon. Resuscitation is followed by resection of bowel with exteriorisation. Then the patient is given vigorous supportive therapy. All such cases are managed in the intensive care unit, as would any patient with toxic megacolon whatever the cause.

An amoeboma that has not regressed after full medical treatment should be managed with colonic resection, particularly if cancer cannot be excluded.

Summary box 6.3

Amoebiasis - treatment

- Medical treatment is very effective
- For large abscesses, repeated aspiration is combined with drug treatment
- Surgical treatment is reserved for complications, such as rupture into the pleural, peritoneal or pericardial cavities
- Acute toxic megacolon and severe haemorrhage are intestinal complications that are treated with intensive supportive therapy followed by resection and exteriorisation: subtotal colectomy with terminal ileostomy and closure of the rectal stump
- When an amoeboma is suspected in a colonic mass, cancer should be excluded by appropriate imaging and biopsy

ROUNDWORM (*ASCARIS LUMBRICOIDES*)

Introduction

Ascaris lumbricoides, commonly called the roundworm, is the commonest intestinal nematode to infect humans and affects a quarter of the world's population. The parasite causes pulmonary symptoms as a larva and intestinal symptoms as an adult worm.

Pathology and life cycle

The eggs can survive in a hostile environment for a long time. The hot and humid conditions in the tropics are ideally suited for the eggs to turn into embryos. The fertilised eggs are present in soil contaminated with infected faeces. Faeco-oral contamination causes human infection.

As the eggs are ingested, the released larvae travel to the liver via the portal system and then through the systemic circulation to reach the lung, the maturation process taking up to 8 weeks. The developed larvae reach the alveoli, are coughed up, swallowed and continue their maturation in the small intestine. Sometimes, the young worms migrate from the tracheobronchial tree into the oesophagus, thus finding their way into the gastrointestinal tract, from where they can migrate to the common bile duct or pancreatic duct. The mature female, once in the small bowel, produces innumerable eggs that are fertilised and thereafter excreted in the stool to perpetuate the life cycle. Eggs in the biliary tract can form a nidus for a stone.

Clinical features

The larval stage in the lungs causes pulmonary symptoms – dry cough, chest pain, dyspnoea and fever – referred to as Loeffler's syndrome. The adult worm can grow up to 45 cm long. Its presence in the small intestine causes malnutrition, failure to thrive, particularly in children, and abdominal pain. Worms that migrate into the common bile duct can produce ascending cholangitis and obstructive jaundice, while features of acute pancreatitis may be caused by a worm in the pancreatic duct.

Small intestinal obstruction can occur, particularly in children, due to a bolus of adult worms incarcerated in the terminal ileum. This is a surgical emergency. Rarely, perforation of the small bowel may occur from ischaemic pressure necrosis from the bolus of worms.

A high index of suspicion is necessary so as not to miss the diagnosis. If a person from a tropical country, or one who has recently returned after spending some time in an endemic area, presents with pulmonary, gastrointestinal, hepatobiliary and pancreatic symptoms, ascariasis should be high on the list of possible diagnoses.

Investigations

As with most parasitic infestations, an increase in the eosinophil count is common. Stool examination may show ova. Sputum or bronchoscopic washings may show Charcot–Leyden crystals or the larvae.

Chest radiograph may show fluffy exudates in Loeffler's syndrome. A barium meal and follow-through may show a bolus of worms in the ileum or lying freely within the small bowel (**Figure 6.4**). Ultrasound may show a worm in the common bile duct (**Figure 6.5**) or pancreatic duct. On magnetic resonance cholangiopancreatography (MRCP), an adult worm may be seen in the common bile duct in a patient presenting with features of obstructive jaundice (**Figure 6.6**). In patients with intestinal obstruction, plain abdominal radiograph may show tubular structures within dilated small bowel, denoting the presence of worms, which would also show up on a contrast CT scan as curvilinear structures.

Wilhelm Loeffler, 1887–1972, Professor of Medicine, Zurich, Switzerland.
Jean Martin Charcot, 1825–1893, Physician, La Salpêtrière, Paris, France.
Ernst von Leyden, 1832–1910, Professor of Medicine, Berlin, Germany.

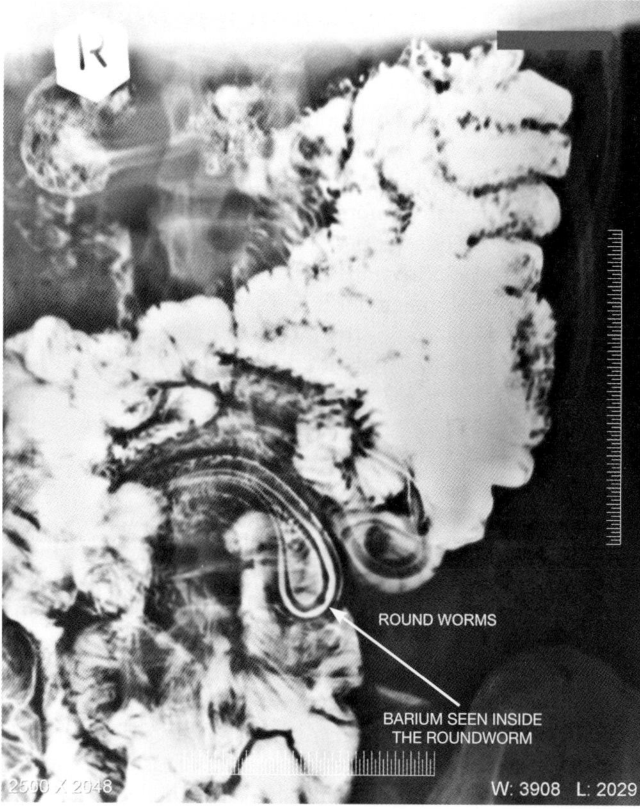

Figure 6.4 Barium meal and follow-through showing roundworms in the course of the small bowel with barium seen inside the worms in an 18-year-old patient who presented with bouts of colicky abdominal pain and bilious vomiting, which settled with conservative management (courtesy of Dr P Bhattacharaya, Kolkata, India).

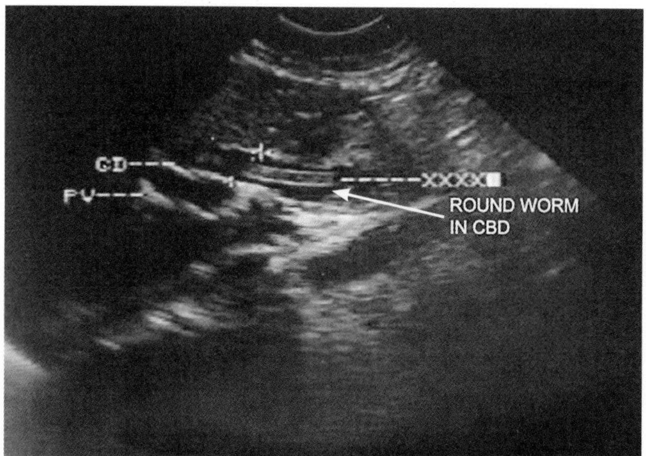

Figure 6.5 Ultrasound scan showing a roundworm in the common bile duct (CBD). The patient presented with obstructive jaundice and had asymptomatic gallstones. On endoscopic retrograde cholangiopancreatography, part of the worm was seen outside the ampulla in the duodenum and was removed through the endoscope. Subsequent laparoscopic cholecystectomy was uneventful.

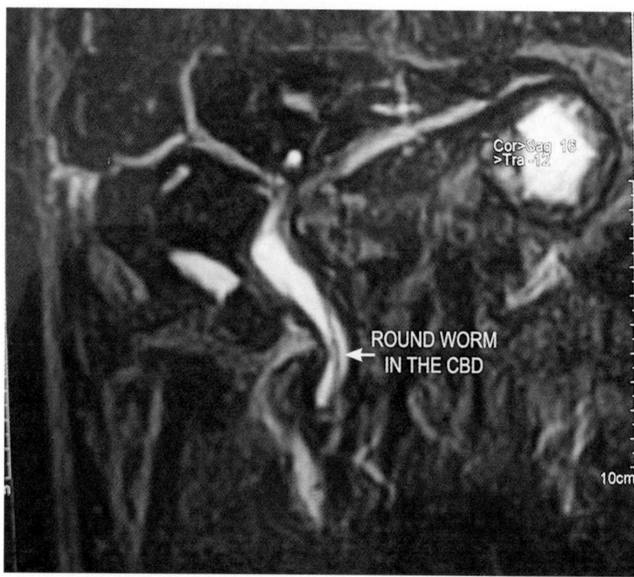

Figure 6.6 Magnetic resonance cholangiopancreatography showing a roundworm in the common bile duct (CBD). The worm could not be removed endoscopically. The patient underwent an open cholecystectomy and exploration of the CBD.

Summary box 6.4

Ascariasis – pathogenesis

- It is the commonest intestinal nematode affecting humans
- Typically found in a humid atmosphere and poor sanitary conditions, hence is seen in the tropics and resource-poor countries
- Larvae cause pulmonary symptoms; adult worms cause gastrointestinal, biliary and pancreatic symptoms
- Distal ileal obstruction is due to a bolus of worms; ascending cholangitis and obstructive jaundice from infestation of the common bile duct
- Acute pancreatitis occurs when a worm is lodged in the pancreatic duct
- Perforation of the small bowel is rare

Treatment

The pulmonary phase of the disease is usually self-limiting and requires symptomatic treatment only. For intestinal disease, patients should ideally be under the care of a physician for treatment with anthelmintic drugs. Certain drugs may cause rapid death of the adult worms and, if there are many worms in the terminal ileum, the treatment may actually precipitate acute intestinal obstruction from a bolus of dead worms. Children who present with features of intermittent or subacute obstruction should be given a trial of conservative management in the form of intravenous fluids, nasogastric suction and hypertonic saline enemas. The last of these helps to disentangle the bolus of worms and also increases intestinal motility.

Surgery is reserved for complications, such as intestinal obstruction that has not resolved on a conservative regime, or when perforation is suspected. At laparotomy, the bolus of worms in the terminal ileum is milked through the ileocaecal valve into the colon for natural passage in the stool.

Postoperatively, hypertonic saline enemas may help in the extrusion of the worms. Strictures, gangrenous areas or perforations need resection and anastomosis. If the bowel wall is healthy, enterotomy and removal of the worms may be performed (**Figure 6.7**).

Rarely, when perforation occurs due to roundworm, the parasites may be found lying free in the peritoneal cavity. It is safer to bring out the site of perforation as an ileostomy because, in the presence of a large number of worms, the closure of an anastomosis may be at risk of breakdown from the activity of the worms.

When a patient is operated upon as an emergency for a suspected complication of roundworm infestation, the actual diagnosis at operation may turn out to be acute appendicitis, typhoid perforation or a tuberculous stricture, and the presence of roundworms is an incidental finding. Such a patient requires the appropriate surgery depending upon the primary pathology.

Common bile duct or pancreatic duct obstruction from a roundworm can be treated by endoscopic removal, failing which laparoscopic or open exploration of the common bile duct is necessary. Cholecystectomy is also carried out. A full course of antiparasitic treatment must follow any surgical intervention.

Summary box 6.5

Ascariasis - diagnosis and management

- Barium meal and follow-through will show worms scattered in the small bowel
- Ultrasound may show worms in the common bile duct and pancreatic duct
- Plain abdominal radiograph and contrast CT scan will show the worms as tubular or curvilinear structures
- Conservative management with anthelmintics is the first line of treatment even in obstruction
- Surgery is a last resort – various options are available

ASIATIC CHOLANGIOHEPATITIS

Introduction

This disease, also called oriental cholangiohepatitis, is caused by infestation of the hepatobiliary system by *Clonorchis sinensis*. It has a high incidence in the tropical regions of South East Asia, particularly amongst those living in the major sea ports and near river estuaries. The organism, which is a type of liver fluke, resides in snails and fish that act as intermediate hosts. Ingestion of infected fish and snails, when eaten raw or improperly cooked, causes the infection in humans and other fish-eating mammals, which are the definitive hosts.

Pathology

In humans, the parasite matures into the adult worm in the intrahepatic biliary radicles where they may reside for many years. The intrahepatic bile ducts are dilated, with epithelial hyperplasia and periductal fibrosis. These changes may lead to dysplasia, causing cholangiocarcinoma – the most serious and dreaded complication of this parasitic infestation.

The eggs or dead worms may form a nidus for stone formation in the gallbladder or common bile duct, which becomes thickened and much dilated in the late stages. Intrahepatic bile duct stones are also caused by the parasite producing mucin-rich bile. The dilated intrahepatic bile ducts may lead to cholangitis, liver abscess and hepatitis.

Diagnosis

The disease may remain dormant for many years. Clinical features are non-specific and include fever, malaise, anorexia and upper abdominal discomfort. The complete clinical picture can consist of fever with rigors due to ascending cholangitis, obstructive jaundice, biliary colic and pruritus from stones in the common bile duct. Acute pancreatitis may occur because of obstruction of the pancreatic duct by an adult worm. Particularly when presenting in non-endemic areas, it should be noted that if a person from an endemic area complains

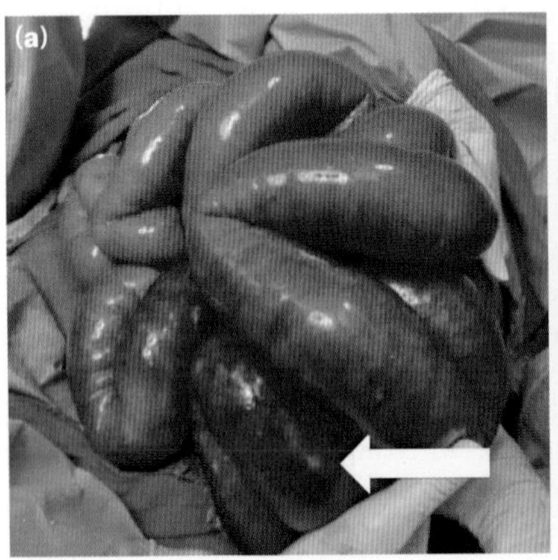

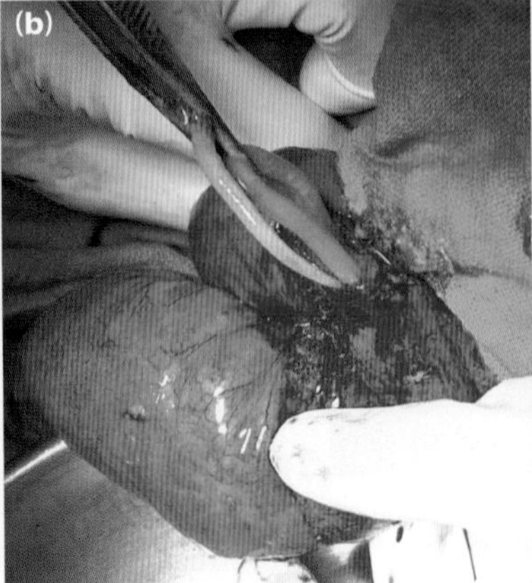

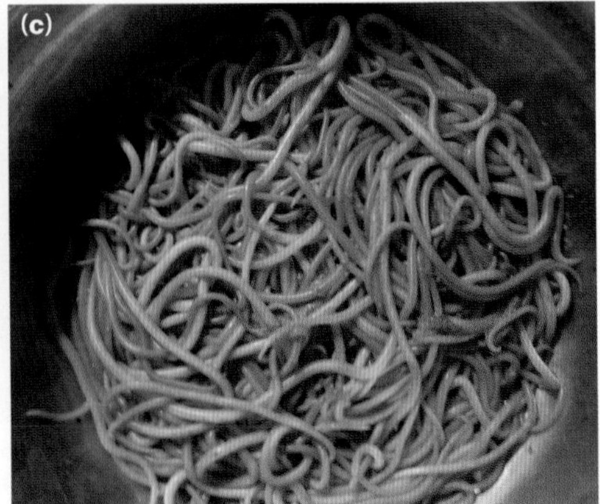

Figure 6.7 **(a)** Roundworms seen through the bowel wall (arrowed). **(b)** Roundworm being removed through enterototomy. **(c)** Removed roundworms.

of symptoms of biliary tract disease, *Clonorchis* infestation should be high in the differential diagnosis.

In advanced cases, liver function tests are abnormal. Confirmation of the condition is by examination of stool or duodenal aspirate, which may show the eggs or adult worms. Ultrasound scan findings may be characteristic, showing uniform dilatation of small peripheral intrahepatic bile ducts with only minimal dilatation of the common hepatic and common bile ducts, although the latter are much more dilated when the obstruction is caused by stones. The thickened duct walls show increased echogenicity and non-shadowing echogenic foci in the bile ducts representing the worms or eggs. Endoscopic retrograde cholangiopancreatography (ERCP) will confirm these findings.

Summary box 6.6

Asiatic cholangiohepatitis – pathogenesis and diagnosis

- Occurs in the Far Eastern tropical zones
- The causative parasite is *Clonorchis sinensis*
- Produces bile duct hyperplasia, intrahepatic duct dilatation and stones
- Increases the risk of cholangiocarcinoma
- May remain dormant for many years
- When active, there are biliary tract symptoms in a generally unwell patient
- Stool examination for eggs or worms is diagnostic
- Ultrasound scan of the hepatobiliary system and ERCP are also diagnostic

Treatment

Praziquantel and albendazole are the drugs of choice. However, the surgeon faces a challenge when there are stones not only in the gallbladder but also in the common bile duct. Cholecystectomy with exploration of the common bile duct is performed when indicated. Repeated washouts are necessary during the exploration, as the common bile duct is dilated and contains stones, biliary debris, sludge and mud. This should be followed by choledochoduodenostomy. As this is a disease with a prolonged and relapsing course, some surgeons prefer to do a choledochojejunostomy to a Roux loop. The Roux loop is brought up to the abdominal wall, referred to as 'an access loop', which allows the interventional radiologist to deal with any future stones.

As a public health measure, people who have emigrated from an endemic area should be offered screening for *Clonorchis* infestation in the form of ultrasound of the hepatobiliary system. This condition can be diagnosed and treated, and even cured, when it is in its subclinical form. Most importantly, the risk of developing the dreadful disease of cholangiocarcinoma is eliminated.

Summary box 6.7

Asiatic cholangiohepatitis – treatment

- Medical treatment can be curative in the early stages
- Surgical treatment is cholecystectomy, exploration of the common bile duct and some form of biliary–enteric bypass
- Prevention – consider offering hepatobiliary ultrasound as a screening procedure to recently arrived migrants from endemic areas

FILARIASIS

Introduction

Filariasis is mainly caused by the parasite *Wuchereria bancrofti* carried by the mosquito. Variants of the parasite called *Brugia malayi* and *Brugia timori* are responsible for causing the disease in about 10% of those infected. The condition affects more than 120 million people worldwide, two-thirds of whom live in India, China and Indonesia. According to the World Health Organization (WHO), after leprosy, filariasis is the most common cause of long-term disability.

Once the host has been bitten by the mosquito, the matured eggs enter the human circulation to hatch and grow into adult worms; the process of maturation takes almost a year. The adult worms mainly colonise the lymphatic system.

Diagnosis

It is mainly males who are affected, because females generally cover a greater part of their bodies with clothing, thus making them less prone to mosquito bites. In the acute presentation, there are episodic attacks of fever with lymphadenitis and lymphangitis.

Occasionally, adult worms may be felt subcutaneously. Chronic manifestations appear after repeated acute attacks over several years. The adult worms cause lymphatic obstruction, resulting in massive lower limb oedema. Obstruction to the cutaneous lymphatics causes skin thickening, not unlike the '*peau d'orange*' appearance in breast cancer, thus exacerbating the limb swelling. Secondary streptococcal infection is common. Recurrent attacks of lymphangitis cause fibrosis of the lymph channels, resulting in a grossly swollen limb with thickened skin, producing the condition of elephantiasis (**Figure 6.8**). Bilateral lower limb filariasis is often associated with scrotal and penile elephantiasis. Early on, there may be a hydrocoele underlying scrotal filariasis (**Figure 6.9**).

Chyluria and chylous ascites may occur. A mild form of the disease can affect the respiratory tract, causing dry cough, and is referred to as tropical pulmonary eosinophilia. The condition of filariasis is clinically very obvious, and thus investigations in the full-blown case are superfluous. Eosinophilia is common, and a nocturnal peripheral blood smear may show

---

Cesar Roux, 1857–1934, Professor of Surgery and Gynaecology, Lausanne, Switzerland, described this method of forming a jejunal conduit in 1908.
Otto Eduard Heinrich Wucherer, 1820–1873, German physician who practised in Brazil, South America.
Joseph Bancroft, 1836–1894, English physician who worked in Australia.
Peau d'orange is French for 'orange skin'.

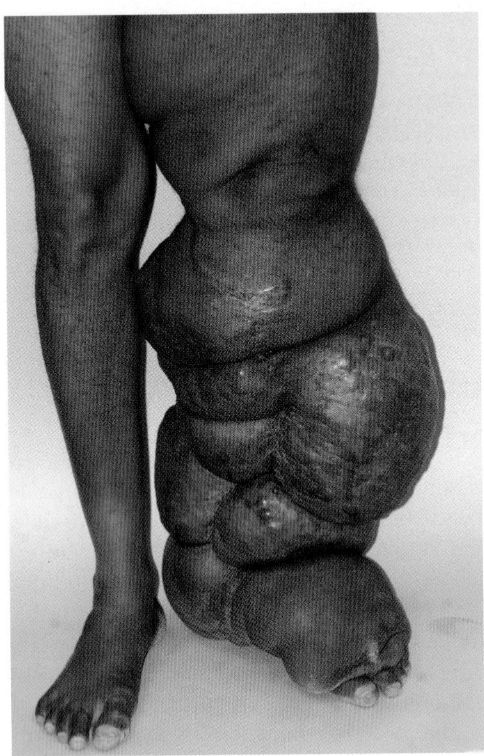

Figure 6.8 Left lower limb filariasis – elephantiasis (courtesy of Professor Ahmed Hassan Fahal, FRCS MD MS, Khartoum, Sudan).

the immature forms, or microfilariae. The parasite may also be seen in chylous urine, ascites and hydrocoele fluid.

Treatment

Medical treatment with diethylcarbamazine is very effective in the early stages before the gross deformities of elephantiasis have developed. In the early stages of limb swelling, intermittent pneumatic compression helps, but the treatment has to be repeated over a prolonged period.

A hydrocoele is treated by the usual operation of excision and eversion of the sac with, if necessary, excision of redundant skin. Operations for reducing the size of the limb are hardly ever done these days because the procedures are so rarely successful.

Summary box 6.8

Filariasis

- Caused by *Wuchereria bancrofti*, which is carried by the mosquito
- Lymphatics are mainly affected, resulting in gross limb swelling
- Eosinophilia occurs; immature worms may be seen in a nocturnal peripheral blood smear
- Gross forms of the disease cause a great deal of disability and misery
- Early cases are very amenable to medical treatment
- Intermittent pneumatic compression gives some relief
- The value of various surgical procedures is largely unproven and hence they are rarely performed

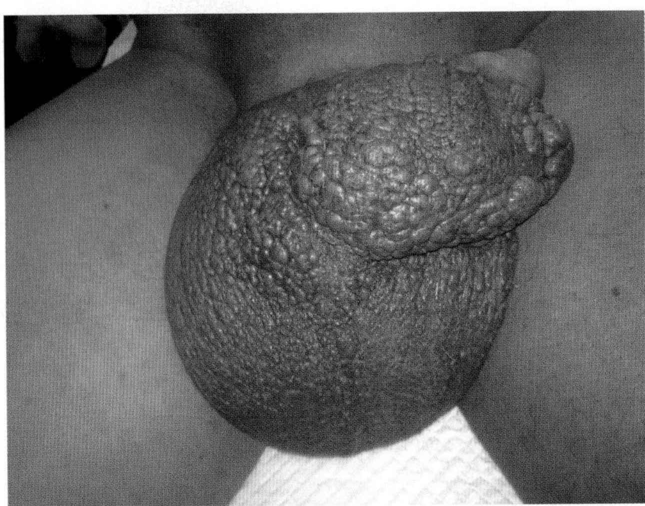

Figure 6.9 Filariasis of the scrotum and penis (courtesy of Professor Ahmed Hassan Fahal, FRCS MD MS, Khartoum, Sudan).

HYDATID DISEASE

Introduction and pathology

Hydatid disease is caused by *Ecchinococcus granulosus*, commonly called the dog tapeworm. The disease is globally distributed and, while it is common in the tropics, it is much less common in other countries; for example, in the UK the occasional patient may come from a rural sheep-farming community.

The dog is the definitive host and is the commonest source of infection transmitted to the intermediate hosts – humans, sheep and cattle. In the dog, the adult worm reaches the small intestine, and the eggs are passed in the faeces. These eggs are highly resistant to extremes of temperature and may survive for long periods. In the dog's intestine, the cyst wall is digested, allowing the protoscolices to develop into adult worms. Close contact with an infected dog causes contamination by the oral route, with the ovum thus gaining entry into the human gastrointestinal tract.

The cyst is characterised by three layers, an outer **pericyst** derived from compressed host organ tissues, an intermediate hyaline **ectocyst**, which is non-infective, and an inner **endocyst** that is the germinal membrane and contains viable parasites which can separate forming daughter cysts. A variant of the disease occurs in colder climates caused by *Echinococcus multilocularis*, in which the cyst spreads from the outset by actual invasion rather than expansion.

Classification

In 2003, the WHO Informal Working Group on Echinococcosis (WHO-IWGE) proposed a standardised ultrasound classification based on the status of activity of the cyst. This is universally accepted, particularly because it helps to decide on the appropriate management. Three groups have been recognised:

- Group 1: Active group – cysts larger than 2 cm and often fertile.

- Group 2: Transition group – cysts starting to degenerate and entering a transitional stage because of host resistance or treatment, but may contain viable protoscolices.
- Group 3: Inactive group – degenerated, partially or totally calcified cysts; unlikely to contain viable protoscolices.

Clinical features

As the parasite can colonise virtually every organ in the body, the condition can be protean in its presentation. When a sheep farmer, who is otherwise healthy, complains of a gradually enlarging painful mass in the right upper quadrant with the physical findings of a liver swelling, a hydatid liver cyst should be considered. The liver is the organ most often affected. The lung is the next most common. The parasite can affect any organ (**Figures 6.10 and 6.11**) or several organs in the same patient (**Figure 6.12**).

The disease may be asymptomatic and discovered coincidentally at postmortem or when an ultrasound or CT scan is done for some other condition. Symptomatic disease presents with a swelling causing pressure effects. Thus, a hepatic lesion causes dull pain from stretching of the liver capsule, and a pulmonary lesion, if large enough, causes dyspnoea. Daughter cysts may communicate with the biliary tree, causing obstructive jaundice and all the usual clinical features associated with it in addition to symptoms attributable to a parasitic infestation (**Figure 6.13**). Features of raised intracranial pressure

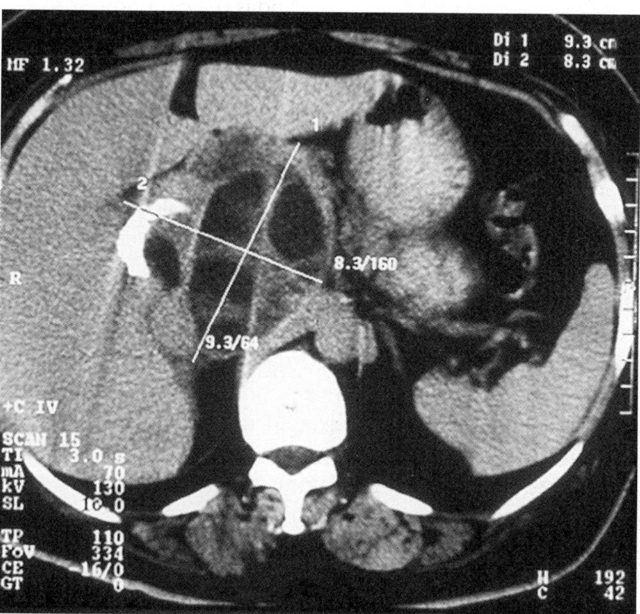

Figure 6.10 Computed tomographic scan showing a hydatid cyst of the pancreas. A differential diagnosis of hydatid cyst or a tumour was considered. At exploration, the patient was found to have a hydatid cyst, which was excised followed by 30 months of treatment with albendazole, and remains free of disease.

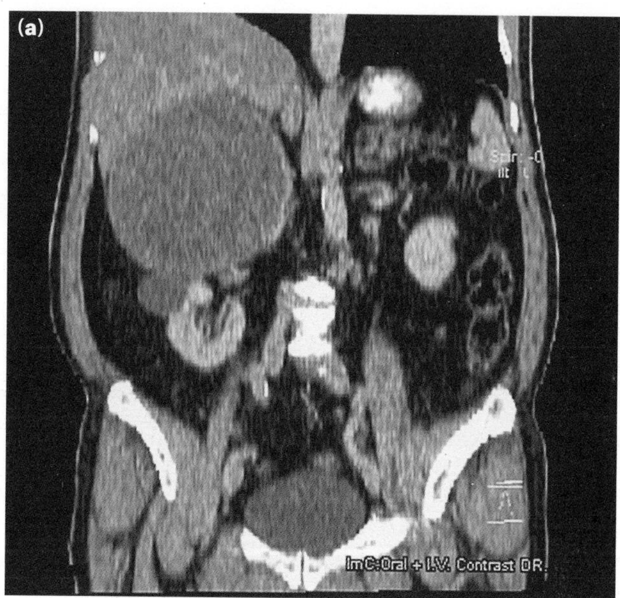

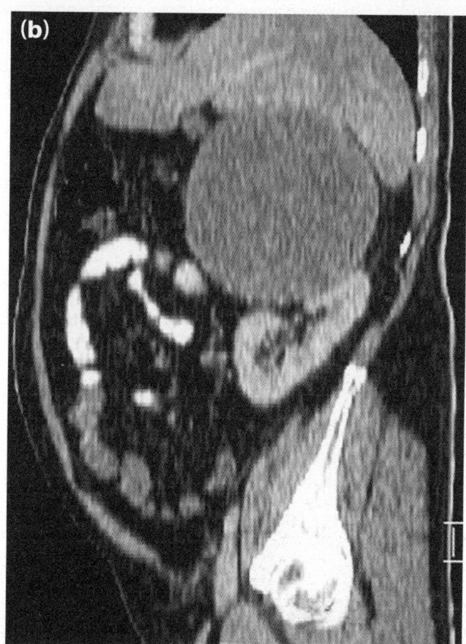

Figures 6.11 Anteroposterior (**a**) and lateral (**b**) views of computed tomographic scans showing a large hydatid cyst of the right adrenal gland. The patient presented with a mass in the right loin and underwent an adrenalectomy (courtesy of Dr P Bhattacharaya, Kolkata, India).

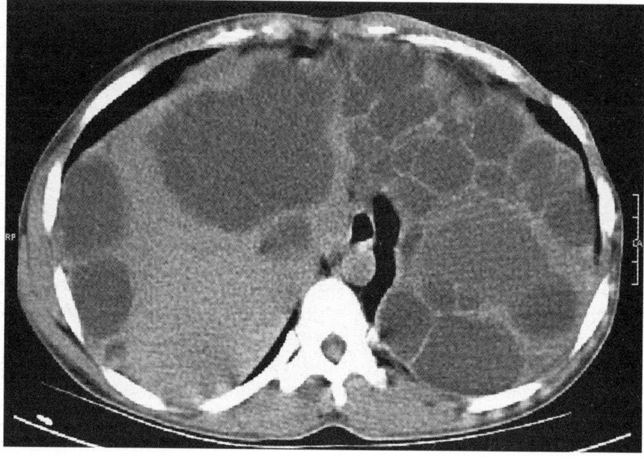

Figure 6.12 Computed tomographic scan showing disseminated hydatid cysts of the abdomen. The patient was started on albendazole but was lost to follow-up (courtesy of Dr P Bhattacharaya, Kolkata, India).

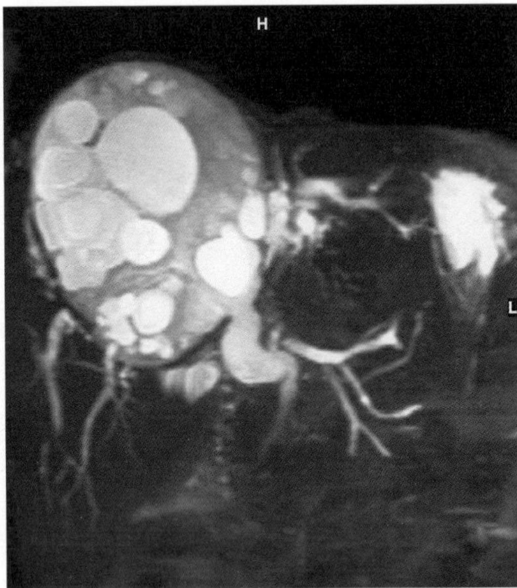

Figure 6.13 Magnetic resonance cholangiopancreatography showing a large hepatic hydatid cyst with daughter cysts communicating with the common bile duct, causing obstruction and dilatation of the entire biliary tree (courtesy of Dr B Agarwal, New Delhi, India).

or unexplained headaches in a patient from a sheep-rearing community should raise the suspicion of a cerebral hydatid cyst.

The patient may present as an emergency with severe abdominal pain following minor trauma, when the CT scan may be diagnostic (**Figure 6.14**). Rarely, a patient may present as an emergency with features of anaphylactic shock without any obvious cause. Such a patient may subsequently cough up white material that contains scolices that have travelled into the tracheobronchial tree from rupture of a hepatic hydatid on the diaphragmatic surface of the liver.

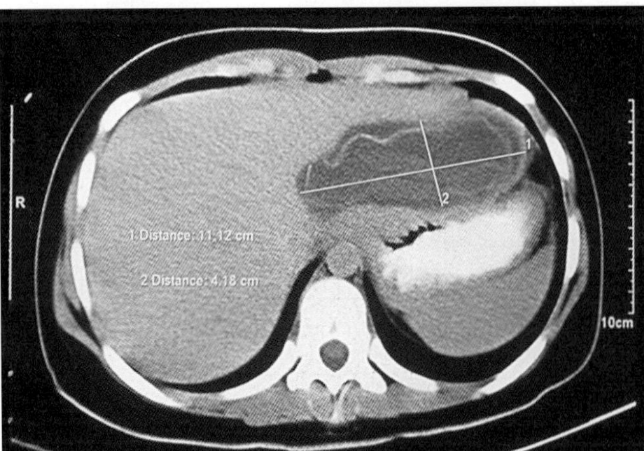

Figure 6.14 Computed tomographic (CT) scan of the upper abdomen showing a hypodense lesion of the left lobe of the liver; the periphery of the lesion shows a double edge. This is the lamellar membrane of the hydatid cyst that separated after trivial injury. The patient was a 14-year-old girl who developed a rash and pain in the upper abdomen after dancing. The rash settled down after a course of antihistamines. The CT scan was performed 2 weeks later for persisting upper abdominal pain.

Diagnosis

There should be a high index of suspicion. Investigations show a raised eosinophil count; serological tests, such as ELISA and immunoelectrophoresis, point towards the diagnosis. Ultrasound and CT scan are the investigations of choice. The CT scan shows a smooth space-occupying lesion with several septa. Ultrasound of the biliary tract may show abnormality in the gallbladder and bile ducts, when hydatid infestation of the biliary system should be suspected. Ultimately, the diagnosis is made by a combination of good history and clinical examination supplemented by serology and imaging.

Summary box 6.9

Hydatid disease - diagnosis

- In the UK, the usual sufferer is a sheep farmer
- While any organ may be involved, the liver is by far the most commonly affected
- Elective clinical presentation is usually in the form of a painful lump arising from the liver
- Anaphylactic shock due to rupture of the hydatid cyst is the emergency presentation
- CT scan is the best imaging technique – the diagnostic feature is a space-occupying lesion with a smooth outline with septa

Treatment

Here, the treatment of hepatic hydatid is outlined because the liver is most commonly affected, but the same general principles apply whichever organ is involved.

These patients should be treated in a tertiary unit where good teamwork between an expert hepatobiliary surgeon, an experienced physician and an interventional radiologist is available. Surgical treatment by minimal access therapy is best summarised by the mnemonic PAIR (puncture, aspiration, injection and reaspiration). This is done after adequate drug treatment with albendazole, although praziquantel has also been used, both of these drugs being available only on a 'named patient' basis.

Whether the patient is treated only medically or in combination with surgery will depend upon the clinical group (which gives an idea as to the activity of the disease), the number of cysts and their anatomical position. Radical total or partial pericystectomy with omentoplasty or hepatic segmentectomy (especially if the lesion is in a peripheral part of the liver) are some of the surgical options. During the operation, scolicidal agents are used, such as hypertonic saline (15–20%), ethanol (75–95%) or 1% povidone iodine (although some use a 10% solution). This may cause sclerosing cholangitis if biliary radicles are in communication with the cyst wall. A laparoscopic approach to these procedures is being tried (see below).

Obviously, cysts in other organs need to be treated in accordance with the actual anatomical site, along with the general principles described. An asymptomatic cyst which is inactive (group 3) may be left alone.

Summary box 6.10

Hydatid cyst of the liver – treatment

- Ideally managed in a tertiary unit by a multidisciplinary team of hepatobiliary surgeon, physician and interventional radiologist
- Leave asymptomatic and inactive cysts alone – monitor size by ultrasound
- Active cysts should first be treated by a full course of albendazole
- Several procedures are available – PAIR, pericystectomy with omentoplasty and hepatic segmentectomy; appropriate management is customised according to the particular patient and organ involved
- Increasingly, a laparoscopic approach is being tried

Laparoscopic management

Currently, surgeons trained in minimal access surgery perform hydatid surgery using minimal access. Laparoscopic marsupialisation of the cyst (de-roofing), consisting of removal of the cyst containing the endocyst along with daughter cysts, is the most common procedure. In the initial steps, the cyst is aspirated, taking care not to spill any contents, using povidone iodine or hypertonic saline as a scolicidal agent. Any communication with the biliary tree is oversewn and pedicled omentum is sutured to the margins of the cyst.

If the cyst is small, superficial and in the left lobe, cysto-pericystectomy is performed at centres experienced enough to do more advanced surgery, removing the entire cyst intact.

Pulmonary hydatid disease

The lung is the second commonest organ affected after the liver. The size of the cyst can vary from very small to a considerable size. The right lung and lower lobes are slightly more often involved. The cyst is usually single, although multiple cysts do occur and concomitant hydatid cysts in other organs, such as the liver, are not unknown. The condition may be silent and found incidentally. Symptomatic patients present with cough, expectoration, fever, chest pain and sometimes haemoptysis. Silent cysts may present as an emergency due to rupture or an allergic reaction.

Uncomplicated cysts present as rounded or oval lesions on chest radiography. Erosion of the bronchioles results in air being introduced between the pericyst and the laminated membrane and gives a fine radiololucent crescent, the 'meniscus or crescent sign' (**Figure 6.15**). This is often regarded as a sign of impending rupture. When the cyst ruptures, the crumpled collapsed endocyst floats in the residual fluid, giving rise to the 'water-lily' sign on CT scan (**Figure 6.16**). Rupture into the pleural cavity results in pleural effusion. CT scan defines the pathology in greater detail.

The mainstay of treatment of pulmonary hydatid is surgery. Medical treatment is less successful and considered when surgery is not possible because of poor general condition or diffuse disease affecting both lungs, or recurrent or ruptured cysts. The principle of surgery is to preserve as much viable lung tissue as possible. The exact procedure can vary: cystotomy, capittonage, pericystectomy, segmentectomy or occasionally pneumonectomy.

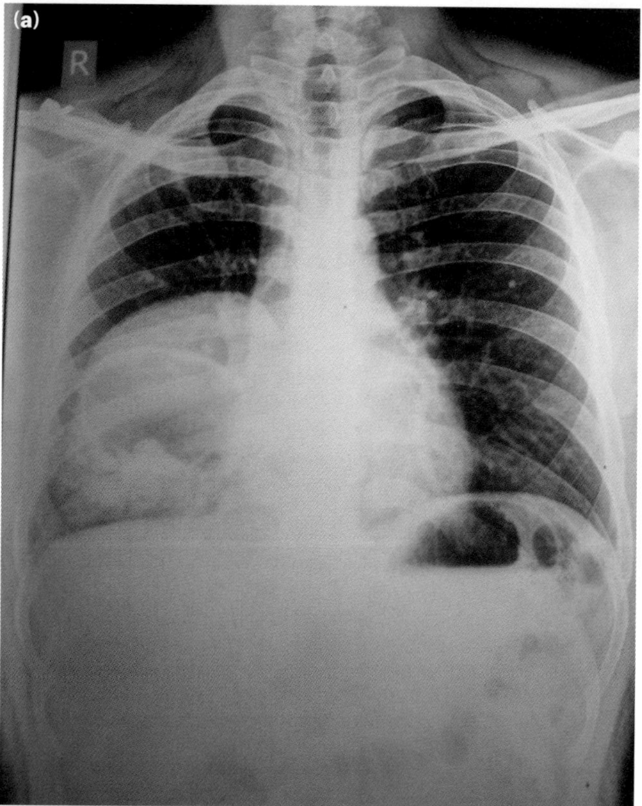

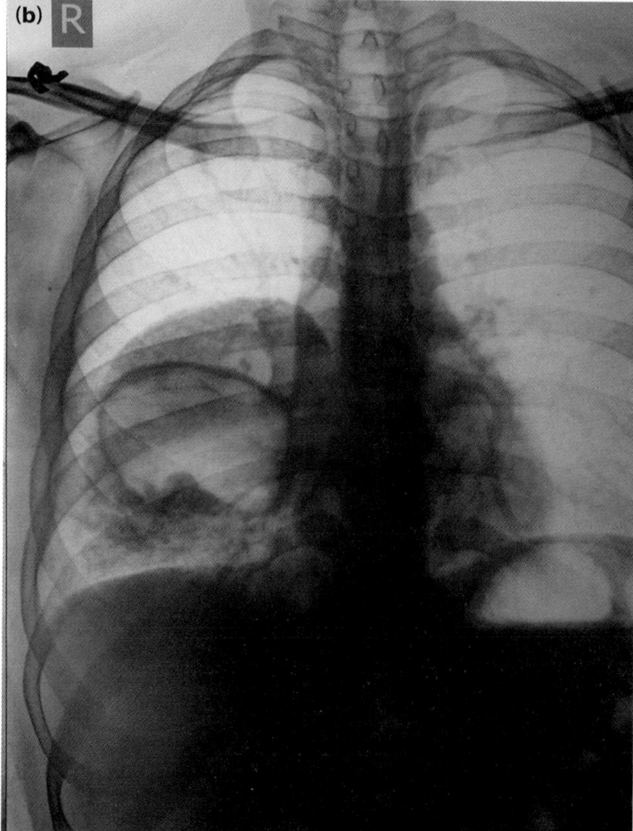

Figures 6.15 Chest radiographs: (**a**) showing a smooth rounded cystic lesion in the right lower lobe; (**b**) showing a 'meniscus or crescent' sign (courtesy of Professor Saibal Gupta, MS, FRCS, Professor of Cardiovascular Surgery, Kolkata, India and Dr Rupak Bhattacharya, Kolkata, India).

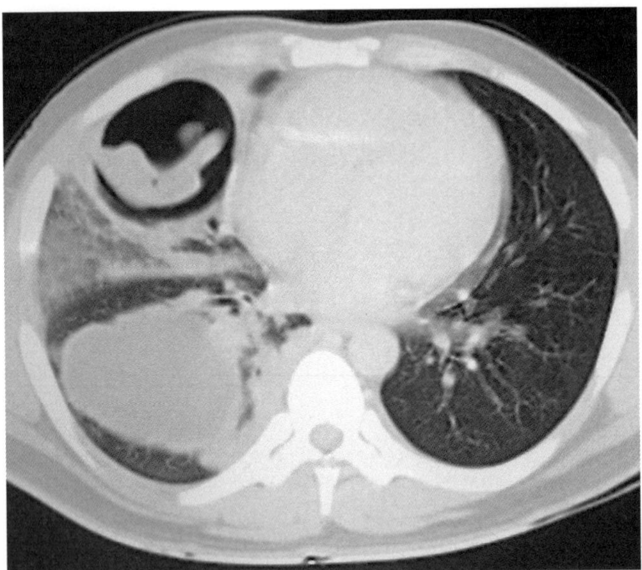

Figure 6.16 Computed tomographic scan showing the 'water-lily' sign. A young mountaineer, while on a high altitude trip, complained of sudden shortness of breath, cough and copious expectoration consisting of clear fluid and flaky material. At first thought to be due to pulmonary oedema, it turned out to be ruptured hydatid cyst, successfully treated by surgery (courtesy of Professor Saibal Gupta, MS, FRCS, Professor of Cardiovascular Surgery, Kolkata, India and Dr Rupak Bhattacharya, Kolkata, India).

Summary box 6.11

Pulmonary hydatid disease

- The second most common organ involved
- Size of the cyst has a wide variation
- May present as an incidental finding
- Clinical presentation may be elective or as an emergency due to rupture
- Plain radiograph shows 'meniscus or crescent' sign; CT shows 'water-lily' sign
- Ideal treatment is surgical – various choices are available

LEPROSY

Introduction

Leprosy, also called Hansen's disease, is a chronic infectious disease caused by an acid-fast bacillus, *Mycobacterium leprae*, that is widely prevalent in the tropics. Globally, India, Brazil, Nepal, Mozambique, Angola and Myanmar account for 91% of all cases; India alone accounts for 78% of the world's disease. Patients suffer not only from the primary effects of the disease but also from social discrimination, sadly compounded by use of the word 'leper' for one afflicted with this disease.

Close contact over a long duration (several years) is required for disease transmission. Ignorance of this fact on the part of the general public results in ostracism and social stigma. History records that in the distant past sufferers were made to wear cow bells so that other people could avoid them. The use of the term 'leper', still used metaphorically to denote an outcast, does not help to break down the social barriers that continue to exist against the sufferer.

Pathology

The bacillus inhabits the colder parts of the body – hence it is found in the nasal mucosa and skin in the region of the ears, thus involving the facial nerve as it exits from the stylomastoid foramen. The disease is transmitted from the nasal secretions of a patient, the infection being contracted in childhood or early adolescence. After an incubation period of several years, the disease presents with skin, upper respiratory or neurological manifestations. The bacillus is acid fast but weakly so when compared with *Mycobacterium tuberculosis*.

The disease is broadly classified into two groups – lepromatous and tuberculoid. In lepromatous leprosy, there is widespread dissemination of abundant bacilli in the tissues, with macrophages and few lymphocytes. This is a reflection of the poor immune response, resulting in depleted host resistance from the patient. In tuberculoid leprosy, on the other hand, the patient shows a strong immune response with scant bacilli in the tissues, epithelioid granulomas, numerous lymphocytes and giant cells. The tissue damage is inversely proportional to the host's immune response. There are various grades of the disease between the two main spectra.

Summary box 6.12

Mycobacterium leprae - pathology

- Leprosy is a chronic curable infection caused by *Mycobacterium leprae*
- It occurs mainly in tropical regions and resource-poor countries
- The majority of cases are located in the Indian subcontinent
- Transmission is through nasal secretions, the bacillus inhabiting the colder parts of the body
- It is attributed to poor hygiene and insanitary conditions
- The incubation period is several years
- The initial infection occurs in childhood
- Lepromatous leprosy denotes a poor host immune reaction
- Tuberculoid leprosy occurs when host resistance is stronger than the virulence of the organism

Clinical features and diagnosis

The disease is slowly progressive and affects the skin, upper respiratory tract and peripheral nerves. In tuberculoid leprosy, the damage to tissues occurs early and is localised to one part of the body, with limited deformity of that organ. Neural involvement is characterised by thickening of the nerves, which are tender. There may be asymmetrical well-defined

Owing to the stigma attached to the word 'leper', RG Cochrane suggested that the best name for **leprosy** is 'Hansen's disease'.
Gerhard Henrik Armauer Hansen, 1841–1912, physician in charge of a leper hospital near Bergen, Norway.
Robert Greenhill Cochrane, 1899–1985, medical missionary who became an international authority on leprosy; he devoted his time to leprosy patients in South East Asia, particularly India.

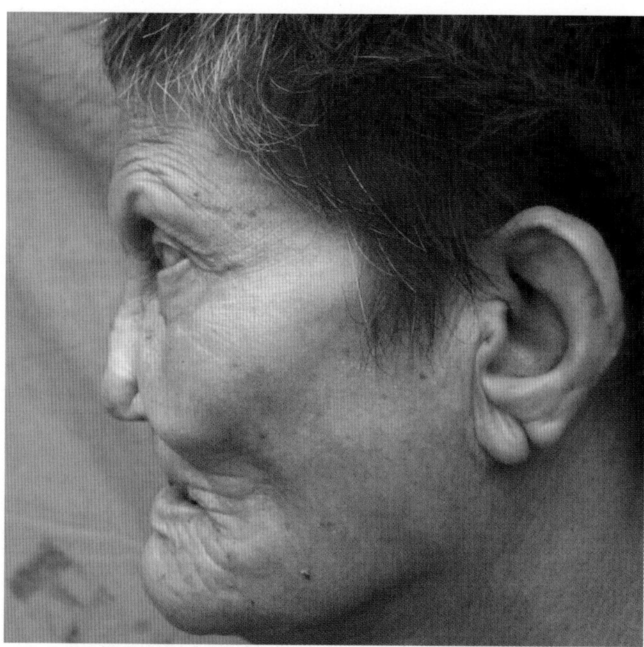

Figure 6.17 Lateral view of the face showing collapse of the nasal bridge due to destruction of nasal cartilage by leprosy.

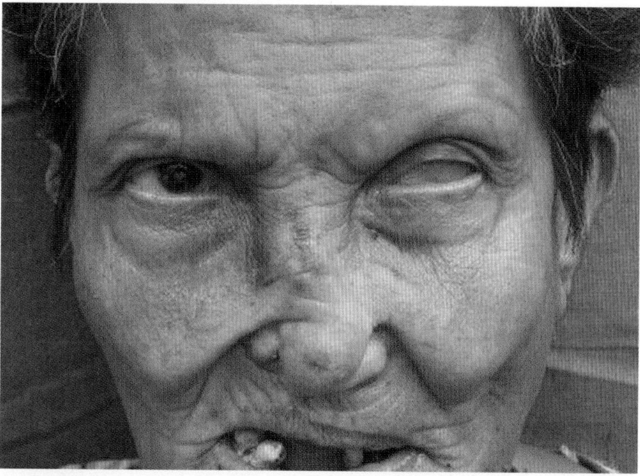

Figure 6.18 Frontal view of the face showing eye changes in leprosy – paralysis of orbicularis oculi and loss of eyebrows.

anaesthetic hypopigmented or erythematous macules with elevated edges and a dry and rough surface – lesions called leprids. In lepromatous leprosy, the disease is symmetrical and extensive. Cutaneous involvement occurs in the form of several pale macules that form plaques and nodules called lepromas. The deformities produced are divided into primary, which are caused by leprosy or its reactions, and secondary, resulting from effects such as anaesthesia of the hands and feet.

Nodular lesions on the face in the acute phase of the lepromatous variety are known as 'leonine facies' (looking like a lion). Later, there is wrinkling of the skin, giving an aged appearance to a young individual. There is loss of the eyebrows and destruction of the lateral cartilages and septum of the nose with collapse of the nasal bridge and lifting of the tip of the nose (**Figure 6.17**). There may be paralysis of the branches of the facial nerve in the bony canal or of the zygomatic branch. Blindness may be attributed to exposure keratitis or iridocyclitis. Paralysis of the orbicularis oculi causes incomplete closure of the eye, epiphora and conjunctivitis (**Figure 6.18**). The hands are typically clawed (**Figure 6.19**) because of involvement of the ulnar nerve at the elbow and the median nerve at the wrist. Anaesthesia of the hands makes these patients vulnerable to frequent burns and injuries. Similarly, clawing of the toes (**Figure 6.20**) occurs as a result of involvement of the posterior tibial nerve. When the lateral popliteal nerve is affected, it leads to foot drop, and the nerve can be felt to be thickened behind the upper end of the fibula. Anaesthesia of the feet predisposes to trophic ulceration (**Figure 6.21**), chronic infection, contraction and autoamputation. Involvement of the testes causes atrophy,

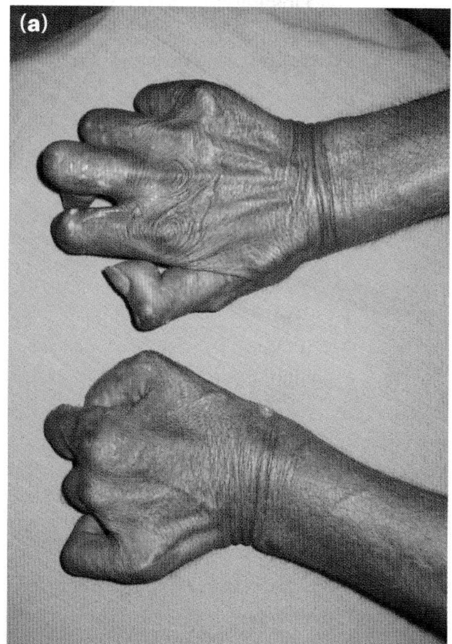

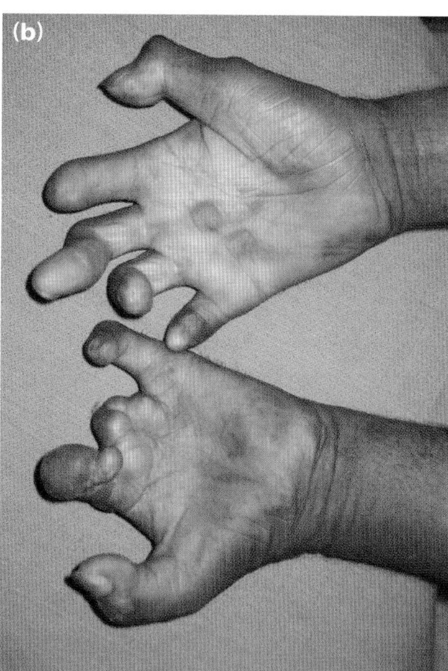

Figures 6.19 **(a, b)** Typical bilateral claw hand from leprosy due to involvement of the ulnar and median nerves.

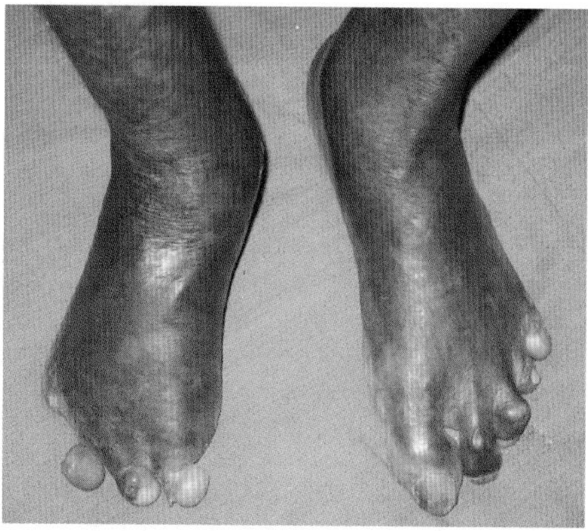

Figure 6.20 Claw toes from involvement of the posterior tibial nerve by leprosy; also note autoamputation of toes of the right foot.

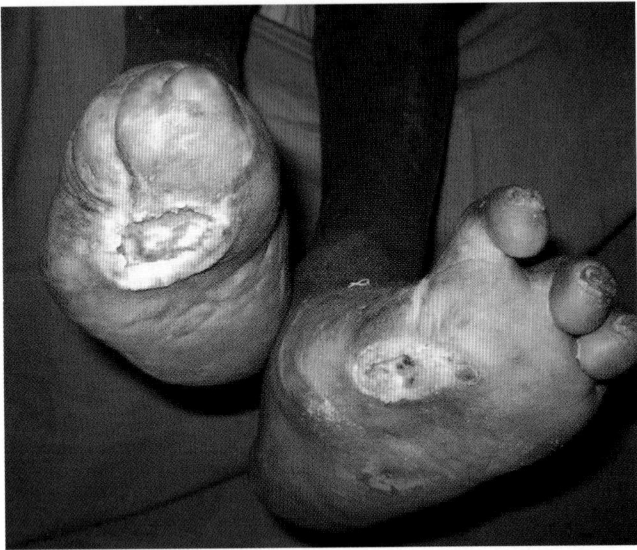

Figure 6.21 Bilateral trophic ulceration of the feet due to anaesthesia of the soles resulting from leprosy; also note claw toes on the left foot.

which in turn results in gynaecomastia (Figure 6.22). Confirmation of the diagnosis is obtained by a skin smear or skin biopsy, which shows the classical histological and microbiological features.

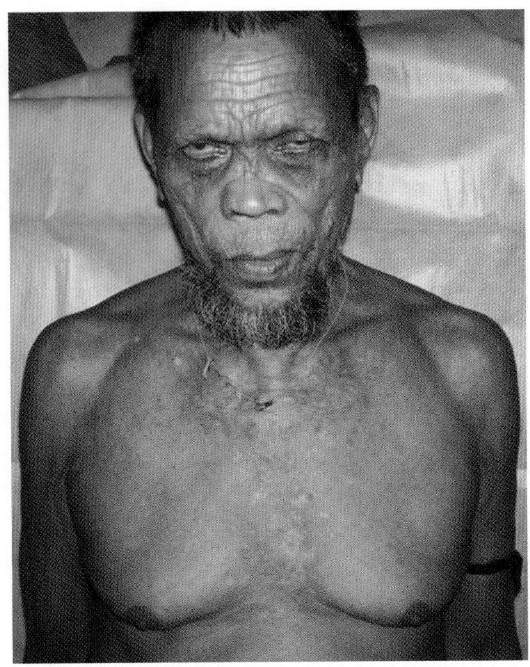

Figure 6.22 Typical leonine facies and gynaecomastia in leprosy.

Summary box 6.13

Leprosy - diagnosis

- Typical clinical features and awareness of the disease should help to make a diagnosis
- The face has an aged look, with collapse of the nasal bridge and ocular changes
- Thickened peripheral nerves, patches of anaesthetic skin, claw hands, foot drop and trophic ulcers are characteristic
- Microbiological examination of the acid-fast bacillus and typical histology on skin biopsy are confirmatory

Treatment

A herbal derivative from the seeds of *Hydrocarpus wightiana* called chalmoogra oil was the mainstay of treatment, with some success, until the advent of dapsone (diamino-diphenyl sulphone). Dapsone, one of the principal drugs, was a derivative of prontosil red (Domagk). This is used according to the WHO guidelines along with rifampicin and clofazimine. During treatment, the patient may develop acute manifestations. These are controlled with steroids. Multiple drug therapy for 12 months is the key to treatment. A team approach between an infectious diseases specialist, plastic surgeon, ophthalmologist, and hand or orthopaedic surgeon is important.

Surgical treatment is indicated in advanced stages of the disease for functional disability of limbs, cosmetic disfigurement of the face and visual problems. These entail major reconstructive surgery, the domain of the plastic surgeon.

Surgery for deformities in the hand is aimed at returning the ability to achieve a grasp and a pinch grip. Tendon transfers are used to recreate the function of the lumbricals which have been lost due to damage to the ulnar nerve. In the foot, damage to the common peroneal nerve leads to a foot drop due to paralysis of tibialis anterior. If a foot-drop splint is not adequate then once again a tendon transfer (tibialis posterior into the dorsum of the foot) will improve function. Ulcers resulting from an insensate foot should be completely debrided followed by protection with a plaster cast.

Gerhard Domagk, 1895–1964, German physician, Lecturer in Pathologic Anatomy, University of Munster, Germany, discovered prontosil in 1935, for which he was awarded the Nobel Prize for Physiology or Medicine in 1939.

Paul Wilson Brand CBE, FRCS, 1914–2003, was born to missionary parents in Southern India, and qualified in London in 1943. He himself was a dedicated missionary who was 'An extraordinary gifted orthopaedic surgeon who straightened crooked hands and unravalled the riddle of leprosy.' As a pioneer in tendon transfer techniques, he established and practised initially in New Life Center, Vellore, South India and Schieffelin Leprosy Research Centre, Karigiri, South India. Initially he trained as a carpenter and builder and maintained that his training as a carpenter helped him in his expertise in tendon transplantation. When he was awarded the CBE, his wife, Margaret, came to know about it when she found a letter from Her Majesty's Government informing him of the award, while emptying the pockets of his trousers before they were put into the wash. He later moved to Louisiana State University, Baton Rouge, LA, where he continued his work, and finally to Seattle as Emeritus Professor of Orthopaedics in the University of Washington, Seattle, USA.

Margaret Brand, alongside her husband, Paul Brand, also contributed immensely to the health of leprosy patients by concentrating on research to prevent blindness in leprosy. She became known as 'the woman who first helped lepers to see'.

Frank Tovey OBE, b.1927, another English surgeon at about the same time (1951–1967), also performed extensive tendon transfers, facial and other reconstructive surgery on leprosy patients in Southern India in the State of Mysore. In this he was helped by his wife, Winifred, who organised the physiotherapy and rehabilitation of the patients and established village diagnostic and treatment centres).

The general surgeon may be called upon to treat a patient when the deformity is so advanced that amputation is required or an abscess needs drainage as an emergency.

All surgical procedures obviously need to be done under antileprosy drug treatment. This is best achieved by a team approach. Educating patients about the dreadful sequelae of the disease so that they seek medical help early is important. It is also necessary to educate the general public that patients suffering from the disease should not be made social outcasts.

Summary box 6.14

Leprosy - treatment

- Multiple drug therapy for a year
- Team approach
- Surgical reconstruction requires the expertise of a hand surgeon, orthopaedic surgeon and plastic surgeon
- Education of the patient and general public should be the keystone in prevention

MYCETOMA

(This section has been contributed by: Professor Ahmed Hassan Fahal MBBS, FRCS, FRCSI, FRCSG, MD, MS, FRCP (London), Professor of Surgery, University of Khartoum, Khartoum, Sudan)

Introduction

Mycetoma is a chronic, specific, granulomatous, progressive, destructive inflammatory disease, which involves the skin, subcutaneous tissues and deeper structures. The causative organism may be true fungi, when the condition is called eumycetoma; when caused by bacteria it is called actinomycetoma. The pathognomonic feature is the triad of painless subcutaneous mass, multiple sinuses and seropurulent discharge. It causes tissue destruction, deformity, disability, and death in extreme cases.

Epidemiology and pathogenesis

The condition predominently occurs in the 'mycetoma belt' that lies between the latitudes 15° south and 30° north, comprising the countries of Sudan, Somalia, Senegal, India, Yemen, Mexico, Venezuela, Columbia, Argentina and a few others. The route of infection is inoculation of the organism that is resident in the soil through a traumatised area. Although in the vast majority there is no history of trauma, the portal of entry is always an area of minor unrecognised trauma in a bare-footed individual walking in a terrain full of thorns. Hence the foot is the commonest site affected. Mycetoma is not contagious.

Once the granuloma forms it increases in size, and the overlying skin becomes stretched, smooth, shiny and attached to the lesion. Areas of hypo- or hyperpigmentation sometimes develop. Eventually it invades the deeper structures. This is usually gradual and delayed in eumycetoma. In actinomycetoma, invasion to deeper tissues occurs earlier and is more extensive. The tendons and nerves are spared until late in the disease. This may explain the rarity of neurological and trophic changes even in patients with long-standing disease. Trophic changes are rare because the blood supply is adequate.

Summary box 6.15

Mycetoma - pathogenesis

- Mostly occurs in the 'mycetoma belt'
- There are two types – eumycetoma and actinomycetoma
- Caused by fungi or bacteria entering through a site of trauma which may not be apparent; hence the foot is most commonly affected
- Produces a chronic, specific, granulomatous, progressive, destructive inflammatory lesion
- Results in tissue destruction, deformity, disability and sometimes death

Clinical presentation

As mycetoma is painless, presentation is late in the majority. It presents as a slowly progressive, painless, subcutaneous swelling commonly at the site of presumed trauma. The swelling is variable in its physical characteristics: firm and rounded, soft and lobulated, rarely cystic, and is often mobile. Multiple secondary nodules may evolve; they may suppurate and drain through multiple sinus tracts. The sinuses may close transiently after discharge during the active phase of the disease. Fresh adjacent sinuses may open while some of the old ones may heal completely. They coalesce and form abscesses, the discharge being serous, serosanguineous or purulent. During the active phase of the disease the sinuses discharge grains, the colour of which can be black, yellow, white or red depending upon the organism. Pain supervenes when there is secondary bacterial infection.

The common sites affected are those that come into contact with soil during daily activities: the foot in 70% (**Figure 6.23**) and the hand in 12% (**Figure 6.24**). In endemic areas the knee (**Figure 6.25**), arm, leg, head and neck (**Figure 6.26**), thigh and perineum (**Figure 6.27**) can

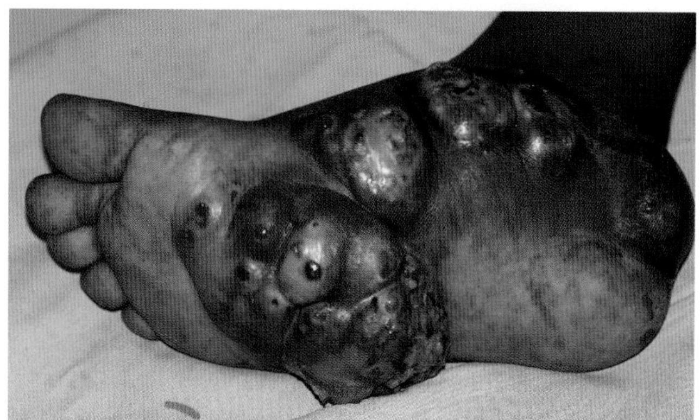

Figure 6.23 Mycetoma of the foot.

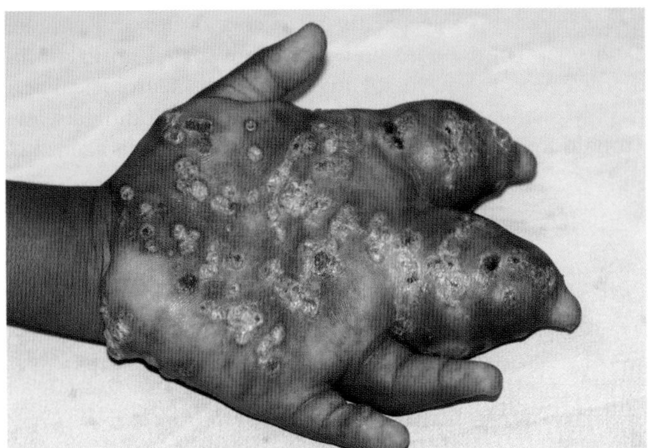

Figure 6.24 Mycetoma of the hand.

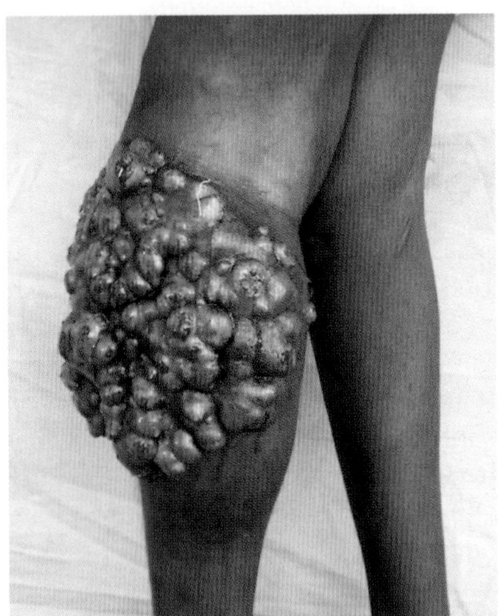

Figure 6.25 Mycetoma of the knee.

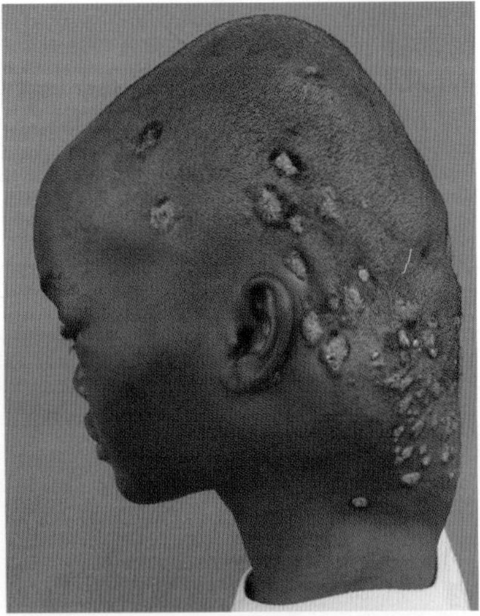

Figure 6.26 Actinomycetoma of the head and neck.

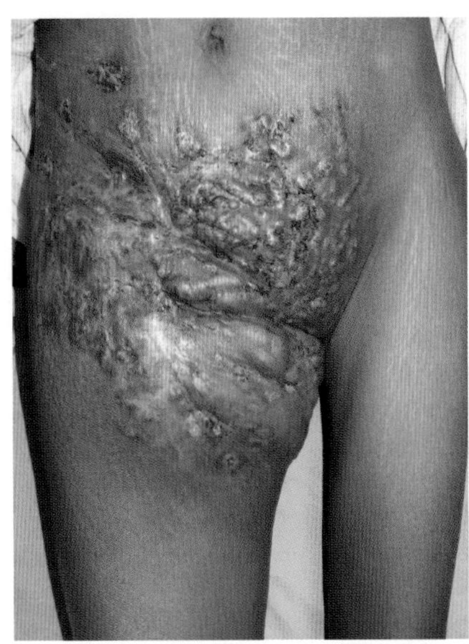

Fibure 6.27 Extensive sattelite inguinal actinomycetoma from a primary foot lesion involving the anterior abdominal wall and perineum.

be involved. Rare sites are the chest, abdominal wall, facial bones, mandible, testes, paranasal sinuses and eye.

In some patients there may be areas of local hyperhidrosis over the lesion. This may be due to sympathetic overactivity or increased local temperature due to raised arterial blood flow caused by the chronic inflammation. In the majority of patients, the regional lymph nodes are small and shotty. Lymphadenopathy is common. This may be due to secondary bacterial infection, lymphatic spread of mycetoma or a local immune response to the disease.

The condition remains localised; constitutional disturbances are a sign of secondary bacterial infection. Cachexia and anaemia from malnutrition and sepsis may be seen in late cases. It can be fatal, especially in cases of cranial mycetoma.

Spread

Local spread occurs predominantly along tissue planes. The organism multiplies to form colonies which spread along the fascial planes to skin and underlying structures. Lymphatic spread, more common in actinomycetoma, occurs to the regional lymph nodes, and increases with repeated inadequate surgical excision procedures. During the active phase of the disease, these lymphatic satellites may suppurate and discharge; lymphadenopathy may also be due to secondary bacterial infection. Spread via the blood stream can occur.

The apparent clinical features of mycetoma are not always a reliable indicator of the extent and spread of the disease. Some small lesions with few sinuses may have many deep connecting tracts, through which the disease can spread quite extensively. Therefore surgery in mycetoma under local anaesthesia is contraindicated.

Differential diagnosis

Mycetoma should be distinguished from Kaposi's sarcoma, malignant melanoma, fibroma and foreign body (thorn) granuloma. A radiograph that demonstrates the presence of bone destruction in the absence of sinuses is suggestive of tuberculosis. The radiological features of advanced mycetoma are similar to those of primary osteogenic sarcoma. Primary osseous mycetoma is to be differentiated from chronic osteomyelitis, osteoclastoma, bone cysts and syphilitic osteitis. In endemic areas the dictum should be 'any subcutaneous swelling must be considered a mycetoma until proven otherwise'.

Diagnosis

Several imaging techniques are available to confirm the diagnosis: plain radiography, ultrasound, CT and magnetic resonance imaging (MRI).

Plain radiograph

In the early stages, soft tissue shadows (often multiple) with calcification and obliteration of the fascial planes may be seen. As the disease progresses, the cortex may be compressed from the outside by the granuloma, leading to bone scalloping. Periosteal reaction with new bone spicules may create a sun-ray appearance and Codman's triangle, not unlike an osteogenic sarcoma (**Figure 6.28**). Late in the disease, there may be multiple punched-out cavities throughout the bone.

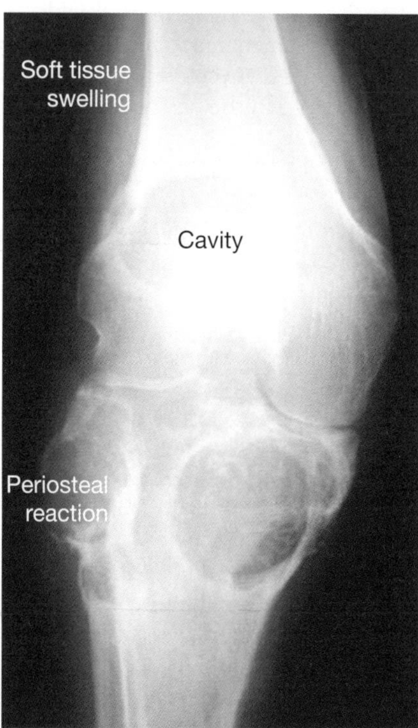

Figure 6.28 Plain x-ray of the knee showing multiple large cavities involving the lower femur, upper tibia and fibula, with well-defined margins and periosteal reaction typical of eumycetoma.

Ultrasound

This can differentiate between eumycetoma and actinomycetoma as well as between mycetoma and other conditions. In eumycetoma, the grains produce numerous sharp bright hyper-reflective echoes. There are multiple thick-walled cavities with absent acoustic enhancement. In actinomycetoma, the findings are similar but the grains are less distinct. The size and extent of the lesion can be accurately determined ultrasonically, a finding useful in planning surgical treatment.

MRI

This helps to assess bone destruction, periosteal reaction, and particularly soft tissue involvement (**Figure 6.29**). MRI usually shows multiple 2–5 mm lesions of high signal intensity, which indicates the granuloma, interspersed within a low-intensity matrix denoting the fibrous tissue. The 'dot-in-circle sign', which indicates the presence of grains, is highly characteristic.

CT scan

CT findings in mycetoma are not specific but are helpful to detect early bone involvement.

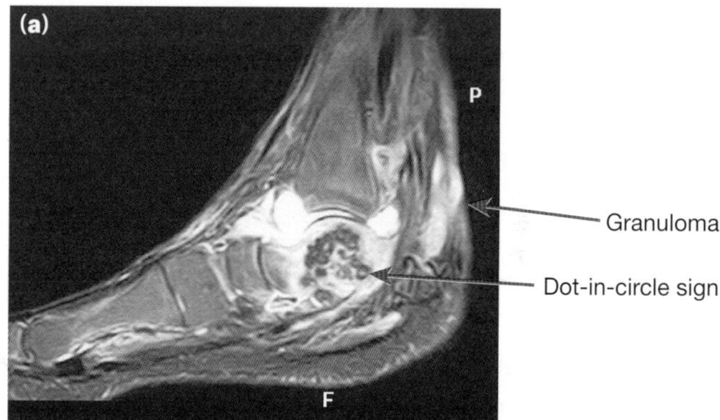

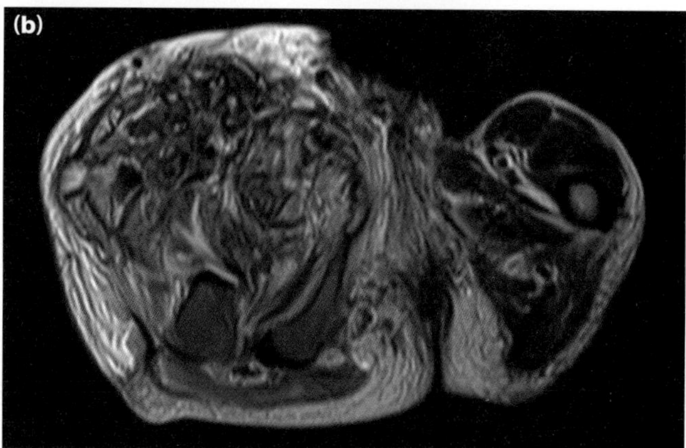

Figure 6.29 (**a**) Magnetic resonance imaging (MRI) of the foot showing multiple lesions of high signal intensity, which indicates granuloma, interspersed within a low-intensity matrix, which is the fibrous tissue and the 'dot-in-circle sign', which indicates the presence of grains. (**b**) MRI showing massive upper thigh and lower abdominal actinomycetoma.

Moritz Kaposi, 1837–1902, Hungarian born, Professor of Dermatology, University of Vienna, Austria, was born to a Jewish family; originally his surname was Kohn. When he converted to Catholicism in 1871, he changed his surname to Kaposi. He described the sarcoma in 1872. The viral cause was discovered in 1994.
Ernest Codman, 1869–1940, American surgeon. Codman's triangle can be seen in osteosarcoma, Ewing's sarcoma and subperosteal abscess and haematoma.

Histopathological diagnosis

Deep biopsy is obtained under general or regional anaesthesia, although the chance of local spread is high. The biopsy should be adequate, contain grains and should be fixed immediately in 10% formal saline.

Three types of host tissue reaction occur against the organism.

- **Type I:** the grains are usually surrounded by a layer of polymorphonuclear leukocytes. The innermost neutrophils are closely attached to the surface of the grain, sometimes invading the grain and causing its fragmentation. The hyphae and cement substance disappear and only remnants of brown pigmented cement are left behind. Outside the zone of neutrophils there is granulation tissue containing macrophages, lymphocytes, plasma cells and few neutrophils. The mononuclear cells increase in number towards the periphery of the lesion. The outermost zone of the lesion consists of fibrous tissue.
- **Type II:** the neutrophils largely disappear and are replaced by macrophages and multinucleated giant cells which engulf grain material. This consists largely of pigmented cement substance although hyphae are sometimes identified.
- **Type III:** this is characterised by the formation of a well organised epithelioid granuloma with Langhan's type giant cells. The centre of the granuloma will sometimes contain remnants of fungal material.

Fine needle aspiration cytology (FNAC)

Fine needle aspiration cytology (FNAC) can yield an accurate diagnosis and helps in distinguishing between eumycetoma and actinomycetoma. The technique is simple, rapid and sensitive.

Culture

A variety of microorganisms are capable of producing mycetoma that can be identified by their textural description, morphology and biological activities in pure culture. Deep surgical biopsy is always needed to obtain the grains which are the source of culture. The grains extracted through the sinuses are usually contaminated and not viable and hence should be avoided. Several media may be used to isolate and grow these organisms.

In the absence of the classical triad of mycetoma, the demonstration of significant antibody titres against the causative organism may be of diagnostic value and aid follow up. The common serodiagnostic tests are immunoelectrophoresis and ELISA.

Summary box 6.16

Mycetoma - diagnosis

- Usually presents late as it is painless
- Triad of painless subcutaneous mass, multiple sinuses and seropurulent discharge
- Clinical picture may be deceptive as there may be deep-seated extension
- May spread to lymph nodes
- Can be confused with Kaposi's sarcoma
- Radiologically can be mistaken for osteosarcoma
- MRI shows typical 'dot-in-circle' sign
- Open biopsy and FNAC are confirmatory

Management

Ideally this should be a combined effort between the physician and the surgeon. In actinomycetoma, combined drug therapy with amikacin sulphate and co-trimoxazole in the form of cycles is the treatment of choice. Amoxicillin–clavulanic acid, rifampacin, sulphonamides, gentamicin and kanamycin are used as a second line of treatment. Long-term drug treatment can have serious side effects.

In eumycetoma, ketoconazole, intraconazole and voriconazole are the drugs of choice. They may need to be used for up to a year. Use of these drugs should be closely monitored for side effects. While not curative, these drugs help to localise the disease by forming thickly encapsulated lesions which are then amenable to surgical excision. Medical treatment for both types of mycetoma must continue until the patient is cured and also in the postoperative period.

Surgical treatment

Surgery is indicated for small localised lesions, resistance to medical treatment or for a better response after medical treatment in patients with massive disease. Excision may need to be much more extensive than suggested at first on clinical appearance because the disease may extend to deeper planes which are not clinically apparent. The surgical options are wide local and debulking excisions and amputations. Amputation, used as a life-saving procedure, is indicated in advanced mycetoma (**Figure 6.30**) refractory to medical treatment with severe secondary bacterial infection.The amputation rate is 10–25%.

Postoperative medical treatment should continue for an adequate period to prevent recurrence. The recurrence rate varies from 25 to 50%. This can be local or distant, to regional lymph nodes. Recurrence is usually due to inadequate surgical excision, use of local anaesthesia, lack of surgical experience, non-compliance with drugs for financial reasons and lack of health education.

Theodor Langhans, 1839–1915, Professor of Pathological Anatomy, University of Berne, Switzerland.

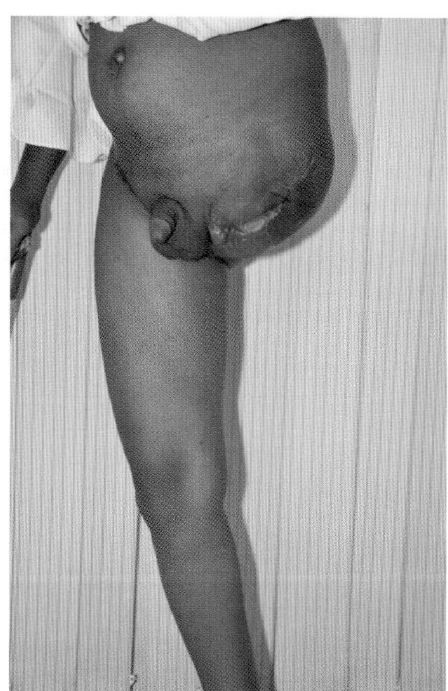

Figure 6.30 Hip disarticulation for a massive thigh eumycetoma.

Summary box 6.17

Mycetoma - management

- Ideally combined management by physician and surgeon
- Medical treatment with appropriate long-term antibiotics
- In large lesions medical treatment to reduce the size followed by excision
- Beware of serious drug side effects
- Surgery in the form of wide excision and amputation as a life-saving procedure
- High recurrence rate

POLIOMYELITIS

Introduction

Poliomyelitis is an enteroviral infection that sadly still affects children in certain parts of the world – this is in spite of effective vaccination having been universally available for several decades. The virus enters the body by inhalation or ingestion. Clinically, the disease manifests itself in a wide spectrum of symptoms – from a few days of mild fever and headache to the extreme variety consisting of extensive paralysis of the bulbar form that may not be compatible with life because of involvement of the respiratory and pharyngeal muscles.

Diagnosis

The disease targets the anterior horn cells, causing lower motor neurone paralysis. Muscles of the lower limb are affected twice as frequently as those of the upper limb (**Figures 6.31 and 6.32**). Fortunately, only 1–2% of sufferers develop paralytic symptoms but, when they do occur, the disability causes much misery (**Figure 6.33**). When a patient develops fever with muscle weakness, Guillain–Barré syndrome needs to be

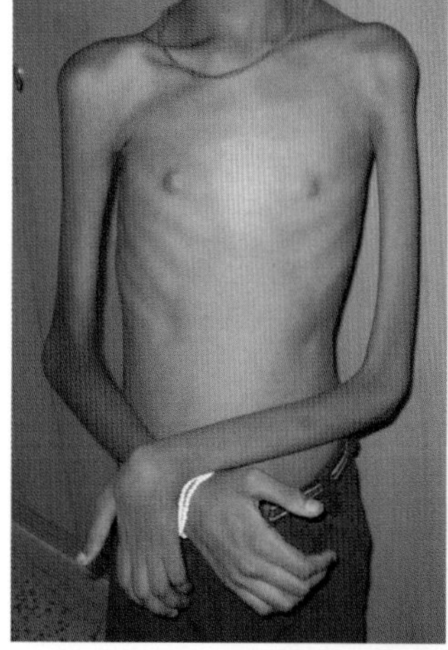

Figure 6.31 Polio affecting predominantly the upper limb muscles with wasting of the intercostal muscles.

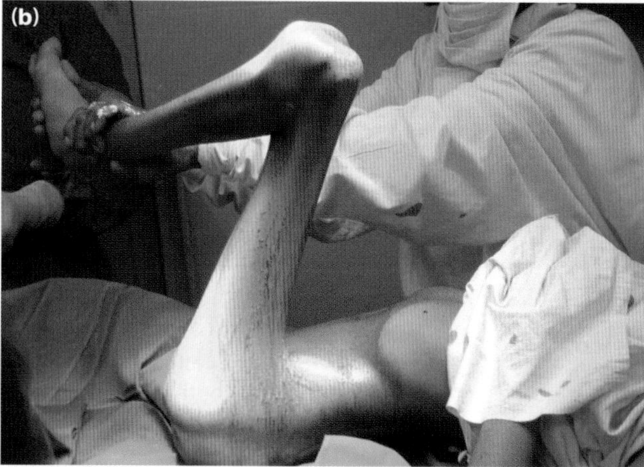

Figure 6.32 (a, b) A 12-year-old patient with polio showing marked wasting of the left upper arm muscles with flexion contractures of the left knee and hip; there is equinus deformity of the foot (courtesy of Dr SM Lakhotia, MS and Dr PK Jain, MD, DA, Kolkata, India).

Georges Guillain, 1876–1961, Professor of Neurology, The Faculty of Medicine, Paris, France.
Jean Alexandre Barré, 1880–1967, Professor of Neurology, Strasbourg, France.
Guillain and Barré described the condition in a joint paper in 1916 whilst serving as Medical Officers in the French Army during the First World War.

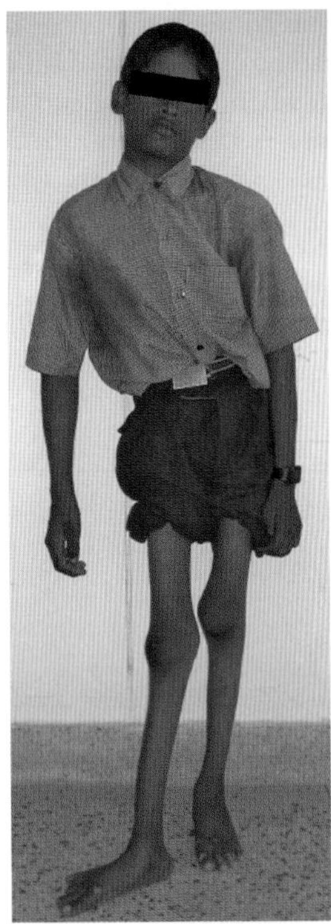

Figure 6.33 A young patient with polio showing paralysis of the lower limb and paraspinal muscles causing marked scoliosis and a deformed pelvis.

excluded. The latter has sensory symptoms and signs. Cerebrospinal fluid (CSF) analysis should help to differentiate the two conditions.

Management

Surgical management is directed mainly towards the rehabilitation of the patient who has residual paralysis, the operations being tailored to the particular individual's disability. Children especially may show improvement in their muscle function for up to 2 years after the onset of the illness. Thereafter, many patients learn to manage their disability by incorporating various manoeuvres ('trick movements') into their daily life. The surgeon must be cautious in considering such a patient for any form of surgery.

Surgical treatment in the chronic form of the disease is the domain of a highly specialised orthopaedic surgeon who needs to work closely with the physiotherapist both in assessing and in rehabilitating the patient. Operations are only considered after a very careful and detailed assessment of the patient's needs. A multidisciplinary team, consisting of the orthopaedic surgeon, neurologist, physiotherapist, orthotist and the family, should decide upon the need for and advisability of any surgical procedure.

A description of the operations for the various disabilities is beyond the scope of this book. The reader should therefore seek surgical details in a specialist textbook. In 2012, WHO declared India a polio-free country.

Summary box 6.18

Poliomyelitis

- A viral illness that is preventable
- Presents with protean manifestations of fever, headache and muscular paralysis without sensory loss, more frequently affecting the lower limbs
- Treatment is mainly medical and supportive in the early stages
- Surgery should only be undertaken after very careful assessment as most patients learn to live with their disabilities
- Surgery is considered for the various types of paralysis in the form of tendon transfers and arthrodesis, which is the domain of a specialist orthopaedic surgeon

TROPICAL CHRONIC PANCREATITIS

Introduction

Tropical chronic pancreatitis is a disease affecting the younger generation from poor socioeconomic strata in resource-poor countries, seen mostly in southern India. The aetiology remains obscure, with malnutrition, dietary, familial and genetic factors being possible causes. Alcohol ingestion does not play a part in the aetiology.

Aetiology and pathology

Cassava (tapioca) is a root vegetable that is readily available and inexpensive and is therefore consumed as a staple diet by people from a poor background. It contains derivatives of cyanide that are detoxified in the liver by sulphur-containing amino acids. The less well-off among the population lack such amino acids in the diet. This results in cyanogen toxicity, causing the disease. Several members of the same family have been known to suffer from this condition; this strengthens the theory that cassava toxicity is an important cause because family members eat the same food.

Macroscopically, the pancreas is firm and nodular with extensive periductal fibrosis, with intraductal calcium carbonate stones of different sizes and shapes that may show branches and resemble a staghorn. The ducts are dilated. Microscopically, intralobular, interlobular and periductal fibrosis is the predominant feature, with plasma cell and lymphocyte infiltration. There is a high incidence of pancreatic cancer in these patients.

Summary box 6.19

Pathology of tropical chronic pancreatitis

- Almost exclusively occurs in resource-poor countries and is due to malnutrition; alcohol is not a cause
- Cassava ingestion is regarded as an aetiological factor because of its high content of cyanide compounds
- Dilatation of pancreatic ducts with large intraductal stones
- Fibrosis of the pancreas as a whole
- A high incidence of pancreatic cancer in those affected by the disease

Diagnosis

The patient, usually male, is almost always below the age of 40 years and from a poor socioeconomic background. The clinical presentation is abdominal pain, thirst, polyuria and features of gross pancreatic insufficiency causing steatorrhoea and malnutrition. The patient looks ill and emaciated.

Initial routine blood and urine tests confirm that the patient has type 1 diabetes mellitus. This is known as fibrocalculous pancreatic diabetes, a label that is aptly descriptive of the typical pathological changes. Serum amylase is usually normal; in an acute exacerbation, it may be elevated. A plain abdominal radiograph shows typical pancreatic calcification in the form of discrete stones in the duct (**Figure 6.34**). Ultrasound and CT scanning of the pancreas confirm the diagnosis. An ERCP, as an investigation, should only be done when the procedure is also being considered as a therapeutic manoeuvre for removal of ductal stones in the pancreatic head by papillotomy.

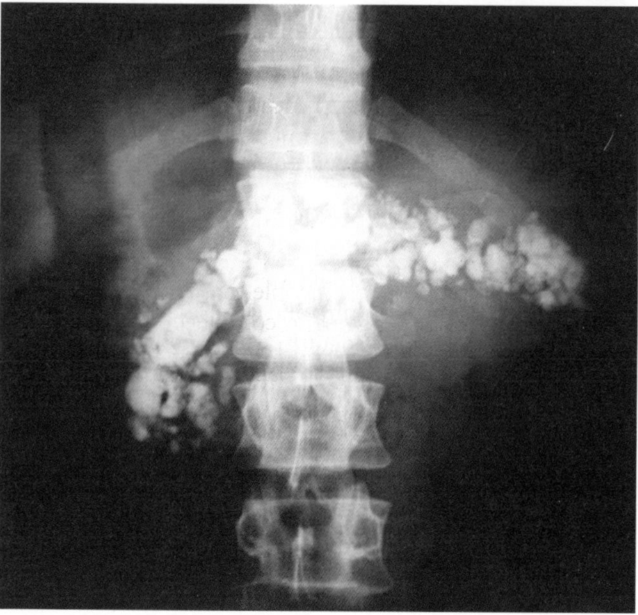

Figure 6.34 Plain radiograph of the abdomen showing large stones along the main pancreatic duct typical of tropical chronic pancreatitis (courtesy of Dr V Mohan, Chennai, India).

Summary box 6.20

Diagnosis of tropical chronic pancreatitis

- The usual sufferer is a type 1 diabetic under 40 years of age
- Serum amylase may be elevated in an acute exacerbation
- Plain radiograph shows stones along the pancreatic duct
- Ultrasound and CT scan of the pancreas confirm the diagnosis
- ERCP should be used as an investigation only when combined with a therapeutic procedure

Treatment

The treatment is mainly medical, with exocrine support using pancreatic enzymes, treatment of diabetes with insulin and the management of malnutrition. Treatment of pain should be along the lines of the usual analgesic ladder: non-opioids, followed by weak and then strong opioids and, finally, referral to a pain clinic.

Surgical treatment is necessary for intractable pain, particularly when there are stones in a dilated duct. Removal of the stones, with a side-to-side pancreaticojejunostomy to a Roux loop, is the procedure of choice. As most patients are young, pancreatic resection is only very rarely considered, and only as a last resort, when all available methods of pain relief have been exhausted.

Summary box 6.21

Treatment of tropical chronic pancreatitis

- Mainly medical – pain relief, insulin for diabetes and pancreatic supplements for malnutrition
- Surgery is reserved for intractable pain when all other methods have been exhausted
- Operations are side-to-side pancreaticojejunostomy; resection in extreme cases

TUBERCULOSIS

Although tuberculosis can affect all systems in the body, in the tropical world the surgeon is most often faced with tuberculosis affecting the cervical lymph nodes and the small intestine. Therefore, in this chapter tuberculous cervical lymphadenitis and tuberculosis of the small bowel will be described.

TUBERCULOUS CERVICAL LYMPHADENITIS

Introduction

This is common in the Indian subcontinent. A young person who has recently arrived from an endemic area, presenting with cervical lymphadenopathy, should be diagnosed as having tuberculous lymphadenitis unless otherwise proven. With acquired immune deficiency syndrome (AIDS) being globally prevalent, this is not as rare in the West in the indigenous population as it used to be.

Diagnosis

Any of the cervical group of lymph nodes (jugulodigastric, submandibular, supraclavicular, posterior triangle) can be involved. The patient has the usual general manifestations of tuberculosis: evening pyrexia, cough (maybe from pulmonary tuberculosis) and malaise; if the sufferer is a child, failure to thrive is a significant finding. Locally there will be regional lymphadenopathy where the lymph nodes may be matted; in late stages a cold abscess may form – a painless, fluctuant, mass which is not warm; significantly there are no signs of inflammation (**Figure 6.35**), hence it is called a 'cold abscess'. This is a clinical manifestation of underlying caseation.

Left untreated, the cold abscess, initially deep to the deep fascia, bursts through into the space just beneath the

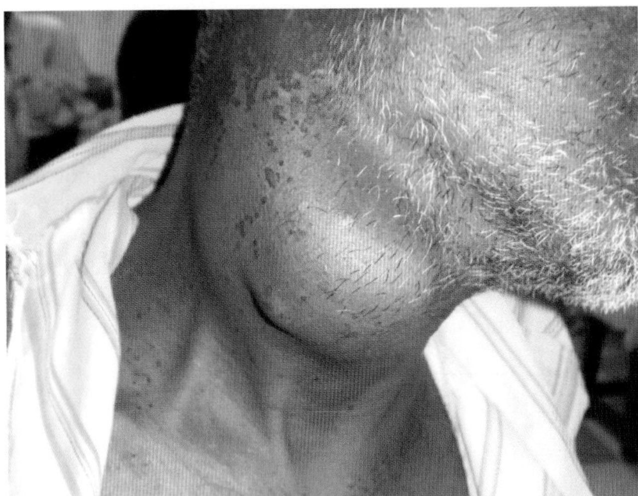

Figure 6.35 Cervical tuberculous: cold abscess about to burst.

superficial fascia. This produces a bilocular mass with cross fluctuation. This is called a 'collar-stud' abscess. Eventually this may burst through the skin, discharging pus and forming a tuberculous sinus (**Figure 6.36**). The latter typically has watery discharge with undermined edges.

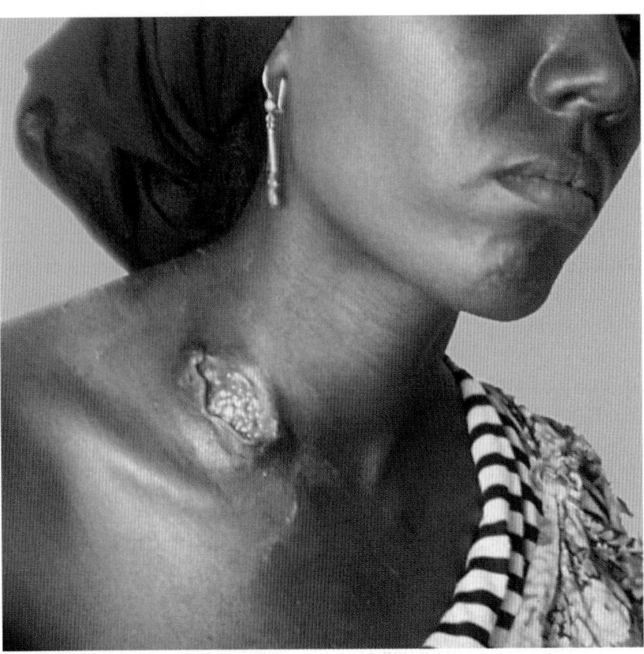

Figure 6.36 Cervical tuberculous sinus with typical overhanging edges (courtesy of Professor Ahmed Hassan Fahal, FRCS MD MS, Khartoum, Sudan).

Summary box 6.22

Tuberculous cervical lymphadenitis

- This is a common condition at any age
- A matted lymph nodal mass is the typical clinical feature
- In later stages the mass may be cystic, denoting an abscess
- The abscess denotes underlying caseation and does not show any features of inflammation – hence called a cold abscess
- Ultimately the abscess may burst, forming a sinus
- Diagnosis is clinched by culture of pus and biopsy of the lymph node
- Involvement of other systems must be excluded
- Treatment is mainly medical

Investigations

Raised ESR and CRP, low haemoglobin and a positive Mantoux test are usual, although the last is not significant in a patient from an endemic area. The Mantoux test (tuberculin skin test), although in use for over a hundred years, has now been superseded by interferon-gamma (IFN-γ) release assays. This is an *in vitro* blood test of cellular immune response. Antigens unique to *Mycobacterium tuberculosis* are used to stimulate and measure T cell release of IFN-γ. This helps to earmark patients who have latent or subclinical tuberculosis and thus will benefit from treatment.

Sputum for culture and sensitivity (the result may take several weeks) and staining by the Ziehl–Neelsen method for acid-fast bacilli (the result is obtained much earlier) should be carried out.

Specific investigations would include aspiration of the pus from a cold abscess for culture and sensitivity. If the mass is still in the early stages of adenitis, excision biopsy should be done. Here, part of the lymph nodes should be sent fresh and unfixed to the laboratory, who should be warned of the arrival of the specimen so that the tissue can be appropriately processed immediately.

Treatment

This must be combined management between the physician and the surgeon. Tuberculous infection at other sites must be excluded and suitably managed. Medical treatment is the mainstay. The reader is asked to look up details of medical treatment in an appropriate source.

TUBERCULOSIS OF SMALL INTESTINE

Introduction

Infection by *Mycobacterium tuberculosis* is common in the tropics. In these days of international travel and increased migration, tuberculosis in general and intestinal tuberculosis in particular are no longer clinical curiosities in non-endemic countries. Any patient, particularly one who has recently

---

A **collar-stud abscess** is so-called because it resembles a collar stud (which has two parts) used in shirts with detachable collars, now largely out of fashion.
Charles Mantoux, 1877–1947, physician, Le Cannet, Alpes Maritimes, France, described the intradermal tuberculin skin test in 1908.
Franz Heinrich Paul Ziehl, 1859–1926, neurologist, Lubeck, Germany.
Friedrich Carl Adolf Neelsen, 1854–1894, pathologist, Prosector, the Stadt-Krankenhaus, Dresden, Germany.

arrived from an endemic area and who has features of generalised ill health and altered bowel habit, should arouse suspicion for intestinal tuberculosis. The increased prevalence of human immunodeficiency virus (HIV) infection worldwide has also made tuberculosis more common.

Pathology

There are two types: ulcerative and hyperplastic. In both types, there may be marked mesenteric lymphadenopathy.

- **Ulcerative type:** When a patient with pulmonary tuberculosis swallows infected sputum, the organism colonises the lymphatics of the terminal ileum, causing transverse ulcers with typical undermined edges. The serosa is usually studded with tubercles. Histology shows caseating granuloma with giant cells **(Figure 6.37)**. This pathological entity, referred to as the ulcerative type, denotes a severe form of the disease in which the virulence of the organism overwhelms host resistance.
- **Hyperplastic type:** This occurs when host resistance has the upper hand over the virulence of the organism. It is caused by drinking infected unpasteurised milk. There is a marked inflammatory reaction causing hyperplasia and thickening of the terminal ileum because of its abundance of lymphoid follicles, thus resulting in narrowing of the lumen and obstruction. Macroscopically, this type may be confused with Crohn's disease. The small intestine shows areas of stricture and fibrosis, most pronounced at the terminal ileum **(Figure 6.38)**. As a result, there is shortening of the bowel with the caecum being pulled up into a subhepatic position.

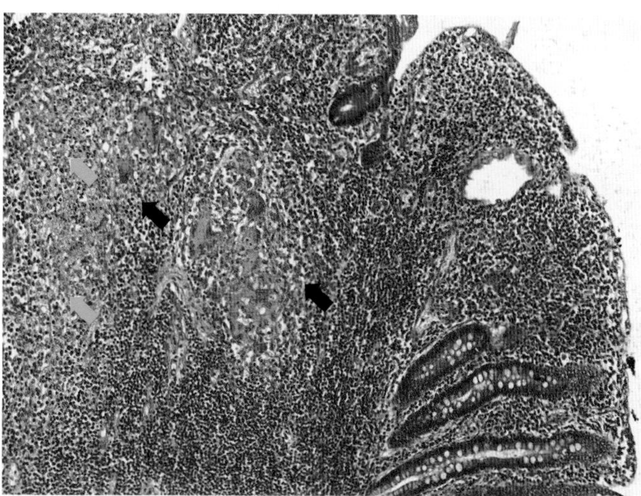

Figure 6.37 Histology of ileocaecal tuberculosis showing epithelioid cell granuloma (black arrows) with caseation (blue arrows) (courtesy of Dr AK Mandal, New Delhi, India).

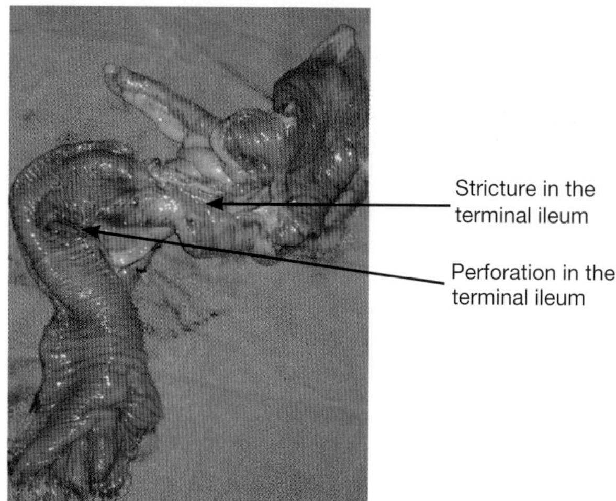

Figure 6.38 Emergency limited ileocolic resection: specimen showing a tuberculous stricture in the terminal ileum and perforation of a transverse ulcer just proximal to the stricture.

Summary box 6.23

Tuberculosis - pathology

- Increasingly being seen in non-endemic areas, mostly among immigrants from endemic areas
- Two types are recognised – ulcerative and hyperplastic
- The ulcerative type occurs when the virulence of the organism is greater than the host defence
- The opposite occurs in the hyperplastic type
- Small bowel strictures are common in the hyperplastic type, mainly affecting the ileocaecal area and presenting with obstructive symptoms
- In the ulcerative type, the bowel serosa is studded with tubercles
- Localised areas of ascites occur in the form of cocoons
- The lungs and other organs, particularly of the genitourinary system, may also be involved simultaneously

Clinical features

Patients present electively with weight loss, chronic cough, malaise, evening rise in temperature with sweating, vague abdominal pain with distension and alternating constipation and diarrhoea. As an emergency, they present with features of distal small bowel obstruction from strictures of the small bowel, particularly the terminal ileum. Rarely, a patient may present with features of peritonitis from perforation of a tuberculous ulcer in the small bowel **(Figure 6.38)**.

Examination shows a chronically ill patient with a 'doughy' feel to the abdomen from areas of localised ascites. In the hyperplastic type, a mass may be felt in the right iliac fossa. In addition, some patients may present with

Burrill Bernard Crohn, 1884–1983, gastroenterologist, Mount Sinai Hospital, New York, NY, USA, described regional ileitis in 1932 along with Leon Ginzburg and Gordon Oppenhiemer.

fistula-in-ano, which is typically multiple with undermined edges and watery discharge.

As this is a disease mainly seen in certain resource-poor countries, patients may present late as an emergency from intestinal obstruction. Abdominal pain and distension, constipation and bilious and faeculent vomiting are typical of such a patient, who is usually *in extremis*.

There may be involvement of other systems, such as the genitourinary tract, when the patient complains of frequency of micturition. Clinical examination does not show any abnormality. The genitourinary tract should then be investigated.

Summary box 6.24

Tuberculosis – clinical features

- Intestinal tuberculosis should be suspected in any patient from an endemic area who presents with weight loss, malaise, evening fever, cough, alternating constipation and diarrhoea and intermittent abdominal pain with distension
- The abdomen has a doughy feel; a mass may be found in the right iliac fossa
- The emergency patient presents with features of distal small bowel obstruction – abdominal pain, distension, bilious and faeculent vomiting
- Peritonitis from a perforated tuberculous ulcer in the small bowel can be another emergency presentation

Investigations

General investigations are the same as those for suspected tuberculosis anywhere in the body. They have been detailed in the previous section.

A barium meal and follow-through (or small bowel enema) shows strictures of the small bowel, particularly the ileum, typically with a high subhepatic caecum with the narrow ileum entering the caecum directly from below upwards in a straight line rather than at an angle (**Figures 6.39 and 6.40a**). Laparoscopy reveals the typical picture of tubercles on the bowel serosa, multiple strictures, a high caecum, enlarged lymph nodes, areas of caseation and ascites. Culture of the ascitic fluid may be helpful. A chest radiograph is essential (**Figure 6.40b**).

If the patient complains of urinary symptoms, urine is sent for microscopy and culture; the finding of sterile pyuria should alert the clinician to the possibility of tuberculosis of the urinary tract, when the appropriate investigations should be done. A flexible cystoscopy would be very useful in the presence of sterile pyuria. A contracted bladder ('thimble' bladder) with ureteric orifices that are in-drawn ('golf-hole' ureter) may be seen; these changes are due to fibrosis.

In the patient presenting as an abdominal emergency, urea and electrolytes show evidence of gross dehydration. A plain abdominal radiograph shows typical small bowel obstruction – valvulae conniventes of dilated jejunum and featureless ileum with evidence of fluid between the loops.

Summary box 6.25

Intestinal tuberculosis – investigations

- Raised inflammatory markers, anaemia and positive sputum culture
- Interferon-γ release assays for subclinical infection
- Ultrasound of the abdomen may show localised areas of ascites
- Chest radiograph shows pulmonary infiltration
- Barium meal and follow-through shows multiple small bowel strictures particularly in the ileum, with a subhepatic caecum
- If symptoms warrant, the genitourinary tract is also investigated

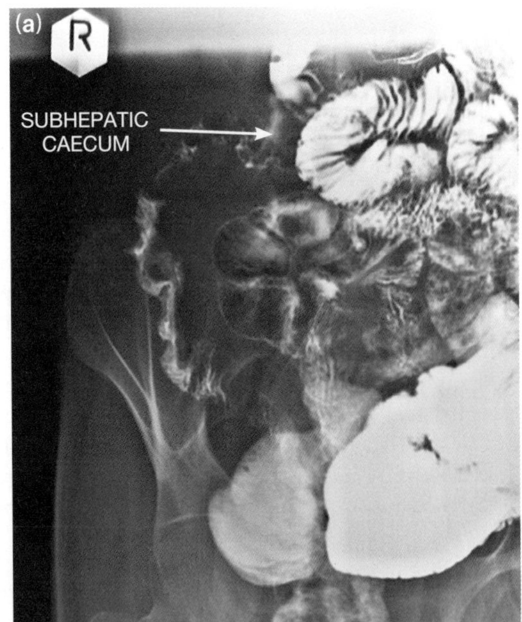

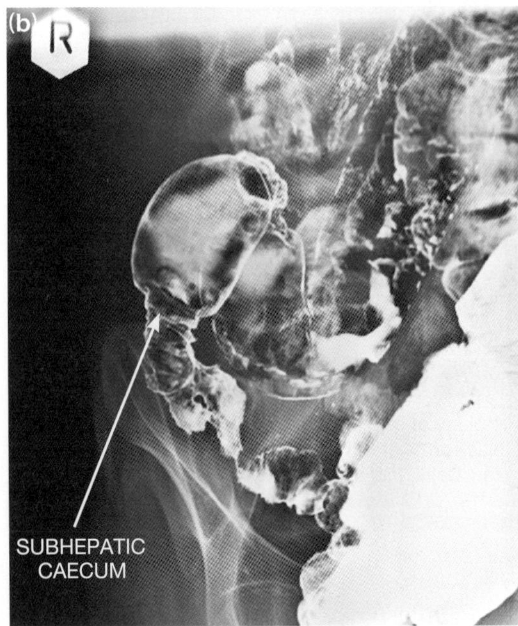

Figures 6.39 (a, b) Series of a barium meal and follow-through showing strictures in the ileum, with the caecum pulled up into a subhepatic position.

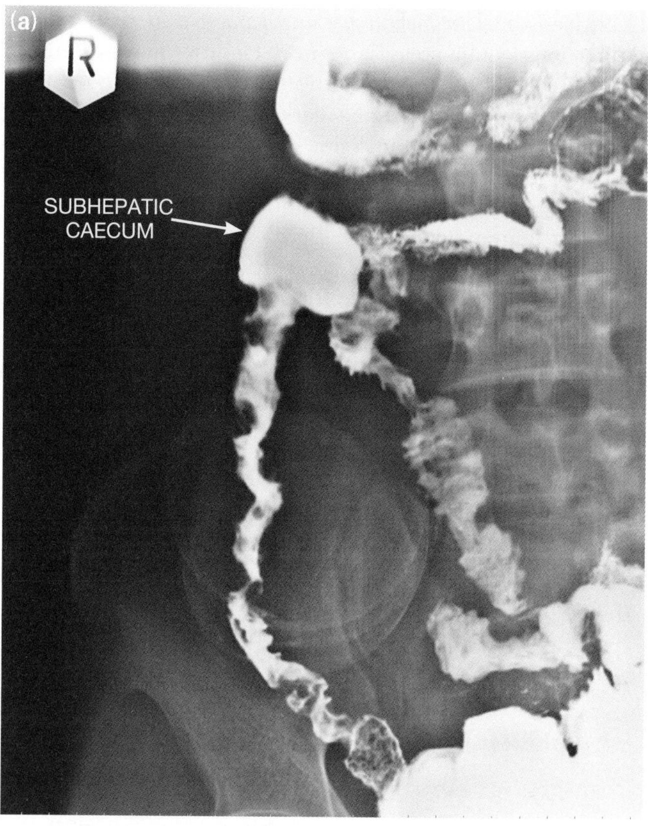

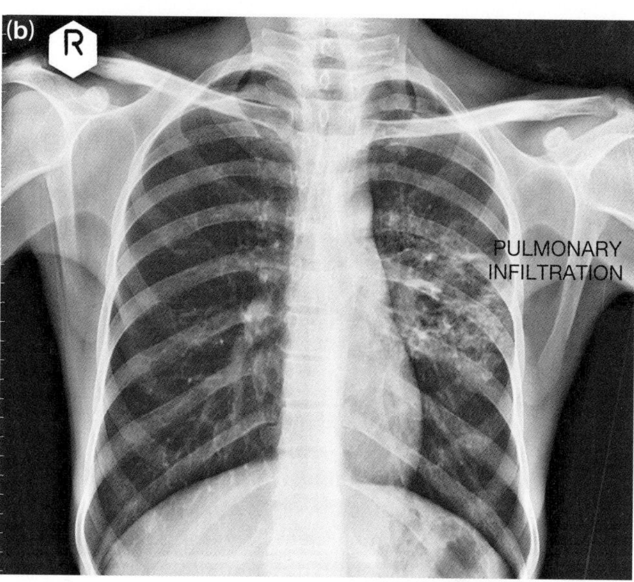

Figures 6.40 Barium meal and follow-through (**a**) and chest radiograph (**b**) in a patient with extensive intestinal and pulmonary tuberculosis, showing ileal strictures with high caecum and pulmonary infiltration.

Treatment

On completion of medical treatment, the patient's small bowel is reimaged to look for significant strictures. If the patient has features of subacute intermittent obstruction, bowel resection, in the form of limited ileocolic resection with anastomosis between the terminal ileum and ascending colon, strictureplasty or right hemicolectomy, is performed as deemed appropriate. The surgical principles and options in the elective patient are very similar to those for Crohn's disease, where resections should be kept as conservative as possible.

The emergency patient presents a great challenge. Such a patient is usually from a poor socioeconomic background, hence the late presentation of acute, distal, small bowel obstruction. The patient is extremely ill from dehydration, malnutrition, anaemia and probably active pulmonary tuberculosis. Vigorous resuscitation should precede the operation. At laparotomy, the minimum life-saving procedure is carried out, such as a side-to-side ileotransverse anastomosis for a terminal ileal stricture. If the general condition of the patient permits, a one-stage resection and anastomosis may be performed.

Thereafter, the patient should ideally be under the combined care of the physician and surgeon for a full course of antituberculous chemotherapy and improvement in nutritional status, which may take up to 3–6 months. The patient who had a simple bypass procedure is reassessed and, when the disease is no longer active (as evidenced by return to normal inflammatory markers, weight gain, negative sputum culture), an elective right hemicolectomy is done to remove the blind loop. This may be supplemented with strictureplasty for short strictures at intervals.

Perforation is treated by thorough resuscitation followed by resection of the affected segment. Anastomosis is performed, provided it is regarded as safe to do so, when peritoneal contamination is minimal and widespread disease is not encountered; otherwise, as a first stage, resection and exteriorisation is done followed by restoration of bowel continuity as a second stage later on after a full course of antituberculous chemotherapy and improvement in nutritional status.

Summary box 6.26

Tuberculosis - treatment

- Patients should ideally be under the combined care of a physician and surgeon
- Vigorous supportive and full drug treatment are mandatory in all cases
- Symptomatic strictures are treated by the appropriate resection, e.g. local ileocolic resection or strictureplasty as an elective procedure once the disease is completely under control
- Acute intestinal obstruction from distal ileal stricture is treated by thorough resuscitation followed by side-to-side ileotransverse bypass
- Once the patient has recovered with medical treatment, then the second-stage definitive procedure of right hemicolectomy is done to remove the blind loop
- One-stage resection and anastomosis can be considered if the patient's general condition permits
- Perforation is treated by appropriate local resection and anastomosis or exteriorisation if the condition of the patient is very poor; this is later followed by restoration of bowel continuity after the patient has fully recovered with antituberculous chemotherapy

TYPHOID

Introduction

Typhoid fever is caused by *Salmonella typhi*, also called the typhoid bacillus, a gram-negative organism. Like most infections occurring in the tropics, the organism gains entry into the human gastrointestinal tract as a result of poor hygiene and inadequate sanitation. It is a disease normally managed by physicians, but the surgeon may be called upon to treat the patient with typhoid fever because of perforation of a typhoid ulcer.

Pathology

Following ingestion of contaminated food or water, the organism colonises the Peyer's patches in the terminal ileum, causing hyperplasia of the lymphoid follicles followed by necrosis and ulceration. The microscopic picture shows erythrophagocytosis with histiocytic proliferation (**Figure 6.41**). If the patient is left untreated or inadequately treated, the ulcers may lead to perforation and bleeding. The bowel may perforate at several sites including the large bowel.

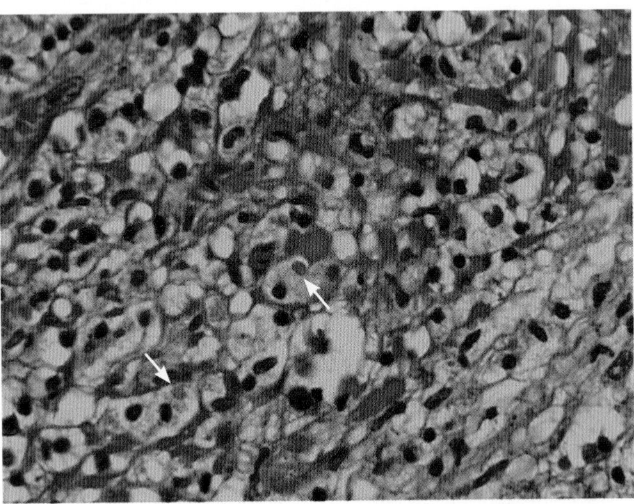

Figure 6.41 Histology of enteric perforation of the small intestine showing erythrophagocytosis (arrows) with predominantly histiocytic proliferation (courtesy of Dr AK Mandal, New Delhi, India).

Diagnosis

A typical patient is from an endemic area or has recently visited such a country and suffers from a high temperature for 2–3 weeks. The patient may be toxic with abdominal distension from paralytic ileus and may have melaena due to haemorrhage from a typhoid ulcer; this can lead to hypovolaemia.

Blood and stool cultures confirm the nature of the infection and exclude malaria. Although obsolete in some parts of the world, the Widal test is still done in the Indian subcontinent. The test looks for the presence of agglutinins to O and H antigens of *Salmonella typhi* and *paratyphi* in the patient's serum. In endemic areas, laboratory facilities may sometimes be limited. Certain other tests have been developed that identify sensitive and specific markers for typhoid fever. Practical and cheap kits are available for their rapid detection that need no special expertise and equipment. These are Multi-Test Dip-S-Ticks to detect immunoglobulin G (IgG), Tubex to detect immunoglobulin M (IgM) and TyphiDot to detect IgG and IgM. These tests are particularly valuable when blood cultures are negative (due to prehospital treatment or self-medication with antibiotics) or facilities for such an investigation are not available.

In the second or third week of the illness, if there is severe generalised abdominal pain, this indicates a perforated typhoid ulcer unless otherwise proven. The patient, who is already very ill, deteriorates further with classical features of peritonitis. An erect chest radiograph or a lateral decubitus film (in the very ill, as they usually are) will show free gas in the peritoneal cavity. In fact, any patient being treated for typhoid fever who shows a sudden deterioration accompanied by abdominal signs should be considered to have a typhoid perforation until proven otherwise.

Summary box 6.27

Diagnosis of bowel perforation secondary to typhoid

- The patient presents in, or has recently visited, an endemic area
- The patient has persistent high temperature and is very toxic
- Positive blood or stool cultures for *Salmonella typhi* and the patient is already on treatment for typhoid
- After the second week, signs of peritonitis usually denote perforation, which is confirmed by the presence of free gas seen on radiograph

Treatment

Vigorous resuscitation with intravenous fluids and antibiotics in an intensive care unit gives the best chance of stabilising the patient's condition. Metronidazole, cephalosporins and gentamicin are used in combination. Chloramphenicol, despite its potential side effect of aplastic anaemia, is still used occasionally in resource-poor countries. Laparotomy is then carried out.

Several surgical options are available, and the most appropriate operative procedure should be chosen judiciously depending upon the general condition of the patient, the site of perforation, the number of perforations and the degree of peritoneal soiling. The alternatives are closure of the perforation (**Figure 6.42**) after freshening the edges, wedge resection of the ulcer area and closure, resection of bowel with or without anastomosis (exteriorisation), closure of the perforation and side-to-side ileotransverse anastomosis, ileostomy or colostomy where the perforated bowel is exteriorised after refashioning the edges.

Daniel Elmer Salmon, 1850–1914, veterinary pathologist, Chief of the Bureau of Animal Industry, Washington, DC, USA.
Johann Conrad Peyer, 1653–1712, Professor of Logic, Rhetoric and Medicine, Schaffhausen, Switzerland, described the lymph follicles in the intestine in 1677.
Georges Fernand Isidore Widal, 1862–1929, Professor of Internal Pathology, and later of Clinical Medicine, The Faculty of Medicine, Paris, France.

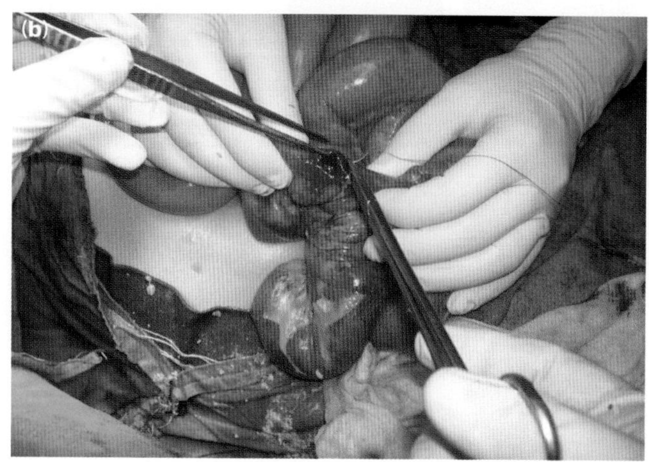

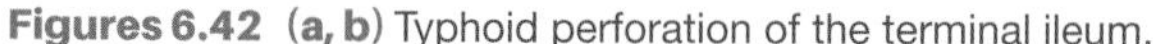

Figures 6.42 **(a, b)** Typhoid perforation of the terminal ileum.

After closing an ileal perforation, the surgeon should look for other sites of perforation or necrotic patches in the small or large bowel that might imminently perforate, and deal with them appropriately. Thorough peritoneal lavage is essential. The linea alba is closed, leaving the rest of the abdominal wound open for delayed closure, as wound infection is almost inevitable and dehiscence not uncommon. In the presence of rampant infection, laparostomy may be a good alternative.

When a typhoid perforation occurs within the first week of illness, the prognosis is better than if it occurs after the second or third week because, in the early stages, the patient is less nutritionally compromised and the body's defences are more robust. Furthermore, the shorter the interval between diagnosis and operation, the better the prognosis.

Summary box 6.28

Treatment of bowel perforation from typhoid

- Manage in intensive care
- Resuscitate and give intravenous antibiotics
- Laparotomy – choice of various procedures
- Commonest site of perforation is the terminal ileum
- Having found a perforation, always look for others
- In the very ill patient, consider some form of exteriorisation
- Close the peritoneum and leave the wound open for secondary closure

FURTHER READING

AMOEBIASIS

Barnes SA, Lillemore KD. Liver abscess and hydatid disease In: Zinner NJ, Schwartz I, Ellis H (eds). *Maingot's abdominal operations*, 10th edn, Vol. 2. New York: Appleton and Lange, McGraw-Hill, 1997, pp. 1527–45.

Bruns BR, Scalea TM. Complex liver abscess. In: *Complications in acute care surgery*. Springer International Publishing, 2017, pp. 189–97.

ASCARIASIS

Das AK. Hepatic and biliary ascariasis. *J Global Infect Dis* 2014; **6**(2): 65.

Steinberg R, Davies J, Millar AJ *et al.* Unusual intestinal sequelae after operations for *Ascaris lumbricoides* infestation. *Paediatr Surg Int* 2003; **19**(1–2): 85–7.

Wani RA, Parray FQ, Bhat NA *et al.* Non-traumatic terminal ileal perforation. *World J Emerg Surg* 2006; **10**: 1–7.

ASIATIC CHOLANGIOHEPATITIS

Choi BI, Han JK, Hong ST, Lee KH. Clonorchiasis and cholangiocarcinoma: etiologic relationship and imaging diagnosis. *Clin Microbiol Rev* 2004; **17**(3): 540–52.

FILARIASIS

Manjula Y, Kate V, Ananthakrishnan N. Evaluation of sequential intermittent pneumatic compression for filarial lymphoedema. *Natl Med J India* 2002; **15**(4): 192–4.

Lim KH, Speare R, Thomas G, Graves P. Surgical treatment of genital manifestations of lymphatic filariasis: a systematic review. *World J Surg* 2015; **39**(12): 2885–99.

HYDATID DISEASE

Barnes SA, Lillemore KD. Liver abscess and hydatid disease. In: Zinner NJ, Schwartz I, Ellis H (eds). *Maingot's abdominal operations*, 10th edn, Vol. 2. New York: Appleton and Lange, McGraw Hill, 1997, pp. 1527–45.

Chiodini P. Parasitic infections. In: Russell RCG, Williams NS, Bulstrode CJK (eds). *Bailey & Love's short practice of surgery*, 24th edn. London: Arnold, 2004, pp. 146–74.

WHO Informal Working Group. International classification of ultrasound images in cystic echinococcosis for application in clinical and field epidemiological settings. *Acta Trop* 2003; **85**(2): 253–61.

LEPROSY

Anderson GA. The surgical management of deformities of the hand in leprosy. *Bone Joint J* 2006; **88**(3): 290–4.

MYCETOMA

Fahal AH. Management of mycetoma. *Expert Rev Dermat* 2010; **5**(1): 87–93.

Hassan MA, Fahal AH. Mycetoma. In: Kamil R, Lumby J (eds). *Tropical surgery*. London: Westminster Publications Ltd, 2004, pp. 786–90.

TROPICAL CHRONIC PANCREATITIS

Barman KK, Premlatha G, Mohan V. Tropical chronic pancreatitis. *Postgrad Med J* 2003; **79**: 606–15.

TYPHOID

Aziz M, Qadir A, Aziz M, Faizullah (2005) Prognostic factors in typhoid perforation. *J Coll Phys Surg Pakistan* 2005; **15**(11): 704–7.

Olsen SJ, Pruckler J, Bibb W *et al.* Evaluation of rapid diagnostic tests for typhoid fever. *J Clin Microbiol* 2004; **42**(5): 1885–9.

Chapter 7

Basic surgical skills and anastomoses

Learning objectives

To understand:

- The principles of patient positioning and operating theatre safety
- The principles of skin and abdominal incisions
- The principles of laparoscopic trocar insertion
- The principles of wound closure

To know the principles in performing:

- Bowel anastomoses
- Vascular anastomoses

To be aware of:

- The principles of drain usage
- The principles of diathermy and advanced energy devices

INTRODUCTION

Successful outcomes in surgery depend on knowledge, skills and judgement. While this chapter concentrates on technical skill, it is important for the modern surgeon to remember that non-technical skills, such as communication, empathy and teamwork, are but a few of the skills required. We used to think of technical skill starting with 'knife to skin'; it is also important to realise that a successful outcome for a patient is dependent on a surgeon who takes responsibility to make sure that the patient reaches that point, with all factors, such as positioning and equipment, considered first. Teamwork includes adherence to modern 'human factors' principles, such as team brief and debrief, and the use of safety checklists.

PATIENT POSITIONING AND SAFETY ON THE OPERATING TABLE

The safety of the patient in the operating theatre is paramount at all times, and is a key responsibility of the surgeon, regardless of grade, experience or seniority. For all cases it is the surgeon's responsibility to make sure the patient is placed on the table to maximise exposure for the procedure itself and to ensure risks of injury are avoided. These are categorised below.

Transfer to and from the operating table

The transfer of the anaesthetised patient is a critical moment where there are significant risks of falls, injuries and, rarely, death, not to mention injury to operating theatre personnel. Staff should all receive regular training in manual handling. Patients at additional risk include the obese, elderly and emaciated. These groups require additional care and specialised equipment.

Positioning on the table

Safe and effective positioning of the anaesthetised patient also requires good training, appropriate equipment and attention to detail. The surgeon should take personal responsibility to maintain safety and to make sure exposure is adequate for the procedure. This includes placement of the passive diathermy electrode ('pad') to minimise the risk of electrosurgical burns and to account for metallic prostheses and pacemakers. The surgeon should also make sure that ancillary equipment, such as energy generators, suction, laparoscopic stack systems and the scrub assistants, is appropriately located around the surgeon and the patient on the operating table. The operating lights should also be placed in an optimal starting position. All these actions need to be undertaken before the surgical team scrubs, including any final checks before the patient is prepped and draped.

Pressure areas

Patients at risk from pressure sores include those with diabetes, immunodeficiency, obesity or malnutrition, and those undergoing prolonged procedures. The areas of the body prone to injury are the heels, sacrum and other bony prominences. These areas should receive particular attention during positioning with additional measures taken in the at-risk groups.

Nerve injury

There are certain areas of the body where an anaesthetised patient can be exposed to neuropraxia (nerve injury) which in some cases can be permanent and disabling. These are the brachial plexus, ulnar nerve and common peroneal nerve. The surgeon should lead the theatre team in ensuring these areas are protected, particularly in high-risk groups and for long procedures.

Compartment syndrome

Acute postoperative compartment syndrome refers, in the context of surgery, to the consequences of increased pressure in a muscle compartment, usually in the lower limb, that can result in permanent disability or amputation. This occurs as a result of underperfusion, usually during prolonged surgery, often with elevation of the leg. Postoperatively, the pressure in the affected compartment rises to the point beyond which irreversible ischaemic damage to muscles and nerves occurs. It manifests with pain, reduced power, swelling, numbness and tingling. Early recognition is essential and prompt surgical fasciotomy is required to avoid the disastrous and permanently disabling sequelae.

Considerations for laparoscopic surgery

Laparoscopic surgery requires some different considerations to open surgery to ensure patient safety and to maximise the ergonomic performance of the procedure. Often, steep angles of tilt to the side, or Trendelenberg (head down) and reverse-Trendelenberg (head up) positions are required to move the abdominal viscera, such as small bowel, away from the operative field. There is significant danger that the patient can slide, or in some cases, fall off the operating table and be injured. It is the surgeon's responsibility to ensure the patient is safely and securely placed on the operating table with appropriate restraints if indicated. So-called 'side boards' or arm restraints are best avoided in laparoscopic surgery as they can interfere with the laparoscopic instruments. Any restraints must be placed in such a way as to avoid or minimise the risk of nerve injury, e.g. the brachial plexus with shoulder supports. Devices such as suction bean bags and antislip mats can be used to help secure placement of the patient. Occasionally, laparoscopic surgery is performed in a lateral position to expose the target organ, e.g. kidney or spleen, with the aid of gravity. Experience and training are required to maintain safety and security for such procedures.

SKIN INCISIONS

Skin incisions should be made with a scalpel, with the blade being pressed firmly down at right angles to the skin and then drawn gently across the skin in the desired direction to create a clean incision, the site and extent of which should have been clearly planned by the surgeon. It is important not to incise the skin obliquely because such a shearing mechanism can lead to necrosis of the undercut edge. The incision is facilitated by tension being applied across the line of the incision by the fingers of the non-dominant hand, but the surgeon must ensure that at no time is the scalpel blade directed at their own fingers as any slip may result in a self-inflicted injury. Blades for skin incisions usually have a curved cutting margin, while those used for an arteriotomy or drain-site insertion have a sharp tip (**Figure 7.1**). Scalpels should at all times be passed in a kidney dish rather than by a direct hand-to-hand process because the latter can lead to injury. Diathermy, laser, harmonic scalpels and combination devices can be used instead of blades when opening deeper tissues, as they can reduce blood loss and save operating time, and may reduce postoperative pain.

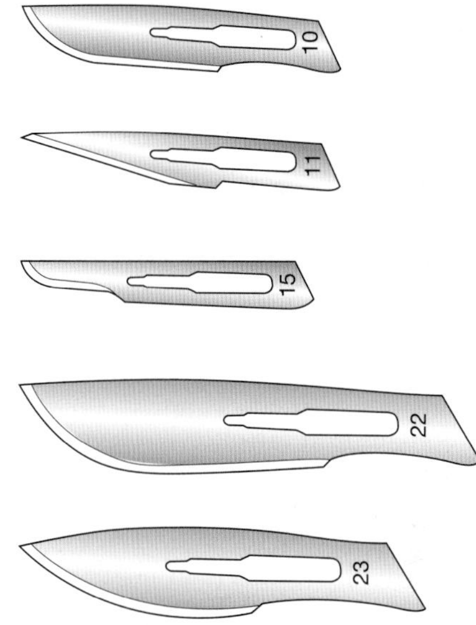

Figure 7.1 Scalpel blade sizes and shapes. The 22-blade is often used for abdominal incisions, the 11-blade for arteriotomy and the 15-blade for minor surgical procedures.

When planning a skin incision, four factors should be considered:

1 **Skin tension lines** (Langer's lines). These lines represent the orientation of the dermal collagen fibres and any incision placed parallel to these lines results in a better scar (**Figure 7.2**).
2 **Anatomical structure**. Incisions should avoid bony prominences and crossing skin creases if possible, and take into consideration underlying structures, such as nerves and vessels.
3 **Cosmetic factors**. Any incision should be made bearing in mind the ultimate cosmetic result, especially in exposed parts of the body, as an incision is the only part of the operation the patient sees.
4 **Adequate access for the procedure**. The incision must be functionally effective for the procedure in hand because any compromise purely on cosmetic grounds may render the operation ineffective or even dangerous.

Occasionally, it may be necessary to excise a skin lesion with a circular incision in an area where the direction of

---

Karl Ritter Von Langer, 1847–1888, Austrian anatomist.

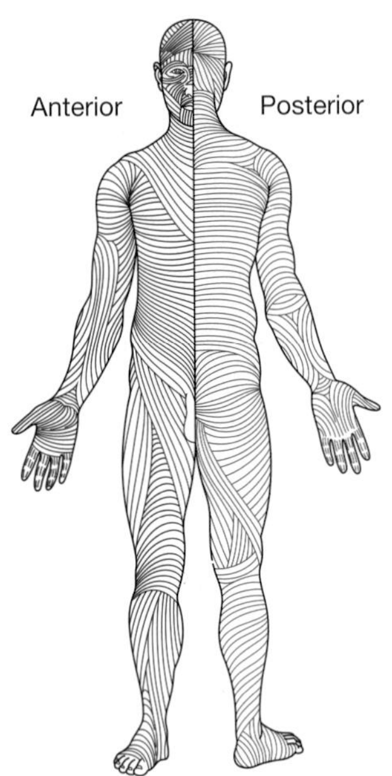

Figure 7.2 Langer's lines. These depict the orientation of the dermal collagen fibres. Reproduced with permission from Thomas WEG, Senninger N (eds). *Short stay surgery*. Berlin: Springer-Verlag, 2008.

Langer's lines is not apparent. However, once the circular incision has been made, it can often be observed that the circular incision is converted to an ellipse, thus indicating the lines of tension. This circular incision should then be formally converted into an elliptical incision, remembering the rule of thumb that 'an elliptical incision must be at least three times as long as it is wide' for the wound to heal without tension. Occasionally, 'dog ears' remain in the corner of elliptical incisions in spite of adequate care having been taken during formation and primary closure of an elliptical wound. In these situations, it is advisable to pick up the 'dog ear' with a skin hook and excise it as shown in **Figure 7.3**. This allows for a satisfactory cosmetic outcome.

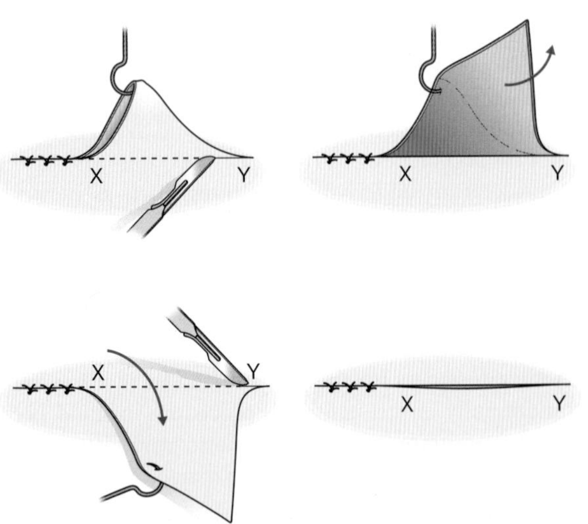

Figure 7.3 Dealing with a 'dog ear' at the corner of an elliptical incision. Reproduced with permission from Thomas WEG, Senninger N (eds). *Short stay surgery*. Berlin: Springer-Verlag, 2008.

Abdominal incisions

As for skin incisions, all abdominal incisions should be planned in advance of surgery and take into consideration access to the relevant organs, surface landmarks, pain control and cosmetic outcome, e.g. transverse incisions tend to be associated with fewer respiratory complications and a better cosmetic outcome. In the past, traditional vertical midline or paramedian incisions were used for the majority of abdominal procedures, but there is a current trend to utilise transverse incisions wherever possible because these minimise postoperative complications. The incision should be carried deeper through the subcutaneous tissues and then, depending on the site of the incision (**Figure 7.4**), the muscle layers should be divided or split, and the peritoneum displayed. This should be picked up between two clips and gently incised to ensure there is no damage to the underlying organs. This is particularly important in the emergency situation when there may be dilatation of the bowel. Every incision should be made with closure in mind, and the layers appropriately delineated. Mass closure of the abdominal wall is usually advocated, using large bites and short steps in the closure technique and either non-absorbable (e.g. nylon or polypropylene) or very slowly absorbable suture material (e.g. polydioxanone suture (PDS)). It has been estimated that, for abdominal wall closure, the length of the suture material should be at least four times the length of the wound to be closed to minimise the risk of abdominal dehiscence or later incisional hernia.

Laparoscopic surgery

Similar attention to detail applies to laparoscopic surgery, where access is of equal importance to open surgery. Correct port site placement and closure are crucial to the success of the operative procedure. Laparoscopic surgery is covered in more detail in Chapter 8.

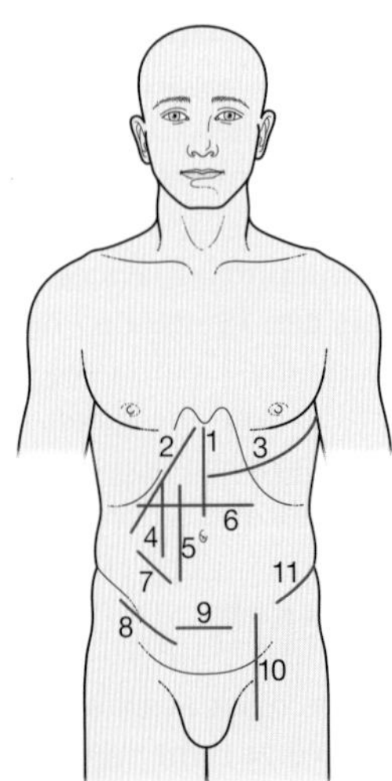

Figure 7.4 Abdominal incisions. Reproduced with permission from Thomas WEG. *Preparation and revision for the MRCS*. London: Churchill Livingstone (Elsevier Limited), 2004. 1, Midline; 2, Kocher's; 3, thoracoabdominal; 4, rectus split; 5, paramedian; 6, transverse; 7, McBurney's gridiron; 8, inguinal; 9, pfannenstiel; 10, McEvedy; 11, Rutherford Morison.

Summary box 7.1

The benefits of laparoscopic surgery

- Less postoperative pain
- Better cosmesis
- Earlier return of normal physiological function
- Shorter hospital stay
- Earlier resumption of normal activities

The basic principles of port (trocar) site placement in laparoscopic surgery are:

1 The umbilicus is a convenient and safe point of insertion of the first (primary) trocar because the skin here is fused to the peritoneum. Care must be taken to avoid bowel regardless of the technique employed. Great care and good technique must be employed to avoid injury to the major vessels (aorta, vena cava and iliac vessels), particularly in thin female patients, who are at greater risk. Elsewhere, the midline is safe for further (secondary) trocars, though care must be taken below the umbilicus to avoid the bladder.
2 An 'open' or 'semi-open' technique is practised by many general surgeons to minimise, if not eradicate, the possibility of injury to an underlying viscus during insertion of the primary trocar.
3 Scars should be avoided as bowel is more likely to be adherent to the undersurface; for midline scars, the primary trocar should be inserted away from the midline with an open cutdown or an optical trocar.
4 All secondary trocars should be inserted under direct vision to avoid damage to bowel, bladder and blood vessels. A 'two-handed' technique should be used to avoid sudden trocar movements that may inadvertently puncture a viscus.
5 Trocars should always be inserted perpendicular to the abdominal wall. Oblique insertion results in increased pressure or torque while instruments are being used, which fatigues the surgeon and causes increased trauma to the patient's abdominal wall. This is of particular relevance in obese patients.
6 A hand's breadth (the patient's hand) either side of the midline is the rectus sheath which contains the epigastric vessels. By placing non-midline trocars lateral to the rectus sheath, usually in the mid-clavicular line, the epigastric vessels can be avoided.
7 Where possible, smaller diameter trocars should be used as they are associated with less postoperative pain, a lower incidence of port-site incisional hernia and better cosmesis. All port sites above 5 mm in diameter should undergo suture closure of the fascial layers to reduce the possibility of port-site hernia in the acute postoperative setting and incisional hernia longer term.
8 All secondary trocars should be removed under direct vision to observe for port site bleeding.
9 Bladed trocars should be avoided near blood vessels to reduce the risk of bleeding.

Summary box 7.2

The principles of safe laparoscopic surgery

- The umbilicus is preferred for primary trocar insertion
- An open or semi-open technique is prefered by most surgeons
- Open insertion away from the umbilicus is safer if there is a midline scar
- Secondary trocars should be inserted and removed under direct vision
- All trocars should be placed perpendicular to the abdominal wall
- All trocar sites above 5 mm in length should undergo closure of the fascial layer

Technique for laparoscopic primary trocar insertion

There are a number of different techniques described for primary trocar insertion. In most cases the umbilicus is the preferred site because the skin is fused to the peritoneum, even in obese patients. The presence of a scar at the umbilicus is a relative contraindication as bowel may be adherent resulting in injury which can be overlooked and result in postoperative peritonitis. The author uses a semi-open technique for a 10–12 mm trocar and this is described here:

1 The umbilical cicatrix is everted with a tissue grasping forceps such as a Littlewood's. It is important to grasp the cicatrix directly as this is closest to the adherent peritoneum. Counter-traction is maintained throughout the subsequent steps until the primary trocar is inserted (**Figure 7.5**).
2 The umbilical stalk is palpated inferior to the everted cicatrix while maintaining cephalad (towards the head) traction.
3 A curved 10–12 mm transverse incision is made inferior to the cicatrix (**Figure 7.6**).
4 The umbilical stalk is exposed with sharp and blunt dissection to reveal the decussation (crossing) of fibres just above its junction with the linea alba (**Figure 7.7**).
5 A 5 mm vertical incision is made through the decussation with an 11-blade, taking care only to incise the fascia at this point and not to enter the peritoneum (**Figure 7.8**).
6 A blunt haemostat is then pushed through the preperitoneal fat and peritoneum; the surgeon will feel a 'pop' as the instrument enters the peritoneal cavity (**Figure 7.9**).
7 A blunt-tipped 10 or 12 mm trocar is pushed through the same point of insertion as the haemostat and in the same direction (**Figure 7.10**).
8 The laparoscopic camera is used to confirm successful placement in the peritoneal cavity before insufflation with CO_2 gas.
9 CO_2 gas insufflation is commenced at low flow (1–4 litres per minute) and increased to a maximum pressure of 15 mmHg and with a maximum flow rate of 20 litres per minute.
10 For patients with scars from previous abdominal surgery, the safest technique is a full open approach at Palmer's

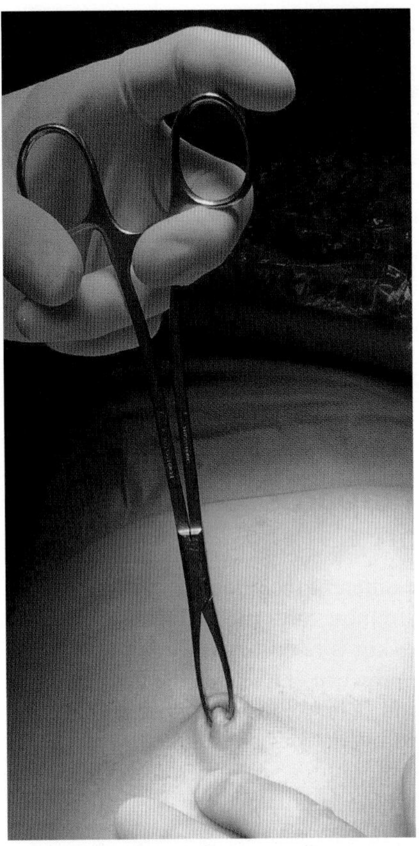

Figure 7.5 The umbilical cicatrix is grasped with a tissue-grasping forceps (e.g. Littlewood's) and everted.

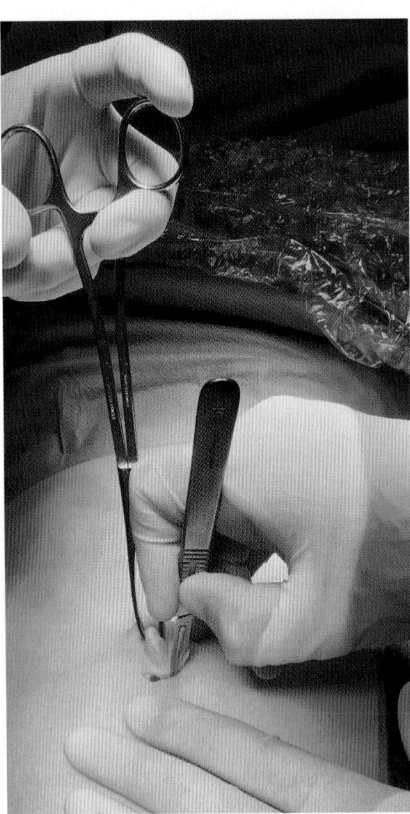

Figure 7.6 A curved subumblilical incision is made.

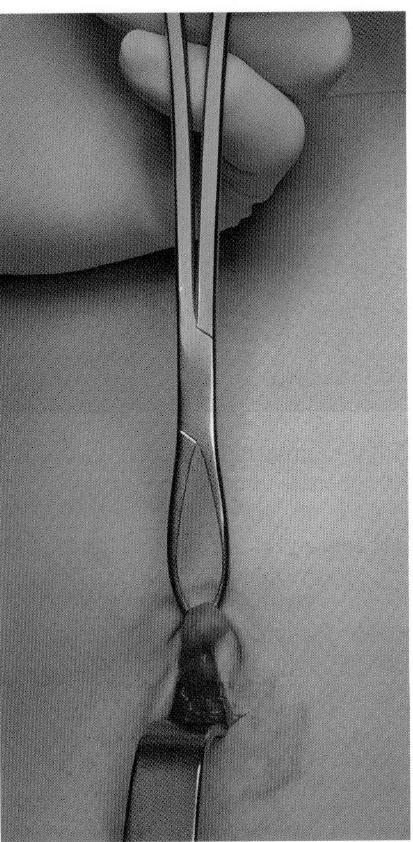

Figure 7.7 The skin is retracted to reveal the junction of the stalk and the linea alba.

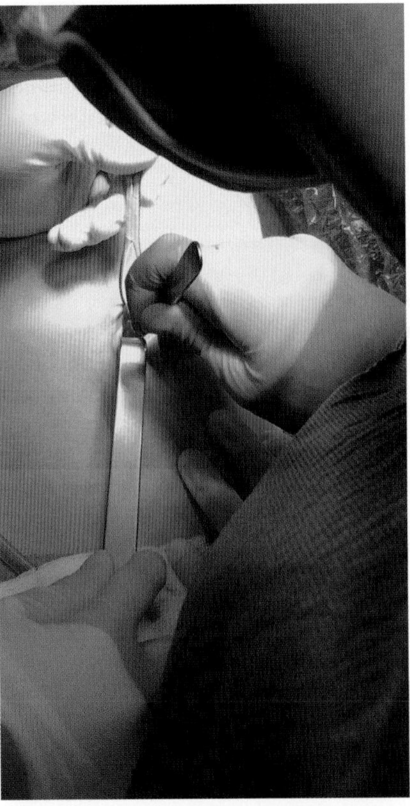

Figure 7.8 A small vertical incision is made in the junction using an 11 bladed scalpel.

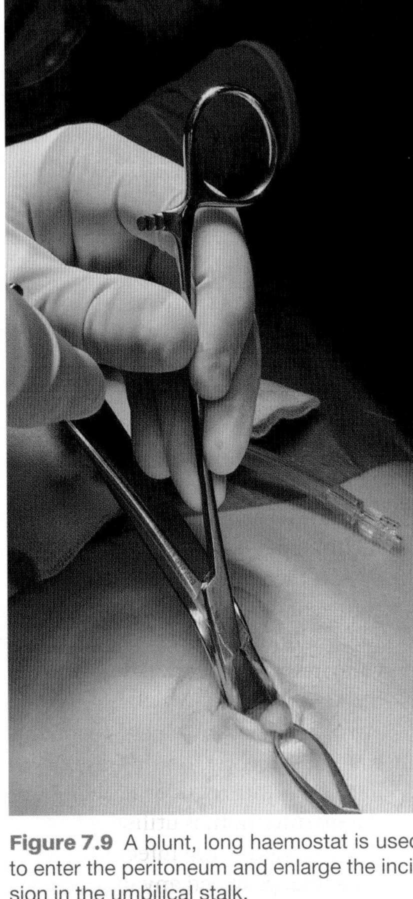

Figure 7.9 A blunt, long haemostat is used to enter the peritoneum and enlarge the incision in the umbilical stalk.

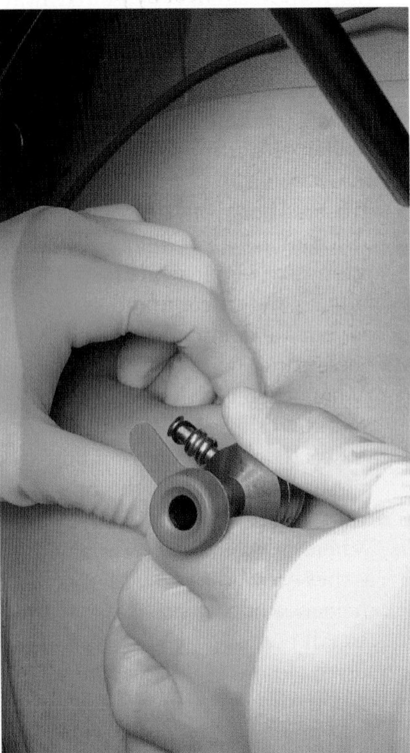

Figure 7.10 A blunt primary trocar and cannula are inserted and their position is confirmed with the laparoscopic camera before insufflation.

point, 3 cm below the left subcostal margin in the midclavicular line. Adequate lighting and good assistance with retraction are essential.

11 In obese patients with scars from previous surgery an optical blunt trocar can be used to enter the peritoneal cavity under vision.

WOUND CLOSURE

The suturing of any incision or wound needs to take into consideration the site and tissues involved, and the technique for closure should be chosen accordingly. There is no ideal wound closure technique that would be appropriate for all situations, and the ideal suture has yet to be produced, although many of the desired characteristics are listed in *Summary box 7.3*. Therefore, the correct choice of suture technique and suture material is vital, but will never compensate for inadequate operative technique, and, for any wound to heal well, there must be a good blood supply and no tension on the closure. Clean uninfected wounds with a good blood supply heal by primary intention and therefore closure simply requires accurate apposition of the wound edges. However, if a wound is left open, it heals by secondary intention through the formation of granulation tissue, which is tissue composed of capillaries, fibroblasts and inflammatory cells. Wound contraction and epithelialisation assist in ultimate healing, but the process may take several weeks or months. Delayed primary closure, or tertiary intention, is utilised when there is a high probability of the wound being infected. The wound is left open for a few days and, provided any infective process has resolved, the wound is closed to heal by primary intention. Skin grafting is another form of tertiary intention healing.

Summary box 7.3

Suture material: desired characteristsics

- Easy to handle
- Predictable behaviour in tissues
- Predictable tensile strength
- Sterile
- Glides through tissues easily
- Secure knotting ability
- Inexpensive
- Minimal tissue reaction
- Non-capillary
- Non-allergenic
- Non-carcinogenic
- Non-electrolytic
- Non-shrinkage

Summary box 7.4

Types of wound healing

- Primary intention
  - Clean wound
- Secondary intention
  - Healthy granulation tissue
  - Overexuberant granulation tissue
  - Infected sloughy wound
  - Black eschar
- Tertiary intention
  - Delayed closure
  - Skin grafting

When choosing suture materials, there are certain specific requirements depending on the tissues to be sutured; for example, vascular anastomoses require smooth, non-absorbable, non-elastic material, while biliary anastomoses require an absorbable material that will not promote tissue reaction or stone formation. When using absorbable material, the time for which wound support is required and maintained will vary according to the tissues in which it is inserted. Furthermore, certain tissues require wound support for longer than others, for example muscular aponeuroses compared with subcutaneous tissues. It is therefore crucial for the surgeon to select the suture material and suture technique that will most effectively achieve the desired objective for each wound closure or anastomosis.

Suture materials

History

> Sutures are best made of soft thread, not too hard twisted that it may sit easier on the tissue, nor are too few nor too many of either of them to be put in.
>
> Aurelius Cornelius Celsus, 25BC–AD50

Multiple examples of early surgery abound, with East African tribes ligating blood vessels with tendon strips, and closing wounds with acacia thorns pushed through the wound with strips of vegetable matter wound round these in a figure of eight. A South American method of wound closure involved using large black ants to bite the wound together with their pincers or jaws acting like skin clips, and then the ant's body was twisted off leaving the head in place keeping the wound apposed. By 1000BC, Indian surgeons were using horsehair, cotton and leather sutures while, in Roman times, linen and silk and metal clips, called fibulae, were commonly used to close gladiatorial wounds. By the end of the nineteenth century, developments in the textile industry led to major advances, and both silk and catgut became popular as suture materials. Lister believed that catgut soaked in chromic acid

Aurelius Cornelius Celsus, Roman physician, 25BC–AD50.
Joseph Lister (Lord Lister), Professor of Surgery in Glasgow, Edinburgh and King's College Hospital, London and Vice President of Royal College of Surgeons of England, 1827–1912.
Alexis Carrel, 1873–1944, surgeon from Lyons in France, worked at the Rockefeller Institute for Medical Research in New York, NY, USA. He received the Nobel Prize for Physiology or Medicine in 1912 'in recognition for his works on vascular suture and the transplantation of blood vessels and organs'.
Gladiators were so called because they fought with a Roman sword called a '*gladius*'.

(a form of tanning) prevented early dissolution in body fluids and tissues, while Moynihan felt that chromic catgut was ideal as it could be sterilised, was non-irritant to tissues, kept its strength until its work was done and then disappeared. However, catgut is no longer in use as it causes an inflammatory cellular reaction with release of proteases and may also carry the risk of prion transmission if of bovine origin.

Suture characteristics

There are five characteristics of any suture material that need to be considered:

1 **Physical structure**. Suture material may be monofilament or multifilament. Monofilament suture material is smooth and tends to slide through tissues easily without any sawing action, but is more difficult to knot effectively. Such material can be easily damaged by gripping it with needle holder or forceps and this can lead to fracture of the suture material. Multifilament or braided sutures are much easier to knot, but have a surface area of several thousand times that of monofilament sutures and thus have a capillary action and interstices where bacteria may lodge and be responsible for persistent infection or sinuses. In order to overcome some of these problems, certain materials are produced as a braided suture, which is coated with silicone in order to make it smooth.

2 **Strength**. The strength of a suture material depends upon its constituent material, its thickness and how it is handled in the tissues. Suture material thickness is classified according to its diameter in tenths of a millimetre (*Table 7.1*), although the figure assigned is also dependent upon the nature of the material, e.g. absorbable material and non-absorbable material, such as polypropylene, may differ in their designations. The tensile strength of a suture can be expressed as the force required to break it when pulling the two ends apart, but is only a useful approximation as to its strength in the tissues, because what matters is the material's *in vivo* strength. Absorbable sutures show a decay of this strength with the passage of time and although a material may last in the tissues for the stated period in the manufacturer's product profile, its tensile strength cannot be relied on *in vivo* for this entire period. Materials, such as catgut (no longer in use in the UK), have a tensile strength that lasts only about a week, while PDS will remain strong in the tissues for several weeks. However, even non-absorbable sutures do not necessarily maintain their strength indefinitely, and may degrade with time. Those non-absorbable materials of synthetic origin, such as polypropylene, probably retain their tensile strength indefinitely and do not change in mass in the tissues, although it is still possible for them to fracture. Non-absorbable materials of biological origin, such as silk, will definitely fragment with time and lose their strength, and such materials should never be used in vascular anastomoses for fear of late fistula formation.

3 **Tensile behaviour**. Suture materials behave differently depending upon their deformability and flexibility. Some may be 'elastic', where the material will return to its original length once any tension is released, while others may be 'plastic', in which case this phenomenon does not occur. Sutures may be deformable, in that a circular cross-section may be converted to an oval shape, or they may be more rigid and have the somewhat irritating capacity to kink and coil. Many synthetic materials demonstrate 'memory', so that they keep curling up in the shape they adopted within the packaging. A sharp but gentle pull on the suture material helps to diminish this memory, but the more memory a suture material has, the lower is the knot security. Therefore, knotting technique also plays a significant role in any suture line's tensile strength and it is important to recognise that sutures lose 50% of their strength at the knot.

4 **Absorbability**. Suture materials may be non-absorbable (*Table 7.2*) or absorbable (*Table 7.3*) and this property must be taken into consideration when choosing suture materials for specific wound closures or anastomoses. Sutures for use in the biliary or urinary tract need to be absorbable in order to minimise the risk of stone production. However, a vascular anastomosis requires a non-absorbable material and it is wise to avoid braided material because platelet adherence may predispose to distal embolisation. Non-absorbable materials tend to be preferred where persistent strength is required and, as an artificial graft or prosthesis never heals fully or integrates into a host artery, persistent monofilament suture materials, such as polypropylene, are almost universally used.

5 **Biological behaviour**. The biological behaviour of suture material within the tissues depends upon the constituent raw material. Biological or natural sutures, such as catgut, are proteolysed, but this involves a process that is not entirely predictable and can cause local irritation, and such materials are therefore seldom used. Synthetic polymers are hydrolysed and their disappearance in the tissues is more predictable. However, the presence of pus, urine or faeces influences the final result and renders the outcome more unpredictable. There is also some evidence that, in

TABLE 7.1 Size of suture material.

Metric (EurPh)	Range of diameter (mm)	USP ('old')
1	0.100–0.149	5-0
1.5	0.150–0.199	4-0
2	0.200–0.249	3-0
3	0.300–0.349	2-0
3.5	0.350–0.399	0
4	0.400–0.499	1
5	0.500–0.599	2

Berkley George Andrew Moynihan (Lord Moynihan of Leeds), 1865–1936, Professor of Clinical Surgery, University of Leeds, Leeds, UK. Moynihan felt that English surgeons knew little about the work of their colleagues both at home and abroad. Therefore, in 1909, he established a small travelling club which in 1929 became the Moynihan Chirurgical Club. It still exists today. He took a leading part in founding the British Journal of Surgery in 1913 and became the first chairman of the editorial committee until his death.

the gut, cancer cells may accumulate at sites where sutures persist, possibly giving rise to local recurrence. For this reason, synthetic materials that have a greater predictability and elicit minimal tissue reaction may have an important non-carcinogenic property.

Barbed sutures

Recently, novel suture materials have helped surgeons to reduce or eradicate the need for knot tying in some situations, such as laparoscopic surgery. These sutures have unidirectional or bidirectional barbs that secure the suture in the tissues.

Suture techniques

There are four frequently used suture techniques.

1 **Interrupted sutures.** Interrupted sutures require the needle to be inserted at right angles to the incision and then to pass through both aspects of the suture line and exit again at right angles (**Figure 7.11**). It is important for the needle to be rotated through the tissues rather than to be dragged through, to avoid unnecessarily enlarging the needle hole. As a guide, the distance from the entry point of the needle to the edge of the wound should be approximately the same as the depth of the tissue being sutured, and each successive suture should be placed at twice this distance apart (**Figure 7.12**). Each suture should reach into the depths of the wound and be placed at right angles to the axis of the wound. In linear wounds, it is sometimes easier to insert the middle suture first and then to complete the closure by successively inserting sutures, halving the remaining deficits in the wound length.

2 **Continuous sutures.** For a continuous suture, the first suture is inserted in an identical manner to an interrupted suture, but the rest of the sutures are inserted in a continuous manner until the far end of the wound is reached (**Figure 7.13**). Each throw of the continuous suture should be inserted at right angles to the wound, and this will mean that the externally observed suture material will usually lie diagonal to the axis of the wound. It is important to have an assistant who will follow the suture, keeping it at the same tension in order to avoid either purse stringing the wound by too much tension, or leaving the suture material too slack. There is more danger of producing too much tension by using too little suture length than there is of leaving the suture line too lax. Postoperative oedema will often take up any slack in the suture material. At the far end of the wound, this suture line should be secured either by using an Aberdeen knot or by tying the free end to the loop of the last suture to be inserted.

3 **Mattress sutures.** Mattress sutures may be either vertical or horizontal and tend to be used to produce either eversion or inversion of a wound edge (**Figure 7.14**). The initial suture is inserted as for an interrupted suture, but then the needle moves either horizontally or vertically, and traverses both edges of the wound once again. Such sutures are very useful in producing accurate approximation of wound edges, especially when the edges to be anastomosed are irregular in depth or disposition.

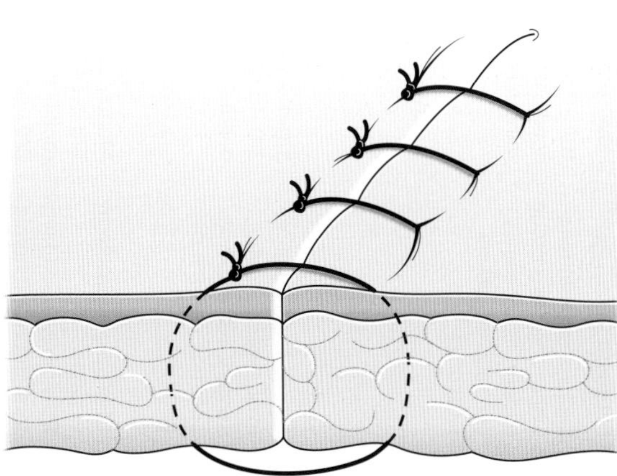

Figure 7.11 Interrupted suture technique. Reproduced with permission from Royal College of Surgeons of England. *The intercollegiate basic surgical skills course participants handbook*, edns 1–4. London: RCS.

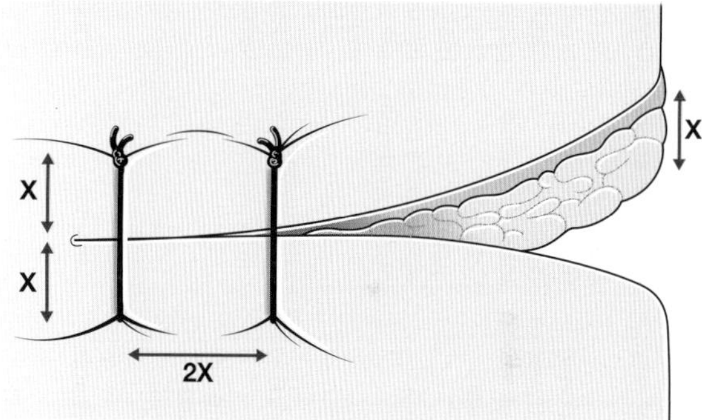

Figure 7.12 The siting of sutures. As a rule of thumb, the distance of insertion from the edge of the wound should correspond to the thickness of the tissue being sutured (X). Each successive suture should be placed at twice this distance apart (2X). Reproduced with permission from Royal College of Surgeons of England. *The intercollegiate basic surgical skills course participants handbook*, edns 1–4. London: RCS.

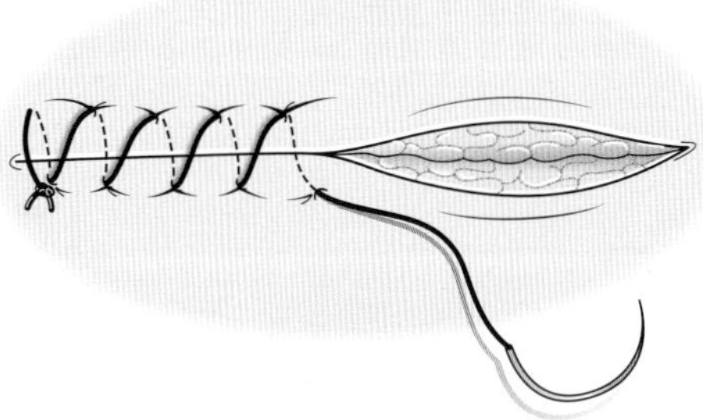

Figure 7.13 Continuous suture technique. Reproduced with permission from Royal College of Surgeons of England. *The intercollegiate basic surgical skills course participants handbook*, edns 1–4. London: RCS.

TABLE 7.2 Non-absorbable suture materials.

Suture	Types	Raw material	Tensile strength	Absorption rate	Tissue reaction	Contraindications	Frequent uses	How supplied
Silk	Braided or twisted multifilament. Dyed or undyed. Coated (with wax or silicone) or uncoated	Natural protein Raw silk from silkworm	Loses 20% when wet; 80–100% lost by 6 months. Because of tissue reactions and unpredictability, silk is increasingly not recommended	Fibrous encapsulation in body at 2–3 weeks Absorbed slowly over 1–2 years	Moderate to high Not recommended Consider suitable absorbable or non-absorbable	Not for use with vascular prostheses or in tissues requiring prolonged approximation under stress Risk of infection and tissue reaction makes silk unsuitable for routine skin closure	Ligation and suturing when long-term tissue support is necessary For securing drains externally	10/0–2 with needles, 4/0–1 without needles
Linen	Twisted	Long staple flax fibres	Stronger when wet Loses 50% at 6 months; 30% remains at 2 years	Non-absorbable Remains encapsulated in body tissues	Moderate	Not advised for use with vascular prostheses	Ligation and suturing in gastrointestinal surgery. No longer in common use in most centres	3/0–1 with needles, 3/0–1 without needles
Surgical steel	Monofilament or multifilament	An alloy of iron, nickel and chromium	Infinite (>1 year)	Non-absorbable Remains encapsulated in body tissues	Minimal	Should not be used in conjunction with prosthesis of different metal	Closure of sternotomy wounds Previously found favour for tendon and hernia repairs	Monofilament: 5/0–5 with needles; multifilament: 5/0–3/0 with needles
Nylon	Monofilament or braided multifilament Dyed or undyed	Polyamide polymer	Loses 15–20% per year	Degrades at approximately 15–20% per year	Low	None	General surgical use, e.g. skin closure, abdominal wall mass closure, hernia repair, plastic surgery, neurosurgery, microsurgery, ophthalmic surgery	Monofilament: 11/0–2 with needles (including loops in some sizes), 4/0–2 without needles; multifilament: 6/0–2 with needles, 3/0–1 without needles
Polyester	Monofilament or braided multifilament Dyed or undyed Coated (polybutylate or silicone) or uncoated	Polyester (polyethylene terephthalate)	Infinite (>1 year)	Non-absorbable: remains encapsulated in body tissues	Low	None	Cardiovascular, ophthalmic, plastic and general surgery	Monofilament: (ophthalmic) 11/10; 10/0 with needles; multifilament: 5/0–1 with needles
Polybutester	Monofilament. Dyed or undyed	Polybutylene terephthalate and polytetramethylene ether glycol	Infinite (>1 year)	Non-absorbable: remains encapsulated in body tissues	Low	None	Exhibits a degree of elasticity. Particularly favoured for use in plastic surgery	7/0–1 with needles
Polypropylene	Monofilament. Dyed or undyed	Polymer of propylene	Infinite (>1 year)	Non-absorbable: remains encapsulated in body tissues	Low	None	Cardiovascular surgery, plastic surgery, ophthalmic surgery, general surgical subcuticular skin closure	10/0–1 with needles

TABLE 7.3 Absorbable suture materials.

Suture	Types	Raw material	Tensile strength retention *in vivo*	Absorption rate	Tissue reaction	Contraindications	Frequent uses	How supplied
Catgut	Plain	Collagen derived from healthy sheep or cattle	Lost within 7–10 days Marked patient variability Unpredictable and not recommended	Phagocytosis and enzymatic degradation within 7–10 days	High	Not for use in tissues that heal slowly and require prolonged support Synthetic absorbables are superior	Ligate superficial vessels, suture subcutaneous tissues Stomas and other tissues that heal rapidly	6/0–1 with needles; 4/0–3 without needles
Catgut	Chromic	Collagen derived from healthy sheep or cattle Tanned with chromium salts to improve handling and to resist degradation in tissue	Lost within 21–28 days Marked patient variability Unpredictable and not recommended	Phagocytosis and enzymatic degradation within 90 days	Moderate	As for plain catgut Synthetic absorbables superior	As for plain catgut	6/0–3 with needles; 5/0–3 without needles
Polyglactin	Braided multifilament	Copolymer of lactide and glycolide in a ratio of 90:10, coated with polyglactin and calcium stearate	Approximately 60% remains at 2 weeks Approximately 30% remains at 3 weeks	Hydrolysis minimal until 5–6 weeks. Complete absorption 60–90 days	Mild	Not advised for use in tissues that require prolonged approximation under stress	General surgical use where absorbable sutures required, e.g. gut anastomoses, vascular ligatures. Has become the 'workhorse' suture for many applications in most general surgical practices, including undyed for subcuticular wound closures. Ophthalmic surgery	8/0–2 with needles; 5/0–2 without needles
Polyglyconate	Monofilament Dyed or undyed	Copolymer of glycolic acid and trimethylene carbonate	Approximately 70% remains at 2 weeks Approximately 55% remains at 3 weeks	Hydrolysis minimal until 8–9 weeks. Complete absorption by 180 days	Mild	Not advised for use in tissues that require prolonged approximation under stress	Popular in some centres as an alternative to Vicryl and PDS	7/0–2 with needles
Polyglycolic acid	Braided multifilament Dyed or undyed Coated or uncoated	Polymer of polyglycolic acid. Available with coating of inert, absorbable surfactant poloxamer 188 to enhance surface smoothness; 87% excreted in urine within 3 days	Approximately 40% remains at 1 week Approximately 20% remains at 3 weeks	Hydrolysis minimal at 2 weeks, significant at 4 weeks. Complete absorption 60–90 days	Minimal	Not advised for use in tissues that require prolonged approximation under stress	Uses as for other absorbable sutures, in particular where slightly longer wound support is required	9/0–2 with needles; 9/0–2 without needles
Polydioxanone (PDS)	Monofilament Dyed or undyed	Polyester polymer	Approximately 70% remains at 2 weeks Approximately 50% remains at 4 weeks Approximately 14% remains at 8 weeks	Hydrolysis minimal at 90 days. Complete absorption at 180 days	Mild	Not for use in association with heart valves or synthetic grafts, or in situations in which prolonged tissue approximation under stress is required	Uses as for other absorbable sutures, in particular where slightly longer wound support is required	Polydioxanone suture (PDS) 10/0–2 with needles
Polyglycaprone	Monofilament	Copolymer of glycolite and caprolactone	21 days maximum	90–120 days	Mild	No use for extended support	Subcuticular in skin, ligation, gastrointestinal and muscle surgery	8/0–2 with needles

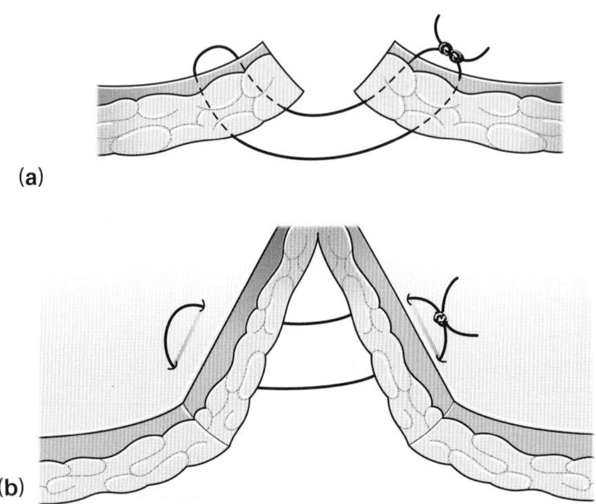

Figure 7.14 (a, b) Mattress suture techniques. Reproduced with permission from Royal College of Surgeons of England. *The intercollegiate basic surgical skills course participants handbook*, edns 1–4. London: RCS.

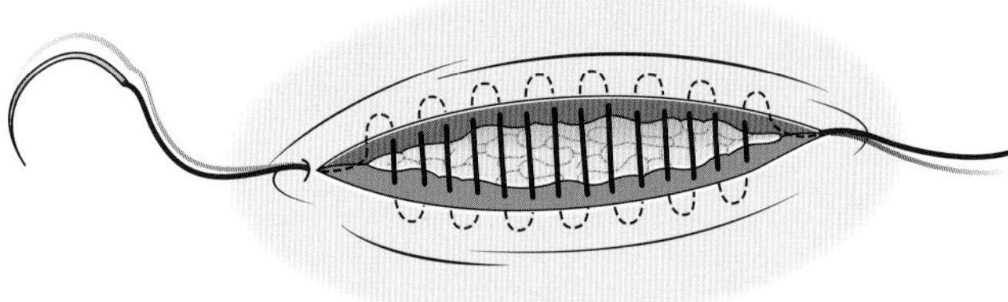

Figure 7.15 Subcuticular suture technique. Reproduced with permission from Royal College of Surgeons of England. *The intercollegiate basic surgical skills course participants handbook*, edns 1–4. London: RCS.

4 **Subcuticular suture**. This technique is used in skin where a cosmetic appearance is important and where the skin edges may be approximated easily (**Figure 7.15**). The suture material used may be either absorbable or non-absorbable. For non-absorbable sutures, the ends may be secured by means of a collar and bead, or tied loosely over the wound. When absorbable sutures are used, the ends may be secured using a buried knot. Small bites of the subcuticular tissues are taken on alternate sites of the wound and then gently pulled together, thus approximating the wound edges without the risk of the cross-hatched markings of interrupted sutures.

Needles

In the past, needles had eyes in them and suture material had to be loaded into them, which was not only time consuming, but it meant that the needle holes in tissues were considerably larger than the suture material being used. Currently, needles are eyeless or 'atraumatic', with the suture material embedded within the shank of the needle. The needle has three main parts:

1 shank;
2 body;
3 point.

The needle should be grasped by the needle holder approximately one-third to one-half of the way back from the rear of the needle, avoiding both the shank and the point. The closer the needle holder is to the tip of the needle, the greater the accuracy of suture placement and the less the degree of rotation of the surgeon's hand required in suturing. The needle should never be grasped nearer than one-third of the way back from the rear of the needle.

The body of the needle is either round, triangular or flattened. Round-bodied needles gradually taper to a point, while triangular needles have cutting edges along all three sides. The actual point of the needle can be round with a tapered end, conventional cutting which has the cutting edge facing the inside of the needle's curvature, or reverse cutting in which the cutting edge is on the outside (**Figure 7.16**). Round-bodied needles are designed to separate tissue fibres rather than cut through them and are commonly used in intestinal and cardiovascular surgery. Cutting needles are used where tough or dense tissue needs to be sutured, such as skin and fascia. Blunt-ended needles are now being advocated in certain situations, such as closure of the abdominal wall, in order to diminish the risk of needle-stick injuries in this era of blood-borne infectious diseases. The choice of needle shape tends to be dictated by the accessibility of the tissue to be sutured, and the more confined the operative space, the more curved the needle. Hand-held straight needles may be used on skin, although today it is advocated that needle holders should be used in all cases to reduce the risk of needle-stick injuries. Half circle needles are commonly utilised in the gastrointestinal tract, while J-shaped needles, quarter circle needles and compound curvature needles are used in special situations, such as the vagina, eye and oral cavity, respectively. The size of the needle tends to correspond with the gauge of the suture material, although it is possible to get similar sutures with differing needle sizes.

Knotting techniques

Knot tying is one of the most fundamental techniques in surgery and yet is often performed poorly. The principles behind a secure knot are poorly understood by many surgeons and sadly a poorly constructed knot may jeopardise an otherwise successful surgical procedure. The general principles behind knot tying include:

- The knot must be tied firmly, but without strangulating the tissues.
- The knot must be unable to slip or unravel.
- The knot must be as small as possible to minimise the amount of foreign material.
- The knot must be tightened without exerting any tension or pressure on the tissues being ligated, i.e. the knot should be bedded down carefully, only exerting pressure against counter-pressure from the index finger or thumb.
- During tying, the suture material must not be 'sawed' as this weakens the thread.
- The suture material must be laid square during tying, otherwise tension applied during tightening may cause breakage or fracture of the thread.
- When tying an instrument knot, the thread should only be grasped at the free end, as gripping the thread with artery forceps or needle holders can damage the material and again result in breakage or fracture.

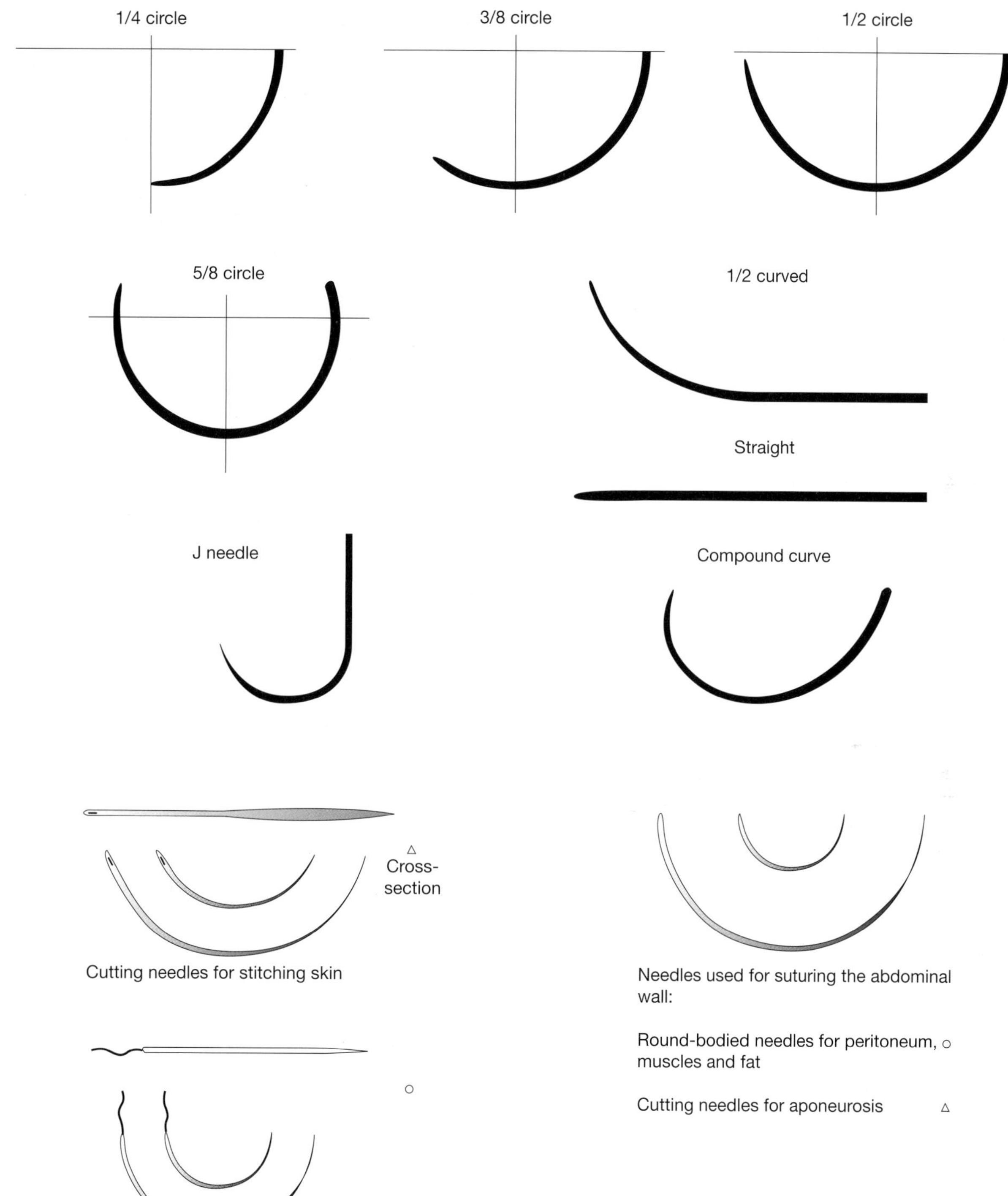

Figure 7.16 Types of needle.

- The standard surgical knot is the reef knot (Figure 7.17), with a third throw for security, although with monofilament sutures, such as used for vascular surgery, six to eight throws are required for security.
- A granny knot involves two throws of the same type of throw and is a slip knot. It may be useful in achieving the right tension in certain circumstances, but must be followed by a standard reef knot to ensure security.
- When added security is required, a surgeon's knot using a two throw technique is advisable to prevent slippage.
- When using a continuous suture technique, an Aberdeen knot may be used for the final knot. The free end of the suture is partially pulled through the final loop several times before being pulled through a final time completely prior to cutting.
- When the suture is cut after knotting, the ends should be left about 1–2 mm long to prevent unraveling. This is particularly important when using monofilament material.

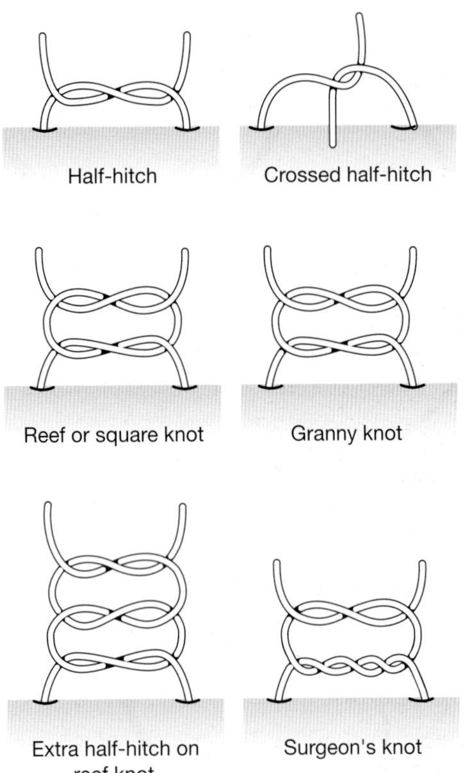

Figure 7.17 Standard knotting formations.

Alternatives to sutures

Many alternatives to standard suture techniques now exist and are in common usage.

Skin adhesive strips

For the skin, self-adhesive tapes or steristrips may be used where there is no tension and not too much moisture, such as after a wide excision of a breast lump. They may also be used to minimise 'spreading' of a scar. Other adhesive polyurethane films, such as Opsite, Tegaderm or Bioclusive, may provide a similar benefit, while such transparent dressings also allow wound inspection and may protect against cross-infection.

Tissue glue

Tissue glue is also available, based upon a solution of *n*-butyl-2-cyanoacrylate monomer. When it is applied to a wound, it polymerises to form a firm adhesive bond, but the wound does need to be clean, dry, with near perfect haemostasis and under no tension. Some specific uses have been described, such as closing a laceration on the forehead of a fractious child in Accident and Emergency, thus dispensing with local anaesthetic and sutures. Although it is relatively expensive, it is quick to use, does not delay wound healing and is associated with an allegedly low infection rate. Other tissue glues involve fibrin and work on the principles of converting fibrinogen to fibrin by thrombin with crosslinking by factor XIII, and the addition of aprotinin to slow the breaking up of the fibrin network by plasmin. This process has good adhesive properties and has been used for haemostasis in the liver and spleen, for dural tears, in ear, nose and throat (ENT) and ophthalmic surgery, to attach skin grafts and also to prevent haemoserous collections under flaps. Fibrin glues have also been used to control gastrointestinal haemorrhage endoscopically, but do not work when the bleeding is brisk.

Laparoscopic wound closure

Laparoscopic wounds are generally 3–12 mm in length. As with all incisions they should be parallel to Langer's lines where possible. Skin closure can be carried out with sutures, using curved or straight needles, or glue, and can be further secured with adhesive strips.

Staples

Mechanical stapling devices were first used successfully by Hümer Hültl in Hungary in 1908 to close the stomach after resection. Today, there is a wide range of mechanical devices with linear, side-to-side and end-to-end stapling devices that can be used both in the open surgery setting and laparoscopically. Most of these devices are disposable and relatively expensive, but their cost is offset by the saving of operative time and the potential increase in the range of surgery possible (see below).

STAPLING DEVICES

In the gastrointestinal tract, stapling devices tend to apply two rows of staples, offset in relation to each other, to produce a sound anastomosis (**Figure 7.18**). Many of them also simultaneously divide the bowel or tissue that has been stapled while other devices merely insert the staples and the bowel has to be divided separately. For all stapling devices, it is crucial for the surgeon to understand the principles behind the device and to know intimately the mechanism and function of the instrument.

- **End-to-end anastomoses.** Circular stapling devices allow tubes to be joined together, and such instruments are in common use in the oesophagus and low rectum. The detached stapling head/anvil is introduced into one end of the bowel, usually being secured within it by means of a purse-string suture. The body of the device is then inserted into the other end of the bowel, either via the rectum for a low rectal anastomosis, or via an enterotomy for an oesophago-jejunostomy, and the shaft is either extended through a small opening in the bowel wall or secured by a further purse-string suture. The head/anvil is reattached to the shaft and the two ends approximated. Once the device is fully closed, as indicated by the green indicator in the window, the device is fired, and, after unwinding, the stapler is gently withdrawn. It is important to assess the integrity of the anastomosis by examining the 'doughnuts' of tissue excised for completeness. It is essential that no extraneous tissue is allowed to become interposed between the two bowel walls on closing the stapler.

Hümer Hültl, surgeon, St Stephen's Hospital, Budapest, Hungary, described his gastric stapler in 1908.

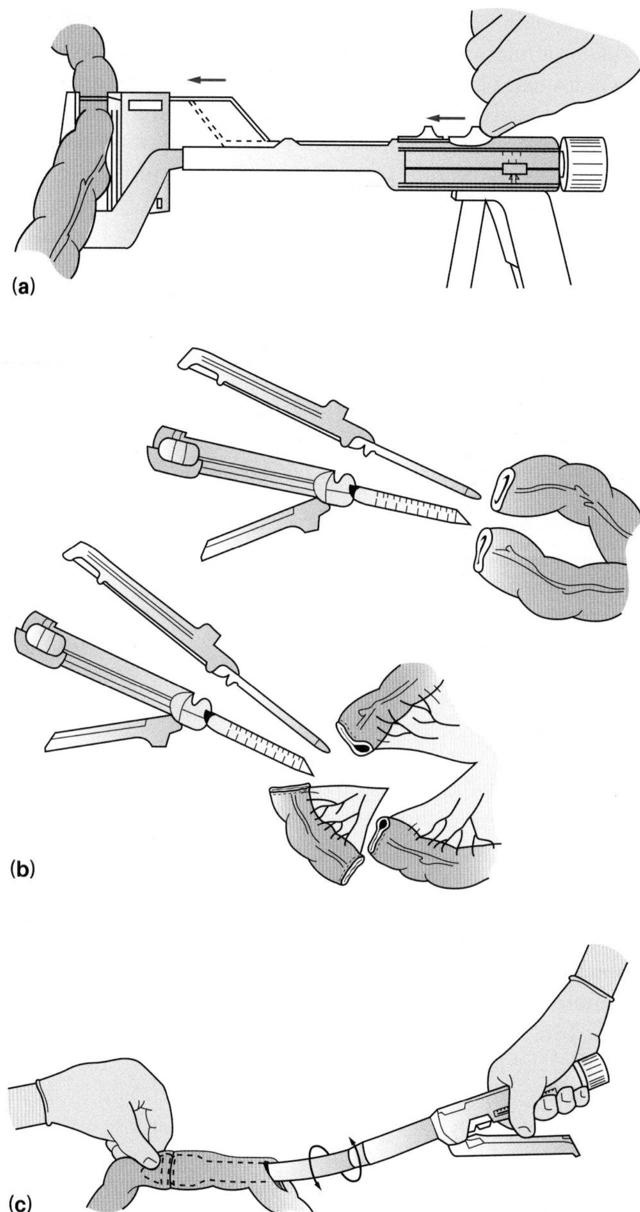

Figure 7.18 (a-c) Standard stapling devices.

- **Transverse anastomoses.** These instruments, which come in different sizes, simply provide two rows of staples for a single transverse anastomosis. They are useful for closing bowel ends, and the larger sizes have been used to create gastric tubes and gastric partitioning. One technical point of importance is that the bowel should be divided before the instrument is reopened after firing, as the instrument is designed with a ridge along which to pass a scalpel to ensure that the cuff of bowel that remains adjacent to the staple line is of the correct length. Down in the pelvis it may be helpful to use such a device with a moveable head (roticulator).
- **Intraluminal anastomoses.** These instruments have two limbs which can be detached. Each limb is introduced into a loop of bowel, the limbs reassembled and the device closed. On firing, two rows of staples are inserted either side of the divided bowel, the division occurring by means of a built-in blade that is activated at the same time as the insertion of staples. Such an instrument may be used in fashioning a gastro-jejunostomy or jejuno-jejunostomy and is used in ileal pouch formation.
- **Other devices.** Other devices are produced that will staple/ligate and divide blood vessels. Skin closure may also be undertaken using hand-held stapling devices rather than individually picking up staples/clips and inserting them as described above.

LAPAROSCOPIC STAPLING DEVICES

Since the early 1990s, increasingly complex surgical procedures have been performed laparoscopically. This revolution in practice has gone hand-in-hand with rapid evolutions in technology to allow existing open instruments and devices to be used laparoscopically, including surgical staplers. Many of the intestinal stapling devices are now adapted to be inserted down trocars during laparoscopic surgery, and although they look very different, the principles of function are identical to their open surgical equivalent. Linear cutting staplers allow bowel and blood vessels to be sealed and divided. Linear and circular staplers also allow intracorporeal anastomoses to be performed. As with open staplers, the surgeon must be trained in their safe use and aware of the principles, including different staple sizes.

THE PRINCIPLES OF ANASTOMOSES

Bowel anastomoses

The word anastomosis comes from the Greek '*ana*', without, and '*stoma*', a mouth, reflecting the join of a tubular viscus (bowel) or vessel (usually arteries) after a resection or bypass procedure. Prior to the nineteenth century, intestinal surgery was limited to exteriorisation by means of a stoma, or closure of simple lacerations. Lembert then described his seromuscular suture technique for bowel anastomosis in 1826, while Senn advocated a two-layer technique for closure. Kocher's method utilised a two-layer anastomosis, first a continuous all-layer suture using catgut, then an inverting continuous (or interrupted) seromuscular layer suture using silk, which became the mainstay of bowel anastomoses for many years (**Figure 7.19**). However, Halsted favoured a one-layer extramucosal closure, and this was subsequently advocated by Matheson as

Antoine Lembert, 1802–1851, surgeon, Hôtel Dieu, Paris, France.
Nicolas Senn, 1844–1908, Professor of Surgery, Rush Medical College, Chicago, IL, USA.
Emil Theodor Kocher, 1841–1917, Professor of Surgery, Berne, Switzerland. In 1909, he was awarded the Nobel Prize for Physiology or Medicine for his work on the thyroid. William Stewart Halsted, 1852–1922, Professor of Surgery, Johns Hopkins Hospital Medical School, Baltimore, MD, USA.
Norman Alistair Matheson, 1907–1966, formerly surgeon, Aberdeen Royal Infirmary, UK.

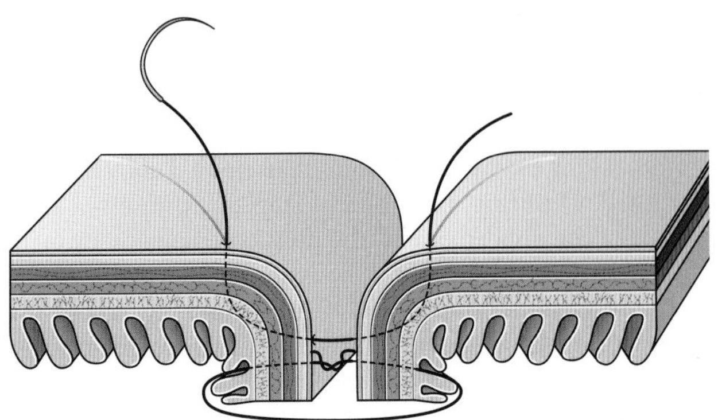

Figure 7.19 Standard two-layer bowel anastomosis. Reproduced with permission from Kocher T, Harder F, Thomas WEG (eds). *Anastomosis techniques in the gastrointestinal tract*, 1st edn. Wollerau: Covidien, 2007.

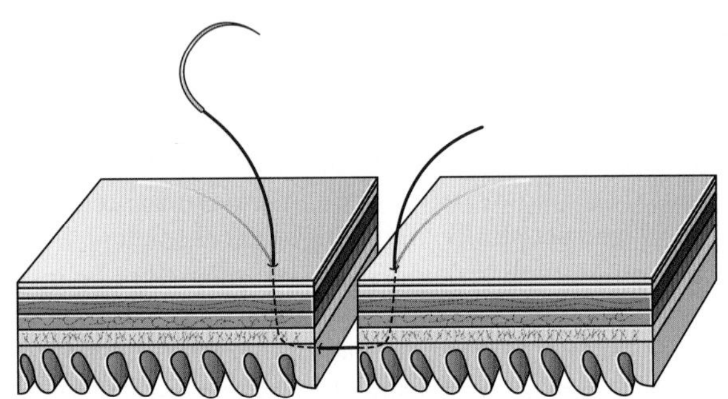

Figure 7.20 Extramucosal technique taking care to include the submucosa. Reproduced with permission from Kocher T, Harder F, Thomas WEG (eds). *Anastomosis techniques in the gastrointestinal tract*, 1st edn. Wollerau: Covidien, 2007.

it was felt to cause the least tissue necrosis or luminal narrowing (**Figure 7.20**). This technique has now become widely accepted, although it is essential that this is not confused with a seromuscular suture technique. The extramucosal suture must include the submucosa because this has a high collagen content and is the most stable suture layer in all sections of the gastrointestinal tract. There are several prospective randomised trials comparing two-layer and single-layer anastomoses demonstrating that there is probably little to choose between these techniques, provided basic essentials as highlighted in *Summary box 7.5* are observed. However, catgut and silk have been replaced by synthetic, usually absorbable, polymers. In the past, great emphasis was placed on good bowel preparation prior to any anastomosis. The rationale was that, with good bowel preparation and an empty bowel, there was less likelihood of faecal contamination and therefore it was probably not necessary to apply bowel clamps (even of the soft occlusion type). However, this tradition is now being challenged, and there is evidence to suggest that conventional bowel preparation provides little benefit, and indeed at times may prove detrimental to the outcome. In spite of this, many surgeons still use some form of bowel preparation, especially for colorectal surgery. Furthermore, if there is any risk of intestinal spillage during anastomosis, when bowel is unprepared or obstructed for example, atraumatic intestinal clamps should be used across the lumen of the bowel. Clamps should not impinge on the mesentery or the vasculature of the bowel for fear of damage to the vessels resulting in ischaemic changes. Ideally, the bowel edges should be pink and bleeding prior to anastomosis. The gold standard for a good blood supply for any anastomosis is the presence of arterial bleeding from the marginal vessel immediately adjacent to the cut end of the bowel and the absence of venous congestion. Excessive bleeding from the bowel wall may need oversewing if natural haemostasis is inadequate.

Summary box 7.5

Intestinal anastomoses

- Ensure good blood supply to both bowel ends before and after formation of anastomosis
- Ensure the anastomosis is under no tension
- Avoid risk to mesenteric vessels by clamps or sutures
- Use atraumatic bowel clamps to minimise contamination
- Interrupted and continuous single-layer suture techniques are adequate and safe
- Stapling devices are an alternative when speed is required or access is a major factor

For all intestinal anastomoses, the bowel ends must be brought together without tension. Stay sutures, which avoid the need for tissue forceps, are invaluable for displaying the bowel ends and help with the accurate alignment of the bowel and the placement of the sutures. If the anastomosis is being undertaken on mobile bowel, the anterior wall layer of sutures can be inserted, either in a continuous or interrupted manner, and then the bowel rotated and the posterior wall sutured in an identical manner to the anterior wall. As the mesenteric edge of the bowel is the most difficult, especially when a fatty mesentery is present, this angle should be dealt with first, with the final sutures being inserted at the antimesenteric border which is far more accessible and visible. The apposition of bowel edges should be as accurate as possible and the suture bites should be approximately 3–5 mm deep and 3–5 mm apart, depending on the thickness of the bowel wall. The suture materials should be of 2/0–3/0 size and made of an absorbable polymer, which can be braided (e.g. polyglactin) or monofilament (e.g. polydioxanone), mounted on an atraumatic round-bodied needle. Braided, coated sutures are the easiest to handle and knot.

It is crucial that only bowel of similar diameter is brought together to form an end-to-end anastomosis. In cases of major size discrepancy, a side-to-side or end-to-side anastomosis may be safer. In cases where the size discrepancy is not marked, a Cheatle split (making a cut into the antimesenteric border) may help to enlarge the lumen of distal, collapsed bowel and allow an end-to-end anastomosis to be fashioned. After all anastomoses, the mesentery should always be closed to avoid the later risk of an internal hernia through a persistent mesenteric defect. Care must be taken during closure of this defect to prevent damage to any mesenteric vessels running in

Sir George Lenthal Cheatle, 1865–1951, surgeon, King's College Hospital, London, UK.

the edge of the mesentery. In certain situations, as indicated above, stapling devices are used to fashion the anastomosis, but as they are expensive, many surgeons reserve them for specific indications, such as oesophageal, rectal and gastric pouch procedures. Several studies have shown them not to be cost effective in routine small bowel surgery, although many surgeons still use them for ease of use and to save time.

Vascular anastomoses

Vascular anastomoses require an extremely accurate closure as they must be immediately watertight at the end of the operation when the vascular clamps are removed. In many cases, some form of prosthetic material or graft may be used which will never be integrated into the body tissues and so the integrity of the suture line needs to be permanent. For this reason, polypropylene is one of the best sutures because it is not biodegradable. It is used in its monofilament form, mounted on an atraumatic, curved, round-bodied needle. Knot security is important, and as polypropylene is monofilament and the anastomosis often depends on one final knot, several throws (between six and eight) of a well-laid reef knot are required. The suture line must be regular and watertight with a smooth intimal surface to minimise the risk of thrombosis and embolus, as well as to avoid any leakage. Suture size depends on vessel calibre: 2/0 is suitable for the aorta, 4/0 for the femoral artery and 6/0 for the popliteal to distal arteries. Microvascular anastomoses are made using a loupe and an interrupted suture down to 10/0 size. All vessel walls must be treated with great care, avoiding causing any damage to the intima. If any significant manipulation is necessary, atraumatic forceps (such as DeBakey's) are utilised. Vascular clamps should be applied with great care, particularly for calcified vessels, and in some cases encircling rubber loops or intraluminal balloon catheters may be less traumatic for control.

Vessels should always be sewn with the needle moving from within to without on the downstream edge of the vessel to avoid creating an intimal flap and to fix any atherosclerotic plaque. The tip of the needle should be inserted at right angles to the surface of the intima and the curve of the needle followed to prevent vessel trauma. The assistant should 'follow' by keeping the suture taut and, once the closure is complete, the distal clamp is released first, before the final watertight knot is made. This allows backflow to clear any clot or air from the anastomosis. The proximal clamp can then be released, a process which minimises the risk of distal embolus. Suture bites should be placed an equal distance apart, with the bite size dependent on the vessel diameter. Care needs to be taken to avoid damaging the suture, which should not be gripped by any surgical instrument. All haemostats that are used to hold any suture material should be shod with soft rubber to prevent suture material damage. A transverse arteriotomy is less likely to stenose following closure than a longitudinal arteriotomy, but may not give adequate access, and a longitudinal arteriotomy is easier to make.

A vein patch can be used if there is any danger of stenosis or doubt about the size of the lumen (**Figure 7.21**). The

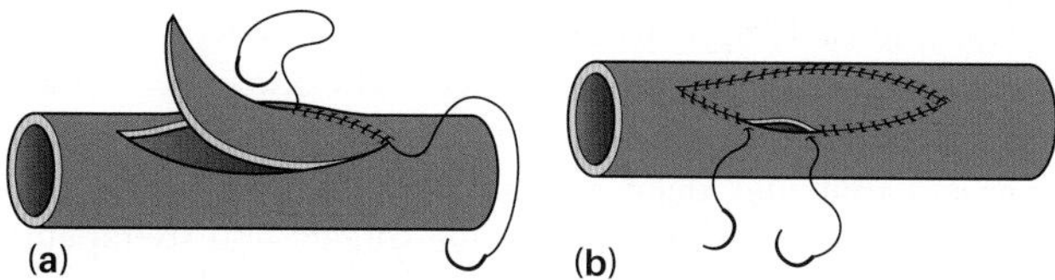

Figure 7.21 **(a, b)** Arteriotomy being closed by vein patch. The technique involves a double armed suture, ensuring that the final knot is half way along one side of the arteriotomy. Reproduced with permission from Royal College of Surgeons of England. *The intercollegiate basic surgical skills course participants handbook*, edns 1–4. London: RCS.

suture line can be started at the apex of the arteriotomy with a double-ended suture, and then carried down each side with the final knot being placed at the midpoint of the vein patch graft, and not at the far end. The suture should go from outside to inside on the graft and from inside to outside on the artery, again to minimise the risk of intimal flap formation. When prosthetic materials or grafts are used, similar non-absorbable monofilament sutures are used with the same in–out technique to ensure eversion of the graft edge and a smooth intimal surface. Again the needle should go from outside to inside on the graft and from inside to outside on the artery. Double-ended sutures make the procedures easier.

Summary box 7.6

Vascular anastomosis

- Non-absorbable monofilament suture material should be used, e.g. polypropylene
- A smooth intimal suture line is essential
- Knots require multiple throws in order to ensure security
- The suture must pass from within outwards on the downflow aspect of the anastomosis

Laparoscopic anastomosis

The same principles apply to laparoscopic anastomosis as to open anastomosis: good blood supply, the avoidance of tension and gentle tissue handling. Both sutured and stapled anastomoses can be performed using laparoscopic needle holders and staplers adapted to laparoscopic surgery. If the ends of the bowel have been adequately mobilised, and there is a specimen extraction site (e.g. right hemicolectomy), an extracorporeal anastomosis can be performed using open surgical techniques. If one or both ends of the bowel to be anastomosed cannot be exteriorised, an intracorporeal anastomosis can be performed. In intra-abdominal surgery, enterotomies are performed in the proximal and distal ends to be anastomosed and a linear stapler is used to join the two ends. The resulting common enterotomy is then closed with a running suture.

DRAINS

Drains are inserted to allow fluid or air that might collect at an operation site or in a wound to drain freely to the surface. The fluid to be drained may include blood, serum, pus, urine,

Michael Ellis DeBakey, b.1908, Professor of Surgery, Baylor University, Houston, TX, USA.

faeces, bile or lymph. Drains may also allow wound irrigation in certain specific circumstances. The adequate drainage of fluid collections prevents the development of cavities or spaces that may delay wound healing. Their use can be regarded as prophylactic in elective surgery and therapeutic in emergency surgery. Three basic principles apply in the use of drains:

1 Open drains that utilise the principle of gravity
2 Semi-open drains that work on the principle of the capillary effect
3 Closed drain systems that utilise suction.

They may be placed through the wound or through a separate incision, although it has been clearly shown that placing them through the wound leads to an increased risk of wound infection. With regard to the indications for drainage, drains were in common use ever since Lawson Tait suggested, in 1887, 'when in doubt drain!' However, this edict has come under strong criticism recently and the value and use of drains has been the subject of close scrutiny; their use remains controversial.

Protagonists suggest that the use of drains may:

- remove any intraperitoneal or wound collection of ascites, serum, bile, chyle, pancreatic or intestinal secretion;
- act as a signal for any postoperative haemorrhage or anastomotic leakage;
- provide a track for later drainage.

However, the antagonists claim that the presence of a drain may:

- increase intra-abdominal and wound infections;
- increase anastomotic insufficiency;
- increase abdominal pain;
- increase hospital stay;
- decrease pulmonary function.

In reality, the use of drains currently tends to depend on a surgeon's individual preference. There are randomised controlled trials suggesting that their use in gastric, duodenal, small bowel, appendix and biliary surgery is unnecessary and may cause more problems than benefits, and this is now reflected in current practice. There are also randomised controlled trials to suggest that they are also not required in colorectal, liver and pancreatic surgery, and yet in today's practice the majority of surgeons will still utilise drains in these forms of surgery. The only area of alimentary tract surgery where drains are still routinely advocated is for oesophageal surgery, although even here the evidence is low, with the level of evidence being only 5 and the level of recommendation being 'D' (i.e. based on expert opinion).

Specialist uses of drains

There are certain clinical situations where specialist forms of drainage are required.

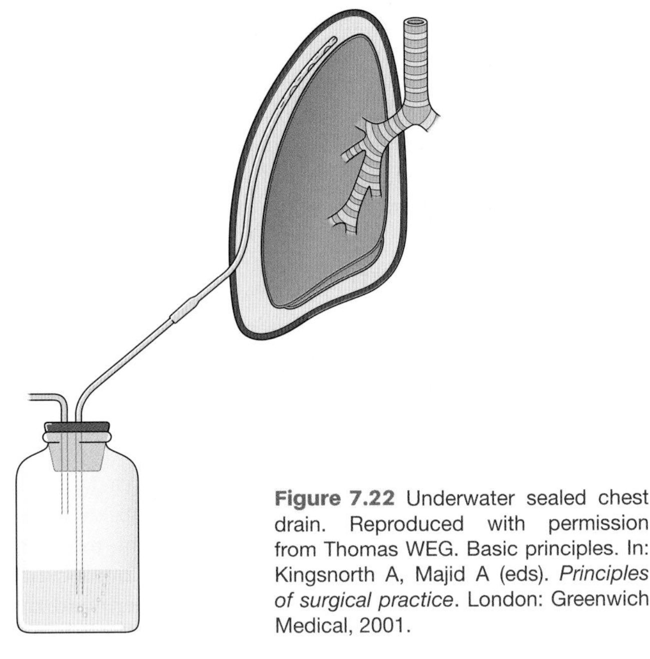

Figure 7.22 Underwater sealed chest drain. Reproduced with permission from Thomas WEG. Basic principles. In: Kingsnorth A, Majid A (eds). *Principles of surgical practice*. London: Greenwich Medical, 2001.

Chest drains

These are indicated for a pneumothorax, pleural effusion, haemothorax or to prevent the collection of fluid or air after thoracotomy. Once the drain has been inserted, it should be connected to an underwater sealed drain (**Figure 7.22**). This system allows air to leave the pleural cavity, but it cannot be drawn back in by the negative pressure that is created in the intrathoracic cavity. During the respiratory process, it should be checked that the meniscus of the fluid is swinging, to ensure that the tube is not blocked. Suction can be applied to the venting tube at the bottle whenever there is significant drainage of fluid or air expected. Between 10 and 20 mm of mercury is adequate to obtain a gentle flow of bubbles from the chest cavity.

T-tube drains

After exploration of the common bile duct, a T-tube (**Figure 7.23**) may be inserted into the duct which allows bile to drain while the sphincter of Oddi is in spasm postoperatively. Once the sphincter relaxes, bile drains normally down the bile duct and into the duodenum. To assist choleresis, it is often advisable to convert the lumen of the limb of the T into a gutter, which also facilitates removal.

Image guided drainage

For many intra-abdominal collections or abscesses, drains may be inserted under ultrasound or computed tomography (CT) control. In order for such drains to remain in site, the end is often fashioned with a pigtail to discourage inadvertent removal. These techniques have been in increasing use as a less invasive method to manage both primary and secondary

---

Robert Lawson Tait, 1845–1899, surgeon, Birmingham, UK.
Ruggero Oddi, 1864–1913, Italian physician.

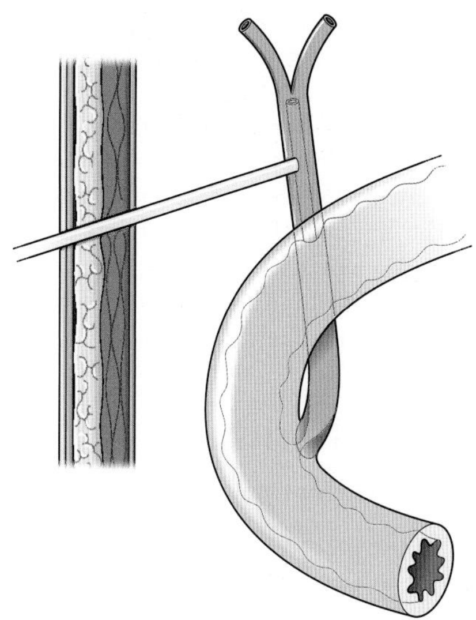

Figure 7.23 T-tube. Reproduced with permission from Thomas WEG. Basic principles. In: Kingsnorth A, Majid A (eds). *Principles of surgical practice*. London: Greenwich Medical, 2001.

(after surgery) collections of fluid. In the context of sepsis they are often used with intravenous or oral antimicrobial therapy.

Removal of drains

A drain should be removed as soon as it is no longer required because, if left in, it can itself predispose to fluid collection as a result of tissue reaction. Indeed there is evidence that by 7 days only 20% of drains are still functioning. It should be stressed how important it is to define the objective of each individual drain and to ensure that once that objective has been met, the drain is removed. If a drain is used at all, the following principles may apply.

- Drains put in to cover perioperative bleeding may usually be removed after 24 hours, e.g. thyroidectomy.
- Drains put in to drain serous collections usually can be removed after 5 days, e.g. mastectomy.
- Drains put in because of infection should be left until the infection is subsiding or the drainage is minimal.
- Drains put in to cover colorectal anastomoses should be removed at about 5–7 days. However, it should be stressed that in no way does a drain prevent any intestinal leakage, but merely may assist any such leakage to drain externally rather than to produce life-threatening peritonitis.
- Common bile duct T-tubes should remain in for 10 days. However, once the T-tube cholangiogram has shown that there is free flow of bile into the duodenum and that there are no retained stones, some surgeons like to clamp the T-tube prior to removal. The 10-day period is required to minimise the risk of biliary peritonitis after removal. T-tubes are traditionally and intentionally made of latex to stimulate fibrosis, which results in the formation of a tract to allow the drainage of bile if required. It is important to use an alternative to latex if the patient is allergic, bearing in mind the decreased potential for fibrosis of silicone-based T-tubes. The increase in less invasive means of intervention for bile duct pathology has resulted in fewer T-tubes being used.
- Any suction drain should have the suction taken off prior to removal of the drain. Even in the absence of suction, a blocked drain may be difficult to remove owing to the creation of a relative vacuum as it is pulled out. This can be released by twisting the drain on removal or flushing with a small volume of sterile saline under aseptic conditions.
- During removal of a chest drain, the patient should be asked to breathe in and hold their breath, thus doing a Valsalva manoeuvre. In this way, no air is sucked into the pleural cavity as the tube is removed. Once the drain is out, a previously inserted purse-string suture should be tied.

Laparoscopic surgery is often accompanied by 'Enhanced Recovery after Surgery' pathways. These pathways comprise a package of pre-, peri- and postoperative care whose objectives are to reduce complications and hospital stay. Such pathways often discourage the use of drains. However the laparoscopic surgeon should always be prepared to use drains where indicated.

THE PRINCIPLES OF DIATHERMY: ELECTROSURGERY

Development of the first commercial electrosurgical device is credited to William T Bovie, who developed the first electrosurgical device while employed at Harvard University. The first use of an electrosurgical generator in an operating room occurred in 1926 at Peter Bent Brigham Hospital in Boston, Massachusetts. The operation – removal of a mass from a patient's head – was performed by Harvey Cushing.

For many years, short wave diathermy has proved a most valuable and versatile aid to surgical technique. Its most common use is in securing haemostasis by means of coagulation, but by varying the strength or wave form of the current produced, it can also result in a cutting effect. Both these effects have been used in open surgery, as well as in laparoscopic surgery or down intraluminal endoscopes, as in transurethral resection of the prostate. However, although diathermy is a valuable surgical tool, many accidents have occurred due to surgeons being unaware of, or not fully understanding, the principles of its use. Most accidents are avoidable if the diathermy or electrocautery is used with care. It is therefore vital for a surgeon to have a sound understanding of the principles and practice of diathermy, and how to avoid complications.

Antonio Maria Valsalva, 1666–1723, Italian physician and anatomist.

Principle of diathermy

When an electrical current passes through a conductor, some of its energy appears as heat. The heat produced depends on:

- the intensity of the current;
- the wave form of the current;
- the electrical property of the tissues through which the current passes;
- the relative sizes of the two electrodes.

There are two basic types of diathermy system in use, monopolar diathermy and bipolar diathermy (**Figure 7.24**). In monopolar diathermy, which is the most commonly used form, an alternating current is produced by a suitable generator and passed to the patient via an active electrode which has a very small surface area. The current then passes through the tissues and returns via a very large surface plate (the passive electrode) back to the earth pole of the generator. As the surface area of contact of the active electrode is small in comparison to the passive electrode, the concentrated powerful current produces heat at the operative site. However, the large surface area electrode of the patient plate spreads the returning current over a wide surface area, so it is less concentrated and produces little heat. In bipolar diathermy, the two active electrodes are usually represented by the limbs of a pair of diathermy forceps. Both forceps ends are therefore active and current flows between them, and only the tissue held between the limbs of the forceps heats up. This form of diathermy is used when it is essential that the surrounding tissues should be free from either the risk of being burned or having current passed through them.

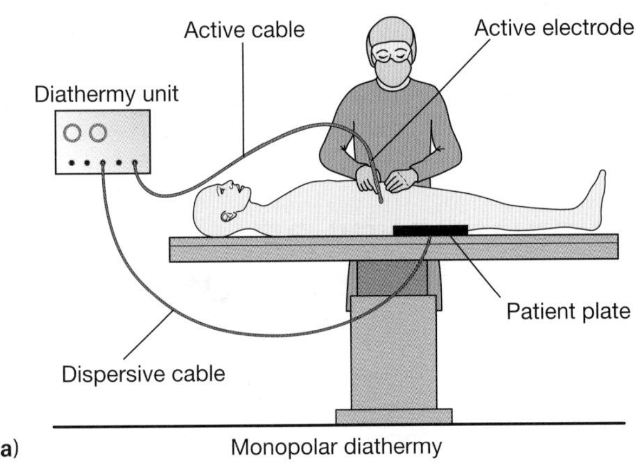

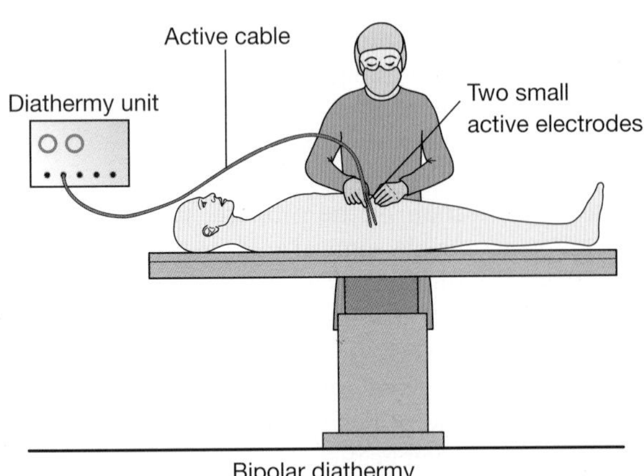

Figure 7.24 The principles of diathermy. (**a**) Monopolar diathermy. (**b**) Bipolar diathermy. Reproduced with permission from Royal College of Surgeons of England. *The intercollegiate basic surgical skills course participants handbook*, edns 1–4. London: RCS.

Effects of diathermy

Diathermy can be used for three purposes:

1. Coagulation: the sealing of blood vessels.
2. Fulguration: the destructive coagulation of tissues with charring.
3. Cutting: used to divide tissues during bloodless surgery.

In **coagulation**, a heating effect leads to cell death by dehydration and protein denaturation. Bleeding is therefore stopped by a combination of the distortion of the walls of the blood vessel, coagulation of the plasma proteins, dried and shrunken dead tissue and stimulation of the clotting mechanism. In an ideal situation, intracellular temperatures should not reach boiling during coagulation, because if this occurs an unwanted cutting effect may be experienced. Cutting occurs when sufficient heat is applied to the tissue to cause cell water to explode into steam. The cut current is a continuous wave form and monopolar diathermy is most effective when the active electrode is held a very short distance from the tissues. This allows an electrical discharge to arc across the gap, creating a series of sparks which produce the high temperatures needed for cutting. In fulguration, the diathermy machine is set to coagulation and a higher effective voltage is used to make larger sparks jump an air gap, thus fulgurating the tissues. This can continue until carbonisation or charring occurs. The voltage and power output can be varied by adjusting the duration of bursts of current, as well the intensity, to give a combination of both cutting and coagulation. This is known as blended current and provides both forms of diathermy activity.

Complications of diathermy

Electrocution

Today, diathermy machines are manufactured to very high safety standards which minimise the risk of any part of the machine becoming live with mains current. However, as with any such instrument, there must be regular and expert servicing.

Explosion

Sparks from the diathermy equipment can ignite any volatile or inflammable gas or fluid within the theatre. Alcohol-based skin preparations can catch fire if they are allowed to pool on or around the patient. Furthermore, diathermy should not be used in the presence of explosive gases, including those which may occur naturally in the colon, especially after certain forms of bowel preparation, such as mannitol, which has now been banned for this use for this very reason.

Burns

These are the most common type of diathermy accidents in both open and endoscopic surgery. They occur when the current flows in some way other than that which the surgeon intended and are far more common in monopolar than bipolar diathermy. Burns may occur as a result of:

- Faulty application of the indifferent electrode with inadequate contact area.
- The patient being earthed by touching any metal object, e.g. the Mayo table, the bar of an anaesthetic screen, an exposed metal arm rest or a leg touching the metal stirrups used in maintaining the lithotomy position.
- Faulty insulation of the diathermy leads, either due to cracked insulation or instruments, such as towel clips, pinching the cable.
- Inadvertent activity, such as the accidental activation of the foot pedal, or accidental contact of the active electrode with other metal instruments, such as retractors, instruments or towel clips.

Channelling

Heat is produced wherever the current intensity is greatest. Normally, this would be at the tip of the active electrode, but if current passes up a narrow channel or pedicle to the active electrode, enough heat may be generated within this channel or pedicle to coagulate the tissues. This can prove disastrous, for example:

- coagulation of the penis in a child undergoing circumcision;
- coagulation of the spermatic cord when the electrode is applied to the testis.

In such situations, diathermy should not be used or, if it is necessary, bipolar diathermy should be employed.

Pacemakers

Diathermy currents can interfere with the working of a pacemaker, with obvious potential danger to the patient's health. Modern pacemakers are designed to be inhibited by high frequency interference, so the patient may receive no pacing stimulation at all while the diathermy is in use. Certain demand pacemakers may revert to the fixed rate of pacing and therefore it is important for the anaesthetist to have a magnet to deactivate the device during surgery.

Laparoscopic surgery

Diathermy burns are a particular hazard of laparoscopic surgery owing to relative lack of visibility of the instrumentation and the actual structure of the instruments used. Such burns may occur by:

- Diathermy of the wrong structure because of lack of clarity of vision or misidentification.
- Faulty insulation of any of the laparoscopic instruments or equipment.
- Intraperitoneal contact of the diathermy with another metal instrument while activating the pedal.
- Inadvertent activation of the pedal while the diathermy tip is out of vision of the camera.
- Retained heat in the diathermy tip touching susceptible structures, such as bowel.
- Capacitance coupling (**Figure 7.25**). This is a phenomenon in which a capacitor is created by having an insulator sandwiched between two metal electrodes. This can be created in situations where there is a metal laparoscopic port and the diathermy hook is passed through it. The insulation of the diathermy hook acts as the sandwiched insulator and, by means of electromagnetic induction, the diathermy current flowing through the hook can induce a current in the metal port, which can potentially damage intraperitoneal structures. In most cases, this current is dissipated from the metal port through the abdominal wall, but if a plastic cuff is used this dissipation of current does not occur and the danger of capacitance coupling is significantly increased. Therefore, metal ports should never be used with a plastic cuff. The danger of capacitance coupling can be prevented by using entirely plastic ports. Reusable instruments are subject to damage and 'wear and tear' through use, cleaning and sterilisation, which can lead to direct coupling that can activate an otherwise passive instrument. Therefore, it is important for the operator, assistants and scrub team to inspect such instruments for damage that may compromise safety.

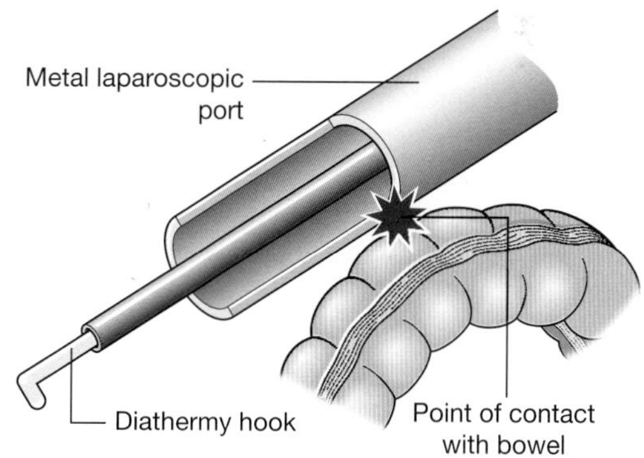

Figure 7.25 Capacitance coupling during laparoscopic surgery. Reproduced with permission from Royal College of Surgeons of England. *The intercollegiate basic surgical skills course participants handbook*, edns 1–4. London: RCS.

PRINCIPLES OF ADVANCED ENERGY DEVICES

Advanced laparoscopic procedures have become widely adopted over the last 25 years. Such 'image based surgery' has driven a parallel explosion in novel technologies which facilitate the performance of such procedures. This is particularly the case for energy devices. Monopolar diathermy still plays a vital and effective role in laparoscopic surgery but has limitations in terms of sealing larger blood vessels and is accompanied by the risks outlined above. Therefore, surgeons have increasingly used advanced energy devices to facilitate dissection and to seal and divide blood vessels up to 7 mm diameter.

There are three main types of advanced energy device: bipolar electrosurgery, harmonic scalpel and combination devices. In all cases the surgeon needs to be aware of the characteristics of these devices and their capacity to cause thermal injury in order to use them safely.

Bipolar electrosurgery devices

Advanced bipolar tissue fusion technology is a vessel sealing system that is used in both open and laparoscopic surgery. It actually fuses the vessel walls to create a permanent seal and is in wide use in a range of surgical specialties, including gynaecology, colorectal, urology and general surgery. It uses a combination of pressure and energy to create vessel fusion which can withstand up to three times the normal systolic pressure. New technology, such as the Ligasure system™ (Medtronic), involves advanced bipolar technology that uses the body's own collagen and elastin to both seal and divide, allowing surgeons to reduce instrument handling when dissecting, ligating and grasping – a valuable asset particularly during laparoscopic surgery. The feedback sensing technology incorporated in the instrument is designed to manage the energy delivery in a precise manner and results in an automatic discontinuation of energy once the seal is complete, thus removing any concern that the surgeon has to use guesswork as to when the seal is complete. The newer instruments actively monitor tissue impedance and provide a real-time adjustment of the energy being delivered. Using this technology, Ligasure can seal vessels of up to 7 mm diameter, with an average seal time of 2–4 seconds, as well as pedicles, tissue bundles and lymphatics, with a consistent controlled and predictable effect on tissue, including less desiccation. Therefore, the new Ligasure Advance™ (Medtronic) can dissect, seal and divide and was designed to be the only tool that a surgeon would need.

Harmonic scalpel devices

The harmonic scalpel is an instrument that uses ultrasound technology to cut tissues while simultaneously sealing them. It utilises a hand-held ultrasound transducer and scalpel which is controlled by a hand switch or foot pedal. During use, the scalpel vibrates in the 20000–50000 Hz range and cuts through tissues, effecting haemostasis by sealing vessels and tissues by means of protein denaturation caused by vibration rather than heat (in a similar manner to whisking an egg white). It provides cutting precision, even through thickened scar tissue, and visibility is enhanced because less smoke is created by this system during use when compared with routine electrosurgery. However, the harmonic scalpel does take longer to cut and coagulate tissues than diathermy, and while diathermy can be used to coagulate a bleeding vessel at any time, the harmonic scalpel can only coagulate as it cuts. It is claimed that patients experience less swelling, bleeding and bruising after the use of the harmonic scalpel than when a conventional scalpel is used, and blood vessels are sealed with a much lower temperature than conventional diathermy and so there is less thermal damage to adjacent tissue, with less charring and desiccation. Furthermore, it is suggested that the use of the harmonic scalpel reduces operative time and recovery is thus enhanced. Currently, the harmonic scalpel is in common use during laparoscopic procedures, as well as in open surgery, such as thyroidectomy, and several plastic surgery operations, e.g. cosmetic breast surgery. There are several such devices on the market, which vary in form and function. Surgeons need to be aware of, and trained in the use of such devices to prevent, complications such as thermal injury of vital structures near to where the energy is activated. There are several manufacturers of harmonic scalpels and the latest versions can seal and divide arteries and veins up to 7 mm in diameter.

Combination energy devices

In the last 5 years, technology has evolved with respect to both harmonic and bipolar advanced energy devices. One product, the Thunderbeat S™ (Olympus), has combined both modalities in a single device. By simultaneously using ultrasonic vibration and bipolar diathermy, this device is able to seal and divide arteries and veins up to 7 mm in diameter. There is also a 'seal only' mode activated by a separate button, which activates bipolar diathermy only.

FURTHER READING

Carol EH Scott-Conner (Ed.) *The Sages manual: Volume 1 basic laparoscopy and endoscopy*. Berlin: Springer, 2012.

Kirk RM. *Basic surgical techniques*, 6th edn. Edinburgh: Churchill Livingstone, 2010.

Pignata G, Bracale U, Fabrizio Lazzara F (Eds.) *Laparoscopic surgery: key points, operating room setup and equipment*. Berlin: Springer, 2016.

Royal College of Surgeons of England. *Intercollegiate basic surgical skills course (participant handbook)*, 4th edn. London: Royal College of Surgeons of England, 2007.

www.websurg.com (website) This is one of the best educational websites for laparoscopic surgery.

Chapter 8

Principles of laparoscopic and robotic surgery

Learning objectives

To understand:

- The principles of laparoscopic and robotic surgery
- The advantages and disadvantages of such surgery
- The safety issues and indications for laparoscopic and robotic surgery
- The principles of postoperative care

DEFINITION

Minimal access surgery is a product of modern technology and surgical innovation that aims to accomplish surgical therapeutic goals with minimal somatic and psychological trauma. This type of surgery has reduced wound access trauma, as well as being less disfiguring than conventional techniques. It can offer cost-effectiveness to both health services and employers by shortening operating times, shortening hospital stays, improving operative precision compared to open surgery in some (but not all) cases and allowing faster recuperation.

EXTENT OF MINIMAL ACCESS SURGERY

The first introduction of an experimental laparoscopic procedure was by Georg Kelling of Dresden in 1901 (he termed it 'celioscopy' and used a Nitze-cystoscope). This was followed by Hans Christian Jacobaeus' successful application in humans in Sweden. Despite the work of these pioneers, it took another 70 years before Patrick Steptoe applied this approach to patients in the United Kingdom in 1980, and Phillipe Mouret's first video-laparoscopic cholecystectomy was performed in Lyon, France in 1987. However, since its mainstream adoption in the mid-1990s, minimal access surgery has crossed all traditional boundaries of specialties and disciplines. Shared, borrowed and overlapping technologies and information are encouraging a multidisciplinary approach that serves the whole patient, rather than a specific organ system.

The core principles of minimal access surgery (independent of procedure or device) can be summarized by the acronym **I-VITROS**:

- **I**nsufflate/create space – to allow surgery to take place in the minimal access setting
- **V**isualise – the tissues, anatomical landmarks and the environment for the surgery to take place
- **I**dentify – the specific structures for surgery
- **T**riangulate – surgical tools (such as port placement) to optimise the efficiency of their action, and ergonomics by minimising overlap and clashing of instruments
- **R**etract – and manipulate local tissues to improve access and gain entry into the correct tissue planes
- **O**perate – incise, suture, anastomose, fuse
- **S**eal/haemostasis.

Broadly speaking, minimal access techniques can be categorised as follows:

Laparoscopy

A rigid endoscope (laparoscope) is introduced through a port into the peritoneal cavity. This is insufflated with carbon dioxide to produce a pneumoperitoneum. Further ports are inserted to enable instrument access and their use for dissection (**Figure 8.1**). It is generally accepted that laparoscopic cholecystectomy has revolutionised the surgical management of cholelithiasis and has become the mainstay of management of uncomplicated gallstone disease. With improved instrumentation, advanced procedures, such as laparoscopic colectomies for malignancy, previously regarded as controversial, have also become fully accepted. There continues to be substantive evidence demonstrating the short-term benefits of laparoscopic surgery over open surgery with regard to postoperative pain, length of stay and earlier return to normal activities; however, the equivalence of the benefits in long-term outcomes, such as oncological quality and cancer-related survival, has not been established.

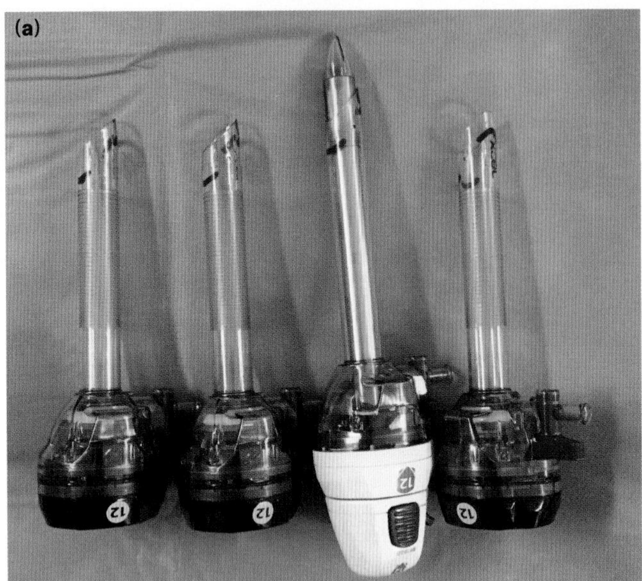

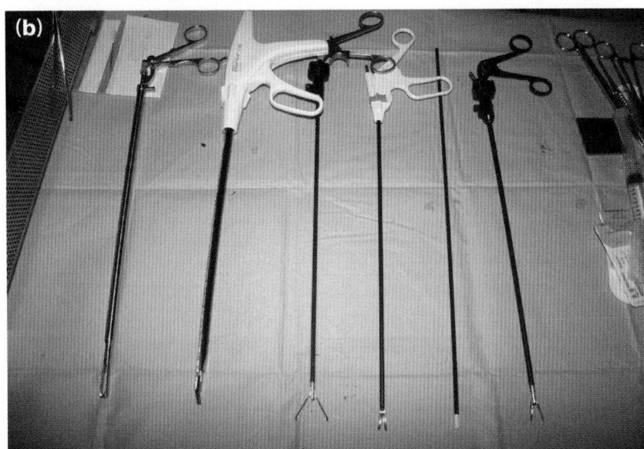

Figure 8.1 (a) Common laparoscopic trocars. (b) Common laparoscopic instruments (photo courtesy of Daniel Leff).

Thoracoscopy

A rigid endoscope is introduced through an incision in the chest to gain access to the thoracic contents. Usually there is no requirement for gas insufflation, as the operating space is held open by the rigidity of the thoracic cavity. In specific cases, such as mediastinal tumour resection and diaphragmatic surgery, gas insufflation at low pressure (5–8 mmHg) may be applied.

Endoluminal endoscopy

Flexible or rigid endoscopes are introduced into hollow organs or systems, such as the urinary tract, upper or lower gastrointestinal tract, and respiratory and vascular systems.

Perivisceral endoscopy

Body planes can be accessed even in the absence of a natural cavity. Examples are mediastinoscopy, retroperitoneoscopy and retroperitoneal approaches to the kidney, aorta and lumbar sympathetic chain. Extraperitoneal approaches to the retroperitoneal organs, as well as hernia repair, are now becoming increasingly commonplace, further decreasing morbidity associated with visceral peritoneal manipulation. Other, more recent, examples include subfascial ligation of incompetent perforating veins in varicose vein surgery.

Arthroscopy and intra-articular joint surgery

Orthopaedic surgeons have applied arthroscopic access to the knee for some time and are applying this modality to other joints, including the shoulder, wrist, elbow and hip.

Combined approach

The diseased organ is visualised and treated by an assortment of endoluminal and extraluminal endoscopes and other imaging devices. Examples include the combined laparoendoscopic approach for the management of biliary lithiasis, colonic polyp excision and several urological procedures, such as pyeloplasty and donor nephrectomy. In some cases the application of this combined approach offers the ability to execute operations via a single incision, thereby better adhering to the minimally invasive approach. The evidence for improved outcomes using these combined approaches remains limited for the majority of procedures.

SURGICAL TRAUMA IN OPEN, MINIMALLY INVASIVE AND ROBOTIC SURGERY

Most of the trauma of an open procedure is inflicted because the surgeon must have a wound that is large enough to give adequate exposure for safe dissection at a target site. The wound is often the cause of morbidity, including infection, dehiscence, bleeding, herniation and nerve entrapment. Wound pain prolongs recovery time and, by reducing mobility, contributes to an increased incidence of pulmonary atelectasis, chest infection, paralytic ileus and deep venous thrombosis.

Mechanical and human retractors cause additional trauma. Body wall retractors can inflict localised damage that may be as painful as the wound itself. In contrast, during laparoscopy, the retraction is provided by the low-pressure pneumoperitoneum, giving a diffuse force applied gently and evenly over the whole body wall, causing minimal trauma.

Exposure of any body cavity to the atmosphere also causes morbidity through cooling and fluid loss by evaporation. There is also evidence that the incidence of postsurgical adhesions has been reduced by the use of the minimally invasive (laparoscopic, thoracoscopic) and robotic approaches, which has been suggested to result from less damage to delicate serosal coverings. In the manual handling of intestinal loops, the surgeon and assistant disturb the peristaltic activity of the gut and provoke adynamic ileus.

Minimal access surgery has many advantages, such as a reduction in the trauma of access and exposure and an improvement in visualisation. While minimal access methods have been an established modality in some elective surgical procedures, they are now also being increasingly applied with success in emergency surgical procedures (including perforated viscus repair, such as omental patch repair of the stomach, and washout of localised perforation of diverticular disease).

Summary box 8.1

Advantages of minimal access surgery

- Decrease in wound size
- Reduction in wound infection, dehiscence, bleeding, herniation and nerve entrapment
- Decrease in wound pain
- Improved mobility
- Decreased wound trauma
- Decreased heat loss
- Improved visualisation

LIMITATIONS OF MINIMAL ACCESS SURGERY

Despite its many advantages, minimal access surgery has its limitations. To perform minimal access surgery with safety, the surgeon must operate remote from the surgical field, using an imaging system that provides a two-dimensional (2D) representation of the operative site. The endoscope offers a whole new anatomical landscape, which the surgeon must learn to navigate without the usual 'open approach' clues that make it easy to judge depth. The instruments are longer and sometimes more complex to use than those commonly used in open surgery. This results in the novice being faced with significant problems of hand–eye coordination. Here there is a well-described learning curve for novice surgeons and experienced 'open' surgeons when adopting the minimally invasive approach.

Some of the procedures performed by these new approaches are more technically demanding and are slower to perform, and they often have a more difficult learning curve as tactile feedback to the surgeon is lost. Indeed, on occasion, a minimally invasive operation is so technically demanding that both patient and surgeon are better served by conversion to an open procedure. Unfortunately, there seems to be a sense of shame associated with conversion, which is quite unjustified. It is vital for surgeons and patients to appreciate that the decision to close or to convert to an open operation is not a complication but, instead, usually implies sound surgical judgement in favour of patient safety.

Another problem occurs when there is intraoperative arterial bleeding. Haemostasis may be very difficult to achieve endoscopically because blood obscures the field of vision and there is a significant reduction of the image quality due to light absorption.

Another disadvantage of laparoscopic surgery is the loss of tactile feedback in the context of some procedures (although many procedures have been successfully performed without 'traditional sense' of tactile feedback). This is an area of ongoing research in haptics and biofeedback systems. Early work suggested that laparoscopic ultrasonography might be a substitute for the need to 'feel' in intraoperative decision-making. The rapid progress in advanced laparoscopic techniques, including biliary tract exploration and surgery for malignancies, has provided a strong impetus for the development of laparoscopic ultrasound. Now more developed, this technique already has advantages that far outweigh its disadvantages.

In more advanced techniques, large pieces of resected tissue, such as the lung or colon, may have to be extracted from the body cavity. Occasionally, the extirpated tissue may be removed through a nearby natural orifice, such as the rectum or the mouth. At other times, a novel route may be employed. For instance, a benign colonic specimen may be extracted through an incision in the vault of the vagina. Several innovative tube systems have been shown to facilitate this extraction. Although tissue 'morcellators, mincers and liquidisers' can be used in some circumstances, they have the disadvantage of reducing the amount of information available to the pathologist. Previous reports of tumour implantation in the locations of port sites raised important questions about the future of the laparoscopic treatment of malignancy, but large-scale trials have shown this claim to be false. Although emerging evidence from large-scale international prospective trials implicates surgical skill as an important aetiological factor, it is important to consider the biological implications of minimally invasive strategies on the tumours. The use of carbon dioxide and helium as insufflants causes locoregional hypoxia and may also change pH. The resultant modulation of the behaviour of spilled tumour cells is increasingly being studied, although the risks of recurrence at port sites seem to be minimised by appropriate tissue handling, separating any tumours by bagging, and washing and protecting the site.

Hand-assisted laparoscopic surgery is a well-developed technique. It involves the intra-abdominal placement of a hand or forearm through a minilaparotomy incision, while pneumoperitoneum is maintained. In this way, the surgeon's hand can be used as in an open procedure. It can be used to palpate organs or tumours, reflect organs atraumatically, retract structures, identify vessels, dissect bluntly along a tissue plane and provide finger pressure to bleeding points, while proximal control is achieved. This approach has been suggested to offer technical and economic efficiency when compared with a totally laparoscopic approach, in some instances, reducing both the number of laparoscopic ports and the number of instruments required. Some advocates of the technique claim that it is also easier to learn and perform than totally laparoscopic approaches, and that there may be increased patient safety.

There has been a continued improvement in dissection techniques in laparoscopic/thoracoscopic surgery beyond that of standard electrosurgery/diathermy and laser technology to improve dissection precision and haemostatic efficacy. Ultrasonic dissection, tissue fusion devices and tissue removal continue to be adopted across specialties and practitioners. This has taken place as a consequence of continuous and incremental technical improvements in devices, increased familiarity with their use and some improvements in cost of access. The adaptation of the technology to minimally invasive surgery grew out of the search for alternative, possibly safer, methods of dissection. Some current units combine the functions of three or four separate instruments, reducing the need for instrument exchanges during a procedure. This flexibility, combined with the ability to provide a clean, smoke-free field, has the potential to improve safety and shorten operating times.

Although dramatic cost savings are possible with laparoscopic cholecystectomy when compared with open cholecystectomy, the position was less clear-cut with other procedures initially. There is another factor that may complicate the computation of the cost–benefit ratio. A significant rise in the rate of cholecystectomy followed the introduction of the laparoscopic approach because the threshold for referring patients for surgery became lower. The increase in the number of procedures performed has led to an overall increase in the cost of treating symptomatic gallstones.

Three-dimensional (3D) imaging systems have been available for some time, but remain expensive and currently are not commonplace, partially because many surgeons feel that 3D technology has not yet offered the ability to perform procedures with significant technical enhancement or to improve safety or outcomes across a range of operations. Stereoscopic imaging for laparoscopy and thoracoscopy is still progressing. Future improvements in these systems carry the potential to enhance manipulative ability in critical procedures, such as knot tying and dissection of closely overlapping tissues. There are, however, some drawbacks, such as reduced display brightness and interference with normal vision because of the need to wear specially designed glasses for some systems. It is likely that brighter projection displays will be developed, at increased cost. However, the need to wear glasses will not be easily overcome.

Looking further to the future, it is evident that the continuing reductions in the costs of elaborate image-processing techniques will result in a wide range of transformed presentations becoming available. It should ultimately be possible for a surgeon to call up any view of the operative region that is accessible to a camera and present it stereoscopically in any size or orientation, superimposed on past images taken in other modalities. Such augmented reality systems have been available for several years but continue to improve. It is for the medical community to decide which of these many potential imaginative techniques will contribute most to effective surgical procedures.

Summary box 8.2

Limitations of minimal access surgery

- Reliance on remote vision and operating
- Loss of tactile feedback
- Dependence on hand–eye coordination
- Difficulty with haemostasis
- Reliance on new techniques
- Extraction of large specimens

ROBOTIC SURGERY

A robot is a mechanical device that performs automated physical tasks according to direct human supervision, a predefined program or a set of general guidelines, using artificial intelligence techniques. In terms of surgery, robots have been used to assist surgeons during procedures. This has been primarily in the form of automated camera systems and telemanipulator systems, thus resulting in the creation of a human–machine interface.

Even though laparoscopic surgery has progressed greatly over the last two decades, owing to its widespread use and dissemination in that time, there are, as discussed above, limitations. To those already mentioned may be added reduced degrees of freedom of movement and ergonomically difficult positions for the surgeon. Such problems undoubtedly affect surgical precision. This has led to interest in robotic surgical systems, which currently exist as two main categories:

- **Teleoperated systems:** a human surgeon performs an operation via a robot and its robotic instruments through a televisual computerised platform, either via onsite connections or remotely through the internet or other digital channels – hence the publicity of 'operating on a patient from another country' (such 'remote' operations are currently rarely performed but their existence is established).
- **Image-guided systems:** A surgical robot completes a preprogrammed surgical task which is guided by preoperative imaging and real-time anatomical constraints and cues through the application of inbuilt navigation systems.

In the current era the concept of the master–slave system prevails (where the surgeon is the master, i.e. the operator, and the robot is the slave). The two are linked by underlying hardware and software components within an advanced computer construction. Such devices have been available for the past 30 years and have become more available during the past two decades. They still remain a relative rarity owing to a multitude of factors including cost, applicability and benefits for a particular operation/pathology, training requirements and the support that is necessary, beyond just that of the individual surgeon but rather at whole institution level.

Since their first clinical use in 1985, with the PUMA 560 being used for a brain biopsy, surgical robots have been considered to offer many benefits, which have arisen as a result of new technology in lenses, cameras and computer software. Just as laparoscopic surgery benefited from advances in light technology, allowing the targeted transmission of light down tubing, robotic surgery benefited from computer integration of mechanical (surgical) arms that paved the way for computer-integrated surgery (CIS). The advantages of robotic surgery are two-fold: first for the patient (as for laparoscopic surgery, see *Summary box 8.1*) and second for the surgeon. The advantages for the surgeon include better visualisation (higher magnification) with stereoscopic views; elimination of hand tremor allowing greater precision; improved manoeuvring as a result of the 'robotic wrist', which in some systems allows up to seven degrees of freedom; and the fact that large external movements of the surgical hands can be scaled down and transformed to limited internal movements of the 'robotic hands', extending the surgical ability to perform complex technical tasks in a limited space. Also, the surgeon is able to work in an ergonomic environment with less stress and to achieve higher levels of concentration. The computer may also be able to compensate for the beating movement of the heart, making it unnecessary to stop the heart during cardiothoracic surgery. There may also be less need for assistance once surgery is under way.

Many surgical specialties have embraced the progression of robot-assisted techniques, including general surgery, cardiothoracic surgery, urology, orthopaedics, ear, nose and throat (ENT) surgery, gynaecology and paediatric surgery. Specialties that use microsurgical techniques also benefit from this technology. Current robotic systems were designed to offer multifunctionality including multi-anatomy and speciality capability in both operating theatre and remote environments. In the current era, however, these devices seem most often applied in pelvic surgery (typically urology, colorectal and gynaecology) within inhouse operating areas.

One major operative barrier to adoption remains the prohibitive costs for many healthcare environments. As a result the current robotic surgical market is dominated by the master–slave da Vinci system (Intuitive Surgical, MenloPark, CA, USA) (**Figure 8.2**), although there are several other commercially available robots and a market open to a small number of new entrants, but also a history of unsuccessful (financially

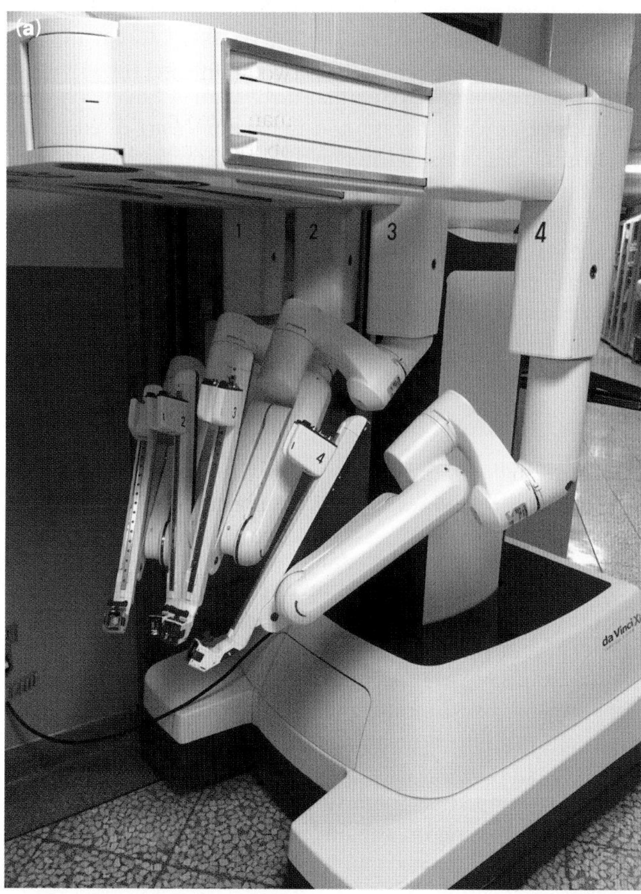

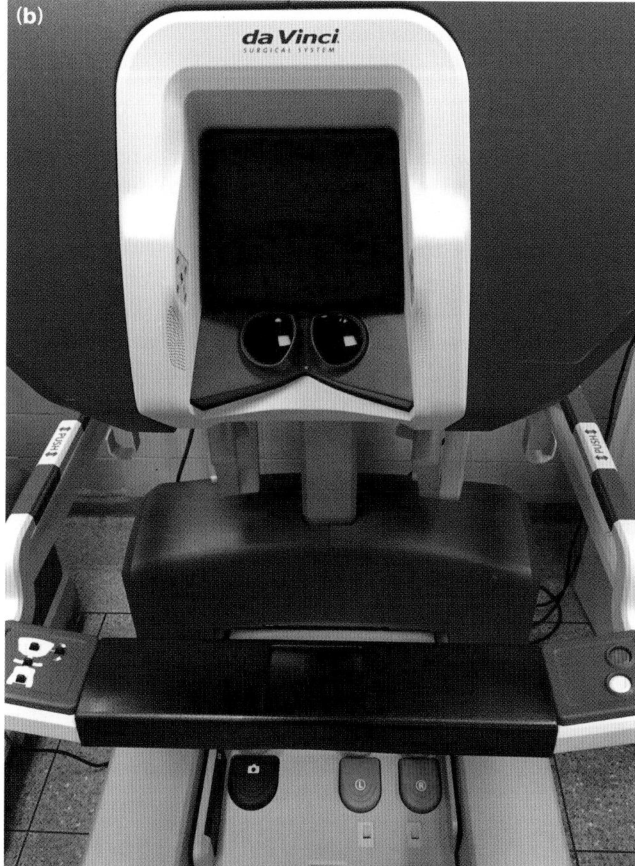

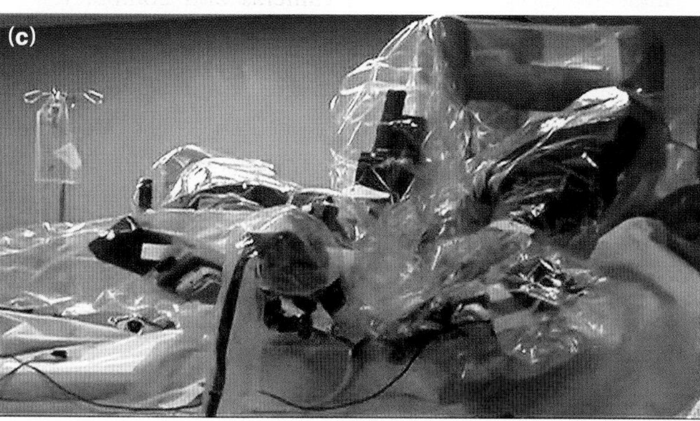

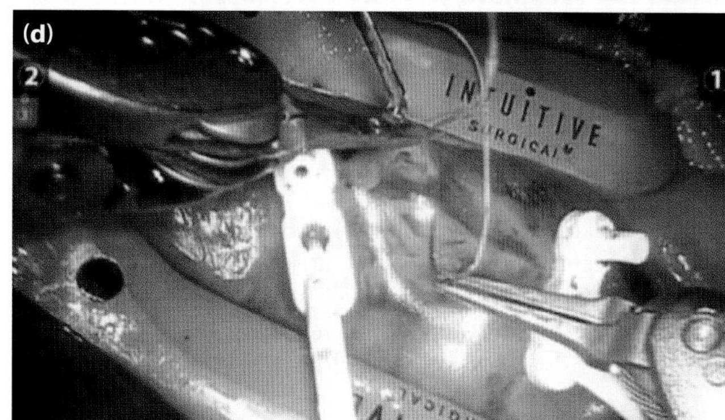

Figure 8.2 **(a)** The DaVinci Xi system. **(b)** The surgical console. **(c)** The robotic arms draped for a robotic coronary artery bypass grafting procedure. **(d)** Robotic distal coronary anastomosis.

or functionally) or withdrawn/ removed devices. This is partly because of the high cost of design and development of new robot technologies and surgical instruments compatible with them, which all require design, translation and intellectual property costs. In addition to the remote master–slave platform design, direct robot systems exist and include:

- tremor suppression robots;
- active guidance systems;
- articulated mechatronic devices;
- force control systems;
- haptic feedback devices.

Each of these systems offers different advantages to the operating surgeon, ranging from reducing the need for assistants and providing better ergonomic operating positions to providing experienced guidance from surgeons not physically present in the operating theatre.

Robotic surgery – the first 30 years

The largest systematic overview of all robot surgical procedures from inception and covering the field's first 30 years revealed only 99 prospective or randomised studies reporting clinical outcomes from over 28000 peer-reviewed research articles that mentioned the term 'robotic surgery'. The 99 studies revealed data from approximately 14500 patients in trials undergoing robotic surgical procedures versus open and minimally invasive operations. The overall pooled results, regardless of specialty, revealed a decrease in blood loss and blood transfusion rate with robotic surgery when compared with both open surgery and minimally invasive surgery. Specifically, when compared with open surgery, robotic procedures demonstrated that there was a reduction in length of hospital stay and overall complication rate. However, robotic procedures did suffer from significantly longer operative times and their cost-effectiveness varied depending on operative site, technique, patient and healthcare setting. While this reveals an overall perspective from the first 30 years of robotics surgery, there remains an incumbent need to offer clearer clinical evidence regarding the most apposite operative method and technology for each individual patient.

PREOPERATIVE EVALUATION

Preparation of the patient

Although the patient may be in hospital for a shorter period, careful preoperative management is essential to minimise morbidity.

History

Patients must be fit for general anaesthesia and open operation if necessary. Potential coagulation disorders (e.g. associated with cirrhosis) are particularly dangerous in laparoscopic surgery. As adhesions may cause problems, previous abdominal operations or peritonitis should be documented.

Summary box 8.3

Preparation for laparoscopic or robotic surgery

- Overall fitness: cardiac arrhythmia, emphysema, medications, allergies
- Previous surgery: scars, adhesions
- Body habitus: obesity, skeletal deformity
- Normal coagulation
- Thromboprophylaxis
- Informed consent

Examination

Routine preoperative physical examination is required as for any major operation. Although, in general, laparoscopic/ thoracoscopic surgery allows quicker recovery, it may involve longer operating times and the establishment of the pneumoperitoneum may provoke cardiac arrhythmias. Severe chronic obstructive airways disease and ischaemic heart disease may be contraindications to the laparoscopic approach. Particular attention should be paid to the presence or absence of jaundice, abdominal scars, palpable masses or tenderness. Moderate obesity does not increase operative difficulty significantly, but massive obesity may make pneumoperitoneum difficult and standard instrumentation may be too short. Access may prove difficult in very thin patients, especially those with severe kyphosis.

Premedication

Premedication is the responsibility of the anaesthetist, with whom coexisting medical problems should be discussed.

Prophylaxis against thromboembolism

Venous stasis induced by the reverse Trendelenburg position during laparoscopic surgery may be a particular risk factor for deep vein thrombosis, as is a lengthy operation and the obesity of many patients. Subcutaneous low molecular weight heparin and antithromboembolic stockings should be used routinely, in addition to pneumatic leggings during the operation. Patients already taking warfarin for other reasons should have this stopped temporarily or converted to intravenous heparin, depending on the underlying condition, as it is not safe to perform laparoscopic surgery in the presence of a significant coagulation deficit.

Urinary catheters and nasogastric tubes

In the early days of laparoscopic surgery, routine bladder catheterisation and nasogastric intubation were advised. Most surgeons now omit these, but it remains essential to check that the patient is fasted and has recently emptied their bladder, particularly before the blind insertion of a Verres needle. However, currently, most general surgeons prefer the direct cut-down technique into the abdomen for the introduction of the first port for the establishment of the pneumoperitoneum (Hasson technique and modified Hasson approaches). More

Janos Verres, 1903–1979, chest physician and chief of the Department of Internal Medicine, The Regional Hospital, Kapuvar, Hungary.
Harrith Hasson, Professor of Gynaecology, Chicago, IL, USA.

recently, direct optical entry has been used, especially in the setting of bariatric surgery.

Informed consent

The basis of many complaints and much litigation in surgery, especially laparoscopic surgery, relates to the issue of informed consent. It is essential that the patient understands the nature of the procedure, the risks involved and, when appropriate, the alternatives that are available. A locally prepared explanatory booklet concerning the laparoscopic procedure to be undertaken is extremely useful.

In an elective case, a full discussion of the proposed operation should take place in the outpatient department with a surgeon of appropriate seniority, preferably the operating surgeon, before the decision is made to operate. On admission, it is the responsibility of the operating surgeon and anaesthetist to ensure that the patient has been fully counselled, although the actual witnessing of the consent form may have been delegated. The patient should understand what laparoscopic surgery involves and that there is a risk of conversion to open operation. If known, this risk should be quantified, for example the increased risk with acute cholecystitis or in the presence of extensive upper abdominal adhesions. The conversion rate will also vary with the experience and practice of the surgeon. Common complications should be mentioned, such as shoulder tip pain and minor surgical emphysema, as well as rare but serious complications, including injury to the bile ducts and visceral injury from trocar insertion or diathermy.

Preparation is very similar to that for open surgery and aims to ensure that:

- The patient is fit for the procedure.
- The patient is fully informed and has consented.
- Operative difficulty is predicted when possible.
- Appropriate theatre time and facilities are available (especially important for robotic cases).

THEATRE SET UP AND TOOLS

Operating theatre design, construction and layout are key to its smooth running on a daily basis. Originally, the video and diathermy equipment and other key tools used in laparoscopic surgery were moved around on stacks, taking up valuable floor space and cluttering up the theatre environment, which was not always ergonomic for the operating team. New theatres are designed with moveable booms that come down from the ceiling; these are easy to place and do not have long leads or wires trailing behind them (**Figure 8.3**). The equipment consists of at least two high-resolution liquid crystal display (LCD) monitors (and, more recently, high definition (HD) monitors for even clearer images), the laparoscopic kit for maintaining pneumoperitoneum and the audiovisual kit. The advent of DVD and other digital recording equipment has also led to these being incorporated into the rigs so that cases can be recorded with ease. This is further facilitated by cameras being inserted into the light handles of the main overhead lights so that open surgery can also be recorded without distracting the surgeons.

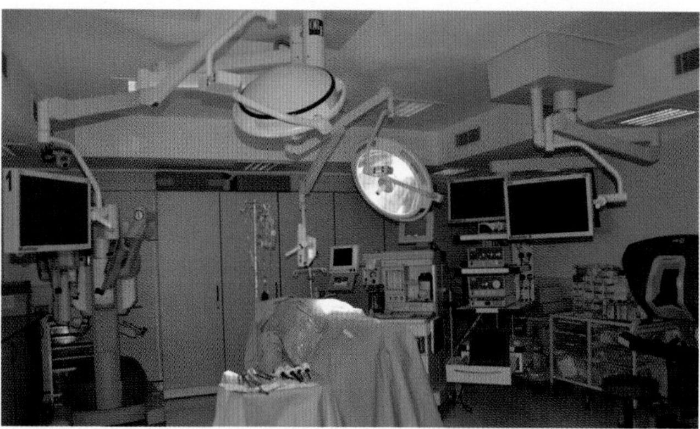

Figure 8.3 Modern laparoscopic theatre set up.

Image quality is vital to the success of laparoscopic surgery. New camera and lens technology allows the use of smaller cameras. Many centres now use 5-mm laparoscopes routinely. Automatic focusing and charge-coupled devices (CCDs) are used to detect different levels of brightness and adjust for the best image possible. Flat panel monitors with HD images are used to give the surgeon the best views possible and 3D technology is now being used for visualisation more routinely in some centres. The usability of the kit has also improved; touch screen panels and even voice-activated systems are now available on the market.

As minimally invasive and robotic procedures have become routine in some institutions, the dedicated theatre team for such procedures has also evolved. Surgeons and anaesthetists, as well as scrub and circulating nurses, have become familiar with working with the equipment and each other. The efficient working of the team is crucial to high-quality surgery and quick yet safe turnover. Laparoscopic tools have also changed. Disposable equipment is more readily available, which does unfortunately increase the cost of the surgery. However, easy to use, ergonomically designed and reliable surgical tools are essential for laparoscopic and robotic surgery. Simple designs for new laparoscopic ports are now being studied, with the aim of reducing the incidence of port-site hernias; see-through (optical) ports that allow the surgeon to cut down through the abdomen while observing the layers through the cameras, and new light sources within the abdomen may be simple ideas that affect surgical technique in the near future.

GENERAL INTRAOPERATIVE PRINCIPLES

Laparoscopic and thoracoscopic principles have specific principles that require careful clinical consideration. As such, they are not purely a less invasive equivalent of an open operation. For example, laparoscopic cholecystectomy is now the 'gold standard' for operative treatment of symptomatic gallstone disease. The main negative aspect of the technique is the increased incidence of bile duct injury compared with open cholecystectomy. Better understanding of the mechanisms of injury, coupled with proper training, will avoid most of these errors. The following sections highlight the important technical steps that should be taken during any form of laparoscopic surgery to avoid complications.

Creating a pneumoperitoneum

There are two methods for creation of a pneumoperitoneum: open and closed.

The closed method involves blind puncture using a Verres needle. Although this method is fast and relatively safe, there is a small but significant potential for intestinal or vascular injury on introduction of the needle or first trocar.

The routine use of the open technique for creating a pneumoperitoneum avoids the morbidity related to a blind puncture. To achieve this, a 1 cm vertical or transverse incision is made at the level of the umbilicus. The umbilicus carries importance as it is a reliable anatomical landmark deriving from the embryological coalescence of the rectus sheath and peritoneum and is devoid of other myofascial planes that could complicate subsequent entry into the peritoneum. Two small retractors are used to dissect bluntly the subcutaneous fat and expose the midline fascia. Two sutures are inserted each side of the midline incision (into the rectus sheath confluence), followed by the creation of a 1 cm opening in the fascia. Free penetration into the abdominal cavity is confirmed by the gentle introduction of a finger. Finally, a Hasson trocar (or other blunt-tip trocar) is inserted and anchored with the fascial sutures (**Figure 8.4**). This is considered the Hasson or 'modified Hasson' approach. The term 'modified' is used here to denote the same principle as the original Hasson with the midline exposure and access, except that the exact technique has been changed to suit an individual surgeon, such as the adoption of a particular angle of retraction of the umbilicus before an incision into the midline is made to get access to the peritoneum.

Rarely, a third, or combination, approach may be employed. Here an open technique is followed with a smaller than usual midline incision. Once access to the peritoneum is visualised, a Verres needle is inserted under direct vision, and then insufflation is carried out. This small open approach then allows the introduction of a laparoscopic port with a view to reducing trauma of the pneumoperitoneum. Such an approach may have benefits for complex cases, such as those for 're-do' procedures, where the risk of umbilical adhesions during pneumoperitoneum may be high.

The open technique may initially appear time consuming and even cumbersome; however, with practice, it is quick, efficient and safe overall. Optical entry to the abdomen under direct vision using optical ports (especially in bariatric surgery) is gaining favour with many laparoscopic surgeons. This allows quick and safe entry to the peritoneal cavity using bladeless see-through trocars that allow the different layers to be dissected through using the laparoscope within an optical port to be inserted into the abdomen.

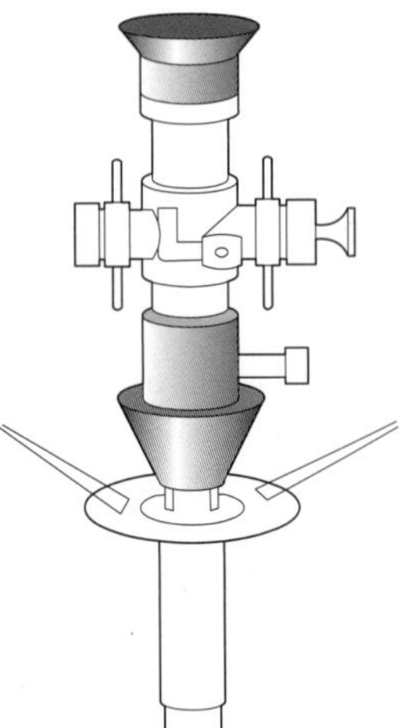

Figure 8.4 Open technique with Hasson port. Apply safe principles of closed technique.

Preoperative problems

Previous abdominal surgery

Previous abdominal surgery is no longer a contraindication to laparoscopic surgery, but preoperative evaluation is necessary to assess the type and location of surgical scars. As mentioned earlier, the open technique for insertion of the first trocar is safer. Before trocar insertion, the introduction of a fingertip helps to ascertain penetration into the peritoneal cavity and also allows adhesions to be gently removed from the entry site. After the tip of the cannula has been introduced, a laparoscope is used as a blunt dissector to tease adhesions gently away and form a tunnel towards the quadrant where the operation is to take place. This step is accomplished by a careful pushing and twisting motion under direct vision. With experience, the surgeon learns to differentiate visually between thick adhesions that may contain bowel and should be avoided and thin adhesions that would lead to a window into a free area of the peritoneal cavity.

Obesity

Laparoscopic and robotic surgery has proved to be safe and effective in the obese population. In fact, some procedures are less difficult than their open counterparts for the morbidly obese patient, e.g. in bariatric surgery. Technical difficulties occur, however, in obtaining pneumoperitoneum, reaching the operative region adequately and achieving adequate exposure in the presence of an obese colon. Increased thickness of the subcutaneous fat makes insufflation of the abdominal cavity more difficult. With the closed technique, a larger Verres needle is often required for morbidly obese patients. Pulling the skin up for fixation of the soft tissues is better accomplished with towel clamps. Only moderate force should be used, to avoid separating the skin farther from the fascia. The needle should be passed at nearly a right angle to the skin and preferably above the umbilicus, where the peritoneum is more firmly fixed to the midline. The open technique of inserting a Hasson trocar is easier and safer for obese patients, but technically demanding in morbidly obese patients, where optical entry is now more commonplace. The main difficulty is reaching the fascia. A larger skin incision (1–3 cm), starting at the umbilicus and extending superiorly, may facilitate this. To reach the operative area adequately, the location of some of the ports has to be modified and, in some instances, larger and longer instruments are necessary. When the length of the laparoscope appears to be insufficient to reach the operative area adequately, the initial midline port should be placed nearer to the operative field. Recently, the use of optical port entry for laparoscopic bariatric surgery has revolutionised port entry for morbid obesity cases.

Operative problems

Intraoperative perforation of a viscus

Perforation of any viscus, such as bowel, solid organs and blood vessels (including the aorta), is a potential hazard of using the laparoscopic approach and these complications may be minimised with surgical experience, education, preparation and patient selection. One example, in a common laparoscopic procedure such as cholecystectomy, includes perforation of the gallbladder. This is more common with the laparoscopic technique than with the open technique (see also Chapter 67). Some authors have reported an incidence of up to up to 30%, but it does not appear to be a factor in increasing the early postoperative morbidity. However, it is well known that bile is not a sterile fluid and bacteria can be present in the absence of cholecystitis. Unless the perforation is small, closure with endoloops or endoclips should be attempted to avoid contamination prior to extraction, which should be with the use of an endobag. Bilious leakage should be suctioned and washed out. If there is stone spillage, every attempt must be made to collect and extract the stones, and if there is a possibility of stones being retained in the peritoneum, then an ultrasound should be arranged 6 weeks postoperatively to assess a collection around a stone and the patient should be informed of this outcome postoperatively.

Antibiotics to manage known sepsis or septicaemia in a patient undergoing surgery

Operating on a patient with established septicaemia or sepsis is not typically recommended unless the operation will contribute to removing or minimising infectious origins. Where necessary pre-, peri- and postoperative antibiotics should be administered, in accordance with local microbiological advice.

Antibiotics to prevent infections and sepsis

A single dose of antibiotics should be administered within 1 hour of skin incision; in contaminated, semi-contaminated or complex procedures, additional doses should be administered, based on local microbiological advice.

Bleeding

In some of the larger series, bleeding has been the most common cause of conversion to an open procedure. Bleeding plays a more important role in laparoscopic surgery because of factors inherent to the technique. These include a limited field that can easily be obscured by relatively small amounts of blood, magnification that makes small arterial bleeding appear to be a significant haemorrhage and light absorption that obscures the visual field.

HOW TO AVOID BLEEDING

As in any surgical procedure, the best way to handle intraoperative bleeding is to prevent it from happening. This can usually be accomplished by identifying patients at high risk of bleeding, having a clear understanding of the laparoscopic anatomy and employing careful surgical technique.

Risk factors that predispose to increased bleeding include:

- cirrhosis;
- inflammatory conditions (acute cholecystitis, diverticulitis);
- patients on clopidogrel and or dipyridamole;
- coagulation defects: these are contraindications to a laparoscopic procedure.

BLEEDING FROM A MAJOR VESSEL

Damage to a large vessel requires immediate assessment of the magnitude and type of bleeding. When the bleeding vessel is identified, a fine-tip grasper can be used to grasp it and apply either electrocautery or a clip, depending on its size. When the vessel is not identified early and a pool of blood forms, compression should be applied immediately with a blunt instrument, a cotton swab (ENT or mastoid swab) or with the adjacent organ. Good suction and irrigation are of utmost importance. Once the area has been cleaned, pressure should be released gradually to identify the site of bleeding. Insertion of an extra port may be required to achieve adequate exposure and at the same time to enable the concomitant use of a suction device and an insulated grasper. Although most bleeding vessels can be controlled laparoscopically, judgement should be used in deciding when not to prolong bleeding, but to convert to an open procedure at an early stage. Surgicel® (absorbable fibrillar oxidized cellulose polymer) or other clot-promoting strips, tissue glues or other haemostatic agent may also be used laparoscopically to aid haemostasis. If at any stage bleeding is difficult to stem laparoscopically, there should be no delay in converting to an open procedure in the interests of patient safety.

BLEEDING FROM ORGANS ENCOUNTERED DURING SURGERY

Intraoperative bleeding from organs can usually be prevented by performing the dissection in the correct plane. As previously mentioned, the common laparoscopic example of a cholecystectomy requires understanding the management of bleeding from the gallbladder bed. When a bleeding site appears during detachment of the gallbladder, the dissection should be carried a little farther to expose the bleeding point adequately. Once this step has been performed, direct application of electrocautery usually controls the bleeding. If bleeding persists, indirect application of electrocautery is useful because it avoids detachment of the formed crust. This procedure is accomplished by applying pressure to the bleeding point with a blunt, insulated grasper and then applying electrocoagulation by touching this grasper with a second insulated grasper that is connected to the electrocautery device. One must be careful to keep all conducting surfaces of the graspers within the visual field while applying the electrocautery current.

BLEEDING FROM A TROCAR SITE

Bleeding from the trocar sites is usually controlled by applying upwards and lateral pressure with the trocar itself. Considerable bleeding may occur if the falciform ligament is impaled with the substernal trocar or if one of the epigastric vessels is injured. If significant continuous bleeding from the falciform ligament occurs, haemostasis is achieved by percutaneously inserting a large, straight needle at one side of the ligament. A monofilament suture attached to the needle is passed into the abdominal cavity and the needle is exited at the other side of the ligament using a grasper (**Figure 8.5**). The loop is suspended and compression is achieved. Maintaining compression throughout the procedure usually suffices. After the procedure has been completed, the loop is removed under direct laparoscopic visualisation to ensure complete haemostasis. When significant continuous bleeding from the abdominal wall occurs, haemostasis can be accomplished either by pressure or by suturing the bleeding site. Pressure can be applied using a Foley balloon catheter. The catheter is introduced into the abdominal cavity through the bleeding trocar site wound, the balloon is inflated and traction is placed on the catheter, which is bolstered in place to keep it under tension. The catheter is left *in situ* for 24 hours and then removed. Although this method is successful in achieving haemostasis, the authors favour direct suturing of the bleeding vessel. This manoeuvre is accomplished by extending the skin incision by 3 mm at both ends of the bleeding trocar site wound. Two figure-of-eight sutures are placed in the path of the vessel at both ends of the wound. Devices such as the EndoClose may also be used to apply transabdominal sutures under direct laparoscopic view to close port sites that bleed.

EVACUATION OF BLOOD CLOTS

The best way of dealing with blood clots is to avoid them. As mentioned, careful dissection and identification of the cystic artery and its branches, as well as identifying and carrying out dissection of the gallbladder in the correct plane, help to prevent bleeding from the cystic vessels and the hepatic bed. Nevertheless, clot formation takes place when unsuspected bleeding occurs or when inflammation is severe and a clear plane is not present between the gallbladder and the hepatic bed. The routine use of 5000–7000 units of heparin per litre of irrigation fluid helps to avoid the formation of clots. When extra bleeding is foreseen, a small pool of irrigation fluid can be kept in the operative field to prevent clot formation. After clots have formed, a large bore suction device should be used for their retrieval. Care should be taken to avoid suctioning in proximity to placed clips.

Principles of electrosurgery during laparoscopic surgery

Electrosurgical injuries during laparoscopy are potentially serious. The vast majority occur following the use of monopolar diathermy. The overall incidence is between one and two cases per 1000 operations. Electrical injuries are usually unrecognised at the time that they occur, with patients commonly presenting 3–7 days after injury with complaints of fever and abdominal pain. As these injuries usually present late, the reasons for their occurrence are largely speculative. The main theories are: (1) inadvertent touching or grasping of tissue during current application; (2) direct coupling between a portion of bowel and a metal instrument that is touching the activated probe (**Figure 8.6**); (3) insulation breaks in the electrodes; (4) direct sparking to bowel from the diathermy probe; and (5) current passage to the bowel from recently coagulated, electrically isolated tissue. Bipolar diathermy is safer and should be used in preference to monopolar diathermy, especially in anatomically crowded areas. If monopolar diathermy is to be used, important safety measures include attainment of a perfect visual image, avoiding excessive current application and meticulous attention to insulation. Alternative methods of performing dissection, such as the use of ultrasonic devices, may improve safety.

POSTOPERATIVE CARE

The postoperative care of patients after laparoscopic surgery is generally straightforward, with a low incidence of pain or other problems. The most common routine postoperative symptoms are a dull upper abdominal pain, nausea and pain

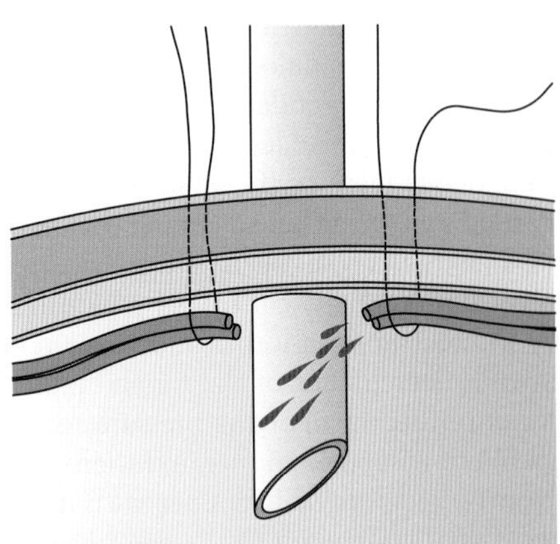

Figure 8.5 Management of bleeding from a surgical trocar site.

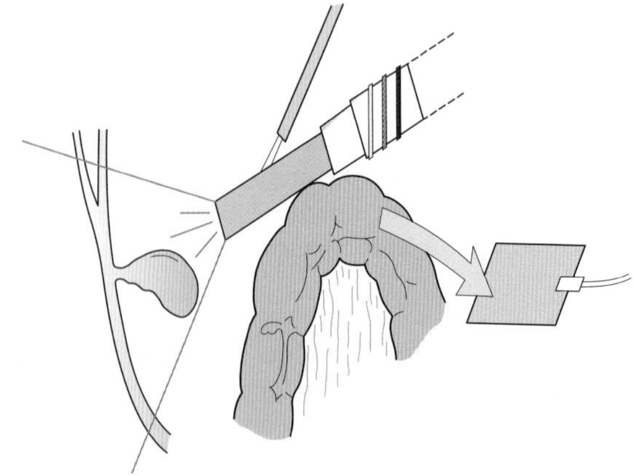

Figure 8.6 Direct coupling between bowel and laparoscope, which is touching the activated probe.

Frederic Eugene Basil Foley, 1891–1966, urologist, Ankher Hospital, St Paul, MN, USA.

around the shoulders (referred from the diaphragm). There has been some suggestion that the instillation of local anaesthetic to the operating site and into the suprahepatic space, or even leaving 1 litre of normal saline in the peritoneum, serves to decrease postoperative pain. It is a good general rule that if the patient develops a fever or tachycardia, or complains of severe pain at the operation site, something is wrong and close observation is necessary. In this case, routine investigation should include a full blood count, C reactive protein (CRP) measurement, liver function tests, an amylase test and, probably, an ultrasound scan of the upper abdomen to detect fluid collections. If bile duct leakage is suspected, endoscopic retrograde cholangiopancreatography (ERCP) may be needed. If in doubt, relaparoscopy or laparotomy should be performed earlier rather than later. Death following technical errors in laparoscopic cholecystectomy has often been associated with a long delay in deciding to re-explore the abdomen.

In the absence of problems, patients should be fit for discharge within 24 hours. They should be given instructions to telephone the unit or their general practitioner and to return to the hospital if they are not making satisfactory progress.

Nausea

About half of patients experience some degree of nausea after laparoscopic surgery and, rarely, this may be severe. It usually responds to an antiemetic, such as ondansetron, and settles within 12–24 hours. It is made worse by opiate analgesics and these should be avoided.

Shoulder tip pain

The patient should be warned about this preoperatively and told that the pain is referred from the diaphragm and not due to a local problem in the shoulders. It can be at its worst 24 hours after the operation. It usually settles within 2–3 days and is relieved by simple analgesics, such as paracetamol.

Abdominal pain

Pain in one or other of the port site wounds is not uncommon and is worse if there is haematoma formation. It usually settles very rapidly. Increasing pain after 2–3 days may be a sign of infection and, with concomitant signs, antibiotic therapy is occasionally required. Occasionally, herniation through a port may account for localised pain and this can sometimes be due to a Richter's hernia, such that the patient exhibits no sign of intestinal obstruction. Successful laparoscopic surgery should not cause a patient increasing or undue pain. If there are any clinical concerns postoperatively due to worsening pain, tachycardia and or pyrexia, senior review with a view to imaging, or increasingly commonly relaparoscopy, should be considered.

Analgesia

A 100-mg diclofenac suppository may be given at the time of the operation (if this medication is not contraindicated). It is important that the patient provides separate consent for this if the suppository is to be administered peroperatively. Suppositories may be administered a further two or three times postoperatively for relief of more severe pain. Otherwise, 500–1000 mg of paracetamol 4-hourly usually suffices (orally or, if more pain, intravenously). Opiate analgesics cause nausea and should be avoided unless the pain is very severe. In this case, suspect a postoperative complication (as above). The majority of patients require between one and four doses of 1 g of paracetamol postoperatively. Severe pain after routine laparoscopic cases should warn the clinician that there may be an iatrogenic or surgical cause of this pain that may need further investigation with blood tests, imaging and even relaparoscopy

Orogastric tube

An orogastric tube may be placed during the operation if the stomach is distended and obscuring the view. It is not necessary in all cases. It should be removed as soon as the operation is over and before the patient regains consciousness. This is more routinely used in bariatrics and oesophagogastric surgery, where a larger (32F or 34F) tube is used.

Oral fluids

There is no significant ileus after laparoscopic surgery, except in resectional procedures, such as colectomy or small bowel resection. Patients can start taking oral fluids as soon as they are conscious; they usually do so 4–6 hours after the end of the operation.

Oral feeding

Provided that the patient has an appetite, a light meal can be taken 4–6 hours after the operation. Some patients remain slightly nauseated at this stage, but almost all eat a normal breakfast on the morning after the operation.

Patients will require advice about what they can eat at home. They should be told that they can eat a normal diet but should avoid excess. It seems sensible to avoid high-fat meals for the first week, although there is no clear evidence that this is necessary.

Urinary catheter

This depends on the operation. If a urinary catheter has been placed in the bladder during an operation with likely short stay, it should be removed before the patient regains consciousness if the procedure has proceeded well. The patient should be warned of the possibility and symptoms of postoperative cystitis and told to ask advice in the unlikely event of this occurring.

Drains

The use of postoperative drains in laparoscopy patients depends on the operation performed. Drains are used to assess postoperative blood loss if this is a clinical concern or to assess the nature of intraperitoneal fluids, depending on procedure and postoperative monitoring needs. Some surgeons drain the abdomen at the end of laparoscopic cholecystectomy, although this is controversial. If a drain is placed to vent the remaining gas and peritoneal fluid, it should be removed within 1 hour of the operation. If it has been placed because of excessive hepatic bleeding or bile leakage it should be removed when that problem has resolved, usually after 12–24 hours. Continued blood loss from a drain is an indication for re-exploration of the abdomen.

Summary box 8.4

Surgical principles

- Meticulous care in the creation of a pneumoperitoneum
- Controlled dissection of adhesions
- Adequate exposure of operative field
- Avoidance and control of bleeding
- Avoidance of organ injury
- Avoidance of diathermy damage
- Vigilance in the postoperative period

DISCHARGE FROM HOSPITAL

Patient discharge is based on clinical indicators and their fitness for recuperating in a non-hospital environment. One of the core drivers for the application of minimally invasive surgery is an earlier recovery and therefore discharge from hospital. For the common laparoscopic procedure of cholecystectomy, most surgeons discharge a significant proportion of their laparoscopic cholecystectomy patients on the day of surgery, but some are kept in overnight and discharged the following morning. Patients should not be discharged until they are seen to be comfortable, have passed urine and are eating and drinking satisfactorily. They should be told that if they develop abdominal pain or other severe symptoms they should return to the hospital or to their general practitioner. Even for more major cases, including procedures such as laparoscopic anterior resection, some units have demonstrated a safe and feasible protocol for a 23-hour stay.

Skin sutures

If non-absorbable sutures or skin staples have been used, they can be removed from the port sites after 7 days.

Mobility and convalescence

Patients can get out of bed to go to the toilet as soon as they have recovered from the anaesthetic and they should be encouraged to do so. Such movements are remarkably pain free when compared with the mobility achieved after an open operation. Similarly, patients can cough actively and clear bronchial secretions, and this helps to diminish the incidence of chest infections. Many patients are able to walk out of hospital on the evening of their operation and almost all are fully mobile by the following morning. Thereafter, the postoperative recovery is variable. Some patients prefer to take things quietly for the first 2–3 days, interspersing increasing exercise with rest. After the third day, patients will have undertaken increasing amounts of activity. The average return to work is about 10 days.

THE PRINCIPLES OF COMMON LAPAROSCOPIC PROCEDURES

The principles of common laparoscopic procedures are described in the appropriate chapters:

- laparoscopic cholecystectomy (Chapter 67);
- laparoscopic inguinal hernia repair (Chapter 60);
- laparoscopic antireflux surgery (Chapter 63);
- laparoscopic appendicectomy (Chapter 72);
- laparoscopic bariatric surgery (Chapter 64);
- laparoscopic colectomy/anterior resection (Chapters 70 and 73);
- laparoscopic upper gastrointestinal (GI) surgery (Chapters 62, 63 and 69)

Other elective minimally invasive (laparoscopic, thoracoscopic) or robotic procedures that are now widely utilised in certain specialist centres include:

- colectomy;
- gastrectomy;
- splenectomy;
- nephrectomy;
- adrenalectomy;
- prostatectomy (typically robotic);
- thyroid and parathyroid surgery;
- aortic aneurysm surgery;
- single-vessel coronary artery bypass surgery;
- video-assisted thorascopic surgery (VATS);
- laparoscopic hernia surgery (inguinal, femoral, paraumbilical, incisional).

Laparoscopy has also been used in certain emergency situations (in stable patients) in the hands of experienced laparoscopic surgeons. These include laparoscopic appendicectomy (typically the most common minimally invasive emergency procedure), repair of a perforated duodenal ulcer, laparoscopic cholecystectomy in severe cholecystitis (so-called 'hot' cholecystectomies), and treatment of intestinal obstruction secondary to adhesions, strangulated hernia repairs and, also, the laparoscopic evaluation of stable trauma patients.

Procedures that have been carried out using robotically assisted minimally invasive surgery include all of those listed above. Currently, robotic surgery still has certain disadvantages:

- increased cost;
- increased set up of the system and operating time;
- socioeconomic implications;
- significant risk of conversion to conventional techniques;
- prolonged learning curve;
- multiple repositioning of the arms can cause trauma;
- haemostasis;
- collision of the robotic arms in extreme positions.

Until these are overcome, by continued development of the technology and the drive of surgeons to progress in the field, robotically assisted surgery will not be commonplace. However, the potential for such systems is immense and continued research and clinical trials will pave the way for future generations of surgeons and patients alike.

FURTHER DEVELOPMENTS THAT HAVE MADE MINIMALLY INVASIVE SURGERY EVEN LESS INVASIVE

Single incision laparoscopic surgery

Laparoscopy has reduced the trauma from surgery, compared with open techniques, and is now used routinely for benign and oncological surgery in many centres. However, there is continued work on how to reduce the trauma and scarring from the incisions used in laparoscopic surgery because multiple port sites are needed for most procedures. Natural orifice transluminal endoscopic surgery (NOTES) (see below) addresses this but, at present, the safety of the transgastric route is not sufficient for the routine use of this approach to surgery. Advanced laparoscopists have therefore turned to focussing on the single incision for open entry via the umbilicus as an alternative. Single incision laparoscopic surgery (SILS) is a technique adopted by some surgeons to insert all the instrumentation via a single incision, through a multiple channel port via the umbilicus, to carry out the procedure. The benefit is that only one incision, through a natural scar (the umbilicus), is made, therefore these procedures are virtually 'scarless'. Second, the use of fewer port sites around the abdomen gives the potential for less pain, less risk of port site bleeding and reduced incidence of port site hernia. This technique has many other synonyms, including laparoendoscopic single site surgery (LESS) and single port access (SPA) surgery among many others, although SILS has gained the most recognition. It does require specially manufactured multichannel ports and often roticulating instruments. There has been an explosion of activity in SILS procedures in the last few years and, in some units, laparoscopic cholecystectomies and hernias are routinely started as SILS cases. The clinical benefit and cost-effectiveness of this technique, which has a difficult and steep learning curve and specific instrument requirements, remain under review, although it has been adopted as a routine approach for some procedures in some units. Early evidence understandably demonstrated better cosmetic outcomes and less pain in the immediate postoperative period; however, this needs to be further corroborated with higher levels of evidence with longer-term follow-up results. Specifically, because the SILS approach was not designed for improving clinical outcomes when compared with standard minimally invasive approaches, any improvements in pain and cosmesis between SILS and standard minimally invasive approaches require further elucidation.

Natural orifice translumenal endoscopic surgery (NOTES)

This technique, whereby surgeons enter the peritoneal cavity via endoscopic puncture of a hollow viscus, has been much publicised in recent years. The NOTES approach has been utilised in nearly every body system and operative speciality addressing the pelvis, abdomen and thorax. Worldwide adoption rates compared to standard open and minimally invasive approaches remain very low. Transvaginal NOTES cholecystectomies have been performed in humans successfully, although hybrid procedures (joint laparoscopy and NOTES) are still employed regularly for safety reasons. The closure of the visceral puncture site is the issue that has prevented widespread uptake of this technique, as transgastric and transcolonic closure of peritoneal entry sites in a routinely safe way remains unperfected for general use. Also, the equipment needed has significant cost and training needs (including surgeons and a large variety of ancillary team members that range from scrub nurses to anaesthetists) and requires a large number of practitioners in the team at present. Nevertheless, it has much promise to be a technique for truly scarless surgery in the future and much research continues in this field, which is less widely adopted at present than SILS.

THE FUTURE

Although there is no doubt that minimal access surgery has changed the practice of surgeons, it has not changed the nature of disease. The basic principles of good surgery still apply, including appropriate case selection, excellent exposure, adequate retraction and a high level of technical expertise. If a procedure makes no sense with conventional access, it will make no sense with a laparoscopic approach. Laparoscopic and robotic surgery training is key to allow the specialty to progress. The pioneers of yesterday have to teach the surgeons of tomorrow not only the technical and dextrous skills required, but also the decision-making and innovative skills necessary for the field to continue to evolve. Training is often perceived as difficult, as trainers have less control over the trainees at the time of surgery and caseloads may be smaller, especially in centres where laparoscopic and robotic procedures are not common. However, trainees now rightly expect exposure to these procedures, and training systems should be adaptable for international exposure so that these techniques can be disseminated worldwide. The predominant video and digital component of these new techniques opens the door for simulation approaches for training in these modalities, which has demonstrated benefits in reducing learning curves and in turn is aimed at improving patient outcomes. The ultimate goal for this educational approach is to develop expert surgeons through the 'totally safe' and 'risk free' environment of simulation before they actually have to operate on patients. The current status for laparoscopic trainees reflects their decreased experience in open approaches so that they feel less comfortable converting cases such as laparoscopic cholecystectomies to open cases. It is important that the 'straight to minimally invasive' trainees continue to have training in open skills so that they can apply both approaches where necessary.

Improvements in instrumentation, the continued progress of robotic surgery and the development of structured training programmes are key to the future of minimal access surgery. The use of robots in surgery has increased dramatically in the last decade. Indeed, robots are now available not only for assisting in surgery, but also for aiding in the perioperative management of surgical patients. The remote presence systems (In Touch Health, Santa Barbara, CA, USA) allow clinicians to assess patients in real time and interact with them while they are not on site or even on a different continent. Applying established devices in different contexts also offers the introduction of innovation; for example, the LABEL procedure (Laser Assisted Bile duct Exploration by Laparoendoscopy for choledocholithiasis) was developed when the concept of laser stone management in urology was applied to laparoscopic biliary tree surgery. Continued advances in related technologies, such as computer science, will allow the incorporation of augmented reality systems alongside robotic systems to enhance surgical precision in image-guided surgery. Endoluminal robotic surgery remains in its infancy, but systems are being developed that will enable navigation within the colon to allow surgery on lesions in spaces that are accessible from the outside without an exterior incision being made. The advent of nanotechnology should also bring about much change in surgery. Miniaturisation may be possible, potentially allowing surgery at a cellular level to be carried out.

At present, work has already started on single-port laparoscopy (see above under Single incision laparoscopic surgery), in which a single port may act as a camera and have unfolding instruments that open up once they are inside the peritoneum to perform the surgery, therefore reducing the number of port sites needed. Extensive research is also being carried out in the field of NOTES. Minimising the potential contamination of the peritoneum and the ability to carry out a safe closure of the peritoneal entry site are the main technical challenges of this type of minimally invasive and essentially 'scarless' or 'incisionless' surgery. It is certain that there is much that is new in minimal access surgery. Only time will tell how much of what is new is truly better.

Specifically, the future evolution of robotic systems includes full integration with next generation technologies such as advanced augmented reality, autobionics, neuromorphic visual processing and real-time diagnostics and theranostics, exemplified by the i-Knife (real-time tissue metabolic profiling and tissue-level diagnosis, developed by Zoltan Takats at Imperial College London). Large master–slave constructions with multiple arms are likely to give way to flexible access bio-inspired (FAB) systems. These will probably offer full robotic arm articulation in much more portable devices with low energy needs. They would be totally modular with integrated imaging and would have platforms to offer multipurpose usage to increase utilisation and cost efficiency. These systems would also result in a smaller physical footprint, with cheaper devices offering more utility, precision and dexterity on platforms that allow both master–slave and direct functionality.

One major obstacle in minimally invasive technology includes the 'Achilles heel' of cost efficiency and device financing in an increasingly rationed global healthcare environment; this is an issue which will require surgical liaison with hospital management and national policy providers. Surgeons need to continue to have a dialogue, discussing their experiences and ideas regarding all the minimally invasive approaches. None of these techniques needs to exist in isolation. The future can offer hybridisation of these approaches, including a vast array of possibilities such as Robotic-SILS, Robotic-NOTES or even endoscopic NOTES-augmented SILS (endoscopes passed through a SILS port). Such cross-fertilisation can offer new innovation and techniques; thus, harvesting the advantages of newer procedures and discarding the individual weaknesses of others can ultimately improve patient outcomes and results.

> The cleaner and gentler the act of operation, the less the patient suffers, the smoother and quicker his convalescence, the more exquisite his healed wound.
>
> Berkeley George Andrew Moynihan (1920)

FURTHER READING

Acharya MN, Ashrafian H, Athanasiou T, Casula R. Is totally endoscopic coronary artery bypass safe, feasible and effective? *Interact Cardiovasc Thorac Surg* 2012; **15**(6): 1040–6.

Antonakis PT, Ashrafian H, Isla AM. Laparoscopic gastric surgery for cancer: where do we stand? *World J Gastroenterol* 2014; **20**(39): 14280–91.

Ashrafian H, Darzi A, Athanasiou T. Autobionics: a new paradigm in regenerative medicine and surgery. *Regen Med* 2010; **5**(2): 279–88.

Ashrafian H, Navarro-Sanchez A, Athanasiou T, Sherman DI, Isla A. Thoracoscopic esophageal repair of a spontaneous Barrett's ulcer perforation. *Ann Thorac Surg* 2015; **99**(1): 331–3.

Athanasiou T, Ashrafian H, Rao C, Yang GZ, Darzi A. The tipping point of robotic surgery in healthcare: from master–slave to flexible access bio-inspired platforms. *Surg Technol Int* 2011; **21**: 28–34.

Athanasiou T, Ashrafian H, Rowland SP, Casula R. Robotic cardiac surgery: advanced minimally invasive technology hindered by barriers to adoption. *Future Cardiol* 2011; **7**(4): 511–22.

Hoeckelmann M, Rudas IJ, Fiorini P, Kirchner F, Haidegger T. Current capabilities and development potential in surgical robotics. *Int J Adv Robot Syst* 2015; 12.

Navarro-Sanchez A, Ashrafian H, Laliotis A, Qurashi K, Martinez-Isla A. Single-stage laparoscopic management of acute gallstone pancreatitis: outcomes at different timings. *Hepatobiliary Pancreat Dis Int* 2016; **15**(3): 297–301.

Navarro-Sanchez A, Ashrafian H, Segura-Sampedro JJ, Martinez-Isla A. LABEL procedure: laser-assisted bile duct exploration by laparoendoscopy for choledocholithiasis: improving surgical outcomes and reducing technical failure. *Surg Endosc* 2017; **31**(5): 2103–8.

Tan A, Ashrafian H, Scott AJ *et al.* Robotic surgery: disruptive innovation or unfulfilled promise? A systematic review and meta-analysis of the first 30 years. *Surg Endosc* 2016; **30**(10): 4330–52.

Bailey & Love Bailey & Love Bailey & Love
Bailey & Love Bailey & Love Bai Chapter 9 ve

Principles of paediatric surgery

Learning objectives

At the end of this chapter, you will be able to:

- Describe clinically important differences between adults and children
- Explain the principles of trauma management in children
- Safely prescribe perioperative fluids in children
- Avoid the pitfalls that often delay the diagnosis of common emergency conditions
- Outline some congenital malformations managed by neonatal surgeons that may present later to general surgeons
- Recognise common safeguarding issues in children and know how to proceed if abuse is suspected

INTRODUCTION

Premature and term neonates differ in their anatomy, physiology, neurology, psychology, pathology and pharmacology, just as infants differ from school-age children and adolescents from adults. These differences underpin the principles of paediatric surgery. As you progress through this chapter and consider children of different ages (*Table 9.1*) you should make your own list of differences and their clinical implications; a few examples appear in *Table 9.2* and in **Figure 9.1** to get you started.

Paediatric surgeons study developmental biology and teratology but because some anomalies first present to adult services (e.g. duplications, malrotation) this knowledge can help adult surgeons. Adult services also need to cater for the transitional needs of those graduating to adulthood, sometimes after complex paediatric surgical care. Most children escape the comorbidities of degenerative diseases but no longer are they free from lifestyle problems. Paediatric bariatric surgery is now developing in a multidisciplinary context with psychologists, dieticians and gastroenterologists.

TABLE 9.1 Common terms.

Preterm	<37 completed weeks of gestation
Full term	Between 37 and 42 completed weeks of gestation
Neonate	Newborn baby up to 28 days after the estimated date of delivery (EDD)
Infant	Up to 1 year of age
Child	All ages up to 16 years (minimum school leaving age), divided into preschool child (usually <5 years), child and adolescent (puberty up to 16 years).
Young person	A popular term referring to anyone under 18 years

TABLE 9.2 Some example differences between adults and children.

Facts	Infants and small children have a wide abdomen, a broad costal margin and a shallow pelvis
	The edge of the liver comes below the costal margin and the bladder is largely intra-abdominal
	The ribs are more horizontal and are flexible
	The umbilicus is relatively low lying
Implications	Transverse supraumbilical incisions give greater access than vertical midline ones for open surgery
	Trauma (including surgical access) can easily damage the liver or bladder
	The geometry of the ribs means that ventilation requires greater diaphragmatic movement. Their flexibility means that rib fractures are rare and often a sign of abuse
	A stoma in the lower abdomen of a neonate must be carefully sited for its bag not to interfere with the umbilicus

We start with three important areas: thermoregulation, airway and fluid management, and then outline trauma, some common problems in older children, a collection of neonatal surgical conditions, oncology and conclude with safeguarding.

MAINTAINING TEMPERATURE

In comparison with older children, infants have less subcutaneous fat, immature vasomotor control, greater heat loss from

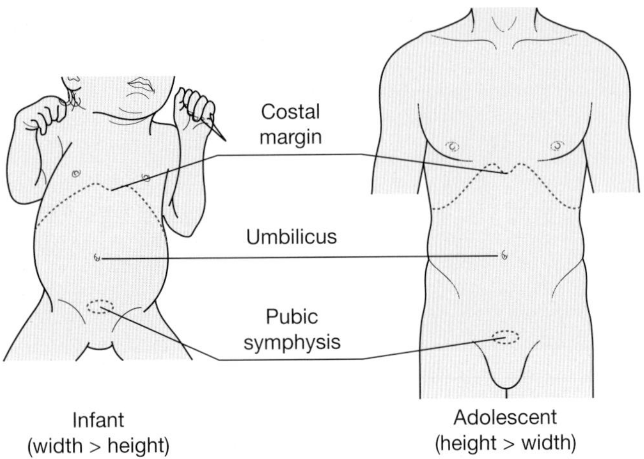

Figure 9.1 Topographical differences in the abdomen.

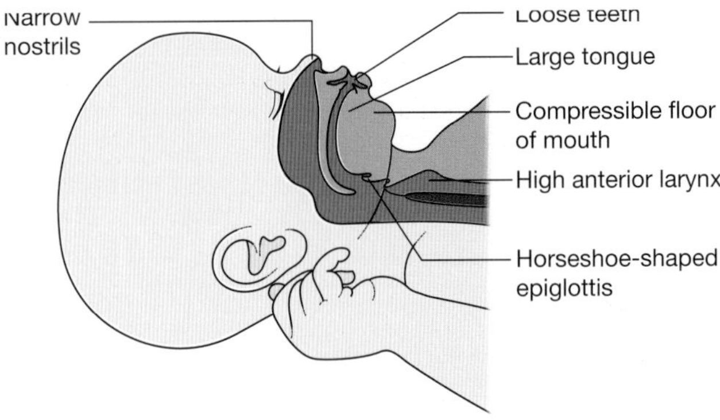

Figure 9.2 Summary of upper airway anatomy in an infant.

pulmonary evaporation and their surface area to weight ratio is higher. Consider these when managing sick children in the Emergency Department, anaesthetic room or theatre. These environments must be warm and the infant's head (20% of surface area, cf. 9% in an adult) should be insulated. Infusions are warmed and respiratory gases both warmed and humidified. Core temperature is monitored and safe direct warming is needed for lengthy operations.

AIRWAY

Anatomical differences in the airway have clinical implications (see **Figure 9.2**). The infant's large head and short neck predispose to flexion. The large tongue can obstruct the airway when the infant is unconscious and impede the airway and laryngoscopy. The epiglottis projects posteriorly and the larynx is high; a straight-bladed laryngoscope is favoured in those under 1 year of age. Uncuffed tubes are preferred as the cricoid ring is the narrowest region (cf. the larynx in an adult) and this is covered in loose epithelium that is easily irritated; damage can result in subglottic stenosis.

PERIOPERATIVE FLUIDS IN CHILDREN

Before prescribing fluids (or drugs), it is important to know the child's weight, their vital signs and their fluid and electrolyte requirements and consider these in relation to normal values and ranges (see *Table 9.3*). Dehydration is difficult to assess: moderate dehydration (5% loss of total body water) may manifest in poor urine output, dry mouth, and sunken eyes and fontanelle; severe dehydration (>10%) in decreased skin turgor, drowsiness, tachycardia and poor capillary refill (>2 seconds) and signs of hypovolaemia.

Children develop hyponatraemic encephalopathy at higher sodium levels than adults because they have a higher brain:skull ratio. A few children have had symptomatic hyponatraemic encephalopathy attributable to poor prescription and monitoring of fluids; some have died and others have permanent neurological disability. Problems have arisen when: (1) hypotonic maintenance fluids (e.g. 0.18% saline) have been inappropriately given to resuscitate or replace loses, or (2) maintenance fluids have been given in excess (3–5 times requirements).

UK National Guidelines are that maintenance fluid administration should contain sodium levels of 131–154 mmol/L.

TABLE 9.3 Basic paediatric data.

(a) Weight

Age	Weight (kg)
Term neonate	3.5
1 year	10
5 years	20
10 years	30

(b) Vital signs

Age (years)	Heart rate (bpm)	Systolic blood pressure (mmHg)	Respiratory rate (b/min)
<1	110–160	70–90	30–40
2–5	90–140	80–100	25–30
5–12	80–120	90–110	20–25

(c) Maintenance fluid requirements

Weight	Daily fluid requirement (mL/kg/day)	mL/kg/hour
Neonate	120–150	5
First 10 kg	100	4
Second 10 kg	50	2
Each subsequent kg	20	1

(d) Maintenance electrolyte requirements

Weight	Sodium (mmol/kg/day)	Potassium (mmol/kg/day)	Energy (kcal/kg/day)
<10 kg	2–4	1.5–2.5	110
>10 kg	1–2	0.5–1.0	40–75

Approximate guide: weight (kg) = 2 × (age in years +4), or use a Broselow tape which estimates the weight from the height.
Systolic blood pressure = 80 + (age in years × 2) mmHg.
Circulating blood volume = 80 mL/kg (90 mL/kg in infants).

Learning objectives for this section are to:

- Know the four reasons for giving intravenous (IV) fluids.
- Be able to calculate fluid rates for children of different weights (see *Table 9.3*).
- Understand the risks of low-sodium containing fluids.
- Understand how the body's response to stress and illness affects fluid balance.
- Know how to recognise and manage hyponatraemia (<135 mmol/L).

Tonicity and osmolarity

The term 'isotonic' is now considered in relation to the tonicity of the electrolyte components of fluids. Thus, isosmolar fluids, such as 0.18% saline with 4% glucose, and hyperosmolar fluids, such as 0.45% saline with 5% glucose, are now considered hypotonic because the glucose is ignored.

Prescribing intravenous fluids.

The four reasons for prescribing fluids are detailed in *Summary box 9.1*. The body's response to stress is to hold on to water, which can promote hyponatraemia. The stresses that drive the non-osmotic retention of water include trauma, head injury, chest infections and the postoperative state. Restricting maintenance fluids to 70% can be appropriate for 24 hours after major surgery. In sick patients, raising the maintenance rate is best guided by the trend in daily electrolyte levels. Urine output often decreases after major surgery without morbidity but a common response can be to increase maintenance fluids inappropriately, leading to hyponatraemia. A postoperative bolus of fluid is appropriate if there is hypovolaemia, hypotension or poor peripheral perfusion but giving it simply because urine output is low can be inappropriate.

Hyponatraemia in the surgical patient is usually a consequence of too much free water and not of insufficient sodium. If mild and asymptomatic (e.g. 135 mmol/L) then fluid restriction is appropriate. If symptomatic with headache, lethargy or seizures and the Na concentration is <125 mmol/L a rapid infusion of 3% hypertonic saline (1 mL/kg over 15 minutes) is needed and paediatric intensive care unit (PICU) admission is required.

Summary box 9.1

Fluids in children

Fluids are given intravenously for four reasons:

- Circulatory support in resuscitating vascular collapse

0.9% saline blood 4.5% albumin colloid	Given as a bolus of 10 or 20 mL/kg over periods up to 20 minutes with close monitoring of the response. Can be repeated up to 40 mL/kg then seek urgent help

- Replacement of previous fluid and electrolyte deficits

0.9% saline + 0.15% KCl Hartmann's solution	Given over a longer period (up to 48 hours) with clinical and biochemical review

- Replacement of ongoing losses

0.9% saline + 0.15% KCl Hartmann's solution	Or a fluid tailored to the losses e.g. 4.5% albumin if protein loss is great. Replace losses mL for mL

- Maintenance outside neonatal period

Plasmalyte 148 Hartmann's ± glucose 0.9% saline + 0.15% KCl ± glucose	Hypotonic 0.18% saline should not be used outside the neonatal period

- Maintenance in the neonate

  In **term** neonates in the first 48 hours of life 10% glucose at 60 mL/kg/day

  Sodium 0.18% and potassium 0.15% are added on day 2

  From day 3 around 4–5 mL/kg/hour or 100–120 mL/kg/day

  Preterm babies or those <2 kg may require 180 mL/kg/day of fluid

  Consider impaired gluconeogenesis: monitor and keep glucose above 2.6 mmol/L

HISTORY AND EXAMINATION

Time, patience and a genuine interest help establish a good rapport with the child and their parents or carers. An opportunistic rather than a systematic approach to the history and examination may be needed but appropriate areas must be covered. Do not forget to explore perinatal problems and the family and social background. Children should be told what to expect from an examination, investigation or surgical procedure in terms that they can understand. Fear, anxiety and pain can be reduced by involving the parents and by looking after the child in an appropriate environment. For elective surgery a preadmission service and anaesthetic review should be considered, with general health concerns being redirected to a paediatrician. Consent for surgery in the young child is obtained from someone with parental responsibility.

OPERATIVE SURGERY

A well-prepared patient who has not been excessively fasted, with appropriate consent, is anaesthetised in a child-friendly anaesthetic room. Surgery benefits from meticulous and gentle technique, strict haemostasis, fine suture materials and magnification. Basic principles apply: maintaining well-vascularised tissues, avoiding tension, minimising tissue necrosis and contamination. The intestine can be anastomosed with single-layer interrupted or continuous extramucosal sutures. Abdominal wounds are closed with absorbable sutures using a layered or a mass closure. Wound dehiscence is rare and usually the result of poor technique. Clean skin incisions are best closed with absorbable subcuticular sutures. Endoscopic minimally invasive approaches can be used at all ages with instruments and insufflation pressures tailored to the size of the child. Postoperatively, children recover swiftly. Analgesia must be adequate and appropriate, recognising the potential for respiratory depression with opioids. Appropriately trained staff monitor the airway, vital signs, oxygen saturation, fluid balance, temperature, pain control and glucose levels during recovery.

Summary box 9.2

Fasting instructions

- Two hours for clear fluids
- Four hours for breast milk
- Six hours for solids

Summary box 9.3

Surgical technique in children

- Gentle tissue handling
- Abdominal incisions can be closed with absorbable sutures
- Bowel can be anastomosed with interrupted or continuous single-layer extramucosal sutures
- Skin can be closed with absorbable subcuticular sutures or glue

Stomas are necessary in some children. A gastrostomy may be required for nutritional support, particularly in the neurologically disabled child (often with a fundoplication). Temporary intestinal stomas are used in the management of anorectal malformations, necrotising enterocolitis and Hirschsprung's disease. Infants with a proximal stoma and high losses frequently require salt or bicarbonate supplements to avoid deficits, which can cause poor weight gain and acidosis. Ileostomies and colostomies are usually spouted but mucous fistulas may be flush.

The long-term outcomes of paediatric surgical conditions should be considered. For example, ileal resection in the neonate may later be complicated by vitamin B12 deficiency, malabsorption of fat-soluble vitamins, gallstones, renal oxalate stones and perianastomotic ulceration. Long-term concerns with other treated anomalies include the impact on continence, fertility, sexual activity, psychosocial adaptation and the potential risk of late malignancy (e.g. undescended testis, choledochal cyst, duplication cysts, oesophageal atresia).

PAEDIATRIC TRAUMA

Trauma remains a leading cause of avoidable death in children and adolescents worldwide. Surgeons should attend the Advanced Trauma Life Support (ATLS) programme which covers trauma in children. Some of the important differences for children follow:

- Avoid overextension of the neck which can obstruct the airway.
- Use a Broselow tape if the weight is not known.
- Blood pressure is often normal until >25% of the circulating blood volume is lost.
- Cardiorespiratory arrest is usually due to hypoxia and not vascular disease.
- Non-operative management is often possible for splenic and liver injuries.

Resuscitation

For fluids see *Summary box 9.1*. High-flow oxygen is required if there is cardiorespiratory compromise, and endotracheal intubation and ventilation are required if oxygenation is inadequate, to control a flail chest or in children with a serious head injury (Glasgow Coma Scale score ≤8). Seriously injured children require two large peripheral intravenous cannulae. The following veins can be used: long saphenous at the ankle, femoral, external jugular and, in babies, scalp veins. Central venous access should only be attempted by an expert. Intraosseous infusion, however, is straightforward and particularly useful in children (**Figure 9.3**).

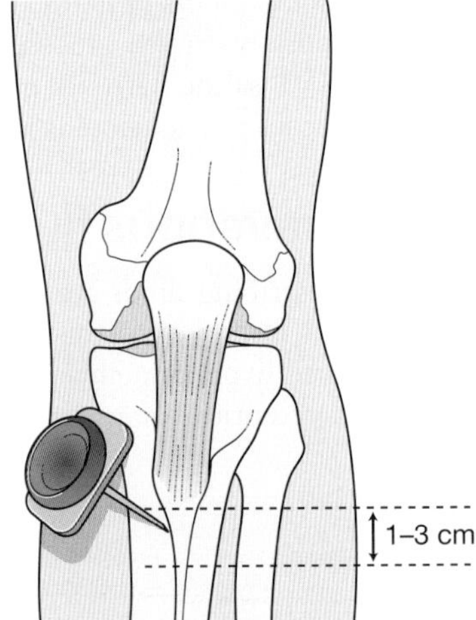

Figure 9.3 The intraosseous needle is inserted into the medullary cavity of the proximal tibia about 1–3 cm below the tibial tuberosity.

A major spinal cord injury can be present in a child without radiographic abnormalities. After major trauma, a cervical spine injury should be assumed and the neck immobilised until cross sectional imaging 'clears' the spine. Other considerations include intravenous analgesia and, in the unconscious or ventilated child or those with major abdominal injuries, a nasogastric tube (orogastric if there is suspicion of a basal frontal skull fracture) and a urethral catheter (if no evidence of a urethral injury).

Secondary survey and emergency management

Chest trauma

Children have elastic ribs that rarely fracture but deformation causes lung contusions. A major thoracic injury may exist despite a normal chest radiograph. The airway is secured, oxygen is given and hypovolaemia is corrected. A tension pneumothorax should be suspected clinically before the chest x-ray (CXR) is requested and immediate needle thoracocentesis (second intercostal space, mid-clavicular line) performed. A chest drain is then placed (fifth intercostal space, mid-axillary

The **Glasgow Coma Scale** was introduced in 1977 by William Bryan Jennet, Professor of Neurosurgery, and Graham Michael Teasdale, a neurosurgeon at the University Department of Neurosurgery at the Institute of Neurological Sciences, The Southern General Hospital, Glasgow, UK. Professor Teasdale was later knighted and became President of the Royal College of Physicians and Surgeons of Glasgow.

line). Massive haemothorax needs a chest drain. Cardiac tamponade may follow blunt or penetrating injury and requires emergency subxyphoid needle pericardiocentesis. The role of emergency department thoracotomy (EDT) in major chest trauma in children remains controversial. Diaphragmatic rupture after blunt abdominal trauma is detected by chest radiography or computed tomography (CT) scan; surgical repair is undertaken once the patient is stable (**Figure 9.4**).

Abdomen

Blunt trauma is more common than penetrating trauma. The liver and spleen are more vulnerable in children, being less well protected by the rib cage. The abdomen is inspected for patterned bruising from seatbelts (**Figure 9.5**) or tyres. Compression will have been against the rigid skeleton. Intra-abdominal or intrathoracic bleeding should be considered promptly in the shocked child if external bleeding has not been profuse. Plasma amylase levels may be normal despite pancreatic injury (**Figure 9.6**).

Imaging

Focused assessment with sonography for trauma (FAST) looks for fluid in the perihepatic and hepatorenal space, the perisplenic area, the pelvis and the pericardium. It has a role in children but it does not detect solid organ injuries or replace CT. In the haemodynamically stable child a CT scan with IV contrast is required (**Figure 9.7**).

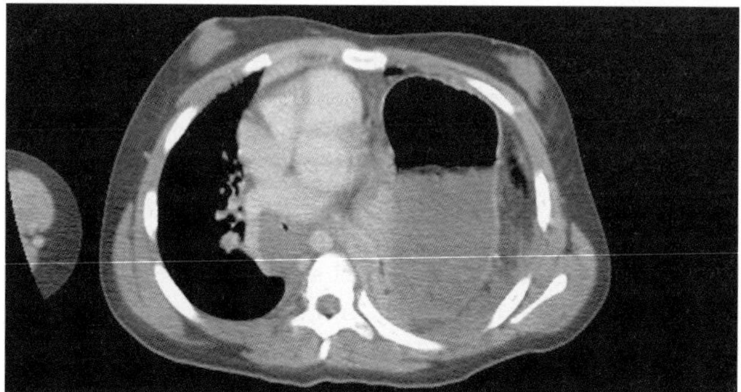

Figure 9.4 Traumatic diaphragmatic rupture.

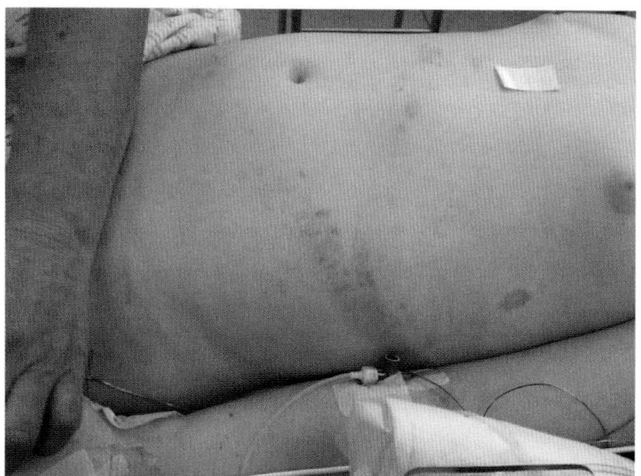

Figure 9.5 Bruises from a lap belt.

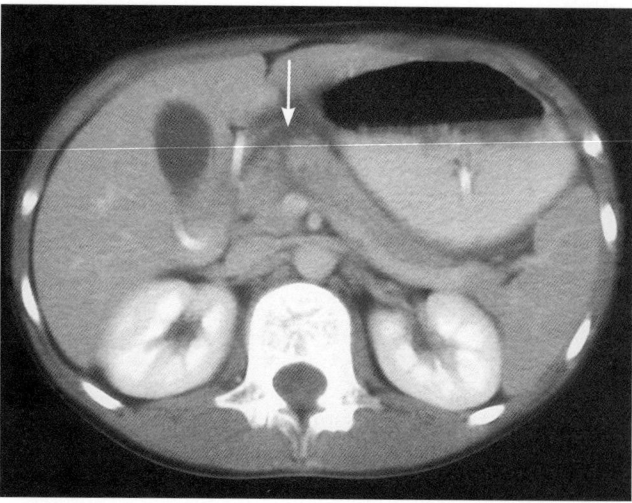

Figure 9.6 Abdominal computed tomographic scan showing a transection through the neck of the pancreas (arrow) from a bicycle handlebar injury.

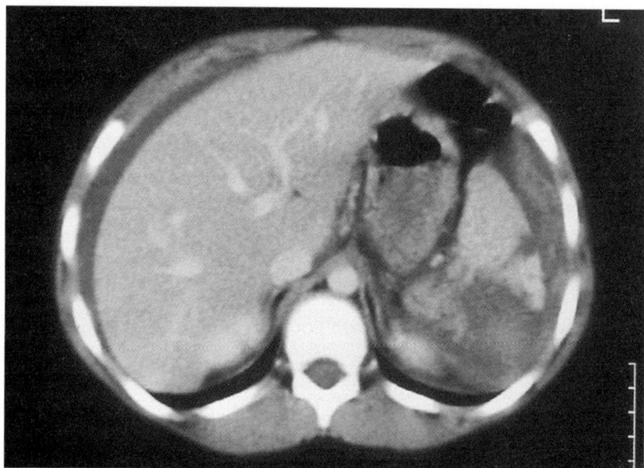

Figure 9.7 Abdominal computed tomographic scan after intravenous contrast in an 11-year-old boy showing a ruptured spleen (successfully managed non-operatively).

Bowel perforation or deep penetrating trauma requires a laparoscopy or laparotomy. Isolated blunt splenic and/or liver injuries identified on a CT scan can be safely and effectively managed non-operatively in the majority of children, so avoiding surgery and the long-term risks of splenectomy (infection from encapsulated bacteria *Streptococcus pneumoniae*, *Haemophilus influenzae* and *Neisseria meningitidis*).

Summary box 9.4

Successful non-operative management of isolated blunt liver or spleen trauma

- Haemodynamic stability after resuscitation with no more than 60 mL/kg of fluid
- A good-quality CT scan
- No evidence of hollow visceral injury
- Close monitoring and the immediate availability of surgical expertise and facilities

Ongoing intra-abdominal bleeding requires a laparotomy, though angiography and arterial embolisation can be useful in some. Bile leaks are uncommon and can usually be managed by an interventional radiological technique. Uncomplicated unoperated cases of liver/spleen trauma can be discharged after 5–7 days but activity is restricted for 3–6 weeks and contact sports avoided for 2–3 months. Blunt renal trauma can be managed conservatively but an acutely non-functioning kidney following abdominal trauma may need urgent exploration with a view to revascularisation.

Patterns of injury

- **Lap belts**: the small intestine or lumbar spine.
- **Bicycle handlebars**: pancreatic, duodenal, mesenteric or liver trauma (**Figure 9.7**).
- **Straddle injuries**: the urethra and pelvis.
- **Run-over injuries**: severe crushing of the chest and/or abdomen.

Summary box 9.5

Paediatric trauma

- Use Advanced Trauma Life Support (ATLS) principles
- Overextension of the neck will compromise the airway
- Cervical spine injury can be present without radiographic signs
- Intraosseous vascular access is helpful in small children
- Lung contusion can occur without rib fractures
- Patterned skin bruising suggests underlying organ injury
- In a stable child, abdominal injuries are best assessed by CT
- Isolated liver or splenic injury can usually be managed non-operatively

COMMON PAEDIATRIC SURGICAL CONDITIONS

Inguinoscrotal disorders

Most genital abnormalities in boys are developmental anomalies. The testis develops from the urogenital ridge on the posterior abdominal wall. Gonadal induction leading to a testis is regulated by genes on the Y chromosome. During abdominal descent the testis migrates towards the internal ring, guided by mesenchymal tissue (gubernaculum). Descent into the scrotum is mediated by testosterone from the fetal testis. A tongue of peritoneum precedes the migrating testis through the inguinal canal and becomes the processus vaginalis. The processus normally becomes obliterated after birth, and failure leads to the development of an inguinal hernia or hydrocoele (**Figure 9.8**).

Inguinal hernias

Inguinal hernias in children are almost always indirect and due to a patent processus vaginalis. Inguinal hernias are common

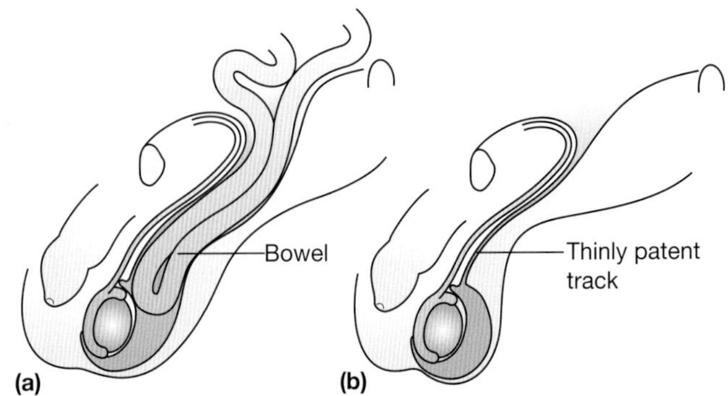

Figure 9.8 (**a**) Inguinal hernia and (**b**) hydrocoele in children are the result of incomplete obliteration of the processus vaginalis.

in boys (1:50), especially if premature, and are more common on the right-hand side (2:1) with 15% being bilateral. Rarely, bilateral inguinal hernias in a phenotypic girl may be the presentation of androgen insensitivity syndrome (testicular feminisation) and the sac may then contain a testis.

An inguinal hernia typically causes an intermittent swelling in the groin or scrotum on crying or straining (**Figure 9.9**). Unless an inguinal swelling is observed, diagnosis relies on the history and the presence of palpable thickening of the spermatic cord (or the round ligament in girls). Some inguinal hernias present as a firm, tender, irreducible lump in the groin or scrotum because of incarceration at the external ring. The infant may be irritable and may vomit. Most incarcerated hernias in children can be successfully reduced by sustained gentle compression ('taxis') aided by cautious analgesia. Repair can be delayed for 24 hours to let the oedema settle. If truly irreducible, emergency surgery is required because of the risk of vascular compromise to the bowel, ovary or testis.

Inguinal herniotomy is performed via an inguinal skin crease incision, opening Scarpa's fascia and then the external oblique. The cremaster is cut and, through an initially small opening, the sac is grasped and gently delivered. The vas and vessels are separated from the sac which is then divided and proximally ligated. Outside the neonatal period inguinal herniotomy is a day-case procedure. A laparoscopic approach is feasible but has a higher recurrence rate.

Summary box 9.6

Inguinal hernias

- More common in premature boys (right > left)
- 15% bilateral
- Indirect with a patent processus vaginalis
- Groin lump that appears on straining or crying
- Incarcerated inguinal hernias can usually be reduced with gentle pressure
- In infants they can transilluminate like a hydrocoele, making the test redundant when the distinction is difficult
- If reduction is impossible emergency surgery is needed
- In infants: repaired promptly to prevent the risk of strangulation
- The hernial sac is isolated, ligated and divided

Hydrocoeles

A patent processus vaginalis may allow peritoneal fluid (but no intestine) to track down to form a hydrocoele. Hydrocoeles are unilateral or bilateral, asymptomatic, non-tender scrotal swellings. Hydrocoeles may be tense or lax but typically transilluminate (**Figure 9.9**). The majority resolve spontaneously as the processus continues to obliterate but ligation and division is recommended in boys over 3 years of age. Rarely, a baby can have a tense painful hydrocoele warranting early repair. A hydrocoele can occasionally extend back up into the canal or abdomen (abdomino-scrotal hydrocoele).

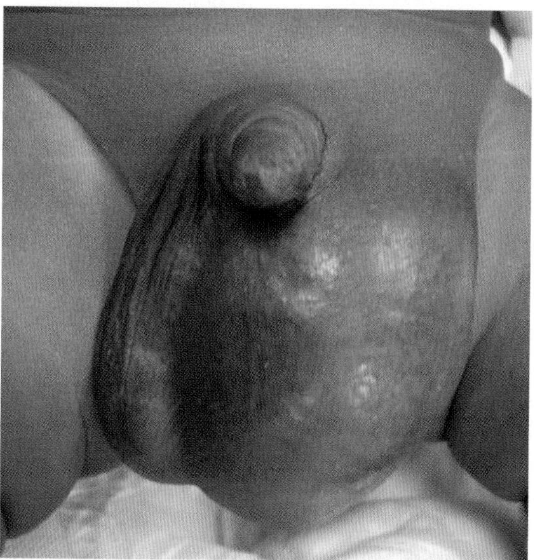

Figure 9.9 A left inguinal swelling. Clinical examination is needed to confidently distinguish a hydrocoele from an inguinal hernia.

Undescended testes are palpable or impalpable

At birth, 4% of full-term boys have unilateral or bilateral undescended testes, but after 3 months of age the incidence is <1% and it changes little thereafter. The incidence is higher in preterm infants, attributed to the testis descending through the canal in the third trimester. A normal testis reaches the base of the scrotum with a good length of cord above it. Testes cannot be palpated in the inguinal canal but can be milked from there into the superficial pouch (**palpable undescended testis**) or in to the scrotum with a good length of cord (normal). A **retractile testis** can be manipulated into the base of the scrotum without tension but is pulled up by the cremaster muscle. With time, retractile testes reside permanently in the scrotum; however, follow-up is advisable because, rarely, the testis ascends back into the inguinal canal. The **ascending testis** needs an orchidopexy. An **ectopic** testis lies outside its normal line of descent, often in the perineum.

A palpable undescended testis ideally requires a day-case orchidopexy between 6 and 12 months of age. The testis is mobilised through an inguinal incision, preserving the vas deferens and testicular vessels. The associated patent processus vaginalis is ligated and divided at the internal ring and the testis is placed in a subdartos scrotal pouch.

Impalpable undescended testes are either absent or located in the abdomen or inguinal canal. There is no benefit from imaging and these are best managed with a laparoscopy (**Figure 9.10**) and usually a staged approach.

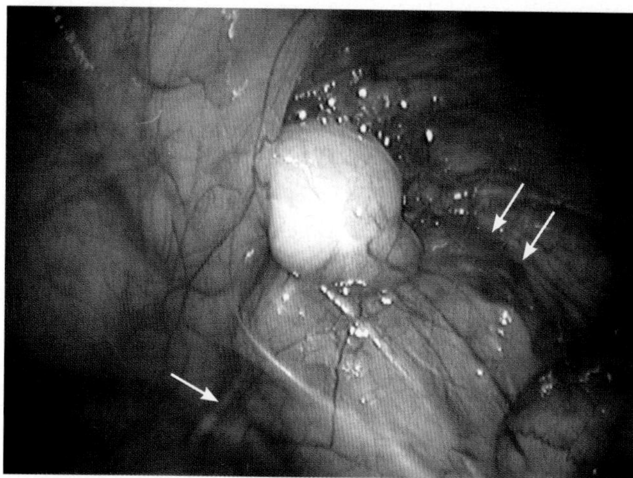

Figure 9.10 Laparoscopic view of a right-sided intra-abdominal testis visible at the internal ring. Vas (single arrow) and testicular vessels (double arrow).

The benefits of orchidopexy include:

- **Fertility.** To optimise spermatogenesis the testis needs to be in the scrotum below core temperature at a young age. Orchidopexy around 6–12 months of age is currently recommended. Fertility after orchidopexy for a unilateral undescended testis is near normal. Men with a history of bilateral intra-abdominal testes are often infertile.
- **Malignancy.** Undescended testes are histologically abnormal and at an increased risk of malignancy. The greatest risk is in patients with bilateral intra-abdominal testes. Early orchidopexy for a unilateral undescended testis may reduce the risk but this is not proven.
- **Cosmetic and psychological.** In an older boy a prosthetic testis can be inserted to replace an absent one.

Summary box 9.7

The undescended testis

- A retractile testis reaches the base of the scrotum but retracts
- An undescended testis may be palpable or impalpable
- An ectopic testis lies outside the normal line of descent
- Palpable undescended testes undergo a single stage orchidopexy
- Impalpable undescended testes undergo a single stage orchidopexy
- Orchidopexy before 1 year of age improves fertility and may reduce the risk of malignancy

The acute scrotum

Testicular torsion is most common in adolescents, but may occur at any age and is usually inside the tunica vaginalis. Perinatal torsion differs and is usually extravaginal. The pain is not always scrotal and may be felt in the groin or lower abdomen. Scrotal oedema and erythema can be absent. Sometimes there is a history of previous transient episodes. Torsion of the testis must be relieved within 6–8 hours of the onset of symptoms for there to be a good chance of testicular salvage. At operation, viability of the testis is assessed after derotation. If salvageable, three-point fixation of both testes with non-absorbable sutures is performed. Expert assessment of testicular blood flow by colour Doppler ultrasound may help in the differential diagnosis but the scrotum must be explored urgently if torsion cannot be excluded.

Torsion of a testicular or epididymal appendage characteristically affects boys just before puberty **(Figure 9.11)**, possibly because of enlargement of the hydatid in response to gonadotrophins. A hydatid of Morgagni is an embryological remnant found on the upper pole of the testis or epididymis. The pain often increases over a day or two. Occasionally, the torted hydatid can be felt or seen (blue dot sign). Excision of the appendage leads to rapid resolution of symptoms. Viral or bacterial **epididymo-orchitis** may cause an acute scrotum in infants and toddlers but this diagnosis is often only made after scrotal exploration. Other conditions can rarely cause acute scrotal symptoms, and signs include idiopathic scrotal oedema (typically painless, erythematous scrotal swelling in a young boy extending off the scrotum into the groin and towards the anus), an incarcerated inguinal hernia, vasculitis or a scrotal haematoma.

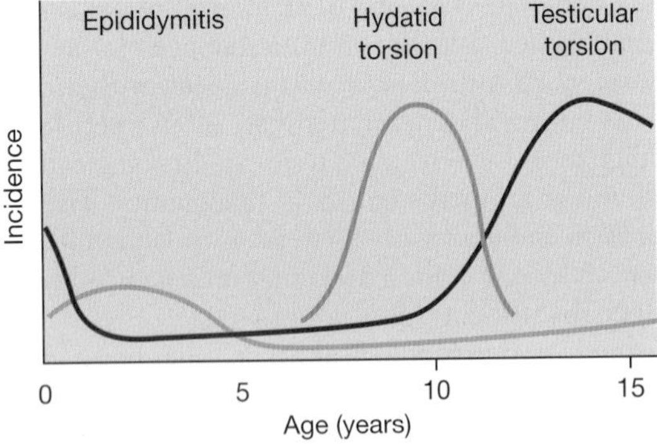

Figure 9.11 Acute scrotal pathology at different ages.

Summary box 9.8

Diagnosis and treatment of the acute scrotum

- Torsion of the testis must be assumed until proven otherwise
- Testicular torsion can present with acute inguinal or abdominal pain
- Urgent surgical exploration is crucial if testicular torsion cannot be excluded
- If torsion is confirmed an orchidopexy should be performed on both sides
- Torsion of a testicular appendage usually occurs just before puberty
- An incarcerated inguinal hernia must be considered in the differential diagnosis

The penis

Hypospadias

In hypospadias, seen in 1:300 boys, the urethra opens proximally and ventrally. Most commonly, the opening is just proximal to the glans but it can open on the penile shaft or onto the perineum. It is attributed to failure of complete urethral tubularisation in the fetus. The foreskin is deficient ventrally **(Figure 9.12)** and there is a variable degree of chordee (a ventral curvature of the penis most apparent on erection). Glanular hypospadias needs correction for cosmetic reasons but more proximal anomalies interfere with micturition and erection. In a newborn with severe hypospadias and bilateral undescended testes disorders of sexual development (DSDs) should be considered. A distal hypospadias is usually repaired before 2 years of age in one or two stages. Proximal varieties require complex staged procedures. Surgery aims to achieve a terminal urethral meatus so that the boy can stand to micturate with a normal stream, a straight erection and a penis that looks normal. Ritual circumcision is contraindicated in infants with hypospadias because the foreskin is often required for the reconstruction.

The foreskin and circumcision

At birth, the foreskin is adherent to the glans penis. These adhesions separate spontaneously with time, allowing the foreskin to become retractile. At 1 year of age, about 50% of boys have a non-retractile foreskin. By 4 years this has declined to 10% and by 16 years to just 1%. Ballooning of the normal non-retractile foreskin on micturition brings many young boys to doctors, and explanation and reassurance are required – but no operation. Gentle retraction of the foreskin

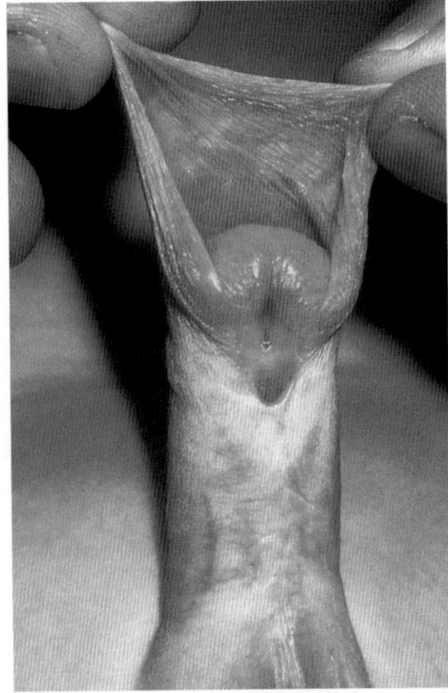

Figure 9.12 Hypospadias: note the hooded foreskin and the ventral meatus.

Giovanni Batista Morgagni, 1682–1771, Professor of Anatomy, Padua, Italy for 59 years, regarded as the founder of morbid anatomy.

at bath times helps to maintain hygiene but forcible retraction should never be attempted. The presence of preputial adhesions, when the foreskin remains partially adherent to the glans, is normal and resolves spontaneously. Smegma pearls accumulating under the foreskin are commonly mistaken for tumours – reassurance is needed.

Circumcision has been an important tradition in Jewish, Muslim and other cultures. Proponents observe that circumcision reduces the incidence of urinary tract infection in infant boys; however, circumcision is not without risk of significant morbidity. The medical indications for circumcision are:

- **Phimosis.** This term is often wrongly applied to describe a normal, non-retractile foreskin. True phimosis is seen as a whitish scarring of the foreskin and is rare before 5 years of age **(Figure 9.13)**. It is caused by the localised skin disease balanitis xerotica obliterans (BXO), which also affects the glans penis and can cause urethral meatal stenosis.
- **Recurrent balanoposthitis.** A single episode of inflammation of the foreskin, sometimes with a purulent discharge, is not uncommon and usually resolves spontaneously; antibiotics are sometimes needed. Recurrent attacks are unusual but may be an indication for circumcision.
- **Recurrent urinary tract infection.** Circumcision is occasionally justified in boys with an abnormal upper urinary tract anomaly and recurrent urinary infection. It may also help boys with spina bifida who need to perform clean intermittent urethral catheterisation.

An emerging but controversial indication for circumcision is in the prevention of sexually acquired human immunodeficiency virus (HIV) infection in communities where this is common; large clinical trials have shown that circumcision reduces the risk of HIV transmission.

Circumcision for medical reasons is best performed under general anaesthesia. A long-acting local anaesthetic regional block can be given to reduce postoperative pain. Circumcision is not a trivial operation; bleeding and infection are well-recognised complications and more serious hazards, such as injury to the glans, may occur if the procedure is not carried out well.

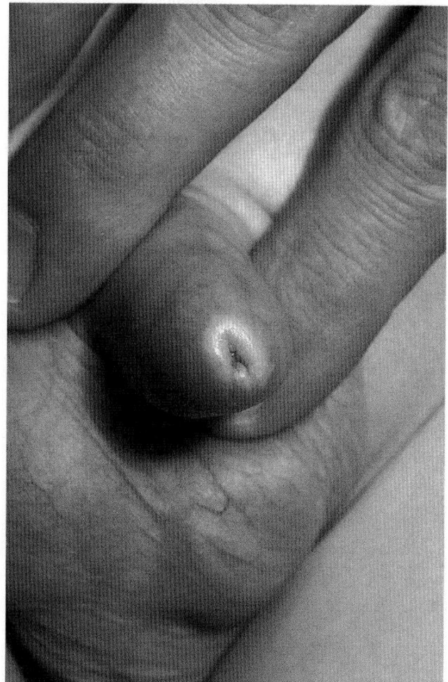

Figure 9.13 True phimosis from balanitis xerotica obliterans.

> **Summary box 9.9**
>
> **Circumcision**
>
> - Medical indications are BXO and recurrent balanoposthitis, paraphimosis, scarring from trauma
> - Circumcision is not indicated for an otherwise healthy non-retractile foreskin
> - Complications include bleeding, poor cosmesis (too much or too little skin removed), and trauma to the glans or urethra

Midline hernias

In the embryo, the umbilical ring is a relatively large defect in the ventral abdominal wall transmitting several structures that connect the fetus to the placenta **(Figure 9.14)**. An umbilical hernia is common and caused by incomplete closure of the umbilical ring; incarceration is very rare. Most umbilical hernias resolve by 4 years of age. Supraumbilical hernias occur through defects in the linea alba just above the umbilical ring and do not close but are still repaired at around 4 years of age. Epigastric hernias are defects higher still that allow a small amount of preperitoneal fat to prolapse. They are repaired if symptomatic.

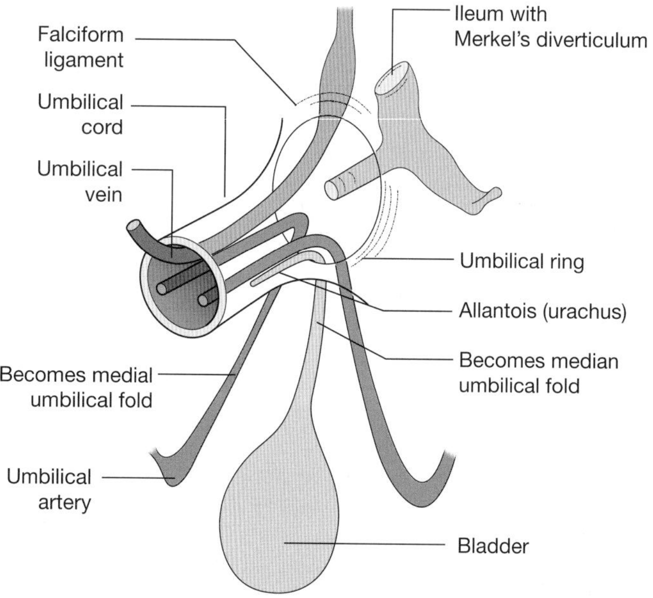

Figure 9.14 Structures at the umbilicus.

Infantile hypertrophic pyloric stenosis (IHPS)

Infantile hypertrophic pyloric stenosis (IHPS) presents with **non**-bilious projectile vomiting between 2 and 8 weeks of age and is only rarely seen after 13 weeks. It is easily distinguished from many other serious causes of vomiting, such as infections, because the baby is particularly hungry. IHPS is a progressive condition and a detailed history helps distinguish it from the more common gastroesophageal reflux (GOR) which is commonly seen in infancy. In the UK it affects 1:300 infants, with a male:female ratio of 4:1. However, if a girl has IHPS her offspring have a high chance of developing it, suggesting a genetic predisposition.

The non-bilious nature is stressed here to contrast the condition with the **bilious vomiting** of the potentially life-threatening malrotation and volvulus seen occasionally in neonates.

IHPS can be diagnosed clinically. During a test feed there is visible gastric peristalsis passing from left to right across the upper abdomen and in a relaxed baby the pyloric 'tumour' is palpable as an 'olive' in the right upper quadrant. The diagnosis can be confirmed by an ultrasound, which shows the thickened pyloric muscle. IHPS is readily treated by surgery but the infant must be adequately rehydrated and the hypochloraemic hypokalaemic alkalosis corrected; this may take 48 hours if the chloride is 85 mmol/L or lower. In most babies, the dehydration and alkalosis can be corrected by giving 150–180 mL/kg/day of 0.9% saline with 0.15% KCl in 5% glucose. Oral feeding is discontinued and the stomach emptied with an 8–10 Fr nasogastric tube; ongoing gastric losses should be replaced intravenously.

Ramstedt's pyloromyotomy is performed by a laparoscopic or open supraumbilical incision. A serosal incision is made and the 'tumour' spread (Figure 9.15). The end result should be an intact bulging submucosa from duodenal fornix to gastric antrum. Perforation of the duodenal fornix is uncommon and not serious provided that it is recognised and repaired immediately.

Postoperatively, intravenous fluids are continued until oral feeding is re-established within 24 hours. Occasionally the baby has small vomits on the first few feeds but this resolves after 72 hours. If it persists then an incomplete myotomy or GOR should be considered. Surgical complications include duodenal perforation, haemorrhage, wound infection and wound dehiscence – all are uncommon and avoidable. Pyloromyotomy has no significant long-term sequelae.

Summary box 9.10

Infantile hypertrophic pyloric stenosis

- Most commonly affects boys aged 2–8 weeks
- Projectile vomiting after feeds
- Test feed or ultrasound to confirm the diagnosis
- Gastric peristalsis can be seen and an 'olive' felt
- Hypochloraemic metabolic alkalosis must be corrected before surgery
- Pyloromyotomy splits the hypertrophied muscle leaving the mucosa intact

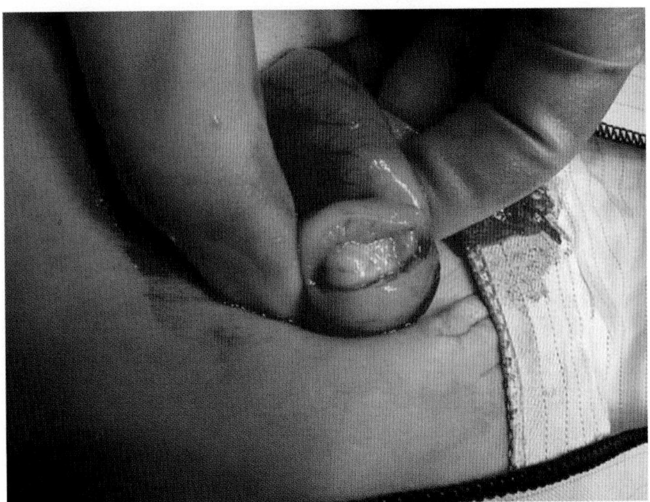

Figure 9.15 Pyloromyotomy for infantile hypertrophic pyloric stenosis.

Other common or serious causes of vomiting in infancy are shown in *Table 9.4*.

Gastro-oesophageal reflux (GOR) is common and tends to resolve spontaneously with maturity. Persistent symptoms respond to thickened feeds and antireflux medication. Complications, such as failure to thrive or respiratory problems, demand further investigation and in some cases laparoscopic fundoplication.

TABLE 9.4 Vomiting in infancy.

Bile-stained	Neonate	Intestinal malrotation with volvulus
		Duodenal atresia/stenosis (Down syndrome, antenatal diagnosis)
		Jejunal/ileal atresia (often isolated anomalies)
		Hirschsprung's disease
		Anorectal malformations
		Meconium ileus (cystic fibrosis)
		Necrotising enterocolitis (an acquired condition in the premature)
		Incarcerated inguinal hernia
	Older infant	Intestinal malrotation with volvulus
		Intussusception (often non-bilious initially)
		Incarcerated inguinal hernia
Non-bilious	Infantile hypertrophic pyloric stenosis	
	Gastro-oesophageal reflux	
	Feeding difficulties (technique/volume)	
	Non-specific marker of illness, e.g. infection (urinary tract infection, meningitis, gastroenteritis, respiratory, metabolic disorder, raised intracranial pressure, congenital adrenal hyperplasia)	

Wilhelm Conrad **Ramstedt**, 1867–1963, surgeon, The Rafaelklinik, Münster, Germany, performed his first pyloromyotomy in 1911.

Intussusception

Most intussusceptions (**Figure 9.16**) in children occur from 2 months to 2 years of age. They are life-threatening. Intussusception typically causes a strangulating bowel obstruction, which can progress to gangrene and perforation. Intussusception is classified according to the site of the intussusceptum and intussuscipiens. In children, more than 80% are ileocolic, beginning several centimetres proximal to the ileocaecal valve with their apex found in the ascending or transverse colon.

In the majority, the cause is hyperplasia of Peyer's patches (lymphoid tissue), which may be secondary to a viral infection. In 10% of children, there is a pathological lead point, such as a Meckel's diverticulum, enteric duplication cyst or even a small bowel lymphoma. Such cases are more likely in children over the age of 2 years and in those with recurrent intussusception.

Classically, a previously healthy infant presents with colicky pain and vomiting (milk then bile). Between episodes, the child initially appears well. Later, they may pass a 'redcurrant jelly' stool. Clinical signs include dehydration, abdominal distension and a palpable sausage-shaped mass in the right upper quadrant. Rectal examination may reveal blood or rarely the apex of the intussusceptum.

Summary box 9.11

Presentation of intussusception

- Bilious vomiting in an infant is a sign of intestinal obstruction until proved otherwise
- Intussusception classically presents with colicky pain and vomiting
- Intussusception should be considered in any infant with bloody stools
- Age range is between 2 and 24 months of age

A plain radiograph is rarely requested but if done it commonly shows signs of small bowel obstruction and a soft-tissue opacity. Diagnosis is confirmed on an abdominal ultrasound.

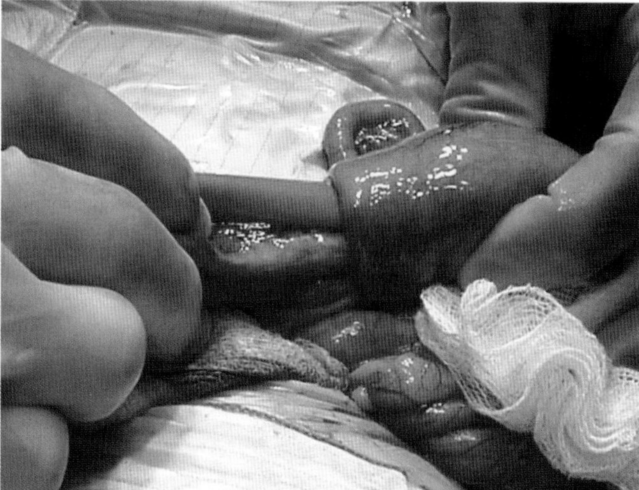

Figure 9.16 Ileocolic intussusception causing small bowel obstruction.

After resuscitation with intravenous fluids, broad-spectrum antibiotics and nasogastric drainage, non-operative reduction is attempted using an air enema (**Figure 9.17**). Successful reduction is recognised if air flows into the small bowel, together with later resolution of symptoms and signs. An air enema is contraindicated if there is peritonitis, perforation or shock. More than 70% of intussusceptions can be reduced non-operatively. Strangulated bowel and pathological lead points are unlikely to reduce. Perforation of the colon during pneumatic reduction is a recognised hazard but is rare. Recurrent intussusception occurs in up to 5% of patients after non-operative reduction.

Operative reduction can be performed open or laparoscopically. The intussusception is milked distally by gentle

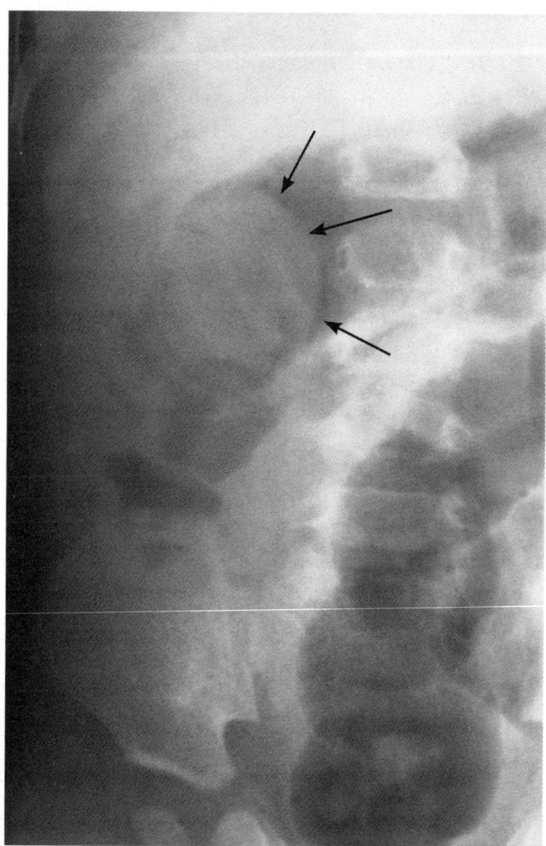

Figure 9.17 Air enema reduction of an intussusception (the arrows mark the soft tissue shadow of the intussusceptum).

Summary box 9.12

Management of intussusception

- Bowel infarction will result without treatment
- Most are ileocolic
- Diagnosis can be confirmed by ultrasound scan
- Fluid and electrolyte resuscitation is essential
- Most intussusceptions can be reduced non-operatively using an air enema
- If there are signs of peritonitis or perforation then an emergency operation is needed

compression from its apex at an open procedure. Both the intussusceptum and the intussuscipiens are inspected for areas of non-viability. An irreducible intussusception or one complicated by infarction or a pathological lead point requires resection and primary anastomosis.

Acute abdominal pain in children over 3 years of age

Between one-third and one-half of children admitted to hospital with acute abdominal pain have non-specific abdominal pain (NSAP). The term mesenteric adenitis is unhelpful and should be dropped. Another one-third have acute appendicitis. Relatively benign conditions, such as constipation and urinary tract infections, account for most of the remainder. A small proportion of children have more serious pathology.

History and examination

Time and patience are required to evaluate the child with acute abdominal pain accurately. The child may be frightened and the parents worried. Young children find it difficult accurately to describe or localise abdominal pain but can often give a good history. The abdomen, genitalia, chest, throat and neck are examined. The abdomen may need reassessment after analgesia and a number of reviews. A gentle abdominal examination of the sleeping toddler, before removing their clothes, may reveal tenderness, guarding or a mass. Rectal examination is only performed if a pelvic appendicitis is suspected and by the surgeon whose decisions will be altered by the findings. **Active observation** acknowledges that a definitive diagnosis is not always possible when the patient is first seen. The surgeon reassesses the child after a few hours while rehydrating with IV fluids or allowing clear fluids and simple analgesics. This approach reduces the need for investigations and can reduce the negative appendicectomy rate to as low as 4%. Ultrasound and CT scans have a role in selected children.

Summary box 9.13

Work-up of children with acute abdominal pain

- A careful history and examination and active observation are paramount
- Routine tests include full blood count (FBC), C-reactive protein (CRP), urine analysis, microscopy and culture
- Abdominal ultrasound scan (not mandated initially but may be useful)
- Other tests may be helpful after a period of observation: abdominal ultrasound scan (can diagnose pelvic and urinary tract pathology)
- Occasionally helpful tests: a plain supine abdominal radiograph (particularly in the preschool child with pain and vomiting), ultrasound or CT scan in complex cases
- Selective specific investigations: blood culture, stool culture, plasma amylase, diagnostic laparoscopy

Acute non-specific abdominal pain (NSAP)

The clinical features of NSAP are similar to those of acute appendicitis but the pain is poorly localised, not aggravated by movement and rarely accompanied by guarding. The site and severity of maximum tenderness often vary during the course of repeated examinations. Symptoms are typically self-limiting within 48 hours. The aetiology of NSAP in children is obscure but viral infections and transient intussusception account for some cases. Viral infections can cause reactive lymphadenopathy, fever and diffuse abdominal pain. In some children, recurrent acute abdominal pain can be organic or sometimes an expression of underlying psychosocial problems or abuse.

Acute appendicitis and its pitfalls

Classically there is anorexia and a few vomits with central abdominal pain which settles in the right iliac fossa. In early acute appendicitis there is a fever of 37.3–38.4°C and localised tenderness. Finding persistent guarding in the right iliac fossa on repeated examination is the key to making the diagnosis and distinguishing it from NSAP, which usually resolves over 24–48 hours. NSAP does not have persistent guarding. Acute appendicitis was principally always a clinical diagnosis but more recently early ultrasound is proving useful. Investigations may help but cannot replace regular expert clinical review. The pitfalls include wrongly making the diagnosis of gastroenteritis when there are loose stools or attributing pain on micturition and pyuria to a urinary tract infection (UTI). Both of these can occur when there is pelvic appendicitis or a pelvic collection. Referred pain from a right lower lobe pneumonia should be considered and it is important to remember that if antibiotics have been given the signs may be reduced and presentation can be delayed. The diagnosis can be difficult in those under 5 years of age. Many under-fives present with a perforated appendix, not because the diagnosis is made late but rather because the omentum is less well developed and inflammation is not well contained. The treatment starts with resuscitation with intravenous fluids, analgesia and broad-spectrum antibiotics. Appendicectomy can be performed laparoscopically or through a muscle-splitting right iliac fossa incision. An appendix mass in a child who is not obstructed may respond to non-operative management with antibiotics, and an interval appendicectomy can be considered 6 weeks later.

Summary box 9.14

Acute appendicitis

- Anorexia, vomiting, low-grade fever
- Tenderness and guarding in the right iliac fossa
- Exclude referred pain from right lower lobe pneumonia
- Surgery is the treatment of choice after resuscitation and antibiotics

Other causes of acute abdominal pain in children

- **Intestinal obstruction.** Consider intussusception, inguinal hernia, adhesions and Meckel's diverticulum.
- **Constipation.** Often over-diagnosed as a cause of acute abdominal pain, particularly as the plain x-ray of a dehydrated ill child frequently shows faecal loading.

- **Urinary tract disorders.** UTI is an uncommon cause of acute abdominal pain. Urinary symptoms, fever and vomiting tend to predominate. Urinalysis, microscopy and culture are useful but a sterile pyuria may accompany acute appendicitis. Children with pelviureteric junction obstruction can present with acute or recurrent abdominal pain and no urinary symptoms.
- **Gastroenteritis.** May cause colicky abdominal pain. Onset of pain before the diarrhoea and the presence of lower abdominal tenderness should raise the suspicion of appendicitis.
- **Tropical diseases.** Ascariasis, typhoid and amoebiasis can cause acute abdominal pain.

There are numerous rarer causes of acute abdominal pain in children including Henoch–Schönlein purpura, sickle cell disease, primary peritonitis, acute pancreatitis, biliary colic, testicular torsion, gynaecological pathology (e.g. ovarian cysts and tumours, pelvic inflammatory disease, haematometrocolpos) and urinary stone disease.

Summary box 9.15

Rare causes of acute abdominal pain in children

- Obstruction from intussusception, adhesions, Meckel's diverticulum or an inguinal hernia
- Constipation
- Urinary tract disorders
- Gastroenteritis
- Ascariasis
- Typhoid

Urinary tract infection

UTIs in children may be due to a urinary tract abnormality which may carry a risk of developing renal scarring from ascending infection. Infection and obstruction are particularly hazardous. Older children complain of dysuria and frequency, whereas infants present with vomiting, fever and poor feeding. Urine specimens from children are easily contaminated during collection and results must be interpreted with care. A proven infection is investigated by an ultrasound scan. Micturating cystography and radioisotope renography are helpful in excluding vesicoureteric reflux and renal scarring. Treatment aims to relieve symptoms, correct causes and preventing renal scarring. Vesicoureteric reflux may resolve spontaneously, some may need antibiotic prophylaxis or in a very small number of cases an endoscopic treatment or a re-implantation of the ureter.

Children with **neuropathic bladders** (e.g. spina bifida) are at risk of secondary upper renal tract complications. Management of these children must take into account their dexterity and motivation. An adequate capacity, low-pressure bladder can frequently be managed by clean intermittent catheterisation but a high-pressure bladder is hazardous and other strategies, such as bladder augmentation, may be necessary. Some of these children empty their bladder via a non-refluxing catheterisable channel fashioned from the appendix, the bowel or a redundant ureter interposed between the abdominal wall and bladder (Mitrofanoff).

Anorectal problems

CONSTIPATION

The passage of hard or infrequent stools is common in children in the West. Severe constipation may be secondary to an anal fissure, Hirschsprung's disease, an anorectal malformation or a neuropathic bowel. A detailed history and examination of the abdomen, anus and spine will identify most causes. Rectal examination and plain abdominal radiography may be helpful in severe cases. In the absence of specific underlying pathology, the child is best managed jointly with a paediatrician, using a combination of diet, extra fluids, reward systems and laxatives.

RECTAL PROLAPSE

Mucosal rectal prolapse can occur in toddlers and is exacerbated by straining or squatting on a potty. It is typically intermittent and frequently self-limiting. Rarely, it may be secondary to cystic fibrosis or spinal dysraphism. The differential diagnosis includes a prolapsing rectal polyp. Underlying factors, such as constipation, should be treated. Recurrent symptomatic prolapse usually responds to injection sclerotherapy. Strapping the buttocks is ineffective.

RECTAL BLEEDING

Unlike in adults, malignancy is an exceptionally rare cause of rectal bleeding. In newborns, the life-threatening causes are malrotation and necrotising enterocolitis, and in older infants and children, intussusception. The quantities of blood loss are small but the conditions are serious. Other causes include anal fissures, juvenile polyps (**Figure 9.18**) and certain gastroenteritides (e.g. *Campylobacter* infection).

The 4-year-old patient who presents with a haemoglobin (Hb) of 40 g/L will most likely have bled profusely from an ulcer adjacent to a Meckel's diverticulum containing ectopic gastric mucosa (**Figure 9.19**). A technetium scan may confirm the presence of ectopic gastric mucosa (**Figure 9.20**).

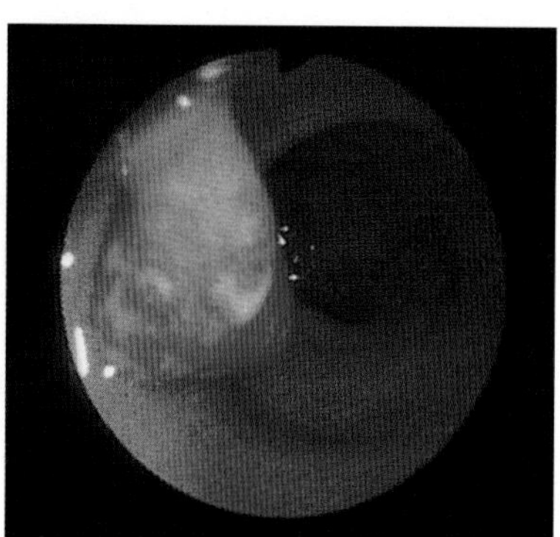

Figure 9.18 Colonic juvenile polyp: these are typically pedunculated.

Eduard Heinrich Henoch, 1820–1910, Professor of Diseases of Children, Berlin, Germany, described this form of purpura in 1868.
Johann Lucas Schönlein, 1793–1864, Professor of Medicine, Berlin, Germany, published his description of this form of purpura in 1837.
Paul Mitrofanoff, b.1934, Professor of Paediatric Surgery, Rouen, France.

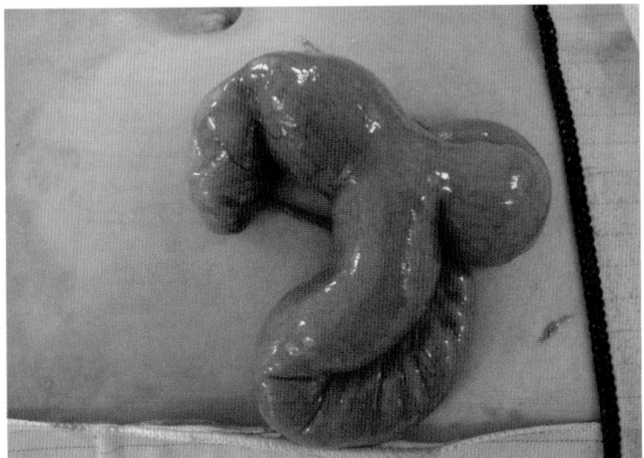

Figure 9.19 Meckel's diverticulum containing ectopic gastric mucosa.

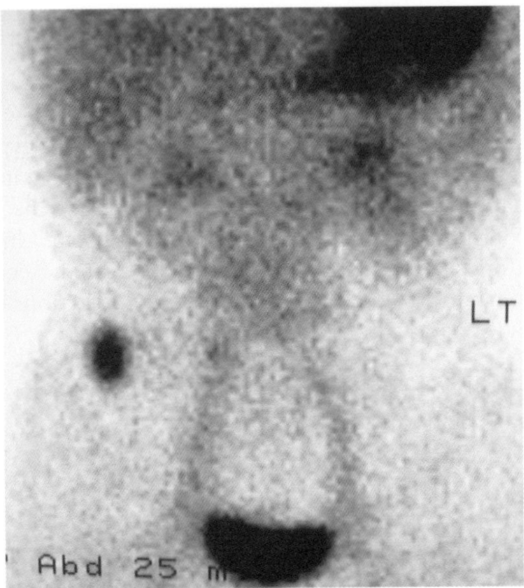

Figure 9.20 A positive Meckel's scan.

A Meckel's diverticulum may also be complicated by an obstructing band between the diverticulum and the umbilicus, diverticulitis, intussusception, intestinal volvulus or perforation.

Swallowed or inhaled foreign bodies

Coins are the most frequently swallowed foreign bodies in children. Once beyond the cardia, they are usually passed in a few days. A plain radiograph of the abdomen, chest and neck should establish the site of radio-opaque objects. Oesophageal objects can be removed endoscopically under general anaesthesia. Button batteries must be removed within hours because if they remain in the oesophagus they can perforate into the trachea or aorta. Batteries in the stomach are either removed urgently or followed very closely with repeat x-rays over a couple of days. The need to remove sharp objects depends on their size, the age of the child and their position in the gut. Ingested magnets can cause entero-enteric fistulae when they fix to one another in adjacent loops of bowel. Battery ingestion in older children and young people may be a manifestation of self-harm.

Inhaled foreign bodies cause sudden-onset coughing and stridor. If there is worsening dyspnoea or signs of hypoxia then the infant should be given back blows in a head-down position. Abdominal thrusts (Heimlich manoeuvre) can be used in older children. A foreign body is suggested by: a unilateral wheeze, decreased transmitted breath sounds and a hyperinflated lung from air trapping on an expiratory CXR (**Figure 9.21**). A rigid bronchoscopy with a ventilating bronchoscope and appropriate optical forceps is needed to assess and remove objects.

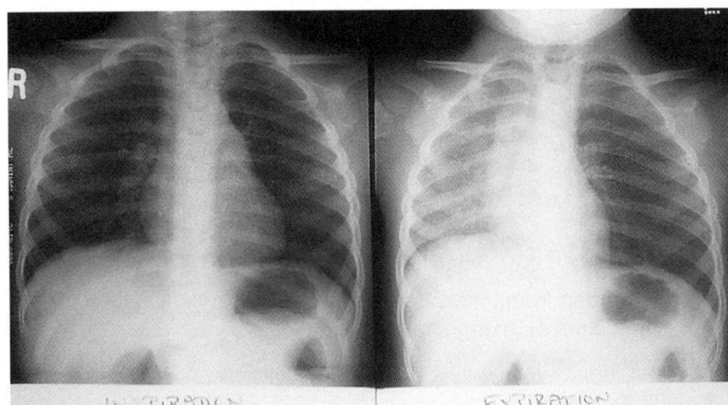

Figure 9.21 An inspiratory (left) and expiratory (right) chest radiograph demonstrating left-sided pulmonary air trapping after inhalation of a radiolucent foreign body.

Summary box 9.16

Swallowed and inhaled objects

- Most swallowed objects pass spontaneously
- Batteries need watching – they must pass quickly if their contents are not to leak
- Objects jammed in the airway or oesophagus need removing promptly

CONGENITAL MALFORMATIONS

Around 2% of babies are born with one or more major structural anomalies caused by genetic defects or teratogenic insults. Some are diagnosed antenatally and surgeons are involved in antenatal counselling. Termination of pregnancy or planned delivery in a specialist centre are options for severe malformations. Prenatal diagnosis may include checking the karyotype (e.g. Down syndrome: trisomy 21) or testing for genetic disorders, such as cystic fibrosis.

The incidence of congenital malformations is variable (*Table 9.5*). Some examples relevant to the general surgeon are briefly outlined in the following sections.

Henry J Heimlich, b.1920, thoracic surgeon, Xavier University, Cincinnati, OH, USA.
John Langdon Haydon Down (sometimes given as Langdon-Down), 1838–1896, physician, The London Hospital, London, UK, published '*Observations on an ethnic classification of idiots*' in 1866.

TABLE 9.5 Incidence of selected malformations.

Abnormality	Incidence
Thoracic	
Congenital diaphragmatic hernia	1:3000
Oesophageal atresia/tracheo-oesophageal fistula	1:3500
Cardiac	
Congenital heart disease	1:150
Gastrointestinal	
Gastroschisis	1:7500
Hirschsprung's disease	1:5000
Anorectal malformations	1:4–5000
Hepatobiliary	
Biliary atresia	1:17 000
Choledochal cyst	1:50 000
Urogenital	
Hypospadias	1:300
Pelviureteric junction dysfunction	1:1000

Oesophageal atresia

A blind proximal pouch with a distal tracheo-oesophageal fistula is the most common type (**Figure 9.22**). Affected infants present soon after birth with drooling and cyanotic episodes on attempting to feed. There may have been polyhydramnios due to failure to swallow amniotic fluid. The diagnosis is confirmed when a nasogastric tube goes no further than the upper oesophageal pouch on the CXR and abdominal gas signifies the tracheo-oesophageal fistula (**Figure 9.22**). Associated anomalies are common and include cardiac, renal and skeletal defects. Repair is usually via a right-sided extrapleural thoracotomy within a day or two of birth – thoracoscopic repair is challenging but feasible, although the magnified view is excellent . The fistula is divided and the tracheal side closed. The oesophageal ends are anastomosed. The blood supply is poor and the anastomosis is under tension.

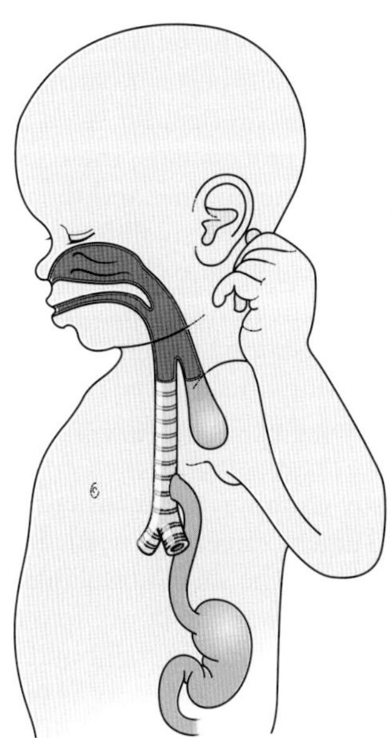

Figure 9.22 Oesophageal atresia with a distal tracheo-oesophageal fistula.

Postoperative complications include anastomotic leak, stricture, recurrent fistula formation and gastro-oesophageal reflux. Infants with pure oesophageal atresia and no tracheo-oesophageal fistula are usually best managed by a temporary gastrostomy and delayed primary repair or an oesophageal replacement. Except for very-low-birth weight babies and those with major congenital heart disease, most infants with repaired oesophageal atresia have a good prognosis.

Congenital diaphragmatic hernia (CDH)

Typically, there is a left-sided posterolateral diaphragmatic defect allowing herniation of abdominal viscera into the chest (**Figure 9.23**). Many are detected antenatally and the prognosis relates to the severity of the associated pulmonary hypoplasia. Despite intensive respiratory support or extracorporeal membrane oxygenation (ECMO), up to 30% of babies with a CDH die from respiratory failure. If the baby can be stabilised, the diaphragmatic defect is repaired. Small diaphragmatic hernias may present with respiratory or gastrointestinal symptoms in later childhood.

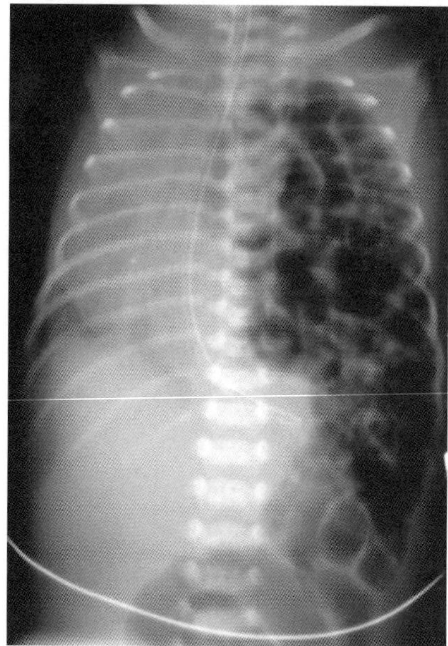

Figure 9.23 Left-sided congenital diaphragmatic hernia.

Intestinal atresias

Duodenal atresia may take the form of a membrane or the proximal and distal duodenum may be completely separated. Prenatal ultrasound finds a 'double bubble' in the fetal abdomen with polyhydramnios. There is an association with Down syndrome. Postnatally, there is bilious vomiting if the atresia is distal to the ampulla. A plain abdominal x-ray also shows the double-bubble (**Figure 9.24**). Repair is by open duodeno-duodenostomy (**Figure 9.25**). Occasionally, there is a duodenal membrane with a modest central perforation, which may delay symptoms until later childhood.

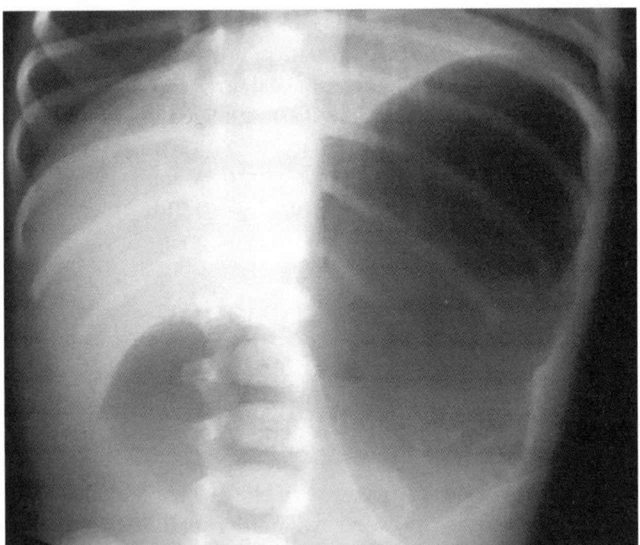

Figure 9.24 Neonatal abdominal x-ray showing the 'double bubble' of duodenal atresia.

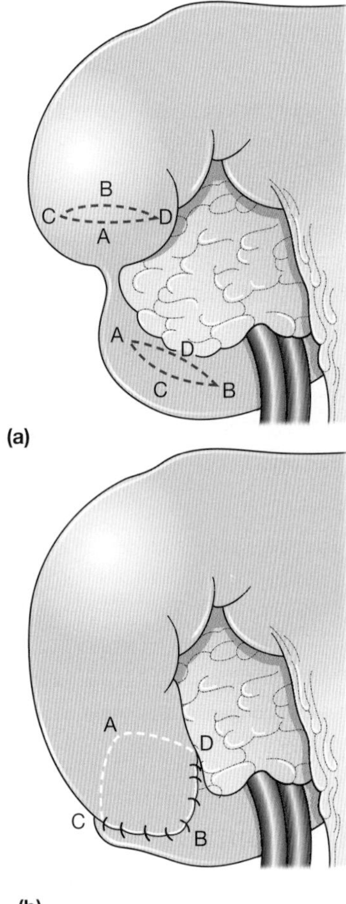

Figure 9.25 (a, b) Duodenal atresia and the incisions used to repair it: a diamond anastomosis is shown.

Jejunal/ileal atresias vary from an obstructing membrane through to widely separated blind-ended bowel ends associated with a mesenteric defect. Small bowel atresias may be single or multiple and are probably secondary to a prenatal vascular or mechanical insult causing sterile infarction of a segment of gut. They present with intestinal obstruction soon after birth. The proximal bowel is often extremely dilated and needs to be tapered prior to anastomosis to the distal bowel (**Figure 9.26**).

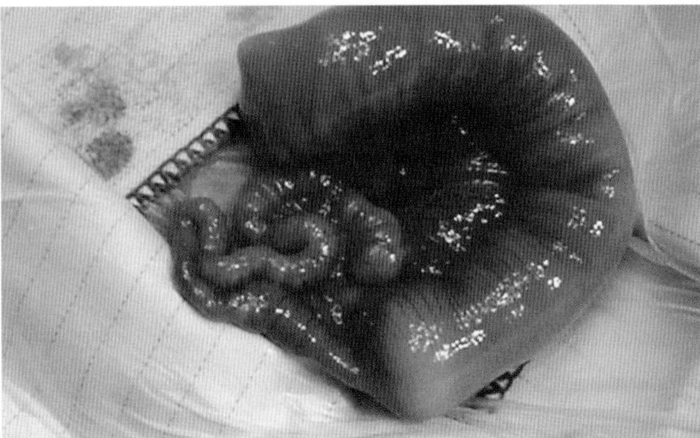

Figure 9.26 Small bowel atresia.

Meconium ileus is a cause of intestinal obstruction from inspissated meconium in the terminal ileum in neonates, most of whom have cystic fibrosis. Meconium is a mixture of epithelial cells, mucin and bile. Babies with uncomplicated meconium ileus (no associated atresia, volvulus or perforation) can sometimes be managed with hyperosmolar contrast enemas to clear the meconium.

Meconium peritonitis is consequent upon a fetal intestinal perforation. The baby is born with a firm, distended, discoloured abdomen and signs of obstruction. An abdominal x-ray shows dilated intestinal loops and areas of calcification. Occasionally, the perforation has resolved spontaneously before birth but most neonates with meconium peritonitis will need surgery. The peritonitic insult is chemical and not bacterial, although in late pregnancy meconium does contain bacteria.

Intestinal malrotation. By the 12th week of gestation, the midgut has returned to the fetal abdomen from the extraembryonic coelom and has begun rotating counterclockwise around the superior mesenteric artery axis. In classical intestinal malrotation, this process fails; the duodenojejunal flexure lies to the right of the midline and the caecum is central, creating a narrow base for the small bowel mesentery, which predisposes to midgut volvulus (**Figure 9.27**). Malrotation with volvulus is life-threatening and typically presents with bilious vomiting. Bile-stained vomiting in the infant is a sign of intestinal obstruction until proved otherwise.

As the gut strangulates, the baby may pass bloodstained stools and becomes progressively sicker. An upper gastrointestinal contrast study confirms the malrotation (**Figure 9.27**). Resuscitation and urgent surgery are needed to untwist the volvulus, widen the base of the small bowel mesentery, straighten the duodenum and position the bowel in a non-rotated position with the small bowel on the right and the colon on the left (Ladd's procedure). The appendix is usually removed to avoid leaving it in an abnormal site within the abdomen.

William Edward Ladd, 1880–1967, Professor of Child Surgery, The University of Harvard, Boston, MA, USA.

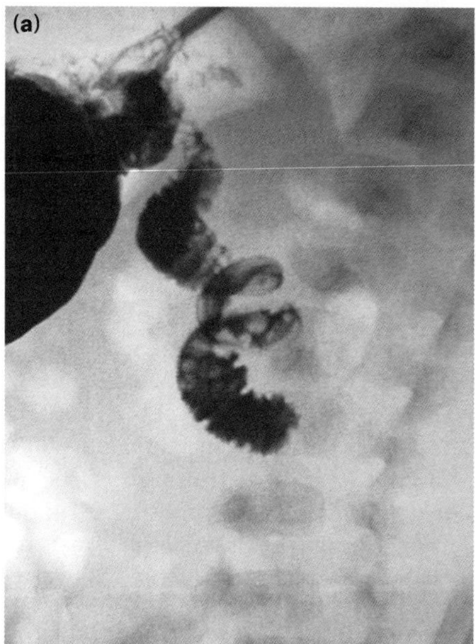

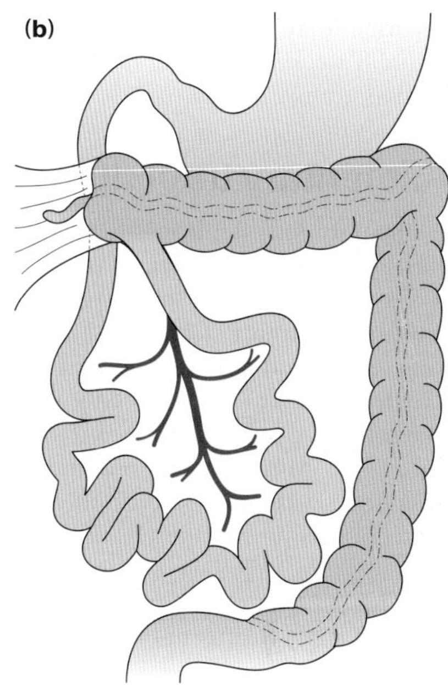

Figure 9.27 (a) Contrast showing malrotation with a volvulus. (b) The narrow origin of the small bowel mesentery predisposes to midgut volvulus.

Abdominal wall defects

Gastroschisis is now the commonest anomaly in babies born to mothers under 20 years of age. The fetal gut prolapses through a defect to the right of the umbilicus. At birth, the bowel is non-rotated, foreshortened and covered by a fibrinous peel (Figure 9.28). After reduction of the bowel, which may need to be staged using a silo, the defect is closed. A silo is a manufactured or hand-sewn plastic or silastic bag attached to the abdominal wall and, containing the herniated viscera, it is gently reduced every 12–24 hours. Gastroschisis has a good prognosis although gut dysmotility delays recovery. Some infants have an intestinal atresia, and some boys have undescended testes but other anomalies are rare.

Exomphalos is a distinctly different anomaly in which the intestines and sometimes the liver are covered with a membranous amniotic sac from which the umbilical cord arises (Figure 9.29). It may be associated with chromosomal or cardiac anomalies.

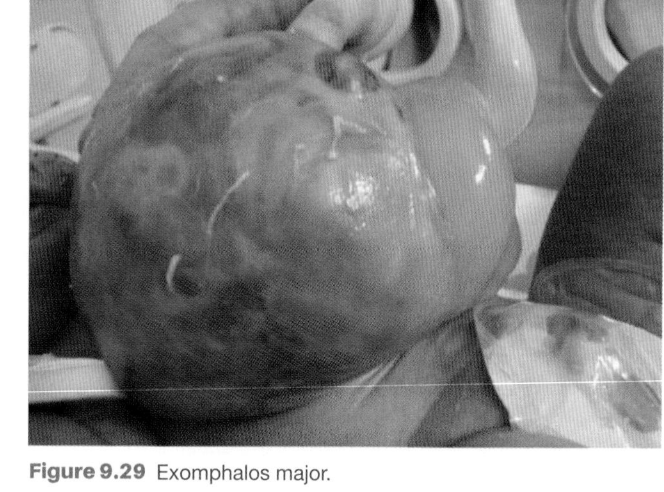

Figure 9.29 Exomphalos major.

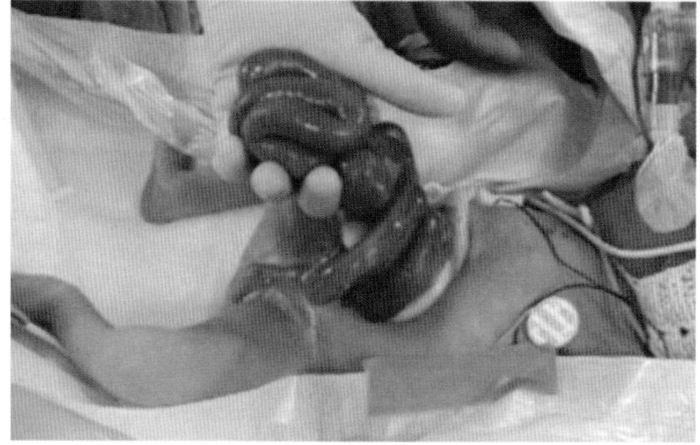

Figure 9.28 A newborn infant with gastroschisis.

Biliary atresia

In biliary atresia the extrahepatic bile ducts are occluded, causing obstructive jaundice (conjugated hyper-bilirubinaemia) and progressive liver fibrosis in early infancy. It should be considered if jaundice persists after 2 weeks of age. Fat malabsorption can lead to a coagulopathy correctable with vitamin K. An abdominal ultrasound scan may show a small or absent gallbladder and no visible bile ducts, and a biliary radionuclide scan may show no excretion. A liver biopsy shows proliferation of small bile ducts. It is treated by a Kasai porto-enterostomy in which the occluded extrahepatic bile ducts are excised and a jejunal Roux loop anastomosed to the

Morio **Kasai**, 1922–2008, formerly Professor of Surgery, The University of Tokyo, Tokyo, Japan.

hepatic hilum. Effective drainage is more likely with surgery before 8 weeks of age and may obviate the subsequent need for liver transplantation.

Alimentary tract duplications

Alimentary tract duplications are rare and are usually single, variable in size and spherical or tubular. Most are located on the mesenteric border of the intestine. Typically, they are lined by alimentary tract mucosa and share a common smooth muscle wall and blood supply with the adjacent bowel, with which they may communicate. Duplications can contain heterotopic gastric mucosa and be associated with spinal anomalies. Most duplications present in infancy or early childhood with intestinal obstruction, haemorrhage, intussusception or perforation (**Figure 9.30**). Rarely, they present in adults and sometimes with a malignancy, which has been reported more often with rectal duplication cysts. Complete excision is the treatment of choice.

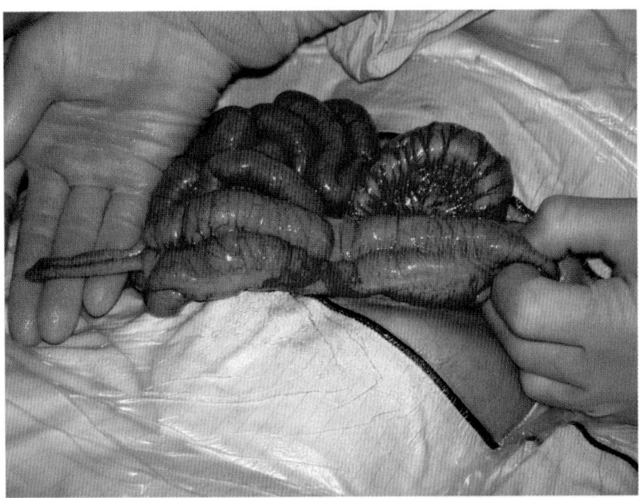

Figure 9.30 A duplicated colon; note the two appendices.

Hirschsprung's disease

Hirschsprung's disease is characterised by the congenital absence of intramural ganglion cells (aganglionosis) and the presence of hypertrophic nerves in the distal large bowel. The absence of ganglion cells is due to a failure of migration of vagal neural crest cells into the developing gut. The affected gut is in spasm, causing a functional bowel obstruction. The aganglionosis is restricted to the rectum and sigmoid colon in 75% of patients (short segment), involves the proximal colon in 15% (long segment) and affects the entire colon and a portion of terminal ileum in 10% (total colonic aganglionosis). A transition zone exists between the dilated, proximal, normally innervated bowel and the narrow, distal aganglionic segment.

Hirschsprung's disease may be familial or associated with Down syndrome or other genetic disorders. Gene mutations have been identified on chromosome 10 (involving the *RET* proto-oncogene) and on chromosome 13 in some patients. Hirschsprung's disease typically presents in the neonatal period with delayed passage of meconium, abdominal distension and bilious vomiting but it may not be diagnosed until later in childhood or even adult life, when it manifests as severe chronic constipation. Enterocolitis is a potentially fatal complication.

The diagnosis requires an adequate rectal biopsy and an experienced pathologist. A contrast enema may show the narrow aganglionic segment, a cone and the dilated proximal bowel (**Figure 9.31**). Surgery aims to remove the aganglionic segment and 'pull-through' ganglionic bowel to the anus (e.g. Swenson, Duhamel, Soave and transanal procedures), and can be done in a single stage or in stages after first establishing a proximal stoma in normally innervated bowel. Most patients achieve good bowel control but a significant minority experience residual constipation and/or faecal incontinence or further enterocolitis.

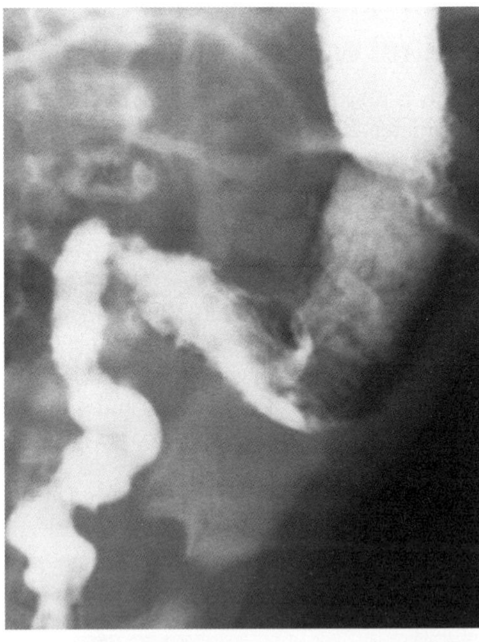

Figure 9.31 Barium enema in an infant, showing a 'transition zone' in the proximal sigmoid colon between the dilated proximal normally innervated bowel and the contracted aganglionic rectum.

Anorectal malformations

The anus is either imperforate or replaced by a fistula which does not pass through the muscle complex and opens away from the specialised skin which represents the true anal site. The sacrum and genitourinary tract are often abnormal. In boys, there may be a rectoperineal fistula but the most common anomaly is an imperforate anus with a rectobulbar urethral fistula (**Figure 9.32**). In girls, the commonest anomalies are a

Harald Hirschsprung, 1830–1916, physician, The Queen Louise Hospital for Children, Copenhagen, Denmark, described congenital megacolon in 1887.
Orvar Swenson, b.1909, Professor of Surgery, Northern University, Chicago, IL, USA.
Bernard George Duhamel, 1917–1996, Professor of Surgery, Hopital St. Denis, Paris, France.
F Soave, twentieth-century Italian paediatric surgeon.

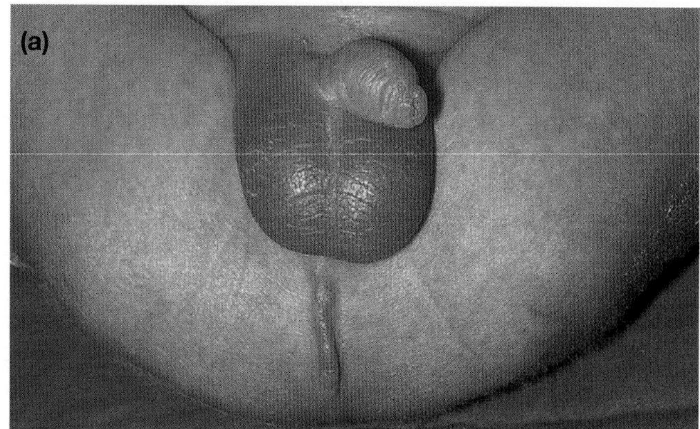

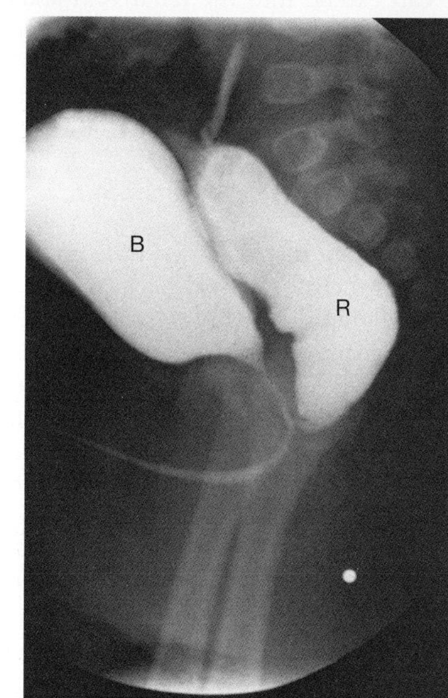

Figure 9.32 (**a**) An imperforate anus in a neonate associated with (**b**) a rectourethral fistula, visible on a contrast study performed via a sigmoid colostomy. The bladder is filled with contrast via the fistula and the radio-opaque dot has been placed on the infant's perineum over the normal site of the anus. B, bladder; R, rectum.

fistula opening in the posterior vestibule behind the vagina or on the perineum. Cloacal malformations, in which the rectum and genitourinary tract share a common outflow channel, are also seen in girls. Where there is a fistula, meconium can be passed and the diagnosis can be delayed for months because the perineum has not been inspected carefully. Most low malformations are treated by an anoplasty soon after birth. Higher, more complex defects need a temporary colostomy, detailed investigation and then reconstructive surgery. Functional outcome is related to the type of malformation and the integrity of the sacrum and pelvic muscles (low defects are associated with constipation, higher defects with faecal incontinence). For children with residual intractable faecal incontinence, antegrade colonic enemas administered via a catheterisable appendicostomy (**Figure 9.33**) (the Malone procedure) enable the child to achieve social continence.

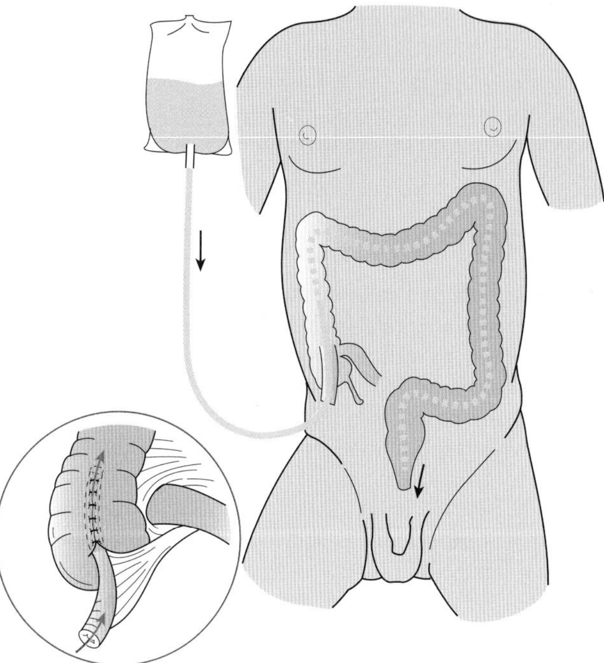

Figure 9.33 Appendicostomy for the delivery of antegrade colonic enemas.

Summary box 9.17

Congenital causes of intestinal obstruction

- Intestinal atresia: may be multiple
- Cystic fibrosis: can present with intestinal obstruction from inspissated meconium
- Intestinal malrotation: predisposes to potentially lethal midgut volvulus
- Alimentary tract duplications: may present with obstruction, haemorrhage or intussusception
- Hirschsprung's disease: typically presents with delay in passing meconium after birth
- Anorectal malformations

Urinary tract malformations

Many of these malformations are now detected by prenatal ultrasound scan. Others present in childhood with urinary infection, obstruction or an abdominal mass. Urinary tract disorders in children are investigated by urine microscopy and culture, ultrasound scan, assessment of renal function and a combination of radioisotope renography (uptake and excretion), contrast radiology and endoscopy.

In many infants, prenatally diagnosed mild to moderate hydronephrosis resolves spontaneously. Those with more significant pelviureteric junction obstruction may be asymptomatic or present in later childhood with urinary tract infection or loin pain. Pyeloplasty is indicated for symptoms or impaired renal function. In boys, partial membranous obstruction in the posterior urethra (valves) can cause a severe prenatal obstructive uropathy. This condition demands urgent investigation and treatment soon after birth to preserve bladder

Patrick Malone, paediatric urologist, Southampton, UK.

and kidney function. Renal failure develops in about one-third of affected boys despite early endoscopic ablation of the obstructing valves. Other congenital urinary tract malformations include ureteric abnormalities (e.g. duplex, ureterocoele, vesicoureteric reflux), multicystic dysplastic kidney and bladder exstrophy.

NECROTISING ENTEROCOLITIS

This is an acquired inflammatory condition of the neonatal gut, mostly affecting premature infants. Immaturity, formula feeds (breast milk is protective), bacterial infection and impaired gut blood flow are implicated in the pathogenesis. The neonate becomes septic, with abdominal distension, bloody stools and bilious aspirates. Patchy or extensive pneumatosis intestinalis progresses to necrosis and perforation (**Figure 9.34**). It commonly affects the terminal ileum and colon. Small intestinal loss can be sufficient to cause severe intestinal failure. Milder cases respond to antibiotics, gut rest and parenteral nutrition but severe cases need an urgent laparotomy. The mortality remains over 30%.

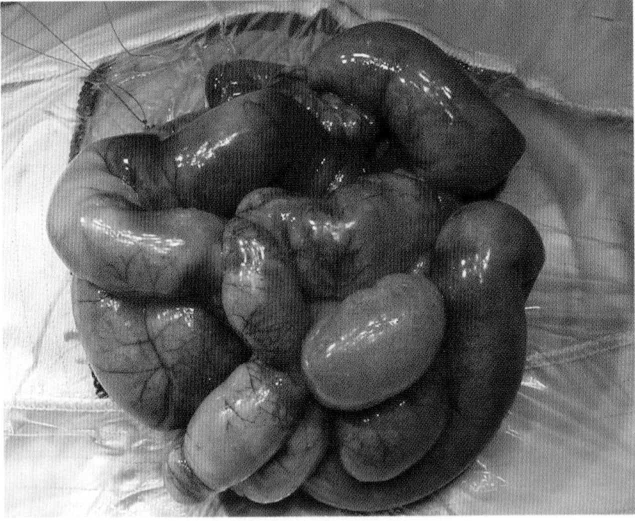

Figure 9.34 Operative appearance of neonatal necrotising enterocolitis.

PAEDIATRIC SURGICAL ONCOLOGY

Neoplasms, though less common in children than in adults, are, with trauma, a leading cause of death in those over 1 year of age. In the West, leukaemia, central nervous system (CNS) tumours, lymphomas, neuroblastomas and nephroblastomas account for most paediatric malignancies. Neuroblastoma and nephroblastoma are among the more common solid abdominal tumours. The prognoses for these cancers have improved after treatments have been refined following numerous multicentre trials.

Neuroblastoma is a malignancy of neuroblasts in the adrenal medulla or sympathetic ganglia and typically presents as an abdominal or paravertebral mass. These cells metastasise to lymph nodes, bone and the liver and raise urinary catecholamine levels. Small localised tumours are excised. Patients with more advanced tumours have surgery after chemotherapy. Survival relates to tumour biology and stage (>90% for small localised tumours, <50% for advanced tumours).

Wilms' tumour (nephroblastoma) is a malignant renal tumour derived from embryonal cells; it typically affects children from 1 to 4 years of age. A mutation in the Wilms' tumour suppressor gene (*WT1*) is responsible for some cases. Wilms' tumours usually present with an abdominal mass. The tumour can extend into the renal vein and vena cava and it metastasises to lymph nodes and lungs. Treatment is with chemotherapy and surgery. Survival depends on tumour spread, completeness of excision and the histological appearance but exceeds 70% even with advanced tumours.

SAFEGUARDING

All staff must be able to recognise abuse and neglect and know the law and their local child safeguarding contacts. In the UK three children die each week from neglect or abuse and half of these deaths are at the hands of the parents. One in a hundred emergency department attendances results from abuse. Consider abuse if any of the following are present: bruises away from bony prominences (face, back, abdomen, arms, buttocks, ears and hands); bruises in clusters or in the pattern of an implement; multiple injuries at different stages of healing; different types of injury (e.g. soft tissue, burns or scalds, cuts and bruises); rib fractures; bite marks (adult bites are difficult to distinguish from child bites, but adult bites are associated with fatal abuse); significant delay between the injury and seeking medical advice; an inconsistent or vague history; or inappropriate parental behaviour.

SERVICE DELIVERY AND SUMMARY

General Paediatric Surgeons working in District General Hospitals in the UK manage the common elective and acute problems of childhood that have been briefly outlined in this chapter for those older than 1 or 2 years. Specialist Paediatric Surgeons and Paediatric Urologists work mainly in regional units, providing a similar service up to age 16, but they also manage infants and neonates with a wide range of conditions. The principles of the speciality arise from the differences that are consequent upon age and development.

FURTHER READING

Carachi R, Grosfeld JL. *The surgery of childhood tumors*. Berlin: Springer, 2016.

Holcomb III GW, Murphy PJ, Ostlie DJ. *Ashcraft's pediatric surgery: expert consult*, 6th edn. London: Elsevier, 2014.

Hutson JM, O'Brien M, Beasley SW, Teague WJ, King SK (eds). *Jones' clinical paediatric surgery*. Oxford: Wiley Blackwell, 2015.

Max Wilms, 1867–1918, Professor of Surgery, Heidelberg, Germany.

Chapter 10

Principles of oncology

Learning objectives

To understand:

- The biological nature of cancer
- That treatment is only one component in the overall management of cancer
- The principles of cancer prevention and early detection
- The principles underlying non-surgical treatments for cancer

To appreciate:

- The principles of cancer aetiology and the major known causative factors
- The likely shape of future developments in cancer management
- The multidisciplinary management of cancer
- The distinction between palliative care and end-of-life care
- The principles of palliative care

WHAT IS CANCER?

History

The name cancer from the Greek word for a crab (καρκινοs), and refers to the claw-like blood vessels extending over the surface of an advanced breast cancer.

The study of cancer has always been a part of clinical medicine: theories have moved from divine intervention, through the humours, and are now firmly based on the cellular origin of cancer. Rudolf Virchow is credited with being first to demonstrate that cancer is a disease of cells and that the disease progresses as a result of abnormal proliferation, encapsulated by his famous dictum '*omnes cellula e cellula*' (every cell from a cell). In 1914, Theodor Boveri pointed out the importance of chromosomal abnormalities in cancer cells and, in the 1940s, Oswald Avery demonstrated that DNA was the genetic material within the chromosomes. In 1953, Watson and Crick described the structure of DNA and this key discovery paved the way for the study of the molecular biology of cancer. We can now investigate, and sometimes even understand, the biochemical mechanisms whereby cancer cells are formed and which mediate their abnormal behaviour.

The psychopath within

Cancer cells are psychopaths. They have no respect for the rights of other cells. They violate the democratic principles of normal cellular organisation. Their proliferation is uncontrolled; their ability to spread is unbounded. Their inexorable, relentless, progress destroys first the tissue and then the person.

In order to behave in such an unprincipled fashion, to become truly malignant, cells have to acquire a number of characteristics. No one characteristic is sufficient and not all characteristics are necessary. These features, based on articles by Hanahan and Weinberg, are summarised in *Summary box 10.1*.

Rudolf Ludwig Carl Virchow, 1821–1902, Professor of Pathology, Berlin, Germany.
Theodor Heinrich Boveri, 1862–1913, Professor of Zoology and Comparative Anatomy, Wurzburg, Germany.
Oswald Theodore Avery, 1877–1955, bacteriologist, Rockefeller Institute, New York, NY, USA.
James Dewey Watson, b.1928, American biologist who worked at Cambridge, UK, and later became Director of the Cold Spring Harbor Laboratory, New York, NY, USA.
Francis Harry Compton Crick, 1916–2004, British molecular biologist who worked at the Cavendish Laboratory, Cambridge, UK and later at the Salk Institute, San Diego, CA, USA. Watson and Crick shared the 1962 Nobel Prize for Physiology or Medicine with Maurice Hugh Frederick Wilkins, 1916–2004, of King's College, London.
Douglas Hanahan, b.1951, American biologist and director of the Swiss Institute for Experimental Cancer Research (ISREC), Lausanne, Switzerland.
Robert A Weinberg, b.1942, The Whitehead Institute of Biomedical Research and Department of Biology, The Massachusetts Institute of Technology, Cambridge, MA, USA.

Summary box 10.1

Features of malignant transformation

- Establish an autonomous lineage
  - Resist signals that inhibit growth
  - Sustain proliferative signalling
- Obtain replicative immortality
- Evade apoptosis
- Acquire angiogenic competence
- Acquire ability to invade
- Acquire ability to disseminate and implant
- Evocation of inflammation
- Evade detection/elimination
- Jettison excess baggage
- Subvert communication to and from the cellular environment
- Develop ability to change energy metabolism

Establish an autonomous lineage

Cells develop independence from the normal signals that control supply and demand. The healing of a wound is a physiological process; the cellular response is exquisitely coordinated so that proliferation occurs when it is needed and ceases when it is no longer required. The whole process is controlled by a series of signals telling cells when, and when not, to divide. Cancer cells escape from this normal system of checks and balances: they grow and proliferate in the absence of external stimuli; they proliferate and grow regardless of signals telling them to desist. Oncogenes, aberrant forms of normal cellular genes, are key factors in this process. They were originally identified as sequences within the genome of viruses that could cause cancer and were thought to be of viral origin but, surprisingly, turned out to be parts of the normal genome that were hitchhiking between cells, using the virus as a vector. Viral oncogenes (*v-onc*) had sequence homology with normal cellular genes (*c-onc*) and are now presumed to be mutated versions of genes concerned with normal cellular husbandry. The implication of this is that we all carry within us the seeds of our own destruction: genetic sequences that, through mutation, can turn into active oncogenes and thereby cause malignant transformation.

Obtain immortality

According to the Hayflick hypothesis, normal cells are permitted to undergo only a finite number of divisions. For humans this number is between 40 and 60. The limitation is imposed by the progressive shortening of the end of the chromosome (the telomere) that occurs each time a cell divides. Telomeric shortening is like a molecular clock and, when its time is up, the lineage will die out. Cancer cells can use the enzyme telomerase to rebuild the telomere at each cell division; there is no telomeric shortening, and the lineage will never die out. The cancer cell has achieved immortality.

Evade apoptosis

Apoptosis is a form of programmed cell death which occurs as the direct result of internal cellular events instructing the cell to die. Unlike necrosis, apoptosis is an orderly and internally driven process. The cell dismantles itself neatly for disposal (**Figure 10.1**). There is minimal inflammatory response. Apoptosis is a physiological process. Cells that find themselves in the wrong place normally die by apoptosis and this is an important self-regulatory mechanism in growth and development: cells in the web space of the embryo die by apoptosis, as do lymphocytes that could react to self. The process was rediscovered in 1972, and named apoptosis from the Greek αποπτωσις, indicating leaf fall. Genes, such as *p53*, that can activate apoptosis function as tumour suppressor genes. Loss of function in a tumour suppressor gene will contribute to malignant transformation. Cancer cells will be able to evade apoptosis, which means that the wrong cells can be in the wrong places at the wrong times.

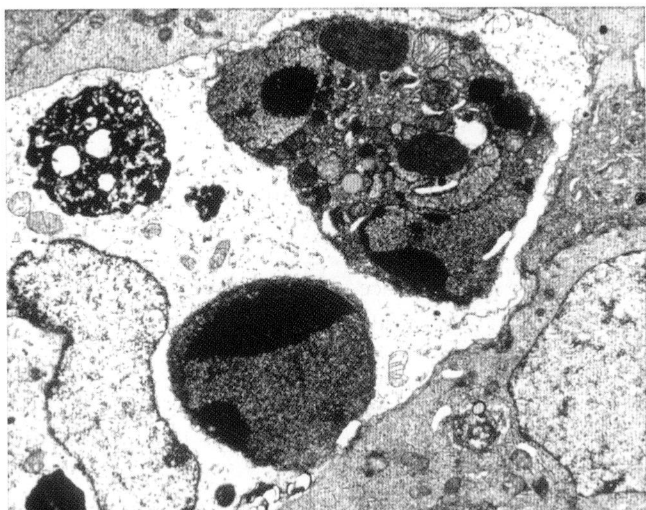

Figure 10.1 Electron micrograph of apoptotic bodies engulfed by a macrophage.

Acquire angiogenic competence

A mass of tumour cells cannot, in the absence of a blood supply, grow beyond a diameter of about 1 mm. This places a severe restriction on the capabilities of the tumour: it cannot grow much larger or spread widely within the body. If, however, the mass of tumour cells is able to attract or to construct a blood supply then it is able to quit its dormant state and behave in a far more aggressive fashion. The ability of a tumour to form blood vessels is termed 'angiogenic competence' and is a key feature of malignant transformation.

Acquire ability to invade

Cancer cells have no respect for the structure of normal tissues. They acquire the ability to breach the basement

---

Leonard Hayflick, b.1928, while working at the Wistar Institute in Philadelphia in 1962, he noted that normal mammalian cells growing in culture had a limited, rather than an indefinite, capacity for self-replication.

membrane and gain direct access to blood and lymph vessels. Cancer cells use three main mechanisms to facilitate invasion: (1) they cause a rise in the interstitial pressure within a tissue; (2) they secrete enzymes that dissolve extracellular matrix; and (3) they become mobile. Unrestrained proliferation and a lack of contact inhibition enable cancer cells to exert pressure directly on the surrounding tissue and push beyond the normal limits. They secrete collagenases and proteases that chemically dissolve any extracellular boundaries that would otherwise limit their spread through tissues and, by modulating the expression of cell-surface molecules called integrins, are able to detach themselves from the extracellular matrix. The abnormal integrins associated with malignancy can also transmit signals from the environment to the cytoplasm and nucleus of the cancer cells ('outside-in signalling') and these signals can induce increased motility. These processes are similar to those involved in normal development, in the migration of the neural crest or the formation of the heart. Epithelial cells behave as if they were mesenchymal cells and the process is termed 'epithelial–mesenchymal transition' (EMT). EMT is a crucial step in malignant transformation and many of the genes and proteins implicated in the formation of cancer control processes are involved in EMT, for example *Src*, *Ras*, integrins, *Wnt /b* –catenin, Notch.

Acquire ability to disseminate and implant, evocation of inflammation

Once cancer cells gain access to vascular and lymphovascular spaces, they have acquired the potential to use the body's natural distribution system. This is not, of itself, sufficient to cause tumours to develop at distant sites. The cells also need to acquire the ability to implant. As Paget pointed out over a century ago, there is a crucial relationship here between the seed (the tumour cell) and the soil (the distant tissue). Most of the cancer cells discharged into the circulation probably do not form viable metastases: circulating cancer cells can be identified in patients who never develop clinical evidence of metastatic disease. Clumping may be important in permitting metastases, the outer cells protecting the inner cells from immunological attack. These outer protective cells may, on occasion, be normal lymphocytes.

Cancer can spread in this embolic fashion but can also spread when individual cells migrate and implant. Whether spread occurs in groups or as individual cells there is still the problem of crossing the vascular endothelium (and basement membrane) to gain access to the tissue itself. Cancer cells probably implant themselves in distant tissues by exploiting, and subverting, the normal inflammatory response. By expressing inflammatory cytokines the cancer cells can fool the endothelium of the host tissue into becoming activated and allowing cancer cells access to the extravascular space. Activated endothelium expresses receptors that bind to integrins and selectins on the surface of cells, allowing them to move across the endothelial barrier.

Evade detection/elimination

Cancer cells are simultaneously both 'self' and 'not self'. Although derived from normal cells ('self') they are, in terms of their genetic make up, behaviour and characteristics, foreign ('not self'). As such, they ought to provoke an immune response and be eliminated, and it is entirely possible that malignant transformation is a more frequent event than the emergence of clinical cancer. The possible role of the immune system in eliminating nascent cancers was proposed by Paul Ehrlich in 1909 and revisited by both Sir Frank McFarlane Burnet and Lewis Thomas in the late 1950s. Cancer cells, or at least those that give rise to clinical disease, appear to gain the ability to escape detection by the immune system. This may be through suppressing expression of tumour associated antigens or it may be through actively co-opting one part of the immune system to help the tumour escape detection by other parts of the immune surveillance system.

Jettison excess baggage

Cancer cells are geared to excessive and remorseless proliferation. They do not need to develop or retain those specialised functions that make them good cellular citizens. They can therefore afford to repress or permanently lose those genes that control such functions. They become leaner and meaner. This may bring some short-term advantages. The longer-term disadvantage is that what is today superfluous may, tomorrow, be essential. This can leave cancer cells vulnerable to external stressors and may, in part, explain why some cancer treatments work.

Subvert communication to and from the environment/milieu

Providing false information is a classic military strategy. Degrading the command and control systems of the enemy is an essential component of modern warfare. Cancer cells almost certainly use similar tactics in their battle for control over their host. Given the complexity of communication between and within cells, this is not an easy statement either to disprove or to prove. Nor does it offer any easy targets for therapeutic manipulation.

Stephen Paget, 1855–1926, surgeon, The West London Hospital, London, UK. Paget's 'seed and soil' hypothesis is contained in his paper 'The distribution of secondary growths in cancer of the breast', in the *Lancet*, 1889.

Paul Ehrlich, 1854–1915, Professor of Hygiene, The University of Berlin, and later Director of The Institute for Infectious Diseases, Berlin, Germany. In 1908, he shared the Nobel Prize for Physiology or Medicine with **Elie Metchnikoff**, 1845–1916, 'in recognition of his work on immunity'. Metchnikoff was Professor of Zoology at Odessa in Russia, and later worked at the Pasteur Institute in Paris, France.

Sir Frank McFarlane Burnet, 1899–1985, Australian virologist, Walter and Eliza Hall Institute, Melbourne, Australia. Burnett shared the 1960 Nobel Prize for Physiology or Medicine with **Sir Peter Brian Medawar**, 1915–1987, Jodrell Professor of Zoology, University College, London, UK, 'for their discovery of acquired immunological tolerance'.

Lewis Thomas, 1913–1993, American pathologist and immunologist, who became President of the Sloan Kettering Memorial Institute, New York, NY, USA.

Develop ability to change energy metabolism

Blood flow in tumours is often sporadic and unreliable. As a result, cancer cells may have to spend prolonged periods starved of oxygen – in a state of relative hypoxia. Compared with the corresponding normal cells, some cancer cells may be better able to survive in hypoxic conditions. This ability may enable tumours to grow and develop despite an impoverished blood supply. Cancer cells can alter their metabolism even when oxygen is abundant; they break down glucose but do not, as normal cells would do, send the resulting pyruvate to the mitochondria for conversion, in an oxygen-dependent process, to carbon dioxide. This is the phenomenon of aerobic glycolysis, or the Warburg effect, and leads to the production of lactate. In an act of symbiosis, lactate-producing cancer cells may provide lactate for adjacent cancer cells which are then able to use it, via the citric acid cycle, for energy production. This cooperation is similar to that which occurs in skeletal muscle during exercise.

Malignant transformation

The characteristics of the cancer cell arise as a result of mutation. Only very rarely is a single mutation sufficient to cause cancer; multiple mutations are usually required. Colorectal cancer provides the classical example of how multiple mutations are necessary for the complete transformation from normal cell to malignant cell. Vogelstein and his colleagues identified the genes required and also postulated not only that it is necessary to have mutations in all the relevant genes, but also that these mutations must be acquired in a specific sequence.

Cancer is usually regarded as a clonal disease. Once a cell has arisen with all the mutations necessary to make it fully malignant, it is capable of giving rise to an infinite number of identical cells, each of which is fully malignant. These cells divide, invade, metastasise and destroy but, ultimately, each is the direct descendant of that original, primordial, transformed cell. There is certainly evidence, mostly from haematological malignancies, to support the view that tumours are monoclonal in origin, but recent evidence challenges the universality of this assumption. Some cancers may arise from more than one clone of cells. Epigenetic modification refers to hereditable changes in DNA that are not related to the nucleotide sequence of the molecule. Epigenetic modification may give rise to distinct cancer cell lineages with differing biological properties. The interactions between cells from each lineage and the tissue within which such cells find themselves may determine the overall clinical behaviour of a tumour.

Two mechanisms may help to sustain and accelerate the process of malignant transformation: genomic instability and tumour-related inflammation.

Genomic instability

A cancer is in a genetic ferment. Cells are dividing without proper checks and balances. Mutations are arising all the time within tumours and some of these mutations, particularly those in tumour suppressor genes, may have the ability to encourage the development and persistence of further mutations. This gives rise to the phenomenon of genomic instability – as it evolves, a cancer contains an increasing variety and number of genetic aberrations. The greater the number of such abnormalities, the greater the chance of increasingly deviant behaviour, and the pace of malignant transformation accelerates.

Tumour-related inflammation

If a tumour provokes an inflammatory response then the cytokines and other factors produced as a result of that response may act to promote and sustain malignant transformation. Growth factors, mutagenic ROS (reactive oxygen species), angiogenic factors and antiapoptotic factors may all be produced as part of an inflammatory process and all may contribute to the progression of a tumour.

A recurring theme in the molecular biology of cancer is that systems and pathways can behave unpredictably – activation may sometimes promote, and sometimes inhibit, growth and transformation. This has important implications for therapy: treatments designed to inhibit the growth and spread of cancer may, occasionally, have precisely the opposite effect. The most consistent feature of cancer is its lack of consistency.

The growth of a tumour

If it is accepted that a cancer starts from a single transformed cell then it is possible, using straightforward arithmetic, to describe the progression from a single cell to a mass of cells large enough to kill the host. The division of a cell produces two daughter cells. The relationship 2^n will describe the number of cells produced after n generations of division. There are between 10^{13} and 10^{14} cells in a typical human being. A tumour 10 mm in diameter will contain about 10^9 cells. Since $2^{30} = 10^9$ this implies that it would take 30 generations to reach the threshold of clinical detectability and, as $2^{45} = 3 \times 10^{13}$, it will take fewer than 15 subsequent generations to produce a tumour that, through sheer bulk alone, would be fatal. This is an oversimplification because cell loss is a feature of many tumours, and for squamous cancers as many as 99% of the cells produced may be lost, mainly by exfoliation. It will, in the presence of cell loss, take many cellular divisions to produce a clinically evident tumour – abundant opportunity for further mutations to occur during the preclinical phase of tumour growth. The growth of a typical human tumour can be described by an exponential relationship, the doubling time of which increases exponentially – so-called Gompertzian growth (**Figure 10.2**). This

Otto Warburg, 1883–1970, chemist, Director of the Kaiser Wilhelm Institute for Cell Physiology, Berlin-Dahlem. Awarded the Nobel Prize for Physiology or Medicine in 1931 for 'his discovery of the nature and mode of action of the respiratory enzyme'.
Bert Vogelstein, b.1949, molecular biologist, Johns Hopkins Hospital, Baltimore, MD, USA.
Benjamin Gompertz, 1779–1865, an insurance actuary who was interested in calculating annuities. To do this, he needed to describe mathematically the relationship between life-expectancy and age. He was able to do this using the function that bears his name. The Gompertzian function provides an excellent fit to data points plotting tumour size against time.

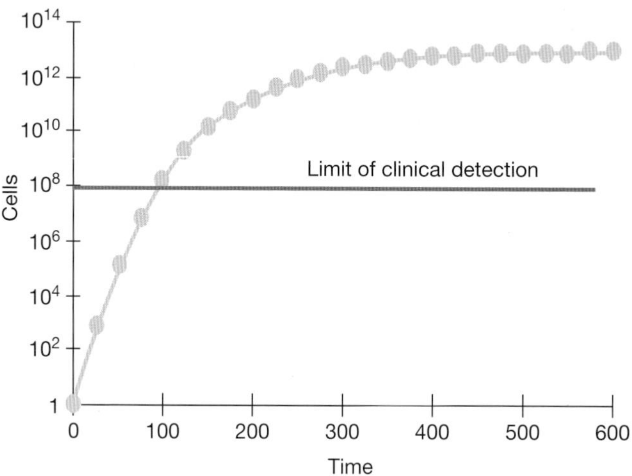

Figure 10.2 The Gompertzian curve describing the growth of a typical tumour. In its early stages, growth is exponential but, as the tumour grows, the growth rate slows. This decrease in growth rate probably arises because of difficulties with nutrition and oxygenation. The tumour cells are in competition: not only with the tissues of the host, but also with each other.

Gompertzian pattern has several important implications for the diagnosis and treatment of cancer.

Summary box 10.2

The implications of Gompertzian growth

- The majority of the growth of a tumour occurs before it is clinically detectable
- By the time they are detected, tumours have passed the period of most rapid growth, that period when they might be most sensitive to antiproliferative drugs
- There has been plenty of time, before diagnosis, for individual cells to detach, invade, implant, and form distant metastases. In many patients cancer may, at the time of presentation, be a systemic disease
- 'Early tumours' are genetically old, yielding many opportunities for mutations to occur, mutations that might confer spontaneous drug resistance (a probability greatly increased by the existence of cell loss)
- The rate of regression of a tumour will depend upon its age (the Norton–Simon hypothesis extends this: chemotherapy results in a rate of regression in tumour volume that is proportional to the rate of growth for an unperturbed tumour of that size)

THE CAUSES OF CANCER

The interplay between nature and nurture

Both inheritance and environment are important determinants of cancer development. Neither influence is totally dominant. Using a familiar example, not all smokers develop lung cancer; lung cancer can occur in people who have never smoked. The debate concerning the relative importance of the two factors has recently become polarised, Tomasetti and Vogelstein claiming that cancer is largely a random process ('bad luck); the contrary view, expressed by Wu, Powers and colleagues, is that extrinsic risk factors make a substantial contribution to the development of cancer. The likelihood is that both sides are correct, but each only partially.

Knowledge about the causes of cancer can be used to design appropriate strategies for prevention or earlier diagnosis. As we find out more about the genes associated with cancer, genetic testing and counselling will play an increasing role in the prevention of cancer. These considerations are incorporated into *Table 10.1*, on the inherited cancer syndromes, and in *Table 10.2*, on the environmental contribution to cancer.

THE MANAGEMENT OF CANCER

Management is more than treatment

The traditional approach to cancer concentrates on diagnosis and active treatment. This is a very limited view that, in terms of the public health, may not have served society well. It implies a fatalistic attitude to the occurrence of cancer and an assumption that, once active treatment is complete, there is little more to be done. Prevention is forgotten and rehabilitation is ignored.

A more comprehensive view considers the management of cancer as taking place along two axes: one is an axis of scale, from the individual to the world population; the other is an axis based on the unnatural history of the disease, from prevention through to rehabilitation or palliative care (**Figure 10.3**).

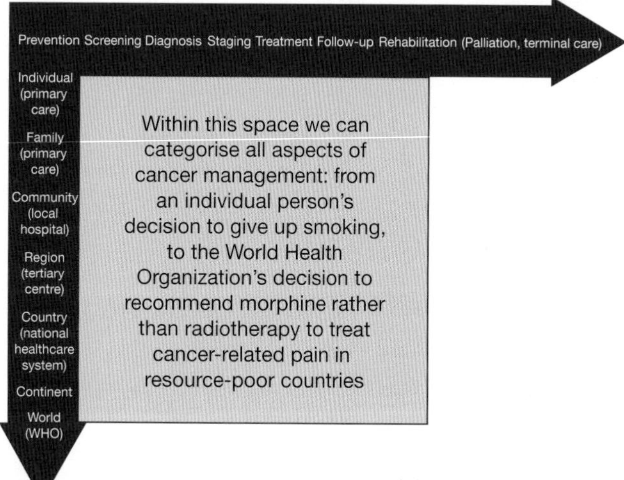

Figure 10.3 The management of cancer spans the natural history of the disease and all humankind, from the individual to the population of the world.

Prevention

The World Cancer Research Fund has published an extensive view of the evidence on the preventable causes of cancer; their conclusion is that many cancers could be prevented if

Larry Norton, b.1947, Valley Stream, New York. Deputy Physician-in-Chief for Breast Cancer Programs, Memorial Sloan-Kettering Cancer Center, New York.
Richard Macey Simon, b.1943, Director, Biometric Research Program Chief, Computational & Systems Biology Branch, National Cancer Institute, Bethesda, Maryland.

TABLE 10.1 Inherited syndromes associated with cancer.

Syndrome	Gene(s) implicated	Inheritance	Associated tumours and abnormalities	Strategies for prevention/ early diagnosis
Familial adenomatous polyposis (FAP)/ Gardner syndrome	*APC* gene	D	Colorectal cancer under the age of 25 Papillary carcinoma of the thyroid Cancer of the ampulla of Vater Hepatoblastomas Primary brain tumours (Turcot syndrome) Osteomas of the jaw CHRPE (congenital hypertrophy of the retinal pigment epithelium)	Prophylactic panproctocolectomy
Hereditary non-polyposis colorectal cancer (HNPCC)	DNA mismatch repair genes (*MLH1*; *MSH2*; *MSH6*)	D	Colorectal cancer (typically in 40s and 50s)	Surveillance colonoscopies / polypectomies Non-steroidal anti-inflammatory drugs
HNPCC1	*MSH2*		Endometrium, stomach, hepatobiliary (Lynch syndrome 1)	
HNPCC2	*MLH1*			
HNPCC3	*PMS1*			
Peutz–Jeghers syndrome	*STK11*	D	Bowel cancer; breast cancer; freckles round the mouth	Surveillance colonoscopy; mammography
Cowden* syndrome	*PTEN*	D	Multiple hamartomas of skin, breast and mucous membranes Breast cancer Neuroendocrine tumours Endometrial cancer Thyroid cancer	Active surveillance
Retinoblastoma	*RB*	D	Retinoblastoma Pinealoma Osteosarcoma	Surveillance of uninvolved eye
Multiple endocrine neoplasia (MEN) Type 1	*Menin*	D	Parathyroid tumours Islet cell tumours Pituitary tumours	Awareness of associations and paying attention to relevant symptoms
MEN Type 2A	*RET*	D	Medullary carcinoma of the thyroid Phaeochromocytoma Parathyroid tumours	Regular screening of blood pressure, serum calcitonin and urinary catecholamines Prophylactic thyroidectomy
MEN2b	*RET*	D	Medullary carcinoma of the thyroid; phaeochromocytoma; mucosal neuromas; ganglioneuromas of the gut	Regular screening of blood pressure, serum calcitonin and urinary catecholamines; Prophylactic thyroidectomy
Li–Fraumeni	*P53*	D	Sarcomas Leukaemia Osteosarcomas Brain tumours Adrenocortical carcinomas	Very difficult, since pattern of tumours is so heterogeneous and varies from patient to patient
Familial breast cancer	*BRCA1; BRCA2*	D	Breast cancer Ovarian cancer Papillary serous carcinoma of the peritoneum Prostate cancer	Screening mammography; pelvic ultrasound; PSA (in males) Prophylactic mastectomy; prophylactic oophorectomy

Continued

Eldon J Gardner, b.1909, Professor of Zoology, Utah State University, Salt Lake City, UT, USA.
Abraham Vater, 1684–1751, Professor of Anatomy and Botany, and later of Pathology and Therapeutics, Wittenburg, Germany.
Jacques Turcot, b.1914, surgeon, Hôtel Dieu de Quebec Hospital, Quebec, Canada.
Henry T Lynch, b.1928, oncologist, Chairman of the Department of Preventive Medicine, Creighton School of Medicine, California, USA.
John Law Augustine Peutz, 1886–1968, Chief Specialist for Internal Medicine, St John's Hospital, The Hague, The Netherlands.
Harold Joseph Jeghers, 1904–1990, Professor of Internal Medicine, The New Jersey College of Medicine and Dentistry, Jersey City, NJ, USA.
Frederick P Li, b.1940, Professor of Medicine, Harvard University Medical School, Boston, MA, USA.
Joseph F Fraumeni, b.1933, Director of Cancer Epidemiology and Genetics, The National Cancer Institute, Bethesda, MD, USA.

TABLE 10.1 Inherited syndromes associated with cancer – *continued*.

Syndrome	Gene(s) implicated	Inheritance	Associated tumours and abnormalities	Strategies for prevention/ early diagnosis
Familial cutaneous malignant melanoma	*CDNK2A; CDK4*	D	Cutaneous malignant melanoma	Avoid exposure to sunlight, careful surveillance
Basal cell naevus syndrome (Gorlin)	*PTCH*	D	Basal cell carcinomas Medulloblastoma Bifid ribs	Careful surveillance, awareness of diagnosis (look for bifid ribs on x-ray)
Von Hippel–Lindau	*VHL*	D	Renal cancer Phaeochromocytoma Haemangiomas of the cerebellum and retina	Urinary catecholamines
Neurofibromatosis type 1	*NF1*	D	Astrocytomas Primitive neuroectodermal tumours Optic gliomas Multiple neurofibromas	A difficult problem; maintain a high index of suspicion concerning any rapid changes in growth or character of any nodule
Neurofibromatosis type 2	*NF2*	D	Acoustic neuromas Spinal tumours Meningiomas Multiple neurofibromas	
Xeroderma pigmentosum	Deficient nucleotide excision repair (*XPA,B,C*)	R	Skin sensitive to sunlight. Early onset of cutaneous squamous or basal cell carcinomas	Avoidance of sun exposure Active surveillance and early treatment Retinoids for chemoprevention
Ataxia–telagiectasia	*AT*	R	Progressive cerebellar ataxia Leukaemia Lymphoma Breast cancer Melanoma Upper gastrointestinal tumours	Active surveillance
Bloom syndrome	*BLM helicase*	R	Sensitivity to ultraviolet light Leukaemia Lymphoma	Active surveillance

D, dominant; PSA, prostate-specific antigen; R, recessive.
* One of the few clinical syndromes named for the patient rather than the clinician. Rachel Cowden was, in 1963, the first patient described with the syndrome. She died from breast cancer at the age of 20.

TABLE 10.2 Environmental causes of cancer (and suggested measures for reducing their impact).

Environmental/behavioural factor	Associated tumours	Strategy for prevention/early diagnosis
Tobacco	Lung cancer Head and neck cancer	Ban tobacco Ban smoking in public places Punitive taxes on tobacco
Alcohol	Head and neck cancer Oesophageal cancer Hepatoma	Avoid excess alcohol Surveillance of high-risk individuals
Ultraviolet exposure	Melanoma Non-melanoma skin cancer	Avoid excessive sun exposure, avoid sunbeds
Ionising radiation	Leukaemia Breast cancer Lymphoma Thyroid cancer	Limit medical exposures to absolute minimum; safety precautions at nuclear facilities; monitor radiation workers

Continued

Robert Gorlin, 1923–2006, Professor of Dentistry, The University of Minnesota, Minneapolis, MN, USA.
Eugen von Hippel, 1867–1939, Professor of Ophthalmology, Göttingen, Germany.
Arvid Lindau, 1892–1958, Professor of Pathology, Lund, Sweden.
David Bloom, b.1892, dermatologist at the Skin and Cancer Clinic, New York University, New York, NY, USA, described the syndrome in 1954.

TABLE 10.2 Environmental causes of cancer (and suggested measures for reducing their impact) – *continued.*

Environmental/behavioural factor			Associated tumours	Strategy for prevention/early diagnosis
Viral infections	Human papillomavirus (HPV)		Cervical cancer Penile tumours	Avoid unprotected sex Vaccination
	Human immunodeficiency virus (HIV)		Kaposi's sarcoma Lymphomas Germ cell tumours Anal cancer	Avoid unprotected sex Antiretroviral therapy
	Hepatitis B		Hepatoma	Avoid contaminated injections/ infusions Vaccination
Other infections	Bilharzia		Bladder cancer	Treatment of infection Cystoscopic surveillance
	Helicobacter pylori		Stomach cancer	Eradication therapy
Inhaled particles	Asbestos		Mesothelioma	Protect workers from inhaled dusts and fibres
	Wood dust		Paranasal sinus cancers	
Chemicals	Environmental pollutants/chemicals used in industry		Angiosarcoma (vinyl chloride) Bladder cancer (aniline dyes, vulcanisation of rubber) Lung, nasal cavity (nickel) Skin (arsenic) Lung (beryllium, cadmium, chromium) All sites (dioxins)	Protection of exposed workers; avoid chemical discharge and spillages
	Medical	Alkylating agents used in cytotoxic chemotherapy	Leukaemia Lymphoma Lung cancer	Avoid over-treatment; only combine drugs with ionising radiation when absolutely necessary
		Immunosuppressive treatment	Kaposi's sarcoma	As low a dose as possible, for as short a period as possible
		Stilboestrol	Adenocarcinoma of vagina in daughters of treated mothers	Use of stilboestrol curtailed
		Tamoxifen	Endometrial cancer	Biopsy if patient on tamoxifen develops uterine bleeding
Fungal and plant toxins	Aflatoxins		Hepatoma	Appropriate food storage, screen for fungal contamination of foodstuffs
Obesity/lack of physical exercise			Breast Endometrium Kidney Colon Oesophagus	Maintain ideal body weight, regular exercise

people ate sensibly and exercised more. This advice supplements the preventative measures outlined in *Table 10.2*.

Screening

Screening involves the detection of disease in an asymptomatic population in order to improve outcomes by early diagnosis. It follows that a successful screening programme must achieve early diagnosis and that the disease in question has a better outcome when treated at an early stage. The criteria which must be fulfilled for the disease, screening test and the screening programme itself are given in *Summary box 10.3*. Merely to prove that screening picks up disease at an early stage, and that the outcome is better for patients with screen-detected disease than for those who present with symptoms, is an insufficient criterion for the success of a screening programme. This is because of inherent biases in screening (lead time bias, selection bias and length bias) which make screen-detected disease appear to be associated with better outcomes than symptomatic disease.

Lead time bias describes the phenomenon whereby early detection of a disease will always prolong survival from the time of diagnosis when compared to disease picked up at a later stage in its development whether or not the screening process has altered the progression of the tumour (**Figure 10.4**). Selection bias describes the finding that individuals who accept an invitation for screening are, in general, healthier than those who do not. It follows that individuals with screen-detected disease will tend to live longer, independently of the condition for which screening is being

Moritz Kaposi (originally Kohn), 1837–1902, Professor of Dermatology, Vienna, Austria, described pigmented sarcoma of the skin in 1872.

Summary Box 10.3

Criteria for screening

The disease:

- Recognisable early stage
- Treatment at early stage more effective than at later stage
- Sufficiently common to warrant screening

The test:

- Sensitive and specific
- Acceptable to the screened population
- Safe
- Inexpensive

The programme:

- Adequate diagnostic facilities for those with a positive test
- High quality treatment for screen-detected disease to minimise morbidity and mortality
- Screening repeated at intervals if disease of insidious onset
- Benefit must outweigh physical and psychological harm

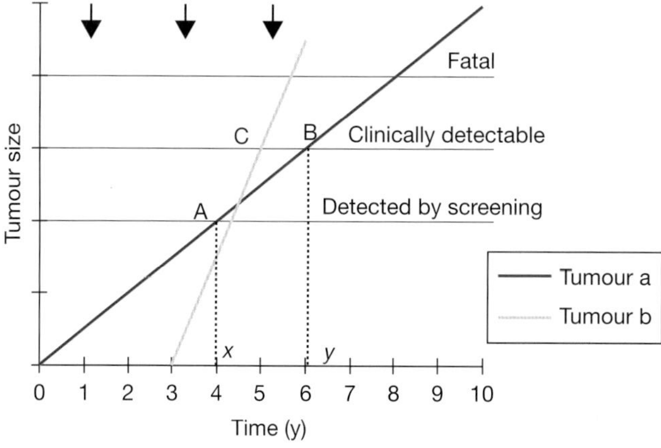

Figure 10.4 An illustration of lead-time and length bias. Tumour a is a steadily growing tumour, its progress is uninfluenced by any treatment. The arrows indicate the timing of tests in a screening programme. The horizontal lines indicate three thresholds: detectability by screening; clinical detectability; and death due to tumour progression. Point A indicates the time at which the tumour would be diagnosed in a screening programme, and point B indicates the time at which the tumour would be diagnosed clinically, that is, in the absence of any screening programme. If the date of diagnosis is used as the start time for measuring survival, then it is clear that, in the absence of any effect from treatment, the screening programme will, artefactually, add to the survival time. The amount of 'increased' survival is equal to $y - x$ years, in this example just over 2 years. This artefactual inflation of survival time is referred to as lead-time bias.

Tumour b is a rapidly growing tumour, again its progress is uninfluenced by treatment. It grows so rapidly that, in the interval between two screening tests, it can cross both the threshold for detectability by screening and that of clinical detectability. It will continue to progress rapidly after diagnosis and the measured survival time will be short. This phenomenon, whereby those tumours that are 'missed' by the screening programme are associated with decreased survival, is called length time bias.

performed. Length bias occurs because slow-growing tumours are likely to be picked up by screening whereas fast-growing tumours are likely to arise and produce symptoms in between screening rounds. Screen-detected tumours will therefore tend to be less aggressive than symptomatic tumours. Because of these biases it is essential to carry out population-based randomised controlled trials and to compare the mortality rate in a whole population offered screening (including those who refuse to be screened and those who develop cancer after a negative test) with the mortality rate in a population which has not been offered screening. This research design has been applied to both breast cancer and colorectal cancer: in both cases there was reduction in disease-specific mortality.

Diagnosis and classification

Accurate diagnosis is the key to the successful management of cancer. Precise diagnosis is crucial to the choice of correct therapy; the wrong operation, no matter how superbly performed, is useless. An unequivocal diagnosis is the key to an accurate prognosis. Only rarely can a diagnosis of cancer be confidently made in the absence of tissue for pathological or cytological examination. Cancer is a disease of cells and, for accurate diagnosis, the abnormal cells need to be seen. Different tumours are classified in different ways: most squamous epithelial tumours are simply classed as well (G1), moderate (G2) or poorly (G3) differentiated. Adenocarcinomas are also often classified as G1, 2 or 3 but prostate cancer is an exception, with widespread use of the Gleason system. The Gleason system grades prostate cancer according to the degree of differentiation of the two most prevalent architectural patterns. The final score is the sum of the two grades and can vary from 2 (1+1) to 10 (5+5) with the higher scores indicating poorer prognosis.

The management of malignant lymphomas is based firmly upon histopathological classification: the first distinction is between Hodgkin's lymphoma (HL) and the non-Hodgkin's lymphomas (NHL). Each of these main types of lymphoma is then subclassified according to a different scheme. The World Health Organization/Revised European–American Lymphoma (WHO/REAL) system classifies Hodgkin's lymphoma into classical HL (nodular sclerosis HL; mixed-cellularity HL; lymphocyte depletion HL; lymphocyte-rich classical HL) and nodular lymphocyte-predominant HL. The WHO/REAL classification of NHL is considerably more complex and recognises 27 distinct pathological subtypes. It is perhaps no coincidence that the non-surgical treatment of lymphomas is, by and large, more successful than the non-surgical treatment of solid tumours. This suggests that precise and accurate subtyping of tumours enables appropriate selection of treatment and, in turn, this is associated with better outcome. The development, over the next decade, of molecular classifiers will profoundly alter our approach. Diseases such as breast cancer and colorectal cancer will become subdivided into a plethora of molecularly distinct entities.

Donald F Gleason, b.1920, pathologist, The University of Minnesota, Minneapolis, MN, USA.
Thomas Hodgkin, 1798–1866, curator of the Museum and demonstrator of Morbid Anatomy, Guy's Hospital, London, UK, described lymphadenoma in 1832.

Investigation and staging

It is not sufficient simply to know what a cancer is; its site and extent must also be known. If it is localised, then locoregional treatments such as surgery and radiation therapy may be curative. If the disease is widespread then, although such local interventions may contribute to cure, they will be insufficient and systemic treatment, for example with drugs or hormones, will also be required.

Staging is the process whereby the extent of disease is mapped out. Staging used to be a fairly crude process based on clinical examination, chest x-ray and the occasional ultrasound; nowadays it is a highly sophisticated process, heavily reliant on the technology of modern imaging. These technological advances bring with them the implication that patients staged as having localised disease in 2017 are not comparable to patients described in 1985 as having localised disease. Many of these latter patients would, had they been imaged using the technology of 2017, have had occult metastatic disease detected. This leads to the paradox of stage shift, also named, by Alvan Feinstein, the Will Rogers phenomenon. A change in staging system, or in the techniques used to provide baseline information concerning staging, can produce 'benefits' to patients in all stages of the disease. These benefits are, however, entirely artefactual and depend simply upon patients in each stage being enriched by patients with improved prognosis. The important cross-check to protect against being misled by stage shift is that the prognosis for the entire group (i.e. all stages pooled) has not been changed. *Table 10.3* shows a worked example of stage shift.

The UICC (International Union against Cancer) is responsible for the TNM (tumour, nodes, metastases) staging system for cancer. This system is compatible with, and relates to, the American Cancer Society (AJCC) system for stage grouping of cancer. Examples of clinicopathological staging systems for colon cancer are shown in *Tables 10.4 and 10.5*.

Therapeutic decision making and the multidisciplinary team

As the management of cancer becomes more complex, it becomes impossible for any individual clinician to have the intellectual and technical competence that is necessary to manage all patients presenting with a particular type of tumour. The formation of multidisciplinary teams represents an attempt to make certain that each and every patient with a particular type of cancer is managed appropriately. Teams should not only be multidisciplinary, they should be multiprofessional. The advantages and disadvantages of multidisciplinary teams are summarised in *Table 10.6*.

Summary box 10.4

The composition of the multidisciplinary team

- Site-specialist surgeon
- Surgical oncologist
- Plastic and reconstructive surgeon
- Clinical oncologist/radiotherapist
- Medical oncologist
- Diagnostic radiologist
- Palliative care physician
- Pathologist
- Speech therapist
- Physiotherapist
- Prosthetist
- Clinical nurse specialist (rehabilitation, supportive care)
- Macmillan nurse (symptom control, palliative care)
- Social worker/counsellor
- Medical secretary/administrator
- Audit and information coordinator

Principles of cancer surgery

For most solid tumours, surgery remains the definitive treatment and the only realistic hope of cure. However, surgery has several roles in cancer treatment including diagnosis, removal of primary disease, removal of metastatic disease, palliation, prevention and reconstruction.

Diagnosis and staging

In most cases the diagnosis of cancer has been made before definitive surgery is carried out but occasionally a surgical

TABLE 10.3 Stage shift: the cure rate improves in both Stage I and Stage IV, and there is no change in cure rates for Stage II and Stage III, after the introduction of a new staging investigation. The overall cure rate is, however, unchanged.

Before new staging test				After new staging test				
Stage	Distribution	Cure rate	Number cured	Stage	Distribution	Cure rate	Number cured	% 'improvement' in cure rate
I	70%	90%	63	I	50%	94%	47	4%
II	10%	80%	8	II	10%	80%	8	0%
III	10%	80%	8	III	10%	80%	8	0%
IV	10%	50%	5	IV	30%	70%	21	20%
All	100%		84	All	100%		84	0%

Alvan Feinstein, 1926–2001, American clinician and epidemiologist.
Will Rogers (properly William Penn Adair Rogers), 1879–1935, American actor, humorist and wit.
There is much confusion about the use of the terms '**multidisciplinary**' and '**multiprofessional**': we use 'multidisciplinary' to imply the presence of various medically qualified specialists (pathologists, radiologists, etc.) and 'multiprofessional' implies the presence of specialists from non-medical backgrounds (nurses, social workers, radiographers).

TABLE 10.4 Staging of colorectal cancer.

TNM	
TX, Primary tumour cannot be assessed	
T0, No evidence of primary tumour	
Tis, Intraepithelial or intramucosal carcinoma	
T1, Tumour invades submucosa	
T2, Tumour invades muscularis propria	
T3, Tumour invades through the muscularis propria into the subserosa or into retroperitoneal (pericolic or perirectal) tissues	a, Minimal invasion: <1 mm beyond muscularis
	b, Slight invasion: 1–5 mm beyond muscularis
	c, Moderate invasion: >5–15 mm beyond muscularis
	d, Extensive invasion: >15 mm beyond muscularis
T4, Tumour directly invades beyond bowel	a, Direct invasion into other organs or structures
	b, Perforates visceral peritoneum
NX, Regional lymph nodes cannot be assessed	
N0, No metastases in regional nodes	
N1, Metastases in 1–3 regional lymph nodes	
N2, Metastases in ≥4 regional lymph nodes	
MX, Not possible to assess the presence of distant metastases	
M0, No distant metastases	
M1, Distant metastases present	

TABLE 10.5 Relationships between staging systems for colorectal cancer.

TNM	AJCC	Dukes	Modified Astler–Coller
TisN0M0	0	–	–
T1N0M0	I	A	A
T2N0M0	I	A	B1
T3N0M0	IIA	B	B2
T4N0M0	IIB	B	B3
T1 or T2 N1M0	IIIA	C	C1
T3 or T4 N1M0	IIIB	C	C2, C3
Any T N2M0	IIIC	C	C1, C2, C3
Any T Any N M1	IV	D	–

procedure is required to make the diagnosis. This is particularly true of patients with malignant ascites where laparoscopy has an important role in obtaining tissue for diagnosis. Laparoscopy is also widely used for the staging of intra-abdominal malignancy, particularly oesophageal and gastric cancer. By this means it is often possible to diagnose widespread peritoneal disease and small liver metastases that may have been missed on cross-sectional imaging. Laparoscopic ultrasound is a particularly useful adjunct for the diagnosis of intrahepatic metastases. Other examples where surgery is central to the diagnosis of cancer include orchidectomy where a patient suspected of testicular cancer and lymph node biopsy in a patient with lymphoma. Recently, sentinel node biopsy in melanoma and breast cancer has attracted a great deal of interest. Here a radiolabelled colloid is injected into or around the primary

TABLE 10.6 The advantages and disadvantages of the multidisciplinary team.

Advantages	Disadvantages
Open debate concerning management	An opportunity for rampant egotism and showing-off
Patient has advantage of many simultaneous opinions from many different specialities	Less confident and less articulate members of the team may not be able to express their views, even though their views may be extremely important
Decision-making is open, transparent and explicit	May degenerate into a rubber-stamping exercise in which the class solutions implied by guidelines are unthinkingly applied to disparate individuals
Team members educate each other	Decisions are made in the absence of patients and their carers: the commodification of the person
A useful educational experience for trainees and students	Clinicians are able to avoid having to take responsibility for their decisions and their actions: the fig-leaf of 'corporate responsibility'
Performance can be monitored by managers	Time-consuming and resource-intensive: takes busy clinicians away from clinical practice for hours at a time

Vernon B Astler, surgeon, The Medical School of the University of Michigan, Ann Arbor, MI, USA.
Frederick A Coller, pathologist, The Medical School of the University of Michigan, Ann Arbor, MI, USA.
Cuthbert Esquire Dukes, 1890–1977, pathologist, St Mark's Hospital, London, UK.

tumour and the regional lymph nodes are then scanned with a gamma camera which will pinpoint the lymph node nearest to the tumour. This lymph node can then be removed for histological diagnosis. Staging laparotomy used to be an important aspect of the staging of lymphomas but with more accurate cross-sectional imaging and the more widespread use of chemotherapy this practice is now largely redundant.

Removal of primary disease

Radical surgery for cancer involves removal of the primary tumour and as much of the surrounding tissue and lymph node drainage as possible in order not only to ensure local control but also to prevent spread of tumour through the lymphatics. Although the principle of local control is still extremely important, it is now recognised that ultra-radical surgery probably has little effect on the development of metastatic disease, as evidenced by the randomised trials of radical versus simple mastectomy for breast cancer. It is important, however, to appreciate that high quality, meticulous surgery taking care not to disrupt the primary tumour at the time of excision is of the utmost importance in obtaining a cure in localised disease and in preventing local recurrence.

Removal of metastatic disease

Under certain circumstances surgery for metastatic disease may be appropriate. This is particularly true for liver metastases arising from colorectal cancer where successful resection of all detectable disease can lead to long-term survival in about one-third of patients. With multiple liver metastases, it may still be possible to take a surgical approach by using *in situ* ablation with cryotherapy or radiofrequency energy. Another situation in which surgery may be of value is pulmonary resection for isolated lung metastases, particularly from renal cell carcinoma.

Palliation

In many cases surgery is not appropriate for cure but may be extremely valuable for palliation. A good example of this is the patient with a symptomatic primary tumour who also has distant metastases. In this case, removal of the primary will increase the patient's quality of life but will have little effect on the ultimate outcome. Other situations where surgical palliation is appropriate include bypass procedures such as an ileo-transverse anastomosis to alleviate symptoms of obstruction caused by an inoperable caecal cancer or bypassing an unresectable carcinoma at the head of the pancreas by cholecysto- or choledocho-jejunostomy to alleviate jaundice.

Principles underlying the non-surgical treatment of cancer

The relationship between dose and response and the principle of selective toxicity

Non-surgical treatments, in common with surgery, have the potential to cause harm as well as benefit. Surgery is difficult to quantify: it is hard to describe a mastectomy in units of measure. Both drugs and radiation can be expressed in reproducible units: milligrams, in the case of drugs; Grays (Gy), in the case of radiation. Thus, in contrast to surgery, it is possible to construct dose–response relationships for both the benefits (such as tumour cure rate) and the harms (such as tissue damage that is both severe and permanent) associated with non-surgical interventions. These curves (see **Figure 10.5**) have the same general shape: they are sigmoidal. The practical consequence of this is that, over a relatively narrow dose range, we move from failure to success, from tolerability to disaster. It is theoretically possible to use dose–response curves to calculate an optimal dose for treating each tumour: the dose is that which is associated with the maximal probability of an uncomplicated cure. Lying behind the concept of the probability of an uncomplicated cure is the principle of selective toxicity: the treatment should be selectively toxic to the tumour and, as far as possible, should spare the normal tissues from damage. It is this simple principle that underpins both the selection of agents used to treat cancer and the schedules used to deliver them. Although the graphical representations of the relationships between, dose, response and the probability of uncomplicated cure are conceptually simple and intuitively appealing they are, in clinical practice, completely impractical. The construction of full dose–response curves for all possible combinations of tumours and normal tissues is neither feasible nor ethical. We have to rely, when it comes to defining optimal doses and schedules, upon incomplete clinical data and a knowledge of the general shape of the relationship between dose and response.

Personalised (precision) medicine

Advances in molecular biology and pharmacogenomics are providing insights into the ways in which tumours and normal tissues might behave in response to treatment. Employing this knowledge, at the level of the individual patient, has become known as **personalised medicine**, or **precision medicine**. *Table 10.7* summarises how a personalised approach, based on knowledge of the relative sensitivities of tumour and normal tissues, might modify therapeutic decisions.

TABLE 10.7 Personalised dose adjustment.

Normal tissue	Tumour	Dose
N	N	Usual dose
N	S	Lower dose
N	R	Use different Rx
S	N	Use different Rx
S	S	Lower dose
S	R	Use different Rx
R	N	Use higher dose
R	S	Usual dose
R	R	Use different Rx

N, normal sensitivity; R, resistant to treatment; Rx, treatment; S, increased sensitivity.

in situ is Latin for 'in the place'.
Louis Harold Gray, 1905–1965, Director, The British Empire Cancer Campaign Research Unit in Radiobiology, Mount Vernon Hospital, Northwood, Middlesex, UK. A Gray (Gy) is the SI unit for the absorbed dose of ionising radiation.

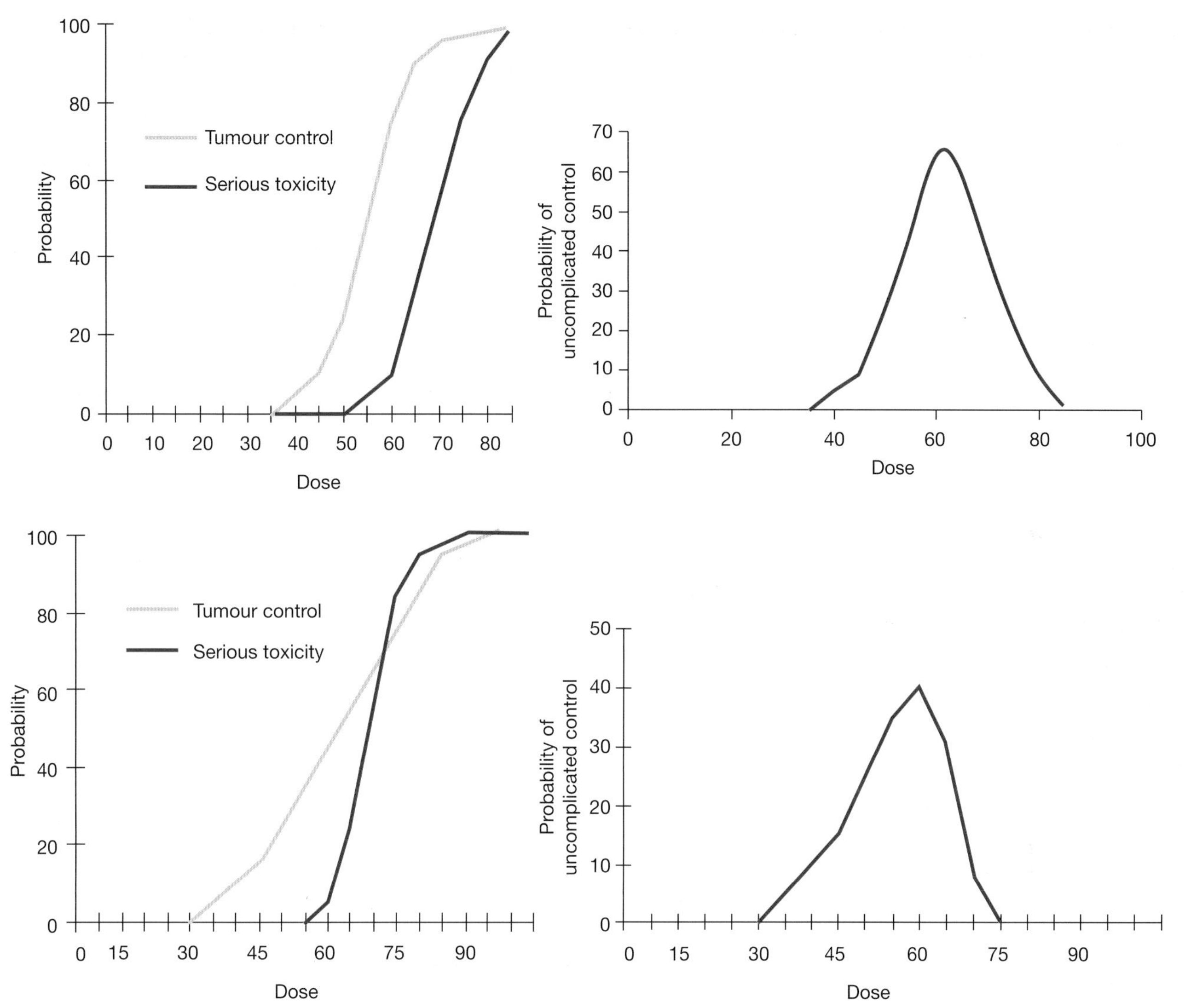

Figure 10.5 A schematic illustration of the relationship between dose, response and the probability of uncomplicated cure. The upper figures show ideal circumstances, with steep dose–response relationships for both normal tissue damage and tumour control. The lower figures show something more like the real world. The dose–response relationship for tumour control is flatter, because tumours are heterogeneous and, consequently, the probability of uncomplicated cure is lower – even for the optimal dose (40% in the lower figure compared with 70% in the upper figure).

General strategies in the non-surgical management of cancer

Curative surgery for cancer is guided by one simple principle: the physical removal of all identifiable disease. The principles underlying the non-surgical management of cancer are more complex. First, the spatial distribution of treatment must be considered: surgery and radiotherapy are local or, at best, locoregional treatments; drugs offer systemic therapy (**Figure 10.6** and *Table 10.8*).

Second, there is the question of the intent underlying the treatment. Radiotherapy, chemotherapy, or the combination of the two, may be used with curative intent. More usually, chemotherapy or radiotherapy is used to lower the risk of recurrence after primary treatment with surgery, so-called adjuvant therapy. Implicit within the concept of adjuvant therapy is the realisation that much of what is done

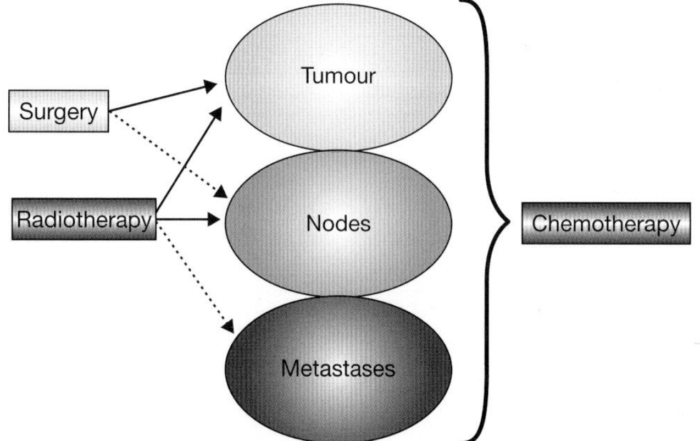

Figure 10.6 Schematic diagram to show the spatial scope of cancer treatments. Chemotherapy is systemic, surgery is mainly a local treatment. Radiotherapy is usually local or locoregional, but can, as in radioiodine therapy for thyroid cancer, be systemic.

TABLE 10.8 Examples of malignancies that may be cured without the need for surgical excision.

Malignancy	Potentially curative treatment
Leukaemia	Chemotherapy (+/– Radiotherapy)
Lymphoma	Chemotherapy (+/– Radiotherapy)
Small cell lung cancer	Chemotherapy (+/– Radiotherapy)
Tumours of childhood (rhabdomyosarcoma, Wilm's tumour)	Chemotherapy (+/– Radiotherapy)
Early laryngeal cancer	Radiotherapy
Advanced head and neck cancer	Chemo-radiation (synchronous chemotherapy and radiotherapy)
Oesophageal cancer	Chemo-radiation (synchronous chemotherapy and radiotherapy)
Squamous cell cancer of the anus	Chemo-radiation (synchronous chemotherapy and radiotherapy)
Advanced cancer of the cervix	Radiotherapy (+/– chemotherapy)
Medulloblastoma	Radiotherapy (+/– chemotherapy)
Skin tumours (BCC, SCC)	Radiotherapy

BCC, basal cell carcinoma; SCC, squamous cell carcinoma.

is unnecessary, or futile, or both. The need for adjuvant therapy, to treat the risk that residual disease might be present after apparently curative surgery, is an acknowledgement of the current inability to detect or predict, with sufficient precision, the presence of residual disease. It also explains why the incremental benefits from adjuvant treatments are so small, and why the existence of these benefits can only be proven using randomised controlled trials including many thousands of patients. As illustrated in **Figures 10.7 and 10.8**,

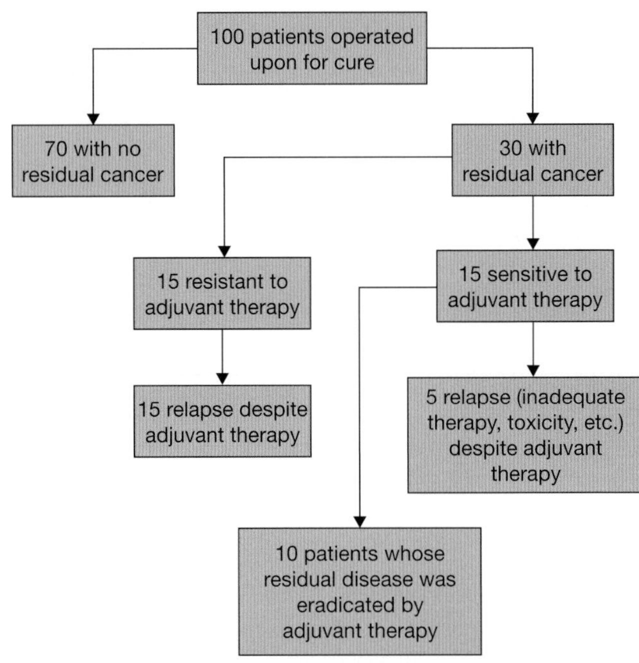

Net benefits		
Futile therapy	20%	90% treated inappropriately
Unnecessary therapy	70%	
Beneficial therapy	10%	10% treated appropriately
No therapy	0%	

Figure 10.7 The concept of adjuvant chemotherapy.

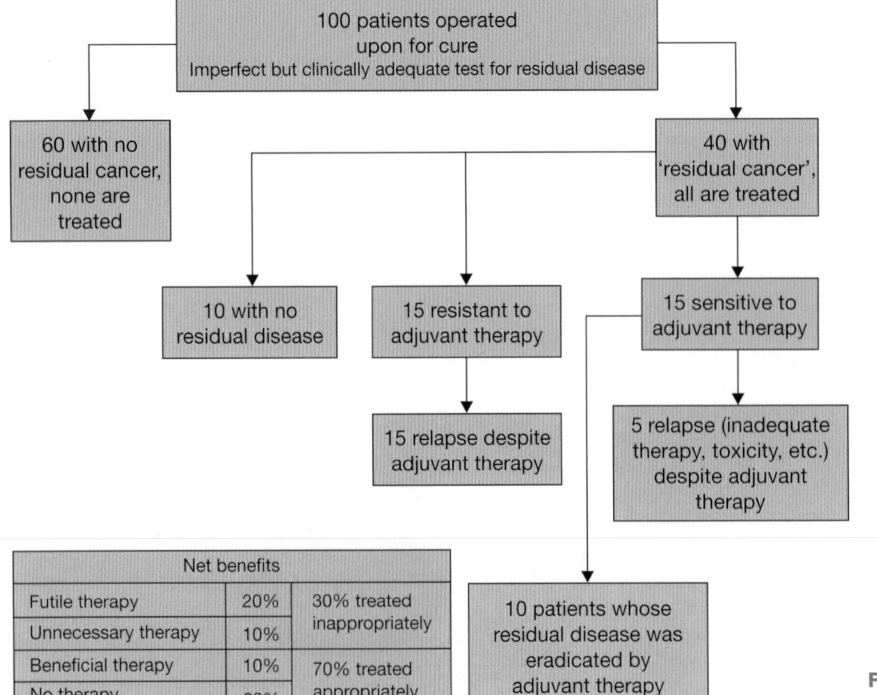

Net benefits		
Futile therapy	20%	30% treated inappropriately
Unnecessary therapy	10%	
Beneficial therapy	10%	70% treated appropriately
No therapy	60%	

Figure 10.8 The concept of adjuvant chemotherapy and testing for minimal residual disease.

Max Wilms, 1867–1918, Professor of Surgery, Heidelberg, Germany.

the current approach to the selection of patients for postsurgical adjuvant treatment is both intellectually impoverished and inefficient. Patients might have been far better off if, rather than so much time and effort being invested in attempting to discover new 'cures' for cancer, equivalent resources had been devoted to devising clinically useful tests to detect residual cancer cells persisting after apparently successful initial therapy. Had this been the case, we might now be better able to distinguish between those patients with systemic disease at presentation and those with truly localised disease.

Radiotherapy

Within a month of their discovery in 1895, x-rays were being used to treat cancer. Despite over 100 years of use, and despite some outstanding clinical achievements, it is still not known how best to use radiation to treat cancer. In part this arises because it is not known precisely how radiation treatment affects tumours and normal tissues. Until about 30 years ago it was assumed that the biological effects of radiation resulted from radiation-induced damage to the DNA of dividing cells. Nowadays it is known that, although this undoubtedly explains some of the biological effects of radiation, it does not provide a full explanation. Radiation can, both directly and indirectly, influence gene expression: over 100 radiation-inducible effects on gene expression have now been described. These changes in gene expression are responsible for a considerable proportion of the biological effects of radiation upon tumours and normal tissues. In this sense, radiotherapy is a precisely targeted form of gene therapy for cancer.

The practicalities of radiation therapy are reasonably straightforward: define the target to treat; design the optimal technical set up to provide uniform irradiation of that target; and choose that schedule of treatment that delivers radiation to that target so as to maximise the therapeutic ratio (**Figure 10.9**). Modern radiotherapy uses sophisticated computer programmes and algorithms to sculpt the shape of the treatment volume. A decade ago it was possible only to treat simple geometric forms, nowadays, with techniques such as intensity-modulated radiation therapy (IMRT) and image-guided radiation therapy (IGRT), it is possible safely to deliver high doses to irregularly shaped target volumes. The ability to give high fractional doses in this way has lead to the development of stereotactic ablative radiotherapy (SABR) in which a small number of fractions can be used to treat primary tumours, or isolated metastases, to curative dose levels.

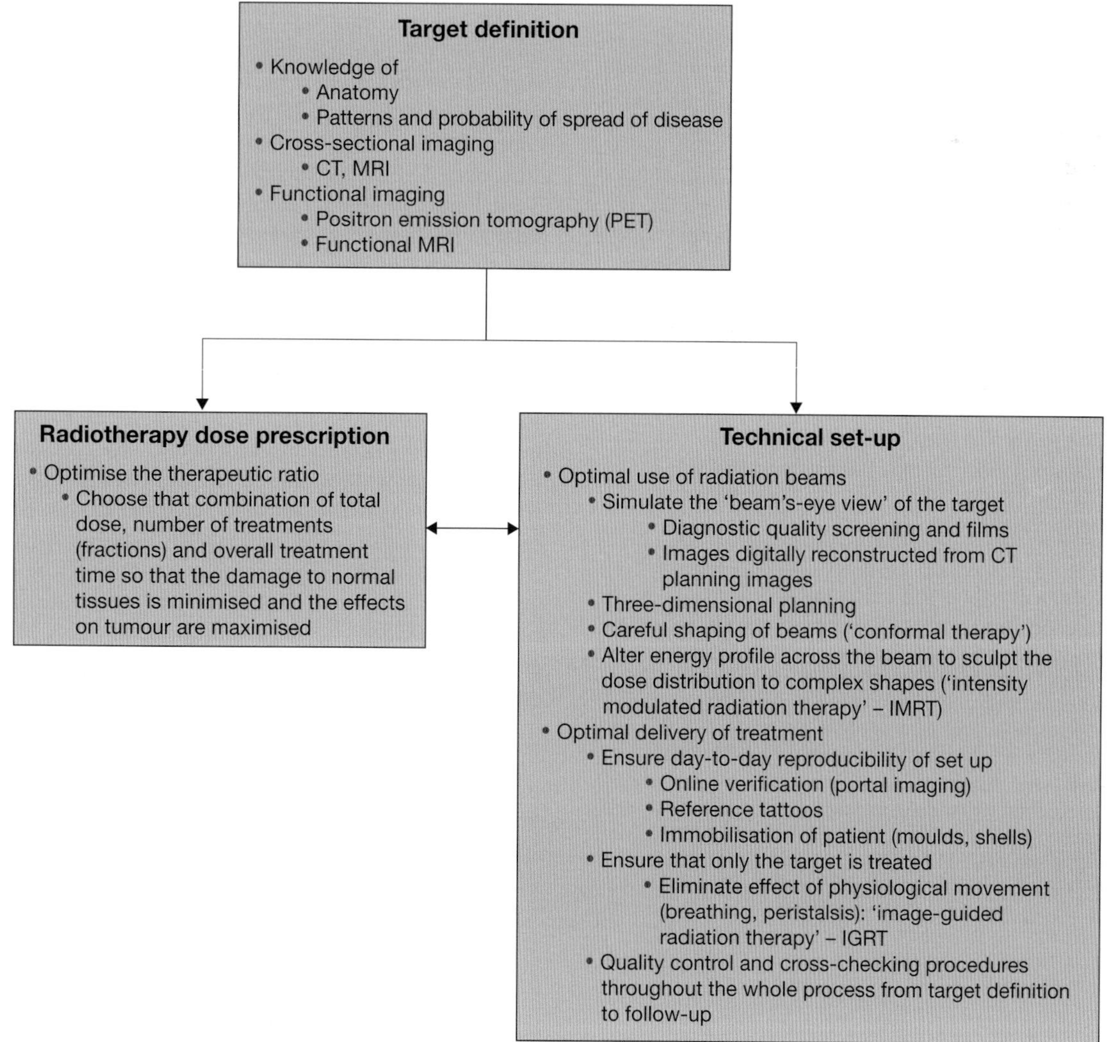

Figure 10.9 The processes involved in clinical radiotherapy. CT, computed tomography; MRI, magnetic resonance imaging.

One of the main problems with assessing a therapeutic ratio for a given schedule of radiation is that there is a dissociation between the acute effects on normal tissues and the late damage. The acute reaction is not a reliable guide to the adverse consequences of treatment in the longer term. Since the late effects following irradiation can take over 20 years to develop, this poses an obvious difficulty: if a radiation schedule is changed it will be known within two or three years whether or not the new schedule has improved tumour control; it may, however, be two decades before it is known, with any degree of certainty, whether or not the new technique is safe. Fractionated radiotherapy selectively spares late, as opposed to immediate, effects. For any given total dose, the smaller the dose per treatment (the larger the number of fractions), the less severe the late effects will be. The problem is that the greater the number of fractions of daily treatment, the longer the overall treatment time, and the greater the opportunity for the tumour to proliferate during treatment. All fractionation is a compromise. Thirty years ago, Withers defined the 4 Rs of radiotherapy; subsequently, a fifth 'R' (intrinsic radiosensitivity) has been added. The clinical practice of radiation oncology operates within the limits defined by these 5 Rs.

Summary box 10.5

The five Rs of radiotherapy

- **Repair**. If given sufficient time between fractional doses of radiation, cells will repair the radiation-induced damage. Repair half-times are typically 3–6 hours. Fractionation offers a means whereby we may be able to exploit any differentials in repair capacity between tumour cells and normal cells.
- **Reoxygenation**. Hypoxic cells are, compared with well-oxygenated cells, relatively radioresistant. Normal tissues are well oxygenated, tumours are often hypoxic. This is an obvious therapeutic disadvantage. The problem may be mitigated if a sequence of daily treatments is used. Cells dying as a result of radiation treatment will not use oxygen; this means that more oxygen is available to the, previously hypoxic, surviving cells. These cells become oxygenated and are therefore more susceptible to the next dose of radiation treatment.
- **Repopulation**. As radiotherapy kills cancer cells within a tumour it may provide a stimulus to rapid proliferation of tumour cells. Thus, during protracted treatment, production of cells by the tumour may equal, or even exceed, radiation-induced cell loss. This provides an argument for keeping the overall treatment time as short as possible.
- **Redistribution**. The sensitivity of cells to radiation varies according to their position within the cell cycle. This may lead to a degree of synchronisation of cellular division within the tumour: ideally, fractions of radiotherapy would be timed to coincide with vulnerable phases of the cell cycle (late G2 and M) in a partially synchronised population of tumour cells.
- **Radiosensitivity**. Experiments using low dose-rate irradiation demonstrate that, for reasons distinct from those summarised above, cells derived from tumours differ in their intrinsic sensitivity to radiation. There may be cells so intrinsically resistant to treatment that no clinically viable schedule of radiation therapy would be able to eliminate them. Conversely, some cells may be so sensitive that virtually any schedule would be successful – the majority of cells will lie somewhere between these extremes.

Chemotherapy and biological therapies

Selective toxicity is the fundamental principle underlying the use of chemotherapy in clinical practice. The importance of the principle is further emphasised by the fact that, by itself, chemotherapy is rarely sufficient to cure cancer. Chemotherapy is often (in effect, if not in intent) a palliative rather than a curative intervention. As such, its use should be influenced by the cardinal principle of palliative treatment: treatment aimed at relieving symptoms should not, itself, produce unacceptable symptoms. The cure of a disease should not be more grievous than its endurance. There are now over 120 different drugs licensed by the US Food and Drug Administration (FDA) for the treatment of cancer; 30 of them were approved between 2013 and 2015. The majority are cytotoxic drugs, hormonal therapies account for around 10%, and an increasing number have been designed to interact with specific molecular targets – so-called targeted therapies. There are now many more options than there were 20 years ago and, perhaps more importantly, lessons have been learned about how better to deploy resources. The classes of chemotherapeutic drugs, their modes of action and clinical indications are summarized in *Table 10.9*.

The newer, 'targeted' therapies (*Tables 10.9* and *10.10*) now available for treating cancer present particular dilemmas. They offer modest prolongation of survival, often with minimal toxicity, but at considerable financial cost. When compared with conventional therapies, these drugs typically cost over £50 000 ($94 000) per quality adjusted life-year gained and, when overall resources are limited, may be considered unaffordable. *Table 10.11* puts into context the cost-effectiveness of various clinical interventions. The current cost of targeted therapies should not obscure their importance: they represent the first attempts to translate advances in molecular biology into clinical practice. The discoveries of the mid-twentieth century are finally bearing fruit. One feature that is emerging is the exquisite selectivity of these treatments – they will only target specific subsets of tumours. The kinase inhibitor vemurafenib will only be effective in patients with melanoma whose tumours have the V600E BRAF mutation; cetuximab is only effective in patients with colorectal cancer who have wild-type (non-mutated) *ras*; imatinib is particularly effective in patients with gastrointestinal stromal tumours (GIST) who have mutations in exon 11 of the *Kit* gene, patients with mutations in exon 9 may still respond to imatinib but will require higher doses, and patients without mutations in *Kit* are far less likely to respond to imatinib.

The next decade will see a major shift in the medical management of cancer – from cell killing to cellular reprogramming. Sophisticated manipulations of the immune system will also become increasingly important. As a result, cancer therapies are likely to become less acutely toxic, but the longer-term consequences of such sophisticated manipulations will be both uncertain and unpredictable.

Hubert Rodney ('Rod') Withers, Professor of Radiation Oncology at the University of California, Los Angeles.

TABLE 10.9 A summary of chemotherapeutic and biological agents currently used in cancer treatment.

Class	Examples	Putative mode of action	Tumour types that may be sensitive to drug
Drugs which interfere with mitosis	Vincristine, Vinblastine	Interfere with formation of microtubules: 'spindle poisons'	Lymphomas Leukaemias Brain tumours Sarcomas
	Taxanes: Taxol, Paclitaxel	Stabilise microtubules	Breast cancer Non-small cell lung cancer Ovarian cancer Prostate cancer Head and neck cancer
Drugs which interfere with DNA synthesis (antimetabolites)	5-Fluorouracil (5-FU)	Inhibition of thymidylate synthase, false substrate for both DNA and RNA synthesis	Breast cancer GI cancer
	Capecitabine	Orally active prodrug which is metabolised to 5-FU. Inhibition of thymidylate synthase, false substrate for both DNA and RNA synthesis	Breast cancer GI cancer
	Methotrexate	Inhibition of dihydrofolate reductase	Breast cancer Bladder cancer Lymphomas Cervical cancer
	6-Mercaptopurine	Inhibits ***de novo*** purine synthesis	Leukaemias
	6-Thioguanine	Inhibits ***de novo*** purine synthesis	Leukaemias
	Cytosine arabinoside	False substrate in DNA synthesis	Leukaemias Lymphomas
	Gemcitabine	Inhibits ribonucleotide reductase	Non-small lung cancer Pancreatic cancer
Drugs which directly damage DNA or interfere with its function	Mitomycin C	DNA cross-linking, preferentially active at sites of low oxygen tension (a bioreductive drug)	Anal cancer Bladder cancer Gastric cancer Head and neck cancer Rectal cancer
	Cis-platinum	Forms adducts between DNA strands and interferes with replication	Germ cell tumours Ovarian cancer Non-small cell lung cancer Head and neck cancer Oesophageal cancer
	Carboplatin	Forms adducts between DNA strands and interferes with replication	Germ cell tumours Ovarian cancer Non-small cell lung cancer Head and neck cancer
	Oxaliplatin	Forms adducts between DNA strands and interferes with replication	Colorectal cancer
	Doxorubicin	Intercalates between DNA strands and interferes with replication	Breast cancer Lymphomas Sarcomas Kaposi's sarcoma
	Cyclophosphamide	A prodrug converted via hepatic cytochrome p450 to phosphoramide mustard. Causes DNA cross links	Breast cancer Lymphomas Sarcomas
	Ifosfamide	Related to cyclophosphamide, causes DNA cross links	Small-cell lung cancer Sarcomas
	Bleomycin	DNA strand breakage via formation of metal complex	Germ cell tumours Lymphomas
	Irinotecan	Inhibits topoisomerase 1 and thereby prevents the DNA from unwinding and repairing during replication	Colorectal cancer
	Etoposide	Inhibits topoisomerase 2, prevents DNA from unwinding and repairing during replication	Small-cell lung cancer Germ cell tumours Lymphomas

Continued

TABLE 10.9 A summary of chemotherapeutic and biological agents currently used in cancer treatment – *continued*.

Class	Examples	Putative mode of action	Tumour types that may be sensitive to drug
Drugs which directly damage DNA or interfere with its function – *continued*	Dacarbazine	A nitrosourea which requires activation by hepatic cytochrome p450. Methylates guanine residues in DNA	Brain tumours Sarcoma Melanoma
	Temozolomide	A nitrosourea but, unlike dacarbazine, does not require activation by hepatic cytochrome p450. Methylates guanine residues in DNA	Glioblastoma multiforme Melanoma
	Actinomycin D	Intercalation between DNA strands, DNA strand breaks	Rhabdomyosarcoma Wilm's tumour
Hormones	Tamoxifen	Blocks oestrogen receptors	Breast cancer
	Anastrazole	An aromatase inhibitor than blocks post-menopausal (non-ovarian) oestrogen production	Breast cancer
	Exemestane	An aromatase inhibitor than blocks post-menopausal (non-ovarian) oestrogen production	Breast cancer
	Letrozole	An aromatase inhibitor than blocks post-menopausal (non-ovarian) oestrogen production	Breast cancer
	Leuprolide	Analogue of gonadotrophin-releasing hormone, continued use produces downregulation of the anterior pituitary with consequent fall in testosterone levels	Prostate cancer
	Goserelin	Analogue of gonadotrophin-releasing hormone, continued use produces downregulation of the anterior pituitary with consequent fall in testosterone levels	Prostate cancer
	Buserelin	Analogue of gonadotrophin-releasing hormone, continued use produces downregulation of the anterior pituitary with consequent fall in testosterone levels	Prostate cancer
	Cabergoline	Blocks prolactin release, a long-acting dopamine agonist	Prolactin-secreting pituitary tumours
	Bromocriptine	Dopamine agonist, blocks stimulation of anterior pituitary	Pituitary tumours
	Cyproterone acetate	Blocks the effect of androgens	Prostate cancer
	Flutamide	Blocks the effect of androgens	Prostate cancer
	Nilutamide	Blocks the effect of androgens	Prostate cancer
	Bicalutamide	Blocks the effect of androgens	Prostate cancer
Inhibitors of receptor tyrosine kinases	Gefitinib	Inhibits EGFR tyrosine kinase	Non-small cell lung lancer
	Imatinib	Blocks ability of mutant BCR–ABL fusion protein to bind ATP	Chronic myeloid meukaemia
		Inhibition of mutant c-KIT	Gastrointestinal stromal tumours (GIST)
	Erlotinib	Inhibits EGFR tyrosine kinase	Non-small cell lung cancer Pancreatic cancer
	Sunitinib, Sorafenib, Regorafenib, Lenvatinib	Promiscuous tyrosine kinase inhibitors (PDGFR, VEGFR, KIT, FLT)	Renal cancer GIST refractory to Imatinib, colorectal cancer, thyroid cancer
	Lapatinib	Inhibits tyrosine kinases associated with EGFR and HER2	Breast cancer
	Axitinib	Inhibits tyrosine kinase associated with VEGF receptor	Renal cancer
Protease inhibitors	Bortezomib	Interferes with proteasomal degradation of regulatory proteins, in particular prevents NF kappa B from preventing apoptosis	Multiple myeloma
Differentiating agents	All ***trans***-retinoic acid	Induces terminal differentiation	Acute promyelocytic leukaemia

Continued

TABLE 10.9 A summary of chemotherapeutic and biological agents currently used in cancer treatment – *continued*.

Class	Examples	Putative mode of action	Tumour types that may be sensitive to drug
Farnesyl transferase inhibitors	Lonafarnib	Inhibition of farnesyl transferase and consequent inactivation of ***ras***-dependent signal transduction	Leukaemia
	Tipifarnib	Inhibition of farnesyl transferase and consequent inactivation of ***ras***-dependent signal transduction	Acute leukaemia Myelodysplastic syndrome
Antibodies directed to cell surface antigens	Trastuzumab	Antibody directed against HER2 receptor	Breast cancer
	Cetuximab	Antibody directed against EGFR receptor	Colorectal cancer Head and neck cancer
	Bevacizumab	Antibody directed against VEGFR	Colorectal cancer
	Rituximab	Antibody against CD20 antigen	Lymphomas
	Alemtuzumab	Antibody against CD52 antigen	Lymphomas
Inducers of apoptosis	Arsenic trioxide	Induces apoptosis by caspase inhibition Inhibition of nitric oxide	Acute promyelocytic leukaemia
Immunological mediators	Ipilumumab	Blocks cytotoxic T lymphocyte-associated protein 4 (CTLA-4) and thus releases the brakes on the activation of T cells	Melanoma
	Pembrolizumab Nivolumab	Block the PD-1 receptor on T lymphocytes and thereby prevents the inhibition of T cell activation	Melanoma
	MEDI6383	OX40 agonist: enhances T cell survival and production of cytokines	In phase I trials
	Interferon alpha-2b	Activates macrophages, increases the cytotoxicity of T lymphocytes, inhibits cell division (and viral replication)	Renal carcinoma Melanoma Hairy-cell leukaemia
	Thalidomide	Anti-inflammatory, stimulates T cells, anti-angiogenic	Myeloma
HDAC inhibitors	Panobinostat Vorinostat	Acetylation of histones is associated with increased transcription of genes; inhibiting deacetylation can decrease expression of mutated or dysregulated genes	Cutaneous T cell lymphoma
	Entinostat		Melanoma
PI3K inhibitors	Idelalisib	Inhibit signalling via the PI3K/AKT/mTOR pathway and thereby switch off stimulus to cellular proliferation	B cell lymphomas
mTOR inhibitors	Temsirolimus	Inhibit the mammalian target of Rapamycin (mTOR) a key component in the PI3K/AKT/mTOR pathway	Renal cancer Neuroendocrine Tumours
	Everolimus		Gastric cancer
MEK inhibitors	Trametinib Selumetinib	Inhibit the mitogen-activated protein kinase pathway (MAPK)	Melanoma
RAF inhibitors	Dabrafenib	Inhibit the mitogen-activated protein kinase pathway (MAPK)	Melanoma
	Vemurafenib		Melanoma

CML, chronic myeloid leukaemia; EGFR, epidermal growth factor receptor; FLT3, FMS-like tyrosine kinase; GI, Gastrointestinal; HDAC, Histone deacetylase; mTOR , mammalian target of rapamycin; NF, nuclear factor; PDGFR, platelet-derived growth factor receptor; PI3K, phosphoinositide 3-kinase; TKI, tyrosine kinase inhibitor; VEGFR, vascular endothelial growth factor receptor.

Principles of combined treatment

Cytotoxic drugs are rarely used as single agents; radiotherapy and chemotherapy are often given together. The rationale behind combination, as opposed to single-agent, drug therapy is straightforward and is somewhat analogous to that used for combined antibiotic therapy: it is a strategy designed to combat drug resistance. By the time of diagnosis many tumours will contain cancer cells that, through spontaneous mutation, have acquired resistance to cytotoxic drugs. Unlike antibiotic resistance, there is no need for previous exposure to the drug. Spontaneous mutation rates are high enough to allow the play of chance to permit the occurrence, and subsequent expansion, of clones of cells resistant to drugs to which they have never been exposed. If drugs were used as single agents then the further expansion of these *de novo* resistant subclones would limit cure. The problem can be mitigated by, from the outset of treatment, combining drugs.

There are three main principles upon which the choice of drugs for combination therapy is based: (1) use drugs active against the diseases in question; (2) use drugs with distinct modes of action; (3) use drugs with non-overlapping toxicities. By using drugs with different biological effects, for

TABLE 10.10 Targeted treatments mapped to the hallmarks of cancer. It is noteworthy that those agents that specifically target the hallmarks of cancer are not widely used in clinical practice. This may simply reflect the novelty of these agents, but could also suggest that an approach based on hallmarks is of more relevance to cancer biologists than to oncologists.

Hallmark	Drug classes	Specific drugs
Resist signals that inhibit growth	Cyclin-dependent kinase inhibitors	Dinaciclib Palbociclib Ronaciclib Seliciclib
Sustaining proliferative signalling	EGFR inhibitors	Trastuzumab Cetuximab
Avoid immune detection/destruction	Immune activators: antagonists of CTLA4, PD1, PD-L1	Ipilumumab Pembrolizumab Nivolumab
	OX40 agonists	MEDI6383
Obtain replicative immortality	Telomerase inhibitors	Imetelstat
Evoke inflammation	Anti-inflammatory drugs	Aspirin
Acquire ability to invade	Inhibition of Wnt/β-catenin	Resveratrol
Acquire ability to disseminate and implant	IGF-1 inhibitors	Linsitinib
Acquire angiogenic competence	Inhibitors of VEGF	Ramucirumab Bevacizumab Aflibercept
Genomic instability	PARP inhibitors	Olaparib Niraparib Rucaparib Veliparib
Evade apoptosis	BH3 mimetics	Navitoclax Venetoclax
Deregulate cellular energy supply & transfer	Aerobic glycolysis inhibitors	Metformin

BH3, B cell lymphoma gene 2 homology region 3; CTLA4, cytotoxic T lymphocyte associated protein 4; EGFR, epidermal growth factor receptor; IGF-1, insulin-like growth factor 1; OX40, also known as CD134, is expressed on activated T cells and is a tumour necrosis factor receptor; PARP, poly ADP ribose polymerase; PD1, programmed death-1 receptor; PD-L1, ligand for programmed death-1 receptor; VEGF, vascular endothelial growth factor.

example by combining an antimetabolite with an agent that actively damages DNA, it may be possible to obtain a truly synergistic effect. It is inadvisable to combine drugs with similar adverse effects: combining two highly myelosuppressive drugs may produce an unacceptably high risk of neutropenic sepsis. Where possible, combinations should be based upon a consideration of the toxicity profiles of the drugs concerned.

In considering the combination of radiotherapy and chemotherapy, radiation could be considered as just another drug. There is, in addition to synergy and toxicity, another factor to consider in the combination of drugs and radiation – the concept of spatial cooperation. Chemotherapy is a systemic treatment, radiotherapy is not. Radiotherapy is, however, able to reach sites, such as the central nervous system and testis, that drugs may not reach effectively. This is why, for example in patients treated primarily with chemotherapy for leukaemias, lymphomas, and small-cell lung cancer, prophylactic cranial irradiation may be part of the treatment protocol.

TABLE 10.11 Comparison of various estimates of cost-effectiveness for selected clinical interventions. Currently, in the United Kingdom, interventions costing less than $60 000 US (2002) are considered 'affordable', that is, they fall below the WTP ('willingness to pay') threshold.

Intervention	Cost (in 2002 US dollars) per quality-adjusted life-year (QALY)
Annual CT chest screening for lung cancer in a 60-year-old male ex-smoker versus no screening	2.4 million
Laparoscopic inguinal hernia repair versus expectant management in adults with inguinal hernia	610
Stroke unit care versus usual care in survivors of acute stroke	1600
Lifetime vitamin D + calcium supplements versus no supplements to prevent/treat osteoporosis in 70-year-old women	8500
Letrazole versus tamoxifen in the first-line management of postmenopausal women with advanced breast cancer	120 000
Erlotinib versus usual care in the treatment of relapsed non-small cell lung cancer	104 000

Data from CEA (Tufts-New England Medical Center) register (accessed via http://www.tufts-nemc.org/cearegistry/ on 15 November 2006) and the UK National Institute for Health and Clinical Excellence (accessed via http://www.nice.org.uk/page.aspx?c=153 on 15 November 2006).

Summary box 10.6

Principles of combined treatment

- Use effective agents
- Use agents with different modes of action (synergy)
- Use agents with non-overlapping toxicities
- Consider spatial cooperation

Palliative therapy

The distinction between palliative and curative treatment is not always clear cut and will become increasingly blurred as professional and public attitudes to towards the management of cancer change. Twenty years ago cancer was perceived as a disease that was either cured or it was not; patients either lived or died. There was little appreciation that, for many patients, cancer might be a chronic disease. Nowadays, it is appreciated that many of the so-called curative treatments are simply elegant exercises in growth delay. Five-year survival is not necessarily tantamount to cure. With the development

A **synergistic effect** is one in which the damage caused by giving the agents together is greater than the damage caused when the drugs are given separately.

of targeted therapies which regulate, rather than eradicate, cancer this state of affairs is likely to continue. The aim of treatment will be growth control rather than the extirpation of every last cancer cell. Patients will live with their cancers, perhaps for years. They will die **with** cancer, but not necessarily **of** cancer. Against this background, the distinction between curative and palliative therapy seems somewhat arbitrary; nevertheless, the control and relief of symptoms is crucial to the successful management of patients with cancer. Much of the fear associated with cancer is due to past failures to control patients' symptoms.

Patients fear the symptoms, distress and disruption associated with cancer almost as much as they fear the disease itself. Palliative treatment has as its goal the relief of symptoms. Sometimes this will involve treating the underlying problem, as with palliative radiotherapy for bone metastases, sometimes it will not. Sometimes it may be inappropriate to treat the cancer itself, but that does not imply that there is nothing more to be done, it simply means that there may be better ways to assuage the distress and discomfort caused by the tumour. Palliative medicine in the twenty-first century is about far more than optimal control of pain: its scope is wide, its impact immense (*Table 10.12*). The most important factor in the successful palliative management of a patient with cancer is early referral. Transition between curative and palliative modes of management should be seamless.

End-of-life care

End-of-life care is distinct from palliative care. Patients treated palliatively may survive for many years; end-of-life care concerns the last few months of a patient's life. Many issues, such as symptom control, are common to both palliative care and to end-of-life care but there are also problems which are specific to the sense of approaching death. These include a heightened sense of spiritual need, profound fear and the specific needs of those who are facing bereavement. The concept of the 'good death' has been embedded in many cultures over many centuries. Healthcare professionals deal with many deaths and sometimes forget that the patient who hopes for a good death has only one chance to get it right. This is why end-of-life care is worth considering in its own right and not as a mere appendage to palliative care.

Summary box 10.7

Issues at the end of life

- Appropriateness of active intervention
- Euthanasia
- Physician-assisted suicide
- Living wills
- Bereavement
- Spirituality
- Support to allow death at home
- The problem of the medicalisation of death

TABLE 10.12 An outline of the domains and interventions included within palliative and supportive care.

Domain	Intervention	
Symptom assessment	Pain, anorexia, fatigue, dyspnoea, etc.	
	Treatment-related toxicity	
Quality of life assessment		
Symptom relief	Drugs	
	Surgery	
	Radiotherapy	
	Complementary therapies:	Acupuncture
		Homeopathy
		Aromatherapy etc.
Psychosocial interventions	Psychological support	
	Relaxation techniques	
	Cognitive behavioural therapy	
	Counselling	
	Group therapy	
	Music therapy	
	Emotional support	
Physical and practical support	Physiotherapy	
	Occupational therapy	
	Speech therapy	
Information and knowledge	Cancer backup	
	Maggie's centres	
Nutritional support	Dietary advice	
	Nutritional supplements	
Social support	Patients	
	Relatives and carers	
Financial support	Ensure uptake of entitlements	
	Grants from charities e.g. Cancer Relief, Macmillan	
Spiritual support		

FURTHER READING

Allison JP. Immune checkpoint blockade in cancer therapy: the 2015 Lasker-DeBakey Clinical Medical Research Award. *JAMA* 2015; **314**(11): 1113–4.

Atun R, Jaffray DA, Barton MB *et al.* Expanding global access to radiotherapy. *Lancet Oncol* 2015; **16**(10): 1153–86.

Bailar JC 3rd, Gornik HL. Cancer undefeated. *N Engl J Med* 1997; **336**(19): 1569–74.

Doll R. The Pierre Denoix Memorial Lecture: nature and nurture in the control of cancer. *Eur J Cancer* 1999; **35**(1): 16–23.

Hanahan, D, Weinberg RA. The hallmarks of cancer. *Cell* 2000; **100**(1): 57–70.

Hanahan, D, Weinberg RA. Hallmarks of cancer: the next generation. *Cell* 2011; **144**(5): 646–74.

Meara JG, Leather AJM, Hagander L *et al.* Global Surgery 2030: evidence and solutions for achieving health, welfare, and economic development. *Lancet* 2015; **386**(9993): 569–624.

Solda F, Lodge M, Ashley S, Whitington A, Goldstraw P, Brada M. Stereotactic radiotherapy (SABR) for the treatment of primary non-small cell lung cancer; systematic review and comparison with a surgical cohort. *Radiother Oncol* 2013; **109**(1): 1–7.

Tomasetti C, Vogelstein B. Cancer etiology. Variation in cancer risk among tissues can be explained by the number of stem cell divisions. *Science* 2015; **347**(6217): 78–81.

Tree AC, Khoo VS, Eeles RA *et al.* Stereotactic body radiotherapy for oligometastases. *Lancet Oncol* 2013; **14**(1): e28–e37.

Weinberg RA. *The biology of cancer*, 2nd edn. New York, London: Garland Science, 2013.

Wu S, Powers S, Zhu W, Hannun YA. Substantial contribution of extrinsic risk factors to cancer development. *Nature* 2016; **529**(7584): 43–7.

Chapter 11

Surgical audit and research

Learning objectives

To understand:

- The planning and conduct of audit and research
- How to write up a project
- How to review a journal article and determine its value

INTRODUCTION

It is essential for a surgeon to understand the educational and legal framework in which he or she works. The agenda for medical education and both clinical and research governance requires surgeons to expand their skills to encompass audit and clinical research capabilities as useful tools for continued outcome measurement, service improvement and innovations for the benefit of patient care.

The aim of this chapter is to enable improvements in patient experience as a result of a successful audit cycle or by recognising the need for clinical research to determine a new and innovative way of treatment. It will also show how to keep track of personal clinical results. In addition, much clinical work is tedious and repetitive. Rigorous evaluation of even the most simple techniques and conditions can help to keep a surgeon stimulated throughout a long career and ensure good outcomes for patients, with cost benefits to the provider and a benefit to society as a whole.

Large numbers of clinical papers appear in the surgical literature every year. Many are flawed, and it is important that a surgeon has the skills to examine publications critically. The best way to develop a critical understanding of the research and audit undertaken by others is to perform studies of one's own. The hardest part of audit and research is writing it up, and the hardest article to write is the first. This chapter contains the information required to write a surgical paper and to evaluate the publications of others.

AUDIT OR RESEARCH?

Health professionals are expected to undertake audit and service evaluation as part of quality assurance. These usually involve minimal additional risk, burden or intrusion for participants. It is important to determine at an early stage whether a project is audit or research, and sometimes that is not as easy as it seems. The decision will determine the framework in which the study is undertaken. In the UK the Health Research Authority (HRA) has developed a decision tool to help decide whether your project is classified as research (http://www.hra-decisiontools.org.uk/research/). The HRA leaflet 'Differentiating clinical audit, service evaluation, research and usual practice/surveillance work in public health' is also helpful (*Table 11.1*).

AUDIT AND SERVICE EVALUATION

Clinical audit is a process used by clinicians who seek to improve patient care. The process involves comparing aspects of care (structure, process and outcome) against explicit criteria and defined standards. Keeping track of personal outcome data and contributing to a clinical database ensures that a surgeon's own performance is monitored continuously and can be compared with a national data set to ensure compliance with agreed standards. It is also an essential component of revalidation for the individual surgeon in the UK. If the care falls short of the criteria chosen, some change in the way that care is organised should be proposed. This change may be required at one of many levels. It might be an individual who needs training or surgical equipment that needs replacing. At times, the change may need to take place at the team level. Sometimes, the only appropriate action is change at an institutional level (e.g. a new antibiotic policy), regional level (provision of a tertiary referral centre) or, indeed, national level (screening programmes and health education campaigns).

Essentially, two types of audit may be encountered: national audits (e.g. in the UK, NHS England) and local/hospital audits. Both are designed to improve the quality of care. In an ideal world, national audits should be driven by needs identified in local and hospital-based audits that are closest to

TABLE 11.1 Research, audit or service evaluation? (Based on information by the National Research Ethics Service.)

Research	Clinical audit	Service evaluation
The attempt to derive generalisable new knowledge including studies that aim to generate hypotheses as well as studies that aim to test them	Designed and conducted to produce information to inform the delivery of best care	Designed and conducted solely to define or judge current care
Quantitative research – designed to test a hypothesis	Designed to answer the question: 'Does this service reach a predetermined standard?'	Designed to answer the question: 'What standard does this service achieve?'
Qualitative research – identifies/explores themes following established methodology;		
Addresses clearly defined questions, aims and objectives	Measures against a standard	Measures current service without reference to a standard
Quantitative research – may involve evaluating or comparing interventions, particularly new ones	Involves an intervention in use ONLY. (The choice of treatment is that of the clinician and patient according to guidance, professional standards and/or patient preference)	Involves an intervention in use ONLY. (The choice of treatment is that of the clinician and patient according to guidance, professional standards and/or patient preference)
Qualitative research – usually involves studying how interventions and relationships are experienced		
Usually involves collecting data that are additional to those for routine care but may include data collected routinely. May involve treatments, samples or investigations additional to routine care	Usually involves analysis of existing data but may include administration of simple interviews or questionnaires	Usually involves analysis of existing data but may include administration of simple interviews or questionnaires
Quantitative research – study design may involve allocating patients to intervention groups	No allocation to interventions: the health professional and patient have chosen intervention before clinical audit	No allocation to intervention: the health professional and patient have chosen intervention before service evaluation
Qualitative research uses a clearly defined sampling framework underpinned by conceptual or theoretical justifications		
May involve randomisation	No randomisation	No randomisation

Although any of the above may raise ethical issues, under current guidance, research requires ethics committee review, whereas audit and service evaluation do not. Advice (in the UK) from National Research Ethics Service (http://www.nres.npsa.nhs.uk/).

the patient. For example, hospital topics are often identified at the departmental morbidity and mortality meetings, where issues related to patient care are discussed. The reporting process might identify a possible national issue, and a national audit could be designed to be completed by the local audit department and surgical teams. The Vascular Society of Great Britain and Ireland is working continually with all its members in an evaluation of process and outcomes for major vascular operations. This is driven through the Vascular Society Quality Improvement Programme (VSQIP), where recently, individual surgeon outcomes for elective aortic aneurysm and carotid surgery are recorded (www.vsqip.org.uk). Audits are formal processes that require a structure. The following steps are essential to establish an audit cycle:

1 define the audit question in a multidisciplinary team;
2 identify the body of evidence and current standards;
3 design the audit to measure performance against agreed standards based on strong evidence. Seek appropriate advice (local audit department in UK) and ensure institutions have agreed to undertake the audit;
4 measure over an agreed interval;
5 analyse results and compare performance against agreed standards;
6 undertake gap analysis:
   a. if all standards are reached, reaudit after an agreed interval;
   b. if there is a need for improvement, identify possible interventions such as training, and agree with the involved parties;
7 reaudit.

Research study

During the design of the audit project, it might become apparent that there is a limited body of evidence available. In this case, the study should be structured as a research proposal. Research is designed to generate new knowledge and might involve testing a new treatment or regimen.

IDENTIFYING A RESEARCH TOPIC

Once an idea has been formed, or a question asked, it needs to be transformed into a hypothesis. It is helpful to approach surgeons who regularly publish articles and who have a special interest in the surgical area being considered. As ideas are suggested, it is important to consider whether the question posed really matters, and to spend some time refining the question (hypothesis) as this is probably the most important part of the process. Choosing the wrong topic at this stage can lead to many wasted hours. Once a topic has been identified, it is also important not rush into the study. The worst possible outcome is to find at the end of a long arduous study that the research has already been done or that the chosen methodology did not support investigation of the primary/secondary outcomes.

The first port of call for information is the internet (with assistance as needed from a medical librarian). Current articles about the proposed research should be retrieved; review articles and meta-analyses can be particularly helpful. At this stage, most clinicians go to an electronic library and perform a database search. It is very important to learn how to do an accurate and efficient search as early as possible. Details are beyond the scope of this chapter, but most librarians will be of assistance. Current techniques involve searching on Medline or other collected databases such as Google Scholar, but as electronic information advances and the world wide web (www) becomes more user friendly, new search strategies may emerge. Collections of reviews are becoming available – the Cochrane Collaboration brings together evidence-based medical information and is available in most libraries (*Table 11.2*).

Once information on the subject has been obtained and the relevent literature identified, it is important that these are carefully perused. It is not sufficient to read the abstract on Medline! If the proposed project is still looking good after some thorough reading, it is worth further discussion with colleagues who have written a paper on a similar subject. All scientists are flattered by interest in their work. It is important to ensure the cooperation of any other specialties or clinicians who will be involved in the study and to agree on the sharing of responsibility for the trial. This will help to prevent disagreement about who takes the credit once a study is ready for presentation and publication.

It is also helpful to seek support from specific networks set up to support health research. In the UK, the National Institute for Health Research Collaboration for Leadership in Applied Health Research and Care (NIHR CLAHRC) works with partner organisations, including the NHS, local authorities and universities, to conduct applied health research and implement research evidence, to improve health and healthcare. There are also a number of training courses in research methodology and application.

Once the forgoing has been completed, it should be possible to start to plan the research project.

PROJECT DESIGN

During the first phase, it is important to keep in the mind some important questions (*Summary box 11.1*).

Summary box 11.1

Questions to answer before undertaking research

- Why do the study?
- Will it answer a useful question?
- Is it practical?
- Can it be accomplished in the available time and with the available resources?
- Will the project benefit from collaboration to increase numbers or make best use of high tech equipment?
- What findings are expected?
- What are the research governance requirments?
- What are the ethical issues?
- What impact could it have?

TABLE 11.2 Electronic information sites.

Database	Producer	Coverage	Availability
Pubmed http://www.ncbi.nlm.nih.gov/pubmed	US National Library of Medicine (NLM)	PubMed comprises more than 25 million citations for biomedical literature from MEDLINE, life science journals, and online books. Citations may include links to full-text content from PubMed Central and publisher web sites	Internet
Pubmed Central http://www.ncbi.nlm.nih.gov/pmc/	U.S. National Institutes of Health (NIH) free digital archive	Full-text archive of biomedical and life sciences journal literature at the U.S. National Institutes of Health's National Library of Medicine	Internet
EMBASE http://embase.com/	EMBASE	Providing extensive coverage of peer-reviewed biomedical literature, along with indexing, searching and information management tools,	Subscription
CINAHL http://www.ebscohost.com/cinahl/	CINAHL is owned and operated by EBSCO Publishing	Cumulated index to nursing and allied health literature	Subscription
Cochrane Collaboration and Library http://uk.cochrane.org/	Global independent network of researchers, professionals, patients, carers and people interested in health to produce credible, accessible health information that is free from commercial sponsorship and other conflicts of interest	Preparing, updating and promoting the accessibility of Cochrane Reviews published online in *The Cochrane Library*	Internet

The **Cochrane Collaboration** was formed in 1993 and named after Archibald Leman Cochrane, 1909–1988, Director of the Medical Research Council Epidemiology Unit, Cardiff, and later the first President of the Faculty of Community Medicine (now the Faculty of Public Health) of the Royal College of Physicians of London, UK.

Time spent carefully designing a potential project is never wasted. There are many different types of scientific study. The design used depends on the study. A randomised controlled trial (RCT) is regarded as one of the best methods of scientific research; however, much surgical practice has been advanced through other different types of study such as those listed in *Table 11.3*. For example, testing a new type of operation often requires a pilot study to assess feasibility, which is then followed by a formal RCT. The introduction of innovative surgical techniques may require novel handling, and recomendations have been made by the IDEAL collaborators (see Further reading).

Research can be qualitative or quantitative. Quantitative research allows hard facts to speak for themselves. A medical condition is analysed systematically using hard, objective endpoints such as death or major complications, which should be clearly defined. For example, surgical complications are now classified using the Dindo–Clavien system. In qualitative research, data often come from patient narratives, and the psychosocial impact of the disease and its treatment are analysed; for example, narratives from patients with breast cancer. These kinds of data are often collected using quality-of-life measurements. A variety of different quality-of-life questionnaires exist to suit several different clinical situations. Much of the best research is both quantitative and qualitative. Recently, the importance of outomes from the patient's perspective has been emphasised; Patient Reported Outcome Measures (PROMs) are now an important component of the evaluation of surgical procedures.

Research should be focused according to institutional, national and international strategies. As finances for health care are always limited, it is important to consider including a cost–benefit analysis in any major area of research so that the value of the proposed intervention or change in treatment can be assessed. The National Institute for Health Research (NIHR) provides the framework through which the Department of Health maintains and manages the research, research staff and research infrastructure of the NHS in England.

TABLE 11.3 Types of study.

Type of study	Definition
Observational	Evaluation of condition or treatment in a defined population
	Retrospective: analysing past events
	Prospective: collecting data contemporaneously
Case–control	Series of patients with a particular disease or condition compared with matched control patients
Cross-sectional	Measurements made on a single occasion, not looking at the whole population but selecting a small similar group and expanding results
Longitudinal	Measurements are taken over a period of time, not looking at the whole population but selecting a small similar group and expanding results
Experimental	Two or more treatments are compared. Allocation to treatment groups is under the control of the researcher
Randomised	Two randomly allocated treatments
Randomised controlled	Includes a control group with standard treatment

Sample size

Calculating the number of patients required to perform a satisfactory investigation is an important prerequisite to any study. An incorrect sample size is probably the most frequent reason for research being invalid. Often, surgical trials are marred by the possibility of error caused by the inadequate number of patients investigated.

- **Type I error.** Benefit is perceived when really there is none (false positive).
- **Type II error.** Benefit is missed when it was there to be found (false negative).

Calculating the number of patients required in the study can overcome this bias. Unfortunately, it often reveals that a larger number of patients is needed for the study than can possibly be obtained from available resources. This often means expanding enrolment by using a multicentre study. There is no point in embarking on a trial if it will never be possible to recruit an adequate population to answer the research question. More patients will need to be randomised than the final sample size to take into account patients who die, drop out or are lost to follow-up.

The following is an example calculation for a study to recruit patients into two groups. In order to calculate a sample size, it is common practice to set the level of power for the study at 80% with a 5% significance level. This means that, if there is a difference between study groups, there is an 80% chance of detecting it. Based on previous studies, realistic expectations of differences between groups should be used to calculate the sample size. The formula below uses the figures of a reduction in event rate from 30% to 10% (e.g. a new treatment expected to reduce the complication rate such as wound infection from 30% = r to 10% = s).

$$8 \times \frac{[r(100 - r) + s(100 - s)]}{(r - s)^2}$$

$$\text{e.g. } 8 \times \frac{[30(100 - 30) + 10(100 - 10)]}{(30 - 10)^2}$$

$$= 60 \text{ needed in each group}$$

Eliminating bias

It is important to imagine how a study could be invalidated by thinking of things that could go wrong. One way to eliminate any bias inherent in the data collection is to have observers or recorders who do not know which treatment has been used (blinded observer). It might also be possible to ensure that the patient is unaware of the treatment allocation (single blind). In the best randomised studies, neither patient nor researcher is aware of which therapy has been used until after the study has finished (double blind). Randomised trials are essential for testing new drugs. In practice, however, in some surgical trials, randomisation may not be possible or ethical.

Study protocol

Now that the question to pose has been decided, and it has been checked that sufficient patients should be available to enrol into the study, it is time to prepare the detail of the trial. At this stage, a study protocol should be constructed to define the research strategy. It should contain a paragraph on the background of the proposed study, the aims and objectives, a clear methodology, definitions of population and sample sizes and methods of proposed analysis. It should include the patient numbers, inclusion and exclusion criteria and the timescale for the work. It is useful to construct a flow diagram giving a clear summary of the research protocol and its requirements (**Figure 11.1**). It is helpful to imagine the paper that will be written about the study, before it is performed. This may prevent errors in data collection.

When a study is planned, sufficient time should be reserved at the beginning for fund-raising and obtaining ethical, regulatory and or other approvals (e.g. HRA). Time for data analysis and preparation of publication needs to be included in funding applications. The cost of any non-routine investigations and extra treatments should be identified and covered by the research grant in line with national guidance (in the UK, the Attributing the costs of health and social care Research and Development (AcoRD) guidance). It is essential to discuss this with institutional leads well in advance of the grant submission date to ensure appropriate authorisation from institutions.

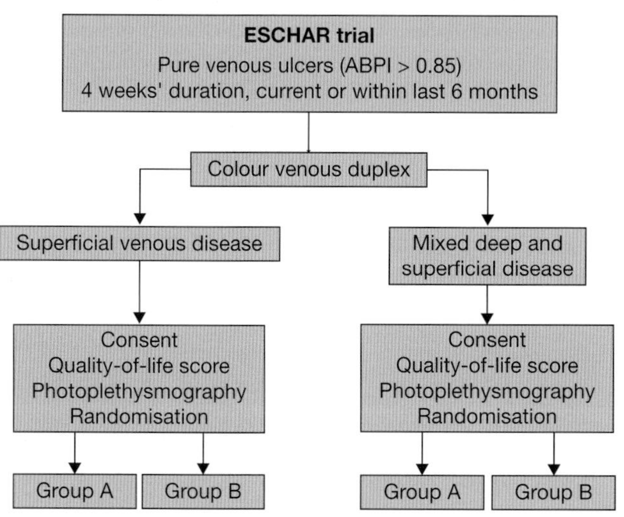

Figure 11.1 ESCHAR trial: completed in Gloucestershire, UK (Gohel MS *et al. British Journal of Surgery 2005*; **92**: 291–7. Copyright British Journal of Surgery Society Ltd. Permission is granted by John Wiley & Sons Ltd on behalf of the BJSS Ltd.) ABPI, ankle–brachial pressure index.

A data collection form should be designed or a computer collection package developed. If data are collected on computer, appropriate safeguards for privacy, confidentiality and data quality will be necessary to comply with legislation. At this stage it is important to consider any validation requirements and needs for open access either in a recognised archive (e.g. the UK Data Archive) or an institutional repository. Any form of data collection needs to be quality assured. The quality assurance process will include training, Standard Operating Procedures as well as monitoring and checking a certain sample of the data. At the end of data collection and analysis, a final data base with all data should be locked and kept for future reference in a safe location. A data archiving policy with a nominated data custodian should be in place.

Research is no longer confined by institutional or even geographical boundaries. Communication by the internet can be a valid way to co-ordinate internalional research. The Global Surgical Outcomes Collaboration (www.globalsurg.org) is a group of young surgeons performing collaborative research with internet data collection.

Some publishers require registration of a study at the time of study set up on a publically available database (e.g. ISRCTN). It is becoming increasingly popular to consider publication of a protocol paper.

Regulatory framework

In the UK, the implementation of the research governance framework by the Department of Health, or its planned successor UK Policy Framework for Health and Social Care, provides a framwork that enhances the integrity of the study and includes requirements for sponsorship by an institution to ensure the following: peer review, independent ethics review, compliance with data protection principles, financial probity, dissemination and management of intellectual property.

Sponsorship is defined by the HRA as the individual, company, institution or organisation that takes on ultimate responsibility for the initiation, management (or arranging the initiation and management) of and/or financing (or arranging the financing) for that research. The sponsor takes primary responsibility for ensuring that the design of the study meets appropriate standards and that arrangements are in place to ensure appropriate conduct and reporting. http://www.hra.nhs.uk/resources/before-you-apply/roles-and-responsibilties/sponsor/

Peer review

Once the protocol is finalised, formal peer review is needed. In the UK, evidence of peer review will be needed before submitting an application to a research ethics committee and for HRA approval.

- If the research is part of a university course, the university (usually the student supervisor) should undertake this review.
- Surgeons working for the NHS can arrange their own peer review by experts who are not connected with the study.

Alternatively, most Research and Development Support Units (NHS) will give guidance through the review process.
- Many funders of research will undertake their own independent peer review. There is usually feedback from this process that can provide valuable advice about the study.

Ethics

In the first instance, common sense is the best guide to whether or not a study is ethical. It is still important to seek advice from an independent research ethics committee whenever research is contemplated.

In the UK the requirement is that a NHS Research Ethics Committee (NHS REC) provides an independent ethical review of all health and social care research if it involves patients and/or carers. The Government arrangment for Research Ethics Commitees (GafREC) provide detailed guidance about NHS REC review requirements. The application for NHS REC review should be made using the Integrated Research Administraion System (IRAS). IRAS is a single system for applying for the permissions and approvals for health and social care/community care research in the UK. It enables entry of information about the project once instead of duplicating information in separate application forms. IRAS captures the information needed for the relevant approvals from the following review bodies:

- Administration of Radioactive Substances Advisory Committee (ARSAC);
- Confidentiality Advisory Group (CAG);
- Gene Therapy Advisory Committee (GTAC);
- Health Research Authority (HRA) for projects seeking HRA approval;
- Medicines and Healthcare products Regulatory Agency (MHRA);
- NHS/HSC R&D offices;
- NHS/HSC Research Ethics Committees;
- National Offender Management Service (NOMS);
- Social Care Research Ethics Committee.

Once all the relevant forms and associated study documentation have been completed, guidance provided by the HRA and the Research Ethics Service should be followed for submission of the request for ethical review and HRA approval. If the study does not require review by an NHS REC, the need for an independent ethical review should still be considered. Universities have developed their own ethical review infrastructure and this will be institute specific and location specific. For collaborative research, local ethical review should be obtained where possible, and developing a local ethics infrastructure should be considered if it does not already exist. Duplicaton of ethical review should be avoided.

Ethics committees prefer to see fully developed trial protocols but it is often possible to get some preliminary advice from the NHS REC Manager. Ethics committee forms may seem long and detailed, but it is important that these are filled in correctly and it helps to prepare the investigators for all practical aspects of the project. All dealings with ethics committees should be intelligent and courteous. It is important to attend the meeting at which the study will be discussed, if invited, as it provides a forum for direct communication in relation to the study. It can save time as possible concerns of the ethics committee can be addressed at the time, avoiding lengthy correspondence.

Regulatory approvals

In the case of interventional clinical or device trials, the European Union Clinical Trial Directives apply, which are regulated by the Medicines and Health Care products Regulatory Agency (MHRA) in the UK. A clinical trial should be registered with the European Clinical Trials Database before applying to the MHRA for a Clinical Trial Authorisation via the common European submission portal. This can be a complicated and trying process, and support should be sought from the investigators' employing institution. Editors of the major surgical journals now agree that all clinical trials should have been registered before an article relating to a trial can be published.

All studies undertaken with NHS patients and/or carers will need HRA approval and confrmation of capacity and capability from NHS sites. Studies involving animals require approval from statutory licensing authorities. Reporting on animal research should employ ARRIVE guidelines (Animal Research: Reporting of In Vivo Experiments).

Research integrity

The principles and responsibilities set out in the Singapore Statement on Research Integrity in 2010 was the first international effort to encourage the development of unified policies, guidelines and codes of conduct, with the long-term goal of fostering greater integrity in research worldwide. The European Code of Conduct followed and in 2012 Universities UK, in collaboration with major funders of research, developed 'the Concordat to support research integrity', which sets out key commitments to ensure a high standard in research. All highlight the principles and professional responsibilities of researchers and research instituions that are fundamental to the integrity of research wherever it is undertaken. These centre around:

- honesty in all aspects of research;
- accountability and transparentcy in the conduct of research;
- professional courtesy and fairness in working with others;
- good stewardship of research.

A study should not under any circumstances commence until the correct approval has been granted and compliance with the principles of research integrity is ensured. Any challenge to the integrity of research can be time-consuming and career-limiting.

STATISTICAL ANALYSIS

Both audit and research commonly require statistical analysis. Many surgeons find the statistical analysis of a project the most difficult part. It is also the most commonly criticised part of papers written by clinicians. There are many useful books about statistics that can be consulted (see Further reading); if in any doubt, a statistician will be pleased to give assistance. Statisticians like to be consulted before research or audit has been conducted rather than being presented with the data at the end; they often give helpful advice over study design and can be an important part of the project team.

The following terms are frequently used when summarising statistical data:

- **Mean:** the result of dividing the total by the number of observations (the average);
- **Median:** the middle value with equal numbers of observations above and below – used for numerical or ranked data;
- **Mode:** the value with the highest frequency observed – used for nominal data collection;
- **Range:** the largest to the smallest value.

The most important decision for analysis is whether the distribution of the data is normal (i.e. parametric or non-parametric). Normally, distributed data have a symmetrical, bell-shaped curve, and the mean, median and mode all lie at the same value. The type of data collected determines which statistical test should be used.

1 Numerical and normally distributed (e.g. blood pressure) – use unpaired *t*-test to compare two groups or paired *t*-test to assess whether a variable has changed between two time points.
2 Numerical but not normally distributed (e.g. tumour size) – use Mann–Whitney *U*-test to compare two groups or a Wilcoxon signed rank test to assess whether a variable has increased/stayed the same/decreased between two time points.
3 Categorical (e.g. admitted or not admitted to an intensive care unit) – can use chi-squared test to compare two groups.

(**Note:** the use of these and any other statistical tests may benefit from professional advice.)

Confidence intervals are the best guide to the possible range in which the true differences are likely to lie. A confidence interval that includes zero usually implies a lack of statistical significance.

Scientists usually employ probability (*P*-values) to describe statistical chance. A *P*-value <0.05 is commonly taken to imply a true difference. It is important not to forget that $P = 0.05$ simply means there is only a 1:20 chance that the differences between the variables would have happened by chance when in fact there is no real difference. If enough variables are examined in any study, significant differences will occur simply by chance. Trials with multiple endpoints or variables require more sophisticated analysis to determine the significance of individual risk factors. Univariable or multivariable logistic regression analysis techniques may be appropriate.

Statistics simply deal with the chance that observations between populations are different and should be treated with caution. Clinical results should show clear differences. If statistics are required to demonstrate differences between results, it is possible that they are unlikely to have major clinical significance.

Computer software packages available

Statistical computer packages offer a quick way of analysing descriptive statistics such as mean, median and range, as well as the most commonly used statistical tests such as the chi-squared test. Various packages are available commercially and are useful tools in data analysis.

ANALYSING A SCIENTIFIC ARTICLE

The simplest way to analyse an article from a scientific journal is to look at the checklist of requirements for good scientific research. A group of scientists and editors developed the CONSORT (Consolidated Standards of Reporting Trials) statement to improve the quality of reporting of RCTs. Looking in detail at the study design is often the best way of deciding whether a trial is any good. The CONSORT document includes a checklist for the conduct of good randomised trials (*Table 11.4*). Often clinicians overlook biases that others

TABLE 11.4 Checklist for authors.

Heading	Sub-heading	Descriptor
Title		Identify as randomised trial
Abstract		Structured format
Introduction		Prospectively defined hypotheses, clinical objective
Methods	Protocol	Study population
		Intervention, timing
		Primary and secondary outcome
		Statistical rationale
		Stopping rules
	Assignment	Unit of randomisation
		Method: allocation schedule
	Masking (blinding)	
Results	Participant flow and follow-up	Trial profile, flow diagram
	Analysis	Estimated effect of intervention
		Summary data with appropriate inferential statistics
		Protocol deviation
Comment		Specific interpretation of study
		Sources of bias
		External validity
		General interpretation

From the CONSORT statement: *Journal of the American Medical Association* 1996; **276**: 637–639.

find obvious to detect, which can have a profound influence on the outcome of any study. Even the randomised design does not always guarantee quality, and a core component of systematic review is the grading of trial quality; several scoring systems have been developed (e.g. Jadad Score). Recent guidelines have been published formalising the methods of systematic review and meta-analysis (PRISMA guidelines), and also many other types of article. These can be found in the instructions to authors of most surgical journals, which will now only accept articles that follow the rules.

PRESENTING AND PUBLISHING AN ARTICLE

There is no point in conducting a research or audit project and then leaving the results unreported. Even when results are negative, they are worth distributing; no project if properly conducted is worthless. Under-reporting of negative outcomes causes a systematic bias in the literature in favour of positive trials. Most studies do not provide dramatic results, and few surgeons publish seminal articles.

The key to both presentation and publication is to decide on the message and then aim for an appropriate forum. Big important randomised studies or national audits merit presentation at national meetings and publication in international journals. Small observational studies and audits are more often accepted for presentation at regional or hospital meetings and for publication in smaller specialist journals. Help and advice from clinicians familiar with presentation and publication are invaluable at this stage. The most important piece of advice is to follow accurately the instructions for journal submission. Most international meetings will accept presentations eagerly (especially by poster) as this increases the attendance at a conference.

Most surgeons publish research in peer-reviewed journals. The work that is submitted is checked anonymously by other surgeons before publication. If in doubt about whether to submit to a journal, many editors will give advice about the suitability of an article for submission to their journal. It is usually free to publish in surgical journals, since the cost of refereeing and editing is born by the journal subscriber. A second model of publication is becoming more prevalent: open access, author pays. This ensures all research is visible to anyone, by pushing the costs of the editorial process onto the study budget. It may well become standard in future.

Convention dictates that articles are submitted in IMRAD form – introduction, methods, results and discussion. Increasingly, electronic publication and the Internet may change the face of scientific publication and, in the next decade, these restrictions on style may disappear. For now, the IMRAD format remains inviolable. The length of an article is important: a paper should be as long as the size of the message. Readers of big randomised multicentre trials wish to know as much detail about the study as possible; reports on small negative trials should be brief.

- **Introduction.** This should always be short. A brief background of the study should be presented and then the aims of the trial or audit outlined.
- **Methods.** The methodology and study design should be given in detail. It is important to own up to any biases. Any new techniques or investigations should be detailed in full; if they are common practice or have been described elsewhere, this should be referenced instead of described.
- **Results.** Results are almost always best shown diagrammatically using tables and figures if possible. Results shown in the form of a diagram need not then be duplicated in the text.
- **Discussion.** It is important not to repeat the introduction or reiterate the results in this section. The study should be interpreted intelligently and any suggestions for future studies or changes in management should be made. It is important not to indulge in flights of fantasy or wild imagination about future possibilities; most journal editors will delete these. Recently, a standard format for the discussion section has been promoted, and journals such as the *British Medical Journal* are keen that authors use it.
- **References.** This section should include all relevant papers recording previous studies on the subject in question. The number should reflect the size of the message and the importance of the work. The reference section does not usually have to be exhaustive, but should include up-to-date articles. Remember to present the references in the style of the journal of submission.

EVIDENCE-BASED SURGERY

Surgical practice has been considered an art: ask 50 surgeons how to manage a patient and you will probably get 50 different answers. There is so much clinical information available that no surgeon can know it all. Evidence-based surgery is a move to find the best ways of managing patients using clinical evidence from collected studies. It was estimated that sufficient evidence to justify routine myocardial thrombolysis for heart attacks was available years before the randomised clinical studies that finally made it clinically acceptable. No one had gathered all the available information together. Centres such as the Cochrane Collaboration have been collecting randomised trials and reviews to provide up-to-date information for clinicians. The Cochrane Library presently includes a database of systematic reviews, reviews of surgical effectiveness and a register of controlled trials. The *BJS* has been collecting surgical randomised trials on its website archive for 10 years (www.bjs.co.uk). There are now almost 1500 annotated references that can be a valuable resource for scientific authors. As evidence accumulates, it is expected that this will gradually smooth out the differences between clinicians as the best way of managing patients becomes more obvious. Collecting published evidence together and analysing it often requires reviews of multiple randomised trials. These meta-analyses involve complex statistical analyses designed to interpret multiple findings and synthesise the results of multiple studies.

FURTHER READING

Altman DG. *Statistics with confidence*. London: BMJ Publishing Group, 2002.

Brown RA, Swanson Beck J. *Medical statistics on personal computers*. Plymouth: BMJ Publishing Group, 1994.
Dindo D, Demartines N, Clavien P-A. Classification of surgical complications: a new proposal with evaluation of a cohort of 6336 patients and the results of a survey. *Ann Surg* 2004; **240**: 205–213.
Greenhalgh T. *How to read a paper: the basics of evidence-based medicine*. London; BMJ Publishing Group, 2010.
Institute of Medicine. *Guidelines for clinical practice: from development to use*. Washington DC; National Academic Press, 1992.
Kelson M. *Promoting patient involvement in clinical audit*. London; London College of Health and the Clinical Outcomes Group, 1998.
Kilkenny C, Browne WJ, Cuthill IC *et al.* (2010) Improving bioscience research reporting: the ARRIVE guidelines for reporting animal research. *PloS Biol* 2010; **8**(6): e1000412.
Kirkwood BR *Essentials of medical statistics*, 2nd edn. Oxford; Blackwell Publishing, 2003.
Lyratzopoulos G, Patrick H, Campbell WB. Registers needed for new interventional procedures. *Lancet* 2008; **371**:1734–1736.
McCulloch P, Altman DG, Campbell WB *et al.* No surgical innovation without evaluation: the IDEAL recommendations. *Lancet* 2009; **374**(9695): 1105–1112.
Moher D, Cooke DJ, Eastwood S *et al.* Improving the quality of reports of meta-analyses of randomised controlled trials: the QUORUM statement. *Lancet* 2009; **354**: 1896–900.
Moher D, Liberati A, Tetzlaff J *et al.*, The PRISMA Group. (2009) Preferred reporting items for systematic reviews and meta-analyses: the PRISMA Statement. *Open Med* **2009; 3**: 123–130.
Morrell C, Harvey G. *The clinical audit handbook*. London; Baillière Tindall, 1999.
Schein M, Farndon JR, Fingerhut A. *A Surgeon's Guide to Writing and Publishing*. Kemberton; TFM Publishing, 2001.
Smith R. *The trouble with medical journals*. London; RSM Press Ltd, 2006.
Swinscow TDV. *Statistics at square one*, 9th edn. London; BMJ Publishing Group, 1996.
Walshe K. Adverse events in health care: issues in measurement. *Qual Health Care* 2000; **9**: 47–52.
Whitman B, Ginham R, Perkins M *et al.* The Human Tissue Act 2004. Reflections on recent changes of regulatory affairs in the United Kingdom. *J Res Admin* 2008; **2**: 91–99.

ON-LINE RESOURCES

AcoRD: https://www.gov.uk/government/publications/guidance-on-attributing-the-costs-of-health-and-social-care-research UK
CLAHRC: http://www.clahrcpp.co.uk/#!clahrcs/cjg9
Clinical Evidence: www.clinicalevidence.com
Cochrane Library: www.cochrane.org/index.htm
Concordat to support research integrity: http://www.universitiesuk.ac.uk/highereducation/Documents/2012/TheConcordatToSupportResearchIntegrity.pdf
Consolidated Standards of Reporting Trials: http://www.consort-statement.org/consort-statement/
Data Archive: http://www.data-archive.ac.uk/
Eudract database: https://www.clinicaltrialsregister.eu/
European Code of Conduct: http://www.esf.org/fileadmin/Public_documents/Publications/Code_Conduct_ResearchIntegrity.pdf
GafREC: http://www.hra.nhs.uk/resources/research-legislation-and-governance/governance-arrangements-for-research-ethics-committees/
Health Research Authority http://www.hra.nhs.uk/
Integrated Research Administration System: https://www.myresearchproject.org.uk/SignIn.aspx
ISRCTN: http://www.isrctn.com/
MHRA: https://www.gov.uk/government/organisations/medicines-and-healthcare-products-regulatory-agency/services-information
National Institute for Health and Care Excellence (NICE): www.nice.org.uk
NHS England audits: https://www.england.nhs.uk/ourwork/qual-clin-lead/clinaudit/
Nice audit information: https://www.nice.org.uk/about/what-we-do/into-practice/audit-and-service-improvement
Research Ethics Service: http://www.hra.nhs.uk/about-the-hra/our-committees/res/
Scottish Intercollegiate Guideline Network (SIGN): www.sign.ac.uk
Singapore Statment: http://www.singaporestatement.org/index.html
Vascular Society: http://www.vascularsociety.org.uk/

Chapter 12

Surgical ethics and law

Learning objectives

To understand:

- The importance of autonomy in good surgical practice
- The moral and legal boundaries and practical difficulties of informed consent
- Good practice in making decisions about the withdrawal of life-sustaining treatment
- The importance and boundaries of confidentiality in surgical practice
- The importance of appropriate regulation in surgical research
- The importance of rigorous training and maintenance of good practice standards

INTRODUCTION

This chapter incorporates references to English common and statute law. Nevertheless, these legal and ethical principles have much in common with many other jurisdictions across the world.

Surgery, ethics and law go hand in hand. In any other arena of public or private life, if someone deliberately cuts another person, draws blood, causes pain, leaves scars and disrupts everyday activity, then the likely result will be a criminal charge. If the person dies as a result, the charge could be manslaughter or even murder. Self evidently, the difference between the criminal and the surgeon is that their intentions differ. While a criminal intentionally (or recklessly) inflicts harm, the surgeon's intention is limited to the treatment of illness. Any harm that ensues is either unintentional, or is necessary (such as an incision), to facilitate treatment.

Patients submit to surgery because they trust their surgeons. What should consent entail in practice and what should surgeons do when patients need help but are unable or unwilling to agree to it? When patients do consent to treatment, surgeons are provided with a wide discretion. The end result may be cure, but disfigurement, disability and death may also result. How should such surgical 'power' be regulated to reinforce the trust of patients and to ensure that surgeons practise to an acceptable professional standard? Are there circumstances, in the public interest, in which it is acceptable to sacrifice the trust of individual patients through revealing information that was communicated in what patients believed to be conditions of strict privacy?

These questions about what constitutes good professional practice concern medical ethics and law relating to consent, confidentiality and the underlying concept of personal autonomy.

In addition, these principles need to be applied to surgical activities, including professional matters relating to governance, regulation and the process of revalidation, in its different guises around the world. Surgical training is starting to embrace the 'basic science' of surgical law, to offer surgeons assistance in the resolution of such ethical dilemmas. This chapter is evidence of that process.

RESPECT FOR AUTONOMY

Surgeons have a duty of care towards their human patients that goes beyond just protecting their life and health. Their additional duty of care is to respect the autonomy of their patients and their ability to make choices about their treatments, and to evaluate potential outcomes in light of other life plans. Such respect is particularly important for surgeons because, without it, the trust between them and their patients may be compromised, along with the success of the surgical care provided. We are careful enough in everyday life about whom we allow to touch us and to see us unclothed. It is hardly surprising that many people feel strongly about exercising the same control over a potentially hazardous activity, such as surgery.

For all these reasons, there is a wide moral and legal consensus that patients have the right to exercise choice over their surgical care. In this context, a right should be interpreted as a claim that can be made on the surgeon. The surgeon, therefore, accepts the strict duty to respect the patient's choice, regardless of personal preferences. Thus, to the degree that patients have a right to make choices about proposed surgical treatment, it then follows that they should be allowed to refuse treatments that they do not want, even when surgeons think that they are wrong. The right to make an unwise decision was exemplified in a recent case[1], where a woman with capacity refused renal replacement therapy. The court reminded doctors that notwithstanding the fact that other citizens might consider her decision unreasonable, illogical or even immoral, none of these criticisms of the decision by themselves provide evidence of a lack of capacity. Patients can refuse surgical treatment that will save their lives, either at present or in the future, the latter through the formulation of advance decisions or lasting powers of attorney specifying the types of life-saving treatments that they do not wish to have, notwithstanding that they may later become incompetent to refuse them.

INFORMED CONSENT

In surgical practice, respect for autonomy translates into the clinical duty to obtain informed consent before the commencement of treatment.

It is easy to underestimate the gap in understanding between a surgeon and his or her patient.[2] How many patients would recognise that unilateral eye surgery might lead to contralateral blindness? The risks and side effects of many operations are not intuitive, and the surgeon is not in the position to guess how the patient's plans for employment, leisure and family life may be inadvertently affected by a forseeable complication. A budding Olympic gymnast might choose to forgo surgery on a quiescent posterior triangle lesion if he or she knew the potentially consequences of division of the accessory nerve. That is why patients need to be informed, beforehand, so they can choose whether to take the risk.

To establish valid consent to treatment, patients need to be given appropriate and accurate information. In England and Wales, the Department of Health's Reference Guide to Consent should be consulted.

Such information, disclosed during a formal and tangible discussion, must include:

- the condition and the reasons why it warrants surgery;
- the type of surgery proposed and how it might correct the condition;
- the anticipated prognosis and expected side effects of the proposed surgery;
- the unexpected hazards of the proposed surgery;
- any alternative and potentially successful treatments other than the proposed surgery;
- the consequences of no treatment at all.

With such information, patients can link their clinical prospects with the management of other aspects of their life and the lives of others for whom they may be morally and/or professionally responsible. Good professional practice dictates that obtaining informed consent should occur in circumstances that are designed to maximise the chances of patients understanding what is said about their condition and proposed treatment, as well as giving them an opportunity to ask questions and express anxieties.

Where possible:

- a quiet venue for discussion should be found;
- written material in the patient's preferred language should be provided to supplement verbal communication, together with diagrams where appropriate;
- patients should be given time and help to come to their own decision;
- the person obtaining the consent should ideally be the surgeon who will carry out the treatment. It should not be – as is sometimes the case – a junior member of staff who has never conducted such a procedure and thus may not have enough understanding to counsel the patient properly.

Good communication skills go hand in hand with properly obtaining informed consent for surgery. It is not good enough just to go through the motions of providing patients with the information required for considered choice. Attention must be paid to:

- whether or not the patient has understood what has been stated;
- avoiding overly technical language in descriptions and explanations;
- the provision of translators for patients whose first language is not English;
- asking patients if they have further questions.

When there is any doubt about their understanding, patients should be asked questions by their surgeon about what has supposedly been communicated to see if they can explain the information in question for themselves.

Surgeons have a legal as well as a moral obligation to obtain consent for treatment based on appropriate disclosure. Failure to do so could result in one of two civil proceedings, assuming the absence of criminal intent. First, in law, intentionally to touch another person without their consent is a battery, remembering that we are usually touched by strangers as a consequence of accidental contact. Surgeons have an obligation to give the conscious and competent patient sufficient information 'in broad terms' about the surgical treatment being proposed and why. If the patient agrees to proceed, no other treatment should ordinarily be administered without further explicit consent.

The second legal action that might be brought against a surgeon for not obtaining appropriate consent to treatment is in the tort (civil wrong) of negligence. Patients may have been given enough information about what is surgically proposed to agree to be touched in the ways suggested. However, surgeons may still be in breach of their professional duty if they do not provide sufficient information about the risks that patients will encounter through such treatment. Although standards of how much information should be provided about risks vary between nations, as a matter of good practice, surgeons should inform patients of the hazards that any reasonable person in the position of the patient would wish to know. In UK law, this level and style of disclosure has been most recently reviewed in the case of *Montgomery v Lanarkshire Health Board*.[2]

Finally, surgeons now understand that, when they obtain consent to proceed with treatment, patients are expected to sign a consent form of some kind. The detail of such forms can differ, but they often contain very little of the information supposedly communicated to the patient who signed it. Partly for this reason, the process of formally obtaining consent can become overly focused on obtaining the signature of patients rather than ensuring that appropriate types and amounts of information have been provided and have been understood.

Both professionally and legally, it is important for surgeons to understand that a signed consent form is not proof that valid consent has been properly obtained. It is simply a piece of evidence that consent may have been attempted. Even when they have provided their signature, patients can and do deny that appropriate information has been communicated or that the communication was effective. Surgeons are therefore well advised to make brief notes of what they have said to patients about their proposed treatments, especially information about significant risks. These notes should be placed in the patient's clinical record, perhaps by referring to the disclosure in the letter to the family doctor, copied to the patient. In addition, information sheets describing the generic risks, benefits and complications associated with the proposed procedure can be provided.

PRACTICAL APPLICATION

Thus far we have examined the moral and legal reasons why the duty of surgeons to respect the autonomy of patients translates into the specific responsibility to obtain informed consent to treatment. For consent to be valid, adult patients must:

- have capacity to give it – be able to understand, remember and deliberate about whatever information is provided to them about treatment choices, and to communicate those choices;
- not be coerced into decisions that reflect the preferences of others rather than themselves;
- be given sufficient information for these choices to be based on an accurate understanding of reasons for and against proceeding with specific treatments.

Surgical care would grind to a halt if it were always necessary to obtain explicit informed consent every time a patient is touched in the context of their care. Fortunately, it is an elementary step merely to ask the patient whether they mind being examined – the usual response will be acceptance. This simple transaction illustrates that the legal and ethical 'rules' that govern a surgeon are often no more than an expression of good clinical practice; in this case, politeness.

Some patients will not be able to give consent because of temporary incapacity. This may result from their presenting illness or intoxication, or an unanticipated situation may be encountered midway through a general anaesthetic. The moral and legal rules that govern such situations are clear. The doctrine of medical necessity enables the surgeon, in an emergency, to save life and prevent permanent disability, operating without consent. This is employed daily, where unconsious emergency patients undergo surgery to save 'life and limb'. No consent has been provided and none is required, providing the treatment is in the patient's best interests.

However, if the patient has made a legally valid advance decision refusing treatment of the specific kind required, their decision must be honoured, providing it is applicable to the current clinical situation. Where possible, surgery on patients who are temporarily incapacitated should be postponed until their capacity is restored and they are able to give informed consent or refusal for themselves.

Surgeons must take care to respect the distinction between procedures that are necessary to prevent death or irremediable harm, and those that are done merely out of convenience. If the patient consents only to a dilatation and currettage, do not consider performing an additional hysterectomy 'in her best interests', simply because she is anaesthetised.

Consent may be made impossible by incompetence of other kinds. In the case of children, parents or someone with parental responsibility are ordinarily required to provide consent on their behalf. This said, surgeons should:

- take care to explain to children what is being surgically proposed, and why;
- always consult with children about their response;
- where possible, take the child's views into account and note that even young children can be competent to consent to treatment provided that they too can understand, remember, deliberate about and believe information relevant to their clinical condition. Plainly, it is almost always appropriate in addition to discuss the treatment with their parents.

When such *Gillick* competence is present, under English law, children can provide their own consent to surgical care, although they cannot unconditionally refuse it until they are 18 years old. These provisions illustrate the importance of respecting as much autonomy as is present among child patients and remembering that, for the purposes of consent to medical treatment, they may be just as autonomous as adults.

If capacity in adults is erased by psychiatric illness or mental handicap, other moral and legal provisions hold. If patients lack the autonomy to choose how to protect themselves as regards the consequences of their illness, then others charged with protecting them must assume the responsibility. However, care must be taken not to abuse this duty. Even when such patients have been legally detained for compulsory psychiatric care, it does not follow that such patients are unable to provide consent for surgical care. Their capacity should be assumed and consent should be sought. Only if it is established with the help of their carers that such patients also lack capacity to provide consent for surgery, and that they are at risk of death or serious and permanent disability, can therapy then proceed in their best interests. However, if treatment can be postponed, then this should be done until, as a result of their psychiatric care, patients become able either to consent or to refuse. If this recovery is not predicted, then legal steps may be taken to make elective surgery lawful. As with children, respect should always be shown for as much autonomy as is present.

Absence of capacity in adults does not vitiate the requirement, where possible, to take into account their sentiments during clinical decision making. In a recent case, a judge declared that an elderly man with a septic leg, although incapacitated by his mental illness, had feelings, beliefs and values that weighed so heavily in the consideration of his best interests that they outweighed the clinical desire to save his life by amputation.[3] Although an unusual judgement in this context, it reflects the growing determination to give incapacitated adults an opportunity to influence their fate, as best they can.

In adult patients who are permanently incapacitated, and thus unable to provide consent for surgery, as noted above, the doctrine of necessity obtains and surgery can proceed in an emergency to save life, to prevent serious and permanent injury. Elective treatment for less grave complaints can also be provided, and in England and Wales is done so under the auspices of the Mental Capacity Act 2005. The associated Code of Practice guides the surgeon in matters of capacity and disclosure, and in dealing with those who have taken steps to influence their treatment, anticipating the time that they will have lost their capacity. These arrangements may manifest either in documentary form, as Advance Decisions, or in person, in the form of persons appointed with a Lasting Power of Attorney.

It is not possible for relatives of incapacitated adult patients to sign consent forms for surgery on their behalf. Indeed, to make such requests can be a disservice to relatives, who may feel an unjustified sense of responsibility if the surgery fails. This said, relatives play a vital role in providing background information about the patient, allowing the clinician to assess and then determine what treatment is in the best interests of the patient.

MATTERS OF LIFE AND DEATH

It has been noted that the right of an adult with capacity to consent to and refuse lawful treatment is unlimited, including the refusal of life-sustaining treatment. Probably the example of this most familiar to surgeons is Jehovah's Witnesses, who may refuse blood transfusions at the risk of their own lives.

There will be some circumstances in which sustaining the life and health of incapacitated adult patients is judged to be inappropriate. They are no longer able to be consulted and may not have expressed a view about what their wishes would be in such circumstances. Here, if possible after discussion and consensus with the next of kin, a decision may be made to withhold or to withdraw life-sustaining treatment on behalf of the incapacitated patient. The fact that such decisions can be seen as omissions to act does not excuse surgeons from morally and legally having to reconcile them with their ordinary duty of care. Ultimately, this can only be done through arguing that such omissions to sustain life are in the patient's best interests.

The determination of best interests in these circumstances will rely on one of three objective criteria, over and above the subjective perception by the surgeon that the quality of life of the patient is poor. There is no obligation to provide or to continue life-sustaining treatment:

- if doing so is futile, when clinical consensus dictates that it will not achieve the goal of extending life. Thought of in this way, judgements about futility exclude considering patient's quality of life, and thus can be difficult to justify as long as treatment might stand even a very small chance of success;
- if a patient is imminently and irreversibly close to death – in such circumstances, it would not be in the patient's best interests to prolong life slightly (e.g. through the application of intensive care) when, again, there is no hope of any sustained success. Declining needlessly to interfere with the process of a dignified death can be just as caring as the provision of curative therapy;
- if patients are so permanently and seriously brain damaged that, lacking awareness of themselves or others, they will never be able to engage in any form of self-directed activity. The argument here is backed up by moral and legal reasoning: that further treatment other than effective palliation cannot be in the best interests of patients as it will provide them with no benefit.

When any of these principles are employed to justify an omission to provide or to continue life-sustaining treatment, the circumstances should be carefully recorded in the patient's medical record, along with a note of another senior clinician's agreement.

Furthermore, the decision to discontinue life-sustaining tretament may go hand in hand with a decision not to attempt cardiopulmonary resuscitation, in the event of cardiorespiratory arrest. In England, it is settled law that before finally making this decision, doctors must discuss it with patients or their relatives.[4] The reason for this insistence is that the patient may have personal circumstances, unbeknown to the surgeon, which might yet influence this final (and for the patient, portentous) decision. The only exclusion to this legal rule is where discussion of this matter with the patient may cause them not merely distress, but harm.

Finally, surgeons will sometimes find themselves in charge of the palliative care of patients whose pain is increasingly difficult to control. There may come a point in the management of such pain when effective palliation is possible at the risk of shortening a patient's life because of the respiratory effects of the palliative drugs. In such circumstances, surgeons can with legal justification administer a dose that might be dangerous, although experts in palliative care are sceptical that this is ever necessary with appropriate training. In any case, the argument employed to justify such action refers to its 'double effect': that both the relief of pain and death might follow from such an action. Intentional killing (active euthanasia) is rejected as unlawful malpractice throughout most of the world. A foreseeably lethal analgesic dose is thus regarded as appropriate only when it is solely motivated by palliative intent, and this motivation can be documented. Recent authority from criminal law indicates that if an analgesic injection is 'virtually certain' also to kill the patient, a court might deduce that the person giving the injection had an intention to kill. The key to the defence of double effect is the absolute absence of such an intention.

A **Jehovah's Witness** is a member of a millenarian fundamentalist Christian sect founded in America in 1884. They have their own translation of the Bible, which they interpret literally.

TRANSPLANTATION

The law and ethics of organ transplantation require more space than this chapter allows. In common with other nations, the UK has a statutory framework for transplantation, but even amongst this small group of nations, there is no unanimity of legislation, thus rules for deceased and live donor transplants differ. In general, the rules for defining a dead donor, for compensating a living donor and for legitimising a market in organs differ widely. It is strongly recommended that you refer to the rules within your own jurisdiction.

CONFIDENTIALITY

Respect for autonomy does not entail only the right of capacitous patients to consent to treatment. Their autonomous right extends to control over their confidential information, and surgeons must to respect their privacy, not communicate information revealed in the course of treatment to anyone else without consent. Generally speaking, such respect means that surgeons must not discuss clinical matters with relatives, friends, employers and others unless the patient explicitly agrees. To do otherwise is regarded by all the regulatory bodies of medicine and surgery as a grave offence, incurring harsh penalties. For breaches of confidentiality are not only abuses of human dignity, they again undermine the trust between surgeon and patient on which successful surgery and the professional reputations of surgeons depend.

Important as respect for confidentiality is, however, it is not absolute. Surgeons are allowed to communicate private information to other professionals who are part of the healthcare team, provided that the information has a direct bearing on treatment. Here, it is argued that patients have given their implied consent to such communication when they explicitly consent to a treatment plan. Whether implied consent can ever be valid is a matter for public debate, as government attempts to apply the doctrine to tissue donation and access to electronic health records. Such examples of implied 'consent' are better viewed as mere aquiescence of patients, ignorant of and not objecting to decisions made about them.

Patients cannot expect strict adherence to the principle of confidentiality if it poses a serious threat to the health and safety of others. There will be some circumstances in which confidentiality either must or may be breached in the public interest. For example, it must be breached as a result of court orders or in relation to the requirements of public health legislation. Confidentiality may be waived in the interests of preventing serious crime or to protect the safety of other known individuals who are at risk of serious harm.

RESEARCH

As part of their duty to protect life and health to an acceptable professional standard, surgeons have a subsidiary responsibility to strive to improve operative techniques through research, to assure themselves and their patients that the care proposed is the best that is currently possible. Yet there is moral tension between the duty to act in the best interests of individual patients and the duty to improve surgical standards through exposing patients to the unknown risks that any form of research inevitably entails.

The willingness to expose patients to such risks may be further increased by the professional and academic pressures on many surgeons to maintain a high research profile in their work. For this reason, surgeons (and physicians, who face the same dilemmas) now accept that their research must be externally regulated to ensure that patients give their informed consent, that any known risks to patients are far outweighed by the potential benefits, and that other forms of protection for the patient are in place (e.g. proper indemnity) in case they are unexpectedly harmed. The administration of such regulation is through research ethics committees, and surgeons should not participate in research that has not been approved by such bodies. Equally, special provisions will apply to research involving incompetent patients who cannot provide consent to participate, and research ethics committees will evaluate specific proposals with great care.

In practice, it is not always clear as to what constitutes 'research' that should be subjected to regulation, as compared with a minor innovation dictated by the contingencies of a particular clinical situation. Surgeons must always ask themselves in such circumstances whether or not the innovation in question falls within the boundaries of standard procedures in which they are trained. If so, what may be a new technique for them will count not as research but as an incremental improvement in personal practice. Nevertheless, major innovations in operative procedure are scrutinised by national regulatory authorities; in the UK by the National Institute for Health and Care Excellence. This process of scrutiny has been designed to ensure that the innovation is safe, efficacous and cost effective. It is regarded (by the NHS) as a mandatory step when introducing a new interventional procedure.

Equally, surgeons know that exigencies of operative surgery sometimes demand a novel and hitherto undecsribed manoeuvre to get the surgeon (and the patient) out of trouble. Providing your solution is necessary, proportionate to the circumstances, performed in good faith and would pass the scrutiny of your peers as reasonable, it is unlikely that any subsequent criticism of your actions could be sustained.

If a proposed innovation passes the criteria for research, it should be approved by a research ethics committee. Such surgical research should also be subject to a clinical trial designed to ensure that findings about outcomes are systematically compared with the best available treatment and that favourable results are not the result of arbitrary factors (e.g. unusual surgical skill among researchers) that cannot be replicated.

MAINTAINING STANDARDS OF EXCELLENCE

To optimise success in protecting life and health to an acceptable standard, surgeons must only offer specialised treatment in which they have been properly trained. To do so will entail sustained further education throughout a surgeon's career in the wake of new surgical procedures. While training, surgery should be practised only under appropriate supervision by someone who has appropriate levels of skill. Such skill can be demonstrated only through appropriate clinical audit, to which all surgeons should regularly submit their results. When these reveal unacceptable levels of success, no further surgical work of that kind should continue unless further training is undergone under the supervision of someone whose success rates are satisfactory. To do otherwise would be to place the interest of the surgeon above that of their patient, an imbalance that is never morally or professionally appropriate.

Surgeons also have a duty to monitor the performance of their colleagues. To know that a fellow surgeon is exposing patients to unacceptable levels of potential harm and to do nothing about it is to incur some responsibility for such harm when it occurs. Surgical teams and the institutions in which they function should have clear protocols for exposing unacceptable professional performance and helping colleagues to understand the danger to which they may expose patients. If necessary, offending surgeons must be stopped from practising until they can undergo further appropriate training and counselling. Too often, such danger has had to be reported by individuals whose anxieties have not been properly heeded and who have then been professionally pilloried rather than acknowleged for their contribution to patient safety. Those who participate in closing ranks, and ostracism, share the moral responsibility for any resulting harm to patients. If something goes wrong with surgical treatment, the UK health regulators unanimously insist that the patient should be told what has happened; in many senses, a similar disclosure to that which occurred during the consent process, but now with the benefit of hindsight. Again, this candid disclosure is designed to put the patient in the same position as the surgeon, with respect to information about their health.[5]

CONCLUSION

Surgeons have combined duties to their patients; to protect life and health and to respect autonomy, both to an acceptable professional standard. The specific duties of surgeons are shown to follow from these: reasonable practice concerning informed consent; confidentiality; decisions not to provide, or to omit, life-sustaining care; surgical research; and the maintenance of good professional standards. The final duty of surgical care is to exercise all these general and specific responsibilities with fairness and justice, and without arbitrary prejudice. Now, at least partly either enshrined in statute or echoed in the English common law, these duties closely reflect the guidance of the General Medical Council.

The conduct of ethical surgery illustrates good citizenship: protecting the vulnerable and respecting human dignity; and equality. To the extent that the practice of individual surgeons is a reflection of such sustained conduct, they deserve the civil respect that they often receive. To the extent that it is not, they should not practise the honourable profession of surgery.

REFERENCES

1 Kings College Hospital v C & V [2015] EWCOP 80
2 Montgomery (Appellant) v Lanarkshire Health Board (Respondent)(Scotland) [2015] UKSC 11
3 Wheeler RA. Tangible Sentiments. Bulletin RCSE, 2016 January 98 44
4 Regina (Tracey) v Cambridge University Hospital NHS Foundation Trust and another [2014] EWCA Civ 822
5 http://www.uhs.nhs.uk/HealthProfessionals/Clinical-law-updates/Clinicallawupdates.aspx

FURTHER READING

Beauchamp T, Childress J. *Principles of biomedical ethics*. London; Oxford University Press, 2001.

British Medical Association. *Medical ethics today*, 2nd edn. London; BMJ Books, 2004.

Department of Constitutional Affairs. *Mental Capacity Act 2005 Code of Practice*. London; The Stationery Office, 2007.

Department of Health. *Reference guide to consent for examination or treatment*, 2nd edn. London; Department of Health, 2009.

Department of Health. *Confidentiality: NHS Code of Practice. Supplementary guidance: public interest disclosures*. London; Department of Health, 2010.

General Medical Council. *Seeking patients' consent: the ethical considerations*. London; General Medical Council, 1998.

General Medical Council. *Withholding and withdrawing life prolonging treatments: good practice in decision making*. London; General Medical Council, 2002.

General Medical Council. *Confidentiality: protecting and providing information*. Available from http://gmc-uk.org/guidance/current/library/confidentiality.asp

General Medical Council. *Good medical practice*. London; General Medical Council, 2006.

General Medical Council. *0–18 years: guidance for all doctors*. London; General Medical Council, 2007.

General Medical Council. *Confidentiality*. London; General Medical Council, 2009.

Mason JK, Laurie GT. *Mason and McCall Smith's law and medical ethics*, 8th edn, Oxford; Oxford University Press, 2011.

McCullough LB, Jones JW, Brody BA (eds). *Surgical ethics*. New York; Oxford University Press, 1998.

Nair, R, Holroyd DJ (eds). *Oxford handbook of surgical consent*. Oxford; Oxford University Press, 2012.

Royal College of Surgeons. *Good surgical practice*. London; Royal College of Surgeons, 2002.

Senate of Surgery of Great Britain and Ireland. *The surgeon's duty of care: guidance for surgeons on ethical and legal issues*. London; Royal College of Surgeons, 1997.

Wheeler RA. Gillick or Fraser? A plea for consistency over competence in children. *Br Med J* 2006; **332**: 807.

Wheeler RA. Presumed or implied; it's not consent. *Clin Risk* 2010; **16**: 1–2

Woodcock T. Surgical research in the United Kingdom. *Ann R Coll Surg Engl* 2009; **91**: 188–191.

Woodcock T. Law and medical ethics in organ transplantation surgery. *Ann R Coll Surg Engl* 2010; **92**: 282–285.

Chapter 13

Human factors, patient safety and quality improvement

Learning objectives

To learn:

- The reasons why contemporary healthcare, despite all its advances, is often less than satisfactory
- The importance of understanding human behaviour if patient care is to improve
- 'Human factors', what they are, and their importance in understanding and rectifying error and working together as teams
- The importance of patient safety and the scale of the problem
- Medical error and its definitions including adverse events and near misses
- Patient safety strategies and solutions
- Applying the science of patient safety into clinical practice
- Patient safety as it relates to the surgeon
- Quality improvement as an overarching activity designed to address gaps in the quality of healthcare delivery
- The different kinds of quality measures
- The patient's surgical journey and its potential for inefficiency and waste
- Some of the methodologies, tools and skills needed for quality improvement
- The need for system thinking and leadership
- The importance of quality improvement, its place in education and as a strategy to address significant healthcare challenges

INTRODUCTION

During the last century improving public health is credited with adding 25 years to the average life expectancy of populations in resource-rich countries. Contributing achievements include immunisation, motor vehicle safety, workplace safety, control of infectious disease, declines in deaths from heart disease and stroke, safer and healthier foods, healthier mothers and babies, family planning and the recognition of tobacco as a health hazard. At the same time the array of surgical, medical, diagnostic and remedial possibilities that can be offered to patients is well illustrated in the chapters of this book with many of the newer innovations developed, not just in the last century, but in the last 20–30 years. This has, in turn, led to greater specialisation. A combination of these three factors presents today's healthcare with two big challenges: greater demand due to greater volumes of patients who are older and have more chronic diseases often requiring multidisciplinary care; and an increasing volume of treatment options often of increasing complexity and cost.

However, the acquisition of newly learnt abilities to manage and treat all these patients and conditions does not mean that these tasks are performed well. Added to this, financial outlay on healthcare is struggling to meet the supply of healthcare providers and this leaves the long-term implications for the quality of patient care uncertain. According to the Institute of Medicine (IoM), patients do not always receive the most suitable care, at the best time or in the best place. Its influential report, '*Crossing the Quality Chasm: A New Health System for the 21st Century*', emphasised the need to redesign healthcare processes and systems in response to this quality gap. It called on providers to ensure more efficient, safe, timely, effective, patient-centred and equitable care.

HUMAN FACTORS

Healthcare largely depends on direct human interventions. It has many goals, which span from preserving life and relieving distress to a wide range of more mundane services all of which society demands must be performed safely and efficiently and achieve broad-based user satisfaction. It is arguably more complex than any other broadly equivalent industry, and because it is extremely resource sensitive, it critically requires a strong evidence base. Even then the return on investment is often difficult to measure. As patient safety and quality improvement are dependent on human behaviour, as well as the systems and processes designed by health care workers, any discussion on these issues is helped by first addressing those 'human factors'.

Human factors (HF) is the study of the interrelationship between humans, the tools they work with and the environment in which they work. A greater understanding of these relationships in healthcare should enhance performance through a better understanding of the effects of teamwork, tasks, equipment, workspace, culture and organisation on human behaviour in clinical settings The SHELL model was designed to help understand these relationships (**Figure 13.1**).

The SHELL concept is named after the initial letters of its components – **S**oftware, **H**ardware, **E**nvironment and two **L**ivewares. In the centre of the model is the human operator, or the first Liveware, represented by 'L'. This may be any individual whose job is relevant to patient care. It is the most flexible component in the system but may be unpredictable due to individual factors such as personality, motivation, stress tolerance, skills, knowledge and attitudes. To overcome these intrinsic limitations the interface with the other components of the SHELL model must be adapted and matched to the Liveware component for optimum performance.

The first interface, Liveware–Hardware, has much to do with the ergonomic design of the tools and medical devices that are used and designed in such a way that they should, for example, make it difficult for the user to make a mistake.

The Liveware–Software interface encompasses the non-physical aspects of the system such as manuals, checklists and computer programs. An adequate Liveware–Software interface should produce a situation where procedural omissions are difficult to make.

The Liveware–Environment interface may include stressors in the physical environment that have to be coped with such as noise, poor acoustics and overcrowding.

The second Liveware–Liveware interface is the interface of interpersonal communication. It embraces concepts such as team coordination, conflict resolution and the continuity of information flow in the care of patients.

In the SHELL model diagram the edges of the blocks are uneven. This is to illustrate the fact that the interdependent components are constantly changing and will never match perfectly. HF are concerned with minimising the mismatch between the different components.

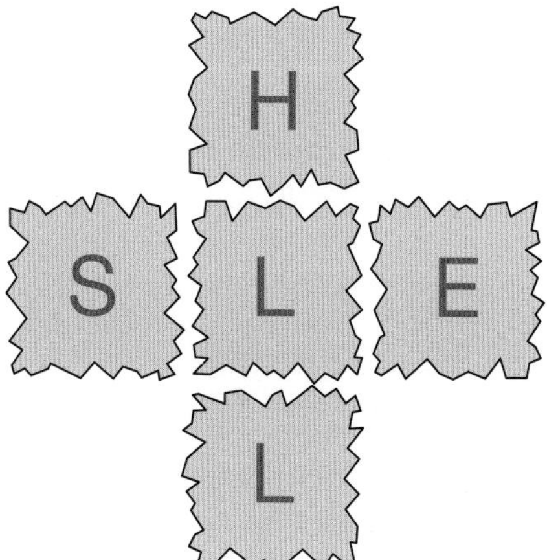

Figure 13.1 SHELL model.

HF was conceived in the 1940s in the aviation industry and is where its principles have been most successfully applied. HF training in healthcare enhances clinical performance through an understanding of the effects of teamwork, tasks, equipment, workspace, culture and organisation on human behaviour in clinical settings. An HF approach to patient safety differs from traditional safety training in that the focus is less with the technical knowledge and skills required to perform specific tasks, but rather with the cognitive and interpersonal skills needed to effectively manage a team-based, high-risk activity.

Crew Resource Management (CRM) training is another term used to describe HF training. In the CRM context, cognitive skills are the mental processes used for gaining and maintaining situational awareness, for solving problems and making decisions. Interpersonal skills are the communications and behavioural activities associated with teamwork. CRM training develops effective communication skills and a cohesive environment among team members, and builds an atmosphere in which all personnel feel empowered to speak up when they suspect a problem. Team members are trained to cross-check each other's actions, offer assistance when needed and address errors in a non-judgmental fashion. Debriefing and providing feedback are also components of CRM training. It also emphasises the role of fatigue, perceptual errors (such as misreading monitors or mishearing instructions) and the impact of management styles and organisational cultures.

It is now widely recognised that HF training, specialist HF groups and the integration of HF into systems, processes and incident investigation is extremely important for achieving the highest standards of patient safety. However, safety is just one aspect of a wider HF systems approach to equipment, task, environment and organisational design. HF training can also significantly contribute to the quality, accessibility and cost of healthcare services.

Summary box 13.1

Acknowledging the gap between medical progress and the delivery of quality patient care

- The need to recognise the things that are wrong
- Understanding that HF among care givers often provides both the causes and the potential solutions
- The different factors that impact on human behaviour can be identified
- Team working is a prerequisite of contemporary healthcare
- The place of CRM training

PATIENT SAFETY

Medicine will never be a risk-free enterprise. From the beginning of training, doctors are taught that errors are unacceptable and that the philosophy of *primum non nocere* (first, do no harm) should permeate all aspects of treatment. Yet, worldwide, despite all the improvements in treatment and investment in technologies, training and services, there remains the challenge of dealing with unsafe practices, incompetent healthcare professionals, poor governance of healthcare service delivery, errors in diagnosis and treatment and non-compliance with accepted standards.

When errors do occur there continue to be inadequate systems in place to ensure that all those affected are informed and cared for, and that there is a process of analysis and learning to uncover the cause and prevent recurrence of such events. Patient safety has become an established healthcare discipline in its own right thus formalising approaches to these inadequacies, directing research and offering solutions for the future.

THE PREVALENCE OF ADVERSE HEALTHCARE EVENTS

The aviation and nuclear industries have a much better safety record than healthcare. This became abundantly clear when, in 1999, the Institute of Medicine of the National Academy of Sciences released a report, *'To Err is Human: Building a Safer Health System'*, that drew widespread attention to the alarming statistics that there were between 44,000 and 98,000 preventable deaths annually due to medical error in American hospitals with some 7,000 preventable deaths related to medication errors alone. This experience has been found to be similar in other resource-rich countries and was emphasised by the Bristol Royal Infirmary Inquiry of 2001 into a series of unacceptable paediatric cardiac surgical deaths. The World Health Organization (WHO) estimates that, even in advanced hospital settings, one in ten patients receiving health care will suffer preventable harm.

The financial burden of unsafe care globally is also compelling, resulting as it does in prolonged hospitalisation, loss of income, disability and litigation costing many billions of dollars every year.

In the years since the Institute of Medicine report there have been many initiatives to improve patient safety. Some interventions have been shown to reduce errors but many have still not been rigorously evaluated. Overall, it remains doubtful whether efforts to reduce errors at national, regional and local levels have yet translated into significant improvements in the safe care of patients. The Francis report (2013) of the Mid Staffordshire NHS Foundation Trust Public Inquiry identified multiple problems relating to that institutions safety culture.

It has also been stated recently that if medical error was a disease it would rank as the third leading cause of death in the United States after heart disease and cancer, although this information is not currently captured or coded on death certificates. This has led to a call for human and system errors to become part of disease coding systems, such as the ICD system – the International Classification of Diseases coding system – that is used by 117 countries for patient administrative purposes.

COMMON CAUSES OF ADVERSE HEALTHCARE EVENTS

Most medical care entails some level of risk to the patient either from their underlying condition or its treatment which, of itself, may lead to recognised complications or side effects. These episodes are different from **patient safety incidents**, which have been described as preventable events or circumstances that could have, or did, result in unnecessary harm to the patient. This might be an adverse event, a near miss or a no-harm event (*Table 13.1*).

The most frequent contributing factors that lead to patient safety incidents are listed in *Table 13.2*. Of these, inadequate communication between healthcare staff, or between medical staff and their patients or family members, ranks highest in frequency.

TABLE 13.1 Patient safety incidents.

Definitions	
An adverse event	An incident that results in harm to the patient
A near miss	An incident that could have resulted in unwanted consequences but did not, either by chance or through a timely intervention preventing the event from reaching the patient
A no-harm event	An incident that occurs and reaches the patient but results in no injury to the patient. Harm is avoided by chance or due to mitigating circumstances

TABLE 13.2 Factors that contribute to patient safety incidents.

Human factors	Inadequate patient assessment; delays or errors in diagnosis
	Failure to use or interpret appropriate tests
	Error in performance of an operation, treatment or test
	Inadequate monitoring or follow-up of treatment
	Deficiencies in training or experience
	Fatigue, overwork, time pressures
	Personal or psychological factors (e.g. depression or drug abuse)
	Patient or working environment variation
	Lack of recognition of the dangers of medical errors
System failures	Poor communication between healthcare providers
	Inadequate staffing levels
	Disconnected reporting systems or over-reliance on automated systems
	Lack of coordination at handovers
	Drug similarities
	Environment design, infrastructure
	Equipment failure due to lack of parts or skilled operators
	Cost-cutting measures by hospitals
	Inadequate systems to report and review patient safety incidents
Medical complexity	Advanced and new technologies
	Potent drugs, their side effects and interactions
	Working environments – intensive care, operating theatres

UNDERSTANDING PATIENT SAFETY INCIDENTS

Understanding the concepts underlying patient safety incidents is useful because it helps to anticipate situations that are likely to lead to errors and highlights areas where preventative action can be taken. The problem of error can be viewed in two ways – from a person approach or from a system approach.

The person approach

Human performance principles tell us that humans are fallible and that errors can occur through doing the wrong thing – errors of commission; failure to act – errors of omission; or errors of execution – doing the right thing incorrectly. These principles also tell us that, by understanding the reasons why adverse events and near misses occur and by applying the lessons learnt from past events, future errors can be prevented. However, for most errors the person approach on its own tends to blame the individual and restricts learning.

The system approach

Health systems add complex organisational structures to human fallibility thus substantially increasing the potential for errors. A systems approach to error recognises that adverse events rarely have a single isolated cause and that they are best addressed by examining why the system failed rather than who made the mistake. James Reason, former Professor of Psychology at Manchester University, has stated that, "We cannot change the human condition but we can change the conditions under which people work so as to make error less provoking."

Heinrich's safety pyramid

Developed in 1931, Heinrich's safety pyramid (**Figure 13.2**) theorised that unsafe acts or near misses lead to minor injuries and, over time, to a major injury. The accident pyramid proposes that for every 300 near misses there are 29 minor injuries and one major injury. **Risk assessment**, which is a step in risk management that calculates the value of risk related to a situation or hazard, has shown us that what prevents patients from being hurt is not only by reducing the number of mistakes but rather by increasing the number of defences set up against the consequences of mistakes. The key message is that near misses provide the best data about the reliability of safety systems. It is, therefore, most important to report near misses as well as adverse events to ensure that defences against adverse events are built and sustained.

Swiss cheese model

Reason's theory of accident causation, often referred to as the Swiss Cheese Model (**Figure 13.3**), is as well known in the aviation and nuclear power industries as it is in healthcare. His model takes Heinrich's concept forward and proposes the notion of **active failures** – acts that are committed by those at the coal face such as slip-ups, lapses or mistakes – and **latent conditions** – created by decisions taken at a higher level within the organisation leading, for example, to staff shortages or time pressures

Reason hypothesised that all organisations operating in potentially harmful environments tend to build up defences against potential damage and that these defences can be broken down by active failures or latent conditions. Although latent conditions are not harmful in themselves, they lie dormant within the system before combining with active failures to bypass the defences.

The defences in this model are represented as slices of Swiss cheese. This is because, instead of being intact, they are, in reality, full of holes or defects that represent either active failures or latent conditions. In addition, these gaps in the defences may not be static but can open and close and change position over time. Danger arises when a set of holes line up for a brief window, allowing a potential hazard to become a fully blown accident. Each slice of cheese or defence is an opportunity to prevent an accident and the more slices there are and the fewer holes the less likely it is that an accident will occur or harm be done to a patient.

While healthcare workers are often at the sharp end of an error they are also often error catchers. It is the clinician's responsibility to observe, discuss and highlight latent conditions before adverse events occur and ensure the appropriate defences are in place.

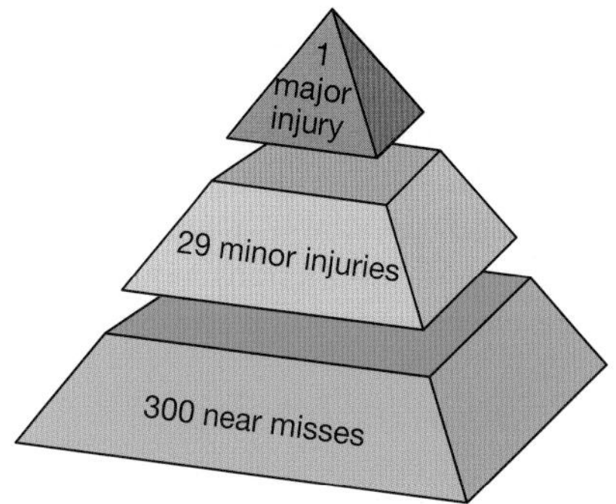

Figure 13.2 Heinrich's pyramid.

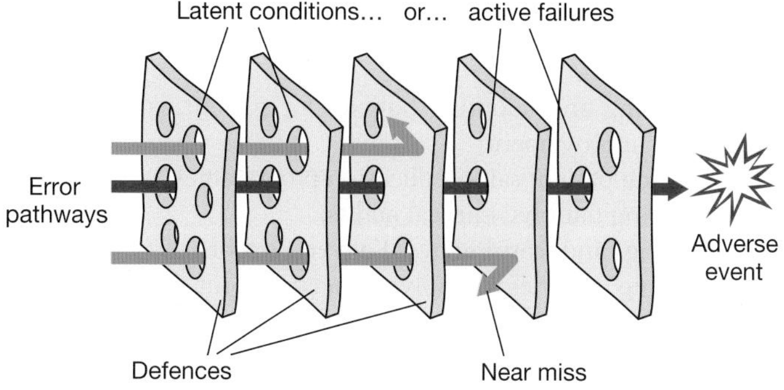

Figure 13.3 Reason's Swiss cheese model.

Herbert William Heinrich, 1886–1962, Assistant Superintendent, Engineering and Inspection Division of Travellers Insurance Co., Hartford, Connecticut, USA. He was a pioneer in industrial safety and developed his pyramid in 1931 when he published the book Industrial Accident Prevention: A Scientific Approach.
James T Reason, contemporary, Professor of Psychology, University of Manchester, proposed in 1990 'The Swiss Cheese Model of Accident Causation'.

Summary box 13.2

Understanding patient safety incidents

- Errors can be viewed from a person-centred or a system approach
- The majority of near misses or adverse events are due to system factors
- Understanding why these errors occur and applying the lessons learnt will prevent future injuries to patients
- It is important to report all near misses or adverse events so that we can constantly learn from mistakes
- Error models can help us understand the factors that cause near misses and adverse events and also direct us to where our defences against harm need to be improved

STRATEGIES FOR PATIENT SAFETY

International

Safety is everybody's business. Since the Institute of Medicine report the WHO has adopted a strong leadership role with many initiatives aimed at addressing safety challenges, notably '*WHO SAVE LIVES: Clean Your Hands campaign*' to ensure sustainable hand hygiene and which has now been adopted by almost 18,000 health facilities in 179 countries, and, '*WHO Guidelines for Safe Surgery 2009*' which includes the Surgical Safety Checklist aimed at decreasing the incidence of operative complications.

In low- and middle-income countries the WHO has also identified priority areas for patient safety such as the Pulse Oximetry Project set up to improve surgical safety and the Global Initiative for Emergency and Essential Surgical Care, a collaboration to reduce death and disability from injuries, pregnancy-related complications, congenital anomalies, disasters and other surgical conditions.

Resource-rich countries

Many governments and national organisations in such countries have developed important strategies aimed at delivering safety and quality in healthcare. These include:

- regulating and licensing of physicians and healthcare institutions;
- developing and adopting policies for patient safety and quality improvement;
- providing patient safety education programmes;
- instituting national clinical audits;
- reporting (and learning from) adverse events;
- setting up agencies to resolve concerns about the practice of doctors by providing case and incident management services.

Resource-poor countries

Resource-poor countries share many of the aspirations and challenges of richer countries. However, they also face issues that are different and require different strategies. The probability of a patient being harmed in hospital is higher with, for example, the risk of healthcare-associated infection being as much as 20 times higher than in richer countries. At least 50% of medical equipment in resource-poor countries is unusable or only partly usable and often the equipment is not used due to lack of parts or necessary skills. In some countries, the proportion of injections given with syringes or needles reused without sterilisation is as high as 70%. Each year, unsafe injections cause 1.3 million deaths, primarily due to transmission of hepatitis viruses and human immunodeficiency virus. Clearly these issues need to be met with a specific range of initiatives.

Institutional or hospital

Team working and training

In order to decrease errors and increase patient safety many medical team training programmes have now been developed internationally, often based on CRM or HF programmes. Some of these programmes are domain-specific (such as in anaesthesia), others are multidisciplinary (emergency department or operating room based), some rely on state-of-the-art simulators (critical care) and others rely primarily on classroom instruction.

Motivated and well prepared healthcare workers who are educated and trained to work together can reduce risks to patients, themselves and their colleagues, especially if they manage incidents positively and make the most of opportunities to learn from adverse events and near misses. Increasingly, healthcare institutions will have to provide this kind of educational support for their workforce.

Teams can work as **clinical microsystems**, which are quality improvement units that can be defined as a small group of people who work together, usually on a regular basis, to provide care. The individuals who receive that care can also be recognised as members of a discrete subpopulation of patients. Clinical microsystems have clinical and business aims, linked processes, a shared information environment and produce services and care that can be measured as performance outcomes. These systems evolve over time and are aimed to become embedded into the larger macrosystems or organisations. As with any living adaptive system, the microsystem must carry out the work, meet the staff needs and maintain its coherence as a clinical unit. Clinical microsystems can be assessed on their evidence base, leadership, patient and staff focus and information systems. In the delivery of healthcare, clinical microsystems invariably come into contact with other microsystems and interactions at their boundaries are common and should be understood and accommodated.

Using information technology

A major barrier to providing quality care to patients is the way health information is collected and stored in paper-based records, often in locations remote from where care is provided. Paper-based record systems are more susceptible to errors and permit fewer checks than electronic systems. There is now good evidence that the routine use of information and communication technology (ICT) will contribute greatly to the use of real time data to support clinical decisions, thereby supporting healthcare workers and patients to more easily access reliable health information and reduce medical errors. Good examples include electronic patient records and physician order entry systems for medication prescribing. However, there are drawbacks to the introduction of these systems including the high capital costs, underestimation of the change management and redesign of clinical processes required, and concern that systems will become obsolete.

Summary box 13.3

Strategies for patient safety

- The WHO has established a number of international initiatives for patient safety
- Various national approaches are being undertaken by countries
- In resource-poor countries patient safety issues are more acute, due to a lack of resource, and face different challenges
- Hospitals or institutions that will offer the greatest patient safety systems in the future will include those that foster team working, maximise the use of information technology and are prepared to realign their systems and processes

PATIENT SAFETY AT THE COAL FACE

Communicating openly with patients and their carers and obtaining consent

A patient-centred approach by medical staff, with involvement of patients and their carers as partners, is now recognised as being of fundamental importance. There are better treatment outcomes and fewer errors when there is good communication while poor communication is a common reason for patients taking legal actions.

Involving patients in and respecting their right to make decisions about their care and treatment is crucial. Explaining risk is a difficult but important part of good communication. It requires skill to explain the potential for harm of a procedure so that it is fully understood because patients vary in their perception and understanding and it is often difficult to assess the trade-offs between harm and benefit.

Obtaining consent for surgery requires that surgeons provide information to help patients to understand the positives and negatives of their various treatment options (*Table 13.3*). If only for the purposes of defending claims, hospitals invariably make signed consent mandatory. However, patients should be allowed to make these informed decisions without coercion or manipulation. Consent should be obtained by someone who is capable of performing the surgery and this should be taken when the patient is fully aware, especially in the non-urgent situation, well before the surgical procedure (see also Chapter 12, Surgical ethics and law).

TABLE 13.3 Information to be provided when seeking consent for surgery.

Details and uncertainties of the diagnosis
The purpose and details of the proposed surgery
Known possible side effects and potential complications
The likely prognosis
Other options for treatment, including the option not to treat
Explanation of the likely benefits and probabilities of success for each option
The name of the doctor who will have overall responsibility
A reminder that the patient can change his or her mind at any time

Communicating honestly with patients after an adverse event, or **open disclosure**, includes a full explanation of what happened, the potential consequences and what will be done to fix the problem. Safe care also involves taking care of the patient after the event, ensuring that the problem does not happen again and sincerely offering regret or an apology, as appropriate. As a consequence of the Francis Report there is now a statutory duty of candour on all healthcare providers who work within the National Health Service.

Professional behaviour and maintaining fitness to practice

Professionalism is an important component of patient safety. This embraces those attitudes and behaviours that serve the patient's best interests above and beyond other considerations. Organisations responsible for maintaining ethical standards include professionalism as one of those standards by which healthcare workers are judged.

Fitness to work or practice – **competence** – refers not just to knowledge and skills but also to the attitudes required to be able to carry out one's duties. Monitoring their own fitness for work is a responsibility of each individual and also their employers and professional organisations. Healthcare workers are now required to have transparent systems in place to identify, monitor and assist them to maintain their competence. **Credentialing** is one way that is used to ensure that clinicians are adequately prepared to safely treat patients with particular problems or to undertake defined procedures.

Reporting adverse events and near misses

Adverse events and near misses go unreported for many reasons including a fear of blame and the potential for litigation. **Clinical risk management** is a specific task, based on risk identification, analysis and control of events, carried out within a 'blame-free' environment. Data collected from these episodes should be collated and learnt both institutionally and by uploading to a national database. Doctors should be familiar with the systems that operate within their own working environment.

Complaints from a patient or carer often highlight a problem that, when analysed, provides opportunities for reducing adverse events and near misses. Poor communication is often the cause and knowing how to manage complaints is an important part of providing better health care. There is wide acceptance for the need for complaints to be made easily and effectively, such that now, more and more **patient advocacy** units provide a range of options for resolving complaints including the provision of information, mediation and the setting up of conciliation meetings between the parties.

Staff communication, understanding the work environment and working well within it

Nowhere is team working more important than in managing the flow of information within healthcare. Poor communication can lead to misinformation to patients and staff, delays in diagnosis, treatment and discharge as well as in failures to follow up on test results. On the other hand, good team work, good communication and continuity of care reduce errors and improve patient care and staff satisfaction within a team.

Stress, tiredness and mental fatigue in the workplace are significant occupational health and safety risks in healthcare. There is good evidence linking tiredness with medical errors. Fatigue can also affect wellbeing by causing depression, anxiety and confusion, all of which negatively impact on clinician performance. Organisations and individuals each bear the responsibility for managing working environments and practices so as to reduce fatigue and stress. This is reflected in the legal restriction of working hours that is now adopted in many countries.

Prescribing safely

Prescribing medication is common to almost all strands of medical practice and patients are vulnerable to mistakes being made in any one of the many steps involved in the ordering, dispensing and administration of medications. Accuracy requires that all steps are correctly executed. Unfortunately, medication errors are common and their many causes include:

- poor assessment or inadequate knowledge of patients and their clinical conditions;
- inadequate knowledge of the medications;
- dosage calculation errors;
- illegible hand writing;
- confusion regarding the name or the mixing up medications.

Summary box 13.4

Patient safety at the coal face

- Communicating well with patients and their carers
- Professionalism, as another essential component of patient safety
- Clinical risk management and patient advocacy and their roles in adverse events and patient complaints
- Team working and information flow as well as managing the work environment
- Recognising the pitfalls to safe prescribing

PATIENT SAFETY AND THE SURGEON

Surgery is one of the most intrusive healthcare interventions that can be visited on patients. More than 100 million people worldwide require surgical treatment every year for different reasons. Problems associated with surgical safety in resource-rich countries account for half of the avoidable adverse events that result in death or disability.

The 'more than one cause' theory of accident causation can be aptly applied to many aspects of surgical patient care during the perioperative period. Cuschieri and others have described **coal-face errors** as those that can potentially be committed by surgeons during the care of their patients and include:

- diagnostic and management errors;
- resuscitation errors,
- prophylaxis errors;
- prescription/parenteral administration errors;
- situation awareness, identification and teamwork errors;
- technical and operative errors.

Situation awareness - identifying teamwork errors

Operating rooms have been described as "among the most complex political, social and cultural structures that exist, full of ritual, drama, hierarchy and too often conflict". In such an environment, systems should seek to prevent error by improving workplace preparedness and by incorporating defences so as to reduce human error or minimise its consequence. Well recognised and potential errors include:

- the wrong patient in the operating room;
- surgery performed on the wrong side or site;
- the wrong procedure performed;
- failure to communicate changes in the patient's condition;
- disagreements about proceeding;
- retained instruments or swabs (**Figure 13.4**).

All these events are catastrophic for the patient and almost invariably occur through a lack of communication (see Never events below). This means that all theatre staff should follow protocols and be familiar with the underlying principles supporting a uniform approach to caring for patients.

Checklists

Checklists in the operating theatre environment are now accepted as standard safety protocols since the '*Safe Surgery Saves Lives*' Study Group at the WHO published their results. The use of a perioperative surgical safety checklist in eight hospitals around the world was associated with a reduction in perioperative mortality from 1.5% to 0.7% and major inpatient complications from 11.0% before, to 7.0% after, the introduction of the checklist. A more recent study from two hospitals in Norway (2015) showed a decrease in complications from 19.9% to 11.5%, a fall in mean length of stay of 2 days and a significant fall in hospital mortality from 1.9% to 0.2% in one hospital.

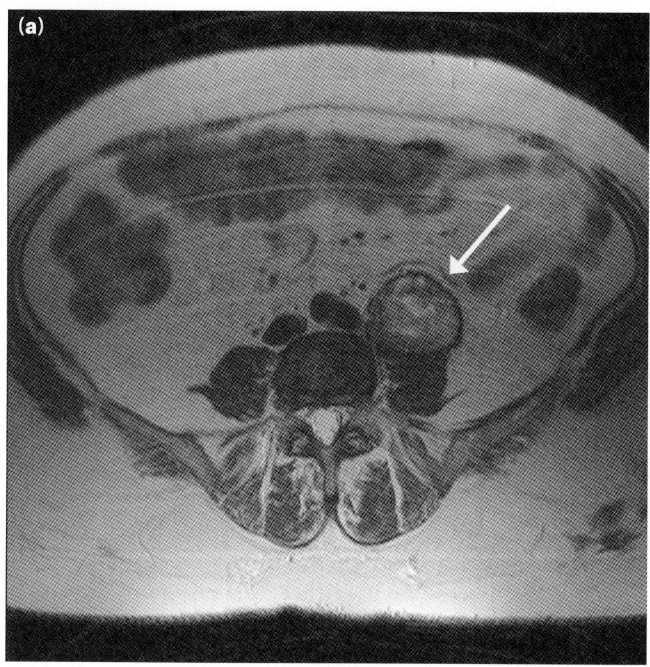

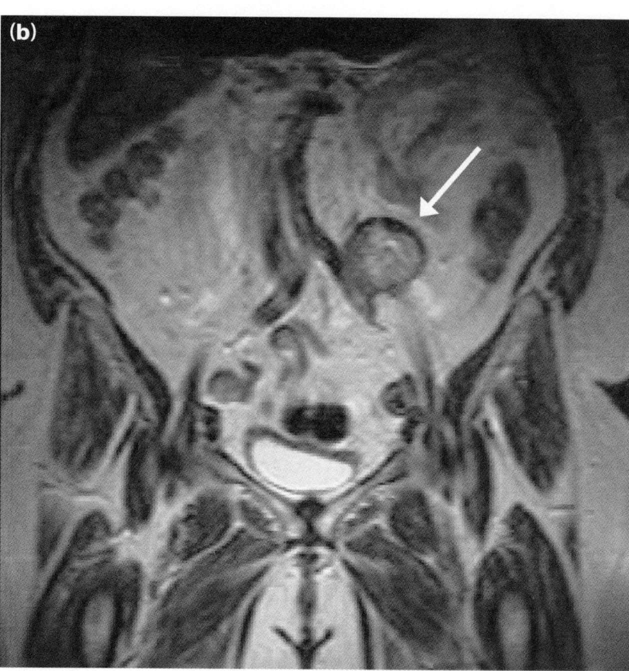

Figure 13.4 Axial (**a**) and coronal (**b**) magnetic resonance images demonstrating a well-defined abdominal mass with whorled stripes in a fluid filled central cavity (arrows). This 60-year-old lady had had an abdominal hysterectomy 10 years previously and presented with pyrexia and flank pain. The cause was due to the late presentation of a retained surgical swab.

The surgical safety checklist identifies specific checks to be carried out at three obligatory time points (Figure 13.5). The checklist items are not intended to be comprehensive and additions and modifications are encouraged.

The benefits of standardisation of surgical processes need not be limited to the operating room. Several studies have shown that the majority of surgical errors (53–70%) occur outside the operating room, before or after surgery, and that a more substantial improvement in safety can be achieved by targeting the entire surgical pathway.

There is no question that checklists are tools that improve outcomes provided they are correctly implemented. However, there are some important considerations. Checklists are suited to solving specific kinds of problems, but not others.

Before induction of anaesthesia

SIGN IN

☐ Patient has confirmed
- Identity
- Site
- Procedure
- Consent

☐ Site marked/not applicable

☐ Anaesthesia safety check completed

☐ Pulse oximeter on patient and fuctioning

Does patient have a:

Known allergy?
☐ No
☐ Yes

Difficult airway/aspiration risk?
☐ No
☐ Yes, and equipment/assistance available

Risk of >500 mL blood loss (7 mL/kg in children)?
☐ No
☐ Yes, and adequate intravenous access and fluids planned

Before skin incision

TIME OUT

☐ Confirm all team members have introduced themselves by name and role

☐ Surgeon, anaesthesia professional and nurse verbally confirm
- Patient
- Site
- Procedure

Anticipated critical events

☐ **Surgeon reviews:** what are the critical or unexpected steps, operative duration, anticipated blood loss?

☐ **Anaesthesia team reviews:** are there any patient-specific concerns?

☐ **Nursing team reviews:** has sterility (including indicator results) been confirmed? are there equipment issues or any concerns?

Has antibiotic prophylaxis been given within the last 60 minutes?
☐ Yes
☐ Not applicable

Is essential imaging displayed?
☐ Yes
☐ Not applicable

Before patient leaves operating room

SIGN OUT

Nurse verbally confirms with the team:

☐ The name of the procedure recorded

☐ That instrument, sponge and needle counts are correct(or not applicable)

☐ How the specimen is labelled (including patient name)

☐ Whether there are any equipment problems to be addressed

☐ Surgeon, anaesthesia professional and nurse review the key concerns for recovery and management of this patient

Figure 13.5 World Health Organisation Surgical Safety Checklist (First Edition).

Even in comparison to aviation, managing patients involves an enormous amount of coordinated, time-pressured decision making and potential delays. Checklists are simple reminders of what to do, and unless they are coupled with attitude change and efforts to remove barriers to actually using them, they will have limited impact. Finally, if one begins to believe that safety is simple and that all it requires is a checklist, there is a danger of abandoning other important efforts to achieve safer, higher quality care.

Technical and operative errors

In surgery, the person rather than systems approach emphasises the accountability of the surgeon who, unlike colleagues in other medical disciplines, when operating, is an instrument of the treatment. During a surgical procedure, for example, there may be a specific action that, of itself, may be the error, such as the inadvertent cutting of the common bile duct during a cholecystectomy (**Figure 13.6**). The practical value of this kind of interpretation is that, provided latent conditions are excluded, it gives a sense of responsibility to the surgeon and it may also help to point to the most effective pathway for remediation, by counselling or retraining, as against reassessing the system and putting in place further safeguards.

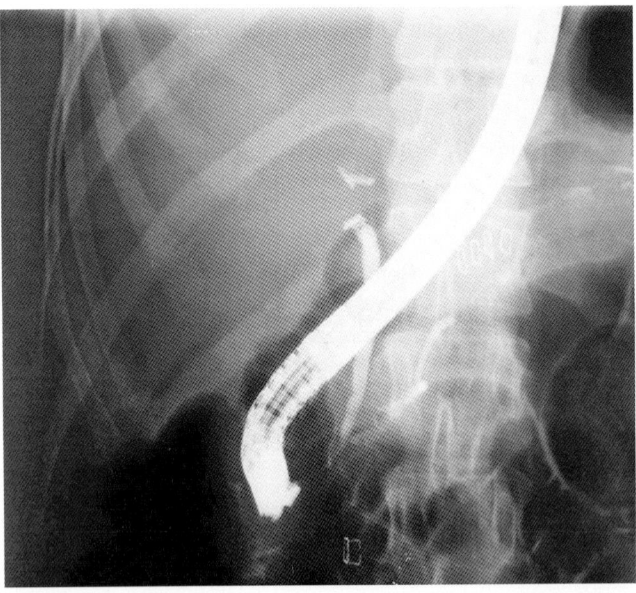

Figure 13.6 Radiograph showing an iatrogenic bile duct injury.

Central to operative performance is proficiency, which is an acquired state, honed by sound teaching, practice and repetition, by which a surgeon consistently performs operations with good outcomes. In cognitive psychology, high surgical proficiency is a state of automatic unconscious processing, with the execution being effortless, intuitive and untiring, as opposed to non-proficient execution which is characterised by conscious control processing requiring constant attention and resulting in slow, deliberate execution and inducing fatigue. The transition from one state to the other is better known as the 'learning curve'. This should not carry negative connotations for trainee surgeons who might be at the conscious processing stage but still perform a perfectly good operation, although it might take longer and be more tiring.

Failures in operative technique include:

- cognitive errors of judgment, such as failure or late conversion of a difficult laparoscopic procedure into an open one;
- procedural, when the steps of an operation are not followed or omitted;
- executional, when, for example, too much force is used which may result in damage that may or may not have consequences;
- misinterpretation, which is unique to minimal access surgery and is a function of the misreading of a two dimensional image;
- misuse of instrumentation, such as with energised dissection modalities (e.g. diathermy);
- missed iatrogenic injury either at the time of surgery or diagnosed late.

Never events

Many national health services and institutions now require that all incidents are managed, reported and investigated. Incidents can be defined as events that could have or did result in unintended and/or unnecessary serious harm.

One subset of serious incidents is a Never or Serious Reportable Event. These events are wholly preventable; for example, a retained abdominal swab or instrument, where guidance providing strong systemic protective barriers should have been implemented, namely checklists. Each Never Event type has the potential to cause serious patient harm or death. However, serious harm or death is not required to have occurred for that incident to be categorised as a Never or Serious Reportable Event.

Newer concepts of approaches to safety

Safety I is the approach to patient safety that has been described so far. It is predicated on identifying errors after the event and aims to prevent them from occurring or recurring in the future. Because healthcare is much more complex than such a linear model suggests, it is felt that that there is a need to switch our efforts to enable getting things to go right more often – a concept called **Safety II**. This acknowledges that healthcare work is resilient and that everyday performance succeeds much more often than it fails. This is because clinicians constantly adjust what they do to match the conditions. Working flexibly, and actively trying to increase their capacity to deliver more care more effectively, is key to this new approach. At its heart, proactive safety management focuses on how everyday performance usually succeeds rather than why it occasionally fails, and actively strives to improve the former rather than simply preventing the latter.

Summary box 13.5

Patient safety and the surgeon and newer concepts on safety

- Errors that can be made by surgeons in their overall management of patients
- Errors that occur in the operating theatre and how they can be mitigated
- The role of checklists in patient safety
- Performance proficiency and understanding technical and operative failures
- Getting things right more often may be a better approach than identifying errors after the event

QUALITY IMPROVEMENT

Quality improvement (QI) comes into play when we need to design or redesign healthcare processes and systems in response to a quality gap in order to ensure more efficient, safe, timely, effective, patient-centred and equitable care. Although safety is just a single aspect, it is self-apparent that improving any one of these components will likely have a beneficial effect on the other. Cost is also an important adjunct to quality improvement. The concept of value – the quotient of what is delivered divided by the cost – is an increasingly important metric in healthcare.

The scope for QI is enormous and can range from redesigning how teams deliver care in clinical microsystems that make up healthcare organisations to large-scale reconfigurations of specialist services such as stroke care and cancer care. It may even extend to redesigning training, budgeting processes and information systems and it requires leadership and cultures that both understand and value quality improvement. Improvements come from the intentional actions of staff equipped with the skills and data needed to bring about changes in patient care either directly or indirectly, and they require substantial and sustained commitment of time and resource.

QUALITY MEASURES

Quality measures are tools that help us measure or quantify healthcare processes, outcomes, patient perceptions and organisational structures or systems that are associated with the ability to provide high-quality health care and/or that relate to one or more quality goals for healthcare. Measurement is important to determine whether changes that are believed to lead to improvements in quality do in fact result in improvements. Improvement efforts require different methods from those used in research, being concerned more with testing of how to introduce best practice rather than determining what that developing best practice should be.

Process measures reflect the procedures and practices implemented by staff in the planning prescribing, delivery and evaluation of care – these may be specific to a clinical process, a service or administrative process. An example of a clinical process might be the starting times of operating lists. Process improvement measures should be associated with better outcomes of care and, ideally, should be important from a patient's perspective – reducing delays in starting times in the example cited.

The patient's surgical journey is a composite of multiple processes. Measurement for improvement less commonly involves comparisons among sites and against thresholds but more commonly involves tracking processes and outcomes in the same site over time.

Outcome indicators are specific, observable and measurable changes that represent the achievement of an outcome of a quality improvement measure. **Clinical outcome measures** refer specifically to outcomes of healthcare interventions whether they are to do with diagnosis, treatment or that care received by service users. Ideally, they should be outcomes that are important to patients rather than to the health provider, and there should be evidence that they reflect the quality of the interventions and their effect. Outcome measures are what are commonly used in **clinical audit** when compared with evidenced-based standards of clinical care.

Patient perception and the principles of patient centred-care should be an important part of QI particularly in those areas that directly affect their care, such as:

- the speed of their access to reliable health advice;
- the effectiveness of their treatment delivered by trusted professionals;
- the continuity of their care and its smooth transitions;
- the involvement of, and support for, their family and carers;
- the availability of clear, comprehensible information and support for self-care;
- their involvement in decisions and the respect for their preferences;
- the emotional support, empathy and respect provided;
- the attention paid to their physical and environmental needs.

Organisational structure and systems refers to the availability of resources required to deliver care. These include the care environment and facilities, the available equipment and the organisation's documented policies, procedures, protocols and guidelines.

The consistent consensus view is that good-quality improvement or clinical audit has to have at least four essential stages of activity to be considered high quality:

- preparation and planning,
- measuring performance;
- implementing change;
- sustaining improvement (including reaudit).

The collection and interpretation of reliable data is of fundamental importance to any QI exercise (*Table 13.4*).

CLINICAL OUTCOMES AND AUDIT

Put simply, clinical audit is that part of clinical governance that finds out if healthcare is being provided in line with standards and it allows care providers and patients know how

TABLE 13.4 Three pioneers of quality improvement and their quotes on data.

William Edwards Denning (1900–1993)	American engineer, statistician, professor, author, lecturer and management consultant. Pioneered the PDSA (Plan, Do, Study, Act) cycle	"In God we trust, all others bring data."
Peter Ferdinand Drucker (1909–2005)	Austrian-born American management consultant and educator	"What gets measured gets improved."
Donald Berwick (Born 1946)	American paediatrician. Former President and Chief Executive Officer of the Institute of Health Care Improvement	Sequence of reactions that challenge data: "The data are wrong." "The data are right but it's not a problem." "The data are right; it is a problem but not my problem." "I accept the burden of improvement."

their service is doing and where there could be improvements. The aim is to allow quality improvement to take place where it will be most helpful and will improve outcomes for patients. Clinical audits can look at care nationwide or locally within hospitals and their departments, in GP practices or anywhere healthcare is provided.

Measuring clinical outcomes as part of the quality improvement cycle aims to:

- improve the quality of clinical care with shorter hospital stays, better outcomes and fewer complications, reduced readmissions and greater patient satisfaction;
- inform the development of national clinical audits, including driving participation, data completeness and accuracy;
- support shared decision making and empowerment of patients, including their treatment options and choice of provider;
- improve the oversight and management of clinicians, their teams and practises and thus reassuring patients that their clinical care is being actively monitored and improved;
- help medical specialty associations to become increasingly transparent and patient focused;
- support team and individual quality improvement including providing information for appraisal and revalidation;
- learn from, spread and celebrate best practice.

'Best practice' dictates that surgeons should not just be aware of their clinical activity and outcomes but also endeavour to benchmark their activity against national and international norms. (Surgical audit is further addressed in Chapter 11.)

There is limited evidence that audit as presently defined and used is meeting health policy makers' aspirations. The alternative, systems-based QI methods, discussed below, although they have produced many successful improvements within healthcare services, have still not yet been scientifically proven to be more impactful.

THE PROCESS OF SURGICAL CARE

The process of QI can perhaps be best illustrated by understanding and optimising the efficiency of the patient journey at each step across the healthcare domains from the patient's home and primary care through the hospital system and then back out into the community. For example, while many illnesses and injuries require hospitalisation, a QI exercise might be the introduction of an admission avoidance policy for selected, appropriate patients attending Emergency Departments who could be better managed at home or in the community, thus providing an overall benefit to those patients in terms of safety, economy and choice.

Patients attend surgeons in many different settings depending on whether they present **electively or urgently** (scheduled or unscheduled). An elective journey is usually predictable and starts out as a referral from primary care and commonly requires an outpatient visit and investigations. If a surgical procedure is required, then we recognise that it is best that the patient is fully assessed from a surgical and anaesthetic perspective prior to admission within a preadmission assessment clinic. Once assessed, the patient should be admitted as a day case, wherever possible, or on the day of surgery or as short a time as possible before surgery as an inpatient. Preoperative checking is followed by the theatre journey, which includes reception, anaesthesia, the surgery itself and recovery – each, in their own way, a series of complex interventions. Returning to the ward and recovery demands another set of skills, procedures and processes followed by a final 'discharge from hospital' process.

The urgent or unscheduled journey is different because it is unpredictable for any single individual, although patterns of presentation do emerge when managing large numbers. The patient commonly presents at the Emergency Department of a hospital either as a self-referral, primary care referral or by ambulance. The journey begins with triage by a team who assess the severity of the illness (using, for example, the Manchester scoring system) and then directing the patient to the appropriate area, which might include, for example, a resuscitation unit, a rapid assessment and treatment unit, an acute surgical assessment unit (or medical assessment for medical patients), a minor injuries unit or an ambulatory care unit. The objective is to be seen as soon as possible by a senior decision maker, so that the patient can be treated or discharged as expeditiously as possible or, if admission and surgery is required, then this too can be expedited. Thereafter the journey follows a similar course to that of an elective admission.

This simple outline of surgical patients' journeys serves to illustrate the very many individual steps or processes in that journey. The scope for errors, delays and inefficiencies from a patient's perspective is almost limitless. Instituting QI aims at their mitigation.

Good surgical practice has, for many years, dictated that surgeons should be aware of their clinical outcomes including their complications, re-admission rates and standardised mortality rates. It is now also incumbent on surgeons and their teams to measure the performance of their surgical processes against best practice. These include the average length of stay of their patients, their day case and day of admission rates, bed occupancy and, as activity-based funding becomes more prevalent, their consumption of institutional costs.

THE QUALITY IMPROVEMENT PATHWAY

QI can be applied to almost any step, process or activity. The Scottish Improvement Hub recommends seven stages that might be undertaken in a QI exercise:

- discovering – is about defining the aims and vision; for example, what the problem is and what data is available;
- exploring – is about defining the present state and visualising the future state;
- designing – is about defining how to move from the present state to the future state and identifying the priorities;
- refining – is about testing change, learning from the data and identifying the benefits;
- introducing – is about managing communications and building the will and culture to change;
- spreading – is about showing the improvements, telling the story and disseminating the message;
- closing – is about capturing and sustaining the learning.

Each step can then be accompanied by any number of established organisational and graphical tools and methodologies appropriate to the design and planning of each step and suitable for the QI improvement exercise being undertaken (*Table 13.5*).

Emergency departments, wards and operating theatres are fertile grounds for process and performance improvement. Bundled educational programmes, such as the Productive Series (for wards and theatres, for example) introduced by the former NHS Institute for Innovation and Improvement, supports teams to redesign and streamline the way they manage and work within specific areas.

TABLE 13.5 Examples of tools used in quality improvement.

Organisational	Graphical
Root cause analysis Benefits realisation planning Demand and capacity planning Process mapping Value stream mapping Kanban and 5 'S'	Driver diagrams Fishbone cause and effect diagrams Spaghetti diagrams Box, frequency and scatter plots Pareto and run charts

Lean

Arguably, the most successful example of system redesign in an industrial setting has been the Toyota Production System from which much of the thinking can be applied to healthcare. 'Kaizen' is the Japanese for improvement. At Toyota, production line personnel are expected to stop the production line when an abnormality is noticed and, along with their supervisor, initiate kaizen. A single cycle of kaizen activity is defined as 'plan, do, study and act', also known as the PDSA cycle. The same application can be used in healthcare, with many sequential cycles growing to 'continuous improvement'.

Lean manufacturing is a management philosophy that is also derived mostly from the Toyota Production System. Defining Lean is difficult; it is in essence the elimination of waste through continuous improvement. Identifying waste leads inevitably to the need to define customer value and reducing waste requires elimination of error. This approach has found widespread application in industry. In medical settings, there is extensive evidence of its benefits in improving efficiency, reducing costs and improving patient satisfaction.

Operating theatres provide a good example of how lean principles can be applied in healthcare. Lean states that, in manufacturing, there are broadly seven types of waste that need eliminating in order to improve productivity: the same could be applied to perioperative care. For example:

- *Overproduction*. Such as: ordering unnecessary preoperative tests. Solution: optimising evidence-based preassessment.
- *Inventory*. Such as: purchasing of excessive drug stock before it is required. Solution: alphabetically ordered drug cupboards with only 1–2 boxes of commonly used drugs.
- *Waiting*. Such as: surgeons waiting for a patient to come down to theatre and sitting in the coffee room doing nothing. Solution: improve communications and, maybe, engage more porters.
- *Waste of transportation*. Such as: wasting time transferring patients from the admitting ward to the theatre or vice versa. Solutions: better design of the theatre complex to optimise patient flow, simplifying mode of transport and better communications and handover.
- *Waste of overprocessing*. Such as: giving patients a nerve block, a spinal and a general anaesthetic for a joint replacement. Solution: general anaesthetic and local infiltration may be equivalent and quicker.
- *Defect*. Such as: patients arrive in theatre with incomplete or inappropriate preoperative paperwork. Solution: more robust checking systems before patients come to theatre.
- *Motion*. Such as: constant repetitive movement around theatre and the anaesthetic room to get drugs, equipment and disposal of waste. Solution: a 'motion efficient' theatre where everything is easily available with minimal movement, and similar layouts in multitheatre complexes.

Six sigma

Six sigma is another scientific business performance methodology that has been adopted for use in healthcare. The fundamental objective of the Six Sigma methodology is the implementation of a measurement-based strategy that focuses on process improvement and variation reduction. One of its sub-methodologies is DMAIC (**D**efine, **M**easure, **A**nalyse, **I**mprove, **C**ontrol), which is an improvement system for existing processes falling below specification and requiring incremental improvement.

Systems thinking and leadership

In a system as fraught with complexity as healthcare, 'systems' thinking allows the whole system to be viewed and the relationships of the parts rather than just the isolated parts. Healthcare is a shared resource with many interdependencies; for surgery these include anaesthesia and critical care and all those specialties we require to work with to manage comorbid patients.

If quality problems exist primarily because of system problems, solutions are more likely in those systems where relationships and integration are considered important, where emphasis is placed on communication, team building, conflict management, behavioural and skill competencies, process management, and education; many of the features discussed under HF. Systems frameworks should never be punitive. They should have leaders who are systems thinkers and foster a culture of continuous QI. Those leaders should be visible at the front line and be champions of a supportive practice environment.

Improvement in the quality of care does not occur by chance. Nor will a programme team, armed with just organisational and graphical tools succeed in producing sustainable change. The underlying, central and agreed principles must include the creation of value for the patient, a constancy of purpose and systems thinking. These should be enabled by the intentional actions of trained staff supported by humble leadership and respect for individuals. Such a culture adjustment also requires integrated and coherent strategies and a sustained commitment of time, patience and resources.

INVESTING IN QI AND ITS EDUCATION

Healthcare as a sector has been late in recognising the important contribution that the theory and practice of QI are able to make in delivering better value care. The experience of a relatively small number of healthcare organisations that have successfully done so, such as the Virginia Mason Medical Centre in Seattle, is a challenge to others to invest in acquiring the necessary skills and capabilities.

A recent report of the Academy of the Medical Royal Colleges of UK and Ireland (2016) has argued that QI should be at the heart of medical training and that there is a pressing need to develop QI learning across the continuum of medical education. Their report sets out to enable education bodies to embed QI education into their curricula while asserting that it is as important as learning anatomy, biochemistry and physiology and a skill as important as CPR.

Summary box 13.6

Understanding QI and its application in healthcare

- The definition of QI and its relationship to clinical audit
- The different kinds of quality measures
- The patient surgical journey and its potential for improvement
- Examples of QI pathways, organisational methodologies and tools
- What system thinking is and its importance alongside leadership
- The requirement for more education and training in QI

FURTHER READING

Academy of Medical Royal Colleges. *Quality improvement – training for better outcomes*. Key Findings, 2016. http://www.aomrc.org.uk/publications/reports-a-guidance

Ham C, Berwick D, Dixon J. *Improving quality in the English NHS – a strategy for action*. The Kings Fund, 2016. http://www.kingsfund.org.uk/publications/quality-improvement

Haugen AS, Softeland E, Almeland SK *et al*. Effect of the World Health Organization checklist on patient outcomes. *Ann Surg*, 2015; **261**: 821–8.

Institute of Medicine. *Crossing the quality chasm: a new health system for the 21st century*. Washington, DC: National Academies Press, 2001.

Kohn LT, Corrigan JM, Donaldson MS (eds). *To err is human – building a safer health system*. Washington, DC: National Academies Press, 2000: 312.

Langley GL, Moen R, Nolan KM, *et al*. *The improvement guide: a practical approach to enhancing organizational performance*, 2nd edn. San Francisco: Jossey-Bass Publishers, 2009.

Makary MA, Daniel M. Medical error – the third leading cause of death in the US. *BMJ* 2016; **353**: i2139.

Neily J, Mills PD, Young-Xu Y, *et al*. Association between implementation of a medical team training program and surgical mortality *JAMA*, 2010; **304**(15): 1693–1700.

NHS Scotland. *Quality improvement hub*. http://www.qihub.scot.nhs.uk/default.aspx

Timmons S, Baxendale B, Buttery A, *et al*. Implementing human factors in clinical practice. *Emerg Med J Online First*, 2014; **32**: 368–72.

PART 2

Investigation and diagnosis

14 Diagnostic imaging 190

15 Gastrointestinal endoscopy 216

16 Tissue and molecular diagnosis 234

Chapter 14

Diagnostic imaging

Learning objectives

To understand:

- The advantages of good working relationships and close collaboration with the imaging department in planning appropriate investigations
- The basic principles of radiation protection and know the law in relation to the use of ionising radiation
- The principles of different imaging techniques and their advantages and disadvantages in different clinical scenarios
- The role of imaging in directing treatment in various surgical scenarios

INTRODUCTION

Appropriate surgical management of the patient relies on correct diagnosis. While clinical symptoms and signs may provide a firm diagnosis in some cases, other conditions will require the use of supplementary investigations including imaging techniques. The number and scope of imaging techniques available to the surgeon have dramatically increased within a generation, from a time when radiographs alone were the mainstay of investigation. The development of ultrasound and colour Doppler, computed tomography (CT) and magnetic resonance imaging (MRI) has enabled the surgeon to make increasingly confident diagnoses and has reduced the need for diagnostic surgical techniques such as explorative laparotomy. Faced with such a plethora of imaging to choose from, it is important that the patient is not sent on a journey through multiple unnecessary examinations.

As a basic principle, the simplest, cheapest test should be chosen that it is hoped will answer the clinical question. This necessitates knowledge of the potential complications and diagnostic limitations of the various methods. For example, in a patient presenting with the clinical features of biliary colic, an ultrasound examination alone may give enough information to enable appropriate surgical management. In more complex cases, it may be more efficient to opt for a single, more expensive investigation, such as CT, rather than embarking on multiple simpler and cheaper investigations that may not yield the answer. The choice of technique is often dictated by equipment availability, expertise and cost, as well as the clinical presentation. However, it must be emphasised that, not infrequently, the most valuable investigation is prior imaging; this not only reduces the cost and the amount of radiation a patient receives but very often improves patient care.

HOW TO REQUEST IMAGING

Best practice depends on close collaboration between the radiologist and the referrer and must take into account local expertise and access to facilities. When requesting imaging, consider what it is that you want to know from the investigation. Give a provisional diagnosis or state the clinical problem. If there is uncertainty over the best method to answer the clinical problem, then discussion with a radiologist is always worthwhile, informally or within the context of a clinicoradiological meeting or a multidisciplinary team (MDT) meeting.

As well as the basic demographic information stored on the radiology information system (RIS), it is important to provide relevant past medical history, e.g. diabetes, epilepsy, renal failure, allergies and anticoagulation, all of which can affect which contrast agent can be given safely, and the date of the last menses in women of childbearing potential.

INTERPRETING IMAGES

While the role of the Imaging department is to provide radiological reports for imaging examinations performed, it is nevertheless good clinical practice to be able to evaluate your patients' examinations, and a systematic approach is encouraged.

The systematic approach to examining a radiograph varies according to the part of the body being imaged. For instance, for a radiograph of an extremity, the alignment, the cortices and the medullary cavity of the individual bones, the joints and the soft tissues all need to be assessed on each view.

Summary box 14.1

A simple system for checking radiographs

Label	Name of patient
Site	Date of examination
Side (check marker)	
	What part is the film centered on?
	Does the film cover the whole area required?
	Is there more than one view?
Quality	Is the penetration appropriate?
Compare	How have the appearances changed from previous images?
Conclude	Is the diagnosis clear?
	Is further imaging needed?

HAZARDS OF IMAGING

Contrast media

There has been a dramatic increase in the use of contrast agents in recent years, mainly related to the increasing use of CT. Potential problems include allergic reaction and nephrotoxicity. Reactions are rare: serious reactions occur in about 1:2500 cases and life- threatening reactions in about 1:25 000 cases. The risk of sudden death, however, has not changed with the new agents. Local policies for dealing with patients at increased risk vary between departments and, indeed, between countries. Advice from the Royal College of Radiologists (RCR) in the UK does not recommend routine steroid prophylaxis for patients at increased risk of allergic reaction, but rather the use of low osmolality contrast media(LOCM) or iso-osmolar media, and observation of the patient for 30 minutes after injection with the intravenous cannula still in situ, since most serious reactions occur shortly after injection. Guidelines from the European Society of Uroradiology (ESUR), however, continue to advocate the use of steroids.

In patients with diabetes or renal impairment, a recent creatinine level should be available. The radiologist should be informed of any history of renal impairment, as all contrast media are nephrotoxic in patients with impaired renal function. The risks and benefits of contrast administration need to be carefully assessed in these patients and, if contrast is given, the patient should be well hydrated and the lowest dose of a LOCM should be given. The British RCR does not recommend the routine use of *N*-acetylcysteine for renal protection.

Concerns about lactic acidosis in patients on metformin receiving contrast led to various recommendations for stopping the metformin. The latest RCR recommendations are that it can be continued in patients with normal renal function. If there is a raised creatinine or reduced estimated glomerular filtration rate (eGFR) below 60 then any decision to stop metformin should be made with the radiologist and the physician managing the patient's diabetes. Gadolinium-containing contrast agents are used in MRI examinations. Allergic reactions to these agents are very rare. However, they can be nephrotoxic in patients with renal failure. In addition, they are associated with a risk of nephrogenic systemic fibrosis (NSF), an extremely rare but serious life-threatening condition whereby connective tissue forms in the skin causing it to become coarse and hard. NSF may also affect other organs, including joints, muscle, liver and heart. High-risk gadolinium-containing contrast agents are contraindicated in severe renal failure, in neonates and in the perioperative period of liver transplantation, and are not recommended in pregnancy. However, lower-risk gadolinium preparations are available that may be used with caution.

Liver-specific contrast agents for MRI, selectively taken up by hepatocytes, are increasingly used to characterise liver lesions and in cancer staging.

HAZARDS OF IONISING RADIATION

The majority of ionising radiation comes from natural sources on the earth and cosmic rays, and this makes up the background radiation. However, medical exposure accounts for around 15% of the total received by humans. The effects of ionising radiation can be broadly divided into two groups. The first group comprises predictable, dose-dependent tissue effects and includes, for example, the development of cataracts in the lens of the eye. These effects are important for those chronically exposed to radiation, including those using image intensifiers regularly. The second group comprises the all-or-nothing effects such as the development of cancer (termed stochastic). These effects are not dose dependent, but increase in likelihood with increased radiation dose.

The risk of radiation-induced cancer for plain films of the chest or extremities is very small, of the order of 1:1 000000. However, that risk rises considerably for high-dose examinations such as CT of the abdomen or pelvis, where the estimated lifetime excess risk of cancer increases to the order of 1:1000. Use of CT has increased dramatically in the last 20 years, with a 12-fold increase in the UK, and it has been estimated that up to 30% of these examinations may be unnecessary. Obviously, the risk of such examinations has to be balanced against the benefit to the patient in terms of increased diagnostic yield, and must also be viewed in the context that the lifetime risk of cancer for people generally is about 1:3. Nevertheless, the increased risk is important since it is iatrogenic and applied to a large population. Therefore, techniques that do not use ionising radiation, such as ultrasound and MRI, should be carefully considered as alternatives, particularly in children and young people.

CURRENT LEGISLATION

In the UK, the Ionising Radiation (Medical Exposure) Regulations (IRMER) introduced in 2000, and amended in 2006, impose on the radiologist the duty to the patient to make sure that all studies involving radiation (plain radiographs, CT and nuclear medicine) are performed appropriately and to the highest standards. Inappropriate use of radiation is a criminal offence, so investigations involving radiation need careful consideration in order to prevent wasteful use of radiology.

Summary box 14.2

Wasteful use of radiology

Results unlikely to affect patient management	
Positive finding unlikely	Do I need it?
Anticipated finding probably irrelevant for management	
Investigating too often	
Before disease could be expected to have progressed or resolved	Do I need it now?
Repeating investigations done previously	
Other hospital (?)	
GP (?)	Has it been done already?
Failing to provide adequate information	
Therefore wrong test performed or essential view omitted	Have I explained the problem?
Requesting wrong investigation	
Discuss with radiologist	Is this the best test?
Over-investigating	Are too many investigations being performed?

After: IRefer gudelines, *Making the best use of radiology*, 7th edition. Royal College of Radiologists, 2012.

Summary box 14.3 gives a summary of the responsibilities of both the radiologist and the referrer.

The RCR produces an evidence-based guidance tool, called iRefer, which is widely available on line. *Table 14.1*, showing the radiation doses for common procedures, is taken from this publication, now in its seventh edition.

Summary box 14.3

Responsibilities

- Radiologists have a legal responsibility to keep imaging as safe as possible
- The referrer has a duty to balance risk against benefit
- The referrer must provide adequate clinical details to allow justification of the examination
- Avoid using portable (mobile) x-ray machines whenever practical
- Take all precautions when using an image intensifier
- The gonads, eyes and thyroid are especially vulnerable to radiation and should be protected

There are special considerations for portable and fluoroscopy units. The longer an operator keeps the fluoroscopy unit running, the higher the dose of radiation to all in the vicinity. Portable x-ray machines and fluoroscopic imaging equipment use much more radiation to achieve the same result. The staff, and patients in the next bed, are at risk

TABLE 14.1 Typical effective doses from diagnostic medical exposure in the 2000s.

Diagnostic procedure	Typical effective dose (mSv)	Equivalent no. of chest radiographs	Approximately equivalent period of natural background radiation[a]
Radiographic examinations			
Limbs and joints (except hip)	<0.01	<0.5	<1.5 days
Chest (single posteroanterior film)	0.02	1	3 days
Skull	0.07	3.5	11 days
Thoracic spine	0.7	35	4 months
Lumbar spine	1.3	65	7 months
Hip	0.3	15	7 weeks
Pelvis	0.7	35	4 months
Abdomen	1.0	50	6 months
Intravenous urography (IVU)	2.5	125	14 months
Barium swallow	1.5	75	8 months
Barium meal	3	150	16 months
Barium follow-through	3	150	16 months
Barium enema	7	350	3.2 years
CT head	2.3	115	1 year
CT chest	8	400	3.6 years
CT abdomen or pelvis	10	500	4.5 years
Radionuclide studies			
Lung ventilation (133Xe)	0.3	15	7 weeks
Lung perfusion (99mTc)	1	50	6 months
Kidney (99mTc)	1	50	6 months
Thyroid (99mTc)	1	50	6 months
Bone (99mTc)	4	200	1.8 years
Dynamic cardiac (99mTc)	6	300	2.7 years
PET head (18F-FDG)	5	250	2.3 years

[a]UK average background radiation = 2.2 mSv per year; regional averages range from 1.5 to 7.5 mSv.
18F-FDG, 18F-2-fluoro-2-deoxy-D-glucose; CT, computed tomography; ^{99m}Tc, ^{99m}technetium; PET, positron emission tomography. From *Making the Best Use of a Department of Clinical Radiology*, 7th edn. Royal College of Radiologists, 2012. By kind permission.

when portable equipment is used. The result is also of lower quality, so portable x-ray machines should not be used unless absolutely necessary.

When using the image intensifier, lead aprons, thyroid shields, lead glasses and radiation badges should always be worn. Pregnancy in the female patient or staff must be excluded.

DIAGNOSTIC IMAGING

Basic principles of imaging methods

Conventional radiography

Although it is over 120 years since the discovery of x-rays by Roentgen in 1895, conventional radiography continues to play a central role in the diagnostic pathway of many acute surgical problems and particularly in chest disease, trauma and orthopaedics.

X-rays emitted from an x-ray source are absorbed to varying degrees by different materials and tissues and therefore cause different degrees of blackening of radiographic film, resulting in a radiographic image. This differential absorption is dependent partly on the density and the atomic number of different substances. In general, higher-density tissues result in a greater reduction in the number of x-ray photons and reduce the amount of blackening caused by those photons. In terms of conventional radiographs, a large difference in tissue structure and density is required before an appreciable difference is manifested radiographically. The different densities visible consist of air, fat, soft tissue, bone and mineralisation, and metal. Different soft tissues cannot be reliably distinguished as, in broad terms, they possess similar quantities of water (**Figure 14.1**). Manipulation of x-ray systems and x-ray energies, as used in circumstances such as mammography, may allow better differentiation between some soft-tissue structures.

Despite this inherent lack of soft-tissue contrast, conventional radiography has many advantages. It is cheap, universally available, easily reproducible and comparable with prior examinations and, in many instances, has a relatively low dose of ionising radiation in contrast to more complex examinations. However, injudicious repeat radiography, particularly of the abdomen, pelvis and spine, can easily result in doses similar to CT.

The lack of soft-tissue contrast allows little assessment of the internal architecture of many abdominal organs. To obviate this problem, techniques employing the administration of contrast material combined with radiography have long been used. These techniques include intravenous urography and barium examinations (**Figure 14.2**). Intravenous urography involves a series of radiographs taken before and after contrast injection, but has been largely superseded by CT urography, which is more accurate in detecting and defining pathology (**Figure 14.3**).

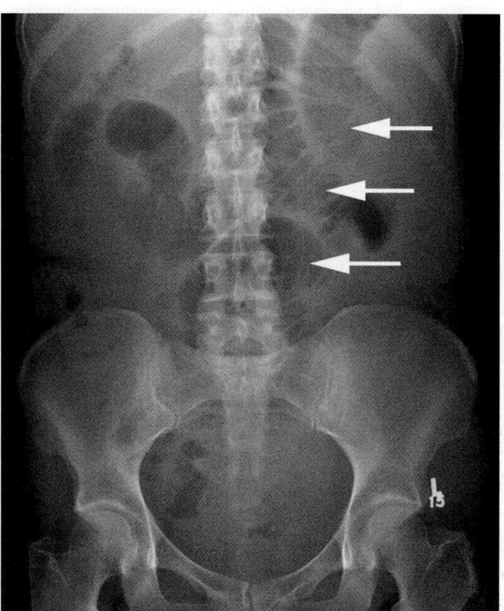

Figure 14.1 Supine abdominal radiograph of a patient with small bowel obstruction demonstrates multiple dilated small bowel loops (arrows). The different densities visible are air (within the bowel), bones, soft tissues and fat. The different soft tissues, subcutaneous and intra-abdominal, cannot be differentiated.

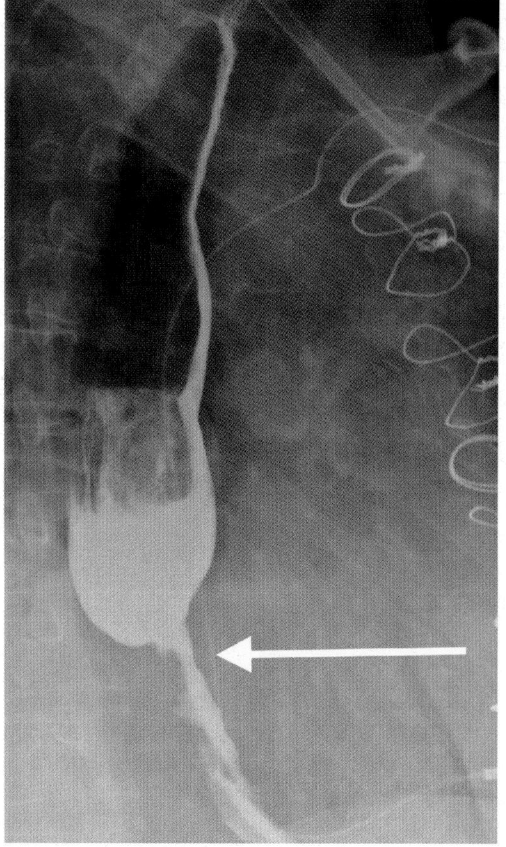

Figure 14.2 Barium swallow examination showing a malignant stricture (arrow) due to an oesophageal carcinoma.

Wilhelm Conrad Roentgen, 1845–1923, Professor of Physics, Wurtzburg (1888–1900), and then at Munich, Germany. He was awarded the Nobel Prize for Physics in 1901 for his work on x-rays.

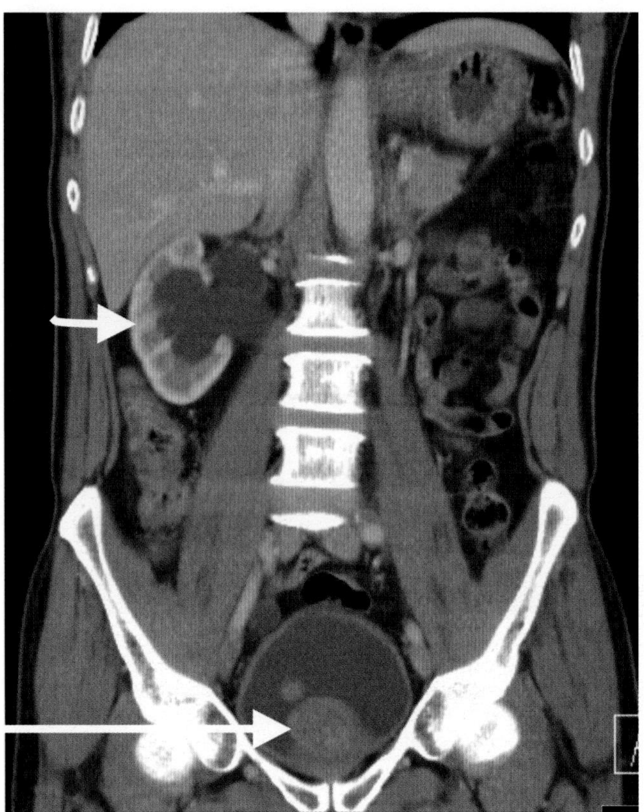

Figure 14.3 Coronal computed tomography intravenous urogram shows a transitional cell carcinoma in the bladder (long arrow) and right hydronephrosis (short arrow).

A further modification of conventional x-rays uses fluorescent screens to allow real-time monitoring of organs and structures as opposed to the 'snapshot' images obtained with radiographs. This is used to follow the passage of barium through the bowel, obtaining dedicated images at specific points of interest only. Motility of the bowel can also be assessed in this way. Fluoroscopy is used extensively in interventional radiology, allowing the operator to guide catheters and wires into the patient while monitoring their position in real time.

Naturally, with the more sustained use of ionising radiation, the cumulative doses tend to be greater than when obtaining a conventional radiograph.

Ultrasound

Ultrasound is the second most common method of imaging. It relies on high-frequency sound waves generated by a transducer containing piezoelectric material. The generated sound waves are reflected by tissue interfaces and, by ascertaining the time taken for a pulse to return and the direction of a pulse, it is possible to form an image. Medical ultrasound uses frequencies in the range 3–20 MHz. The higher the frequency of the ultrasound wave, the greater the resolution of the image, but the less depth of view from the skin. Consequently, abdominal imaging uses transducers with a frequency of 3–7 MHz, while higher-frequency transducers are used for superficial structures, such as musculoskeletal and breast ultrasound. Dedicated transducers have also been developed for endocavitary ultrasound, such as transvaginal scanning and transrectal ultrasound of the prostate, allowing high-frequency scanning of organs by reducing the distance between the probe and the organ of interest (**Figure 14.4**). A further application of dedicated probes has been in the field of endoscopic ultrasound, allowing exquisite imaging of the wall of a hollow viscus and the adjacent organs such as the biliary tree and pancreas.

Reflection of an ultrasound wave from moving objects such as red blood cells causes a change in the frequency of the ultrasound wave. By measuring this frequency change, it is possible to calculate the speed and direction of the movement. This principle forms the basis of Doppler ultrasound, whereby velocities within major vessels, as well as smaller vessels in organs such as the liver and the kidneys, can be measured. Doppler imaging is widely used in the assessment of arterial and venous disease, in which stenotic lesions cause an alteration in the normal velocity. Furthermore, diffuse parenchymal diseases, such as cirrhosis, may cause an alteration in the normal Doppler signal of the blood vessels of the affected organ.

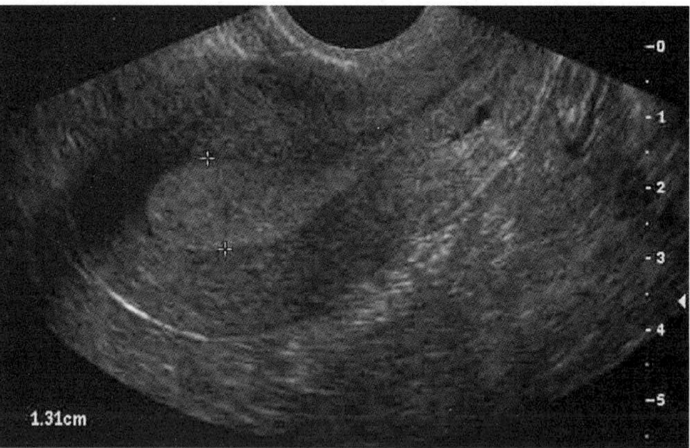

Figure 14.4 Longitudinal transvaginal ultrasound scan of the uterus demonstrates thickening of the endometrium in a patient during the secretory phase of the menstrual cycle.

The advantages of ultrasound are that it is cheap and easily available. It is the first-line investigation of choice for assessment of the liver, the biliary tree and the renal tract (**Figures 14.5 and 14.6**). Ultrasound is also the imaging method of choice in obstetric assessment and gynaecological disease. High-frequency transducers have made ultrasound the best imaging technique for the evaluation of thyroid and testicular disorders, in terms of both diffuse disease and focal mass lesions. It is also an invaluable tool for guiding needle placement in interventional procedures such as biopsies and drainages, allowing direct real-time visualisation of the needle during the procedure.

Christian Johann Doppler, 1803–1853, Professor of Experimental Physics, Vienna, Austria, enunciated the 'Doppler Principle' in 1842.

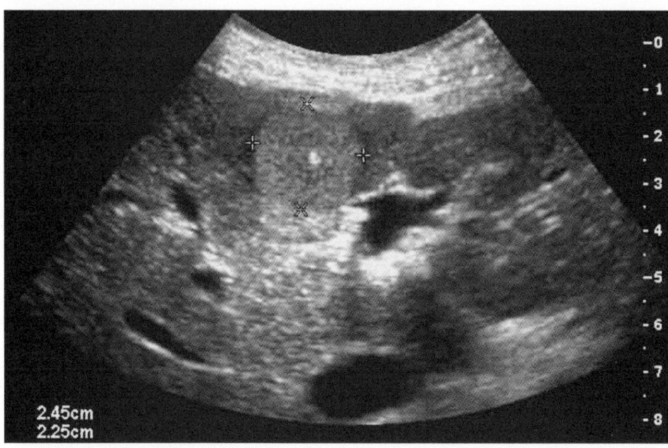

Figure 14.5 Transverse ultrasound image of the liver in a patient with colorectal cancer shows a solitary liver metastasis.

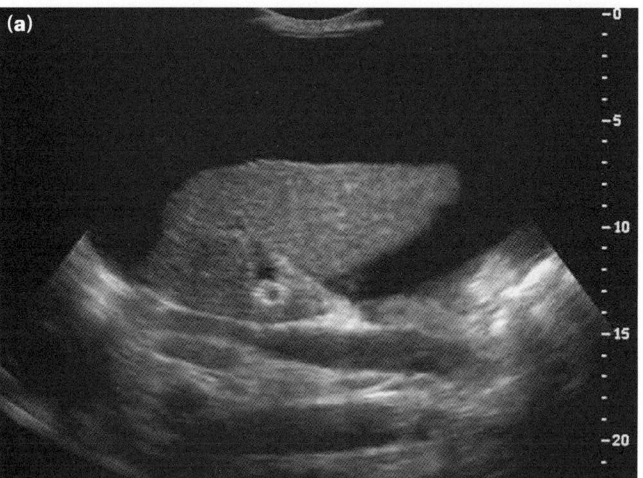

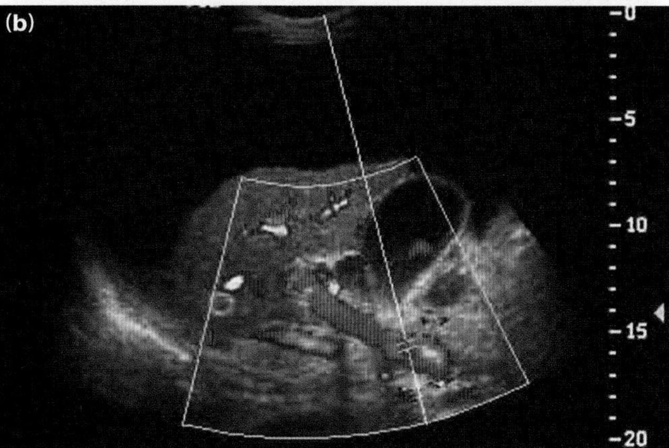

Figure 14.6 Sagittal ultrasound image of the liver (**a**) in a patient with cirrhosis demonstrates nodularity of the liver surface and extensive ascites. Doppler ultrasound (**b**) illustrates portal vein flow with a normal direction.

Ligament, tendon and muscle injuries are also probably best imaged in the first instance by ultrasound (**Figure 14.7**). The ability to stress ligaments and to allow tendons to move during the investigation gives an extra dimension, which greatly improves its diagnostic value. The use of 'panoramic' or 'extended field of view' ultrasound (**Figure 14.8**) provides

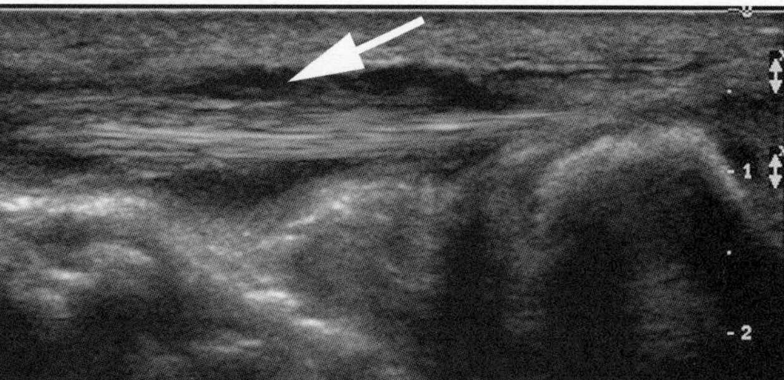

Figure 14.7 Ultrasound of the dorsal surface of the wrist shows the normal fibrillar pattern of the extensor tendons. There is increased fluid (arrow) within the tendon sheath in this patient with extensor tenosynovitis.

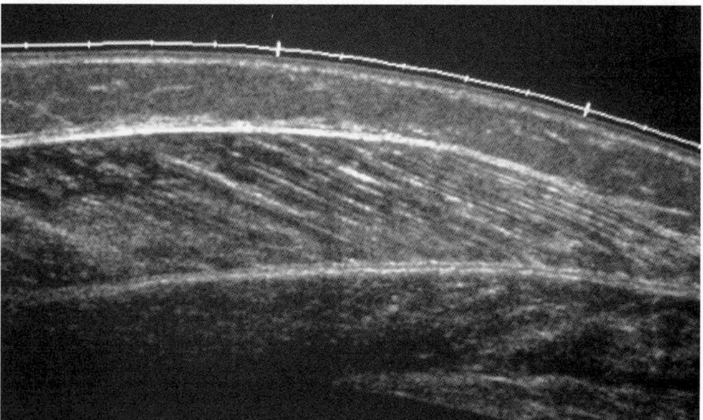

Figure 14.8 Panoramic ultrasound of the calf. The normal muscle fibres and the fascia can be identified over an area measuring approximately 12 cm.

images that are more easily interpreted by an observer not performing the examination, and are of particular assistance to surgeons planning a procedure. Ultrasound will demonstrate most foreign bodies in soft tissues, including those that are not radio-opaque.

The disadvantages of ultrasound are that it is highly operator dependent, and most of the information is gained during the actual process of scanning as opposed to reviewing the static images. Another drawback is that the ultrasound wave is highly attenuated by air and bone and, thus, little information is gained with regard to tissues beyond bony or air-filled structures; alternative techniques may be required to image these areas.

Computed tomography

There has been a great deal of development in CT technology over the last 30 years from the initial conventional CT scanners through to helical or spiral scanners and the current multidetector machines. CT scanners consist of a gantry containing the x-ray tube, filters and detectors, which revolve around the patient, acquiring information at different angles and projections. This information is then mathematically reconstructed to produce a two-dimensional grey-scale image of a slice through the body. This technique overcomes the problem of superimposition of different structures, which is inherent in conventional radiography. Improvements in

Summary box 14.4

Ultrasound

Strengths

- No radiation
- Inexpensive
- Allows interaction with patients
- Superb soft-tissue resolution in the near field
- Dynamic studies can be performed
- First-line investigation for hepatic, biliary and renal disease
- Endocavitary ultrasound for gynaecological and prostate disorders
- Excellent resolution for breast, thyroid and testis imaging
- Good for soft tissue, including tendons and ligaments
- Excellent for cysts and foreign bodies
- Doppler studies allow assessment of blood flow
- Good real-time imaging to guide interventional biopsies and drainages

Weaknesses

- Interpretation only possible during the examination
- Long learning curve for some areas of expertise
- Resolution dependent on the machine available
- Images cannot be reliably reviewed away from the patient

gantry design, advances in detector technology using more sensitive detectors and an increase in the number of detectors have resulted in an increase in spatial resolution, as well as the speed at which the images are acquired. In early CT scanners, the table on which the patient was positioned moved in between the gantry revolution to allow imaging of an adjacent slice. Modern scanners allow for continuous movement of the table and the patient during the gantry revolution, thus greatly reducing the scan time. With modern equipment, it is now not only possible to obtain images of the chest, abdomen and pelvis in under 20 seconds, but these axial images can be reformatted in multiple planes with practically no degradation in image quality.

In addition, CT has a far higher contrast resolution than plain radiographs, allowing the assessment of tissues with similar attenuation characteristics. As with radiographs, the natural contrast of tissues is further augmented by the use of intravenous contrast medium. Rapid scanning of a volume of tissue also allows the scans to be performed at different phases of enhancement, which is advantageous in identifying different diseases. For instance, very early scanning during the arterial phase is ideally suited to the examination of the arterial tree and hypervascular liver lesions, whereas scanning performed after a delay may be better suited to the identification of other solid organ pathology such as renal masses. Furthermore, it is possible to obtain scans during several phases including the arterial and venous phases in the same patient, which may aid in the identification and characterisation of lesions.

CT is widely used in thoracic, abdominal (**Figure 14.9**), neurological (**Figure 14.10**), musculoskeletal (**Figure 14.11**) and trauma imaging. The thinner collimation and improved spatial resolution have also resulted in the development of newer techniques such as CT angiography, virtual colonoscopy and virtual bronchoscopy. Furthermore, three-dimensional images can be reconstructed from the raw data to aid in surgical planning. The disadvantage of CT compared with ultrasound and conventional radiography lies largely in the increased costs and the far higher doses of ionising radiation. For instance, a CT scan of the abdomen and pelvis has a radiation dose equivalent to approximately 500 chest radiographs.

Summary box 14.5

Computed tomography

Strengths

- High spatial and contrast resolution
- Contrast resolution enhanced by ability to image in multiple phases, including arterial, venous and delayed
- Rapid acquisition of images in one breath-hold
- Imaging of choice for the detection of pulmonary masses
- Allows global assessment of the abdomen and pelvis
- Excellent for liver, pancreatic, renal and bowel pathology
- Three-dimensional reconstruction allows complex fracture imaging
- Multiplanar reconstruction and three-dimensional imaging,
- e.g. CT angiography and colonoscopy
- Ability to guide intervention such as percutaneous biopsy and drainage

Weaknesses

- High radiation dose
- Poor soft-tissue resolution of the peripheries and superficial structures
- Patient needs to be able to lie flat and still

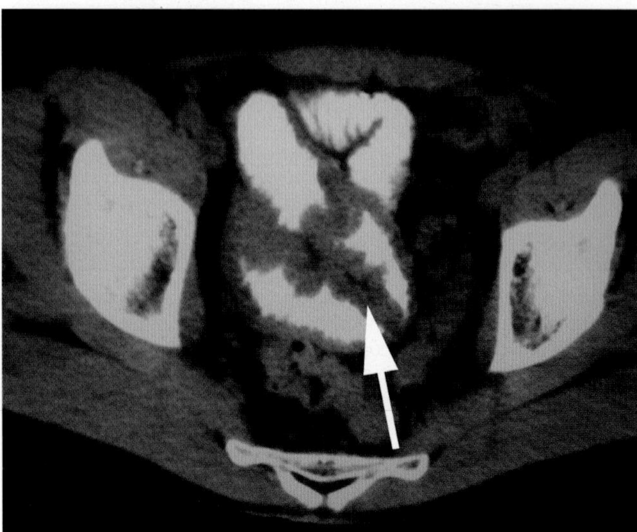

Figure 14.9 Axial computed tomography scan through the pelvis with oral contrast administration illustrates loops of distal ileum with mural thickening in a patient with Crohn's disease (arrow).

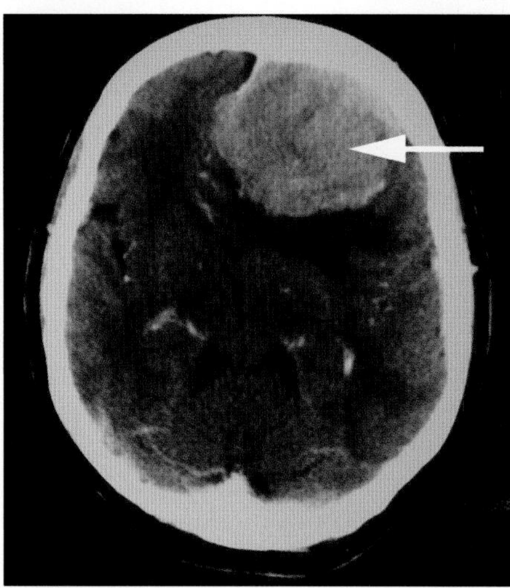

Figure 14.10 Axial computed tomography scan of the head following intravenous contrast demonstrates a large mass lesion in the left frontal region (arrow) in a patient with a large left frontal meningioma.

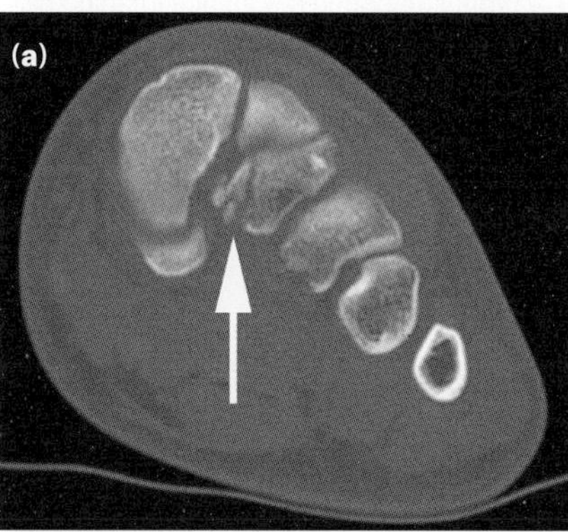

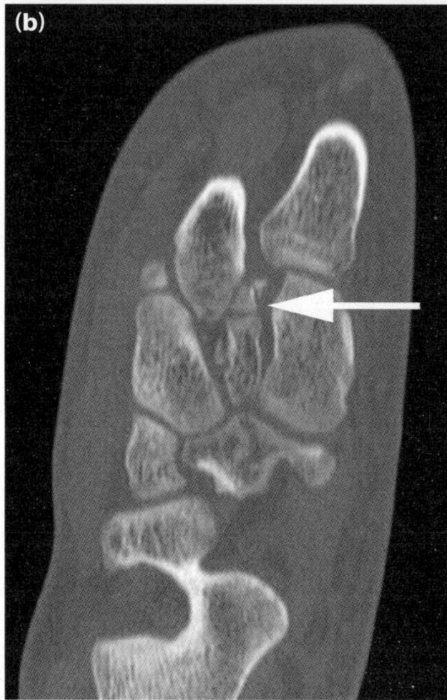

Figure 14.11 Coronal computed tomography **(a)** and axial reformats **(b)** of the foot in a patient involved in a road traffic accident demonstrates Lisfranc fracture dislocation with a comminuted fracture of the base of the second metatarsal (arrows).

Magnetic resonance imaging

Over the last 20 years, MRI has become an integral part of the imaging arsenal with ever-expanding indications. MRI relies on the fact that nuclei containing an odd number of protons have a characteristic motion in a magnetic field (precession) and produce a magnetic moment as a result of this motion. In a strong uniform magnetic field such as an MRI scanner, these nuclei align themselves with the main magnetic field and result in a net magnetic moment. A brief radiofrequency pulse is then applied to alter the motion of the nuclei. Once the radiofrequency pulse is removed, the nuclei realign themselves with the main magnetic field (relaxation) and in the process emit a radiofrequency signal that can be recorded, spatially encoded and used to construct a grey-scale image. The specific tissue characteristics define the manner and rate at which the nuclei relax. This relaxation is measured in two ways, referred to as the T1 and T2 relaxation times. The relaxation times and the proton density determine the signal from a specific tissue.

There are a large number of imaging sequences that can be used by applying radiofrequency pulses of different strengths and durations. The image characteristic and signal intensity from different tissues are governed by the pulse sequence employed and whether it is T1 weighted or T2 weighted. For instance, fat, methaemoglobin and mucinous fluid are bright on T1-weighted images, whereas water and thus most pathological processes, which tend to increase tissue water content, are bright on T2-weighted images. Cortical bone, air, haemosiderin and ferromagnetic materials are of very low signal on all pulse sequences. In general, T1-weighted images are superior in the delineation of anatomy, while T2-weighted images tend to highlight pathology better. For added tissue contrast, intravenous gadolinium may be administered. Other more specific contrast media are also available for liver, bowel and lymph node imaging.

MRI's exquisite contrast resolution, coupled with a lack of ionising radiation, is very attractive in imaging, particularly of tissues that have relatively little natural contrast. MRI also has the advantage of multiplanar imaging, as images can be acquired in any plane prescribed. It has traditionally been used extensively in the assessment of intracranial, spinal and musculoskeletal disorders (**Figures 14.12, 14.13 and 14.14**), allowing a global assessment of bony and soft-tissue structures. More recent developments have resulted in new indications and applications. Today, MRI is commonly used in oncological imaging, such as staging of rectal carcinoma and gynaecological malignancies, identification and characterisation of hepatic masses and assessment of the biliary tree (magnetic resonance cholangiopancreatography (MRCP) (**Figure 14.15**)). MRI has become increasingly important in imaging of the small bowel, for example in Crohn's disease, where repeated imaging with ionising radiation can incur a significant radiation dose over time.

MR angiographic techniques allow non-invasive angiographic assessment of the cranial and peripheral circulation (**Figure 14.16**), and cardiac imaging.

Jacques Lisfranc de St. Martin, 1790–1847, Professor of Surgery and Operative Medicine, Paris, France.

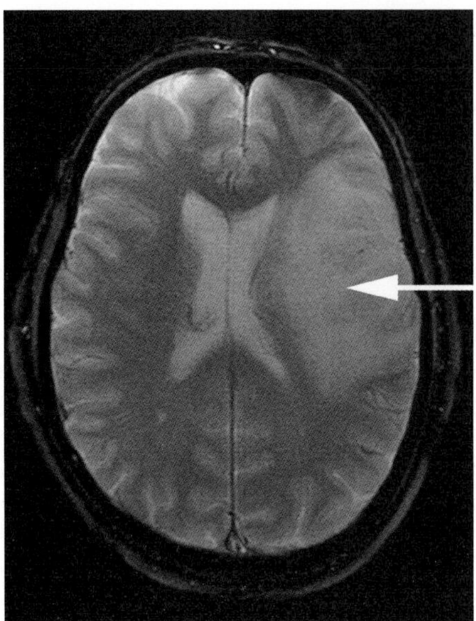

Figure 14.12 T2-weighted axial magnetic resonance imaging scan of the head in a patient with a large left-sided oligodendroglioma (arrow).

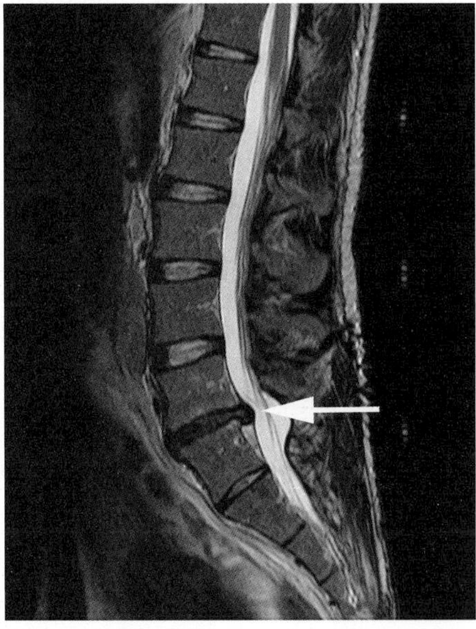

Figure 14.13 Sagittal T2-weighted magnetic resonance imaging scan of the lumbar spine demonstrates disc herniation (arrow) in a patient with acute back pain.

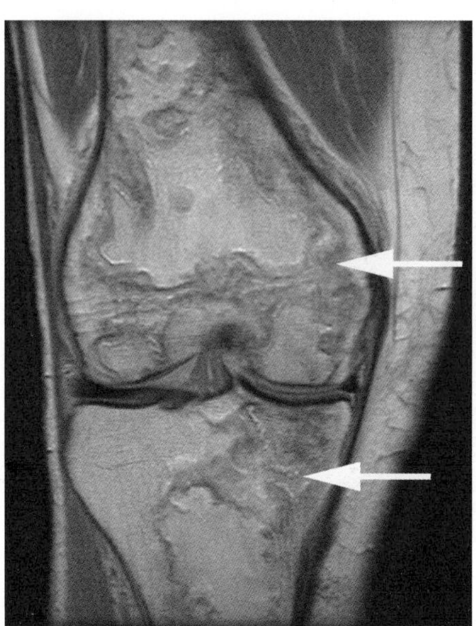

Figure 14.14 Coronal magnetic resonance imaging scan of the knee demonstrates extensive serpiginous areas of altered signal intensity in the distal femur and proximal tibia (arrows) in a patient with bone infarcts secondary to oral corticosteroids.

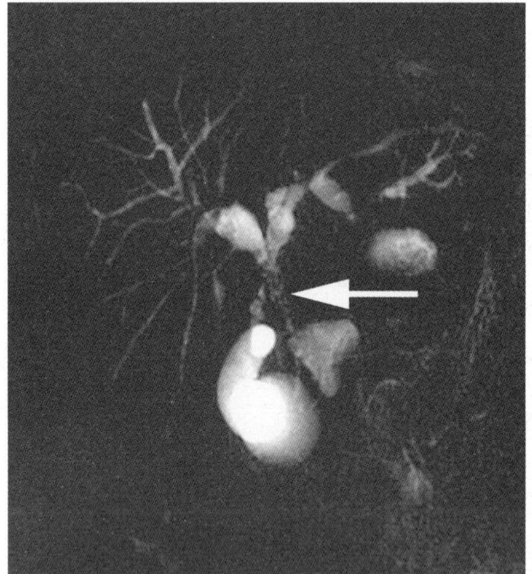

Figure 14.15 Magnetic resonance cholangiopancreatography demonstrates dilated central intrahepatic bile ducts and a stricture of the common bile duct (arrow) in a patient with obstructive jaundice and cholangio-carcinoma.

Diffusion weighted imaging is a relatively new type of MRI sequence that exploits the different rates of Brownian motion between different tissues. Tissues with greater cellular density have lower rates of diffusion of water molecules, and this difference can be exploited to distinguish benign and malignant lesions in a variety of organs as malignant lesions tend to have greater density of cells.

However, the availability of MRI is still relatively limited in comparison with other imaging techniques, and it is time-consuming with respect to image acquisition and interpretation. Images are easily degraded by motion, including respiratory and cardiac motion. The use of respiratory and cardiac gating can minimise this, although bowel peristalsis can still be a problem. The long acquisition times require a cooperative patient who can lie very still, which can be difficult especially in claustrophobic individuals or those in pain. Furthermore, because of the use of high-strength magnetic fields, patients with some metallic implants, such as some aneurysm clips and prosthetic heart valves, and those with implanted electronic devices, such as pacemakers and defibrillators, cannot be examined. Some newer implants may, however, be MRI compatible, and patients with joint replacements can be studied safely.

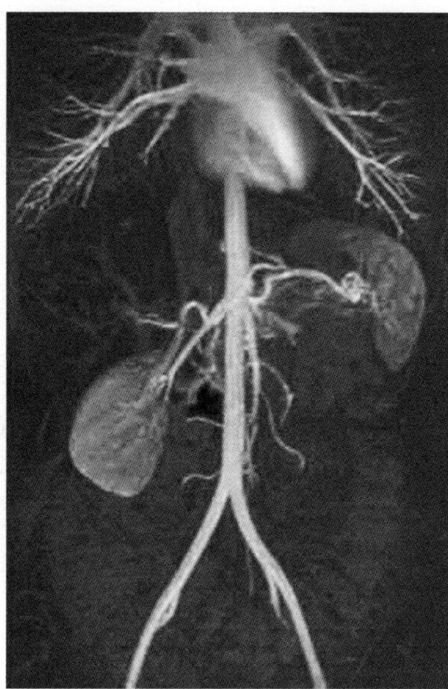

Figure 14.16 Maximum intensity projection image from a magnetic resonance angiogram demonstrates the abdominal aorta, common and external iliac arteries as well as parts of the pulmonary, mesenteric and renal vasculature.

Summary box 14.6

Magnetic resonance (MR) imaging

Strengths

- No ionising radiation
- Excellent soft-tissue contrast
- Best imaging technique for
  - Intracranial lesions
  - Spine
  - Bone marrow and joint lesions

Evolving use

- Staging
- MRCP
- MR angiography
- Breast malignancy
- Pelvic malignancy
- Cardiac imaging
- MR enterography
- Diffusion-weighted imaging

Weaknesses

- Absolute contraindications
  - Ocular metallic foreign bodies
  - Pacemakers
  - Cochlear implants Cranial aneurysm clips
- Relative contraindications
  - First trimester of pregnancy
  - Claustrophobia
- Long scan times so patients may not be able to keep still, especially if in pain
- Limited availability
- Expensive

Nuclear medicine

In other imaging techniques using ionising radiation such as CT and conventional radiography, the individual is exposed to ionising radiation from an external source and the radiation transmitted through the patient is recorded. In nuclear medicine, however, a radioactive element or radionuclide such as technetium, gallium, thallium or iodine is administered to the patient as part of a radiopharmaceutical agent, and a detector such as a gamma camera is then used to record and localise the emission from the patient, thus forming the image. The radionuclide is chosen and coupled with other compounds such that it is distributed and taken up in the tissues of interest. Therefore, a variety of radionuclides are required for imaging of different tissues. Nuclear medicine also differs from other means of imaging, which are largely anatomically based, as it also provides functional information.

Radionuclide imaging is widely used in bone imaging with very high sensitivity for assessing metastatic disease, metabolic bone disease, established arthropathies and occult infection and traumatic injuries (**Figure 14.17**), although many of these applications are being replaced by MRI. In

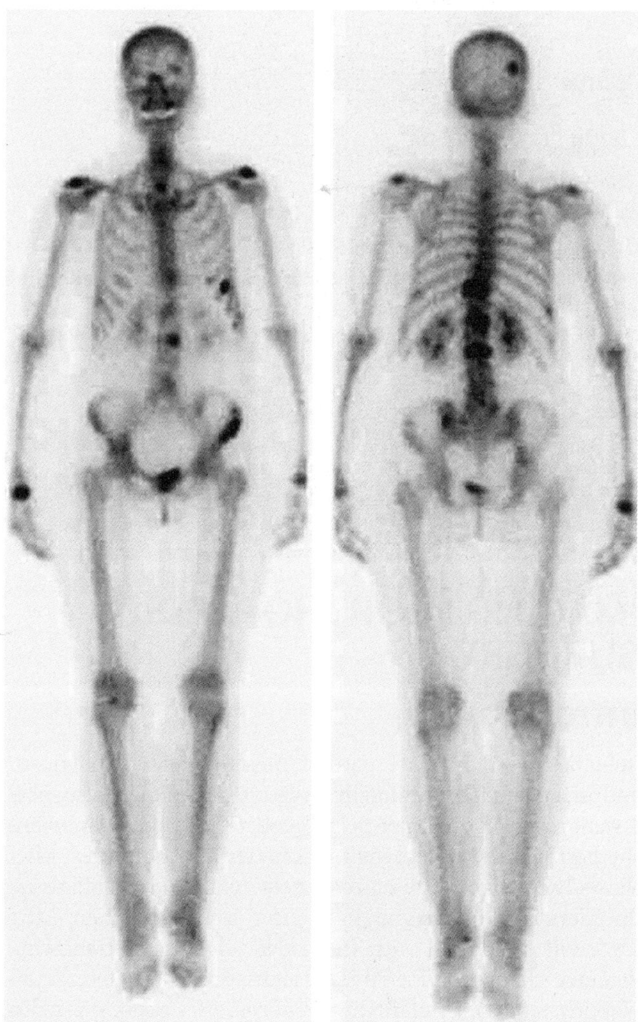

Figure 14.17 Bone scintigraphy in a patient with carcinoma of the breast illustrates bony metastatic deposits involving multiple vertebrae, the skull, pelvis and ribs.

genitourinary disease, dynamic imaging can be performed to assess renal perfusion and function including obstruction, investigate renovascular hyper- tension and evaluate renal transplants. Radionuclide imaging is also commonly used in thyroid and parathyroid disorders, ischaemic cardiac disease, detection of pulmonary emboli and assessment of occult infection and inflammatory bowel disease.

Positron emission tomography (PET) is an extension of nuclear medicine, in which a positron-emitting substance such as 18F is tagged and used to assess tissue metabolic characteristics. The most commonly used radiolabelled tracer is 18F-2-fluoro-2-deoxy-D-glucose (FDG), although other tracers can also be used in order to assess metabolic functions such as oxygen and glucose consumption and blood flow. Radioisotope decay causes the emission of a positron, which subsequently, within a few millimetres, collides with and annihilates an electron to produce a pair of annihilation photons. The drawbacks have been high cost, very limited availability and relatively low spatial resolution. The last of these has been addressed by PET/CT systems combining simultaneous PET imaging and CT, allowing the two sets of images to be registered so that the anatomical location of the abnormality can be localised more precisely.

Summary box 14.7

Radionuclide imaging

Strengths

- Allows functional imaging
- Allows imaging of the whole body
- Bone scan has a high sensitivity for metastatic bone disease, fractures and infection
- PET scanning is valuable in the detection of metastatic cancer

Weaknesses

- Specific agents are required for specific indications
- Often non-specific and an abnormal result may require further imaging
- Generally poor spatial resolution

IMAGING IN ORTHOPAEDIC SURGERY

Introduction

Imaging is an intricate part of musculoskeletal diagnosis, and image-guided, minimally invasive techniques also play a major role in treatment. In broad terms, radiographs are the best method of looking for bony lesions or injuries, MRI shows bone marrow disease, muscle tendon and soft-tissue disorders and ultrasound has better resolution than MRI for small structures, with the added advantage of showing dynamic changes. CT enables visualisation of the fine detail of bony structures, clarifying abnormalities seen on plain radiographs.

There are occasions when a combination of techniques will be important, and due consideration should be given to reducing the ionising radiation burden to the patient, using ultrasound and MRI as primary investigations whenever appropriate.

Summary box 14.8

Types of imaging

- Radiographs are the best first-line test for bone lesions and fractures
- MRI is good for diagnosing bone marrow disease, occult fractures and tendon and soft-tissue disorders
- CT enables visualisation of the fine detail of bony structures
- CT gives the best three-dimensional information on fractures
- Ultrasound has better resolution in accessible soft tissues and can be used dynamically
- Ultrasound is the best method of distinguishing solid from cystic lesions
- Ultrasound is the only method for locating non-metallic foreign bodies
- Ultrasound is the best method for detecting muscle hernias

Skeletal trauma

Musculoskeletal trauma is best imaged by an initial plain radiograph. All skeletal radiographs should be taken from two different angles, usually at right angles to each other. This is important in trauma because a fracture or dislocation may not be visible on a single view (**Figure 14.18**). Occasionally, and in specific locations such as the scaphoid, more than two views are routinely performed. If this fails to make a clear diagnosis, or if there is suspicion of soft-tissue injuries, then cross-sectional studies are indicated.

Increasingly in the assessment of spinal trauma, CT is replacing radiographs as the first-line investigation for two main reasons: the first is that the sensitivity of CT is superior, the second is that it is quicker, enabling treatment to commence sooner).

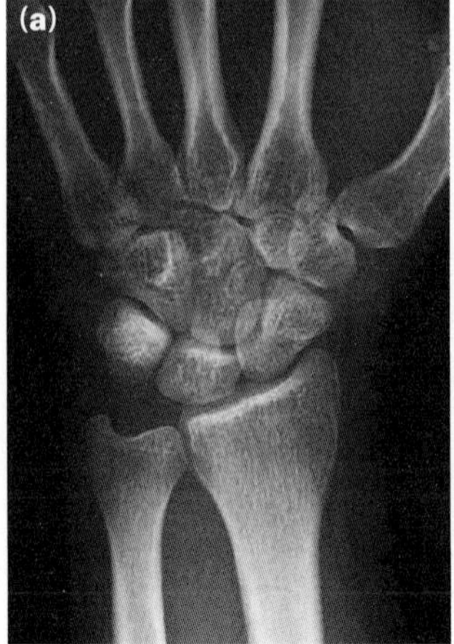

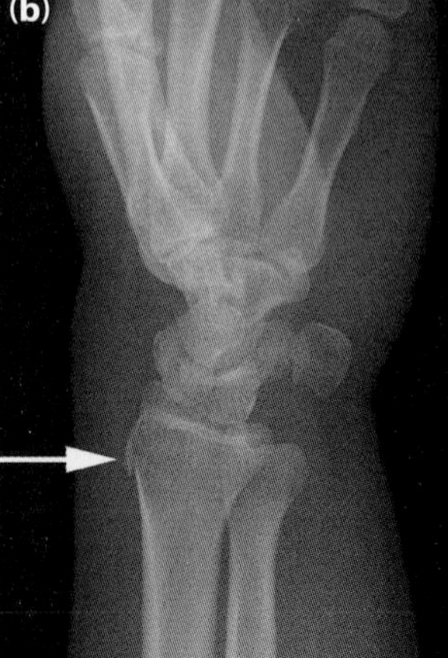

Figure 14.18 Anteroposterior radiograph of the wrist (**a**) in a patient following a fall does not show an acute bony injury. It is only on the second view (**b**) that a fracture of the dorsal cortex of the distal radius is visualised (arrow).

Summary box 14.9

Trauma imaging

- Initial imaging is either radiography or CT
- At least two views are needed for radiographs
- Use CT for spine, intra-articular or occult fractures

Axial CT images alone may fail to diagnose some fractures, so three-dimensional reformatting is important to prevent errors. Sections should be thin, but care must be taken not to cover too wide an area, as the radiation burden may be excessive, particularly with multislice CT.

Degenerative disease

Synovitis

Radiographs are usually the first-line imaging investigation performed for the examination of joints. Typical changes of a degenerative or an erosive arthropathy are well known and understood. However, early arthropathy will be missed on radiographs and, with the advent of disease-modifying drugs, it is important to detect early synovitis before it is even apparent on clinical examination. Gadolinium diethyl triamine penta-acetic (DTPA)-enhanced MRI is the most sensitive method for detecting synovial thickening of numerous joints, but ultrasound is also sensitive, albeit more laborious to perform. Ultrasound shows effusions and synovial thickening clearly, and shows the increased blood flow around the affected joints without the use of contrast agents (**Figures 14.19 and 14.20**).

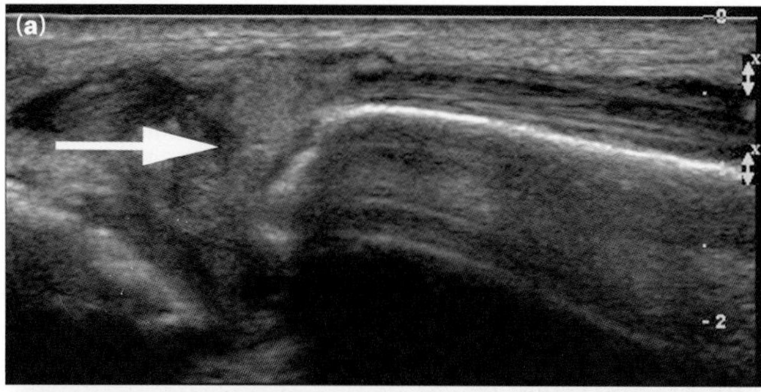

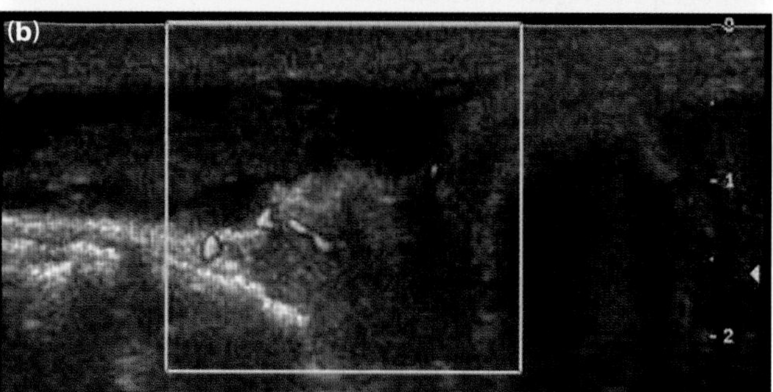

Figure 14.20 Ultrasound of the wrist (**a**) shows thickening of tissues on the dorsal aspect of the radiocarpal joint (arrow). (**b**) There is increased flow on power Doppler ultrasound in this patient with wrist synovitis and rheumatoid arthritis.

Articular cartilage damage

Articular surface disease is difficult to detect using non-invasive techniques. MRI is probably the best method, although it is not sensitive to early chondral changes (**Figure 14.21**). Higher field strength magnets (3 Tesla and above) with dedicated surface coils provide more precise assessment; however, MR arthrography

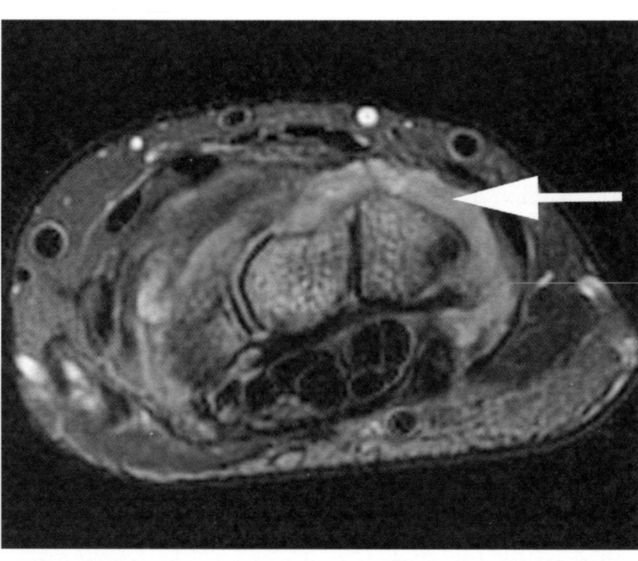

Figure 14.19 Axial T2-weighted fat-suppressed image of the wrist in a patient with rheumatoid arthritis demonstrates synovitis manifested as increased signal dorsal to the carpal bones (arrow).

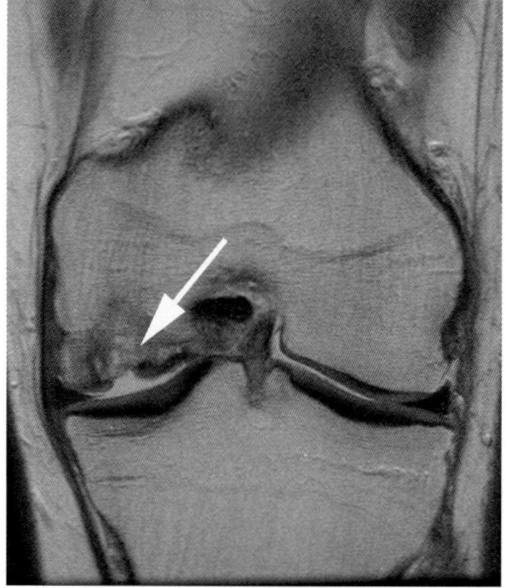

Figure 14.21 Coronal magnetic resonance imaging of the knee demonstrates a focal osteochondral abnormality of the medial femoral condyle, with full-thickness loss of the articular cartilage and abnormality of the subchondral bone (arrow).

Nikola Tesla, 1856–1943, American physicist and electrical engineer who worked for the Westinghouse Company. A Tesla is the SI unit of magnetic flux density.

is currently the imaging 'gold standard'. Saline mixed with a dilute quantity of gadolinium DTPA is introduced into the joint by needle puncture, which is followed by an MRI examination. Using this technique, more subtle changes in the articular surface can be seen, including thinning, fissuring and ulceration. However, early softening of articular cartilage will not be visible. MR arthrography is also useful for detecting labral tears in the shoulder or hip, and in the assessment of patients who have undergone a previous meniscectomy. The triangular fibrocartilage of the wrist is also difficult to assess fully without MR or CT arthrography (**Figure 14.22**).

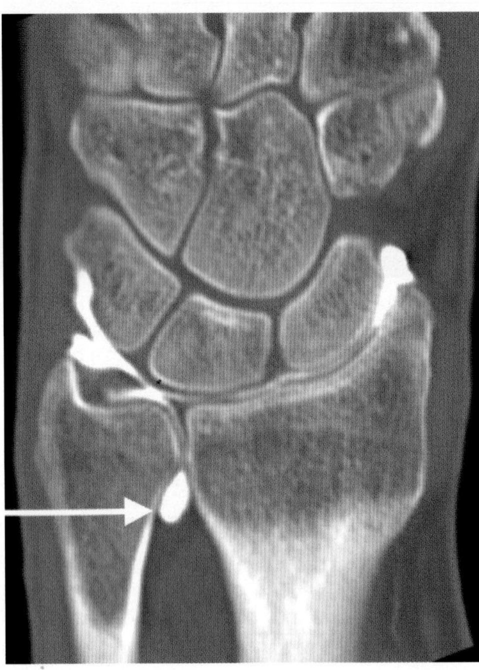

Figure 14.22 Coronal CT arthrogram of the wrist showing a central perforation of the triangular fibrocartilage with contrast extending into the distal radioulnar joint and radiocarpal articulation (arrow).

In the shoulder, rotator cuff trauma and degenerative changes can be studied using ultrasound or MRI. In experienced hands, ultrasound has a higher accuracy rate, because image resolution is better and because the mechanical integrity of the cuff can be tested by dynamically stressing it (**Figure 14.23**). MRI has the advantage of being able to show abnormalities in the subcortical bone.

In the majority of arthropathies and degenerative disorders, serial imaging is useful. Changes in films taken weeks or months apart are far easier to see and interpret than a single snap-shot study.

Aggressive bone disease

The radiograph is the first imaging technique for destructive lesions in bones. There is considerable experience required in the interpretation of these films, especially with regard as to whether the lesion is benign or malignant (**Figure 14.24**).

Summary box 14.10

Imaging techniques for joint disease

- Radiographs are good for assessing established articular disease
- Synovitis can be detected using ultrasound or contrast-enhanced MRI
- Early damage to articular cartilage is difficult to image by conventional methods
- Rotator cuff lesions are best studied using ultrasound or MRI
- Destructive lesions are best studied first on plain radiographs
- MRI is best for staging tumours
- Biopsy can be guided by fluoroscopy, CT or ultrasound

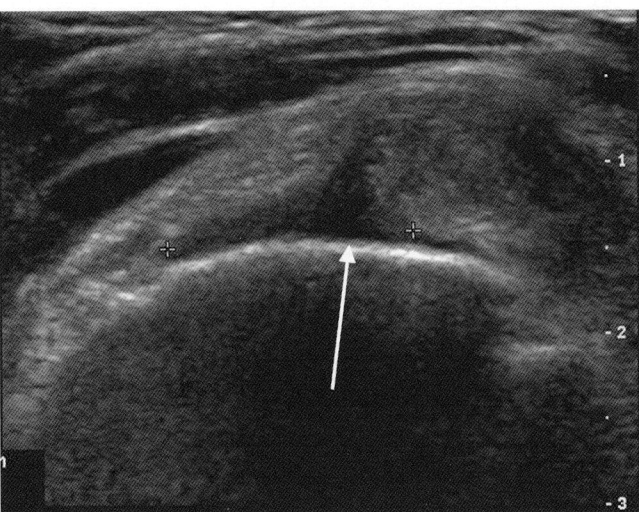

Figure 14.23 Ultrasound of the supraspinatus tendon identifies a partial tear of the tendon (arrow), which is predominantly articular sided but with a component that is nearly full thickness.

Radiographs are also vital in the assessment of soft-tissue calcification in tumours of muscle, tendon and subcutaneous fat. When a lesion is detected, there needs to be an early decision as to whether this is benign or malignant. If there is a suspicion of malignancy on the radiograph, or any uncertainty, then local staging is indicated. This is best performed by MRI for both bone and soft-tissue lesions (**Figure 14.25**). At this stage, it is likely that a biopsy will be indicated, and preferably under image guidance. Soft-tissue and bone biopsy needles may be guided by CT, ultrasound or interventional MRI systems. The route of puncture should avoid vital structures and must be agreed with the surgeon, who will perform local excision if the lesion proves to be malignant. Care should be taken to avoid contaminating other compartments. In all circumstances, samples are best sent for both histopathological and microbiological examination. It may be difficult to tell on imaging whether or not a lesion is infected, and histology often provides a clear diagnosis in inflammatory conditions. Bone scintigraphy is useful in detecting whether a lesion is solitary or multiple, although whole-body MRI is becoming available.

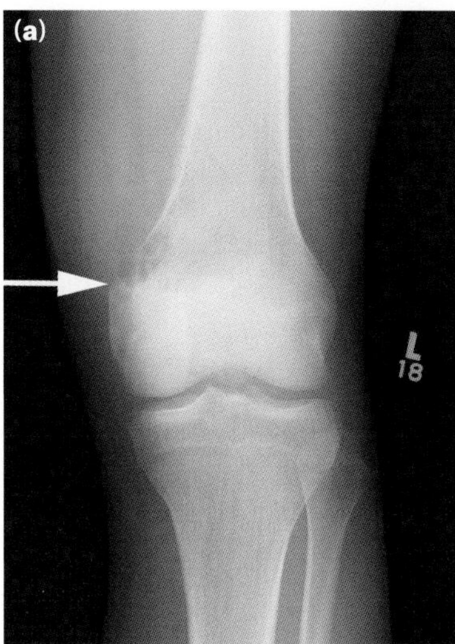

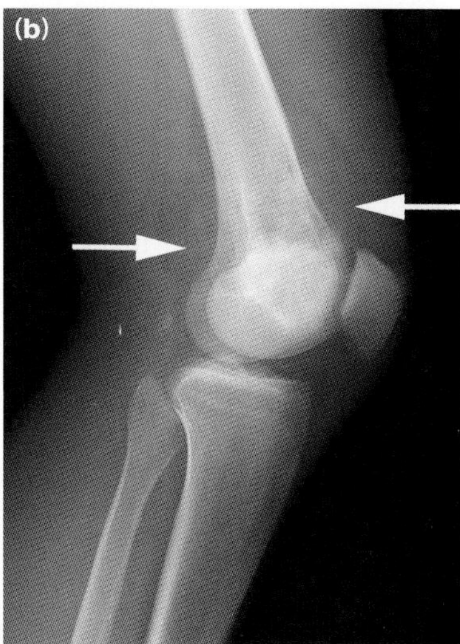

Figure 14.24 Anteroposterior (**a**) and lateral (**b**) radiographs of the left knee in a young patient with knee pain. There is a mixed lucent and sclerotic lesion of the distal femur with breach of the cortex medially and soft-tissue extension seen anteriorly and posteriorly (arrows). The location and appearances are consistent with osteosarcoma.

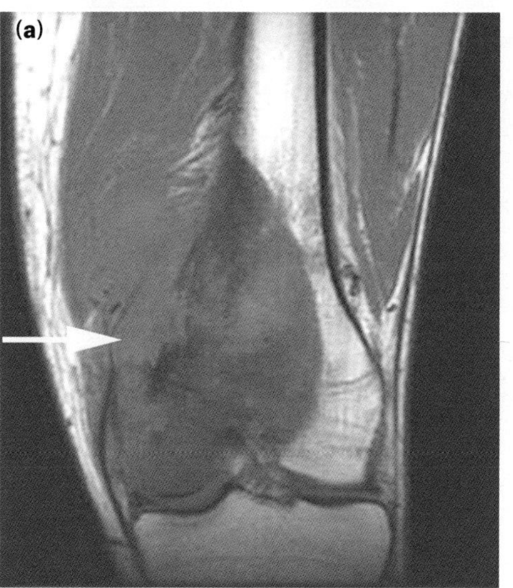

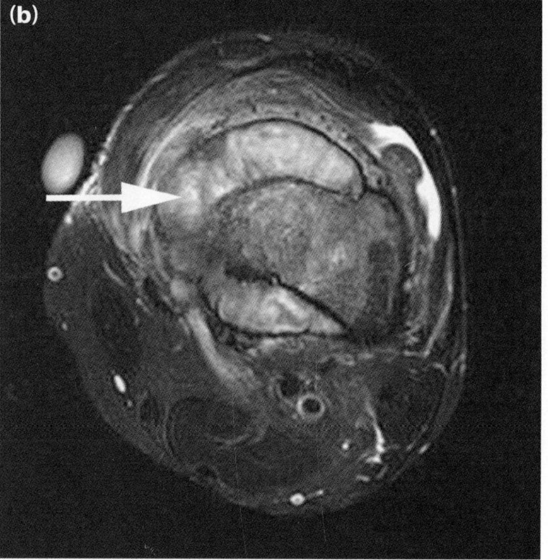

Figure 14.25 Coronal T1- (**a**) and axial T2-weighted fat-suppressed (**b**) images through the distal femur of the patient in Figure 14.24 illustrates the bony area involved, the soft-tissue extent of the tumour and the relationship of the neurovascular structures to the mass (arrows).

Summary box 14.11

Imaging of aggressive lesions in bone

- Plain radiographs are important as a first investigation
- MRI is best for local staging
- Bone scintigraphy or whole-body MRI for solitary or multiple lesion determination
- CT detects lung metastases
- Fluoroscopy, CT, MRI or ultrasound can be used to guide the biopsy

Mass lesions

Mass lesions in muscle and soft tissue are examined by ultrasound, which can be diagnostic in the majority of cases, thereby avoiding the need for further imaging. This is most often the case when a lesion is purely cystic and, as most soft-tissue masses are cysts, ultrasound is a very effective screening test. There are occasions when no mass lesion is found at the site of concern, and then reassurance can be offered. If the ultrasound examination is normal, this effectively excludes soft-tissue neoplasia. A reasonable protocol is to perform ultrasound on all palpable 'lesions' to exclude cysts, and on patients without any identifiable mass, and to proceed to MRI only when there is a solid or partly solid element to an unidentifiable lesion. Tumour vascularity is best assessed by Doppler ultrasound. It can be studied by intravenous gadolinium DTPA-enhanced MRI; however, this is a more expensive and invasive technique, providing no more information than Doppler ultrasound.

Summary box 14.12

Imaging of soft-tissue lesions

- Ultrasound is the best for screening; it is often the only imaging required
- MRI is best for local staging and follow-up
- Doppler ultrasound can assess vascularity cheaply and effectively
- Ultrasound is useful for biopsy

Infection

In the early stages of joint infection, the plain films may be normal, but they should still be performed to exclude bony erosions, in case a painful joint is the first sign of an arthropathy. Ultrasound examination is the easiest and most accurate method of assessing joint effusions, although, when an effusion is identified, it is not possible to discriminate between blood and pus. Aspiration guided by ultrasound is the best method of making this distinction. MRI may be required to assess early articular cartilage and bone involvement.

Radiographs should also be used to examine patients with suspected osteomyelitis. Although they may not detect early infection, they will demonstrate or exclude bony destruction, calcification and sequestrum formation. CT may be needed to give a cross-sectional view, in order to assess the extent of bony sequestrum.

MRI is perhaps the most sensitive method for detecting early disease and is the preferred technique to define the activity and extent of infection, as it shows not only the bony involvement but also the extent of oedema and soft-tissue involvement (**Figure 14.26**). Abscesses may be detected or excluded, and subperiosteal oedema is readily visible. MRI can be used as a staging procedure to plan treatment, including surgical intervention. Serial examinations can be used to follow the response to intravenous antibiotics and are very useful in the management of complex osteomyelitis. In cases of negative or equivocal MRI, nuclear medicine techniques such as bone scintigraphy can be very sensitive, and specialised studies using tracers such as gallium citrate or indium-labelled white cells increase specificity.

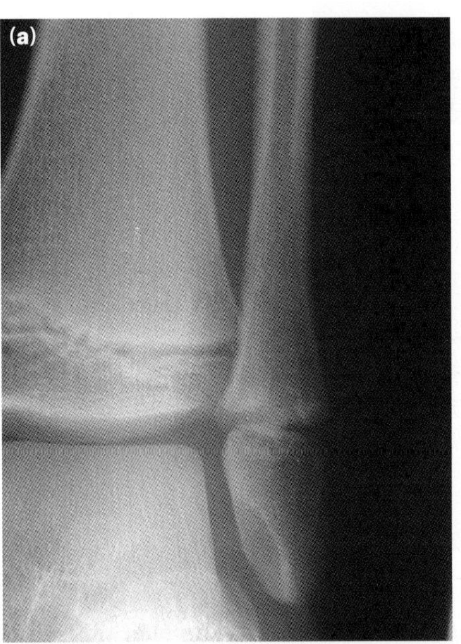

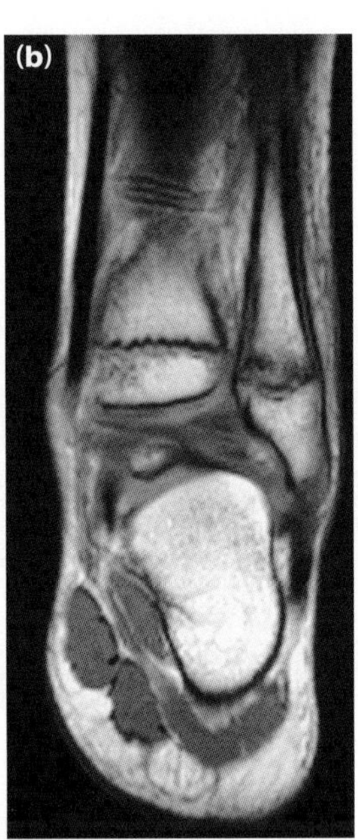

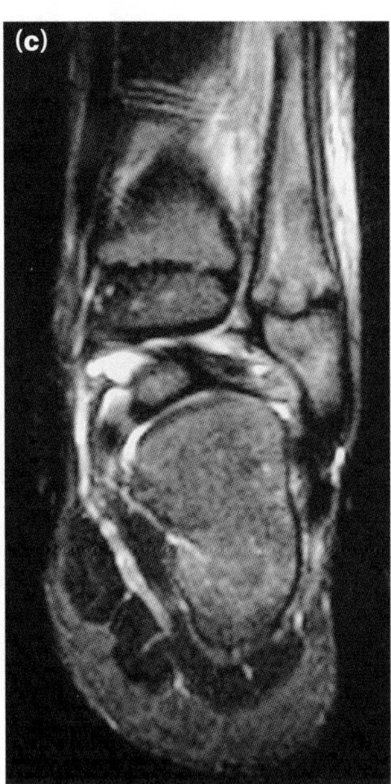

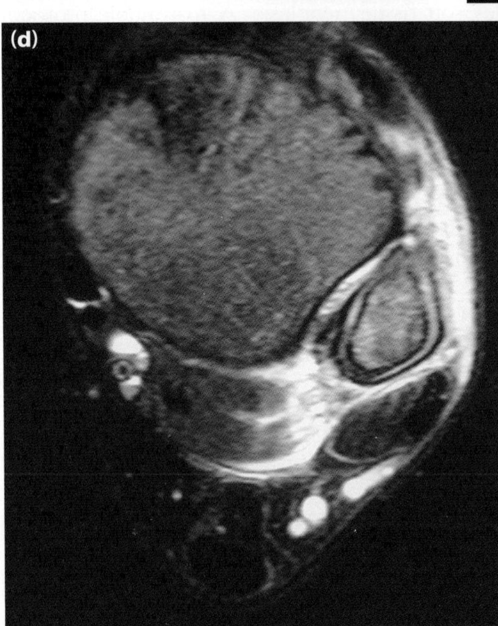

Figure 14.26 (**a**) The plain films of this 13-year-old are close to normal. On close inspection, there is a fine periosteal reaction on the fibula. (**b**) The coronal T1-weighted magnetic resonance image shows little more, but (**c**) the coronal fast STIR (short tau inversion recovery) images and (**d**) axial T2 fast spin echo with fat suppression show the oedema in bone as white and the extensive periosteal fluid with soft-tissue inflammation. The diagnosis is acute osteomyelitis.

Summary box 14.13

Imaging of potentially infected bone and joint

- Plain radiographs may be needed to exclude bone erosion
- Ultrasound is sensitive for an effusion, periosteal collections and superficial abscesses and can be used for guided aspiration
- CT is useful in established infection to look for sequestrum
- MRI is useful to define the activity of osteomyelitis, early infection and soft-tissue collections
- Bone scans are sensitive but of low specificity
- Complex nuclear medicine studies are useful in negative MR examinations or equivocal cases

Metabolic bone disease

Plain radiographs should be the first images of patients with metabolic bone disease. They may detect the subperiosteal erosions in hyperparathyroidism or, more commonly, the osteopenia in osteoporosis, but they cannot be used to quantify osteoporosis. The apparent density of the bone on the film is linked to the penetration of the rays, among other variables, as well as to the bone density. If a quantitative method is needed, however, bone mineral density using dual x-ray absorptiometry (DEXA) is the most accurate and practical. However, fractures will cause erroneously high readings, and they tend to occur in the vertebrae used for DEXA measurements. Quantitative CT is an alternative technique, although this is less readily available. Ultrasound transmission measurement in the extremities has its advocates, as it arguably measures factors that better represent the strength of bone rather than its density. Its limitations are that it cannot be used to study the vertebrae or hip, and these are the sites where osteoporotic fractures occur most frequently. MRI may be useful in detecting fractures and is an essential prerequisite to percutaneous vertebroplasty.

IMAGING IN MAJOR TRAUMA

Introduction

Trauma remains a major cause of mortality and morbidity in all age groups. Presented with a multiply injured patient, rapid and effective investigation and treatment are required to maximise the chances of survival and to reduce morbidity. Imaging plays a major role in this assessment and in guiding treatment. As with the clinical assessment, imaging is carried out according to the principles of primary and secondary surveys, identifying major life-threatening injuries of the airway, respiratory system and circulation before a more detailed and typically time-consuming assessment of other injures. At no point should imaging delay the treatment of immediately life-threatening injuries. As in other settings, the quickest and least invasive examinations should be performed first. A radiologist present in the trauma room at the time of patient assessment is able to evaluate the radiographs rapidly, relay this information back to the team and guide further imaging, which may include further plain films, CT, ultrasound and MRI.

Plain radiographs

Conventional radiography allows rapid assessment of the major injuries and can be carried out in the trauma room while the patient is clinically assessed and treated. Despite the time constraints, the number of staff involved and the restricted mobility of the patient, high-quality images can be routinely obtained with due care and attention.

There is no routine set of radiographs to be obtained, and the decision is based on the mechanism of injury, the stability of the patient's condition and whether the patient is intubated. The most commonly performed initial radiographs are a chest radiograph, a single anteroposterior view of the pelvis and a cervical spine series.

The supine chest radiograph should encompass an area from the lung apices to the costophrenic recesses and include the ribs laterally. Chest radiographs give valuable information in both blunt and penetrating trauma. Evaluation of the radiograph should be undertaken in a systematic manner to minimise the chances of missing an injury. In the first instance, the position of line and tubes, including the endotracheal tube, should be assessed followed by assessment of the central airways. Following this, the lungs should be evaluated for abnormal focal areas of opacification, which may represent aspiration, haemorrhage, haematoma or oedema, as well as more diffuse opacification reflecting a pleural collection. Alternatively, relative focal or unilateral lucency may reflect a pneumothorax in the supine position. Evaluation of the mediastinum should include its position, which may be altered by tension pneumothoraces or large collections, as well as its contour, an alteration of which may reflect a mediastinal haematoma due to aortic or spinal injury. Finally, the skeleton and the soft tissue should be carefully examined for rib, vertebral, scapular and limb fractures, as well as evidence of surgical emphysema and paraspinal haematomas (**Figure 14.27**).

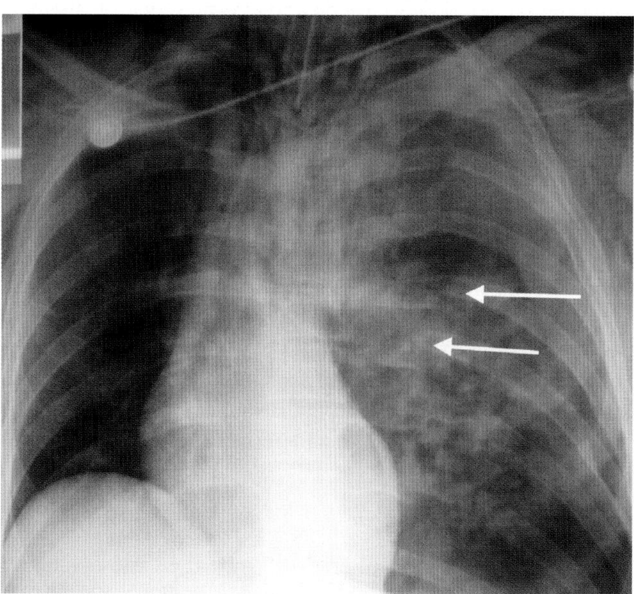

Figure 14.27 Supine chest radiograph of a patient involved in a road traffic accident. The patient is intubated. There are multiple left-sided rib fractures (arrows) and extensive surgical emphysema. Depression of the left hemidiaphragm and mediastinal shift to the right suggest that there is a tension pneumothorax present.

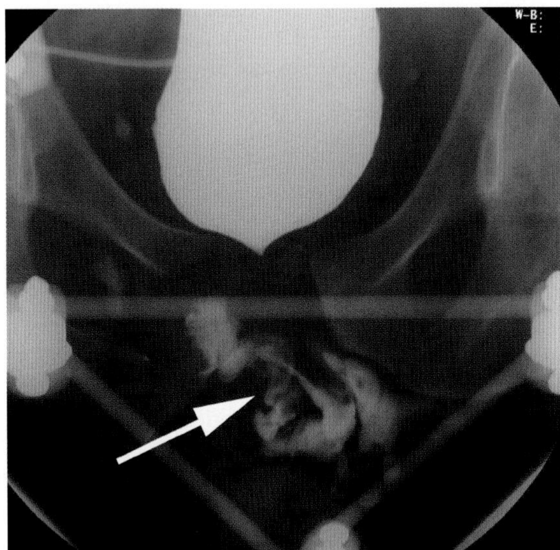

Figure 14.28 Retrograde urethrogram in a patient who sustained extensive pelvic fractures following a fall. The pelvic injuries have been stabilised using an external fixation device. The urethrogram identifies extensive injury to the urethra with extravasation of contrast (arrow).

Pelvic radiographs are also commonly performed to screen for, and assess, fractures of the bony pelvis. The image should include the iliac crests in their totality and extend inferiorly to below the lesser trochanters. When assessing the film, the alignment of the sacroiliac joints and the symphysis pubis should be carefully examined, as some fractures, especially those of the sacral arcades, can be very subtle on the pelvic radiograph. The presence of pubic fractures raises the possibility of urethral injury and should alert clinicians to exercise caution with bladder catheterisation (Figure 14.28).

The utility of cervical spine x-rays depends on the consciousness level of the patient and the presence of distracting injuries. In fully conscious patients with an isolated neck injury, clinical assessment can be used to guide the need for x-rays. In patients with distracting injuries and/or altered consciousness, including intubated patients, CT is preferred (Figure 14.29).

Further radiographs of the thoracic and lumbar spine and the peripheral skeleton may be required, depending on the clinical setting. As with all skeletal radiographs, two perpendicular views are required for adequate assessment. However, with the increasing use of CT in assessment of the torso the need for plain films is diminishing.

Radiographs of the skull or facial bones have no role in the immediate assessment of the multitrauma individual, except for immediate localisation of a penetrating object.

Ultrasound

Ultrasound has an evolving role in the assessment of acutely traumatised patients. The main current roles of ultrasound include the assessment of intraperitoneal fluid and haemo-pericardium (focused assessment with sonography for trauma, FAST), the evaluation of pneumothoraces in supine patients and in guiding intervention.

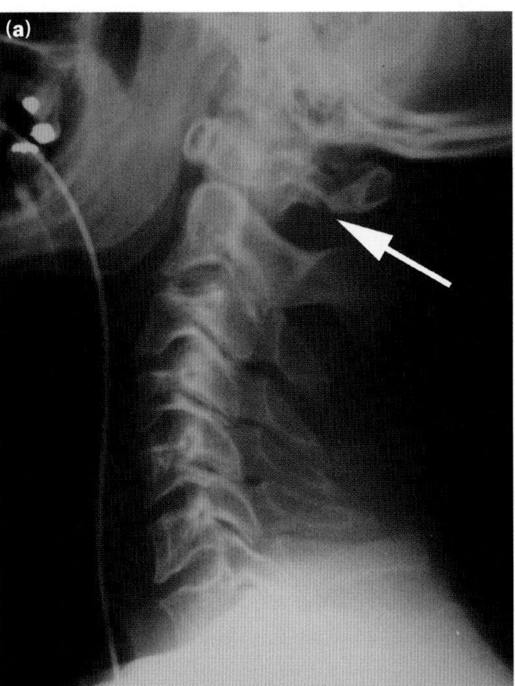

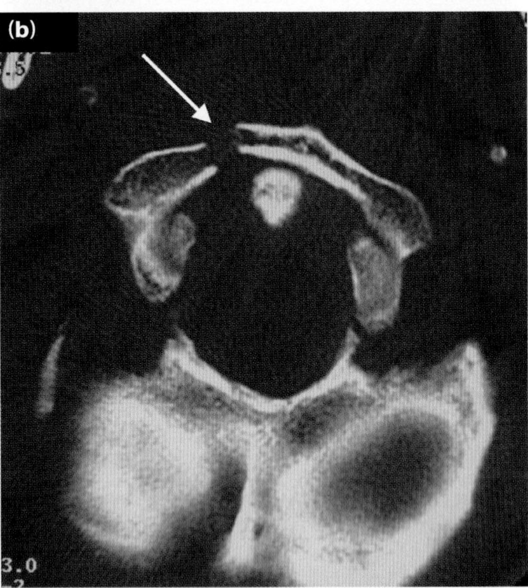

Figure 14.29 Lateral view of the cervical spine (**a**) fails to demonstrate the cervicothoracic junction. In addition, there appears to be a break in the posterior arch of C1 (arrow). Computed tomography of the cervical spine (**b**) demonstrates a fracture of the anterior arch as well as the posterior arch of C1 (arrow).

FAST ultrasound is a limited examination directed to look for intraperitoneal fluid or pericardial injury as a marker of underlying injury. This avoids the invasiveness of diagnostic peritoneal lavage. In the presence of free intraperitoneal fluid and an unstable patient, the ultrasound allows the trauma surgeon to explore the abdomen as a cause of blood loss. In the presence of fluid and a haemodynamically stable individual, further assessment by way of CT can be performed. However, it is important to realise that ultrasound has limitations in the identification of free fluid. This includes obscuration of fluid by bowel gas or extensive surgical emphysema. More organised haematoma may be more difficult to visualise. It must also be emphasised that the principal role of ultrasound is not to identify the primary solid organ injury, although this may be visualised. Occasionally, a second ultrasound scan may show free fluid in the presence of an initially negative FAST scan.

The detection of a pneumothorax on a supine radiograph can be very difficult. Ultrasound examination may be used to identify a radiographically occult pneumothorax. With a high-resolution linear probe, the pleura can be visualised as an echogenic stripe, and its motion with respiration can also be assessed. In the presence of a pneumothorax, the sliding motion of the pleura is lost. Ultrasound may also be used to detect a haemothorax or haemopericardium.

Finally, ultrasound may be of value in guiding the placement of an intravascular line by direct visualisation of the vessels. This can be especially advantageous in shocked patients.

Computed tomography

CT is the main imaging method for the investigation of intracranial and intra-abdominal injuries and vertebral fractures. With current multidetector scanners a comprehensive examination of the head, spine, chest, abdomen and pelvis can be completed in less than 5 minutes. However, much more time is taken up in transferring the patient and the associated monitoring equipment onto the scanner. Therefore, the total time can be in excess of 30 minutes, and CT should be reserved for individuals whose condition is stable.

CT examination of the head is accurate in identifying treatable intracranial injuries (**Figures 14.30 and 14.31**) and should not be delayed by radiography of peripheral injuries, as there is declining success in cases of intracranial collection when treated after the initial 3–4 hours. In comparison, identification of more widespread injuries, such as diffuse axonal injury, is relatively poor. Examination of facial injuries and cervical spine fractures can also be carried out at the same time as this only adds seconds to the examination. There is evidence that CT of the abdomen and pelvis is of benefit in multiple trauma when there is a head injury, as it often shows unexpected abnormalities, and this may affect the immediate management, especially if the patient deteriorates.

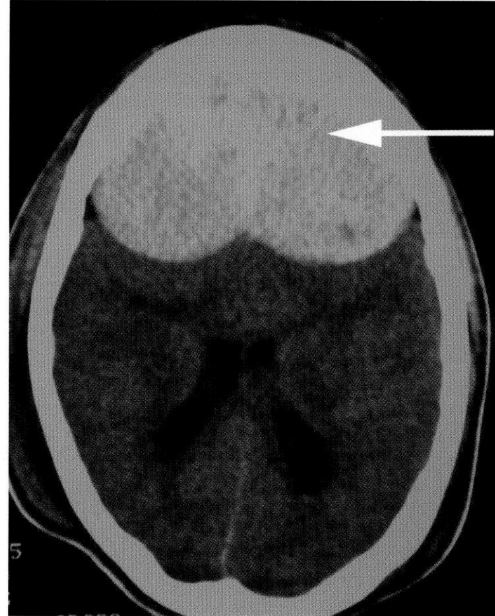

Figure 14.30 Computed tomography of the head in a patient with head injury shows bilateral large frontal extradural collections (arrow).

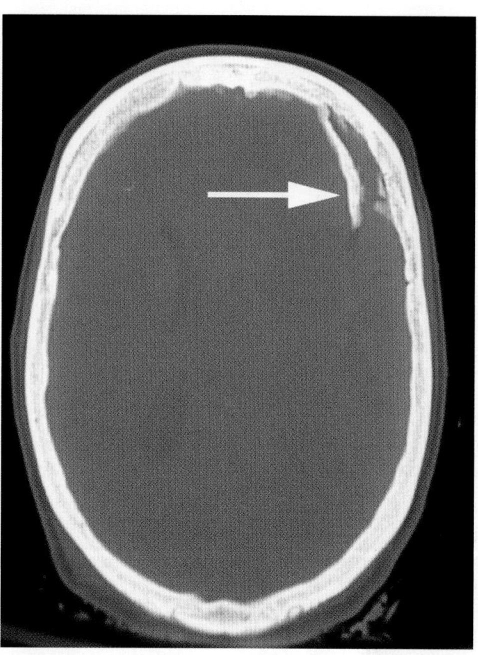

Figure 14.31 Computed tomography of the head following head trauma shows a skull fracture with a large depressed component (arrow).

Chest CT with intravenous contrast agent is valuable in identifying vascular and lung injuries and is the most accurate way of demonstrating haemothorax and pneumothorax. The position of chest drains can be identified, allowing adjustment of position if necessary. Abdominal and pelvic CT is usually undertaken as an extension to the chest CT. If an abdominal examination is performed, the pelvis should be included to avoid missing pelvic injuries and free pelvic fluid. CT is an excellent means of identifying hepatic, splenic (**Figure 14.32**) and renal injuries. Delayed examination after the administration of intravenous contrast agents allows assessment of the pelvicalyceal system in cases of renal trauma. Pancreatic and duodenal injuries may also be identified, but detection of these injuries may be more problematic. Using CT, the accuracy of detection of bowel or mesenteric injuries is less than it is for solid organ injury, and these injuries should be suspected when there is free intraperitoneal fluid without an identifiable cause (**Figure 14.33**).

The image data may be reconstructed into thinner slices for the diagnosis of injuries to the thoracic and lumbar spine and for the better delineation of pelvic and acetabular fractures. Complex intra-articular fractures of the peripheral skeleton, such as calcaneal and tibial plateau fractures, may be usefully examined by dedicated thin-section studies provided this does not delay the treatment of other more serious injuries (**Figure 14.34**). CT angiography may be used to demonstrate vascular injuries in the limbs in those with penetrating injuries or complex displaced fractures.

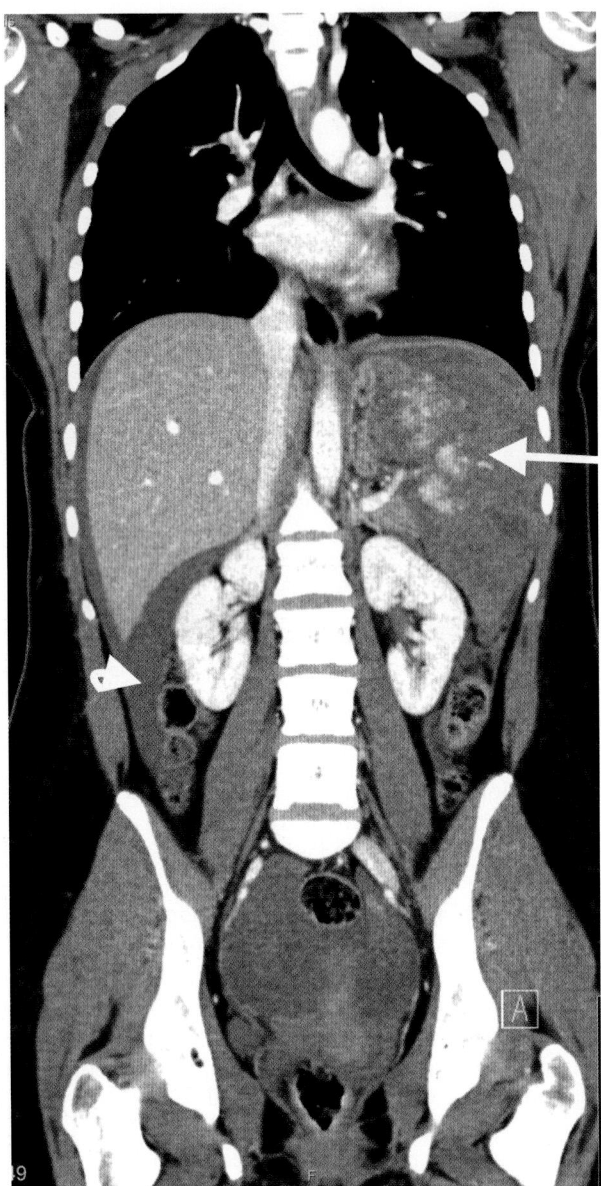

Figure 14.32 Coronal computed tomography image of the body shows a grade V splenic injury ('shattered spleen', arrow) with vascular injury at the hilum and free fluid around the spleen and liver (arrowhead).

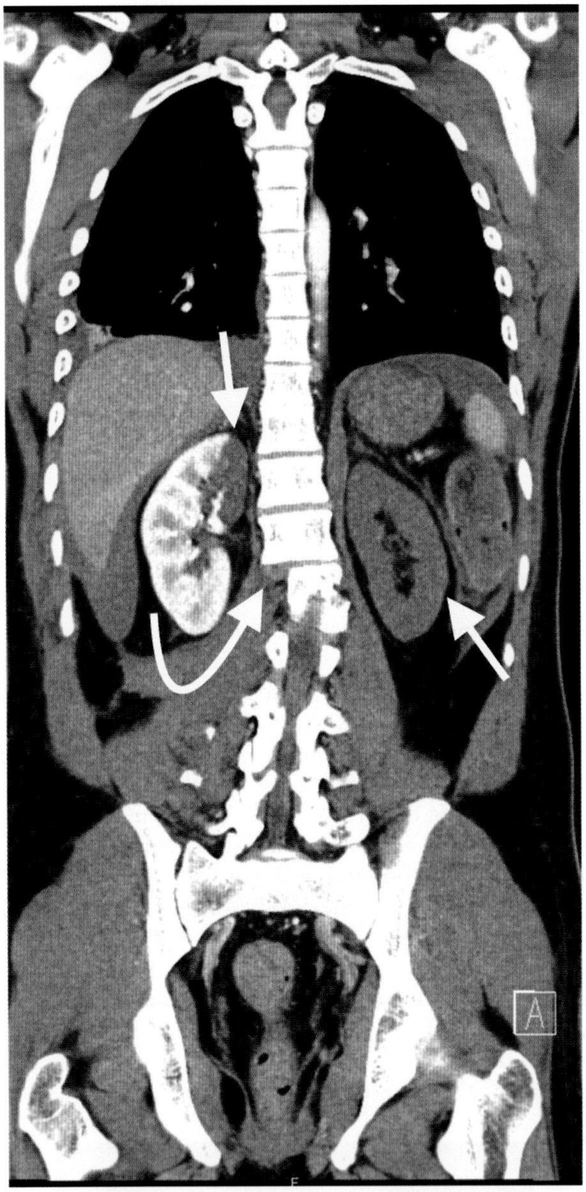

Figure 14.33 Coronal computed tomography demonstrating free fluid around the liver. The upper pole of the right kidney and left kidney demonstrate no contrast uptake in keeping with acute vascular injury (arrows). In addition there is a distraction injury with lateral dislocation of the T11–T12 intervertebral junction (curved arrow).

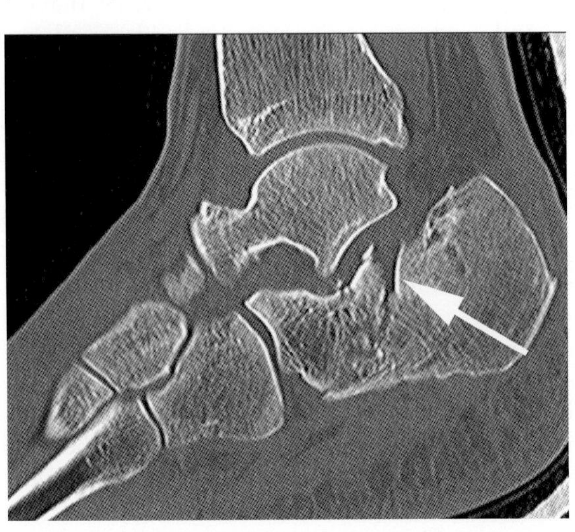

Figure 14.34 Sagittal reformats of computed tomography of the calcaneus in a patient following a fall illustrate a comminuted calcaneal fracture with intra-articular extension into the posterior facet of the subtalar joint (arrow).

Magnetic resonance imaging

The value of immediate MRI in trauma is relatively limited and is largely confined to the imaging of spinal injuries (Figure 14.35).

Access to urgent MRI is not widely available, and there are major practical problems in imaging patients who require ventilation or monitoring. MRI is therefore only practical in stable patients. All monitoring equipment must be MRI compatible, and ventilation support should be undertaken by staff skilled and experienced in these techniques as applied to the MRI environment. MRI may be used to diagnose injuries of the spinal cord and associated perispinal haematomas in patients with neurological signs or symptoms. MRI can supplement CT in spinal injuries by imaging soft-tissue injuries to the longitudinal and interspinous ligaments. MRI is mandatory in patients in whom there is facetal dislocation if surgical reduction is being considered, to minimise the risk of displacing soft-tissue or disc material into the spinal canal during reduction procedures. Subtle fractures may be difficult to identify, particularly if they are old, but an acute injury is normally identified by the surrounding oedema. Bony abnormalities should be reviewed using CT, as fracture lines are hard to identify with MRI and unstable injuries may be overlooked. In the less acute setting, MRI may also be used to assess diffuse axonal injuries, with an accuracy exceeding CT.

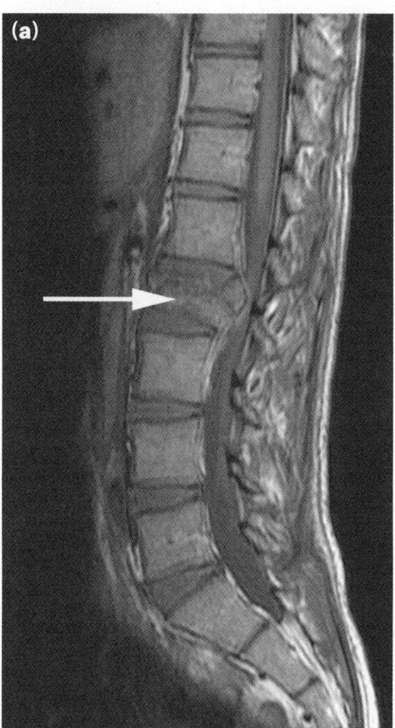

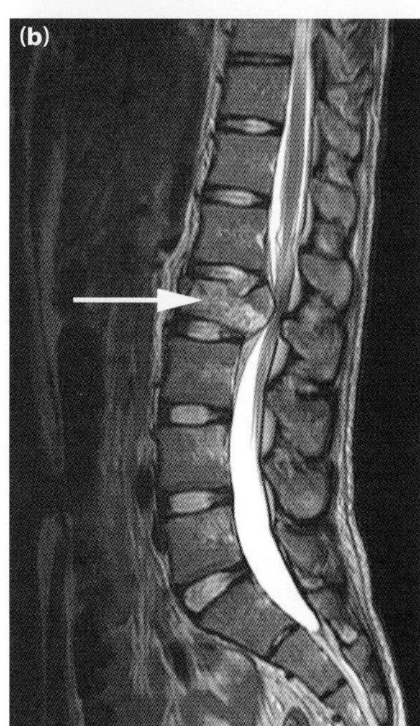

Figure 14.35 Sagittal T1-weighted (**a**) and T2-weighted (**b**) magnetic resonance imaging of the spine demonstrate a burst fracture of L2 causing neural compression (arrows).

Vascular interventional radiology

With the development and refinement of CT angiography techniques, the diagnostic role of formal angiography has become limited. CT angiography is the first-line investigation for aortic trauma and for penetrating and non-penetrating peripheral vascular trauma.

Endovascular techniques play an important role in the treatment of acute solid organ injuries, and the interventional radiologist should be consulted early in the decision-making process. Using coaxial catheter systems and a variety of available embolic agents such as soluble gelatine sponge and microcoils, selective embolisation and reduction of blood flow to the injured segment can be achieved without causing infarction. Selective embolisation techniques are also suitable for the treatment of patients with pelvic fractures with ongoing blood loss and volume issues. With penetrating and non-penetrating extremity trauma, balloon occlusion and embolisation may be employed to control haemorrhage, while the application of stent grafts can aid in re-establishing the circulation to the affected extremity.

IMAGING IN ABDOMINAL SURGERY

The acute abdomen

The term 'acute abdomen' encompasses many diverse entities.

IMAGING IN COMMON SURGICAL CLINICAL SCENARIOS

In this section the roles of different radiological modalities in common surgical scenarios are discussed, with a brief rationale behind their use and typical appearances of various pathological processes.

Bowel obstruction

The plain abdominal radiograph is a useful tool in diagnosing bowel obstruction. Small bowel obstruction can generally be distinguished from large bowel obstruction by virtue of the following: small bowel lies centrally in the abdomen while large bowel lies peripherally; the valvulae conniventes (folds) of the small bowel traverse the entire width of the lumen while the haustra of the large bowel do not; and the calibre of the small bowel is typically less than the large, even when obstructed (typical measurements in obstruction: small bowel 3.5–5 cm, large bowel 5–8 cm).

However, it must be stressed that a normal plain radiograph does not exclude an obstruction and if there is persistent concern, further imaging is indicated; CT is the modality of choice having largely superseded the contrast follow-through or enema, particularly in the acute setting. The key to diagnosis of a mechanical obstruction of either small or large bowel on CT, and differentiation from paralytic ileus, is identification of a transition zone from dilated proximal bowel to collapsed distal bowel. In small bowel obstruction if no obvious cause such as a mass, volvulus or intussusception is identified, then the most likely aetiology is adhesional. There is no need to give oral contrast for a suspected bowel obstruction CT as fluid in the lumen is a natural contrast agent and, in any case, oral contrast may well not reach the point of obstruction by the time of the scan. CT is also invaluable to diagnose complications of bowel obstruction such as perforation and ischaemia.

Closed loop obstruction, where the bowel is obstructed at two points, often in close proximity to each other and frequently related to an internal hernia or adhesional band, is a particular type of small bowel obstruction prone to developing ischemia, and should be suspected at CT if the bowel is dilated distal to a transition point with a further transition point more distally (**Figure 14.36**).

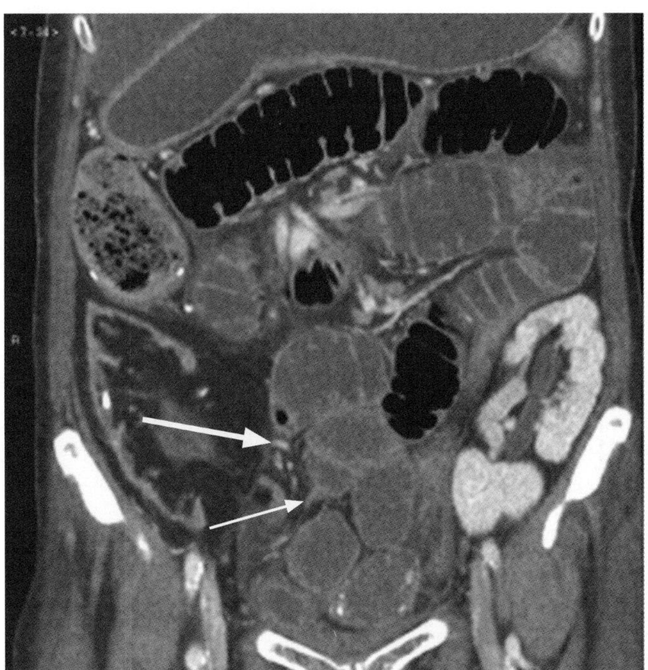

Figure 14.36 Coronal computed tomography showing a failed renal transplant in the right iliac fossa and second transplant in the left iliac fossa. There has also been a right hemicolectomy. There is proximal small bowel obstruction with dilated fluid filled small bowel loops. Distal to the first point of obstruction (large arrow) there are dilated thick walled fluid filled loops in the pelvis with some adjacent free fluid, which could be followed to a second point of obstruction (small arrow). The patient was taken to surgery, which confirmed a closed loop obstruction secondary to an adhesive band with ischaemia in the segment of small bowel between the points of obstruction.

Perforation

The erect chest x-ray (CXR) is the ideal first test for hollow organ perforation and as little as 10–20 mL of free air can be detected under the diaphragm, with the following caveats (**Figures 14.37 and 14.38**): about 10 minutes should be left between sitting the patient upright to allow air time to rise; the free air must be sought under the right hemidiaphragm to prevent misinterpretation of the gastric air bubble; and the reviewer must be able to recognise Chilaiditi's syndrome, the harmless and asymptomatic interposition of large bowel between the liver and diaphragm. Caution must also be exercised in interpreting any free air in the context of recent abdominal surgery, as air can persist for up to 5–7 days in the peritoneal cavity.

If the erect CXR is equivocal or a possible walled-off perforation is suspected, a CT is the optimal modality, which may show tiny quantities of free air but may also show the cause, e.g. peptic ulcer, diverticulitis or a neoplastic lesion. As with suspected obstruction, oral or rectal contrast is unnecessary if perforation is suspected as making the diagnosis should prompt appropriate management even if the precise site of perforation is not identified. Also, it cannot be overstressed that if there is any possibility of a leak from the gastrointestinal tract (including an anastomotic leak after surgery), then the use of barium is absolutely contraindicated as it can induce a serious and potentially fatal peritonitis.

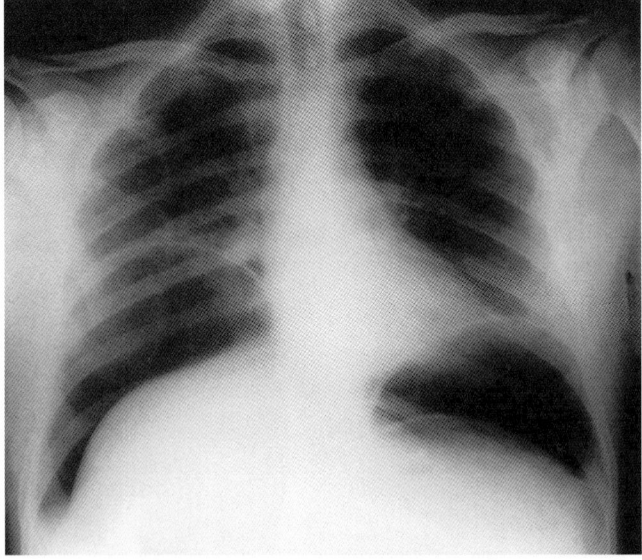

Figure 14.37 Erect chest radiograph showing marked bilateral elevation of the hemidiaphragms with a large volume of subdiaphragmatic free gas.

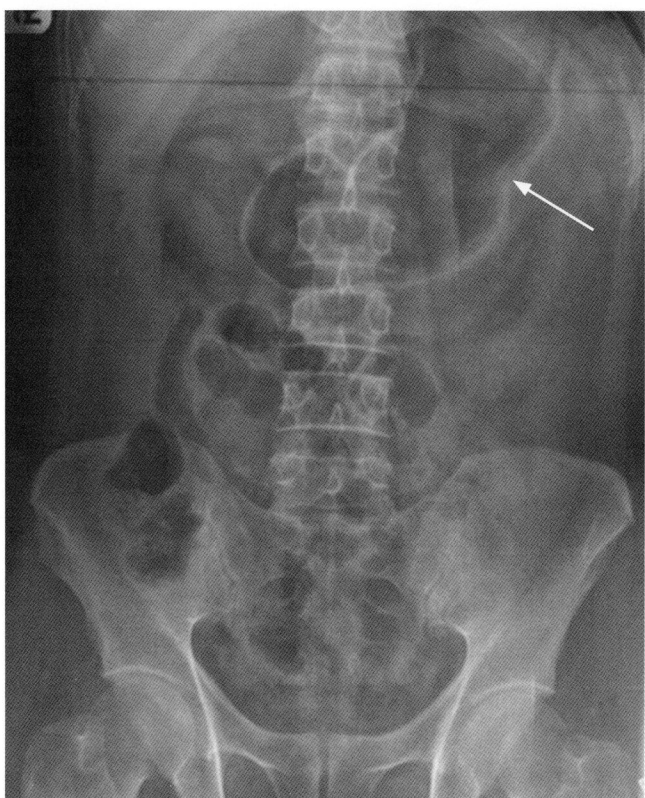

Figure 14.38 Plain abdominal radiograph showing an abnormal appearance to the gastric wall, which is very clearly visualised due to the presence of gas both inside the lumen and also outside the lumen (arrow). This is Rigler's sign of hollow organ perforation, in this case due to a duodenal ulcer.

Ischaemia/infarction

The most useful test when bowel ischaemia or infarction is suspected is a CT scan. Intravenous contrast administration is essential to look for thrombus/embolus in the mesenteric vessels, though ischaemia due to low flow states can still occur in their absence. Ischaemia can be a difficult diagnosis to make radiologically but is suspected, in the appropriate clinical context, by bowel wall thickening, submucosal oedema and free fluid between the folds of the mesentery (particularly if haemorrhagic). Ischaemia must be strongly suspected if these findings are seen in association with a closed loop obstruction or strangulated hernia. Ischaemic colitis typically affects the 'watershed area', which is the junction of the areas supplied by the superior and inferior mesenteric arteries, typically in the region of the splenic flexure.

When bowel wall ischaemia proceeds to transmural infarction, the diagnosis is usually more straightforward with evidence of pneumatosis (air in the bowel wall) typically identified. The air in the bowel wall can then track into mesenteric veins and thence to the portal vein, a CT sign of grave prognostic significance in an adult as it implies widespread and relatively long-standing bowel infarction.

Gastrointestinal haemorrhage

The aetiology of acute gastrointestinal haemorrhage varies between the upper gastrointestinal tract (GIT) (common causes including peptic ulcer disease, varices and Mallory Weiss tears) and the lower GIT (common causes including angiodysplasia, diverticular haemorrhage and neoplastic lesions). While endoscopy is a useful first-line investigation for both, in refractory or occult gastrointestinal (GI) haemorrhage radiology can also contribute to diagnosis and management. Nuclear medicine scans using radioisotope-labelled red blood cells are useful when bleeding is intermittent, but for patients suspected of active bleeding the best investigation is a CT mesenteric angiogram. Non-contrast scans to look for bright blood in the bowel lumen should be supplemented with scans in the arterial phase to assess for a blush due to active extravasation, and portal venous phase to optimise detection of wall thickening and masses and to look for sites of venous bleeding. If non-invasive imaging is effective, catheter angiography can be used to embolise a bleeding point.

Inflammatory processes

Appendicitis

Historically, a straightforward clinical diagnosis of appendicitis obviated any need for imaging, but with the proven accuracy of available modalities imaging has become increasingly popular to reduce negative appendicectomy rates and to make alternative diagnoses. While a plain radiograph may demonstrate a calcified appendicolith in the right iliac fossa, it is insufficiently sensitive or specific to be reliable. In children ultrasound is the best test, to reduce radiation exposure and due to typically favourable body habitus. This also applies to females of childbearing age, again to reduce radiation exposure, but also as the symptoms may be mimicked by gynaecological pathology, such as ectopic pregnancy, haemorrhagic ovarian cyst and tubo-ovarian abscess, all diagnoses best made with ultrasound. The definitive exclusion of appendicitis, however, hinges on the identification of a normal appendix, measuring less than 6 mm diameter. Retrocaecal appendicitis can readily escape detection with ultrasound, and thus CT is the next modality of choice and indeed frequently the first requested in most adults (**Figure 14.39**). The diagnosis of appendicitis on CT requires the identification of a thickened appendix (>7 mm), with periappendiceal inflammatory change as evidenced by stranding in the surrounding fat. Other signs that may be sought include free fluid, thickening of the caecal pole, possible localised small bowel ileus and right iliac fossa lymphadenopathy. Both CT and ultrasound can also identify collections if an inflamed appendix ruptures, and can be used to guide percutaneous drainage as a bridge to definitive surgery.

Diverticulitis

Inflammation of an obstructed diverticulum typically presents with left iliac fossa pain and pyrexia (**Figure 14.40**). While some authors have promoted the use of focused ultrasound

---

Leo George Rigler, 1896–1979, American radiologist, described the double wall sign in pneumoperitoneum.

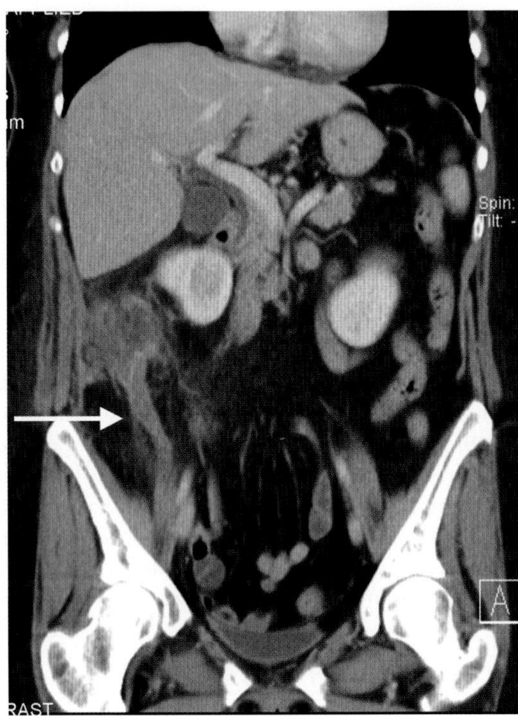

Figure 14.39 Acute appendicitis. Contrast enhanced CT scan reconstructed in the coronal plane demonstrates a thickened appendix in the right iliac fossa (arrow) with inflammatory changes in the surrounding fat and reactive thickening of the caecal pole.

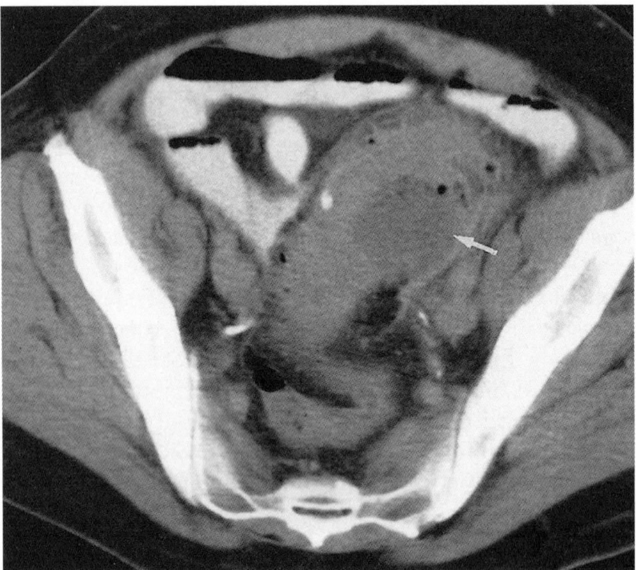

Figure 14.40 Computed tomography scan showing a segment of thickened sigmoid colon with a paracolic abscess (arrow) in a patient with diverticulitis.

for this indication, in general it is best diagnosed with a CT scan. The typical CT appearance is of pericolic inflammatory change around a diverticulum, most commonly in the sigmoid colon. Complications of diverticulitis include perforation, abscess formation, fistulation to adjacent structures and strictures in the bowel; CT is also the modality of choice to identify these, and as with appendicitis can be used to guide percutaneous abscess drainage as a bridge to definitive surgery.

Inflammatory bowel disease

The diagnosis of inflammatory bowel disease is made histologically, though a barium study of the small bowel, either a follow-through (where barium is ingested orally) or enteroclysis (where dilute barium is infused via a nasojejunal (NJ) tube) is often used as a screening tool if symptoms are vague. If the diagnosis of Crohn's disease is established, barium studies are useful to demonstrate the extent of disease, particularly to demonstrate the length and number of strictures if surgery is planned, although increasingly this role is being superseded by MRI enterography, which entails an abdominopelvic MRI scan after ingestion of an agent such as lactulose or mannitol to distend the small bowel. The other obvious advantage of MRI is the lack of radiation, particularly relevant in young patients with Crohn's disease who often undergo multiple imaging studies over their lifetime, and for this reason it is gaining in popularity for inflammatory bowel disease follow-up.

An acute flare up may also require imaging, and an ultrasound is usually a good first test to look for dilated bowel loops and any abscess, though CT may ultimately be required as gas-filled bowel loops can obscure visualisation of an abscess on ultrasound. MRI is the imaging modality of choice to assess perianal fistulae and abscesses.

Acute pancreatitis

As with acute appendicitis, when the diagnosis is straightforward clinically there may be no need for imaging, though increasingly it is used to confirm the diagnosis, to assess the severity of the process and to look for complications. While ultrasound may show gallstones and can demonstrate an enlarged pancreas with peripancreatic fluid and inflammatory changes, the optimal modality is CT. CT performed too early in the course of the attack, e.g. in the first 12 hours, can be equivocal and the optimal timing of imaging is 48–72 hours.

In mild acute pancreatitis, CT may be normal or may show an enlarged oedematous gland, but in more severe attacks other findings which should be sought include peripancreatic fluid collections, vascular complications such as arterial pseudo- aneurysm formation or venous thrombosis and necrosis either of the gland itself or of the surrounding fat. Necrosis typically develops 48–72 hours after the onset of symptoms, and is manifest on CT as lack of enhancement of the necrotic areas. CT with intravenous contrast is therefore essential to look for necrosis, which is potentially catastrophic particularly if it becomes infected. While CT is not always reliable to diagnose infected necrosis, it is suggested by bubbles of air in the necrotic segment. As with other intra-abdominal inflammatory processes, either ultrasound or more usually CT can be used to guide percutaneous drainage of inflammatory fluid collections.

Acute cholecystitis/biliary colic/jaundice

While acute cholecystitis is usually due to mechanical obstruction of the cystic duct or gallbladder neck by a gallstone, acute acalculous cholecystitis can occur in critically ill patients from a number of causes. In any case ultrasound is the modality of choice should this diagnosis be suspected, and the classic diagnostic features are of gallbladder distension with wall thickening (>3 mm). A gallstone obstructing the gallbladder neck or cystic duct may be visualised; alternatively, in acalculous cholecystitis sludge may be seen layering in the gallbladder lumen. Associated signs include pericholecystic fluid and hyperaemia on Doppler examination. Ultrasonographic Murphy's sign refers to tenderness over the gallbladder when pressure is applied while scanning and is a supportive finding in making the diagnosis. As a second-line investigation CT is also accurate for this condition, demonstrating similar signs of gallbladder distension and wall thickening with surrounding inflammatory changes. CT is also useful to diagnose complications such as gangrenous cholecystitis, gallbladder perforation and emphysematous cholecystitis, which may necessitate emergency cholecystectomy. If cross-sectional studies are equivocal, hepatobiliary scintigraphy can be useful, with the diagnosis of acute cholecystitis suggested by non-visualisation of the gallbladder 3 hours after radioisotope administration.

A frequent limitation of ultrasound is failure to visualise the common bile duct throughout its length due to overlying bowel gas, and elective cholecystectomy was typically accompanied by bile duct exploration to look for duct calculi. Increasingly, however, MRCP has been shown to be highly accurate in excluding bile duct calculi before surgery.

Ultrasound is also a useful first-line investigation for jaundice of unknown cause as it can demonstrate duct dilatation and gallstones. If a definitive cause is not shown with ultrasound, or a mass is identified but its precise nature and extent is uncertain, CT is indicated to look for common causes including stones, cholangiocarcinoma and pancreatic carcinoma. CT can not only identify malignant lesions but can also demonstrate the extent of local infiltration and the presence of metastases to determine potential resectability. If the ducts are of normal calibre in a jaundiced patient, liver biopsy should be considered.

Renal colic

The historical methods of imaging for renal colic all have their limitations. Plain film radiography may not demonstrate all calculi, will not show renal tract obstruction and is unreliable for alternative diagnoses. Intravenous urography (IVU) necessitates the administration of intravenous contrast and, if a level of obstruction is sought, delayed films up to 8 hours after injection may be required; it also will not provide alternative diagnoses. Ultrasound will demonstrate hydronephrosis and hydroureter, and calculi in the kidneys and either the proximal or distal ureters can usually be identified as echogenic foci with posterior acoustic shadowing; however, the ureter from just below the kidneys to the pelvis is usually obscured by bowel gas, which significantly impairs stone detection.

For these reasons the optimal investigation is now CT KUB, a non-contrast, low dose (2–3 MSv if a low mA scan is performed, equivalent to the dose from a limited IVU series) scan from the upper poles of the kidneys to the pubic symphisis. Contrast administration, either orally or intravenously, is not employed as it does not aid stone detection and may even impair it. Stones are readily identified as high attenuation (typically calcific) foci, and the secondary signs of acute ureteric obstruction may also be seen, including hydronephrosis and hydroureter, renal enlargement and perinephric fat stranding. The most common sites for stones to be seen are at the areas of ureteric narrowing, namely the pelvi-ureteric junction, the pelvic brim and vesico-ureteric junction. CT also offers unrivalled capability for making alternative diagnoses when compared with other modalities.

Abdominal aortic aneurym

If a pulsatile mass is felt in the abdomen and the diagnosis of a possible abdominal aortic aneurysm (AAA) is suspected, ultrasound is a useful modality and provided the aorta is not obscured by bowel gas an aneurysm can usually reliably be excluded. If, however, ultrasound visualisation is suboptimal and the diagnosis is as a result equivocal, or if an aneurysm is identified and information regarding the extent and exact size is required, for example for surgical or endovascular repair planning, CT angiography is indicated, with the aorta typically scanned from the arch to the pubic symphisis in the arterial phase after intravenous contrast. MR angiography is a useful alternative if iodinated contrast is contraindicated.

In the case of suspected aneurysm rupture, provided the patient is sufficiently haemodynamically stable to undergo CT, CT angiography should be urgently performed; a supplementary non-enhanced initial scan is useful to look for retroperitoneal haematoma, which is typically of relatively high attenuation compared to the blood in the lumen on a non-contrast scan.

IMAGING IN ONCOLOGY

Modern surgical treatment of cancer requires an understanding of tumour staging systems, as in many instances the tumour stage will define appropriate management. The development of stage-dependent treatment protocols involving neoadjuvant chemotherapy and preoperative radiotherapy relies on the ability of imaging to determine stage accurately before surgical and pathological staging. Once a diagnosis of cancer has been established, often by percutaneous or endoscopic biopsy, new imaging techniques can considerably improve the ability to define the extent of tumour, although the pathological specimen remains the 'gold standard'. Many staging systems are based on the tumour–node–metastasis (TNM) classification.

Tumour

In most published studies, cross-sectional imaging techniques (CT, ultrasound, MRI) are more accurate in staging advanced (T3, T4) than early (T1, T2) diseases, and the staging of early disease remains a challenge. In gut tumours, endoscopic ultrasound is more accurate than CT or MRI in the local staging of early disease (T1 and T2) by virtue of its ability to demonstrate the layered structure of the bowel wall and the depth of tumour penetration (**Figure 14.41**). Developments in MRI may also improve the staging accuracy of early disease. MRI is extremely valuable in bone and soft-tissue tumour staging and in intracranial and spinal disease.

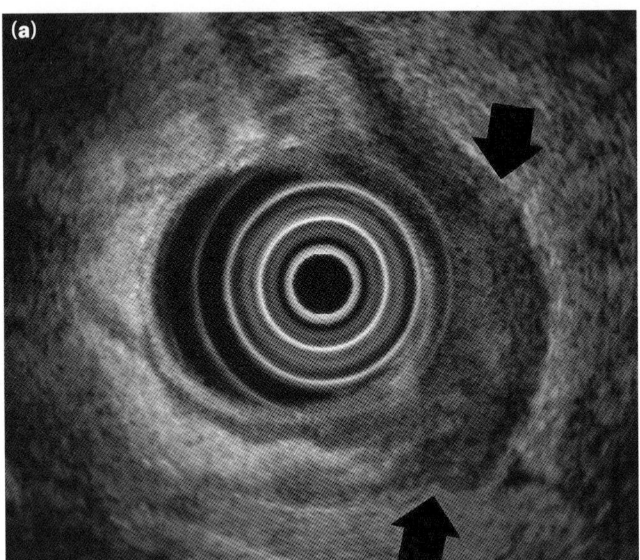

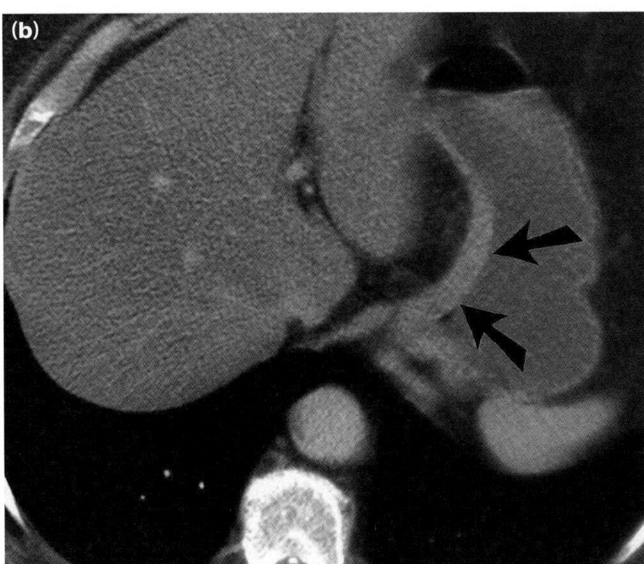

Figure 14.41 (**a**) Echo endoscopy in gastric cancer. The hypoechoic tumour (arrows) is destroying the layered structure of the gastric wall and extending out beyond the serosa. (**b**) Computed tomography scan demonstrates thickening and enhancement of the gastric wall in the same area (arrows). The stomach is distended with water to provide low-density contrast.

Nodes

Accurate assessment of nodal involvement remains a challenge for imaging. Most imaging techniques rely purely on size criteria to demonstrate lymph node involvement, with no possibility of identifying micrometastases in normal-sized nodes. A size criterion of 8–10 mm is often adopted, but it is not usually possible to distinguish benign reactive nodes from infiltrated nodes. This is a particular problem in patients with intrathoracic neoplasms, in whom enlarged benign reactive mediastinal nodes are common. The echo characteristics of nodes at endoscopic ultrasound have been used in many centres to increase the accuracy of nodal staging, and nodal sampling is possible via either mediastinoscopy or transoesophageal biopsy under endoscopic ultrasound control. PET-CT is of increasing use in detecting nodal metastases from a wide range of malignancies, with the capacity to coregister the area of increased FDG uptake with a precise anatomical location. Novel MRI contrast agents may help in the identification of non-enlarged tumour-infiltrated nodes.

Metastases

The demonstration of metastatic disease will usually significantly affect surgical management. Modern cross-sectional imaging has greatly improved the detection of metastases, but occult lesions will be overlooked in between 10% and 30% of patients. CT is the most sensitive technique for the detection of lung deposits, although the decision to perform CT will depend on the site of the primary tumour, its likelihood of intrapulmonary spread and the effect on staging and subsequent therapy of the demonstration of intrapulmonary deposits.

Ultrasound and CT are most frequently used to detect liver metastases. Contrast-enhanced CT can detect most lesions greater than 1 cm, although accuracy rates vary with the technique used and range from 70% to 90%. Recent studies suggest that MRI may be more accurate than CT in demonstrating metastatic disease. Preoperative identification of the segment of the liver involved can be determined by translation of the segmental surgical anatomy, as defined by Couinaud, to the cross-sectional CT images (**Figure 14.42**).

The technique of PET/CT with FDG, an analogue of glucose, is becoming a powerful tool in oncological imaging. This functional and anatomical imaging technique reflects tumour metabolism and allows the detection of otherwise occult metastases. The most common indications for PET/CT have been staging of lymphoma, lung cancer, particularly non-small cell lung cancer, and preoperative assessment of potentially resectable liver metastases, such as colorectal carcinoma metastases (**Figure 14.43**).

Intraoperative ultrasound is an additional method of staging that provides superb high-resolution imaging of subcentimetre liver nodules that may not be palpable at surgery. This is often used immediately prior to resection of liver metastases.

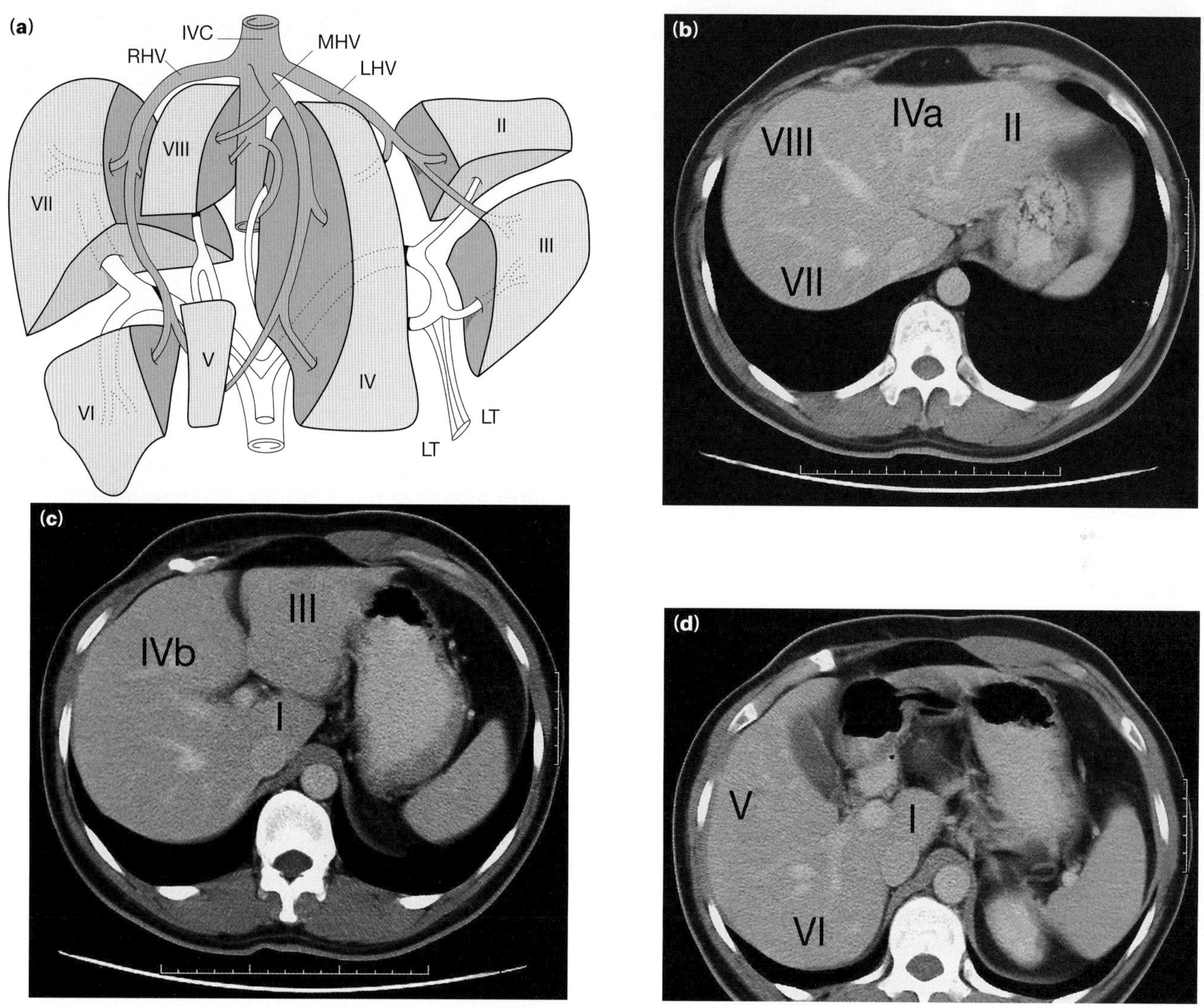

Figure 14.42 **(a)** Surgical lobes of the liver (after Couinaud). IVC, inferior vena cava; LHV, left hepatic vein; LT, ligamentum teres; MHV, middle hepatic vein; RHV, right hepatic vein. **(b)** Segmental anatomy on computed tomography scan at the level of the hepatic veins. **(c)** Segmental anatomy at the level of the portal veins. **(d)** Segmental anatomy below the level of the portal veins.

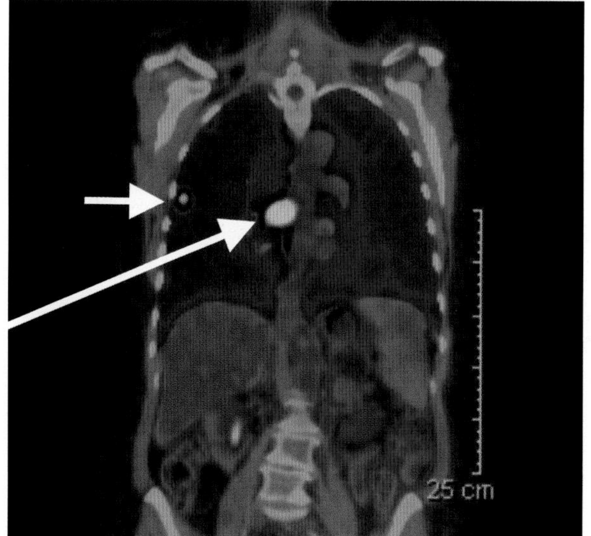

Figure 14.43 Positron emission tomography shows fluorodeoxyglucose uptake in a carcinoma of the lung (short arrow) and mediastinal lymph nodes (long arrow).

FURTHER READING

Adam A, Dixon AK (eds). *Grainger and Allison's diagnostic radiology: a textbook of medical imaging*, 6th edn. London: Elsevier, 2014.

iRefer Guidelines. *Making the best use of clinical radiology*, 8th edition. London: Royal College of Radiologists, 2017.

Krishnam MS, Curtis J (eds). *Emergency radiology*. New York: Cambridge Medicine, 2010.

Pope T, Bloem HL, Beltran J *et al. Musculoskeletal imaging*, 2nd edn. Oxford: Saunders, 2015.

Rockall AG, Hatrick A, Armstrong P, Wastie M. *Diagnostic imaging*, 7th edn. Oxford: Wiley-Blackwell, 2013.

Chapter 15

Gastrointestinal endoscopy

Learning objectives

To gain an understanding of:

- The role of endoscopy as a diagnostic and therapeutic tool
- The basic organisation of an endoscopy unit and its equipment
- Consent and safe sedation
- Special situations: the key points in managing endoscopy in at-risk patients
- The indications for diagnostic and therapeutic endoscopic procedures including endoscopic ultrasound
- The recognition and management of complications
- Novel techniques for endoscoping the small bowel
- Advances in diagnostic ability

INTRODUCTION

The gastrointestinal tract has a myriad of functions, such as digestion, absorption and excretion, as well as the synthesis of an array of hormones, growth factors and cytokines. In addition, a complex enteric nervous system has evolved to control its function and communicate with the central and peripheral nervous systems. Finally, as the gastrointestinal tract contains the largest sources of foreign antigens to which the body is exposed, it houses well-developed arms of both the innate and acquired immune system. Therefore, it is not surprising that malfunction or infection of this complex organ results in a wide spectrum of pathology. However, its importance in disease pathogenesis is matched only by its inaccessibility to traditional examination.

Few discoveries in medicine have contributed more to the practice of gastroenterology than the development of diagnostic and therapeutic endoscopy. Although spectacular advances in radiology have occurred recently with the introduction of multislice spiral computed tomography (CT) and magnetic resonance imaging (MRI), the ability to take targeted mucosal biopsies remains a unique strength of endoscopy. Historically, radiological techniques were required to image areas of jejunum and ileum inaccessible to the standard endoscope; however, the introduction of both capsule endoscopy and single/double-balloon enteroscopy allows both diagnostic and therapeutic access to the entire gastrointestinal tract. Image enhancement with techniques such as chromoendoscopy, magnification endoscopy and narrow band imaging allows increased resolution at the mucosal level and increases diagnostic yield. Endoscopic ultrasound can examine all layers of the intestinal wall as well as extraintestinal structures. Finally, experimental techniques such as confocal laser endomicroscopy give resolution at a level compatible with standard histology. The advances in the diagnostic accuracy of endoscopy lend themselves to disease surveillance for specific patient groups as well as population screening for gastrointestinal malignancy. Likewise, there has been a rapid expansion in the therapeutic capability of endoscopy with both luminal and extraintestinal surgery being performed via endoscopic access.

As in all areas of interventional practice, competent endoscopists must match a thorough grounding in anatomy and physiology with a clear understanding of the capabilities and limitations of the rapidly advancing techniques available. Perhaps most importantly they must appreciate all aspects of patient care including preprocedural management, communication before and during the procedure and the management of endoscopic complications. This chapter aims to guide the reader through these areas in addition to providing an introduction to the breadth of procedures that are currently performed.

HISTORY OF ENDOSCOPY

Over the last 50 years, endoscopy has become a powerful diagnostic and therapeutic tool. However, its development required two obvious but formidable barriers to be overcome. First, the gastrointestinal tract is rather long and tortuous and, second, no natural light shines through the available orifices! Therefore, successful visualisation of anything beyond the distal extremities requires a flexible instrument with an intrinsic light source that can transmit images to the operator. The illumination issue was solved in 1879 by

Thomas Edison, but 25 years elapsed before a light source was incorporated into the primitive rigid endoscopes available at that time. The first approach to gastrointestinal tortuosity was an instrument with articulated lenses and prisms, proposed by Hoffmann in 1911. Again, approximately two decades elapsed before this concept was incorporated into a semiflexible gastroscope by Wolf, a fabricator of medical instruments, and Schindler, a physician.

The real breakthrough was the discovery that images could be transmitted using flexible quartz fibres. Although this was first described in the late 1920s, it was not until 1954 that Hopkins built a model of a flexible fibre imaging device. The availability of highly transparent optical quality glass led to the development in 1958 of the first flexible fibreoptic gastroscope by Larry Curtiss, a graduate student in physics, and Basil Hirschowitz, a trainee in gastroenterology. Over the next 30 years, the fibrescope evolved to allow examination of the upper gastrointestinal tract, the biliary system and the colon. In parallel with advances in diagnostic ability, a range of therapeutic procedures was developed (*Table 15.1*). Although the fibreoptic endoscope has been the workhorse of many endoscopy units over the last three decades, its obsolescence was guaranteed by the invention of the charge coupled device (CCD) in the 1960s, which allowed the creation of a digital electronic image, permitting endoscopic images to be processed by a computer and transmitted to television screens. Thus, the modern endoscope was born (**Figure 15.1**).

History does not sit still, and endoscopic evolution will continue with the replacement of much diagnostic endoscopy with capsule endoscopy and virtual imaging. Enhanced resolution using chromoendoscopy and even histological grade images have increased the diagnostic yield of surveillance procedures. Endoscopic ultrasound allows diagnosis and therapy to extend beyond the mucosal surface of the intestine.

TABLE 15.1 Historical landmarks of gastrointestinal endoscopy.

1958	Development of fibreoptic gastroscope
1968	Endoscopic retrograde pancreatography
1969	Colonoscopic polypectomy
1970	Endoscopic retrograde cholangiography
1974	Endoscopic sphincterotomy (with bile duct stone extraction)
1979	Percutaneous endoscopic gastrostomy
1980	Endoscopic injection sclerotherapy
1980	Endoscopic ultrasonography
1983	Electronic (charge coupled device) endoscope
1985	Endoscopic control of upper gastrointestinal bleeding
1990	Endoscopic variceal ligation
1996	Introduction of self-expanding metal stents
2008	Endomicroscopy delivers histological mucosal definition

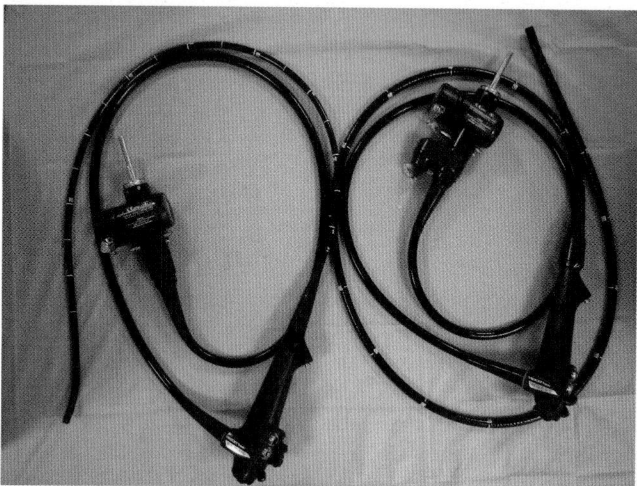

Figure 15.1 Photograph of standard gastroscope and colonoscope.

Traditional endoscopy will therefore become increasingly therapeutic and historical divisions between medicine, radiology and surgery will become progressively blurred. As the complexity of the procedures increase, the distinction between specialist and general endoscopists will become more definite. This reinforces the need for all endoscopic practitioners to have a detailed understanding of the units in which they work and the instruments that they use.

THE MODERN ENDOSCOPY UNIT

Organisation

A well-designed endoscopy unit staffed by trained endoscopy nurses and dedicated administrative staff is essential to support good endoscopic practice and training. Clinical governance with regular appraisal and assessment of performance should be a routine process embedded within the unit philosophy. Endoscopist training demands particular attention, with a transparent process of skills- and theory-based education centred on practical experience and dedicated training courses. Experienced supervision of all trainee endoscopists is essential until competency has been obtained and assessed by an appropriately validated technique, such as direct observation of practical skills (DOPS) and review of procedure logbooks. However, all endoscopists should keep an on-going log to record diagnostic and therapeutic procedure numbers and markers of competency such as colonoscopy completion rates, polyp detection rates, mean sedation use and complication rates. Central to this is an efficient data management system that provides outcome analysis for all aspects of endoscopy including adherence to guidelines, near misses, patient satisfaction, decontamination processes and scope tracking, as well as the more obvious completion and complication rates.

In the UK the Joint Advisory Group (JAG) provide guidance for endoscopist competence assessment and operate a

Thomas Alva Edison, 1847–1931, American physicist and inventor of Menlo Park, New Jersey, NJ, USA, produced the first carbon filament electric light bulb in 1879.

Harold Horace Hopkins, 1918–1994, Professor of Applied Optics, The University of Reading, Reading, UK.

Basil I. Hirschowitz, Professor of Medicine, Birmingham, AL, USA.

certification system of individual endoscopic competencies, based on procedure numbers, key performance indicators (e.g. caecal intubation rate, adenoma detection, sedation levels, complications), course attendance and peer assessment.

Equipment

A full description of all available endoscopic equipment is beyond the scope of this chapter. However, each unit should have a sufficient range of endoscopes, processors and accessories as dictated by the local case mix and sufficient endoscope numbers to ensure smooth service provision. These should include both forward- and lateral-viewing gastroscopes, an enteroscope for proximal small bowel visualisation and a range of adult and paediatric colonoscopes to aid examination of both redundant and fixed colons. Dedicated small bowel centres require capsule endoscopy and a single/double-balloon enteroscope for ileojejunal visualisation and therapeutics. Larger centres will require linear and radial endoscopic ultrasound, particularly if they specialise in gastrointestinal and hepatobiliary malignancy. An electrosurgical unit is the cornerstone of many therapeutic procedures and this may be supplemented by an argon plasma coagulation (APC) unit and laser units for advanced therapeutics in specialised centres.

Instrument decontamination

Endoscopes will not withstand steam-based autoclaving and therefore require high-level disinfection between cases to prevent transmission of infection. Although accessories may be autoclaved, best practice requires the use of disposable single-use items whenever possible. All equipment should be decontaminated to an identical standard whether for use on immunocompromised/infected patients or not. This process involves two equally important stages: first, removal of physical debris from the internal and external surfaces of the instrument and, second, chemical neutralisation of all microbiological agents. A variety of agents are available and endoscopists should familiarise themselves with the agent in use in their department. In 2014 the British Society of Gastroenterology has updated guidelines for decontamination of endoscopes (http://www.bsg.org.uk/images/stories/docs/clinical/guidelines/endoscopy/decontamination_2014_v2.pdf). Particular care should be applied to the decontamination of duodenoscopes due to reports of transmission of multiresistant bacteria.

Key points in endoscope decontamination are shown in *Summary box 15.1*.

There are currently no reliable means of decontaminating scopes from contact with prion-associated conditions such as variant Creutzfeldt–Jakob disease (vCJD), although risk of transmission of this is considered very low. If an 'invasive' procedure (where gut mucosa is breached and an unsheathed accessory withdrawn through the endoscope working channel) is conducted in a patient with known or possible vCJD, the endoscope needs to be quarantined after use. The performance of an invasive procedure in a patient at risk of vCJD due to receipt of pooled plasma concentrates is no longer deemed to confer a high risk of endoscope contamination. A single quality assured decontamination cycle is considered sufficient, but the endoscope should be decontaminated separately from others with a single-use disinfectant. There is no longer a requirement to quarantine the endoscope provided that routine traceability data can be demonstrated.

Summary box 15.1

Disinfection of endoscopes

- All channels must be brushed and irrigated throughout the disinfection process
- All instruments and accessories should be traceable to each use, patient and cleaning cycle
- All staff should be trained and protected (particularly if glutaraldehyde is used in view of its immune-sensitising properties)
- Regular monitoring of disinfectant power and microbiological contamination should be performed

CONSENT IN ENDOSCOPY

Approximately 1% of medical negligence claims in the USA relate to the practice of endoscopy. Many of these could have been avoided by a careful explanation of the procedure, including an honest discussion of the risks and benefits. Therefore, obtaining informed consent is a cornerstone of good endoscopic practice. It preserves a patient's autonomy, facilitates communication and acts as a shield against future complaints and claims of malpractice.

The most important aspect of the consent procedure is that a patient understands the nature, purpose and risk of a particular procedure. Current guidelines would suggest that a patient should be informed of minor adverse events with a risk of more than 10% and serious events with an incidence of more than 0.5%. The key risks of endoscopy are summarised in *Summary box 15.2*. The 2008 British Society of Gastroenterology Guidelines for consent can be found using the link http://www.bsg.org.uk/images/stories/docs/clinical/guidelines/endoscopy/consent08.pdf.

Summary box 15.2

The risks of endoscopy

- Sedation-related cardiorespiratory complications
- Damage to dentition
- Aspiration
- Perforation or haemorrhage after endoscopic dilatation/therapeutic endoscopic ultrasound
- Perforation, infection and aspiration after percutaneous endoscopic gastrostomy insertion
- Perforation or haemorrhage after flexible sigmoidoscopy/colonoscopy with polypectomy
- Pancreatitis, cholangitis, perforation or bleeding after endoscopic retrograde cholangiopancreatography

Hans Gerhard Creutzfeldt, 1885–1964, neurologist, Kiel, Germany.
Alfons Marie Jakob, 1884–1931, neurologist, Hamburg, Germany.

SAFE SEDATION

If performed competently the majority of diagnostic endoscopy and colonoscopy can be performed without sedation or with pharyngeal anaesthesia alone. However, therapeutic procedures may cause pain and patients are often anxious; thus, in most countries sedation and analgesia are offered to achieve a state of conscious sedation (not anaesthesia). Medication-induced respiratory depression in elderly patients or those with comorbidities is the greatest cause of endoscopy-related mortality and, therefore, safe sedation practices are essential. The involvement of anaesthetists to advise on appropriate protocols is recommended. Endoscopy in certain situations (particularly paediatric endoscopy) requires a general anaesthetic – this should only be undertaken by appropriately trained staff with adequate equipment available.

Summary box 15.3

Sedation in endoscopy

- Pharyngeal anaesthesia may increase the risk of aspiration in more heavily sedated patients
- Comorbidities must be identified so that sedation can be individualised
- All sedated patients require secure intravenous access
- Benzodiazepines reach their maximum effect 15–20 min after administration – doses should be titrated carefully, particularly in the elderly or those with comorbidities
- Coadministration of opiates and benzodiazepines has a synergistic effect – opiates should be given first and doses need to be reduced
- The use of supplementary oxygen is essential in all sedated patients
- Sedated patients require pulse oximetry to monitor oxygen saturation; high-risk patients or those undergoing high-risk procedures also require blood pressure and electrocardiogram monitoring
- A trained assistant should be responsible for patient monitoring throughout the procedure
- Resuscitation equipment and sedation reversal agents must be readily available
- The use of anaesthetic agents such as propofol for complex procedures requires specialist training
- The halflife of benzodiazepines is 4–24 hours – appropriate recovery and monitoring is essential. Postprocedural consultations may not be remembered, and patients must be advised not to drink alcohol or drive for 24 hours

ENDOSCOPY IN DIABETIC PATIENTS

As approximately 2% of the population is diabetic, managing glycaemic control before and after endoscopy is an essential aspect of endoscopic practice. Each unit should develop a policy for managing diabetic control during endoscopy. Factors influencing management include the type of diabetes, the procedure that is planned, the preparation/recovery time, and the history of diabetic control in the individual patient. Thus, a poorly controlled insulin-dependent diabetic undergoing colonoscopy will require more input than a type 2 diabetic on oral hypoglycaemic medication undergoing upper gastrointestinal endoscopy. All patients should bring their own medication to the unit and should be advised not to drive in case there is an alteration in their glycaemic control. The majority of patients can be managed using clear protocols on an outpatient basis; however, elderly patients and those with brittle control should be admitted. In general, diabetic patients should be endoscoped first on the morning list. In complex cases the diabetic team should be involved.

ANTIBIOTIC PROPHYLAXIS

The majority of endoscopy can be performed safely without the need for routine antibiotic prophylaxis. However, given that certain endoscopic procedures are associated with a significant bacteraemia (*Table 15.2*), there are several specific situations where antibiotic cover is required to prevent either bacterial endocarditis, infection of surgical prostheses or systemic sepsis. In general, the risk of infection relates to the level of bacteraemia and the risk of the underlying medical condition. Traditionally, patients with a previous history of endocarditis or a metallic heart valve received antibiotic prophylaxis for all endoscopic procedures, and some national guidelines still reflect this. However, in 2009 UK guidelines changed in response to the low reported incidence of infective endocaritis in this patient group undergoing endoscopy (http://www.bsg.org.uk/images/stories/docs/clinical/guidelines/endoscopy/prophylaxis_09.pdf). Patients with severe neutropenia may also require antibiotic prophylaxis for

TABLE 15.2 Approximate incidence of bacteraemia in immunocompetent individuals following various procedures involving the gastrointestinal tract.

Procedure	Incidence of bacteraemia (%)[a]
Rectal digital examination	4
Proctoscopy	5
Barium enema	11
Tooth brushing	25
Dental extraction	30–60
Colonoscopy	2–4
Diagnostic upper gastrointestinal endoscopy	4
Sigmoidoscopy	6–9
ERCP (no duct occlusion)	6
ERCP (duct occluded)	11
Oesophageal varices band ligation	6
Oesophageal varices sclerotherapy	10–50[b]
Oesophageal dilatation/prosthesis	34–54
Oesophageal laser therapy	35
EUS +/– fine needle aspirate	0–6

[a] Summary of published data.
[b] Higher after emergency than after elective management. ERCP, endoscopic retrograde cholangiopancreatography; EUS, endoscopic ultrasound.

endoscopy. The antibiotic regime used will depend on local guidelines. Procedures such as endoscopic percutaneous gastrostomy are associated with a significant incidence of wound or stoma infection, particularly if inserted for malignancy. There is excellent evidence that antibiotic prophylaxis reduces this complication and a single intravenous injection of coamoxiclav should be administered before the procedure. Ciprofloxacin is routinely used during endoscopic manipulation of an obstructed biliary tree in which it is unlikely that complete drainage will be achieved or there is significant comorbidity. When cystic cavities are aspirated at endoscopic ultrasound, a one-off dose of broad spectrum antibiotic (e.g. co-amoxiclav) is recommended to prevent cyst infection. Patients with chronic liver disease and ascites undergoing variceal sclerotherapy should receive antibiotic prophylaxis to prevent bacterial peritonitis.

ANTICOAGULATION IN PATIENTS UNDERGOING ENDOSCOPY

Many patients undergoing endoscopy may be taking medication that interferes with normal haemostasis, such as warfarin, heparin, direct oral anticoagulants, clopidogrel or aspirin. The key points to remember when managing anticoagulants in patients undergoing endoscopy are given in *Summary box 15.4*.

Summary box 15.4

Managing anticoagulants in patients undergoing endoscopy

It is important to recognise and understand:

- The risk of complications related to the underlying gastrointestinal disease from anticoagulant therapy
- The risk of haemorrhage related to an endoscopic procedure in the setting of anticoagulant therapy
- The risk of a thromboembolic/ischaemic event related to interruptions of anticoagulant therapy

Urgent endoscopy for gastrointestinal bleeding in the anticoagulated patient

The risk of clinically significant gastrointestinal bleeding in patients on warfarin is increased, particularly in patients with a past history of similar events, if the international normalised ratio (INR) is above the therapeutic range or if they are taking concomitant aspirin/non-steroidal anti-inflammatory drugs (NSAIDs). In these situations the risk of reversing the anticoagulation must be weighed against the risk of on-going haemorrhage. If complete reversal is not appropriate, correction of the INR to approximately 1.5 is usually sufficient to allow endoscopic diagnosis and therapy. Anticoagulation can often be resumed 24 hours after successful endoscopic therapy. If rapid resumption of anticoagulation is required, intravenous heparin should be used.

Elective endoscopy in patients on anticoagulants and antiplatelet agents

Endoscopic procedures vary in their potential to produce significant or uncontrolled bleeding. Diagnostic oesophagogastroduodenoscopy (OGD), colonoscopy, enteroscopy, diagnostic endoscopic ultrasound and endoscopic retrograde cholangiopancreatography (ERCP) without sphincterotomy are considered low risk, as is mucosal biopsy. High-risk procedures include colonoscopic polypectomy (1–2.5%), gastric polypectomy (4%), laser ablation of tumour (6%), endoscopic sphincterotomy (2.5–5%), EMR and ESD, stent placement and procedures with the potential to produce bleeding that is inaccessible or uncontrollable by endoscopic means, such as dilatation of benign or malignant strictures, percutaneous gastrostomy insertion and endoscopic ultrasound (EUS)-guided fine-needle aspiration. Likewise, the probability of a thromboembolic complication during temporary cessation of anticoagulant or antiplatelet therapy depends on the underlying medical condition (*Table 15.3*).

TABLE 15.3 The risk of a thromboembolic event varies according to the underlying medical condition.

Condition	Risk
Atrial fibrillation with valvular heart disease	High
Mechanical mitral valve	High
Mechanical valve and previous thromboembolic event	High
Deep vein thrombosis	Low
Uncomplicated atrial fibrillation	Low
Bioprosthetic valve	Low
Mechanical aortic valve	Low

Summary box 15.5

Recommendations concerning P2Y12 antiplatelet drugs (clopidogrel, prasugrel, ticagrelor)

Low-risk procedures

- Continue therapy

High-risk procedures, low-risk indication for antiplatelet therapy

- Stop 5 days before procedure (continue aspirin if taken)

High-risk procedures, high-risk indication for antiplatelet therapy (e.g. coronary artery stent)

- Liaise with cardiologist (consider stopping for 5 days if drug-eluting stent older than 12 months or bare metal stent older than 1 month)

Summary box 15.5 - *contd*

Recommendations concerning warfarin anticoagulant management

Low-risk procedures

- No adjustment to anticoagulation required
- Check INR within the week before procedure
- Avoid elective procedures when anticoagulation is above the therapeutic range

High-risk procedure in a patient with a low-risk condition

- Discontinue warfarin 5 days before the procedure
- Check INR on day of procedure to ensure <1.5
- Restart warfarin on evening after procedure if uncomplicated and recheck INR in 1 week

High-risk procedure in a patient with a high-risk condition

- Discontinue warfarin 5 days before the procedure
- Start low molecular weight heparin (LMWH) 2 days after stopping warfarin
- Check INR on day of procedure to ensure <1.5
- Omit LMWH on day of procedure
- Warfarin may be resumed the night of the procedure
- LMWH should be continued until INR adequate
- The decision to administer intravenous heparin should be individualised

Recommendations concerning direct oral anticoagulants (e.g. dabigatran, rivaroxaban, apixaban)

Low-risk procedures

- Omit on the morning of procedure

High-risk procedures

- Take last dose ≥48 h before procedure (for dabigatran ≥72 h before if estimated glomerular filtration rate (eGFR) 30–50 mL/min)

Aspirin

Aspirin and NSAIDs inhibit platelet cyclo-oxygenase resulting in suppression of thromboxane A_2-induced platelet aggregation. Limited published data do not suggest an increased bleeding risk in patients taking standard doses and, therefore, there is no need to discontinue therapy before endoscopic procedures.

UPPER GASTROINTESTINAL ENDOSCOPY

OGD is the most commonly performed endoscopic procedure. Excellent visualisation of the oesophagus, gastrooesophageal junction, stomach, duodenal bulb and second part of the duodenum can be obtained (**Figure 15.2**). Retroversion of the gastroscope in the stomach is essential to obtain complete views of the gastric cardia and fundus (**Figure 15.2**). Traditional forward-viewing endoscopes do not adequately visualise the ampulla, and a side-viewing scope should be used if this is essential. Likewise, although it is possible to reach the third part of the duodenum with a standard 120 cm instrument, a longer enteroscope is required if views beyond the ligament of Treitz are required. In addition to clear mucosal views, diagnostic endoscopy allows mucosal biopsies to be taken, which may either undergo processing for histological examination or be used for near-patient detection of *Helicobacter pylori* infection using a commercial urease-based kit. In addition, brushings may be taken for cytology and aspirates for microbiological culture.

Indications for oesophagogastroduodenoscopy

A full assessment of the role of OGD is outside the scope of this chapter. It will vary with local circumstances and the availability of alternative diagnostic techniques. OGD is usually appropriate when a patient's symptoms are persistent despite appropriate empirical therapy or are associated with warning signs such as intractable vomiting, anaemia, weight loss, dysphagia or bleeding. It is also part of the diagnostic work-up for patients with anaemia, symptoms of malabsorption and chronic diarrhoea. However, increasing ease of access to OGD with the availability of 'open access' endoscopy has resulted in a significant number of unnecessary procedures being performed in young patients with dyspepsia or gastro-oesophageal reflux disease (GORD). This has led to a number of international gastroenterology societies proposing guidelines for the management of dyspepsia and GORD, including the empirical use of acid suppression and non-invasive *H. pylori* tests, such as urease breath tests and stool antigen assay (e.g. the National Institute for Health and Care Excellence guidelines on dyspepsia: https://www.nice.org.uk/guidance/cg184/chapter/1-recommendations). In addition to the role of OGD in diagnosis, it is also commonly used in the surveillance of neoplasia development in high-risk patient groups. Whereas there is consensus about its role in genetic conditions such as familial adenomatous polyposis and Peutz–Jeghers syndrome, controversy remains about the role and frequency of endoscopic surveillance in premalignant conditions such as Barrett's oesophagus and gastric intestinal metaplasia (although ongoing studies will hopefully answer some of these uncertainties).

Therapeutic oesophagogastroduodenoscopy

Increasing technological advances have revolutionised the therapeutic applications of upper gastrointestinal endos-

Wenzel Treitz, 1819–1872, Professor of Pathology, Prague, The Czech Republic.
John Law Augustine Peutz, 1886–1968, Chief Specialist for Internal Medicine, St. John's Hospital, The Hague, The Netherlands.
Harold Joseph Jeghers, 1904–1990, Professor of Internal Medicine, New Jersey College of Medicine and Dentistry, Jersey City, NJ, USA.
Norman Rupert Barrett, 1903–1979, surgeon, St. Thomas's Hospital, London, UK.

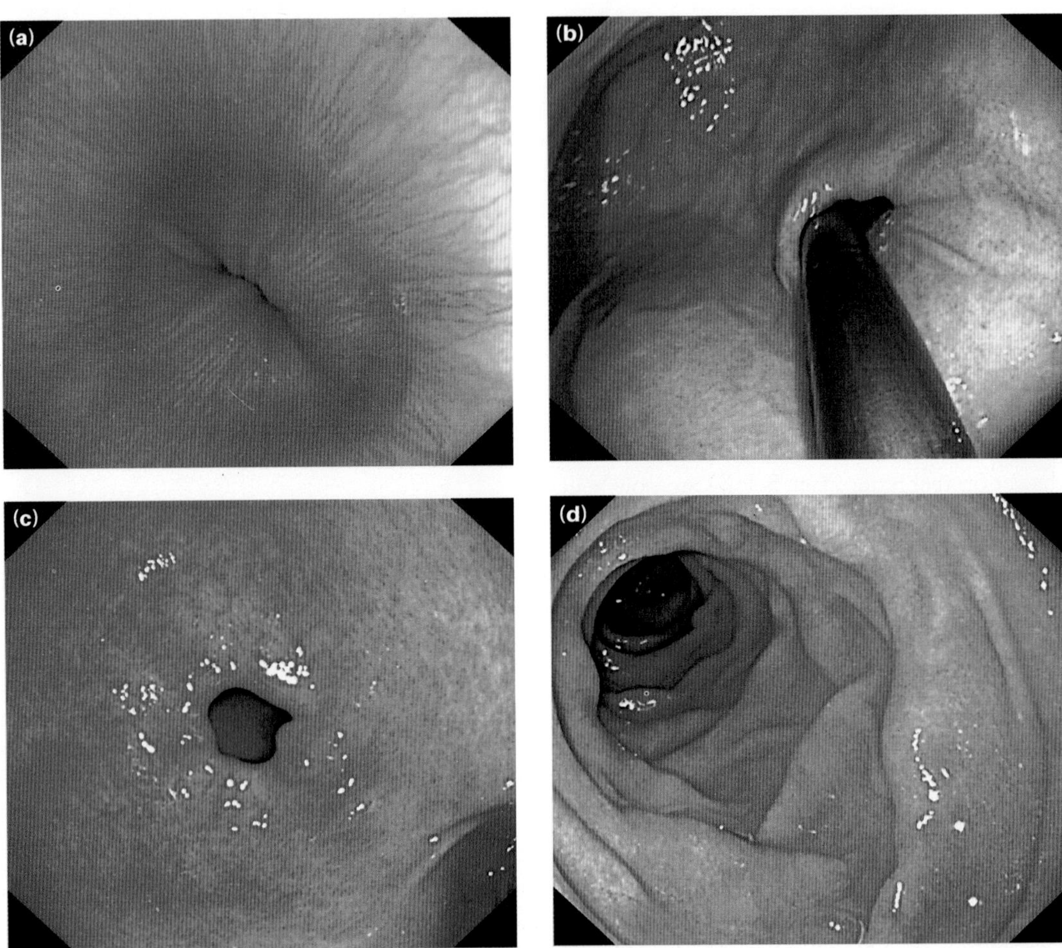

Figure 15.2 A normal upper gastrointestinal endoscopy showing the gastro-oesophageal junction (**a**), the gastric fundus in the 'J' position (**b**), the gastric antrum (**c**) and the second part of the duodenum (**d**).

copy. However, appropriate patient selection and monitoring is essential to minimise complications. The most common therapeutic endoscopic procedure performed as an emergency is the control of upper gastrointestinal haemorrhage of any aetiology. Band ligation has replaced sclerotherapy in the management of oesophageal varices (Figure 15.3), whereas sclerotherapy using thrombin-based glues can be used to control blood loss from gastric and duodenal varices. Injection sclerotherapy with adrenaline coupled with a second haemostatic technique such as heater probe vessel obliteration or haemoclip application, remains the technique of choice for a peptic ulcer with an active arterial spurt or high-risk stigmata

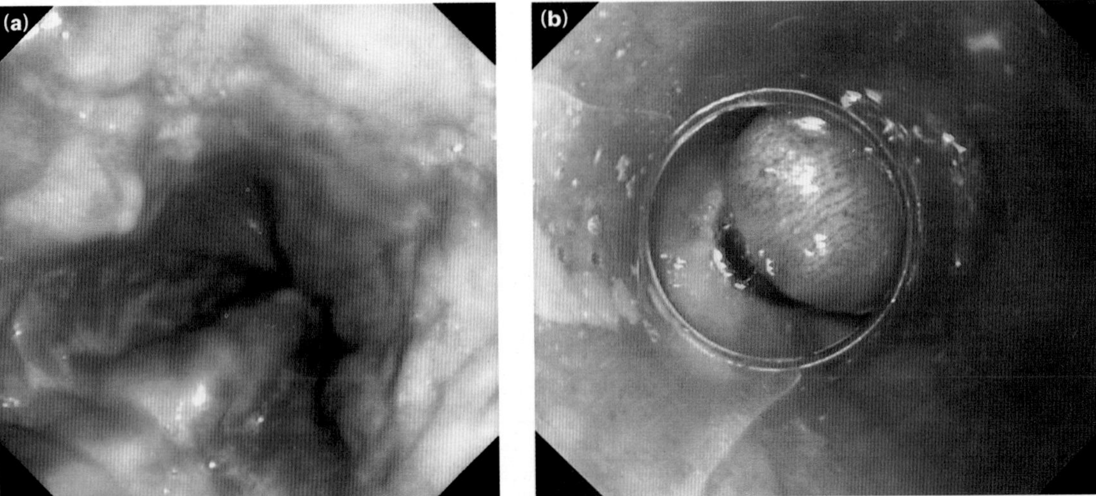

Figure 15.3 Grade 2 oesophageal varices (**a**), which can be treated by the application of bands to ligate the vessel and reduce blood flow (**b**).

of haemorrhage (Figure 15.4). Such high-risk bleeds should be followed by 72 hours of intravenous proton pump inhibition in all cases. Chronic blood loss from angioectasia is most safely treated with APC because of the controlled depth of burn compared with alternative thermal techniques (Figure 15.5).

Benign oesophageal and pyloric strictures may be dilated under direct vision with 'through-the-scope' (TTS) balloon dilators or the more traditional guidewire-based systems such as Savary–Guillard bougie dilators (Figure 15.6). On occasion, more difficult benign strictures can be treated by the insertion of a fully-covered removable stent, or with a biodegradeable stent. Likewise, the non-relaxing lower oesophageal sphincter associated with achalasia can be treated by pneumatic balloon dilatation with a 30–40 mm balloon. Endoscopic dissection techniques (see below) are now being employed to treat achalasia by natural orifice myotomy (peroral endoscopic myotomy, POEM) with good early follow-up results. An alternative in patients unfit to suffer endoscopic complication is the injection of botulinum toxin into the lower oesophageal sphincter, although this has a limited (3–6 month) duration of benefit.

There are a limited number of endoscopic techniques available to reduce gastro-oesophageal reflux, which rely on tightening the loose gastro-oesophageal junction by plication or by the application of radial thermal energy. These techniques may have a role in some patients, but are yet to demonstrate benefit over surgical fundoplication. Likewise, endoscopic techniques to tackle obesity, such as gastric balloon insertion, have not been associated with evidence of long-lasting benefit. In contrast, there is clear evidence that the insertion of a percutaneous endoscopic gastrostomy (PEG) tube enhances nutritional and functional outcome in patients unable to maintain oral nutritional intake (Figure 15.7). PEG insertion is often a prelude to treatment of

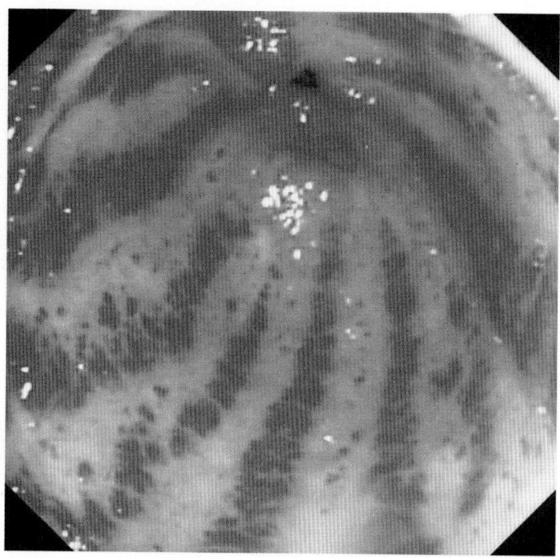

Figure 15.5 The classic appearance of gastric antral vascular ectasia (GAVE), which is often treated with argon plasma coagulation.

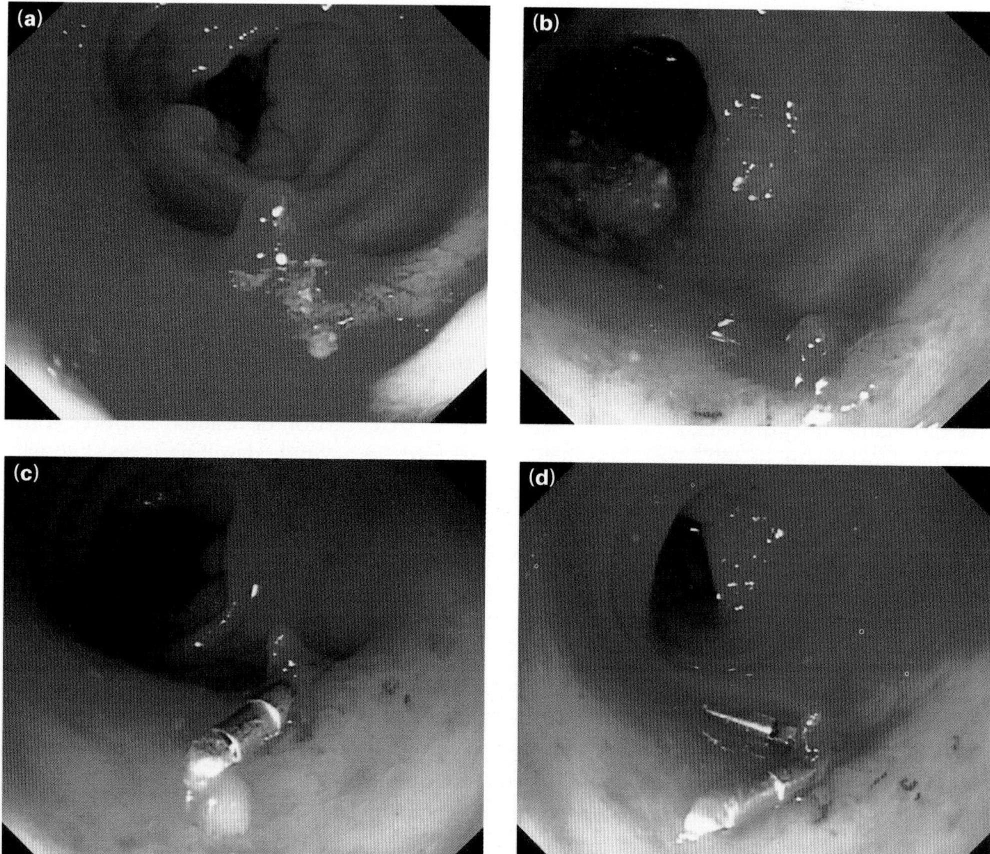

Figure 15.4 A gastric ulcer with active bleeding (**a**) is initially treated with adrenaline injection to achieve haemostasis (**b**). Two haemoclips are then applied to prevent rebleeding (**c and d**).

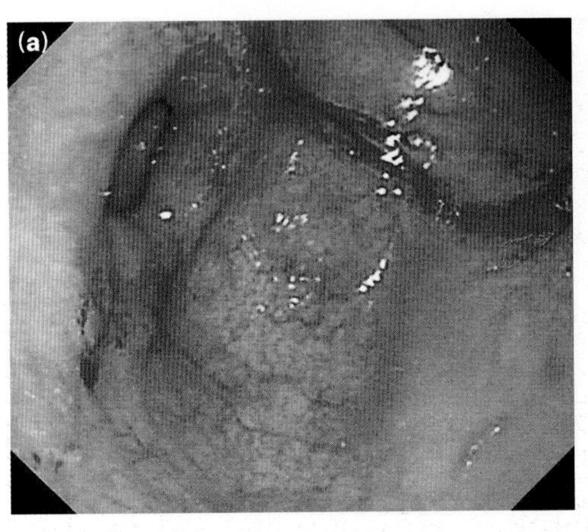

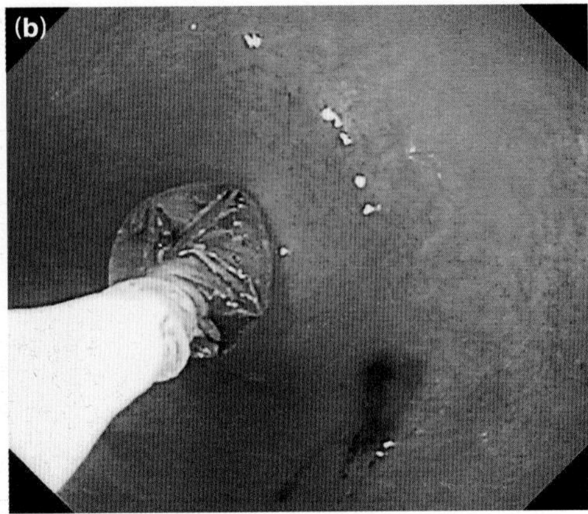

Figure 15.6 A pyloric stricture (**a**) can be dilated using a 'through-the-scope' balloon under direct vision to minimise complications (**b**).

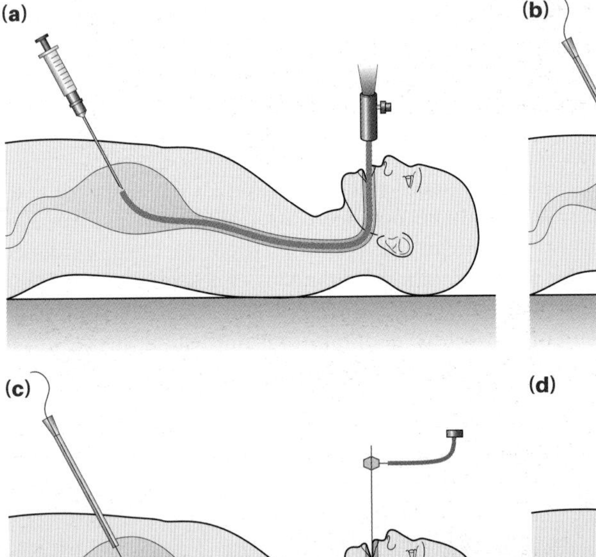

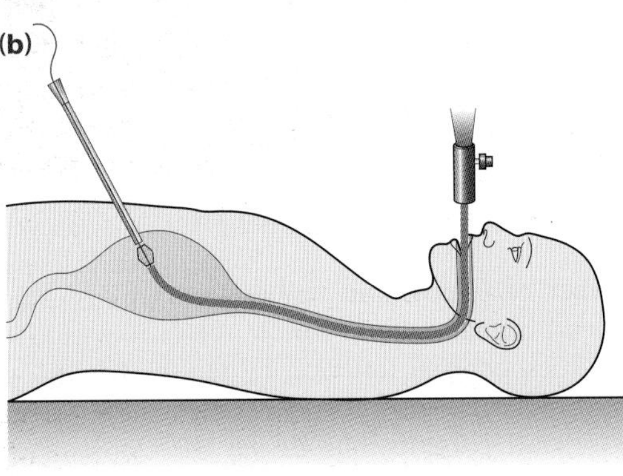

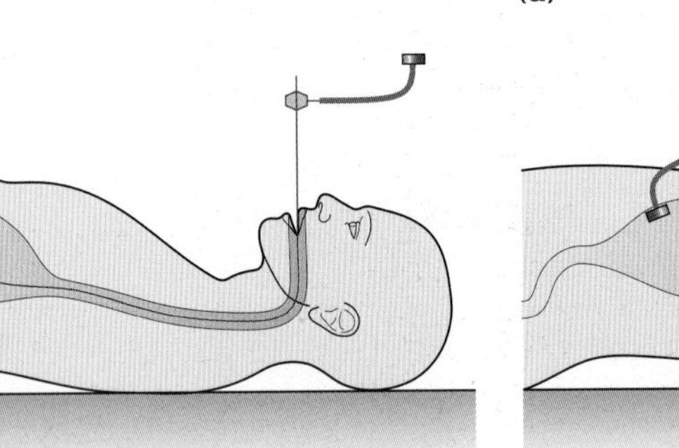

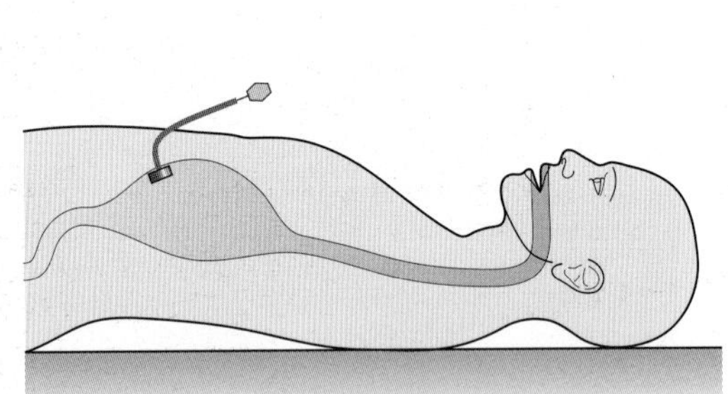

Figure 15.7 A schematic diagram of percutaneous endoscopic gastrostomy insertion. A standard endoscopy is performed to ensure that there are no contraindications to gastrostomy insertion. The stomach is insufflated with air and a direct percutaneous needle puncture made at a point where the stomach abuts the abdominal wall. Lignocaine is infused on withdrawal (**a**). A trochar is inserted and a wire passed into the stomach, which can be caught with a snare (**b**). The scope is withdrawn, pulling the wire out through the mouth, at which point it is attached to the gastrostomy tube (**c**). The gastrostomy is pulled through into the stomach and out through the track created by the trochar insertion (**d**).

complex orofacial malignancy, and may be used to support nutrition in patients with alternative malignant, degenerative or inflammatory diseases.

The deployment of self-expanding metal stents with or without a covering sheath inserted over a stiff guidewire leads to a significant improvement in symptomatic dysphagia and quality of life in patients with malignant oesophageal and gastric outlet obstruction (**Figure 15.8**). Covered stents are the mainstay of treatment for benign or malignant tracheo-oesophageal fistulae.

Perhaps the area of greatest progress over recent years has been in the endoscopic management of early oesophageal and gastric neoplasia with endoscopic mucosal resection (EMR) or endoscopic submucosal dissection (ESD). These techniques require specialist training, but have allowed endoscopic management of mucosal lesions that were previously subject to surgical intervention (**Figure 15.9**). A prime example has been improved endoscopic treatment of Barrett's high-grade dysplasia and early oesophageal adenocarcinoma. Destruction of residual Barrett's epithelium in cases of low- or high-grade dysplasia is possible with endoscopic ablation, and has been shown to reduce risk of progression to cancer. The most commonly used technique for this purpose is radiofrequency ablation, where 360° ablation can be achieved with a balloon catheter, or more focused ablation with smaller probes. Cryotherapy and APC can also be used for ablation, but photodynamic therapy is now used much less often.

Complications of diagnostic and therapeutic oesophagogastroduodenoscopy

Diagnostic upper gastrointestinal endoscopy is a safe procedure with minimal morbidity as long as appropriate patient

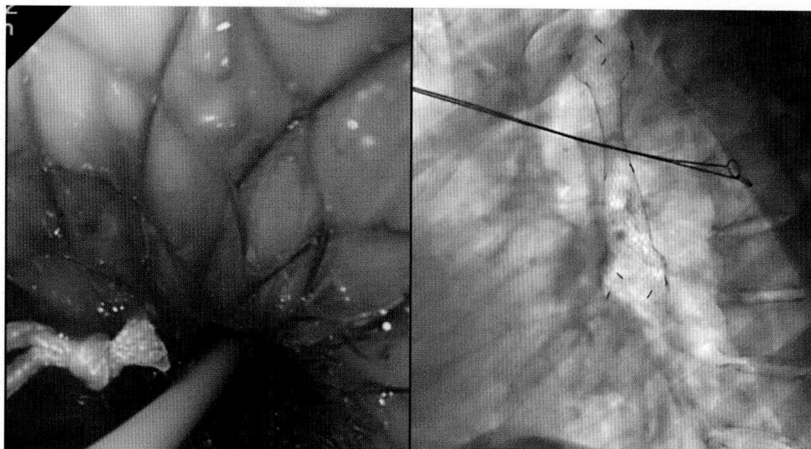

Figure 15.8 A self-expanding metal stent may alleviate symptoms relating to malignant oesophageal strictures. The left panel shows an endoscopic view of a deployed stent, and the right panel shows the radiographic image.

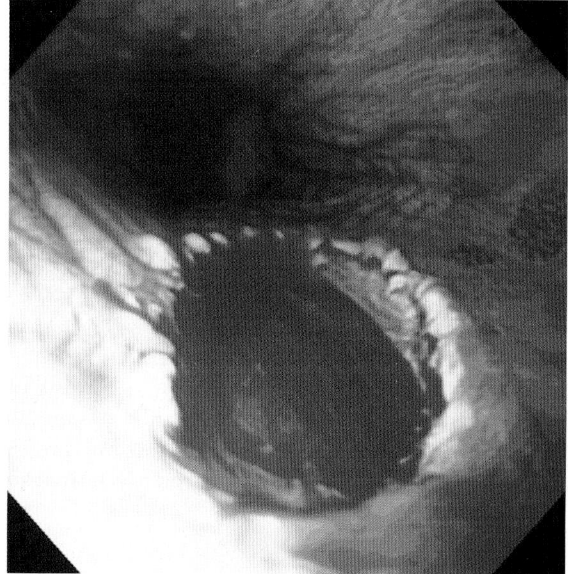

Figure 15.9 Novel upper gastrointestinal therapeutic uses of oesophagogastroduodenoscopy include the use of endoscopic mucosal resection to remove early gastric cancer leaving a clean base.

selection and safe sedation practices are embedded in the unit policy. The mortality rate is estimated to be less than 1:10 000, with a complication rate of approximately 1:1000. As mentioned above, the majority of adverse events relate to sedation and patient comorbidity. Particular caution should be exercised in patients with recent unstable cardiac ischaemia and respiratory compromise. Perforation can occur at any point in the upper gastrointestinal tract, including the oropharynx. It is rare during diagnostic procedures and is often associated with inexperience. Perforation is more common in therapeutic endoscopy, particularly oesophageal dilatation and EMR/ESD for early malignancy. Early diagnosis significantly improves outcome and thus all staff must be alert to the symptoms.

Prompt management includes radiological assessment using CT/water-soluble contrast studies, strict nil by mouth, intravenous fluids and antibiotics and early review by an experienced upper gastrointestinal surgeon.

Summary box 15.6

Symptoms of endoscopic oesophageal perforation

- Neck/chest pain
- Dysphagia/drooling saliva
- Abdominal pain
- Increasing tachycardia
- Hypotension
- Surgical emphysema

ENDOSCOPIC ASSESSMENT OF THE SMALL BOWEL

Introduction and indications

The requirement to visualise, biopsy and treat the small bowel is far less than in the stomach, biliary tree or colon, resulting in a time lag in technological advances. The most frequent indication is the investigation of gastrointestinal blood loss, which may present with either recurrent iron deficiency anaemia (occult haemorrhage) or recurrent overt blood loss per rectum (cryptic haemorrhage) in a patient with normal OGD (with duodenal biopsies) and colonoscopy. Other indications include the investigation of malabsorption; the exclusion of cryptic small bowel inflammation such as Crohn's disease in patients with diarrhoea/abdominal pain and evidence of an inflammatory response; targeting lesions seen on radiological investigations; and surveillance for neoplasia in patients with inherited polyposis syndromes.

A standard enteroscope is able to reach and biopsy lesions detected in the proximal small bowel; however, even in the most experienced hands this is limited to approximately 100 cm distal to the pylorus, although the use of a stiffening overtube may increase this somewhat. The procedure takes approximately 45 min and may be uncomfortable, requiring high doses of sedation with the attendant increased risk of perforation and sedation-related morbidity. Sonde endoscopy, in theory, has the potential to examine the entire small bowel. In this procedure a long thin endoscope is inserted transnasally into the stomach and pushed through the pylorus with a gastroscope passed through the mouth. It is carried distally by peristalsis, which propels a balloon inflated at the tip. The technique has several limitations including a long examination time (6–8 hours),

Burrill Bernard Crohn, 1884–1983, gastroenterologist, Mount Sinai Hospital, New York, NY, USA, described regional ileitis in 1932.

patient discomfort, the danger of perforation and the inability to perform therapeutic procedures. For these reasons it is not widely performed and will soon become obsolete.

Therefore, until recently, barium follow-through or enteroclysis were the most effective imaging modalities to visualise the distal duodenum, jejunum and ileum. Obviously these techniques do not give true mucosal views, and outside specialist centres their decreasing use has led to diminished expertise and a reduced diagnostic yield. There have been rapid advances in axial radiological techniques such as MRI and CT enteroclysis, which demonstrate excellent diagnostic accuracy in this area (see Chapter 14). However, although these techniques may yield information about vascularity and bowel wall thickening, they do not allow direct mucosal views, have no biopsy capability and have limited scope in terms of therapeutics. Historically, if an area of interest was outside the reach of a standard enteroscope, direct access via enterotomy under either laparoscopic or open surgery was required. Two major clinical advances over the last decade have revolutionised small bowel diagnosis and therapeutics. First, the development of the capsule endoscope allows diagnostic mucosal views of the entire small bowel to be obtained with minimal discomfort in unsedated patients. Second, the novel technique of single/double-balloon enteroscopy allows endoscopic access to the entire small bowel for biopsy and therapeutics (*Table 15.4*).

TABLE 15.4 Comparison of the advantages and disadvantages of the currently available modalities to endoscope the small intestine.

Technique	Advantages	Disadvantages
Traditional enteroscopy	Simple technique with wide availability Full range of therapeutics available Performed under sedation	Some discomfort Can only access proximal small bowel
Capsule endoscopy	Able to visualise the entire small bowel Preferable for patients No sedation Painless	No biopsies Not controllable and no accurate localisation Variable transit Incomplete studies due to battery life Not suitable for patients with strictures Large capsule to swallow
Double/single-balloon enteroscopy	Able to visualise the entire small bowel Full range of therapeutics	Requires sedation/general anaesthesia Patient discomfort May take 3–4 hours; may require admission Specialist centres only Complications include perforation

Capsule endoscopy

The prototype capsule endoscope was developed at the Royal London Hospital in the UK by Professor Paul Swain. Several companies have developed different systems for routine clinical use, but the basic principles remain identical. The technique requires three main components: an ingestible capsule, a portable data recorder and a workstation equipped with image-processing software. The capsule consists of an optical dome and lens, two light-emitting diodes, a processor, a battery, a transmitter and an antenna encased in a resistant coat the size of a large vitamin pill (**Figure 15.10**). It acquires

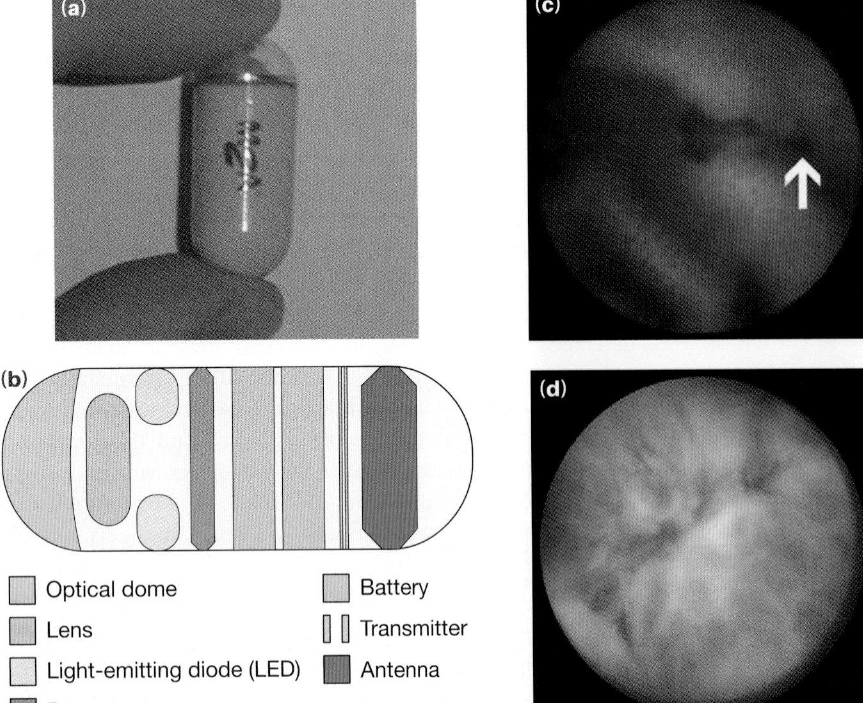

Figure 15.10 Complete diagnostic visualisation of the small bowel can be achieved with capsule endoscopy (**a**). The structure of the capsule is shown in (**b**). Clear mucosal pictures can be achieved here showing angioectasias (arrow) (**c**) and small bowel Crohn's disease (**d**).

Christopher Paul Swain, Professor of Gastroenterology, The Royal London Hospital, London, UK.

video images during natural propulsion through the digestive system that it transmits via a digital radiofrequency communication channel to the recorder unit worn outside the body; this also contains sensors that allow basic localisation of the site of image capture within the abdomen. Upon completion of the examination, the physician transfers the accumulated data to the workstation for interpretation via a high-capacity digital link. The workstation is a modified personal computer required for off-line data storage, interpretation and analysis of the acquired images and report generation.

The small bowel capsule provides good visualisation from mouth to colon with a high diagnostic yield. It compares favourably with the 'gold standard' techniques for the localisation of cryptic and occult gastrointestinal bleeding and the diagnosis of small bowel Crohn's disease. Use of the capsule endoscope is contraindicated in patients with known small bowel strictures in which it may impact, resulting in acute obstruction requiring retrieval at laparotomy or via laparoscopy. Severe gastroparesis and pseudo-obstruction are also relative contraindications to its use. Some units advocate a barium follow-through or small bowel MRI to exclude stricturing disease in all patients before capsule endoscopy. However, there are well-reported episodes of capsule impaction in a stricture that was not visualised on prior imaging. Therefore, a 'dummy' patency capsule that can be tracked via a handheld device or conventional radiology as it passes through the intestine should be used in all patients where there is a possibility of stricturing disease. The patency capsule will dissolve after 40 hours if it becomes impacted. Technology in this field is rapidly advancing, with capsule systems designed to image the oesophagus and colon nearing the market. Prototype capsules that can be directed, take biopsies and deliver thermal therapy to angioectasia are in development.

Single/double-balloon enteroscopy

This technique allows the direct visualisation of and therapeutic intervention for the entire small bowel and may be attempted via either the oral or rectal route. Double-balloon enteroscopy was developed in 2001 in Japan; it involves the use of a thin enteroscope and an overtube, which are both fitted with a balloon. The procedure is usually carried out under general anaesthesia, but may be undertaken with the use of conscious sedation. The enteroscope and overtube are inserted through either the mouth or anus and steered to the proximal duodenum/terminal ileum in the conventional manner. Following this the endoscope is advanced a small distance in front of the overtube and the balloon at the end is inflated. Using the assistance of friction at the interface between the enteroscope and intestinal wall, the small bowel is accordioned back to the overtube. The overtube balloon is then deployed and the enteroscope balloon is deflated.

The process is then continued until the entire small bowel is visualised (**Figure 15.11**). In single-balloon enteroscopy, developed more recently, an enteroscope and overtube are used, but only the overtube has a balloon attached. A full range of therapeutics including diagnostic biopsy, polypectomy, APC and stent insertion are available for balloon enteroscopy. Some experts advocate routine capsule endoscopy before balloon enteroscopy in an attempt to localise any lesions and plan whether oral or rectal access is more appropriate. The indications for single/double-balloon endoscopy are given in *Summary box 15.7*.

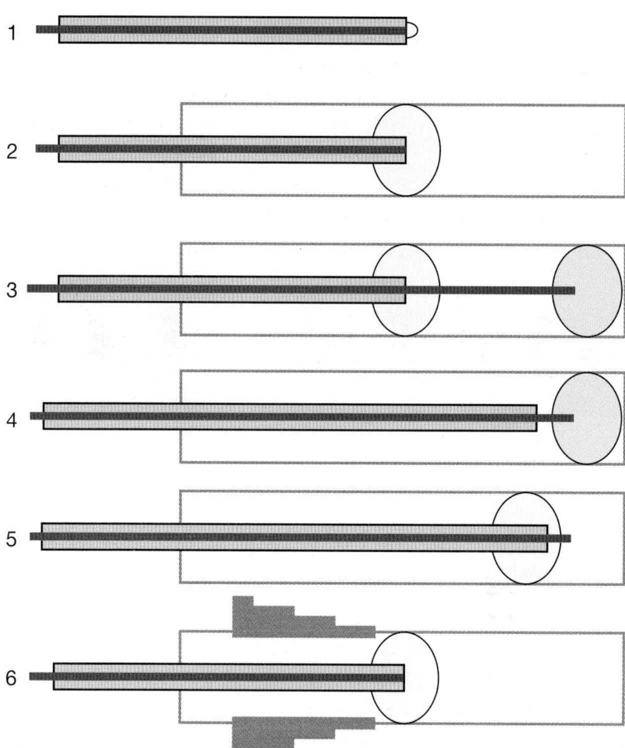

Figure 15.11 The technique of double-balloon enteroscopy is performed with an adapted enteroscope and overtube, both of which have inflatable balloons at their tip.

Summary box 15.7

Current established indications for single/double-balloon endoscopy

- Bleeding from the gastrointestinal tract of obscure cause
- Iron deficiency anaemia with normal colonoscopy and gastroscopy
- Visualisation of and therapeutic intervention for abnormalities seen on traditional small bowel imaging/capsule endoscopy

ENDOSCOPIC RETROGRADE CHOLANGIOPANCREATOGRAPHY

This procedure involves the use of a side-viewing duodenoscope, which is passed through the pylorus and into the second part of the duodenum to visualise the papilla. This is then cannulated, either directly with a catheter or with the help of a guidewire (**Figure 15.12**). Occasionally a small precut is required to gain access. By altering the angle of approach one can selectively cannulate the pancreatic duct or biliary tree, which is then visualised under fluoroscopy after contrast injection. The significant range of complications associated with this procedure and improvements in radiological

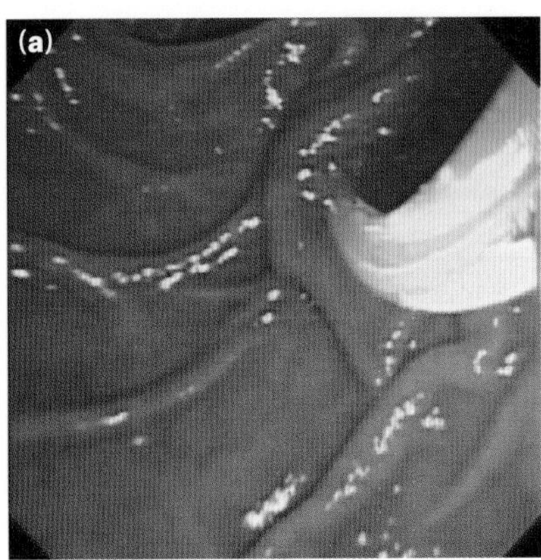

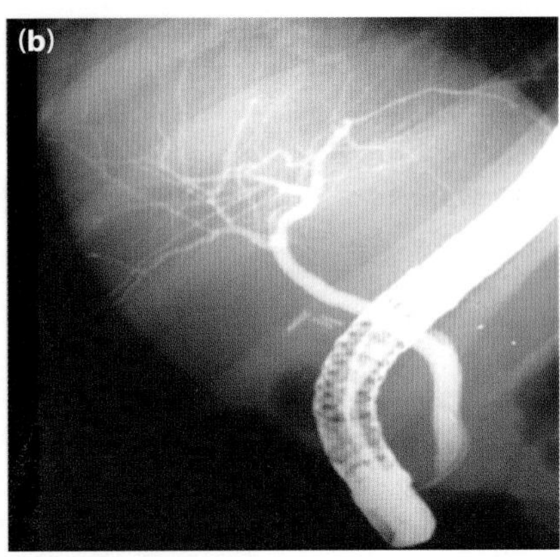

Figure 15.12 During endoscopic retrograde cholangiopancreatography a side-viewing duodenoscope is positioned opposite the papilla, which can then be cannulated using either a catheter or a guidewire (**a**). Contrast is injected to achieve a cholangiogram (**b**).

imaging using magnetic resonance cholangiopancreatography (MRCP) have rendered much diagnostic ERCP obsolete, and thus most procedures are currently performed for therapeutic purposes. There is still a role for accessing cytology/biopsy specimens.

Therapeutic endoscopic retrograde cholangiopancreatography

It is essential to ensure that patients have appropriate assessment prior to therapeutic ERCP, which is associated with a significant morbidity and occasional mortality. All patients require routine blood screening including a clotting screen. Assessment of respiratory and cardiovascular comorbidity is essential. The use of supplementary oxygen and both cardiac and oxygen saturation monitoring during the procedure are essential because of the high level of sedation that is often required.

The most common indication for therapeutic ERCP is the relief of biliary obstruction due to gallstone disease and benign or malignant biliary strictures. The preprocedural diagnosis can be confirmed by contrast injection, which will clearly differentiate the filling defects associated with gallstones and the luminal narrowing of a stricture. If there is likely to be a delay in relieving an obstructed system, percutaneous drainage may be required.

The cornerstone of gallstone retrieval is an adequate biliary sphincterotomy, which is normally performed over a well-positioned guidewire using a sphincterotome connected to an electrosurgical unit. Most gallstones less than 1 cm in diameter will pass spontaneously in the days and weeks following a sphincterotomy, but most endoscopists prefer to ensure duct clearance at the initial procedure to reduce the risk of impaction, cholangitis or pancreatitis. This can be achieved by trawling the duct using a balloon catheter or by extraction using a wire basket. If standard techniques fail, large or awkwardly placed stones can be crushed using mechanical lithotripsy. If adequate stone extraction cannot be achieved at the initial ERCP it is imperative to ensure biliary drainage with the placement of a removable plastic stent while alternative options are considered. These include surgery, endoscopically directed shockwaves under direct choledochoscopic vision (see below) and extracorporeal shockwave lithotripsy with subsequent ERCP to remove stone fragments.

Dilation of benign biliary strictures uses balloon catheters similar to those used in angioplasty inserted over a guidewire under fluoroscopic control. It is traditional to insert a temporary plastic stent to maintain drainage as several attempts at dilatation may be required. Self-expanding metal stents are most commonly used for the palliation of malignant biliary obstruction and are also normally inserted after a modest sphincterotomy. Correct stent placement can normally be confirmed by a flow of bile after release and by the presence of air in the biliary tree on follow-up plain abdominal radiographs. Stent malfunction, associated with recurrent or persistent biochemical cholestasis, may be due to poor initial stent position, stent migration, blockage with blood clot or debris or tumour ingrowth. A repeat procedure is required to assess the cause, which can usually be remedied by the insertion of a second stent through the original one.

In addition to the standard techniques discussed above, ERCP is also used for pancreatic disease and the assessment of biliary dysmotility (sphincter of Oddi dysfunction) using manometry in specialist centres. Indications include pancreatic stone extraction, the dilatation of pancreatic duct strictures and the transgastric drainage of pancreatic pseudocysts. To minimise the risks of subsequent pancreatitis, pancreatic sphincterotomy is most safely performed after the placement of a temporary pancreatic stent to prevent stasis within the pancreatic duct.

Visualisation and sampling of biliary lesions is becoming easier and more effective with the development of newer through-the-duodenoscope cholangioscopes that allow direct visualisation and instrumentation of the biliary and pancreatic ducts.

Complications associated with endoscopic retrograde cholangiopancreatography

The same risks associated with other endoscopic procedures also apply to patients undergoing ERCP, but risks may be increased because of the increased patient frailty and high sedation levels required. Complications specific to ERCP

Ruggero Oddi, 1845–1906, physiologist, Perugia, who later worked in Rome, Italy.

include duodenal perforation (1.3%)/haemorrhage (1.4%) after scope insertion or sphincterotomy, pancreatitis (4.3%) and sepsis (3–30%); the mortality rate approaches 1%. It is important to remember that postsphincterotomy complications may be retroperitoneal and, therefore, CT scanning is essential in patients with pain, tachycardia or hypotension postprocedure. Although normally mild, post-ERCP pancreatitis can be severe with extensive pancreatic necrosis and a significant mortality rate (*Table 15.5*). Many trials have assessed pharmacological strategies to reduce the incidence of pancreatitis. It is now recommended that, where there is no contraindication, all patients undergoing ERCP should be administered per-rectal indomethacin or diclofenac immediately before or after the procedure to reduce the risk of post-ERCP pancreatitis.

TABLE 15.5 Risk factors for post-ERCP pancreatitis.

Definite	Suspected SOD
	Young age
	Normal bilirubin
	Prior ERCP-related pancreatitis
	Difficult cannulation
	Pancreatic duct contrast injection
	Pancreatic sphincterotomy
	Balloon dilatation of biliary sphincter
Possible	Female sex
	Low volume of ERCPs performed
	Absent CBD stone

CBD, common bile duct; ERCP, endoscopic retrograde cholangiopancreatography; SOD, sphincter of Oddi dysfunction.

COLONOSCOPY

Early attempts at colonoscopy were hindered by poor technique and the limitations of the available instruments. The ability to steer an endoscope around the entire colon and into the terminal ileum was made possible by the development of fully flexible colonoscopes with greater than 90° angulation of the tip. Advances in bowel preparation have enhanced mucosal visualisation during the examination. Two key revelations about the practical performance of colonoscopy have allowed skilled operatives to achieve a greater than 95% caecal intubation rate and frequent ileal intubation with minimal discomfort using light sedation. The first is that continued inward pressure of the endoscope results in the formation of loops within the mobile sigmoid and transverse colon, decreasing angulation control at the tip and removing the beneficial effect of shaft torque to aid steering around acute bends. The second is that pulling back the scope regularly with appropriate torque to ensure a straight passage through the sigmoid colon and around the splenic flexure greatly aids the completion of right-sided examination. Targeted abdominal hand pressure to prevent loops in a mobile colon and regular patient position change to enhance mucosal views and remove residual bowel content are also important aids to successful colonoscopy. It is essential that caecal intubation is confirmed to avoid missing pathology by incorrectly assuming that the caecal pole has been reached. The landmarks may not be clear and, therefore, visualisation of the appendix orifice or preferably terminal ileal intubation is necessary to confirm a complete colonoscopy (**Figure 15.13**).

Mucosal biopsies may either be targeted to areas of abnormality or random to exclude microscopic colitis in a patient

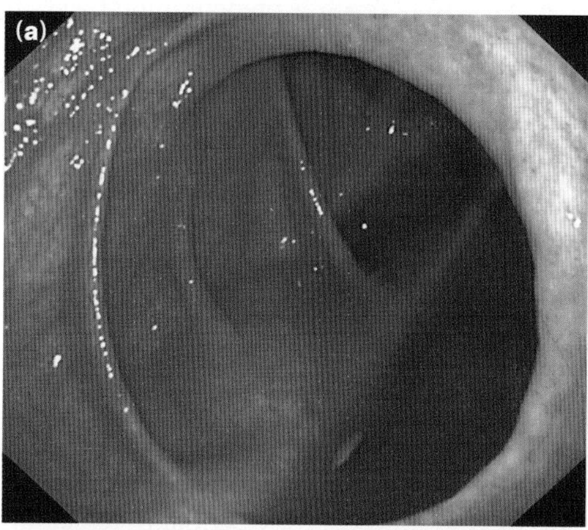

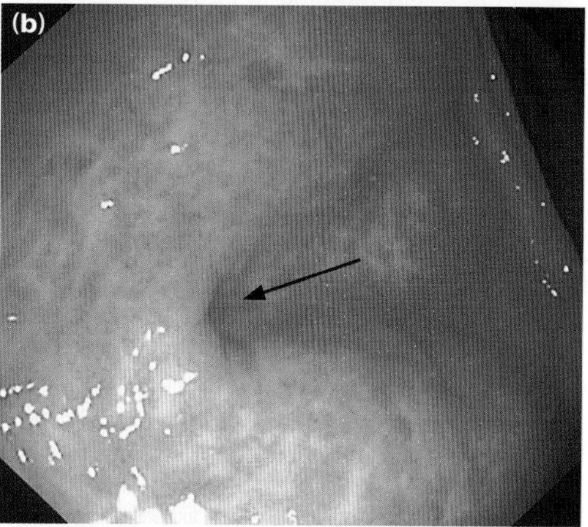

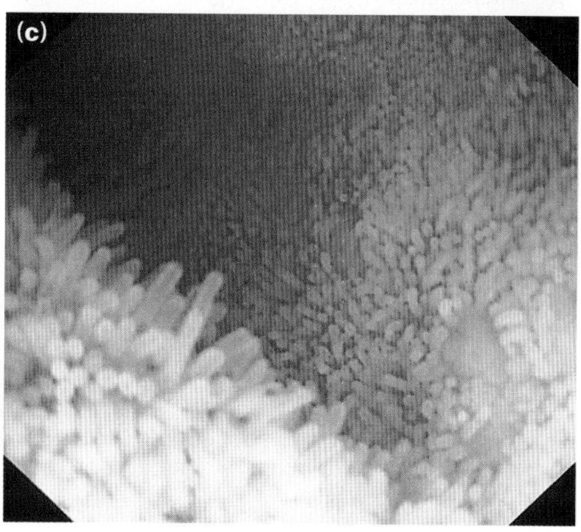

Figure 15.13 The caecal pole may not be easy to identify (**a**) and, therefore, the endoscopist should confirm complete colonoscopy by visualising the appendix orifice (**b**) (arrow) or preferably intubating the terminal ileum (**c**), which demonstrates villi and Peyer's patches.

Johann Conrad Peyer, 1653–1712, Professor of Logic, Rhetoric and Medicine, Schaffhausen, Switzerland, described the lymph follicles in the intestine in 1677.

with chronic watery diarrhoea but a macroscopically normal mucosa. Despite the increasing sophistication of radiological techniques to assess the colon, such as CT colonography, the ability to biopsy areas of abnormality and resect polyps will ensure that colonoscopy remains the most appropriate investigation for the majority of patients. Several countries including the USA and the UK have recently introduced colorectal cancer (CRC) screening programmes in the asymptomatic population once they reach a predetermined age. The goal is to increase the number of early-stage CRCs detected and hence decrease mortality, as well as to identify and remove adenomatous polyps and prevent the onset of disease. Increased polyp detection rates are associated with a longer period of colonoscope withdrawal, optimal bowel preparation and retroversion of the colonoscope in the right colon to visualise both sides of colonic folds. Current research is assessing whether polyp detection rates are also increased by the use of devices such as a 'third eye' and an endocuff. There is ongoing debate about the relevant benefits of different screening modalities including colonoscopy, CT colonography, flexible sigmoidoscopy and biannual/one-off faecal occult blood testing with colonoscopy only in positive patients. Whichever modality is used, colonoscopy is essential to resect any polyps identified and biopsy unresectable lesions.

Summary box 15.8

Indications for colonoscopy

- Rectal bleeding with looser or more frequent stools +/− abdominal pain related to bowel actions
- Iron deficiency anaemia (after biochemical confirmation +/− negative coeliac serology): oesophagogastroduodenoscopy and colonoscopy together
- Right iliac fossa mass if ultrasound is suggestive of colonic origin
- Change in bowel habit associated with fever/elevated inflammatory response
- Chronic diarrhoea (>6 weeks) after sigmoidoscopy/rectal biopsy and negative coeliac serology
- Follow-up of colorectal cancer and polyps
- Screening of patients with a family history of colorectal cancer
- Assessment/removal of a lesion seen on radiological examination
- Assessment of ulcerative colitis/Crohn's extent and activity
- Surveillance of inflammatory bowel disease
- Surveillance of acromegaly/ureterosigmoidostomy

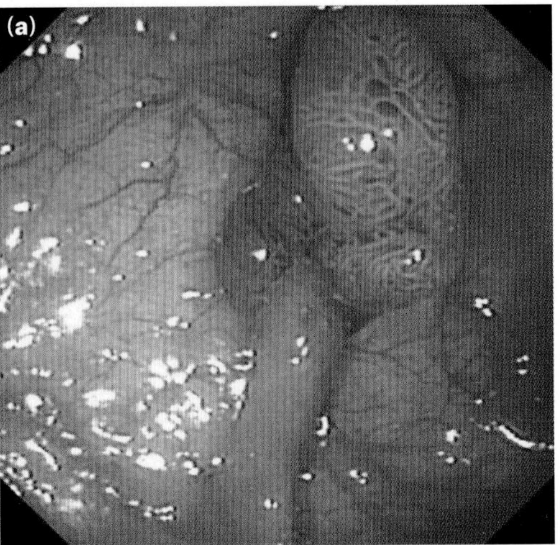

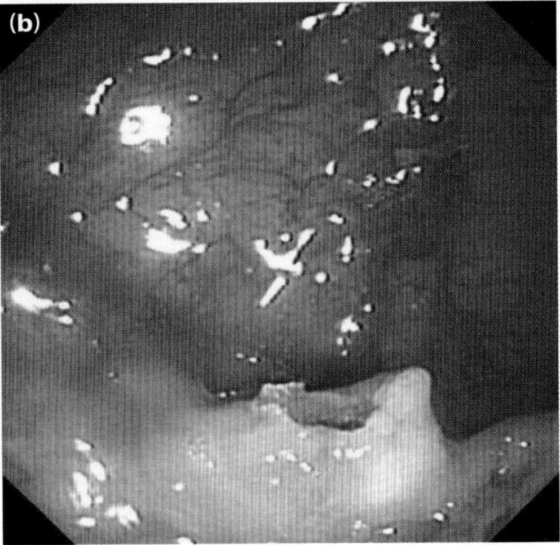

Figure 15.14 Colonoscopy is the most appropriate investigation to detect colonic polyps (**a**), which can be removed by snare polypectomy during the same procedure leaving a clean polyp base (**b**).

Therapeutic colonoscopy

The most common therapeutic procedure performed at colonoscopy is the resection of colonic polyps (Figure 15.14). Retrieved specimens can be assessed for risk factors for neoplastic progression and an appropriate surveillance strategy determined (http://www.bsg.org.uk/images/stories/docs/clinical/guidelines/endoscopy/ccs_10.pdf). Small polyps up to 5 mm should be removed by cheese-wiring with a 'cold' snare. Hot biopsy is a technique in which the tip of a small pedunculated polyp is grasped between diathermy biopsy forceps and tented away from the bowel wall. A brief burst of monopolar current is used to coagulate the stalk, allowing the polyp to be removed. This is rarely performed in current practice due to an increased risk of immediate and delayed thermal damage to the bowel wall, particularly in the right colon. Larger polyps with a defined stalk can be resected using snare polypectomy with coagulating current either *en bloc* (French for 'in a block') or piecemeal depending on their size (Figure 15.14). Postpolypectomy bleeding can be prevented by the application of haemoclips or an endoloop to the polyp stalk. Sessile polyps extending over several centimetres can be removed by endoscopic mucosal resection, which involves lifting the polyp away from the muscularis propria with a submucosal injection of saline to prevent iatrogenic perforation (Figure 15.15). Any residual polyp is obliterated with APC. Care should be taken with all polypectomies in the right colon where the wall may only be 2–3 mm thick. Removal of large or extensive flat polyps should only be attempted by appropriately trained endoscopists. Endoscopic submucosal dissection (ESD) can be used to remove large flat lesions which are not amenable to EMR.

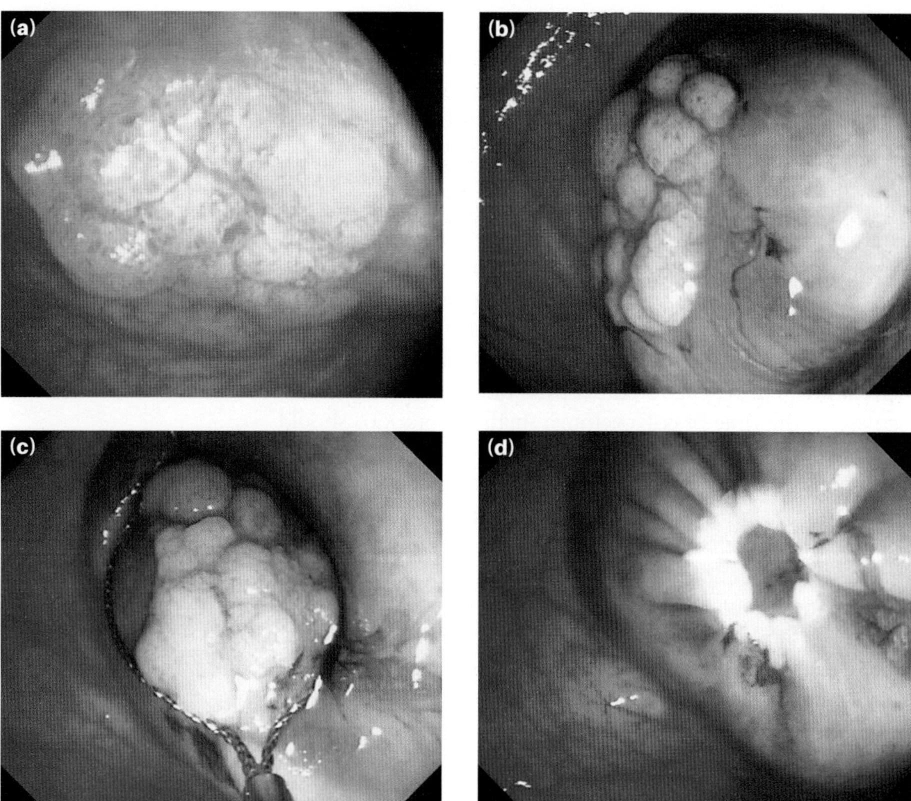

Figure 15.15 Large sessile polyps (**a**) can be removed by endoscopic mucosal resection. First the polyp is raised on a bed of injected saline containing dye (**b**). This ensures that there is no submucosal invasion and protects from transmural perforation. A snare is closed around the polyp (**c**), which is then resected leaving a clean excision base (**d**).

APC and alternative thermal therapies such as heater probes are also used in the treatment of symptomatic angioectasias of the colon (Figure 15.16). Laser photocoagulation may be used to debulk colonic tumours not suitable for resection. As with benign oesophageal strictures, through-the-scope (TTS) balloons can be used to dilate short (less than 5 cm) colonic strictures. The dilatation of surgical anastomoses gives the most durable benefit as inflammatory strictures tend to recur even if intramucosal steroids are injected at the time of the dilatation. Finally, the colonoscopic placement of self-expanding metal stents may provide excellent palliation of inoperable malignant strictures (Figure 15.17) and may also play an invaluable role in decompressing an obstructed colon to allow planned as opposed to emergency surgery.

Complications of colonoscopy

Complications during routine diagnostic colonoscopy by an experienced colonocopist are rare, although perforations have been reported as a result of excessive shaft tip pressure and with excessive air insufflation in severe diverticular disease.

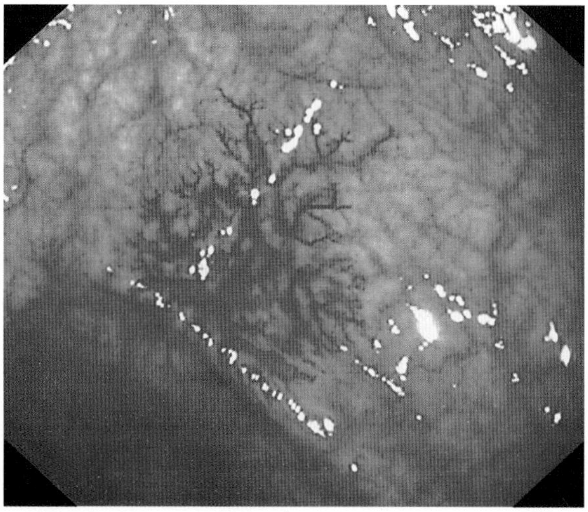

Figure 15.16 A large angioectasia of the colon. If this results in symptomatic anaemia, it should be obliterated with argon plasma coagulation.

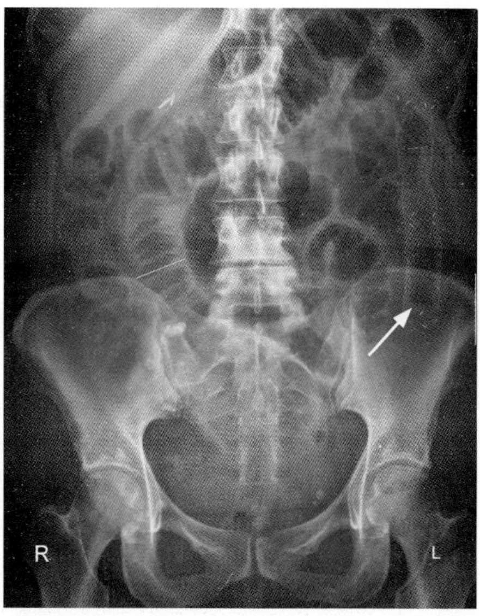

Figure 15.17 Malignant colonic obstruction can be palliated or temporarily relieved by insertion of a self-expanding metal stent (arrow).

Total colonoscopy is contraindicated in the presence of severe colitis; a limited unprepped examination and careful mucosal biopsy only should be performed. Polypectomy is associated with a well-documented rate of perforation (approximately 1%) and haemorrhage (1–2%). Immediate haemorrhage should be managed by re-snaring the polyp stalk where possible and applying tamponade for several minutes followed by careful coagulation if this is unsuccessful. Submucosal adrenaline injection and the deployment of haemoclips are alternatives if this is not possible. Delayed haemorrhage may occur 1–14 days postpolypectomy and can normally be managed by conservative observation. Transfusion may occasionally be required, but repeat colonoscopy is rarely necessary. If recognised at the time of polypectomy, small perforations should be closed using clips and the patient admitted for observation. Symptoms of abdominal pain and cardiovascular compromise after a polypectomy should alert one to the risk of delayed perforation. Patients should be kept nil by mouth and receive intravenous resuscitation and antibiotics. Prompt assessment with plain radiography and a CT scan will often distinguish between a frank perforation and a transmural burn with associated localised peritonitis (the postpolypectomy syndrome). Assessment by an experienced colorectal surgeon is essential, as surgery is often the most appropriate course of action.

ENDOSCOPIC ULTRASOUND

One key disadvantage of conventional endoscopy is that the views are limited to the mucosal surface and it is therefore not possible to diagnose submucosal or extraintestinal pathology. These limitations can be overcome using endoscopic ultrasound (EUS), which combines the traditional mucosal image with a separate ultrasound view that clearly depicts the intestinal layers and proximate extraintestinal structures. Its use has revolutionised the staging and management of upper gastrointestinal and hepatobiliary malignancy.

There are two main types of echoendoscope: the radial echoendoscope has a radially arranged ultrasound probe and a forward-viewing lens. This is used for diagnostic work such as local tumour staging in the oesophagus and stomach. The linear echoendoscope is a side-viewing scope with a working channel much like an ERCP scope, and a linearly arranged ultrasound probe. This conformation allows ultrasound assessment and ultrasound-guided sampling of tissues to be performed (**Figures 15.18 and 15.19**). It allows sampling of paraoesophageal and coeliac lymph nodes, sampling of pancreatic, biliary and other solid abdominal lesions and drainage of peripancreatic abscess or pseudocysts. Using TTS cystotomes it is possible to perform EUS cystgastrostomy and stent placement, and increasingly biliary interventional procedures are being performed with EUS assistance.

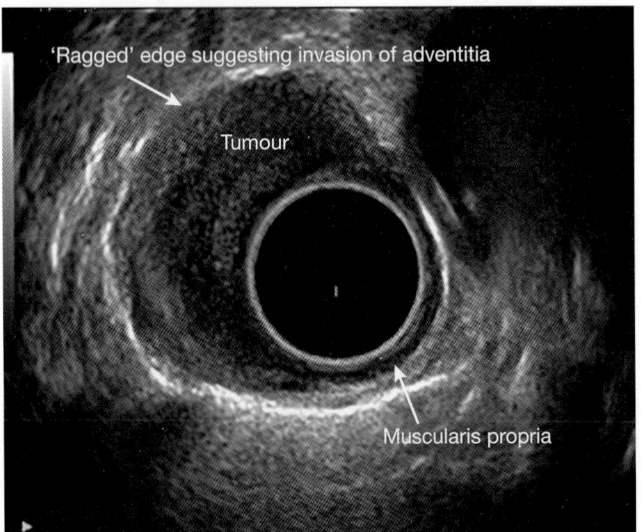

Figure 15.18 Endoscopic ultrasound image of an oesophageal tumour invading into the wall.

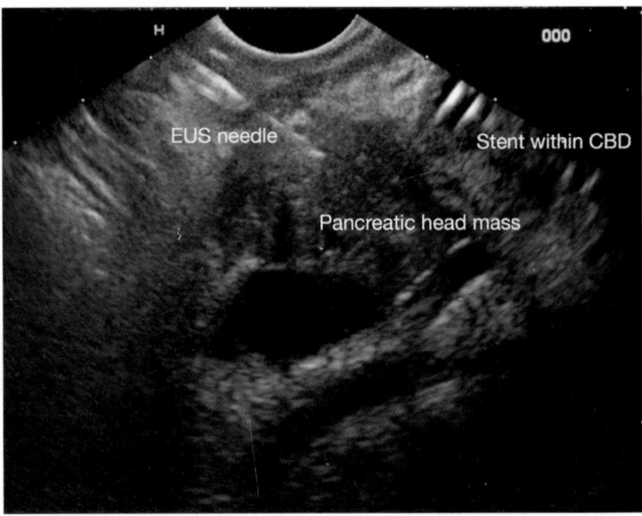

Figure 15.19 Endoscopic ultrasound-guided fine needle aspiration of a pancreatic head mass.

EUS requires dedicated training, both in scope manipulation and radiographic interpretation. Due to the width and lack of flexibility of the endo-ultrasound scope as well as the duration of complex therapeutic procedures, sedation is normally required, and some units perform tests using propofol-based anaesthesia. The main indications for endoscopic ultrasound are listed in *Table 15.6*. All patients undergoing therapeutic endoscopic ultrasound require a normal coagulation screen. Complications include over-sedation and oesophageal perforation during diagnostic procedures and haemorrhage/perforation during therapeutic procedures.

TABLE 15.6	Indications for endoscopic ultrasound.
Diagnostic:	Staging of oesophageal/gastric malignancy
	Staging of hepatobiliary malignancy
	Diagnosis of choledoccal microlithiasis
Therapeutic	Biopsy of paraoesophageal lymph nodes
	Biopsy of submucosal upper GI lesions
	Biopsy of pancreaticobiliary mass
	Biopsy of portal lymphadenopathy
	Biopsy of left adrenal and left liver masses
	Transgastric drainage of pancreatic pseudocyst
	Coeliac plexus block

IMPROVED ENDOSCOPIC IMAGING

Chromoendoscopy, narrow band imaging and high resolution magnification endoscopy

The ability to enhance lesion detection and achieve near-patient discrimination of pathology without the need for histology is a common theme of several active areas of endoscopic development. The goal is to allow accurate discrimination of dysplasia grade in areas of Barrett's oesophagus or quiescent ulcerative colitis and to aid polyp detection and the recognition of early gastric and colorectal cancer. The most widely available technique is chromoendoscopy, which involves the topical application of stains or pigments to improve tissue localisation, characterisation or diagnosis. Several agents have been described, which can broadly be categorised as absorptive (vital) stains such as methylene blue; contrast (reactive) stains, such as indigo carmine; and those used for tattooing, such as India ink. Acetic acid can be used to improve dysplasia detection in Barrett's oesophagus and Lugol's iodine can be useful in detecting early squamous cell carcinoma.

Narrow band imaging (NBI) relies on an optical filter technology that radically improves the visibility of capillaries, veins and other subtle tissue structures by optimising the absorbance and scattering characteristics of light. NBI uses two discrete bands of light: one blue at 415 nm and one green at 540 nm. Narrow band blue light displays superficial capillary networks, whereas green light displays subepithelial vessels; when combined they offer an extremely high contrast image of the tissue surface. Autofluorescence images can also be used to increase lesion discrimination. Finally, high-resolution magnifying endoscopy may be used alone or in combination with one of the above techniques to achieve near-cellular definition of the mucosa (**Figure 15.20**), and is of particular use in neoplasia surveillance. New directions for the future include the increased use of confocal endomicroscopy to achieve histological images at the time of the endoscopic procedure.

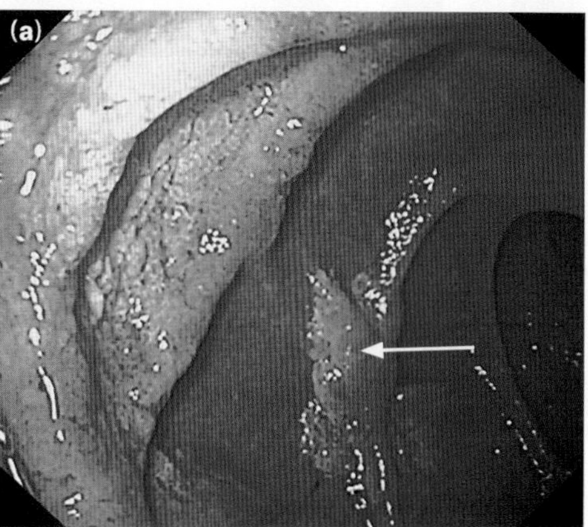

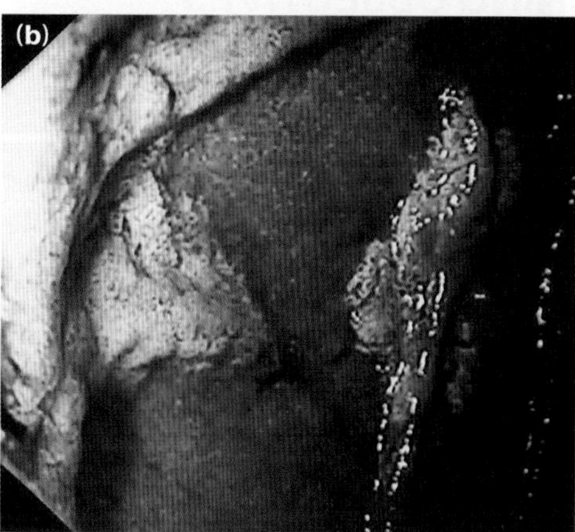

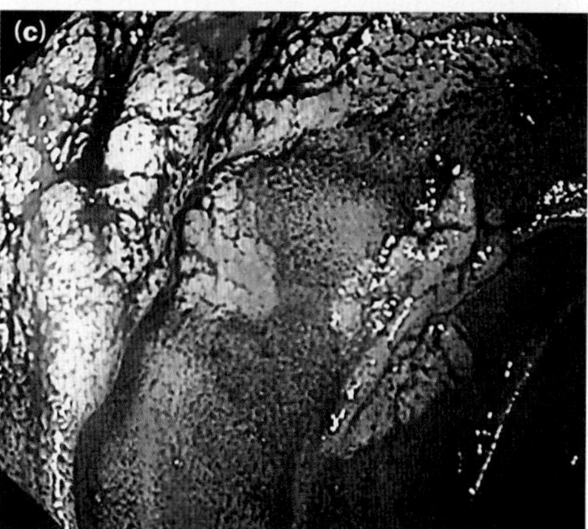

Figure 15.20 Endoscopic diagnostic accuracy can be improved by novel endoscopic techniques. This duodenal adenoma can be seen with conventional white light (**a**) (arrow), but its full extent is more clearly delineated using narrow band imaging (**b**) or chromoendoscopy with indigo carmine (**c**).

CONCLUSIONS

Over the last 30 years endoscopy has become an integral part of the diagnostic work-up of patients with gastrointestinal disease. Whereas advances in radiology may obviate the need for some diagnostic procedures (routine OGD and ERCP), the ability to take mucosal biopsies will ensure that it retains a vital role. Moreover, on-going advances in technology such as magnifying endoscopy and chromoendoscopy are able to give near-histological quality definition to allow near-patient diagnosis. There have also been major advances in the range of conditions that are amenable to endoscopic therapy; such therapy may have substantially lower associated morbidity rates than traditional surgical approaches. However, as the scope of procedures widens and the age range/comorbidities of the patients increases it is beholden to the endoscopist to ensure that he or she adheres to appropriate governance/consent and sedation practice to minimise complications.

FURTHER READING

Hawes RH, Fockens P, Varadarajulu S. *Endosonography*, 3rd edn. Philadelphia: Saunders, 2014.

Haycock A, Cohen J, Saunders BP *et al. Cotton and Williams' practical gastrointestinal endoscopy*, 7th edn. Oxford: Wiley-Blackwell, 2014.

Veitch AM, Vanbiervliet G, Gershlick AH *et al.* Endoscopy in patients on antiplatelet or anticoagulant therapy, including direct oral anticoagulants: British Society of Gastroenterology (BSG) and European Society of Gastrointestinal Endoscopy (ESGE) guidelines. *Gut* 2016; **65**: 374–89.

Chapter 16

Tissue and molecular diagnosis

LEARNING OBJECTIVES

To understand:

- The value and limitations of tissue diagnosis
- How tissue samples are processed
- The role of histology and cytology

To be aware of:

- The role of additional techniques used in clinical practice, including special stains, immunohistochemistry and molecular pathology
- The principles of microscopic diagnosis, including the features of neoplasia
- The importance of clinicopathological correlation
- Management issues

INTRODUCTION

In the past, tissue diagnosis was restricted to macroscopic examination of autopsy material and of a limited range of surgical specimens. In the nineteenth century, microscopic examination of human tissue from autopsies and surgical procedures was introduced, and its value was accepted eventually by physicians and surgeons. Tissue analysis is now an integral and routine element of clinical management. It is heavily dependent on microscopy and is usually the responsibility of a histopathologist, who is a medically qualified practitioner. The specialty variably known as Histopathology, Anatomic Pathology or Cellular Pathology, encompasses histopathology, cytopathology, autopsy work and molecular pathological tissue diagnosis.

Cellular pathology has changed considerably over the past few decades. There has been a steady increase in biopsy numbers, partly because of the widespread introduction of flexible endoscopy and also because of an ageing population with a higher risk of cancer. Screening programmes (breast, bowel and cervical) have had a major impact on volume and practice. New techniques have improved the quality and clinical value of histological assessment, while autopsies have steadily diminished in number. Adherence to national or international reporting standards, e.g. for cancer, is increasingly expected, as is participation by pathologists in multidisciplinary clinical management meetings. Tissue analysis has sometimes been replaced by newer less invasive methods, e.g. human papilloma virus (HPV) testing rather than cytological assessment of cervical smears for cervical cancer screening, while newer forms of radiology and imaging may be so informative that tissue analysis is not needed.

A modern cellular pathology department is usually located in a medium-sized or large hospital or in a purpose-built laboratory. Typically, more than 80% of specimens are from the gastrointestinal tract, gynaecological tract, urological system or skin. In line with clinical services, highly specialised work such as neuropathology is largely confined to major regional centres.

REASONS FOR ASSESSMENT OF TISSUE

There are several reasons for tissue analysis. These include diagnosis, staging of disease, prediction of clinical outcome, selection of therapy and audit. These reasons are often interrelated.

A new diagnosis may be made or a known diagnosis confirmed. Often, tissue analysis confirms or refines a suspected or suggested clinical diagnosis. There may be clues to a cause, e.g.

Summary box 16.1

Reasons for tissue analysis

- To make a new diagnosis
- To confirm a suspected or established clinical diagnosis
- To exclude additional diagnoses
- To assist with prognosis
- To stage tumours
- To help select therapy and plan management
- To assess response to treatment
- Audit

granulomas. Additional diagnoses, either expected or unexpected, may be made. For example, an appendix removed for appendicitis could contain an incidental carcinoid tumour, polyp or carcinoma, while biopsies from a patient with inflammatory bowel disease may be taken to confirm the diagnosis and to exclude dysplasia but might reveal additional findings, e.g. cytomegalovirus or lymphoma.

Tissue analysis also helps, increasingly, to determine or refine treatment and prognosis. For example, the assessment of a cancer resection specimen confirms the diagnosis but perhaps more importantly provides information about features such as tumour stage, vascular invasion and resection margin involvement, which in turn predict clinical outcome and help determine postoperative treatment. More recently, pathologists have been asked to assess the degree of tumour regression after neoadjuvant therapy. Increasingly, molecular pathological analysis of cancer tissue contributes to various aspects of management, including diagnostic categorisation, prognostic predictions and selection of targeted drug therapy.

Additionally, the pathologist's assessment of resection specimens helps surgeons and radiologists to audit their performance.

It is worth remembering that a tissue sample does not represent the entire patient. The interpretation of microscopic and molecular changes is enhanced considerably by correlation with the clinical picture and the macroscopic findings. Accordingly, a request form with adequate clinical details should accompany all specimens. Essential details include site of biopsy, date of birth, gender, medications, relevant risk factors, past medical and surgical history and details of neoadjuvant therapy in cancer cases.

TISSUE SPECIMENS

Routine tissue specimens received by a histopathology department include those intended for histopathological analysis and those for cytopathological assessment. These two areas may overlap.

Summary box 16.2

Common types of tissue sample

- Histology
  - Formalin-fixed tissue
    - Biopsy
      - Mucosal
      - Punch
      - Needle (core)
      - Curettings
      - Excision
    - Resection
  - Fresh tissue (usually for frozen section)
- Cytology
  - Cervical
  - Washings, brushings, scrapes
  - Fine-needle aspirate (FNA)
  - Fluids/sputum

Histology

Specimens for histology are arbitrarily classified as biopsies and resections. Biopsies are taken for diagnosis and assessment rather than treatment. A resection is usually done to remove a lesion (e.g. a tumour) or to manage a related problem (e.g. sleeve gastrectomy for obesity), but may also have other uses including diagnosis, staging, and determination of further management. Types of small biopsy include punch biopsy, needle core biopsy and mucosal biopsy. An excision biopsy is larger and serves as both a diagnostic biopsy and a limited resection.

All samples for routine histology are immediately placed in a fixative, usually formalin (10% formaldehyde), to preserve morphology. Ultrasound-guided and computed tomography (CT)-guided biopsies of focal and less accessible lesions have become more common and may pose challenges to the pathologist because of limited sample size.

Cytology

Cytological specimens can be obtained from many sites using a variety of approaches. Some are easy to obtain, e.g. urine and sputum, whereas others require more intervention. A conventional cervical smear is obtained by sampling the cervical transformation zone with a brush/broom. Bronchial aspirates, washings and brushings and gastrointestinal and biliary brushings sample a relatively wide area and may therefore be useful for the diagnosis of neoplasia.

Fine-needle aspiration (FNA) cytology may sample accessible sites such as the breast, thyroid and superficial lymph nodes, while FNA from deeper and less accessible structures, e.g. liver, pancreas, kidney and lung, is usually assisted by ultrasound or CT guidance. Ultrasound-guided transbronchial FNA may be used for mediastinal masses and transmucosal FNA for submucosal gastrointestinal lesions or perivisceral lesions. FNA cytology samples may be accompanied by a biopsy taken at the same procedure.

Fluids may be submitted directly to the laboratory for cytological assessment.

Fresh tissue

The most common indication for submission of a fresh tissue sample (i.e. without fixative) is rapid frozen section diagnosis, usually done intraoperatively. Other indications are microbiological assessment, electron microscopy, chemical analyses (e.g. quantification of iron) and some types of molecular pathological analysis. Before fixing a histology or cytology specimen, the operator should consider whether any of these investigations might be useful.

Risk management

Safety and risk management are priorities in the laboratory. Any risk of contamination by transmissible infection, e.g. hepatitis B virus, human immunodeficiency virus (HIV), must be minimised by the use of warning labels, especially when fresh tissue is being submitted. Formalin kills many microorganisms, but any risk of infection should still be notified. Also, formalin itself is toxic to the eyes and skin. Accordingly, leaking or faulty specimen containers should be discarded. Containers must be labelled with the patient's details to avoid errors of identity (**Figure 16.1**).

Figure 16.1 Sections on glass slides stained with haematoxylin and eosin (H&E). Each slide has a unique specimen identifying number (06S022081), a letter corresponding to the biopsy site (A1–F1) and a site label (e.g. DUOBX for duodenal biopsy).

SPECIMEN PROCESSING

Histology specimen

On arrival in the histopathology department, specimens are given a unique number and submitted for macroscopic assessment and sampling ('cut up'). The largest specimens are opened (e.g. bowel) or sliced (e.g. uterus) and left to fix in formalin for at least 1 day (**Figure 16.2**). When they are fixed and, accordingly, in a suitable condition for cutting and sampling, a text description of the specimen and any abnormality is made. Small specimens such as biopsies are processed in their entirety. Representative samples are taken from any specimen too large to be processed whole (**Figure 16.3**). This is traditionally done by a histopathologist, but increasingly may be done by specifically trained non-medical staff. In the UK, a local or national protocol for sampling is often followed. For example, samples from most types of cancer should include resection margins, tumour, lymph nodes, non-neoplastic tissue and any other abnormal areas. Coloured inks help to identify resection margins and surfaces as they are also visible under the microscope (**Figure 16.4**).

Specimens, or samples from specimens, are placed in plastic cassettes (**Figure 16.5**) and then embedded in paraffin wax while in the cassette to make a tissue block (**Figure 16.6**). Sections with a thickness of approximately 5 μm (microns) are cut from the block using a microtome (**Figure 16.7**). The sections are placed on a glass slide and stained with haematoxylin and eosin (H&E) (**Figure 16.1**). This work is done by expert trained staff, known in the UK as biomedical scientists (BMSs). High standards are necessary because a poorly cut section may have various artefacts, such as lines and folds, which impede accurate assessment. H&E as the first-line stain has stood the test of time, probably because it is inexpensive, safe, fast, reliable, familiar and informative.

The stained sections are examined with a microscope (**Figure 16.8**) and the histological features are correlated with the clinical details and the macroscopic description. After completion of any further studies, the pathologist writes a report that is usually entered onto a computer system.

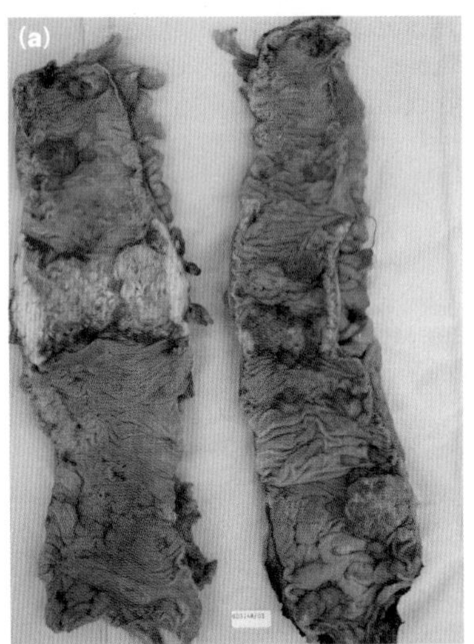

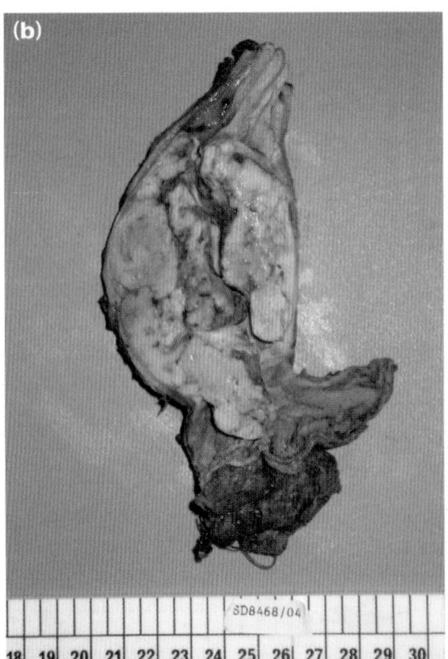

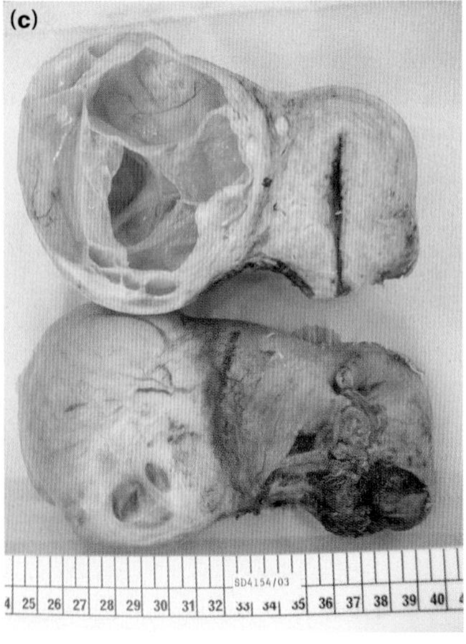

Figure 16.2 (**a**) A colon from a patient with familial adenomatous polyposis has been opened longitudinally to allow fixation. Multiple polyps and a carcinoma are seen. (**b**) An oesophagogastrectomy containing a distal oesophageal tumour has been opened and sliced to allow fixation. (**c**) A uterus and an adjacent cystic lesion have been bisected with a knife to allow fixation (all figures courtesy of Dr J Chin Aleong, Barts Health NHS Trust, London, UK).

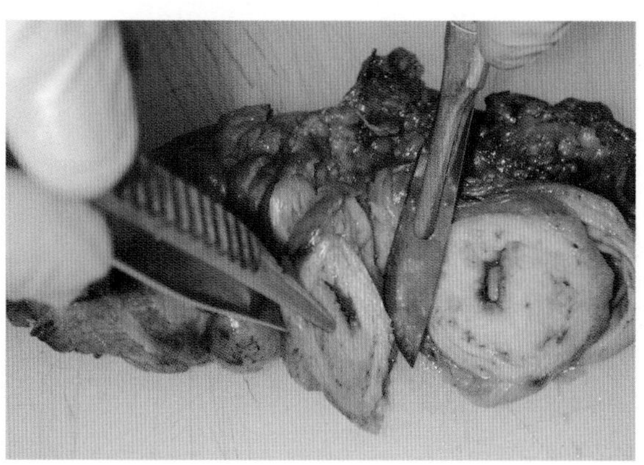

Figure 16.3 A scalpel is used to take a sample from a resection specimen.

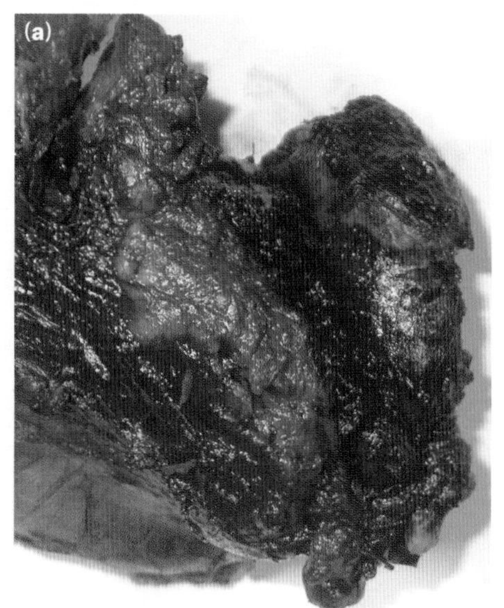

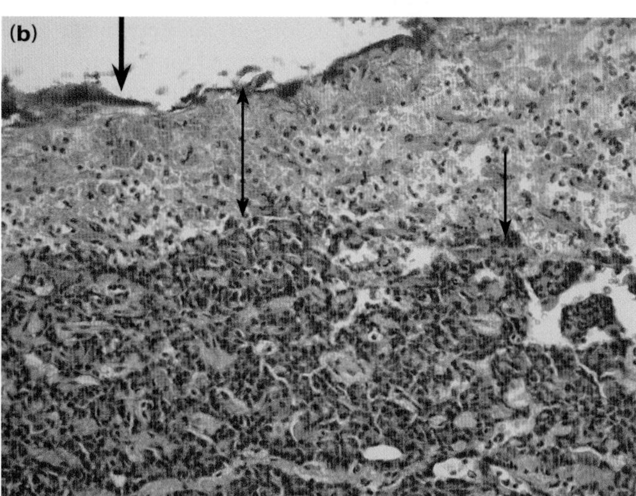

Figure 16.4 (**a**) An unopened pancreatoduodenectomy specimen (posterior view). Four inks of different colours have been painted onto various resection margins and external surfaces. (**b**) Yellow ink on the edge of a histology section (thick arrow). Tumour (thin arrow) lies close to the surface. The distance between the tumour and a surface or a resection margin can be measured (double-headed arrow).

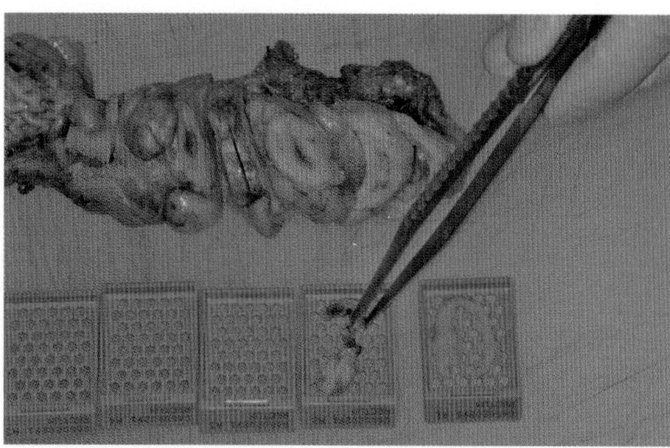

Figure 16.5 A tissue sample from a resection specimen is placed in a cassette.

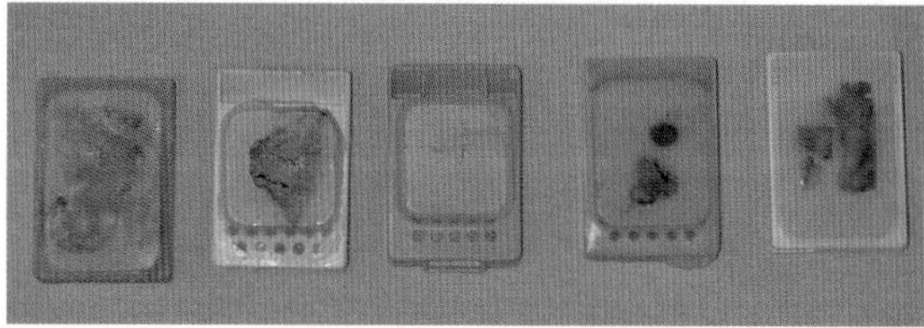

Figure 16.6 Paraffin wax blocks. Cassettes of different colours allow specimens to be organised into groups.

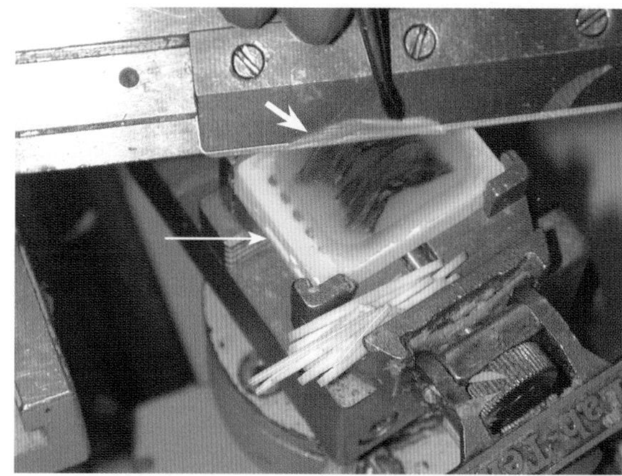

Figure 16.7 A section (thick arrow) being cut from a paraffin wax block (thin arrow) with a microtome.

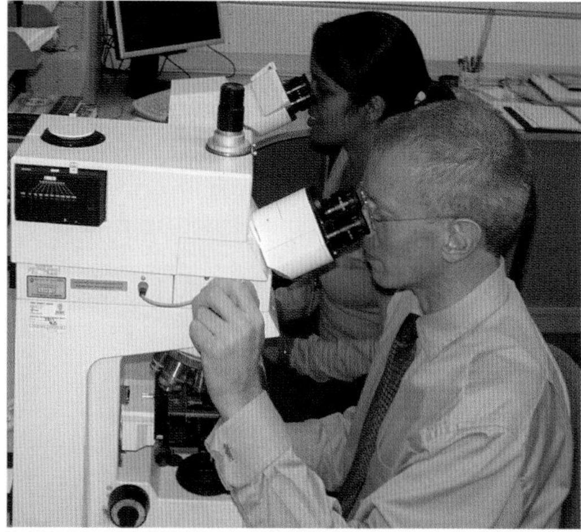

Figure 16.8 A double-headed microscope allows a consultant histopathologist and a trainee to view a slide simultaneously.

Summary box 16.3

Histological processing: sequence of events

- Biopsy or resection specimen received
- Macroscopic (gross) description made
- Specimen sampled (unless small enough to submit in its entirety)
- Specimen or samples placed in cassette(s)
- Paraffin wax block(s) made
- 5-μm sections cut
- Sections put on glass slides
- Sections stained with H&E
- Histopathologist examines slides
- Histology compared with clinical and macroscopic findings
- Further studies if necessary
- Report entered onto computer system
- Report authorised or signed

Frozen section specimen

Frozen section diagnosis is useful when a very rapid answer is necessary for diagnosis or management. Surgeons are the main users of this service. A representative fresh tissue sample of the area of interest is supplied by the surgeon and frozen quickly in the pathology laboratory, and sections are cut and stained within several minutes. There are a few disadvantages: fresh tissue carries a higher risk of infection than fixed tissue; the quality of a frozen section slide is inferior to that of routinely processed material, reducing the accuracy and precision of diagnosis; small samples are required; certain types of tissue (e.g. fat) are difficult to deal with; and the process is time-consuming and disruptive for the histopathology department.

Cytology specimen

Many samples for cytology can be smeared immediately onto glass slides, fixed (usually in alcohol) or air dried and stained immediately or later. Several slides are usually produced, some of which are stained with a Papanicolaou (Pap) stain and some with another method such as May–Grünwald–Giemsa (MGG) or Romanowsky. Pap stain is regarded as the preferred stain for fixed specimens while MGG is better for air-dried material. Often the sample will be stained with both. Cervical smears are usually stained with a Pap stain only (**Figure 16.9**). There has been a move to liquid-based thin-layer technology for many samples, particularly cervical. For liquid-based cytology, the sampling device is usually washed in a liquid medium and the material obtained is then processed in the laboratory using purpose-built equipment.

Summary box 16.4

Frozen section: advantages and disadvantages

Advantages:

- Quick diagnosis

Disadvantages:

- Labour intensive
- Disruptive
- Risk of infection
- Poorer quality sections
- Small sample required
- Some tissue types difficult to process

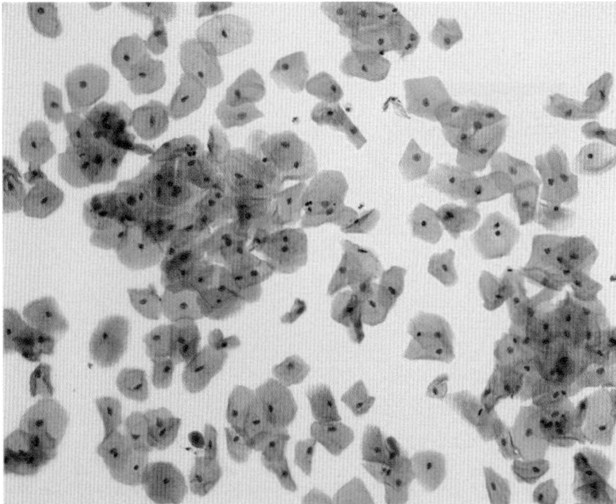

Figure 16.9 A cervical smear stained with a Papanicolaou stain. Numerous cells are present (courtesy of Professor MT Sheaff, Barts Health NHS Trust).

Storage

Resection specimens are generally stored for about 4–6 weeks. Tissue blocks are retained for as long as space permits, e.g. 30 years, while glass slides might be retained for a shorter time, e.g. 10 years. Fresh tissue can be frozen and stored. Stored tissue may be useful for future clinical review, teaching, audit or research. In many countries, the subsequent use of stored tissue for non-clinical purposes is now subject to legal constraints.

PRINCIPLES OF MICROSCOPIC DIAGNOSIS

Diagnosis of malignancy

Neoplasia is a broad term that includes benign and malignant tumours. Classification of a neoplasm or tumour as malignant

---

George Nicholas Papanicolaou, 1883–1962, Professor of Anatomy, Cornell University, New York, NY, USA, reported on the value of cervical smears in the diagnosis of carcinoma of the uterus in 1941.
Richard May, b.1863, physician, Münich, Germany.
Ludwig Grünwald, b.1863, otolaryngologist, Münich, Germany.
Gustav Giemsa, 1867–1948, bacteriologist who became Privatdozent in Chemotherapy, at The University of Hamburg, Hamburg, Germany.
Dmitri Leonidovich Romanowsky, 1861–1921, Professor of Medicine, St. Petersburg, Russia.

Summary box 16.5

Microscopic features of malignancy

- Metastasis
- Invasion
  - Of surrounding tissue
  - Vascular
  - Perineural
- Architectural abnormalities
- Necrosis
- Numerous mitotic figures
- Atypical mitotic figures
- Nuclear abnormalities
  - Pleomorphism
  - Enlargement
  - Hyperchromaticity
  - Chromatin clumping
- Nucleolar enlargement and multiplicity

(or as 'cancer') usually implies that it has the potential to behave aggressively. The main histological features of malignancy are metastasis, invasion, architectural changes and cytological features, but the criteria for a diagnosis of malignancy differ between anatomical sites and between tumour types.

Microscopic evidence of aggressive behaviour by the tumour is usually sufficient for a malignant label. For example, metastasis to another organ such as lymph nodes or liver is virtually always diagnostic of malignancy. Invasion of surrounding structures, perineural invasion (**Figure 16.10**) and vascular invasion (**Figure 16.11**) strongly suggest malignancy.

Other microscopic features that are typical of malignancy include derangement of the usual architecture, an increased number of mitotic figures, atypical mitoses and necrosis (tissue death) (**Figure 16.12**). Microscopic changes at the cellular level (cytological changes) include nuclear enlargement, an increased nuclear:cytoplasmic ratio, nuclear pleomorphism (variation in shape) and nuclear hyperchromasia (dark colour) (**Figure 16.13a**). Multiplicity, irregularity and enlargement of nucleoli may also be seen (**Figure 16.13b**).

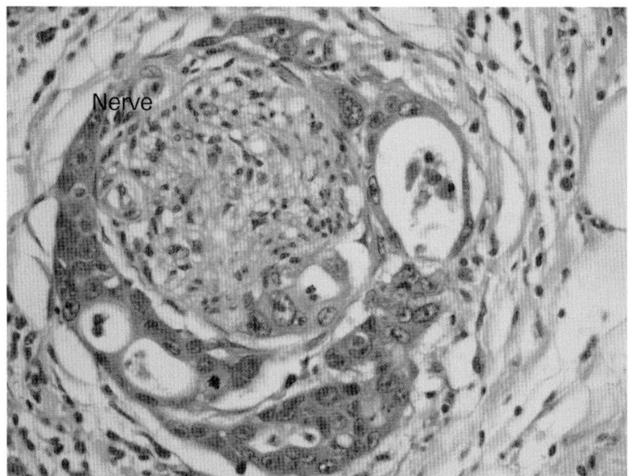

Figure 16.10 Perineural invasion. A nerve is almost completely surrounded by adenocarcinoma.

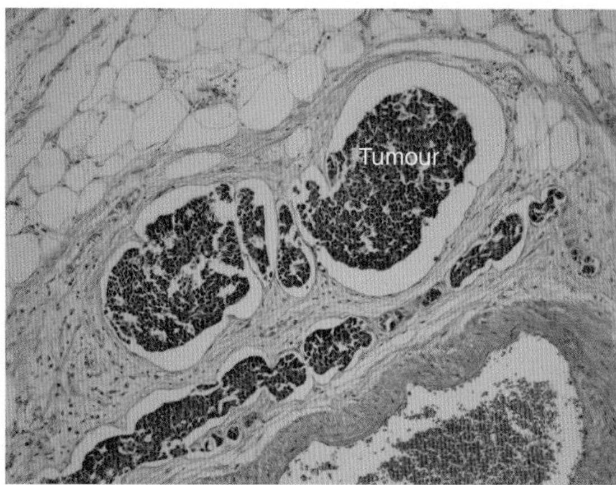

Figure 16.11 Vascular invasion. Aggregates of carcinoma cells are present within blood vessels. The tumour is poorly differentiated.

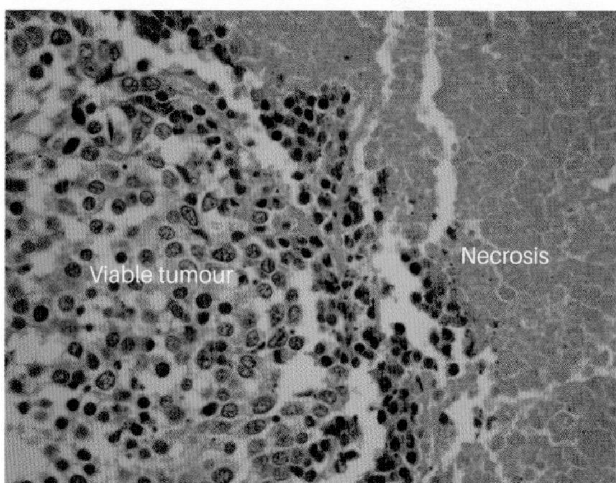

Figure 16.12 An area of necrosis in a poorly differentiated carcinoma.

The criteria for a histological diagnosis of malignancy are modified by the site and type of tissue. Carcinoma is the most common type of malignancy, and is typically diagnosed when epithelial cells invade beyond their normal boundaries. However, the categorisation of some types of non-epithelial proliferations (e.g. lymphoid, mesenchymal) as malignant may rely on cytological and architectural features rather than on invasiveness. In some cases, e.g. certain endocrine tumours, histological distinction between benign and malignant may be impossible. In other cases, e.g. gastrointestinal stromal tumours (GIST) and neuroendocrine tumours, there may be risk categories rather than benign and malignant designations. The risk categories are based on combinations of histological features that help predict the likelihood of aggressive behaviour.

Additional techniques such as immunohistochemistry and clonality studies may help to confirm neoplasia or malignancy (see below).

The term 'dysplasia' usually indicates that microscopic features of carcinoma, or similar to those of carcinoma, are present but that invasion has not occurred, e.g. cervical intraepithelial neoplasia (CIN), colorectal dysplasia (**Figure 16.14**).

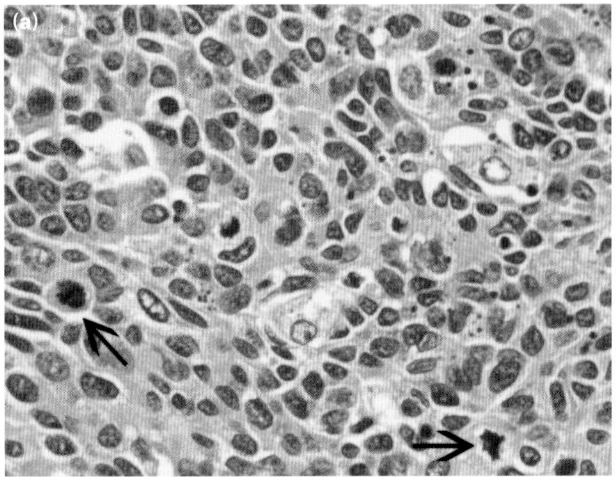

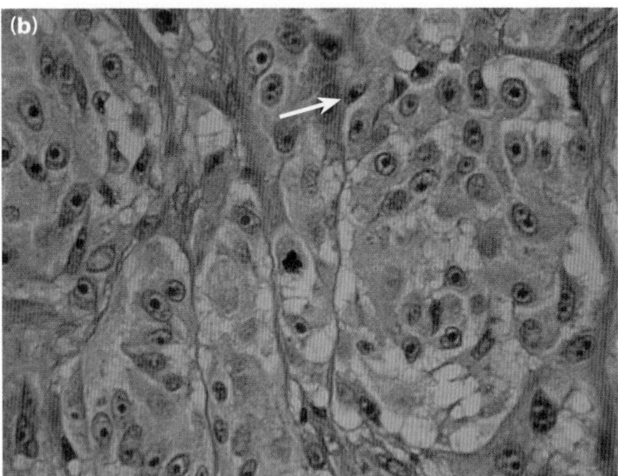

Figure 16.13 Cytological features of malignancy. (**a**) A high-grade neuroendocrine carcinoma showing nuclear pleomorphism (variation in shape) and variation in nuclear size. There are several mitotic figures (arrows). (**b**) A malignant melanoma showing nuclear pleomorphism and prominent nucleoli (arrow) (courtesy of Dr E Husain, Aberdeen Royal Infirmary, United Kingdom).

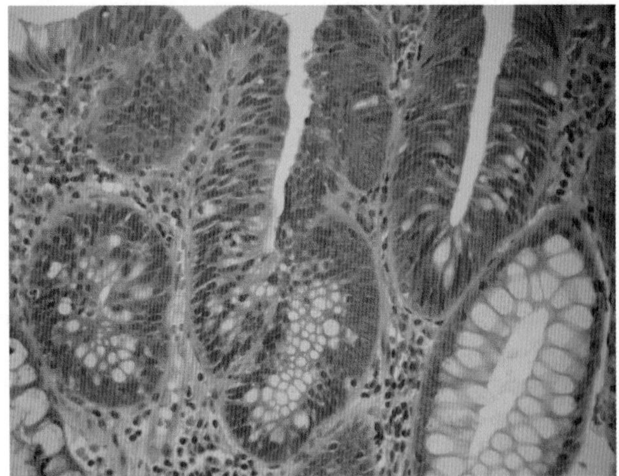

Figure 16.14 A colonic biopsy from a tubular adenoma with low-grade dysplasia. There is one non-dysplastic crypt (lower right corner). The remaining crypts show features of dysplasia, including nuclear stratification (multilayering) and nuclear hyperchromaticity (dark colour).

There are various causes of a false-positive diagnosis of malignancy. These include contamination of a specimen with tumour from elsewhere, interchanging of specimens and observer error. Several conditions can mimic malignancy histologically. For example, radiation effect on a mucosal layer can mimic malignancy, as can the histological changes in regenerating tissue adjacent to an ulcer. Additional studies may also be misleading, particularly if interpreted in isolation. The risk of interpretative error by the histopathologist is reduced by thorough training, regular updating, discussion of difficult cases with colleagues and avoidance of excessive workloads. The surgeon also helps to minimise such errors by supplying good clinical details, e.g. a history of radiotherapy.

A false-negative diagnosis, i.e. failure to diagnose malignancy when present, may reflect absence of tumour in the specimen or failure of the pathologist to recognise the changes as neoplastic.

Summary box 16.6

Causes of false-positive diagnoses of malignancy

- Interchanged samples
- Contamination
- Interpretative error
- Treatment-induced change
- Ulceration

Histological types of malignancy

A malignant tumour showing features of epithelial differentiation, and typically arising in an epithelial layer, is a carcinoma. Other important types of malignancy include malignant melanoma (melanocytes) (**Figure 16.13b**), lymphoma (lymphoid cells) and sarcoma (mesenchymal cells). Further subclassification is usually possible. For example, a carcinoma can be classified as squamous cell carcinoma if it shows evidence of keratinisation (**Figure 16.15**), adenocarcinoma if it shows evidence of glandular differentiation (in the form of tubule formation and/or mucin production) (**Figure 16.16**), neuroendocrine carcinoma/small cell carcinoma (**Figure 16.13a**) (usually requiring immunohistochemical confirmation), clear cell carcinoma (**Figure 16.17**) or one of many other types.

Prognostic factors for malignant tumours

Tissue assessment is important for cancer prognosis. Stage is generally the most important prognostic factor for carcinomas. The commonly used and internationally accepted UICC (Union internationale contre le cancer)/AJCC (American Joint Committee on Cancer) staging schemes depend heavily on the histopathological TNM (**T**umour **N**ode **M**etastasis) category (pTNM), although the M category is usually evaluated clinically and the final stage is derived from a combination of clinical, imaging, pathological and other assessments. Degree of differentiation may also be prognostic and is usually determined microscopically. Well-differentiated tumours recapitulate some of the features of their non-neoplastic

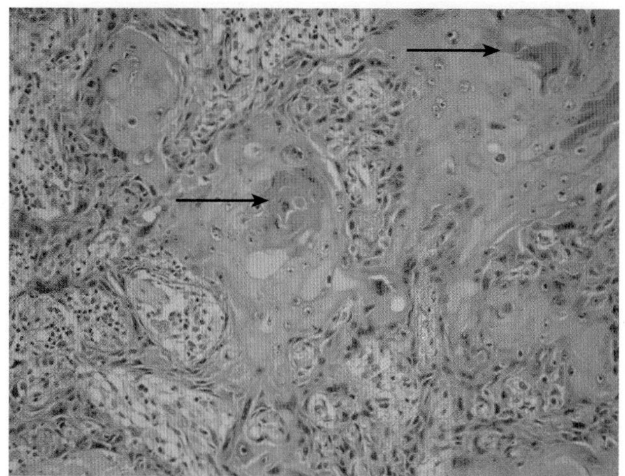

Figure 16.15 A well-differentiated squamous cell carcinoma. Irregular nests of squamous cells with foci of keratinisation (arrows).

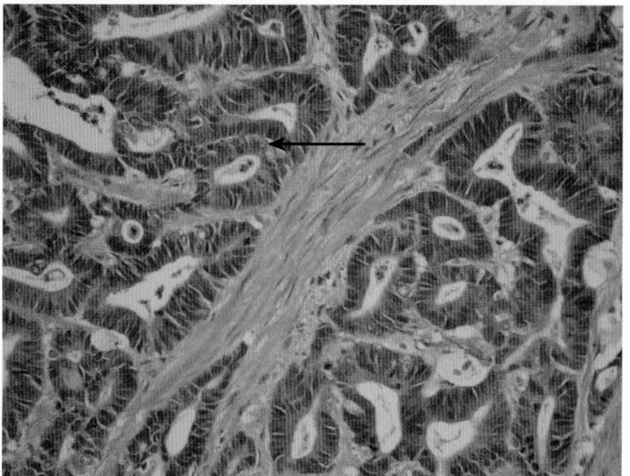

Figure 16.16 A well-differentiated adenocarcinoma. Gland formation (arrow) is obvious.

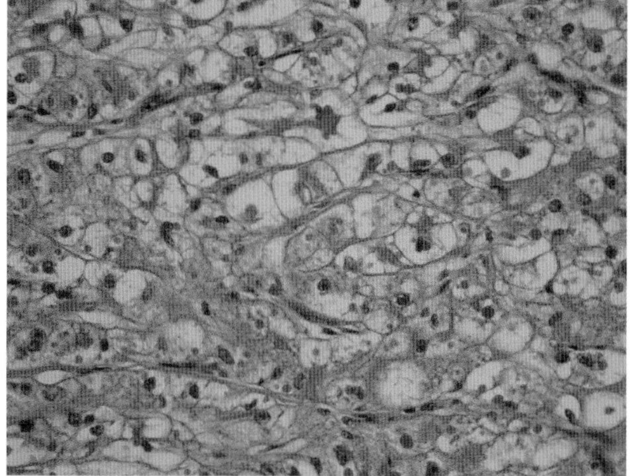

Figure 16.17 A metastatic clear cell carcinoma, composed of sheets of cells with clear cytoplasm. A tumour with this appearance is most likely to be of renal origin.

tissue counterparts (**Figures 16.15** and **16.16**), whereas poorly differentiated tumours do not (**Figures 16.11** and **16.12**). Other histological features associated with a worse prognosis include vascular invasion (**Figure 16.11**), perineural invasion (**Figure 16.10**) and positive resection margins. The prognostic value of these factors differs between tumour types and sites.

Non-neoplastic and inflammatory conditions

Some of the commonest surgical specimens in the pathology laboratory are taken for the management of non-neoplastic disease. These include appendectomies for appendicitis, cholecystectomies for gallstone disease, hysterectomies for fibroids, partial gastrectomies for obesity, skin lesions such as sebaceous cysts and chippings from prostate glands with hyperplasia. All specimens are examined thoroughly in order to confirm the suspected clinical diagnosis and also to exclude other conditions that are not necessarily apparent to the surgeon, e.g. dysplastic and malignant lesions of the gallbladder, sarcomatous change within uterine fibroids or adenocarcinoma in prostatic chippings. Correlation with the clinical picture may be particularly important if a biopsy is taken specifically for non-neoplastic disease. For example, full clinical details are essential for meaningful interpretation of inflammatory bowel disease biopsies, inflammatory skin biopsies, renal biopsies and medical liver biopsies.

Microscopic features of inflammation

Acute inflammation is characterised by neutrophils (polymorphonuclear leucocytes) (**Figure 16.18**), and chronic inflammation by lymphocytes and plasma cells. Other inflammatory cells include eosinophils (**Figure 16.19**), mast cells and histiocytes. Granulomas (i.e. collections of epithelioid histiocytes) (**Figure 16.20**) raise the possibility of mycobacterial infection, fungal infection, sarcoid, Crohn's disease or a reaction to foreign material, among numerous possible causes. Eosinophils in large numbers may reflect parasitic infection or allergy. Interpretation depends heavily on the site and clinical setting.

Other terms

Other specific tissue abnormalities are also detectable by microscopy. Histopathologists may use specific terms for these changes. For example, hyperplasia means an increase in cell number while hypertrophy refers to an increase in cell size. Atrophy encompasses a reduction in cell number and/or cell size. Metaplasia describes the change from one mature cell type to another, e.g. columnar metaplasia in the oesophagus (known as Barrett's oesophagus) where squamous epithelium is

Norman Rupert Barrett, 1903–1979, surgeon, St Thomas's Hospital, London, UK.

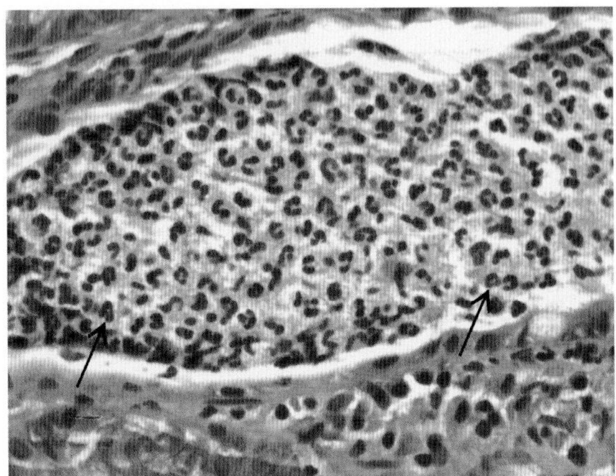

Figure 16.18 An acute inflammatory process characterised by numerous neutrophils. Note the typical multilobated nuclei in many cells (arrows).

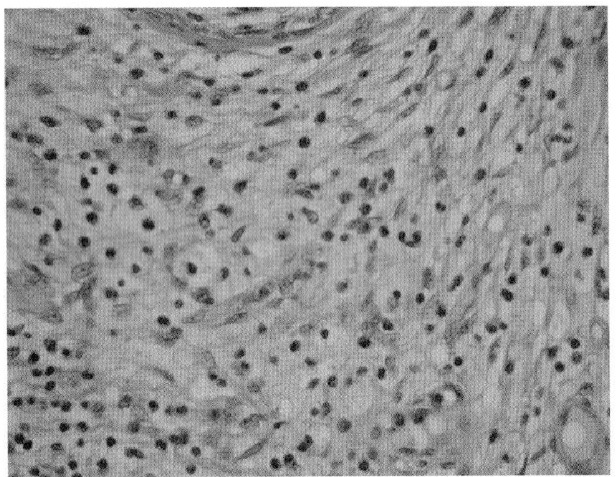

Figure 16.19 An inflammatory lesion in which eosinophils, characterised by bright red cytoplasm, are predominant.

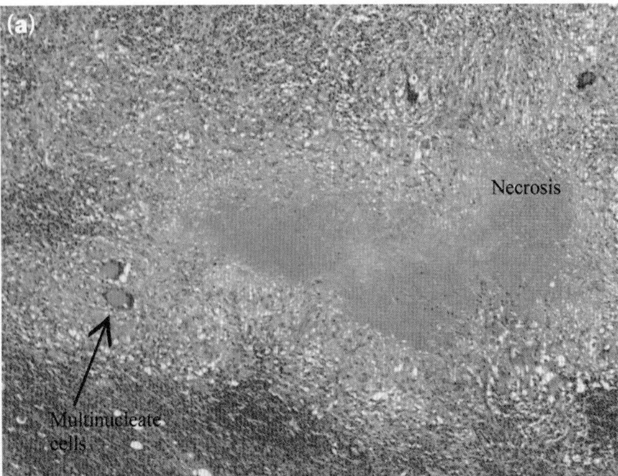

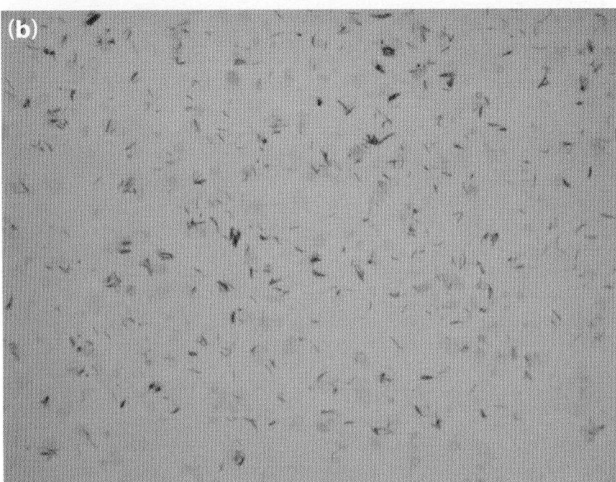

Figure 16.20 (**a**) A granuloma with necrosis, suggesting tuberculosis. Multinucleate giant cells of Langhan's type are also present (arrow). (**b**) A Ziehl–Neelsen stain (different case) shows numerous acid-fast bacilli.

replaced by gastric or intestinal type epithelium. Necrosis refers to cell or tissue death, typically as a result of external factors, and is often associated with cell swelling and inflammation. Apoptosis is a process of programmed cell death that occurs in normal cells as a result of internal signals, and typically causes cell shrinkage and nuclear chromatin condensation.

ASSESSMENT

Light microscopy

Most tissue assessment depends on conventional light microscopy. Microscopes have several lenses with various powers of magnification, typically ranging from ×20 to ×400 or more. A low-power lens allows a sample to be scanned and its overall architecture to be assessed, while a high-power lens allows a closer and more detailed view (**Figure 16.21**). A teaching arm and a camera can be attached to most microscopes (**Figure 16.8**). Polarisation can be used to detect foreign material (e.g. sutures) or to assess a special stain (e.g. Congo red).

Histological assessment

In a histological preparation, the microscopic structure of the tissue is preserved, allowing direct visualisation of architecture. Accordingly, the pathologist can see not only the characteristics of the cells that form the tissue, but also the way in which these cells are related to one another and the way in which different tissue compartments are arranged.

Cytological assessment

A cytological preparation consists of a sample of cells. Architecture cannot be determined, because intact tissue is absent or sparse (**Figures 16.9 and 16.22**). Therefore, assessment relies mainly on the characteristics of the cells themselves. Accordingly, it may be difficult to diagnose malignancy because many of the criteria, particularly invasiveness, cannot be assessed. However, cytology has several potential advantages over histology. A wider area may be sampled, and obtaining a specimen may be easier and less traumatic. Processing times are usually shorter and costs lower. Also, non-medical staff can be trained to report the cases, particularly cervical smears (**Figure 16.9**).

Congo red is sodium diphenylbisazobisnaphthylamine sulphonate.

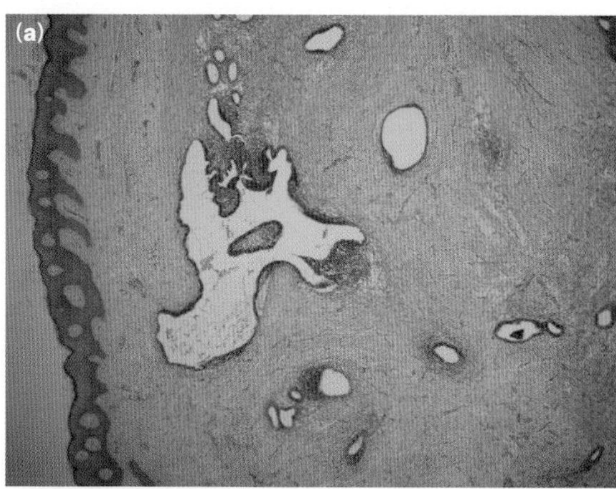

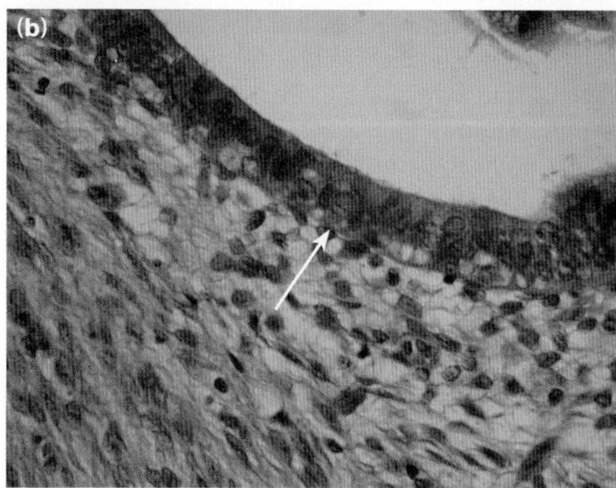

Figure 16.21 (**a**) Low-power view of an umbilical nodule. Glands are distributed irregularly through the tissue. (**b**) High-power view shows benign columnar epithelium lining the glands (arrow), favouring endometriosis over carcinoma.

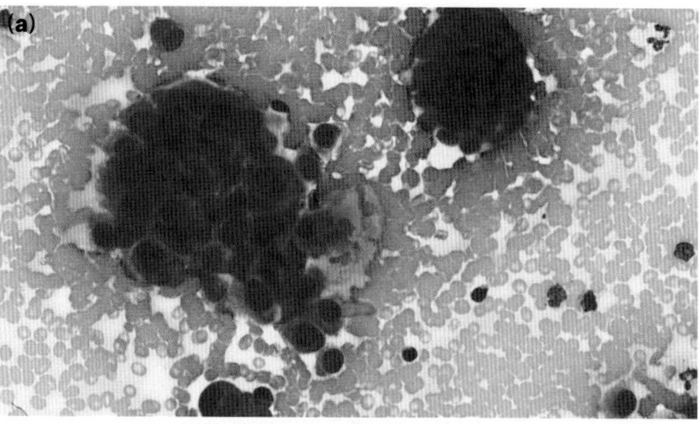

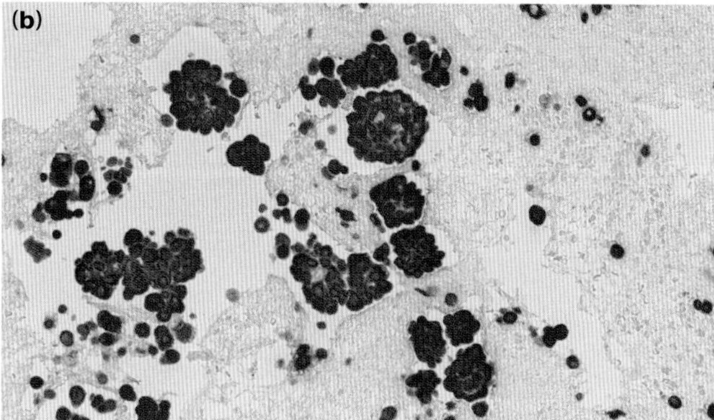

Figure 16.22 (**a**) A cytology preparation of a pleural effusion. Numerous cells with atypical features are present. (**b**) Immunohistochemistry shows positive staining for carcinoembryonic antigen (CEA), favouring carcinoma over mesothelioma

Summary box 16.7

Cytology compared with histology

Advantages:

- Wider area may be sampled
- Sampling may be less invasive
- Fast
- Cheap

Disadvantages:

- Cannot assess tissue architecture
- Less amenable to further studies

Screening

Screening programmes aim to detect and treat premalignant tissue changes, e.g. dysplasia, or early stage malignancy (rather than advanced disease). They may rely on cytology, histology or both. The largest is the cervical cancer programme, which currently uses cytology initially, with biopsy and histology follow-up if appropriate. The breast cancer screening programme may use cytology and/or histology, while the bowel cancer screening programme relies initially on a non-tissue-based test followed, if appropriate, by endoscopy and, where required, biopsy and histology. Screening for cancer in ulcerative colitis relies on endoscopic assessment and histology.

Specimen adequacy

There are several possible reasons for an inadequate specimen. The operator may fail to sample the intended organ or lesion, or may take too few samples to detect a heterogeneous abnormality. A sample from the centre of a necrotic or ulcerated lesion might include no viable tissue. Superficial biopsies from a carcinoma may fail to distinguish dysplasia (Figure 16.14) from invasive carcinoma. Cautery and crush artefact are sometimes severe enough to impede assessment.

Summary box 16.8

Reasons for an inadequate sample

Histology and cytology:

- Failure to sample the intended organ or lesion
- Sample too limited
- Non-viable tissue

Histology:

- Sample too superficial
- Cautery artefact
- Crush artefact

Deeper levels and extra blocks

The pathologist may request 'deeper levels', whereby the BMS cuts further into the paraffin block to obtain further sections. For example, deeper levels of a histologically atypical but non-invasive epithelial lesion might show foci of invasion, allowing carcinoma to be diagnosed. Extra blocks may be taken from a resection specimen if it has been sampled inadequately, e.g. if insufficient lymph nodes have been retrieved from a cancer case.

Summary box 16.9

Additional techniques

- Special stains
- Immunohistochemistry
- Electron microscopy
- Molecular pathology
- *In situ* hybridisation, including fluorescence *in situ* hybridisation (FISH)
- PCR-based techniques

FURTHER WORK

Further diagnostic work is performed on a significant minority of histology specimens, and includes special stains, immunohistochemistry and various molecular pathology techniques such as *in situ* hybridisation and polymerase chain reaction (PCR)-based methods. Electron microscopy is used less often. Some techniques can also be applied to cytology specimens (**Figure 16.22**).

Special stains

A 'special stain' is a stain that is not routine, i.e. not an H&E stain. Immunohistochemical stains are conventionally excluded from this category. Some special stains demonstrate normal substances in increased quantities or in abnormal locations. The periodic acid–Schiff (PAS) stain demonstrates both glycogen and mucin, whereas a diastase PAS (D-PAS) stain demonstrates mucin, e.g. in an adenocarcinoma. Perls Prussian blue stain demonstrates iron accumulation (**Figure 16.23**), e.g. in haemochromatosis. A reticulin stain helps to demonstrate fibrosis (**Figure 16.24**). Elastic stains also show fibrosis and can highlight blood vessels by outlining their elastic laminae. Special stains can also reveal the accumulation of abnormal substances, e.g. a Congo red stain for amyloid.

(a)

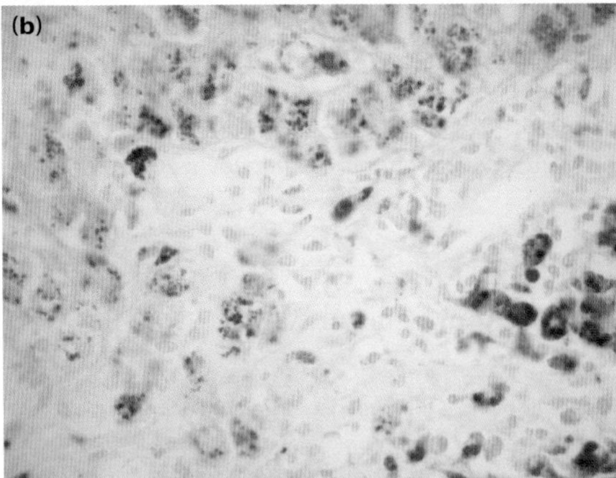

Figure 16.23 **(a)** Brown pigment in a biopsy. **(b)** A Perls stain is positive, indicating that the pigment is iron.

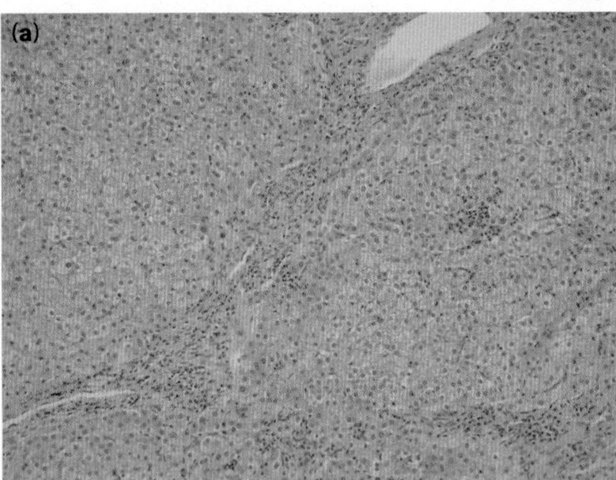

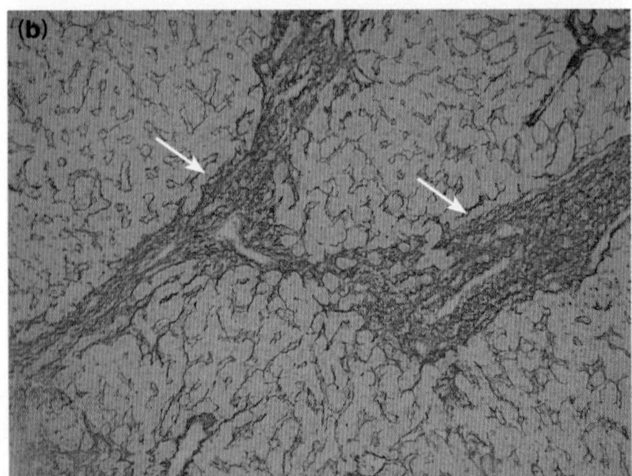

Figure 16.24 **(a)** A liver biopsy stained with haematoxylin and eosin (H&E) in which the severity of fibrosis cannot be determined. **(b)** A reticulin stain demonstrates fibrous bridges (arrows).

Hugo Schiff, 1834–1915, German biochemist who worked in Florence, Italy.
Max Perls, 1843–1881, pathologist, Giesen, Germany.

Summary box 16.10

Common special stains

- PAS: glycogen, fungi
- D-PAS: mucin
- Perls Prussian blue: iron
- Reticulin: reticulin fibres, fibrosis
- van Gieson: collagen
- Congo red: amyloid
- Ziehl–Neelsen: mycobacteria

Special stains are also useful for the diagnosis of infection. For example, a Ziehl–Neelsen stain demonstrates acid-fast bacilli, particularly mycobacteria, by staining them bright red in a blue background (**Figure 16.20**). Mycobacteria cannot be seen on H&E slides. Other microorganisms that may be detectable on H&E but are easier to see with a special stain include fungi (PAS or Grocott stain), protozoa (Giemsa stain) and spirochaetes (Warthin–Starry stain).

Electron microscopy

Electron microscopy allows tissue to be visualised at very high magnification, e.g. ×1000 to ×500 000. It may help to decide the lineage of a non-neoplastic or neoplastic cell in difficult cases and may help to determine the nature of abnormal deposits, e.g. in renal disease. Unfortunately, it is time-consuming, labour intensive and expensive, and is now used very selectively.

Immunohistochemistry

Immunohistochemistry was introduced in the 1970s and has had a major impact on histopathological diagnosis. This technique detects a specific antigen using an antibody. The antibody is labelled with a dye and when bound to its target antigen is seen in the tissue section as a coloured stain, often brown (**Figure 16.25**). This allows the presence, tissue distribution and cellular localisation of an antigen to be determined. It can also be used to quantify expression: for example, Ki67 is a cell cycle marker that allows a proliferative index to be calculated, which in turn has prognostic value for neuroendocrine tumours and other neoplasms. Immunohistochemistry can be applied to fixed and frozen tissue and to cytological preparations (**Figure 16.22b**). It is specific, safe, quick and relatively inexpensive. However, false-positive results can result from non-specific staining or from cross-reaction with similar antigens. Over-reliance on immunohistochemistry by clinicians and pathologists should be avoided.

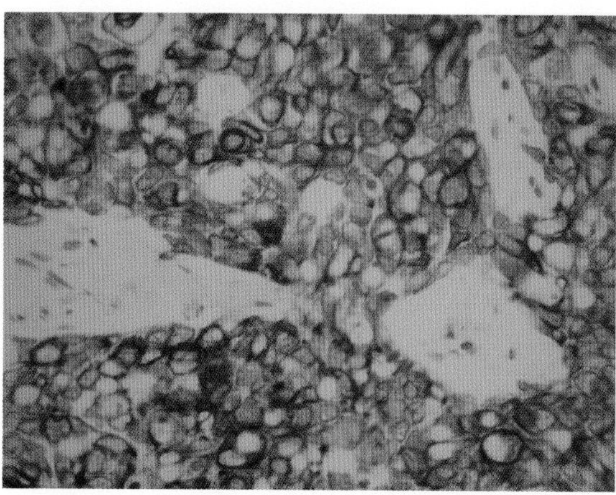

Figure 16.25 Diffuse immunohistochemical staining (brown) for a pancytokeratin marker in a malignancy, favouring carcinoma over other tumours.

Immunohistochemistry: tumour pathology

Immunohistochemistry has multiple applications in tumour pathology, including elucidation of site of origin and determination of cell type/direction of differentiation. Immunohistochemistry may also help to confirm neoplasia, determine the selection of treatment, refine prognostic predictions and screen for known underlying genetic changes.

Various immunohistochemical stains are used to detect cell type. Cytokeratins are expressed by epithelial cells. Cytokeratin positivity favours carcinoma (**Figure 16.25**) over

Summary box 16.11

Some immunohistochemical stains used for tumours

- Cell type/site of origin:
  - Epithelial (carcinoma): cytokeratins
  - Lymphoid (lymphoma): CD45, CD3, CD20
  - Melanocytic (melanoma): S100, HMB45, Melan A
  - Neuroendocrine: synaptophysin, chromogranin
  - Vascular: CD31
  - Myoid: desmin, actin
- Site of origin/cell type:
  - Prostate: prostate-specific antigen (PSA)
  - Lung: thyroid transcription factor-1 (TTF-1)
  - Thyroid: thyroglobulin
  - Colorectum: cytokeratin 20 (CK20), CDX2
  - Liver: HepPar
  - Gastrointestinal stromal tumour (GIST): CD117, DOG-1
- Prognosis and treatment:
  - Breast and gastric carcinomas: HER2
  - Neuroendocrine tumours: Ki67 labelling index
- Screening for mutations
  - Colorectal carcinoma: mismatch repair genes (MLH1, MSH2, MSH6, PMS2)

Ira Thompson van Gieson, 1866–1913, American neuropathologist, described this stain in 1889.
Franz Heinrich Paul Ziehl, 1859–1926, neurologist, Lübeck, Germany.
Friedrich Carl Adolf Neelsen, 1854–1894, pathologist, prosector, the Stadt-Krankenhaus, Dresden, Germany.
Aldred Scott Warthin, 1866–1931, Professor of Pathology, The University of Michigan, Ann Arbor, MI, USA.

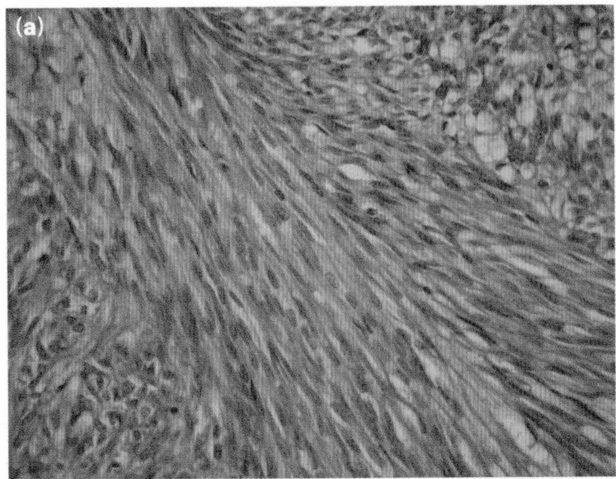

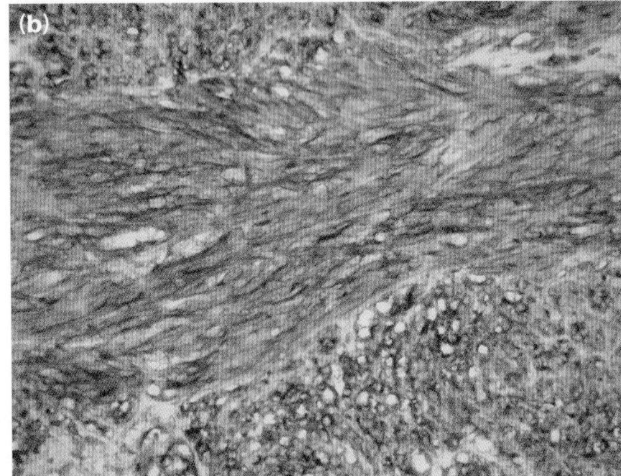

Figure 16.26 (**a**) A metastatic tumour composed of spindle cells. Gastrointestinal stromal tumour (GIST) was suspected. (**b**) Positive immunohistochemistry for CD117, confirming GIST.

other malignancies. Lymphoid markers include the panlymphoid marker CD45, the T-cell marker CD3 and the B-cell marker CD20. Markers of melanocytic differentiation include S100, MelanA and HMB45. Chromogranin, synaptophysin and CD56 stain neuroendocrine tumours such as carcinoid and small cell carcinoma. A gastrointestinal stromal tumour (GIST) typically expresses CD117 (**Figure 16.26**) and DOG-1. Endothelial cell markers include CD31, which may highlight vascular invasion or confirm a diagnosis of vascular neoplasia.

The site of origin of a metastatic tumour may be suggested by H&E appearances. For example, an adenocarcinoma has several possible sources. A clear cell carcinoma (**Figure 16.17**) is often of renal origin. Immunohistochemical stains may provide further information. Some are highly specific for an anatomical site, e.g. prostate-specific antigen (PSA) and thyroglobulin. Others are somewhat less specific, but still useful, e.g. thyroid transcription factor-1 (TTF-1), a marker of bronchogenic origin; HepPar, that suggests hepatocellular origin; and cytokeratin 20 and CDX2, typically expressed by colorectal carcinoma. Carcinoembryonic antigen (CEA) is seen in several types of carcinoma (**Figure 16.22b**). However, some malignancies, especially poorly differentiated examples, do not conform to the typical patterns. Therefore, the clinical picture and imaging results should always be taken into account.

Less often, immunohistochemistry is used to help confirm malignancy. For example, kappa or lambda light chain restriction (expression of only one immunoglobulin light chain) in lymphoid proliferations suggests clonality and, in turn, neoplasia rather than a reactive process. Strong expression of p53 may support a diagnosis of dysplasia or neoplasia in specific settings.

Immunohistochemistry also plays a role in the selection of treatment and in predicting prognosis. For example, carcinomas of the breast are routinely assessed for oestrogen receptor (ER) and human epidermal growth factor receptor-2 (HER2) status, while lymphomas are typically subjected to a comprehensive panel of markers that help determine treatment and prognosis. Ki67 proliferative index is an important prognostic factor for neuroendocrine tumours and for some other neoplasms (**Figure 16.27**).

Immunohistochemistry: infections and other applications

There are antibodies to many infective agents, including cytomegalovirus (CMV), Epstein–Barr virus (EBV), herpes simplex virus, human herpes virus 8 (HHV8), hepatitis B virus and *Helicobacter pylori*. Some of these organisms, e.g. *H. pylori* and CMV, can be seen or suspected on H&E slides, while others, e.g. EBV and HHV8, require immunohistochemistry or other techniques for their detection.

Immunohistochemistry can also be used to study immunoglobulin and complement expression (e.g. in lymphomas or renal biopsies); to assess the abnormal accumulation of various proteins such as alpha-1-antitrypsin (A1AT); to characterise amyloid; and to screen for mismatch repair gene mutations. As molecular pathological techniques progress, further immunohistochemical markers that detect specific

Summary box 16.12

Uses of immunohistochemistry

- Cell type
- Neoplasia:
  - Differentiation
  - Determination of site of origin
  - Confirmation of neoplasia
  - Selection of treatment
  - Screening for mutations
  - Prognosis
- Microorganisms
- Other:
  - Amyloid
  - Immunoglobulins
  - Complement

Michael Anthony Epstein, b.1921, formerly Professor of Pathology, the University of Bristol, Bristol, UK.
Yvonne Barr, b.1931, virologist who emigrated to Australia. Epstein and Barr discovered this virus in 1964.

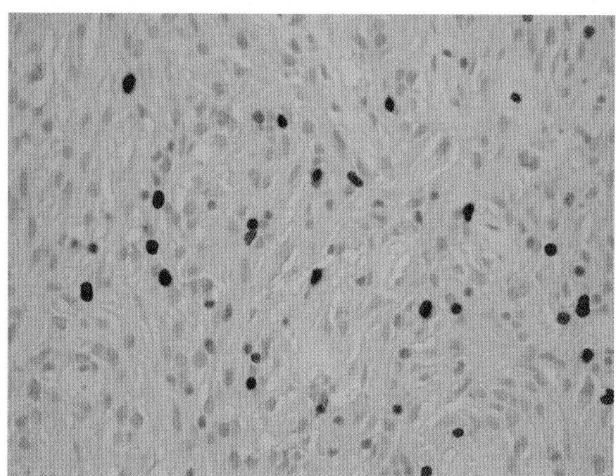

Figure 16.27 Immunohistochemistry for Ki67. The proliferative index is approximately 10%.

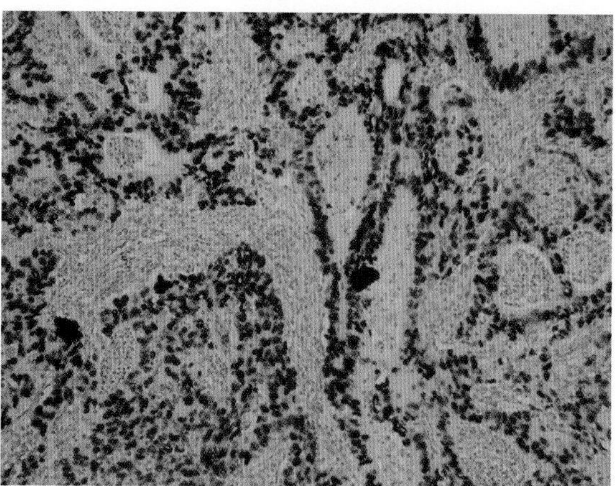

Figure 16.28 *In situ* hybridisation for Epstein–Barr virus (EBV) showing extensive nuclear positivity (black nuclei) in a gastric adenocarcinoma.

gene mutations are being developed and may become useful in clinical practice in the future.

DIAGNOSTIC MOLECULAR PATHOLOGY

The broad heading of diagnostic molecular pathology refers to multiple tests that assess molecules (proteins, ribonucleic acid [RNA] and deoxyribonucleic acid [DNA]) in tissue. The information that they provide may be useful for diagnosis, prognostic predictions, identifying patients with a hereditary cancer risk, determining treatment and identifying residual disease after treatment. Immunohistochemistry is conventionally excluded from this category.

Methods

In situ hybridisation

In situ hybridisation (ISH) uses a labelled oligonucleotide probe targeted at a specific sequence of RNA or DNA. It can be performed on fixed or fresh tissue sections, allowing the presence or absence of a particular sequence and its location to be seen *in situ*. Autoradiography, fluorescence microscopy or immunohistochemistry can be used for visualisation. Chromogenic *in situ* hybridisation (CISH) combines ISH and immunohistochemistry for the detection of DNA regions and it is widely and routinely used in pathology laboratories for the detection of HER2 amplifications. Viral genomes, e.g. EBV (**Figure 16.28**), CMV and human papillomavirus, can be detected using this approach. ISH plays an important role in the management of tumours (see below).

Polymerase chain reaction

The polymerase chain reaction (PCR) amplifies DNA, yielding millions of copies from a single copy of a selected target. RNA also may be amplified, using the technique of reverse transcriptase PCR (RT-PCR). PCR is fast and safe and can be performed on homogenised fresh or formalin-fixed tissue. PCR-based methods have many applications in oncology (see below), including mutational analysis (**Figures 16.29 and 16.30**), testing for clonality (**Figure 16.31**), detection of transcripts resulting from cytogenetic changes, detection of amplifications, demonstration of microsatellite instability and detection of gene hypermethylation. PCR-based methods can also be used to detect microorganisms.

Cytogenetics and FISH

Cytogenetics is the microscopic study of chromosomal changes in individual cells. Conventional cytogenetics is complemented, and is increasingly being replaced, by newer techniques including interphase cytogenetics and RT-PCR. Interphase cytogenetics relies mainly on FISH, although other forms of ISH may be used. Cytogenetic tests seek alterations such as gene amplification (e.g. HER2 in breast and upper gastrointestinal cancer; MDM2 in liposarcoma and atypical lipomas),

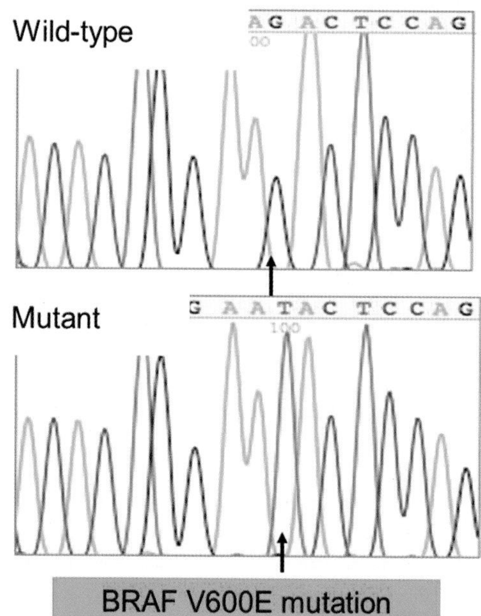

Figure 16.29 Sanger sequencing showing wild type BRAF (above) and a BRAF V600E mutation (below) (courtesy of Dr M Rodriguez-Justo, UCL-AD, Cancer Institute, London, United Kingdom).

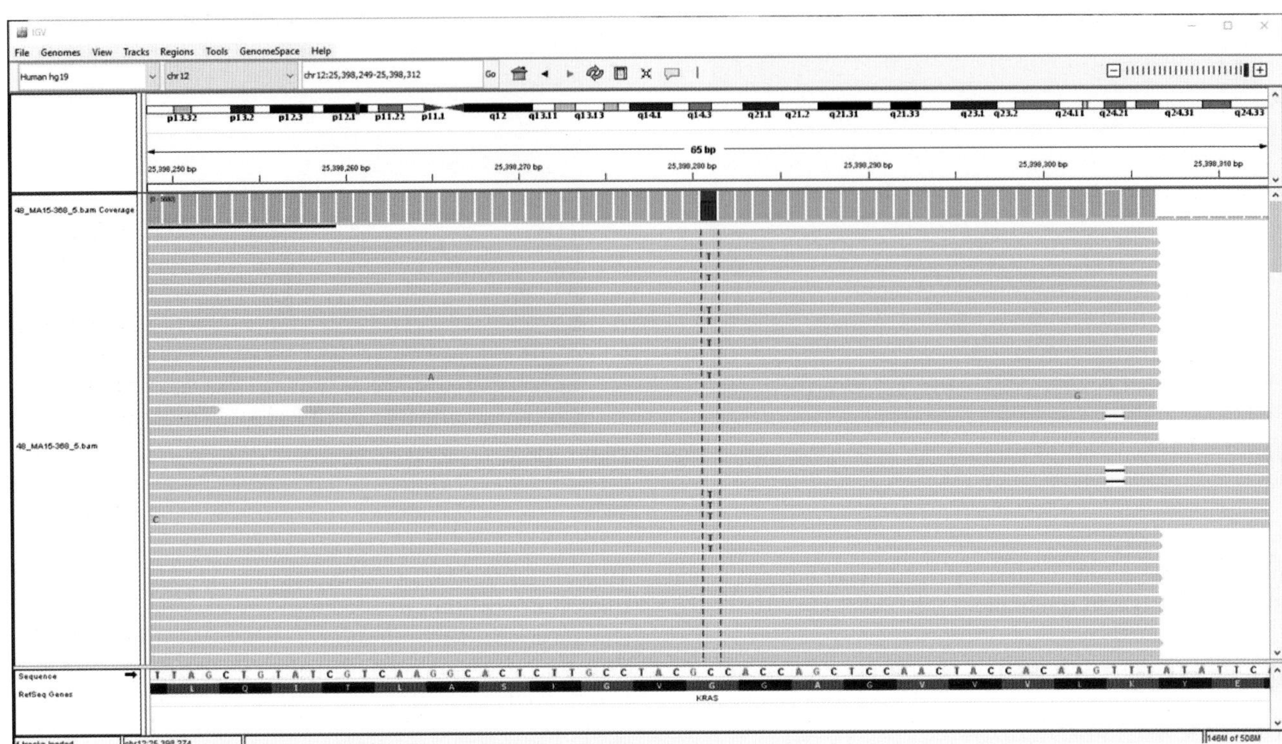

Figure 16.30 KRAS mutation detected using next generation sequencing (Ion Torrent, Life Technologies) (courtesy of Dr M Rodriguez-Justo).

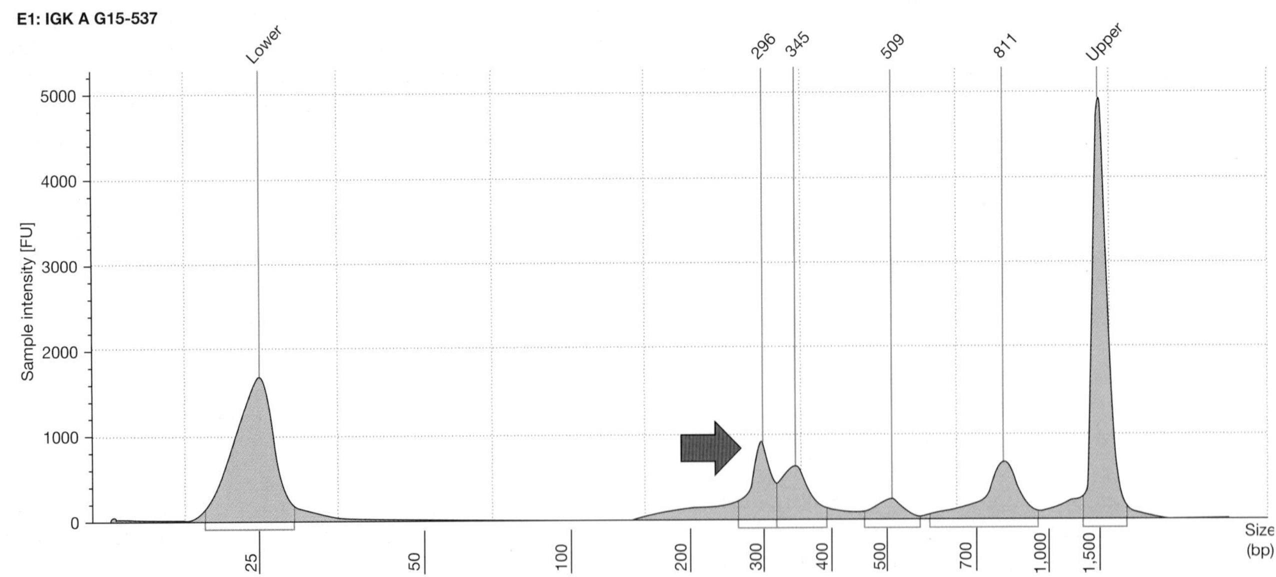

Figure 16.31 Clonality analysis showing a reproducible clonal peak (296) consistent with IG-kappa gene/clonal rearrangement (IG-Kappa Gene clonality assay, Invivoscribe) (courtesy of Dr M Rodriguez-Justo).

loss of segments of chromosomal material, loss of whole chromosomes (e.g. renal cell carcinoma) and translocations and fusion genes (e.g. haematological and soft tissue tumours).

Flow cytometry

Flow cytometry (FC) is a laser- or impedance-based technique used for cell counting, cell sorting, biomarker detection and protein engineering. Cells are suspended in a stream of fluid and passed by an electronic detection apparatus. It is useful for detecting antigens in haematological neoplasms, usually in blood samples, and for determining ploidy, i.e. the number of sets of chromosomes in the nucleus of a cell. Although traditional FC is of limited value for tissue analysis, new applications on image cytometric DNA analysis (ICDA) have been developed that allow detection of aneuploidy in tissue sections of gastrointestinal cancers.

Gene changes in tumours

In normal circumstances, the division and proliferation of cells is carefully controlled. For example, various growth factors influence division by binding to specific cell surface tyrosine kinase receptors resulting in the initiation of an intracellular cascade of changes. Damaged cells may undergo apoptosis, a carefully regulated process of programmed cell death.

Tumours occur as a consequence of uncontrolled cell proliferation. Abnormalities of numerous genes can affect cell proliferation and favour tumour development. The genes that are involved fall into two main categories. Those that stimulate cell proliferation are known as proto-oncogenes (often referred to as oncogenes), while those that inhibit proliferation are called tumour suppressor genes. Inappropriate activation of proto-oncogenes may accelerate cell proliferation, while inhibition of tumour suppressor genes may remove the controls that retard cell growth and division.

Several types of gene or nucleic acid abnormality can occur during tumorigenesis. Mutations are a very common type of abnormality. They are changes in the sequence of nucleic acids, usually DNA. Mutations can be either germline, i.e. inherited from a parent and accordingly present in every cell in the body; or somatic, i.e. acquired at some point during life and affecting only some cells in the body. Mutations are of several types. Point mutations are single nucleotide changes, where one base pair is replaced by another. Other types of mutation include deletions and insertions (indels). Examples of clinically relevant mutations include p53 tumour suppressor gene mutations, causing production of an abnormal p53 protein that lacks suppressor function; and mutation of the KIT gene, causing ligand-independent activation of a growth factor receptor.

Other abnormalities of genes include amplification, e.g. HER2, resulting in over-expression of the growth factor; translocations, e.g. t14:18 in follicular lymphoma that results in juxtaposition of the anti-apoptotic bcl-2 gene to a regulatory region of an immunoglobulin heavy chain gene, with subsequent bcl-2 overexpression; and loss of one of the two copies of a particular gene, or loss of heterozygosity.

Gene defects may ultimately interfere with the function of proteins involved in various regulatory processes, such as cell cycle control (e.g. p53); apoptosis (e.g. bcl-2); and signal transduction pathways. The latter can be affected by abnormalities of growth factor receptors or of intracellular components such as KRAS (**Figure 16.30**) and NRAS. DNA mismatch repair (MMR) genes can also be affected, causing instability of repeated sequences of DNA called microsatellites (known as microsatellite instability or MSI).

Epigenetic changes

Epigenetic factors are external to the gene and can switch it on or off. The latter is known as epigenetic silencing and can result from DNA methylation (addition of a methyl group to DNA with alteration of its structure), modifications of histones (components of chromatin) and RNA-associated silencing. Loss of methylation with gene activation can occur in tumours. Conversely, hypermethylation of tumour suppressor genes or of the mismatch repair gene MLH1 can reduce their activity, favouring malignancy. The importance and high frequency of epigenetic changes in tumours is increasingly being recognised.

Detection of mutations

There are two broadly related areas of clinical practice that rely on mutational analysis. Firstly, tumour tissue DNA can be analysed for mutations to improve diagnostic precision, enhance treatment plans and help predict clinical outcome. Secondly, a sample (usually blood) may be submitted for detection of germline mutations that are characteristic of an inherited disease. This is referred to as genetic testing and can be used to confirm non-neoplastic conditions, such as cystic fibrosis, or to diagnose a hereditary predisposition to cancer, e.g. Lynch syndrome (see below). Genetic testing may be offered to those who have a strong family history of cancer or whose clinical presentation suggests a family history of cancer, e.g. diagnosis before the age of 50.

Mutational analysis is based on PCR and requires extraction of DNA from tissue (or from other sources such as blood). It includes sequencing-based screening methods (e.g. Sanger sequencing, pyrosequencing) (**Figure 16.29**), screening methods comparing mutated with normal DNA and targeted mutation detection methods.

Next-generation sequencing (NGS or NextGen) (**Figure 16.30**) has emerged relatively recently and has already changed cancer management profoundly. The term NGS encompasses several methods, each of which performs massively parallel sequencing, allowing millions of fragments of DNA to be examined simultaneously for mutations. It is quicker and potentially cheaper than older methods and is applicable to formalin-fixed tissue. Targeted NGS is capable of identifying multiple known and novel mutations and other variants in genes of interest in a single test. In addition, NGS is able to detect low-frequency alleles with higher sensitivity towards low-frequency mutations compared with traditional Sanger sequencing.

New powerful platforms have been developed recently, designed to detect simultaneously not only mutations but also copy number variants (CVN) and gene fusions in more than 100 genes involved in human oncogenesis with minimal nuclear acid (DNA and RNA) sample input (Oncomine cancer Panel).

NGS has several applications, including prediction of tumour response to therapy, prediction of clinical behaviour and, increasingly, diagnosis.

Adequate amounts of tumour DNA must be present in the tissue sample for these techniques to be successful. Many

Summary box 16.13

Indications for molecular pathology testing of tissue

- Diagnosis and classification of tumours
- Confirmation of neoplasia: clonality
- Staging
- Prognosis
- Selection of therapy
- Monitoring disease burden

samples include both non-neoplastic tissue and tumour. If necessary, microdissection of the area of interest can be done using conventional techniques or laser-assisted approaches.

Molecular testing: examples of clinical settings

Lymphoma

The distinction between benign and malignant lymphoid proliferations relies initially on morphology, immunohistochemistry and the clinical setting, but is sometimes difficult. Clonal immunoglobulin heavy chain (IgH) gene rearrangements in B-cell proliferations and clonal T-cell receptor gene rearrangements in T-cell proliferations favour lymphoma over reactive proliferations, although clonality is not synonymous with malignancy. Clonality is typically detected using PCR-based methods (**Figure 16.31**). Also, identification of characteristic cytogenetic abnormalities plays a very important role in diagnosis, classification and management of various lymphomas and other haematological neoplasms.

Soft tissue tumours

The diagnosis of many types of soft tissue tumour/sarcoma is assisted by molecular testing. Examples include Ewing's sarcoma, alveolar rhabdomyosarcoma and leiomyosarcoma. Characteristic cytogenetic changes are usually detected by FISH.

Gastrointestinal stromal tumour

Most GISTS have either a KIT gene mutation or a PDGFRA gene mutation, more often the former. Identification of known mutations helps confirm the diagnosis of GIST in difficult cases. Mutational profile may also help predict clinical outcome and response to chemotherapy (e.g. imatinib, a tyrosine kinase inhibitor).

Treatment of advanced colorectal carcinoma (CRC), lung cancer and malignant melanoma

An increasingly common reason for molecular testing is the prediction of response to drug therapy for advanced carcinomas and other malignancies ('theranostics'). In CRC, the anti-EGFR monoclonal antibodies cetuximab and panitumumab are used in combination with chemotherapy for metastatic disease. This drug is less likely to be effective if KRAS or NRAS mutations are present than if a tumour is 'wild-type' (i.e. has no RAS mutation). In lung cancer, response to the anti-EGFR tyrosine kinase inhibitor Gefitinib is confined to a minority of lesions and is predicted by specific EGFR mutations, while response to the anaplastic lymphoma kinase (ALK) inhibitor crizotinib is predicted by ALK gene rearrangement. In metastatic malignant melanoma, response to the BRAF kinase inhibitor vemurafenib is predicted by specific BRAF mutations.

HER2 gene amplification in breast and gastric cancer

The management of breast cancer, and more recently of untreated metastatic gastric adenocarcinoma, is influenced by the tumour's HER2 status. Patients whose tumours overexpress HER2 are offered treatment with the monoclonal antibody trastuzumab. Screening for HER2 overexpression relies on immunohistochemistry. Confirmation or exclusion of underlying gene amplification in equivocal cases depends on FISH testing or PCR.

Mismatch repair genes

CRC and endometrial carcinoma can harbour germline or sporadic abnormalities of mismatch repair (MMR) genes (MLH1, MSH2, MSH6 and PMS2). Lynch syndrome, characterised by germline MMR gene defects, predisposes to CRC and other tumours that may occur at a relatively young age. Immunohistochemistry is a common screening method for MMR mutations. Loss of immunohistochemical staining by neoplastic cells is a marker for a genetic defect and an indication for considering genetic testing of patients and their families for Lynch syndrome (**Figure 16.32**). In addition, MMR gene defects in CRC predict lower recurrence rates, later recurrence, a better response to 5-FU-based chemotherapy and better survival rates.

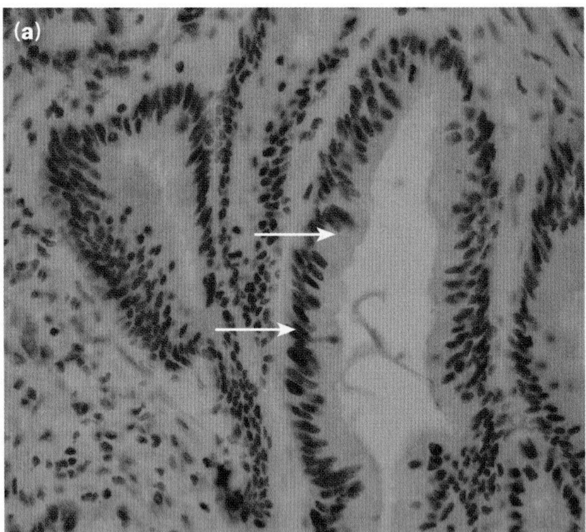

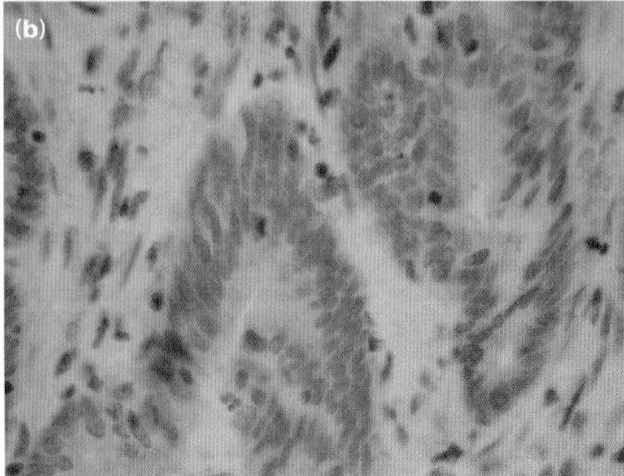

Figure 16.32 Immunohistochemical screening for mismatch repair gene mutations in a carcinoma. (**a**) Nuclear MLH1 expression is retained (arrows showing positively staining brown neoplastic nuclei). (**b**) In contrast, MSH2 expression is lost, suggesting a mismatch repair gene abnormality.

Staging and response to treatment

Tests can be used to confirm the presence or absence of a tumour at a particular anatomical site, thus refining staging. Similarly, they can help to assess the response to anti-cancer therapy. This has been particularly useful for haematological neoplasms such as myeloid leukaemias, where the presence of minimal residual disease can be detected by PCR-based methods.

Prognosis

Tests that help determine the selection of therapy for tumours may also have prognostic value, additional to that of established prognostic factors, e.g. BRAF in CRC. Some genetic changes have prognostic value in one type of tumour but not another, e.g. MMR gene defects are more predictive for CRC than for endometrial cancer. Of course, the outcome of many tumours now depends to some extent on their response to drug therapy, and accordingly a molecular test predicting response to therapy is at the same time prognostic. Packages of tests with additional prognostic value are also available, e.g. Oncotype DX, which analyses multiple genes in breast cancer tissue.

Cancer 'precision medicine'

This refers to the development of individualised cancer care plans, on the basis of molecular abnormalities. Germline and somatic mutations may be taken into consideration, so as to tailor treatments precisely and to target the cancer cells as effectively as possible. With the advent of NGS, analysis of a single sample of tumour tissue for multiple known and novel mutations that may predict treatment response is possible. In addition, mutations affecting as few as 5% of neoplastic cells can be detected. Other techniques may be used at the same time to detect abnormalities in the proteome (protein), transcriptome (mRNA), metabolome (metabolites) or epigenome, sometimes referred to as 'omics' assays. Such plans may, inevitably, be very complex.

Summary: diagnostic molecular pathology

Progress in molecular pathology is undoubtedly improving patient management. There is justifiable enthusiasm for the potential of emerging techniques. However, factors such as tumour heterogeneity, development of resistance to treatment and the genetic plasticity of many cancers could limit the development of precision medicine. Cost is also a consideration. Furthermore, the results of molecular studies should be interpreted not in isolation but with the clinical setting and basic tumour morphology in mind. For example, several types of tumour, including melanoma, CRC and papillary carcinoma of the thyroid, may have the same BRAF mutation, but the response to specific anti-BRAF therapy depends on the histology and the anatomical site. Similarly, the clinical implications of MMR gene defects in CRC and endometrial cancer are dissimilar. Finally, it is worth remembering that an H&E stained slide is inexpensive, easy to produce and a good summary of the genetic complexity of cells.

AUTOPSY

In the past, advances in medical knowledge were sometimes based on autopsy findings. Autopsies remain very useful for medical education and audit, as well as identifying the cause of death. In the UK there are two types of autopsy. The first is the coroner's postmortem, when the coroner decides that there is a need, or is obliged, to establish the cause of death. No consent from relatives is required. The second is the hospital autopsy, which requires relatives' consent. Valuable information may be revealed through both of these routes, especially in the unusual event of death following surgery.

FINAL COMMENTS

Analysis of tissue has played an increasingly important role in clinical management over the past few decades, and there has been rapid recent progress in the field of diagnostic molecular pathology. Pathologists need to work more closely with clinicians than ever before in order to optimise management, and to ensure that the value and limitations of tissue diagnosis and of new technologies are appreciated.

ACKNOWLEDGEMENTS

The author is very grateful to the following contributors: Professor MT Sheaff, for assistance with the sections of this chapter that discuss cytology and autopsy; Dr M Rodriguez-Justo, for reviewing and improving the section on diagnostic molecular pathology.

FURTHER READING

Kumar V, Abbas AK, Aster JC. In: *Robbins and Cotran. Pathologic basis of disease*, 9th edn. Philadelphia: Elsevier Saunders, 2015.

Rosai J (ed). *Rosai and Ackerman's surgical pathology*, 10th edn. Philadelphia: Mosby Elsevier, 2011.

PART 3

Perioperative care

17 Preoperative care including the high-risk surgical patient 254
18 Anaesthesia and pain relief 269
19 Nutrition and fluid therapy 278
20 Postoperative care 290
21 Day case surgery 301

Chapter 17

Preoperative care including the high-risk surgical patient

Learning objectives

To be able to organise the preoperative care and the operating list

To understand preoperative preparation for surgery:

- Surgical, medical and anaesthetic aspects of assessment
- How to optimise the patient's condition
- How to identify and optimise the patient at higher risk
- Importance of critical care in management
- How to take consent
- How to organise an operating list

INTRODUCTION

The stress of major surgery can lead to increased oxygen demand by about 40%. Changes such as cytokine release-related inflammatory changes, endocrine responses, hypercoagulability and redistribution of fluid between compartments may last several postoperative days. The purpose of careful preoperative planning is to minimise the unwanted effects of these physiological changes.

Systematic history taking, examination and ordering of investigations at the preoperative clinic should include not only an assessment of functional reserve but also the formulation of advice on optimisation, to best cope with the anticipated operative stress. General practitioner (GP) records and hospital notes are useful sources of baseline information. GPs can help by monitoring chronic conditions, adjusting medications, and facilitating in weight reduction, exercise and the cessation of smoking.

A simple questionnaire, working within agreed guidelines, can identify high-risk patients undergoing high-risk surgery needing specific tests and optimisation (see later). Patients with severe comorbidities or undergoing high-risk surgery should be referred to specialists to quantify and to reduce perioperative risks. Risks of surgery, anaesthesia and the effects of comorbid conditions should be discussed so that the patient can make an informed decision. Patients should be given advice on 'nil by mouth' (NBM) and regular medication and premedication at the preoperative visit.

A plan for the operating list should be drawn-up and all those involved in making the list run smoothly should be informed. The World Health Organization (WHO) checklist, which is started just prior to induction of anaesthesia and continued during and after the surgery, aims to improve the safety of anaesthesia and surgery.

Summary box 17.1

Preoperative plan for the best patient outcomes

- Gather and record all relevant information
- Optimise patient condition
- Choose surgery that offers minimal risk and maximum benefit
- Anticipate and plan for adverse events
- Adequate hydration, nutrition and exercise are advised

PATIENT ASSESSMENT

Evidence suggests that correction of anaemia, better diabetes control, preoperative exercises and better nutrition leads to better patient outcomes and fewer postoperative complications. Based on population statistics, associated comorbidities and the type of surgery, one can estimate risks for an individual undergoing surgery and various tools and scores (see later) can be used as risk predictors.

History taking

Each organ system problem should be noted with dates, aetiology and treatment delivered (*Table 17.1*). Screening questions will reveal 'fitness' for surgery and anaesthesia. Patients with recent chest infections should be assessed for anaesthetic risks and postoperative surgical infection. Increasing severity of symptoms generally indicates worsening of the condition and possible need for a change in medication. Inability to achieve four metabolic equivalents, e.g. climbing a flight of stairs, increases cardiac risk after major surgery. Some factors leading to these findings may be amenable to treatment preoperatively such as anaemia, angina, palpitations or obesity.

The history of past surgery and anaesthesia can reveal the problems one may face during current hospitalisation (e.g. intra-abdominal adhesions for planned laparoscopic surgery, suxamethonium apnoea). The use of recreational drugs and alcohol consumption should be noted as they are known to be associated with adverse outcomes. Check for allergies and risk factors for deep vein thrombosis (DVT). Social history, ability to communicate and mobility are important in planning rehabilitation after surgery.

Summary box 17.2

Principles of history-taking

- Listen. What is the problem? (Open questions)
- Clarify. What does the patient expect? (Closed questions)
- Narrow. Differential diagnosis (Focused questions)
- Fitness. Comorbidities (Fixed questions)

TABLE 17.1 Key topics in past medical history.

Cardiovascular
- Ischaemic heart disease – angina, **myocardial infarction**
- **Hypertension**
- Heart failure
- Dysrhythmia
- Peripheral vascular disease
- Deep vein thrombosis and pulmonary embolism

Respiratory
- Chronic obstructive pulmonary disease
- Asthma
- Respiratory infections

Gastrointestinal
- Peptic ulcer disease and gastro-oesophageal reflux
- Liver disease

Genitourinary tract
- Urinary tract infection
- Renal dysfunction

Neurological
- Epilepsy
- Cerebrovascular accidents and transient ischaemic attacks
- Psychiatric disorders
- Cognitive function

Endocrine/metabolic
- Diabetes
- Thyroid dysfunction
- Phaeochromocytoma
- Porphyria

Locomotor system
- Osteoarthritis
- Inflammatory arthropathy such as rheumatoid arthritis

Other
- Human immunodeficiency virus
- Hepatitis
- Tuberculosis
- Malignancy
- Allergy

Previous surgery
- **Problems encountered**
- Family history of problems with anaesthesia

Entries in bold need to be recorded even when negative.

Examination

Patients should be treated with respect and dignity, receive a clear explanation of the examination undertaken and be kept as comfortable as possible (*Table 17.2*). A chaperone should be present, especially for intimate examinations. This is will often be part of a local guideline or policy.

In symptomatic patients one should look specifically for evidence of cardiac failure (raised jugular venous pressure (JVP), fine pulmonary crackles, gallop rhythm), peripheral vascular disease (loss of peripheral pulses, ulcerations) and valvular heart disease with characteristic murmurs (e.g. ejection systolic murmur in aortic stenosis, pansystolic murmur in tricuspid regurgitation and mid-diastolic murmur in mitral stenosis heard at respective areas on auscultation). When possible, the medical or surgical treatments for these conditions should be started and the patient stabilised before elective surgery. UK statistics show that patients with cardiac failure or cirrhosis even though on treatment have a high (8%) '30-day mortality' after major surgery.

The presence of a rapid respiratory rate, reduced air entry, crepitations and rhonchi may indicate respiratory problems. A history of dyspnoea along with examination findings of tachycardia, raised JVP, tricuspid regurgitation, hepatomegaly and oedematous feet will indicate severe respiratory disease with pulmonary hypertension and right ventricular failure.

Summary box 17.3

Examination

- General. Positive findings even if not related to the proposed procedure should be explored further
- Surgery related. Type and site of surgery, complications occurred due to underlying pathology
- Systemic. Comorbidities and extent of limitation of each organ function
- Specific. For example, suitability for positioning during surgery

TABLE 17.2 Medical examination.

General	Anaemia, jaundice, cyanosis, nutritional status, sources of infection (teeth, feet, leg ulcers)
Cardiovascular	Pulse, blood pressure, heart sounds, bruits, peripheral oedema
Respiratory	Respiratory rate and effort, chest expansion and percussion note, breath sounds, oxygen saturation
Gastrointestinal	Abdominal masses, ascites, bowel sounds, hernia, genitalia
Neurological	Consciousness level, cognitive function, sensation, muscle power, tone and reflexes
Airway assessment	

Examination specific to surgery

At preoperative assessment, the clinical findings, site, side, specific imaging or investigation findings related to the pathology for which the surgery is proposed should be noted. Suitability of the patient for the proposed surgical option and vice versa should also be assessed. For example, laparoscopic procedures are less invasive and are therefore preferred in most; however, not all patients can tolerate pneumoperitoneum and positioning.

The type of surgery along with patient comorbidities determine perioperative risks, for example perioperative mortality in major surgery such as that of open aortic aneurysm repair in the UK is 3% and that with endovascular repair is 1%.

Sources of potential bacteraemia can compromise surgical results especially if artificial material is implanted, such as in joint replacement surgery or arterial grafting. Check for and treat infections in the preoperative period, e.g. infected toes, pressure sores, teeth and urine; screen the patients for methicillin-resistant *Staphylococcus aureus* colonisation.

Investigations

The National Institute of Health and Care Excellence, UK (NICE) guidelines lay out the investigations needed for various categories of surgery.

Summary box 17.4

Investigations needed

- Type of surgery. Major surgery can lead to organ system dysfunction needing most investigations
- Patient. For example, sickle cell test for patients of Afro-Caribbean origin with family history of sickle cell disease
- Comorbidities. For example, peak flow rates for severe asthmatics

- Full blood count. A full blood count (FBC) is needed for major operations, in the elderly and in those with anaemia or pathology with ongoing blood loss and chronic disease. In case of suspicion or history of sickle crisis, a sickle cell test is needed in patients of Afro-Caribbean and Indian subcontinent origin.
- Urea and electrolytes. Urea and electrolytes (U&Es) are needed before all major operations, in most patients over 65 years of age especially with cardiovascular, renal and endocrine disease, or if significant blood loss is anticipated. It is also needed in those on medications that affect electrolyte levels, e.g. steroids, diuretics, digoxin, non-steroidal anti-inflammatory drugs, intravenous fluid or nutrition therapy and endocrine problems.
- Electrocardiography. Electrocardiography (ECG) is required for those patients over 65 years of age and symptomatic patients with a history of rheumatic fever, diabetes, cardiovascular, renal and cerebrovascular disease, with and without severe respiratory problems. It will also depend on if the surgery is minor/intermediate or major.
- Chest radiograph. Cost-effectiveness and risks of radiation exposure mean that chest radiographs should be restricted to specific patients, such as those with cardiac failure, severe chronic obstructive pulmonary disease (COPD), acute respiratory symptoms, pulmonary cancer, metastasis or effusions or those who are deemed to be at risk of active pulmonary tuberculosis.
- Clotting screen. If a patient has a history suggestive of a bleeding diathesis, liver disease, eclampsia, cholestasis or has a family history of bleeding disorder, or is on antithrombotic or anticoagulant agents then coagulation screening will be needed. However, the effects of antiplatelet agents, low molecular weight heparins and newer agents affecting factor Xa cannot be measured by routine laboratory tests.
- Urinalysis. Dipstick testing of urine should be performed on all patients to detect urinary infection, biliuria, glycosuria and inappropriate osmolality.
- β-Human chorionic gonadotrophin. Women of child-bearing age should be asked sensitively about their pregnancy status. If in doubt a laboratory test or a reliable pregnancy kit (low cost) can be used, after obtaining consent from the patient, to avoid danger of exposure to surgery and anaesthesia on the foetus.
- Blood glucose and HbA1c. Poor control of diabetes can lead to perioperative infection and slow recovery in patients with diabetes mellitus and endocrine problems. HbA1C indicates how well diabetes has been controlled over a longer duration. Early mobilisation, oral intake and return to routine medication should be the goals in management of diabetes.
- Arterial blood gases. A low-cost tool that can give quick and vital information in acute or chronic severe respiratory conditions, acid–base disturbances and conditions where there is changing milieu, e.g. immediately before kidney transplant.
- Liver function tests. These are indicated in patients with jaundice, known or suspected hepatitis, cirrhosis, malignancy or in patients with poor nutritional status.
- Other investigations. Specialist radiological views and recent imaging are sometimes required. If imaging is going to be needed during surgery, then this needs to be planned in advance.

SPECIFIC PREOPERATIVE PROBLEMS AND MANAGEMENT

Specific medical problems encountered during preoperative assessment should be corrected to the best possible level. Many patients with severe disease (see later) will need to be referred to specialists; the referral letter should include all the details including history, examination and investigation results.

Cardiovascular disease

Perioperative cardiovascular complications are frequent. Patients who can climb a flight of stairs without getting short of breath or chest pain or needing to stop are likely to

Summary box 17.5

Preoperative management of patients with systemic disease

- Capacity. Baseline organ function capacity should be assessed
- Optimisation. Medication, lifestyle changes, specialist referral will improve organ capacity
- Alternative. Minimally impacting procedure, appropriate postoperative care will improve outcomes
- Theatre preparations. Timing, teamwork, special instruments and equipment

tolerate a wide range of surgeries with an acceptable risk of perioperative cardiovascular morbidity and mortality. However, at preoperative assessment it is important to identify the patients who have a high perioperative risk of major adverse cardiovascular events (MACE) including myocardial infarction (MI), and make appropriate arrangements to reduce this risk. Patients at high risk are those with ischaemic heart disease (IHD), congestive cardiac failure (CCF), arrhythmias, severe peripheral vascular disease, cerebrovascular disease or significant renal impairment, especially if they are undergoing major intra-abdominal or intra-thoracic surgery.

In patients with ischaemic heart disease the cardiac and coronary reserve can be evaluated using a stress test (stress ECG, stress echocardiogram, myocardial scintigraphy). The tests have a high negative predictive value but a relatively low positive predictive value. If the test is negative, the patient is unlikely to have IHD; conversely, if it is positive the chances of the patient actually having IHD is not necessarily very high, but there is a need for further investigation such as coronary angiography. Recently, measurement of the fractional coronary flow reserve (FFR) during coronary angiography using a pressure wire, has made it possible to identify coronary lesions that have the largest impact on myocardial perfusion.

In patients with any suggestion of valvular heart disease or poor left ventricular function, an echocardiogram should be obtained. Pressure gradients across the valves, dimensions of the chambers and contractility can be determined using echocardiography; an ejection fraction of less than 30% is associated with poor patient outcomes.

Cardiopulmonary exercise testing provides a non-invasive assessment of combined pulmonary, cardiac and circulatory function.

The patient should be referred to a cardiologist if:

- A murmur is heard and the patient is symptomatic.
- The patient is known to have poor left ventricular function or cardiomegaly.
- Ischaemic changes can be seen on ECG even if the patient is not symptomatic (silent ischaemia, silent MIs are frequent).
- There is an abnormal rhythm on the ECG, for example tachy-/bradycardia or heart block.

Hypertension, ischaemic heart disease (IHD) and coronary stents

Prior to elective surgery blood pressure should be controlled to near 160/100 mmHg. If a new antihypertensive agent is introduced, a stabilisation period of at least 2 weeks should be allowed.

Patients with angina, that is not well controlled, should be investigated further by a cardiologist. The indications for coronary revascularisation in these patients before major surgery are the same as the medical indications. Pharmacological protection is indicated. Patients on β-blockers and on statins should be maintained on their medication. Initiating statins preoperatively should be considered. Most long-term cardiac medications should be continued over the perioperative period. Angiotensin-converting enzyme (ACE) inhibitors and receptor blockers are often omitted 24 hours prior to surgery and reintroduced gradually in the postoperative period.

After a proven myocardial infarction (Figure 17.1), elective surgery should be postponed for 3–6 months to reduce the risk of perioperative reinfarction. As primary percutaneous intervention is the treatment of choice for acute coronary syndromes, many patients receive stents and are on dual antiplatelet therapy for 12 months. If surgery is absolutely necessary within the period of dual antiplatelet therapy, the management strategy should be decided jointly by surgeon, cardiologist, anaesthetist and patient, as it is essential to consider the balance of risk of continuing antiplatelet agents (with the risk of increased bleeding) and stopping them (with the risk of stent thrombosis).

The risk of stent thrombosis with consequences of MI and death is reduced if elective surgery is delayed until after dual antiplatelet therapy is no longer needed (about 6 weeks after bare metal and 12 months after drug-eluting stent insertion, although with the newest drug-eluting stents 6 months dual antiplatelet therapy may be enough).

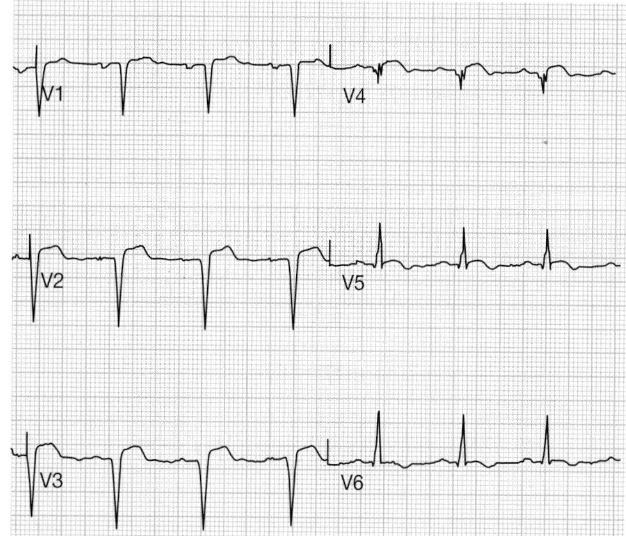

Figure 17.1 Preoperative electrocardiogram of a patient who complained of chest pain the previous day, showing recent transmural anterior myocardial infarction with Q waves and ST elevation.

If surgery cannot be postponed and the risk of significant perioperative bleeding is low, dual antiplatelet therapy can be continued during surgery. If the benefits of surgery can be negated by bleeding in closed cavities (spinal, intracranial, cardiac, posterior chamber of the eye and prostate surgery) clopidogrel or ticagrelor therapy may have to be stopped and, if possible, aspirin continued. However, a cardiology opinion should be sought.

Dysrhythmias

In patients with atrial fibrillation, β-blockers, digoxin or calcium channel blockers should be started preoperatively (or continued if the patient is already on such medication) in order to control rate and possibly rhythm. Cardiac output can increase by 15% if sinus rhythm is restored. Warfarin in patients with atrial fibrillation (AF) should be stopped 5 days preoperatively to achieve an international normalised ratio (INR) of 1.5 or less, which is safe for most surgery. The newer anticoagulants such as dabigatran (direct thrombin inhibitor) or rivaroxaban, apixaban and edoxaban (direct factor Xa inhibitors) do not have antagonists and must be stopped preoperatively, generally for 2–3 days in patients with normal renal function and longer when renal function is impaired. Alternative anticoagulation is not required in the perioperative period unless the risk of stroke is high (high CHA2DS2-VACs score). Bridging therapy with unfractionated heparin or low molecular weight heparin (LMWH) is recommended for patients with AF and a mechanical heart valve undergoing procedures that require interruption of warfarin. Decisions on bridging therapy should balance the risks of stroke and bleeding.

Implanted pacemakers and cardiac defibrillators

Checks and appropriate reprogramming should be done preoperatively by specialists. Monopolar diathermy activity during surgery may be sensed by the pacemaker as ventricular fibrillation. Therefore, cardioversion and overpace modes must be turned off (and switched on after surgery) or converted to 'ventricle paced, not sensed with no response to sensing' (VOO) mode. Bipolar diathermy should be made available at surgery.

Symptomatic heart blocks and asymptomatic second- (Mobitz II) and third-degree heart blocks, if discovered at preoperative assessment clinic, will need cardiology consultation and temporary or permanent pacemaker insertion.

Figures 17.2 and 17.3 illustrate ECGs from two cases requiring preoperative optimisation.

Valvular heart disease

While anaesthetic management is altered to achieve haemodynamic stability in moderate valvular diseases, the patients with severe aortic and mitral stenosis may benefit from valvuloplasty before elective non-cardiac surgery. Appropriate referral to anaesthetist and cardiologist should be made.

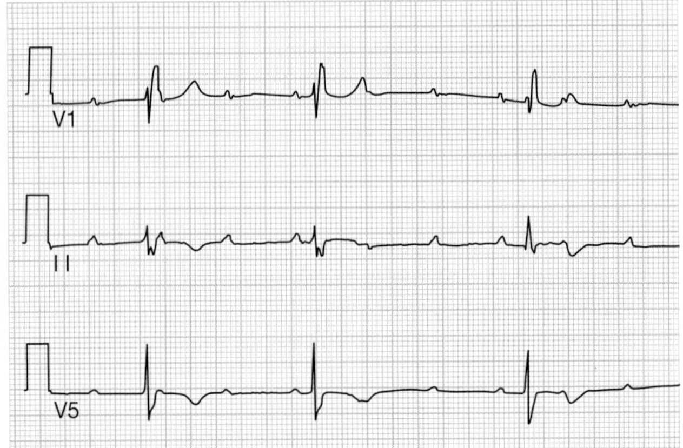

Figure 17.2 Routine preoperative electrocardiogram in an 83-year-old patient with no symptoms other than lethargy for the last 3 months. This shows complete heart block with dissociated P waves and QRS complexes, requiring preoperative pacing.

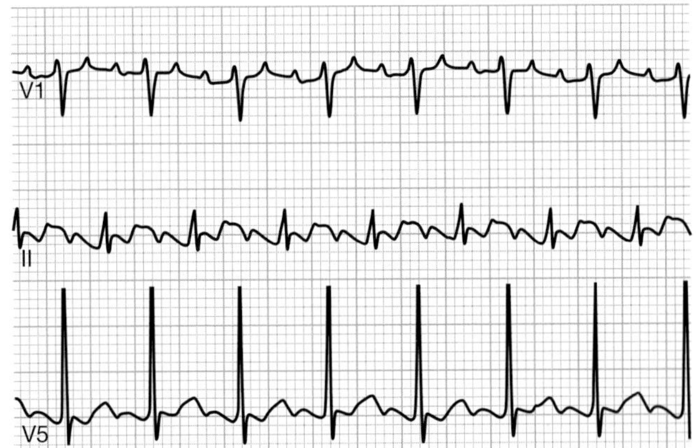

Figure 17.3 Atrial flutter.

In patients with mechanical heart valves, warfarin needs to be stopped for 5 days before surgery, and an infusion of unfractionated heparin started when the INR falls below 1.5. The activated partial thromboplastin time (APTT), should be monitored to keep it at 1.5 times normal and the infusion is then stopped 2 hours before surgery. Heparin and warfarin should be started in the postoperative period, and heparin is stopped when the full effect of warfarin takes effect. Thrombin inhibitors and factor Xa inhibitors are not licensed and should not be used in patients with mechanical valves.

Anaemia and blood transfusion

Patients found to be anaemic at preoperative assessment should be investigated for the cause of their anaemia. They should be treated with iron and vitamin supplements. Chronic anaemia is well tolerated in the perioperative period; however, if the patient is undergoing a major procedure preoperative transfusion may be considered. If excessive bleeding is expected, then a preoperative 'group and save' should be performed and an appropriate number of units of blood crossmatched.

Some patients may refuse blood transfusion, for example a Jehovah's witness. In such a case, during the consent process (see later) discussion should include which blood product and/or device system (e.g. cell salvage, reinfusion from drains) is acceptable. The discussion should extend to other areas, for example whether refusal of transfusion would apply in life-threatening situations. As in all consent processes, the discussion and outcome should be clearly documented (see Further reading; RCS 2016).

Respiratory disease

Postoperative respiratory complications, such as pneumonia, are a major cause of morbidity and mortality especially after major abdominal and thoracic surgery. A patient's current respiratory status should be compared with their 'normal state'. Make a note of the severity of the asthma and COPD, such as past hospital admissions for treatment of the condition, records of pulmonary function tests, use of oral steroids, home oxygen, non-invasive ventilation support and evidence of right heart failure.

A preoperative chest radiograph or scan is useful in a patient with known emphysematous bullae, pulmonary cancer, metastasis or effusions.

Patients on oral steroid treatment, oxygen therapy or who have a forced expiratory volume in the first second (FEV_1) less than 30% of predicted value (for age, weight and height), or $PaCO_2$ level of greater than 6kPa, have severe disease and are at risk of pneumonia and respiratory failure in the postoperative period.

Patients should continue to use their regular inhalers until the start of anaesthesia. Brittle asthmatics may also need extra steroid cover. Encourage the patients to be compliant with the medications, take a balanced diet and stop smoking. Information should be provided to indicate perioperative risks associated with smoking. Stopping smoking reduces carbon monoxide levels and offers the patient a better ability to clear sputum. Evidence suggests that preoperative inspiratory muscle training significantly improves respiratory (muscle) function in the early postoperative period, reducing the risk of pulmonary complications.

Regional anaesthetic techniques and less invasive surgical options should be considered in severe cases. Elective surgery should be postponed until acute exacerbations are treated.

The patient should be referred to a respiratory physician if:

- There is a severe disease or significant deterioration.
- Major surgery is planned in a patient with significant respiratory comorbidities.
- Right heart failure is present – dyspnoea, fatigue, tricuspid regurgitation, hepatomegaly and oedematous feet.
- The patient is young and has severe respiratory problems (indicates a rare condition).

Gastrointestinal disease

Nil by mouth and regular medications

Patients are advised not to take solids within 6 hours and clear fluids (isotonic drinks and water) within 2 hours before anaesthesia to avoid the risk of acid aspiration syndrome. These restrictions are further reduced in infants, as keeping hydrated reduces discomfort and is known to improve postoperative outcomes.

If the surgery is delayed, oral intake of clear fluids should be allowed until 2 hours before surgery or intravenous fluids should be started, especially in vulnerable groups of patients, e.g. children, the elderly and diabetics.

Patients can continue to take their specified routine medications with sips of water in the NBM period.

Regurgitation risk

Patients with hiatus hernia, obesity, pregnancy and diabetes are at high risk of pulmonary aspiration, even if they have been NBM before elective surgery. Clear antacids, H2-receptor blockers, e.g. ranitidine, or proton pump inhibitors, e.g. omeprazole, may be given at an appropriate time in the preoperative period.

Liver disease

In patients with liver disease, the cause of the disease needs to be known, as well as any evidence of clotting problems, renal involvement and encephalopathy. Elective surgery should be postponed until any acute episode has settled (e.g. cholangitis). The blood tests that need to be performed include liver function tests, coagulation, blood glucose and U&Es. The presence of ascites, oesophageal varices, hypoalbuminaemia and sodium and water retention should be noted, as all can influence the choice and outcome of anaesthesia and surgery.

Genitourinary disease

Renal disease

Underlying conditions leading to chronic renal failure such as diabetes mellitus, hypertension and ischaemic heart disease, should be stabilised before elective surgery. Appropriate measures should be taken to treat acidosis, hypocalcaemia and hyperkalaemia of greater than 6 mmol/L. Arrangements should be made to continue peritoneal or haemodialysis until a few hours before surgery. After the final dialysis before surgery, a blood sample should be sent for FBC and U&Es.

Chronic renal failure patients often suffer chronic microcytic anaemia that is well tolerated; therefore, preoperative blood transfusion is often not necessary.

Acute kidney injury can present with an acute surgical problem, for example bowel obstruction needing emergency surgery. In these patients, medical treatment should be started at the earliest opportunity and carried on through surgery and through into the critical care unit.

Urinary tract infection

Uncomplicated urinary infections are common in women, while outflow uropathy with chronically infected urine is common in men. These infections should be treated before embarking on elective surgery where infection carries dire consequences, e.g. joint replacement. For emergency procedures, antibiotics should be started and care taken to ensure that the patient maintains a good urine output before, during and after surgery.

Endocrine and metabolic disorders

Malnutrition

Body mass index (BMI) is weight in kilograms divided by height in metres squared. A BMI of less than 18.5 indicates nutritional impairment and a BMI below 15 is associated with significant hospital mortality. Nutritional support for a minimum of 2 weeks before surgery is required to have any impact on subsequent morbidity.

If a patient is unlikely to be able to eat for a significant period, arrangements should be made by the preoperative assessment team to start nutritional support in the immediate postoperative phase.

Obesity

Morbid obesity can be defined as BMI of more than 35 (other definitions exist) and is associated with increased risk of postoperative complications. Patients should be made aware of risks involved and advised on healthy eating and taking regular exercise.

Associated sleep apnoea can be predicted by using a clinical scoring system, the perioperative sleep apnoea prediction (P-SAP) score or sleep apnoea studies. There is evidence to suggest that patient outcomes improve with more than 6 weeks of use of a continuous positive airway pressure (CPAP) device preoperatively, and cholesterol reducing agents in the perioperative phase.

If possible surgery should be delayed until the patient is more active and has lost weight. If this fails, prophylactic measures need to be taken (such as preventative measures for acid aspiration and DVT) and associated risks need to be explained prior to the surgery.

Diabetes mellitus

Diabetes and associated cardiovascular and renal complications should be controlled to as near normal level as possible before embarking on elective surgery. Any history of hyper- and hypoglycaemic episodes, and hospital admissions, should be noted. HbA1c levels should be checked. For elective surgery, HBA1c of <69 mmol/mol is recommended. Lipid-lowering medication should be started in patients who are in a high-risk group for cardiovascular complications of diabetes.

Patients with diabetes should be first on the operating list and, if the operation is in the morning, advised to omit the morning dose of medication and breakfast. Though tight control of blood sugar is not needed, the patient's blood sugar levels should be checked 2 hourly. For those on the afternoon list, breakfast can be given with half their regular dose of intermediate-acting insulin (or full dose oral antidiabetic agents) and then managed with regular blood sugar checks as above. An intravenous insulin sliding scale should be started for insulin-dependent diabetes mellitus patients undergoing major surgery, or if blood sugar is difficult to control for other reasons.

Adrenocortical suppression

Patients receiving oral adrenocortical steroids should be asked about the dose and duration of the medication in view of supplementation with extra doses of steroids perioperatively, to avoid an Addisonian crisis.

Coagulation disorders

Thrombophilia

Patients with a strong family history or previous personal history of thrombosis should be identified (*Table 17.3*). They will need thromboprophylaxis in the perioperative period.

The progesterone-only contraceptive pill should be continued; however, the risks of continuing the combined pill (slight increase risk of significant thrombosis) should be weighed against the risks of an unplanned pregnancy. Consider stopping oestrogen-containing oral contraceptives or hormone replacement therapy 4 weeks before surgery (NICE guidance; see Further reading). The reader is advised to use an appropriate resource for precise formulation information and current guidance.

Patients with a low risk of thromboembolism can be given thromboembolism-deterrent stockings to wear during the perioperative period. High-risk patients with a history of recurrent DVT, pulmonary embolism and arterial thrombosis will be on warfarin. This should be stopped before surgery and replaced by low molecular weight heparin or factor Xa inhibitors. Local or national guidelines advise what type of DVT prophylaxis should be used for each type of surgery.

Neurological and psychiatric disorders

In patients with a history of stroke, pre-existing neurological deficit should be recorded. These patients may be on anti-

TABLE 17.3 Risk factors for thrombosis.

- Age >60 years
- Obesity BMI >30 kg/m^2
- Trauma or surgery (especially of the abdomen, pelvis and lower limbs), anaesthesia >90 minutes
- Reduced mobility for more than 3 days
- Pregnancy/puerperium
- Varicose veins with phlebitis
- Drugs, e.g. oestrogen contraceptive, HRT, smoking
- Known active cancer or on treatment, significant medical comorbidities, critical care admission
- Family/personal history of thrombosis, e.g. deficiencies in antithrombin III, protein S and C

Thomas Addison, 1795–1860, physician, Guy's Hospital, London, UK, described the effects of disease of the suprarenal capsules in 1849.

platelet agents or anticoagulants. If it is felt that the neurological and cardiovascular thrombotic risks are low, antiplatelet agents should be withdrawn (7 days for aspirin, 10 days for clopidogrel). If the thrombotic risks are perceived to be high and the patient is undergoing surgery with a high risk of bleeding, aspirin alone should be continued.

Anticonvulsants and anti-Parkinson medication is continued perioperatively to help early mobilisation of the patient.

Lithium should be stopped 24 hours prior to surgery; blood levels should be measured to exclude toxicity. The anaesthetist should be informed if patients are on psychiatric medications such as tricyclic antidepressants or monoamine oxidase inhibitors, as these may interact with anaesthetic drugs.

Musculoskeletal disorders

Rheumatoid arthritis can lead to an unstable cervical spine with the possibility of spinal cord injury during intubation. Therefore, flexion and extension lateral cervical spine radiographs should be obtained in symptomatic patients (Figures 17.4 and 17.5).

Assessment of the severity of renal, cardiac valvular and pericardial involvement as well as restrictive lung disease, should be carried out. Rheumatologists will advise on steroids and disease-modifying drugs so as to balance immunosuppression (chance of infections) against the need to stabilise the disease perioperatively (stopping disease modifying drugs can lead to flare-up of the disease).

In ankylosing spondylitis patients, in addition to the problems discussed above, techniques of spinal or epidural anaesthesia are often challenging. Patients with systemic lupus erythematosus may exhibit a hypercoagulable state along with airway difficulties.

With certain types of orthopaedic operations, such as joint replacement, antibiotic prophylaxis will be required, and will usually follow specific local or national guidelines.

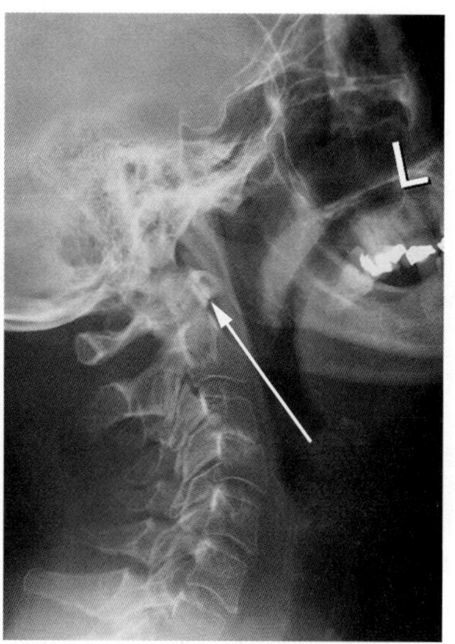

Figure 17.4 Extension view of cervical spine in patient with rheumatoid arthritis.

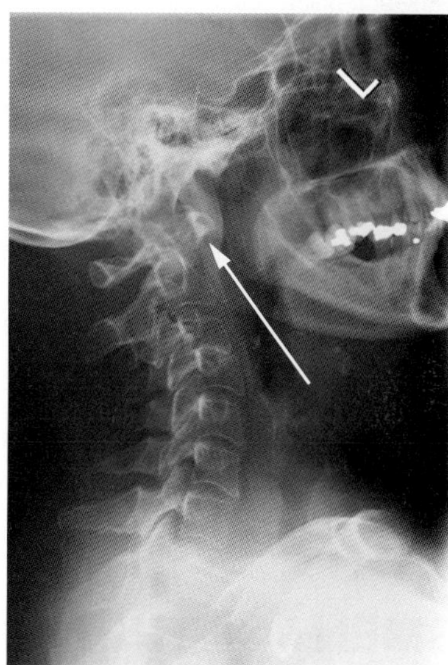

Figure 17.5 Flexion view in the same patient as in Figure 17.4. Note the large increase in the atlantodens interval, implying significant instability at this level.

Airway assessment

The ability to intubate the trachea and oxygenate the patient are basic and crucial skills of the anaesthetist. The ease or difficulty encountered when performing airway manoeuvres can be predicted by simple examination findings of full mouth opening (modified Mallampati class), jaw protrusion, neck movement and thyromental distance. The anaesthetist should look for loose teeth, obvious tumours, scars, infections, obesity, thickness of the neck, etc., which will indicate difficulty in visualising the airway. When more than one of the above tests are positive, the chances of experiencing difficulty in obtaining and securing the airway become greater. To obtain the modified Mallampati class, the anaesthetist sits in front of the patient who is asked to open their mouth and protrude the tongue (Figure 17.6). The higher the grade, the higher the risk in obtaining and securing an airway (Table 17.4).

Preoperative assessment in emergency surgery

In urgent or emergency surgery the principles of preoperative assessment should be the same as in elective surgery, except that the opportunity to optimise the condition is limited by time constraints. Medical assessment and treatments should be started (e.g. as per Advanced Trauma Life Support guidelines) even if there is no time to complete them before the start of the surgical procedure. Some risks may be reduced but some may persist and, whenever possible, these need to be explained to the patient.

SR Mallampati published the original article suggesting that the size of the base of the tongue is an important factor determining the degree of difficulty of direct laryngoscopy in the *Canadian Anaesthetists' Society Journal* in 1985. The original Mallampati classifications was modified from a total of three to four classes by **GLT Sampsoon** and **JRB Young** after reviewing a series of obstetric and general surgical patients who had had difficult intubations.

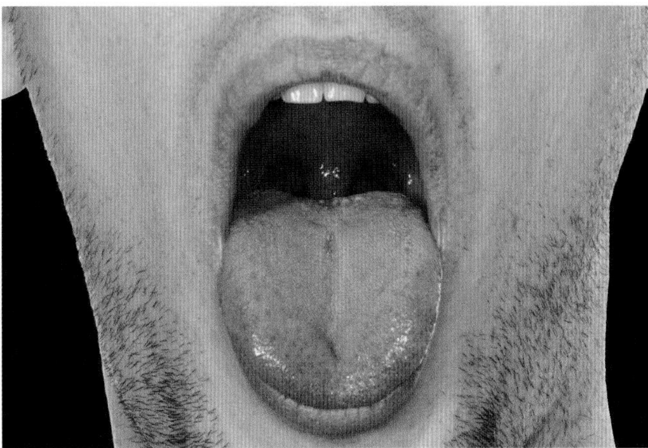

Figure 17.6 Normal mouth opening view.

TABLE 17.4 Airway assessment (Samsoon and Young modified Mallampati test).

• Fauces, pillars, soft palate and uvula seen	Grade 1
• Fauces, soft palate with some part of uvula seen	Grade 2
• Soft palate seen	Grade 3
• Hard palate only seen	Grade 4

Summary box 17.6

Preoperative assessment for emergency surgery

- Start. Similar principles to that for elective surgery
- Constraints. Time, facilities available
- Consent. May not be possible in life-saving emergencies
- Organisational efforts. For example, local/national algorithms for treatment of the patient with multiple injuries

ASSESSMENT OF THE HIGH-RISK PATIENT

Despite higher-risk patients presenting for surgery, the perioperative mortality has decreased significantly over the last half a century, especially in resource-rich countries. In a published systematic review in *The Lancet* (Bainbridge *et al.*, 2012), perioperative mortality has declined from 10 603 per million (95% CI: 10 423–10 784) in the 1970s to 1176 per million (1148–1205) in the 1990s–2000s ($p<0{\cdot}0001$). However, there remains a subgroup of patients who are at higher risk of morbidity and mortality after surgery. By identifying high-risk patients in the preoperative phase and planning their perioperative management, morbidity and mortality can be reduced.

Patients who have a predicted mortality ≥5% should be considered as 'high risk'. It is estimated that although the high-risk group accounts for less than 15% of all surgical procedures, they contribute to more than 80% of all perioperative deaths in UK.

What causes these patients to be at a high risk of death and complications after surgery? After surgery tissue destruction, blood loss, fluid shifts, changes in temperature, pain and anxiety result in increased demands for oxygen delivery to the tissues. This demand increases from an average of 110 mL/min/m^2 at rest to 170 mL/min/m^2 in the postoperative period. Most patients meet this increase in demand by increasing their cardiac output and tissue oxygen extraction. Patients who are unable to meet these demands, as a result of a limited cardiorespiratory reserve, are at a risk of oxygen debt.

Occult hypovolemia resulting from fluid shift or blood loss can further impair oxygen delivery. Splanchnic vasoconstriction to compensate for this may result in gut ischaemia. Those with coronary or cerebrovascular disease are also at a higher risk of myocardial ischaemia or stroke.

Factors contributing to risk

Risk is a complex interaction of multiple factors that can be classified into patient and surgical factors. Patient factors are listed in *Table 17.5*. The elderly, though not independently at higher risk, not only suffer more cardiac, pulmonary and renal disease but also require surgery four times as often as the rest of the population. Around 10% of the population over 65 have frailty with increasing incidence with age. Frailty is a distinctive state that is related to ageing. Multiple body systems lose their in-built reserves in the elderly.

The type of surgery contributes independently and is listed in *Table 17.6*. This risk increases if the surgery is performed as an emergency. Often, the underlying condition necessitating surgery itself may be associated with an increased risk of complications. For example, a patient with severe peripheral vascular disease resulting from heavy smoking, may need a femoral-popliteal bypass graft and can be expected also to have significant COPD and IHD.

Moreover, when mortality by type of surgery is adjusted for patient risk factors, the apparent hierarchy of surgical risk may change. The average mortality risk for an individual patient undergoing thoracic surgery, for example, is likely to be higher than the average risk for that same patient undergoing vascular surgery. Complications associated with the latter are nevertheless more frequent because vascular patients have greater medical risk factors (*Table 17.7*).

TABLE 17.5 Patient factors that predispose to high risk of morbidity and mortality.

Previous severe cardiorespiratory illness, e.g. acute myocardial infarction, COPD or stroke
Late stage vascular disease involving aorta
Age >70 years with limited physiological reserve in one or more vital organs
Extensive surgery for carcinoma
Acute abdominal catastrophe with haemodynamic instability (e.g. peritonitis)
Acute massive blood loss >8 units
Septicaemia
Positive blood culture or septic focus
Respiratory failure: PaO_2 <8 kPa or FiO_2 >0.4 or mechanical ventilation >48 h
Acute renal failure: urea >20 mmol or creatinine >260 mmol/L

(Based on clinical criteria used by Shoemaker and colleagues modified by Boyd.)

TABLE 17.6 Surgery specific estimates of risk

High risk (cardiac risk >5%)	Intermediate risk (cardiac risk 1–5%)	Low risk (cardiac risk <1%)
Open aortic Major vascular Peripheral vascular Urgent body cavity	Elective abdominal Carotid Endovascular aneurysm Head and neck Major neurosurgery Arthroplasty Elective pulmonary Major urology	Breast Dental Thyroid Ophthalmic Gynaecological Reconstructive Minor orthopaedic Minor urology

(From Eagle *et al. J Am Coll Cardiol* 2002; **39**(3): 542–53.)

TABLE 17.7 The effect of adjustment for patient factors on surgery-specific operative mortality.

Type of surgery	Unadjusted 30-day mortality (% (rank))	Adjusted 30-day mortality (%(rank))
Vascular	5.97 (1)	0.98 (5)
Thoracic	3.40 (2)	2.28 (1)
Abdominal	2.73 (3)	1.83 (2)
Cardiac	2.70 (4)	1.13 (4)
Neurosurgery	1.74 (5)	1.60 (3)
Orthopaedic	1.25 (6)	0.49 (7)
ENT	0.85 (7)	0.68 (6)
Urology	0.81 (8)	0.38 (8)
Gynaecology	0.13 (9)	0.17 (9)
Breast	0.07 (10)	0.08 (10)

(Modified from Noordzij *et al*. 2010.)

In summary, the typical high-risk patient is the elderly patient with coexisting conditions such as IHD and/or COPD undergoing major surgery. The risk will increase if the surgery is performed as an emergency.

Management of risk

The key to managing patients effectively is the identification and accurate quantification of the risk, and subsequent measures taken to minimise it.

Realistic estimates of risk are the cornerstone of informed patient consent and shared decision making. The patient and the surgeon may choose a less extensive or even a non-surgical option where risks of the definitive procedure are deemed to be too high or unacceptable. The Royal College of Surgeons (RCS) of England has recommended that the patients who are predicted to have greater than 5% mortality risk should have active consultant input in all stages of their management.

Surgical procedures in those with predicted mortality of >10% should be conducted under the direct supervision of consultant surgeon or anaesthetist, unless the consultants are satisfied with the seniority and competence of the staff managing these patients. Moreover, those with a mortality >10% should be managed in the critical care facility.

Depending on particular comorbidities, it may be possible for a patient's underlying conditions to be improved by optimising their medical therapy. Additional physiological optimisation may take the form of measures to minimise myocardial ischaemia or measures to improve oxygen delivery to the other major organs, depending on the prevailing risks.

Optimisation before surgery can be more effective in a critical care environment and patients may need to be admitted to a high dependency unit (HDU) or intensive therapy unit (ITU) preoperatively. The likelihood of the high-risk patient requiring postoperative critical care should be planned preoperatively and discussed with the duty critical care physician.

The identification of patients who will benefit the most from these interventions is important, not only for the improvement of outcomes but also the effective allocation of resources. As discussed above, emergency surgery is associated with higher risks because by its very nature there is less time and opportunity to organise these additional levels of care.

Summary box 17.7

A practical approach to the care for the high-risk patient

- Identify the high-risk patient
- Assess the level of risk
- Detailed preoperative assessment
- Adequate resusciatation
- Optimise medical management
- Investigation to define the underlying surgical problem
- Immediate and definitive treatment of underlying problems
- Consider admission to a critical care facility postoperatively

Identification of the high-risk patient

A number of scoring systems have been developed over the years with the aim of identifying high-risk patients (*Table 17.8*).

American Society of Anaesthesiologists system

The American Society of Anaesthesiologists (ASA) scoring system is widely used. Although not designed to be used as a risk prediction score, it has a quantitative association with the predicted percentage of postoperative mortality (*Table 17.9*). However, it does not account for age or nature of surgery and the term 'systemic disease' in ASA grading introduces an element of 'subjectivity'.

Metabolic equivalent

As discussed earlier, overall functional physical fitness can be judged by the ability to tolerate metabolic equivalent tasks (METs) (*Table 17.10*). One MET is equivalent to the oxygen consumption of an adult at rest (~3.5 mL/kg/min). Different tasks are assigned a number of METs. If the patient is able to perform >4 METs (e.g. climbing at least one flight of stairs) they are considered suitable candidates for major surgery. However, once again this depends on a subjective assessment of the ability of a patient and may be overestimated by them.

Objective indices based on weighted scores pertaining to surgery and comorbidity, have been created to stratify cardiac risk. Examples include the Goldman cardiac risk index and

TABLE 17.8 Surgical risk scores classified by outcome measures and need for intraoperative information.

	Scores predicting mortality	Scores predicting morbidity
Scores not requiring operative information	ASA APACHE-II Donati score Hardman index Glasgow aneurysm score Sickness assessment Boey score Hacetteppe score Physiological POSSUM ACS NSQIP surgical risk score	ASA APACHE-II Goldman cardiac risk index Veltkamp score VA respiratory failure score VA pneumonia prediction index ACS NSQIP surgical risk score
Scores requiring operative information	Mannheim peritonitis index Reiss index Fitness score POSSUM P-POSSUM Cleveland colorectal model Surgical risk scale	POSSUM P-POSSUM

APACHE-II, Acute Physiology and Chronic Health Evaluation II; VA, Veterans Affairs; P-POSSUM, Portsmouth-POSSUM; see text for additional abbreviations. (Modified from Rex TE, Bates T. *World J Emerg Surg* 2007; **2**: 16.)

TABLE 17.9 Operative mortality by ASA grade.

ASA Grade	Description	30 day mortality (%)
I	Healthy	0.1
II	Mild systemic disease, no functional limitation	0.7
III	Severe systemic disease, definite functional limitation	3.5
IV	Severe systemic disease, constant threat to life	18.3
V	Moribund patient unlikely to survive 24 hours with or without operation	93.3
E	Emergency operation	–

(From Boyd O, Jackson N. *Crit Care* 2005; **9**: 390–6.)

TABLE 17.10 Metabolic equivalent of task (MET).

- 1 MET = 3.5 mL O_2/kg/min (oxygen consumption by 40-year-old,70 kg man at rest)
- 1 MET = eating and dressing
- 4 MET = climbing 2 flights of stairs
- 6 MET = short run
- >10 MET = able to participate in strenuous sport
- Patients who can exercise at 4 METS or above have lower risk of perioperative mortality

the revised cardiac risk index (RCRI) of Lee (*Table 17.11*). Although they can predict risk of cardiac complications, they are not designed to predict mortality.

POSSUM score

The POSSUM score (Physiologic and Operative Severity Score for the enUmeration of Mortality and Morbidity) and its modifications (P-POSSUM, CR-POSSUM) are used to predict all-cause mortality in postoperative critical care patients as well as non-cardiac morbidity.

TABLE 17.11 The revised cardiac risk index (RCRI) of Lee.

Risk factors	Risk of major cardiac complications (%)
History of ischaemic heart disease	Number of factors
History of compensated or prior heart failure	0 = 0.4
History of cerebrovascular disease	1 = 0.9
Diabetes mellitus	2 = 7.0
Renal insufficiency (creatinine >177 μmol/L)	3+ = 11.0
High-risk surgery	

ACS NSQIP score

The American College of Surgeons (ACS) National Surgical Quality Improvement Programme (NSQIP) surgical risk score estimates the chance of a complication or death after surgery for more than a thousand different surgical procedures. It compares the patient's risk with an average person's risk. It is a web based tool done preoperatively. The risk is calculated based on surgical procedure and 19 patient-specific preoperative risk factors.

Cardiopulmonary exercise testing

Cardiopulmonary exercise testing (CPET) can be used as a screening tool to identify high-risk patients. The oxygen (O_2) consumption and carbon dioxide (CO_2) production of the patient are measured while they undergo a 10 minute period of incrementally demanding exercise (usually on a cycle ergometer) up to their maximally tolerated level (**Figure 17.7**).

CPET is based on the principle that when a subject's delivery of O_2 to active tissues becomes inadequate, anaerobic metabolism begins; lactate is buffered by bicarbonate and the resulting CO_2 increases out of proportion to the escalation in physical difficulty and O_2 consumption. The 'anaerobic threshold' (AT) is the O_2 consumption in mL/kg/min above

Lee Goldman, b.1948, Dean of Health Sciences and Medicine, Columbia University, New York, NY, USA, since 2006. He developed his Index in 1977.
Thomas H Lee, Professor of Medicine, Harvard Medical School, Professor of Health Policy and Management, Harvard School of Public Health, Boston, MA, USA.

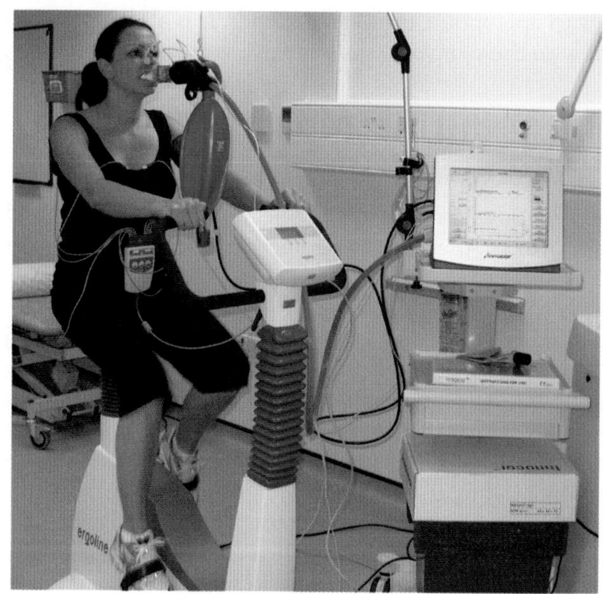
Figure 17.7 Cardiopulmonary exercise testing (CPET).

which this occurs. Peak oxygen consumption (VO_2) is also measured. They are the end product of a subject's combined respiratory, cardiac, vascular and musculoskeletal fitness, and subjects with either an AT above a somewhat arbitrary cut-off of 11 and a VO_2 below 15 mL/kg/min are at higher risk of morbidity and mortality after surgery.

When CPET is not available, a simple walk test, such as the 6-minute walk test (6MWT) and the incremental shuttle walk test (ISWT), can be used to assess the functional capacity of the patient. They depend on the patient's ability to walk for a fixed 6 minute period or at increasing speed over a flat surface.

Optimisation of the high-risk patient

As discussed above, all coexisting disease processes should be reviewed and optimised. Simple measures include stopping smoking (maximal benefit only seen if stopped for 8 weeks prior to surgery), reducing alcohol intake, losing weight, improving nutrition and/or haemoglobin levels.

In the high-risk group there may a need for more complex investigations, review of medication or even consideration of further surgery. Patients scheduled for abdominal aortic aneurysm (AAA) repair surgery for example, frequently require carotid duplex scans. If the scans reveal a significant blockage and a high risk of perioperative stroke, a carotid endarterectomy may be indicated prior to AAA repair.

All high-risk patients benefit from multidisciplinary team care and the involvement of experienced physicians in the perioperative period. The impact and management of the comorbidities that commonly contribute to risk are outlined below.

Ischaemic heart disease

Perioperative myocardial infarction (MI) is associated with a high mortality (15–25%). Ischaemia, and ultimately MI, occur when the supply of oxygen to the myocardium is exceeded by its demand. This situation can be precipitated by hypotension, tachycardia and procoagulant states (of which the inflammatory response to surgery is an example).

Preparation of these patients for surgery should aim to optimise myocardial oxygen supply and demand ratio and so minimise the risk of myocardial ischaemia developing. This work may involve further investigations or even the decision to postpone non-cardiac surgery for 3–6 months after an MI. Some patients may require preoperative revascularisation, using either a coronary artery bypass grafting (CABG) or percutaneous coronary intervention (PCI) with a stent or angioplasty.

Minimising myocardial ischaemia

Anaesthesia techniques that dampen the stress response to surgery (especially minimising pain) and provide a good degree of cardiac stability should be used. Anaesthesia should avoid tachycardia, systolic hypertension and diastolic hypotension, and may be facilitated by the use of invasive arterial blood pressure monitoring. Blood loss must be accurately monitored and haemoglobin maintained at a level suitable for the patient's cardiac risk factors. Perioperative use of β-blockers may be considered but this is controversial.

Troponin testing allows early diagnosis of perioperative MIs, but there are limited reperfusion options due to risk of bleeding from the surgical site. Admission to HDU should be considered for patients with IHD and supplemental oxygen therapy continued for 3–4 days.

Cardiac failure

Left ventricular failure is the end result of several conditions including IHD, hypertension, cardiomyopathies and valve dysfunction. Decompensated heart failure puts the patient at risk of multiorgan failure. Those with ejection fractions of less than 35%, and in whom the failure is undiagnosed or its severity underestimated, are at the highest risk. The patient's functional capacity needs to be assessed and surgery may have to be delayed for investigations such as an echocardiogram and/or for optimisation of medical therapy. Drugs used in chronic heart failure have significant implications for perioperative care, and β-blockers and probably ACE inhibitors (unless renal perfusion is to be significantly affected) should be continued. Anaesthesia should ensure minimal myocardial depression and change in afterload during surgery. Arrhythmias must be rapidly brought under control, particularly AF, and correcting any electrolyte imbalance is crucial in this respect. Invasive monitoring of trends in central venous and arterial pressure monitoring may help management, particularly when large fluid shifts are expected to occur.

Respiratory failure

Around 1.5% of patients develop lower respiratory tract infection after surgery with a 30-day mortality over 20%. Surgery, particularly open abdominal procedures under general anaesthesia, result in changes to respiratory physiology. The functional residual capacity of the lungs is reduced. This combined with the respiratory depressant effect of residual anaesthetic agents, the patient's limited mobility and pain from surgery causes atelectasis (failure of gas exchange due to alveolar collapse) and predisposes patients to postoperative respiratory infection. Other complications including bronchospasm, pneumothorax and acute respiratory distress syndrome (ARDS) contribute as much to morbidity and length of hospital stay as cardiac complications. Respiratory failure defined as a PaO_2 <8 kPa in air, PaO_2/FiO_2 <40 kPa or inability to extubate a patient 48 hours after surgery, is by far the most significant of these and is associated with a mortality of 27–40%.

Again, as with cardiac risk management, it may be necessary to postpone surgery to allow medical optimisation or consider a non-operative option. Preoperatively, bronchodilator therapy will be required in those with reversible obstructive airway disease and steroids may need to be started or increased. Nutritional status should be optimised and albumin levels corrected. Physiotherapy for postural drainage, and deep breathing exercises or incentive spirometry should be considered for patients at increased risk of respiratory complications. General anaesthesia is associated with more respiratory complications and so regional techniques should be considered where possible in these patients. Hypoxemia and CO_2 retention leading to the need for reintubation is better avoided in those at risk, by delaying extubation until analgesia, hydration and acid–base status have been corrected. Patients may benefit from ITU admission and this needs planning. Application of non-invasive respiratory support (Figure 17.8) may allow certain patients to be extubated earlier.

Other comorbidities

Acute kidney injury, chronic kidney disease, diabetes, peripheral vascular disease and liver dysfunction are some of the medical conditions that contribute to risk and need to be optimised.

Sepsis

Sepsis needs urgent identification and treatment, as if not treated early it can lead to either a prolonged admission to a critical care unit or death. Early resuscitative measures in sepsis include administering broad spectrum antibiotics and treating hypotension, hypovolemia and elevated lactate levels with appropriate intravenous fluids. It is also important to deal with the source of sepsis as early as possible.

Minimising the impact of surgery in the high-risk patient

There are situations where the selection of one surgical technique over another may be significantly influenced by patient risk factors. Some procedures are not primarily high-risk but may become so in unsuitable patients. Laparoscopic surgery, for example, has come of age as a preferred technique for patients predisposed to postoperative respiratory complications, but its effect on cardiac physiology means the same may not apply to patients at risk of cardiac complications. The expanding demand and indications for minimal access surgery are now pushing the boundaries of intraoperative physiological tolerance. Robotic prostatectomy and some laparoscopic colorectal procedures require a pneumoperitoneum with steep Trendelenburg (head down) positioning for several hours (Figure 17.9). This can be associated with adverse cardiovascular and neurological complications, such as myocardial ischaemia and increased intracranial pressure in the high risk group. This risk may be minimised by attention to patient selection.

Role of critical care and outreach services

Optimal care in the high-risk group should be extended to include postoperative support, which for a majority of these patients means admission to a critical care bed. Reports from the National Confidential Enquiry into Surgical Deaths (NCEPOD) show that the majority of postoperative deaths

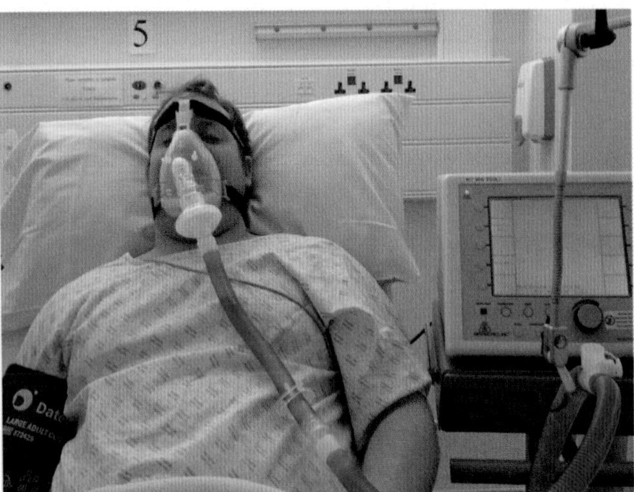

Figure 17.8 Non-invasive ventilation.

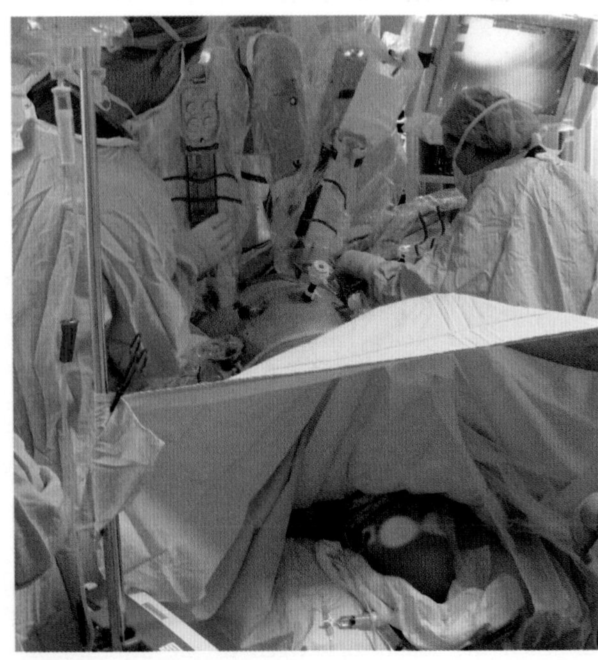

Figure 17.9 Robotic surgery.

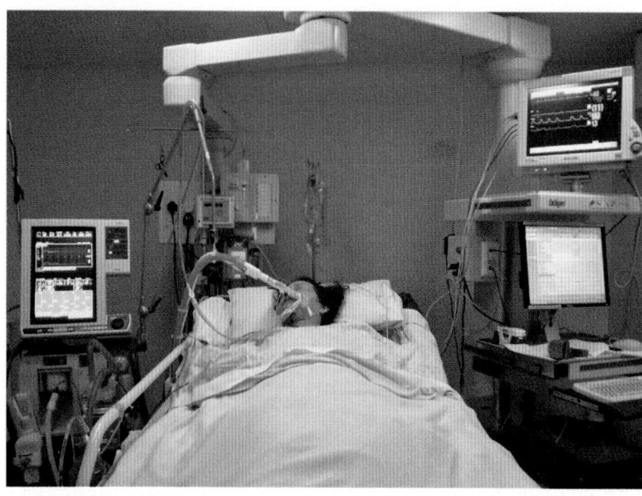

Figure 17.10 A high-risk patient admitted to the intensive care unit postoperatively.

in the UK occur more than 5 days after surgery. Admission to a critical care unit allows for early intervention and a level of care that is difficult to deliver in the ward environment during this crucial period (Figure 17.10). The high-risk surgical population accounts for 80% of postoperative deaths but only about 15–30% of high-risk surgical patients are admitted to a critical care unit at any time following surgery. One study that compared surgical mortality in the UK and the USA found an observed mortality of 9.95 % in the UK as compared to 2.1% in USA. It is suggested that the difference may be related to the provision of critical care services, with 8.6 critical care beds per 100 000 population in the UK compared to 30.5 in the USA.

In the last decade, the role of critical care has been expanded to the concept of 'critical care without walls'. The intensive care outreach services (ICORS) grew from a recognition that there were many patients in the hospital who are at risk of being critically ill, and early identification of these patients using 'early warning scores' could allow for early intervention. The outreach team functions to bridge the gap between critical care unit and ward.

CONSENT

Consent should be both voluntary and informed. The process of consent has evolved over the years and in the UK, following a recent legal judgement, new guidance has been published (see Further reading; RCS). This describes the importance of supported decision-making concerning a treatment or operation. The guidance outlines the key principles of consent and how the discussion should:

- give the patient the information required to make a decision;
- be tailored to the individual patient;
- explain all reasonable treatment options;
- discuss all material* risks.

Furthermore, the guide explains that consent:

- should be written and recorded on a form;
- the key points of the discussion should be recorded in the case notes.

**Material risk: "whether, in the circumstances of the particular case, a reasonable person in the patient's position would be likely to attach significance to the risk, or the doctor is or should reasonably be aware that the particular patient would likely attach significance to it" (Source RCS 2016).*

Clearly in certain emergency situations, it may not be possible to follow all of the key principles. For consent to be given, the patient must have capacity, which includes the ability to understand the information provided, to retain and use the information to make a decision and to indicate what that decision is (see Further reading; RCS). The surgeon should presume the patient has capacity for consent (Mental Capacity Act, 2005) unless during the process it is demonstrated that this is not the case. Generally, children are presumed to have capacity at 16 and for those under that age, capacity can be assessed (GMC guidance, 2007).

The person obtaining consent must be appropriately experienced to do so.

Summary box 17.8

Consent

- Consent should be voluntary and informed
- Supported decision-making is considered good practice
- Explain all treatment options and material risks
- Capacity is needed for a patient to give their consent

ARRANGING THEATRE LIST

The date, place and time of operation should be matched with availability of personnel. Appropriate equipment and instruments should be made available. The operating list should be distributed as early as possible to all staff who are involved in making the list run smoothly (*Table 17.12*). If this is done electronically, familiarity with the computer system is required.

Prioritise patients, e.g. children and diabetic patients should be placed at the beginning of the list; life- and limb-threatening surgery should take priority; cancer patients need to be treated early.

TABLE 17.12 Perioperative teams.
• Ward, theatre and specialist nursing staff
• Anaesthetic and surgical teams
• Radiology, pathology involvement
• Rehabilitation and social care workers
• Specific personnel in individual cases

FURTHER READING

Bainbridge D1, Martin J, Arango; Task Force on Practice Guidelines (Committee to Update the 1996 Guidelines on perioperative cardiovascular M, Cheng D; Evidence-based Perioperative Clinical Outcomes Research (EPiCOR) Group. Perioperative and anaesthetic-related mortality in developed and developing countries: a systematic review and meta-analysis. *Lancet* 2012; **380**(9847): 1075–81.

Boyd O, Jackson N. How is risk defined in high-risk surgical patient management? *Crit Care* 2005; **9**: 390–6.

Fleisher LA, Beckman JA, Buller CE *et al.* ACCF/AHA focused update on perioperative beta blockade. *J Am Coll Cardiol* 2009; **54**: 2102–28.

Giglio MT, Marucci M, Testini M, Brienza N. Goal-directed haemodynamic therapy and gastrointestinal complications in major surgery: a meta-analysis of randomised controlled trials. *Br J Anaesth* 2009; **103**: 637–46.

Eagle KA, Berger PB, Calkins H *et al.*; American College of Cardiology; American Heart Association. ACC/AHA guideline update for perioperative cardiovascular evaluation for noncardiac surgery: executive summary: a report of the American College of Cardiology/ American Heart Association evaluation for noncardiac surgery. *J Am Coll Cardiol* 2002; **39**(3): 542–53.

European Society of Anaesthesiology, Task Force on preoperative evaluation of the adult noncardiac surgery patient. Preoperative evaluation of the adult patient undergoing non-cardiac surgery: guidelines from the European Society of Anaesthesiology. *Eur J Anaesthesiol* 2011; **28**: 684–722.

Fleisher LA, Beckman JA, Brown KA *et al.* ACC/AHA 2007 Guidelines on perioperative cardiovascular evaluation and care for noncardiac surgery: executive summary: a report of the American College of Cardiology/American Heart Association Task Force on practice guidelines (Writing Committee to Revise the 2002 Guidelines on perioperative cardiovascular evaluation for noncardiac surgery): developed in collaboration with the American Society of Echocardiography, American Society of Nuclear Cardiology, Heart Rhythm Society, Society of Cardiovascular Anesthesiologists, Society for Cardiovascular Angiography and Interventions, Society for Vascular Medicine and Biology, and Society for Vascular Surgery. *Circulation* 2007; **116**: 1971–96.

General Medical Council. GMC guidance 0–18 years: Guidance for all doctors. 2007.

Lee TH, Marcantonio ER, Mangione CM *et al.* Derivation and prospective validation of a simple index for prediction of cardiac risk of major noncardiac surgery. *Circulation* 1999; **100**: 1043–9.

Mental Capacity Act (2005) UK.

Minto G, Biccard B. Assessment of the high-risk perioperative patient. *BJA Education* 2014; **14**(1): 12–17.

National Confidential Enquiry into Patient Outcome and Death. Knowing the risk. A review of the peri-operative care of surgical patients. 2011. Available from www.ncepod.org.uk/2011report2/downloads/POC_fullreport.pdf.

National Institute for Health and Care Excellence. CG3 preoperative tests: NICE guideline, June 2003.

National Institute for Health and Care Excellence. Venous thromboembolism: reducing the risk for patients in hospital. Clinical guideline (CG92), 2010, updated 2015.

Noordzij PG1, Poldermans D, Schouten O *et al.* Postoperative mortality in The Netherlands: a population-based analysis of surgery-specific risk in adults. *Anesthesiology* 2010; **112**(5): 1105–15.

Pearse RM1, Holt PJ, Grocott MP. Managing perioperative risk in patients undergoing elective non-cardiac surgery. *BMJ* 2011; **343**: d5759.

Poldermans D, Bax JJ, Boersma E *et al.* Guidelines for preoperative cardiac risk assessment and perioperative cardiac management in non-cardiac surgery: the Task Force for preoperative cardiac risk assessment and perioperative cardiac management in non-cardiac surgery of the European Society of Cardiology (ESC) and European Society of Anaesthesiology (ESA). *Eur Heart J* 2009; **30**: 2769–812.

Ramachandran SK, Kheterpal S, Consens F *et al.* Derivation and validation of a simple perioperative sleep apnea prediction score. *Anesth Analg* 2010; **110**: 1007–15.

Rix TE, Bates T. Preoperative risk scores for the prediction of outcome in elderly people who require emergency surgery. *World J Emerg Surg* 2007; **2**: 16.

Royal College of Surgeons of England/Department of Health. The higher risk general surgical patient: towards improved care for a forgotten group. 2011.

Royal College of Surgeons. Caring for patients who refuse blood. 2016.

Royal College of Surgeons. Consent: Supported Decision Making. 2016.

Sanon S, Rihal CS. Non-cardiac surgery after percutaneous intervention. *American Journal of Cardiology* 2014; **114**: 1613–20.

Shoemaker WC, Appel PL, Kram HB *et al.* Prospective trial of supranormal values of survivors as therapeutic goals in high-risk surgical patients. *Chest* 1988; **94**: 1176–86.

Stonelake S, Thomson P, Suggett N. Identification of the high-risk emergency surgical patient: which risk prediction model should be used? *Ann Med Surg (Lond)* 2015; **4**(3): 240–7.

van Veen JJ, Spahn DR, Makris M. Routine preoperative coagulation test: an outdated practice? *Br J Anaesth* 2011; **106**: 1–3.

Chapter **18**

Anaesthesia and pain relief

Learning objectives

To gain an understanding of:
- Techniques of anaesthesia and airway maintenance
- Methods of providing pain relief
- Local and regional anaesthesia techniques
- The management of chronic pain and pain from malignant disease

HISTORY

Anaesthesia, as we know it today, was first successfully demonstrated by William Morton, a local dentist, at the Massachusetts General Hospital Boston, USA on 16th October 1846 when he administered ether to Gilbert Abbot for operation on a vascular tumour on his neck. Earlier Horace Wells had successfully used nitrous oxide in 1844 for painless extraction of teeth.

Simpson at Edinburgh University overcame some of the technical difficulties of ether administration by introducing chloroform. The benefits of anaesthesia were then universally recognised and antagonism by religious leaders was countered when Queen Victoria accepted chloroform from John Snow during the birth of Prince Leopold in 1853.

KEY PRINCIPLES OF ANAESTHESIA

Optimum patient care is dependent on a collaborative approach from anaesthetic and surgical teams, together with the other perioperative care providers. The importance of multidisciplinary collaboration has been clearly demonstrated by national audits such as the *Confidential Enquiries in Perioperative Deaths (CEPOD)* and *Enquiries into Maternal Deaths UK*. These audits have led to changes in clinical and non-clinical practice to improve morbidity and mortality.

The use of a set of safety checklists in the operating theatre in the form of the *World Health Organisation's Surgical Safety Checklist* has shown a reduction in incidence of perioperative untoward events.

The role of the modern anaesthetist has evolved from just being responsible for the patient in the operating suite into a 'perioperative physician' who optimises the patient for surgery, assessing and minimising risk, cares for them during the operation, and then manages both pain and homeostasis in the postoperative period (*Table 18.1*).

TABLE 18.1 Key features of commonly used intravenous anaesthetic agents.
Propofol (di-isopropyl phenol) Smooth induction, better haemodynamic stability, blunting of autonomic reflexes and ability to use as a continuous infusion
Thiopentone (barbiturate) Rapid induction, myocardial depression. Reduced metabolic rate and lowering of intracranial pressure is useful in neurosurgical patients but drop in blood pressure can give detrimental effects
Etomidate (steroid derivative) Good haemodynamic stability, brief duration of action, but concern over adrenocortical depression
Ketamine (phencyclidine derivative) Preservation of blood pressure and respiratory reflexes together with excellent analgesia makes it an ideal choice for field anaesthesia. Emergence delirium is associated with administration of ketamine

Anaesthesia; the name was suggested by Oliver Wendell-Homes and first appeared in Bailey's English Dictionary in 1751.
Humphrey Davy, 1800, suggested that nitrous oxide inhalation might be used to relieve pain of surgical operations and named it 'laughing gas'.
Henry Edmund Gaskin Boyle in 1917 obtained his gas-oxygen machine which became the first 'Boyle apparatus'.
William Thomas Gren Morton, 1819–1868, dentist who practised in Boston, MA, USA.
Sir James Young Simpson, 1811–1870, Professor of Midwifery, Edinburgh, UK.
Alexandrina Victoria, Queen of the United Kingdom of Great Britain and Ireland, 1837–1901.
John Snow, 1813–1858, general practitioner, London, UK, was one of the pioneers of anaesthesia.
Prince Leopold, 1853–1884, who later became Duke of Albany, was the eighth of Queen Victoria's nine children, and her fourth son.

Summary box 18.1

Ground rules for anaesthesia

- Safe surgery is achieved by close teamwork between surgeon, anaesthetist and perioperative care providers
- Safety checklists make sure that things are not forgotten
- Risk assessments allow the best strategy to be chosen
- Anaesthetists are extending their care into the pre- and postoperative phase

PREPARATION FOR ANAESTHESIA

In the previous chapter, the preoperative preparation for anaesthesia was discussed in detail, and its importance is emphasised (Chapter 17). Moreover, a careful preassessment, multidisciplinary approach, standardised care pathway with a carefully chosen anaesthetic and analgesic technique form the cornerstone of 'enhanced recovery programmes' being introduced recently across the surgical specialities (see Chapter 20).

GENERAL ANAESTHESIA

General anaesthesia is commonly described as the triad of unconsciousness, analgesia and muscle relaxation.

Summary box 18.2

The general anaesthetic triad

- Amnesia: loss of awareness
- Analgesia: pain relief
- Muscle relaxation

Induction of general anaesthesia is most frequently done by intravenous agents. Propofol has replaced thiopentone as the most widely used induction agent and can be used for maintenance of anaesthesia. Other infrequently used intravenous agents include etomidate and ketamine. Newer agents based on benzodiazepine receptor agonists, etomidate derivatives and fospropofol are still in the experimental stage.

Inhalational induction using agents such as non-pungent sevoflurane is useful in children, needle-phobic adults and those in whom a difficult airway is anticipated. These patients will have a higher risk of developing airway obstruction (Figure 18.1).

Rapid sequence induction (RSI) using a predetermined dose of intravenous anaesthetic agent together with rapidly acting muscle relaxant is used in those with high risk of regurgitation in order to secure the airway quickly. Commonly needed in emergency surgery it is also a technique of choice in any non-emergency surgery in a patient with delayed emptying of stomach.

Total intravenous anaesthesia (TIVA) is becoming popular following the introduction of propofol and the ultra-short-acting opioid remifentanil. The lack of a cumulative effect,

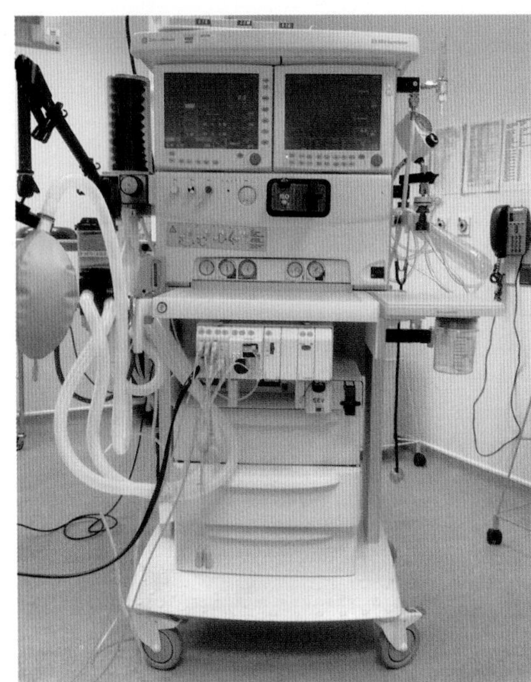

Figure 18.1 Anaesthetic machine.

better haemodynamic stability, excellent recovery profile and concerns over environmental effects of inhalational agents have made TIVA an attractive choice. TIVA is routinely used in neurosurgery, airway laser surgery, during cardiopulmonary bypass and for day-case anaesthesia (Figure 18.2).

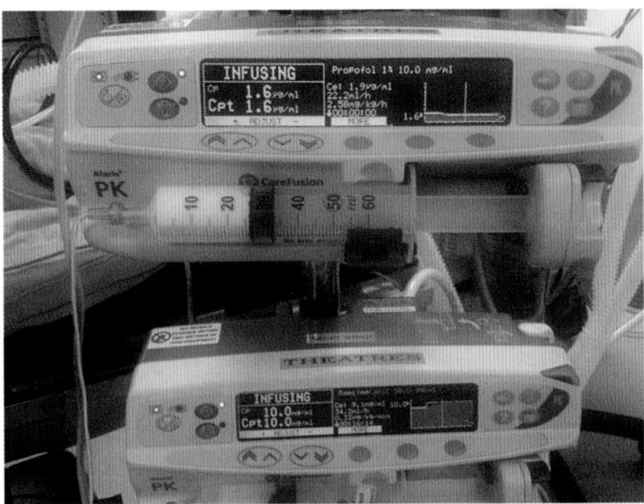

Figure 18.2 Total intravenous anaesthesia pumps in use.

Summary box 18.3

Special terms in anaesthesia

- Rapid sequence induction (RSI) is a technique that allows the airway to be rapidly secured. It is used when there is a high risk of regurgitation that may lead to pulmonary aspiration
- Total intravenous anaesthesia (TIVA) is becoming increasingly popular

Maintenance of anaesthesia, on the other hand, can be done using continuous infusion of intravenous agent (propofol) or inhaled vapour such as isoflurane, sevoflurane or desflurane.

The use of nitrous oxide is declining despite its analgesic and weak anaesthetic properties due to concerns over postoperative nausea and vomiting. It also increases the size of the air bubble causing adverse effects, for example in eye, ear and abdominal surgery. Finally, it is possibly mutagenic and is a powerful greenhouse gas.

Management of airway during anaesthesia

Loss of muscle tone as a result of general anaesthesia means that the patient can no longer keep their airway open. Therefore, the patients need their airway maintained for them. The use of muscle relaxants will mean that they will also be unable to breathe for themselves and so will require artificial ventilation. Head tilt, chin lift and jaw thrust manoeuvres, along with adjuncts such as oropharyngeal airways, are used to facilitate bag-mask ventilation while induction agents exert full effect. Laryngeal mask airway or endotracheal tube are then inserted and the patient is allowed to breathe spontaneously or is ventilated during the procedure.

The addition of a cuff to the endotracheal tube facilitates positive pressure ventilation and protects the lungs from aspiration of regurgitated gastric contents.

Supraglottic airways

- **Laryngeal mask airway (LMA).** Developed by Dr Archie Brain in the UK, the original LMA is a first-generation supraglottic airway. The mask with an inflatable cuff is inserted via the mouth and produces a seal around the glottic opening, providing a very reliable means of maintaining the airway. Its placement is less irritating and less traumatic to a patient's airway than endotracheal intubation. The technique can be easily taught to non-anaesthetists and paramedics and can be used as an emergency airway management tool. Several varieties of first generation LMAs are available, including the classic LMA and the flexible LMA. Further advancement has led to the development of second-generation supraglottic devices such as the ProSeal LMA, the i-Gel and LMA Supreme (Figure 18.3). These devices usually have an in-built 'bite-block' and an oesophageal drain tube; they can be used for ventilation of the lungs at higher inflation pressures and are more suitable for patients with a higher body mass index. There are also modified versions of the LMA including the intubating LMA (ILMA) that allow a blind technique in aiding insertion of a tracheal tube in difficult conditions. There is increasing evidence that second-generation devices have a good safety and efficacy profile and should be replacing all first-generation devices.

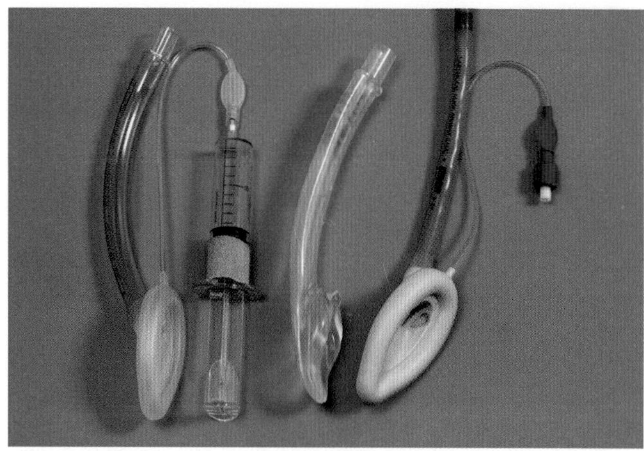

Figure 18.3 The laryngeal mask airway. The laryngeal mask airway (left), i-Gel airway (centre) and reinforced laryngeal mask airway (right).

- **Difficult intubation.** Endotracheal intubation is feasible in most patients, but in a certain proportion of patients this may be difficult or impossible; if compounded by inability to ventilate the patient by bag-mask, consequences can be catastrophic hypoxia. Many devices have been developed to aid intubation if difficulty is anticipated and protocols created by specialised societies to deal with such situations. One specialised method for intubation in difficult situations is the use of the fibreoptic intubating bronchoscope facilitated by topical local anaesthetic in awake patients or using general anaesthesia. The anaesthetist places the endotracheal tube in the trachea by threading the tube over the bronchoscope, and so places the tube in the trachea under direct bronchoscopic vision. An awake intubation requires careful patient selection, as it may not be a suitable technique for all patient groups (Figures 18.4, 18.5 and 18.6).

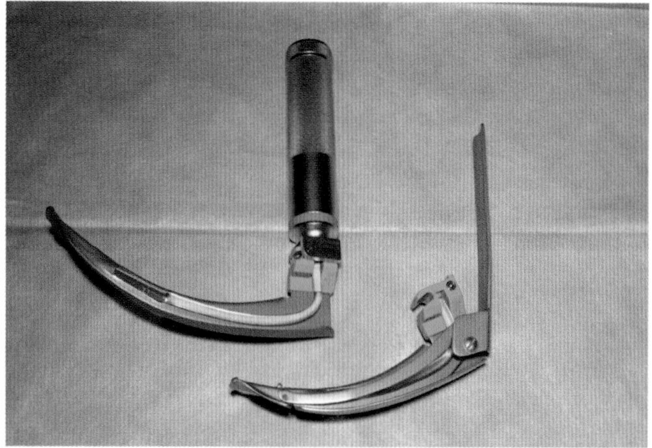

Figure 18.4 The Macintosh laryngoscope with a standard blade (left) and McCoy's modification of the Macintosh blade (right).

Archibald Ian Jeremy Brain, formerly anaesthetist, The Royal Berkshire Hospital, Reading, UK.
Sir Robert Reynolds Macintosh, 1897–1989, Nuffield Professor of Anaesthetics, The University of Oxford, Oxford, UK. First Chair in anaesthesia in 1937. First Chair in anaesthesia in USA: Ralph Waters, Wisconsin, USA in 1933. First examination for the Diploma in anaesthesia was held in London in 1935.
Sir Ivan Whiteside Magill, 1888–1986, anaesthetist, The Westminster Hospital, London, UK. During the First World War Sir Ivan Magill and Stanley Rowbotham, while working with Harold Gillies (pioneer of plastic surgery), developed tracheal intubation. Sir Magill is also remembered for his laryngoscope, Magill attachment and laryngeal forceps.

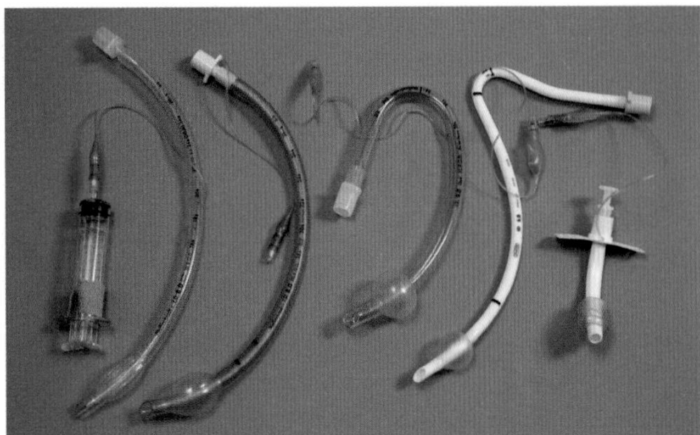

Figure 18.5 Endotracheal devices. From left to right: an uncut orotracheal tube; reinforced orotracheal tube; oral version of a Ring, Adair and Elwyn (RAE) preformed tube; nasal version of an RAE preformed tube; tracheostomy tube.

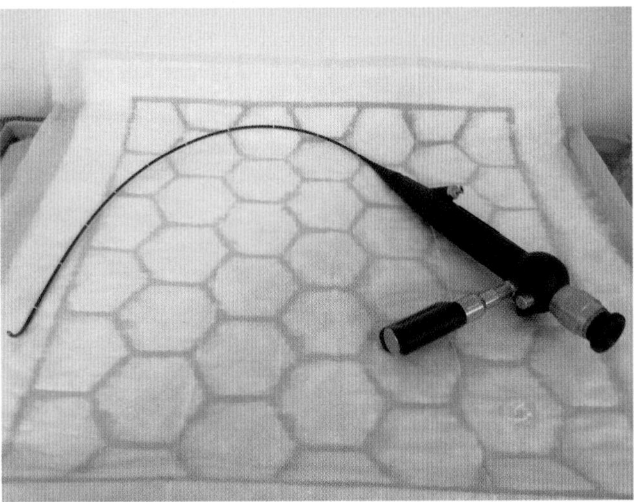

Figure 18.6 Fibreoptic intubating bronchoscope.

Double lumen tubes and endobronchial tubes are used in procedures such as thoracoscopic, pulmonary and oesophageal surgery to allow collapse of one lung (while ventilating the other) for ease of surgery. Their use is also essential to isolate the healthy lung in pyopneumothorax and in the case of a bronchopleural fistula.

Ventilating bronchoscopes and endobronchial catheters can be used to maintain oxygenation during laryngo-tracheal surgery or bronchoscopy by using intermittent jets of oxygen.

Summary box 18.4

Techniques for maintaining an airway

- Chin lift and jaw thrust: suitable for short term when no aid available
- Guedel airway: holds tongue forward but does not prevent aspiration
- Supraglottic device: easy insertion, reliable airway, allows ventilation
- Endotracheal intubation: secure and protected airway

Summary box 18.5

Complications of intubation

- Failed intubation
- Accidental bronchial intubation
- Trauma to teeth, pharynx, larynx
- Aspiration of gastric contents during intubation
- Disconnection, blockage, kinking of tube
- Delayed tracheal stenosis

Muscle relaxation and artificial ventilation

Pharmacological blockade of neuromuscular transmission provides relaxation of muscles allowing easy surgical access, but the patient requires artificial ventilation.

Neuromuscular blocking agents are broadly classified into depolarising and non-depolarising groups according to their mode of action.

Suxamethonium is the most commonly used depolarising agent. It binds to the nicotinic acetylcholine receptors, resulting in opening of the cation channel leading to depolarisation and rapid relaxation of muscles. Despite its adverse effects such as hyperkalaemia, muscle pain, anaphylaxis and potentially life-threatening malignant hyperthermia, suxamethonium is still widely used because of its quick onset and short duration of action. These properties are useful where rapid endotracheal intubation is necessary to protect the patient's airway or short-duration surgery is performed.

Non-depolarising muscle relaxants act by competitive blockade of postsynaptic receptors at the neuromuscular junction. They provide longer, predictable activity, but require careful monitoring, appropriate timing and reversal of their action by agents such as neostigmine and sugammadex at the end of the procedure. A peripheral nerve stimulator is routinely used to monitor the depth of neuromuscular block and also to confirm satisfactory recovery of muscle power prior to extubation (*Table 18.2*). With the increasing availability and evidence of the use of sugammadex, the non-depolarising muscle relaxant rocuronium is an alternative to suxamethonium in the 'rapid-sequence' induction, as it allows reversal of its actions with sugammadex in a rapid manner.

Ventilation during anaesthesia

Mechanical ventilation is required when the patient's spontaneous ventilation is inadequate or when the patient is not breathing because of the effects of the anaesthetic, analgesic agents or muscle relaxants.

In volume control ventilation, a preset volume is delivered by the machine irrespective of the airway pressure. The pressure generated will be in part dependent on the resistance and compliance of the airway. In laparoscopic surgery requiring the Trendelenburg position (the patient is positioned

The RAE tube takes its name from the initials of the surnames of the people who introduced it, Wallace Harold Ring, John Adair and Richard Elwyn.
Arthur Ernest Guedel, 1883–1956, Clinical Professor of Anaesthesiology, University of Southern California, Los Angeles, CA, USA.

TABLE 18.2 Properties of commonly used muscle relaxants.

Suxamethonium	Quickest onset, very short duration, spontaneous recovery. Ideal for rapid intubation and for short procedures	Muscle pain, hyperkalaemia, prolonged apnoea and life-threatening malignant hyperthermia
Vecuronium	Long acting, minimal cardiovascular effect and less allergic reaction	Dependent on hepatic metabolism and renal clearance, hence caution if hepatic and renal impairment
Atracurium	Intermediate acting. Non-enzymatic Hoffmann degradation. Suitable in renal and hepatic failure	Histamine release and allergic reactions
Rocuronium	Rapid onset, intermediate action. Suitable for rapid intubation. Rapid reversal possible using sugammadex	Allergic reactions. Excreted unchanged via bile and urine

head down), and in morbidly obese patients and those with lung disease, this may result in excessive pressures being developed, which may lead to barotrauma (pneumothorax).

In pressure control mode, the ventilator generates flow until a preset pressure is reached. The actual tidal volume delivered is variable and depends on airway resistance, intra-abdominal pressure and the degree of relaxation.

Positive end expiratory pressure (PEEP) is often applied to help maintain functional residual capacity (FRC). This avoids lung collapse by opening collapsed alveoli, and maintains a greater area of gas exchange so reducing vascular shunting.

Summary box 18.6

Intermittent positive pressure ventilation

- Volume controlled, which ensures adequate gas entry but risks high pressure damage
- Pressure controlled, which avoids high pressure damage but risks inadequate ventilation
- Positive end expiratory pressure (PEEP) reduces alveolar collapse and reduces vascular shunting so improving perfusion

Monitoring and care during anaesthesia

A minimum basic monitoring of cardiovascular parameters is required during surgery. This includes:

- Vascular:
  - electrocardiogram (ECG);
  - blood pressure;
- Adequacy of ventilation:
  - inspired oxygen concentration;
  - oxygen saturation by pulse oximetry;
  - end tidal carbon dioxide concentration.

Monitors of temperature, ventilation parameters and delivery of anaesthetic agents are also routinely used, while measurement of urine output and central venous pressure are recommended for major surgery.

Anaesthesia for day case surgery

This is discussed in Chapter 21.

LOCAL ANAESTHESIA

Local anaesthetic drugs may be used to provide anaesthesia and analgesia as a sole agent or as adjuncts to general anaesthesia. Available techniques include topical anaesthesia, local infiltration, regional nerve blocks and central neuroaxial blocks (spinal and epidural anaesthesia) (*Table 18.3*).

TABLE 18.3 The common local anaesthetic drugs.

Name	Maximum dose	Comments
Lignocaine	3 mg/kg (7 mg/kg with adrenaline)	Early onset, short acting, good sensory block
Bupivacaine	2 mg/kg	Long lasting, more cardiotoxic, must never be used intravenously
Prilocaine	6 mg/kg (9 mg/kg with adrenaline)	Least systemic toxicity, causes methaemoglobinaemia
Ropivacaine	3–4 mg/kg	Less cardiotoxic, greater sensory–motor separation
Levobupivaciane	2 mg /kg	Isomer of bupivacaine with fewer cardiotoxic properties

Local anaesthesia techniques can lead to complications that may be local, such as infection or haematoma, or systemic due to overdose or accidental intravascular injection. The systemic effects of local anaesthetic agents are dose dependent and manifest as cardiovascular (cardiac arrhythmia, cardiac arrest) or neurological (depressed consciousness, convulsions). Prilocaine overdose causes methaemoglobinaemia while bupivacaine overdose causes treatment-resistant ventricular arrhythmia and cardiac arrest.

The addition of adrenaline to local anaesthetic solutions hastens onset, prolongs duration of action and permits a higher upper dose limit. The use of adrenaline is contraindicated in patients with cardiovascular disease, those taking tricyclic and monoamine oxidase inhibitors and in end-arterial locations.

Appropriately skilled personnel, resuscitation equipment and oxygen should always be available with local anaesthetic use because of the potential risks of life-threatening complications.

Regional anaesthesia

Regional anaesthesia involves central neuroaxial or peripheral nerve or plexus blocks. It has a clear advantage where general anaesthesia carries a higher risk of morbidity and mortality, such as in patients with debilitating respiratory and cardiovascular disease and obstetric cases. It also provides excellent pain relief in the postoperative period, reducing the need for analgesics such as opioids.

As with general anaesthesia obtaining venous access, monitoring vital parameters should be performed during regional anaesthesia.

Localising nerves using anatomical landmarks and eliciting paraesthesia alone carries a high risk of nerve damage, intravascular injection and has lower success rate. The use of nerve stimulators to localise nerves improves success rate and reduces risks. Ultrasound-guided regional anaesthesia allows the visualisation of nerves and the spread of local anaesthetics, enabling the use of a smaller dose of local anaesthetic agents, with improved success rates and safety.

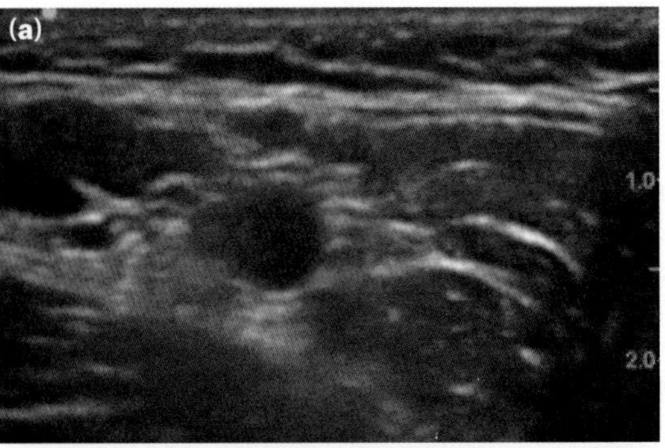

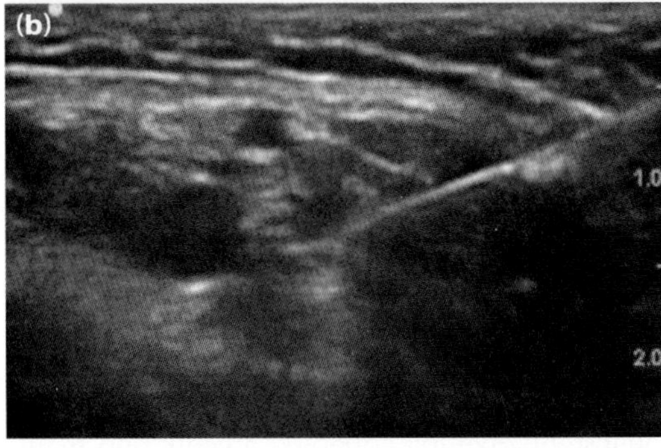

Figure 18.7 (a, b) Ultrasound scans of brachial plexus block.

> **Summary box 18.7**
>
> **Types of anaesthesia**
>
> - General anaesthesia may be more acceptable to the patients
> - Regional anaesthesia has major advantages in obstetrics and patients with respiratory compromise
> - Local blocks have been transformed by nerve stimulators and ultrasound guidance
> - All require full resuscitation and monitoring equipment to be available

TRANSVERSUS ABDOMINIS PLANE BLOCK

Transversus abdominis plane block (TAP) is growing rapidly in popularity. The technique has been shown to provide effective analgesia after a wide range of abdominal surgery. The T6–L1 segmental nerves enter the triangle of Petit just medial to the anterior axillary line. Injection of local anaesthetic into the fascial plane between the internal oblique and transversus abdominis muscles allows a block of all these nerves, and excellent anaesthesia of the anterior abdominal wall (Figure 18.8).

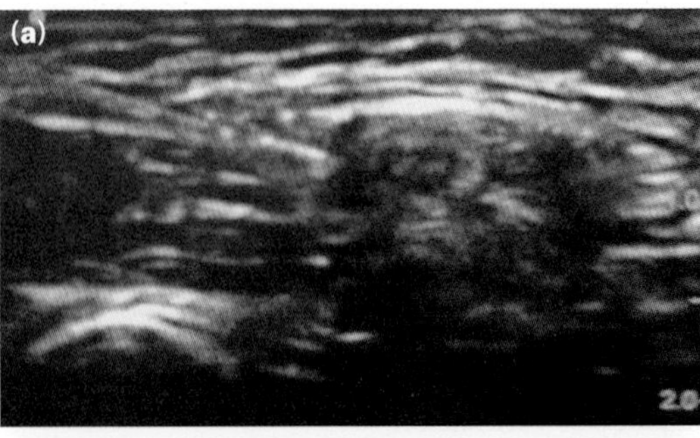

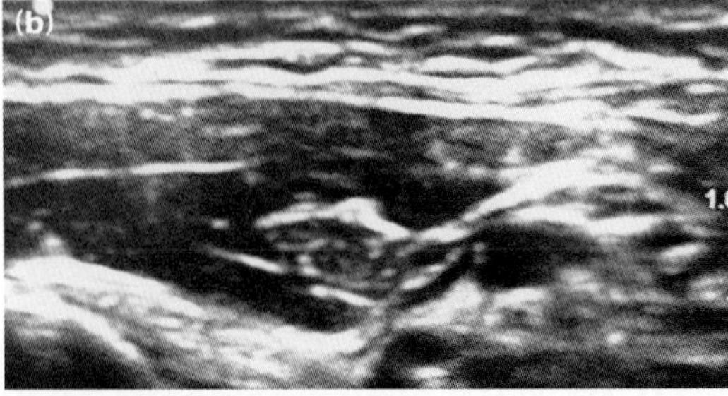

Figure 18.8 (a, b) Ultrasound scans of lateral abdominal wall and the spread of local anaesthetics.

Common local anaesthesia techniques

Topical anaesthesia

- **EMLA (eutectic mixture of local anesthetics)**. This is a mixture of lignocaine and prilocaine for application to the skin for venepuncture in children.
- **Cocaine**. It may be called Mofatt's solution (with an added mixture of adrenaline and sodium bicarbonate) and used in nasal surgery for anaesthesia and vasoconstriction.
- **Lignocaine 2/4/10%**. Spray to anaesthetise the airway during awake fibreoptic intubation.

Nerve blocks

- Interscalene block for shoulder surgery produces excellent postoperative analgesia. Complications include phrenic nerve block, Horner's syndrome, as well as accidental intravascular and spinal injection.
- Axillary brachial plexus block can be used as the sole anaesthetic technique for upper limb surgery (Figure 18.7).
- Femoral and sciatic nerve blocks are often used for anaesthesia and analgesia for lower limb surgery.

INTRAVENOUS REGIONAL ANAESTHESIA (BIER'S BLOCK)

Bier's block produces excellent anaesthesia for short surgery, particularly for the upper limb (e.g. carpal tunnel release). Exsanguination using an Esmarch bandage, inflation of proximal cuff of the double tourniquet is followed by intravenous injection of prilocaine into the vein on the back of the hand that is being operated on. After 5–10 minutes the distal cuff of the tourniquet is inflated and then the proximal one deflated. Even if surgery is finished, the tourniquet should be left inflated until the local anaesthetic has bound to tissues (20 minutes), so that release of local anaesthetic into the systemic circulation does not occur. Lignocaine can be used with caution (consider safe dose and time of tourniquet inflation) but bupivacaine should never be used for Bier's block.

Spinal anaesthesia

Spinal anaesthesia alone, and in combination with general anaesthesia or sedation is used extensively for lower limb, obstetric and pelvic surgery. Injection of a 'single shot' local anaesthetic agent intrathecally produces intense and rapid block for surgery. Addition of opioids provides prolonged postoperative analgesia but carries the risk of late respiratory depression.

Autonomic sympathetic blockade produces hypotension, particularly if the level of block is above T10. Caution is needed in patients with hypovolemia and cardiovascular disease.

The incidence of dural puncture headache can be minimised by limiting the number of punctures and use of fine bore pencil tip needles designed to split rather than cut the dura.

Epidural anaesthesia

Epidural anaesthesia is slower in onset than spinal, but has the advantage of prolonged analgesia by multiple dosing or continuous infusion through a catheter placed in the epidural space. Being slower in onset, the resulting hypotension from sympathetic blockade can be better controlled and can reduce blood loss.

Continuous infusion (with a patient-controlled bolus) of weak local anaesthetic combined with opioids (such a fentanyl) is routinely used for postoperative analgesia. Placement of an epidural catheter in the high thoracic region provides excellent analgesia for a wide variety of upper abdominal and thoracic surgical operations, enabling early mobilisation and reducing respiratory complications.

Epidural anaesthesia is technically more difficult than spinal anaesthesia, with a higher failure rate and carries the risk of nerve damage, spinal injuries, accidental spinal injection of large volume of local anaesthetics and risk of infection and epidural haematoma (Figure 18.9).

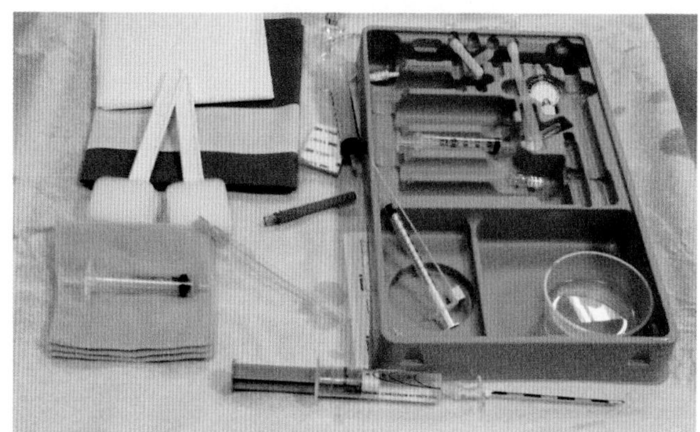

Figure 18.9 Equipment for epidural/spinal anaesthesia.

Summary box 18.8

Local anaesthetics

- EMLA cream for children needing injections
- Regional and nerve blocks for limb surgery
- Spinal anaesthesia offers quick onset and short duration of anaesthesia
- Epidurals are more difficult but can then be topped-up postoperatively and used as continuous infusion

Chronic pain management

In surgical practice, the patient with chronic pain may present for treatment of the cause (e.g. pancreatitis, malignancy), or concomitant benign pathology. Acute pain after surgery may progress to chronic pain and is believed to be due to inadequate treatment of acute pain itself.

Chronic pain may be of several types:

- **Nociceptive pain** may result from musculoskeletal disorders or cancer activating cutaneous nociceptors (pain receptors). Prolonged ischaemic or inflammatory processes result in sensitisation of peripheral nociceptors and altered activity in the central nervous system, leading to exaggerated responses in the dorsal horn of the spinal cord. The widened area of hyperalgesia and increased sensitivity (allodynia) has been attributed to the increased transmission in the central nervous system.
- **Neuropathic (or neurogenic) pain** is dysfunction in peripheral or central nerves (excluding the 'physiological' pain due to noxious stimulation of the nerve terminals). It is classically of a 'burning', 'shooting' or 'stabbing' type and may be associated with allodynia, numbness and diminished thermal sensation. It is poorly responsive to opioids. Examples include trigeminal neuralgia, postherpetic and diabetic neuropathy. Monoaminergic, tricyclic inhibitors and anticonvulsant drugs are the mainstay of treatment.
- **Psychogenic pain** is associated with depressive illness; chronic pain and the illness may exacerbate each other.

August Karl Gustav Bier, 1861–1949, Professor of Surgery, Bonn (1903–1907) and Berlin, Germany (1907–1932).

Summary box 18.9

Types of pain

- Nociceptive pain arises from inflammation and ischaemia
- Neuropathic pain arises from a dysfunction in the central nervous system
- Psychogenic pain is modified by the mental state of the patient

Chronic pain control in benign disease

Surgical patients may present with chronic persistent pain (more than 3 months' duration) from a variety of disorders including postoperative neuropathic pain, chronic inflammatory disease, recurrent infection, degenerative bone or joint disease, nerve injury and sympathetic dystrophy. This may result from persistent excitation of the nociceptive pathways causing spontaneous firing of pain signals at N-methyl-D-aspartate receptors in the ascending pathways. This pain does not respond to opiates or neuroablative surgery and would merit neuropathic pain management.

Amputation of limbs may result in phantom limb pain; the likelihood is increased if the limb was painful before surgery. Continuous regional local anaesthetic blockade (epidural or brachial plexus) established before operation and continued postoperatively for a few days, is believed to effectively reduce the risk of phantom limb pain.

- **Local anaesthetic and steroid injections** can be effective around an inflamed nerve and they reduce the cycle of constant pain transmission with consequent muscle spasm. Transforaminal selective root blocks in the epidural space are used for the pain of nerve root irritation associated with or without minor disc prolapse, followed by active physiotherapy and rehabilitation to promote mobility.
- **Nerve stimulation procedures** such as acupuncture and transcutaneous nerve stimulation, increase the endorphin production in the central nervous system. Nerve decompression craniotomy rather than percutaneous coagulation of the ganglion is now performed for trigeminal neuralgia. Spinal cord stimulation by dorsal column stimulation is now a recognised and effective management of intractable neuropathic pain. This involves placement of electrodes in the posterior epidural space to allow dorsal column stimulation through an implantable pulse generator inserted in the body.

Summary box 18.10

Pain control in benign disease

- Bring pain under control before amputation to avoid phantom pain
- Local anaesthetic and steroid injected around a nerve may reduce muscle spasm
- Transcutaneous nerve stimulators (TNS) modifies pain by increasing endorphin production
- Trigeminal neuralgia responds to decompression of the nerve

Drugs in chronic non-malignant pain

Paracetamol and the non-steroidal anti-inflammatory drugs (NSAIDs) are the mainstay of musculoskeletal pain treatment. The tricyclic antidepressant drugs and anticonvulsant agents are often useful for the pain of nerve injury, although side effects can prove troublesome and reduce compliance. Both pregabalin and gabapentin reduce spontaneous neuronal activity by their action on the alpha-2-delta subunit of calcium channels, and are now used for managing neuropathic chronic pain. In more severe and debilitating non-malignant chronic pain, opioid analgesic drugs are used in slow release oral preparations of morphine and oxycodone, and transcutaneous patches delivering fentanyl and buprenorphine. Tapentadol with its dual action on opioid and noradrenaline selective reuptake inhibition pathways may provide relief in patients with pain of both neuropathic and nociceptive elements. Combinations of drugs often prove useful to achieve the optimum of efficacy with minimal side effects.

Treatment of pain dependent on sympathetic nervous system activity

Even minor trauma and surgery, (often of a limb) can provoke chronic burning pain, allodynia, trophic changes and resultant disuse due to excessive sympathetic adrenergic activity inducing vasconstriction and abnormal nociceptive transmission.

Management includes antineuropathic pain medications (pregabalin, gabapentin, amitriptyline) as part of multimodal analgesia with a multidisciplinary pain management approach including considerable input of psychological, targeted physiotherapy and counselling. Interventional treatment may include local anaesthetic injection of stellate ganglion for upper limb symptoms. Percutaneous chemical lumbar sympathectomy with local anaesthetic is used for relief of rest pain in advanced ischaemic disease of the legs.

Pain control in malignant disease

Pain is a common symptom associated with cancer, more so during the advanced stages. In intractable pain, the underlying principle of treatment is to encourage independence of the patient and an active life in spite of the symptom. The World Health Organisation's booklet advises use of a 'pain stepladder':

- First step. **Simple analgesics**: aspirin, paracetamol, non-steroidal anti-inflammatory agents, tricyclic drugs or anticonvulsant drugs.
- Second step. **Intermediate strength opioids**: codeine, tramadol or dextropropoxyphene.
- Third step. **Strong opioids**: morphine (pethidine has now been withdrawn).

Oral opiate analgesia is necessary when the less powerful analgesic agents no longer control pain on movement, or enable the patient to sleep. Fear that the patient may develop an addiction to opiates is usually not justified in malignant disease. It is also important to distinguish between the addiction and dependence; the former being a psychosocial phenomenon while the latter is a pure physiological response to a given drug. Some patients experience 'breakthrough pain' (acute, excruciating and incapacitating), which occurs either spontaneously or in relation to a specific predictable or unpredictable trigger, experienced by patients who have relatively stable and adequately controlled background pain.

Oral morphine, often used for chronic pain, can be prescribed in short-acting liquid or tablet form and should be administered regularly every 4 hours until an adequate dose of drug has been titrated to control the pain over 24 hours. Once this is established, the daily dose can be divided into two separate administrations of enteric-coated, slow-release morphine tablets (MST morphine) every 12 hours. Additional short-acting opioids (morphine/fentanyl) can then be used to cover episodes of 'breakthrough pain'. Nausea treated using antiemetic agents does not usually persist, but constipation is frequently a persistent complication requiring regular prevention by laxatives.

Infusion of subcutaneous, intravenous, intrathecal or epidural opiate drugs

The infusion of opiate is necessary if a patient is unable to take oral drugs. Subcutaneous infusion of diamorphine is simple and effective to administer. Epidural infusions of diamorphine with an external pump can be used on mobile patients. Intrathecal infusions with pumps programmed by external computers are used; however, there is a possibility of developing infection with catastrophic effects. Intravenous narcotic agents may be reserved for acute crises, such as pathological fractures.

Neurolytic techniques in cancer pain

These should only be used if the life expectancy is limited and the diagnosis is certain. The useful procedures are:

- Subcostal phenol injection for a rib metastasis.
- Coeliac plexus neurolytic block with alcohol for pain of pancreatic, gastric or hepatic cancer.
- Intrathecal neurolytic injection of hyperbaric phenol.
- Percutaneous anterolateral cordotomy divides the spinothalamic ascending pain pathway. It is a highly effective technique in experienced hands, selectively eliminating pain and temperature sensation in a specific limited area.

Alternative strategies include:

- The development of antipituitary hormone drugs, such as tamoxifen and cyproterone, enables effective pharmacological therapy for the pain of widespread metastases instead of pituitary ablation surgery.
- Palliative radiotherapy can be most beneficial for the relief of pain in metastatic disease.
- Adjuvant drugs such as corticosteroids to reduce cerebral oedema or inflammation around a tumour may be useful in symptom control. Tricyclic antidepressants, anticonvulsants and flecainide are also used to reduce the pain of nerve injury.

In the management of chronic pain, a multidisciplinary approach by a team of medical and nursing staff working with psychologists, physiotherapists and occupational therapists can often achieve much more benefit than the use of powerful drugs. 'Pain Management Programmes' lay out a logical structure for this.

Summary box 18.11

Options for controlling severe pain in malignant disease

- Oral morphine using slow-release enteric-coated tablets
- Slow infusion of opiates subcutaneously, by epidural or intrathecally
- Neurolysis for patients with limited life expectancy
- Palliative hormone, radiotherapy, or steroids control pain from swelling

FURTHER READING

Aitkenhead AR, Moppett IK, Rowbotham DJ, Thompson J. *Smith and Aitkenhead's textbook of anaesthesia*, 6th edn. Edinburgh: Churchill Livingstone Elsevier, 2013.

McLeod G, McCartney C, Wildsmith T (eds). *Principles and practice of regional anaesthesia*, 4th edn. Edinburgh: Churchill Livingstone, 2012.

Rawal N (ed.). *Management of acute and chronic pain*. London: BMJ Books, 1998.

Sneyd JR. Recent advances in intravenous anaesthesia. *Br J Anaesth* 2004; **93**: 725–36.

Chapter 19

Nutrition and fluid therapy

Learning objectives

To understand:

- The causes and consequences of malnutrition in the surgical patient
- Fluid and electrolyte requirements in the pre- and postoperative patient
- The nutritional requirements of surgical patients and the nutritional consequences of intestinal resection
- The different methods of providing nutritional support and their complications

INTRODUCTION

Malnutrition is common. It occurs in about 30% of surgical patients with gastrointestinal disease and in up to 60% of those in whom hospital stay has been prolonged because of postoperative complications. It is frequently unrecognised and consequently patients often do not receive appropriate support. There is a substantial body of evidence to show that patients who suffer starvation or have signs of malnutrition have a higher risk of complications and an increased risk of death in comparison with patients who have adequate nutritional reserves.

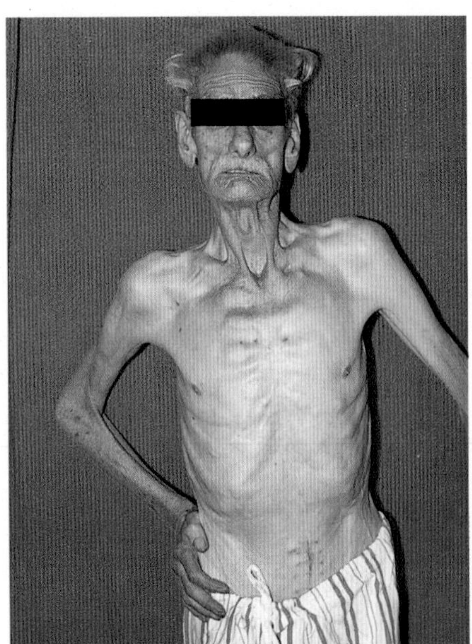

Figure 19.1 Severely malnourished patient with wasting of fat and muscle.

Long-standing protein–calorie malnutrition as seen in cachexia or general frailty is easy to recognise (Figure 19.1). Short-term undernutrition, although less easily recognised, frequently occurs in association with critical illness, major trauma, burns or surgery, and also impacts on patient recovery. The aim of nutritional support is to identify those patients at risk of malnutrition and to ensure that their nutritional requirements are met by the most appropriate route and in a way that minimises complications.

PHYSIOLOGY

Metabolic response to starvation

After a short fast, lasting 12 hours or less, most food from the last meal will have been absorbed. Plasma insulin levels fall and glucagon levels rise, which facilitates the conversion of liver glycogen (approximately 200 g) into glucose. The liver, therefore, becomes an organ of glucose production under fasting conditions. Many organs, including brain tissue, red and white blood cells and the renal medulla, can initially utilise only glucose for their metabolic needs. Additional stores of glycogen exist in muscle (500 g), but these cannot be utilised directly. Muscle glycogen is broken down (glycogenolysis) and converted to lactate, which is then exported to the liver where it is converted to glucose (Cori cycle). With increasing

Carl Ferdinand Cori, 1896–1984, Professor of Pharmacology and later Biochemistry, Washington University Medical School, St Louis, MI, USA and his wife Gerty Theresa Cori, 1896–1957, also Professor of Biochemistry at the Washington University Medical School. In 1947, the Coris were awarded a share of the Nobel Prize for Physiology or Medicine for their discovery of how glycogen is catalytically converted.

duration of fasting (>24 hours), glycogen stores are depleted and *de novo* glucose production from non-carbohydrate precursors (gluconeogenesis) takes place, predominantly in the liver. Most of this glucose is derived from the breakdown of amino acids, particularly glutamine and alanine as a result of catabolism of skeletal muscle (up to 75 g per day). This protein catabolism in simple starvation is readily reversed with the provision of exogenous glucose.

With more prolonged fasting, there is an increased reliance on fat oxidation to meet energy requirements. Increased breakdown of fat stores occurs, providing glycerol, which can be converted to glucose, and fatty acids, which can be used as a tissue fuel by almost all of the body's tissues. Hepatic production of ketones from fatty acids is facilitated by low insulin levels and, after 48–72 hours of fasting, the central nervous system may adapt to using ketone bodies as their primary fuel source. This conversion to a 'fat fuel economy' reduces the need for muscle breakdown by up to 55 g per day.

Another important adaptive response to starvation is a significant reduction in the resting energy expenditure, possibly mediated by a decline in the conversion of inactive thyroxine (T4) to active tri-iodothyronine (T3). Despite these adaptive responses, there remains an obligatory glucose requirement of about 200 g per day, even under conditions of prolonged fasting.

Summary box 19.1

Metabolic response to starvation

- Low plasma insulin
- High plasma glucagon
- Hepatic glycogenolysis
- Protein catabolism
- Hepatic gluconeogenesis
- Lipolysis: mobilisation of fat stores (increased fat oxidation) – overall decrease in protein and carbohydrate oxidation
- Adaptive ketogenesis
- Reduction in resting energy expenditure (from approximately 25–30 kcal/kg per day to 15–20 kcal/kg per day

Metabolic response to trauma and sepsis

This is described in full in Chapter 1 and summarised in *Summary box 19.2*.

From a nutritional point of view, two factors deserve emphasis. First, in contrast to simple starvation, patients with trauma have impaired formation of ketones, and the breakdown of protein to synthesise glucose (gluconeogenesis) cannot be entirely prevented by the administration of glucose. Second, although it is generally accepted that the metabolic response to trauma and sepsis is always associated with 'hypermetabolism' or hypercatabolism', these terms are ill defined and do not indicate the need for very high-energy intakes. There is no evidence to show that the provision of high-energy intake is associated with an amelioration of the catabolic process and it may indeed be harmful; there is mounting evidence for the benefits of permissive underfeeding in critically ill surgical patients.

Summary box 19.2

Metabolic response to trauma and sepsis

- Increased counter-regulatory hormones: adrenaline, noradrenaline, cortisol, glucagon and growth hormone
- Increased energy requirements (up to 40 kcal/kg per day)
- Increased nitrogen requirements
- Insulin resistance and glucose intolerance
- Preferential oxidation of lipids
- Increased gluconeogenesis and protein catabolism
- Loss of adaptive ketogenesis
- Fluid retention with associated hypoalbuminaemia

NUTRITIONAL ASSESSMENT

Laboratory techniques

There is no single biochemical measurement that reliably identifies malnutrition. Albumin is not a measure of nutritional status, particularly in the acute setting. Although a low serum albumin level (<30 g/L) is an indicator of poor prognosis, hypoalbuminaemia invariably occurs because of alterations in body fluid composition and because of increased capillary permeability related to ongoing sepsis. Malnutrition is associated with defective immune function, and measurement of lymphocyte count and skin testing for delayed hypersensitivity frequently reveal abnormalities in malnourished patients. Immunity is not, however, a precise or reliable indicator of nutritional status, nor is it a practical method in routine clinical practice.

Body weight and anthropometry

A simple method of assessing nutritional status is to estimate weight loss. Measured body weight is compared with ideal body weight obtained from tables or from the patient's usual or premorbid weight. Unintentional weight loss of more than 10% of a patient's weight in the preceding 6 months is a good prognostic indicator of poor outcome. Body weight is frequently corrected for height, allowing calculation of the body mass index (BMI, defined as body weight in kilograms divided by height in metres squared). A BMI of less than 18.5 indicates nutritional impairment and a BMI below 15 is associated with significant hospital mortality. Major changes in fluid balance, which are common in critically ill patients, may make body weight and BMI unreliable indicators of nutritional status.

Anthropometric techniques incorporating measurements of skinfold thicknesses and mid-arm circumference permit estimations of body fat and muscle mass, and these are indirect measures of energy and protein stores. These mea-

de novo is Latin for 'from the beginning'.

surements are, however, insufficiently accurate in individual patients to permit planning of nutritional support regimens. Similarly, use of bioelectrical impedence analysis (BIA) permits estimation of intra- and extracellular fluid volumes. These techniques are only useful if performed frequently on a sequential basis in individual patients; in this respect, trends are much more important than absolute impedance figures. All of these techniques are significantly impaired by the presence of oedema.

Clinical

The possibility of malnutrition should form part of the workup of all patients. A clinical assessment of nutritional status involves a focused history and physical examination, an assessment of risk of malabsorption or inadequate dietary intake and selected laboratory tests aimed at detecting specific nutrient deficiencies. This is termed 'subjective global assessment' and encompasses historical, symptomatic and physical parameters. Recently, the British Association of Parenteral and Enteral Nutrition introduced a malnutrition universal screening tool (MUST), which is a five-step screening tool to identify adults who are malnourished or at risk of undernutrition (Figure 19.2).

FLUID AND ELECTROLYTES

Fluid intake is derived from both exogenous (consumed liquids) and endogenous (released during oxidation of solid foodstuffs) fluids. The average daily water balance of a healthy adult is shown in *Table 19.1*.

TABLE 19.1 Average daily water balance of a healthy adult in a temperate climate (70 kg).

Output	Volume (mL)	Intake	Volume (mL)
Urine	1500	Water from beverage	200
Insensible losses	900	Water from food	1000
Faeces	100	Water from oxidation	300

Fluid losses occur by four routes:

1 **Lungs**. About 400 mL of water is lost in expired air each 24 hours. This is increased in dry atmospheres or in patients with a tracheostomy, emphasising the importance of humidification of inspired air.

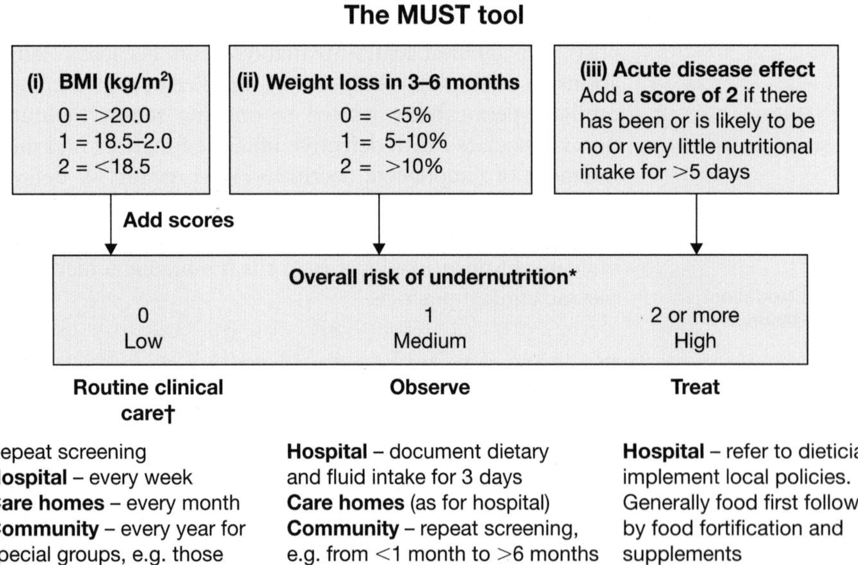

***If height, weight or weight loss cannot be established**, use documented or recalled values (if considered reliable). When measured or recalled height cannot be obtained, use knee height as a surrogate measure.
If neither can be calculated, obtain an overall impression of malnutrition risk (low, medium, high) using the following:
(i) Clinical impression (very thin, thin, average, overweight);
(iia) Clothes and/or jewellery have become loose fitting;
(iib) History of decreased food intake, loss of appetite or dysphagia up to 3–6 months;
(iic) Disease (underlying cause) and psychosocial/physical disabilities likely to cause weight loss.

† Involves treatment of underlying condition, and help with food choice and eating when necessary (also applies to other categories).

Figure 19.2 The malnutrition universal screening tool (MUST) for adults (adapted from Elia M (ed.). *The MUST Report. Development and use of the 'malnutrition universal screening tool' (MUST) for adults*. A report by the Malnutrition Advisory Group of the British Association for Parenteral and Enteral Nutrition. Report No. 152, 2003, ISBN 1 899467 70X).

Marinos Elia, contemporary, Head of the Adult Clinical Nutrition Group, The Medical Research Council, Cambridge, UK.

2 **Skin**. In a temperate climate, skin (i.e. sweat) losses are between 600 and 1000 mL/day.
3 **Faeces**. Between 60 and 150 mL of water are lost daily in patients with normal bowel function.
4 **Urine**. The normal urine output is approximately 1500 mL/day and, provided that the kidneys are healthy, the specific gravity of urine bears a direct relationship to volume. A minimum urine output of 400 mL/day is required to excrete the end products of protein metabolism.

Maintenance fluid requirements are calculated approximately from an estimation of insensible and obligatory losses. Various formulae are available for calculating fluid replacement based on a patient's weight or surface area. For example, 30–40 mL/kg gives an estimate of daily requirements.

The following are the approximate daily requirements of some electrolytes in adults:

- sodium: 50–90 mM/day;
- potassium: 50 mM/day;
- calcium: 5 mM/day;
- magnesium: 1 mM/day.

The nature and type of fluid replacement therapy will be determined by individual patient needs. The composition of some commonly used solutions is shown in Table 19.2.

Note that Hartmann's solution also contains lactate 29 mmol/L. Dextrose solutions are also commonly employed. These provide water replacement without any electrolytes and with modest calorie supplements (1 litre of 5% dextrose contains 400 kcal). A typical daily maintenance fluid regimen would consist of a combination of 5% dextrose with either Hartmann's or normal saline to a volume of 2 litres.

There has been much controversy in the literature regarding the respective merits of crystalloid versus colloid replacement. There is no consensus on this topic and the usual advice is to replace like with like. If the haematocrit is below 21%, blood transfusion may be required. There is increasing recognition, however, that albumin infusions are of little value.

In addition to maintenance requirements, 'replacement' fluids are required to correct pre-existing deficiencies and 'supplemental' fluids are required to compensate for anticipated additional intestinal or other losses. The nature and volumes of these fluids are determined by:

- A careful assessment of the patient including pulse, blood pressure and central venous pressure, if available. Clinical examination to assess hydration status (peripheries, skin turgor, urine output and specific gravity of urine), urine and serum electrolytes and haematocrit.
- Estimation of losses already incurred and their nature: for example, vomiting, ileus, diarrhoea, excessive sweating or fluid losses from burns or other serious inflammatory conditions.
- Estimation of supplemental fluids likely to be required in view of anticipated future losses from drains, fistulae, nasogastric tubes or abnormal urine or faecal losses.
- When an estimate of the volumes required has been made, the appropriate replacement fluid can be determined from a consideration of the electrolyte composition of gastrointestinal secretions. Most intestinal losses are adequately replaced with normal saline containing supplemental potassium (Table 19.3).

TABLE 19.3 Composition of gastrointestinal secretions (mmol/L).

	Na	K	Cl	HCO_3
Saliva	10	25	10	30
Stomach	50	15	110	–
Duodenum	140	5	100	–
Ileum	140	5	100	30
Pancreas	140	5	75	115
Bile	140	5	100	35

NUTRITIONAL REQUIREMENTS

Total enteral or parenteral nutrition necessitates the provision of the macronutrients, carbohydrate, fat and protein, together with vitamins, trace elements, electrolytes and water. When planning a feeding regime, the patient should be weighed and an assessment made of daily energy and protein requirements. Standard tables are available to permit these calculations.

Daily needs may change depending on the patient's condition. Overfeeding is the most common cause of complications, regardless of whether nutrition is provided enterally or parenterally. It is essential to monitor daily intake to provide an assessment of tolerance. In addition, regular biochemical monitoring is mandatory (Table 19.4).

TABLE 19.2 Composition of crystalloid and colloid solutions (mmol/L).

Solution	Na	K	Ca	Cl	Lactate	Colloid
Hartmann's	131	5	2	111	29	
Normal saline (0.9% NaCl)	154			154		
Dextrose saline (4% dextrose in 0.18% saline)	30	30				
Gelofusine	150	150				Gelatin 4%
Haemacel	145	5.1	<1	145		Polygelin 75 g/L
Hetastarch						Hydroxyethyl starch 6%

Alexis Frank Hartmann, 1898–1964, paediatrician, St Louis, MO, USA.

TABLE 19.4 Monitoring feeding regimes.

Daily	Body weight Fluid balance Full blood count, urea and electrolytes Blood glucose Electrolyte content and volume of urine and/or urine and intestinal losses Temperature
Weekly (or more frequently if clinically indicated)	Urine and plasma osmolality Calcium, magnesium, zinc and phosphate Plasma proteins including albumin Liver function tests including clotting factors Thiamine Acid–base status Triglycerides
Fortnightly	Serum vitamin B12 Folate Iron Lactate Trace elements (zinc, copper, manganese)

Macronutrient requirements

Energy

The total energy requirement of a stable patient with a normal or moderately increased need is approximately 20–30 kcal/kg per day. Very few patients require energy intakes in excess of 2000 kcal/day. Thus, in the majority of hospitalised patients in whom energy demands from activity are minimal, total energy requirements are approximately 1300–1800 kcal/day.

Carbohydrate

There is an obligatory glucose requirement to meet the needs of the central nervous system and certain haematopoietic cells, which is equivalent to about 2 g/kg per day. In addition, there is a physiological maximum to the amount of glucose that can be oxidised, which is approximately 4 mg/kg per minute (equivalent to about 1500 kcal/day in a 70-kg person), with the nonoxidised glucose being primarily converted to fat. However, optimal utilisation of energy during nutritional support is ensured by avoiding the infusion of glucose at rates approximating physiological maximums. Plasma glucose levels provide an indication of tolerance. Avoid hyperglycaemia. Provide energy as mixtures of glucose and fat. Glucose is the preferred carbohydrate source.

Fat

Dietary fat is composed of triglycerides of predominantly four long-chain fatty acids. There are two saturated fatty acids (palmitic (C16) and stearic (C18)) and two unsaturated fatty acids (oleic (C18 with one double bond) and linoleic (C18 with two double bonds)). In addition, smaller amounts of linolenic acid (C18 with three double bonds) and medium-chain fatty acids (C6–C10) are contained in the diet.

The unsaturated fatty acids, linoleic and linolenic acid, are considered essential because they cannot be synthesised *in vivo* from non-dietary sources. Both soybean and sunflower oil emulsions are rich sources of linoleic acid and provision of only 1 litre of emulsion per week avoids deficiency. Soybean emulsions contain approximately 7% alpha-linolenic acid (an omega-3 fatty acid). The provision of fat as a soybean oil-based emulsion on a regular basis will obviate the risk of essential fatty acid deficiency.

Safe and non-toxic fat emulsions based upon long-chain triglycerides (LCTs) have been commercially available for over 30 years. These emulsions provide a calorically dense product (9 kcal/g) and are now routinely used to supplement the provision of non-protein calories during parenteral nutrition. Energy during parenteral nutrition should be given as a mixture of fat together with glucose. There is no evidence to suggest that any particular ratio of glucose to fat is optimal, as long as under all conditions the basal requirements for glucose (100–200 g/day) and essential fatty acids (100–200 g/week) are met. This 'dual energy' supply minimises metabolic complications during parenteral nutrition, reduces fluid retention, enhances substrate utilisation (particularly in the septic patient) and is associated with reduced carbon dioxide production.

Concerns have been expressed about the possible immunosuppressive effects of LCT emulsions. These are more likely to occur if the recommended infusion rates (0.15 g/kg per hour) are exceeded. Nonetheless, these concerns have prompted the development of newer emulsions based upon medium-chain triglycerides, omega-3 fatty acids and, most recently, structured triglycerides, which combine long and medium-chain triglycerides in the same emulsion. The evidence of clinical benefit for these emulsions compared with conventional LCTs is tenuous, particularly if infusion rates are appropriate and hypertriglyceridaemia is avoided.

Protein

The basic requirement for nitrogen in patients without pre-existing malnutrition and without metabolic stress is 0.10–0.15 g/kg per day. In hypermetabolic patients the nitrogen requirements increase to 0.20–0.25 g/kg per day. Although there may be a minority of patients in whom the requirements are higher, such as after acute weight loss when the objective of therapy is longterm repletion of lean body mass, there is little evidence that the provision of nitrogen in excess of 14 g/day is beneficial.

Vitamins, minerals and trace elements

Whatever the method of feeding, these are all essential components of nutritional regimes. The water-soluble vitamins B and C act as coenzymes in collagen formation and wound healing. Postoperatively, the vitamin C requirement increases to 60–80 mg/day. Supplemental vitamin B12 is often indicated in patients who have undergone intestinal resection or gastric surgery and in those with a history of alcohol dependence. Absorption of the fat-soluble vitamins A, D, E and K is reduced in steatorrhoea and the absence of bile.

Sodium, potassium and phosphate are all subject to significant losses, particularly in patients with diarrhoeal illness.

---

in vivo is Latin for 'in a living thing'.

Their levels need daily monitoring and appropriate replacement.

Trace elements may also act as cofactors for metabolic processes. Normally, trace element requirements are met by the delivery of food to the gut and so patients on long-term parenteral nutrition are at particular risk of depletion. Magnesium, zinc and iron levels may all be decreased as part of the inflammatory response. Supplementation is necessary to optimise utilisation of amino acids and to avoid refeeding syndrome.

FLUID AND NUTRITIONAL CONSEQUENCES OF INTESTINAL RESECTION

Up to 50% of the small intestine can be surgically removed or bypassed without permanent deleterious effects. With extensive resection (<150 cm of remaining small intestine), metabolic and nutritional consequences arise, resulting in the disease entity known as short bowel syndrome. The clinical presentation of patients with short bowel syndrome is dependent upon the site and extent of intestinal resection.

Small bowel motility

Small bowel motility is three times slower in the ileum than in the jejunum. In addition, the ileocaecal valve may slow transit. The adult small bowel receives 5–6 litres of endogenous secretions and 2–3 litres of exogenous fluids per day. Most of this is reabsorbed in the small bowel. In the jejunum, the cellular junctions are leaky and jejunal contents are always isotonic. Fluid absorption in this region of bowel is inefficient compared with the ileum. It has been estimated that the efficiency of water absorption is 44% and 70% of the ingested load in the jejunum and ileum, respectively. The corresponding figures for sodium are 13% and 72%, respectively. It can be seen, therefore, that the ileum is critical in the conservation of fluid and electrolytes.

Ileum

The ileum is the only site of absorption of vitamin B12 and bile salts. Bile salts are essential for the absorption of fats and fat-soluble vitamins. The enterohepatic circulation of bile salts is critical to maintain the bile salt pool. Following resection of the ileum, the loss of bile salts increases and is not met by an increase in synthesis. Depletion of the bile salt pool results in fat malabsorption. In addition, loss of bile salts into the colon affects colonic mucosa, causing a reduction in salt and water absorption, which increases stool losses.

Colon

Transit times in the colon vary between 24 and 150 hours. The efficiency of water and salt absorption in the colon exceeds 90%. Another important colonic function is the fermentation of carbohydrates to produce short-chain fatty acids. These have two important functions: first, they enhance water and salt absorption from the colon and, second, they are trophic to the colonocyte.

Effects of resection

Resection of proximal jejunum results in no significant alterations in fluid and electrolyte levels as the ileum and colon can adapt to absorb the increased fluid and electrolyte load. Absorption of nutrients occurs throughout the small bowel, and resection of jejunum alone results in the ileum taking over this lost function. In this situation, there is no malabsorption.

Resection of ileum results in a significant enhancement of gastric motility and acceleration of intestinal transit. Following ileal resection, the colon receives a much larger volume of fluid and electrolytes and it also receives bile salts, which reduce its ability to absorb salt and water, resulting in diarrhoea. Even the loss of 100 cm of ileum may cause steatorrhoea, which can necessitate the administration of oral cholestyramine to bind bile salts. With larger resections (>100 cm) dietary fat restriction may be necessary. Regular parenteral vitamin B12 is required.

The most challenging patients are those with short bowel syndrome who have had in excess of 200 cm of small bowel resected together with colectomy. These patients will usually have a jejunostomy. They are conveniently divided into two groups termed 'net absorbers' and 'net secretors'. Absorbers characteristically have more than 100 cm of residual jejunum and they absorb more water and sodium from the diet than passes through the stomach. These patients can be managed without supplementary parenteral fluids.

Secretors usually have less than 100 cm of residual jejunum and lose more water and sodium from their stoma than they take by mouth. These patients require supplements. Their usual daily jejunostomy output may exceed 4 litres per 24 hours. The sodium content of jejunostomy losses or other high-output fistulae is about 90 mmol/L. Jejunal mucosa is leaky and rapid sodium fluxes occur across it. If water or any solution with a sodium concentration of less than 90 mmol/L is consumed, there is a net efflux of sodium from the plasma into the bowel lumen. It is therefore inappropriate to encourage patients with high-output jejunostomies (secretors) to drink large amounts of oral hypotonic solutions. Treatment begins with restricting the total amount of hypotonic fluids (water, tea, juices, etc.) consumed to less than 1 litre a day. Patients should be encouraged to take glucose and saline replacement solutions, which have a sodium concentration of at least 90 mmol/L. The World Health Organization (WHO) cholera solution has a sodium concentration of 90 mmol/L and is commonly used.

Complications of short bowel syndrome include peptic ulceration related to gastric hypersecretion, cholelithiasis because of interruption of the enterohepatic cycle of bile salts and hyperoxaluria as a result of the increased absorption of oxalate in the colon predisposing to renal stones. Some patients with short bowel syndrome develop a syndrome of slurred speech, ataxia and altered affect. The cause of this syndrome is fermentation of malabsorbed carbohydrates in the colon to d-lactate and absorption of this metabolite. Treatment necessitates the use of a low carbohydrate diet.

Anti-secretory drugs reduce the amount of fluid secreted from the stomach, liver and pancreas. These include H2-receptor antagonists, proton pump inhibitors and the somatostatin analogue octreotide. Octreotide also reduces gastrointestinal motility, while proton pump inhibitors lower gastric pH sufficiently to decrease the need for neutralisation of acid in the duodenum and proximal jejunum. This results in significant lowering of high jejunostomy outputs and dosage should be titrated against stoma effluent pH for optimal results. Anti-motility drugs include loperamide and codeine phosphate, which also decrease water and sodium output from the stoma by about 20%.

ARTIFICIAL NUTRITIONAL SUPPORT

The indications for nutritional support are simple. Any patient who has sustained 5 days of inadequate intake or who is anticipated to have no or inadequate intake for this period should be considered for nutritional support. The periods may be less in patients with pre-existing malnutrition. This concept is important because it emphasises that the provision of nutritional support is not specific to certain conditions or diseases. Although patients with Crohn's disease or pancreatitis, or those who have undergone gastrointestinal resections, may frequently require nutritional support, it is the fact that they have had inadequate intakes for defined periods that is the indication rather than the specific disease process.

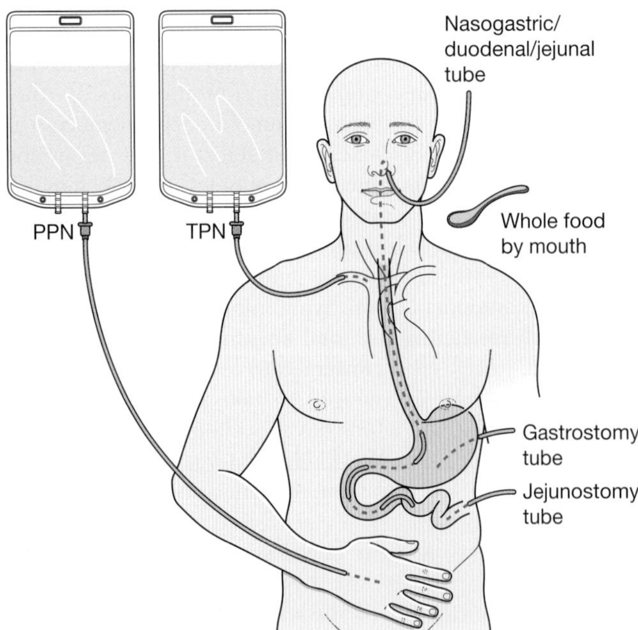

Figure 19.3 Techniques used for adjuvant nutritional support. PPN, partial parenteral nutrition; TPN, total parenteral nutrition. Redrawn with permission from Rick Tharp, rxkinetics.com.

Enteral nutrition

The term 'enteral feeding' means delivery of nutrients into the gastrointestinal tract. The alimentary tract should be used whenever possible. This can be achieved with normal food, oral supplements (sip feeding) or with a variety of tube-feeding techniques delivering food into the stomach, duodenum or jejunum.

A variety of nutrient formulations are available for enteral feeding. These vary with respect to energy content, osmolarity, fat and nitrogen content and nutrient complexity; most contain up to 1–2 kcal/mL and up to 0.6 g/mL of protein. Polymeric feeds contain intact protein and hence require digestion, whereas monomeric/elemental feeds contain nitrogen in the form of either free amino acids or, in some cases, peptides. These are less palatable and are used much less frequently than in previous years. Newer feeding formulations are available that include glutamine and fibre to optimise intestinal nutrition, or immunonutrients such as arginine and fish oils, but these are expensive and their use is controversial.

Sip feeding

Commercially available supplementary sip feeds are used in patients who can drink but whose appetites are impaired or in whom adequate intakes cannot be maintained with *ad libitum* intakes. These feeds typically provide 200 kcal and 2 g of nitrogen per 200 mL carton. There is good evidence to demonstrate that these sip-feeding techniques are associated with a significant overall increase in calorie and nitrogen intakes without detriment to spontaneous nutrition. The evidence that these techniques improve patient outcomes is less convincing.

Tube-feeding techniques

Enteral nutrition can be achieved using conventional nasogastric tubes (Ryle's), fine-bore feeding tubes inserted into the stomach, surgical or percutaneous endoscopic gastrostomy (PEG) or, finally, postpyloric feeding utilising nasojejunal tubes or various types of jejunostomy (Figure 19.3). The choice of method will be determined by local circumstances and preference in many patients. Whichever method is adopted, it is important that tube feeding is supervised by an experienced dietician who will calculate the patient's requirements and aim to achieve these within 2–3 days of the instigation of feeds. Conventionally, 20–30 mL are administered per hour initially, gradually increasing to goal rates within 48–72 hours. In most units, feeding is discontinued for 4–5 hours overnight to allow gastric pH to return to normal. There is some evidence that this might reduce the incidence of nosocomial pneumonia and aspiration. There is good evidence to confirm that feeding protocols optimise the tolerance of enteral nutrition. In these, aspirates are performed on a regular basis and if they exceed 200 mL in any 2-hour

ad libitum is Latin for 'freely or as much as you wish'.
John Alfred Ryle, 1889–1950, Regius Professor of Medicine, Cambridge University and later Professor of Social Medicine, Oxford University, Oxford, UK, introduced the Ryle's tube in 1921.

period, then feeding is temporarily discontinued or the rate of feed administration is diminished.

Tube blockage is common. All tubes should be flushed with water at least twice daily. If a buildup of solidified diet occurs, instillation into the tube of agents such as chymotrypsin may salvage a partially obstructed tube. Guidewires should not be used to clear blockages as these may perforate the tube and cause contiguous damage.

Nasogastric tubes are appropriate in a majority of patients. If feeding is maintained for more than a week or so, a fine-bore feeding tube is preferable and is likely to cause fewer gastric and oesophageal erosions. These are usually made from soft polyurethane or silicone elastomer and have an internal diameter of <3 mm.

Fine-bore tube insertion

The patient should be semi-recumbent. The introducer wire is lubricated and inserted into the fine-bore tube (Figure 19.4). The tube is passed through the nose and into the stomach via the nasopharynx and oesophagus. The wire is withdrawn and the tube is taped to the patient. There is a small risk of malposition into a bronchus or of causing pneumothorax. The position of the tube should be checked using plain abdominal radiography (Figure 19.5). Confirmation of position by pH testing is possible but limited by the difficulty of obtaining a fluid aspirate with narrow lumen tubes.

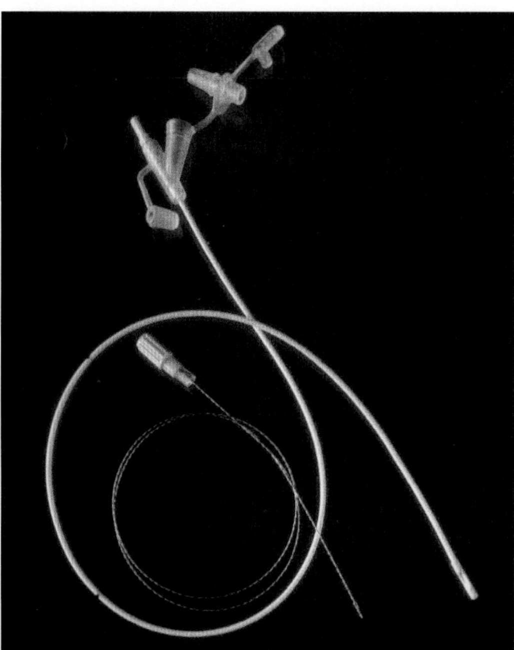

Figure 19.4 A fine-bore feeding tube with its guidewire.

Gastrostomy

The placement of a tube through the abdominal wall directly into the stomach is termed 'gastrostomy'. Historically, these were created surgically at the time of laparotomy. Today, the majority are performed by percutaneous insertion under endoscopic control using local anaesthesia, known as PEG (percutaneous endoscopic gastrostomy) tubes (Figure 19.6).

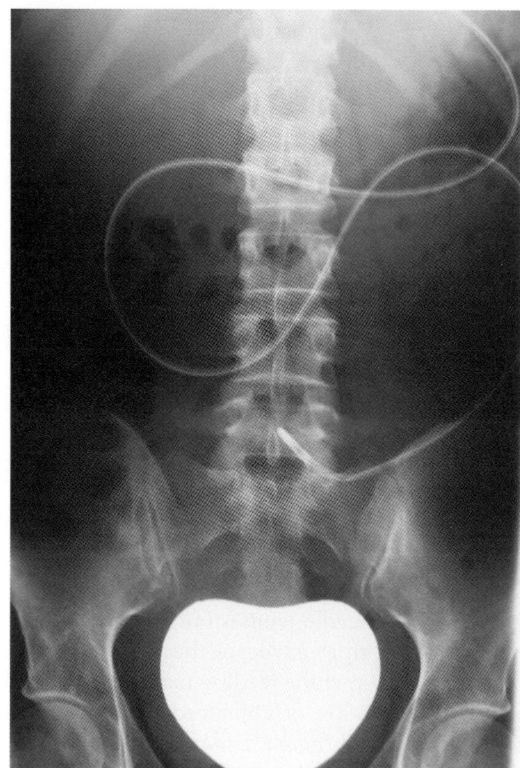

Figure 19.5 Radiograph of a tube similar to that in Figure 19.4 inserted beyond the duodenojejunal flexure.

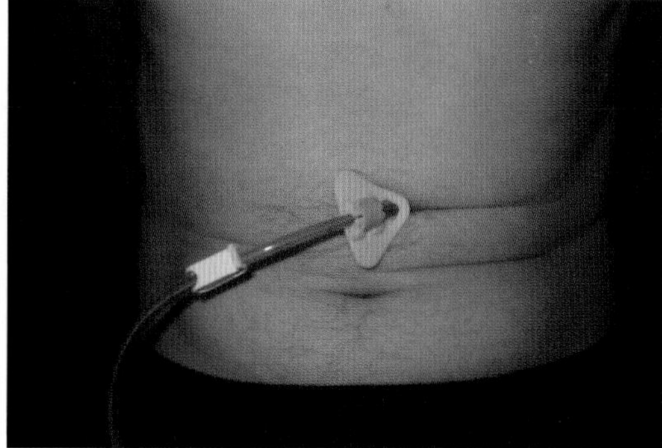

Figure 19.6 Percutaneous endoscopic gastrostomy tube.

Two methods of PEG are commonly used. The first is called the 'direct-stab' technique in which the endoscope is passed and the stomach filled with air. The endoscopist then watches a cannula entering the stomach having been inserted directly through the anterior abdominal wall. A guidewire is then passed through the cannula into the stomach. A gastrostomy tube (commercially available) may then be introduced into the stomach through a 'peel away' sheath. The alternative technique is the transoral or push-through technique, whereby a guidewire or suture is brought out of the stomach by the endoscope after transabdominal percutaneous insertion and is either attached to a gastrostomy tube or the tube is pushed over a guidewire. The abdominal end of the wire is then pulled, advancing the gastrostomy tube through the oesophagus and into the stomach. Continued pulling abuts it up against the abdominal wall.

If patients require enteral nutrition for prolonged periods (4–6 weeks), then PEG is preferable to an indwelling nasogastric tube; this minimises the traumatic complications related to indwelling tubes. PEG does have procedure-specific complications, although these are uncommon. Necrotising fasciitis and intra-abdominal wall abscesses have been recorded. Sepsis around the PEG site is more common and may necessitate systemic antibiotics or repositioning. A persistent gastric fistula can occur on removal of a PEG if it has been in place for prolonged periods and epithelialisation of the tract has occurred. This necessitates surgical closure.

Jejunostomy

In recent years, the use of jejunal feeding has become increasingly popular. This can be achieved using nasojejunal tubes or by placement of needle jejunostomy at the time of laparotomy. Some authorities advocate the use of jejunostomies on the basis that postpyloric feeding may be associated with a reduction in aspiration or enhanced tolerance of enteral nutrition. In particular, there are many advocates of jejunostomies in patients with severe pancreatitis, in whom a degree of gastric outlet obstruction may be present, related to the oedematous head of pancreas. In most patients it is appropriate to commence with conventional nasogastric feeding and progress to postpyloric feeding if the former is unsuccessful.

Nasojejunal tubes often necessitate the use of fluoroscopy or endoscopy to achieve placement, which may delay commencement of feeding. Surgical jejunostomies, even using commercially available needle-insertion techniques, do involve creating a defect in the jejunum, which can leak or be associated with tube displacement; both of these complications result in peritonitis.

Complications

Most complications of enteral nutrition can be avoided with careful attention to detail and appropriate infusion rates. Patients should be nursed semi-recumbent to reduce the possibility of aspiration. Complications can be divided into those resulting from intubation of the gastrointestinal tract and those related to nutrient delivery. The former are more frequent with more invasive means of gaining access to the intestinal tract (see above under Enteral nutrition). The latter include diarrhoea, bloating and vomiting. Diarrhoea occurs in more than 30% of patients receiving enteral nutrition and is particularly common in the critically ill. Up to 60% of patients in intensive care units may fail to receive their targeted intakes. There is no evidence that the incidence of diarrhoea and bloating is reduced by the use of half-strength feeds. It is important to introduce normal feeds at a reduced rate according to patient tolerance. Metabolic complications associated with excessive feeding are uncommon in enterally fed patients. There have been reports of nosocomial enteric infections associated with contamination of feeds, which should be kept in sealed containers at 4°C and discarded once opened. In all patients, it is essential to monitor intakes accurately as target intakes are often not achieved with enteral nutrition.

The complications of enteral nutrition are summarised in *Summary box 19.3*.

Summary box 19.3

Complications of enteral nutrition

- Tube-related
  - Malposition
  - Displacement
  - Blockage
  - Breakage/leakage
  - Local complications (e.g. erosion of skin/mucosa)
- Gastrointestinal
  - Diarrhoea
  - Bloating, nausea, vomiting
  - Abdominal cramps
  - Aspiration
  - Constipation
- Metabolic/biochemical
  - Electrolyte disorders
  - Vitamin, mineral, trace element deficiencies
  - Drug interactions
- Infective
  - Exogenous (handling contamination)
  - Endogenous (patient)

Parenteral nutrition

Total parenteral nutrition (TPN) is defined as the provision of all nutritional requirements by means of the intravenous route and without the use of the gastrointestinal tract.

Parenteral nutrition is indicated when energy and protein needs cannot be met by the enteral administration of these substrates. The most frequent clinical indications relate to those patients who have undergone massive resection of the small intestine, who have intestinal fistula or who have prolonged intestinal failure for other reasons.

Route of delivery: peripheral or central venous access

TPN can be administered either by a catheter inserted in the central vein or via a peripheral line. In the early days of parenteral nutrition, the only energy source available was hypertonic glucose, which, being hypertonic, had to be given into a central vein to avoid thrombophlebitis. In the second half of the last century, there were a number of important developments that have influenced the administration of parenteral nutrition. These include the identification of safe and non-toxic fat emulsions that are isotonic; pharmaceutical developments that permit carbohydrates, fats and amino acids to be mixed in single containers; and a recognition that the provision of energy during parenteral nutrition should be a mixture of glucose and fat and that energy requirements are rarely in excess of 2000 kcal/day (25–30 kcal/kg per day). These changes enabled the development of peripheral parenteral nutrition.

Peripheral

Peripheral feeding is appropriate for short-term feeding of up to 2 weeks. Access can be achieved either by means of a dedicated catheter inserted into a peripheral vein and manoeuvred into the central venous system (peripherally inserted central venous catheter (PICC) line) or by using a conventional short cannula in the wrist veins. The former method has the advantage of minimising inconvenience to the patient and clinician. PICC lines have a mean duration of survival of 7 days. The disadvantage is that when thrombophlebitis occurs, the vein is irrevocably destroyed. In the alternative approach, intravenous nutrients are administered through a short cannula in wrist veins, infusing the patient's nutritional requirements on a cyclical basis over 12 hours. The cannula is then removed and resited in the contralateral arm. Peripheral parenteral nutrition has the advantage that it avoids the complications associated with central venous administration, but suffers the disadvantage that it is limited by the development of thrombophlebitis (Figure 19.7). Peripheral feeding is not indicated if patients already have an indwelling central venous line or in those in whom long-term feeding is anticipated.

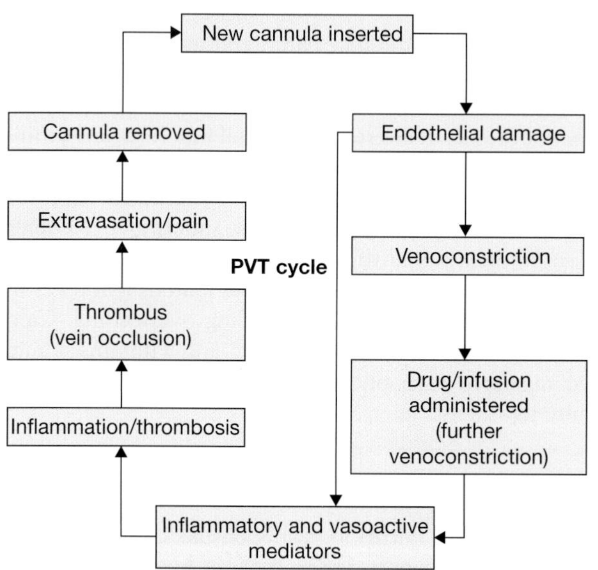

Figure 19.7 Cycle of causes of peripheral vein thrombophlebitis (PVT) (after Payne-James J, Grimble G, Silk D (eds). *Artificial nutrition support in clinical practice*, 2nd edn. London, Greenwich Medical Media, 2001).

Central

When the central venous route is chosen, the catheter can be inserted via the subclavian or internal or external jugular vein. There is good evidence to show that the safest means of establishing central venous access is by insertion of lines under ultrasound guidance; however, this will not be practicable for all cases. Most intensive care physicians and anaesthetists favour cannulation of internal or external jugular veins as these vessels are easily accessible. They suffer the disadvantage that the exit site is situated inconveniently on the side of the neck, where repeated movements result in disruption of the dressing with the attendant risk of sepsis. The infraclavicular subclavian approach is more suitable for feeding as the catheter then lies flat on the chest wall, which optimises nursing care (Figure 19.8).

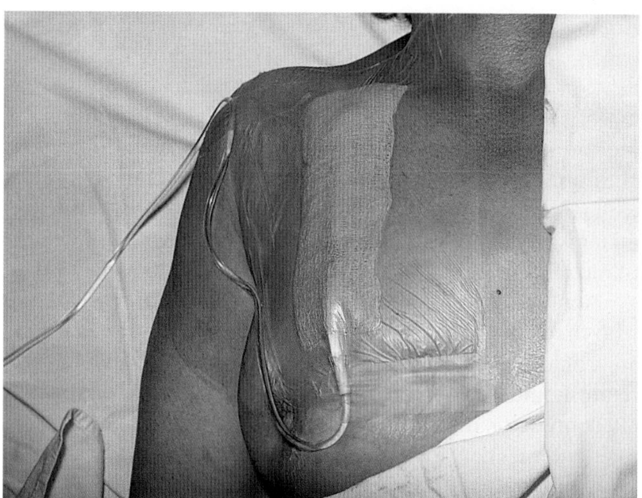

Figure 19.8 Infraclavicular subclavian line.

For longer-term parenteral nutrition, Hickman lines are preferable. These are often inserted by a radiologist with fluoroscopic guidance or ultrasound. They incorporate a small cuff, which sits at the exit site of a subcutaneous tunnel. This is thought to minimise the possibility of line dislodgement and reduce the possibility of line sepsis. Whichever technique is employed, a postinsertion chest x-ray is essential before feeding is commenced to confirm the absence of pneumothorax and that the catheter tip lies in the distal superior vena cava, to minimise the risk of central venous or cardiac thrombosis. Multilumen catheters can be used for the administration of TPN; one port should be employed for that sole purpose and strict protocols of aseptic care employed.

An alternative technique for central intravenous access allows the PICC technique under ultrasound guidance to cannulate the cephalic vein in the arm, which facilitates passage of a catheter into the bracheocephalic vein or superior vena cava. This has many advantages as it minimises the risks of insertion and ensures distance between the site of skin entry and the tip of the catheter. Thrombophlebitis, however, can occur.

Complications of parenteral nutrition

The commencement of TPN may precipitate or accentuate underlying nutrient deficiency by encouraging anabolism.

John Jason Payne-James, contemporary forensic physician and medical writer, Leigh-on-Sea, Essex, UK.
Robert O Hickman, b.1929, formerly paediatric nephrologist, Seattle Childrens' Hospital, Seattle, WA, USA.

Common metabolic complications include fluid overload, hyperglycaemia, abnormalities of liver function and vitamin deficiencies. Fluid overload can be avoided by daily weighing of the patient. A weight change of >1 kg/day normally indicates fluid retention. Hyperglycaemia is common because of insulin resistance in critically ill patients. Even modest rates of glucose administration may be associated with hyperglycaemia. Hyperglycaemic patients undergoing surgery are known to run a substantially higher risk of infectious complications.

Abnormalities of liver enzymes are common in patients who are receiving TPN. Although the precise mechanisms are unclear, intrahepatic cholestasis may occur and hepatic steatosis and hepatomegaly have been reported. Reducing the fat content or infusion of fat-free TPN may be required. If liver enzymes continue to deteriorate, TPN should be temporarily discontinued. In addition, overfeeding is a major factor in hepatic and other metabolic complications associated with TPN. Supplemental parenteral glutamine during parental nutrition should be considered, particularly in the critically ill patient.

Catheter-related sepsis occurs in 3–14% of patients. It may occur at the time of line insertion or afterwards by migration of skin bacteria along the external catheter surface. Some studies suggest that manoeuvring of the catheter hub due to frequent manipulation is a common cause. Contamination of the infusate is rare. Seeding on the catheter at the time of bacteraemia from a remote source may also cause catheter infection.

Diagnosis of catheter-related sepsis requires that the same organism is grown from the catheter tip as is recovered from blood and that the clinical features of infection resolve on removal of the catheter. Traditional methods of confirming line sepsis have necessitated removal of the line with subsequent bacteriological assessment. An alternative approach is to use an endoluminal brush passed down the catheter and withdrawn into a polythene sheath. The brush tip is cultured at the same time as performing blood cultures. Catheter sepsis is confirmed if identical organisms are cultured from brush and blood. A second alternative is to culture blood withdrawn through the catheter and compare this with peripheral blood cultures. If the colony count from the catheter sample is five or more times higher than that from peripheral blood, then line sepsis is probable.

Some of the complications of TPN may not be a direct result of the provision of nutrients by the intravenous route, but rather a consequence of the absence of luminal nutrients. This may cause a shift in the mucosa-associated intestinal microbiome, an increased mucosal proinflammatory state and the loss of epithelial barrier function leading to bacterial translocation of enteric organisms. The gut origin of sepsis, mediated by bacterial translocation, may be significant in critical illness and multiorgan failure.

The complications of parenteral nutrition are summarised in *Summary box 19.4*.

Summary box 19.4

Complications of parenteral nutrition

- Related to nutrient deficiency
  - Hypoglycaemia/hypocalcaemia/ hypophosphataemia/ hypomagnesaemia (refeeding syndrome)
  - Chronic deficiency syndromes (essential fatty acids, zinc, mineral and trace elements)
- Related to overfeeding
  - Excess glucose: hyperglycaemia, hyperosmolar dehydration, hepatic steatosis, hypercapnia, increased sympathetic activity, fluid retention, electrolyte abnormalities
  - Excess fat: hypercholesterolaemia and formation of lipoprotein X, hypertriglyceridaemia, hypersensitivity reactions
  - Excess amino acids: hyperchloraemic metabolic acidosis, hypercalcaemia, aminoacidaemia, uraemia
- Related to sepsis
  - Catheter-related sepsis
  - Possible increased predisposition to systemic sepsis
- Related to line
  - On insertion: pneumothorax, damage to adjacent artery, air embolism, thoracic duct damage, cardiac perforation or tamponade, pleural effusion, hydromediastinum
  - Long-term use: occlusion, venous thrombosis

Refeeding syndrome

This syndrome is characterised by severe fluid and electrolyte shifts in malnourished patients undergoing refeeding. It can occur with either enteral or parenteral nutrition, but is more common with the latter. It results in hypophosphataemia, hypocalcaemia and hypomagnesaemia. These electrolyte disorders can result in altered myocardial function, arrhythmias, deteriorating respiratory function, liver dysfunction, seizures, confusion, coma, tetany and death. Patients at risk include those with alcohol dependency, those suffering severe malnutrition, anorexics and those who have undergone prolonged periods of fasting. Treatment involves matching intakes with requirements and assiduously avoiding overfeeding. Calorie delivery should be increased slowly and vitamins administered regularly. Hypophosphataemia and hypomagnesaemia require treatment.

Nutrition support teams

Multidisciplinary nutrition teams ensure cost-effective and safe nutritional support, irrespective of how this is administered. The incidence of catheter-related sepsis is significantly reduced.

SUMMARY

Fluid therapy and nutritional support are fundamental to good surgical practice. Accurate fluid administration demands an understanding of maintenance requirements and an appreciation of the consequences of surgical disease on fluid losses. This requires knowledge of the consequences of surgical intervention and, in particular, intestinal resection. Malnutrition is common in hospital patients. All patients who have sustained or who are likely to sustain 5 days of inadequate oral intake should be considered for nutritional support. This may be dietetic advice alone, sip feeding or enteral or parenteral nutrition. These are not mutually exclusive. The success or otherwise of nutritional support should be determined by tolerance to nutrients provided and nutritional end points, such as weight. It is unrealistic to expect nutritional support to alter the natural history of disease. It is imperative that nutrition-related morbidity is kept to a minimum. This necessitates the appropriate selection of feeding method, careful assessment of fluid, energy and protein requirements, which are regularly monitored, and the avoidance of overfeeding.

ACKNOWLEDGEMENTS

With thanks to Marcel Gatt and Clare McNaught.

FURTHER READING

British Association Parenteral and Enteral Nutrition. BAPEN. Available from: (www.bapen.org.uk/res_pub.html).

Elia M, Ljungqvist O, Stratton R, Lanham SA (eds). *Nutrition Society textbook: clinical nutrition*, 2nd edn. Oxford: Wiley-Blackwell, 2012.

Nice guideline: Nutrition support for adults: oral nutrition support, enteral tube feeding and parenteral nutrition. Clinical guidelines (CG32). Feb 2006.

Chapter 20

Postoperative care

Learning objectives

To understand:

- What is required to deliver immediate postoperative care
- What are the common postoperative problems seen in the immediate postoperative period
- How to predict and prevent common postoperative complications
- How to recognise and treat common postoperative complications
- The principles of enhanced recovery
- A system for discharging patients

INTRODUCTION

The aim of postoperative care is to provide the patient with as quick, painless and safe a recovery from surgery as possible. This requires the appropriate knowledge and skills to manage medical, as well as surgical, postoperative problems.

Standards of postanaesthesia care in the immediate postoperative period

Both the American Society of Anaesthesiologists (ASA) and Association of Anaesthetists of Great Britain and Ireland (AAGBI) have set standards for the provision of immediate postoperative care of patients who have undergone a procedure requiring a general anaesthetic or central neuraxial blockade. In brief, they both specify that care should be undertaken in a dedicated postanaesthetic care unit (PACU) with staff trained in the management of patients in the immediate postoperative care period. Standards for equipment (including resuscitation, difficult airway and monitoring), drugs and schedules of measurement of patient vital signs are described, as well as the discharge criteria each patient must satisfy prior to transfer out.

Immediate postoperative care

In many settings around the world, the process starts with a 'sign out' as part of the World Health Organization check list. The theatre team should then formally hand over the care of the patient to the PACU staff. The information provided should include the patient's name, age, the surgical procedure, existing medical problems, allergies, the anaesthetic and analgesics given, fluid replacement, blood loss, urine output, any surgical and anaesthetic problems encountered or expected and a plan for the management of pain and nausea or vomiting.

Postoperative observations

The patient's vital signs (including pulse, blood pressure and pulse oximetry reading), level of consciousness, pain and hydration status are monitored in the recovery room and supportive treatment is given. In recent years, patient observations have been collated in recording systems designed to provide an early warning of clinical deterioration (Figure 20.1).

Surgery-specific observations such as Doppler flow for a free flap, regular neurological evaluation and laboratory tests, such as blood gas analysis, should also be performed when necessary.

The patient can be discharged from PACU when they fulfil the following criteria:

- Patient is fully conscious.
- Respiration and oxygenation are satisfactory.
- Patient is normothermic, not in pain and not nauseous.
- Cardiovascular parameters are stable.
- Oxygen, fluids and analgesics have been prescribed.
- There are no concerns related to the surgical procedure.

Christian Johann Doppler, 1803–1853, Professor of Experimental Physics, Vienna, Austria, enunciated the 'Doppler Principle' in 1842.

NEWS KEY 0 1 2 3	NAME:	D.O.B.	ADMISSION DATE:

Parameter	Value	Score	Value
	DATE		DATE
	TIME		TIME
RESP. RATE	≥25	3	≥25
	21-24	2	21-24
	12-20		12-20
	9-11	1	9-11
	≤8	3	≤8
SpO2	≥96		≥96
	94-95	1	94-95
	92-93	2	92-93
	≤91	3	≤91
Inspired O2%	%	2	%
TEMP	≥39°	2	≥39°
	38°	1	38°
	37°		37°
	36°	1	36°
	≤35°	3	≤35°
BLOOD PRESSURE (NEW SCORE uses Systolic BP)	230		230
	220	3	220
	210		210
	200		200
	190		190
	180		180
	170		170
	160		160
	150		150
	140		140
	130		130
	120		120
	110		110
	100	1	100
	90	2	90
	80	3	80
	70		70
	60		60
	50		50
HEART RATE	>140		140
	130	3	130
	120	2	120
	110		110
	100	1	100
	90		90
	80		80
	70		70
	60		60
	50		50
	40	1	40
	30	3	30
Level of Consciousness	Alert		Alert
	V / P / U	3	V / P / U
BLOOD SUGAR			Bl'd Sugar
TOTAL NEW SCORE			TOTAL SCORE
Additional Parameters	Pain Score		Pain Score
Urine Output			Urine Output
Monitoring Frequency			Monitor Freq
Escalation Plan Y/N n/a			Escal Plan
Initials			Initials

National Early Warning Score: July 2012

Figure 20.1 An example of an early warning system using patient observations; the National Early Warning System from the Royal College of Physicians.

Summary box 20.1

Postoperative period

- All anaesthetised patients should be recovered in a dedicated PACU
- All vital parameters should be monitored and documented according to local protocols
- Treat pain and nausea/vomiting
- Observe for complications

SYSTEM-SPECIFIC POSTOPERATIVE COMPLICATIONS

Postoperative complications are an important cause of morbidity, mortality, extended hospital stay and increased costs. Most patients at increased risk of developing postoperative complications can be identified prior to surgery at the preoperative assessment clinic using a variety of scoring systems (for example the American College of Surgeons National Surgical Quality Improvement Programme risk stratification for perioperative myocardial infarction and cardiac arrest (NSQiP) surgical risk calculator, see Chapter 17). Early identification of risk allows for targeted, appropriate, anticipatory and supportive medical care, which will reduce both the incidence and severity of such complications when they occur.

Classification of postoperative complications

There are three common approaches for the classification of postoperative complications of surgery:

1. Linked to time after surgery:
   - immediate (within 6 h of procedure);
   - early (6–72 h);
   - late (>72 h).
2. Generic and surgery specific.
3. Clavian-Dindo: this system relates to surgical complications only and is used to objectively and reproducibly measure the impact of the surgical complication on the outcome of the procedure. It is included here for completeness and will be discussed no further.

Respiratory system

Early detection of respiratory complications is facilitated by periodic assessment of airway patency, respiratory rate and routine oxygen saturation measurement, performed during emergence and recovery as described earlier.

Immediate respiratory complications

AIRWAY

Upper airway obstruction is one of the commonest immediate postoperative complications and can be due to laryngospasm, persisting relaxation of airway muscles, soft tissue oedema, haematoma, vocal cord dysfunction or foreign body. Vigilance and early intervention are necessary to prevent harm to the patient. Most interventions are simple and involve manual support of the jaw or insertion of an oral or nasal airway.

RESPIRATION

The residual effects of anaesthetic drugs (neuromuscular blockers, anaesthetic agents, opioids) can contribute to reduced or impaired adequacy of ventilation postoperatively. Continuous pulse oximetry and respiratory rate evaluation can identify respiratory compromise and consequent hypoxia early. Supplemental oxygen should be given to all patients in PACU until adequate respiration and oxygenation are restored.

HYPOXAEMIA

This may occur, in addition to the situations already described above, as a consequence of acute pulmonary oedema (fluid overload, cardiac failure, postobstructive), bronchospasm, pneumothorax (Figure 20.2), aspiration and, rarely, pulmonary embolism (Figure 20.3). *De novo* pneumonia is very

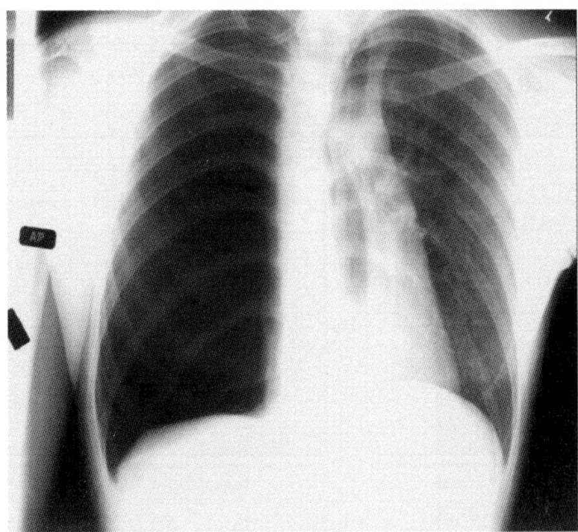

Figure 20.2 Radiograph showing a right tension pneumothorax with tracheal deviation to the left (courtesy of Professor Stephen Eustace, Dublin).

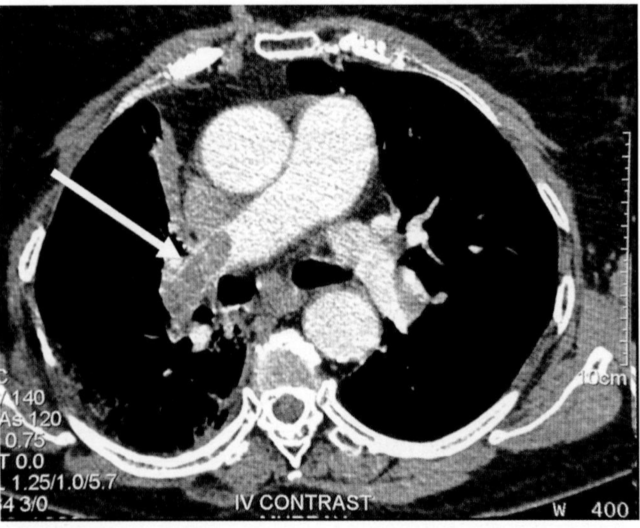

Figure 20.3 Computed tomography (CT) scan showing pulmonary artery blood embolism (arrow) (courtesy of Professor Stephen Eustace, Dublin).

unusual in the immediate postoperative period. Hypoxaemia develops most quickly in patients with obstructive sleep apnoea, lung disease and obesity, who should therefore be closely observed.

Patients with hypoxaemia should be treated urgently. If the patient is breathing spontaneously, oxygen should be administered at 15 L/min using a non-rebreathing mask. A head tilt, chin lift or jaw thrust should relieve obstruction related to reduced muscle tone. Suctioning of any blood or secretions and insertion of an oropharyngeal airway may be needed. Early anaesthetic intervention may be required.

SURGERY-SPECIFIC

Vocal cord palsy (as a consequence of recurrent laryngeal nerve injury), neck haematoma and post-tonsillectomy bleeding are recognised and life-threatening complications of head and neck surgery, which need immediate medical attention for safe resolution.

Early and late respiratory complications

Early and late postoperative pulmonary complications are a significant cause of postoperative morbidity and mortality (figures vary between 5% and 70%). Complications include fever (due to microatelectasis), cough, dyspnoea, bronchospasm, hypercapnoea, atelectasis (Figure 20.4), pneumonia (Figure 20.5), pleural effusion, pneumothorax and respiratory failure. The risk of each varies with the patient and the type of surgery being performed. Thoracic or abdominal surgery carries the highest risk. The majority of patients at risk (obese, smokers, chronic lung disease, obstructive sleep apnoea, poor nutritional status) can be identified preoperatively, facilitating the development of strategies that will reduce the impact of surgery on the individual patient.

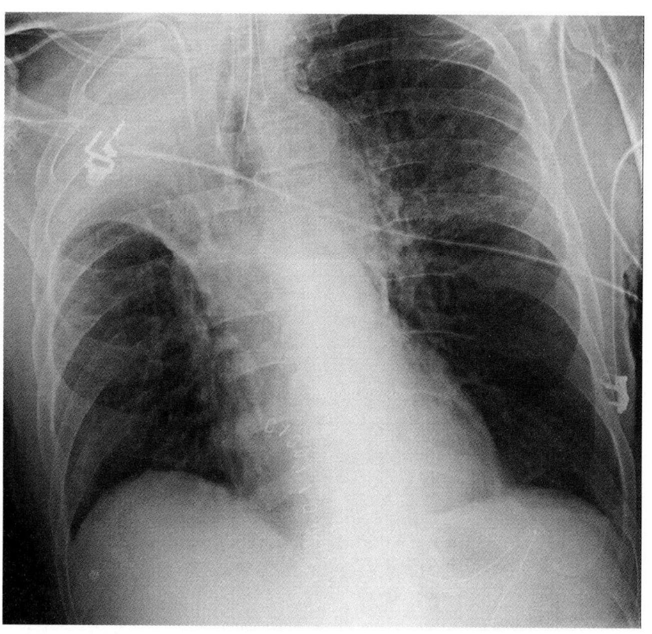

Figure 20.4 Radiograph showing right upper lobe atelectasis (courtesy of Professor Stephen Eustace, Dublin).

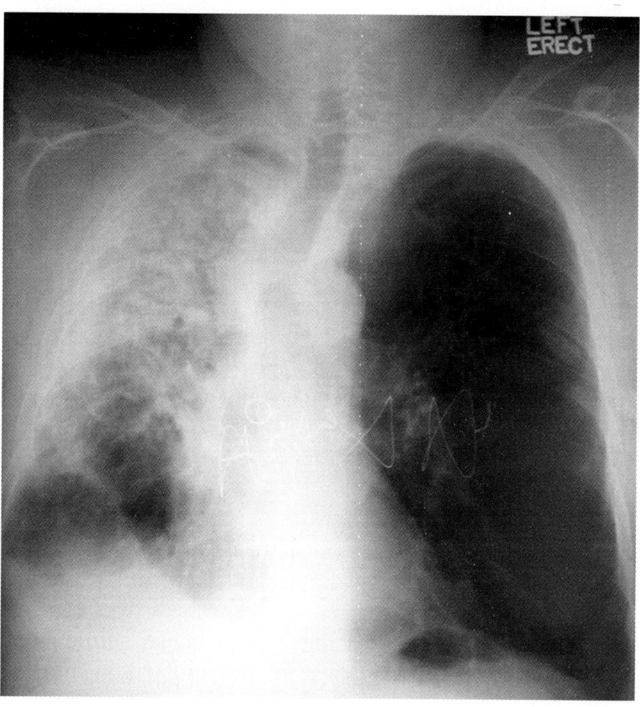

Figure 20-.5 Radiograph showing classical *Staphylococcus aureus* pneumonia (courtesy of Professor Stephen Eustace, Dublin).

Summary box 20.2

Respiratory complications

- Respiratory complications can occur either immediately or a few days later on the ward
- Obesity, smoking, chronic lung disease, poor nutritional status and obstructive sleep apnoea predispose to a higher risk of respiratory complications
- Early intervention and multidisciplinary involvement can prevent life-threatening respiratory complications

Cardiovascular system

Cardiovascular complications are the leading cause of death within 30 days after non-cardiac surgery. Recent trials, reported in the *New England Journal of Medicine*, have identified ways to improve safety and therefore outcome (see Further reading).

Routine pulse, blood pressure, and electrocardiographic (ECG) monitoring detect cardiovascular complications, reduce adverse outcomes and should be recorded during emergence from, and recovery after, anaesthesia. There are certain categories of patient and procedure for which routine cardiovascular monitoring may be required for upwards of 24 hours, usually in a PACU or high-dependency unit.

Immediate cardiovascular complications

HYPOTENSION

In the immediate postoperative period this is associated with adverse outcomes. Multivariable analysis from the POISE-2 trial showed that clinically important hypotension was an independent predictor of the subsequent risk of myocardial infarction (see Further reading).

Hypotension may be due to hypovolaemia, myocardial impairment or vasodilatation from subarachnoid and epidural anaesthesia. Other causes of hypotension such as surgical bleeding, sepsis, arrhythmias, tension pneumothorax, pulmonary embolism, pericardial tamponade and anaphylaxis should also be considered in the differential diagnosis.

Treatment should be aimed at the cause. Postoperative hypotension leading to end-organ dysfunction, (e.g. decreased urine output <0.5 mL/kg/h, decreased level of consciousness, myocardial ischaemia, capillary refill >2 seconds) needs immediate management with fluid and may require the use of vasopressors and inotropes.

HYPERTENSION

Hypertension is also common. It may be due to pain, agitation, anxiety, bladder spasm secondary to urinary catheterisation or pre-existing poorly-controlled hypertension. Consequences include bleeding from vascular suture lines, cerebrovascular haemorrhage and myocardial ischaemia or infarction.

MYOCARDIAL ISCHAEMIA

Patients with a history of cardiovascular disease or with known cardiac risk factors undergoing major surgery are at risk of major adverse cardiac events. This risk can be predicted preoperatively using the ACS National Surgical Quality Improvement Programme (NSQIP) risk stratification for perioperative myocardial infarction and cardiac arrest (MICA). Symptoms can include retrosternal pain radiating into the neck, jaw or arms, nausea, dyspnoea or syncope, but many events in the perioperative period are silent.

ECG changes can include ST-elevation in two continuous leads, new left bundle branch block or an arrhythmia. In the case of a non-ST segment MI, only a rise in serial troponin levels will clarify the diagnosis. Cardiologists should be involved early and may start coronary reperfusion therapy in the form of primary percutaneous coronary intervention or thrombolysis. These should be discussed with the surgical team due to the risk of bleeding after major surgery.

ARRHYTHMIAS

When they occur in the postoperative period, arrhythmias can cause hypotension, myocardial ischaemia and cardiac arrest. Treatment should be guided by the Resuscitation Council periarrest guidelines.

Tachycardia (sinus or supraventricular) may occur due to anxiety, pain, myocardial ischaemia or infarction, hypovolaemia, sepsis or hypoxia in the postoperative period. Consideration should be given to correction of the underlying causes and rate controlled with β-blockers, amiodarone or cardioversion, depending on the state of the patient.

Sinus bradycardia may be normal in athletes but it may also be associated with hypoxia, preoperative β-blockers, digoxin and increased intracranial pressure. Pharmacological options include glycopyrrolate or atropine intravenously.

STROKE

Stroke is a recognised complication of carotid endarterectomy surgery both early (secondary to emboli) and later (secondary to cerebral hyperperfusion syndrome). It is also a recognised consequence of both hypotension and hypertension. Thrombolysis may be indicated but the neurology and surgical teams must discuss together the risks and benefits of such a treatment plan.

Early and late cardiovascular complications

Major postoperative cardiac complications account for at least one-third of postoperative deaths, resulting in substantial rates of complications, prolonged length of stay and increased medical costs.

MI, congestive heart failure, arrhythmias and stroke need to be identified and treated early. Recent studies advocate shared postoperative care of patients at high risk, in order that the signs of deterioration may be identified early and treated (see Further reading).

Summary box 20.3

Cardiovascular complications

- Hypotension and hypertension in the postoperative period can be multifactorial and result in serious morbidity
- Arrhythmias can be prevented and corrected by treating hypotension and electrolyte imbalance
- Arrhythmias, myocardial ischaemia/infarction and stroke will need management with the help of cardiologists and neurologists

Renal and urinary system

Acute kidney injury

About one-quarter of cases of hospital-acquired renal failure occur in the perioperative period and are associated with high mortality, especially after cardiac and major vascular surgery. Patients with known chronic renal disease, diabetes, liver failure, peripheral vascular disease and cardiac failure are at high risk (*Table 20.1*).

According to national guidance (National Institute for Health and Care Excellence, NICE) based on several definitions, acute kidney injury can be detected by the following criteria (see Further reading):

- a rise in serum creatinine of 26 μmol/L or greater within 48 hours;

TABLE 20.1 Common causes of acute kidney injury.

Prerenal	Hypotension Hypovolaemia
Renal	Nephrotoxic drugs (gentamicin, diuretics, non-steroidal anti-inflammatory drugs) Surgery involving renal vessels Myoglobinuria Sepsis
Postrenal	Ureteric injury Blocked urethral catheter

- a ≥50% rise in serum creatinine known or presumed to have occurred within the past 7 days;
- a fall in urine output to less than 0.5 mL/kg/h for more than 6 hours in adults and more than 8 hours in children and young people;
- a ≥25% fall in estimated glomerular filtration rate in children and young people within the past 7 days.

Urinary retention

Inability to void after surgery is common with pelvic and perineal operations, or after procedures performed under spinal anaesthesia. Pain, hypovolaemia, problems with access to urinals and bed pans and a lack of privacy on wards may contribute to the problem of urine retention. The diagnosis of retention may be confirmed by clinical examination and by using ultrasound imaging. Catheterisation should be performed prophylactically when an operation is expected to last 3 hours or longer, or when large volumes of fluid are administered.

Urinary infection

Urinary infection is one of the most commonly acquired infections in the postoperative period. Patients may present with dysuria and/or pyrexia. Immunocompromised patients, diabetics and those patients with a history of urinary retention are known to be at higher risk. Treatment involves adequate hydration, proper bladder drainage and antibiotics depending on the sensitivity of the microorganisms.

Summary box 20.4

Renal and urinary complications

- Postoperative renal failure is associated with high mortality
- Prophylactic measures to prevent renal failure should be taken in high-risk cases
- Urinary retention and infection are common problems postoperatively

Central nervous system

Postoperative delirium

With an increasingly frail and elderly population presenting for elective surgery, the incidence of postoperative delirium (POD) is increasing. POD is frequently recognised late and has significant postoperative sequelae.

POD can occur during recovery from anaesthesia or a few days after surgery. The overall incidence of POD is 5–50%. It occurs more frequently in the elderly orthopaedic patient and those undergoing emergency surgical procedures. Delirium is associated with increased all-cause morbidity, mortality and discharge to a nursing home. There are two types of delirium – hyperactive (restlessness, incoherent speech, agitation, hallucinations) and hypoactive (withdrawn, poorly responsive to the environment, depressed). Preoperative risk factors for POD include pre-existing cognitive impairment, dementia, frailty, Parkinson's disease, severe illness, renal impairment and depression. Precipitating factors include surgery, intraoperative administration of narcotics and benzodiazepines, change of medications, electrolyte and fluid abnormalities, constipation, catheterisation and an unfamiliar environment (*Table 20.2*).

Correcting any reversible cause, involving relatives or friends whom the patient knows and pain control can all contribute to reducing the impact and duration of delirium. As a last option, haloperidol may be given in titrated doses according to local protocols.

TABLE 20.2 Causes of delirium.

Renal	Renal failure/uraemia Hyponatraemia and electrolyte disorders Urinary tract infection Urinary retention
Respiratory	Hypoxia, e.g. chest infection Atelectasis
Cardiovascular	Pulmonary embolism Dehydration Septic shock Myocardial infarction Chronic heart failure Arrhythmia
Drugs	Opiates including heroin Hypnotics Cocaine Alcohol withdrawal Hypoglycaemia
Neurological	Epilepsy Encephalopathy Head injury Cerebrovascular accident
Idiopathic (rare)	Hypothyroidism Hyperthyroidism Addison's disease

Stroke – has been discussed above.

Seizures – are uncommon except in those patients with known poorly-controlled epilepsy. They may occur as a complication of neurosurgery.

GENERAL POSTOPERATIVE COMPLICATIONS

Bleeding

Postoperative haemorrhage is most common in the immediate postoperative period. It may be caused by an arterial or venous leak, but also by a generalised ooze or a coagulopathy. Slow bleeds may go undetected for hours and then the patient suddenly decompensates. All patients must have their vital signs (pulse rate, blood pressure, oximetry, central venous pressure, if available, and urine output) monitored regularly. Dressings and drains should be inspected regularly in the first 24 hours after surgery. If haemorrhage is suspected, blood samples should be taken for a full blood count, coagulation profile and cross match. A large bore intravenous cannula should be sited

Thomas Addison, 1795–1860, physician, Guy's Hospital. London, UK, described the effects of disease of the suprarenal capsules in 1849.

and fluid resuscitation commenced. If the source of bleeding is in doubt and the patient is stable, an ultrasound or computed tomography (CT) scan may be required to determine the nature of the bleed (most commonly if a haematoma is suspected in the days following surgery). If the patient's cardiovascular system is unstable or compromised in any way (for example neck haematoma or bleeding tonsil) they should be taken back to the operating theatre immediately.

The treatment of haemorrhage is both to stop the bleeding and supportive. Supportive treatment includes oxygen and fluid resuscitation. It may require correction of coagulopathy. All patients will require close observation. Blood transfusion carries risks (acute haemolytic transfusion reaction, sensitisation, fluid overload, hyperkalaemia, transfusion-related lung injury and transmission of blood-borne infection). There is much published about what is the right transfusion trigger and how to balance the need for adequate tissue perfusion and the risks of transfusion. The decision about when to transfuse should be based on the individual patient; in general, however, the accepted transfusion trigger is 75 g/L except in the presence of known or suspected coronary artery disease when a higher trigger is acceptable.

All hospitals should have a 'major haemorrhage protocol' in place. The consultant surgeon, anaesthetist and haematologist should all be involved early on in the care of unstable patients.

Summary box 20.5

Postoperative bleeding

- All hospitals should have a major haemorrhage protocol in place
- Need to transfuse blood in absence of continued bleeding in patients with haemoglobin >75 g/L should be weighed against the risks

Deep vein thrombosis

Deep vein thrombosis (DVT) is a well-known and, when complicated by pulmonary embolus, potentially fatal complication of surgery (*Table 20.3*). All hospitals must have a process for screening all surgical patients to identify those at risk and for implementing prophylactic measures. There is international agreement on risk and therapeutic options. Methods of prevention are guided by the risk score and include the use of compression stockings, calf pumps and pharmacological agents, such as low molecular weight heparin.

The symptoms and signs of DVT include calf pain, swelling, warmth, redness and engorged veins. However, most will show no physical signs. On palpation the muscle may be tender and there may be a positive Homans' sign (calf pain on dorsiflexion of the foot), but this test is neither sensitive nor specific.

Duplex Doppler ultrasound and venography can be used to assess flow and the presence of a thrombosis. Other investigations include D-dimer. If a significant DVT is found (one that extends above the knee), treatment with parenteral anticoagulation initially, followed by longer-term warfarin or new oral anticoagulant (refer to national guidance, e.g. NICE; see Further reading). In some patients with a large DVT, a caval filter may be required to decrease the possibility of pulmonary embolism.

TABLE 20.3 Stratification surgical procedure and the associated risk of deep vein thrombosis.

Risk	Procedures
Low	• Maxillofacial surgery • Neurosurgery • Cardiothoracic surgery
Medium	• Inguinal hernia repair • Abdominal surgery • Gynaecological surgery • Urological surgery
High	• Pelvic elective and trauma surgery • Total knee and hip replacement

Pulmonary embolus

Pulmonary embolism (PE) is not usually an immediate complication, but can present in the early postoperative period. Thrombus can arise from DVT in the legs/pelvis, venae cavae or the right atrium. Signs and symptoms depend on the size of the embolus and may range from dyspnoea, cough, and pleuritic chest pain to sudden cardiovascular collapse. Diagnosis of PE begins with history (including risk factors and recent surgery) and physical examination (which may include signs of DVT). Investigations may include, depending on the presentation, ECG, chest radiograph, blood tests (arterial blood gas and d-dimer) and radiological tests (usually CT pulmonary angiography). If the presentation includes cardiovascular collapse, resuscitation will be needed. Thrombolysis can be considered with massive PE causing cardiovascular collapse, but this should include senior clinical opinion and would generally follow appropriate guidelines. The patient may need inotropes and admission to the intensive care unit. In less severe cases of PE, supportive measures include oxygen therapy and analgesia. After initial resuscitation, the patient will need anticoagulation, initially parenteral anticoagulation, followed by long-term oral anticoagulation (refer to national guidance, e.g. NICE; see Further reading). A vena cava filter may be needed if anticoagulation is not possible or if the patient has an embolism while anticoagulated (see Further reading).

Fever

About 40% of patients develop pyrexia after major surgery; however, in most cases no cause is found. The inflammatory response to surgical trauma may manifest itself as fever, and so pyrexia does not necessarily imply sepsis. However, in all patients with a pyrexia, a focus of infection should be sought.

John Homans, 1877–1954, Professor of Clinical Surgery, Harvard Medical School, Boston, MA, USA.

The causes of a raised temperature postoperatively include:

- atelectasis of the lung;
- superficial and deep wound infection;
- chest infection, urinary tract infection and thrombophlebitis;
- wound infection, anastomotic leakage, intracavitary collections and abscesses.

The possible causes of pyrexia of a non-infective origin include:

- DVT;
- transfusion reactions;
- wound haematomas;
- atelectasis;
- drug reactions.

Patients with a persistent pyrexia need a thorough review. Relevant investigations include full blood count, urine culture, sputum microscopy and blood cultures.

Summary box 20.6

Fever

- A very common problem postoperatively
- Consider infection in the lung, urine and wound

Wound dehiscence

Wound dehiscence is disruption of any or all of the layers in a wound. Dehiscence may occur in up to 3% of abdominal wounds and is very distressing to the patient.

Wound dehiscence most commonly occurs from the fifth to the eighth postoperative day when the strength of the wound is at its weakest. It may herald an underlying abscess and usually presents with a serosanguinous discharge. The patient may have felt a popping sensation during straining or coughing. Most patients will need to return to the operating theatre for resuturing. In some patients it may be appropriate to leave the wound open and treat with dressings or vacuum-assisted closure (VAC) pumps.

Summary box 20.7

Risk factors in wound dehiscence

General

- Malnourishment
- Diabetes
- Obesity
- Renal failure
- Jaundice
- Sepsis
- Cancer
- Treatment with steroids

Local

- Inadequate or poor closure of wound
- Poor local wound healing, e.g. because of infection, haematoma or seroma
- Increased intra-abdominal pressure, e.g. in postoperative patients suffering from chronic obstructive airway disease, during excessive coughing

Pressure sores

Patients undergoing surgery for a prolonged period of time are vulnerable to the development of a pressure sore or to worsening of a pre-existing sore. Careful positioning and padding of the patient is standard practice intraoperatively to reduce risk. Pressure sores occur as a result of friction or persisting pressure on soft tissues. They particularly affect the pressure points of a recumbent patient, including the sacrum, greater trochanter and heels. Risk factors are poor nutritional status, dehydration and lack of mobility and nerve block anaesthesia technique. Early mobilisation prevents pressure sores. High-risk patients may be nursed on an air mattress, which automatically relieves the pressure areas.

Summary box 20.8

Preventing pressure sores

- Recognise patients at risk
- Address nutritional status
- Keep patients mobile or regularly turned if bed-bound

SURGERY-SPECIFIC COMPLICATIONS

Abdominal surgery

The abdomen should be examined daily for excessive distension, tenderness or drainage from wounds or drain sites. In certain operations, such as those for intestinal obstruction, oesophageal and gastric procedures, a nasogastric tube may be required. It is of particular value in those patients suffering from ileus or a marked level of altered consciousness, who are therefore liable to aspirate.

Paralytic ileus

Paralytic ileus may present with nausea, vomiting, loss of appetite, bowel distension and absence of flatus or bowel movements. Following laparotomy, gastrointestinal motility temporarily decreases. Treatment is usually supportive, with maintenance of adequate hydration and electrolyte levels. However, intestinal complications may present as prolonged ileus and so should be actively sought and treated.

Return of function of the intestine occurs in the following order: small bowel, large bowel and then stomach. This pattern allows the passage of faeces despite continuing lack of stomach emptying and, therefore, vomiting may continue even when the lower bowel has already started functioning normally.

Localised infection

An abscess may present with persistent abdominal pain, focal tenderness and a spiking fever. The patient may have a prolonged ileus. If the abscess is deep-seated these symptoms may be absent. The patient will have a neutrophilic leucocytosis and may have positive blood cultures. An ultrasound or CT scan of the abdomen should identify any suspicious collection and will identify a subphrenic abscess, which can otherwise be difficult to find.

Summary box 20.9

The main complications after abdominal surgery

- Paralytic ileus
- Bleeding or abscess
- Anastomotic leakage

Orthopaedic surgery

Neurovascular supply to the extremity

Patients who have undergone extremity surgery, for example open reduction and internal fixation of a fracture, require regular neurovascular observations, both in recovery and on the ward (this will usually follow a local or national guideline). Moreover, if a tourniquet has been used, the restoration of the distal neurovascular supply should be established. Careful documentation of findings before and after surgery will allow comparison. Concern about the neurovascular status requires urgent and experienced surgical review and further management. Circumferential casts can be split and dressings cut down to skin.

Compartment syndrome

Raised pressure in an osseofascial compartment can prevent adequate tissue perfusion and present after surgery. Patients with compartment syndrome complain of pain out of proportion to that expected, pain that is increasing and pain on passive stretching of the muscles in the affected compartment. Other symptoms that relate to pressure on nerves (paralysis, paraesthesia) and blood vessels (pallor and pulselessness) occur late. When suspected, prompt senior input is required. In terms of initial management, circumferential casts can be split, dressings cut down to skin and the limb elevated. Further management will require experienced judgement and may include compartment pressure monitoring and/or fasciotomies. Compartment syndrome is considered more extensively in Chapter 28.

Summary box 20.10

Compartment syndrome symptoms and signs

- Pain out of proportion to that expected
- Pain that is increasing
- Pain on passive stretching of the muscles in the affected compartment
- Paralysis, paraesthesia, pallor and pulselessness generally occur late

Neck surgery

Patients having neck surgery, e.g. thyroid surgery, must be observed for accumulation of blood in the wound, which may cause rapid asphyxia. Another potential complication is damage to the recurrent laryngeal nerve, which can produce voice change.

Thoracic surgery

Careful fluid management is important in patients undergoing a lobectomy or pneumonectomy as they are susceptible to fluid overload in the first 24–48 hours postoperatively. Chest drains require regular review. If the fluid in a chest drain swings then the drain has been correctly inserted into the pleural cavity. If the chest drain continues to bubble then a bronchopleural fistula probably exists. A haemothorax or pleural effusion will reveal itself as a prolonged loss of blood or fluid, respectively, into the drain. Cardiac patients require continuous ECG monitoring postoperatively.

Neurosurgery

Postoperatively the patient should be kept under close observation. A rise in intracranial pressure may be signalled by a deterioration in the state of consciousness, as well as by neurological signs. Some patients may have an intracranial monitoring device to allow for more sensitive monitoring.

Vascular surgery

The patency of grafts and anastomoses, for example femoropopliteal bypasses and abdominal aneurysmal, needs to be checked by regular clinical assessment of the limbs and by Doppler ultrasound in the postoperative phase.

Plastic surgery

The viability of flaps is crucial and the perfusion needs to be monitored regularly. The blood supply may be compromised by position, dressings or collection of fluids or blood beneath the flap.

Urology

Catheter patency must be checked regularly following urological surgery. In patients who have undergone transurethral resection of the prostate (TURP), continuous bladder irrigation may be used. More generalised complications can occur, for example transurethral resection syndrome, and are discussed further in the appropriate section.

GENERAL POSTOPERATIVE PROBLEMS AND MANAGEMENT

When considering postoperative problems, the importance of pain control and fluid management should be appreciated, and the reader is directed to Chapters 18 and 19.

Nausea and vomiting

Postoperative nausea and vomiting (PONV) are unpleasant for patients, can delay recovery and prolong length of stay.

They can lead to more serious complications including aspiration pneumonia, precipitation of bleeding and dehiscence of wounds by dislodging the clots and bursting suture lines. In neurosurgical patients PONV may precipitate raised intracranial pressure with disastrous effects.

Risk factors for PONV include female gender, non-smoking, and a history of PONV, motion sickness or migraine. Use of volatile anaesthetic agents, opioids and nitrous oxide add to the risk. Duration and type of surgery also affect the incidence of PONV.

The risk of PONV can be estimated by using validated risk scores such as the Apfel (*Table 20.4*) or Koivuranta scores and appropriate preoperative strategies applied to high-risk individuals.

Treatment of PONV includes adequate treatment of pain, anxiety, hypotension and dehydration. Antiemetics can be administered both prophylactically and for treatment. A multimodal pharmacological approach, using drugs that work at different sites, such as HT3 receptor antagonists (e.g. ondansetron), steroids (e.g. dexamethasone), phenothiazines (e.g. prochlorperazine) and antihistamines (e.g. cyclizine), is the most effective.

TABLE 20.4 Apfel score to predict postoperative nausea and vomiting (PONV).

Characteristics	Points
Female sex	1
History of motion sickness or PONV	1
Non-smoker	1
Postoperative opioid treatment is planned	1
Total:	___

Score	Probability of PONV (%)
0	10
1	21
2	39
3	61
4	78

Hypothermia and shivering

Anaesthesia induces loss of thermoregulatory control. Exposure of skin and organs to a cold operating environment, antiseptic skin preparation (that cools by evaporation), and the infusion of cold intravenous fluids all lead to hypothermia. This in turn can lead to shivering, with imbalance of oxygen supply and demand (risking cardiac morbidity), a hypocoagulable state and immune function impairment, with the possibility of wound infection, dehiscence and anastomotic breakdown. It is now expected that temperature is monitored intraoperatively and the incidence of postoperative hypothermia has decreased significantly as a consequence. Active warming devices should be used to treat hypothermia as appropriate.

Drains

Drains are used to prevent accumulation of blood, serosanguinous or purulent fluid or to allow the early diagnosis of a leaking surgical anastomosis. In clean surgery, such as joint replacement, blood collected in drains can be transfused back into the patient provided that an adequate volume is collected rapidly and that a specifically-designed drain and filter system is used.

The use of surgical drains has decreased in recent years as the evidence for their benefits has been questioned. Complications of drains include trauma to surrounding tissues and infection. The quantity and character of drain fluid can be used to identify an abdominal complication such as fluid leakage (e.g. bile or pancreatic fluid) or bleeding.

Drains should be removed as soon as possible and certainly once the drainage has stopped or become less than 25 mL/day.

Wound care

Within hours of the wound being surgically closed, the dead space fills up with an inflammatory exudate. Within 48 hours of closure a layer of epidermal cells from the wound edge bridges the gap. Consequently, sterile dressings applied in theatre should not be removed before this time.

Wounds should be inspected only if there is a concern about their condition or the dressing needs changing. Inspection of the wound should be performed under sterile conditions. If the wound looks inflamed, a wound swab can be taken and sent for microbiological examination, but this can be unreliable. Infected wounds and haematomata may need treatment with antibiotics or even wound washout. If a surgical procedure is performed it gives an opportunity to collect samples for bacteriology (before any antibiotics, if the patient's general condition allows), to excise dead tissue and to control any bleeding. Depending on location, the wound may require packing if it is contaminated or if non-viable tissue remains. The dressing should then be changed regularly until the wound is clean.

Skin sutures or clips are usually removed between 6 and 10 days after surgery. The period can be shorter in wounds on the face or neck, and are left longer if the incision has been closed under tension. Wound healing is delayed in patients who are malnourished, or have vitamin A and C deficiency. Steroids also inhibit the adequate healing of wounds as they inhibit protein synthesis and fibroblast proliferation. Poorly-controlled diabetes delays wound healing and increases the risk of infection at the surgical site.

ENHANCED RECOVERY

Enhanced recovery is an approach to the perioperative care of patients undergoing surgery. It is designed to speed clinical recovery of the patient and reduce both the cost and the length of stay of the patient in the hospital. It is achieved by optimising the health of the patient before surgery through prehabilitation and then delivering evidence-based best care in the perioperative period.

Postoperative strategies advocated by enhanced recovery protocols include:

- Early planned physiotherapy and mobilisation.
- Early oral hydration and nourishment.
- Opioid-sparing analgesia regimens that include the use of regional blocks, regular non-steroidal anti-inflammatory drugs and paracetamol.
- Discharge planning is started before the patient is admitted to hospital and involves support from stoma care nurses, physiotherapists and other community care workers.

Early mobilisation is encouraged to reduce the risks of DVT, urinary retention, atelectasis, pressure sores and faecal impaction. Telephone follow-up is carried out to make sure that the patient is recovering well.

DISCHARGE OF PATIENTS

Patients discharged home need a 'discharge letter' detailing the postoperative plan. The discharge letter should include details of the final diagnosis, the treatment and any complications that may have occurred. There should be advice for referring the patient back to hospital and indications for readmission if specific problems do occur. The general practitioner (GP) should be informed of the subsequent care plan, including follow-up, physiotherapy and other support needed. Pathology results should be included if available, and the basis of these in the subsequent care plan should be described along with the prognosis if appropriate.

Summary box 20.11

Discharge letter

Diagnosis
Treatment
Laboratory results
Complications
Discharge plan
Support needed
Follow-up

Follow-up in clinic

Patients should only be reviewed in clinic when a key decision on management needs to be made. The findings and the care plan agreed with the patient at the clinic appointment should be included in a letter to the patient's GP, as well as in a clear entry in the notes or electronic patient record. This should include advice on how to recognise the onset of complications and what to do if there is concern. Patients should be discharged from clinic as soon as their GP or they themselves, can manage their care.

FURTHER READING

American Society of Anesthesiologists. Practice guidelines for postanesthetic care. *Anesthesiology* 2013; **118**(2): 291–307.

Devereaux PJ, Sessier DI. Cardiac complications in patients undergoing major non-cardiac surgery. *N Engl J Med* 2015; **373**: 2258–69.

Devereaux PJ, Sessler DI, Leslie K, *et al.*; POISE-2 Investigators. Clonidine in patients undergoing noncardiac surgery. *N Engl J Med* 2014; **370**(16): 1504–13.

Gan TJ, Meyer TA, Apfel CC *et al.* Society for ambulatory anesthesia guidelines for the management of postoperative nausea and vomiting. *Anesth Analg* 2007; **105**(6): 1615–28.

Gupta PK, Gupta H, Sundaram A *et al.* Development and validation of a risk calculator for prediction of cardiac risk after surgery. *Circulation* 2011; **124**: 381.

http://riskcalculator.facs.org/RiskCalculator/

http://www.aagbi.org/publications/guidelines/immediate-post-anaesthesia-recovery-2013

Intensive care society website: http://www.ics.ac.uk/intensive_care_professional/standards_and_guidelines/levels_of_critical_care_for_adult_patients

National Institute for Health and Care Excellence. Venous thromboembolic diseases: diagnosis, management and thrombophilia testing. Clinical guideline (CG144), June 2012, updated November 2015.

National Institute for Health and Care Excellence. Acute kidney injury: prevention, detection and management. Clinical guideline (CG169), August 2013.

Chapter 21

Day case surgery

Learning objectives

To understand:

- The concept of the day surgery pathway
- The importance of patient selection and preoperative assessment
- Basic principles of anaesthesia for day surgery
- The spectrum of surgical procedures suitable for day surgery
- Postoperative management and discharge arrangements

DAY SURGERY

The delivery of a surgical procedure on a day case basis offers advantages in providing significant benefits for both patient and healthcare providers. The removal of an overnight stay causes less disruption to the patient's domestic and social situation, and provides significant financial savings to the hospital. In resource-rich countries, day surgery is now an integral component of healthcare delivery, while in resource-poor countries, day surgery is increasing in popularity due to patient preference and healthcare reorganisation.

Day surgery is defined as the admission and discharge of a patient for a specific procedure within the 12-hour working day. Where a patient requires an overnight admission, then the term '23 hour stay' should be used.

Day surgery is a patient pathway, not a surgical procedure, and extends from first patient contact to final discharge (Figure 21.1). Success in day surgery requires each component of the pathway to be safe and efficient and to be performed in sequence. Unplanned overnight admissions are minimised by ensuring that:

- the patient is informed and fit for the procedure;
- the procedure itself is achievable as a day case;
- the procedure is scheduled early on the operating list to allow safe recovery and discharge; and
- the home environment can support a postoperative ambulatory patient.

Summary box 21.1

Definition of terms used in ambulatory surgery

- Outpatient surgery: not admitted to a ward facility
- Procedure room surgery: surgery not requiring full sterile theatre facilities
- Day or same-day surgery: admitted and discharged within the 12-hour day
- Overnight stay: 23-hour admission with early morning discharge
- Short-stay surgery: admission of up to 72 hours

MODELS OF CARE

Office-based care

This model, common in North America and Europe, where diagnostics and ambulatory interventions are performed in

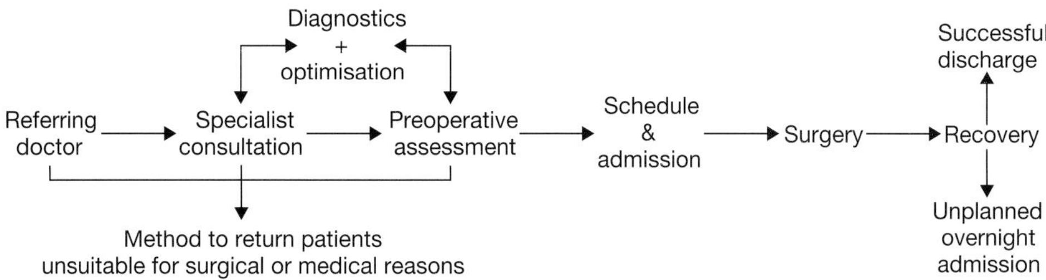

Figure 21.1 Elective day surgery pathway.

James H Nicoll, 1864–1921, paediatric surgeon, Glasgow, Scotland, specialised in pyloric stenosis and spina bifida and pioneered the 'Glasgow dispensary', where his work earned him the title of 'father of Day Surgery'. He was made Legion of Honour France.

consultation premises, allows patients ready access to 'high street' care. The downside is that the practice is usually limited to procedures under local anaesthesia, with or without conscious sedation. The use of general anaesthesia is limited, as this requires additional equipment and personnel, and raises safety issues in an isolated facility.

Stand-alone day surgery facilities

Where day case procedures are performed in isolated facilities, either on a remote site, or in the campus of the parent hospital, the workload is free from interference by emergency admissions. The spectrum of procedures performed is, by necessity, limited to those under local or regional anaesthesia or minor to intermediate procedures under general anaesthesia, to avoid unplanned overnight admissions and the requirement to transfer the patient to the parent hospital, which may be some distance away.

Self-contained integrated day surgery facilities

Though structurally part of a hospital, self-contained units have their own reception, ward, theatre and recovery areas and are functionally separate from the main hospital and potential disruption by emergency admissions. The back-up facilities of the main hospital are readily available if required, so these units can undertake a full spectrum of day surgery procedures. The growing demand for day surgery can lead to capacity issues and there may be duplication of costly capital equipment where procedures are performed on both a day case and inpatient basis.

Integrated day and short-stay surgery facilities

This type of unit allows complete flexibility in the delivery of day and short-stay surgery, with the ability to embark on more challenging day surgery procedures or consider day surgery on less fit patients. The availability of overnight beds has its downside: the preassessment team may convert fewer patients from overnight stay to day surgery by adopting the easy option of keeping the more challenging patient in overnight. Moreover, the availability of beds rather than day surgery recovery trolleys, puts these ambulatory beds at risk from emergency admissions.

While dedicated day surgery facilities are welcome, regardless of model, they are not mandatory for the successful delivery of the day surgery pathway. Success *does* require a dedicated day ward facility, where the staff can concentrate on the timely recovery and discharge of the day case patient. In mixed wards of day cases and inpatients, nursing and medical staff naturally prioritise the care of the less fit patient, and it may be easier to keep the day case patient overnight, rather than ensuring an optimum discharge process.

SELECTION CRITERIA

Medical criteria

Age

There is no upper age limit. The physiological health of the patient is a superior determinant of day surgery success.

Summary box 21.2

Selection criteria for day surgery

- Medical: use physiological rather than chronological age
  - ASA status over 2 requires careful review
  - Provided that the BMI is under 40, this alone is not a contraindication
- Social: a responsible adult carer must be available for the first 24 hours, for the elderly and patients at risk of covert bleeding
  - home conditions need to be suitable
  - ability to contact hospital in an emergency
- Surgical: operations up to 2 hours
  - recognised day surgery procedures
  - ability to eat and drink within a reasonable timescale

Comorbidity

Day surgery units traditionally use the American Society of Anaesthesiologists (ASA) Classification, which is a crude evaluation of chronic health (*Table 21.1*). Stand-alone units often confine their criteria to ASA 1 and 2 patients, while ASA 3 patients are more suitable for hospital-integrated units. Patients with significant respiratory or cardiovascular disease should be reviewed by an anaesthetist before being accepted for day surgery (see Chapter 17). Many patients who are fit but hypertensive are incorrectly excluded from day surgery. There is no evidence to support cancellation when blood pressure is below 180/110 mmHg.

Diabetes

The incidence of diabetes is increasing worldwide. Patients with well-controlled Type 1 and Type 2 diabetes are good candidates for the well-managed day surgery pathway. Control can be assessed by measuring their HBA1c, with a level of below 8.5% indicating good control. Diabetes is associated with potentially severe comorbidities, such as renal disease,

TABLE 21.1 The American Society of Anaesthesiologists (ASA) Physical Status Classification (American Society of Anaesthesiologists 1963).

ASA 1	A normal healthy patient
ASA 2	A patient with mild systemic disease
ASA 3	A patient with severe systemic disease
ASA 4	A patient with severe systemic disease that is a constant threat to life
ASA 5	A moribund patient who is not expected to survive without the operation

autonomic neuropathy and cardiovascular disease, and so these patients must be assessed carefully preoperatively and managed by an experienced team. It is important to have protocols for the care of diabetic patients that have been agreed with the local diabetic team and to involve them in the care of more complex patients. Success depends on ensuring these patients return to normal eating and drinking and managing their own diabetes as quickly as possible in the postoperative period.

Traditional care, with placing the patient first on the list and providing them with instructions on management of their medication preoperatively, works well. Those on morning lists can simply miss their morning dose of oral hypoglycaemic medication or insulin, though they must be instructed to bring their medications with them and to manage any hypoglycaemia as they would normally. Those on afternoon lists and those patients who are on more complex therapy, such as continuous subcutaneous infusions, can still be managed with input from the anaesthetic or diabetic team.

Epilepsy

A diagnosis of epilepsy does not contraindicate day surgery. Patients who have well-controlled epilepsy should be managed as normal patients, though it is important to ensure that their regular medication is not omitted in the preoperative period. Patients who are on medication but remain poorly controlled need careful review and discussion with their medical and anaesthetic teams. However, if they have suitable home support and the proposed surgery does not put them at risk, then they too are suitable for day surgery.

Obesity

The body mass index (BMI) is calculated as weight in kilograms divided by the square of height in metres (kg/m^2) and obesity is defined as a BMI >30 (Figure 21.2). Traditional guidelines are conservative about obesity due to fears of intra- and postoperative complications. Although there is an increased incidence of non-serious respiratory complications intraoperatively and in the immediate postoperative recovery

Weight in kilograms

Height in metres	40	45	50	55	60	65	70	75	80	85	90	95	100	105	110	115	120	125	130	135	140	Height in metres
1.92	11	12	14	15	16	18	19	20	22	23	24	26	27	28	30	31	33	34	35	37	38	1.92
1.90	11	12	14	15	17	18	19	21	22	24	25	26	28	29	30	32	33	35	36	37	39	1.90
1.88	11	13	14	16	17	18	20	21	23	24	25	27	28	30	31	33	34	35	37	38	40	1.88
1.86	12	13	14	16	17	19	20	22	23	25	26	27	29	30	32	33	35	36	38	39	40	1.86
1.84	12	13	15	16	18	19	21	22	24	25	27	28	30	31	32	34	35	37	38	40	41	1.84
1.82	12	14	15	17	18	20	21	23	24	26	27	29	30	32	33	35	36	38	39	41	42	1.82
1.80	12	14	15	17	19	20	22	23	25	26	28	29	31	32	34	35	37	39	40	42	43	1.80
1.78	13	14	16	17	19	21	22	24	25	27	28	30	32	33	35	36	38	39	41	43	44	1.78
1.76	13	15	16	18	19	21	23	24	26	27	29	31	32	34	36	37	39	40	42	44	45	1.76
1.74	13	15	17	18	20	21	23	25	26	28	30	31	33	35	36	38	40	41	43	45	46	1.74
1.72	14	15	17	19	20	22	24	25	27	29	30	32	34	35	37	39	41	42	44	46	47	1.72
1.70	14	16	17	19	21	22	24	26	28	29	31	33	35	36	38	40	42	43	45	47	48	1.70
1.68	14	16	18	19	21	23	25	27	28	30	32	34	35	37	39	41	43	44	46	48	50	1.68
1.66	15	16	18	20	22	24	25	27	29	31	33	34	36	38	40	42	44	45	47	49	51	1.66
1.64	15	17	19	20	22	24	26	28	30	32	33	35	37	39	41	43	45	46	48	50	52	1.64
1.62	15	17	19	21	23	25	27	29	30	32	34	36	38	40	42	44	46	48	50	51	53	1.62
1.60	16	18	20	21	23	25	27	29	31	33	35	37	39	41	43	45	47	49	51	53	55	1.60
1.58	16	18	20	22	24	26	28	30	32	34	36	38	40	42	44	46	48	50	52	54	56	1.58
1.56	16	18	21	23	25	27	29	31	33	35	37	39	41	43	45	47	49	51	53	55	58	1.56
1.54	17	19	21	23	25	27	30	32	34	36	38	40	42	44	46	48	51	53	55	57	59	1.54
1.52	17	19	22	24	26	28	30	32	35	37	39	41	43	45	48	50	52	54	56	58	61	1.52
1.50	18	20	22	24	27	29	31	33	36	38	40	42	44	47	49	51	53	56	58	60	62	1.50
1.48	18	21	23	25	27	30	32	34	37	39	41	43	46	48	50	53	55	57	59	62	64	1.48
	40	45	50	55	60	65	70	75	80	85	90	95	100	105	110	115	120	125	130	135	140	

Weight in kilograms

Key	
21	BMI 20–25
25	BMI 25–30
32	BMI 30–35
37	BMI 35–40
41	BMI >40

Figure 21.2 Body mass index calculator.

Adolphe Quetelet, 1796–1874, Belgian mathematician, astronomer and statistician, the pioneer in establishing the criteria of obesity that became known as the Quetelet Index. In 1972 Ancel Keys (1904–2004), an American scientist from the University of Minnesota and an expert on human nutrition, public health and epidemiology, named it the body mass index.

period, the course of these patients is otherwise uneventful. They should however, be managed by experienced medical and nursing staff. Hypertension, congestive cardiac failure and sleep apnoea are all more common in patients with morbid obesity, but in selected and optimised patients, a BMI up to 40 for surface procedures and 38 for laparoscopic procedures are acceptable and achievable in advanced units. Patients established on nasal positive airway pressure for obstructive sleep apnoea can be managed successfully.

Anticoagulants

Patients are generally on oral anticoagulants due to atrial fibrillation, previous thromboembolism or because they have a metal heart valve. It is therefore important to review these patients carefully before deciding to discontinue their anticoagulant for their operation. When it is felt that surgery will require its discontinuation, this should be discussed with their cardiologist and the risks involved explained to the patient.

Social criteria

Safe and comfortable discharge home requires the patient to be accompanied by a responsible and physically able adult. A journey time to home of 1 hour or less is advocated, but the comfort of the journey rather than the time involved is more relevant. Home circumstances require appropriate toilet facilities and the means of contacting the hospital should complications occur.

Surgical criteria

Patients undergoing procedures up to 2 hours in duration can safely undergo day surgery with modern anaesthetic techniques. The degree of surgical trauma is an important determinant of success, with entry to abdominal and thoracic cavities confined to minimal access techniques. Whatever the procedure, the main requirement is that there is suitable control of pain and the ability to drink and eat in a reasonable timescale. With day surgery now applicable to more major and prolonged procedures, patients should undergo a venous thromboembolism risk assessment and have prophylaxis provided if required.

PREOPERATIVE ASSESSMENT

The evaluation and optimisation of a patient's fitness for surgery is known as preoperative assessment (see Chapter 17) and is best performed by a specialist nursing team with support from an anaesthetist with an interest in day surgery. All elective surgical patients should be initially regarded as suitable for day surgery until proved otherwise. The assessment should be performed early in the pathway to allow time to optimise health problems before surgery The consultation consists of a basic health screen to include the measurement of BMI, blood pressure and an assessment of past medical history with current medication recorded. Appropriate investigations are performed to ensure the patient is fit for surgery. The patient and/or their carer should be given verbal and written information regarding admission, operation and discharge.

Summary box 21.3

Preoperative assessment

- On all day surgery patients
- Early in the patient pathway
- By a specialist nursing team with anaesthetic support

PERIOPERATIVE MANAGEMENT

Scheduling

With dedicated day surgery lists, major procedures should be scheduled early on morning lists to allow maximum recovery time. When the list is in the afternoon, the allocation of local or regional anaesthetic cases later in the day helps reduce unplanned overnight admissions. When mixed lists of day and inpatient cases are planned, then day cases are scheduled first. The mixing of day and complex inpatient cases is not advisable. The complex case may be inappropriately delayed if the day case is scheduled first and, conversely, if the day case patient is scheduled later, there is a risk of cancellation or unplanned overnight admission for the day case.

Anaesthesia and analgesia

Successful day surgery anaesthesia requires a multimodal approach to analgesia, while ensuring patients are given optimal dosages of anaesthetic agent (see Chapter 18). The agents used matter less than the skill of the person providing anaesthesia.

Multimodal analgesia starts in the preoperative period and unless contraindicated, patients should receive full oral doses of paracetamol and a non-steroidal anti-inflammatory drug, such as ibuprofen. Intraoperative anaesthesia can be maintained by any of the traditional inhalational agents. Total intravenous anaesthesia (TIVA) techniques using propofol are also popular and offer the advantage of reduced postoperative nausea and vomiting (PONV). The use of intraoperative analgesia will depend on the procedure being performed. When available, the anaesthetist should use short-acting opioids (fentanyl, alfentanil). Careful use of these agents can minimise the incidence of PONV. Where the choice is limited to morphine, this should be used in small doses (<0.1 mg/kg) to minimise sedation and PONV. Wherever possible, a long-acting local anaesthetic agent such as bupivacaine should be injected into wounds by the surgeon.

Pain levels should be routinely assessed in the postoperative recovery area. Further doses of paracetamol, fentanyl or low doses of morphine can be used to ensure that patients are comfortable prior to return to the ward.

Postoperative complications

The range of postoperative complications is no different from inpatient surgery. However, the fact that the patient is discharged home within a few hours of surgery requires proactive monitoring in the immediate postoperative period.

Summary box 21.4

Optimal analgesia and anaesthesia

- Multimodal analgesia with paracetamol and NSAIDs (if not contraindicated) should be given preoperatively
- Use long-acting local anaesthetic infiltration of the surgical wound
- Careful dosing of inhalational or intravenous agents should be used to maintain anaesthesia
- Avoid long-acting opiates such as morphine, to reduce the incidence of sedation and PONV

Reactionary haemorrhage is uncommon but requires careful consideration following tonsillectomy and laparoscopic procedures. Reactionary haemorrhage following tonsillectomy occurs within the first 6 hours and these patients should be monitored for this period. The danger in laparoscopic surgery is covert haemorrhage, especially in young fit patients who can lose over 15% of their blood volume before showing any cardiovascular signs of hypovolaemia (tachycardia and hypotension). These patients require a high index of suspicion as the first signs can often be as subtle as slow recovery and mobilisation or uncontrolled abdominal pain. When problems do occur, there should be clear escalation policies to ensure the patient is reviewed by the surgical team as soon as possible. Nausea and vomiting is not uncommon and should be managed actively to maximise successful discharge (Figure 21.3).

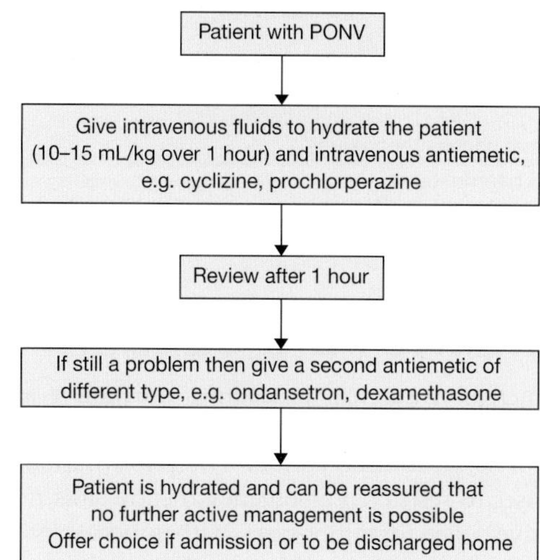

Figure 21.3 Active management of postoperative nausea and vomiting (PONV).

Summary box 21.5

Surgical haemorrhage

- Reactionary: occurs 4–6 hours after surgery and is caused by ligature slippage, clot displacement or cessation of vasospasm after mobilisation or coughing
- Secondary: occurs more than 24 hours after surgery and is due to infection eroding a vessel

ELECTIVE DAY SURGERY

For some surgical specialties, over 90% of their elective workload can be achieved in day surgery. As a result, teaching and training now routinely occurs on day surgery lists but requires structure and close supervision. As the spectrum of procedures has increased and become more challenging, many surgeons have increased their involvement in day surgery. This is important because safe and efficient day surgery demands the competence and skill of an experienced surgeon. Some surgeons have concerns regarding patient safety after discharge. The risk of postoperative haemorrhage occurring once the patient has returned home is often stated as a major reason to keep the patient in hospital overnight, especially where the abdominal or thoracic cavities have been entered. Reactionary haemorrhage commonly occurs in the first 4–6 hours after surgery, but the patient is unlikely to have been discharged home within this time period. It may be caused by slippage of a ligature or displacement of blood clot, precipitated by a rise in blood pressure, coughing or increased mobility. Postoperative monitoring of vital signs should alert the recovery team to any underlying bleed. Secondary haemorrhage is defined as occurring at least 24 hours after surgery but usually presents several days later, as it is due to postoperative infection. Thus, even if the patient had stayed overnight, these postoperative bleeds are still likely to occur once the patient has returned home.

Good surgical technique requires minimal tissue traction or tension and good haemostasis. In day surgery these attributes are even more important. The number and variety of surgical procedures performed on a day case basis is increasing year on year. Volume procedures in general surgery where the British Association of Day Surgery considers at least 40% of procedures can be performed on a day case basis, are shown in *Table 21.2*.

TABLE 21.2 Volume procedures where 40% or more should be performed on a day case basis.

Abdominal	Excisional/treatment of anal lesions, haemorrhoidectomy, primary and recurrent inguinal/femoral herniae, laparoscopic cholecystectomy, laparoscopic fundoplication, pilonidal sinus surgery
Breast	Excision/biopsy breast lesion, sentinel node excision
Genitourinary	Laser prostatectomy, orchidectomy, circumcision, excision of hydrocoele/varicocoele/epididymis
Orthopaedic	Dupuytren's fasciectomy, carpal tunnel release, therapeutic arthroscopy of knee or shoulder, bunion operations, removal of metalwork
Vascular	Varicose vein procedures, thoracoscopic sympathectomy

British Association of Day Surgery 2012.

Summary box 21.6

Successful day surgery requirements

- Minimal access techniques
- Good haemostasis
- Avoidance of unnecessary tissue handling or tension

EMERGENCY DAY SURGERY

Many emergency surgical procedures are minor and non-life threatening, and traditionally have been considered low priority for surgical intervention. The prioritisation of more urgent cases to restricted emergency theatre slots may result in extensive delays for minor cases, with unnecessary bed stays and preoperative starvation. Many of these cases, such as incision and drainage of abscesses, can be safely discharged home after their initial evaluation in the emergency department. They are provided with adequate analgesia and scheduled to return to the hospital at an appointed time the following day, suitably starved for their operation. This allows same-day discharge for minor emergency procedures.

If performed early in the day, the surgery rather than the pathway, may be defined as 'day case'. Some patients may, by chance, achieve a true day case pathway with admission, operation and discharge in the same day, provided they are admitted early in the day, there is no diagnostic delay and a theatre slot is available. Others may only achieve day case surgery, but not a day case pathway, if there has been diagnostic or clinical delay on admission (Figure 21.4). Common procedures suitable for the emergency day surgery pathways are shown in *Table 21.3*.

TABLE 21.3 Common procedures suitable for the emergency day surgery pathway.

Arthroscopy
Biopsy (temporal, lymph node)
Evacuation retained products of conception
Irreducible or strangulated hernia (inguinal, femoral, paraumbilical)
Incision and drainage of abscess (axillary, groin, neck, perianal, pilonidal)
K-wiring (finger or wrist)
Laparoscopic appendicectomy
Laparoscopic ovarian cystectomy
Reduction and internal fixation
Tendon repair

The success of an emergency day surgery pathway is dependent on the identification of unallocated theatre slots. These may be planned where there is reasonable predictability of emergency cases or may arise on elective lists, either day case or inpatient, due to patient cancellations. Emergency facilities may also be underutilised when there are delays in getting the more seriously ill patient to surgery. There is therefore an opportunity, providing staff are available, to utilise the empty theatre for a minor case before bringing the optimised sick patient to operation. This allows the ambulatory patient to be discharged on the day of surgery, provided discharge protocols are in place. This balance between clinical and managerial priority can be difficult to achieve without surgical experience, but forethought can permit a positive outcome for the quality of emergency patient care and the managerial requirement to shorten duration of stay.

When designing an emergency day surgery pathway, traditional day surgery selection criteria are ignored, with clinical judgement used to determine whether patients are appropriate for day surgery. The only absolute contraindications are systemic sepsis, unstable diabetes, major comorbidities and if parenteral, rather than oral, analgesia is required.

DISCHARGE

The assessment of when a patient is fit for discharge is best performed by trained day surgery nurses using strict discharge criteria (*Table 21.4*). While postoperative review by the surgical team is encouraged, the discharge should not be delayed by failure of their timely attendance. A suitable supply of analgesics for the management of pain should be provided. Paracetamol, NSAIDs and codeine form the basis of the drugs available in many countries.

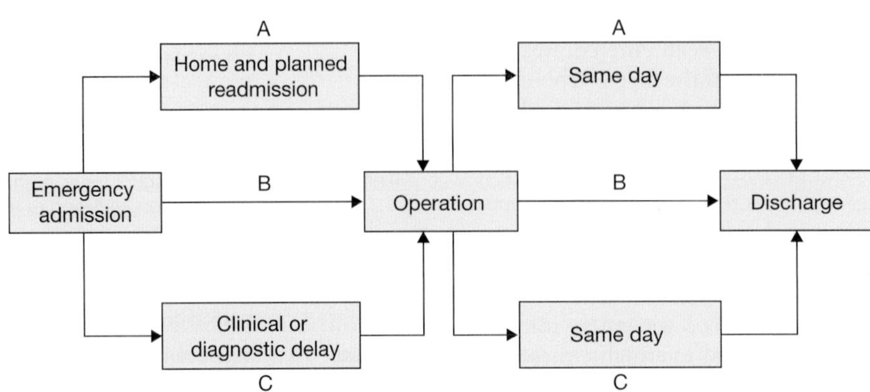

Figure 21.4 Emergency day surgery pathways. A, Planned preoperative discharge home with imminent return for day surgery. B, 'True' emergency day surgery with the entire pathway of admission, surgery and discharge on the same day. C, Preoperative delay, but surgery and discharge on a day case basis.

TABLE 21.4 Discharge criteria.
Vital signs stable for at least 1 hour
Correct orientation as to time, place and person
Adequate pain control with supply of oral analgesia
Understands how to use oral analgesia supplied
Ability to dress and walk where appropriate
Minimal nausea, vomiting or dizziness
Has taken oral fluids
Minimal bleeding or wound drainage
Has passed urine (if appropriate)
Has a responsible adult to take them home
Written and verbal instructions given about postoperative care
Knows when to come back for follow-up (if appropriate)
Emergency contact number supplied

FURTHER READING

McWhinnie D, Jackson I, Smith I, Skues M. *Patient safety in the ambulatory pathway*. British Association of Day Surgery Handbook Series. London: BADS, 2013.

McWhinnie D, Skues M, Thompson D, Richards S, Connolly V. *Ambulatory emergency care*. British Association of Day Surgery Handbook Series. London: BADS, 2016.

Smith I, McWhinnie D, Jackson I. *Day case surgery*. Oxford Handbook Series. Oxford: Oxford Medical Publications, 2012.

PART 4

Trauma

22	Introduction to trauma	310
23	Early assessment and management of severe trauma	322
24	Traumatic brain injury	328
25	Neck and spine	338
26	Maxillofacial trauma	355
27	Torso trauma	364
28	Extremity trauma	381
29	Disaster surgery	409
30	Conflict surgery	424

Chapter 22

Introduction to trauma

Learning objectives

- Become familiar with the timeline concept in trauma management
- Understand how to assess a trauma problem
- Learn how to respond to a trauma problem
- Understand how to select early total care and damage control surgical strategies

DEFINITION OF TRAUMA

Trauma originates from the Greek word meaning 'wound'. It implies that a physical force exerted on a person has led to a physical injury. External energy forms and forces that can lead to injury include chemical, thermal, ionising radiation and, most frequently, those of mechanical origin. The degree and severity of trauma sustained can vary substantially and depend upon the magnitude of force exerted.

Major trauma denotes injuries to more than one body region and organ system. In the next group of chapters, trauma will be examined from a variety of viewpoints, interconnected to different specialties. In this section we will examine the facets that bind the whole topic together.

THE MAGNITUDE OF THE PROBLEM

Trauma remains the most common cause of death and disability in children and young adults in the resource-rich countries. Globally, approximately 10 000 people die daily as a result of an injury. Road traffic accidents (RTA), falls and intentional violence have been identified as the major vectors of traumatic injury. It is notable that the major burden of injury is increasingly occurring in middle- and low-income countries as they industrialise and adopt motorised transportation.

In terms of the annual incidence and trends over time there is variation from country to country. Information is usually obtained from national statistics organisations that use the International Classification of Disease, a system that can be limited in providing accurate descriptions of injury severity. However, the Abbreviated Injury Scale (AIS) dictionary consists of a greater level of detail (including more than 2000 injury codes) and assigns to every injury a severity score between 1 (mild) and 6 (maximum). This can be summated into the so called Injury Severity Score (ISS), providing an image of the anatomical severity of injury suffered by the individual patient. Major trauma is defined as an ISS greater than 15, which can be written as >15. The majority of hospital admissions with injury have low ISS values, ranging between the values 4 and 8, and are secondary to single isolated limb fractures and isolated mild head injury. Overall, major trauma affects approximately 15% of all injured patients.

The total number of casualties from RTA alone reported to the police in Great Britain during 2015 was 186 189, which was around 4% lower when compared with 2014. Of these, 21 657 people were seriously injured, among whom 1730 lost their lives, representing a 3% decrease compared with 2014. Across Europe, according to the data presented by the European Transport Safety Council's Performance Index (PIN) report, it appears that fatalities rose in the majority of countries. Of the 32 countries covered, 21 had an increase in the number of fatalities in 2015, ten had a decrease, and one remained unchanged. Since countries do not use the same definition of serious injury, international comparisons are based on road deaths per million inhabitants (Figure 22.1). The United Kingdom as a whole had 27.7 deaths per million inhabitants in 2015. The only European countries with a better rate than this in 2015 were Sweden with 26.6, Malta with 25.6 and Norway with 22.6. The UK and Sweden have been consistently at the head of this table for a number of years.

A large proportion of the severely injured survivors experience long-term or permanent disability as a result of their injuries. Almost 30% of them are no longer able to return to their previous occupation and a great deal of time is lost from work. These individuals end up having profound changes in their lifestyle, with long-term pain and suffering. It should be emphasised that an injury not only affects the injured person but also affects everyone who is involved in the injured person's life. The impact of the modern epidemic of road traffic

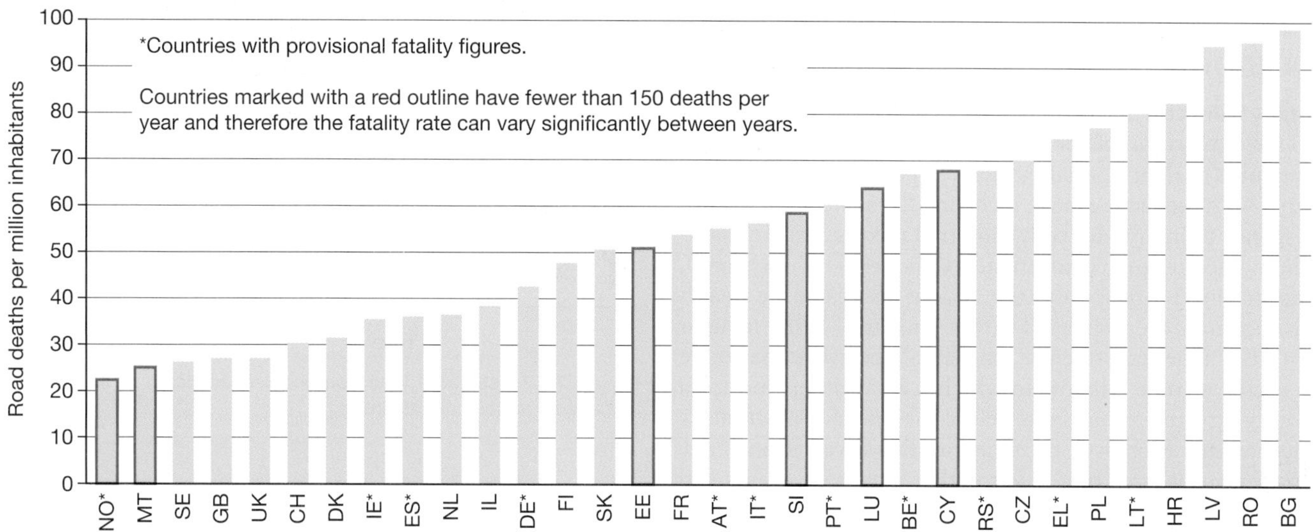

Figure 22.1 Number of road deaths per million inhabitants.

accidents on the universal epidemic of violent injury cannot be overstated. The annual direct medical cost of injuries treated in hospitals and additional care facilities is estimated to be £3.7 billion. Moreover, additional costs, due to loss of earnings, loss of productivity and quality of life damage, increase the total sum significantly.

While young patients are involved in road traffic accidents characterised by high energy transfer, older patients may sustain injuries from falls (low energy transfer). The most common group to be admitted to hospital in the UK are older patients who have sustained a 'fragility' fracture. Approximately 65 000 to 70 000 patients are admitted annually with proximal femoral fractures, among whom 30% over the age of 65 will die within a year of the incident. Most of the rest will end up having diminished independence and functional capacity. It is therefore no surprise that this particular cohort of patients, which will increase in the coming years owing to the anticipated increase in life expectancy, is thought to represent a huge burden on healthcare services and society in general.

In general terms, the vast majority of injuries sustained are not limb threatening or life threatening. They are straightforward and most patients are expected to recover fully and return to their preinjury status. Nonetheless, the challenge remains to appreciate and diagnose the injuries at an early stage, with an awareness of important features that may influence the outcome.

For instance, we must be vigilant not to miss non-accidental injury (NAI) in children (see Chapter 39) and injuries in other age groups related to an underlying disease process rather than the injury itself, for example pathological fractures. Of note, it has been shown that in 66% of cases when children die as a result of abuse, there has been some previous interaction with a health professional or social services but the seriousness of the situation was not fully appreciated.

Summary box 22.1

Trauma: the magnitude of the problem

- The vast majority of injuries are not life or limb threatening
- Severe trauma continues to be a major cause of death in young patients
- Older patients with fragility fractures pose an additional burden to the healthcare system
- Look for important features of injuries that could influence the outcome

THE MANAGEMENT OF TRAUMA

From the moment that injury is sustained, every aspect of decision making and management is essential in terms of the survival of the victim. Our initial assessment and concepts of management have specific objectives and are usually based on knowledge acquired over a long period of time in practice. A better understanding of the physiological processes underpinning the host responses to an acute threat to our homeostatic mechanisms, together with protocols formulated to allow clinicians to use standardised measures and to speak a common language, have revolutionised the way we manage patients. All of the above help to reduce delays, particularly when under pressure to make a decision. However, it remains crucial to understand the reasoning as to why we are carrying them out.

In trauma, as in other acute conditions, the patient is particularly reliant upon the clinician. A patient with a chronic condition is familiar with the nature of their problem and the way in which it is progressing. The surgeon may offer a remedy and the patient may consider the potential benefits and choose appropriately whether to accept it. The injured patient does not know what will happen without treatment and so relies on their surgeon to inform them of both the natural history and the potential benefits of any intervention. The implication is that as surgeons we have a duty to be aware of both.

The significance of time in the outcome

Injury can occur in the blink of an eye. In the seconds prior to the application of the external injury force or vector, the patient is at their normal baseline, which can be called time zero. All subsequent events, including the acute physiological response to injury, the body's internal mechanisms to maintain homeostasis (to compensate for the sequelae of trauma), the healing processes and the actions instigated by health professionals, are associated with a 'timeline'. Being familiar with the 'timeline principle', one should be aware that there is a critical time window in which we can intervene for a positive treatment outcome, before the loss of compensatory mechanisms. Moreover, the timeline allows evaluation of any progress made from time zero to other important events and to reflect on whether a specific course of action could have been performed better.

Overall, interventions can be distinguished as emergency (life saving), acute (restoring haemodynamic stability) and delayed or semielective, focusing on the treatment of post-fracture fixation complications (non-union, infection and malunion from the orthopaedic trauma point of view).

It is essential to appreciate that the physiological crisis initiated in the immediate aftermath of trauma will continue to evolve and the risk of mortality is substantial unless the correct and timely interventions are performed. For instance, conditions such as airway obstruction, tension haemothorax and haemopericardium can progress very rapidly if left untreated and should be given priority in terms of our initial medical response to the injured patient. Thus, the seriousness and the immediate impact of a specific clinical condition should be prioritised and treated in a systematic approach (what kills first should be managed first). This concept of the hierarchy of medical responses can only be applied and become effective when we are in a position to diagnose early the underlying clinical conditions (Figure 22.2).

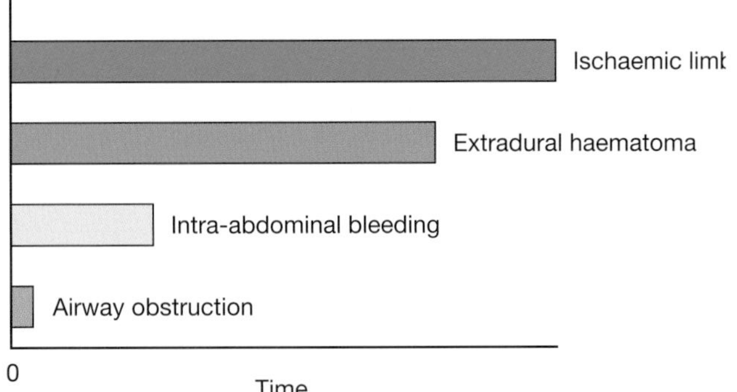

Figure 22.2 Estimated time from incident to death or irretrievable damage for various conditions.

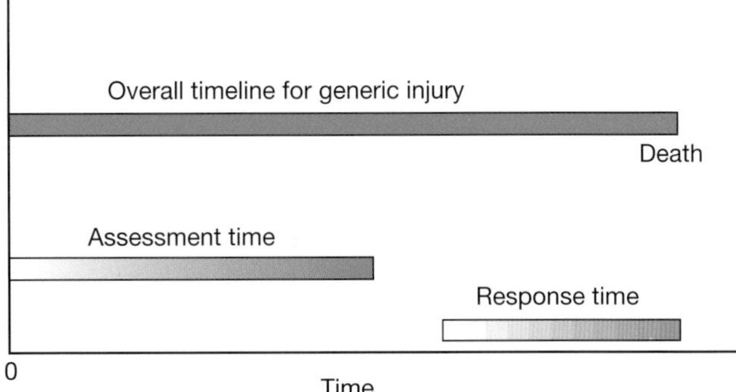

Figure 22.3 Diagrammatic representation of the relationship between assessment and response times. In this example, there is time to assess and respond effectively before death.

The ATLS (Advanced Trauma Life Support) system delineates an order of priorities set by ABCD; that is, **a**irway, **b**reathing, **c**irculation and **d**isability (neurology). This hierarchy of priorities is instituted upon the 'time dependence' principle. The clinician should bear in mind that a successful management plan is dependent on, first, the time needed to evaluate and diagnose the nature of the problem and, second, the time taken to respond effectively to the condition discovered (Figure 22.3).

Evaluating and diagnosing a condition can be challenging, as the initial clinical signs may be non-specific. The clinical condition will continue to evolve as the time progresses, but by the time the diagnosis has been made it may be too late to prevent mortality. Taking into consideration the mechanism of the accident and promptly requesting special investigations, for example computed tomography (CT), the underlying diagnosis can be made punctually, thus allowing intervention in a timely fashion.

A patient presenting following a road traffic accident with a scalp laceration and a reduced Glasgow Coma Scale (GCS) score of 13/15 represents an example of such a scenario, where a drop in the GCS could be related to a head injury or to the presence of shock and hypoxia. An injury to the brain can deteriorate with the development of an expanding haematoma, which can be diagnosed with a head CT prior to the presentation of clinical signs. Surgical decompression can be organised speedily, reducing the risk of morbidity and mortality. In this situation, if the time taken to make the diagnosis was prolonged and the clinical signs had presented prior to treatment intervention, it may be too late to prevent the death of the patient (Figure 22.4). This clinical case scenario demonstrates the principle that we need to introduce a treatment response even before we have made the definitive diagnosis if we want to save the patient's life. It is clear, therefore, that the 'timeline concept' is critical in the safe management of trauma patients.

Reducing the diagnosis time and response time of our interventions is dependent not only on the clinical staff but also on the availability of resources. Recently, the 24/7 availability of the trauma team and the designation of regional hospitals to operate as Level I Trauma Centres, with the availability of all disciplines and appropriate equipment on site, has provided the necessary foundation for the development of a unified trauma care system in England. Indeed, the first reports published on its effectiveness in saving lives have been very positive.

The 'timeline concept' that has been discussed in the management of patients with multiple trauma can be applied

Summary box 22.2

The importance of time

- The 'timeline concept' is an essential component of trauma management
- Assessment should be completed within a set time
- The time to respond is limited
- Both assessment and response should take place in the time window prior to irreversible damage or death

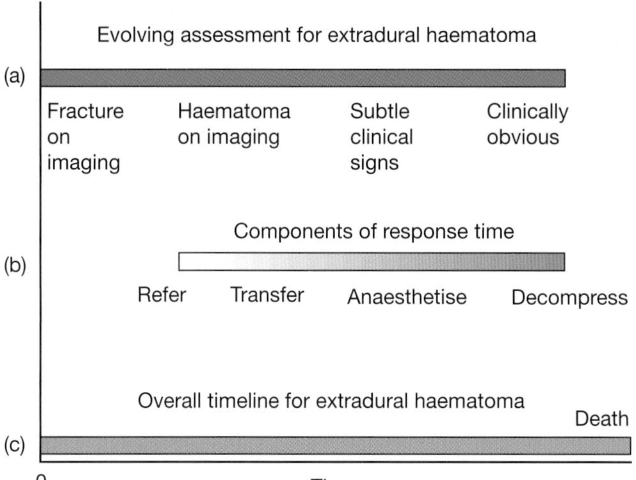

Figure 22.4 Diagrammatic representation of the relationship between assessment and response times for extradural haematoma: **(a)** the stages of assessment, **(b)** the components of the response and **(c)** the overall time from incident to death. It can be seen that relying on obvious clinical signs gives insufficient time to respond effectively.

to patients with isolated injuries. The key issue, irrespective of the type of patient managed, with or without multiple injuries, is to reduce unnecessary delays in making the diagnosis and initiating appropriate treatment. Such a global approach would save lives, minimise morbidity and would make the healthcare system more efficient in terms of resource utilisation, as well as cost-effectiveness.

Finally, it should not be forgotten that all clinical conditions are characterised by a dynamic process. This implies that our observations and analysis of the situation can change rapidly and to an extent that interventions would have to be modified accordingly. Ongoing evaluation of the patient is therefore essential in order to identify and respond to the changes noted in a timely fashion (as previously discussed). The initial primary survey, applied according to the ATLS protocol in trauma patients, should be followed by secondary and tertiary clinical assessment, even after the acute phase of treatment has been completed successfully. Ongoing monitoring of vital organ activity, ordering of the necessary biochemical and radiological investigations and recording of all the findings in a single place can allow easier evaluation and identification of trends over time to facilitate prompt intervention. Such a strategy may reduce the risk of having undiagnosed injuries and delays in their treatment. A number of studies have been published reporting on missed injuries and making some recommendations on how to avoid this.

The timeline following an injury is continuous, and the accumulated documentation may become voluminous, complex and confusing. It is helpful periodically to make the effort to stand back and summarise the situation. The UK National Institute for Health and Care Excellence (NICE), in their recent Trauma Guidelines, recognise this and advise that a plain language summary of the situation directed at the patient's family doctor, but intelligible and available to the patient or carers, should be available within 24 hours.

ASSESSMENT AND RESPONSE

The assessment of trauma

The initial assessment of the trauma patient, besides the clinical examination, should include analysis of the interactions between the patient, the mechanism of injury and the extent of the injury sustained. Being able to synthesise the inter-relationships among these parameters is essential to addressing the pressures of the 'timeline concept' previously discussed. The associations among these three factors are usually very clear, but can be hidden.

For instance, a 50-year-old male restrained passenger in a car involved in a head-on collision with another vehicle may sustain rib fractures, a sternal fracture, thoracic spine fracture and possibly cardiac contusion. Abdominal injuries could also be suspected but, overall, the clinician, knowing the mechanism, can proceed quickly in making the diagnosis and initiating treatment. However, in cases where no association can be synthesised (between the mechanism of the accident, the patient's condition and the clinical signs observed) the reasons behind this 'picture' should be sought, for example the reported mechanism may have been underestimated. We will now analyse how the clinician can make best use of the information available.

Summary box 22.3

The assessment of trauma

- Include the information formula: mechanism + patient = injury
- Look for both obvious and less obvious features
- Identify more reasons when the above formula does not make sense

Mechanisms

Mechanisms may be blunt, penetrating or even of a combined nature (*Table 22.1*). Blunt trauma can be categorised as direct or indirect, and continues to be the most common mechanism. In a direct mechanism, the damage is localised to the site of injury. In contrast, in an indirect mechanism the damage occurs at a distant site after transmission of the force

TABLE 22.1 Examples of patterns of injury.

Mechanism	Obvious features	Covert injuries
Left-sided impact from road traffic accident	Lateral compression of the pelvis	Splenic rupture
	Left-sided pneumothorax	Extradural haematoma
Flexion distraction (lap belt)	Chance fracture of the lumbar spine	Duodenal rupture
	Dislocated knee	Popliteal artery disruption
	Head injury	Cervical spine fracture
Electrocution	Burn on hand and collapse	Posterior dislocation of the shoulder
Dashboard impact	Knee wound	Posterior dislocation of the hip

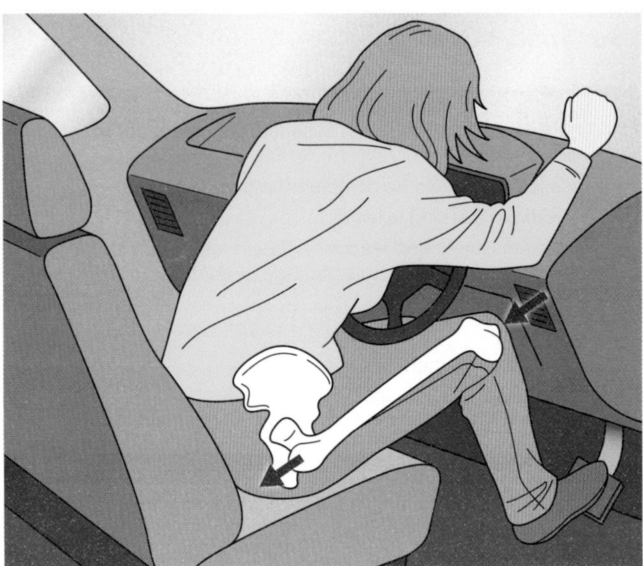

Figure 22.5 The injury force in a car accident can be transmitted from the dashboard, to the knee and then to the hip, which is the site of injury.

exerted. For example, a direct kick to the medial aspect of the mid-shaft of the tibia in a footballer by an opponent will induce an isolated tibial fracture. Such an injury represents a direct mechanism with bruising and ecchymosis at the area of the force exertion. On the other hand, a fall from a height of 1 metre with a twisting moment as the foot hits the ground can lead to a spiral fracture of the distal tibia. In this situation, the vector of the force was transmitted through the body's tissues to a location some distance away from its original point of application. In this case, other injuries should also be looked for, such as a fibular fracture or even an ipsilateral tibial plateau fracture, around the knee joint area. Similarly, a motor vehicle crash associated with direct trauma of the knee joint of the driver on the dashboard of the car could induce a fracture dislocation of the acetabulum and hip joint (transmission of force from the knee joint to the hip socket – an indirect blunt mechanism) (Figure 22.5).

The 'timeline concept' previously discussed may or may not be urgent, depending on the location and type of injury sustained. For instance, a minimally displaced tibial fracture that a footballer has sustained can be treated satisfactorily for some time after the moment of injury but, in contrast, a fracture of the acetabulum with a hip dislocation (as described above) represents an emergency owing to the potential development of neurovascular complications (damage to sciatic nerve; avascular necrosis of the femoral head). Therefore, the clinician's decision-making process should take into account both the peculiarities of the type of injury sustained and the anatomical location involved.

Moreover, it should be appreciated that the conduction of energy in an indirect mechanism, which is transferred via the soft tissues or fluid, can be difficult both to understand and to diagnose (accurately and promptly). For example, the rise in pressure secondary to a lower abdominal force could be passed to the vascular tree (aorta), leading to unexpected haemorrhage and death. All in all, one can argue that the effects of direct mechanisms are easier to comprehend than those of indirect ones.

Penetrating mechanisms can be divided into those caused by sharp objects and those induced by firearms (see Chapter 30). With regard to injuries caused by sharp objects, it is necessary to take into account the length of the sharp object, its surface area and the size of the entry point. The sharp object, for example a pair of scissors, will cause damage to the underlying tissues that it contacts (skin, subcutaneous fat, fascia, etc.). Local examination will confirm the extent of the injury and the need for wound exploration. Being familiar with the relevant anatomy of the area involved allows assessment of the peripheral nerve function, and tendon and muscle integrity. Here again the 'timeline concept' of prompt assessment and response (treatment) can be crucial in cases where there is vascular injury, a compartment syndrome due to internal bleeding or even joint penetration that could lead to septic arthritis. Knowledge of the anatomical structures at risk is essential to making the right decision in a timely fashion. This is particularly critical for penetrating wounds over the torso (see Chapter 27), because it is not always easy to establish the track that the sharp object has followed. In this context, it should not be forgotten that the abdominal structures extend higher than anticipated, and as high as the level of the fifth rib in expiration.

Summary box 22.4

Sharp object injuries

- Think about the length of the sharp object involved
- Knowledge of the local anatomy is essential
- Remember that abdominal structures at risk of injury extend high into the chest

Firearms induce penetrating injuries, which are more difficult to comprehend than incisional injuries caused by sharp objects. For instance, a high velocity projectile (bullet) causes extensive damage to the tissues as it travels, inducing lateral acceleration far from the point of impact, and producing either a permanent or a temporary cavity (see Chapter 30). The importance of the temporary cavity is that it lasts only for milliseconds and usually is not evident during the clinical examination. It is important to be aware that this temporary cavity usually extends far from the boundaries of the apparent injury (Figure 22.6). Awareness of this phenomenon will ensure that the surgeon carries out sufficient exploration and wound excision.

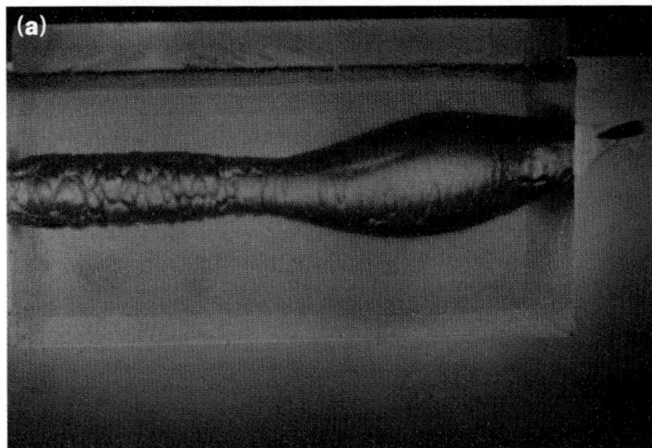

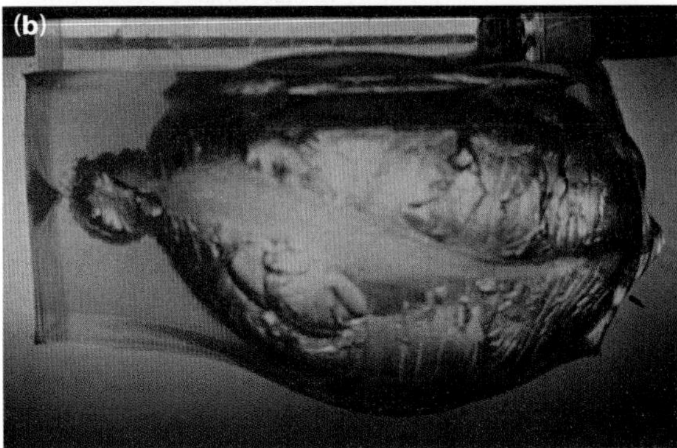

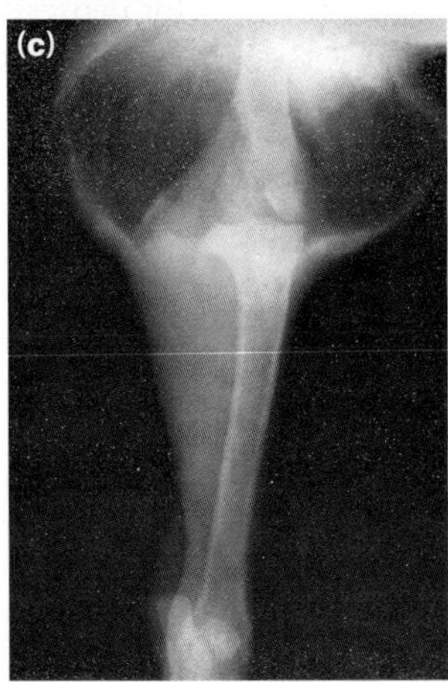

Figure 22.6 A projectile passing through a gelatin block: (a) low energy transfer; (b) high energy transfer; (c) the effect of high energy transfer on tissues (courtesy of Professor J Ryan).

Summary box 22.5

Firearm injuries

- High velocity bullets induce permanent and temporary cavitation
- Temporary cavitation can contain foreign material
- Low velocity bullets induce similar damage to knives

Patient factors

All patients possess a unique profile and medical history and so will react and respond differently to a given traumatic incident. Children and adults of different ages will sustain different injuries as a result of the same mechanism. For instance, a car hitting a pedestrian will induce different injuries in an adult, compared with a child (Figure 22.7). It is important to consider the other aspects of the patient's history. Past medical history, medication and allergy risk will direct not only the clinical assessment but also the treatment.

Obvious injuries

Some injuries are very obvious and can be identified before details of the mechanism or patient are known. One can take advantage of this, as the presence of an obvious injury can inform and lead to the identification of another which is less obvious. Obvious injuries are usually visible externally. It is therefore no surprise that at the end of the ABCD protocol there is also an E, referring to **e**xposure and the need to look for other signs of injury. Bruising to the scrotum of a motorcyclist following a collision with a car suggests a pelvic fracture. Contusion over the greater trochanter of the proximal femur in an older patient experiencing difficulty with straight leg raise points to a neck of femur fracture. Finger-shaped bruises on a child's arms or thighs suggest NAI. The presence of a seat belt mark on the lower abdomen of a patient involved in a car crash and who has substantial abdominal pain points to damage inside the abdomen. Thus, exposure of the trauma patient should be routine practice in order to avoid missing the 'obvious'.

Hidden factors

MECHANISMS

When analysis of the relationship of the formula 'mechanism + patient = injury' does not seem to add up, then the hidden information may be contained in the mechanism. Occasionally, it is observed that there has been a deliberate attempt to misinform. While the majority of alert and orientated patients tell the truth, others, in order to protect themselves or others, may fabricate a mechanism. This may mislead the clinician and lead them to look for the wrong pattern of injuries. For instance, a young patient with a calcaneal fracture may report that this was the result of a fall into a hole in the road, when in fact it had occurred during a burglary, following a fall from a height of 10 metres. This can delay the accurate diagnosis of the specific injury and may prevent the diagnosis of other important injuries, such as a lumbar spine fracture. Although the patient should be given the chance to tell their

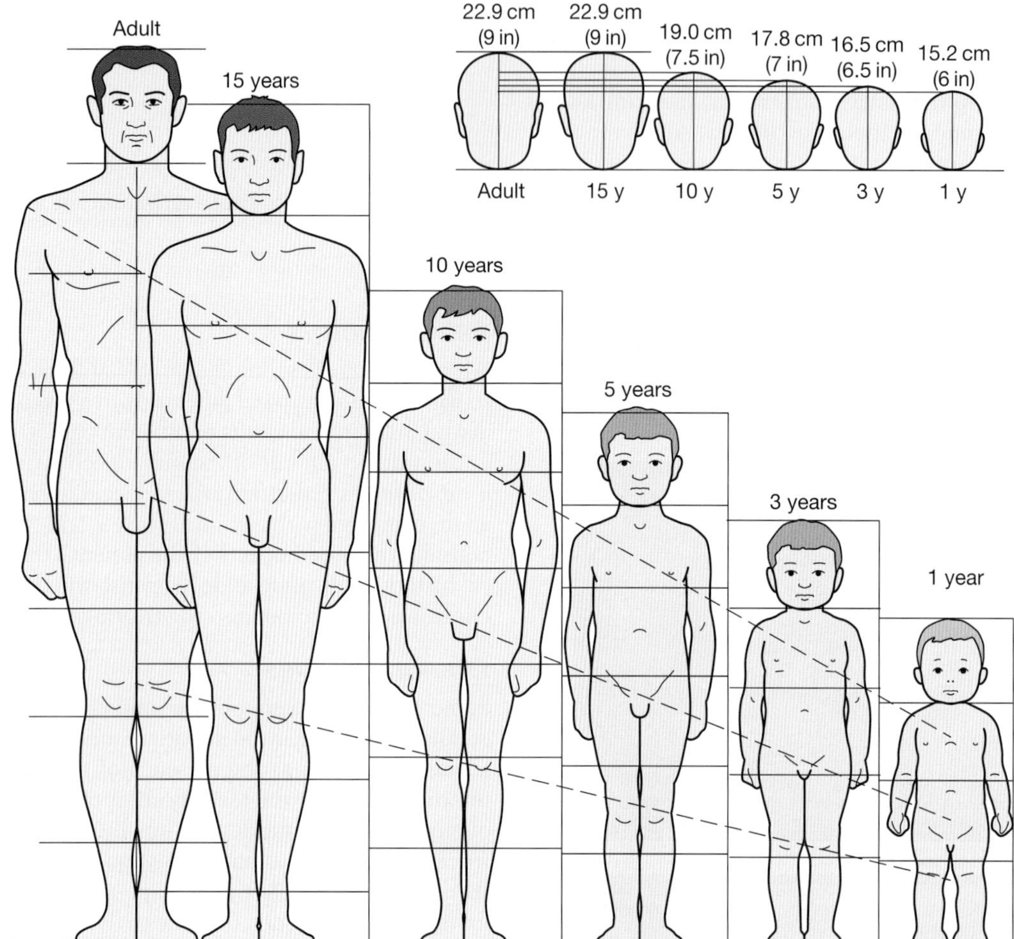

Figure 22.7 Body proportions at various ages and anatomical location of injuries when hit by a car.

story, it should not always be believed, particularly if there are inconsistencies.

A hidden mechanism can also arise when the patient is unable to give their history of events, for instance patients who are unconscious. The physically and mentally vulnerable include older patients, perhaps with dementia, and very young children. The difficulty or inability to report the injury is compounded by the fact that it might relate to criminal activity (e.g. NAI). Parameters that should alert the clinician and raise suspicion of NAI include:

- external signs of injuries not consistent with the mechanism reported;
- long bone fractures in a preambulatory child;
- inconsistent or changing history;
- aggressive or unusual behaviour of carers at interview;
- posterior rib injuries.

It must be emphasised that the clinician, in addition to diagnosis and treatment, must also protect the patient from further harm. This is of paramount importance when dealing with vulnerable individuals (children and the elderly). If the early signs of abuse are ignored or not taken seriously, it may not be possible to prevent later episodes, where serious harm may occur. While NAI is a serious issue to address, mechanisms are usually in place and can be followed by passing on the problem to the appropriate team and professionals (see Chapter 39).

Another important issue is the fact that any obvious injuries may provide important evidence regarding the mechanism, which may be important to a criminal investigation. We must endeavour, without compromising treatment, not to affect such evidence by our medical actions and bear in mind that forensic evidence may be needed for a conviction at a later stage. Furthermore, the importance is made more apparent if we consider that the victim of an attack may subsequently be a murder victim.

Summary box 22.6

Hidden mechanisms

- The vast majority of conscious patients will tell the truth
- Patients involved in criminal activity may not tell the truth
- Fear of abuse may prevent vulnerable patients from telling the truth
- Clinicians have the responsibility to take action when NAI is suspected

PATIENTS

In circumstances where the injury and mechanism are inconsistent, one should consider the possibility that the patient may have an unknown pre-existing condition. For example, an apparently healthy middle-aged woman who bends to lift a box and sustains a fracture at the thoracolumbar junction of her spine may have pathological weakness of the vertebral bone, such as advanced osteoporosis. Treatment should not be confined to the local injury, but should extend to appropriate investigation and treatment of the underlying fragility of the skeleton, thus reducing the risk of further fracture. Similarly, fractures may be secondary to an undiagnosed or poorly controlled medical condition. For example, a patient presenting with a scalp laceration and a wrist fracture may have fallen as a result of a transient ischaemic attack (a hidden patient factor). In this situation, it is essential to include a medical secondary survey to identify the real cause of the injuries sustained and prevent further trauma.

INJURIES

When analysis of the formula 'mechanism + patient = injury' has failed to identify hidden injury, there are two other approaches:

1 the look everywhere approach;
2 the focused exclusion approach.

Look everywhere approach. This represents the secondary and tertiary elements of the ATLS system and involves a detailed secondary survey, from top to bottom and at different time points: soon after the initial treatment phase when measures relating to saving the patient's life have been completed, the day after injury, e.g. during a ward round, or several days after injury, e.g. when the patient first wakes up in the intensive care environment. The implementation of whole body CT (WBCT) (scanning the whole body) in all major trauma centres has allowed the clinical team to pick up injuries early. Such injuries would have been missed in the past when reliance was made on the initial radiographs of the chest, pelvis and cervical spine. The threshold for using more WBCT has been lowered substantially. There is no doubt that WBCT scan algorithms have been shown to accelerate diagnostic work-up, but their effect on survival is controversial. Moreover, concerns have been voiced about the overexposure of patients to radiation with the increasing and often uncritical use of this type of scan. The effective radiation dose to all organs from a single full-body CT is 12–16 millisieverts (mSv). Survivors of the atomic bomb whose radiation dose ranged 5–100 mSv had a statistically significant increase in the risk of solid cancers. Overall, the risks associated with one scan are relatively modest, approximately 1 in 1250, or 0.08%. However, it has been reported that widespread liberal CT use is responsible for 1.5–2.0% of all cancers in the USA. Of interest, WBCT equates to 76 chest x-rays or 6 months of background radiation. It has been suggested that it should be requested wisely and that developing a triaging protocol can minimise the critisim of its overuse.

Focused exclusion approach. This is based on the knowledge that some specific injuries are missed on a remarkably regular basis. Such injury patterns include metatarsal and metacarpal fractures, scaphoid fractures, perilunate dislocations and posterior shoulder dislocations. When such injuries are suspected, a detailed focused history, clinical examination and appropriate investigations should be carried out to either confirm or exclude them.

Summary box 22.7

Trauma assessment

- Knowledge of timelines for important diagnoses is essential
- Initial assessment should focus on what kills first
- Screen high-risk patients before clinical signs become apparent, as it may be too late to intervene once signs develop

THE RESPONSE TO TRAUMA

Completion of the initial assessment according to the formula (patient + mechanism = injury) should provide the necessary information to formulate and execute a 'response' (treatment). During this stage of care, the response to injury will continue to evolve and decompensation may occur unexpectedly. Vigilance is required throughout management to identify the potential exhaustion of reserve mechanisms.

The patient's response to injury

From the time of the accident, a cascade of physiological responses will be upregulated to maintain survival. All such responses are part of homeostatic mechanisms that alter with the time elapsed following injury. The timing and nature of interventions should be altered accordingly. Important patient responses that require prompt attention, in order to avoid a subsequent negative impact on the patient's haemodynamic condition, include the body temperature, oxygenation and organ perfusion. A decline in body temperature is a frequent finding after injury and may be due to exposure, blood loss and inactivity. Measures should be taken not only to prevent further reduction in temperature but also to restore it. Covering the patient with appropriate blankets during transportation, resuscitation and in the theatre environment will minimise the risk of hypothermia, coagulation disturbances and ongoing bleeding.

Patient oxygenation can be optimised with the administration of inspired oxygen or ventilation if needed.

Blood loss can give rise to an altered level of consciousness, low blood pressure, reduced perfusion of the extremities (skin discolouration) and tachycardia. By way of response, endogenous clotting factors are activated to stop the bleeding and to maintain adequate circulatory volume. A further consideration is that traumatised lung parenchyma cannot tolerate surplus fluid. Therefore, the latest resuscitation guidelines advocate a reduction in crystalloid administration and the early transfusion of blood products. Furthermore, there is a need to quickly identify and stop the source of bleeding.

Another important part of the response to injury is the activation of the immune–inflammatory system. Acute phase mediators are released systemically, stimulating cellular elements (polymorphonuclear leukocytes) to interact with the endothelium. Under certain circumstances, extravasation of leukocytes may take place, with possible autodestruction. Clinical decisions should aim to minimise the risk of an exaggerated immune–inflammatory reaction. Surgical procedures, which can act as a second hit, where injury is considered the first hit, should be carefully timed and selected.

The medical response to injury

Initial management

Where resources are available, a patient found to have sustained serious injuries at the scene of the accident will lead the paramedics to activate 'the trauma team on call', allowing personnel to await the patient's arrival in the resuscitation room. The team leader, according to the ATLS protocol, will assign trained nurses and doctors to specific tasks. Protective clothing, such as gloves and lead aprons, is required to protect the personnel from fluids and radiation exposure. Following the ATLS protocol should be a routine process, involving experienced team members and ideally avoiding careless delays, which may compromise the response time. Potential problems can be predicted. The involvement of different disciplines in assessing and planning treatment of injuries in different body areas may lead to issues around priority, which can lead to confusion and uncertainty: 'Who should go first?' 'What investigation should be next?' It is the role of the team leader to ensure that this is avoided and that decisions which may be critical for the patient's wellbeing are executed smoothly.

In situations where the system operates according to locally developed protocols, someone should have the responsibility of overruling the protocol if this would be to the best interest of the patient, in order to keep the process rolling.

Following common pathways to manage patients can save time and reduce errors. The management of hip fractures in older age groups has improved in the UK with the regulated and monitored involvement of surgeons, geriatricians and anaesthetists. However, early labelling can also be misleading and troublesome. For instance, an older female patient with multiple medical problems might, after falling down a step, sustain an ankle fracture and be given the label 'ankle fracture'. Once the label is given the 'pathway' is set and she may be placed in a plaster of Paris back slab and be admitted for fixation under the care of someone who thinks primarily about mechanical matters. The so-called 'accidental benign falls' may be associated with more severe pathology and injuries. Furthermore, a patient may fall as a result of a medical condition (e.g. a mini stroke) and, in addition to an ankle fracture, may sustain other injuries including fractures of the pubic ramus and ribs. The wrong label may disguise the seriousness of the injuries sustained and the fact that the patient's condition may rapidly deteriorate, putting their life at risk. The first person in the diagnostic chain has disproportionate responsibility. Early labelling after inappropriate assessment can be incorrect and direct the patient to the wrong care pathway. In general terms, all patients, and particularly vulnerable patients, should undergo physiological triage to reduce the risk of being wrongly assigned.

Beyond the first hour

Following the initial assessment and management according to the ATLS protocol, and when the end points of resuscitation have been accomplished, further interventions are necessary in a patient with multiple injuries. The presence of an open book pelvic fracture, a lumbar spine fracture, a femoral fracture, a liver laceration and a tarsometatarsal dislocation are examples of outstanding injuries waiting treatment. The timing of the initiation of fixation, the type of fixation to use and the priority of various injuries have been points of discussion for some years.

The original work by Bone *et al.* in the 1980s, demonstrating the benefits of early fracture fixation of all injuries, led to the acceptance and wide application of the so called 'early total care' (ETC) philosophy. This practice became the gold standard of treatment for patients with multiple injuries. However, in some specific patient groups, for example those with severe chest and/or head injuries or those in an extreme physiological state (with ongoing bleeding from different sources such as abdomen, pelvis and chest), it was observed that the ETC concept led to early complications and mortality.

Knowledge acquired at the molecular level related to the immune–inflammatory response to injury and the concepts of the phenomena of the first hit (the impact exerted on the homeostatic mechanisms as a result of the original trauma sustained) and the second hit (the additional physiological stress induced by surgical procedures) led to the acceptance and implementation of the so call 'damage control orthopaedics' (DCO) philosophy, which is called damage control surgery (DCS) in more generalised settings (see later chapters). The stages of DCO are:

- resuscitation;
- haemorrhage control;
- decompression;
- decontamination;
- fracture splintage.

In the DCO concept, initially any long bone fractures and the pelvis are temporarily stabilised with the use of external fixators. Definitive stabilisation of the fractures (conversion of the external fixators to intramedullary (IM) nailing for the femur and plating of the pelvis) would take place usually 4 days later, when the physiological state of the patient has been stabilised. In contrast, a patient with similar injuries who has stable physiology throughout would be managed with IM nailing of the femoral fracture and plating of the pelvis within the first 24–36 hours: the ETC approach. The two strategies of fracture fixation, the ETC and DCS, are currently practised on the basis of some specific criteria. The vast majority of polytrauma patients are suitable for ETC (80–90%). Specific criteria are shown in Table 22.2.

TABLE 22.2 Criteria for damage control surgery (DCS) and early total care (ETC).

Criteria for DCS	Criteria for ETC
Hypothermia: <34°C	Stable haemodynamics
Acidosis: pH <7.2	No need for vasoactive/ inotropic stimulation
Serum lactate >5 mmol/L	No hypoxaemia, no hypercapnia
Coagulopathy	Serum lactate <2 mmol/L
Blood pressure <70 mmHg	Normal coagulation
Transfusion approaching 15 units	Normothermia
Injury severity score >36	Urinary output >1 mL/kg/hour

It is important for the clinician to appreciate that the physiology of the patient can change rapidly. Patients with a high injury severity score, the so called 'patient at risk' can decompensate quickly. Ongoing evaluation of the patient is therefore paramount to allow the clinician to choose the right strategy for the right patient. ETC and DCS should complement, rather than compete with, each other. The decision regarding 'who should go first, what is to be fixed first and with what type of implant' is, most of the time, straightforward. Nonetheless, the clinician should always be prepared for the unexpected and have a bail out solution ready to be implemented.

Consequently, a plan should always be made available to the trauma team to inform them about the details of treatment, particularly in the operating room environment. The plan can be recorded on a whiteboard with clear guidance on the alternative pathway to be implemented should the patient's condition deteriorate. Ongoing monitoring of such parameters as core temperature, lactate, base excess, coagulation, etc. will give knowledge of the patient's condition at any time point during care. Appropriate decisions can then be taken to ensure that the safety of the patient has not been compromised. For instance, if the ETC concept has been applied and a polytrauma patient with a head injury and chest trauma is on the operating table, waiting to have a femoral fracture stabilised with IM nailing, and their condition deteriorates the ETC plan can be changed to DCO (an external fixator can be applied quickly to stabilise the femoral fracture temporarily). This allows prompt transfer of the patient to the intensive care unit (ICU) where resuscitation can continue within a safe environment with ongoing monitoring of vital organ function (lungs and brain).

When injuries involve the input of different disciplines in terms of surgical intervention, for instance a general surgeon for a liver laceration, a neurosurgeon for an intracranial haematoma, an orthopaedic surgeon for a pelvic and femoral fracture and a maxillofacial surgeon for a depressed orbital fracture, the most important intervention should go first. Clearly, communication and prioritisation among the team members is essential. As each procedure nears its completion, communication with the anaesthetist will allow a decision as to whether it is safe to go on to the next procedure. Not infrequently, and assuming that it is technically possible, two teams can work simultaneously to significantly shorten the time the patient will spend in the operating theatre environment and allow subsequent prompt transfer to the ICU for optimisation and ongoing monitoring.

LOCAL PROTOCOLS AND GUIDELINES

While the ATLS protocol has become the standard of care for the initial management of patients with multiple injuries, other protocols and guidelines have also been developed to allow the treatment of patients in a more standardised way. It is not uncommon for each trauma centre to develop its own local guidelines, although national guidelines may also exist. Regional guidelines may refer to smaller areas of practice, such as antibiotic prophylaxis for open fractures, mass transfusion, pharmacotherapy for coagulation disturbances, steroids for spinal cord injuries, clearance of the cervical spine and angiographic embolisation of pelvic fractures. These protocols can facilitate quicker decision making, eliminating delays and benefiting the patient. They also protect the clinician and care provider with regard to medicolegal issues. An example referring to angiographic embolisation of pelvic fractures is shown in Figure 22.8.

Local policies focusing on the creation of single charts facilitating daily input of patients' vital signs and biochemical results are useful in allowing sequential observation of the results, which can demonstrate important trends. These trends can be useful in identifying early a clinical condition which can be treated within the timeline frame concept and prior to the establishment of irreversible damage to the affected organ, at which point any form of intervention will be meaningless. For instance, the clinical evolution of respiratory insufficiency in an individual without pre-existing lung disease secondary to pulmonary embolism is easier to identify by evaluating the trend in the oxygen saturation of inspired oxygen.

Planning an individual operation

Operative procedures in a polytrauma patient struggling for survival are critical in the acute phase. Their outcome can

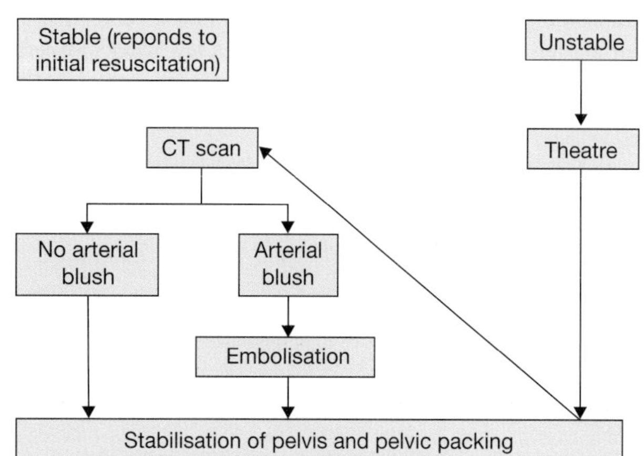

Figure 22.8 Pelvic fracture: angiography protocol.

Summary box 22.8

The response to trauma

- Rationalise patient management with development of protocols and guidelines
- Avoid unnecessary delays
- Observe trends and identify promptly evolving conditions

affect morbidity and mortality. For this reason, it is **essential** to get it right the first time. It is therefore also essential that there is adequate study of the problem to be solved, followed by the appropriate planning and execution. Analysing the fracture pattern, and deciding about patient positioning, the surgical approach to be used to get adequate access to the bone for reduction, the type of implant to be used, the correct positioning of the implant, the soft tissue handling and the type of rehabilitation, are just some of the parameters for consideration.

The surgeon should answer questions such as: Is it the optimum time to carry out the procedure? Am I the most appropriate person to carry out the procedure? Have I made a contingency plan should the procedure become difficult to complete? What is my plan A, B, or C so I am able to successfully finish the procedure? Recording all the important issues on a piece of paper, or suitable alternative, will ensure that no parameter of importance will be left out of the planning. In order that the procedure runs smoothly in theatre, documentation of the plan can be made on the white board. Such a practice will allow every member of the surgical team to be aware of the potential issues to be addressed and the plan of action that has been decided. The appropriate surgical equipment for plans A, B and C can be clearly identified and kept in close proximity to the operating theatre. The above strategy will eliminate unnecessary detail and ensure that there will be no surprises, for instance required equipment found to be unavailable.

The response to the mechanism of injury (injury prevention)

Not infrequently, patients are seen who have been injured at the same geographical area with the same mechanism. A possible scenario is that, over a period of a few weeks, several patients are noted to present with a fall of 2–3 metres, in the same location, from a particular bridge. Further investigation might establish that the bridge is easy to access, perhaps because of damage to safety measures. With appropriate steps the damage can be rectified and the access to the bridge limited, preventing further harm. In this example, the surgeon is involved in both the treatment and the prevention of injury. Therefore, when a mechanism of injury becomes more frequent and is associated with serious life-threatening trauma, it is essential to take steps either to eliminate the mechanism or to lessen the consequences.

The issue of injury prevention is not only an important consideration for clinicians but also for other stakeholders, for example politicians (developing appropriate legislation relevant to road safety), manufacturers (optimising the safety of cars) and the construction industry. This accounts for the improvements in safety that can be achieved.

Summary box 22.9

Planning an individual operation

- Adequate preoperative planning is essential to eliminate unnecessary delays
- Document the plan to ensure no important parameter is left out
- A whiteboard can be used to demonstrate the order of plan execution and act as a means of communication with the staff

Summary box 22.10

Response to the mechanism of injury

- Be alert to identify frequent patterns of injury
- Many stakeholders, including clinicians, should engage in injury prevention
- Legislation and education are essential

The response to patient factors

Injuries presenting with increased frequency in an individual patient require special attention. Older patients, perhaps with multiple medical problems, can represent such a vulnerable group. The reduced bone mineral density making their skeletons 'fragile' is associated with an increased risk of fracture. Hip fractures, wrist fractures, spinal fractures and pelvic fractures are just some of the many results following minimal trauma. The risk of fracture is increased with the presence of comorbidities such as visual impairment, parkinsonism or transient ischaemic heart attacks. Consequently, knowing the parameters associated with a particular group of patients, attempts can be made to reduce the number of patients requiring treatment. For instance, prescription of bone protection therapy and addressing early the medical comorbidities (e.g. cataract surgery) may help to reduce the number and severity of injuries sustained. Development of specific guidelines and protocols can facilitate the much needed implementation of unified measures allowing easy patient access and treatment.

Summary box 22.11

Response to patient factors

- Older patients may be vulnerable to injury, owing to poor bone stock and other comorbidities
- Bone protection treatment is essential
- Development of local and national guidelines to respond to patient factors is desirable

CONCLUSION

Trauma can affect all patient age groups. The severity of injury depends on the type and nature of the mechanical force applied. The formula 'patient + mechanism = injury' should be kept in mind when dealing with trauma patients. There is a connection among the three components of the formula, all of which should fit together in a coherent way. When no relationship can be made, examine for pre-existing pathology and hidden injuries, or consider whether the history given by the patient is at fault (including deliberate attempts to mislead).

Be aware of the timeline concept because there is a minimum response time to initiate and complete treatment in order to deal with a specific condition successfully.

Early assessment and management of patients with multiple injuries is carried our using the ATLS protocol and other guidelines developed either locally or at a national level. Subsequent treatment for definitive stabilisation can be personalised by one of two of the existing fracture fixation strategies, ETC or DCO. Specific criteria can assist the clinician to make the right decision for the right patient. Different groups of patients, such as older patients and children, have different demands and should be managed accordingly. While we, as clinicians, are focusing on treating the injury sustained, we have other responsibilities including our active involvement in preventive measures. Preventive measures should be commissioned when particular mechanisms can be identified as being common or important causes of injury.

Summary box 22.12

Conclusion

- Look for hidden injuries
- Remember the timeline concept
- Specific criteria will decide the fixation strategy: ETC or DCO

FURTHER READING

Bone LB, Johnson KD, Weigelt J, Scheinberg R. Early versus delayed stabilization of femoral fractures: a prospective randomized study. *Clin Orthop Relat Res* 2004; **422**: 11–16.

Department for Transport. *Reported road casualties in Great Britain. Main results 2015.* Available at: https://www.gov.uk/government/statistics/reported-road-casualties-in-great-britain-main-results-2015 (accessed on 11/11/16).

Giannoudis PV, Giannoudis VP, Horwitz DS. Time to think outside the box: 'Prompt-Individualised-Safe Management' (PR.I.S.M.) should prevail in patients with multiple injuries. *Injury* 2017; **48**(7): 1279–82.

Hajibandeh S, Hajibandeh S, Idehen N. Meta-analysis of the effect of tertiary survey on missed injury rate in trauma patients. *Injury* 2015; **46**(12): 2474–82.

Huber-Wagner S, Lefering R, Qvick LM *et al.*; Working Group on Polytrauma of the German Trauma Society. Effect of whole-body CT during trauma resuscitation on survival: a retrospective, multicentre study. *Lancet* 2009; **373**(9673): 1455–61.

Hui CM, MacGregor JH, Tien HC, Kortbeek JB. Radiation dose from initial trauma assessment and resuscitation: review of the literature. *Can J Surg* 2009; **52**(2): 147–52.

Kehoe A, Smith JE, Edwards A, Yates D, Lecky F. The changing face of major trauma in the UK. *Emerg Med J* 2015; **32**(12): 911–5.

Lozano R, Naghavi M, Foreman K *et al.* Global and regional mortality from 235 causes of death for 20 age groups in 1990 and 2010: a systematic analysis for the Global Burden of Disease Study 2010. *Lancet* 2012; **380**(9859): 2095–128.

Palmer CS, Gabbe BJ, Cameron PA. Injury. Defining major trauma using the 2008 Abbreviated Injury Scale. *Injury* 2016; **47**(1): 109–15.

Roberts CS, Pape HC, Jones AL *et al.* Damage control orthopaedics: evolving concepts in the treatment of patients who have sustained orthopaedic trauma. *Instr Course Lect* 2005; **54**: 447–62.

Shore R, Walsh L, Azizova T, Rühm W. Risk of solid cancer in low dose-rate radiation epidemiological studies and the dose-rate effectiveness factor. *Int J Radiat Biol* 2017; **15**: 1–15.

Tammelin E, Handolin L, Söderlund T. Missed injuries in polytrauma patients after trauma: tertiary survey in trauma intensive care unit. *Scand J Surg* 2016; **105**(4): 241–7.

Chapter 23

Early assessment and management of severe trauma

Learning objectives

- How to identify and assess the severely injured patient
- Early treatment goals for multiply injured patients
- Understand the role of permissive hypotension, tranexamic acid and massive transfusion protocols
- Understand the principles of damage control surgery (DCS) versus early total care (ETC)

IDENTIFICATION OF SEVERE TRAUMA

The severely injured patient, with multiple injuries to different body systems, poses unique diagnostic and treatment challenges. The early assessment and management of severe trauma begins in the prehospital environment. Many of these patients will be easily identified at the scene of injury and forewarning the receiving hospital allows the activation of the trauma team to prepare for the patient's arrival. Key information in the pre-alert includes basic demographic information (age and gender), mechanism of injury, injuries identified and vital signs, including respiratory rate, pulse, blood pressure and Glasgow Coma Scale (GCS).

Patients that are identified prehospital as sustaining, or at high risk of sustaining, severe multisystem trauma should generate trauma team activation in the receiving hospital. It should be noted that not all patients with severe multisystem trauma are immediately obvious. An elderly patient falling down a few steps can easily sustain a hip fracture, multiple rib fractures and a small subdural haemorrhage. At first glance the patient can appear well, but their injury severity score (ISS) and potential mortality could easily exceed those of the younger patient with multiple open long bone fractures. Both patients are critically injured and should be managed with the same principles in mind.

ROLE OF THE TRAUMA TEAM

All hospitals managing severe trauma should have a dedicated trauma team, who are available immediately to attend and manage patients presenting with severe trauma. The composition of the team will depend on local policies but it will invariably involve doctors from the emergency department, anaesthetics and/or critical care, orthopaedics and general surgery. Increasingly, radiology and haematology doctors are contributing to the trauma team, as part of the patient's initial assessment and management. Hospitals managing large volumes of cases of severe multisystem trauma are recognising the need for an enhanced trauma team activation for the most severely injured patients – the so called 'code-red trauma call'. Patients identified prehospital as being haemodynamically unstable or with acute airway compromise may initiate 'code-red', triggering the automatic attendance of the most senior clinicians from each discipline prior to the patient's arrival and prehospital activation of massive transfusion protocols.

The role of the trauma team is to apply the principles of Advanced Trauma Life Support (ATLS) to rapidly identify and treat life-threatening injuries during the primary survey. The principle advantage of a trauma team is that this activity can occur concurrently instead of sequentially; while the anaesthetist may be assessing and managing the patient's airway, another team member can be assessing and managing the patient's breathing, etc. The importance of the trauma team leader cannot be overemphasised: they brief and prepare the team, coordinate these sequential activities, manage time, interpret findings and plan the next move. Increasing recognition of the importance of this role has led to the development of postgraduate training courses designed to teach both the technical and non-technical skills required. Generally, the trauma team leader and most senior clinicians should be standing back from the patient, looking at the bigger picture, in order to anticipate the next key decisions.

Summary box 23.1

The role of the trauma team

- Allows the simultaneous and efficient application of ATLS principles to rapidly identify and treat life-threatening pathologies
- Should be led by the most senior clinician
- The most senior clinicians from each specialty should attend 'code red trauma calls'
- The team leader should be trying constantly to anticipate the next move

PRIMARY SURVEY

The primary survey aims to identify and manage the most immediately life-threatening pathologies first and follows **cABCDE**.

c: Exsanguinating external haemorrhage

Experience from war zones over the past 20 years has shown that exsanguinating external haemorrhage from massive arterial bleeding needs to be controlled even before the airway is managed (see Chapter 30). Most of these injuries are due to gunshot wounds or blasts and are mainly seen in military practice. However, they are encountered in civilian practice. Bleeding must be controlled immediately by the application of packs and pressure directly onto the bleeding wound and artery. Haemostatic dressings that contain agents that augment local coagulation are now available. Failure to control bleeding in the limb by direct pressure should be followed by the application of a tourniquet proximal to the wound. In the field, simple tourniquets can be improvised if pneumatic tourniquets are not available. It is vital to appreciate that once a tourniquet is applied the limb becomes ischaemic – the time for which the tourniquet is applied must be recorded on the patient and the patient requires **urgent** surgical control of the bleeding in order to reperfuse the limb.

A: Airway with cervical spine control

All trauma patients should have their cervical spine immobilised and protected throughout. An immediate assessment of the patient's airway is made. A compromised airway requires a stepwise progression, first clearing the airway by suctioning secretions or blood, followed by simple airway manoeuvres such as a jaw thrust, chin lift and insertion of an oropharyngeal or nasopharyngeal airway. Advanced airway manoeuvres necessitate the insertion of a cuffed endotracheal tube. This may require an anaesthetic with rapid sequence induction or a surgical airway. Emergency intubation of the severely injured trauma patient is a difficult and demanding skill – standardised and rehearsed procedures should be in place for failure to intubate (**Figure 23.1**). Equipment and expertise for achieving a surgical airway must be readily available.

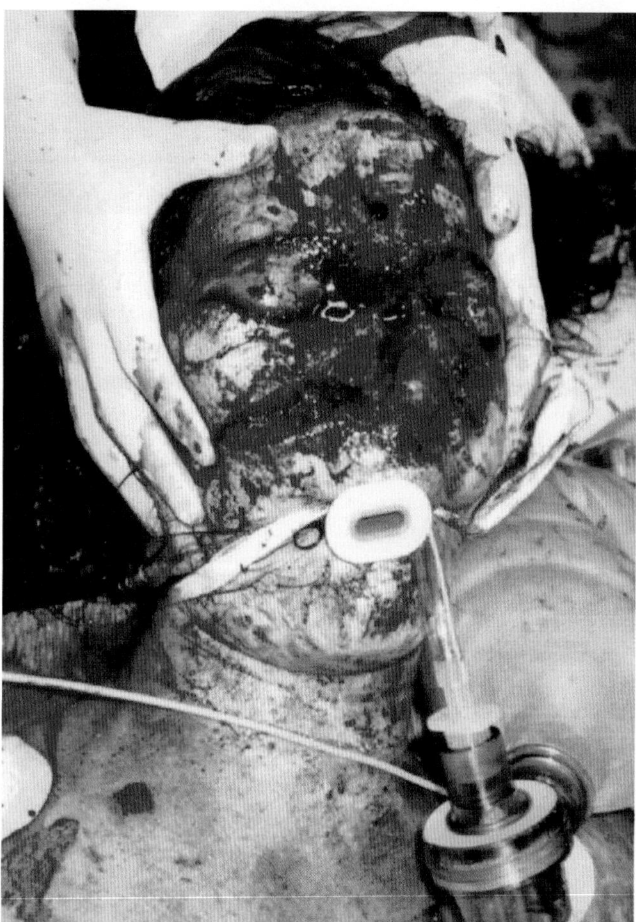

Figure 23.1 Unrestrained driver with severe craniofacial injury (courtesy of Johannesburg Hospital Trauma Unit).

B: Breathing and ventilation

All patients should receive high-flow oxygen. Life-threatening chest pathology such as tension pneumothorax, massive haemothorax and flail segment should be diagnosed and managed immediately. Equipment and expertise for rapid insertion of intercostal chest drains should be available.

C: Circulation and haemorrhage

All patients require adequate intravenous access with at least two large-bore intravenous (IV) cannulae. Equipment and expertise for insertion of central or intraosseous venous access should be available where peripheral access is not easily obtainable. Blood should be taken for cross-match and laboratory assessment, including haemoglobin and venous lactate. An assessment of the haemodynamic status should be made to identify shocked patients: the skin may be pale, cool and sweaty, the pulse rate raised to over 100 per minute and the blood pressure low. A pelvic binder should be applied to all haemodynamically unstable patients following blunt trauma and not removed until after a pelvic fracture has been excluded. Hypotensive trauma patients are treated as hypovolaemic until proven otherwise. The priority is now simultaneous fluid resuscitation and identification of the source of the haemorrhage.

Permissive hypotension, massive transfusion protocols and tranexamic acid

The initial aim of resuscitation is to maintain the blood supply to the vital organs: the brain, heart and kidneys. For a short time, this can be achieved with a target systolic blood pressure of 70–90 mmHg, although a higher pressure of >90 mmHg should be the target if a head injury is suspected. Small boluses of IV fluids (e.g. 250 mL of O negative blood, or normal saline if blood is not immediately available) should be administered to achieve this target, which should result in a palpable radial pulse. Excessive intravenous crystalloid or colloid solutions should be avoided because they cause haemodilution, increase coagulopathy and increase the risk of adult respiratory distress syndrome (ARDS). However, the key to this approach of permissive hypotension is that it is time limited. The primary source of haemorrhage must be identified and controlled as soon as possible.

Severely injured hypovolaemic patients should be resuscitated with blood and blood products, not crystalloid/colloid fluids. These must be warmed. All hospitals managing severe trauma should have a massive transfusion protocol which aims to provide blood and blood products in a ratio of 1 packed red cells:1 fresh frozen plasma:1 platelets.

TRANEXAMIC ACID

Tranexamic acid is an antifibrinolytic drug that reduces the risk of mortality from bleeding in both blunt and penetrating trauma. One gram is given intravenously over 10 minutes, followed by a further 1 g dose over 8 hours. Tranexamic acid should be given to all trauma patients suspected to have significant haemorrhage, including those with a systolic blood pressure of <110 mmHg or a pulse of over 110 per minute. It needs to be administered within 3 hours of injury and in the UK it is normally given by paramedics in the prehospital environment.

Summary box 23.2

Severe hypovolaemia

- Tranexamic acid reduces mortality after trauma
- All traumatised patients with signs of shock should receive tranexamic acid as soon as possible after injury
- All trauma centres should have an established massive transfusion protocol
- Severely hypovolaemic trauma patients should be resuscitated using blood and blood products
- The only role for crystalloids in the initial management of severely hypovolaemic patients is for the administration of small quantities to maintain blood pressure while waiting for blood products to arrive

Identification and management of haemorrhage

The sites of major haemorrhage in trauma patients are the chest, abdomen, pelvis, long bones and external haemorrhage (Figure 23.2). Blunt trauma patients frequently have multiple sources of haemorrhage. Clinical examination and investigations should aim rapidly to confirm or exclude significant bleeding from each of these sites. Computed tomography (CT) from the head to pelvis with IV contrast, the so called 'whole body CT' (WBCT) is the gold standard investigation in patients with signs or symptoms of multiple injury or deranged physiology, but note that WBCT should not be performed on the basis of the mechanism of injury alone (see Further reading). There is no role for scanning selective body systems in the severely injured trauma patient. Wherever possible, WBCT should be performed as soon as possible during the patient's resuscitation. A provisional 'hot report' can be issued within minutes to identify immediate life-threatening pathology to the trauma team. A more detailed definitive report should be available within 30–60 minutes.

Traditionally, chest and pelvis radiographs have been obtained early in the assessment of patients with polytrauma but these investigations are increasingly omitted in favour of obtaining a rapid CT scan, as described above. Most trauma centres now have rapid access to CT scanners located within, or immediately adjacent to, the resuscitation area. This has allowed haemodynamically unstable patients to have a WBCT with resuscitation by the trauma team continuing simultaneously during CT. Identifying which patients are too haemodynamically unstable to scan safely is a difficult decision for the trauma team leader and will be influenced by local factors and facilities.

Some patients will be so haemodynamically unstable on arrival that they need immediate surgical control of their haemorrhage before a CT scan. The most likely sources are abdominal or pelvic bleeding. An immediate chest radiograph will exclude catastrophic intrathoracic haemorrhage. An immediate pelvic radiograph is essential but should not delay transfer to the operating room. A focused abdominal sonography for trauma (FAST) scan (if immediately available) may also be useful in this scenario to locate the major source of haemorrhage. All patients undergoing immediate laparotomy in the operating room should have a pelvic binder applied **and not removed**. A correctly positioned pelvic binder at the level of the greater trochanters does not obstruct trauma laparotomy. These patients will invariably require a WBCT scan after surgical control of haemorrhage has been achieved.

Summary box 23.3

'Whole body CT' (WBCT)

- WBCT from the head to pelvis with IV contrast is the gold standard investigation of the severely injured adult blunt trauma patient
- There is no role for selective scanning of body systems in these patients
- WBCT scan is a time-critical investigation and should be obtained as early as possible in resuscitation of the severely injured patient
- Any patient undergoing immediate trauma laparotomy after blunt trauma without a WBCT scan should have a pelvic binder applied and not removed until a pelvic fracture is excluded. Such patients should have an immediate pelvic radiograph either in the emergency department, or as they arrive in the operating room

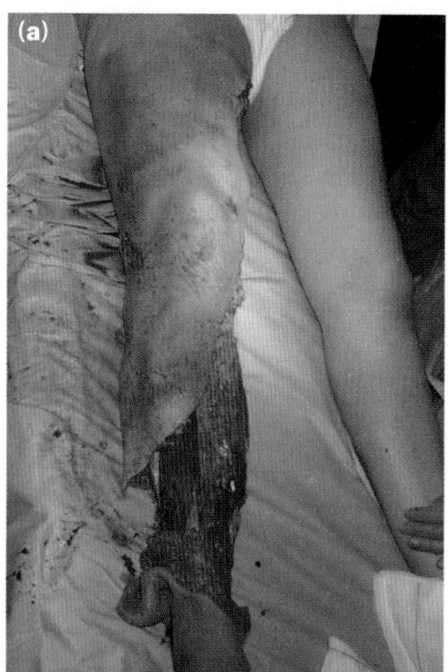

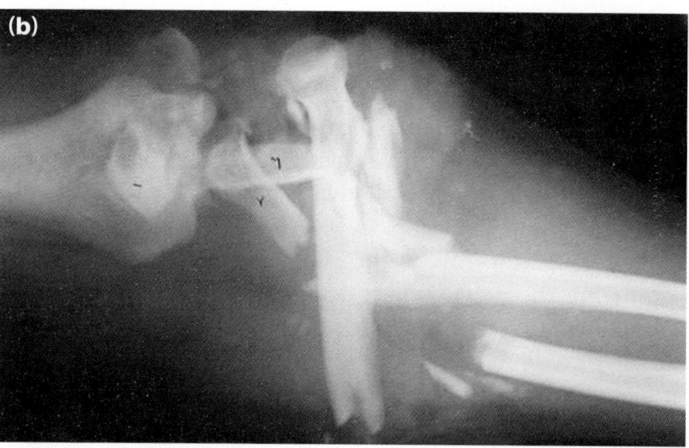

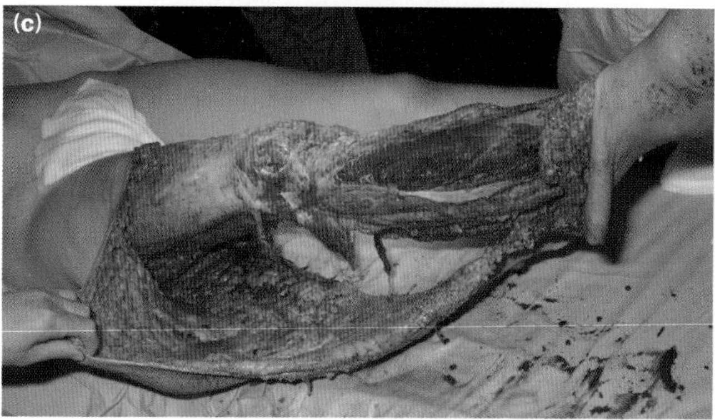

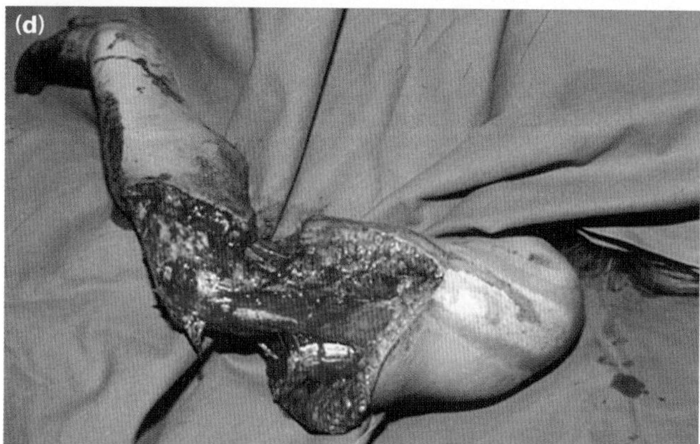

Figure 23.2 (a-d) Severe degloving injuries to the upper and lower limbs following a high-speed road traffic accident. The initial appearance and severity of the injury should not detract from following the important Advanced Trauma Life Support (ATLS) sequence in evaluating and treating immediate life-threatening injuries.

D: Disability and E: Exposure

On admission, the GCS score should be calculated (*Table 23.1*), the pupils assessed for size and reaction to light and the patient observed to determine whether they are moving all four limbs. The core temperature must be recorded. Patients are managed with cervical spine protection (cervical collar and blocks) and protection of the thoracolumbar spine using standard log roll techniques until a spinal injury has been excluded. Early WBCT scan will rapidly identify the majority of intracranial and spinal pathology.

The patient must be adequately exposed to allow a thorough and systematic clinical examination during the secondary survey but they must be kept warm. Trauma patients are frequently hypothermic and this will further increase coagulopathy. Every effort should be made to maintain normal temperature by minimising unnecessary exposure of the patient, and by using warmed blankets and trolleys and warmed fluids during resuscitation.

Log-rolling patients with severe pelvic fractures may harm the patient by disturbing established blot clots. Log-rolling should not occur until a pelvic fracture has been radiographically excluded. If patients need to be moved during their primary survey, such as when moving on to the CT scanning gantry, a 20° roll with inline spinal stabilisation should be used. Modern 'Scoop Stretchers' mean that there is no requirement to roll any patient more than 20° until a pelvic fracture has been excluded.

TABLE 23.1 Glasgow Coma Scale

Best eye response (E)	Best verbal response (V)	Best motor response (M)
4 Eyes opening spontaneously	**5** Oriented	**6** Obeys commands
3 Eye opening to speech	**4** Confused	**5** Localises to pain
2 Eye opening in response to pain	**3** Inappropriates words	**4** Withdraws from pain
1 No eye opening	**2** Incomprehensible sounds	**3** Flexion in response to pain
	1 None	**2** Extension to pain
		1 No motor response

Formal log-rolling of the blunt trauma patient to examine the back during the primary survey adds minimal useful clinical information, delays the WBCT scan and may cause harm to a patient with a pelvic fracture. It should be deferred until after the primary survey, with the exception of patients with penetrating trauma, where it is important to identify the presence of a posterior torso wound.

Mechanical testing of the pelvis in the emergency room ('springing the pelvis') adds no useful clinical examination and will disrupt any blot clot that has formed around a pelvic fracture. It should never be performed – a pelvic fracture should always be diagnosed radiographically.

Summary box 23.4

The cABCDE of trauma care

- c – Control of massive external haemorrhage
- A – Airway with cervical spine protection
- B – Breathing and ventilation
- C – Circulation and haemorrhage control: apply a pelvic binder and do not remove until a pelvic fracture is excluded
- D – Disability (neurological status)
- E – Exposure (assess for other injuries)

SECONDARY SURVEY

All severely injured patients require a detailed top to toe examination after life-threatening injuries have been identified and managed during the primary survey. Patients may be intubated and unresponsive at this point, limiting the accuracy of clinical examination. Such patients should have a 'tertiary survey' when extubated and alert, to identify any missed 'minor' injuries such as a scaphoid fracture in the wrist or a rotator cuff tear in the shoulder. These injuries have the potential to cause significant long-term disability. It is essential that the findings of the primary, secondary and tertiary surveys are clearly recorded in the patient case notes.

DAMAGE CONTROL SURGERY VERSUS EARLY TOTAL CARE

As discussed in Chapter 22, the concept of damage control surgery (DCS) was developed because severely traumatised patients with impaired physiology have poor outcomes after lengthy and complex surgical reconstructive procedures performed shortly after their trauma. Prolonged procedures result in additional trauma and further immune and physiological derangement; the 'triad of death', a cycle of acidosis, coagulopathy and hypothermia, may develop and result in multiorgan failure and death.

Consequently, surgical interventions in the trauma patient with physiological abnormality are limited to rapid life- and limb-saving procedures: control of haemorrhage, decompression of cavities (e.g. craniotomy), revascularisation of ischaemic organs and limbs and removal of contamination. This damage control approach aims to rapidly achieve these objectives and then move the patient to a critical care environment and continue with resuscitation.

Subsequent definitive reconstructive procedures are deferred until the patient is adequately resuscitated and physiologically optimised. DCS in the abdomen is limited to packing and control of haemorrhage, debridement and resection of devitalised tissue and removal of contamination by foreign bodies or faeces. Damage control orthopaedic surgery is limited to debridement of severe open fractures, rapid temporary splintage or stabilisation of long bone fractures and decompression of limb compartment syndrome where required.

Revascularisation of a limb following arterial injury may be appropriate for isolated injuries but in the patient with severe multiple system trauma it may increase the threat to life and therefore amputation may be the better option. Such patients are then transferred to critical care for further resuscitation and physiological stabilisation before definitive surgical procedures can be planned.

The majority of trauma patients respond well to resuscitation and are not physiologically compromised after appropriate resuscitation. A number of physiological indices are used to evaluate the response to resuscitation, including a pulse rate less than 100 per minute, normal blood pressure and respiratory rate, as well as urine output >30 mL per hour. The patient should not have hypothermia (temperature <35°C) nor evidence of acidosis on arterial blood gases and should have a normal coagulation screen.

Lactate levels are also a good indicator of tissue perfusion and should rapidly return to normal. In this situation, it is usually safe for the surgeon to proceed with definitive repair or reconstruction of injured organs.

For musculoskeletal injuries, early total care allows definitive fixation of all unstable long bone, spinal and pelvic fractures within 36 hours of injury. This facilitates nursing care, allows early mobilisation of the patient and reduces pulmonary complications and length of stay on intensive care.

If a sequence of fracture fixations is required, at the conclusion of each procedure the surgeon and anaesthetist should determine whether the patient's physiological status has been maintained sufficiently to allow the next procedure, or whether the patient should return to critical care for a further period of resuscitation.

Summary box 23.5

Early total care versus damage control surgery

- Early total care describes the definitive management of a patient's injuries within 36 hours of injury after a period of initial resuscitation
- Damage control surgery describes simultaneous resuscitation with early rapid life- and limb-saving surgery. Time-consuming definitive surgery is deferred until the patient's physiological status allows
- An early total care approach can be changed to a damage control approach if the patient's physiology deteriorates during definitive surgery

Venous lactate

Venous lactate is a useful marker of resuscitation and physiological state. A normal lactate (<2 mmol/L) is a sign that the patient is probably resuscitated and suitable for early total care. An elevated lactate (>3 mmol/L) suggests the patient is under-resuscitated and should either have a period of further resuscitation, or DCS if surgery is urgent. If a patient's lactate is 2–3 mmol/L then the trend (upwards or downwards) should be noted and the other physiological markers considered, to determine whether the patient is suitable for definitive surgical procedures.

The identification of patients suitable for ETC versus DCS should be made by senior surgeons and anaesthetists/critical care doctors. This may be an easy decision, for example the haemodynamically unstable patient with intra-abdominal bleeding will always undergo rapid damage control laparotomy. In other cases a careful review of the patient's physiology and coagulation state will be required.

Summary box 23.6

Venous lactate is an essential marker of resuscitation

- <2 mmol/L – Early total care
- 2–3 mmol/L – Look at the trend (increasing or decreasing)
- >3 mmol/L – May be under-resuscitated; should either have further resuscitation or damage control surgery (DCS) if surgery is urgent
- >5 mmol/L – DCS (see Chapters 22 and 27)

SUMMARY

The early assessment and management of trauma patients should follow established ATLS principles.

A WBCT scan, from the head to the pelvis, with IV contrast is the gold standard investigation for major trauma patients and should be performed early and whenever possible.

Warmed blood and blood products in a 1:1:1 ratio should be used with tranexamic acid in the early resuscitation of haemodynamically unstable trauma patients.

Trauma patients requiring surgery should have an early decision made whether a damage control or ETC approach is required. Surgical procedures in physiologically compromised patients should be limited to those required to save the life and/or limb of the patient, while simultaneous resuscitation is continued.

FURTHER READING

Sierink HJC, Treskes K, Edwards MJR *et al.*, for the REACT-2 study group. Immediate total-body CT scanning versus conventional imaging and selective CT scanning in patients with severe trauma (REACT-2): a randomised controlled trial. *Lancet* 2016; **388**: 673–83.

Chapter 24

Traumatic brain injury

Learning objectives

To understand:

- The physiology of cerebral blood flow and the pathophysiology of raised intracranial pressure
- The classification and assessment of head injury
- Management and sequelae of minor and mild traumatic brain injury
- Medical and surgical management of moderate and severe traumatic brain injury

INTRODUCTION

Head injury accounts for 3–4% of emergency department attendances, with around 1500 cases per 100 000 population per year in the UK. Annual mortality attributable to head injury is estimated at 9 per 100 000, and it remains the leading cause of death and disability from childhood to early middle age, with an estimated 2% of the US population suffering long-term disability as a result of head injury. Road traffic accidents are the leading cause of head injury, being responsible for up to 50% of cases. Other common mechanisms of injury include falls and assault. There is significant geographical variation, for example firearms are the third leading cause in the US.

Significant traumatic brain injury can be considered a combination of the primary injury sustained on impact, and secondary injury developing in the following hours and days. Understanding the importance of intracranial pressure and related parameters is key to minimising secondary injury and improving outcomes.

INTRACRANIAL PRESSURE

Intracranial pressure and cerebral blood flow

The brain depends on continuous perfusion for oxygen and glucose delivery, and hence survival. Normal cerebral blood flow (CBF) is about 55 mL per minute for every 100 grams of brain tissue. Ischaemia results when this rate drops below 20 mL per minute, and even lower levels will result in infarction unless promptly corrected.

Flow depends on cerebral perfusion pressure (CPP), the difference between mean arterial pressure (MAP) and intracranial pressure (ICP).

Summary box 24.1

Intracranial pressure (ICP)

- A continuous supply of oxygenated blood is essential for brain survival
- Raised ICP can compromise cerebral perfusion, resulting in a cycle of secondary brain injury and swelling

CPP (75–105 mmHg) = **MAP** (90–110 mmHg) – **ICP** (5–15 mmHg)

Typical normal values are given in parentheses. In fact, in the normal brain, variations in vascular tone maintain a constant CBF across a range of MAP between 50 and 150 mmHg (or higher in the setting of chronic hypertension), and a corresponding range of CPP, the process of cerebral autoregulation.

The Monro Kellie doctrine and herniation syndromes

Alexander Monro observed in 1783 that the cranium is a 'rigid box' containing a 'nearly incompressible brain'. Any expansion in the contents, especially haematoma and brain swelling, may be initially accommodated by exclusion of fluid components, venous blood and cerebrospinal fluid (CSF). Further expansion is associated with an exponential rise in ICP (Figure 24.1)

Uncontrolled increases in ICP result in cerebral herniation (Figure 24.2). Typically, herniation of the uncus of the temporal lobe over the tentorium results in pupil abnormalities (see *Pupils* below), usually occurring first on the side of any expanding haematoma. Cerebellar tonsillar herniation through the foramen magnum compresses medullary vasomotor and respiratory centres, classically producing **Cushing's**

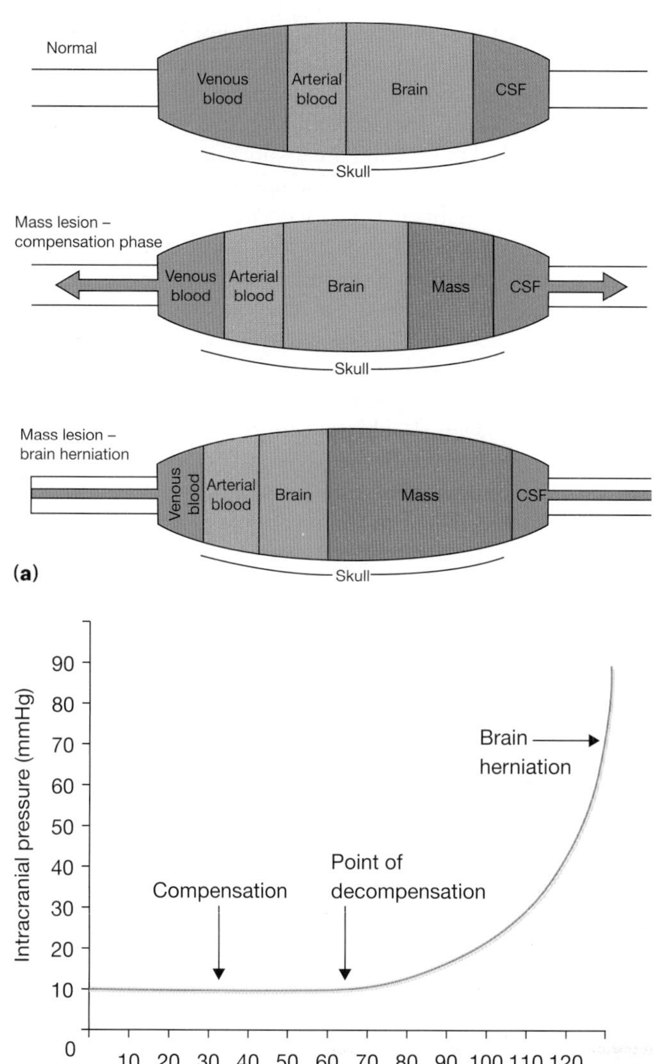

Figure 24.1 The Monro Kellie doctrine accounts for the ability of the intracranial compartment to accommodate expanding mass lesions, primarily by excluding venous blood and cerebrospinal fluid (CSF), and the rapid rise in pressure associated with exhaustion of this compensation.

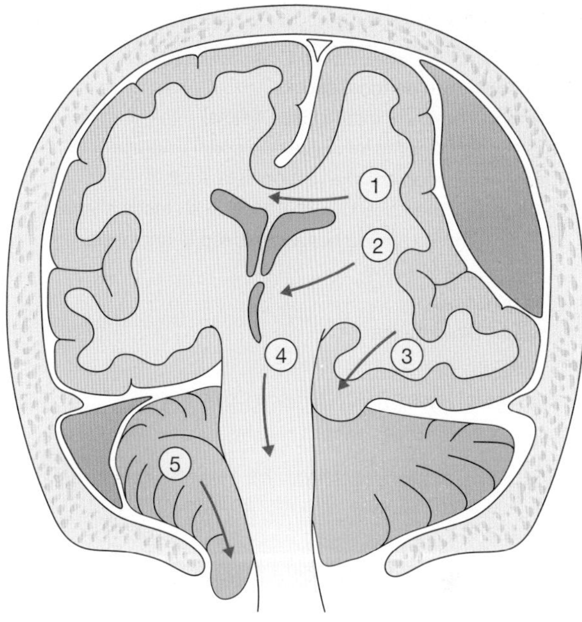

Figure 24.2 Brain herniation. Herniation of the cingulate gyrus under the falx cerebri is termed subfalcine herniation (1). (2) Midline shift is evident. (3) Uncal herniation: the temporal lobe is herniating over the tentorium cerebelli where it can compress the third nerve. (4) Central herniation and (5) tonsillar herniation result in brainstem compromise, manifesting as Cushing's triad.

triad – hypertension, bradycardia and irregular respiration. The patient is then said to be 'coning', and brainstem death will result without immediate intervention.

CLASSIFICATION OF HEAD INJURY

Severity of head injury is classified according to the postresuscitation Glasgow Coma Scale (GCS) (*Table 24.1*), as it is the GCS score, and in particular the motor score (see *Table 24.4*), that is the best predictor of neurological outcome. In broad terms, significantly obtunded patients have moderate injuries and comatose patients have severe injuries; alcohol and drug effects often complicate the classification.

TABLE 24.1 Head injury classification using the Glasgow Coma Scale (GCS) score.

Minor head injury	GCS 15 with no loss of consciousness (LOC)
Mild head injury	GCS 14 or 15 with LOC
Moderate head injury	GCS 9–13
Severe head injury	GCS 3–8

MINOR AND MILD HEAD INJURY

After exclusion of associated cervical spine injury, the major concern for these patients is to avoid discharge during the 'lucid interval' that may precede delayed deterioration due to an expanding intracranial haematoma. In general, patients with isolated head injuries and without ongoing deficits can safely be discharged from the emergency department, provided they meet suitable criteria, for instance those provided by the UK National Institute for Heath and Care Excellence (*Table 24.2*).

Summary box 24.2

Minor and mild head injury

- Decisions on imaging and discharge are best made guided by published criteria
- In preverbal children and other vulnerable groups, non-accidental injury must be considered
- Amnesia, confusion, headaches and somnolence are typical features of concussion

TABLE 24.2 National Institute for Health and Care Excellence discharge criteria in minor and mild head injury.

- GCS 15/15 with no focal deficits
- Normal CT brain if indicated (see below)
- Patient not under the influence of alcohol or drugs
- Patient accompanied by a responsible adult
- Verbal and written head injury advice: seek medical attention if:
  - Persistent/worsening headache despite analgesia
  - Persistent vomiting
  - Drowsiness
  - Visual disturbance
  - Limb weakness or numbness

CT, computed tomography; GCS, Glasgow Coma Scale.

TABLE 24.3 National Institute for Health and Care Excellence guidelines for computed tomography (CT) in head injury.

Indications for CT imaging within 1 hour
GCS <13 at any point
GCS <15 at 2 hours
Focal neurological deficit
Suspected open, depressed or basal skull fracture
More than one episode of vomiting
Post-traumatic seizure
Indications for CT imaging within 8 hours
Age >65 years
Coagulopathy (e.g. aspirin, warfarin or rivaroxaban use)
Dangerous mechanism of injury (e.g. fall from a height, road traffic accident)
Retrograde amnesia >30 minutes

Patients who do not meet all the discharge criteria will need admission for a further period of observation, and/or brain imaging. Early computed tomography (CT) imaging is desirable in patients with a persistent reduced conscious level, focal deficits, suspected fractures or risk factors for intracranial bleed (*Table 24.3*). Significant clinical or radiological abnormalities should be discussed with the neurosurgical service. Many of these patients will struggle with features of concussion for a period after their injury, with headaches and somnolence typical. Follow-up by a head injury specialist nurse or equivalent is therefore desirable.

Non-accidental injury

Head injury in children and vulnerable adults may be due to abuse. Significant findings include delayed presentation, injuries of disparate age, retinal haemorrhages, bilateral chronic subdural haematomas, multiple skull fractures and neurological injury without external signs of trauma.

Concussion, second impact syndrome and postconcussive syndrome

Concussion is defined as alteration of consciousness as a result of closed head injury, but is generally used in describing mild head injury without imaging abnormalities; loss of consciousness (LOC) at the time of injury is not a prerequisite. Key features include confusion and amnesia. The patient may be lethargic, easily distractable, forgetful, slow to interact or emotionally labile. Gait disturbance and incoordination may be seen. It is claimed that while symptomatic following a head injury, patients may be especially vulnerable to repeat impacts. It is proposed that in the context of disordered cerebral autoregulation, a second minor injury may trigger a form of malignant cerebral oedema refractory to treatment. Although the existence of the syndrome is disputed, and it is certainly rare, it should be considered in advice to individuals engaged in sports or activities carrying a risk of further injury: symptomatic players should not return to play.

Postconcussive syndrome is a loosely defined constellation of symptoms, persisting for a prolonged period after injury, and exacerbated in some patients by the potential for secondary gain (compensation). Patients may report somatic features such as headache, dizziness and disorders of hearing and vision. They may also suffer a variety of neurocognitive and neuropsychological disturbances, including difficulty with concentration and recall, insomnia, emotional lability, fatigue, depression and personality change.

MODERATE AND SEVERE TRAUMATIC BRAIN INJURY

Resuscitation and evaluation

Resuscitation is performed according to Advanced Trauma and Life Support (ATLS) guidelines, beginning with management of the airway and cervical spine control, and proceeding to assess and manage breathing and circulation. History obtained in parallel is key to shaping ongoing management.

History

Mechanism

In moderate and severe traumatic brain injury (TBI), history must be obtained from witnesses and paramedics. High-energy mechanisms of injury, including fall from a height or high-speed road traffic accident (RTA), will require careful clinical and radiological exclusion of associated multisystem

Summary box 24.3

History

Bystanders and paramedics may give vital information on the:

- preinjury state (fits, alcohol, chest pain)
- mechanism and energy involved in the injury (speed of vehicles, height fallen)
- conscious state and haemodynamic stability of the patient after the accident
- length of time taken for extrication

Check the medication history especially anticoagulants and antiplatelet agents and spinal injury (see Chapter 25). In the case of RTAs in particular, extraction time and evidence of hypoxia or haemodynamic instability at the scene is important information to obtain from the paramedics. Falls and crashes are often caused by a primary medical problem such as myocardial infarction, hypoglycaemia or subarachnoid haemorrhage, with implications for management.

Neurological progression

A specific check should be made for any loss of consciousness at the time of injury, and its duration. The GCS and pupil responses at the scene and on arrival in the emergency department should be obtained and documented. They should also be checked regularly thereafter; deterioration in GCS is an important index of developing, and potentially reversible, secondary injury. It is also useful to assess the extent of amnesia, retrograde (events prior to the injury) and anterograde (events afterwards). If the patient was intubated at the scene of the accident it is valuable to know whether the patient was moving all four limbs before this.

Past medical history

Details of the patient's medical background should be obtained, including allergies and normal medications. Of particular note here, are antiplatelet agents, potentially requiring platelet transfusion especially if surgery is required, and anticoagulants, which may need reversal.

Examination: primary survey

ATLS guidelines address a fundamental priority, ensuring uninterrupted perfusion of the brain with oxygenated blood. This is especially important after a head injury given the disturbance to intracranial autoregulation and the sensitivity of the primary injured brain tissue to further insult. Bleeding from scalp lacerations may require management as part of the primary survey, as the blood loss can be substantial and ongoing. Check the responsiveness of the pupils, conscious level and for any gross focal neurological deficits. Blood glucose level should also be measured as early as possible as hypoglycaemia is very dangerous and easily reversible.

Summary box 24.4

Primary survey

- Ensure adequate oxygenation and circulation
- Exclude hypoglycaemia
- Check pupil size and response and Glasgow Coma Scale score as soon as possible
- Check for focal neurological deficits before intubation, if possible

Pupils

The pupil size should be recorded in millimetres, and reactivity documented as present, sluggish or absent. Uncal herniation (Figure 24.2) can compress the third nerve, compromising the parasympathetic supply to the pupil. Unopposed sympathetic activity produces a sluggish enlarged pupil, progressing to fixed and dilated under continued compression. Established pupil changes may reflect pathology anywhere in the eye or the reflex loop made up by the optic nerve, the oculomotor nerve and the brainstem. Direct ocular trauma or nerve injury in association with a skull base fracture can cause mydriasis (dilated pupil) present from the time of injury. Pre-existing discrepancy in pupil size (anisocoria), as a result of Holmes–Adie pupil or cataracts for example, may also complicate assessment.

Glasgow Coma Scale score

The GCS is the sum of scores on three components as detailed in *Table 24.4*. The breakdown of the GCS into eye opening, verbal and motor components should always be recorded and used when communicating the status to other doctors. Remember that the score represents the best performance elicited, so a patient flexing in response to a painful stimulus on the left and localising on the right scores 'M5'. A sternal or supraorbital rub, or trapezius squeeze represents an appropriate painful stimulus.

Neurological deficit

Gross focal neurological deficits, such as paraplegia, may be evident at the primary survey, and an assessment to exclude such deficit should be carried out, especially if the patient is to

TABLE 24.4 Glasgow Coma Scale score for head injury.

Eyes open	Spontaneously	4
	To verbal command	3
	To painful stimulus	2
	Do not open	1
Verbal	Normal oriented conversation	5
	Confused	4
	Inappropriate/words only	3
	Sounds only	2
	No sounds	1
	Intubated patient	T
Motor	Obeys commands	6
	Localises to pain	5
	Withdrawal/flexion	4
	Abnormal flexion	3
	Extension	2
	No motor response	1

Sir Gordon Morgon Holmes, 1876–1965, physician, The National Hospital for Nervous Diseases, Queen's Square, London, UK.
William John Adie, 1886–1935, physician, The National Hospital for Nervous Diseases, Queen's Square, London, UK.

be intubated so that subsequent examination will be impossible. Detailed neurological examination is included in the secondary survey.

Examination: secondary survey

A full secondary survey will be required. Particular attention must be paid to head, neck and spine.

Head

Examination of the head should include inspection and palpation of the scalp for evidence of subgaleal haematoma and scalp lacerations, which may bleed profusely, and potentially overlie fractures. Examine the face for evidence of fractures, especially to the orbital rim, zygoma and maxilla. Clinical evidence of a skull base fracture may include Battle's sign (Figure 24.3), and 'racoon' or 'panda' eyes (bilateral periorbital bruising). Haemotympanum, or overt bleeding from the ear if the tympanic membrane has ruptured, and CSF rhinnorrhoea or otorrhoea are also highly suggestive of a fracture of the base of the skull.

A complete examination of the cranial nerves will reveal, for example, facial or vestibulo-cochlear nerve damage associated with skull base fracture. Midbrain or brainstem dysfunction may produce gaze paresis (inability of eye to look across beyond the midline), dysconjugate gaze (inability of the eyes to work together) or roving eye movements. Inspect the conjunctiva and cornea of the eyes, and the retina using an ophthalmoscope, looking for hyphaema (blood in the anterior chamber of the eye), papilloedema or retinal detachment. Blood in the mouth may be due to tongue-biting at seizure. The GCS and pupil status, assessed as part of the primary survey, require re-evaluation at the secondary survey and regularly thereafter.

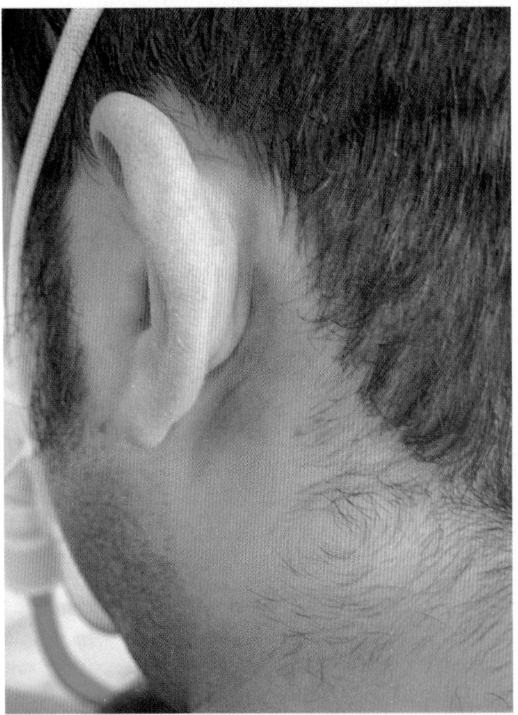

Figure 24.3 Battle's sign. A skull base fracture may be associated with bruising over the mastoid process.

Neck and spine

Studies have demonstrated an incidence of cervical fracture of up to 10% in association with moderate and severe TBI. Cervical spine injury must be presumed in the context of head injury until actively excluded. In a high-energy mechanism such as RTA or fall from a height, thoracic and lumbar spine injuries must also be excluded. Plain radiographs can be of limited value in excluding significant cervical spine injury. Even CT imaging does not exclude the possibility of significant ligamentous injury. Therefore, whenever feasible, these patients should be managed in a hard collar until the neck can be cleared clinically.

A peripheral nerve examination with documentation of limb tone, power, reflexes and sensation needs to be performed early to identify spinal pathology. This is especially important in patients who may subsequently be intubated and ventilated, when this assessment will no longer be possible. Obtunded patients should move all four limbs in response to an appropriate painful stimulus.

The patient will need to be log-rolled to palpate for thoracic or lumbar deformity, and any cervical collar should be removed at this stage to allow palpation of the cervical spine, before it is replaced. If there is associated spinal injury, a thoracic sensory level is much more easily established by sensory examination on the back. A per rectal examination is also performed at log-roll, assessing for anal tone, sensation in the awake patient and anal wink (sphincter seen to contract in response to a pinprick stimulus). Priapism is a strong predictor of severe cord injury even in intubated patients.

Summary box 24.5

Secondary survey

- Battle's sign, periorbital bruising and blood in ears/nose/mouth may point to base of skull fracture
- Cervical spine fractures are common and must be actively excluded
- Log-roll to check whole spine for steps and tenderness, and for per rectum exam

Surgical management

Fractures: skull vault

Closed linear fractures of the skull vault are managed conservatively. Open or comminuted fractures should be considered for debridement and prophylactic antibiotic therapy.

William Henry Battle, 1855–1936, surgeon, St Thomas's Hospital, London, UK.
A racoon is a small mammal native to North and Central America that has a pale face with dark rings round its eyes.

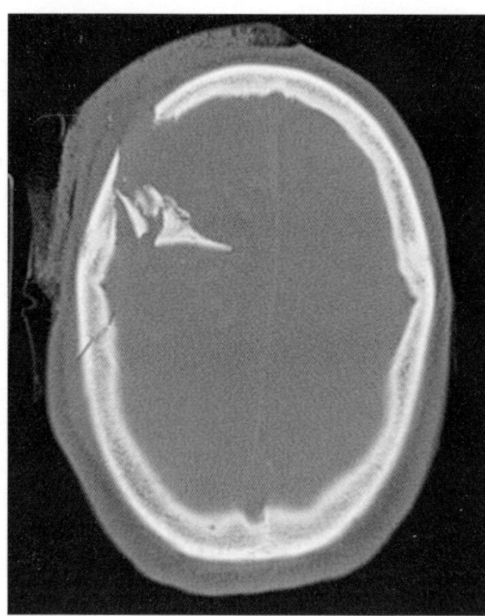

Figure 24.4 A right frontal comminuted depressed skull fracture, with a linear undisplaced fracture of the right parietal bone visible posteriorly.

Depressed skull fractures involve inward displacement of a bone fragment by at least the thickness of the skull (Figures 24.4 and 24.5). They occur when small objects hit the skull at high velocity. They are usually compound (open) fractures, and are associated with a high incidence of infection, neurological deficit and late-onset epilepsy. These fractures require exploration and elevation, especially where intracranial air is present pointing to a breach in the dura mater. Fractures that involve the air sinuses should generally be managed as open fractures, using broad spectrum antibiotics with or without exploration.

Fractures: skull base

Clinical signs of skull base fracture include bleeding or CSF leak from the ears (otorrhoea) or nose (rhinnorrhea), and bruising behind the ear (Figure 24.3) or around the eyes. Skull base fractures may be complicated by pituitary dysfunction, arterial dissection or cranial nerve deficits, with anosmia, facial palsy or hearing loss typical. CSF leak will generally resolve spontaneously but persistent leak can result in meningitis so repair may be required. Blind nasogastric tube placement is contraindicated in these patients.

Extradural haematoma

Extradural haematoma (Figure 24.6) is a neurosurgical emergency. It results from rupture of an artery, vein or venous sinus, in association with a skull fracture. The classical injury is a fracture to the thin squamous temporal bone, with associated damage to the middle meningeal artery. Transient loss of consciousness is typical, and the patient may then present in the subsequent lucid interval with headache but without any neurological deficit. As the haematoma expands, compensation is exhausted (see Monro Kellie doctrine above), with rapid deterioration. There is contralateral hemiparesis, reduced conscious level and ipsilateral pupillary dilatation, the cardinal signs of brain compression and herniation.

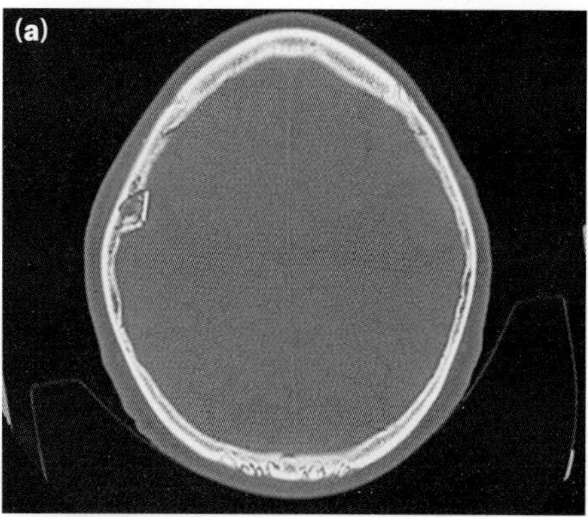

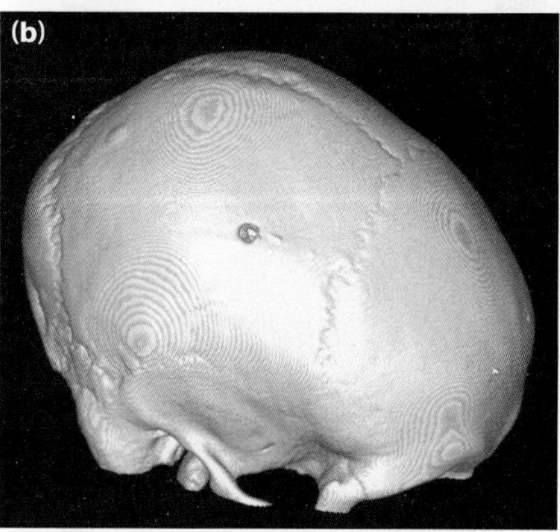

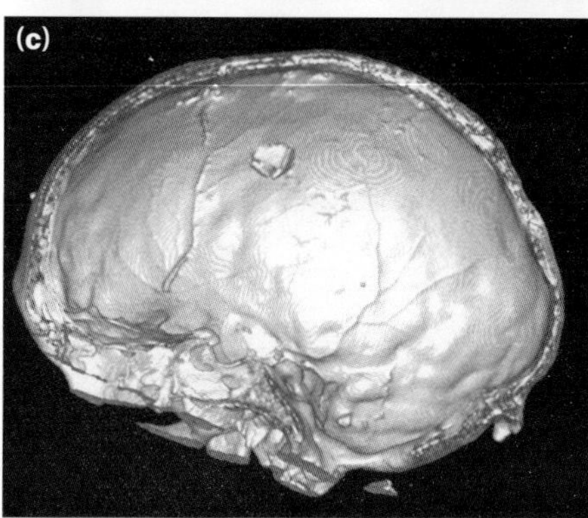

Figure 24.5 A small depressed skull fracture of the parietal bone visible on axial bone windows (a), visualised on bone vault reconstructions (b) and with an underlying breach of dura (c).

> **Summary box 24.6**
>
> **Extradural haemorrhage**
>
> - Can follow relatively minor trauma with brief loss of consciousness
> - Followed by a lucid interval and then sudden deterioration
> - Lentiform lesion on computed tomography
> - Require immediate transfer to a neurosurgical unit for decision on evacuation

Although this classical presentation occurs in only one-third of cases, it emphasises the potential for rapid avoidable

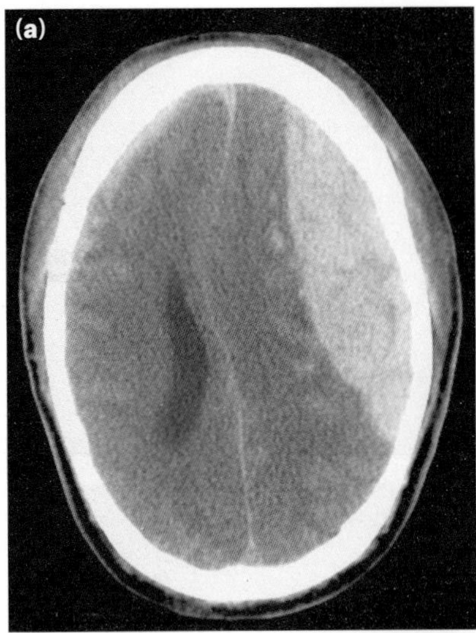

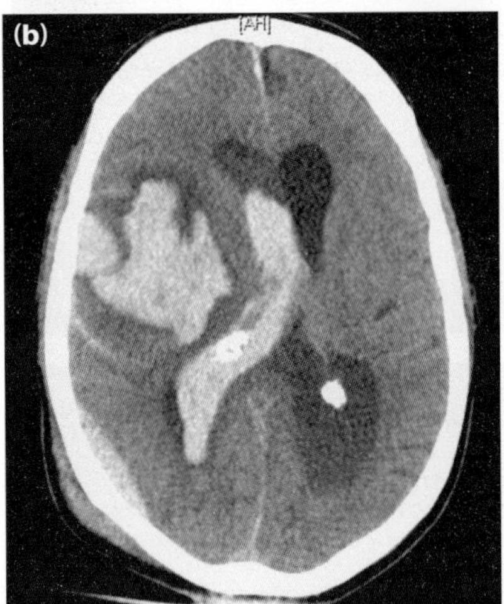

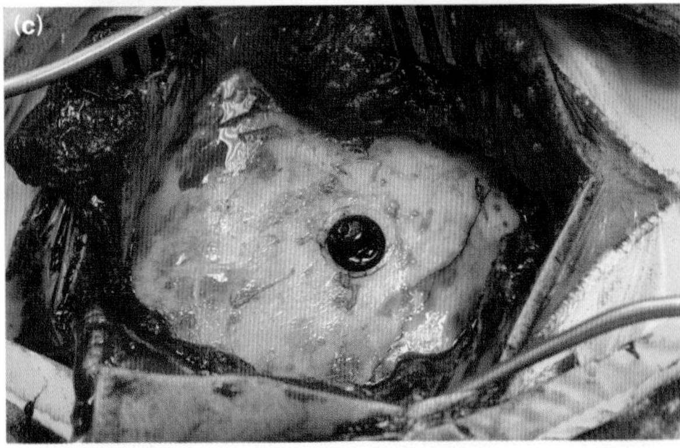

Figure 24.6 (a) A large left extradural haematoma (note the biconvex shape) exerts mass effect; a smaller right acute subdural haematoma is also evident. (b) Right frontal intracerebral haematoma extending into the lateral ventricle is evident. There is a small right posterior extradural haematoma and traumatic subarachnoid bleeding in the sulci of the right hemisphere. (c) A surgical temporal bone exposure showing a linear skull fracture with underlying extradural haematoma visible through a burr hole.

secondary brain injury in patients with minimal primary injury.

On CT, extradural haematomas appear as a lentiform (lens-shaped or biconvex) hyperdense lesion between skull and brain, constrained by the adherence of the dura to the skull. Mass effect may be evident, with compression of surrounding brain and midline shift. Areas of mixed density suggest active bleeding. A skull fracture will usually be evident. Extradural haematoma mandates urgent transfer to the most accessible neurosurgical facility, for immediate evacuation in deteriorating or comatose patients or those with large bleeds, and for close observation with serial imaging in other cases. The prognosis for promptly evacuated extradural haematoma, without associated primary brain injury, is excellent.

Acute subdural haematoma

Acute subdural haematoma (Figure 24.7a) is encountered in two broadly distinct contexts. Firstly, high-energy injury mechanisms can result in the rupture of cortical surface vessels with significant associated primary brain injury. This results in expanding haematoma with rapid deterioration and

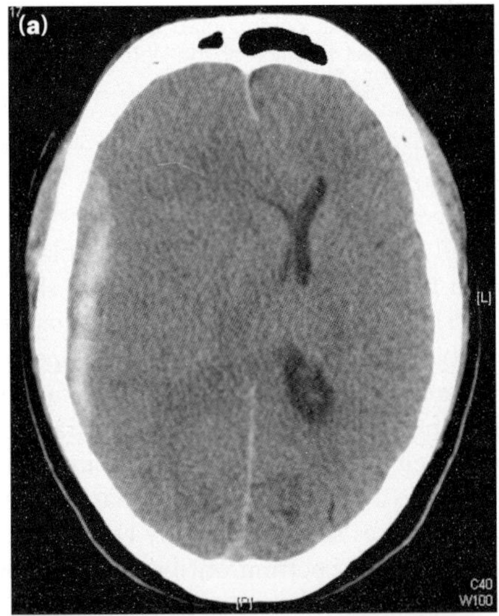

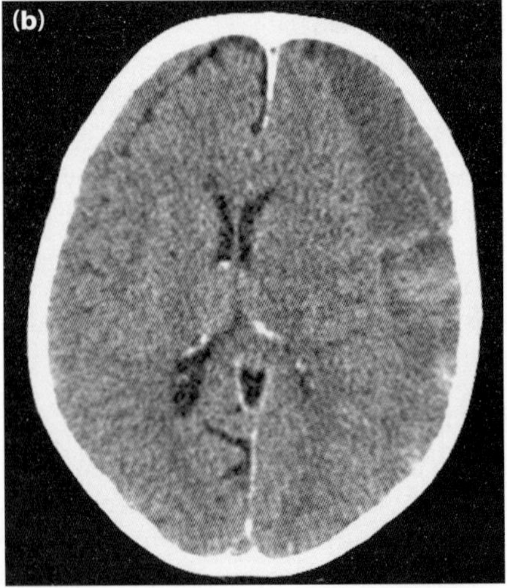

Figure 24.7 (a) Right-sided acute subdural haematoma (hyperdense). The substantial midline shift reflects brain swelling as well as bleeding; this is a high-energy injury. (b) Bilateral chronic subdural haematomas: the left is mixed density, the hypodense material representing old blood and the higher density indicating more recent bleeding, probably loculated so requiring a craniotomy to evacuate. The bleed on the right is isodense, indicating intermediate age.

developing signs of raised ICP, reminiscent of extradural haematoma without the lucid interval. These collections require prompt evacuation, typically by craniotomy or craniectomy.

In a second group of patients, older and often anticoagulated, a lower-energy injury leads to venous bleeding around the brain. Depending on the total volume of bleeding, the resulting haematoma may present early as acute subdural haematoma, after delay and osmotic expansion as chronic subdural haematoma or may even remain clinically silent. This latter group may present much later with a further 'acute-on-chronic' subdural haematoma. On diagnosis, clotting function should be corrected wherever possible. Bleeds of significant size, with significant associated midline shift or with deteriorating neurology, require urgent evacuation. Smaller bleeds in neurologically stable patients may be managed conservatively, at least initially: liquefaction of the clot over 7–10 days after the bleed may allow for a much less invasive evacuation through burr holes.

Summary box 24.7

Acute subdural haemorrhage

- High-energy injury, or elderly/anticoagulated
- Generally requires urgent evacuation by craniotomy/craniectomy

Since the dura is not adherent to the brain as it is to the skull, subdural blood is free to expand across the brain surface giving a diffuse concave appearance.

Chronic subdural haematoma

Chronic subdural haematoma (Figure 24.7b) is a common cause of acute neurological deterioration in the elderly. Cerebral atrophy in this age group results in stretching of cortical–dural bridging veins, which are then vulnerable to rupture. The resulting haematoma can expand over days or weeks by osmosis, ultimately producing symptoms of raised ICP or focal deficits. There is usually a history of recent injury, but especially in the context of antiplatelet or anticoagulant medication even apparently trivial impacts may be responsible.

Summary box 24.8

Chronic subdural haemorrhage

- Common in the elderly especially those on anticoagulants
- Clinical deficits result from osmotic expansion of a degrading clot over days/weeks
- Diffuse hypodense lesion on computed tomography
- Burr hole drainage is usually preferred.

On presentation, it is important to exclude coexisting electrolyte disturbance and infections, which may contribute to clinical impairment. Imaging reveals diffuse hypodensity overlying the brain surface. Recent bleeding may be isodense or hyperdense, and mixed density can indicate an acute-on-chronic subdural haematoma.

Anticoagulation should be reversed, either by administration of vitamin K, or urgently by transfusion of recombinant clotting factors in patients who have deteriorated acutely. Conservative management, sometimes with administration of corticosteroids, can be considered for small bleeds without symptoms or with headache alone. For the majority, drainage is performed using burr holes. Urgency is dictated by the clinical condition of the patient and imaging evidence of mass effect. If clinically stable, a delay of 7–10 days may be considered to allow platelet function to normalise after withdrawal of aspirin/clopidogrel.

Traumatic subarachnoid haemorrhage

Trauma is the commonest cause of subarachnoid haemorrhage (Figures 24.6b, 24.8), and this is managed conservatively. It is not usually associated with significant vasospasm, which characterises aneurysmal subarachnoid haemorrhage (see later). The possibility of spontaneous subarachnoid haemorrhage leading to collapse and so causing a head injury needs to be borne in mind, and formal or CT angiography may be required to exclude this.

Summary box 24.9

Specific head injuries

- Traumatic vs. primary subarachnoid haemorrhage is an important distinction
- Cerebral contusions arise adjacent to rough bone surfaces
- Diffuse axonal injury results from extreme accelerations of the skull contents
- Arterial dissection is associated with fractures of the skull base

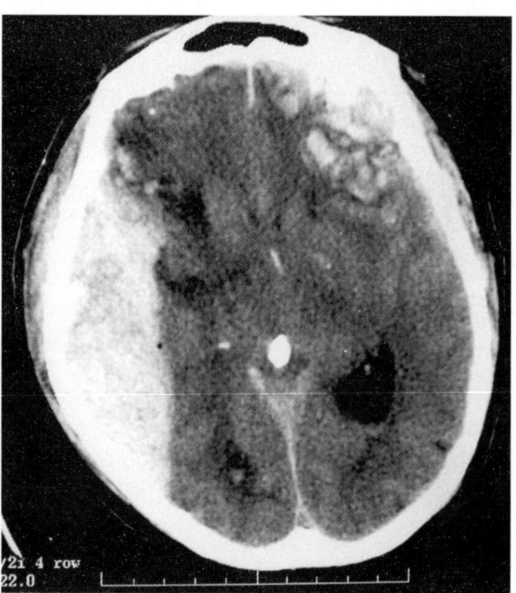

Figure 24.8 A large right extradural haematoma is evident. There are widespread cerebral contusions most prominent in the left frontal lobe. There is traumatic subarachnoid blood in the third and lateral ventricles.

Cerebral contusions

Contusions are common and are found predominantly where brain is in contact with the irregularly ridged inside of the skull, i.e. at the inferior frontal lobes and temporal poles. 'Coup contre-coup' contusions are brain injury at the site of impact and where the brain is struck by the inside of the skull on the far side, as the skull and brain accelerate and then decelerate out of synchrony with each other. Contusions appear heterogenous on CT, reflecting their composition of injured brain matter interspersed with acute blood (**Figure 24.8**). Contusions rarely require surgical intervention, but may warrant delayed evacuation to reduce mass effect.

Diffuse axonal injury

This is a form of primary brain injury, seen in high-energy accidents, and which usually renders the patient comatose. It is strictly a pathological diagnosis made at postmortem, but haemorrhagic foci in the corpus callosum and dorsolateral rostral brainstem on CT may be suggestive, although the CT often appears normal.

Arterial dissection

Cerebral arterial dissection occurs spontaneously or in the context of trauma. In the hours after significant trauma, dissection of the carotid extracranially, or at the skull base in association with fractures, is most common. It presents with headache, neck pain and focal ischaemic deficits, due to occlusion by mural haematoma, thrombus and thromboembolism. Intracranial dissection often affects the vertebral artery and may result in subarachnoid bleeding.

Medical management

From initial resuscitation, through surgical intervention and into the subsequent phase of intensive care management, medical management strategies aim to minimise secondary brain injury, through avoidance of hypoxia and hypotension and control of ICP. Unchecked, secondary injury leads to a further cycle of deterioration (**Figures 24.2 and 24.9**).

Summary box 24.10

Medical management of head injury

- First-line ICP control involves optimising sedation, ventilation and serum sodium levels
- Paralysis and external ventricular CSF drainage are important adjuncts
- There is little evidence for benefit with therapeutic hypothermia, barbiturate coma or decompressive craniectomy
- Check pituitary function, consider seizure prophylaxis, commence enteral nutrition within 72 hours

The role of neurosurgical centres

Early discussion of patients and imaging with the regional neurosurgical service is advisable. UK trauma audit and research network data show higher mortality in patients with severe TBI managed in non-neurosurgical centres, and this is reflected in NICE guidelines, which recommend early transfer irrespective of the need for surgery.

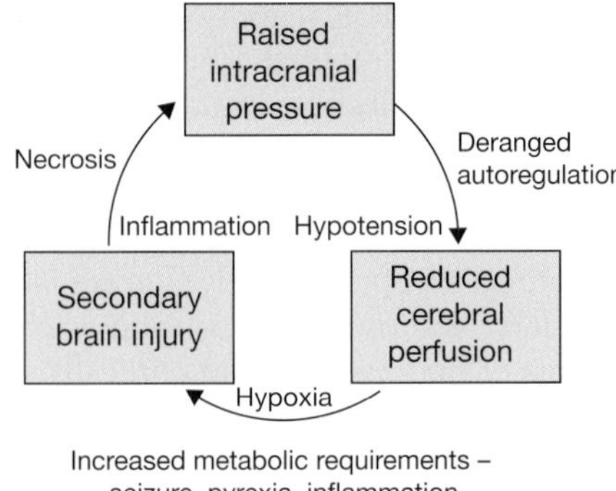

Figure 24.9 Brain swelling and mass lesions contribute to a raised intracranial pressure, which compromises perfusion, leading to secondary brain injury and further swelling.

Control of intracranial pressure

Intubation and ventilation is required early in the management of severe brain injury for airway control. It is often required in moderate brain injury to facilitate the safe management and transfer of unstable and frequently agitated patients and in order to control ICP. UK trauma audit and research network data indicate that severe TBI survival is better in a neurosurgical centre, irrespective of the need for surgery. Where there is evidence of raised ICP, for example pupil changes, a bolus of mannitol may be administered to control pressure temporarily while scanning and transferring the patient.

Management of the intubated patient, following evacuation of any focal haematomas, is guided by ICP monitoring using a bolt ICP monitor, or else an external ventricular drain inserted into the lateral ventricle, which can also contribute to ICP control by permitting CSF drainage. A sustained rise of ICP over 20–25 mmHg above normal is associated with a poor outcome, and maintenance of a cerebral perfusion pressure of at least 60 mmHg is important in preventing secondary injury.

ICP can be controlled by simple measures including raising the head of the bed and loosening the collar to improve venous drainage. Seizures and pyrexia should be actively controlled. Medical management titrated to ICP includes escalating doses of sedatives, analgesics and ultimately muscle relaxants. Target ventilatory and circulatory parameters are set out in *Table 24.5*.

Where these measures fail, neurointensivists may seek to control brain swelling using mannitol or hypertonic saline infusions. Where autoregulation is preserved, inducing high cerebral perfusion pressure may reduce ICP through vasoconstriction. A range of further interventions are effective in controlling ICP, but evidence for long-term outcome benefit is limited or absent. These include induction of therapeutic hypothermia or thiopentone coma and surgical decompressive craniectomy.

TABLE 24.5 Key parameters to maintain in head-injured patients in neurointensive care.
pCO_2 = 4.5–5.0 kPa
pO_2>11 kPa
MAP = 80–90 mmHg
ICP <20 mmHg
CPP >60 mmHg
[Na^+] >140 mmol/L
[K^+] >4 mmol/L

Pituitary dysfunction

Electrolyte imbalance is common in TBI, and contributes to brain swelling and to causing seizures. Diverse mechanisms are involved. Cerebral salt wasting, a poorly understood form of excretory dysregulation in association with brain insult, leads to volume depletion and hyponatraemia. The syndrome of inappropriate antidiuretic hormone (SIADH) leads to a water retention and hyponatraemia in the context of pituitary damage. This is of particular concern in head injury since low serum osmotic pressure can contribute to brain swelling, so hypotonic fluids are avoided in this setting. Conversely, ADH secretion may be compromised in the context of trauma, producing diabetes insipidus resulting in hypernatraemia.

All aspects of pituitary function may be compromised in the setting of TBI. Routine screening of pituitary hormone levels and liaison with endocrinology is an important aspect of optimal medical management. Note that routine, rather than directed, administration of corticosteroids in severe head injury is associated with increased mortality and is not recommended.

Seizures

Seizures may occur early (within 7 days) or late. The cumulative probability is between 2% (mild TBI) and 60% (severe TBI with exacerbating features). Risk factors include injury severity, especially the presence of intracerebral haemorrhage, and depressed skull fractures and tears of the dura. Antiepileptics, typically phenytoin, are administered prophylactically to patients at high risk of seizures.

Nutrition

Enteral nutrition is preferred to intravenous parenteral nutrition on grounds of cost and associated complications, and should be commenced within 72 hours of injury. Prokinetics (e.g. metaclopramide, erythromycin) can be administered to promote absorption.

Outcomes and sequelae

The long-term sequelae of moderate and severe traumatic brain injury include headache, memory and cognitive impairments, contributing to the postconcussive syndrome described above. Rehabilitation represents a complex and prolonged multidisciplinary challenge. The Glasgow outcome score is used to quantify the degree of recovery achieved after head injury, especially for research purposes, and is detailed in *Table 24.6*. Good recovery implies independence and potential to return to work rather than a full return to previous capacity.

TABLE 24.6 Glasgow outcome score (GOS).	
Good recovery	5
Moderate disability	4
Severe disability	3
Persistent vegetative state	2
Dead	1

FURTHER READING

Greenberg MS. *Handbook of neurosurgery*, 8th edn. Stuttgart: Thieme Medical Publishers, 2016.

Samandouras G (ed). *The neurosurgeon's handbook*. Oxford: Oxford University Press, 2010.

Chapter 25

Neck and spine

Learning objectives

To be familiar with:

- The accurate assessment of spinal trauma
- The basic management of spinal trauma and the major pitfalls
- The pathophysiology and types of spinal cord injury
- The prognosis of spinal cord injury, factors affecting functional outcome and common associated complications

ANATOMY OF THE SPINE AND SPINAL CORD

Spinal column anatomy

The vertebral column is composed of a series of motion segments (Figure 25.1). A motion segment consists of two adjacent vertebrae, their intervertebral disc and ligamentous restraints (Figure 25.2).

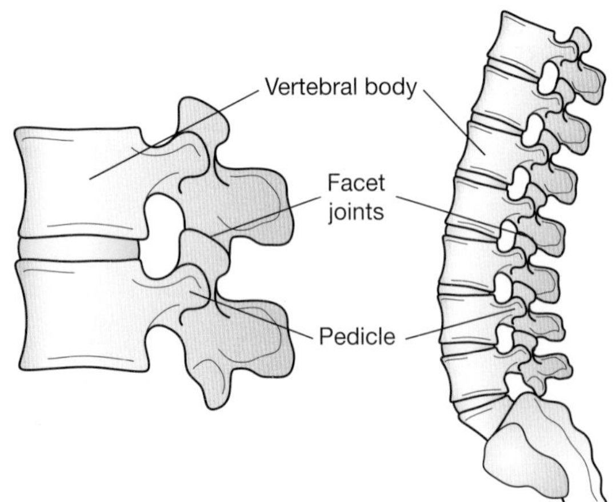

Figure 25.1 The spinal motion segment.

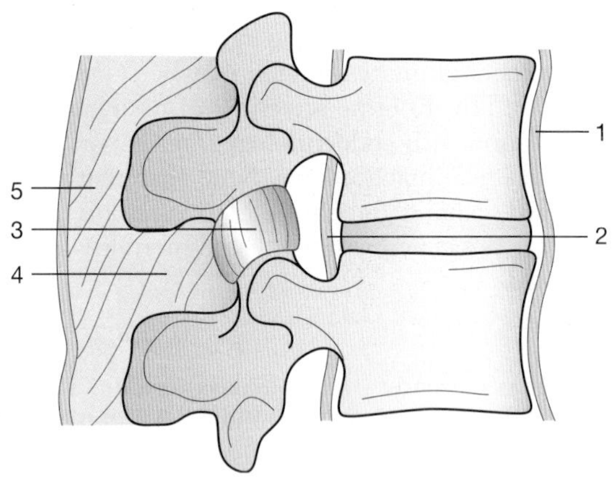

Figure 25.2 Ligamentous spinal restraints. (1) Anterior longitudinal ligament, (2) intervertebral disc and posterior longitudinal ligament, (3) facet joint capsule, (4) interspinous ligament, (5) supraspinous ligament.

Regional variations

Upper cervical spine anatomy is designed to facilitate motion (Figure 25.3), and stability here is dependent on ligamentous restraints (Figure 25.4). Vertebral anatomy from C3 to C7 is similar. The cervicothoracic (Figure 25.5) and thoracolumbar junctions (Figure 25.6) are transitional zones where the

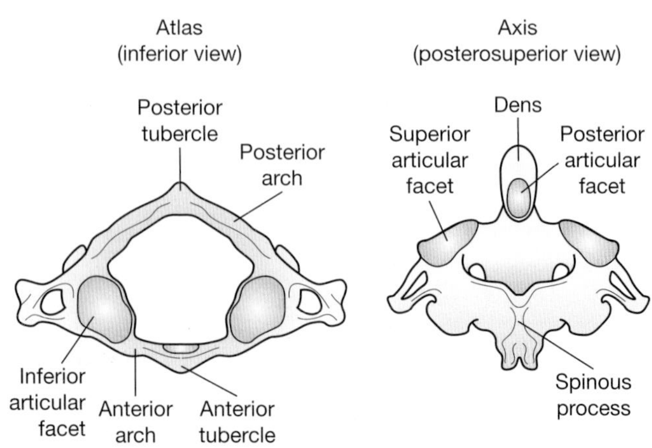

Figure 25.3 Atlantoaxial bony anatomy.

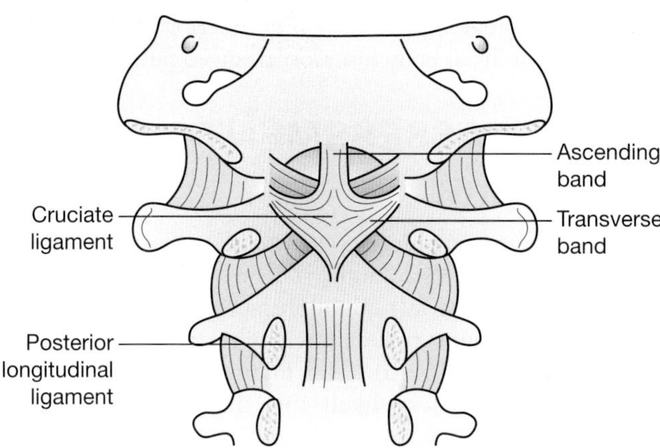

Figure 25.4 Atlantoaxial ligaments.

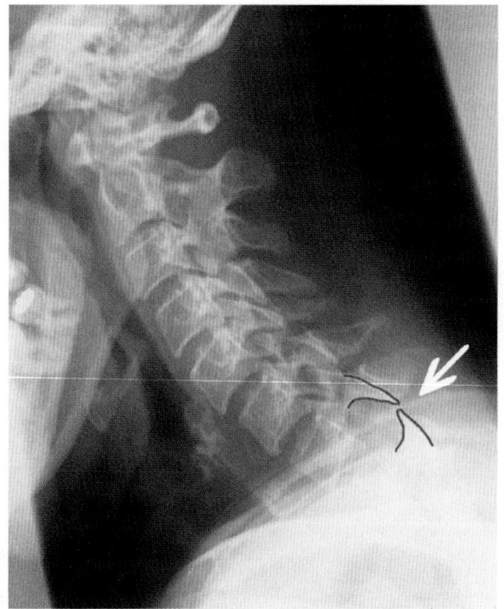

Figure 25.5 Cervicothoracic facet subluxation (arrow) (easily missed with inadequate x-rays).

spine changes from a mobile section (cervical and lumbar) to a more fixed one (thoracic). These two areas are common sites of injury.

Spinal stability

Spinal stability is the ability of the spine to withstand physiological loads with acceptable pain, avoiding progressive deformity or neurological deficit. The spinal column can be divided into three columns: anterior, middle and posterior (Figure 25.7) If two or more columns of the spine are injured the spine is considered unstable. The AO classifications (Magerl and AO Spine Subaxial Classification System) are based on the mechanism of injury and used to assess spinal stability.

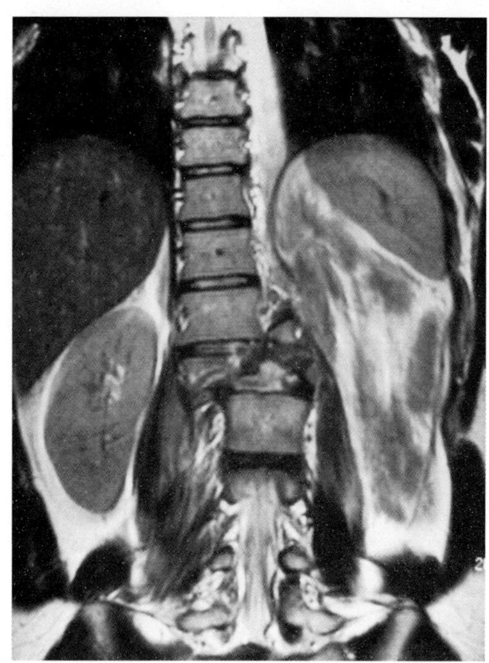

Figure 25.6 Coronal T2-weighted magnetic resonance image demonstrating a fracture dislocation at the thoracolumbar junction.

Summary box 25.1

Spinal column anatomy

- Upper cervical spine stability is dependent on ligamentous restraints
- The cervicothoracic and thoracolumbar junctions are common sites of injury

Spinal neuroanatomy

The spinal cord extends from the foramen magnum to the L1/L2 level, where it ends as the conus medullaris in adults (lower in children) (Figure 25.8). Below this level lies the cauda equina. Figure 25.9 illustrates a cross-section of the spinal

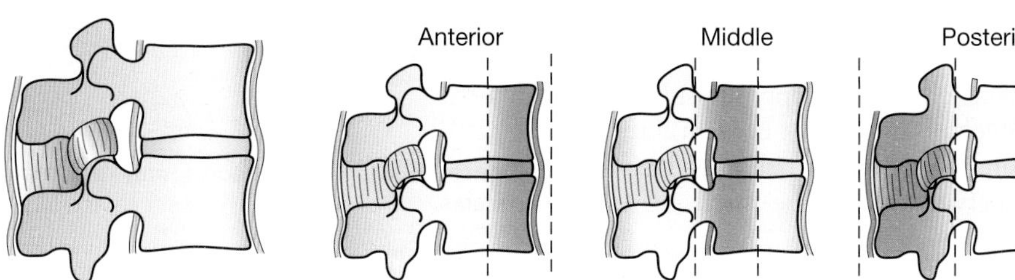

Figure 25.7 The three-column model of spinal stability.

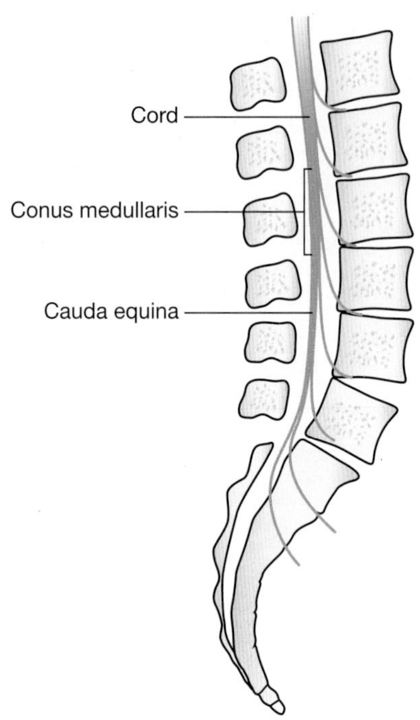

Figure 25.8 The spinal cord ends at T12/L1 at the conus medullaris, which gives rise to the cauda equina.

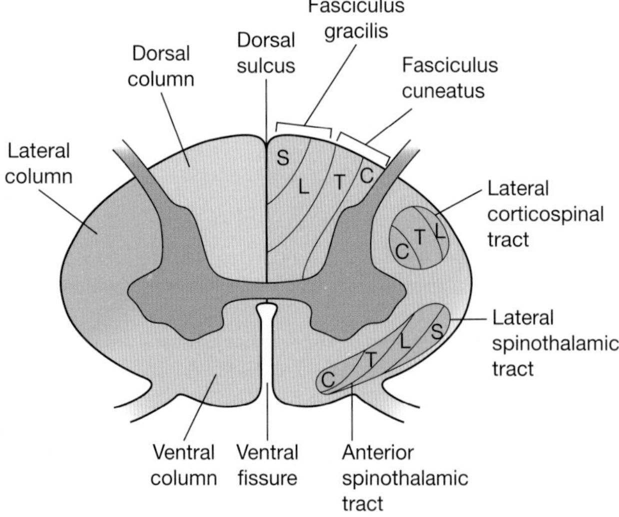

Figure 25.9 A cross-section of the spinal cord.

cord. The lateral spinothalamic tracts transmit the sensations of pain and temperature, the lateral corticospinal tracts are responsible for motor function and the posterior columns transmit position, vibration and deep pressure sensation.

The spinothalamic tracts cross to the opposite side of the spinal cord within three levels of entering the cord. In contrast, the corticospinal tracts and the posterior columns decussate proximally at the craniocervical level. The tracts are topographically arranged; proximal body function is represented centrally, with distal body function arranged peripherally.

PATIENT ASSESSMENT

Basic points

The advanced trauma life support (ATLS) principles apply in all cases (see Chapters 22 and 23). The spine should initially be immobilised using full spinal precautions, on the assumption that every trauma patient has a spinal injury until proven otherwise (Figure 25.10). The finding of a spinal injury makes it more (not less) likely that there will be a second injury at another level.

Spinal boards lead to skin breakdown in insensate patients, and are very uncomfortable for those with normal sensation (Figure 25.11). They should only be used for transferring patients.

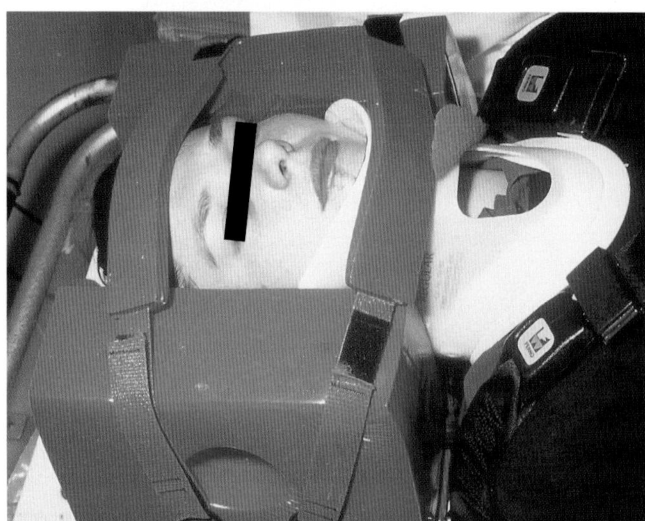

Figure 25.10 Spinal immobilisation.

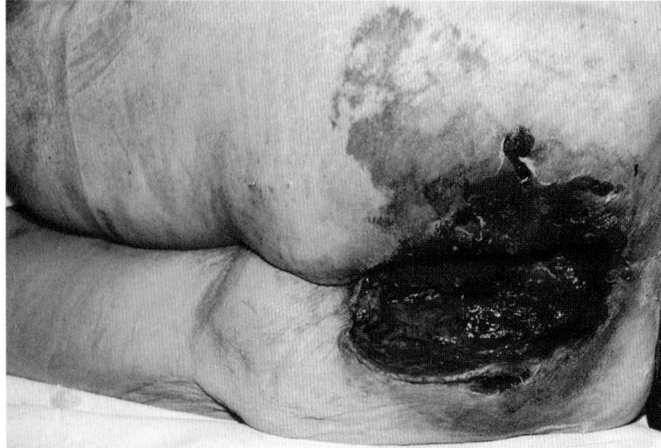

Figure 25.11 Pressure sores may develop rapidly in insensate patients.

The unconscious patient

Definitive clearance of the spine may not be possible in the initial stages and spinal immobilisation should then be maintained, until MRI or equivalent can be used to rule out an unstable spinal injury.

> **Summary box 25.2**
>
> Patient assessment
>
> - Use ATLS principles in all cases of spinal injury
> - In polytrauma cases suspect a spinal injury
> - A second spinal injury at a remote level may be present in 10% of cases
> - Spinal boards cause pressure sores

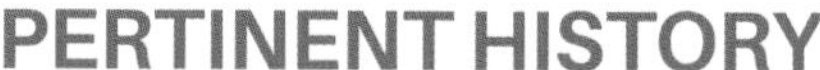

PERTINENT HISTORY

The mechanism and velocity of injury should be determined at an early stage. A check for the presence of spinal pain should be made. The onset and duration of neurological symptoms should also be recorded.

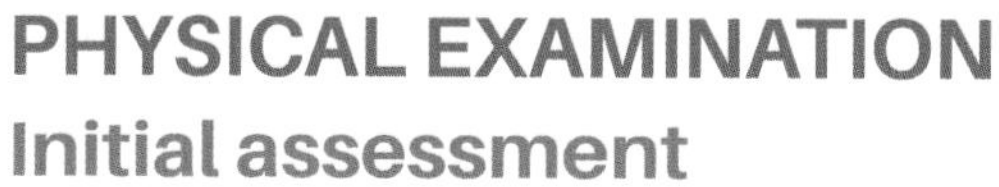

PHYSICAL EXAMINATION

Initial assessment

The primary survey always takes precedence, followed by a careful systems examination paying particular attention to the abdomen and chest. Spinal cord injury may mask signs of intra-abdominal injury.

Spinal examination

The overlying skin should be inspected (e.g. for possible penetrating wounds) and the entire spine must be palpated. A formal spinal log roll must be performed to achieve this (Figure 25.12). Significant swelling, tenderness, palpable steps or gaps suggest a spinal injury. A rectal examination should be undertaken to assess anal tone and perianal sensation (see Neurological examination). Seatbelt marks on the abdomen and chest must be noted, as these suggest a high-energy accident.

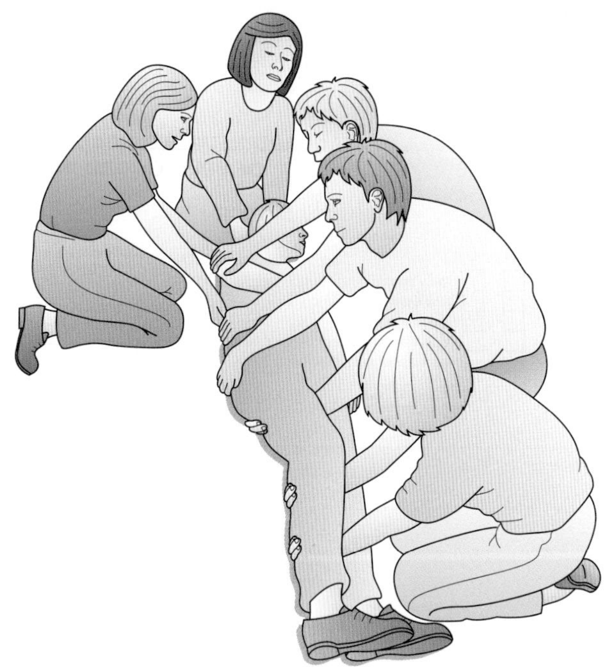

Figure 25.12 Spinal log roll.

Neurological examination

The American Spinal Injury Association (ASIA) neurological evaluation system (Figure 25.13) is an internationally accepted method of neurological evaluation.

Motor function is assessed using the Medical Research Council (MRC) grading system (0–5) in key muscle groups (Figure 25.13). A motor score can then be calculated (maximum 100).

Sensory function (light touch and pin prick) is assessed using the dermatomal map (Figure 25.13). A total sensory score is then calculated.

Rectal examination is performed to assess anal tone, voluntary anal contraction and perianal sensation.

Level of neurological impairment

The ASIA Neurological Impairment Scale is based on the Frankel classification of spinal cord injury:

- **A**: complete spinal cord injury;
- **B**: sensation present, motor absent;
- **C**: sensation present, motor present but not useful (MRC grade $<3/5$);
- **D**: sensation present, motor useful (MRC grade $\geq 3/5$);
- **E**: normal function.

> **Summary box 25.3**
>
> Physical examination
>
> - There are three types of shock following spinal cord injury
> - The ASIA neurological scoring system should be used
> - Functional motor power is grade 3/5 or higher

Hans Ludwig Frankel, formerly Clinical Director, The National Spinal Injuries Centre, Stoke Mandeville, Buckinghamshire, UK.

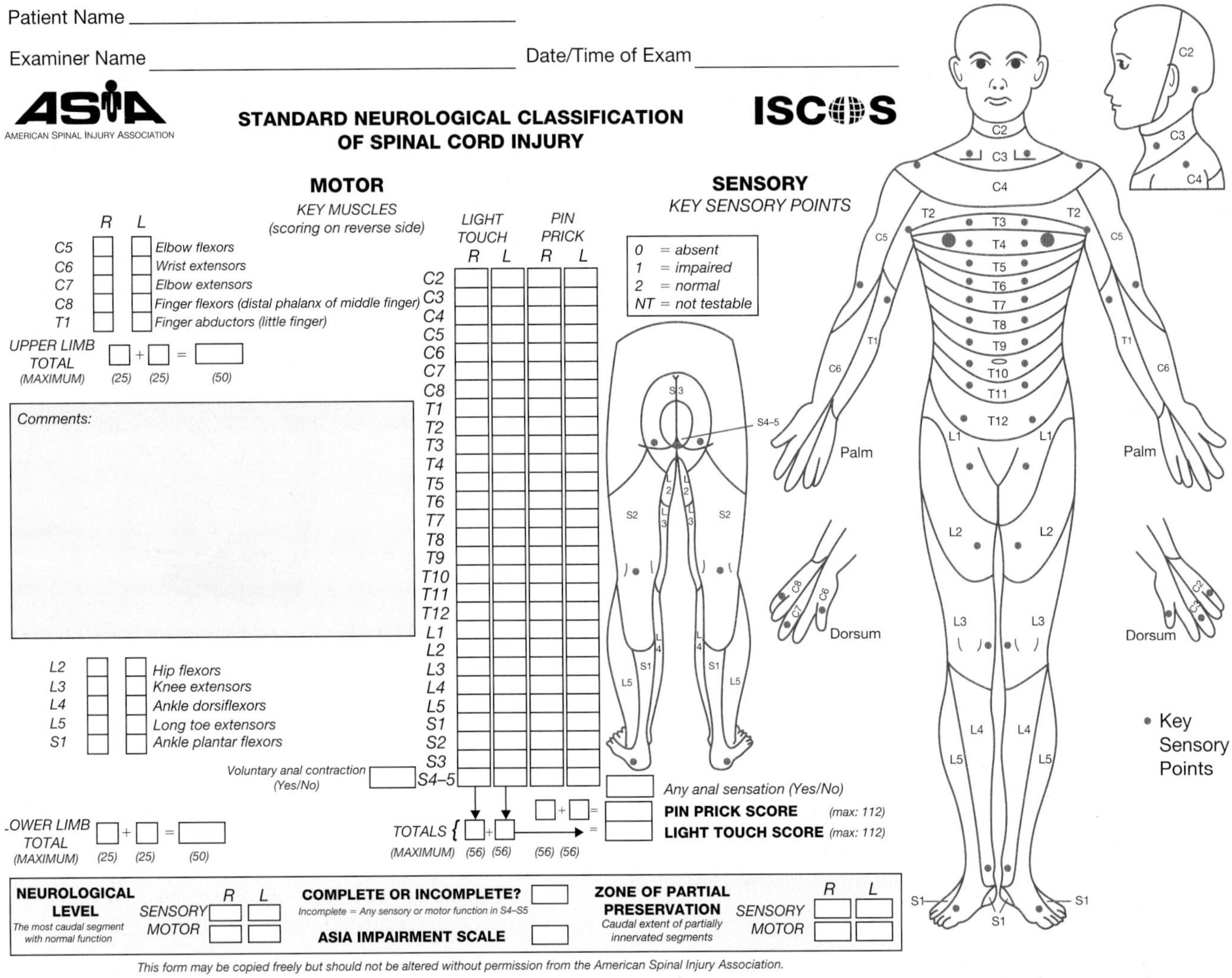

Patient Name ______________________

Examiner Name ______________________ Date/Time of Exam ______________

ASIA — AMERICAN SPINAL INJURY ASSOCIATION

STANDARD NEUROLOGICAL CLASSIFICATION OF SPINAL CORD INJURY

ISCOS

MOTOR
KEY MUSCLES (scoring on reverse side)

R L
C5 Elbow flexors
C6 Wrist extensors
C7 Elbow extensors
C8 Finger flexors (distal phalanx of middle finger)
T1 Finger abductors (little finger)

UPPER LIMB TOTAL (MAXIMUM) (25) + (25) = (50)

Comments:

L2 Hip flexors
L3 Knee extensors
L4 Ankle dorsiflexors
L5 Long toe extensors
S1 Ankle plantar flexors

Voluntary anal contraction (Yes/No)

LOWER LIMB TOTAL (MAXIMUM) (25) + (25) = (50)

SENSORY
KEY SENSORY POINTS

LIGHT TOUCH R L — PIN PRICK R L

C2, C3, C4, C5, C6, C7, C8, T1, T2, T3, T4, T5, T6, T7, T8, T9, T10, T11, T12, L1, L2, L3, L4, L5, S1, S2, S3, S4–5

0 = absent
1 = impaired
2 = normal
NT = not testable

TOTALS (MAXIMUM) (56) (56) (56) (56)

Any anal sensation (Yes/No)
PIN PRICK SCORE (max: 112)
LIGHT TOUCH SCORE (max: 112)

• Key Sensory Points

NEUROLOGICAL LEVEL — The most caudal segment with normal function — SENSORY R L / MOTOR R L

COMPLETE OR INCOMPLETE? — Incomplete = Any sensory or motor function in S4–S5

ASIA IMPAIRMENT SCALE

ZONE OF PARTIAL PRESERVATION — Caudal extent of partially innervated segments — SENSORY R L / MOTOR R L

This form may be copied freely but should not be altered without permission from the American Spinal Injury Association.

Figure 25.13 American Spinal Injury Association neurological evaluation.

DIAGNOSTIC IMAGING

Plain radiographs

A full cervical spine series includes anteroposterior and lateral radiographs of the whole cervical spine, and open mouth views. Clear visualisation of the cervicothoracic junction is essential in all cases of suspected spinal injury, as this is a common site for injury and often not seen on a plain radiograph. If a spinal fracture is identified then further imaging of the whole spine is required because there is a 15% incidence of a further spinal fracture.

A system for evaluation of the lateral cervical spine radiograph

1. Assess prevertebral soft tissue swelling (Figure 25.14).
2. Assess sagittal alignment using three imaginary lines (Figure 25.15).
3. Assess for instability (Figure 25.16):
   a. 3.5 mm of sagittal translation;
   b. Sagittal angulation of >11° (compared to adjacent level).

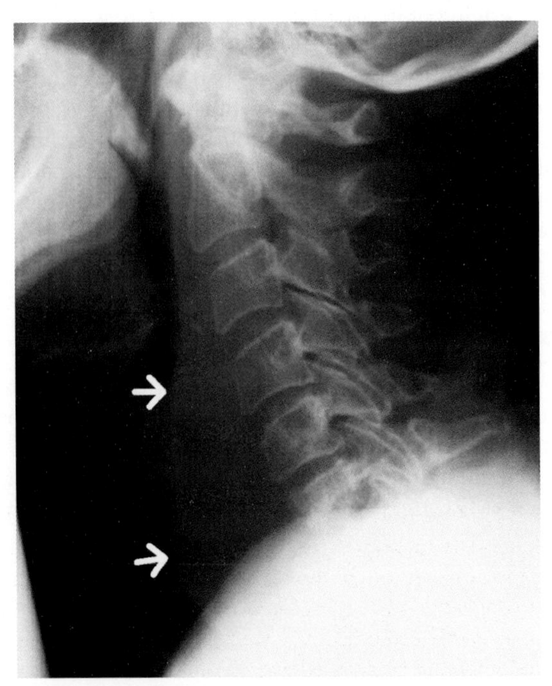

Figure 25.14 Large prevertebral haematoma (arrows).

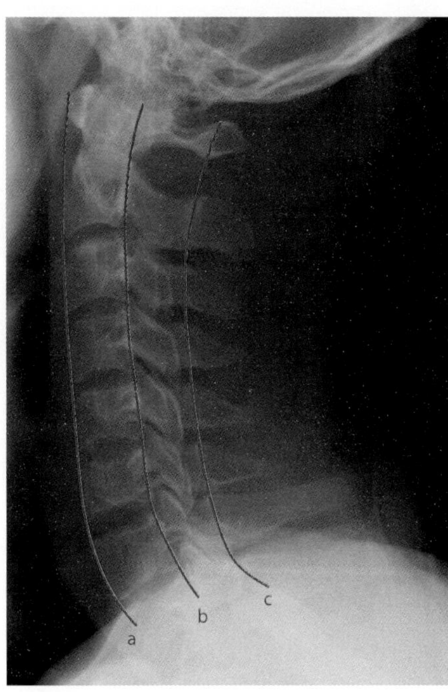

Figure 25.15 The anterior (**a**), posterior (**b**) and spinolaminar (**c**) lines are useful in identifying anterior translation on lateral x-rays of the neck.

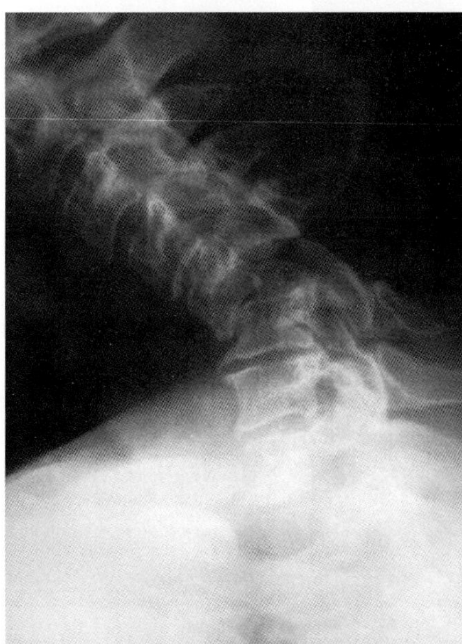

Figure 25.16 Lateral cervical spine x-ray showing obvious spinal instability with marked sagittal angulation and translation. This patient walked into the outpatient department.

Computed tomography

Computed tomography (CT) scanning with two-dimensional (2D) reconstruction remains the gold standard in spinal trauma and is indicated for patients with suspected or visible injuries on plain radiographs (Figure 25.17). Patients undergoing a head CT scan for closed head injury should also have a cervical screening CT. Often CT scans of the chest and abdomen are performed as part of the assessment of polytrauma patients and will usually include the spine.

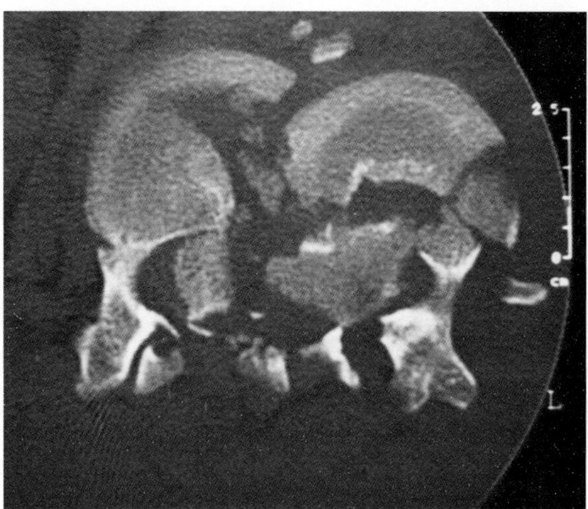

Figure 25.17 Axial computed tomography demonstrating a thoracolumbar fracture dislocation.

Magnetic resonance imaging

Magnetic resonance imaging (MRI) is indicated in all cases with neurological deficit and where assessment of ligamentous structures is important (Figure 25.18).

Dynamic imaging

Lateral flexion–extension radiographs of the cervical spine should not be undertaken acutely although they can have a role in assessing spinal stability in the longer term.

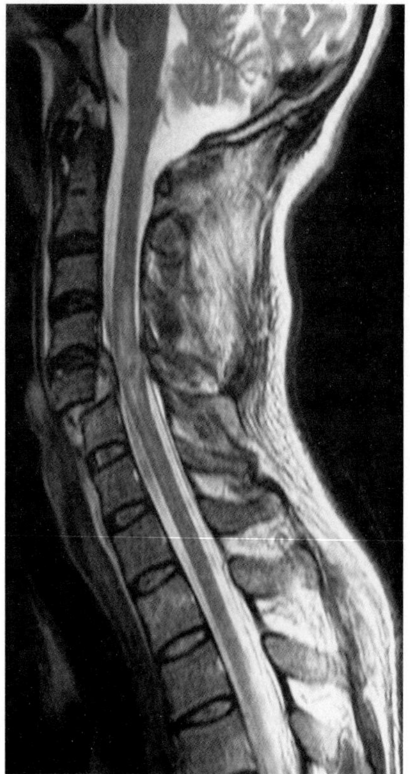

Figure 25.18 Sagittal T2-weighted magnetic resonance imaging scan demonstrating a cervical spine subluxation and spinal cord contusion.

Summary box 25.4

Diagnostic imaging of spinal injuries

- Clear visualisation of the cervicothoracic junction is mandatory
- Plain cervical spine radiographs fail to identity 15% of injuries

CLASSIFICATION AND MANAGEMENT OF SPINAL AND SPINAL CORD INJURIES

Basic management principles

Spinal realignment

In cases of cervical spine subluxation or dislocation, skeletal traction is necessary to achieve anatomical realignment. This is done using skull tongs (Figure 25.19).

In many cases of spinal trauma, formal open reduction and stabilisation using internal fixation is also required (Figure 25.20).

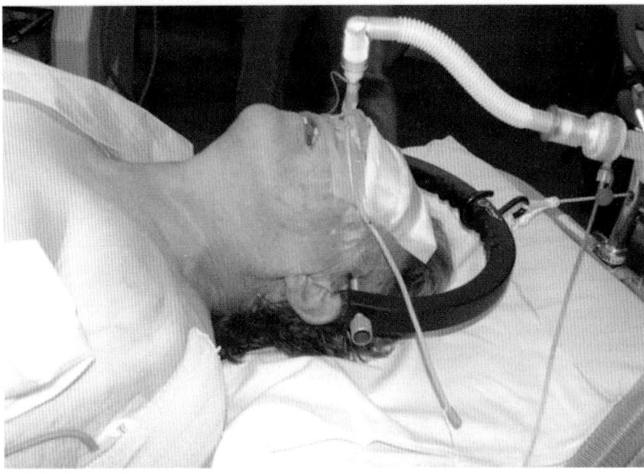

Figure 25.19 Skeletal traction using skull tongs.

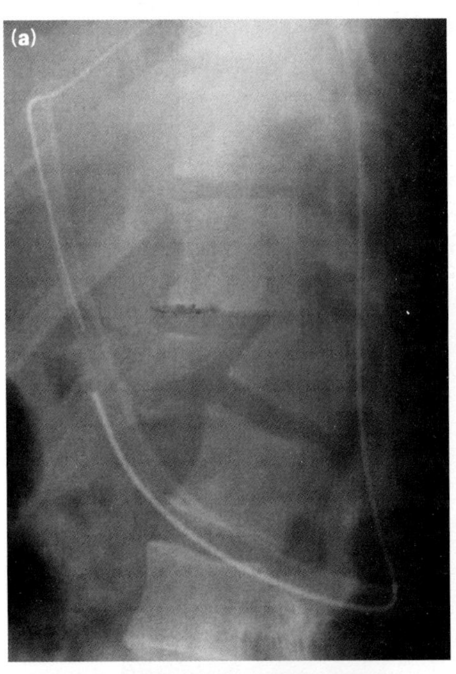

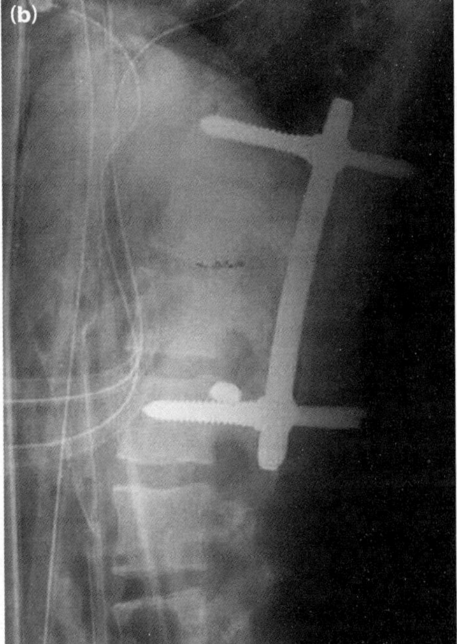

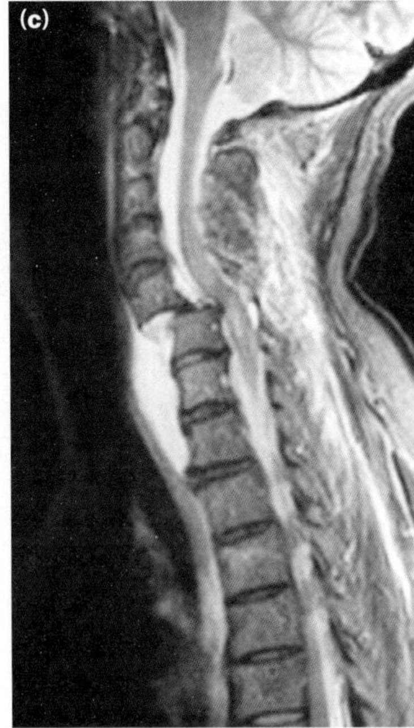

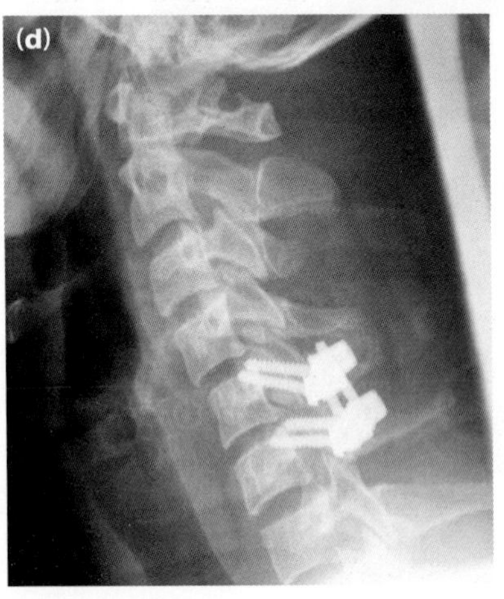

Figure 25.20 (a) Thoracolumbar fracture dislocation, (b) treated with open reduction and posterior fixation. (c) Bifacetal cervical spine dislocation. (d) Posterior stabilisation following closed reduction.

A halo brace can be used to perform a closed realignment and immobilisation of cervical fractures (Figure 25.21).

Stabilisation

The indication for operative intervention is influenced by the injury pattern, level of pain, degree of instability and the presence of a neurological deficit. The only absolute indication for surgery in spinal trauma is deteriorating neurological function.

Decompression of the neural elements

Realignment of the spine and correction of the spinal deformity may achieve an indirect decompression. A direct decompression of the neural elements may also be indicated if there are bone fragments causing residual compression or a significant haematoma (Figure 25.22). The timing of surgery in spinal cord trauma remains controversial.

Corticosteroids

Corticosteroids are no longer indicated in acute spinal cord injury because of a lack of evidence to support efficacy. Steroids do have a role in non-traumatic spinal cord compression e.g. malignant spinal cord compression (MSCC).

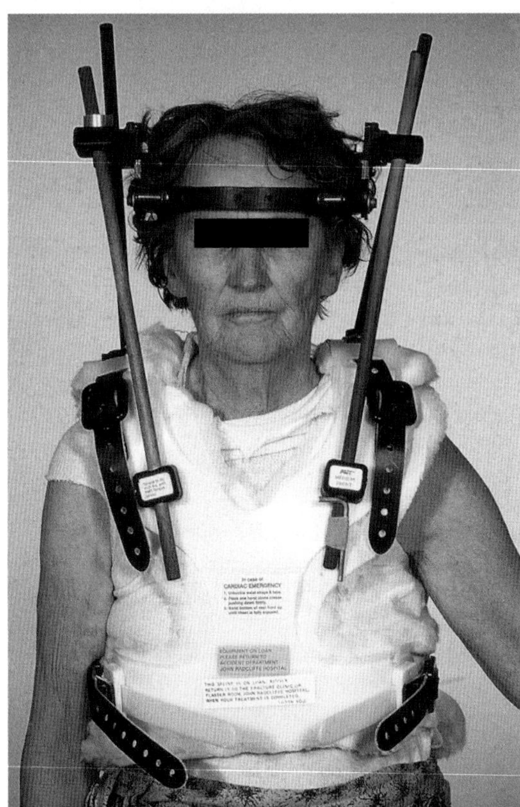

Figure 25.21 External immobilisation using a halo jacket.

> **Summary box 25.5**
>
> Management of spinal trauma
> - Neurological deficit determines management
> - Deteriorating neurological status requires surgical intervention
> - Corticosteroids are ineffective

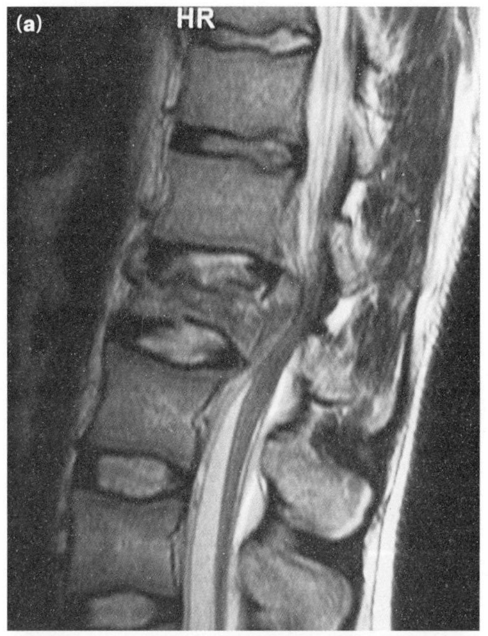

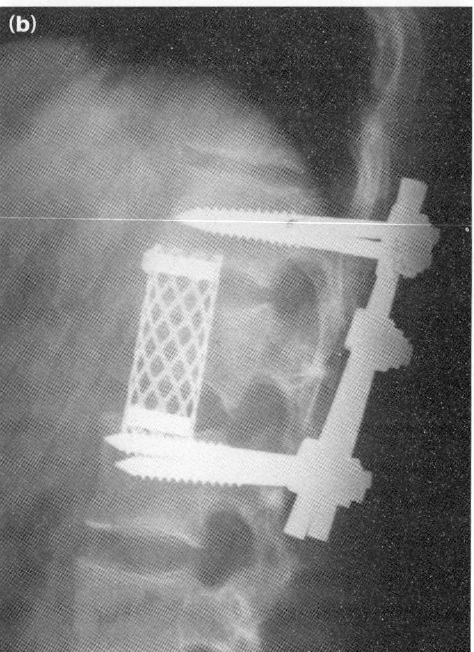

Figure 25.22 (a) Sagittal T2-weighted magnetic resonance imaging scan showing an L1 burst fracture and neural compression; (b) treated with combined anterior and posterior surgery.

SPECIFIC SPINAL INJURIES

Upper cervical spine (skull-C2)

Occipital condyle fracture

This is a relatively stable injury often associated with head injuries and is best treated in a hard collar for 6–8 weeks.

Occipitoatlantal dislocation

This injury is usually caused by high energy trauma and is often fatal. The dislocation may be anterior, posterior or vertical (Figure 25.23). Power's ratio (Figure 25.24) is used to assess skull translation. Treatment is with a halo brace or occipitocervical fixation.

Atlas fracture (Jefferson fracture)

Fracture of the C1 ring is associated with axial loading of the cervical spine and may be stable or unstable (Figure 25.25a, b). Associated transverse ligament rupture may occur (Figure 25.25c). Most are treated non-operatively in a cervical collar or halo brace.

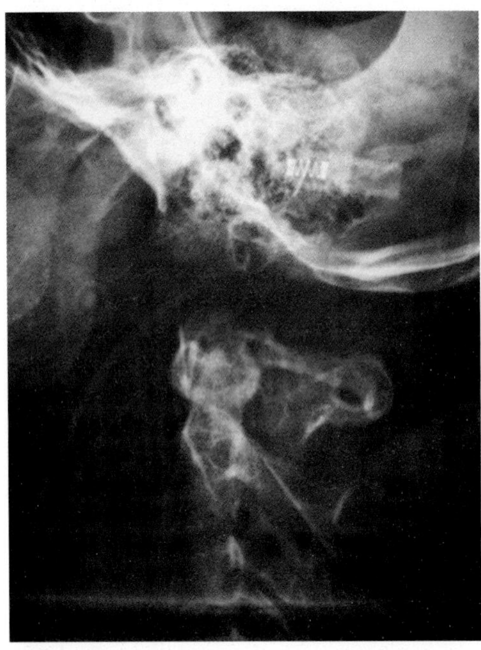

Figure 25.23 Vertical occipitocervical dislocation.

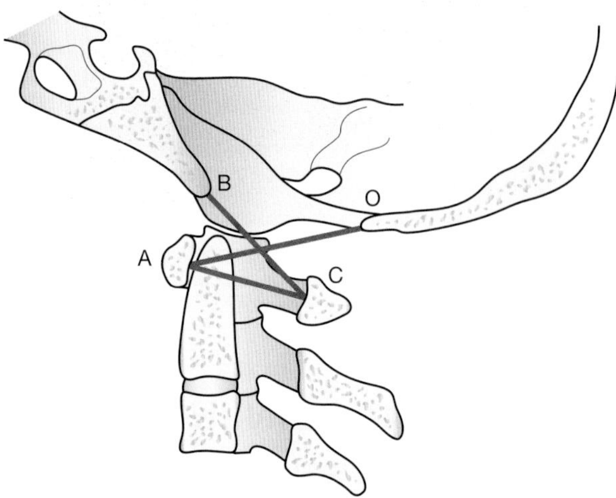

Figure 25.24 Power's ratio. BC/OA ≥1 indicates anterior translation, ≤0.75 indicates posterior translation.

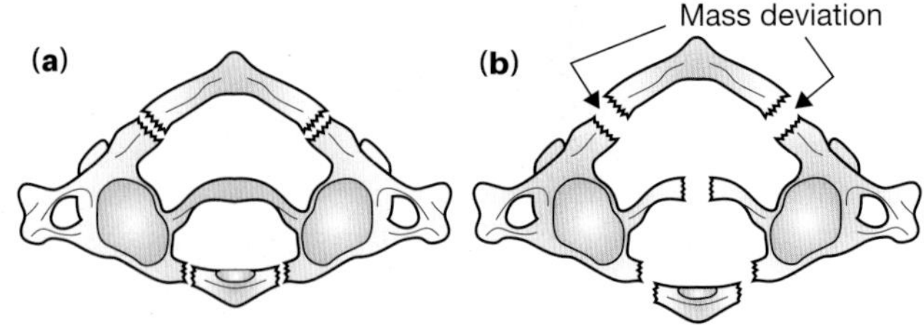

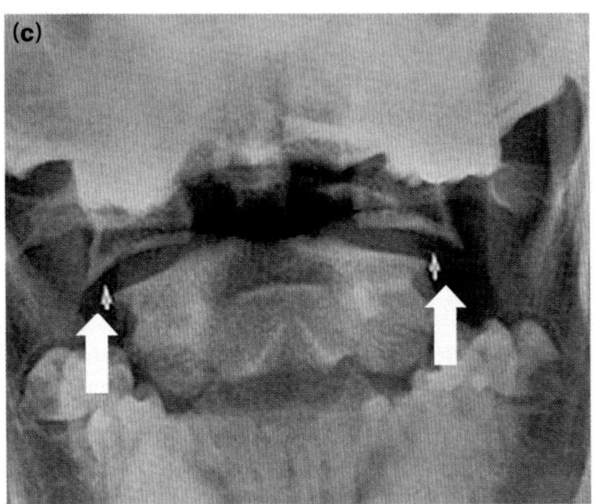

Figure 25.25 Stable (a) versus unstable (b) Jefferson's fracture of C1. (c) Open mouth view of C1/2 demonstrating C1 lateral mass deviation (arrows). Rupture of the transverse ligament is present when the combined lateral mass deviation exceeds 6.9 mm.

Atlantoaxial instability

This is defined as non-physiological movement between C1 and C2. It can be translational or rotatory and resolves either spontaneously or with traction followed by a cervical collar. Isolated, traumatic transverse ligament rupture leading to C1/2 instability is uncommon and is treated with posterior C1/2 fusion (Figure 25.26).

Odontoid fractures

There are three types of odontoid peg fracture (Figure 25.27). Neurological injury is rare. The majority of acute injuries are treated non-operatively in a hard collar or halo jacket for 3 months. Internal fixation with an anterior compression screw is indicated for displaced fractures (Figure 25.28), and a posterior C1/2 fusion is considered in cases of non-union. In the elderly, treatment in a soft collar should be considered on the basis that a relatively stable pseudarthrosis will occur.

Barry Powers, contemporary, Chief and Clinical Professor of Radiology, Duplin General Hospital, Kenansville, NC, USA, described his ratio in 1979.
Sir Geoffrey Jefferson, 1886–1961, Professor of Neurosurgery, University of Manchester, UK, became the UK's first Professor of Neurosurgery in 1939. In 1947 he was elected a Fellow of the Royal Society, a rare distinction for a practising surgeon. Although he became a neurosurgeon, he performed the first successful embolectomy in England in 1925 at Salford Royal Hospital.

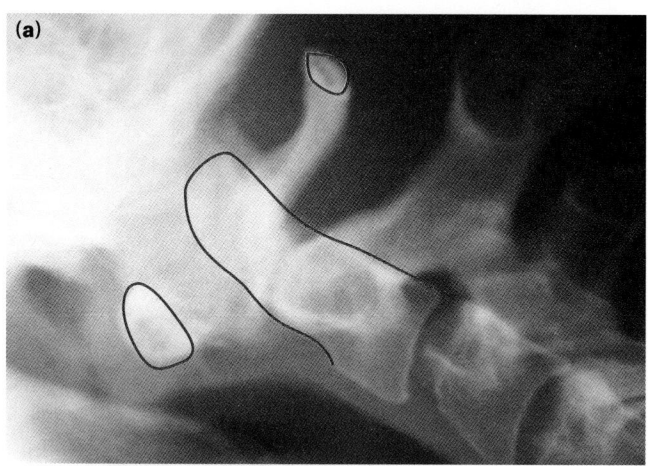

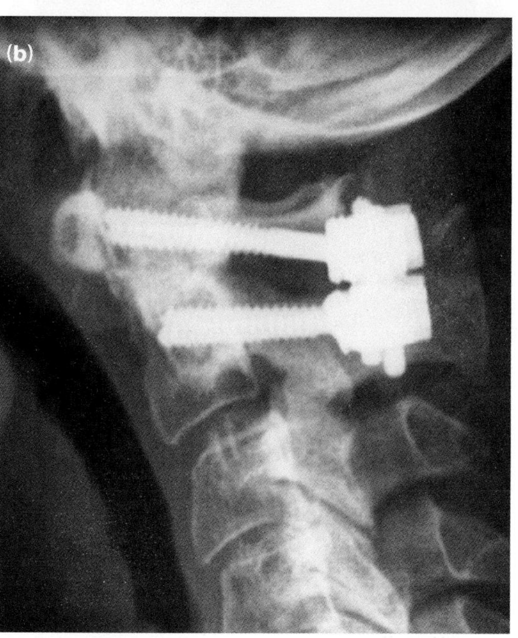

Figure 25.26 (a) Atlantoaxial subluxation. (b) C1/2 posterior fusion using C1 lateral mass and C2 pedicle screws.

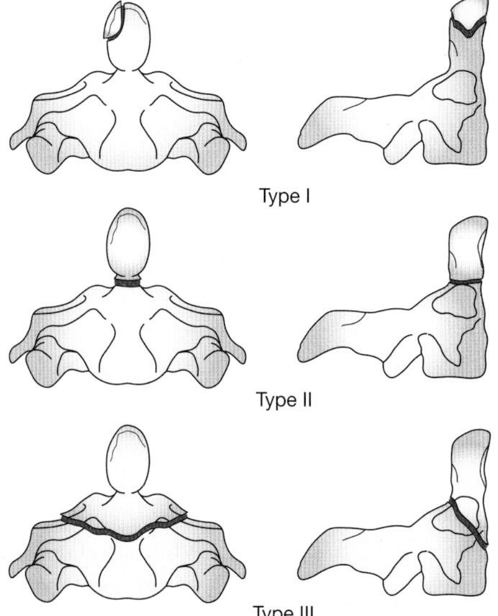

Figure 25.27 Types of odontoid fracture.

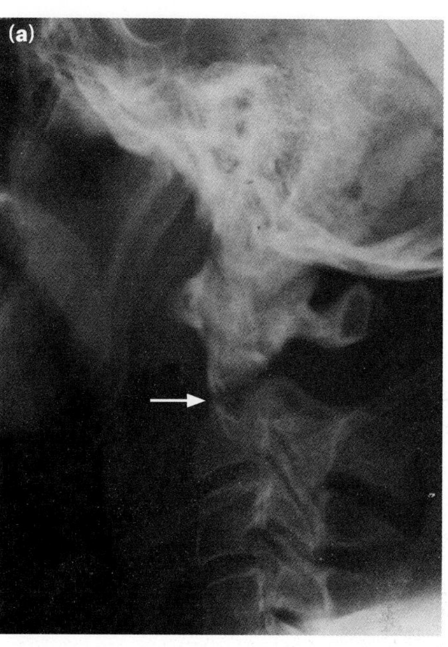

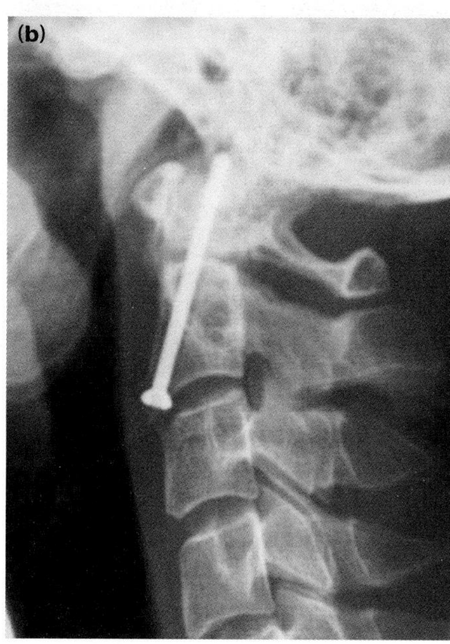

Figure 25.28 (a) Type II odontoid fracture (arrow); (b) treated with an anterior compression screw.

Traumatic spondylolisthesis of the axis (hangman's fracture)

This is a traumatic spondylolisthesis of C2 on C3. There a four types with varying degrees of instability (Figure 25.29). Those with significant displacement or associated facet dislocation are treated operatively, usually with posterior stabilisation.

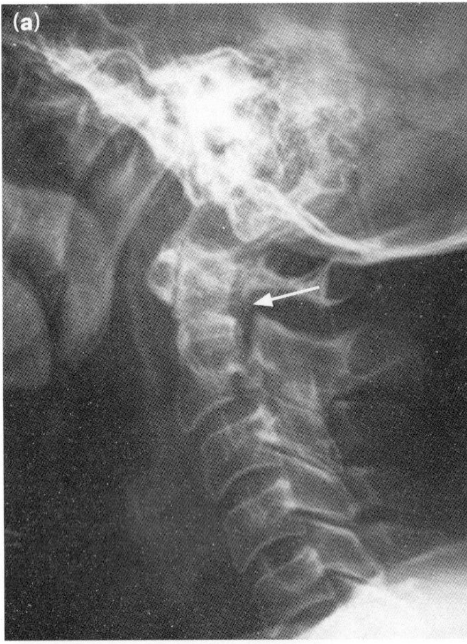

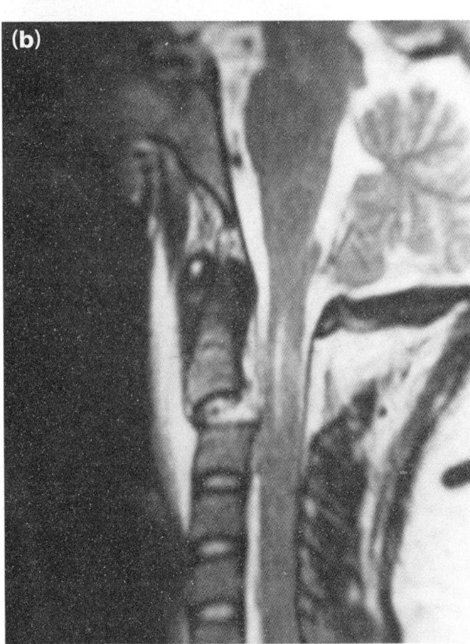

Figure 25.29 (a) Hangman's fractures of C2 with minimal forward translation (arrow). (b) C2/3 subluxation with spinal cord contusion.

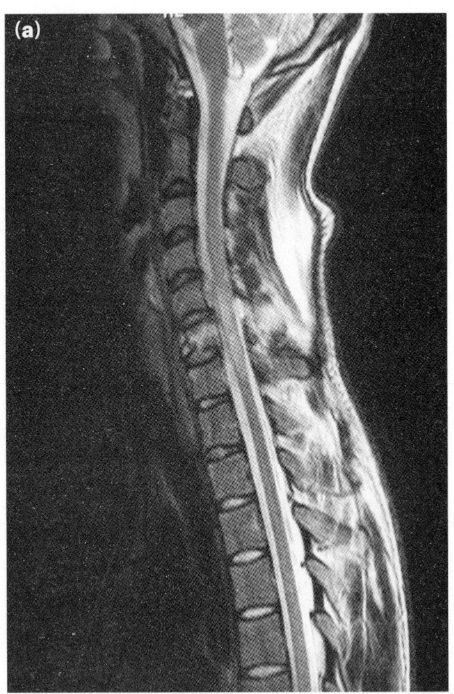

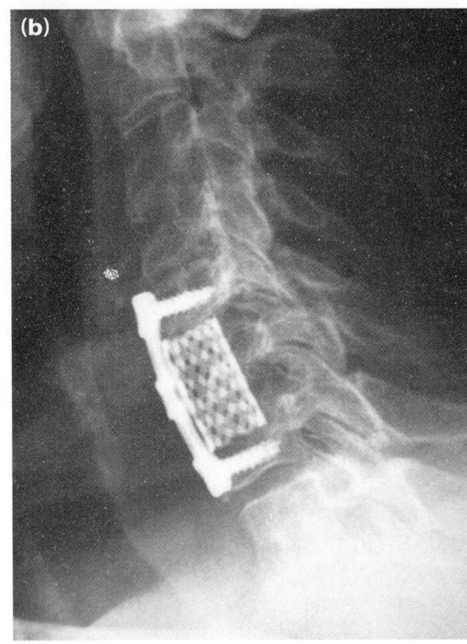

Figure 25.30 (a) Cervical burst fracture with spinal cord contusion; (b) treated by anterior decompression and reconstruction.

Subaxial cervical spine (C3-C7)

The pattern of lower cervical spine injury depends on the mechanism of trauma. These include compression fractures (hyperflexion), burst fractures (axial compression) and facet subluxation/dislocation injuries (distraction–flexion), teardrop fractures (hyperextension) and fracture of posterior elements. The more severe injuries are accompanied by spinal cord injury (Figure 25.30a). Operative intervention may be required to decompress the spinal cord, and to stabilise the spine with internal fixation (Figure 25.30b).

Facet subluxation/dislocation ranges in severity from minor instability to complete dislocation with spinal cord injury (Figure 25.31).

Fractures in patients with ankylosing spondylitis

Ankylosing spondylitis is a seronegative inflammatory disorder that causes autofusion of the spine. These patients have a higher risk of spinal fractures and spinal cord injury than the normal population. Senior advice should be obtained, because application of a cervical collar may be contraindicated, and patients should be managed instead in a position of comfort. Surgical stabilisation is commonly indicated.

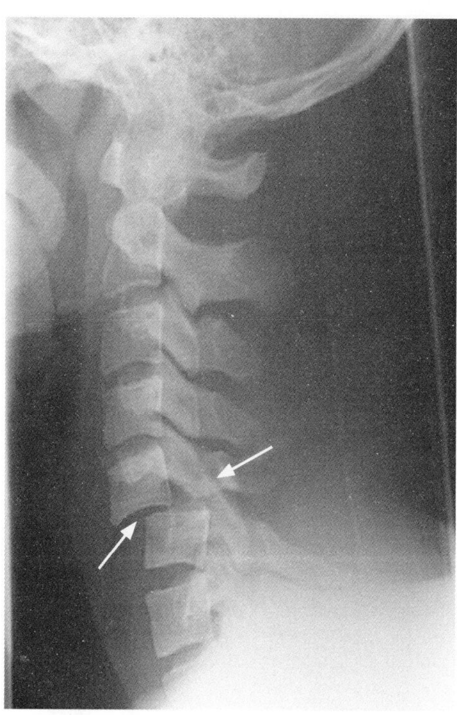

Figure 25.31 C5/6 bifacetal dislocation (arrows).

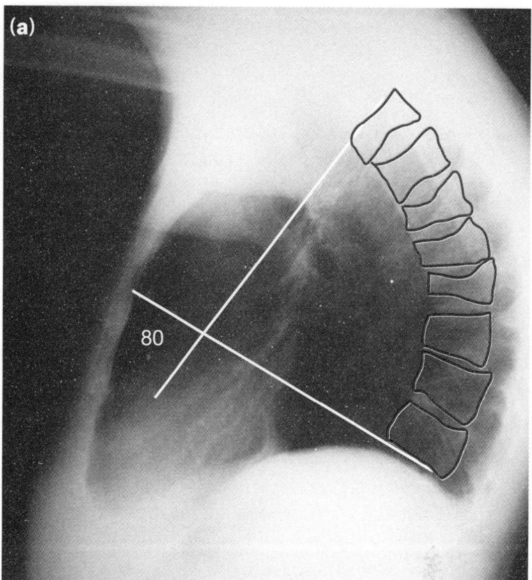

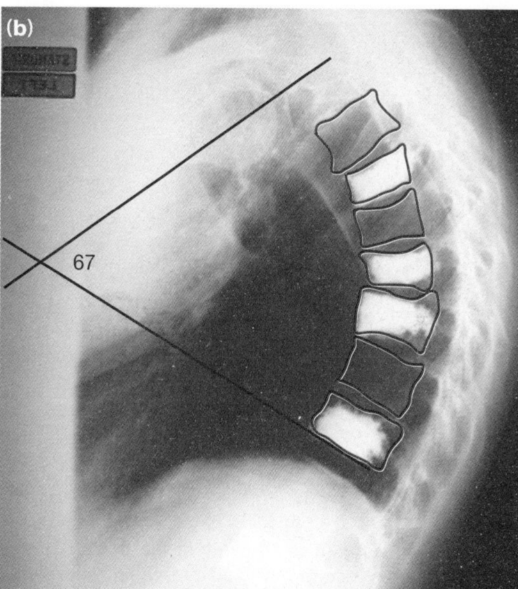

Figure 25.32 (a) Lateral x-ray showing multiple osteoporotic compression fractures. (b) Reduction in thoracic kyphotic deformity following four-level kyphoplasty.

Summary box 25.6

Cervical spine injuries

- The majority of upper cervical spinal injuries are treated non-operatively
- Spinal cord injury is more commonly associated with subaxial cervical spinal injuries

Thoracic and thoracolumbar fractures

The system developed by the AO (Arbeitsgemeinschaft für Osteosynthesefragen) can be used to classify these fractures. There are three main injury types, A, B and C, with increasing instability and risk of neurological injury.

Type A fractures are vertebral body compression fractures. Type B injuries involve distraction of the anterior or posterior elements and type C injuries are rotational and often coexist with Type A or Type B injuries. The majority of type B and type C injuries require surgical stabilisation.

Thoracic spine (T1–T10)

Osteoporotic wedge compression fractures in the elderly are the commonest injury in this group. Most of these fractures heal, but symptomatic fractures can be treated with percutaneous bone cement augmentation, known as vertebroplasty or kyphoplasty (Figure 25.32).

In trauma cases, unstable fractures are associated with significant energy transfer to the patient and may be associated with major internal injuries, such as pulmonary contusion and spinal cord injury. The combination of thoracic spine disruption and a sternal fracture (Figure 25.33) also carries a significant risk of aortic rupture. Multiple posterior rib fractures and rib dislocations above and below a thoracic spinal injury signify a major rotational injury to the chest and can be associated with vascular injury and significant pulmonary contusion (Figure 25.34). Multimodality diagnostic imaging is recommended. Surgery is appropriate for most thoracic injuries if unstable.

AO, *Arbeitsgemeinschaft für Osteosynthesefragen*, may be translated from the German as 'Working Party on Problems of Bone Repair'.

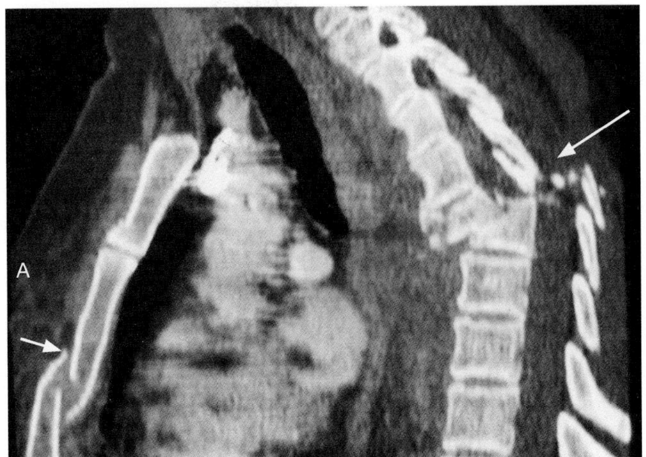

Figure 25.33 Sagittal CT reconstruction showing an upper thoracic spine fracture dislocation (long arrow) and associated sternal fracture (short arrow).

Thoracolumbar spinal fractures (T11-L2)

The thoracolumbar junction is especially prone to injury. This can vary from a from minor wedge fracture to spinal dislocation (Figure 25.35). Burst fractures are comminuted fractures of the vertebral body. They are characterised by widening of the distance between the pedicles, and can be associated with retropulsion of bone fragments into the spinal canal (Figure 25.36). Anterior surgery for this type of fracture is now very rarely used and the current treatment principles involve posterior fixation (Figure 25.37). Chance fractures

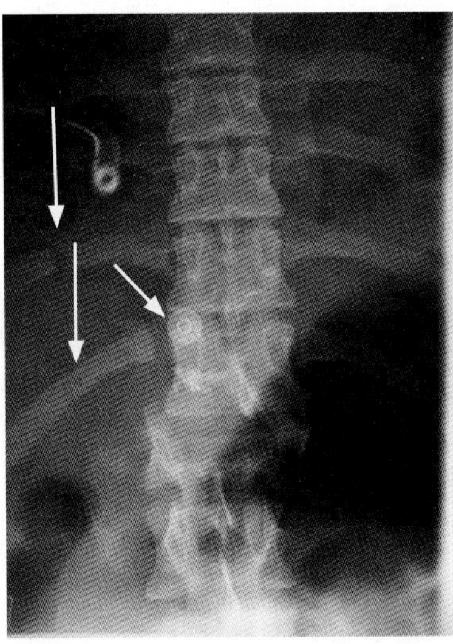
Figure 25.34 Rotational (type C) injury at the thoracolumbar junction. Note rib fractures (long arrows) and dislocation (short arrow), and presence of chest tube.

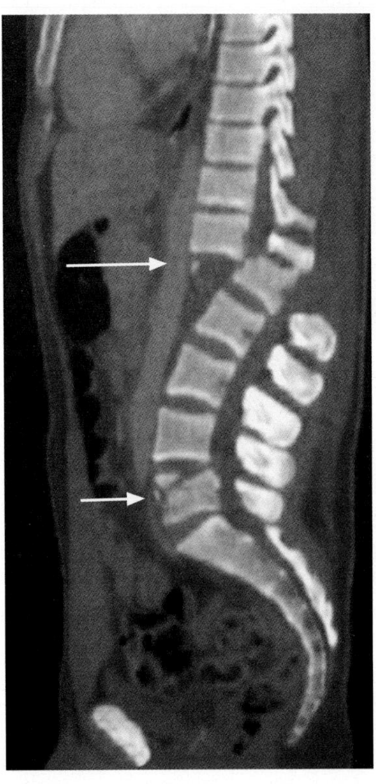
Figure 25.35 Total spinal sagittal computed tomography reconstruction demonstrating a thoracolumbar fracture dislocation (long arrow) and fracture of L5 (short arrow).

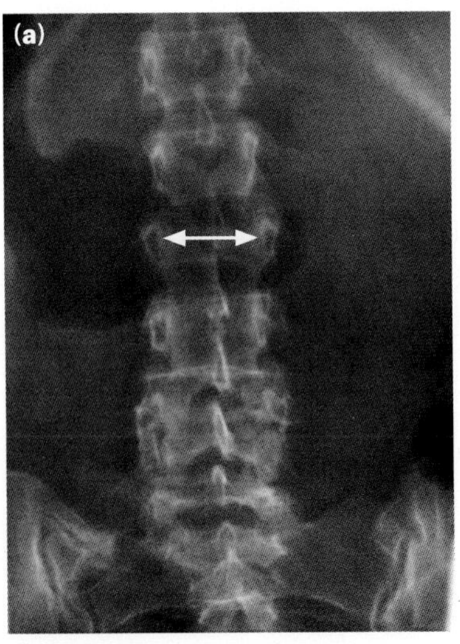

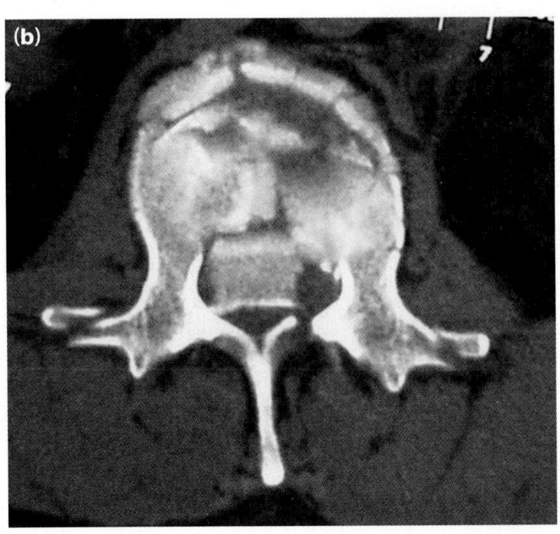

Figure 25.36 Lumbar burst fracture with increase in interpedicular distance (a) (arrow) and spinal canal compromise (b).

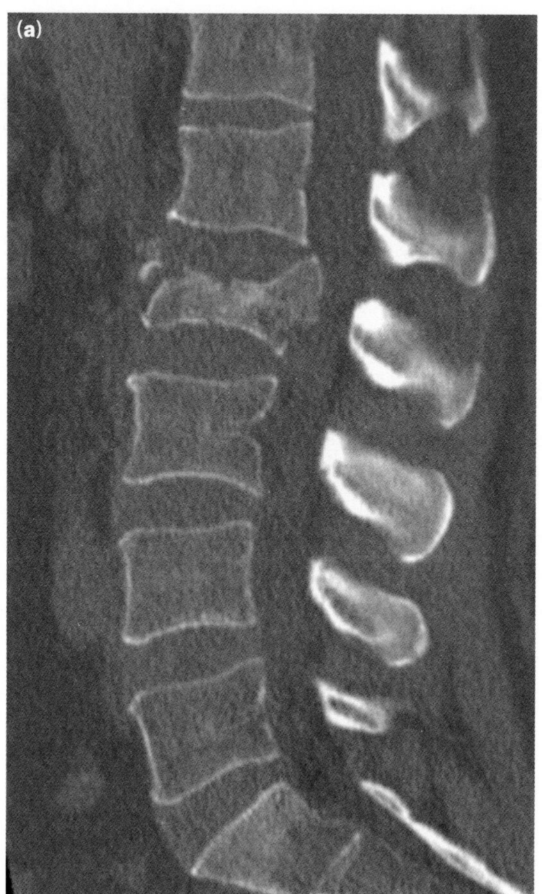

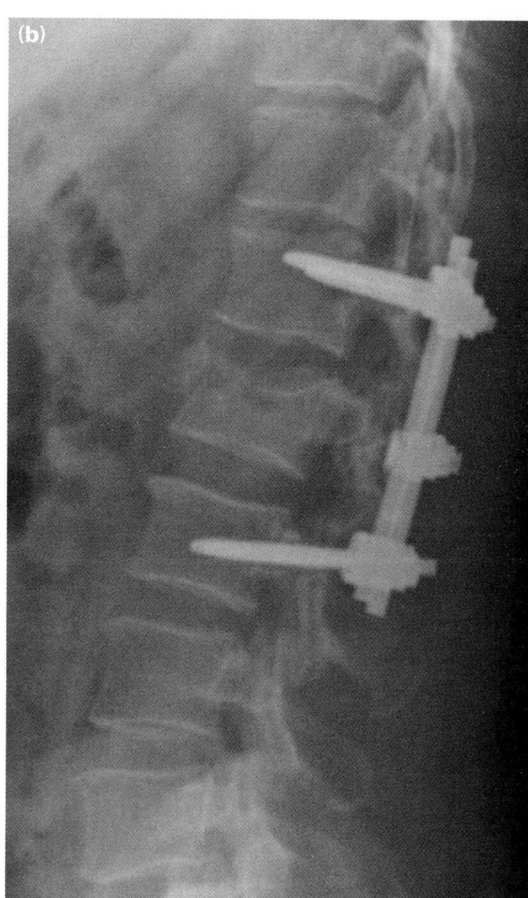

Figure 25.37 Lumbar burst fracture at L2 (a), and posterior instrumentation with indirect reduction (b).

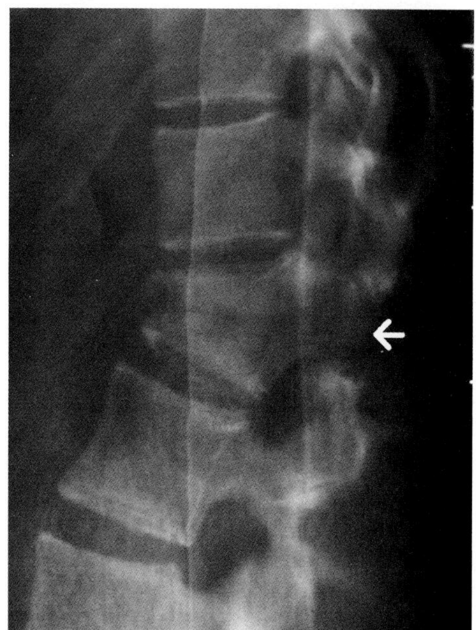

Figure 25.38 A bony Chance fracture at the thoracolumbar junction (arrow) secondary to a lap-belt injury.

are flexion–distraction injuries of the thoracolumbar junction and are classically associated with the use of lap-belts (Figure 25.38). Duodenal, pancreatic and/or aortic ruptures are also associated with these injuries.

Lumbar spinal fractures (L3-S1)

Most fractures of the lower lumbar spine can be treated non-surgically because the incidence of neurological injury is lower. The neural canal is more capacious at this level (the spinal cord terminates at L1/L2). Owing to the lumbar lordosis, patients with these injuries are less likely to develop a kyphotic deformity than those with injuries at the thoracolumbar junction.

Summary box 25.7

Thoracic and thoracolumbar fractures

- Unstable thoracic spine fractures and thoracolumbar flexion–distraction injuries are commonly associated with vascular and/or visceral injuries

George Quentin Chance, formerly Director of Diagnostic Radiology, The Derby Group of Hospitals, Derbyshire, UK.

EPIDEMIOLOGY OF SPINAL CORD INJURY

The incidence and causation of spinal cord injury (SCI) vary globally and reflect the demographics and industrialisation of society. The worldwide annual incidence is 15–40 cases per million (according to the National Spinal Cord Injury Statistical Center, University of Alabama at Birmingham: spinal cord injury facts and figures, April 2009). Road traffic accidents remain the leading cause of spinal cord injuries worldwide. Males in the third decade of life are the most likely group to sustain serious spinal cord injury.

EVOLUTION OF THE MANAGEMENT OF SPINAL CORD INJURY

The development of specialised SCI centres has dramatically improved the survival rates, health and functional outcomes of individuals with SCI. The first SCI centre was established in the USA in 1936 by Dr Donald Munro. In 1944 The National Spinal Injuries Centre was established at Stoke Mandeville, England, by Sir Ludwig Guttmann.

Summary box 25.8

Spinal cord injury

- The incidence of spinal cord injury remains constant
- The outcome is improved in regional/national spinal cord injury centres

PATHOPHYSIOLOGY OF SPINAL CORD INJURY

The primary injury

This is the direct insult to the neural elements and occurs at the time of the initial injury.

The secondary injury

Haemorrhage, oedema and ischaemia result in a biochemical cascade that causes the secondary injury. This may be accentuated by hypotension, hypoxia, spinal instability and/or persistent compression of the neural elements. Management of spinal cord injury must focus on minimising secondary injury.

Summary box 25.9

Pathophysiology of spinal cord injury

- The spinal cord contains various tracts that are topographically arranged
- Spinal cord injury involves both primary and secondary phases
- Therapeutic strategies are directed at reducing the secondary injury

Identification of shock

Three categories of shock may occur in spinal trauma

- **Hypovolaemic shock**. Hypotension with tachycardia and cold clammy peripheries. This is most often due to haemorrhage. It should be treated with appropriate resuscitation.
- **Neurogenic shock**. This presents with hypotension, a normal heart rate or bradycardia and warm peripheries. This is due to unopposed vagal tone resulting from cervical spinal cord injury at or above the level of sympathetic outflow (T1/T5). It should be treated with inotropic support, and care should be taken to avoid fluid overload.
- **Spinal shock**. Spinal shock is a temporary physiological disorganisation of spinal cord function that starts within minutes following the injury. The length of effect is variable, but it can last 6 weeks or longer. It is characterised by paralysis, decreased tone and hyporeflexia. Once it has resolved the bulbocavernosus reflex (Figure 25.39) returns.

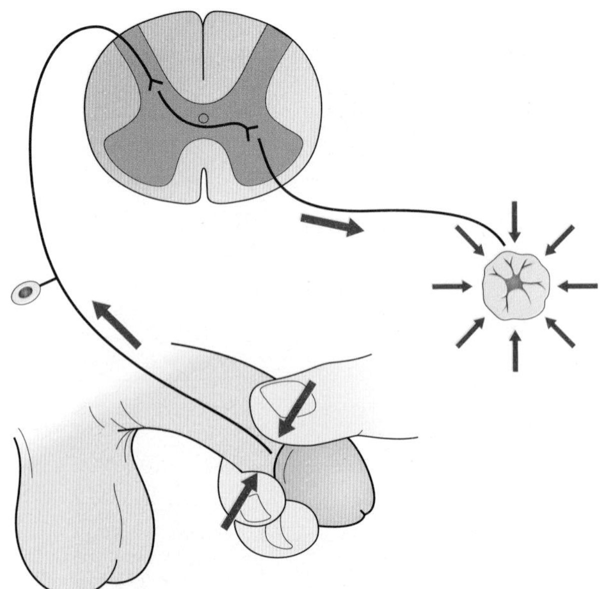

Figure 25.39 The bulbocavernosus reflex (this can be elicited in females by traction on the Foley catheter).

Sir Ludwig Guttmann is considered by many to be the father of spinal cord medicine. He was a leading neurosurgeon in Germany, working at the Jewish Hospital in Breslau. He fled to England in 1939.

Level of neurological injury

The level of neurological injury is simply the most caudal neurological level with normal neurological function.

Complete versus incomplete spinal cord injury

A spinal cord injury is incomplete when there is preservation of perianal sensation.

Types of incomplete spinal cord injury

There are several types of incomplete spinal cord injuries. These include:

- central cord syndrome;
- Brown-Séquard syndrome (hemisection);
- anterior spinal syndrome;
- posterior cord syndrome;
- cauda equina syndrome.

REHABILITATION AND PATIENT OUTCOME

The goal of spinal cord injury rehabilitation is based on a multidisciplinary approach. There is a focus on goal-setting, maximising remaining neurological function and reintegration into employment and society. The level of neurological impairment determines the functional outcome (*Table 25.1*).

Prognosis of spinal cord injury

Despite continuing improvements in patient care, life expectancy remains below normal following SCI. The median life expectancy is 33 years, but varies considerably (*Table 25.2*).

The prognosis for neurological recovery is strongly influenced by factors such as the level and completeness of the injury, ventilator dependence and the age at presentation.

TABLE 25.1 Expected functional outcome versus level of cervical spinal cord injury.

Level of injury	Functional goal
C3–C4	Power wheelchair with mouth or chin control. Verbalise care, communicate through adaptive equipment. May be ventilator dependent
C5	Power wheelchair, dress upper body, self-feed with aids, wash face with assistance
C6	Propel power wheelchair, possibly push manual wheelchair, transfer with assistance, dress upper body (lower body with assistance), self-groom with aids, bladder/bowel care with assistance, self-feed with splints, able to drive
C7	Manual wheelchair, independent transfer, dressing (with aids), feeding, bathing, self-care. Bladder and bowel care with assistance
C8–T4	Independent with most activities of daily living, and bowel and bladder care
T5–T12	As above but with more ease. Independent with all self-care
L1–L5	Independent. Walk with short or long leg braces
S1–S5	Independent, able to walk if able to push off (S1) (may need brace). Bladder, bowel and sexual function may remain compromised

TABLE 25.2 Life expectancy (years) post injury by severity of injury and age at injury.

Age at injury	No SCI	Motor functional at any level	Para	Low tetra (C5–C8)	High tetra (C1–C4)	Ventilator-dependent at any level
(a) For people who survive the first 24 hours						
20	58.4	52.8	45.6	40.6	36.1	16.6
40	39.5	34.3	28.0	23.8	20.2	7.1
60	22.2	17.9	13.1	10.2	7.9	1.4
(b) For people surviving at least 1 year post injury						
20	58.4	53.3	46.3	41.7	37.9	23.3
40	39.5	34.8	28.6	24.7	21.6	11.1
60	22.2	18.3	13.5	10.8	8.8	3.1

SCI, spinal cord injury.

Charles Edward Brown-Séquard, 1817–1894, physiologist and neurologist who held a number of academic posts, amongst them Physician, The National Hospital for Nervous Diseases, Queen's Square, London, UK (1860–1864), Professor of Medicine at Harvard University, Boston, MA, USA (1864–1878) and at the College de France, Paris, France (1878–1894). He described his syndrome in 1851.

Complications associated with spinal cord injury

Pressure ulcers

Many are preventable. Patients should be turned regularly on an appropriate mattress to minimise the risk of skin break-down

Pain and spasticity

Neurogenic pain is common. Once reflex activity returns following cord injury, spasticity may occur and can be problematic. Intrathecal infusion of baclofen may be required in resistant cases.

Autonomic dysreflexia

This is a paroxysmal syndrome of hypertension, hyperhydrosis (above level of injury), bradycardia, flushing and headache in response to noxious visceral and other stimuli. It is most commonly triggered by bladder distension or rectal loading from faecal impaction.

Neurological deterioration

Post-traumatic syringomyelia (PTS) may occur in up to 28% of SCI patients up to 30 years following injury. Approximately 30% of cases are symptomatic. Clinically, patients present with segmental pain at or above the level of injury, sensory loss, progressive asymmetrical weakness or increased spasticity. This warrants early MRI assessment. Expanding cavities require neurosurgical intervention.

Thromboembolic events

Deep vein thrombosis (DVT) occurs in 30% of patients with SCI. Fatal pulmonary embolus is reported in 1–2% of cases. Thomboprophylaxis with compression stockings and low molecular weight heparin is indicated, provided there are no contraindications.

Osteoporosis, heterotopic ossification and contractures

Disuse osteoporosis is an inevitable consequence of SCI and fragility fractures may occur. Heterotopic ossification may affect the hips, knees, shoulders and elbows. It occurs in 25% of spinal cord injured patients. Surgery is appropriate in selected cases. Soft tissue contractures around joints may occur due to spasticity but can be avoided by appropriate physical therapy, positioning and splinting.

FURTHER READING

Aebi M, Thalgott JS, Webb JK. *AO ASIF principles in spine surgery*. Berlin, Heidelberg: Springer-Verlag, 1998.

Bridwell KH, DeWald RL (eds). *The textbook of spinal surgery*, 3rd edn. Philadelphia: Lipponcott, Williams and Wilkins, 2011, pp.1377–473.

British Orthopaedic Association. The initial care and transfer of patients with spinal cord injuries, 2006. Available from: www.sbns.org/rcsed/RCSEdDocuments/DocumentsView.aspx?tabID=0&ItemID=31562&MId=4607&wversion=Staging

Cotler JM, Simson MJ, An HS *et al.* (eds). *Surgery of spinal trauma*. Philadelphia: Lippincott, Williams and Wilkins, 2000.

Denis F. The three column spine and its significance in the classification of acute thoracolumbar spinal injuries. *Spine* 1983; **8**(8): 817–31.

Dimar JR. Early versus late stabilisation of the spine in the polytrauma patient. *Spine* 2010; **35**(21S): S187–S192.

Fardon DF, Herzog RJ, Mink JH *et al.* (eds). *Orthopaedic knowledge update – spine*. Rosemont, IL: American Academy of Orthopaedic Surgeons, 1997.

Fehlings MG. *Essentials of spinal cord injury. Basic research to clinical practice*. Stuttgart: Thieme, 2013.

Focus issue. Spinal trauma. *Spine* 2006; **31**(11S): S1–104.

Panjabi M, White A. *Functional anatomy of the spine*. Oxford: Butterworth-Heinemann Ltd, 1990.

Chapter 26

Maxillofacial trauma

Learning objectives

To be able to:
- Identify and understand the significance of potentially life-threatening injuries to the face, head and neck

To have:
- A systematic methodology for examining facial injuries

To know:
- The classification of facial fractures

To understand:
- The diagnosis and management of fractures of the middle third of the facial skeleton and the mandible
- The principles of the diagnosis and management of facial soft tissue injuries

To appreciate:
- The management of dental injuries

EMERGENCY ASSESSMENT AND TREATMENT

The management of a patient with facial trauma must begin with an immediate assessment of the airway, breathing and circulation in keeping with the advanced trauma life support (ATLS) principles (see Chapter 23). If the patient has facial or midface bleeding they may sit forward or be placed on their side (Figure 26.1) to minimise the risk of blood and/or dental fragments obstructing the airway. The use of good light and high volume suction is often helpful.

The midface, when fractured, is displaced downwards and backwards (Figure 26.2), and if this occurs in combination with a mandibular fracture, particularly if the anterior mandible is comminuted, the tongue is also displaced downwards and backwards, adding to the airway compromise and creating the risk of obstruction (Figure 26.3). In these circumstances intubation is indicated, but emergency procedures can be employed to buy time. In the obtunded or unconscious patient the maxilla can be grasped by hand, disimpacted and pulled forwards. In addition, the tongue can be pulled forwards and held forwards, with a large suture or towel clip, to help clear the airway. If intubation is not possible a surgical airway is indicated.

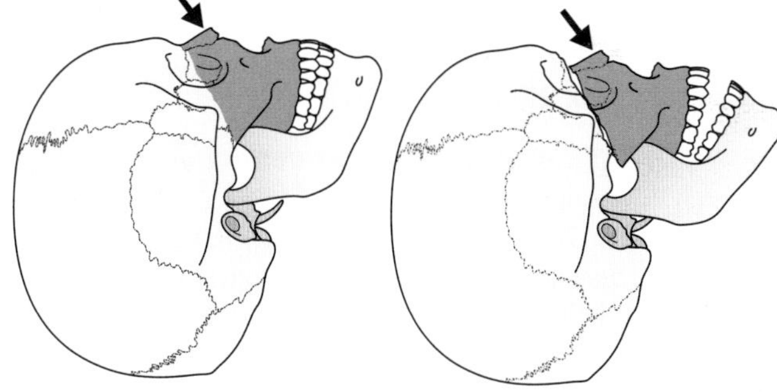

Figure 26.2 A blow from the front of the face may separate the facial skeleton from the base of the skull and thrust it downwards and backwards.

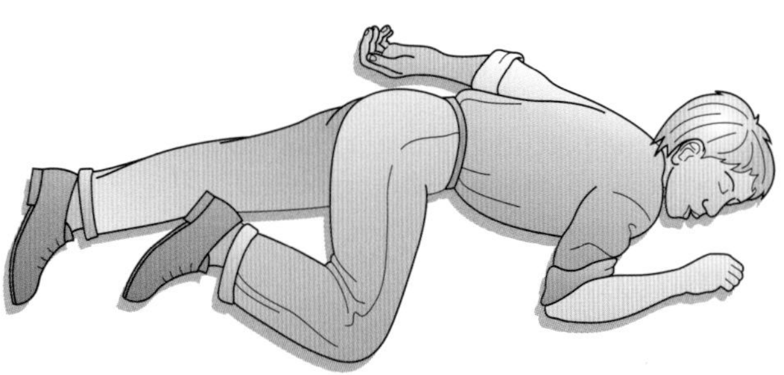

Figure 26.1 The patient should be nursed in the semiprone position to allow secretions, blood and foreign bodies to fall from the mouth.

Massive, life-threatening bleeding is usually only seen in the context of major trauma, lacerations, blast, ballistic, penetrating or gunshot injuries. Significant bleeding, usually from the pterygoid venous plexus and/or the rich blood supply of the nose, can be seen in central midface injuries.

Management of massive midface bleeding may require intubation and the placement of anterior and or posterior nasal packs. There are specific inflatable nasal balloons that can facilitate the immediate management, however Foley catheters may also be utilised.

Once the patient has been stabilised a more formal assessment may be performed.

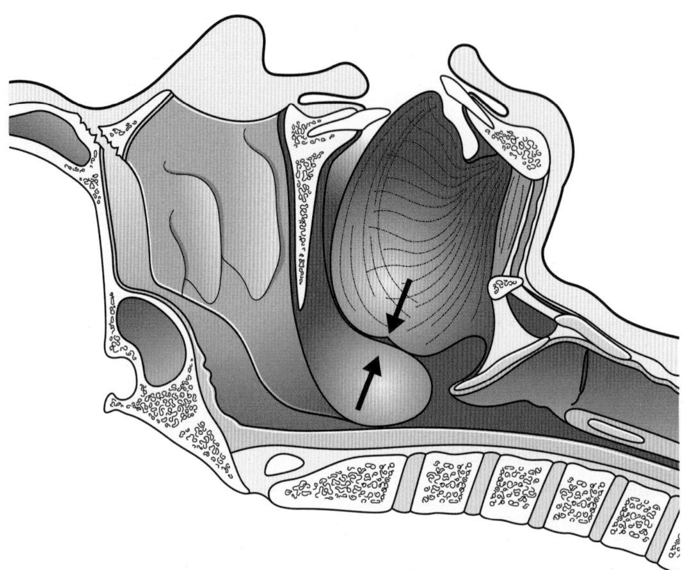

Figure 26.3 Loss of nasopharyngeal space and oedema of the soft palate and tongue (arrows) may close off the airway in severe maxillofacial injuries, 2–3 hours after injury.

Where skull fractures occur in combination with facial fractures or the fractures extend into the frontal or ethmoidal sinuses, they are classified as craniofacial, and a joint neurosurgical and maxillofacial approach is necessary.

If fractures occur at all levels of the face the term panfacial is utilised. This does not necessarily alter the management of the individual fracture components, however it does imply a significant degree of force and one must be suspicious of other injuries, especially head injuries. As with all trauma patients, associated injuries, including chest and abdominal trauma, must be actively excluded.

In considering the bony injuries, the fractures may be displaced or undisplaced and comminuted or non-comminuted. In the past, and with particular reference to mandibular fractures, stability was also considered, however with modern treatment methods this is a less important factor.

Soft tissue injuries and lacerations

Lacerations are crushing injuries where the soft tissues are compressed between the underlying bone and some form of blunt object. Incised wounds are caused by a cutting implement, such as a knife or glass. Often the injuries are a combination of the two. Either type of wound can occur with or without tissue loss. Where the injury results in a communication between the skin and the mucosa of the oral cavity the wound is termed 'through and through'.

Summary box 26.1

Emergency assessment

- Airway, breathing, circulation with cervical spine control is the starting point
- Do not let dramatic facial injuries distract from other potentially life-threatening injuries

Summary box 26.2

Classification of facial injuries

- Divide the face into thirds
- Assess orbit independently
- Assess bony and soft tissue injuries

CLASSIFICATION OF FACIAL INJURIES

Bony injuries and fractures

The facial skeleton can be divided into thirds vertically:

- upper face (from level of canthi upwards);
- midface (from maxillary teeth to canthi);
- lower face (mandible and mandibular teeth).

In addition, the midface can be divided into central and lateral portions. The central midface is the naso-orbital–ethmoidal complex and the lateral portion comprises the cheekbones (Malar bones, zygomatic bones or zygomatic–maxillary complex).

The eye socket can be considered as a separate entity, because orbital fractures can occur in isolation or as part of a constellation of multiple fractures. Orbital fractures can affect the orbital floor, medial and/or lateral walls and the roof of the orbit.

CLINICAL ASSESSMENT

History

As with all aspects of surgical diagnosis, the history is paramount. As much information as possible should be obtained about the mechanism of injury, the past medical history and the postinjury course. This will be directly from the patient, friends, family, witnesses and emergency services.

Knowledge of the mechanism of injury will often help to identify the potential occult injuries that are not obvious on first inspection. As the craniofacial region is so richly vascularised, the often dramatic appearance seen in major facial trauma has the potential of distracting the unwary clinician from potentially more important injuries.

Examination

Primary survey

Initially, the primary survey is aimed at the airway: controlling bleeding, restoring and maintaining the circulation and assessing for neurological deficits, with cervical spine control. The more detailed secondary survey is aimed at a definitive examination, with the clear expectation that this will need to be repeated on several occasions.

The face, head and neck should be inspected and wounds cleaned and assessed for tissue loss, and then dressed to control any bleeding not addressed in the primary survey. Their size, location and depth should be carefully recorded in the case notes. Large and obvious foreign bodies should be removed but care should be exercised with penetrating wounds involving large fragments or blades which potentially penetrate deep structures. These should be removed in the operating theatre, in more controlled conditions, after imaging (note also glass that may injure the assessing surgeon). On occasions it is helpful to administer local anaesthetic for the examination and (temporary) repair of facial lacerations, particularly if a single vessel continues to bleed. In these circumstances it is very helpful to perform a thorough examination of the key sensory and motor nerves that may have been injured, before the local anaesthetic makes this assessment meaningless.

This principle also applies to the management of those patients for whom intubation is imminent. While this may be difficult, a brief assessment of Glasgow Coma Scale (GCS) score, eye function (motility and acuity), facial and trigeminal nerves and cervical spine pain and function prior to the induction of anaesthesia can be very helpful in ongoing management.

Secondary survey

The secondary survey examination should be systematic because it is easy to be distracted and miss potentially important injuries that leave only a small external sign, e.g. a small entry wound from a stabbing to the back of the neck. The surface inspection should include the back of the neck, the whole scalp and then move to the frontal view. At this time it is helpful to perform a formal cranial nerve examination; of particular importance are cranial nerves II, III, IV, VI, V and VII.

Further examination

Examination of the eyes should then take place to exclude globe or retinal injury, as well as to assess acuity, test for diplopia and assess motility. This is possible even in the most swollen of eyes because one can gently prise the eyelids apart with cotton wool buds (or microbiology swabs). These are held parallel to the eyelids and gently pushed into the oedematous tissue close to the eyelashes, rotating the swabs to open the eye. A colleague can then examine the eye.

The position of the globe – whether there is proptosis or enophthalmos – and visual acuity (utilising a Snellin chart) in each eye, and whether there is diplopia in all nine positions of gaze, should be recorded.

The intraoral examination is facilitated by the use of good light (a headlight is helpful) and suction to allow removal of blood and saliva. The teeth should be examined and their presence or absence noted. Dental injuries should be classified. Teeth may be knocked out in an injury (termed avulsion), displaced but still attached to soft tissues and/or bone (termed subluxation) or fractured. If a tooth is mobile it may be subluxated or have a root fracture (detected on a radiograph). It is important to account for all missing teeth or tooth fragments as aspiration of an avulsed tooth or tooth fragment is a major risk. If there is any doubt about the location of missing teeth a chest radiograph should be obtained.

If there is a fracture of the mandible, the overlying mucosa is often torn and there may be an associated haematoma in the floor of the mouth (Figure 26.4). A key assessment is that of the dental occlusion (the way in which the teeth bite together). Patients are able to discriminate tiny alterations in their occlusion. These occlusal changes may represent dental injuries or, more commonly, displaced fractures of the maxilla and/or mandible.

Palpation of the bony contours of the facial bones should identify sites of tenderness, steps and asymmetry. This can start at the supraorbital margins, move around the infraorbital margins and then along the zygomatic arches, moving onto the condylar heads of the mandible and then running along the lower border of the mandible.

Investigations

The investigations required fall into two major categories: first, those required to confirm the provisional and specific clinical diagnosis with regard to the facial injuries and, second, those to assess and manage the systemic condition of the patient.

Systemic investigations will be governed by the general state of the patient and the past medical history. Typically, they will include routine laboratory (haematological and biochemical) investigations and radiological (for example the cervical spine) and other imaging.

Specific head and neck investigations are utilised and the general trend is away from plain radiology towards computed tomography (CT) scanning. If the clinical picture suggests an isolated mandibular fracture, plain radiographs at right angles to each other (rotational tomograph, orthopantomogram (Figure 26.5) and a posteroanterior (PA) mandible) may suffice, but clinicians should have a low threshold for cross-sectional imaging, particularly if a head or cervical spine CT

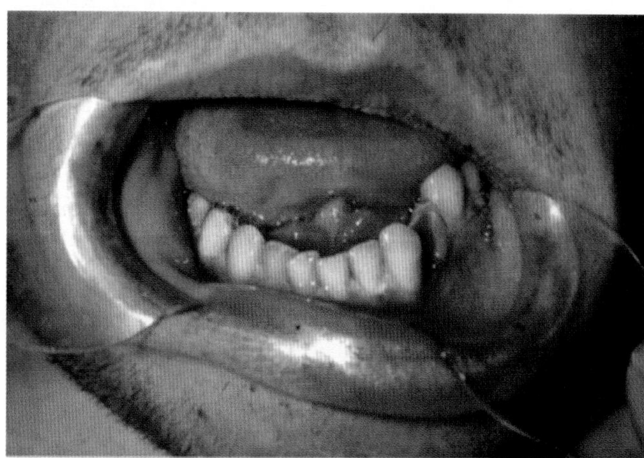

Figure 26.4 A fracture of the right parasymphysis of the mandible, demonstrating a tear of the gingivae in the lower right lateral incisor/canine region.

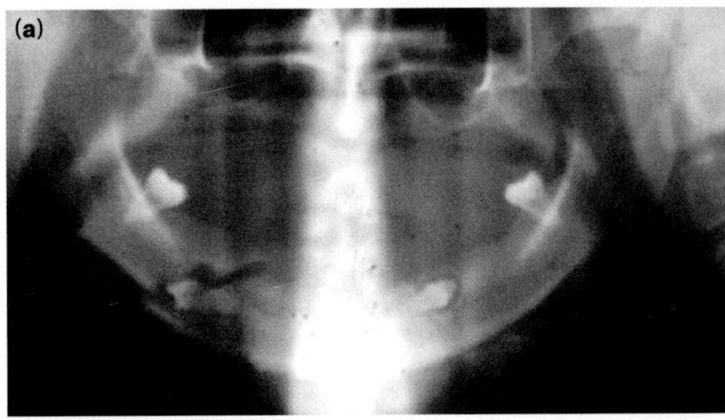

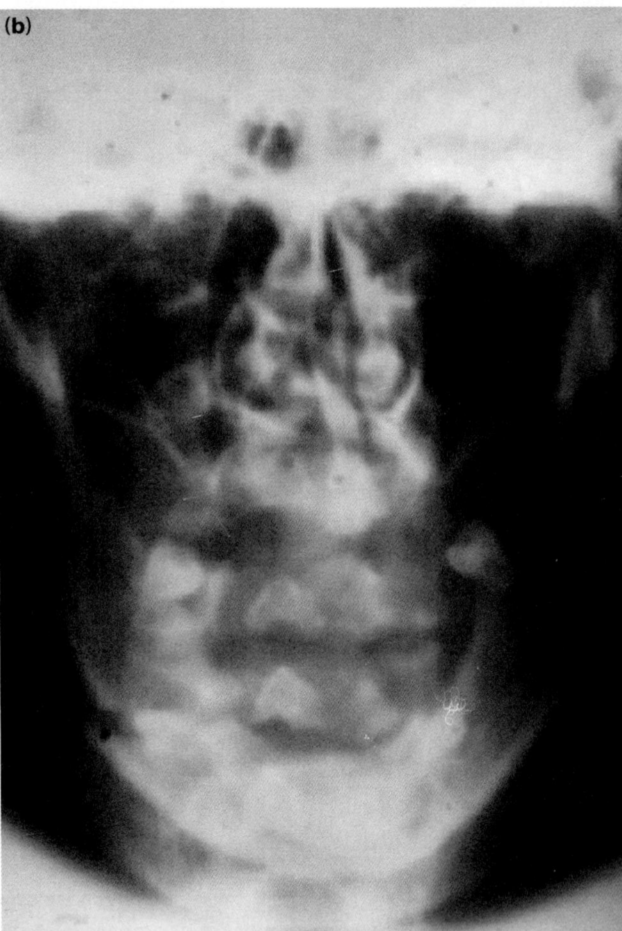

Figure 26.5 (a) Rotational tomogram showing a right mandibular body fracture. (b) Posterioanterior (PA) mandible showing the same mandibular body fracture.

is indicated. The additional information from 1 mm imaging cuts through the facial skeleton is worth the additional radiation dose, especially if plain radiography has been avoided.

Summary box 26.3

History, examination and investigation

- The history, particularly the mechanism of injury, is vital
- For simple injuries radiographs in two planes are required, but increasingly cross-sectional imaging is the norm: CT scanning

SPECIFIC INJURIES

Mandibular fractures

Mandibular fractures typically occur at specific sites (Figure 26.6). As with all fractures the principles of reduction, fixation, immobilisation and then rehabilitation apply to facial fractures. In previous years the reduction and immobilisation was often achieved by wiring the teeth together, known as intermaxillary fixation (IMF). However, in recent years this technique has largely been superseded by the use of open reduction and internal fixation (ORIF) techniques (Figure 26.7) utilising titanium fixation plates secured with screws. In general, the facial bones heal well and undisplaced fractures or those treated with ORIF heal after about 4 weeks. If the patient has had IMF a liquid diet is required and those who have had an ORIF procedure must also remain on a very soft sloppy diet for the same period.

In general, straightforward mandibular fractures treated with ORIF techniques have 2 mm diameter screws engaging a single bone cortex (monocortical). These small plates are said to be load sharing, in that the fractures are reduced and load is shared between the native bone and the plate. With more complex or comminuted fractures, larger plates and screws (up to 2.7 mm diameter) may be utilised; these are termed fracture or reconstruction plates. They are regarded as load bearing, and bicortical fixation may also be utilised.

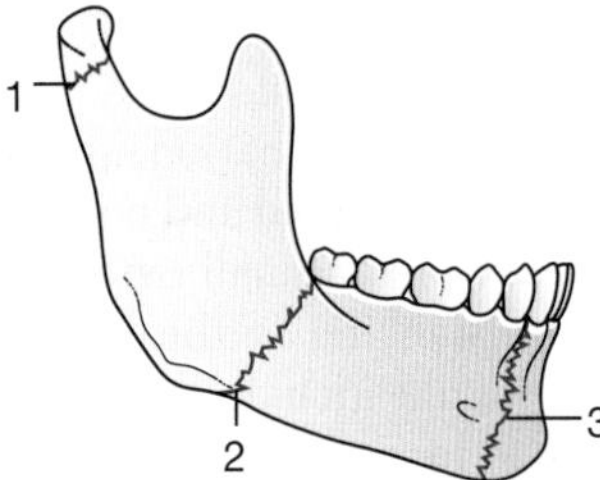

Figure 26.6 The patterns of fracture of the mandible. (1) The neck of the condyle is the most common site, followed by (2) the angle of the mandible through the last tooth. (3) The third point of weakness is in the region of the canine tooth.

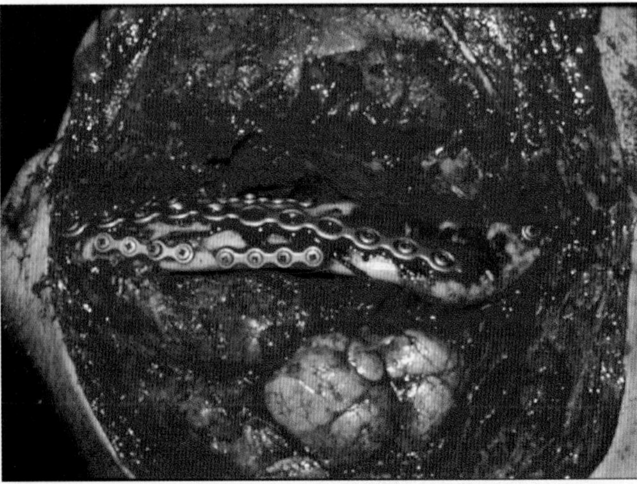

Figure 26.7 Intraoperative photograph showing a comminuted mandibular fracture reduced and fixed with a combination of 2 mm mini plates (monocortical) and a larger fracture plate with bicortical screws.

The timing of the definitive treatment of mandibular fractures is dependent on the general state of the patient; however, optimal timing is for treatment within 24–48 hours post injury.

Condylar neck fractures are increasingly being treated with open reduction and internal fixation techniques, with better technology and the use of endoscopically assisted surgery. This can be done via intraoral approaches. Undisplaced or minimally displaced condylar neck fractures can be treated non-operatively or with elastic IMF.

Summary box 26.4

Mandibular fractures

- Mandibular fractures are diagnosed clinically, often because of deranged dental occlusion
- Numbness over the distribution of the mental nerve is common
- Treatment is primarily with open reduction and internal fixation

Fractures of the zygomatico-orbito complex (ZMC)

ZMC (malar/cheekbone) fractures are the commonest facial fractures and have been classified in a variety of different ways. However, from a clinical perspective, considering the cheekbone as a four-legged stool is helpful – the four legs are comprised of the zygomatic arch running anteroposteriorly, the zygomatic process running vertically (to join the frontozygomatic process of the frontal bone at the frontozygomatic (FZ) suture), the infraorbital rim running horizontally and the maxillary buttress running vertically (Figure 26.8).

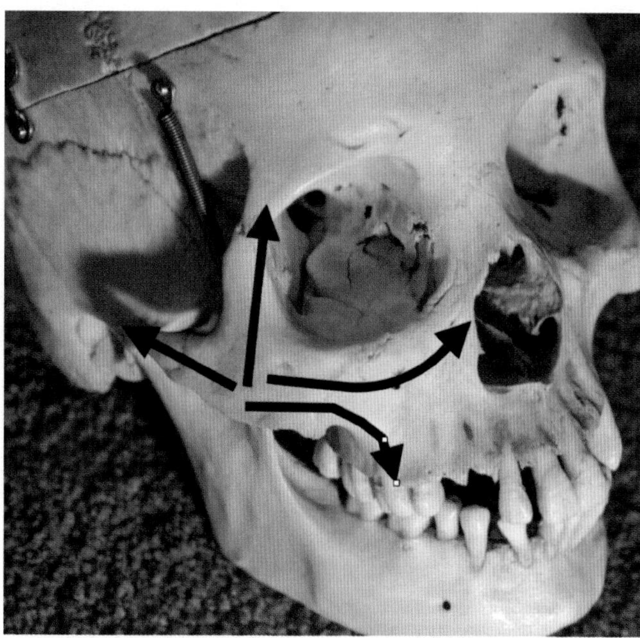

Figure 26.8 The 'four legs of the stool'.

With the exception of isolated zygomatic arch, isolated infraorbital rim and extensively comminuted fractures, if the ZMC is fractured then all four legs of the stool are fractured and displacement occurs about two axes, running vertically through the line from the FZ suture to the maxillary buttress or running anteroposteriorly along the zygomatic arch.

All ZMC fractures (with the exception of isolated zygomatic arch and isolated infraorbital rim fractures) involve the bony orbit, and careful assessment of ocular position and function is necessary.

On examination there is often periorbital bruising and swelling and subconjunctival haemorrhage with no posterior limit is often seen (Figure 26.9). On palpation (or inspection), bowing or depression of the zygomatic arch may be detected. Bony steps and tenderness at the frontozygomatic suture, the infraorbital rim or the zygomatic buttress may also be detected. Altered sensation over the distribution of the infraorbital nerve is common, as a result of either direct trauma or crushing of the nerve as it exits the maxilla or runs along the orbital floor.

As with mandibular fractures, the role of plain radiography is diminishing and cross-sectional imaging utilising CT scanning is the standard investigation except for the simplest fractures.

In terms of management, the mainstay of treatment is ORIF with fixation at one of the four 'legs of the stool', namely the frontozygomatic suture, the buttress region, the infraorbital rim or the zygomatic arch. The necessity for single, double, triple or four-point fixation will depend on the stability of the fracture post reduction and the degree of comminution. Uncomplicated ZMC fractures are generally treated within 10 days of injury.

Summary box 26.5

Fractures of the ZMC

- Fractures of the zygomatico-orbital complex are common
- Eye injuries should be actively excluded
- CT scanning is the investigation of choice

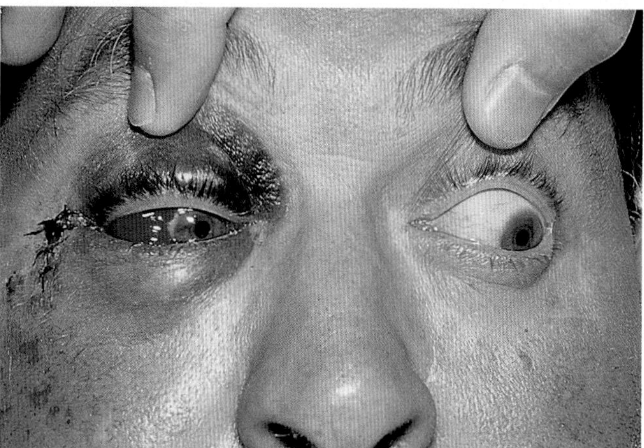

Figure 26.9 Fractures of the zygoma may often be associated with subconjunctival haemorrhage. This example shows no posterior border to the haemorrhage as the patient looks away from the side of the fracture.

Maxillary fractures

Maxillary fractures are traditionally classified after René Le Fort's work, in which he recreated the maxillary fractures utilising cadavers and a sandbag. Interestingly, the numbering, in modern usage, has become reversed from the original: the Le Fort I fracture being inferior and the Le Fort III being superior (Figure 26.10). While the classification is simple, real life presentations are often not. CT scanning and the use of open surgical techniques have demonstrated that the described patterns are not often adhered to and that comminution is the norm.

Midface fractures are often accompanied by significant facial swelling and this makes palpation of the skeleton difficult. The characteristic finding is of a mobile maxilla which tends to be displaced backwards and inferiorly. This can compromise the airway (see above) and results in an anterior open bite (inability to close the front teeth together). There is often infraorbital nerve injury resulting in altered sensation and, with upper level (Le Fort II and III) fractures, the orbit is involved to a greater or lesser degree.

The treatment of maxillary fractures, in all but the entirely undisplaced fractures, involves ORIF techniques utilising a variety of miniplates (1.5/1.7 mm diameter screws) and/or microplates (1.0/1.2 mm diameter screws). Fixation is usually placed along the main facial buttresses (the 'four legs of the stool') for optimal strength and bone quality to be able to hold the screws (Figure 26.11).

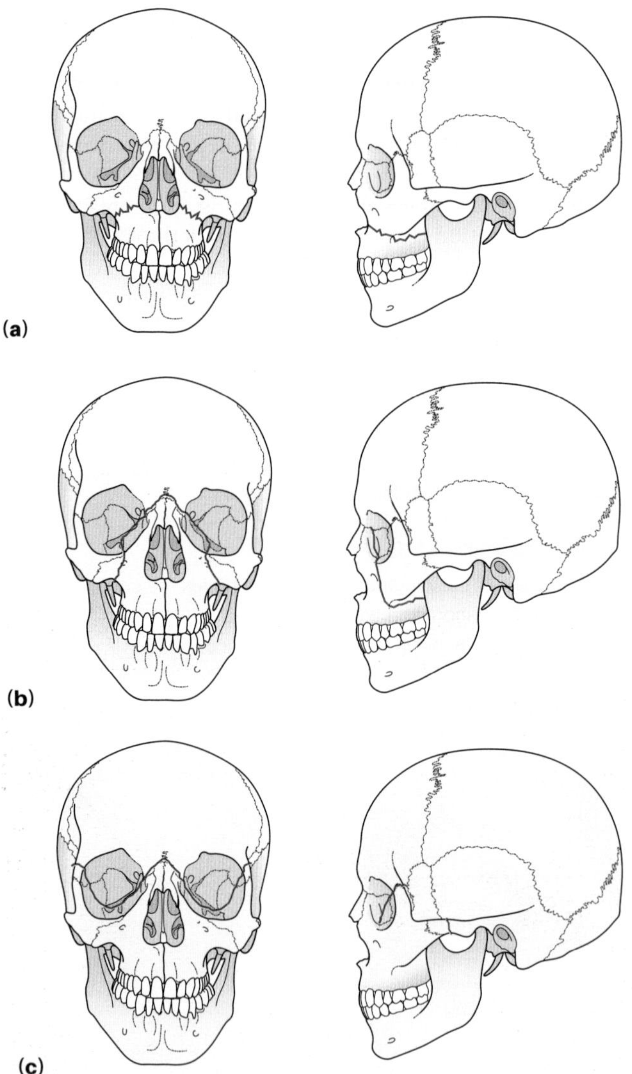

Figure 26.10 Maxillary fractures as classified by Le Fort. **(a)** Le Fort I; **(b)** Le Fort II; **(c)** Le Fort III.

Summary box 26.6

Maxillary fractures

- Maxillary fractures indicate significant force transfer – other associated injuries should be excluded
- Bleeding from the pterygoid venous plexus may be occult

Orbital fractures

The bones that comprise the orbit can be fractured and, in order of frequency, the floor, medial wall, lateral wall and roof may be disrupted either in combination or as isolated injuries. The mechanism of this is unclear and, particularly with isolated injuries, it may be that a rapid increase in pressure within the confined space of the orbit, typically, for example, when a squash ball hits the eye, results in fracture of the very thin floor and/or medial wall. Alternatively, forces are transmitted from the outer bony orbital rim, which is possibly

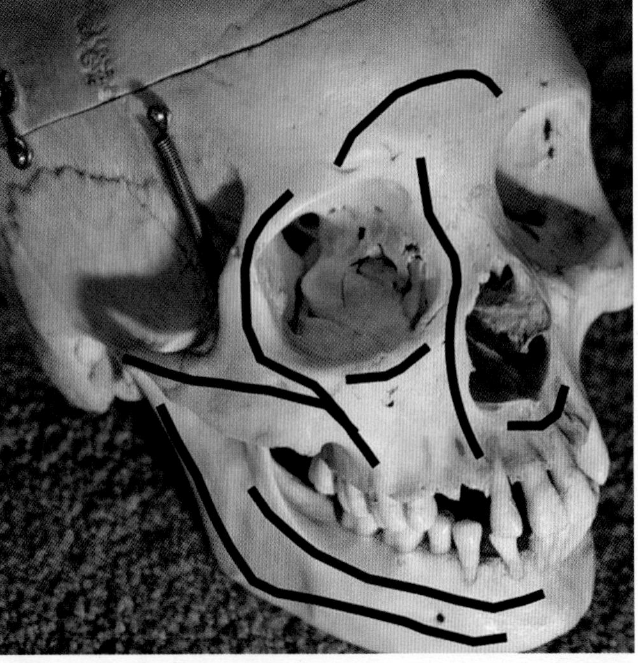

Figure 26.11 The buttresses of the face.

René Le Fort, 1869–1951, French surgeon, classified facial fractures after macabre research in which he dropped rocks and other heavy objects on the faces of cadavers.

temporarily deformed, causing the buckling and fracturing of the thin, vulnerable walls. It is likely that both of these mechanisms have a role in the genesis of orbital fractures.

In any orbital injury the eye must be examined carefully, even if there is significant swelling. Pupillary response, visual acuity (utilising a pinhole to correct for missing glasses), ocular motility and the results of careful ophthalmoscopy (including the anterior chamber, lens and fundus) should be documented. Binocular diplopia indicates a motility issue; however, monocular diplopia suggests a problem within the globe such as a dislocated lens or retinal detachment.

In general, orbital floor fractures lead to ocular motility problems, primarily restriction of upgaze due to trapping of the orbital fat and associated fibrous septae. However, on occasion the inferior rectus or inferior oblique muscles may also be trapped. Inferior rectus entrapment is much more common in children and this needs to be treated as an emergency because muscle necrosis can occur, leading to irreversible damage. In these cases the orbital floor appears, on imaging, undisplaced, i.e. a trap door defect has opened and then closed again, entrapping the muscle. In addition to motility problems, orbital wall fractures can lead to changes in globe position, with dropping of the globe (hypoglobus) or sinking in of the globe (enophthalmos) (Figure 26.12). In many cases such changes in globe position are masked in the immediate postinjury phase by oedema and only become obvious as this resolves.

A retrobulbar haemorrhage is a surgical emergency because when left untreated it can lead to blindness. It presents with decreasing visual acuity, increasing pain, loss of pupillary response and a tense proptosis. Should this diagnosis be suspected medical management should be initiated with acetazolamide, mannitol and steroids; however, the main treatment is surgical, with lateral canthotomy and cantholysis forming the initial intervention.

Investigation of orbital injuries requires CT scanning (Figure 26.13) but if a retrobulbar haemorrhage is suspected treatment should be given prior to scanning.

With the exception of retrobulbar haemorrhages and paediatric orbital fractures, the definitive treatment can be delayed for 7–10 days (Figure 26.14). This allows oedema to settle and globe motility and position to be assessed more accurately. Reconstruction of the orbital rim is usually accomplished with ORIF techniques and the orbital walls repaired with autologous materials such as cranial bone or rib grafts, but proving more popular are preformed titanium implants or patient-specific custom-made implants.

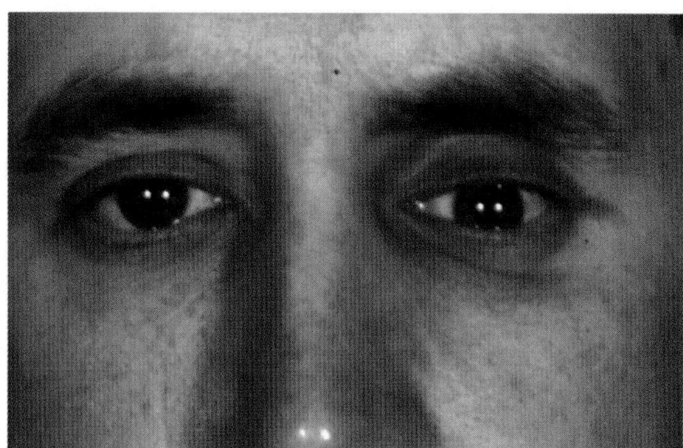

Figure 26.12 Previously undiagnosed left orbital blow-out fracture, presenting 3 months after the initial injury. Enophthalmos and lowered pupillary level are evident.

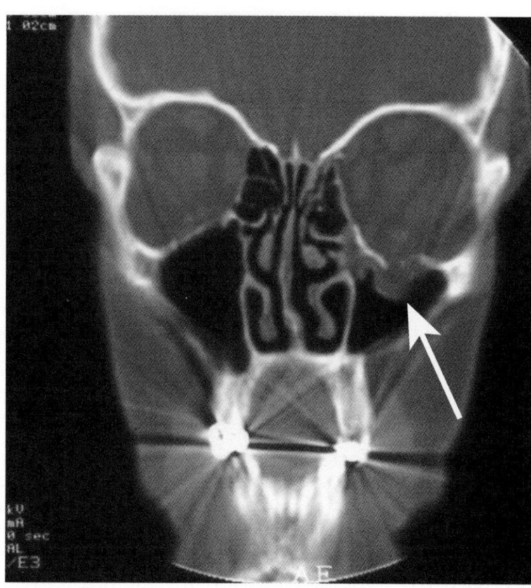

Figure 26.13 Coronal computed tomography scan showing a left orbital blow-out fracture, with evident soft tissue herniation into the maxillary antrum (arrrow).

Summary box 26.7

Orbital fractures

- Visual acuity and motility must be assessed
- In children, orbital floor injuries should be assessed and treated as emergencies because muscle injury may be permanent, resulting in reduced ocular motility

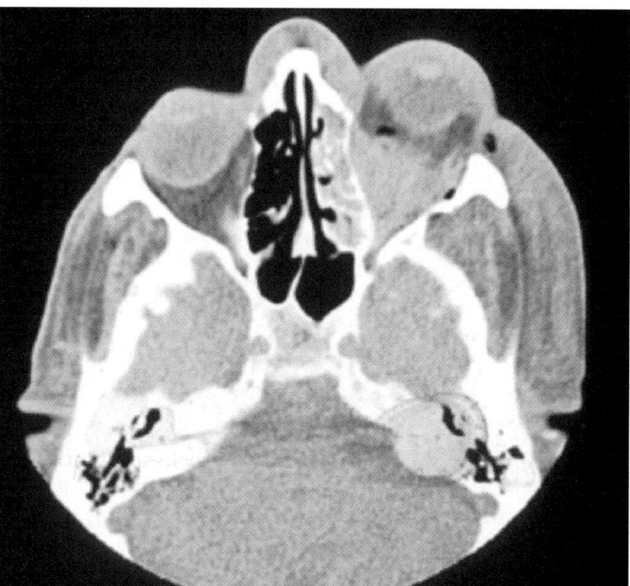

Figure 26.14 Computed tomography scan showing retrobulbar haemorrhage and severe proptosis.

Naso-orbito ethmoidal fractures

These central upper midface fractures can range from simple undisplaced nasal bone fractures to complex comminuted fractures, impacted into the anterior cranial fossa, in the region of the cribriform plate. Typically they are caused by a blow to the bridge of the nose. The more severe fractures present with periorbital ecchymosis, swelling and nasal bleeding with the bridge of the nose depressed and the nasal tip rotated upwards, allowing the nostrils to be seen straight on ('piggy nose'). The nasal septum is often disrupted and should be inspected for haematomas. Cerebrospinal fluid (CSF) may be seen to be leaking. However, in the initial assessment it is often difficult to make this diagnosis with any certainty.

Disruption of the attachment of the medial canthal ligaments can result in traumatic telcanthus – this is due to traumatic detachment of the ligament from its bony insertion or, more commonly, comminution of the naso-orbital ethmoidal complex with the canthal insertion intact, but with a small fragment of displaced bone.

Investigation is necessary with CT scanning (Figure 26.15) for all but the simplest nasal bone fractures. Treatment is usually delayed for 7–10 days post injury and generally necessitates ORIF and repositioning of the fragments with the medial canthi attached. If a formal canthopexy is required, this can be achieved with stainless steel wires or specialised canthopexy wires.

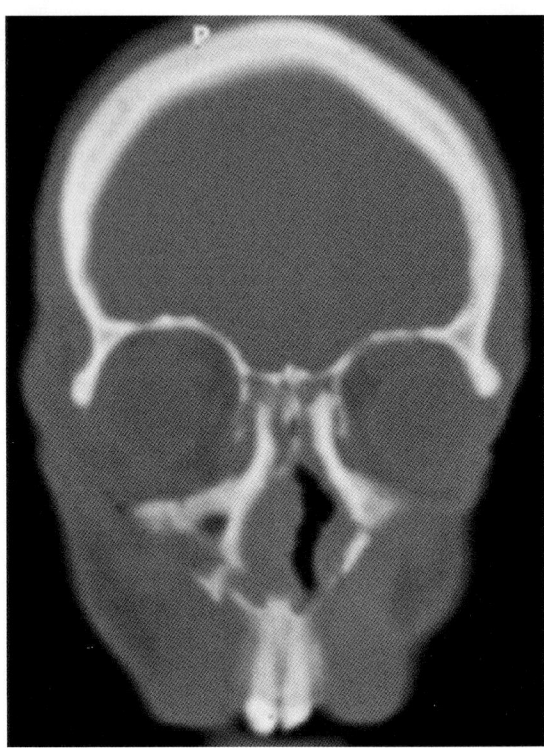

Figure 26.15 Coronal computed tomography scan showing posteriosuperior impaction of the naso-orbito complex.

Summary box 26.8

Naso-orbito ethmoidal fractures

- Naso-orbito ethmoidal injuries indicate significant force transfer
- Other associated injuries should be excluded, particularly craniofacial/anterior cranial fossa injuries

Craniofacial fractures

These are fractures that involve the cranial cavity and the facial bones in continuity. In many cases they involve the frontal and ethmoidal sinuses, creating a communication between the cranial cavity and the nasal air sinuses. If this is combined with a dural tear, CSF will leak into the nose and is detected as CSF rhinorrhoea with or without a salty taste. In these circumstances antibiotics are not indicated and the threshold for surgical intervention is quite variable between surgeons. The most common site of injury is the posterior wall of the frontal sinus, however fractures of the ethmoid and sphenoid sinus can also cause CSF leaks.

Most surgeons would treat persistent leaks lasting 10 days with surgical intervention, and mostly this is done with an open anterior fossa repair (necessitating a frontal craniotomy). In a limited number of cases the CSF leak can be repaired endoscopically. In most patients the treatment involves cranialisation of the frontal sinus with obliteration of the frontonasal duct. Although some surgeons advocate reconstruction of the posterior sinus wall, others will obliterate the sinus with fat or bone. Unless there are other pressing imperatives treatment is usually delayed for 7–14 days.

Summary box 26.9

Craniofacial fractures

- Usually managed by a multispecialty team involving neurosurgery, ear, nose & throat (ENT) and oral & maxillofacial surgery
- Significant head injuries are common

Panfacial fractures

In cases where there are fractures at all levels of the facial skeleton (upper, mid and lower face) the term panfacial fracture is used, and these fractures can present particular management challenges. First, multiple-level fractures indicate a significant amount of force and therefore energy transfer, hence associated injuries to the brain, cervical spine and other organs are much more common. Second, reconstruction of the multiple fractures is much more difficult because there is little normal anatomy to act as a guide. Each component of the panfacial fracture is treated in the same way as an isolated fracture would be, but sequencing the repair is challenging. The options are top down (craniofacial, zygomatico-orbital, maxillary and finally mandibular), bottom up, inside out (starting centrally and working laterally) or outside in. Most surgeons experienced in managing this type of injury would tailor the sequence to the particular fracture pattern to optimise the use of normal or near normal anatomy as a guide.

There are some particular pitfalls: obtaining adequate cheekbone projection anteroposteriorly while making the zygomatic arch too prominent, over-impacting the anterior maxilla, and an anterior mandibular fracture being fixed with the mandibular angles flared outwards.

Dental injuries

The primary (deciduous) dentition is usually fully erupted by 2.5 years, and the first permanent teeth (lower incisors) usually erupt at about the age of 6. Between the ages of 5 and 13 the primary dentition is shed and replaced by the secondary teeth.

If an adult whole tooth is avulsed it should be cleaned gently in saline and reimplanted; the sooner that this can happen the better the prognosis (avulsed deciduous teeth are not reimplanted). This is best achieved under local anaesthesia and after irrigation and debridement of the socket. The patient should then be referred urgently to a dentist for ongoing care; in many cases the tooth may need to be splinted to immobilise it and ensure that it is protected from the dental occlusion.

Fractures of the teeth may involve the enamel only, the enamel and dentine or the enamel, dentine and pulp. Once the dentine is exposed the fractured tooth can be exquisitely painful and benefits from a simple dental dressing – in the first instance local anaesthetic infiltrated in the region of the apex of the root is helpful in reducing pain pending a specialist dental assessment. If the pulp is exposed, local anaesthetic applied topically to the exposed pulp can also give some pain relief.

Summary box 26.10

Dental injuries

- It is important to account for all missing teeth and/or dental fragments – a chest radiograph may be indicated
- Exposed dentine and pulp can be exquisitely painful and referral for emergency dental treatment can be very helpful
- Avulsed teeth should be reimplanted as soon as possible

Soft tissue injuries

Lacerations and wounds

Facial lacerations and incised wounds often bleed quite profusely as a result of the excellent blood supply. This has the benefit of excellent healing and therefore wounds should only be debrided of frankly necrotic tissue.

In assessing facial soft tissue wounds it is important to check the function of the facial nerve and the patency of the parotid duct because both of these structures require repair should they be involved in the injury.

Uncomplicated wounds with no tissue loss should be cleaned and closed in layers under either local or general anaesthesia. If the skin is contaminated with dirt it should be scrubbed clean with a brush to prevent dirt tattooing. Usually, absorbable sutures are utilised intraorally and for the deep layers. It is important for good closure that the muscle layers are accurately opposed. The final skin layer should be closed with a monofilament suture (in children this can be absorbable). For some small linear incised wounds cyanoacrylate glue can be utilised.

Wounds involving the eyelid margins and crossing the vermillion of the lip need special attention to detail and very careful approximation of all the involved layers such that referral to a specialist should be considered by the inexperienced surgeon.

Where there has been skin loss the management depends on the size of the defect, the elasticity of the surrounding skin and the circumstances. Small defects can be closed with direct closure, but for larger defects the mobilisation of local skin flaps may be necessary. When there is greater tissue loss, skin grafting and/or free tissue transfer may be required.

Parotid duct

The parotid duct may be damaged as a result of an incised wound or a crushing injury. This is usually obvious as saliva leaking into the wound and should this be the case the buccal branch of the facial nerve is often injured at the same time. If the duct is transected or damaged this should be repaired over a cannula inserted into the parotid papilla. This is usually best achieved with magnification (loupes or microscope) under the controlled conditions of general anaesthetic.

Facial nerve

Facial nerve injuries are best repaired primarily, and the biggest challenge to achieving this is not identifying the motor deficit at presentation. In general, injuries that lie behind a line from lateral canthus or the eye to the angle of the mouth are repairable and this should be attempted. Again, this is best achieved under microscope magnification and a nerve stimulator/monitor is very helpful in identifying the cut nerve ends.

Animal and human bites

Unlike those elsewhere on the body, facial bites should be closed primarily and not left open. The abundant blood supply renders this normal precaution unnecessary. All bites should be debrided carefully and closed in the usual way; however, antibiotics, in accordance with local protocols, should be prescribed. If there is significant tissue loss consideration should be given to a staged reconstruction.

Summary box 26.11

Soft tissue injuries

- Examination of both motor and sensory nerve function should be conducted prior to the administration of local anaesthetic
- Tissue loss can occur and usually warrants specialist referral
- Careful cleaning (debridement) with removal of all dirt minimises the chances of wound tattooing

FURTHER READING

Brennan P, Schliephake H, Ghali GE, Cascarini L. *Maxillofacial surgery*, 3rd edn. London: Churchill Livingstone, 2017.

Fonseca R, Barber HD, Powers M, Frost DE. *Oral and maxillofacial trauma*, 4th edn. Philadelphia: Saunders, 2012.

Perry M, Holmes S. *Atlas of operative maxillofacial trauma surgery: primary repair of facial injuries*. Berlin: Springer, 2014.

Chapter 27

Torso trauma

Learning objectives

To understand:

- That the management of trauma is based on physiology as well as anatomy (as in general surgery)
- The gross and surgical anatomy of the chest and abdomen
- The pathophysiology of torso injury
- The strength and weaknesses of clinical assessment in the injured patient
- The use of special investigations and their limitations
- The operative approaches to the thoracic cavity
- The special features of an emergency room thoracotomy for haemorrhage control
- The indications for and techniques of the trauma laparotomy
- The philosophy of damage control surgery
- The management of trauma to the pelvis

INTRODUCTION

Because injury does not respect anatomical boundaries, division of the body into abdomen and thorax is artificial, and injury to the torso, with its associated physiological consequences, is more appropriate. The torso is generally regarded as the main part of the human body, primarily made up of the chest, abdomen and pelvis, not including the head, neck, arms and legs. About 42% of all deaths are the result of brain injury, but some 39% of all trauma deaths are caused by major haemorrhage, usually from torso injury (Figure 27.1).

Although initially, injury was treated on an anatomical basis, it has become clear that physiology should be the over-riding consideration, and the driver of successful resuscitation is therefore the preservation of normal physiology. Techniques such as 'damage control resuscitation' and 'damage control surgery' have dramatically improved survival through an understanding of the best techniques required to restore physiological stability (see Chapters 1, 22 and 23).

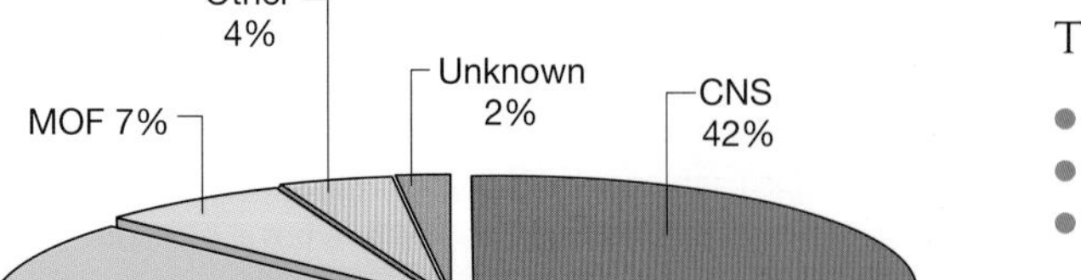

Figure 27.1 Causes of death in trauma. CNS, central nervous system; MOF, multiple organ failure.

INJURY MECHANISMS ASSOCIATED WITH TORSO TRAUMA

Injury often traverses different anatomical zones of the body, affecting structures on both sides of traditional anatomical zones. These zones are known as junctional zones.

Junctional zones

The key junctional zones are:

- between the neck and the thorax;
- between the thorax and the abdomen;
- between the abdomen, the pelvic structures and the groin.

These zones represent surgical challenges in terms of both the diagnosis of the area of injury and the surgical approach, which have to be balanced against the physiological stability of the patient.

Root of the neck

Most injuries affecting the base of the neck also affect the upper mediastinum and thoracic inlet. Choice of access is determined by the need for surgical control of the vascular structures contained within.

The mediastinum

The zone overlying the mediastinum with its major vessels and the heart is also an extremely high-risk area for penetrating wounds. Any wound in this region should immediately raise the suspicion of a major vascular or an associated cardiac injury, even in the absence of initial gross physical signs.

Diaphragm

The thorax and abdomen are separated by the diaphragm, which is mainly responsible for breathing, and moves during breathing between the fourth and eighth interspace. Any penetrating injury of the lower half of the chest may therefore have penetrated the diaphragm and entered the abdomen. Injuries in this junctional zone, therefore, should be investigated as if both cavities had been penetrated (Figure 27.2). In blunt trauma, rupture of the diaphragm can result in migration of abdominal viscera into the chest.

Pelvic structures

The pelvis contains a large plexus of vessels, both venous and arterial. Should injury occur, control of haemorrhage can prove to be exceptionally difficult and may require control of both arterial inflow and venous outflow. Angioembolisation can be a very useful adjunct to treatment, especially with deep pelvic injuries.

Summary box 27.1

Junctional zones

- Between neck and the thorax
- Between thorax and the abdomen
- Between the abdomen, the pelvic structures and the groin

CRITICAL PHYSIOLOGY

Resuscitation of all injuries to the chest and abdomen should follow traditional ATLS® principles (*Table 27.1* and Chapters 22 and 23).

Bleeding is the major problem. This may be obvious at the time of evaluation; however, in the young physically fit individual, bleeding may only produce subtle changes in vital measures and therefore be difficult to assess (*Table 27.2*). Although obvious injury may be present, traditional indicators (such as pulse rate), in isolation, are unreliable.

TABLE 27.1 ATLS® principles of resuscitation.

A	Airway
B	Breathing
C	Circulation
D	Disability (neurology)
E	Environment and Exposure

Bleeding occurs from five major sites – **'one on the floor and four more':**

- external – 'floor';
- chest;
- abdomen (including the retroperitoneum);
- pelvis;
- extremities.

THORACIC INJURY

Thoracic injury accounts for 25% of all severe injuries. In a further 25%, it may be a significant contributor to the subsequent death of the patient. In most of these patients, the cause of death is haemorrhage. About 80% of patients with chest injury can be managed non-operatively. The key to a good outcome is early physiological resuscitation followed by a correct diagnosis.

TABLE 27.2 Clinical indicators of potential ongoing bleeding in torso trauma.

Physiological	Increasing respiratory rate
	Increasing pulse rate
	Falling blood pressure
	Rising serum lactate
Anatomical	Visible bleeding
	Injury in close proximity to major vessels
	Penetrating injury with a retained missile

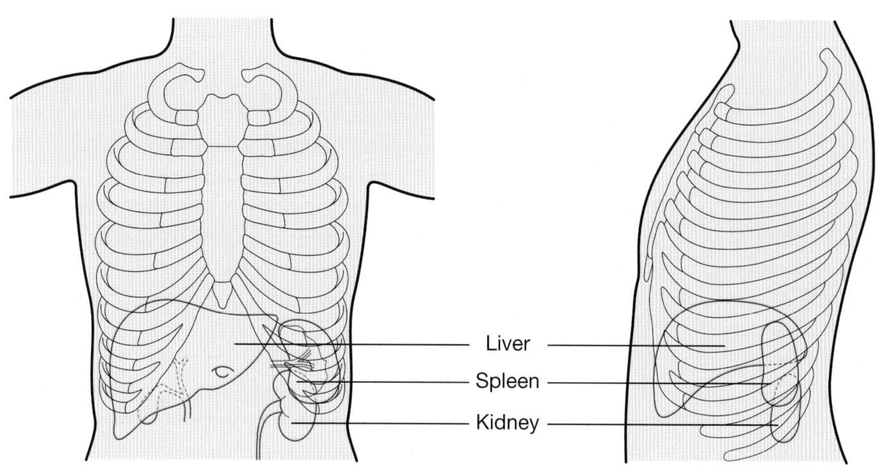

Figure 27.2 The anatomical extent of the abdomen.

Investigation

Routine investigation in the emergency department of injury to the chest is based on clinical examination, supplemented by chest radiography.

Ultrasound - extended focused assessment with sonar for trauma

Ultrasound can be used to differentiate between contusion and the actual presence of blood. Extended focused assessment with sonar for trauma (eFAST) is becoming the most common investigation. The technique uses sonar assessment in the chest, looking for a cardiac tamponade or free blood and air in the hemithorax on each side, and assessment for blood in the abdominal cavity, in the paracolic gutters, subdiaphragmatic spaces and pelvis.

Underwater chest drain

In the physiologically grossly unstable patient, where physical examination is inconclusive and there is no time for radiological investigations, insertion of an underwater chest drainage tube can be a diagnostic procedure as well as a therapeutic one, and the benefits of insertion often outweigh the risks.

Chest radiograph

In those cases where the patient is haemodynamically unstable or the spine is at risk, an anteroposterior (AP) supine chest radiograph is usually the simplest initial investigation, and will provide good information regarding tracheal deviation, lung and mediastinal pathology, as well as skeletal injury.

In penetrating injury, it may be more helpful for the radiograph to be performed with the patient positioned erect, as this will best reveal a small pneumothorax, fluid meniscus, air–fluid level or the presence of free gas under the diaphragm, indicating the presence of a hollow abdominal viscus perforation. Note that up to 300 mL of blood may pool behind the domes of the diaphragm, and may not be visible even in the erect view.

The presence of thoracic skeletal injury should alert the clinician to the possibility of adjacent thoracic or abdominal visceral injury. Rupture of the thoracic aorta can be related to fractures of the first and second rib, bilateral clavicular fracture and fracture of the sternum, thoracic spine or scapula. Fracture of the lower ribs can be related to injury of liver or spleen. Fracture of ribs, irrespective of site, can be related to injury to the lung parenchyma or thoracic wall vasculature, causing pneumothorax, haemothorax or lung contusion.

Computed tomography scan

The computed tomography (CT) scan with contrast allows for three-dimensional reconstruction of the chest and abdomen, as well as of the bony skeleton. It has become the principal and most reliable examination for major injury in thoracic trauma. In blunt chest trauma, the CT scan will allow the definition of fractures, as well as showing haematomas, pneumothoraces and pulmonary contusion. In penetrating trauma, the scan may show the track or presence of the missile and allow the proper planning of definitive surgery. However, although the presence of an isolated rupture of the diaphragm with migration of abdominal contents into the chest can be detected by CT scan, in injury without migration the diagnosis will not be obvious. CT scanning has replaced angiography as the diagnostic modality of choice for the assessment of the thoracic aorta and mediastinal vessels.

The pitfalls of investigation are:

- failure to assess tracheal shift immediately above the sternal notch clinically (deviation of the trachea occurs **away** from the affected side in tension pneumothorax, and **towards** the affected side in lung collapse);
- failure to percuss and auscultate both front and back in a supine patient (an inflated lung will 'float' on a haemothorax, so auscultation from the front may sound normal);
- failure to pass a nasogastric tube if rupture of the diaphragm is suspected; a chest radiograph will show the nasogastric tube apparently within the chest cavity;
- a supine chest radiograph can show a haemothorax as a homogenous increase in opacity of the hemithorax; this can cause confusion between the darker side and the lighter side, as to which may be a haemothorax (less radiolucent), or a pneumothorax (more radiolucent). Look carefully for lung markings, and don't drain the wrong side;
- pursuing radiological investigation (radiography or CT scan) instead of resuscitation in the unstable patient.

Summary box 27.2

Investigation of chest injuries

- Directly or indirectly involved in >50% of trauma deaths
- 80% can be managed non-operatively
- A chest radiograph is the investigation of first choice
- A chest drain can be diagnostic as well as therapeutic
- A spiral CT scan provides rapid diagnoses in the chest and abdomen

Management

In penetrating injury, most patients who have suffered injury to the chest can be managed with appropriate resuscitation and insertion of an intercostal drain.

If a sucking chest wound is present, this should not be fully closed but should be covered with a piece of plastic, closed on three sides, to form a one-way valve, and thereafter an underwater chest drain should be inserted remote from the wound. No attempt should be made to close a sucking chest wound until controlled drainage has been achieved, in case a stable patient with an open pneumothorax is converted into an unstable patient with a tension pneumothorax.

In blunt injury, most bleeding occurs from the intercostal or internal mammary vessels and it is relatively rare for these to require surgery. If bleeding does not stop spontaneously, the vessels can be tied off or encircled. In blunt chest compressive injury, particularly in the presence of a flail chest, there can be an associated lung contusion.

The patient *in extremis* with exsanguinating chest haemorrhage will be discussed in the section on Emergency department thoracotomy (EDT) later in the chapter.

Summary box 27.3

Closed management of chest injuries

- About 80% of chest injuries can be managed with the insertion of an intercostal drain only
- Do not close a sucking chest wound until a drain is in place
- If bleeding persists, the chest will need to be opened and direct haemostatic control is obtained

Life-threatening injuries can be remembered as the '**deadly dozen**'. Six are immediately life threatening and should be sought for and managed during the primary survey and six are potentially life threatening and should be detected during the secondary survey (*Table 27.3*). A high index of suspicion must be maintained thereafter to diagnose the potential threats to life, as their symptoms and signs can be very subtle. Early consultation and referral to a trauma centre is advised in cases of doubt.

Immediate life-threatening injuries

Airway obstruction

Early intubation is very important, particularly in cases of neck haematoma or possible airway oedema. Airway distortion can be insidious and progressive and can make delayed intubation more difficult if not impossible.

Tension pneumothorax

A tension pneumothorax develops when a 'one-way valve' air leak occurs either from the lung or through the chest wall. Air is sucked into the thoracic cavity without any means of escape, completely collapsing then compressing the affected lung. The mediastinum is displaced to the opposite side, decreasing venous return and compressing the opposite lung.

The most common causes are penetrating chest trauma, blunt chest trauma with a parenchymal lung injury and air leak that did not spontaneously close, iatrogenic lung injury (e.g. due to central venepuncture) and mechanical positive pressure ventilation.

TABLE 27.3 The 'deadly dozen' threats to life from chest injury.

Immediately life threatening	Airway obstruction
	Tension pneumothorax
	Pericardial tamponade
	Open pneumothorax
	Massive haemothorax
	Flail chest
Potentially life threatening	Aortic injuries
	Tracheobronchial injuries
	Myocardial contusion
	Rupture of diaphragm
	Oesophageal injuries
	Pulmonary contusion

The clinical presentation is dramatic. The patient is increasingly restless with tachypnoea, dyspnoea and distended neck veins (similar to pericardial tamponade). Clinical examination may reveal tracheal deviation; this is a late finding and is not necessary to clinically confirm diagnosis. There will also be hyper-resonance and decreased or absent breath sounds over the affected hemithorax. Tension pneumothorax is a **clinical** diagnosis and treatment should never be delayed by waiting for radiological confirmation (**Figure 27.3**).

Treatment consists of immediate decompression, initially by rapid insertion of a large-bore cannula into the second intercostal space in the mid-clavicular line of the affected side, then followed by insertion of a chest tube through the fifth intercostal space in the anterior axillary line.

Pericardial tamponade

Pericardial tamponade needs to be differentiated from a tension pneumothorax in the shocked patient with distended neck veins. It is most commonly the result of penetrating trauma. Accumulation of a relatively small amount of blood into the non-distensible pericardial sac can produce compression of the heart and obstruction of the venous return, leading to decreased filling of the cardiac chambers during diastole. All patients with penetrating injury anywhere near the heart plus shock must be considered to have a cardiac injury until proven otherwise. Classically, the presentation consists of central venous pressure elevation, decline in arterial pressure with tachycardia and muffled heart sounds. However, in cases in which major bleeding from other sites has taken place, the neck veins may be flat. A central line should be inserted, checking for a rising central venous pressure. A high index of suspicion and further diagnostic investigations will be needed to make the diagnosis is those cases that are not clinically obvious. These include an eFAST showing fluid in the pericardial sac. This is the most expeditious and reliable diagnostic tool, or chest radiography looking for an enlarged heart shadow.

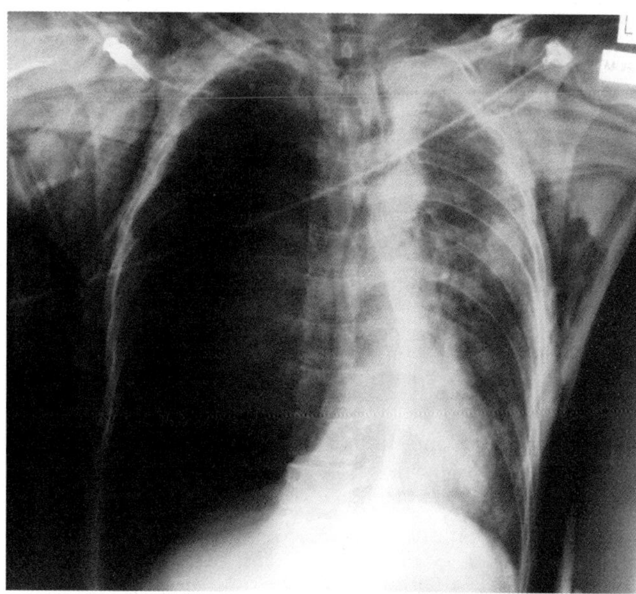

Figure 27.3 Radiological appearance of a tension pneumothorax.

Needle pericardiocentesis has been suggested. However, in penetrating injury to the heart there is usually a substantial clot in the pericardium, which may prevent aspiration. A dry pericardiocentesis proves only that there is a 'clot' on both ends of the needle! Pericardiocentesis has a high potential for iatrogenic injury to the heart and it should, at the most, be regarded as a desperate temporising measure in a transport situation (under electrocardiogram (ECG) control). The correct immediate treatment of tamponade is operative, either via a subxiphoid window, or by open surgery (sternotomy or left thoracotomy), with repair of the heart in the operating theatre if time allows or otherwise in the emergency room.

Summary box 27.4

Pericardial tamponade

- The presentation is similar to a tension pneumothorax – deteriorating cyanosis, tachycardia and agitation
- eFAST is diagnostic and may also detect free fluid in the abdomen or pericardium
- The central venous pressure may not be elevated if the circulating volume is depleted, e.g. because of other injuries
- Pericardiocentesis is a temporising measure only, with a high complication rate and is not a substitute for immediate operative intervention

Open pneumothorax ('sucking chest wound')

This is due to a large open defect in the chest (>3 cm), leading to immediate equilibration between intrathoracic and atmospheric pressure. If the opening in the chest wall exceeds about two-thirds of the diameter of the trachea, then with each inspiratory cycle, air will be preferentially drawn through the defect, rather than through the trachea. Air accumulates in the hemithorax (rather than in the lung) with each inspiration, leading to profound hypoventilation on the affected side and hypoxia. If there is a valvular effect, increasing amounts of air in the pleura will result in a tension pneumothorax (see above).

Initial management consists of promptly closing the defect with a sterile occlusive plastic dressing (e.g. Opsite®), taped on three sides to act as a flutter-type valve. A chest tube is inserted as soon as possible in a site remote from the injury site.

Massive haemothorax

The most common cause of massive haemothorax in blunt injury is continuing bleeding from torn intercostal vessels or occasionally from the internal mammary artery secondary to fractures of the ribs. In penetrating injury, a variety of viscera, both thoracic and abdominal (with blood leaking through a hole in the diaphragm from the positive pressure abdomen into the negative pressure thorax) may be involved.

Accumulation of blood in a haemothorax can significantly compromise respiratory efforts, compressing the lung and preventing adequate ventilation. Presentation is with haemorrhagic shock, flat neck veins, unilateral absence of breath sounds and dullness to percussion. The initial treatment consists of correcting the hypovolaemic shock, insertion of an intercostal drain and, in some cases, intubation. Initial drainage of more than 1500 mL of blood or ongoing haemorrhage of more than 200 mL/h over 3–4 hours is generally considered an indication for urgent thoracotomy.

Blood in the pleural space should be removed as completely and rapidly as possible to prevent ongoing bleeding, an empyema or fibrothorax later. Clamping a chest drain to tamponade a massive haemothorax is not helpful.

The following points are important in the management of an open pneumothorax/haemothorax:

- a common problem is using too small a tube – a 28FG or larger tube should be used in an adult;
- if the lung does not reinflate, the drain should be placed on low-pressure (5 cm water) suction;
- clot occlusion of a chest drainage tube may result in 'no' drainage, even in the presence of ongoing bleeding;
- a second drain is sometimes necessary (but see Tracheobronchial injuries);
- a chest radiograph can help identify the presence of blood;
- physiotherapy and active mobilisation should begin as soon as possible.

Flail chest

This condition usually results from blunt trauma associated with multiple rib fractures, and is defined as three or more ribs fractured in two or more places. The blunt force typically also produces an underlying pulmonary contusion. The diagnosis is made clinically in patients who are not ventilated, not by radiography. To confirm the diagnosis the chest wall can be observed for paradoxical motion of a chest wall segment. On inspiration, the loose segment of the chest wall is displaced inwards and therefore less air moves into the lungs. On expiration, the segment moves outwards (paradoxical respiration). Voluntary splinting of the chest wall occurs as a result of pain, so mechanically impaired chest wall movement and the associated lung contusion all contribute to the hypoxia. There is a high risk of developing a pneumothorax or haemothorax. The CT scan, with contrast to display the vascular structures and a 3-D reconstruction of the chest wall, is the gold standard for diagnosis of this condition.

Traditionally, mechanical ventilation was used to 'internally splint' the chest, but had a price in terms of intensive care unit resources and ventilation-dependent morbidity. Currently, treatment consists of oxygen administration, adequate analgesia (including opiates) and physiotherapy. If a chest tube is *in situ*, topical intrapleural local analgesia introduced via the tube, can also be used. Ventilation is reserved for cases developing respiratory failure despite adequate analgesia and oxygen. Surgery to stabilise the flail segment using internal fixation of the ribs may be useful in a selected group of patients with isolated or severe chest injury and pulmonary contusion.

in situ is Latin for 'in place'.

Potentially life-threatening injuries

Thoracic aortic disruption

Traumatic aortic rupture is a common cause of sudden death after an automobile collision or fall from a great height. The vessel is relatively fixed distal to the ligamentum arteriosum, just distal to the origin of the left subclavian artery. The shear forces from a sudden impact disrupt the intima and media. If the adventitia is intact, the patient may remain haemodynamically stable. For this subgroup of immediate survivors, salvage is frequently possible if aortic rupture is identified and treated early. Aortic disruption should be clinically suspected in patients with gross asymmetry in systolic blood pressure (between the two upper limbs, or between upper and lower limbs), widened pulse pressure and chest wall contusion. Erect chest radiography can also suggest thoracic aortic disruption, the most common radiological finding being a widened mediastinum (**Figure 27.4**). The diagnosis is confirmed by a CT scan of the mediastinum (**Figure 27.5**), or possibly by transoesophageal

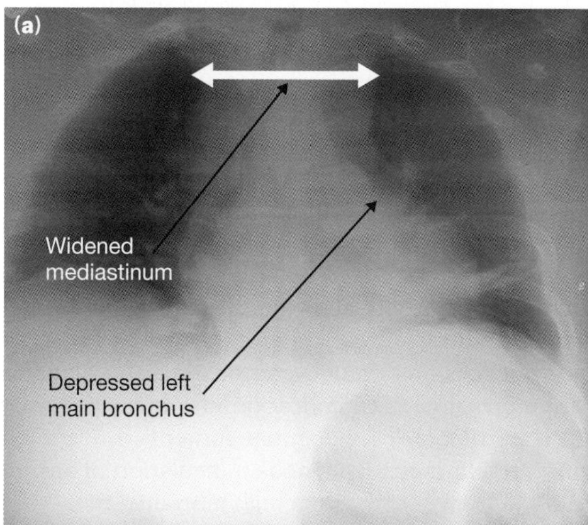

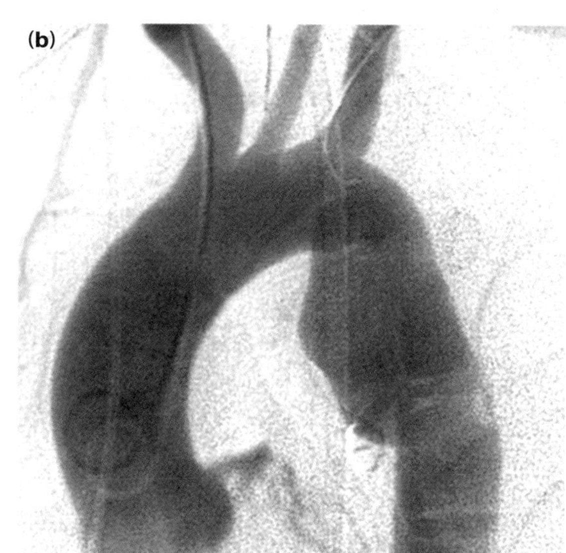

Figure 27.4 (**a**) Chest radiograph showing a widened mediastinum. (**b**) Aortogram showing aortic disruption.

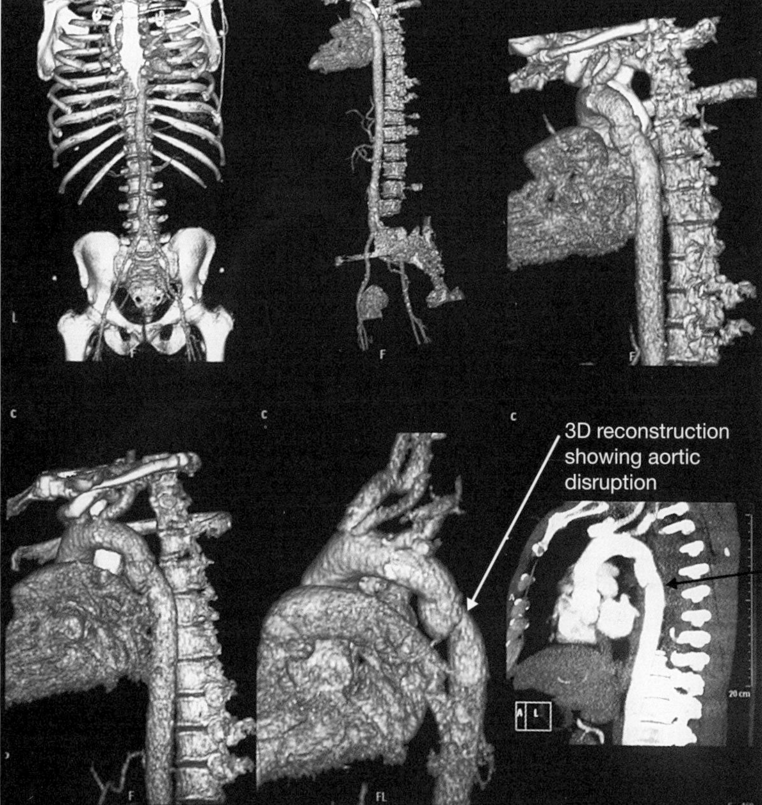

Figure 27.5 Computed tomography scans showing aortic disruption.

echocardiography, in unstable patients who cannot be moved to the scanner.

Initially, management consists of control of the systolic arterial blood pressure (to less than 120 mmHg). Thereafter, an endovascular intra-aortic stent (Figure 27.6) can be placed, or the tear can be operatively repaired by direct repair or excision and grafting using a Dacron graft.

Tracheobronchial injuries

Severe subcutaneous emphysema with respiratory compromise can suggest tracheobronchial disruption. A chest drain placed on the affected side will reveal a large air leak and the collapsed lung may fail to re-expand. Bronchoscopy is diagnostic. Treatment involves intubation of the unaffected bronchus followed by operative repair. Referral to a trauma centre is advised.

Blunt myocardial injury

Significant blunt cardiac injury that causes haemodynamic instability is rare. Blunt myocardial injury should be suspected in any patient sustaining blunt trauma who develops early ECG abnormalities.

Two-dimensional echocardiography may show wall motion abnormalities. A transoesophageal echocardiogram may also be helpful. There is very little evidence that enzyme estimations have any place in diagnosis.

All patients with myocardial contusion diagnosed with conduction abnormalities are at risk of developing sudden dysrhythmias and should be closely monitored.

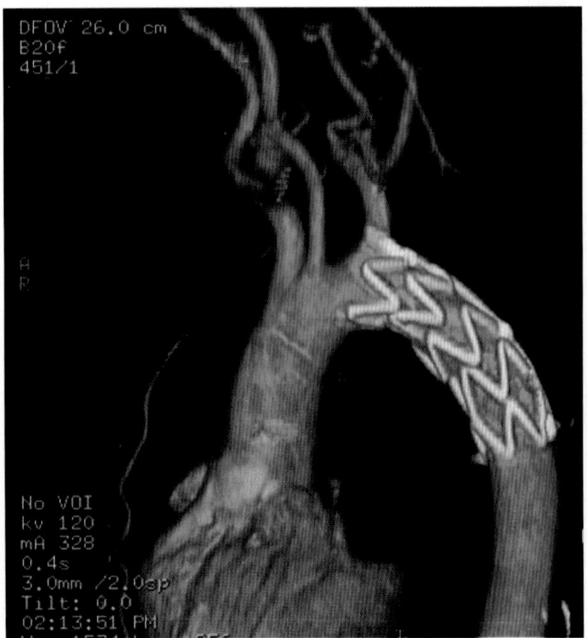

Figure 27.6 Aortic tear showing the presence of a stent.

Diaphragmatic injuries

Any penetrating injury below the fifth intercostal space should raise suspicion of diaphragmatic penetration and, therefore, injury to abdominal contents.

Blunt injury to the diaphragm is usually caused by a compressive force applied to the pelvis and abdomen. The diaphragmatic rupture is usually large, with herniation of the abdominal contents into the chest. Diagnosis of diaphragmatic rupture can easily be missed in the acute phase, and may only be discovered at operation, or through the presentation of complications.

Most diaphragmatic injuries are silent and the presenting features are those of injury to the surrounding organs. There is no single standard investigation. Chest radiography after placement of a nasogastric tube may be helpful (as this may show the stomach herniated into the chest). Contrast studies of the upper or lower gastrointestinal tract, CT scan, ultrasound and diagnostic peritoneal lavage all lack positive or negative predictive value. The most accurate evaluation is by video-assisted thoracoscopy (VATS) or laparoscopy, the latter offering the advantage of allowing the surgeon to proceed to a repair and additional evaluation of the abdominal organs.

The thorax is at negative pressure and the abdomen is at positive pressure. A complication of a breach of the diaphragm is herniation of abdominal contents into the chest. This may present much later, and strangulation of any of the contents can then occur, with a high mortality rate.
Operative repair is recommended in all cases. All penetrating diaphragmatic injury must be repaired via the abdomen and not the chest, to rule out penetrating hollow viscus injury.

Oesophageal injury

Most oesophageal injuries result from penetrating trauma; blunt injury is rare. A high index of suspicion is required. The patient can present with odynophagia (pain on swallowing saliva, foods or fluids), subcutaneous or mediastinal emphysema, pleural effusion, air in the perioesophageal space and unexplained fever. Mediastinal and deep cervical emphysema are evidence of an aerodigestive injury until proven otherwise.

The mortality rate rises exponentially if treatment is delayed. A combination of oesophagogram in the decubitus position and oesophagoscopy confirm the diagnosis in the great majority of cases. The treatment is operative repair of any defect and drainage.

Pulmonary contusion

Pulmonary contusion occurs more frequently following blunt trauma, usually associated with a flail segment or fractured ribs. This is a very common, potentially lethal injury and the major cause of hypoxaemia after blunt trauma. Following gunshot wounds, there is an area of contusion from the shock wave of the bullet.

The natural progression of pulmonary contusion is worsening hypoxaemia for the first 24–48 hours. Chest radiographic

Charles Thomas Stent, 1805–1885, dentist, Brighton, UK.

findings may be typically delayed. Contrast CT scanning can be confirmatory. Haemoptysis or blood in the endotracheal tube is a sign of pulmonary contusion.

In mild contusion, the treatment is oxygen administration, pulmonary toilet and adequate analgesia. In more severe cases mechanical ventilation is necessary. Normovolaemia is critical for adequate tissue perfusion and fluid restriction is not advised.

EMERGENCY THORACIC SURGERY

Emergency thoracic surgery is an essential part of the armamentarium of any surgeon dealing with major trauma. A timely surgical intervention for the correct indications can be the key step in saving an injured patient's life.

It is important to make a distinction between:

- immediate thoracotomy in the ED for the control of haemorrhage, cardiac tamponade or internal cardiac massage;
- emergency sternotomy for anterior mediastinal structures and heart;
- planned thoracotomy for definitive correction of the problem – this usually takes place in the more controlled environment of the operating theatre.

The clinical decision as to whether a patient requires ED surgery or can be transferred to the operating room can be complex. It is far better to perform a thoracotomy in the operating room, either through an anterolateral approach or a median sternotomy, with good light and assistance and the potential for autotransfusion or bypass, than it is to attempt heroic emergency surgery in the resuscitation area. However, if the patient is *in extremis* with a falling systolic blood pressure, there is no choice but to proceed immediately with a left anterolateral thoracotomy. In certain circumstances, when care is futile, it may not need to be performed at all. A resuscitation room thoracotomy following blunt trauma has limited indications and is rarely successful.

Emergency department thoracotomy or sternotomy

EDT should be reserved for those patients suffering **penetrating** injury **in whom signs of life are still present.** Patients who have received cardiopulmonary resuscitation (CPR) in the prehospital phase of their care are unlikely to survive, and electrical activity must be present.

In certain situations, EDT is considered futile:

- CPR in the absence of endotracheal intubation for more than 5 minutes;
- CPR for more than 10 minutes (despite endotracheal intubation);
- blunt trauma when there have been no signs of life at the scene (see above).

The survival rates for EDT in patients with penetrating trauma in whom the blood pressure is falling despite adequate resuscitation are shown in *Table 27.4*.

TABLE 27.4 Survival rates for thoracotomy in patients with penetrating trauma.

Blood pressure despite resuscitation	Survival (%)
>60 mmHg	60%
>40 mmHg	30%
<40 mmHg	3%

The aim of EDT is to perform:

- internal cardiac massage;
- control of haemorrhage from injury to the heart or lung;
- control of intrathoracic haemorrhage from other sources;
- control of massive air leak;
- clamping of the thoracic aorta to preserve the blood supply to the heart and brain, and cutting off the arterial supply distally, in a moribund patient with a major distal penetrating injury.

Planned emergency thoracotomy

Planned emergency thoracotomy implies an emergency thoracotomy performed as a planned procedure in the operating room, directed at the management of a specific injury. As such, the approach chosen is dependent on the indication for surgery and the organ injured (*Table 27.5*). Some organs are best approached through a median sternotomy. Otherwise the thoracotomy may be right- or left-sided, and these may be joined, producing the so called 'clamshell incision'. This gives excellent exposure for any surgeon who is not routinely entering the chest.

Posterolateral thoracotomy is not used in the emergency situation because of the difficulties in positioning of the patient, except for specific access to certain posterior mediastinal organs.

TABLE 27.5 Different approaches to the contents of the chest cavity.

Approach	Best for
Left anterolateral thoracotomy	Left lung and lung hilum Thoracic aorta Origin of left subclavian artery Left side of heart Lower oesophagus
Right anterolateral thoracotomy	Right lung and lung hilum Azygos veins Superior vena cava Infracardiac inferior vena cava Upper oesophagus Thoracic trachea
Median sternotomy	Anterior aspect of heart Anterior mediastinum Ascending aorta and arch of aorta Pulmonary arteries Carina of the trachea

ABDOMINAL INJURY

Patients who have suffered abdominal trauma can generally be classified into the following categories based on their physiological condition after initial resuscitation:

- haemodynamically 'normal' – investigation can be completed before treatment is planned;
- haemodynamically 'stable' – investigation is more limited. It is aimed at establishing whether the patient can be managed non-operatively, whether angioembolisation can be used or whether surgery is required;
- haemodynamically 'unstable' – investigations need to be suspended as immediate surgical correction of the bleeding is required.

A trauma laparotomy is the final step in the pathway to delineate intra-abdominal injury. Occasionally it is difficult to determine the source of bleeding in the shocked, multiple injured patient. If doubt still exists, especially in the presence of other injuries, a laparotomy may still be the safest option.

The patient's physiology must be assessed at regular intervals and, if there is an indication that the patient is still actively bleeding, then the source must be identified, unless the patient is unstable, requiring immediate surgery. Blood loss into the abdomen can be subtle and there may be no clear clinical signs. Blood is not an irritant and does not initially cause any abdominal pain. Distension is subjective, and a drop in the blood pressure may be a very late sign in a young fit patient. Examination in unstable patients should take place either in the ED or in the operating theatre if the patient is deteriorating rapidly.

Investigation

Investigations are driven by the cardiovascular status of the patient. In torso trauma, the best and most sensitive modality is a CT scan with intravenous contrast; however, in the unstable patient, this is generally not possible.

In patients with penetrating injury, metal markers (e.g. bent paper clips) should be placed on all external wounds before plain films are taken, irrespective of the area being radiographed, as this allows an assessment of the trajectory and helps to correlate the number of holes and the number of missiles that can be seen within the patient. This will help determine whether two holes are indicative of one missile passing through the patient, or two missiles, both retained internally (Figure 27.7). A single hole implies that the projectile has been retained.

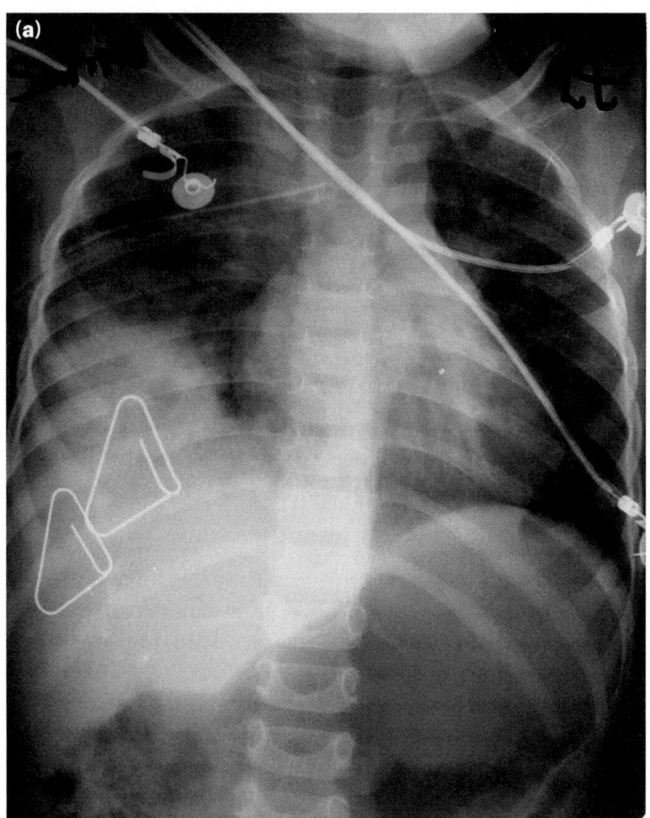

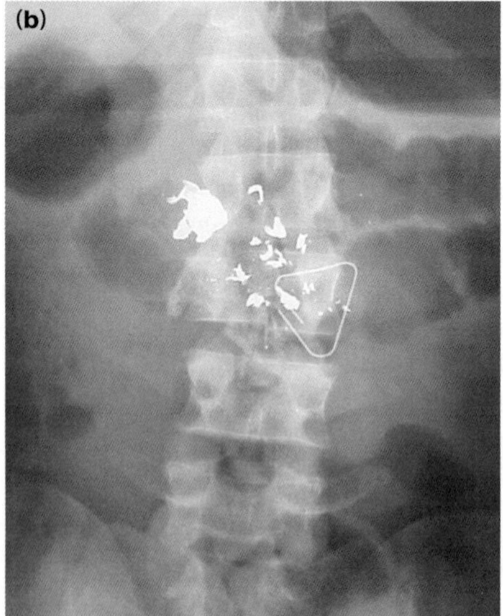

Figure 27.7 (a) Chest radiograph showing a gunshot wound with bullet markers. (b) Abdominal radiograph of a gunshot wound showing bullet markers.

Focused abdominal sonar for trauma and extended FAST

Focused abdominal sonar for trauma (FAST) is a technique whereby ultrasound (sonar) imaging is used to assess the torso for the presence of free fluid, either in the abdominal cavity, and is extended into the thoracic cavities and pericardium (eFAST). There should be no attempt to determine the nature or extent of the specific injury. eFAST is usually a rapid, reproducible, portable and non-invasive bedside test and can be performed at the same time as resuscitation. eFAST is accurate at detecting >100 mL of free blood; however, it is very operator dependent and, especially if the patient is very obese or the bowel is full of gas, it may be unreliable. Hollow viscus injury and solid organ injury are difficult to diagnose, even in experienced hands, as small amounts of gas or fluid are difficult to assess, and eFAST a low sensitivity (29–35%) for organ injury without haemoperitoneum. eFAST is also unreliable for excluding injury in penetrating trauma. If there is doubt, the eFAST examination can be repeated.

Summary box 27.5

Utilisation of eFAST

- Detects free fluid in the abdomen or pericardium
- Will not reliably detect less than 100 mL of free blood
- Does not directly identify injury to hollow viscus
- Cannot reliably exclude injury in penetrating trauma
- May need repeating or supplementing with other investigations
- Is unreliable for assessment of the retroperitoneum

Diagnostic peritoneal lavage

Diagnostic peritoneal lavage (DPL) is a test used to assess the presence of blood or contaminants in the abdomen. A gastric tube is placed to empty the stomach and a urinary catheter is inserted to drain the bladder.

A cannula is inserted below the umbilicus, directed caudally and posteriorly. The cannula is aspirated for blood (>10 mL is deemed as positive) and, following this, 1000 mL of warmed Ringer's lactate solution is allowed to run into the abdomen and is then drained out via the same route. The presence of >100 000 red cells/μL or >500 white cells/μL is deemed positive (this is equivalent to 20 mL of free blood in the abdominal cavity), as is the presence of vegetable fibre or a raised amylase level. In penetrating trauma, a minimum of one-tenth of the above would be regarded as evidence of peritoneal penetration or intraperitoneal injury. In the absence of laboratory facilities, a urine dipstick may be useful. Drainage of lavage fluid via a chest drain indicates penetration of the diaphragm.

Although DPL has largely been replaced by eFAST (see above), it remains the standard in many institutions where eFAST is not available or is unreliable. DPL is especially useful in the hypotensive, unstable patient with multiple injuries as a means of excluding intra-abdominal bleeding.

Computed tomography scan

CT has become the 'gold standard' for the intra-abdominal diagnosis of injury in the stable patient. The scan can be performed using intravenous contrast. CT is sensitive for blood and individual organ injury, as well as for retroperitoneal injury. An entirely normal abdominal CT is usually sufficient to exclude intraperitoneal injury.

The following points are important when performing CT:

- it remains an inappropriate investigation for unstable patients;
- if duodenal injury is suspected from the mechanism of injury, oral contrast may be helpful;
- if rectal and distal colonic injury is suspected in the absence of blood on rectal examination, rectal contrast may be helpful.

Laparoscopy

Laparoscopy or thoracoscopy may be a valuable screening investigation in stable patients with penetrating trauma, to detect or exclude peritoneal penetration and/or diaphragmatic injury.

Laparoscopy may be divided into:

- **Screening**: used to exclude a penetrating injury with breach of the peritoneum.
- **Diagnostic**: finding evidence of injury to viscera.
- **Therapeutic**: used to repair the injury.

In most institutions, evidence of penetration requires a laparotomy to evaluate organ injury, as it is difficult to exclude all intra-abdominal injuries laparoscopically. When used in this role laparoscopy reduces the non-therapeutic laparotomy rate. There is no place for laparoscopy in the unstable patient.

INDIVIDUAL ORGAN INJURY

Liver

Blunt liver trauma occurs as a result of direct injury. The liver is a solid organ and compressive forces can easily burst the liver substance (Figure 27.8). The liver is usually compressed between the impacting object and the rib cage or vertebral column. Most injuries are relatively minor and can be managed non-operatively.

Penetrating trauma to the liver is relatively common. Bullets have a shock wave and when they pass through a solid structure such as the liver they cause significant damage some distance from the actual track of the bullet. Not all penetrating wounds require operative management and may stop bleeding spontaneously.

In the stable patient, CT is the investigation of choice. It provides information on the liver injury itself, as well as on injuries to the adjoining major vascular and biliary structures.

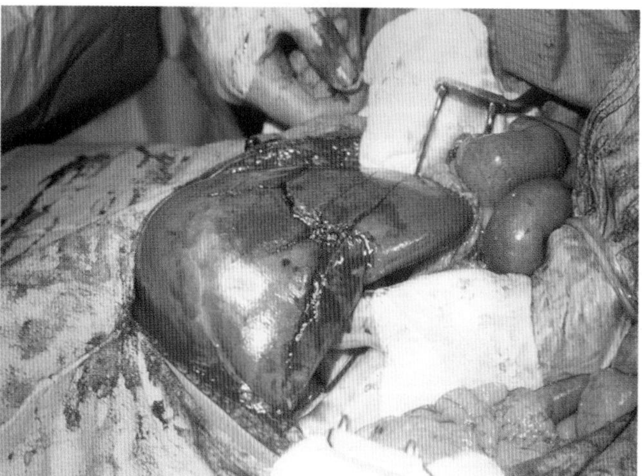

Figure 27.8 Compression injury to the liver, bursting the liver substance.

Sydney Ringer, 1835–1910, Professor of Clinical Medicine, University College Hospital, London, UK.

Injury in which there is a suggestion of a vascular component should be reimaged, as there is a significant risk of the development of subsequent ischaemia, false aneurysms, arteriovenous fistulae or haemobiliary fistula. It is advised that all patients should be rescanned prior to discharge.

Liver injury can be graded and managed using the American Association for the Surgery of Trauma (AAST) Organ Injury Scale (OIS) (www.aast.org/injury).

Management

The operative management of liver injuries can be summarised as 'the four Ps':

- push;
- Pringle;
- plug;
- pack.

At laparotomy the liver is reconstituted and bleeding is controlled by direct bimanual compression to achieve its normal architecture as best as possible (push). The inflow from the portal triad is controlled by a Pringle's manoeuvre, with direct compression of the portal triad, either digitally or using a soft clamp (Figure 27.9). This has the effect of reducing arterial and portal venous inflow into the liver, although it does not control the backflow from the inferior vena cava and hepatic veins. Any holes due to penetrating injury can be plugged directly using silicone tubing or a Sengstaken–Blakemore tube, and, after controlling any arterial bleeding, the liver can then be packed (see Damage control surgery, below).

Bleeding points should be controlled locally when possible, and such patients if required, subsequently undergo subsequent angioembolisation. It is not usually necessary to suture penetrating injuries of the liver, unless haemostasis cannot be controlled by other means. If there has been direct damage to the hepatic artery, it can be tied off. Damage to the portal vein must be repaired, as tying off the portal vein carries a greater than 50% mortality rate. If it is not technically feasible to repair the vein at the time of surgery, it should be shunted and the patient referred to a specialist centre. A closed suction drainage system must be left *in situ* following hepatic surgery. Finally, the liver can be definitively packed, restoring the anatomy as closely as possible. Placing omentum into cracks in the liver is not recommended.

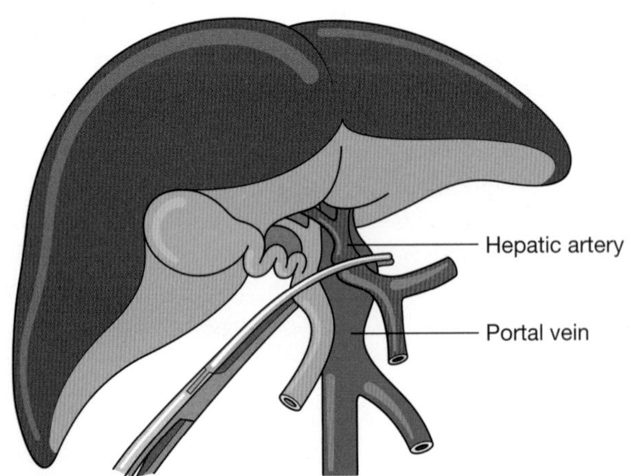

Figure 27.9 The Pringle manoeuvre.

Summary box 27.6

Liver trauma

- Blunt trauma occurs as the result of direct compression
- Penetrating trauma of the upper abdomen or lower thorax can damage the liver
- CT scanning is the investigation of choice in the stable patient
- Surgical management consists of push, Pringle, plug and pack
- The hepatic artery can be tied off but not the portal vein (which should be stented)
- Closed suction drainage should always be used

Biliary injuries

Isolated traumatic biliary injuries are rare and occur mainly from penetrating trauma, often in association with injuries to other structures that lie in close proximity. The common bile duct can be repaired over a T-tube or drained and referred to appropriate care as part of damage control, or even ligated.

Spleen

Splenic injury occurs from direct blunt trauma. Most isolated splenic injuries, especially in children, can be managed non-operatively. However, in adults, especially in the presence of other injury or physiological instability, laparotomy should be considered. The spleen can be packed, repaired or placed in a mesh bag. Splenectomy may be a safer option, especially in the unstable patient with multiple potential sites of bleeding. In certain situations, selective angioembolisation of the spleen can play a role.

Following splenectomy there are significant, though transient, changes to blood physiology. The platelet and white count rise and may mimic sepsis. Innoculation against *Pneumococcus* is advisable within 2–3 weeks, by which time the patient's immune system has recovered.

James Hogarth Pringle, 1863–1941 (Australian born), surgeon, The Royal Infirmary, Glasgow, UK.
Robert William Sengstaken, 1923–1978, surgeon, Garden City, NY, USA and **Arthur Hendley Blakemore**, 1897–1970, Associate Professor of Surgery, The College of Physicians and Surgeons, Columbia University, New York, NY, USA, designed a tube with two in-built balloons for the treatment of oesophageal varices. The tube was passed and the distal balloon inflated. The tube was drawn backwards until the distal balloon was held at the oesophageal hiatus. The proximal balloon was inflated, allowing the tamponade of any varices in the distal oesophagus.

Pancreas

Most pancreatic injury occurs as a result of blunt trauma. The major problem is that of diagnosis, because the pancreas is a retroperitoneal organ. CT remains the mainstay of accurate diagnosis. Amylase or lipase estimation is insensitive. In penetrating trauma, injury may only be detected during laparotomy.

Classically the pancreas should be treated with conservative surgery and closed suction drainage. Injuries are treated according to the OIS system of the AAST. Injuries to the pancreatic body to the left of the superior mesenteric vessels and to the tail are treated by closed suction drainage alone, with distal pancreatectomy if the duct is involved. Proximal injuries (to the right of the superior mesenteric artery) are treated as conservatively as possible, although partial pancreatectomy may be necessary. The pylorus can be temporarily closed (pyloric exclusion) in association with a gastric drainage procedure, to minimise pancreatic enzyme stimulation by gastric juice or distension. A Whipple's procedure (pancreaticoduodenectomy) is rarely needed and should not be performed in the emergency situation because of the very high associated mortality rate. A damage control procedure with packing and drainage should be performed and the patient referred for definitive surgery once stabilised.

Stomach

Most stomach injuries are caused by penetrating trauma. Blood presence is diagnostic if found in the nasogastric tube, in the absence of bleeding from other sources.

Surgical repair is required but great care must be taken to examine the stomach fully, as an injury to the front of the stomach can be expected to have an 'exit' wound elsewhere on the organ.

Duodenum

Duodenal injury is frequently associated with injuries to the adjoining pancreas. Like the pancreas, the duodenum lies retroperitoneally and so injuries are hidden, discovered late or at laparotomy performed for other reasons. CT is the diagnostic modality of choice. The only sign may be gas or a fluid collection in the periduodenal tissue, and leakage of oral contrast, administration of which may improve accuracy of diagnosis.

Smaller injuries can be repaired primarily. The first, third and fourth parts of the duodenum behave like small bowel, and can be repaired in the same fashion. The second part of the duodenum is fixed to the head of the pancreas with a common blood supply, and may have a poorer blood supply compared to the remainder. Major trauma, especially if the head of the pancreas is simultaneously injured, should be treated as part of a damage control procedure and be referred for definitive care.

Small bowel

The small bowel is frequently injured as a result of blunt trauma. The individual loops may be trapped, causing high-pressure rupture of a loop or tearing of the mesentery. Penetrating trauma is also a common cause of injury.

Small bowel injuries need urgent repair. Haemorrhage control takes priority and these wounds can be temporarily controlled with simple sutures. In blunt trauma with mesenteric vessel damage, the bowel ischaemia that results will dictate the extent of a resection. Resections should be carefully planned to limit the loss of viable small bowel, but should be weighed against an excessive number of repairs or anastomoses. Haematomas in the small bowel mesenteric border need to be explored to rule out perforation. With low-energy wounds, primary repair can be performed, whereas more destructive wounds associated with military type weapons require resection and anastomosis. Damage control 'clip and drop' of damaged or resected bowel may be necessary.

Colon

Injuries to the colon from blunt injury are relatively infrequent, and are more frequently a penetrating injury. If relatively little contamination is present and the viability is satisfactory, such wounds can be repaired primarily. If, however, there is extensive contamination, the patient is physiologically unstable or the bowel is of doubtful viability, then the bowel can be closed off ('clip and drop'). A defunctioning colostomy can be formed later or the bowel reanastomosed once the patient is stable.

Rectum

Only 5% of colon injuries involve the rectum. These are generally from a penetrating injury, although occasionally the rectum may be damaged following fracture of the pelvis. Digital rectal examination will reveal the presence of blood, which is evidence of intestinal or rectal injury. These injuries are often associated with bladder and proximal urethral injury.

With intraperitoneal injuries, the rectum is managed as for colonic injuries. Full-thickness extraperitoneal rectal injuries should be managed with either a diverting end-colostomy and closure of the distal end (Hartmann's procedure) or a loop colostomy. Presacral drainage is no longer used.

Renal and urological tract injury

In the stable patient, CT scanning with contrast is the investigation of choice.

For assessment of bladder injury a cystogram should be performed. A minimum of 300 mL of contrast is instilled into the bladder via a urethral catheter. The large volume is

---

Allen Oldfather Whipple, 1881–1963, Valentine Mott Professor of Surgery, The College of Physicians and Surgeons, Columbia University, New York, NY, USA.
Henri Albert Charles Antoine Hartmann, 1860–1952, Professor of Clinical Surgery, Faculty of Medicine, The University of Paris, Paris, France.

essential because a small volume may not distend the bladder enough to produce a leak from a small bladder injury once the cystic muscle is contracted. It is important to assess the films as follows:

- two views – AP and lateral (and sometimes oblique);
- two occasions – full and postmicturition.

Generally, renal injury is managed non-operatively unless the patient is unstable. The kidney can be angioembolised if required.

Ureteric injury is rare and is generally due to penetrating trauma. Most ureters can be repaired or diverted if necessary, or may even be ligated as part of Damage control procedures.

Intraperitoneal rupture of the bladder, usually from direct blunt injury, will require surgical repair. Extraperitoneal rupture is usually associated with a fracture of the pelvis and will heal with adequate urine drainage via the transurethral route. Suprapubic drainage is reserved for when this is not possible.

Summary box 27.7

Injuries to structures in the abdomen

- In children, splenic injury can be managed non-operatively in most cases, but not if haemodynamically unstable
- Duodenal injuries are often associated with pancreatic trauma
- Bowel injuries need urgent definitive repair, or isolation using resection or by stapling
- Rectal injuries may be best managed initially with a diverting colostomy
- Kidney and urinary tract injury is best diagnosed with enhanced CT scanning
- Intraperitoneal bladder tears need formal repair and drainage

Retroperitoneum

Injury to the retroperitoneum is often difficult to diagnose, especially in the presence of other injury, when the signs may be masked. Diagnostic tests (such as ultrasound and DPL) may be negative. The best diagnostic modality is CT, but this requires a physiologically stable patient. The retroperitoneum is divided into three zones (Figure 27.10) for the purposes of intraoperative management:

In blunt trauma:

- Zone 1 (central): central haematomas should always be explored, once proximal and distal vascular control has been obtained.
- Zone 2 (lateral): lateral haematomas should only be explored if they are expanding or pulsatile. They are usually renal in origin and can be managed non-operatively, though they may sometimes require angioembolisation.
- Zone 3 (pelvic): as with zone 2, these should only be explored if they are expanding or pulsatile. Pelvic haematomas are exceptionally difficult to control and, whenever possible, should not be opened; they are best controlled with compression or extraperitonea packing, and if the bleeding is arterial in origin, with angioembolisation.

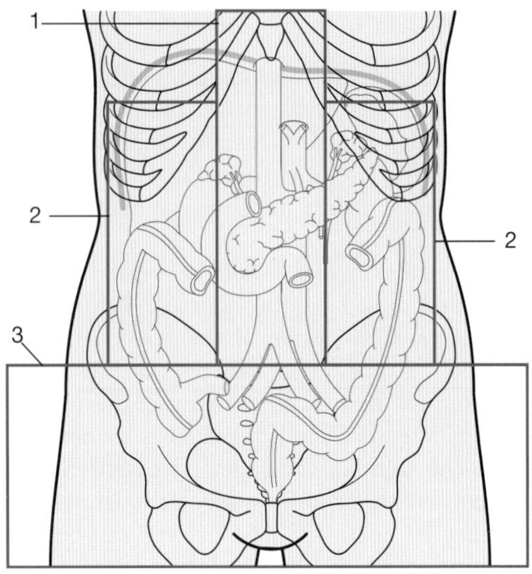

Figure 27.10 The zones of the retroperitoneum. Zone 1: central; zone 2: lateral; zone 3: pelvic.

In penetrating trauma, every injury should be explored for damage to structures along the wound track (e.g. ureter), unless preoperative investigation allows non-surgical management of the injury.

THE PELVIS

Although mortality following severe pelvic fractures has decreased dramatically with better methods of controlling haemorrhage, these patients still represent a significant challenge to every link of the treatment chain. Mortality rates exceeding 40% have recently been reported. Further, pelvic bleeding as one of the 'hidden bleeding sources' is still underestimated or missed, as retrospective chart analyses of potentially preventable deaths have revealed. Extreme force is required to disrupt the pelvic ring, and associated injuries and extrapelvic bleeding sources are common (up to 50% of cases). The haemodynamically unstable patient with severe pelvic fracture has a 90% risk of associated injuries, and a 30% risk of intra-abdominal bleeding.

To save these patients, three questions need to be addressed:

- Is the patient at high risk of massive bleeding?
- Where is the source of the bleeding?
- How to stop the bleeding?

Anatomy

The surgical anatomy of the pelvis is a key to the understanding of pelvic injuries.

- The pelvic inlet is circular, a structure that is immensely strong, but routinely gives way at more than one point should sufficient force be applied to it. Therefore, isolated fractures of the anterior or posterior pelvic ring are uncommon.
- The forces required to fracture the pelvic ring do not respect the surrounding organ systems.

- The pelvis has a rich collateral blood supply, especially across the sacrum and posterior part of the ileum. The cancellous bone of the pelvis also has an excellent blood supply. Most pelvic haemorrhage emanates from venous injury and fracture sites. However, in the haemodynamically unstable patient with severe pelvic injury, arterial bleeding is more frequent. Important for the treatment is that the surgeon has to deal both with arterial and venous bleeding.
- Postmortem examination has shown that the extrapelvic peritoneal space can accommodate more than 3000 mL. However, in the case of a severe pelvic fracture where the retroperitoneal compartment is disrupted and the external bony barrier is not stable, haematoma may extend upwards towards the mediastinum ('chimney effect') or downwards into the medial thigh in case of rupture of the pelvic floor.
- All iliac vessels, the sciatic nerve roots (including the lumbosacral nerve) and the ureters cross the sacroiliac joint; disruption of this joint may cause severe haemorrhage and sometimes cause arterial obstruction of the internal iliac artery and sciatic nerve palsy. Injuries to the ureters are rare.
- The pelvic viscera are suspended from the bony pelvis by condensations of the endopelvic fascia. Shear forces acting on the pelvis will transmit these to pelvic viscera, leading to avulsion and shearing injuries.
- The pelvis also includes the acetabulum, a major structure in weight transfer to the leg. Inappropriate treatment will lead to severe disability.

Classification

Pelvic ring fractures can be classified into three types, using the Tile classification (for subtypes and other classifications see Further reading), based on the severity of the fracture (and reflecting the energy required to cause it) (Figure 27.11). However, no fracture pattern can exclude significant haemorrhage.

Type A

Type A are the most common fractures and are completely stable. They result from lateral compression, which causes compression fractures of the pubic rami or compression fracture of the sacrum posteriorly.

Type B

These fractures are partially stable, and there is disruption of the anterior pelvis and partial disruption of the posterior pelvis. The pelvis can open and close 'like a book', but because the sacroiliac ligaments remain intact, there is no vertical displacement. Internal or external stabilisation is required. Blood loss can be significant.

Type C

This fracture is completely unstable. Both anterior pelvis and the entire posterior pelvic complexes are disrupted and the disrupted pelvic bones are free to displace horizontally and vertically. In both type B and type C pelvic injuries, there is a high risk of associated abdominal injuries (bowel perforation or mesenteric laceration) and rupture of the diaphragm.

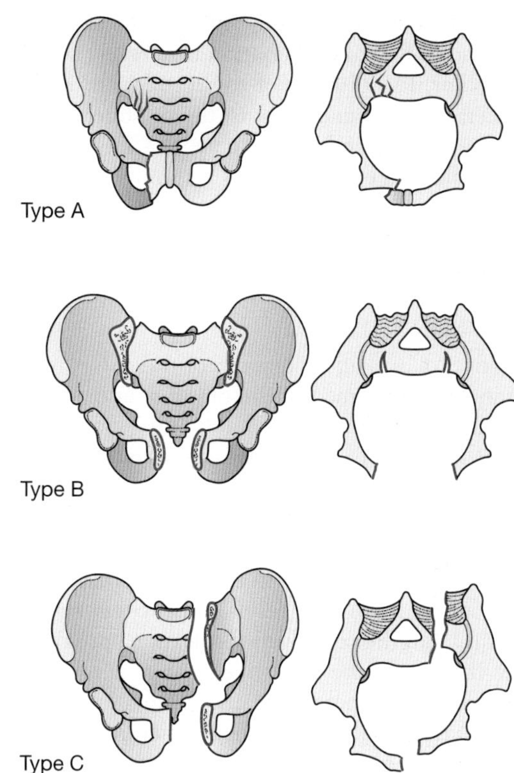

Figure 27.11 Tile classification of fractures of the pelvis.

Clinical examination

Pelvic fractures should be easily identified if ATLS guidelines are followed (i.e. clinical palpation and compression of the pelvic brim from sacroiliac joint to pubic symphysis, and a routine chest and pelvic radiograph for any blunt injury in a patient unable to walk). Clinical examination may reveal instability. Any instability felt indicates the presence of major pelvic fracture, associated with life-threatening blood loss, and requires appropriate measures. The absence of clinical instability does not, however, preclude an unstable pelvic fracture. One-third of such trauma victims with pelvic ring fractures present with circulatory instability on arrival.

Inspection of the skin may reveal lacerations in the groin, perineum or sacral area, indicating an open pelvic fracture, the result of gross deformation. Evidence of perineal injury or haematuria mandates radiological evaluation of the urinary tract from below upwards (retrograde urethrogram followed by cystogram or CT cystogram and an excretory urogram, as appropriate) when the physiology allows. Inspection of the urethral meatus may reveal a drop of blood, indicating urethral damage.

Marvin Tile, b.1933, orthopaedic surgeon, Sunnybrook Medical Centre, Toronto, Canada.

Inspection of the anus may reveal lacerations to the sphincter mechanism. Rectal examination may reveal blood in the rectum and/or discontinuity of the rectal wall, indicating a rectal laceration. In male patients, the prostate is palpated; a high-riding prostate indicates a complete urethral avulsion. A full neurological examination is performed of the perineal area, sphincter mechanism and femoral and sciatic nerves.

Diagnosis

Radiograph

Examination of a plain radiograph of the pelvis requires an understanding of the mechanism of injury and a decision on the stability of the pelvic rim.

An open book type mechanism causes one or both ilea to rotate externally (opening, like a book). A lateral compression mechanism causes the pelvis to collapse. An 'open-book fracture' is seen as a widening of the pubic symphysis or widening at the site of a fracture in the pubic ramus. Not only is there disruption of the bony pelvis, but also tearing of the pelvic floor and thus the pelvic venous plexus is at risk. The more unstable the pelvis, the more likely the structures are to be damaged. When the pelvis collapses from a lateral compression injury, the pubic bones usually fracture. Displacement of the anterior pelvis by greater than 2 cm indicates at least partial instability. A vertical shear disruption of the sacroiliac joint, with apparent shortening of the limb on the affected side implies significant energy of injury.

FAST may be unreliable as it does not localise intra-abdominal bleeding in these patients.

CT is the diagnostic modality of choice in the haemodynamically stable patient, and CT angiography is particularly helpful to provide details of both the anatomy of the facture, as well as details of the origin of the bleeding (venous or arterial).

Management

The treatment of bleeding is to stop the bleeding!

The priorities for resuscitating patients with pelvic fractures are no different from the standard. These injuries can produce a real threat to the circulation, and management is geared toward controlling this threat. Initial management requires the use of a compression binder or a sheet, applied around the true pelvis at the level of the greater trochanters ('reduce the pelvic volume'), a potentially lifesaving procedure that has to be done in the emergency room.

85% of bleeding originating from the pelvis is of venous origin and can be controlled by non-operative means, including compression either by binding or external fixator, or by extraperitoneal packing (i.e. packing the loose space between the bony wall of the pelvis and the peritoneum) to compress the pelvic veins. If other sources of bleeding have been ruled out, the extraperitoneal pelvic packing is done without entering the peritoneal cavity. This may be combined with external fixation.

If the bleeding is of arterial origin, interventional angioembolisation is the next choice for bleeding control. The techniques for bleeding control (compression, packing, fixation and angioembolisation) do not exclude each other but rather may complement each other. Persistent bleeding after packing may require angioembolisation and vice versa.

Severe pelvic injuries require a multidisciplinary team approach. If adequate orthopaedic experience is unavailable, consideration should be given towards early transfer of this patient to an institution with the necessary expertise.

If the source of the bleeding is in doubt or FAST/CT results are positive, showing a significant amount of blood in the peritoneal cavity, concurrent intra-abdominal injury cannot be excluded, and it is wise to perform an exploratory laparotomy to treat or rule out intra-abdominal bleeding.

Summary

In summary, a haemodynamically normal patient can be safely transferred for stabilisation of unstable fractures within hours after injury and following control of the associated damage.

Summary box 27.8

Pelvic injury

- Associated injuries can only be managed once the patient is haemodynamically stable
- Decision on the stability is of paramount importance
- Procedures for damage control may be the only available option
- External stabilisation of the pelvic ring is the basis of all treatment
- If necessary, further bleeding control can be achieved either by angioembolisation or extraperitoneal packing
- Most associated injuries can be managed once the patient is haemodynamically stable

DAMAGE CONTROL

Following major injury, protracted surgery in the physiologically unstable patient can in itself prove fatal. Patients with the 'deadly triad' (hypothermia, acidosis and coagulopathy) are those at highest risk. 'Damage control' or 'damage limitation surgery' is a concept that originated from naval shipbuilding strategy, whereby ships were designed so that the damage was kept 'local' and which allowed only the minimal repairs needed to prevent it from sinking, while definitive repairs waited until it had reached port. The technique has been adopted following major trauma, and includes initial care and resuscitation (damage control resuscitation) and the surgical correction of the injury (damage control surgery).

The minimum amount of surgery needed to stabilise the patient's condition may be the safest course until the physiological derangement can be corrected. Damage control surgery is restricted to only two goals:

- stopping any active surgical bleeding;
- controlling any contamination.

Once these goals have been achieved then the operation is suspended and the abdomen temporarily closed. The patient's resuscitation then continues in the intensive care unit, where other therapeutic interventions can take place.

Once the physiology has been corrected, the patient warmed and the coagulopathy corrected, the patient is returned to the operating theatre for any definitive surgery.

Damage control resuscitation

The concept of damage control has been broadened to include the techniques used in resuscitation as well as in surgery. The time in the ED is minimised and the majority of resuscitation of the patient is carried out in the operating room and not in the resuscitation bay (*Table 27.6*). The resuscitation is individualised through repeated point of care testing, of haemoglobin, acidosis (pH and lactate) and clotting, and is therefore directed towards the early delivery of biologically active colloids, clotting products and whole blood in order to buy time. The physiological disturbances that are associated with the downward spiral of acidosis, coagulopathy and hypothermia in these serious injuries are predicted and attempts are made to avoid them rather than react to them.

Damage control surgery

The decision whether damage control surgery is the appropriate course should be made early (*Table 27.7*) and allows the whole surgical and anaesthetic team to work together to limit the time in surgery and the earliest possible admission of the patient to the intensive care unit. Damage control is a staged process.

The initial focus is haemorrhage control, followed by control and limitation of contamination, achieved using a range of abbreviated techniques including simple ligation of bleeding vessels, shunting of major arteries and veins, drainage, temporary stapling of bowel and therapeutic packing.

Following the above, the abdomen is closed in a temporary fashion using a sheet of plastic (e.g. Opsite®) over the bowel, an intermediate pack to allow suction and a further sheet of adherent plastic drape to the skin to form a watertight and airtight seal. Suction is applied to the intermediate pack area to collect abdominal fluid. This technique is known as the 'Vacpac' or 'Opsite® sandwich' (**Figure 27.12**). As soon as control has been achieved the patient is transferred to the intensive care unit where resuscitation is continued.

The next stage following damage control surgery and physiological stabilisation is definitive surgery. The team should aim to perform definitive anastomoses, vascular reconstruction and closure of the body cavity within 24–72 hours of injury. However, this must be individualised to the patient, the response to critical care resuscitation and the progression of injury complexes.

TABLE 27.6 The stages of damage control surgery.

Stage	
I	Patient selection
II	Control of haemorrhage and control of contamination
III	Resuscitation continued in the intensive care unit
IV	Definitive surgery
V	Abdominal closure

TABLE 27.7 Indications for damage control surgery.

Anatomical	Inability to achieve haemostasis
	Complex abdominal injury, e.g. liver and pancreas
	Combined vascular, solid and hollow organ injury, e.g. aortic or caval injury
	Inaccessible major venous injury, e.g. retrohepatic vena cava
	Demand for non-operative control of other injuries, e.g. fractured pelvis
	Anticipated need for a time-consuming procedure
Physiological (decline of physiological reserve)	Temperature <34°C
	pH <7.2
	Serum lactate >5 mmol/L (normal: <2.5 mmol/L)
	Prothrombin time (PT) >16 s
	Partial thromboplastin time (PTT) >60 s
	>10 units blood transfused
	Systolic blood pressure <90 mmHg for >60 min
Environmental	Operating time >60 min (core temperature loss in usually 2°C/h)
	Inability to approximate the abdominal incision
	Desire to reassess the intra-abdominal contents (directed relook)

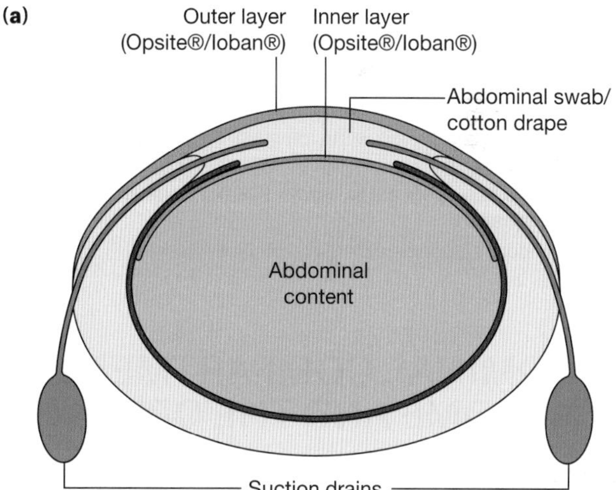

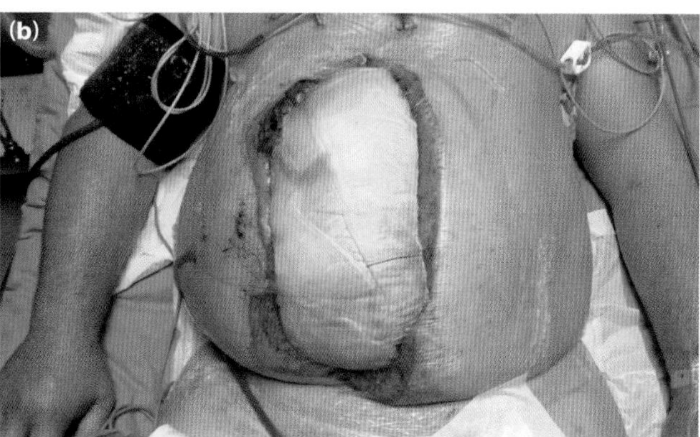

Figure 27.12 (a) Diagram showing temporary skin closure in damage control. (b) Abdominal closure following damage control surgery showing an Opsite® closure.

The abdomen is closed as soon as possible, bearing in mind the risks of abdominal compartment syndrome (ACS). The closure is not without its own morbidity. Successful closure may require aggressive off-loading of fluid and even haemofiltration to achieve this if the patient will tolerate it. The best situation is closure of the abdominal fascia, or, if this cannot be achieved, then skin closure only. Occasionally, mesh closure can be used, with skin grafting over the mesh and subsequent abdominal wall reconstruction.

Thoracic damage control is conceptually based on the same philosophy. This is that haemorrhage control and focused surgical procedures minimise further surgical insult and lead to improved survival in the unstable trauma patient. The aim is to control bleeding and limit air leaks using the fastest procedures available, such as staplers, to minimise the operative time. Often, damage control surgery **is** the definitive surgery.

The indications and techniques for emergency thoracic surgery have already been described.

Damage control applies equally to the extremities. In this case, it is shunting of blood vessels, identifying and marking damaged structures such as nerves, fasciotomy and removal of contaminated tissue that are the main tasks. Subsequent definitive management can be carried out at a later stage.

Summary box 27.9

Damage control

- Resuscitation is carried out in the operating room using biologically active fluids (i.e. blood) – damage control resuscitation (DCR)
- The surgery performed is the minimum needed to stabilise the patient
- The aims of surgery are to control haemorrhage and limit contamination
- Secondary surgery is aimed at definitive repair

ABDOMINAL COMPARTMENT SYNDROME AND THE OPEN ABDOMEN

Raised intra-abdominal pressure has far-reaching consequences for the patient; the syndrome that results is known as ACS. ACS is a major cause of morbidity and mortality in the critically ill patient and its early recognition is essential (*Table 27.8*).

In all cases of abdominal trauma in which the development of ACS in the immediate postoperative phase is considered a risk, the abdomen should be left open and managed as for damage control surgery.

TABLE 27.8 Effect of raised intra-abdominal pressure on individual organ function.

Organ	Effect
Renal	Increase in renal vascular resistance leading to a reduction in glomerular filtration rate and impaired renal function
Cardiovascular	Decrease in venous return resulting in decreased cardiac output because of both a reduction in preload and an increase in afterload
Respiratory	Increased ventilation pressures because of splinting of the diaphragm, decreased lung compliance and increased airway pressures
Visceral perfusion	Reduction in visceral perfusion
Intracranial effects	Severe rises in intracranial pressures

INTERVENTIONAL RADIOLOGY

Interventional radiology can be useful in the management of torso trauma as both an investigative and a therapeutic tool for patients with vascular injury. Angioembolisation following demonstration of ongoing bleeding in splenic and renal injury is a valuable technique.

NON-OPERATIVE MANAGEMENT

Non-operative management is generally preferred for the management of solid organ injury in haemodynamically stable children. Non-operative management of solid abdominal organ injury has rapidly gained acceptance in the management of adults as well. A stable patient and accurate CT imaging are prerequisites for this approach. Failure of non-operative management is uncommon and typically occurs within the first 12 hours after injury. Therefore, if correctly selected, the vast majority of these patients will avoid surgery, require less blood transfusion, and sustain fewer complications than operated patients.

ANTIBIOTICS IN TORSO TRAUMA

There is no level 1 evidence to recommend the use of antibiotics for the insertion of chest drains. However, prophylactic antibiotics prior to surgery should be used in all cases of penetrating abdominal trauma. Unless there is major contamination, a single dose is sufficient.

FURTHER READING

American Association for the Surgery of Trauma. Organ Injury Scaling System. Available online at: http://www.aast.org (accessed February 2016).

American College of Surgeons. *Advanced trauma life support course manual for doctors*, 9th edn. Chicago: American College of Surgeons, 2015.

Boffard KD (ed). *Definitive surgery of trauma care*, 4th edn. London: Taylor and Francis, 2015.

Eastern Association for the Surgery of Trauma. Guidelines for practice management: evidence-based guidelines. Available online at: http//:www.east.org (accessed February 2016).

Mattox LK, Moore EE, Feliciano DV (eds). *Trauma*, 7th edn. New York: McGraw Hill, 2013.

Tornetta P, Court-Brown CM, Heckman JD *et al. Rockwood and Green's fractures in adults*, 8th edn. Lippincott Williams and Wilkins, 2014.

World Society for Abdominal Compartment Syndrome. Abdominal compartment syndrome. Available online at: http//:www.wsacs.org (accessed February 2016).

Chapter 28

Extremity trauma

Learning objectives

To gain an understanding of:

- How to identify whether an injury exists
- The important injuries not to miss
- The principles of the description and classification of fractures
- The range of available treatments
- How to select an appropriate treatment

INTRODUCTION

In several chapters the importance of life-threatening trauma is emphasised, but numerically for every patient that dies following a traumatic event, there are three that are left with a lifelong functional impairment.

Appropriate treatment of extremity trauma is important to return the patient to optimal function as quickly and as safely as possible. The management of extremity trauma is step-wise and involves initially saving the patient's life by the identification and treatment of life and limb threatening injuries first, according to the Advanced Trauma Life Support (ATLS) principles.

Treatment depends on injury specific factors, patient factors and surgeon factors, including the resources available.

It is imperative for the clinician to involve the patient in the decision making process when it comes to the choice of treatment for that individual. Moreover, treatment priorities, functional demands and risk versus benefit vary from individual to individual.

DIAGNOSIS

The diagnosis of extremity trauma begins with the taking of a pertinent history followed by focussed physical examination and appropriate special tests.

History

It is important to ascertain the mechanism of injury and the amount of force involved in the injury. Take time to gather sufficient detail in order to do this. Certain injury mechanisms result in classical injury patterns; for example, electrocution or seizure activity may lead to a posterior dislocation of the shoulder. In your mind translate the mechanism of injury into the common anatomical injury patterns. For example, a head on collision between two cars each travelling at 40 miles per hour coming to a dead stop should be interpreted by the history taker as a rapid deceleration injury, which then allows anticipation of likely injuries, such as rupture of the aortic arch. Similarly, a fall on the outstretched hand might be associated with wrist, elbow, shoulder and clavicular injuries.

Following the history of the presenting complaint, it is important to collect information beyond that of the injury and the AMPLE mnemonic is an abbreviated system taught in ATLS.

A: Allergies
M: Medication – important to ask about anticoagulant and antiplatelet therapies, corticosteroid use and any possible immunosuppressive treatment
P: Past medical and surgical history – has the patient had an anaesthetic in the past and were there any complications
L: Last time – something to eat or drink
E: Events – events that led to the injury

In the multiply injured patient or patients with altered levels of consciousness, gain as much collateral history as possible. Listen to the account of pre-hospital personnel; for example, the amount of cabin intrusion in a vehicle or whether a collision was head on or a side on.

Examination

An initial general examination, including vital signs and general assessment, should be conducted. Is this an isolated injury or do you need to start right at the beginning, considering the A, B, C approach as advocated by ATLS? Examination of the individual extremity only begins once you are sure the patient is stable and life- and limb-threatening conditions have been excluded.

It is crucial to undertake a thorough top to toe evaluation in the secondary survey. Often the minor extremity injuries are missed (**Figure 28.1**) and can cause significant long-term problems (*Table 28.1*).

A top to toe evaluation is is achieved by a systematic approach (see Chapter 31 and *Apley's system of orthopaedics and fractures* [Further reading]) to the injured extremity:

- look;
- feel;
- move (active and passive);
- special tests;
- special investigations.

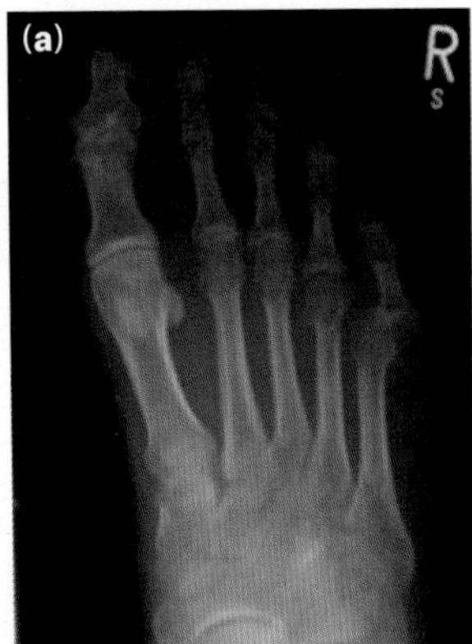

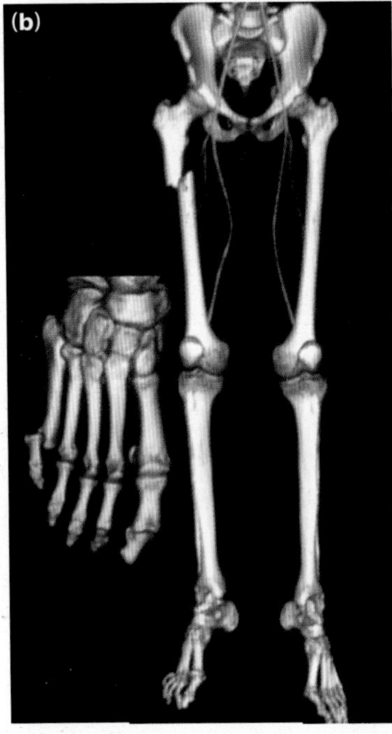

Figure 28.1 **(a)** Missed dislocation of metatarsophalangeal joint of the little toe, picked up at 8 weeks. **(b)** Initial trauma computed tomography angiogram. In retrospect, on close inspection the dislocation is visible on the angiogram; do not be distracted by the obvious femoral shaft fracture.

TABLE 28.1 Extremity injuries that are notorious for being missed.
Posterior dislocation of the shoulder
Lateral condylar mass fracture of the distal humerus
Perilunate dislocation
Scaphoid fracture
Tarsometatarsal fracture dislocation
Compartment syndrome
Vascular injury with knee dislocation
Talar neck fracture
Slipped upper femoral epiphysis
Achilles tendon rupture

Ensure you examine the joint above and the joint below the site of injury. Consider the events and mechanism of injury and examine the areas that could possibly be affected. For example, a patient who falls from a height may fracture the calcaneus, which is an obvious diagnosis with a very swollen hindfoot and extremely tender heel. The concomitant lumbar spine fracture may not become evident until a few days later when the distracting pain in the heel starts to subside.

Look

It is important to look at the whole limb, back and front, noting any localised swelling, bruising and any obvious deformity. A shortened externally rotated leg in an older patient suggests a fracture of the proximal femur. A slightly flexed, adducted internally rotated leg might suggest a posterior dislocation of the hip.

Any break in the skin or abrasion needs to be noted and the treating orthopaedic surgeon informed, even if you do not think it communicates with the fracture. A graze over the knee in a closed tibial fracture may preclude intramedullary nailing until the wound has healed over, or perhaps an alternative treatment may have to be considered.

Ideally a photograph (with appropriate consent) should be taken to document the injury and obviate the need for repeated manipulation of the dressings (see Open fractures).

Note the colour of the limb and the degree of general swelling. A compartment syndrome may still be present even when a limb does not appear to be very swollen (see Compartment syndrome), but if it is grossly swollen, note, document and pass on the information.

Look for pre-existing scars; a scar at the back of the elbow or over the cubital tunnel might signify an anterior transposition of the ulna nerve. Scars might signify previous metalwork that remains in situ or has been removed in the past.

Feel

Start gently examining the limb away from the zone of obvious injury, gaining the patients trust and gathering as much information as possible before and without causing the patient pain or discomfort. Feel for bony tenderness and note

---

Achilles, the Greek hero was the son of Peleus and Thetis. When he was a child, his mother dipped him in the Styx, one of the rivers of the Underworld so that he should be invulnerable in battle. The heel by which she held him did not get wet, and was, therefore, not protected. Achilles died from a wound in the heel received at the seige of Troy.

the degree of swelling and tenseness of the compartments. It should be noted that it is not possible to exclude a compartment syndrome based on how tense the limb feels. The deep posterior compartment of the lower leg cannot be felt when palpating the skin.

The characteristic crepitus of subcutaneous air can be felt in the setting of open fractures, air jet injuries and around the chest in the presence of a pneumothorax.

The examiner should feel for pulses and assess capillary return (see Neurovascular examination) as well as feeling for temperature changes.

Move

Movement as part of the examination should once again be approached carefully and without causing the patient pain and discomfort. Two types of movement can be assessed:

1 active – active movement is movement initiated and maintained by the patient;
2 passive – passive movement is when the examiner moves the limb.

Special tests

There are often special tests to detect injury in precise anatomical locations and many are described elsewhere in the book; for example, looking for a ruptured Achilles tendon by placing the patient prone with the foot over the edge of the bed and squeezing the calf; plantarflexion of the foot and ankle then suggests the Achilles tendon is intact.

The examiner should be aware of gravity simulating active movements. For example, a leg lying flat, fully extended on the couch does not mean the extensor mechanism of the knee is intact. In all knee injuries make sure the patient can actively straight leg raise and get their leg off the couch.

Similar pitfalls exist in the upper limb with gravity straightening the elbow. In order to assess triceps function and elbow extension, ensure the patient can actively extend against resistance from the examiner or against gravity.

Beware of trick movements. Patients with a complete rupture of the quadriceps can still walk with the leg locked in full to slight hyperextension by using the iliotibial band. Patients with complete rupture of the Achilles tendon can still actively plantar flex the foot and ankle using the long toe flexors.

Neurovascular examination

This is an important part of extremity examination and summary terms such as 'neurovascularly intact' are best avoided. It is preferable to clearly document the examination performed and its findings, along with a conclusion about the function of the particular neurological or vascular anatomy tested. On occasion you may not be able to examine all movements due to injury or casts.

It is important to examine and document findings before and after any manipulation or cast application, to ensure no change. A radial nerve palsy in association with a humeral shaft fracture that occurs at the time of injury may be treated expectantly. If, however, radial nerve function is lost after application of a cast or brace, the nerve should be explored. Most peripheral nerves have a motor and sensory component; document both sensibility and motor function.

Laceration or rupture of major vessels may result in life- and limb-threatening injury and should be dealt with as an emergency (see ATLS guidelines). Complete laceration or occlusion of a major vessel is obvious and seldom missed. In contrast, occult vessel injuries must be considered and actively excluded. In 30% of knee dislocations (tibio–femoral dislocation) a vascular injury will occur (Figure 28.2).

The presence of palpable pulses does not exclude a significant vascular injury and an intimal flap may develop, progress and thrombose over time. Repeated evaluation is necessary, before and after any intervention (manipulation/cast).

In injuries commonly associated with vascular injury, such as knee dislocations, occult injury should be actively excluded with an angiogram. If an angiogram is not performed, repeated thorough vascular evaluation of the limb should be undertaken for the first 24–48 hours.

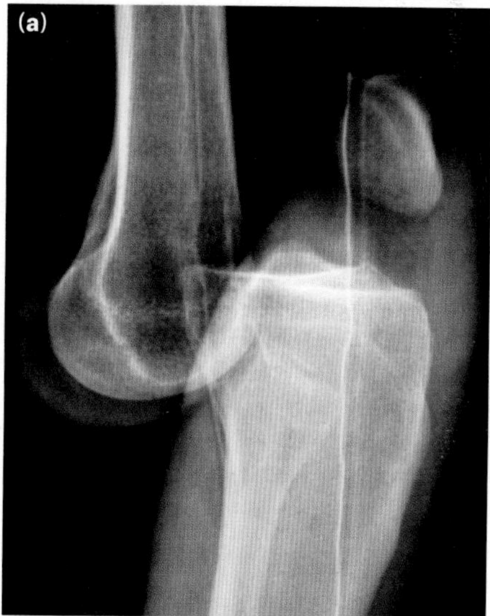

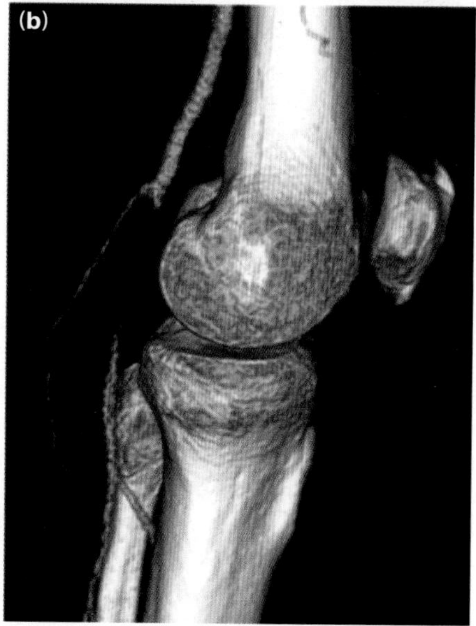

Figure 28.2 (a) Initial anterior tibio–femoral dislocation. (b) Post-reduction computed tomography angiogram showing complete blockage of the popliteal artery with reconstitution distally from a collateral blood supply.

Investigations

The mainstay of extremity trauma investigation remains radiography of the affected limb to see if there is a bony injury. However, this is not the sole investigation available.

Haematological investigations

Simple haematological investigations are seldom useful in the evaluation of single limb injury. In the polytrauma patient a full blood count, serum biochemistry, clotting factor and creatinine kinase may be useful. A blood gas, including PH, base excess and lactate, can be useful to show the severity of the injury and the response to resuscitation.

Ultrasound

Ultrasound is very useful to define soft tissue injuries. Fractures of the bones can be visualised on ultrasound but generally it is reserved for the soft tissues. One limitation of ultrasound is the variability depending on the experience of the sonographer.

Radiography

Radiographs are the mainstay in the initial evaluation of suspected extremity trauma. The rule of 2's should be remembered:

- 2 views – ensure acquisition of 2 views in orthogonal planes to avoid missing a fracture out of plane on the first radiograph view. For shoulder injuries ensure at least an AP and axillary or modified axillary view (Figure 28.3);
- 2 joints – radiographs are required of the joint above and the joint below the fracture;
- 2 occasions – sometimes the fracture may not be initially visible; a second series of radiographs should be undertaken after 10–14 days if suspicion of bony injury persists. The classic injury here is a scaphoid fracture. If initial scaphoid views are normal, consider repeating them 10–14 days later, if pain and tenderness in the anatomical snuff box persists;
- 2 sides – in paediatric injuries it can be useful to consider a radiograph from the opposite and uninjured side if doubt exists. With improved access to atlases of normal variants this is less important.

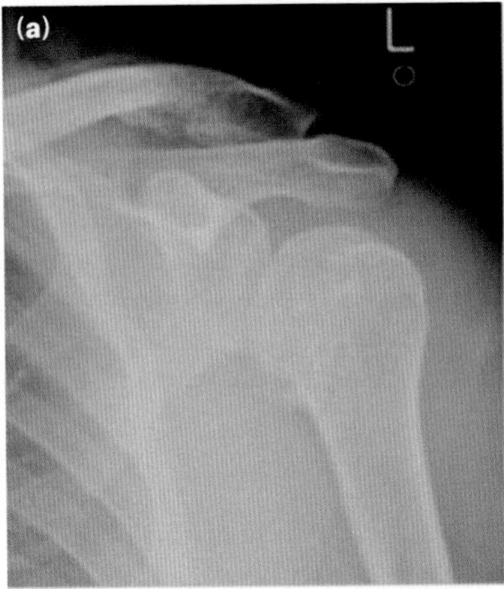

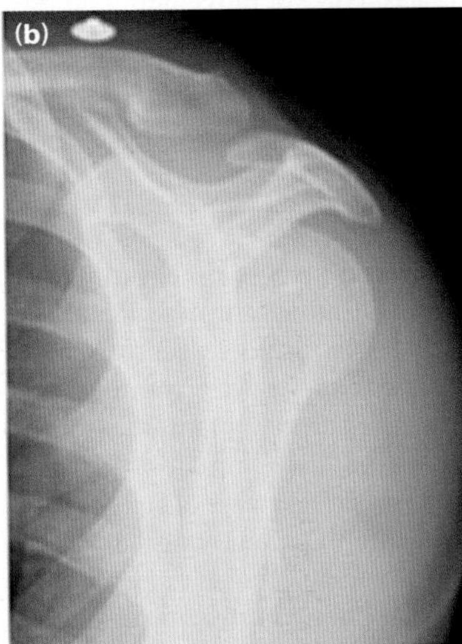

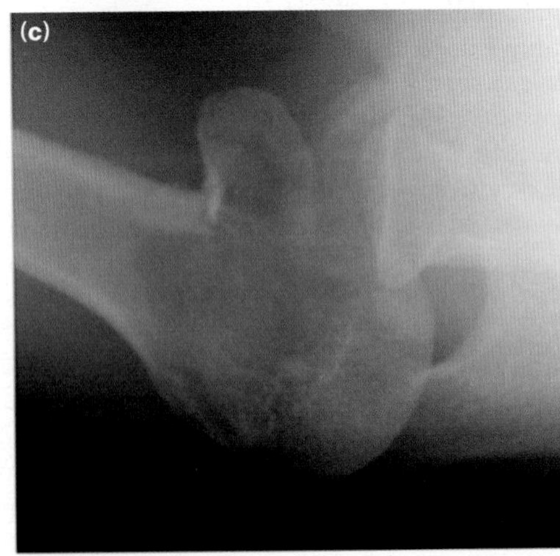

Figure 28.3 Radiographic series of the same patient demonstrating the value of 2 views in 2 planes and the true value of the axillary view in shoulder trauma. (a) Anteroposterior radiograph of the shoulder, initially reported as normal. (b) Lateral scapula radiograph, initially reported as normal; humeral head slightly posteriorly directed. (c) Axillary view – true value of axillary view shown with obvious posterior dislocation of the glenohumeral joint.

Computed axial tomography

Computed axial tomography (CT) is very good for characterising the bony anatomy of injuries, allowing for multiplanar reconstruction of injury anatomy and providing other 3D information. It is very useful for periarticular injuries, where the exact characterisation of the bony injury is essential.

Surface volume rendering is a useful addition allowing for easier visualization of the injury (see Figure 28.1b). CT angiography (see Figure 28.2b) may be added, providing information on the vascular anatomy. One disadvantage of CT is the dose of radiation involved.

Magnetic resonance imaging

Magnetic resonance imaging (MRI) provides 3D information without the radiation involved in CT. It provides useful information, particularly about the soft tissues. MRI can provide information on the blood supply to the bone; for example, avascular necrosis of the proximal pole of the scaphoid.

One disadvantage of MRI is the time taken to acquire the image; patients suffering from claustrophobia find the experience traumatic. Another issue is that the magnetic field may be disrupted by non-ferrous metal and the presence of ferrous metal contraindicates an MRI.

MRI angiography can also be performed providing information about the vascular anatomy.

Nuclear medicine scans

Technetium 99 nuclear medicine scans register osteoblastic activity and may be used to demonstrate occult fractures; for example, an undisplaced scaphoid fracture.

Summary box 28.1

History, examination and investigations

- Follow a systematic approach
- History requires sufficient detail of injury
- History can be organised in the AMPLE format
- Examination follows look, feel, move, special tests approach
- Investigations will include radiographs with rule of 2s observed
- Selective use of special investigations can help diagnosis

DESCRIPTION AND CLASSIFICATION OF THE INJURY

Soft tissue injury

There are several classification systems for soft tissue injuries, the Tscherne classification for closed injuries, the Gustilo and Anderson for open injuries (*Table 28.2*) and the Ganga classification of severe open injuries.

The first step of soft tissue injury characterisation is to decide if this is an open or closed fracture. An open fracture being any fracture where the fracture haematoma communicates with a breach in the epithelial lining, not just skin. For example, an open pelvic fracture may communicate with the vagina or rectum and a mandibular fracture through the mucosa of the mouth (see Open fractures).

Consider all the soft tissues crossing the zone of injury, as it is possible to get a closed rupture or avulsion of tendons without a break in the skin. Consider the possibility of a neurovascular injury. (see Neurological injury). Severe soft tissue injury in the presence or absence of a fracture may still lead to compartment syndrome (see Compartment syndrome).

TABLE 28.2 Gustilo and Anderson open fracture classification.

Type	
I	A low energy open fracture with a wound less than 1 cm long and clean
II	An open fracture with a laceration more than 1 cm long without extensive soft tissue damage, flaps or avulsion
III	Characterised by high energy injury irrespective of the size of the wound. Extensive damage to soft tissues, including muscles, skin, and neurovascular structures, and a high degree of contamination. Multifragmentary and unstable fractures
Subgroups of type III	
A	Adequate soft tissue cover of a fractured bone after stabilisation
B	Inadequate soft tissue cover of a fractured bone after stabilisation (i.e. flap coverage required)
C	Open fracture associated with an arterial injury requiring repair

Source: Gustilo RB, Mendoza RM, Williams DN. Problems in the management of type III (severe) open fractures: a new classification of type III open fractures. *J Trauma* 1984; **24**: 742–6.

Neurological injury

Seddon classified nerve injuries into neurapraxia, axonotmesis and neurotmesis:

- neurapraxia – no loss of nerve sheath continuity or peripheral Wallerian degeneration. Recovery potential good may take months if the pressure is removed from the nerve;
- axonotmesis – nerve sheath remains intact, with internal nerve fibre damage with Wallerian degeneration. The neural tube (endoneurium) can guide the regenerating nerve fibres to their target. Good potential for recovery; nerve fibre regrowth is at 1 mm per day;
- neurotmesis – complete division of the nerve, nerve sheath and nerve fibre. Functionally poor outcome without surgical intervention to restore continuity of the nerve sheath.

Although the Seddon classification is useful in understanding the pathoanatomy, the critical discriminator in defining recovery, and need for possible surgical intervention, is the presence or lack of continuity of the enveloping nerve sheath.

Bony injury

Description

Describing the bony injury depends on several characteristics and includes the:

- name of the bone that has been injured;
- region of bone injured;
- pattern of fracture line: transverse, oblique, spiral, segmental or multifragmentary (**Figure 28.4**);

Ramon Balgoa Gustilo, surgeon, Hennepin County Medical Center, Minneapolis, MN, USA.
John T Anderson, surgeon, Hennepin Medical Center, Minneapolis, MA, USA.
Sir Herbert J Seddon, trained at St Barts, London University, and the Royal National Orthopaedic Hospital, Stanmore, UK. He became the second Nuffield Professor of Orthopaedic Surgery in Oxford.

- presence of compression; compression fractures occur when cancellous bone collapses; vertebral wedge compression fracture;
- presence of displacement of the fracture fragments, undisplaced or displaced;
- type and degree of displacement (Figure 28.4):
  - angulation;
  - translation;
  - rotation (Figure 28.5);
  - shortening;
- presence of pre-existing pathology;
- associated joint pathology, dislocation or subluxation.

In children and adolescents the fracture line may be incomplete due to the plastic, less brittle nature of their bones (Figure 28.6) These incomplete fractures are called greenstick fractures, where one tension cortex fails. If the compression cortex buckles, they are called torus or buckle fractures. Paediatric bone may also simply undergo plastic deformation without a visible fracture line.

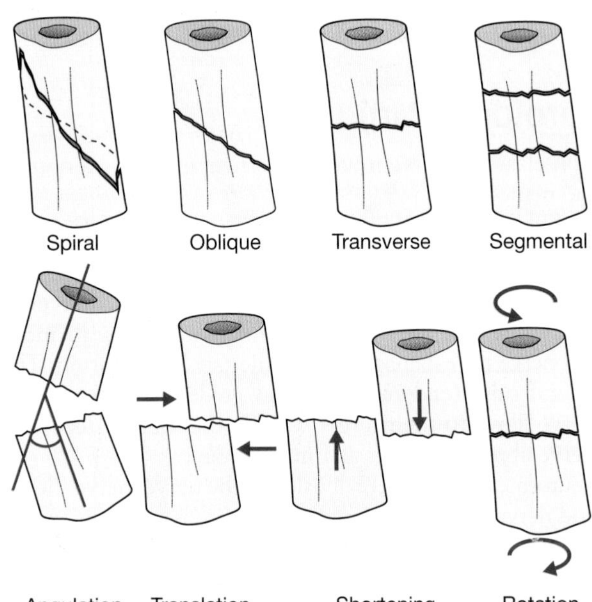

Figure 28.4 Descriptive terms for fractures.

> **Summary box 28.2**
>
> **Describing an injury**
>
> Use plain language to describe:
> - Location
> - Soft tissue component
> - Bony injury

Classification

For each specific bony injury there may be several injury specific classification systems.

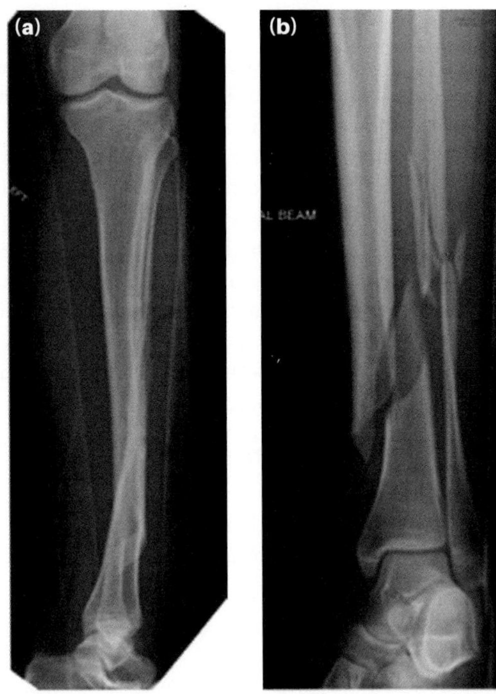

Figure 28.5 Describing fractures: the importance of rotation. (a) Anteroposterior (AP) view of the knee seen at the top of the radiograph and lateral view of the ankle at the bottom, showing a spiral fracture at the junction of the middle and distal thirds of the tibia. (b) AP radiograph of the ankle on the same patient. Note the varied diameter of the fracture fragments; this implies rotational deformity. The distal fragment has translated laterally by 50%. There is no significant angulation on this view.

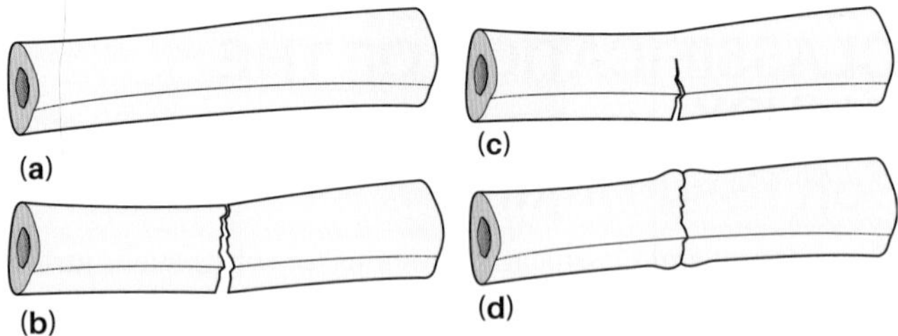

Figure 28.6 Types of bony injury: (a) uninjured bone; (b) adult transverse fracture failure across the whole bone; (c) greenstick fracture; the bone has failed on the tension side; (d) torus or buckle fracture; the bone has failed on the compression side.

AO CLASSIFICATION

The AO (*Arbeitsgemeinschaft fur Osteosynthesefragen)* system provides a comprehensive classification of all fractures (Figure 28.7). The first number defines the bone injured and the second number the segment of bone injured: proximal metaphysis, diaphysis, distal metaphysis. The letter and number that follows further defines the nature of the injury (Figure 28.8). For example, the previously described humeral fracture would be 12-A1 (1 humerus, 2 diaphysis, A simple, 1 spiral). (For more detail see Further reading.)

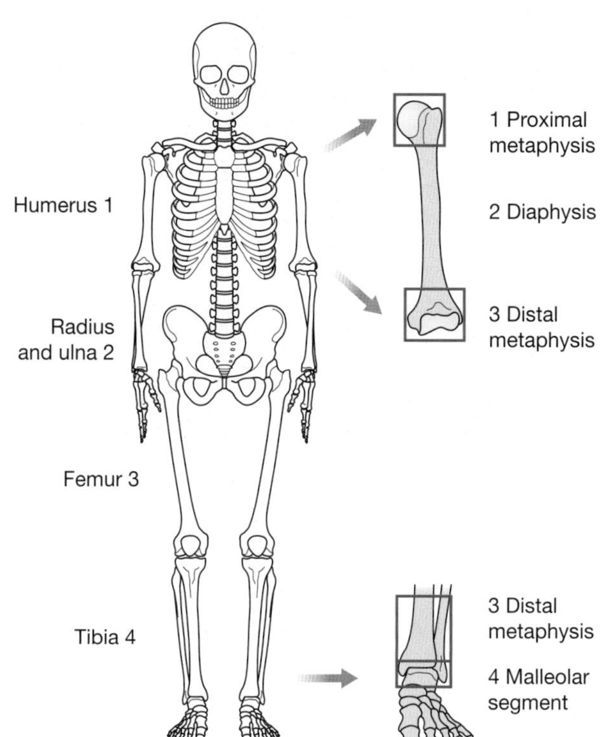

Figure 28.7 The AO classification system: the first two numbers specify the site of the fracture.

GROWTH PLATE INJURY CLASSIFICATION

In children and adolescent injuries involvement of the growth plate (physis) can lead to abnormal growth or growth arrest, either complete or partial. Complete growth arrest will result in length abnormalities and partial growth arrest might result in angular deformities. The severity of injury to the physis is classified in the Salter–Harris classification which considers whether the fracture line passes through the epiphysis, physis, metaphysis or combinations of all above. Salter–Harris described five and Mercer Rang added the sixth (**Figure 28.9**):

- Type I – simple fracture line just involving the physis. Seldom affects growth.
- Type II – fracture line through the physis exiting through the metaphysis, producing a metaphyseal fragment. Seldom affects growth.
- Type III – fracture line through the physis exiting through the epiphysis (intra-articular). Seldom affects growth, but intra articular affecting joint surface.
- Type IV – fracture line across epiphysis, cross physis and across metaphysis. This injury can cause focal fusion of the physis leading to abnormal growth.
- Type V – a crush injury of the physis. Growth disturbance is common and may be the first radiological sign of an injury.
- Type VI – injury to perichondral structures by direct trauma. Rare injury, high chance of abnormal growth.

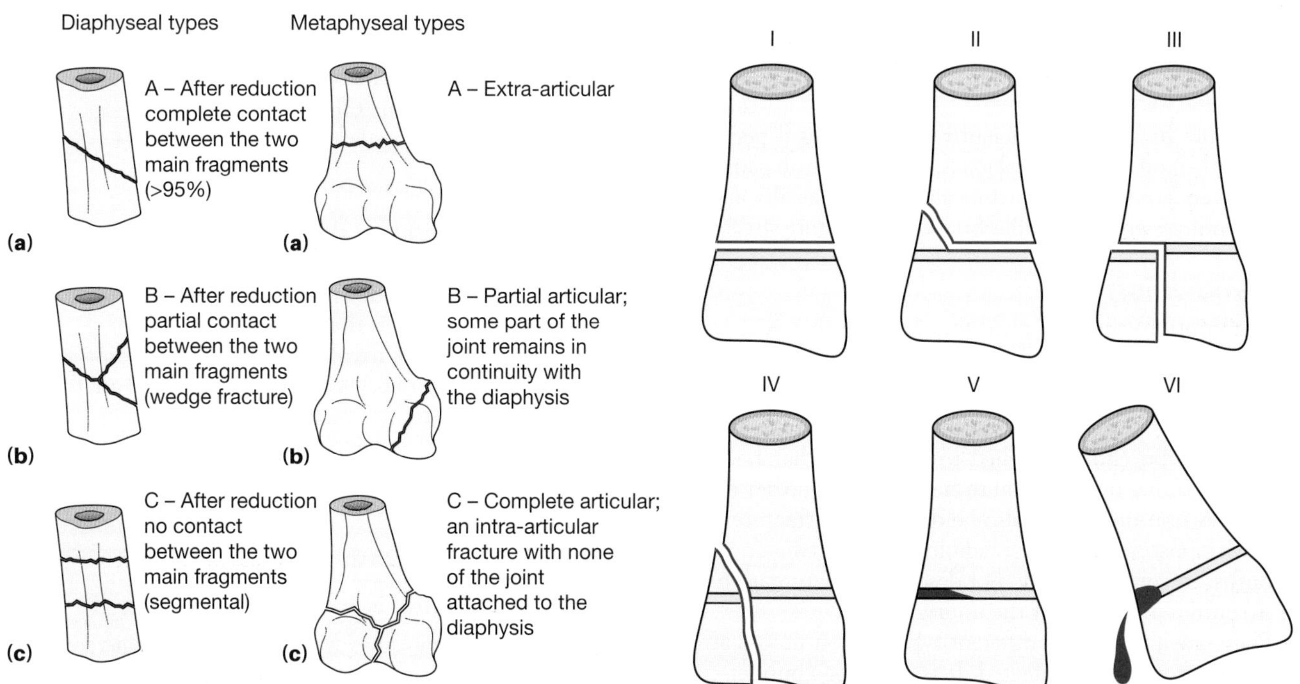

Figure 28.8 The AO classification system: the letter defines the nature of the fracture.

Figure 28.9 The Salter–Harris classification of growth plate injuries.

Robert Bruce Salter, 1924–2010, Professor of Orthopaedic Surgery, The University of Toronto, Ontario, Canada. A pioneer in the field of paediatric orthopaedic surgery, he received international awards for medical science and the Distinguished Achievement for Orthopaedic Research award.

W Robert Harris, 1922–2005, formerly Professor, University of Toronto, President Canadian Orthopaedic Foundation (1968) and President of the Canadian Orthopaedic Association (1975 and 1976).

FRACTURE HEALING

It is useful to review fracture healing, as it relates to treatment and outcome. Following a fracture, bone can heal in two different ways: direct (primary) bone healing or indirect (secondary) bone healing:

- **Direct bone healing**, as the name implies, heals directly with bone and without callus formation. It happens in an environment of cortical apposition and absolute stability with no movement or gap between the fracture fragments. The normal osteoclastic-mediated remodelling of bone is directed across the fracture interface. Osteoclastic cutting cones cut across the fracture line, with following osteoblasts laying down lamellar bone across the fracture.
- **Indirect bone healing** involves a transition from one tissue to another with callus formation. It is the most common form of bone healing. Following the injury, haematoma fills the gap at the fracture site. In response to a varying strain and under the influence of bone stimulating factors, the tissue undergoes differentiation, from haematoma to fibrous tissue and then to soft callus, followed by mineralisation and formation of mature bone. The amount of strain determines the nature of tissue it differentiates into; under 100% leads to fibrous tissue, under 10% soft callus, less than 2% hard callus and progressive mineralisation. Hence a little movement is good, too much movement is bad.

Terminology of bone healing after fracture

Union

The fracture has healed sufficiently from a clinical perspective to withstand physiological loads, with very little pain and minimal tenderness at the fracture site. Radiologically a fracture has united when the callus bridges the fracture site.

Delayed union

This description can be applied to a fracture that is slow to heal and which has not healed in the expected time frame.

Non-union

This description can be applied to a fracture that has not healed and shows no potential to heal without further intervention. A non-union can also be defined as a fracture that fails to demonstrate clinical or radiological improvement over 3 months. In general, you do not describe a fracture as 'non-union' until 6 months after the injury.

There are a number of different types of non-union: atrophic, hypertrophic and infected. It is useful to consider certain factors with regard to the non-union; the biology of the fracture, the mechanical environment and the host (patient factors like diabetes and smoking).

In an atrophic non-union, the problem is generally a biological one, with a lack of stimulus or blood supply. A hypertrophic non-union generally occurs when there is too much movement at the fracture site.

Consolidation

Follows union and demonstrates that the bone has returned to normal strength. Radiologically it is demonstrated by the return of the normal cortical pattern.

Remodelling

In children, and to a lesser degree in adults, bone remodels based on the forces passing through it.

Summary box 28.3

Fracture healing

- Direct - cortical apposition and absolute stability
- Indirect – secondary bone healing, requires some movement

TREATMENT

The main principle of extremity fracture management builds on the classical concept of reduction and stabilisation of the fracture. Treatment can be considered under the following headings (see *Apley's system of orthopaedics and fractures* [Further reading]):

- reduce;
- hold;
- heal;
- rehabilitate.

The main objective of any treatment is to return the patient to normal function as soon and as safely as possible. Broadly speaking, treatment may be operative or non-operative, with differing risks and benefits (*Table 28.3*).

Reduce

The first thing to consider is the degree of displacement of the fracture fragments. It is useful to ask the following question: if the bone were to heal in this position, would it be compatible with optimum function in the short and long term?

In general, fractures involving the articular joint surface need to be reduced perfectly back to their original anatomical

TABLE 28.3 Risks and benefits of fracture treatment.

Benefits	Risks
Pain relief	Anaesthesia
Prevention of infection	Introduction of infection
Restoration of anatomy	Damage to soft tissues and neurovascular structures
Early movement of the limb	
Early movement of the patient	Devitalising bone
Improved function	Need for implant removal
Reduced risk of secondary arthritis	Financial cost (cost of treatment)
Financial cost (time off work)	

position, to restore normal joint movement in the short term and avoid degenerative joint disease in the long term – **intra-articular fracture = anatomical reduction**.

Fractures that do not involve the joint surface generally require restoration of mechanical alignment of the joints above and below. The fracture fragments do not need to be reduced perfectly. Focus on acceptable alignment, length and rotation – **extra-articular fracture = mechanical alignment**.

In children an extra articular fracture has the ability to remodel, and therefore an increased degree of displacement can be accepted.

If a fracture requires reduction, it can be reduced open or closed. A closed reduction is where the bones are manipulated and moved without exposing the bone. Often the best way to reduce a fracture is to reverse the sequence of injury, without tearing or further damaging the intact soft tissues and periosteum. On occasion this may mean exaggerating the deformity (Figure 28.10).

Open reduction is utilised if an acceptable closed reduction is not achieved or likely to succeed. A combination of closed and open methods can be used to reduce a fracture. Care should be taken during an open reduction not to unduly devitalise the fracture fragments by stripping intact periosteum. A balance between maintaining a blood supply to the fracture fragments (biology) and achieving anatomical reduction needs to be maintained.

Adequacy of reduction is complex and depends on many factors. If intra-articular, the joint surface involved needs to be considered. By way of an example, 2 mm of residual displacement of the articular surface may be accepted in the patella and tibial plateau and may be acceptable in fractures involving the distal radius, but is not acceptable in the condylar joints of the fingers. In general consider the relative thickness of the articular surface involved.

On occasion consideration on how you intend to subsequently hold the fracture may affect the primary form of reduction.

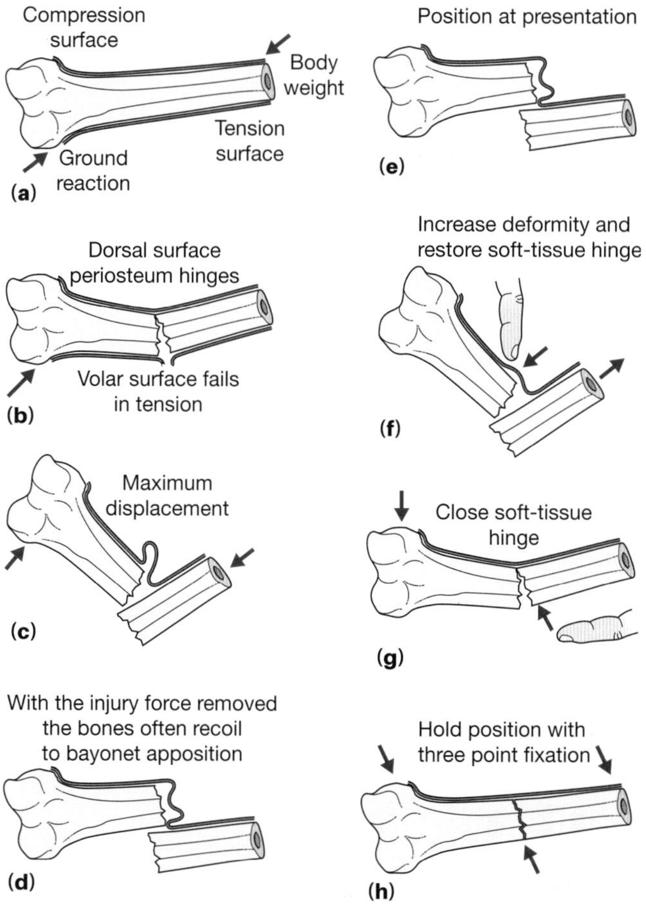

Figure 28.10 (a-d) Representation of how the mechanism of injury causes the bony and soft-tissue injury. (e-h) Representation of how the residual mechanical properties of the tissues may be used to effect and hold a reduction.

Summary box 28.4

Reduction

- Reduction has two components: reducing the fragments and assessing adequacy of reduction
- Reduction can be performed open or closed
- The principle is to reverse the movement which created the fracture
- Over-angulation allows the intact periosteum to guide the fragments into position

Hold

If the fracture fragments are in an acceptable position, or have been reduced into an acceptable position, they then need to be held in that position until they heal. When choosing a method to hold a fracture the aim is to:

- optimise the biological and mechanical environment to create the most favourable conditions possible for fracture healing;
- minimise the period of disability by speeding up the healing process or providing enough stability to return to normal function while the fracture heals.

There are several methods of holding fracture fragments in place:

- plaster cast/ splints;
- traction;
- Kirschner (K-) wires;
- external fixation;
- plates and screws
- intramedullary nails.

Note: Arthroplasty may be used where fragments cannot be held together.

On occasion a combination of holding methods may be used; for example, K-wires and a moulded cast in the case of a simple extra-articular distal radial fracture. It is important to consider the way of holding the reduction in terms of outcome and ensure this is part of the overarching goal to optimise the patient's return to function as safely and fast as possible.

For example, a displaced clavicle fracture in a 10 year old has a 99% chance of sound union within a few months if treated non-operatively. In contrast, a displaced multifragmentary mid-third clavicle in a 35-year-old female will carry a 35% chance of going on to a non-union at 6 months. Therefore, even though this fracture may heal with non-operative treatment, with appropriate explanation and shared decision making, a patient may choose to have surgery early in order to get back to normal function as soon as possible.

Stability can be absolute or relative:

- **Absolute stability.** Implies no displacement or movement and is achieved by accurate anatomical reduction with compression across the fracture fragments to optimise the environment for direct bone healing. This is desirable in intra-articular fractures, where callus at the fracture site might inhibit movement. Intra-articular fractures require an anatomical reduction and absolute stability.
- **Relative stability.** Allows a little movement at the fracture site, optimising the environment for callus formation and indirect bone healing.

Selected examples of achieving absolute and relative stability are shown in **Figure 28.11**.

Plaster cast and splints

Plaster casts and splints are generally used to hold stable fractures or supplement the fixation of unstable fractures (e.g. below elbow cast applied to a distal radial fracture after K-wire fixation [see below]).

Plaster casts come in two forms: plaster of Paris and synthetic casting materials. Plaster of Paris is the preferred method in acute fractures and, where more support is needed, it is easier to mould plaster of Paris than a synthetic cast. In acute injuries, where there is a risk of swelling and compartment syndrome, a backslab will often be applied. A backslab is not always positioned on the dorsal surface as the name suggests, but is a partial cast where a layer of plaster of Paris or synthetic cast is applied along roughly half the circumference. An alternative to a backslab includes a full cast that is split along its full length to allow for swelling. The use of an incomplete cast does not remove the risk of swelling and compartment syndrome and must always be accompanied by close clinical observation.

Moulding of the cast is an art form requiring appropriate skill to achieve the desired effect. Three point moulding is used to control the position, often using the intact dorsal periosteal hinge to mould against (see **Figure 28.11**). Often, a correctly moulded cast will look crooked, leading to the adage 'Bent casts make straight bones' **(Figure 28.12)**.

Commercially available upper limb and lower limb splints provide comfort, support and social protection to stable fractures. Ease of application and the ability to remove make them very useful for patients to return to activities of daily living including bathing and showering.

The advantages and disadvantages of plaster cast and splint usage are described in *Table 28.4*.

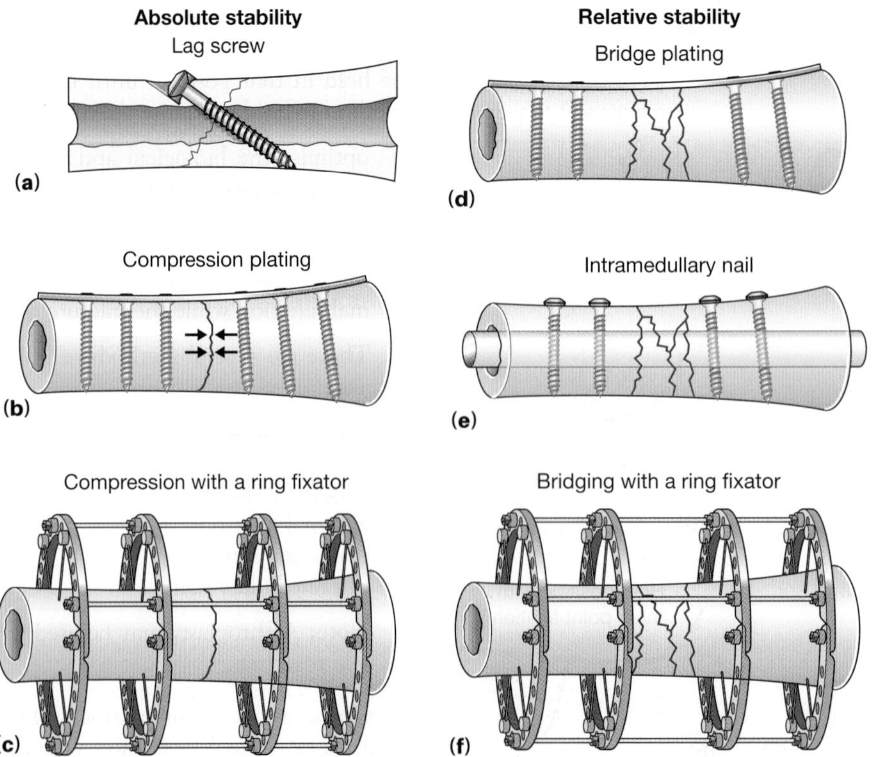

Figure 28.11 (a-f) How absolute and relative stability can be achieved. The same implants may be used to achieve different mechanical effects.

Plaster of Paris is a white crystalline powder, calcium sulphate hemihydrate $CaSO_4$-$0.5H_2O$, which sets hard when water is added to it.

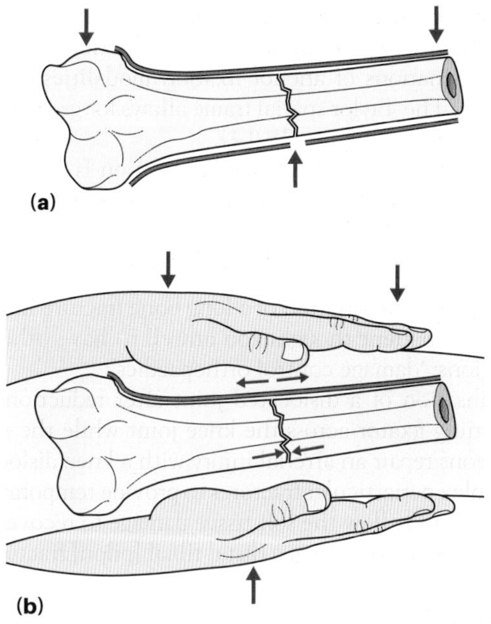

Figure 28.12 (a) The position achieved at the end of the manipulation described in Figure 28.10. (b) Demonstration of how by moulding the cast the intact periosteum is kept under tension and the bone under compression; thus, the remaining mechanical properties are used to achieve stability.

TABLE 28.4 Advantages and disadvantages of casting and splinting.

Advantages	No wound
	No interference with fracture site
	Cheap
	Adjustable
	No implants to remove
Disadvantages	Limited access to the soft tissues
	Cumbersome (particularly in the elderly)
	Interferes with function
	Poor mechanical stability
	'Plaster disease' – joint stiffness and muscle wasting

Traction

Traction is defined as a stretching force on a limb to pull a fracture straight. After appropriate pain control, simply pulling on the limb using manual traction will help realign fracture fragments, returning overall length and alignment. If the fracture is simple and off ended, it may require more than simply pulling to reduce it (see reduction in Figure 28.10). Once reduced, however, continued longitudinal traction will often hold it reduced.

A traction force can be applied and maintained by a variety of systems and techniques. It is easy to apply traction to any extremity; however, it is cumbersome and requires a fixed point to pull on. This can require the patient to be fixed to one place and limit return to normal function. (See *Table 28.5* for advantages and disadvantages.)

TABLE 28.5 Advantages and disadvantages of traction.

Advantages	No wound in zone of injury
	No interference with fracture site
	Materials cheap
	Adjustable
Disadvantages	Restricts mobility of patient
	Expensive in hospital time
	Skin pressure complications
	Pin site infection
	Thromboembolic complications

Traction is often used in the treatment of femoral shaft fractures in adults as a temporary measure for comfort and to allow transfer of the patient, until definitive fixation can be undertaken. A Thomas splint is applied to the limb initially in a static fashion (Figure 28.13a) and then, once in bed, balanced traction is applied to help pull the leg out to length and pull the splint off the ischial tuberosity (Figure 28.13b).

The anchor point on the limb may be either skin, by applying an adhesive or non-adhesive bandage, or skeletal traction, where a pin is placed in the proximal tibia or distal femur.

A common everyday example of traction is the use of a collar and cuff in proximal humeral fractures. When the patient is upright, the lower part of the arm, under the action

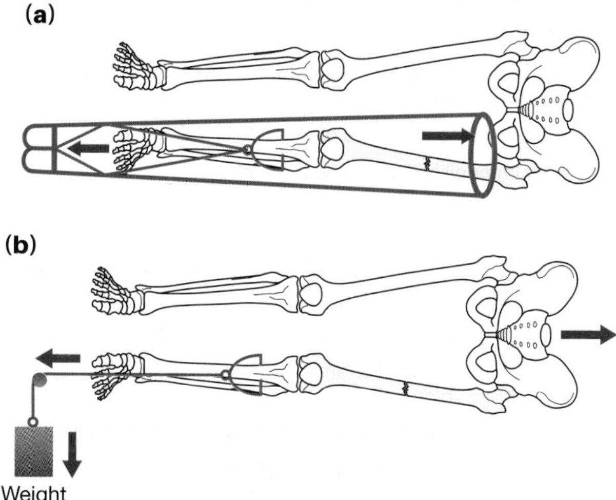

Figure 28.13 (a) Static traction with a Thomas splint. The force and counterforce are contained within a static system. The load is applied to the patient through the tibial traction pin via a cord tightened with a Spanish windlass. The counterforce is applied through pressure by the splint on the ischial tuberosity. (b) A dynamic system in which the load is applied by weights suspended from the tibial pin and the counterforce is the patient's own weight.

Hugh Owen Thomas, 1834–1891, general practitioner of Liverpool, UK, is regarded as the 'founder of orthopaedic surgery', although never holding a hospital appointment preferring to treat patients in their own homes. He introduced the Thomas splint in 1875.

of gravity, provides longitudinal traction, thus aligning the fracture fragments.

Kirschner wires

Kirschner wires (also called K-wires) are smooth, non-threaded, thin flexible wires often between 0.9 and 2.5 mm in diameter. They are used to hold small fragments in place. They may be used in a temporary fashion intraoperatively to hold fracture fragments in place until definitive fixation with plates and screws can be performed. They are inexpensive and simple to use. Moreover, they are extensively used for definitive fixation of injuries around the hand and wrist. The flexible nature of the wires can often require supplementation, as a hybrid construct of K-wires and plaster cast fixation.

In distal radial fractures the wires are placed percutaneously after closed reduction, the trailing end of the wire is left proud of the skin and the end bent to limit wire migration. K-wires around the distal radius can be removed in the clinic setting 4–6 weeks after insertion. Complications of K-wires include pin site infection, wire breakage, loss of fixation and wire migration. Wire migration may be a potentially serious problem in certain locations. It is not advisable to use non-threaded K-wires around the shoulder girdle and clavicle as migration into the thoracic cavity and heart has been reported (*Table 28.6*).

External fixation

External fixation involves percutaneous placement of metal rods or fine wires into bone to anchor a metal frame on the outside (*Table 28.7*). The frame construct itself may be comprised of tubular rods with connectors, or circular ring constructs 'ilizarov' type of frame. Hybrid variations are infinite, with combinations of anchor fixation modalities and frame constructs. The Taylor spatial frame allows for gradual correction of deformity (**Figure 28.14**).

The major drawback of external fixation is that they can be cumbersome to the patient and pin site infection can be a problem (*Table 28.7*).

Specific indications for external fixators include:

- emergency stabilisation of a long bone fracture in the polytrauma patient thought too unwell to have other interventions; 'damage control orthopaedics';
- stabilisation of a dislocated joint after reduction (e.g. a spanning fixator across the knee joint while the vascular surgeons repair an arterial injury with a knee dislocation);
- complex periarticular fractures to provide temporary stabilisation and allow the soft tissue damage to recover before definitive fixation (e.g. a distal tibial [pilon] fracture);
- fractures associated with infection;
- treating fractures with bone loss.

TABLE 28.6 Indications for K-wire insertion.

Temporary fixation
Definitive fixation – with small fracture fragments (e.g. wrist fractures and hand injuries)
Tension band wiring (fractures of the patella and olecranon)
Temporary immobilisation of a small joint

TABLE 28.7 Advantages and disadvantages of external fixation.

Advantages	No interference with fracture site
	Adjustable after application: alignment; biomechanics
	Soft tissues accessible for plastic surgery
	Rapid stabilisation of fracture
	Hardware easy to remove
Disadvantages	Pin site infection
	Interferes with plastic surgical procedures
	Soft-tissue tethering
	Cumbersome for the patient

Plates and screws

Plates and screws can be used in many different ways. A 'lag screw' can be used to generate compression across a fracture site, optimising the environment for direct bone healing. Similarly, compression can be achieved using a dynamic compression plate. A plate might also be used simply to neutralise forces, buttress a fracture or work as an internal external fixator (see **Figure 28.11**).

In general, plates and screws are used where possible in articular and periarticular fractures where an anatomical reduction is required, often via open means, followed by the application of the plate and screws to achieve a rigid construct. In extra-articular fractures, where mechanical alignment is required together with relative stability, one option is the use of locking plate technology. This allows a closed reduction and percutaneous placement of the plate with locking screws to create an internal construct, which behaves like an external fixator. Injury-specific plating systems have revolutionised the ability to treat certain injuries, with plates pre-bent and pre-shaped for specific anatomical regions and specific injury patterns. (See *Table 28.8* for the advantages and disadvantages of plate fixation.)

Intramedullary nails

Diaphyseal fractures are best suited for intramedullary nailing. Where mechanical alignment is required together with relative stability, they allow for indirect bone healing. After nail insertion, mechanical alignment is checked particularly for length, alignment and rotation. Locking screws are then placed proximally and distally to maintain length and alignment. Intramedullary nailing of metaphyseal and articular fractures is a challenge. However, with improved implant

Martin Kirschner, 1879–1942, Professor of Surgery, Heidelberg, Germany, introduced the use of skeletal traction wires in 1909.
Gavriil Abramovich Ilizarov, 1921–1993, orthopaedic surgeon, Kurgan, Western Siberia, Russia. He did not attend school until he was 11 years old as his family was too poor to buy him shoes.

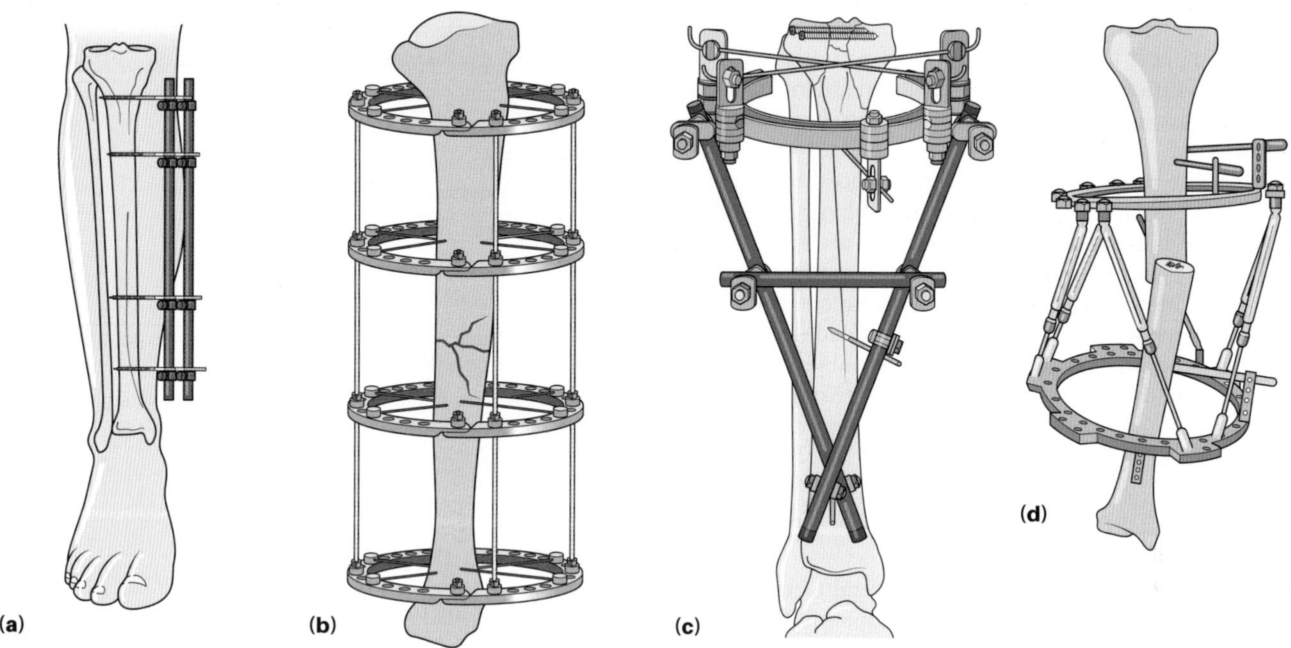

Figure 28.14 (a) Monolateral tubular frame with metal rod (half pin anchorage to bone. (b) Circular ring fixator with fine wire anchorage to bone. (c) Hybrid circular/tubular rod frame construct with combination of half pin and fine wire anchorage to bone. (d) Taylor spatial frame; allows for gradual correction of deformity.

TABLE 28.8 Advantages and disadvantages of plate and screw fixation.

Advantages	Can be used when anatomical reduction is required
	Allows early mobilisation
	Can provide absolute or relative stability
Disadvantages	May interfere with fracture site
	Periosteal/soft-tissue damage
	Does not normally allow for immediate load-bearing
	Potential for infection
	Metalwork complications
	Possible need for plate removal

TABLE 28.9 A comparison of reamed versus unreamed nailing (an assumption is that nails used unreamed are usually thinner than those used reamed).

	Reamed IMN	Unreamed IMN
Insertion time	Longer	Quicker
Time to union	Shorter	Longer
Size of implant	Larger	Smaller
Reduction of distal fractures	Easier	More difficult
Strength of construct	More	Less

IMN, intramedullary nail.

design and the ability to lock the nails very distally and in multiple directions, the indications for intramedullary nailing is expanding.

Intramedullary nails may be placed in an unreamed or reamed fashion. Reaming is the process whereby the intramedullary canal is widened slightly to allow passage of a larger diameter nail, relating to the last reamer size used. Table 28.9 compares reamed to unreamed nails.

Intramedullary nailing can be a technically demanding procedure. The advantages and disadvantages are summarised in Table 28.10.

TABLE 28.10 Advantages and disadvantages of intramedullary nailing.

Advantages	Minimally invasive
	Early weight-bearing
	Less periosteal damage than open reduction and internal fixation
	Seldom need removal
Disadvantages	Increased risk of fat emboli/chest complications
	Infection difficult to treat
	Difficult to remove if broken

Arthroplasty

Arthroplasty is indicated in certain acute circumstances: articular fractures that are not reconstructible, or injuries where the vascularity of the articular segment is compromised (e.g. displaced intracapsular femoral neck fracture in an older patient).

The patient demographics and functional demands need to be considered in choosing arthroplasty as a treatment option. Implant longevity and level of activities following implant insertion need to be matched. Traditionally, arthroplasty for trauma was limited to hip and shoulder hemi-arthroplasty.

Total hip replacement, acute distal femoral replacement, radial head replacement, total and hemi-elbow arthroplasty, and reverse polarity shoulder arthroplasty are current treatment options for older patients with osteoporotic periarticular fractures. The selection of a particular technique will depend on clinical evidence and our previously stated aim to return patients to optimal function as soon as possible. It should be considered in the context that it can be expensive and require considerable other resources to make the procedure safe and long lasting.

Heal

Time to fracture healing depends on several factors: patient co-morbidities, the age of the patient, bone involved (upper limb or lower limb), patient factors (diabetes), choice of treatment. Well known factors that slow down bone healing include diabetes mellitus (doubles time to union), diminished blood supply (peripheral vascular disease, vascular injury at time of injury), smoking, non-steroidal anti-inflammatory drugs and infection at the fracture site.

Several chemical and mechanical methods have been attempted to enhance fracture healing, including bone marrow injections into the fracture site and other orthobiologics such as bone morphogenic proteins. Mechanical methods include controlled axial micromotion (using an external fixator), electromagnetic stimulation and low intensity pulsed ultrasound. There is good basic scientific evidence to support their theoretical benefit; however, to date there is little clinical evidence for their use in the primary treatment of closed fractures.

Rehabilitate

The main aim of treatment is to return the patient to a similar level of pre-morbid function as quickly as possible. Rehabilitation begins as soon as feasible. It is often not necessary to wait until bone union before beginning rehabilitation. It is important to move the affected joints and the joints in close proximity to the fracture (e.g. elbow and shoulder exercise while in a cast for a distal radial fracture), limiting global stiffness and wasting of the muscles on that limb.

TREATMENT BY FRACTURE LOCATION

In general, the principles of treatment described above are dependent on the fracture location: diaphyseal, metaphyseal and intra-articular.

Table 28.11 outlines some indications for operative stabilisation.

TABLE 28.11 Indications for surgery in limb trauma. The main indication is that operation will produce a better outcome; the principles are given below.
A fracture requiring treatment that is unsuitable for non-operative measures
Open fractures
Failed non-operative management
Multiple injuries
Pathological or impending pathological fractures
Displaced intra-articular fractures
Fractures through the growth plate, where arrest is possible (Salter–Harris type III–V)
Avulsion fractures that compromise the functional integrity of a ligament/tendon around a joint (e.g. olecranon fracture)
Established non-unions or malunions

Diaphyseal fractures

Extra articular fractures do not require an anatomical reduction, but rather a mechanical restoration by correction of length, alignment and rotation (Figure 28.15).

Angular malunion of a diaphyseal fracture of the weight-bearing long bones will lead to abnormal joint forces on the joint above and below, leading to pain and secondary degenerative joint disease.

Diaphyseal fractures are generally well suited to intramedullary fixation techniques, as previously discussed.

Summary box 28.5

Diaphyseal fractures

- Restore length, alignment and rotation
- Consider whether primary or secondary bone healing is the objective
- Radius and ulna need precise reduction to function

Metaphyseal fractures

In the AO classification metaphyseal fractures are classified into A type – extra-articular, B type – partial articular, and C type – complete articular.

In A type fractures, joint congruity is not an issue and as such the principles of mechanical alignment, length and rotation need to be considered. Fixation of metaphyseal fractures is less predictable with intramedullary nailing, therefore plate and screw fixation, external fixation or, in the smaller joints, K-wire fixation is used. Metaphyseal fractures are close to the joint and so consideration is given to stable fixation to allow early joint movement and rehabilitation.

Intra-articular fractures

AO type B and type C fractures are intra-articular and as such the principles of treating intra-articular fractures need to be respected; namely, anatomical reduction of the articular sur-

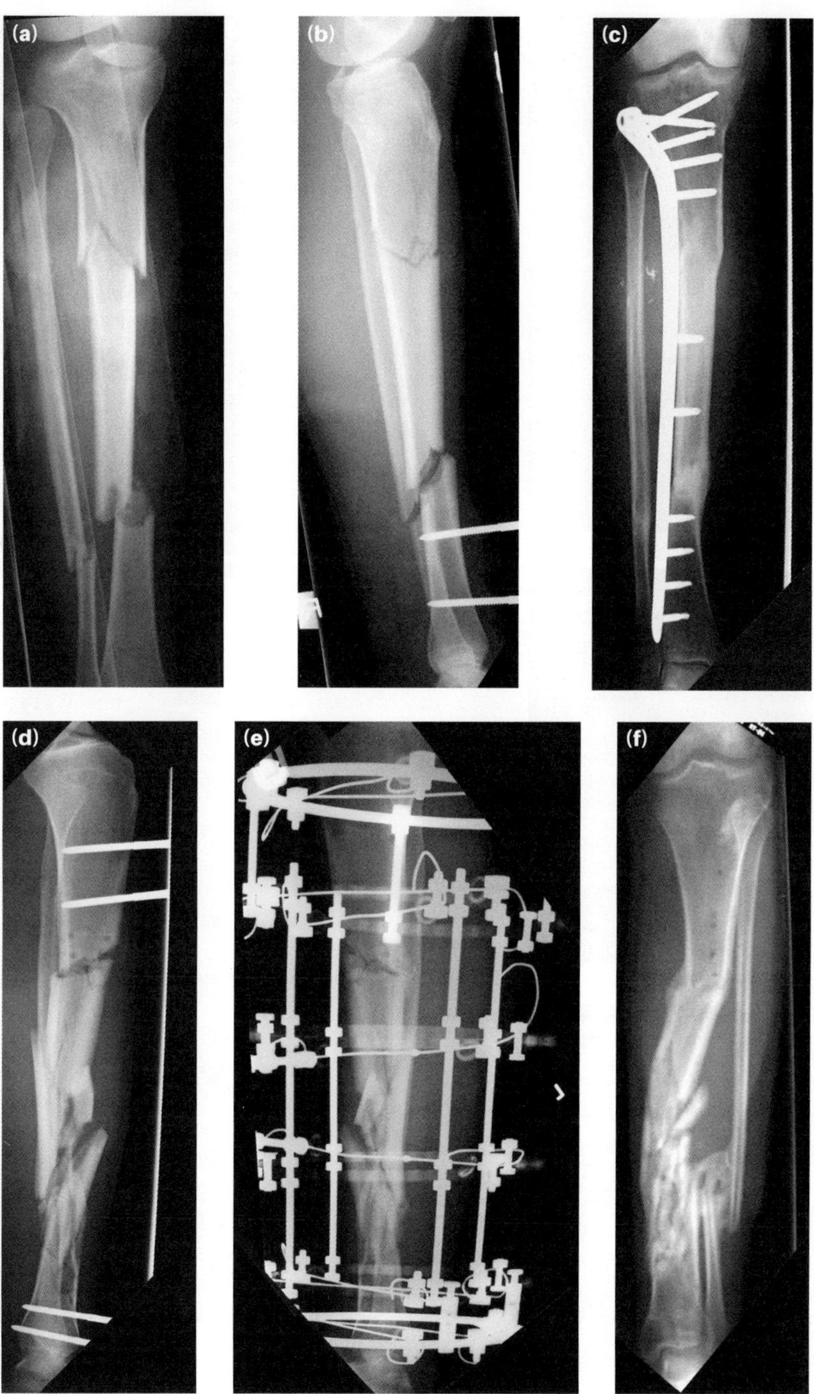

Figure 28.15 (a) and (d) are C-type or segmental tibial fractures. Each was a high-energy injury; (b) and (e) show a temporary spanning external fixator applied in each case; (c) and (f) show definitive relative stability was achieved with different methods of bridging fixation. Healing was by indirect means in both cases. Despite irregularities at the fracture sites the overall position was satisfactory and function was good.

face and rigid stabilisation to allow early joint movement and avoidance of degenerative joint disease (Figure 28.16). However, these principles have to be balanced with the increased wound complications of open surgery and devitalising bone fragments with excessive exposure of the bone.

Osteoporotic intra-articular fractures are a considerable challenge. Although anatomical reduction may be achieved, rigid fixation devices may cut out of soft bone. Injectable bone substitutes may be used to fill bone voids and augment fixation. If stable fixation is not possible, then consideration might be given to non-operative treatment and delayed joint replacement or, on occasion, primary joint replacement may be undertaken.

In type C fractures where the articular surface has separated from the metaphysis, the articular surface is initially anatomically reduced with temporary K-wires or lag screws and then the articular block is reattached to the shaft (Figure 28.17).

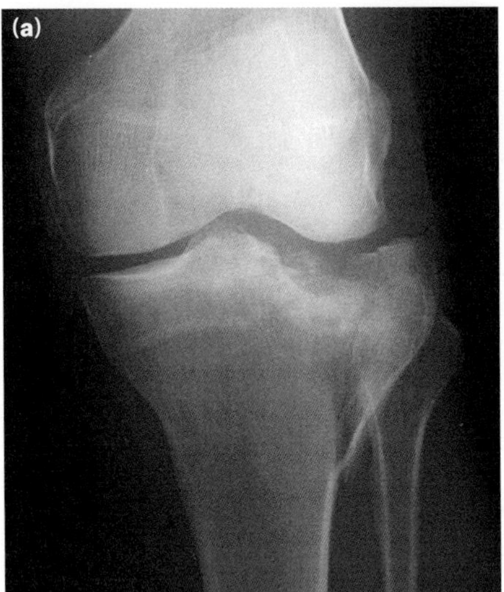

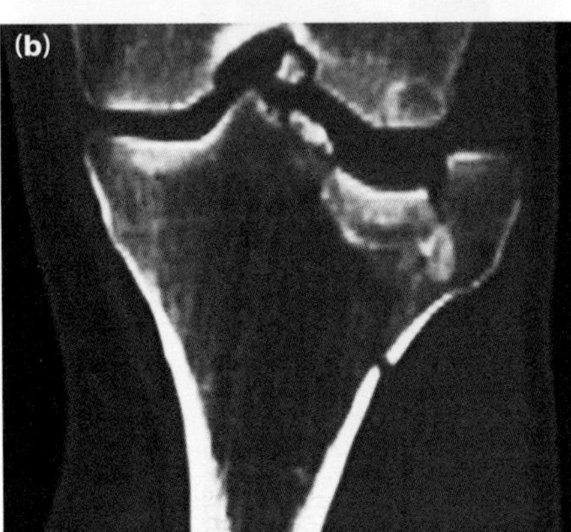

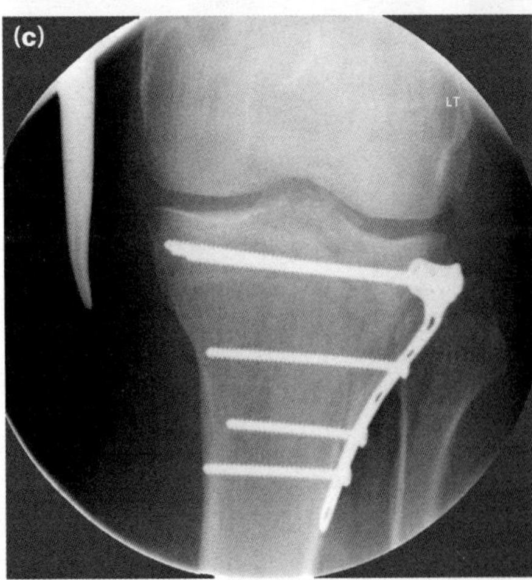

Figure 28.16 A B-type or partial articular fracture. (a) Plain radiograph; (b) computed tomography clarifies the injury; (c) fixation with plate and screws achieving compression across a previously reduced fracture.

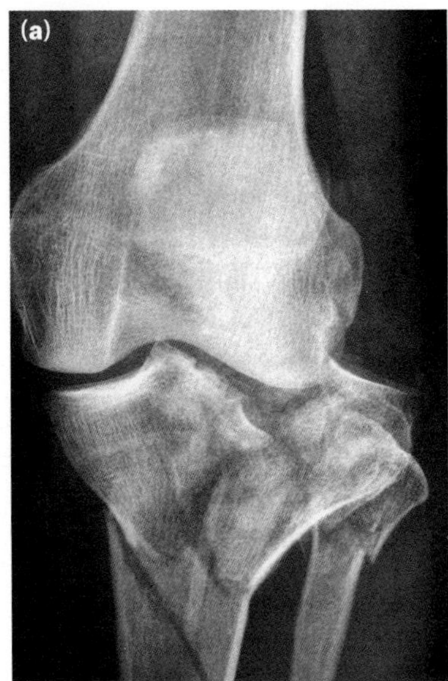

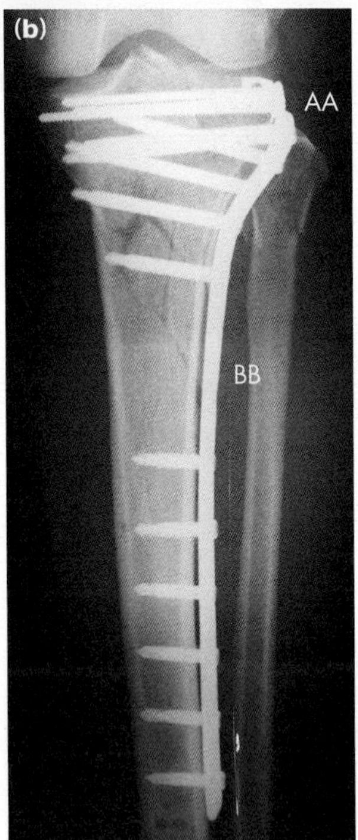

Figure 28.17 (a) A C-type proximal tibial articular fracture (i.e. none of the joint remains attached to the diaphysis). (b) The small plate and screws (AA) are used to compress the joint fragments, aiming for absolute stability. The heavy duty fixed angled device (BB) spans the fracture and provides relative stability

TREATMENT BY REGION (FROM TOP TO TOE)

Scaphoid fracture

The blood supply to the scaphoid enters distally and supplies the scaphoid in a retrograde fashion. As such, a displaced waist of scaphoid fracture interrupts the blood supply to the proximal pole, leading to avascular necrosis. An undisplaced fracture of the scaphoid may not be visible on the initial radiographs. If a patient is tender in the anatomical snuff box following a fall on the outstretched hand, special scaphoid view radiographs should be requested (Figure 28.18).

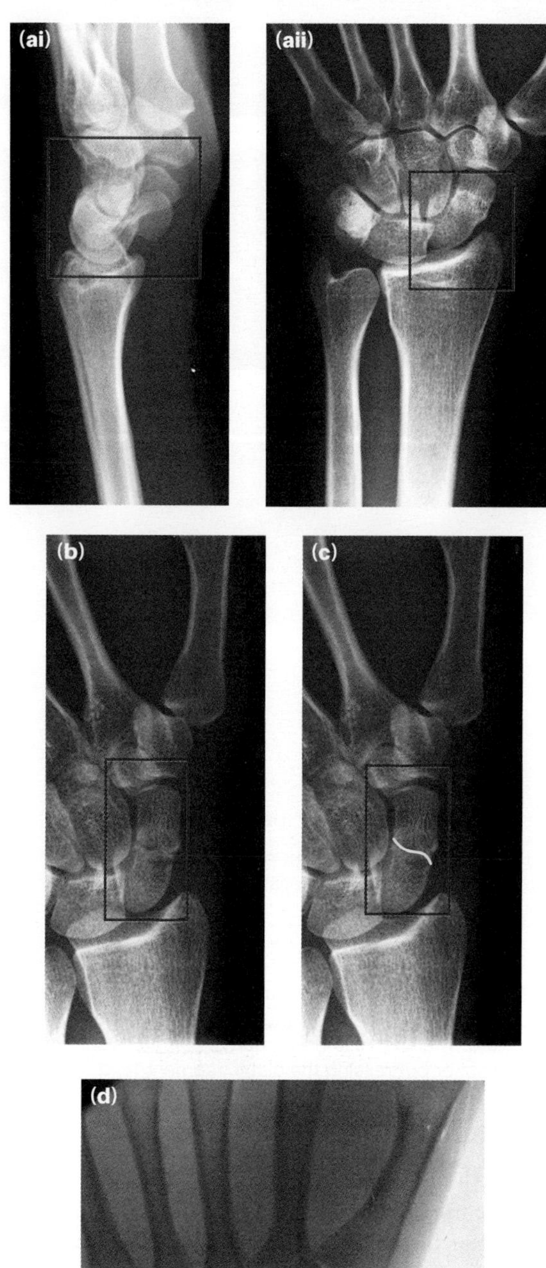

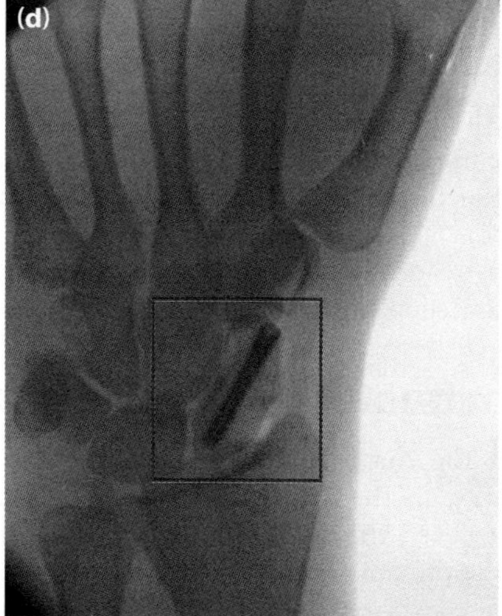

Figure 28.18 Scaphoid fracture. (ai, aii) Anteroposterior and lateral views in which the injury is difficult to see; (b, c) oblique views with the fracture line highlighted; (d) in this case of a young patient, the fracture was treated with early fixation.

If a fracture is not evident on the initial radiographs and the patient remains tender in the anatomical snuff box, then treat as a suspected scaphoid fracture until a fracture is actively excluded. The standard protocol of a suspected scaphoid fracture is to immobilise the wrist and examine again 10–14 days later. If tenderness remains, repeat the scaphoid views. If facilities and resources allow, an earlier diagnosis may be made with a bone scan, MRI or CT.

Undisplaced fractures can be treated non-operatively in a below elbow cast. It is not necessary to include the thumb as a routine. In displaced or unstable fractures (>1 mm) consideration should be given to open reduction and rigid fixation with a headless compression screw. Complications of scaphoid fractures include: non-union, avascular necrosis, malunion and carpal instability.

Carpal instability

The most commonly involved carpal bone is the lunate. A lunate dislocation is where the lunate bone dislocates out of the radiocarpal joint. In a perilunate dislocation the lunate remains in the radiocarpal joint and the rest of the carpus dislocates around the lunate. Lunate and perilunate dislocations are easily missed unless careful attention is paid to carpal alignment on the lateral radiograph (Figure 28.19). Review of the radiographs should particularly ensure the anatomical location of the lunate in the radiocarpal fossa and that the capitate in the 'cup' of the lunate is maintained.

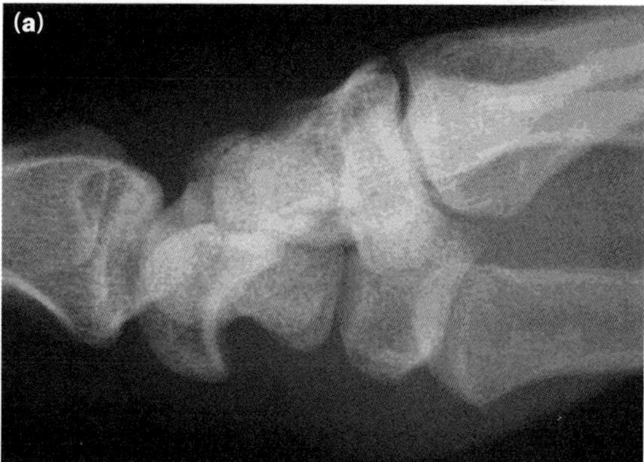

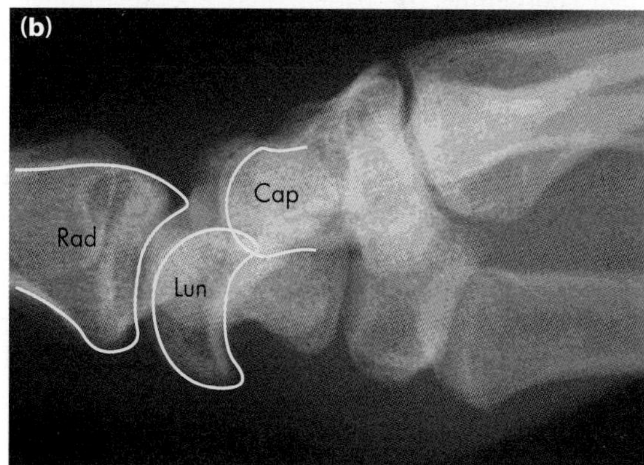

Figure 28.19 Perilunate dislocation. (a) A plain lateral radiograph of the wrist; (b) the outline of the perilunate dislocation is highlighted. Cap, capitate; Lun, lunate; Rad, radius.

Acute injuries should be reduced closed initially to remove pressure from the median nerve. Anatomical carpal alignment is difficult to hold and therefore surgical reconstruction of damaged intrinsic ligaments, together with K-wire fixation of the carpal bones, is often undertaken. Ligamentous healing is slow and may be incomplete. K-wires are kept in place for 8 weeks and the wrist casted or splinted for 3 months.

Thumb metacarpophalangeal ulnar collateral ligament.

Injury to the thumb metacarpal ulnar collateral ligament is a unique injury often termed 'game keepers' thumb or 'skiers' thumb. Due to the unique anatomical arrangement of adductor policis, if the ligament undergoes complete rupture the aponeurosis may become interposed, inhibiting ligament to bone healing. A rupture of the ulnar collateral ligament should be suspected when an ulnar directed force is directed across the metacarpophalangeal (MCP) joint. A tender swelling on the ulna side of the MCP joint may signify the 'Stener' lesion. Increased laxity may be clinically evident, and if there is uncertainty, stress radiographs can demonstrate the degree of injury. Complete ruptures with a Stener lesion (interposed aponeurosis) require open reduction of the ligament to restore bone contact, with a suture anchor repair of the associated ulnar collateral ligament.

Distal radial fractures

Extra-articular (type A) fractures of the distal radius may displace in a volar or dorsal direction. It is possible to reduce volar displaced fractures (Smith's fracture) of the distal radius with a closed technique. However they tend to be unstable and displace if held in a cast. Hence most volar displaced extra articular distal radial fractures are reduced and held with a volar buttress plate (Figure 28.20).

Most dorsally displaced fractures (Colles' fracture) can be addressed with closed reduction and held in a cast. However, some will slip or collapse with cast treatment, and so close review for the first few weeks is advocated.

Fractures with significant initial displacement and dorsal comminution are at risk of early and late collapse. After thorough counselling the patient may choose to have the fracture reduced and then held surgically with K-wires, plate and screw fixation (volar or dorsal) or external fixation. The K-wires may be placed across the fracture fragments or intrafocally, going through the fracture site. The latter can be used to help reduce the fracture and then used to lock the fracture fragments in place (Figure 28.21)

Treatment is individualised based on patient and fracture pattern factors. Intra-articular fractures (types B and C) of the distal radius require anatomical reduction of the joint surface; a gap or step of less than 2 mm can be accepted in the radius. The distal radius fails fairly predictably with splitting of the lunate fossa fragment in the coronal plane and separation of the radial styloid.

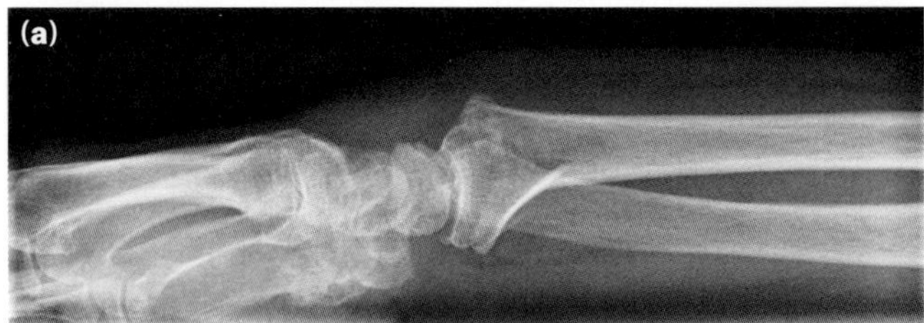

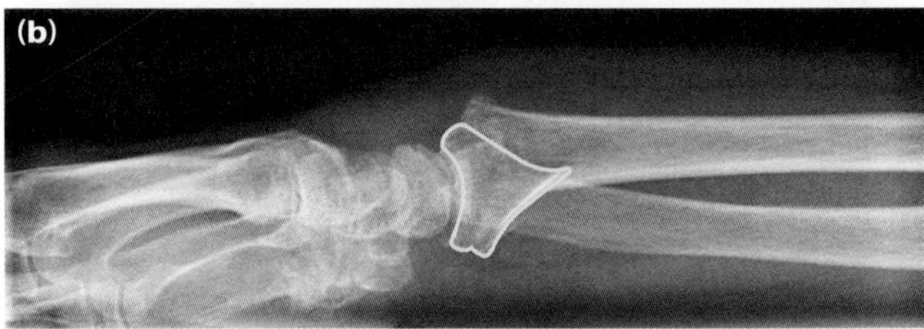

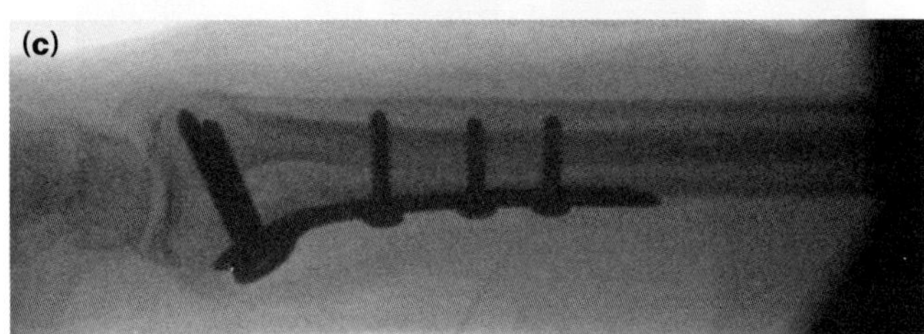

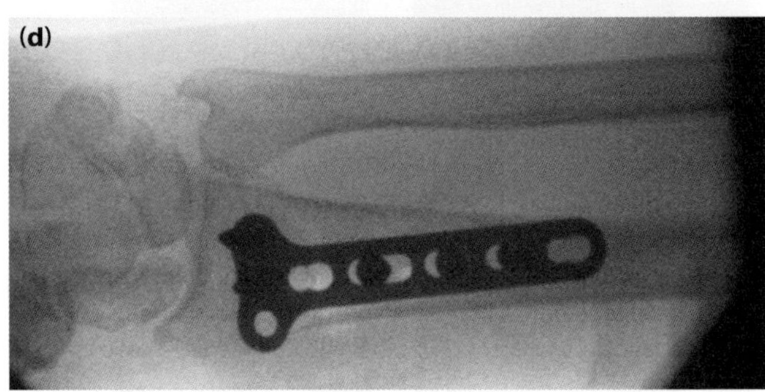

Figure 28.20 An A-type or extra-articular metaphyseal fracture. A plain lateral radiograph of this Smith-type fracture (**a, b**). Fracture fixed to a plate. There is no interfragmental compression. The plate is pushing against or buttressing the distal fragment (**c, d**).

If a closed reduction can be achieved with manipulation, the fracture fragments can subsequently be held with K-wires, plate and screw fixation or external fixation. The most common form of treatment is closed reduction and percutaneous K-wire fixation, supplemented with a plaster cast for 4–6 weeks.

Forearm fractures (radius and ulna)

Fractures of the diaphyseal shaft of the radius and ulna are technically, in the anatomic sense of the word, extra-articular. However, the forearm bones work together, being coupled at the proximal and distal radioulnar joints to allow

---

Robert William Smith, 1807–1873, Professor of Surgery, Trinity College, Dublin, Ireland, described the reverse Colles fracture in 1847.
Abraham Colles, 1773–1843, President of the Royal College of Surgeons of Ireland (1802), Professor of Anatomy Physiology and Surgery (1804) and described distal radial fracture in 1814.

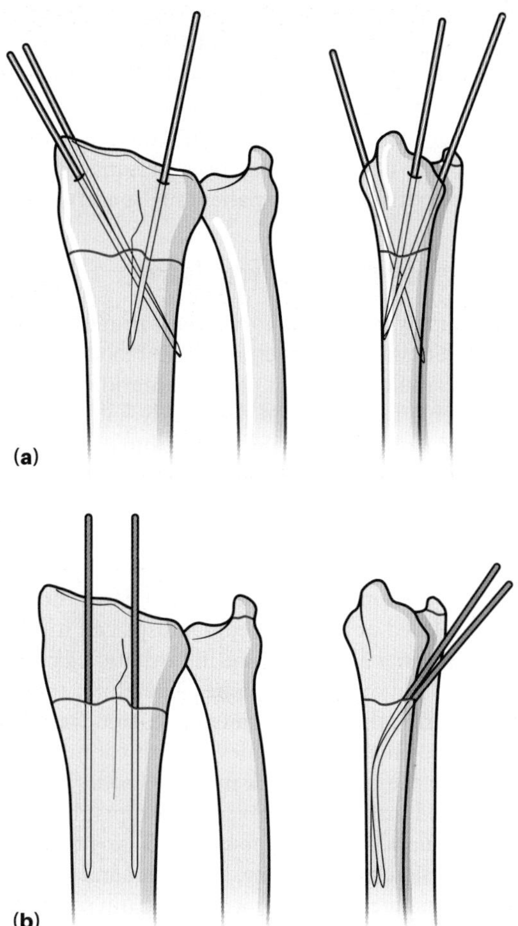

Figure 28.21 (a) K-wires placed across fracture fragments; (b) intrafocal K-wire used to help reduce the fracture.

for forearm pronation and supination. Therefore, when considering treatment the principles that apply to intra-articular fractures need to be considered: anatomic reduction and rigid fixation to allow for early joint motion. Most fractures that involve both radius and ulna in adults require open reduction, anatomic alignment and rigid plate fixation.

Isolated fractures of the ulna, the so-called nightstick fracture, are a little more controversial, as non-operative management is possible but in this location risks delayed union and non-union, hence treatment depends on patient factors. Operative fixation with plate and screw fixation is technically simple and allows early predictable return to function.

Olecranon fractures

Olecranon fractures may be displaced or undisplaced. Undisplaced fractures <2 mm gap or step at the articular surface can be treated non-operatively. In displaced fractures the extensor mechanism is interrupted and the articular surface requires anatomical reduction and stable fixation to allow early movement. Fixation may comprise K-wire and figure-of-eight tension band wiring or plate fixation. In multifragmentary fractures or fractures associated with an elbow dislocation, increased stability is required with the use of a plate and screws.

Humeral fractures

Fractures of the diaphyseal portion of the humeral shaft are extra-articular fractures and as such require mechanical alignment. Non-operative treatment with functional bracing will achieve union in an acceptable position within 12 weeks in over 80% of cases. Gravity can provide traction on the arm and in conjunction with a humeral brace help to hold alignment and allow early range of motion of the elbow. Active shoulder abduction is avoided until fracture union, to prevent varus deformity.

Shoulder movement must not be absent during treatment and so gravity assisted pendulum exercises are instituted early on to prevent shoulder stiffness. As the fracture approaches the metaphyseal region of the humerus it becomes more difficult to control with humeral bracing. Distal third extra-articular fractures of the humerus can be treated non-operatively in a humeral brace but have a tendency to go into varus. Articular fractures of the distal humerus require anatomical reduction and stable fixation to allow early joint movement.

Internal fixation is indicated for displaced intra-articular fractures, non-union or delayed union, open fractures, multiple injuries and those fractures not held in an acceptable position with brace treatment. Fixation of diaphyseal fractures can be achieved with intramedullary nailing or plate and screw fixation. Plate fixation is associated with higher union rates and lower rates of reintervention. (Figure 28.22).

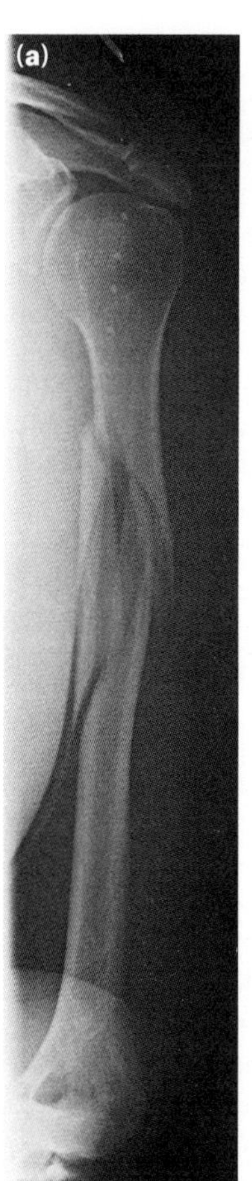

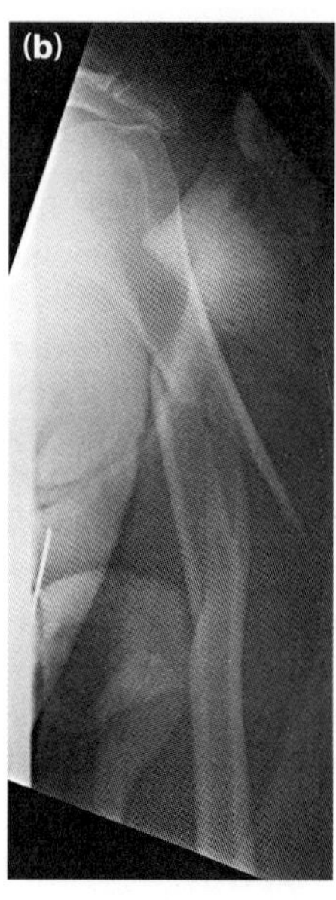

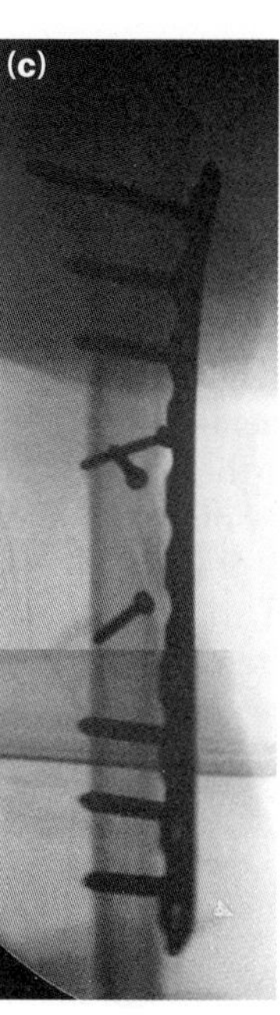

Figure 28.22 (a-c) A B-type humeral shaft fracture. This fracture could not be controlled by non-operative means and was treated with lag screws protected by a plate.

The radial nerve is the most commonly injured nerve in humeral shaft fractures. Treatment of a humeral shaft fracture with a concomitant radial nerve palsy remains topical. Most will recover spontaneously. In general, if the nerve injury occurs at the time of the original injury, non-operative treatment can be considered. If it occurs after the injury, for example at the time of brace application, then it should be explored. When exploring the radial nerve, plate and screw fixation is then undertaken to stabilise the humerus.

Fractures of the proximal humerus

In fractures of the proximal humerus consideration is given to the vascularity of the humeral head. The most common classification of the proximal humerus is the Neer classification looking at the four individual pieces of the proximal humerus (articular head fragment, lesser tuberosity, greater tuberosity and the shaft).

If a fragment is displaced by more than 1 cm or angulated by more than 45 degrees in respect of another fragment, it is considered a part. As such, based on the fracture pattern, it may be undisplaced, 2 part, 3 part or 4 part. Consideration is then given to potential joint dislocation, anterior or posterior. The greater the number of parts, the higher the chances of interruption of the vascularity to the humeral head and the more complex the injury.

Three factors can be used to predict avascularity of the humeral head:

- fracture through the anatomical neck;
- loss of the medial hinge;
- less than 8 mm of bone along the medial calcar.

With displaced fractures, where the head is avascular, occurring in older patients who may have osteoporosis and other co-morbidities, consideration may be given to replacing the humeral head. This may take the form of an anatomical hemi-arthroplasty. One of the limitations of trauma hemi-arthroplasty for proximal humeral fractures involves reliable healing of the tuberosities and the rotator cuff. Increasingly, a primary reverse polarity shoulder prosthesis is being used. This implant does not rely on tuberosity healing, as it functions under the power of the deltoid muscle.

In younger patients reduction and fixation may be considered. A variety of fixation methods are available: percutaneous fixation, intramedullary nails and plate fixation.

Clavicle fractures

Diaphyseal fractures of the middle third of the clavicle have traditionally been treated non-operatively with a broad arm sling for comfort and social protection, followed by increasing use of the arm.

Most mid-third fractures of the clavicle will unite with non-operative treatment. There is, however, a subset of clavicle fractures that may be slow to heal and that do impact on shoulder girdle function. Displaced, comminuted fractures show a propensity to be slow to heal and increasing age and female gender further negatively impact on fracture healing. It has been shown that 2 cm of shortening of the clavicle impacts on shoulder girdle function, with weakness and fatigability when working above shoulder height.

Internal fixation with an intramedullary device or plate and screw construct can restore length, alignment and rotation. This can improve the speed and amount of functional restoration, but carries all the risks of surgical treatment. Treatment is individualised to patient needs and expectations.

Proximal femoral fractures

The blood supply to the femoral head is a prime consideration in treating femoral neck fractures. The blood supply comes via the hip capsule. The joint capsule anteriorly inserts along the intertrochanteric line and posteriorly half way along the femoral neck. Fractures proximal to the hip capsule are intracapsular and those distal to the capsule are extracapsular fractures.

Intracapsular femoral neck fractures

Intracapsular fractures are further broken down into whether they are displaced or undisplaced. Undisplaced intracapsular fractures are generally stable and interruption of the blood supply to the femoral head is rare. Therefore, treatment is aimed at ensuring the head fragment does not displace during rehabilitation. This can be achieved with cannulated screws inserted along the femoral neck into the head.

A displaced intracapsular fracture disrupts the blood supply to the femoral head and risks avascular necrosis. If the patient is physiologically young, reduction and internal fixation with cannulated screws or a dynamic hip screw might be attempted to preserve the native head.

If the patient is older and would benefit from a single operation, then the head may be sacrificed and replaced with a prosthetic head. Arthroplasty of the proximal femur may take the form of hemi-arthroplasty or total hip replacement, depending on patient's functional demands and surgical expertise available.

Extracapsular femoral neck fractures

If the fracture is extracapsular, vascularity of the head is not an issue. Extracapsular femoral neck fractures are subdivided into stable or unstable. Unstable fractures include a reverse oblique pattern or where the medial calcar is comminuted (lesser trochanter) fracture. Stable extracapsular fractures simply require connection of the head to the shaft, often using a dynamic hip screw (Figure 28.23).

In unstable fractures a dynamic hip screw can also be used, but due to the unfavourable mechanical environment relating to the loss of the medial calcar or a reverse oblique pattern, an intramedullary device might be considered.

Femoral shaft fractures

It is possible to treat diaphyseal fractures of the femoral shaft non-operatively. The fracture can be reduced and held in position until union with traction; however, it takes 3 months. This is a long time to be in hospital and carries all the potential risks of prolonged bed rest. Most femoral shaft fractures are treated with a locked intramedullary nail.

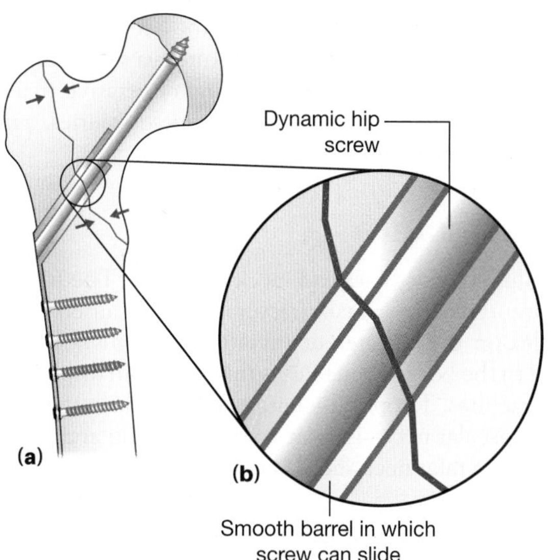

Figure 28.23 **(a)** A dynamic hip screw for fixing a trochanteric proximal femoral fracture. This allows for compression at the fracture site on load-bearing and protects the femoral head from penetration by the screw when the osteoporotic bone settles; **(b)** insert to show the sliding screw in the barrel.

With modern locked intramedullary implants, the patient will be up and out bed the following day and, if it is an isolated injury, home within a few days. Weight bearing depends on the fracture pattern and implant used. If there is a simple fracture pattern with cortical apposition, it will be possible to mobilise with crutches, weight bearing as comfort allows. Although it may still take 3 months or more for the fracture to unite, the implant will be able to carry the load until union, allowing earlier return to function out of the hospital.

Distal femoral fractures

Metaphyseal osteoporotic fractures of the distal femur are amenable to internal fixation with locked intramedullary nails or plate and screw fixation. If the fracture extends into the articular surface, reconstruction may be undertaken with cannulated screws augmented with intramedullary nailing or injury specific locking plates for the distal femur. More recently, arthroplasty has been considered in these situations, to allow early mobilisation.

Patellar fractures

Similar to olecranon fractures, undisplaced fractures where the extensor mechanism is intact can be treated non-operatively. Displaced fractures require anatomical reduction of the articular surface and reconstitution of the integrity of the extensor mechanism. The cartilage on the patella is very thick and as such increased amounts of displacement compared with other joints may be accepted.

Surgical treatment of simple displaced fractures can be achieved with two K-wires and figure-of-eight tension band wiring.

Multifragmentary patellar fractures can be very challenging. Patellar excision is an option but significantly reduces the mechanical advantage of the extensor apparatus. A tension band construct may be augmented by using circumferential wiring of the patella.

Tibial plateau fractures

Intraarticular fractures of the tibial plateau are common. Injuries may involve the lateral or medial side, or both. The joint articular surface may be split, depressed or a combination of both. A CT scan should be performed to see the full extent of the injury. Undisplaced fractures may be treated non-operatively with a hinged knee brace and progressive protected weight bearing over 8–12 weeks.

Displaced fractures require reduction and stabilisation. The articular surface once reduced is often held with plate and screw fixation or fine wire external fixation.

Tibial shaft fractures

For an undisplaced non-comminuted fracture of the tibial shaft, closed reduction and above knee cast is a safe and inexpensive treatment. At 4–6 weeks this may be converted to a patellar tendon below knee cast to allow knee movement. Prolonged casting can lead to stiffness of the knee and the subtalar joint. Cast treatment requires close and constant monitoring of the position of the fracture site. To correct minor angular deformities the cast can be wedged.

A patient may choose to have an intramedullary nail to allow free knee and ankle movement. This, however, risks infection of the implant and anterior knee pain. This is another situation where information and shared decision making can allow the patient to select the most appropriate treatment option.

For comminuted and complex fractures of the tibial shaft, although cast treatment is possible, intramedullary nailing is preferred despite the potential complications of infection and anterior knee pain. Fractures at the diaphyseal metaphyseal junction at the knee and ankle are difficult to hold with an intramedullary nail and as such may be held with a plate and screws.

Tibial fractures are also very amenable to external fixation with either a monolateral frame or fine wire circular construct, particularly where surgical skills and implants are not available for intramedullary nailing.

Ankle fractures

Ankle fractures are very common. As with all intra-articular fractures one should strive for an anatomical reduction. Due to the biconvex saddle shape of the articular surface, small amounts of talar shift significantly increase joint surface contact pressures.

It is useful to think of the ankle mortise as having two columns, a medial and lateral. Each column has a bony and a soft tissue component. On the lateral side there are the lateral malleolus, lateral collateral ligament and syndesmotic ligaments. On the medial side there are the medial malleolus and medial collateral ligament (deltoid ligament).

If only one column (either bony or soft tissue component) has been injured, then it is considered a stable injury and can be treated non-operatively with cast or splint protection for 6–8 weeks.

If both columns are involved or there is evidence of talar shift, it is an unstable injury. Depending on patient age and risk factors for wound complications, in general unstable fractures are treated with open reduction and rigid fixation to hold the fracture anatomically.

Non-operative treatment may be used for unstable fractures in elderly patients or patients with poor skin and unfavourable soft tissues, but this approach requires close observation and careful attention to casting technique.

Calcaneal fractures

The os calcis injury is most frequently caused by a fall from a height. It is important to exclude associated injuries to the lumbar spine that occur in 20% of cases. Most os calcis fractures involve the posterior facet of the subtalar joint. The severity of the injury is often best appreciated with CT scans (**Figure 28.24**). Treatment depends on the severity of injury to the subtalar joint and widening of the heel leading to peroneal impingement. An os calcis fracture is a significant injury and outcomes following surgical or non-operative treatment are unpredictable. On occasion in severe injuries, primary fusion of the subtalar joint may be considered.

Talus fracture

The talus consists of a head, neck and body. The most common injury is a talar neck fracture. This is caused by forced dorsiflexion of the forefoot (aviator's astralgus). The blood supply to the body of the talus is interrupted in displaced talar neck fractures. To optimise outcome and reduce the possibility of avascular necrosis, anatomical reduction and stable fixation of the talar neck should be performed.

Tarsometatarsal (Lisfranc) joint injuries

Injuries to the mid-foot are associated with significant morbidity ranging from a mid-foot sprain to complete rupture of the ligaments connecting the forefoot to the mid-foot. Injury

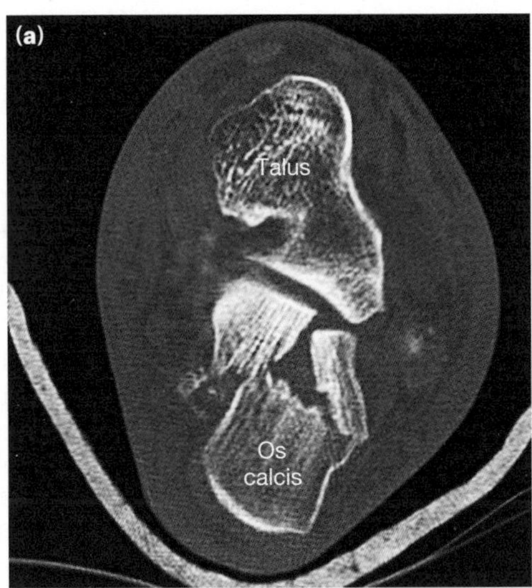

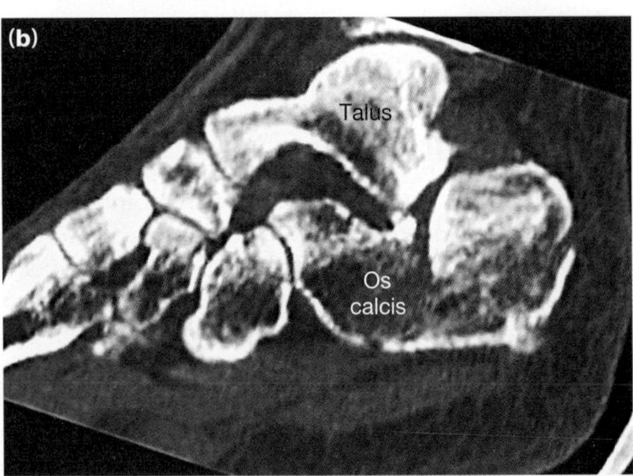

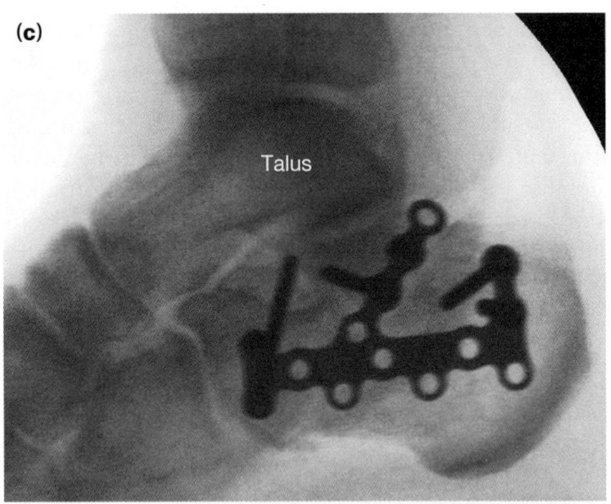

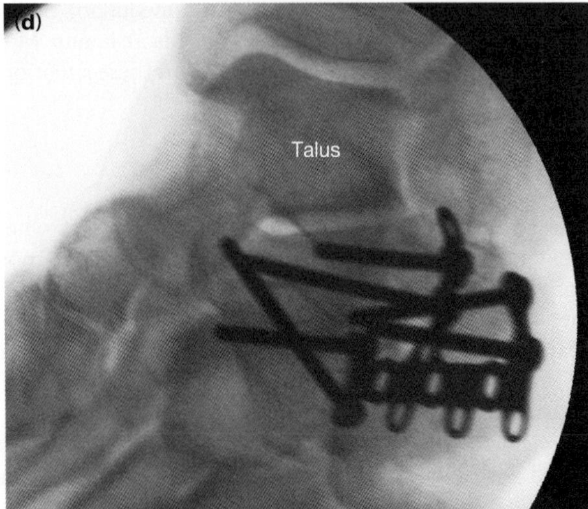

Figure 28.24 Axial (**a**) and sagittal (**b**) views of a displaced intra-articular fracture of the os calcis. (**c, d**) Intraoperative views of the reconstruction. Both the overall shape and the articular surface have been restored.

classically follows forced plantar flexion of the mid-foot. An alternative mechanism of injury are crush injuries where the foot is forced flat by a heavy weight. Lisfranc's ligament connects the second metatarsal to the medial cuneiform. Poorly treated injuries to the mid-foot lead to significant morbidity and if suspected, a CT of the foot should be undertaken. Treatment options range from closed reduction and plaster cast application to K-wire fixation. In severe cases primary tarsometatarsal fusion may be considered.

Achilles tendon rupture

Complete rupture of the tendo Achilles is a common injury; 20% of acute injuries are missed. Active plantar flexion of the ankle is still possible, although weak, through the use of the toe plantar flexors.

A classic history is a feeling as if kicked in the heel and feeling something go. The most common activity leading to Achilles tendon rupture is badminton or squash following sudden forced contraction of the calf.

On examination a palpable gap may be felt. The diagnosis is confirmed by placing the patient prone on the examination couch, feet off the edge of the bed; squeezing the calf fails to elicit passive plantar flexion of the foot. If doubt exists, an ultrasound can confirm the diagnosis.

Treatment of acute Achilles tendon rupture involves surgical repair or functional management. There is an increasing trend to functional management as opposed to direct surgical repair.

TREATMENT OF FRACTURES IN THE SKELETALLY IMMATURE

The treatment principles that were described for the adult, are equally applicable to the child (i.e. reduce, hold, heal, rehabilitate).

A major difference to consider is that in extra-articular fractures there is a remodelling potential, which means increased degrees of deformity may be accepted. Remodelling happens best in the plane of the joint and the closer the injury to the growth plate. Rotational and joint surface remodelling are poor. Fractures occurring near the site of greatest longitudinal growth will remodel the most (e.g. fractures around the distal femur have a greater remodelling potential than the proximal femur). The younger the patient the greater the remodelling potential. Significant remodelling essentially ceases when the growth plates have closed.

A further difference is that paediatric fractures heal more rapidly and as such do not need to be held as long as in the adult counterpart. Similarly, fixation does not need to be as rigid, as fracture union is more rapid.

Growth plate injuries require special mention (see Salter–Harris classification, Figure 28.9). In general, growth plate injuries should be anatomically reduced to minimise the potential for growth disturbance. However, in the process of reducing the fracture, further injury to the growth plate should be avoided.

Repeated manipulation of physeal injuries should be avoided. Injury to the perichondral ring and placing metal work across the physis (where possible) should similarly be avoided. If fixation necessitates crossing the physis, consider limited damage by using the smallest smooth K-wires with a single pass in the middle of the physis if possible.

The paediatric periosteum is often thick and very strong; this needs to be considered when reducing the fracture, requiring an exaggeration of the deformity and pushing the fracture back into place instead of just applying longitudinal traction. The perisosteal hinge should be preserved as it also allows for better holding of the fracture if it remains intact as previously described (see Figure 28.9).

Always consider the possibility of non-accidental injury, as discussed in Chapters 22 and 39.

SPECIFIC PAEDIATRIC INJURIES

Distal radial fractures

Fractures of the distal radius are very common in children. The bone either fails at the physis, leading to Salter–Harris type 2 fractures of the distal radius, or the metaphysis fails. The treatment principle of physeal fractures is to achieve an anatomical reduction. This can often be achieved with closed manipulation and the fracture held in position until healing with a below elbow plaster cast. Growth arrest is rare after physeal fractures of the distal radius.

Complete metaphyseal fractures of the distal radius require close attention (Figure 28.25). In most cases an acceptable closed reduction can be achieved, but holding the distal fragment in an acceptable position can be challenging with cast immobilisation. Brachioradialis, which is attached to the radial styloid, is a continual deforming force. If non-operative treatment using a cast application is chosen, the position should be checked with radiographs weekly for the first 3 weeks, and if re-displacement occurs, then repeat manipulation and K-wire fixation may be required.

Distal humerus (supracondylar fracture)

Supracondylar humeral fractures are very common injuries in children. The distal humerus may go into flexion or extension, extension being by far the most common. Treatment depends on the degree of displacement. Undisplaced fractures may be protected in a collar and cuff or backslab for 3 weeks and then progressive mobilisation.

If displaced, the fracture can often be reduced with closed manipulation. If the dorsal periosteal hinge is intact, then above elbow cast immobilisation is often sufficient to hold the fracture until union in 4–6 weeks. If the periosteal hinge is broken, then percutaneous K-wires are used to hold the fracture, supplemented with an above elbow cast.

Jacques Lisfranc de St Martin, 1790–1847, Professor of Surgery and Operative Medicine, Paris, France.

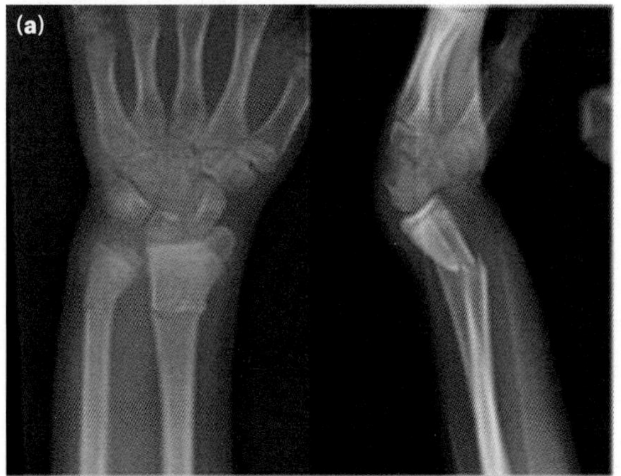

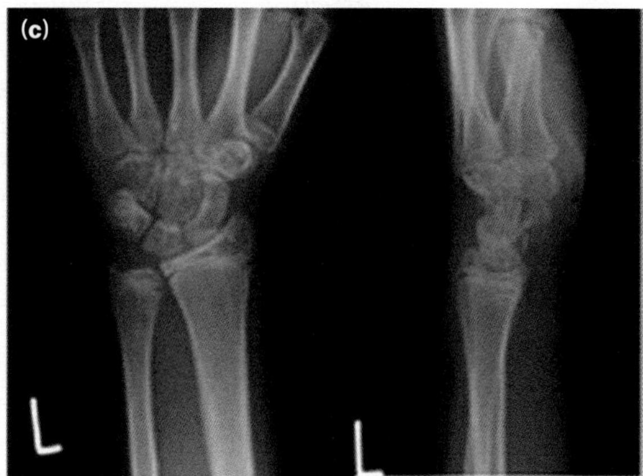

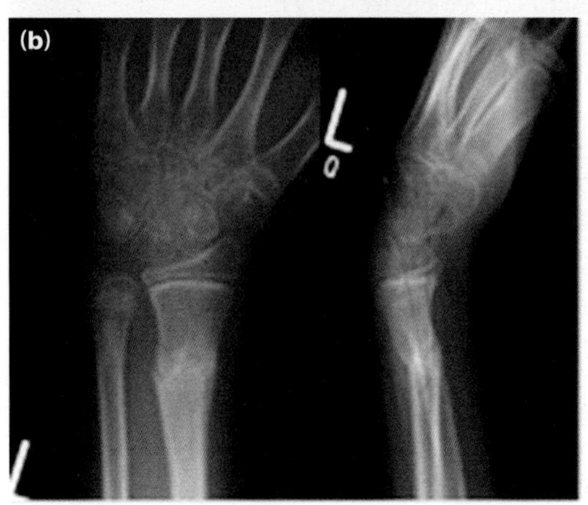

Figure 28.25 (a) AP and lateral radiographs of a 10-year-old showing a dorsally angulated metaphyseal fracture of the radius and undisplaced fracture of the ulna. (b) Injury treated with closed manipulation and cast application. Eight weeks' post-injury radiograph out of cast. Fracture is united, with residual 11 degree dorsal angulation. (c) Radiograph of the wrist following repeat injury 2 years later at age 12, showing complete remodelling. No residual deformity.

A very rare but feared complication of paediatric supracondylar fractures is Volkmann's ischaemic contracture. This is due to excessive swelling and missed compartment syndrome in the forearm. It is particularly important not to put the elbow into deep flexion if there is a lot of swelling. If deep flexion is the only way to hold the fracture, then K-wire fixation should be considered.

Neurovascular injury at the time of a supracondylar fracture is not uncommon. Careful attention should be paid to the neurovascular status of the limb. The white pulseless hand is a surgical emergency and requires emergent reduction. If the pulse does not return with reduction, then the vessels should be explored by appropriately trained surgeons.

The pink pulseless hand is more controversial and requires early senior decision making. If there is satisfactory perfusion of the limb, no suggestion of compartment syndrome and no neurological injury, then reduction and stabilisation of the fracture is warranted and a more expectant approach to the vascular injury can be taken. Often the pulse will return within 24–48 hours.

Neurological injury is common, most often a neuropraxia. They often resolve on fracture reduction, stabilisation and resolution of the swelling.

Malunion in varus or valgus remains a problem. Often the elbow will remodel the deformity in the anteroposterior flexion extension plane, but varus and valgus malunion remodels less. Careful attention needs to be paid to the adequacy of the reduction and K-wire placement to hold the fracture to avoid angular malunion.

Lateral condylar mass fracture of the elbow

Lateral condylar mass fractures of the elbow are easily missed and often considered benign as there is often only a small flake of bone visible. This thin sliver of metaphyseal bone on the lateral side of the elbow is very deceptive. Do not underestimate the significance of this injury (Figure 28.26).

Treatment depends on the stability of the lateral mass fragment. If stable, non operative treatment is acceptable. If unstable, anatomical reduction and fixation should be attempted to avoid complications.

Unstable fractures are suggested by significant soft tissue swelling, by fracture displacement of more than 2 mm or by the fracture being visible on both anteroposterior and lateral views of the elbow.

Unstable fractures require anatomical reduction and rigid fixation with K-wires or screw fixation to avoid displacement and complications. Avascular necrosis of the capitellum and non-union of the lateral condyle lead to the so- called 'fish tail' deformity.

Slipped upper femoral epiphysis

A slipped upper femoral epiphysis classically occurs in a child approaching puberty. It is easily missed as symptoms may be mild and the predominant symptom may be knee pain referred from the hip. A history of trauma may be offered and the child may limp.

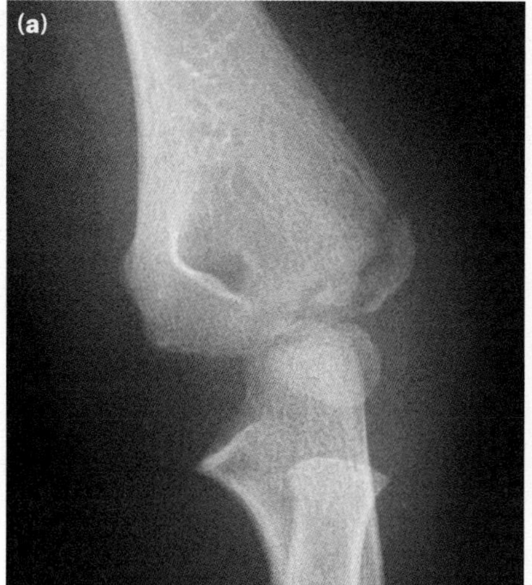

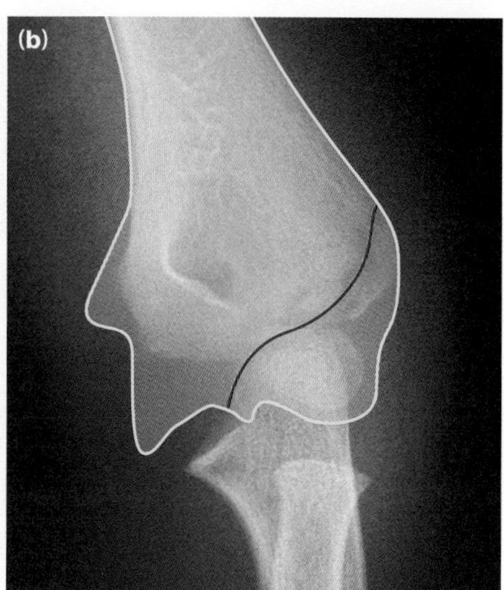

Figure 28.26 Lateral condylar mass fracture. (a) Plain radiograph showing the metaphyseal fracture. (b) The yellow shows the shape of the distal humerus including the cartilaginous analogue, and the red shows the true extent of the injury (i.e. a significant intra-articular fracture).

Examination of the limb reveals a hip that flexes into external rotation. Radiographs should include a good lateral view of the femoral head and neck (Figure 28.27). If the radiographs are normal, consider MRI, looking for a pre-slip, and prophylactic fixation. If treated in the early stages, the prognosis is very good. A severely displaced slipped upper femoral epiphysis might lead to avascular necrosis of the femoral head and chondrolysis. This is a very difficult condition to treat effectively in young patients.

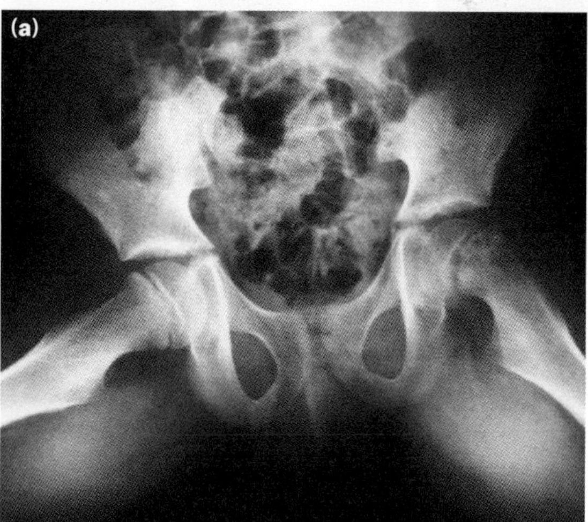

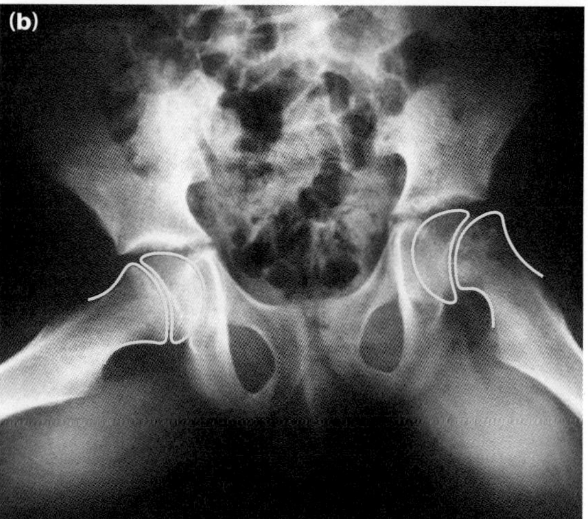

Figure 28.27 Slipped left upper femoral epiphysis. (a) Plain radiograph; (b) the injury highlighted.

Femoral shaft fractures

Femoral shaft fractures in children are treated based on the age and size of the child:

- infants (0–18 months);
- toddlers and small children (18 months–4 years);
- children (4–12 years);
- older children/adolescents.

In infants (0–18 months), ensure there is no evidence of non-accidental injury. In infants under 12–15 kg, gallows traction is acceptable. This traction involves suspension of the legs vertically with the buttocks just off the bed. In toddlers and small children treatment is by traction initially followed by hip spica application. Shortening of up to 1 cm and angulation of 15–20 degrees can be accepted depending on the age of the child due to extensive remodelling potential.

As the child gets older and time to union increases, so the non-operative measures of traction and hip spica become more cumbersome.

In children from 4 to 12 years several treatment options exist from traction and hip spica, elastic stable intramedullary nailing (ESIN), external fixation or plate fixation. Definitive treatment depends on surgeon skills, facilities and patient and parent needs.

In older children and adolescents, non-operative treatment with traction and hip spica cast application becomes less tolerable. Depending on patient size and build, operative treatment may include ESIN (Figure 28.28), external fixation or plate fixation. In larger overweight adolescents,

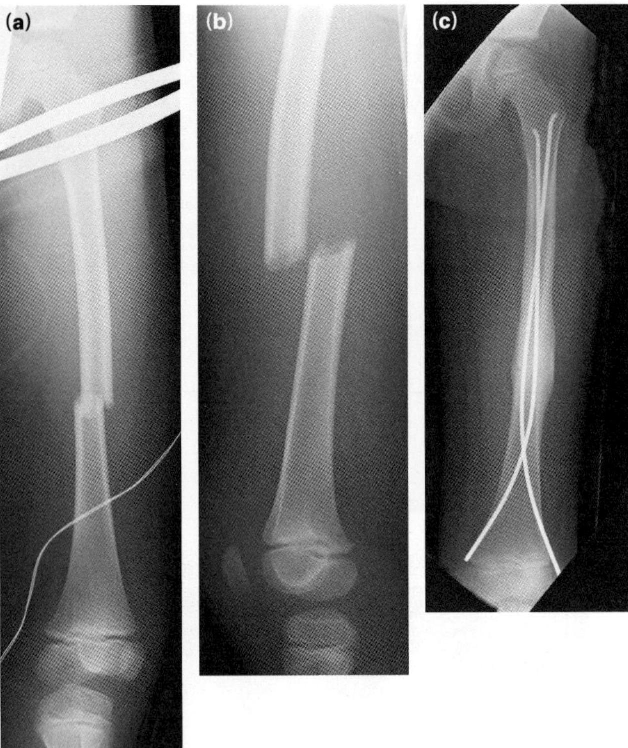

Figure 28.28 (a-c) Femoral shaft fracture in a child, which has been stabilised with elastic nails.

Summary box 28.6

Fractures in the skeletally immature

- Do not forget non-accidental injury
- Be reluctant to remanipulate a physeal injury
- Elastic nails are a significant step forward in fracture treatment in children
- Not many fractures require operative intervention in children

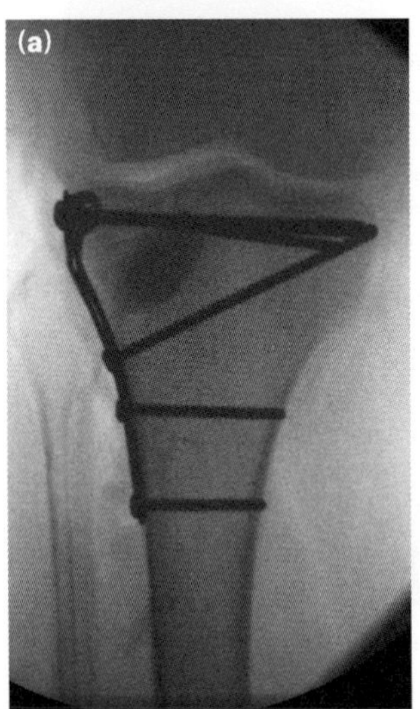

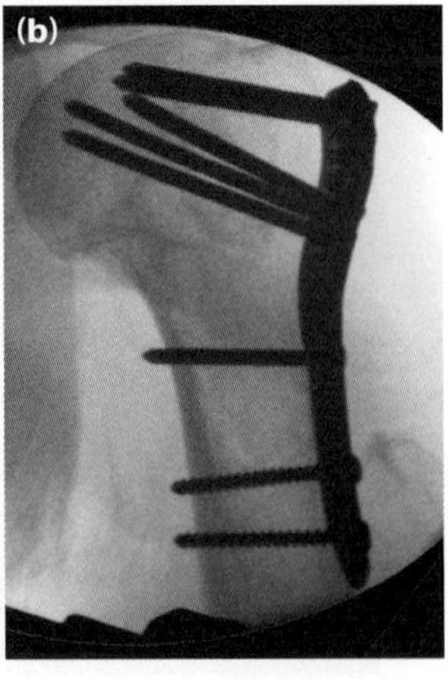

Figure 28.29 Variations in fixation technique suited to osteoporotic bone. (a) Norian bone substitute has been injected to support the lateral tibial plateau in the partial articular fracture. (b) A locking plate in a proximal humerus. The screws are threaded into the plate to make a fixed-angle device.

titanium elastic nails may not be strong enough to resist bending forces and locked intramedullary nailing may be considered.

It is important, however, to remember that there is a 1–2% chance of avascular necrosis of the femoral head if an antegrade intramedullary nail is used prior to or just after physeal closure. This is a rare but devastating complication in this age group. Far lateral entry point nails on the greater trochanter have been developed to limit the effect on the blood supply to the femoral head; however, the risk of avascular necrosis persists.

Tibial shaft fractures

Tibial fractures in children are often very amenable to nonoperative treatment, starting with an above knee cast, followed by conversion to a Sarmiento patellar tendon below knee cast at 4–6 weeks. Remodelling in the tibia is somewhat limited and as such less angular deformity can be accepted, no rotational deformity and only 10–15 degrees of angular deformity. Some shortening of the tibia can be accepted as the tibia is expected to overgrow by 0.5 cm in response to injury. If it is not possible to hold the fracture in an acceptable position with a cast, then external fixation, ESIN TENS or plating is an option.

SPECIAL CONSIDERATIONS

Special consideration needs to be given to osteoporotic and pathological fractures, for example the ability to hold the fracture until union. Furthermore, open fractures require urgent appropriate treatment to ensure bone healing in the absence of infection.

Osteoporotic fractures

Osteoporosis is a condition characterised by low bone mineral density and reduced strength. Osteoporotic bone is liable to fracture with low energy injuries (e.g. a fall from standing height). Treatment of lower limb osteoporotic fractures in older patients are challenging. As there may be additional and pre-existing mobility problems, such patients are unable to partially weight bear and so fixation should be strong enough to allow immediate weight bearing and to hold the position until union. Locking plate technology improves fixation in osteoporotic bone, and bone void fillers can be utilised (Figure 28.29).

Pathological fractures

When abnormal bone fails under normal load this is referred to as a pathological fracture. Depending on the cause of the pathological fracture the bone may not heal and consideration should be given to a load-bearing device not load sharing. If involving the joint surface or close to the joint surface, the affected area may be excised *en bloc* and a joint replacement performed.

The bone may be weakened by a primary bone tumour, secondary metastatic deposits, haematological malignancy (myeloma, lymphoma, leukaemia), osteomyelitis and metabolic bone disease (osteomalacia, Paget's disease, osteoporosis).

A pathological fracture should be suspected if the history is not consistent with the severity of the injury. The patient may give a history of low energy injury that normally would not cause a fracture. If a pathological fracture is suspected, the cause should be actively sought. Where a primary bone tumour is suspected, treatment should be planned to prevent disseminating the disease (see Chapter 37).

In patients with metastatic bone disease, the primary source should be sought if multiple metastatic deposits are identified. If life expectancy is poor, then stabilisation with a load bearing device may be considered. If an isolated metastasis is identified and an overall good prognosis is offered by the oncologists, then a more aggressive curative approach may be taken with en-bloc excision of the primary and the isolated secondary deposit.

If a metastatic deposit is identified prior to fracture, prophylactic fixation should be considered if impending fracture is likely. Prophylactic stabilisation with a load-bearing device is once again advocated. If life expectancy is good and the deposit periarticular, an en-bloc excision and joint arthroplasty may be considered to optimise return to near normal function as soon as possible.

Open fractures

Any fracture with an overlying wound should be considered an open fracture. The term previously used was a compound fracture. Open fractures require particular mention because adequate stabilisation of the bony injury and appropriate management of the soft tissue injury is paramount to ensure a good outcome with a low complication rate. The treatment of bone and joint infection is expensive, laborious and time-consuming for the professional as well as the patient. An infected femoral shaft fracture following intramedullary nailing will typically take 3 years and five operations to clear the infection and achieve union.

The Gustilo and Anderson classification of open fractures is the most frequently used classification (see *Table 28.2*). The definitive grade is determined intraoperatively after thorough debridement. It is not based on size of wound alone but takes into account several factors; a farmyard or heavily contaminated wound of under 1 cm may still be considered a grade III injury.

The aim of open fracture management is to achieve bony union, optimum function and avoid infection. The treatment of open fractures should be considered in two phases: the emergency department pre-surgical phase and the surgical phase.

Pre-surgical phase

1. Take a photograph to document the severity of the injury and limit the need for repeated opening of dressings. (Do not delay steps below unduly.)
2. Assess neurovascular status and if compromised and the fracture displaced, quickly remove any macroscopic dirt and reduce the fracture/dislocation. It is not essential to achieve an anatomical reduction; simply remove the pressure from the soft tissues (make a leg look like a leg and an arm look like an arm). If the bone was out of the skin and is reduced under the skin, then document clearly and inform the surgical team.
3. Once overall alignment is achieved, splint the affected limb; treatment of an open fracture is treatment of the soft tissues.
4. Apply a moist saline dressing to the wound. It is acceptable to irrigate the wound with saline in the emergency department to remove any macroscopic dirt, but definitive debridement and wash out of the wound should be undertaken in a theatre environment.
5. Administer intravenous antibiotics according to local protocols. It has been shown that early administration of intravenous antibiotics is one of the most important steps. A broad-spectrum antibiotic should be chosen covering gram-positive, gram-negative and if severe contamination, anaerobic organisms.
6. Obtain a tetanus immunisation history and treat accordingly.
7. Inform senior orthopaedic surgeon of the injury as soon as possible and make preparations for surgical phase.

Surgical phase

In the past an open fracture was considered a contraindication to internal fixation. It is increasingly evident that stable fixation of the bony injury is very important to prevent deterioration of the soft tissues, allowing recovery and healing.

Fracture stabilisation may come in the form of external fixation, internal fixation with screws/plates/intramedullary nails – depending on the setting.

Management of the soft tissues is critical to prevent the zone of injury spreading. Thorough debridement of any contaminated or non-vital soft tissue is important. Any loose or devitalised bone fragments should be discarded. Bone defects are easier to deal with than an infected non-union.

Summary box 28.7

Special considerations

- Osteoporotic fractures in the older patients may require specialised fixation techniques with locking screw/plate technology and injectable bone cement augmentation
- Pathological fractures may not heal and require load-bearing not load-sharing implants
- Arthroplasty in suitable patients bypasses the problems of blood supply, weak bone and allows early full weight bearing and return to function
- Open fractures require prompt debridement, stabilisation and adequate soft tissue cover to prevent infection.

Sir James Paget, 1814–1899, surgeon, St Bartholomew's Hospital, London, UK.

Soft tissue reconstruction may involve primary or delayed primary closure of the wound, or more sophisticated soft tissue reconstruction options including microvascular free tissue transfer.

Continue intravenous antibiotics until 48 hours after definitive wound closure.

COMPARTMENT SYNDROME

Compartment syndrome is raised pressure in an osseofascial compartment to a level that compromises tissue perfusion. There are several causes of compartment syndrome, fractures being the most common (70%), followed by soft tissue contusions (23%). Rarer causes include: bleeding disorders including anticoagulation, burns (particularly circumferential 3rd degree burns); post-ischaemic swelling (reperfusion injury); tight casts/dressings; and extravasation of intravenous infusions (contrast under pressure).

The pathophysiology involves increased tissue pressure, which leads to reduced microperfusion resulting in tissue ischaemia and irreversible muscle damage from cellular anoxia.

Compartment syndrome is a clinical diagnosis characterised by pain out of proportion, increasing pain and pain on passive stretch. Paralysis, paraesthesia and pallor are late signs and pulselessness is an extremely late sign.

Compartment pressure monitoring may be useful in cases of diagnostic uncertainty and in patients with altered levels of consciousness (intubated, head injury).

Measure multiple sites near but not in the fracture site, in all the compartments of the affected limb. Generally accepted pressure thresholds include an absolute pressure greater than or equal to 30 mmHg or pressure difference (diastolic pressure – compartment pressure) less than or equal to 30 mmHg.

Emergency treatment involves splitting casts and or dressings to the skin and elevating the extremity. Senior input should be sought and arrangements put in place to perform definitive treatment with fasciotomies.

There are some common pitfalls to remember. The incidence of compartment syndrome associated with high and low energy injuries is nearly equal. Compartment syndrome can occur in open fractures. Have a high index of suspicion and be particularly vigilant in patients with an altered level of consciousness.

CONCLUSION

The correct identification of extremity trauma, combined with timely and appropriate treatment, is essential to return patients to normal function as safely and as quickly as possible. The same injury may be treated in different ways based on patient factors, age, functional demands and co-morbidities. Surgeon and resource based factors also need to be considered.

Summary box 28.8

Summary of extremity trauma

- Realise that an injury exists
- Find the characteristics of the injury, describe and classify it
- Consider the natural history of the injury
- Treatment is guided by outcome if known or by principle if not
- Beware of injuries that are 'easily missed'

FURTHER READING

Bone LR, Johnson KD, Weight J, Scheinberg RJ. Early versus delayed stabilization of femoral fractures. *J Bone Joint Surg* 1989; **71A**: 336–40.

Charnley J. *The closed treatment of common fractures*. Edinburgh: E&S Livingstone, 1950.

Court-Brown CM, Heckman JD, McQueen MM *et al.* (eds). *Rockwood and Green's fractures in adults*, 8th edn. Wolters Kluwer, 2014.

Gustilo RB, Anderson JT. Prevention of infection in the treatment of 1025 open fractures of long bones. *J Bone Joint Surg* 1976; **8A**: 453–8.

Mast J, Jakob R, Ganz R. *Planning and reduction technique in fracture surgery*. Berlin: Springer-Verlag, 1989.

Muller ME, Nazarian S, Koch P. *The AO classification of fractures*. Schatzker J (trans). Berlin: Springer-Verlag, 1988.

Solomon L, Warwick D, Nayagam S. *Apley's system of orthopaedics and fractures*, 9th edn. Boca Raton: CRC Press, 2010.

Chapter 29

Disaster surgery

Learning objectives

To recognise and understand:
- The common features of various disasters
- The principles behind the organisation of the relief effort and of triage in treatment and evacuation
- The role and limitations of field hospitals in disaster
- The features of conditions peculiar to disaster situations and their treatment

INTRODUCTION

Natural disasters provide a constant reminder of the power and capricious nature of our planet. The depletion of the ozone layer and global warming mean that the future may hold in store calamitous events with even greater magnitude than those experienced before. National conflicts and ideological differences have not lessened and the resultant 'unnatural disasters' have the potential to rival the natural ones in enormity (see Chapter 30). Disasters by their very nature are unpredictable and no two are alike. Nevertheless, there are numerous common elements and it has been shown that countries that invest in disaster preparedness are better equipped to cope with such catastrophes. Recent wars and disasters have highlighted the increasingly crucial role of surgeons in these scenarios.

COMMON FEATURES OF MAJOR DISASTERS

Any event that results in the loss of human life is disastrous, but most accidents, such as aeroplane and train crashes, are limited in the number of people involved. Conversely, natural disasters, such as earthquakes and tsunamis, leave in their wake massive destruction over large areas that can transcend national boundaries. All the apparatus of a society that responds to such disasters (the civil administration, emergency services, fire brigades and hospitals) may itself be involved and unable to respond (Figure 29.1). Large numbers of people may require immediate shelter, clean water and food, in addition to any medical needs.

A breakdown of communication is inevitable and can be accompanied by widespread panic and a disruption of civil order. Access to the disaster area may be limited because of the destruction of bridges, affecting road and rail links.

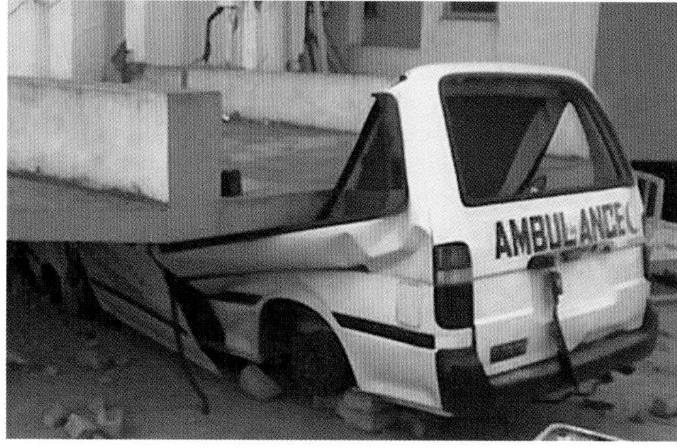

Figure 29.1 Damage to emergency medical services.

Summary box 29.1

Common features of major disasters
- Massive casualties
- Damage to infrastructure
- A large number of people requiring shelter
- Panic and uncertainty among the population
- Limited access to the area
- Breakdown of communication

FACTORS INFLUENCING RELIEF EFFORTS AND PROVISION OF MEDICAL AID

Good communication is critical for the authorities to respond quickly to a disaster. Wireless technology and satellite imag-

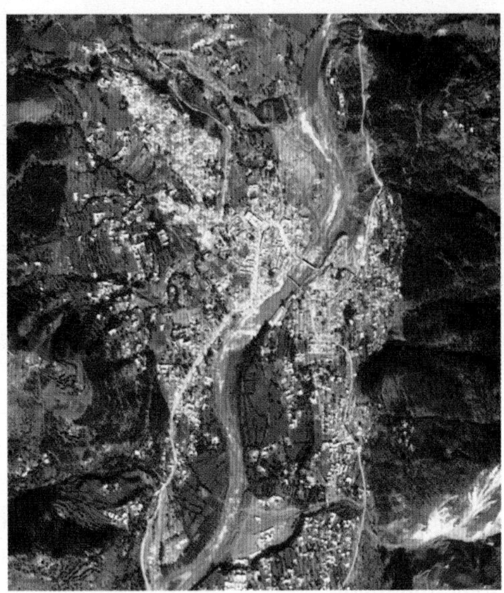

Figure 29.2 Satellite image showing destruction of a bridge as a result of flooding.

ery have revolutionised the way in which real-time information can be obtained (Figure 29.2). Nonetheless, there is an inevitable lag period between the occurrence of the disaster and the response from the establishment.

The location of the disaster area has a bearing on relief efforts. In large cities emergency and medical services are better developed. However, these areas are densely populated and may have limited access by road and air. Disasters in remote areas can be particularly difficult to manage because relief efforts are hampered by geographical isolation and the lack of infrastructure.

Summary box 29.2

Factors influencing rescue and relief efforts

- Status of communications
- Location, whether rural or urban
- Accessibility of the location
- Time-frame in which disaster occurs
- Economic state of development of the area

The time-frame in which a disaster occurs also impacts on the relief efforts. Earthquakes can unleash havoc in seconds but floods and hurricanes may continue for several days. Another important factor is the state of resources of the country; disasters in poorer countries can seldom be managed without significant outside assistance.

SEQUENCE OF RELIEF EFFORTS AFTER A DISASTER

Establishing a chain of command

Many countries have dedicated organisations that deal with disasters. In others, an administrative hierarchy is established to coordinate the efforts of the teams participating in relief efforts (Figure 29.3).

Damage assessment

The first objective in disaster management is an assessment of the damage and the number of casualties. All sources of information must be employed. The 24-hour news services

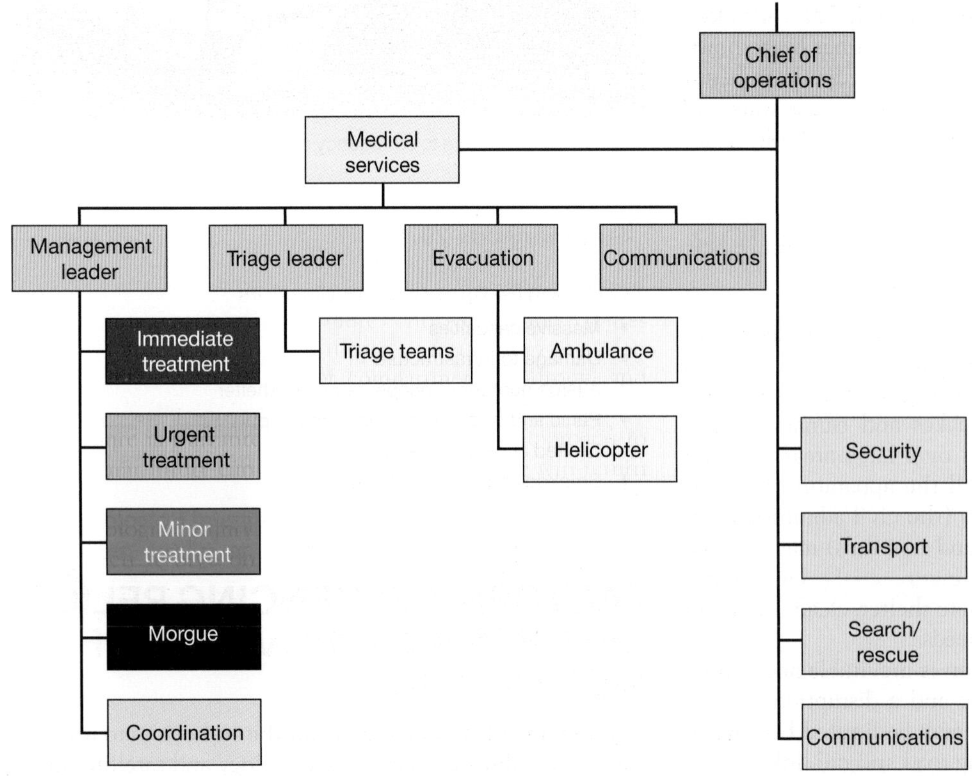

Figure 29.3 Organisation chart for disaster management.

are frequently the first on the scene and can be an important source of information.

Mobilising resources

The next step is mobilisation of human and material resources appropriate to the extent of the disaster. Although all modes of transport need to be considered, helicopters provide the quickest access for the first responders (Figure 29.4). The teams who make up the initial response must include experienced staff who can assess the situation and who have the authority to take immediate decisions.

Rescue operation

Early coordination of the rescue effort allows optimal use of resources. The first priority is to prevent further damage from occurring, both to people and to the infrastructure. The types of injuries encountered by rescue workers depends on the delay between the onset of the disaster and their arrival. Patients with head injuries and abdominal and thoracic trauma will either have been treated or have succumbed to their injuries within 48–72 hours of a disaster. After the first week, the only casualties requiring treatment are those with complex limb trauma and infected wounds (Figure 29.5).

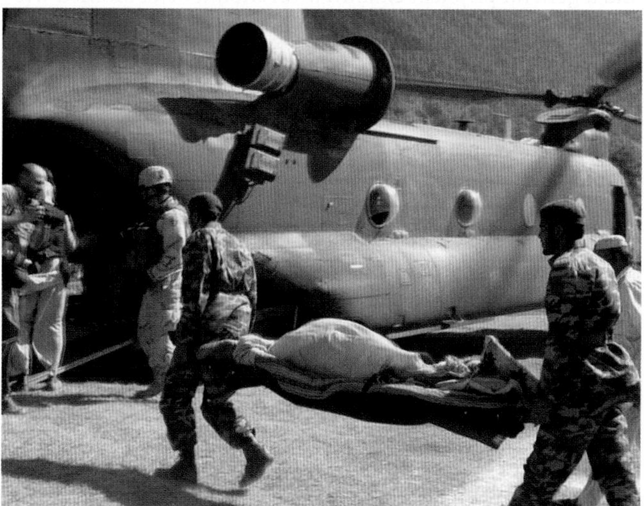

Figure 29.4 Heli-evacuation.

Coordination with relief agencies

A laudable aspect of globalisation is the outpouring of help from governments and non-governmental organisations (NGOs) in response to a disaster. Some, like Rescue and Preparedness in Disasters (RAPID), deal with search and rescue whereas others, like the International Committee of the Red Cross (ICRC) and Oxfam, provide general disaster-related relief (Figure 29.6). The various United Nations (UN) agencies deal with medical care, food provision and refugees. Coordinating the efforts of these organisations is essential for optimal results, as medical aid in isolation is inadequate without the simultaneous provision of safe drinking water, food, clothing and shelter.

Summary box 29.3

Sequence of the relief effort in major disasters

- Establish chain of command
- Set up lines of communication
- Carry out damage assessment
- Mobilise resources
- Initiate rescue operation
- Triage casualties
- Start emergency treatment
- Arrange evacuation
- Start definitive management

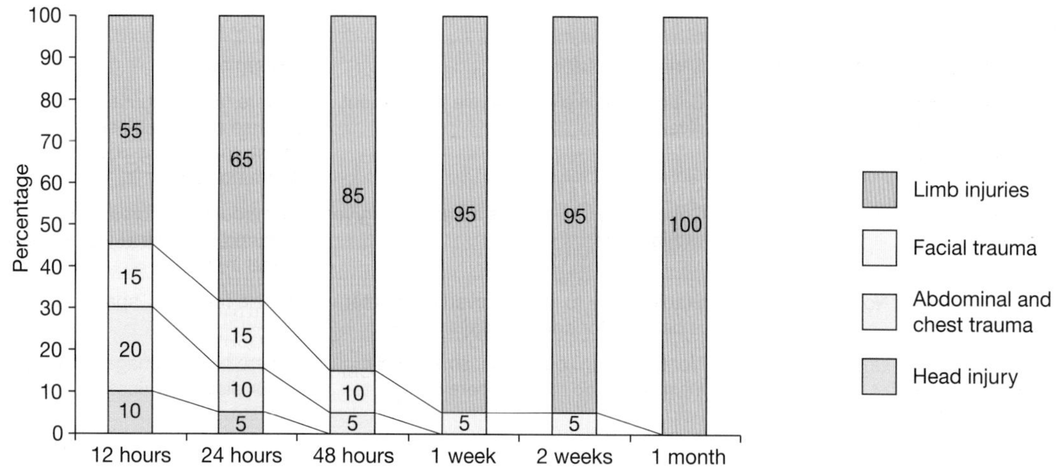

Figure 29.5 Time-line showing the type of injuries encountered at different times in a disaster.

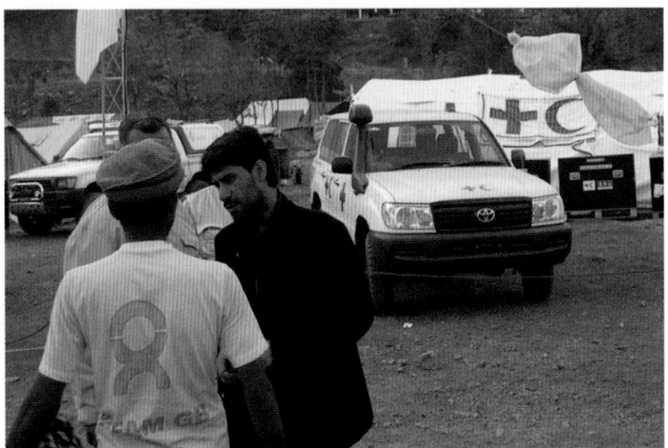

Figure 29.6 Oxfam and the International Committee of the Red Cross provide generalised relief.

Dealing with the media

Disasters act like a magnet for the media which, in today's world of 24-hour news coverage, plays an important part in shaping public opinion. It is essential to establish a working relationship between the media and the rescue teams. With careful handling the media can become a powerful ally and play a constructive role in identifying problems, galvanising aid and keeping the public informed.

Triage

Derived from the French verb 'trier', triage means 'to sort' and is the cornerstone of the management of mass casualties. It aims to identify the patients who will benefit the most by being treated the earliest, ensuring 'the greatest good for the greatest number'. Numerous studies show that only 10–15% of disaster casualties are serious enough to require hospitalisation. By sorting out the minor injuries, triage lessens the immediate burden on medical facilities. Deciding who receives priority when faced with hundreds of seriously injured victims is a daunting prospect. Triage should be undertaken by someone senior, who has the experience and authority to make these critical decisions. To keep pace with the changing clinical picture of an injured person, triage needs to be undertaken in the field, before evacuation and at the hospital.

Triage areas

For efficient triage the injured need to be brought together into any undamaged structures that can shelter a large number of wounded. A good water supply, lighting and ease of access are useful. Separate areas should be reserved for patient holding, emergency treatment and decontamination (in the event of discharge of hazardous materials).

Practical triage

Emergency life-saving measures should proceed alongside triage and can actually help the decision-making process. The assessment and restoration of airway, breathing and circulation are critical and are discussed in Chapter 23. Vital signs and a general physical examination should be combined with a brief history taken by a paramedic or by a volunteer worker if one is available.

Documentation for triage

Accurate documentation is an inseparable part of triage and should include basic patient data, vital signs with timing, brief details of injuries (preferably on a diagram) and treatment given. A system of colour-coded tags attached to the patient's wrist or around the neck should be employed by the emergency medical services. The colour denotes the degree of urgency with which a patient requires treatment (**Figure 29.7**).

Triage categories

All methods of triage use simple criteria based on vital signs. A rapid clinical assessment should be made taking into account the patient's ability to walk, their mental status and the presence or absence of ventilation or capillary perfusion. A commonly used four-tier system is presented in *Table 29.1*.

TABLE 29.1 Triage categories.

Priority	Colour	Medical need	Clinical status	Examples
First (I)	Red	Immediate	Critical, but likely to survive if treatment given early	Severe facial trauma, tension pneumothorax, profuse external bleeding, haemothorax, flail chest, major intra-abdominal bleed, extradural haematomas
Second (II)	Yellow	Urgent	Critical, likely to survive if treatment given within hours	Compound fractures, degloving injuries, ruptured abdominal viscus, pelvic fractures, spinal injuries
Third (III)	Green	Non-urgent	Stable, likely to survive even if treatment is delayed for hours to days	Simple fractures, sprains, minor lacerations
Last (0)	Black	Unsalvageable	Not breathing, pulseless, so severely injured that no medical care is likely to help	Severe brain damage, very extensive burns, major disruption/loss of chest or abdominal wall structures

Triage is the earliest example of clinical risk management. This is done on the basis of need so that resources can be allocated by good prioritisation. The process was first used in 1792 by Baron Dominique Jean Larrey, Surgeon in Chief to Napoleon's Imperial Guard. The concept of triage emerged from the French Service de Sante so that resources could be used to the optimum – "most for the most".

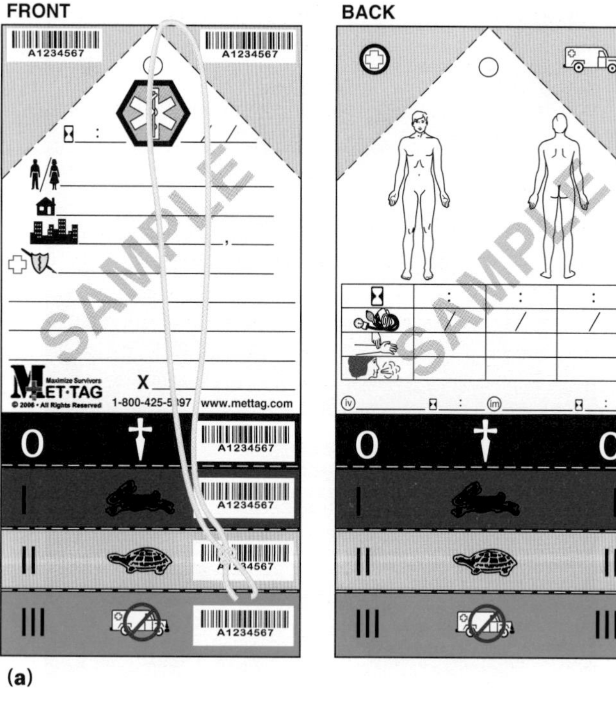

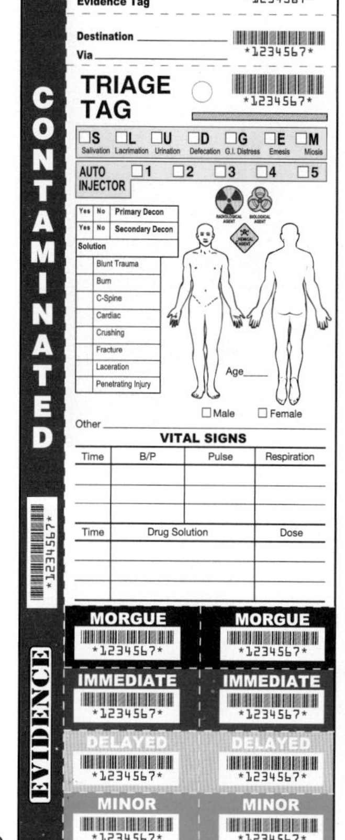

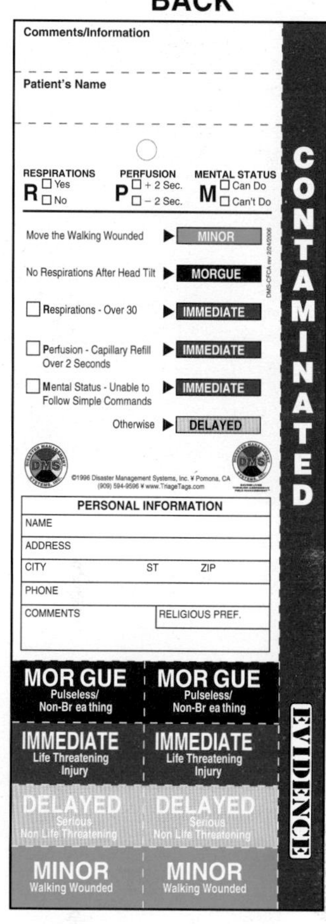

Figure 29.7 Triage tags. **(a)** Courtesy of TACDA & METTAG products, American Civil Defense Association. **(b)** Courtesy of Disaster Management Systems.

Evacuation of casualties

Decisions regarding the best destination for each patient need to be based on how far it is safe for them to travel and whether the facilities that they need for definitive treatment will be available. A quick retriage is very useful in this situation. The paramedics accompanying the casualties should be resolved to prevent the 'second accident' (damage caused inadvertently by transport and treatment). An adequate supply of essentials such as intravenous fluids, dressings, pain medication, and oxygen must be arranged (see Chapter 30).

Field hospitals

The decision to deploy field hospitals depends on the location, the number of casualties and the speed with which evacuation can be organised (**Figure 29.8**). Whether the traditional tented structure or the modular type housed in containers is employed, the facility must be equipped with radiograph capability, operating rooms, vital signs monitors, sterilising equipment, a blood bank, ventilators and basic laboratory facilities.

> **Summary box 29.4**
>
> **Essentials of casualty evacuation**
>
> - Retriage to upgrade priorities amongst the injured
> - Select appropriate medical facilities for transfer
> - Choose appropriate means of transport
> - Prevent the 'second accident' during transfer
> - Ensure an adequate supply of materials to accompany the patient

Management in the field

Field hospitals principally function in three main areas (*Table 29.2*).

First aid

Care for patients with minor injuries involves cleaning and dressing wounds, suturing lacerations and splinting simple fractures. Most of these 'walking wounded' can be sent away with antibiotics and simple pain relief.

DAMAGE CONTROL SURGERY

Damage control surgery (DCS) is the concept that only life- and limb-saving surgery be performed in field hospitals to allow safe transfer of a patient to a definitive treating facility. This will include ensuring that the airway is secure, haemorrhage is under control and compartments are decompressed in the chest, skull, abdomen and the limbs. Devitalised tissue should be removed and any contamination prevented from

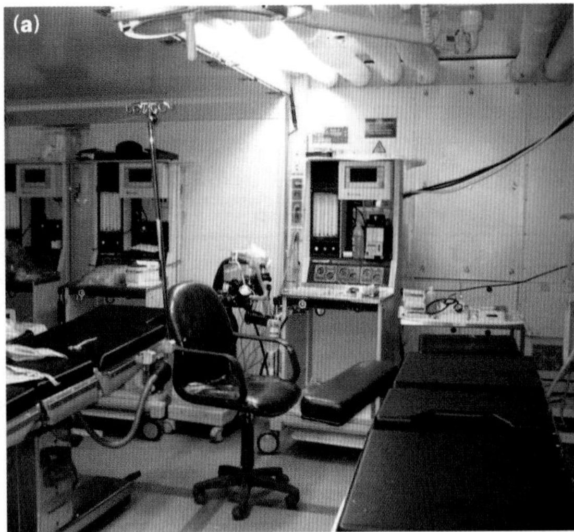
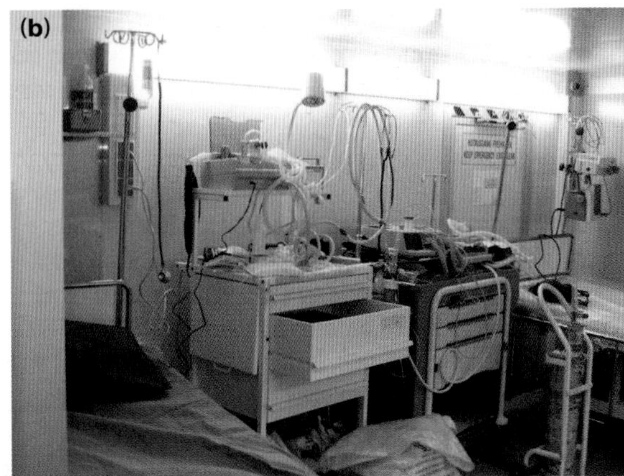
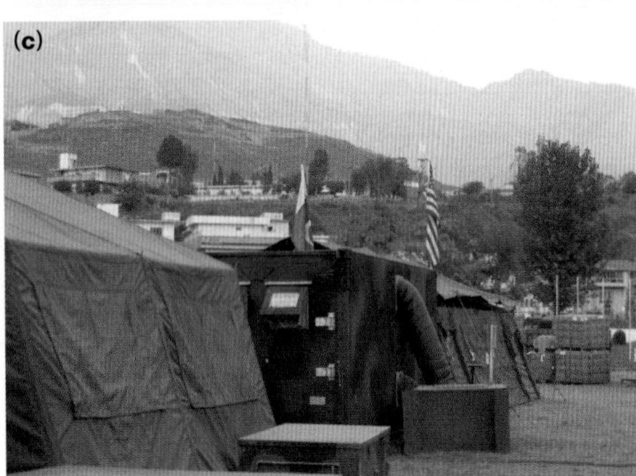
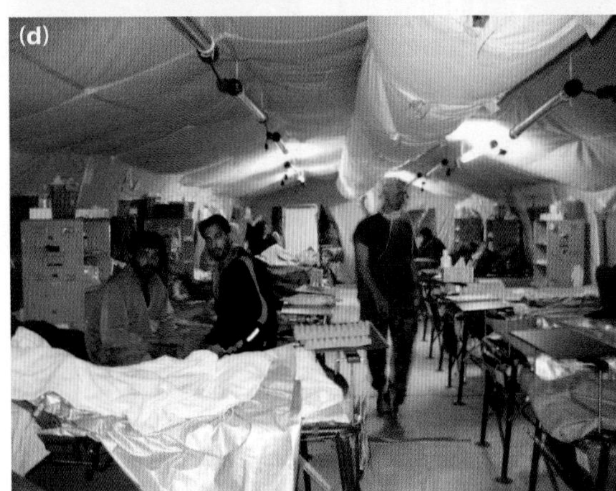

Figure 29.8 Field hospitals: (a, b) modular type; (c) tented structure; (d) interior of a tented field hospital.

TABLE 29.2 Type of treatment given in field hospitals.

	Examples	Further
First aid	Suturing cuts and lacerations, splinting simple fractures	Review at local hospital
Emergency care for life-threatening injuries	Endotracheal intubation, tracheotomy, relieving tension pneumothorax, stopping external haemorrhage, relieving an extradural haematoma, emergency thoracotomy/laparotomy for internal haemorrhage	After damage control surgery, transfer patients to base hospitals once stable
Initial care for non-life-threatening injuries	Debridement of contaminated wounds, reduction of fractures and dislocations, application of external fixators, vascular repairs	Transfer patients to base hospitals for definitive management

developing into infection. DCS is explained in more detail, in the context of early management and other settings, throughout the chapters in the trauma section (see Part 4: Trauma).

Emergency care for immediate life-threatening injuries

There are many patients who may be saved by relatively simple measures, provided that these are taken urgently. Endotracheal intubation and tracheotomy may be needed to provide a secure airway. A needle thoracocentesis will relieve a tension pneumothorax and a chest drain will be needed before a patient with a significant chest injury is transferred by air. An open pneumothorax should be closed. Damaged major vessels to limbs should be repaired if possible. Fasciotomies will be

Summary box 29.5

Principles of damage control surgery

- Do the minimum needed to allow safe transfer to a definitive facility
- Take actions that prevent deterioration of that patient during transfer
- Secure the airway – may require tracheostomy
- Control bleeding – may require craniotomy, laparotomy, thoracotomy, repair of major limb vessels
- Prevent pressure build up – may require burr holes, chest drain, laparotomy, fasciotomy
- Prevent infection by extensile exposure and removing dead and contaminated tissue

needed for muscle compartments that are swelling from injury or from reperfusion. Amputation for clearly devitalised limbs and gas gangrene should be undertaken at field hospitals as delay will be fatal.

Specific aspects of care are discussed in the relevant chapters elsewhere in this book.

Initial care for non-life-threatening injuries

Many patients sustain serious injuries that require prolonged care. These include compound limb fractures, degloving injuries, dislocations of major joints, major facial injuries and complex hand injuries. These patients will need specialised care requiring transfer to the appropriate facility. Replantations of amputated limbs and other extensive procedures should not be attempted in field hospitals as they are time-consuming and divert resources and personnel to the treatment of a few patients.

Debridement

Taken from the French, meaning to 'unleash or cut open', debridement plays a crucial part in the management of trauma. Wounds sustained in disasters are often heavily contaminated, containing foreign bodies and non-viable tissues (Figure 29.9). Debridement reduces the chances of anaerobic and necrotising infections and can prevent systemic sepsis. The following principles of debridement apply to all contaminated wounds:

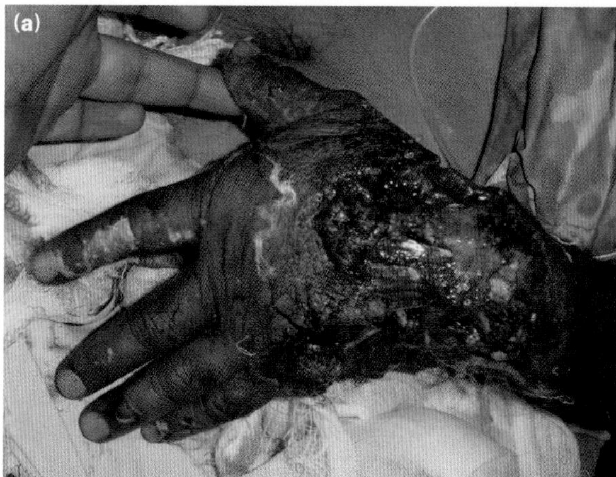

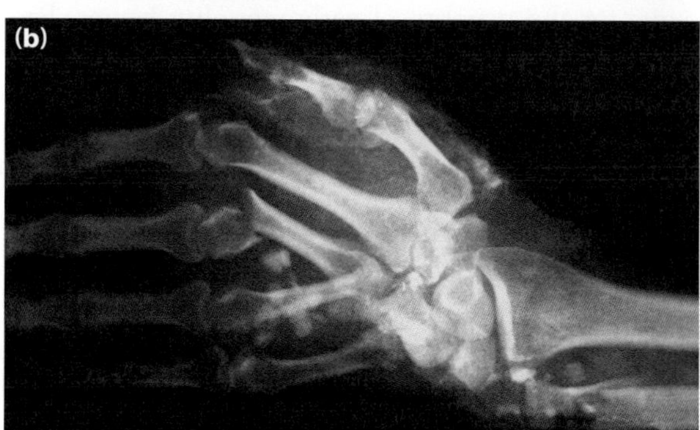

Figure 29.9 (a, b) Gross contamination typically seen in wounds sustained in disasters. The radiograph shows numerous radiopaque foreign bodies in the soft tissues.

- After the administration of anaesthesia, the injured area is copiously irrigated with normal saline. Lavage using a pressurised system is controversial, with concerns over tissue trauma and spread of debris (Figure 29.10). The wound is palpated and all foreign matter removed. Dirt and debris enmeshed in soft tissues can only be removed by excision of those tissues. Open joints should be thoroughly irrigated and all foreign material removed.
- Wounds with extensive cavitation should be enlarged longitudinally to gain better access and allow full decompression of the underlying muscles. This should be carried out under tourniquet. This helps to visualise the damaged structures, and allow the surgeon to gain proximal and distal control of vascular injuries, and to identify severed ends of major nerves and tendons.
- The next step is excision of all dead and devitalised tissue. At this stage the tourniquet is let down to check the vascularity of the tissues. Skin excision is kept to a minimum and only the margins of the wound need be trimmed back to healthy bleeding edges. Excision of devitalised muscle should be undertaken generously. Muscle that is pale or dark in colour, does not contract on pinching and does not bleed on cutting must be removed. In patients with traumatic amputations, the bone ends are tidied, the skin and muscle edges trimmed to the lowest level possible and the wound left open.
- In patients with associated fractures, skeletal stabilisation should be obtained before embarking on any repairs. External fixators are invaluable for this and make wound management much easier (Figure 29.11).

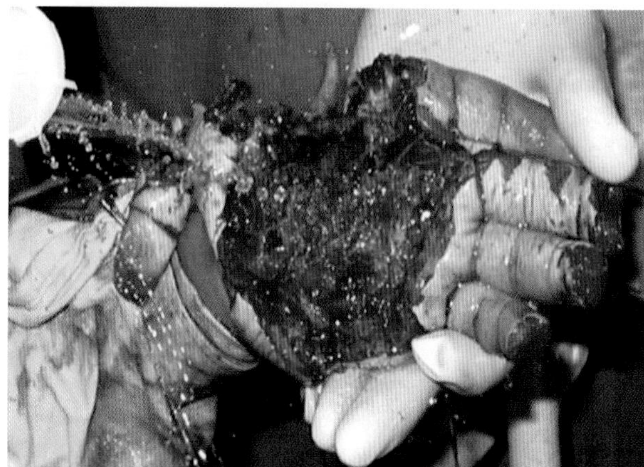

Figure 29.10 Lavage with normal saline to decontaminate a wound.

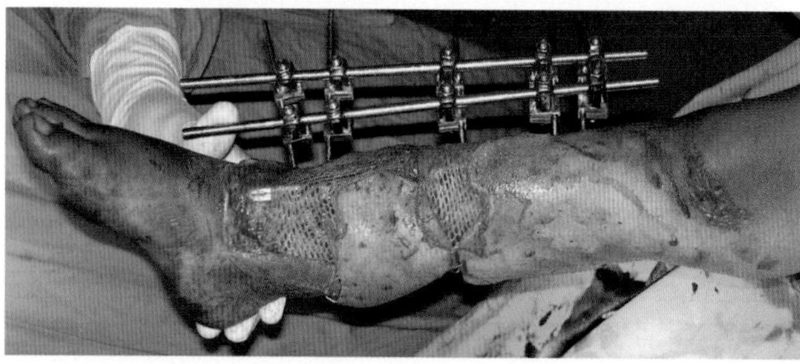

Figure 29.11 External fixators provide skeletal stabilisation and allow easy management of the soft tissues.

- In the acute setting, only vascular repairs are justified. For lacerated vessels the ends are trimmed and an anastomosis performed. In the case of loss of substance of the vessel wall, a vein patch or reversed vein graft may be employed. Silicone tubing may be used as a temporary bypass (stent) while vascular repair is being carried out in patients with critically compromised distal circulation.
- Nerves and tendons should not be dissected out nor should any attempt be made at definitive repair in wounds with tissue devitalisation, as this leads to poor results. The key structures should be identified and the edges trimmed and tagged with non-absorbable sutures to facilitate repair during subsequent exploration.
- Wounds sustained in disasters are heavily contaminated and are not suitable for primary closure. However, blood vessels and exposed joint surfaces need to be covered. This can be achieved by loosely tacking adjoining muscle over the exposed area. The wound is then covered with fluffed gauze and sterile cotton and the extremity splinted with a plaster of Paris slab. For extremity injuries, elevation is critical to reduce oedema.
- Broad-spectrum antibiotics, such as third-generation cephalosporins, are started prophylactically and continued for 5–7 days.
- The wound is reinspected at 24–48 hours to assess the viability of the tissues. Wounds are closed between the fourth and sixth day if there is no infection. Tension should be avoided and one should not hesitate to use skin grafts to obtain cover.
- In wounds with gross infection no attempt at closure is made until infection is eradicated. These wounds are re-explored to make sure that there are no residual foreign bodies or devitalised tissue. Tissue should be taken for microbiological culture. Vacuum-assisted closure (Vac-Pac) has emerged as a very useful tool for deeply cavitating wounds. It utilises low-pressure suction to evacuate exudate, promote granulation tissue and reduce the size of the wound (Figure 29.12). Once the wounds are free from infection secondary closure can be undertaken.

DEFINITIVE MANAGEMENT

The hospitals designated to undertake definitive management should be selected on the basis of the facilities available and

Summary box 29.6

Principles of debridement and initial wound care

- Obtain generous exposure through skin and fascia
- Identify neurovascular bundles
- Excise devitalised tissue
- Remove foreign bodies
- Repair major vessels
- Obtain skeletal stabilisation with external fixators
- Only tag tendons and nerves that have been cut
- Leave the wound open and delay primary closure
- Avoid tight dressings
- Elevate the injured limb

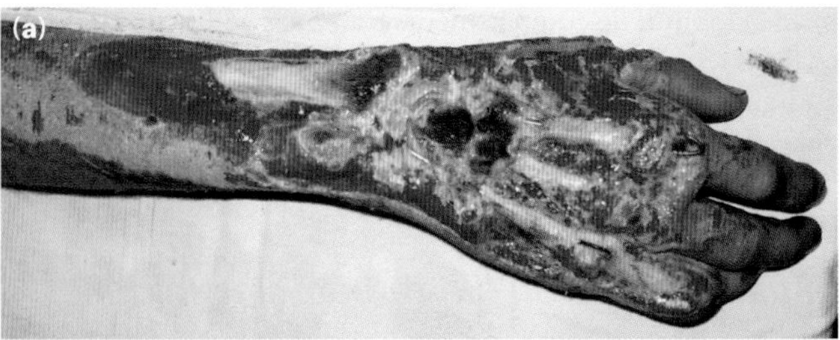

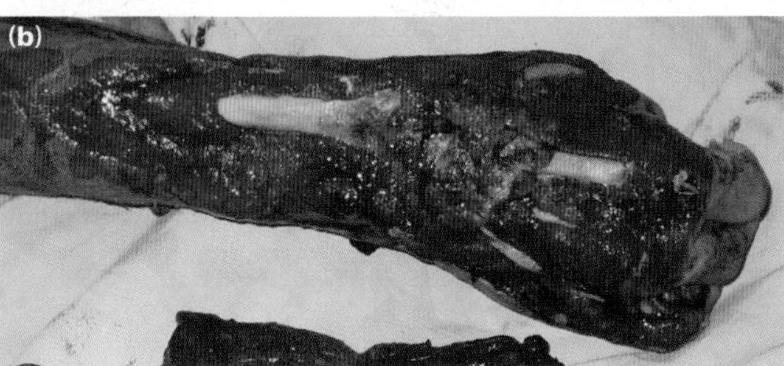

Figure 29.12 (a, b) Use of low-pressure vacuum therapy in preparing a wound for secondary closure.

the number of injured that they can handle. The resources required for trauma patients are more than the typical case mix of a hospital. A rule of thumb is that only half the bed strength of a hospital can be utilised to provide optimum trauma care in an emergency situation.

Hospital reorganisation

In hospitals receiving mass casualties some reorganisation of services is unavoidable. This includes transferring patients with non-urgent conditions to other facilities, augmenting surgical services, reorganising the specialist rota and redesignating medical wards as surgical care areas. An appeal for blood donations should be broadcast.

SPECIFIC ISSUES

There is no injury that is peculiar to disasters and the whole spectrum of external injuries from minor cuts, compound fractures and amputations is seen. Internal organ damage is frequent and, unless immediate help is available, this accounts for the majority of early mortality figures. People trapped under fallen buildings may suffer crush injuries and crush syndrome if the duration is prolonged. Crush injuries and missile injuries cause extensive tissue damage and gross contamination, both favourable conditions for anaerobic and micro-aerophilic infections.

Limb salvage

The Mangled Extremity Severity Score (MESS) and its modifications are useful in deciding about limb salvage. Extensive tissue loss, neurovascular damage and loss of long fragments of bone are traditionally indications for amputation. Currently, wounds of any dimension can be covered with microvascular flaps and distraction osteogenesis and vascularised bone can be used to restore bony continuity. If performed in time, vascular repairs can salvage most acutely ischaemic limbs. Because of these developments the indications for amputation in trauma have undergone a paradigm shift and the majority of patients who reach a tertiary-care facility within 24 hours are candidates for limb salvage (Figure 29.13). This assumes that debridement and, if required, vascular repairs have been performed in a field medical facility. A limb is unlikely to survive if the vascular repair of major limb vessels has been delayed for more than 4–6 hours.

Facial injuries

The management of facial injuries follows the same general principles of debridement and delayed closure as already outlined. Because of the functional and cosmetic importance of facial structures, skin and soft-tissue excisions are kept to a minimum. The face has a robust vascularity and a high ability to counter infection. Even in patients who present late with gross contamination, careful debridement followed by delayed primary closure can lead to good results (Figure 29.14).

Tetanus

This potentially fatal condition, also called 'lockjaw', is caused by *Clostridium tetani*, a gram-positive spore-forming bacillus occurring naturally in the intestines of humans and in the soil. It enters the body through a wound and replicates, thriving on the anaerobic conditions present in devitalised tissues. It produces tetanospasmin, an exotoxin that binds to the neuromuscular junctions of the central nervous system neurones, rendering them incapable of neurotransmitter release. This leads to failure of inhibition of motor reflex responses to sensory stimulation and generalised contractions of agonist and antagonist muscles produce tetanic spasms. The median incubation period is 7 days, ranging from 4–14 days.

Early symptoms are painful spasms of the facial muscles resulting in risus sardonicus (Figure 29.15). The spasms spread to involve the respiratory and laryngeal musculature. Spasms of the paravertebral and extensor limb musculature produce opisthotonus, an arching of the whole body. Laryngeal muscle spasm leads to apnoea and, if prolonged, to asphyxia and respiratory arrest. The spasms can be brought on by the slightest of sensory stimulus.

The diagnosis is obvious once it is fully manifest. There are three aspects of management:

- **Prevention.** Wounds contaminated with soil can harbour tetanus spores, and active immunisation is indicated by administering 0.5 mL of tetanus toxoid intramuscularly. Patients with gross contamination of cavitating wounds should also receive 250–500 U of human anti-tetanus globulin (ATG) intramuscularly to provide passive immunisation and to neutralise the circulating toxin. In full-

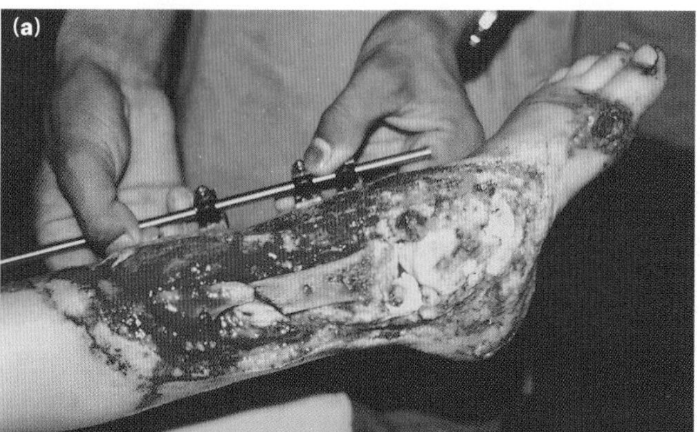

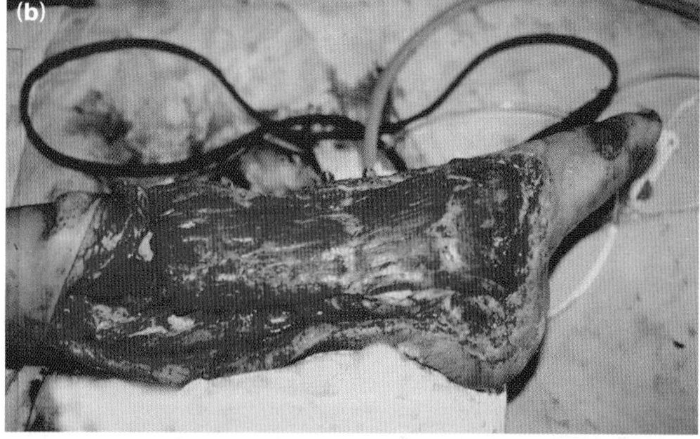

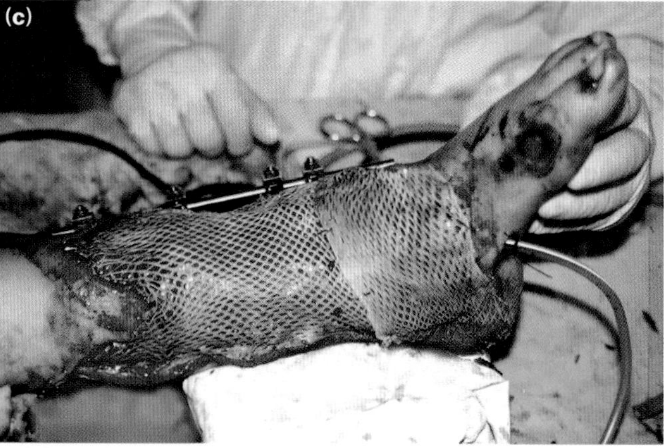

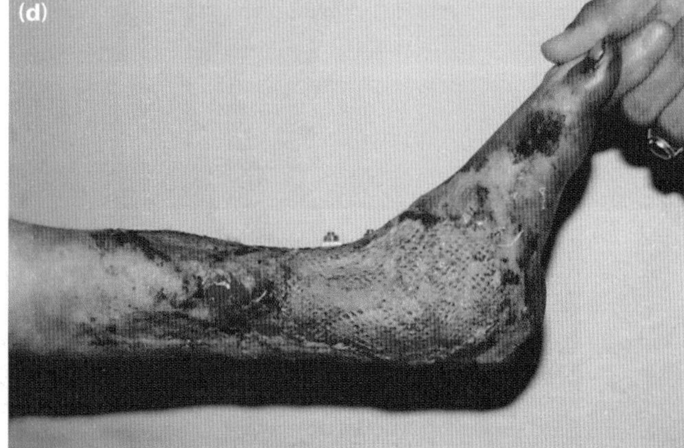

Figure 29.13 (a-d) Badly traumatised lower limb. Reconstruction has been performed using a microvascular rectus abdominis flap covered with a skin graft.

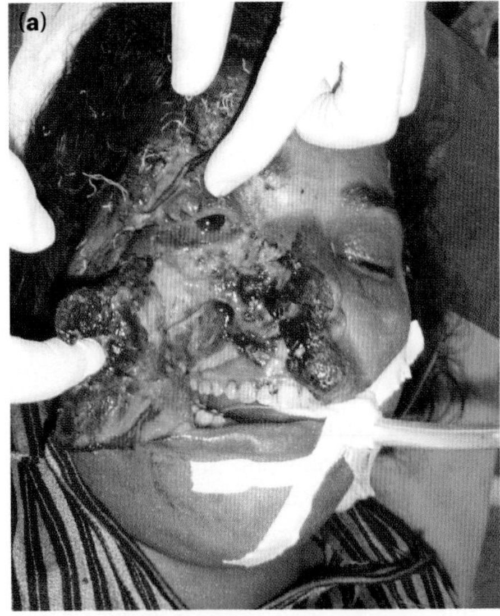

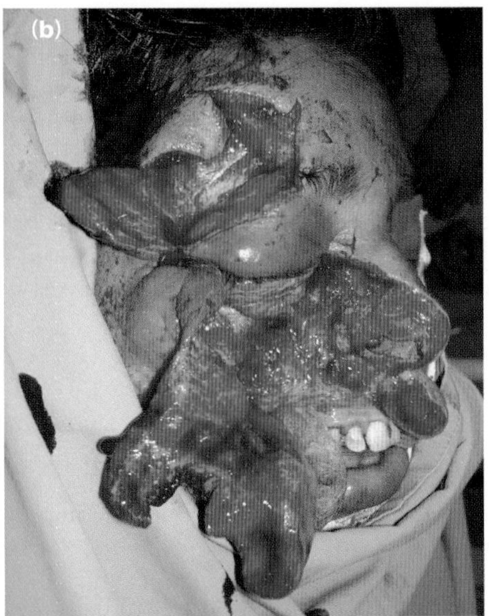

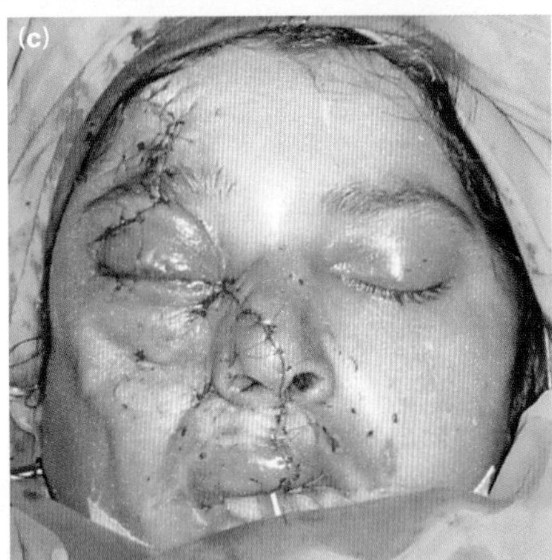

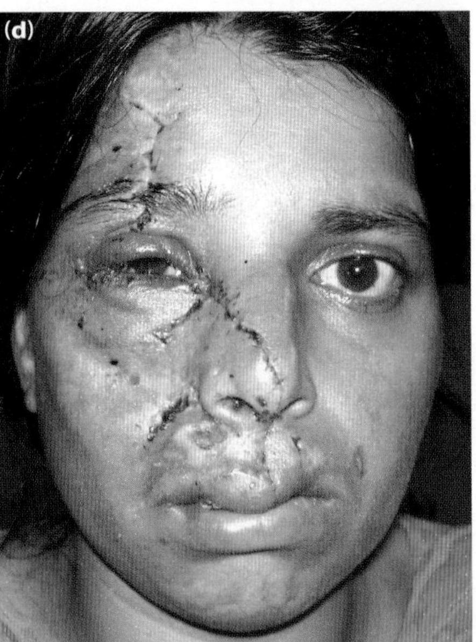

Figure 29.14 (a-d) Late-presenting facial injury with gross contamination. A thorough debridement followed by delayed primary closure has yielded good results.

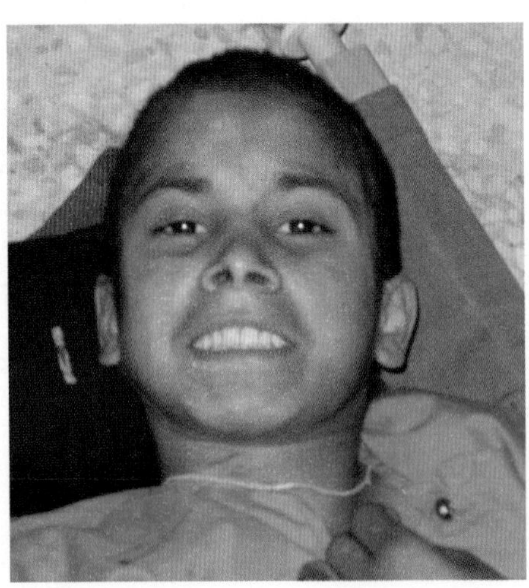

Figure 29.15 Risus sardonicus of 'lockjaw' (courtesy of Dr Samira Ajmal, FRCS).

blown clinical tetanus, 3000–10 000 U of ATG should be administered. Wound manipulation should be avoided for 2–3 hours after ATG administration to minimise tetanospasmin release.

- **Local wound care.** This includes a thorough wound debridement to eliminate the anaerobic environment. Intravenous administration of 10–24 × 10^6 U per day of penicillin G should be continued for 10–14 days. The wound should be closed using the delayed primary or secondary closure techniques.
- **Supportive care for established disease.** These patients are nursed in an intensive care unit (ICU) environment, free from strong sensory stimuli. Diazepam is useful in preventing the onset of spasms but if these become sustained, the patient is paralysed, intubated and placed on a ventilator. The patient is then gradually weaned off the ventilator under cover of anticonvulsants. The overall mortality rate is around 45%, prognosis being determined by the

Summary box 29.7

Tetanus

- Caused by *Clostridium tetani*
- Spores are present in the soil
- Thrives in dead or contaminated tissue
- Produce tetanospasmin an exotoxin
- Produces spasm of muscles
- Make sure patients are immunised
- For heavily contaminated wounds give anti-tetanus globulin

incubation period and the time from the first symptom to the first tetanic spasm. In general, shorter intervals indicate a poorer prognosis.

Necrotising fasciitis

Necrotising fasciitisis is a rapidly spreading infection that produces necrosis of the subcutaneous tissues and overlying skin. It is caused by β-haemolytic streptococci and, occasionally, *Staphylococcus aureus* but may take the form of a polymicrobial infection associated with other aerobic and anaerobic pathogens, including *Bacteroides*, *Clostridium*, *Proteus*, *Pseudomonas* and *Klebsiella*. It is termed Fournier's gangrene when it affects the perineal area and Meleney's gangrene when it involves the abdominal wall. The underlying pathology includes acute inflammatory infiltrate, extensive necrosis, oedema and thrombosis of the microvasculature. The area becomes oedematous, painful and very tender. The skin turns dusky blue and black secondary to the progressive underlying thrombosis and necrosis (Figure 29.16). The area may develop bullae and progress to overt cutaneous gangrene. It spreads contiguously but occasionally produces skip lesions that later coalesce. It is accompanied by fever and severe toxicity. Renal failure may occur as a result of hypovolaemia and cardiovascular collapse caused by septic shock. The rate of progression is dramatic and unless aggressively treated it leads to serious consequences with mortality approaching 70%.

The diagnosis is made on clinical grounds. Creatinine kinase levels may show enormous elevation and biopsy of the fascial layers will confirm the diagnosis. Patients should be admitted to the ICU and treated with careful monitoring of volume derangements and cardiac status. Oxygen supplementation is beneficial and endotracheal intubation is required in patients unable to maintain their airway.

High-dose penicillin G along with broad-spectrum antibiotics, such as third-generation cephalosporins and metronidazole, are given intravenously. The cornerstone of management is surgical excision of the necrotic tissue. The devitalised tissue is removed generously, going beyond the area of induration. The wound is lightly packed with gauze and dressed. This process is repeated daily as the necrosis is prone to spread beyond the edges of the excised wound. In patients who survive, this results in a large wound, which will require skin grafting or flap coverage.

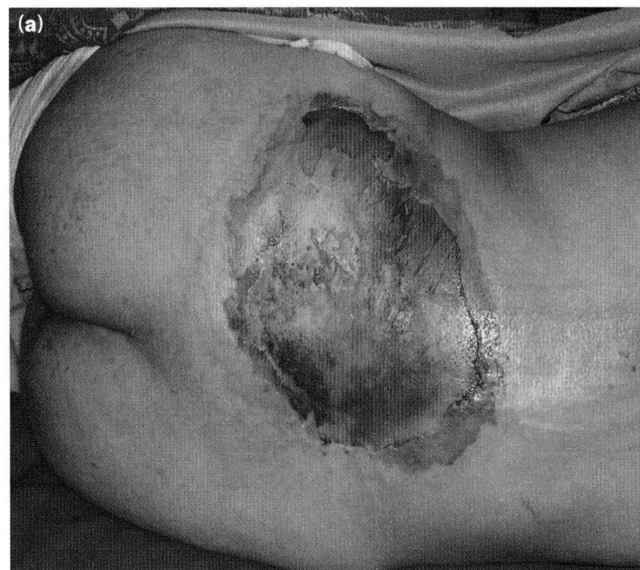

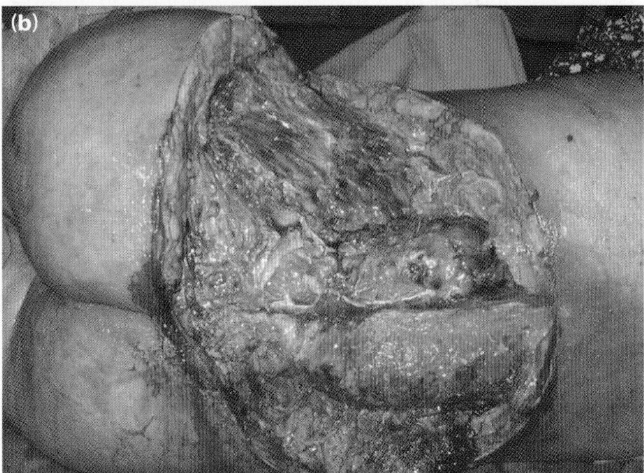

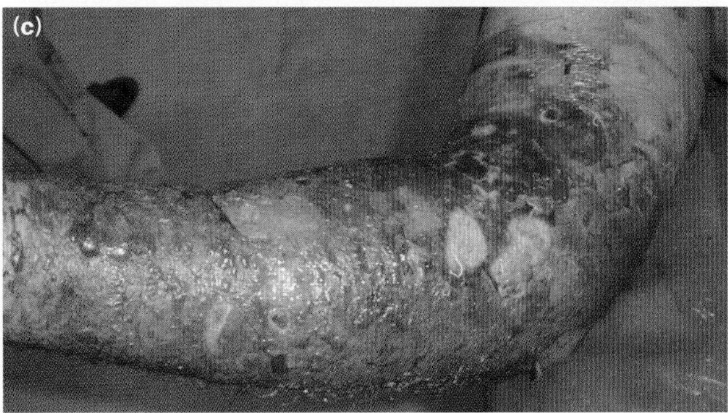

Figure 29.16 (a) Necrotising fasciitis at presentation and (b) rapid progression seen after 24 hours. (c) Typical bullae and induration.

Theodor Albrecht Edwin Klebs, 1834–1913, Professor of Bacteriology successively at Prague, Czechoslovakia, Zurich, Switzerland and then the Rush Medical College, Chicago, USA.
Jean Alfred Fournier, 1832–1915, syphilologist, the Founder of the Venereal and Dermatological Clinic, Hospital St. Louis, Paris, France.
Frank Lamont Meleney, 1889–1963, Professor of Clinical Surgery, Coumbia University, New York, USA.

Summary box 29.8

Necrotising fasciitis

- Caused by β-haemolytic strep or is polymicrobial
- Also called Fournier's or Meleney's gangrene
- Progress is rapid and renal failure is an early complication
- Treat with radical surgical excision repeated every 24 hours
- Give oxygen and penicillin

Recently, the role of hyperbaric oxygen (HBO) has become more established with a reduction in mortality in patients treated with HBO (9–20%) compared with patients who did not receive HBO (30–50%).

Gas gangrene

Gas gangrene is a dreaded consequence of late presenting missile wounds and crushing injuries. It is a rapidly progressive, potentially fatal condition characterised by widespread necrosis of the muscles and soft-tissue destruction. The common causative organism is *Clostridium perfringens*, a spore-forming, gram-positive saprophyte that flourishes in anaerobic conditions. Other organisms implicated in gas gangrene include *C. bifermentans*, *C. septicum* and *C. sporogenes*. Non-clostridial gas-producing organisms such as coliforms have also been isolated in 60–85% of cases of gas gangrene.

C. perfringens produces many exotoxins but their exact role is unclear. Alpha-toxin, the most important, is a lecithinase, which destroys red and white blood cells, platelets, fibroblasts and muscle cells. The phi-toxin produces myocardial suppression while the kappa-toxin is responsible for the destruction of connective tissue and blood vessels.

Devitalised tissue or premature wound closure provides the anaerobic conditions necessary for spore germination. The usual incubation period is <24 hours but ranges from 1 hour to 6 weeks. A vicious cycle of tissue destruction is initiated by rapidly multiplying bacteria and locally and systemically acting exotoxins. This causes spreading necrosis of muscle and thrombosis of blood vessels. The typical feature of this condition is the production of gas that spreads along the muscle planes. Systemically, the exotoxins causes severe haemolysis and, combined with the local effects, this leads to the rapid progression of the disease, hypotension, shock, acute kidney injury and acute respiratory distress syndrome.

Pain that rapidly increases in severity is the earliest symptom. The limb swells up and the wound exudes a serosanguineous discharge. The skin is involved secondary to muscle necrosis, turning brown and progressing to a blue–black colour with haemorrhagic bullae (Figure 29.17). The characteristic sickly sweet odour and soft tissue crepitus appear with established infection but their absence does not exclude the diagnosis. These local signs are accompanied by pyrexia, tachycardia, tachypnoea and altered mental status.

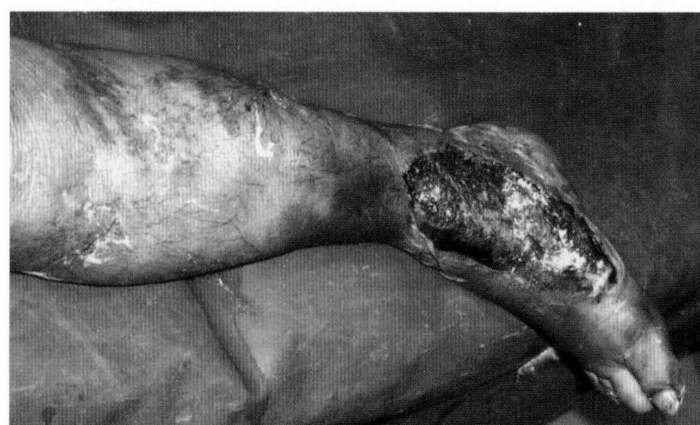

Figure 29.17 Typical picture of spreading gas gangrene caused by a crush injury.

The diagnosis is made on the basis of history and clinical features: a peripheral blood smear may suggest haemolysis; a Gram stain of the exudate reveals large gram-positive bacilli without neutrophils; and the biochemical profile may show metabolic acidosis and renal failure. Radiography can visualise gas in the soft tissues and is particularly useful in patients with chest and abdominal involvement.

Patients should be admitted to the ICU and treated aggressively with careful monitoring. High-dose penicillin G and clindamycin, along with third-generation cephalosporins, should be given intravenously. Surgical treatment is the same as for necrotising fasciitis (see above). In established gas gangrene with systemic toxicity, amputation of the involved extremity is life saving and should not be delayed. No attempt is made at closure, amputation stumps are left open and the wound is lightly packed with saline-soaked gauze and then dressed.

The role of HBO is not as clear as in necrotising fasciitis, but it is recommended in severe cases if the facilities are available.

Crush injury and syndrome

A crush injury occurs when a body part is subjected to a high degree of force or pressure, usually after being squeezed between two heavy or immobile objects. Damage related to a

Summary box 29.9

Gas gangrene

- Caused by *Clostridium perfringens*
- Spores are present in the soil
- Thrives in anaerobic conditions and produces many exotoxins
- Treat with radical and regular surgical excision
- Give oxygen and penicillin
- Early amputation may be life-saving

Hans Christian Joachim Gram, 1853–1938, Professor of Pharmacology (1891–1900) and of Medicine (1900–1923), Copenhagen, Denmark, described this method of staining bacteria in 1884.

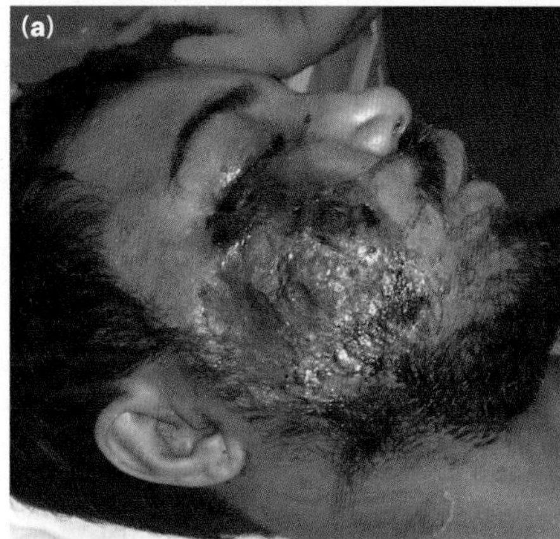

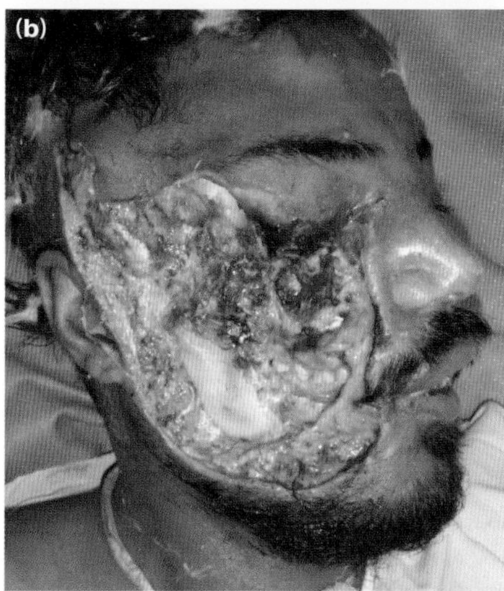

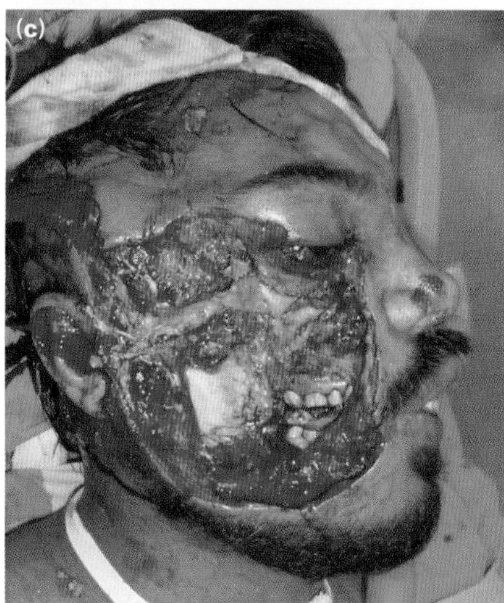

Figure 29.18 (a-c) Extensive crush injury in a man trapped in a fallen house. The depth to which the soft tissues have been devitalised is seen clearly.

crush injury includes lacerations, fractures, bleeding, bruising, compartment syndrome and crush syndrome (Figure 29.18).

Crush syndrome

The association between crush injury, rhabdomyolysis and acute kidney injury was first reported in victims trapped during the 'London Blitz'. It is seen in earthquake and mining accident survivors and in battlefield casualties. Prolonged crushing of muscle leads to a reperfusion injury when the casualty is rescued. This releases myoglobin and vasoactive mediators into the circulation. It also sequesters many litres of fluid, reducing the intravascular volume and resulting in renal vasoconstriction and ischaemia. The myoglobinuria leads to renal failure from tubular obstruction.

The treatment of crushed casualties should begin as soon as they are discovered. Rescuers must be alert to the presence of associated injuries (Figure 29.19). Aggressive volume-loading of patients, preferably before extrication, is the best treatment. After provision of first aid and starting intravenous fluids the patient should be catheterised to measure urine output. In adults, a saline infusion of 1000–1500 mL per hour should be initiated. This should be continued until myoglobin is no longer detectable in the urine. Mannitol administration can reduce the reperfusion component of this injury. Once a flow of urine is observed, a mannitol–alkaline diuresis of up to 8 litres per day should be maintained, keeping the urinary pH greater than 6.5. A late fasciotomy, when it is obvious that the muscles of that compartment must be dead, is only likely to cause a massive release of myoglobin, as well as potentially introducing infection into dead tissue. It therefore best not to perform a fasciotomy in cases where entrapment has been for over 12 hours.

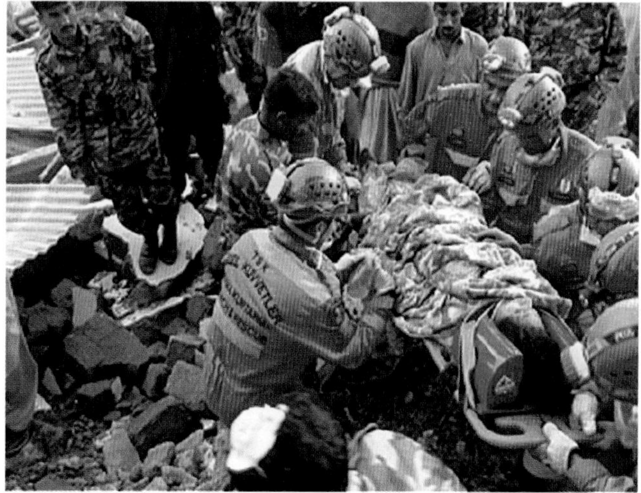

Figure 29.19 Rescuers must be prepared for injuries to the spine. Treatment of crush syndrome should start before extrication.

The London Blitz is the name given to the German air raids on London between the 7th of September 1940 and the 17th of May 1941, during which it is estimated that more than 15 000 people were killed. Blitz is short for Blitzkrieg, the German for 'lightning war'.

Summary box 29.10

Crush syndrome

- Arises as a result of reperfusion
- Acute kidney injury and renal failure from myoglobinuria is a complication
- A late fasciotomy may make things worse not better

Intensive care is required with close attention to fluid balance and renal dialysis if required.

Compartment syndrome

A compartment syndrome develops when the pressure within a muscle compartment starts to rise as a result of trauma (see Chapter 28). This occurs in muscles enclosed in a fascia such as the calf and forearm muscles and the intrinsic muscles of the hand and foot. A tight bandage or plaster, haemorrhage from a fracture or severe blunt trauma leads to a rise in pressure in the compartment until it exceeds venous drainage pressure. If the pressure rises further, it will cut off perfusion of the muscle. Passive stretching of the affected muscle will cause extreme pain and this is diagnostic of the condition. If the condition is left unrelieved, then nerves passing through the compartment will cease to function and the muscle will die and then undergo fibrosis and shortening, producing a Volkmann's ischaemic contracture. Removal of any constricting agent and, if necessary, a fasciotomy will relieve the pressure and muscle perfusion will restart. Pressure studies are not reliable and if in doubt, perform a fasciotomy.

Summary box 29.11

Compartment syndrome

- Commonest in a closed fracture or soft-tissue crush injury
- Pain on passive extension of the muscles is diagnostic
- Intra-compartmental pressure studies are not reliable
- If there is any suspicion, then fasciotomy must be performed early

Frost bite and immersion injuries (trench foot)

Frost bite occurs when a part of the body freezes. The cells are disrupted and the tissue dies. It is in effect a 'cold' burn and can be categorised according to the depth that it affects in the same way as a conventional burn. Other mechanisms at play include vasoconstriction caused by cold, capillary sludging and reperfusion injury with the release of free radicals, which occurs on rewarming the part. It commonly involves the fingers, toes, cheeks, the tip of the nose and the ears. When frozen the tissue feels hard and cannot be indented. Immersion injury is a cold injury, which does not involve actual freezing of the tissue and is commonly caused by prolonged immersion in cold water (hence trench foot). The patient may also be hypothermic. Warming should be gentle as the heat used may actually cause a burn! Rehydration with warm fluids and use of non-steroidal anti-inflammatory drugs like ibuprofen are beneficial. Demarcation will occur between dead and viable tissue and at this stage no surgery should be undertaken as there is often considerable deep recovery. The injured area should be kept clean and dry and efforts made to prevent further injury, as well as to prevent infection. Definitive surgery to excise dead tissue can be left for many months. Recent developments, such as the use of tissue plasminogen activator (TPA) and nerve blocks, show promising results in reducing amputations, but have to be started within 24 hours and are seldom possible in the field.

Summary box 29.12

Frostbite

- Can be superficial or deep like a burn
- Rewarm gently
- Allow demarcation to occur naturally
- Protect against further trauma and infection

HANDING OVER

Follow-up and secondary problems

The medical aspect of disaster management does not involve a single short-term effort. It requires a long-term commitment and involvement of various disciplines. Because of the large numbers of casualties, the initial treatment is directed towards the anatomical restoration of damaged structures. There are therefore numerous patients who will need secondary procedures for functional restoration. This second wave of patients is encountered 3–6 months following a major catastrophe and arrangements should be made to deal with this.

Designated centres

Initially, the casualties may be scattered amongst many hospitals. After the first few weeks most of the acute problems have been dealt with and only those patients who require longer-term treatment remain. At this point it is advisable to designate a particular hospital as a centre for these patients. It concentrates resources and expertise and makes to follow up easier.

DISASTER PLANS

Disasters are unforeseen events and planning for them may seem paradoxical. It has, however, been shown that disaster planning not only works but also saves lives. Disaster planning is a wide field but a résumé of the important aspects follows.

Establishment of a national disaster management organisation

This is the first step in the planning for disasters. Most resource-rich countries already have such an agency, which can formulate policy at the national level and has the infrastructure to react quickly when the need arises.

Anticipating disasters

Areas near active volcanoes and geological fault lines are at risk from seismic disturbances, whereas regions along major rivers are liable to flooding. The urban centres of all countries are now potential targets for terrorist attacks. It is important to not only carry out threat assessments but also, if possible, set up an early warning system.

Evacuation planning

Evacuation of large population centres as a prelude to, or in the wake of, an impending disaster is a complex exercise. Yet it may be the most prudent course of action to remove as many people as possible from harm's way. Clear identification of exit routes must be determined and communicated to the populations at risk.

Organisation of emergency services

Emergency services such as the fire brigade, police and ambulance service must have defined roles and areas of responsibility to ensure a coordinated response during a crisis. Members of these teams must be included in the planning phase to ensure that the final plan is practicable and reflects the situation on the ground.

Summary box 29.13

Disaster planning

- Disaster can be anticipated and should be prepared for
- Evacuation of a whole population may be a best option
- Coordination between military, police,fire, ambulance and medical services is important

Medical planning

Identification of hospitals able to take large numbers of casualties and the location of areas that can be used for patient holding and triage in case of mass casualties is important. Hospitals that offer specialised services should be identified and their role during a major crisis defined. Suitable hospitals in the surrounding areas must be designated as overflow hospitals in the eventuality of a very large volume of patients.

FURTHER READING

Ciottone GR, Biddinger PD, Darling RG *et al*. *Ciottone's disaster medicine*, 2nd edn. Philadelphia: Elsevier, 2016.

Hogan DE, Burstein JL. *Disaster medicine*, 2nd edn. Philadelphia: Lipincot Wiliams & Wilkins, 2007.

Partridge RA, Proano L, Marcozzi D *et al*. *American handbook of disaster medicine*. New York: Oxford University Press, 2012.

World Health Organisation. *Emergency surgical care in disaster situations*. WHO Integrated Management on Emergency and Essential Surgical Care (IMEESC) tool kit. (CD)

Chapter 30

Conflict surgery

Learning objectives

To understand and appreciate:

- Fundamental differences of war surgery
- Injury patterns of modern warfare
- Principles of war surgical management
- Blast and ballistic injury

INTRODUCTION

'He who wishes to be a surgeon must first go to war.'
Hippocrates, (c. 460–377 BC)

The treatment of war wounds is as ancient as warfare itself. The Edwin Smith papyrus has been dated to between 1600 BC and is the oldest known treatise on trauma surgery and anatomy.[1] The history of battlefield surgery is the history of surgical advancement and the importance of the medical lessons learned from war have long been recognised.

While almost every conflict has served to increase our knowledge of the treatment of war injuries, and many individuals have played significant parts is the development of war surgery, Dominque Jean Larrey is considered by many to be the first modern military surgeon. Larrey, a French battlefield surgeon and favourite of Napoleon, devised some of the first systems of triage and casualty care that still form the fundamentals of modern military medicine.

HOW IS WAR SURGERY DIFFERENT?

While civilian trauma surgery bears some of the hallmarks of the battlefield, there are fundamental contrasts in environment and injury pattern that must be appreciated:

- The environment of war is likely to be austere. While recent long-term deployment has led to the establishment of some well-equipped field hospitals, logistical and personnel restrictions mean that sophisticated diagnostic and therapeutic techniques may not be available.
- War is hostile and potentially dangerous. Necessary workforce protection must be considered to ensure safety of medical personnel and patients alike. Modern fighting forces employ physician-led resuscitation, along with forward surgical teams. Moving medical personal closer to the fighting may increase their personnel risk.
- War injuries are different to civilian trauma. Modern weapons may deliver such amounts of energy that the tissue destruction and patterns of injury seen are unlike all but the most extreme of civilian trauma practice.
- War is a mass casualty situation. Although casualty numbers vary between treatment facilities, triage is an important aspect of military surgery. The dictum 'do the best for the most, not everything for everyone' is important and may require a change in thinking for many used to civilian practice.
- War surgery is usually delivered in stages. The principles of damage control are often applied to allow transfer of patients between echelons of care. Careful planning, coordination and communication is essential.

ETHICAL AND LEGAL CONSIDERATIONS

International Humanitarian Law (IHL) regulates humanitarian issues during armed conflict. Modern IHL is derived from a variety of sources, notably the Geneva Conventions and its additional protocols, along with further specific regulations from the United Nations and The Hague. IHL provides medical personnel with rights in times of armed war, but also assigns duties to them surrounding the rights of protected personnel under their care.

The papyrus is named after Edwin Smith, the Egyptologist who discovered it in 1866 and held at the New York Academy of Medicine.
Dominique Jean Larrey, 1766–1842, French surgeon in Napoleon's Grand Armée.

Importantly, medical personnel are bound by medical ethics and IHL to treat patients solely based on need and without regard for their nationality, race and class, religious or political beliefs.

Along with providing medical support to deployed forces, treatment is offered to both home nation and enemy combatants. The treatment of such patients may require a change in the approach to the definitive care. Evacuation of these personnel to certain categories of subsequent facility (see below) may not be possible and the staged approach to care may need modification. Transfer to host nation medical facilities may be possible but dependent on local capability.

This scenario may require an adaption to clinical thinking. As an example, consider the ethical and logistical dilemma in performing revascularisation and orthoplastic procedures for a local patient in a country without rehabilitation facilities.

Medical personnel and facilities are protected under IHL and should not be attacked. However, the nature of modern conflict is unconventional; guerrilla warfare and the inability of deployed forces to define the enemy combatant requires security of facilities and personnel to be of the highest priority.

MEDICAL SUPPORT ROLES

The term 'role' is used to designate the tiers of medical support that integrate into a modern military operation. An appreciation of the capabilities and limitations of these roles is essential to improving the care of casualties at each stage. Different nations and forces will have medical support configured with some variability but overall, systems are similar in order to ensure those basic treatment, supply and evacuation needs that are essential for a military operation.

- **Role 1** medical support provides for routine primary health care, specialised first aid, triage, resuscitation and stabilisation. It is integrated within a small unit. The capabilities of role 1 care will depend greatly on the size of the unit and the training of the personnel within it.
- **Role 2** provides an intermediate capability for the reception and triage of casualties, as well as being able to perform resuscitation and treatment of shock to a higher technical level than role 1. It is prepared to provide evacuation from role 1 facilities. It has capability for damage control surgery (DCS) and may include a limited holding facility for the short-term holding of casualties until they can return to duty or evacuated.
- **Role 3** medical support is deployed hospital care and the elements required to support it. This includes a mission-tailored variety of clinical specialties including primary surgery and diagnostic support. In recent conflicts role 3 facilities grew and evolved into sophisticated hard-built hospitals.
- **Role 4** provides the full spectrum of definitive medical care that cannot be deployed to theatre or is too time-consuming to be conducted there. It is normally provided in the country of origin or an allied nation depending on the location of deployment and time-lines of transfer.

Summary box 30.1

Medical support roles

- R1– unit level medical care including first aid and primary health care
- R2 – intermediate unit for resuscitation, damage control and stabilisation
- R3 – deployed hospital care with multi-speciality capability
- R4 – definitive hospital care within home or allied nation

It is important to appreciate that these roles are highly variable both within and between different nations. The size and scale of the operations as a whole, along with predictions of both civilian and military medical requirements, will dictate the structure of the medical support.

MEDICAL EVACUATION

Medical evacuation refers to the movement and en-route care of casualties within a conflict zone. The evacuation may be the initial movement from a battlefield or between other more sophisticated echelons of care, up to and including repatriation to a home nation.

Aeromedical evacuation using either fixed or rotary wing aircraft has had a major impact on the evacuation timelines. Certain considerations must be made prior to and during aeromedical evacuation:

- the patient should be sufficiently stabilised for the anticipated mode and duration of travel;
- the patient's airway and breathing are adequate for movement;
- intravenous access, surgical drains, urinary catheters and any other tubes should be firmly secured;
- patients at high risk for thoracic barotrauma should be considered for prophylactic chest tube placement before prolonged aeromedical evacuation;
- blankets and/or warmers should cover the patient securely to mitigate against hypothermia.

The capability of different evacuation platforms may vary from highly sophisticated mobile critical care units to the simple transportation of casualties by non-medical personnel. These capabilities, along with the time-lines and distances involved in casualty movement should be major considerations for the planning of medical support operations.

PATTERNS OF MODERN WAR SURGERY

Modern warfare has changed over recent decades. Cause of injury is particular to individual conflict, nation and armed service.[2] Historically, the predominance of penetrating trauma was sustained by combat infantry, while naval and air personnel sustained more blunt injuries (*Table 30.1*).

Improvements in trauma scoring systems and the development of a concise system for the recording of injuries and casualty care have increased the ability of modern armed

TABLE 30.1 Historical causes of injury amongst US service personnel. Adapted from Champion *et al.*[2]

	Service			
Mechanism	Infantry (%)	Armoured (%)	Sea (%)	Air (%)
Ballistic	90	50	25	5
Blunt	2–3	5	10	50
Blast	2–3	5	10	<10
Thermal	2–3	25	30	25
Combined	<5	15	25	10

services to analyse the injury patterns of their deployed personnel.

A cohort analysis of combat injuries sustained by US forces[3] showed significant differences in injury patterns sustained in the most recent Afghanistan and Iraq conflicts compared with World War 2, Korea and Vietnam. Head and neck injuries were far more common in recent conflict while thoracic and extremity injuries were less so. This is probably due to increased use of body armour and similar personnel protective equipment.

Mechanism of injury has also changed. While ballistic injuries remain an important contributor to battlefield trauma, injuries due to explosions (which includes improvised explosive devices [IEDs], landmines, mortars, grenades and rockets) have become increasingly common and are now the predominant mode of wounding and fatality. The relative proportions of injuries caused by explosive and ballistic weapons is shown in *Table 30.2*.

The emergence of explosive patterns of injury is due to the increasing use of IEDs within conflict. IEDs have been the signature weapon within operations in Afghanistan and Iraq; however, their use has not been limited to these regions. The relative low cost, ease of production and widespread expertise means that IEDs will likely play significant roles in most contemporary and future conflicts.

PRINCIPLES OF WAR SURGERY

Battlefield death occurs early (or immediately) due to devastating central nervous system injury and haemorrhage, or late due to infection. Some of the injuries causing immediate death (including brain, heart and great vessel injury) are non-survivable[4] and may only be managed with prevention.

TABLE 30.2 Relative proportion of injuries caused by gunshot wounds and explosions amongst US personnel. Adapted from Owens *et al.*[3]

	Gunshot wound	Explosion
US Civil War	91	9
World War I	65	35
World War II	27	73
Korea	31	69
Vietnam	35	65
Iraq/Afghanistan	19	81

Treatment of haemorrhage is therefore the mainstay of military trauma medicine. Bleeding should be recognised and managed from point of wounding.[5] Tourniquets are indicated for the control of catastrophic extremity bleeding. Non-compressible torso haemorrhage carries a poor prognosis,[6] although it may be amenable to methods of endovascular control not yet commonly used.[7]

An approach to surgery must be employed to stop bleeding, to remove necrotic tissue and foreign material and to reduce contamination. In addition to life-saving surgery, procedures to salvage limbs, including revascularisation (or temporary shunting) and fasciotomy, should be considered early, when physiology allows.

DAMAGE CONTROL SURGERY

DCS was first formerly described by Rotondo *et al*[8], although the idea of an abbreviated laparotomy for the unwell patient was not totally novel. The concepts of DCS were initially applied to complex trauma patients with combined vascular and visceral injuries. Improved outcomes were seen following DCS principles compared with conventional definitive surgery.

The DCS approach is to restore physiology over anatomy and is typically divided into several phases:

- **Phase 1**. Recognition of injury severity and need for damage control principles, both surgical and resuscitative. Features of phase 1 include rapid-sequence induction of anaesthesia and intubation, early rewarming and prompt movement to the operating theatre.
- **Phase 2**. Immediate laparotomy with rapid control of bleeding and contamination, abdominal packing and temporary wound closure.
- **Phase 3**. Movement to the intensive care unit (ICU) for ongoing resuscitation with normalisation of biochemical and physiological parameters.
- **Phase 4**. Re-exploration in theatre to perform definitive repair of all injuries. Multiple procedures on multiple occasions may be required. Even at this stage, non-essential procedures may be truncated or delayed if physiology deteriorates.

Selection of patients for damage control management may not be straightforward. While various physiological and biochemical markers of injury have been suggested, there is no validated threshold. Hypothermia, coagulopathy, acidosis, blood loss and anticipated operative time should all be considered (see Chapters 22 and 23).

The benefits of a DCS approach to those patients that need it has been repeatedly shown, but liberal, and perhaps overzealous use of DCS is unlikely to be beneficial to those who would tolerate definitive repair. DCS puts a heavy toll on theatre and ICU resources. In addition, multiple trips to theatre may increase the likelihood of morbidity including abdominal wall hernias, fistulae and infection.

Damage control resuscitation (DCR) should be concurrent with DCS. The principles of DCR include permissive hypotension, avoidance of crystalloid with haemostatic resuscitation, and recognition and management of acute traumatic coagulopathy (ATC). The application of these principles to military patients is uncertain because of longer time-lines. Prolonged periods of permissive hypotension are likely to be harmful[9] while haemostatic resuscitation and management of ACT is ineffectual in the absence of haemorrhage control.[10]

MASSIVE TRANSFUSION

While haemorrhage control prior to the need for massive transfusion is ideal, this is often not the case. The degree of injury and associated massive blood loss associated with war injuries may necessitate large volume transfusion. The use of crystalloids to resuscitate exsanguinating patients is strongly discouraged, but the optimal ratio of blood products has not yet been ascertained. Massive Transfusion Protocols exist within most deployed units. Use of such a protocol at a UK role 3 facility, along with aggressive resuscitation and use of blood products, has been associated with improved trauma outcomes.[11] The success of such a protocol is highly dependent on a steady stream of blood products and reflects the sophisticated transfusion infrastructure that should be woven into a deployed capability,

Blood transfusion is increasingly administered in a more forward location (within both role 1 and role 2 environments) with limited volumes of blood transported to the point of wounding by aeromedical response teams. The future will almost certainly include more alternatives to conventional blood components, which can combine adequate oxygen carriage with positive or neutral effects on patient coagulation.

DECISION-MAKING WITHIN THE DEPLOYED ENVIRONMENT

The damage control approach is vital in a proportion of war injuries, but thought must be given to available resources. Within a well-established role 3 unit, both DCS and definitive procedures are likely to be possible. Blood and blood products are also likely to be available and restocked regularly. In this scenario, patient physiology is the major determinant of mode of care.

In contrast, decision-making becomes more crucial within the austere environment. Theatre space, intensive care beds, equipment and blood products may be limited. Long evacuation times may contraindicate permissive hypotension.

Limited resources, such as blood, may need to be divided between casualties. Within a role 1 or role 2 facility, immediate evacuation may be undertaken in preference to a more thorough stabilisation.

Decision-making of this nature is complex and difficult and requires practice in the context of simulation, exercises and courses.

WEAPON EFFECTS

Ballistics

The ability to manage conflict injuries relies on an understanding of the underlying mechanism of wounding, which is likely to be different to civilian trauma. As stated, while ballistic injuries are no longer the most common cause of battlefield injury, firearms remain a common element in all conflict. Civilian trauma practice, depending on local firearm laws, may well encompass a significant volume of gunshot wounds, although patterns of injury with war wounds may well differ due to the weapons used. An understanding of the mechanism of ballistic wounding is required to treat these wounds effectively.

The earliest recorded depiction of a firearm is from 1326, but firearms became ubiquitous on the battlefield during the 17th century.[12] Ballistic weapons all work with the same principles – an explosion is used to propel a projectile along and out of a straight tube – but have evolved considerably from rudimentary cannons to sophisticated modern day firearms. The explosive force within a modern firearm comes from propellant encased within a cartridge. The basic design of a cartridge is shown in Figure 30.1.

Internal ballistics describes the characteristics of a projectile, while inside the hammer mechanism of the weapon strikes a primer at the base of the cartridge, which ignites the propellant. Hot gas produced by the explosion expands and forces the bullet away from the cartridge and along the barrel. Spiral grooves, or rifling, imparts spin on the bullet, which aids in accuracy and stabilisation.

While the basic principles apply to nearly all firearms, advances in firearm design have served predominantly to improve accuracy, reliability and rate of fire. Ammunition is normally held within a magazine or belt that loads directly into the chamber of the weapon. The loading mechanism determines the rate of fire. In a semi-automatic or fully automatic system, the recoil forces of the spent cartridge eject the

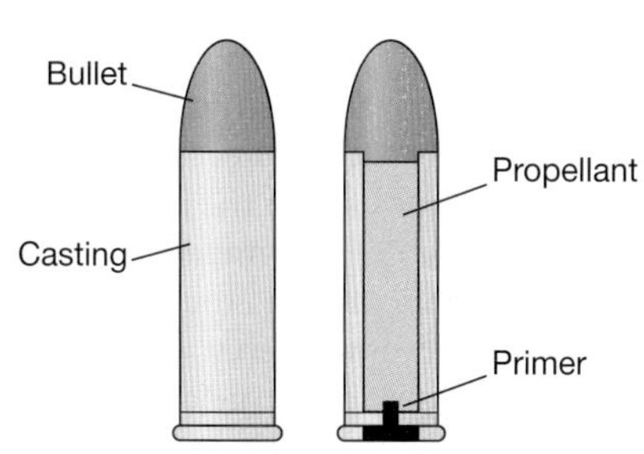

Figure 30.1 Diagram of basic cartridge structure.

cartridge while resetting the chamber and accepting a new cartridge from the magazine, such that the process may be repeated rapidly.

Shotguns utilise a similar mechanism except that a collection of smaller projectiles – 'shot' – are expelled rather than a single bullet. These smaller projectiles disperse away from one another after leaving the barrel. The degree of dispersal is dependent on the relative length of the barrel.

External ballistics describe the characteristics of a projectile in free flight. It may be influenced by ammunition type and ambient conditions. Ammunition differs widely with the most pronounced difference between pistol and rifle ammunition. Rifles are expected to be accurate at ranges up to and beyond 1000 metres, while pistols are intended for far shorter ranges. Rifle cartridges are longer and typically have a greater proportion of propellant to projectile. The characteristics of ammunition that determine wound effects are the size or calibre (which describes the internal diameter of the weapon barrel) and the material components of the bullet:

- full metal jacket ammunition has an outer coating of harder metal around a softer core. This reduces breakdown of the bullet along the barrel and improves accuracy, reliability and target penetration;
- soft tip and hollow point ammunition have a degree of exposed lead that flattens and deforms on impact. These bullets have less penetrating ability but rapidly transfer energy to the impacted tissue and cause large wounds.

Ballistic injuries

Terminal ballistics (or wound ballistics) describes the interaction between projectiles and target tissue. This interaction and subsequent transfer of energy cause injury. The kinetic energy of the bullet is related to the mass and velocity of the impacting projectile. Both the mass and velocity of military firearms may be considerably greater than those commonly seen in civilian trauma, leading to higher energies and more severe wounds. While the weapon and ammunition type may be a determinant in the potential injury caused, many other factors, including range, angle, clothing, armour and anatomical variation, will determine the actual wound pattern. Although an understanding of ballistic science may allow a surgeon to anticipate possible injuries, each should be evaluated and managed individually.

In consideration of the damage done, tissue may be described by the areas of disruption caused by the projectile – the permanent and temporary wound cavity, which are illustrated in Figure 30.2.

The permanent cavity is the localised area of definitive tissue injury caused by contact with the projectile. This area of cell necrosis is the result of direct contact, crushing and laceration of tissues in the path of the projectile. The size and trajectory of the projectile determines the cavity size. This type of cavity is the predominant wound effect of pistol bullets that have relatively low energy. Higher energy projectiles, including military rifle and machine gun bullets, may be subject to greater degrees of deformation and tumbling as they travel through tissue. This increases the effective cross-sectional area of the projectile and may lead to a larger and less regular permanent wound cavity.

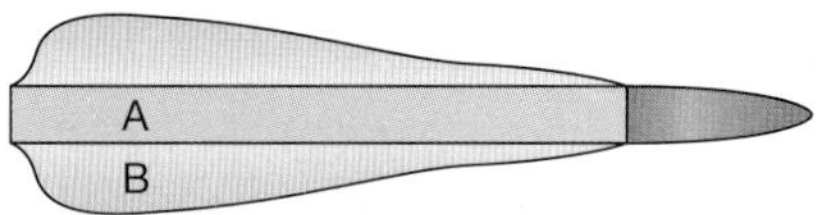

Figure 30.2 Diagram showing permanent wound cavity (A) and temporary wound cavity (B). This relatively large temporary cavity would be more typical of a higher-energy weapon.

In contrast, the temporary wound cavity is created by lateral displacement of tissue that has not been in direct contact with the bullet. The degree of damage in this area is dependent on the amount of energy transferred by the bullet and the material properties of the tissue itself. Individual tissues have an elastic strength that resists the stretching caused by a projectile. As the energy increases, the tissue is no longer able to rebound and above certain thresholds, contusion, laceration and permanent damage may occur. Skin, muscle, lung and bowel wall tissues have good elastic strength and may rebound well following stretch, with minimal damage within the temporary wound cavity. In contrast, liver, brain and spleen have poor elasticity and are more likely to shatter when stretched. Incompressibility of fluids within hollow organs (bowel and bladder) means that they are vulnerable to stretch despite favourable properties of the tissue wall itself.

Summary box 30.2

Ballistics

- Internal ballistics – characterise projectile within weapon during firing
- External ballistics – characterise projectile in free flight
- Terminal ballistics – characterise projectile/tissue interaction

MANAGEMENT OF GUNSHOT WOUNDS

The management of gunshot wounds in a conflict setting may differ to civilian practice. The typical low energy wounds caused by pistols are sometimes managed conservatively in civilian trauma centres with adequate wound care, cleaning and antibiotics. Military wounds are associated with higher energies, higher rates of infection and more severe injury. The extent of these injuries, including the size of the wound cavities, may not be adequately assessed without thorough surgical examination (Figure 30.3). As such, most penetrating wounds in the military setting are explored under anaesthetic. The extent and capacity for recovery of the temporary wound cavity may not be appreciated at the time of the first operation. A damage control approach should be adopted if the physiology of the patient dictates so. An interval period may also allow for adequate appreciation of the permanent wound cavity, along with response of the surrounding structures and demarcation of non-viable tissue.

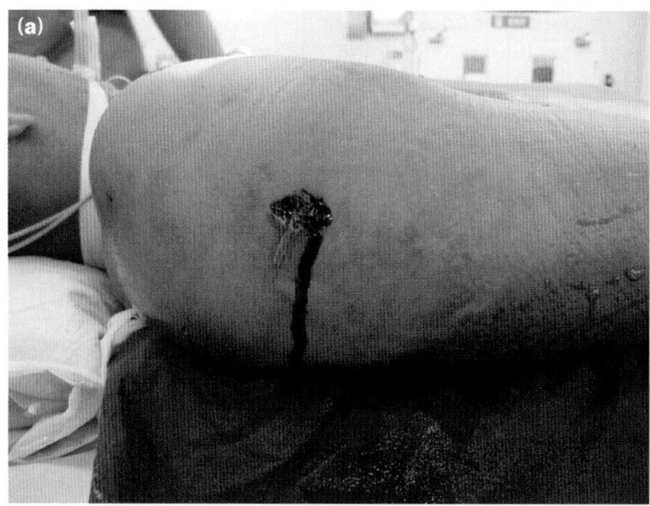

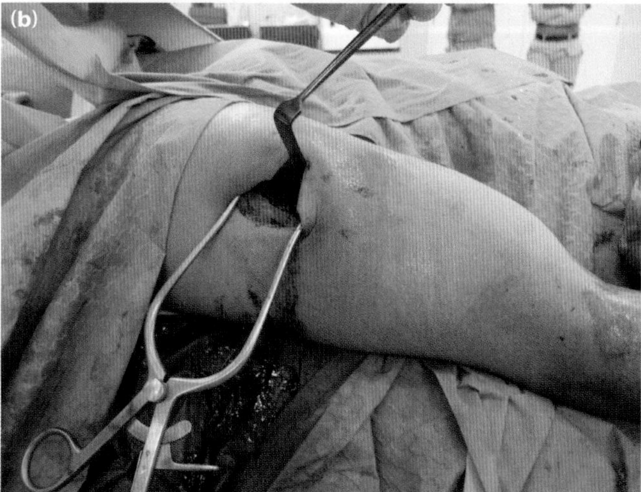

Figure 30.3 Entry wound to the right shoulder **(a)** with the wound extended in order to assess adequately **(b)**.

BLAST

As previously discussed, blast has become the predominant mechanism of injury in recent conflict. Unfortunately, terrorist attacks within urban centres mean that these injuries are increasingly encountered within civilian practice.

While explosives come in many forms and their effects vary as a result, fundamental principles underlie all blast events.

An explosive may be defined as 'a substance that can be made to undergo a rapid chemical reaction that will transform a liquid or solid into gas, liberating a large amount of energy'.[13] The explosive properties of such a material are determined by the chemical composition of the material and the speed at which energy is expelled. Low explosives react by a process called deflagration whereby the reaction is propagated by flame passing through the material at a rate significantly slower than the speed of sound. They are made up of a combustible material and an accompanying oxidant. Low explosives include gunpowder, gasoline and pyrotechnics such as fireworks and flares. Low explosives more commonly cause burns than typical blast injuries and will not be discussed further.

In contrast, high explosives degrade via detonation. Shockwaves are passed through the material at supersonic speeds and the resultant energy is expelled at very high rates. High explosives include plastic explosive and trinitrotoluene (TNT). The input of a relatively small amount of energy results in the production of a very large volume of gas, at high speed and pressure. The outward expansion causes a wave of compressed air that moves away from the point of detonation at supersonic speeds and in a uniform sphere (within a free field).

The change in surrounding pressure is described as the blast overpressure. Following detonation within a free field, there is a near instantaneous pressure rise, which falls exponentially. This is classically described by the Friedlander curve (Figure 30.4).

This characteristic pressure peak is only seen during a truly free (almost theoretical) scenario. Enclosure of the blast or reflection of blast waves by people, vehicles or buildings is likely to change the overpressure profile such that high pressures may be sustained for longer periods and have a greater propensity to cause injury. For this reason, blasts within enclosed spaces are notable for causing a greater range and severity of injury.

In addition to expanding gases, detonation of explosives may result in the expulsion of fragments. These fragments may be part of a device casing, separate material deliberately added with the intention of fragmentation, or environmental material flung by the blast.

Blast winds are generated by the displacement of surrounding air. The direction of these winds may change as the blast overpressure drops transiently beneath ambient pressure and creates a partial vacuum.

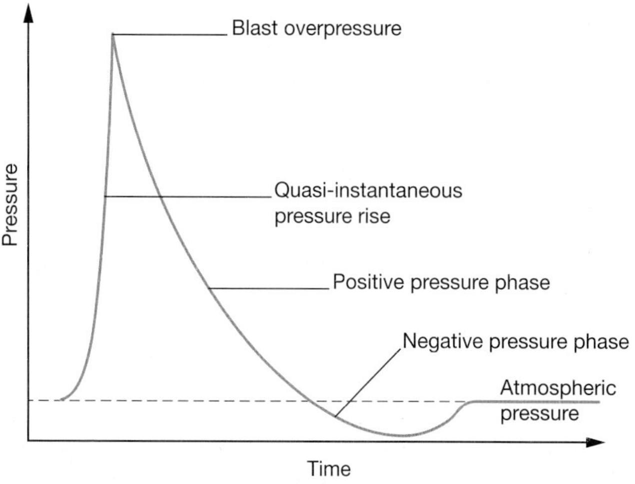

Figure 30.4 Theoretical blast overpressure changes within a free field.

Improvised explosive devices

The characteristic weapon of modern warfare has been the IED, which was the leading cause of death amongst coalition troops in Iraq and Afghanistan.[14] These devices may range from rudimentary homemade explosives to sophisticated devices containing high explosives. Within this broad range of devices are further categories including roadside explosives and blast mines, suicide bombers, and explosive formed projectiles (EFPs). EFPs are a particular form of device with a deformable plate on the uppermost surface. The detonation of the device and expansion of the explosive products deforms this plate into a missile shape, while simultaneously accelerating it upwards to very high velocities. Alternatively, copper plates may melt to create a high-speed molten jet (a shaped charge). Upon contact with a target (typically a vehicle), the missile impacts the hull of the vehicle with a degree of penetration dependent on the device and vehicle armour. Huge amounts of kinetic energy are dispersed through the vehicle and occupants. Injuries may be caused by both direct impact of the deforming hull and gross upwards acceleration, followed by downwards deceleration of the whole vehicle.

BLAST INJURIES

Blast injuries are classified by the blast mechanism (*Table 30.3*).

Primary blast injury

Primary blast injuries result from the overpressure and are, as such, unique to blast. The effect of blast overpressure is most marked at the interface between air and tissue or liquid.

Tympanic membrane (TM) rupture is the most common primary blast injury. Patients may be asymptomatic or have a degree of transient hearing loss and otorrhoea. Previously, the presence of TM rupture was used as a marker for other occult blast injuries. This has been challenged recently by findings that show TM injury is not ubiquitous in the presence of more severe primary blast injury. The blast environment and orientation of the ear canal to the shockwave are likely to determine the chance of injury.

TABLE 30.3 Classification of blast injuries.

Classification	Injury type	Examples
Primary blast	Overpressure	Tympanic membrane injury, blast lung, intestinal blast injury
Secondary blast	Penetrating/ fragmentation	All penetrating injuries
Tertiary blast	Blunt	Blunt and crush injuries. Traumatic amputation.
Quaternary blast	Miscellaneous	Burns, inhalation injury
Quinary blast	Effect of device additions	Radiation sickness, infection

Primary blast lung injury, or blast lung, is the most widely researched blast phenomenon. The exact mechanism of blast lung remains contested but it depends on the propagation of energy from the shockwave into the lung tissue, where it causes disruption. Proposed mechanisms of injury include spalling (disruption of tissues at air–liquid interfaces), implosion (compression and re-expansion of air-filled structures) and rapid acceleration of tissues of different densities. Large animal models have demonstrated that the level of injury is related to the rate of chest wall displacement, rather than the maximal depth of deflection.[15] Severity of injury is dependent on strength of the blast, range from detonation and surrounding environment.

Those working closely with explosives may wear personal armour that assists in decoupling the effect of primary blast. Current examples of such armour tend to be cumbersome. More common varieties of torso body armour provide protection against penetrating injury but probably do little to mitigate the effects of primary blast.

The pathophysiology of blast lung includes both immediate and delayed responses. There is an immediate bradycardia and apnoea of variable length, which is a likely to be a vagally mediated reflex.[16] The lung injury itself is typified by alveolar capillary rupture with subsequent intrapulmonary bleeding and oedema. The extent of this injury is proportional to the blast exposure and may range from microscopic petechial injury to areas of frank haemorrhage.

While rarely seen in isolation, primary blast may leave little external evidence of injury since the skin itself is rarely affected. Clinical features of blast lung include progressive hypoxia, which may not be apparent at time of injury and is related to the inflammatory response to intrapulmonary haemorrhage and worsening oedema.

Other structural lung injuries are associated with primary blast, although the prediction of these injuries by blast conditions is not consistent and likely complicated by tertiary impact. Pneumothoraces may occur due to pleural rupture in the absence of penetrating injury. Injury to the larger vessels may lead to haemothoraces and the formation of alveolar-venous or bronco-venous fistulae. Air embolism due to such fistulae may cause acute hypoxia with cardiovascular collapse and is a leading cause of death in those who do not survive until treatment.

Diagnosis of blast lung is clinical with findings of hypoxia following blast exposure. Typical 'bat-wing' pulmonary infiltrates are seen on chest radiograph and computed tomography may discriminate these injuries from the more peripheral contusions seen in blunt trauma. Imaging may be useful in detecting associated structural lung injuries.

Treatment of blast lung is largely supportive. Mechanical ventilation may be required but consideration should be given to the possibility of air embolism and pneumothorax that may be exacerbated. Some centres advocate the use of prophylactic bilateral pleural decompression, although there is little evidence to suggest an effect on outcomes. Patients with significant blast lung injury are highly likely to have sustained other blast related injuries and any management plan should consider their overall condition.

The abdomen may also be subject to primary blast. The incidence of abdominal injury due to air blast has not been extensively examined, although a recent review of multiple incidents, including a variety of blast conditions, showed that abdominal injury is not common – seen in around 3% of incidents.[17]

Damage is dependent on coupling of the blast overpressure and shockwave to a stress wave that travels through the abdomen. The effect of shockwave dispersal is most marked at tissue–air interfaces. As such, the hollow organs are those most commonly injured. The caecum segment is probably most sensitive to intestinal blast injury. Conversely, the small bowel and its extensive mesentery may be more susceptible to large shear waves causing mesenteric tearing.

Presentation of primary blast injury to the bowel may be delayed relative to the acute onset of blast lung. Abdominal symptoms may be absent initially with progression to pain and frank peritonitis should perforation and contamination occur. Given the lack of external injury, indications for operative intervention are largely clinical, as with conventional blunt abdominal trauma. The patient should be assessed anaesthetically with particular consideration to the effect of anaesthesia and ventilation on any concomitant blast lung injury.

The most common operative findings of intestinal blast are subserosal haemorrhage.[17] Tearing of the mucosal surface with bleeding into the lumen of the tract may occur following repeated exposure to relatively lower blast overpressures. As in blunt injury, there is a propensity for mural haematomata to progress to perforation due to tissue necrosis. Full-thickness injuries to the bowel with immediate perforation can occur with a greater exposure to blast overpressure.

The surgical management of blast bowel injury is that of any penetrating and blunt trauma, with primary repair or resection as indicated. Surgical judgment is essential regarding the findings of non-perforated but contused bowel. A damage control approach to such injuries may allow for repeat assessment later, but in a physiologically well patient, in whom a relook would not be justified, the surgeon must decide to resect a segment or risk future progression of these lesions to perforation.

The solid organs are more resistant to primary blast. Parenchymal disruption due to the shockwave has been described at very high levels of overpressure, although the experimental data for these injuries are sparse. Injury, with subsequent bleeding, may result from rapid distractions of organ attachments and mesenteries. These blast conditions are more likely encountered in enclosed conditions and differentiation of primary from tertiary injuries is difficult.

Secondary blast injury

Secondary blast injury refers to the effect of fragments that are accelerated away from the device following detonation. Sources of fragments include:

- the casing of the device;
- purposefully placed fragments within the device. These may include nails, bolts or ball bearings and are embedded within the device or adherent to the exterior;
- nearby objects including glass and stones;
- biological material including bone may be expelled, particularly following a suicide bomb or anti-personnel mine attack.

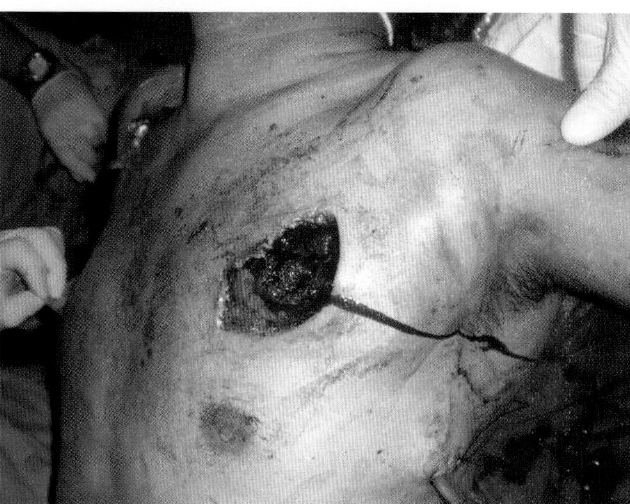

Figure 30.5 Large anterior fragmentation injury.

Shrapnel is often used to describe explosive fragments, although the term more strictly applied to a specific from of artillery shell.

The energy of a primary blast wave disperses quickly in proportion to the distance from the blast; it is subject to the inverse cube law. As such, only those within a reasonably small radius of the blast are affected. Conversely, the velocity and wounding potential of an energised fragment is subject to the inverse square law. Secondary blast injuries may occur at long range from the detonation. Fragments may be accelerated up to very high velocities. As with ballistics, injuries are dependent on the range and energy of the fragment.

In contrast to bullet wounds, the variability of fragments produces a wide range of wounds and no two wounds will be the same (Figure 30.5). The irregular surfaces of fragments cause complex patterns of yaw and tumble. Both permanent and temporary wound cavities may be unpredictable and irregular.

The management of fragment wounds is similar to ballistic and conventional penetrating trauma. Wounds should be adequately debrided. Fragment wounds should be considered dirty and principles of septic surgery applied. Where possible, serial debridement and delayed primary closure should be attempted.

The fragments should be removed at time of surgery if easily accessible. Other indications for early removal include fragments within joint spaces or adjacent to structures with danger of erosion and further injuries. Late indications for fragment removal include ongoing sepsis, pain or lack of function.

Tertiary blast injury

Tertiary blast injury is the result of gross movement of personnel, objects or infrastructure by blast wind. Tertiary injury is analogous to conventional blunt trauma and may cause a wide variety of injuries to all organ systems. Traumatic amputation is typically included within this category, although primary blast and the shattering or 'brissiance' effect on bone may play a part.

Quaternary and quinary injury

Quaternary blast injury refers to a miscellaneous group of injuries that do not fall within other categories. These include burns, inhalational injuries and late-onset respiratory problems. Quinary injury, a more novel concept, refers to injury caused by the intentional addition of either biologically or radioactively active material to an explosive device.

Environmental effects

As already alluded to, the shockwave of blast overpressure is modified by an enclosed or partially enclosed space. Environmental differences may make marked differences to injury rates and clinical presentations following blast. Higher rates of blast lung and TM rupture are seen following enclosed blast (in which both casualty and blast are enclosed). In contrast, secondary blast injuries may be lower in number as more people are protected from energised fragments. Tertiary injury is difficult to predict based on blast characteristics but a higher proportion of blunt injuries have been seen following enclosed blast.

A distinct pattern of injury has been described following underbody blast against military vehicles. Underbody blast casualties have a greater range of injuries and are overall more severely injured.[18] In addition to blunt injury sustained from displacement within the vehicle, the effect of blast is manifested both by propagation of the shockwave through a solid, with upwards deformation of the floor and a rapid upwards acceleration of the whole vehicle and subsequent deceleration following impact with the ground. The solid blast injury burden includes severe foot and ankle[19] and pelvic injury.[20] Mortality from underbody blast is most commonly caused by head injury and non-compressible torso haemorrhage including aortic disruption and liver laceration.

In contrast, the dismounted IED casualty may sustain a characteristic pattern of injuries including lower limb amputation, pelvic fracture and genital, perineal and rectal injuries (**Figure 30.6**).

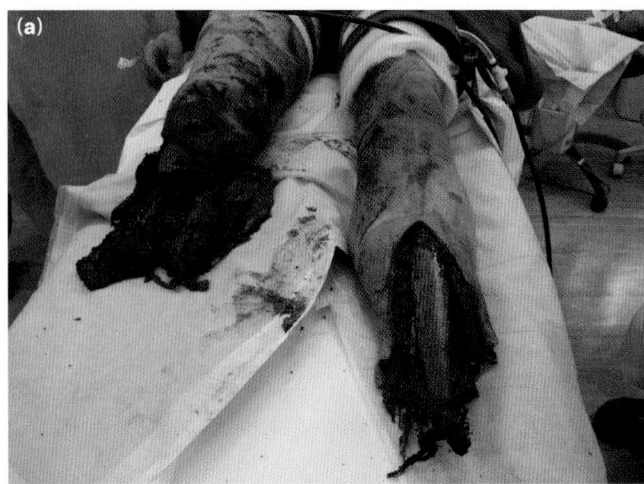

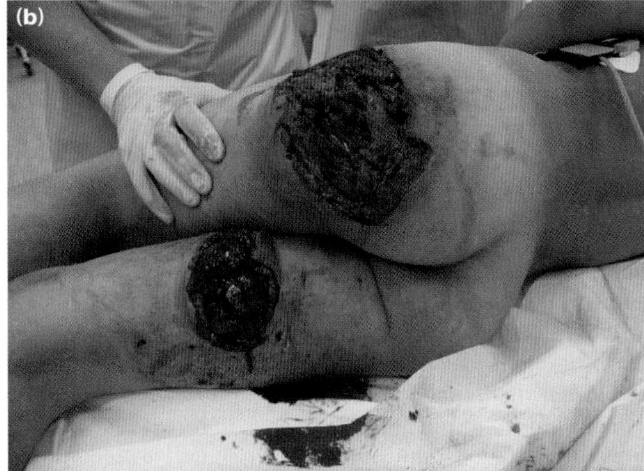

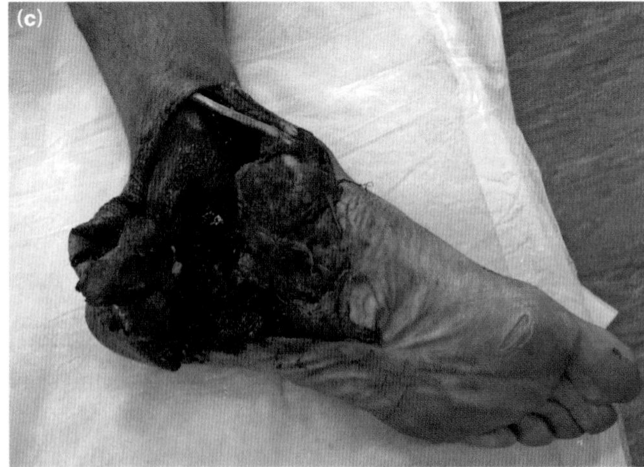

Figure 30.6 Blast injuries including bilateral lower limb amputation (**a**), buttock and thigh soft tissue injury (**b**) and complex hind foot injury (**c**). The need for extensive debridement is evident from the level of wound contamination and non-viable tissue.

INFECTION

Battlefield wounds are by their very nature grossly contaminated and the treatment and prevention of infection is one of the basic functions of war surgery. Wounds sustained during warfare are high-energy wounds with large areas of devitalised tissue. Wounding agents are all non-sterile and highly likely to be contaminated by bacteria. Both large calibre ballistic wounds and blast wounds may contain dirty clothing or contaminated fragments. Multiple steps in casualty evacuation and substantial delays before treatment may allow progression of contamination to clinically significant infection.

Specific organism patterns will depend on endemic flora, but commonly seen bacteria include:[21]

- Gram-positive cocci including staphylococci, streptococci and enterococci;
- Gram-negative rods including *Escherichia coli*, *Proteus* and *Klebsiella*;

- *Pseudomonas*, *Enterobacter*, *Acinetobacter* and *Serratia* are common nosocomial pathogens usually expected among casualties following long periods of hospitalisation;
- *Salmonella*, *Shigella* and *Vibrio* should be suspected in cases of bacterial dysentery.

Fungal infection including *Candida* should be considered in casualties hospitalised for prolonged periods, those malnourished or immunosuppressed, or those who have received broad-spectrum antibiotics, adrenocortical steroids or parenteral nutrition.

Techniques to reduce the infectious burden are part of every aspect of war surgery. At point of wounding, sterile dressings should be applied. Antibiotics, if available, should be administered if evacuation and further treatment is likely to be delayed.

Empirical antibiotic therapy should be commenced or continued following movement to a medical facility. The mainstay of treatment is prompt surgical control of the infectious cause with adequate debridement of non-viable tissue and drainage of infective material. Extensive irrigation should be employed to remove dead tissue and foreign bodies. High-pressure wound lavage has been shown to increase bacterial propagation into soft tissue and is not indicated.

With few exceptions (such as facial wounds), closure of contaminated war wounds should not be performed at time of first operation. The open wound should be left with clean, moist dressings. Negative pressure wound therapy should be considered for larger wounds.

Antibiotic therapy should be tailored to specific wounds with empirical antibiotic choice dependant on the injured body region or cavity. Microbial culture will aid the guidance of therapy for more established infection. Contaminated war wounds should be considered tetanus prone and appropriate tetanus prophylaxis administered.

Clinical experience and judgement are essential in the assessment of war wounds. Adequate exposure, often with extension of the wound, is mandated to ensure debridement of all devitalised tissue. Serial operations may be required. Early consideration should be given to soft tissue coverage. The skin is often remarkably resilient to injury and conservative debridement of it may facilitate more successful reconstruction.

REFERENCES

1 Atta HM. Edwin Smith Surgical Papyrus: the oldest known surgical treatise. *Am Surg* 1999; **65**(12): 1190–2.

2 Champion HR, Bellamy RF, Roberts P, Leppaniemi A. A profile of combat injury. *J Trauma* 2003; **54**(5 Suppl): S13–19.

3 Owens BD, Kragh JF, Wenke JC, Macaitis J, Wade CE *et al.* Combat wounds in operation Iraqi Freedom and operation Enduring Freedom. *J Trauma* 2008; **64**(2): 295–99.

4 Eastridge BJ, Hardin M, Cantrell J, Oetjen-Gerdes L, Zubko T *et al.* Died of wounds on the battlefield: causation and implications for improving combat casualty care. *J Trauma (other)* 2011; **71**(1 supplement): S4–8.

5 Hodgetts TJ. ABC to <C>ABC: redefining the military trauma paradigm. *Emerg Med J* 2006; **23**(10): 745–46.

6 Morrison JJ, Stannard A, Rasmussen TE, Jansen JO, Tai NRM *et al.* Injury pattern and mortality of noncompressible torso hemorrhage in UK combat casualties. *J Trauma Acute Care Surg* 2013; **75**(2 Suppl 2): S263–68.

7 Morrison JJ, Ross JD, Rasmussen TE, Midwinter MJ, Jansen JO. Resuscitative endovascular balloon occlusion of the aorta: a gap analysis of severely injured UK combat casualties. *Shock* 2014; **41**(5): 388–93.

8 Rotondo MF, Schwab CW. 'Damage control': an approach for improved survival in exsanguinating penetrating abdominal injury. *J Trauma* 1993; **35**(3): 375–82.

9 Garner J, Watts S, Parry C, Bird J, Cooper G *et al.* Prolonged permissive hypotensive resuscitation is associated with poor outcome in primary blast injury with controlled hemorrhage. *Ann Surg* 2010; **251**(6): 1131–39.

10 Khan S, Brohi K, Chana M, Raza I, Stanworth S *et al.* Hemostatic resuscitation is neither hemostatic nor resuscitative in trauma hemorrhage. *J Trauma Acute Care Surg* 2014; **76**(3): 561–67; discussion 567–68.

11 Jansen JO, Morrison JJ, Midwinter MJ, Doughty H. Changes in blood transfusion practices in the UK role 3 medical treatment facility in Afghanistan, 2008–2011. *Transfus Med* 2014; **24**(3): 154–61.

12 Brooks AJ, Clasper J, Midwinter M, Hodgetts TJ, Mahoney PF. (eds.) *Ryan's ballistic trauma.* London: Springer London, 2011.

13 Stuhmiller J, Phillips Y, Richmond DR. The physics and mechanisms of primary blast injury. In: Bellamy RF, Zajtchuk R (eds) *Conventional warfare ballistic, blast and burn injuries.* Washington DC: Department of the Army, Office of the Surgeon General, 1991, pp. 241–70.

14 Ramasamy A, Hill AM, Clasper JC. Improvised explosive devices: pathophysiology, injury profiles and current medical management. *J R Army Med Corps* 2009; **155**(4): 265–72.

15 Cooper GJ, Taylor DE. Biophysics of impact injury to the chest and abdomen. *J R Army Med Corps* 1989; **135**(2): 58–67.

16 Guy RJ, Kirkman E, Watkins PE, Cooper GJ. Physiologic responses to primary blast. *J Trauma* 1998; **45**(6): 983–87.

17 Owers C, Morgan JL, Garner JP. Abdominal trauma in primary blast injury. *Br J Surg* 2011; **98**(2): 168–79.

18 Singleton JA, Gibb IE, Hunt NC, Bull AM, Clasper JC. Identifying future 'unexpected' survivors: a retrospective cohort study of fatal injury patterns in victims of improvised explosive devices. *BMJ Open* 2013; **3**(8): e003130–e003130.

19 Ramasamy A, Hill AM, Masouros S, Gibb I, Bull AMJ *et al.* Blast-related fracture patterns: a forensic biomechanical approach. *J R Soc Interface* 2011; **8**(58): 689–98.

20 Webster C, Masouros S, Gibb I, Clasper JC. Fracture patterns in pelvic blast injury: a retrospective analysis and implications for future preventative strategies. *Bone Joint J* 2015; **97-B**(Supp 8): 14.

21 Cubano, MA, and MK Lenhart. 'Emergency war surgery.' 2014. https://scholar.google.co.uk/scholar?q=emergency+war+surgery+2014&btnG=&hl=en&as_sdt=0%2C5#2.

PART 5

Elective orthopaedics

31	History taking and clinical examination in musculoskeletal disease	436
32	Sports medicine and sports injuries	463
33	The spine	471
34	Upper limb	488
35	Hip and knee	511
36	Foot and ankle	524
37	Musculoskeletal tumours	534
38	Infection of the bones and joints	549
39	Paediatric orthopaedics	561

Chapter 31

History taking and clinical examination in musculoskeletal disease

Learning objectives

To understand how to:

- Take a comprehensive musculoskeletal history
- Perform a structured and systematic musculoskeletal examination
- Use and interpret special tests
- Use findings to understand the impact on a patient's pain and function

INTRODUCTION

The components of the musculoskeletal (MSK) system include the bones, joints, ligaments, muscles and tendons as well as the neurological and vascular structures. A simple system allows a concise yet comprehensive history to be taken and a reliable examination to be performed. This will permit diagnosis of the common, the rare and the clinically urgent musculoskeletal problems that are likely to be encountered in clinical practice.

HISTORY

Introduction

- Introduce yourself and check the patient's name and date of birth.
- Explain what you are going to do, obtain verbal consent and ensure that the patient is comfortable.

Take a history

- **Presenting complaint**. Start with an open-ended question. Ask the patient to 'explain what the problem is' in their own words, and ask the patient what their hopes and expectations are from the interview.
- **History of the presenting complaint** ('the three Ws'). When did you first notice the problem? What were you doing when it started? Was the onset sudden or did it develop gradually?
- **Associated symptoms**. Ask about the following: pain; swelling; instability – 'giving way'; mechanical symptoms (e.g. locking, clicking, clunking); loss of power; altered sensation.
- **Functional impairment**. Ask whether the patient is having difficulties performing activities of daily living: upper limb, e.g. personal hygiene, feeding; lower limb, e.g. putting on shoes and socks, standing, walking and climbing stairs.
- **Past medical history (PMH)**. Check for comorbid conditions which may contribute to the presenting problem or affect the patient's fitness for an anaesthetic, e.g. diabetes, asthma, previous heart attack or stroke. Check for any previous problems with anaesthetics.
- **Past surgical history**: relevant surgical procedures.
- **Drug history**. Ask about all medication and the following in particular: anticoagulants, steroids, aspirin, immunosuppressant therapy, oral contraceptive pill and hormone replacement therapy.
- **Social history**. Tailor questions to the patient's condition: patient's age; hand dominance; employment status; dependents; alcohol; smoking; hobbies; home help; accommodation – own house, residential or nursing home; use of walking aids; mental test score assessment.
- **Family history**. This may reveal a history of MSK disease.

Summary box 31.1

Taking a history

- Introduce yourself and put the patient at ease
- Explain what you are doing and ensure that the patient agrees
- Start with an open question to understand the presenting complaint
- Check for history of presenting complaint and associated symptoms
- Ask about functional impairment
- Check past medical history and relevant surgical and family history
- Check drug and social history

MUSCULOSKELETAL EXAMINATION

General principles

Apley described a useful and systematic approach to clinical examination. This approach is divided into three parts:

1 look;
2 feel;
3 move.

Look

The inspection begins as soon as you enter the examination room. Look for any walking aids. Remember to look at the whole patient and not just at the joint of interest. For example:

- look at the hands for rheumatoid arthritis;
- look at the eyes for Horner's syndrome;
- look for any obvious upper or lower limb or spinal deformity.

Gait

The gait cycle is all of the activity between the initial contact of the foot with the ground and the succeeding initial contact of the same limb. There are two main stages: the stance phase (60%) and the swing phase (40%). Ask the patient to stand, and inspect from the front, side and back. Then, ask the patient to walk using any walking aids. Some of the types of limp that might be present are described in *Table 31.1*.

Focused inspection

Adequately expose the joint above and below. Expose the opposite limb for comparison. Make sure that the patient is comfortable. It may be easier for you and the patient if they remain standing for the first part of the examination. When a couch is used, make sure that it is in the centre of the room (not against the wall) so that you can work on both sides of the patient. Remember that all joints are covered by an envelope of soft tissues and skin. Look at the skin for:

- surgical scars (arthroscopy scars may be difficult to see);
- bruising (may indicate recent injury or a bleeding disorder);
- erythema (e.g. cellulitis);
- ulcers (e.g. arterial, vascular or neuropathic);
- rashes;
- sinuses (e.g. secondary to osteomyelitis);
- hair loss and the presence or absence of sweating;
- pigmentations or raised lesion (e.g. café-au-lait spots or neurofibromas).

Look at the soft tissues for:

- swelling (e.g. may indicate a joint effusion);
- lumps (consider which tissue layer they are arising from);
- muscle wasting (e.g. may be secondary to disuse atrophy, neuropathy);
- muscle fasciculation (lower motor neurone pathology).

Look at the bones for:

- abnormal limb alignment – comparison with the other side may be helpful;
- deformity.

TABLE 31.1 Types of limp.

Cause	Pathogenesis	Presentation
Long	Osteoarthritis (in other leg)	Head dips. Cadence dash/dash
Incoordinated	Cerebral palsy	Head movement lacks coordination. No regular cadence
Muscle weakness	Osteoarthritis hip	Head moves from side to side (windscreen wiper)
Pain	Osteoarthritis hip	Head dips. Cadence dot/dash
Stiff	Arthrodesis hip	Head rocks too and fro
Limp	**Pathology**	
Antalgic	Hip joint arthritis	
Trendelenburg	Weakness of hip abductors	
High-stepping gait	Foot drop secondary to common peroneal nerve palsy	
Spastic	Cerebral palsy	
Ataxic	Cerebellar pathology	

Alan Graham Apley, 1914–1996, Director of Orthopaedic Surgery, St Thomas' Hospital, London, UK. As a consultant also at Rowley Bristow Orthopaedic Hospital, he conducted the most popular orthopaedic postgraduate course for the FRCS examination in Pyrford, Surrey, which became internationally known as the 'Pyrford Orthopaedic Course'.
Johann Friedrich Horner, 1831–1886, Professor of Ophthalmology, Zurich, Switzerland, described this syndrome in 1869.
Friedrich Trendelenburg, 1844–1924, Professor of Surgery successively at Rostock (1875–1882), Bonn (1882–1895), Leipzig (1895–1911), Germany. The Trendelenburg position was first described in 1885.

Feel

Ask the patient if they have any areas of tenderness. Ensure that you do not cause the patient pain – watch their face as you feel. It may be easier (especially with children) to feel the normal side first.

Skin

The aim of sensory testing is to establish a pattern of sensory loss. Look for a dermatomal (may indicate spinal root or peripheral nerve pathology) or glove and stocking distribution (may indicate a neuropathy, e.g. diabetes). Perform a screening test by lightly stroking both limbs. Record whether the patient feels a difference. If none is noticed there is no need to spend more time on the neurological examination. If there is a difference, then a full neurological examination should now be performed.

Soft tissues

- **Tenderness.** Try to determine the actual anatomical structure from which the pain arises (e.g. subcutaneous fat, bursae, nerves, arteries).
- **Lumps and effusions.** Determine the characteristics of any lump or effusion using *Table 31.2* as a guide.
- **Pulses.** Palpate the distal pulses (or capillary return) of the limb. Recording distal neurovascular status both before and after surgery is important. Absence of distal pulses is an absolute contraindication to elective surgery in that limb. Acute loss of circulation to a limb is a surgical emergency.

Bone

Palpate the contours of the joint and assess for tenderness. For superficial joints, such as the knee, the joint line can be felt and checked for lumps and tenderness.

Move

There are three stages to assessing movement. The words used to describe a particular movement are shown in *Table 31.3*.

- **Active.** Ask the patient to move the joint within the limits of their pain.

TABLE 31.2 Swelling – an acronym for history and examination of a lump.

Start	Did it appear after trauma or gradually on its own?
Where	Anatomical site and layer (skin, fat, muscle); does it move in relation to these?
External features	Size, surface and definition of margins
Lymph nodes	Are the local ones enlarged?
Liquid	Is it fluctuant? Can it be transilluminated?
Internal features	Is it hard? Is it tender?
Noise	Is there a thrill? Is there a bruit?
General	Examination of the whole patient for general lumps

TABLE 31.3 Terminology used to describe the direction of movement.

Flexion	Forward or anterior movement of the trunk or limb
Lateral flexion	Bending of the forward-facing head and trunk to either side
Extension	Backward or posterior movement
Abduction	A movement away from the midline of the body
Adduction	A movement towards the midline of the body
Internal rotation	Rotation towards the midline of the body
External rotation	Rotation away from the midline
Supination	Movement of the forearm so that the palm faces anteriorly
Pronation	Movement of the forearm so that the palm faces posteriorly
Circumduction	A combination of flexion, abduction, extension and adduction without rotation
Inversion	Movement of the foot that directs the sole of the foot medially
Eversion	Movement of the foot that directs the sole of the foot laterally
Retraction	Backwards movement of the head, jaw or shoulders

- **Passive.** Move the limb or joint yourself. Record the range of movement in 'degrees' (a goniometer may be helpful). Comparison of active and passive range allows the three causes of loss of range of movement to be distinguished. In limitation caused by pain or stiffness the ranges are the same but one is painful. In weakness passive range is greater than active.
- **Stability.** Stability has a static and a dynamic component: static tests assess the integrity of the ligaments and joint (bone) surfaces; dynamic tests assess the integrity and functions of the muscles and tendons. Ask the patient to move the joint actively through its range of motion while you try to stop the movement. Record power using the Medical Research Council (MRC) grading system as illustrated in *Table 31.4*. Consider the muscles that drive each movement, the peripheral nerves that supply them and the nerve root values (*Table 31.5*).

TABLE 31.4 The Medical Research Council grading system of muscle power.

Grade	Description
0	No movement
1	Flicker of movement
2	Active movement with gravity elimination
3	Active movement against gravity
4	Active movement against resistance but power less than full
5	Normal power

TABLE 31.5 Peripheral nerves.

Root level	Sensation	Motor	Reflex
C5	Lateral upper arm	Deltoid	Biceps
C6	Lateral forearm	Wrist extension	Brachioradialis
C7	Middle finger	Triceps	Triceps
C8	Little finger	Finger flexors	–
T1	Medial forearm	Interossei	–
L1	Anterior thigh	Psoas	–
L2	Anterior thigh/groin	Quadriceps	–
L3	Anterior and lateral thigh	Quadriceps	–
L4	Medial leg and foot	Tibialis anterior	Knee jerk
L5	Lateral leg and first dorsal web space	Extensor hallucis longus	–
S1	Lateral and plantar foot	Gastrocnemius/perineals	Achilles
S2–S4	Perianal	Bladder and foot intrinsics	–

In the following sections, in addition to the approach of 'Look, Feel, Move', we have included details of special tests for each joint as well as neurological examination of the limb. The peripheral nerve examination comprises sensory and motor testing, reflexes, tone and coordination and proprioception.

Summary box 31.2

Musculoskeletal examination

- Introduce yourself and put the patient at ease
- Assess the gait
- Look
- Feel
- Move
- Special tests
- Neurological examination
- Pulses

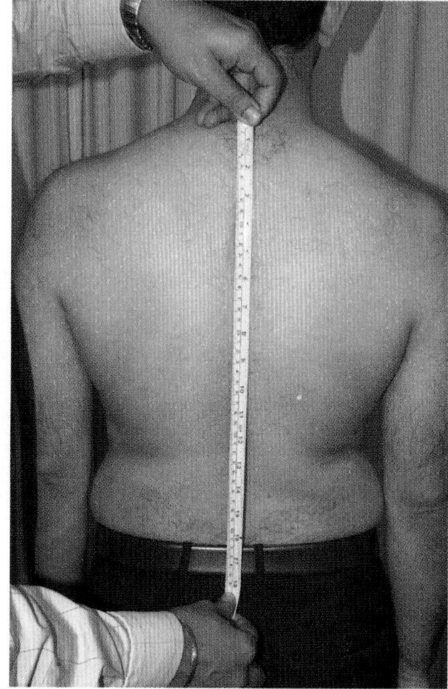

Figure 31.1 Plumb line.

CLINICAL EXAMINATION OF THE SPINE

The spinal column consists of 33 vertebrae with 23 intervertebral discs. This is supported by numerous ligaments and paraspinal muscles.

When observed from the front (coronal plane) with the patient standing and the hips and knees fully extended, the head should be centred over the sacrum. A 'plumb line' dropped from the spinous process of C7 should fall through the gluteal crease (Figure 31.1). If it falls to either side of the cleft, lateral tilt of the spine is present. The ear, shoulder and greater trochanter of the hip should lie in the same vertical plane. When the patient is observed from the side, assess the four physiological sagittal plane curves (cervical and lumbar lordosis, and thoracic and sacral kyphosis) (Figure 31.2).

Cervical spine

Look

Ensure that the shoulders, back muscles and scapulae can be seen. Look for muscle wasting and asymmetry of the neck creases and check that the shoulders are level and that there is a normal cervical lordosis (range 20–40°).

Feel

Stand behind the patient and support the patient's chin.

- **Soft tissues.** Feel for spasm of the paraspinal muscles.
- **Bone.** Palpate the spinous processes (tenderness and alignment); the spinous processes of C7 (vertebra prominens) and T1 are usually large and are easily palpable at the base of the neck.

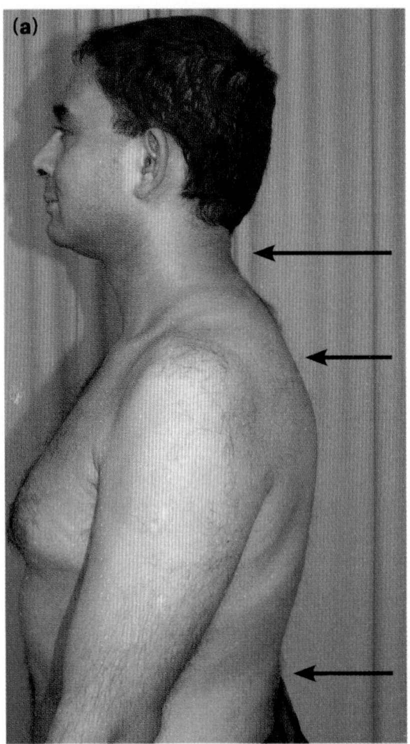

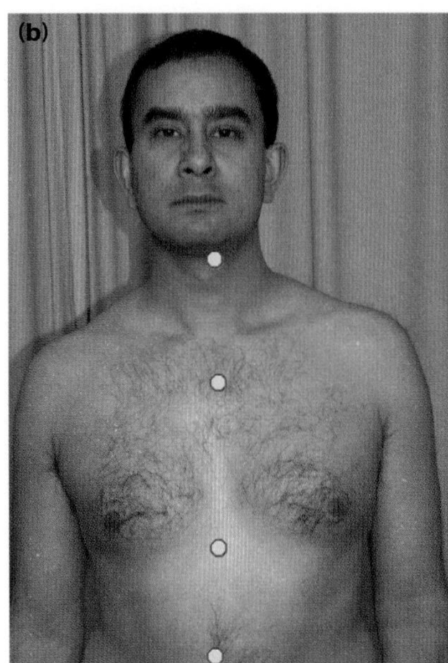

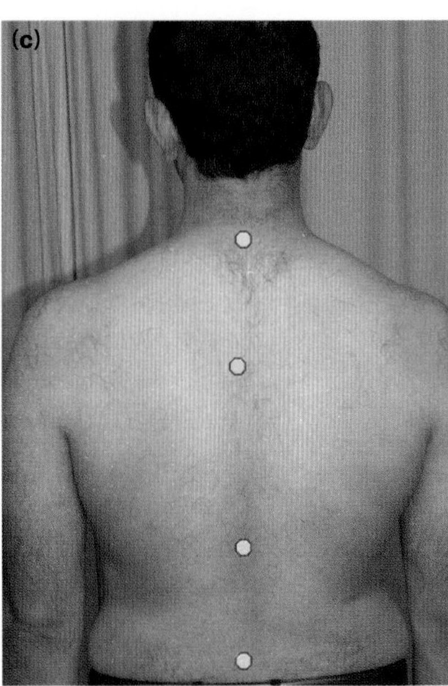

Figure 31.2 Standing sagittal profile of cervical and lumbar lordosis (**a**), and thoracic (**b**) and sacral (**c**) kyphosis.

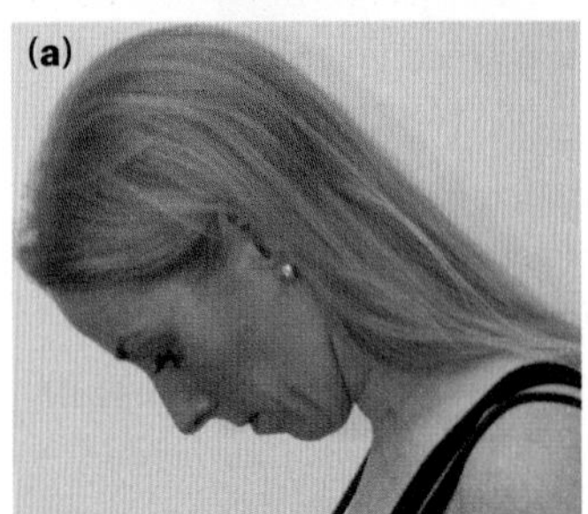

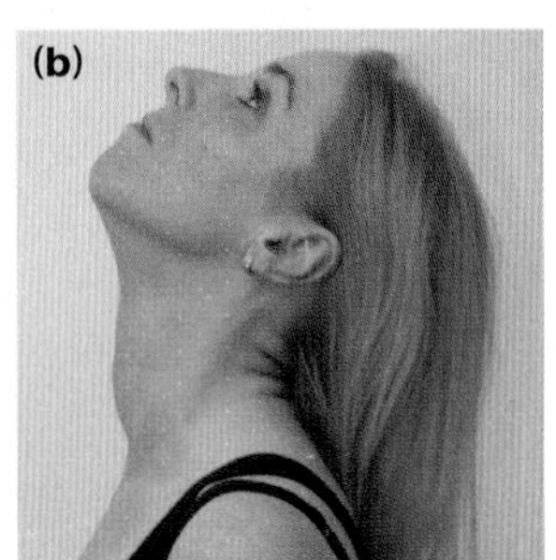

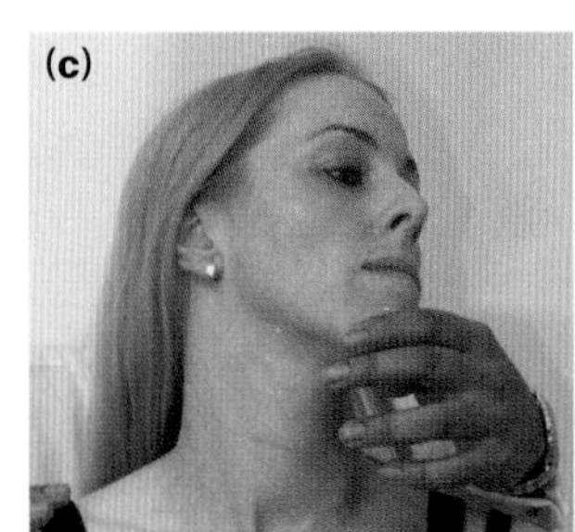

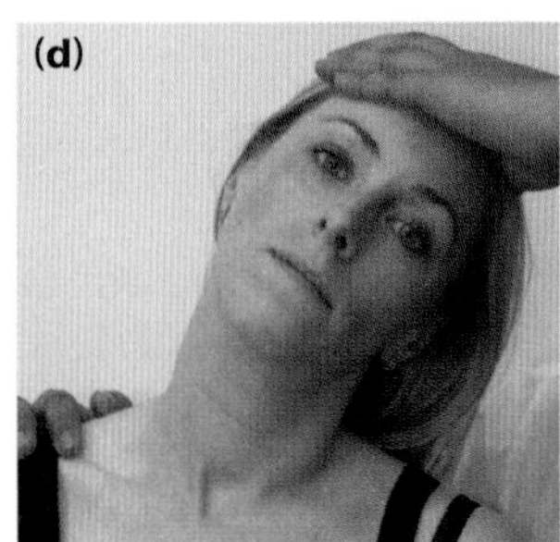

Figure 31.3 Cervical spine flexion/extension (**a, b**), rotation (**c**) and bending (**d**).

Move

Motion occurs in three planes: flexion/extension, bending and rotation (**Figure 31.3**).

- **Flexion (45°)/extension (55°)**. Ask the patient to bend their neck forwards – place the chin on the chest. Measure the distance from the chin to the sternum. Ask the patient to extend their neck by looking up at the ceiling.
- **Right/left rotation (70°)**. Ask the patient to look over each shoulder while not moving the chest wall.
- **Right/left bending (40°)**. Ask the patient to lay their ear on their ipsilateral shoulder.

Neurological

Focus your examination on the C5 to T1 nerve roots. These supply the upper extremities (**Figure 31.4**).

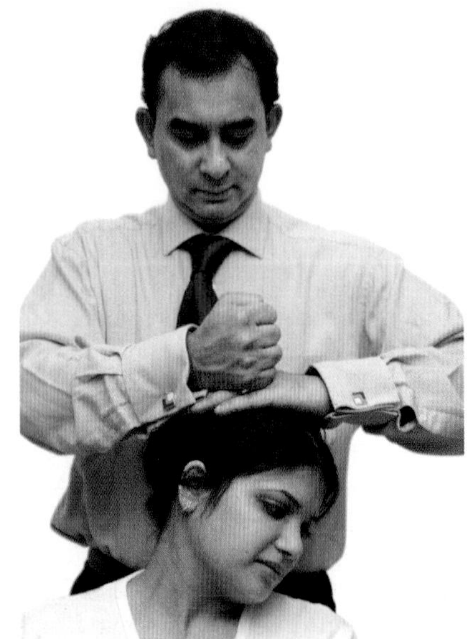

Figure 31.4 Spurling's test for cervical spine nerve root entrapment. Extend the cervical spine and rotate the head to each shoulder in turn. The presence of a shooting pain down the arm may indicate cervical nerve root compression.

Thoracic spine

Pathology commonly presents with pain and deformity. The thoracic spine is normally convex with a gentle kyphosis (normal range 20–45°).

Look

Ensure that the front and the back from the neck to the gluteal cleft can be visualised. Note skin markings (e.g. café-au-lait spots, hairy patches). These may suggest occult neurology or bony pathology.

- **Front.** Check for asymmetry of the shoulder and rib cage suggesting scoliosis.
- **Back.** Look for a difference in the height of the iliac crests (pelvic tilt). Assess for coronal plane deformity, such as scoliosis (lateral curvature of the thoracic spine with rotation). A rib hump suggesting a structural scoliosis may be visible.
- **Side.** Assess for sagittal plane deformity, such as an increased kyphosis.

Feel

Palpate, with one hand supporting the patient's pelvis.

Move

Range of motion is limited in the thoracic spine:

- **Forward bending test** (Figure 31.5). Ask the patient to bend forwards to touch their toes:
  - *structural scoliosis:* a rib hump will increase in size (bulge posteriorly on the thoracic convex side) as the patient bends forwards; this is diagnostic of idiopathic thoracic scoliosis (rotatory deformity);
  - *functional scoliosis*: the spine straightens as the patient bends forwards and no rib hump is visible; this flexible deformity is secondary to other abnormalities such as abnormal leg lengths and muscle spasm in the lumbar region.
- **Lateral bending.** This can be used to assess the flexibility of a scoliosis. Radiographs are taken in this position to supplement the assessment.

Lumbar spine

Examination should include the pelvis, hips, lower limbs, gait and peripheral vascular system as well as the lumbar region. Irritation of nerves in the lumbar spine can mimic problems in the lower limb. Always consider referred pain.

Look

- **Back.** Check the skin at the base of the spine for hairy tufts and dimples (underlying spina bifida). Prominence of the spinal muscles on one side may be the result of muscle spasm secondary to pain.
- **Side.** The lumbar spine has a smooth concavity known as the lumbar lordosis (normal range is 40–60°). Muscle spasm is a cause of loss of the normal lordosis.

Feel

Feel for any 'step-off' in the spinous processes. This may indicate forward slippage of one of the vertebrae on another.

Move

Movement occurs in flexion, extension, lateral bending and rotation (Figure 31.6). Record the motion in each plane in degrees. Remember that a significant portion of lumbar flexion is achieved through the hip joint.

- **Forward flexion.** This is a measure of lumbar flexibility. The skin of the lumbar spine stretches as the patient bends forwards. To measure flexion, place the tip of your thumb over the T12–L1 junction and the tip of your index finger of the same hand over the lumbosacral junction. Ask the patient to bend forwards and touch the toes (normal range 40–60°). Measure the distance by which your thumb and the tip of your index finger separate.
- **Lateral bending.** Ask the patient to slide their right hand down the outer side of their right leg and then their left hand down the outside of their left leg. Note the distance that each hand moves down that side of the thigh.
- **Rotation.** Stand behind the patient and hold their pelvis still with both hands. Ask the patient to twist around and Look over their shoulder. Note the angle that the shoulder girdle forms with the pelvis (range 3–18°).

Special tests

- **Lasègue's straight leg raise test** (Figure 31.7). This test increases tension along the sciatic nerve (L5 and S1 nerve roots). With the patient supine, elevate the leg with the knee bent to check pain-free movement of the hip. Then,

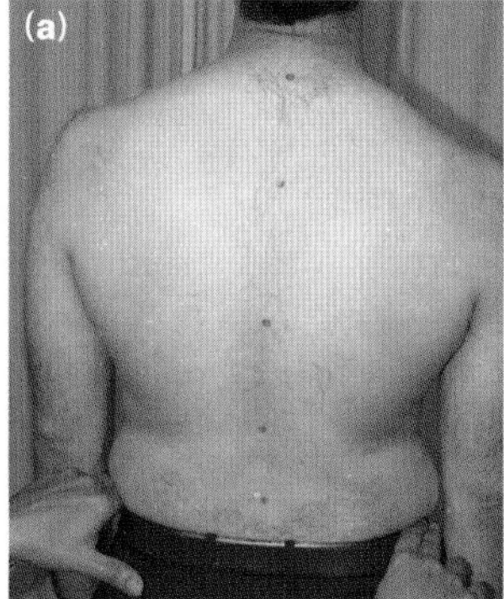

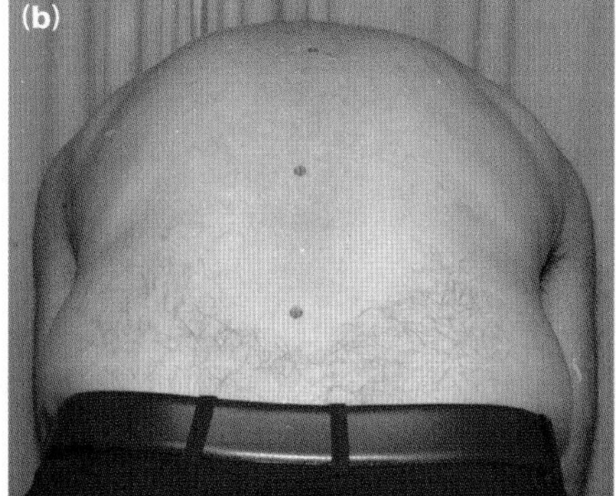

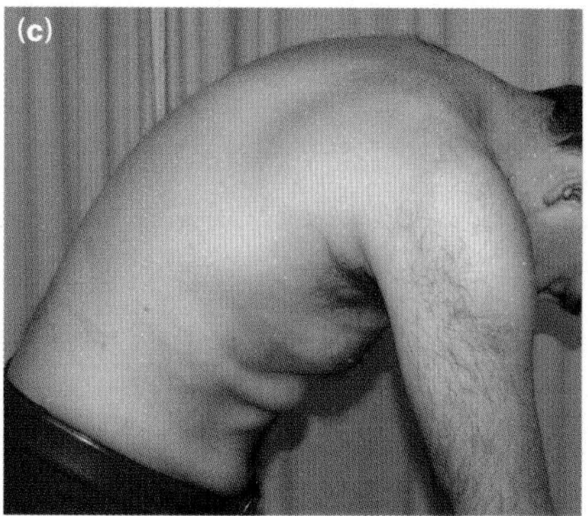

Figure 31.5 (a-c) Forward bending test.

Charles Ernest Lasègue, 1816–1863, Professor of Medicine, The University of Paris, and Physician, La Salpêtrière, Paris, France. This test was described by Lasègue's student, who named it after his teacher.

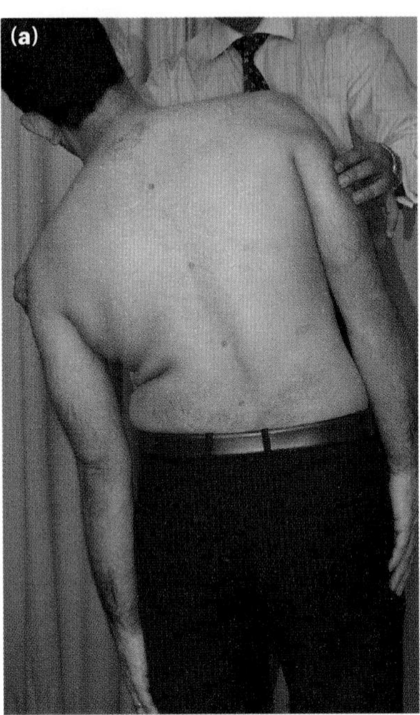

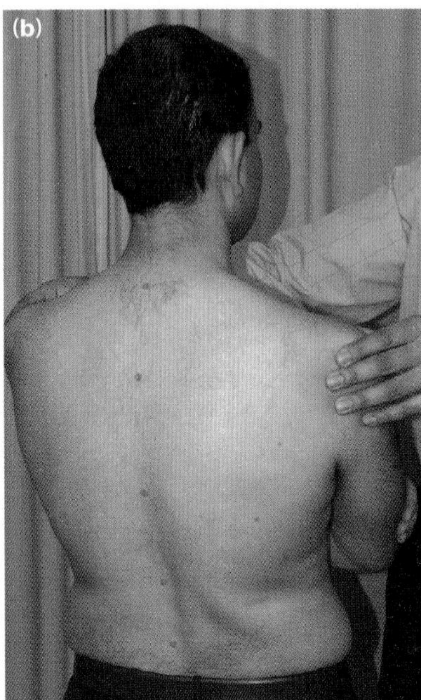

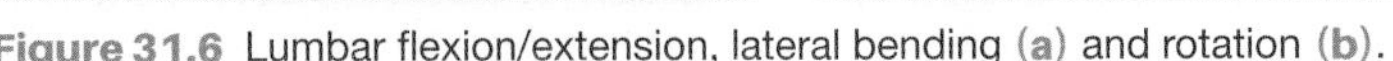
Figure 31.6 Lumbar flexion/extension, lateral bending (a) and rotation (b).

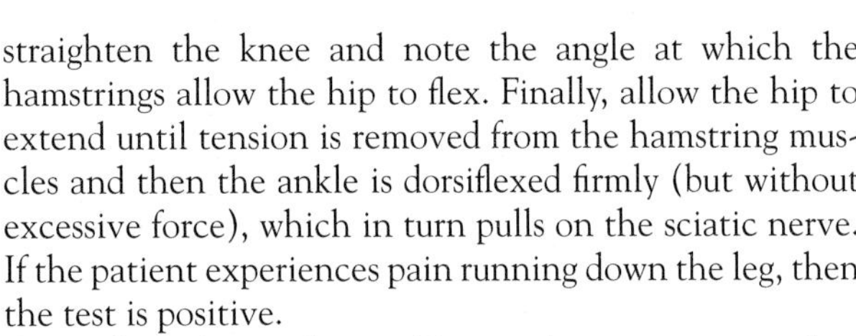
straighten the knee and note the angle at which the hamstrings allow the hip to flex. Finally, allow the hip to extend until tension is removed from the hamstring muscles and then the ankle is dorsiflexed firmly (but without excessive force), which in turn pulls on the sciatic nerve. If the patient experiences pain running down the leg, then the test is positive.

- **Contralateral stretch test**. Elevate the asymptomatic leg; if pain is reproduced in the other leg the test is considered positive.

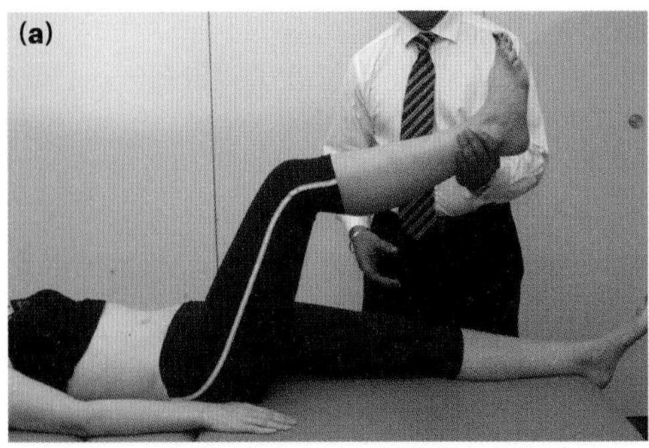

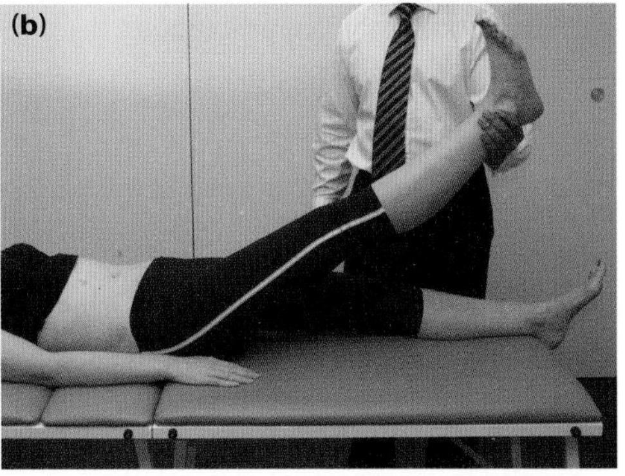

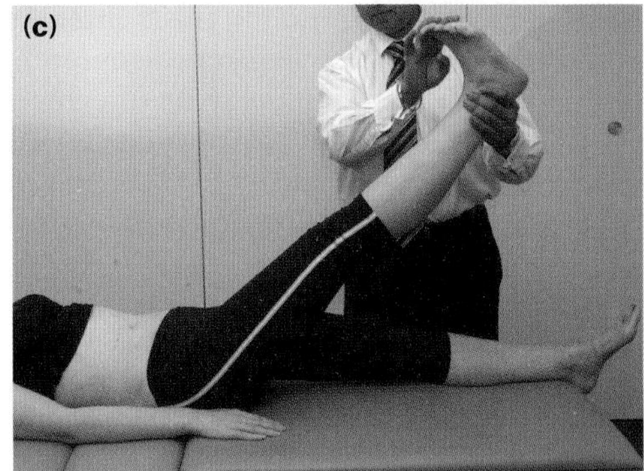

Figure 31.7(a-c) Lasègue's straight leg test.

Summary box 31.3

Spine examination

Inspection of the standing patient
- From the front and back (coronal plane)
- From the side (saggittal plane)
- Palpation
- Palpation of the posterior bony elements and the paraspinal muscles
- Move
- Assess flexion, extension, lateral rotation and bending

Neurological
- Assess sensation, tone, power, reflexes, proprioception and coordination

Special tests
- Spurling's test
- Forward bending test
- Lasègue's straight leg test
- Contralateral stretch test

CLINICAL EXAMINATION OF THE HAND AND WRIST

The hand and wrist should be thought of as one functional unit. The muscles may be divided into extrinsic (the muscle bellies in the forearm) and intrinsic (origins and insertions within the hand alone). The 'flexors' (volar side) flex the wrist and fingers and the 'extensors' (dorsal surface) extend the digits and fingers.

Look

Inspect the posture of both hands. A nerve lesion will produce a specific resting position (e.g. an ulnar nerve lesion will produce clawing of the little and ring fingers).

- **Skin**. Assess for scars, discolouration (café-au-lait spots, erythema) and loss of hair. The nails may reveal systemic disease (e.g. psoriatic pitting). Look for tight bands in the palm (Dupuytren's contracture). Loss of sweating is seen in complex regional pain syndrome.

- **Soft tissue**. Centrally located swellings at the wrist may indicate a ganglion arising from the wrist joint itself; de Quervain's tenosynovitis may present with a swelling around the radial styloid.
- **Muscle wasting**. Check for thenar, hypothenar (Figure 31.8) and intrinsic muscle wasting. To assess thenar eminence wasting, place the hands side by side with the thumbs upwards and look down and compare the thenar regions. Patterns of muscle wasting are shown in *Table 31.6*.
- **Bones**. Look for bony deformity (dinner fork deformity, Colles' fracture). Typical bony deformities are described in *Table 31.7*.

TABLE 31.6 Patterns of muscle wasting in the hand.

Thenar wasting	Median nerve palsy (C8)
Hypothenar wasting	Ulnar nerve palsy (T1)
Intrinsic wasting	Ulnar nerve palsy (T1)

(a)

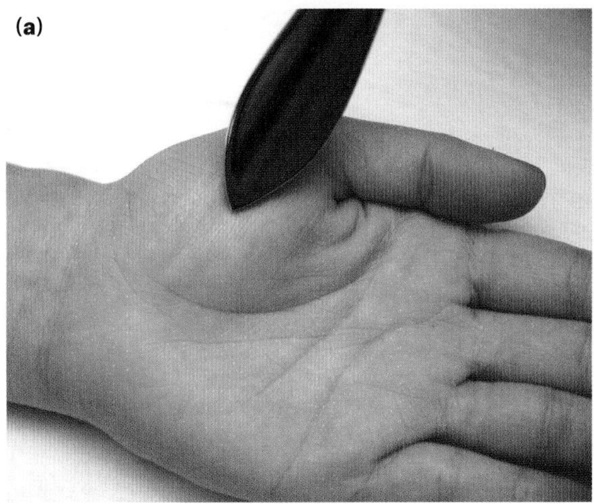

(b)

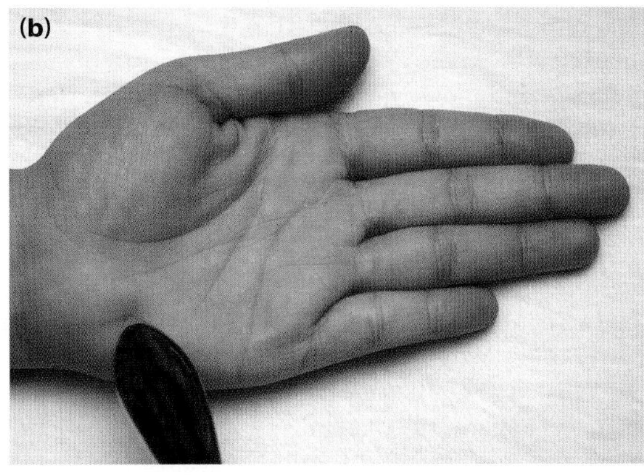

Figure 31.8 Thenar (a) and hypothenar (b) wasting.

TABLE 31.7 Bony deformities of the hand.

Anatomical site	Name	Association
Distal interphalangeal joint (DIPJ)	Heberden's nodes	Osteoarthritis
Proximal interphalangeal joint (PIPJ)	Bouchard's node	Osteoarthritis
Hyperextension of the metacarpophalangeal joint (MCPJ), flexion of the PIPJ and hyperextension of the DIPJ	Boutonnière deformity	Rheumatoid arthritis
Hyperextension of the MCPJ and PIPJ and flexion of the DIPJ	Swan neck deformity	Rheumatoid arthritis
Flexion of the MCPJ with hyperextension of the interphalangeal joint	Z deformity of the thumb	Rheumatoid arthritis
Subluxation of the MCPJ	Ulnar drift	Rheumatoid arthritis

Feel

- **Skin**. If there is any question of abnormal sensation on a simple stroke test comparing both sides, proceed to the two-point discrimination test using the sharp ends of a paper clip. Record the minimum distance between the tips of the paper clip at which the patient is able to recognise two points. *Table 31.8* describes the anatomical regions supplied by the median, ulnar and radial nerves.
  - *Pen sliding test*. To assess the absence or presence of sweating, slide a pen along the radial border of the index finger. If the pen slides smoothly, this may indicate loss of sweating.
- **Soft tissue**. Feel for muscle bulk and tendon thickening. Feel bony prominences, radial styloid, ulnar styloid, anatomical snuff box. Feel for sensation using two-point discrimination of medial nerve (radial aspect of index finger), radial nerve (in anatomical snuff box) and ulnar nerve (ulnar aspect of little finger).
  - *Blood vessels:* check the radial and ulnar artery pulses; assess the capillary refill time, which is normally less than 2 seconds; Allen's test should also be performed before surgery (*Table 31.9* and **Figure 31.9**).
  - *Nerves:* compressive neuropathies are most commonly seen affecting the median nerve (see Tinel's (**Figure 31.10a**) and Phalen's (**Figure 31.10b**) tests in *Table 31.9*).

TABLE 31.8 Sensory distribution of the nerve supply to the hand.

Nerve	Sensory distribution
Ulnar	Little finger and ulnar half of the ring finger
Median	Thumb, index, middle and radial half of the ring finger
Radial	Base of the thumb on the dorsum of the hand

Baron Guillaume Dupuytren, 1777–1835, surgeon, Hôtel Dieu, Paris, France, described the condition in 1831.
Friedrich Joseph de Quervain, 1868–1940, Professor of Surgery, Berne, Switzerland, described this form of tenosynovitis in 1895.
William Heberden (Snr.), 1710–1801, physician, practised first in Cambridge and later in London, UK.
Charles Jacques Bouchard, 1837–1915, physician, Dean of the Faculty of Medicine, Paris, France.
Boutonnière is French for 'button-hole'.

TABLE 31.9 Special hand tests.

Test	Technique	Significance
Allen's test	Elevate the hand and apply digital pressure on the radial and ulnar arteries to occlude them. Ask the patient to make a fist several times. The tips of the finger should go pale. Release each artery in turn and observe the return of colour	Tests the adequacy of the blood supply to the hand from the radial and ulnar arteries and the arcade between them
Tinel's test	Tap over the nerve of interest. Tingling may indicate nerve compression	Identifies compression of a peripheral nerve
Phalen's test	Place the wrist in maximum flexion with the elbows extended	Compression of the medial nerve causes paraesthesia
Froment's sign	Ask the patient to grip a sheet of paper between the index finger and thumb of both hands. Grip the paper yourself similarly. Ask the patient to resist as you attempt to pull the paper away	A positive test indicated by flexion of the thumb interphalangeal joint suggests weakness of the adductor pollicis muscle supplied by the ulnar nerve. Recruitment of the median nerve-innervated flexor pollicis brevis explains the thumb posture

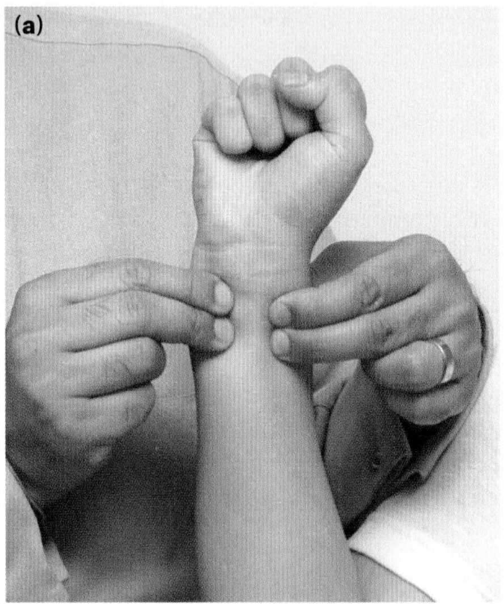

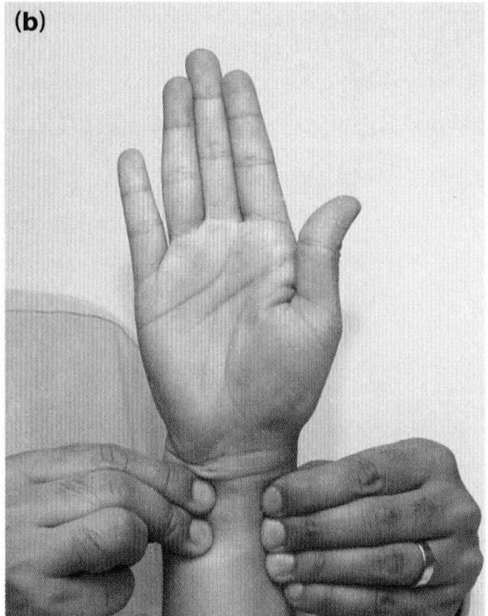

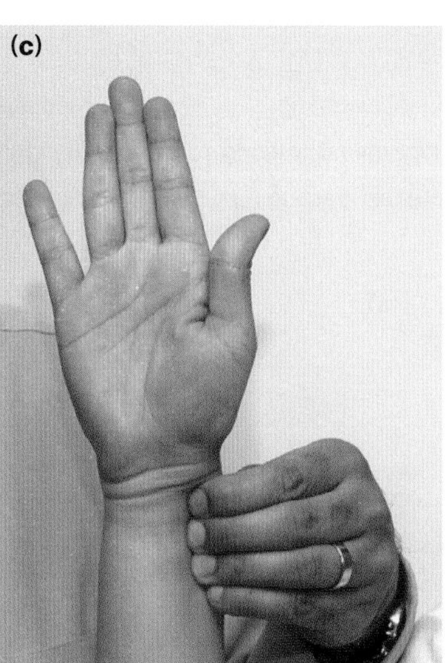

Figure 31.9 (a-c) Performing Allen's test.

- *Palmar fascia:* feel for palmar thickening and skin pits; long finger-like structures (cords), most commonly affecting the ring and little fingers, are suggestive of Dupuytren's disease.
- **Bones.** Palpate from the radial to the ulnar side of the wrist joint. In the trauma setting, palpate the anatomical snuff box (Figure 31.11). A fracture of the scaphoid may cause tenderness. The scaphoid tubercle, pisiform and the hook of hamate are all palpable on the volar aspect of the wrist.

Move

The wrist can be moved into flexion and extension, and ulnar and radial deviation.

- **Wrist.** Extension is tested by asking the patient to push the hands together into a 'prayer' position (Figure 31.12a). If there is loss of extension, the palms will not meet and/or one forearm will be dropped. Palmar flexion is tested in a similar fashion but with the hands pointing down and the back of the hands in contact (Figure 31.12b). Ulnar and radial deviation are tested by taking the patient's hand in your own and moving the hand into these directions.
- **Hand.** A general screening assessment is to ask the patient to roll up their fingers from full extension to full flexion. This will reveal a trigger finger.

Extensors and flexors

Asking the patient to grip two of your fingers in their fist tests the power of the extensors of the wrist (radial nerve) because they are needed to brace the wrist. It also tests the power of the flexors in the forearm (median nerve). Asking the patient then to extend and spread their fingers apart against resistance tests the intrinsic muscles of the hand (mainly the ulnar nerve).

Edgar van Nuys Allen, 1900–1961, Professor of Medicine, The Mayo Clinic, Rochester, MN, USA.
Jules Tinel, 1879–1952, Physician, Hôpital Beaujon, Paris, France.
George S Phalen, contemporary orthopaedic surgeon and Chief of Hand Surgery, The Cleveland Clinic, Cleveland, OH, USA. He helped to establish the American Society for Surgery of the Hand.
Jules Froment, 1878–1946, Professor of Clinical Medicine, Lyons, France.

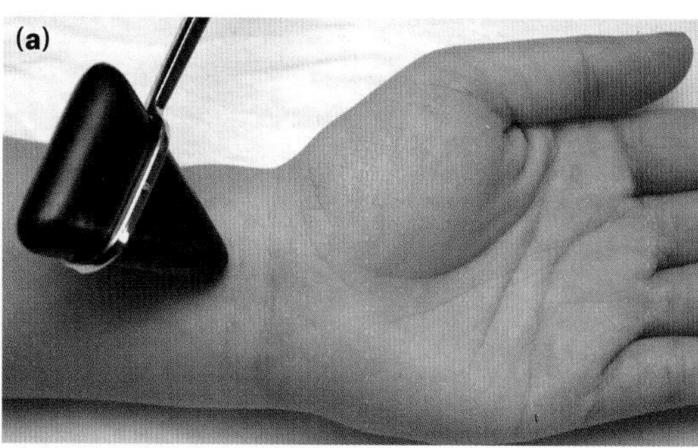
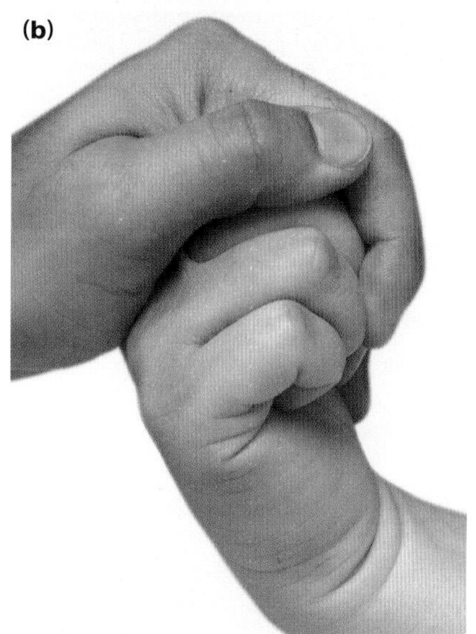

Figure 31.10 (a) Tinel's test; (b) Phalen's test.

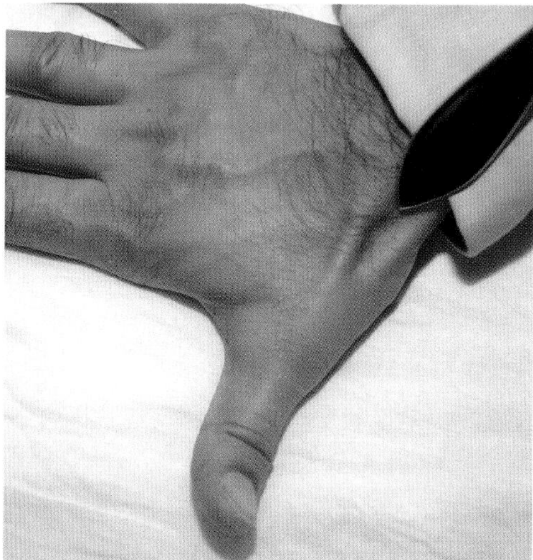

Figure 31.11 Palpating the anatomical snuff box between the tendons of extensor pollicis longus and abductor pollicis brevis.

Finger flexors

- **Superficialis tendon test**. The flexor digitorum profundus (FDP) usually has one muscle belly from which tendons to all of the fingers arise. The FDP can be immobilised by holding all of the fingers (except the one being examined) in extension; this allows the superficialis tendon to be tested in isolation. If the test finger is able to flex, despite profundus being immobilised, then the superficialis tendon to that finger is working. Repeat the test for the other fingers individually (Figure 31.13).

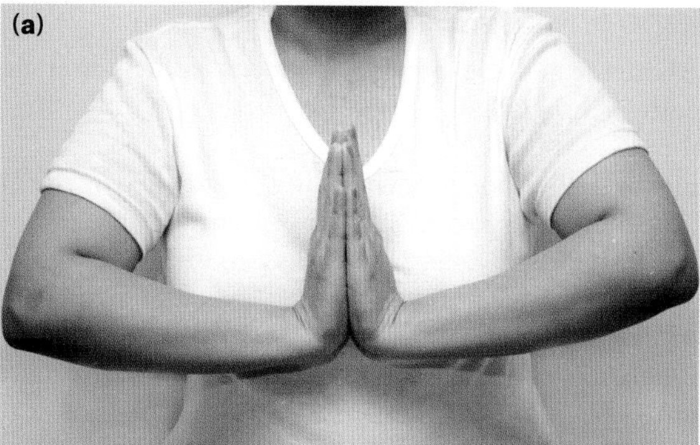
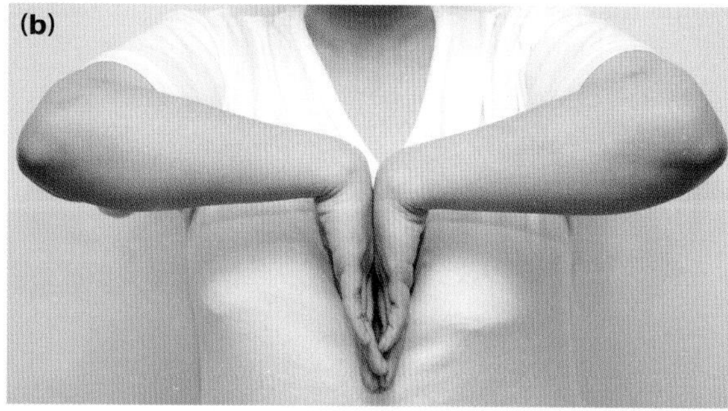

Figure 31.12 Testing the range of (a) wrist extension; (b) wrist flexion.

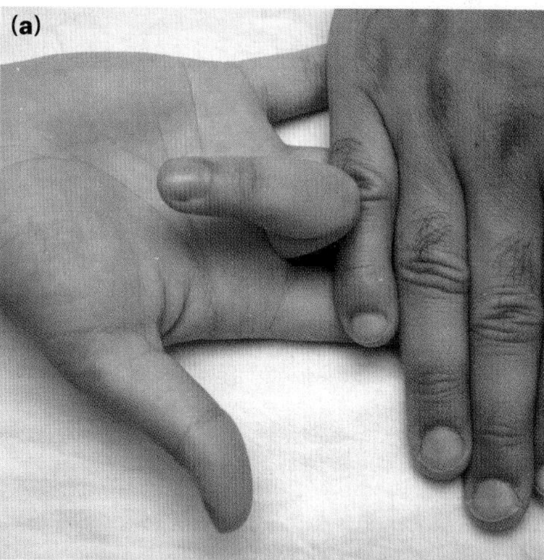
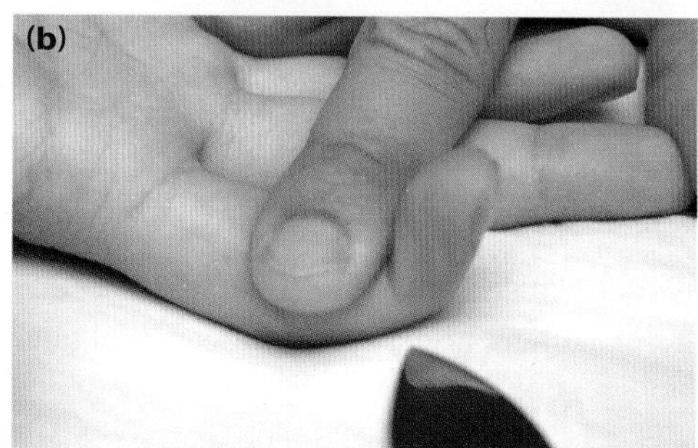

Figure 31.13 Testing the (a) flexor digitorum superficialis; (b) flexor digitorum profundus.

Thumb and thenar eminence

- **Abductor pollicis brevis, opponens pollicis and flexor pollicis brevis** can be tested together by opposing the thumb to the little finger.
- **Flexor pollicis longus.** The muscle is supplied by the anterior interosseus nerve (branch of the median nerve) and can be tested by asking the patient to bring the tips of the thumb and index finger together (the 'OK' sign – Figure 31.14).
- **Extensor pollicis longus.** The integrity of the tendon is tested by asking the patient to lift the thumb off a table with the palm flat on the table (Figure 31.15).
- **Adductor pollicis.** Test using Froment's sign (see *Table 31.9* and Figure 31.16).

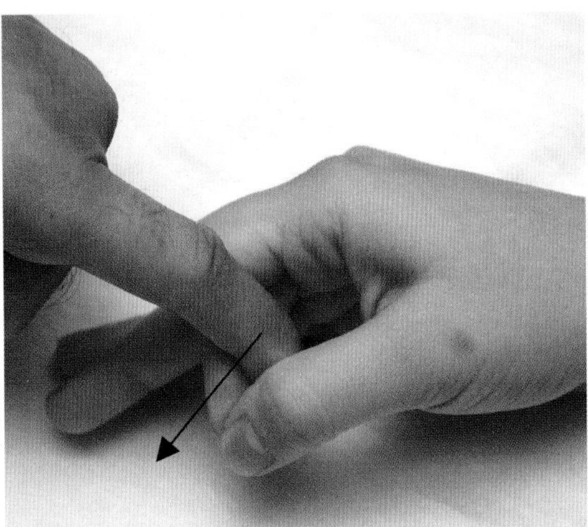

Figure 31.14 Test for flexor pollicis longus supplied by the anterior interosseus nerve.

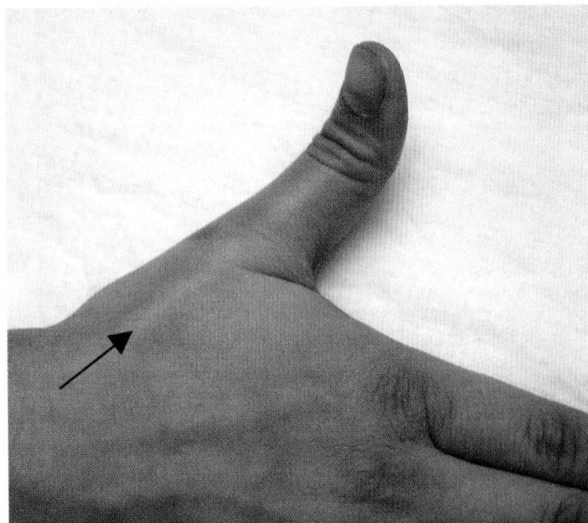

Figure 31.15 Testing the integrity of extensor pollicis longus.

- **Abductor pollicis brevis.** This muscle is supplied by the median nerve. With the hand lying flat on a table with the palm facing upwards, ask the patient to raise the thumb towards the ceiling. Ask the patient to resist as you push the thumb back towards the palm (Figure 31.17) .

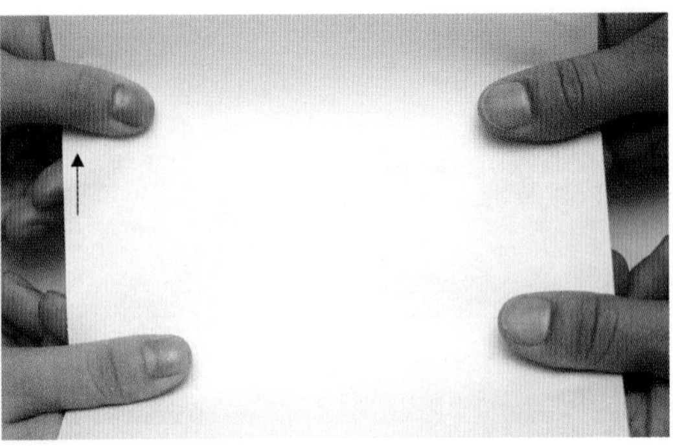

Figure 31.16 Froment's sign; the arrow illustrates the flexed posture of the thumb interphalangeal joint, indicating weakness of the ulnar nerve-innervated adductor pollicis muscle.

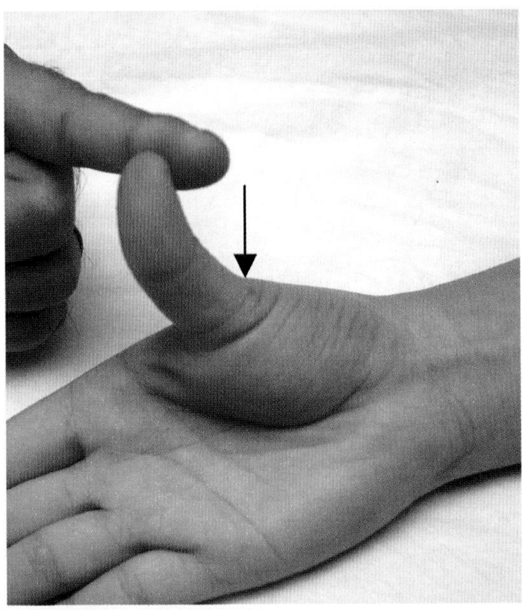

Figure 31.17 Testing the power of the abductor pollicis brevis supplied by the median nerve.

Summary box 31.4

Hand and wrist examination

Inspection of the standing patient

- Dorsum and palm – asymmetry, deformity, muscle wasting
- Inspection of the supine patient
- Skin, scars, soft tissues
- Palpation of bony structures and joints of the hand

Movements

- Wrist – flexion and extension, ulnar and radial deviation
- Hand – thumb movements, metatarsophalangeal joints and small joints of the hand

Special tests

- Allen's test
- Tinel's and Phalen's tests for the median nerve
- Froment's sign
- Finkelstein's test

CLINICAL EXAMINATION OF THE ELBOW

The elbow is a hinge joint formed by the articulation of the ulna and radius with the humerus.

Look

- **Skin**. Check the extensor surface for signs of psoriasis.
- **Soft tissues**. Look for any swellings, e.g. olecranon bursa, rheumatoid nodules, gouty tophi.
- **Muscle wasting**. Examine the biceps and triceps muscle bulk. Note that compression of the ulnar nerve at the elbow leads to wasting distally in the hypothenar eminence and intrinsic muscles of the hand – assess the hand for the presence of clawing and wasting.
- **Bone**. With the elbow in extension, look at the axis between the upper arm and forearm. There is a physiological valgus ('carrying angle') of 9–14° (2–3° greater in women) (Figure 31.18). This angle allows the elbow to be tucked into the waist depression above the iliac crest:
  - *cubitus varus* (gun-stock deformity): the carrying angle is reversed, secondary to a malunited supracondylar fracture;
  - *cubitus valgus:* the carrying angle is increased, caused by malunion of a distal humeral fracture;
  - *hyperextension:* there is normally a physiological hyperextension of the elbow (5°).

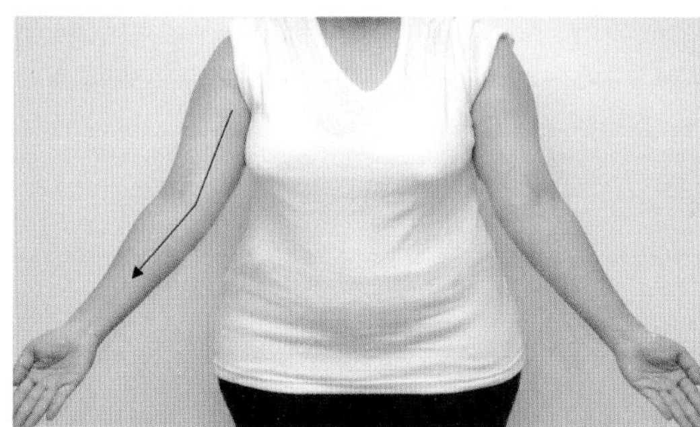

Figure 31.18 Carrying angle of the elbow illustrating the normal cubitus valgus.

Feel

- **Soft tissues**. An effusion may be detected by performing a cross fluctuation test. The ulnar nerve can be rolled under your fingers placed between the medial epicondyle and the olecranon. Test the distal sensation in the hand (especially in the distribution of the ulnar nerve) and assess the vascular status.
- **Bones**. The three palpation landmarks are the medial and lateral epicondyles and the apex of the olecranon. These form an equilateral triangle when the elbow is flexed to 90°. The radial head is palpated with the examiner's thumb while the other hand pronates and supinates the forearm. On the medial side, palpate the medial epicondyle. Posteriorly, palpate the olecranon fossa.

Move

- **Flexion–extension**. The normal range is from −5° (slight hyperextension) to 150°. Ask the patient to bend the elbow from the fully straight position (Figure 31.19).
- **Pronation and supination.** With the elbows at 90° and the palms facing upwards (full supination), ask the patient to turn the forearm so that the dorsum of the hand faces upwards (full pronation) (Figure 31.20). The normal values are 70° pronation and 90° supination.

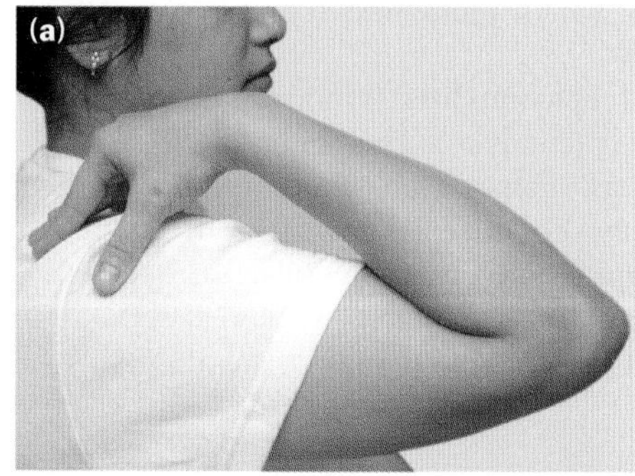

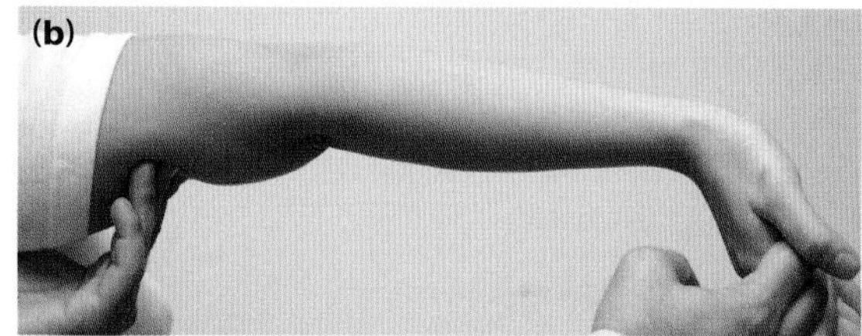

Figure 31.19 (a) Elbow flexion; (b) elbow extension.

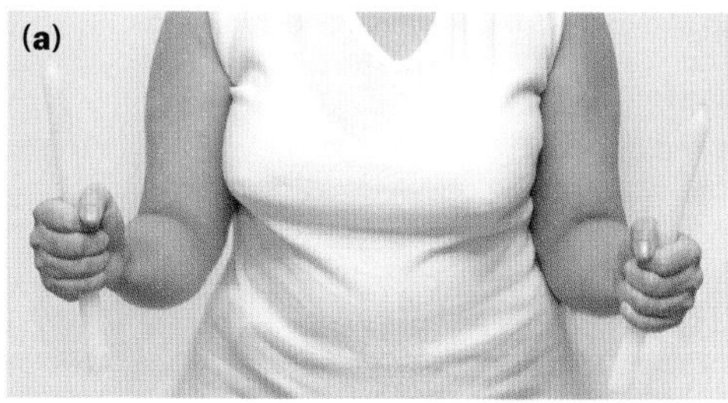

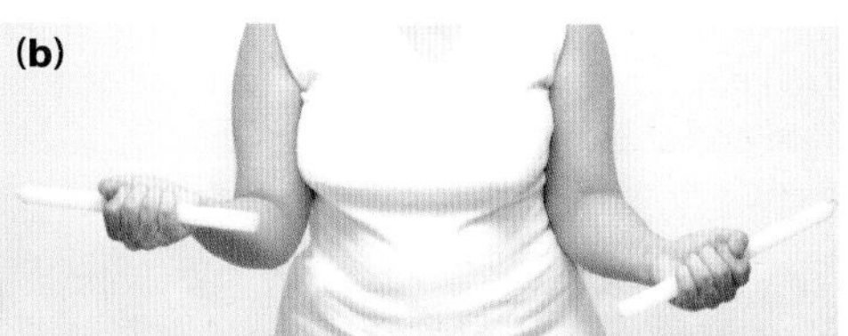

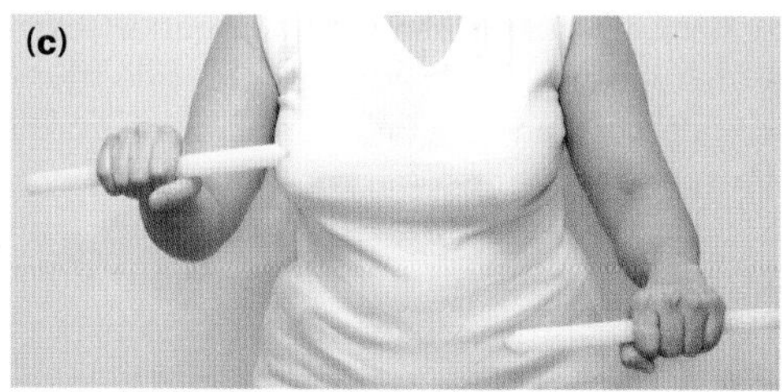

Figure 31.20 Testing forearm rotation: (a) mid-prone position; (b) full supination; (c) full pronation.

Special tests and diagnoses

Tennis elbow and golfer's elbow

Both conditions are inflammatory processes of the tendons that attach the large muscle mass of the forearm to the lateral or medial epicondyle.

- **Medial epicondylitis** (synonym = golfer's elbow). The medial epicondyle is the common origin of the forearm flexors and the pronator muscle. Palpate the medial epicondyle for tenderness. The diagnostic test is resisted wrist flexion, which reproduces the pain over the medial epicondyle.
- **Lateral epicondylitis** (synonym = tennis elbow). The lateral epicondyle is the common origin of the forearm extensors. Palpate for tenderness – usually just distal (5–10 mm) to the epicondyle near the origin of the extensor carpi radialis brevis muscle. Wrist extension against resistance with the elbow extended should provoke the patient's symptoms.

Summary box 31.5

Elbow examination

Inspection of the standing patient

- Front – asymmetry, carrying angle, deformity
- Back – olecranon fossa

Inspection of the supine patient

- Skin, scars, soft tissues, deformity
- Palpation of bony structures

Movements

- Flexion and extension, pronation and supination

Special tests

- Tennis and golfer's elbow

CLINICAL EXAMINATION OF THE SHOULDER

Pain arising from the shoulder joint may be felt anterolaterally. Referred pain may present from the cervical spine, heart, mediastinum and the diaphragm.

Look

Assess the attitude of the limb.

- **Skin**. Check for surgical scars. An anterior scar is used for the deltopectoral approach. At the side, the deltoid splitting approach and lateral arthroscopic portals may be seen. Posteriorly, arthroscopic portal sites can be seen.
- **Soft tissues**. Wasting of the deltoid muscle is commonly seen after shoulder dislocation when there is a temporary loss of function of the axillary nerve that supplies it. The rotator cuff comprises four muscles: supraspinatus, infraspinatus, subscapularis and teres minor. Wasting of these muscles may occur following a rotator cuff problem.
- **Bone**. Look for any obvious deformity or prominence. A fracture of the middle third clavicle is the most common cause. A dislocation may be suspected by a loss of normal shoulder contour. The more common anterior dislocation often presents with an anterior bulge and a squared-off shoulder.

Feel

Generalised pain in the shoulder may arise from the neck or the shoulder joint itself. More localised pain is often indicative of acromioclavicular joint pathology.

- **Skin**. Test sensation in the upper part of the lateral aspect of the arm ('regimental badge area') (Figure 31.21). Loss may indicate damage to the axillary nerve (following shoulder dislocation).
- **Bones**. Palpate the acromioclavicular and sternoclavicular joints and the clavicle.

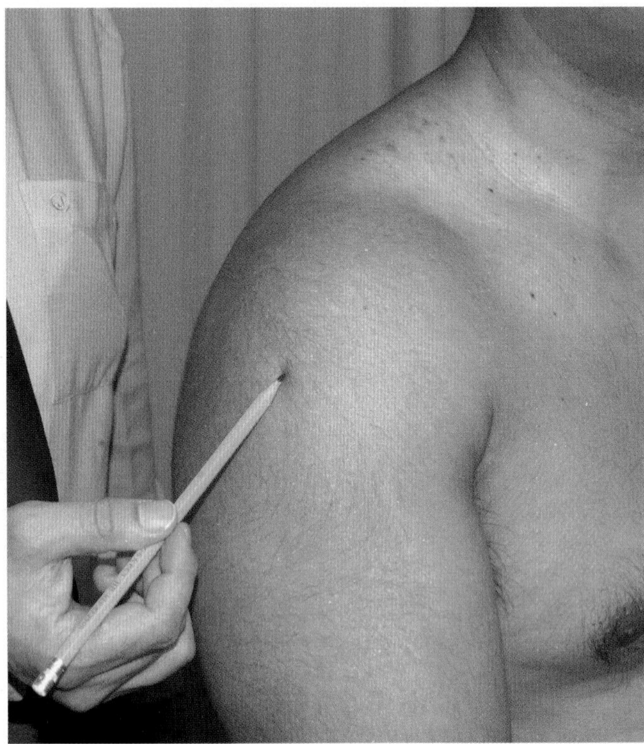

Figure 31.21 The area of skin supplied by the axillary nerve – the 'regimental badge area'.

Move

Differentiate between movements of the shoulder joint and scapulothoracic movement of the scapula on the chest wall. Patients with a painful shoulder will commonly move from the scapulothoracic joint. Stabilise the scapula by placing the thumb over the coracoid process and the fingers of the same hand over the spine of the scapula. Start in the 'neutral position' with the arms by the sides, elbows extended and the palms facing forwards. Note any pain throughout the range of movement (Figure 31.22).

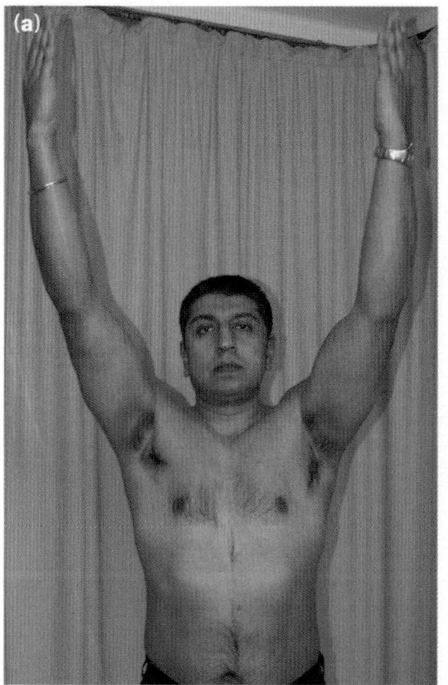
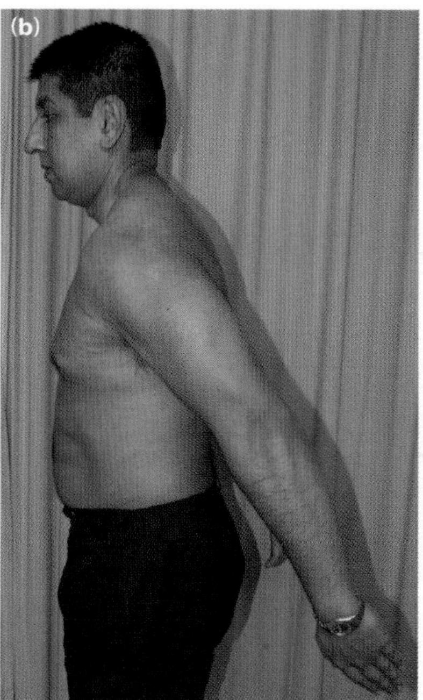
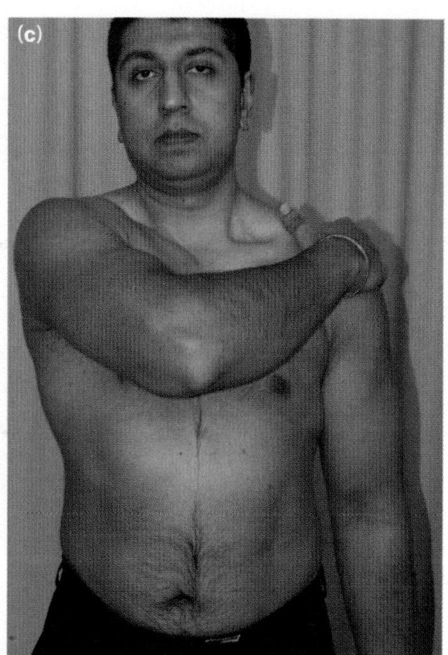
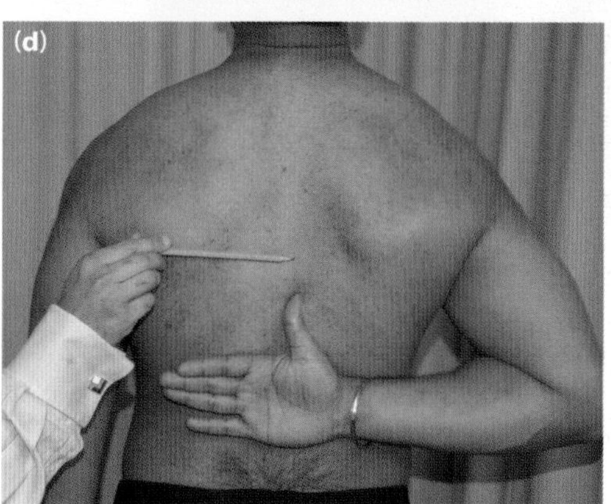
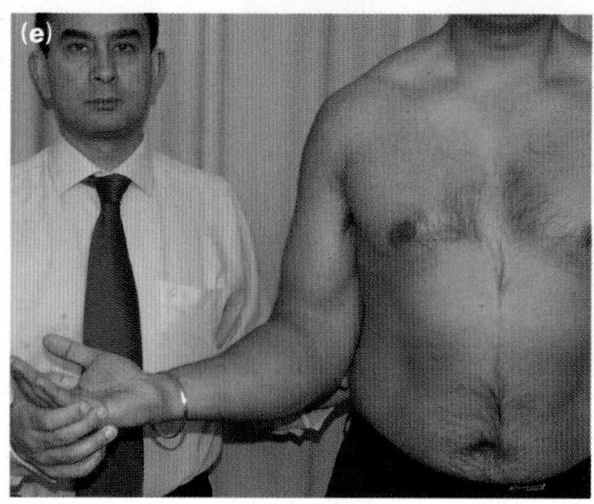

Figure 31.22 Movements of the shoulder: (**a**) forward flexion; (**b**) extension; (**c**) adduction; (**d**) internal rotation; (**e**) external rotation.

- **Forward flexion**. Ask the patient to raise their hands in front to touch the ceiling while keeping the elbows extended (0–180°).
- **Extension**. Ask the patient to extend both arms behind (0–30°).
- **Abduction**. Shoulder abduction involves the glenohumeral joint and scapulothoracic movement. The first 60° of movement is mainly at the glenohumeral joint. Beyond this the scapula begins to rotate on the thorax and final movements are almost entirely scapulothoracic. Raise the arms sideways until the fingers point to the ceiling (180°).
- **Adduction**. Ask the patient to touch their other shoulder tip.
- **Internal rotation**. Ask the patient to touch their back with the dorsum of the hand and to raise their hand up the back as high as possible (normal range is thoracic spine level T7–9).
- **External rotation**. With the arms by the sides, bend the elbows to 90° and rotate the forearms to the mid-prone position. Ask the patient to separate their hands as much as possible (0–40°).

Special tests and diagnoses

Impingement syndrome

This is impairment of rotator cuff function within the subacromial bursa. It may lead to inflammation (tendinitis) or a partial or full-thickness tear. Impingement is characterised by pain and weakness on abduction and internal rotation.

- **Painful arc test** (Figure 31.23). Ask the patient to abduct their arms from their sides. The presence of pain from 60° to 120° is positive.
- **Jobe's test** (empty can) (**Figure 31.24**). Ask the patient to abduct the arm to 90° elevation in the scapular plane with full internal rotation (empty can position). Ask the patient to resist downward pressure. The presence of pain is a positive test.

Shoulder instability

Instability may be defined as a shoulder that slips in and out of joint (dislocation) more than once or twice, or frequently slips partially out of joint and then returns on its own. Instability can be anterior, posterior, inferior or multidirectional.

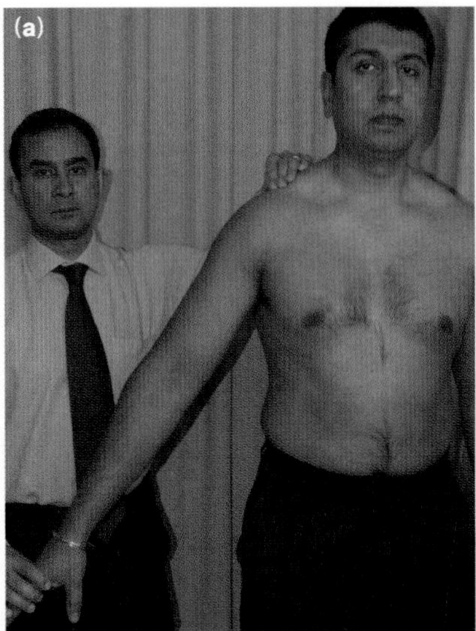

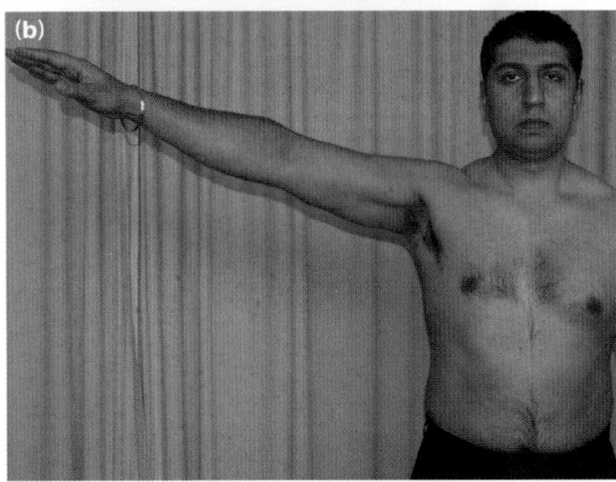

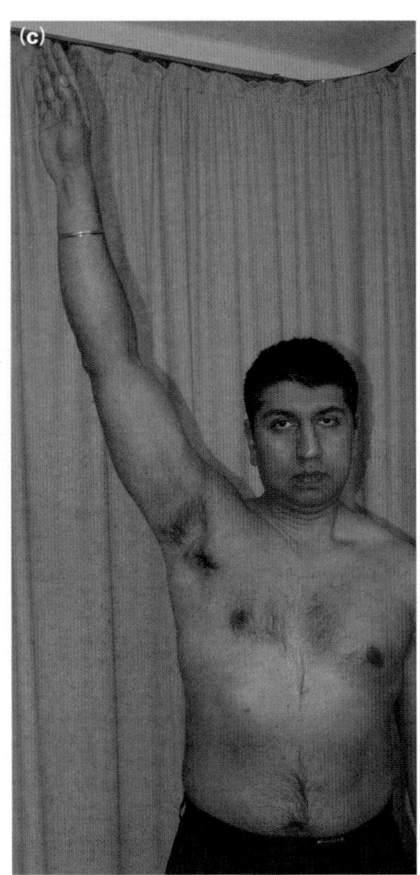

Figure 31.23 (a-c) Painful arc test for rotator cuff impingement.

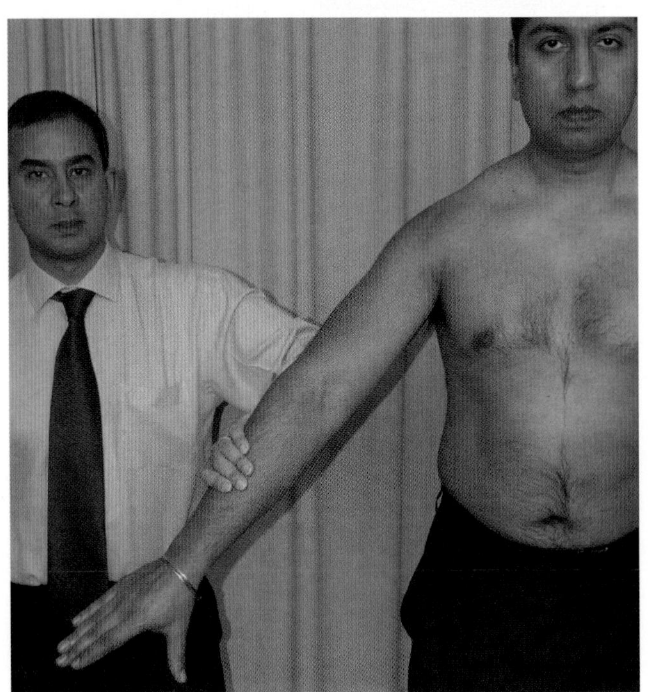

Figure 31.24 Jobe's test for rotator cuff impingement.

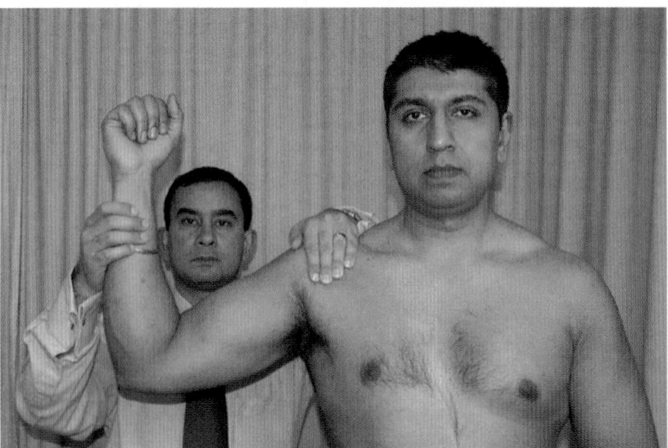

Figure 31.25 Anterior apprehension test for anterior shoulder instability.

- **Apprehension test** (Figure 31.25). With the patient supine or standing, flex the elbow to 90° and abduct the shoulder to 90°. Now externally rotate the shoulder. Apprehension indicates anterior instability.

Summary box 31.6

Shoulder examination

Inspection of the standing patient
- Front – asymmetry, deformity
- Side – muscle wasting
- Back – muscle wasting, scapula

Inspection of the supine patient
- Skin, scars, soft tissues, deformity
- Palpation of shoulder girdle (sternum to scapula)

Movements
- Flexion and extension, abduction and adduction, internal and external rotation

Special tests
- Impingement syndrome – painful arc, Jobe's test, Hawkins' test (see also Chapter 34)
- Shoulder instability – apprehension, relocation test, sulcus sign
- Rotator cuff assessment
- Acromioclavicular joint pathology
- Frozen shoulder versus glenohumeral osteoarthritis

CLINICAL EXAMINATION OF THE HIP JOINT

The hip is a synovium-lined ball and socket joint. Typical clinical diseases of the hip that may be encountered in children and adults are shown in *Table 31.10*. A patient complaining of hip pain should undergo a careful examination of the spine, abdomen, pelvis, groin and thigh. In addition, consider a gynaecological examination in women.

TABLE 31.10 Common clinical diseases of the hip in children and adults.

Children	Adults
Developmental dysplasia of the hip	Primary osteoarthritis
Transient synovitis of the hip	Secondary osteoarthritis
Perthe's disease	Inflammatory arthritis
Septic arthritis and osteomyelitis	Avascular necrosis
Slipped capital femoral epiphysis	Labral tears
Juvenile idiopathic arthritis	Referred pain

Look

With the patient standing, look at the front, side and back of the hip. Look around the room for walking aids and heel raises in the shoes.

- **Skin**. Look for scars and sinuses.
- **Soft tissues**. Muscle wasting may be present as a consequence of hip arthritis or primary muscle or neurological disease.
- **Bone**. Look at the posture of the limb and assess for adduction deformity; fixed adduction may be present in severe osteoarthritis and cerebral palsy, and makes the leg appear short because the pelvis is tilted (apparent shortening).

Feel

- **Soft tissues**. Tenderness overlying the greater trochanter may suggest trochanteric bursitis or an abductor enthesopathy.
- **Bone**. Bony landmarks can be palpated; these include the anterior superior iliac spine (ASIS), iliac crest and the greater trochanter of the femur.

Other areas for palpation include the inguinal ligament, which may have a local hernia or lymphadenopathy. The femoral artery can be palpated as it passes under the inguinal ligament at its midpoint halfway between the ASIS and the pubic tubercle.

Move

The hip joint can be moved into flexion, extension, abduction and adduction, and internal and external rotation (Figure 31.26). True hip movement ends when the pelvis begins to move. To detect true hip movement, simultaneously place a finger/hand on the anterior superior iliac spine (ASIS) contralateral to the hip being examined. Remember to compare both sides.

Passive movement

HIP FLEXION (120–0°) WHEN LYING SUPINE

The patient is asked to lie on their back and then roll themselves into a ball, flexing the hips and the spine fully. A comparison of the flexion of the two hips can be made in this position. The patient is then asked to hold onto the knee of the 'bad' leg with both hands (thereby fixing the pelvis in flexion) and the other leg is allowed to extend down onto the couch. A note is made of any fixed flexion deformity (inability of the thigh to come down onto the couch). This 'good' hip is then returned to full flexion and the patient grasps that knee while dropping the other, 'bad', hip into extension. This modified Thomas's test is the most comfortable and accurate way of measuring flexion and extension of the hip, minimising movement of the painful hip (Figure 31.27).

HIP EXTENSION (0–10°) WHEN LYING IN A PRONE POSITION

Hip extension can be measured by asking the patient to roll onto their front and extend the hip.

ROTATION

- **Internal rotation (45°)**. With the hip flexed to 45° and the knee in 90° of flexion, hold the front of the knee with one hand and the foot with the other. Internally rotate the hip (the foot goes outwards), then externally rotate

Hugh Owen Thomas, 1834–1891, general practitioner, Liverpool, UK. He is regarded as the founder of orthopaedic surgery although never holding a hospital appointment, preferring to treat patients in their own homes. He introduced the Thomas splint in 1875.

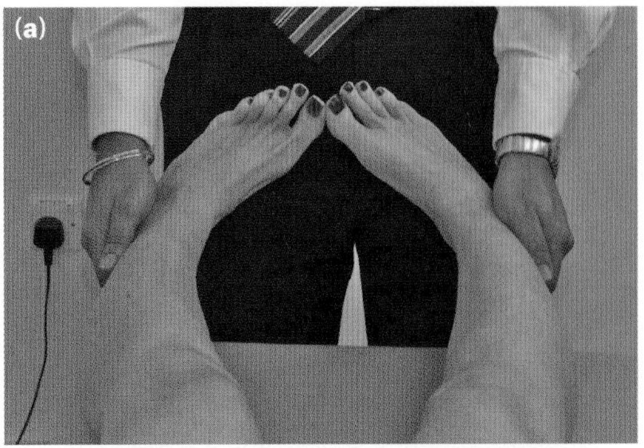

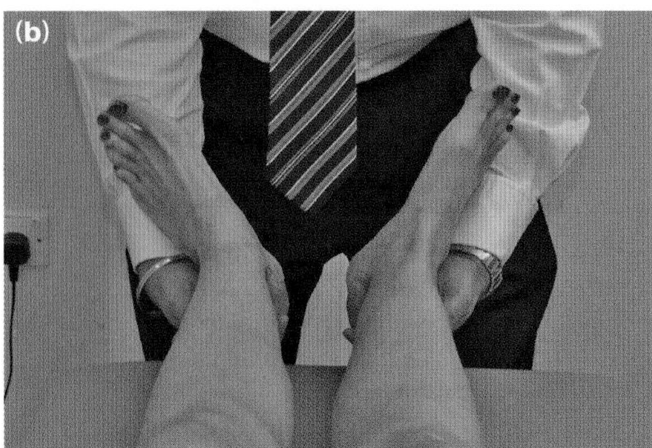

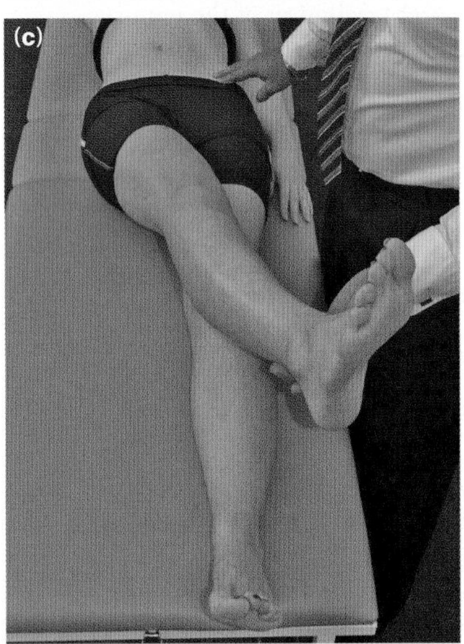

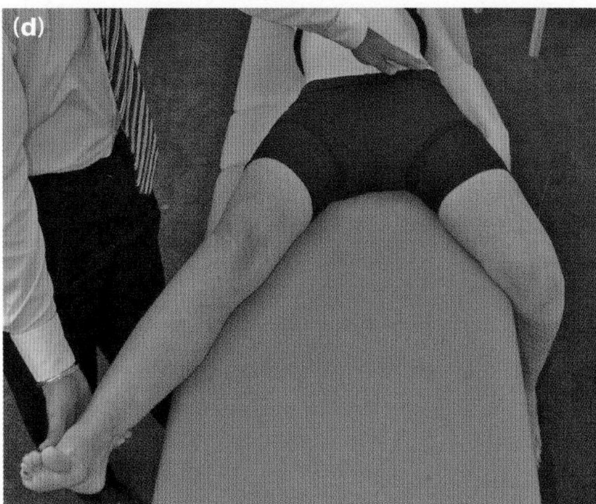

Figure 31.26 Hip movements: (**a**) internal rotation; (**b**) external rotation; (**c**) adduction; (**d**) abduction.

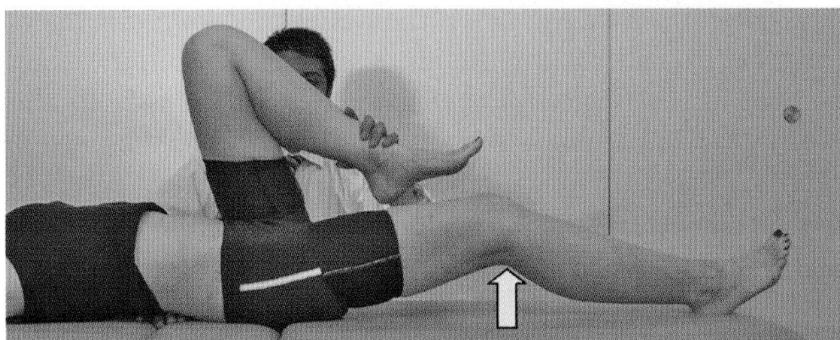

Figure 31.27 Modified Thomas's test for assessing a fixed flexion deformity. A fixed flexion deformity of the right hip is indicated by an inability to fully straighten the right leg (arrow).

the hip (the foot goes in). The angle that the tibia makes with the vertical indicates the range of movement. Pain at the extremes of movement suggests inflammation in the hip.

- **Abduction (40°)**. The hip should be abducted by moving the leg away from the midline with the other hand on the patient's pelvis to detect any tilt in the pelvis.

Special tests

- **Trendelenburg test** (Figure 31.28). Face the patient and ask them to place their hands on the palm of your hands for support. Then ask them to stand first on one leg, then the other. Increased pressure from the opposite hand as they take weight through the weak hip indicates a positive Trendelenburg test.
- **Leg length discrepancy (LLD)**. The inequality may be in the hip joint, femur, tibia, ankle or foot or a combination of these. The pathology may be from the bone being too short or too long. When assessing LLD, square the pelvis. If that is not possible then place both legs in the same position. For example, if there is an adduction deformity present in the affected leg, place the good leg in the same degree of adduction. LLD can be caused by a real difference in the leg lengths (the bones are different lengths) or by a deformity that makes the leg appear short because the pelvis must be tilted to get the leg onto the ground. The first is called 'real' LLD, measured ASIS to medial malleolus. The second is called 'apparent' LLD, measured midline, e.g. xiphisternum to medial malleolus. Each differs in

Summary box 31.7

Common causes of limb length inequality in the hip

- Osteoarthritis
- Hip fracture
- Hip dislocation
- Hip dysplasia
- Avascular necrosis
- Fixed flexion deformity

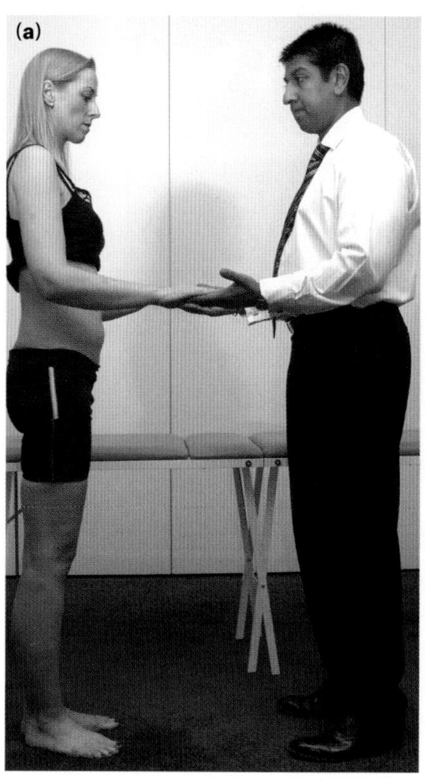

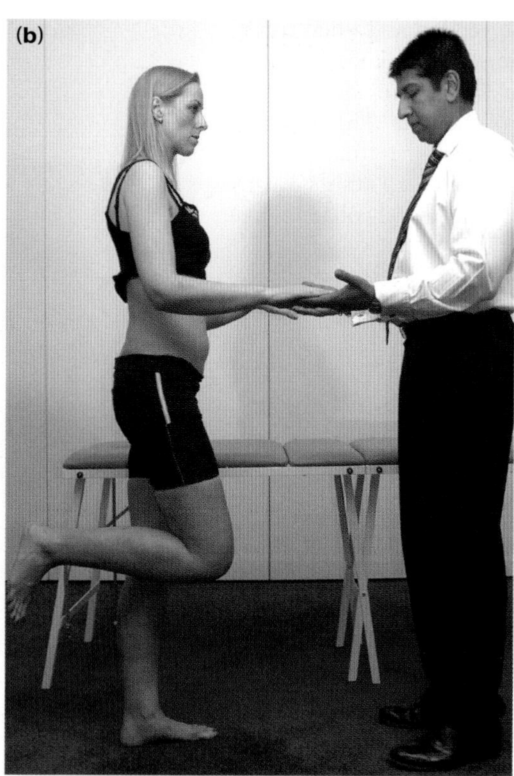

Figure 31.28 (**a, b**) Trendelenburg test.

cause and therefore treatment. The LLD apparent to the patient can also be measured using wooden blocks placed under the patient's 'short' leg until the patient feels level.

- **Gait**. Hip disease can present with an altered gait pattern. The common types of abnormal gait are described in *Table 31.11* (also see *Summary box 31.8*).
- **Impingement test**. To assess for femoroacetabular impingement, perform two tests: first, hip flexion at greater than 90° combined with some adduction and internal rotation (FADIR test). The second test is placing the hip into flexion, full adduction and internal rotation. A positive test is indicated by pain.

TABLE 31.11 Common limps observed in hip disease.

Gait pattern	Description
Weak: Trendelenburg	May lead to pelvic sway or tilt. The patient swings the body over the weak hip to stay in balance when it is weight bearing
Painful: antalgic	The rhythm is dot–dash, with a short period spent on the painful limb
Unbalanced: broad-based	May be caused by ataxia, e.g. cerebellar pathology. The rhythm also tends to be disordered
Loss of muscle control: high-stepping	May be due to loss of proprioception or a drop foot. This leads to difficulty in clearing the toes during the swing phase: the patient compensates by externally rotating the leg and flexing the hip and knee
Deformity: in-toeing	Can be caused by persistent femoral anteversion. The foot may catch on the back of the calf of the weight-bearing leg, tripping the patient

Summary box 31.8

Hip examination

Inspection of the standing patient

- Front – pelvic tilt, rotational deformity
- Side – lumbar lordosis
- Back – pelvic tilt, scoliosis, gluteal wasting
- Gait – Trendelenburg, antalgic

Inspection of the supine patient

- Skin, scars, soft tissues, deformity
- Palpation of the anterior joint line, adductor origin, greater trochanter, ischial tuberosity

Movements

- Flexion and extension
- Abduction and adduction
- Internal and external rotation

Special tests

- Thomas's test
- Leg length assessment – real/apparent
- Trendelenburg test
- Snapping hip
- Impingement tests

CLINICAL EXAMINATION OF THE KNEE

The knee is a synovial hinged joint. There are three compartments: medial, lateral and patellofemoral. The quadriceps,

quadriceps tendon, patella, patellar tendon and tibial tuberosity comprise the extensor mechanism of the knee.

The anterior cruciate ligament (ACL) provides primary restraint to anterior displacement of the tibia. The posterior cruciate ligament (PCL) provides posterior restraint of the tibia. The medial collateral ligament (MCL) resists valgus and external rotation forces whereas the lateral collateral ligament (LCL) resists varus forces.

Look

Look at the front, sides and back of both knees and for any walking or mobility aids or external appliances.

- **Skin**. Check for scars.
- **Soft tissues**. Look for wasting of the quadriceps and swelling in front of and behind the knee.
- **Bone**. Look for overall alignment (varus or valgus deformity). Measure the intermalleolar distance if a valgus deformity is present. With varus deformity, measure the distance between the medial aspects of the knees. From the side of the knee, look for fixed flexion or recurvatum hyperextension).

Gait

Look for antalgic gait (osteoarthritis) and varus thrust (collapse of the knee into more varus as weight is taken on that leg).

Feel

- **Soft tissue**. Feel the tendons for quadriceps and patellar tendon rupture.
- **Fluid displacement or stroke test**. First empty the medial side of the knee by stroking any fluid up from the medial side into the suprapatellar pouch. Then place your hand on the superior aspect of the suprapatellar pouch and move it inferiorly, attempting to displace any fluid into the knee joint. Maintain your hand at the level of the superior pole of the patella. Now look to see whether the normal gutters on either side of the knee are less noticeable because of fluid distension. Stroke the back of your hand over each gutter in turn. Look at the opposite gutter to see if there is cross-filling.
- **Patellar tap test**. This test is used when a large effusion is present. Place one hand on either side of the patella and, with the other hand, push down on the patella. With an effusion, fluctuance is present as the patella moves towards the joint.
- **Bone**. Feel the tibial tuberosity, inferior pole of the patella, patellar facets, origin and insertion of the knee ligaments and joint line (medial and lateral). Remember to palpate for any popliteal swellings. Note the height of the patella.

Move

The knee moves principally in flexion (0–135°) and extension (from 0 to −10°) (**Figure 31.29**). Assess hyperextension by placing one of your hands on the anterior aspect of the distal femur. Now lift the distal tibia with the other hand. Measure the angle or the height that the heel can be lifted off the couch before the knee starts to move.

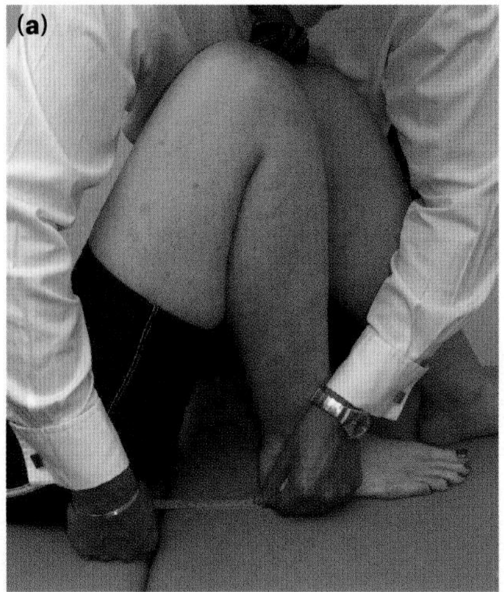

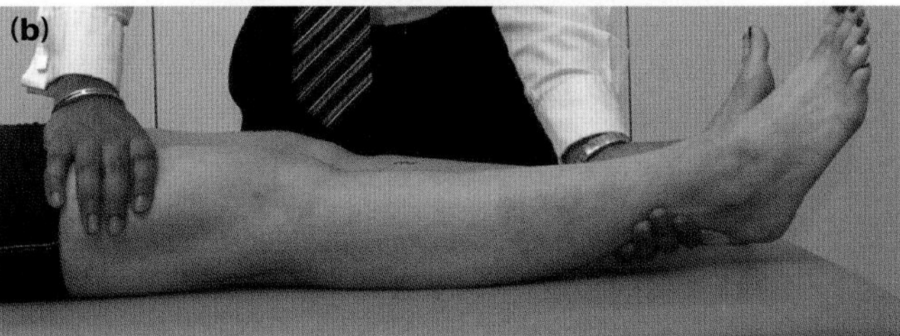

Figure 31.29 (**a**) Knee flexion and (**b**) extension.

Perform a lag test to assess the integrity of the extensor mechanism. The patient is asked to lift the whole leg up off the bed (10°) with the knee straight. They are then asked to bend the knee and then try to straighten it again with the leg still held in the air. If they are unable to re-straighten the knee they have a positive lag. This indicates significant weakness of the quadriceps mechanism.

In the presence of an apparent fixed flexion deformity of the knee (seen in osteoarthritis), decide whether this is arising from the knee or the hip joint. To differentiate, sit the patient up with the knees hanging over the edge of the couch; this obliterates the effect of any hip flexion deformity. Passively try to extend the knee fully. With a flexion deformity of the knee, this is not possible.

Special tests

Collateral ligaments

To assess the ligaments, place the leg under your arm. Flex the knee to 10° (not more) to relax the posterior capsule (the MCL and LCL are taut in full extension and lax in flexion). Stress each ligament in turn by applying a valgus or varus force. With your index fingers simultaneously palpate over the collateral ligaments. Assess for signs of instability (excessive opening of the joint). The quality of the end point should be noted (is it firm or spongy?). Compare both sides (**Figure 31.30**).

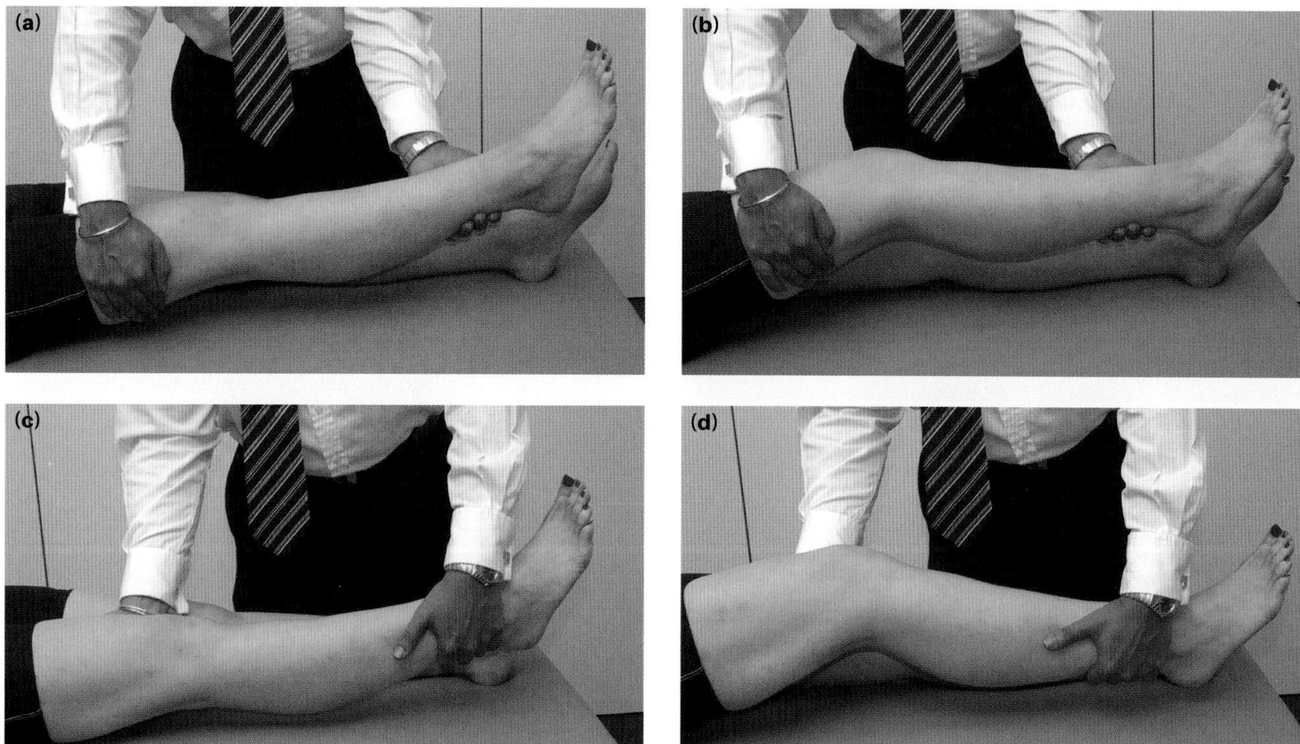

Figure 31.30 Assessing the medial (a, b) and lateral (c, d) collateral ligaments.

- **Medial collateral ligament**. A lax MCL or deficient lateral compartment may cause knee instability when applying a valgus stress. It is important to note that the valgus stress test should be applied with the knee in 30° of flexion. Valgus instability in full extension (0°) should alert you to a possible posterior structure injury (e.g. posterior capsule, posterior cruciate ligament).
- **Lateral collateral ligament**. A lax LCL or deficient medial compartment may cause knee instability when applying a varus stress in 10° of flexion. Instability in full extension (0°) suggests injury to the posterior structures. In a suspected lateral injury, evaluation of the peroneal nerve must be performed.

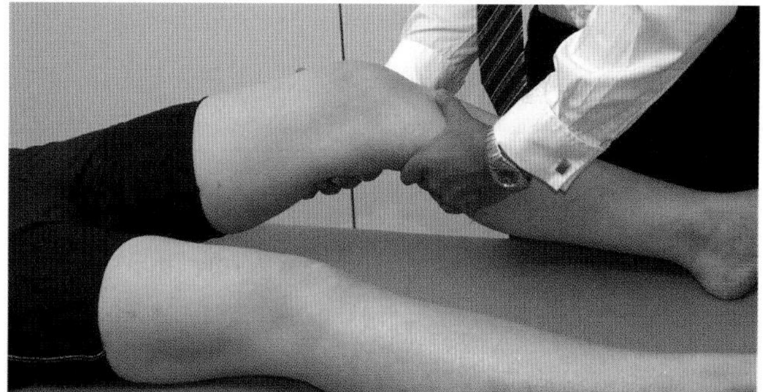

Figure 31.31 Lachmann's test: flex the knee to 15–30° and pull the proximal tibia forwards.

Anterior cruciate ligament

The most sensitive test for evaluation of the ACL is the Lachmann test.

- **The Lachmann test** (Figure 31.31). Flex the knee to 15–30° and pull the proximal tibia gently forwards. Excessive laxity may indicate rupture of the ACL. Anterior translation of the tibia associated with a soft or no end point is a positive test. The test may be negative in chronic ruptures because the ACL stump can scar to the PCL.
- **Anterior draw test** (Figure 31.32a). Flex both knees to 90° and look for a posterior sag (compare the height of the tibial tuberosities looking from the side). This may indicate an injury to the PCL. Stabilise the feet by sitting on them. Now place your hands around the proximal and posterior aspect of the tibia. With your index fingers, push up the hamstrings to encourage them to relax. Now draw the tibia gently forwards and measure any laxity, comparing it with the other knee. The degree of laxity can be graded: grade I (0–5 mm), grade II (5–10 mm) and grade III (>10 mm).

Posterior cruciate ligament

The PCL is the primary restraint to posterior tibial translation between 30 and 90° of knee flexion. At 90°, the PCL accepts 95% by the degree of posterior translation of the tibia with the knee in 90° of flexion. Look for a posterior sag with the knees flexed to 90°. The posterior draw test is the most reliable clinical test for a PCL injury.

- **Posterior draw test** (Figure 31.32b). Perform the test with the knee flexed to 90°. Push the anterior aspect of

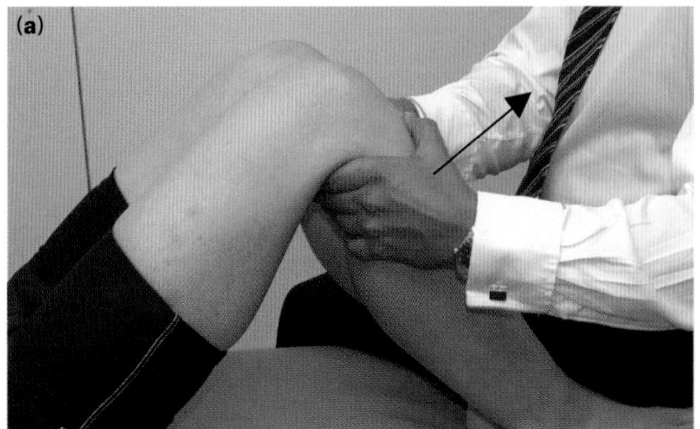

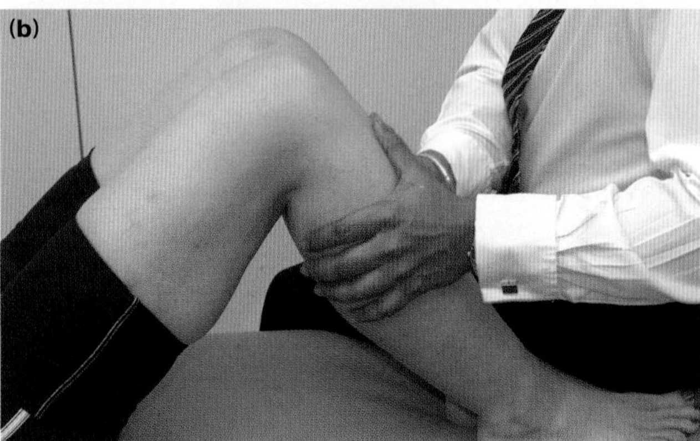

Figure 31.32 **(a)** Anterior draw test for anterior cruciate ligament stability; **(b)** posterior draw test for posterior cruciate ligament stability.

the proximal tibia posteriorly and compare any laxity with the other side. If more than 10 mm of posterior tibial translation is noted at 30 and/or 90° of knee flexion, a combined PCL and posterolateral corner injury may be present. An evaluation of the competency of the posterolateral corner is necessary.

Menisci

The presence of palpable joint line tenderness is the most sensitive clinical examination test for a meniscal tear. Flex the knee to 90° and palpate the joint line using your thumb and index finger. Note any areas of tenderness. Tests for meniscal damage are not very reliable but, combined with a history of mechanical symptoms, locking, catching and pain, may be helpful. With posterior medial meniscal tears patients suffer pain on high flexion or squatting. The well-known test for meniscal tears is McMurray's test. The patient lies supine with their knee flexed to 45° and hip flexed to 45°. The examiner braces the lower leg: one hand holds the ankle; the other hand holds the knee. For assessment of the medial meniscus, palpate the medial joint line with knee flexed. A 'click' may be felt suggesting meniscus relocation. A valgus stress is applied to the flexed knee. Externally rotate the leg (toes point outward), and slowly extend the knee while it is still in valgus.

Patellofemoral joint

The patella normally enters the trochlea from a lateral position and becomes centralised with increasing knee flexion, travelling in a 'J' pattern.

- **Patellar tracking** (Figure 31.33). Sit the patient and ask them to let their legs hang off the end of the couch with the knees flexed to 90°. Ask the patient to extend the knee slowly to full extension. Towards the end of extension, look for lateral subluxation of the patella ('J' sign). This indicates maltracking.
- **Patellar apprehension** (Fairbank's) test (for instability). Attempt to displace the patella laterally with the knee in

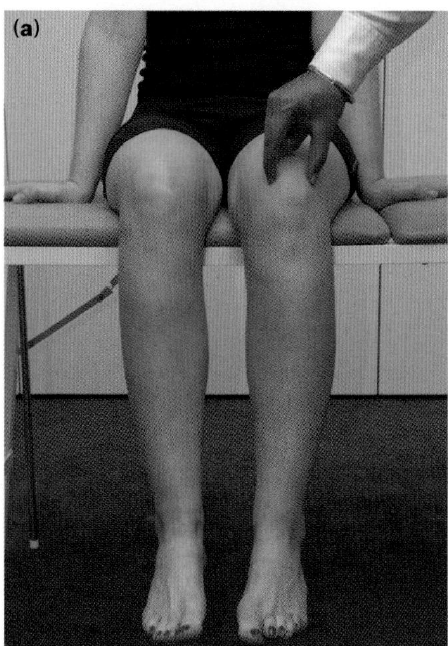

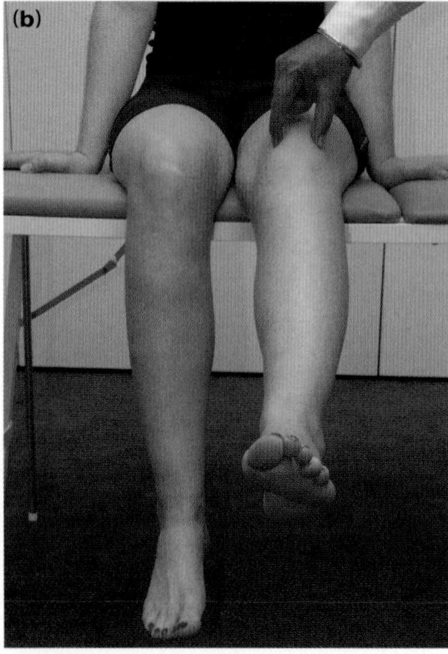

Figure 31.33 **(a, b)** Patellar tracking.

Thomas Porter McMurray, 1887–1949, Professor of Orthopaedic Surgery, Liverpool University, Liverpool, UK.
Sir Harold Arthur Thomas Fairbank, 1876–1961, orthopaedic surgeon, King's College Hospital, London, UK.

extension. Patients with instability contract their quadriceps muscle or complain of pain. With the patient supine and the quadriceps relaxed, flex the knee to 30° while trying to push the patella laterally. With instability the patient may react with apprehension. In addition, the quadriceps muscle may contract in an attempt to realign the patella.

Patellar tendon

The patellar tendon serves as the distal limit of the extensor mechanism. Rupture usually occurs at the osseotendinous junction. This results in an inability actively to perform and maintain full knee extension. A rupture presents with diffuse swelling in the anterior knee. A high-riding patella (patella alta) is present secondary to the unopposed pull of the quadriceps muscle. A defect in the tendon is usually palpable. When the rupture extends through the medial and lateral retinaculae, active extension is lost.

Summary box 31.9

Knee examination

Inspection of the standing patient

- Front – alignment (varus/valgus/rotational deformity), muscle bulk
- Side – fixed flexion deformity
- Back – popliteal swellings, hamstrings
- Gait – antalgic, high stepping gait (foot drop), varus thrust

Inspection of the supine patient

- Skin, scars, soft tissues, deformity
- Palpation of the extensor mechanism, medial and lateral joint lines and collateral ligaments, hamstrings, tibial tuberosity, fibular head

Movements

- Flexion and extension

Special tests

- Patellar apprehension test and extensor mechanism
- Cruciate ligaments
- Collateral ligaments
- Menisci

CLINICAL EXAMINATION OF THE FOOT AND ANKLE

The foot can be divided into three parts: the hindfoot (calcaneus, talus), the midfoot (navicular, cuboids, cuneiforms) and the forefoot (metatarsals and phalanges).

Look

Ask the patient to stand, and assess the overall limb alignment. Assess pelvic obliquity, limb length discrepancy (and its level), valgus/varus deformities of the knee and rotational alignment. Check for contractures of the hips and knees. Now focus your attention on the foot itself:

- **Foot shape**. Assess the overall shape of the forefoot from the front. From the side, look for the normal medial arch (**Figure 31.34a**). The hindfoot is best appreciated from behind. Now look at the vertical relationship between the Achilles tendon and the calcaneus (normal heel valgus of 5–7°). Look from behind and count the number of toes that can be seen. The 'too many toes' sign demonstrates increased forefoot abduction (pes planus (flat foot)) and a splayed forefoot. Foot shapes that may be encountered include neutral foot (no overall deformity), skew foot (hindfoot valgus and forefoot adduction), metatarsus adductus (neutral hindfoot and adduction of the metatarsus), pes planus (collapse of the medial arch) and pes cavus or high arch (increased medial arch). The possible causes of pes planus and pes cavus are shown in *Summary boxes 31.10* and *31.11*, respectively.

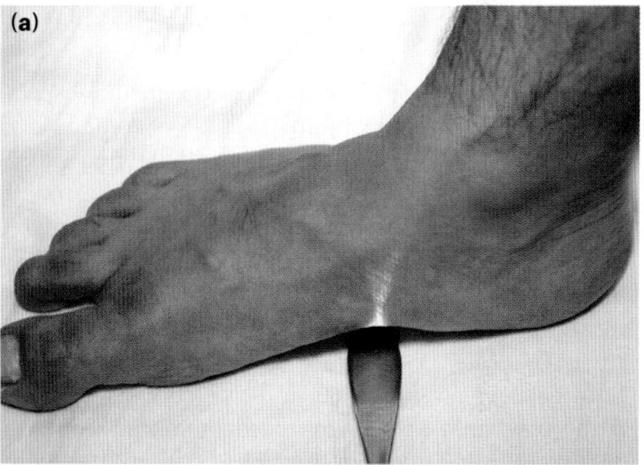

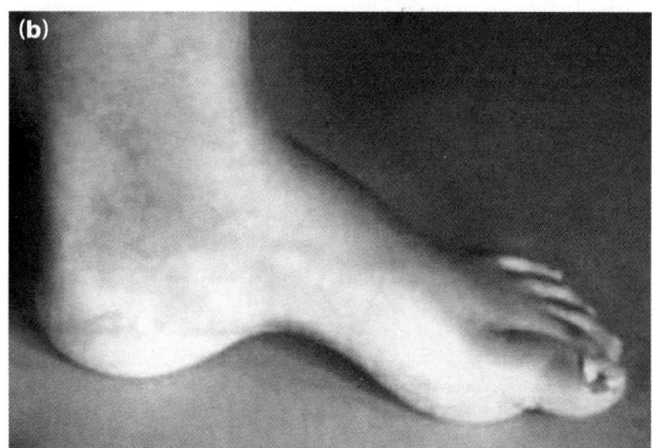

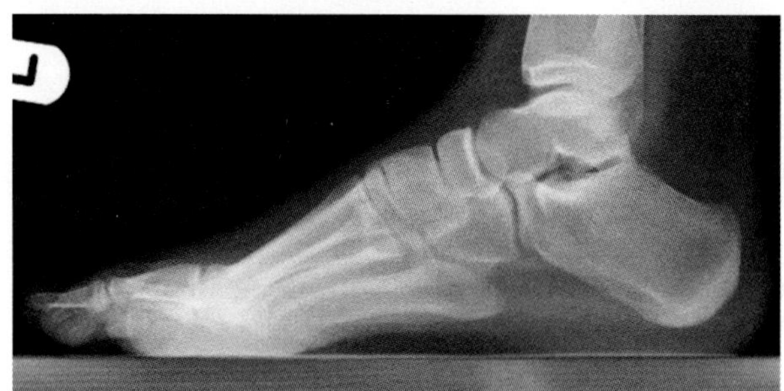

Figure 31.34 (a) Normal medial longitudinal arch of the foot. (b) Clinical and radiological appearance of pes cavus.

Summary box 31.10

Causes of pes planus

- Normal variant
- Hyperlaxity syndrome, e.g. Marfan's syndrome
- Tarsal coalition – rigid and painful flat foot (see **Figure 31.39a**)
- Tibial posterior dysfunction

Summary box 31.11

Causes of pes cavus (Figure 31.34b)

- Spinal anomalies, e.g. spina bifida
- Hereditary sensorimotor neuropathies, such as Charcot–Marie–Tooth disease
- Charcot foot (e.g. neuropathic foot)
- Post-compartment syndrome (e.g. Volkmann's ischaemic contracture)

- **Skin**. A bunion or red swelling on the medial aspect of the metatarsophalangeal joint (MTPJ) is common. This is an area of inflamed skin with an underlying subcutaneous bursa and a joint osteophyte. Systemic manifestations include gouty tophi and thin fat pads under the metatarsal heads as seen in rheumatoid arthritis. Corns are callosities which form where toes rub against the inside of shoes. Remember to assess the appearance of the nails.
- **Soft tissues**. Swelling may indicate soft tissue or joint pathology. Muscle wasting is most commonly seen on the dorsum of the foot and in the clefts between the metatarsals. If this is present, a full neurological examination of the upper and lower limbs should be performed, including the spine.
- **Bones**. Look for any bony prominences or exostoses. Common forefoot deformities are shown in *Table 31.12*.

Gait

Look for a high stepping gait (foot drop), painful (antalgic) gait (ankle and foot joint pain) and a short propulsive phase (forefoot pain).

Footwear

Inspect the footwear. This may reveal areas of abnormal weight bearing. With normal wear of the sole, a corner is typically worn off the posterolateral aspect of the heel (heel strike). In addition, there may be a circular wear pattern under the ball of the big toe (toe-off phase).

- **External appearance**. Look at the materials used, the metal supports and heel raise, depth and width.
- **Internal appearance**. Look at the insoles, arch supports and heel cups.

Feel

- **Skin**. Reduced sensation in a glove and stocking distribution is seen with diabetes.
- **Soft tissues**. The posterior tibial and the dorsal pedis pulses should be identified (**Figure 31.35**). Palpate the tibialis anterior tendon and the long extensor tendons on the dorsum of the foot. From the back, palpate the Achilles tendon. Palpate the peroneal tendons from the lateral side and the tibialis posterior tendon from the medial side. The sinus tarsi can be assessed. This is an anatomical space bounded by the talus and calcaneus and is recognisable as a soft-tissue depression anterior to the lateral malleolus. It is filled with fat and the extensor digitorum brevis muscle. Sinus tarsi syndrome may occur. This may be caused by injury to the interosseous talocalcaneal ligament or the subtalar joint. There is pain and tenderness over the sinus tarsi with subjective hindfoot instability. The pain is characteristically relieved by local anaesthetic injection.
- **Bones**. Feel for deformity, bony prominences and loose bodies:
  - ankle joint: the medial and lateral malleoli, anterior and posterior joint line, lateral gutter and ligament complex, the syndesmosis (front of the ankle), medial gutter and medial ligament complex;
  - subtalar joint: palpate each facet;
  - midtarsal joints: the talonavicular and calcaneocuboid joints;
  - tarsometatarsal joints (TMTJ): note that the second TMTJ is several millimetres proximal to the others; movement is minimal in the second ray, limited in the

TABLE 31.12 Common forefoot deformities.

Deformity	Metatarsophalangeal joint	Proximal interphalangeal joint	Distal interphalangeal joint
Claw toe	Hyperextension	Flexion	Flexion
Hammer toe	Normal	Flexion	Flexion
Mallet toe	Normal	Normal	Flexion
Hallux valgus or varus	Valgus or varus position	Normal	–

Antoine Bernard-Jean Marfan, 1858–1942, physician, Hôpital des Infants-Malades, Paris, France, described this syndrome in 1896.
Jean Martin Charcot, 1825–1893, physician, La Salpêtrière, Paris, France.
Pierre Marie, 1853–1940, neurologist, Hospice de Bicêtre, Paris, France, later became Professor of Pathological Anatomy in the Faculty of Medicine, and finally, in 1918, Professor of Neurology.
Howard Henry Tooth, 1856–1925, physician, St Bartholomew's Hospital and the National Hospital for Nervous Diseases, Queen's Square, London, UK, described peroneal muscular atrophy in 1886, independently of Charcot and Marie.

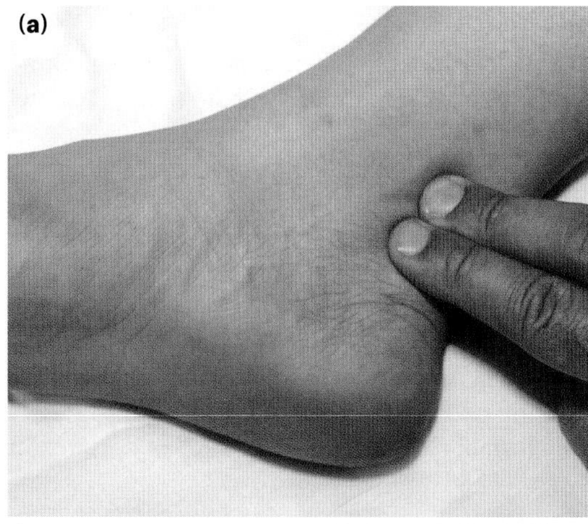

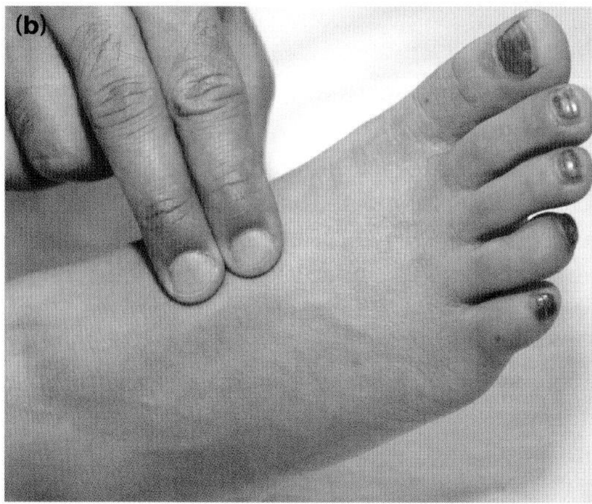

Figure 31.35 (a) Palpation of the posterior tibial pulse. (b) Palpation of the dorsalis pedis pulse.

third ray, moderate in the fourth and fifth rays and very variable in the first ray.

- **Specific structures** to palpate:
  - calcaneus (heel bone): the most common cause of pain is plantar fasciitis; this may present with numbness, burning and electric shock sensations, which are worse in the morning and improve as the day goes on; identify the exact point of tenderness;
  - tendons: examine for contracture of the Achilles tendon insertion and the peroneal or tibialis posterior tendons;
  - head of talus: invert and evert the patient's foot;
  - sustentaculum tali: palpate one fingerbreadth below the medial malleolus; this important structure serves as an attachment for the spring ligament;
  - cuneiforms (medial, middle and lateral), MTPJs, web spaces and all the forefoot bones.

Move

The movements of the foot and ankle are linked via the ankle, subtalar and midfoot joints. Remember the acronyms PAED – pronation, abduction, eversion and dorsiflexion – and SAPI – supination, adduction, plantarflexion and inversion. These are the two common general foot deformities.

Ankle (Figure 31.36)

- **Dorsiflexion**. Test dorsiflexion with the knee both flexed and extended. If restriction is greater with the knee extended than flexed, the contracture is principally in the gastrocnemius. Restriction that is equal in all knee positions is caused by a contracture principally of the soleus.
- **Plantarflexion**. Ask the patient to touch the floor with their foot (15°). Weakness suggests injury to the Achilles tendon or pathology affecting the S1 nerve root.

Subtalar joint (Figures 31.37 and 31.38)

Hold the talar neck and ask the patient to move their heel from side to side. Repeat using a hand on the heel to move the joint and apply a varus and valgus stress while feeling for movements of the talus. Holding the talus as opposed to the tibia isolates subtalar from ankle motion. (Normal range is 5° in each direction.)

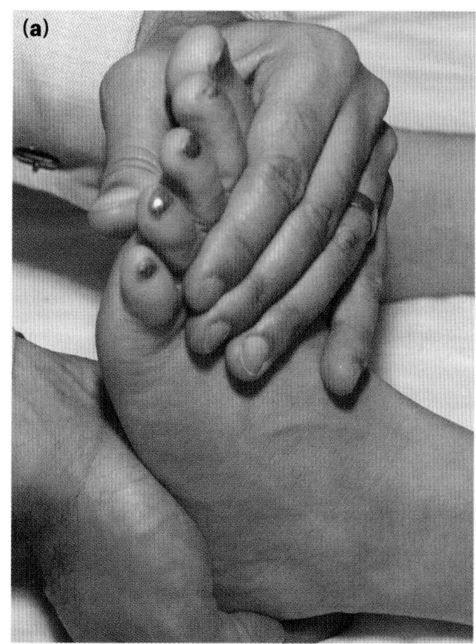

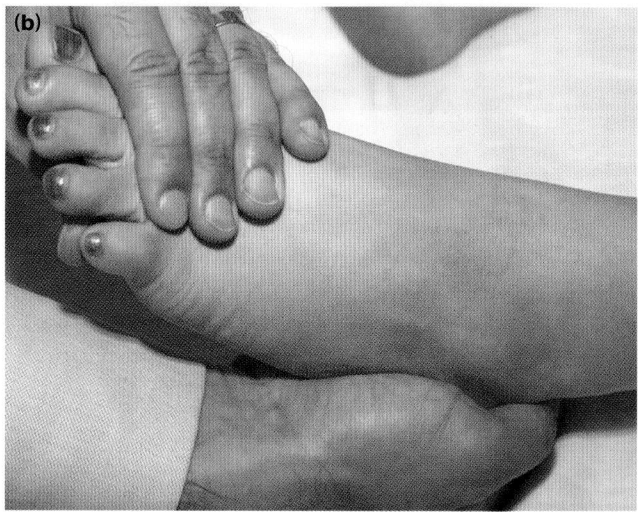

Figure 31.36 (a) Ankle dorsiflexion and (b) ankle plantarflexion.

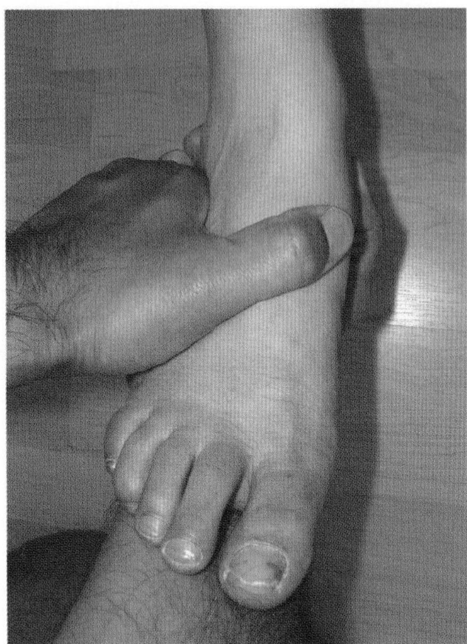

Figure 31.37 Testing subtalar joint motion.

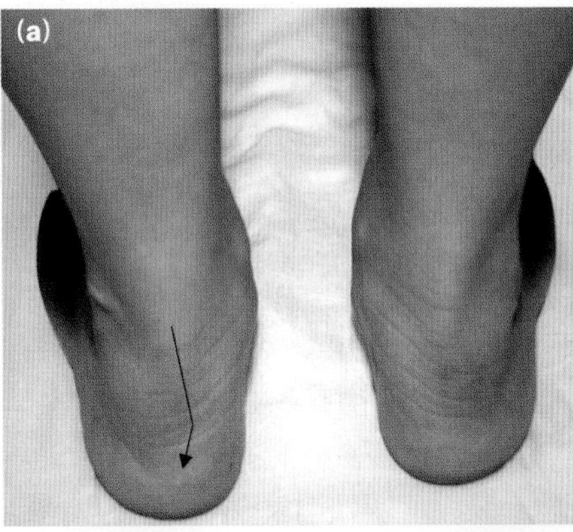

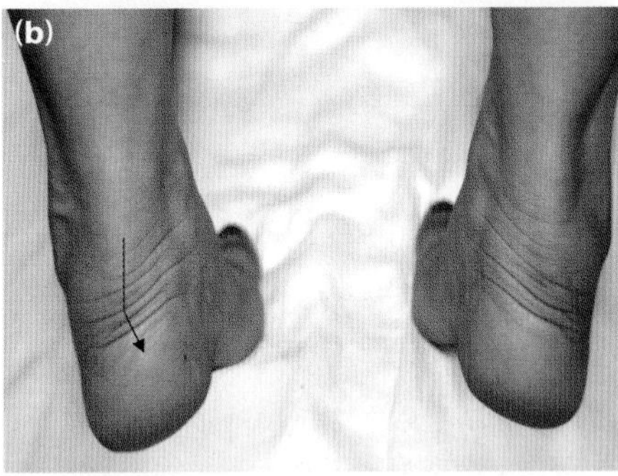

Figure 31.38 (a, b) Testing subtalar joint flexibility.

- Inversion. Ask the patient to move their foot in towards them.
- Eversion. Ask the patient to move their foot out to the side.

Midtarsal joint

Hold the heel with one hand and move the forefoot medially (adduction = 20°) and laterally (abduction = 10°) with the other hand.

Tarsometatarsal joint

Hold the midfoot and manipulate each metatarsal up and down to estimate the passive range of movement.

Metatarsophalangeal joint

Test extension (70–90°) by asking the patient to lift the toes to the ceiling and test flexion (45°) by pointing the toes to the floor. Normal toe-off requires 35–40° of dorsiflexion.

Special tests

Achilles tendon

Feel the gastrocnemius and soleus bellies and the whole length of the tendon for gaps (rupture), tenderness or swelling. Also identify the posterolateral (Haglund's) prominence of the calcaneus and palpate the retro-Achilles bursa.

The test for integrity of the tendon is the Thompson's or Simmonds' test. Do not be misled by the patient's ability to stand on tiptoes – some people can do this using their long toe flexors alone. Lie the patient prone and allow their calves to rest on your forearms. Squeeze each calf in turn and watch for movement at the ankle joint. Lack of movement may indicate a rupture.

Subtalar joint flexibility

Ask the patient to stand on their toes and observe the heel from behind; the heel moves normally from valgus to varus, indicating flexibility. The Coleman's block test is used to assess the flexibility of the subtalar joint. Ask the patient to stand on a 2-cm block with the great toe over the medial edge, resting on the floor. Now look from behind. If the hindfoot varus remains, the subtalar joint is fixed. If it corrects to valgus, the joint is mobile (**Figure 31.38**).

Flat foot flexibility

Use the Windlass and Jack's tests to distinguish a flexible from a fixed flat foot (**Figure 31.39**).

- **Windlass test**. Ask the patient to stand on their toes, and observe the arch of the foot on the medial aspect. As soon as the patient stands on their toes, the arch forms. Failure of this indicates a fixed flat foot.
- **Jack's test**. With the patient standing, lift up the great toe. The arch should form in the flexible flat foot.

Ankle stability

Trauma to the ankle is a common cause of instability. Accurate assessment may be difficult in the acute setting because of pain.

Patrik Haglund, 1870–1937, Swedish orthopaedic surgeon.
Frankin Adin Simmonds, 1911–1983, orthopaedic surgeon, The Rowley Bristow Hospital, Pyrford, Surrey, UK.

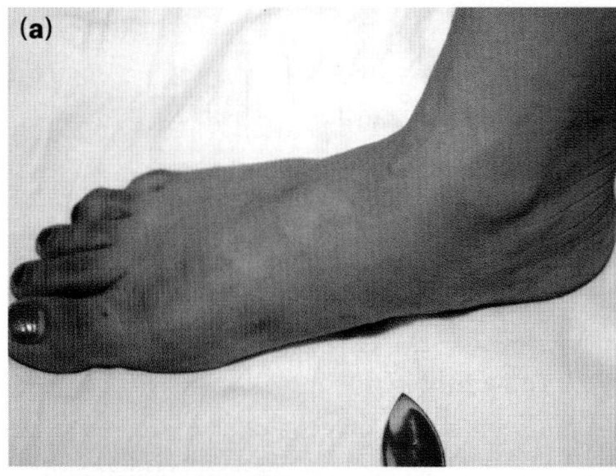

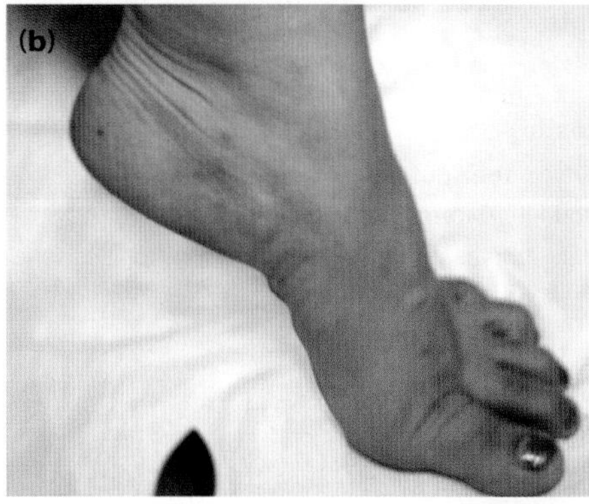

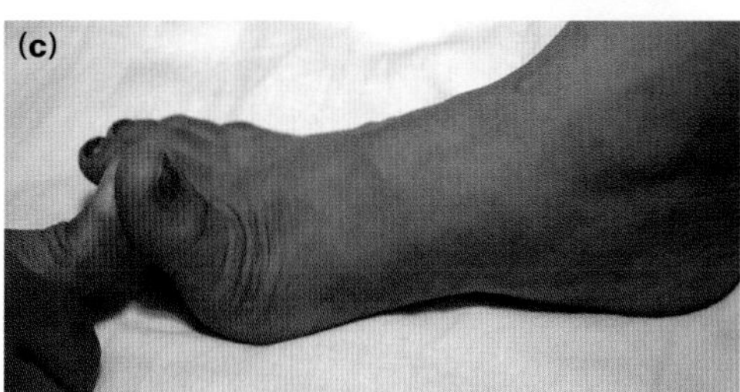

Figure 31.39 (**a**) Flat foot appearance with a reduced medial longitudinal arch; (**b**) Windlass test; (**c**) Jack's test.

- **Anterior draw test**. With the foot resting over the bed, hold the heel with one hand and the front of the tibia with the other. Move the heel forwards on the fixed tibia. Compare with the other side. Instability of the syndesmosis may be palpable (**Figure 31.40**).

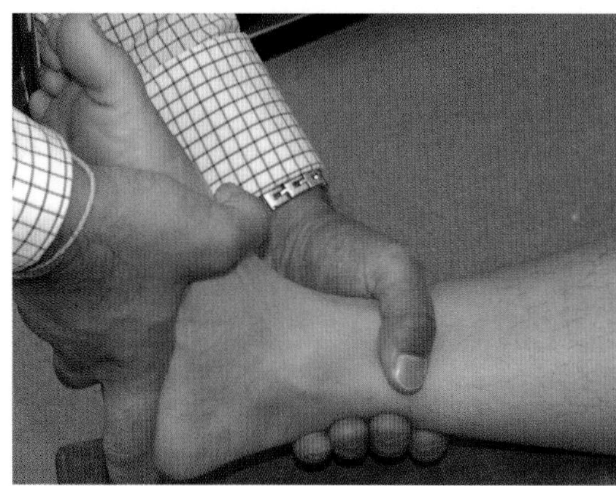

Figure 31.40 Anterior draw test.

- **Squeeze test for distal tibiofibular stability**. Compress the proximal calf. Pain at the ankle may indicate separation of the distal fibula from the tibia.
- **Tilt test**. Hold the talus at the neck rather than the heel so that you can be sure that any tilt is in the ankle and not the subtalar joint.

Tarsometatarsal joint stability

Stability can be assessed by pushing each joint up and down. Standing lateral radiographs may be used in addition.

Tibialis anterior

Ask the patient to walk on their heels with their feet inverted; the tibialis anterior tendon can be seen. With the patient's feet resting over the edge of the couch, ask the patient actively to dorsiflex and invert their foot to reach your hand. Palpate the tibialis anterior muscle.

Tibialis posterior

Pathology of the tibialis posterior typically presents with posteromedial ankle pain, swelling and gradual onset of a flat foot. When assessing the tendon, look for swelling along its course, a flat foot with heel valgus, the 'too many toes' sign and prominence of the talar head. Palpate for tenderness, swelling or gaps in the tendon.

- **To test integrity**, ask the patient to perform a single foot tiptoe test on both sides. The inability to lift the affected heel off the ground is suggestive of a tibialis posterior tendon injury or insufficiency.
- **To test strength**, position the foot in the plantarflexed and inverted position. Ask the patient to hold this position while you push against their foot.

Dorsiflexors

Tendinitis of the long toe dorsiflexors usually presents in athletes. Pain affects gait in the early contact phase. Palpate for swelling, gaps or any tenderness. Ask the patient to move the foot into dorsiflexion and to hold this position while you push the foot down.

Inability to dorsiflex the foot is referred to as foot drop. Causes include stroke, spinal injury, spinal stenosis or disc prolapse, peripheral nerve injury (e.g. sciatic, common and deep peroneal) or a peripheral neuropathy.

Peroneal tendons

Peroneal tendon pathology presents with swelling and/or pain of the lateral hindfoot or midfoot. There may be a history of the ankle 'giving way'. Presentations of peroneal tendon pathology include:

- **'peroneal spasm'**: may be seen in tarsal coalition; here, the muscles are usually contracted secondary to the hindfoot valgus;
- **peroneal tendon dislocation**: attempt to dislocate the tendons by dorsiflexing and everting the foot.

The peroneus longus may be palpated just before it crosses under the foot to insert onto the base of the first metatarsal. Ask the patient to plantarflex the first metatarsal. Test strength and integrity by active and resisted eversion while you palpate the tendons for swelling, tenderness or gaps.

Morton's neuroma

This condition represents thickening of the tissue that surrounds the digital nerve leading to the toes as the nerve passes under the ligament connecting the metatarsals in the forefoot. It is most frequent between the third and fourth toes. A neuroma presents with burning pain in the ball of the foot that radiates to the involved toes. The condition is difficult to diagnose and requires a high index of suspicion. Palpate in the web space between the symptomatic toes for a mass. Compression of the metatarsals may elicit a 'click' between the bones (Molders' click).

FURTHER READING

Ellenbecker TS, Nirschl R, Renstrom P. Current concepts in examination and treatment of elbow tendon injury. *Sports Health* 2013; **5**(2): 186–94.

Guosheng Y, Chongxi R, Guoqing C, Junling X, Hailong J. The diagnostic value of a modified Neer test in identifying subacromial impingement syndrome. *Eur J Orthop Surg Traumatol* 2017. (Epub ahead of print.)

Martin HD, Palmer IJ. History and physical examination of the hip: the basics. *Curr Rev Musculoskelet Med* 2013; **6**(3): 219–25.

Rossi R, Dettoni F, Bruzzone M, Cottino U, D'Elicio DG, Bonasia DE. Clinical examination of the knee: know your tools for diagnosis of knee injuries. *Sports Med Arthrosc Rehabil Ther Technol* 2011; **3**: 25.

Summary box 31.12

Ankle and foot examination

Inspection of the standing patient

- Front – alignment, foot shape and deformity
- Side – medial arch
- Back – heel position
- Gait – antalgic, high stepping gait (foot drop)

Inspection of the supine patient

- Skin, scars, soft tissues, bony deformity
- Palpation of the ankle, subtalar, midfoot and forefoot joints

Movements

- Dorsiflexion, plantarflexion, inversion, eversion

Special tests

- Flexibility of the subtalar joint and a flat foot
- Joint stability, Morton's neuroma
- Tendons – tibialis posterior and anterior, Achilles tendon, peroneals and dorsiflexors

---

Thomas George Morton, 1835–1903, surgeon, The Pennsylvania Hospital, Philadelphia, PA, USA.

Chapter 32

Sports medicine and sports injuries

Learning objectives:

- To understand the important issues behind a patient's sporting injury in the context of taking a history
- To know the common sports injuries
- To know the appropriate ways of imaging to confirm or refute a diagnosis
- To assess the patient and offer treatment and rehabilitation plans

INTRODUCTION

Regular physical exercise is integral to the body staying healthy. However, stressing the human body to its limits may lead to injury. Sports medicine is the science of understanding how these injuries can be avoided, recognised when they do occur, and then treated appropriately. Sports injuries are, in principle, the same as other injuries. The major difference can be in the expectations of the patients. The injuries can be classified into three broad groups. Acute extrinsic injuries are those which arise from a direct external blow. These are commonly wounds, bruises and fractures. Acute intrinsic injuries result from failure of the patient's anatomical structures as a result of excessive loading. Examples are tendon ruptures, avulsion fractures and ligament injuries. Chronic injuries are those with an insidious or unknown onset and commonly involve degeneration or failure secondary to repetitive loading. Examples are tendinosis of the Achilles tendon and stress fractures.

Summary box 32.1

Types of sports injury

- Acute extrinsic – caused by direct external blow (bruises)
- Acute intrinsic – internal failure secondary to excessive external force (ligament tear)
- Chronic – repetitive and stress injuries

DIAGNOSIS OF SPORTS INJURIES

There are some additional questions that need to be asked in the history when treating a patient with a sports injury:

1. How was the injury sustained?
2. What type of training are they undertaking: mixed training or only one type of sport?
3. How many hours of training are they doing and has this changed recently?
4. Have they had previous injury? When did they sustain the injury and what rehabilitation have they had?
5. What are they aiming for in the way of competitions or level of sport that they perform?
6. Do they want to compete again or are they worried about competing?

The examination should follow the system described in Chapter 31.

TENDON DISEASE

Tendons can become weak and/or painful because of physical damage or as a result of inflammation of the tendon sheath around them (peritendonitis). Tendon injury is either due to overload (the strength of the tendon being exceeded by the force applied) or to overuse, where there is repetitive load leading to fatigue and failure. In this case the patient may present with tendinosis rather than rupture.

Current opinion now accepts that both tendinopathy and tenosynovitis are predominantly degenerative but do contain an inflammatory response on histology so the word 'tendinitis' can still be used.

Overuse injuries

Internal factors

Overuse injury can be precipitated in a tendon by decreased oxygen supply, decreased nutrition, hormonal changes, chronic inflammation and ageing.

External factors

A change in the environment (new running surface) or worn out equipment (old running shoes) may both bring about an overuse injury, as can excessive training when the patient is not fit enough to tolerate it.

In younger patients, the weakest area of a tendon is the apophyseal attachment. In adults, the musculotendinous junction is more liable to injury. In adolescents, the common sites of injury are tendon insertions. Examples are the anterior superior iliac spine (origin of sartorius), the anterior inferior iliac spine (rectus femoris), the lesser trochanter of the femur (iliopsoas), and the ischial tuberosity (hamstrings).

Summary box 32.2

Problems with tendons

- Rupture due to excessive loads and internal delamination
- Pain and degeneration due to repetitive or abnormal loading

MUSCLE INJURY

Muscle injuries or strains can be classified into a sprain, partial tear, complete tear or re-tear (if there has been previous injury). Most will heal spontaneously but may leave a painless defect in the muscle belly (*Table 32.1*). Muscle injuries leave an area of weakness that can re-tear in 30% of athletes. Despite extensive research we cannot predict the return to sport after such an injury but if the injury is large and involves the myotendinous junction it is more significant and likely to take longer.

TABLE 32.1 Muscle injuries graded according to severity.

Grade	Description
0	Normal muscle
1	Subtle muscle abnormality/sprain
2	Definite muscle disruption without muscle retraction
3	Complete muscle tear with retraction

LIGAMENTS

Ligament injuries are acute intrinsic injuries and can be graded according to their severity (*Table 32.2*).

In the acute phase it may be difficult to assess the ligament injury thoroughly. Once the acute injury has settled, any difference in laxity when comparing the two sides is diagnostic. However, the laxity of ligaments varies dramatically between patients and with age so absolute measurements are not reliable. When the diagnosis remains in doubt, imaging can be useful, for example ultrasound or magnetic resonance imaging (MRI). Grade 1 and 2 ligament injuries can be treated with pain relief, splinting and gentle mobilisation to avoid stiffness. Grade 3 injuries may require surgical repair to bring together the torn ends of the ligament, or another reconstructive procedure. The treatment depends on the site of the ligament and joint stability. For example, in ankle inversion injuries, the patient will recover without anterior talofibular ligament reconstruction.

TABLE 32.2 Ligament injuries graded according to severity.

Grade	Description
0	Normal ligament
1	No increase in joint laxity but there is tenderness around the injured ligament
2	Partial disruption of the ligament fibres with increased joint laxity, and a soft end point
3	Complete disruption of the ligament; there is a marked increase in joint laxity with no end point clinically

Summary box 32.3

Ligament injuries

- Difficult to assess clinically in the acute phase
- Use the opposite side for comparison
- If doubt, use imaging (ultrasound or MRI) to assess further
- Surgical repair may be needed for complete disruption, in a small percentage
- The stability of the joint is the most important factor in making this decision

BURSAE

Bursae are found between the joints and overlying tissues or muscles and tendons and are small fluid-filled endothelium-lined sacks. They decrease frictional forces between structures, but can become inflamed. The most commonly affected sites are over the first metatarsophalangeal joint (bunion), in front of the patella (housemaid's knee), behind the elbow (olecranon bursa) and the shoulder (subdeltoid subacromial bursitis). They can become inflamed or even infected. On the rare occasion that they fail to settle with appropriate treatment, they can be surgically excised.

BONE FRACTURES AND STRESS FRACTURES

True fractures can be encountered in any sport, but the fracture type found more commonly in sportsmen and -women is a stress fracture. This is caused by multiple repetitions of moderate loads that would not be expected to cause fracture in a single application. Clinically these lesions give poorly localised pain, which is worse on exercise. They are more common in runners, especially women who may have reduced bone density. The most common sites for stress fractures are the metatarsals and the tibia.

INJURIES ASSOCIATED WITH INDIVIDUAL SPORTS

Golf

The shoulder and the back are the commonest site of overuse injuries. Golfer's elbow or medial epicondylitis is due to a common flexor origin tendinosis. It does not just occur in golfers. Tennis elbow is, however, more common in golfers than golfer's elbow.

Tennis

Tennis elbow is tendinosis of the common extensor origin. It occurs in novice tennis players but not the elite.

Partial ruptures of the calf muscles, especially the medial head of the gastrocnemius, are also found in tennis players (called tennis leg), and in other sports requiring sudden extreme acceleration.

Rowing

The common problems with rowing (Figure 32.1) are rib fractures and intercostal muscle tears (Figure 32.2), and tendon problems such as tenosynovitis at the wrist, which is more common than intersection syndrome (a tendinosis where the first and second extensor tendon compartments of the forearm cross)

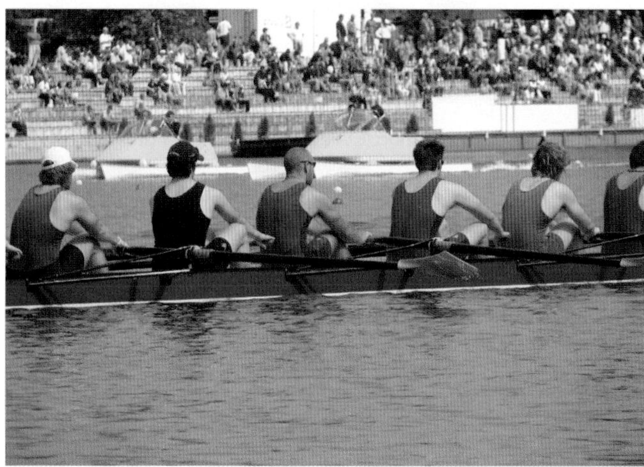

Figure 32.1 Rowers in action at an English regatta (© Vladislav Gagic–Fotolia).

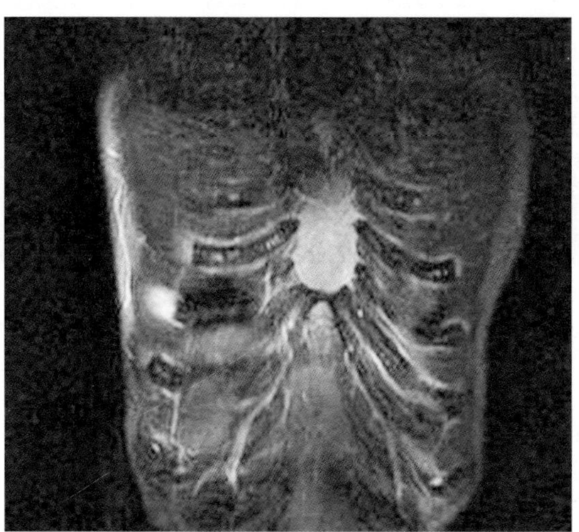

Figure 32.2 Coronal magnetic resonance imaging scan of the chest showing an intercostal muscle injury in a rower.

Football

The main injuries are fractures, groin injuries, muscle tears and twisting injuries to the knees and ankles leading to ligament tears (Figures 32.3 and 32.4). Injuries specific to football include turf toe and neuromas to the deep peroneal nerve on the dorsum of the foot due to repetitive trauma from kicking the football. Goalkeepers get wrist and hand injuries, including occult scaphoid fractures.

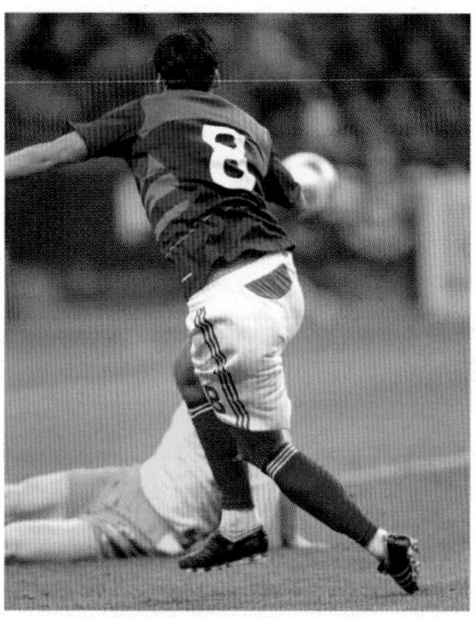

Figure 32.3 A footballer in action (© lilufoto–Fotolia).

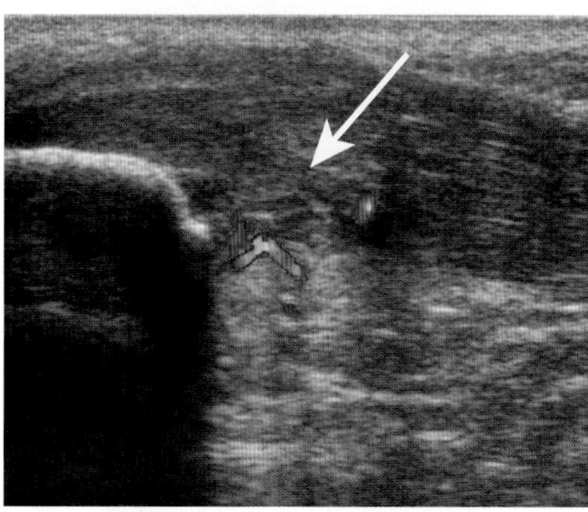

Figure 32.4 Ultrasound showing a patellar tendinosis with neovascularisation in a footballer (arrow).

Rugby

This is a high intensity contact sport so injuries include concussion due to head trauma, neck injuries including fractures to the cervical spine, muscle tears, shoulder, acromioclavicular joint and finger injuries, including dislocation of the phalanges, and tendon injuries e.g. rugger jersey finger where there is injury to the flexor profundus tendon.

Javelin

Javelin throwers get injuries due to abnormal stresses on the elbow similar to those seen in baseball. This causes abnormalities of the ulnar collateral ligament and capitellum.

Swimming

Shoulder injuries are more common in swimmers, especially in those performing the crawl or the butterfly stroke because these can lead to impingement syndromes (rotator cuff tendinosis and tears).

Volleyball, netball and basketball

Hand injuries are common, as is patellar tendinopathy and internal derangements of the ankle and knee.

Ballet dancing

Ballet dancers (**Figure 32.5**) have problems with posterior impingement of the ankle and tendinopathy of the flexor hallucis longus tendon when working on pointe (tip-toe). Stress fractures are also found in female dancers due to the abnormal stresses (**Figure 32.6**). Male ballet dancers are prone to back and shoulder injuries due to carrying ballerinas. Young dancers often complain of clicking and pain around the hip which may be due to iliopsoas tendinopathy.

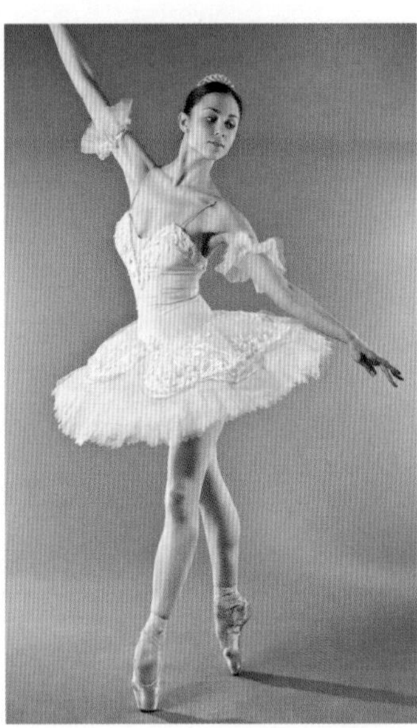

Figure 32.5 Ballet dancer on pointe (© Zoja–Fotolia).

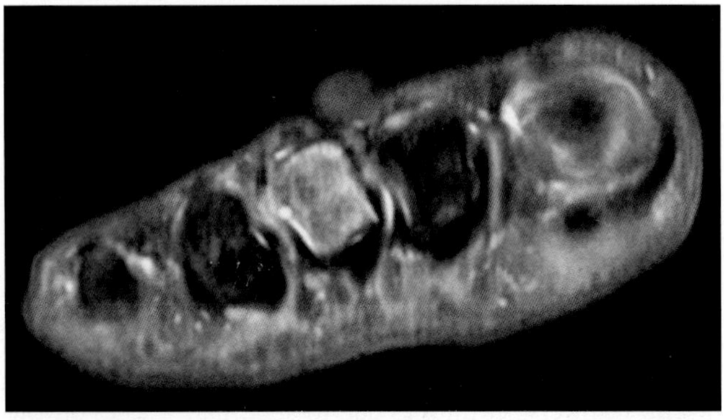

Figure 32.6 Magnetic resonance imaging short T1 inversion recovery (MRI STIR) sequence showing a stress injury to a metatarsal.

Snowboarding and skiing

Participants in both sports (**Figure 32.7**) have the full range of injuries associated with a high-speed sport. The rigid high boots used by skiers protect the ankle, but increase the loads transmitted up the limb, risking fracture of the tibia and ligament disruption of the knee (especially the anterior cruciate) (**Figure 32.8**). Novice snowboarders tend to get wrist fractures, whilst all levels of snowboarder can injure the acromioclavicular joint.

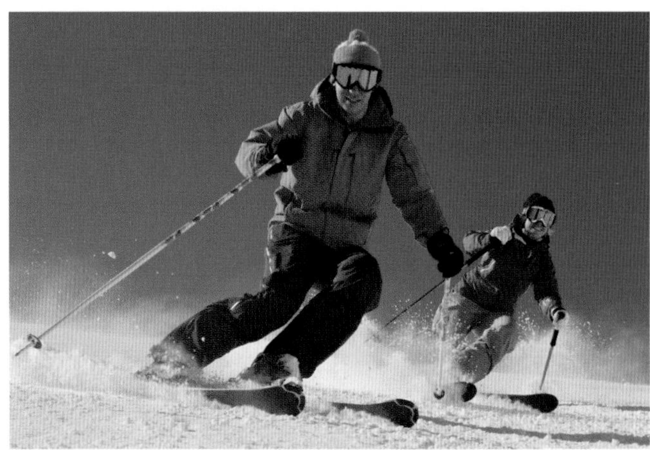

Figure 32.7 Skiers in action (©Alexander Rochau–Fotolia).

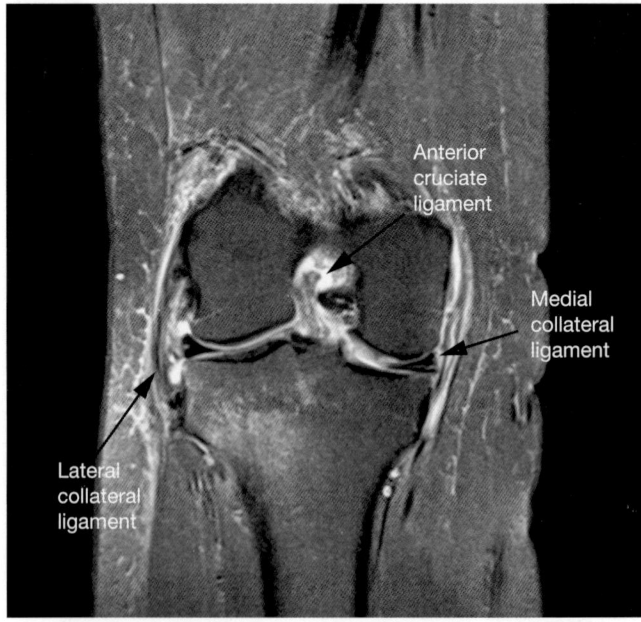

Figure 32.8 A knee magnetic resonance imaging scan showing a significant skiing injury with tears of the anterior cruciate ligament, medial collateral ligament and lateral collateral ligament.

Martial arts: judo, karate and taekwondo

All are associated with acute extrinsic injuries (direct blows) and acute intrinsic injuries (failure of ligaments and other structures due to sudden excessive loads).

Weight training

Weight training tends to produce the third type of sports injury (chronic), for example problems with the shoulders, including pectoralis major tears, carpal tunnel syndrome and the spine.

Kayaking

This causes problems with the forearm, including posterior interosseous nerve compression at the level of the elbow.

Marathon running

Problems include iliotibial band syndrome and stress fractures in the feet and shins.

INJURIES ACCORDING TO REGION OF SYMPTOMS

Pelvis, hip and thigh injuries

- **Thigh bruise** (Charley Horse, corked thigh or helmet thigh): These occur in all contact sports and can be both large and painful. They require prolonged rest as they are slow to settle and can rebleed. A pseudo-tumour may develop. Surgical drainage should be avoided if possible as it can lead to infection of the haematoma. Percutaneous aspiration of the liquefied haematoma under antibiotic cover is being performed by some groups to speed recovery with good results.
- **Quadriceps tears**: these most commonly occur in the rectus femoris muscle. They may be due to a direct blow, but more commonly they are due to twisting injury and occur along the aponeurosis of the rectus femoris, which is a weak point where the two muscle bellies join.
- **Complete quadriceps rupture**: this is less common, but may occur when kicking balls or in older patients. The patient can often perform a straight leg raise due to trick manoeuvres. However, they cannot restraighten the raised leg (quadriceps lag). Surgical repair is not usually needed in the elderly but is necessary in athletes.
- **Hamstring injury**: this commonly occurs due to twisting injuries following sudden and maximal muscle contraction. The injuries most commonly occur in the biceps femoris tendon, but can occur in the semimembranosus and to a lesser degree semitendinosus.

Groin pain

This is a very difficult area to assess as referred pain to the groin can come from many sources.

These include:

- the hip (labral tears and osteoarthritis);
- adductor tendon injuries;
- stress fractures of the femur, especially femoral neck and pubis;
- hernias (these may be small and include femoral and obturator hernias);
- tumours;
- sexually transmitted diseases;
- gynaecological and urinary problems;
- referred pain from the lumbar spine.

Adductor tendon injuries produce localised tenderness over the adductor origin.

A labral tear of the hip may cause clicking and pain; characteristically, on examination this occurs in internal rotation and adduction – the impingement sign (see Chapter 31).

Knee injury

Acute

Knee injuries are common in contact sports because of studded boots applying excessive loads to the knee in rapid turning. It is also a common site of injury in skiers. If the patient cannot play on and the knee swells immediately then there is likely to be blood in the knee (haemarthrosis). The most likely causes are a tear of the anterior cruciate ligament, dislocation of the patella (which usually relocates again immediately), and an intra-articular fracture (when there will be marrow fat globules visible in the aspirate).

If the patient plays on and the knee swells later then the diagnosis is more likely to be a tear of a meniscus and the fluid aspirated will be clear. The early diagnosis of a knee injury is very difficult as the knee is too painful to examine. Aspiration of any effusion, using full sterile precautions, followed by early physiotherapy to maintain quadriceps strength, will allow most acute injuries to settle.

Patellar dislocation is more common in the hypermobile patient and in contact sports. If it has not already relocated, straightening the knee allows it to relocate.

Subsequent diagnosis

Patients who have had a patellar dislocation will have a patellar apprehension sign (see Chapter 31). True locking is caused by a loose body in the knee (osteochondritis dissecans), or a torn meniscus. The patient will be moving normally at the time (unlike pseudo-locking) and will suddenly find that they are unable to straighten or even bend the knee. After a period of 'jiggling' the knee they may be able to release the block and move normally again. Thessaly's test is said to have high sensitivity and specificity for this condition. Imaging should be performed on locked knees because clinical assessment is difficult and an arthroscopy may not be needed.

If a meniscal tear is diagnosed but is peripheral (where there is a blood supply providing an environment for healing) then meniscal repair should be undertaken.

Giving way can be caused by weakness, pain or instability. Weakness will usually be the result of quadriceps wasting secondary to the injury and is best treated with physiotherapy.

Patellofemoral pain can arise spontaneously in adolescents, but can also arise after a knee injury when the vastus medialis wastes rapidly, and the patella starts to mal-track. Clinically the patient will give a history of finding it difficult to descend stairs and experience severe pain and giving way when trying to move the knee after a period when it has been held still (pseudo-locking). Once again physiotherapy is the treatment of choice.

Instability may be the result of disruption of the anterior cruciate ligament with or without medial collateral ligament damage. The knee will give way on twisting or turning, and on examination the Lachmann test (see also anterior draw test) may be positive (see Chapter 31).

If physiotherapy fails to build the patient's muscles enough to stabilise the knee (it often does) then reconstruction of the cruciate ligament must be considered, using a synthetic graft or a length of tendon transferred from elsewhere.

If there is a posterolateral corner ligamentous injury in addition to the anterior cruciate ligament rupture, then surgery is mandatory to regain stability.

Iliotibial band syndrome is due to a friction injury of the iliotibial band both proximally over the greater trochanter and distally over the tibia. It occurs most commonly in long distance runners, such as marathon runners, and occurs proximally in females and distally as it extends over the lateral femoral epicondyle in males. If it does not respond to stretching and rest then sometimes a steroid injection in the adjacent bursae can help.

Summary box 32.4

Knee injuries

- Very difficult to examine in the acute stage clinically
- Effusions should be aspirated and early physiotherapy started
- Patellar dislocations will have a positive apprehension sign
- Anterior cruciate reconstruction should only be undertaken once the patient has been given a trial of physiotherapy in non-complex injuries (i.e. when there is an isolated anterior cruciate ligament rupture)

Ankle injury

Ankle sprains are a common cause of morbidity. Most occur due to a predominant inversion when the lateral ligament complex and the fibula and lateral talus can be injured. There is usually an eversion component to this injury. Isolated eversion or abduction injuries are much less common and will cause trauma to the medial ligament complex.

The ankle should only have radiographs taken if the Ottawa ankle rules are fulfilled (*Table 32.3*) as otherwise the likelihood of a fracture is very low.

Ankle dislocations should be reduced immediately as otherwise necrosis of the tented skin will occur, and ischaemia of the foot.

TABLE 32.3 Ottawa ankle rules.

- Bone tenderness along the distal 6 cm of the posterior margin or at the tip of the lateral malleolus
- Bone tenderness along the distal 6 cm of the posterior margin or at the tip of the medial malleolus
- Inability to bear weight at the time of the accident or at the time of examination

Sprains of the ankle should be treated with analgesia (but not non-steroidal anti-inflammatories because they decrease soft tissue healing) and PRICE (protection, rest, ice, compression and elevation) until the swelling has subsided, and then a physiotherapy programme should be started to reintroduce proprioception to the ankle. If this is not done, repeat injuries are more likely.

If there is diastasis of the distal tibiofibular joint then surgery may be required to regain stability of the ankle.

In adolescents, the peroneal tendon retinaculum can be torn. This leads to a subluxating peroneal tendon, with a painful flicking sensation over the lateral malleolus. In younger patients, this is best treated by immobilisation for a month, but if this does not resolve the problem then surgical intervention may be needed.

The Achilles tendon is a common site for tendinosis due to repetitive trauma. There is a fusiform swelling of the central tendon.

Tendon rupture classically occurs in middle-aged squash and badminton players. Simmonds or Thompson test is usually diagnostic (see Chapter 31). If there is the classic history of a feeling of a 'kick to the calf' and Simmonds test is negative, then ultrasound or MRI examination is mandatory as the Achilles rupture may be masked by the presence of a plantaris tendon. The Achilles tendon (see Chapter 36) can be allowed to heal in plaster with the foot plantar flexed to bring the tendon ends into contact. This takes several months. Alternatively, a surgical repair can be attempted. This opposes the ends and so should speed return to function, but risks compromising the blood supply to the tendon ends and so delays healing if the incision for access is large. In small-incision surgery, the risks are markedly reduced.

Summary box 32.5

Ankle injuries

- Dislocated ankles should be reduced immediately
- Radiographs should only be performed if the Ottawa ankle rules are fulfilled
- Physiotherapy to rebuild proprioception reduces the risk of recurrence of ankle sprains
- In Achilles tendon rupture, Simmonds–Thompson test is often positive (when there is no movement of the foot on squeezing the calf)

Foot injuries

Turf toe is pain, swelling and stiffness in the first metatarsophalangeal joint due to rupture of the plantar plate and injury to the joint capsule following hyperextension of the toe. Treatment is symptomatic.

Stress fractures are a common source of pain in marathon runners. These cause localised pain over a metatarsal on pressure and running. They can be identified by MRI or ultrasound. Navicular stress fractures are difficult to detect clinically and MRI should be performed if there is unexplained pain. Prolonged rest is the best treatment.

Shoulder and upper limb injuries

Shoulder dislocations occur in contact sports such as rugby. Almost all are anterior. Those who dislocate for the first time should be treated with intensive physiotherapy and rehabilitation. However, over half will have significant anatomical damage (tear of the labrum) (**Figure 32.9**) and 60% will go on to become recurrent dislocators. In these cases, surgical stabilisation (either open or arthroscopic) is the only treatment.

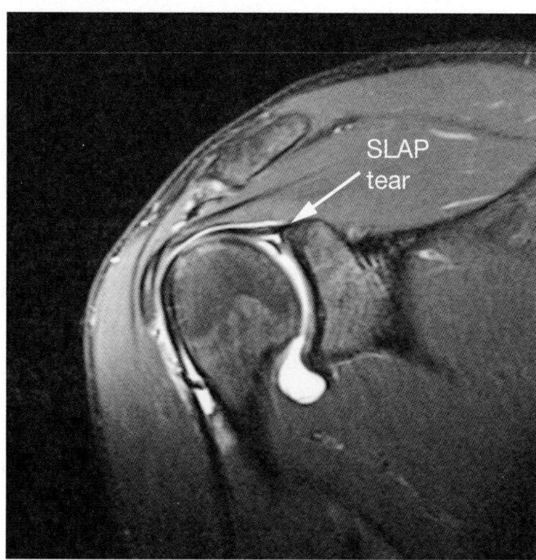

Figure 32.9 A magnetic resonance arthrogram of the shoulder showing a labral (superior labrum anterior posterior; SLAP) tear in a rugby player.

Shoulder instability can also result from overuse. This happens with throwing sports and also during sports such as gymnastics, and while serving in tennis and squash.

Tendinosis of the rotator cuff can also occur with overuse in patients who perform overhead sports repetitively, such as tennis players and cricket bowlers. Overload leads to impingement and then inflammation and tendinosis. Subacromial subdeltoid bursitis will cause pain radiating down the arm and to the wrist. This can be worse at night. Impingement can be significant in the overhead position and the patient may have difficulty combing their hair. The supraspinatus tendon can also tear, either secondary to impingement or after an acute injury. In the younger athlete this should be repaired surgically.

The acromioclavicular joint can be injured by direct impact in wrestlers, rugby players and cyclists. Treatment is usually symptomatic as surgical repair is not easy. If osteoarthritis develops in the joint, the distal end of the clavicle can be excised.

Summary box 32.6

Shoulder injuries

- Anterior dislocations are initially treated with physiotherapy
- Recurrent dislocations will require surgical stabilisation
- Overuse injuries are common in throwing sports
- Rotator cuff impingement is common
- Torn rotator cuffs should be repaired in young patients

Biceps injuries can occur in the long head of biceps proximally and the distal biceps tendon in weightlifters, wrestlers and gym users on anabolic steroids, but can also occur as part of a significant rotator cuff injury proximally where the rotator cuff can be torn from the supraspinatus across the anterior interval and into the subscapularis tendon. There is no treatment needed in proximal injuries.

Arm and hand injuries

Medial and lateral epicondylitis are discussed above (**Figure 32.10**). Treatment should commence with physiotherapy and an epicondyle support. Percutaneous interventions should then be tried before surgical treatment.

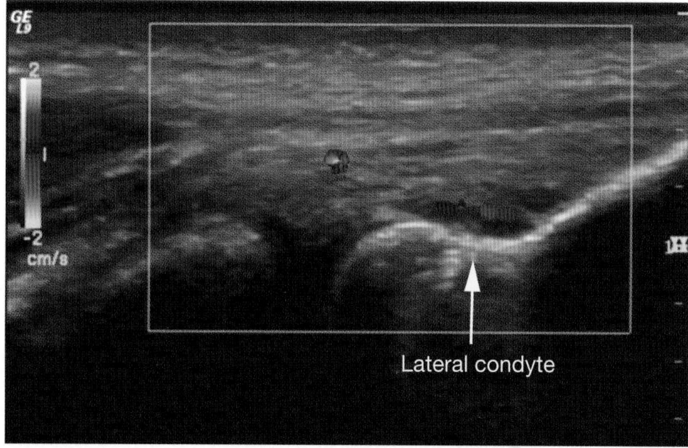

Figure 32.10 An ultrasound scan of the common extensor origin at the elbow showing a tendinosis with neovascularisation.

De Quervain's tenosynovitis occurs in repetitive injuries involving the fingers. This can be treated effectively with physiotherapy and steroid injections into the tendon sheath.

Skiers (or gamekeeper's) thumb occurs where the proximal phalanx of the thumb is forced radially in a fall. The ulnar collateral ligament of the thumb at the level of the metacarpophalangeal joint is damaged. If it is avulsed, the aponeurosis of the abductor pollicis brevis can become interposed (a Stener lesion) and so surgical intervention in this scenario is the only option if this lesion is to repair.

Mallet fingers or baseball fingers occur when there is a rupture of the distal insertion of the extensor tendon into the distal phalanx. This can be treated conservatively with a mallet splint.

The radial slips of the extensor tendon can be torn at the level of the metacarpophalangeal joints in boxing injuries and here the retinaculum needs reattaching surgically.

Disruption of the flexor tendon pulleys in the hand occurs in climbers, and leads to bow stringing of the flexor tendons. If this occurs, surgical intervention is needed.

All of these hand injuries can be assessed by the use of ultrasound examination using dynamic stress, which is better in resolution and specificity than MRI.

Summary box 32.7

Arm and hand injuries

- Medial and lateral epicondylitis should be treated symptomatically
- Ulnar collateral ligament injuries of the thumb may require surgical repair if a Stener lesion is present
- Flexor tendon pulley injuries require surgical repair

TREATMENT OF INJURIES

Initial care

In the acute phases of a sports injury PRICE describes the treatment plan (*Table 32.4*).

TABLE 32.4 PRICE for the nonoperative management of the acute sports injury.
• Protection
• Rest
• Ice
• Compression
• Elevation

Analgesia

In the initial phase of an injury, non-steroidal anti-inflammatory drugs are thought to slow healing, but may reduce pain and oedema. This is especially true for fracture healing. Paracetamol and codeine have less of an effect on injury healing and can also help with pain relief.

When prescribing any drugs it is important to be aware of the World Anti-Doping Agency (WADA) guidelines on doping for athletes as some substances are banned in competition and training. Spot checks are performed on athletes so they need to adhere to this throughout the year. A prohibited list is available on their website (http://www.wada-ama.org).

If steroids are needed to help with continued rehabilitation, then a TUE or temporary use exemption certificate needs to be given to the athlete so that if they are spot checked for drugs they will not be disqualified.

Rehabilitation

After an initial period of rest, passive movements should be started, followed by more active movements as healing occurs. Physiotherapy is an essential part of rehabilitation and close liaison between the sports doctor and the coach are needed in getting an athlete back to their sport. Steroid treatment should not be used around the Achilles tendon (according to advice from the National Institute for Health and Clinical Excellence and the British National Formulary).

Some patients develop myositis ossificans after a muscle haematoma. This presents itself as increasing swelling and pain. It can be treated with indomethacin, which helps prevent further formation, but it will resolve naturally.

FURTHER READING

Brukner P, Clarsen B, Cook J *et al*. *Brukner & Khan's clinical sports medicine*, vol 1, 5th edn. McGraw-Hill, New York, 2017.

MacAuley D. *Oxford handbook of sport and exercise medicine*, 2nd edn. Oxford: Oxford University Press, 2012.

Chapter 33

The spine

Learning objectives

To learn:
- The salient features relating to the history and examination of the spine
- The investigations commonly used in the field of spinal disorders
- The treatment principles for common conditions affecting the spine
- The global issues in spinal surgery

EPIDEMIOLOGY

The lifetime prevalence of low back pain has been reported at between 60 and 80%. By contrast, the lifetime prevalence of true sciatica is between 2 and 4%. It is generally accepted that 90% of acute low back pain episodes settle, allowing return to work within 6 weeks. However, some 5–7% of the population aged between 45 and 64 years will report back problems as a 'chronic sickness'. Up to 70% of acute episodes of sciatica resolve within 3 months.

Summary box 33.1

Epidemiology
- Low back pain is extremely common
- 90% of acute low back pain episodes settle within 6 weeks
- Sciatica is much less frequent
- 70% of acute sciatic episodes settle within 3 months

CLINICAL ANATOMY

The normal cervical lordosis measures between 35° and 45°. The normal lumbar lordosis is between 40° and 80° (mean 60°) and decreases with age. Most lumbar lordosis occurs between L4 and S1. The normal thoracic kyphosis is between 20° and 50° (mean 35°) and increases with age. When standing, the normal sagittal vertical axis (sagittal plumb-line) falls from the odontoid process through the C7–T1 disc space and crosses the spinal column at the T12–L1 disc space, before reaching the posterosuperior corner of the S1 vertebral body. For an energy efficient posture, cervical and lumbar lordosis will balance thoracic kyphosis.

The spinal canal is formed behind the articulated vertebral body by the posterior elements of the vertebral column and can be divided into a **central** portion and two **lateral** portions. The central portion is occupied by the thecal sac containing the spinal cord which terminates behind the body of L1. The lateral portions contain the nerve roots.

The spinal nerve roots comprise 8 cervical, 12 thoracic, 5 lumbar, 5 sacral and 1 coccygeal. Dorsal and ventral roots join to form spinal nerves. The ventral root and the dorsal root ganglion lie within the intervertebral foramen. This foramen is bounded superiorly and inferiorly by pedicles, anteriorly by the disc and posteriorly by the facet joint. Degenerative changes in these structures may lead to neural compromise. Laminar overlap within the lumbar spine decreases from L1 to S1 so that, at the L5–S1 level, access to the intervertebral disc requires less bone removal than at a more proximal level.

The blood supply of the spinal cord is derived from the vertebral, deep cervical, intercostal and lumbar arteries. The arteries of the spinal cord include the anterior spinal artery and two posterior spinal arteries, with the anterior spinal artery supplying the majority of the vascular supply to the spinal cord. The radicular artery of Adamkiewicz makes a major contribution to the anterior spinal artery, supplying the lower spinal cord. It originates on the left in 80% of people, usually accompanying the ventral root of T9, T10 or T11, but can originate anywhere from T5 to L5. Ligation of this important artery may lead to critical ischaemia of the spinal cord. Ligating segmental vessels over the midpoint of the vertebral body will minimise the risk of injury to this important artery during anterior approaches to the spine.

Albert Adamkiewicz, 1850–1921, Professor of Pathology, the University of Krakow (Cracow), Poland, described the arterial supply to the spinal cord in 1882.

PATIENT HISTORY

The commonest reasons for referral to a spinal clinic include **pain** and **spinal deformity**. A detailed history of the pain including site, type, severity, duration, frequency and aggravating factors should be sought. Has there been any history of trauma? Is the pain present at night? Is there associated pain in the upper limbs (brachalgia) or lower limbs (sciatica)? Is there associated numbness, tingling, weakness or difficulty with gait? Is there a family history of ankylosing spondylitis or rheumatoid arthritis? Are there concurrent medical conditions such as diabetes, peripheral vascular diseases, osteoarthritis of the hip or previous malignancies? Are there systemic symptoms such as unexplained weight loss, chills or fever? *Table 33.1* lists the commonly accepted 'red flags' that allow diagnostic triage into those with serious pathology of the spine (such as fractures, tumours, infection or cauda equina syndrome) and those without serious pathology.

TABLE 33.1 'Red flags': when present in patients with back pain, red flags suggest the likelihood of serious underlying pathology.
• Age <20 years or >50 years
• Recent significant trauma
• History of malignant disease
• Unexplained weight loss
• Constitutional symptoms (fever, chills)
• Immunosuppression (intravenous drug abuse, prolonged corticosteroid use)
• Severe or progressive sensory alteration or motor weakness
• Acute difficulty with micturition (painless retention)
• Numbness in perineum or buttocks and/or faecal incontinence

Pain may arise from the spine, but non-spinal causes of pain must also be considered (*Table 33.2*). Patients should always be asked about the presence of perineal numbness (saddle area) and/or difficulties passing urine or faeces, as these symptoms may indicate a cauda equina syndrome (*Table 33.3*).

TABLE 33.2 Non-spinal causes of low back pain: referred pain.
• Respiratory, e.g. mesothelioma
• Vascular, e.g. abdominal aortic aneurysm
• Renal, e.g. pyelonephritis
• Gastrointestinal, e.g. peptic ulcer, pancreatitis
• Urogenital, e.g. testicular, ovarian or prostatic cancinoma

Patients should be asked whether the pain is interfering with their ability to work. What treatment has the patient already tried and how effective were these treatments (e.g. analgesics, exercise, physiotherapy or spinal injections)? Pending litigation or worker's compensation claims may have a negative prognostic effect on future treatments and therefore should be enquired about.

Spinal deformities, e.g. scoliosis and excessive kyphosis (>50°), are generally painless in children, but may be symptomatic in adult life. How quickly has the spinal deformity progressed? It is important to assess skeletal maturity and whether the child has gone through a recent growth spurt. Has menstruation commenced in the female or has the voice dropped in the male, indicating the onset of puberty?

TABLE 33.3 Cauda equina syndrome presentation.
• Low back pain
• Uni- or bilateral sciatica
• Saddle anaesthesia
• Motor weakness in the lower extremities
• Variable rectal and urinary symptoms

PHYSICAL EXAMINATION

The patient should be undressed and posture should be evaluated in both the frontal and sagittal planes. Shoulder or waist asymmetry suggests the presence of scoliosis. The Adam's forward bend test will accentuate trunk asymmetry and allow appreciation of rib or loin prominence on the convex side of each curve. The skin should be examined for cutaneous neurofibromata, café-au-lait patches or axillary freckling commonly present in neurofibromatosis. Neurological examination should include abdominal reflexes. Leg lengths should be measured. In the case of kyphosis, the sagittal alignment and forward gaze should be assessed.

William Adams described the forward bending test for scoliosis in 1865. His understanding of the nature of the rotational element of scoliosis was given by a postmortem examination he performed on an eminent surgeon and geologist, Gideon Mantell. The clinical history of Dr Mantell is well documented.

Palpation is useful to locate specific areas of tenderness. Ranges of motion should be assessed. The normal range of motion in the cervical spine is 45° of flexion, 55° of extension, 70° of rotation and 40° of lateral bend. The normal range of motion in the lumbar spine is 40–60° of flexion, 20–35° of extension, 15–20° of lateral bending and 3–18° of rotation. Schober's test is a simple clinical test to evaluate spinal mobility. A tape measure is used to mark the skin midway between the posterior superior iliac spines and at points 10 cm proximal and 5 cm distal to this mark while the patient is standing. The patient is then asked to bend forward as far as possible and the distance between the two points is measured with the patient in the flexed position. Normally one would expect to see an increase of at least 5 cm between the two points in the erect and flexed positions. A distance of less than 5 cm between these points may indicate ankylosing spondylitis.

Neurological examination of the upper and lower limbs will focus on tone, power, coordination, reflexes, sensation and gait (*Tables 33.4* and *33.5*). A rectal examination should be performed if there is any concern about cauda equina integrity. The superficial abdominal reflex is an upper motor neurone reflex. It is performed by stroking one of four abdominal quandrants in succession. The umbilicus should move toward the quandrant that was stroked. The reflex should be symmetrical from side to side. Absent or asymmetrical abdominal

TABLE 33.4 Neurological evaluation of the upper limb.

Neurological level	Motor	Sensation	Reflexes
C5	Deltoid	Lateral arm	Biceps (C5–C6)
C6	Wrist extensors	Lateral forearm	Brachioradialis (C5–C6)
C7	Triceps	Middle finger	Triceps (C7–C8)
C8	Long finger flexors	Medial forearm	No reflex
T1	Interosseus muscles	Medial arm	No reflex

TABLE 33.5 Neurological evaluation of the lower limb.

Neurological level	Motor	Sensation	Reflex
L2	Hip flexion	Anterior thigh, groin	No reflex
L3	Knee extension	Anterior and lateral thigh	Patellar (L3–L4)
L4	Ankle dorsiflexion	Medial leg and foot	Patellar (L3–L4)
L5	Extensor hallucis longus	Lateral leg and foot	No reflex
S1	Ankle plantarflexion	Lateral foot and little toe	Achilles (S1–S2)

reflexes may indicate intraspinal pathology such as syringomyelia or spinal cord injury.

Myelopathy or upper motor neurone (UMN) lesions are suggested by spasticity, motor weakness, hyper-reflexia, positive Hoffmann's sign (forceful flexion of the distal phalanx of the middle finger results in flexion of the thumb and index finger), upgoing Babinski response, and patellar and ankle clonus.

Summary box 33.2

Upper motor neurone lesions are characterised by:

- Increased tone – spastic
- Hyper-reflexia
- Muscle spasms
- Motor weakness
- Disuse atrophy
- Positive Hoffman's sign
- Ankle and patellar clonus
- Upgoing plantar response

Typical signs of radiculopathy (lower motor neurone (LMN) lesion) include sensory loss, motor weakness, flaccid paralysis, muscle atrophy, loss of reflexes and muscle fasciculation.

The straight leg raise (SLR) test is performed with the patient in the supine position. The leg is elevated with the knee straight to increase tension along the L5 and S1 nerve roots. The test is positive if the leg elevation provokes radicular pain. The crossed SLR test is carried out by elevating the asymptomatic leg, and produces sciatic symptoms in the opposite leg. A positive test is associated with a herniated disc in 97% of patients. Lasègue's sign denotes radicular pain aggravated by ankle dorsiflexion.

The femoral nerve stretch test is performed with the patient in the prone position by extending the hip and flexing the knee. This creates tension on the L2, L3 and L4 nerve roots. The femoral nerve stretch test is considered positive if radicular pain occurs in the anterior thigh region during the test.

The examination should include, where appropriate, examination of the shoulder, hip, knee, sacroiliac joint and vascular system, as dual pathology is common in the ageing community.

In 1979, Waddell and colleagues developed and validated a series of signs and tests that have proved helpful in identifying individuals who are magnifying or exaggerating symptoms, possibly for secondary gain (*Table 33.6*).

TABLE 33.6 Non-organic physical signs in low back pain.

- *Tenderness*: superficial or non-anatomical
- *Simulation tests*: axial loading or rotation
- *Distraction tests*: variable straight leg raises
- *Regional disturbances*: non-anatomical sensory or motor loss
- *Over-reaction*: grimacing, muscle tremor, etc.

Summary box 33.3

Lower motor neurone lesions are characterised by:

- Decreased tone – flaccid
- Hyporeflexia
- Denervation fasciculations
- Motor weakness
- Sensory loss
- Severe atrophy
- Downgoing plantar response

Johann Hoffmann, 1857–1919, Professor of Neurology, Heidelberg, Germany.
Joseph Francis Felix Babinski, 1857–1932, neurologist, Hôpital de la Pitie, Paris, France.
Charles Ernest Lasègue, 1816–1863, Professor of Medicine, University of Paris, and physician, La Salpêtrière, Paris, France.

INVESTIGATIONS

The most common diagnostic imaging tests used to evaluate spinal disorders include plain radiographs, computed tomography (CT), magnetic resonance imaging (MRI), CT myelography and isotope bone scanning. These investigations are extremely sensitive, but relatively non-specific. For example, at least one-third of asymptomatic patients have been noted to have 'abnormalities' on MRI scans. All investigations must therefore be carefully correlated with the clinical findings.

Plain radiographs

It is not appropriate to order spine radiographs for every patient presenting with neck or low back pain. Patients with red flag signs or symptoms and those who have not responded to conservative treatment require imaging, with most units in resource-rich countries utilising MRI (no radiation penalty) in this situation. Standing radiographs of the whole spine are important for the assessment of scoliosis. Radiographs cannot diagnose early-stage tumour or infection, because significant bone destruction (between 40% and 60% of bone mass) must occur before a radiographic abnormality is detected

Computed tomography

This investigation is the best test for assessing bone anatomy. Three-dimensional reconstructions are often useful for the assessment of congenital spinal deformity. However, one should remember that a typical CT of the lumbar spine will expose the patient to an effective dose of 5–10 milliseiverts (mSv), which would be equivalent to 2.5–5 years of background radiation.

Magnetic resonance imaging

This allows detailed visualisation of the spinal cord, thecal sac, epidural space, intervertebral discs, nerve roots, paraspinal soft tissues and bone marrow. It is contraindicated for patients with certain pacemakers and coronary stents, intracranial metal clips, metallic bodies in the eye, spinal cord stimulators and certain drug pumps.

Bone scintigraphy

Isotope bone scans are highly sensitive, but non-specific, tests useful for screening the skeletal system for metastatic disease, discitis or vertebral body osteomyelitis, or to assess the relative activity of bone lesions such as osteoid osteoma, osteoblastoma, defects in the pars interarticulares or a pseudarthrosis (incomplete fusion). In the case of multiple myeloma or purely lytic metastases, the bone scan may not show increased activity as these tumours may not stimulate a significant **osteoblastic** response.

Bone densitometry

Bone density and osteoporosis can be measured using dual-energy x-ray absorptiometry (DEXA) of the hip, wrist and spine.

Provocative discography

This investigation involves the placement of a 24-gauge needle into the centre of the intervertebral disc in a conscious patient. One to 3.5 mL of radio-opaque contrast agent is then injected into the disc. The contrast pattern will allow the discrimination of different degrees of disc degeneration; cottonball or lobular would be considered normal whereas irregular, fissured or ruptured would be considered degenerate (**Figure 33.1**). The patient is asked if they are experiencing their 'usual type of back pain'. To diagnose discogenic low back pain one must document evidence of disc degeneration and concordant pain during the injection. Treatment options may include spinal fusion or disc replacement

Facet joint injections

For patients with facet joint arthropathy, x-ray-guided local anaesthetic and steroid injections may be both diagnostic and therapeutic for 4–6 weeks. Longer-term relief may be obtained by facet joint rhizolysis. This percutaneous procedure denervates the facet joint using heat.

Foraminal epidural steroid injections

For patients with radiculopathy due to a prolapsed intervertebral disc or lateral recess stenosis, a targeted foraminal epidural steroid injection of local anaesthetic and steroid may provide important diagnostic information and have a lasting therapeutic effect.

Spinal biopsy

Either CT-guided or open biopsy is often performed to obtain tissue for diagnostic study in cases of suspected tumour and/or infection.

DEGENERATIVE CONDITIONS OF THE SPINE

Cervical radiculopathy

Patients present with neck and arm pain (brachalgia), paraesthesia and motor weakness in the distribution of the compromised nerve root (radiculopathy). This may be caused by disc herniation or degenerative stenosis. Symptoms often respond to conservative treatment including physiotherapy and medication for neuropathic pain (amitriptyline, gabapentin or pregabalin) or CT-guided foraminal epidural steroid injections of local anaesthetic and steroid. Intractable pain and/or functional neurological deficit are indications for surgical intervention. Surgical options include anterior cervical discectomy and fusion (using a cage packed with bone graft and plate), cervical total disc replacement (**Figure 33.2**) or posterior laminoforaminotomy. Randomised controlled trials have compared anterior cervical discectomy and fusion to cervical disc replacement. Similar clinical outcomes have been observed in both groups. However, cervical disc replacements preserve motion in the operated level, and may protect against adjacent segment disease in the longer term.

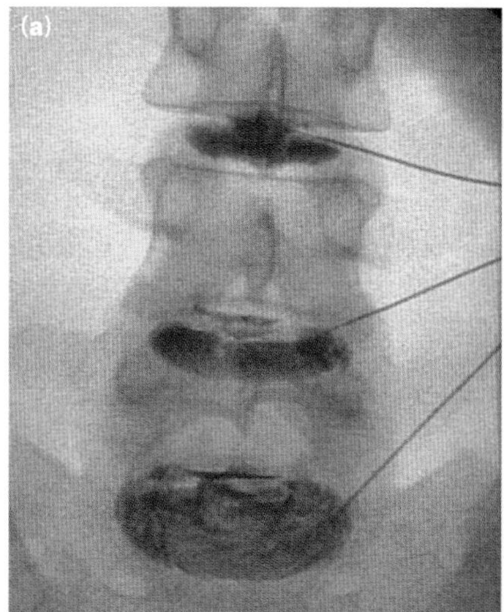

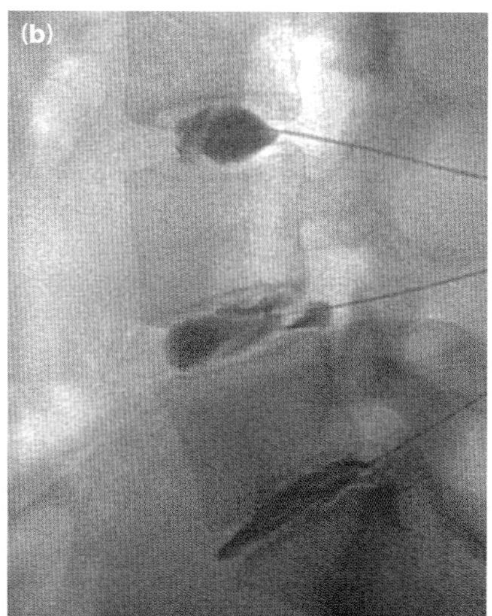

Figure 33.1 Lumbar discography. Anteroposterior (**a**) and lateral (**b**) radiographs following injection of contrast media into the lower three lumbar discs. Morphology: L3/4 cottonball, L4/5 fissured, L5/S1 ruptured. Concordant low back pain was reproduced when injecting the L4/5 and L5/S1 discs. No pain was experienced when the L3/4 disc was injected. The patient underwent a posterolateral fusion L4 to S1.

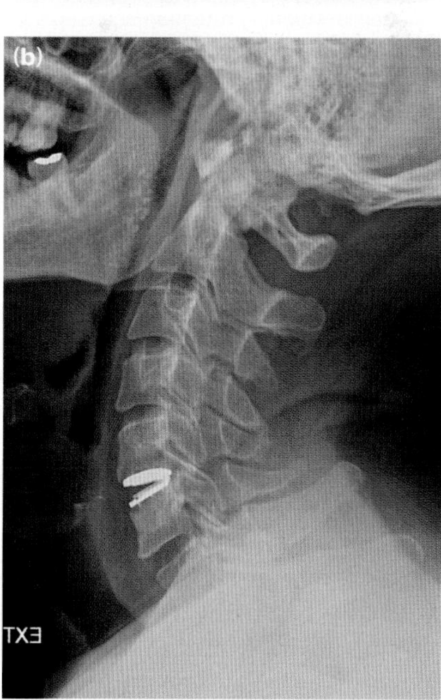

Figure 33.2 Cervical total disc replacement. The patient presented with severe left-sided C6 radiculopathy. MRI scan confirmed a left C5/6 disc herniation. The patient underwent a C5/6 discectomy and decompression of the left C6 nerve root, followed by insertion of a cervical disc replacement. Lateral radiographs in flexion (**a**) and extension (**b**) show restored motion to the C5/6 level.

Cervical myelopathy

Degenerative change in the cervical spine leading to spinal cord compression is the commonest cause of cervical myelopathy in patients over 55 years of age. Lower motor neurone changes occur **at the level** of the lesion, with atrophy of the upper extremity muscles, particularly the intrinsic muscles of the hands. Upper motor neurone findings are noted **below** the level of the lesion and may involve both upper and lower extremities. If surgery is considered appropriate then an anterior or posterior decompression may be required.

Thoracic disc herniation

Thoracic disc herniations that require surgical intervention are rare, accounting for less than 2% of all discectomy procedures. Typically, the patient presents with axial pain, radiculopathy or myelopathy. Conservative treatment including non-steroidal anti-inflammatory drugs, physiotherapy and general fitness improvement should be considered initially. If required, thoracic discectomy may be performed via a thoracotomy or, for a soft disc prolapse, via a thoracoscopic approach.

Cauda equina syndrome

Cauda equina syndrome (CES) is rare, accounting for only 2–6% of all lumbar disc herniations. It presents most commonly in the 20–45-year age group, with some or all of the following symptoms: low back pain, unilateral or bilateral sciatica, lower limb motor weakness, sensory abnormalities including saddle anaesthesia, bladder dysfunction (painless retention in early stages, overflow incontinence in later stages), sexual and bowel dysfunction. CES may result from acute or chronic compression of the cauda equina nerve roots. The most frequent cause is a massive central lumbar disc protrusion at L4/5; other causes include lumbar fractures, postoperative epidural haematoma, spinal stenosis, spinal tumours and occlusion of the lumbar arteries by dissection or aneurysm of the abdominal aorta.

Cauda equina nerve roots lack epineurium and perineurium, and only have a thin endoneurium root sheath, making them more susceptible to compression forces when compared with peripheral nerves. The syndrome can result in permanent motor deficit, and bladder, bowel and sexual dysfunction. It represents a true spinal emergency and requires urgent surgical decompression. The outcome for patients who undergo surgical decompression within 24 hours of the onset of loss of bladder or bowel control is significantly better than that of those who undergo surgery beyond this 24-hour period.

Summary box 33.4

Cauda equina syndrome

- Commonest presenting symptoms: perineal numbness, painless urinary retention and faecal incontinence
- Urgent investigation with MRI is required for all suspected cases
- Confirmed CES requires surgical decompression within 24 hours to achieve optimum outcomes

Lumbar disc herniation

Symptomatic lumbar disc herniation occurs during the lifetime of approximately 2–4% of the population. Risk factors include family history, male gender, age (30–50 years), heavy lifting or twisting, stressful occupation, lower income and cigarette smoking.

Over 90% of lumbar disc herniations occur at the L4/5 or L5/S1 levels. A posterolateral disc protrusion will affect the **traversing** root, e.g. an L4/5 disc protrusion will affect the L5 nerve root. A far-lateral disc protrusion (extraforaminal) will affect the **exiting** nerve root, e.g. a far-lateral L5/S1 disc protrusion will affect the L5 nerve root. Symptoms typically commence with a period of back pain followed by sciatica. There may be paraesthesia, motor weakness, loss of reflexes and a reduction in straight leg raise.

For simple sciatica, a period of 6–12 weeks of conservative treatment is advised. Up to 70% of patients will settle within this period. A trial of pregabalin (GABA analogue) and/or a transforaminal epidural steroid injection maybe helpful. Microdiscectomy is the standard surgical intervention for those in whom conservative treatment has failed. The procedure is carried out in the prone position with radiographic confirmation of the correct level. Loupes with a headlight or use of the operating microscope greatly facilitate the procedure. A 3–5 cm incision is made with a unilateral take down of the multifidus. The spinal canal is entered via removal of the ligamentum flavum under the lamina. The thecal sac and traversing nerve root are identified. The dura and nerve root are retracted medially and the offending disc prolapse incised via a transverse annulotomy. The disc fragment is removed and the disc space cleared of any remaining nuclear material with rongeurs and multiple washouts of the disc space. The wound is closed. Patients are generally discharged the next morning.

Spinal stenosis

Spinal stenosis may be defined as any type of narrowing of the spinal canal, nerve root canal or intervertebral foramen. The resultant nerve root compression leads to nerve root ischaemia, presenting with back, buttock or leg pain provoked by exercise. Spinal stenosis may be congenital, as is the case in achondroplasia, or acquired, as is the case for degenerative types (commonly presenting between 50 and 70 years of age). The narrowing is caused by facet joint hypertrophy, disc bulging and ligamentum flavum thickening.

Symptoms of spinal claudication can be distinguished from vascular claudication because they are frequently associated with neurological symptoms, are often worse in extension, and pedal pulses are present on clinical examination. Symptoms progress in approximately 20–33% of patients who receive no treatment. The condition may be treated successfully by surgical decompression alone with preservation of the facet joints.

Summary box 33.5

Spinal stenosis

- Extremely common condition in the 50–70-year age group
- Classic symptoms: back, buttock, thigh and calf pain
- Provoked by walking and extended posture
- Relieved by flexed posture
- Symptoms progress in up to one-third of untreated patients

Discogenic low back pain

Discogenic low back pain has been defined as a continuum of diagnostic categories (internal disc disruption, degenerative disc disease, segmental instability) reflecting various stages of degenerative pathology affecting the intervertebral disc. Not all degenerate discs are painful. Patients typically present with chronic relapsing episodes of low back pain between the ages of 40 and 60 years.

A recent study has compared rehabilitation with spinal fusion for discogenic pain. Both groups reported reductions in disability, with the authors strongly recommending a course of rehabilitation **before** surgical intervention. For those who fail to improve with conservative measures, provocative lumbar discography (see **Figure 33.1**) may help to identify the source of pain, and surgery in the form of a lumbar spinal fusion (**Figure 33.3**) or lumbar disc replacement (**Figure 33.4**) may be considered.

SPONDYLOLYSIS AND SPONDYLOLISTHESIS

Spondylolysis

This is a unilateral or bilateral defect in the pars interarticularis without vertebral slippage. The incidence is reported at approximately 6% by the age of 14 years, but is much higher in the young athletic population. Many cases remain

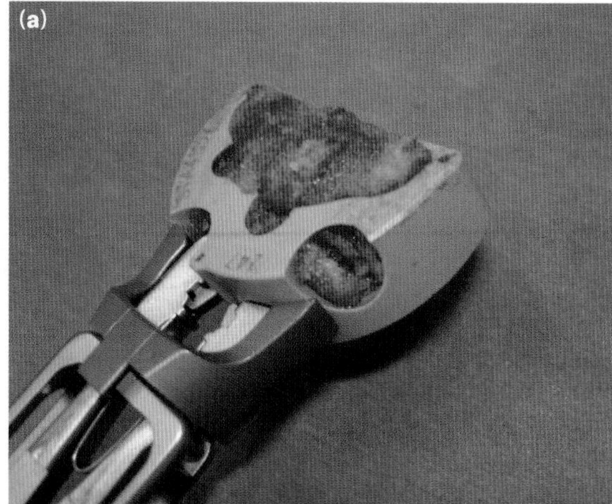

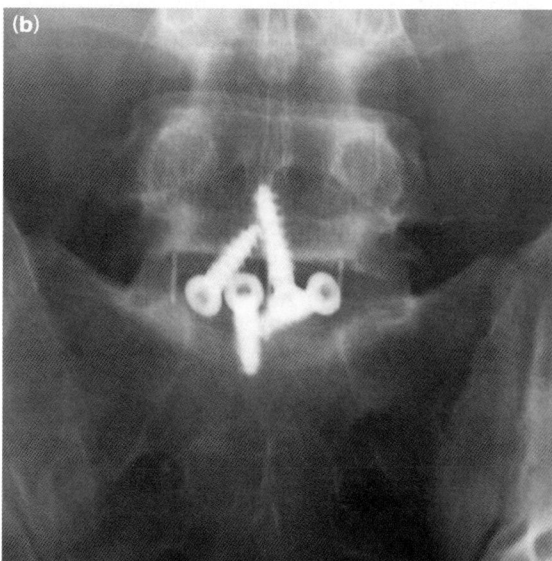

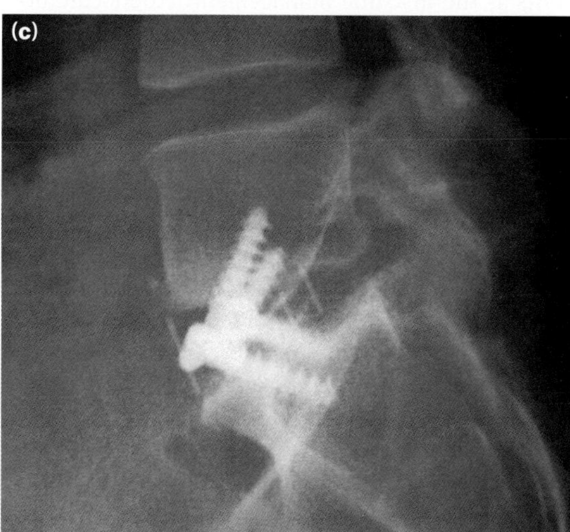

Figure 33.3 Anterior lumbar interbody fusion. (**a**) The PEEK (poly-ethyl-ethyl-ketone) cage has been packed with bone graft prior to insertion; (**b**) and (**c**) show the anteroposterior and lateral postoperative radiographs, respectively.

asymptomatic. The diagnosis is difficult to confirm with plain radiographs. Reverse gantry CT, MRI and single photon emission computed tomography (SPECT) are very useful investigations for this condition. Treatment involves rest, nonsteroidal anti-inflammatory medication, activity modification and a lumbosacral orthosis. For patients who remain symptomatic despite an adequate trial of non-operative care, surgery in the form of a direct repair of the pseudarthrosis by a Buck's fusion may be indicated.

Summary box 33.6

Spondylolysis

- Incidence in general population 6% by 14 years
- Incidence in athletic population 15–47%
- May be completely asymptomatic/incidental finding on radiograph
- Difficult to image, but MRI proving more useful
- Conservative treatment: activity modification, antilordotic brace
- Surgical treatment: direct repair preserving motion or spinal fusion if associated disc degeneration

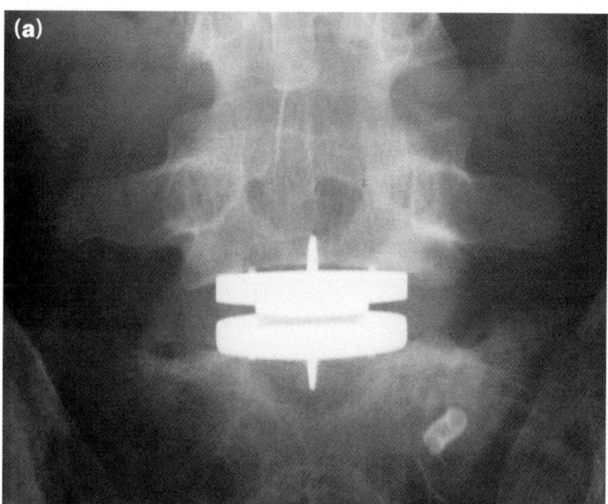

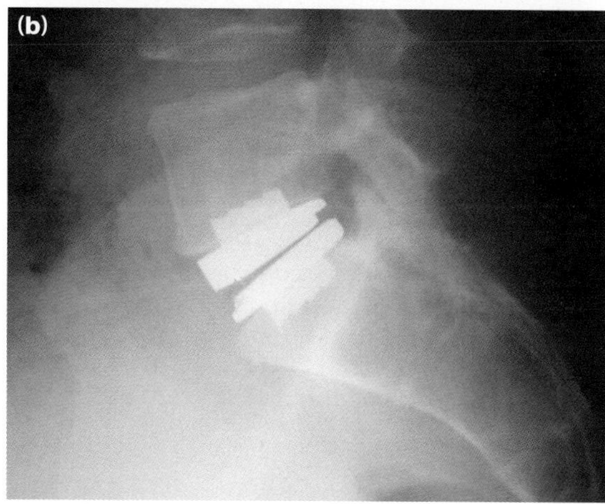

Figure 33.4 Lumbar total disc replacement. (**a**) Anteroposterior radiograph with 30° of cranial inclination. (**b**) Lateral radiograph with the implant appropriately positioned.

Spondylolisthesis

Spondylolisthesis is a forward slippage of the vertebral body engendered by a break in the continuity or elongation of the pars interarticularis and presents in 4% of the adult population. Spondylolisthesis can be classified into six types by causation (*Table 33.7*), or by the degree of slip (*Table 33.8*).

For skeletally immature patients (<18 years old) who have progressive slips in the spine, and in individuals with intractable low back or radicular pain, or neurological symptoms, surgery may be indicated. For low-grade slips (Meyerding Grade I and II) fusion-*in-situ* is the procedure of choice. If there is **objective** evidence of neural compression (e.g. weakness of extensor hallucis longus), a spinal decompression should be performed at the same time. For high-grade slips (Meyerding Grade III or IV) (**Figure 33.5**), opinion is divided on whether to reduce the slip first and then fuse, or simply to fuse *in situ*.

TUMOURS OF THE SPINE

Metastatic tumours

These are the most common tumours affecting the spine, accounting for 98% of all spine lesions. The commonest malignancies that metastasise to the spine are shown in *Table 33.9*. Red flags picked up on history or examination will alert the clinician to this possible diagnosis.

Over 80% of patients with spinal metastases present with progressive pain, and only 20% present with spinal cord compression. Relevant investigations include full blood count (FBC), urea and electrolytes, liver function tests, calcium, erythrocyte sedimentation rate (ESR), C-reactive protein (CRP), prostate-specific antigen (PSA), serum protein electrophoresis, thyroid function tests (where a thyroid mass has been palpated) and nutritional indices. Plain radiographs may show an absent pedicle ('winking owl' sign), vertebral cortical erosion and/or vertebral collapse. MRI of the whole spine will detect most metastases. Most metastases are **osteoblastic** and will show up on bone scintigraphy; however, osteolytic lesions such as multiple myeloma and renal cell carcinoma may not show up on an isotope bone scan. Metastases from the prostate may be sclerotic. Biopsies may be obtained via a percutaneous CT-guided method or open biopsy.

Treatment options include orthotics, steroids (dexamethasone), radiotherapy, chemotherapy, hormonal therapy, surgery or a combination of any of the above. Radiotherapy promotes reossification of the vertebral body and reduces tumour load. It can be very effective for reducing 'bone pain'. Lymphoma, breast, lung and prostate metastases are highly radiosensitive. Gastrointestinal adenocarcinoma, metastatic melanoma, thyroid and renal carcinoma are radioresistant. Small cell carcinoma of the lung, Ewing's sarcoma, thyroid carcinoma, breast carcinoma and neuroblastoma are usually sensitive to chemotherapy and should have chemotherapeutic agents as the first-line management. Adenocarcinoma of the lung is resistant to chemotherapy. Prostate metastases may respond well to antiandrogenic hormone medication.

Extensive reconstructive tumour surgery should be reserved for those patients whose life expectancy exceeds 3–6 months. For patients with malignant spinal cord compression, the combination of decompressive surgery with stabilisation and postoperative radiotherapy has been shown to be superior in outcome when compared with radiotherapy alone. In one randomised trial, surgery and radiotherapy permitted most patients to remain ambulatory for the remainder of their lives, whereas patients treated with radiotherapy alone spent a large portion of their remaining time as paraplegics.

TABLE 33.7 Wiltse classification of spondylolisthesis.

Type 1	Dysplastic	Associated with congenital deficiency of the L5–S1 articulation
Type 2	Isthmic	Associated with a lesion of the pars interarticulares Three subtypes: 2A: lytic defect of the pars 2B: elongated or attenuated pars 2C: acute pars fracture
Type 3	Degenerative spondylolisthesis	Segmental instability due to disc degeneration/facet arthrosis
Type 4	Traumatic	Acute fracture in the region of the posterior elements, other than the pars interarticulares
Type 5	Pathological	Generalised bone disease resulting in attenuation of the pars (e.g. metabolic, neoplastic)
Type 6	Postsurgical	After decompression of the lumbar spine

TABLE 33.8 The Meyerding classification for the degree of slip of spondylolisthesis.

Grade I	1–25%
Grade II	26–50%
Grade III	51–75%
Grade IV	76–100%

TABLE 33.9 Commonest malignancies that metastasise to the spine and their frequency.

• Breast	21%
• Lung	14%
• Prostate	7.5%
• Renal	5%
• Gastrointestinal	5%
• Thyroid	2.5%

Summary box 33.7

Metastatic tumours of the spine

- Commonest presentation is progressive spinal pain
- Whole spine MRI will detect most metastases
- Surgery is indicated for instability, pain, progressive deformity or neurological deficit

James Ewing, 1866–1943, Professor of Pathology, Cornell University Medical College, New York, NY, USA, described this type of sarcoma in 1921.

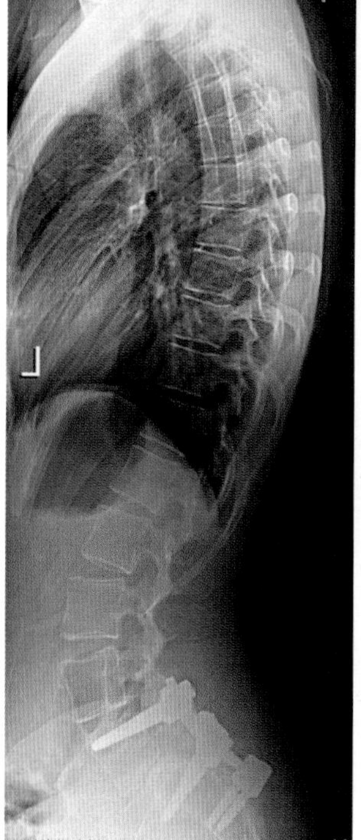

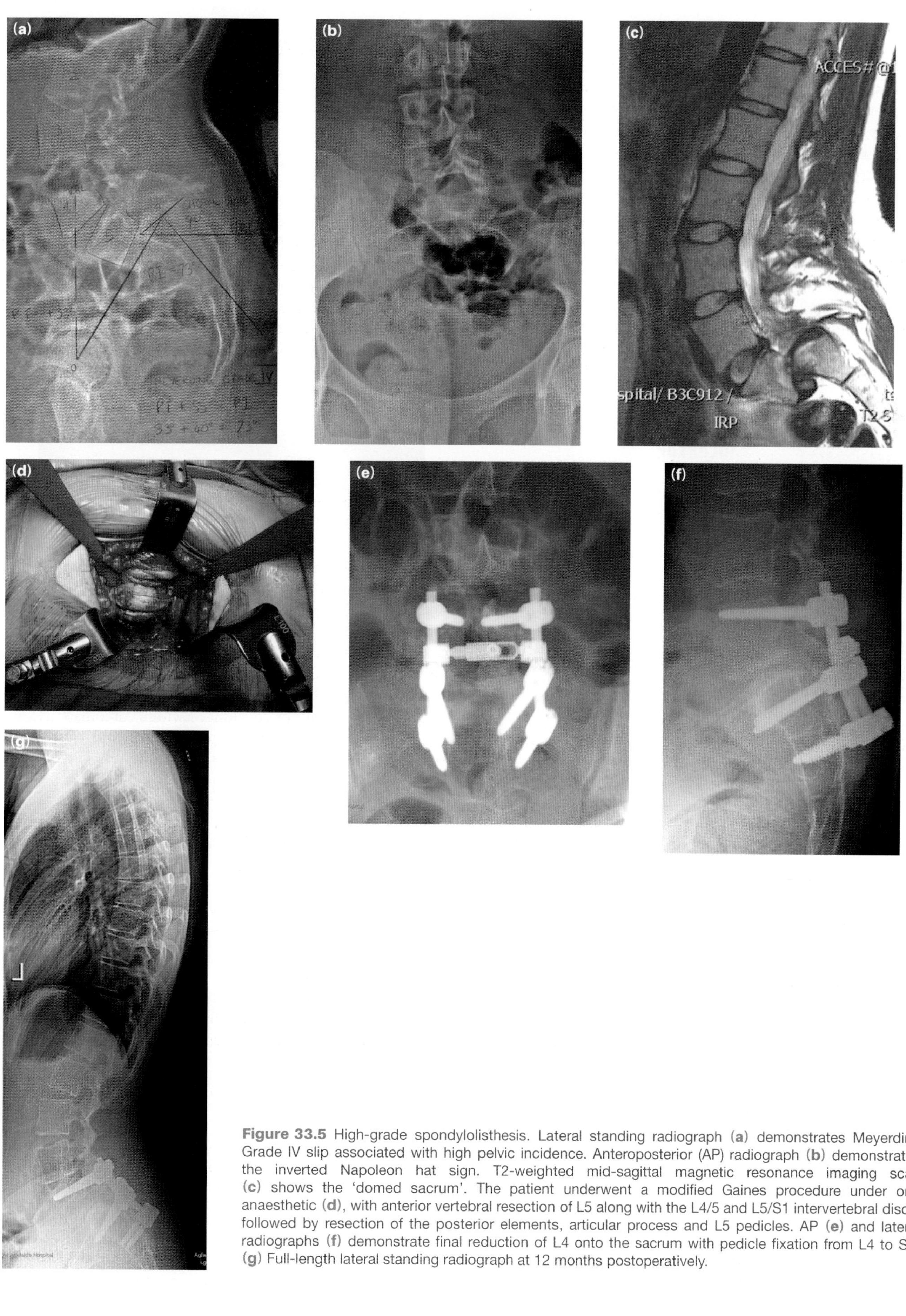

Figure 33.5 High-grade spondylolisthesis. Lateral standing radiograph (**a**) demonstrates Meyerding Grade IV slip associated with high pelvic incidence. Anteroposterior (AP) radiograph (**b**) demonstrates the inverted Napoleon hat sign. T2-weighted mid-sagittal magnetic resonance imaging scan (**c**) shows the 'domed sacrum'. The patient underwent a modified Gaines procedure under one anaesthetic (**d**), with anterior vertebral resection of L5 along with the L4/5 and L5/S1 intervertebral discs, followed by resection of the posterior elements, articular process and L5 pedicles. AP (**e**) and lateral radiographs (**f**) demonstrate final reduction of L4 onto the sacrum with pedicle fixation from L4 to S2. (**g**) Full-length lateral standing radiograph at 12 months postoperatively.

Primary tumours of the spine

Primary bone tumours of the spine account for only 2% of all spinal tumours. They arise *de novo* in the bone, cartilage, neural or ligamentous structures of the spine. They may be benign, intermediate or malignant. Benign primary spine tumours include osteoid osteoma, osteoblastoma (Figure 33.6), chondroma, chondroblastoma, chondromyxoid fibroma, giant cell tumours, haemangioma, lymphangioma and lipoma. Intermediate primary spine tumours include aggressive osteoblastoma, haemangiopericytoma, haemangioendothelioma and chordoma. Malignant primary spinal tumours include osteosarcoma, chondrosarcoma, Ewing's sarcoma, neuroectodermal tumours, malignant lymphoma, myeloma, angiosarcoma, fibrosarcoma and liposarcoma. The reader is referred to Chapter 37 for more specific aspects of orthopaedic oncology.

In patients less than 18 years of age, 68% of all tumours are benign. For those patients who present over 18 years of age, more than 80% of tumours are malignant. Benign tumours tend to occur in the posterior elements; malignant tumours tend to involve the vertebral body.

Intradural tumours

These are rare. They may be intramedullary (within the substance of the cord) or extramedullary (outside the cord). Most are extramedullary and benign; the commonest are meningiomas and neurofibromas.

Meningiomas are usually benign and arise from the meninges. They are generally slow growing and often warrant radiological surveillance. If the lesion is large and impinges on the spinal cord or nerve roots, steroids and early surgery may be indicated.

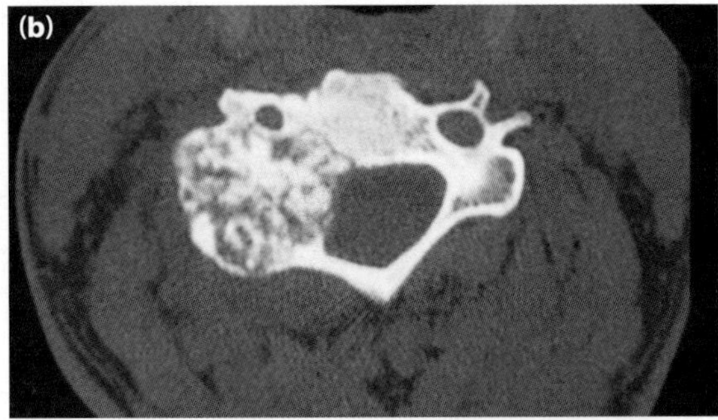

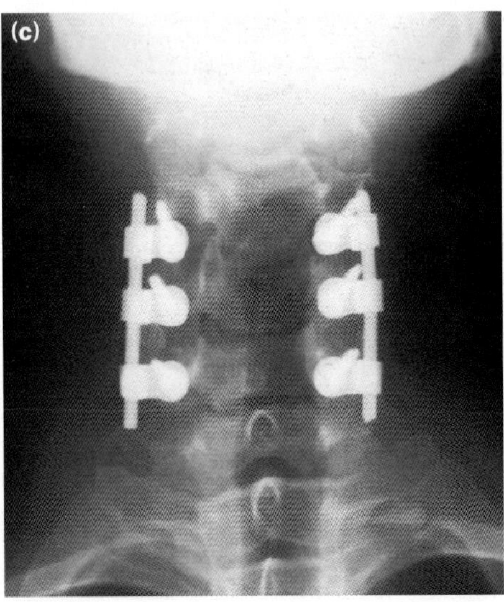

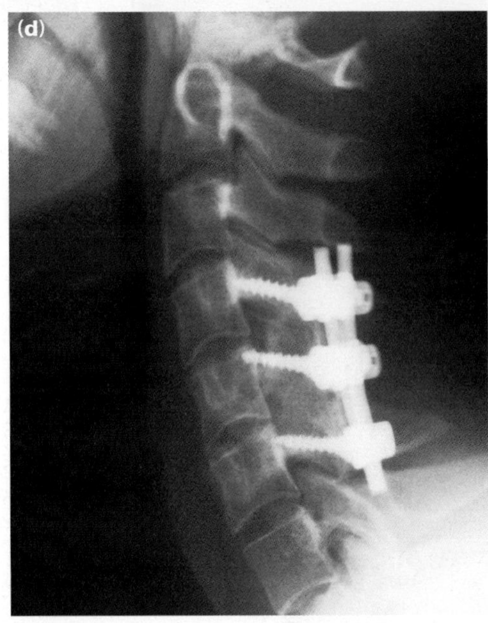

Figure 33.6 Osteoblastoma arising from the posterior elements of C5. This 21-year-old man presented with severe unremitting neck pain. Isotope bone scan (**a**) demonstrated increased uptake in C5. An axial CT scan (**b**) further delineated the expansive lesion. The tumour was successfully removed with the aid of an intraoperative gamma probe to confirm complete excision; (**c**) and (**d**) show the postoperative anteroposterior and lateral radiographs, respectively, following reconstruction with a tricortical bone graft, lateral mass screws and rods.

Neurofibromas are benign tumours that arise from the nerve sheath. There are three major types of neurofibroma: cutaneous, spinal and plexiform. In 90% of cases they present as solitary lesions, with the remainder presenting in patients with neurofibromatosis type 1 (NF1), an autosomal dominant genetically inherited disease. NF1 occurs in 1 in 3000 births and has been referred to as peripheral neurofibromatosis or von Recklinghausen disease. Diagnosis of NF1 is confirmed when an individual has two or more of the following: at least six café-au-lait macules >5 mm diameter before puberty, or six café-au-lait macules >15 mm after puberty, two or more neurofibromas of any type or one plexiform neurofibroma, multiple freckles in the axillary or inguinal regions, a distinctive bone abnormality involving the eye socket or arm/leg bones, optic glioma in the brain, two or more Lisch nodules in the eye, and a parent, sibling or child with NF1. Neurofibromatosis type 2 (NF2) is a genetically determined disorder which affects 1 in 40000 individuals worldwide. A diagnosis of NF2 is made when an individual has the following findings: schwannomas on both 8th cranial (vestibular) nerves or a parent, sibling or child with NF2 plus one vestibular schwannoma in a person less than 30 years of age, or any two of the following: meningioma, glioma, schwannoma, juvenile cataracts.

INFECTIONS OF THE SPINE

Pyogenic infections

Pyogenic vertebral osteomyelitis is primarily a lesion of the disc and its osseous margins. The most common method by which an organism spreads to the spine is via the haematogenous route. The disc is nearly always involved in pyogenic vertebral infection. In contrast, granulomatous infection, such as tuberculosis, typically does not involve the disc space.

Risk factors for pyogenic vertebral osteomyelitis include advancing age, intravenous drug abuse, diabetes, renal failure, recent infections and trauma. *Staphylococcus aureus* accounts for 30–55% of the infections. Gram-negative organisms such as *Escherichia coli*, *Pseudomonas* species and *Proteus* species are associated with recent genitourinary infections and intravenous drug abuse. Anaerobic infections are uncommon, but may be seen in diabetic patients and after penetrating trauma.

Operative intervention should be considered for:

- open biopsy (when a closed biopsy has failed);
- failure of medical management (persistent pain, elevated ESR, CRP);
- drainage of abscesses;
- decompression of spinal cord compression;
- correction of progressive spinal deformity;
- stabilisation of progressive spinal instability.

Epidural abscess

This condition is often a surgical emergency. The majority of cases occur within the thoracic spine. Without treatment, neurological deficit including paralysis may develop.

Tuberculosis

This is discussed in Chapters 6 and 38.

INFLAMMATORY SPONDYLOARTHROPATHY

Rheumatoid arthritis

Between 33% and 50% of patients develop atlantoaxial subluxation (AAS) within 5 years of the diagnosis of rheumatoid arthritis. Some 2–10% of patients with AAS develop myelopathy over the next 10 years. Once diagnosed with myelopathy, 50% of patients die within 1 year. Approximately 20% of patients develop symptomatic subaxial disease. Neurological symptoms may occur as a result of direct compression by bone or soft tissue or from neural ischaemia. Care needs to be taken with these patients whenever they require surgery. The degree of subluxation may need to be checked by performing flexion and extension radiographs, and the theatre staff (especially the anaesthetist) need to be warned to take special care especially with intubation. The indications for surgery to stabilise the cervical spine are given in *Table 33.10*.

TABLE 33.10 Recommendations for spinal surgery in rheumatoid arthritis.
• AAS with a PADI of 14 mm or less
• AAS with at least 5 mm of basilar invagination
• Subaxial subluxation with a sagittal canal diameter of 14 mm or less

AAS, atlantoaxial subluxation; PADI, posterior atlantodental interval.

Ankylosing spondylitis

Should a patient with ankylosing spondylitis (AS) present following trauma, a high index of suspicion for occult fractures should be present. It is common for patients with AS to develop epidural haematomas with subtle neurological deficit.

Patients with a significant fixed flexion deformity at the cervicothoracic junction ('chin-on-chest' deformity), limited forward gaze, eating and swallowing difficulties may be treated with a closing wedge osteotomy at the cervicothoracic junction (**Figure 33.7**). Extension osteotomies can also be performed in the thoracic and lumbar spine.

Freidrich Daniel von Recklinghausen, 1833–1910, Professor of Pathology, Strasbourg, France, described generalised neurofibromatosis in 1882.
Hans Christian Joachim Gram, 1853–1938, Professor of Pharmacology (1891–1900) and of Medicine (1900–1923), Copenhagen, Denmark, described this method of staining bacteria in 1884.
Theodor Escherich, 1857–1911, Professor of Paediatrics, Vienna, Austria, discovered the *Bacterium Coli Commune* in 1886.

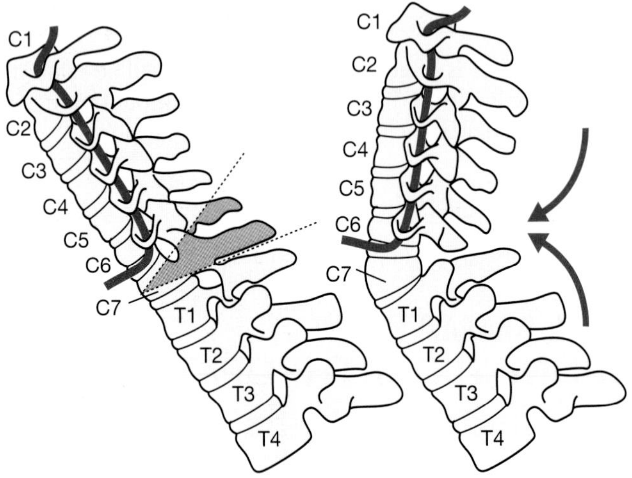

Figure 33.7 C7 closing wedge osteotomy for correction of cervicothoracic kyphosis in patients with ankylosing spondylitis. Planned resection lateral view (left) and lateral view after closure of the osteotomy (right).

SPINAL DEFORMITY

Spinal deformity may be categorised into a coronal plane deformity (scoliosis) or a sagittal plane deformity (kyphosis and lordosis). Further classification may be made on the basis of aetiology into congenital, neuromuscular, idiopathic or syndromic. Appropriate radiographs for the assessment of scoliosis include a full posteroanterior and lateral standing spine. When surgery is contemplated, supine lateral bending radiographs are obtained to assess the flexibility of the curve(s). Curve magnitude is measured in degrees and is known as the Cobb angle. The criterion for diagnosis of scoliosis is a Cobb angle of 10° or more. The causes of scoliosis are given in *Table 33.11*.

TABLE 33.11 Aetiology of scoliosis.

- Idiopathic
- Neuromuscular
- Congenital
- Syndrome-related

Idiopathic scoliosis

Idiopathic scoliosis accounts for 70% of presentations. It can be classified into **early onset** (before 8 years of age) (Figure 33.8) and **late onset** (after 8 years of age; typical adolescent idiopathic scoliosis). The distinction is important, as the number of alveoli in the lung does not increase after the age of 8 years. Patients with severe curves in the early-onset group may develop cor pulmonale and right ventricular failure resulting in premature death. Adolescent idiopathic scoliosis is associated with a normal or near-normal life expectancy.

The prevalence of curves with a Cobb angle >10° is between 0.5% and 3%. The prevalence of curves >30° is between 1.5 and 3 per 1000. Risk factors for progression include female gender, remaining skeletal growth, curve location and curve magnitude. Not all curves stabilise when skeletal maturity is reached. In long-term studies, 68% experienced curve progression; the most marked progression of 1° per year was observed in patients with thoracic curves between 50 and 75°.

Idiopathic curves of less than 25° are monitored with clinical and radiographic examination. In growing children (premenarchal) with curves between 20° and 29°, a brace may be indicated. Bracing is used to **prevent** curve progression and generally does not lead to permanent curve correction. Curves beyond 45° are not amenable to brace treatment.

Surgery in the form of corrective instrumentation and spinal fusion is indicated for curve progression beyond 40°, truncal imbalance and unacceptable cosmesis. During surgery, continuous spinal cord monitoring is used in the form of somatosensory evoked potentials (SSEP), motor-evoked potentials (MEP) and free-run and stimulated electromyographic (EMG) activity to minimise the risk of neurological damage. The risk of neurological injury is 0.4% (1 in 250).

Neuromuscular scoliosis

This may be due to neuropathic disorders, such as cerebral palsy, spinocerebellar degeneration, syringomyelia, tetraplegia (Figure 33.9), spinal muscular atrophy and poliomyelitis, or **myopathic** disorders, such as Duchenne muscular dystrophy and myotonic dystrophy. There is good evidence that stabilisation of the spine in children with Duchenne muscular dystrophy who are able to walk (before respiratory compromise is too severe to preclude a general anaesthetic) may increase their lifespan by several years.

Congenital scoliosis

This is caused by vertebral anomalies that produce a frontal plane growth asymmetry. The anomalies are present at birth, but the curvature may take years to be clinically evident. Close observation of spinal growth is required until skeletal maturity is reached. Brace treatment is ineffective for the primary structural curves, which are often short and rigid, but it may have a role in the control of compensatory curves. For progressive curves, surgical options include growing rod constructs such as magnetically controlled growing rod (MCGR) procedures, hemivertebra excision, correction and fusion or posterior instrumented correction and fusion.

Summary box 33.8

Spinal deformity

- Early onset idiopathic scoliosis (<8 years old) has potential to impair lung function
- Neuromuscular scoliosis: timely surgery may prolong life
- Congenital scoliosis: rigid curves do not respond to brace treatment

John R. Cobb, American surgeon, wrote a paper in 1948 on how to measure the angle on an x-ray in scoliosis.
Guillaume Benjamin Amand Duchenne, 1806–1875, neurologist, worked successively in Boulogne and Paris, France, but who never held a hospital appointment.

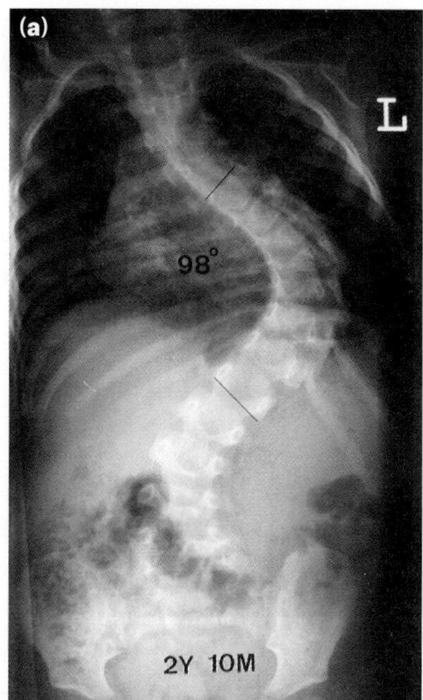

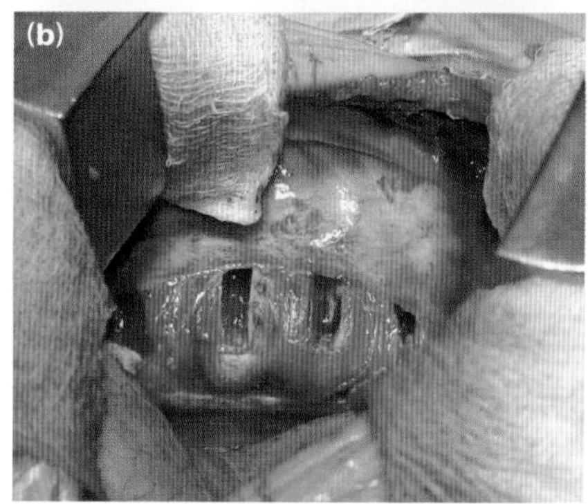

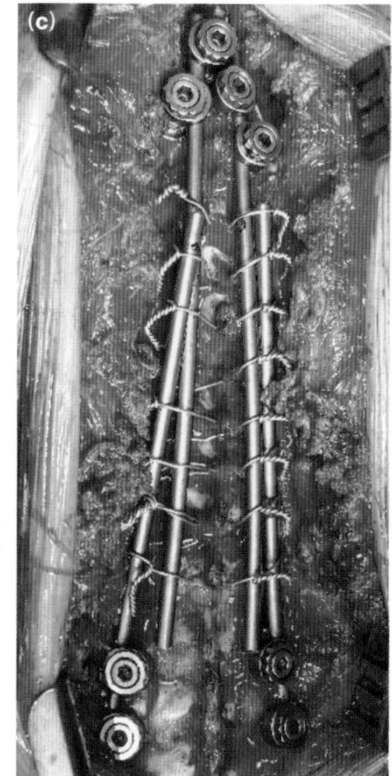

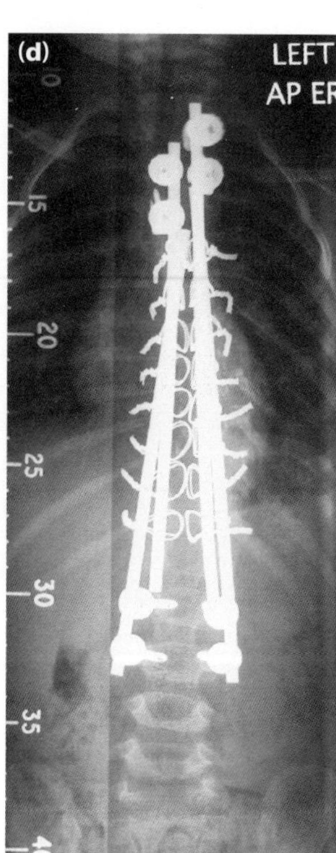

Figure 33.8 Early-onset idiopathic scoliosis. The anteroposterior standing radiograph (**a**) demonstrates a Cobb angle of 98° and dextrocardia. This 34-month-old boy underwent a convex hemiepiphysiodesis over the apical four discs (**b**), followed by posterior Luque trolley instrumentation **without** fusion to correct the spinal deformity and allow continued growth (**c, d**).

Scheuermann's kyphosis

Typically, in this condition, there is wedging of the 7th to 10th thoracic vertebrae. The patient presents with both apical pain and low back pain (due to attempts by lumbar musculature to compensate for the thoracic hyperkyphosis). The incidence has been estimated at 1–8% of the population, and it is more common in males. Physiotherapy may be useful. Bracing for skeletally immature patients with kyphosis up to 65° may be effective in arresting progression. Indications for surgery include pain (apical or low back pain produced by compensatory hyperlordosis), progressive deformity greater than 70°, unacceptable cosmesis and neurological and/or cardiopulmonary compromise. If surgery is contemplated, it may require anterior release followed by posterior correction and fusion. Increasingly, posterior chevron osteotomies carried out at the time of posterior instrumentation may prevent the need for the initial anterior release.

DEVELOPMENTAL ABNORMALITIES

Developmental abnormalities of the spine and spinal cord can be divided into primary bony disorders (e.g. congenital scoliosis, as discussed above) and primary neurological disorders (e.g. spina bifida, Arnold–Chiari malformation and spinal dysraphism).

Spina bifida

Spina bifida is caused by a failure of fusion of the vertebral arches and possibly the underlying neural tube. Spina bifida cystica has an incidence of 1 in 300 live births and is associated with hydrocephalus. It is now decreasing as a consequence of folic acid supplementation, antenatal ultrasound and the measurement of α-fetoprotein (AFP) levels. There are two basic types:

Holger Weriel Scheuermann, 1877–1960, radiologist, the Municipal Hospital, Sundby, Copenhagen, Denmark, described juvenile kyphosis in 1920.
Julius Arnold, 1835–1915, Professor of Pathological Anatomy, the University of Heidelberg, Heidelberg, Germany, described this condition in 1894.
Hans Chiari, 1851–1916, Professor of Pathological Anatomy, Strasbourg, Germany (Stragbourg was returned to France in 1918 after the end of the First World War), gave his account of this condition in 1891.

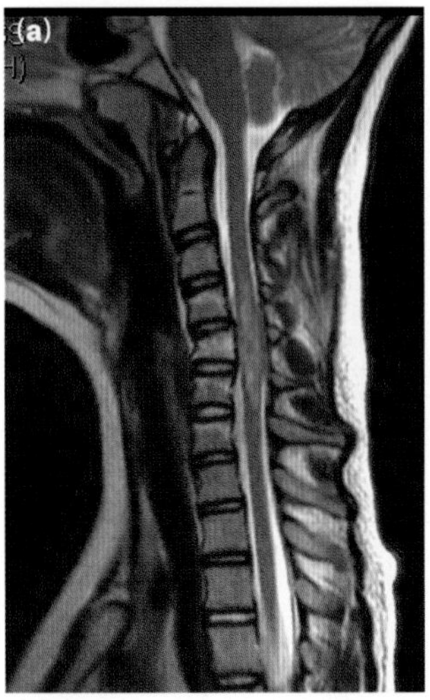
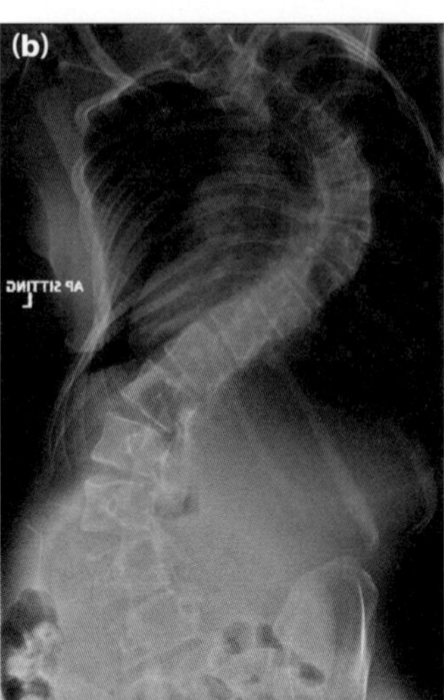

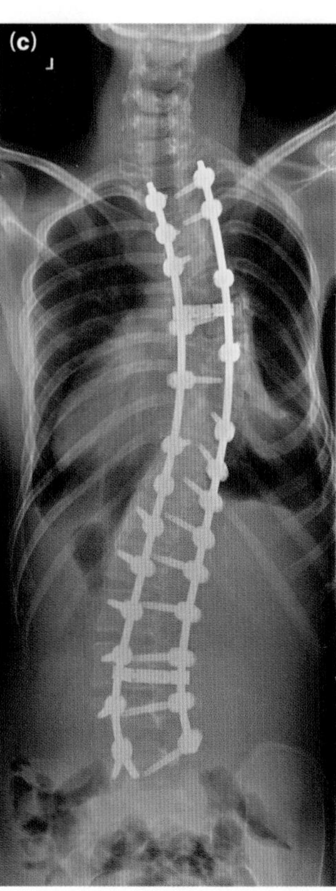
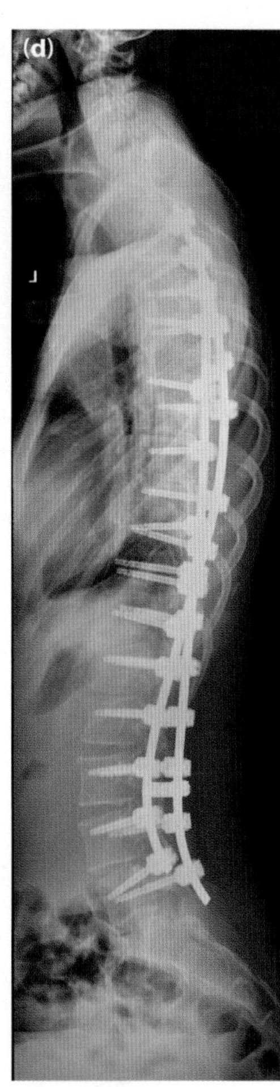

Figure 33.9 Neuromuscular scoliosis. This 13-year-old girl sustained a cervical spinal cord injury (C5 ASIA B) following a dive into a swimming pool. The T2 sagittal MRI scan (**a**) demonstrated signal change maximal at the level of C5. The patient developed significant scoliosis. The AP sitting radiograph (**b**) demonstrates a right thoracic curve with Cobb angle of 104° and a left lumbar curve with a Cobb angle of 82°. Following pedicle screw instrumentation, correction and fusion from T2 to L5, the right thoracic curve corrected to 40° and the left lumbar curve corrected to 38°, as noted on the AP (**c**), with restoration of sagittal balance (**d**).

- **Meningocoele**: the meninges herniate through the bony defect and are covered by skin.
- **Myelomeningocoele**: the roof of the defect is formed by exposed neural tissue, with 75% of cases developing hydrocephalus.

A meningocoele with good-quality skin over the defect may be treated conservatively. A meningocoele with a more prominent sac can be excised at 3–6 months. The management of myelomeningocoele is more controversial. Enthusiasm for closing all defects has been replaced by a more selective approach with the recognition that it was inappropriate to operate on children with severe hydrocephalus, a large open defect and no distal neurological function. The majority of these children die in their first year if closure is not attempted. With antibiotics, early surgical closure and shunts to prevent hydrocephalus, half the children who survive the first 24 hours will reach school age, but long-term problems remain, including skin problems, neuromuscular scoliosis, bone and joint deformity and the complications associated with a neuropathic bladder.

Arnold-Chiari malformation

Arnold–Chiari malformation occurs when the medulla oblongata and the cerebellar tonsils extend through the foramen magnum into the cervical spinal canal, causing pressure on the lower medulla. Hydrocephalus and impaired neurological function are common, and there is a strong association with spina bifida and syringomyelia. Symptoms may include headache, vomiting, visual disturbances, mental impairment, cerebellar ataxia, sensory disturbances or paralysis. Management consists of decompressing the foramen magnum and, usually, the posterior arch of the atlas to restore normal cerebrospinal fluid flow.

Spinal dysraphism

This is a group of disorders arising from abnormal embryological formation of tissues; all are associated with a progressive neurological deficit as the result of spinal cord tethering and traction or cord compression. There is a strong association with spina bifida.

In diastematomyelia, there is an abnormal bony or cartilaginous spur projecting across the middle of the vertebral canal, dividing the dural tube and spinal cord in two. Between 50% and 70% of patients are seen to have a skin naevus, dimple or hairy patch when the spine is examined. Surgical release of the tethering has variable results.

Syringomyelia

Patients may present with sensory disturbance, weakness of the hands, loss of pain and temperature sensation, asymmetrical abdominal reflexes or progressive kyphoscoliosis. It is associated with Arnold–Chiari malformation and spinal cord tumours. Where syringomyelia is associated with an Arnold–Chiari malformation and scoliosis, a posterior cranial fossa decompression should be carried out first to resolve the syringomyelia. The scoliosis may then be corrected at a later date.

METABOLIC BONE DISEASES AFFECTING THE SPINE

Osteoporosis

Patients with osteoporosis may present with pain following minimal trauma, loss of height and exaggerated thoracic kyphosis. Medications used to prevent and treat osteoporosis include calcium, vitamin D, bisphosphonates (alendronate, risedronate, once-yearly intravenous zoledronic acid), denosumab, strontium ranelate, selective oestrogen receptor modulators (SERMS) such as raloxifene, hormone replacement therapy and teriparatide.

Patients with painful thoracic fractures may be treated with short-term bed rest, analgesics and a spinal orthosis. If the back is still painful 6 weeks after the injury, patients may be considered for vertebroplasty or kyphoplasty. Vertebroplasty involves the injection of polymethylmethacrylate bone cement (PMMA) under pressure into the vertebral body with fluoroscopic guidance. The goals of the procedure are to **stabilise the spine** and **decrease the pain** associated with compression fractures. Kyphoplasty, on the other hand, involves inserting bilateral bone tamps with balloons into the vertebral body. These are inflated under fluoroscopic control with the bone tamp re-expanding the body, and elevating the end plates to reduce the fracture deformity. The balloons are then deflated and removed, and PMMA is placed in the cavity created by the balloons. The goals of kyphoplasty are **spinal stabilisation, pain relief and restoration of vertebral body height**. Significant complications have been reported, including nerve root injury and spinal cord injury resulting from cement extravasation, along with cement embolism, infection and hypotension.

GLOBAL ISSUES IN SPINE SURGERY

It is important that the information presented in this chapter, which is widely used throughout the world for teaching and training, outlines the very best evidence-based treatment that is available for surgical conditions. The text has covered the essentials of spine surgery and has very rightly demonstrated current techniques which involve up-to-date equipment. It is, however, an inescapable fact that the majority of the world's population does not have access to state-of-the-art spinal surgery. There are two main reasons for this: first, the cost of spinal surgery and, second, the lack of trained surgeons.

Cost implications of modern spinal surgery

There have been dramatic advances in spinal surgery due to modern imaging, modern instruments and implants, and advanced spinal cord monitoring equipment. The widespread availability of MRI in high-income countries such as the USA, UK and most of Europe has meant that diagnostic accuracy is available to the whole population in these countries. This is not, however, the case for most of the world, where there is no free or state-sponsored MRI service, and a private scan costing US$500 is unaffordable to most. If a family cannot afford a scan, then they also cannot afford the cost of an operation, the spinal implants, spinal cord monitoring and the use of expensive disposable instruments such as high-speed burrs.

The lack of trained spinal surgeons

In the last 20 years high income countries have seen the rapid development of spinal surgery, and the rapid development of spinal surgery as a complete career. It is now normal in such countries for spine surgeons to practise only in the field of spinal surgery and no longer to undertake general orthopaedic or neurosurgical operations. This has inevitably led to refinement of skills and increasing subspecialisation. In low-income countries, where there may be a single orthopaedic surgeon for 1 million people, doing 'just spinal surgery' is not an option, and a much more general approach is needed. In the map shown in **Figure 33.10**, each country in the world is represented with an area proportional to the number of people in the population per active surgeon. This represents surgeons of all types, but it shows that, in many parts of Africa, there are more than half a million people per surgeon. The map showing the population covered by each **spine** surgeon would be even more striking.

Can good spine care be given without modern imaging and equipment?

The key to good surgery in all disciplines is a surgeon who is dedicated to the care of his or her patient, who takes a good history and examination, then offers the best treatment that is available under the circumstances. In a high-income country this will often involve MRI scanning, dissection under microscope control and expensive titanium implants. In a resource-poor, low-income country it may involve just as much time and skill, but often a much more conservative approach. When surgery is needed the surgeon may have to do the best that he or she can with the equipment available. The case in **Figure 33.11** illustrates this point well. Note the lateral cervical spine radiograph with a fracture/dislocation at C2/C3 sustained by a patient living in a low-income country. The pedicles of C2 are fractured, allowing C2 to subluxate forwards on C3 and compress the spinal cord. The patient was admitted several days after a car crash, holding his head with his hands for stability. In a high-income country where there was imaging and fluoroscopic-guided pedicle screw fixation available, the fracture could easily have been fixed. In the low-income country, there was no cervical spine instrumentation available and the surgeon used a low-risk, low-technology technique of wiring the arch of C1 to the spine of C2 with a

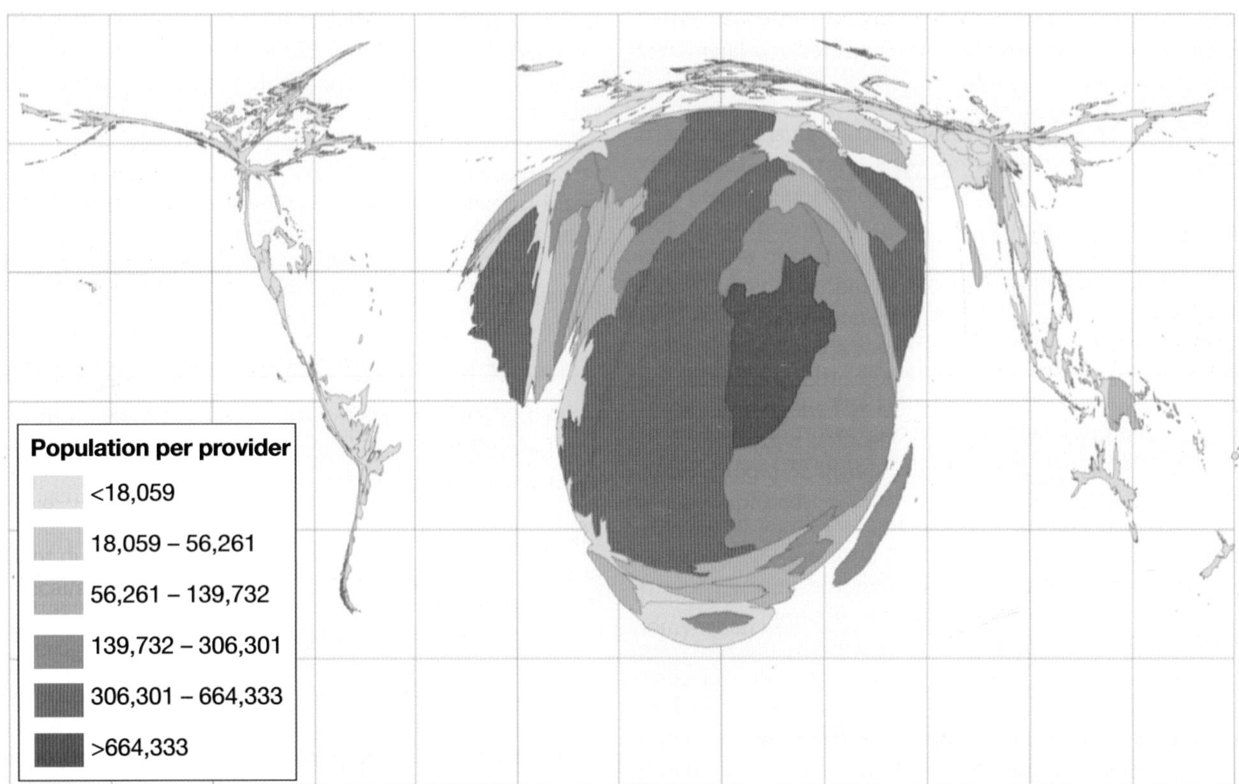

Figure 33.10 Global distribution of surgeons, anaesthesiologists and obstetricians. Each country in the world is represented with an area proportional to the number of people in the population per active surgeon. With permission from Holmer H *et al.*, *The Lancet Global Health*, 2015; 3, pp.S9–S11.

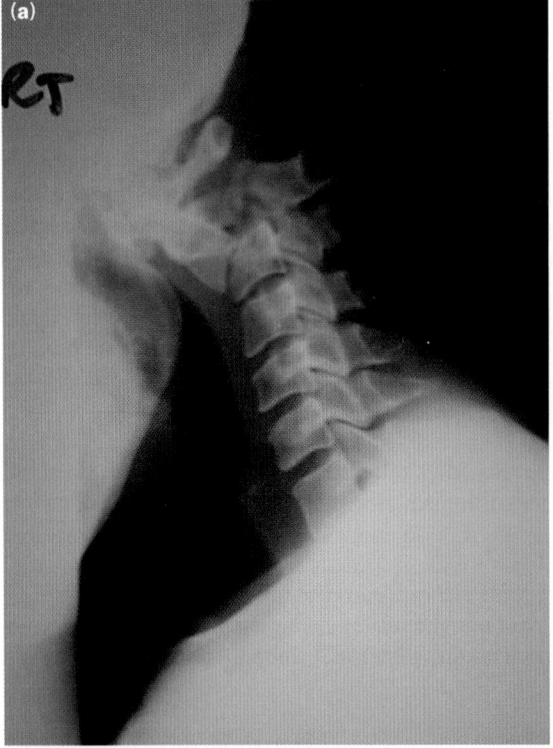

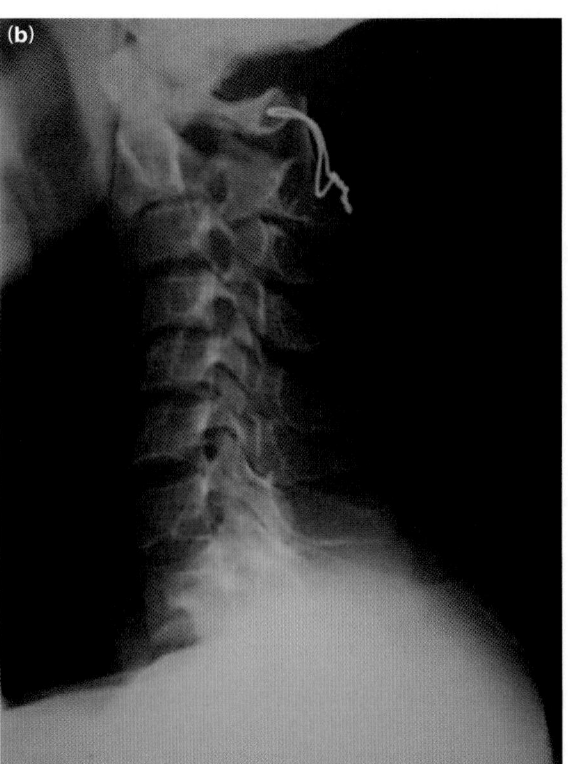

Figure 33.11 **(a)** Lateral cervical spine radiograph with a fracture/dislocation at C2/C3 sustained by a patient living in a low-income country. **(b)** The surgeon used a low-risk, low-technology technique, wiring the arch of C1 to the spine of C2 with a piece of stainless steel wire, then laying on corticocancellous bone graft.

piece of stainless steel wire, then laying on corticocancellous bone graft. The reduction was stable, the graft incorporated and the patient was thankful. It is not appropriate to say that this was inadequate treatment compared to the best that the world has to offer, because the best that the world has to offer was not available.

FURTHER READING

Debnath UK, Freeman BJ, Gregory P *et al*. Clinical outcome and return to sport after the surgical treatment of spondylolysis in young athletes. *J Bone Joint Surg Br* 2003; **85**(2): 244–9.

Fairbank J, Frost H, Wilson-McDonald J *et al*. Randomised controlled trial to compare surgical stabilisation of the lumbar spine with an intensive rehabilitation programme for patients with chronic low back pain: The MRC spine stabilisation trial. *BMJ* 2005; **330**: 1233–8.

Fritzell P, Hägg O, Wessperg P *et al*. Volvo Award in clinical science: lumbar fusion versus non-surgical treatment for chronic low back pain. A multi-centre randomised controlled trial from the Swedish lumbar spine study group. *Spine* 2001; **26**: 2521–34.

Gardner A, Gardner E, Morley T. Cauda equina syndrome: a review of the current clinical and medico-legal position. *Eur Spine J* 2011; **20**(5): 690–7.

Holmer H, Lantz A, Kunjuman T *et al*. Global distribution of surgeons, anaesthesiologists, and obstetricians. *Lancet Global Hlth* 2015; **3**: S9–11.

Janssen ME, Zigler JE, Spivak JE *et al*. ProDisc-C total disc replacement versus anterior cervical discectomy and fusion for single-level symptomatic cervical disc disease. Seven-year follow-up of the prospective randomized U.S. Food and Drug Administration investigational device exemption study. *J Bone Joint Surg Am* 2015; **97**(21): 1738–47.

Meara JG, Leather AJ, Hagander L *et al*. Global Surgery 2030: evidence and solutions for achieving health, welfare, and economic development. *Lancet* 2015; **386**: 569–624.

Patchell RA, Tibb PA, Regine WF *et al*. Direct decompressive surgical resection in the treatment of spinal cord compression caused by metastatic cancer: A randomised trial. *Lancet* 2005; **366**: 643–8.

Tokala DP, Lam KS, Freeman BJ *et al*. C7 decancellisation closing wedge osteotomy for the correction of fixed cervico-thoracic kyphosis. *Eur Spine J* 2007; **16**(9): 1471–8.

Waddell G, McCulloch JA, Kummel ED *et al*. Volvo Award in clinical science: non organic physical signs in low-back pain. *Spine* 1979; **5**: 117–25.

Wiltse LL, Newman PH, Macnab I. Classification of spondylosis and spondylolisthesis. *Clin Orthop* 1976; **117**: 23–9.

Chapter 34

Upper limb

Learning objectives

To understand:

- Anatomy and physiology relevant to upper limb pathology

To be able to explain:

- The diagnosis and treatment of common upper limb conditions

SHOULDER GIRDLE

Anatomy and function

The shoulder girdle (scapula and clavicle) is controlled and supported by muscles crossing between the spine, thorax, scapula and humerus. The sternoclavicular joint is the only synovial joint between the upper limb and the axial skeleton. The glenohumeral joint is most closely controlled by the deltoid and rotator cuff muscles (subscapularis, supraspinatus, infraspinatus and teres minor). The scapula is integral to shoulder motion, both gliding and rotating on the posterior surface of the thorax (**Figure 34.1**).

Congenital abnormalities

Sprengel's shoulder

The commonest congenital abnormality is due to abnormal scapular descent from its embryonic midcervical position. The typical presentation is a high, small, rotated scapula which remains connected to the cervical spine by a bony bar, fibrous band or an omovertebral body (**Figure 34.2**). Other

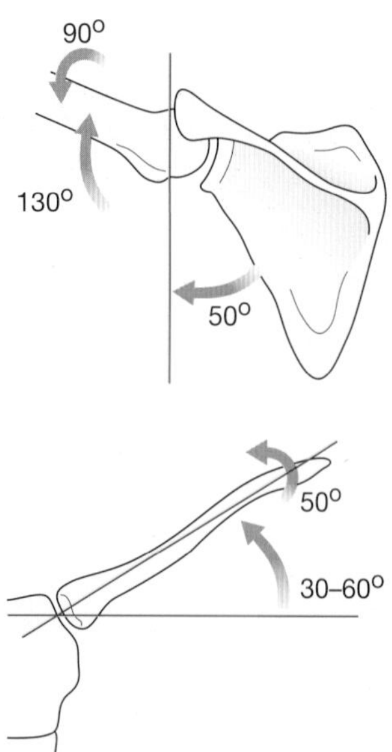

Figure 34.1 Relative motion of the elements of the shoulder girdle.

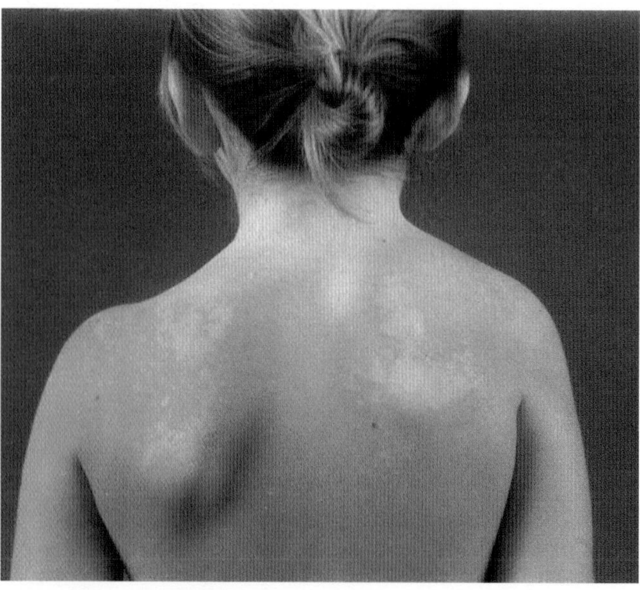

Figure 34.2 Sprengel's shoulder (right) of a 4-year-old girl.

Otto Gerhard Karl Sprengel, 1852–1915, surgeon, Grossherzogliches Krankenhaus (the Grand Ducal Hospital), Brunswick, Germany, described congenital high scapula in 1891.

congenital deformities are rib abnormalities, and cervical or thoracic abnormalities including scoliosis and Klippel–Feil syndrome (congenital fusion of cervical vertebrae).

Acquired abnormalities

History

Patients usually associate the onset of their symptoms with an unusual event (trauma or excessive activity) even though the causation may not be as clear as the patient thinks. Even so, the onset (sudden or gradual) and duration are important, as is the age of the patient, and their occupation. Pain presenting in the shoulder (or anywhere in the upper limb) can arise from the nerves of the neck, so the history should include questions about neck problems.

Examination

If the patient can localise the source of the pain to an exact point around the shoulder, then the problem is unlikely to be referred from the neck. Tests for inflammation and impingement involve trying to reproduce the pain by loading the limb in the position that creates the problem (Hawkin's test for impingement, **Figure 34.3**). Tests for tears in structures such as the rotator cuff look specifically for weakness, while apprehension tests check for instability (such as may predispose to recurrent shoulder dislocation).

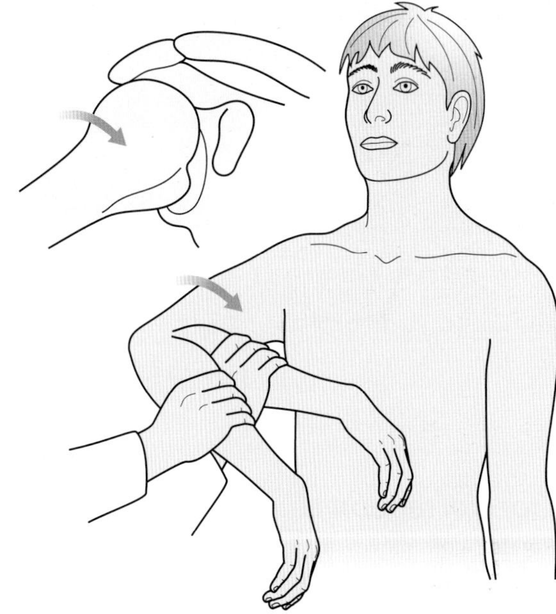

Figure 34.3 Hawkin's impingement test. Impingement pain is reproduced when the shoulder is internally rotated with 90° of forward flexion, thereby locating the greater tuberosity underneath the acromion.

Investigations

Radiographs are of limited value because most lesions in the shoulder involve damage to the soft tissues. However, a reduced subacromial space may be clearly visible in full thickness rotator cuff tears (**Figure 34.4a**). The appearance of a typical subacromial spur can be seen on the radiograph in **Figure 34.4b** and morphological variants are shown in **Figure 34.5**. The appearance of a spur is usually due to calcification within the coracoacromial ligament and it may be a secondary consequence of degenerative cuff disease rather than a primary event.

Both ultrasound and magnetic resonance imaging (MRI) allow the integrity and health of the rotator cuff to be checked, and MR arthrography also gives information on the integrity of the labrum of the glenohumeral joint (**Figure 34.6**).

Local anaesthetic injections may help to localise the source of inflammation and pain.

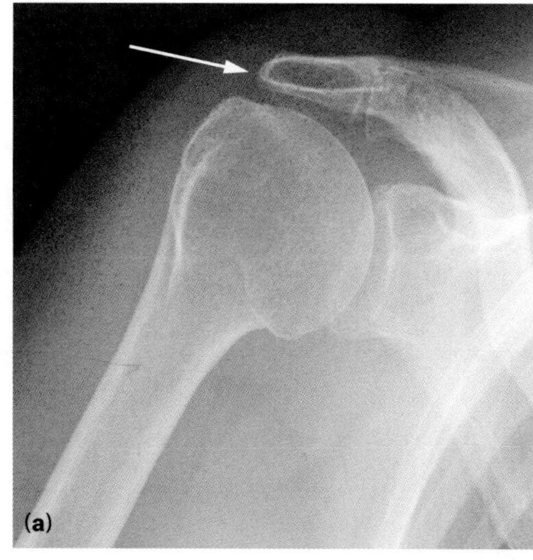

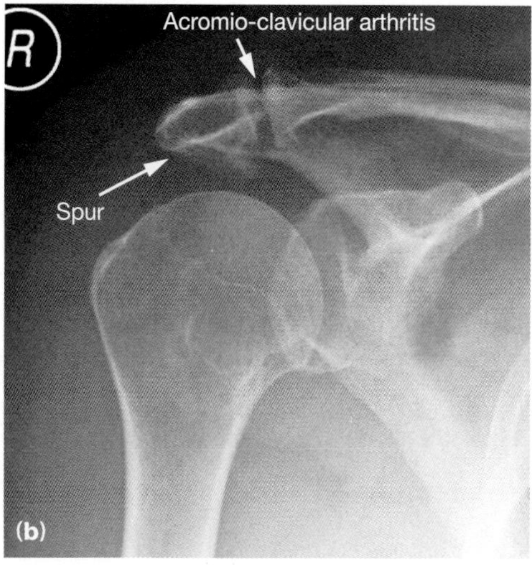

Figure 34.4 (**a**) Radiograph showing sclerosis on the undersurface of the acromion and the greater tuberosity, with reduced subacromial space. (**b**) Radiograph showing an acromial spur and arthritis of the acromioclavicular joint.

Maurice Klippel, 1858–1942, neurologist, Hôpital Tenon, Paris, France.
André Feil, 1889–?, neurologist, Paris, France. **Klippel and Feil** described this condition in a joint paper in 1912.

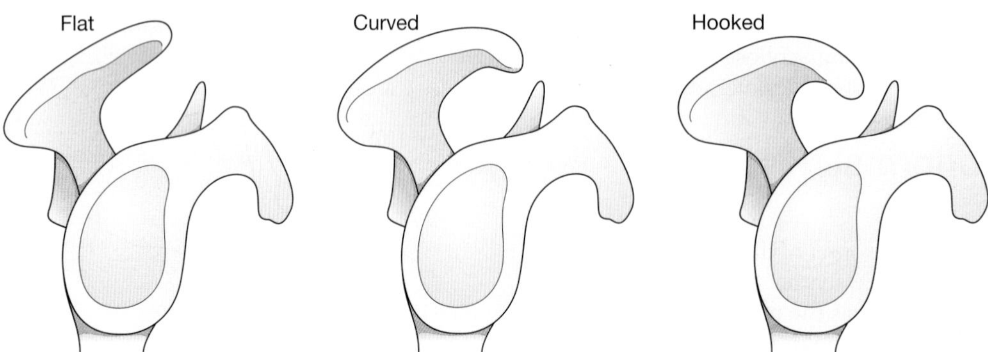

Figure 34.5 The three commonest acromial morphologies.

Rotator cuff tendonitis

The rotator cuff moves in a confined space between the humeral head, the acromion and the coracoacromial ligament (CAL). Even a trivial injury can start a progression of inflammation, swelling and pain, which in turn causes subacromial pain, termed impingement, felt to be attributable to abrasion of the cuff and bursa on the undersurface of the acromion. The impingement then causes further swelling and pain and a vicious circle is set up. The likelihood of tendonitis developing is increased in patients with a spur beneath the acromion, which is seen increasingly commonly with age (Figure 34.5) and may be an effect rather than a cause of painful subacromial degeneration, as described above. The result is a painful arc of movement for the patient, which corresponds to the position where the inflamed segment of the supraspinatus tendon jams under the anterior acromial spur. The examiner may find that, although the patient cannot lift their arm through this segment (because of the pain), passively lifting the arm for the patient enables them to continue with pain-free movement once the area of impingement is past (Figure 34.7).

TREATMENT

Injection of steroid into the inflamed area may break the cycle of inflammation and impingement (Figure 34.8), but arthroscopic removal of the subacromial spur, anteroinferior acromion and the CA ligament (if it is impinging) should give good relief of symptoms (Figure 34.9).

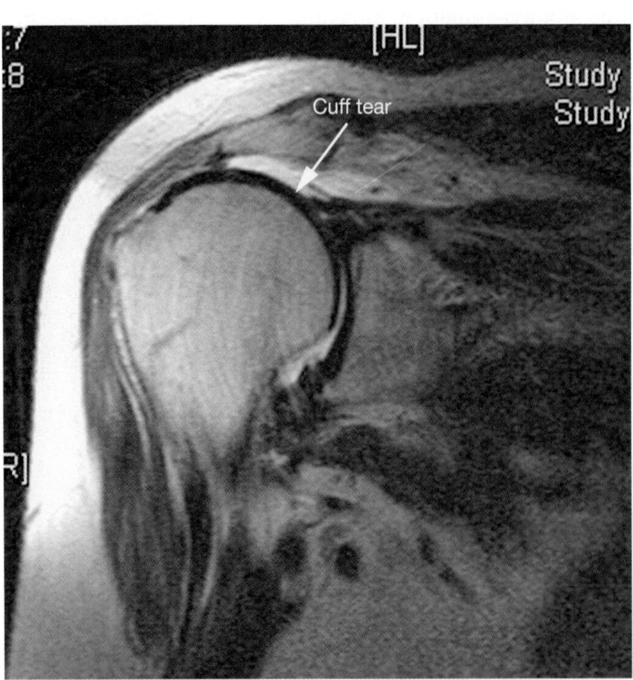

Figure 34.6 Magnetic resonance imaging scan showing a retracted cuff tear.

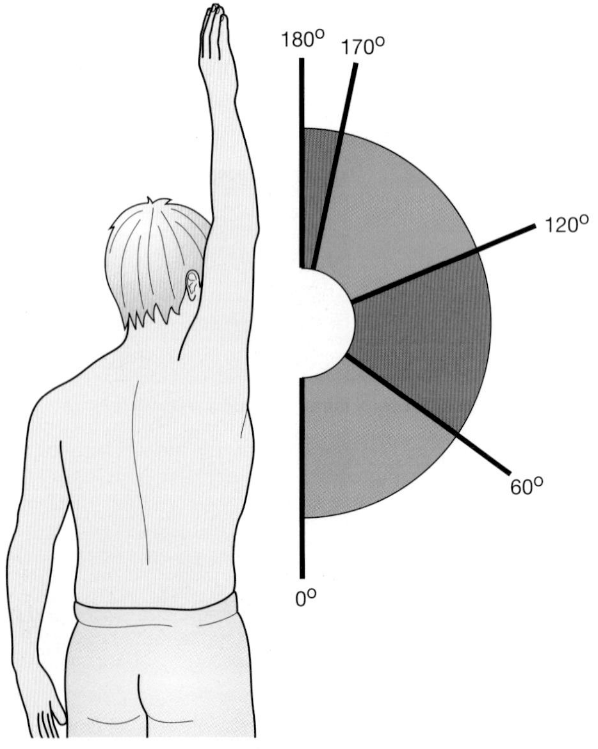

Figure 34.7 Arcs of shoulder girdle motion with subacromial impingement pain between 60° and 120° of abduction, and acromioclavicular joint pain between 170° and 180°.

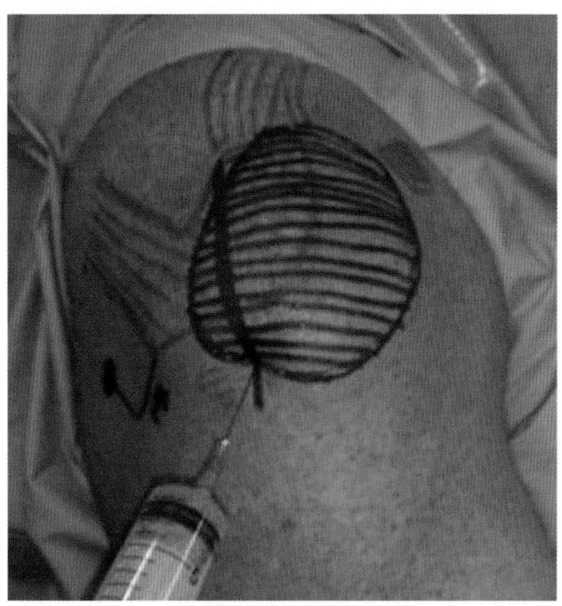

Figure 34.8 Technique of administering an injection into the subacromial bursa.

Summary box 34.1

Rotator cuff tendonitis

- Tendonitis produces weakness secondary to pain (often a painful arc)
- A tendon tear produces weakness which is only secondarily painful
- Injection of local anaesthetic and retesting can be diagnostic

Summary box 34.2

Treatment of subacromial impingement

- Non-operative treatment includes injections and rotator cuff rehabilitation
- Surgery indicated if symptoms persist beyond 3 to 6 months
- Surgery decompresses the rotator cuff

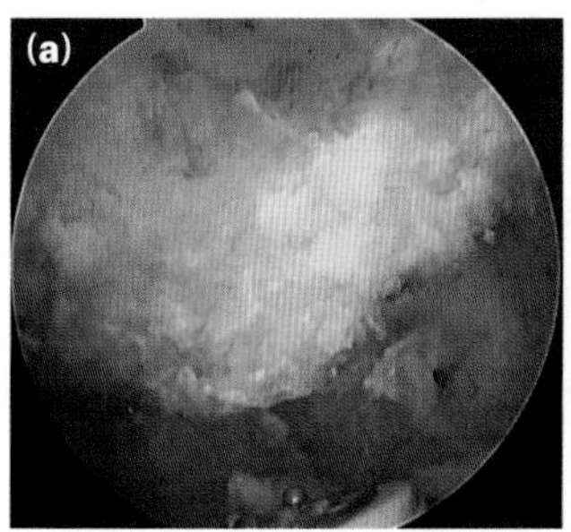

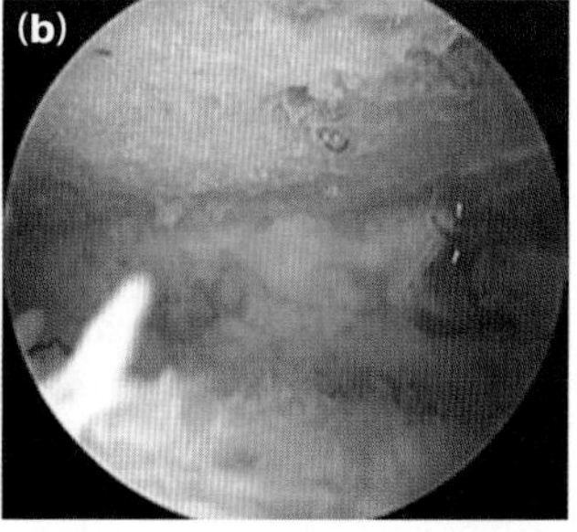

Figure 34.9 (a) Arthroscopic view of an acromial spur. (b) Arthroscopic view after the acromial spur has been removed and the cuff decompressed.

Rotator cuff tears

The rotator cuff has a poor blood supply in the segment that glides between the humeral head and acromion and is subject to degenerative changes, which weaken it with age. The cuff thins and eventually develops defects that are termed tears, whether or not there has been any trauma involved in their appearance. This means that tears are more common in the elderly, and at any age they do not heal spontaneously. Tears usually begin at the anterolateral edge of the supraspinatus, and progress posteriorly to involve the infraspinatus and teres minor tendons. This creates a bare area over the greater tuberosity, as the torn cuff retracts medially (Figure 34.10).

HISTORY

In the younger patient with a healthier cuff the onset often requires relatively major trauma, e.g. avoiding a fall by hanging onto the rung of a ladder, but in the elderly the onset may

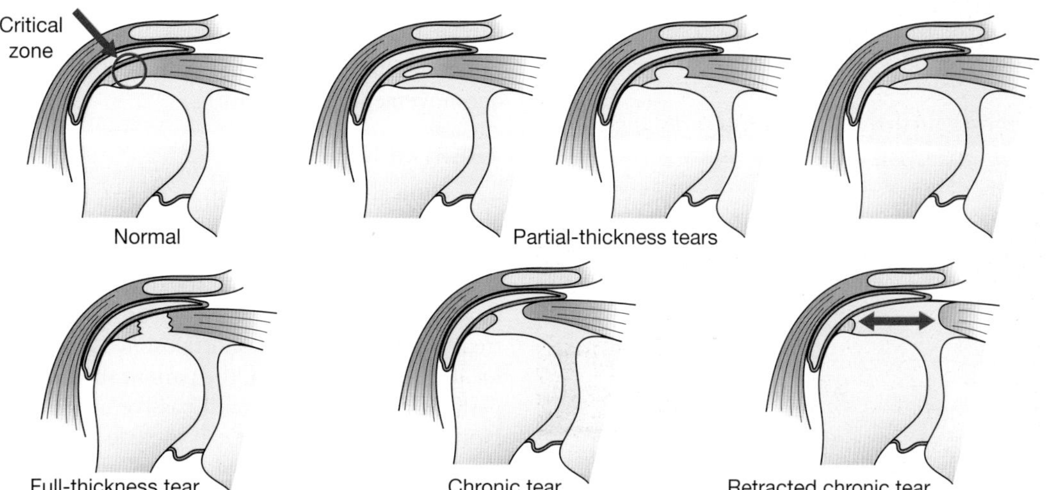

Figure 34.10 Various stages of rotator cuff tear. Initial partial-thickness tears have the potential to progress to full-thickness and retracted tears.

follow a painful period of tendonitis or the condition may apparently occur spontaneously.

EXAMINATION

The patient may have a mixed picture of tendonitis and a tear, but if the pain is removed by injection of local anaesthetic the weakness will persist. Symptomatic tears are associated with pain, weakness, limited active abduction, cuff muscle wasting and hunching of the shoulder when attempting abduction (Figure 34.11).

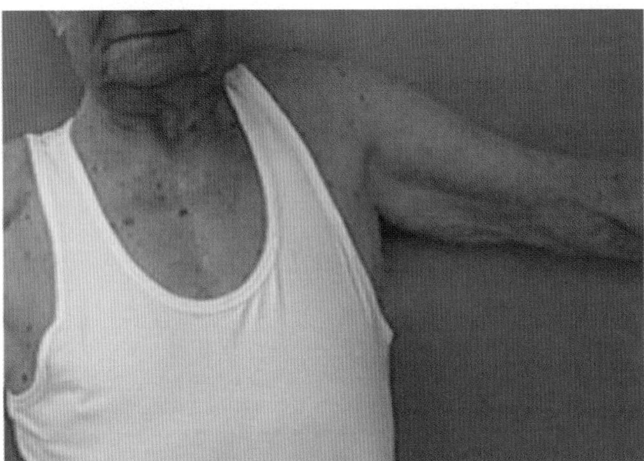

Figure 34.11 A 75-year-old man with a >5 cm retracted cuff tear attempting to abduct his shoulder, which is limited, by lack of balanced motor power, below 60°.

INVESTIGATION

Tears are classified as small (less than 1 cm), intermediate (2–4 cm) and large (more than 5 cm).

TREATMENT

Treatment depends on the patient's age, lifestyle and severity of symptoms. Arthroscopic or open repair with subacromial decompression can be considered for all tears, but is likely to give a better outcome in the young (see characteristics above) than in the old. It may not be possible to suture large tears owing to their size, or the attempt at repair may be fruitless because of fatty atrophy of the rotator cuff and loss of muscle contractility, in which case complex surgery e.g. tendon transfers, patch grafts or reverse joint replacement (**Figure 34.12**) will need to be considered.

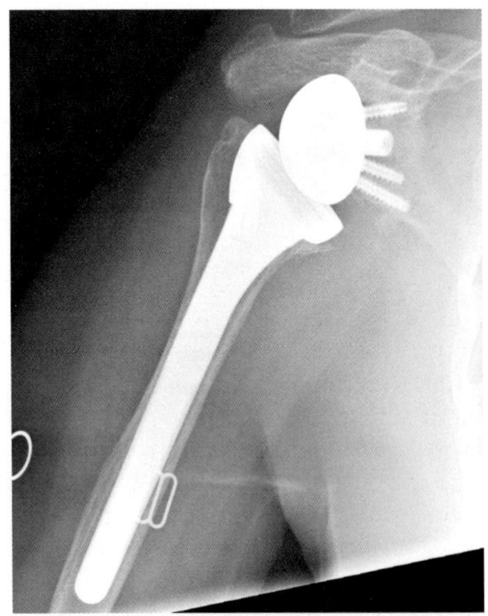

Figure 34.12 Reverse geometry total shoulder replacement.

Summary box 34.3

Rotator cuff tears

- Occur more commonly in older age groups
- 4–20% of 40–50 year olds have asymptomatic rotator cuff tears
- Up to 50% of 70 year olds have an asymptomatic tear
- Subacromial decompression is carried out to facilitate pain relief at cuff repair
- Acute tears may present with little pain but profound weakness
- Earlier repair after traumatic onset gives better results

Frozen shoulder (adhesive capsulitis, contracted shoulder)

This is an idiopathic painful and stiff condition most commonly affecting females in their 50s. It is also associated with diabetes, heart or thyroid disease.

HISTORY AND EXAMINATION

Frozen shoulder is characterised by the onset of severe pain and may follow minor trauma. The differential diagnosis includes infection, fractures and rotator cuff tears. Initially there is severe pain but this improves with time. However, there is global loss of active and passive movement, limited by pain. The pathognomonic sign is loss of external rotation active. Radiographs are normal and distinguish it from the other condition that can globally and painfully affect shoulder movement: osteoarthritis.

TREATMENT

The clinical course can run over 1–2 years, often considerably longer in diabetic individuals, and is divided into painful, stiffening and thawing phases. If untreated, frozen shoulder will resolve, and the majority of patients are left with no functional problems. In the first phase of the condition, treatment is pain relief. Corticosteroids can also be injected locally. Despite the pain, the patient should be encouraged to perform as much active and passive movement as they can. Non-operative treatment can include distension injection of the glenohumeral joint with local anaesthetic and steroid. Operative options include manipulation under anaesthesia or arthroscopic release of the tight capsule, which usually produce pain relief and are indicated for prolonged stiffness.

Summary box 34.4

Frozen shoulder (adhesive capsulitis)

- Most commonly occurs in females in their 50s
- Spontaneous onset
- Produces severe pain followed by reduced shoulder motion
- Spontaneous resolution can occur over 1–2 years
- Differential diagnoses: calcific tendonitis and rotator cuff tear
- Injections, distension with saline, manipulation and surgical release may all help

Calcific tendinitis

Calcium deposition within the supraspinatus tendon is believed to be part of a degenerative process, or the consequence of a partial degenerative tear of the tendon.

HISTORY AND EXAMINATION

There is severe, rapid onset shoulder pain with painful, restricted motion. However, in contrast to adhesive capsulitis, external rotation is possible. Subacromial calcific deposits can be seen on plain radiographs (Figure 34.13).

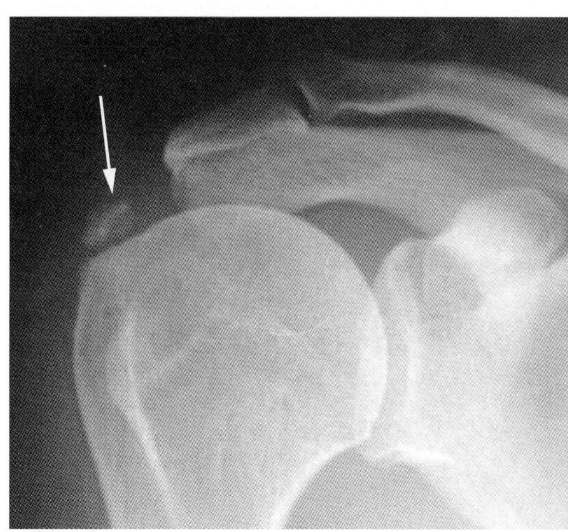

Figure 34.13 Radiograph demonstrating calcific tendonitis.

TREATMENT

Subacromial corticosteroid injections may help and can be accompanied by needling, aspiration or flushing of the deposits (barbotage). The condition is often self-limiting, with resorption of the calcium deposits. Surgery for resistant cases includes arthroscopic or open subacromial decompression and excision of the calcific deposits if they are prominent.

Arthritis of the shoulder

Rheumatoid arthritis

The glenohumeral joint is commonly involved in rheumatoid arthritis (Figure 34.14). As is typical of this condition, there is osteoporosis, destruction of the articular cartilage and synovial proliferation with pannus formation. The rotator cuff is weakened and frequently tears. Arthroscopic synovectomy may slow the progress of the joint destruction and lead to a reduction in pain and improvement in range of movement, though it is needed much less frequently since the introduction of biological therapies for rheumatoid disease. Intra-articular steroid injections may also be helpful. Shoulder replacement is complicated by poor bone stock and damage to the stabilising structures around the shoulder, especially the rotator cuff. The patient should only expect a reduction in pain. Any increase in range of movement is a bonus.

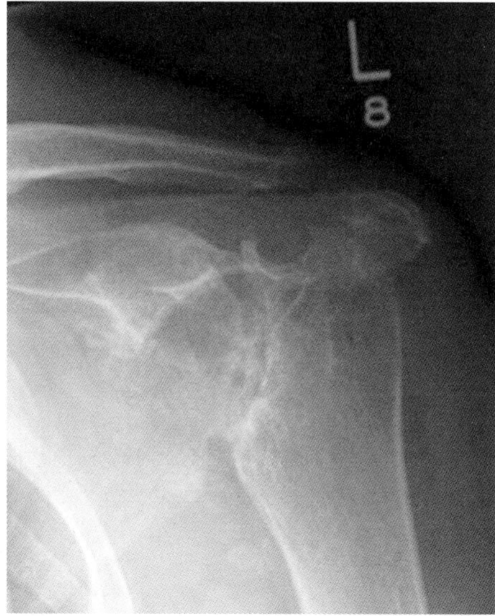

Figure 34.14 Rheumatoid arthritis of the shoulder.

Summary box 34.5

Shoulder problems in rheumatoid arthritis

- Arthroscopic synovectomy may be effective
- Rotator cuff tears are common
- Glenohumeral joint replacement improves pain but motion depends on rotator cuff involvement

Osteoarthritis of the shoulder

Glenohumeral joint osteoarthritis is either primary (Figure 34.15), secondary to trauma (Figure 34.16) or end-stage rotator cuff disease i.e. cuff arthropathy (Figure 34.17).

TREATMENT

If medical treatment has failed, the surgical options are arthroscopic debridement or joint arthroplasty. Debridement is not predictable, but both total shoulder replacement (Figure 34.18) and hemiarthroplasty (Figure 34.19) have good results in appropriate patients. A standard total shoulder arthroplasty can be performed if the rotator cuff is intact. However, in most rheumatoid patients and all patients with cuff tear arthropathy, the cuff is deficient and either a hemiarthroplasty or a reverse polarity total shoulder arthroplasty (see Figure 34.12) should be used. Shoulder arthroplasty is an effective pain-relieving procedure, but less predictable in restoring motion, especially above shoulder level.

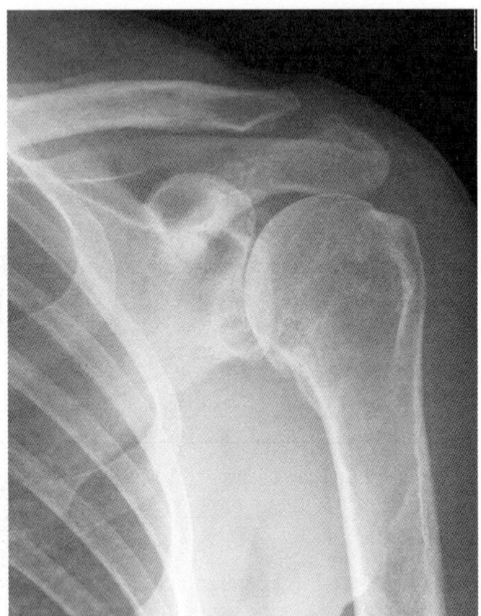

Figure 34.15 Osteoarthritis of the glenohumeral joint.

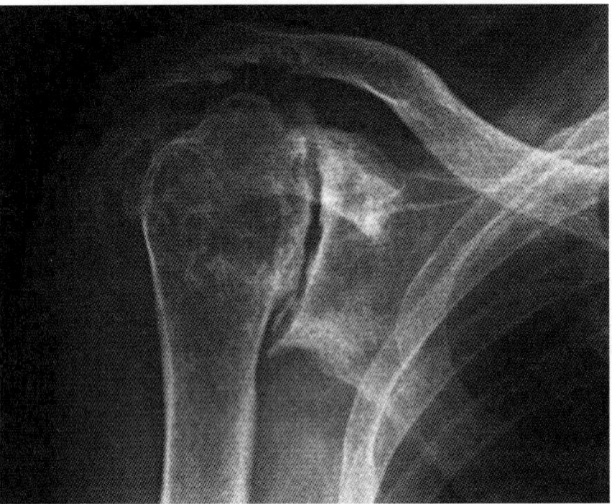

Figure 34.16 Post-traumatic arthritis with malunion of the proximal humerus, collapse of the humeral head, subchondral sclerosis and osteophytes.

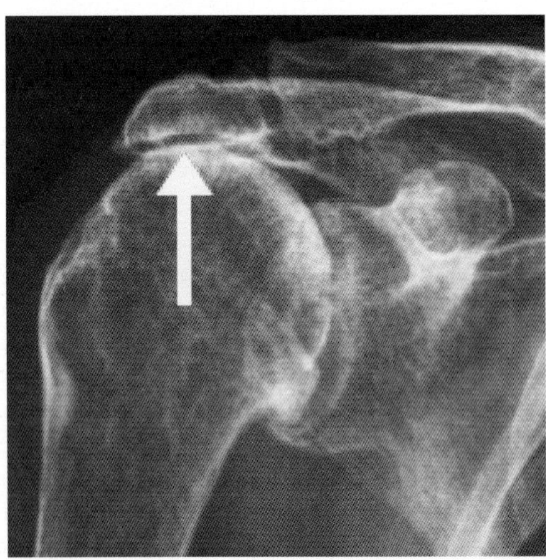

Figure 34.17 A massive cuff tear that has led to superior migration of the humeral head and secondary osteoarthritis of the glenohumeral joint.

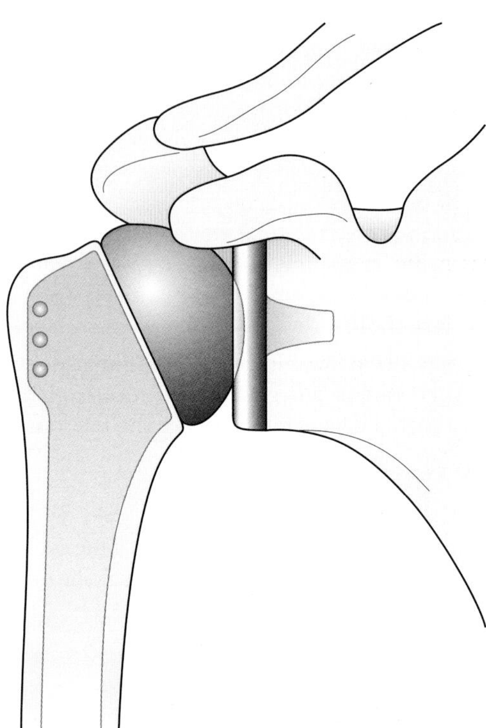

Figure 34.18 Total shoulder replacement performed for osteoarthritis. An intact rotator cuff is essential.

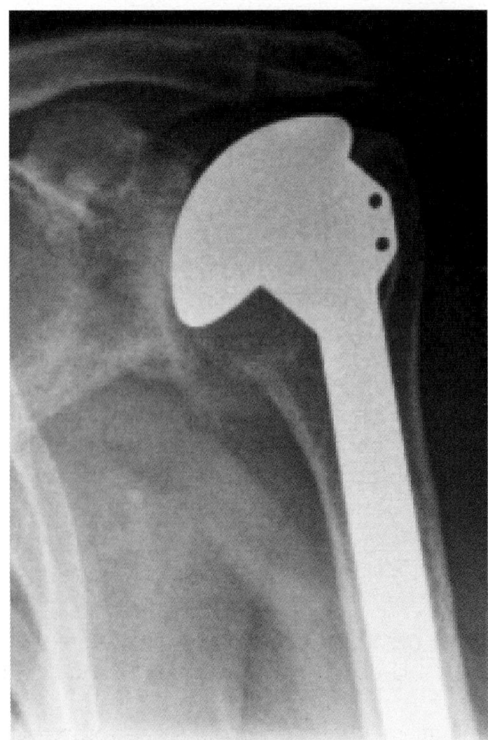

Figure 34.19 Shoulder hemiarthroplasty is performed for arthritis if there is a deficient rotator cuff.

Arthrodesis of the joint is an alternative in younger patients with a history of sepsis or neurological problems (Figure 34.20). It is also used after brachial plexus injury, when nerve repairs restore hand and elbow function but the shoulder remains flail because of loss of the C5 supply. Good scapulothoracic control, tested by the ability to shrug the shoulder powerfully, is a prerequisite to successful arthrodesis. Patients retain a moderate range of movement at the shoulder girdle, as a result of scapulothoracic motion, which normally makes up one-third of apparent shoulder elevation, the remaining two-thirds being glenohumeral movement, which is lost in arthrodesis.

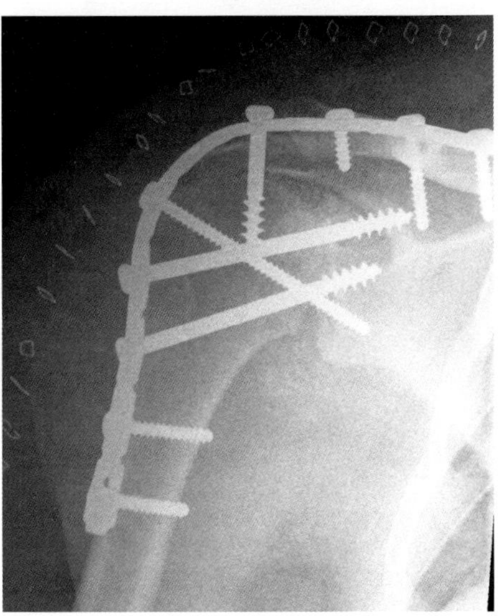

Figure 34.20 Arthrodesis of the shoulder.

> **Summary box 34.6**
>
> Arthritis of the shoulder
> - Severe cases are treated with hemiarthroplasty or total shoulder arthroplasty
> - Total shoulder replacements should not be performed if the rotator cuff is deficient
> - Pain relief is good following arthroplasty, though improvement in range of motion is less predictable
> - Glenohumeral arthrodesis is an option in the young or those with a history of sepsis
> - Post arthrodesis, motion is fair but is entirely scapulothoracic

Acromioclavicular joint arthritis

Acromioclavicular joint (ACJ) arthritis is common and is often asymptomatic, noted as an incidental finding on radiographs (see Figure 34.4b). Symptoms typically arise in males aged 20–50 years. Inferior osteophytes can impinge on the underlying rotator cuff.

HISTORY AND EXAMINATION

There may be a history of trauma to the ACJ. Pain is activity related. There is prominence of the lateral end of the clavicle. The joint line is tender. Flexing and adducting the arm to place the hand behind the opposite shoulder reproduces pain. If symptoms are related to inferior osteophytes, impingement symptoms and signs are also present.

TREATMENT

An intra-articular corticosteroid injection will usually help, and even if the effect is short lived it localises the problem accurately. Surgery involves arthroscopic or open excision of the lateral 0.5–1 cm of the clavicle (Figure 34.21). This gives good pain relief. In patients with symptoms that are predominantly those of impingement, arthroscopic removal of the inferior osteophytes with subacromial decompression should be performed.

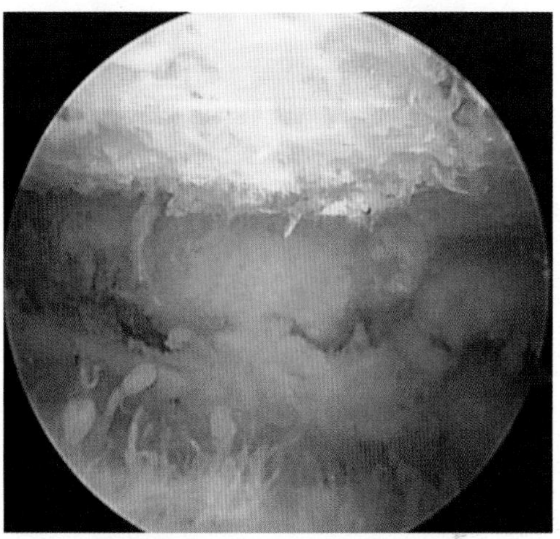

Figure 34.21 Arthroscopic end-on view of the clavicle after excision of its distal end.

> **Summary box 34.7**
>
> Acromioclavicular joint problems
> - AC joint arthritis is common and may be asymptomatic
> - It may become symptomatic secondary to trauma or repetitive overload
> - Inferior clavicular osteophytes can impinge on the cuff
> - Intra-articular steroid and local anaesthetic injection may relieve symptoms
> - Excision of the lateral end of the clavicle gives good results

Long head of biceps tendon rupture

Rupture of the long head of biceps usually occurs in the elderly and is due to abrasion of the tendon in the bicipital groove, especially at the superior end, beneath the anterior acromion. It is associated with rotator cuff tears. Most patients present with few symptoms, although they often seek advice because of the bulge they notice in their arm.

HISTORY AND EXAMINATION

Patients feel a sense of 'something giving way' in front of the shoulder, sometimes with relief of pain if there was any present beforehand due to biceps tendinitis. The upper arm is bruised and elbow flexion produces a swelling in the front and middle of the arm (**Figure 34.22**). The lump will be permanent and is initially tender. Power is slightly diminished in the early stages, when there may also be cramping pains on use of the arm.

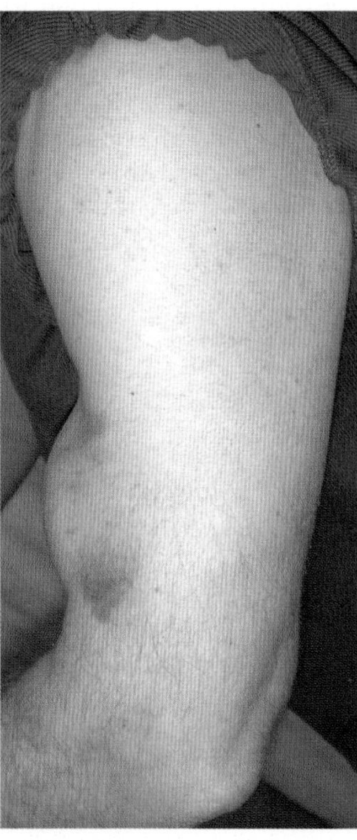

Figure 34.22 Bruising and change in the upper arm shape due to rupture of the long head of biceps.

TREATMENT

Reassurance that pain and bruising will resolve is sufficient. Power improves over several months and surgery (biceps tenodesis) is not needed for function, though it may help the cosmetic appearance.

Dislocation of the shoulder and instability of the glenohumeral joint

Three broad groups of shoulder instability exist.

Classification of glenohumeral instability

- **Traumatic**: unidirectional; involuntary; surgery is usually successful.
- **Atraumatic**: multidirectional, painful; involuntary; responds to surgery.
- **Habitual**: voluntary, with ligament laxity, painless; surgery usually contraindicated.

Recurrent traumatic instability

HISTORY

Traumatic shoulder dislocation is the commonest of all dislocations, usually first presenting in patients under 25. Usually the shoulder dislocates anteroinferiorly. Initially there is a notable traumatic event. Subsequent dislocations require less force. The shoulder may subluxate or actually dislocate (complete separation of the joint surfaces).

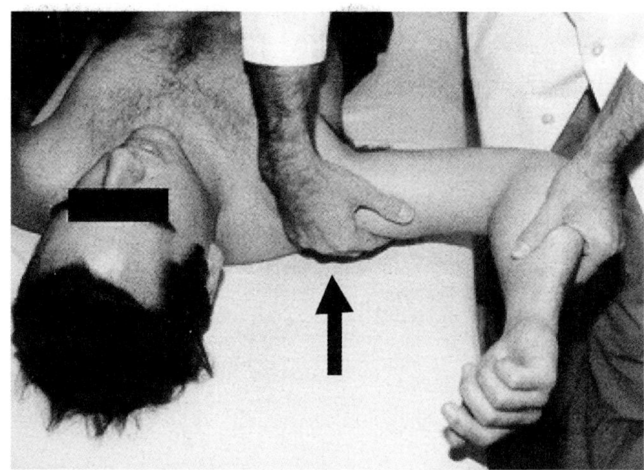

Figure 34.23 Apprehension test for anterior instability.

EXAMINATION

On examination the shoulder has a full range of motion, but with forced abduction and external rotation the patient experiences apprehension (a sense of impending doom!) (**Figure 34.23**).

INVESTIGATIONS

On computed tomography (CT) or MR arthrography (**Figure 34.24**), detachment of the anteroinferior labrum (Bankart's lesion) (**Figures 34.25 and 34.26**) and damage to the humeral head (Hill–Sach's lesion) can often be seen.

TREATMENT

The relative indications for surgery are repeated dislocations, or symptoms of instability that persist after reduction of the first dislocation, that are interfering with the patient's quality of life. Anterior instability can be treated with arthroscopic or open repair of the Bankart defect with tightening of the capsule, which prevents further dislocations in up to 90–95% of patients. Bony defects of the glenoid, and occasionally large Hill–Sachs lesions, may have to be grafted. For the less common recurrent posterior instability, repair of the damaged labrum and tightening of the posterior capsule is needed.

Arthur Sydney Blundell Bankart, 1879–1951, orthopaedic surgeon, The Middlesex Hospital, London, UK.

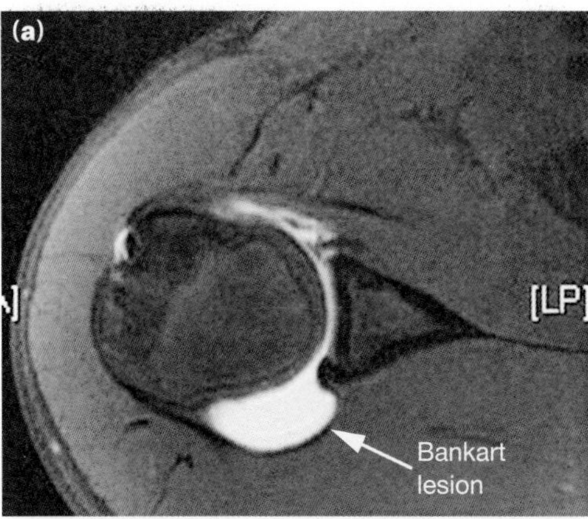

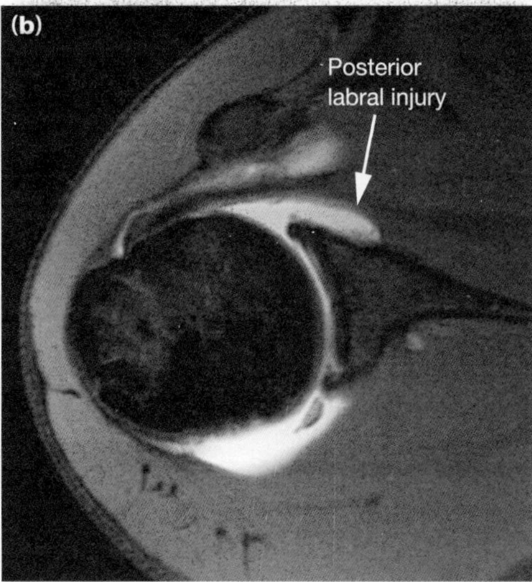

Figure 34.24 (**a**) Magnetic resonance (MR) arthrogram showing anterior Bankart lesion. (**b**) MR arthrogram showing posterior labral injury.

> **Summary box 34.8**
>
> **Recurrent traumatic shoulder instability**
>
> - An appreciable force leads to the first dislocation or subluxation
> - Subsequent dislocations/subluxations require less force
> - The commonest direction of dislocation is anteroinferior
> - There is a positive apprehension sign
> - Surgical treatment repairs the labral lesion and tightens the capsule

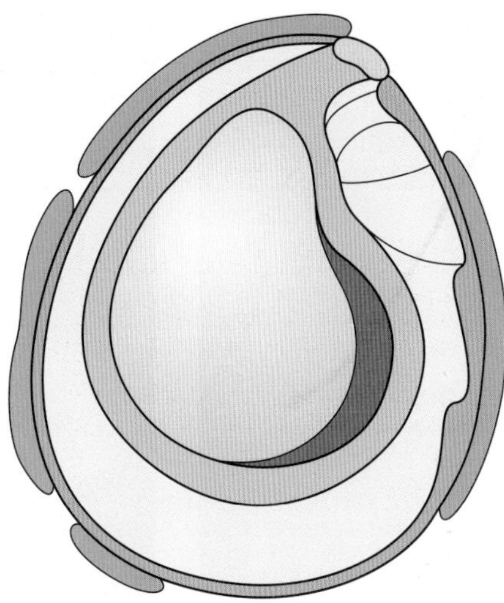

Figure 34.26 An end-on view of the glenoid labrum, demonstrating anteroinferior labral detachment (red) with the rotator cuff muscles (brown), long head of biceps tendon and labrum (grey).

Posterior dislocation of the shoulder

This is a rare event but is easy to miss. The clue is often in the history, as the patient will have either had an electric shock, had an epileptic fit, or have been subject to severe restraint when their arm has been forced up their back (a half-Nelson) – all mechanisms producing forced internal rotation of the glenohumeral joint.

The patient will be in severe pain and can be difficult to examine e.g. if they are psychotic and if this is why they are being restrained. For the same reason, the radiographer may only be able to get an anteroposterior (AP) view of the shoulder and, on this view, the shoulder may look normal to the unwary (Figure 34.27). It is the high 'index of suspicion' from the history which gives the best chance of making the diagnosis.

TREATMENT

This dislocation may be difficult to reduce if the posterior margin of the glenoid is embedded in the humeral head (a 'locked' posterior dislocation), so that open reduction is needed.

Atraumatic instability

HISTORY

There is usually no history of an initial injury. Instability may be multidirectional and the shoulder is usually associated with

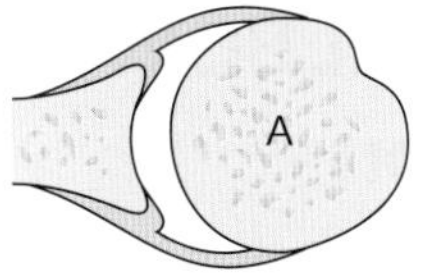

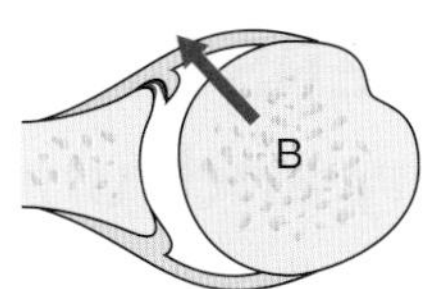

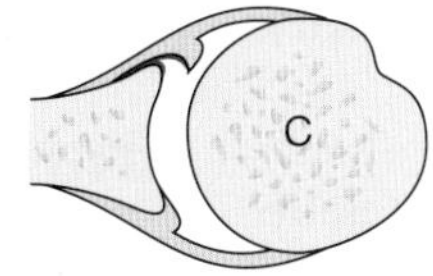

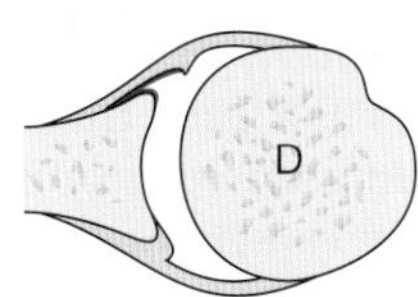

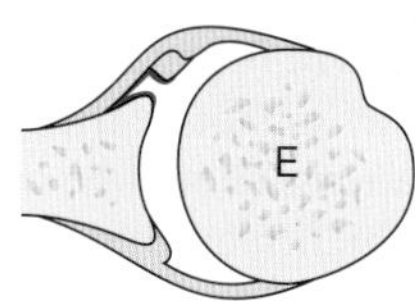

Figure 34.25 Schematic representation of Bankart's lesion, which forms a spectrum of pathology from minor labral detachment (B) to large detachments with glenoid rim fractures (bony Bankart; E).

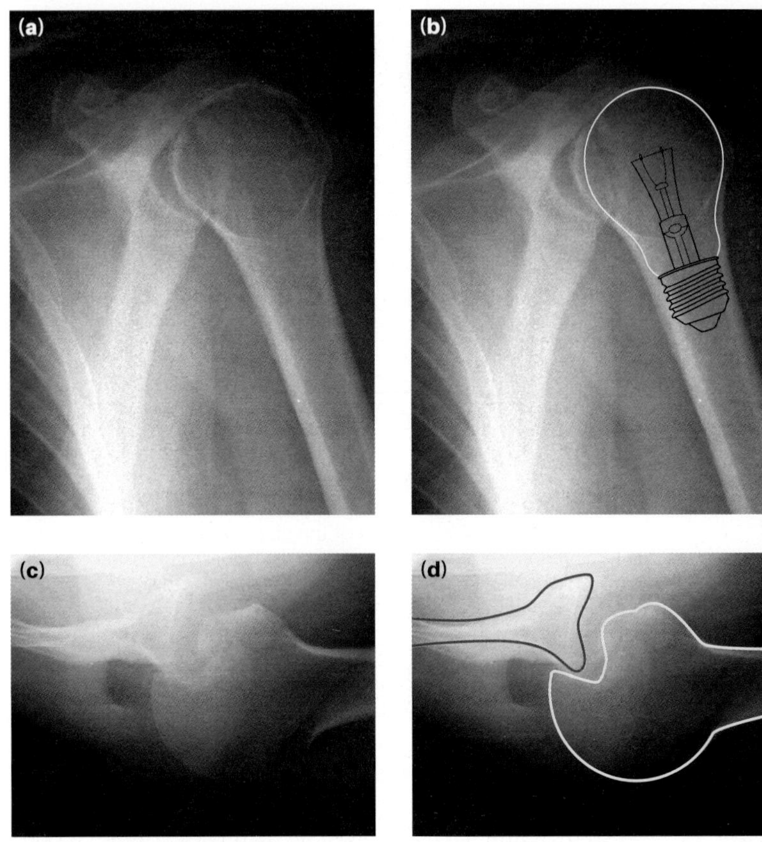

Figure 34.27 Posterior dislocation of the shoulder. (**a**) Anteroposterior view; (**b**) origin of the light bulb sign; (**c**) axial projection demonstrating how much easier it is to visualise the injury on this view; (**d**) axial projection highlighting this joint and further demonstrating the impacted fracture in the humeral head, or Hill–Sachs lesion.

subluxation rather than dislocation. The patient is often able to reduce the shoulder without assistance.

EXAMINATION

Generalised ligament laxity is common. Apprehension tests are positive, but often in more than one direction. Anterior and posterior drawing of the humeral head allows laxity to be tested (Figure 34.28). Overactivity of muscle groups such as pectoralis major should be sought, as this gives an avenue of treatment through rehabilitation.

TREATMENT

Specialist physiotherapy should be tried first in these patients, aiming to improve both the proprioception and firing patterns of the muscles around the shoulder (for instance biofeedback to control an overactive pectoralis major, or strengthening of underactive muscle groups). If this fails then surgery may be considered, by way of capsular tightening.

Habitual dislocation

Habitual dislocators are patients who can sublux the shoulder at will, usually either anteroinferiorly or posteriorly. The manoeuvre is painless. Patients have generalised joint laxity and may subluxate the shoulder as a 'party trick'.

Patients should be advised to stop subluxating the shoulder, which may then allow the capsule to tighten naturally with age. They may benefit from assessment and advice from a specialist physiotherapist. Surgery is associated with a high failure rate and should be avoided.

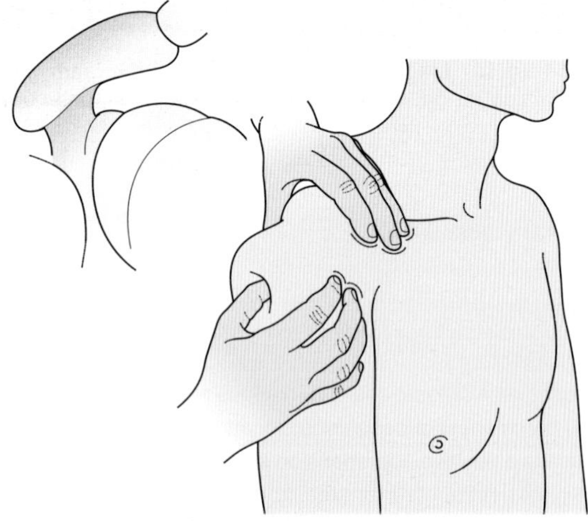

Figure 34.28 Generalised laxity can be appreciated by drawing the humeral head in anterior and posterior directions and feeling it slide up to, and possible even over, the glenoid rim. A sulcus will be produced under the acromion if the humerus is drawn inferiorly (sulcus sign).

DISORDERS OF THE ELBOW

Anatomy and function

The elbow joint allows flexion and extension as well as making up the proximal part of the radioulnar joint, which permits pronation and supination of the forearm. The brachial artery passes immediately in front of the joint, while the ulnar nerve passes lateral to the medial epicondyle, immediately behind it.

Tennis elbow (lateral epicondylitis) and golfer's elbow (medial epicondylitis)

These are discussed in Chapters 31 and 32.

Arthritis of the elbow

Rheumatoid arthritis

Surgery may be required, especially in end-stage disease (Figure 34.29). Arthroscopic or open radial head excision and synovectomy is effective for painful, restricted pronation and supination. Elbow arthroplasty is effective in the earliest stages for pain relief and functional restoration.

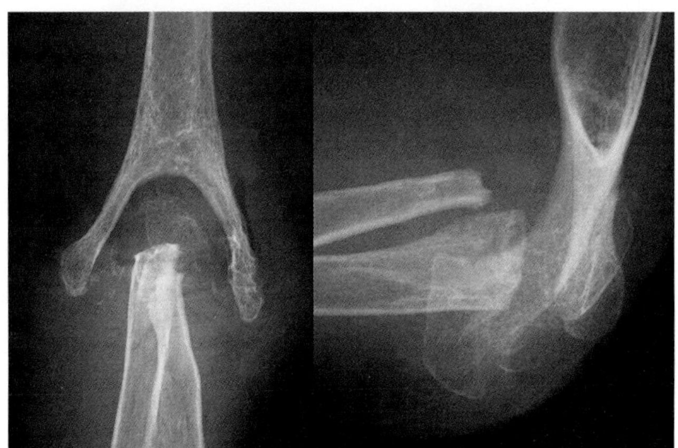

Figure 34.29 Typical end-stage unstable and destroyed rheumatoid elbow.

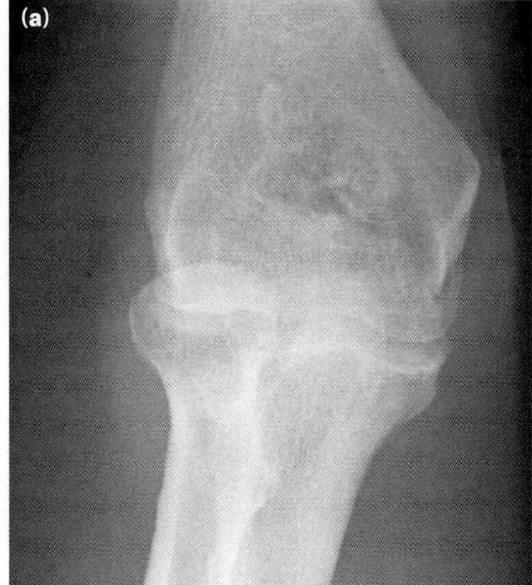

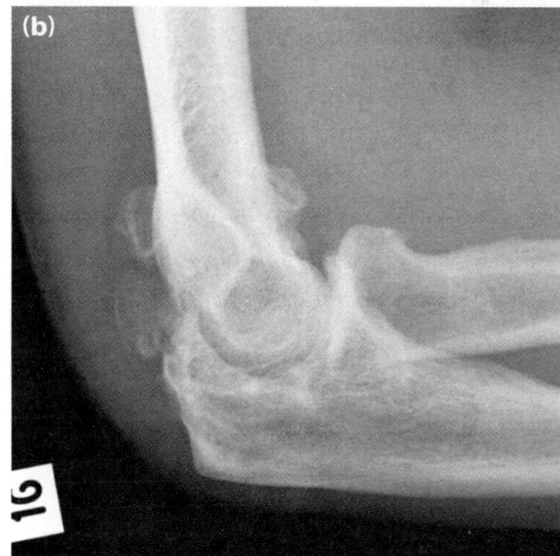

Figure 34.30 (a, b) Radiographs showing osteoarthritis of the elbow joint.

Osteoarthritis

Osteoarthritis of the elbow is usually primary (Figure 34.30) or secondary to trauma.

HISTORY

Typical patients are middle-aged males in manual occupations. Symptoms are pain, locking, crepitus and painful motion with loss of extension. Ulnar nerve entrapment symptoms may be present.

EXAMINATION

There is usually loss of extension and restriction of flexion. Pronation and supination tend to be spared in comparison with rheumatoid arthritis.

TREATMENT

Surgery should be considered only if medical treatment fails. Arthrodesis may be offered for those performing heavy manual work (Figure 34.31), but is associated with significant residual functional loss, as a joint replacement will not survive long under heavy loading. Surgical debridement alleviates pain and increases range of motion in earlier stages. Interposition arthroplasty (for example Achilles tendon allograft) may be considered in younger patients though it can be associated

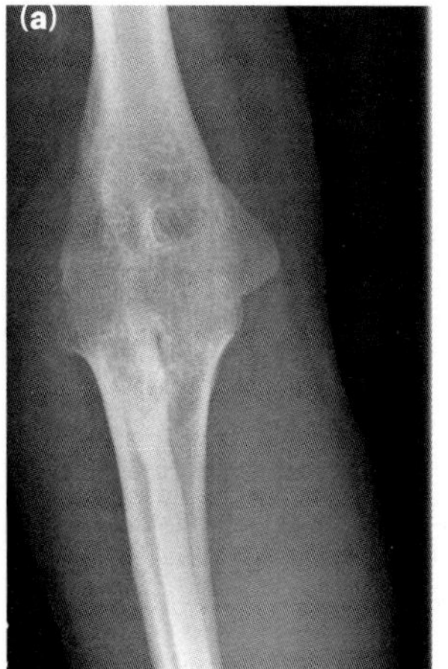

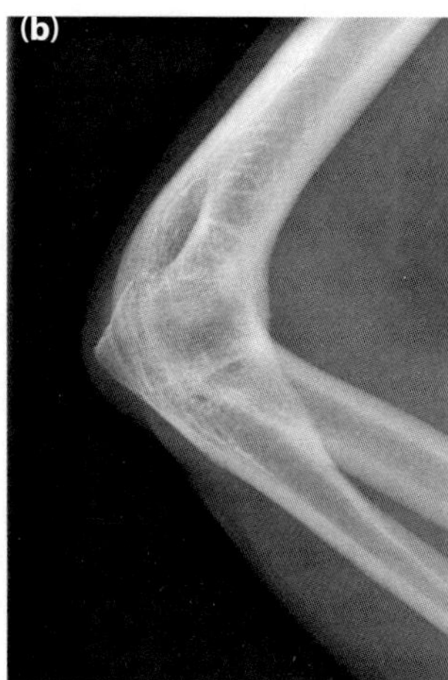

Figure 34.31 (a, b) Ankylosed elbow after tuberculosis. Arthrodesis is a surgical procedure to achieve the same end result, by excising the articular surfaces and compression plating across the joint.

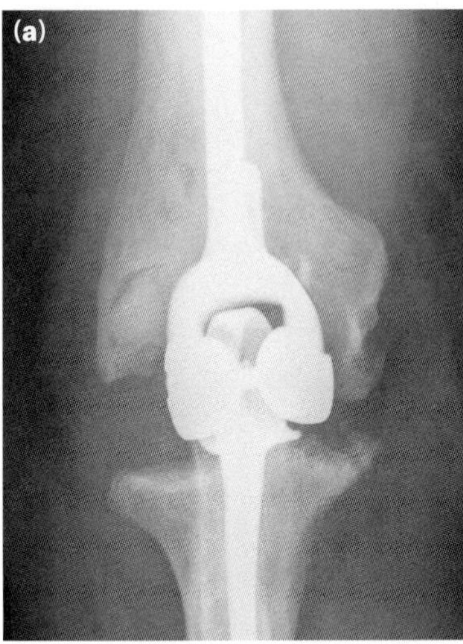

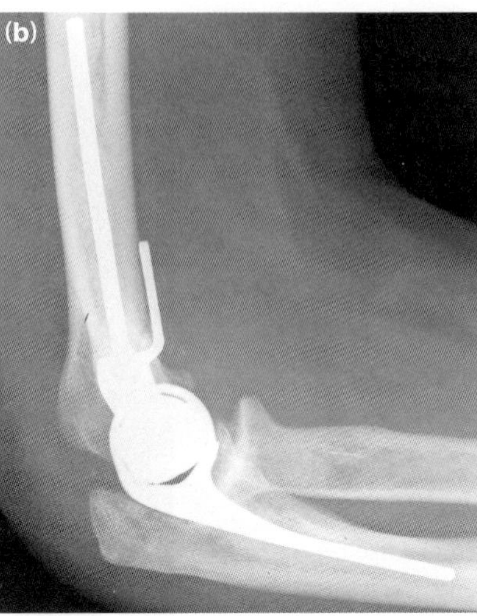

Figure 34.32 (a, b) Linked total elbow replacement.

with significant bone loss with time, possibly restricting future treatments). Prosthetic joint arthroplasty provides more predictable symptomatic relief (**Figure 34.32**) but high activity levels are associated with early loosening.

Summary box 34.9

Arthritis of the elbow

- Excision of the radial head improves pain and pronation–supination in rheumatoid arthritis
- Total elbow replacement gives good results in rheumatoid and low demand patients
- Arthrodesis may be the only surgical option in a high demand manual labourer

Figure 34.33 Osteochondritis dessicans of the capitellum (Panner's disease).

Loose bodies in the elbow

The common causes are osteoarthritis, osteochondritis dissecans in the young (**Figure 34.33**) and synovial chondromatosis (**Figure 34.34**). Patients describe sudden pain and locking, and the need to manipulate the elbow for relief. Plain radiographs will usually confirm the diagnosis (**Figure 34.35**). Arthroscopic clearance of the joint produces good results (**Figure 34.36**).

Olecranon bursitis

This is a relatively common disorder in which the elbow becomes red, warm, swollen and painful. Initially, septic arthritis may be suspected. However, on examination signs and symptoms are confined to the back of the elbow (**Figure 34.37**) and movement within an arc of 30–130° is possible. Most cases settle with anti-inflammatories. If the patient is pyrexial antibiotics should be given. Formal drainage of the bursa is indicated if purulent material is present.

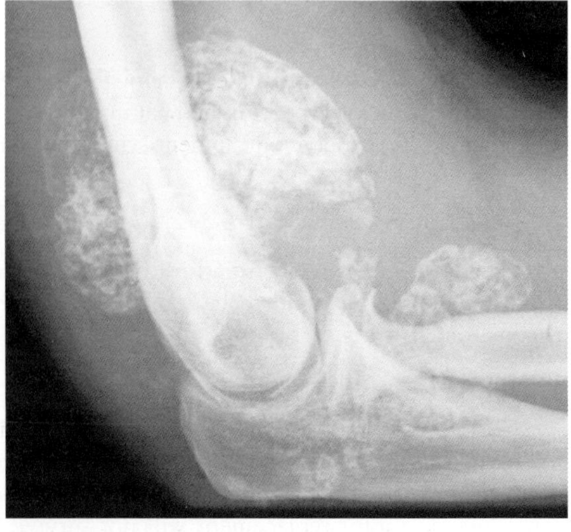

Figure 34.34 Synovial chondromatosis.

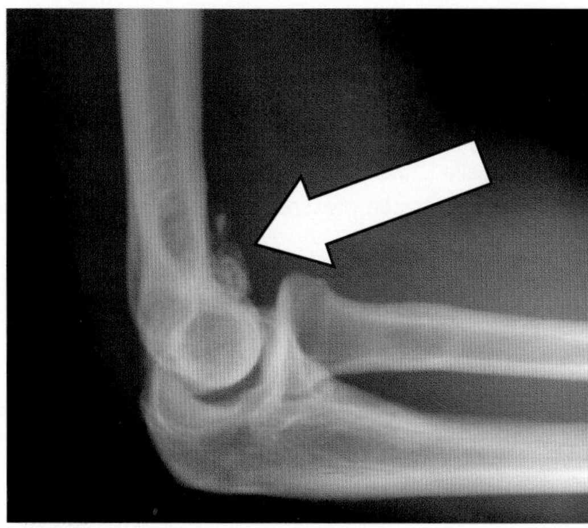

Figure 34.35 Radiographs showing loose bodies in the elbow (arrow).

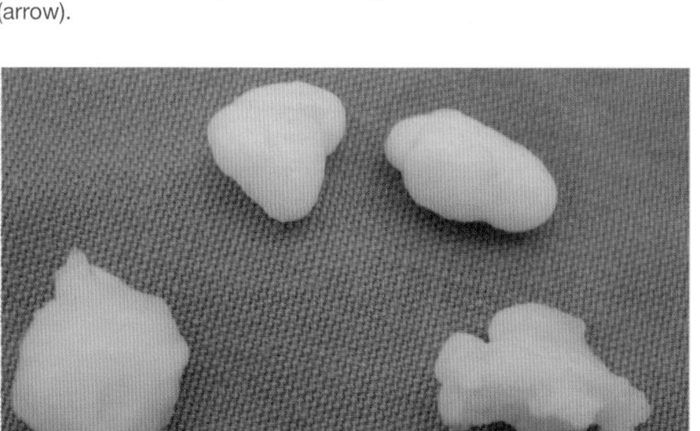

Figure 34.36 Loose bodies removed arthroscopically from the patient in Figure 34.35.

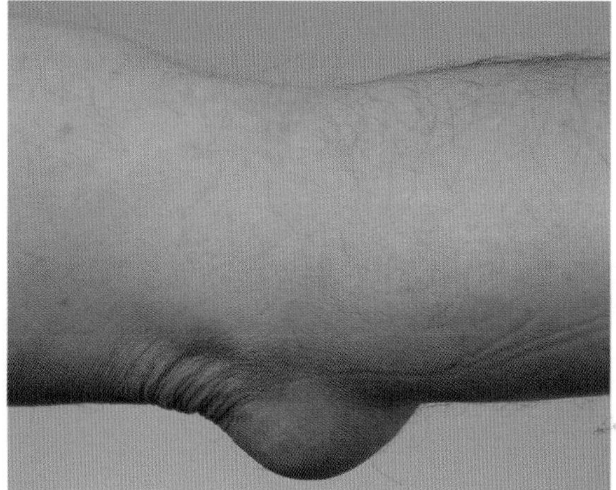

Figure 34.37 Olecranon bursitis.

Chronic bursitis may be associated with calcific nodules of the bursal lining (Figure 34.38). These can be excised if they prove troublesome.

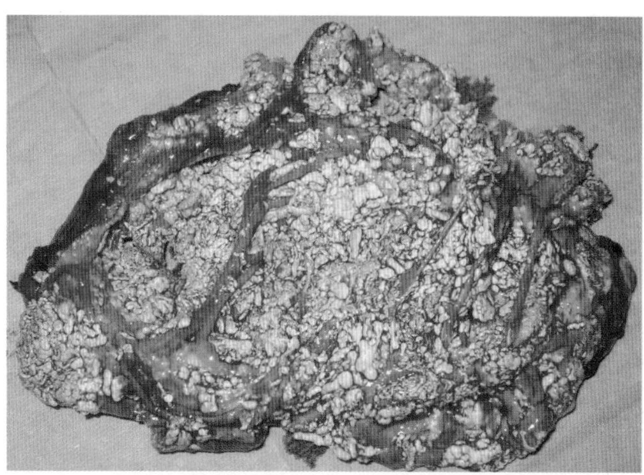

Figure 34.38 Large chronic olecranon bursa with dense calcific deposit.

Ulnar nerve compression

Compression of the ulnar nerve occurs in the cubital tunnel (behind the medial epicondyle), at the junction of the arcade of Struthers, and also at the medial intermuscular septum, as the nerve passes into the posterior compartment of the distal humerus. It can also occur as the nerve passes between the heads of the flexor carpi ulnaris (Figure 34.39).

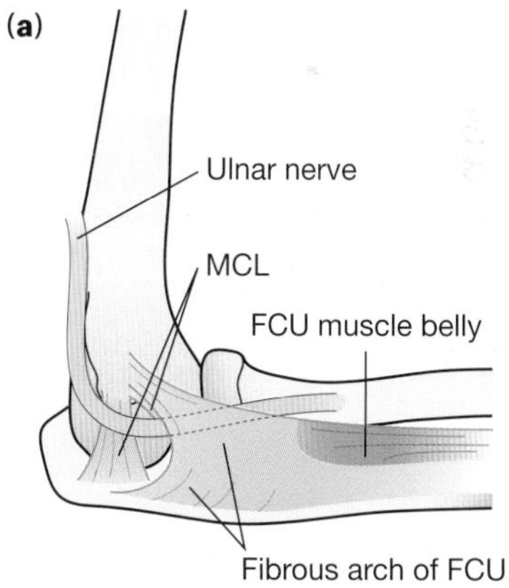

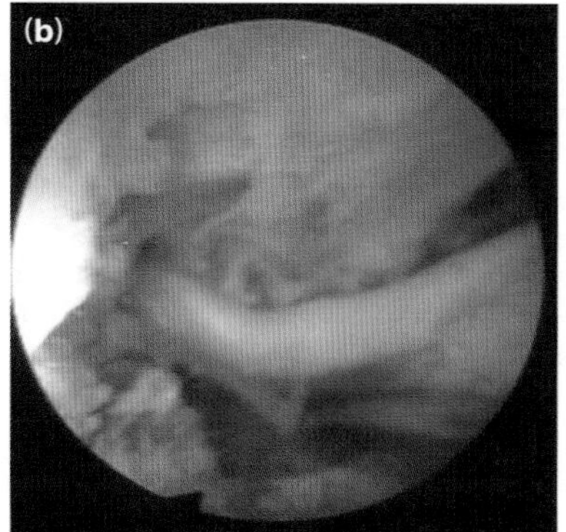

Figure 34.39 (a) Anatomy of the cubital tunnel site for ulnar nerve compression, with (b) a view of arthroscopic ulnar nerve decompression (inset). FCU, flexor carpi ulnaris; MCL, medial collateral ligament.

Sir John Struthers, 1823–1899, Professor of Anatomy, University of Aberdeen, Aberdeen, UK.

HISTORY AND EXAMINATION

Patients describe tingling/numbness in the little and ring fingers. A positive Tinel's sign is usually present at the compression site, with wasting and weakness of the intrinsic muscles of the hand (**Figure 34.40**). Froment's sign will be positive, due to weakness of the adductor pollicis (**Figure 34.41**). Nerve conduction studies have an unpredictable diagnostic value in the early stages. Radiographs may confirm medial osteophytes if compression is secondary to arthritis.

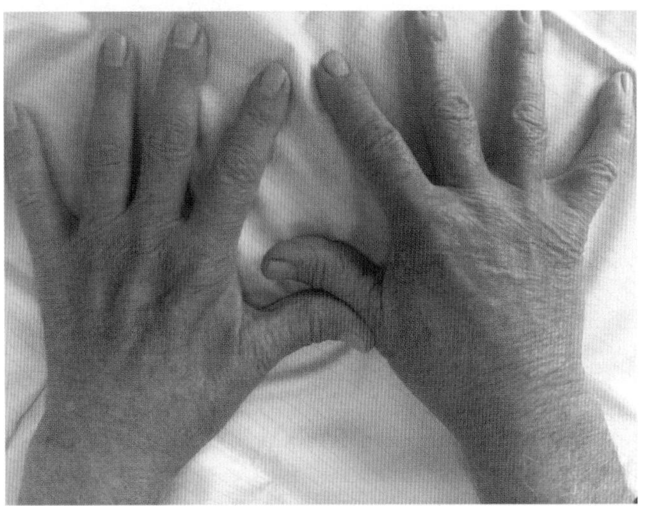

Figure 34.40 Intrinsic muscle wasting on the left due to ulnar neuropathy.

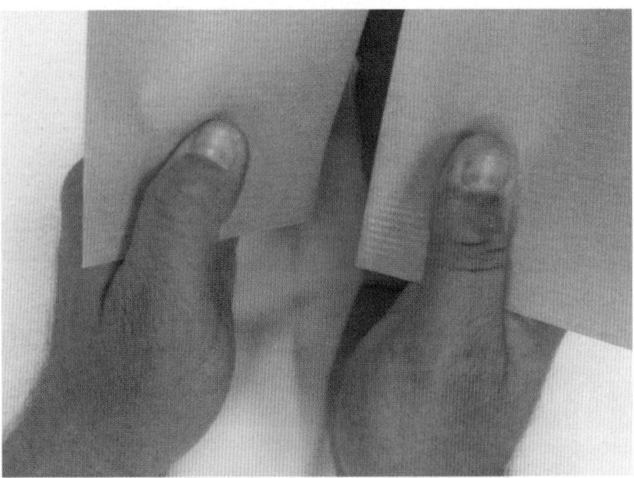

Figure 34.41 Froment's sign tests the adductor pollicis. The patient is asked to hold a piece of paper in a side pinch between the thumb and the index finger. The examiner attempts to pull the paper out. Owing to weakness of the adductor pollicus, the patient will compensate by flexing the flexor pollicis longus, which is supplied by the anterior interosseous nerve.

TREATMENT

Splints preventing elbow flexion at night may be useful. If symptoms persist, surgery can be performed, including simple nerve decompression (most cases), partial medial epicondylectomy and/or anterior transposition of the nerve. Transposition is necessary in cases of valgus deformity or if the nerve is unstable after decompression.

Summary box 34.10

Other common elbow problems

- Loose bodies cause locking and can be removed arthroscopically
- If the ulnar nerve is compressed, weakness and wasting will be seen in the hands
- Simple decompression is usually successful

TUMOURS OF THE UPPER LIMB

Tumours are discussed in Chapter 37.

HAND

The index finger works against the thumb for fine pinch grip; the thumb can press against the side of the flexed index finger for a key grip; the tips of the thumb, index and middle fingers provide a tripod pinch; all fingers curl for hook grip while the little and ring fingers provide the most power when making a fist. A stable wrist is required to allow good hand function.

Clinical history and physical examination

History

The occupation, sport and recreational activities (especially music) and hand dominance are all important items of information needed when treating a hand problem.

Examination

The examination of the hand should assess perfusion, sensation, movement, power and coordination. A check should also be made for rotational malalignment of the digits (**Figure 34.42**). There are also a number of special tests (which are beyond the scope of this chapter) relevant to different conditions.

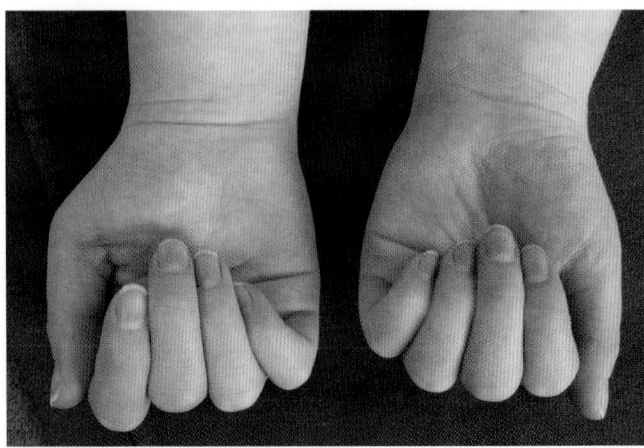

Figure 34.42 Rotational deformity of the little finger.

Investigations

Radiographs can be used to assess for arthritis or tumours. Electrophysiological studies may be required to assess nerve function. MRI is useful for diagnosing avascular necrosis, ligament injuries or soft tissue tumours.

Hand swelling and stiffness

Swelling followed by stiffness is the arch enemy of hand rehabilitation. The hand will swell after injury, surgery or infection. In response, the wrist flexes and then there is compensatory metacarpophalangeal joint (MCPJ) extension and interphalangeal joint (IPJ) flexion. If action is not taken this position will become permanent, as collateral ligaments shrink and tissues fibrose. Hand elevation to reduce swelling, splintage in the position of safety to prevent collateral shortening (Edinburgh position: wrist extension, MCPJ flexion, IPJ extension) and early mobilisation prevent permanent stiffness.

Summary box 34.11

General principles of treatment

Avoid swelling and stiffness by:

- Elevation – reduce swelling
- Splintage – avoid contractures
- Movement – pump away swelling and encourage suppleness

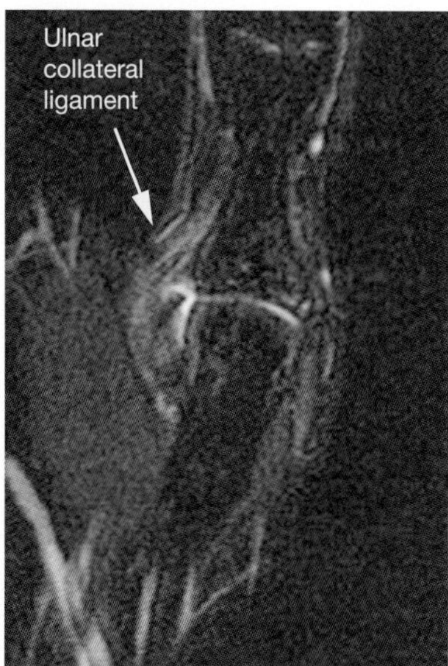

Figure 34.43 Magnetic resonance imaging showing rupture of the ulnar collateral ligament of the thumb (skier's thumb).

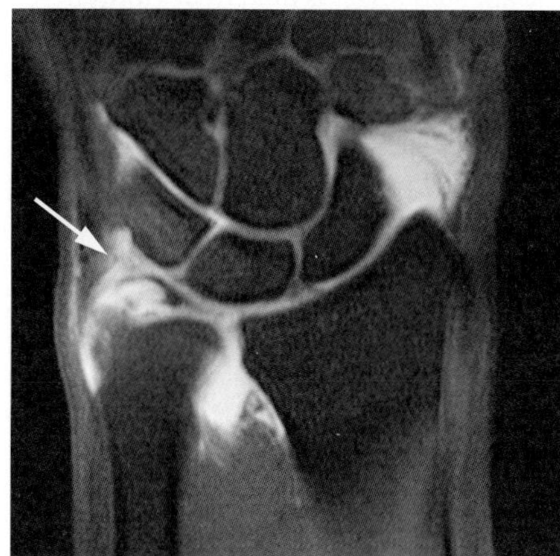

Figure 34.44 Magnetic resonance arthrogram showing peripheral detachment of the triangular fibrocartilage complex.

Thumb ulnar collateral ligament injury

Chronic thumb overuse leads to stretching of the ulnar collateral ligament and instability (gamekeeper's thumb). The ligament can also rupture acutely if the thumb is forcibly abducted (skier's thumb). If valgus stress causes significant opening of the joint on the ulnar side then the ligament needs to be repaired surgically, as the adductor aponeurosis interposes between the torn end of the ligament and its insertion (**Figure 34.43**), preventing healing and causing chronic instability.

Triangular fibrocartilage complex (TFCC)

The triangular fibrocartilage is a complex consisting of the ulnocarpal ligaments, extensor carpi ulnaris tendon sheath and a meniscus-like structure between the distal ulna and the carpus. It is continuous with the dorsal and volar wrist capsules and stabilises the distal radioulnar joint. It can undergo traumatic or degenerative tears, presenting with ulna-sided wrist pain and distal radioulnar instability. An MR arthrogram or wrist arthroscopy aids diagnosis (**Figure 34.44**). Peripheral tears of the TFCC can be repaired (open or arthroscopically), while central degenerative tears can be arthroscopically debrided.

Infections

Paronychia

Nail bed infection is the commonest hand infection (**Figure 34.45**). After initial inflammation, pus accumulates beside the nail. It is best treated with incision, drainage and appropriate antibiotic therapy. This is sometimes, but not always, facilitated by partial nail removal to allow full drainage of the collection.

Felon

A felon is an abscess between the specialised fibrous septae in the fingertip pulp. It causes intense pain and may lead

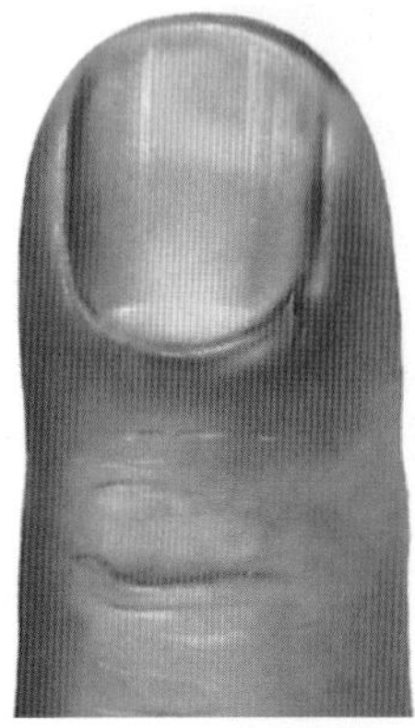

Figure 34.45 Acute paronychia.

to terminal phalangeal osteomyelitis. Incision and drainage through the midline of the pulp of the finger in the location of maximal swelling, followed by intravenous antibiotics, are recommended.

Flexor tendon sheath infection

Flexor tendon sheath infections present with Kanavel's cardinal signs: the affected finger is held in flexion; there is uniform swelling over the tendon and digit; it is tender to touch; and the patient experiences pain on passive extension of the finger. Treatment is by tendon sheath irrigation using catheters inserted through small wounds at the proximal and distal ends of the affected sheath or by an open approach if the viability of the digit is threatened. This is followed by what is often an extended course of intravenous antibiotics. If infection is untreated tendon adhesions and necrosis occur. Infection can spread proximally, damaging the whole hand.

Summary box 34.12

Treatment of hand infections

- Elevate, splint and give intravenous antibiotics
- Surgical drainage should include tendon sheath irrigation
- Early mobilisation

Mycobacterial infections

Tuberculosis may involve the tenosynovium, joints or bone. The most dramatic form is a compound palmar ganglion, with synovial swelling proximal and distal to the transverse carpal ligament, occasionally causing symptoms of carpal tunnel syndrome. The diagnosis is made by taking a biopsy. Synovectomy should be performed and the patient treated with the appropriate antibiotics.

Deep fascial space infections

These infections occur in the palm but may be limited to a web space. The whole hand becomes swollen and tender as pus collects on either side of the septum. Treatment is incision and drainage with thorough washout of the wound. It is important that all deep spaces are opened: incision on both dorsal and volar sides of the hand may be needed. If in doubt an ultrasound scan or MRI can delineate the extent of the collections within the deep palmar spaces.

Arthritis

Rheumatoid arthritis

Rheumatoid arthritis presents with classic symptoms: morning stiffness, symmetrical arthritis, hand deformities and rheumatoid nodules. Diagnostic criteria include seropositive rheumatoid factor and radiographic changes (*Table 34.1*). The inflamed rheumatoid synovium (pannus) destroys ligaments, tendons and joints, producing pain, deformity and loss of function. Typical rheumatoid deformities in the hand include boutonnière (**Figure 34.46**), swan neck (**Figure 34.47**) and radial drift of the wrist (due to supination of the

TABLE 34.1 Radiographic differences between rheumatoid and osteoarthritis.

Rheumatoid arthritis	Osteoarthritis
Periarticular osteoporosis/ subchondral erosions	Subchondral sclerosis and cysts
Periarticular soft-tissue swelling	Less pronounced swelling
Joint space narrowing	Joint space narrowing
Marginal erosions	Marginal osteophytes
Joint deformity/malalignment	Less pronounced deformities
Ankylosis	Less common ankylosis

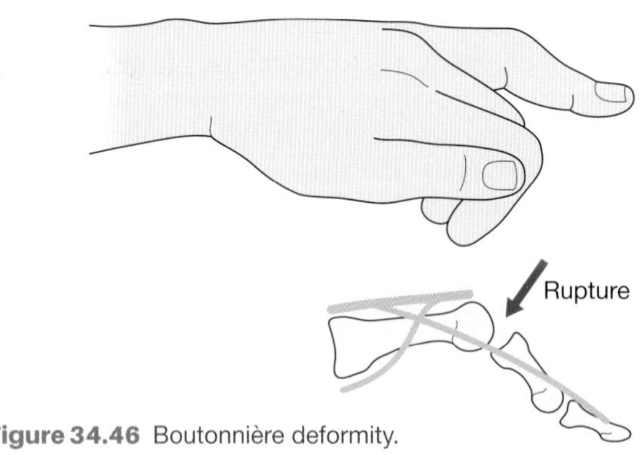

Figure 34.46 Boutonnière deformity.

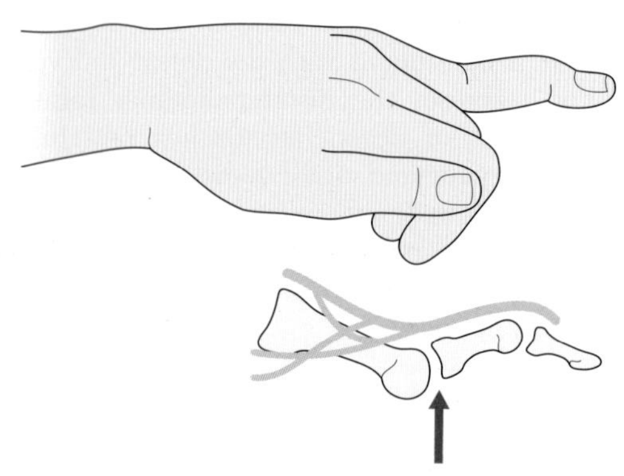

Figure 34.47 Swan neck deformity.

carpus), with compensatory ulnar deviation of the metacarpophalangeal joints (**Figure 34.48**). Pannus can cause extensor tendon ruptures, classically starting with the little finger and progressing stepwise in a radial direction (Vaughan Jackson syndrome). With progressive deformity and instability of the wrist and hand, activities such as key pinch and the opening of jars become impossible to perform. The treatment should be dictated by the patient's levels of pain and disability, not purely on the basis of deformity.

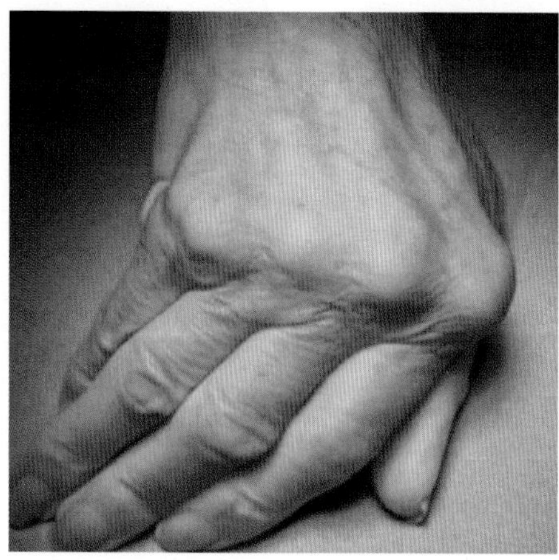

Figure 34.48 Rheumatoid hand showing ulnar drift at the metacarpophalangeal joints.

Summary box 34.13

Manifestations of rheumatoid arthritis in the hand

- Swan neck, Boutonnière finger deformities
- Extensor tendon ruptures (Vaughan–Jackson syndrome)
- Flexor tendon synovitis or rupture
- Metacarpophalangeal joints: flexion, ulnar deviation, subluxation, dislocation
- Wrist: radial deviation, carpal supination, prominent ulnar head (caput ulnae), extensor tenosynovitis

MANAGEMENT

The primary indications for surgery are: (1) pain relief; (2) functional improvement; (3) to prevent disease progression; (4) cosmesis. Patients may require many surgical procedures over time and a helpful axiom is to start proximally and work distally, alternating between motion-sacrificing and -sparing procedures. The various procedures which can be considered are:

1. Synovectomy: improves pain, increases function and prevents tendon rupture.
2. Trigger finger releases and nerve decompression surgery (carpal tunnel syndrome).
3. Distal ulna excision: reduces pain, prevents extensor tendon rupture or protects repaired extensor tendons. Distal ulna excision leads to instability and so, in the young patient, a constrained ulnar head arthroplasty is preferred.
4. Arthrodesis of the wrist, thumb and some of the smaller joints: gives good pain relief and creates a stable axis against which other parts can function.
5. Metacarpophalangeal and interphalangeal joint replacements: provide pain relief and functional improvement. Total wrist arthroplasty will also provide good pain relief and some motion (**Figure 34.49**).
6. Tendon reconstructions: some ruptured tendons can cause significant morbidity (**Figure 34.50**) and are often treated either by a tendon transfer or a local joint fusion

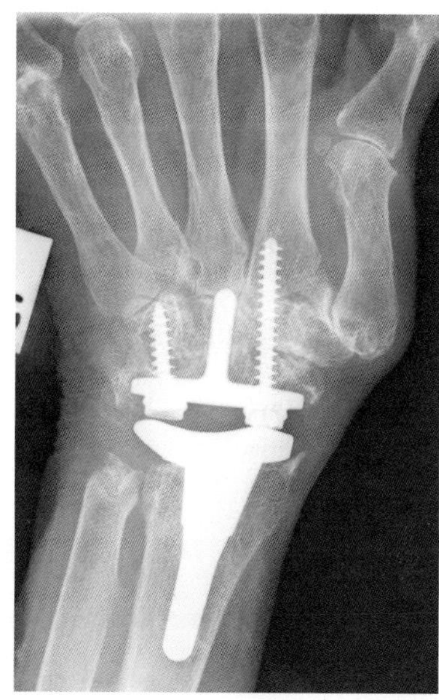

Figure 34.49 Total wrist replacement.

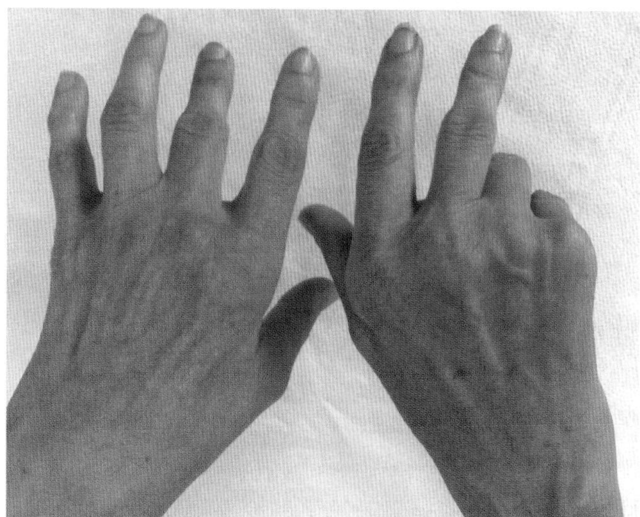

Figure 34.50 Rupture of the extensor tendons to the little and ring fingers.

Boutonnière is French for 'button-hole'.

Osteoarthritis

WRIST

The radiocarpal joint can develop primary or secondary osteoarthritis (after intra-articular trauma and infection). If conservative measures have failed then operative management includes limited or total wrist arthrodesis and total wrist replacement.

HAND

Females are more commonly affected than males. The commonly affected joints are the distal interphalangeal (Heberden's nodes), proximal interphalangeal (Bouchard's nodes) and the thumb carpometacarpal joints (Figure 34.51). Symptoms rarely correlate with the appearance, either clinically or radiographically. Treatment includes splinting, physiotherapy and steroid injections. Surgical options include arthrodesis for distal (DIP) and proximal interphalangeal (PIP) joints (Figure 34.52), joint replacement (PIP and metacarpophalangeal (MCP) joints) and excision arthroplasty (excision of the trapezium for thumb carpometacarpal joint arthritis). Joint arthrodesis eliminates pain at the expense of motion, but function is often well preserved.

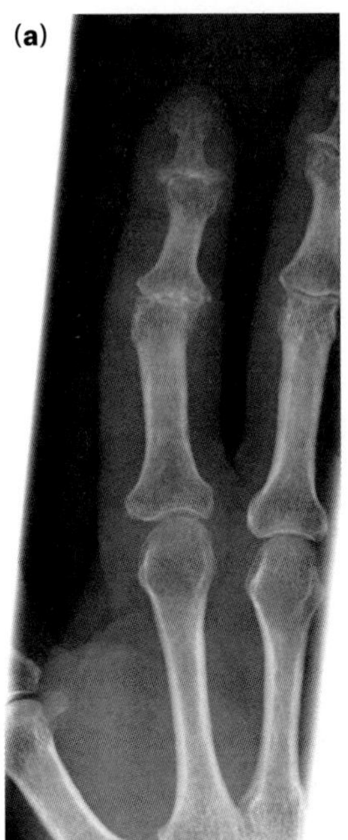

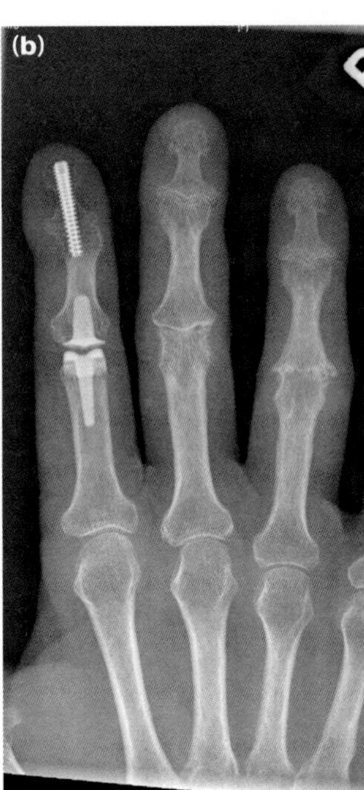

Figure 34.52 Radiographs of the distal interphalangeal and proximal interphalangeal joints treated with arthrodesis (a) and joint replacement (b).

Other forms of arthritis in the hand

Psoriasis particularly affects the interphalangeal joints, but is asymmetrical in nature and causes fusiform swelling of the digits along with nail changes. Gout causes pain, joint redness, occasionally tophi, and can be difficult to differentiate from septic arthritis. Serum urate is not always raised in acute attacks but finding negatively birefringent sodium urate crystals on microscopy of aspirated joint fluid is diagnostic.

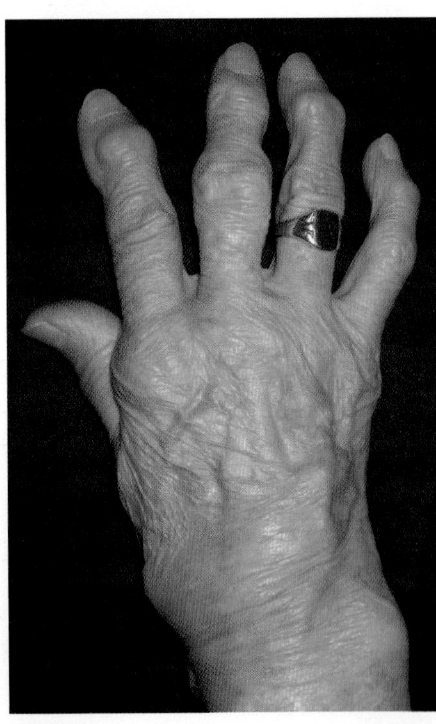

Figure 34.51 Hand deformities secondary to osteoarthritis.

Dupuytren's contracture

Dupuytren's contracture is most often characterised as an autosomal dominant condition, common in northern Europe, predominantly in men in the 5th–7th decades of life. Four out of seven cases occur in those with a family history but there are also many sporadic cases. It is associated with smoking, trauma, epilepsy, AIDS, hypothyroidism and alcoholic cirrhosis. It also appears very frequently as a clinical case in postgraduate exams! The characteristic features are palmar nodules, skin puckering, cords of the palm and digits and flexion contractures of the digits (Figure 34.53). It is commonest on the ulnar side of the hand. Garrod's knuckle pads (thickened skin on the dorsum of the PIP joint) are another feature visible on examination and seen in more severe forms of the disease (Figure 34.54). The condition can also produce cords in the penis, causing it to become curved (Peyronie's disease) and may also produce plantar thickening (Ledderhosen disease). Intervention is indicated when the patient cannot put the affected hand flat on the table owing to fixed deformity, or when any flexion contracture develops in the PIP joint. Milder cases may be treated by needle fasciotomy or

---

William Heberden (Snr.), 1710–1801, physician, who practised first in Cambridge and from 1748 in London, UK, described these nodes in 1802.
Charles Jacques Bouchard, 1837–1915, physician, Dean of the Faculty of Medicine, Paris, France.
Baron Guillaume Dupuytren, 1777–1835, surgeon, Hôtel Dieu, Paris, France, described this condition in 1831.

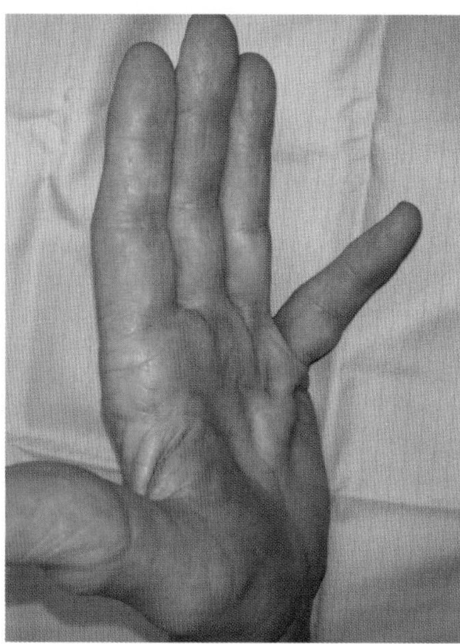

Figure 34.53 Dupuytren's contracture.

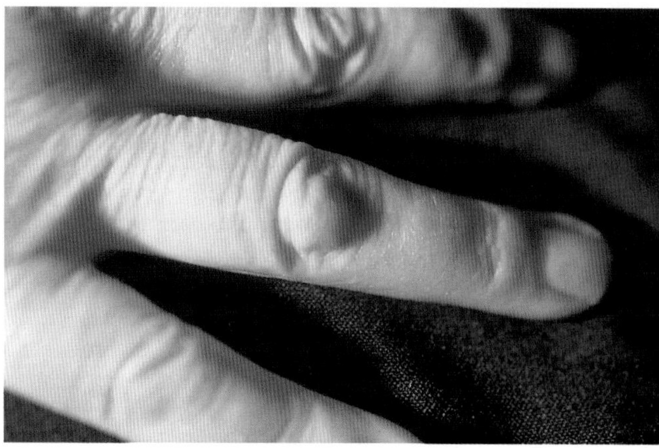

Figure 34.54 Garrod's knuckle pads.

collagenase injections, while more severe cases are managed surgically. Great care should be taken during surgery to avoid damage to the digital nerves, which may be trapped in the fibrous tissue. At the end of surgery, it may not be possible to obtain primary closure of the skin, so one should consider performing Z-plasties to lengthen the skin, full thickness skin grafting taken from the anteromedial proximal forearm (hairless) or occasionally leaving an open wound to heal by secondary intention.

In late stage disease a fixed contracture of the MCP and PIP joints may develop. In these cases, excision of the fibrous bands may produce no improvement in the condition, and if the contracted finger is preventing useful function of the hand then amputation may have to be considered.

Summary box 34.14

Dupuytren's contracture

- Autosomal dominant inheritance but many sporadic cases
- Fibroblastic hyperplasia with resultant skin nodules, cords and deformities
- Intervention is indicated if hand cannot be placed flat
- Severe fixed flexion deformities may mean that amputation is the only surgical option

Tendon disorders

Trigger digit

Triggering occurs in the fingers or in the thumb as a result of a size mismatch between the flexor tendon and the sheath (usually at the A1 pulley) in which it glides.

The patient complains of painful locking or snapping of the finger, usually when attempting to straighten a bent finger. Occasionally, it may present as a finger that is too painful to bend, associated with pain and tenderness at the A1 pulley. There is often a palpable nodule in the tendon. Management is a steroid injection into the sheath, and if this fails then surgical tendon sheath (A1 pulley) release should be performed under local anaesthesia, taking care not to cut too much of the pulley and create bowstringing of the flexor tendon. Trigger digits, especially the thumb, can occur in infants and usually resolve spontaneously.

De Quervain's disease

De Quervain's disease is caused by tenosynovitis of the abductor pollicis longus (APL) and extensor pollicis brevis (EPB) in the first dorsal wrist extensor compartment (1st EC). It is predominantly seen in middle-aged females and is associated with pregnancy (new mother's wrist) and inflammatory arthritis. The clinical features are radial wrist pain, tenderness, swelling (Figure 34.55) and a positive Finkelstein's test

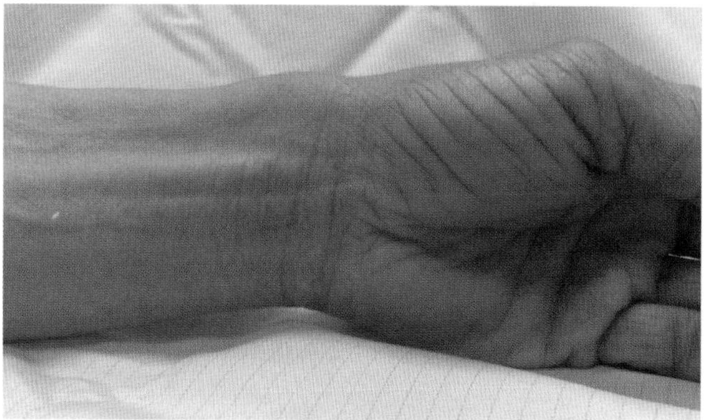

Figure 34.55 De Quervain's disease.

Sir Archibald Edward Garrod, 1857–1936, Regius Professor of Medicine, the University of Oxford, Oxford, UK, described this condition in 1893.
Francois de la Peyronie, 1678–1747, surgeon to King Louis XIV of France and founder of the Royal Academy of Surgery, Paris, France.
Georg Ledderhose, 1855–1925, German surgeon, described this disease in 1894.
Fritz de Quervain, 1868–1940, Professor of Surgery, Berne, Switzerland, described this form of tenosynovitis in 1895.

(pain over the 1st EC associated with ulnar deviation of the wrist when the thumb is clasped in the palm). The management options are non-steroidal anti-inflammatories, splintage, steroid injections and surgical release of the extensor retinaculum of the first dorsal compartment. If surgery is considered, careful attention should be paid to fully releasing the APL and EPB, which frequently consist of bundles of separate tendon slips that lie in separate sheaths.

Compressive neuropathies

Median nerve (carpal tunnel syndrome)

The majority of cases of carpal tunnel syndrome are idiopathic. It is however, associated with diabetes, thyroid disorders, alcoholism, amyloidosis, inflammatory arthritis, pregnancy and obesity.

HISTORY

The patient presents with tingling and infrequently numbness of the volar aspects of the radial three and a half digits. Patients also complain of being woken at night by pain and tingling, and that hanging their hand out of the bed provides relief. They may also complain of clumsiness when picking up small objects or when carrying heavy ones. Symptoms and signs are often bilateral.

EXAMINATION

Wasting of the thenar eminence is visible (**Figure 34.56**) in chronic severe cases, and there is sometimes weakness of the abductor pollicis brevis. The tests for carpal tunnel compression are described in Chapter 31 but the most reliable are: (1) Tinel's – percussion over the carpal tunnel and (2) Phalen's test – reproduction of paraesthesia with full wrist flexion. More recently, Durkin's compression test, in which digital pressure over the carpal tunnel reproduces the symptoms, has been shown to be highly sensitive and specific. Electrophysiological studies may confirm the diagnosis, with evidence of slowing of nerve conduction through the carpal tunnel. Non-operative treatment includes night splintage of the wrist in extension and steroid injections. If surgery is required the median nerve is surgically decompressed by incising the roof of the tunnel (transverse carpal ligament), as either an open or an endoscopic percutaneous procedure.

Summary box 34.15

Carpal tunnel syndrome

- Night pain is common and relieved by shaking the hand
- Thenar wasting is an advanced sign
- Tinel's, Phalen's and Durkin's tests are useful
- Treatment includes splints and surgical decompression

Ulnar nerve (Guyon's tunnel syndrome)

Ulnar nerve compression in Guyon's canal can lead to tingling and numbness in the ring and little fingers with hypothenar wasting. There is preservation of dorsal sensation over the little and ring fingers, because although these areas are innervated by the ulnar nerve the dorsal branches do not pass through Guyon's canal. Compression is usually due to a ganglion, ulnar artery aneurysm or a fracture of the hook of hamate.

Avascular necrosis of carpal bones

Idiopathic avascular necrosis of the lunate (Kienböck's disease, **Figure 34.57**) or scaphoid (Preiser's disease) can occur. The clinical presentation is of wrist pain and the diagnosis

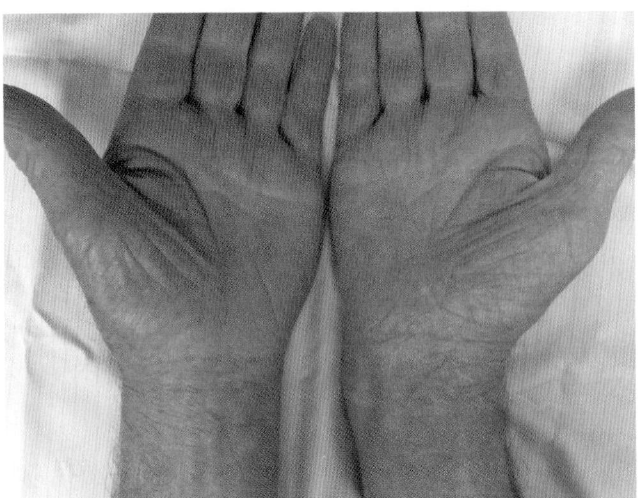

Figure 34.56 Thenar muscle wasting in carpal tunnel syndrome.

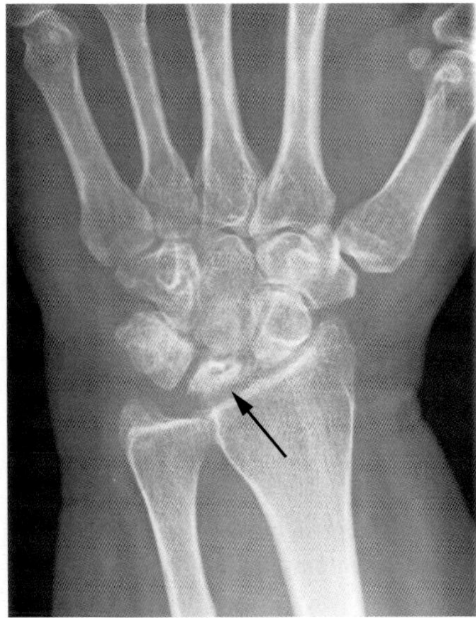

Figure 34.57 Avascular necrosis of the lunate (Keinbock's).

Jean Casimir Felix Guyon, 1831–1920, Professor of Genito-urinary Surgery, Paris, France.
Robert Keinböck, 1871–1953, Professor of Radiology, Vienna, Austria, described this condition in 1910.

can be confirmed with radiographs and MRI. The natural history of the condition is that it leads to collapse of the avascular carpal bones and subsequent arthritis of the carpus, which may be best treated with a partial or complete fusion of the wrist. This will at least give a strong and painless wrist. The limitation in movement caused by arthrodesis procedures is not as great as might be expected.

Ganglion cysts

Ganglion cysts are the commonest cause of a swelling in the hand and they are found most often on the dorsal (**Figure 34.58**) and volar (**Figure 34.59**) surfaces of the wrist, over the dorsum of the DIP joint (digital mucous cyst) or within the flexor tendon sheath at the base of the finger (seed ganglion). Dorsal and volar wrist ganglions can cause discomfort. The swellings are smooth, fluctuant and transilluminate brightly. Mucous cysts can frequently discharge and cause nail changes (**Figure 34.60**). Seed ganglions can be painful when gripping. Aspiration or surgical excision can be considered. Patients should be informed regarding possible recurrence.

Congenital malformations

There are many congenital malformations of the upper limb and these are discussed in Chapter 39. A classification summarising the main congenital defects and based on aetiology appears as Table 34.2

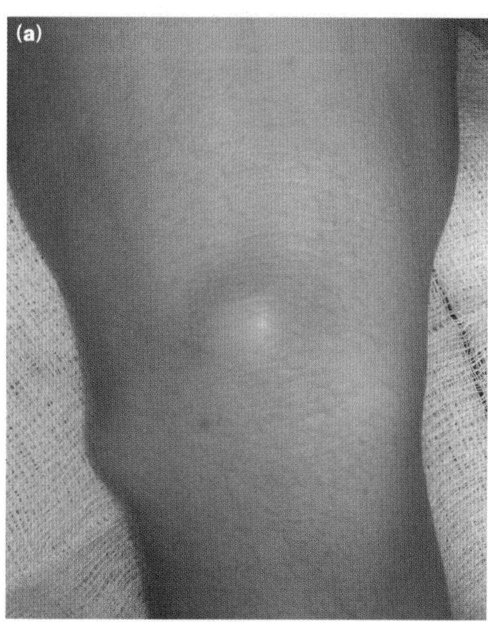

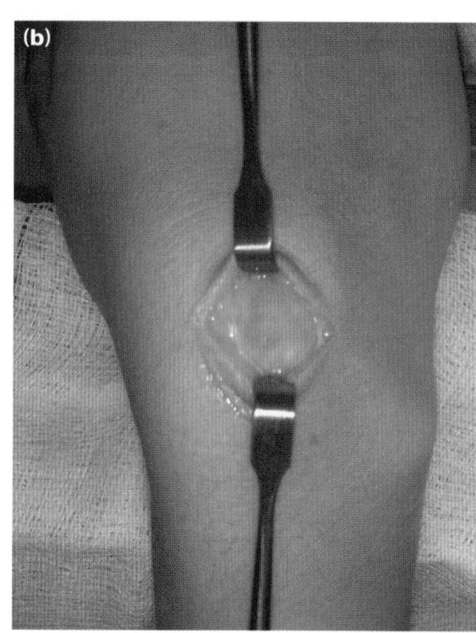

Figure 34.58
(**a**) Clinical and (**b**) surgical appearance of a dorsal wrist ganglion.

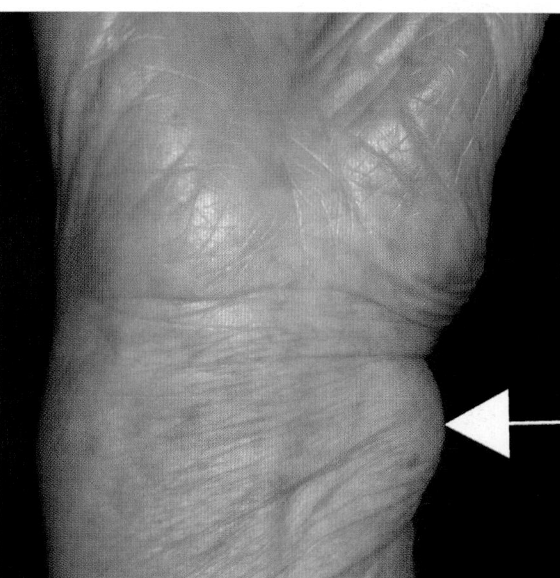

Figure 34.59 Volar wrist ganglion.

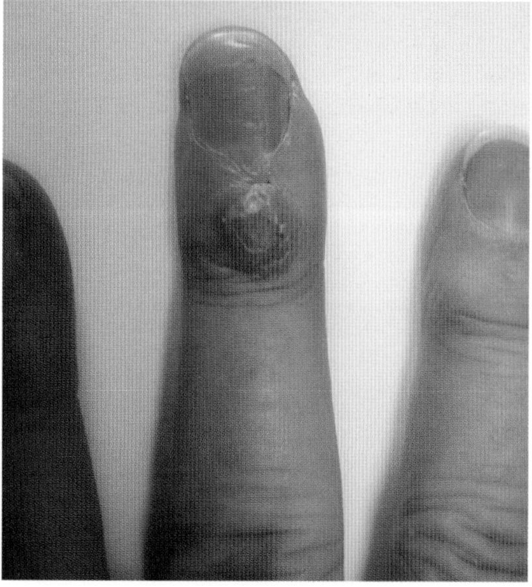

Figure 34.60 Myxoid cyst with changes in the nail.

TABLE 34.2 Congenital malformations (hand and wrist)

A Defects in formation due to arrested development	1 Transverse agenesis 2 Longitudinal agenesis (a) radial ray aplasia; (b) median ray aplasia; (c) ulnar ray aplasia 3 Thumb aplasia/hypoplasia
B Defects in differentiation/separation	1 Syndactyly 2 Camptodactyly 3 Clinodactyly 4 Kirner's deformity 5 Radioulnar synostosis
C Duplications	1 Supernumerary phalanges 2 Supernumerary digits (polydactyly)
D Excess development/hyperplasia	Macrodactyly
E Insufficient development/hypoplasia	Thumb hypoplasia
F Constricting (amniotic) bands	Simple amniotic band syndrome
G Generalised skeletal anomalies	Marfan, Turner and Down syndromes

FURTHER READING

Carr AJ, Cooper CD, Campbell AK *et al.* Clinical effectiveness and cost-effectiveness of open and arthroscopic rotator cuff repair [the UK Rotator Cuff Surgery (UKUFF) randomised trial]. *Health Technol Assess* 2015; **19**(80): 1–218.

Constant CR, Murley AH. A clinical method of functional assessment of the shoulder. *Clin Orthop* 1987; **214**: 160–4.

Dawson J, Rogers K, Fitzpatrick R, Carr A. The Oxford shoulder score revisited. *Arch Orthop Trauma Surg* 2009; **129**(1): 119–23.

Gill DR, Morrey BF. The Coonrad-Morrey total elbow arthroplasty in patients who have rheumatoid arthritis. A ten to fifteen-year follow-up study. *J Bone Joint Surg Am* 1998; **80**: 1327–35.

Mizuno N, Denard PJ, Raiss P *et al.* Long-term results of the Latarjet procedure for anterior instability of the shoulder. *J Shoulder Elbow Surg* 2014; **23**(11); 1691–9.

Neer CS. Anterior acromioplasty for the chronic impingement syndrome in the shoulder: a preliminary report. *J Bone Joint Surg [Am]* 1972; **54-A**: 41–50.

O'Driscoll SW, Bell DF, Morrey BF. Posterolateral rotatory instability of the elbow. *J Bone Joint Surg Am* 1991; **73**: 440–6.

Poppen NK, Walker PS. Normal and abnormal motion of the shoulder. *J Bone Joint Surg [Am]* 1976; **58-A**: 195–201.

Rowe CR, Patel D, Southmayd WW. The Bankart procedure: long-term end-result study. *J Bone Joint Surg [Am]* 1978; **60-A**: 1–16.

Singh JA, Sperling JW, Schleck S *et al.* Periprosthetic infections after total shoulder arthroplasty: A 33-year perspective. *J Shoulder Elbow Surg.* 2012; **21**(11): 1534–41.

Chapter 35

Hip and knee

Learning objectives

To understand:

- The anatomy and biomechanics of the hip and knee and their clinical implications
- The clinical presentation, aetiology and management of common hip and knee pathologies
- The principles of joint replacement including important complications
- The advances in surgical practice in this field

THE HIP JOINT

Applied anatomy

The hip is a ball and socket joint formed by the head of the femur and the cup-shaped acetabulum (Latin: little vinegar cup) (Figure 35.1). The joint allows a considerable range of movement in different planes, and is still inherently stable because of its bony anatomy and the static and dynamic stabilisers. The static stabilisers are composed of the ligaments (iliofemoral and pubofemoral ligaments anteriorly and the ischiofemoral ligament posteriorly), the joint capsule and the labrum. The muscles running across the joint (short external rotator muscles posteriorly, the iliopsoas anteriorly and the hip abductors laterally) constitute the dynamic stabilisers. The acetabular labrum is a fibrocartilagenous structure that is triangular in cross-section and attaches to the rim of the acetabulum except at its base, where it is replaced by the transverse ligament. It helps in deepening the socket, thereby enhancing stability. It also acts as a fluid seal and thereby helps to improve joint lubrication.The femoral head derives its blood supply mainly from the retinacular branches of the medial circumflex femoral artery and there is a small contribution from the artery of the ligamentum teres.

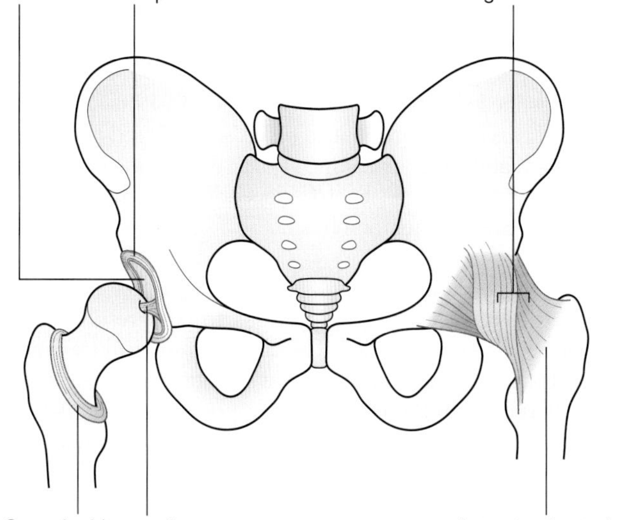

Figure 35.1 Anatomy of the hip joint.

Summary box 35.1

Anatomy

- The hip joint is a ball and socket joint, stabilised by static and dynamic stabilisers
- Static stabilisers include the capsule, ligaments and labrum
- Dynamic stabilisers consist of the muscles acting across the joint
- Blood supply to the femoral head is mainly derived from the medial circumflex femoral artery

Biomechanics of the hip joint

Kinetic analysis reveals that forces as high as three times body weight can be exerted across the hip joint during activities of daily living, and eight times body weight during physically demanding activities. This is primarily the result of contraction of muscles crossing the joint. The abductors, because of their insertion at the greater trochanter, help in supporting the pelvis when the patient stands on one leg and thereby form the basis of a Trendelenburg test (**Figure 35.2**).

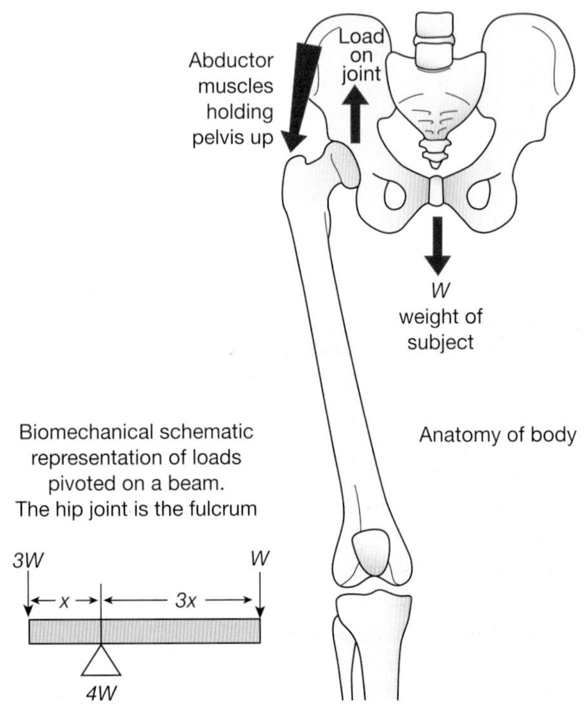

Figure 35.2 Load on the hip joint when a subject weighing W stands on one leg. Hopping increases the load from 4 to 10W.

Summary box 35.2

Forces going through the hip joint

- Lifting leg from bed – one and a half times body weight
- Standing on one leg – three times body weight
- Running and jumping – ten times body weight

Conditions affecting the hip joint

Common hip pathologies in the paediatric age group and secondary to trauma are covered in Chapters 39, 27 and 28. This chapter focuses on the acquired pathological conditions in the adult.

Avascular necrosis

Avascular necrosis (AVN), or osteonecrosis of the femoral head, occurs because of an interruption in the blood supply to the femoral head that causes bone death. This leads to collapse of the femoral head, and subsequent secondary osteoarthritis. AVN can be primary (idiopathic) or secondary to other pathology (*Table 35.1*).

TABLE 35.1 Aetiology of avascular necrosis of the femoral head.
Sickle cell disease
Haemoglobinopathies
Caisson disease ('the bends' in divers)
Hyperlipidaemia
Systemic lupus erythematosus
Gaucher's disease
Chronic liver disease
Antiphospholipid antibody syndrome
Radiotherapy
Chemotherapy
Human immunodeficiency virus
Hypercoagulable states (protein C and protein S deficiency)
Steroids
Alcohol excess
Idiopathic (see Perthes' disease, Chapter 39)

CLINICAL FEATURES

AVN usually affects men aged from 35 to 45 and is bilateral in over 50% of patients. The patient is frequently asymptomatic in the early stages. As the disease progresses the patient may complain of an ache in the groin and walk with a limp; clinical examination may reveal limitation of movement.

INVESTIGATIONS

A weight-bearing anteroposterior (AP) radiograph of the pelvis along with a lateral radiograph will show the classical features of AVN including increased sclerosis in the early stages, and the crescent sign indicating subchondral bone resorption. In the late stages there may be flattening indicating a segmental head collapse (**Figure 35.3**). However, radiographs may be normal in the early stages of the disease and, therefore, the most sensitive and specific way of investigating these patients is with magnetic resonance imaging (MRI). MRI allows accurate assessment of the extent of involvement and can also identify associated bone marrow changes. This helps in early diagnosis and prediction of prognosis (**Figure 35.4**). In 1985, Ficat classified the disease into five stages. In 1995, Steinberg modified this classification into seven stages based upon both radiograph and MRI appearance (*Table 35.2*). Stages I–IV are further divided into A, B or C depending on the extent of involvement of the femoral head.

TREATMENT

Conservative treatment usually leads to poor results and is therefore not recommended. The choice of surgical treatment depends on whether the head has collapsed or not. In the pre-collapse group the principle is to preserve and preferably encourage revascularisation of the femoral head, whereas in

Friedrich Trendelenburg, 1844–1924, Professor of Surgery successively at Rostock (1875–1882), Bonn (1882–1895) and Leipzig (1895–1911), Germany. The Trendelenburg position was first described in 1885.
A caisson is a watertight chamber used to protect construction workers during the building of underwater structures by means of pressurised air introduction.
Philippe Charles Ernest Gaucher, 1854–1918, physician, Hôpital St. Louis, Paris, France, described familial splenic anaemia in 1882.

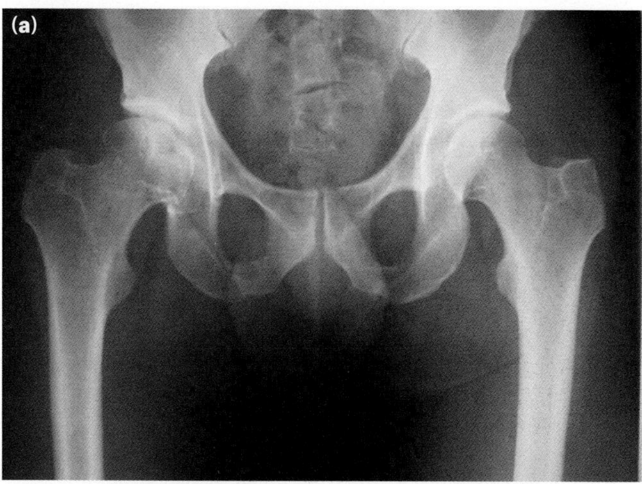

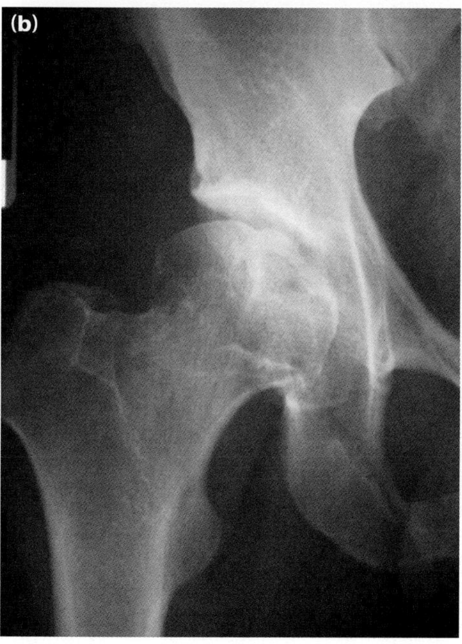

Figure 35.3 (**a, b**) Radiological appearance of avascular necrosis of the femoral head.

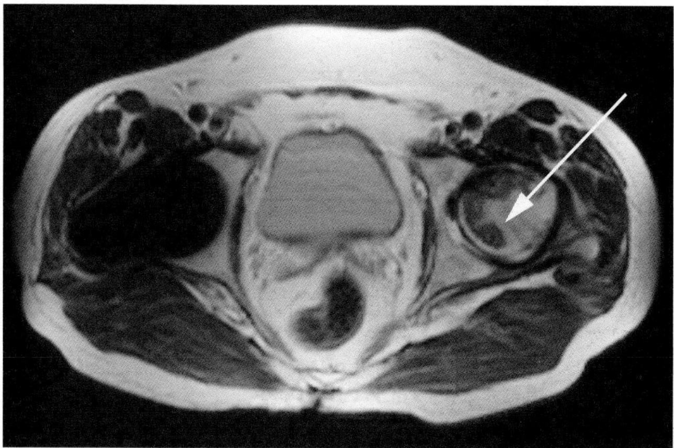

Figure 35.4 Magnetic resonance imaging scan of the hip joint showing avascular necrosis and the extent of involvement of the femoral head (arrrow).

TABLE 35.2 Steinberg's classification of avascular necrosis of the femoral head based on the type of radiological change on radiography and magnetic resonance imaging (MRI).

Stage	Description
0	Normal or non-diagnostic radiograph, bone scan or MRI
I	Normal radiograph, abnormal MRI or bone scan
II	Sclerosis and cysts
III	Subchondral collapse, crescent sign
IV	Flattening of the head, normal acetabulum
V	Acetabular involvement
VI	Obliteration of joint space

the collapse group the aim is to bring the undamaged parts of the femoral head into the load-bearing area.

The surgical treatment for the pre-collapse stage includes core decompression, which is aimed at relieving intravascular congestion in the femoral head, and thereby pain. This can be achieved with or without bone grafting; a vascularised bone graft can also be used to stimulate bone formation. Once the femoral head has collapsed, either a femoral osteotomy (which aims to transfer the weight-bearing area of the femoral head and thereby protect the collapsed segment) or a joint replacement (if degenerative changes have set in) is the preferred option (see later).

Summary box 35.3

Avascular necrosis of the femoral head

- Patients can be asymptomatic in the early stages and therefore a high index of suspicion is necessary for initial diagnosis
- MRI scans are needed for early diagnosis
- Treatment is based on whether the patient presents before or after the femoral head has collapsed
- In the pre-collapse stage, treatement focuses on revascularisation
- In the collapsed stage, the aim is to replace the damaged joint surface
- Prognosis is dependent upon the extent of femoral head involvement

Osteoarthritis (OA)

OA is referred to as primary when no predisposing cause can be found and secondary (including traumatic) when it develops after an insult to the hip joint. A multitude of factors including genetic, biochemical and mechanical influences have been implicated in the development of primary OA. The exact mechanism for the development of primary OA remains unknown and it is therefore termed idiopathic. Femoroacetabular impingement (FAI) has been proposed as an aetiological factor responsible for the development of OA. Secondary OA develops following trauma, AVN, dysplasia, slipped capital femoral epiphysis, inflammatory arthropathy or other known predisposing cause. The causes of OA of the hip are given in *Table 35.3*.

TABLE 35.3 Aetiology of osteoarthritis.
Primary
Cause unknown, termed idiopathic
Associations: for example, genetics, gender, obesity
Secondary
Trauma
Avascular necrosis
Inflammatory arthropathy (e.g. rheumatoid arthritis)
Perthes' disease
Developmental dysplasia of the hip
Slipped capital femoral epiphysis
Septic arthritis
Femoroacetabular impingement implicated as a possible cause

CLINICAL FEATURES

Osteoarthritis of the hip affects 10–25% of those over the age of 65 years. The most consistent symptoms are groin pain and limitation of movement. The pain may also radiate down to the knee joint, and in some cases the only presenting feature may be a painful knee. In the early stages of the disease, pain is activity related but as the disease progresses the patient also complains of pain at rest. The patient frequently complains of night pain and may also find it difficult to get into a comfortable position while sleeping. Functionally, most have difficulty in putting on their shoes and socks, and getting into and out of a bath or a car. As the pain increases the joint gradually loses its movement because of muscle spasm, capsular contracture and osteophyte formation.

Clinical examination may reveal gluteal muscle wasting. There may also be a limp, with a positive Trendelenburg's test. Leg length discrepancy, usually shortening, and limitation of movement, particularly internal rotation, are consistent features. Many patients present with a fixed flexion deformity that is best elicited by a modified Thomas' test (see Chapter 31).

INVESTIGATIONS

The characteristic features on radiograph are (1) a reduction of joint space, (2) sclerosis in the subchondral bone, (3) subchondral cysts and (4) osteophyte formation (**Figure 35.5**). Eventually, a collapsed femoral head may also be evident.

TREATMENT

There is no specific pharmacological therapy for OA; however, conservative treatment with non-steroidal anti-inflammatories, regular exercise, physiotherapy and modification of lifestyle with loss of weight does help. Patients should also be encouraged to use walking aids (usually a walking stick in the opposite hand to offload the affected joint).

The indications for surgery are relentless pain, limitation of lifestyle and activities of daily living, and failure of conservative treatment. The surgical options include an arthrodesis (fusion), an osteotomy (re-alignment) or a joint replacement (**Figure 3.6**). More and more joint replacements are now being performed. The indications are based on limitation of lifestyle and individual needs, thereby making it a truly life-improving operation.

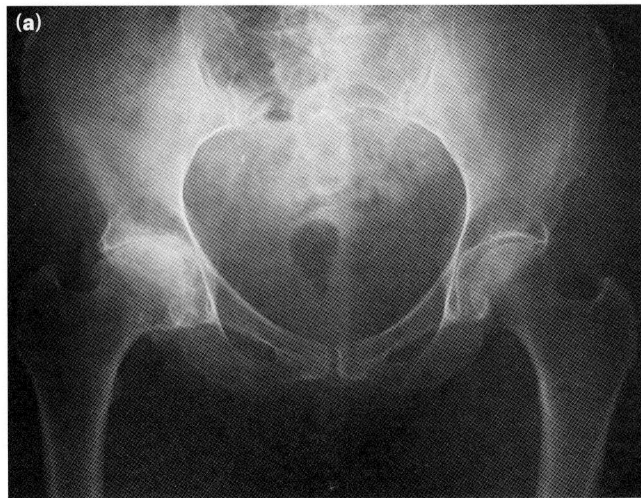

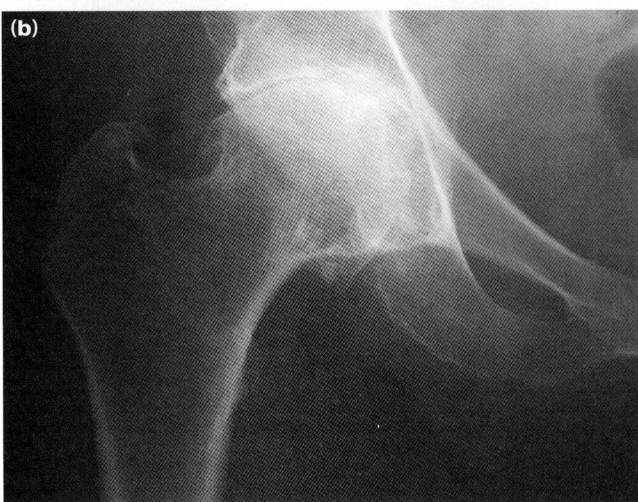

Figure 35.5 Anteroposterior (**a**) and enlarged anteroposterior (**b**) radiographs of the hip joint showing osteoarthritis.

Summary box 35.4

Osteoarthritis of the hip

- Osteoarthritis is a non-inflammatory and low-grade inflammatory condition leading to progressive damage to the articular cartilage and other joint structures
- The most consistent clinical features are groin pain and limitation of movement
- Characteristic radiological findings include reduction of joint space, subchondral sclerosis, subchondral cysts and osteophyte formation
- Conservative treatment includes walking aids, non-steroidal analgesics, physiotherapy and weight loss
- Surgical options include osteotomy, arthrodesis or a joint replacement

Georg Clemens Perthes, 1869–1927, Professor of Surgery, Tubingen, Germany, described osteochondritis of the femoral capital epiphysis in 1910.

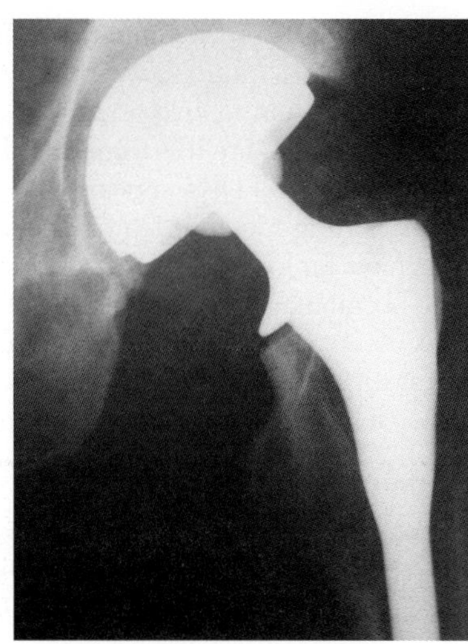

Figure 35.6 Radiograph showing an uncemented total hip replacement *in situ*.

Inflammatory arthritis

The hip joint can also be affected by inflammatory arthritides, however these are not as common as OA. This group includes rheumatoid arthritis, ankylosing spondylitis, gout and chondrocalcinosis, juvenile rheumatoid arthritis and systemic lupus erythematosus.

Femoroacetabular impingement (FAI)

Femoroacetabular impingement has recently been recognised as a cause of hip pain in the young adult and may lead to secondary hip OA. The non-spherical portion of the femoral head is assumed to exert abnormal shear and compressive forces on the corresponding portion of the acetabular cartilage during deep hip flexion with internal rotation. Patients typically present with groin pain, and MRI-arthrograms typically reveal acetabular rim lesions and aberrant femoral head morphology.

Two distinct types of FAI have been described – cam and pincer – although many patients have a mixed picture with both morphologies occuring simultaneously. Pincer impingement is a result of anterior overcoverage or retroversion of the acetabulum, while cam impingement is secondary to abnormal morphology of the femoral head and neck junction. Treatment options for FAI depend on the patient's symptoms and vary from conservative treatment to hip arthroscopic procedures that aim to address labral and bone pathology, or osteotomy.

Surgical procedures

Arthroscopy of the hip

The hip joint presents challenges to arthroscopy in terms of access and instrumentation of the deeply recessed femoral head in the acetabulum and the surrounding thick fibrocapsular and muscular envelope. Technical advances, including an improved ability to manage the capsule and gain exposure, have led to an expanding list of applications, including the treatment of symptomatic labral tears, femoroacetabular impingement and the removal of loose bodies, e.g. synovial chondromatosis. Arthroscopy allows a clear view of the femoral and acetabular articular surfaces, the labrum, the ligamentum teres and the head–neck junction, along with the surrounding synovium and its folds and the peritrochanteric space. Advantages include minimally invasive access to all these structures coupled with rapid recovery, in comparison with open surgery.

Arthrodesis of the hip

Arthrodesis or fusion of the hip is an uncommon operation. It is generally reserved for young patients with severe osteoarthritis who have heavy manual jobs and in whom joint replacements would fail early. The aim is to achieve a painless joint by fusing it in a functional position, which is about 30° of flexion, 15° of external rotation and 5° of abduction. This can be achieved by an intra-articular dynamic hip screw or by an extra-articular plate with screws.

Several problems can occur following an arthrodesis, including altered gait and excessive loading of the ipsilateral knee, the contralateral hip and the spine. Degenerative change in these joints in the long term is the rule rather than the exception.

Osteotomies around the hip

The goal of an osteotomy around the hip is to redistribute forces evenly across the joint, thereby eliminating excessive point loading. This can be achieved by performing an osteotomy on the femoral or the acetabular side, depending upon the desired goal, e.g. an excessive valgus neck–shaft angle and an uncovered femoral head on the lateral aspect can be corrected by carrying out a varus femoral osteotomy. Similarly, a redirection osteotomy on the acetabular side can also be performed to improve coverage of the femoral head. The common indications for an osteotomy around the hip include:

- developmental dysplasia of the hip;
- Perthes' disease;
- OA in a young patient;
- slipped capital femoral epiphysis;
- AVN.

Ideally, an osteotomy should be considered in a young patient who maintains a good range of movement of the hip and whose radiographs show a reasonable amount of joint space. Thorough preoperative planning is essential to assess whether the desired position can be achieved. Three-dimensional computed tomography (CT) scans are helpful for appropriate preoperative planning.

Total hip replacement

Over 80 000 primary total hip replacements are performed annually in the UK. The results of surgery are encouraging. With evidence-based technique and selection of prosthesis, up to 95% of patients will have a well-functioning hip replacement at 10 years after surgery. In the best series, 85% will still be functioning at 20 years, although some are still in place because the patient may have increasing comorbidities, preventing revision. Following surgery, pain is reduced, mobility increases and sleep, as well as social and sexual function, is improved. Nevertheless, with the ever-increasing number of patients with joint replacements, the number of patients whose replacement has failed and come to the point of revision, or even re-revision, is rising.

PRINCIPLES AND DESIGN OF HIP REPLACEMENTS

Any joint replacement should be biocompatible and made of inert materials. It should be well fixed to the host tissue and the design should incorporate features that allow a good range of movement and stability. The bearing surfaces should produce minimal friction to prevent early loosening, and the material released from the bearing surface should be non-toxic. It should remove the minimum amount of the patient's bone so that revision is possible, and it should create a biomechanically stable joint. Finally, any implanted joint should ideally outlive the patient and be cost effective.

Summary box 35.5

Features of an ideal joint replacement

- Biocompatible
- Well fixed to the host tissue, stable and allowing a good range of movement
- Bearing surfaces should be designed to minimise friction
- Material released from the bearings should be non-toxic
- Remove the minimum amount of bone
- Produce mechanical stability
- Should ideally outlive the patient

MATERIALS FOR THE FEMORAL COMPONENT

Most of the implants available currently are made of cobalt–chrome alloy, but stainless steel and titanium are also used. Metal implants are able to withstand high loads, are relatively inert and can be manufactured easily. However, they do pose problems in terms of ion release if they are used as bearing surfaces. Also, corrosion can be a cause for concern if two dissimilar metals are used.

BEARING SURFACES

The total hip replacement (THR) designed by Charnley used a bearing surface of metal on high-density polyethylene. This is described as a hard-on-soft bearing surface and has a low coefficient of friction. High-density polyethylene has good shock-absorbing properties but does wear slowly over the years, producing small particles that can stimulate an inflammatory response in the joint, which then leads to aseptic loosening of the implants. The activated macrophages resorb bone and may also stimulate osteoclasts to do the same. There has therefore been a move towards using bearing surfaces with a lower wear rate, such as ceramic on ceramic. With metal on metal bearing surfaces, although the wear rate is lower, the wear particles are smaller (nano rather than micro) and there is increasing evidence that these implants are less forgiving than conventional metal on polyethylene THRs, appearing to require more precise implant positioning. Ceramic femoral heads bearing on polyethylene cups have far lower friction, but ceramic femoral heads on ceramic acetabular cups have the lowest friction of all. However they are expensive to manufacture and produce small-sized wear particles. A summary of the advantages and disadvantages of each bearing surface is provided in *Table 35.4*.

FIXATION OF IMPLANTS

Artificial joints must be securely fixed to the bone on each side of the joint so that the implant does not work loose. This can be achieved with the help of cement or biological interdigitation between the prosthesis and bone (*Table 35.5*).

Traditionally, hip replacements were fixed into a bed of polymethylmethacrylate (PMMA) cement (**Figure 35.7a**). The cement acts as a grout (spacer) and not as a glue between

TABLE 35.4 Bearing surfaces for hip replacements.

Type of bearing	Advantages	Disadvantages
Metal on polyethylene	Proven efficacy; easy to manufacture; cheap	Comparatively high friction; high wear rates; wear particles excite an inflammatory response that leads to osteolysis
Ceramic on polyethylene	Lower wear rate	Expensive; ceramic fracture can be a problem
Metal on metal	Lower wear rate	Published examples of failure requiring early revision; implant recalls; metal ion release is a problem; expensive
Ceramic on ceramic	Lowest wear rate	Very expensive; ceramic can fracture; squeaking

TABLE 35.5 Fixation of implants.

Method of fixation	Advantages	Disadvantages
Cemented	Implant does not need to fit cavity exactly; well-proven results	Cement polymerisation is exothermic with possibility of thermal injury; fragments may cause third-body wear and stimulate aseptic loosening; difficult to remove at revision
Uncemented	No cement needed; fixation more secure; dynamic and biological fixation	Risk of fracture; fit must be perfect; osseous integration may not be established; expensive

Sir John Charnley, 1911–1982, Professor, Wrightington Hospital, UK, pioneer in hip replacment design, particularly the concept of low friction arthroplasty.

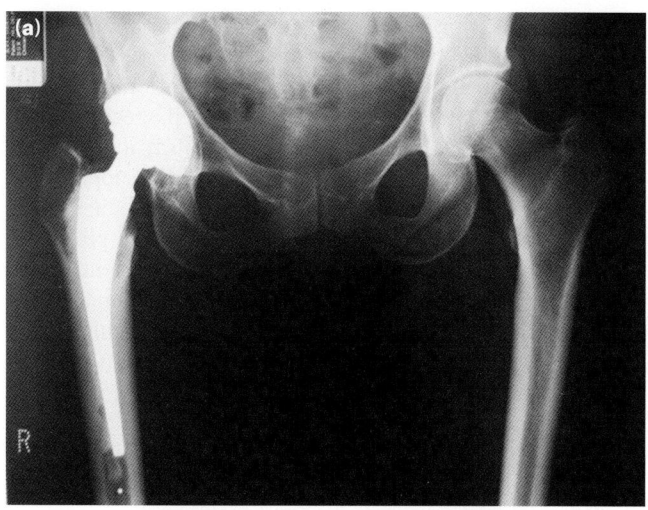

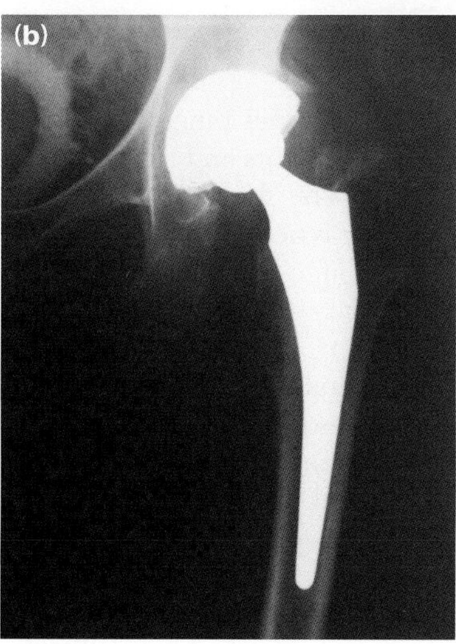

Figure 35.7 Radiographs of a cemented (**a**) and non-cemented (**b**) femoral component.

the implant and the bone. In the majority of cases it gives an excellent outcome as shown by the data in the national joint registries. However, it can cause potential problems: cement pressurisation can result in release of cement and marrow contents into the patient's blood stream. This can cause a drop in blood pressure.

On the other hand, this problem can be obviated by using an uncemented prosthesis where biological fixation can be achieved by providing a rough surface on the prosthesis for bone to grow into the prosthesis or by coating the surface of the prosthesis with hydroxyapatite, an osteoconductive agent, to encourage bone to bond to the prosthesis (**Figure 35.7b**). These uncemented devices have also shown good long-term outcomes, although they can be associated with higher implant costs, increased risk of intraoperative fracture and difficulty in removing them if revision surgery is needed.

Surgical approaches to the hip, postoperative course and complications

The operation can be performed via a posterior approach, a trochanteric osteotomy, an anterolateral or Hardinge approach or an anterior approach (*Table 35.6*). Each approach has its own advantages and disadvantages. Minimally invasive surgery has been described that shortens the size of the incision and attempts to lessen soft tissue damage. Specialised instruments have been developed to facilitate this as access can be restricted. Although the concept is attractive, no long-term benefits have been conclusively shown in hip surgery over the conventional technique. Eventually, whichever approach is used, it is essential to be able to implant a prosthesis that has the correct offset, is at the correct centre of rotation with the correct component orientation, that restores leg length and carries minimal risk of complications.

The postoperative course generally involves a 3–5 day stay in hospital, where the physiotherapist encourages the patient to mobilise safely and independently, avoiding any movements which might lead to a dislocation (**Figure 35.8**). Before discharge, the occupational therapist assesses the patient's home circumstances and arranges for any modifications that may be required to assist the patient e.g. a raised toilet seat. Follow-up visits are arranged at 6 weeks and at 1 year post surgery. Although hip replacement is a generally a successful and safe procedure, it does have associated complications. A comprehensive list of complications is given in *Table 35.7*. Deep vein thrombosis is relatively common if no precautions are taken to reduce this risk, for which the use of regional anaesthesia and early postoperative mobilisation are invaluable. In additon, either mechanical devices

TABLE 35.6 Surgical approaches to the hip.

Surgical approach	Anatomical interval and muscle
Posterior	Along the fibres of the gluteus maximus, and dividing the short external rotators
Trochanteric	A trochanteric osteotomy is required
Anterolateral/ Hardinge	Parts of the gluteus medius and minimus are reflected off the greater trochanter
Anterior	The interval is developed between the sartorius and rectus femoris and the tensor fascia lata

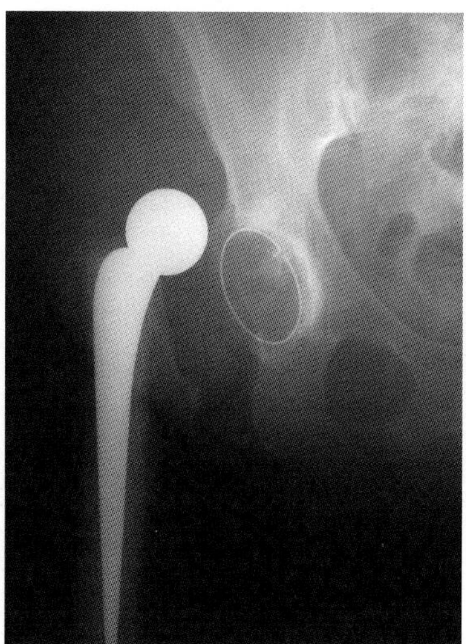

Figure 35.8 Dislocation of the hip.

TABLE 35.7 Complications of total hip replacement.

Intraoperative complications
Nerve injury – sciatic, femoral and obturator
Vascular injury – femoral vein and artery
Femoral fracture
Fragments of cement left in joint
Postoperative complications
Deep vein thrombosis and pulmonary embolism
Leg length inequality
Dislocation
Infection
Aseptic loosening
Heterotopic ossification

(thromboembolic deterrent (TED) stockings, foot pumps or intermittent pneumatic calf compression devices) and medication (low molecular weight heparin, warfarin or oral anticoagulants) are commonly prescribed for a period of 4–6 weeks after surgery to reduce the risk of DVT (this will depend on local and national guidelines).

Revision total hip replacement

Revision of a total hip replacement is required if the patient is symptomatic secondary to failure of the implant by loosening (Figure 35.9), recurrent dislocations or a periprosthetic fracture. Loosening of the implant can occur because of an infection or as a result of aseptic osteolysis caused by an inflammatory response secondary to particle wear.

In the initial stages of loosening the patient complains of pain, which is experienced mainly on weight bearing. A history of infection in the immediate postoperative period may suggest infection as a cause of premature implant loosening. The infection can be low-grade, with *Staphylococcus epidermidis* multiplying slowly within a glycocalyx coating, and therefore normal measures of infection such as a raised C-reactive protien (CRP) may be equivocal (see Chapter 38).

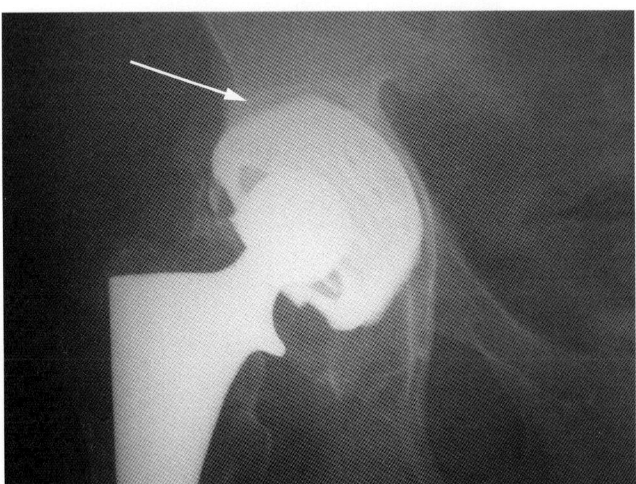

Figure 35.9 Acetabular loosening (arrow).

If the loosening is secondary to infection, a two-staged revision is usually preferred. The first stage consists of implant removal, thorough debridement and implantation of an antibiotic loaded cement spacer. Multiple deep specimens are sent for bacteriology to determine the organism and its sensitivity. The patient is subsequently prescribed an appropriate antibiotic regime (see Chapter 38). At the second stage of the procedure, the cement spacer is removed and a new prosthesis implanted. In the case of aseptic loosening, revision is performed as a single-stage procedure. If there has been a significant amount of bone loss, bone grafting or trabecular metal augments may be required. The results following a revision hip replacement are not as good as those following a primary THR and the rate of complications, especially dislocation, is also higher.

THE KNEE

Applied anatomy

The knee joint is a synovial hinge joint. It consists of two condyloid tibiofemoral joints and a sellar (or saddle shaped) patellofemoral joint. The shape makes the joint inherently unstable, but stability is achieved by a combination of static (ligaments) and dynamic (muscles) stabilisers acting across the joint.

Interposed between the tibial and femoral condyles are the medial and lateral menisci. These fibrocartilaginous structures aid shock absorption, increase the area over which load is dissipated and have a role in anteroposterior stability (Figure 35.10). Medial meniscal tears are three times more

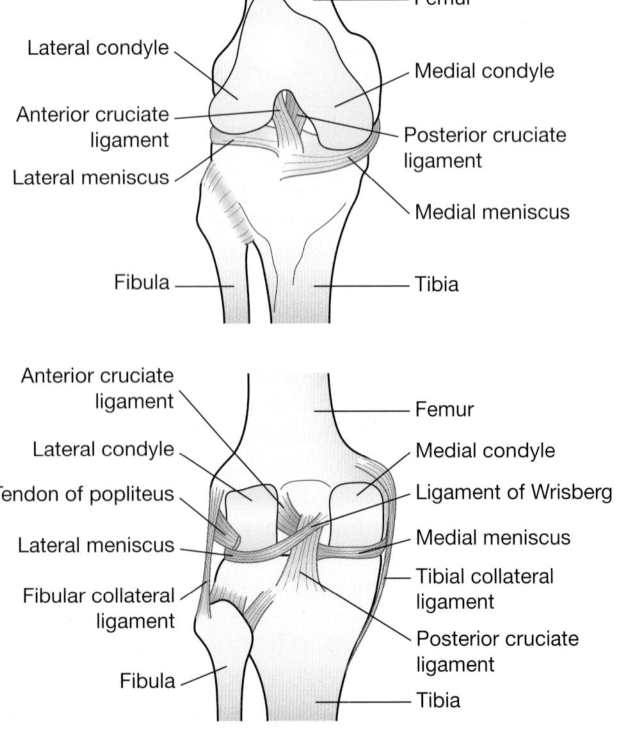

Figure 35.10 Anatomy of the knee joint.

common than those in the more mobile lateral meniscus. The outer third of the meniscus is vascular and so tears can be repaired with the prospect of healing.

The medial and lateral collateral ligaments are the primary restraints to valgus and varus stress, respectively. The medial collateral ligament is a broad, flat ligament composed of a superficial and a deep layer. The deep layer is attached to the medial meniscus. The lateral collateral ligament is a simple cord-like structure.

The cruciate ligaments are vital for anteroposterior stability. Each cruciate ligament comprises two bundles. The anterior cruciate ligament (ACL) is composed of an anteromedial bundle that is tight in flexion and a posterolateral bundle that is tight in extension. The posterior cruciate ligament (PCL) has an anterolateral bundle (tight in flexion) and a posteromedial portion (tight in extension). The ACL and PCL prevent anterior and posterior translation of the tibia on the femur respectively.

The knee has bursae surrounding it that can become inflamed and infected.

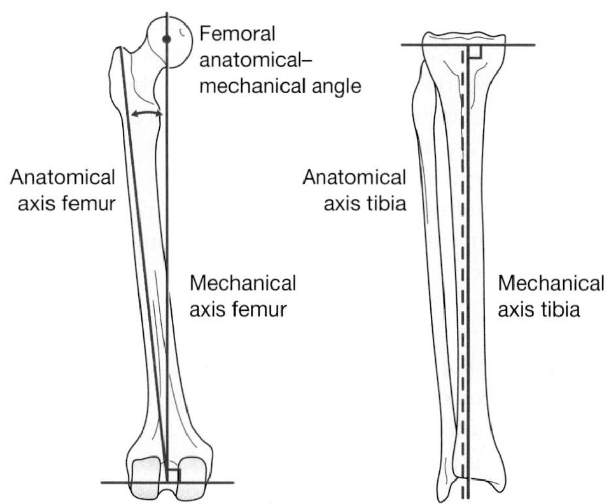

Figure 35.11 Axes of the lower limb. Anatomical and mechanical axes are coincident. Adapted from Miller, M. *Review of Orthopaedics*, 4th edn. 2004, Elsevier, Philadelphia. By kind permission of the publishers.

Summary box 35.6

Anatomy of the knee joint

- Complex synovial hinge joint
- The shape of the joint surfaces make it inherently unstable
- The static stabilisers are the joint capsule, menisci, cruciate and collateral ligaments
- The dynamic stabilisers are the quadriceps and hamstrings muscles

Biomechanics

Axes of the lower limb

The anatomical axes of the femur and tibia are defined by their medullary canal. The mechanical axis of the lower limb runs from the centre of the femoral head, through the intercondylar notch of the knee to the centre of the ankle joint. The angle between the anatomical and mechanical axes of the femur is usually between 5 and 7° (often called the valgus cut angle in arthroplasty) (Figure 35.11). An artificial knee joint must have the joint surface parallel with the ground, and with the load transmitted equally between the condyles. This is achieved by cutting the femur perpendicular to the mechanical axis, by measuring the valgus cut angle off the anatomical axis. The tibia is cut perpendicular to its anatomical and mechanical axes.

Kinematics and kinetics

Knee motion is predominately in the sagittal plane. A limited degree of rotation also occurs and increases as knee flexion increases. The normal range of motion is between 5° of hyperextension and 135° of flexion. MRI of cadaveric knees has revealed that, during knee flexion, a combination of rolling and sliding of the femur on the tibia occurs but there is also internal rotation of the tibia with flexion. This is because the larger medial femoral condyle rolls back less than the smaller lateral femoral condyle.

The biomechanical role of the patella is to function as a pulley for the quadriceps. It increases the power of the quadriceps by increasing the lever arm. It has the thickest articular cartilage in the body and is designed to withstand loads as high as 20 times body weight when jumping.

Summary box 35.7

Biomechanics of the knee joint

- The anatomical–mechanical angle of the femur is the angle between the anatomical and mechanical axes of the femur
- Knee motion is mainly in the sagittal plane with some rotation
- The patella acts as a pulley, increasing the lever arm of the quadriceps
- Loads of up to 20 times body weight are transmitted across the patella when jumping

Conditions affecting the knee joint

Osteoarthritis

OA commonly affects the knee joint. Females are affected more often than their male counterparts and more than 3% of women aged over 75 years are affected. Osteoarthritis can be either primary (idiopathic) or secondary. Secondary osteoarthritis may occur following a previous intra-articular fracture, meniscectomy, osteonecrosis or in a neuropathic joint.

CLINICAL FEATURES

Pain is the main symptom, made worse with use. With patellofemoral involvement, pain is worse on stairs. As the disease progresses, exercise tolerance diminishes, pain becomes constant, often disturbing sleep, and patients become increasingly reliant on walking aids. In severe cases, patients may even become housebound.

Clinical examination reveals an antalgic gait where the patient limps, spending a short time on the painful limb, and moves their centre of gravity to minimise the weight that they are taking through this limb. In osteoarthritic patients the deformity is usually varus, with bone loss on the medial side, while in rheumatoid patients valgus deformity is commonplace. An effusion is frequently present and movement is restricted, particularly extension. Crepitus can be both palpable and audible.

INVESTIGATIONS

The radiographic features are joint space narrowing, subchondral sclerosis, osteophytes and subchondral cysts (**Figure 35.12**). MRI can be used to judge both articular cartilage involvement and the integrity of the ACL, with a view to guiding future surgical intervention.

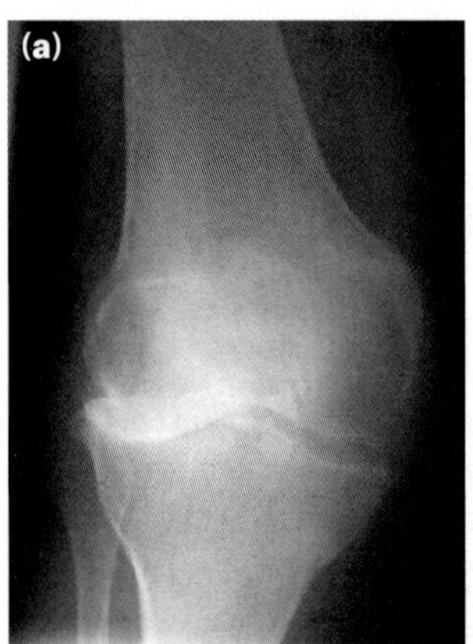

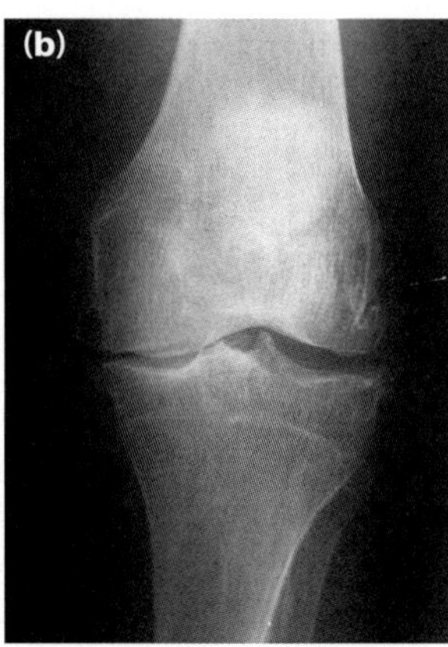

Figure 35.12 (a, b) Osteoarthritis of the knee.

TREATMENT

Non-operative methods are the first line of treatment. Patients should be encouraged to lose weight, undertake regular exercise to prevent joint stiffness and use anti-inflammatory medication. Walking aids, e.g. a stick, may be beneficial. Intra-articular steroid injections can provide long-term pain relief, although may actually cause more rapid degeneration of the joint cartilage.

Surgical options include osteotomy, arthrodesis or knee replacement. These are all discussed below.

> **Summary box 35.8**
>
> **Knee osteoarthritis**
>
> - More common in females
> - Can be primary (idiopathic) or secondary (e.g. post traumatic)
> - The main symptom is pain made worse by use
> - Examination reveals swelling, and reduced range of motion with or without deformity
> - The key radiographic features are joint space narrowing, subchondral sclerosis and cysts, and osteophytes
> - Treatment is non-operative initially. Knee replacement is reserved for end-stage disease

Soft tissue knee problems

Knee problems, in the case of injury, can present acutely or some time after the event (see Chapter 32). Problems can be associated with degenerative changes, in which case a more chronic presentation can be encountered. Specific structures commonly involved are the ligaments, tendons and menisci. Ligamentous injuries may involve the cruciate and collateral ligaments and can be combined with injury to stabilising structures, e.g. the posterolateral corner. Tendon problems include injuries to the quadriceps tendon and the patellar tendon. The pattern of meniscal injury or degeneration is variable, affecting either the medial or lateral meniscus (or both). There are several patterns of injury within a meniscal structure, some relating to blood supply and healing potential. Furthermore, soft tissue problems can be associated with chondral or osteochondral lesions.

ANTERIOR CRUCIATE LIGAMENT

The ACL is the most commonly injured ligament in the knee and injury most frequently results from pivoting injuries in high-energy contact sport. It may be associated with an audible 'pop', immediate swelling, and the need to be 'carried-off' the field.

The injury risk is higher among females, thought to be due to smaller ligaments, smaller femoral notches and different landing biomechanics.

Some controversy exists concerning the incidence of secondary osteoarthritis in ACL-deficient versus reconstructed knees. However, chronic ACL deficiency is clearly linked with an increased incidence of complex meniscal tears and chondral injury.

INVESTIGATION

MRI of the knee is useful for the identification of ligamentous and meniscal injuries, and any associated chondral lesions. An ultrasound scan is more commonly used to identify the more superficial tendon injuries.

TREATMENT

Isolated ligament injuries are generally initially managed non-operatively in a knee brace. Surgical repair, augmentation and reconstruction are considered in multiligament injuries, and in cases of chronic instability after non-operative management of isolated ligament injuries. Meniscal injuries that are associated with mechanical symptoms, e.g. catching, locking and giving way, generally respond well to arthroscopic treatment. This can include either a repair or debridement depending on the location, morphology and chronicity of the tear. Chondral lesions do not breach the subchondral bone and make no spontaneous attempt to heal. These lesions, if appropriate, are commonly managed with microfracture to stimulate bone marrow cells to form fibrocartilage repair tissue.

Some patients with ACL injuries may decide that they have adequate stability in the knee once they have been through a full rehabilitation programme. If, however, they continue to experience instability, particularly with twisting activities, they should be considered for surgical reconstruction. Surgical reconstruction of the ACL should only be undertaken in those patients who have a full range of knee motion and good hamstring and quadriceps function preoperatively, as otherwise results are poor.

Surgical procedures

Arthroscopy of the knee

Knee arthroscopy is used in the diagnosis and treatment of injuries, e.g. ligamentous and meniscal injuries and articular cartilage defects. There are a number of other indications for knee arthroscopy summarised in *Table 35.8*.

TABLE 35.8 Indications for knee arthroscopy.
Torn meniscus resection or repair
Anterior/posterior cruciate ligament reconstruction
Loose body removal
Cartilage regeneration techniques including microfracture
Septic arthritis washout
Inflammatory arthritis – synovectomy
Diagnosis of unexplained knee pain
Tibial plateau fractures – allows intraoperative assessment and reduction of the articular surface

Cruciate reconstruction

An isolated ACL injury is most commonly treated with an arthroscopic intra-articular reconstruction. The graft can be bone–patella, tendon–bone or four-strand hamstring autograft. Postoperative rehabilitation programmes are crucial to a favourable outcome. Complications following ACL surgery are usually a result of incorrect tunnel placement (placing the femoral tunnel too far anteriorly limits knee flexion) and early surgery. The graft re-rupture rate is approximately 1% per year.

Osteotomy

Osteoarthritis can lead to varus or valgus deformity of the knee. This results in excessive stresses on the affected compartment, leading to premature degenerative change in that compartment. Osteotomy aims to divide the bone, correct the deformity and alter the load-bearing mechanics of the joint.

The most commonly performed operation is a high tibial osteotomy (HTO) for a varus knee. Realignment is achieved with either an opening-wedge medial HTO or a closing-wedge lateral HTO. In valgus knees with relatively mild deformity (less than 12°) a varus-producing HTO on the medial side can be performed. A deformity of 12° or more requires distal femoral varus osteotomy.

The ideal patient for osteotomy is a young and active, well-motivated individual with disease limited to one compartment.

Knee arthrodesis

The most common indication for knee arthrodesis is a failed total knee replacement. Other indications include uncontrollable sepsis, a neuropathic joint, post-traumatic arthritis in a young patient and disruption of the extensor mechanism. The ideal position of fusion is 7° of valgus and 15° of flexion. Arthrodesis is performed using either a custom-made intramedullary nail or an extramedullary technique such as an external fixator.

Knee joint replacement

There are three compartments within the knee: medial and lateral tibiofemoral, and patellofemoral. Osteoarthritis may affect these individually or collectively. The medial compartment is most commonly affected, producing a varus deformity. For single-compartment disease a unicompartmental replacement may be used, while in tricompartmental disease a total knee replacement (TKR) is indicated (**Figure 35.13**).

Knee replacement can be regarded as a resurfacing procedure in which the femoral articular surface is replaced with metal and the tibial articular surface is replaced by a tough polyethylene insert.

The main indication for knee replacement is pain, especially when combined with deformity and instability. Knee replacement should be reserved until a patient's quality of life is significantly impaired.

Natural knee motion is complex. It involves translation and rotation about each of the *x*, *y* and *z* axes (six degrees of freedom). It has proven very difficult to reproduce this natural

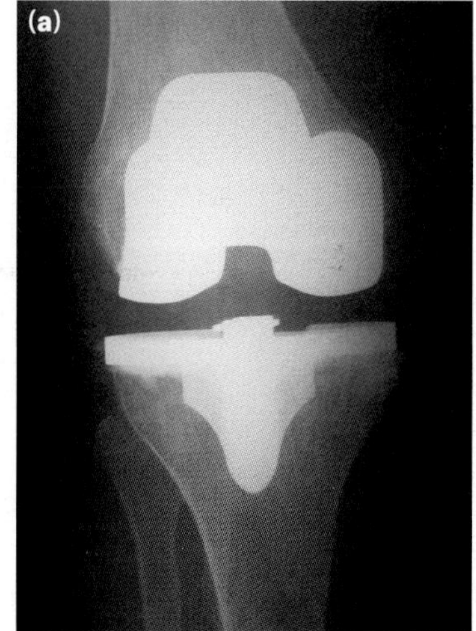

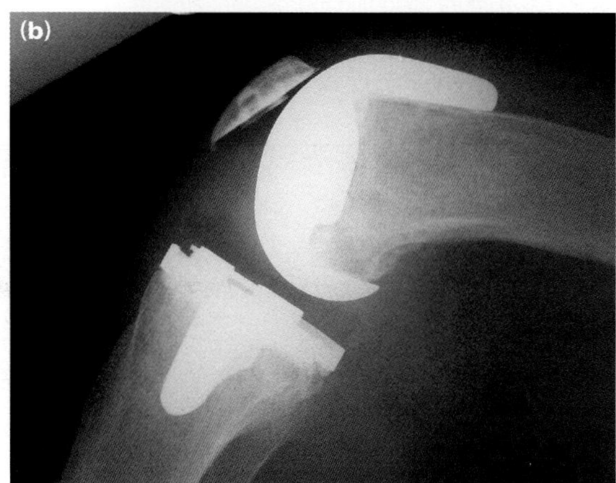

Figure 35.13 (a, b) Total knee replacement.

motion in TKRs. In comparison to THR, patients with TKR find it hard to forget they have a knee replacement. Consequently, patient satisfaction is lower with TKR.

There are three types of TKR currently used: unconstrained, constrained–non-hinged and constrained–hinged. Almost all primary TKR are unconstrained while the constrained types are used in revision TKR when there may be significant bone loss and ligament deficiency.

The more constrained the implant the greater the force transmitted to the implant–cement–bone interfaces, therefore increasing the risk of loosening.

The main aim of TKR is to create a mechanical axis (weight-bearing line) that passes through the centre of the femoral head, knee and ankle. The joint line should then be perpendicular to the mechanical axis. It should also be parallel with the ground. If implants of the correct size are used and exactly the right amount of bone is cut away from both the tibia and the femur, the new joint surface will be placed exactly where the patient's original surface had been before disease supervened.The collateral ligaments will then provide stability without constraint and ensure that the patella will track correctly on the femur.

Postoperatively, patients require physiotherapy to regain quadriceps strength and to achieve full extension. In addition they need at least 90° knee flexion to enable them to sit comfortably. The average length of hospital stay is between 3 and 5 days. Complications following TKR can be broadly classified into intraoperative and postoperative (*Table 35.9*).

Summary box 35.9

Aims of total knee replacement

- Mechanical axis through centre of knee
- Joint line perpendicular to mechanical axis
- Balance collateral ligaments
- Ensure patellofemoral joint tracks normally

TABLE 35.9 Complications of total knee replacement.
Intraoperative
Poor placement of implants leading to instability or stiffness, or pain
Nerve or vessel injury including tourniquet damage
Fracture
Patellar tendon avulsion
Malalignment
Fat embolism
Postoperative
Infection
Deep vein thrombosis/pulmonary embolism
Pain/stiffness
Instability
Osteolysis
Component loosening
Dislocation

Unicompartmental knee replacement (UKR)

The natural history of osteoarthritis reveals that, in up to 92% of cases, the disease begins in the medial compartment alone. This was the basis for the development of the UKR, which is available in either fixed or mobile bearing forms (**Figure 35.14**). Although generally the longevity of the implants is not as good as with TKRs, a number of series report 10-year survival figures over 90% for medial UKRs.

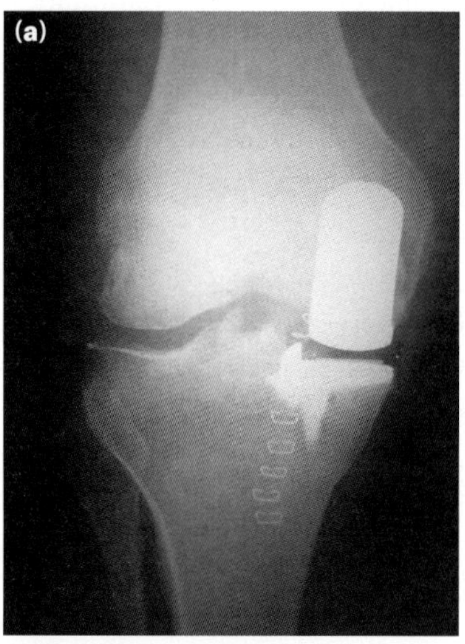

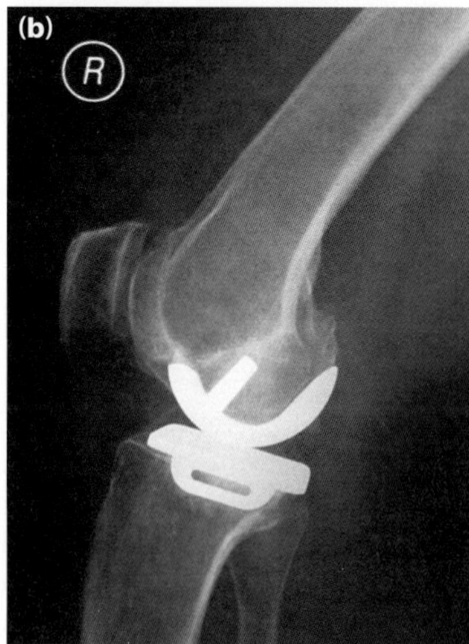

Figure 35.14 **(a, b)** Unicompartmental knee replacement.

Prerequisites to undertaking medial UKR include intact ligaments (especially the ACL), disease limited to one compartment and varus/flexion deformities of not more than 15°. As it is a less invasive procedure than a TKR, it is associated with a more rapid recovery, shorter hospital stay and preservation of knee kinematics. It is a bone preserving procedure, and therefore revision is generally to a TKR rather than to more constrained implants.

Lateral UKR is performed for lateral compartment disease; this is far less common than medial UKR, partly owing to a reported dislocation rate of 10%.

Patellofemoral replacement is also performed but again the longevity of the implants is not as good, and the numbers are low in view of the scarcity of patients with isolated patellofemoral disease.

Revision knee replacement

Implant loosening secondary to either infection or polyethylene-induced osteolysis is the main reason for revising TKR. Other indications include periprosthetic fracture, malalignment, instability, stiffness and patellar maltracking. Regardless of the indication, as with any type of revision procedure it is important to exclude infection because this often warrants a two-stage rather than a single-stage procedure. Although it is more technically challenging, the aims of revision TKR are no different from those of primary TKR. That is to provide a well-aligned, stable and pain-free knee (Figure 35.15).

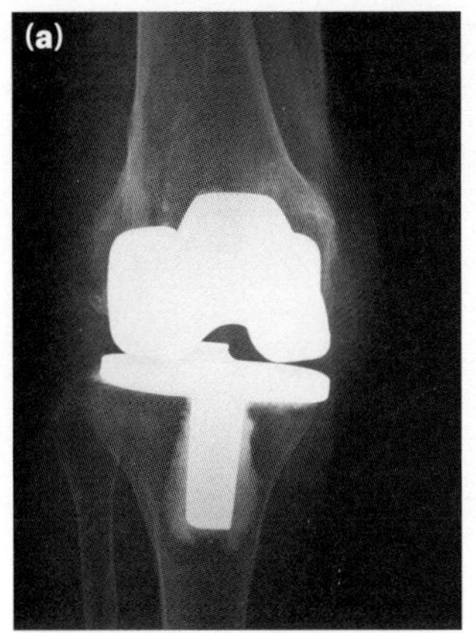

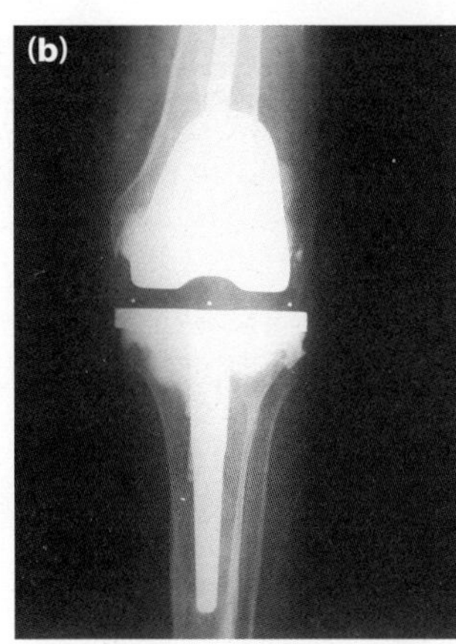

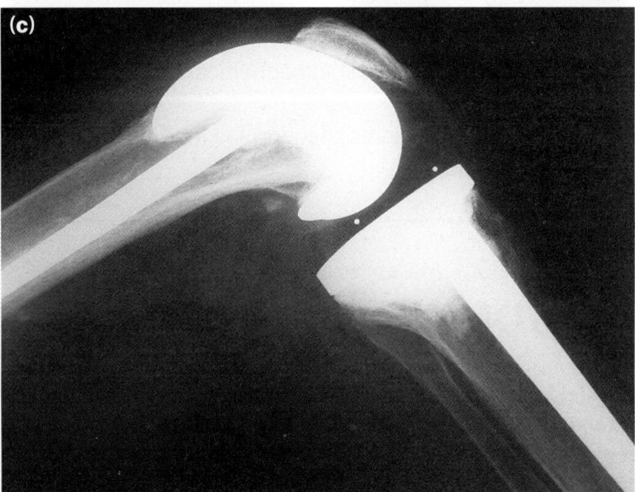

Figure 35.15 Radiographs of a malaligned knee (**a**) and a well-aligned revised knee (**b, c**).

FURTHER READING

Bulstrode C, Wilson MacDonald J, Eastwood D *et al. Oxford textbook of trauma and orthopaedics*, 2nd edn. Oxford: Oxford University Press, 2017.

Miller MD, Thompson SR. *Miller's review of orthopaedics*, 7th edn. Philadelphia: Elsevier, 2016.

Solomon L, Warwick, DJ, Nayagam S. *Apley & Solomon's concise system of orthopaedics and trauma*, 4th edn. Boca Raton: CRC Press, 2014.

Chapter 36

Foot and ankle

Learning objectives

To understand:

- The basic anatomy and biomechanics of the foot and ankle
- The common problems affecting the foot and ankle in each age group
- The principles behind the treatment of each condition, be it conservative or surgical
- The significance of progressive neurological diseases

ANATOMY

There are 26 (25 with variant) main bones in the foot (seven tarsal bones, five metatarsals and 14 phalanges; 13 in the biphalangeal fifth toe varient) plus the two sesamoids of the hallux and a variable number of other sesamoid and accessory bones.

Movements at the ankle joint are mainly dorsiflexion and plantarflexion, but are more complex than this. The joint is actually a truncated section of a cone, meaning the motion is not simply a hinge and, in addition, movement of the ankle leads to rotation of the fibula at the syndesmosis. This means that the foot externally rotates with dorsiflexion and internally rotates with plantarflexion.

Stability is conferred upon the ankle by the congruence of the mortice and the integrity of principally the medial, lateral and the inferior tibiofibular ligaments.

The subtalar joint is divided into anterior, middle and posterior facets and, along with the talonavicular and calcaneocuboid joints, makes up the triple joint complex. These joints are responsible for inversion and eversion of the hind and midfoot. The joints are codependent such that limitation of one affects movement at the others. Fusion of the triple complex slightly affects movement at the ankle and vice versa.

The second tarsometatarsal joint is recessed relative to the first and third and acts as a 'keystone'. Disruption of this joint (Lisfranc's injury) leads to loss of the transverse arch and an acquired flat foot.

The lower leg is divided into four compartments:

- the superficial posterior – gastrocnemius, soleus and plantaris;
- the deep posterior – tibialis posterior, flexor digitorum longus and flexor hallucis longus;
- the lateral – peroneus brevis and peroneus longus;
- the anterior – tibialis anterior, extensor hallucis longus, extensor digitorum longus and peroneus tertius.

There is only one muscle on the dorsum of the foot, the extensor digitorum brevis. The muscles on the plantar aspect of the foot are divided into four layers, the first being the most superficial, and the course of the neurovascular structures is a favourite exam topic. The plantar fascia is a very important structure that takes its origin from the heel and inserts into the bases of the proximal phalanges of the toes. At toe-off, the fascia tightens and accentuates the medial plantar arch and helps provide a rigid lever arm, the so-called 'windlass mechanism'. This is essential in the preservation of the integrity of the arch of the foot and function of the toes.

The blood supply of the foot is from the anterior tibial, the posterior tibial and the peroneal arteries. The following nerves supply sensation to the foot: posterior tibial, saphenous, sural, superficial and deep peroneal (**Figure 36.1**).

Summary box 36.1

Anatomy of the foot

- There are 26 major bones in the foot
- There are four layers of muscles in the sole of the foot
- The blood supply of the foot is from the anterior and posterior tibial arteries plus the peroneal artery

Jacques Lisfranc, 1790–1847, Professor of Surgery and Operative Medicine, Paris, France.

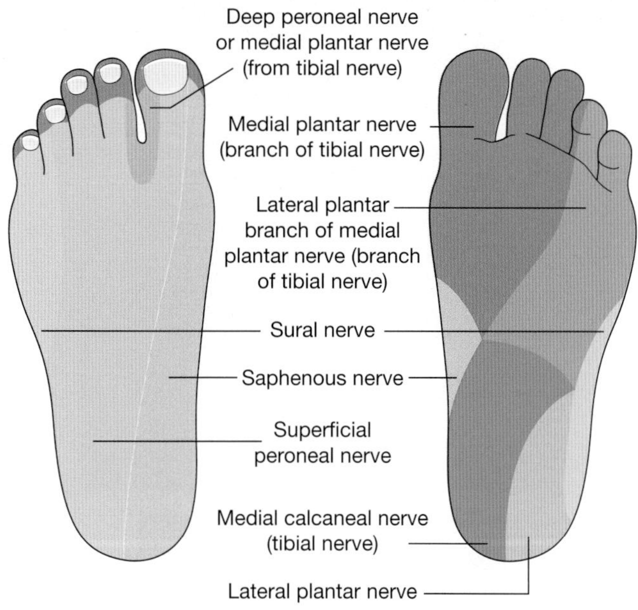

Figure 36.1 Cutaneous nerve supply of the foot (courtesy of Bartleby.com).

BIOMECHANICS

The walking cycle is divided into the stance (60%) and swing (40%) phases. The stance phase is divided into three intervals: (1) heel strike to foot flat; (2) foot flat until the body passes over the ankle; and (3) ankle joint plantarflexion to toe-off. During walking up to 12% of the gait cycle is spent with both feet in the stance phase but with running there is a period when neither foot is in contact with the ground, the 'float' phase. During running the cycle time is shortened but the forces generated are very much increased.

Summary box 36.2

Biomechanics

- The gait cycle is divided into swing and stance phases
- Running generates increased forces, shortens the gait cycle and has a float phase when neither foot touches the ground

Examination

The examination of the foot is described in Chapter 31. The patient should be watched walking, and both the foot and the footwear of the patient need examining when looking for abnormal load and wear.

PAEDIATRIC CONDITIONS

These are discussed in Chapter 39.

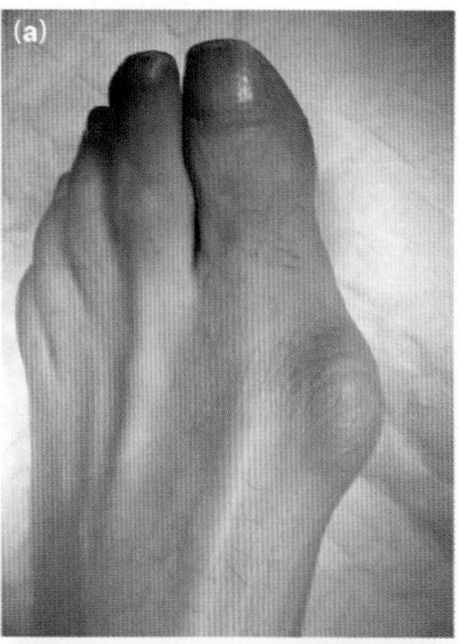

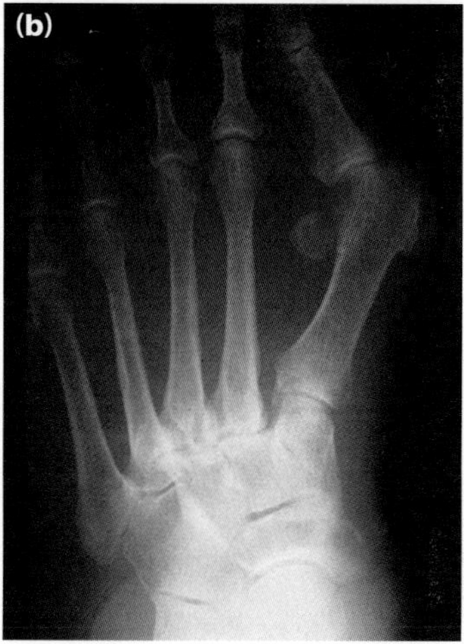

Figure 36.2 (a, b) Hallux valgus and bunion.

PATHOLOGY IN THE ADULT

The forefoot

Hallux valgus

Hallux valgus is deviation of the big toe away from the midline, i.e. towards the lesser toes, and is usually associated with a bunion, a swelling made up of both bone and bursa on the medial aspect of the first metatarsal head (**Figure 36.2**). It is a common condition that affects women more than men, and which is often bilateral. It is believed that the tendency to hallux valgus is inherited and that fully enclosed shoes accelerate the development of the condition.

With increasing deformity the first ray becomes defunctional and elevated, and overload of the second metatarsophalangeal (MTP) joint often results in pain, swelling and eventually plantar plate disruption and dislocation. This can present with a prominent callosity beneath the second MTP joint and eventually hammering of the second toe.

Non-operative treatment of hallux valgus includes a wider toe box and pressure relief. Surgical intervention is commonly offered, but has a 10% rate of dissatisfaction.

For mild deformities a distal osteotomy (e.g. chevron) is usually adequate. For moderate deformities the surgeon is more likely to use a shaft e.g. Scarf (**Figure 36.3**) or Ludloff,

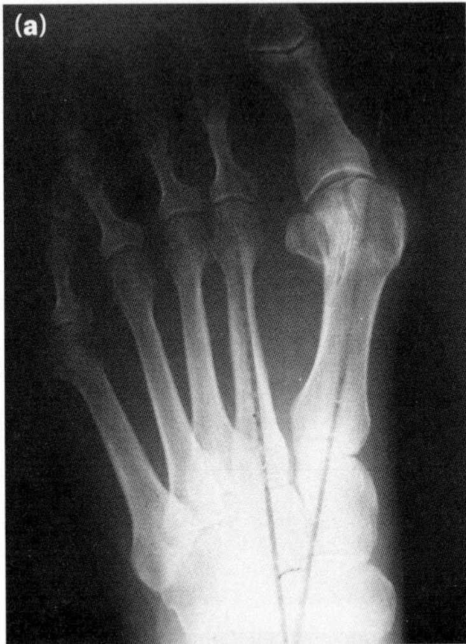

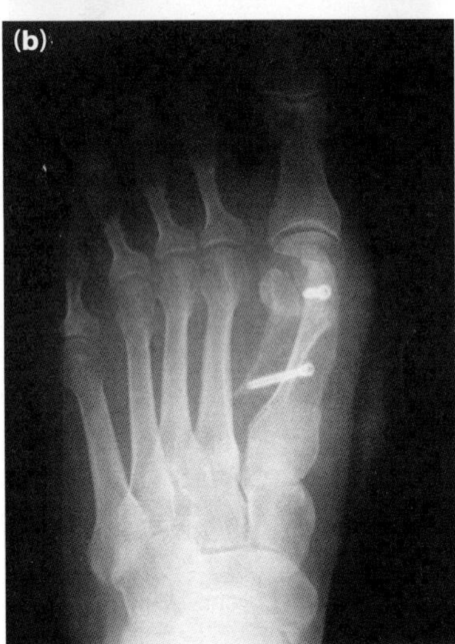

Figure 36.3 Pre- (a) and postoperative (b) radiographs of a Scarf osteotomy.

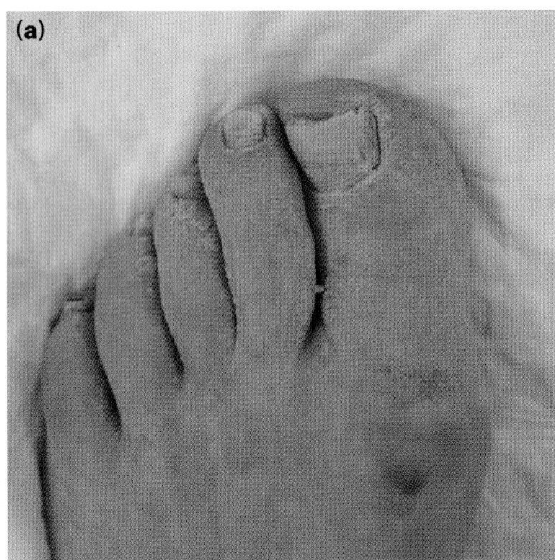

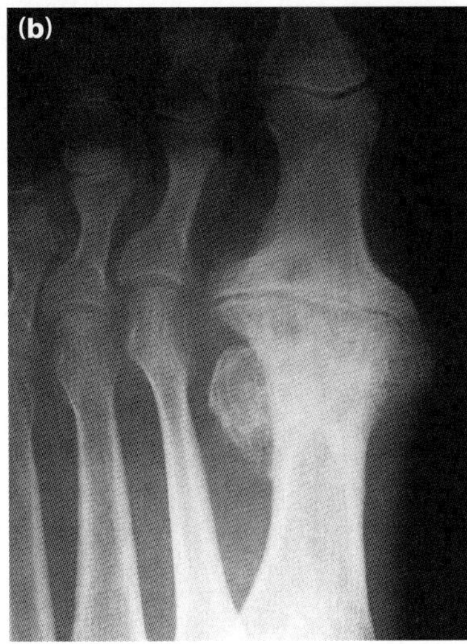

Figure 36.4 Clinical (a) and radiographic (b) appearance of hallux rigidus.

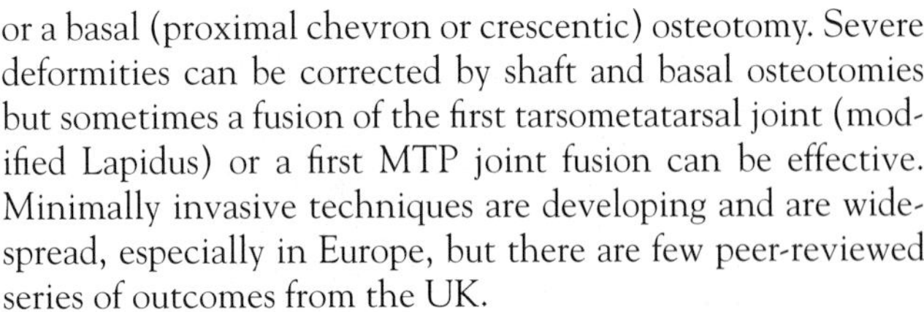

or a basal (proximal chevron or crescentic) osteotomy. Severe deformities can be corrected by shaft and basal osteotomies but sometimes a fusion of the first tarsometatarsal joint (modified Lapidus) or a first MTP joint fusion can be effective. Minimally invasive techniques are developing and are widespread, especially in Europe, but there are few peer-reviewed series of outcomes from the UK.

Basal osteotomies and fusions have a higher risk of abnomal elevation or depression of the rays, resulting in overload of the rest of the forefoot. However, they do allow a massive correction. They are best stabilised using plates.

Operations such as a Keller's excision arthroplasty, where the proximal third of the proximal phalanx is excised, serve to defunction the toe and sesamoids and are reserved for low-demand high-risk patients where there is a high risk that healing of an osteotomy might fail.

The complications of bunion surgery are infection, cutaneous nerve damage, recurrence or overcorrection of deformity, stiffness and overload of the second MTP joint (transfer lesion), and 10% of patients have reservations about their outcome. Occasionally patients develop early arthritis following surgery and require revision to fusion.

Summary box 36.3

Hallux valgus

- Bunions affect women more often than men
- Patients with hallux valgus have inherited a tendency to develop the condition
- Not all patients need surgery
- The choice of operation is determined by the severity of the deformity and presence or absence of any arthritis

Hallux rigidus

Hallux rigidus is a painful condition of the hallux MTP joint characterised by loss of motion especially in dorsiflexion and osteophyte formation on the dorsum and sides of the joint (Figure 36.4).

William Lordan Keller, 1874–1959, Head of the Department of Surgery, the Walter Reed Hospital, Washington, DC, USA, described this operation in 1904.

In adults there is often a history of trauma or repetitive microtrauma (sport) but, occasionally, there is a strong family history of the condition. Gout and rheumatological conditions may present in this way. Patients complain of stiffness and pain on weight bearing.

The most effective non-operative treatment is provision of a stiff-soled shoe with a deep toe box or a rocker-soled shoe, which are now available on the high street.

The mainstays of surgical management are injection/manipulation, cheilectomy (a radical debridement and excision of the part of the joint blocking movement), fusion, and interpostion arthroplasty (Keller's-type procedure or silicon interposition). Prosthetic arthroplasty, with hemi-, total, interposition or spacer arthroplasty, is available but many prostheses have been withdrawn for high failure rates and few series extend beyond 9 years.

Fusion is for the severely affected and is an effective means of abolishing pain, but affects the biomechanics and some patients are left with intractable pain beneath the sesamoids. A fusion will still usually allow sports participation.

Summary box 36.4

Hallux rigidus

- Hallux rigidus can affect adolescents as well as adults
- Stiff-soled shoes with a deep toe box are the most comfortable type of shoe
- Cheilectomy and fusion are the mainstays of surgical treatment

Sesamoid problems

Acute injuries (turf toe) can be managed non-operatively or surgically depending on the grade of the injury and the occupation of the patient. Grade 4 acute fracture may require surgery.

Chronic conditions are indistinguishable and range from stress fracture to avascular necrosis and sesamoiditis but are probably all the same phenomenon. Management includes offloading with orthotics and injections of steroids and, rarely, shaving/excison. Excision surgery carries a high risk.

Lesser toe deformities

Hammer, mallet, and claw toes are frequent and are usually non-indicative but may be secondary to other deformities in the foot or to underlying neurological disease. Non-operative treatment involves appropriate padding and footwear modification. For symptomatic flexible deformities soft-tissue surgery such as flexor/extensor tenotomies +/– capsulotomy is usually adequate, but for fixed deformities bony procedures are required such as interposition arthroplasty, fusion or excision arthroplasty.

Isolated lesser toe MTP extension/subluxation may result from a ruptured plantar plate, and repair techniques have evolved recently.

Freiberg's disease

Freiberg's disease (Figure 36.5) is an ischaemic necrosis of the epiphysis, resulting in pain and swelling of the joint. It will often settle with rest. Re-shaping osteotomies are described, or excision of the proximal phalangeal head for severe adult cases with joint destruction. Excision of the whole metatarsal head should never be performed.

Morton's neuroma and metatarsalgia

Metatarsalgia usually occurs secondary to joint problems, overload or irritation of a nerve. Morton's neuroma is a painful condition which in most cases arises from compression of the common digital nerve between the third and fourth metatarsal heads and is usually secondary to other forefoot pathology.

The diagnosis is confirmed by ultrasound or magnetic resonance imaging (MRI). Non-operative treatments include advice about footwear, an orthosis (premetatarsal dome) to splay the metatarsal heads or an injection of steroids.

Surgery involves resection (the affected toes will be permanently partly hemi-numb if the nerve is removed) but this is not without risk of patient dissatisfaction, pain and recurrence.

Summary box 36.5

Morton's neuroma

- Morton's neuroma most commonly affects the second or third web space
- Surgical excision of a neuroma is often successful but has a risk of pain syndrome and recurrence; guided injections form the mainstay of treatment for most

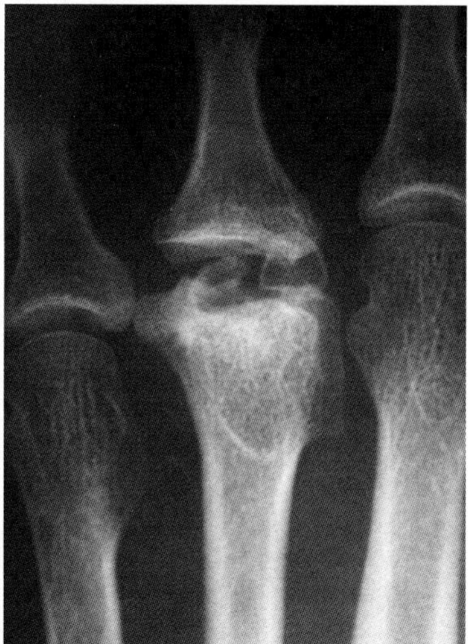

Figure 36.5 Freiberg's disease.

Albert Henry Freiberg, Professor of Orthopaedic Surgery, University of Cincinnati, Cincinnati, OH, USA, gave his account of this condition in 1926.
Thomas George Morton, 1835–1903, surgeon, the Pennsylvania Hospital, Philadelphia, PA, USA, described this condition in 1876.

Stress fracture

May be post sport or incipient. Usually presents in the forefoot and may mimic Morton's or metatarsalgia. A unexplained aetiology might require biochemical or biomechanical evaluation. Forefoot fractures can usually be managed non-operatively.

Stress fractures may occur in any bone. Those of the navicular, talus and tibial sesamoid often present with vague symptomatology but early diagnosis with MRI and management are essential, with early fixation if required.

The midfoot

The midfoot comprises the cuneiforms and the cuboid and related joints.

Midfoot arthritis

The aetiology is usually not known but the risk factors include microtrauma, rheumatological causes, flat foot, Lisfranc or similar injuries (which may have been missed), Charcot and cavus foot. Patients are best managed non-operatively with orthotics, shoes, analgesia and modifications of their lifestyle.

Pain, often with palpable dorsal osteophytes, is the commonest finding.

Injections and orthotics are the mainstay of treatment, with surgery high risk and having moderate outcomes. Fusion of the lateral two tarsometatarsal (TMT) joints has a universally poor outcome. Arthroplasty, similarly, has little evidence to support its use and has poor outcomes in the hands of most.

Charcot

An acute hot, red swollen foot (which may or may not be painful) may be indicative of Charcot (often secondary to diabetes which may as yet be undiagnosed) or other neuropathy. Immediate offloading in plaster and urgent management are indicated, and National Institute of Health and Care Excellence (NICE) guidelines are available in the UK.

Tendinopathy

Rarely, dorsal pain may be due to tibialis anterior tendinosis at its insertion; management is usually non-operative.

Ganglions

Midfoot ganglions are common and may cause neuralgia over dorsal bosses. Injection/aspiration should be attempted. Surgery may be required but recurrence is high and secondary neuralgia not infrequent.

The hindfoot and ankle

Ankle arthritis

The definitive operative treatment for arthritis of the ankle will usually be in the form of total ankle replacement (TAR) or more commonly arthrodesis (fusion); the latter is often carried out via an open approach but arthroscopic techniques have better outcomes, more rapid recovery and fewer complications. Such techniques are mandatory in the presence of poor soft-tissue envelope or in the presence of a clotting diathesis. A UK National trial is currently underway to evaluate the relative outcomes of TAR versus arthrodesis (the TARVA trial), which are as yet undefined.

The advantage of fusion is it has a known track record, good outcomes (over 90% do well) and minimal morbidity, especially with modern arthroscopic techniques, but not all do well with fusion. Function following isolated fusion is virtually normal for most patients and this is probably due to increased mobility at other joints. However, this may precipitate arthralgia elsewhere.

Total ankle replacements (TARs) are usually three-component devices (except in the USA) that allow preservation of joint mobility but at the expense of larger incisions and possible eventual failure. Revision rates of <1% to 7% per annum are reported. Two of the most widely used TARs have been withdrawn in recent years, one due to massive osteolysis.

Hindfoot (excluding ankle) arthritis

The triple complex refers to the subtalar (talocalcaneal), calcaneocuboid and talonavicular joints. These joints are often affected by arthritis. Treatment options are limited and, if simple measures have failed, a fusion should be performed. Smokers and diabetics have a massively increased non-union rate for all foot fusion procedures and should be warned of this when they give consent. Late presentation of coalitions usually requires fusion.

Ankle combined with other hindfoot arthritis

If surgical input is required, one option is to treat one set of joints and then see how the patient fares. For example, offer the patient an ankle fusion or replacement and then assess the outcome. Secondary surgery to the other joints can then be performed if required. The alternative is to treat all joints at once.

Modern techniques now use third-generation hindfoot fusion nails which fuse both ankle and subtalar joints and are inserted with an open or arthroscopic fusion technique.

A pantalar fusion is quite disabling but may be necessary in rheumatological patients with deformities/stress fractures, patients with a failed arthroplasty with subtalar joint involvement, pantalar arthritis or avascular necrosis (AVN) with collapse of the talus.

Summary box 36.6

Midfoot and hindfoot

- Joint disorders are degenerative or inflammatory
- The mainstay of surgical treatment remains fusion although ankle replacements are becoming more successful
- Rheumatoid arthritis must be medically controlled as well as possible before surgery
- Knee deformities should be corrected before tackling foot problems

Jean Martin Charcot, 1825–1893, physician, La Salpêtrière, Paris, France.

Rheumatological presentations in the foot

The early presentations of rheumatological disease may include synovitis of the lesser MTP joints and widespread small joint disease, often in association with enthesopathy such as plantar fasciitis or Achilles tendonosis. However, the classic deformity is of hallux valgus with or without hallux rigidus deformity and subluxation or even dislocation of the lesser MTP joints in the forefoot, and arthritis and deformity in the mid/hindfoot.

The patient may present with a bunion and prominent lesser metatarsal heads which can often be felt to be dislocated on clinical examination, and are painful to palpation. Joint-sparing surgery is preferred, with preservation of the metatarsal (MT) heads if possible, often shortening and relocating the MTP joints. Destruction of the joints can be treated with proximal phalangeal partial excisions. Fusion of the first MTP is the usual requirement. Late recurrence can be managed with excision arthroplasty.

Excision of the metatarsal heads produces an almost instantaneous and gratifying relief of pain. If a plantar approach is used an ellipse of skin can be excised to move the metatarsal padding back over the end of the metatarsal. While most surgeons avoid scars on the plantar aspect of the foot wherever possible, this is one procedure where the results are good. However, such surgery leaves no room for revision in later years.

The requirement for rheumatoid forefoot correction has fallen dramatically in the last 10 years with the advent of disease-modifying drugs.

MIDFOOT

Rheumatological disease may also affect the midfoot and here the outcome is usually just pain and stiffness. Options are limited to injections and fusion surgery if non-operative measures have failed.

HINDFOOT AND ANKLE

Rheumatological disease also affects the hindfoot and ankle. Many patients require surgical hindfoot fusions and the options for the ankle are discussed in the arthritis section.

The rheumatological diseases also affect soft tissues. Patients are more prone to developing enthesopathy, tendinitis and tendonosis, and even tendon rupture. The Achilles tendon should never be injected with steroid for fear of rupture and, similarly, the tibialis anterior and tibialis posterior tendons are risky for injection.

Tendon disorders

Tenosynovitis occurs as a result of injury, overuse or is secondary to inflammatory joint conditions. Rest, anti-inflammatory medication and physiotherapy are often helpful but, in inflammatory conditions, tenosynovectomy may be required.

The tendons most commonly affected by degeneration are the Achilles (Figure 36.6), tibialis posterior and peroneii (brevis more than longus).

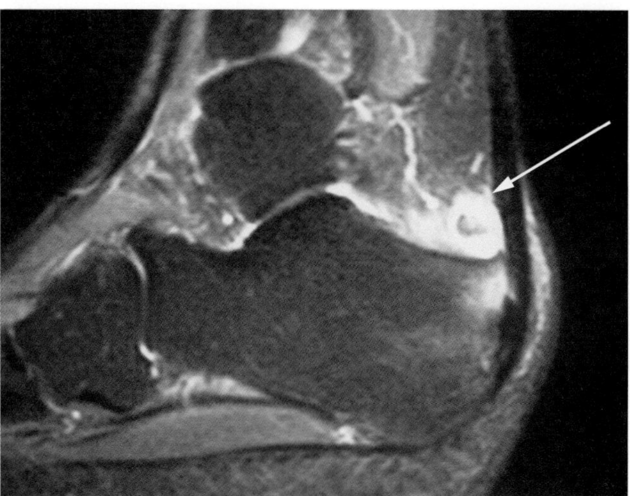

Figure 36.6 Insertional Achilles tendinitis (arrow).

Ruptured Achilles tendon

The Achilles tendon rupture is relatively frequent in the 40- to 50-year-old age group who are undertaking vigorous sport after a long period away from such activities. Management of acute rupture is more frequently non-operative nowadays, provided ultrasound has shown closure of the gap in plantarflexion, and many protocols are described for non-operative management. Surgical fixation is an alternative.

Many patients do not suffer the acute rupture classically described in all textbooks and many seem to have a series of micro tears that gradually lead to total rupture. Studies have shown that elderly patients with Achilles rupture regained 70–90% of the normal power with no treatment whatsoever when reviewed at 1 year; for many patients, this is enough to allow them to return to normal function.

Non-operative options for a missed rupture include a sprung ankle–foot orthotic (AFO) ankle brace, while operative options involve reconstructive surgery with or without flexor hallucis longus (FHL) tendon augmentation.

Achilles tendinosis

Non-insertional and insertional tendinosis are frequent, often related to overuse and are usually managed non-operatively. Shockwave therapy is a recent addition to the armoury. Steroid injections may rupture the Achilles and are discouraged, but high volume saline, dry-needling and sclerosant injections have all been described. Surgery for non-insertional tendinosis has moderate success. Minimally invasive excision of the prominent posterolateral corner of the calcaneum or reshaping osteotomy forms the mainstay of modern surgical techniques for insertional problems but both conditions have a high failure rate with surgery.

Peroneal tendon problems

The peroneal tendons may develop tendinosis, may subluxate or may become involved in an inflammatory process with or without bony overgrowth at the inferior retinaculum (**Figure 36.7**). An associated varus heel will amplify the problem and will need addressing with an appropriate reconstruction/osteotomy or fusion.

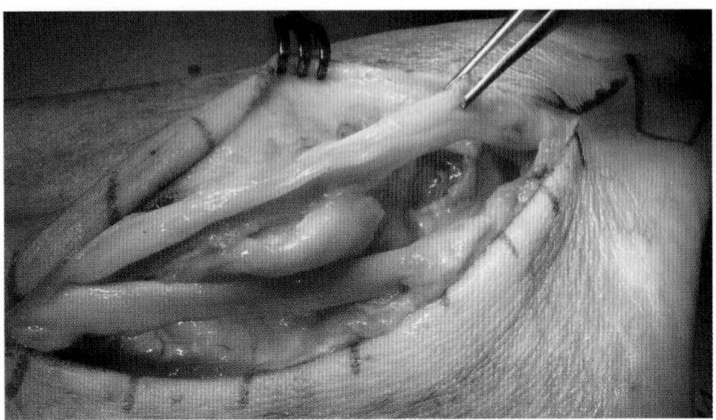

Figure 36.7 Split and degenerate peroneus brevis.

Peroneal tendon subluxation can occur spontaneously or after injury. It may be associated with the groove at the back of the fibula being too shallow to contain the peroneal tendons, but may just be secondary to a superior retinaculum tear. The patient may be able to demonstrate a tendon subluxation over the fibula. Surgical repair is usually required and involves deepening of the groove.

Tendinosis/itis can be managed non-operatively, although injections have occasionally caused rupture. Surgical debridement or repair of splits/tears/ruptures is well described but has only moderate success.

Acquired flat foot

There is a wide range of normal appearance of adult feet. Pathological causes of a flat foot include:

- tibialis posterior tendon dysfunction;
- tarsometatarsal arthritis/injury (Figure 36.8);
- Charcot neuroarthropathy, e.g. diabetes (see later);
- inflammatory/degenerative arthritis of the subtalar/talonavicular/naviculocuneiform joints;
- spring ligament rupture;
- tarsal coalition.

Summary box 36.7

Acquired flat foot

- Tibialis posterior tendon dysfunction and tarsometatarsal osteoarthritis are common causes of an acquired flat foot
- Orthoses, rest and non-steroidal anti-inflammatory drugs (NSAIDs) can help with symptomatic relief
- Surgery is a major undertaking but often highly successful at achieving symptomatic relief

The tibialis posterior tendon tends to fail in overweight individuals and those who have flat feet. Often, after unaccustomed exercise, the tendon swells and is painful. The diagnosis is rarely made early. The condition occurs mainly in women and the key test is that the patient cannot stand on tiptoe on that leg alone. Many individuals will require surgical treatment in the form of a medial displacement calcaneal osteotomy, flexor digitorum longus or FHL tendon transfer and spring ligament repair. Failure to treat this condition can lead to spectacular deformity (Figure 36.9).

An acute traumatic flat foot may develop in young athletes and military recruits after traumatic injury; here the injury is an isolated spring ligament tear and early surgery is needed to effect a repair.

Ankle instability

Most people who sustain an ankle sprain will recover, particularly if they receive prompt physiotherapy. However, some individuals develop significant instability. On examination an unstable ankle due to ligament disruption will show a marked 'anterior drawer' sign.

If physiotherapy is unsuccessful at resolving the problem, a reconstruction may be needed with ligament augmentation. Anatomical techniques such as the Brostrum procedure are favoured and may be augmented with synthetic augments for early mobilisation.

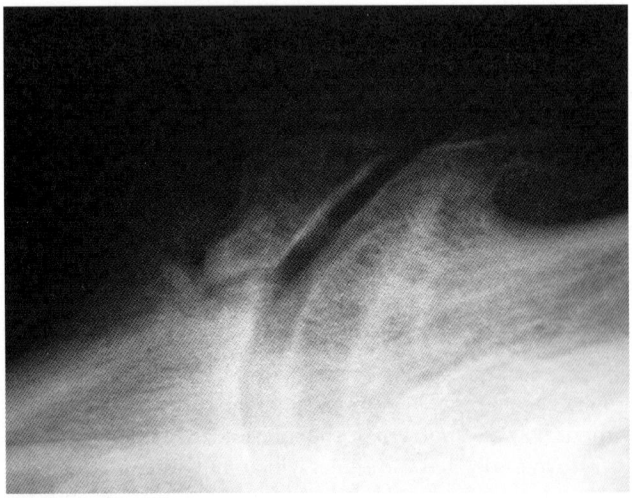

Figure 36.8 Tarsometatarsal arthritis.

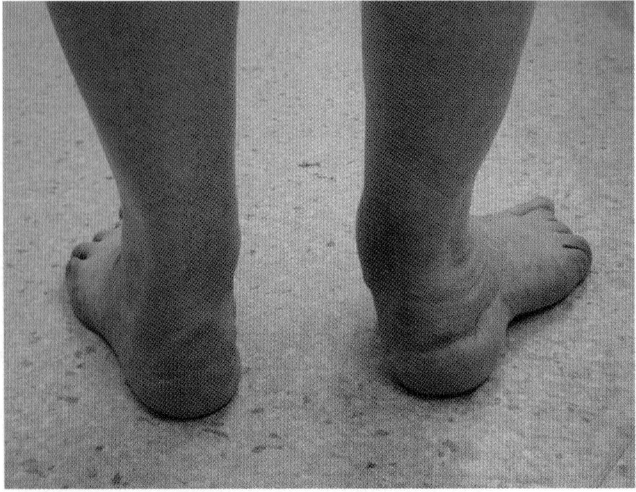

Figure 36.9 A tibialis posterior tendon-deficient foot.

Osteochondral lesion of the talus

Patients with persistent pain in the ankle following an injury should be suspected of having an osteochondral lesion, with MRI or computed tomography (CT) usually required for diagnosis.

Repair of cartilage is not yet possible and large meta-analyses of experimental techniques such as grafting, cell culture, implants and stem cells have not yet shown any statistical benefit. Debridement and microabrasion/microfracture form the mainstay of treatment. Large fragments seen early might benefit from early fixation. Juveniles seem to have a high spontaneous recovery rate and surgery should not be necessary.

Synovitis

Many patients have ongoing pain following ankle injury that is simply due to synovitis within the ankle joint, prominence of the syndesmotic ligament into the joint, impaction injury or undiagnosed fracture or osteochondritis dissecans (OCD) lesion. MRI is mandatory for these cases. Synovitis may be treated non-operatively, with an injection of steroid. Persistent symptoms may require arthroscopic debridement.

Neurological foot conditions

Pes cavus

The development of unilateral pes cavus is likely to be arising from an upper motor neurone lesion so an appropriate neurological examination should be performed.

Pes cavus is usually bilateral and most cases will be associated with an underlying neurological condition, the most common being Charcot–Marie–Tooth disease. These patients may present with characteristic progressive small muscle wasting, thin calf musculature, hand symptoms, aches and pains, and cavo-varus feet. Examination may show early loss of vibration sense. Precise diagnosis is confirmed with nerve conduction studies and genetic testing.

The key deforming force is always relative preservation of the tibialis posterior (tib post) tendon. Surgical correction of the deformity is often required. The principle goal of treatment is to obtain a foot which can be placed flat on the ground, and with the power of the muscles around the ankle in balance. It will be necessary to transfer or release the tib post tendon. The most commonly performed procedure is to transfer the tib post to the dorsolateral side of the foot, followed by lateralising of the heel with an osteotomy and dorsiflexion osteotomy of the first ray with or without a Jones procedure to the great toe.

Summary box 36.8

Pes cavus

- Pes cavus needs neurological investigation
- About 80% of cases of pes cavus are associated with a neurological disease
- The commonest cause is Charcot–Marie–Tooth disease
- Unilateral pes cavus – think diastematomyelia/ tumour

Tumours

The most common benign tumours of the foot are ganglia, giant cell tumour and angioleiomyomas (**Figure 36.10**); these tumours may need surgical excision.

Pigmented villonodular synovitis (PVNS) is a locally aggressive condition found in the ankle and is diagnosed by MRI or at histology. Surveillance for recurrence is mandatory.

The most common 'tumour' seen in the foot is the plantar fibroma or 'ledderhosens disease', which presents as a painful often growing lump in the sole along the plantar fascia. The condition is linked to Dupytren's and Peyronie's disease. Surgery should be avoided. Ultrasound or MRI will confirm the multifocal nature of the disease and exclude other pathology.

Any large or growing lump in the foot needs formal work-up along tumour guidelines, especially in the presence of night pain.

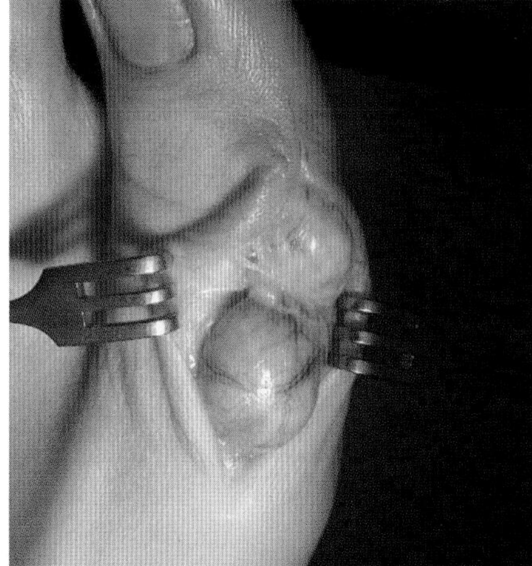

Figure 36.10 Angioleiomyoma of the hallux.

Infection

Septic arthritis in the foot or ankle is rare except in diabetic patients and constitutes a surgical emergency; when it occurs it usually follows a surgical procedure but it can also arise

---

Pierre Marie, 1853–1940, neurologist, Hospice de Bicêtre, Paris, France, later becoming Professor of Pathological Anatomy in the Faculty of Medicine, and finally, in 1918, Professor of Neurology.
Howard Henry Tooth, 1856–1925, physician, St Bartholomew's Hospital, and the National Hospital for Nervous Diseases, Queen Square, London, UK, described peroneal muscular atrophy in 1886 independently of Charcot and Marie.

as a result of haematogenous spread. Treatment is immediate surgical drainage and administration of appropriate high-dosage antibiotics once cultures are obtained. The most common causative organism is *Staphylococcus aureus* with methicillin-resistant *S. aureus* (MRSA) becoming more common. Even with prompt treatment chondrolysis often occurs and subsequent degenerative changes develop rapidly.

In immunocompromised patients opportunistic infections can arise and, in diabetics, failure to treat with debridement can lead to amputation. It is important to realise that radiographs in the early stages of infection are usually normal and that diagnosis is made on clinical suspicion and with blood tests and more sophisticated imaging such as MRI or bone scanning.

Tuberculosis can affect the foot and is associated with major bony damage; it responds surprisingly well to debridement and appropriate antituberculous therapy (Figure 36.11).

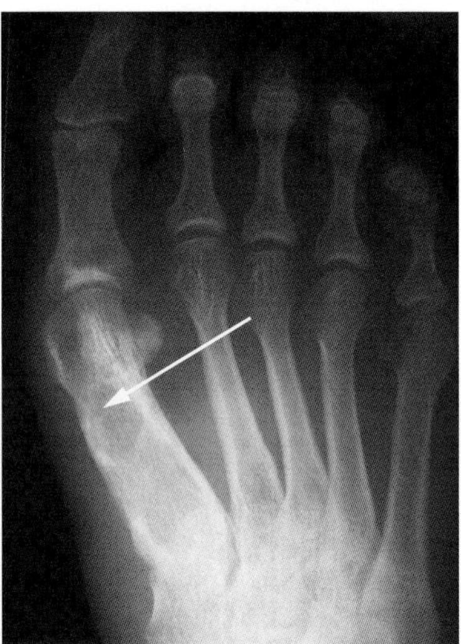

Figure 36.11 Tuberculosis of the foot (arrow).

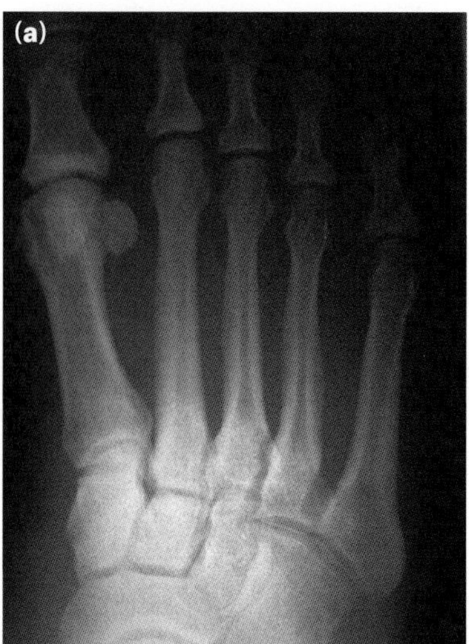

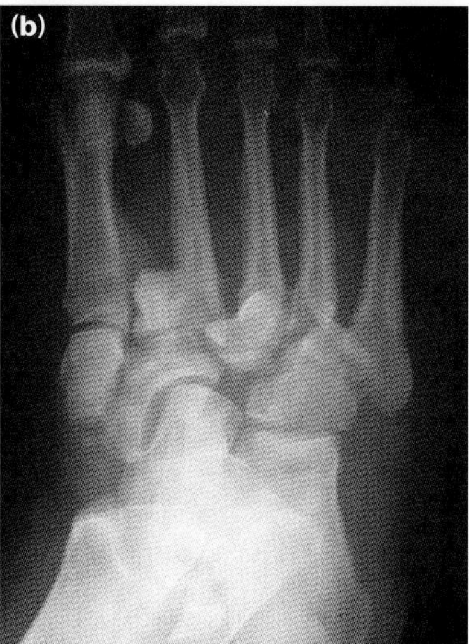

Figure 36.12 Charcot foot: radiographs taken at the time of a trivial injury (**a**) and 6 weeks later (**b**).

Diabetes

Diabetic patients have foot problems secondary to neuropathy and microvascular changes. They are at increased risk of infection and ulceration, and trauma (sometimes trivial) can lead to collapse of the foot, also known as Charcot neuroarthropathy (Figure 36.12).

Ulceration and amputation

Ulceration can lead to major morbidity and amputation (Figure 36.13). Ulcers need to be treated urgently, and when ulcer healing has occurred the aim should be to keep the foot ulcer free. NICE guidelines detail optimal management pathways with urgent admission, radiological and clinical assessment, followed by debridement, antibiotics if required and formal offloading. Ulceration is a surgical emergency.

Most amputations are preceeded by ulceration.

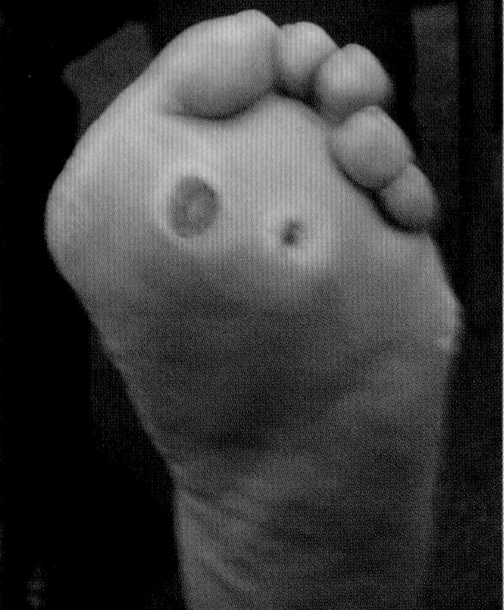

Figure 36.13 Diabetic foot ulcer.

Charcot

Charcot is a condition in which patients develop a neuropathic destruction of the joints. It is often described as painless but actually the majority of patients have some pain. In the Western world diabetes is the biggest cause but in the rest of the world leprosy is also important. However, any other neurological condition can cause this disease.

Charcot often presents with a hot, swollen, red extremity. It is often misdiagnosed as cellulitis, gout, fracture or deep vein thrombosis (DVT), and many present late because of the difficulty in diagnosis.

If there is no history of skin damage, infection is unlikely, but MRI and even biopsy can help differentiate between infection and Charcot. From initiation through to bone consolidation may take up to 18 months. The principle of treatment throughout is to maintain a foot-shaped foot to prevent late pressure ulcers. The acute Charcot foot requires appropriate splintage in a Charcot retaining orthotic walker (CROW) or a total contact cast (TCC), but many surgeons offer an aggressive early surgical approach if bony prominence ulceration is thought to be inevitable. Surgical options include early stabilisation to prevent deformity, or late reconstruction or removal of bony prominences to prevent ulceration. Failure results in ulceration and amputation.

Summary box 36.9

Diabetes

- Diabetics are prone to infection because of:
  - Peripheral neuropathy
  - Peripheral vascular disease
  - Impaired resistance to infection
- A Charcot foot is often misdiagnosed but is a surgical emergency and requires urgent admission and management
- An ulcer in a diabetic foot is a surgical emergency and requires urgent admission and management

Entrapment neuropathies

Any nerve supplying the foot can become entrapped and result in pain, and treatment often requires surgical decompression. Tarsal tunnel syndrome is much rarer than carpal tunnel syndrome.

Heel pain

The commonest cause of heel pain is plantar fasciitis. Pain is located inferomedially within the heel and is worst first thing in the morning and after periods of rest. The majority of cases settle within 18 months and surgery is rarely required or successful. Ultrasound-guided injection forms the mainstay of treatment for the non-resolving cases. The differential diagnosis list includes calcaneal stress fracture, tarsal tunnel, seronegative arthropathy and lederhosens disease.

FURTHER READING

Bulstrode C, Wilson MacDonald J, Eastwood D *et al. Oxford textbook of trauma and orthopaedics*, 2nd edn. Oxford: Oxford University Press, 2017.

Miller MD, Thompson SR. *Miller's review of orthopaedics*, 7th edn. Philadelphia: Elsevier, 2016.

Solomon L, Warwick DJ, Nayagam S. *Apley & Solomon's concise system of orthopaedics and trauma*, 4th edn. Boca Raton: CRC Press, 2014.

Chapter 37

Musculoskeletal tumours

Learning objectives

- List the symptoms and signs associated with a musculoskeletal tumour
- Understand why a patient with a suspected musculoskeletal tumour should be referred to a specialist centre for staging, biopsy and multidisciplinary management
- Understand why staging should be completed before biopsy
- Explain why a diagnosis is required before treatment
- Understand the principles of biopsy
- Describe the principles of surgical treatment of musculoskeletal tumours
- List the aims of surgical treatment for metastatic bone disease
- Understand how to manage patients with an impending or completed pathological fracture
- Evaluate the risk of pathological fracture

INTRODUCTION

Musculoskeletal tumours include primary and secondary benign and malignant tumours of bone and soft tissue. The most common malignant bone tumours are secondary metastatic carcinomas (**Figure 37.1**). Advances in oncological treatment mean that the number of patients living with metastatic bone disease is increasing. The most common carcinomas that metastasise to bone originate in the breast, prostate, lung, kidney and thyroid (**Figure 37.2**).

Haematopoietic tumours may also arise in bone: multiple myeloma (**Figure 37.3**) is a malignant neoplasm arising from plasma cells in the bone marrow, leading to multiple lesions in the skeleton. When solitary, this type of tumour is called a plasmacytoma.

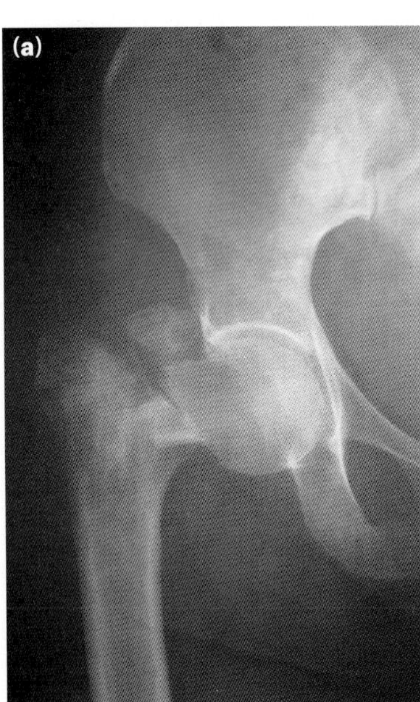

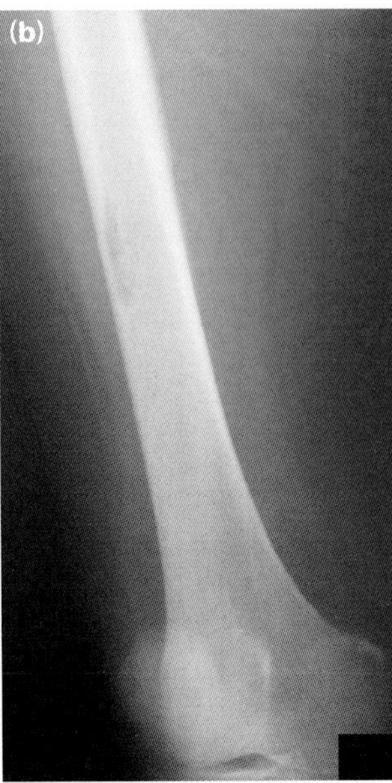

Figure 37.1 (a) Pathological fracture of the proximal femur through metastatic breast carcinoma. **(b)** Radiographs of the whole femur show a further, more distal metastatic deposit.

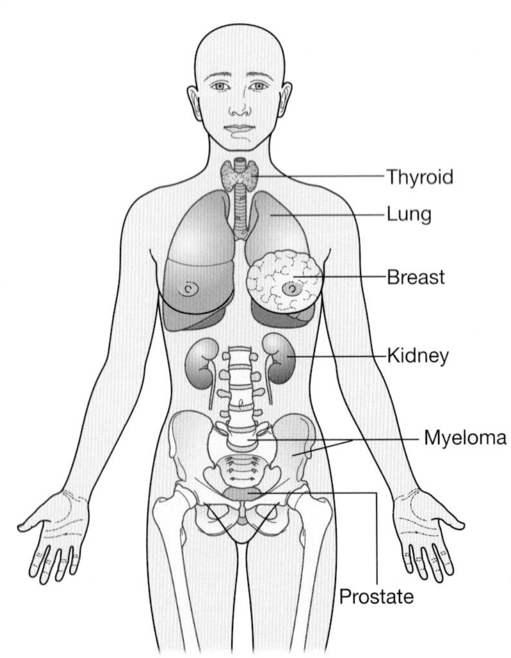

Figure 37.2 Malignant tumours that commonly metastasise to bone.

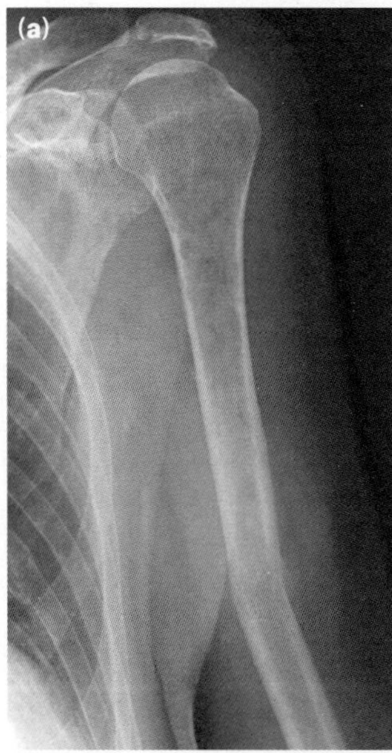
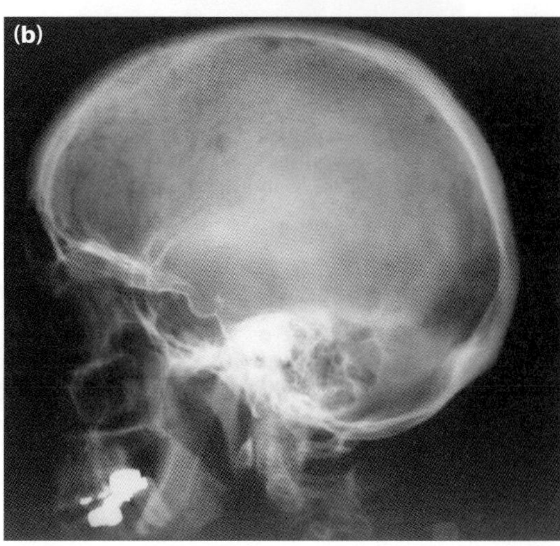

Figure 37.3 (a) Multiple myeloma affecting the left humerus with a pathological fracture. (b) Multiple myeloma with multiple deposits in the skull.

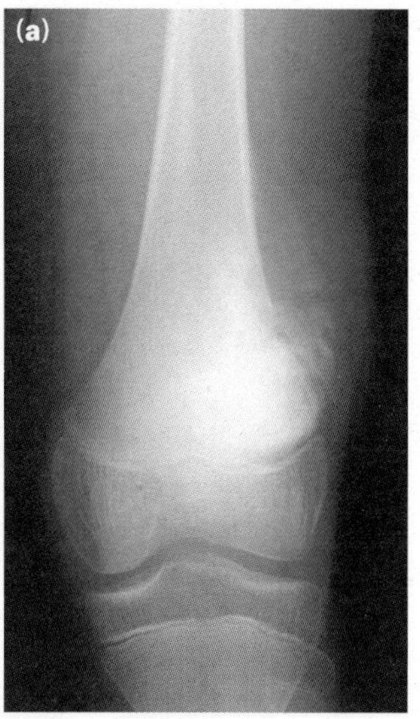
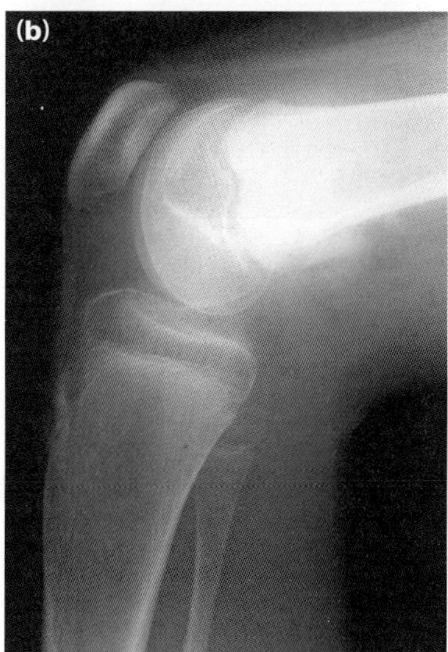

Figure 37.4 (a, b) Sclerotic osteosarcoma of the distal femur in a child.

Malignant primary bone tumours (sarcomas) are very rare, but notably can occur in children and young adults. The most common of these are osteosarcoma (Figure 37.4), chondrosarcoma (Figures 37.5, 37.6 and 37.7) and Ewing's sarcoma (Figure 37.8).

Soft tissue tumours are common. However, only one in a hundred is malignant (Figure 37.9).

BONE TUMOURS

Tumours found in bone are classified according to the tissue of origin. These include:

- metastatic carcinomas – may show histological features of their tissue of origin;
- haematopoietic tumours – e.g. myeloma;
- osteogenic tumours – e.g. osteosarcoma;
- chondrogenic tumours – e.g. chondrosarcoma;
- others – e.g. Ewing's sarcoma.

Osteosarcoma has two age incidence-peaks, one in adolescence and the other later in life. Osteosarcomas in older patients usually arise in association with Paget's disease or after radiotherapy treatment. Ewing's sarcoma occurs in adolescence, whilst the incidence of chondrosarcoma increases from middle age onwards.

Some conditions are associated with an increased likelihood of developing malignant tumours in bone and/or cartilage (*Table 37.1*).

James Ewing, 1866–1943, Professor of Pathology, Cornell University Medical College, New York, NY, USA, described this type of sarcoma in 1921.
Sir James Paget, 1814–1899, surgeon, St Bartholomew's Hospital, London, UK, described osteitis deformans in 1877.

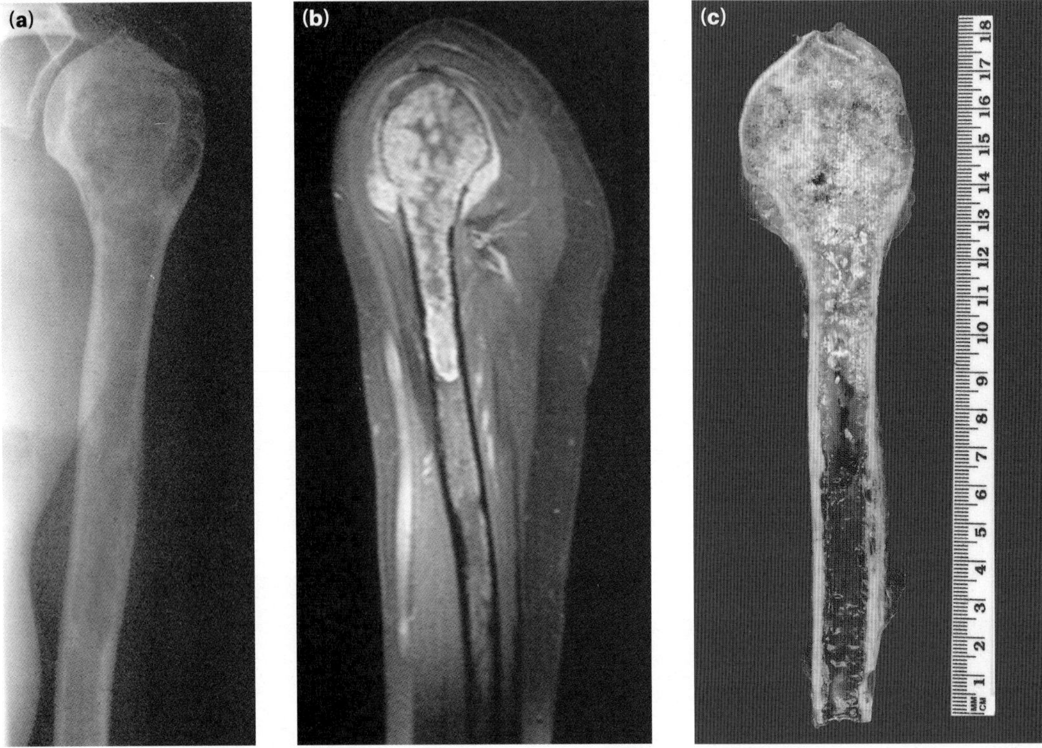

Figure 37.5 (**a**) Chondrosarcoma of the proximal humerus with multiple calcifications. (**b**) Magnetic resonance imaging scan showing extensive involvement. (**c**) Excised chondrosarcoma of the proximal humerus.

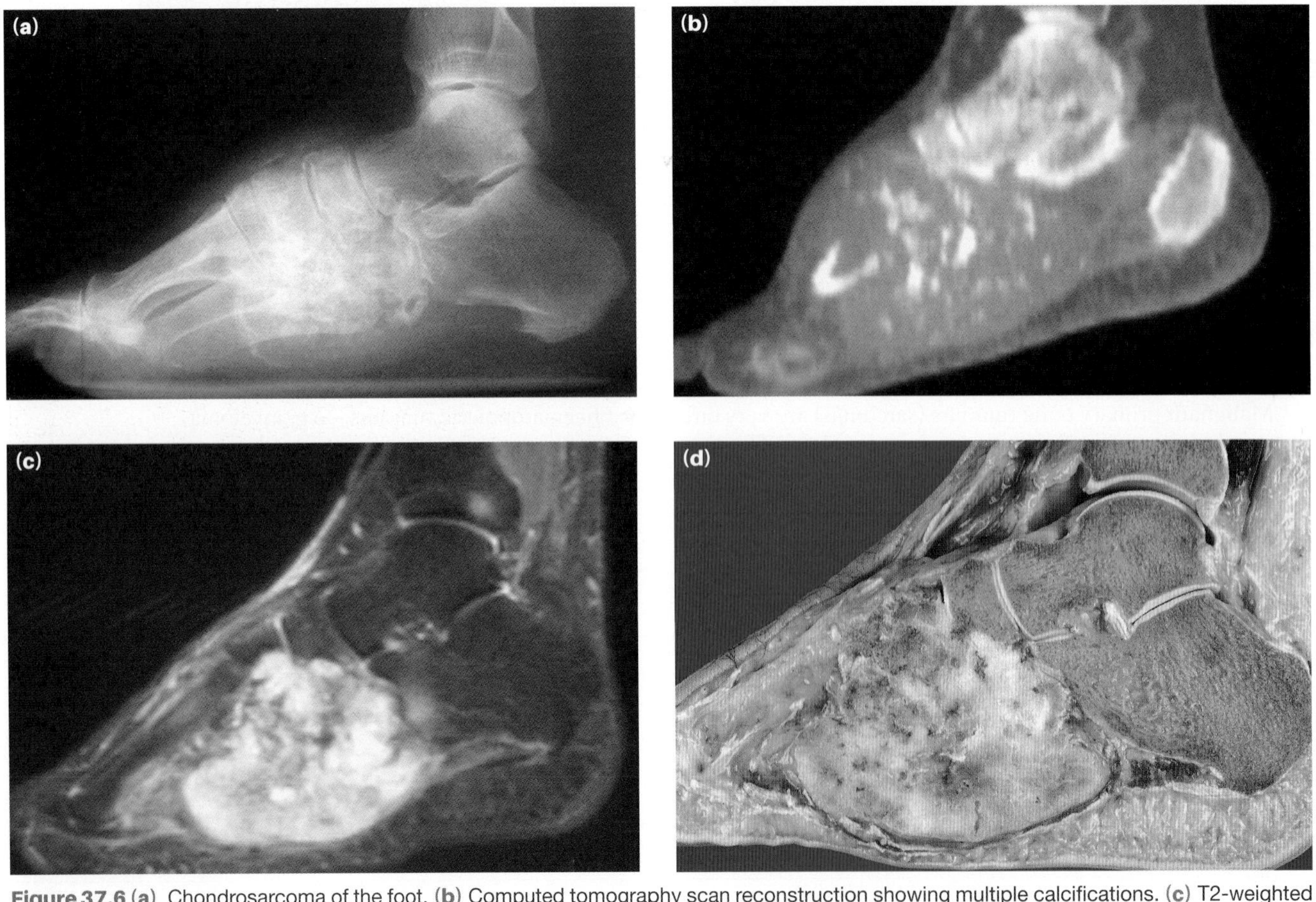

Figure 37.6 (**a**) Chondrosarcoma of the foot. (**b**) Computed tomography scan reconstruction showing multiple calcifications. (**c**) T2-weighted magnetic resonance imaging scan shows high signal in chondrosarcoma. (**d**) Excised chondrosarcoma of the foot.

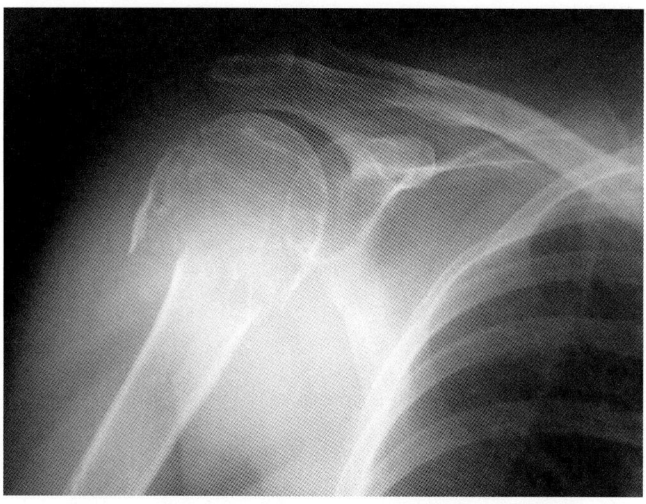

Figure 37.7 Pathological fracture through a primary chondrosarcoma of the proximal humerus.

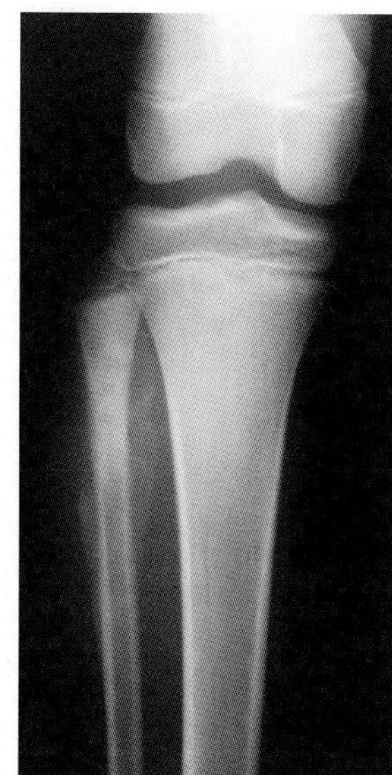

Figure 37.8 Ewing's sarcoma of the proximal fibula. The tumour is metadiaphyseal in location with a periosteal reaction and subtle onion-skinning.

TABLE 37.1 Conditions associated with an increased risk of malignant disease in bone and cartilage.

High risk	Moderate risk	Low risk
Maffucci syndrome (enchondromatosis and angiomas of soft tissue)	Hereditary multiple exostoses	Chronic osteomyelitis
Ollier disease (enchondromatosis)	Polyostotic Paget's disease	Osteonecrosis
Familial retinoblastoma syndrome	Radiation osteitis	Fibrous dysplasia, osteogenesis imperfecta, osteoblastoma and chondroblastoma

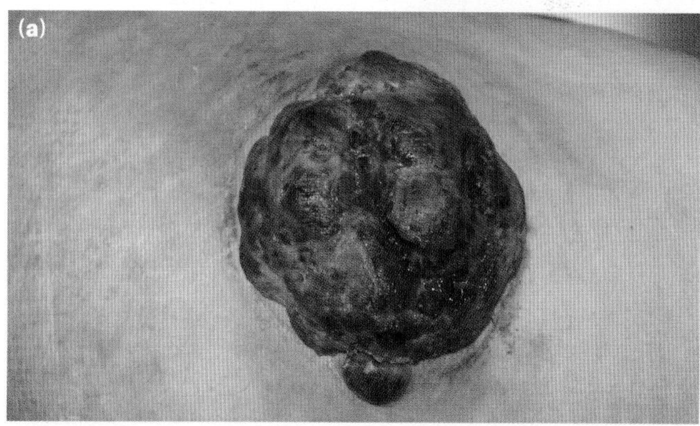

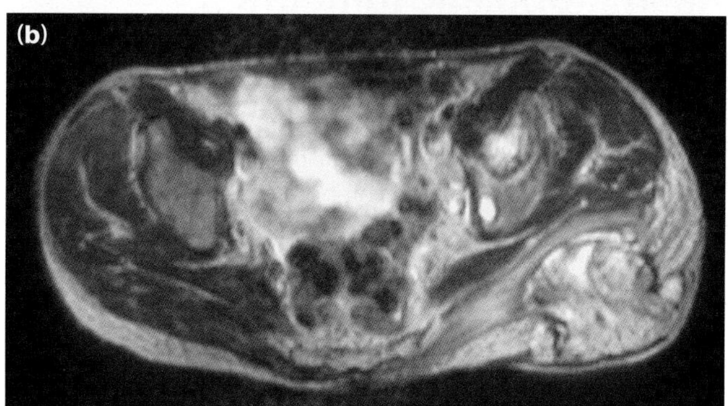

Figure 37.9 **(a)** Large, fungating soft-tissue sarcoma of the buttock. **(b)** Magnetic resonance imaging scan showing a large fungating sarcoma of the buttock.

Metastatic bone disease

Most tumours which metastasise to bone are carcinomas. Not infrequently the primary tumour is never found despite further investigation: these patients are described as having 'carcinoma of unknown primary'.

Carcinomas usually spread to bone by the haematogenous route: the spine is the third most common site for metastases, after the lung and liver. Although most patients with metastatic cancer will have bone metastases in the spine before they die, only 10% are symptomatic.

Tumour cells metastasise to the spine via Batson's venous plexus. These retroperitoneal veins have no valves and allow retrograde embolic spread to the spine and proximal long bones (**Figure 37.10**).

Bone metastases can be lytic, sclerotic or mixed. Lytic metastases are usually highly vascular or locally aggressive such that there is no healing response from the bone. Metastases from prostate cancer may appear sclerotic.

Metastases are rare in children, but bone metastases can occur from neuroblastoma, rhabdomyosarcoma and clear cell carcinoma of the kidney.

Summary box 37.1

Most common tumours metastasising to bone (93%)

- Breast
- Prostate
- Lung
- Renal
- Thyroid

Oscar V Batson, 1894–1979, American otolaryngologist.

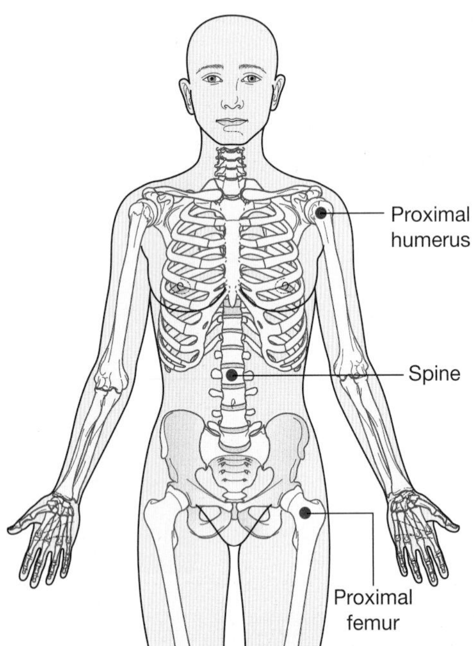

Figure 37.10 Common sites of metastatic bone disease.

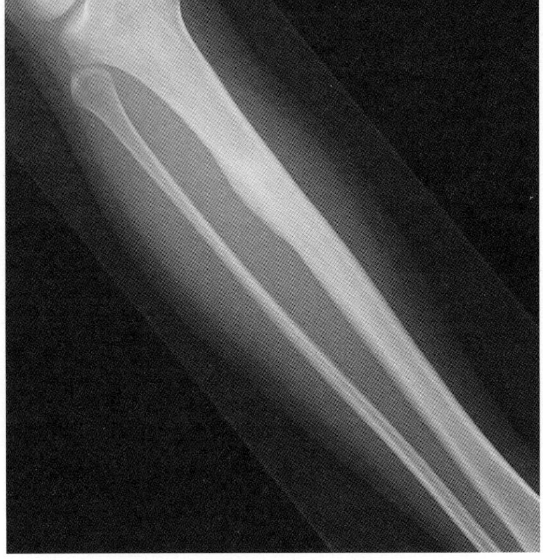

Figure 37.11 Radiograph showing an osteoid osteoma of the tibial diaphysis with reactive bone formation.

Summary box 37.2

Most common sites of bone metastases

- Spine
- Proximal femur
- Proximal humerus

Haematopoietic tumours

There are no benign neoplasms of the haematopoietic system. Malignant haematopoietic tumours, that commonly present in orthopaedic clinic, are either solitary plasmacytoma/ multiple myeloma (arising from plasma cells, see Figure 37.2) or lymphomas (arising from lymphoid cells).

Summary box 37.3

Malignant bone tumours

- Plasmacytoma – solitary form of multiple myeloma
- Osteosarcoma – often secondary to Paget's disease and radiotherapy
- Chondrosarcoma
- Ewing's sarcoma

Osteogenic tumours

These tumours characteristically produce osteoid or bony matrix which may be seen on imaging studies or on histological examination.

Osteoid osteoma (Figures 37.11 and 37.12) is a benign bone-forming lesion which is small but very painful. Usually, pain occurs at night and is typically relieved by non-steroidal anti-inflammatory medication. Osteoid osteomas usually occur in children and adolescents. They arise in any bone, particularly

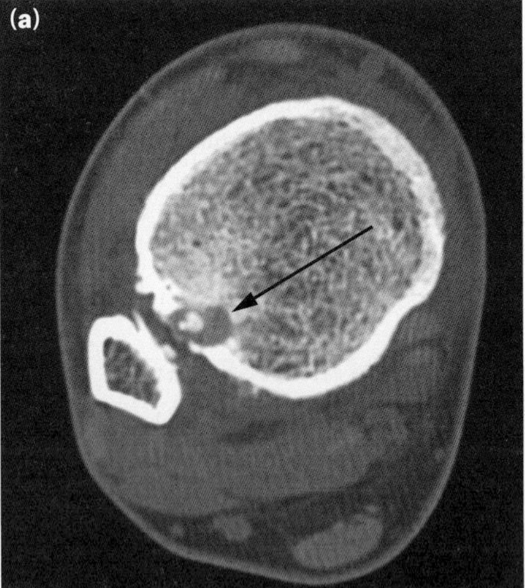

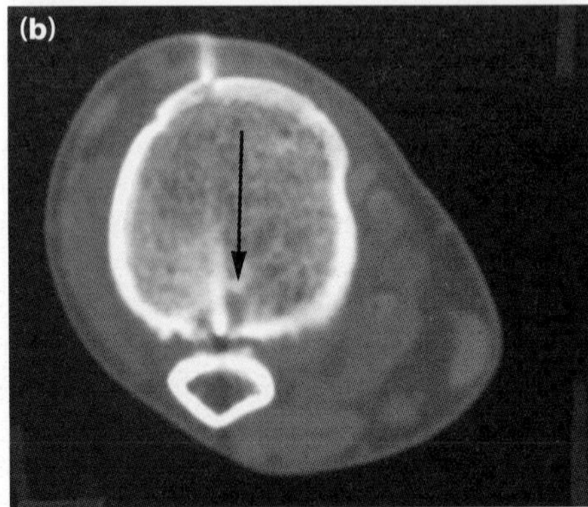

Figure 37.12 (a) Axial computed tomography (CT) scan showing an osteoid osteoma nidus in the distal tibia (arrow). (b) CT-guided radiofrequency thermocoagulation of an osteoid osteoma of the distal tibia. The scan shows the electrode *in situ* (arrow).

the proximal femur, and cause a dense cortical reaction in the centre of which is a nidus (Figure 37.12). Osteoid osteomas can cause irritation and effusions if they occur close to a joint.

Osteoblastoma is the larger (>2 cm), more aggressive counterpart of osteoid osteoma that more typically occurs in the spine.

Osteosarcoma (see Figure 37.4) is a malignant bone-forming tumour, most common in the distal femur, followed by the proximal tibia, proximal humerus and distal tibia. The radiological and histological classification of osteosarcomas includes sclerotic (Figure 37.4), chondroblastic, telangiectatic and other more unusual forms. Usually, osteosarcomas are intraosseous, but they can also arise from the surface of bones. Parosteal osteosarcoma (Figure 37.13) is a low-grade osteosarcoma that arises from the surface of the bone, typically of the distal femur or proximal tibia. Symptoms are often mild and longstanding.

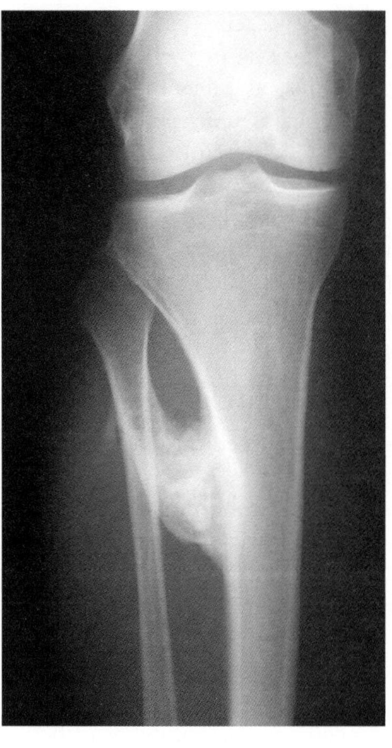

Figure 37.14 Pedunculated osteochondromas of the proximal fibula with pseudoarthrosis. Osteochondromas always grow away from the physis and are in continuity with the intramedullary cavity of the bone they arise from.

Summary box 37.4

Tumours producing bone

- Osteoid osteoma – small, painful; produce dense cortical reaction
- Osteoblastoma – larger and more aggressive than osteoid osteoma
- Osteosarcoma – malignant; commonest in lower femur and upper tibia

Chondrogenic tumours

These tumours produce chondroid matrix and include a wide range of benign and malignant tumours.

Osteochondroma (Figures 37.14 and 37.15) is a benign cartilage-capped bony projection, thought to originate from the physis. The bony projection always grows away from the joint towards the diaphyseal region of the bone. It has no structures attached to it. Osteochondromas can be pedunculated (with a stalk) or sessile (without a stalk). The stalk or base is always continuous with the intramedullary cavity of the bone, and the continuity of the cortex of the bone into an osteochondroma is a characteristic radiological feature. They are usually solitary, but some patients have multiple osteochondromas (hereditary multiple exostoses, autosomal dominant inheritance) (Figure 37.16). Osteochondromas can cause local irritation and complications include mechanical

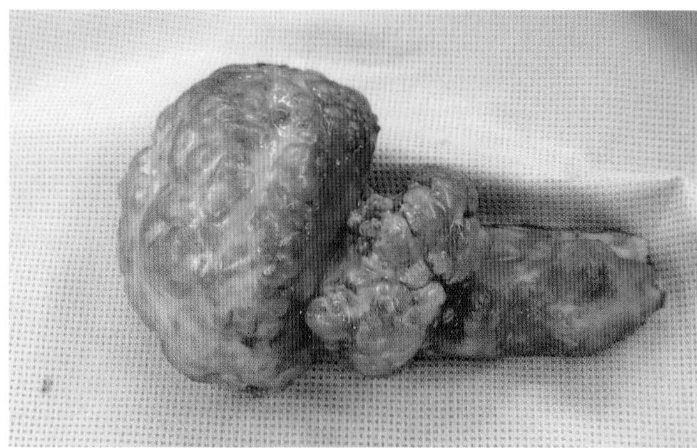

Figure 37.15 Excised pedunculated osteochondroma showing cartilage cap.

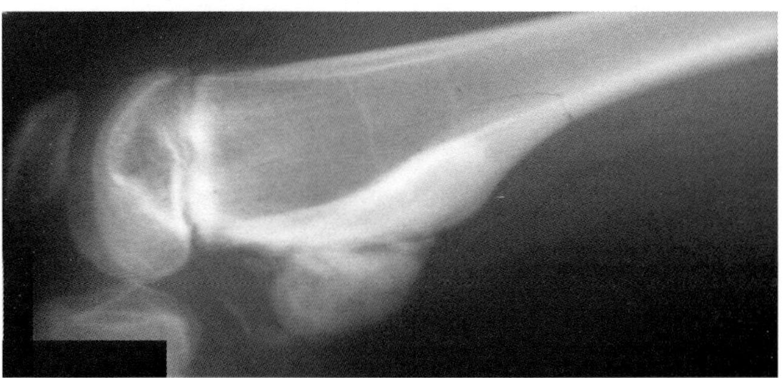

Figure 37.13 Paraosteal osteosarcoma of the distal femur in an unusually young patient. There is no continuity between the tumour and the intramedullary cavity of the femur.

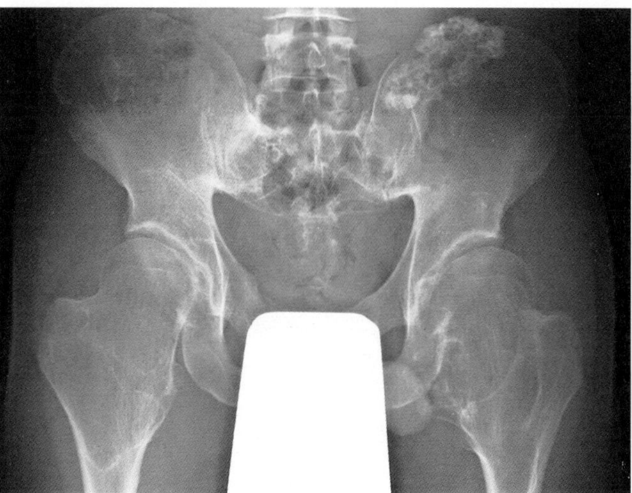

Figure 37.16 Multiple osteochondromas in hereditary multiple exostoses.

symptoms, nerve impingement, vascular pseudoaneurysm, fracture and infarction. Increasing size or pain, particularly after skeletal maturity, is concerning and may indicate malignant transformation. The incidence of malignant transformation is less than 1% in solitary osteochondromas and 1–3% in patients with multiple osteochondromas.

Enchondroma (Figure 37.17) is a benign cartilaginous neoplasm within the intramedullary cavity of bone. Approximately 50% are in the hands and feet: enchondromas are the most common bone tumours in the hand. Although they can present with pain, swelling or pathological fracture, many are entirely asymptomatic and are detected incidentally. Patchy calcification, expansion and scalloping can be visible on radiographs, but some are only diagnosed on magnetic resonance imaging (MRI) scan.

Ollier disease is a developmental condition characterised by multiple enchondromas. In Maffucci syndrome, multiple enchondromas are associated with multiple angiomas. Malignant transformation to chondrosarcoma can occur in approximately 20% of patients with Ollier disease and is almost inevitable in patients with Maffucci syndrome.

Chondroblastoma (Figure 37.18) is a benign cartilage-producing tumour that occurs in the epiphyses of bones

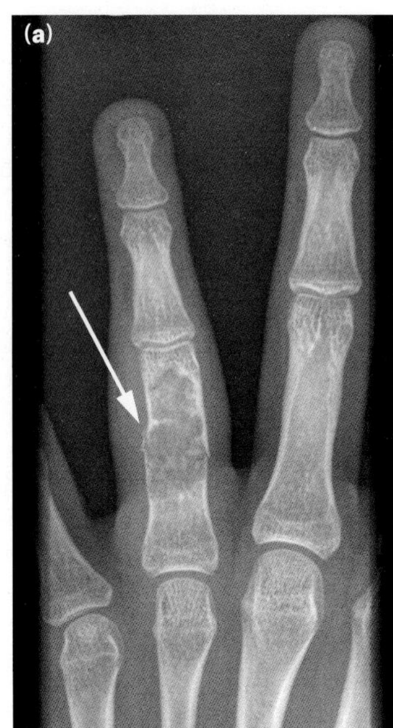
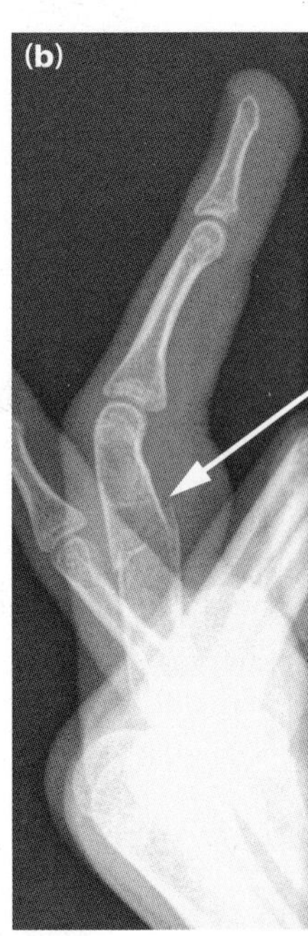

Figure 37.17 **(a, b)** Calcification and pathological fracture in a benign enchondroma of the proximal phalanx of the ring finger (arrows).

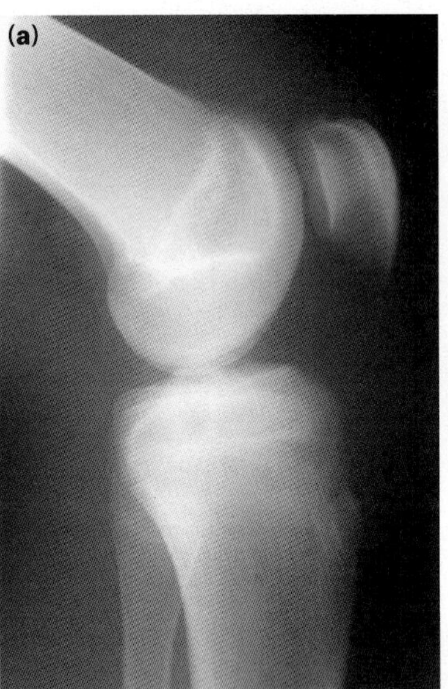
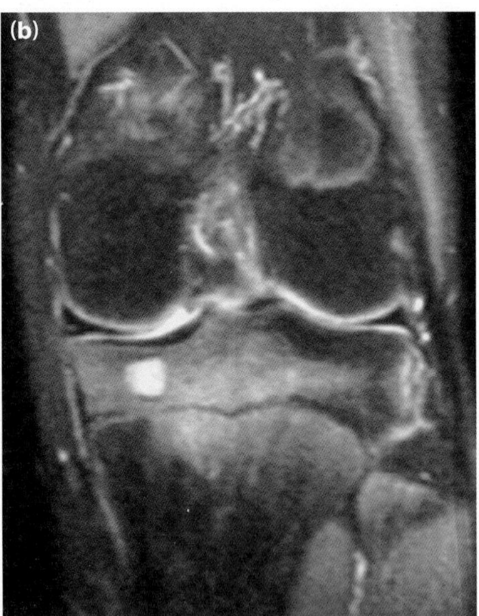
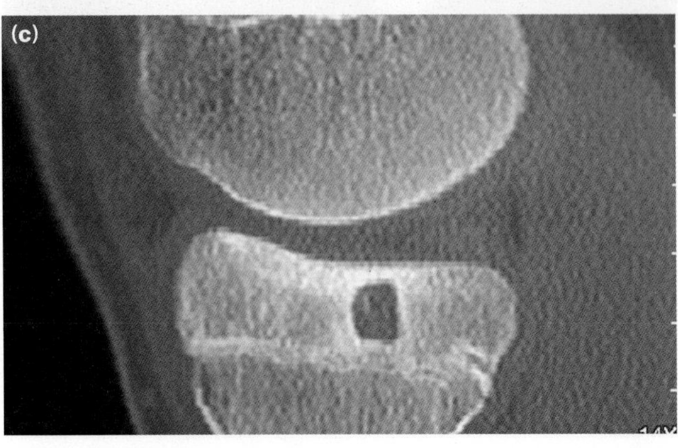

Figure 37.18 **(a)** Lateral radiograph with barely visible chondroblastoma in the epiphysis of the proximal tibia. **(b)** Coronal T2-weighted magnetic resonance imaging scan showing chondroblastoma in the epiphysis of the proximal tibia with surrounding oedema. **(c)** Sagittal computed tomography reconstruction showing calcification within a chondroblastoma of the proximal tibial epiphysis.

Angelo Maffucci, 1845–1903, Professor of Surgery, Lyons, France, described enchondromatosis in 1899.

in children. It is most common around the knee. Pain is often severe, with associated inflammation and possibly joint effusion. Radiologically, there is an often barely visible lytic lesion in the centre of the epiphysis. The diagnosis is often missed, and isotope bone scan can help identify the lesion.

Chondrosarcoma (see Figures 37.5, 37.6 and 37.7) is a malignant tumour with cartilage differentiation. The biological behaviour ranges from very low-grade lesions to highly aggressive dedifferentiated tumours. Patients usually present with pain and/or swelling and symptoms may be longstanding. Many chondrosarcomas arise in pre-existing lesions such as osteochondromas or enchondromas. Diagnosis of a chondrosarcoma requires clinical, radiological and pathological correlation. Clear cell chondrosarcoma is a rare form of chondrosarcoma that occurs in the epiphysis (Figure 37.19).

Summary box 37.5

Tumours producing cartilage

- Osteochondroma – cartilage capped; grows away from physis
- Enchondroma – inside bone; commonest in hands and feet
- Chondroblastoma – in epiphyses of adolescents
- Chondrosarcoma – of varying malignancy

Others

Simple (unicameral) bone cyst (Figure 37.20) is a membrane-lined cavity filled with serous fluid within a bone. It usually occurs in the proximal long bones of children. Associated thinning of the cortex of the bone can lead to fracture. Such fractures usually heal with conservative treatment, but the cyst may only partially resolve.

Aneurysmal bone cyst (Figure 37.21) is a benign cystic lesion of bone consisting of blood-filled spaces separated by fibrous septa. The lesion is more aggressive than a simple bone cyst and often presents with pain and swelling. Plain radiographs commonly show aggressive features with eccentric expansion of the cortex and an open physis. Scans often show multiple fluid levels (Figure 37.21b).

Giant cell tumour of bone (Figure 37.22) is a locally aggressive tumour with large osteoclast-like giant cells. It usually occurs between the ages of 20 and 45, after the physes have closed. Giant cell tumour of bone typically affects the epiphysis of long bones and erodes bone under the articular cartilage, especially around the knee, proximal humerus and distal radius. Metastases are rare.

Eosinophilic granuloma is a rare neoplasm of Langerhans cells (Figure 37.23). It can be unifocal (eosinophilic granuloma), multifocal (Hand–Schuller–Christian disease) or disseminated (Letterer–Siwe disease). There is a predilection for the skull and the diaphyses of long bones. In the spine it can present with collapse, known as *vertebra plana*. Radiographs can appear aggressive and similar to Ewing's sarcoma.

Fibrous dysplasia (Figure 37.24) is a benign fibro-osseous lesion that can be mono- or polyostotic. It usually affects the long bones, ribs and skull. Patients can present with pain, swelling and/or fracture, but many lesions are

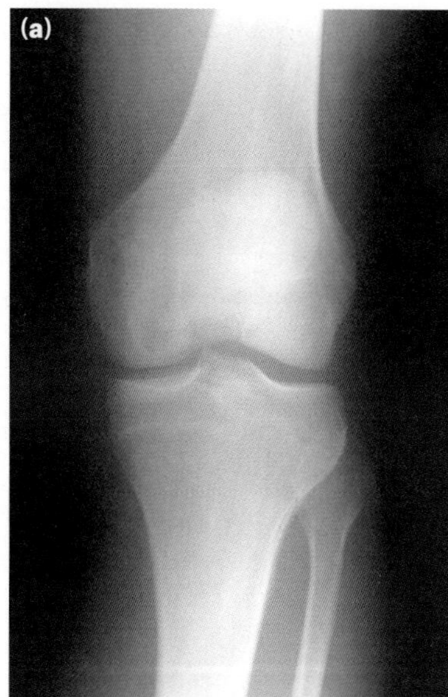

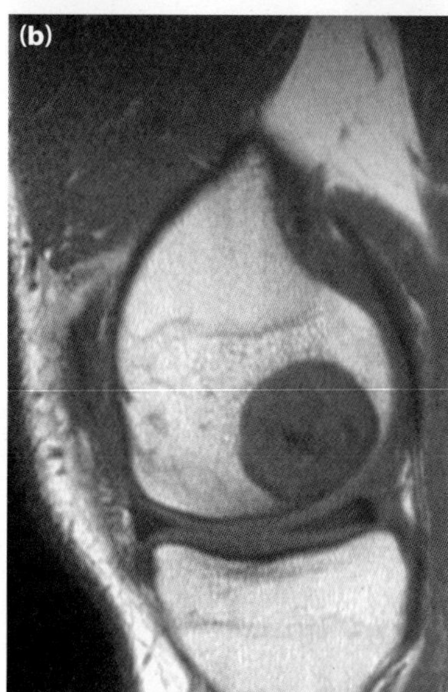

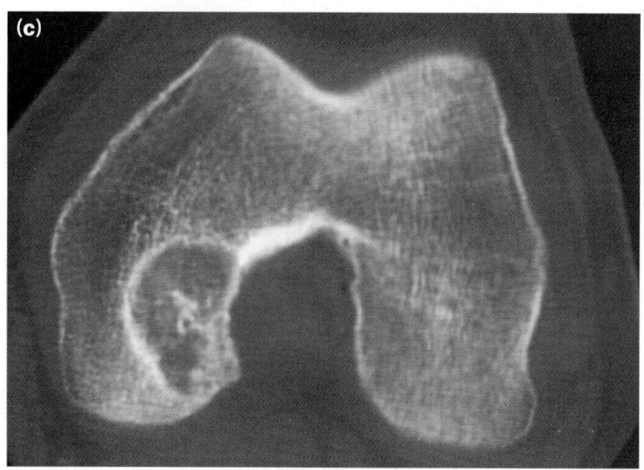

Figure 37.19 (**a**) Clear cell chondrosarcoma of the medial femoral condyle. (**b**) Sagittal T1-weighted magnetic resonance imaging scan showing clear cell chondrosarcoma in the medial femoral condyle. (**c**) Computed tomography scan reconstruction shows calcification within the lesion.

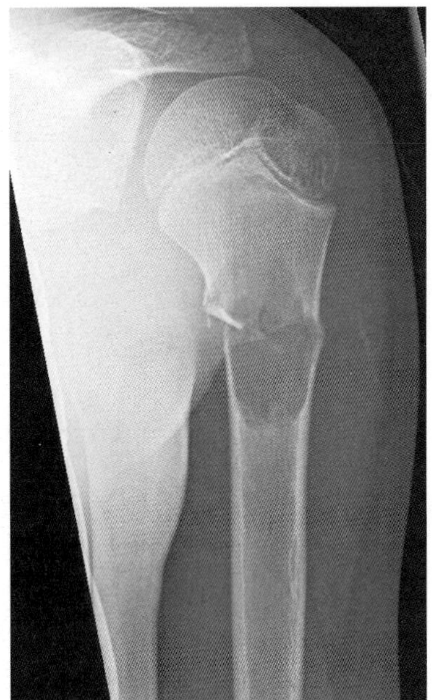

Figure 37.20 Pathological fracture through a simple bone cyst with the pathognomonic fallen leaf sign. The fracture healed and the cyst consolidated without operative intervention.

detected incidentally. Hip fractures can produce a 'shepherd's crook' deformity of the proximal femur. Radiologically there is often expansion and a ground glass appearance, sometimes with cystic change.

Ewing's sarcoma (see Figure 37.8) is a malignant round cell sarcoma of bone in which cells usually have a characteristic 11:22 translocation. It tends to arise in the diaphysis of a long bone or the pelvis. Patients usually present with a painful mass and may have systemic symptoms including fever, anaemia and increased erythrocyte sedimentation rate (ESR). Radiologically the bone appears moth-eaten and may show an 'onion-skin' periosteal reaction. MRI may show a large extraosseous soft tissue mass as well as significant inflammation with oedema.

Bone tumours usually occur in characteristic anatomical locations (*Table 37.2*), and epiphyseal tumours are likely to be benign (*Table 37.3*).

TABLE 37.2 Classification of bone tumours by site.

Tumour and site		
Diaphyseal	**Metaphyseal**	**Epiphyseal**
Eosinophilic granuloma	Most	Chondroblastoma
Osteoid osteoma		Intra-articular osteoid osteoma
Fibrous dysplasia		Giant cell tumour (physis closed)
Adamantinoma		Clear cell chondrosarcoma
Ewing's sarcoma		

TABLE 37.3 Common diaphyseal bone tumours according to age.

Age and most common diaphyseal tumour	
<10 years	Eosinophilic granuloma
Teenage	Ewing's sarcoma
Adult	Lymphoma
>60 years	Metastasis/myeloma

Summary box 37.6

Other bone tumours

- Simple bone cyst – proximal long bones of children
- Aneurysmal bone cyst – more aggressive, expanding
- Giant cell tumour – found in epiphyses around the knee
- Fibrous dysplasia – may be multiple; long bones, ribs and skull
- Ewing's – round cell sarcoma; patients may have fever and anaemia

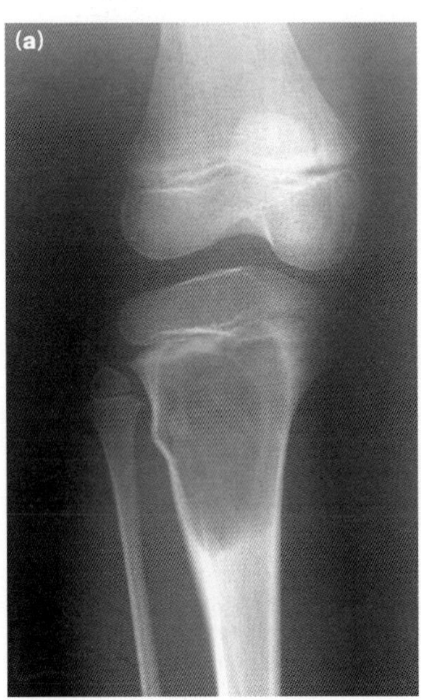

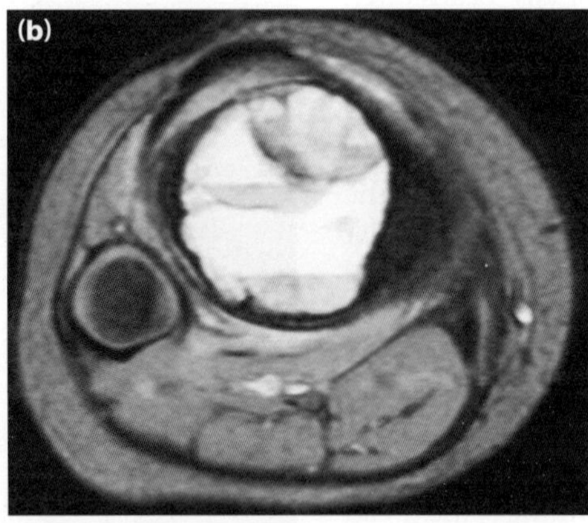

Figure 37.21 (**a**) Aneurysmal bone cyst with pathological fracture of the proximal tibia. (**b**) Magnetic resonance imaging scan shows multiple fluid levels.

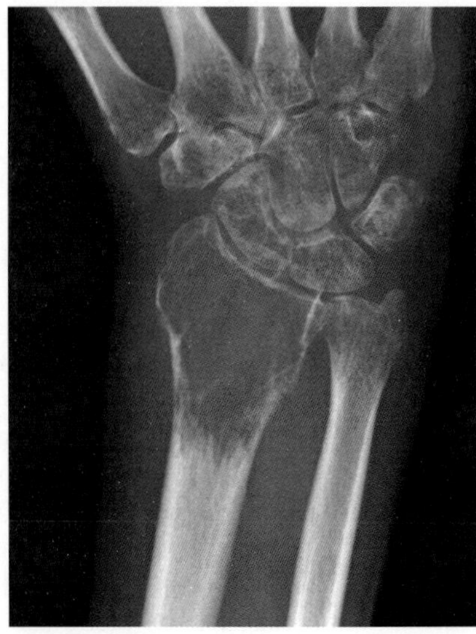

Figure 37.22 Giant cell tumour of the distal radius.

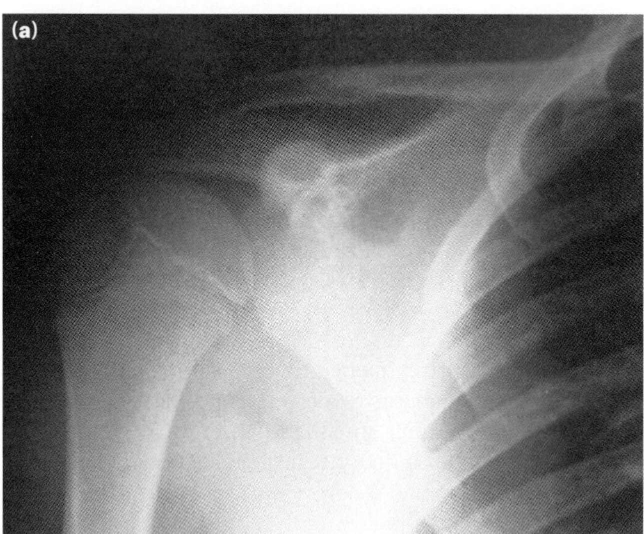

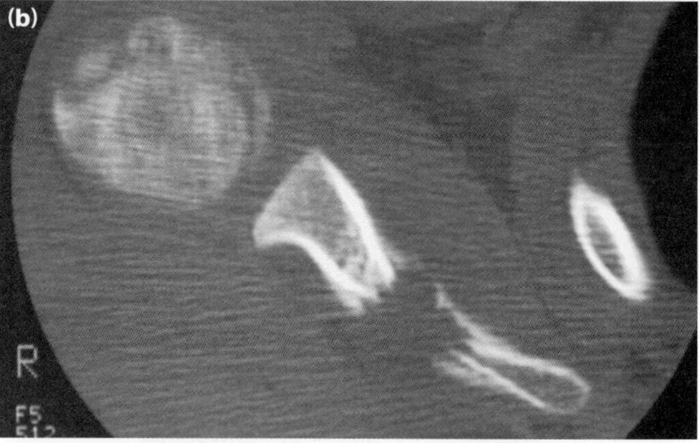

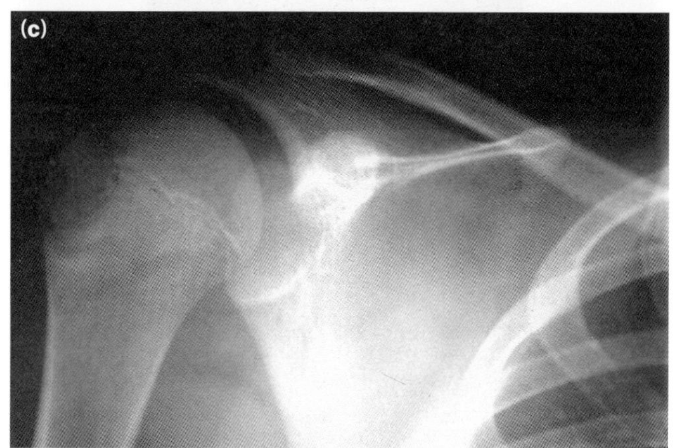

Figure 37.23 (**a**) Eosinophilic granuloma of the scapula. (**b**) Computed tomography scan shows a 'punched-out' lesion. (**c**) Spontaneous resolution.

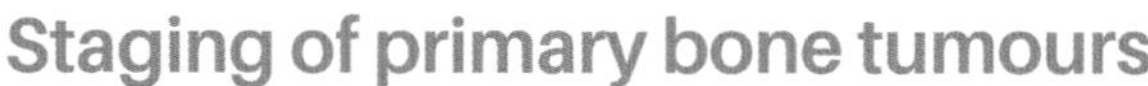

Staging of primary bone tumours

In the Enneking system, benign tumours are staged as:

- latent (e.g. osteochondroma);
- active (e.g. osteoid osteoma);
- aggressive (e.g. giant cell tumour).

Latent lesions are usually asymptomatic and often discovered incidentally. Active lesions, such as osteoid osteoma, present with mild symptoms and continue to grow. Aggressive lesions tend to grow rapidly and destroy bone.

The Enneking staging system for malignant tumours combines the local extent of the tumour and the histological grade (*Table 37.4*). The compartment is the bone in which the tumour arises. A tumour is extracompartmental when it has breached the cortex of the bone. Most primary malignant bone tumours are Enneking stage 2B at diagnosis, meaning they have extended outside the bone of origin but metastases are not detectable. The American Joint Committee on Cancer (AJCC) staging system is also widely used.

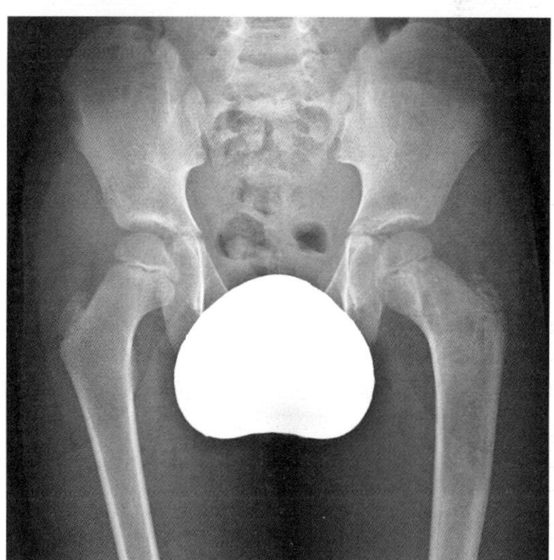

Figure 37.24 Fibrous dysplasia affecting the left proximal femur. There is expansion of the bone with a ground glass appearance.

TABLE 37.4 The Enneking staging system for bone tumours.

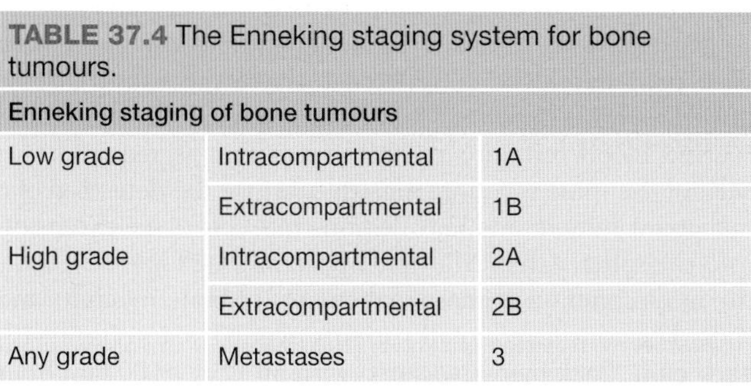

Enneking staging of bone tumours		
Low grade	Intracompartmental	1A
	Extracompartmental	1B
High grade	Intracompartmental	2A
	Extracompartmental	2B
Any grade	Metastases	3

Summary box 37.7

Warning signs - bone tumour

- Non-mechanical bone pain
- Especially around the knee in young adolescents
- Concerning radiographs

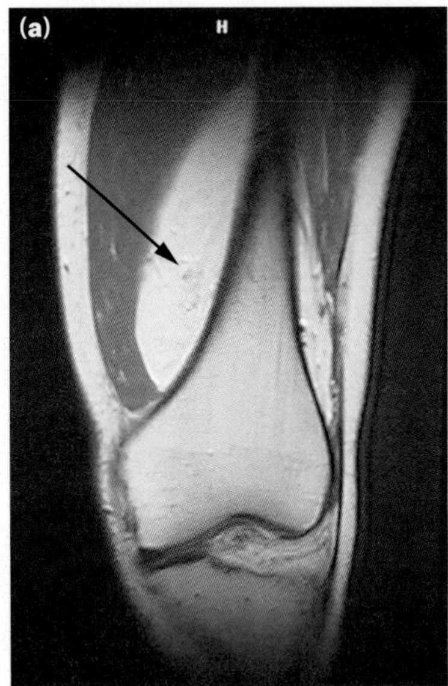

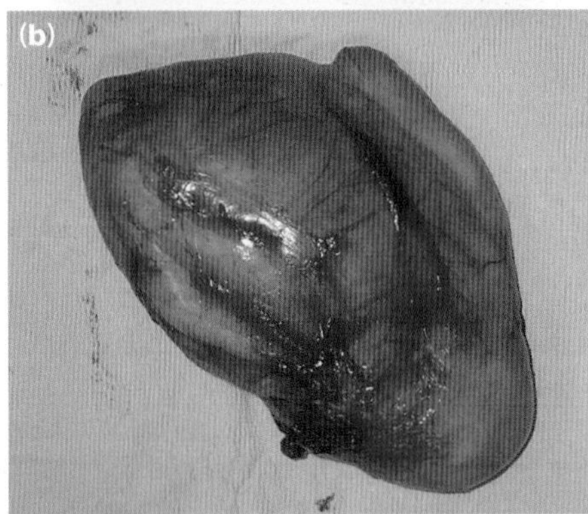

Figure 37.25 (**a**) Coronal T1-weighted magnetic resonance imaging scan showing a benign lipoma deep to the quadriceps muscle (arrow). (**b**) Excised benign lipoma.

SOFT TISSUE TUMOURS

Soft tissue tumours have also historically been classified according to their morphological appearance and presumed cell of origin. The range of biological behaviours is wide and most morphological types have a benign and malignant counterpart, for example lipoma (**Figure 37.25**) and liposarcoma. Other more frequent types include undifferentiated pleomorphic sarcoma and synovial sarcoma. Patients with suspected or confirmed soft tissue sarcomas should be assessed and managed in a specialist centre.

Summary box 37.8

Warning signs - soft tissue tumour

- Larger than 5 cm
- Increasing in size
- Painful
- Deep to the fascia
- Recurrence after previous excision

The Trojani system, based on tumour differentiation, mitotic count and tumour necrosis, is the standard for grading malignant soft tissue tumours. The Enneking and AJCC systems can also be used to stage malignant soft tissue tumours.

EVALUATION AND INVESTIGATION OF THE PATIENT WITH A SUSPECTED BONE OR SOFT TISSUE TUMOUR

The diagnosis and treatment of patients with primary bone and/or soft tissue tumours requires a high index of suspicion, appropriate and prompt investigation, and early referral to a specialist multidisciplinary team for diagnosis, biopsy and appropriate treatment. When a musculoskeletal tumour is suspected, clinicians should:

- stop;
- think;
- investigate.

The assessment and investigation of any patient with a bone or soft tissue tumour can be divided into three phases. The first two phases can be performed at the referring hospital, but the third phase may be best done in a specialist centre (*Table 37.5*).

TABLE 37.5 The three phases of assessment of lesions.

Phase 1 (within 24 hours)	Phase 2 (within first week)	Phase 3 (at specialist centre)
History and examination	Bone scan	CT-scan lesion
Bloods	Ultrasound scan abdomen	MRI-scan lesion
Radiograph whole bone	CT-scan chest	Biopsy
Chest radiograph		

CT, computed tomography; MRI, magnetic resonance imaging.

History and examination

It is important to take a thorough history, including a pain history. Non-mechanical and/or night pain, particularly in the young adolescent, are concerning symptoms and a primary bone tumour should be suspected. Relief with non-steroidal anti-inflammatory drugs may suggest an osteoid osteoma.

Patients with a history of malignancy who present with back pain should be considered to have metastatic disease until proven otherwise. Plain radiographs of the spine and routine blood tests are the minimum that is required. An MRI of the spine is a more sensitive test for the detection of a malignant tumour and may demonstrate soft tissue extension into the spinal canal. Multiple myeloma (see **Figure 37.3**) is the most common primary malignancy of bone in adults and should be considered in all patients over 65 years of age with back pain. Back pain associated with an ESR >100 mm/hour indicates multiple myeloma until proven otherwise. Monoclonal gammopathy or elevated urinary and serum Bence Jones proteins are diagnostic.

Great care should be taken when managing a patient with an apparently 'solitary' bone metastasis. This could be a primary bone tumour, and further investigation including biopsy is required.

Soft tissue tumours are common and the vast majority are benign. However, a soft tissue mass meeting any of the following criteria may be malignant and the patient should be referred to a specialist centre:

- painful;
- increasing in size;
- more than 5 cm in diameter.

In addition, tumours which have recurred after previous excision and tumours located deep to the fascia are more likely to be malignant.

Investigation

The investigation of a patient with a suspected primary bone or soft tissue tumour should include the following.

- Local investigations:
  - ultrasound scan (for soft tissue tumours only);
  - plain radiographs of the whole affected bone or soft tissue lesion (see **Figure 37.1**);
  - MRI of the whole affected bone or soft tissue mass;
  - Computed tomography (CT) scan may be helpful in addition to or instead of MRI scan.
- Distant:
  - blood tests; including full blood count, ESR, urea and electrolytes, bone profile and protein electrophoresis;
  - plain radiographs or CT scan of the chest (more sensitive);
  - whole body isotope bone scan (for suspected primary or metastatic bone tumours);
  - ultrasound or CT scan of abdomen (if renal metastasis is a possibility).

Plain radiographs are usually the most useful imaging investigations in determining the diagnosis of a primary bone tumour, but further appropriate scans are usually required for confirmation and staging. Imaging should always include the whole of the affected bone to look for satellite lesions and skip metastases. Satellite lesions occur within, whilst skip lesions occur beyond, the reactive zone of the tumour.

Both primary bone and soft tissue sarcomas metastasise to the lungs, and a CT scan of the chest is an essential part of staging.

Patients who present with a lytic bone lesion could have a primary renal carcinoma and an ultrasound or CT scan of the abdomen is advised. Biopsy of a renal metastasis can lead to significant blood loss.

Summary box 37.9

Staging

- Plain radiography is most informative for bone tumours
- Always image the whole bone in case of skip lesions
- CT of the lung detects lung metastases
- Lytic lesions require ultrasound of the abdomen to check for a renal primary

Biopsy

A biopsy is performed only when staging investigations have been completed. Because removal of the biopsy track is an important principle in the treatment of sarcomas, biopsies should be performed either in, or after consultation with, the specialist centre where the definitive surgical procedure will be performed.

Image-guided biopsies (usually ultrasound- or CT-guided) have a higher diagnostic accuracy because areas of radiological concern can be targeted. If image-guided biopsy is performed, close discussion between radiologist and surgeon is required to ensure an appropriate biopsy route is used (**Figures 37.26 and 37.27**).

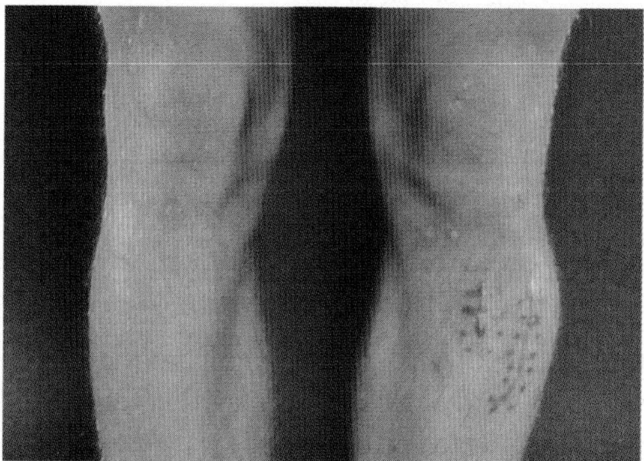

Figure 37.26 Poorly placed biopsies, making subsequent surgical excision of the track impossible.

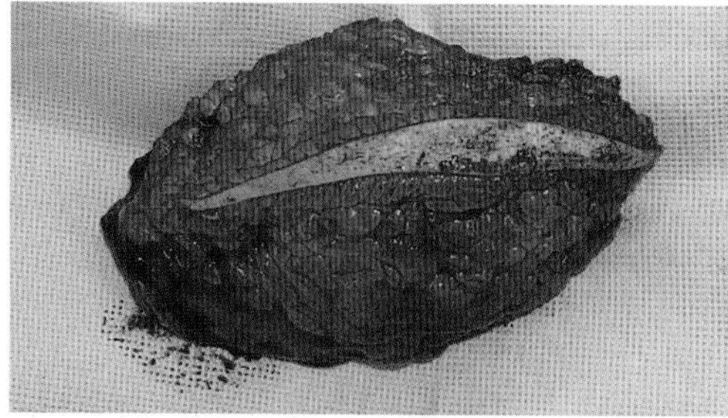

Figure 37.27 *En bloc* excised tumour and biopsy track.

Henry Bence Jones, 1813–1873, physician, St George's Hospital, London, UK.
en bloc is French for 'in a block'.

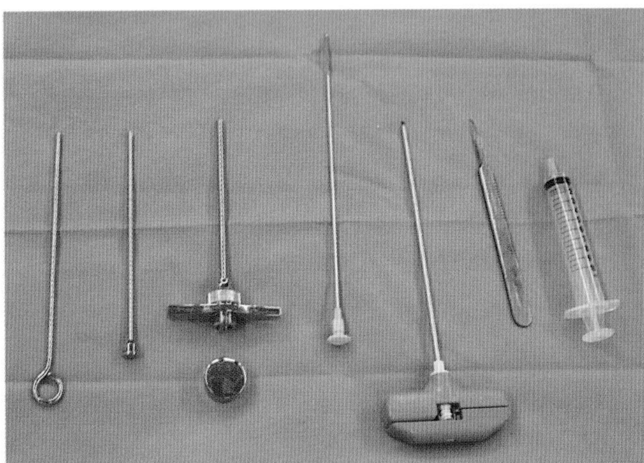

Figure 37.28 Bone biopsy instruments.

Summary box 37.10

Biopsy

- Only biopsy once staging is completed
- Biopsy should be performed at the institution undertaking the main surgery
- Imaging-guided biopsy is more reliable
- The biopsy track must be excised at definitive surgery
- Jamshidi needles for bone, Trucut needles for soft tissues

Biopsies for bone tumours are usually taken using a Jamshidi or other hollow needle (Figure 37.28), while Trucut needles are preferred for soft tissue tumours.

Although most biopsies are performed with a needle, sometimes an open biopsy is required, which should be performed according to the following principles.

- A tourniquet can be used; but exsanguination by compression should be avoided as this may theoretically disseminate the tumour locally or into the circulation.
- Use longitudinal incisions that are part of an extensile approach.
- Do not cross anatomical compartments or contaminate critical anatomical structures (e.g. nerves or blood vessels).
- Use a biopsy track that can be excised at the time of definitive surgery.
- Ensure specimens are sent for microbiology as well as histopathology.
- Some specimens should be sent fresh to the laboratory for cytogenetic studies.

PRINCIPLES OF TREATMENT

Primary bone tumours

Benign

Most latent and active benign bone tumours are treated by intralesional curettage. Packing of the cavity with a graft or bone substitutes is usually not required.

Simple bone cysts usually heal following pathological fracture and an initial conservative approach following fracture is best. If the cyst persists following union of the fracture, and the risk of further fracture is deemed to be high, then a variety of treatments including injection with steroid or bone marrow and surgical curettage have been described.

Osteoid osteomas can resolve spontaneously. However, symptoms are often pronounced and most patients are treated by CT-guided thermocoagulation. Surgical removal (which usually requires burring down onto the surface of the nidus and removing it) is seldom required.

Large or more rapidly growing benign bone tumours may require more extensive surgical excision and reconstruction. Giant cell tumours of bone are associated with a high local recurrence rate and are usually treated with radical curettage or, when very extensive, surgical resection of the affected bone. The RANK-ligand antibody denosumab has an evolving role in treating these tumours.

Malignant tumours

Malignant primary bone tumours require a multidisciplinary approach which may include chemotherapy and radiotherapy as well as surgery. Osteosarcoma and Ewing's sarcoma are treated with neoadjuvant (before surgery) chemotherapy and surgery. Chondrosarcomas are not sensitive to chemotherapy or radiotherapy and treatment is surgical excision where possible.

The aim of surgery for a primary malignant bone tumour is to remove it completely (usually with a layer of normal tissue around it and the biopsy track) and then to reconstruct the limb to maximise physical function.

Following excision the surgical margins can be classified as shown in *Table 37.6*.

TABLE 37.6 Classification of surgical resection margins.

Surgical margins	
Intralesional	Resection through the tumour
Marginal	Resection through the reactive zone of the tumour
Wide	Resection outside the reactive zone of the tumour
Radical	Resection of the whole anatomical compartment

In most cases, limb salvage with excision and reconstruction is possible (Figure 37.29). Only a minority of patients (10–15%) require primary amputation, either because of neurovascular invasion or because the reconstructed limb may be less functional than an amputation (e.g. for some tumours in the foot and ankle). Limb salvage is associated with a slightly higher rate of local recurrence than amputation. However, no difference in overall survival has been demonstrated. The surgical options for malignant primary bone tumours include:

- amputation or van Ness rotationplasty;
- excision alone (for dispensable bones or areas where reconstruction is difficult, e.g. in parts of the pelvis);
- excision and replacement with graft or massive endoprosthesis.

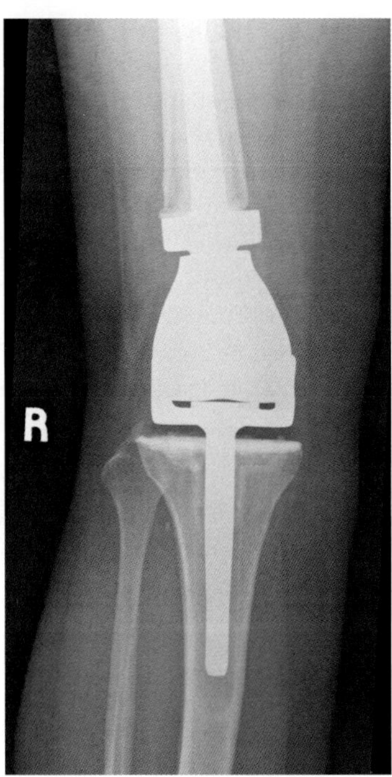

Figure 37.29 Endoprosthetic replacement of the distal femur.

The complications of massive endoprosthetic reconstruction of a limb include infection and wear or loosening of the prosthesis.

Summary box 37.11

Treatment of benign bone tumours

- Benign lesions can be simply curetted
- CT-guided thermocoagulation is used for osteoid osteoma
- Large benign tumours may require reconstruction

Summary box 37.12

Treatment of malignant bone tumours

- Osteosarcomas and Ewing's sarcoma require neoadjuvant chemotherapy
- Chondrosarcomas are insensitive to radiotherapy or chemotherapy
- Most malignant tumours can be treated with limb salvage
- There is no difference in survival between amputation and limb salvage

Metastatic bone disease

Patients with confirmed metastatic bone disease may require resuscitation for electrolyte imbalance, anaemia, cardiorespiratory problems or hypercalcaemia before surgical treatment can be considered. Hypercalcaemia can be treated effectively with fluid resuscitation and bisphosphonate infusion.

Surgical treatment in patients with metastatic bone disease is usually palliative; although radical resection of solitary metastases in selected patients may confer some survival benefit, the evidence for this is not strong.

Surgery of the spine may be required for stabilisation and/or decompression when tumour extension puts the spinal cord at risk. Surgery in the peripheral skeleton is mainly for treatment of (impending) pathological fracture.

Renal metastases tend to be very vascular and massive blood loss can be encountered during surgery. Therefore, preoperative embolisation should be considered just before surgery to prevent blood loss (Figure 37.30).

Treatment of myeloma is mainly haematological. Non-surgical treatments including radiotherapy can lead to healing of bone lesions in some cases. Surgical treatment is only required for complications such as fracture and spinal cord compression.

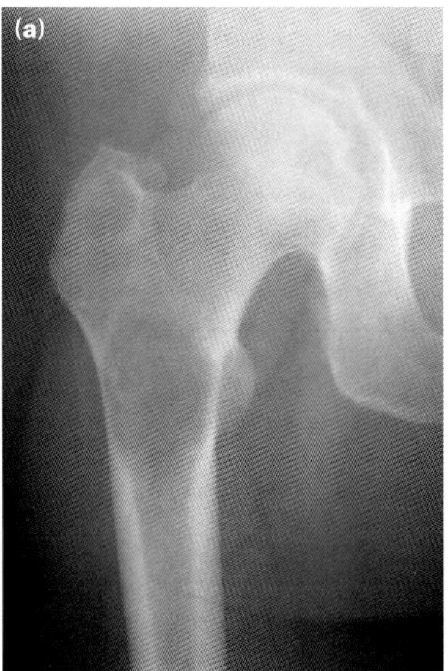

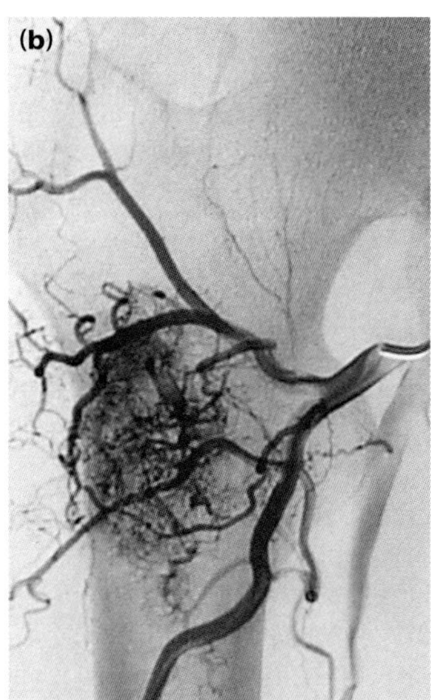

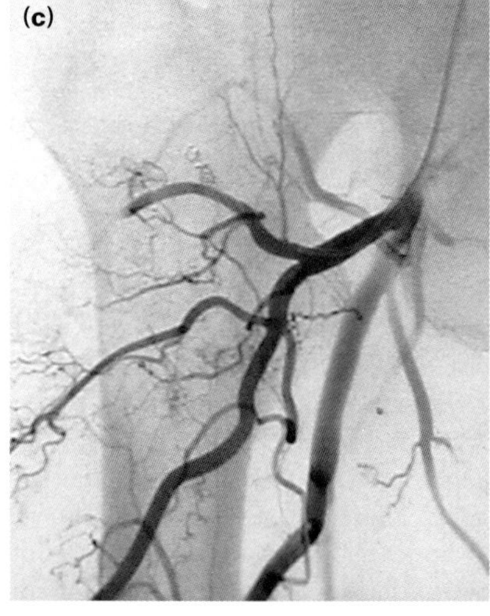

Figure 37.30 (**a**) Lytic metastasis of renal cell carcinoma. (**b**) Angiogram shows increased vascularity. (**c**) Following embolisation.

The following factors should be considered when contemplating surgical treatment for patients with metastatic bone disease:

- likely survival (**Figure 37.31**) – consider the primary diagnosis and performance status;
- quality of life;
- fitness for anaesthesia and surgery;
- fracture risk;
- single or multiple bone lesions;
- response to adjuvant treatment such as radiotherapy and hormonal treatment;
- radiotherapy can be administered pre- or postoperatively.

The risk of pathological fracture can be assessed using the Mirels score (*Table 37.7*).

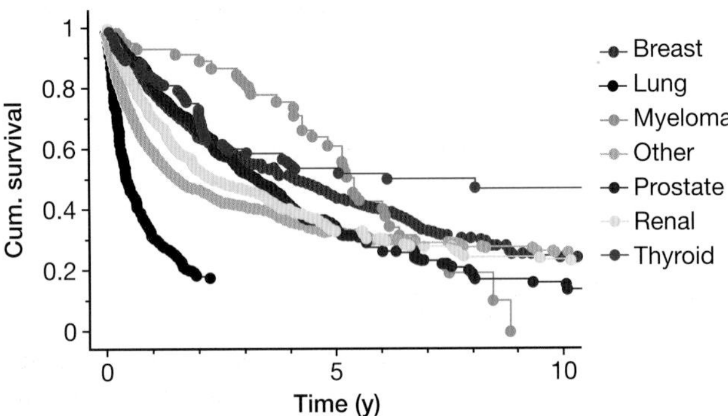

Figure 37.31 Cumulative survival curves of patients who present with bony metastasis.

TABLE 37.7 The Mirels scoring system for risk of pathological fracture.

	Score		
	1	2	3
Site	Upper limb	Lower limb	Peritrochanteric
Pain	Mild	Moderate	Functional
Size	<1/3	1/3–2/3	>2/3
Lesion	Blastic	Mixed	Lytic

Score ≥8, high risk of fracture – urgent prophylactic fixation should be considered; score <8, low risk of fracture – orthopaedic intervention may not be required.

Bone healing following a fracture through a metastasis is unpredictable and there can be local recurrence of the tumour after treatment. The approach is therefore different from the treatment of other fractures. The aim of surgery should be to improve pain and maintain mobility. Approaches which require prolonged protected weight bearing to allow healing are not appropriate in this group of patients with reduced life expectancy. Therefore, as a general rule, prosthetic replacement of bones is preferred, particularly for epiphyseal and metaphyseal lesions. Metastases in the diaphysis may be most appropriately treated with an intramedullary nail. In the shoulder, prosthetic replacements have a poor function and internal fixation may give better physical functioning. However, for hip lesions, the best treatment is often a joint replacement.

Patients with solitary breast and renal metastases can have prolonged disease-free survival so excision and replacement rather than fixation should be the treatment of choice.

Summary box 37.13

Treatment of bone metastases

- Surgery cannot lengthen life but may shorten it
- The spine may need stabilising and nerves or the cord decompressing
- Long bones will need stabilising if a pathological fracture is imminent
- Patients who have a possibility of long-term survival may need a prosthesis
- Radiotherapy relieves pain

Soft tissue tumours

The treatment of soft tissue tumours should take account of tumour type and the response to other treatments including radiotherapy. Large low-grade or benign lipomatous tumours may be excised in a deliberately marginal or close but complete fashion. Soft tissue sarcomas should however be excised with a margin of normal tissue around them wherever possible, and usually including the biopsy track (see **Figure 37.27**). Skin involvement may require resection of the skin and reconstruction with a split skin graft or skin flap.

Following surgical excision of high-grade soft tissue sarcomas, adjuvant radiotherapy should be considered. Preoperative radiotherapy can also have good results, but there is a risk of wound healing problems following surgery. Chemotherapy has a limited role in the treatment of soft tissue sarcomas.

FURTHER READING

British Orthopaedic Oncology Society and British Orthopaedic Association. *Metastatic bone disease. A guide to good practice*. 2015 Revision.

Cool P, Grimer R. Pathological fractures of the extremities. *Trauma* 2000; **2**: 101–11.

Cool P, Grimer R, Rees R. Surveillance in patients with sarcoma of the extremities. *Eur J Surg Oncol* 2005; **31**(9): 1020–4.

Dangoor A, Seddon B, Gerrand C *et al.* UK guidelines for the management of soft tissue sarcomas. *Clin Sarcoma Res* 2016; **6**: 20.

Enneking WF, Spanier SS, Goodman MA. A system for the surgical staging of musculoskeletal sarcoma. *Clin Orthop Relat Res* 1980; **153**: 106–20.

Gerrard C, Athanasou N, Brennan B *et al.* on behalf of the British Sarcoma Group. UK guidelines for the management of bone sarcomas. *Clin Sarcoma Res* 2016; **6**: 7.

Mankin HJ, Lange TA, Spanier SS. The hazards of biopsy in patients with malignant primary bone and soft tissue tumors. *J Bone Joint Surg* 1982; **64-A**: 1121–7.

Mirels H. Metastatic disease in long bones. *Clin Orthop* 1989: **249**: 256–64.

Wedin R, Bauer HC. Surgical treatment of skeletal metastatic lesions of the proximal femur: endoprosthesis or reconstruction nail? *J Bone Joint Surg Br* 2005; **87**(12): 1653–7.

World Health Organization, International Agency for Research on Cancer. *WHO classification of tumours of soft tissue and bone*, 4th edition. Lyon: IARC Press, 2013.

Chapter 38

Infection of the bones and joints

Learning objectives

To understand:

- Characteristic features in the history and examination of infection of bone and joint
- Diagnostic principles in bone and joint infection
- Treatment of infection of native bone and joint
- Treatment of implant-associated orthopaedic infection

INTRODUCTION

Osteomyelitis is an old disease, identified in dinosaur bones, early hominids and skeletons from ancient civilisations. While infections of native bones and joints persist as a relevant problem in the twenty-first century, implant-associated infection has progressively emerged as a new and major challenge to healthcare systems.

Orthopaedic infection can present acutely with major systemic upset, local inflammation and purulence, or insidiously, with gradual bone destruction leading to loss of function and slowly evolving local symptoms, in the presence or absence of systemic features.

Bone and joint infection causes a substantial burden of complex morbidity. Acute infections can be life or limb threatening, while undiagnosed or incompletely treated infection can persist for decades, causing pain and interfering with activities of daily living. In turn, this has the potential for complicated psychosocial impact on patients and their families.

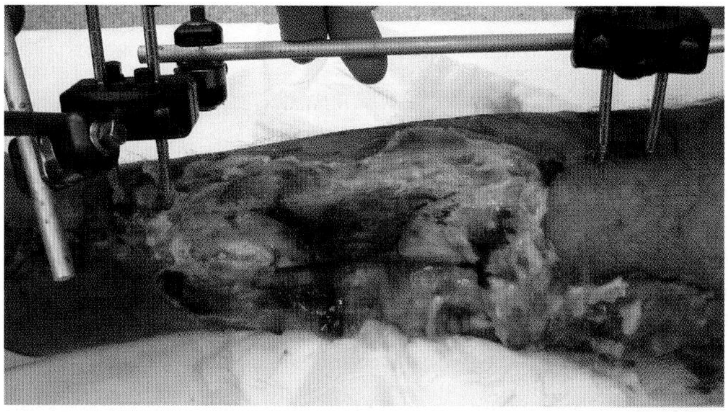

Figure 38.1 An infected open fracture of the tibia that has been stabilised with an external fixator. The central fracture fragment is dead.

EPIDEMIOLOGY

The pattern of bone infection is changing. Worldwide, childhood acute haematogenous osteomyelitis and septic arthritis are common, with chronic disease following inadequate initial management. In resource-rich countries, bone infection is now mostly seen after injury or surgery (contiguous focus osteomyelitis) and is often implant-related (**Figure 38.1**). The high number of patients with comorbidities (diabetes, peripheral vascular disease, immunocompromise), more frequent bone and joint surgery and longer population survival contribute to a group of patients with increased susceptibility to infection. In the UK, the number of prosthetic joint replacements (hip, knee) has doubled in 15 years. It is projected that, in the USA, there will be around 65 000 new infected joints in 2020. Although the incidence of infection after fracture has decreased, the increased use of internal fixation has increased the prevalence of post-traumatic bone infection overall. This will produce a significant economic burden for healthcare providers in the future.

Summary box 38.1

Epidemiology of bone infection

- Bone and joint infections from haematogenous spread remain common worldwide
- The increased use of implants for joint replacement and fracture fixation is an important source of new infections
- Immunocompromised patients are another increasing source (e.g. diabetes, cancer treatment)

GENERAL PRINCIPLES OF ORTHOPAEDIC INFECTION

Pathology

Acute osteomyelitis occurs when pathogenic organisms cause infection, leading to inflammation in the bone and surrounding tissues. The medullary bone may form abscesses and the infection may track through the cortex to form periosteal elevation and soft-tissue extension. This process will devascularise the bone, causing bone death – the characteristic feature of chronic osteomyelitis.

Bacteria can adhere to dead bone or implant surfaces, forming a complex community enveloped in a polysaccharide matrix, known as a biofilm. These bacteria alter their metabolic state, making them more resistant both to the host immune system and to antibiotics. Toxins and lytic enzymes from bacteria cause early damage to articular cartilage.

The infected bone reacts to the infection by separating dead fragments of bone (sequestration) and forming sinuses to drain pus and discharge small bone fragments. New bone is laid down around the infection from the periosteum (involucrum) (**Figure 38.2**).

In septic arthritis, infection may follow direct ingress of bacteria after injury or surgery, or may result from discharge of an adjacent acute osteomyelitis into the joint. Particularly in neonates or the elderly, bacteraemia may infect a previously normal joint.

Microbiology

Virulent gram-positive organisms, particularly *Staphylococcus aureus*, are the most common cause of bone or joint infection in native tissue. However, once prosthetic material is implanted, a wide range of organisms can be involved. This includes organisms with low virulence that are usually considered skin commensals, such as coagulase-negative staphylococci, alpha-haemolytic streptococci and propionibacteria (*Table 38.1*).

TABLE 38.1 Organisms most commonly involved in bone and joint infection.

Classification of infection	Group(s) of organisms	Examples of specific organisms and context in which infection occurs
Gram positive	Staphylococci	*Staphylococcus aureus* (commonest across all settings) Coagulase-negative staphylococci (common in implant-associated infection)
	Streptococci	Alpha-haemolytic streptococci, including *S. pneumoniae*, *S. milleri* group and *S. viridans* (in implant-associated infection)
		Beta-haemolytic streptococci (e.g. *S. pyogenes*, *S. agalactiae*)
	Propionibacteria	Increasingly recognised in implant-associated infection and septic arthritis of the shoulder
Gram negative	Enterobacteriaceae	*Escherichia coli* (especially at extremes of age)
		Klebsiella species
		Salmonella species (particularly associated with sickle cell disease)
	Pseudomonas species	Associated with diabetic foot infections, osteomyelitis underlying chronic wounds/ulcers, patients heavily exposed to hospital environment and/or prior antibiotics
	Haemophilus species	*H. influenzae* (consider in non-immunised children)
	Neisseria species	*N. meningitidis*
		N. gonorrhoeae (consider risk factors for sexually transmitted infection)
Others	Anaerobes	
	Fungi	(Cause infection in immunocompromised and/or heavily antibiotic-exposed hosts)
	Mycobacteria	*Mycobacterium tuberculosis*
		Atypical mycobacteria (may be a component of disseminated infection in HIV-infected patients; also cause postsurgical infection in immunocompetent hosts)
Mixed	Any combination of the above organisms	More common after trauma, recurrent surgery, with poor wound healing and sinuses, or resulting from contiguous spread from an infected source (e.g. skin, gastrointestinal tract)
'Culture negative'	No growth from cultures, but diagnosis of infection made on clinical/radiological/histopathological grounds	Most common in patients who have had recent antimicrobial exposure prior to surgical sampling

HIV, human immunodeficiency virus.

Summary box 38.2

Pathology of bone infection

- Bacteria infecting bone form a resistant biofilm on dead bone and implant surfaces
- Infected bone dies and forms a sequestrum
- The periosteum around lays down new bone – an involucrum

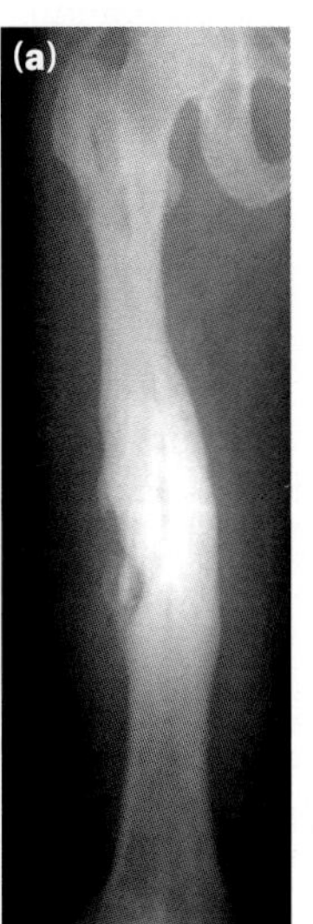

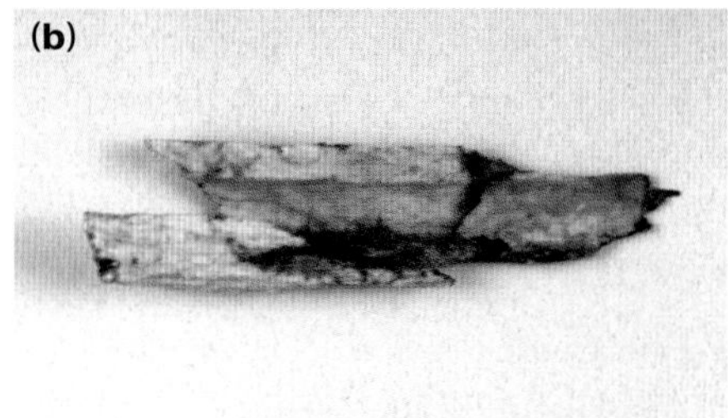

Figure 38.2 (a) Radiograph of chronic infection of the femur with a large central sequestrum and well developed involucrum. (b) The sequestrum removed from the mid-femur at surgery.

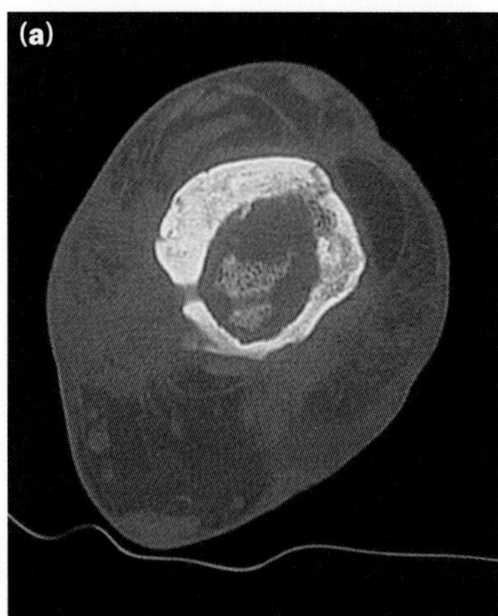

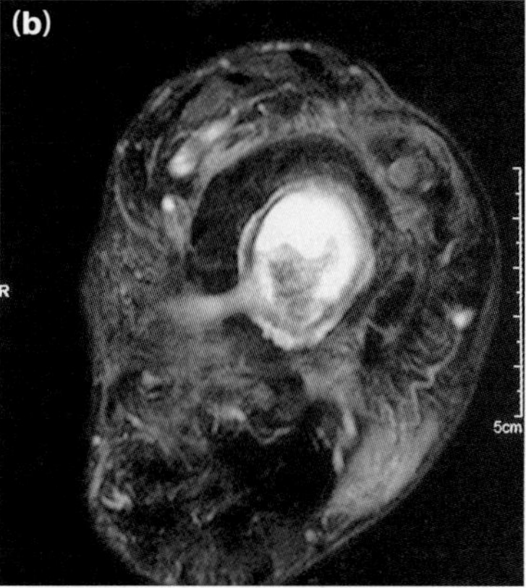

Figure 38.3 (a) Transverse computed tomography scan of femur with central sequestrum, sinus and cortical bone erosion. (b) Magnetic resonance imaging scan of the same femur with better resolution of medullary infection and soft-tissue involvement.

Diagnosis

Clinical

Diagnosis is predominantly clinical with confirmation using other tests, as outlined below.

Biomarkers

Raised inflammatory markers (erythrocyte sedimentation rate (ESR), C-reactive protein (CRP) and white cell count (WCC)) are characteristic of acute infection, but they are insufficiently sensitive or specific to rule infection in or out.

Imaging

Plain radiographs can demonstrate dead bone, periosteal reaction, involucrum formation and loosening of implants. However, in the early stages of acute infection, plain radiographs may be normal and should not be used to exclude infection. Serial radiography is most useful in charting the onset of implant loosening, bone lysis or progression of chronic osteomyelitis.

Ultrasonography is ideal for identifying soft-tissue collections and joint effusions and can be used to guide bone biopsy and aspiration.

Computed tomography (CT) scans are helpful in assessing bone union of infected fractures. Small sequestra and cortical erosions are best seen with CT and these scans can be used to plan surgery for excision of dead bone (Figure 38.3a).

Isotope bone scans are of very limited value as they are non-specific and give no information which may guide diagnosis or treatment. The combination of ^{18}F-fluorodeoxyglucose positron-emission tomography (^{18}FDG-PET) with a CT scan allows localisation of active infection in chronic osteomyelitis and may facilitate planning of surgery. However, ^{18}FDG-PET/CT is not specific for infection and so cannot reliably distinguish infective from aseptic loosening in implants.

Magnetic resonance imaging (MRI) scanning is the investigation of choice. It is highly sensitive and specific, showing all components of the disease (Figure 38.3b). However, it can be adversely affected by metal implants and can overestimate the extent of infection when there is widespread reactive oedema.

Culture and susceptibility

Superficial samples from wounds or spontaneously draining pus are unreliable for culture, because the organisms colonising the surface may bear no relation to those causing the invasive infection in the deeper tissues. Microbiological samples may be falsely negative if antibiotics are given first. Synovial tissue samples are particularly important in producing a higher diagnostic yield for infection with mycobacteria or fungi.

In complex infections, particularly those involving prosthetic material, multiple biopsy samples are needed to help determine whether organisms such as coagulase-negative staphylococci are likely to be the causative pathogens, or whether they are simply contaminants from the skin. This distinction cannot be made on a single sample, but the growth of an indistinguishable organism from three or more culture samples is 94% specific for infection.

It is also possible to culture organisms from removed implants which have been subjected to ultrasonic vibration to disrupt biofilm (sonication).

Histopathology

The histological diagnosis of infection (rather than other sources of inflammation) depends on identifying organisms on a Gram stain, or the presence of a neutrophilic infiltrate. However, such an infiltrate may be patchy and so histological studies are incompletely sensitive. Histology is valuable in confirming the presence of infection in culture-negative cases.

Summary box 38.3

Principles of diagnosis

- ESR and CRP are neither sensitive nor specific in making a diagnosis of bone infection
- Plain radiographs may be normal in the early phase
- Ultrasound is valuable for identifying fluid/pus collections
- MRI is usually the investigation of choice
- Superficial swabs are of no value in identifying the organism causing deep infection
- If the patient is on antibiotics, cultures may be falsely negative
- Multiple biopsy specimens should be obtained to optimise microbiological diagnosis
- A neutrophil infiltrate on histology is strongly indicative of infection

Management

Successful treatment relies on the careful multidisciplinary delivery of a package of care, summarised as follows:

- Preoperative:
  - Patient assessment and clinical staging of disease.
  - Full discussion of all treatment options with potential complications.
  - Diagnostic tests for general health.
  - Optimisation of patients and treatment of comorbidities.
- Operative:
  - Exposure for multiple, deep bone sampling.
  - Excision of all non-viable tissue.
  - Intravenous antibiotics after sampling.
  - Bone stabilisation, if necessary.
  - Dead space management.
  - Soft-tissue cover which may include plastic surgery.
- Postoperative:
  - Functional rehabilitation.
  - Continued antimicrobial therapy guided by culture results, with regular clinical monitoring.

Patients with bone and joint infections should be treated in centres which have the facilities to manage all aspects of this care. With the exception of those who are acutely ill with sepsis, there is usually time to optimise comorbidities and improve general health prior to surgical treatment of the infection. Attention to diabetes control, peripheral vascular disease, nutrition and smoking cessation is essential. Many patients will benefit from psychological support or at least good counselling around the difficulties of eradicating infection and the components of treatment.

For patients requiring long courses of intravenous antibiotics, outpatient parenteral antibiotic therapy (OPAT) services can facilitate discharge from hospital. They must be delivered by a dedicated team with experience in supervising and supporting all aspects of intravenous therapy in the community, including surveillance and care of a long-line, monitoring for side effects and toxicity, management of complications and accessing appropriate psychosocial support.

Antibiotic therapy

Patients with septic shock, or with rapidly advancing local or systemic signs of infection, should receive prompt empirical antibiotic therapy. When delay in antibiotics would be unsafe, blood cultures, local aspiration of pus or radiologically guided biopsy may give valuable culture material immediately prior to starting antibiotics.

In the majority of cases, it is safe to delay antibiotics until definitive operative microbiological samples have been taken; this is particularly important when prosthetic material is involved. For patients who have already been started on antibiotics, a clinical assessment should be made, and – if safe to do so – antibiotics should be stopped at least 2 weeks before biopsy or surgery.

Local guidelines should be followed, but most hospitals recommend a 'community acquired' level of cover using an agent such as co-amoxiclav. Additional antibiotics to cover resistant gram-positive organisms (e.g. vancomycin for methicillin-resistant *Staphylococcus aureus* (MRSA)) are considered if there has been significant prior hospital exposure or if the patient is known to be colonised with these organisms. Cover for resistant gram-negative organisms (e.g. meropenem for *Pseudomonas*) is considered in certain settings, including severe diabetic foot infection.

Prolonged intravenous antibiotic courses (i.e. 4–6 weeks of treatment) are usually recommended for bone infection, although there is little evidence to support this.

Summary box 38.4

Antibiotics for osteomyelitis

- Septic shock needs treatment without delay, with antibiotics chosen empirically based on local guidelines
- In clinically stable patients, antibiotics should be delayed until specimens have been taken
- In elective surgery for osteomyelitis, antibiotics should be stopped at least 2 weeks in advance
- Agents such as co-amoxiclav or ceftriaxone are appropriate for most community acquired infections
- Vancomycin provides cover for MRSA
- Meropenem may be needed for *Pseudomonas* species and other resistant gram-negative organisms

NATIVE JOINT SEPTIC ARTHRITIS

Epidemiology

Bacterial infection of native joints occurs at an estimated incidence of 4–10 per 100 000 population per year in Western Europe, with higher rates in association with socioeconomic deprivation and in resource-poor countries. The condition most characteristically affects patients at extremes of age, and in the context of an underlying joint abnormality or immunocompromise (*Table 38.2*).

Joint infection may arise as a result of haematogenous dissemination of bacteria from another focus (e.g. endocarditis), or may occur as a result of direct inoculation or local extension from an infected source (e.g. traumatic wound).

TABLE 38.2 Risk factors for native joint septic arthritis.

- Extremes of age
- Underlying joint abnormality, especially rheumatoid arthritis
- Immunocompromise (e.g. diabetes mellitus, human immunodeficiency virus infection, immunosuppressive therapy)
- Joint instrumentation (e.g. steroid injection, arthroscopy)
- Intravenous drug abuse
- Indwelling central venous catheter
- Bacteraemia (especially *Staphylococcus aureus*)

Clinical features

Most patients present with an acute or subacute history of a single hot, swollen, painful joint. In children, there is often a history of recent minor trauma. The joint is held immobile in the 'position of comfort', and there is severe pain if any attempt is made to move the affected joint actively or passively. In children and adults, the knee joint is most frequently affected; in neonates, the hip. Fever and other systemic signs are usually present, but their absence does not rule out the diagnosis, especially in adults, where there may be no fever or only a low-grade one.

Diagnosis

Aspiration and/or biopsy of intra-articular fluid or tissue will allow a Gram stain to be performed (although this is positive in only about one-third of infected cases), and then culture of a causative organism (positive in 80–90%). However, results are delayed by the time taken to grow and identify the organism in the laboratory. A high WCC in joint fluid (e.g. 50–150 000 cells/mm^3), with a neutrophil predominance, is characteristic of infection. However, other inflammatory conditions can also cause a raised cell count, and crystals may be seen in infected joints as well as gout or pseudo-gout. The limited sensitivity and specificity of direct microscopy and Gram stain, and the time taken to obtain a positive culture result, should not delay early treatment for the infection. The decision to perform a surgical washout and give antibiotics should therefore be based on the clinical picture.

Summary box 38.5

Presentation of septic arthritis

- Children may be toxic and febrile but adults may only have a low-grade fever
- The joint is swollen and held in a characteristic 'position of comfort'
- Any movement causes extreme pain

Management

Surgical management

Medical treatment alone is rarely indicated in joint sepsis. Prompt surgical drainage is a priority in order to avoid further damage to the joint. In general, open washout is preferred to arthroscopic washout, depending on the joint involved. Inadequate clearance may lead to chronic infection with destruction of the joint (**Figure 38.4**). Treatment

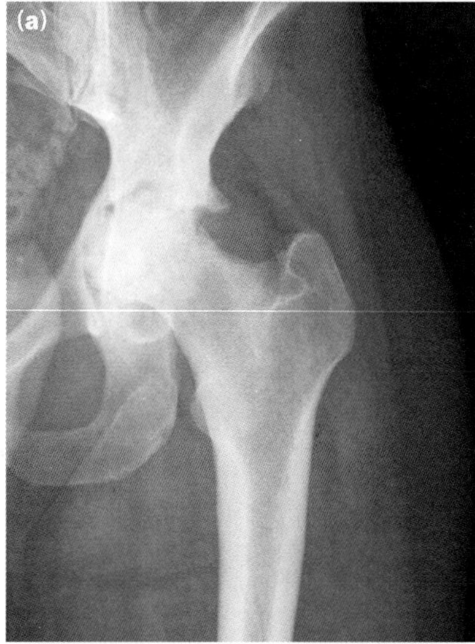

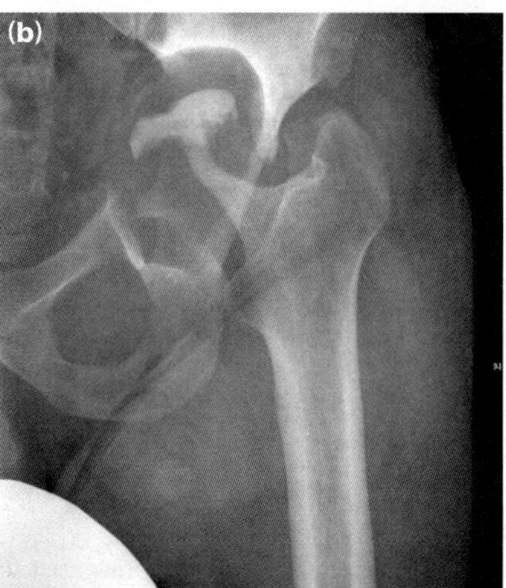

Figure 38.4 (a) Septic arthritis of the hip in an intravenous drug user. This was untreated for several weeks, resulting in destruction of the joint surface. **(b)** The same hip after 9 months without treatment. The proximal femur and acetabulum have been grossly eroded by infection.

may then require joint excision, joint fusion or staged joint replacement.

Medical management

Antibiotics are usually given for 4–6 weeks (of which at least the first 2 weeks are commonly given intravenously). There are sparse data to guide duration; in general, longer courses should be considered if the infection is slow to resolve, if more than one washout is required, if the patient is bacteraemic and/or if the infection is caused by *Staphylococcus aureus*. Choice of antibiotics can be summarised as above (see *Summary box 38.4*).

Summary box 38.6

Native joint septic arthritis

- Most common at extremes of age, in patients with rheumatoid arthritis and in association with immunocompromise
- Most commonly affects hips in neonates, and knees in adults and children
- The commonest pathogen is *Staphylococcus aureus*
- Joints should be aspirated for microbiology before starting antibiotics if safe to do so
- Management is prompt surgical joint washout, followed by 4–6 weeks of antibiotics
- Joint fluid Gram stain and WCC are poorly predictive of infection

IMPLANT-RELATED INFECTION

Epidemiology

The incidence of prosthetic joint infection in the UK is now <1% per joint per year, with hips at slightly higher risk than knees. These rates have fallen with improved operative practice and the recent introduction of surgical 'care bundles'. Risk factors include obesity, skin disease, comorbidity, prolonged or complicated surgery, revision surgery, fracture and postoperative wound infection or haematoma.

Infection complicates around 3–5% of all fracture fixations. Open tibial fractures are a high-risk group with up to 15% becoming infected after fixation. Calcaneal fractures and ankle fracture fixation in the elderly also have high infection rates.

Clinical features

Implant-related infections may present early (within 2 weeks of injury or surgery), in a delayed manner (3–10 weeks from surgery) or late (after 10 weeks).

Early infections are acquired at surgery or injury and are usually caused by virulent organisms (e.g. *Staphylococcus aureus*). They present with a discharging wound, cellulitis, pain, inflammation and swelling.

Delayed infections are more characteristically due to low-virulence organisms (e.g. coagulase-negative staphylococci or propionibacteria).

Late infections are more likely to present with an indolent clinical syndrome of joint discomfort or mechanical dysfunction ('start-up' symptoms are particularly characteristic), with or without a discharging sinus. Late presentations may represent a new haematogenous infection of a previously uninfected joint and can occur years after implantation. More often, they are due to a recurrence of a previously inadequately treated early or delayed infection.

Diagnosis

Infection should be suspected in any patient with a leaking wound over an implant, unresolved pain or new pain around a previously pain-free implant. Routine blood tests may be helpful in acute infection but are often falsely reassuring.

Plain radiographs may show features of loosening of a chronically infected prosthesis, and ultrasound may identify associated collections. Nuclear scans cannot distinguish aseptic loosening from infection. The gold standard for diagnosis is the culture of microorganisms from clean, deep samples (see above, under 'Diagnosis'). These should be taken at the time of revision surgery or open debridement.

Summary box 38.7

Implant-associated infection

- Good centres should have an infection rate of <1% per joint per year
- Internal fixation of open fractures remains a high infection risk
- Late infection may present with low-grade symptoms (grumbling pain and start-up stiffness)
- Radiographs may show lucency around the implant
- Multiple specimens need to be taken at surgery for reliable diagnosis

Management

A multidisciplinary approach is required, including orthopaedics, plastic surgery, infectious diseases/microbiology, pharmacy, nursing, occupational therapy and physiotherapy, centred on the patient's understanding and wishes regarding their condition. Many of these patients have other medical comorbidities which should also be addressed and optimised. Implant-associated infections can be associated with a range of emotional, psychological and mental health issues, ranging from anger about surgical complications to depression arising from chronic symptoms, lack of function and prolonged hospitalisation.

The choice of surgical strategy for prosthetic joints can be categorised as:

- salvage of an infected implant;
- removal of the infected implant with or without reimplantation.

Some groups have used the timing of presentation to determine this (i.e. salvage for early infection, versus removal and revision for late infection). Others regard any firmly fixed implant as potentially salvageable, irrespective of the timing (and there are now several case series suggesting that this is feasible). However, it is agreed that loose infected implants should always be removed (Figure 38.5). Furthermore, it is essential to achieve soft-tissue cover of bone and prosthetic material. This may be difficult around the knee, requiring local muscle flaps and the involvement of a plastic surgical team.

Management options can be divided into the following broad approaches:

- Debridement, antibiotics and implant retention, 'DAIR': This can only be undertaken if the prosthesis is well-fixed. The surrounding infected soft tissue and bone must be fully excised and modular components exchanged. This cannot be achieved by arthroscopic surgery. Good soft-tissue cover is essential. Following debridement, the patient is treated with long-term antibiotics (frequently 6 weeks of intravenous therapy followed by 6 months or more of oral antibiotics). Prolonged infection-free intervals will be achieved in 80% of patients but success with this strategy may be lower in infections caused by *Staphylococcus aureus*.
- Two-stage joint revision surgery: A thorough excision is undertaken and all cement and loose foreign material is removed. An antibiotic-impregnated spacer may be implanted (which may be articulating). This is a temporary measure and cannot withstand full weight bearing. The patient is treated with oral or intravenous antibiotics, most commonly for 6 weeks. A new prosthesis is implanted after the course of antibiotics has been completed. Re-revision surgery for infection has a higher failure rate than a first revision, and so early referral to a specialist centre should be considered.
- Single-stage joint revision surgery: the procedure is the same as above, but removal and reimplantation are undertaken in the same operating session. Healthy soft tissues around the new implant are essential to prevent reinfection. Some centres consider single-stage revisions when less florid signs of infection are present (i.e. absence of collections or sinus tracts), or for frail patients for whom the risk of a second operation is higher. There are no adequate trial data comparing outcomes with the two-stage approach.
- Joint removal or fusion: For patients who have intolerable symptoms (either pain or profuse discharge), but for whom the surgical strategies outlined above are technically not possible or are ruled out by comorbid conditions, removal of the prosthesis without reimplantation may palliate symptoms. An example is the Girdlestone hip arthroplasty. In prosthetic infections of the knee, ankle or wrist, it may be possible to create a joint fusion after prosthesis removal. This is complex surgery, which may involve major bone reconstruction. Amputation may be necessary for knee or ankle implants.
- Suppressive therapy with antibiotics: In patients who are not medically fit for any operative intervention, or who choose to decline all surgical options, long-term treatment with antibiotics may help to suppress the symptoms of infection. There are limited data, but anecdotally the success rate of this approach seems low.

Antimicrobial therapy for implant-associated infection

Following surgical sampling, it is frequently routine practice to institute broad-spectrum antibiotic therapy (e.g. vancomycin and meropenem) and then to rationalise this in the subsequent

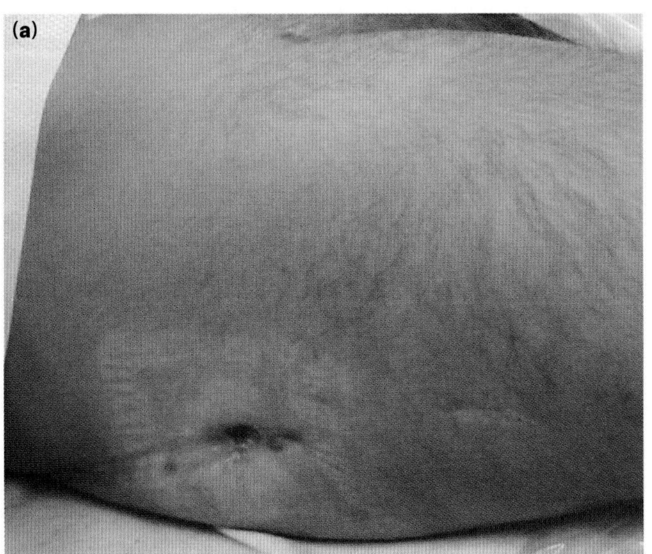

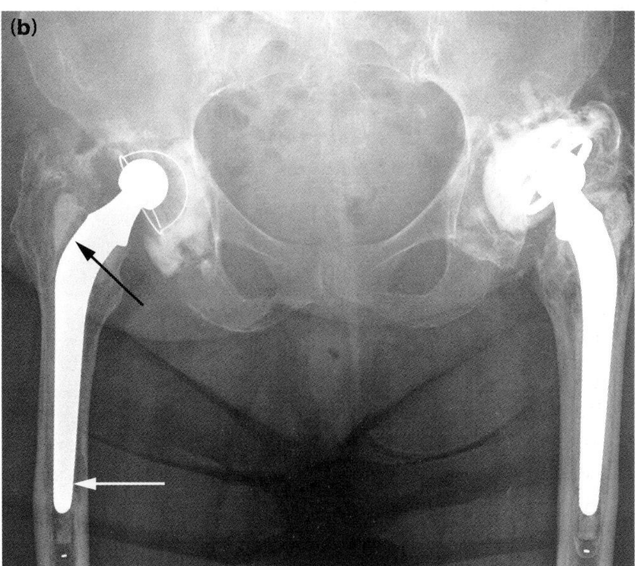

Figure 38.5 **(a)** Sinus draining from a scar over the lateral side of the hip. This patient had a total hip replacement 14 years before that had been complicated by a wound haematoma and infection. **(b)** Radiograph of both hips of the same patient. Both hips are loose but only the right side has definite infection (arrows).

Gathorne Robert Girdlestone, 1881–1950, Nuffield Professor of Orthopaedics, University of Oxford, UK, described excision arthroplasty of the hip for septic arthritis.

48–72 hours according to culture results. In culture-negative cases, ongoing therapy to cover the most likely pathogens should be instituted.

The duration of therapy is determined according to the surgical approach, with 6 weeks for those in whom prosthetic material is completely removed, versus 6 months for patients undergoing a 'DAIR' strategy, and prolonged (occasionally life-long) treatment for patients in whom all other options are contraindicated or intolerable. In a small subset of patients, the best therapy is no intervention, when chronic low-grade symptoms are well controlled and preferable to the risks of either surgery or long-term antibiotic therapy.

The antibiotic regimen should be planned with the advice of a microbiologist, and supervised carefully to promote compliance, and to detect and manage side effects. Monitoring of the joint is largely on clinical grounds; biomarkers including CRP are not predictive of treatment failure.

Serial radiographs are helpful to detect progressive bone loss, which may be an indicator of recurrent active infection and can predispose to periprosthetic fracture and implant loosening.

Summary box 38.8

Prosthetic joint Iinfection

- Well-fixed prostheses may be debrided, treated with antibiotics and the implant retained ('DAIR' approach)
- Loose prostheses must be removed
- Replacement can be made at the initial surgery (one-stage) or after a delay to allow infection to be eradicated with a course of antibiotics (two-stage)
- Multiple surgical samples are crucial for identifying a pathogen
- Thorough excision of infected tissue is a key determinant of outcome
- Long-term antibiotics may be used for patients who are not suitable for major revision surgery

INFECTION FOLLOWING FRACTURE FIXATION

Many of the principles outlined above can be applied to infections associated with metalwork used to fix fractures.

There may be several clinical scenarios which must be addressed:

- Unhealed fracture with stable fixation: This is usually seen early after fixation and can be managed with deep sampling, debridement of infected tissues and management of dead spaces (often with local antibiotic carriers). It is extremely important to provide good soft tissue cover over the fracture. In the tibia, this will most often require a plastic surgical reconstruction. After surgery, systemic antibiotics must be given to suppress infection until bone union, followed by removal of the implant.
- Healed fracture with infected implant: In these cases, the implant can be removed, but there should still be a careful debridement, deep sampling, dead space management and soft tissue cover.
- Unhealed fracture with unstable fixation: Stability is essential for bone healing and eradiation of infection. If the implant is not stable, it should be removed and replaced by an external fixator. Radical excision of the infected fracture is needed and the resulting defect may present a major reconstructive challenge (**Figure 38.6**). Recently, antibiotic-coated implants have been used to stabilise infected fractures with some success.

ACUTE OSTEOMYELITIS

This presents like septic arthritis with a short history of pain, loss of function and systemic upset. In adults, the vertebral column is the commonest site; in children, long bones are most frequently affected and there may be swelling of the affected limb. In young children, a fever and refusal to bear weight may be the only clues.

Diagnosis

In the early phase (2–3 days) radiographs may be normal but MRI will show bone oedema and periosteal elevation. After 5–7 days, plain radiographs may show subtle abnormality with osteopenia and periosteal new bone formation. The WCC and CRP are often abnormal in the early phase. Treatment should not be delayed pending investigations.

Management

Acute osteomyelitis can be treated with antibiotics alone when the diagnosis is made within 2–3 days of onset of symptoms, there is no dead bone on imaging and there is no adjacent septic arthritis. Culture results help to guide therapy, so blood cultures should be taken, and radiologically guided sampling should be considered. Prompt intravenous antibiotics, active against community-acquired pathogens, should then be started (see *Summary box 38.4*).

The limb should be splinted and good analgesia given. Intravenous antibiotics may be converted to oral therapy, depending on clinical progress and the results of cultures, and therapy is continued for a total of at least 4 weeks. If the patient does not respond rapidly, the limb deteriorates or there is imaging evidence of progression of disease, surgery is indicated to prevent bone destruction and the onset of chronic osteomyelitis.

With prompt treatment, acute bone infection has a good prognosis with a 90% cure rate. Failure to treat adequately produces chronicity, with recurrent infection over many years. In children, the adjacent growth plates and joints may be affected with subsequent deformity and joint destruction.

CHRONIC OSTEOMYELITIS

This is a serious condition which may affect the patient for decades. Chronic bone infection is best treated by a dedicated multidisciplinary team, who have the skills to deal with all aspects of the condition, the associated comorbidities and the range of surgical reconstructive options.

Summary box 38.9

Acute osteomyelitis

- Presents in children with toxaemia, fever and unwillingness to move the limb
- May affect the vertebral column in adults, where back pain may be the only symptom
- Radiographs may be normal for up to 1 week so are of limited value in early diagnosis
- WCC and CRP are usually raised
- Early diagnosis is treated with high dose intravenous antibiotics, started empirically and modified with culture results
- Late diagnosis and/or failure of medical treatment requires surgical debridement

Diagnosis

Plain radiographs can delineate soft-tissue swelling, subperiosteal reaction, bone destruction and sequestra. CT scans are good for cortical bone imaging and for planning surgical excision. MRI is the imaging test of choice (see 'General principles' section). Blood tests are often normal in chronic osteomyelitis.

Management

The Cierny and Mader classification helps to define the features of the infection in the bone (four stages) and to relate this to the general condition of the patient (three groups). Patients can be divided into three physiological 'host types'

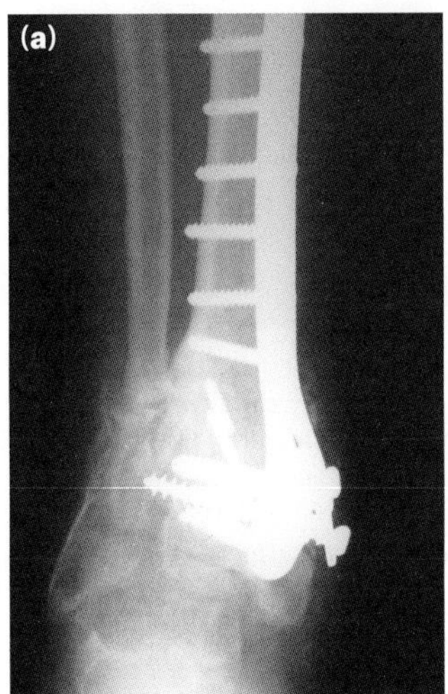

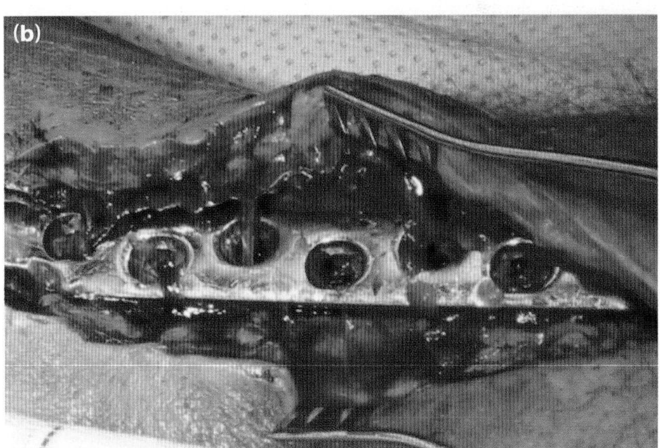

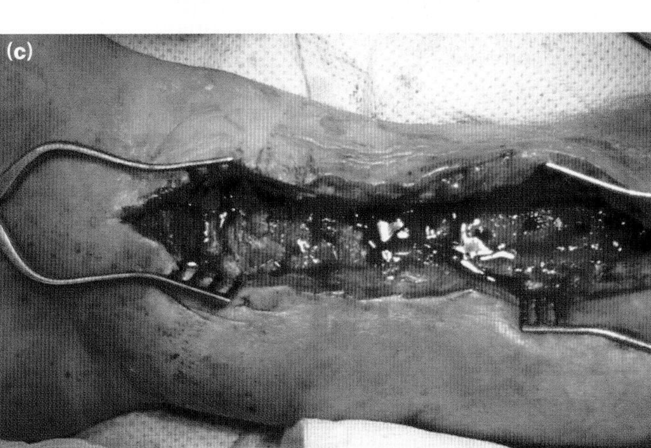

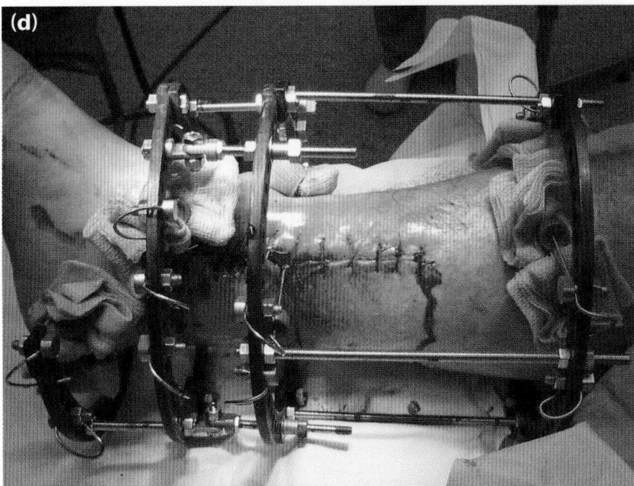

Figure 38.6 **(a)** Radiograph of a complex distal tibia fracture that was internally fixed but complicated by deep infection. **(b)** At operation, the plate was loose and grossly infected. **(c)** The plate was removed and all infected tissue was excised. Deep samples were sent for microbiology and histology. The defect at the lower end was filled with an absorbable antibiotic carrier. **(d)** The bone was stabilised with an Ilizarov circular external fixator and the skin primarily closed.

Goerge Cierny III, 1947–2013, osteomyelitis surgeon, San Diego, California, USA.
Jon T Mader, 1944–2002, Department of the Marine Biomedical Institute, Division of Infectious Diseases, the University of Texas Medical Branch, Galveston, USA.
Cierny and Mader described the classification in: G Cierny, JT Mader, JJ Pennick. A clinical staging for adult osteomyelitis. *Contemp Orthop* 1985; 10: 17–37. They appreciated the importance of treating the whole patient alongside the infected bone.

(A, no active concurrent disease; B, compromised host; C, severe comorbidity preventing surgery). The interaction between the patient's health status and the extent of the bone infection greatly affects the outcome after surgery. In chronic infection, it is helpful to address medical conditions which may impair wound healing (e.g. smoking, peripheral vascular disease, diabetes, steroid use) prior to surgery. This approach has been shown to improve cure rates.

Stage 1 (medullary)

Only cancellous bone is involved. Excision of the dead bone can be carried out by intramedullary reaming or by windowing the cortex. The resulting defect may be filled with antibiotic-loaded cement beads or absorbable pellets. Structural stability is rarely affected (Figure 38.7).

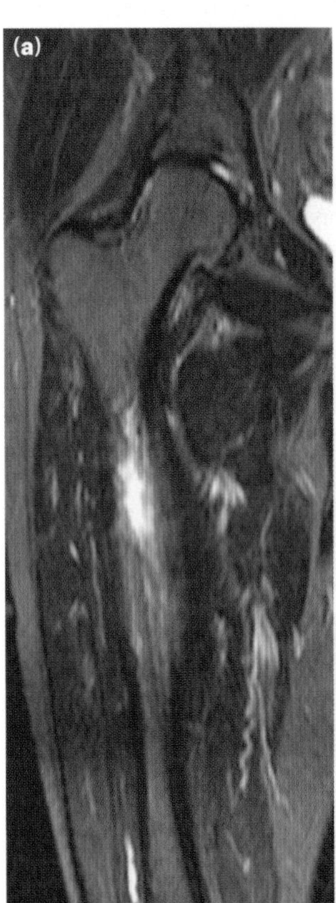

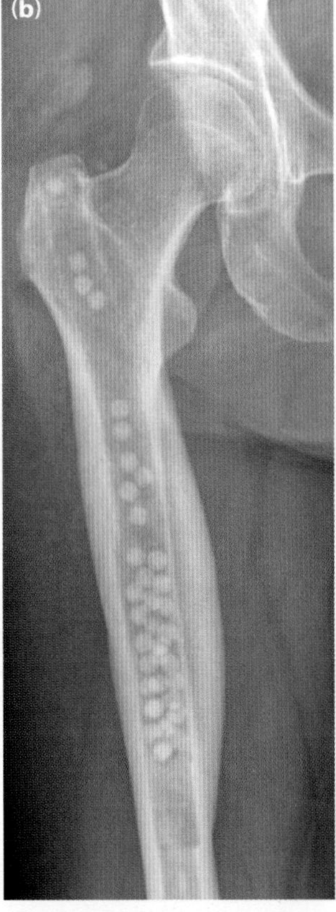

Figure 38.7 **(a)** Magnetic resonance imaging scan showing a typical medullary osteomyelitis of the femur, in a patient with human immunodeficiency virus. **(b)** The infected bone has been removed by reaming and the central defect filled with absorbable calcium sulphate pellets with gentamicin.

Stage 2 (superficial)

Only the cortical bone is involved and this requires excision. It often follows skin ulceration and there may be large skin defects which require complete excision and local or free muscle flaps. If more than one-third of the cortical circumference is excised, splintage is essential, usually with external fixation to prevent fracture. Secondary bone grafting may be needed.

Stage 3 (localised)

There is a limited area of dead cortical bone with medullary infection. Radical excision is required, and filling the defect and providing soft-tissue cover may be a challenge. Staged reconstruction may be necessary with cancellous bone grafting (Figure 38.8).

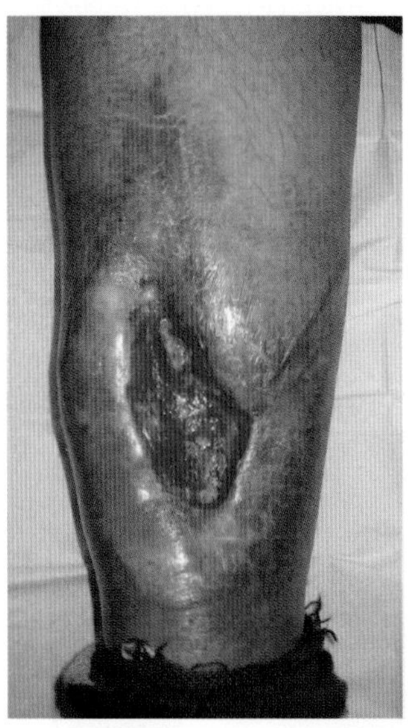

Figure 38.8 This large ulcer had been present for 30 years with underlying Stage 3 chronic osteomyelitis. Biopsy of the skin edge revealed a squamous cell carcinoma; a rare complication of a long-standing sinus (Marjolijn's ulcer).

Stage 4 (diffuse)

This involves the entire circumference of the bone and surrounding soft tissue. All infected non-unions are Stage 4. Resection must be segmental and stabilisation in an external fixator will be required. Reconstruction will involve the introduction of new bone and healthy soft tissue. The Ilizarov method, which uses distraction osteogenesis to fill bone defects, is a powerful and successful technique. It can be combined with free tissue transfer. This allows reconstruction to proceed in parallel with rehabilitation.

After surgery, patients should be given antibiotics. After total segmental excision of infection a short course may be indicated, but in most chronic infections, 6–12 weeks is often advised. If there is any doubt about the adequacy of clearance of infection, a long antibiotic course will be needed and recurrence may be more likely. In infected fractures, antibiotics should continue until fracture union.

There is now increasing interest in the use of local antibiotics with absorbable carriers. These can deliver high doses of antibiotics into the bone, without systemic effects. Some biocomposite materials (with hydroxyapatite) can form new bone in the defect, avoiding the need for secondary bone grafting.

Gavril Abramovich Ilizarov, 1921–1992, pioneered this eponymous approach to bone reconstruction in Siberia in the 1960s for the management of osteomyelitis.

Summary box 38.10

Chronic osteomyelitis

- Chronic disease requires specialist surgery with excision, stabilisation and reconstruction
- Host status should be optimised before surgery
- Following surgery, antibiotic therapy is typically continued for at least 6 weeks

DIABETIC FOOT INFECTION

The global prevalence of diabetes has increased exponentially in recent years. Foot infections are a leading cause of hospital admissions in this group, with an annual incidence of foot complications of 1–2% per year, due to the combined influence of macro- and microvascular insufficiency, mechanical disruption, peripheral and autonomic neuropathy, immune defects and impaired tissue healing. Ulceration of the calcaneum and bones of the forefoot, especially the great toe and first metatarsal head, is common, potentially leading to deep extension and osteomyelitis (**Figure 38.9**).

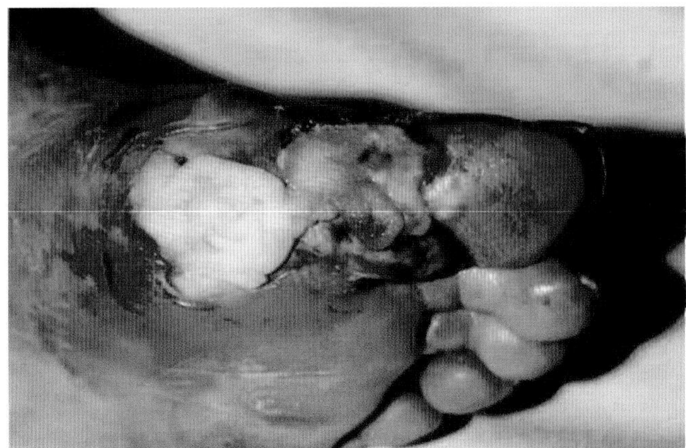

Figure 38.9 A severe diabetic foot infection, with marked infection, necrosis and soft-tissue loss. The patient was neuropathic but not ischaemic and it was possible to salvage a functional foot by 'filleting' the hallux and using the soft tissues to cover the defect.

Fever and systemic symptoms are relatively unusual in diabetic foot infections but, if present, should be acted on promptly, as they may herald rapidly advancing infection, bacteraemia or necrotising fasciitis. In unwell patients, blood cultures, imaging, careful clinical assessment with optimisation of organ function and prompt empirical antibiotics are essential.

Blood tests are frequently unhelpful, as inflammatory markers may be normal or only mildly raised. Plain radiographs may show evidence of osteomyelitis, but can be normal (particularly early in infection). MRI is the most sensitive imaging modality for diagnosis of bone involvement. Limited disease has a good prognosis, and in the absence of risk factors for resistant organisms (including prior treatment), empirical treatment can be justified. In extensive or complicated infections, antibiotic therapy should be guided by the results of culture of deep bone or tissue samples obtained surgically or radiologically. Superficial swabs or cultures from ulcers or sinus tracts are not reliable in determining the organisms responsible for underlying deep-seated infection.

The aetiological agents of diabetic foot infection are the same as for bone infection in non-diabetic individuals, namely *Staphylococcus aureus*, beta-haemolytic streptococci and aerobic gram-negative bacilli. *Pseudomonas* is over-represented, and empirical therapy for severe infections should include cover for this organism. Anaerobes may also be present, and the addition of metronidazole (particularly for abscesses and/or devitalised tissue) should be considered.

Surgical debridement is required for collections, necrotic areas or more extensive osteomyelitis. Thought should be given to distinguishing superficial osteitis (stage 2 disease) resulting from loss of soft tissue cover (often in association with vascular compromise) from more extensive bone involvement. In the former, biopsy and antibiotic therapy may be of limited importance and optimising glycaemic control, improving vascular supply and relieving pressure with appropriate footwear are much more important. This approach may avoid more extensive tissue loss or later amputation.

Vascular compromise should be considered a relative contraindication to a surgical approach. In patients with poor peripheral pulses, a full vascular assessment is mandatory. Proximal angioplasty or bypass surgery may improve distal vascularity to a level where infection surgery in the foot may be more successful.

Amputation is not an easy option in diabetic foot disease, and wound healing can be problematic. In general, excision should be adequate to remove all infected material, and excess bone may need to be resected to allow tension-free skin closure. If there is extensive peripheral neuropathy, a below-knee amputation in an area with better sensation may be appropriate.

Summary box 38.11

Diabetic foot infection

- The most important risk factor for osteomyelitis is the presence of a foot ulcer
- Ulcer swabs are not reliable in determining the pathogens responsible for osteomyelitis
- Bone biopsy for culture should be considered in extensive/complex infection, but may not be necessary in mild disease
- In severe disease, surgical debridement of collections and/or necrotic tissue is required, followed by antibiotics tailored according to culture results

MUSCULOSKELETAL INFECTION CAUSED BY MYCOBACTERIA

Tuberculous arthritis/osteomyelitis had become uncommon in the UK, but remains prevalent in resource-poor countries. There is now a resurgence in higher-income countries as a consequence of immigration and immunocompromise (including human immunodeficiency virus [HIV]). The most common organism is *Mycobacterium tuberculosis*. Around half of all cases affect the spine, typically manifesting as paradiscal infection but also causing discitis and vertebral osteomyelitis. Native joint infection typically presents with monoarticular pain in a weight-bearing joint.

Surgery may be crucial to facilitate synovial biopsy for diagnosis by culture and histopathology, as well as to decompress the spinal cord and debride infected tissue.

For optimal management of tuberculosis, the patient must be referred to a specialist multidisciplinary team, for input that includes the following components.

- Baseline screening for HIV and other blood-borne viruses.
- Assessment for other sites of mycobacterial infection.
- Measurement of baseline renal and liver function, to be repeated at intervals throughout treatment. Drug-induced hepatitis is the commonest serious side effect that may require temporary withdrawal or alteration of therapy.
- Baseline and follow-up testing of hearing (if injectable agents to be used) and colour vision (if ethambutol to be used).
- Consideration of any potential drug interactions (rifampicin is a potent inducer of the cytochrome P450 system; it can interact with many classes of drug including anticonvulsants, antiretroviral therapy, anticoagulants, antibiotics and antifungals).
- Institution of appropriate infection control precautions and contact tracing.
- Appropriate education and support to optimise adherence to therapy.
- Prescription of an appropriate combination of drug therapy.
    - For fully sensitive *Mycobacterium tuberculosis*, the preferred regimen is oral rifampicin, isoniazid, pyrazinamide and ethambutol for 2 months, followed by rifampicin and isoniazid for a further 4 months.
    - Worldwide, there is an increase in the prevalence of drug-resistant tuberculosis, classified as multidrug resistant (MDR) and extensively drug resistant (XDR). Infection with these organisms requires a treatment regimen that includes an injectable agent (typically amikacin, kanamycin or capreomycin) together with oral agents selected according to the susceptibility profile of the isolate (these may include cycloserine, ethionamide, p-aminosalicylic acid (PAS), fluoroquinolones and linezolid). Prolongation of therapy is required, and side effects and toxicity are common.

Non-tuberculous mycobacteria are ubiquitous environmental organisms. They are best recognised as agents of disease in patients with underlying immunocompromise (including HIV, diabetes and organ transplantation), or other risk factors for introduction of infection (such as penetrating trauma or the presence of a prosthesis). However, they may occasionally also cause infection in hosts without obvious risk factors.

Treatment can be difficult. These organisms are resistant to the standard agents used for first-line antituberculous therapy; surgery to debride and drain sites of infection can therefore be particularly important to reduce the bacterial burden. There is no single standardised drug regimen or duration, so choice of therapy depends on the *in vitro* susceptibility of the organism, and length of treatment depends on the location of disease, extent of surgical debridement, the identification and phenotypic characteristics of the organism, the patient's underlying condition, presence of immunocompromise and response to therapy. As for treatment of *Mycobacterium tuberculosis*, expert medical oversight is crucial throughout treatment.

ACKNOWLEDGEMENT

Dr Philip Bejon contributed to an earlier version of this chapter, and we remain grateful for his previous input.

FURTHER READING

Barrett L, Atkins B. The clinical presentation of prosthetic joint infection. *J Antimicrob Chemother* 2014; **69**(Suppl 1): i25–7.
Bejon P, Berendt A, Atkins BL *et al.* (2010) Two-stage revision for prosthetic joint infection: predictors of outcome and the role of reimplantation microbiology. *J Antimicrob Chemother* 2010; **65**: 569–75.
Bose D, Kugan R, Stubbs D, McNally M. Management of infected nonunion of the long bones by a multidisciplinary team. *Bone Joint J* 2015; 97-B: 814–17.
Byren I, Bejon P, Atkins BL *et al.* (2009) One hundred and twelve infected arthroplasties treated with 'DAIR' (debridement, antibiotics and implant retention): antibiotic duration and outcome. *J Antimicrob Chemother* 2009; **63**: 1264–71.
Ferguson JY, Riley N, Dudareva M *et al.* The use of a biodegradable antibiotic-loaded calcium sulphate carrier containing tobramycin for the treatment of chronic osteomyelitis. *Bone Joint J* 2014; 96-B: 829–36.
Mathews CJ, Weston VC, Jones A, Field M, Coakley G. Bacterial septic arthritis in adults. *Lancet* 2010; **375**: 846–55.
Matthews PC, Berendt AR, McNally MA, Byren I. Diagnosis and management of prosthetic joint infection *BMJ* 2009; **338**: 1378–83.
McNally MA, Ferguson JY, Diefenbeck M *et al.* Single-stage treatment of chronic osteomyelitis with a new absorbable, gentamicin-loaded, calcium sulphate/hydroxyapatite biocomposite. A prospective series of 100 cases. *Bone Joint J* 2016; 98-B: 1289–96.
McNally MA, Nagarajah K. Osteomyelitis. *Orthop Trauma* 2010; **24**(6): 416–29.
Uçkay I, Gariani K, Dubois-Ferrière V, Suvà D, Lipsky BA. Diabetic foot infections: recent literature and cornerstones of management. *Curr Opin Infect Dis* 2016; **29**(2): 145–52.

Chapter 39

Paediatric orthopaedics

Learning objectives

To be familiar with:

- Normal and abnormal development of the musculoskeletal system
- Normal variants versus pathological deformity
- Diagnosis and treatment of developmental hip dysplasia
- Presentation and management of other childhood hip conditions
- Management of clubfoot
- Problems associated with musculoskeletal infection in childhood

INTRODUCTION

Immature skeletons heal rapidly and can remodel with growth but physeal injury or muscle imbalance may lead to progressive deformity. The conservative treatment of common conditions, such as developmental dysplasia of the hip (DDH) combines the child's remodelling ability with an understanding of the Heuter–Volkmann principle and Wolff's law (*Table 39.1*): improving the biomechanical environment may reverse abnormal growth. In contrast, in conditions such as Blount's disease, a poorly functioning growth plate leads to asymmetrical growth and deformity. Advances in genetics and molecular science are improving our understanding of certain conditions and may lead to potential new avenues of treatment.

DEVELOPMENT OF THE MUSCULOSKELETAL SYSTEM

The upper limb bud forms on the lateral wall of the embryo 4 weeks after fertilisation, followed promptly by the lower limb bud. By 2 months' gestation, differentiation of the limb elements is complete. Most congenital limb anomalies arise during this second month.

TABLE 39.1 Laws governing the remodelling of bone.

Heuter–Volkmann principle
• Compressive forces inhibit growth
• Tensile forces stimulate growth
Wolff's Law
• Bone deposition and resorption depend on the stresses applied

Three coordinated signalling centres control limb development. The **apical ectodermal ridge** (AER) guides mesodermal differentiation (in the progress zone) in a proximal to distal direction and controls digit formation via the production of several fibroblast growth factors (FGFs). The mesodermal **zone of polarising activity** (ZPA) directs anteroposterior limb development via the sonic hedgehog protein which is itself sustained by the FGFs. The ectodermal driven **wingless-type** (Wnt) signalling centre develops dorsoventral axis configuration and limb alignment.

Certain limb anomalies are directly related to alterations in these centres. In experiments it is found that removal of the AER leads to a truncated limb, similar to a congenital amputation, and prevents interdigital necrosis. This results in syndactyly. An additional ZPA results in a mirror duplication of the distal limb, while the Wnt signalling system is critical for the transcription factor Lmx1b in the distal mesenchyme, such that absence of this gene affects the development of dorsal limb structures in the nail patella syndome.

An error during fetal limb development may disturb the formation of other organs. Thus some limb anomalies are associated with systemic disorders which may be life-threatening.

Summary box 39.1

Development of the musculoskeletal system

- Occurs 4–8 weeks after fertilisation
- AER controls proximal to distal differentiation and interdigital necrosis
- ZPA directs posterior to anterior differentiation
- Wnt influences dorsal to ventral differentiation

Richard von Volkmann, 1830–1889, Professor of Surgery, Halle, Germany.
Julius Wolff, 1836–1902, Professor of Orthopaedic Surgery, Berlin, Germany.

NORMAL VARIANTS

The many normal variants of growth and development can cause significant parental concern. The common problems are related to an intoeing gait, tripping and falling, bowlegs, knock-knees and flatfeet. In general, if they are symmetrical, symptom-free and supple and in an otherwise normal child, they require no intervention. There is often a family history of similar complaints. If the child fails to achieve their developmental milestones or there are functional problems, further investigation and help may be required.

Intoeing gait

Intoeing is defined as a negative foot progression angle. It can result from one or more lower limb torsional anomalies (Figure 39.1 and *Table 39.2*).

Persistent anteversion of the femoral neck presents clinically with excessive internal rotation at the hip joint which is best measured with the patient prone (Figure 39.2a). All femurs are anteverted at birth but as the femur lengthens it also rotates, leading to spontaneous improvement in the degree of anteversion. If, by 10–12 years, a significant deformity persists associated with functional difficulties, corrective osteotomy may be justified. In such cases, the child has usually lost the ability to externally rotate the extended hip. In other cases, compensatory external tibial torsion may have developed, in which case the foot progression angle will be normal but the child may have symptoms of the miserable malalignment syndrome, which include anterior knee pain and feelings of instability.

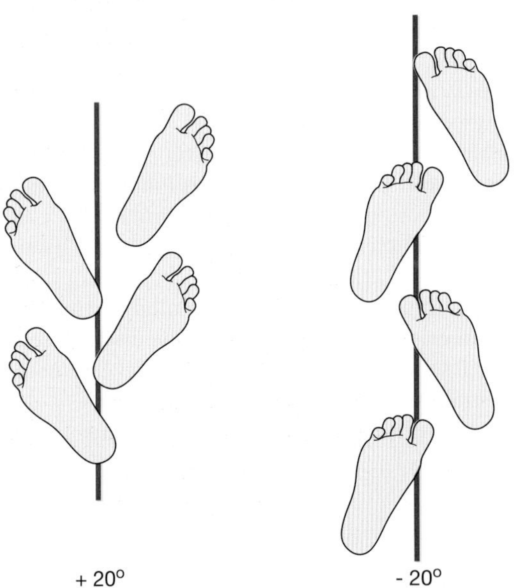

Figure 39.1 Foot progression angle: a positive angle is caused by an extoeing gait, a negative angle by an intoeing gait.

TABLE 39.2 Common sites and causes of intoeing gait in childhood.

Site	Cause
Femur/hip	Persistent femoral neck anteversion
Tibia	Internal tibial torsion
Foot	Metatarsus adductus

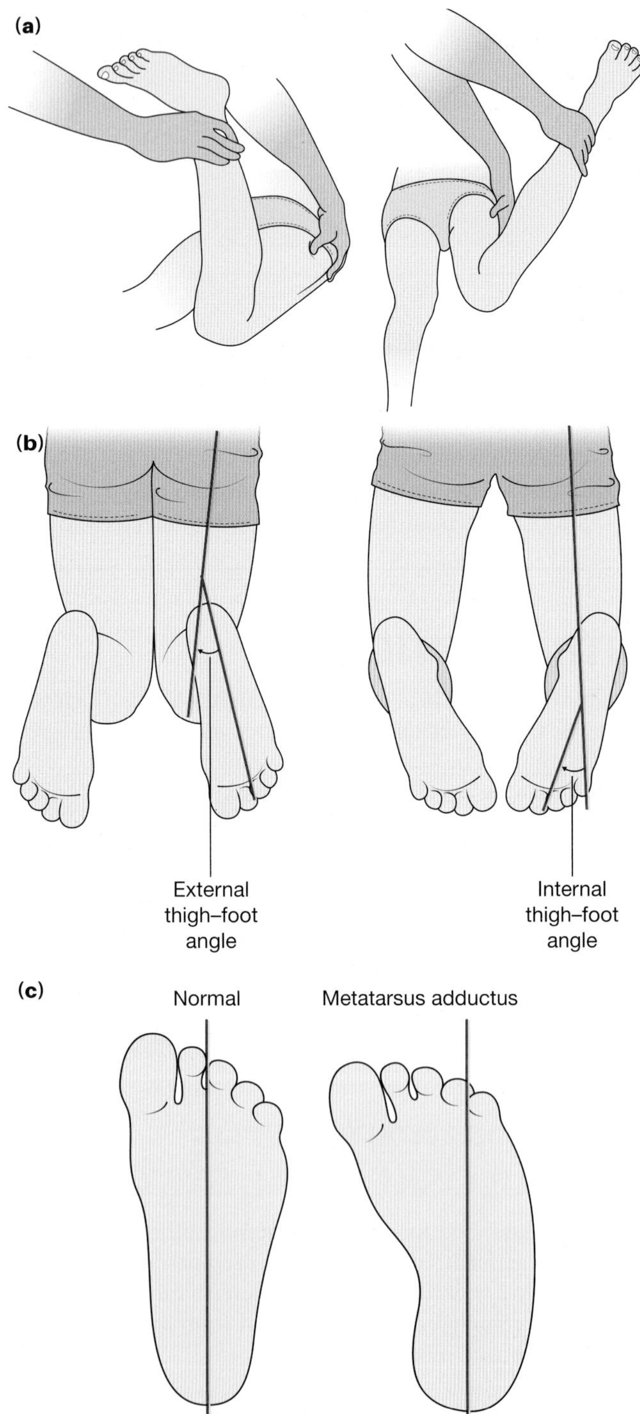

Figure 39.2 Line diagrams illustrating assessment of the torsional profile: all assessments are done with the child prone. **(a)** Femoral neck anteversion measured as the range of internal hip rotation with the child prone, the hip extended and the knee flexed. Craig's test measures the degree of internal rotation present when the greater trochanter is at its most prominent (also called the Trochanteric Prominence Test). **(b)** The thigh–foot angle (TFA) measures the angle between the relaxed hindfoot and the thigh (also measured with the child prone). **(c)** The bean-shaped foot of metatarsus adductus viewed from above: a curved lateral border with/without a medial crease. This deformity may be passively correctable.

Internal tibial torsion is assessed by the thigh–foot angle and is commonly associated with physiological tibia vara in infants (Figure 39.2b). Spontaneous correction can be expected by age 4, as the tibia also rotates as it grows.

Metatarsus adductus (Figure 39.2c) is usually flexible; spontaneous correction occurs in 90% of children by the age of 2–4 years. For the more rigid foot, stretching, with or without plaster casts or straight-last shoes, may help. Surgical release is rarely indicated.

Other abnormalities of gait

Extoeing is less common than intoeing but may result from relative femoral retroversion, external tibial torsion or flexible flat feet. The young child may be late walking because of poor balance associated with the foot posture and the overall alignment. This condition improves with growth/time.

Toe-walking is a phase in normal gait development. If the gait does not mature to a heel–toe pattern by 3 years, physiotherapy may help, and older children benefit from surgical lengthening of a contracted gastrocsoleus complex, if it is present. If toe walking starts after walking age, a spinal or neuromuscular aetiology such as a tethered cord or a muscular dystrophy must be considered and in the unilateral case, an orthopaedic cause for a short leg, such as fibula hemimelia or a dislocated hip, needs to be considered and excluded.

Knock-knees and bowlegs

In the normal child, leg shape changes dramatically over time. All children start life with bowlegs, often accompanied by internal tibial torsion. By the age of 2–3 years they have developed knock-knees, which regress towards the normal adult tibiofemoral angle of 7° valgus by the age of 7 (Figure 39.3).

Traditionally, the intercondylar or intermalleolar distance is used to quantify the deformity, rather than measuring the angle. This is not very accurate. Further investigation is needed when the deformity is severe, asymmetrical or symptomatic. The most common pathological causes are previous trauma, rickets or a skeletal dysplasia.

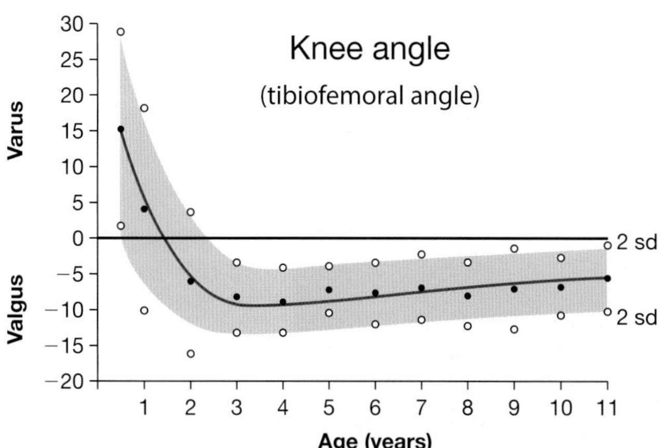

Figure 39.3 Graph to show the normal tendency of limb alignment to change from varus to valgus with growth; normal is slight valgus after the age of 7–8 years.

Flat foot

Before development of the medial longitudinal arch, all children (<3 years) have flat feet, often with a fat pad obscuring the arch. Only 15% of adults have flat feet so the natural history is for improvement, influenced by both familial and racial factors.

The painless, flexible flat foot needs no treatment. Orthoses **do not** alter the natural history but can alleviate symptoms **if** they are present. All flat feet have a flattened medial arch with a valgus heel but two major types must be distinguished (*Table 39.3*).

The symptomatic, rigid flat foot is usually the result of inflammation or a tarsal coalition and requires appropriate investigation followed by medical or surgical management (Figure 39.4).

TABLE 39.3 Flat feet.

Types	Characteristics
Flexible	On tiptoe the arch is restored and the heel corrects into varus; subtalar joint movements are full and pain free
Rigid	On tiptoe the arch fails to return and the heel remains in valgus; subtalar joint movements are restricted and often painful

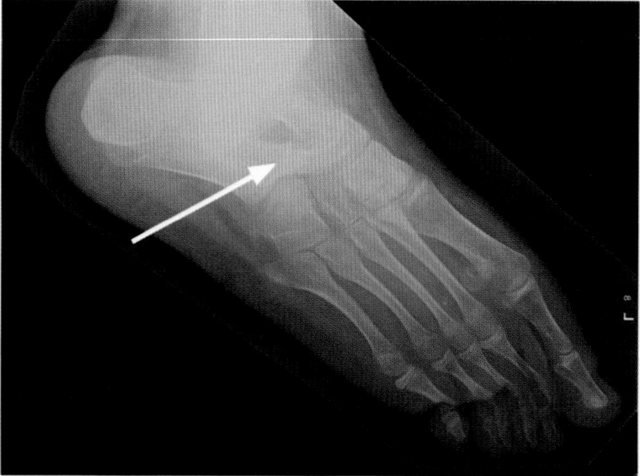

Figure 39.4 Oblique radiograph of the foot that shows the most common form of tarsal coalition, a calcaneonavicular bar (arrow).

Summary box 39.2

Normal variants

- Children's legs are often bowed until age 2 years and then knock-kneed until age 6 or 7 years
- Neuromuscular pathology must be excluded in toe walkers, particularly when the onset is late
- Intoeing or extoeing may be caused by excessive femoral or tibial torsion or foot deformity
- Flexible, pain-free flat feet do not need treatment

Postural abnormalities

Many babies are subjected to moulding pressures *in utero*. At birth they exhibit 'postural abnormalities' such as torticollis, calcaneovalgus feet and plagiocephaly, which improve with time and/or stretching exercises.

CONGENITAL AND DEVELOPMENTAL ABNORMALITIES OF THE SKELETON

Although many skeletal abnormalities are identified antenatally or at birth, others only become apparent with growth. Skeletal disorders are often linked to soft-tissue abnormalities which may be generalised or focal; the presence of a skin dimple or a vascular malformation should be a warning sign as should the 'featureless' limbs of a child with arthrogryposis multiplex congenita (AMC) (*Table 39.4*, **Figure 39.5**).

Many anomalies require little treatment and cause minimal functional disability whereas others, such as proximal femoral focal deficiency (PFFD) and radial club hand, pose considerable challenges to both the patient and their doctors. In these cases the functional and cosmetic needs of the child and family must be balanced against available resources and expertise (**Figure 39.6**). Despite advances in limb reconstruction techniques there is little high-quality evidence-based data from skeletally mature patients to support their widespread use. Concurrently, considerable advances are occurring with amputation prosthetics which may result in better patient-reported quality of life outcome scores, particularly in certain regions.

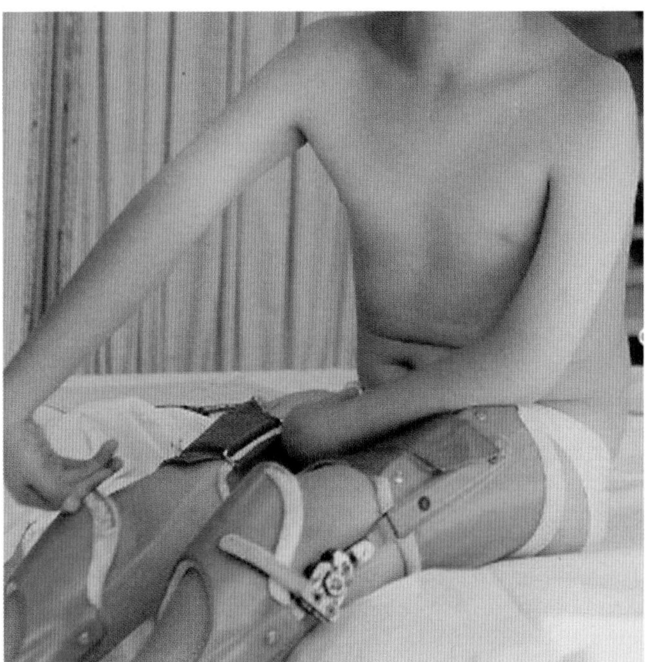

Figure 39.5 Clinical photograph of a child with arthrogryposis multiplex congenita and featureless upper limbs (no skin creases or muscle definition). He mobilises with the help of knee–ankle–foot orthoses.

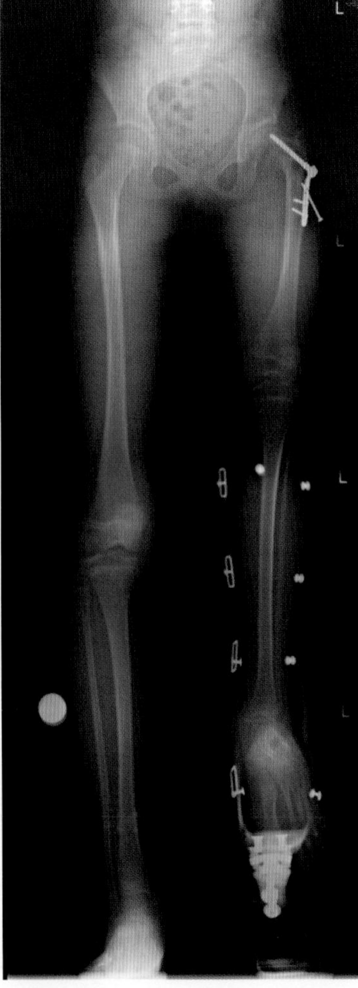

Figure 39.6 Radiograph of a child born with proximal femoral focal deficiency. A proximal femoral osteotomy improved her hip mechanics and stabilty (a screw has come loose from the plate). She opted to keep her foot and not to undergo leg lengthening. She functions well with an extension prosthesis.

Generalised skeletal dysplasias

Achondroplasia

Achondroplasia is caused by a gain in function mutation in the *FGFR3* (fibroblast growth factor receptor 3) gene, located on the short arm of chromosome (Chr) 4, which affects

TABLE 39.4 Classification of congenital limb malformations.

Category	Example
Failure of formation of parts	
Transverse	Congenital amputation of the forearm/lower limb
Longitudinal	Fibular hemimelia
Failure of differentiation	Radioulnar synostosis; vertebral body fusion
Duplication	Extra digits
Overgrowth	Gigantism; macrodactyly
Undergrowth	
Congenital constriction band syndrome	Often affects hands/feet with poor formation of the digits distally
Generalised skeletal abnormalities	Skeletal dysplasia, e.g. achondroplasia

enchondral bone formation. It is an autosomal dominant condition. Patients present with disproportionate short stature where the limbs are shorter than the trunk, together with classical clinical and radiographic features (**Figure 39.7**).

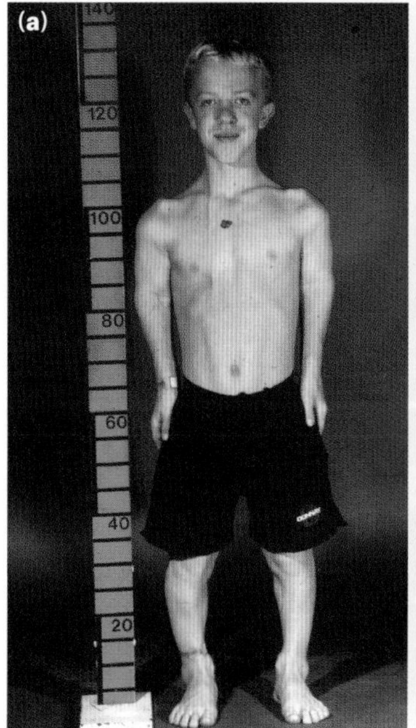

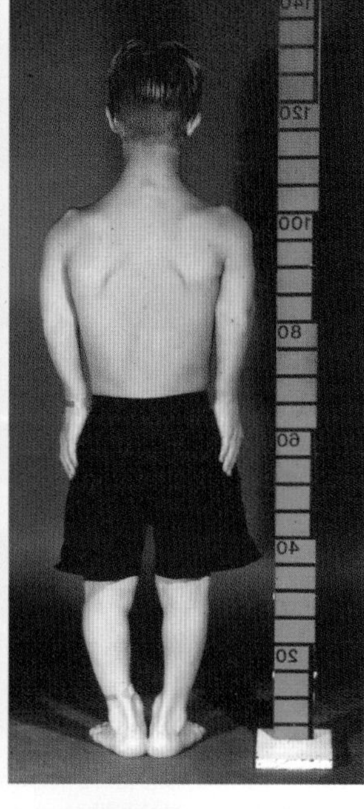

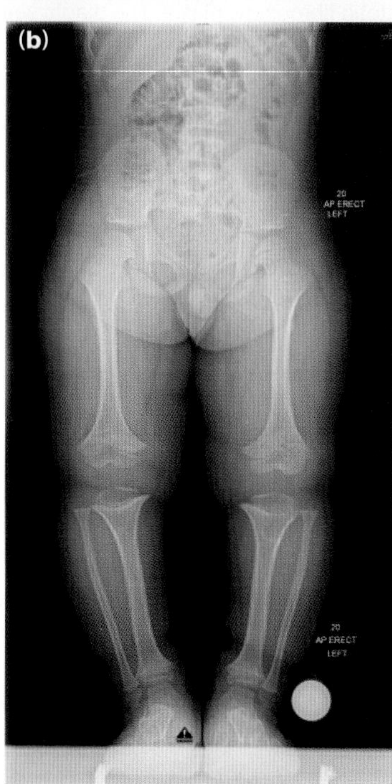

Figure 39.7 Achondroplasia. (**a**) Clinical photograph of a child with achondroplasia. (**b**) Standing leg length/alignment radiograph of a different child with achondroplasia showing short limbs, flared/widened metaphysis, an overlong fibula and slight bowing, The acetabulum is very horizontal and the pelvic wings seem square: all classical features of this condition.

Underdevelopment of the foramen magnum and spinal stenosis can cause neurological difficulties. Correction of limb alignment may be necessary and limb lengthening techniques are used in some countries.

Hereditary multiple exostoses - diaphyseal aclasis

This is an autosomal dominant condition usually related to a loss of function mutation in either the *EXT 1* (on Chr 8q) or *EXT 2* gene (Chr 11p), although it is unclear how this defect leads to the disregulated growth which results in an exostosis. Exostoses consisting of a cartilaginous cap on a bony stalk may be sessile or pedunculated. They grow as the child grows and may cause cosmetic or functional difficulties that justify excision. Differential growth between the paired bones of the forearm and lower leg can lead to joint deformity and dislocation of the radial head, exacerbated by the disorded physeal growth secondary to altered mechanical forces. Such growth abnormalities are predictable and treatment is designed to prevent deformity from developing (**Figure 39.8**). Continued growth after skeletal maturity may represent malignant transformation of a previously benign osteochondroma: a rare but recognised problem (see Chapter 37).

Enchondromatosis

This non-hereditary skeletal dysplasia is also called Ollier's disease. Enchondromas arise from rests of chondrocytes located within the medullary canal of tubular bones: they consist of mature hyaline cartilage (**Figure 39.9**). Larger lesions may show calcification on radiographs, and vertical streaks of lucency (representing cartilage columns) may run the length of the metaphysis. Pathological fractures are common. If there are also soft tissue haemangiomas and lymphangiomas, the condition is called Maffucci's syndrome (see Chapter 37).

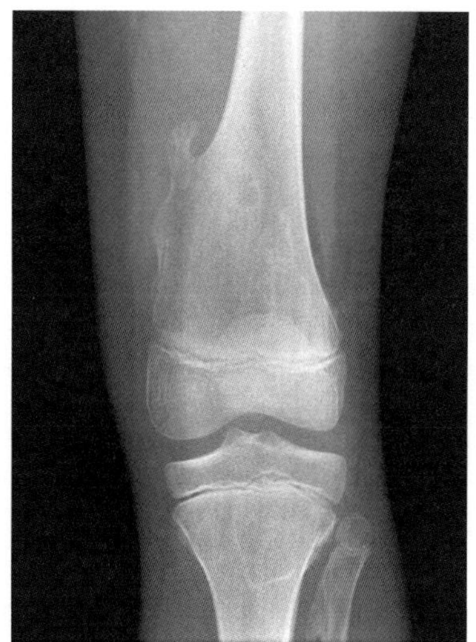

Figure 39.8 Radiograph of the knee showing multiple broad-based osteochondromas.

Louis Xavier Edouard Léopold Ollier, 1830–1900, Professor of Surgery, Lyons, France, described enchondromatosis in 1899.
Angelo Maffucci, 1845–1903, Professor of Pathological Anatomy, Pisa, Italy, described enchondromatosis in association with soft tissue haemangiomas in 1881.

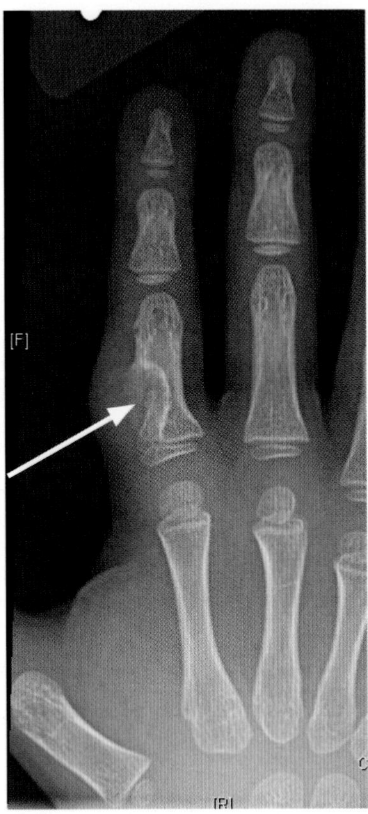

Figure 39.9 Anteroposterior radiograph of the index finger of a child showing a solitary enchondroma (arrow): note the opacity in the soft tissues that represents the extent of the cartilaginous lesion.

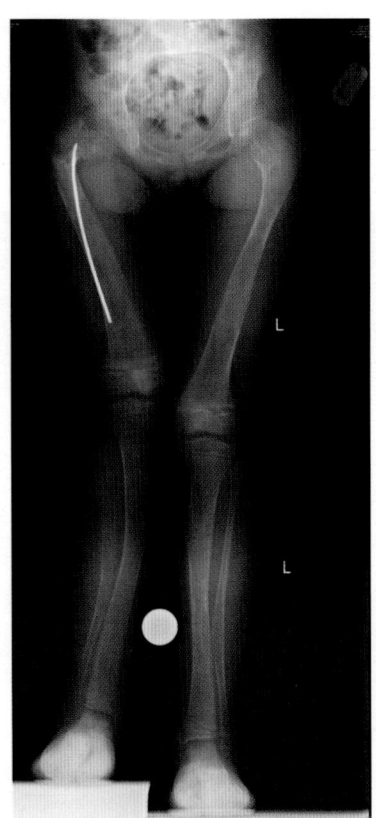

Figure 39.10 Standing leg length and alignment radiograph of a child with polyostotic fibrous dysplasia. The diaphyseal lesions classically have a 'ground glass' appearance. The bones are often deformed and the limb may be short, as seen particularly on the right. The femur has fractured previously and one intramedullary nail remains in place.

Fibrous dysplasia

This common disorder is often a chance finding on radiographs, particularly in its monostotic form. It is a localised defect in osteoblastic differentiation and maturation where normal bone is replaced by fibrous stroma. With polyostotic fibrous dysplasia, limb deformity and pathological fractures are common. In patients with precocious puberty and Coast of Maine café-au-lait spots, the diagnosis is McCune Albright's syndrome (Figure 39.10).

Summary box 39.3

Congenital and developmental abnormalities of the skeleton

- Achondroplasia affects enchondral ossification and presents with disproportionate short stature
- Exostoses may cause functional and/or cosmetic problems
- Patients with Ollier's disease (multiple enchondromatosis) often have lesions in the hands and feet

METABOLIC BONE DISEASE

Rickets

In all types of rickets, the primary problem is inadequate mineralisation of growing bone (*Table 39.5*). In severe cases, skeletal deformities, with classic radiographic features, affect every physis (Figure 39.11). Medical treatment improves mineralisation. Correction of the deformity then occurs with growth. Once the medical condition has been stabilised, surgery may be necessary for the management of any residual limb deformity. Guided growth techniques are often used in preference to osteotomies.

TABLE 39.5 Common causes of rickets.

Nutritional	Reduced intake of vitamin D and calcium
Environmental	Inadequate exposure to sunlight
Gastrointestinal disease	Crohn's disease, gluten-sensitive enteropathy
Genetic	X-linked hypophosphataemia
Renal disease	End-stage renal failure, renal tubular anomalies; changes related to secondary hyperparathyroidism may be present

Osteogenesis imperfecta (OI) (brittle bone disease)

OI represents a spectrum of conditions linked by a qualitative and/or quantitative malfunction of collagen production. Many specific genetic defects have been identified, most caused by mutations in the collagen genes. The bone may break easily but it heals promptly and well. All structures that

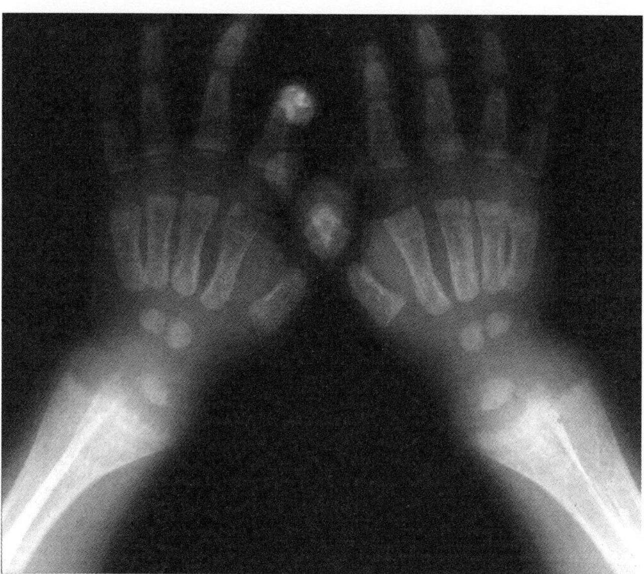

Figure 39.11 Radiographs in cases of rickets demonstrate widened physes with cupped, flared metaphyses.

contain collagen may be affected. This accounts for the ligamentous laxity, blue sclerae and poor teeth found in some phenotypes.

Cyclical bisphosphonate treatment decreases bone resorption and bone turnover. This reduces bone pain and the fracture rate, which in turn improves weight-bearing mobility and bone strength (Figure 39.12).

Following fracture, care must be taken to minimise disuse osteoporosis and to maintain bone alignment. Treatment options range from simple casting techniques to more specialised surgical procedures to correct/maintain limb alignment while allowing growth. Intramedullary techniques for reduction and stabilisation of fractures or osteotomies are preferred to plate fixation because of the associated problems with stress risers. Immobilisation must be minimised and rehabilitation commenced promptly.

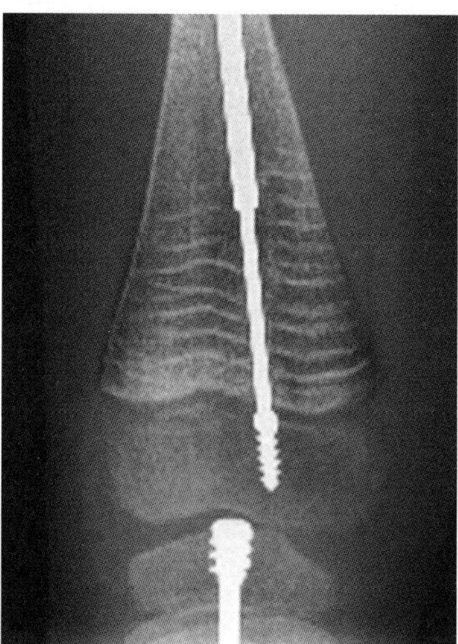

Figure 39.12 Radiograph of a child with osteogenesis imperfecta who has been treated with cyclical bisphosphonates. Multiple growth lines are visible in addition to intramedullary devices in both the femur and tibia.

Summary box 39.4

Metabolic bone disease

- Rickets, from nutritional or other causes, is characterised by a failure of bone mineralisation
  - X-linked hypophosphataemic rickets is transmitted in a dominant fashion, therefore affecting both boys and girls
- In osteogenesis imperfecta:
  - There is defective type I collagen production
  - In severe forms frequent fractures lead to progressive deformity
  - Systemic treatment with bisphosphonates reduces the fracture rate

ABNORMALITIES OF THE HIP

Developmental dysplasia of the hip (DDH)

DDH defines the spectrum of hip instability, ranging from the hip that is in joint but has a shallow (dysplastic) acetabulum and may be 'pushed out' (Barlow positive) to the dislocated hip that is irreducible (Ortolani negative). These tests are described below. The associated clinical picture varies with the pathology and the age at presentation: neonatal hips may be unstable, a toddler may limp, adolescents may experience exercise-induced pain and an adult may have pain secondary to degenerative arthritis.

Incidence

The incidence of neonatal instability is ~20 per 1000 live births whereas that of true dislocation is ~2 per 1000 live births; many hips stabilise spontaneously.

Aetiology of DDH

- **Gender**. DDH is 4–5 times more common in girls than in boys, possibly related to hormonal factors causing temporary joint laxity.
- **Breech presentation**. DDH is more common in breech babies, particularly with the extended breech position.
- **Birth order**. DDH is more common in firstborns and in the left hip because of the common fetal position (LOA – left occipitoanterior) in a tight primigravid uterus where movement is restricted.
- **Oligohydramnios**. Restricts fetal movement. The presence of other postural deformities (torticollis and metatarsus adductus) raises the possibility of DDH.
- **Family history**. A positive family history significantly increases the risk of DDH. This may reflect faulty acetabular development or excessive ligamentous laxity.
- **Regional and racial variation**. DDH is more common in certain regions and in certain races, probably because of a combination of genetic, environmental and cultural factors. Swaddling the legs together will exacerbate an unstable hip whereas carrying the baby astride the carer's hip or back encourages a position of hip flexion and abduction that will help stability.

Hip dislocation is often found in association with generalised syndromes or neuromuscular conditions. These teratological hips are often resistant to the simpler surgical procedures and a holistic approach to the child's overall condition and prognosis must be taken when planning treatment.

Diagnosis

NEONATES

Clinical assessment and screening. In many countries, all neonates are screened for limitation of hip abduction and hip joint instability. In the UK, as part of the newborn and infant physical examination (NIPE) guidelines, the hips are examined again at 6 weeks. The knees and hips are flexed and the thigh held by the examiner with the thumb along the medial aspect and a finger behind the greater trochanter. The hips are abducted gently: if abduction is limited, the hip may be dislocated. The examiner's finger then lifts the greater trochanter upwards; a soft clunk – the Ortolani test – with improved hip abduction signifies hip reduction (**Figure 39.13a**). If the hip does abduct fully, then the leg is brought back up to neutral and then adducted while downward pressure is applied to the knee with the examiner's thumb and palm: an unstable hip may dislocate or subluxate – the Barlow test (**Figure 39.13b**). With an irreducible hip there is no clunk of reduction but there will be limitation of abduction. Bilateral dislocation may be missed because abduction is symmetrical and abduction may be normal when there is low muscle tone and joint laxity. In a dislocated hip, the femoral head may be palpable in the buttock.

Ultrasound assessment. Ultrasonography defines the anatomy and the stability of the hip joint. It is used to monitor early treatment (**Figure 39.14**) or as a screening tool (universally or just for 'at risk' patients). Ideally, screening scans should be performed between 4 and 6 weeks of age and treatment, when necessary, by 6 weeks. The sonographic appearance of most hips improves (both in terms of hip stability and acetabular dysplasia) spontaneously as the child grows.

Radiography. Plain radiographs are used to evaluate DDH from 4–5 months of age, but are of limited value in the newborn because no ossific nucleus is visible within the cartilaginous femoral head so its relationship to the acetabulum is difficult to judge. The appearance of the femoral ossific nucleus is also often delayed in DDH (**Figure 39.15**).

Summary box 39.5

The neonatal clinical examination must ask and answer the following questions:

- Is the hip dislocated?
  - If so is it reducible (Ortolani postive) or not (Ortolani negative)?
- If the hip is not dislocated, is it dislocatable (or subluxable)?
  - If so, it is Barlow positive.
- If the hip is not dislocated or dislocatable, is it clinically normal?
  - If so, do the risk factors in the history still demand further assessment with an ultrasound scan (USS) or plain radiograph?

INFANTS

Hip checks, looking for limitation of abduction in >90° of flexion and limb shortening, are part of routine developmental monitoring.

CHILD

Children present with a limp and sometimes with unilateral tiptoeing, because the affected leg is short. It is also externally rotated. Abduction in flexion is limited and there may be an extra thigh crease. The signs may be subtle and easily missed in an unsteady toddler. If both hips are affected there will be a waddling gait and a lumbar lordosis.

ADOLESCENT/ADULT

Discomfort after exercise is common but the pain may be in the knee. Radiographs show dysplasia, subluxation or degenerative change.

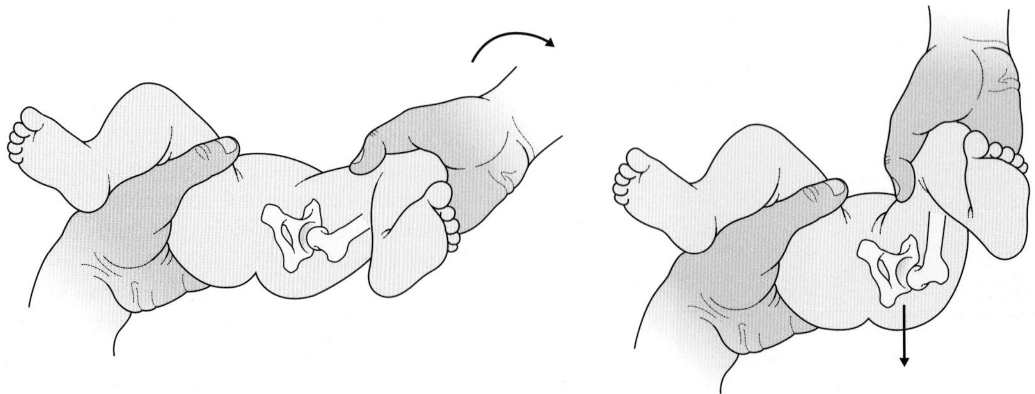

Figure 39.13 Line diagram illustrating the **(a)** Ortolani and **(b)** Barlow tests for developmental dysplasia of the hip. For the Barlow test the femur must be at 90° to the bed.

Marius Ortolani, orthopaedic surgeon, Instituto Provinciale Per L'Infanzia di Ferrara, Italy, described this test in 1937.
Thomas Geoffrey Barlow, 1915–1975, orthopaedic surgeon, the Salford Royal Hospital, Salford, UK.

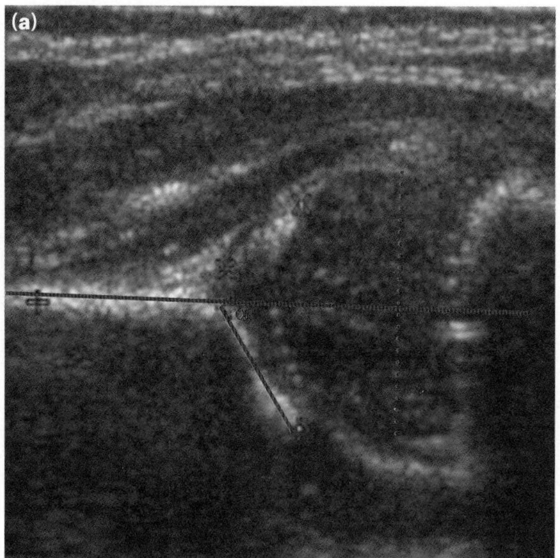

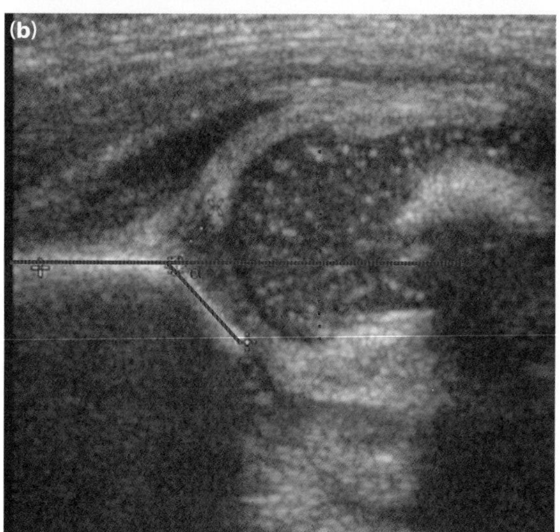

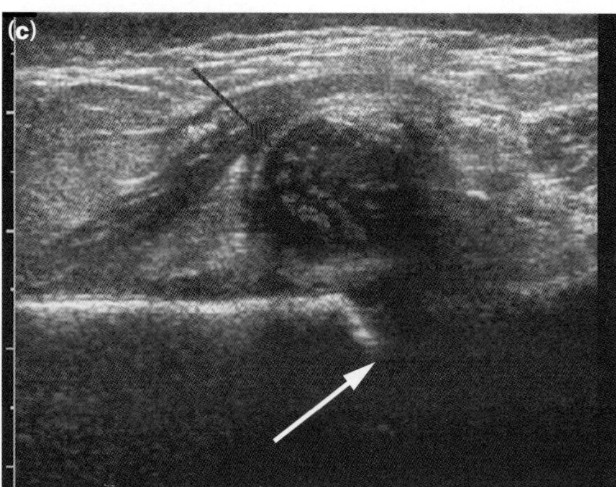

Figure 39.14 Ultrasound images of an infant hip. **(a)** Normal hip with a high α angle and a Morin index of 50% (defined as the percentage of the femoral head covered by the acetabulum, i.e. the portion lying below the horizontal red line). **(b)** Grossly dysplastic hip with a low α angle and a Morin index of <50%. This hip is likely to be unstable on dynamic ultrasound scanning, i.e. Barlow positive. **(c)** A dislocated hip joint (dislocated femoral head, red arrow; 'empty' acetabulum, white arrow).

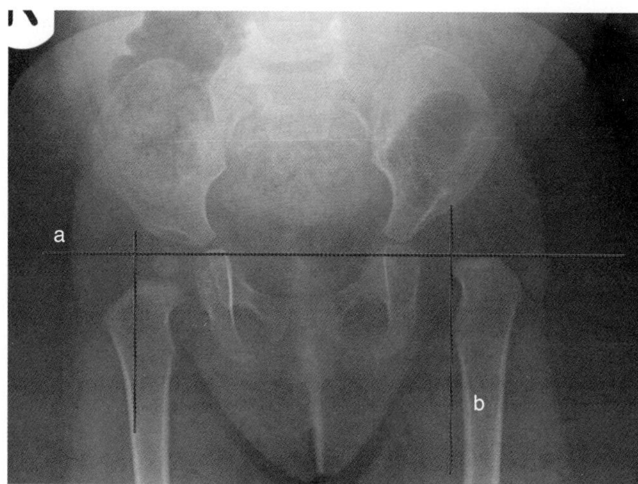

Figure 39.15 Anteroposterior pelvic radiograph showing Hilgenreiner's line **(a)** and Perkins' line **(b)**. The femoral head (ossific nucleus) of a normal hip lies in the inner lower quadrant. The right hip is normal, the left hip has developmental dysplasia of the hip.

Summary box 39.6

Diagnosis of developmental dysplasia of the hip

- Is always based on the history and clinical examination and then confirmed by appropriate investigations
- All neonates are screened clinically (Barlow and Ortolani tests), at birth and at 6 weeks
- Ultrasound is used to monitor hip stability/anatomy and often as a screening test in 'at-risk' babies
- Radiography is useful from 4 months onwards
- Older children present with a limp and/or tiptoeing.

Management

When diagnosed early, conservative treatment is usually successful, but after walking age surgery is required. The objective is to obtain a stable, congruous reduction of the femoral head into the acetabulum while avoiding damage to the capital epiphysis (avascular necrosis) or to the growth plate, which causes stiffness, coxa vara and shortening.

NEONATE

Owing to the hormonal effects in play during the perinatal period many hips are unstable initially. Most stabilise within the first few weeks of life and do **not** need treatment.

Hips that remain unstable at 6 weeks or that are dislocated at rest, are treated with harnesses or splints that obtain and then maintain hip reduction in the position of abduction and flexion. Most harnesses (**Figure 39.16**) allow controlled movement while splints hold the hips more rigidly and so may carry a greater risk of avascular necrosis (AVN). If the hips fail to relocate or stabilise then non-operative treatment should be discontinued.

INFANT

Successful treatment using a harness is unusual after the age of 4–6 months. For the late-presenting hip or the hip that

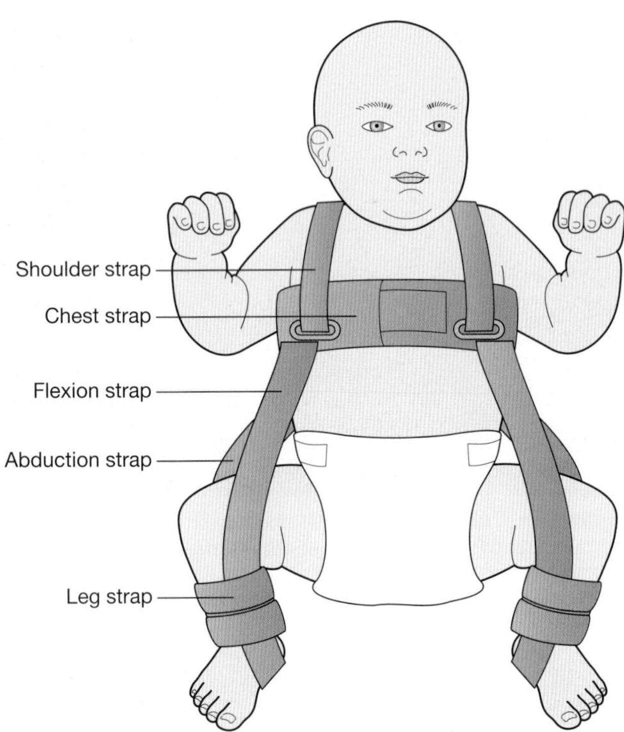

Figure 39.16 The anterior strap of the Pavlik harness controls hip flexion, whereas the posterior strap limits adduction and encourages abduction.

fails conservative treatment, an examination under anaesthetic may result in a closed reduction. The arthrogram shows whether a concentric reduction is present and, if not, it will indicate which structures are blocking reduction. A psoas/adductor release can be performed as necessary. Following a closed reduction, the hip will need to be held reduced with a hip spica cast for several months.

If the hip is irreducible or can only be held reduced in an extreme position with a small safe zone then treatment must be abandoned and an open reduction considered via a medial or anterior approach.

Summary box 39.7

Management of early developmental dysplasia of the hip

- Many hips that are unstable in the first few days/weeks of life do not need treatment as they improve spontaneously
- Up to age 4–6 months, a harness or splint is effective treatment
- In older babies, closed reduction is often possible and preferable to an open reduction
- For failed closed treatment, open surgical reduction is required

YOUNG CHILD OR TODDLER

The older the child, the less likely it is that reduction by closed methods will succeed (Figure 39.17) The traditional approach is then to carry out open reduction via an anterior approach around the age of 9–12 months. A pelvic osteotomy

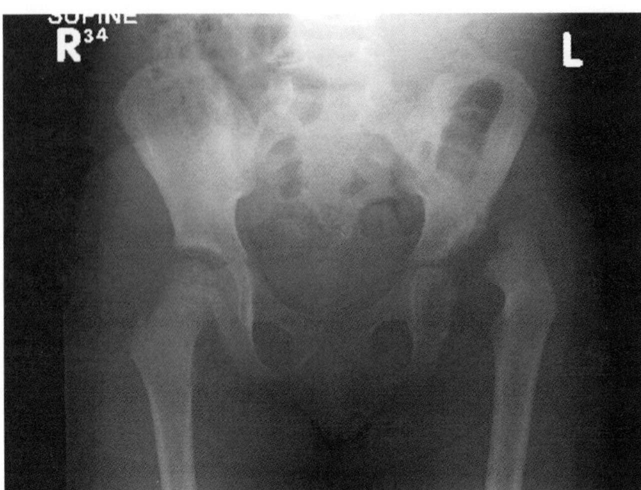

Figure 39.17 Anteroposterior pelvic radiograph showing acetabular dysplasia with subluxation (developmental dysplasia of the hip) of the left hip. This child presented at the age of 4 years.

may be required to reorientate or close down the acetabulum, and femoral shortening or derotation osteotomies are often required to improve stability. Earlier surgery via the medial approach can be considered but no additional surgery such as capsulorraphy or bony realignment can be performed through that incision.

OLDER CHILD

In the older child a similar approach is necessary but pelvic and femoral realignment will always be needed, and the results tend to be less rewarding. Surgery is often avoided in children over the age of 6–8 years (bilateral cases) and the age of 8–10 in unilateral cases (Figure 39.18).

ADOLESCENT AND YOUNG ADULT

These hips are often subluxated rather than truly dislocated. On investigation, the hip may be reducible and the joint can be recreated with a combination of pelvic and femoral osteotomies. For the irreducible hip, acetabular augmentation may reduce symptoms and delay the onset of degenerative change.

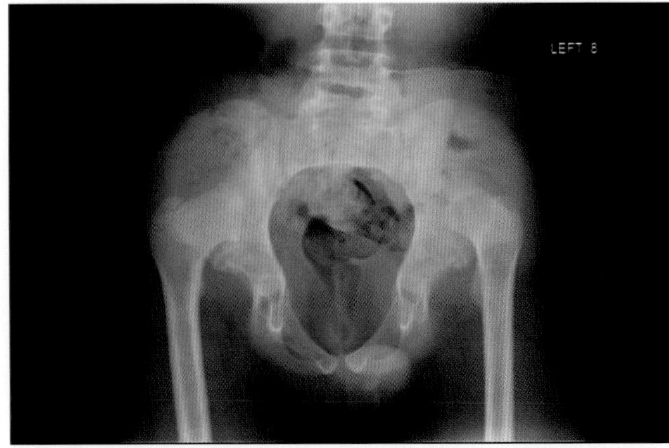

Figure 39.18 Anteroposterior pelvic radiograph showing bilateral true dislocations in a 9-year-old child; the decision was made not to offer an operation. The pathology in these hips is different from that shown in Figure 39.17.

Summary box 39.8

Management of late-presenting DDH

- The older the child, the more likely it is that they will require surgery
- Femoral osteotomy can stabilise the hip and reduce pressure on the femoral head
- Pelvic osteotomy redirects or reshapes the acetabulum
- The potential for acetabular remodelling decreases after the age of 3–4 years
- Avascular necrosis is a risk with all DDH treatment

SECONDARY PROCEDURES AND COMPLICATIONS

Regular follow-up ensures that the hip development is monitored. Acetabular remodelling may be assessed objectively by measuring the acetabular index or the centre–edge angle (Figure 39.19).

If the acetabulum does not improve, a variety of pelvic osteotomies can be considered. AVN with overgrowth of the greater trochanter can cause a Trendelenburg limp and distal transfer of the trochanter may help (Figure 39.20). Occasionally, a leg length difference needs treatment. There is also an increased risk of osteoarthritis which may need arthroplasty later in life.

Legg-Calvé-Perthes' (LCP) disease

Incidence and aetiology

This rare condition, characterised by the development of avascular necrosis (AVN) of the proximal femoral epiphysis, affects boys predominantly between the ages of 4 and 7 years; 10% develop bilateral disease. Although the aetiology is unclear, several factors have been implicated (*Table 39.6*). There are also other causes of AVN of the femoral head (*Table 39.7*). Overall, the incidence appears to be declining.

TABLE 39.6 Factors implicated in the pathogenesis of Perthes' disease.

- Low birth weight
- Delayed bone age
- Short stature with rostral sparing
- Associated with congenital urogenital anomalies
- Socioeconomic deprivation

TABLE 39.7 Causes of avascular necrosis of the femoral head.

- Steroids
- Infection/surgery/previous injury or fracture
- Perthes' disease
- Sickle cell disease
- Hypothyroidism
- Skeletal dysplasia – classically multiple epiphyseal dysplasia

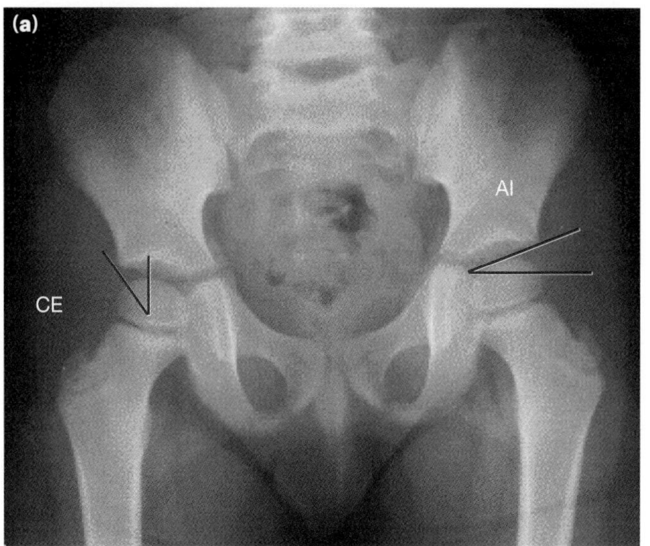

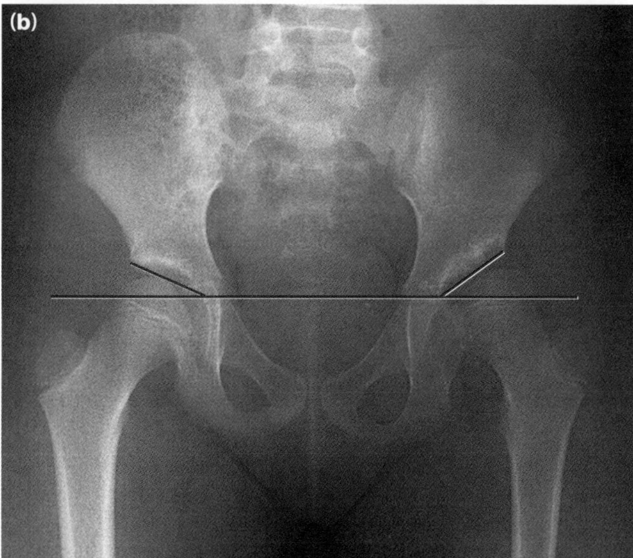

Figure 39.19 Anteroposterior pelvic radiographs demonstrating the acetabular index (AI) and the centre–edge (CE) angle: (**a**) normal hips; (**b**) the left hip shows residual dysplasia. The AI is increased when compared with the normal right hip. The left CE angle would be smaller than the right too but it has not been measured on this radiograph.

Pathology

Once established the process follows a well-described course. The avascular change may affect all or part of the femoral epiphysis. The avascular bone may collapse. This is followed by revascularisation, resorption and fragmentation of the dead ossific nucleus within the cartilaginous femoral head, and finally by reossification and regeneration ('healing') of the bony epiphysis. In this respect, Perthes' disease is a self-limiting condition but, during the collapse and fragmentation phases, femoral head deformity occurs as the cartilage 'follows' the shape of the newly reossified epiphysis. This change in

Legg, Calvé and Perthes all described osteochondritis of the head of the femur independently in 1910.
Arthur Thornton Legg, 1874–1939, orthopaedic surgeon, The Children's Hospital, Boston, MA, USA.
Jacques Calvé, 1875–1927, orthopaedic surgeon, La Fondation Franco-Americaine, Berck Plage, Pas-de-Calais, France.
Georg Clemens Perthes, 1869–1927, Professor of Surgery, Tubingen, Germany.

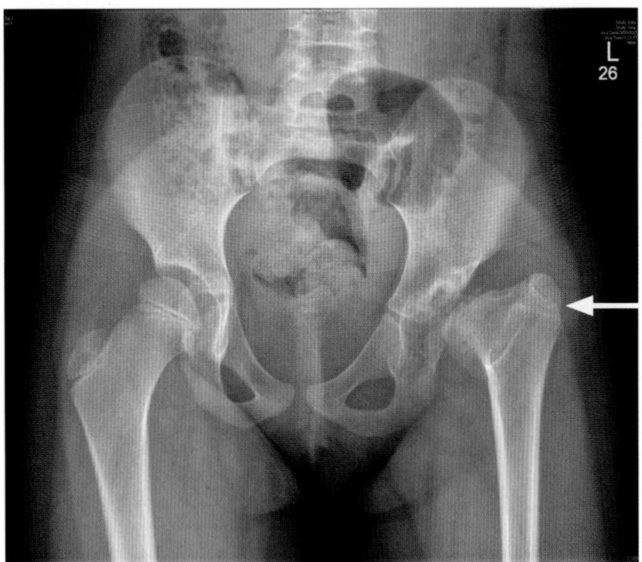

Figure 39.20 Anteroposterior pelvic radiograph of a 7-year-old girl who developed avascular necrosis secondary to a postoperative wound infection following a closed reduction of her dislocated left hip. Note the destruction of the femoral head and the proximal femoral physis, so that the femoral neck is short and the greater trochanter relatively high (arrow).

shape is not reversible and has a permanent effect on the health of the hip joint.

Diagnosis

The history, clinical examination and anteroposterior and 'frog' lateral radiographs of the pelvis make the diagnosis. An intermittently painful hip (or knee) with a limp and irritability or restriction of hip movements requires investigation. The radiographic features vary with the disease stage and may not correlate with the clinical condition (**Figure 39.21**).

AVN of the femoral head may be due to other causes and a differential diagnosis should be considered, particularly when changes are bilateral.

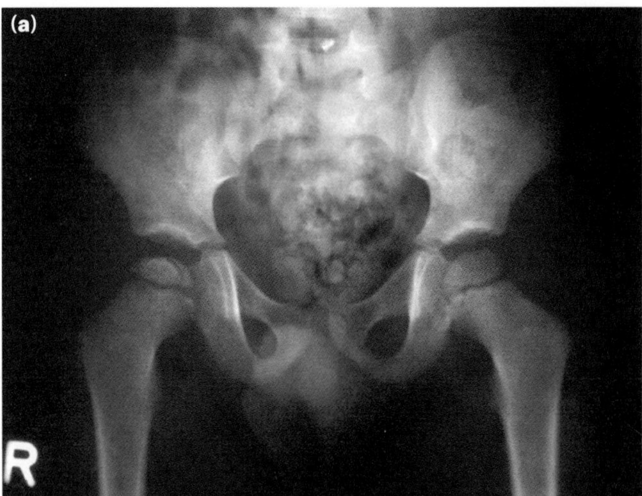

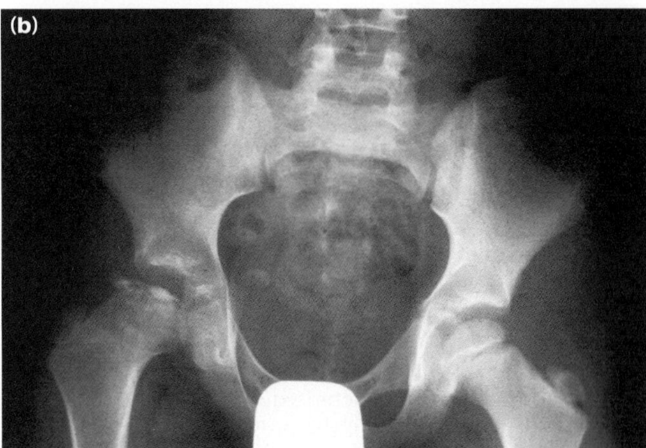

Figure 39.21 Anteroposterior pelvic radiographs of Perthes' disease demonstrating whole head involvement: (**a**) right-sided disease; the process is in an early phase and the area of dense necrotic bone is visible; (**b**) there has been collapse and fragmentation. The Catterall classification relates to how much of the epiphysis has been affected and the Herring classification relates to the height of the lateral pillar (lateral portion of the epiphysis) in the fragmentation phase of the disease.

Management

The prognosis, and hence the management, is influenced by the extent of AVN and the degree of collapse. Traditionally, LCP disease has been classified with the Catterall classification but currently the popular system in use is the Herring classification; however, this can only be applied when the head is in the fragmentation phase. In both systems, if the anterolateral portion is preserved, the prognosis is good.

Treatment aims to minimise femoral head deformity and thus the likelihood of secondary acetabular dysplasia. This is achieved by maintaining a good range of joint movement, with some restriction in activity level, and using analgesia and physiotherapy as required. The routine use of crutches and/or wheelchairs is discouraged because they promote a flexion/adduction posture. Recent evidence suggests that brace management on its own does not alter the natural history of the condition.

The role of operative treatment is controversial. Surgery can be performed early to prevent deformity secondary to femoral head collapse or late to 'salvage' a poor mechanical situation when deformity is limiting movement (*Table 39.8*). Joint distraction (arthrodiastasis) may preserve joint movement and maintain femoral head height but has not gained popularity.

Not all hips with deformity require 'salvage' surgery: young children, with more time to remodel, have a better prognosis as the acetabular changes (in response to the changed shape of the femoral head) result in an aspherical but congruent joint. Long-term follow-up may be required to deal with mechanical symptoms caused by loose osteochondral fragments, a Trendelenburg gait secondary to trochanteric overgrowth or a short-leg gait. Degenerative change may occur in adult life.

Other conditions (all eponymous) also show radiographic changes of AVN (*Table 39.9*). Again, the radiographic changes 'heal' but the change in shape of the affected bone may lead to secondary joint stiffness and loss of function.

TABLE 39.8 A guide to some of the surgical options available for the management of Perthes' disease.

Timing	Type of procedure	Comments	Aim
Early	Femoral osteotomy	Varus and derotation Consider an opening wedge osteotomy to maintain length	To cover ('contain') the vulnerable femoral head
	Innominate osteotomy		
	Shelf acetabuloplasty		
Intermediate	Arthrodiastasis	Hinged distraction to allow movement, primarily flexion/extension	To reduce deforming pressures on the femoral head
Late	Femoral osteotomy	Valgus With extension to undo a fixed flexion deformity or flexion to remove the anterior bump from impinging on the acetabulum	To improve joint congruity and hence function; to improve joint mechanics
	Arthrotomy	To remove osteochondral fragments	
	Head-neck osteoplasty	After physeal closure	To improve head shape by reducing femoroacetabular impingement and increasing head/neck offset.
	Trochanteric epiphyseodesis or distal transfer	Epiphyseodesis probably not effective after age 7–8 years	To improve lever arm function
Contralateral limb	Distal femoral epiphyseodesis		To improve leg length discrepancy and reduce effects on hip joint mechanics

TABLE 39.9 Other conditions (commonly called osteochondroses) in which the radiographic appearance is of avascular necrosis.

Condition	Affected bone
Kienbock's disease	Lunate
Panner's disease	Capitellum of the humerus
Freiberg's disease	Metatarsal head – usually the second
Köhler's disease	Navicular

Summary box 39.9

Legg-Calvé-Perthes' disease

- Most common in boys aged 4–7 years
- AVN leads to femoral head collapse; the return of the blood supply heralds the resorption and reossification phases that allow the femoral head to 'heal'
- The prognosis is better in younger children (and in boys), who have more remodelling potential before skeletal maturity
- Management aims to maintain femoral head sphericity
- Treatment may be non-surgical (to maximise range of movement) or surgical (early for containment or late for 'salvage')

Slip of the upper (capital) femoral epiphysis (SUFE/SCFE)

The physis connects the proximal femoral epiphysis (the femoral head) to the metaphysis (femoral neck). In certain physiological or pathological conditions a 'stress fracture' through the physis allows the epiphysis to displace as it would with an intracapsular femoral neck fracture, so the leg lies short and externally rotated. There is painful limitation of hip movement. Hilton's law, which states that a joint is supplied by the same nerves as the muscles that move the joint, explains why many children present with knee pain although the pathology is in the hip.

Incidence and aetiology

SUFE or SCFE is rare, with an incidence of ~5 per 100 000 population. Boys are affected most commonly; the peak incidence is related to the start of puberty, hence it is earlier in girls. As a result of growth stimulated by hormonal changes, the strength of the growth plate, its resistance to shear and its orientation are reduced. The hip is therefore 'at risk' and normal forces, exacerbated by obesity and repetitive minor trauma, precipitate a slip. Other conditions such as hypothyroidism, renal failure and previous radiotherapy treatment (local or to the pituitary region) also increase the risk.

Diagnosis

The diagnosis is suggested by the history and examination and confirmed on plain radiograph (**Figure 39.22**). Displacement is often more obvious on a lateral view. Indeed, it can easily be missed by the unwary clinician if only the AP view is checked.

Classification

A SCFE can be classified according to three parameters: timing, severity and stability. The onset of symptoms divides

Robert Kienbock, 1871–1953, Professor of Radiology, Vienna, Austria, described this condition in 1910.
Hans Jessen Panner, 1871–1930, radiologist, of Copenhagen, Denmark, described this condition in 1927.
Albert Henry Freiberg, 1869–1940, Professor of Orthopaedic Surgery, The University of Cincinnati, Cincinnati, OH, USA, described this disease in 1926.
Alban Köhler, 1874–1947, radiologist, of Wiesbaden, Germany, described this disease in 1908.
John Hilton, 1805–1878, surgeon, Guy's Hospital, London, UK.

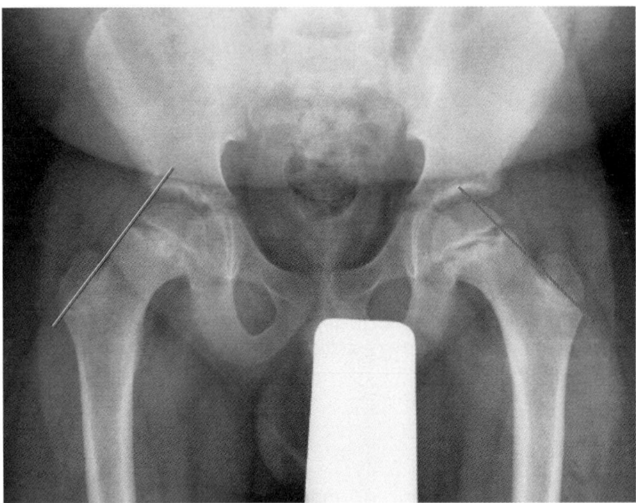

Figure 39.22 Anteroposterior pelvic radiograph demonstrating a mild slip of the upper (capital) femoral epiphysis on the right side. A line drawn along the upper margin of the femoral neck should transect the femoral head (left side) – if it does not do so (right side) a slip is present. There are many other radiographic features that help confirm the diagnosis but the changes are often subtle and may be seen first on the frog lateral view.

slips into those that are acute, chronic, or acute on chronic. Slip severity is assessed on the lateral radiograph in terms of percentage uncovering of the metaphysis (*Table 39.10*) or by measuring the slip angle of Southwick (**Figure 39.23**). An unstable slip is defined by Loder as one where the patient can not bear weight on the limb.

Management

Following an **acute** episode the patient is often completely unable to bear weight and the slip is considered to be **unstable**.

TABLE 39.10 Grading of the severity of slip of the upper (capital) femoral epiphysis.

Slip severity	Metaphysis uncovered (%)
Mild	<33
Moderate	33–66
Severe	>66

Displacement is often **moderate** or **severe**. This situation is essentially equivalent to a displaced intracapsular femoral neck fracture. This means that an acute unstable SUFE is an emergency. The AVN risk is considerable but is reduced by prompt screw fixation that stabilises the 'fracture' (**Figure 39.24**).

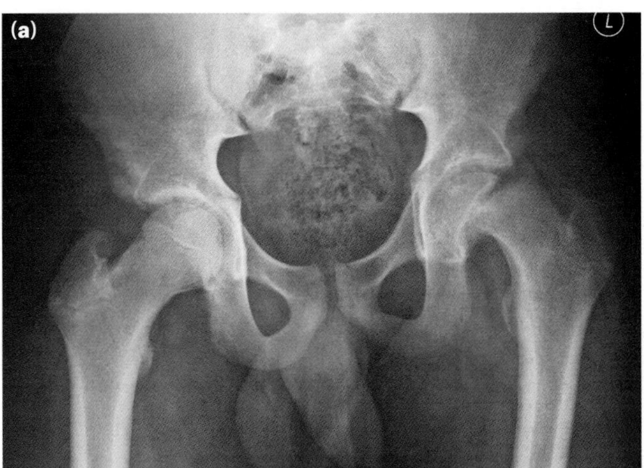

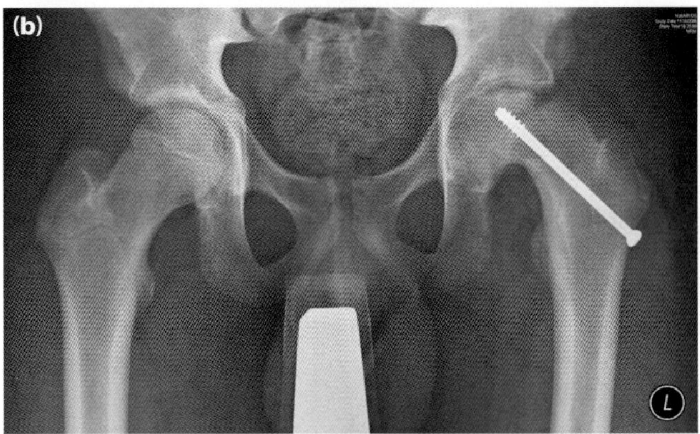

Figure 39.24 Anteroposterior pelvic radiograph showing a left-sided acute severe unstable slip of the upper (capital) femoral epiphysis: (**a**) at presentation; (**b**) following partial repositioning and fixation with a cannulated screw. When this heals, because of the incomplete reduction it is likely that the metaphysis will impinge on the acetabulum (FAI, femoroacetabular impingement) during movement, causing pain and leading to degenerative change.

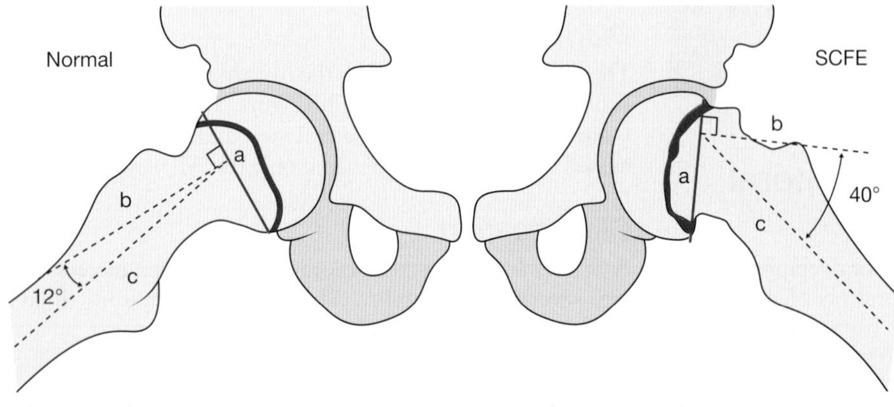

Figure 39.23 The Southwick slip angle is measured on a lateral radiograph and denotes how far the epiphysis has slipped off the metaphysis. The value on the normal side must be subtracted from the value on the abnormal side to get the true value. (SCFE, slip of the capital femoral epiphysis.)

Randall Loder, Professor of Orthopaedic Surgery, Philadelphia, PA, USA.

With the reduction in muscle spasm that accompanies a general anaesthetic, a gentle repositioning of the femoral epiphysis takes place as the externally rotated limb is lifted into the neutral position; no force must be used with this maneouvre. A capsulotomy also helps reduce the tamponade effect on the vessels to the epiphysis. To be effective such treatment must take place within 24 hours of injury. If delayed, the AVN rate increases.

With **chronic** slips the patient is usually able to bear weight, albeit with pain, and the slip is considered stable. Screw or pin fixation *in situ* relieves pain and often improves the range of movement but permanent reduction in abduction, flexion and internal rotation will be present (Figure 39.25). The leg will also always be slightly short.

In the **acute-on-chronic** case, repositioning of the acute element of the slip may be feasible.

In the **chronic severe** slip it may be impossible to place a screw in a satisfactory position in the epiphysis, even by starting anteriorly on the neck. In addition, once healed, there may be significant, persistent deformity leading to restriction of joint movement. In these cases a realignment osteotomy may be considered. As with all osteotomies, the closer the correction is to the site of deformity, the better the outcome. However, in this situation the centre of rotation of angulation (CORA) for the deformity is at the level of the physis; the risk of AVN or chondrolysis may be unacceptably high with an osteotomy at this level, and so an intertrochanteric osteotomy could be considered. The slipped epiphysis is associated with a 'cam' type of femoroacetabular impingement and this may require treatment with a head-neck osteoplasty to restore the offset between the head and neck.

Bilateral slips do occur and prophylactic pinning of the normal but 'at-risk' hip may be indicated.

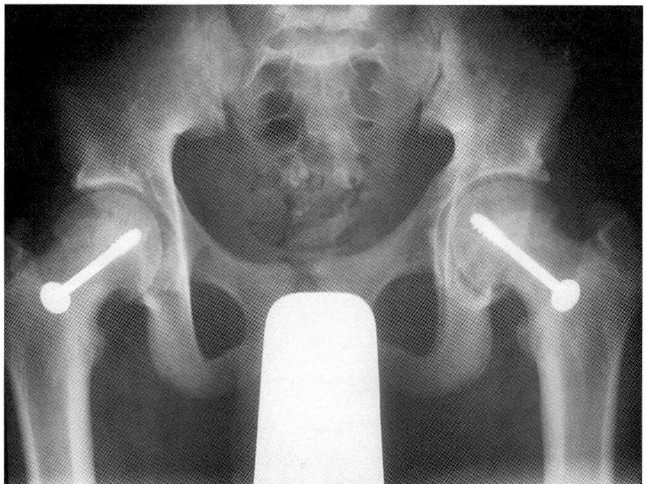

Figure 39.25 Anteroposterior radiograph showing screw fixation *in situ* of a case of bilateral chronic slip of the upper (capital) femoral epiphysis. Note the position of the screw: the more severe the slip, the more proximal and more anterior the screw entry point has to be on the femoral neck.

Summary box 39.10

Slip of the upper (capital) femoral epiphysis

- Occurs in prepubertal children, boys more commonly than girls
- Often presents with knee pain, and the leg may be short and externally rotated
- Classification systems relate to timing, severity and stability– all affect the prognosis
- Most slips are pinned *in situ* with a single screw into the centre of the epiphysis
- AVN is the most feared complication of both the condition and its treatment

ABNORMALITIES OF THE KNEE AND LOWER LEG

Many knee problems in children or adolescents are self-limiting. Others require surgical consideration to reduce the risk of later degenerative change.

Osteochondritis dissecans (OCD)

OCD most commonly affects the lateral aspect of the medial femoral condyle of the distal femur (but also the talus and the humerus). An osteochondral fragment becomes partially or completely separated from the joint surface. Magnetic resonance imaging (MRI) is the best method for demonstrating the site, extent and stability of the lesion. In mild cases, the osteochondral fragment remains attached and heals, particularly if treated early with rest and activity modification. If it detaches, partially or completely, mechanical symptoms necessitate treatment either to encourage bone healing via fixation of the fragment or to remove a loose body. Younger children have a better prognosis.

Discoid meniscus

This invariably affects the lateral meniscus, which is abnormally thick and covers most of the tibial plateau. The child presents with a painful clunk on knee extension. MRI is usually diagnostic. Surgery is indicated for relief of pain or mechanical symptoms.

Anterior knee pain

In adolescents the extensor mechanism of the knee is a common site of knee pain.

Osgood–Schlatter disease is a traction apophysitis of the patellar tendon insertion. Pain, tenderness and swelling at the tibial tubercle, exacerbated by exercise, are diagnostic and radiographs are unnecessary (except in unilateral cases, where it is important to exclude a diagnosis such as a malignancy). Treatment is relative rest and analgesia, and the condition resolves once the apophysis has fused.

Robert Bailey Osgood, 1873–1956, Professor of Orthopaedic Surgery, Harvard University Medical School, Boston, MA, USA.
Carl Schlatter, 1864–1934, Professor of Surgery, Zurich, Switzerland. Osgood and Schlatter described osteochondritis of the tibial tubercle independently in 1903.

Patellofemoral pain is common and often attributed to an adolescent growth spurt: symptoms are exacerbated either by activity or by rest with the knee in the flexed position. Alterations to activity levels and sitting position, physiotherapy to stretch and strengthen both the hamstrings and the quadriceps muscles and time usually result in a return to normal within a few months.

Anterior knee pain may be associated with a degree of patellar maltracking and/or instability. Treatment starts with physiotherapy to develop the quadriceps muscles, particularly the vastus medialis oblique (VMO) and to counteract any wasting secondary to the pain. There are a multitude of operations described to improve patellar tracking and these include options for realignment of the extensor mechanism both proximally and distally.

Fibular hemimelia

In fibular hemimelia there is a congenital failure of formation of the lateral 'column' of the lower leg (**Figure 39.26** and *Table 39.11*).

Management is tailored to the severity of the deficiency. Treatment options range from a shoe raise, through multiple episodes of limb equalisation surgery, to amputation for the worst cases. An early prediction of the leg length discrepancy at maturity allows a realistic treatment plan to be devised for the patient, which should include consideration of a contralateral epiphysiodesis.

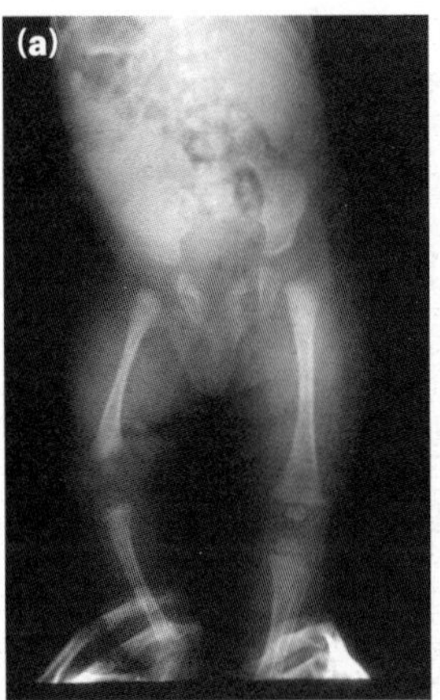

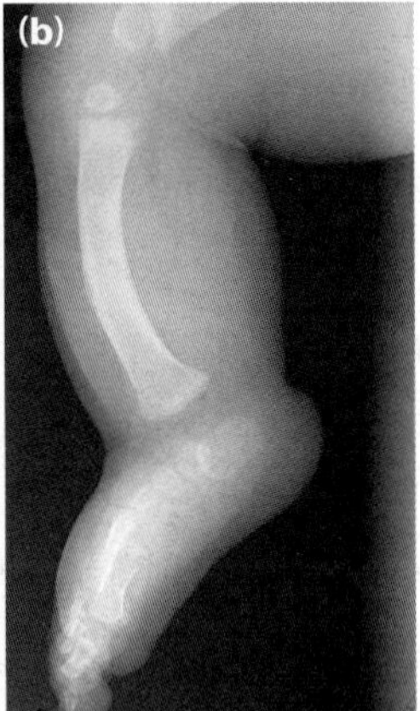

Figure 39.26 Anteroposterior (**a**) and lateral (**b**) radiographs of two lower limbs showing some of the features of a fibular hemimelia: absent 5th ray in the foot, absent fibula and deformed tibia.

TABLE 39.11 Classical radiographic features of fibular hemimelia.

Foot and ankle	Absent lateral rays; tarsal coalition; ball and socket ankle joint
Lower leg	Absent or deficient fibula; short bowed tibia
Knee	Absent tibial spine (no cruciate ligament); deficient lateral femoral condyle
Femur	Relative hypoplasia
Limb length and alignment	Short; external rotation ± valgus

Blount's disease

The aetiology of this disordered growth in the posteromedial proximal tibial physis is unknown. The infantile form is more common in Afro-Caribbeans but the adolescent-onset disease affects all ethnic origins. The child presents with progressive and often severe tibia vara with significant intoeing. The radiographic features are diagnostic (**Figure 39.27**).

Treatment is surgical: following correction of limb alignment via an osteotomy, an epiphyseodesis of the remaining physis may be necessary to prevent recurrence. In unilateral cases, the limb once straightened is short and concomitant tibial lengthening with an external fixator is often an attractive option.

Congenital pseudarthrosis of the tibia

This rare condition presents clinically with an anterolateral bow of the tibia with or without a fracture. Classic radiographic changes are noted and 50% are associated with neurofibromatosis. Once fractured the tibia is reluctant to heal. Long-term orthotic treatment may be necessary, with subsequent surgical procedures designed to obtain bony union and restore leg length (**Figure 39.28**).

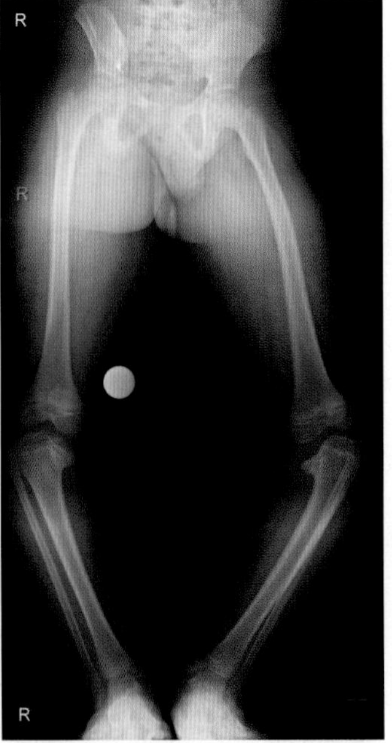

Figure 39.27 Standing leg length and alignment radiograph of a child with bilateral asymmetrical bow legs. Both proximal and medial tibial physes/epiphyses are abnormal: this is bilateral Blount's disease.

Walter Putnam Blount, 1900–1992, Professor of Orthopaedic Surgery, Marquette University, Milwaukee, WI, USA, described this condition in 1937.

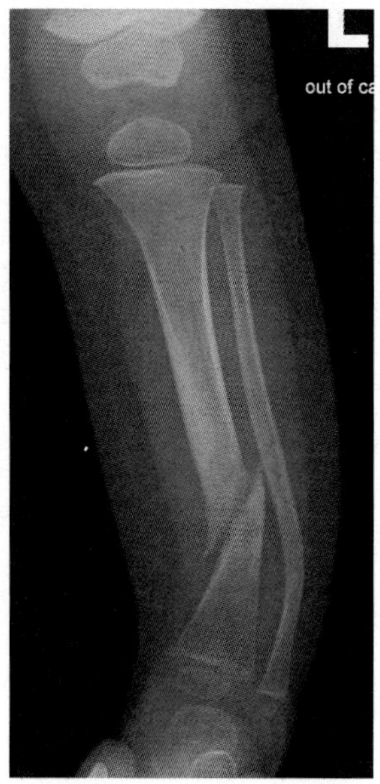

Figure 39.28 Anteroposterior radiograph of a child showing a congenital tibial pseudarthrosis. She was actually born with a bowed lower leg that subsequently fractured. She has a family history of neurofibromatosis.

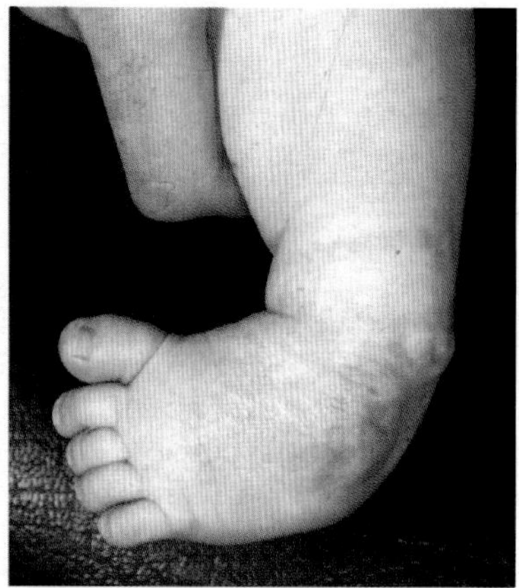

Figure 39.29 Anteroposterior photograph of a foot showing the classic deformities associated with a clubfoot. The hindfoot is in equinus and varus, there is midfoot cavus and the forefoot lies adducted and apparently supinated, although actually pronated relative to the hindfoot.

Summary box 39.11

Abnormalities of the knee and lower leg

- Osteochondritis dissecans – better prognosis in children than adults
- Discoid meniscus – usually lateral, may require surgery
- Anterior knee pain – treatment almost always conservative
- Fibular hemimelia – associated with abnormalities from the foot proximally (foot worse than hip), the tibial bow has an anteromedial apex
- Blount's disease – clinically, a sharp proximal tibial angulation
- Congenital pseudarthrosis of the tibia – the tibial bow has an anterolateral apex
- Posteromedial apex tibial bow – largely physiological, the bow improves with time but the limb may be short

ABNORMALITIES OF THE FOOT AND ANKLE

Parents are often concerned that minor foot abnormalities will cause their child to be clumsy or slow. This is rarely the case, so reassurance is a cornerstone in the management of abnormalities of the foot and ankle in children.

Congenital talipes equinovarus (CTEV) (the 'club foot')

The club foot is deformed in three planes (Figure 39.29). In true CTEV the deformity is fixed. Intrauterine moulding can cause an identical pattern of deformity that is postural and therefore correctable.

Incidence and aetiology

The reported incidence varies from 1 to 6 per 1000 live births, depending on racial differences. It is more common in boys and bilateral in approximately 50% of cases. A family history is common but inheritance is multifactorial. The diagnosis of CTEV may be made during an antenatal ultrasound: the sensitivity is higher in bilateral cases, and these patients are statistically more likely to have a syndromic association. In some countries, the detection of such an abnormality leads to consideration of a termination of the pregnancy but the parents can be reassured that with treatment their child will walk, run and play with his/her peers.

Most cases are idiopathic but because the outcome varies with the aetiology it is important to consider the cause when planning treatment (*Table 39.12*). Many of the idiopathic cases will have some weakness of the evertor muscles.

Pathology

The talonavicular joint is subluxated, with the navicular displaced medially with respect to a deformed talar head and neck. Ligaments, particularly the calcaneofibular ligament, and tendon sheaths, such as the posterior tibial tendon sheath, are shortened and thickened and contain contractile myofibroblasts. The gastrocsoleus and posterior tibial muscles are smaller than normal, with reduced myofibrils and increased connective tissue, possibly because of a local neuromuscular abnormality. The vascular supply via the dorsalis pedis may be diminished. It remains unclear which abnormalities are primary and which occur as the deformity develops.

Clinical assessment

It should be possible to distinguish the postural clubfoot from the structural (rigid) foot soon after birth. The postural clubfoot may benefit from physiotherapy stretches but, by

TABLE 39.12 Several different types of clubfoot are recognised.

Type	Example
Postural	
Idiopathic	
Neuromuscular	Spina bifida; arthrogryposis;
Syndromic	Trisomy 15

definition, it must be completely normal by 3 months of age with 45° of forefoot abduction, full ankle dorsiflexion with the calcaneus well down in the heel pad, no significant medial crease and only shallow/multiple posterior creases.

In contrast, the structural idiopathic clubfoot has fixed deformity with elements of hindfoot equinus and varus, midfoot adductus and pronation of the first ray, giving the appearance of forefoot cavus. The heel feels 'empty' as the calcaneus is held up by the shortened tendo Achilles. There is a deep medial and a single posterior crease.

All children with structural clubfoot deformity will have a small calf and foot and some tibial shortening but this may not be apparent until later in childhood. Children should be examined carefully for neurological signs of intraspinal pathology.

Both Pirani and Dimeglio have developed scoring systems, based on the appearance of the foot in its position of maximal correction, which predict treatment response and hence outcome.

Summary box 39.12

Clubfoot

- Multiplanar deformity: hindfoot equinus and varus, midfoot adductus and forefoot cavus
- Incidence is 1–6 per 1000 live births, more common in boys and with a familial tendency
- Most cases are idiopathic but neuromuscular causes include spina bifida and arthrogryposis
- Scoring systems (Pirani/Dimeglio), are used to assess the severity

Treatment

PONSETI METHOD

The method described by Ponseti corrects foot deformity in 95% of idiopathic cases without the need for a formal surgical release and has now become the treatment of choice for all such feet. Treatment commences within a few days of birth. A specific series of manoeuvres, followed by a series of well-moulded above-knee plaster casts, results in gradual correction of the deformity (Figure 39.30). The head of the talus is the fulcrum around which the rest of the foot rotates. After the forefoot has been corrected, most feet (about 80%) require a percutaneous Achilles tenotomy (performed under local anaesthetic in the clinic setting) in order to dorsiflex the foot satisfactorily.

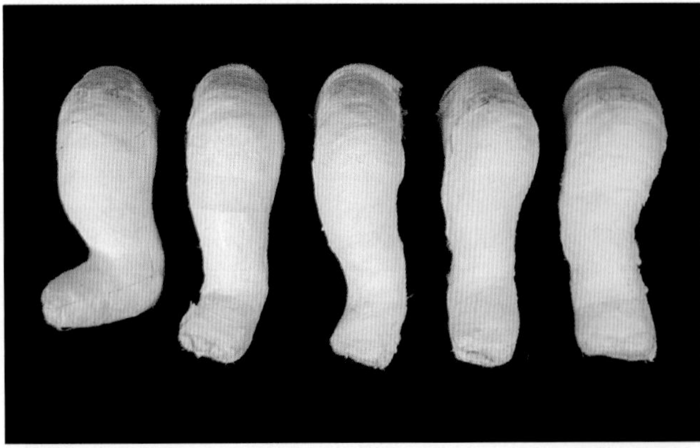

Corrected ◄——— Uncorrected

Figure 39.30 A photograph of a series of casts documenting the stepwise correction of the foot deformity with the Ponseti method of serial manipulation and casting.

Once corrected the foot position is maintained by a foot abduction orthosis (FAO) that holds the feet in external rotation and slight dorsiflexion. The FAO is worn full-time for 3 months and at 'night and nap-time' for up to 4 years. Poor compliance with the FAO is associated with a higher relapse rate. Recurrent deformity can be treated with further plasters, but a tibialis anterior tendon transfer may be required around the age of 2.5–4 years for persisting dynamic supination.

Feet treated with the Ponseti method are less stiff, less likely to be painful and less subject to overcorrection than those treated surgically. The Ponseti method is significantly better than other reported conservative regimes. It also works reasonably well in non-idiopathic feet but both the failure and relapse rates are higher.

SURGICAL TREATMENT

When conservative treatment fails, surgical intervention is required, ideally before walking age.

Surgical release is generally performed 'à la carte', with sequential release of the pathologically tight structures via either a Turco incision or the Cincinnati incision (*Table 39.13*) to reduce the subluxated joints. Stabilisation may require the use of temporary Kirschner wires. Deformity correction should not be compromised by wound closure and the Cincinnati incision can be left to heal by secondary intention if necessary.

TABLE 39.13 The four stages of a peritalar release that may be required for the correction of a severe clubfoot deformity.

Site	Structures requiring lengthening or release
Posterior	Tendo Achilles
	Ankle and subtalar joints
	Calcaneofibular ligament
	Posterior elements of the peroneal tendon sheaths
Medial	Abductor hallucis
	Tibialis posterior
	Talonavicular joint
	Toe flexors
Lateral	Calcaneocuboid joint
Plantar	Plantar ligaments
	Plantar fascia
Protect	*Neurovascular bundle*
	Talocalcaneal interosseous ligament (if possible)

Martin Kirschner, 1879–1942, Professor of Surgery, Heidelberg, Germany, introduced the use of skeletal traction wires in 1909.

Postoperative casting is followed by splinting and physiotherapy as required. Good or excellent results are reported in 60–80% of children treated surgically but stiffness and over- or undercorrection are common complications.

Surgery for residual or recurrent deformity is often difficult and requires a careful assessment of the forefoot, hindfoot and tibial torsion. Surgical procedures may involve further soft-tissue releases or tendon transfers but, in the presence of fixed deformity, bony correction is often necessary. The foot becomes progressively stiffer with each surgical intervention.

Summary box 39.13

Treatment of clubfoot

- The Ponseti method of serial casting is successful in 95% of feet when defined as avoiding formal surgical release
    - The standard sequence of manipulations is:

      C – correction of the apparent forefoot **cavus** by elevation of the first ray

      A – gradual forefoot **abduction** to 60°, and simultaneous

      V – correction of the hindfoot **varus**

      E – correction of hindfoot **equinus** which usually follows a percutaneous Achilles tenotomy, which is an integral part of this treatment method
- Tibialis anterior tendon transfer (TATT) can be used to correct dynamic supination in older children

If the Ponseti method fails:

- Surgical release may be needed to address posterior, medial, plantar and lateral structures, and will result in a stiffer foot than one treated conservatively

Other foot and ankle conditions

Most postural deformities such as metatarsus adductus and calcaneovalgus feet improve spontaneously.

Congenital vertical talus (CVT) is rare and often associated with neuromuscular conditions such as arthrogryposis and spinal dysraphism. Clinically, there is a stiff 'rocker-bottom' foot with dorsal dislocation of the navicular on the talus (Figure 39.31). Correction is surgical although a 'reverse' Ponseti method with a limited surgical approach to reduce the talonavicular joint and a percutaneous Achilles tenotomy is showing some good early results.

In **tarsal coalition** there is failure of segmentation of adjacent tarsal bones. School-age children present with hindfoot pain and recurrent ankle sprains. The stiff subtalar joint cannot accommodate uneven ground. The most common coalitions are talocalcaneal and calcaneonavicular (see Figure 39.4). Radiographs, computed tomography (CT) or MRI may be required to confirm the diagnosis. Treatment is initially conservative but if the coalition requires surgical excision, this should be carried out before significant degenerative changes develop.

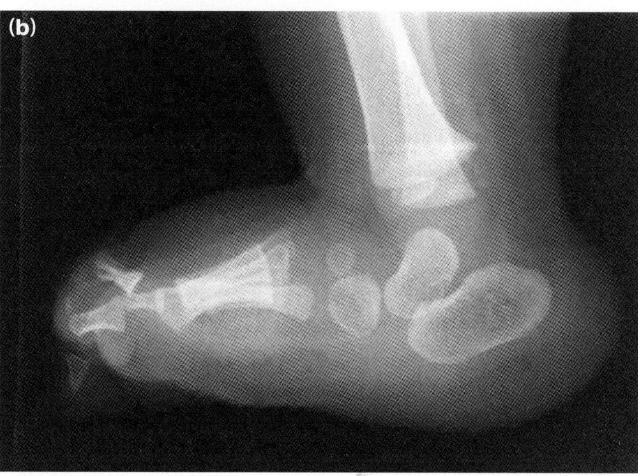

Figure 39.31 Congenital vertical talus: **(a)** lateral photograph demonstrating a 'rocker-bottom foot'; **(b)** lateral radiograph showing hindfoot equinus and suggesting dorsal subluxation of the non-ossified navicular and forefoot with respect to the head of the talus.

Curly toes that are flexed and medially deviated are common, often familial and rarely need treatment. Strapping is ineffective. Flexor tenotomy is used when there are symptoms or cosmetic concerns.

Other causes of foot pain in children include osteochondroses:

- **Freiberg's osteochondrosis** presents with forefoot pain and avascular change in the second metatarsal head. It may be asymptomatic and present as an incidental finding on a radiograph. Symptomatic bony spurs and osteochondral fragments may need excision.

Summary box 39.14

Other foot and ankle conditions

- Congenital vertical talus – presents as 'rocker-bottom' foot
- Tarsal coalition – presents as a stiff, painful flat foot
- Curly toes are common – most do not need treatment
- Osteochondroses – almost always self-limiting

Ignacio Ponseti, 1914–2009, faculty member of the University of Iowa, USA. Born in Menorca, fled Spain during the Civil War because of the political situation, worked as a general practitioner in Mexico and then went to Iowa to train in orthopaedics. The technique that bears his name only became popular years after he retired – but it brought him back to work for another 20 years.

- **Köhler's disease** presents with dorsal forefoot pain and swelling in young children. The navicular becomes avascular and there is alteration in the ossification process. The alarming radiological appearance resolves spontaneously and without sequelae.
- **Sever's disease** (enthesopathy of the calcaneal apophysis) presents with heel pain related to activity. Tightness in the calf muscle complex may be a contributing factor. The 'features' on a radiograph are, in fact, part of normal growth and development.

ABNORMALITIES OF THE UPPER LIMB

Minor finger abnormalities are common (*Table 39.14*) but not all require surgical intervention. Comfort and function are more important than appearance.

Function is also the most important consideration when managing more extensive upper limb abnormalities. Treatment is often delayed until hand dominance is established and it is clear what problems a specific deformity is causing a given child. Children are very adaptable and cope with disabilities much more readily than their parents/doctors expect.

Radial club hand

This longitudinal failure of formation is commonly associated with other malformations, for example as part of the VACTERL syndrome (abnormal **v**ertebrae, **a**nus, **c**ardiovascular system, **t**rachea, **o**esophagus, **r**enal system and **l**imb buds). The clinical problem depends, most specifically, on whether the thumb is present and functional (**Figure 39.32**). Treatment is a balance of conservative measures, including physiotherapy and splinting, and judicious surgery to centralise and stabilise the hand and wrist on the single bone forearm.

TABLE 39.14 Common minor congenital anomalies affecting the hand.

Anomaly	Definition	Treatment
Extra/accessory digits		Excise/amputate when necessary
Syndactyly	Failure of separation of digits	Separation with/without skin grafting for functional or cosmetic reasons
Trigger thumb (digit)		Release of the A1 pulley of the flexor tendon sheath
Clinodactyly (usually the fifth digit)	Abnormal angulation of the digit in the radioulnar plane	Surgical treatment of the delta phalanx if deformity progressive or interfering with hand function
Camptodactyly (usually the fifth digit)	Fixed flexion deformity of proximal interphalangeal joint	Splinting/physiotherapy; surgery rarely indicated

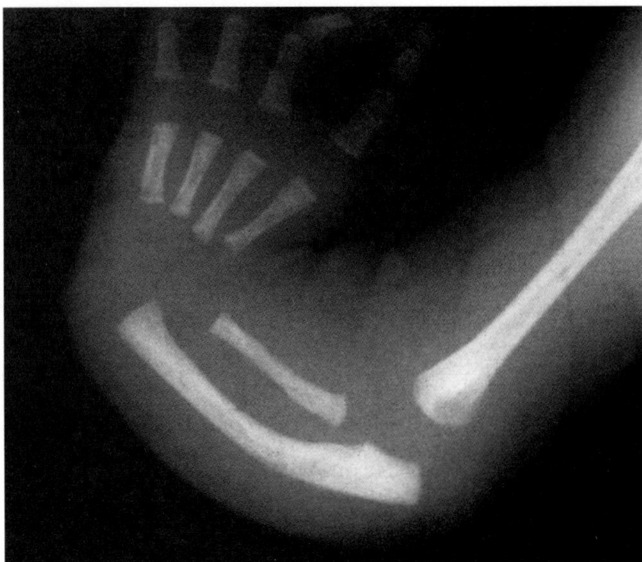

Figure 39.32 Anteroposterior radiograph of a radial club hand demonstrating a short radius, a deformed ulna and an absent thumb.

Thumb reconstruction may be technically challenging. In later childhood, forearm lengthening may be considered.

Radioulnar synostosis

Failure of proximal separation of the embryonic radius and ulna means that the forearm never develops the ability to pronate or supinate. The hand, on the end of the forearm, is therefore in a fixed position somewhere along the arc from full pronation–neutral–full supination and the child presents if this fixed position results in a functional problem. Osteotomy of the forearm bones can change the fixed position (for example, from pronation to neutral) but does not restore movement. Attempts at undoing the synostosis are not successful. If surgery is comtemplated, the choice of the position post surgery will depend on hand dominance, cultural considerations and functional demands.

Congenital radial head dislocation

The dislocation is usually posterolateral, compared with the classic traumatic anterior dislocation (**Figure 39.33**). Some restriction of elbow joint movement and forearm rotation is noted along with discomfort on activity. Radial head excision may be required after skeletal maturity.

Summary box 39.15

Upper limb abnormalities

- Radial club hand is frequently associated with other congenital anomalies, for example the VACTERL or Holt–Oram syndromes
- Radioulnar synostosis presents with a fixed forearm position in childhood
- Congenital radial head dislocation is usually posterolateral

James Warren Sever, 1878–1964, orthopaedic surgeon, The Children's Hospital, Boston, MA, USA, described apophysitis of the os calcis in 1912.

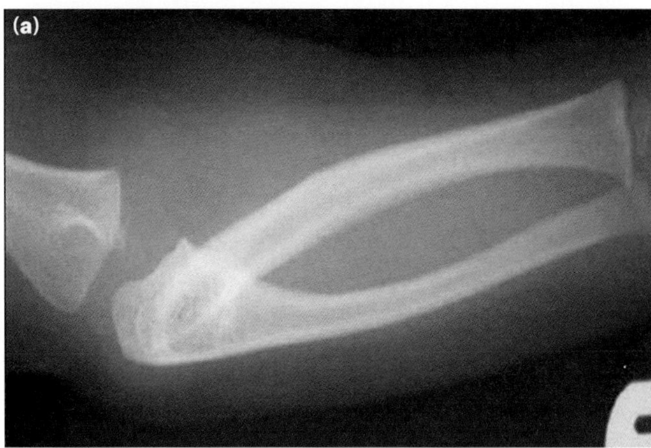

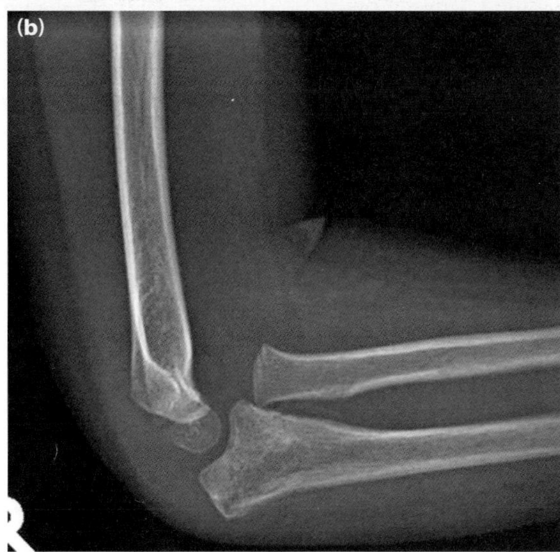

Figure 39.33 Radial head dislocation: (**a**) lateral radiograph of a forearm showing a proximal radioulnar synostosis with a congenital posterolateral dislocation of the radial head. Note the underdeveloped radial head and neck and compare with (**b**), a lateral radiograph of a traumatic anterior dislocation of the radial head with a normal appearance to the head and neck and a deformity in the proximal ulna.

SPINAL DEFORMITIES AND BACK PAIN

Congenital deformities

Congenital vertebral deformities are failures either of formation (a hemivertebra) or of segmentation (unilateral or bilateral fusions or bars). The clinical result is usually a scoliosis (Figure 39.34). Treatment should be based on the potential for curve progression. When a kyphosis develops, progressive neurological deficit is common. Bracing is ineffective for congenital vertebral deformities.

Scoliosis

The term 'scoliosis' describes spinal deformity in three planes: lateral curvature is the most obvious deformity while the rotational component is most apparent in forward flexion when

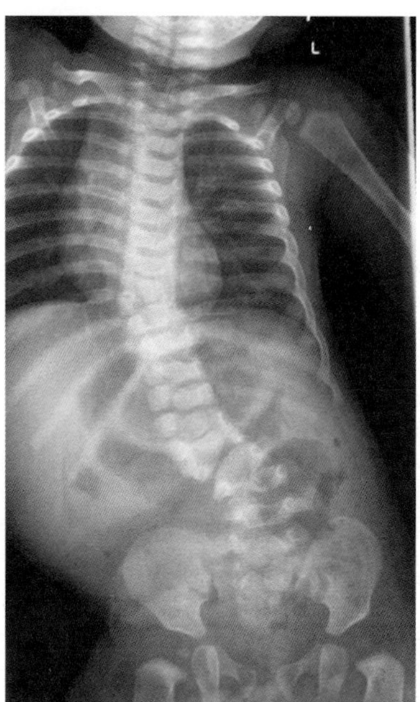

Figure 39.34 Anteroposterior radiograph of the spine demonstrating multiple congenital vertebral anomalies including hemivertebrae.

the rib asymmetry creates a 'rib hump' (Figure 39.35). The cause may be idiopathic, neuromuscular, syndrome-related or congenital. Both the aetiology and the age of onset affect the natural history (*Table 39.15*). In general, the earlier the onset, the more likely the deformity is to be progressive. As so much lung development occurs in early childhood, the management of early-onset scoliosis must preserve growth: casting techniques or the use of 'growing rods' may be appropriate.

The adolescent idiopathic curve is the most common, affecting girls more than boys. Idiopathic scoliosis is generally not painful and, therefore, in the presence of significant pain

TABLE 39.15 Classification of idiopathic scoliosis.

Type	Age at onset
Early onset	<10 years
Adolescent	11–18 years
Adult	Onset at maturity

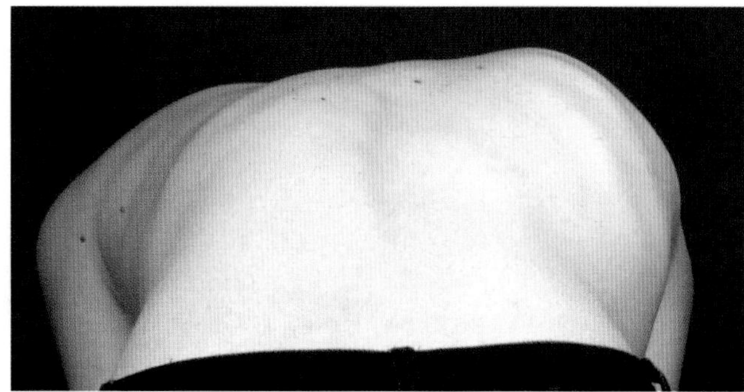

Figure 39.35 Clinical photograph of the Adams forward bend test that demonstrates the presence of a rib hump and the level of the curve.

tumour and infection must be excluded. The Cobb angle is a radiological measurement that defines severity and helps to guide treatment (Figure 39.36). Curves <20° do not need treatment, progressive curves of 25–40° may be braced, and those >40° are considered for surgery, which involves instrumenting the spine and fusing it (see also Chapter 33).

Summary box 39.16

Scoliosis

- Multiplanar deformity includes an unsightly rotational component
- Aetiology may be congenital (underlying bony malformation), neuromuscular, syndromic or idiopathic
- A leg length discrepancy causes a postural scoliosis
- Adolescent idiopathic scoliosis is the most common structural scoliosis
- Back pain associated with scoliosis may be due to infection or tumour
- Treatment depends on the severity and likelihood of curve progression – it varies from observation, through bracing, to surgery

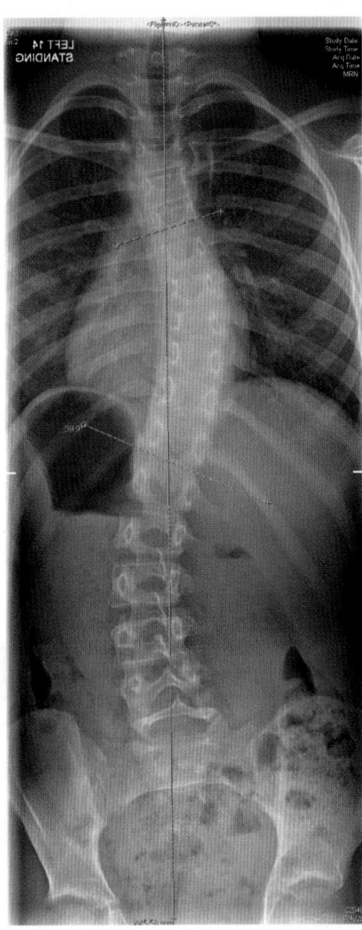

Figure 39.36 Anteroposterior radiograph of a spine with a scoliosis (right thoracic), with a Cobb angle of 40°.

Kyphosis

When a kyphosis exceeds the normal 20–50° the cause may be postural or structural. Structural kyphosis is commonly secondary to **Scheuermann's disease**, presenting as a progressive adolescent kyphosis characterised radiologically by ≥5° vertebral wedging at three adjacent levels and end-plate changes. The aetiology is unknown. Treatment ranges from physiotherapy and bracing to surgery, depending on severity, progression and symptoms.

Spondylolisthesis

Spondylolysis defines a defect in the pars interarticularis of the vertebra. There are six types: congenital (dysplastic facet joints), isthmic (weak or elongated pars), degenerative, post-traumatic, pathological and post-surgical. **Spondylolisthesis** occurs when the upper vertebra slips forward on the lower; it is graded according to the percentage slip, measured by relating the slipped vertebra to the one below (*Table 39.16*).

Mild slips are often asymptomatic and do not require treatment. Treatment (physiotherapy, bracing and surgery) depends on the degree of slip and symptoms; mechanical back pain may respond to conservative methods but neurological involvement usually requires surgical intervention.

Torticollis

In torticollis the head is tilted towards and rotated away from the tight sternocleidomastoid muscle.

Congenital torticollis is usually secondary to intrauterine moulding but may present with fixed sternocleidomastoid contracture or with a palpable 'tumour' within the muscle. There is a strong correlation with DDH. Most cases resolve with stretching but persistent cases develop facial asymmetry and require surgical release of the sternocleidomastoid at one or both ends.

Acquired torticollis is less common and may be caused by gastro-oesophageal reflux, posterior fossa tumour/other regional abnormality, inflammation/infection, ocular problems or atlantoaxial rotatory subluxation.

TABLE 39.16 Classification of spondylolisthesis according to severity of the slip.

Grade	Percentage slip
0	No slip
1	<25%
2	26–50%
3	51–75%
4	>75%
Spondyloptosis	>100% – complete translation

Holger Werfel Scheuermann, 1877–1960, radiologist, The Municipal Hospital, Sundby, Copenhagen, Denmark, described juvenile kyphosis in 1920.

Back pain

Children report back pain less frequently than adults, although >50% will have had an episode by late adolescence. Back pain in a child is a 'red flag' for serious spinal pathology but if mild, intermittent or occurring only on strenuous activity, it is usually self-limiting: many children do suffer posture related discomfort. Physiotherapy designed to improve core strength and stability leads to a reduction in symptoms, if exercises are performed regularly.

Summary box 39.17

'Red flag' symptoms and signs for spinal pathology

- Systemic illness, fever or weight loss
- Progressive neurological deficit
- Unrelenting or night pain
- Spinal deformity

All 'red flag' signs require urgent further investigation with a full blood count (FBC), erythrocyte sedimentation rate (ESR) and C-reactive protein (CRP), plain radiograph and MRI or other appropriate imaging. Other causes of back pain include intra-abdominal, renal and systemic pathology; all must be considered.

Summary box 39.18

Other spinal conditions

- Excessive kyphosis may be caused by Scheuermann's disease
- Spondylolisthesis is forward slip of one vertebra on another; it may cause mechanical and, rarely, neurological symptoms
- Torticollis may be congenital and usually responds to stretching of the fibrosed sternocleidomastoid muscle
- Acquired torticollis may be due to one of several significant pathologies
- Back pain with red flag symptoms and signs requires urgent investigation

NEUROMUSCULAR CONDITIONS

Joint stability and limb function rely on the complex integration of the musculoskeletal and neurological systems. Damage to either leads to one of several conditions linked only by the fact that they are incurable and often progressive, particularly during the period of skeletal growth. Management is directed at helping the child cope with their disability, minimising further deterioration and maximising function. It is important to have an understanding of what the damage is and what the future holds (*Table 39.17*).

Spina bifida and polio are classic lower motor neurone lesions, whereas cerebral palsy and head injuries affect upper motor neurones and the higher centres. There are often other disabilities such as blindness, epilepsy and intellectual difficulties to consider.

TABLE 39.17 Factors to be considered in the assessment of a neuromuscular disability.

Is the insult to the neurological system progressive or nonprogressive?
Is it located centrally or peripherally?
Is it general or focal?
Is it associated with other abnormalities or not?
If the insult is not neurological, is is myopathic?

In children, even if the initial insult to the neuromuscular system is non-progressive, the effects of the insult change with growth. Damage at any level of the neuromuscular system leads to an alteration in tone and muscle imbalance associated with decreased control of movement. Abnormal muscle pull, particularly in combination with the effects of gravity, alters bone growth, leading to deformity and joint contracture. Muscles are relatively weak and, with body growth and a weight increase, they are no longer strong enough to control a heavier limb, particularly when deformity means they are working at a mechanical disadvantage.

A multidisciplinary approach to management is essential. Good physiotherapists and orthotists will reduce the need for surgical intervention and in the postoperative period they help ensure that the surgical benefits are maximised. In conditions such as Duchenne muscular dystrophy there is substantial evidence for the benefits of certain surgical procedures; however, in other conditions (cerebral palsy) there are fewer such long-term validated studies.

In general, it is important to maintain a full range of joint movement, muscle length and tendon excursion. This is easier to achieve in patients with a flaccid paralysis or low tone. The maintenance of muscle strength is also important. The use of splints, positioning techniques, seating and sleeping systems is common with the aim of preventing fixed contractures.

Surgery has a valuable role in the management of selected patients (*Table 39.18*).

The surgeon must understand that altering ankle posture may affect knee and hip posture/function and vice versa. The patient must have the intellectual ability and motivation to recover from the surgical procedure. Some of the factors mentioned previously (see *Table 39.17*) must be considered in any holistic approach to the patient.

Summary box 39.19

Principles of treatment of neuromuscular conditions

- A neurological defect, whether progressive or not, may cause progressive deformity as the skeleton grows
- A multidisciplinary approach is essential
- Primary therapy aims to maintain range of movement and prevent fixed contractures with an emphasis on managing tone and position
- Surgery has a limited role in the management of neuromuscular conditions

Guillaume Benjamin Amand Duchenne (Duchenne de Boulogne), 1806–1875, neurologist, worked successively in Boulogne and Paris, France, but who never held a hospital appointment.

TABLE 39.18 General types of surgical procedure that may be considered in the management of a patient with a neuromuscular condition.

Surgical procedure	Aim of treatment
Lengthening of the muscle–tendon unit	Restores joint range (but results in relative muscle weakness)
Tendon transfer	Improves functional movement; rebalances muscle forces, after correction of fixed deformity
Release of joint contracture; correction of bony deformity	Restores mechanical alignment, and allows muscles to work in a more efficient manner
Fuse/stabilise/relocate joints	Improves posture/function; reduces pain
Neurological procedures: • selective dorsal rhizotomy (SDR) • intrathecal baclofen pumps (ITB)	Reduce spasticity (not primarily useful in dystonia)
Leg equalisation procedures	Improve lower limb mechanics

Cerebral palsy

Cerebral palsy is caused by a non-progressive insult to the developing brain in the perinatal period; in most cases only risk factors, such as prematurity, rather than specific causes, such as hypoxia (HIE, hypoxic ischaemic encephalopathy), can be identified. The effects of cerebral palsy may only become apparent as the child grows and fails to reach expected developmental milestones. At this stage investigations may help with aetiology and may predict the pattern of the cerebral palsy: premature babies may show evidence of periventricular leucomalacia (PVL) on a brain MRI, which is associated with the development of spastic diplegia with relative preservation of intellectual function.

In general, the pattern of involvement can be classified according to the anatomical site involved and the effect on muscle tone (*Table 39.19*). The prognosis for walking can be predicted by identifying evidence of neurological development, i.e. gaining motor skills with the loss of primitive reflexes. The age related Gross Motor Function Classification System (GMFCS) has five categories which also relate to mobility and prognosis (GMFCS I – near normal versus GMFCS V – wheelchair based). Many children with GMFCS V cerebral palsy have multiple associated problems and 40% will die before they reach their mid-20s.

An important aspect of management is the control of high tone. Tone can be reduced with drugs such as diazepam and baclofen. Alternatively, neuromuscular blockers such as botulinum toxin can bring about a focal reduction in tone by preventing acetylcholine release at the neuromuscular junction The effect is temporary, giving a 'window' during which the physiotherapists can stretch agonists and strengthen antagonists. It is important to differentiate between dynamic and fixed contractures; the latter will not respond to tone management or splinting.

The classic cerebral palsy gait patterns demonstrate flexor spasticity. The child with spastic diplegia has problems at all levels of the lower limb. Single event multilevel surgery (SEMLS) is popular, and gait analysis (both observational and computerised) contributes to the selection of an appro-

TABLE 39.19 Classification of cerebral palsy with respect to muscle tone and site of involvement.

	Characteristics
Tone	
Spastic ('high')	Commonest type of abnormality; due to damage to the pyramidal system Velocity-dependent increased muscle tone and brisk reflexes
Dyskinetic • Dystonic • Choreoathetoid	Increased tone but reduced activity – stiff movements Low tone but increased activity – uncoordinated jerky movements • Due to damage in the extrapyramidal system
Ataxia	Generalised low tone, loss of muscle coordination • Due to damage in the cerebellum
Mixed	No one tone/movement disorder predominates • Combination of spasticity and dystonia is common
Hypotonia	Usually a phase (which may last years) before the features of spasticity develop
Site	
Unilateral	
• Hemiplegia	Arm more affected than leg
Bilateral • Diplegia	Legs more affected than arms
• Total body involvement	Often significant intellectual impairment and associated difficulties

priate management plan for an individual patient. Computerised analysis provides objective evidence of joint movement and mechanics in multiple planes (Figure 39.37). Appropriate bone and soft-tissue procedures can then be planned. Botulinum toxin helps with postoperative pain and spasm.

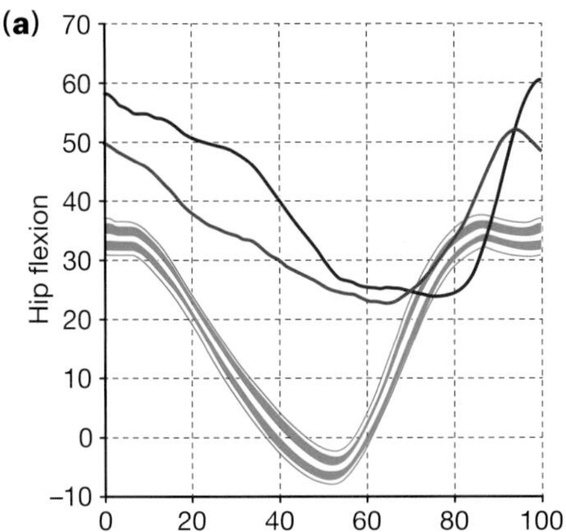

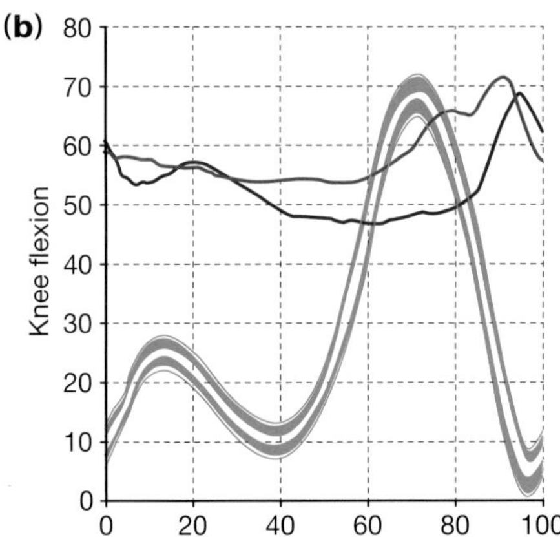

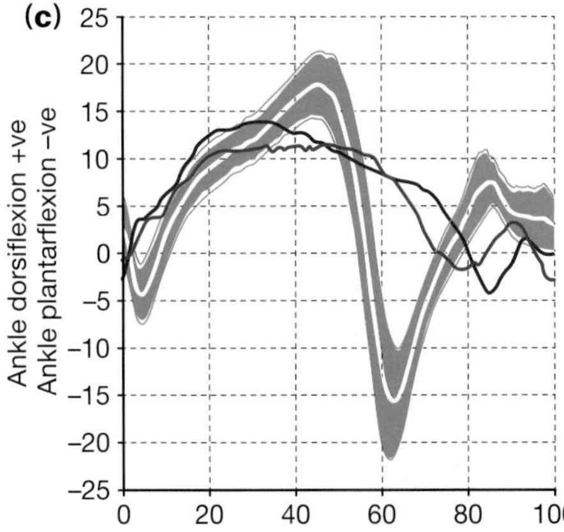

Figure 39.37 Gait analysis graphs such as these demonstrate the normal range of joint movements (green band) at hip (**a**), knee (**b**) and ankle (**c**) during the stance and swing phases of the gait. The abnormal joint ranges are shown in red (right leg) and blue (left leg) and demonstrate the excessive hip flexion and lack of knee extension and abnormal ankle mechanics associated with the 'crouch' gait of a child with cerebral palsy.

In the child with total body involvement (TBI) and high muscle tone, hip subluxation and eventual dislocation are common but often relatively asymptomatic (Figure 39.38). Current thinking is that symmetry and pelvic position are important so the hips should be kept in joint by the simplest means possible, with early surgical intervention if necessary. Aggressive management of a spinal deformity will initially concentrate on seating position and subsequently emphasise spinal bracing or surgery.

Overall, it is important to remember what the child's needs will be once they have reached adulthood. Independent mobility and an effective means of communication are two of the most important requirements. Hence, it may not be appropriate to invest time and effort in gaining an upright posture if mobility will be achieved via an electric wheelchair and a hand-controlled car and life expectancy is limited.

Summary box 39.20

Cerebral palsy

- Brain injury is non-progressive
- Classified as unilateral or bilateral involvement: hemiplegia, diplegia or TBI
- Tone may be high, low or variable but there is always a generalised, relative muscle weakness
- In ambulant children, gait analysis may be used to plan surgery or botulinum toxin injections
- In TBI, primary concerns are hip subluxation and spinal deformity

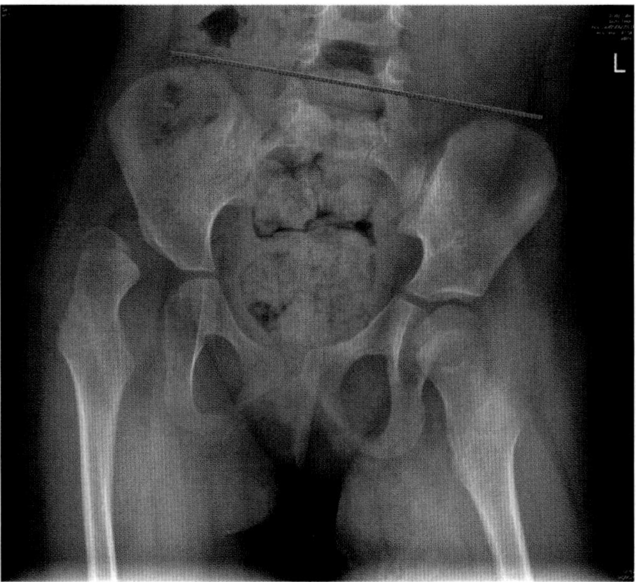

Figure 39.38 Anteroposterior pelvic radiograph of a child with spastic cerebral palsy. The right hip is essentially dislocated: none of the head lies medial to the vertical Perkins line. The acetabulum is dysplastic and the leg lies in slight adduction. The left leg is in abduction. There is often this 'windswept' appearance with one leg stiff in abduction and the other stiff in adduction. The line demonstrates the pelvic obliquity; many children also have a scoliosis.

Polio

Despite an effective polio vaccine, this disease still occurs. About 1–2% of patients develop neurological problems when the virus affects the anterior horn cells. Muscle weakness is proportionate to the number of motor units destroyed. Patients often develop trick movements to cope with their muscle weakness and minor joint contractures may actually improve function (for example, ankle equinus in the presence of weak quadriceps muscles). Careful assessment before surgery is essential and both the surgeon and the patient must understand the goals of treatment.

Spina bifida

The extent of the disability varies with the level of the lesion: upper motor neurone involvement will produce spasticity while the more classic lower motor neurone lesion will merely produce a flaccid paralysis. Hydrocephalus may contribute to the complexity of the situation. Muscle imbalance leads to secondary joint deformity but the, often profound, accompanying sensory disturbance may affect the choice of surgical and non-surgical options. Many children require a ventriculoperitoneal (VP) shunt to drain the hydrocephalus that develops following closure of the myelocoele. A tethered cord may develop, with growth adversely influencing the neurological picture.

Muscular dystrophy

Many types of muscular dystrophy exist that vary in terms of severity and distribution of involvement. Surgical intervention aims to improve quality of life. This is best achieved by operating early to release joint contractures and facilitate the maintenance of walking abilities and good spinal posture.

Brachial plexopathy

The neonatal brachial plexus injury is still common, with a devastating effect on upper limb function, particularly if antigravity motor activity has not recovered by 6 months. Physiotherapy is the mainstay of early treatment to maintain muscle length and joint range of movement and thus reduce the risk of glenohumeral dislocation. Neural repair may be necessary in the infant. Later surgical interventions aim to release joint/muscle contractures and improve function, perhaps with tendon transfers.

INFECTION

Worldwide, osteoarticular infection remains a frequent cause of significant morbidity.

Septic arthritis

Joint infection is usually secondary to haematogenous spread but direct inoculation can occur, for example during a neonatal venepuncture. Diagnosis can be difficult in the very young and in those presenting with overwhelming sepsis. Neonates, children with immunocompromise and those with sickle cell disease are at increased risk. At the other end of the spectrum the differentiation between joint sepsis and transient synovitis of the hip can also be difficult.

Classically, the child presents with pain, fever and a reluctance to use the joint; in the lower limb this implies a reluctance to weight bear. On examination, local tenderness and painful restriction of movement are apparent and in superficial joints inflammation may be obvious, with a hot, swollen joint.

Investigations include FBC, ESR, CRP and blood cultures. Plain radiographs help to exclude other diagnoses and may identify osteomyelitis. Ultrasound scans of deep seated joints, such as the hip, will identify joint effusions (Figure 39.39). Increasingly, MRI is considered the investigation of choice but this resource is not available to all (in a timely manner) and, in young children, it requires a general anaesthetic if useful information is to be obtained. Good clinical skills, regular patient review and a high index of suspicion are still the most valuable tools. Four clinical predictors can differentiate between septic arthritis and transient synovitis (*Table 39.20*).

Pus in a joint is destructive: the proteases produced by leukocytes destroy both the bacteria and the collagen matrix of the articular cartilage. AVN may occur secondary to pressure effects or ischaemic infarction. The treatment of a presumed septic arthritis therefore requires the prompt removal of pus from the joint and appropriate adequate antibiotic therapy. Pain relief and rest are also important, as are the general health and nutrition of the patient. The joint is aspirated and, if pus is confirmed, a formal washout is mandatory; standard teaching states that the joint must be opened, irrigated and free drainage encouraged via the capsulotomy. Recent literature supports repeated aspiration/irrigation via a large-bore cannula or a small arthroscope for all joints except the hip joint. Antibiotic usage is guided by the local hospital policy, the source of the infection, the Gram stain and, in due course,

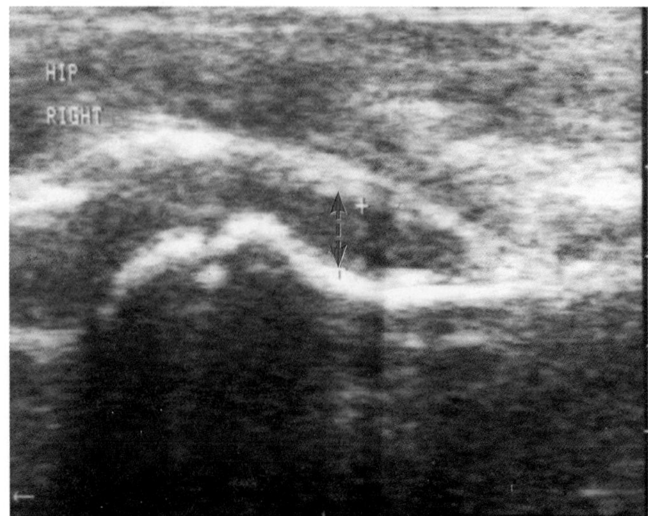

Figure 39.39 Ultrasound scan of a hip joint. A large effusion is distending the joint capsule. The dotted line represents the distance between the femoral neck and the joint capsule.

TABLE 39.20 Septic arthritis.

(a) The clinical predictors of Kocher *et al.* for the diagnosis of septic arthritis:

- History of fever >38.5°C
- Non-weight bearing
- Erythrocyte sedimentation rate >40 mm/hour
- White cell count >12 × 10^9/L

(b) The value of the clinical predictors of Kocher *et al.* in determining the likelihood of a joint being septic:

Number of positive predictors	Predicted probability of joint sepsis
0	2.0%
1	9.5%
2	35.0%
3	72.8%
4	93.0%

the culture and sensitivity of the organism identified. Joint instability, particularly in the hip joint (**Figure 39.40**), may require the joint to be splinted in the reduced position while the inflammatory process settles.

The most frequently identified organism is *Staphylococcus aureus*. Streptococcal infection is also common and other organisms are more prevalent in certain age groups, e.g. the neonate, in certain conditions, e.g. sickle cell disease, or in certain countries. The *Haemophilus influenzae* type B (Hib) vaccine has essentially eliminated *H. influenzae* as a cause of infection, but in some countries *Kingella kingae* has taken its place.

Improvement is judged clinically and by monitoring the inflammatory markers. Reaccumulation of pus does occur and must be suspected and treated promptly if the child fails to improve.

Summary box 39.21

Septic arthritis

- Diagnosis is difficult in neonates and the immunocompromised
- Typical presentation is pain, fever and a reluctance to move the joint or weight bear
- Investigations should include FBC, ESR, CRP, blood cultures and appropriate imaging studies, combined with astute clinical skills
- Pus in a joint can destroy articular cartilage and cause avascular necrosis
- Treatment is prompt removal of pus, appropriate antibiotic therapy, pain relief and splintage

Osteomyelitis

As with septic arthritis, bone infection is usually caused by haematogenous spread. Infection often occurs in the metaphyses of long bones where the slow flow through the looped vessels combined with microtrauma is believed to encourage seeding of infection during a bacteraemia (**Figure 39.41a**). Inflammation follows and, if purulent material forms, the pressure effects secondary to the formation of an abscess will lead to

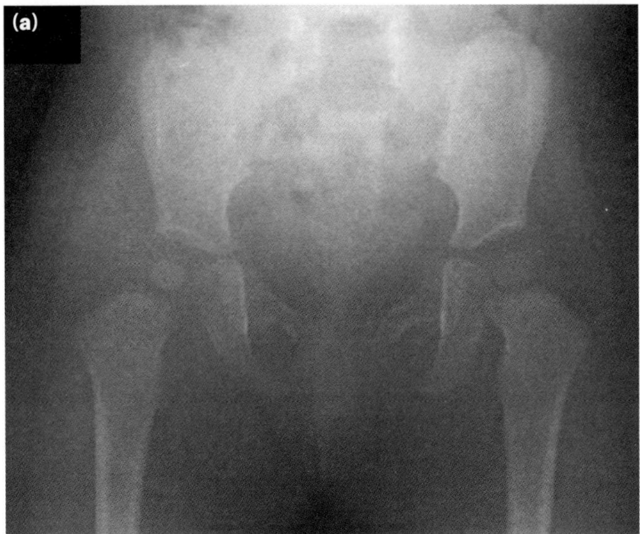

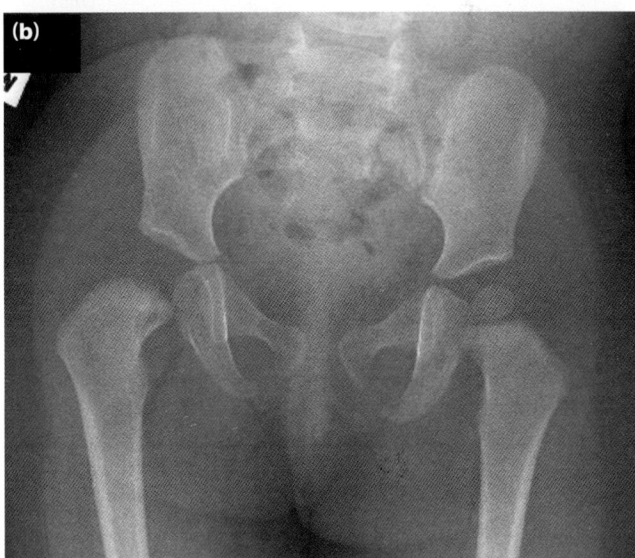

Figure 39.40 Septic arthritis of the right hip: (**a**) anteroposterior pelvic radiograph with subtle signs of right hip subluxation; (**b**) anteroposterior pelvic radiograph 6 months later showing destruction of the femoral head secondary to late treatment of a septic joint.

progressive bony destruction. Pus can pass through cortical bone and when it does so it elevates the strong periosteum, which may render the cortical bone avascular. As in cases of trauma or tumour, the periosteal elevation is a potent stimulus for new bone formation. In cases of untreated or chronic infection this new bone or involucrum may surround the dead bone, the sequestrum, leading to a 'bone-within-a-bone' appearance (**Figure 39.41b**).

The presentation and investigation of osteomyelitis can be similar to those for joint sepsis. The differentiation between the two may be difficult and a sympathetic joint effusion may occur with metaphyseal osteomyelitis. Thus, if there are no organisms seen on microscopy of a joint aspirate, the possibility of a coexisting osteomyelitis must be considered. The metaphysis of a long bone may be intracapsular and infection may spread easily into the joint once the periosteum is breached. In the neonate, proximal femoral osteomyelitis

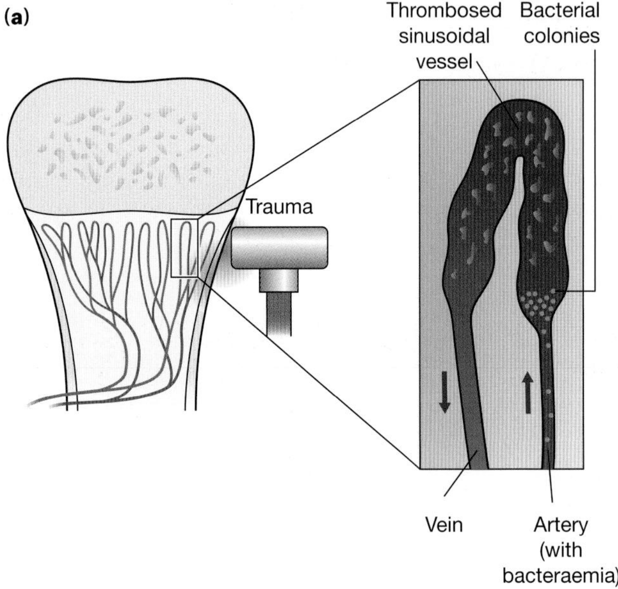

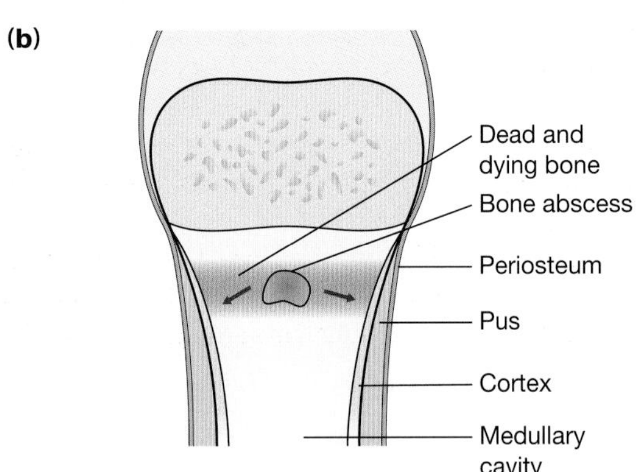

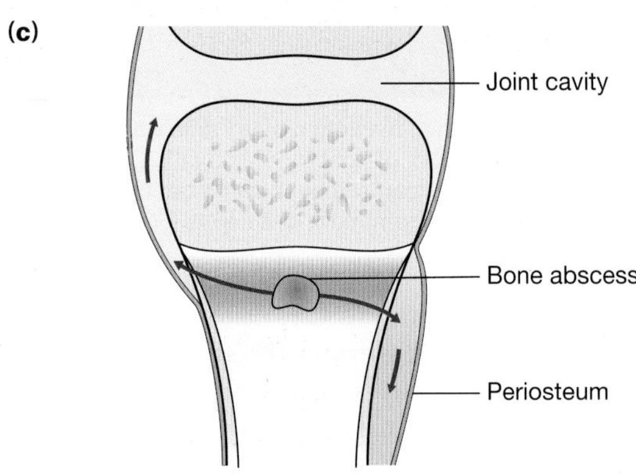

Figure 39.41 (a-c) Diagrams illustrating the pathology underlying the development of osteomyelitis. The longer the infection goes untreated the greater the destruction, with the possibility of sequestrum formation and secondary joint infection.

and septic arthritis are essentially the same condition (**Figure 39.41c**).

General principles for the management of infection should be followed. Pus needs to be drained but otherwise the treatment is medical. Debate continues over the duration of treatment and indeed whether antibiotics should be parenteral or oral: management varies from region to region and relates to the local bacteriological prevalences. Methicillin-resistant *Staphylococcus aureus* (MRSA) is common in some areas and not in others: the *Staphylococcus aureus*-associated *Panton Valentine leucocidin* gene significantly alters the morbidity associated with *S. aureus* infection.

It must be noted that the reduced intravenous and oral treatment times published recently are for **uncomplicated** cases of osteomyelitis and septic arthritis only, and only for those patients who are improving promptly both clinically and haematologically.

Summary box 39.22

Occurence and treatment principles for bone and soft tissue infection

- Occurs by haematogenous spread, enhanced by microtrauma
- In untreated and/or chronic osteomyelitis, new involucrum envelops dead sequestrum
- In addition to antibiotics, treatment consists of:
  - Rest/splintage of affected limb
  - Analgesia
- A joint effusion may be sympathetic or caused by direct spread from the adjacent metaphysis
- Treatment involves drainage of pus when present
- Appropriate and often prolonged antibiotic therapy: parenteral and then oral
- Treatment of the underlying condition, e.g. nutritional deficiency, sickle cell disease

Complications of bone and joint sepsis

Treated appropriately, most cases of bone and joint sepsis resolve with no sequelae. However, significant complications can occur, particularly in terms of chronic infection and in cases in which there has been damage to the joint and/or the physis and the epiphyseal growth centres. In the neonate, vascular channels pass through the physis, connecting the metaphysis with the epiphysis, and a poorer outcome may ensue (see **Figure 39.40b**). Orthopaedic follow-up should be continued until normal growth patterns are documented.

Meningococcal sepsis

The often debilitating, late orthopaedic sequelae of meningococcal septicaemia are secondary to endotoxin-induced microvascular injury and ischaemic physeal damage (**Figure 39.42**).

Tuberculosis

Tuberculosis is still common. The clinical presentation is often insidious, with malaise and weight loss combined with a boggy joint swelling, muscle wasting and joint contractures. Spinal deformity and neurological symptoms are particular problems.

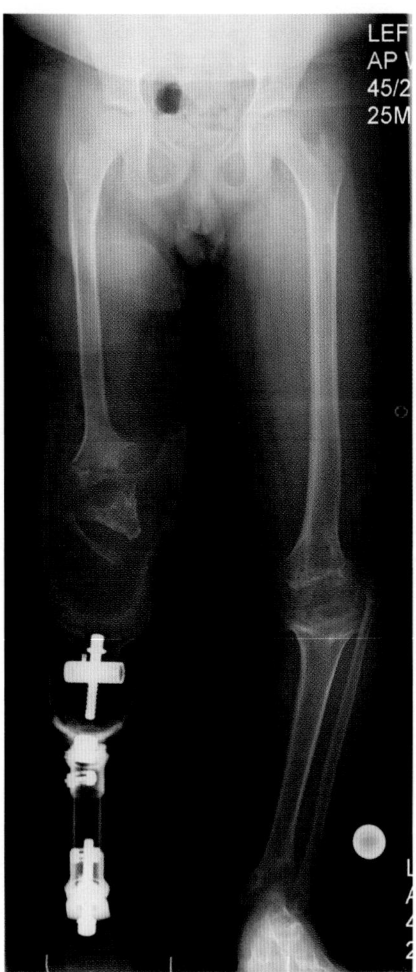

Figure 39.42 Anteroposterior leg length and alignment radiograph of a child who had meningococcal septicaemia as a child; he was left with multiple problems. He has a below-knee amputation of the right leg. Many of his lower limb physes are not growing well so he has deformity of his remaining right proximal tibia, a very short left tibia and an overgrown fibula. His right femur is also short.

Chronic relapsing/recurrent multifocal osteomyelitis

The radiographic features suggest subacute or chronic osteomyelitis (or tumour) but laboratory and histopathological findings are usually non-specific and cultures negative. This is probably an inflammatory rather than an infective condition.

Discitis

Children who refuse to weight bear and complain of back pain may have discitis. The aetiology of this condition may be infective or inflammatory but if vertebral bodies are involved, infection is assumed.

Brodies's abscess

Chronic infections may present with radiographic features of a sclerotic walled cyst.

CLINICAL DILEMMAS

The limping child

Children may limp because of pain, weakness, deformity or to gain attention; the causes vary from sepsis to a spinal tumour and from a leg length discrepancy to a shoe that rubs. Serious causes must be excluded and the 'surgical sieve' helps identify the most likely diagnoses. See *Table 39.21*.

TABLE 39.21 A guide to the clinical assessment of the limping child.

Symptom onset: sudden or gradual?
Symptom duration
Concurrent events: recent viral infection, trauma, new shoes, new sport?
General health: is the child well?

The examination must include all joints and soft tissues and, in addition, a brief neurological examination, measurement of leg length and an assessment of pain at rest or on weight bearing.

Many conditions, such as sepsis and juvenile arthritis, can present at any age but certain hip conditions are more likely in particular age groups (*Table 39.22*).

Plain radiographs should usually include both anteroposterior and 'frog' lateral views of the pelvis. Always bear in mind the possibility of a tumour; further imaging such as MRI may be required.

TABLE 39.22 Age at presentation of certain hip conditions.

Age (years)	Diagnosis
1–3	Late presenting developmental dysplasia of the hip; sepsis
3–10	Transient synovitis; Perthes' disease
11–15	Slipped upper femoral epiphysis

Non-accidental injury (NAI)

No child is exempt but some children are at particular risk, including those under 3 years of age and those with disabilities in a family who are suffering socioeconomic deprivation. A careful clinical assessment is required (**Figure 39.43** and *Table 39.23*). Characteristic patterns should warn the clinician to consider the possibility of NAI (*Table 39.24*).

Child abuse occurs in different forms: emotional, physical, sexual and neglect. When suspected it should be discussed with the relevant child safeguarding team. All injuries should be documented carefully. It may be prudent to admit the child until further checks have been made.

Sir Benjamin Collins Brodie, 1783–1862, surgeon, St. George's Hospital, London, UK, described 'Brodie's abscess' in 1828.

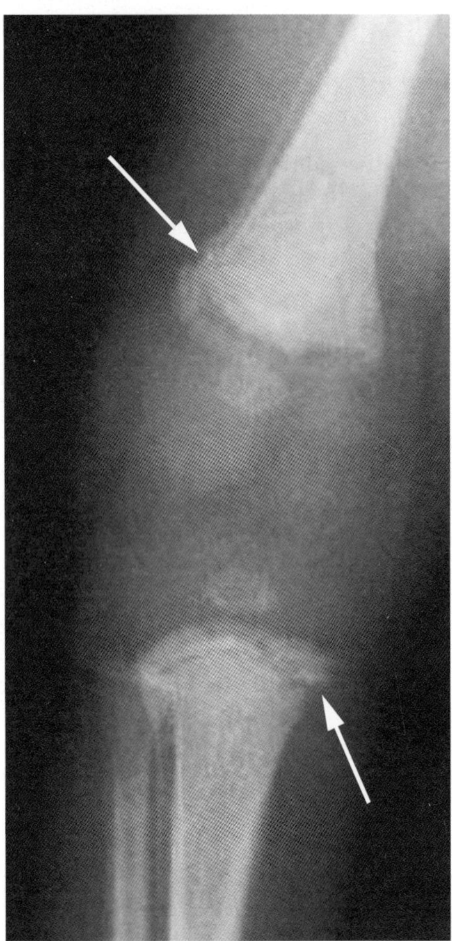

Figure 39.43 Anteroposterior radiograph of a knee showing metaphyseal corner fractures that are often considered to be pathognomonic of non-accidental injury. Non-accidental injury must also be considered in any fracture that presents late or without an adequate explanation.

TABLE 39.23 Factors that raise concern in the clinical assessment of suspected non-accidental injury.

History
Delay in seeking medical advice
Variable story
Mechanism inconsistent with injury pattern
Examination
Unexpected bruising to the buttocks/back of legs
'Finger-mark' bruises
Bruises of various ages
Burns, deep scratches, etc.

TABLE 39.24 Fracture patterns with a high specificity for non-accidental injury.

Multiple fractures at different stages of healing/old fractures
Posterior rib fractures
Corner or bucket-handle metaphyseal fractures
Scapular fractures
Any fracture in a child below walking age

FURTHER READING

Benson MKD, Fixsen JA, MacNicol MF (eds). *Children's orthopaedics and fractures*, 3rd edn. London, Harcourt, 2010.

Dartnell J, Ramachandran M, Katchburian M. Haematogenous acute and subacute paediatric osteomyelitis: a systematic review of the literature. *J Bone Joint Surg Br* 2012; **94**(5): 584–95.

Kocher MS, Mandiga R, Zurakowski D, Barnewolt C, Kasser JR. Validation of a clinical prediction rule for the differentiation between septic arthritis and transient synovitis of the hip in children. *J Bone Joint Surg Am* 2004; **86-A**(8):1629–35.

Sewell MD, Eastwood DM, Wimalasundera N. *Managing common symptoms of cerebral palsy in children*. BMJ 2014; **349**: g5474.

Weinstein, SL, Flynn JM (eds). *Lovell and Winter's pediatric orthopaedics*, Vols 1 and 2, 7th edn. Philadelphia, PA: Lippincott, Williams and Wilkins, 2014.

PART 6

Skin and subcutaneous tissue

40 Skin and subcutaneous tissue 592

41 Burns 617

42 Plastic and reconstructive surgery 633

Chapter 40

Skin and subcutaneous tissue

Learning objectives

To understand:

- The structure and functional properties of skin
- The classification of vascular skin lesions
- The cutaneous manifestations of generalised disease as related to surgery
- The classification of benign skin tumours
- The management of malignant skin tumours

FUNCTIONAL ANATOMY AND PHYSIOLOGY OF SKIN

Skin can be divided into two layers: the outer epidermis and the inner dermis. Deep to the dermis lies subcutaneous fat and remnants of the panniculus carnosus.

Epidermis

The epidermis is 5% of the skin and is composed of five layers of keratinised, stratified squamous epithelium; the strata: basalis (deep), spinosum, granulosum, lucidum and corneum (superficial).

Most epidermal cells are keratinocytes arranged in layers. The basal epidermis (stratum basalis) also contains melanocytes. Keratinocytes are classified according to their depth in the epidermis and their degree of differentiation. Keratinocytes grow and are replaced via mitoses in the cells of the stratum granulosum as they progress from deep to superficial, losing their nuclei and organelles as they ascend, before forming the stratum corneum. The other keratinocyte layers in the skin (strata lucidum; granulosum and spinosum) are variably thick according to body site – for instance all three are thick in the glabrous skin of the palms and soles of the feet and almost absent in eyelid skin.

Melanocytes are dendritic cells of neural crest origin, usually located in the basal epidermis. Each melanocyte synthesises melanin, a brown-black pigment, which is transferred via membrane processes to the keratinocytes in the strata granulosum and spinosum. Melanin provides protection against ultraviolet radiation. Ethnic differences in skin colour are determined by variations in the amount, combination and distribution of melanin within the keratinocytes, not by differences in the number of melanocytes.

Dermis

Dermis comprises 95% of skin and is structurally divided into a superficial papillary layer; composed of delicate collagen and elastin fibres in ground substance, into which a capillary and lymphatic network ramifies and a deeper reticular layer; composed of course branching collagen, layered parallel to the skin surface (**Figure 40.1**).

The epidermis and dermis meet at the dermo-epidermal junction in a three-dimensional wave-like arrangement in which epidermal rete ridges project down, interdigitating with upward-pointing, dermal papillae containing vascular and lymphatic plexi.

The skin also contains specialised cells such as Langerhan's cells, whose role is to engulf antigens and present them to T cells. Merkel cells, Meissner's and Pacinian corpuscles have roles in mechano-sensation.

Skin adnexa

Adnexal structures such as hair follicles, sebaceous and sweat glands span both the epidermal and dermal layers and contain some keratinocytes in their ducts. In injuries where epidermis is lost, re-epithelialisation occurs from these structures as well as from the wound margins.

Paul Langerhans, 1847–1888, Professor of Pathological Anatomy, Freiberg, Germany.
Filippo Pacini, 1812–1883, Professor of Anatomy and Physiology, Florence, Italy.

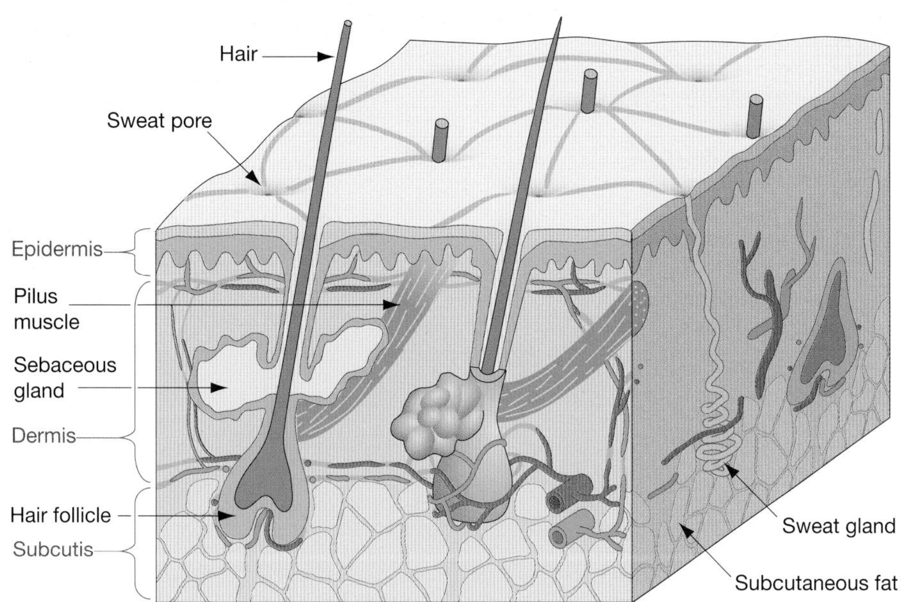

Figure 40.1 Three-dimensional diagram of the structural layers of the skin and its adnexal structures. (Reproduced from Simonsen T, Aarbakke J, Kay I *et al*. *Illustrated pharmacology for nurses*. London: Hodder Arnold, 2006 with kind permission of the illustrator Roy Lysaa.)

Hair follicles

Hair follicles are tubular invaginations of the epidermis, from which grow hair shafts (dead keratinised tissue). Strips of smooth muscle (arrector pili) are inserted into the wall of the hair follicle and lead to hair elevation in times of stress and cold.

Sebaceous glands

Sebaceous glands are hair follicle appendages situated between each hair follicle and the associated arrector pili muscle. When the arrector pili muscle contracts to elevate the hair, it compresses the gland and sebum is released (holocrine secretion).

Sweat glands

Simple eccrine and apocrine sweat glands open into pores in hair follicles. Eccrine glands are distributed throughout the entire body surface, except the lips. They secrete sweat in response to emotion or during thermoregulation. Apocrine glands are found in the axillae and groins and become active at puberty. Their secretion, characteristically malodourous after bacterial degradation, is in response to emotion and hormone secretion.

Skin thickness

Skin thickness varies with age, location and sun damage, but in any given region it is thinner in children than adults. The dermis is between 15 and 40 times thicker than the epidermis, but starts to thin during the fourth decade. The epidermis is thickest on the palms, soles, back and buttocks and thinnest on eyelids (0.5–1 mm on the sole of the foot, 0.05–0.09 mm on the eyelid).

Blood supply of the skin

The body can be envisaged as three-dimensional segments of tissue called angiosomes, each with an arterial supply and a venous drainage. Blood equilibrates and flows between neighbouring angiosomes via 'choke' vessels, which tend to be situated within muscles. Cutaneous arteries, direct branches of segmental arteries (concentrated at the dorsoventral axes and intermuscular septae), perforate the underlying muscles or run directly within fascial layers to the skin from the deep tissues (**Figure 40.2**).

The blood supply to the skin anastomoses in subfascial, fascial, subdermal, dermal and subepidermal plexi. The epidermis contains no blood vessels so cells there derive nourishment by diffusion.

The venous drainage of the skin is via both valved and unvalved veins. Unvalved veins allow oscillating flow in the subdermal plexus between cutaneous territories, equilibrating flow and pressure. The valved cutaneous veins drain via plexi to the deep veins.

Anomalies of skin metabolism

Blood flow to the skin can vary between 5 and 100 mL/100 g/min in the temperature range 20–40°C. Thus, skin has the potential for a blood supply 20–100 times greater than its metabolic and thermoregulatory requirements. This apparent excess enables restitution of mechanical integrity after the myriad trivial injuries (scratching, stretching, compressing, thermal) to which skin is subjected; however, blood supply is inadequate to support full-thickness wound healing, which requires primary closure or granulation tissue.

Skin functions optimally at temperatures below body core temperature and can tolerate long periods of ischaemia (allowing it both to be grafted and/or expanded for use in reconstruction (see Chapter 42 on plastic surgery).

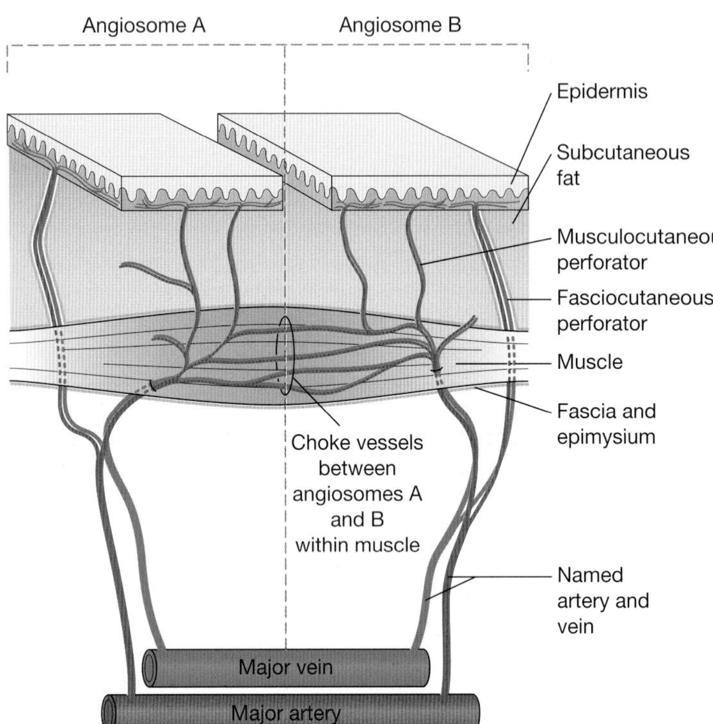

Figure 40.2 Schematic showing two neighbouring angiosomes. Note the choke vessels within the muscle spanning the two cutaneous territories of angiosome A and B; two common examples of myocutaneous flaps that utilise this physiology include the rectus abdominus and the latissimus dorsi flaps.

FUNCTION OF THE SKIN

Human skin and subcutaneous tissue have several important functions:

- Barrier to the environment enveloping the body and protecting against trauma, radiation and pathogens.
- Regulates temperature and water homeostasis.
- Organ of excretion for urea, sodium chloride, potassium and water, as well as sulphur-containing metabolites from drugs (e.g. dimethyl sulphoxide) or food (garlic, cumin).
- The skin has significant endocrine and metabolic functions and interactions. Skin cells contain receptors for and respond to: peptides, steroid sex hormones, thyroid hormones and neurotransmitters and they both produce (cholecalciferol) and metabolise (androgens) hormones and precursors to activate, potentiate and inactivate their functions.
- Sensory organ with multiple receptors for pain, pressure and movement.

PATHOPHYSIOLOGY OF THE SKIN AND SUBCUTANEOUS TISSUES

Radiation damage

Ultraviolet radiation (UVR) and ionising radiation (IR) damage cellular deoxyribonucleic acid (DNA) via the tumour suppressor gene *p53*, inhibiting cellular repair and apoptotic mechanisms. There is also evidence that efferent immune responses are impaired after skin exposure to UVR, facilitating neoplasia.

Ultraviolet radiation

UVR is divisible into A, B and C according to wavelength. UVR is the principal cause of skin cancer in all skin types. Its effects are attenuated by melanin and there is an inverse relationship between melanin content and skin susceptibility to UV-induced neoplasia. Some protection is afforded by the stratum corneum, which reflects and refracts UVR, and by clothing, protective creams, cloud cover, particulate air pollution and buildings.

Ionising radiation

The effects of IR are dose, wavelength and time dependent. The skin with its rapid cellular turnover exhibits signs soon after exposure. High-frequency rays cause electron coupling at the molecular level, damaging proteins, polysaccharides and lipids.

Infrared radiation

Infrared radiation generates heat; cumulative exposure can cause thermal burns.

Congenital/genetic disorders

Neurofibromatosis

There are two distinct neurofibromatosis (NF) syndromes, where Schwann cells form tumours (**Figure 40.3**). Each is

Friedrich Theodor Schwann, 1810–1882, Professor of Anatomy successively at Louvain (1839–1848) and Liege, Belgium (1849–1880). Original researches before the age of 27 laid the foundation of physiology of nerve and muscle. The first to deal with problems related to living matter on a purely physical and chemical basis, and to recognise the cell as the unit of living matter. Discoverer of pepsin, and role of living organisms in fermentation.

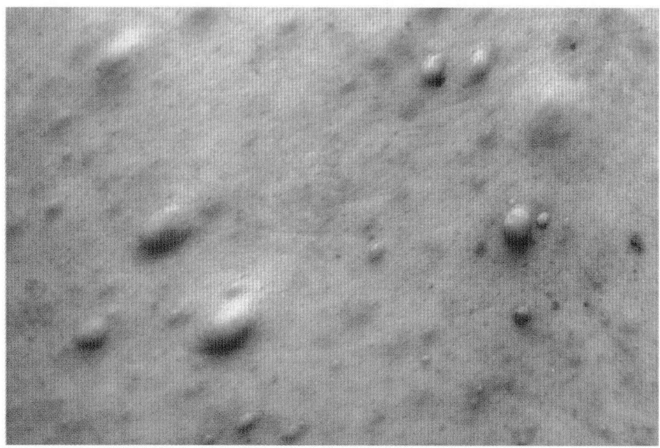

Figure 40.3 Neurofibromatosis (courtesty of St John's Institute for Dermatology, London, UK).

caused by different genes on different chromosomes. 70% are autosomal dominant and 30% arise from sporadic mutations. NF 1 (Von Recklinghausen's disease) is the commoner variant, affecting approximately 1:4000 births. It arises from a gene mutation on chromosome (Ch.) 17. Skin manifestations appear in early life, with the development of more than five smooth surfaced café-au-lait spots, subcutaneous neurofibromata, armpit or groin freckling and Lisch nodules.

Naevoid basal cell carcinoma (Gorlin's) syndrome

This is an autosomal dominant inherited condition caused by an abnormal tumour suppressor gene on Ch. 9q 22-31 coding the 'patched' protein. 90% of patients develop multiple basal cell carcinomas (BCCs). Patients may exhibit specific phenotypical characteristics including: over-developed supraorbital ridges; broad nasal roots; hyperteliorism; bifid ribs; scoliosis; brachymetacarpalism; palmar pits and molar odontogenic cysts.

Xeroderma pigmentosum

This syndrome is caused by an abnormality on the 'patched' gene of Ch. 9q resulting in aberrant nucleotide repair during cellular DNA maintenance. It confers a >2000-fold increase in skin cancer risk and has autosomal recessive inheritance. Sufferers are intolerant of UVR, leading to premature skin ageing and development of multiple neoplasms. Most affected individuals die in early adulthood from metastatic disease (60% mortality by 20 years of age).

Gardner's syndrome

This syndrome is an autosomal dominant disease variant of familial adenomatous polyposis (FAP) caused by an abnormal gene on Ch. 5. Gardner's syndrome can cause the development of cutaneous pathology such as multiple epidermoid cysts and lipomata.

Ferguson-Smith syndrome

This is a rare, autosomal-dominantly inherited abnormality on Ch. 9q in which affected individuals develop multiple self-healing squamous cell carcinomas (SCC).

Cutaneous manifestations of generalised disease

Many diseases have cutaneous manifestations that present in surgical practice. These include: necrobiosis lipoidica, granuloma annulare in diabetes mellitus and pyoderma gangrenosum in inflammatory bowel disease. Their management should be sought in appropriate texts.

Hyperhydrosis

This involves excessive eccrine sweating of the palms, soles of the feet, axillae and groins, causing functional and social problems. It can be treated with antiperspirants or periodic local injections with botulinum toxin A. More resistant cases are treated by laparoscopic cervical sympathectomy.

Lipodystrophy

Lipodystrophy (lipoatrophy) is a localised or generalised loss of fatty tissue, which can be primary or secondary. It can be a complication of long-term administration of insulin, following treatment of human immunodeficiency virus (HIV) with protease inhibitors or in transplant recipients.

It can be treated in selected cases by autologous fat grafting, injections of poly-L-lactic acid and free tissue transfer.

Inflammatory conditions

HIDRADENITIS SUPPURATIVA (HS)

Follicular occlusion followed by folliculitis and secondary infection with skin flora (usually *Staphylococcus aureus* and *Propionibacterium acnes*) culminates in chronic suppurative, painful, skin abscesses, sinus tracts and scarring. HS occurs in skin containing apocrine glands, commonly in the axillae and groins; but also the scalp, breast, chest and perineum (**Figure 40.4**). It appears to have a genetic predisposition with variable penetrance, and is strongly associated with obesity and smoking. It affects four women for every man.

Management Patients should stop smoking and lose excess weight. Symptoms can be reduced by the use of antiseptic soaps, tea tree oil and wearing non-compressive and aerated underwear. Medical treatments include topical and oral antibiotics and antiandrogen drugs. In selected cases, patients require radical excision of the affected skin and subcutaneous tissue. Reconstruction after excision avoids contracture and functional impairment.

Friedrich Von Recklinghausen, 1833–1910, German Professor of Pathology, also described haemochromatosis.
Karl Lisch, 1907–1999, ophthalmologist, Wörgl, Austria.
Robert J Gorlin, 1923–2006, American dentist and Professor of Oral Pathology, published over 400 articles on craniofacial syndromes.
John Ferguson-Smith, 1888–1978, Glaswegian dermatologist.

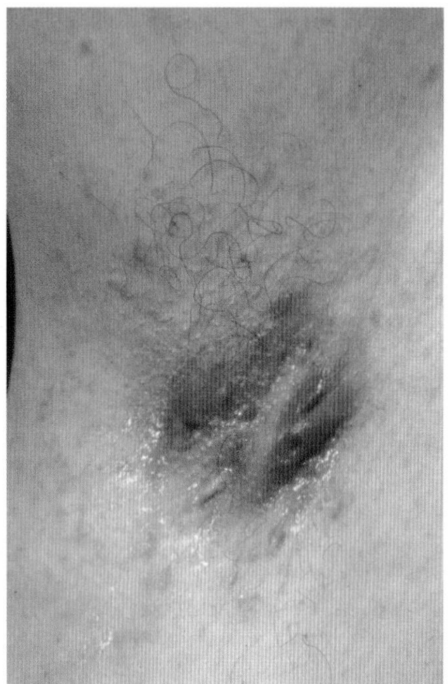

Figure 40.4 Hidradenitis suppurativa affecting the axilla (courtesy of St John's Institute for Dermatology, London, UK).

PYODERMA GANGRENOSUM (PG)

Characterised by cutaneous ulceration with purple undermined edges, PG is secondary to heightened immunological reactivity, usually from another disease process, such as inflammatory bowel disease, rheumatoid arthritis, non-Hodgkin's lymphoma or Wegener's granulomatosis (**Figure 40.5**). Ulcers generally respond to steroids; surgery is rarely indicated and may exacerbate the condition.

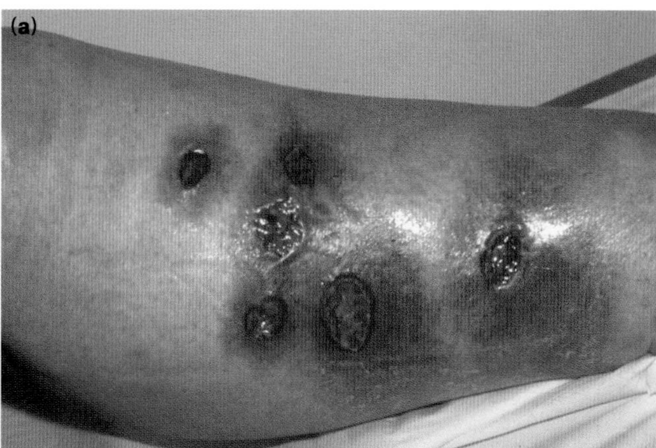

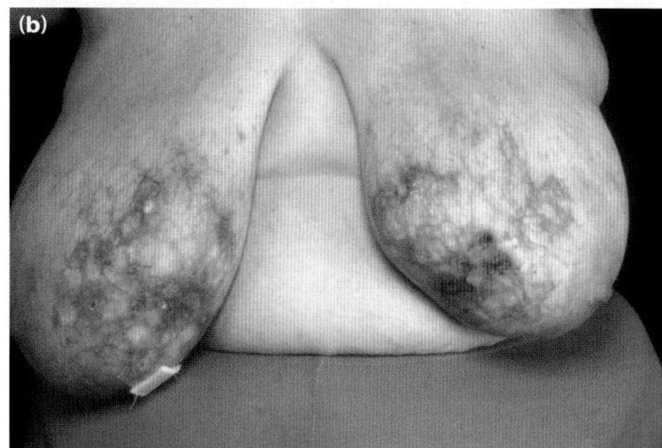

Figure 40.5 Pyoderma gangrenosum affecting the legs (**a**) and the breasts (**b**) (courtesy of St John's Institute for Dermatology, London, UK).

Infections

Skin and soft tissue infections can be localised or spreading, necrotising or non-necrotising. Localised or spreading, non-necrotising infections usually respond to broad spectrum antibiotics. Localised necrotising infections need surgical debridement as well as antibiotic therapy. Spreading, necrotising soft-tissue infection constitutes a life-threatening surgical emergency, requiring immediate resuscitation, intravenous antibiotic therapy and urgent surgical intervention with radical debridement.

Impetigo

Impetigo is a superficial infection of skin with staphylococci, streptococci or both (**Figure 40.6**). It is highly infectious, characterised by blisters that rupture and coalesce to form a honey-coloured crust and usually affects children. Treatment is directed at washing the affected areas and applying topical antistaphyloccocal treatments, and broad spectrum oral antibiotics if streptococcal infection is also implicated.

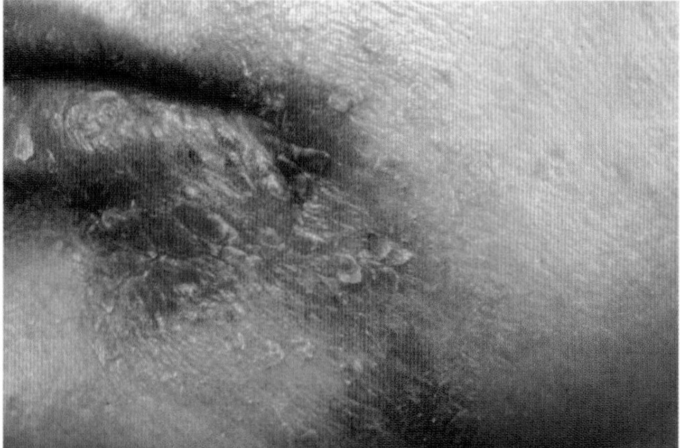

Figure 40.6 Impetigo. Note the honey-coloured crust (courtesy of St John's Institute for Dermatology, London, UK).

Erysipelas

Erysipelas is a sharply demarcated streptococcal infection of the superficial lymphatics, usually associated with broken skin on the face (**Figure 40.7**). The area affected is erythematous

Thomas Hodgkin, 1798–1866, curator of the Museum and demonstrator of Morbid Anatomy, Guy's Hospital, London, UK.

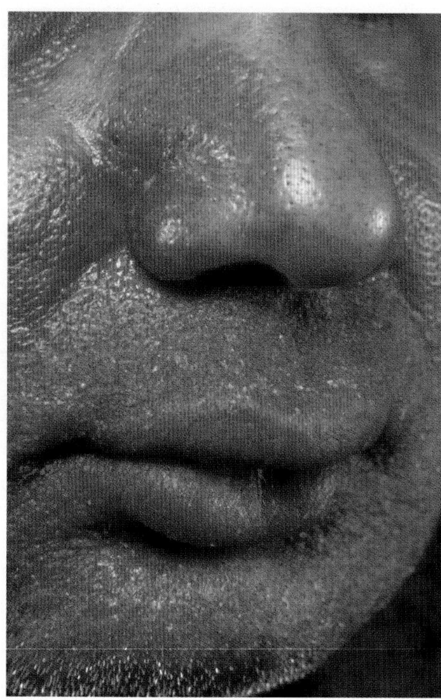

Figure 40.7 Erysipelas (courtesy of St John's Institute for Dermatology, London, UK).

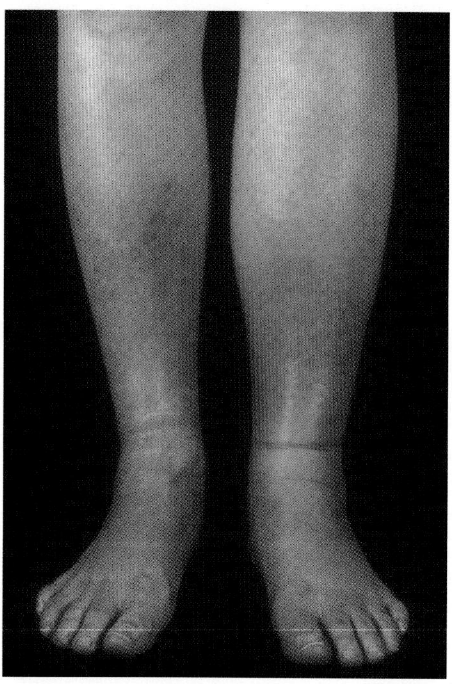

Figure 40.8 Cellulitis affecting the left leg (courtesy of St John's Institute for Dermatology, London, UK).

and oedematous. The patient may be febrile and have a leucocytosis. Prompt administration of broad spectrum antibiotics after swabbing the area for culture and sensitivity is usually all that is necessary.

Cellulitis/lymphangitis

This is a bacterial infection of the skin and subcutaneous tissue that is more generalised than erysipelas. It is usually associated with broken skin or pre-existing ulceration. It is characterised by an expanding area of erythematous, oedematous tissue that is painful, in association with fever, malaise and leucocytosis. Erythema tracking along lymphatics may be visible (lymphangitis) (**Figure 40.8**). The commonest causative organism is *Streptococcus*. Blood and skin cultures for sensitivity should be taken before prompt administration of broad spectrum, intravenous antibiotics and elevation of the affected extremity.

Necrotising fasciitis

Meleney's synergistic gangrene and Fournier's gangrene are variants of a similar disease process.

Necrotising fasciitis results from synergistic, polymicrobial infection; most commonly a streptococcal species (Group A β-haemolytic) in combination with *Staphylococcus*, *Escherichia coli*, *Pseudomonas*, *Proteus*, *Bacteroides* or *Clostridia*. 80% have a history of previous trauma/infection and over 60% commence in the lower extremities. Predisposing conditions include: diabetes mellitus; smoking; penetrating trauma; pressure sores; immunosuppression; intravenous drug abuse; perineal infection (perianal abscess, Bartholin's cysts); and skin damage/infection (abrasions, bites, boils).

Summary box 40.1

Necrotising fasciitis

- Surgical emergency
- Polymicrobial synergistic infection
- 80% history of previous trauma or infection
- Rapid progression to septic shock
- Urgent resuscitation, antibiotics and surgical debridement
- Mortality 30–50%

Classical clinical signs include: oedema stretching beyond visible skin erythema; a woody-hard texture to the subcutaneous tissues; an inability to distinguish fascial planes and muscle groups on palpation; disproportionate pain in relation to the affected area, with associated skin vesicles and soft-tissue crepitus (**Figure 40.9**). Lymphangitis tends to be absent. Early on, patients may be febrile and tachycardic, with a very rapid progression to septic shock. Radiographs, that should not have delayed urgent treatment, may demonstrate air in the tissues.

Management should commence with urgent fluid resuscitation, monitoring of haemodynamic status and administration of high-dose, intravenous broad spectrum, antibiotics.

Frank Meleney, 1889–1963, American surgeon in the First World War, then became a Professor at Columbia Medical School in New York.
Jean Fournier, 1832–1914, French dermatologist, also described tertiary syphilis.

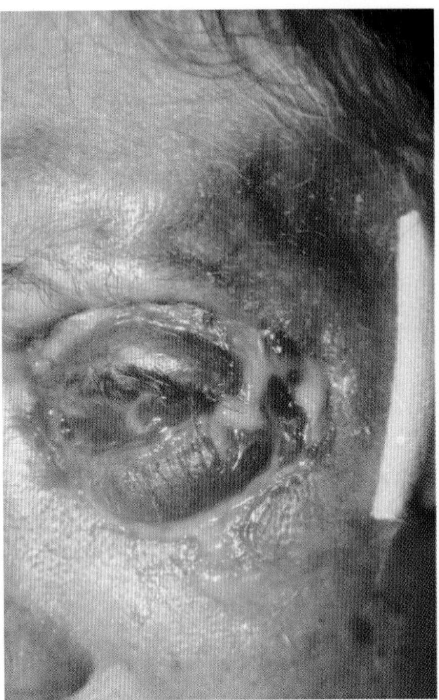

Figure 40.9 Necrotising fasciitis affecting the left orbit and facial skin (courtesy of St John's Institute for Dermatology, London, UK).

This is a surgical emergency and the diseased area should be debrided as soon as possible until viable, healthy, bleeding tissue is reached. Early surgical review and further debridement is advisable, together with the use vacuum-assisted dressings. Early skin grafting in selected cases may minimise protein and fluid losses. Mortality of between 30% and 50% can be expected, even with prompt with operative intervention.

Purpura fulminans

This is a relatively rare condition in which intravascular thrombosis produces rapid skin necrosis and haemorrhagic infarction, which progresses rapidly to septic shock and disseminated intravascular coagulation. Usually seen in children, it can occur in adults and may be subdivided into three types based on aetiological mechanism: 'acute infectious'; 'neonatal' and 'idiopathic' purpura fulminans.

Acute infectious is the commonest form. It is associated with a mortality rate of 40–50%, usually from multiorgan failure and is secondary to either an acute bacterial (*Neisseria meningitidis*) or viral infection (varicella). It is most common in children under 7 years, following an upper respiratory tract infection, or in asplenia. Endotoxins produce an imbalance in procoagulant and anticoagulant endothelial activity, producing protein C deficiency; this gives the clinical picture of an initial petechial rash developing into confluent ecchymoses and haemorrhagic bullae, which necrose to form well-demarcated lesions that form hard eschars. Extensive tissue loss is common, which often culminates in limb amputation (Figure 40.10).

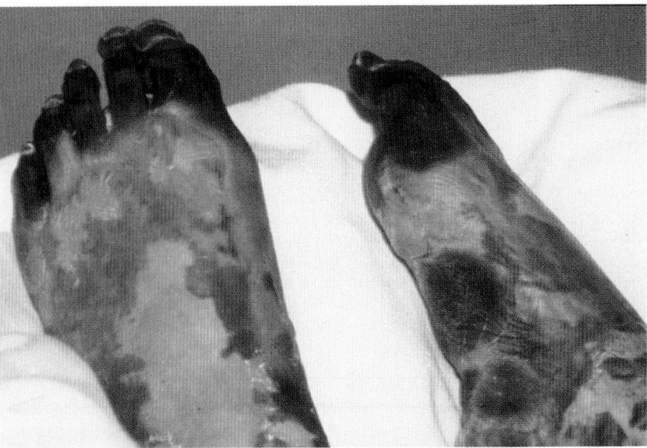

Figure 40.10 Acute infectious purpura fulminans caused by meningococcal septicaemia. Note the sharply demarcated necrotic areas distal to the affected end or perforating arteries with surrounding normal skin (courtesy of St John's Institute for Dermatology, London, UK).

Skin and soft tissue cysts

Milia

Milia are small, hard, keratin retention cysts seen both in babies and, after chronic sun exposure, in the elderly (Figure 40.11).

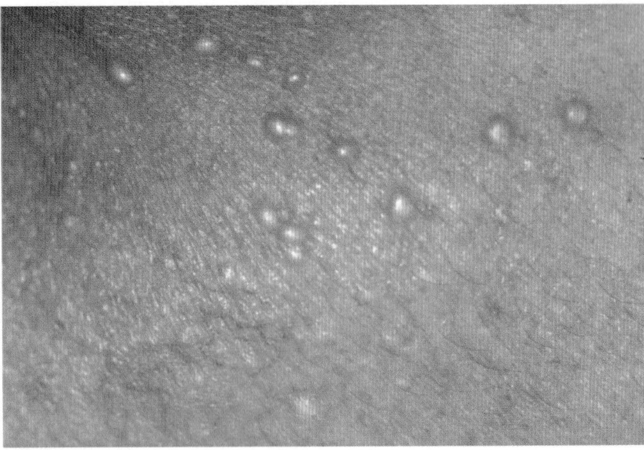

Figure 40.11 Milia (courtesy of St John's Institute for Dermatology, London, UK).

Epidermal cysts

These cysts are lined with true, stratified-squamous epithelium, derived from hair follicle infundibuli or traumatic inclusion. Commonly known as sebaceous cysts, they can occur anywhere. They are fixed to the skin and usually have a central punctum (Figure 40.12).

Treatment depends on the clinical state of the cyst. When inflamed or infected, they should be incised and drained initially, and removed later once the inflammation and

Albert Ludwig Seigmund Neisser, 1855–1916, Director of the Dermatological Institute, Breslau, Germany (now Wroclaw, Poland).

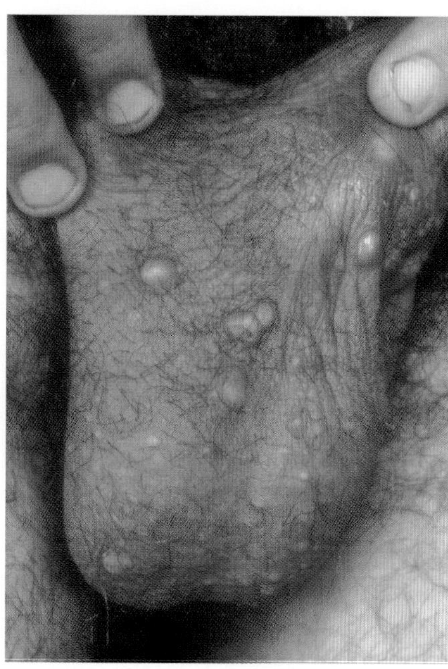

Figure 40.12 Multiple scrotal epidermal cysts (courtesy of St John's Institute for Dermatology, London, UK).

induration has subsided. It is important to excise the cyst in its entirety as failure to do so usually results in recurrence.

Meibomian cysts are epidermal cysts found on the free edge of the eyelid. Tricholemmal (pilar/pilosebaceous) cysts are derived from the epidermis of the external root sheath of the hair follicle. 90% are found in the scalp and 70% are multiple; they are usually distinguished from epidermal cysts by pathologists, rather than clinically.

SKIN TUMOURS

Benign lesions

Basal cell papilloma (seborrhoeic keratosis, senile keratosis, verruca senilis)

These vary from macular to soft, excrescent, warty lesions, which are often pigmented and hyperkeratotic. They are formed from the basal layer of epidermal cells and contain melanocytes.

Papillary wart (verruca vulgaris)

This is a benign skin tumour arising from infection with the human papilloma virus (HPV), which is also responsible for plantar warts and condylomata acuminata.

Freckle (ephelis)

A freckle is an area of skin that contains a normal number of melanocytes, producing an abnormally large number of melanin granules.

Lentigo

These are small, circumscribed pigmented macules, which stem from sun damage and some systemic syndromes. Solar lentigos are commoner in fairer skins.

Moles/naevi

Melanocytes migrate from the neural crest to the basal epidermis during embryogenesis. When melanocytes aggregate in the dermis or at the dermo-epidermal junction, they are called naevus cells.

Junctional naevus

A junctional naevus is a dermo-epidermal proliferation of naevus cells, visible as deeply pigmented macules or papules that occur commonly in childhood or adolescence, usually progressing to form compound or intradermal naevi with advancing age. Benign mucosal lesions tend to be junctional naevi (**Figure 40.13**).

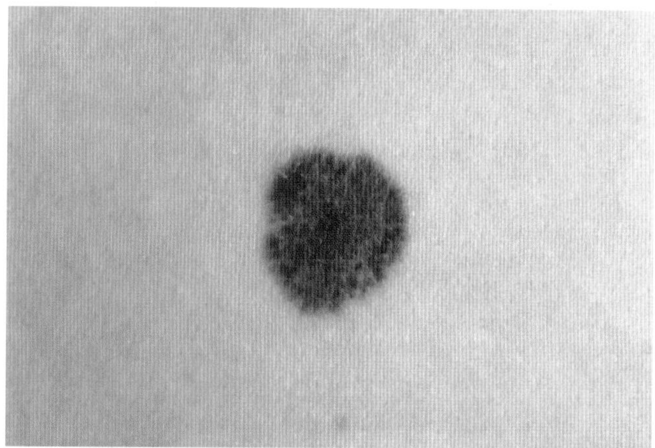

Figure 40.13 Junctional naevus (courtesy of St John's Institute for Dermatology, London, UK).

Compound naevus

This is a maculopapular, pigmented lesion that becomes most prominent during adolescence (**Figure 40.14**). It represents a junctional proliferation of naevus cells, with nests and columns in the dermis.

Intradermal naevus

Intradermal naevi are faintly pigmented papules in adults showing no junctional proliferation, but a cluster of dermal melanocytes (**Figure 40.15**).

Spitz naevus

These are reddish brown (occasionally deeply pigmented) nodules, previously termed 'juvenile melanoma' (**Figure**

Heinrich Meibom (Meibomius), 1638–1700, Professor of Medicine, History and Poetry, Helmstadt, Germany, described these glands in 1666.
Sophie Spitz, 1910–1956, American dermatopathologist at Sloan-Kettering Cancer Center, published the first case series of 'juvenile melanoma' in 1948. Died at the age of 46 from carcinoma of the colon.

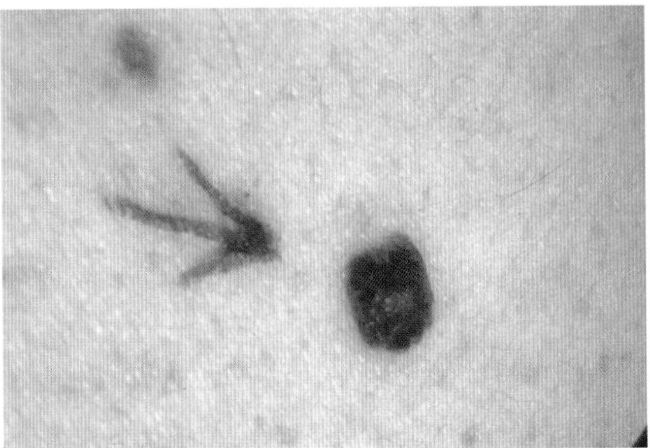

Figure 40.14 Compound naevus (courtesy of St John's Institute for Dermatology, London, UK).

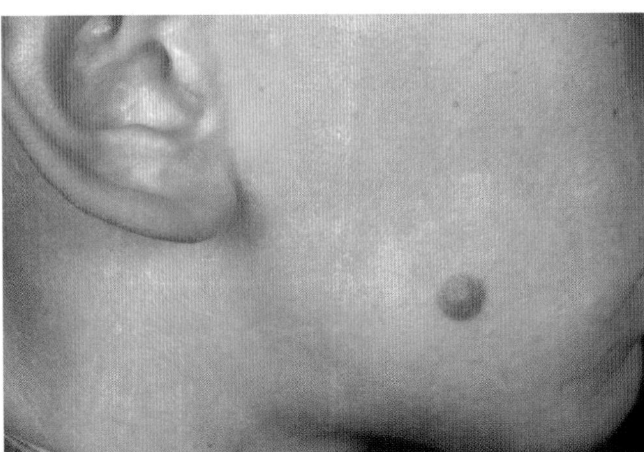

Figure 40.16 Spitz naevus (courtesy of St John's Institute for Dermatology, London, UK).

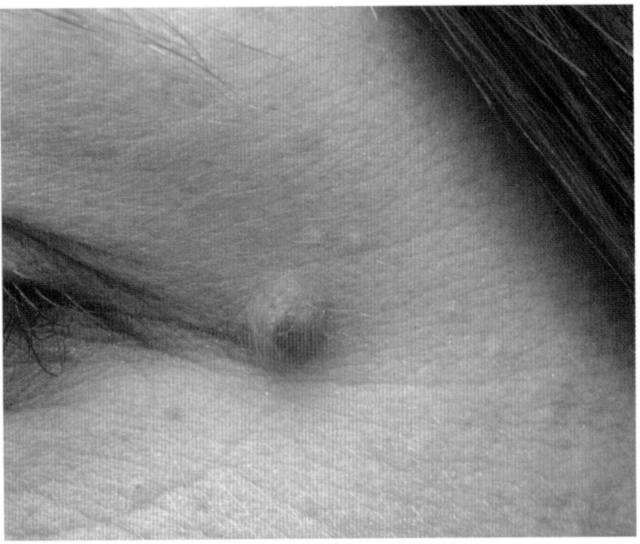

Figure 40.15 Intradermal naevus (courtesy of St John's Institute for Dermatology, London, UK).

40.16). They most commonly occur on the face and legs, growing rapidly initially then remaining static or regressing. The differential diagnosis is melanoma and excision biopsy is warranted if there is doubt as to the diagnosis.

Spindle cell naevus

Spindle cell naevi are dense black lesions, which contain spindle cells and atypical melanocytes at the dermo-epidermal junction. They are commonly seen on the thighs and affect women more frequently. They may have malignant potential.

Halo naevus

The halo of depigmentation around any benign naevus represents an antibody response to melanocytes. Depigmentation may also be a feature of a malignant melanoma. Halo naevi are associated with vitiligo (**Figure 40.17**).

Café-au-lait spots

These are coffee-coloured macules of variable size (from a few mm to 10 cm) (**Figure 40.18**). Multiple lesions are associated with NF 1 and McCune–Albright syndromes. They are more common in dark-skinned races.

Naevus spilus (speckled lentiginous naevus)

These are similar in appearance to a café-au-lait spots, but with hyperpigmented speckles throughout (**Figure 40.19**). They are benign lesions that are associated with various cutaneous diseases, but whose speckled appearance can be confused with malignant change. The mainstay of management is observation and serial photography as malignant transformation is rare.

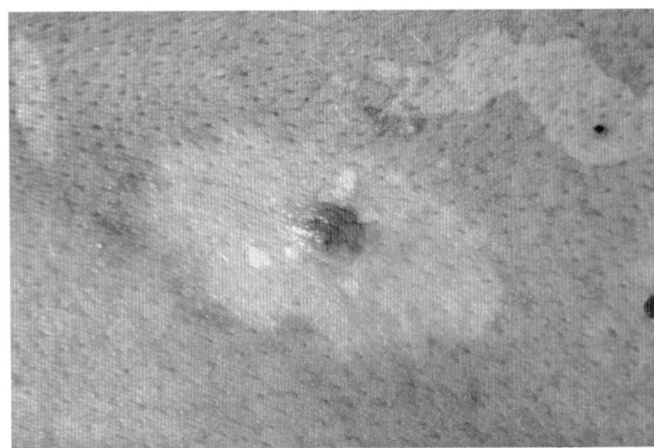

Figure 40.17 Halo naevus (courtesy of St John's Institute for Dermatology, London, UK).

Donovan James McCune, 1902–1976, American paediatrician.
Fuller Albright, 1900–1969, physician, Massachusetts General Hospital, Boston, MA, USA.

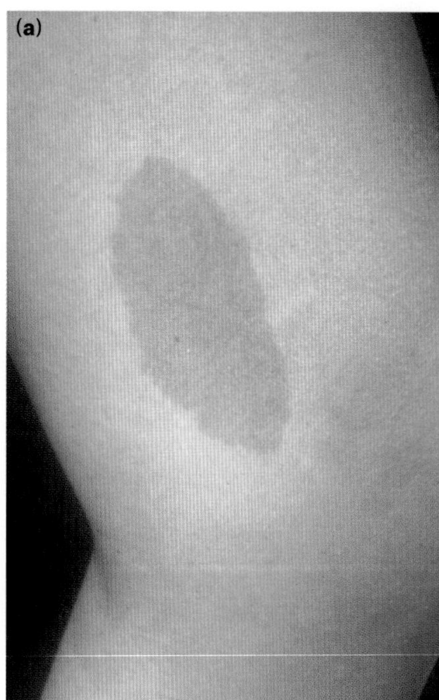

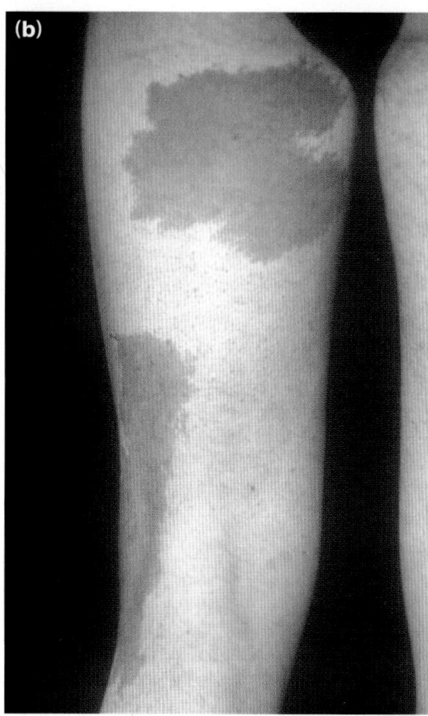

Figure 40.18 Café-au-lait spots. Note the two topographical variants: in (**a**) the spot has a smooth 'coast of California' border, whereas the upper spot in (**b**) has an irregular 'coast of Maine' border. Multiple smooth-bordered lesions are commonly associated with syndromes (courtesy of St John's Institute for Dermatology, London, UK).

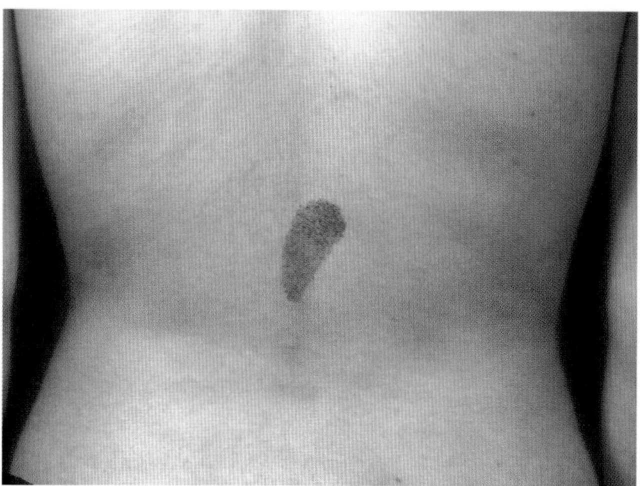

Figure 40.19 Naevus spilus (courtesy of St John's Institute for Dermatology, London, UK).

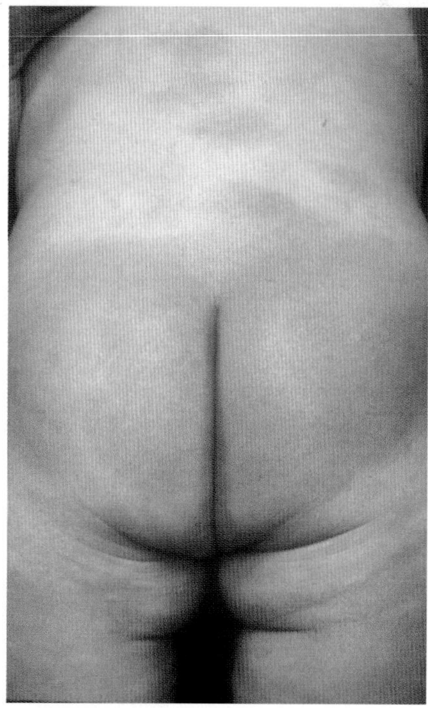

Figure 40.20 Mongolian spot (courtesy of St John's Institute for Dermatology, London, UK).

Mongolian spot

A Mongolian spot is a congenital blue grey macule found on the sacral skin (Figure 40.20). Pigmentation initially deepens and then regresses completely by age 7 years.

Blue naevus

This is a benign skin lesion that is four times more common in children, typically affecting the extremities and face (Figure 40.21).

Naevi of Ota and Ito

A naevus of Ota is a dermal, melanocytic hamartoma visible as a blue or grey macule in the trigeminal V1 and V2 dermatomes. It is four times more common in women and most frequently seen in Oriental and African races (Figure 40.22).

Minoru Ito, 1892–1986, Professor of Dermatology, Tohoko University, Sendai, Honshu, Japan.

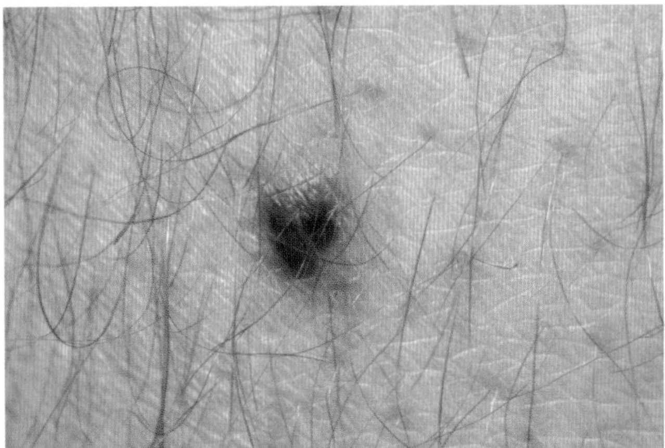

Figure 40.21 Blue naevus (courtesy of St John's Institute for Dermatology, London, UK).

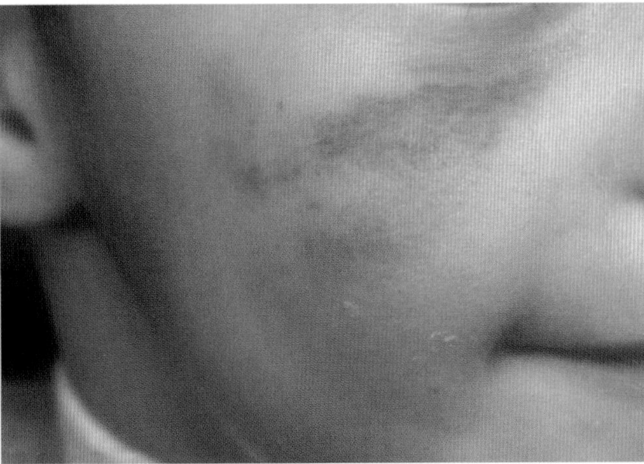

Figure 40.22 Naevus of Ota (courtesy of St John's Institute for Dermatology, London, UK).

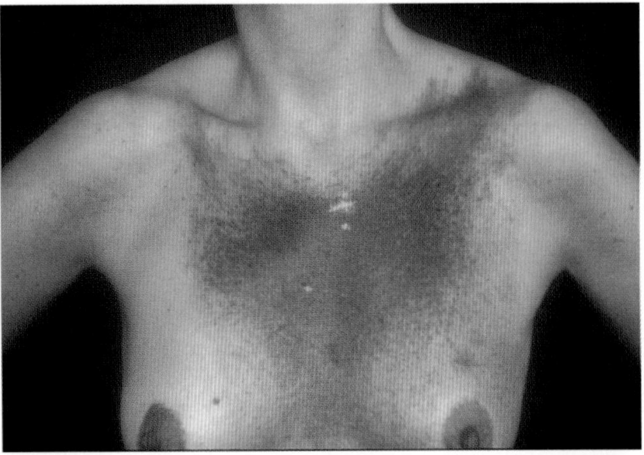

Figure 40.23 Naevus of Ito (courtesy of St John's Institute for Dermatology, London, UK).

A naevus of Ito is characterised by dermal melanocytosis in the shoulder region and can occur simultaneously in patients with naevus of Ota (Figure 40.23).

Hair follicles

Trichoepithelioma

These are small skin-coloured nodules, found most often in the nasolabial folds. It is clinically and histologically similar to a basal cell carcinoma.

Pilomatrixoma (calcifying epithelioma of Malherbe)

These are benign hair matrix cell tumours that often calcify. 40% are found in the under-10 age group.

Tricholemmoma (naevus sebaceous of Jadassohn)

Tricholemmoma is a congenital hamartoma with the appearance of a linear verrucous naevus. 10% form a BCC life-long (Figure 40.24).

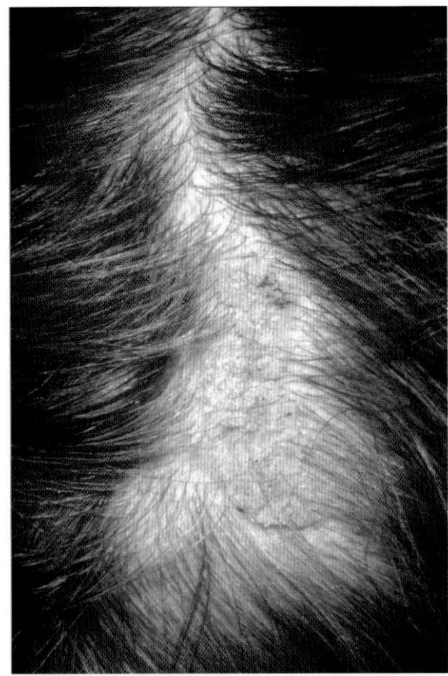

Figure 40.24 Naevus sebaceous of Jadassohn (courtesy of St John's Institute for Dermatology, London, UK).

Adenoma sebaceum (tuberous sclerosis, Bourneville disease)

These are typically red, facial papules (angiofibromas), usually on the nasolabial folds, cheek and chin. They usually appear in children before 10 years of age and increase in size and

Josef Jadassohn, 1863–1936, dermatologist, Breslau, Germany (now Wroclaw, Poland).
Desire M Bourneville, 1840–1909, physician, Le Bicêtre, Paris, France.

number until adolescence. Cosmetic removal by argon or pulse dye lasers or scalpel is indicated (Figure 40.25).

Rhinophyma

Rhinophyma is the end-stage sequela of nasal acne rosacea (Figure 40.26). It is nasal sebaceous gland hypertrophy and hyperplasia and tends to affect elderly men (M:F12:1). Occult BCCs exist in 3%. Treatment by dermabrasion or laser resurfacing produces good results.

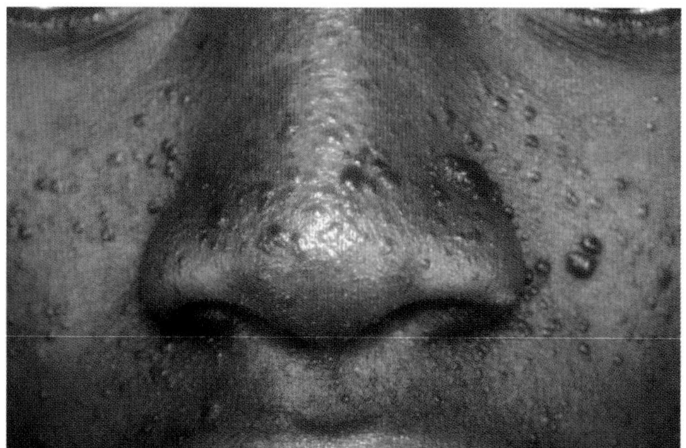

Figure 40.25 Adenoma sebaceum (courtesy of St John's Institute for Dermatology, London, UK).

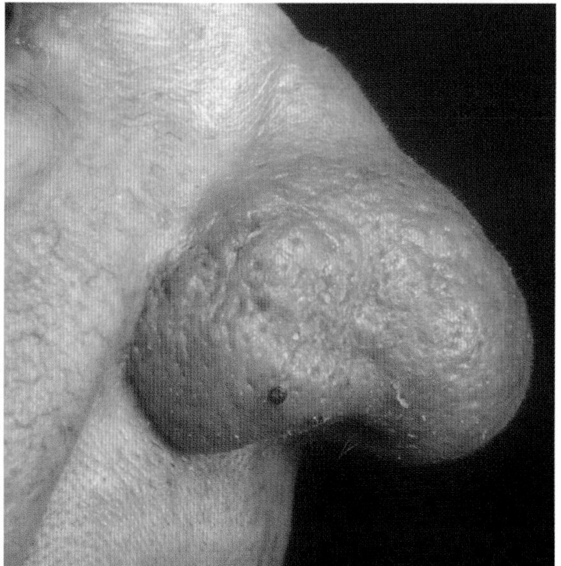

Figure 40.26 Rhinophyma (courtesy of St John's Institute for Dermatology, London, UK).

Sweat glands

Cystadenoma (hydrocystadenomas, hidradenomas)

These are 1–3 cm translucent blue cystic nodules.

Eccrine poroma (papillary syringoma)

These are single raised or pedicled lesions found most often on the palm or sole.

Cylindroma (turban tumour)

A variant of eccrine spiradenoma, which coalesce when multiple on the scalp, forming a 'turban tumour'.

Premalignant lesions

Extramammary Paget's disease (intraepidermal adenocarcinoma)

This occurs in cutaneous sites rich in apocrine glands such as the axillae, genital and perianal regions. Approximately 25% are associated with an underlying *in situ* or invasive adenocarcinoma. Early skin changes are subtle and may present as an eczematous lesion or intertrigo. Surgical excision forms the basis of treatment, with up to 20% demonstrating invasive disease after pathology assessment (Figure 40.27).

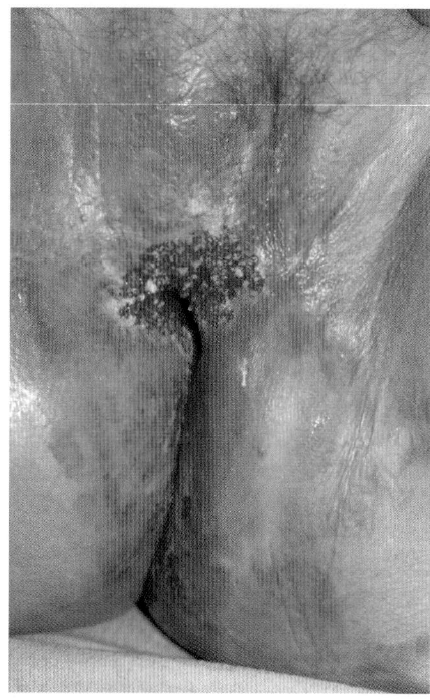

Figure 40.27 Extramammary Paget's disease involving the perineum (courtesy of St John's Institute for Dermatology, London, UK).

Giant congenital pigmented naevus (GCPN) or giant hairy naevus

This naevus causes a great deal of confusion as its definition and management is contentious. It is a hamartoma of naevo-melanocytes that has a tendency to dermatomal distribution (Figure 40.28). It has a similar histology to compound naevi, but the naevus cells are distributed variably from the epidermis throughout all layers and into the subdermal fat and muscle. GCPNs are precursors of melanoma, but the magnitude of this risk is unclear, largely due to the lack of well-conducted studies and variable classification of the naevus. A 3–5% lifetime risk of melanoma is quoted. 1 in 3 childhood malignant melanomas (MM) arise in patients with GCPN, but the risk decreases with age: 15% of MMs present at birth; 62% present by puberty and 99% by 45 years of age.

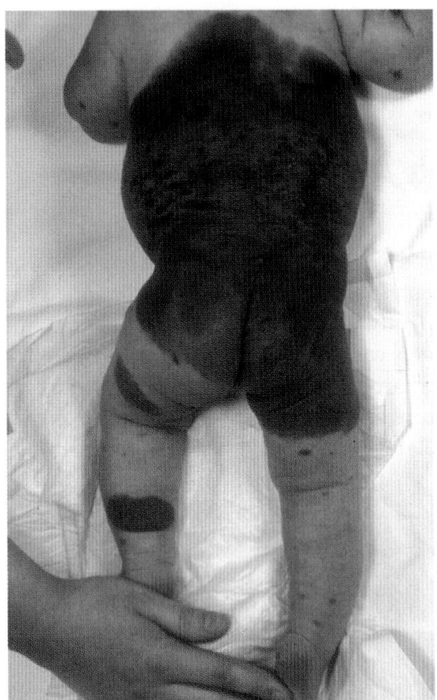

Figure 40.28 Giant congenital pigmented naevus (courtesy of St John's Institute for Dermatology, London, UK).

A multidisciplinary management approach is advocated, with initial investigations examining for neurocutaneous melanosis as there may be leptomeningeal involvement. Removal of GCPN should be considered for both aesthetic and oncological reasons.

Atypical (dysplastic) naevus

To be 'atypical naevi', lesions must have three of the following characteristics: variegated pigmentation; ill-defined borders; undulating irregular surfaces; or measure >5 mm. Histologically, they are irregular proliferations of melanocytes at the basal layer of epidermis. They can be sporadic or familial (familial atypical multiple mole-melanoma (FAMMM) syndrome). Possession of more than five confers a relative risk of melanoma six times greater than usual; within FAMM syndrome, they confer a life-long 10% risk of MM (**Figure 40.29**).

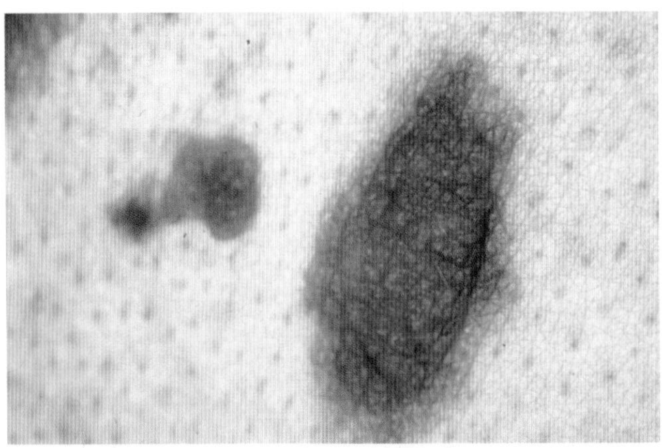

Figure 40.29 Dysplastic naevus (courtesy of St John's Institute for Dermatology, London, UK).

Malignant lesions

WHO data suggest both non-melanoma and melanoma skin cancers continue to increase in incidence, despite educational programmes and wide-ranging changes in uptake of sun protective measures and improvements in sun-screens. Annually, global figures reveal 33% of all recorded malignancy affects the skin, with 2–3 million new non-melanoma skin cancers and 132 000 new malignant melanomas diagnosed each year.

Basal cell carcinoma

This is usually a slow-growing, locally-invasive, malignant tumour of pluripotential epithelial cells arising from basal epidermis and hair follicles; hence, it affects the pilo-sebaceous skin.

Summary box 40.2

Basal cell carcinoma

- Slow growing
- Risk factor – ultraviolet radiation
- 90% nodular/nodular cystic
- High- and low-risk basal cell carcinoma

EPIDEMIOLOGY

The strongest predisposing factor to BCC is UVR. It occurs in the elderly or the middle-aged after excessive sun exposure, with 95% occurring between the ages of 40 and 80 years. The incidence of BCC rises with proximity to the equator, although 33% arise in parts of the body not usually sun-exposed. Other predisposing factors include exposure to arsenical compounds, coal tar, aromatic hydrocarbons, ionising radiation and genetic skin cancer syndromes. White-skinned people are almost exclusively affected. BCC is more common in men than women.

PATHOGENESIS

BCCs have no apparent precursor lesions and their development is proportional to the initial dose of the carcinogen, but not duration of exposure. The most likely model of pathogenesis for BCCs involves mesodermal factors as intrinsic promoters coupled with an initiation step.

BCCs metastasise extremely rarely.

MACROSCOPIC

BCC can be divided into localised (nodular; nodulocystic; cystic; pigmented and naevoid) and generalised (superficial: multifocal and superficial spreading; or infiltrative: morphoeic, ice pick and cicatrizing). Nodular and nodulocystic variants account for 90% of BCC.

MICROSCOPIC

Twenty-six histological subtypes have been described. The characteristic finding is of ovoid cells in nests with a single 'palisading' layer. It is only the outer layer of cells that actively divide, explaining why tumour growth rates are slower than their cell cycle speed would suggest, and why incompletely excised lesions are more aggressive. Morphoeic BCCs synthesize type 4 collagenase and so spread rapidly (Figure 40.30).

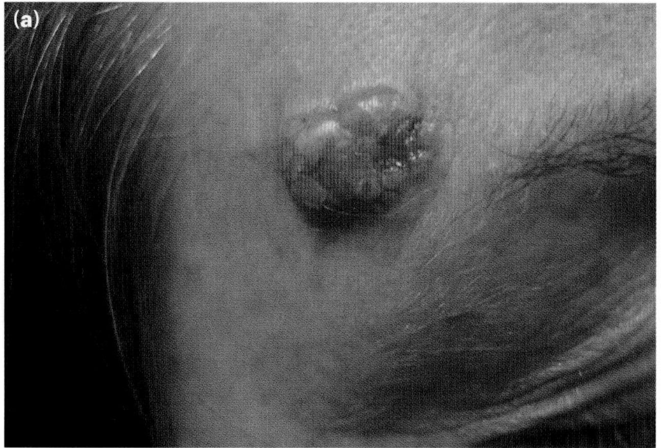

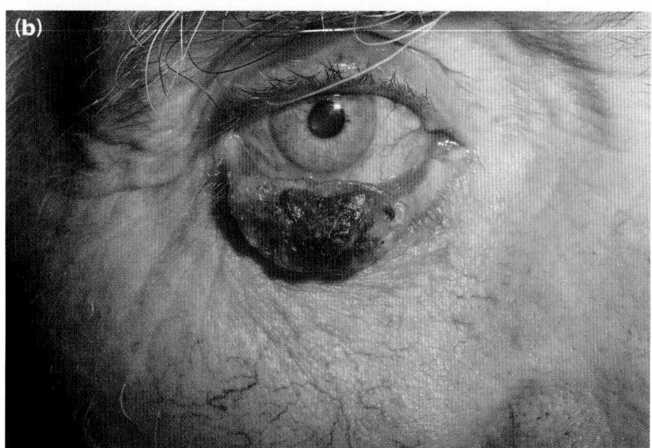

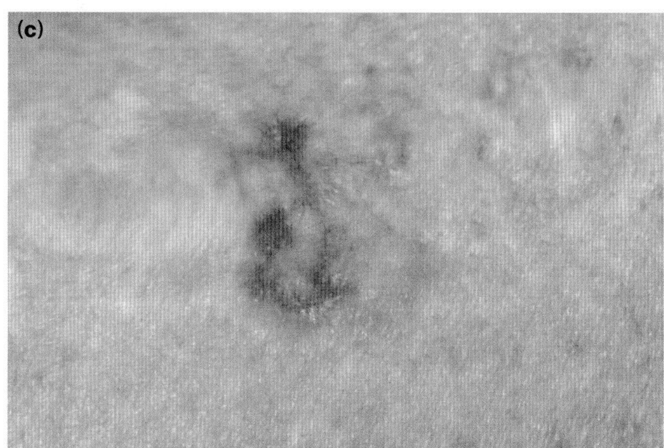

Figure 40.30 (a) A nodulocystic basal carcinoma (BCC). Note the characteristic pearly surface with telangectasia. (b) An ulcerating BCC on the lower eyelid. (c) A recurrent morphoeic BCC. ((a) and (b) courtesy of Mr AR Greenbaum; (c) courtesy of St John's Institute for Dermatology, London, UK.)

PROGNOSIS

There are 'high-risk' and 'low-risk' BCCs. High-risk BCCs are: large (>2 cm); located at sites where direct invasion gives access to the cranium (near the eye, nose and ear); recurrent tumours; tumours forming in the presence of immunosuppression; or that have micronodular or infiltrating histological subtypes.

MANAGEMENT

Treatment can be surgical or non-surgical. Tumour and surrounding surgical margins should always be assessed and marked under loupe magnification; the latter varying between 2 and15 mm, depending on the macroscopic variant. Where margins are ill-defined, or tissue at a premium (nose, eyes) then either a two-stage surgical approach with subsequent reconstruction after confirmation of clear margins, or Mohs' micrographic surgery is advisable. The histological sample must be orientated and marked for pathological examination.

Mohs' micrographic surgery is a method used by dermatological surgeons (dermatologists who have undergone extra training in techniques of cutaneous surgery and histopathology) to excise skin cancer under microscopic control.

In the elderly or infirm patients, radiotherapy produces similar recurrence rates to surgery; but with the risk of generating further malignancy after 1–2 decades. Biopsy-proven, superficial tumours can be treated with topical treatments (5-fluorouracil, imquimod).

Unless excision of a BCC is complete, there is a 67% recurrence rate if margins are grossly involved and a 33% recurrence rate within 2 years with microscopic involvement or when reported 'close'.

Patients with uncomplicated, completely-excised lesions can be discharged. Follow-up is reserved for patients with tumours in high-risk areas; with globally, sun-damaged skin; with syndromes; and for those who decline further surgery after incomplete excisions.

Cutaneous squamous cell carcinoma

SCC is a malignant tumour of keratinising cells of the epidermis or its appendages. It arises from the stratum basalis of the epidermis and expresses cytokeratins 1 and 10.

EPIDEMIOLOGY

Four BCCs occur for every SCC, which is the second most common form of skin cancer. It is strongly-related to cumulative sun exposure and damage, especially in white skinned individuals living nearer the equator. In the northern hemisphere it affects the elderly, whereas it is not uncommon in sun-damaged, middle-aged, white people in the southern hemisphere. Everywhere, it is more common in men than women. SCC is also associated with chronic inflammation (chronic sinus tracts, pre-existing scars, osteomyelitis, burns, vaccination points) and immunosuppression. When a SCC appears in a scar it is known as a Marjolin's ulcer.

Frederic E Mohs, 1910–2002, twentieth century American physician and general surgeon, University of Wisconsin, Madison, WI, USA, developed the Mohs micrographic surgical technique in 1938 for cutaneous malignant lesions.

Jean-Nicholas Marjolin, 1780–1850, surgeon, Paris, France, described the development of carcinomatous ulcers in scars in 1828.

Summary box 40.3

Squamous cell carcinoma

- Associated with ultraviolet radiation, chronic inflammation and chemical carcinogens
- High- and low-risk squamous cell carcinoma
- Metastasis in 2% cases

IR causes SCC, as do chemical carcinogens (arsenicals, tar) and infection with HPV 5 and 16. There is also evidence that current and previous tobacco use doubles the relative risk of SCC.

In the past, actinic (solar) keratoses (AK), i.e. cutaneous horns and keratoacanthomas, were considered to be premalignant lesions leading to SCC. Current thinking is to classify these lesions on a continuum of lesions, some of which can improve, as with other squamous cell tumours such as cervical intraepithelial neoplasia.

AKs are areas of permananent sun damage in which there is dyskeratosis and partial-thickness, cellular atypia, subepidermal inflammation, but an intact basement membrane (Figure 40.31). They 'wax and wane' macroscopically between macular and papular, with and without, keratinous surfaces. Most improve after moisturisation and remain as erythematous macules; however, up to 20% form SCC.

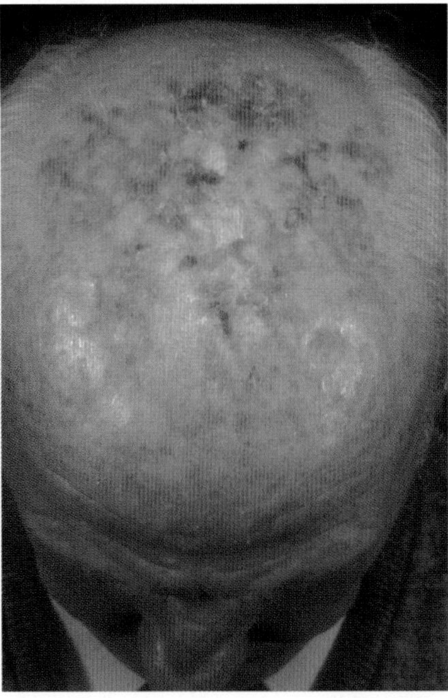

Figure 40.31 Actinic keratosis (courtesy of St John's Institute for Dermatology, London, UK).

When an AK has a keratinous surface with a height greater than its base diameter, it is termed a keratin horn. 10% will have an underlying SCC (**Figure 40.32**).

Keratoacanthomas are rapidly-growing, nodular tumours, exhibiting symmetry around a central, keratin-filled crater. Current thought is that rather than being separate premalignant entities, they are better considered as self-healing SCCs and as such, are often reported by pathologists as 'keratoacanthoma-like SCCs' (**Figure 40.33**). Keratoacanthomas are twice as common in men than women and usually found on the face or limbs of chronically, sun-damaged 50–70-year-old white-skinned individuals. They may be caused by HPV in a hair follicle during growth phase and are also associated with smoking and chemical carcinogen exposure. Excision is recommended, rather than observation, as the differential diagnosis includes anaplastic SCC and the excision scar is often better than that which remains after resolution.

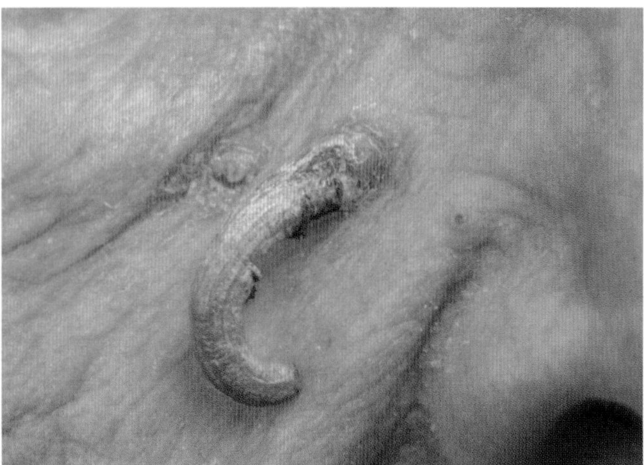

Figure 40.32 Cutaneous horn (courtesy of St John's Institute for Dermatology, London, UK).

Bowen's disease is SCC *in situ* and often develops as full-thickness dysplasia in hypertrophic AKs (**Figure 40.34**). SCC in situ usually presents as a slowly enlarging, erythematous scaly plaque and may occur anywhere on the mucocutaneous surface of the body. On the glans penis, it is called erythroplasia of Queyrat (**Figure 40.35**). Topical therapy with 5-fluorouracil or imiquimod are effective treatments. Alternatives include surgical excision with a 4 mm margin, or Mohs' micrographic surgery for larger or recurrent lesions.

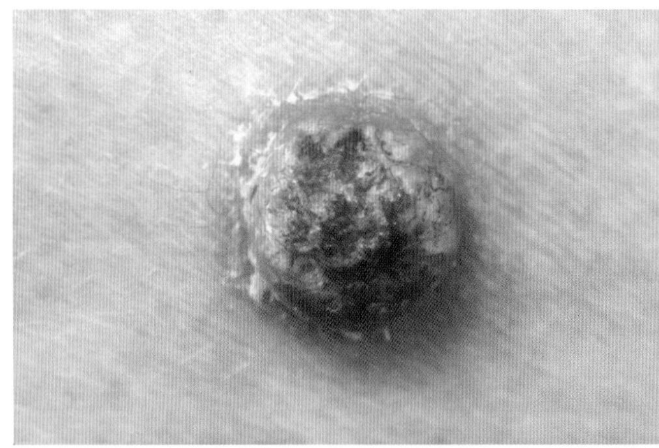

Figure 40.33 Keratocanthoma (courtesy of St John's Institute for Dermatology, London, UK).

John T Bowen, 1857–1940, Professor of Dermatology at Harvard, USA.
August Queyrat, 1856–1933, dermatologist, Paris, France, described this condition in 1911.

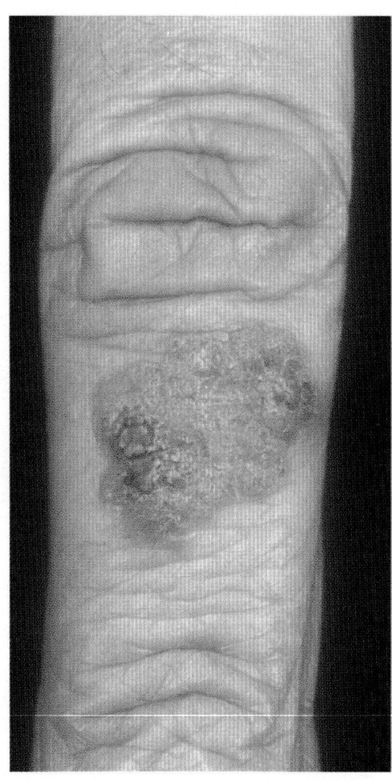

Figure 40.34 Bowen's disease – squamous cell carcinoma *in situ* (courtesy of St John's Institute for Dermatology, London, UK).

MACROSCOPIC

The appearance of SCC may vary from smooth nodular, verrucous, papillomatous to ulcerating lesions. All ulcerate eventually, as they grow. The ulcers have a characteristic everted edge and are surrounded by inflamed, indurated skin. Differential diagnoses of SCC include: AK; BCC; pyoderma gangrenosum; warts; and lichen simplex chronicus (Figure 40.36).

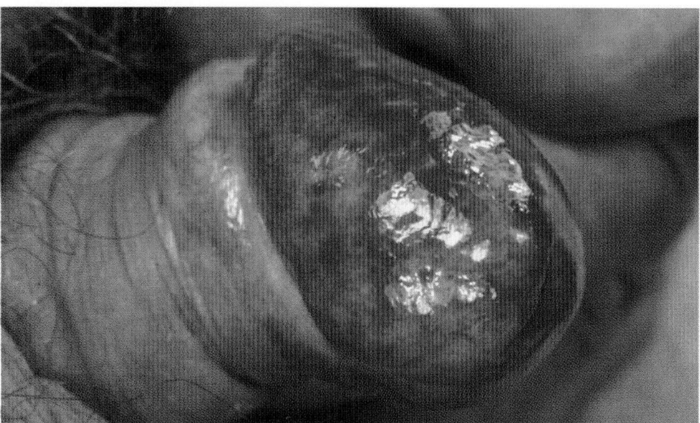

Figure 40.35 Erythroplasia of Queyrat – squamous cell carcinoma *in situ* on the glans penis; also called Paget's disease of the penis (courtesy of St John's Institute for Dermatology, London, UK).

MICROSCOPIC

Characteristic irregular masses of squamous epithelium are noted to proliferate and invade the dermis from the basal layer. The tumour stains positive for cytokeratins 1 and 10. SCC can be graded histologically according to Broder's grading, which describes the proportion of dedifferentiated cells in the tumour. *Table 40.1* presents tumour classification and staging.

PROGNOSIS

There are several independent prognostic variables for SCC:

- Depth: the deeper the lesion, the worse the prognosis. For SCC <2 mm, metastasis is highly unlikely; whereas if >6 mm, 15% of SCC will have metastasised.

TABLE 40.1 TNM Classification and staging.

Size	Nodes	Mets	Stages
TX Primary tumour cannot be assessed	NX Nodal involvement cannot be assessed	M0 No metastatic disease	Stage 0 Tis, N0, M0
T0 No evidence of primary tumour	N0 No regional nodes	M1 Metastatic disease present	Stage I T1, N0, M0
Tis In situ (confined to full thickness epidermal) disease	N1 Spread to 1 ipsilateral, nearby node that is <3 cm diameter		Stage II T2, N0, M0
T1 Primary <2 cm	N2a Spread to 1 ipsilateral nearby node that is 3–6 cm diameter		Stage III T3, N0, M0 or T1–T3, N1, M0
T2 Primary >2 cm	N2b Spread to >1 ipsilateral, nearby nodes, but none >6 cm diameter		Stage IV T1–T3, N2, M0 or any disease that is N3, or T4 or M1
T3 Primary invasion of a facial bone	N2c Spread to contralateral node(s), but none are >6 cm diameter		
T4 Invasion of muscle, base of skull or other bones	N3 Spread to any node >6 cm diameter		

Albert Compton Broders, 1885–1964, American pathologist of Minnesota, USA and Chairman of the Department of Surgical Pathology, The Mayo Clinic, Rochester, Minnesota, MN, USA; for 1 year in 1935 Professor of Surgical Pathology and Director of Cancer Research, University of Virginia, VA, USA. Broders graded rectal cancer in the USA in a manner that Cuthbert Dukes classified them in the UK. A combination of Broders' grading and Dukes' classification gave a more accurate prognosis for rectal carcinoma than either method alone.

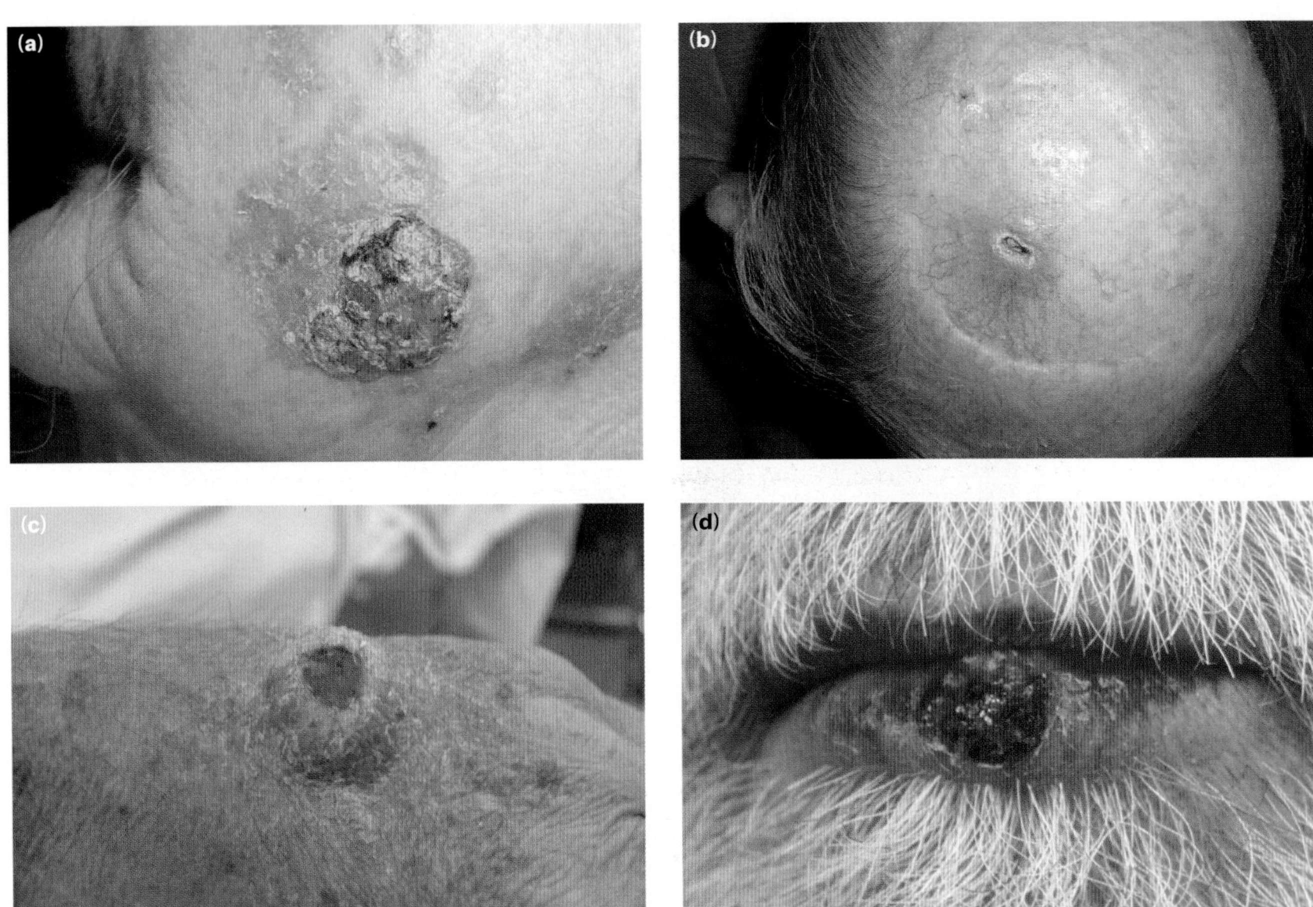

Figure 40.36 (a) A squamous cell carcinoma (SCC) on the face. (b) A recurrent SCC arising in a previously skin-grafted area of the scalp. (c) SCC arising on the dorsum of the hand in a renal transplant recipient on immunosuppressive therapy. (d) SCC arising on the lip of a smoker who worked outside on a farm. ((a–c) courtesy of Mr AR Greenbaum; (d) courtesy of St John's Institute for Dermatology, London, UK.)

- Surface size: lesions >2 cm have a worse prognosis than smaller ones.
- Histological grade: the higher the Broder's grade, the worse the prognosis.
- Microscopic invasion of lympho-vascular spaces or nerve tissue carries a high risk of metastatic disease.

Therefore, as well as information on pathological pattern, cellular morphology and Broder's grade, any histopathology report for SCC should include the depth of invasion, the presence of perineural or lymphovascular invasion and the deep and peripheral margin clearance.

- Site: SCCs on the lips and ears have higher local recurrence rates than lesions elsewhere, and tumours at the extremities fare worse than those on the trunk.
- Aetiology: SCCs that arise in burn scars, osteomyelitis skin sinuses, chronic ulcers and areas of skin that have been irradiated have a higher metastatic potential.
- Immunosuppression: SCCs will invade further in those with impaired immune response.

The overall rate of metastasis is 2% for SCC (usually to regional nodes) with a local recurrence rate of 20%.

MANAGEMENT

SCC is a heterogeneous tumour with a malignant potential that varies between subtypes. Management must address the tumour's tendency for lymphatic metastasis and the possibility of in-transit metastasis.

Surgical excision is the only means of providing accurate information on histology and clearance. The margins for primary excision should be tailored to surface size in the first instance. This should ideally be assessed using surgical loupe magnification. A 4 mm clearance margin should be achieved if the SCC measures <2 cm across, and a 1-cm clearance margin if >2 cm. 95% of local recurrence and regional metastases occur within 5 years, thus follow-up beyond this period is not indicated.

Cutaneous malignant melanoma

Melanoma is a cancer of melanocytes and can, therefore, arise in skin, mucosa, retina and the leptomeninges.

EPIDEMIOLOGY

Cutaneous melanoma is caused by exposure to UVR. Its rise in incidence reflects increased recreational activity in the sun and emigration among white skinned races, not suited to sun exposure. Although it accounts for less than 5% of skin malignancy (and 1.6% of all malignancy worldwide), it is responsible for over 75% of skin malignancy-related deaths.

It is the commonest cancer in young adults (20–39 years) and the most likely cause of cancer-related death.

Distribution between the sexes varies around the world and reflects occupational and recreational exposure to sunlight. Likewise, geographical distribution reflects exposure of white-skinned individuals to sunlight: Taranaki in New Zealand, a country with a predominantly white-skinned, immigrant population, currently reports the highest (and rising) incidence per capita. 5% of all patients with MM will develop a second primary melanoma. 7% of MM presents as occult metastasis from an unknown primary.

PATHOPHYSIOLOGY

Cumulative UV exposure favours the development of lentigo maligna melanoma (LMM) and later onset of disease, whereas 'flash fry' exposure, typical of rapidly-acquired, holiday tans, favours the other morphological variants and early onset of disease.

A small proportion of MM is genetically-mediated and develops at an earlier age. People at most risk of developing MM include: those with genetic syndromes; a past history of MM or with first-degree relatives who have MM; those who have more than 30 sun-acquired naevi or a history of five significant sun-burns before the age of 16; fair-skinned/red-haired people living close to the equator; anyone with excessive UVR exposure (environmental or salon-delivered); or anyone with immunosuppression (which increases MM incidence 20–30-fold).

Summary box 40.4

Malignant melanoma

- Rising incidence
- Genetic and acquired risk factors
- Superficial spreading form the most common
- Breslow thickness most important prognostic indicator
- Sentinel node biopsy useful for staging

MACROSCOPIC

Only 10–20% of MM form in pre-existing naevi, with the remainder arising *de novo* in previously normally pigmented skin. The most likely naevi to form MM are atypical naevi, atypical junctional lenitiginous naevi (usually facial) and giant pigmented congenital naevi.

Macroscopic features in a pre-existing naevus that suggest malignant change are listed in *Summary box 40.5*.

There are four common macroscopic variants of MM and several other notable, but rarer forms:

Summary box 40.5

Macroscopic features in naevi suggestive of malignant melanoma

- Change in size
- Shape
- Colour
- Thickness (elevation/nodularity or ulceration)
- Satellite lesions (pigment spreading into surrounding area)
- Tingling/itching /serosanguinous discharge (usually late signs)

Superficial spreading melanoma (SSM) This is the most common presentation (70%), usually arising in a pre-existent naevus after several years of slow change, followed by rapid growth in the preceding months before presentation (**Figure 40.37**). Nodularity within SSM heralds the onset of the vertical growth phase.

Nodular melanoma (NM) Nodular melanoma accounts for 15% of all MM and tends to be more aggressive than SSM, with a shorter clinical onset. These lesions often arise *de novo* in skin and are more common in men than women, often presenting in middle age and usually on the trunk, head or neck (**Figure 40.38**). They typically appear as blue/black papules, 1–2 cm in diameter, and because they lack the horizontal growth phase, they tend to be sharply demarcated. Up to 5% are amelanotic.

Lentigo maligna melanoma LMM was previously also known as Hutchinson's melanotic freckle. This variant

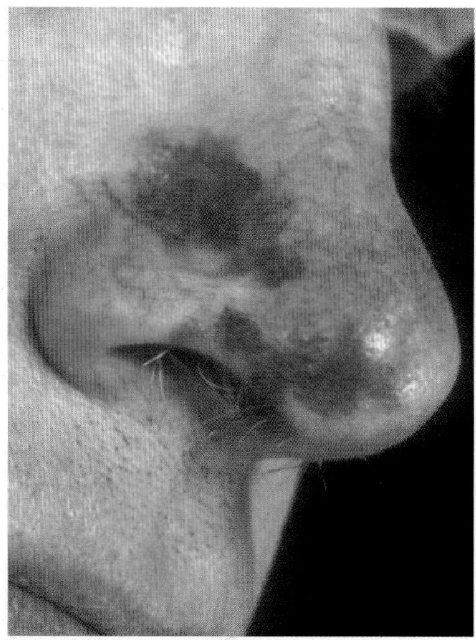

Figure 40.37 Superficial spreading melanoma (courtesy of St John's Institute for Dermatology, London, UK).

Sir Jonathan Hutchinson, 1828–1913, surgeon, St Bartholomew's Hospital, London, UK.

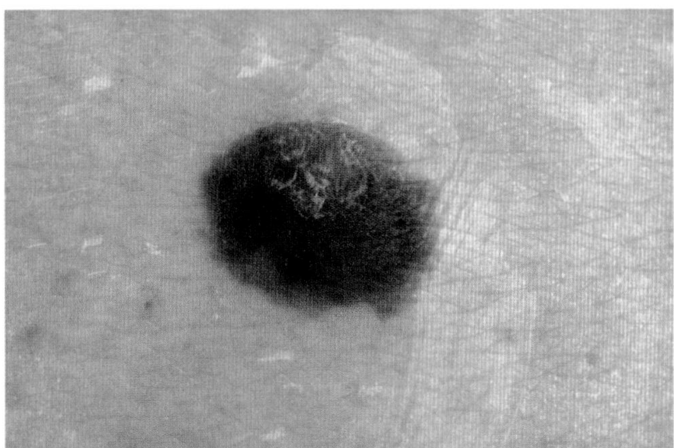

Figure 40.38 Nodular melanoma (courtesy of St John's Institute for Dermatology, London, UK).

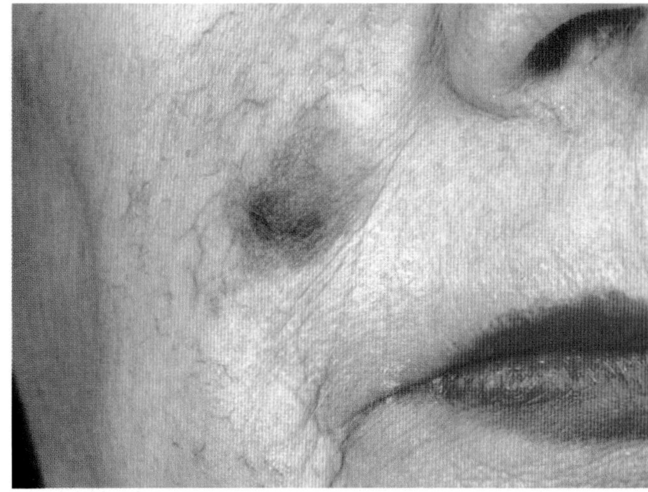

Figure 40.39 Lentigo maligna melanoma (courtesy of St John's Institute for Dermatology, London, UK).

presents as a slow-growing, variegated brown macule on the face, neck or hands of the elderly (Figure 40.39). They are positively correlated with prolonged, intense sun exposure, affecting women more than men. They account for between 5% and 10% of MM.

LMM are thought to have less metastatic potential than other variants as they take longer to enter a vertical growth phase. Nonetheless, when they have entered the vertical growth phase their metastatic potential is the same as any other melanoma.

Acral lentigious melanoma (ALM) ALM affects the soles of feet and palms of hands. It is rare in white-skinned individuals (2–8% of MM) but more common in the Afro-Caribbean, Hispanic and Asian population (35–60%). It usually presents as a flat, irregular macule in later life. 25% are amelanotic and may mimic a fungal infection or pyogenic granuloma.

MM under the finger nail are usually SSM rather than ALM. For finger or toe nail lesions it is vital to biopsy the nail matrix, rather than just the pigment on the nail plate. A classical feature of a subungual melanoma is Hutchinson's sign: nail fold pigmentation that widens progressively to produce a triangular pigmented macule with associated nail dystrophy. The differential diagnosis is 'benign racial melanonychia', which produces a linear dark streak under a nail in a dark-skinned individual. Malignancy is unlikely if the nail fold is uninvolved (Figure 40.40).

Miscellaneous

- Amelanotic melanoma may present as a flesh-coloured, skin lesion; as a metastasis from an unknown skin primary; or, in the gastrointestinal tract, with obstruction or intussusception.
- Desmoplastic melanoma is mostly found on the head and neck region. It has a propensity for perineural infiltration and often recurs locally if not widely excised. It may be amelanotic clinically.

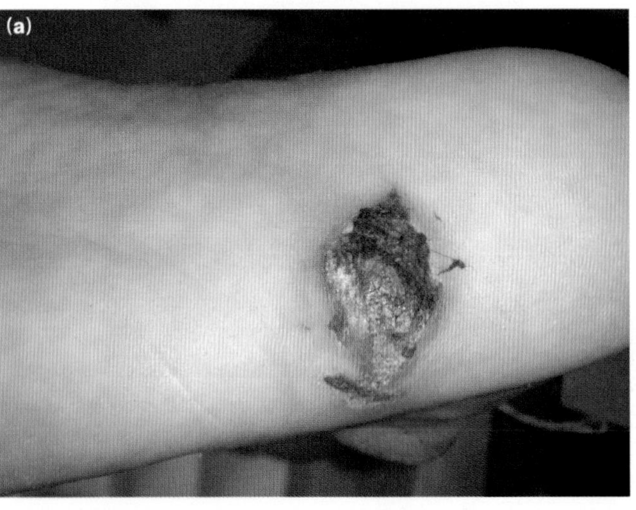

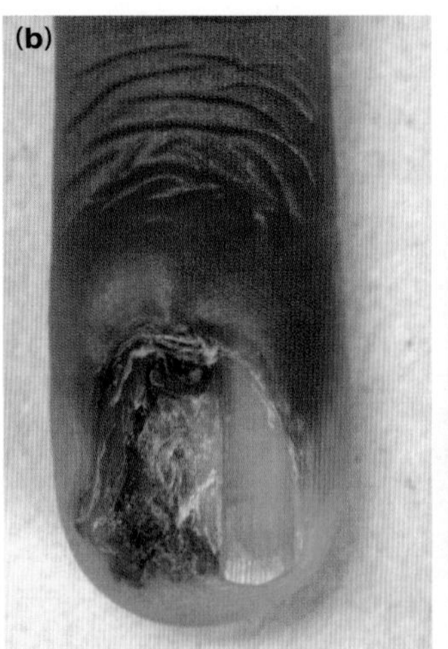

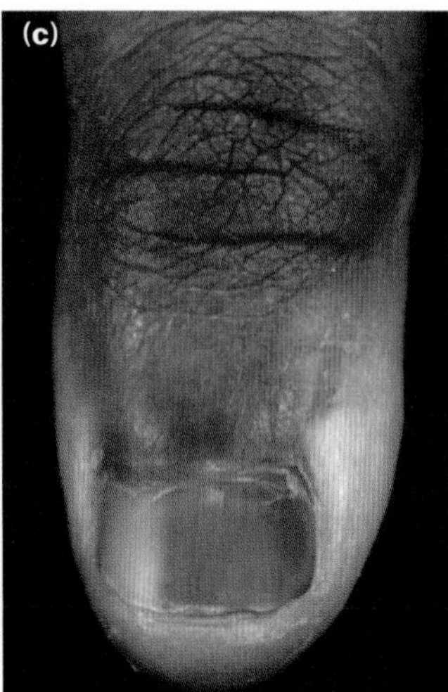

Figure 40.40 **(a)** Acral lentiginous melanoma on the sole of the foot (courtesy of Mr AR Greenbaum). **(b)** Subungual melanoma – probably a superficial spreading melanoma. Note the swelling proximal to the nail fold. **(c)** Benign racial melanonychia. ((**b**) and (**c**) courtesy of St John's Institute for Dermatology, London, UK.)

MICROSCOPIC

Malignant change occurs in the melanocytes in the basal epidermis, while *in situ*, atypical melanocytes are limited to the dermo-epidermal junction and show no evidence of dermal involvement. During the horizontal growth phase, cells spread along the dermo-epidermal junction and although they may breach the dermis, their migration is predominantly radial. During the vertical growth phase, the dermis maybe invaded. The greater the depth of invasion, the greater is the metastatic potential of the tumour.

MANAGEMENT

History and clinical examination should be directed at discovering the primary lesion and identification of local, regional or distant spread.

An excision biopsy with 2–3 mm margin of skin and a cuff of subdermal fat is acceptable. Incision biopsy is occasionally indicated: for instance, in large lesions on the face where an excision biopsy of the whole lesion would be disfiguring.

In experienced hands, observation and review every 2 months may avoid biopsies in equivocal cases, but serial clinical and dermoscopic photography by a clinician with expertise in dermoscopy is mandatory when observation is chosen, rather than excision biopsy, for definitive histopathological diagnosis.

Biopsy and pathological examination provide the first step towards staging melanoma. The Breslow thickness of a melanoma (measured to nearest 0.1 mm from granular layer to base of tumour) is the most important prognostic indicator in the absence of lymph node metastases. The American Joint Committee on Cancer (AJCC) staging system then takes lymph node and distant metastases into account (*Table 40.2*).

INVESTIGATIONS

Guidelines for staging are controversial. The authors suggest investigations should be directed towards detecting occult disease, so as to upstage patients and treat them accurately and appropriately, the only cure for MM currently being appropriate surgery. Thus, offering sentinel node biopsy to patients with T2a disease and greater is prudent and investigations for T3a disease and greater should be directed to individual clinical presentation.

LOCAL TREATMENT

The treatment for melanoma is surgery. Lentigo maligna (melanoma *in situ*) should be excised completely in most clinical situations because of the risk of it entering the vertical growth phase to become LMM. A complete excision requires no further treatment.

For *in situ* melanoma a wide excision of 5 mm is sufficient; for melanoma <1 mm deep, a 1 cm margin is sufficient; and for deeper lesions, a 2 cm only margin is recommended, as there is no evidence that wider margins make a difference.

TABLE 40.2 AJCC 2009 melanoma staging.

Primary tumour		Regional nodes		Distant metastases
Tx Primary tumour cannot be assessed (has been curettage or severely regressed)		NX Patients in whom nodes cannot be assessed (e.g. previous excision)		
T0 No evidence of primary tumour		N0 No node involvement		M0 No detected distant metastases
Tis melanoma in situ				
T1 ≤1.0 mm	a: no ulceration or mitoses b: with ulceration, or >1 mitosis/mm2	N1 1 node	a: micrometastasis b: macrometastasis	M1a Skin, subcutaneous, or distant lymph node metastases (normal serum LDH levels)
T2 1.01–2.0 mm	a: no ulceration b: with ulceration	N2 2–3 nodes	a: micrometastasis b: macrometastasis c: in transit mets/ satellite(s), without metastatic node(s)	M1b Lung metastases (normal serum LDH levels)
T3 2.01–3.0 mm	a: no ulceration b: with ulceration	N3	≥4 nodes, or matted nodes, or in transit mets/ satellite(s), with metastatic node(s)	M1c All other visceral metastases or any distant metastases with elevated serum LDH levels
T4 >4 mm	a: no ulceration b: with ulceration			
Clinical staging of melanoma				
Stage 0: Tis, N0, M0 Stage Ia: T1a, N0, M0 Stage Ib: T1b or T2a, N0, M0		Stage IIa: T2b or T3a, N0, M0 Stage IIb: T3b or T4a, N0, M0 Stage IIc: T4b, N0, M0		Stage III: any T, ≥ N1, M0 Stage IV: any T, Any N1, M1

LDH, lactate dehydrogenase.

Alexander Breslow, 1928–1980, American pathologist. George Washington University, Washington DC, USA, first reported in 1970 that the prognosis depends upon the thickness of the tumour.

REGIONAL LYMPH NODES

The likelihood of metastatic spread to regional lymph nodes is proportional to the Breslow thickness of the melanoma. Management of regional lymph nodes has been a contentious topic for well over a century. Some advocated simultaneous elective lymph node clearance at the time of wide excision of the primary melanoma. Others favoured a therapeutic lymphadenectomy if regional metastases became clinically evident. Evidence from retrospective studies demonstrate that patients with thick melanomas had better survival after elective lymphadenectomy, while data from prospective randomized studies were less convincing, except in specific subgroups. Ideally, one would like to be able to select for treatment those patients with the highest risk of metastatic spread. Sentinel node biopsy (SNB), an investigation based on the fact that lymphatic metastases proceed in an orderly fashion and can be predicted by mapping the lymphatic drainage from a primary tumor to the first or 'sentinel' node in the regional lymphatic basin, offered that potential; but extensive studies show no survival benefit, so SNB in melanoma is currently a staging investigation for patients with tumours of Breslow thickness >1 mm.

ADJUVANT THERAPY

Since the last edition of this book, great advances have occurred in treatment for unresectable and metastatic MM.

When mutation locks B-RAF protein signalling to 'on', it affects the mitogen-activated protein kinase (MAPK) cellular pathway, promoting initiation, malignant transformation, tumour progression and metastasis in the 50% of MM with B-RAF V600 mutations. Targeted therapy in stage IV melanoma using dabrafenib or vemurafenib, which block B-RAF action has shown promising results with metastatic melanoma. Trametinib has a different action on the MAPK pathway: stopping cell growth and promoting apoptosis. Combined use with dabrafenib to counter acquired tumour resistance via MAPK pathway reactivation, shows promising results in stage 4 disease. Also, selective immune checkpoint inhibitors ipilimumab or nivolimumab demonstrate benefit in metastatic or unresectable melanoma.

PROGNOSIS

The Breslow thickness of the primary tumour offers the best correlation with survival in stage I disease. The higher the mitotic index, the poorer is the prognosis of the primary tumour. This has greater significance than the presence or absence of ulceration.

The presence of lymph node metastases is the single most important prognostic index in melanoma, outweighing both tumour and host factors. The number of affected nodes and the presence of extranodal extension are also significant outcome predictors. Once regional nodes are clinically involved, 70–85% of patients will have occult distant metastases.

Merkel cell (dermal mechanoreceptor) tumour

This is an aggressive malignant tumour of Merkel cells and usually affects the elderly. It is four times more common in women than men (**Figure 40.41**). Treatment is with wide local excision aiming for a 25–30 mm margin, followed by radiotherapy.

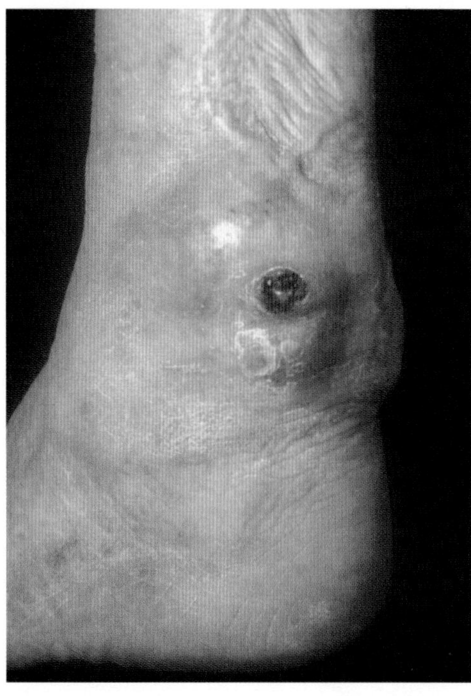

Figure 40.41 Merkel cell tumour (courtesy of St John's Institute for Dermatology, London, UK).

VASCULAR LESIONS

Congenital: haemangiomata and vascular malformations

These can be subclassified *biologically* into vascular tumours or vascular malformations based on their endothelial characteristics, or *radiologically* into haemangiomata, vascular and lymphatic malformations based on their vascular dynamics.

Haemangiomata

These are benign endothelial tumours that affect three girls for every boy. 30% have a herald patch at birth, which then grows rapidly in the first year of life and slowly involutes over several years, with 70% having resolved by 7 years of age. Large hamangiomata can trap platelets leading to thrombocytopenia (Kasabach–Merritt syndrome).

Friedrich Sigmud Merkel, 1845–1919, Professor of Anatomy successively at Rostock, Koningsberg (now Kaliningrad in Russia) and Göttingen, Germany.
Haig H Kasabach, 1898–1943, radiologist, the Presbyterian Hospital, New York, NY, USA.
Katharine K Merritt, b.1886, American paediatrician, Department of Paediatrics, the Babies Hospital, Columbia University College of Physicians and Surgeons, New York, NY, USA. Kasabach and Merritt described the condition as a joint paper in 1940.

Vascular malformations

Vascular malformations affect boys and girls equally and are associated with numerous syndromes. They are invariably present at birth, but may be missed if deep to the skin. Vascular malformations subsequently grow in proportion to the child's growth (other than in response to sepsis or hormonal stimulation). Stasis can lead to a localised, consumptive coagulopathy in large venous malformations. Low-flow malformations may cause skeletal hypoplasia, while high-flow malformations can cause hypertrophy.

Common vascular birthmarks

Salmon patch

A salmon patch is a haemangioma that presents as a pinkish macule, usually at the nape of neck (Figure 40.42). It is caused by an area of persistent fetal dermal circulation, which usually disappears at 1 year.

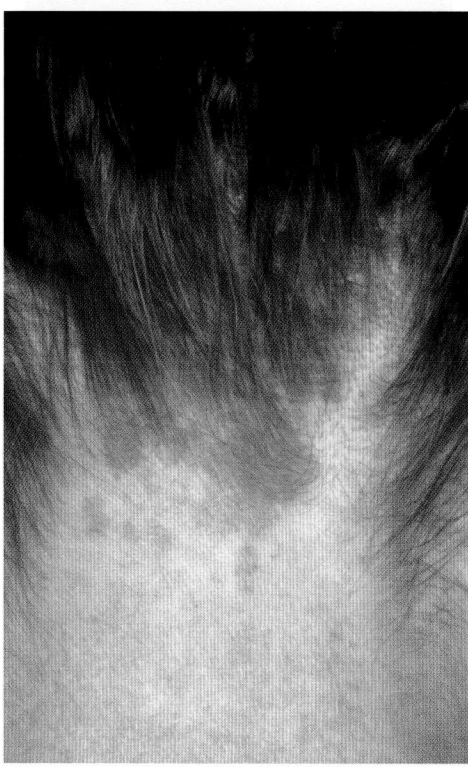

Figure 40.42 Salmon patch (courtesy of St John's Institute for Dermatology, London, UK).

Capillary haemangioma (strawberry naevus)

This is the commonest 'birth mark', occurring most commonly on the head and neck (Figure 40.43). 90% appear at birth, and, as a consequence of intravascular thrombosis, fibrosis and mast cell infiltration, 10% resolve each subsequent year, with 70% resolved by 7 years old.

Whites skin is affected most commonly and girls are affected three times more than boys.

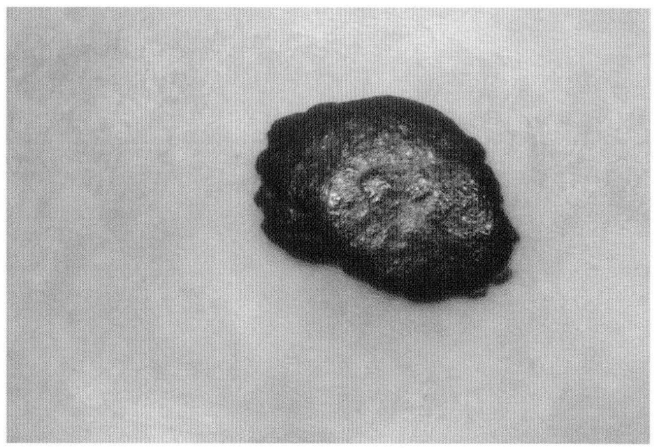

Figure 40.43 Capillary haemangioma (courtesy of St John's Institute for Dermatology, London, UK).

Capillary vascular malformations 'port-wine' stains

Capillary vascular malformations ('port-wine stains' (PWS)) are 20 times less common than capillary haemangiomata and result from defective maturation of cutaneous sympathetic innervation during embryogenesis, leading to localised intradermal capillary vasodilatation (Figure 40.44). They appear at birth as flat, smooth, intensely purple-stained areas, most frequently on the head and neck, often within the maxillary and mandibular dermatomes of the trigeminal nerve.

Treatment with intense pulsed light and pulse dye laser are successful. PWS may be associated with various syndromes.

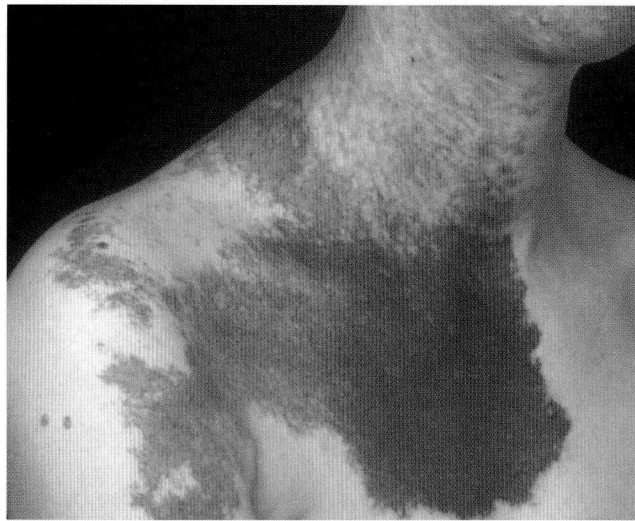

Figure 40.44 'Port-wine' stain (courtesy of St John's Institute for Dermatology, London, UK).

Acquired

Campbell de Morgan spots

These are arteriovenous fistulae at the dermal capillary level in sun-exposed skin of older patients (Figure 40.45).

Campbell Greig de Morgan, 1811–1876, surgeon, the Middlesex Hospital, London UK.

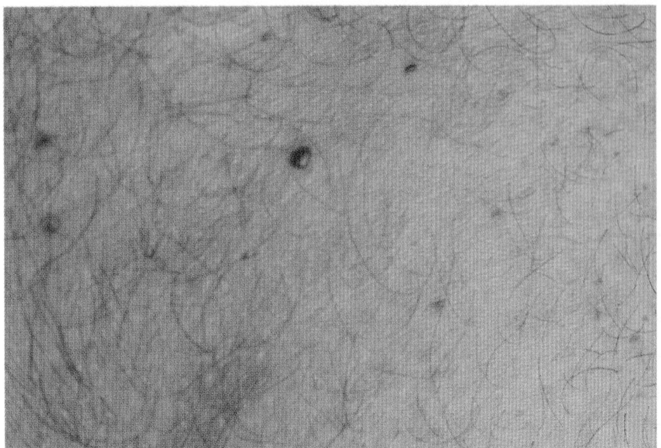

Figure 40.45 Campbell de Morgan spot (courtesy of Mr AR Greenbaum).

Spider naevi

These are angiomata that appear (and may disappear) spontaneously at puberty or in two-thirds of pregnant women, usually disappearing in the puerperium (Figure 40.46). Spider naevi are also associated with chronic liver disease. They can be treated with intense pulsed light or pulse dye laser.

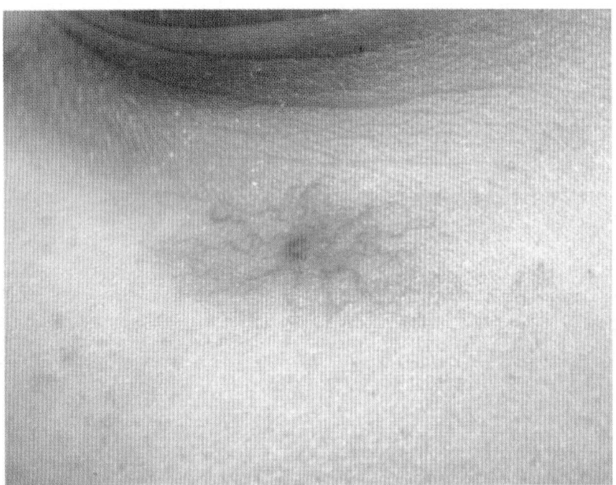

Figure 40.46 Spider naevus (courtesy of St John's Institute for Dermatology, London, UK).

Pyogenic granuloma

These share many histological characteristics of haemangiomas and are probably a subtype thereof (Figure 40.47). Most are small (0.5–1.5 cm), raised, pedunculated, soft red nodular lesions showing superficial ulceration and a tendency to bleed after trivial trauma. They should be excised with a minimal margin.

Glomus tumour

These arise from a subcutaneous arteriovenous shunt (Sucquet–Hoyer canals), especially in the corium of the nail bed. Typically, it is a small, purple nodule measuring a few millimetres in size, which is disproportionately painful in response to insignificant stimuli, including cold exposure (Figure 40.48). Subungual varieties may be invisible causes of paroxysmal digital pain.

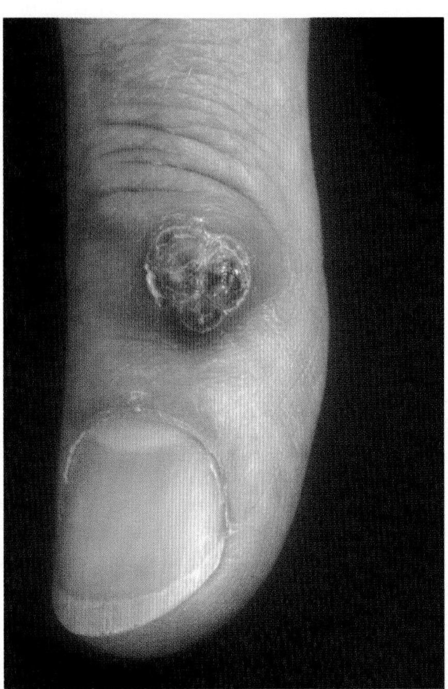

Figure 40.47 Pyogenic granuloma (courtesy of St John's Institute for Dermatology, London, UK).

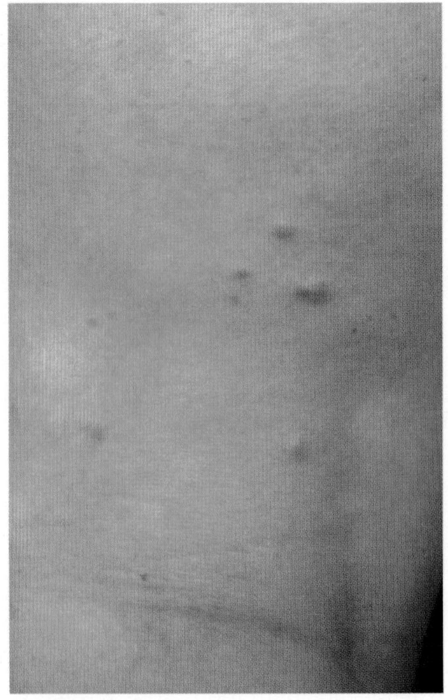

Figure 40.48 Glomus tumour (courtesy of St John's Institute for Dermatology, London, UK).

JP Sucquet, 1840–1870, anatomist, Paris, France.
Heinrich Hoyer, 1834–1907, Professor of Histology, Embryology and Anatomy, the Central Medical School, The Polish University, Warsaw, Poland.

Angiosarcoma ('malignant angioendothelioma')

A rare, highly malignant tumour arising from the endothelial cells (Figure 40.49). The lymphangiosarcoma variant arises from lymphatic endothelium and can develop in lymphoedematous tissue, particularly an extremity. Proliferation is rapid with early systemic spread.

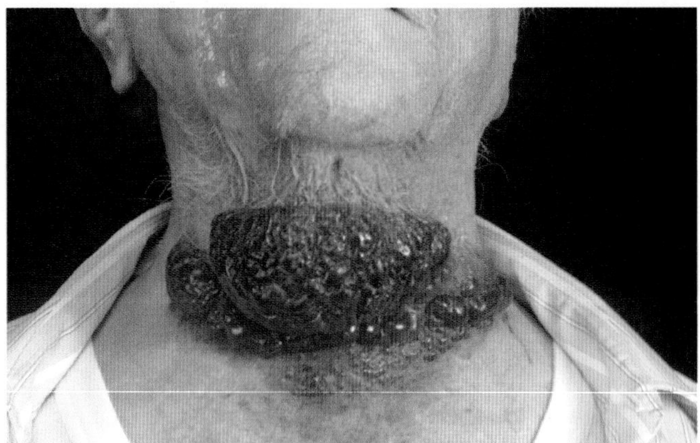

Figure 40.49 Angiosarcoma (courtesy of St John's Institute for Dermatology, London, UK).

Kaposi's sarcoma

Kaposi's sarcoma is a malignant, proliferative tumour of vascular endothelial cells, which was first described in elderly Jewish men but is now most commonly associated with immune compromise after transplantation or HIV infection (Figure 40.50). There appears to be a causal link with infection by human herpes virus 8. Kaposi's sarcoma usually starts as a red brown, indurated, plaque-like, skin lesion that becomes nodular and then ulcerates. Treatment is with radiotherapy.

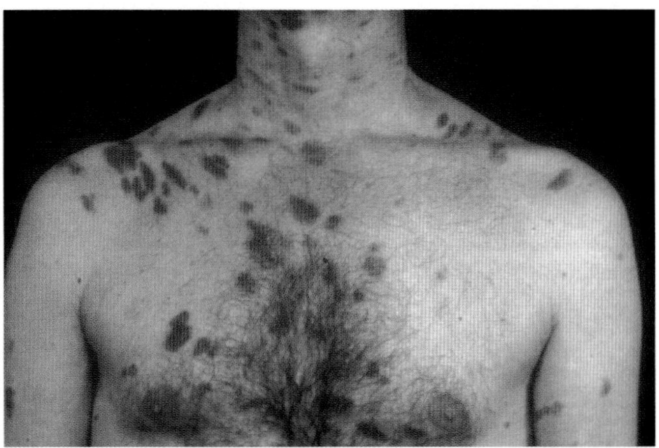

Figure 40.50 Kaposi's sarcoma (courtesy of St John's Institute for Dermatology, London, UK).

WOUNDS

Congenital

Cutis aplasia congenita

This is a rare condition characterised by the congenital absence of epidermis, dermis and, in some cases, subcutaneous tissues, with underlying bony defects in 20%. Treatment depends on the severity of the presentation, but usually involves plastic surgery.

Parry-Romberg disease

Parry–Romberg disease is an uncommon and poorly understood progressive, hemifacial atrophy of skin, soft tissue and bone. Its incidence is unknown and its inheritance uncertain, but it affects women more commonly than men.

The disease commonly starts in a patient's late 20s, but can present in childhood, when the resulting deformity is worse because it is magnified by differential growth elsewhere. The condition is self-limiting, usually by 5–10 years after onset. Once stable, plastic surgical techniques can be employed alone or in combination to reconstruct an aesthetic contour.

Spina bifida

Failure of closure of the caudal neuropore during the 4th week *in utero* results in incomplete development of some or all of the structural elements posterior to the spinal cord. This can occur anywhere, but is commonest in lumbar vertebrae and presents as gross variants: spina bifida occulta, in which there is a bony defect without neural protrusion and spina bifida cystica, in which there is herniation of the meninges (meningocoele), spinal cord (myelocoele) or, most commonly, both (menigomyelocoele) and is therefore asymptomatic. Management ideally involves a multidisciplinary approach and is directed towards protecting the spinal cord, preventing cerebrospinal fluid contamination and secondary hydrocephalus and meningitis.

Acquired

Pressure sores

These begin with tissue necrosis at a pressure point and develop into a cone-shaped volume of necrotic loss. As many as 10% of acute hospital in-patients will suffer some degree of pressure sore. The majority affect the elderly and patients with spinal injury or decreased sensibility; 80% of paraplegics will get a pressure sore and 8% die as a result.

The pathogenesis of pressure sores revolves around unrelieved pressure: an increase in local tissue pressure above that of perfusion pressure produces ischaemic necrosis that is directly proportional to the duration and degree of pressure and inversely proportional to the area over which it is applied. Muscle and fat are more susceptible to pressure than skin.

Moricz K Kaposi, 1837–1902, Austrian dermatologist, described xeroderma pigmentosum in 1874. He also described a rare cutaneous sarcoma in Ashkenazi Jews, now more often an AIDS-defining condition.
Caleb Hillier Parry, 1755–1822, physician, The General Hospital, Bath, UK.
Moritiz Heinrich Romberg, 1795–1873, German neurologist, Director of the University Hospital, Berlin, Germany.

In a patient who has no predisposing factors management is aimed at debridement and repair of the defect, on the assumption that recurrence will not occur once normal function and sensibility returns. In the paraplegic patient recurrence is likely, so management should involve a multidisciplinary approach. Primary treatment involves relieving pressure (special mattress; nursing care; relief of muscle spasm and contractures); optimising nutrition; correcting anaemia; and preventing infection and dressings. Surgery involves thorough debridement to promote healing and plastic surgery to reconstruct the defect.

Ulcers

An ulcer is a discontinuity of an epithelial surface. It is characterised by destruction of the surface epithelium and a granulating base. Ulcers can be classified as non-specific, specific and malignant (Figure 40.51).

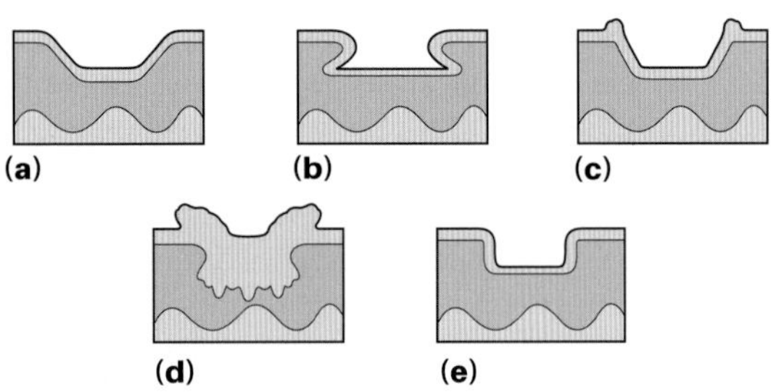

Figure 40.51 Some characteristic shapes of the edges of ulcers. (**a**) Non-specific ulcer: note the shelving edge. (**b**) Tuberculous ulcer: note the undermined edge. (**c**) Basal cell carcinoma (rodent ulcer): note the rolled edge, which may exhibit small blood vessels. (**d**) Epithelioma: note the heaped-up, everted edge and irregular thickened base. (**e**) Syphilis: note the punched-out edge and thin base, which may be covered with a 'wash-leather' slough.

Sinus

A sinus is a blind-ending tract connecting a cavity lined with granulation tissue (often an abscess cavity) to an epithelial surface (Figure 40.52a). Sinuses may be congenital or acquired. Congenital sinuses arise from the remnants of persistent embryonic ducts. Acquired sinuses can result from: a retained foreign body (ingrown hair or suture material); chronic infection (tuberculosis, osteomyelitis or actinomycosis); chronic inflammation (Crohn's disease); malignancy; or inadequate surgical drainage of the cavity.

Treatment of a sinus is directed at removing the underlying cause. Biopsies should always be taken from the wall of a sinus to exclude malignancy or specific infection. For specific management of the disease conditions, please refer to the appropriate chapter.

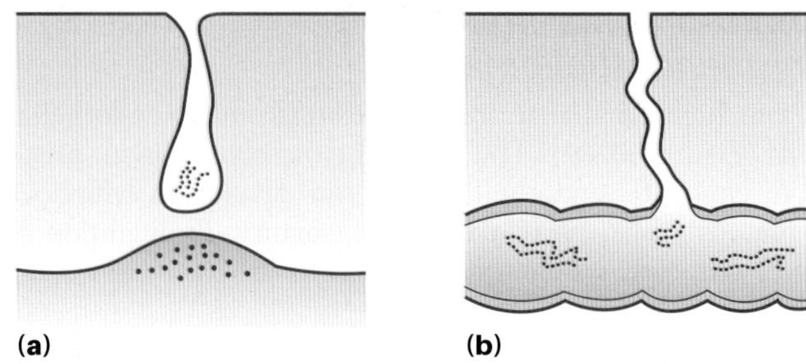

Figure 40.52 A sinus (**a**) and a fistula (**b**); both usually arises from a preceding abscess. (**a**) This is a blind track, in this case a pilondial abscess. (**b**) This is a track connecting two epithelium-lined surfaces, in this case a colocutaneous fistula from colon to skin.

Fistula

A fistula is an abnormal communication between two epithelial-lined surfaces (Figure 40.52b). This communication or tract may be lined by granulation tissue, but may become epithelialised in chronic cases. Fistulas may be congenital (for example, tracheo-oesophageal and branchial fistulas) or acquired (for example, enterocutaneous complicating Crohn's disease or surgery, or arteriovenous). Management of a fistula is directed at the underlying aetiology (see the appropriate chapters).

FURTHER READING

Balch CM, Gershenwald,JE, Soong SJ *et al*. Final version of the American Joint Committee on Cancer staging system for cutaneous melanoma. *J Clin Oncol* 2009; **27**(36): 6199–206.

Calonje JE, Brenn T, Lazar A, McKee PH. *Pathology of the skin*, 4th edn. Elsevier, 2011.

Patterson J. *Weedon's skin pathology*, 4th edn. Elsevier, 2015.

Soyer HP, Argenziano G, Hoffmann-Wellenhof R, Zalaudek I. *Dermoscopy: the essentials*, 2nd edn. Elsevier, 2011.

WEBSITE ADDRESSES

The American Joint Committee on Cancer: https://cancerstaging.org

Dermnet New Zealand – a reliable online educational resource run by a community of dermatologists and other health specialists: https://www.dermnetnz.org/

International Dermoscopy Society. Free to join, this society is run by dermatologists to promote clinical research and education in dermoscopy: https://dermoscopy-ids.org/

Chapter 41

Burns

Learning objectives

To assess:

- The area and depth of burns

To understand:

- Methods for calculating the rate and quantity of fluids to be given
- Techniques for treating burns and the patient
- The pathophysiology of electrical and chemical burns

INTRODUCTION

The incidence of burn injury varies greatly between cultures. In the United Kingdom (with its population of 65 million), each year around 175 000 people visit accident and emergency (A&E) departments suffering from burns, of whom about 13 000 need to be admitted. About 1000 have severe burns requiring fluid resuscitation, and half of the victims are under 16 years of age.

The majority of burns in children are scalds caused by accidents with kettles, pans, hot drinks and bath water. Among adolescent patients, the burns are usually caused by young males experimenting with matches and flammable liquids. In adults, scalds are not uncommon, but are less frequent than flame burns. Most electrical and chemical injuries occur in adults. Cold and radiation are very rare causes of burns. Associated conditions in adults, such as mental disease (attempted suicide or assault), epilepsy and alcohol or drug abuse, are underlying factors in as many as 80% of patients with burns admitted to hospital in some populations.

Legislation, health promotion and appliance design have reduced the incidence of burns, with regulations regarding flame-retardant clothes and furniture, the promotion of smoke alarms, the design of cookers and gas fires, the almost universal use of cordless kettles and the education of parents to keep their hot water thermostat to 60°C all playing their part.

The last 50 years have seen great strides made to reduce both morbidity and mortality from burn injuries. The coming years will see a better understanding of the control of physiology along with improvements in reconstruction and rehabilitation.

A large burn injury will have a significant effect on the patient's family and friends and the patient's future. The importance of multidisciplinary care needs to be stressed for the adequate and effective care of the burn patient.

Summary box 41.1

Prevention of burns

A significant proportion of burns can be prevented by:

- Implementing good health and safety regulations
- Educating the public
- Introducing of effective legislation

THE PATHOPHYSIOLOGY OF BURN INJURY

Burns cause damage in a number of different ways, but by far the most common organ affected is the skin. However, burns can also damage the airway and lungs, with life-threatening consequences. Airway injuries occur when the face and neck are burned. Respiratory system injuries usually occur if a person is trapped in a burning vehicle, house, car or aeroplane and is forced to inhale the hot and poisonous gases.

Summary box 41.2

Warning signs of burns to the respiratory system

- Burns around the face and neck
- A history of being trapped in a burning room
- Change in voice
- Stridor

INJURY TO THE AIRWAY AND LUNGS

Physical burn injury to the airway above the larynx

The hot gases can physically burn the nose, mouth, tongue, palate and larynx. Once burned, the linings of these structures will start to swell. After a few hours, they may start to interfere with the larynx and may completely block the airway if action is not taken to secure an airway.

Summary box 41.3

Dangers of smoke, hot gas or steam inhalation

- Inhaled hot gases can cause supraglottic airway burns and laryngeal oedema
- Inhaled steam can cause subglottic burns and loss of respiratory epithelium
- Inhaled smoke particles can cause chemical alveolitis and respiratory failure
- Inhaled poisons, such as carbon monoxide, can cause metabolic poisoning
- Full-thickness burns to the chest can cause mechanical blockage to rib movement

Physical burn injury to the airway below the larynx

This is a rare injury as the heat exchange mechanisms in the supraglottic airway are usually able safely to absorb the heat from hot air. However, steam has a large latent heat of evaporation and can cause thermal damage to the lower airway. In such injuries, the respiratory epithelium rapidly swells and detaches from the bronchial tree. This creates casts, which can block the main upper airway.

Metabolic poisoning

There are many poisonous gases that can be given off in a fire, the most common being carbon monoxide, a product of incomplete combustion that is often produced by fires in enclosed spaces. This is the usual cause of a person being found with altered consciousness at the scene of a fire. Carbon monoxide binds to haemoglobin with an affinity 240 times greater than that of oxygen and therefore blocks the transport of oxygen. Levels of carboxyhaemoglobin in the bloodstream can be measured. Concentrations above 10% are dangerous and need treatment with pure oxygen for more than 24 hours. Death occurs with concentrations around 60%.

Another metabolic toxin produced in house fires is hydrogen cyanide, which causes a metabolic acidosis by interfering with mitochondrial respiration.

Inhalational injury

Inhalational injury is caused by the minute particles within thick smoke, which, because of their small size, are not filtered by the upper airway, but are carried down to the lung parenchyma. They stick to the moist lining, causing an intense reaction in the alveoli. This chemical pneumonitis causes oedema within the alveolar sacs and decreasing gaseous exchange over the ensuing 24 hours (**Figure 41.1**), and often gives rise to a bacterial pneumonia. Its presence or absence has a very significant effect on the mortality of any burn patient.

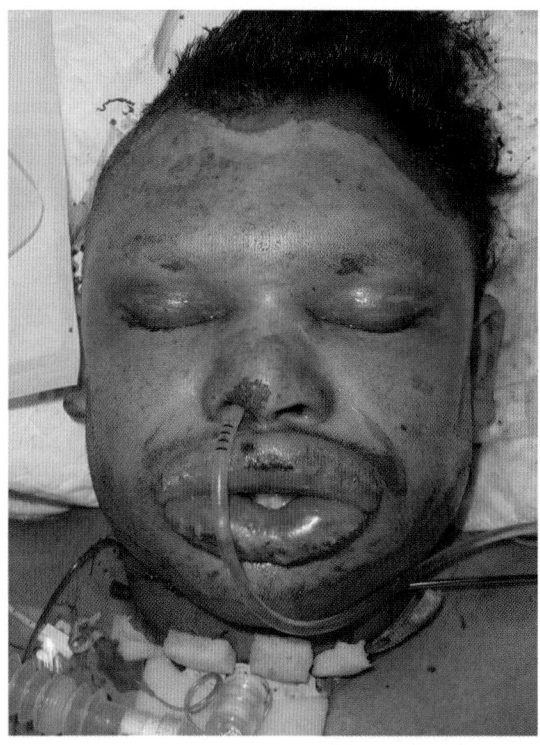

Figure 41.1 The swelling that occurs with inflammation due to burns.

Mechanical block on rib movement

Burned skin is very thick and stiff, and this can physically stop the ribs moving if there is a large full-thickness burn across the chest.

INFLAMMATION AND CIRCULATORY CHANGES

The dangers to the airway and respiration described above are readily apparent, but the cause of circulatory changes following a burn are more complex. The changes occur because burned skin activates a web of inflammatory cascades. The release of neuropeptides and the activation of complement are initiated by the stimulation of pain fibres and the alteration of proteins by heat. The activation of Hageman factor

John Hageman was a 37-year-old railroad brakeman in whom this factor deficiency was discovered by Dr Oscar Ratnoff in 1955.

initiates a number of protease-driven cascades, altering the arachidonic acid, thrombin and kallikrein pathways.

At a cellular level, complement causes the degranulation of mast cells and coats the proteins altered by the burn. This attracts neutrophils, which also degranulate, with the release of large quantities of free radicals and proteases. These can, in turn, cause further damage to the tissue. Mast cells also release primary cytokines such as tumour necrosis factor alpha (TNF-α). These act as chemotactic agents to inflammatory cells and cause the subsequent release of many secondary cytokines. These inflammatory factors alter the permeability of blood vessels such that intravascular fluid escapes. The increase in permeability is such that large protein molecules can also now escape with ease. The damaged collagen and these extravasated proteins increase the oncotic pressure within the burned tissue, further increasing the flow of water from the intravascular to the extravascular space (Figure 41.2).

The overall effect of these changes is to produce a net flow of water, solutes and proteins from the intravascular to the extravascular space. This flow occurs over the first 36 hours after the injury, but does not include red blood cells. In a small burn, this reaction is small and localised but, as the burn size approaches 10–15% of total body surface area (TBSA), the loss of intravascular fluid can cause a level of circulatory shock. Furthermore, once the area increases to 25% of TBSA, the inflammatory reaction causes fluid loss in vessels remote from the burn injury. This is why such importance is attached to measuring the TBSA involved in any burn. It dictates the size of inflammatory reaction and therefore the amount of fluid needed to control shock.

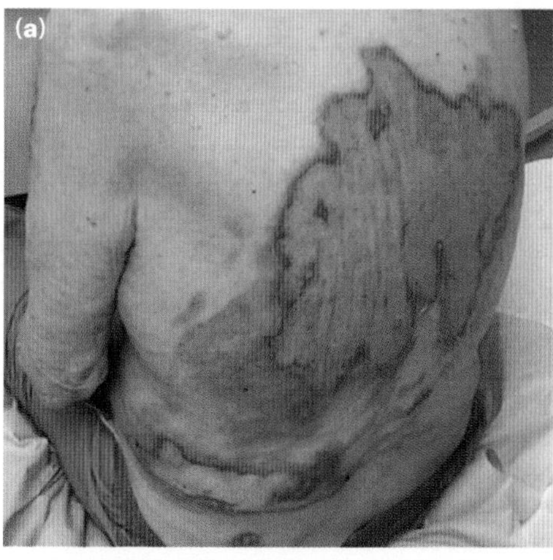

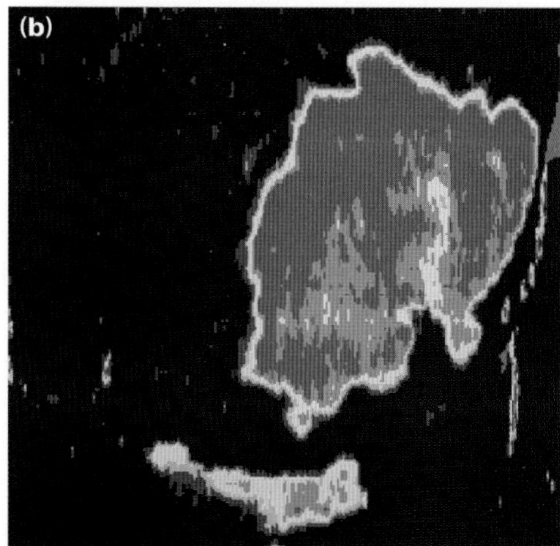

Figure 41.2 A scald burn (**a**) and its laser doppler image (**b**) showing burn depth. Red and pink areas are superficial burns, which should heal with conservative dressings.

Summary box 41.4

The shock reaction after burns

- Burns produce an inflammatory reaction
- This leads to vastly increased vascular permeability
- Water, solutes and proteins move from the intra- to the extravascular space
- The volume of fluid lost is directly proportional to the area of the burn
- Above 15% of surface area, the loss of fluid produces shock

OTHER LIFE-THREATENING EVENTS WITH MAJOR BURNS

The immune system and infection

The inflammatory changes caused by the burn have an effect on the patient's immune system. Cell-mediated immunity is significantly reduced in large burns, leaving them more susceptible to bacterial and fungal infections. There are many potential sources of infection, especially from the burn wound and from the lung if this is injured, but also from any central venous lines, tracheostomies or urinary catheters present.

Changes to the intestine

The inflammatory stimulus and shock can cause microvascular damage and ischaemia to the gut mucosa. This reduces gut motility and can prevent the absorption of food. Failure of enteral feeding in a patient with a large burn is a life-threatening complication. This process also increases the translocation of gut bacteria, which can become an important source of infection in large burns. Gut mucosal swelling, gastric stasis and peritoneal oedema can also cause abdominal compartment syndrome, which splints the diaphragm and increases the airway pressures needed for respiration.

Danger to peripheral circulation

In full-thickness burns, the collagen fibres are coagulated. The normal elasticity of the skin is lost. A circumferential full-thickness burn to a limb acts as a tourniquet as the limb swells. If untreated, this will progress to limb-threatening ischaemia.

Summary box 41.5

Other complications of burns
- Infection from the burn site, lungs, gut, lines and catheters
- Malabsorption from the gut
- Circumferential burns may compromise circulation to a limb

Summary box 41.6

Major determinants of the outcome of a burn
- Percentage surface area involved
- Depth of burns
- Presence of an inhalational injury

IMMEDIATE CARE OF THE BURN PATIENT

Prehospital care

The principles of prehospital care are:

- **Ensure rescuer safety**. This is particularly important in house fires and in the case of electrical and chemical injuries.
- **Stop the burning process**. Stop, drop and roll is a good method of extinguishing fire burning on a person.
- **Check for other injuries**. A standard ABC (airway, breathing, circulation) check followed by a rapid secondary survey will ensure that no other significant injuries are missed. Patients burned in explosions or even escaping from fires may have head or spine injuries and other life-threatening problems.
- **Cool the burn wound**. This provides analgesia and slows the delayed microvascular damage that can occur after a burn injury. Cooling should occur for a minimum of 10 minutes and is effective up to 1 hour after the burn injury. It is a particularly important first aid step in partial-thickness burns, especially scalds. In temperate climates, cooling should be at about 15°C, and hypothermia must be avoided.
- **Give oxygen**. Anyone involved in a fire in an enclosed space should receive oxygen, especially if there is an altered consciousness level.
- **Elevate**. Sitting a patient up with a burned airway may prove life-saving in the event of a delay in transfer to hospital care. Elevation of burned limbs will reduce swelling and discomfort.

Hospital care

The principles of managing an acute burn injury are the same as in any acute trauma case:

- A, Airway control.
- B, Breathing and ventilation.
- C, Circulation.
- D, Disability – neurological status.
- E, Exposure with environmental control.
- F, Fluid resuscitation.

The possibility of injury additional to the burn must be sought both clinically and from the history, and treated appropriately. The major determinants of severity of any burn injury are the percentage of TBSA that is burned, the presence of an inhalation injury and the depth of the burn.

Not all burned patients will need to be admitted to a burns unit, but the main criteria are given in *Table 41.1*.

TABLE 41.1 The criteria for acute admission to a burns unit.
Suspected airway or inhalational injury
Any burn likely to require fluid resuscitation
Any burn likely to require surgery
Patients with burns of any significance to the hands, face, feet or perineum
Patients whose psychiatric or social background makes it inadvisable to send them home
Any suspicion of non-accidental injury
Any burn in a patient at the extremes of age
Any burn with associated potentially serious sequelae, including high-tension electrical burns and concentrated hydrofluoric acid burns

Airway

The burned airway creates problems for the patient by swelling and, if not managed proactively, can completely occlude the upper airway. The treatment is to secure the airway with an endotracheal tube until the swelling has subsided, which is usually after about 48 hours. The symptoms of laryngeal oedema, such as change in voice, stridor, anxiety and respiratory difficulty, are very late symptoms. Intubation at this point is often difficult or impossible owing to swelling, so acute cricothyroidotomy equipment must be at hand when intubating patients with a delayed diagnosis of airway burn. Because of this, early intubation of suspected airway burn is the treatment of choice in such patients. The time-frame from burn to airway occlusion is usually between 4 and 24 hours, so there is time to make a sensible decision with senior staff and allow an experienced anaesthetist to intubate the patient.

Summary box 41.7

Initial management of the burned airway
- Early elective intubation is safest
- Delay can make intubation very difficult because of swelling
- Be ready to perform an emergency cricothyroidotomy, if intubation is delayed

The key in the management of airway burn is the history and early signs, rather than the symptoms. The history is of inhalation of hot gases such as in a house or car fire. Clues on examination include blisters on the hard palate, burned nasal mucosa and loss of all the hair in the nose (the anterior hairs are often burned), but perhaps the most valuable signs are the presence of deep burns around the mouth and in the neck.

Summary box 41.8

Recognition of the potentially burned airway

- A history of being trapped in the presence of smoke or hot gases
- Burns on the palate or nasal mucosa, or loss of all the hairs in the nose
- Deep burns around the mouth and neck

Breathing

Inhalational injury

Time is also a factor; anyone trapped in a fire for more than a couple of minutes must be observed for signs of smoke inhalation. Other signs that raise suspicion are the presence of soot in the nose and the oropharynx and a chest radiograph showing patchy consolidation.

The clinical features are a progressive increase in respiratory effort and rate, rising pulse, anxiety and confusion and decreasing oxygen saturation. These symptoms may not be apparent immediately and can take 24 hours to 5 days to develop.

Treatment starts as soon as this injury is suspected and the airway is secure. Physiotherapy, nebulisers and warm humidified oxygen are all useful. The patient's progress should be monitored using respiratory rate, together with blood gas measurements. If the situation deteriorates, continuous or intermittent positive pressure may be used with a mask or T-piece. In the severest cases, intubation and management in an intensive care unit will be needed.

The key, therefore, in the management of inhalational injury is to suspect it from the history, institute early management and observe carefully for deterioration.

Thermal burn injury to the lower airway

These rare injuries can occur with steam injuries. Their management is supportive and the same as that for an inhalational injury.

Metabolic poisoning

Any history of a fire within an enclosed space and any history of altered consciousness are important clues to metabolic poisoning. Blood gases must be measured immediately if poisoning is a possibility. Carboxyhaemoglobin levels raised above 10% must be treated with high inspired oxygen for 24 hours to speed its displacement from haemoglobin. Metabolic acidosis is a feature of this and other forms of poisoning.

Once again, the key to diagnosing these injuries is suspicion from the history. Blood gas measurement will confirm the diagnosis. The treatment is oxygen.

Mechanical block to breathing

Any mechanical block to breathing from the eschar of a significant full-thickness burn on the chest wall is obvious from the examination. There will also be carbon dioxide retention and high inspiratory pressures if the patient is ventilated. The treatment is to make some scoring cuts through the burned skin to allow the chest to expand (escharotomy). The nerves have been destroyed in the skin, and this procedure is not painful for the patient.

ASSESSMENT OF THE BURN WOUND

Assessing size

Burn size needs to be formally assessed in a controlled environment. This allows the area to be exposed and any soot or debris washed off. Care should be taken not to cause hypothermia during this stage. In the case of smaller burns or patches of burn, the best measurement is to cut a piece of clean paper the size of the patient's whole hand (digits and palm), which represents 1% TBSA, and match this to the area. Another accurate way of measuring the size of burns is to draw the burn on a Lund and Browder chart (**Figure 41.3**), which maps out the percentage TBSA of sections of our anatomy. It also takes into account different proportional body surface area in children according to age. The 'rule of nines', which states that each upper limb is 9% TBSA, each lower limb 18%, the torso 18% each side and the head and neck 9%, can be used as a rough guide to TBSA outside the hospital environment.

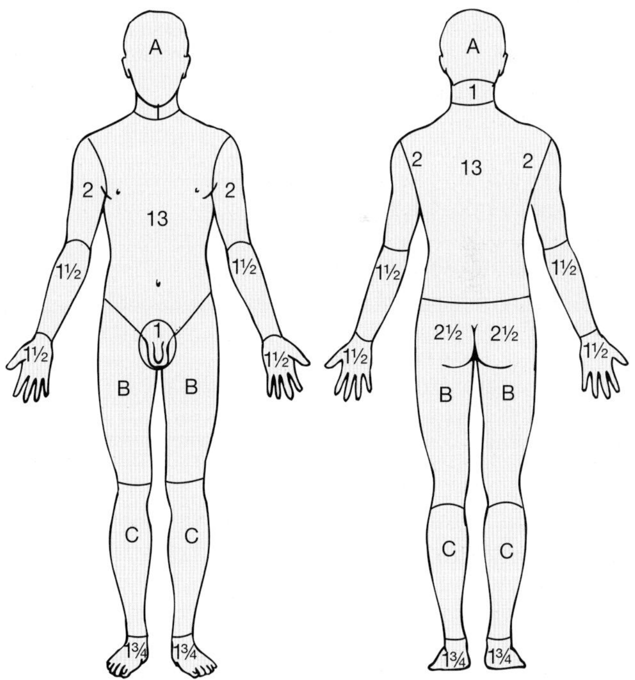

Relative percentage of area affected by growth

Age in years	0	1	5	10	15	Adult
A Head	9	8	6	5	4	3
B Thigh	2	3	4	4	4	4
C Leg	2	2	3	3	3	3

Figure 41.3 The Lund and Browder chart.

Summary box 41.9

Assessing the area of a burn

- The patient's whole hand is 1% TBSA, and is a useful guide in small burns
- The Lund and Browder chart is useful in larger burns
- The 'rule of nines' is adequate for a first approximation only

Assessing depth from the history

The first indication of burn depth comes from the history (*Table 41.2*). The burning of human skin is temperature- and time-dependent. It takes 6 hours for skin maintained at 44°C to suffer irreversible changes, but a surface temperature of 70°C for 1 s is all that is needed to produce epidermal destruction. Taking an example of hot water at 65°C: exposure for 45 s will produce a full-thickness burn, for 15 s a deep partial-thickness burn and for 7 s a superficial partial-thickness burn.

TABLE 41.2 Causes of burns and their likely depth.

Cause of burn	Probable depth of burn
Scald	Superficial, but with deep dermal patches in the absence of good first aid. Will be deep in a young infant
Fat burns	Deep dermal
Flame burns	Mixed deep dermal and full thickness
Alkali burns, including cement	Often deep dermal or full thickness
Acid burns	Weak concentrations superficial; strong concentrations deep dermal
Electrical contact burn	Full thickness

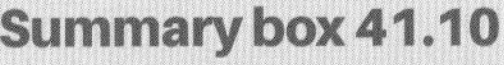

Summary box 41.10

Assessing the depth of a burn

- The history is important – temperature, time and burning material
- Superficial burns have capillary filling
- Deep partial-thickness burns do not blanch, but have some sensation
- Full-thickness burns feel leathery and have no sensation

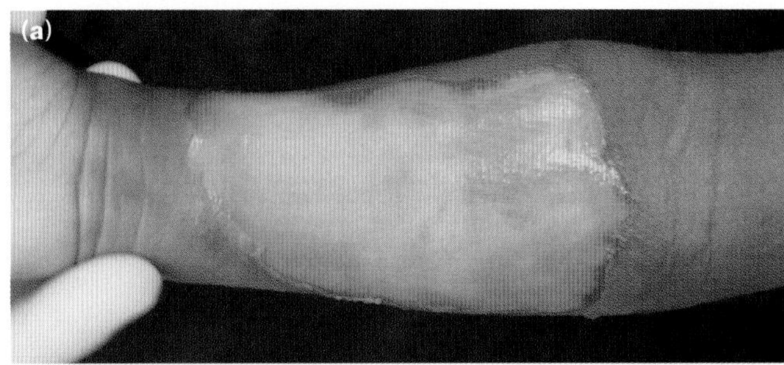

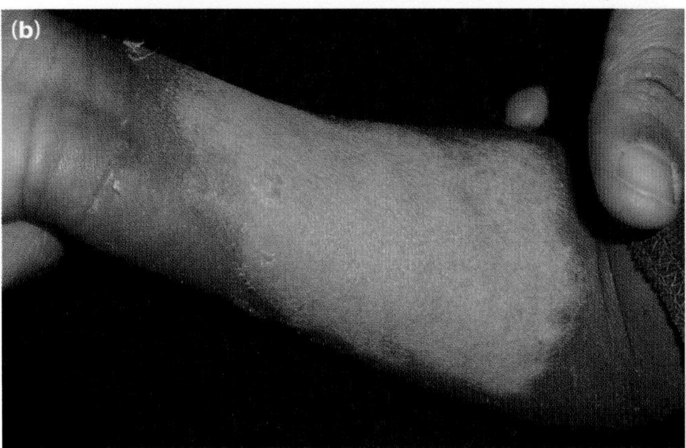

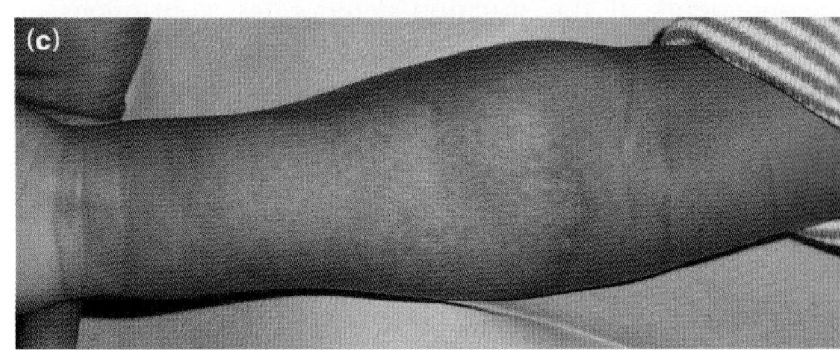

Figure 41.4 (a) A superficial partial-thickness scald 24 hours after injury. The dermis is pink and blanches to pressure. (b) At 2 weeks, the wound is healed but lacks pigment. (c) At 3 months, the pigment is returning.

Superficial partial-thickness burns

The damage in these burns goes no deeper than the papillary dermis. The clinical features are blistering and/or loss of the epidermis. The underlying dermis is pink and moist. The capillary return is clearly visible when blanched. There is little or no fixed capillary staining. Pinprick sensation is normal. Superficial partial-thickness burns heal without residual scarring in 2 weeks. The treatment is non-surgical (**Figure 41.4**).

Deep partial-thickness burn

These burns involve damage to the deeper parts of the reticular dermis (**Figure 41.5**). Clinically, the epidermis is usually lost. The exposed dermis is not as moist as that in a superficial burn. There is often abundant fixed capillary staining, especially if examined after 48 hours. The colour does not blanch with pressure under the examiner's finger. Sensation is reduced, and the patient is unable to distinguish sharp from blunt pressure when examined with a needle. Deep dermal burns take 3 or more weeks to heal without surgery and usually lead to hypertrophic scarring (**Figure 41.6**).

Full-thickness burns

The whole of the dermis is destroyed in these burns (**Figure 41.7**). Clinically, they have a hard, leathery feel. The appearance can vary from that similar to the patient's normal skin to charred black, depending upon the intensity of the heat. There is no capillary return. Often, thrombosed vessels can be seen under the skin. These burns are completely anaesthetised: a needle can be stuck deep into the dermis without any pain or bleeding.

FLUID RESUSCITATION

The principle of fluid resuscitation is that the intravascular volume must be maintained following a burn, in order to provide sufficient circulation to perfuse not only the essential visceral organs such as the brain, kidneys and gut, but also the peripheral tissues, especially the damaged skin.

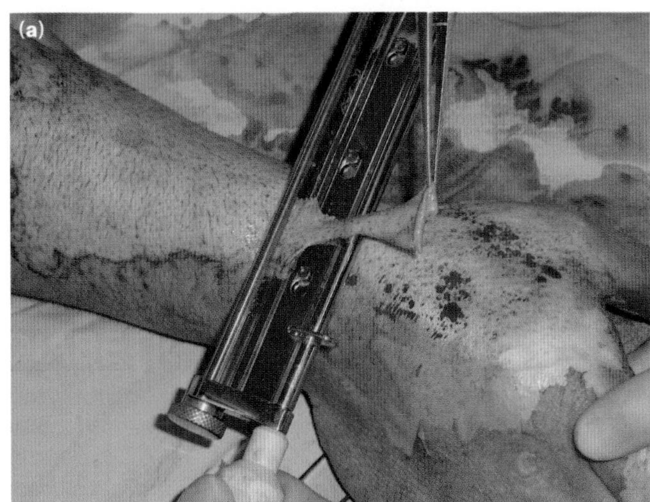

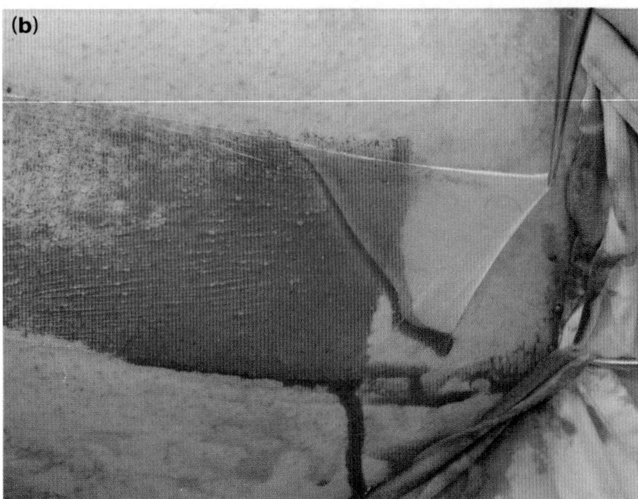

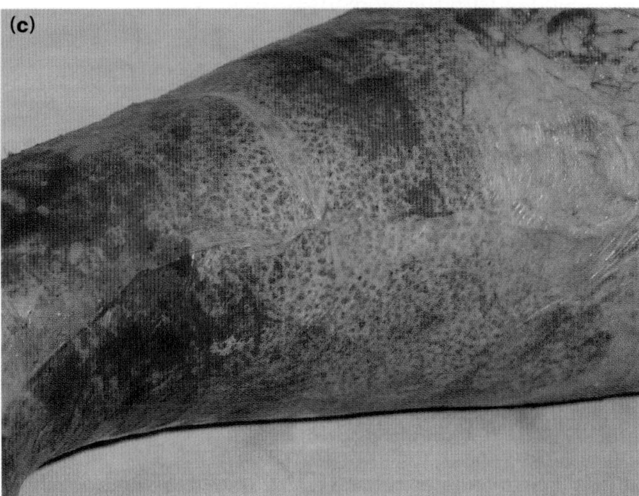

Figure 41.5 (**a**) A deep dermal burn undergoing tangential shaving. The dead dermis is removed layer by layer until healthy bleeding is seen. The burn is pale because it was dressed with silver sulphadiazine cream, but no blanching was visible under this layer. The patient was unable to differentiate between pressure from the sharp and blunt ends of a needle. (**b**) A thin, split-thickness graft harvested from the thigh. (**c**) The thin graft is placed in the dermal remnants. The rete pegs can be seen between the remnants of the dermis through the graft.

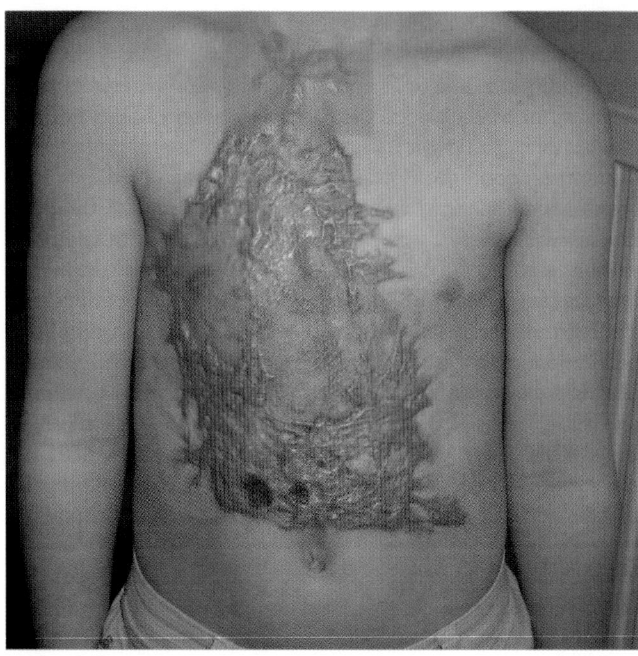

Figure 41.6 Hypertrophic scarring following a deep dermal burn.

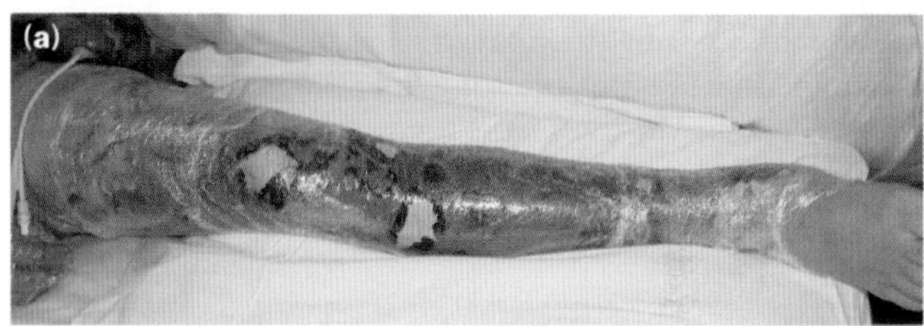

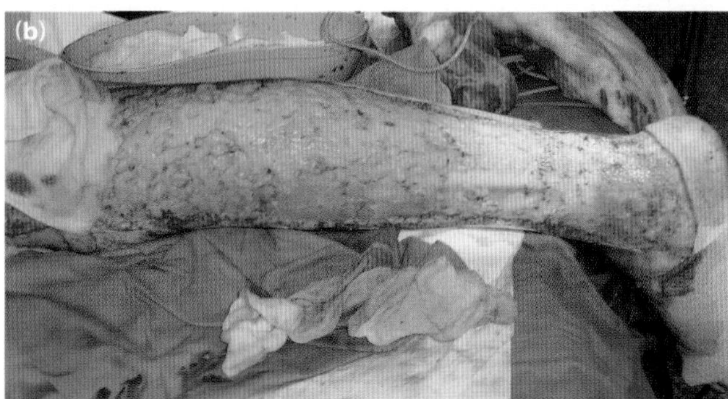

Figure 41.7 (**a**) A full-thickness burn on admission just prior to escharotomy. The wound is wrapped in cling film while in transit. The patient's facial burn is shown in Figure 41.10. (**b**) Excision of the same full-thickness burn, down to healthy fat.

Summary box 41.11

Fluids for resuscitation

- In children with burns over 10% TBSA and adults with burns over 15% TBSA, consider the need for intravenous fluid resuscitation
- If oral fluids are to be used, salt must be added
- Fluids needed can be calculated from a standard formula
- The key is to monitor urine output

Intravenous resuscitation is appropriate for any child with a burn greater than 10% TBSA. The figure is 15% TBSA for adults. In some parts of the world, intravenous resuscitation is commenced only with burns that approach 30% TBSA. If oral resuscitation is to be commenced, it is important that the water given is not salt free. It is rarely possible to undergo significant diuresis in the first 24 hours in view of the stress hormones that are present. Hyponatraemia and water intoxication can be fatal. It is therefore appropriate to give oral rehydration with a solution such as Dioralyte®.

The resuscitation volume is relatively constant in proportion to the area of the body burned and, therefore, there are formulae that calculate the approximate volume of fluid needed for the resuscitation of a patient of a given body weight with a given percentage of the body burned. These regimes follow the fluid loss, which is at its maximum in the first 8 hours and slows, such that, by 24–36 hours, the patient can be maintained on his or her normal daily requirements.

There are three types of fluid used. The most common is Ringer's lactate or Hartmann's solution; some centres use human albumin solution or fresh-frozen plasma; and some centres use hypertonic saline.

Perhaps the simplest and most widely used formula is the Parkland formula. This calculates the fluid to be replaced in the first 24 hours by the following formula: total percentage body surface area × weight (kg) × 4 = volume (mL). Half this volume is given in the first 8 hours and the second half is given in the subsequent 16 hours.

Crystalloid resuscitation

Ringer's lactate is the most commonly used crystalloid. Crystalloids are said to be as effective as colloids for maintaining intravascular volume. They are also significantly less expensive. Another reason for the use of crystalloids is that even large protein molecules leak out of capillaries following burn injury; however, non-burnt capillaries continue to sieve proteins virtually normally.

In children maintenance fluid must also be given. This is normally dextrose–saline given as follows:

- 100 mL/kg for 24 hours for the first 10 kg;
- 50 mL/kg for the next 10 kg;
- 20 mL/kg for 24 hours for each kilogram over 20 kg body weight.

Hypertonic saline

Hypertonic saline has been effective in treating burns shock for many years. It produces hyperosmolarity and hypernatraemia. This reduces the shift of intracellular water to the extracellular space. Advantages include less tissue oedema and a resultant decrease in escharotomies and intubations.

Colloid resuscitation

Human albumin solution (HAS) is a commonly used colloid. Plasma proteins are responsible for the inward oncotic pressure that counteracts the outward capillary hydrostatic pressure. Without proteins, plasma volumes would not be maintained as there would be oedema. Proteins should be given after the first 12 hours of burn because, before this time, the massive fluid shifts cause proteins to leak out of the cells.

The most common colloid-based formula is the Muir and Barclay formula:

- 0.5 × percentage body surface area burnt × weight = one portion;
- periods of 4/4/4, 6/6 and 12 hours, respectively;
- one portion to be given in each period.

Monitoring of resuscitation

The key to monitoring of resuscitation is urine output. Urine output should be between 0.5 and 1.0 mL/kg body weight per hour. If the urine output is below this, the infusion rate should be increased by 50%. If the urine output is inadequate and the patient is showing signs of hypoperfusion (restlessness with tachycardia, cool peripheries and a high haematocrit), then a bolus of 10 mL/kg body weight should be given. It is important that patients are not over-resuscitated and urine output in excess of 2 mL/kg body weight per hour should signal a decrease in the rate of infusion.

Other measures of tissue perfusion such as acid–base balance are appropriate in larger, more complex burns, and a haematocrit measurement is a useful tool in confirming suspected under- or over-hydration. Those with cardiac dysfunction, acute or chronic, may well need more exact measurement of filling pressure, preferably by transoesophageal ultrasound or with the more invasive central line.

TREATING THE BURN WOUND

Escharotomy

Circumferential full-thickness burns to the limbs require emergency surgery (**Figure 41.8**). The tourniquet effect of this injury is easily treated by incising the whole length of full-thickness burns. This should be done in the mid-axial line, avoiding major nerves (*Table 41.3*). One should remember that an escharotomy can cause a large amount of blood loss; therefore, adequate blood should be available for transfusion if required.

Thereafter, the management of the burn wound remains the same, irrespective of the size of the injury. The burn needs to be cleaned, and the size and depth need to be assessed. Full-thickness burns and deep partial-thickness burns that will require operative treatment will need to be dressed with an antibacterial dressing to delay the onset of colonisation of the wound.

Alexis Frank Hartmann, 1898–1964, paediatrician, St Louis, MO, USA.
Thomas Laird Barclay, d.2007, formerly plastic surgeon, The Royal Infirmary, Bradford, UK.
Ian Fraser Kerr Muir, 1921–2008, formerly plastic surgeon, Aberdeen Royal Infirmary, Aberdeen, UK, referred to as 'a gentle giant of plastic surgery'.

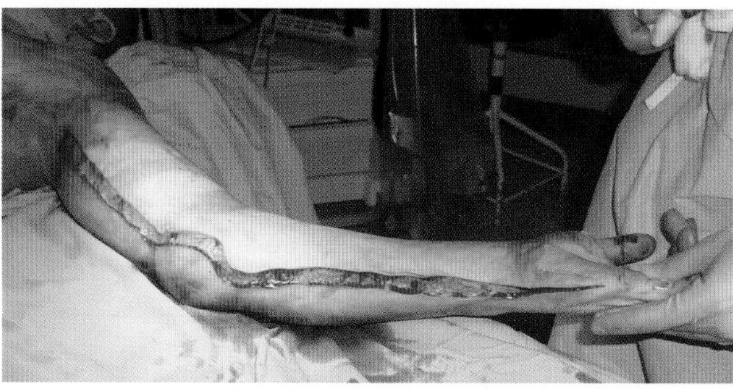

Figure 41.8 A full-thickness burn to the upper limb with a mid-axial escharotomy. The soot and debris have been washed off.

TABLE 41.3 Key features of escharotomy placement.

Upper limb	Mid-axial, anterior to the elbow medially to avoid the ulnar nerve
Hand	Midline in the digits. Release muscle compartments if tight. Best done in theatre and with an experienced surgeon
Lower limb	Mid-axial. Posterior to the ankle medially to avoid the saphenous vein
Chest	Down the chest lateral to the nipples, across the chest below the clavicle and across the chest at the level of the xiphisternum
General rules	Extend the wound beyond the deep burn Diathermy any significant bleeding vessels Apply haemostatic dressing and elevate the limb postoperatively

Full-thickness burns and obvious deep dermal wounds

The four most common dressings for full-thickness and contaminated wounds are listed in *Table 41.4*.

TABLE 41.4 Options for topical treatment of deep burns.

1% silver sulphadiazine cream
0.5% silver nitrate solution
Mafenide acetate cream
Serum nitrate, silver sulphadiazine and cerium nitrate

Dressings with nanocrystalline silver

- **Silver sulphadiazine cream (1%)**. This gives broad spectrum prophylaxis against bacterial colonisation and is particularly effective against *Pseudomonas aeruginosa* and also methicillin-resistant *Staphylococcus aureus*.
- **Silver nitrate solution (0.5%)**. Again, this is highly effective as a prophylaxis against *Pseudomonas* colonisation, but it is not as active as silver sulphadiazine cream against some of the gram-negative aerobes. The other disadvantage of this solution is that it needs to be changed or the wounds resoaked every 2–4 hours. It also produces black staining of all the furniture surrounding the patient.
- **Mafenide acetate cream**. This is popular, especially in the United States, but is painful to apply. It is usually used as a 5% topical solution, but has been associated with metabolic acidosis.
- **Silver sulphadiazine and cerium nitrate**. This is also a very useful burn dressing, especially for full-thickness burns. It induces a sterile eschar on the burned skin and has been shown in certain instances, especially in elderly patients, to reduce some of the cell-mediated immunosuppression that occurs in burns. Cerium nitrate forms a sterile eschar and is especially useful in treating burns when a conservative treatment option has been chosen. Cerium nitrate has also been shown to boost cell-mediated immunity in these patients.

Superficial partial-thickness wounds and mixed-depth wounds

Around the world, a wide variety of substances are used to treat these wounds, from honey or boiled potato peel to synthetic biological dressings with live cultured fibroblasts within the matrix. This is testament to the fact that superficial partial-thickness burns will heal almost irrespective of the dressing. Thus, the key lies with dressings that are easy to apply, non-painful, reduce pain, simple to manage and locally available. The choice of dressings does, however, become crucial in the case of burns that border on being deep dermal (**Figure 41.9**). Here, the choice of dressing can make the difference between scar and no scar and/or operation and no operation. Some of the options for dressing choice are described below.

If the wound is heavily contaminated as a result of the accident, then it is prudent to clean the wound formally under a general anaesthetic. With more chronic contamination, silver sulphadiazine cream dressing for 2 or 3 days is very effective and can be changed to a dressing that is more efficient at promoting healing after this period.

The simplest method of treating a superficial wound is by exposure. The initial exudate needs to be managed by frequent changes of clean linen around the patient but, after a few days, a dry eschar forms, which then separates as the wound epithelialises. This is often used in hot climates and for small burns on the face. However, this method is painful and requires an intensive amount of nursing support. A variation on this theme is to cover the wound with a permeable wound dressing, such as Mefix® or Fixamol®. This allows the wounds to dry but, because it is a covering, it avoids the problems of the wound adhering to the sheets and clothes. A similar method of managing these types of burn is to place a Vaseline-impregnated gauze (with or without an antiseptic, such as chlorhexidine) over the wound. An alternative is a fenestrated silicone sheet (e.g. Mepitel®). These can then be backed with swabs to absorb the exudate. The Vaseline gauze or silicone layer is used to prevent the swabs adhering to the wound and reduces the stiffness of the dry eschar, preventing it from cracking so easily. The swabs need to be changed after the first 48 hours as they are often soaked. After that, they can be left for longer.

More interactive dressings include hydrocolloids and biological dressings. Hydrocolloid dressings need to be changed

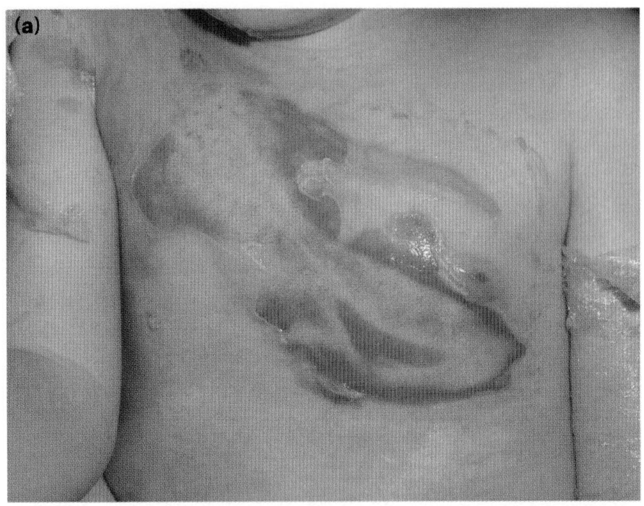

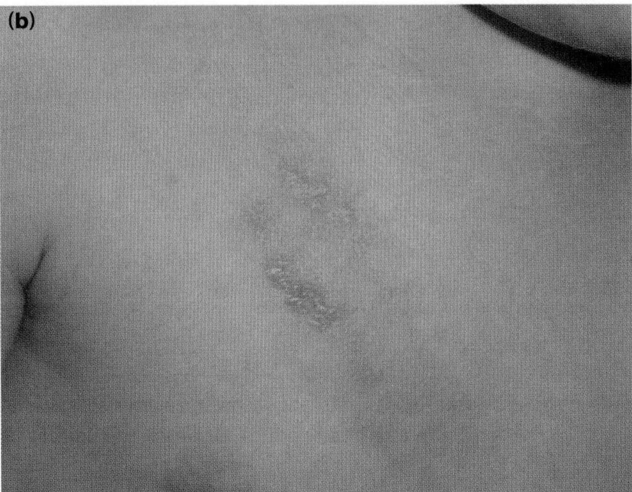

Figure 41.9 (a) A scald to the chest from boiling water, mainly superficial but in some areas close to being deep dermal. This was treated with a hydrocolloid dressing. (b) There are two tiny areas of hypertrophy indicating how close the burn was to being deep dermal. The good first aid this patient received probably made a difference to the outcome.

every 3–5 days. They are particularly useful in mixed-depth burns as the high protease levels under the occlusive dressings aid with the debridement of the deeper areas of burn. They also provide a moist environment, which is good for epithelialisation. Duoderm® is a hydrocolloid dressing. There is good evidence for its value in burns.

Biological, synthetic (e.g. Biobrane®) and natural (e.g. amniotic membranes) dressings also provide good healing environments and do not need to be changed. They are ideal for one-stop management of superficial burns, being easy to apply and comfortable. However, they will become detached if applied to deep dermal wounds as the eschar needs to separate. They are therefore not as useful in mixed-depth wounds.

Early debridement and grafting is the key to effectively treating deep partial- and full-thickness burns in a majority of cases.

Summary box 41.12

Principles of dressings for burns

- Full-thickness and deep dermal burns need antibacterial dressings to delay colonisation prior to surgery
- Superficial burns will heal and need simple dressings
- An optimal healing environment can make a difference to outcome in borderline depth burns

ADDITIONAL ASPECTS OF TREATING THE BURNED PATIENT

Analgesia

Acute

Analgesia is a vital part of burns management. Small burns, especially superficial burns, respond well to simple oral analgesia, paracetamol and non-steroidal anti-inflammatory drugs. Topical cooling is especially soothing. Large burns require intravenous opiates. Intramuscular injections should not be given in acute burns over 10% of TBSA, as absorption is unpredictable and dangerous.

Subacute

In patients with large burns, continuous analgesia is required, beginning with infusions and continuing with oral tablets, such as slow-release morphine. Powerful, short-acting analgesia should be administered before dressing changes. Administration may require an anaesthetist, as in the case of general anaesthesia or midazolam and ketamine, or less intensive supervision, as in the case of morphine and nitrous oxide.

Energy balance and nutrition

One of the most important aspects in treating burns patients is nutrition. Any adult with a burn greater than 15% (10% in children) of TBSA has an increased nutritional requirement. All patients with burns of 20% of TBSA or greater should receive a nasogastric tube. (Feeding should start within 6 hours of the injury to reduce gut mucosal damage.) A number of different formulae are available to calculate the energy requirements of patients.

Burn injuries are catabolic in the acute episode. Successful management of the patient's energy balance involves a

Summary box 41.13

Nutrition in burns patients

- Burns patients need extra feeding
- A nasogastric tube should be used in all patients with burns over 15% of TBSA
- Removing the burn and achieving healing stops the catabolic drive

number of strategies. The catabolic drive continues while the wound remains unhealed and, therefore, rapid excision of the burn and stable coverage of the wound are the most significant factors in reversing this. Obligatory energy utilisation must be reduced to a minimum by keeping the patient warm with good environmental control. The excess energy requirements must be provided for and the nutritional balance monitored by measuring weight and nitrogen balance (*Table 41.5*).

TABLE 41.5 Commonly used feeding formulae.

Curreri formula	Age 16–59 years: (25)W + (40)TBSA Age 60+ years: (20)W + (65)TBSA
Sutherland formula	Children: 60 kcal/kg + 35 kcal%TBSA Adults: 20 kcal/kg + 70 kcal%TBSA
Protein needs	Greatest nitrogen losses between days 5 and 10 20% of kilocalories should be provided by proteins
Davies formula	Children: 3 g/kg + 1 g%TBSA Adults: 1 g/kg + 3 g%TBSA

TBSA, total body surface area; W, weight.

Monitoring and control of infection

Patients with major burns are immunocompromised, having large portals of entry to pathogenic and opportunistic bacteria and fungi via the burn wound. They have compromised local defences in the lungs and gut due to oedema, and usually have monitoring lines and catheters, which themselves represent portals for infection.

Summary box 41.14

Infection control in burns patients

- Burns patients are immunocompromised
- They are susceptible to infection from many routes
- Sterile precautions must be rigorous
- Swabs should be taken regularly
- A rise in white blood cell count, thrombocytosis and increased catabolism are warnings of infection

Control of infection begins with policies on hand-washing and other cross-contamination prevention measures. Bacteriological surveillance of the wound, catheter tips and sputum helps to build a picture of the patient's flora. If there are signs of infection, then further cultures need to be taken and antibiotics started. This is often initially on a best guess basis, hence the usefulness of prior surveillance; close liaison with a bacteriologist is essential. In patients with large burns that remain catabolic, the core temperature is usually reset by the hypothalamus above 37°C. Significant temperatures are those above 38.5°C, but often other signs of infection are more useful to the clinician. These include significant rise or fall in the white cell count, thrombocytosis, increasing signs of catabolism and decreasing clinical status of the patient.

Nursing care

Burns patients require particularly intensive nursing care. Nurses are the primary effectors of many decisions that directly affect healing. Bandaged hands and joints that are stiff and painful need careful coaxing. Personal hygiene, baths and showers all become time-consuming and painful, but are vital parts of the patient's physiotherapy. Their success or failure has a powerful psychological impact on the patient and his or her family.

Physiotherapy

All burns cause swelling, especially burns to the hands. Elevation, splintage and exercise reduce swelling and improve the final outcome. The physiotherapy needs to be started on day 1, so that the message can be reinforced on a daily basis.

Psychological

A major burn is an overwhelming event, outside the normal experience, which stretches the patient's coping ability, suspends the patient's sense of safety and causes post-traumatic reactions. These are normal and usually self-limiting, receding as the patient heals. The features of this intensity of experience are of intrusive reactions, arousal reactions and avoidance reactions.

SURGERY FOR THE ACUTE BURN WOUND

Any deep partial-thickness and full-thickness burns, except those that are less than about 4 cm^2, need surgery. Any burn of indeterminate depth should be reassessed after 48 hours. This is because burns that initially appear superficial may well deepen over that time. Delayed microvascular injury is especially common in scalds.

The essence of burns surgery is control. First and foremost, the anaesthetist needs good control of the patient. A wide-bore cannula should be used and the patient's blood pressure must be monitored adequately. If a large excision is considered, then an arterial line (to monitor blood pressure) and a central venous pressure monitor are needed. The anaesthetist also needs measurements and control of the acid–base

Summary box 41.15

Surgical treatment of deep burns

- Deep dermal burns need tangential shaving and split-skin
- grafting
- All but the smallest full-thickness burns need surgery
- The anaesthetist needs to be ready for significant blood loss
- Topical adrenaline reduces bleeding
- All burnt tissue needs to be excised
- Stable cover, permanent or temporary, should be applied at once to reduce burn load

balance, clotting time and haemoglobin levels. The core temperature of the patient must not drop below 36°C, otherwise clotting irregularities will be compounded.

For most burn excisions, subcutaneous injection of a dilute solution of adrenaline 1:1 000 000 or 1:500 000 and tourniquet control are important for controlling blood loss.

In deep dermal burns, the top layer of dead dermis is shaved off until punctate bleeding is observed and the dermis can be seen to be free of any small thrombosed vessels (**Figure 41.5a**). A topical solution of 1:500 000 adrenaline also helps to reduce bleeding, as does the application of the skin graft. The use of a tourniquet during burn excisions in the limbs helps to decrease blood loss and maintain control.

Full-thickness burns require full-thickness excision of the skin (**Figure 41.7b**). In certain circumstances, it is appropriate to go down to the fascia but, in most cases, the burn excision is down to viable fat. Wherever possible, a skin graft should be applied immediately. With very large burns, the use of synthetic dermis or homografts provides temporary stable coverage and will allow complete excision of the wound and thus reduce the burn load on the patient.

Postoperative management of these patients obviously requires careful evaluation of fluid balance and levels of haemoglobin. The outer dressings will quickly be soaked through with serum and will need to be changed on a regular basis to reduce the bacterial load within the dressing.

Physiotherapy and splints are important in maintaining range of movement and reducing joint contracture. Elevation of the appropriate limbs is important. The hand must be splinted in a position of function after grafting, although the graft needs to be applied in the position of maximal stretch. Knees are best splinted in extension, axillae in abduction. Supervised movement by the physiotherapists, usually under direct vision of any affected joints, should begin after about 5 days.

Delayed reconstruction and scar management

Delayed reconstruction of burn injuries is common for large full-thickness burns. In the early healing period, acute contractures around the eye need particular attention. Eyelids must be grafted at the first sign of difficulty in closing the eyelids, and this must be done before the patient has any symptoms of exposure keratitis (**Figure 41.10**). Other areas that require early intervention are any contracture causing significant loss of range of movement of a joint. This is particularly important in the hand and axilla.

An established contracture can be treated in a number of ways. Burn alopecia is best treated with tissue expansion of the unburned hair-bearing skin. Tissue expansion is also a useful technique for isolated burns and other areas with adjacent normal skin. Z-plasty is useful where there is a single band and a transposition flap is useful in wider bands of scarring (**Figure 41.11**). In areas of circumferential or very broad areas of scarring, the only real treatment is incision and replacement with tissue. By far the best tissue for replacement is from either a full-thickness graft or vascularised tissue as in a free flap. Occasionally, the situation requires the less ideal covering of split skin, possibly with an artificial dermis, such as Integra® (**Figure 41.12**). These last two options require prolonged scar management after their use.

Hypertrophy of many scars will respond to pressure garments. These need to be worn for a period of 6–18 months. Where it is difficult to apply pressure with pressure garments, or with smaller areas of hypertrophy, silicone patches will speed scar maturation, as will intralesional injection of steroid. Itching and dermatitis in burn scar areas are common. Pharmacological treatment of itch is an essential adjunct to therapy.

Summary box 41.16

Delayed reconstruction of burns

- Eyelids must be treated before exposure keratitis arises
- Transposition flaps and Z-plasties with or without tissue expansion are useful
- Full-thickness grafts and free flaps may be needed for large or difficult areas
- Hypertrophy is treated with pressure garments
- Pharmacological treatment of itch is important

MINOR BURNS/OUTPATIENT BURNS

Local burn wound care

Blisters

Whether to remove blisters or leave them intact has been the subject of much debate. Proponents of blister removal quote laboratory studies that show that blister fluid depresses immune function, slowing down chemotaxis and intracellular killing and also acting as a medium for bacterial growth.

Conversely, other authors advocate leaving blisters intact as they form a sterile stratum spongiosum. Leaving a ruptured blister is not advised.

Initial cleaning of the burn wound

Washing the burn wound with chlorhexidine solution is ideal for this purpose.

The Guinea Pig Club. Sir Archibald McIndoe (1900–1960), born in New Zealand, was appointed in 1938 as Consultant Plastic Surgeon to the Royal Air Force. He trained with his cousin, **Sir Harold Gillies**, another internationally reputed plastic surgeon. McIndoe became world famous for his pioneering work on Battle of Britain pilots who were badly burnt. His work on these airmen, who needed several operations, and using his innovative technical and psychological methods, was the start of a life-long service. The young fighter pilots were therefore referred to as 'guinea pigs' – thus was formed The Guinea Pig Club. McIndoe referred to his patients as 'the boys' who in turn called him 'the boss' or 'the maestro'. To this day, some of the members of the Guinea Pig Club from all over the world still meet on an annual basis in Sussex. McIndoe founded the British Association of Plastic Surgeons (BAPS).

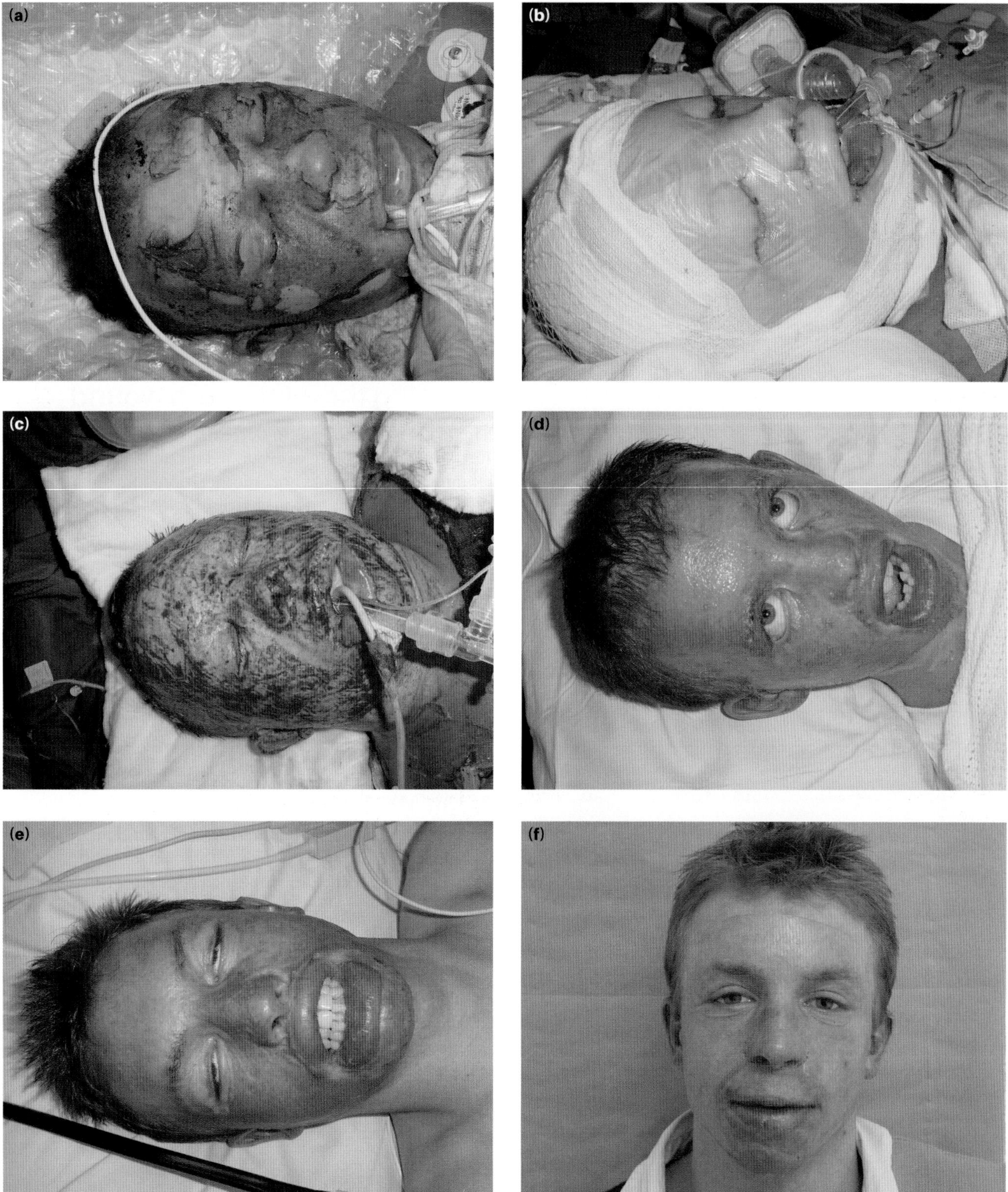

Figure 41.10 (a) A mixed superficial and deep burn to the face after a petrol explosion. The patient's airway was protected prior to transfer. He has an orogastric tube and feeding has commenced. (b) The face dressed with a hydrocolloid dressing. The endotracheal tube is wired to the teeth. (c) Day 6, the swelling is still present. (d) Six weeks after injury. With the mouth wide open, the lower eyelids are pulled down, demonstrating the intrinsic and extrinsic shortening of the eyelids. (e) Three months after injury. The eyelids have been grafted but note the contracture of the lips. (f) Six months after injury. The patient has had grafts to the upper and lower lips.

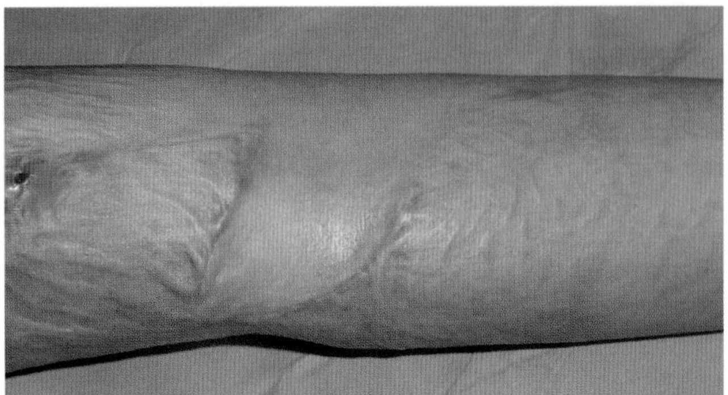

Figure 41.11 A transposition flap bringing normal skin across a scarred elbow.

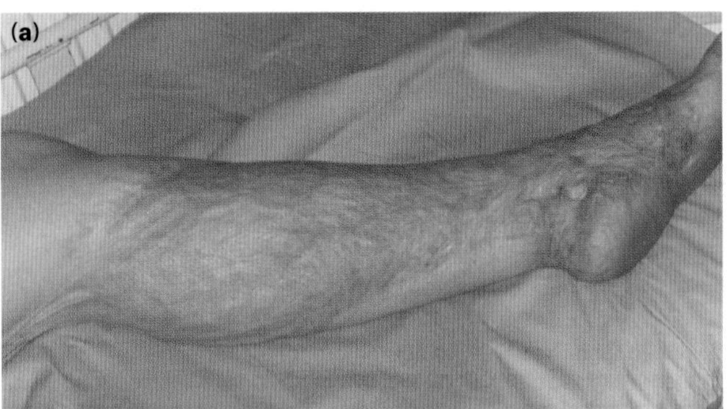

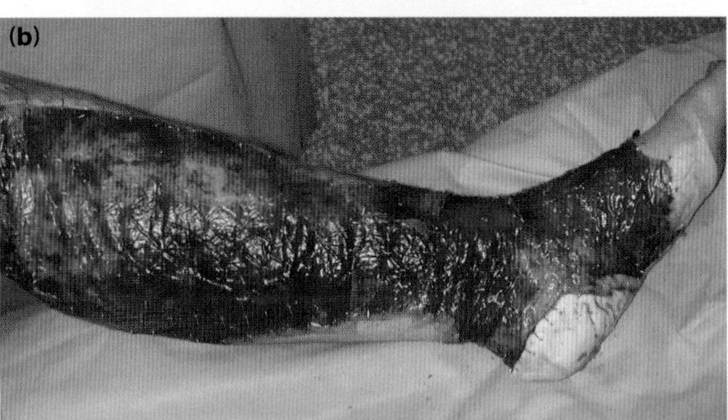

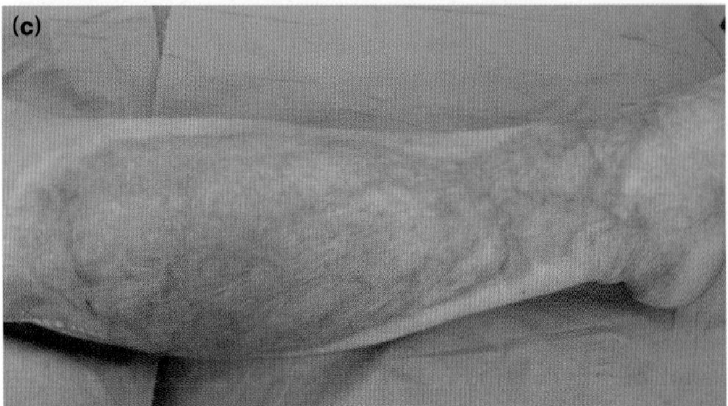

Figure 41.12 (**a**) A healed full-thickness leg burn prior to resurfacing with Integra. (**b**) The burn scar has been excised and Integra applied prior to split-thickness skin grafting. (**c**) Six months after Integra resurfacing. The skin is smoother and more supple and the scar has faded.

Topical agents

For initial management of minor burns that are superficial or partial thickness, dressings with a non-adherent material, such as Vaseline-impregnated gauze or Mepitel are often sufficient. These dressings are left in place for 5 days. These burns, by definition, should be healed after 7–10 days. Various topical creams and ointments have been used for the treatment of minor burns. All published comparative data show no advantage of these agents over petroleum gauze.

Silver sulphadiazine (1%) or Flamazine® is the most commonly used topical agent. However, it should be avoided in pregnant women, nursing mothers and infants less than 2 months of age because of the increased possibility of kernicterus in these patients.

Dressing the minor burn wound

The aims of dressing are to decrease wound pain and to protect and isolate the burn wound. The small superficial burn requires Vaseline gauze or another non-adherent dressing, such as Mepitel, as the first layer. Following this, gauze or Kerlix® is wrapped around with sufficient tightness to keep the dressing intact, but not to impede the circulation. This is further wrapped with bandage. It is important to realise that bulkiness of dressings in the minor burn wound depends upon the amount of wound discharge. A special case is burns of the hands where dressings should be minimised so as not to impede mobilisation and physiotherapy.

Synthetic burn wound dressings are popular as they:

- decrease pain associated with dressings;
- improve healing times;
- decrease outpatient appointments;
- lower overall costs.

Biobrane® is a bilaminar dressing made up of an inner layer of knitted nylon threads coated with porcine collagen and an outer layer of rubberised silicone impervious to gases, but not to fluids and bacteria. Wounds to be dressed with Biobrane should be carefully selected. Burn wounds should be fresh (less than 24 hours), sensate, show capillary blanching and refill. Biobrane should be applied to the wound after removal of all blisters. It should be checked at 48 hours for adherence and any signs of infection. It should be removed if any sign of infection is found.

Duoderm® or hydrocolloid dressings are not bulky, help in healing and can be kept in place for 48–72 hours. They provide a moist environment, which helps in re-epithelialisation of the burn wound.

Healing of burn wounds

Burns that are being managed conservatively should be healed within 3 weeks. If there are no signs of re-epithelialisation in this time, the wound requires debridement and grafting.

Infection

Infection in the minor burn should be tackled very aggressively as it is known to convert a superficial burn to a partial-thickness burn and a partial- to a deep partial-thickness burn, respectively. It should be managed using a combination of topical and systemic agents. Debridement and skin grafting should also be considered.

Itching

Most burn patients have itchy wounds. Histamine and various endopeptides are said to be the causative factors of itching. Antihistamines, analgesics, moisturising creams, aloe vera and antibiotics have all been tried with varying degrees of success. Sometimes gabapentin has been used in patients with severe itch. Examples of therapeutic agents described include cyproheptadine, loratidine and topical doxepin cream.

Traumatic blisters

The healed burn wound is prone to getting traumatic blisters because the new epithelium is very fragile. Non-adherent dressings usually suffice; regular moisturisation is also useful in this condition.

NON-THERMAL BURN INJURY

Electrical injuries

Electrical injuries are usually divided into low- and high-voltage injuries, the threshold being 1000 v.

Summary box 41.17

Electrical burns

- Low-voltage injuries cause small, localised, deep burns
- They can cause cardiac arrest through pacing interruption without significant direct myocardial damage
- High-voltage injuries damage by flash (external burn) and conduction (internal burn)
- Myocardium may be directly damaged without pacing interruption
- Limbs may need fasciotomies or amputation
- Look for and treat acidosis and myoglobinuria

Low-tension injuries

Low-tension or domestic appliance injuries do not have enough energy to cause destruction to significant amounts of subcutaneous tissues when the current passes through the body. The resistance is too great. The entry and exit points, normally in the fingers, suffer small deep burns; these may cause underlying tendon and nerve damage, but there will be little damage between. The alternating current creates a tetany within the muscles, and thus patients often describe how they were unable to release the device until the power was turned off. The main danger with these injuries is from the alternating current interfering with normal cardiac pacing. This can cause cardiac arrest. The electricity itself does not usually cause significant underlying myocardial damage, so resuscitation, if successful, should be lasting.

High-tension injuries

High-tension electrical injuries can be caused by one of three sources of damage: the flash, the flame and the current itself.

When a high-tension line is earthed, enormous energy is released as the current travels from the line to the earth. It can arc over the patient, causing a flash burn. The extremely rapid heating of the air causes an explosion that often propels the victim backwards. The key here is that the current travelled from the line to the earth directly and not through the patient. The flash, however, can go on to ignite the patient's clothes and so cause a normal flame burn.

In accidents with overhead lines, the patient often acts as the conduction rod to earth. In these injuries, there is enough current to cause damage to the subcutaneous tissues and muscles. The entry and exit points are damaged but, importantly, the current can cause huge amounts of subcutaneous damage between these two points. These can be extremely serious injuries.

The damage to the underlying muscles in the affected limb can cause the rapid onset of compartment syndrome. The release of the myoglobins will cause myoglobinuria and subsequent renal dysfunction. Therefore, during the resuscitation of these patients, efforts must be made to maintain a high urine output of up to 2 mL/kg body weight per hour. Severe acidosis is common in large electrical burns and may require boluses of bicarbonate. These patients are also at risk of myocardial damage as a result of direct muscle damage, rather than by interference with cardiac pacing. This gives rise to significant electrocardiogram changes, with raised cardiac enzymes. If there is significant damage, there is rapid onset of heart failure. In the case of a severe injury through a limb, primary amputation is sometimes the most effective management (**Figure 41.13**).

Chemical injuries

There are over 70 000 different chemicals in regular use within industry. Occasionally, these cause burns. Ultimately, there are two aspects to a chemical injury. The first is the physical destruction of the skin and the second is any poisoning caused by systemic absorption.

The initial management of any chemical injury is copious lavage with water. There are only a handful of chemicals for which water is not helpful, for example phosphorus, which is a component of some military devices, and elemental sodium, which is occasionally present in laboratory explosions. These substances need to be physically removed with forceps; however, it is extremely rare that any medical practitioner will encounter these in his or her lifetime. The more common injuries are caused by either acids or alkalis. Alkalis are usually the more destructive and are especially dangerous if they have come into contact with the eyes. After copious lavage, the next step in the management of any chemical injury is to identify the chemical

Summary box 41.18

Chemical burns

- Damage is from corrosion and poisoning
- Copious lavage with water helps in most cases
- Then identify the chemical and assess the risks of absorption

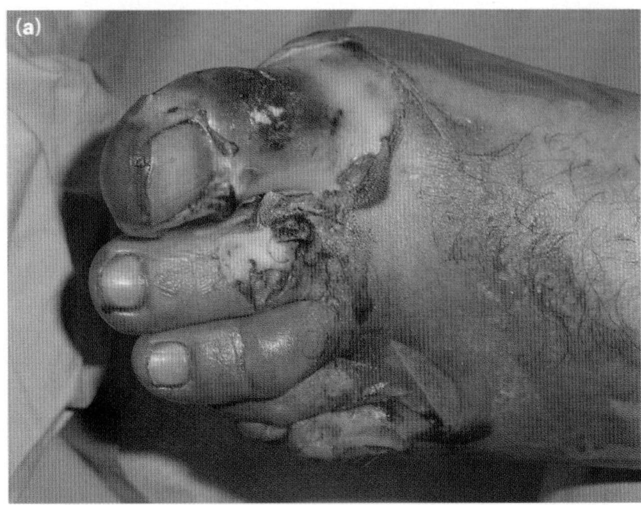

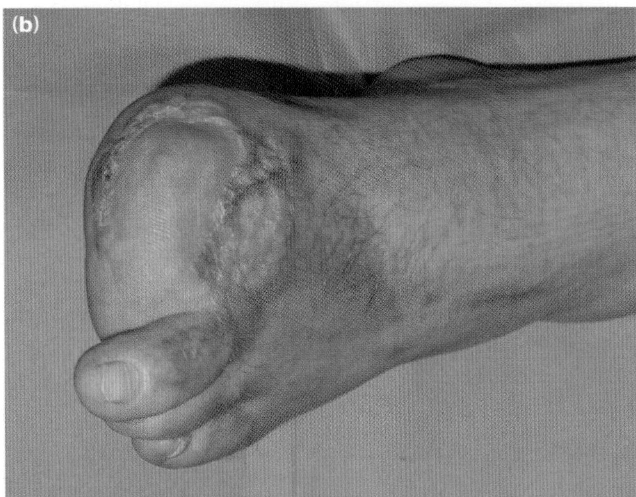

Figure 41.13 (**a**) An exit wound of a high-tension injury, with a dead big toe and significant damage to the medial portion of the second toe. (**b**) Amputation and cover with the lateral portion of the second toe.

and its concentration and to elucidate whether there is any underlying threat to the patient's life if absorbed systemically.

One acid that is a common cause of acid burns is hydrofluoric acid. Burns affecting the fingers and caused by dilute acid are relatively common. The initial management is with calcium gluconate gel topically; however, severe burns or burns to large areas of the hand can be subsequently treated with Bier's blocks containing calcium gluconate 10% gel. If the patient has been burnt with a concentration greater than 50%, the threat of hypocalcaemia and subsequent arrhythmias then becomes high, and this is an indication for acute early excision. It is best not to split-skin graft these hydrofluoric acid wounds initially, but to do this at a delayed stage.

Ionising radiation injury

These injuries can be divided into groups depending on whether radiation exposure was to the whole body or localised. The management of localised radiation damage is usually conservative until the true extent of the tissue injury is apparent. Should this damage have caused an ulcer, then excision and coverage with vascularised tissue is required.

Whole-body radiation causes a large number of symptoms. The dose of radiation either is, or is not, lethal. A patient who has suffered whole-body irradiation and is suffering from acute desquamation of the skin has received a lethal dose of radiation, which can cause a particularly slow and unpleasant death. Non-lethal radiation has a number of systemic effects related to the gut mucosa and immune system dysfunction. Other than giving iodine tablets, the management of these injuries is supportive.

Summary box 41.19

Radiation burns

- Local burns causing ulceration need excision and vascularised flap cover, usually with free flaps
- Systemic overdose needs supportive treatment

Cold injuries

Cold injuries are principally divided into two types: acute cold injuries from industrial accidents and frostbite.

Exposure to liquid nitrogen and other such liquids will cause epidermal and dermal destruction. The tissue is more resistant to cold injury than to heat injury, and the inflammatory reaction is not as marked. The assessment of depth of injury is more difficult, so it is rare to make the decision for surgery early.

Frostbite injuries affect the peripheries in cold climates. The initial treatment is with rapid rewarming in a bath at 42°C. The cold injury produces delayed microvascular damage similar to that of cardiac reperfusion injury. The level of damage is difficult to assess, and surgery usually does not play a role in its management, which is conservative, until there is absolute demarcation of the level of injury.

RECENT ADVANCES

Advanced technology, newer drugs and skin substitutes are the major advances in burn care. An intelligent use of these modalities is essential to make an effective case for cost–benefit ratios.

The introduction of new modalities needs to be carried out within critically reviewed and controlled clinical protocols, working towards building appropriate clinical evidence.

FURTHER READING

British Burns Association. *Emergency management of burns*, 8th edn. UK Course Pre-reading. British Burns Association, 2004.

Herndon D (ed.). *Total burn care*, 4th edn. Philadelphia, PA: Saunders and Elsevier, 2012.

Pape S, Judkins K, Settle J. *Burns: the first five days*, 2nd edn. Romford: Smith and Nephew, 2000.

August Karl Gustav Bier, 1861–1949, Professor of Surgery, Berlin, Germany.

Chapter 42

Plastic and reconstructive surgery

Learning objectives

To understand:

- The spectrum of plastic surgical techniques used to restore bodily form and function
- The relevant anatomy and physiology of tissues used in reconstruction
- The various skin grafts and how to use them appropriately
- The principles and use of flaps
- How to use plastic surgery to manage difficult and complex tissue loss

HISTORICAL CONTEXT

Reconstructive plastic (from the ancient Greek *plassein*, to mould or shape – which is also the stem for our modern use of the materials termed 'plastics') surgery involves using various techniques to restore form and function to the body when tissues have been damaged by injury, cancer or congenital loss. Its origins can be traced back to ancient Egypt, with wound care depicted in hieroglyphs on papyrus, to India in the sixth century BC, where Sushruta described using the forehead flap to reconstruct a nose, and to Al-Zahrawi, the tenth-century Islamic surgical scholar from Cordoba. Modern techniques were developed after the First World War, especially with Sir Harold Gillies' work on reconstructing facial injuries (**Figure 42.1**), which was enabled by new safe anaesthetic intubation (Sir Ivan Magill). Later in the twentieth century, renewed understanding of detailed soft tissue anatomy led to an explosion in the use of new flaps, which with microsurgical methods, craniofacial surgery and tissue expansion resulted in an entirely new set of techniques becoming available to surgeons for reconstructing parts.

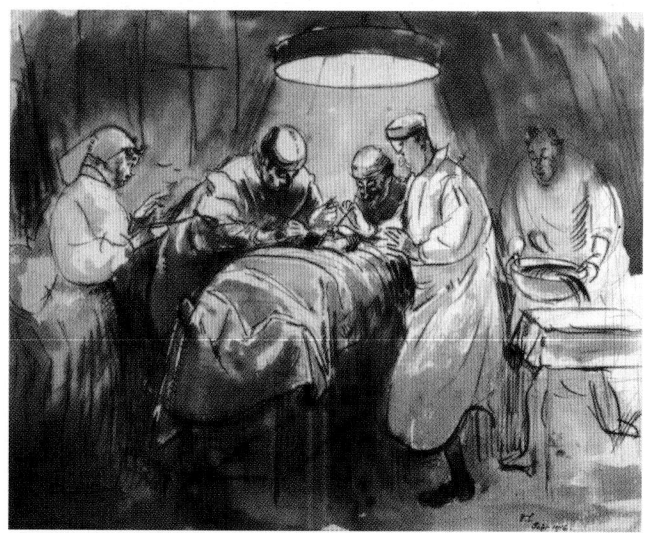

Figure 42.1 Sir Harold Gillies operating during the First World War – 'the birth of plastic surgery'. Picture by Henry Tonks (by kind permission of the Royal College of Surgeons of England).

Today, the need for reconstructive plastic surgery, especially in resource-poor countries, has never been greater. Road, war and domestic injury inflict life-diminishing effects, which plastic surgery can reduce. The reconstructive surgeon's 'toolbox' is now very diverse and will continue to grow in order to address problem wounds and tissue defects, which arise as modern medical care is more successful in treating cancer, preserving life into old age and salvaging victims of trauma.

Sushruta, regarded as the father of modern surgery, lived in the Indian city of Kashi (now called Banaras) in 600BC (while the exact period is unclear, most scholars maintain that he practised between 600 and 1000BC). A large part of his practice was plastic surgery in the form of rhinoplasty carried out on criminals who had their noses amputated as a punishment for their crimes. His medical pursuits were recorde d in 'Sushsruta Samhita (compendum)'.
Sir Harold Delf Gillies, 1882–1960, born New Zealand, studied medicine at the University of Cambridge, pioneer of plastic surgical techniques during and after World War 1.
Sir Ivan Whiteside Magill, 1888–1986, anaesthetist, Westminister Hospital, London, UK.
Henry Tonks, 1862–1937, commenced a career in surgery, but abandoned it for art and became, from 1917 to 1930, Slade Professor at the Westminster School of Art, London, UK.

ANATOMY RELATED TO RECONSTRUCTIVE SURGERY

Skin

The surface of the skin is important as a biological layer for homeostasis. Restoring the skin surface is therefore critical, even if the underlying structures can await later reconstruction. Epidermis regenerates from deeper follicular elements, with the most superficial layer losing vascularity and acting as a barrier to fluid loss and providing important protection against invasion by microorganisms. (Epidermal keratinocytes can be artificially cultured *in vitro* and are used in some wound management systems.)

The depth of the dermis and the amounts of elastin and skin adnexal elements, such as sweat glands and hair follicles, vary depending on the functional requirements of the area concerned. This means that some areas are much more vulnerable to injury than others, e.g. the fine flexible elastic skin of the eyelid rapidly suffers a full-thickness burn after a flash burn, whereas thick back skin suffers only a partial loss after the same flash burn.

Skin vascularity is derived from fine perforating vessels that run through underlying muscles or through fascial septal layers, and then horizontally in a subcutaneous plane from which capillaries branch (**Figure 42.2**). Nerves run axially out from major trunks and are less well defined than most perforating blood vessels.

When local, random-pattern skin flaps are raised, they are lifted at the subcutaneous level and are nourished by the subdermal plexus of blood vessels. However, this plexus can only survive a limited distance from the more substantial arterial branches running in the fascial, septal or muscle-perforating planes. Understanding the detailed anatomy of different parts of the skin and tissues to be moved is a key element of successful plastic surgery.

Without skin, wounds heal by **secondary intention** with fibrosis and contracture (**Figure 42.3**), and underlying structures are vulnerable to necrosis, chronic infection and dysfunction.

Graft anatomy

Split-thickness skin grafts

Split-thickness skin grafts are harvested by taking all of the epidermis together with some dermis, leaving the remaining dermis behind to heal the donor site. The thicker the dermis that is taken (seen by more brisk punctate bleeding at the donor site; **Figure 42.4**), the more durable will be the graft once healed (although it might take longer and require more care), but also the more difficult will be donor site healing.

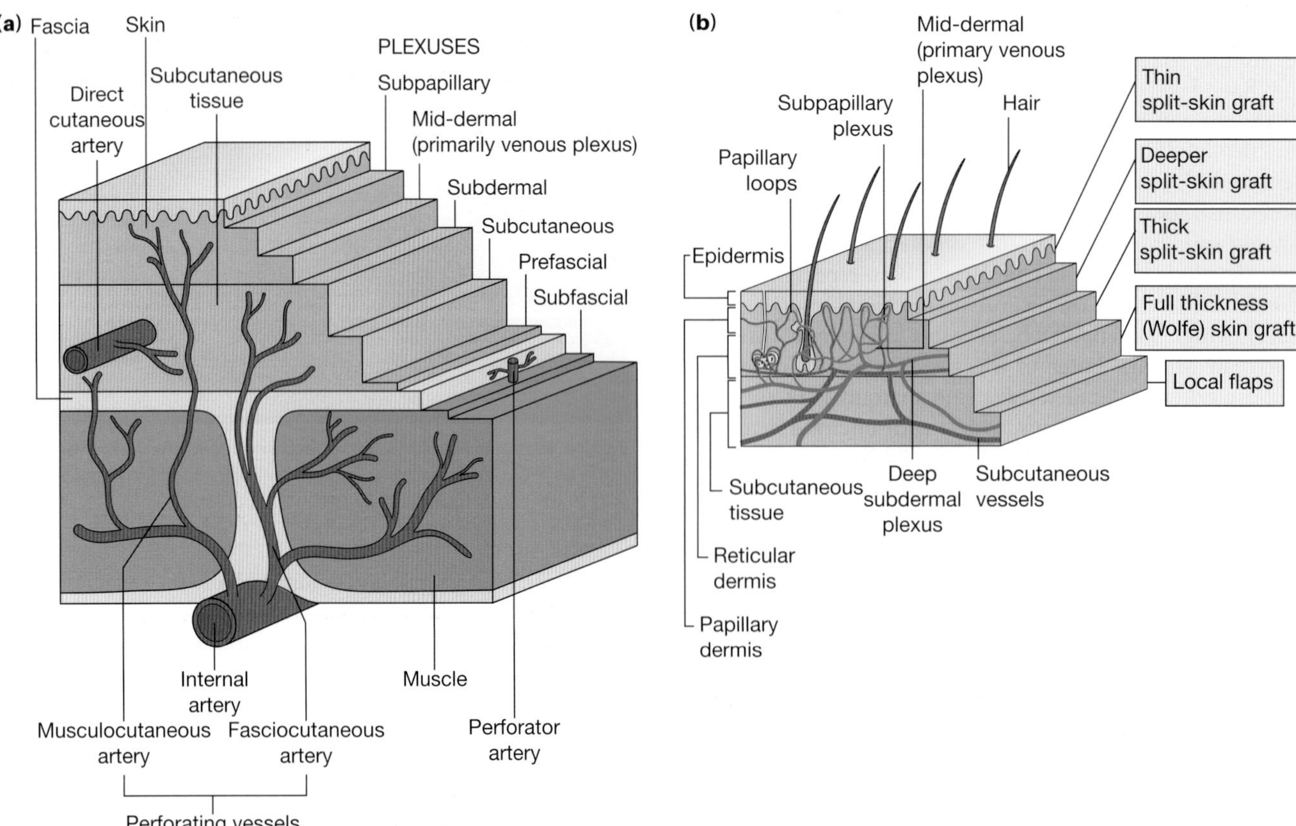

Figure 42.2 Diagram of skin anatomy with vascular plexus.

in vitro is Latin for 'in the glass'.

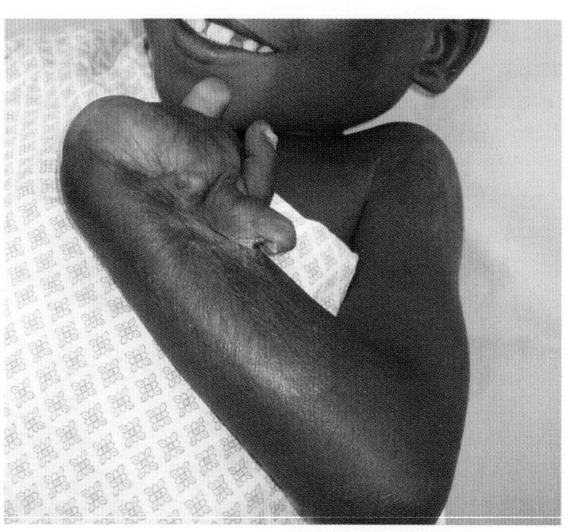

Figure 42.3 A severely contracted hand following burn to the dorsal aspect.

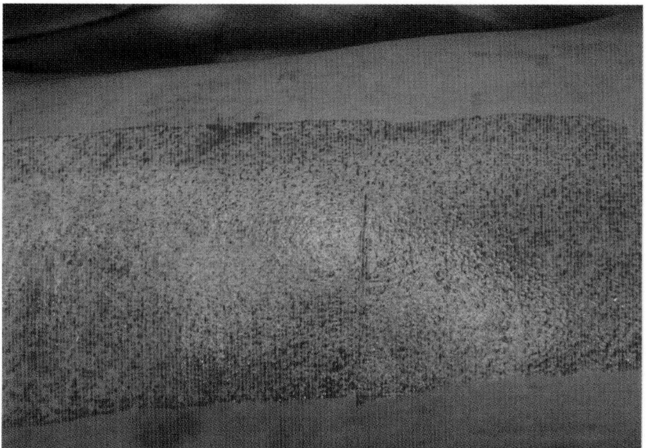

Figure 42.4 Fine punctate bleeding from a split-thickness skin graft donor site.

Summary box 42.1

Split-thickness skin grafts

- Thicker knife-gap settings give rise to fewer but brisker bleeding points on the donor site.
- Thicker grafts heal with less contracture and are more durable.
- Thinner donor sites heal better.
- Grafts are hairless and do not sweat (these structures are not transferred).

Full-thickness skin grafts

Full-thickness grafts are harvested to incorporate the whole dermis, with the underlying fat trimmed away – unless elements of fat (or even cartilage as well) are deliberately left attached to form a **composite graft**. Full-thickness and composite grafts require the most careful handling and postoperative nursing to help ensure that they 'take' in their transplanted site.

How does a skin graft survive?

Split-thickness skin grafts survive initially by **imbibition** of plasma from the wound bed; after 48 hours, fine anastomotic connections are made, which lead to **inosculation** of blood. Capillary ingrowth then completes the healing process with fibroblast maturation. Because only tissues that produce granulation will support a graft, it is usually contraindicated to use grafts to cover exposed tendons, cartilage or cortical bone.

Skin grafts inevitably contract, with the extent of contracture determined by the amount of dermis taken with the graft and the level of postoperative splintage and physiotherapy applied to the grafted site.

CLASSIFICATION

The reconstructive toolbox

Plastic surgery offers a variety of techniques to address clinical problems. Sometimes, a problem is managed using a 'ladder' approach, with the simplest methods being used first and only moving to more complex methods when absolutely necessary. However, this is frequently not the ideal approach for best outcomes. If resources permit, it is often more cost-effective and better functionally for the patient to begin with a more complex treatment, with other easier management options held in reserve as 'lifeboats'. Plastic surgeons now prefer to think of the range of options available as a toolbox from which they can take the most appropriate method to solve a problem, taking into account available skill, resources and the consequences of failure.

The scope of plastic surgery

The tools of reconstruction are used for a wide range of conditions:

- trauma:
  - soft-tissue loss (skin, tendons, nerves, muscle);
  - hand and lower limb injury;
  - faciomaxillary;
  - burns;
- cancer:
  - skin, head and neck, breast, soft tissue sarcoma;
- congenital:
  - clefts and craniofacial malformations;
  - skin, giant naevi, vascular malformations;
  - urogenital;
  - hand and limb malformations;
- miscellaneous:
  - Bell's (facial) palsy;
  - pressure sores;
  - aesthetic surgery;
  - chest wall reconstruction.

Sir Charles Bell, 1774–1842, surgeon, Middlesex Hospital, London, UK and from 1835 until his death, Professor of Surgery, the University of Edinburgh, Edinburgh, UK.

A few key principles that can also be applied to other surgical specialties should be observed. In many reconstructions, success depends upon good rapid wound healing, which itself depends upon attention to detail from the surgeon. Adequate debridement, careful technique, gentle handling of tissues and consideration of blood supply are all key factors that influence outcome (*Table 42.1*).

The placement of incisions can be critical, especially in reducing the appearance of scars on the face and in areas of tension. When possible, incisions should lie in the lines of minimal tension (described by Langer, but frequently different from those originally noted) **(Figure 42.5)**.

TABLE 42.1 Plastic surgery principles.
Optimise wound by adequate debridement or resection
Wound or flap must have a good blood supply to heal
Place scars carefully – 'lines of election'[a]
Replace defect with similar tissue – 'like with like'[b]
Observe meticulous surgical technique
Remember donor site 'cost'

[a]Lines of election – analogous to Langer's lines of minimal skin tension.
[b]Millard DR. *Principalization of plastic surgery*. Boston: Little & Brown, 1986.

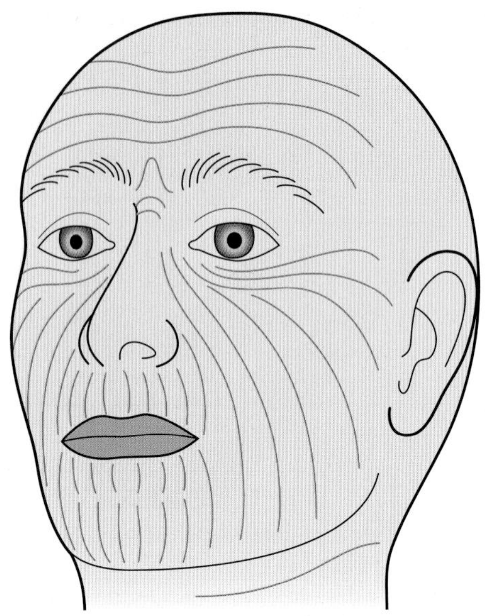

Figure 42.5 Lines of relaxed skin tension.

Grafts

Grafts are tissues that are transferred without their blood supply, which therefore have to revascularise once they are in a new site. They include the following:

- **Split-thickness skin grafts (of varying thickness).** These are sometimes called Thiersch grafts. They are used to cover all sizes of wound, are of limited durability and will contract. They may be used to provide valuable temporary wound closure before better cosmetic secondary correction after rehabilitation.
- **Full-thickness skin grafts (Wolfe grafts).** Used for smaller areas of skin replacement where good elastic skin that will not contract is required (such as fingers, eyelids, facial parts).
- **Composite skin grafts (usually skin and fat, or skin and cartilage).** Often taken from the ear margin and useful for rebuilding missing elements of nose, eyelids and fingertips.

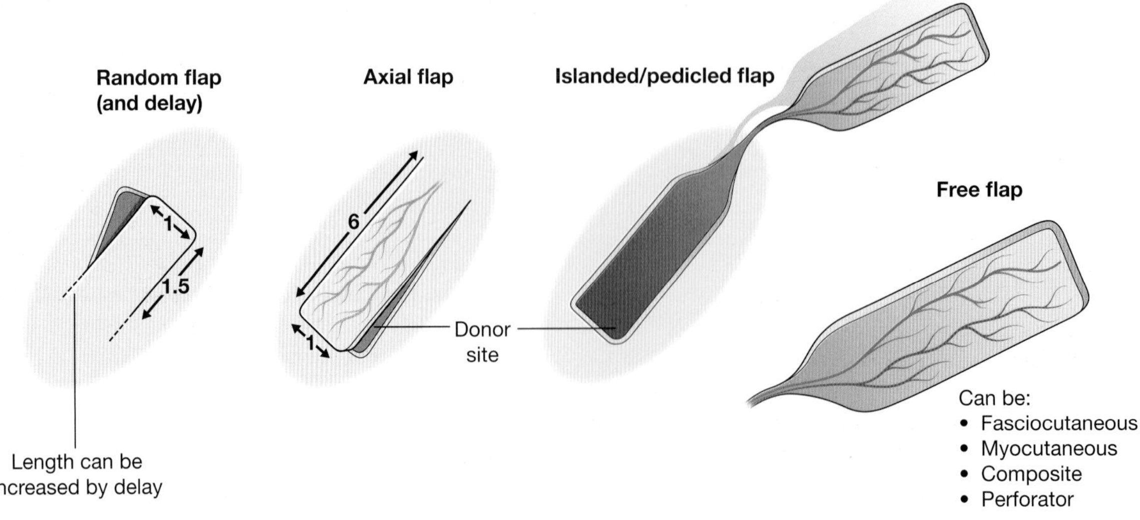

Figure 42.6 Skin flaps, from simple to complex.

Karl Ritter von Edenberg Langer, 1819–1887, Professor of Anatomy, Vienna, Austria described these lines in 1862.
Karl Thiersch, 1822–1895, Professor of Surgery, Leipzig, Germany, pioneer of free skin grafts and described his method of skin grafting in 1874.
John Reissburg Wolfe, 1824–1904, ophthalmic surgeon, Glasgow, UK, described full thickness skin grafts in 1875 and in the same year used forearm skin to construct an eyelid.

- **Nerve grafts**. Usually taken from the sural nerve, but smaller cutaneous nerves may be used.
- **Tendon grafts**. Usually taken from the palmaris longus or plantaris tendon (runs just anteromedial to the Achilles tendon) and used for injury loss or nerve damage correction.

Flaps

Flaps are tissues that are transferred with a blood supply. They therefore have the advantage of bringing vascularity to the new area. Flaps can be raised to consist of any specific tissue; for skin the following will illustrate the types that exist (Figure 42.6):

- **Random flaps**. Three sides of a rectangle, bearing no specific relationship to where the blood supply enters; the length to breadth ratio is no more than 1.5:1. This pattern can be lengthened by 'delaying' the flap, a process in which the cuts are partially made and the flap is part lifted at a first operation; it is then replaced, thus 'training' the blood supply from a single border of the rectangle. At a second procedure, it is raised further and finally transferred.
- **Axial flaps**. Much longer flaps, based on known blood vessels supplying the skin. This technique was rediscovered in the 1960s and 1970s and enables many long thin flaps to be safely moved across large distances.
- **Pedicled/islanded flaps**. The axial blood supply of these flaps means that they can be swung round on a stalk or even fully 'islanded' so that the business end of the skin being transferred can have the pedicle buried (Figure 42.7).
- **Free flaps**. The blood supply has been isolated, disconnected and then reconnected using microsurgery at the new site (Figure 42.8).
- **Composite flaps**. Various tissues are transferred together, often skin with bone or muscle (osseocutaneous or myocutaneous flaps, respectively).
- **Perforator flaps**. This description refers to a whole new subgroup of axial flaps, in which tissues are isolated on small perforating vessels that run from more major blood vessels to supply the surface.

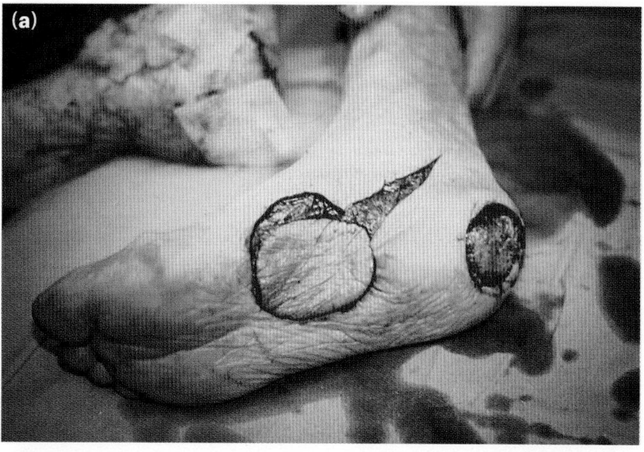

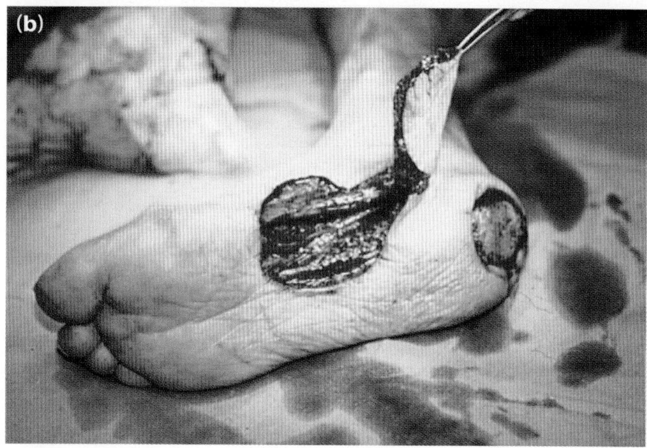

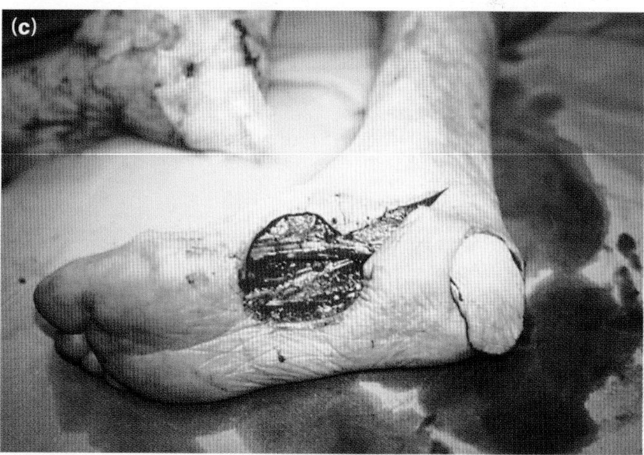

Figure 42.7 (a-c) Islanded pedicled flap used from the instep to resurface a heel defect.

Skin substitutes

One solution to the problem presented by major skin loss with inadequate skin donor sites has been to use artificially engineered skin substitutes. These vary from thin sheets of autologous keratinocytes, to artificial collagen matrices with embedded fibroblasts and a keratinocyte sheet covering. They are costly, but are becoming widely used, and it is likely that tissue-engineered products will continue to be developed in an attempt to solve difficult reconstructive problems.

Tissue expansion

This technique is valuable in using 'local' tissue for reconstruction. The natural ability of tissue to expand has been harnessed clinically since the experiments of Austad and the clinical work of Radovan in the 1970s. It is a technique borrowed from nature, and it is observed during pregnancy when skin expands over the underlying mass. It involves placing a device – usually an expandable balloon constructed from silicone – beneath the tissue to be expanded, and progressively enlarging the volume with fluid while the overlying tissue accommodates to the changed vascular pressure (Figure 42.9). The fluid (usually sterile saline coloured blue in Figure 42.9) is introduced via a self-sealing port attached to a filling tube that enters the balloon. It may be introduced as frequently as can be tolerated by the patient until the tissues are

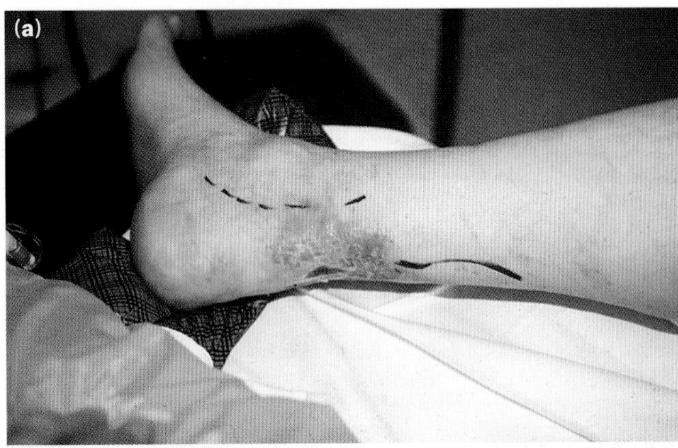

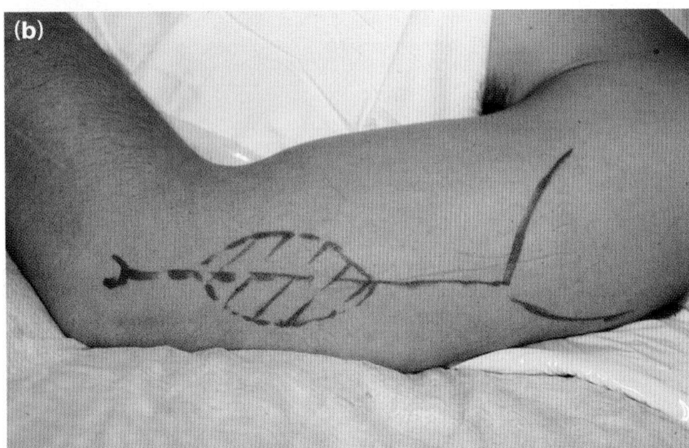

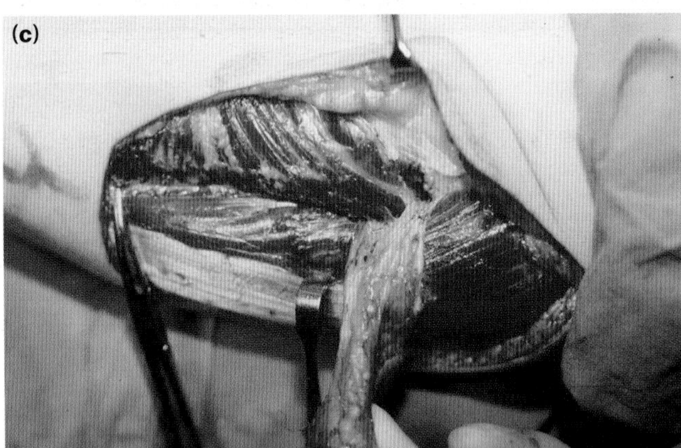

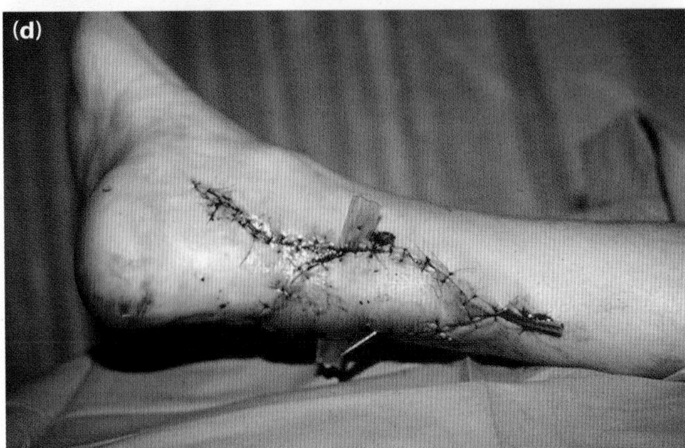

Figure 42.8 (a-d) Free lateral arm fasciocutaneous flap used to resurface a tendo Achilles defect.

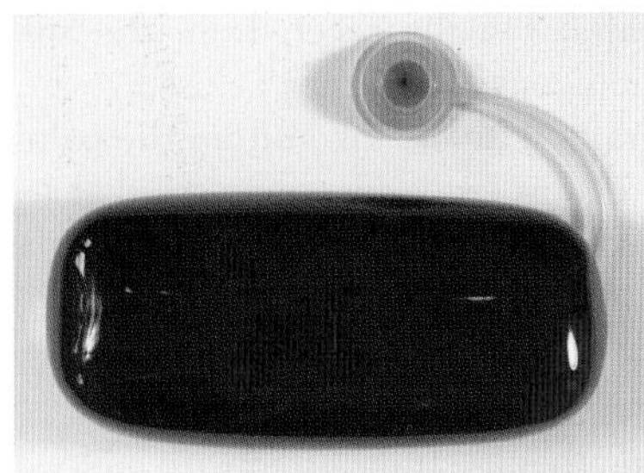

Figure 42.9 Tissue expander.

stretched enough to be used for reconstruction. The tissues expanded do not hypertrophy, but there are major changes in the collagen structure.

The process is time-consuming, although it can be very valuable in problematic cases. It is invaluable for sharing remaining areas of scalp hair after severe burns, removing major congenital skin naevi and restoring full-thickness skin over previously grafted limb wounds.

It must never be used under irradiated tissues (such as mastectomy sites), which will not expand but necrose.

Summary box 42.2

Tissue expansion

Advantages

- Well-vascularised tissue
- Tissue next to defect, so likely to be of similar consistency
- Good colour match

Disadvantages

- Multiple expansion episodes (sometimes painful)
- Cost of device
- High incidence of infection and extrusion (especially limbs)

Vacuum-assisted closure

The use of negative pressure applied to a tissue defect has positive effects on wound closure, as well as making difficult and complex wounds more manageable during the early stages of granulation.

Exudate is removed and the suction pressure affects angiogenesis and tissue regeneration. The technique can be applied as part of early wound management before definitive surgical closure has been planned, or in some cases to avoid the need for surgery altogether. The foam sponge dressing is connected by a tube to a negative pressure pump that can be controlled to give intermittent suction (Figure 42.10).

Implants and prosthetics

Many tissue deficiencies cannot be adequately reconstructed with autologous tissue, however sophisticated the technique used. In such circumstances, implants are part of the reconstructive surgical 'toolbox'; they include solid and soft

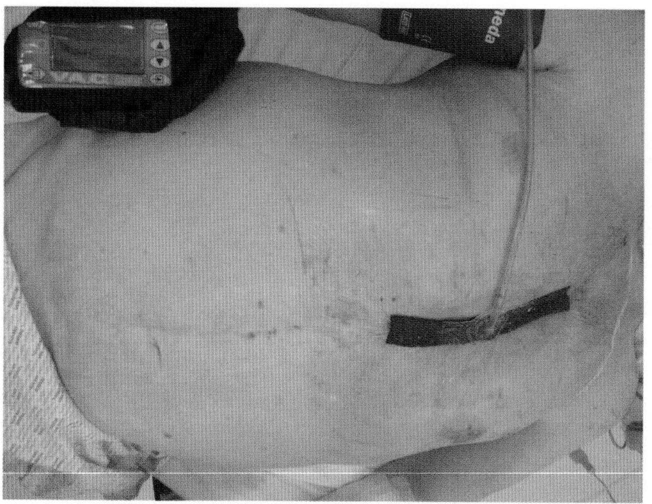

Figure 42.10 VAC™ device used to temporarily close a sternal dehiscence prior to definitive debridement and flap cover.

silicone materials, many forms of filler including collagen and polymers, and osseointegratable anchor points for prosthesis fixation.

Lipofilling and transfer

The use of fat as a reconstructive tissue is longstanding, but has recently become a well-established tool in the armamentarium of plastic surgery. It follows the systematisation of the technique for harvesting and subsequent management of the fat by Sydney Coleman in the late 20th century. Early scepticism for the value of the technique has given way to a recognition that a proportion (variable) of transferred fat can indeed survive injection, and the high volume of stromal and stem cells within fat give it possible advantages for whatever area it is used to manage. Current debate surrounds the best method for each stage in harvesting and preparation, including what preliminary infiltration to use, what dimension cannula is least destructive, whether centrifugation of the aspirate is of value and how best to place the transferred liquid.

The main use for small-volume fat transfer to date has been to provide autologous permanent filling of facial defects and scars. Such small volumes can be harvested and transferred under local anaesthesia, and should be used with care to avoid intravascular escape of fat that can produce emboli and associated injury. Larger volumes of fat have been used to 'lipo-fill' residual defects after conventional breast reconstruction as well as postinjury subcutaneous fat deformities. There is also some evidence that such transfers, rich in stromal and stem cells, have a beneficial effect on the adverse tissue damage induced by radiotherapy, and advances in this area are anticipated.

ASSESSMENT AND DIAGNOSTIC PLANNING

Formation of a definitive treatment plan, carefully considering all available options for care with the whole of the patient's needs in mind, is a vital component of wise plastic surgical practice. This is never more so than when managing major trauma cases in the acute setting or when planning major cancer management, which might be staged over a period of treatments and procedures. If the reconstructive surgeon can be involved in early wound debridement and incisions, vital flap pedicles can be protected and the functional and cosmetic outcome made optimal. This pattern of shared team care has become the norm in many units demonstrating good outcomes from major trauma salvage.

The initial assessment of wounds involves adequate removal of devitalised tissue, assessment of which vital structures will need reconstruction immediately and which might be better reconstructed later, and assessment of the degree of contamination involved, which will require further cleaning. Further planning will include the definitive soft-tissue cover of the wound and functional rehabilitation with full psychosocial rehabilitation.

TREATMENT AND COMPLICATIONS

Split-thickness skin grafts

Split-thickness skin grafts are taken with either hand-held (Figure 42.11) or powered skin knives (Figure 42.12). The most used donor site is the thigh, with the buttock preferable in children and cosmetically sensitive individuals. For larger grafts, almost any flat surface can be harvested, including the scalp if shaved (a very good and useful donor site). The thickness of the graft harvested, ease of graft 'take' and donor site healing must be weighed against the lack of durability of thin split-thickness skin grafts.

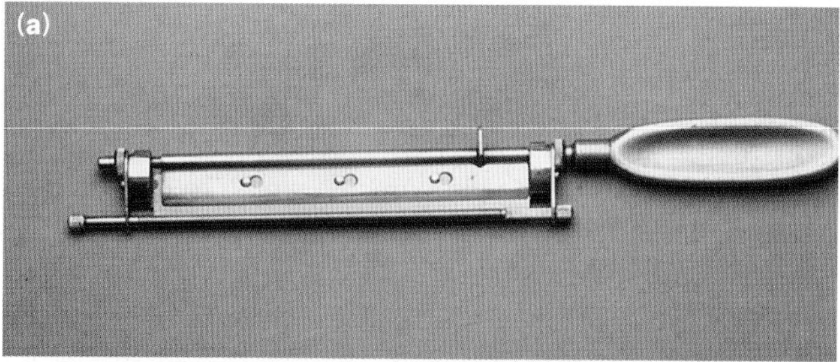

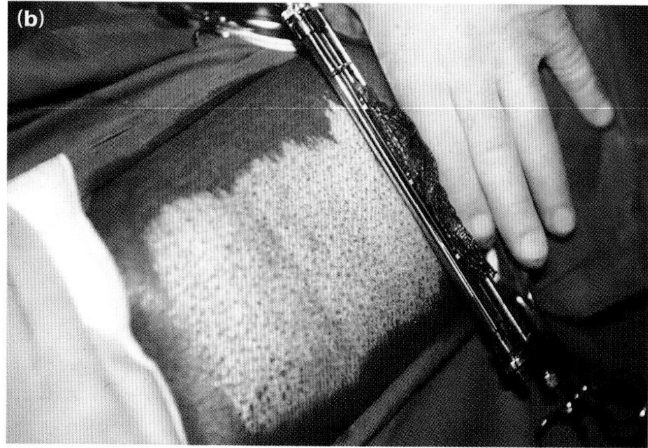

Figure 42.11 Hand-held skin knife (**a**) and harvesting skin with a hand-held knife (**b**).

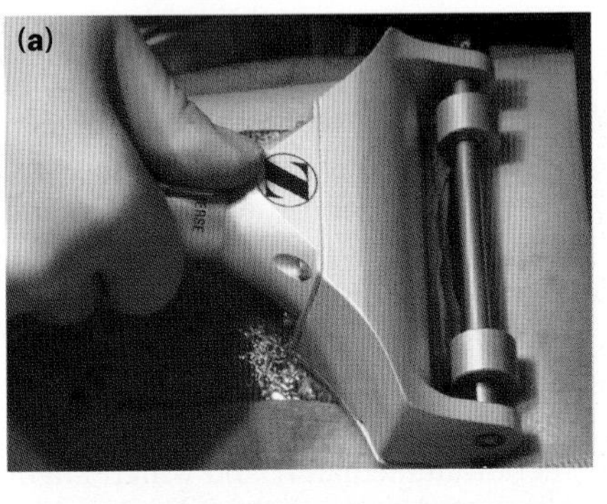
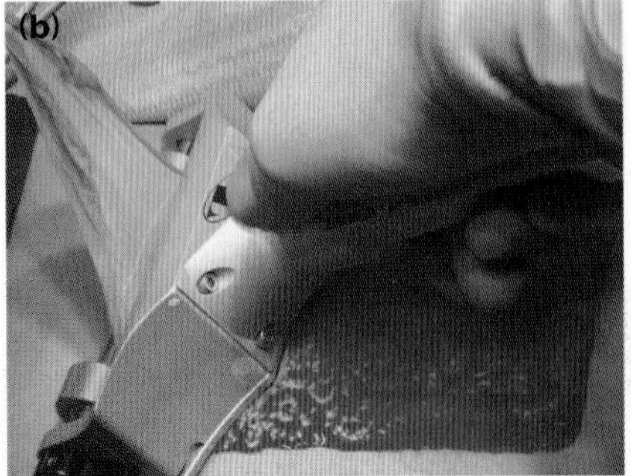
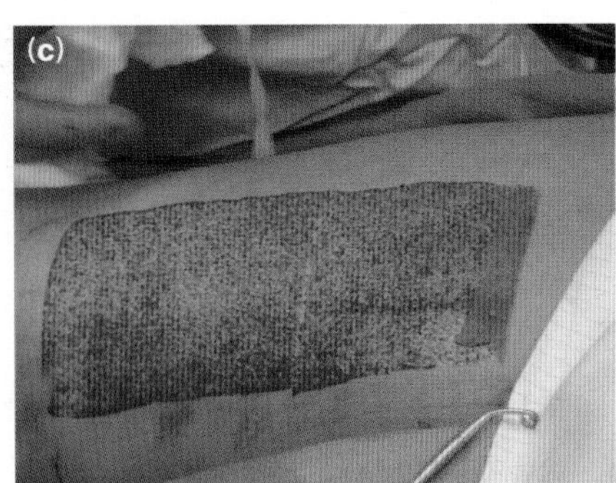
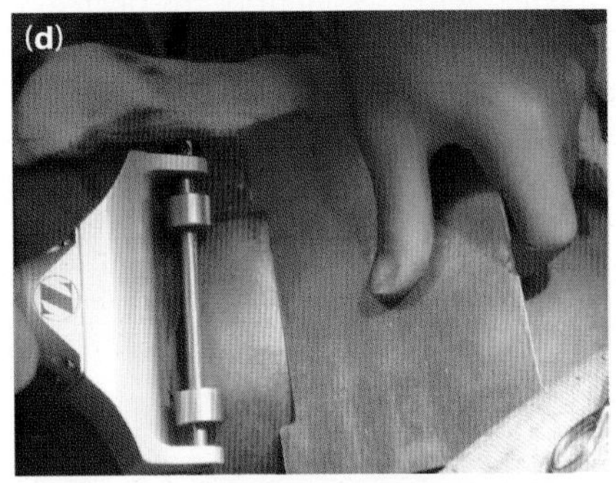
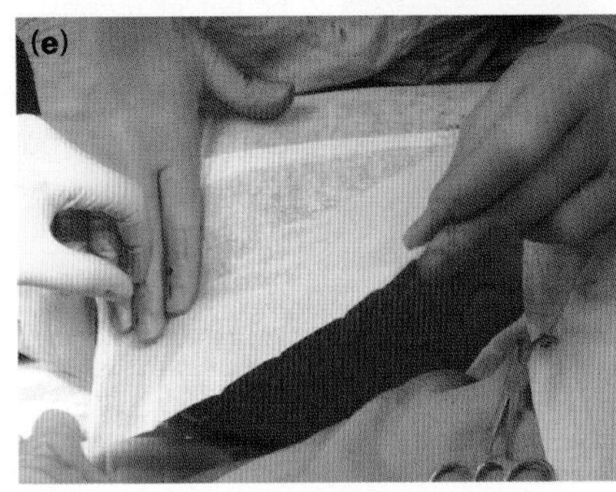

Figure 42.12 Power dermatome harvest of a split-thickness skin graft, with the correct method of providing skin tension (**a–d**), and dressing of the donor site with adhesive material (**e**).

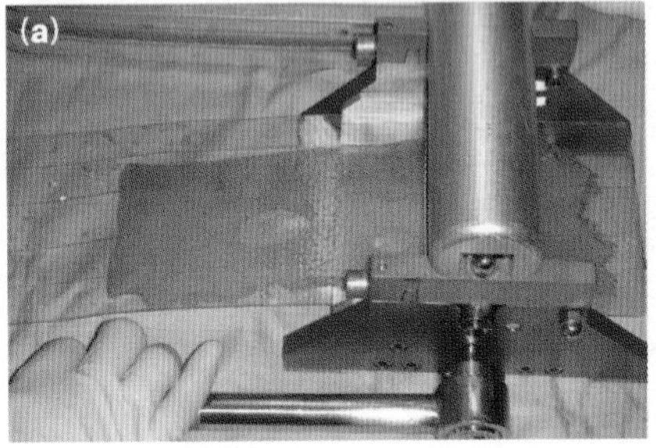
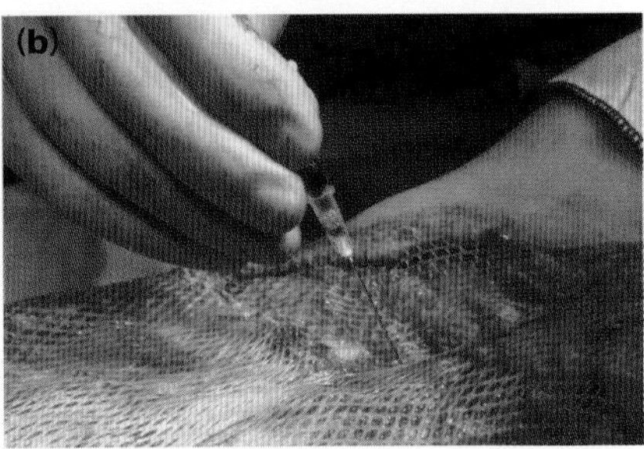

Figure 42.13 Split-thickness skin graft mesher (**a**) and meshed skin applied to the wound (**b**).

Split grafts can be perforated to allow exudates to escape and improve 'take'; they can be further meshed to allow expansion (**Figure 42.13**). This is carried out on a device that cuts a series of slits along the skin, allowing it to expand from a ratio of anything from 1:1.5 to about 1:6.

Grafts will only take on a bed on which they can become vascularised. Preparation of the wound bed is therefore an essential part of a successful graft (**Figure 42.14**). Graft failure is commonly caused by pus, exudate or residual dead tissue beneath the skin, haematoma or shearing forces. A clean healthy wound bed with a meshed graft tied in place to stop movement will encourage success. The group A β-haemolytic *Streptococcus* can destroy split grafts completely (and also convert a donor site to a full-thickness defect) and so the presence of this microorganism is a contraindication to grafting.

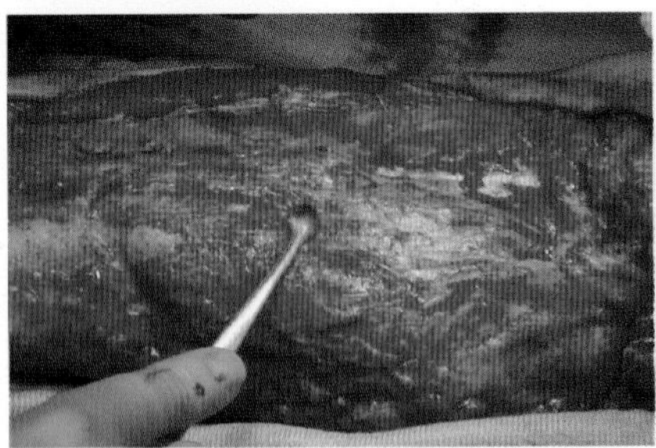

Figure 42.14 Cleaning a wound of excessive granulation tissue before grafting.

Full-thickness skin grafts

Small dermal grafts (Wolfe grafts) can be taken from behind the ear, the groin creases and the neck, with easy direct closure of the donor site. Older people can sustain larger harvests because of skin laxity. Large full-thickness skin graft use is uncommon and requires great care to obtain a good take. Large donor sites require secondary split-thickness skin grafting. Major secondary burn contractures of the face and flexion creases can achieve remarkable functional and cosmetic improvement using such large grafts, particularly as the remaining facial muscle function can still produce a more natural appearance than when covered by a bulky full-thickness skin flap. Smaller full-thickness grafts are useful for contracture release around sensitive facial and extremity structures.

Technique

The shape of the graft needed is drawn and copied onto a small template (paper or cloth), which is used to transfer the same shape to the donor site. Full-thickness skin is cut; grafts take best if additional underlying fat is removed, after which the graft is applied with normal skin tension and tied down with a pressure dressing. The graft will remain vulnerable to shearing forces for several weeks after application.

Flaps

Local flaps

A local flap is raised next to a tissue defect in order to reconstruct it. Basic patterns include (**Figure 42.15**):

- **Transposition flap**. The most basic design, leaving a graftable donor site (**Figure 42.16**);
- **Z-plasty**. For lengthening scars or tissues;
- **Rhomboid flap**. For cheek, temple, back and flat surface defects;
- **Rotation flap**. For convex surfaces;
- **Advancement flap**. For flexor surfaces; may need triangles excised at the base to make it work (commonly called Burow's triangles);
- **V-to-Y advancement**. Commonly used for fingertips and extremities;
- **Bilobed flap**. For convex surfaces, especially the nose (**Figure 42.17**);
- **Bipedicle flap**. For eyelids, rarely elsewhere.

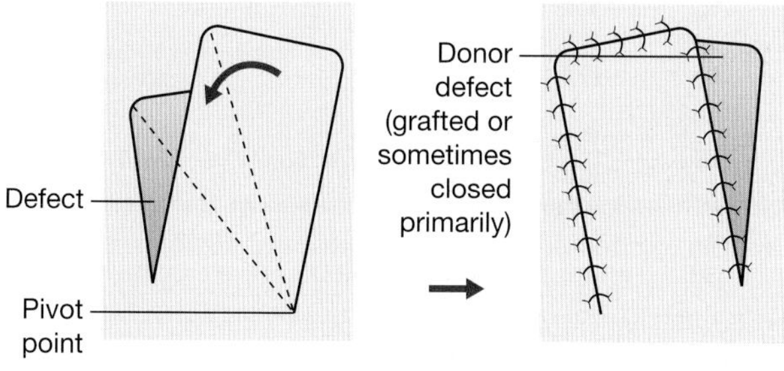

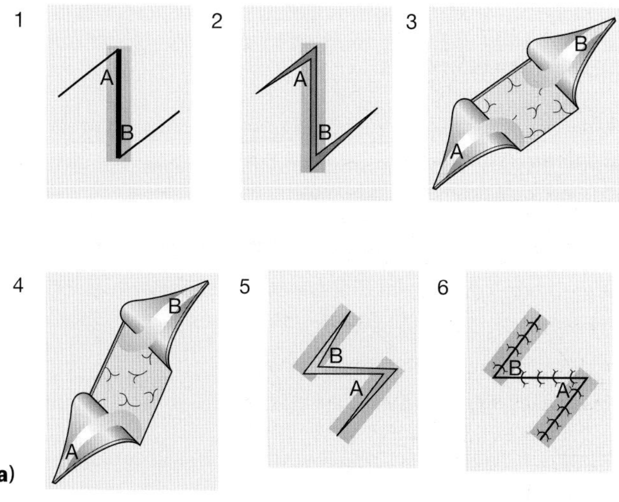

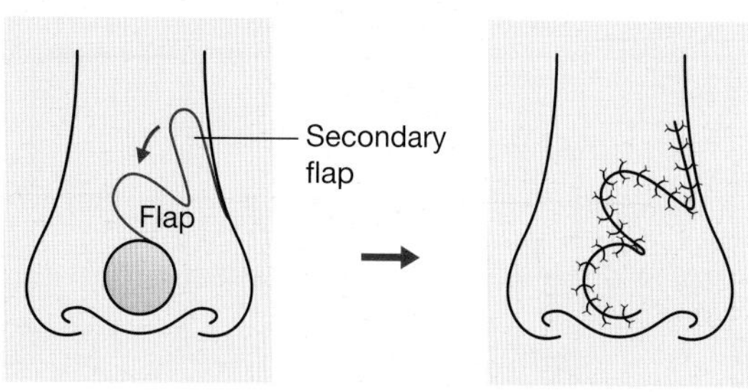

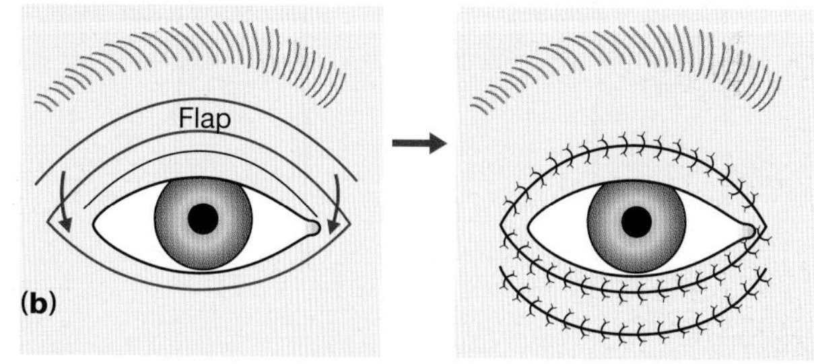

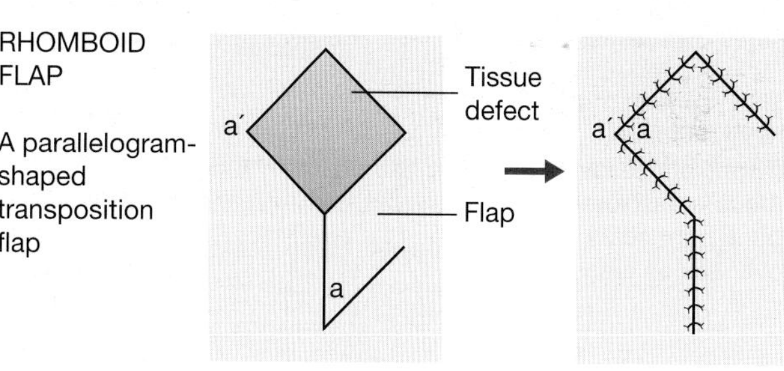

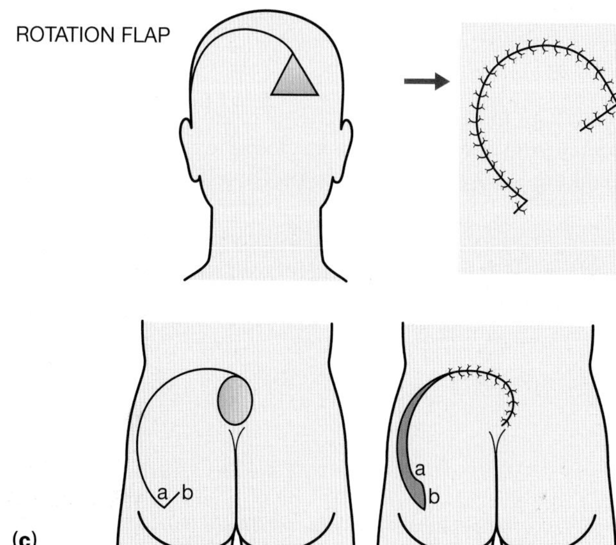

Figure 42.15 Local flap diagrams: (**a**) transposition and Z-plasty flaps; (**b**) bilobed and bipedicled flaps; (**c**) rhomboid and rotation flaps. *(continued overleaf)*

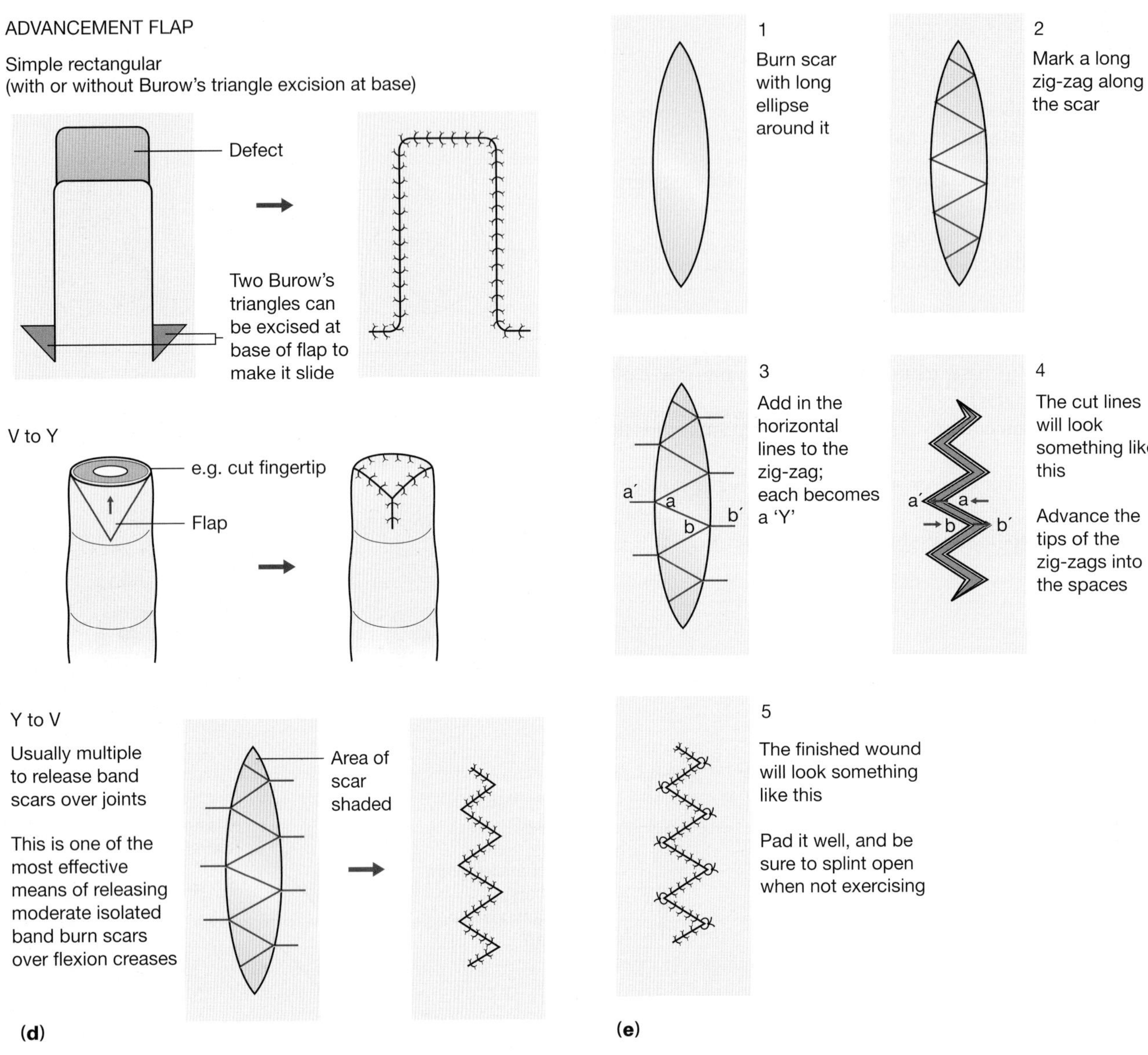

Figure 42.15 (*continued*) Local flap diagrams: (**d**) advancement flaps; (**e**) multiple Y-to-V plasty for burn scar.

All flaps must be raised in the subcutaneous plane. Gentle undercutting of margins helps to close the donor site. The art of making local flaps work is to pull available local spare lax skin into the defect, so that the scar when closed sits in a good 'line of election'. Local flaps are usually not based on specific blood vessels, but are very useful in head and neck and smaller defect reconstructions. Good planning is essential to gain the best result from these flaps.

Summary box 42.3

Local flaps

Benefits

- Best local cosmetic tissue match
- Often a simple procedure
- Local or regional anaesthesia option

Disadvantages

- Possible local tissue shortage
- Scarring may exacerbate the condition
- Surgeon may compromise local resection

Karl August von Burow, 1809–1974, surgeon, Konigsberg, Germany.

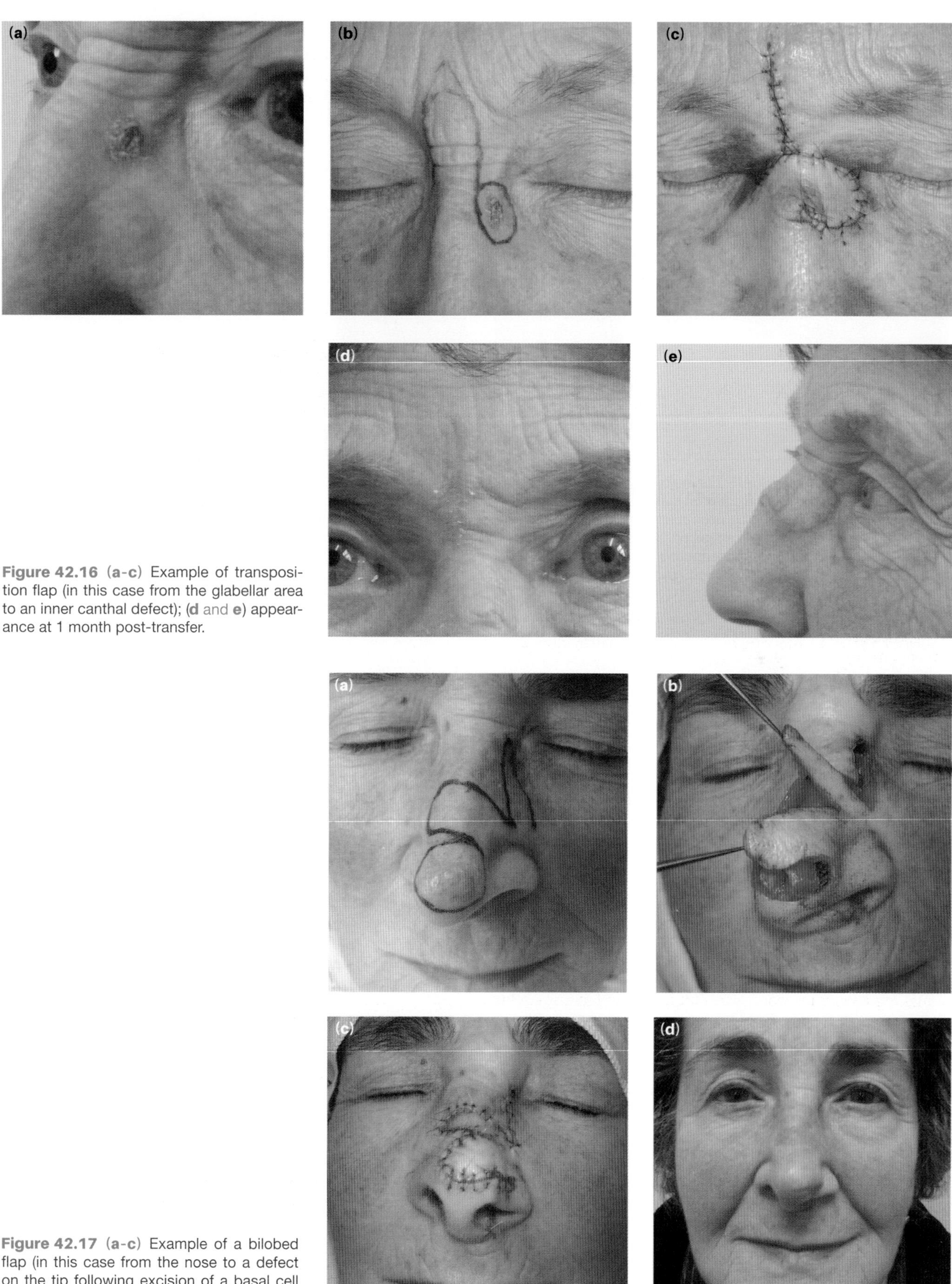

Figure 42.16 (a-c) Example of transposition flap (in this case from the glabellar area to an inner canthal defect); (d and e) appearance at 1 month post-transfer.

Figure 42.17 (a-c) Example of a bilobed flap (in this case from the nose to a defect on the tip following excision of a basal cell carcinoma); (d) appearance at 6 weeks post-transfer.

Combined local flaps

In some circumstances, such as burn contracture release, local flaps can usefully be combined to import surplus tissue from a wide area adjacent to a scar or defect that needs removal. Examples are the W-plasty and the multiple Y-to-V plasty, which is a very versatile means of releasing an isolated band scar contracture over a flexion crease (**Figure 42.18**).

Distant flaps

To repair defects in which local tissue is inadequate, distant flaps can be moved on long pedicles that contain the blood supply. The pedicle may be buried beneath the skin to create an island flap or left above the skin and formed into a tube.

The most common means of moving flaps long distances while still attached are with a long muscular pedicle that contains a dominant blood supply (a myocutaneous flap) (**Figure 42.19**) or with a long fascial layer that likewise contains a major septal blood supply (a fasciocutaneous flap) (**Figure 42.20**). These flaps can carry large composite skin parts for reconstruction very great distances, e.g. from the abdomen to the chest (for breast reconstruction), from the chest to the face (for oral cancer reconstruction) and from the calf to the knee.

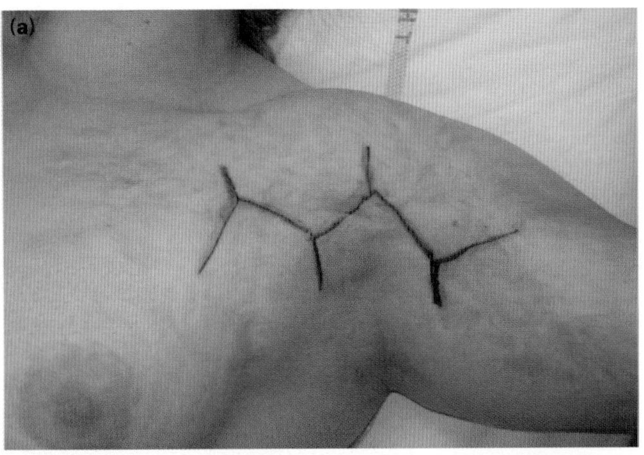
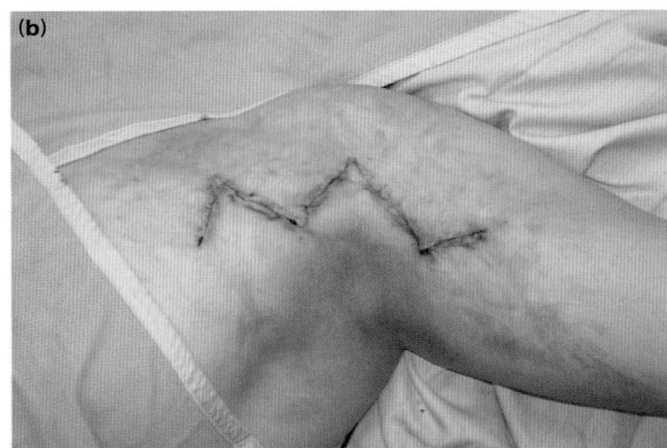

Figure 42.18 **(a, b)** Y-to-V flap to release axillary contracture.

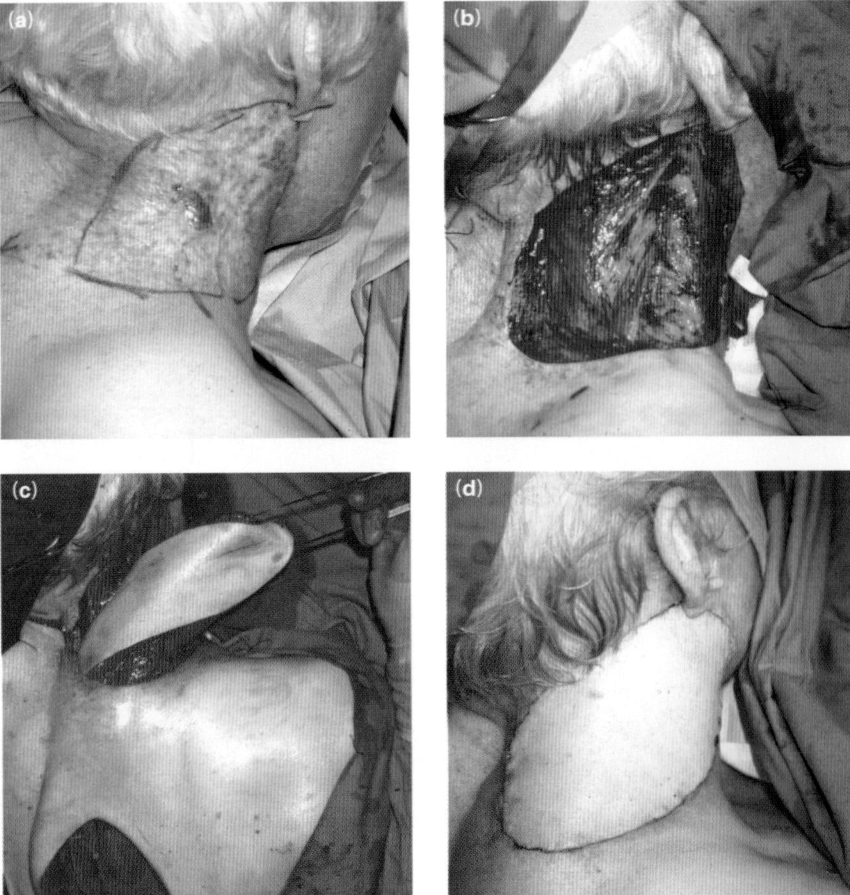

Figure 42.19 **(a–d)** Trapezius pedicled myocutaneous flap to an area of recurrent squamous carcinoma in the neck.

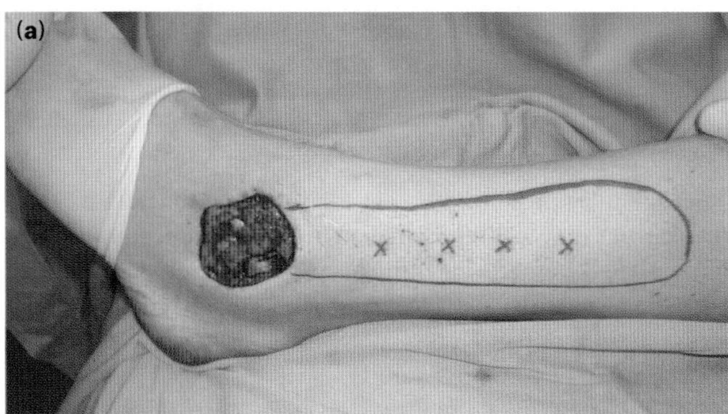

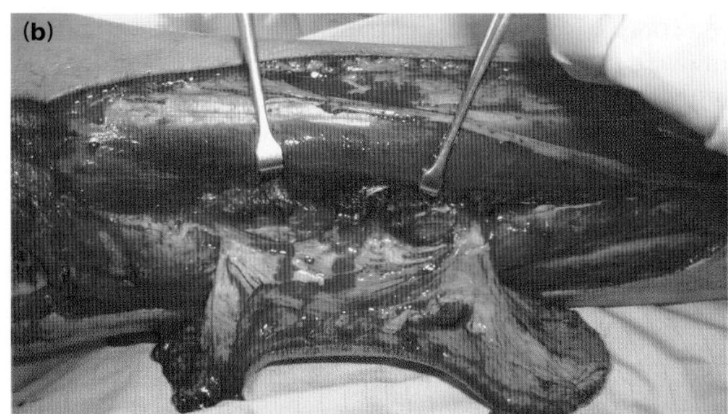

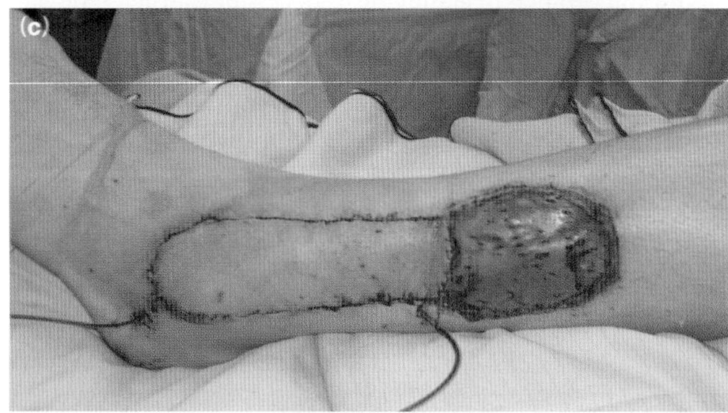

Figure 42.20 (**a**) Defect at the ankle with the flap to be transferred outlined and the position of the perforating vessels (identified with hand-held Doppler device) marked with crosses; (**b**) flap raised with preserved septal perforators to skin paddle clearly visible; (**c**) flap rotated into position to cover the defect; proximal donor defect covered with a split- thickness skin graft (case courtesy of Mr David Johnson FRCS(Plast)).

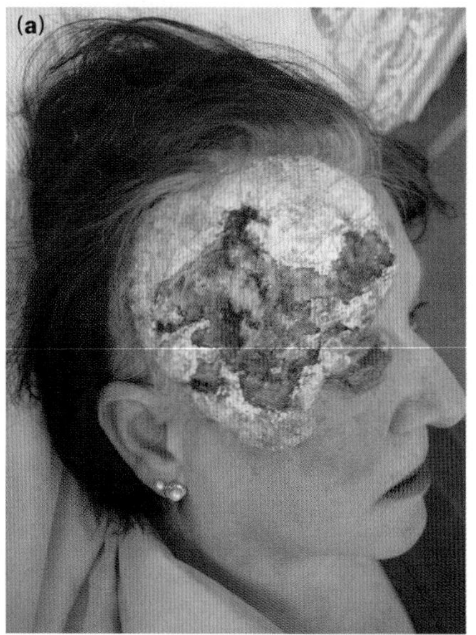

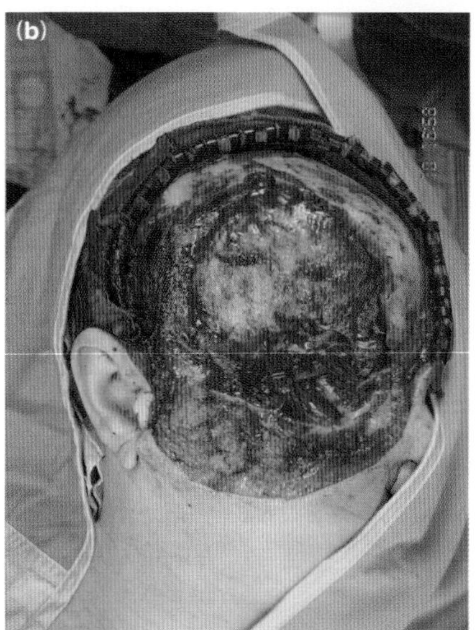

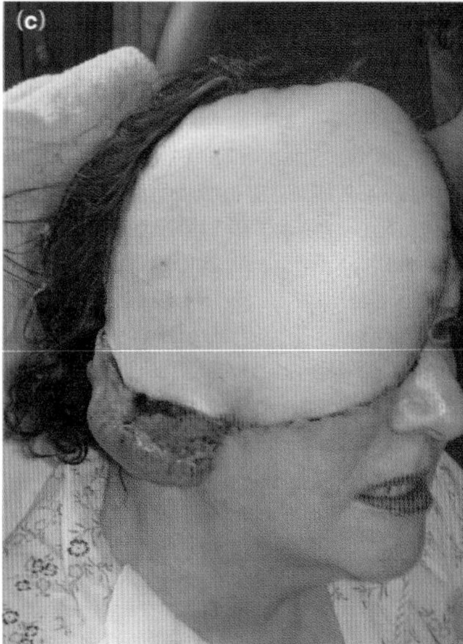

Figure 42.21 (**a–c**) Large myocutaneous free flap (latissimus dorsi) to cover an exposed cranial defect following the excision of advanced basal cell carcinoma (case courtesy of Mr David Johnson FRCS(Plast)).

There are a vast number of carefully described myocutaneous and fasciocutaneous flaps throughout the body, all of which are based on known blood vessels. They are reliable when the anatomy of the blood supply is known by the surgeon and the skin is raised carefully in continuity with the underlying fascia or muscle, through which the small perforating vessels run to supply the piece of skin that is being transferred. They are the 'workhorse' of plastic surgery worldwide because they do not require complex equipment to raise them and they can solve the majority of reconstructive problems.

Microsurgery and perforator flaps

With fine instruments and materials, it has become commonplace to be able to disconnect the blood supply of the flap from its donor site and reconnect it in a distant place using the operating microscope.

The free tissue transfer is now the best means of reconstructing major composite loss of tissue in the face, jaws, lower limb and many other body sites, as long as resources allow it (**Figure 42.21**). The operative procedure is similar whether the defect is newly produced from a recent injury or cancer resection or whether it is to be used for the secondary correction of a deformity, such as rebuilding a mastectomy deformity. At the site of the defect, the surgeon must be sure that all contaminated and dead tissue has been thoroughly cleared and cleaned, a process commonly described as debridement, although that term strictly refers to the release of constricting tissue. If this removal of poorly viable tissue is in doubt, then consideration should be given to delaying the reconstruction.

The surgeon must then find a suitable blood supply for the tissue transfer at the site to be reconstructed. A good arterial flow in and venous return out, without external tissue pressure (such as from surrounding wound induration), is of paramount importance in achieving a successful transfer. The flap is then raised (*Table 42.2*) and transferred using magnification (**Figure 42.22**). Free muscle transfers should be reanastomosed within 1–2 hours if possible; fasciocutanous flaps are more robust and can survive slightly greater ischaemic times.

TABLE 42.2 Common free tissue transfer donor sites.

Muscle only	Latissimus dorsi Rectus abdominis Gracilis
Myocutaneous	Latissimus dorsi Transverse rectus abdominis
Fasciocutaneous	Radial forearm flap Scapular Lateral arm Anterolateral thigh Groin
Osseous	Fibula (may be cutaneous as well) Forearm (taking sliver of radius bone) Iliac crest
Fascial	Temporoparietal
Miscellaneous	Jejunum – for oesophageal reconstruction Pectoralis minor – for facial reanimation Omentum – for chest wall and limb defects

Summary box 42.4

Free tissue transfer (or free flap)

Advantages

- Being able to select exactly the best tissue to move
- Only takes what is necessary
- Minimises donor site morbidity

Disadvantages

- More complex surgical technique
- Failure involves total loss of all transferred tissue
- Usually takes more time unless the surgeon is experienced

Further developments have led to surgeons dissecting distant flaps free from the carrier muscle or fascia, to reduce the donor morbidity further. These distant 'perforator' flaps increase the flexibility of the use of the flap tissue while reducing donor site problems. Flap design has moved towards delivering individualised tissue transfers that are customised to cater for the specific reconstructive and aesthetic requirements of treatment. This has led to numerous combinations of tissue raised on common vascular pedicles (**Figure 42.23**).

Combined flaps

The difficulty presented by defects needing multiple parts to reconstruct is now often managed using various forms of 'combined flap'. These use parts fully separated (but blood supplied by a single vascular pedicle) in order to make reconstruction more flexible and therefore not only better functioning but also cosmetically more accurate.

'Conjoined' flaps have two or more 'territories' of tissue supplied by separate pedicles. These may be conjoined by skin in continuity at the extremes of each pedicle's reach (such as the raising of a latissimus dorsi flap in continuity with a groin flap with a pedicle at each end), or be separate perforator-based territories on the same 'mother' blood supply.

'Chimeric' flaps again have multiple flap territories, each with an independent vascular supply, but are independent of any physical connection except when they are linked by a common feeder vascular pedicle (**Figure 42.22**). Such flaps have become amongst the most widely used, in circumstances when several elements of soft tissue need reconstructing, along with perhaps a bony element as well as a functional muscle transfer. The antero-lateral thigh flap is very amenable to separation into several parts and muscle elements, as is the scapular/subscapular array of flaps.

The chimeric principle can be extended yet further by the joining of additional flaps to the main flap-feeding vessels using microsurgical anastomosis. This is to prefabricate the most suitable tissue element for the reconstructive purpose in hand, which although requiring considerable technical expertise to accomplish, can achieve excellent outcomes in single-staged procedures.

Supermicrosurgery

In the last decade, Koshima's description of anastomosing vessels with a diameter of 0.8 mm or less has been utilised to improve on perforator flap donor site morbidity, as well as speed of flap harvest. So-called 'perforator to perforator' anastomoses can make reconstruction very accurate in skilled hands. It begins to make the previously constrained selection of flap donor sites and recipient vessels redundant, with terms such as 'free style free flap' being coined to describe such versatility in reconstructive work.

The technique has also been used to advance the art of lymphatico-venous anastomosis to treat lymphoedema. In correctly selected cases and with good facilities, such surgery has begun to offer new therapeutic options to those with chronically morbid conditions.

Care of flaps and monitoring

After a flap has been moved, it should be observed for tissue colour, warmth and turgor, and be pressed to assess blanching and capillary refill time. Loss of arterial inflow results in pale, cold, flaccid tissue; loss of venous outflow results in blue congestion, increased turgor, rapid capillary refill and initially a warm flap. In a pedicled flap, such venous congestion may be relieved by releasing suture tension; applying leeches to suck out excess venous blood is a last resort when no other means of restoring venous drainage can be obtained.

The most common causes of flap failure are:

- poor anatomical knowledge when raising the flap (such that the blood supply is deficient from the start);
- flap inset with too much tension;
- local sepsis or a septicaemic patient;
- the dressing applied too tightly around the pedicle;
- microsurgical failure in free-flap surgery (usually caused by problems with surgical technique);
- tobacco smoking by patient.

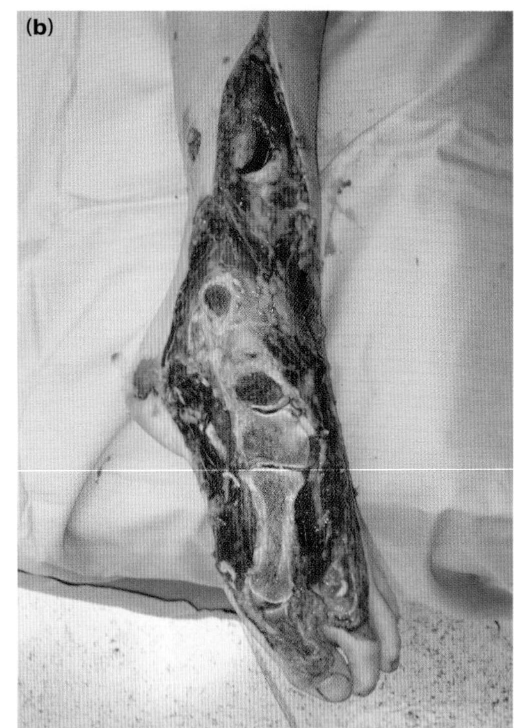

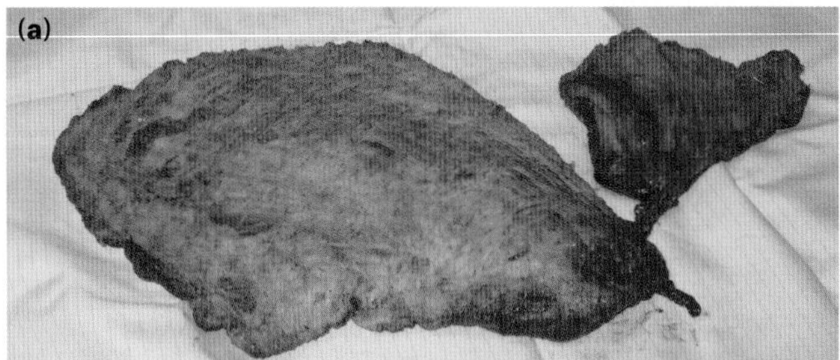

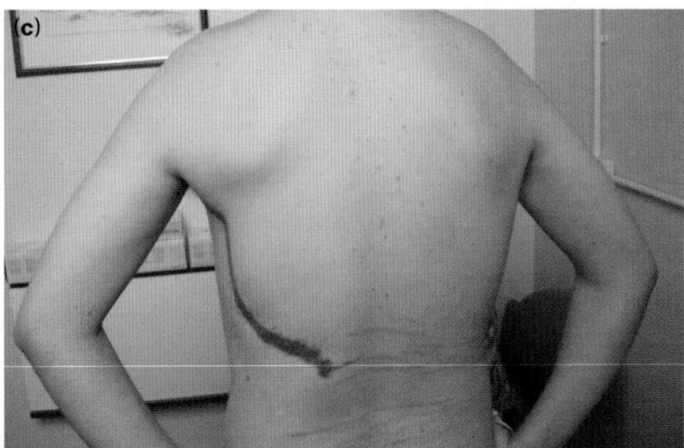

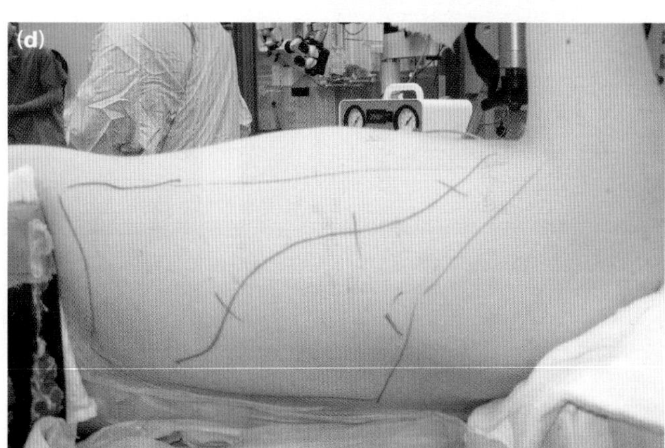

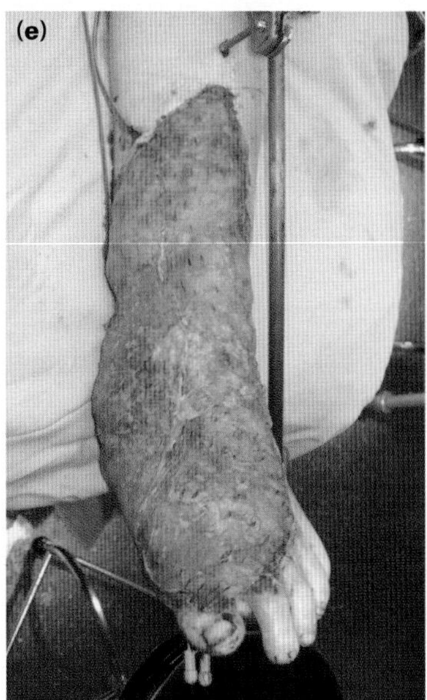

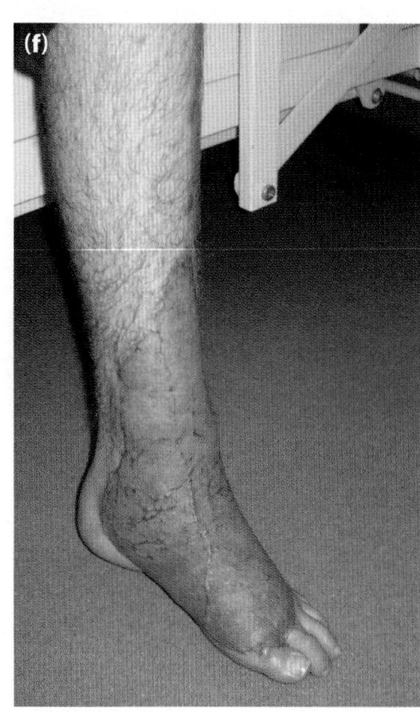

Figure 42.22 Large 'chimeric flap' of latissimus dorsi and serratus anterior muscles (**a**), to cover a complex open wound of the foot and ankle (**b**), illustrating the donor site (**c, d**) and fully covered defect (**e, f**) (case courtesy of Mr David Johnson FRCS(Plast)).

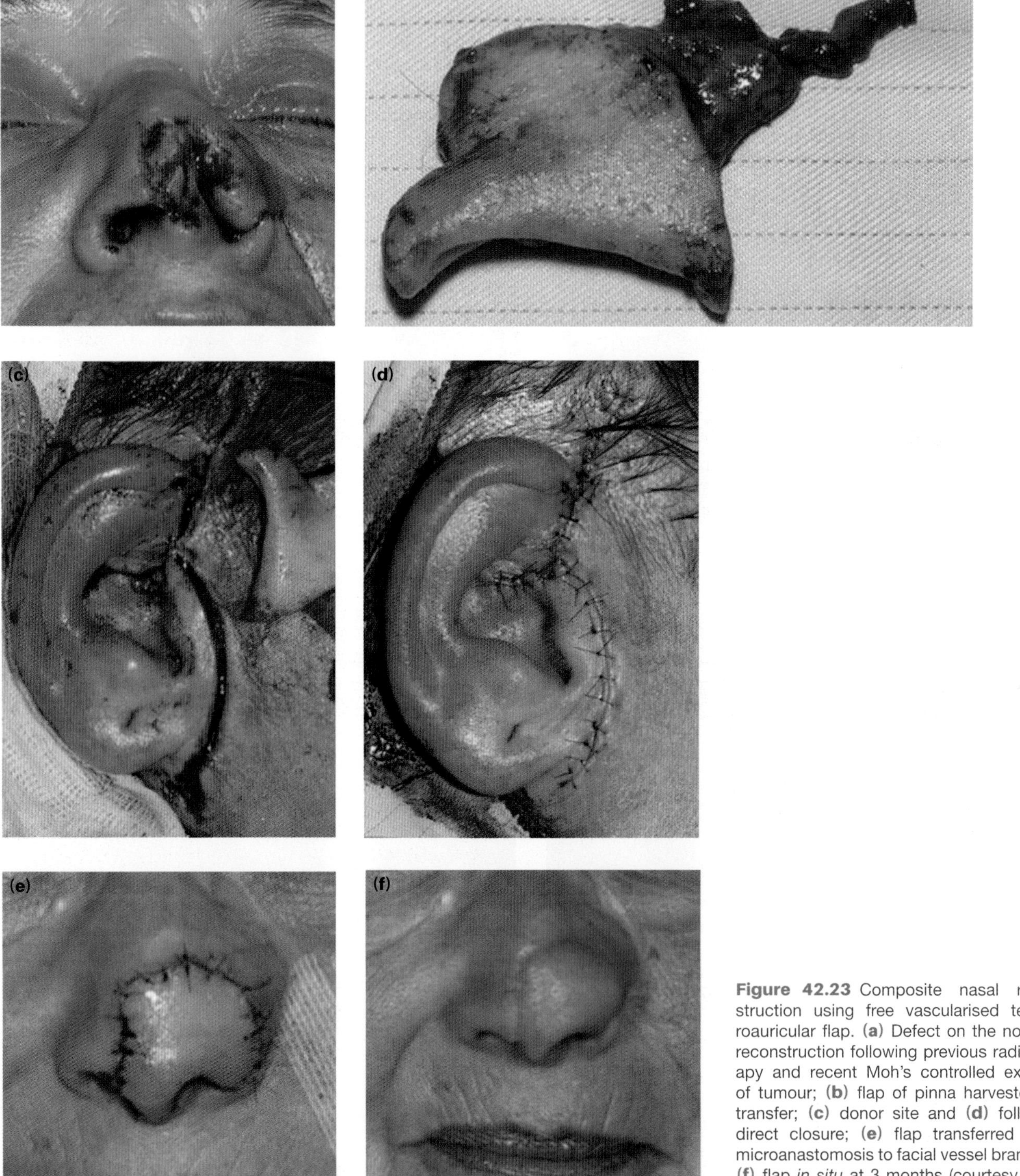

Figure 42.23 Composite nasal reconstruction using free vascularised temporoauricular flap. **(a)** Defect on the nose for reconstruction following previous radiotherapy and recent Moh's controlled excision of tumour; **(b)** flap of pinna harvested for transfer; **(c)** donor site and **(d)** following direct closure; **(e)** flap transferred using microanastomosis to facial vessel branches; **(f)** flap *in situ* at 3 months (courtesy of Mr Henk Giele, FRACS).

'Wet, warm and comfortable'

The best advice for postoperative flap care for major tissue transfers is to keep the patient 'wet, warm and comfortable'. This means that the patient should be well hydrated with a hyperdynamic circulation, a very warm body temperature and well-controlled analgesia to reduce catecholamine output.

Reconstructing complex areas

Certain areas, such as the eyelids, nose, lips, ears, genitalia, fingers, breast and intraoral structures, often require a combination of methods to produce the most functional and acceptable outcome for the patient. Planning such reconstruction involves considering each cosmetic subunit involved in the defect and bringing the best tissue to rebuild it. An example is the Indian forehead rhinoplasty of Sushruta, which involves transposition of a pedicled fasciocutaneous flap from forehead to nose, with the donor site usually thin skin grafted, but occasionally closed primarily in small flaps. It remains the finest means of transporting cosmetically correct tissue to the nose.

FUTURE TRENDS

Vascularised composite allografting (VCA)

Plastic surgeons have long sought to use transplanted tissue to solve the problems posed by the most severe tissue defects. Esser, in the early twentieth century, pioneered much innovative surgery and urged research into this area. Later, Joe Murray, a plastic surgeon in the United States, undertook the first kidney transplant and was awarded the Nobel Prize for his work. Improved understanding of immunology and means of tolerance induction are now leading to the use of transplanted composite tissues for the most intractable cases of loss of tissue following injury and cancer.

In the latter part of the 20th century, the constraints of total systemic immunosuppression alongside the difficulties in overcoming the inherent problems of cutaneous immunosensitivity led to transplants being confined predominantly to solid organs in clinical practice.

Recent refinements in immune suppression therapy and anticipated advances in tolerance induction strategies have opened the door to the use of more complex transplants including skin for non-life-threatening disorders. The first hand transplant was performed in Lyon, France in 1998, and limb transplantation now has an established place in reconstructive plastic surgery. Other composite allografts have followed, including facial tissue and abdominal wall reconstruction (Figure 42.24).

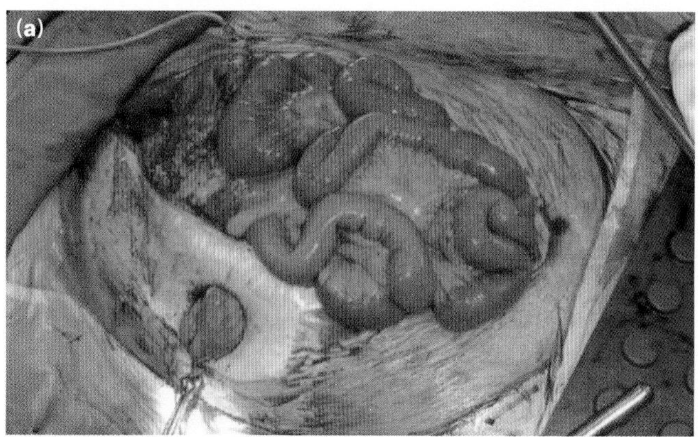

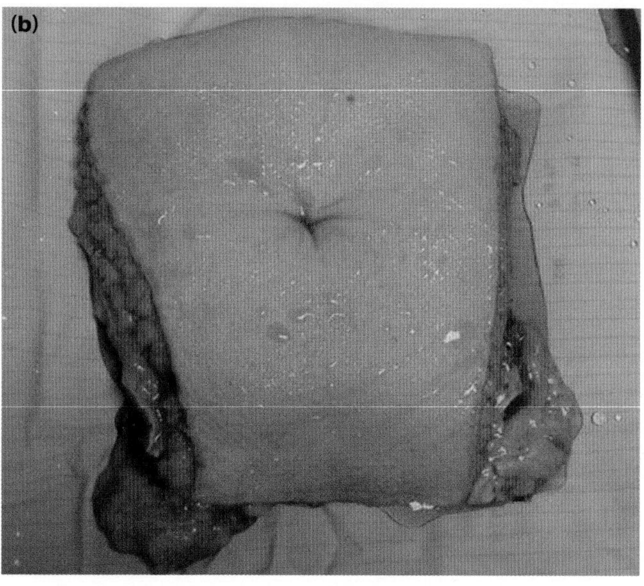

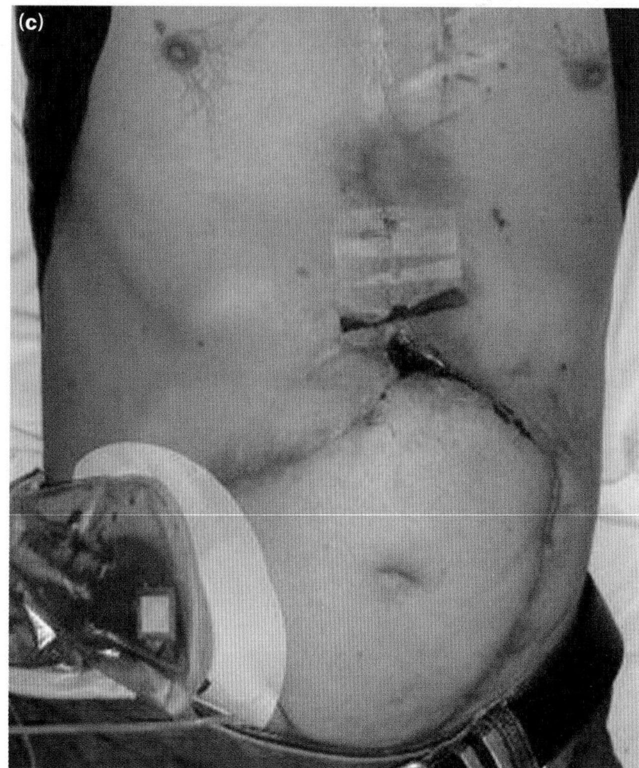

Figure 42.24 Abdominal wall transplant: **(a)** open abdomen with transplanted small bowel that cannot be closed using the patient's own skin cover; **(b)** donor transplant abdominal wall element harvested; **(c)** abdominal wall with transplant *in situ* (courtesy of Mr Henk Giele, FRACS).

Johannes Fredericus Samuel Esser, 1877–1946, born in Leyden, Netherlands. He was a Dutch plastic surgeon who pioneered reconstructive surgery on soldiers wounded in the First World War and is thought to have coined the term 'stent' in 1917 to describe his use of a dental impression compound invented in 1856 by the English dentist Charles Stent (1807–1885) to create a form for facial reconstruction.

Joseph E Murray, b.1919, Professor Emeritus of Plastic Surgery, Harvard University Medical School, Boston, MA, USA, shared the 1990 Nobel Prize for Physiology or Medicine with E Donnall Thomas for his work on organ and cell transplantation. Murray's interest in transplantation began during his military service in the Second World War. The early experiences with skin transplantation for burns in pilots formed the basis for Murray's interest in solid organ transplantation. He performed the world's first kidney transplantation in identical twins in Peter Brent Brigham Hospital, Boston in 1954.

As immunotolerance strategies develop (especially the probable use of TReg cell therapy in some form or other) it is likely that there will be a burgeoning of microsurgically transferred VCAs to facilitate complex reconstruction throughout the body. This will precede the development of more sophisticated tissue engineered substitutes that are decades away from use for more complex composite tissue reconstructions.

Tissue and bioengineering

Improved understanding of tissue behaviour is leading to numerous innovations in wound manipulation using biological mechanisms. Tissue-engineered biological substitutes for tendon, nerve, larynx and other vital structures are becoming established, and will greatly influence the spectrum of reconstructive procedures in the coming years (see Chapter 4).

Novel polymers and biologically tolerated materials are also being developed to act as nerve conduits, facial muscle substitutes and self-inflating expansion devices. The interface of new material science with reconstructive surgery is still in its infancy.

FURTHER READING

Achauer BM, Erikson E, Guruyon R *et al.* (eds). *Plastic surgery indications, operations and outcomes*, vols 1–5. St Louis: Mosby, 2000.

Cormack GC, Lamberty BGH. *The arterial anatomy of skin flaps*. Edinburgh: Churchill Livingstone, 1986.

Geddes CR, Morris SF, Neligan PC. Perforator flaps: evolution, classification, and applications. *Ann Plastic Surg* 2003; **50**: 90–9.

Koshima I, Soeda S. Inferior epigastric artery skin flaps without rectus abdominis muscle. *Br J Plastic Surg* 1989; **42**: 645–8.

MacGregor AD, MacGregor IA. *Fundamental techniques in plastic surgery*, 10th edn. Edinburgh: Churchill Livingstone, 2000.

Mustarde JC, Jackson IT. *Plastic surgery in infancy and childhood*. Edinburgh: Churchill Livingstone, 1988.

Nabri IA. El Zahrawi (936–1013), the father of operative surgery. *Ann R Coll Surg Engl* 1983; **65**: 132–4.

Neligan P C (ed). *Plastic surgery, 3rd edn*, vols 1–6. Philadelphia: Saunders, 2012.

Wei F-C, Mardini S. *Flaps and reconstructive surgery, 1st edn*. Philadelphia: Saunders, 2010. ISBN 978-0721605197.

Weinzweig J. *Plastic surgery secrets plus*. St Louis: Mosby, 2010.

PART 7

Head and Neck

43	Cranial neurosurgery	652
44	The eye and orbit	672
45	Cleft lip and palate: developmental abnormalities of the face, mouth and jaws	686
46	The ear, nose and sinuses	703
47	Pharynx, larynx and neck	725
48	Oral cavity malignancy	760
49	Disorders of the salivary glands	776

Chapter 43

Cranial neurosurgery

Learning objectives

- To recognise the features of raised intracranial pressure, hydrocephalus and infection typical to acute neurosurgical presentations.
- To be familiar with aneurysmal subarachnoid haemorrhage and other causes of intracranial haemorrhage.
- To recognise common brain tumours, their presentation, investigation and treatment.
- To be aware of common developmental and other pathologies encountered in paediatric neurosurgical practice.
- To understand the indications and approaches available for the management of epilepsy, pain syndromes and movement disorders.
- To note key practical and ethical issues relating to consent and risks, Creutzfeldt–Jacob disease (CJD) precautions and diagnosis of brainstem death.

RAISED INTRACRANIAL PRESSURE

The importance of intracranial pressure (ICP) management in the context of head injury has been discussed elsewhere (Chapter 24). Likewise, intracranial pressure is key to presentation and management across the spectrum of cranial neurosurgery.

Clinical features of raised ICP

Symptoms of raised ICP include a 'high pressure headache', worse on coughing or bending forward; low pressure headaches, encountered after excessive cerebrospinal fluid (CSF) drainage, are typically worse on standing. High pressure headaches may be accompanied by nausea and vomiting, blurred vision and double vision; cranial nerve compression can result in eye movement and pupil abnormalities. Fundoscopy can detect papilloedema (Figure 43.1), but this takes time to develop so may be absent in the acute phase.

In infants, the fontanelle is tense and bulging, with an increase in head circumference and bulging scalp veins. As pressure rises, conscious level is impaired. In children Parinaud's syndrome results from dorsal midbrain compression, with a loss of upgaze known as sunsetting (Figure 43.2).

Raised ICP requires urgent evaluation and management: delay risks progression to cerebral herniation (see Chapter 24) resulting in cardiovascular instability, neurological deficit and death. Vision may also deteriorate rapidly and irreversibly.

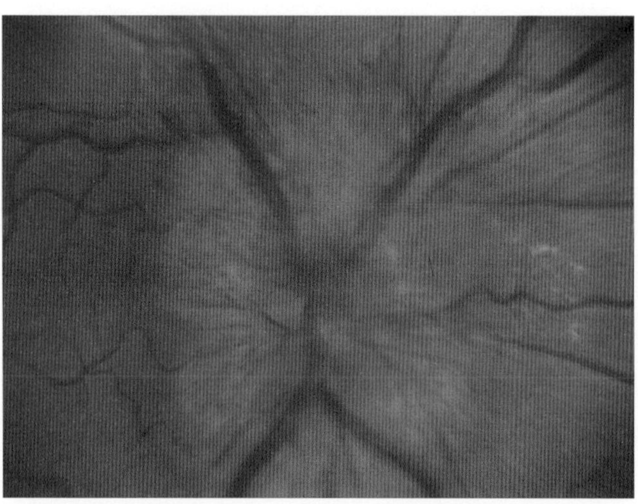

Figure 43.1 Papilloedema. The optic disc is swollen with blurred margins.

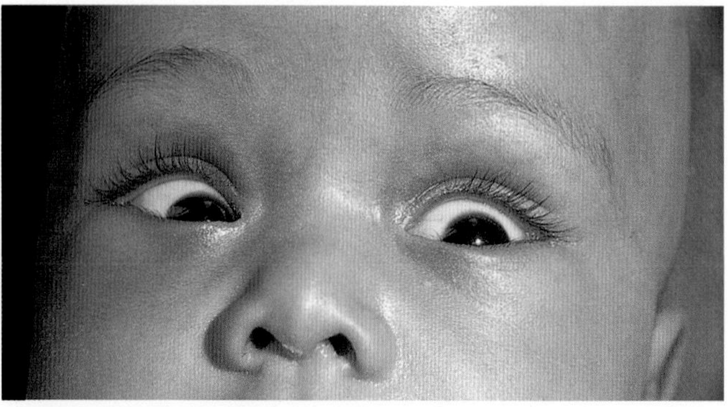

Figure 43.2 Parinaud's syndrome with sunsetting.

Investigation of raised ICP

Causes of raised ICP include mass lesions, cerebral oedema and hydrocephalus. Where raised ICP is suspected, computed tomography (CT) is a first line investigation to demonstrate these and other pathologies, and to evaluate the degree of mass effect and the patency of the basal cisterns, the spaces surrounding the brainstem. This is key to management since lumbar puncture in the setting of raised ICP can result in downward herniation of brain structures. Many pathologies, as well as the anatomy relating to potential treatments such as third ventriculostomy, may be better visualised on magnetic resonance imaging (MRI). Where high pressure is suspected but not clearly demonstrated by imaging, ICP monitoring by placement of a transducer in the brain substance allows continuous monitoring over hours or days (Figure 43.3).

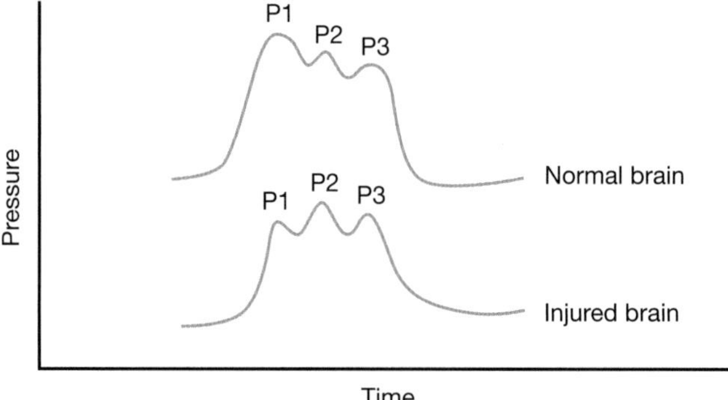

Figure 43.3 The intracranial pressure waveform. The P1 percussion wave corresponds to arterial pulsation. Reduced brain compliance in the setting of traumatic brain injury among others is associated with a prominent P2 tidal wave. The P3 dicrotic wave represents venous pulsation.

Summary box 43.1

Raised intracranial pressure

Acutely raised ICP is a neurological emergency. The presentation includes:

- Headache
- Nausea and vomiting
- Diplopia and blurred vision
- Drowsiness then coma

HYDROCEPHALUS

The total CSF volume is normally about 150 mL. Production from the walls of the ventricles and the choroid plexus is about 20 mL per hour. Hydrocephalus refers to an increase in CSF volume with ventricular enlargement, often presenting symptoms of raised ICP.

Physiology of CSF flow

CSF flows from the lateral ventricles through the foramen of Monro to the third ventricle, then down the cerebral aqueduct to the fourth ventricle, where it exits to the subarachnoid space via the midline foramen of Magendie and the lateral foramina of Luschka (Figure 43.4). CSF is reabsorbed into the arachnoid villi along the superior sagittal sinus.

Obstructive and communication hydrocephalus

Hydrocephalus almost always reflects obstruction to circulation (an obstructive hydrocephalus) or failure of reabsorption (a communicating hydrocephalus) (*Table 43.1*) (Figures 43.5–43.7). The distinction is important since obstructive hydrocephalus especially can cause very

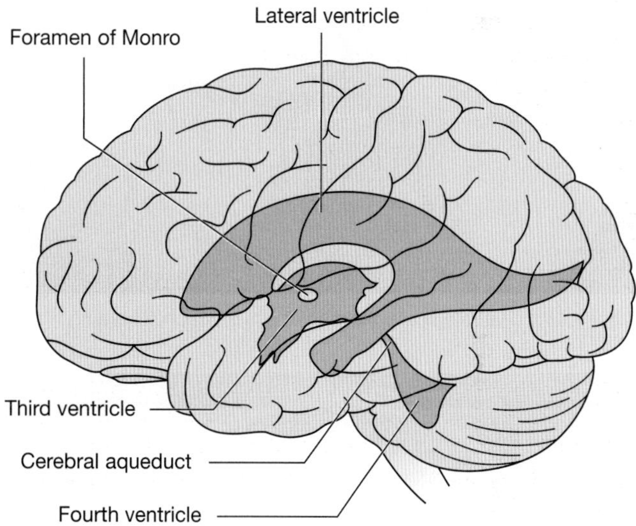

Figure 43.4 'CSF pathways'. Cerebrospinal fluid (CSF) is produced by the choroid plexus of the lateral ventricles and flows through the ventricular system to exit into the subarachnoid space through the foramina of Magendie and Luschka in the fourth ventricle.

TABLE 43.1 Aetiology of hydrocephalus.

Obstructive hydrocephalus	Lesions within the ventricle
	Lesions in the ventricular wall
	Lesions distant from the ventricle but with a mass effect
Communicating hydrocephalus	Post haemorrhagic
	CSF infection
	Raised CSF protein
Excessive CSF production (rare)	Choroid plexus papilloma/ carcinoma

CSF, cerebrospinal fluid.

Alexander Monro, 1733–1817, Professor of Anatomy at Edinburgh University, a post also held by his father, Alexander Monro (primus), and son, Alexander Monro (tertius)

Francois Magendie, 1783–1855, physician and Professor of Pathology and Physiology, Paris, also described the Magendie sign, a downward and inward rotation of the eye due to a cerebellar lesion.

sudden deterioration with coma and death, and because lumbar puncture in this context carries a risk of herniation of the brainstem and cerebellar tonsils due to the resulting differential pressure changes (sometimes termed 'coning'). For communicating hydrocephalus, lumbar puncture is of diagnostic value, deriving an opening pressure and assessment of the CSF contents. It is also therapeutic; drainage of typically between 10 and 30 mL of CSF, with the goal of halving the opening pressure, can relieve the hydrocephalus at least temporarily.

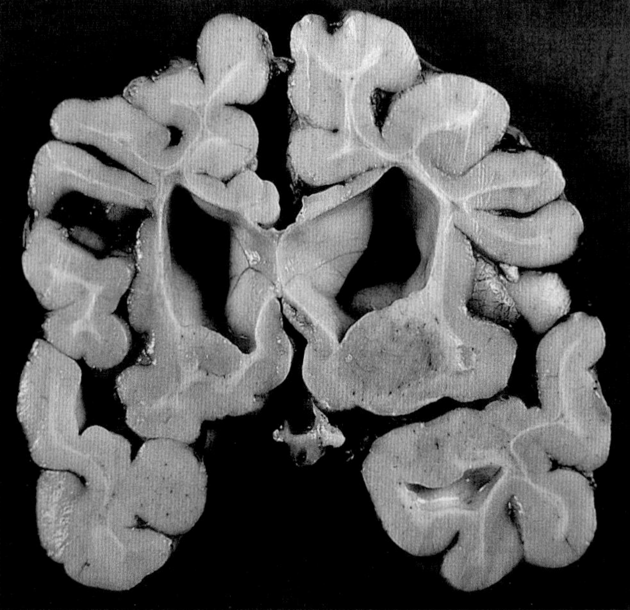

Figure 43.5 Pathological specimen of a hydrocephalic brain.

Treatment of hydrocephalus in the emergency setting usually involves CSF diversion, for example using an external ventricular drain. Management is discussed further under Treatment of hydrocephalus. Disorders of CSF flow with poorly understood mechanisms manifest in two syndromes: normal pressure hydrocephalus and idiopathic intracranial hypertension (IIH).

Normal pressure hydrocephalus

This is an important cause of dementia since it is readily reversible. It typically presents with the triad of gait disturbance, incontinence and cognitive decline. It may occur de novo or on a background of previous brain insults including subarachnoid haemorrhage (SAH), head injury, meningitis and tumour. Ventriculomegaly is evident on imaging, although this is also seen in the context of cortical atrophy due to other dementia pathologies. The CSF pressure at lumbar puncture (LP) is typically normal, but it is believed that intermittent elevations in pressure may be involved in the aetiology. Lumbar infusion testing involves insertion of a fine drain at LP, followed by measurement of the CSF pressure changes associated with a fluid challenge administered through this. This allows evaluation of the likely benefit from definitive treatment by shunt insertion.

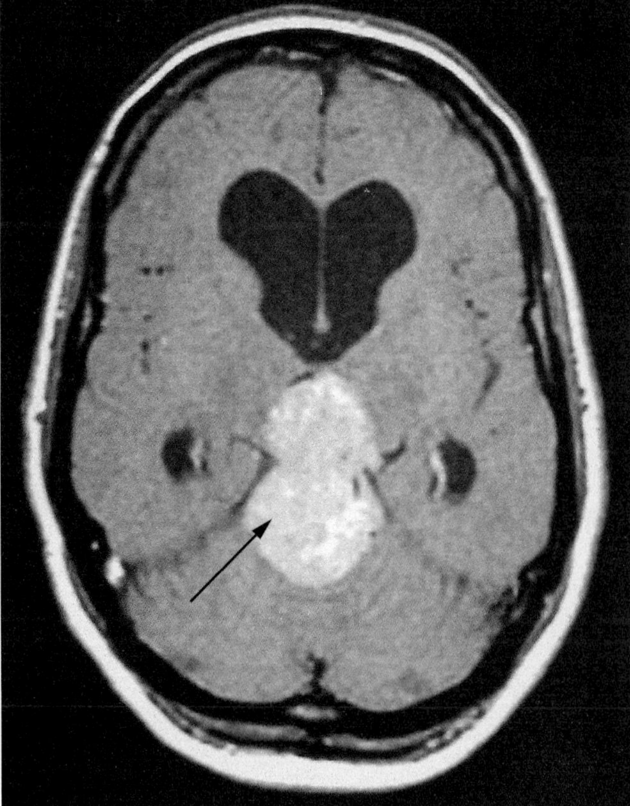

Figure 43.6 Pineal region tumour (arrow) causing obstructive hydrocephalus.

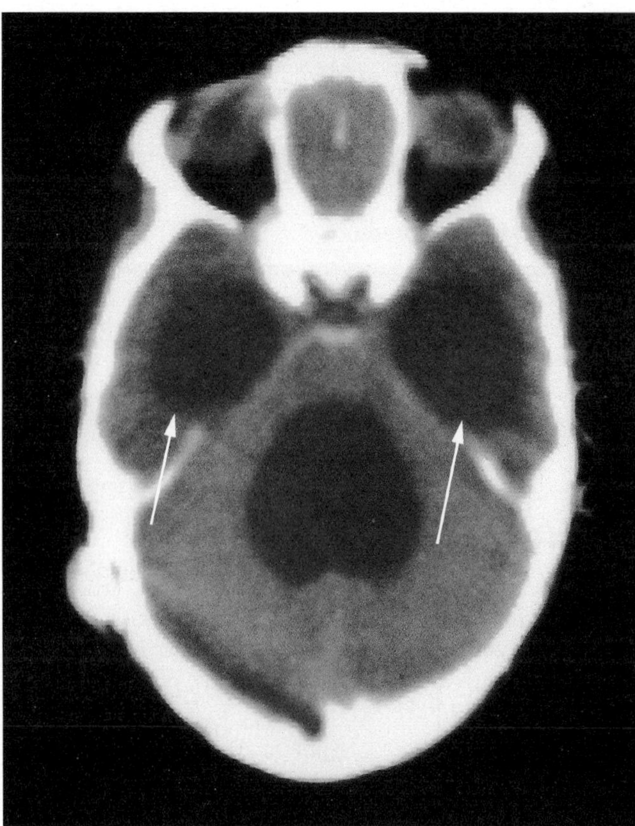

Figure 43.7 Gross hydrocephalus in a neonate with very prominent temporal horns (arrows) and fourth ventricle.

Idiopathic intracranial hypertension

This condition presents with features of raised ICP without an underlying tumour, explaining the old terms for the condition, pseudotumour cerebri or benign intracranial hypertension. This description is misleading, since IIH can progress rapidly to blindness. The patient, typically a young overweight female, describes a headache typical of raised pressure, and visual deterioration. Examination may reveal papilloedema, and occasionally cranial nerve palsies. Imaging is unremarkable, but LP demonstrates a raised opening pressure >25 mm Hg. The diagnosis is one of exclusion and the aetiology is not well understood. Impaired CSF resorption may reflect raised venous pressure, either as a result of sinus thrombosis or secondary to raised intra-abdominal pressure in obese patients. Weight loss and cessation of certain medications including the oral contraceptive pill is often effective. This is combined with medical therapy using acetazolamide to reduce CSF production. For patients with visual field loss or visual failure, despite medication, lumboperitoneal or ventriculoperitoneal shunting is offered. Optic nerve sheath fenestration by an ophthalmologist may also be employed.

Summary box 43.2

Hydrocephalus and disorders of CSF flow

- Obstructive or communicating hydrocephalus may occur as a result of neurosurgical pathology or its treatment
- CT is the first line of investigation. For communicating hydrocephalus, LP can confirm raised CSF pressure and relieve it temporarily
- Idiopathic intracranial hypertension results in symptomatic raised CSF pressure without ventricular enlargement, typically in young, overweight women. CSF diversion may be necessary to prevent permanent visual loss
- Normal pressure hydrocephalus is a potentially reversible cause of dementia, presenting with gait disturbance, incontinence and cognitive decline

Treatment of hydrocephalus

Acute obstructive hydrocephalus is an emergency because of the risk of rapid progression to coma and death, sometimes with very sudden deterioration, a 'hydrocephalic attack'. It may be relieved by addressing the underlying pathology, for example by excision of a tumour responsible for an obstructive hydrocephalus. Most often, however, temporary ventricular drainage is required, either as an emergency in an obtunded or deteriorating patient or as a precaution during definitive surgery considering the possibility for postoperative swelling.

External ventricular drain

External ventricular drains (EVDs) are an effective temporary measure to relieve hydrocephalus. Most commonly they are inserted to the right of midline, anterior to the coronal suture, so that the catheter tip rests adjacent to the foramen of Monro in the lateral ventricle. The catheter is then connected to a drain set such that CSF drains when the ventricular pressure exceeds a threshold typically set at 10–20 mm Hg. Intrathecal antibiotics may also be delivered through the EVD. Lumbar drains are an alternative means of temporary CSF diversion, often used to manage CSF leaks resulting from communicating hydrocephalus.

Ventriculoperitoneal shunts

Ventriculoperitoneal shunting comprises insertion of a ventricular catheter into the frontal or occipital horn of the lateral ventricle, while a distal catheter is tunnelled subcutaneously to the abdomen. Ventriculoatrial and ventriculopleural shunting is also possible, and lumbar-peritoneal shunts may be used in communicating hydrocephalus or IIH. A shunt valve, with an opening pressure that may be high, medium or low, is inserted at the junction of these catheters (Figure 43.8). Selection of the shunt valve is a balance and must be tailored to each patient: high pressure valves may fail to allow adequate CSF drainage, whereas low pressure valves can overdrain (see below). An anti-siphon system may be incorporated to prevent excessive drainage in the standing position. Programmable valves offer variable opening pressures, adjusted magnetically using a device applied externally over the valve. The valve system will also typically incorporate a CSF reservoir, which allows for percutaneous sampling.

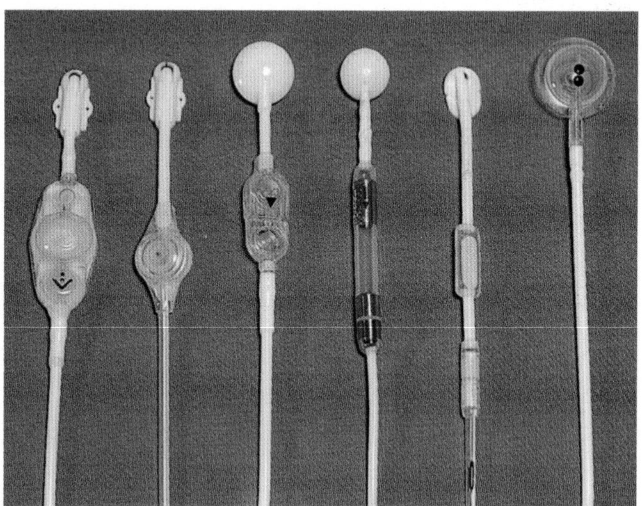

Figure 43.8 Examples of ventriculoperitoneal shunt valves.

Shunt complications

Overdrainage can result in low-pressure headaches, which are typically worse on standing. Collapse of the ventricles can cause accumulation of fluid or blood in the subdural space, resulting in subdural hygroma or subdural haematoma. The **slit ventricle syndrome** describes the situation in children treated with shunts, whose ventricles and subarachnoid spaces are underdeveloped, resulting in poor brain compliance. In these patients normal fluctuations in ICP are exaggerated so that coughing and straining may cause symptoms of raised ICP. Any shunt blockage may not be evident on scan, as the ventricles fail to enlarge.

Shunts are vulnerable to disconnection, infection and blockage, with the result that 15–20% require replacement within 3 years. Seventy five per cent of infections present within 1 month, reflecting introduction at the time of insertion. Risk factors include very young patients, open myelomeningocoele, long operation time and staff movement in and out of theatre. The shunt is removed, and external CSF drainage or serial lumbar puncture instituted to cover a course of antibiotic therapy. Once CSF sampling confirms resolution of the infection and a normal protein concentration, a shunt can be inserted at a new site.

The majority of blockages are attributable to cellular and proteinaceous debris, especially due to infection, but choroid plexus adhesion, blood clot or failure of the valve mechanism may also be responsible.

Endoscopic third ventriculostomy

This procedure is especially useful in obstructive hydrocephalus due to aqueduct stenosis. A neuroendoscope is inserted into the frontal horn of the lateral ventricle and then into the third ventricle via the foramen of Monro. The floor of the ventricle is then opened between the mammillary bodies and the pituitary recess. Free drainage between the third ventricle and the adjacent subarachnoid cisterns is then possible, without the infection risk posed by implanted tubing. Reblockage of this route is common, however, and many patients will subsequently require a shunt. Rare but serious complications include damage to the basilar artery, or fornicial damage resulting in permanent memory impairment.

Summary box 43.3

Treating hydrocephalus

- Temporary CSF diversion can be achieved with an EVD
- In the long term a shunt, usually connecting the lateral ventricles with the peritoneal cavity in the abdomen (VP shunt), is the mainstay of management
- Shunt blockage and infection are common complications

INTRACRANIAL INFECTION

Meningitis

Meningitis describes inflammation of the meninges of the brain and spinal cord, most commonly and most seriously due to bacterial infection. The clinical features of meningeal irritation or meningism are fever, headache, neck stiffness and photophobia. Community-acquired bacterial meningitis can progress rapidly without antibiotic treatment to subpial encephalopathy, venous thrombosis, cerebral oedema and death. Meningitis as a complication of head injury or surgery typically follows a more insidious course, but nonetheless remains a feared complication requiring prompt intervention. Typical organisms are *Staphylococcus aureus*, Enterobacteriaceae, *Pseudomonas* and pneumococci.

Meningitis after head injury is common, affecting 25% of patients with base of skull fracture and CSF leak. Repair of the CSF leak may be required, and empirical antibiotics should have activity against commensal nasal organisms including gram-positive cocci and gram-negative bacilli in the presence of symptoms/signs of clinical meningitis.

Summary box 43.4

Meningitis

- A feared complication of neurosurgery and of head injury
- CT head allows exclusion of raised ICP prior to LP
- CSF should be sent for microscopy and culture, and for assay of protein and glucose levels
- Treatment, pending identification of an organism, is with broad-spectrum antibiotics including anaerobic cover

Brain abscess and empyema

Abscesses arise when the brain is exposed directly, for example as a result of fracture or infection of an air sinus, or at surgery. They also result from haematogenous spread, typically in association with respiratory and dental infections, or endocarditis. In 25% of cases, no underlying primary infection is found. The organisms involved are normally bacteria, but immunocompromised hosts in particular are vulnerable to a broad range of pathogens (Box 43.1).

Box 43.1 Common causative organisms.

- Sinus/mastoid infection: aerobic and anaerobic streptococci; bacteroides; enterobacteria; staphylococci; *Pseudomonas*
- Haematogenous spread: bacteroides; streptococci
- Penetrating trauma: *Staphylococcus aureus*; clostridia; bacillus; enterobacteria
- Food contamination: *Toxoplasma*, pork tapeworm (producing neurocysticercosis)
- Immunocompromise (e.g. HIV/AIDS): protozoal (e.g. *Toxoplasma*), fungal (e.g. *Cryptococcus*), viral (e.g. JC virus producing multifocal leukoencephalopathy) and mycobacterial abscesses are encountered

Typical presenting features include low-grade fever, confusion, seizures and focal deficits, often with equivocal blood markers of inflammation; blood cultures should be obtained at an early stage. CT scan with contrast is the initial imaging modality of choice. Hypodense oedematous brain representing early cerebritis is visible in the first few days (Figure 43.9). The classic appearances of a smooth-walled, well-defined, ring-enhancing mass develop as the abscess matures (Figure 43.10). The distinction between abscess and tumour can be difficult and has important management implications, since abscesses generally require urgent drainage. Diffusion-weighted MRI is a valuable tool in this context (Figure 43.11).

Early surgical drainage of abscesses is the mainstay of management, helping to prevent dangerous complications: mortality for these patients is about 4%, but is greater than 80% in the case of ventriculitis due to rupture of an abscess into the ventricles. Intravenous antibiotic therapy is administered, broad spectrum initially and then according to sensitivities of the organisms responsible once identified. Treatment should last at least 6 weeks, but a switch to oral therapy may be appropriate after an interval and in consultation with microbiology. Up to 50% of patients with brain abscess will develop seizures at some stage, therefore prophylactic anticonvulsants should be considered.

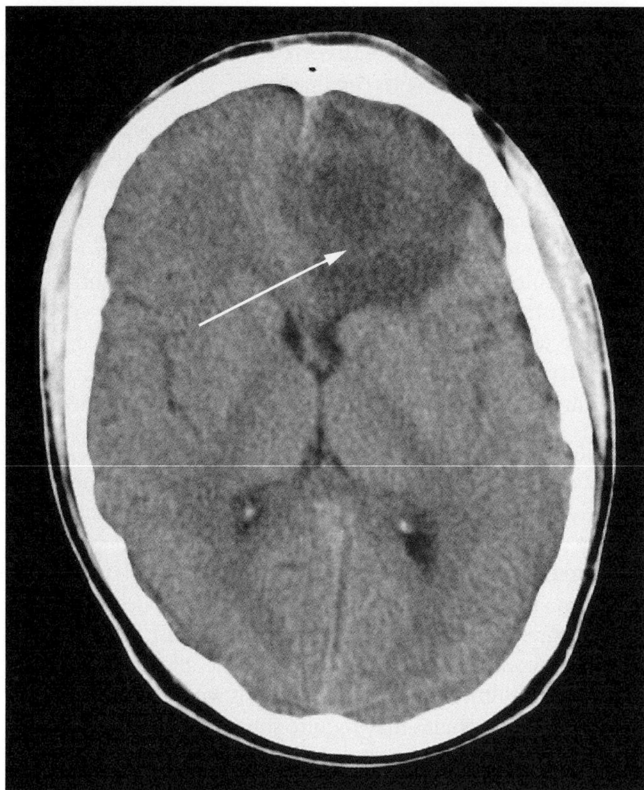

Figure 43.9 Axial computed tomography scan with contrast of a patient with frontal sinusitis presenting with seizures. Early cerebritis is evident in the left frontal region (arrow).

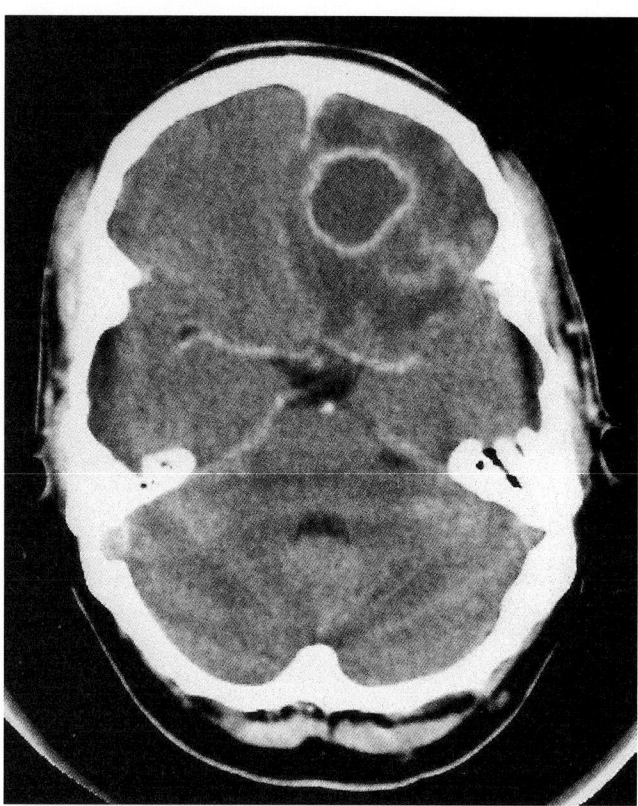

Figure 43.10 Axial computed tomography scan with contrast of the same patient as in Figure 43.9 2 weeks later. A ring-enhancing smooth-walled lesion is evident, an abscess suitable for image-guided drainage.

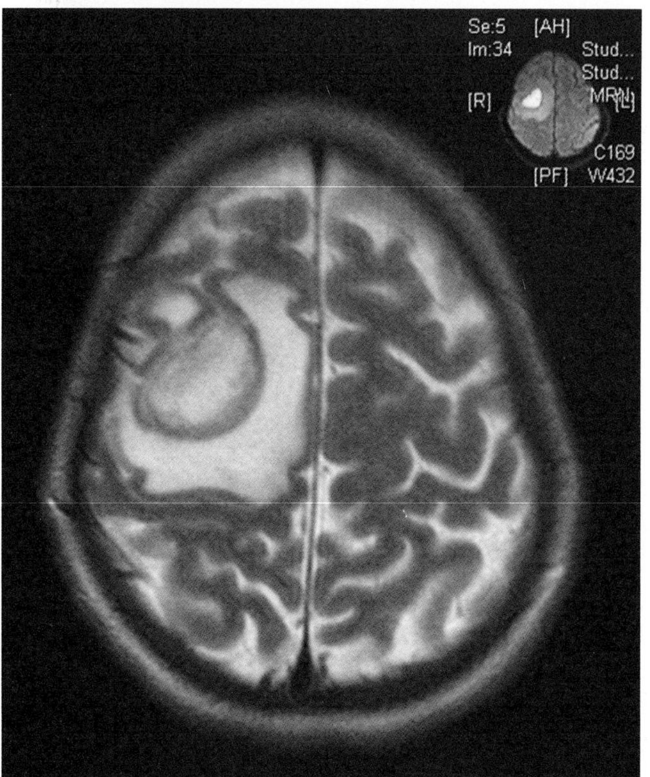

Figure 43.11 The right frontal lesion evident on T2-weighted magnetic resonance imaging (MRI) (main image) exhibits high signal on diffusion-weighted MRI sequences (top right inset) indicative of brain abscess.

Summary box 43.5

Brain abscesses

- Presenting features are those of infection and of intracranial mass lesion
- Imaging reveals a 'ring-enhancing lesion', with tumour usually the main differential
- Early diagnosis, usually followed by drainage, is key for good outcome.

Subdural empyema

Subdural empyema refers to an infective collection in the subdural space. This may develop as a result of sinusitis, mastoiditis or meningitis, and can complicate trauma or surgery. Figure 43.12 shows a subdural empyema associated with osteomyelitis of the frontal bone and associated scalp swelling (Pott's puffy tumour). In empyema, pus will generally collect in the parafalcine region and over the convexity, triggering inflammation and thrombosis in the cortical veins, which helps to explain the high mortality of 8–12%. Presentation mimics that of meningitis and cerebral abscess; typical CT appearances are of hypodense or isodense subdural collection, with contrast enhancement at the margins, and a degree of swelling and midline shift. The empyema may be difficult to visualise especially on non-contrast CT. LP should not be performed given the risk of herniation.

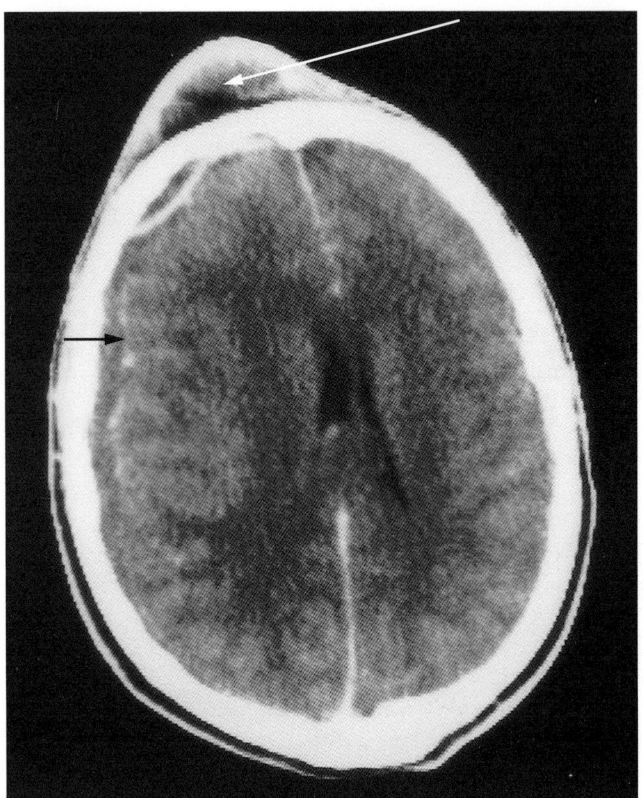

Figure 43.12 Axial computed tomography scan with contrast showing a right hemisphere subdural empyema (short arrow) and a right frontal Pott's puffy tumour (long arrow) (osteomyelitis of the frontal bone).

Craniotomy or craniectomy allows drainage of the collection and relieves raised ICP and is the treatment of choice. Burrhole drainage, and occasionally IV antibiotics without surgical intervention, may also be considered.

Summary box 43.6

Subdural empyema

- Presenting features are similar to those of meningitis or cerebral abscess
- Typically a crescentic collection with a contrast-enhancing rim is evident on CT
- Drainage is the mainstay of treatment

Tuberculosis

Tuberculosis (TB) infection of the central nervous system (CNS) represents haematogenous spread from primary pulmonary foci. A high index of suspicion is required, especially when population or individual risk factors are present. TB can result in a diverse but overlapping spectrum of pathology, including in the head:

- tuberculous meningitis – this commonly affects young children; CT demonstrates intense meningeal enhancement, and hydrocephalus is a common sequela;
- tuberculoma – discrete tumour-like granulomas at the base of the cerebral hemispheres, presenting with mass effect;
- tuberculous abscess – seen predominantly in immunocompromised hosts, this represents progression of a tuberculoma with prominent central caseating necrosis;
- miliary tuberculosis – describes a diffuse distribution of multiple small tuberculomas through brain substance.

Where the meninges are involved, lymphocytes can be expected to predominate in the CSF, rather than the polymorphs seen with other bacterial meningitides. The increase in protein content and reduction in glucose concentration are also less marked. Ziehl–Neesen staining for myobacteria is frequently negative, and polymerase chain reaction testing offers relatively rapid diagnosis compared to culture for acid-fast bacilli which may take weeks. A 20–30 mL CSF sample allows spinning to increase the culture yield. Management is with anti-tuberculous therapy; hydrocephalus may require shunt insertion.

VASCULAR NEUROSURGERY

Subarachnoid haemorrhage

'Spontaneous' subarachnoid haemorrhage (SAH) is usually the result of bleeding from a ruptured aneurysm (~80% of SAH) or an arteriovenous malformation (AVM). Most ruptured aneurysms are located in the circle of Willis, at branch points in the arterial tree associated with turbulent blood flow (Figure 43.13). A distinct subgroup of SAH patients suffer bleeds confined to the basal cisterns anterior to the midbrain and pons, without an underlying lesion evident on angiogram. This is termed **perimesencephalic SAH**, is believed to represent venous bleeding and has an excellent prognosis. Aneurysms may also develop as a result of infective infiltration of arterial walls in the context of bacteraemia (mycotic aneurysm), often in the setting of intravenous drug use or infective endocarditis. Pseudoaneurysms may also develop after trauma or after surgery.

Aneurysmal bleeding has an incidence of 10–15 per 100 000 population per year. Risk factors include age, female sex, hypertension, smoking, cocaine abuse and a family history with two first-degree relatives affected. A range of genetic disorders, in particular adult polycystic kidney disease, fibromuscular dysplasia, neurofibromatosis type 1, Ehlers–Danlos and Marfan's syndromes, are known to predispose patients to this condition.

Percival Pott, 1714–1788, surgeon, St Bartholomew's Hospital, London, UK, described the 'Puffy Tumour' in 1760. In 1756 he sustained a broken leg after a fall from his horse. As he lay on the ground, he sent a servant to buy a door which acted as a stretcher. While his surgeons were contemplating amputating his leg, he persuaded them to splint the leg instead as a result of which he recovered completely. Although some think that Pott's fracture of the ankle was described after this injury of his, it is not so. He sustained a compound fracture of the femur. Pott was the first to link an environmental factor to the aetiology of cancer when he demonstrated that chimney sweeps developed squamous cell scrotal cancer.

Thomas Willis, 1621–1675, Sedleian Professor of Natural Philosophy at Oxford, was the first anatomist to number the cranial nerves in the order used today.

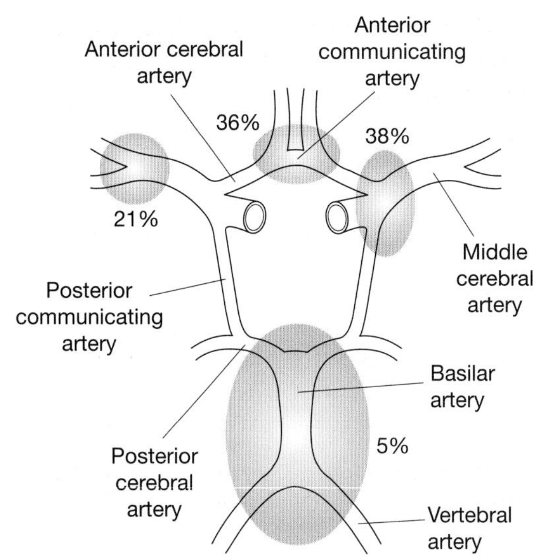

Figure 43.13 Common sites of aneurysm in the circle of Willis.

History and examination

The typical presentation of a SAH includes a 'thunderclap' headache, which is both sudden and severe and is outside the patient's normal experience. Some patients describe prodromal headaches preceding the event, potentially representing aneurysm growth or subclinical bleeds. The sudden onset occurs commonly but not exclusively during exertion, and may be associated with seizure (10%), unresponsiveness (50%) and vomiting (70%). Sometimes it is difficult to establish whether SAH has caused a fall, or whether a fall with head injury is responsible for the SAH. Approximately one-third of SAHs are incorrectly diagnosed at initial presentation. They are then at high risk of succumbing to early complications, especially a rebleed.

Neurological examination may be normal ('good clinical grade') or the patient may have focal deficits and an impaired conscious level ('poor grade'). The World Federation of Neurological Surgeons (WFNS) grading of SAH is measured against the condition of the patient after resuscitation rather than at the time of ictus (*Table 43.2*). A painful third nerve palsy is typically the result of compression from a posterior communicating artery aneurysm. Meningitic features of neck stiffness and photophobia often develop over hours. Intraocular haemorrhages, classically subhyaloid, may be visible on fundoscopy. The combination of SAH and vitreous haemorrhage is known as Terson's Syndrome and occurs in 15–20% of patients. Papilloedema should be sought, but may not be evident early in the course of a developing hydrocephalus.

TABLE 43.2 World Federation of Neurological Surgeons (WFNS) grading of subarachnoid haemorrhage.

Grade	Glasgow Coma Scale	Focal deficits[a]
I	15	–
II	13–14	–
III	13–14	+
IV	7–12	±
V	3–9	±

[a]Focal deficit = dysphasia or limb weakness.

Investigation

CT scan is the imaging of first choice, and, when performed within 12 hours of ictus, will confirm bleeding in more than 98% of cases. This makes a diagnostic LP unnecessary (**Figure 43.14**).

The sensitivity of a CT scan, however, deteriorates to less than 50% at 1 week after a bleed. In light of this, patients with a suggestive history and negative CT scan will require LP, especially where presentation is delayed. The CSF supernatant should be analysed by spectrophotometry (visual inspection is not reliable) for the spectra of haemoglobin breakdown products oxyhaemoglobin and bilirubin. These are clearly detectable in samples taken at least 6 and preferably 12 hours after SAH, but not in CSF mixed with fresh blood due to traumatic puncture, and analysed immediately. Failure to exclude SAH with an appropriate delayed LP may necessitate formal cerebral angiography, and the risks this entails.

Catheter angiography generally involves access to both vertebral and carotid arteries through the femoral artery under local anaesthetic. This allows visualisation of the vascular anatomy by injection of contrast medium with simultaneous screening (**Figures 43.15 and 43.16**). The serious potential risks include ischaemic stroke or arterial dissection (1–2%), and renal failure or allergic reactions attributable to contrast.

Surgical/interventional management

CT angiography has a high sensitivity for aneurysms and AVMs, but digital subtraction angiography remains the gold standard.

Aneurysms demonstrated may be removed from the circulation surgically by craniotomy and 'clipping' or by endovascular embolisation, also known as 'coiling'. Sometimes mesh stents may also be used to help secure the metal coils within the aneurysm sac as part of this procedure. Class 1 evidence suggesting a lower risk of poor outcomes, at least for small anterior circulation aneurysms, has driven the uptake of coiling. However, a surgical approach remains necessary or

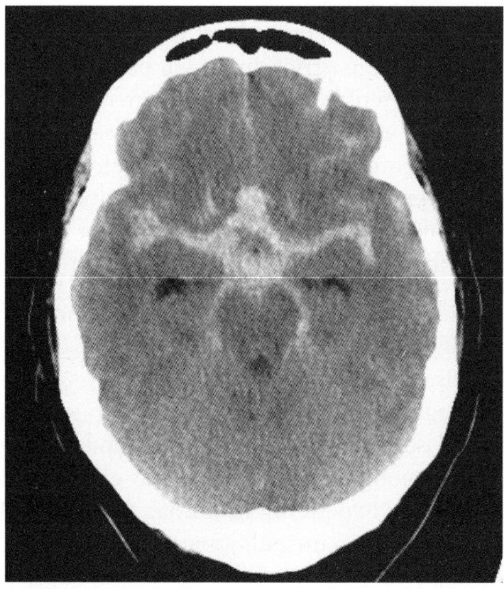

Figure 43.14 Diffuse subarachnoid bleeding from a ruptured anterior communicating artery aneurysm extends to the prepontine and ambient cisterns around the brainstem, and into both Sylvian fissures.

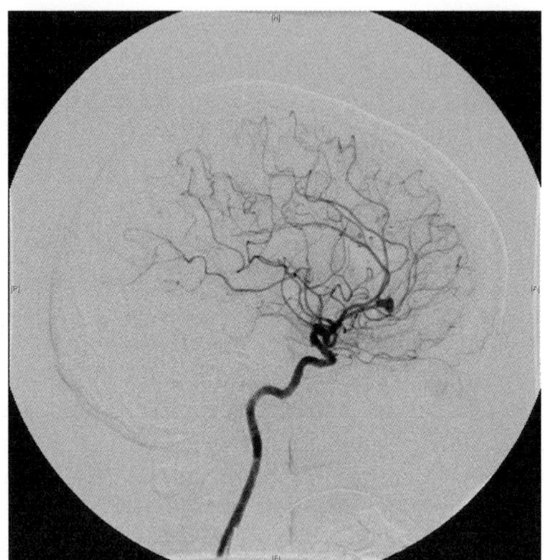

Figure 43.15 There is a small saccular aneurysm of the pericallosal branch of the anterior cerebral artery.

preferable in many cases. A rebleed risk of 4% in the first 24 hours, then 1.5% per day thereafter is quoted for aneurysms, and 80% of patients who rebleed have an eventual poor outcome. For this reason, and to permit optimal management of vasospasm, the current consensus favours early intervention, despite the surgical challenges presented by brain swelling and blood load.

Overall survival of SAH is about 50%, and one-third of survivors remain dependent. Only 50% of WFNS grade 1 patients return to work. Treated aneurysms can regrow and rebleed, especially after coiling, so that a programme of surveillance is necessary.

Unruptured aneurysms represent a thorny management problem: incidentally detected small anterior circulation aneurysms represent a minimal bleeding risk. Screening, even in high risk groups, is therefore of questionable benefit.

Medical management

Patients should be placed on bed rest with hourly neuro observations. They require strict input–output monitoring and intravenous fluid replacement with normal saline initially. Oral nimodipine at a dose of 60 mg every 4 hours reduces the rate of poor outcome (see Vasospasm below). Analgesics, laxatives, anti-emetics, gastric protection and compression stockings are also likely to be necessary. After resuscitation, the priorities in subarachnoid haemorrhage are:

1. to prevent rebleeding by identifying and controlling any underlying lesion;
2. to recognise and manage:
   - neurological complications, especially vasospasm (or delayed ischaemic neurologic deficit) and hydrocephalus;
   - systemic complications, including electrolyte imbalance, severe hypertension, cardiac infarct and arrhythmia, and neurogenic pulmonary oedema.

These goals are best served by early transfer of the patient to a neurosurgical centre. In elderly patients with a poor WFNS grade, a decision to offer only supportive management may be appropriate.

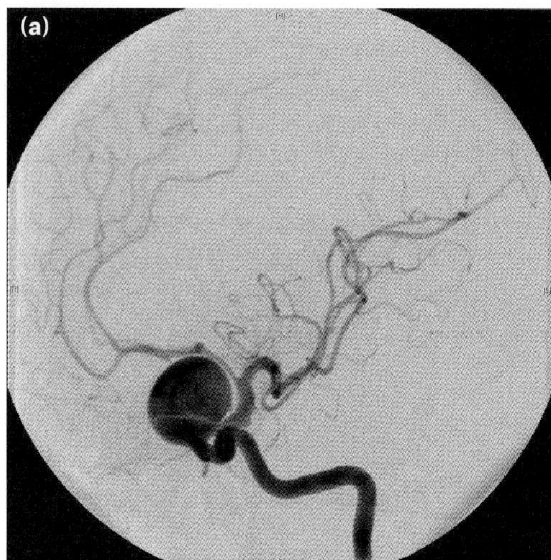

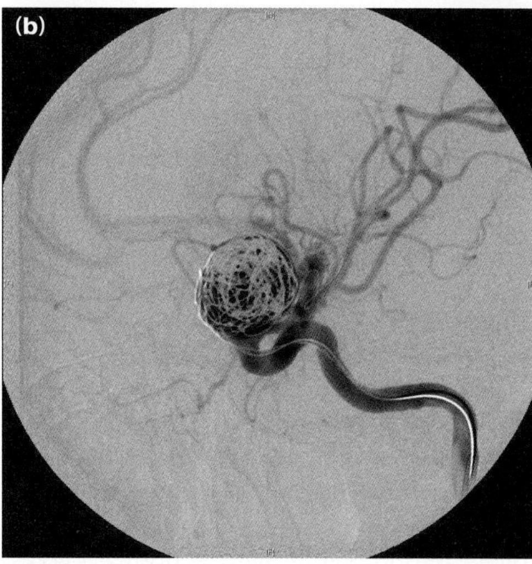

Figure 43.16 (a) A giant aneurysm of the internal carotid artery. (b) Angiographic embolisation (coiling) of the giant aneurysm. Note the single displaced coil passing into the distal internal carotid artery and then the middle cerebral artery.

Neurological deterioration should prompt a repeat scan to exclude evidence of rebleeding and of hydrocephalus. This is typically the communicating type, which is a common sequela of haemorrhage. Where these complications are not demonstrated, deterioration is often attributable to **delayed ischaemic neurological deficit** (DNID), which commonly develops 3 to 10 days after aneurysmal haemorrhage and can progress rapidly to infarction. The process is attributed to cerebral vasospasm in response to, and correlating with, the blood load. This process can be visualised angiographically, and the velocity of bloodflow in the cerebral vasculature, measured using transcranial Doppler ultrasound, provides an indirect assessment of the degree of stenosis. Outcomes are optimised by the prophylactic administration of nimodipine and maintenance of fluid volume, typically with 2.5–3 litres per day of normal saline. In established vasospasm, the goal is to maintain cerebral perfusion by administration of fluid and inotropes.

Hyponatraemia is a frequent complication of SAH, attributed to cerebral salt wasting in the context of fluid depletion, and otherwise to the syndrome of inappropriate antidiuretic hormone secretion. This is associated with a higher incidence of DNID, and practical management, irrespective of the underlying pathology, is based on sodium replacement, with hypertonic infusions if necessary. Fluid restriction is not appropriate in these patients since this risks further compromising perfusion.

Summary box 43.7

Subarachnoid haemorrhage

- Most result from rupture of an aneurysm of the circle of Willis
- Plain CT and LP are first line investigations
- Even 'good grade' patients treated promptly have a significant morbidity due to vasospasm, cardiac arrhythmias, neurogenic pulmonary oedema, etc.

Intracerebral haemorrhage

Spontaneous intracerebral haemorrhage accounts for 10–15% of strokes and has a mortality of 40% at 1 year. The majority occur in the context of hypertension or amyloid angiopathy, or as a complication of ischaemic stroke. Coagulation disorders, especially patients being treated with warfarin, are a major risk factor.

Patients typically present with sudden focal deficit and reduced conscious level. Following initial resuscitation, these patients will require CT scan to establish the diagnosis, and the size and position of the bleed (Figure 43.17). They require reversal of anticoagulation, ongoing hourly neuro observations and blood pressure monitoring. High blood pressure may be longstanding and associated with adaptations to autoregulation, so attempts at lowering it acutely with intravenous antihypertensives should be made only if the values are very high (e.g. mean arterial pressure >130 mm Hg).

Craniotomy and evacuation may be used to alleviate raised ICP, just as it can be in a subgroup of patients with ischaemic strokes in the posterior fossa or in the middle cerebral artery territory. Importantly, this surgery may be life-saving but cannot reverse focal deficits. Young patients with haematomas close to the cortical surface, demonstrating progressive neurological deterioration, represent good surgical candidates. Posterior fossa clot is also a strong indication for surgery because of the potential for rapid deterioration due to brainstem compression and hydrocephalus. A substantial minority of intracerebral bleeds are attributable to focal vascular lesions (see above). This must be considered when planning any surgery, and may be an indication for acute vascular imaging in discussion with neurovascular specialists. Delayed follow-up imaging is often recommended to exclude underlying tumour as a cause for bleed.

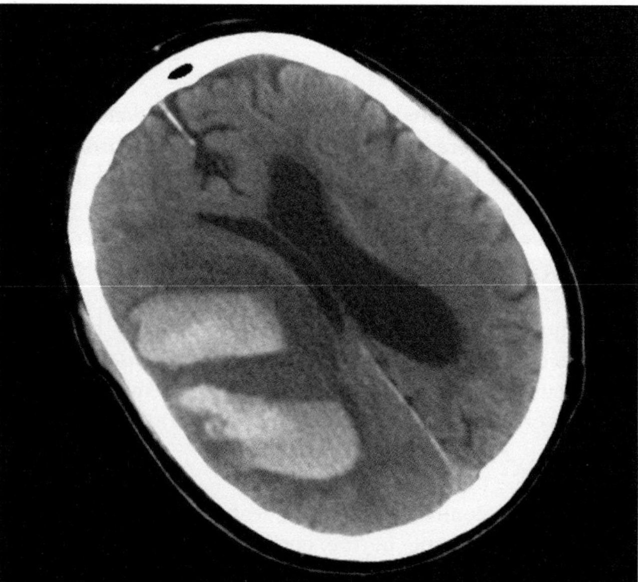

Figure 43.17 Large acute intracerebral haemorrhages in the right frontal and parietal lobes are evident, with surrounding oedema and midline shift.

Summary box 43.8

Intracerebral haemorrhage

- These account for 10–15% of strokes
- Presentation is with headache, focal deficits and signs of raised ICP
- High blood pressure may be chronic so should only be reduced with care
- Anticoagulants should be reversed
- In fit patients, clot evacuation is an option to relieve raised ICP but not reverse deficits
- Further imaging may be required to exclude an underlying vascular or neoplastic lesion

Vascular malformations

Vascular malformations are usually congenital in origin, with certain key exceptions discussed below. They may present with headaches, pulsatile tinnitus, seizures or focal deficit, or else acutely with rupture and haemorrhage.

AVMs are responsible for a small proportion of subarachnoid and intracerebral haemorrhages. Vessels and calcification may be apparent on CT or MRI, and the lesion is confirmed on angiography (Figure 43.18)

When AVMs present with bleeding, there is an approximately 4% risk of rebleed per annum. The risk is particularly high in the first 6 weeks and where the bleed is from an aneurysm related to the AVM. Surgery is the generally preferred treatment, but this may not be possible for some lesions which are large, in eloquent brain or with deep venous drainage. Radiosurgery and endovascular embolisation with tissue glue are options here.

Vein of Galen malformations are AVMs feeding into an embryological venous remnant dorsal to the brainstem presenting in childhood. High-flow malformations may cause cardiac failure. They may be treated by embolisation.

Dural arteriovenous fistulae (DAVFs) are shunts between dural arteries and veins or sinuses. They are proposed to arise as a result of vessel remodelling in response to dural sinus thrombosis and subsequent recanalisation. They may present with subarachnoid, intracerebral or subdural bleeding, or with headache and pulsatile tinnitus. A carotid cavernous fistula is a spontaneous or traumatic DAVF between the internal carotid artery and surrounding cavernous sinus, typically

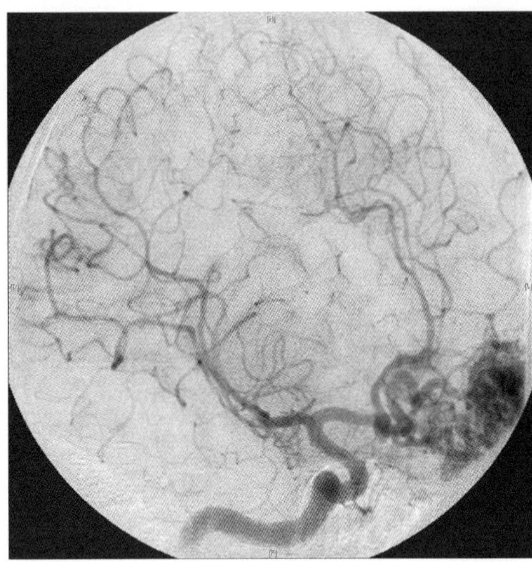

Figure 43.18 An arteriovenous malformation supplied by the anterior cerebral, middle cerebral and middle meningeal arteries is demonstrated at the 4 o'clock position in this angiogram.

producing eye pain, ocular muscle palsies and exophthalmos. Angiography is diagnostic.

Cavernomas (Figure 43.19) are venous anomalies, demonstrated on MRI but not with angiography, which may require operation if they cause progressive deficits, intractable epilepsy or recurrent bleeding.

Related lesions, usually clinically silent, include developmental venous anomalies and capillary telangectasia.

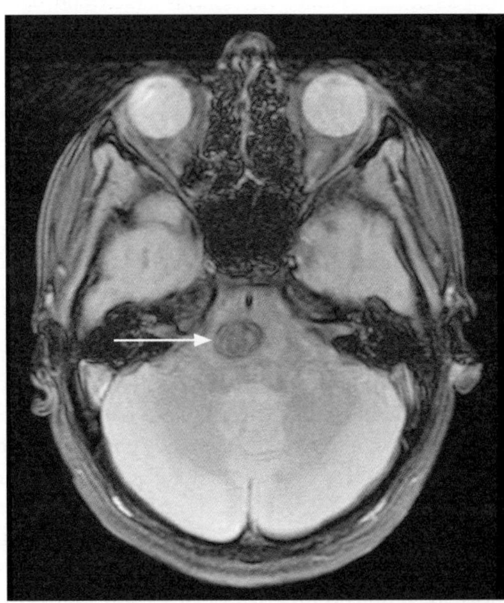

Figure 43.19 A brainstem cavernoma (arrow).

Occlusive vascular disease

In a subgroup of young patients with completed posterior fossa or non-dominant middle cerebral artery territory infarcts, there is a role for decompressive craniectomy in the acute setting to manage the brain swelling and raised ICP associated with the infarct.

There is class 1 evidence for the role of carotid endarterectomy in reducing the risk of stroke in patients with symptomatic carotid stenosis, and a debatable role for the procedure in patients with no previous transient ischaemic episodes.

Moya moya disease describes the progressive obliteration of one or both internal carotid arteries, thought to represent an autoimmune process. The development of external carotid circulation collaterals produces the angiographic 'puff of smoke' appearance responsible for this Japanese-derived name. It presents in youth or early middle age with ischaemia or haemorrhage. Untreated, the majority of patients suffer major deficit or die within 2 years. Ischaemia may be addressed by a variety of bypass techniques, for example by anastomosing the superficial temporal artery (arising from the external carotid) to the middle cerebral artery.

BRAIN TUMOURS

The term 'brain tumour' applies to a wide array of pathologies detailed in the World Health Organisation (WHO) classification. Many are malignant, but even histologically benign tumours may carry a grave prognosis where they encroach on key structures that also limit surgical access. The commonest brain tumour is a metastasis. Primary brain tumours represent 1.5% of all cancers, with an incidence of 19 per 100 000 person years. Nevertheless, many, especially glial tumours, present commonly in younger age groups and are incurable, so they account for disproportionate morbidity and mortality.

Classification

The WHO classifies primary brain tumours on the basis of cell of origin and histological grade. A simplified classification is shown in Figure 43.20.

Common adult primary brain tumours include gliomas, meningiomas (15–20% of total), pituitary adenomas (10–15% of total) and vestibular schwannomas. Grade 1 is applied to 'benign' lesions, while grade 4 implies high-grade malignancy.

Aetiology

The common primary brain tumours mentioned above occur sporadically. There is no proven risk due to environmental factors, except for radiation exposure, but genetic abnormalities may also predispose (*Table 43.3*).

Presentation

Most tumours present with one or more features belonging to three cardinal categories: these are seizure, raised ICP and focal neurological deficit. Pituitary adenomas may also present with endocrine disturbance.

Seizures

Seizures are a common presenting feature, especially of low-grade gliomas arising in the cortical hemispheres. Simple partial seizures, involving focal twitching or similar with preserved consciousness, are the rule, but temporal location will commonly produce complex partial seizures, and any seizure may progress to a secondary generalized tonic-clonic fit.

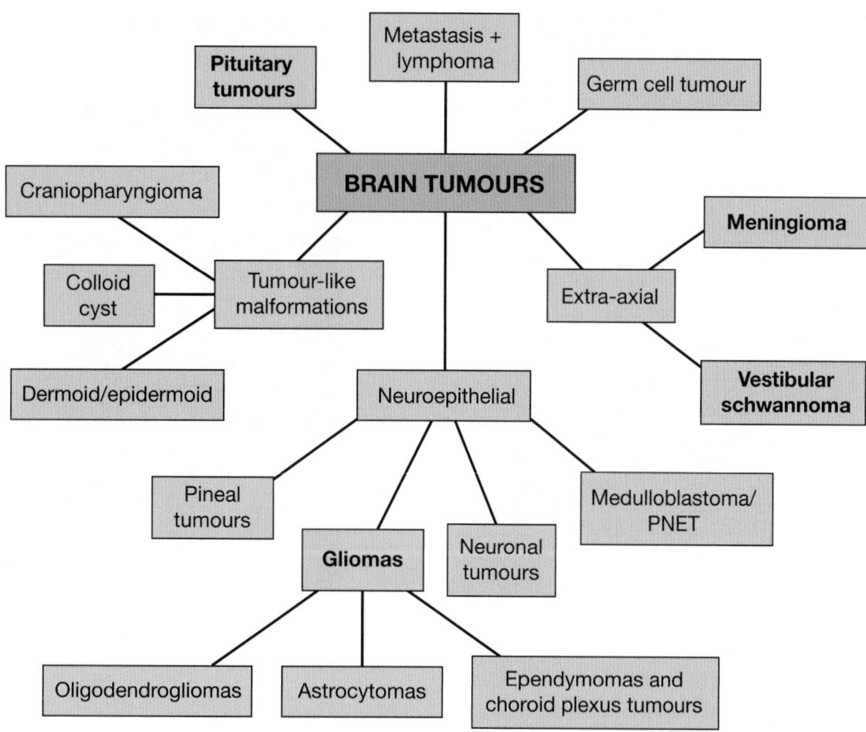

Figure 43.20 Brain tumour classification. A simplified schema encompassing some of the key brain tumour categories. Highlighted in bold are the pathologies discussed in more detail in this chapter.

TABLE 43.3 Chromosomal abnormalities associated with brain tumours.

Syndrome	Gene defect	Tumour
Neurofibromatosis type 1	*Neurofibromin* (Chr 17)	Astrocytomas; neurofibromas
Neurofibromatosis type 2	*Schwannomin* (Chr 22)	Acoustic neuromas (bilateral); meningiomas
Cowden's disease	*PTEN* (Chr 10)	Astrocytomas
Hereditary non-polyposis colorectal cancer	Multiple	Astrocytomas
Li–Fraumeni syndrome	*p53* (Chr 17)	Astrocytomas

Patients who have had a seizure should be started on an antiepileptic drug, usually phenytoin, levetiracetam or carbamazepine. Therapeutic levels of phenytoin can be achieved rapidly with intravenous loading, but its enzyme-inducing effect can complicate the administration of chemotherapy. Routine prophylaxis in patients with tumours who have no history of seizures is not recommended, although a short course at the time of craniotomy for tumour excision may be warranted.

Raised intracranial pressure

Headache is a presenting feature in only about 50% of patients. It is classically worse in the morning and on straining, and accompanied by nausea and vomiting. Pressure effect develops due to tumour mass effect and surrounding oedema, especially in fast growing metastases and high-grade gliomas (see Raised intracranial pressure). Where the differential diagnosis of abscess can be confidently excluded (see Brain abscess), mass effect is controlled initially using high-dose glucocorticoids (e.g. dexamethasone) to reduce swelling. Acute deterioration in this group may represent a developing obstructive hydrocephalus due to compression of CSF drainage pathways (see Hydrocephalus), a neurosurgical emergency.

Focal neurological deficit

A focal deficit progressive over time, as opposed to the sudden onset of a vascular accident, is suspicious of tumour. Lesions generally produce characteristic deficits due to local pressure effect, and reflecting location (*Table 43.4*).

Common brain tumours

Cerebral metastases

Cerebral metastases (Figure 43.21) are the most common intracranial tumours, and affect about one quarter of cancer sufferers, a proportion that is increasing with extended survival associated with more effective treatment of primary cancers. The tumours of origin and their contribution to the burden of cerebral metastases is detailed in *Table 43.5*. In general patients with multiple cerebral metastases are not suitable for surgery. Occasionally, diagnostic biopsy may be warranted where the primary is unknown. In patients with good functional status and well controlled systemic disease, craniotomy for resection of a single metastasis, and exceptionally up to three metastases, may be considered.

TABLE 43.4 Patterns of deficit generally associated with certain tumours.

Tumour location	Expected deficit
Pituitary (e.g. pituitary adenoma)	Bitemporal hemianopia; gaze palsies
Cerebellopontine angle (e.g. vestibular schwannoma)	Hearing loss; balance disturbance; tinnitus
Anterior skull base (e.g. olfactory groove meningioma)	Anosmia; ipsilateral optic atrophy; contralateral papilloedema (Foster-Kennedy syndrome)
Occipital (e.g. glioma, metastasis)	Homonymous hemianopia with central sparing
Parietal (dominant hemisphere)	Acalculia; agraphia; left-right disorientation; finger agnosia (Gerstmann syndrome)
Parietal (e.g. glioma)	Sensory inattention; dressing apraxia; astereognosis
Temporal (e.g. glioma)	Memory disturbance; contralateral superior quadrantanopia; dysphasia (dominant hemisphere)
Frontal (e.g. glioma)	Personality change; gait disturbance; urinary incontinence
Brainstem (e.g. brainstem glioma)	Multiple cranial nerve deficits; long tract signs; nystagmus
Posterior fossa (e.g. medulloblastoma)	Ataxia; hydrocephalus

Summary box 43.9

Brain tumours

- Most brain tumours will present with one or more feature related to the following triad:
  - Raised ICP
  - Seizures
  - Focal deficit

Glioma

These are tumours of glial cell origin, with subtypes including astrocytomas, oligodendrogliomas, ependymomas and mixed tumours. The diagnosis is histological, but imaging often predicts both a glial origin and the grade of tumour (Figure 43.22): MRI of the head with and without contrast is the preferred modality, generally combined with CT of the chest/abdomen/pelvis to exclude an extracranial primary, since metastasis is usually the main differential diagnosis. Diffusion-weighted MRI sequences are valuable in excluding another differential diagnosis, brain abscess, which is associated with prominent restricted diffusion in these images.

Initial management of these tumours should generally include high-dose steroids to alleviate any mass effect, combined with a proton pump inhibitor to address the potential steroid side effect of stomach ulcers. Antiepileptics are administered where seizures are a presenting feature, or are likely in

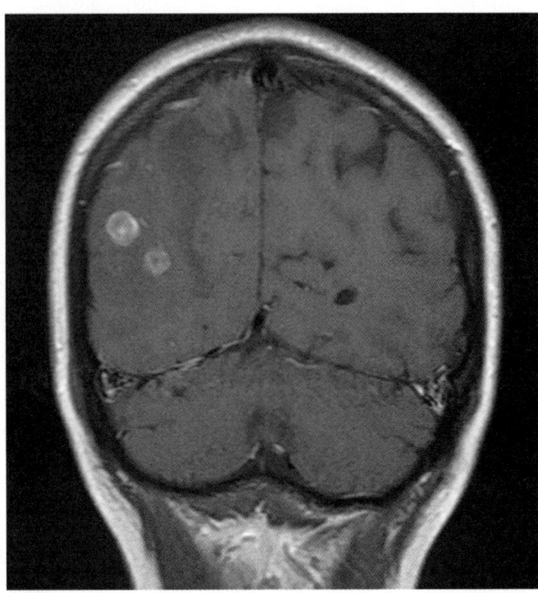

Figure 43.21 T1-weighted magnetic resonance imaging with contrast. Two right occipital lung metastases are demonstrated. They are well demarcated and enhance with gadolinium contrast.

TABLE 43.5 Tissue of origin for brain metastases (approximate).

Origin	Percentage
Lung	40
Breast	15
Melanoma	10
Renal/genitourinary	10
Other/unknown	25

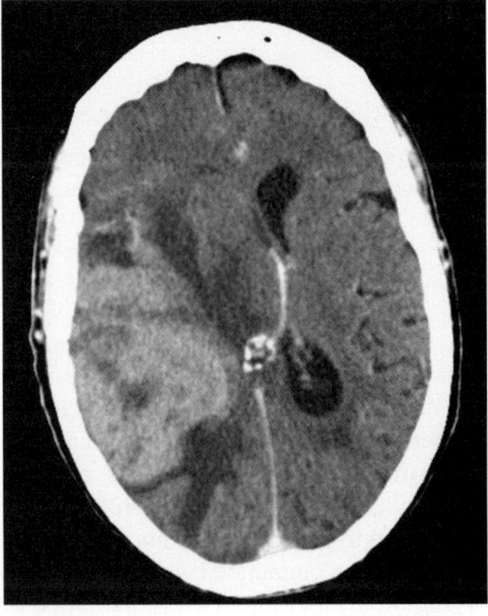

Figure 43.22 Computed tomography with contrast demonstrates a heterogeneous right frontoparietal lesion with mass effect and midline shift, almost certainly a glioblastoma multiforme. A magnetic resonance imaging scan with and without contrast will aid evaluation.

Robert Foster Kennedy, British neurologist, awarded the Chevalier de la Legion d'honneur for his service in French front line field hospitals in World War 1.
Josef Gerstmann, Austrian neurologist who fled to America in 1938 to escape the Nazis.

view of temporal location. Surgical resection is usually the primary treatment, aiming to reduce disease burden and to obtain tissue for diagnosis. Except for the grade I pilocytic astrocytoma, which typically occurs in children, gliomas are notable for their diffuse infiltration into surrounding brain, so that recurrence after even macroscopically complete resection is the rule.

Low-grade gliomas (WHO grade II) have a peak incidence in the fourth decade of life, and commonly present with seizures initially. Where tumours encroach on eloquent cortex, especially the speech areas of the dominant hemisphere, awake craniotomy allows mapping of function with surface electrodes at operation, to limit resection and minimise postoperative deficit. High-grade gliomas include anaplastic astrocytoma (WHO grade III) and glioblastoma (WHO grade IV), the commonest glial tumour (Figure 43.23). They typically present *de novo* with peak incidence in the fifth and sixth decades of life, respectively, or they may represent transformation of previously diagnosed, or clinically silent, low-grade gliomas. Active treatment consists of maximal resection, high-dose focused radiation therapy, and chemotherapy administered locally as carmustine wafers at the time of resection and/or systemically with oral temozolomide. Median survival for glioblastoma remains just over 12 months.

Meningioma

Meningiomas are usually benign lesions, although anaplastic variants do occur. They arise from the meninges, and typically present due to mass effect from the tumour, compounded by vasogenic oedema in the adjacent brain and obstructive hydrocephalus where CSF drainage is impaired. Imaging will demonstrate a contrast-enhancing mass distinct from the brain with a dural base (Figure 43.24).

These are generally slow-growing lesions. Smaller lesions, perhaps detected incidentally in an elderly patient, may well warrant a 'watch-and-wait' approach. If the lesion is large or positioned so as to impinge on key structures, the patient may require steroids and early surgery. The degree of resection predicts recurrence, with rates of 10% at ten years for total excision with a clear dural margin and 30% at ten years for subtotal excision. Lesions that are difficult to approach surgically may be managed with radiotherapy or stereotactic radiosurgery.

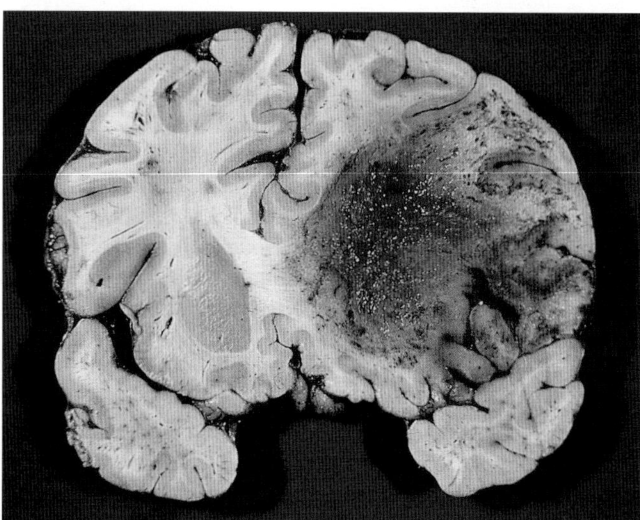

Figure 43.23 Pathological specimen of glioblastoma multiforme.

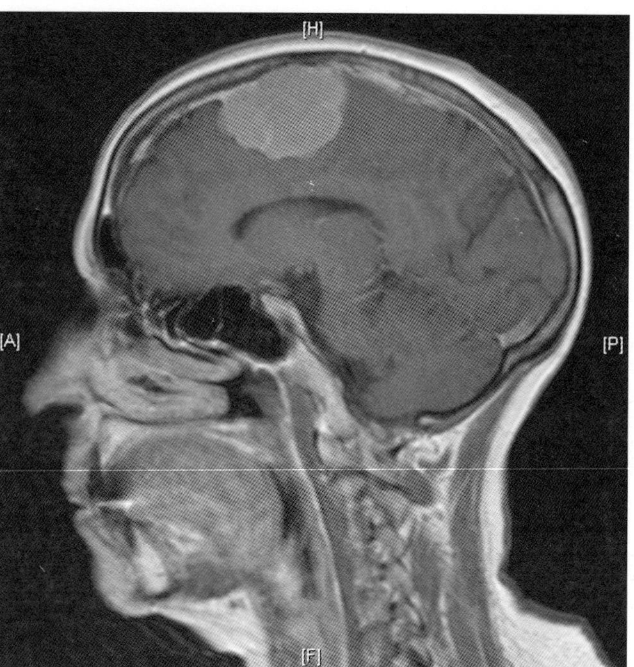

Figure 43.24 On T1-weighted magnetic resonance imaging an extra-axial, durally-based lesion is seen to arise in the region of the falx. This is a meningioma.

Summary box 43.10

Common supratentorial brain tumours

- Metastases and gliomas are common tumours arising within brain substance, appearing as 'ring-enhancing' lesions on contrast CT. Surgery is usually life-extending rather than curative
- Meningiomas arise from the meninges around the brain and typically enhance uniformly on contrast CT. Most are benign and amenable to curative resection
- MRI is usually the best modality for evaluating brain tumours. Diffusion-weighted sequences help to exclude abscess when glioma or metastasis is suspected
- Metastasis is the main differential diagnosis, and CT of the body is useful in identifying extracranial primary tumours
- Steroids with proton-pump inhibitor cover are administered to control swelling and mass effect in the short term

Pituitary tumours

Most tumours in the sellar region are benign pituitary adenomas, but pathology in this region can also include malignant variants, craniopharyngioma, meningioma, aneurysm and Rathke's cleft cyst (Figure 43.25).

Microadenomas are less than 10 mm in size and usually present incidentally or with endocrine effects. Macroadenomas are larger than 10 mm, and often present with visual field deficits. Thirty per cent of adenomas are prolactinomas, 20%

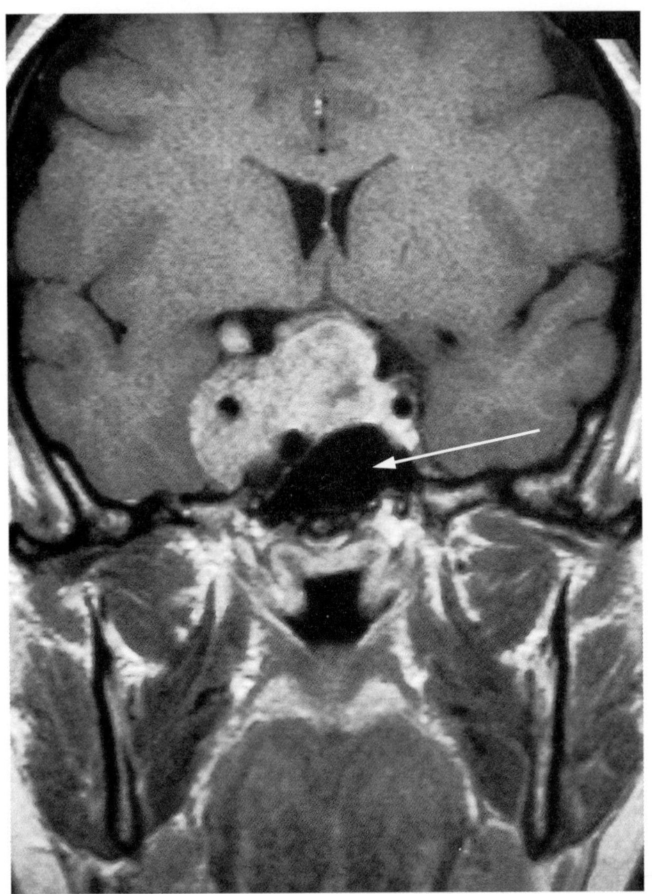

Figure 43.25 Non-functioning pituitary macroadenoma (arrow) compressing the optic chiasm superiorly, extending into the right cavernous sinus and encasing the right carotid artery.

are non-functioning, 15% secrete growth hormone and 10% secrete ACTH.

Features of note in the initial assessment include any history of galactorrhoea (suggestive of prolactinoma), and Cushingoid or acromegalic features pointing to ACTH- or growth hormone-secreting tumours, respectively. Baseline assessment of pituitary function should include serum prolactin, follicle-stimulating hormone and luteinising hormone together with testosterone in males or oestradiol in females, thyroid function tests and fasting serum growth hormone and cortisol. Preoperative prolactin levels are crucial since prolactinomas may be managed without the need for surgery. Prolactinomas are managed initially with dopamine agonists such as bromocryptine and cabergoline. Growth hormone-secreting tumours may also respond to dopamine agonists or to somatostatin analogues such as octreotide. The cortisol level is also important, since deficiency must be corrected, especially in the perioperative period. Diagnosis of ACTH-secreting tumours can be difficult and may require the use of specialised tests such as petrosal sinus sampling and the dexamethasone suppression test.

Effective treatment requires close cooperation between the neurosurgical team and an endocrinologist. Compression of the chiasm with any evidence of visual compromise is the main indication for urgent surgical intervention.

Surgical resection is usually performed by a transsphenoidal approach through the nose, using a microscope or endoscope. Sometimes large tumours also require a craniotomy. After operation patients are at risk of CSF leak (3%), and pituitary insufficiency. Diabetes insipidus resulting from manipulation of the pituitary stalk is common in the immediate postoperative period and usually resolves spontaneously. Where it is suspected, the patient will require hourly measurement of urine output, and blood and urine samples for calculation of sodium concentration and osmolality. If confirmed, the condition can be managed with DDAVP in consultation with endocrinology.

Pituitary apoplexy is the syndrome associated with haemorrhagic infarction of a pituitary tumour. It presents with sudden headache, visual loss and ophthalmoplegia with or without impaired conscious level. Endocrine resuscitation with intravenous steroids is the priority, and surgical decompression may be required.

Vestibular schwannoma

These are nerve sheath tumours arising in the cerebellopontine angle, which present with hearing loss, tinnitus and balance problems. Facial numbness and weakness are less common, while large tumours may present with features of brainstem compression or hydrocephalus. The differential diagnosis includes meningioma, metastasis and epidermoid cyst (Figure 43.26).

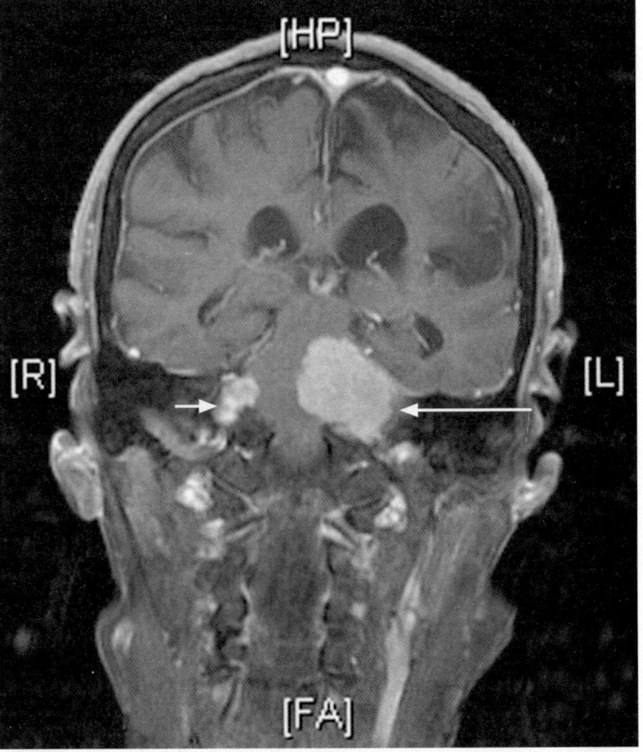

Figure 43.26 The appearances of a meningioma in the left cerebellopontine angle (CPA) (long arrow), with a coexisting vestibular schwannoma in the right CPA (short arrow).

Harvey Williams Cushing, 1869–1939, Professor of Surgery at Harvard University Medical School, credited as the father of modern neurosurgery, and described the eponymous disease, but also pioneered new techniques in bacteriology, blood pressure measurement and electrocautery.

Small intracanalicular tumours (within the internal auditory canal) may be managed with surveillance. For intermediate size tumours, radiosurgery is an alternative to operation. Large lesions (>4 cm), especially with brainstem compression, will require excision and consideration of ventriculoperitoneal shunt to relieve hydrocephalus. Translabyrinthine, retrosigmoid and middle fossa approaches are possible, the latter options offering potential preservation of hearing in smaller tumours with some intact function at presentation. In removing larger tumours, it is often impossible to preserve hearing, or indeed facial nerve function.

Brain tumours in children

Brain tumours are the most common solid tumours in children.

Neonates develop predominantly neuroectodermal tumours in supratentorial locations:

- teratoma;
- primitive neuroectodermal tumour (PNET);
- high-grade astrocytoma;
- choroid plexus papilloma/carcinoma.

Older children tend to suffer infratentorial tumours, especially:

- medulloblastoma (an infratentorial PNET);
- ependymoma;
- pilocytic astrocytoma.

Summary box 43.11

Skull base and paediatric tumours

- Pituitary tumours typically present with endocrinological disturbance (microadenomas) or visual deficits due to compression (macroadenomas). Some of these tumours are managed surgically, in close cooperation with endocrinologists
- Vestibular schwannomas (acoustic neuromas) are benign nerve sheath tumours, usually presenting with hearing loss, tinnitus and balance problems. Their proximity to the brainstem allows them to cause significant morbidity and mortality, and can present a major surgical challenge
- A large variety of mostly neuroectodermal brain tumours represent the most common solid organ tumours in children

PAEDIATRIC NEUROSURGERY

Paediatric neurosurgery presents a wide range range of isolated and syndrome-associated developmental abnormalities including cysts, neural tube defects and posterior fossa malformations. In general these present with combinations of developmental delay, seizures and macrocephaly or hydrocephalus. Early fusion of one or more cranial sutures, craniosynostosis, is also a common neonatal presentation.

Cysts

These benign fluid-filled intracranial lesions typically present incidentally or with mass effect or hydrocephalus. Treatment of symptomatic or enlarging lesions is usually surgical, involving excision, endoscopic fenestration into a cistern or ventricle, or shunting for hydrocephalus. Cyst types include:

- arachnoid cyst: typically middle fossa, CSF enclosed in an envelope of arachnoid mater;
- colloid cyst: occur in the roof of the third ventricle, believed to represent embryonic endoderm remnants;
- dermoid and epidermoid cysts: epithelial lined structures arising from displaced ectodermal remnants, typically in the posterior fossa (midline) and cerebellopontine angle respectively;
- porencephalic cysts: brain cavities lined with gliotic white matter, containing CSF in communication with the ventricles or subarachnoid space.

Neural tube defects

Failure of closure of the neural tube is associated with folate deficiency, family history and some anticonvulsants. Prenatal screening, using serum alphaprotein levels and ultrasound, and diagnostic testing, using amniocentesis, are possible. The spectrum of conditions associated with failed closure of the posterior neuropore includes the conditions described below.

Spina bifida occulta

A congenital absence of a spinous process, without exposure of meninges or neural tissue, but presenting a characteristic shallow hair-covered hollow at the base of the spine. This is common and rarely clinically significant. Sometimes it may be associated with **tethered cord syndrome**, which involves thickening of the filum terminale, resulting in traction on the cord. Presentation is with progressive deficits, spasticity, bladder dysfunction or scoliosis, and treatment involves surgical exploration and untethering of the cord.

Meningocoele

A sac of meninges, covered by skin and containing CSF alone, herniates through an anterior or posterior bony defect.

Myelomeningocoele

A herniating sac of meninges without covering skin contains spinal cord, nerves or both. This is always associated with Chiari II malformation (see below). Open myelomeningocoele presents a high infection risk and requires early surgical repair.

Lipomyelomeningocoele

Adipose tissue adherent to the spinal cord herniates through a bony defect to the sacrolumbar soft tissue. This may be associated with bladder dysfunction and require surgical relief of the resultant cord tethering.

Failure of closure of the anterior neuropore produces anencephaly, which is uniformly fatal; the spectrum of spinal dysraphisms, however, is replicated in the skull. Cranium bifidum is a failure of fusion, often in the occipital region. This may be associated with herniation of meninges and CSF (meningocoele) and, potentially, also brain substance (encephalocoele) (Figure 43.27).

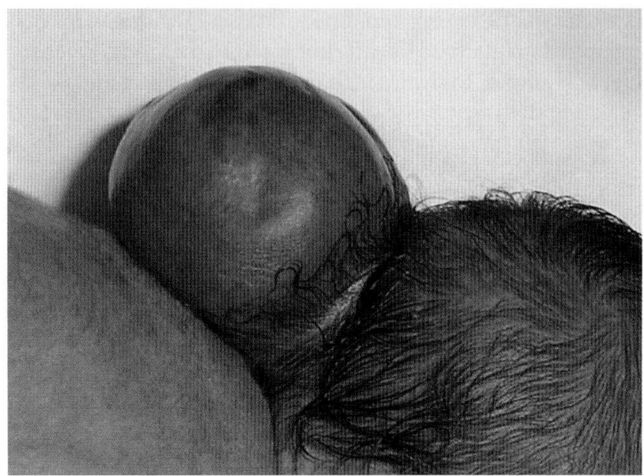

Figure 43.27 An occipital encephalocoele.

Posterior fossa malformations

Chiari malformations involve cerebellar herniation through the foramen magnum:

- Normal: up to 5 mm of cerebellar tonsillar descent through the foramen magnum;
- Chiari I: >5 mm of tonsillar descent: presents typically in young adults with cough headaches and neurological disturbance reflecting brainstem/cerebellar compression and/or formation of a fluid-filled syrinx in the spinal cord as a result of disordered CSF flow. Shunting and foramen magnum decompression are the mainstay of treatment;
- Chiari II: descent of the tonsils and vermis associated with myelomeningocoele and hydrocephalus, so clinically apparent in infancy.

Dandy Walker malformations present in infancy with macrocephaly, developmental delay and hydrocephalus; most patients have associated abnormalities in the CNS and other organ systems. Imaging demonstrates a hypoplastic cerebellar vermis, with the posterior fossa occupied by a large thin-walled cyst. Treatment usually involves shunt placement.

Craniosynostosis

Normal fusion of the coronal, lambdoidal, squamosal and sagittal sutures occurs between 6 and 12 months of age; others such as the frontal suture fuse later. Craniosynostosis is the premature fusion of one (simple craniosynostosis) or more (complex craniosynostosis) cranial sutures, preventing growth perpendicular to the suture. This results in a range of skull deformities (*Table 43.6*; **Figures 43.28 and 43.29**) and hydrocephalus. Syndromic craniosynostosis, often associated with abnormalities of the fibroblast growth factor receptor genes, is accompanied by developmental delay and other abnormalities. The surgical treatment aims to correct deformity and prevent development of raised ICP.

TABLE 43.6 Types of craniosynostosis.

Type	Suture involved	Clinical features
Scaphocephaly	Sagittal suture	Narrow boat-shaped head
Brachycephaly	Coronal suture	Shortened/ broad forehead
Microcephaly	All sutures involved	Small head
Plagiocephaly	Unilateral coronal/ lambdoid suture	Asymmetric skull
Trigonocephaly	Metopic suture	Pointed narrow forehead

Summary box 43.12

Paediatric neurosurgery

Children manifest a range of developmental pathologies requiring neurosurgical management including:

- Cysts
- Neural tube defects
- Posterior fossa abnormalities
- Craniosynostosis
- In general intracranial pathologies present with features including developmental delay, seizures, macrocephaly and hydrocephalus

FUNCTIONAL NEUROSURGERY

Where most neurosurgery seeks to avoid disruption of neural tissue as far as possible, functional procedures aim to relieve epilepsy, movement disorders or pain by ablation or stimulation of brain tissue and nerves.

Epilepsy

Up to 10% of the population will suffer a seizure at some point in their lives, and epilepsy, a syndrome of recurrent unprovoked seizures, represents the most common neurological disorder. About 20–30% of patients fail to achieve adequate seizure control with drugs, and many of these focal epilepsies may benefit from surgery. Where a primary lesion such as a tumour, AVM or cavernoma is present, lesionectomy alone may be appropriate. In other cases the clinical picture, including seizure type, focal features and investigation results, can be used to identify the seizure focus. Dual pathology refers to the presence of an extrahippocampal lesion plus hippocampal atrophy, important because removal of both the lesion and the atrophic hippocampus will be necessary to achieve seizure control.

Investigation

MRI is a mainstay, demonstrating for example reduced hippocampal volume and distorted architecture in mesial temporal sclerosis. Nuclear medicine modalities including single-photon emmision CT and positron emission tomography are sometimes used to demonstrate ictal and inter-ictal metabolic abnormalities.

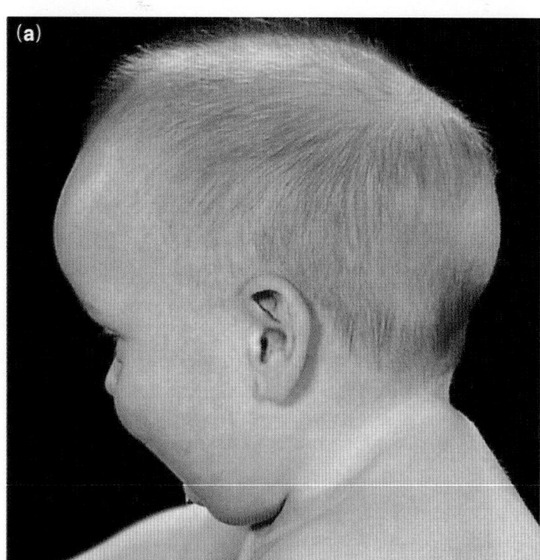

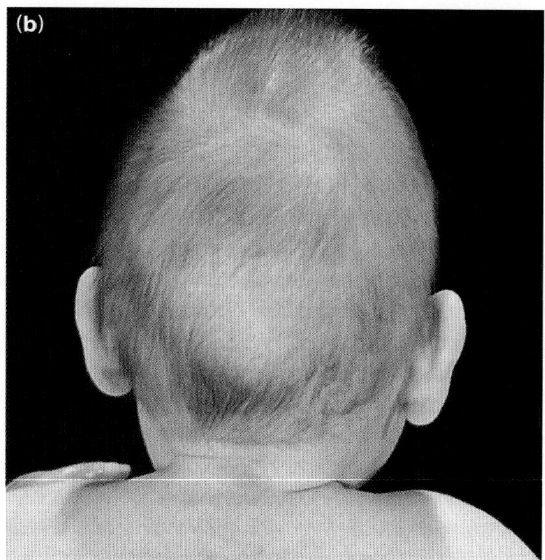

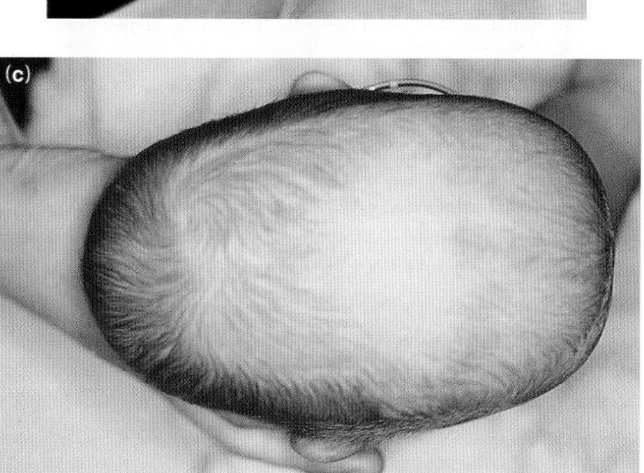

Figure 43.28 (a–c) Characteristic appearance of scaphocephaly due to sagittal suture synostosis.

Electroencephalography entails recording from an array of scalp electrodes, and comparison between ictal and inter-ictal recordings. This is especially helpful in lateralising the focus of complex partial seizures in temporal lobe epilepsy, and is combined with video monitoring of the seizure in a videotelemetry suite. A more detailed localisation may be achieved invasively by the preoperative placement of subdural or depth electrodes or by intraoperative electrocorticography.

Neuropsychological evaluation is used to evaluate the patient's preoperative function looking for concordant focal impairments, and, using the Wada test (Box 43.2), to assess the risk of postoperative language and memory deficits in temporal lobe epilepsy surgery.

Box 43.2

Wada test. Sodium amytal is injected into each internal carotid artery in turn, with simultaneous speech and memory testing to localise function. The aim is to confirm language laterality that resection on the side of the lesion will not significantly impair verbal memory functions.

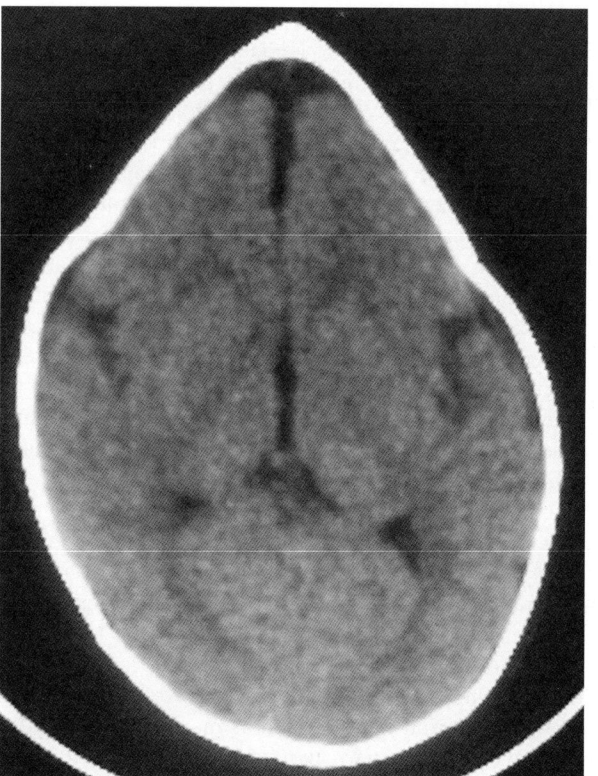

Figure 43.29 Axial computed tomography scan showing severe trigonocephaly due to premature fusion of the metopic suture.

Juhn Atsushi Wada, b.1924 Tokyo, appointed as Professor of Neurology, University of British Columbia, Vancouver, Canada, in 1956. The test is also known as 'intracarotid sodium amobarbitol' procedure.

Surgical management

The seizure focus may be resected, generally where it is in non-eloquent brain, or otherwise a disconnection can be performed. Awake craniotomy, allowing mapping particularly of speech centres, is increasingly employed.

Mesial temporal epilepsy is commonly medically refractory and can be addressed surgically by amygdalohippocampectomy or resection of the temporal lobe including the mesial structures. The extent of resection is limited by the potential for damage to the optic tracts and to speech areas in the dominant hemisphere. With careful patient selection, cure rates of up to 70% or greater can be achieved.

Functional or, rarely, anatomical hemispherectomy (Figure 43.30) may be performed for specific epilepsy syndromes associated with hemiplegia, such as infantile hemiplegia syndrome. This is usually considered in the early years of life when plasticity and potential for functional recovery is greatest.

Disconnection procedures include corpus callosotomy, used for patients suffering drop attacks, and subpial transections to isolate a seizure focus in eloquent brain from the surrounding cortex.

Vagal nerve stimulators can be implanted in severe drug refractory epilepsy, with electrodes applied to the vagus nerve in the carotid sheath in the neck. This option can achieve effective seizure control, especially in children, although the mechanism is not clear.

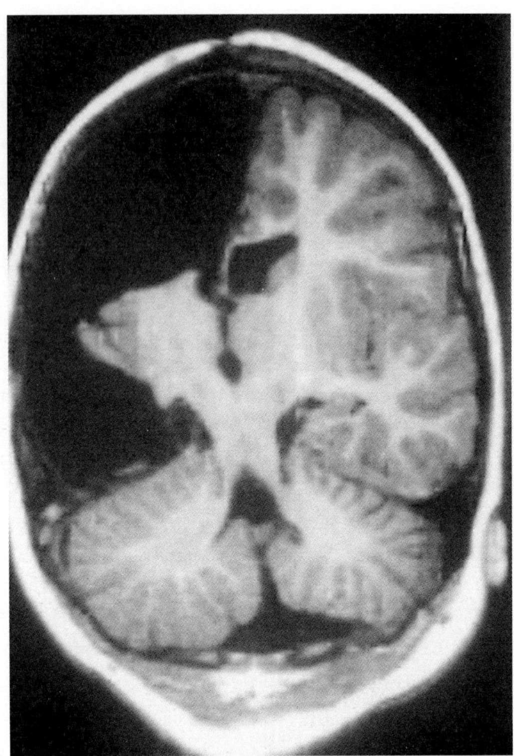

Figure 43.30 Coronal T2-weighted magnetic resonance image following anatomical hemispherectomy.

Movement disorders

Prior to the development of levodopa drug therapy, surgical ablation of the subthalamic nucleus or globus pallidus interna (GPi) was a mainstay of management for Parkinson's. Inhibition of the action of these centres remains a valuable tool later in the course of the disease as the therapeutic window using levodopa narrows, but this is now generally achieved using deep brain stimulation with electrodes. This offers the advantage of an adjustable and reversible effect, and can be performed bilaterally where equivalent lesioning surgery would likely result in deficits.

Deep brain stimulation is also an option for other movement disorders where less invasive approaches are ineffective. These include dystonias, which may be amenable to bilateral GPi stimulation, and essential tremor where the Vim nucleus of the thalamus is the target.

Pain syndromes

Neurosurgical approaches to the relief of pain may address the underlying aetiology directly or may seek to interrupt or modulate the transmission responsible for the pain. The contrasting approaches are demonstrated in the management of trigeminal neuralgia. This manifests, generally in middle age or later, with paroxysmal lancinating pain in the distribution of one or more divisions of the trigeminal nerve. The pain occurs without other neurological disturbance, and may be triggered by trivial stimuli such as eating or brushing the teeth. The pain is often attributable to impingement on the nerve by the superior cerebellar artery or other vessels, as first postulated by Walter Dandy. Occasionally another primary lesion is responsible; for example bilateral trigeminal neuralgia in younger patients is suggestive of multiple sclerosis. Where medications such as gabapentin and carbamazepine cannot achieve control, surgical options include:

- **Craniotomy and microvascular decompression**: this is designed to address the proposed origin of the neuropathic pain, by applying material between the nerve and adjacent vessel to prevent direct contact and stimulation. It achieves long-lasting relief of symptoms in about 80% of patients, but is associated with the standard risks of craniotomy and a significant incidence of cranial nerve deficit.
- **Peripheral nerve injections** can achieve good short-term relief of pain restricted to small areas supplied by terminal branches of the trigeminal.
- **Percutaneous Gasserian rhizolysis**: this involves needle placement under radiological guidance at the Gasserian ganglion in Meckel's cave. This permits lesioning of the ganglion by glycerol injection, radiofrequency thermocoagulation or balloon compression, with the aim of disrupting aberrant pain transmission. A similar effect can also be achieved using stereotactic radiosurgery. Facial numbness and late recurrence of pain are common after these procedures.

James Parkinson, 1755–1824, general practitioner, Shoreditch, London, UK.

Treatment of pain elsewhere may also be based on lesioning of nerve tracts. For example, pain related to brachial plexus infiltration or injury, may be treated by sectioning the spinothalamic tract (cordotomy) or the dorsal root entry zone (DREZ operation). These approaches are limited by the potential for producing deficits, and especially by the occurrence of deafferentation ('phantom limb') pain syndromes, which are particularly unpleasant and difficult to treat.

Electrical stimulation is used to modulate pain transmission: for example spinal cord stimulators can be applied to a range of pain syndromes especially associated failed spinal surgery. Deep brain stimulation targeting the periaqueductal grey and sensory thalamic nuclei has a role in chronic pain arising in the context of thalamic stroke. Implanted devices may also be used for intrathecal delivery of opiates for pain control, or baclofen to alleviate spasticity.

Summary box 43.13

Functional neurosurgery

- Intractable epilepsy can be treated surgically by implantation of a vagal nerve stimulator or by resection of one or more seizure foci
- Deep brain stimulation using implanted electrodes has largely replaced lesioning of these structures for management of drug-refractory Parkinson's disease
- Microvascular decompression is offered for trigeminal neuralgia, and other neuropathic pain syndromes may respond to lesioning of nerve tracts

PRACTICAL AND ETHICAL ISSUES

Creutzfeldt-Jakob disease

Creutzfeldt–Jakob disease (CJD) is a rare transmissible spongiform encephalopathy producing a rapidly progressive dementia, and is uniformly fatal. The causative agent seems to be a misfolded protein, a prion, which is not destroyed by conventional sterilisation techniques. UK practice involves undertaking preoperative checks to exclude any risk factors for CJD infection. These include family history, receipt of pituitary-derived human growth hormone, cadaveric dura mater grafts and previous brain or spinal surgery prior to 1997. Where risk factors are present, instruments must be quarantined or destroyed postoperatively.

Risks of craniotomy

The risks associated with craniotomy are important to appreciate in discussing operations with patients and family, and in evaluating patients who deteriorate postoperatively. Specific risks depend on the anatomy of each approach and the figures quoted in brackets will vary significantly between individual procedures and even between centres:

- infection (5%) and wound breakdown;
- intracerebral haemorrhage;
- seizures;
- CSF leak;
- permanent neurological deficit;
- death (1%).

Brainstem death

This is defined as the irreversible loss of cerebral and brainstem function. Brainstem death is legally equivalent to death, and is a precondition for the harvesting of organs for transplant from heart-beating donors.

Diagnosis requires:

- identification of the cause of irreversible coma;
- exclusion of reversible causes of coma;
- clinical demonstration of the absence of brainstem function.

In the UK, this entails testing twice, by two clinicians, to demonstrate the absence of:

- response to pain;
- respiratory drive (apnoea despite a pCO_2 >6.7 kPa);
- pupillary light reflex;
- corneal reflex;
- vestibulo-ocular reflex;
- oculo-cephalic reflex;
- gag reflex.

FURTHER READING

Greenberg MS. *Handbook of neurosurgery*, 8th edn. New York: Thieme, 2016. The accepted everyday reference handbook for trainee neurosurgeons.

Patton J. *Neurological differential diagnosis*, 2nd edn. New York: Springer, 1998. Clear explanations of neurological and neurosurgical pathology supported by the best illustrations available in the field.

Samandouras G. *The neurosurgeon's handbook*. Oxford: Oxford Publishing, 2010. A more concise and readable handbook offering a good overview of core material.

Chapter 44

The eye and orbit

Learning objectives

To understand and appreciate:

- The anatomy of the eye and orbit
- The common ocular disorders and their symptoms and specific signs
- The value of special investigations
- When specialist referral is appropriate
- Recent advances in ocular surgery

OCULAR ANATOMY

Adnexae

The lids comprise skin, connective tissue, the orbicularis oculi (cranial nerve VII) and the tarsal plate, with multiple meibomian glands opening posterior to the lashes and lined with conjunctiva, which is reflected onto the sclera. The upper lid is elevated by the levator muscle (cranial nerve III) and has a horizontal strip of sympathetically innervated Müller's muscle, giving rise to 2 mm of ptosis in Horner's syndrome. The frontalis muscle may also contribute to eyelid elevation, particularly when the levator muscle is weak. Both lids are attached to the orbital rim by the medial and lateral canthal tendons. Both have a rich vascular supply and are innervated by the V1 division of the trigeminal nerve (cranial nerve V) above and the V2 division below.

Lacrimal system

The almond-shaped lacrimal gland lies under the upper outer orbital rim and opens into the upper conjunctival fornix through 10–15 ducts. Tears are swept across the globe by the lids and evaporate or pass into the upper and lower lid puncta, and then into the canaliculi to join the common canaliculus, which passes into the lacrimal sac under the medial canthal tendon. The sac is drained by the nasolacrimal duct into the nose, opening in the inferior meatus under the inferior turbinate.

The globe

The cornea is the 12 mm-diameter window of the eye, 550 micrometres thick centrally on average; its clarity is due to the regular arrangement of collagen bundles and relative dehydration. It merges into the sclera at the corneoscleral junction (the limbus), the insertion of the bulbar conjunctiva. The sclera, which is 1 mm thick, comprises four-fifths of the wall of the eye, and gives attachment to the extraocular muscles (Figure 44.1). It is perforated by the long and short posterior ciliary arteries and the vortex veins and is contiguous with the optic nerve sheath. The uvea comprises iris,

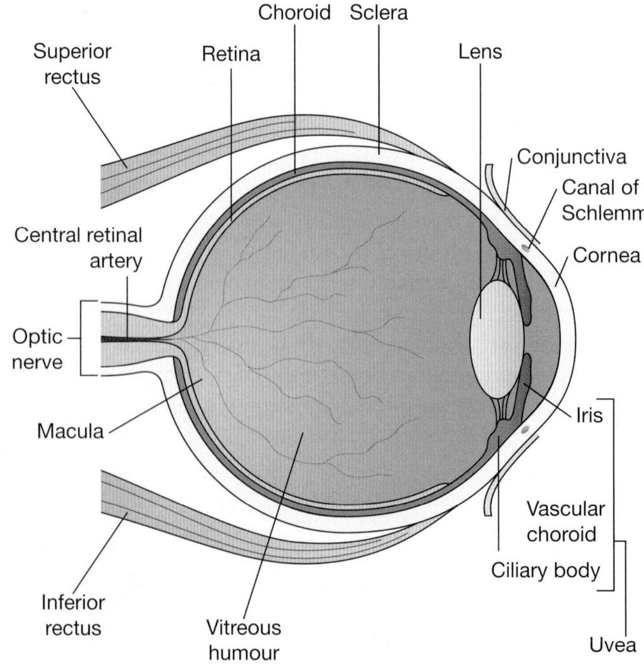

Figure 44.1 Anatomy of the eye.

Johannes Peter Müller, 1801–1858, Professor of Anatomy and Physiology, Berlin, Germany.
Johan Friedrich Horner, 1831–1886, Professor of Ophthalmology, Zurich, Switzerland, described this syndrome in 1869.

ciliary body and vascular choroid. Photoreceptor cells in the outer retina sense light and send impulses to retinal ganglion cells in the inner retina via bipolar cells. The retinal pigment epithelium underlies the photoreceptors and is responsible for reprocessing of photopigments. The optic nerve conveys the axons of retinal ganglion cells from the eye to the brain. The most high-resolution part of the retina, the macula, lies at the posterior pole within the vascular arcade. The biconvex lens and capsule are suspended by the lens zonules, over 300 tiny fibres attached to the ciliary muscle. Aqueous humour arises from the ciliary processes, hydrates the vitreous gel, passes through the pupil into the anterior chamber between the iris and the cornea and then drains out through the trabecular meshwork into Schlemm's canal in the drainage angle and from there to the episcleral venous circulation. The balance between production and drainage of aqueous humour determines the intraocular pressure, which in most normal eyes is regulated at a level of 10–21 mmHg. The inner retina is supplied by the central retinal artery and drained by the central retinal vein.

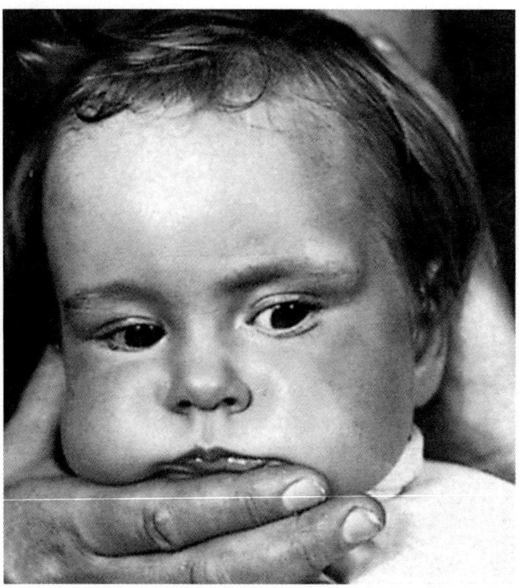

Figure 44.2 External angular dermoid.

Orbit

The orbit is four-sided and pyramidal in structure, housing the globe, optic nerve, the four rectus and two oblique muscles, the lacrimal gland, orbital fat, the cranial nerves III, IV, V and VI, the ophthalmic artery with its tributaries and the ophthalmic veins, which anastamose anteriorly with the face and posteriorly with the cranial cavity. Above is the frontal lobe of the brain, temporally the temporal fossa, inferiorly the maxillary sinus and nasally the lacrimal sac and ethmoidal and sphenoidal air sinuses. The optic nerve passes through the optic canal to the chiasm, with other nerves and vessels passing through the superior ophthalmic fissure.

PERIORBITAL AND ORBITAL SWELLINGS

Swellings related to the supraorbital margin

Dermoid cysts

Dermoid cysts are benign congenital choristomas of the orbit that originate from fetal bone suture lines during development, most commonly the frontozygomatic suture (Figure 44.2) although they may also occur more medially. Dermoid cysts account for about half of childhood orbital neoplasms and consist of keratinised epithelium and adnexal structures such as sweat glands and hair follicles. They often cause a bony depression and they may have a dumbbell extension into the orbit, which is of particular importance should they need to be excised. Dermoid cysts can also erode the orbital plate of the frontal bone to become attached to dura and for this reason it is important to image the area by computed tomography (CT) before excision.

Neurofibromatosis

Neurofibromatosis may also produce swellings above the eye. The diagnosis can usually be confirmed by an examination of the whole body, as there are often multiple lesions. Proptosis can also result (Figure 44.3). Other ophthalmic features may be present.

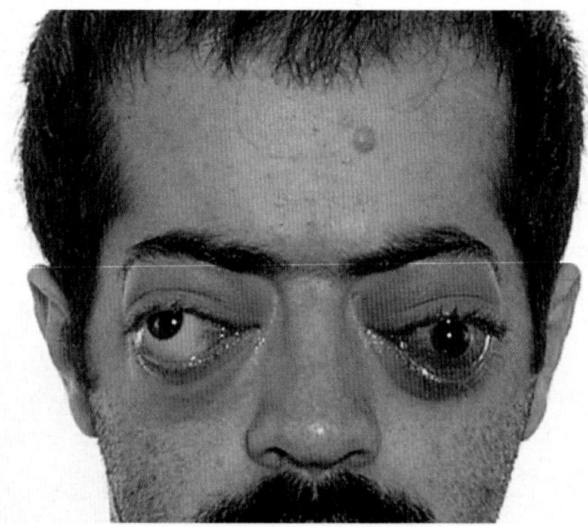

Figure 44.3 Neurofibroma in the orbit with proptosis, and also similar lesions in the forehead.

Swellings of the lids

Meibomian cysts (chalazion)

These are the most common lid swellings (Figure 44.4). A meibomian cyst is a chronic granulomatous inflammation of a meibomian gland. It may occur on either upper or lower lids and presents as a smooth, painless swelling. It can be felt by rolling the cyst on the tarsal plate. It can be distinguished

Friedrich Schlemm, 1795–1858, Professor of Anatomy, Berlin, Germany.
Heinrich Meibom (Meibomius), 1638–1700, Professor of Medicine, History and Poetry, Helmstadt, Germany, described these glands in 1666.

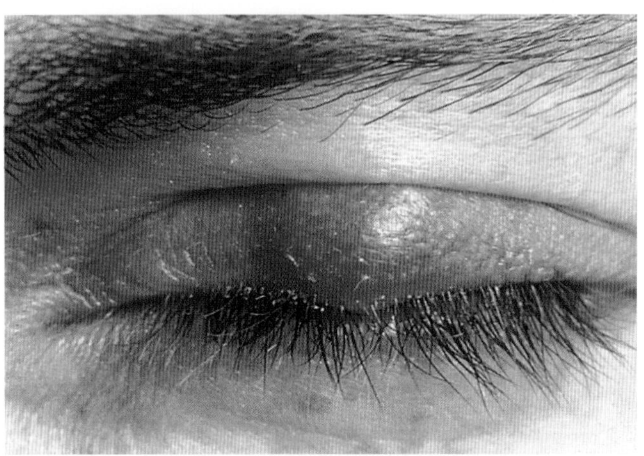

Figure 44.4 Meibomian cyst (courtesy of Mr D Spalton, FRCS).

from a stye (hordeolum), which is an infection of a hair follicle and is usually painful. Persistent meibomian cysts that do not resolve with conservative treatment (hot compresses) are treated by incision and curettage from the conjunctival surface. Styes are treated by antibiotics and local heat.

Basal cell carcinoma (rodent ulcer)

This is the most common malignant tumour of the eyelids (Figure 44.5). Basal cell carcinomas may be locally invasive but do not tend to metastasise. They are more common on the lower lids, often start as a small pimple that ulcerates and has raised edges ('rodent ulcer') and are usually easily excised in the early stages. Histological confirmation that the excision is complete is required. More extensive lesions may require specialist techniques such as Mohs' micrographic surgical excision controlled by frozen section. Local radiotherapy or cryotherapy can be carried out; however, recurrence is more common, more aggressive and more difficult to detect.

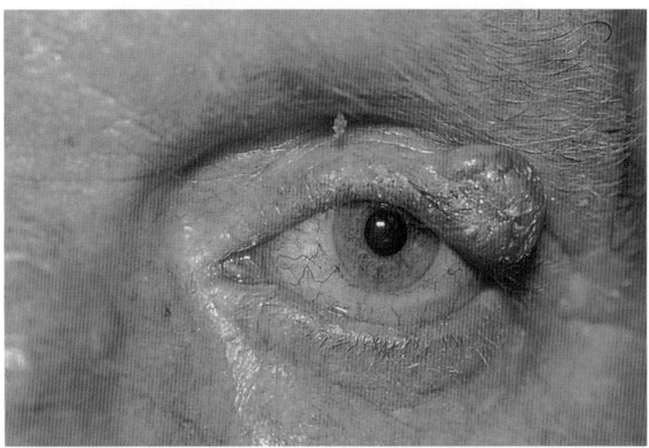

Figure 44.5 Rodent ulcers (courtesy of Mr J Beare, FRCS).

Summary box 44.1

Basal cell carcinomas

- Basal cell carcinomas are the most common malignant eyelid tumour
- Treatment is by wide local excision with careful histopathological margin control
- All unusual eyelid lesions (especially in the elderly) should be biopsied

Other lid swellings

Other types of lid swelling are less common. They include squamous cell carcinoma and malignant melanoma, sebaceous cyst, papilloma, keratoacanthoma, cyst of Moll (sweat glands) (Figure 44.6) or Zeis (sebaceous glands) and molluscum contagiosum. When molluscum contagiosum occurs on the lid margin, it can give rise to a mild viral chronic keratoconjunctivitis and should be curetted or excised.

Carcinoma of the meibomian glands and rhabdomyosarcomas are rare lesions; they need to be treated by radical excision. Atypical or meibomian cysts that recur should be biopsied to exclude sebaceous gland carcinoma.

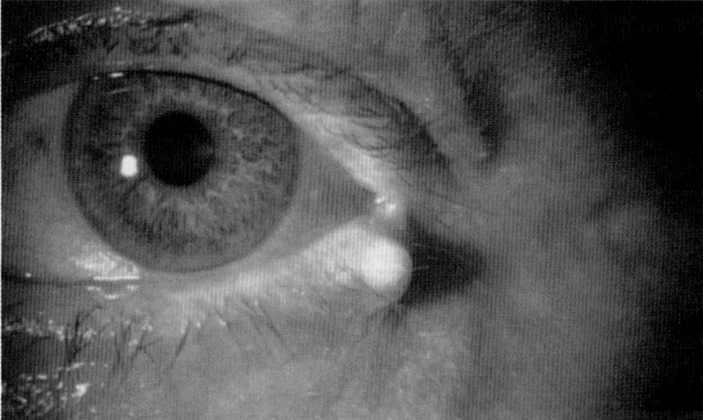

Figure 44.6 Cyst of Moll.

Swellings of the lacrimal system

Lacrimal sac mucocoele

This occurs from obstruction of the lacrimal duct beyond the sac and results in a fluctuant swelling that bulges out just below the medial canthus. It can become infected to give rise to a painful tense swelling (acute dacryocystitis). If untreated, it may give rise to a fistula. Treatment is by performing a bypass operation between the lacrimal sac and the nose (a dacryocystorrhinostomy). Watering of the eye can also occur due to eversion of the lower lid (ectropion), which causes loss of contact between the lower punctum and the tear film, or

Frederic E. Mohs, 1910–2002, developed the technique of micrographic surgical excision while a medical student at University of Wisconsin, USA.
Jacob Antonius Moll, 1832–1913, ophthalmologist of The Hague, The Netherlands.
Edward Zeis, 1807–1868, Professor of Surgery, Marburg, (1844–1850), who later worked at Dresden, Germany, described these glands in 1835.

from reflex hypersecretion as a result of irritation, for example by inturning lashes in entropion, and these must be distinguished from a mucocoele.

Lacrimal gland tumours

These are swellings of the lacrimal glands, which lie in the upper lateral aspect of the orbit. Eventually they lead to impairment of ocular movements and displacement of the globe forwards, downwards and inwards. Pathologically the tumours resemble parotid tumours and they can be pleomorphic adenomas with or without malignant change, carcinomas or mucoepidermoid tumours.

Orbital swellings

Orbital swellings result in displacement of the globe and limitation of movement. A full description of orbital swellings is outside the realm of this text, but some of the most common causes include the following:

- **Pseudoproptosis**. This results from a large eyeball, as seen in congenital glaucoma or high myopia.
- **Orbital inflammatory conditions** that result in orbital cellulitis (Figure 44.7).
- **Haemorrhage** after trauma or retrobulbar injection.
- **Neoplasia** affecting the lacrimal gland, the optic nerve, the orbital walls or the nasal sinuses (e.g. glioma [neurofibromatosis, Figure 44.3], meningioma and osteoma (Figure 44.8).
- **Thyroid eye disease** (Figures 44.9–44.11). This is the most common cause of unilateral and bilateral proptosis in adults and may occur in the absence of active thyroid disease or after thyroidectomy. Management of severe thyroid eye disease may require large doses of systemic steroids, radiotherapy or even orbital lateral wall decompression if the eyeball is threatened by exposure or optic nerve compression. The disease is often more severe in smokers and those with poorly controlled thyroid function. CT

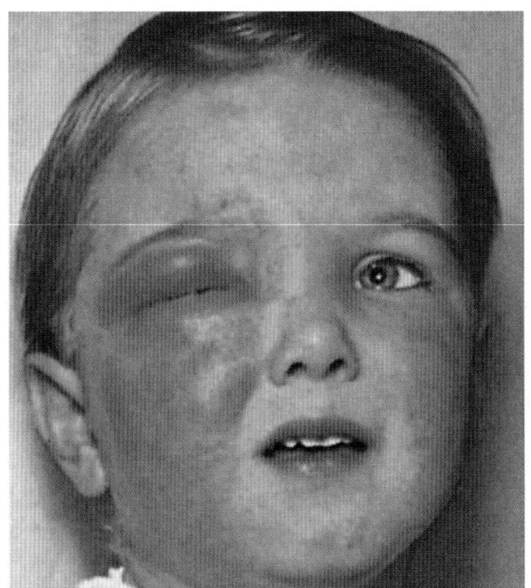

Figure 44.7 Orbital cellulitis.

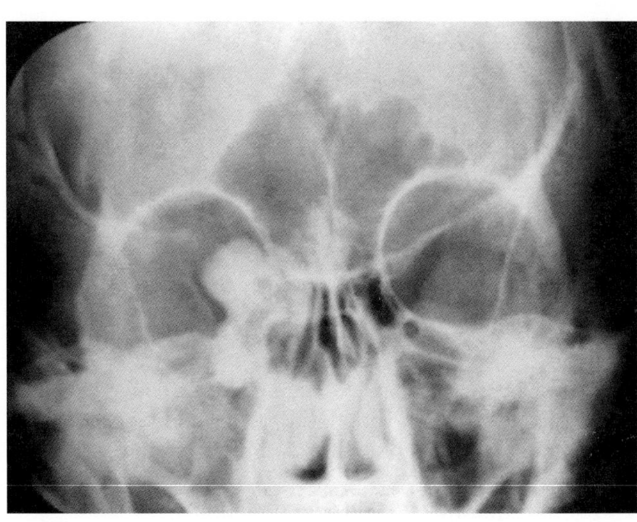

Figure 44.8 Radiograph showing an osteoma on the nasal side of the orbit giving rise to proptosis.

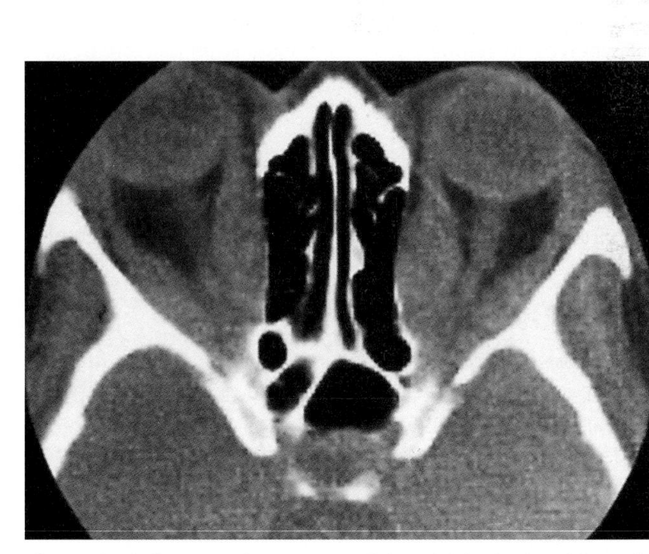

Figure 44.9 Computed tomogram of the orbit in dysthyroid exophthalmos, showing swollen muscles (courtesy of Dr Glyn Lloyd).

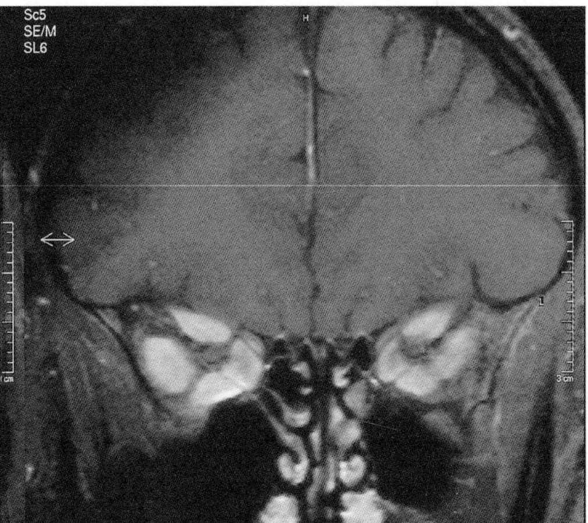

Figure 44.10 Magnetic resonance imaging scan of a coronal view of the orbit, showing enlarged muscles in thyroid disease (courtesy of Dr Juliette Britton).

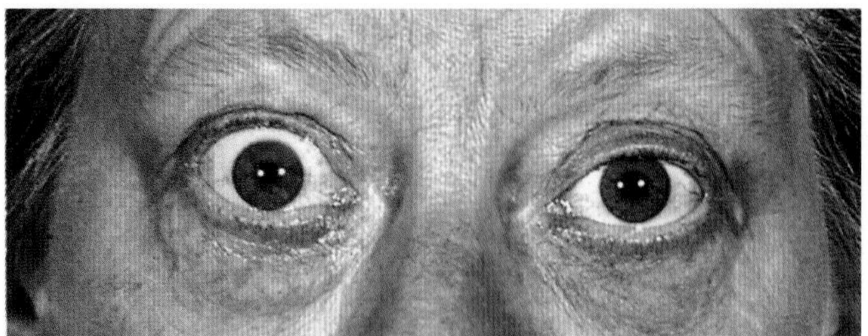

Figure 44.11 Exophthalmos in dysthyroid eye disease.

and magnetic resonance imaging (MRI) scans are useful in diagnosis. MRI with STIR sequences is particularly useful for identification of active inflammation within the orbital tissues.
- **Pseudotumour**, or malignant lymphoma.
- **Haemangiomas** of the orbit (Figure 44.12).
- **Tumour metastases**. These are rare. In children they usually arise from neuroblastomas of the adrenal gland, whereas in adults the oesophagus, stomach, breast and prostate can be sites of primary lesions.

Diagnostic aids

Diagnostic aids include radiography, CT, MRI, ultrasonography and, less commonly, tomography and orbital venography.

Treatment

Treatment is directed to the cause of the lesion taking care to prevent exposure of the eye, diplopia or visual impairment from optic nerve compression.

INTRAOCULAR TUMOURS

Children

Retinoblastoma, the most common ocular malignancy of childhood, is a malignant tumour of the retina that can be bilateral in around one-third of cases. Half of cases are hereditary (autosomal dominant) due to mutation of the RB1 gene on chromosome 13 and children with a family history should be carefully monitored from birth. Remaining cases occur sporadically. Inherited retinoblastoma is more likely to be bilateral. Retinoblastoma is often not spotted until the tumour fills the globe and presents as a white reflex in the pupil or as a squint (Figure 44.13). The differential diagnosis includes retinopathy of prematurity, primary hyperplastic vitreous and intraocular infections. If the tumour is large, enucleation may be required, but radiotherapy, cryotherapy, chemotherapy or laser treatment can cure small lesions. Liaison with a paediatric oncologist is essential.

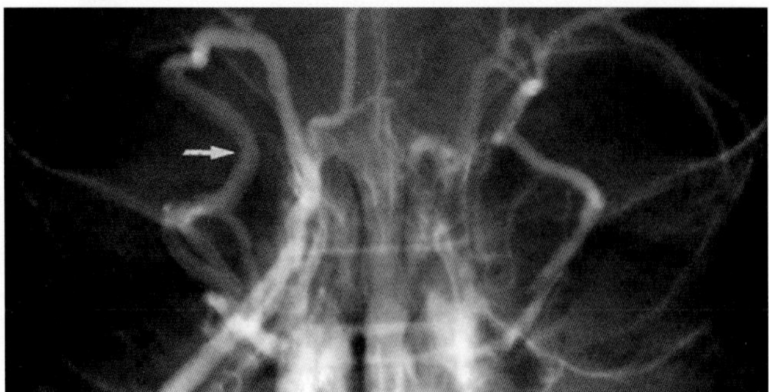

Figure 44.12 Capillary haemangioma in a child. An orbital venogram demonstrates displacement of the second part of the superior ophthalmic vein (arrow) (courtesy of Dr Glyn Lloyd).

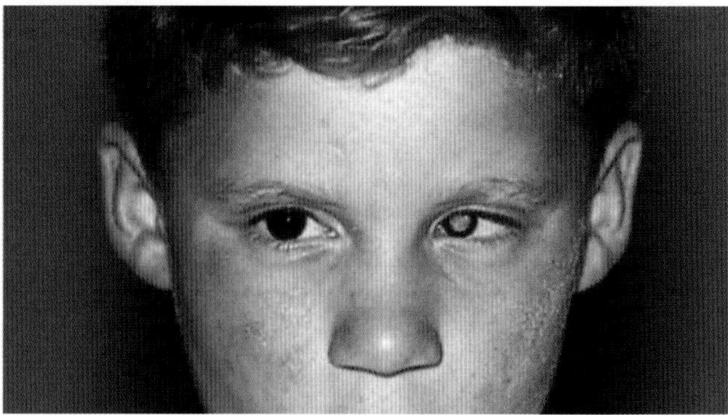

Figure 44.13 Retinoblastoma giving rise to a white pupillary reflex. This child was first seen with a convergent squint and discharged without a fundus examination. He was next seen many years later with a 'white reflex' and died soon after diagnosis (courtesy of MA Bedford, FRCS).

Summary box 44.2

Intraocular tumours

- Any child with a white pupil (leukokoria) should be referred to an ophthalmologist to exclude retinoblastoma, although congenital carataracts may also cause this sign
- A blind painful eye may hide a melanoma or other ocular tumour

Adults

Malignant melanoma is the most common primary malignant tumour of the eye and originates in the pigmented cells of the choroid (Figure 44.14), ciliary body or iris. It can present with a reduction in vision, a vitreous haemorrhage or by the chance finding of an elevated pigmented lesion in the eye. Tumour growth is variable but, as a general rule, the more posterior the lesion, the more rapidly progressive it is likely to be. Spread may be delayed for many years; however, the liver is frequently involved, hence the advice 'beware of the patient with a glass eye and an enlarged liver'. Treatment options vary by size and location of the tumour but include laser photocoagulation, radioactive plaque, radiotherapy/proton beam therapy, enucleation and, in selected cases, local excision. Diagnosis is made by direct observation and/or ultrasound, which shows a solid tumour, often with low internal reflectivity on ultrasound (Figure 44.15).

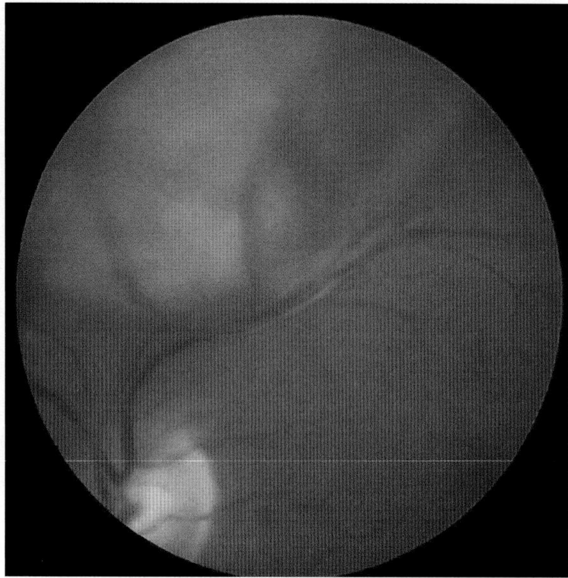

Figure 44.14 Choroidal melanoma.

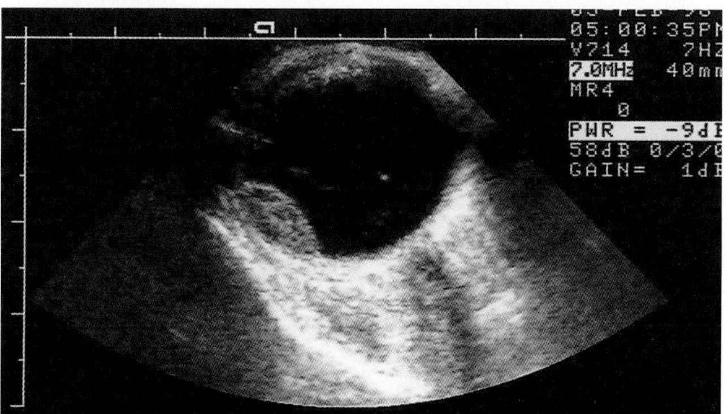

Figure 44.15 B-scan showing choroidal melanoma (courtesy of Dr Marie Reston).

INJURIES INVOLVING THE EYE AND ADJACENT STRUCTURES

Corneal abrasions and ulceration

The cornea is frequently damaged by direct trauma or by foreign bodies (Figure 44.16). Ulceration can occur with infection, exposure (for example in severely ill patients with incomplete eye closure) or after damage to the facial nerve. Post-herpetic ulceration is common and serious if not treated. Fluorescein instillation illuminated by blue light shows up corneal ulceration at an early stage, with areas of epithelial loss fluorescing green.

Treatment of sterile corneal abrasions or exposure is by topical lubrication or padding of the eye. If bacterial infection is suspected, a swab or scrape may be performed for microbiological diagnosis and topical antibiotics such as 0.5% chloramphenicol or ofloxacin eye drops are commonly used. The eye is made more comfortable by the use of mydriatics such as cyclopentolate to reduce photophobia. Herpes simplex dendritite ulcers are treated with aciclovir ointment.

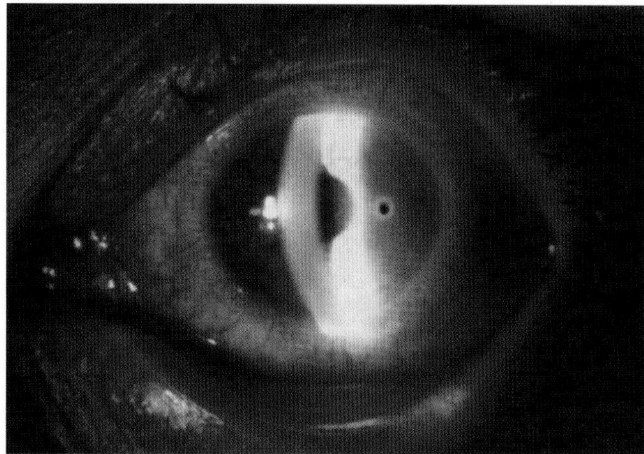

Figure 44.16 Corneal foreign body.

In countries in the Far and Middle East, chronic infection with trachoma can cause corneal opacification and blindness, although the worldwide incidence of this condition is falling. Corneal grafting is the only cure for an opaque cornea. Until recently, full-thickness penetrating keratoplasty was the only corneal graft technique. For some conditions this has largely been replaced by lamellar or partial-thickness graft surgery, in a technique termed DSEK or 'Descamets stripping endothelial keratoplasty'. However, penetrating keratoplasy remains the treatment of choice for severe corneal damage due to infection or injury. Rarely, osteo-odonto keratoprosthesis can be attempted in very severe cases of opaque corneas that are not suitable for grafting. Artifical corneal prostheses have also been developed. Acanthamoeba is a rare serious cause of corneal infection. This infection usually follows the use of contact lenses. Specialist management and treatment is recommended.

Summary box 44.3

Corneal abrasions

- A drop of fluorescein dye illuminated by a blue light reveals even the smallest corneal abrasion
- Corneal ulcers are often more serious in contact lens wearers and require prompt assessment and treatment
- Development of white infiltate in/around a corneal abrasion is a sign of infection

Blunt injuries to the eye and orbit

The floor of the orbit is its weakest wall and in blunt trauma, such as a blow from a fist, it is often fractured without fractures of the other walls. This is called a blow-out fracture. Clinical signs are enophthalmos, bruising around the orbit, maxillary hypoaesthesia, limitation of upward gaze due to entrapment of the inferior rectus muscle leading to vertical diplopia. This occurs when the extraocular muscles or orbital septa become trapped in the fracture and can be identified as a soft-tissue mass in the antrum on a radiograph (Figure 44.17), although CT scans or tomograms may be necessary.

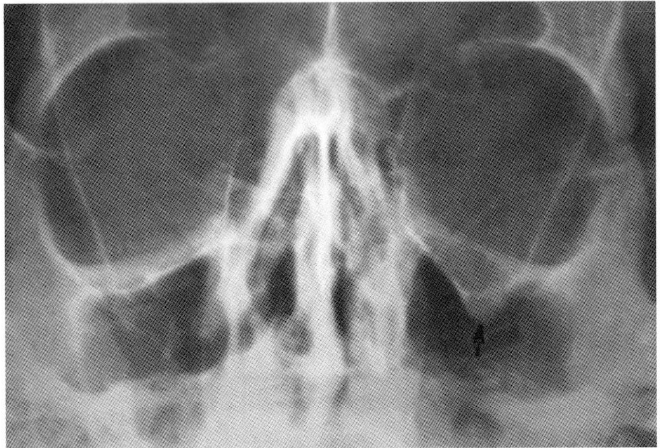

Figure 44.17 Radiograph showing a blow-out fracture of the orbit (left) with soft tissue in the antrum (courtesy of Dr Glyn Lloyd).

Surgical repair of the orbital floor with freeing of the trapped contents may be necessary if troublesome diplopia persists or enophthalmos is marked. A child with an orbital floor fracture requires urgent assessment, particularly if upgaze is restricted, as trapping of the inferior rectus muscle may cause ischaemia and require urgent surgery. If an orbital haemorrhage is too extensive to examine the eye, it may be necessary to examine the eye under anaesthesia because there may be a hidden perforation of the globe. Injuries to the lids and lid margins must be repaired, and if the lacrimal canaliculi are damaged, they should be repaired if possible, especially the lower canaliculus, as 75% of tear drainage goes through it.

Blunt injuries can also cause damage to the optic nerve, which can result in blindness and a total afferent nerve defect (Figures 44.18 and 44.19).

Blunt ocular injuries

Blunt injuries to the eye can give rise to several problems, which include the following:

- **Iritis**. Inflammation; treated with topical steroids.
- **Hyphaema** (blood in the anterior chamber) (Figure 44.20). Rest and sedation, particularly in children, are advised because the main danger in this condition is secondary bleeding, resulting in an acute rise in intraocular pressure and blood staining of the cornea. The use of anti-fibrinolytic agents (ε-aminocaproic acid) has been advocated and, if the pressure rises, surgery to wash out the blood may be necessary.
- **Subluxation of the lens**. This is suspected if the iris, or part of the iris, 'wobbles' on movement (iridodonesis).
- **Secondary glaucoma**. This is often associated with recession of the iridocorneal drainage angle.
- **Retinal and macular haemorrhages and choroidal tears** (Figure 44.21).
- **Retinal dialysis**. This may lead to a retinal detachment and permanent damage to vision (Figure 44.22).

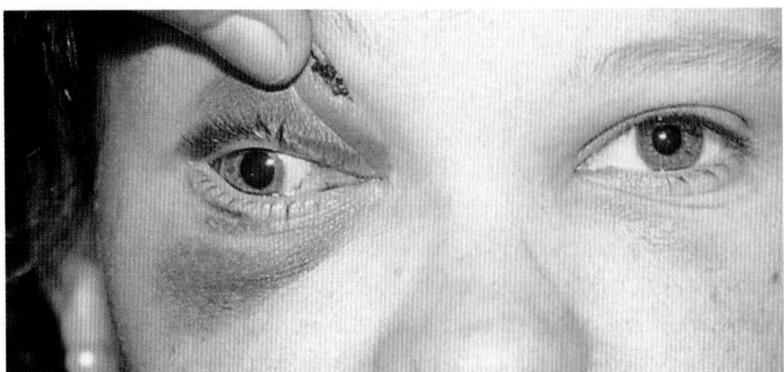

Figure 44.18 Injury from a ski pole into the right brow. Vision reduced to 'no perception of light' (courtesy of J Beare, FRCS).

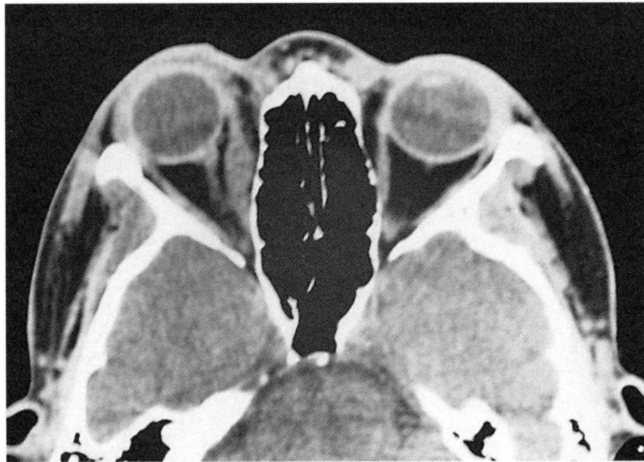

Figure 44.19 Scan of orbit from Figure 44.18 showing a massive swelling of the medial rectus (courtesy of J Beare, FRCS).

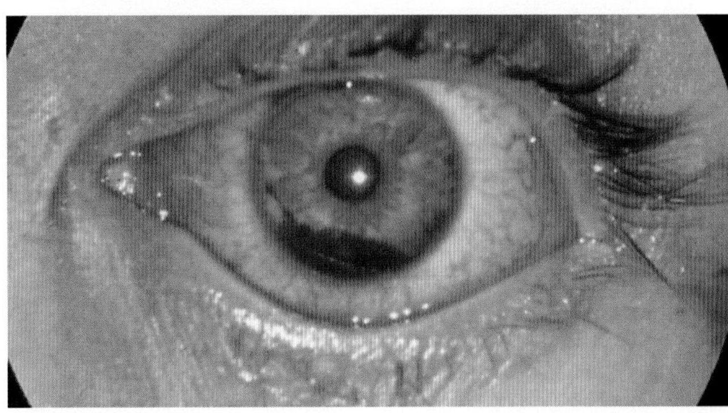

Figure 44.20 Hyphaema. Blood in the vitreous chamber after a concussional injury.

Penetrating eye injuries

These occur when the globe is penetrated, often in road traffic and other major accidents (Figure 44.23), and also in injuries from sharp instruments. The compulsory wearing of seat belts in motor vehicles has substantially reduced the incidence of this type of eye injury, by up to 73% in the UK. The presence of an irregular pupil suggests prolapse of the iris and should arouse suspicion of a penetrating injury. Treatment is prompt primary repair to restore the integrity of the globe. If a perforation is suspected, extensive eye examination should not be attempted before anaesthesia because this may lead to further extrusion of the intraocular contents. If the fundal view is poor, ultrasonography and orbital imaging are

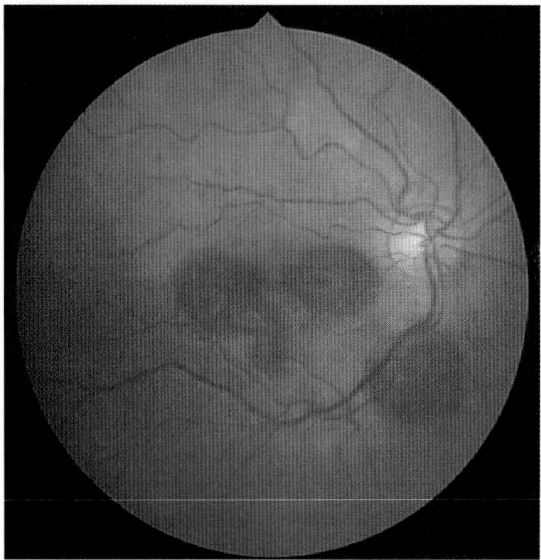

Figure 44.21 Retinal haemorrhage from a cricket bat injury (courtesy of J Beare, FRCS).

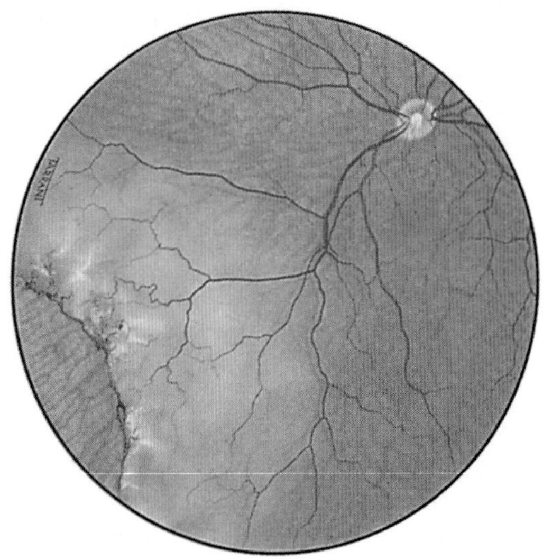

Figure 44.22 Retinal dialysis after a concussional injury.

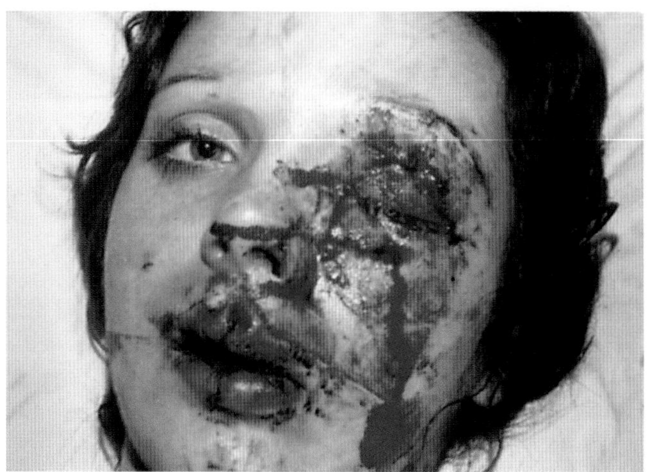

Figure 44.23 Facial lacerations from a windscreen injury. Beware of a perforating eye injury.

indicated. Secondary corneal grafting, lensectomy and vitrectomy have considerably improved the visual prognosis; these must be done by an experienced eye surgeon. Injuries to the optic nerves must also be excluded in severe accidents.

Intraocular foreign bodies

Intraocular foreign bodies must always be excluded when patients attend the accident and emergency department with an eye injury and a history of working with a hammer and chisel or a history of a potentially high-velocity injury. Radiography of the orbits must be performed. Ferrous and copper foreign bodies should always be removed, sometimes requiring the use of a magnet. B-scan ultrasonography can also assist in localising foreign bodies when a vitreous haemorrhage or cataract is present. CT can be used, but MRI is contraindicated if a ferrous intraocular foreign body is suspected.

Summary box 44.4

Penetrating eye injuries

- A distorted and irregular pupil warrants the careful exclusion of a penetrating eye injury
- Avoid extensive eye examination if globe rupture is suspected to avoid worsening the injury prior to surgical repair

Burns

Radiation burns

Corneal injury may occur after exposure to ultraviolet radiation, for example after arc welding or excessive sunlight (snow blindness) and sun lamps. Such burns cause intense gritty burning pain and photophobia as a result of keratitis (corneal inflammation), which starts some hours after exposure. Mydriatic and local steroids with antibiotic drops ease the condition, and healing usually occurs after 24 hours.

Thermal burns

If these involve the full thickness of the lids, corneal scarring may occur from exposure, and immediate corneal protection is necessary. A splash of molten metal may cause marked local necrosis and may lead to permanent corneal scarring. Treatment is to remove any debris by irrigation and to instill local atropine, antibiotics and steroids to prevent superadded infection and scarring. Lid reconstruction may be necessary.

Chemical burns

Chemical burns, and especially alkali burns, can be serious because ocular penetration occurs quickly and ischaemic necrosis can result (Figure 44.24). Immediate copious irrigation until the pH is neutral will ensure that the chemical is diluted as much as possible, and all particles should be removed from the fornices. Treatment can then be continued as with thermal burns. Well-fitting goggles should prevent such injuries.

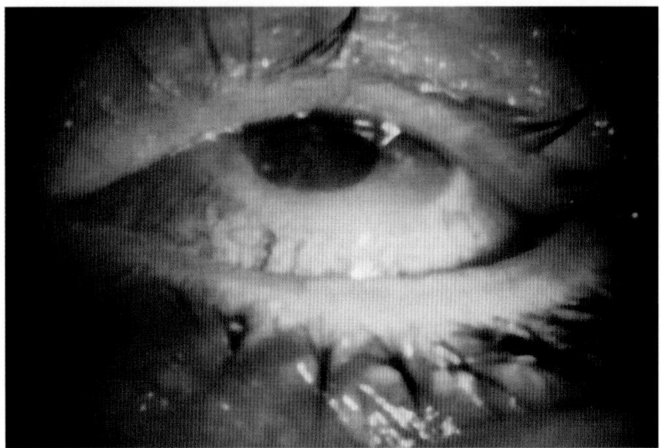

Figure 44.24 Chemical burn showing conjunctival necrosis.

DIFFERENTIAL DIAGNOSIS OF THE ACUTE RED EYE

This is important in the management of minor ocular complaints and the recognition of conditions that require expert attention. Possible causes of the acute red eye include:

- subconjunctival haemorrhage;
- conjunctivitis;
- keratitis;
- uveitis;
- episcleritis and scleritis;
- acute glaucoma.

Any condition with pain, visual impairment or a pupil abnormality suggests a more serious diagnosis.

Subconjunctival haemorrhage

This presents as a bright red eye, often noticed incidentally with only minimal discomfort and normal vision. Causes include coughing, sneezing, minor trauma, hypertension and, rarely, a bleeding disorder. Subconjunctival haemorrhages are more common in those receiving antiplatelet or anticoagulation therapy. Reassurance and treatment of the underlying cause are required. Most settle within a week, but can recur.

Conjunctivitis

Symptoms are grittiness, redness and discharge. Causes are infective, chemical, allergic or traumatic. In the newborn it can be serious; gonococcal and chlamydial infection must be excluded. Bacterial conjunctivitis is purulent, usually self-limiting and treated with topical broad-spectrum antibiotics. Chlamydial and adenovirus infections must be considered. Adenoviral infections are common and usually affect one eye much more in severity and onset, tending to be more watery than sticky, and are often associated with a palpable preauricular gland.

Vernal conjunctivitis (Figure 44.25) is a form of allergic conjunctivitis, characterised by itchy eyes, usually worse in the spring and early summer and often associated with other allergic problems such as hay fever. Clinically, most signs are under the upper lid, which may have a cobblestone appearance instead of a smooth surface.

Giant pupillary conjunctivitis with large papillae under the upper lid may be seen in soft contact lens wearers. This is usually caused by an allergy to the sterilising solutions and lens protein and may be helped by either using a preservative-free solution or using daily-wear disposable lenses.

Kaposi's sarcoma, often associated with HIV infection, can rarely present like a subconjunctival haemorrhage (Figure 44.26).

Considerable conjunctival and corneal irritation can be caused by the lids turning in (entropion) (Figure 41.27) or turning out (ectropion) (Figures 41.28 and 41.29), and by ingrowing lashes. The lids should be repaired surgically to their normal position.

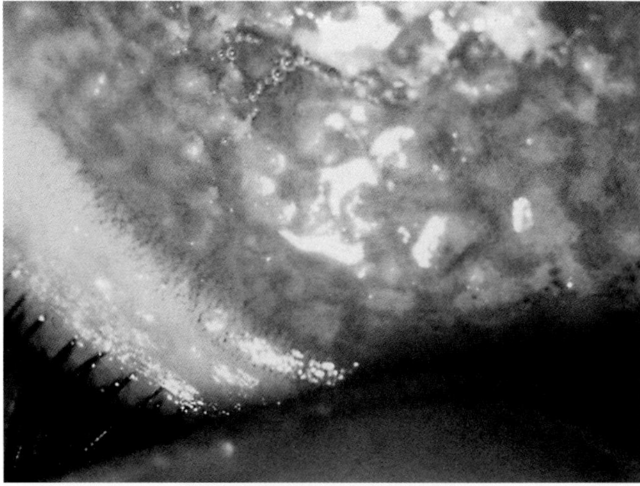

Figure 44.25 Vernal conjunctivitis (spring catarrh) showing cobblestone appearance under the upper lid.

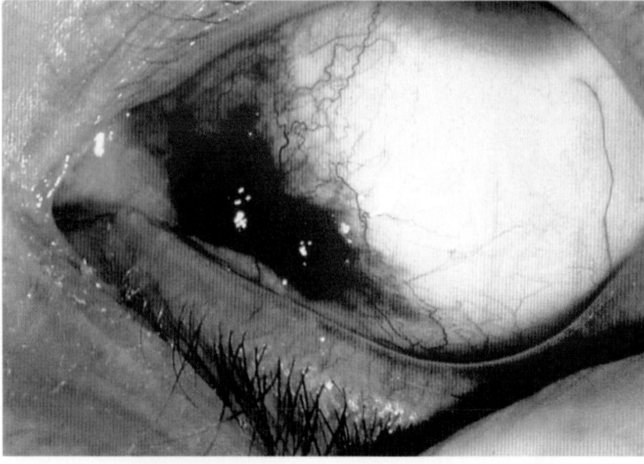

Figure 44.26 Kaposi's sarcoma of conjunctiva.

Moritz Kaposi, 1837–1902, Professor of Dermatology, Vienna, Austria, described pigmented sarcoma of the skin in 1872.

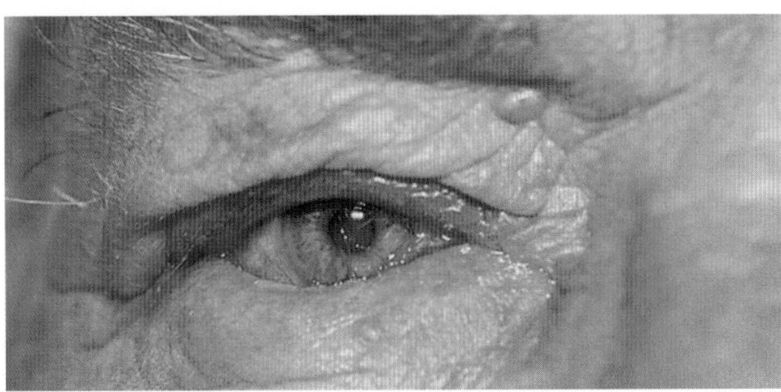

Figure 44.27 Entropion (courtesy of J Beare, FRCS).

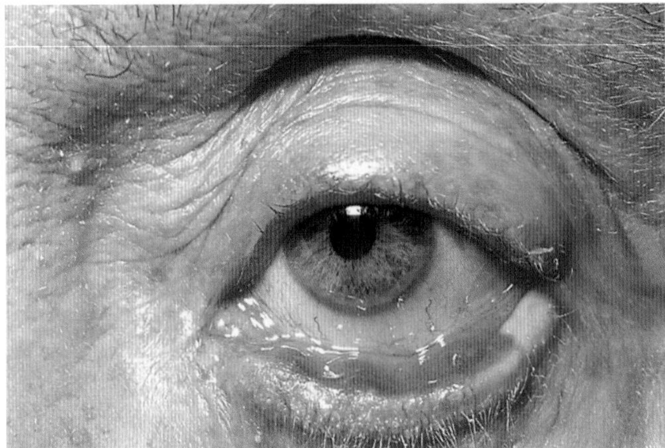

Figure 44.28 Ectropion, lower lid (courtesy of J Beare, FRCS).

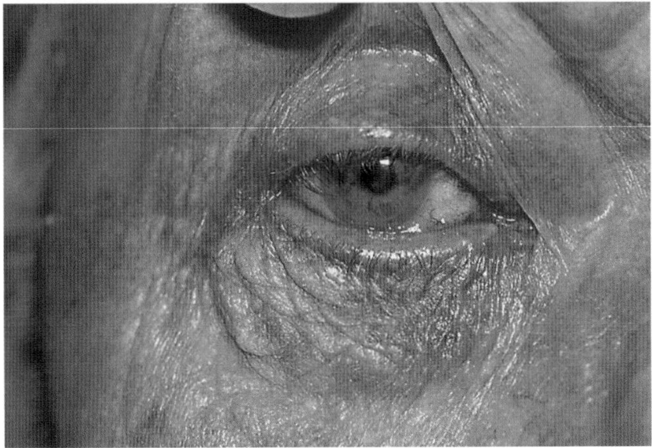

Figure 44.29 Ectropion, upper lid – chronic staphylococcal infection (courtesy of J Beare, FRCS).

Vision is not commonly affected in conjunctivitis but, with some viral infections, a keratitis may be present and result in visual impairment and pain. All of the other conditions below are painful and usually affect vision.

Keratitis (inflammation of the cornea)

Herpes simplex infection presents as a dendritic (branching) ulcer, shown easily by staining with fluorescein or Bengal Rose. It is treated with aciclovir ointment five times per day. The use of steroid drops must be avoided as this can make the condition much worse (Figure 44.30).

Corneal ulceration may occur as a result of ingrowing lashes or corneal foreign bodies, marginal ulceration and infected abrasions. Infected ulcers can occur in patients wearing soft contact lenses or elderly immunocomprimised individuals. Herpes zoster (shingles) may affect the ophthalmic division of cranial nerve V and can give rise to a keratitis and uveitis. It is important to avoid the use of steroid drops until a diagnosis has been made. Local anaesthetic drops should also not be given on a regular basis.

Uveitis

This can be anterior (iritis) or, more rarely, posterior. In anterior uveitis, the pupil is sometimes small and/or irregular due to formation of posterior synechiae (adhesions between the iris and the lens). There is often circumcorneal injection and there may be keratic precipitates present on the posterior surface of the cornea. Pain, photophobia and some visual loss are usually present. Posterior uveitis can present with a white eye and blurred vision. It usually takes a chronic course. Granulomatous diseases, Behçet's disease, Reiter's syndrome, toxoplasmosis and cytomegalovirus infection should be excluded. Topical systemic steroids and, sometimes, immunosuppressive drugs are useful in treating these conditions; management should be under the care of an ophthalmologist.

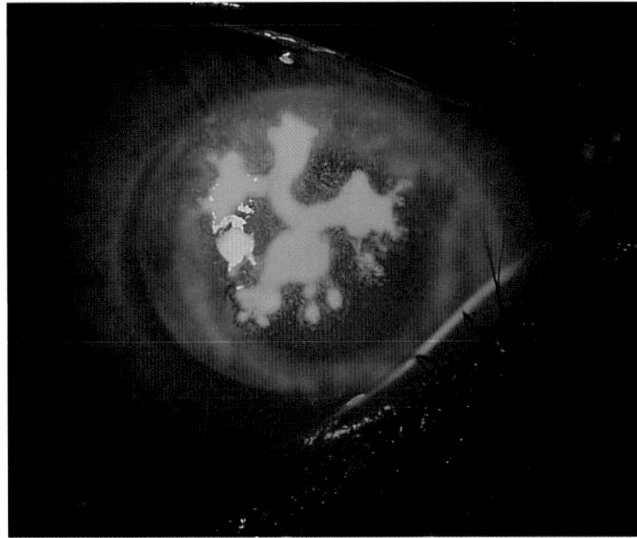

Figure 44.30 Dendritic staining caused by herpes keratitis.

Bengal Rose (or Rose Bengal) is dichlortetraiodofluorescein.

Hulusi Behçet, 1889–1948, Professor of Dermatology, Istanbul, Turkey, described this disease in 1937.

Hans Conrad Julius Reiter, 1881–1968, President of the Health Service and Honorary Professor of Hygiene at the University of Berlin, Germany, described this disease in 1916.

Episcleritis and scleritis

Episcleritis or inflammation of the episcleral tissue often occurs as an idiopathic condition (Figure 44.31). Scleritis is a less common, more serious, condition in which the deeper sclera is involved. There is often an associated uveitis and severe pain. Thinning of the sclera may result. Systemic nonsteroidal anti-inflammatory drugs or steroids/other immunomodulatory agents may be required to treat the condition adequately. Appoximately half of patients with scleritis have an underlying systemic disorder.

Scleritis is often associated with severe rheumatoid conditions. The presence of scleritis suggests that there is active systemic disease and this requires systemic work-up including renal function tests.

Acute angle closure glaucoma

This usually occurs in older, often hypermetropic, patients. The prevalence is much higher in some Asian populations. The cornea becomes hazy, the pupil oval, dilated and nonreacting, the vision poor and the eye feels hard. In severe cases pain may be accompanied by vomiting and the condition can be mistaken for an acute abdominal problem. Tonometry (intraocular measurement) and examination of the iridocorneal angle by gonioscopy (using a prism placed on the cornea) is diagnostic. Urgent treatment to reduce the pressure with pilocarpine eyedrops, oral acetazolamide and, if refractory, mannitol should be started, followed by YAG laser iridotomy, laser iridoplasty, anterior chamber paracentesis or surgical iridectomy. The condition is usually bilateral and the second eye usually needs a prophylactic iridotomy at the same time.

Except for a simple conjunctivitis and subconjunctival haemorrhage, which are self-limiting, the management of an acute red eye requires expert treatment and a specialist opinion should be sought. A painful eye with a cranial nerve III palsy (ptosis, dilated pupil, globe down and out) often signifies an intracranial aneurysm and should be investigated immediately.

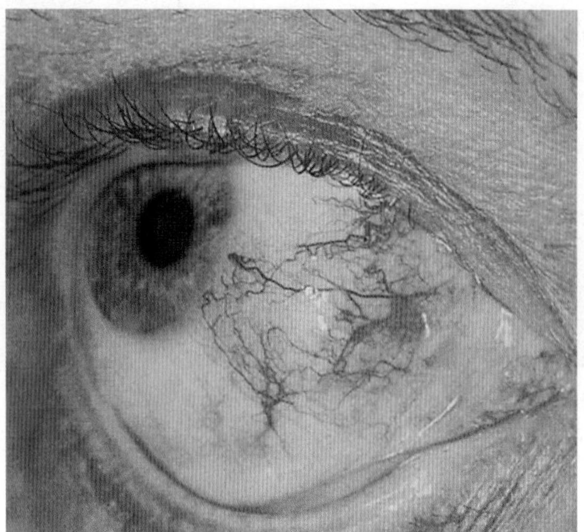

Figure 44.31 Episcleritis.

PAINLESS LOSS OF VISION

This may occur in one or both eyes, and the visual loss may be transient or permanent. Possible causes are:

- Acute:
  - obstruction of the central retinal artery (Figure 44.32);
  - obstruction of the central retinal vein (Figure 44.33);
  - ischaemic optic neuropathy;
  - migraine and other vascular causes;
  - vitreous and retinal haemorrhages;
  - retinal detachment (Figure 44.34);
  - macular hole, cyst or haemorrhage;
  - cystoid macular oedema, often after surgery;
  - hysterical blindness.
- Chronic:
  - cataract;
  - glaucoma;
  - macular degeneration.
  - diabetic retinopathy.

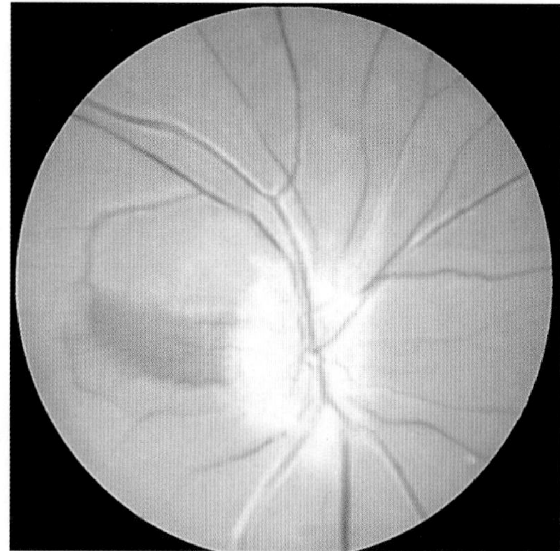

Figure 44.32 Retinal artery occlusion.

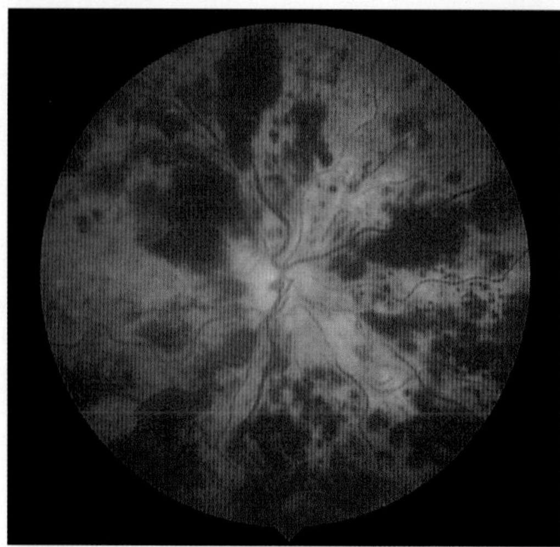

Figure 44.33 Central retinal vein occlusion.

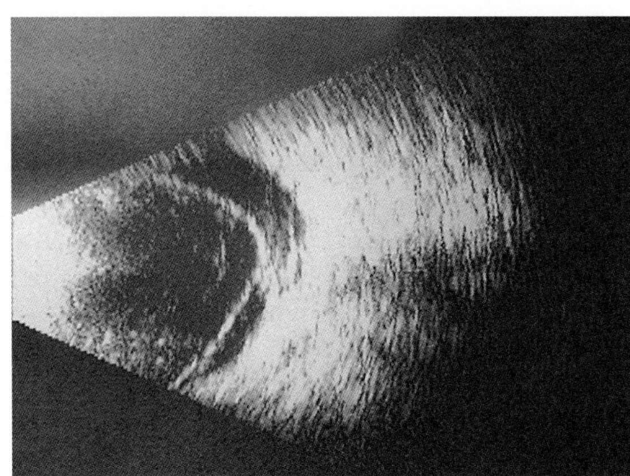

Figure 44.34 B-scan of a retinal detachment.

Specialist help should be sought in any case of loss of vision. The possibility of temporal arteritis should always be considered in the differential diagnosis of sudden visual loss, as prompt treatment of this condition is extremely important. Elderly patients with sudden visual loss should be specifically asked for symptoms of scalp tenderness and jaw claudication and temporal arteries should be palpated for pulsation and tenderness. The erythrocyte sedimentation rate and C-reactive protein should be measured immediately if temporal arteritis is suspected, and the carotid system should be examined for bruits and other signs of arteriosclerosis in cases of ischaemic optic neuropathy and central retinal artery occlusion. Glaucoma, hypertension, hyperviscosity syndromes and diabetes should be looked for in cases of central vein thrombosis.

RECENT DEVELOPMENTS IN EYE SURGERY

In the last three decades, eye surgery has become a microsurgical specialty. Cataract surgery has been transformed by changes in local anaesthesia, implants, phacoemulsification and small-incision surgery, which allows compressible/foldable silicone or acrylic implants to be inserted through a 2-mm incision. The implant power can be more accurately measured by new formulae and the use of A-scan ultrasonography or laser wavefront biometry, and multifocal and accommodative lenses are now available. An even more recent advance in cataract surgery is the development of femtosecond laser technology, which allows extremely controlled corneal incisions, lens capsule opening and lens fragmentation to be achieved automatically together with the facility to adjust the shape of the cornea at the time of surgery to improve visual outcome for some patients. The extent to which this technology improves long-term visual outcomes remains to be seen.

There are new treatments for eye disorders that involve abnormal growth of blood vessels in the back of the eye, such as the wet form of age-related macular degeneration. Anti-vascular endothelial growth factor (VEGF) antibodies, such as the drug ranibizumab, may be injected directly into the vitreous cavity to reduce new vessel proliferation. Intravitreal steroid injections or anti-VEGF agents are now also being used to treat patients with macular oedema caused for example by diabetic retinopathy or retinal vein occlusion.

Developments in vitreous surgery have enabled membranes to be peeled off the retina and macular holes to be repaired, and have also increased success rates in retinal detachment surgery with the additional use of gases and silicone oil or heavy liquid inserted into the vitreous cavity to tamponade the retina. Advances in technology have also led to to the development of photosensitive chips and camera systems that can be implanted into the eye to restore some vision in patients with severe and otherwise untreatable macular diseases.

Some paralytic squints can be helped by the use of adjustable sutures or injections of botulinum toxin into the overacting muscles.

Refractive errors can be treated by the excimer laser. These can be combined with laser *in situ* keratomeilusis (LASIK) surgery, which involves cutting a corneal flap (by femto second laser or surgery) and performing the laser surgery at a deeper level. There have been some concerns about defective contrast sensitivity and problems with night vision after laser correction of myopia. Phakic implants have also been used to correct high refractive errors. Corneal topography aids the accuracy of corneal and refractive surgery and the increased use and quality of CT and MRI scans has revolutionised the diagnosis of orbital and intracranial lesions involving the optic pathways (Figures 44.35–44.37).

Fluorescein angiography and ocular coherence tomography (OCT) are invaluable in the diagnosis and treatment of macular conditions. OCT angiography has recently been developed; this allows assessment of the retinal microvasculature without the need for systemically-administered agents. This technology may reduce the need for fluroscein angiography in the future. OCT as well as scanning laser polarimetry of the retinal nerve fibre layer and Heidelberg retinal tomography (HRT) are widely used in the diagnosis and management of glaucoma. Surgical glaucoma management is also developing rapidly. Trabeculectomy surgery, where eye pressure is reduced by creating a fistula between the anterior chamber

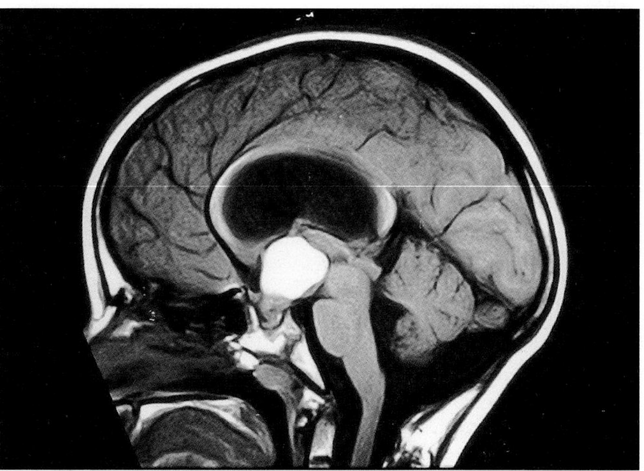

Figure 44.35 Magnetic resonance imaging scan, sagittal view. Craniopharyngioma. The mass in the suprasellar cistern is of high signal intensity because of the proteinaceous fluid that the cyst contains (courtesy of Dr Juliette Britton).

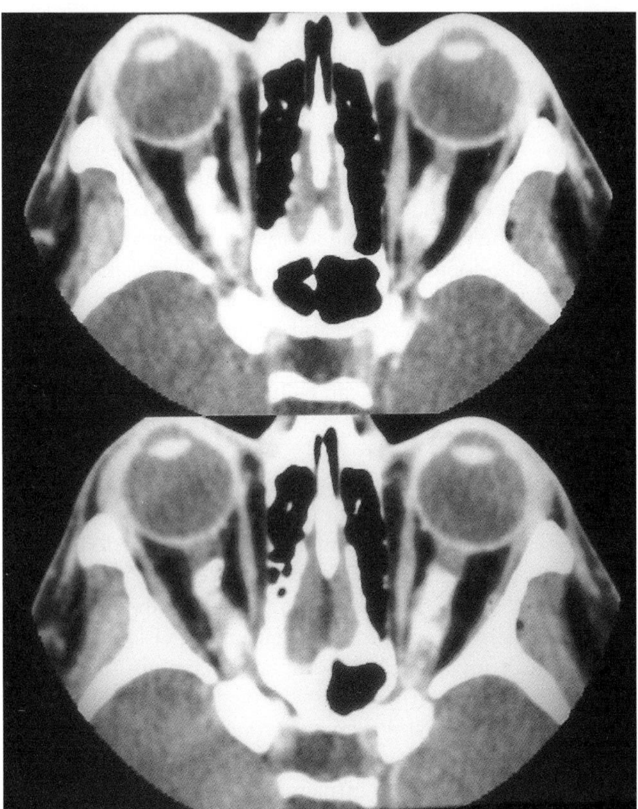

Figure 44.36 High-resolution computed tomography through the orbits showing dense calcification of the optic nerve sheaths typical of optic nerve meningioma (courtesy of Dr Juliette Britton).

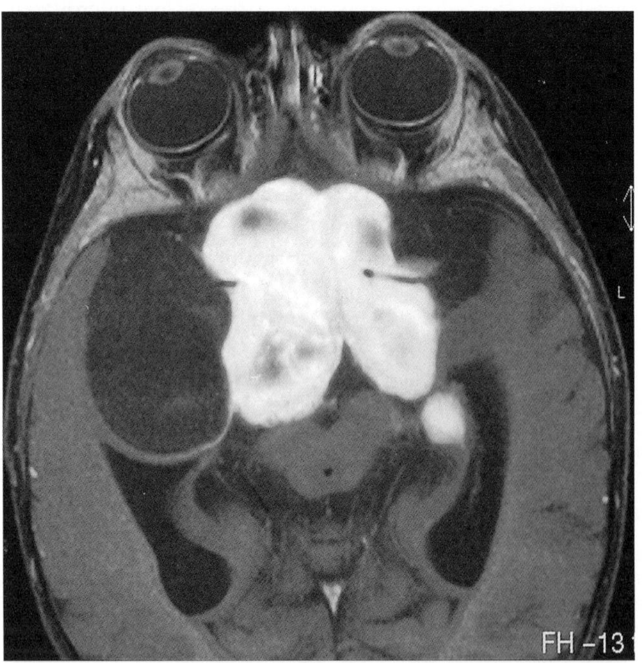

Figure 44.37 Axial enhanced magnetic resonance imaging scan showing a mass involving the optic chiasma and extending down the optic nerves and tracts.

and the subconjunctival space, remains widely used and has become more refined in recent years, with better control of wound healing using topical application of anti-scarring drugs such as mitomycin C. Alternatives to trabeculectomy have been developed using devices such as Baerveldt and Ahmed shunts that drain aqueous from the eye to lower the pressure. A new revolution is also underway using minimally invasive glaucoma surgical techniques, with a variety of tiny devices now available to shunt aqueous and reduce eye pressure.

LASERS IN OPHTHALMOLOGY

Blue-green lasers (argon or frequency-doubled YAG) or diode lasers are used to treat the retina in diabetic retinpoathy (pan-retinal photocoagulation for proliferative disease or focal treatment for leaky microaneurysms) and may also used to close retinal tears or breaks that might lead to retinal detachment.

Argon laser or selective laser trabeculoplasty can be used to open the drainge angle to control elevated intraocular pressure in open angle glaucoma. Trans-scleral diode photocoagulation of the ciliary body is used to treat refactory secondary glaucoma with uncontrolled ocular pressure.

Laser iridotomy with the Nd-Yag laser is used to treat both the affected and fellow eye in acute angle closure glaucoma. The Nd-Yag laser is also used to photodisrupt and clean an opaque posterior capsule, which occurs in 5–10% of cases following cataract surgery.

SURGICAL PROCEDURES

Excision of an eyeball/ enucleation

Indications include a blind, painful eye, a blind, cosmetically poor eye/intraocular neoplasm and, in cadavers, for use in corneal grafting.

The operation

The speculum is introduced between the lids and opened. The conjuctiva is picked up with toothed forceps and divided completely all round as near as possible to the cornea. Tenon's capsule is entered and each of the four rectus and two oblique muscle tendons is hooked up on a strabismus hook and divided close to the sclera. The speculum is now pressed backwards and the eyeball projects forwards. Blunt scissors, curved on the flat, are insinuated on the inner side of the globe, and these are used to sever the optic nerve. The eyeball can now be drawn forwards with the forceps, and the oblique muscles, together with any other strands of tissue that are still attaching the globe to the orbit, are divided. A swab, moistened with hot water and pressed into the orbit, will control the haemorrhage. If an orbital implant is inserted to give better eye movement, the muscles are sutured to the implant at the appropriate sites. The subconjunctival tissues and conjunctiva are closed in layers.

George G Baerveldt, contemporary, ophthalmologist, Emeritus Professor of Ophthalmology, UC Irvine, CA, USA.
Ike K Ahmed, contemporary, ophthalmologist, Toronto, Canada.
Jacques Rene Tenon, 1724–1816, surgeon, La Salpêtrière, Paris, France.

Evisceration of an eyeball

Evisceration is preferred to excision in endoophthalmitis, minimising the risk of orbital and intracranial spread with meningitis. The sclera is transfixed with a pointed knife a little behind the corneosclerotic junction, and the cornea is removed entirely by completing the encircling incision in the sclera. The contents of the globe are then removed with a curette, care being exercised to remove all of the uveal tract. At the end of the operation the interior must appear perfectly white. A ball orbital implant made of acrylic or hydroxyapatite may be placed within the orbit behind the sclera to improve the appearance when the artificial eye is fitted.

Incision and curettage of chalazion (meibomian cyst)

The lid margin is everted to allow the application of a meibomian clamp. The ring of the clamp is placed on the palpebral conjunctiva with the granuloma in the centre. An incision is made with a small blade in the axis of the gland. The herniating granulomatous tissue is removed with a curette and the cavity is scraped clean. Recurrent cysts may have to have the cyst wall dissected away with scissors. A biopsy may be necessary in atypical or recurrent cysts to exclude malignant change.

FURTHER READING

Bowling B. *Kanski's Clinical ophthalmology: a systematic approach*, 8th edn. Philadelphia: Saunders, 2015.

Denniston A, Murray P. *Oxford handbook of ophthalmology*, 3rd edn. Oxford: Oxford University Press, 2014.

Jackson TL. *Moorfields manual of ophthalmology*, 2nd edn. London: JP Medical Ltd, 2014.

Olver J, Cassidy L. *Ophthalmology at a glance*. Oxford: Blackwell Publishing, 2005.

Wills Eye Hospital. *The Wills eye manual: office and emergency room diagnosis and treatment of eye disease*, 6th edn. Philadelphia: Lippincott Williams & Wilkins, 2012.

Chapter 45

Cleft lip and palate: developmental abnormalities of the face, mouth and jaws

Learning objectives

To understand:

- The aetiology and classification of developmental abnormalities of the face, mouth and jaws
- Perinatal and early childhood management
- The principles of reconstruction of cleft lip and palate
- The key features of perioperative care
- The management of complications associated with cleft lip and palate

INTRODUCTION

Developmental abnormalities of the face, mouth and jaws are relatively rare and because of the complexity of developmental abnormalities an ideal classification system is not available. Consequently, there are a number of different systems available, some purely descriptive (e.g. Tessier's classification of clefts), while others apply only to single conditions, such as the OMENS (O, orbital alteration; M, mandibular deformity; E, ear deformity; N, nerve involvement; and S, soft tissue alterations) classification of hemifacial (craniofacial) microsomia, which has utility in instituting treatment protocols.

Van der Meulen and his colleagues proposed a classification that has significant utility in helping to understand the variety and complexity of craniofacial malformations. This classification considered the embryological development of the craniofacial region firstly in terms of the formation and fusion of the processes (branchial arches) – the failure of the fusion of these processes leading to clefting disorders, thus the failure of fusion between the frontonasal process and the maxillary process resulting in a cleft lip, either unilaterally or bilaterally; secondly in relation to the formation of bone and cartilage. If this is abnormal, it is termed dysostosis or dyschondrosis; and thirdly in relation to the formation and growth at the sutures between the various bones of the craniofacial skeleton – premature fusion leading to synostosis. Superimposed on this concept is the consideration of the development of the central nervous system. This leads to a number of types of abnormality, as outlined in Table 45.1.

TABLE 45.1 Types of developmental abnormalities of the face, mouth and jaws.

Type	Examples
Cerebrocranial dysplasias	Anencephaly, microcephaly
Cerebrofacial dysplasias	Rhinencephalic and oculo-orbital dysplasias
Craniofacial dysplasias with clefting	Latero-naosmaxillary, medionasomaxillary, intermaxillary, maxilomandibular clefting
Craniofacial dysplasias with dysostosis	Sphenoidal, sphenoidal frontal, frontal, fronto-frontal, fronto-nasoethmoidal, internasal, nasal, premaxillo-maxillary, nasomaxillary, maxillo-zygomatic, zygomatic, zygo-auro madibular, temporoauromandibular, mandibular, intermandibular
Craniofacial dysplasias with synostosis	Craniosynostosis: lambdoid and sagittal. Craniofaciosynostosis: metopic, coronal, bicoronal Faciosynostosis: vomeropremaxillary (Binder syndrome)
Craniofacial dysplasias with dysostosis and synostosis	Crouzon, Apert and Pfiffer syndromes
Craniofacial dysplasias with dyschondrosis	Achondroplasia

After van der Meulen JC, Mazzola R, Vermey-Keers C, Stricker M *et al*. A morphogenetic classification of craniofacial malformations. *Plast Reconstr Surg* 1983; **71**(4): 560–72.

Jacques van der Meulen, b.1929, Professor in Plastic and Reconstructive Surgery, Erasmus University, Rotterdam, The Netherlands.

In addition and in common with all classification systems, there is another large group of conditions that does not sit within the system outlined above.

EPIDEMIOLOGY

The incidence of congenital craniofacial anomalies varies in different parts of the world and is often not easy to quantify. *Table 45.2* outlines the various incidences of the more common craniofacial abnormalities.

DIAGNOSIS

The diagnosis of the craniofacial anomalies has, in recent years, undergone a massive change on two fronts. Firstly, advances in ultrasonography have increased the rate of prenatal diagnosis and impacted significantly on management. Secondly, the rapid expansion in genetic understanding has led to many more mutations being linked to particular phenotypes. Despite these advances the diagnosis of the majority of these conditions is clinical.

MANAGEMENT

In considering the management of this vast range of heterogeneous congenital abnormalities it is very difficult to generalise about management protocols. In the majority, management is delivered by multidisciplinary teams within specialist centres.

Prenatal management

Should a diagnosis be made or suspected prenatally there have been a few reported case of prenatal surgery; however, these procedures at present remain experimental and in general the options open are for termination or best supportive care in preparation for the birth. This can often provide the parents a period of time to adjust to the impending birth of a child with additional demands and needs. The opportunity to meet parents, adults and children who have experienced the same condition is often very valuable. Termination and its therapeutic uses is obviously a contentious and very personal issue; however, some parents may request this for very treatable conditions (e.g. isolated cleft lip) and in these circumstances the local ethics board must be involved and ultimately on occasions the advice of the courts must also be sought.

TABLE 45.2 Approximate incidence data from multiple sources.

Condition	Incidence
Apert syndrome	1 in 100 000
Pfeiffer syndrome	1 in 100 000
Crouzon syndrome	1 in 62 500
Treacher Collins syndrome	1 in 50 000
Unicoronal synostosis	1 in 10 000
Metopic synostosis	1 in 7000
Sagittal synostosis	1 in 5000
Hemifacial microsomia	1 in 3500
Neurofibromatosis	1 in 2600
Cleft lip and palate	1 in 600

Neonatal management

In the neonatal period management is aimed at addressing the urgent issues relating to the airway, breathing, eye protection and establishing feeding.

In many craniofacial conditions, the airway can be affected and either fully or partially obstructed due to a retropositioned hypoplastic maxilla with the tongue falling back to close off the upper airway, often compounded by a hypoplastic mandible. The trachea itself may also be abnormal and tracheomalacia can also lead to respiratory problems. Neonates are obligate nasal breathers and some forms of nasal obstruction can also precipitate airway symptoms. In the most severe cases intubation is not possible as a result of the abnormal anatomy and a tracheostomy may be necessary. In emergency situations it may be helpful to nurse the baby prone, allowing the tongue to fall forward.

In some cases, particularly the syndromic craniosynostoses such as Apert syndrome, Pfeiffer syndrome or Crouzon syndrome, the combination of the midface retrusion and the brachycephalic forehead shape can lead to severe exorbitism. In the worst cases this can cause ocular dislocation with the eyelids closing behind the globe. In severe exorbitism, the eyelids do not close adequately to moisturise and protect the cornea and without intervention this may lead to irreversible corneal damage.

In neonates with airway embarrassment, even without anatomical abnormalities, the effort of breathing can be exhausting and this can significantly compromise the ability to feed. Structural anomalies can also affect the ability to feed and expert input from a specialist feeding nurse is often helpful. The use of specialised teats may be helpful, but in some cases naso- or orogastric feeding may be necessary.

Management in infancy (0–12 months)

At this age treatment falls into two categories: first, that directed at major functional issues as a continuum of neonatal care; and second, skull surgery in cases of craniosynostosis.

Craniosynostosis results in premature fusion of one or more of the skull sutures. The condition may be isolated or part of a syndrome. This can result in abnormalities of both the skull and, particularly in syndromic cases, the facial skeleton.

Eugene Apert, 1868–1940, physician L'Hôpital des Infants Malades, Paris, France, described this syndrome in 1906.
Rudolf Arthur Pfeiffer, 1931–2012, geneticist, Münster, Germany, described this syndrome in 1964.
Louis Edouard Octave Crouzon, 1874–1938, neurologist, Paris, France, described this syndrome in 1912.

In 10–20% of single suture cases and a higher proportion of syndromic multisuture cases the infants develop raised intracranial pressure, which presents with episodes of distress, listlessness and disturbed sleep. This may be associated with papilloedema and untreated, can lead to visual failure. The diagnosis is confirmed with intracranial pressure monitoring.

Some congenital lesions may obstruct the vision of one or both eyes and this needs to be addressed to minimise the chances of amblyopia developing. An example of this would be the development of a large true haemangioma of the eyelids threatening to obscure the child's vision out of one eye.

In the older child the indications for surgery remain the same; however, there is the possibility of surgery to advance the mandible in the severely retrognathic patient. This can be used to obviate the need for a tracheostomy or allow for early decannulation. The most effective technique is distraction osteogenesis (or distraction histogenesis), which utilises the same basic principles as in limb lengthening. The bone is cut and a device placed across the osteotomy site and after a short latent period the bone ends gradually separate, distracting the callus. In the mandible, unlike the long bones, it is not necessary to limit the bone cut to the cortex (corticotomy) and a complete osteotomy is used. The technique allows for a lengthening of approximately 1 mm per day, after which there is a retention period to allow for consolidation of the callus.

Management in early childhood (1–12 years)

In early childhood management should be aimed at dealing with functional problems, airway obstruction, speech and feeding issues, but there is an increasing imperative for surgery to address the appearance of the child. There is no doubt that visible differences can affect the development, socially and emotionally; however, there is a significant role for psychological and emotional support for the whole family and in some cases for the school community to help the child, family and school understand and deal with the additional pressures that visible difference makes. Surgery can make a significant difference for some cases, but for many surgery should be delayed as long as possible for an optimal outcome in the long term.

In the older child airway issues can become a problem and their identification is more difficult. The usual presentation is of sleep apnoea, which often has an insidious onset and the history should be actively sought; parents are used to noisy snoring and daytime tiredness in the child and may not consider it abnormal. Initial investigation is with a home overnight oxygen saturation monitor, which if abnormal should trigger a comprehensive sleep study. The management of obstructive sleep apnoea includes the use of tonsillectomy/adenoidectomy, midface advancement and mandibular distraction as well as a variety of ventilator support devices.

Management in late childhood to maturity

Airway and other functional issues are usually stabilised by this time and interventions are aimed at optimising the overall appearance. The transition from primary school to secondary school is often a period of distress for patients with visible differences and their families and if there are pressing psychological reasons, corrective surgery can be offered, although usually this is best postponed until growth is complete. In general, a comprehensive integrated corrective plan should be developed within the multidisciplinary team. This would usually address the skeletal and dental abnormalities first and secondarily address the soft tissues. The majority of the major craniofacial abnormalities should be managed by a formal multidisciplinary team.

CLEFT LIP AND PALATE

Clefts of the lip, alveolus and hard and soft palate are the most common congenital abnormalities of the orofacial structures. They frequently occur as isolated deformities but can be associated with other medical conditions, particularly congenital heart disease. They are also an associated feature in over 300 recognised syndromes.

All children born with a cleft lip and palate need a thorough paediatric assessment to exclude other congenital abnormalities. In certain circumstances genetic counselling must be sought if a syndrome is suspected.

Incidence

The incidence of cleft lip and palate is 1:600 live births and of isolated cleft palate is 1:1000 live births. The incidence increases in Oriental groups (1:500) and decreases in the black population (1:2000). The highest incidence reported for cleft lip and palate occurs in the Indian tribes of Montana, USA (1:276).

Although cleft lip and palate is an extremely diverse and variable congenital abnormality, several distinct sub-groups exist, namely cleft lip with/without cleft palate (CL/P), cleft palate (CP) alone and submucous cleft palate (SMCP).

The typical distribution of cleft types is:

- cleft lip alone: 15%;
- cleft lip and palate: 45%;
- isolated cleft palate: 40%.

Cleft lip/palate predominates in males, whereas cleft palate alone appears to be more common in females. In unilateral cleft lip the deformity affects the left side in 60% of cases.

Aetiology

Contemporary opinion on the aetiology of cleft lip and palate is that cleft lip and palate and isolated cleft palate have a genetic predisposition and a contributory environmental component. A family history of cleft lip and palate in which the first-degree relative is affected increases the risk to 1:25 live births. Genetic influence is more significant in cleft lip/palate than cleft palate alone, in which environmental factors exert a greater influence.

Environmental factors implicated in clefting include maternal epilepsy and drugs (e.g. steroids, diazepam and phenytoin). The role of antenatal folic acid supplements in preventing cleft lip and palate remains equivocal.

Although most clefts of the lip and palate occur as an isolated deformity, Pierre Robin sequence is an important association. This sequence comprises isolated cleft palate, retrognathia and a posteriorly displaced tongue (glossoptosis), which is associated with early respiratory and feeding difficulties.

Isolated cleft palate is more commonly associated with a syndrome than cleft lip/palate and cleft lip alone. Over 150 syndromes are associated with cleft lip and palate, although Stickler (ophthalmic and musculoskeletal abnormalities), Shprintzen (cardiac anomalies), Down, Apert and Treacher Collins syndromes are most frequently encountered.

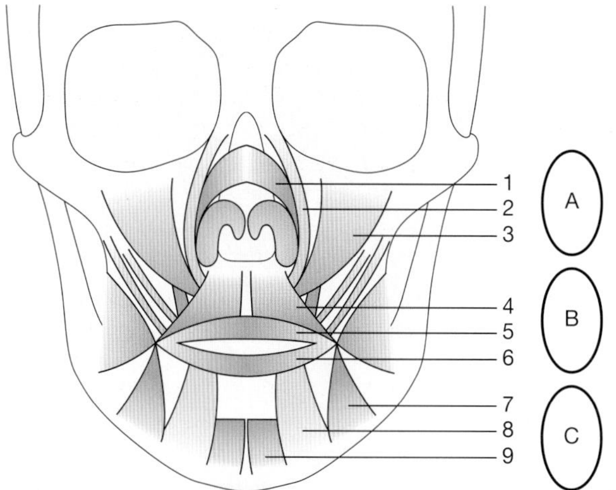

Figure 45.1 The muscle chains of the face: frontal view. The nasal cartilages are represented in blue. A, nasolabial (muscles 1–3); B, bilabial (muscles 4–6); C, labiomental (muscles 7–9); 1, transverse nasalis; 2, levator labii superioris alaeque nasi; 3, levator labii superioris; 4, orbicularis oris (oblique head) – upper lip; 5, orbicularis oris (horizontal head) – upper lip; 6, orbicularis oris – lower lip; 7, depressor anguli oris; 8, depressor labii inferioris; 9, mentalis.

Summary box 45.1

Cleft lip and palate

- Associated with other congenital abnormalities
- Incidence varies between 1:300 to 1:2000
- Aetiology is both genetic and environmental

ANATOMY OF CLEFT LIP AND PALATE

Cleft lip

The abnormalities in cleft lip are the direct consequence of disruption of the muscles of the upper lip and nasolabial region. The facial muscles (Figure 45.1) can be divided into three muscular rings of Delaire: the nasolabial muscle ring surrounds the nasal aperture; the bilabial muscle ring surrounds the oral aperture; and the labiomental muscle ring envelops the lower lip and chin regions.

Unilateral cleft lip

In the unilateral cleft lip, the nasolabial and bilabial muscle rings are disrupted on one side, resulting in an asymmetrical deformity involving the external nasal cartilages, nasal septum and anterior maxilla (premaxilla) (Figure 45.2). These deformities influence the mucocutaneous tissues causing a displacement of nasal skin onto the lip and a retraction of labial skin, as well as changes to the vermilion and lip mucosa. All these changes need to be considered in planning the surgical repair of the unilateral cleft lip.

Bilateral cleft lip

In the bilateral cleft lip the deformity is more profound but symmetrical. The two superior muscular rings are disrupted on both sides, producing a flaring of the nose (caused by lack of nasolabial muscle continuity), a protrusive premaxilla and an area of skin in front of the premaxilla devoid of muscle, known as the prolabium (Figure 45.3). As in the unilateral cleft lip, the muscular, cartilaginous and skeletal deformities influence the mucocutaneous tissues, which must be respected in planning the repair of the bilateral cleft lip.

Cleft palate

Embryologically, the **primary** palate consists of all anatomical structures anterior to the incisive foramen, namely the alveolus and upper lip. The **secondary** palate is defined as the remainder of the palate behind the incisive foramen, divided into the hard palate and, more posteriorly, the soft palate.

Cleft palate results in failure of fusion of the two palatine shelves. This failure may be confined to the soft palate alone or involve both hard and soft palate. When the cleft of the hard palate remains attached to the nasal septum and vomer, the cleft is termed **incomplete**. When the nasal septum and vomer are completely separated from the palatine processes, the cleft palate is termed **complete**.

Soft palate

In the normal soft palate, closure of the velopharynx, which is essential for normal speech, is achieved by five different muscles functioning in a complete but coordinated fashion.

Pierre Robin, 1867–1950, Professor, The French School of Dentistry, Paris, France, described this syndrome in 1929.
Gunnar B Stickler, 1925–2010, born in Germany, Chair of Section of Paediatrics and later Paediatric Cardiology, The Mayo Clinic, Rochester, MN, USA.
Robert J Shprintzen, b.1946, surgeon, Syracuse, NY, USA.
John Langdon Haydon Down (sometimes given as Langdon-Brown), 1828–1896, physician, The London Hospital, UK, published 'observations on the ethnic classification of idiots' in the London Hospital Reports in 1866.
Edward Treacher Collins, 1862–1932, ophthalmic surgeon, the Royal London Ophthalmic Hospital, and Charing Cross Hospital, London, UK, described this syndrome in 1900.

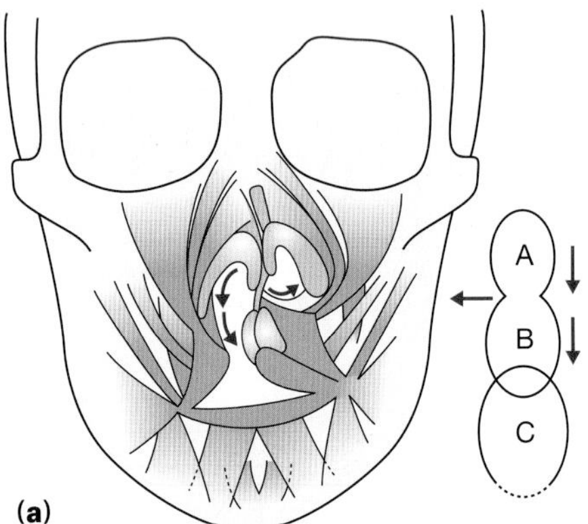

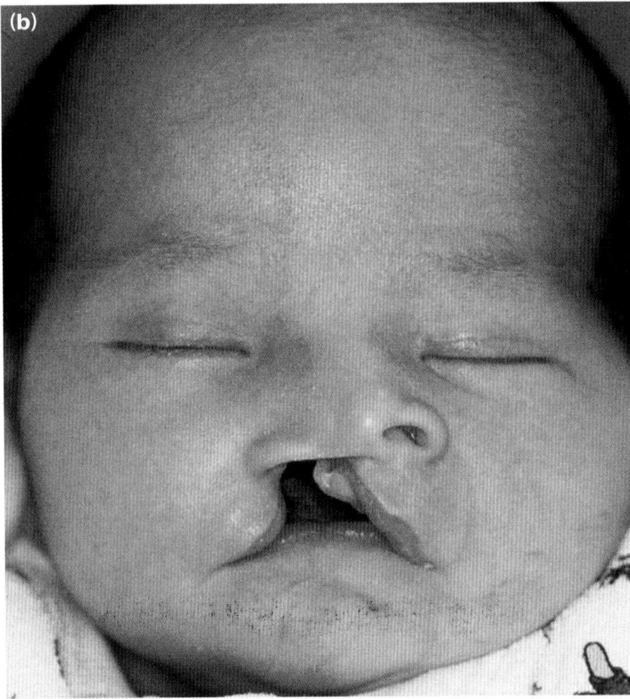

Figure 45.2 (a) Schematic representation of disruption of the nasolabial and bilabial muscle chains in unilateral (left) cleft lip. A, nasolabial; B, bilabial; C, labiomental. (b) Unilateral cleft lip before muscular reconstruction.

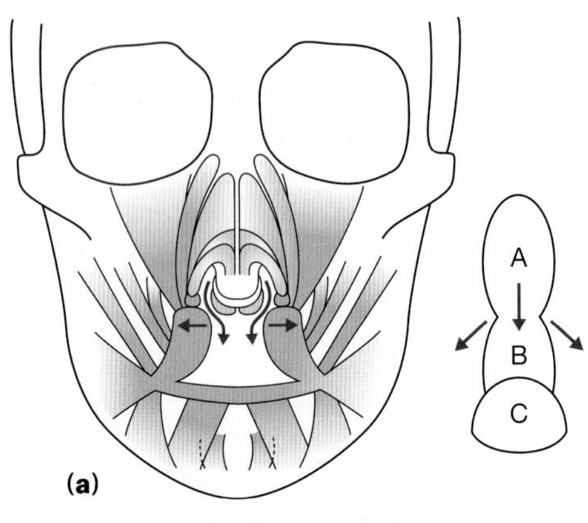

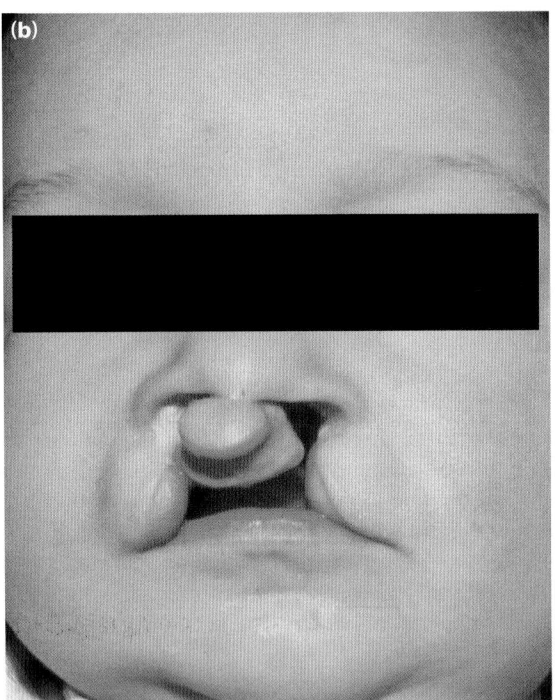

Figure 45.3 (a) Schematic representation of disruption of the nasolabial and bilabial muscle chains in bilateral cleft lip. A, nasolabial; B, bilabial; C, labiomental. (b) Bilateral cleft lip before muscular reconstruction.

Summary box 45.2

Types of cleft palate

- May involve the soft palate or the soft and hard palate
- It is complete when nasal septum and vomer are separated from the palatine process

In general, the muscle fibres of the soft palate are orientated transversely with no significant attachment to the hard palate.

In a cleft of the soft palate (Figure 45.4a) the muscle fibres are orientated in an anteroposterior direction, inserting into the posterior edge of the hard palate (Figure 45.4b).

Hard palate

The normal hard palate can be divided into three anatomical and physiological zones (Figure 45.5). The central **palatal fibromucosa** is very thin and lies directly below the floor of nose. The **maxillary fibromucosa** is thick and contains the greater palatine neurovascular bundle. The **gingival fibromucosa** lies more lateral and adjacent to the teeth.

In performing surgical closure of cleft palate the changes associated with the cleft must be understood to obtain an anatomical and functional repair. In complete cleft palate the median part of the palatal vault is absent and the palatal fibromucosa is reduced in size. The maxillary and gingival fibromucosa are not modified in thickness, width or position.

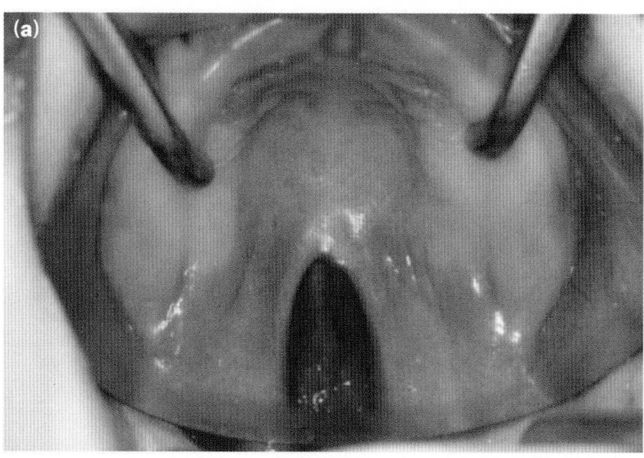

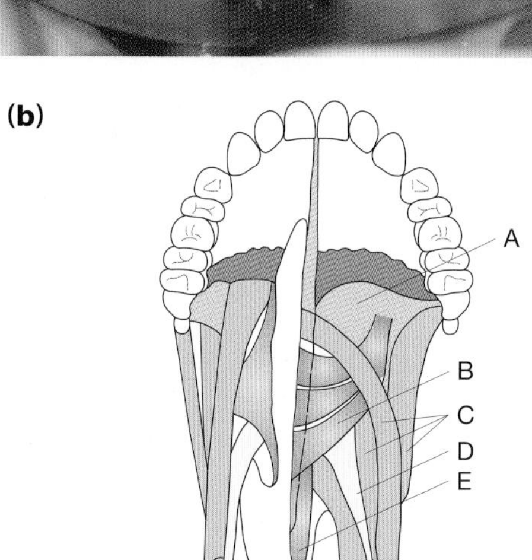

Figure 45.4 (a) Cleft of soft palate and incomplete cleft of hard palate. (b) Muscles of the soft palate: left, cleft palate; right, normal anatomy. A, tensor palati; B, levator palati; C, palatopharyngeus; D, palatoglossus; E, musculus uvulae.

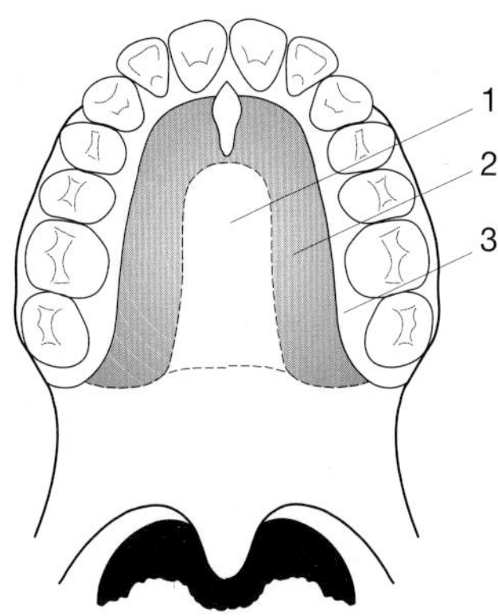

Figure 45.5 The three mucosal zones of the hard palate. 1, palatal fibromucosa; 2, maxillary fibromucosa; 3, gingival fibromucosa.

PRIMARY MANAGEMENT

Antenatal diagnosis

An antenatal diagnosis of cleft lip, whether unilateral or bilateral, is possible by ultrasound scan after 18 weeks of gestation. Isolated cleft palate cannot be diagnosed by antenatal scan. When an antenatal diagnosis is confirmed, referral to a cleft surgeon is appropriate for counselling to allay fears. Photographs of cleft lip shown to parents 'before and after' surgery are invaluable. Introduction to a parent support group and meeting parents of a child with a similar cleft who has undergone surgery may also be extremely helpful.

Summary box 45.3

Antenatal diagnosis and counselling

- All but isolated cleft palate can be diagnosed by ultrasound after 18 weeks' gestation
- Parents need counselling and support

Feeding

Most babies born with cleft lip and palate feed well and thrive, provided that appropriate advice is given and support is available. Some mothers are successful in breast-feeding, particularly when the cleft is incomplete and confined to the lip. Good feeding patterns can be established with soft bottles (e.g. Mead Johnson) and modified teats (orthodontic, Nuyk). Simple measures such as enlarging the hole in the teat often suffice. Feeding plates, constructed from a dental impression of the upper jaw, are rarely necessary to improve feeding. Some babies are provided with an active plate that aims not only to improve feeding but also reduce the width of the cleft lip and palate prior to surgery. The long-term benefit of such a regime remains unproven.

Airway

Major respiratory obstruction is uncommon and occurs exclusively in babies with Pierre Robin sequence. Hypoxic episodes during sleep and feeding can be life-threatening. Intermittent airway obstruction is more frequent and is managed by nursing the baby prone. More severe and persistent airway compromise can be managed by 'retained nasopharyngeal intubation' to maintain the airway. Surgical adhesion of the tongue to the lower lip (labioglossopexy) in the first few days after birth is an alternative but less commonly practised method of management. Early mandibular surgery, in the form of distraction osteogenesis, is indicated for a proportion of cases and may avoid the need for a tracheostomy.

Summary box 45.4

Problems immediately after birth

- Some babies are able to feed normally but others require assistance
- Breathing problems in Pierre Robin sequence may be life threatening

PRINCIPLES OF CLEFT SURGERY

The ultimate goal in cleft lip and palate management is a patient with a normal appearance of lip, nose and face, whose speech is normal and whose dentition and facial growth fall within the range of normal development.

Surgical techniques are aimed at restoring normal anatomy. With the exception of rare conditions such as holoprosencephaly, there is no true hypoplasia of the tissues involved on either side of the cleft. There is, however, displacement, deformation and underdevelopment of the muscles and facial skeleton. Emphasis is placed on muscular reconstruction of the lip, nose and face as well as muscles of the soft palate. Normal or near-normal anatomy promotes normal function, thereby encouraging normal growth and development of lip, nose, palate and facial skeleton. An in-depth understanding of the anatomy of the cleft is invaluable if the surgeon is to achieve normal, or near-normal, anatomical reconstruction.

Summary box 45.5

Surgical anatomy

- Normal lip, face and nose
- Underdevelopment and displacement of muscles
- Restoration of normal anatomy encourages normal facial growth and function

TABLE 45.3 Timing of primary cleft lip and palate procedures (after Delaire).

Cleft lip alone		
Unilateral (one side)	One operation at 5–6 months	
Bilateral (both sides)	One operation at 4–5 months	
Cleft palate alone		
Soft palate only	One operation at 6 months	
Soft and hard palate	Two operations	Soft palate at 6 months
		Hard palate at 15–18 months
Cleft lip and palate		
Unilateral	Two operations	Cleft lip and soft palate at 5–6 months
		Hard palate and gum pad with or without lip revision at 15–18 months
Bilateral	Two operations	Cleft lip and soft palate at 4–5 months
		Hard palate and gum pad with or without lip revision at 15–18 months

Surgical techniques

There have been many different surgical techniques and sequences advocated in cleft lip and palate management, leading to considerable debate between surgeons regarding surgical regime and philosophy; however, all modern approaches have functional muscle reconstruction as their core principle. Cleft lip repair is commonly performed between 3 and 6 months of age, whereas cleft palate repair is frequently performed between 6 and 18 months.

The Delaire technique and sequence (*Table 45.3*) is one of the many regimes currently practised.

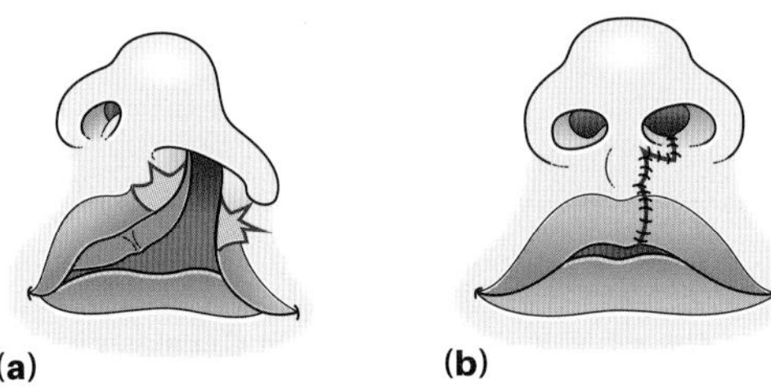

Figure 45.6 (a, b) Skin incisions (highlighted in red) for left unilateral complete cleft lip (after Delaire).

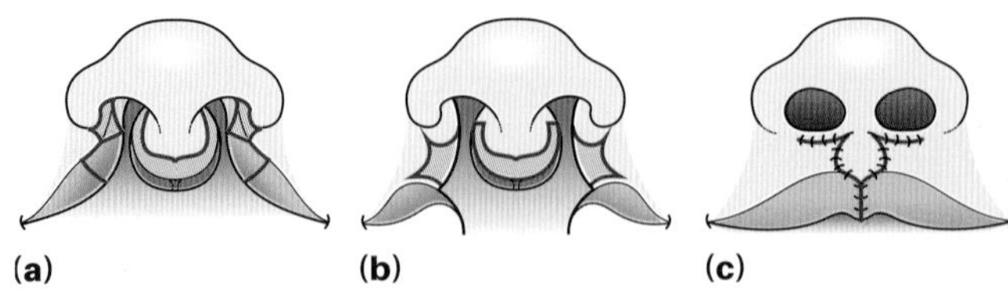

Figure 45.7 (a–c) Skin incisions for bilateral complete cleft lip shown in red. Areas for excision shown in grey: mucosa (a) or skin (b) (after Delaire).

Cleft lip surgery

Skin incisions (Figures 45.6 and 45.7) are developed to restore displaced tissues, including skin and cartilage, to their normal position, while gaining access to the facial, nasal and lip musculature.

Muscular continuity is achieved by subperiosteal undermining over the anterior maxilla. Nasolabial muscles are anchored to the premaxilla with non-resorbable sutures. Oblique muscles of orbicularis oris are sutured to the base of the anterior nasal spine and cartilaginous nasal septum. Closure of the cleft lip is completed by suturing the horizontal fibres of orbicularis oris to achieve a functioning oral sphincter (Figures 45.8 and 45.9).

When the cleft lip is incomplete (Figures 45.10a and 45.11a), meticulous assessment of the cleft deformity is of paramount importance, as complete muscle disruption may be present leading to nasal and skeletal deformity. Full muscular exposure and reconstruction is imperative in many incomplete clefts if facial symmetry is to be achieved (Figures 45.10b and 45.11b).

Cleft palate surgery

Cleft palate closure can be achieved by one- or two-stage palatoplasty. The surgical principle is mobilisation and

Jean Delaire, Professor of Stomatology and Maxillofacial Surgery, University of Nantes, Nantes, France, 1960–1991.

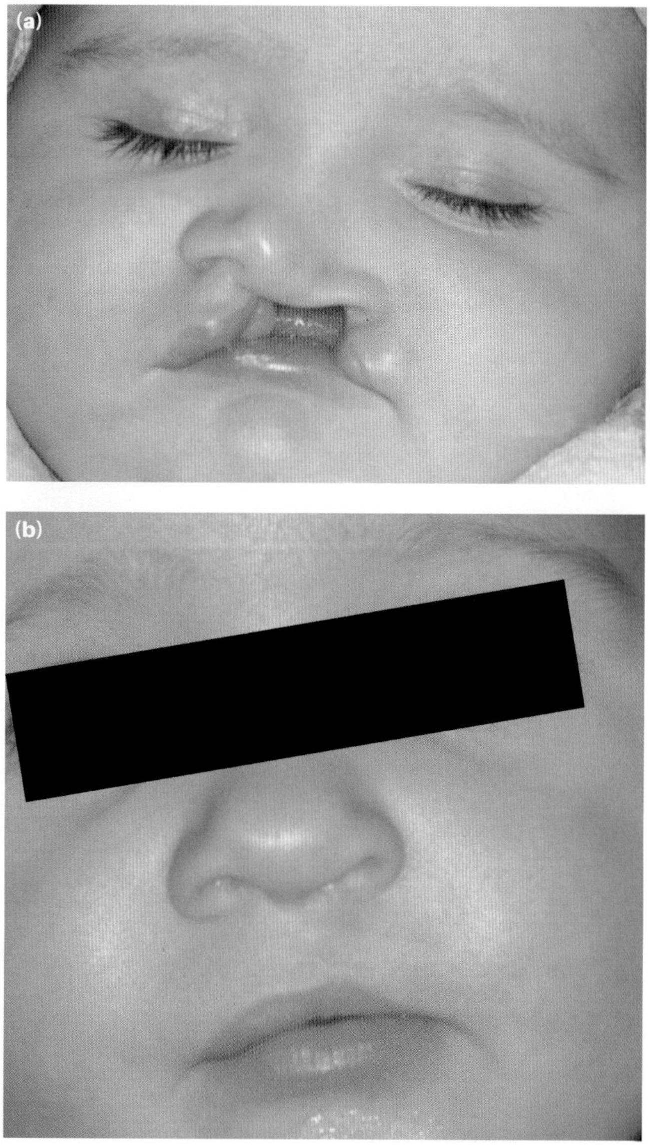

(a)

(b)

Figure 45.8 Unilateral complete cleft lip before (a) and after (b) muscular reconstruction.

(a)

(b)

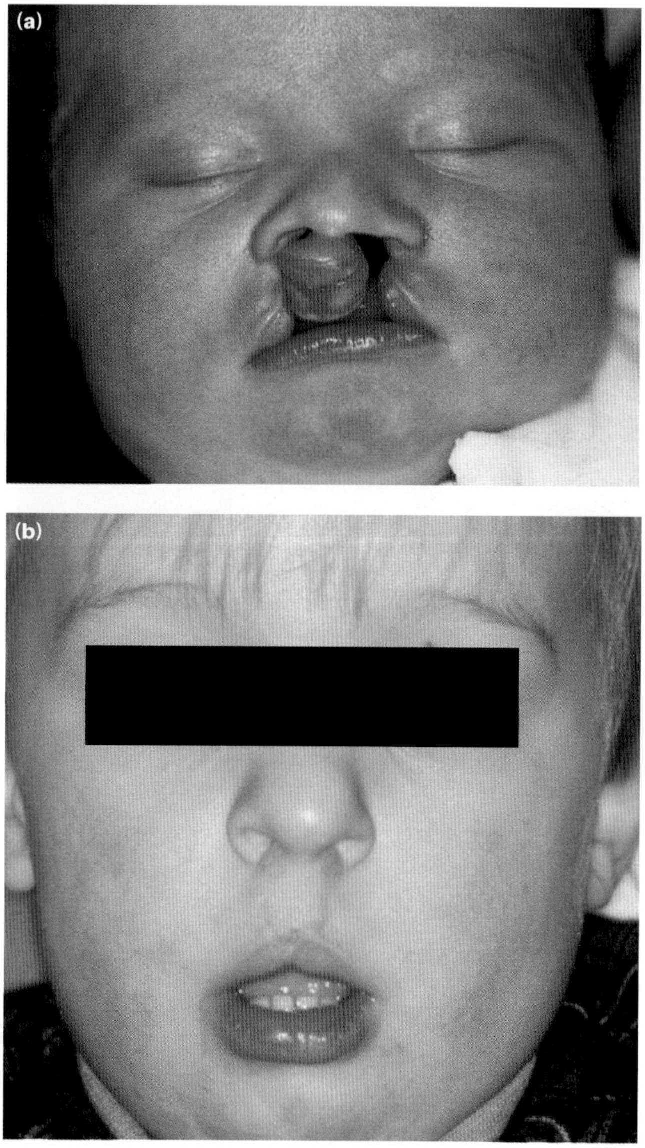

Figure 45.9 Bilateral cleft lip before (a) and after (b) muscular reconstruction.

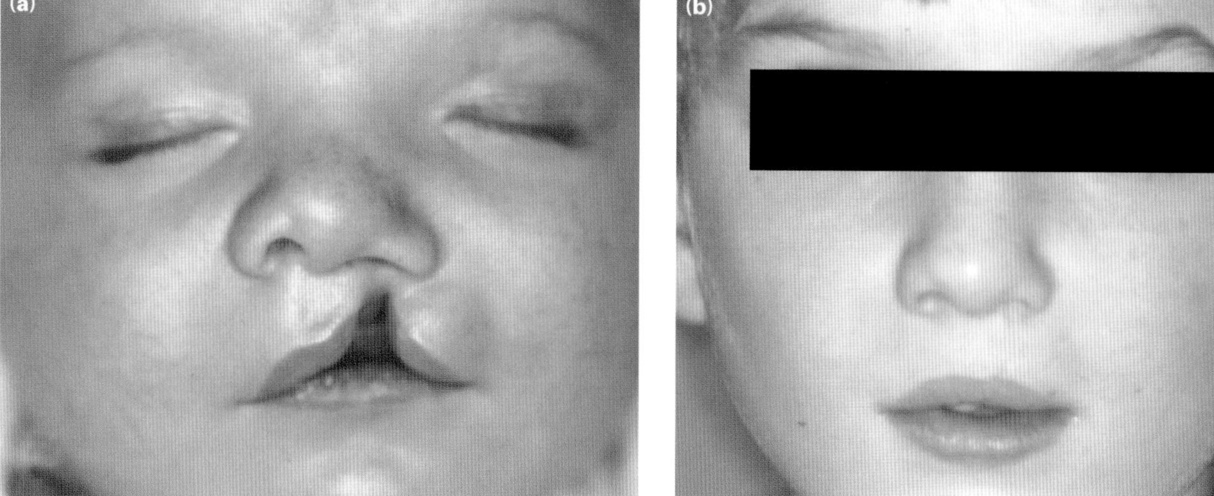

Figure 45.10 Unilateral incomplete cleft lip before (a) and after (b) muscle reconstruction.

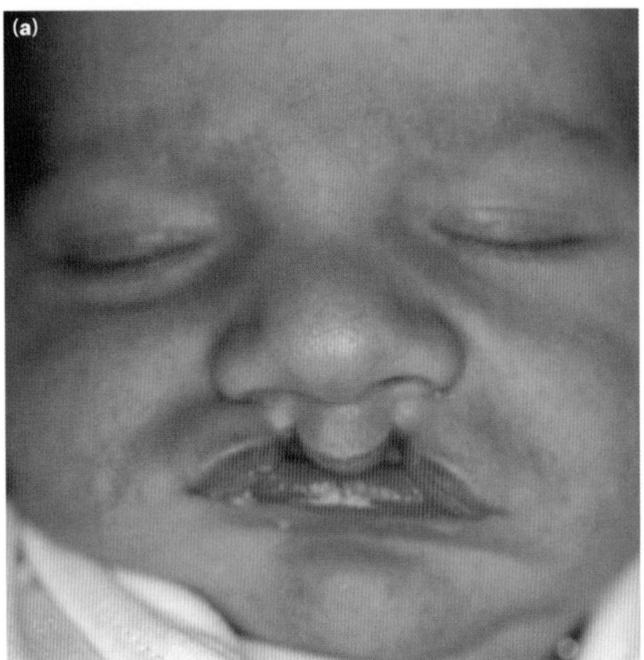

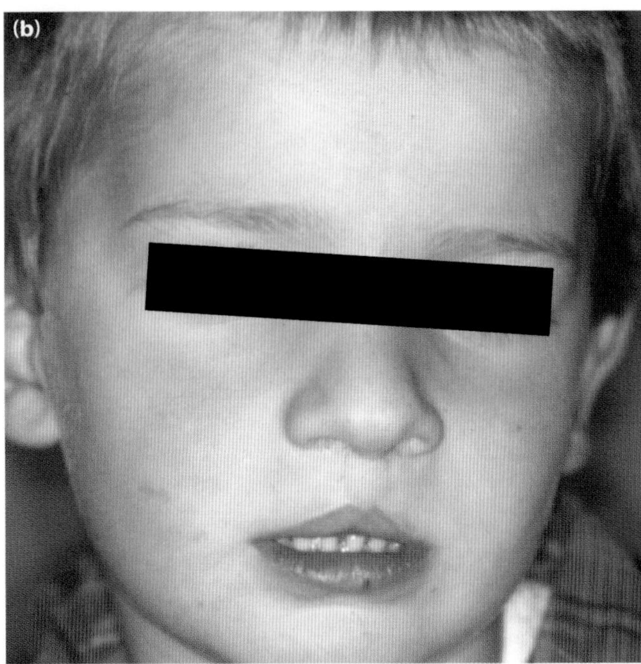

Figure 45.11 Bilateral incomplete cleft lip before (a) and after (b) muscular reconstruction.

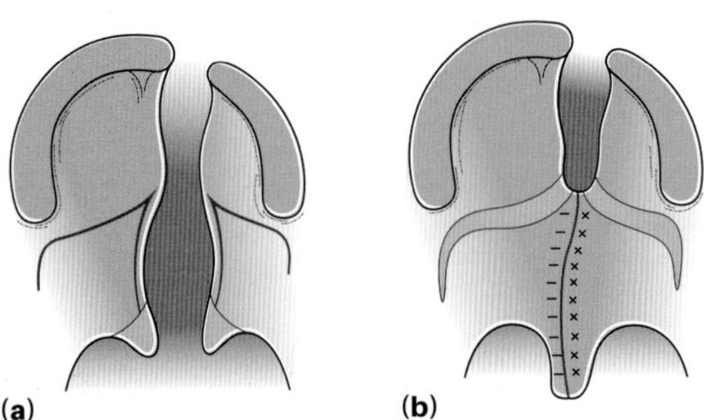

Figure 45.12 (a, b) Method of repair of cleft palate. First-stage palatoplasty to reconstruct muscles of the soft palate. Red lines represent incisions and orange areas raw surfaces.

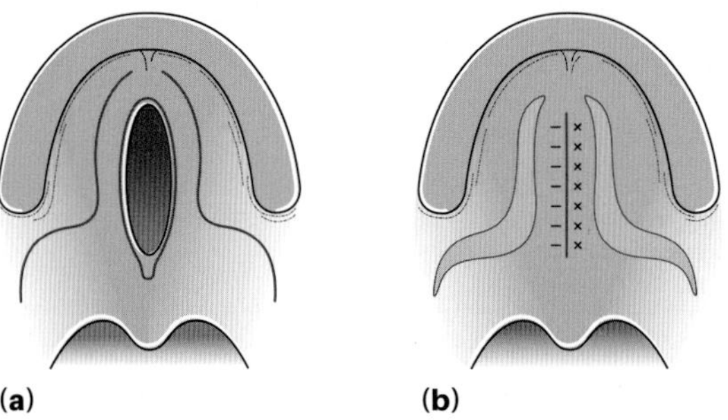

Figure 45.13 (a, b) Schematic representation of closure of the hard palate. Second-stage palatoplasty achieved with two-layered closure. Red lines represent incisions and orange areas raw surfaces.

reconstruction of the aberrant soft palate musculature (Figure 45.12) together with closure of the residual hard palate cleft by minimal dissection and subsequent scar formation (Figure 45.13). Excess scar formation in the palate adversely affects growth and development of the maxilla. The philosophy of two-stage closure encourages a physiological narrowing of the hard palate cleft to minimise surgical dissection at the time of the second procedure.

Summary box 45.6

Principles of surgery

- Cleft lip surgery attaches and reconnects the muscles around the oral sphincter
- Cleft patate surgery aims to bring together mucosa and muscles with minimal scarring
- Two-stage procedures minimises dissection

SECONDARY MANAGEMENT

Following primary surgery, regular review by a multidisciplinary team is essential. Many aspects of cleft care require long-term review:

- hearing;
- speech;
- dental development;
- facial growth.

Hearing

Eustachian tube dysfunction plays a central role in the pathogenesis of otitis media, with effusion in babies and children born with a cleft palate. Children with a cleft lip alone exhibit the same frequency of otitis media as their age-matched non-cleft counterparts; however, a child with a craniofacial anomaly, including cleft lip and palate, is at increased risk of a sensorineural hearing deficit. All children born with a cleft lip and palate should undergo assessment before 12 months of age for **sensorineural and conductive hearing loss** by auditory brainstem responses and tympanometry, respectively.

Sensorineural hearing loss is managed with a hearing aid whereas the management of secretory otitis media remains more controversial. Early (6–12 months) prophylactic myringotomy and grommet insertion temporarily eliminates middle ear effusion. Regular audiological testing may be as appropriate, reserving surgery for established secretory otitis media with infection. No firm evidence is available to support the interventional approach over the conservative regime. Nevertheless, the relationship between hearing loss and potential speech problems remains important. Regular audiological assessment during childhood is of utmost importance.

Speech

Initial speech assessment should be performed early (18 months) and repeated regularly to ensure that problems are identified early and managed appropriately.

Common speech problems associated with cleft lip and palate are:

- **Velopharyngeal incompetence**. This is associated with increased nasal airflow and resonance producing a nasal or 'hypernasal' quality to speech. It frequently reflects poor function of the soft palate associated with inadequate muscle repair.
- **Articulation problems**. These arise either as a compensatory mechanism to overcome velopharyngeal incompetence or, less commonly, are caused by jaw/dental and occlusal abnormalities. Videofluoroscopy, nasal airflow studies (aerophonoscopy) and nasendoscopy are helpful in defining the exact mechanism of the problem, aiding management.
- **Speech problems**. These are managed by speech and language therapy; secondary palatal surgery, either intravelar veloplasty (muscular reconstruction of soft palate) or pharyngoplasty; and speech training devices .

Summary box 45.7

Associated hearing and speech problems

- Higher incidence of sensineural and conductive hearing loss
- Regular hearing tests are important if speech is to develop normally
- Speech problems may result from airflow problems

Dental

Dental anomalies are common findings in children with cleft lip and/or palate. Various phenomena including delayed tooth development, delayed eruption of teeth and morphological abnormalities are well documented. The number of teeth may be reduced (hypodontia) or increased (hyperdontia), occurring most commonly in the region of the cleft alveolus involving the maxillary lateral incisor tooth. These abnormalities can occur in both primary and secondary dentition.

All children with cleft lip and palate should undergo regular dental examination. Dental management should also include preventive measures such as dietary advice, fluoride supplements and fissure sealants.

A well-maintained and disease-free dentition in childhood is an absolute prerequisite for orthodontic treatment.

Summary box 45.8

Dental problems

- Too many/too few teeth or problems with eruption of teeth are common
- Good dentition is essential for successful reconstructive surgery

Orthodontic management

Many children with cleft lip and palate require orthodontic treatment. Orthodontic treatment is commonly carried out in two phases:

- Mixed dentition (8–10 years) – to expand the maxillary arches as a prelude to alveolar bone graft.
- Permanent dentition (14–18 years) – to align the dentition and provide a normal functioning occlusion. This phase of treatment may also include surgical correction of a malpositioned/retrusive maxilla by maxillary osteotomy (Figure 45.14).

Secondary surgery for cleft lip and palate

Good outcome in cleft lip and palate is directly attributable to the quality of the primary surgery. Secondary cleft procedures include:

- cleft lip revision (unilateral and bilateral);
- alveolar bone graft;
- simultaneous lip revision and alveolar bone graft;
- secondary palate procedures (e.g. veloplasty and pharyngoplasty, closure of a palatal fistula);
- dentoalveolar procedures, including transplantation of teeth/insertion of osseo-integrated dental implants;
- orthognathic surgery;
- rhinoplasty.

Cleft lip revision

Indications for revisional surgery to a previously repaired cleft lip are dependent on the site and severity of the residual deformity.

Revisional surgery should be delayed for 2 years after primary lip closure unless the surgeon is of the opinion that the initial procedure was inadequate, particularly with respect to muscular reconstruction.

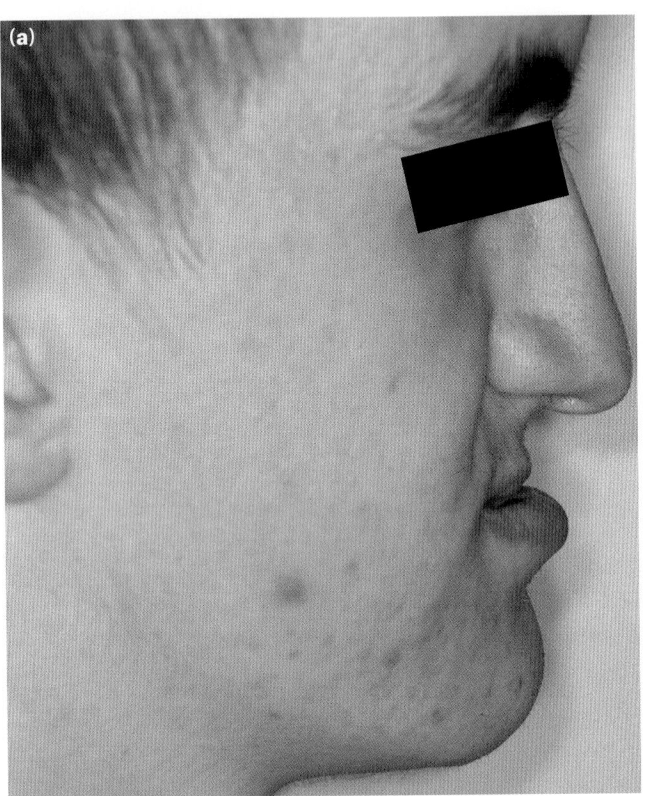

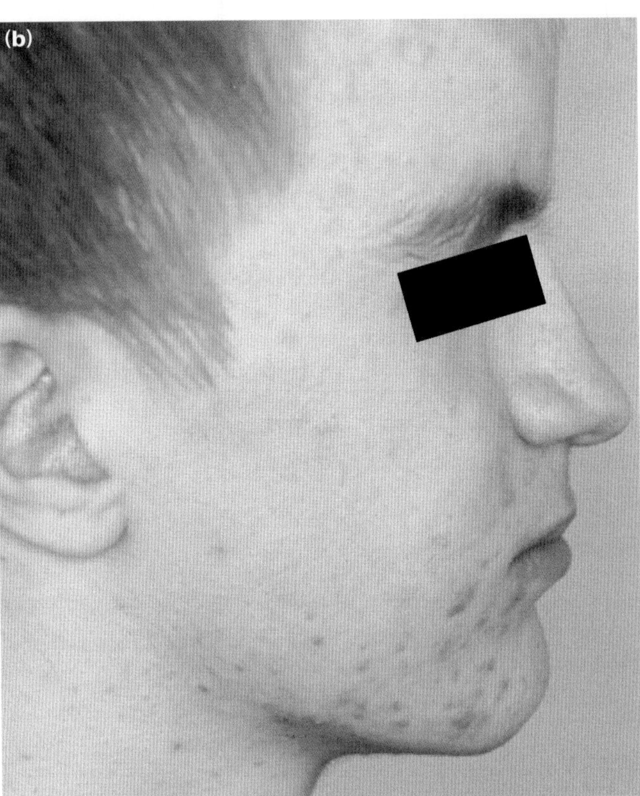

Figure 45.14 Correction of midface retrusion by maxillary advancement osteotomy, before (a) and after (b) surgery.

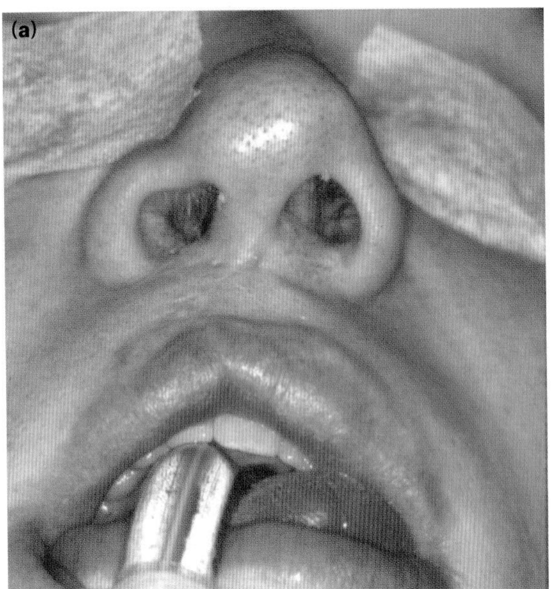

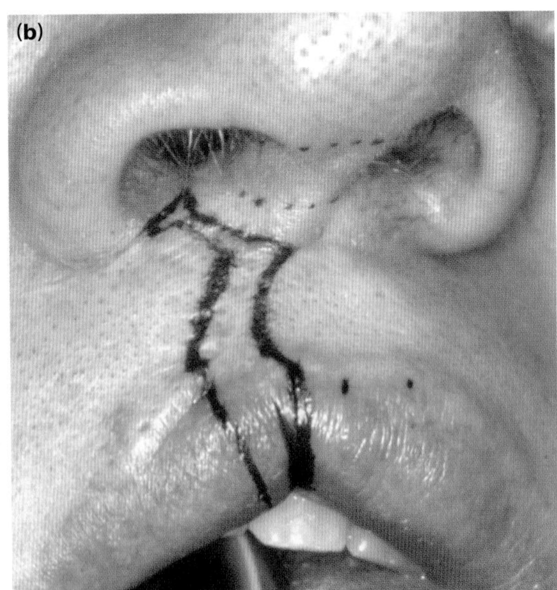

Figure 45.15 (a) Revision of unilateral complete cleft lip, seen from below. (b) Skin incisions. (c) Wide exposure of nasolabial and orbicularis oris muscle. (d) Lip closure highlighting improved nasal symmetry.

Indications for revision include:

- lip deformity:
  - malaligned vermilion;
  - asymmetrical Cupid's bow;
  - muscle discontinuity or malalignment;
- nasal deformity:
  - lateral drift of alar base;
  - poor nasal tip projection;
  - deviation of cartilaginous nasal septum into the non-cleft nostril.

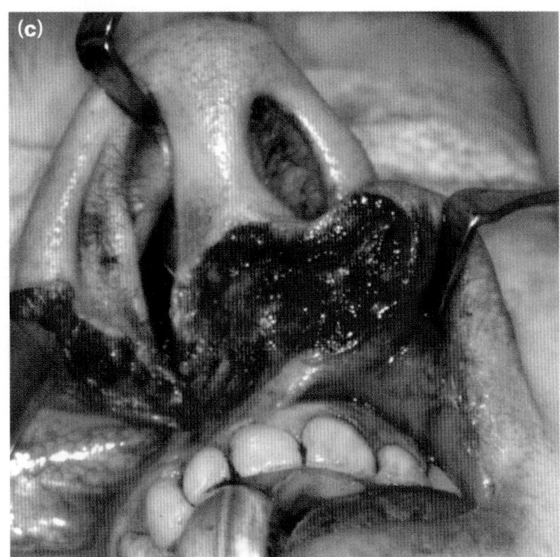
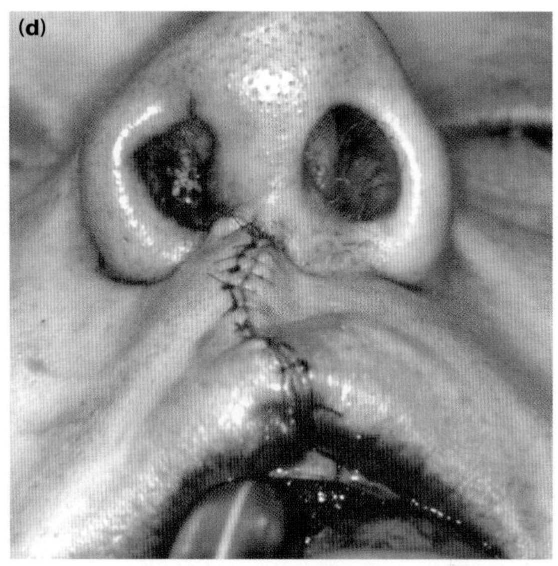

Figure 45.15 (*Continued*)

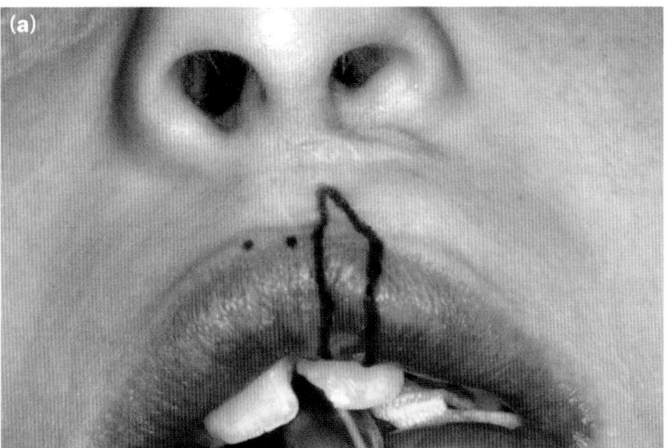
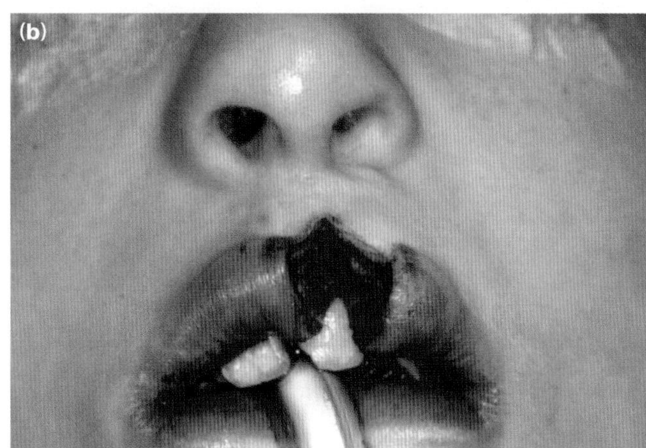
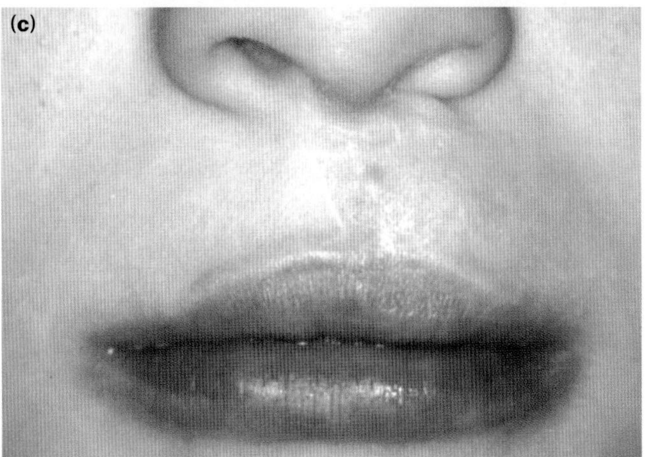

Figure 45.16 (a) Asymmetrical Cupid's bow. Revision of unilateral cleft lip – skin markings. (b) Identification and realignment of orbicularis oris muscle. (c) Postoperative appearance.

Residual nasal deformity is an external manifestation of incomplete reconstruction of the nasolabial muscle ring.

Examples of lip revision are shown in Figures 45.15–45.18.

Summary box 45.9

Cleft lip revisional surgery

- Should be delayed for at least 2 years after primary surgery
- Aims to improve incomplete primary reconstruction

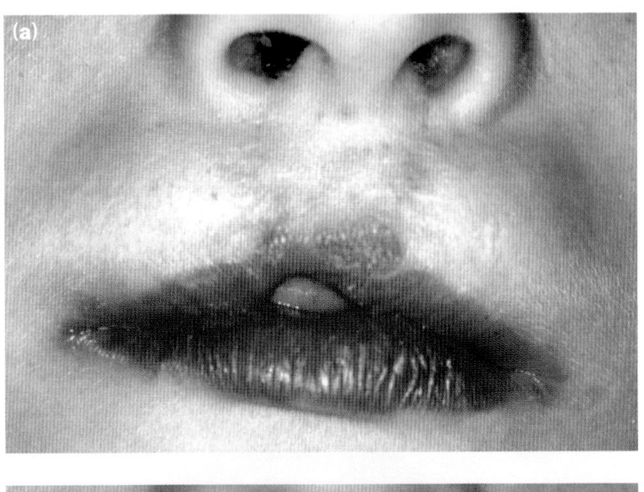

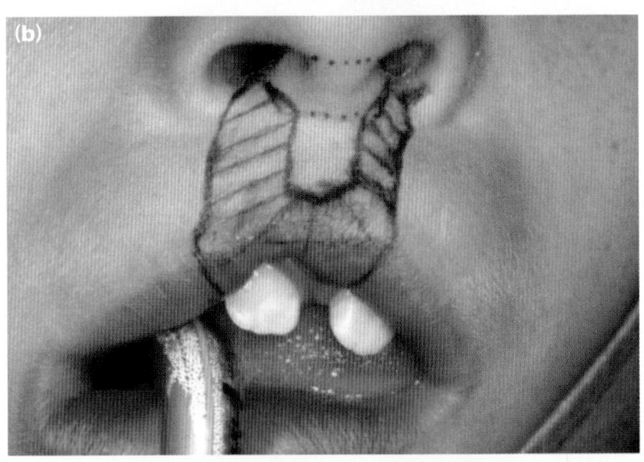

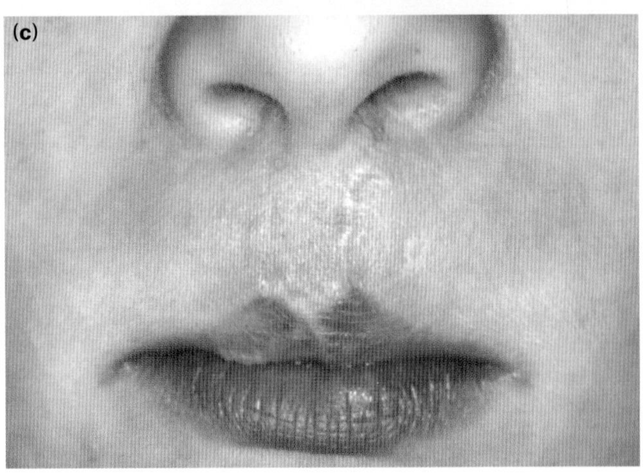

Figure 45.17 (a) Revision of bilateral cleft lip with reconstruction of nasolabial muscles. (b) Skin incisions and development of philtrum. (c) Postoperative view – improved nasal and lip symmetry.

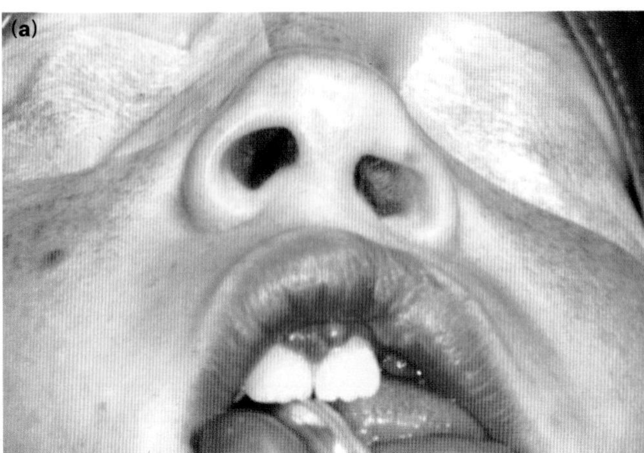

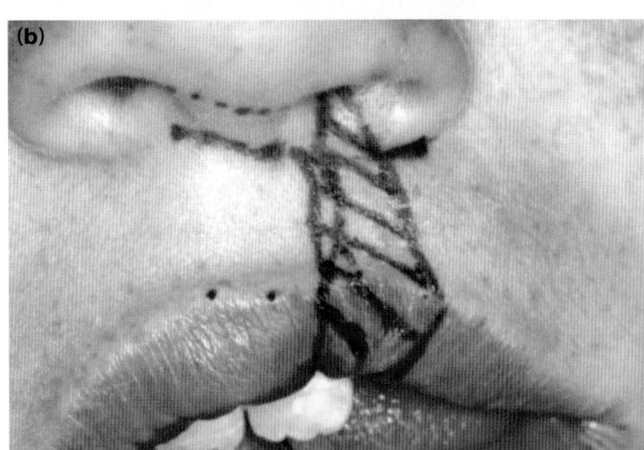

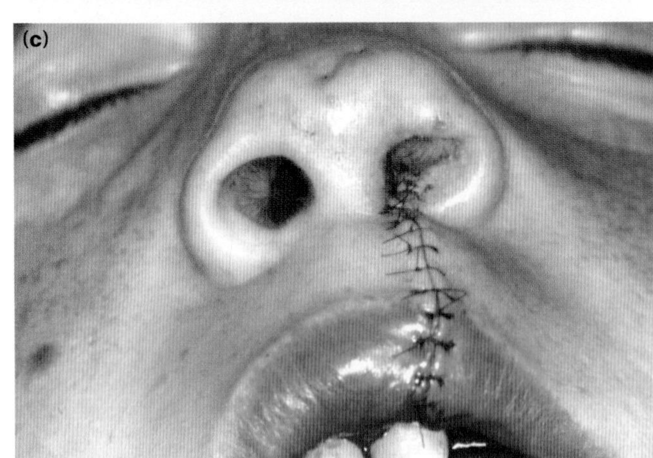

Figure 45.18 (a) Revision of left unilateral cleft lip to correct a nasal deformity. (b) Skin incision. (c) Postoperative view.

Alveolar bone grafting

Alveolar bone grafting in a mixed dentition is a well-established procedure for patients with a residual alveolar cleft associated with cleft lip and palate. The rationale for performing alveolar bone grafting includes:

- stabilisation of maxillary segments;
- to promote eruption of the canine tooth into the cleft site;
- to enhance bony support of the teeth adjacent to the cleft alveolus;
- to promote closure of the oronasal fistula;
- to close residual fistula of the anterior palate;
- to provide adequate bone stock to receive an osseo-integrated dental implant where a tooth is congenitally absent.

Normally patients undergo a period of orthodontic treatment prior to bone grafting. The maxillary segment is expanded orthodontically (if necessary) to widen the cleft alveolus. The surgery is best performed before the canine tooth erupts (between 8 and 11 years of age). Earlier bone grafting may be beneficial not only for the unerupted canine tooth but also to promote eruption and bony support to the adjacent central and lateral incisor when present. Alveolar bone grafting can also be performed simultaneously with secondary lip revision (Figure 45.19).

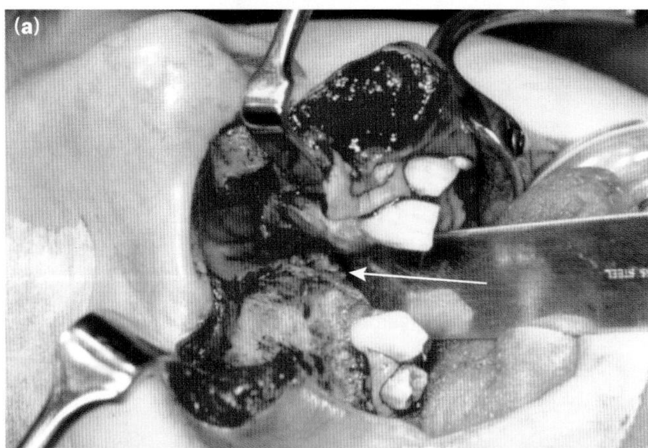

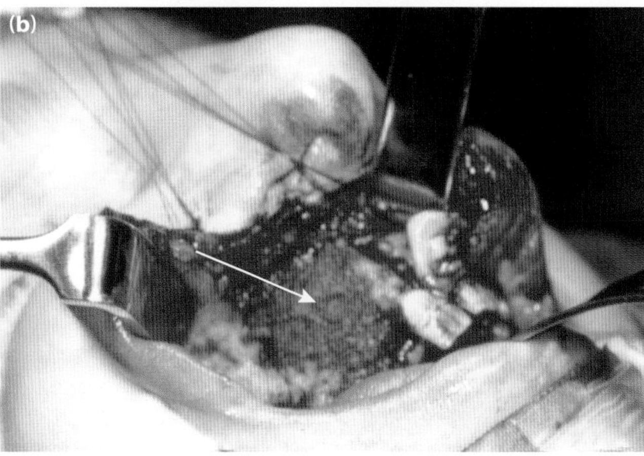

Figure 45.19 (a) Peroperative view of alveolar bone graft demonstrating defect in alveolus (arrow) (simultaneous lip revision). (b) Cancellous bone graft (arrow) packed into the defect.

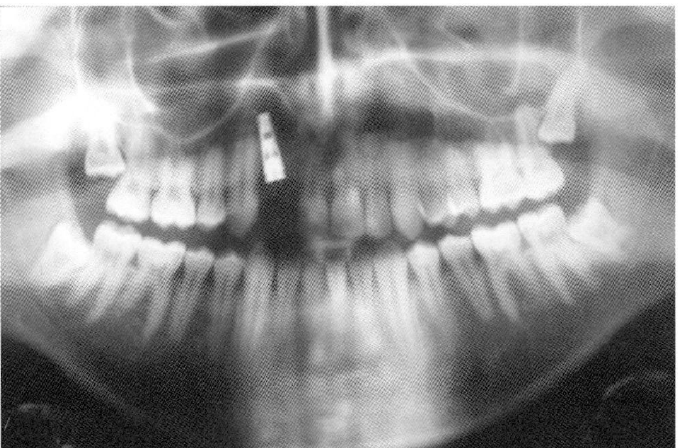

Figure 45.20 Radiographic appearance of an implant in an alveolar bone graft site.

Bone grafting is a highly successful procedure when carried out in experienced hands, with over 90% of patients achieving acceptable interdental alveolar bone height, but it does require the interaction of surgeon and orthodontist. When the lateral incisor is absent and the canine tooth fails to erupt, surgical exposure of the canine tooth may be required to aid its eruption. It is a fundamental principle that, following alveolar bone grafting, efforts should be made to ensure that a tooth erupts into the alveolar bone graft site. Failure to provide a tooth in the alveolar bone graft site usually results in bony resorption in the long term. This can be overcome by the insertion of an osseo-integrated implant into the grafted site, thereby preserving bone stock (Figure 45.20)

Orthognathic surgery

Impaired growth of the midface (maxilla) is now attributed to poor primary surgery. Surgical techniques must endeavour to minimise scarring, although in many cases patients also have a genetic predisposition to poor midfacial growth. Elective maxillary advancement or bimaxillary surgery is often indicated to restore aesthetics and dental occlusal harmony. Orthognathic surgery is usually performed when facial growth is complete (16–17 years in female patients, 17–19 years in male patients).

The principal dentofacial deformity associated with cleft lip and palate is underdevelopment in both the horizontal and vertical direction of the maxilla. This jaw size discrepancy can be corrected with orthognathic surgery (Figure 45.21)

Open septorhinoplasty

Following revisional cleft lip and palate surgery, orthognathic surgery and alveolar bone grafting, many patients still require definitive surgical nasal correction. In patients with cleft lip and palate, open rhinoplasty is preferred to gain access to the external cartilaginous framework, which is frequently deformed (Figure 45.22). The principal deformity is a collapse of the lower lateral cartilage on the cleft side together with a dislocation of the cartilaginous septum into the noncleft nostril. The open method ensures adequate access and repositioning of the cartilaginous framework as a tertiary procedure to improve nasal tip projection, correct septal deformity and relocate alar cartilages. A postauricular onlay graft to the middle crus of the cleft nostril lower lateral cartilage may be required to enhance good nasal tip projection and symmetry.

Summary

The management of children with cleft lip and palate is complex, requiring the skill of a multidisciplinary team. Each team should include professionals who are appropriately qualified with specialist training, treating an adequate number of patients per year in centralised units. Meticulous record keeping of photography, radiology, dental casts and speech recordings are indispensable to permit regular audits and improve outcomes.

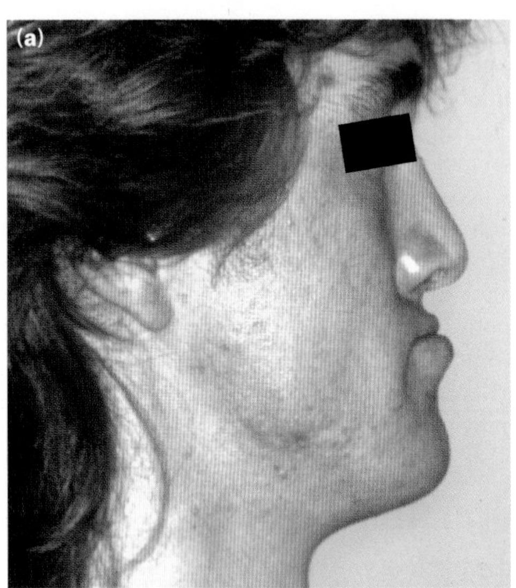
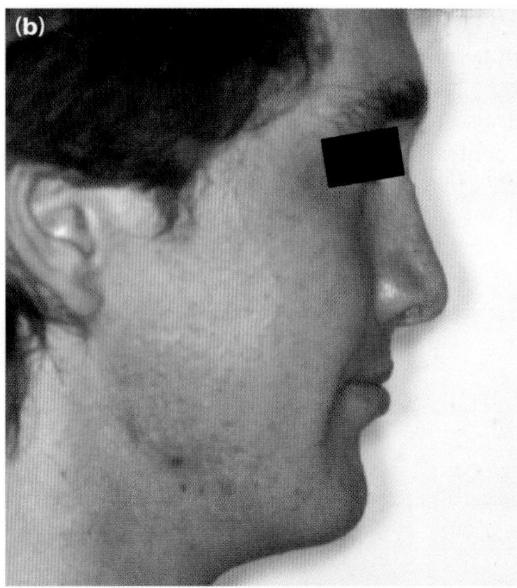

Figure 45.21 (a) Lateral view of an adult a with previously repaired cleft lip and palate demonstrating mandibular prognathism and maxillary retrusion. (b) Postoperative appearance following maxillary advancement and mandibular setback surgery.

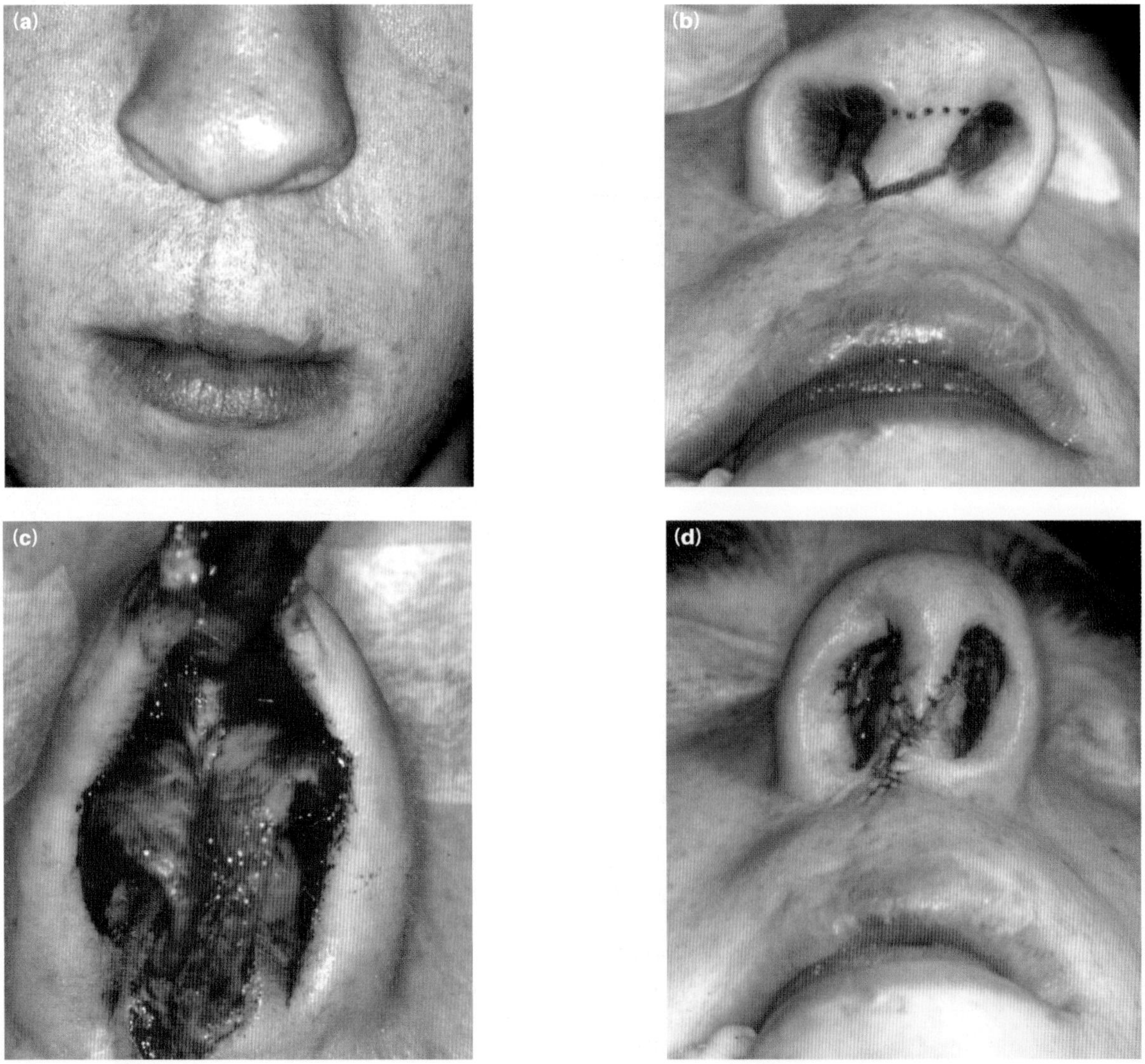

Figure 45.22 (a) Characteristic nasal deformity of a non-functional unilateral cleft lip repair. (b) Incisions for open rhinoplasty. (c) Exposure of the cartilaginous skeleton of the external nose. (d) Repositioning of the external nasal cartilages to improve nasal tip projection.

DEVELOPMENTAL ABNORMALITIES OF THE JAWS

Jaws

Disproportionate growth between the maxilla and mandible can occur, which results in derangement of the dental occlusion. The dental occlusion (the way in which the teeth bite and mesh together) can be classified into three different subtypes:

- class I: a normal relationship of upper and lower incisors and molar dentition;
- class II: the mandibular teeth are placed posterior to the maxillary teeth;
- class III: the mandibular teeth are placed anterior to the maxillary teeth.

This classification is usually, but not invariably, the consequence of aberrant skeletal development of the maxilla and mandible, such that in a class II condition there is usually underdevelopment of the mandible (mandibular retrognathia), whereas in a class III condition there may be simultaneous overgrowth of the mandible (mandibular prognathism) and underdevelopment of the maxilla (maxillary hypoplasia).

In the Caucasian population the most common deformity of the facial skeleton is underdevelopment of the mandible (retrognathia), producing a class II relationship often associated with excessive vertical growth of the maxilla. Bimaxillary protrusion is rare but is a characteristic of African races.

Condylar hyperplasia is an idiopathic condition seen in patients between 15 and 30 years of age, more common in women than men, in which there is hyperplasia or overgrowth of the neck of the mandibular condyle. This gives an asymmetrical growth to the jaw in both a vertical and horizontal plane.

Facial disproportionate growth is also a characteristic of many syndromes. Examples include:

- Treacher Collins syndrome;
- Crouzon syndrome;
- Apert syndrome;
- Pierre Robin sequence.

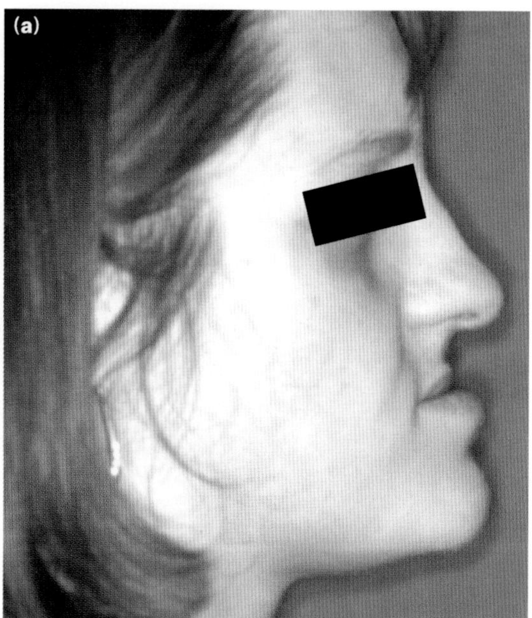

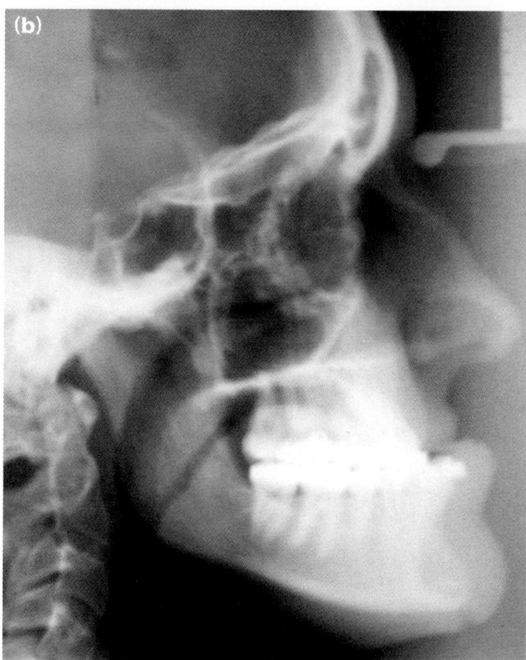

Figure 45.23 (a) Profile of class III skeletal relationship and maxillary hypoplasia and mandibular prognathism. (b) Lateral skull radiograph. (*Continued*)

Orthognathic surgery

Orthognathic surgery is the term given to the surgical correction of deformities of the jaw. It is usually undertaken in close cooperation between orthodontic and maxillofacial surgeons. Surgery is directed at simultaneously changing the position of both maxilla and mandible at the end of the growth period. This is termed bimaxillary osteotomy. Treatment planning usually commences at the age of 12–13 years, in which the orthodontist aligns the dental arches in correct relation for each jaw. This frequently results in an accentuation of the facial deformity at the end of the orthodontic phase of treatment. Treatment normally takes 2 years, in which orthognathic surgery is performed towards the end of orthodontic treatment, although orthodontic treatment in the form of fixed appliances usually continues postoperatively for up to 6 months after surgery. Surgical planning should be meticulous and involves clinical examination and cephalometric assessment in the form of radiograph analysis, as well as study model analysis, working in close cooperation with maxillofacial technologists.

Orthognathic surgery is generally carried out through intraoral incisions, in which the upper and lower jaws are mobilised by achieving osteotomy cuts with saws and drills (Figure 45.23). Following mobilisation of the mandible and maxilla, the jaws are repositioned and held with titanium

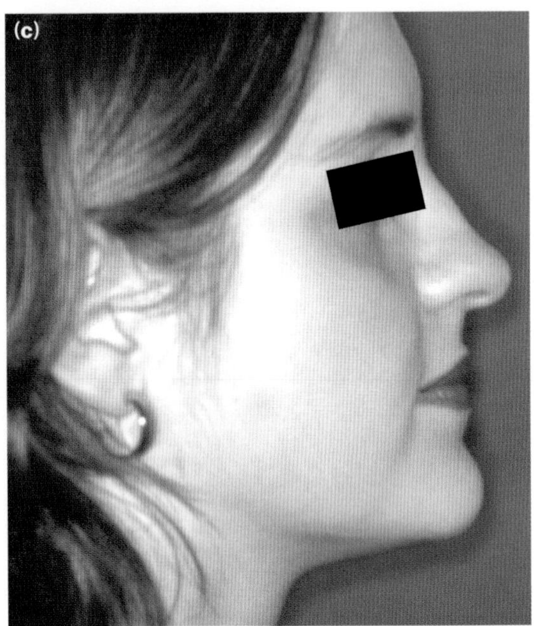

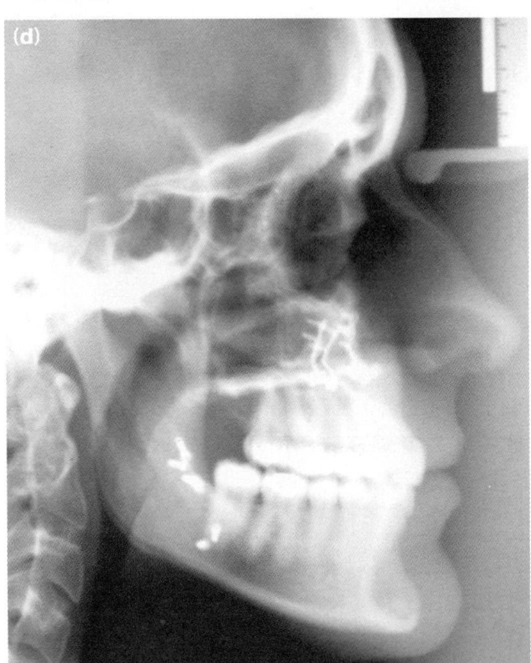

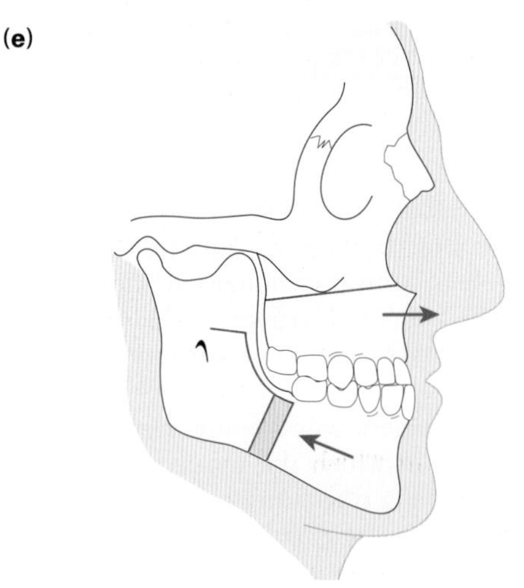

plates and screws placed through an intraoral approach. This frequently avoids the use of intermaxillary fixation and allows earlier function of the jaws as well as improved early dietary intake.

Patients with syndromic conditions such as hemifacial microsomia and Crouzon syndrome and Treacher Collins syndrome require the services of a craniofacial surgeon. As these syndromes are extremely rare, management and surgery should only be carried out in designated centres. The principal treatment is to correct the deformity from the cranium downwards, with correction of the cranial deformity within the first 3 years of life and correction of the residual midfacial and lower facial deformity in childhood and adolescence.

The use of distraction osteogenesis in the management of craniofacial deformity has reduced the requirements for major orthognathic surgery in patients with severe facial deformity.

Summary box 45.10

Principles of orthognathic surgery

- Orthodontist aligns the dental arches
- Surgery then corrects the jaw deformity

FURTHER READING

Brennan P, Schliephake H, Ghali GE, Cascarini L. *Maxillofacial surgery*, 3rd edn. St. Louis: Elsevier, 2017.

Hayward R, Jones B, Dunaway D, Evans R. *The clinical management of craniosynostosis*. London: MacKeith Press, 2004.

Sitzman TJ, Marcus JR. Cleft lip and palate: current surgical management. *Clin Plast Surg* 2004: **41**(2): xi–xii.

van der Meulen JC, Mazzola R, Vermey-Keers C, Stricker M *et al*. A morphogenetic classification of craniofacial malformations. *Plast Reconstr Surg* 1983; **71**(4): 560–72.

Figure 45.23 *(Continued)* (c) Profile following bimaxillary osteotomy. (d) Postoperative radiograph following bimaxillary osteotomy demonstrating internal fixation. (e) Schematic representation of bimaxillary osteotomy with maxillary advancement and mandibular retrusion.

Chapter 46

The ear, nose and sinuses

Learning objectives

To be familiar with:

- The anatomy of the ear
- The conditions of the outer, middle and inner ear
- The examination of the ear including hearing tests
- The basic anatomy of the nose and paranasal sinuses
- The principles of managing post-traumatic nasal and septal deformity
- The causes and management of epistaxis

To understand that:

- The outer layer of the tympanic membrane migrates outwards
- The facial nerve can be damaged by trauma and ear disease
- Chronic ear disease can lead to intracranial sepsis
- There are two types of hearing loss: conductive and sensorineural
- The clinical features of sinus infection, its treatment and potential complications
- The diagnosis and management of chronic rhinosinusitis with and without nasal polyposis
- The common sinonasal tumours, their presentation, investigation and principles of treatment

INTRODUCTION

Disorders affecting the ear, nose and sinus are common reasons for primary care attendance; however, few surgeons will encounter such diseases in day to day practice. Nonetheless, traumatic, infective and neoplastic processes can impact on these organs and their anatomical proximity to critical anatomical structures demands a basic understanding in order to efficiently diagnose, refer and treat conditions. A full and detailed review of the management of ear and nose conditions is beyond the scope of this text. Instead, the aim of this chapter is to familiarise the reader with the basic anatomy and pathology relevant to patients who present with conditions affecting the ear, nose and sinuses.

THE EAR

The mammalian ear is an evolutionary masterpiece. Its highly complex 'three-dimensional anatomy' is best learnt by dissecting cadaver temporal bones.

The external ear

The external and middle ear develop from the first two branchial arches. The external ear canal is 3 cm in length; the outer two-thirds is cartilage and the inner third is bony. The skin on the lateral surface of the tympanic membrane is highly specialised and migrates outwards along the ear canal. As a result of this migration most people's ears are self-cleaning. The external canal is richly innervated and the skin is tightly bound down to the perichondrium so that swelling in this region results in severe pain.

The lymphatics of the external ear drain to the retroauricular, parotid, retropharyngeal and deep upper cervical lymph nodes.

The tympanic membrane and middle ear

The anatomy of the tympanic membrane and ossicles is shown in (Figure 46.1). The relations of the middle ear are important (Figure 46.2). The tympanic membrane and ossicles act as a transformer of vibrations in the air to vibrations within the fluid-filled inner ear.

The inner ear

The inner ear comprises the cochlea and vestibular labyrinth (saccule, utricle and semicircular canals). These structures are embedded in dense bone called the otic capsule.

The cochlea is a coiled shell of two and three-quarter turns. Within the cochlea is a spiral structure called the cochlear duct (Figure 46.3) containing endolymph that is partitioned by Reissner's membrane from the perilymph of the scala vestibuli, which joins the round window and the basement membrane from the perilymph of the scala tympani, which joins the oval window and stapes footplate. The endolymph has a

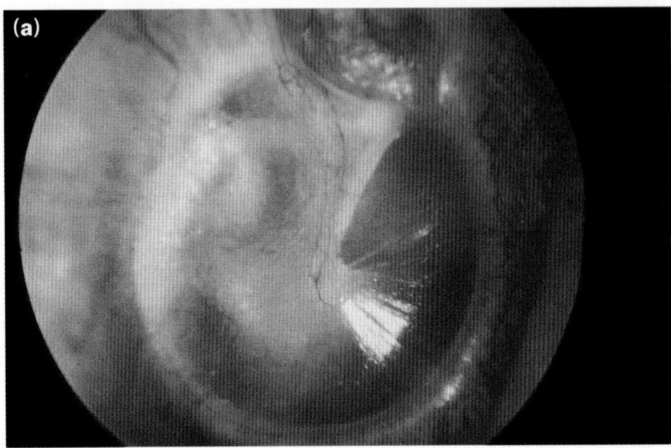

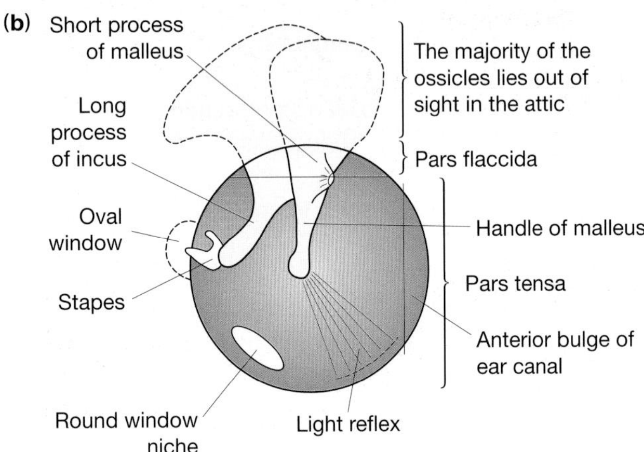

Figure 46.1 (a) Right tympanic membrane and (b) diagram to illustrate the anatomy of the tympanic membrane and ossicles (courtesy of Dr Christian Deguine).

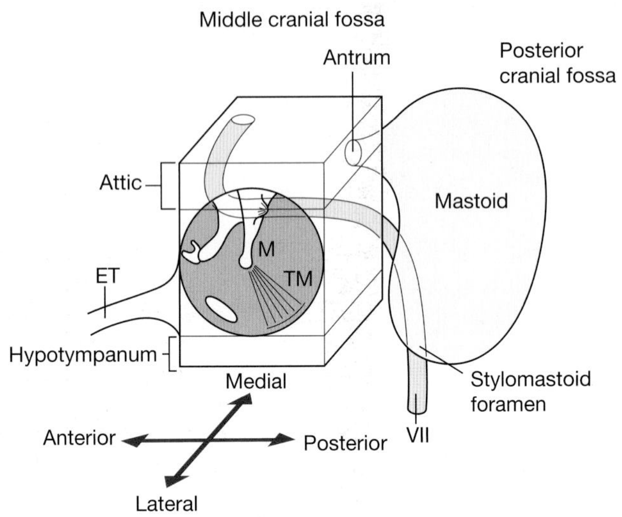

Figure 46.2 Diagram to show the relationships of the middle ear (courtesy of Dr Christian Deguine). ET, Eustachian tube; M, malleus; TM, tympanic membrane; VII, facial nerve.

high concentration of potassium, similar to intracellular fluid, and the perilymph has a high sodium concentration and communicates with the cerebrospinal fluid (CSF). Maintenance of the ionic gradients is an active process and is essential for neuronal activity.

There are approximately 15 500 hair cells in the human cochlea. They are arranged in rows of 3500 inner and 12 000 outer hair cells. The inner hair cells act as mechanicoelectric transducers, converting the acoustic signal into an electric impulse. The outer hair cells contain contractile proteins and serve to tune the basilar membrane on which they are positioned.

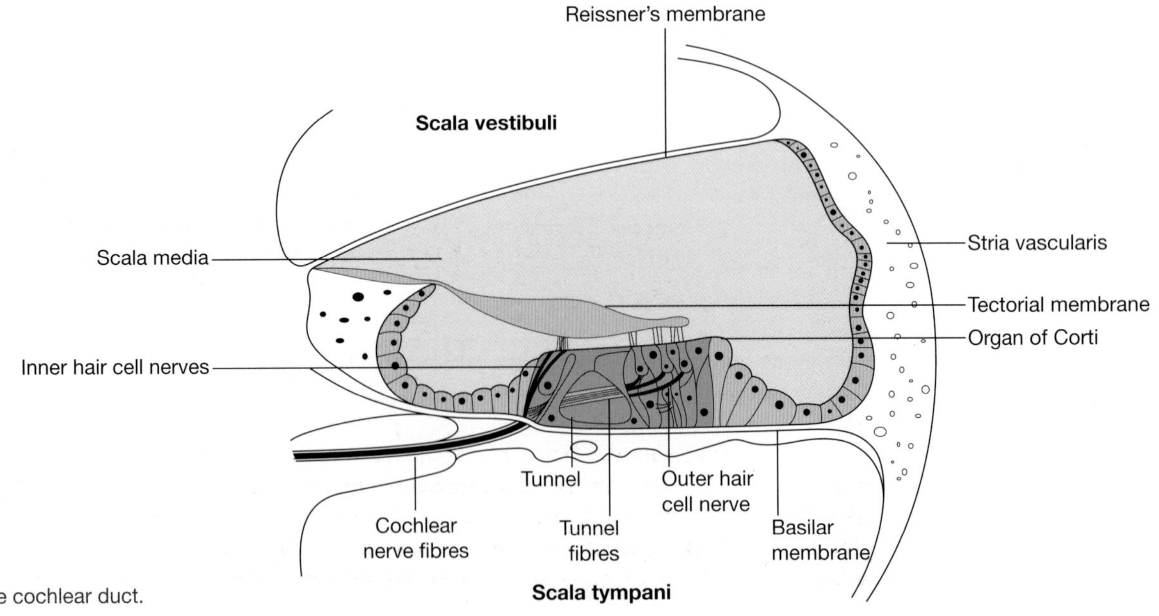

Figure 46.3 The cochlear duct.

Ernst Reissner, 1824–1878, Professor of Anatomy at Dorpat and later at Breslau, Germany (now Wroclaw, Poland), described the vestibular membrane of the cochlea in 1851.

Each inner hair cell responds to a particular frequency of vibration. When stimulated, it depolarises and passes an impulse to the cochlear nuclei in the brainstem.

The vestibular labyrinth consists of the semicircular canals, utricle and saccule and their central connections. The three semicircular canals are arranged in the three planes of space at right angles to each other. Like the auditory system, hair cells are present. In the lateral canals, the hair cells are embedded in a gelatinous cupula. Shearing forces, caused by angular movements of the head, produce hair cell movements and generate action potentials. In the utricle and saccule the hair cells are embedded in an otoconial membrane, which contains particles of calcium carbonate. These respond to changes in linear acceleration and the pull of gravity.

Impulses are carried centrally by the vestibular nerve and connections are made to the spinal cord, cerebellum and external ocular muscles. Its function is to record the position and movements of the head.

The sensory nerve supply

The external ear is supplied by the auriculotemporal branch of the trigeminal nerve (cranial nerve [CN] V) and the greater auricular nerve (C2/3), together with branches of the lesser occipital nerve (C2.) CNs VII, IX and X also supply small sensory branches to the external ear. The middle ear is supplied by the glossopharyngeal nerve (CN IX).

This complicated and rich sensory innervation means that referred otalgia is common and may originate from the normal area of distribution of any of the above nerves. A classic example is the referred otalgia caused by cancer of the larynx.

Taking a thorough history is the most important part of the assessment; the symptoms that need to be enquired after are listed in *Table 46.1*.

Summary box 46.1

Applied anatomy

- The skin on the outer surface of the eardrum migrates outwards so that the ear canal is 'self-cleaning'
- Infection of the middle ear and mastoid can easily spread to the cranial cavity
- The facial nerve pursues a tortuous course through the middle ear
- The ear has a rich sensory innervation so that 'referred otalgia' is common
- Cancer of the larynx can present with otalgia

TABLE 46.1 History taking.

Ask about:
Earache, pain and itch
Hearing loss
Discharge: type, quantity and smell
Tinnitus
Vertigo
Facial weakness
Speech and development (in children)
Past history: head injury, baro- or noise trauma, ototoxics, family history and previous ear surgery

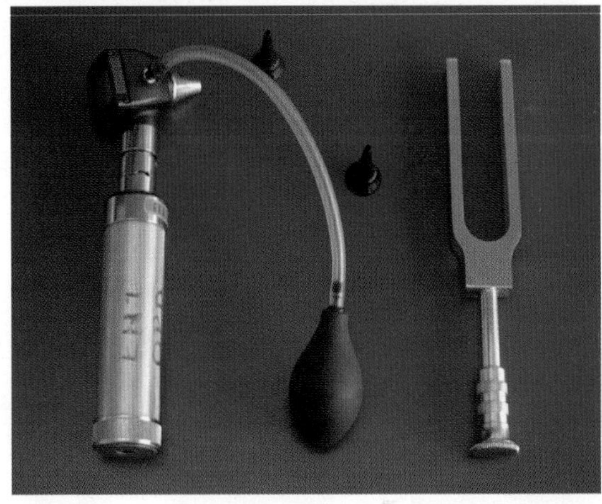

Figure 46.4 Tools of the trade: a fibreoptic otoscope, with pneumatic attachment and a selection of specula. Also a 512 Hz tuning fork.

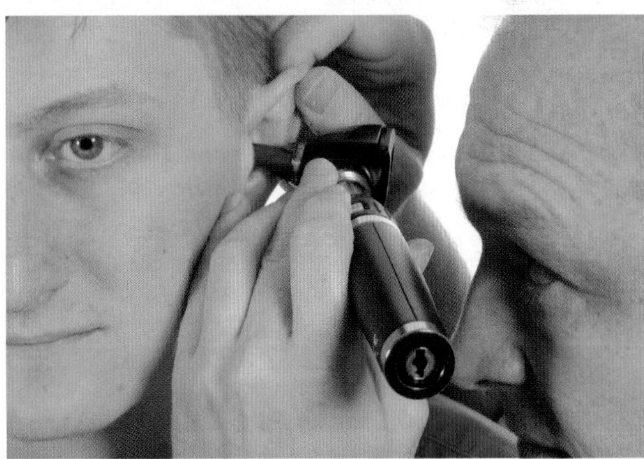

Figure 46.5 The correct method of holding the otoscope. Note the pinna is retracted to straighten the ear canal. Hold the barrel of the otoscope so that the examiner's little finger is balanced on the patient's cheek; this prevents the speculum impinging on the tympanic membrane in case of sudden movement.

EXAMINATION OF THE EAR

The instruments required for examination are shown in Figure 46.4. Examination of the ear is part of the general ear, nose and throat (ENT) examination. Rinne and Weber tuning fork tests are used to distinguish between a conductive and a sensorineural hearing loss. The correct way to hold an otoscope is shown in Figure 46.5.

The CNs and especially the function of the facial nerve should be examined. Although conversational testing can

Friedrich Heinrich Adolf Rinne, 1819–1868, otologist, Gottingen, Germany, described his test in 1855.
Friedrich Eugen Weber-Liel, 1832–1891, otologist, University of Berlin and Jena, Germany, described the operation of tenotomy of the tensor tympani used for certain forms of partial deafness.

give a useful guide to the level of hearing, pure tone audiometry in a soundproof booth is the best way of establishing the air and bone hearing levels (Figure 46.6). Other common audiological tests include speech audiometry, tympanometry, stapedial reflexes, electric response audiometry, otoacoustic emissions, caloric testing and electronystagmography (see Further reading).

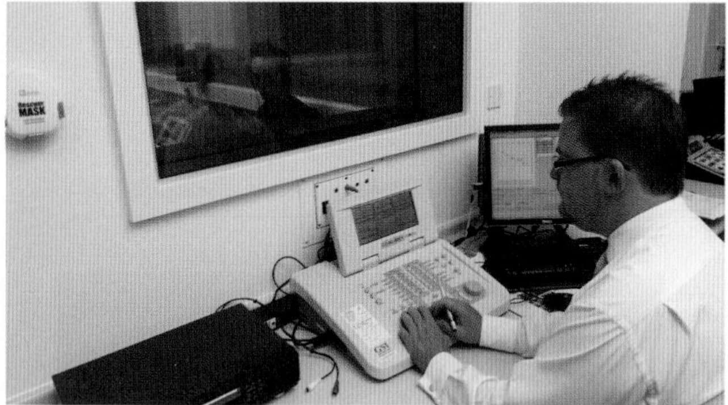

Figure 46.6 Audiometry. The patient sits in a soundproof room and the audiologist presents sounds at different thresholds and records the responses.

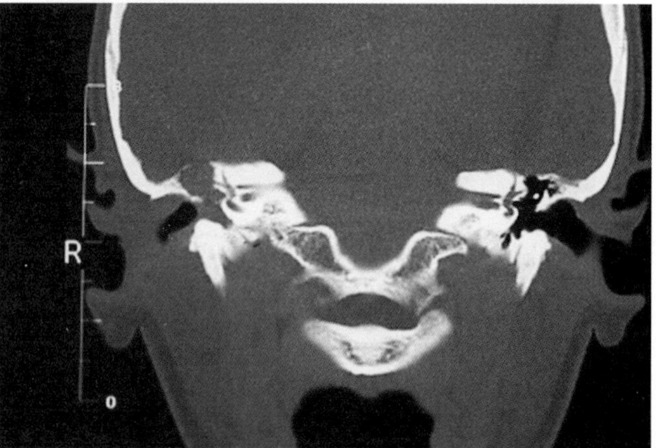

Figure 46.7 Computed tomography scan showing a normal left ear. The air-filled middle ear and the incus and stapes and the lateral and semicircular canals and internal acoustic meatus can be seen. In the right ear the entire middle ear and mastoid is opaque and filled with soft tissue. This is the typical appearance of a cholesteatoma.

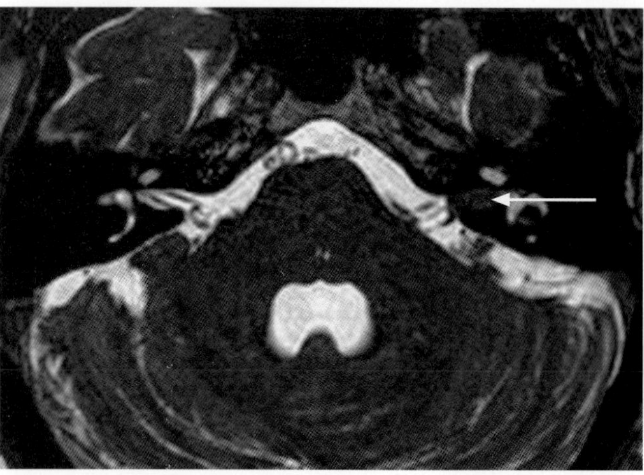

Figure 46.8 Computed tomography scan showing a vestibular schwannoma occluding the left internal acoustic meatus (arrow).

Radiological investigation

Computed tomography (CT) scanning of the temporal bones is commonly performed before mastoid surgery to show detailed individual anatomy, as well as alerting the surgeon to anatomical variants. Pus, bone and air are shown well on high-resolution CT (Figure 46.7).

Magnetic resonance imaging (MRI) is better than CT at imaging soft tissue (e.g. facial and auditory nerve) and is the best method for imaging tumours of the acoustic nerves (Figure 46.8). Diffusion-weighted MRI is also commonly used to detect recurrent cholesteatoma.

CONDITIONS OF THE EXTERNAL EAR

Congenital anomalies

The external and middle ear originate from the first and second branchial arches, but the cochlea is neuroectodermal in origin. An individual can have a congenital abnormality of the pinna and middle ear with a normal cochlea and therefore the potential for normal hearing.

Trauma

A haematoma of the pinna occurs when blood collects under the perichondrium. The cartilage receives its blood supply from the perichondrial layer and will die if the haematoma is not evacuated, resulting in a so-called cauliflower ear. A generous incision under anaesthetic, with a pressure dressing or compressive sutures and antibiotic cover, is recommended (Figure 46.9).

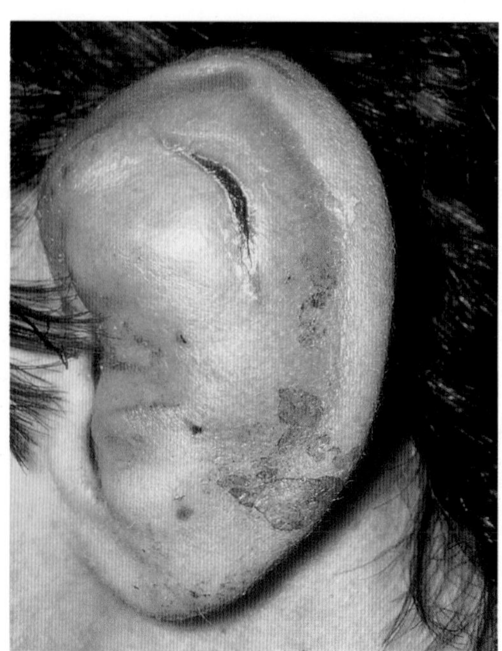

Figure 46.9 Haematoma of the pinna.

Foreign bodies in the ear canal are most easily removed at the first attempt by an experienced practitioner with the aid of a microscope. General anaesthesia may be required in children and those with learning difficulties. Batteries need to be removed within the hour (Figure 46.10).

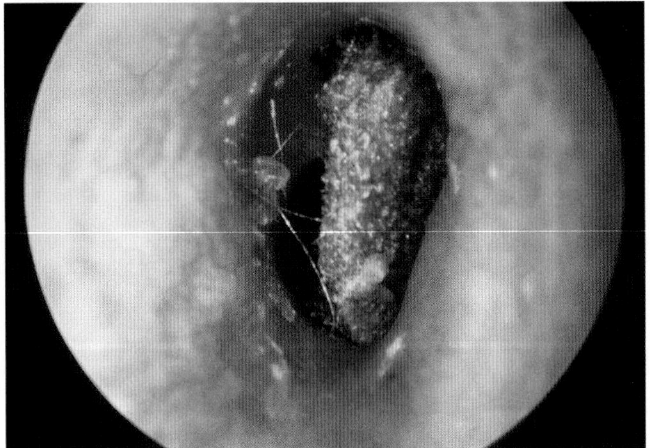

Figure 46.10 Removal of a foreign body from the ear canal can be a challenge (courtesy of Dr Christian Deguine).

Summary box 46.2

Trauma of the external ear

- A haematoma of the pinna requires thorough drainage, antibiotics and a compressive dressing or sutures
- Foreign bodies in the ear canal are most easily removed at the first attempt with the aid of a microscope
- Batteries need to be removed urgently

Inflammation and infection

Otitis externa is very common and consists of generalised inflammation of the skin of the external auditory meatus. The cause is often cotton bud use, moist enviroment, immunocompromise, allergies or skin disorders, such as psoriasis and eczema. Common pathogens are *Pseudomonas* and *Staphylococcus* bacteria, *Candida* and *Aspergillus*. Once the skin of the ear canal becomes oedematous, skin migration stops and debris collects in the ear canal. This acts as a substrate for the pathogens. Movement of the pinna elicits pain, which distinguishes it from otitis media.

The initial treatment is with a topical antibiotic and steroid ear drops together with analgesia. If this fails, meticulous removal of the debris with the aid of an operating microscope is required. Fungal infection can be recognised by the presence of hyphae within the canal (Figure 46.11). Fungal infection causes irritation and itch. The treatment is meticulous removal of the fungus and any debris, as well as stopping any concurrent antibiotics. Systemic antibiotics are rarely required for otitis externa but should be used if cellulitis of the pinna occurs (Figure 46.12).

Necrotising otitis externa is a rare but important condition. It presents as a severe, persistent, unilateral otitis

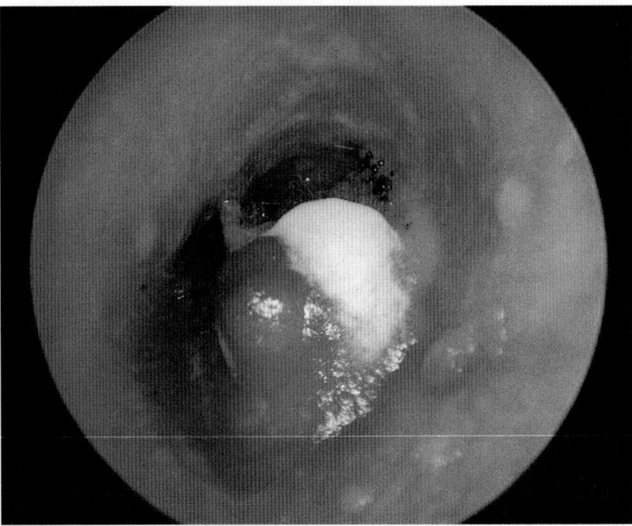

Figure 46.11 Fungal otitis externa. Note the spores.

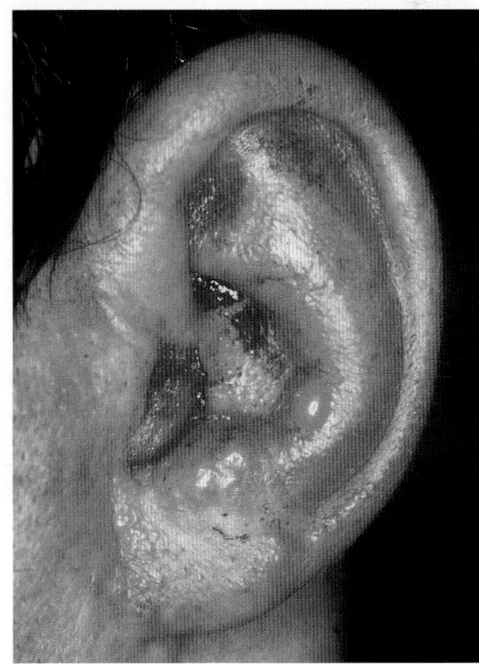

Figure 46.12 Cellulitis of the pinna.

Summary box 46.3

Types of otitis externa

- Acute bacterial otitis externa is very common and painful; treat with topical steroid and antibiotic drops
- Systemic antibiotics should be reserved for cellulitis of the pinna
- Chronic otitis externa needs the underlying dermatitis to be treated
- Fungal otitis externa itches and can be diagnosed by the presence of hyphae and spores; treat with meticulous cleaning and stop antibiotics
- Necrotising otitis externa is a progressive skull base infection that occurs in immunocompromised individuals and can be life-threatening; intensive long-term antibiotic treatment is required

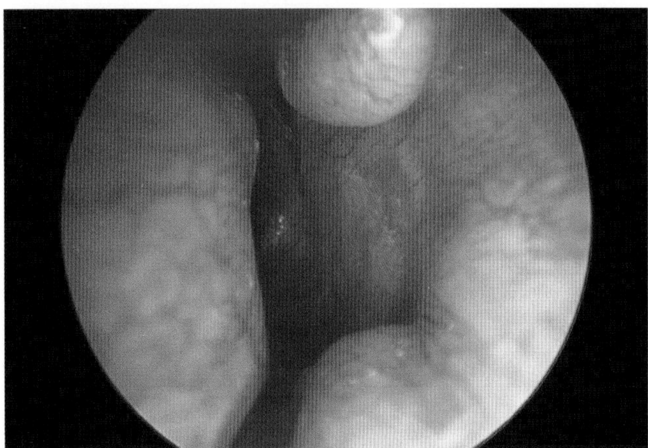

Figure 46.13 Exostoses grow from the bony part of the ear canal in response to cold and so are found in swimmers, surfers and divers. Treatment is only required if the exostoses occlude the ear canal.

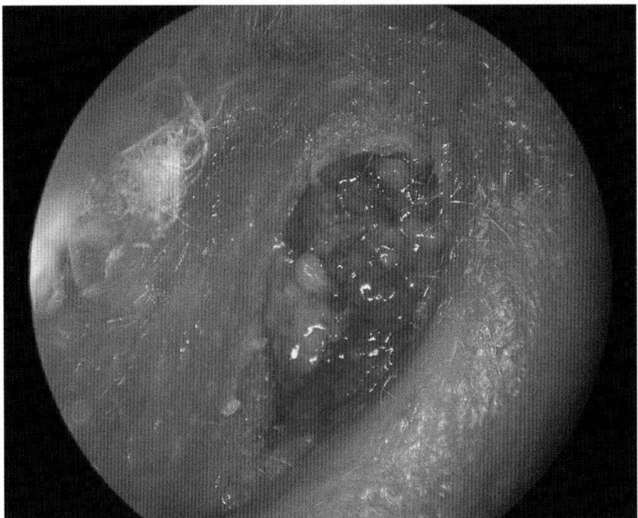

Figure 46.14 Squamous cell carcinomas of the external ear usually originate from the pinna. In this case the tumour is growing from the canal (courtesy of Mr P Beasley).

externa possibly with facial weakness in an immunocompromised individual (e.g. elderly diabetic patient). Usually the infecting organism is *Pseudomonas aeruginosa*. Osteomyelitis of the skull base may result in lower CN palsy (VII–XII). Intensive systemic antibiotics are required and the disease process should be monitored by high-resolution imaging.

Neoplasms

Exostosis is an area of hyperostosis rather than a neoplasm that arises from the bone of the ear canal in individuals who swim in cold water (syn: 'surfer's ear') (Figure 46.13). No treatment is required unless the exostosis obstructs the canal. Osteomas are true neoplasms, often singular and more lateral than exostosis. Other benign tumours include papillomas and adenomas.

Malignant primary tumours of the external ear are either basal cell or squamous cell carcinomas (Figure 46.14). Both may present as ulcerating or crusting lesions that grow slowly and may be ignored by elderly patients. Squamous cell carcinomas metastasise to the parotid and/or neck nodes. The ear canal may be invaded by tumours from the parotid gland and postnasal space carcinomas, which 'creep' up the Eustachian tube. All resectable malignant tumours of the ear are treated primarily with surgery, with or without the addition of radiation therapy.

CONDITIONS OF THE MIDDLE EAR

Congenital anomalies

Aural atresia and congenital anomalies of the middle ear occur in 1/10000 to 1/20000 births and are typically unilateral and nonsyndromal but may be associated with other branchial arch syndromes (e.g. Pierre Robin, craniofacial dysostosis, Down's and Treacher Collins syndromes).

Trauma

Trauma to the middle ear can result in a perforated tympanic membrane (Figure 46.15a). 90% of such perforations heal spontaneously with 6 weeks (Figure 46.15b). Trauma can also result in ossicular discontinuity and it is usually the incus that is displaced. Damaged ossicular chain and tympanic membrane are repaired by ossiculoplasty or tympanoplasty, respectively.

Summary box 46.4

Congenital anomalies and trauma of the middle ear

- Congenital anomalies may be isolated or associated with general congenital deformities
- Traumatic perforations of the tympanic membrane usually heal spontaneously but explosive and welding injuries do not
- A myringoplasty is an operation that repairs the tympanic membrane
- With severe head trauma the incus can be displaced, which leads to a conductive hearing loss

Acute otitis media

Acute otitis media (AOM) occurs in 70% of children by the age of 2 and 90% by the age of 6. It is characterised by purulent fluid in the middle ear. The tympanic membrane bulges

Bartolomeu Eustachio (Eustachius), 1513–1574, Professor of Anatomy, appointed physician to the Pope in 1547.
John Langdon Haydon Down, (sometimes given as Langdon-Brown), 1828–1896, physician, The London Hospital, London, UK, published the classification of ailments in 1866.
Edward Treacher Collins, 1862–1932, ophthalmic surgeon, The Royal London Ophthalmic Hospital and Charing Cross Hospital, London, UK, described this syndrome in 1900.

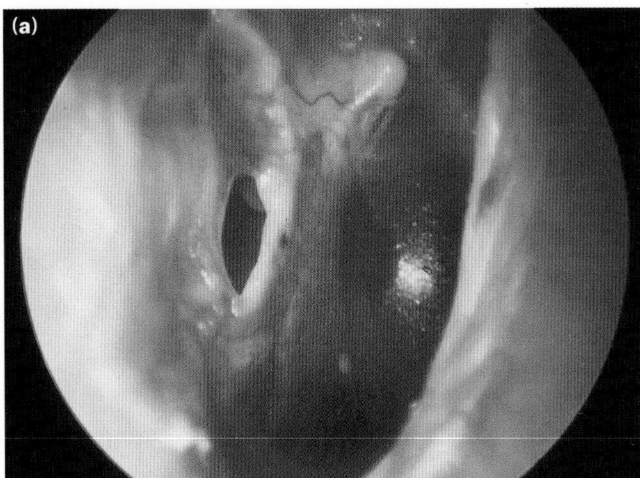

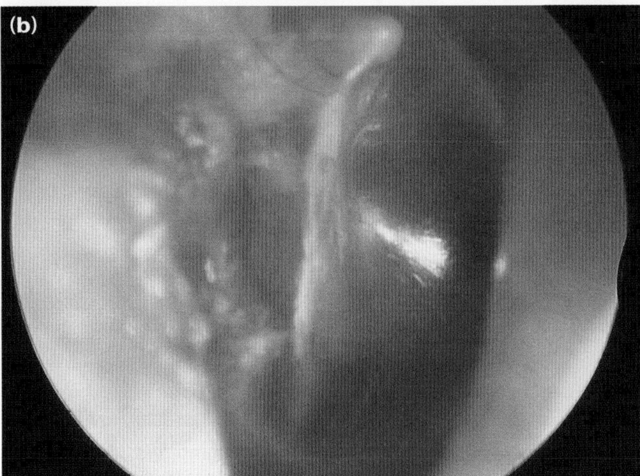

Figure 46.15 (a) Traumatically perforated tympanic membrane. (b) The same tympanic membrane 2 days later (courtesy of Dr Christian Deguine). (Reproduced from O'Donoghue GM, Bates GJ, Narula A (1991) *Clinical ENT*, with permission from Oxford University Press, Oxford.)

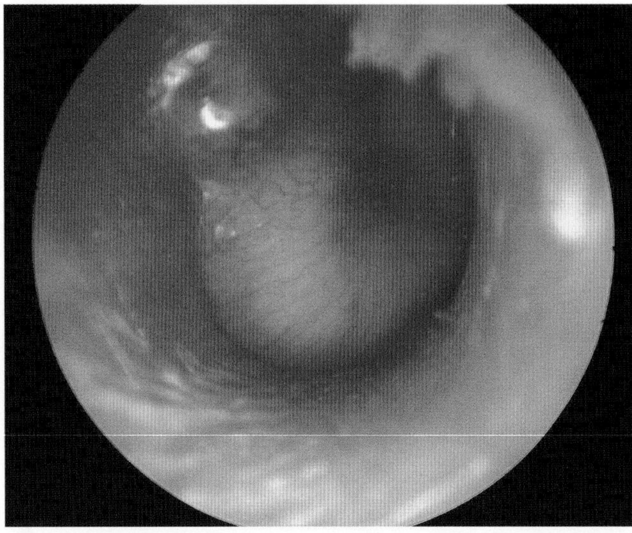

Figure 46.16 Acute otitis media of the left ear. Note the bulging tympanic membrane.

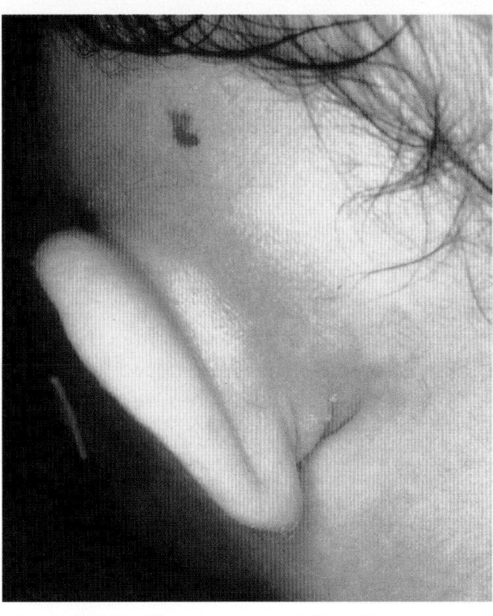

Figure 46.17 Child with acute mastoiditis whose tympanic membrane is shown in Figure 46.16.

because of pressure from the pus in the middle ear (Figure 46.16). The child suffers extreme pain until the tympanic membrane bursts. The most common infecting organisms are *Streptococcus pneumoniae* and *Haemophilus influenzae*. Treatment is with analgesics and antipyretics. Systemic antibiotics should be reserved for children under 2 with bilateral disease or those with other risk factors for complications

Complications are rare, but can be categorised as: intratemporal – otitis media with effusion, chronic otitis media, mastoiditis, facial palsy and labyrinthitis; extratemporal extradural such as abscess; extratemporal intradural such as meningitis, intracranial abcess and sigmoid sinus thrombosis.

The most common complication is mastoiditis because the mastoid air cells connect freely with the middle ear space. Mastoiditis (Figure 46.17) requires hospital admission for intravenous antibiotics and to monitor for complications. If complications arise or the infection does not resolve quickly, a cortical mastoidectomy is required, which decompresses the mastoid cavity, together with a myringotomy and grommet insertion to ventilate the middle ear space.

Otitis media with effusion (glue ear)

Otitis media with effusion (OME) is a middle ear effusion with no evidence of infection. It has a bimodal incidence affecting 40% of 2 year olds and 20% of 5 year olds mainly in the winter months, suggesting an infective aetiology. Infection and inflammation of the immature Eustachian tube results in poor middle ear ventilation, negative pressure and the transudation of fluid.

The following symptoms may be associated with glue ear:

- hearing impairment, which often fluctuates;
- delayed speech;
- behavioural problems;
- recurrent ear infections (the exudate is an ideal culture medium for microorganisms);
- reading and learning difficulties at school.

Otoscopic findings with glue ear

The otoscopic findings of exudative glue ear are of a dull drum that is immobile on pneumatic otoscopy. The tympanic membrane is retracted and radial blood vessels may be present (Figure 46.18).

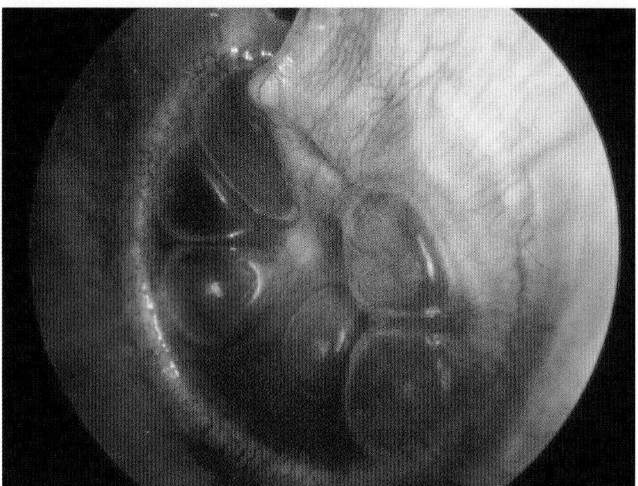

Figure 46.18 The initial serous transudate of glue ear, left ear (courtesy of Dr Christian Deguine). (Reproduced from O'Donoghue GM, Bates GJ, Narula A (1991) *Clinical ENT*, with permission from Oxford University Press, Oxford.)

In children first presenting with bilateral glue ear, 50% will be better within 12 weeks, therefore a 'wait and watch' policy is appropriate. If a bilateral conductive hearing loss persists, there is some evidence of reduced IQ and behaviour changes. However, speech delays are reversed by age 8.

Medical treatment is of limited value. Valsalva manouvres and the Otovent® device (Figure 46.19) are worth trying for patients old enough to comply in an attempt to improve Eustachian tube function. Surgical insertion of ventilation tubes (grommets) (Figure 46.20) and adenoidectomy are effective and should be discussed if there is no resolution after a period of watchful waiting. A middle ear effusion in adults is often associated with an upper respiratory tract infection. A persistent unilateral effusion in an adult requires examination of the postnasal space to exclude obstructive nasopharyngeal carcinoma, which is the most common carcinoma in men in southern China.

Summary box 46.5

Acute otitis media and otitis media with effusion

- Acute otitis media is very common but rarely associated with severe complications such as mastoiditis
- OME is very common in children and usually resolves without treatment
- Persistent OME and/or recurrent AOM is best treated with grommets and/or adenoidectomy
- A persistent middle ear effusion in an adult may be caused by a cancer of the postnasal space, especially in Chinese and Asian races

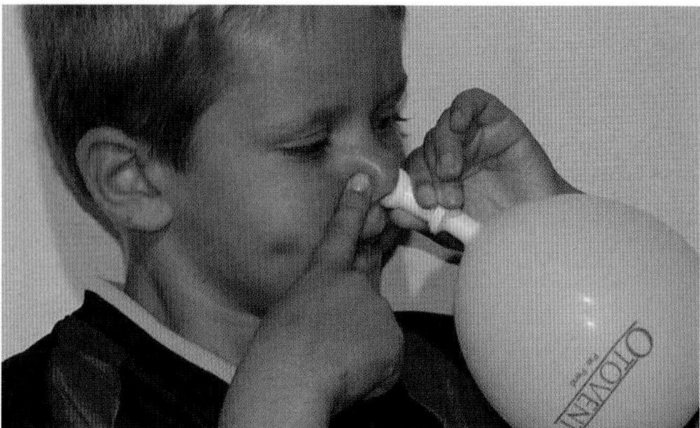

Figure 46.19 Otovent® device.

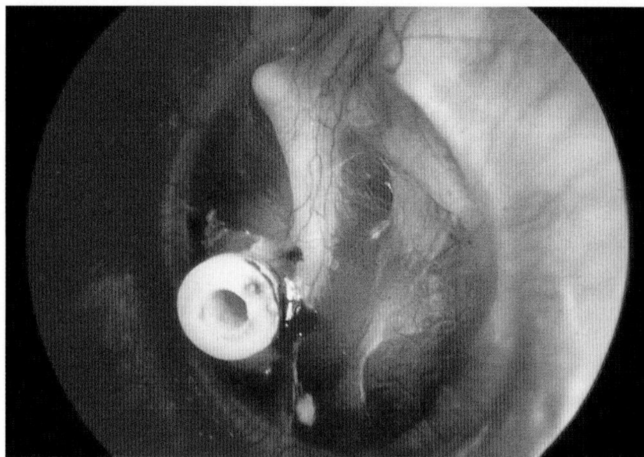

Figure 46.20 Ventilation tube in tympanic membrane, left ear (courtesy of Dr Christian Deguine).

Chronic otitis media

Chronic otitis media (COM) is a permenant abnormality of the tympanic membrane from previous recurrent AOM and/or OME. It is classified as active (i.e. inflamation and pus present) or inactive. Active and passive are then further subclassified as mucosal or squamous (Figure 46.21)

Active mucosal COM implies a perforation with otorrheoa (ear discharge) due to inflamed middle ear mucosa with or without granulation tissue. Inactive mucosal COM implies a dry perforation without inflamation. Surgery in the form

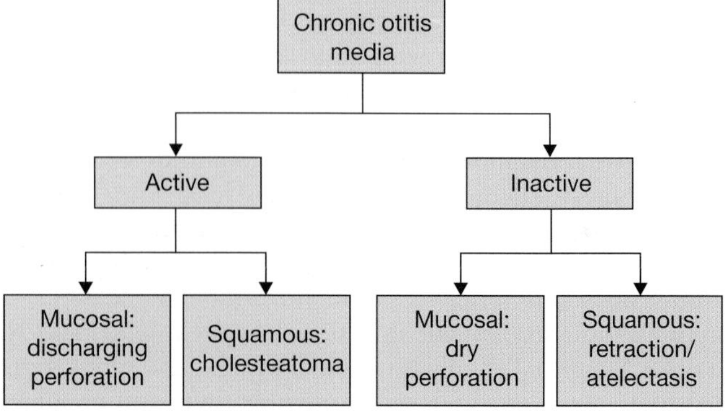

Figure 46.21 Classification of chronic otitis media.

of tympanoplasty (repair of the perforation) is indicated in patients getting recurrent infection (to reduce symptoms of otorrheoa and prevent further deterioration of the hearing due to the ototoxic effects of infection) and where there is a likelyhood that it will restore hearing in the operated ear to 30 dB or better or to within 15 dB of the contralateral ear (this is known as the Belfast rule of thumb).

Active squamous COM is otherwise known as cholesteatoma and usually presents with persistent otorrheoa and hearing loss as a result of keratinising squamous epithelium within the middle ear. The cholesteatoma matrix destroys the structures in its path through the release of lytic enzymes, inflammatory mediators and pressure necrosis. If left, there is a risk of all the complications attributable to AOM. The lifetime risk of intracerebral abscess is 1/200 in a 30-year-old patient. The recommended treatment is mastoid surgery using a drill under microscopic or endoscopic guidence to access and remove the cholesteatoma. Often the ossicles are involved or eroded so an ossiculoplasty (to restore hearing by reconstructing the ossicular chain) is performed at the same time.

Otosclerosis

This is an autosomal dominant condition of variable penetrance in which excess bone is laid down around the footplate of the stapes, impeding mobility of the stapes and resulting in a conductive hearing loss (Figure 46.22). A diagnosis should be suspected in any patient with a conductive hearing loss and a normal tympanic membrane.

The treatment options are simple reassurance, a convetional hearing aid, a stapedotomy operation or bone conduction hearing aid (Figure 46.23).

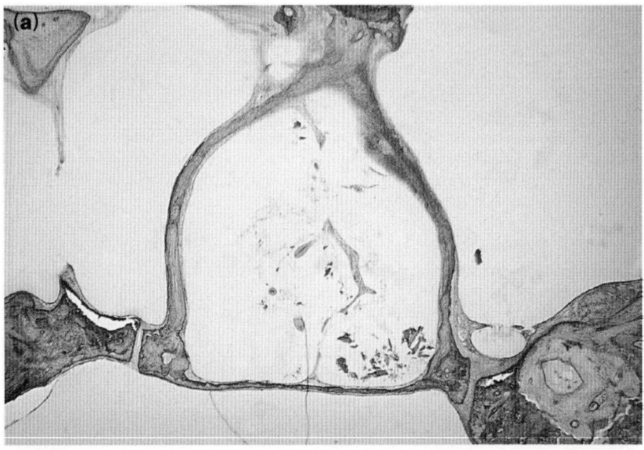

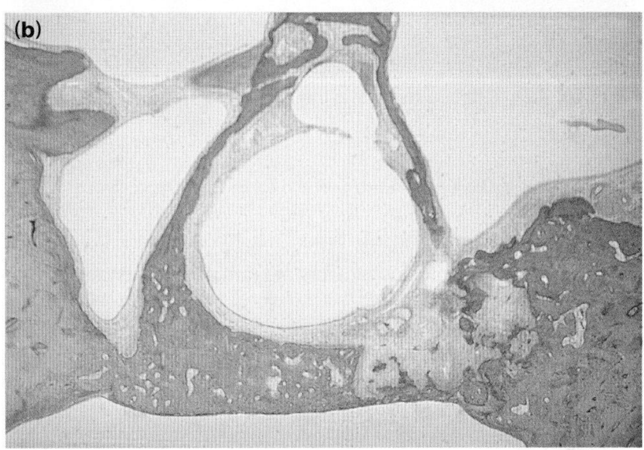

Figure 46.22 Section of normal stapes (a) and section of stapes affected by otosclerosis (b).

Neoplasms

Middle ear tumours are rare with the most common being a glomus tumour (Figure 46.24). Glomus tumours arise from nonchromaffin paraganglionic tissue. The carotid body tumour arising in the neck is an example of this type of tumour. In the temporal bone, three types of glomus tumour are recognised and classification depends on the location: glomus tympanicum (arising in the middle ear), glomus jugularae (arising next to the jugular bulb) and glomus vagale (skull base).

Symptoms include pulse synchronous tinnitus, conductive and sensorineural hearing loss, and lower cranial nerve palsies. Palsies of CNs VII, IX, X, XI and/or XII may occur. The classic sign is a cherry-red mass lying behind the tympanic membrane. The treatment of choice is preoperative embolisation followed by surgical excision. Radiotherapy is also effective.

Squamous cell carcinoma may also occur within the middle ear. It usually presents with deep-seated pain and a blood-stained discharge. Facial paralysis often occurs. Squamous carcinomas usually arise in a chronically discharging ear and can arise in a chronically infected mastoid cavity. Radical surgical excision with or without radiotherapy provides the only chance of cure.

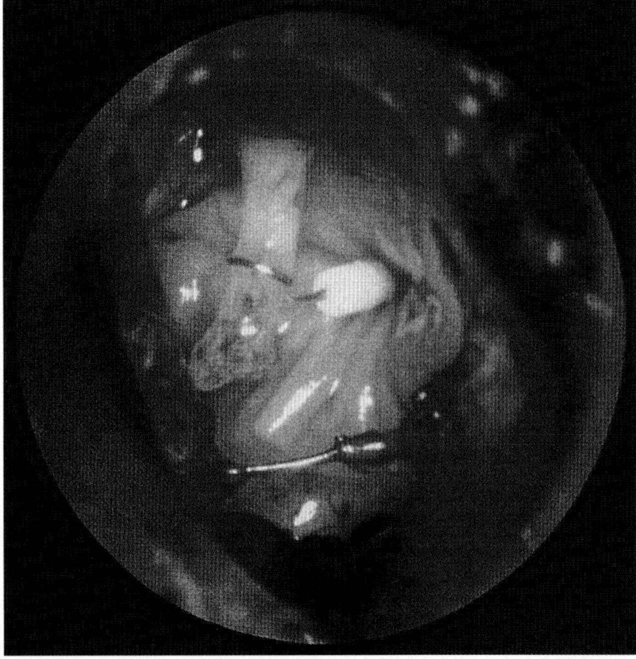

Figure 46.23 The stapedotomy operation showing the piston linking the incus to the vein graft, left ear.

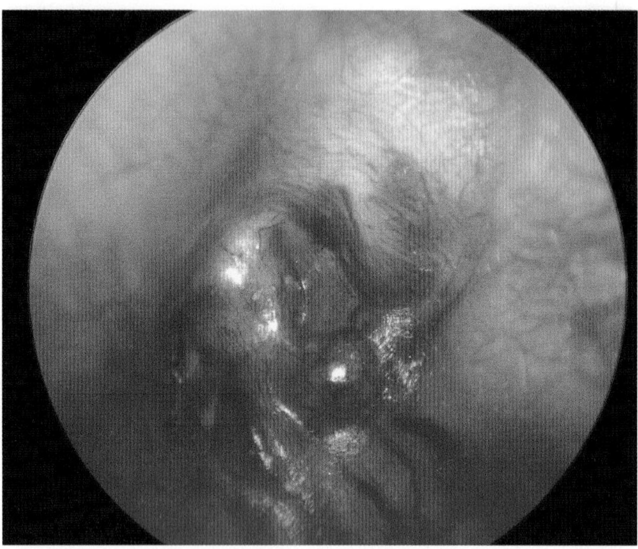

Figure 46.24 Glomus tumour in the middle ear, left ear.

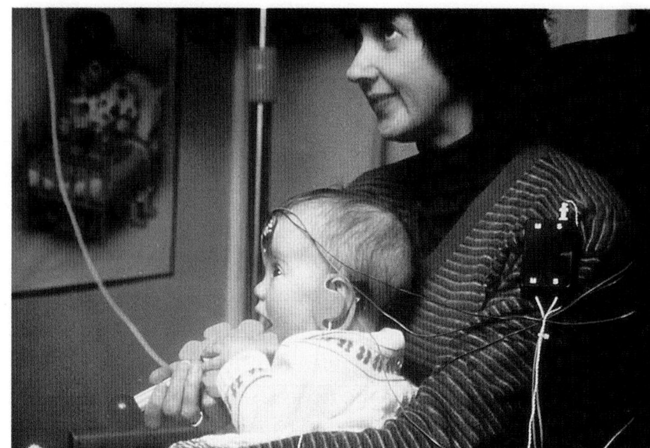

Figure 46.25 Evoked-response audiometry. A simple non-invasive objective test of hearing thresholds. (Reproduced from O'Donoghue GM, Bates GJ, Narula A (1991) *Clinical ENT*, with permission from Oxford University Press, Oxford.)

Summary box 46.6

Neoplasms of the middle ear

- Highly vascular glomus tumours are rare and may present with pulsatile tinnitus
- Squamous cell cancer usually presents with pain and facial paralysis

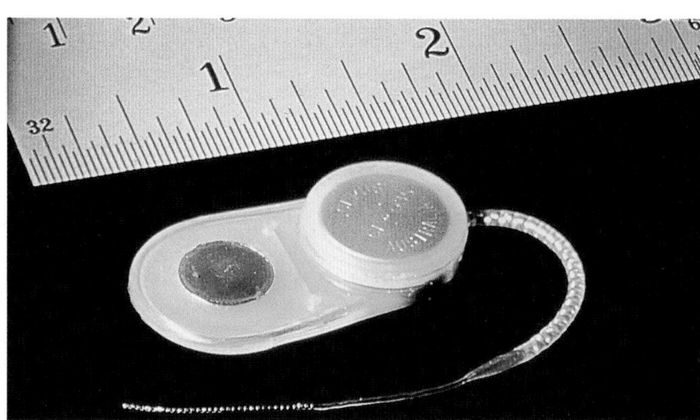

Figure 46.26 Multichannel cochlear implant (Cochlear Corporation).

CONDITIONS OF THE INNER EAR

Congenital sensorineural hearing loss

Half of congenital sensorineural hearing loss is genetic and half is aquired. Of the genetic hearing loss 75% is non-syndromic, of which the most common is a connexin 26 gene mutation. Syndromic causes include Usher, Pendred, Jervell and Lange-Nielsen, Waardenberg, Treacher Collins, Alport, Stickler neurofibromatosis type 2 and branchio-oto-renal syndromes.

Aquired causes are intrauterine infections, including rubella, toxoplasmosis and cytomegalovirus infection; perinatal hypoxia, jaundice and prematurity; and postnatal meningitis

All newborn babies in the UK are now screened at birth for deafness by measuring otoacoustic emisions in response to 'clicks' in the ear. Children failing this are referred for auditory brainstem response to establish hearing thresholds (Figure 46.25). If some hearing is present, the early fitment of hearing aids can maximise the neural plasticity that is present in the developing brain. If a child has a profound hearing loss, early intervention with a cochlear implant is essential for the development of the auditory cortex (Figure 46.26). Most cases of profound sensorineural hearing loss are due to loss of cochlear hair cells, so an implant inserted through the round window can selectively stimulate the cochlear neurones, which usually remain intact.

Presbycusis

Presbycusis is characterised by a gradual loss of hearing in both ears, with or without tinnitus. The hearing loss usually affects the higher frequencies and a classical audiogram is shown in Figure 46.27. The consonants of speech lie within the high-frequency range, which makes speech discrimination difficult.

Many patients with presbycusis are concerned that they may lose their hearing completely and they need reassurance.

Charles Howard Usher, 1865–1942, ophthalmologist Aberdeen Royal Infirmary, Aberdeen, UK.
Vaughan Pendred, 1869–1946, general practitioner, Durham, UK.
Anton Jervell, 1901–1987, physician, University of Oslo, Norway.
Fred Lange-Nielsen, 1919–1989, physician and jazz musician, Oslo, Norway.
Petrus Johannes Waardenburg, 1886–1979, ophthalmologist, Utrecht, Nederlands.
Arthur Cecil Alport, 1880–1959, Professor of Medicine, King Faud I Hospital, University of Cairo, Egypt.
Gunnar B Stickler, 1925–2010, paediatrician, Mayo Clinic, USA.

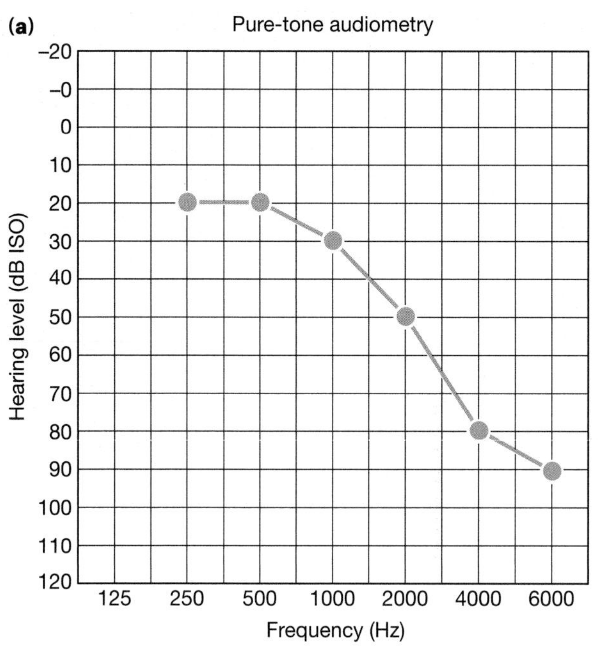

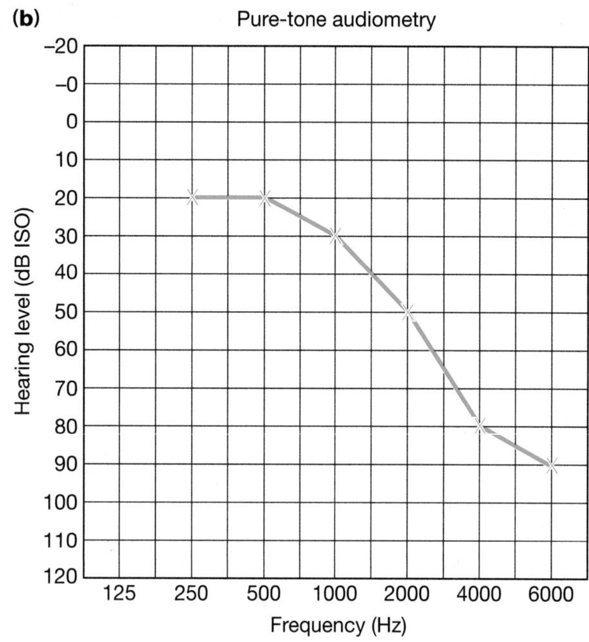

Figure 46.27 Typical audiogram of presbycusis: (a) right ear; (b) left ear.

Hearing aid technology has improved dramatically over recent years and most patients can derive benefit (Figure 46.28).

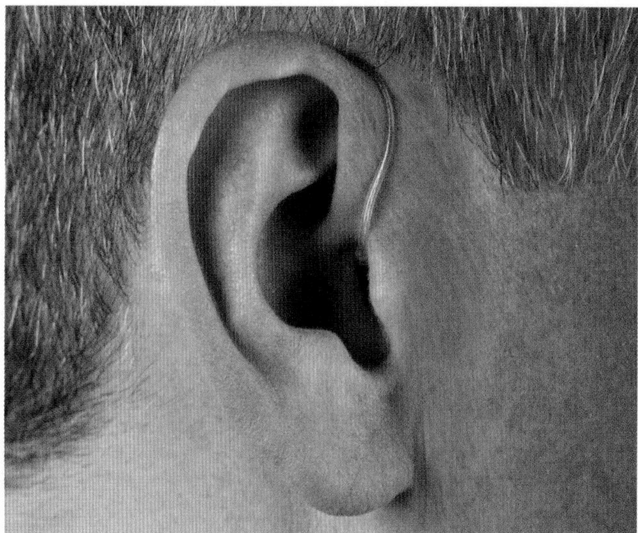

Figure 46.28 Modern hearing aid.

Tinnitus

Tinnitus is the perception of sound when no external sound source is present. It may have an extrinsic cause; for example, the pulsatile tinnitus of a glomus tumour. Usually, however, the tinnitus is generated within the internal auditory pathway. Thirty per cent of people will experience tinnitus at some time in their lives. Tinnitus frequently accompanies presbycusis, as well as any other condition that affects hearing. Most individuals habituate to the presence of tinnitus but in some patients it proves intrusive. Treatment is with reassurance, masking and hearing aids (for patients with hearing loss).

Sudden sensorineural hearing loss

Defined as >30 dB sensorineural hearing loss at 3 frequencies within 3 days. History and examination should focus on a cause, which may be infective, neoplastic, traumatic, ototoxic, neurological or autoimmune. Investigations such as MRI are important (1% of acoustic neuromas present as sudden sensorineural hearing loss) but screening blood tests are of low yield where there is nothing in the history to suggest a cause. Sixty per cent are idiopathic and the recommended treatment is oral +/- intratympanic steroids with salvage intratympanic steroids for those that do not recover after a month.

Trauma

Noise exposure

Hair cells within the cochlea are damaged by sudden acoustic trauma (blast injury or gunfire) or prolonged exposure to excessive noise. The sensorineural hearing loss that results is greatest between 3 and 6 KHz and is often accompanied by tinnitus (Figure 46.29). The law in the UK requires that workers are protected from noise

Head injury

The otic capsule is the hardest bone in the body but, if trauma to the head is severe, temporal bone fractures may occur. These are traditionally described as either longitudinal (80%) or transverse (20%); however, the majority have longitudinal and transverse components. Longitudinal fractures may lead to fracture of the external auditory canal, conductive hearing loss and CSF otorrhoea. Transverse fractures may involve the

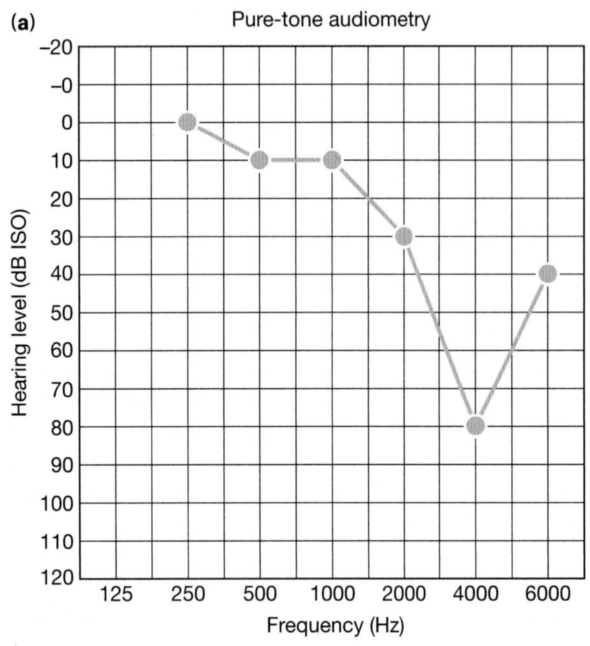

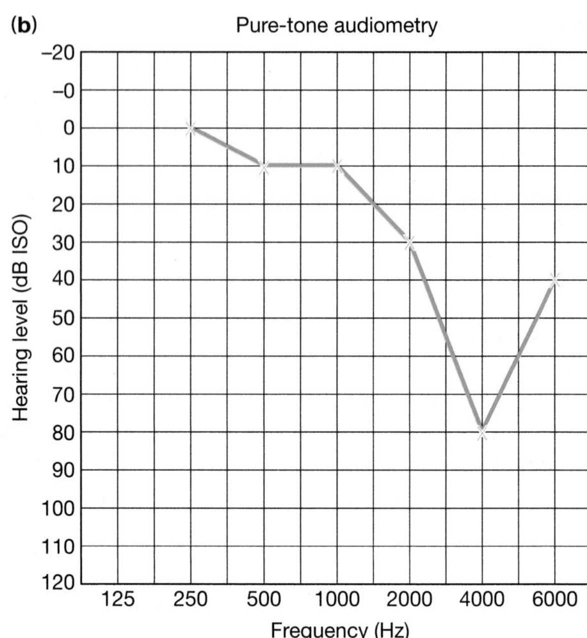

Figure 46.29 A typical audiogram of noise damage: (a) right ear; (b) left ear.

facial nerve leading to palsy and labyrinth leading to a sensorineural hearing loss that is permanent. Profound vertigo occurs initially, followed by gradual compensation.

Drug ototoxicity

Antibiotics such as aminoglycosides, vancomycin and erythromycin, loop diuretics such as frusemide, chemotherapy agents such as cisplatin and carboplatin, and salicylates such as aspirin and quinine are all ototoxic. Recognition of risk factors, such as poor renal function in patients being treated with aminoglycosides, is therefore important. Although many topical ear drops contain aminoglycosides, there is little evidence that short periods of topical treatment cause sensorineural hearing loss

Balance disorders

Vertigo is the halucination of movement.

Benign paroxysmal positional vertigo

Benign paroxysmal positional vertigo (BPPV) is the most common form of vertigo. It is caused by otoliths (calcium carbonate crystals) within the posterior semicircular canal abnormally triggering the ampullary hair cells. Typically, the vertigo is triggered by turning, only lasts for a few seconds and is not associated with other otological symptoms. A positive Hallpike test confirms the diagnosis. The condition is usually self-limiting but recovery may be expediated by an Epley manoeuvre.

Vestibular neuronitis

Infection or inflamation of the supererior vestibular nerve, often caused by a upper respiratory or chest infection, results in persistent vertigo lasting a few days. If the hearing is also affected, this is known as labrinthitis. Treatment is supportive with vestibular sedatives such as prochlorperazine in the first week followed by early mobilisation. There is emerging evidence for systemic steroids as well.

Menière's disease

It has been said that not only can clinicians not agree on the cause of Menières disease, they cannot even agree on the spelling. There is certainly evidence of endolymphatic hydrops (long-standing high pressure changes within the inner ear) in pathological specimens of patients who have had the condition. The condition is characterised by a triad of symptoms: intermittent attacks of vertigo, a unilateral fluctuating sensorineural hearing loss and tinnitus. The patient often has a sensation of pressure in the affected ear before an attack. The hearing loss typically affects the lower frequencies. The vertigo characteristically lasts between 30 minutes and 6 hours and is often accompanied by nausea and vomiting. The investigations include pure tone audiometry and an MRI scan to exclude an acoustic neuroma. The only evidence-based treatment is intratympanic therapy whereby repeated injections of dexamethasone or gentamicin are given into the middle ear. Traditional medical treatment starts with a low salt diet, betahistadine and diuretics, but this is not evidence based

Charles Skinner Hallpike, 1900–1979, aural surgeon, National Hospital for Neurology and Neurosurgery, Queen Square, London, UK.
John W Epley, contemporary, Director, Portland Otology Clinic, Portland, Oregon, USA, established his clinic in 1975; he developed the Epley manoeuvre for treating benign paroxysmal positional vertigo (BPPV).
Prosper Menière, 1799–1862, physician, The Institute of Deaf Mutes, Paris, France, described this condition in 1861.

Vestibular migraine

Five times more prevalent than Menière's disease, this condition presents with similar symptoms but without the hearing loss or tinnitus. It is thought that the migrainous process affects the labyrinth and therfore treatment is along the lines of migraine management, with attention paid to risk factors such as dietary triggers, and prophlatic medication such as propranolol, tricyclic antidepressants and antiepileptic medication.

Facial paralysis

Seventy-five per cent of all facial palsies are due to Bell's palsy. This probably results from a herpes simplex viral infection of the facial nerve. The nerve swells and is compressed within the temporal bone. Early treatment with high-dose steroids and eye protection is mandatory. Not all facial nerve palsies are due to viral infection and a thorough otoneurological examination is required. The facial nerve can be damaged at the cerebellopontine angle, within the internal auditory meatus, within the middle ear, at the skull base and within the parotid gland. It is essential to consider these potential sites of facial nerve damage in any patient with CN VII paralysis and perform an MRI scan if appropriate.

Summary box 46.7

Facial paralysis

- The facial nerve passes through the middle ear and mastoid
- When considering a paralysis, think 'complete' or 'partial'
- Protect the eye: carry out a full otoneurological examination to find the cause
- If acute, consider steroids

Ramsay Hunt syndrome

This is caused by herpes zoster virus and is characterised by facial paralysis, pain and the appearance of vesicles on the tympanic membrane, ear canal, pinna or inside of the cheek (Figure 46.30). It ay be accompanied by vertigo and sensorineural hearing loss (CN VIII). Treatment with aciclovir is effective if given early.

Neoplasms

These are uncommon but can present with sensorineural hearing loss, tinnitus and vertigo. Acoustic neuromas, which are actually schwannomas of the vestibular division of CN VIII, are the most common, followed by meningiomas. Acoustic

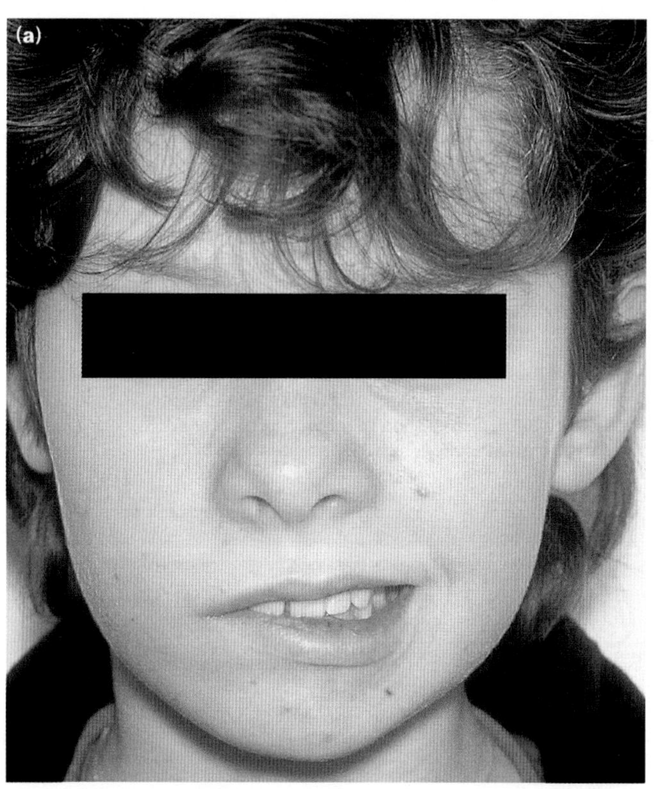

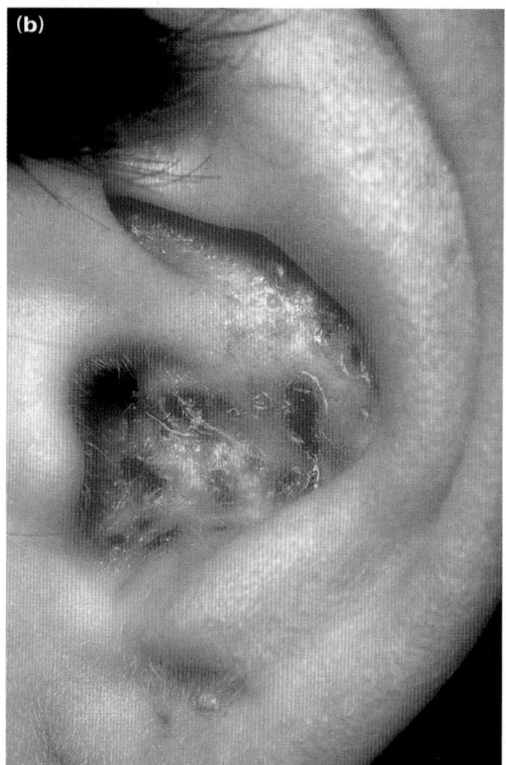

Figure 46.30 Herpes zoster infection of cranial nerve (CN) VII (a) and CN VIII (b) with vesicles on the pinna.

Sir Charles Bell, 1774–1842, surgeon, The Middlesex Hospital, London, UK, and from 1835 until his death, Professor of Surgery, The University of Edinburgh, Edinburgh, UK
James Ramsay Hunt, 1874–1937, Professor of Neurology, The Columbia College of Physicians and Surgeon, New York, USA.

neuromas grow slowly and somewhat unpredictably and as they expand can cause CN palsies, brainstem compression and raised intracranial pressure. The early symptoms are a unilateral sensorineural hearing loss or unilateral tinnitus, or both. Therefore, it is essential to perform an MRI on all patients with persistent unilateral sensorineural hearing loss or tinnitus. Relatively asymptomatic acoustic neuromas that are less than 2 cm in diameter and growing less than 2 mm a year (70%) are generally treated with a 'watch, wait and rescan' policy or occasionally stereotactic radiotherapy. Tumour volumes greater than 2 cm in diameter are often best treated by skull base surgery in the form of a translabyrinthine, retrolabyrinthine or middle fossa approach.

Summary box 46.8

Conditions of the inner ear

- Presbycusis is the bilateral high-frequency loss associated with ageing
- Unilateral tinnitus or sensorineural hearing loss needs to be investigated to exclude acoustic neuroma
- Sudden sensorineural hearing loss needs immediate treatment with steroids and routine MRI to exclude acoustic neuroma
- Menière's disease presents with the triad of sensorineural hearing loss, tinnitus and vertigo

THE NOSE AND SINUSES

BASIC ANATOMY OF THE NOSE AND PARANASAL SINUSES

The supporting structures of the nose are shown in Figure 46.31. The septum consists of the anterior quadrilateral cartilage, the perpendicular plate of the ethmoid and the vomer (Figure 46.32). The lateral wall of the nasal cavity contains the superior, middle and inferior turbinates, which warm and moisten nasal airflow (Figure 46.33). There are paired frontal, sphenoid, maxillary and anterior and posterior ethmoid sinuses. The anterior nasal sinuses (frontal, maxillary and anterior ethmoid) drain into the middle meatus (between the middle turbinate and lateral wall of nose). The posterior ethmoid and sphenoid sinuses drain into the superior meatus and sphenoethmoidal recess (between the superior turbinate and nasal septum), respectively (Figures 46.34 and 46.35).

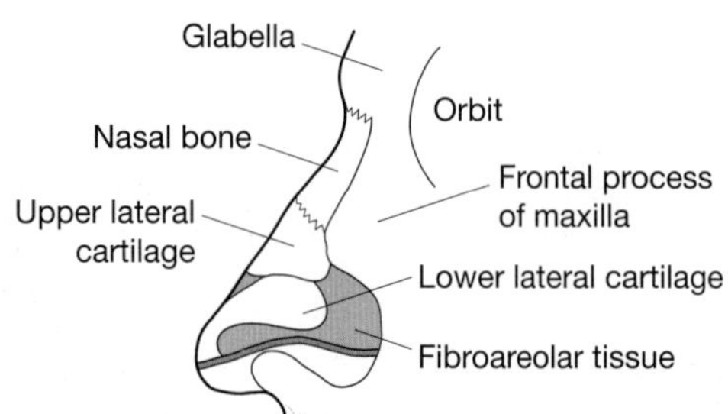

Figure 46.31 The nasal skeleton.

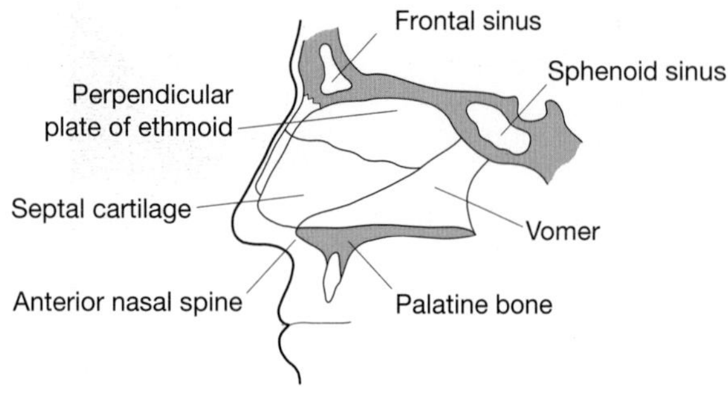

Figure 46.32 The left side of the nasal septum.

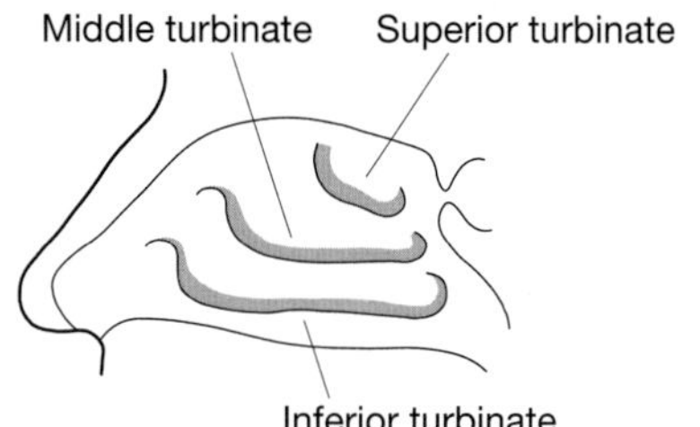

Figure 46.33 The right lateral nasal wall.

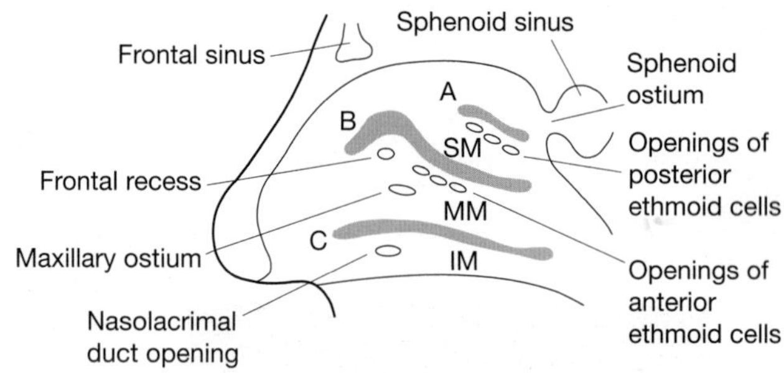

Figure 46.34 The right lateral nasal wall with turbinates removed to show the sinus ostia. A, insertion of superior turbinate; B, insertion of middle turbinate; C, insertion of inferior turbinate; IM, inferior meatus; MM, middle meatus; SM, superior meatus.

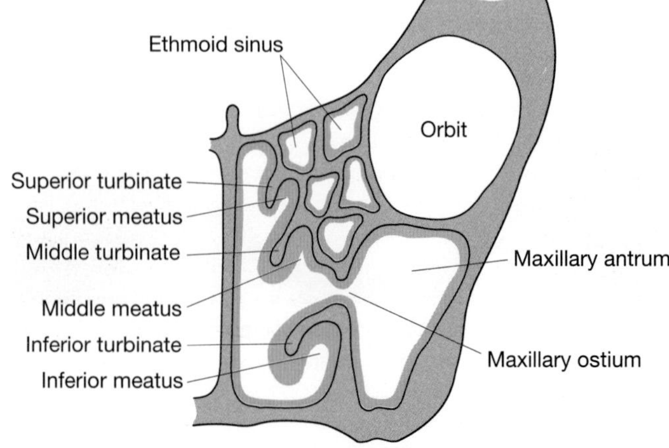

Figure 46.35 Coronal section through the left maxillary and ethmoid sinuses.

The nasal fossae and sinuses receive their blood supply via the external and internal carotid arteries. The external carotid artery supplies the interior of the nose via the maxillary and sphenopalatine arteries. The greater palatine artery supplies the anteroinferior septum via the incisive canal. The contribution from the internal carotid artery is via the anterior and posterior ethmoidal arteries, which are branches of the ophthalmic artery (Figure 46.36). All of these arteries anastomose to form a plexus of vessels (Kiesselbach's plexus) on the anterior part of the nasal septum. Venous drainage is via the ophthalmic and facial veins and the pterygoid and pharyngeal plexuses. Intracranial drainage into the cavernous sinus via the ophthalmic vein is of particular clinical importance because of the potential for intracranial spread of nasal sepsis.

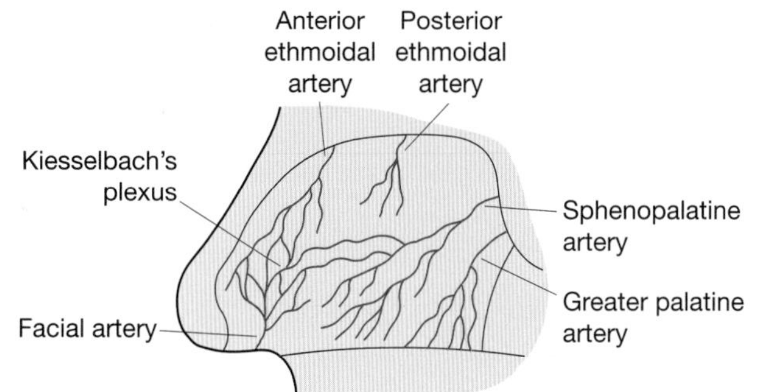

Figure 46.36 Arterial blood supply to the left side of the nasal septum.

EXAMINATION OF THE NOSE AND PARANASAL SINUSES

Internal inspection of the nasal fossae can be achieved to a limited extent with the use of a Thudichum's speculum. The anterior nasal septum, nasal vestibule and anterior inferior turbinate can be assessed. A more detailed examination of the nose is possible with the use of either rigid or flexible endoscopes.

IMAGING OF PARANASAL SINUSES

Plain radiographs are of limited value in the assessment of sinus disease. CT is far superior in demonstrating sinus pathology and to assess bony anatomy to plan any surgical intervention. CT scans are acquired and reconstructed to produce images in axial, coronal and sagittal planes. The three planes allow the drainage of the frontal sinus to be identified and important surgical landmarks can be reviewed preoperatively, including the cribiform plate, anterior skull base, lamina papyracea and location of the anterior ethmoid artery. MRI is useful in sinus pathology to assess any intracranial or orbital extension of disease.

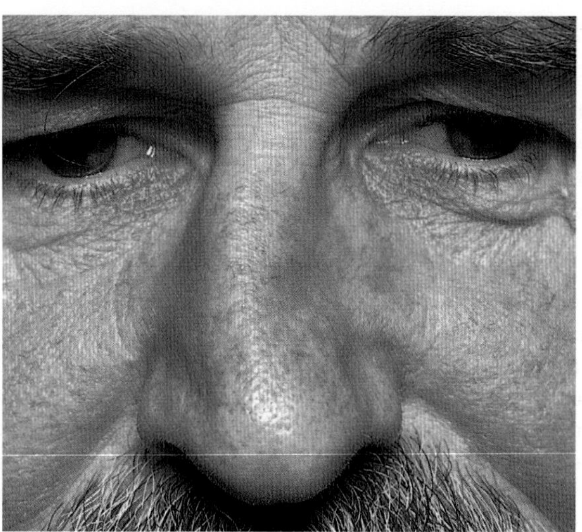

Figure 46.37 Fracture of the nasal bones with displacement of the bony nasal complex to the right side.

TRAUMA TO THE NOSE AND PARANASAL SINUSES

Fracture of the nasal bones

Blunt injury to the nose may fracture the nasal bones (Figure 46.37). The fracture line can extend into the lacrimal bone and tear the anterior ethmoidal artery, producing catastrophic haemorrhage. This may be delayed, occurring only as the soft-tissue swelling subsides, reducing the tamponade effect on the torn vessel.

Violent trauma to the frontal area of the nose can result in a fracture of the frontal and ethmoid sinuses with potential extension into the anterior cranial fossa. Dural tears and brain injuries, either open or closed, are then at risk from sinonasal ascending infection, which may progress to meningitis or brain abscess. CSF rhinorrhoea is a certain sign of a dural tear. CSF rhinorrhoea can be confirmed by collecting a sample of the fluid and sending for beta-2 transferrin. A bony defect in the anterior skull base following trauma can be identified on high-resolution CT. The CSF leak will often settle with conservative management but if persistent, can be repaired endoscopically.

Management of fractured nasal bones

Fractured nasal bones are normally accompanied by extensive overlying soft-tissue swelling and bruising, which may hinder the assessment of any underlying bony deformity. Reviewing after 4–5 days when the soft-tissue swelling has diminished will allow a better assessment of any deformity. If there is a significant degree of nasal deformity, then this can be corrected by manipulation of the nasal bones under local or general anaesthesia. This should be carried out within 3 weeks of the injury while the bony fragments are still mobile. After this period, if there is significant cosmetic or functional issues, a septorhinoplasty can be performed at least 6 months following the injury.

Wilhelm Kiesselbach, 1839–1902, Professor of Otology, Erlangen, Germany.
Johann Ludwig Wilhelm Thudichum, 1829–1901, biochemist and general practitioner, London, UK.

Septal injury

A blunt injury of moderate force may lead to lateral displacement or deformity of the septal cartilage, restricting the nasal airway. Unlike the nasal bones the nasal septum cannot be manipulated back into position and requires a formal septoplasty procedure to restore the anatomy and the patency of the nasal airways.

Bleeding under the mucoperichondrium of the septum will cause a septal haematoma and nasal obstruction. Untreated, a septal haematoma will progress to abscess formation and ultimately result in necrosis of the septal cartilage, septal perforation and nasal collapse. A septal haematoma should be treated by incision and drainage of the blood clot, insertion of a small silicone drain and packing of the nasal fossa. A broad-spectrum prophylactic antibiotic should be prescribed.

Summary box 46.9

Nasal trauma

- Do not overlook a septal haematoma
- Displaced nasal bone fractures should be reduced within 3 weeks of injury
- Severe persistent epistaxis after trauma suggests lacrimal bone fracture and injury to the anterior ethmoid artery
- CSF rhinorrhoea indicates a fracture involving the anterior skull base with a dural tear

THE NASAL SEPTUM

Septal deformity

Deviation of the nasal septum may occur naturally or arise as a result of nasal trauma and is readily apparent on anterior rhinoscopy (Figure 46.38). Surgical correction can be achieved by a submucous resection (SMR) of the septum where the deformed septal cartilage is excised while preserving a caudal and dorsal strut for support (Figure 46.39). The alternative is a septoplasty procedure during which the septal cartilage is preserved but the anatomical abnormalities giving rise to its deformity, such as a twisted maxillary crest or inclination of the bony septum posteriorly, are corrected.

Complications of septal surgery include septal perforation. If too much cartilage is excised in the SMR procedure, loss of support to the dorsum of the nose may result in a supra-tip depression or drooping of the tip of the nose.

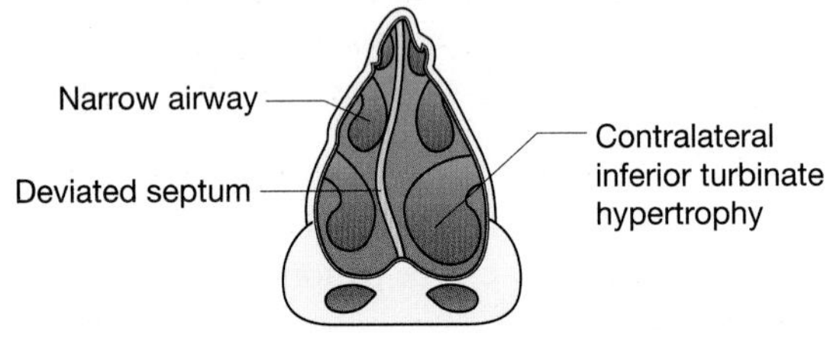

Figure 46.38 Coronal section through the anterior nasal fossae with deviated nasal septum to the right side.

Septal perforation

A hole in the nasal septum causes a turbulent airflow through the nose and a resulting sensation of nasal blockage, extensive nasal crusting, bleeding and whistling. The causes of septal perforation are listed in *Summary box 46.10*.

Septal perforations seldom heal spontaneously. A great variety of operations have been described to close septal perforations but none has met with universal success. These have included closing the perforation using cartilage or synthetic material and covering with local flaps. Alternatively, the perforation may be occluded by inserting a Silastic biflanged prosthesis or 'septal button' (Figures 46.40 and 46.41). In some cases, particularly those patients with significant

Summary box 46.10

Causes of septal perforations

- Trauma
  - Iatrogenic following septal surgery
  - Nose picking
  - Following a septal haematoma from nasal injury
- Infection
  - Syphilis
  - Tuberculosis
- Vasculitis
  - Granulomatosis with polyangiitis
- Tumours
- Toxins
  - Chrome salts
  - Cocaine
- Idiopathic

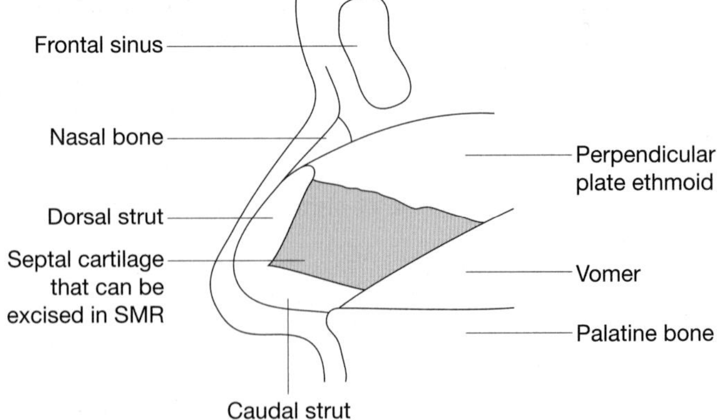

Figure 46.39 Area of cartilage that can be removed in submucous resection (SMR) leaving dorsal and caudal strut for support.

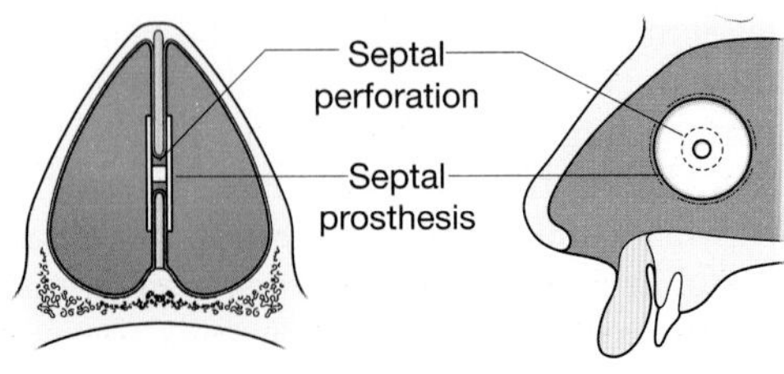

Figure 46.40 Anterior and lateral views of septal perforation occluded with prosthesis.

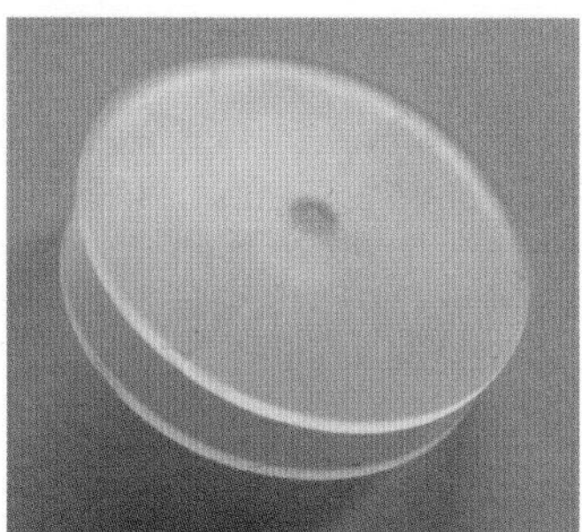

Figure 46.41 Silastic prosthesis for septal perforation.

whistling and bleeding from the posterior edge, the perforation can be enlarged and mucosa folded around the posterior edge to stabilise it.

Granulomatosis with polyangiitis is a systemic idiopathic autoimmune disease affecting the nose, lungs and kidneys. Mucosal granulations on the nasal septum destroy cartilage, producing a septal perforation with saddle deformity of the nose. Laboratory findings include a high erythrocyte sedimentation rate, impaired creatinine clearance and antineutrophil cytoplasmic antibodies (c-ANCA) in most cases.

EPISTAXIS

The causes of epistaxis are listed in *Table 46.2*. The most common site of bleeding is from Kiesselbach's plexus in Little's area of the anterior portion of the septum (see Figure 46.36). Anterior bleeding is common in children and young adults as a result of nose blowing or picking. In the elderly, anticoagulants and hypertension are the underlying causes of arterial bleeding from the posterior part of the nose.

Hereditary haemorrhagic telangiectasia (Osler's disease) gives rise to recurrent multifocal bleeding from thin-walled vessels deficient in muscle and elastic tissue (Figure 46.42).

Juvenile angiofibroma is an uncommon condition that affects adolescent boys and may lead to massive life-threatening episodes of bleeding. Diagnosis is made with contrast CT or MRI. Anterior bowing or indentation of the posterior antral wall (Holman–Miller or antral sign) is the classical finding, but may be seen in other expansive lesions in this area. It is a very vascular tumour, which should not be biopsied because of the risk of uncontrollable haemorrhage. Excision is best carried out by an experienced surgeon and is usually performed endoscopically often using image guidance (Figure 46.43). Preoperative embolisation of the feeding blood vessels may help to reduce blood loss during surgery.

TABLE 46.2 Causes of epistaxis.

Local	Nose picking
	Nasal trauma
	Nasal foreign bodies
	Tumours
	Infection
	Granulomatous disorders
	Juvenile angiofibroma
Systemic	Hypertension
	Warfarin therapy
	New anticoaglants (rivaroxaban)
	Aspirin, clopidogrel therapy
	Haemophilia
	von Willebrand's disease
	Leukaemia
	Haemorrhagic telangiectasia

Management of epistaxis

Anterior bleeding from Kiesselbach's plexus may be controlled by silver nitrate cautery under local anaesthesia. Even in more posterior epistaxis, the bleeding point can often be identified using rigid nasendoscopy and controlled with the use of a topical vasoconstrictor, and then dealt with directly using electrocautery. However, posterior bleeding, as seen in the elderly, may require anterior nasal packing either with

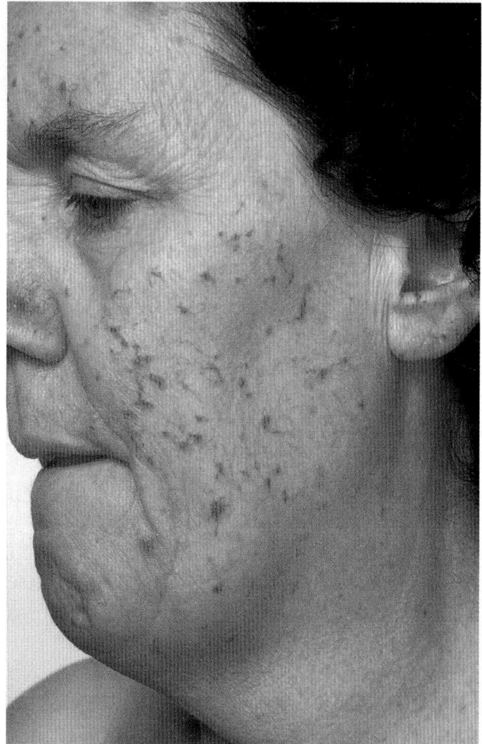

Figure 46.42 Osler's disease showing multiple telangiectasia.

James Laurence Little, 1836–1885, Professor of Surgery, The University of Vermont, Montpelier, VT, USA.

Erik Adolf von Willebrand, 1870–1949, physician, Diakonissanstaltens Hospital, Helsinki, (Helsingfors), Finland, described hereditary pseudohaemophilia in 1926.

Sir William Osler, 1849–1919, Professor of Medicine successively at McGill University, Montreal, Canada, The University of Philadelphia, Pennsylvania, PA, and The Johns Hopkins University, Baltimore, MD, USA, finally becoming Regius Professor of Medicine at Oxford University, Oxford, UK, in 1904.

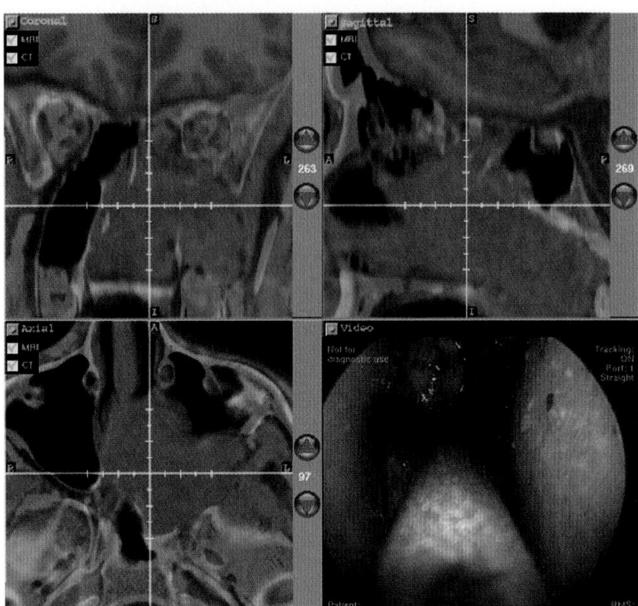

Figure 46.43 Endoscopic resection of juvenile angiofibroma using image-guidance (merged computed tomography and magnetic resonance imaging scans).

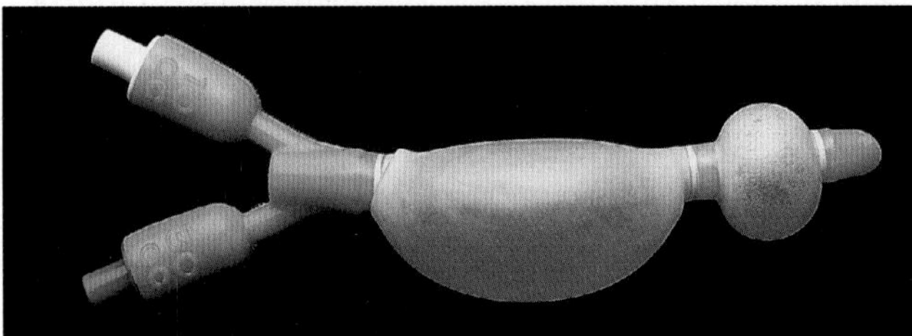

Figure 46.44 Epistaxis balloon catheter.

Vaseline-impregnated ribbon gauze or a non-absorbable sponge. There are also many haemostatic, absorbable materials that can be used to pack the nose to help control bleeding. An alternative to anterior packing is the use of an inflatable epistaxis balloon catheter (Figure 46.44). The catheter is passed into the nose and the distal balloon is inflated in the nasopharynx to secure it. The proximal balloon, which is sausage shaped, is then inflated within the nasal fossa to compress the bleeding point. Although usually effective, they can be uncomfortable.

Postnasal packing may be required in refractory cases whereby a gauze pack is positioned in the nasopharynx under general anaesthesia. Endoscopic sphenopalatine artery clipping is an effective treatment for significant epistaxis not responding to direct cautery or nasal packing.

For uncontrolled life-threatening epistaxis in which the above methods have proved ineffective, haemostasis is secured by vascular ligation. Depending on the origin of bleeding it may be necessary to ligate the internal maxillary artery in the pterygopalatine fossa (which can be accessed endoscopically) and the anterior and posterior ethmoidal arteries. An alternative measure is external carotid artery ligation above the origin of the lingual artery. Another option is to involve the interventional radiologist for possible embolisation. It is also important to recognise, and if possible treat, any factors contributing to the epistaxis, such as clotting or platelet abnormalities.

In Osler's disease, anterior nasal packing is best avoided if at all possible because it is most likely to lead to further mucosal trauma and bleeding. High-dose oestrogen induces squamous metaplasia of the nasal mucosa and has been used effectively in treating this condition.

Summary box 46.11

Epistaxis

- The most common causes are nose picking, hypertension and anticoagulant therapy
- Young people bleed from the anterior septum – Kiesselbach's plexus
- Elderly people bleed from the posterior part of the nose
- Epistaxis is ideally treated with direct cautery to bleeding point under endoscopic guidance
- Silver nitrate cautery can be used to control anterior bleeding
- Moderate bleeding may require anterior nasal packing
- Severe bleeding may require anterior and posterior nasal packing
- Persistent bleeding may require endoscopic sphenopalatine artery ligation

RHINOSINUSITIS

Rhinosinusitis is inflammation of the sinonasal mucosa and is defined as the presence of nasal congestion or nasal discharge and at least one of facial pain or hyposmia with endoscopic and/or CT changes to confirm the diagnosis. It can be divided into acute rhinosinusitis (ARS) and chronic rhinosinusitis (CRS) depending on the timing of symptoms. Symptoms are present for less than 12 weeks in ARS and more than 12 weeks in CRS.

Acute rhinosinusitis

ARS is thought to result from bacterial superinfection of virally damaged mucosa. The commonest bacteria involved are *Streptococcus pneumoniae*, *Haemophilus influenzae* and *Moraxella catarrhalis*. Upper dental sepsis may also predispose to acute maxillary sinusitis. Patients with maxillary sinusitis have a mucopurulent discharge, facial pain and nasal obstruction. Irritation of the superior alveolar nerve may give rise to referred upper toothache. In ARS nasendoscopy reveals inflammed and swollen nasal mucosa with mucopurulent secretions in the middle meatus. Dental sepsis from anaerobic organisms causes around 10% of cases of maxillary sinusitis. The resultant mucopurulent nasal secretion has a foul taste and smell. Plain sinus radiographs may show a fluid level in the antrum or complete opacity (Figure 46.45). However, plain radiographs are now seldom used and have been superceded by CT scans to investigate ARS. CT scans confirm opacifiction and mucosal thickening of the maxillary sinus as well as providing anatomical detail prior to endoscopic surgical intervention (Figure 46.46).

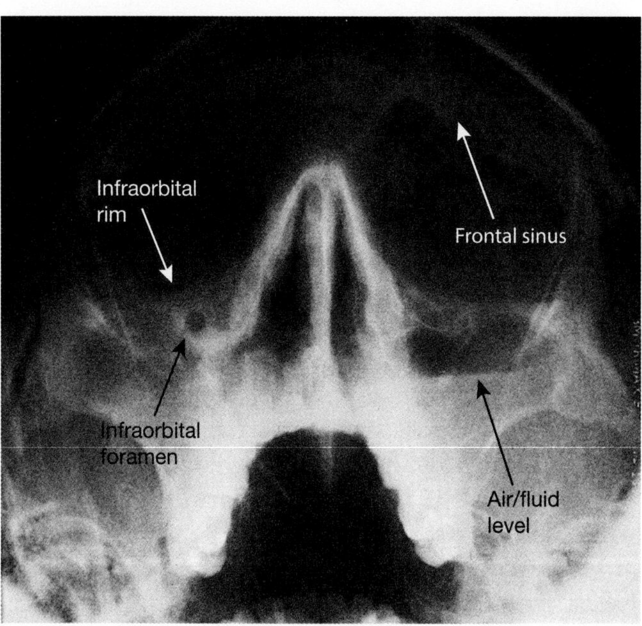

Figure 46.45 Plain radiograph showing the fluid level in the left maxillary antrum and total opacity of the right antrum.

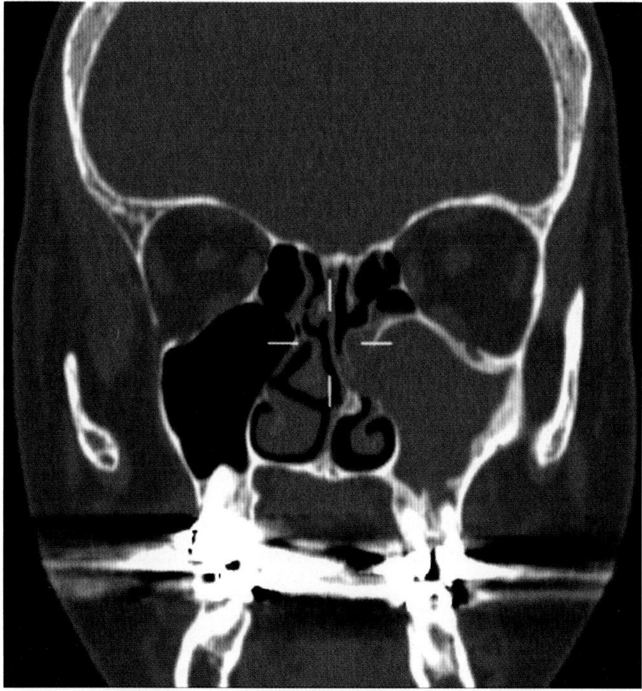

Figure 46.46 Coronal computed tomography scan showing left-sided maxillary sinus opacification due to maxillary sinusitis.

Acute frontoethmoidal sinusitis can also occur and presents with mucopurulent discharge, facial pain (including frontal headache), nasal congestion and hyposmia. Again, mucopus is seen on endoscopy in the middle meatus and is investigated with CT.

Treatment

Penetration of antibiotics into chronically inflamed sinus mucosa is reduced and, therefore, treatment may need to be prolonged. Topical nasal decongestants, such as ephedrine nasal drops, will often encourage the sinus to drain and topical corticosteroids are used to reduce inflammation. Saline douches can also be beneficial.

Antral lavage under local or general anaesthesia was previously used to confirm the diagnosis and provided the opportunity to obtain samples for bacteriology. Nowadays, pus in the middle meatus can simply be sampled endoscopically in clinic and antral lavage is rarely performed. Endoscopic sinus surgery allows a more functional approach to diseases of the paranasal sinuses and enables the drainage pathways of the paranasal sinuses to be opened. Most cases of ARS can be treated conservatively with antibiotics and topical treatment. Surgery is used for those patients unresponsive to medical management or with complications. The majority of patients with ARS who require surgery are treated endoscopically. However, in some cases an open surgical approach may be necessary.

> **Summary box 46.12**
>
> Acute rhinosinusitis
>
> - The most common causative organisms are *Streptococcus pneumoniae, Haemophilus influenzae, Moraxella cattarhalis*
> - Anaerobic infection of the maxillary sinus may result from dental sepsis
> - Acute infection should be treated with antibiotics, topical decongestants and corticosteroids
> - Endoscopic sinus surgery may be required

Complications

Complications as a result of ARS include orbital and intracranial problems. The spread of infection from the sinuses occurs either through diploic veins or directly through bone erosion. This can result in epidural, subdural or cerebral abscesses, or meningitis/encephalitis. Cavernous sinus thrombosis may also result and can present with bilateral ptosis, proptosis, retro-ocular pain, opthalmoplegia, papilloedema and spiking fevers.

Orbital complications of ARS are more common. Most often this is related to ethmoid sinus infection (Figure 46.47). An opthalmology review is essential due to the threat to vision and IV antibiotics covering aerobic and anaerobic organisms are used. If there are any concerns regarding the eye, including proptosis, chemosis, opthalmoplegia, or reduced visual acuity, then CT with contrast is required

> **Summary box 46.13**
>
> Complications
>
> - Orbital – cellullitis, abscess
> - Orbital infections may threaten sight
> - Intracranial spread may cause meningitis, cerebral abscess or cavernous sinus thrombosis
> - Osteomyelitis of the bones, particularly frontal, may occur

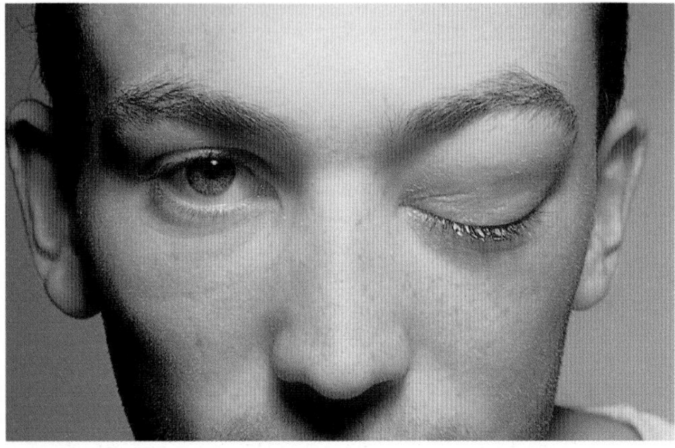

Figure 46.47 Left periorbital cellulitis complicating acute left ethmoiditis.

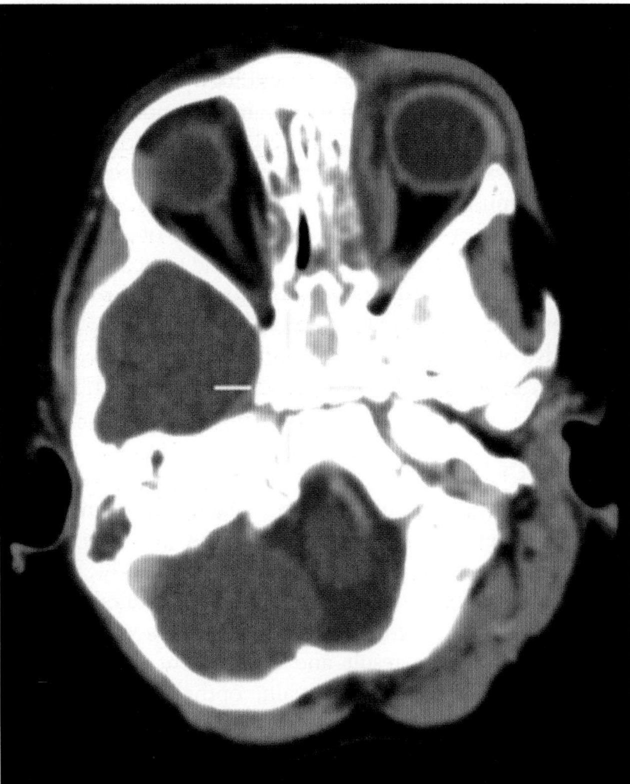

Figure 46.48 Axial computed tomography scan showing a subperiosteal abscess in the left orbit.

Summary box 46.14

Chandler classification of orbital complications of sinusitis

- I – preseptal cellulitis
- II – orbital cellulitis
- III – subperiosteal abscess
- IV – orbital abscess
- V – cavernous sinus thrombosis

(Figure 46.48). If an abscess is identified, then this should be drained (endoscopically or open).

Osteomyelitis of the frontal bones can also occur as a result of ARS. If the anterior table of the frontal sinus is involved, it can present with significant swelling of the skin of the forehead and a mass (Pott puffy tumour).

Chronic rhinosinusitis

CRS is common affecting around 11% of the population. The cause is unknown but a number of factors have been linked to CRS including ciliary dyskinesia, allergy, asthma, bacteria (*Staphylococcus aureus*) and fungi, and a number of host factors including anatomical variations (deviated septum, concha bullosa of the middle turbinates). CRS can be divided into CRS with nasal polyps (CRSwNP) and without (CRSsNP).

Pathology

Nasal polyps are benign swellings of the sinus mucosa of unknown origin. Histologically, the polyps contain an oedematous stroma infiltrated with inflammatory cells and eosinophils. Inflammatory polyps tend to be bilateral and extend into the middle meatus. A single large polyp arising from the maxillary antrum is referred to as an antrochoanal polyp (Figure 46.49). This usually fills the nose and eventually prolapses posteriorly down into the nasopharynx.

Clinical features

CRSwNP patients present with nasal obstruction, watery rhinorrhoea, postnasal drip and often hyposmia/anosmia. Pain does not tend to be a significant feature. Polyps are easily identifiable within the nose as pale semitransparent grey masses, which are mobile and insensitive when palpated with a fine probe. This allows them to be distinguished from hypertrophied turbinates (Figure 46.50). In CRSsNP the middle meatus is often congested, with mucopus present.

Malignancy should be considered in adults with unilateral nasal polyps whereas in children such polyps must be distinguished from a meningocoele or encephalocoele by high-resolution CT scanning of the anterior cranial fossa. Nasal polyps are unusual in children; however, they do occur in conjunction with cystic fibrosis in 10% of cases.

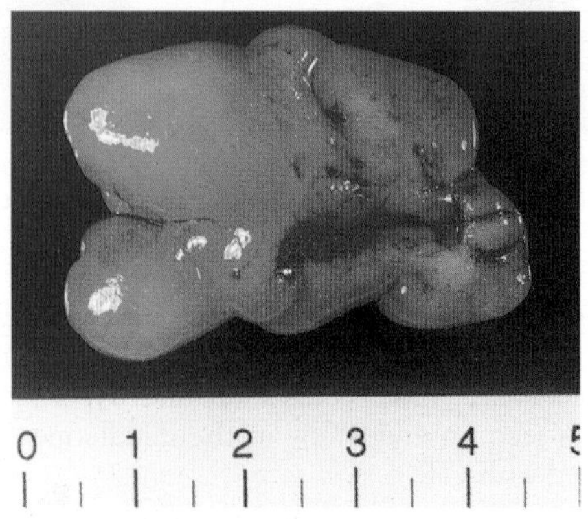

Figure 46.49 Antrochoanal polyp.

Percivall Pott, 1714–1788, surgeon, London, UK.

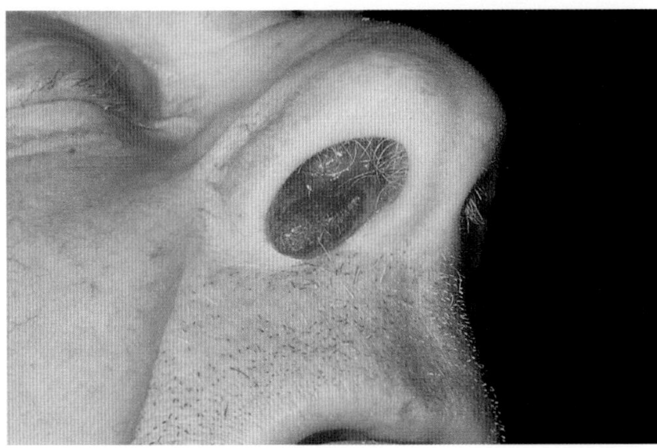

Figure 46.50 Nasal polyp in the right nasal vestibule.

Management

Medical treatment for CRSwNPs with systemic steroids will often reduce the size of the nasal polyps and give short-term relief of nasal blockage. Unfortunately, the polyps tend to recur when the treatment stops. Topical corticosteroid drops and sprays are also used along with saline douching. In CRSsNP, in addition to topical treatments a long course of low-dose antibiotics (macrolides) can be used in those patients with a normal IgE. Surgical treatment is indicated in patients that do not respond to medical treatment. Endoscopic nasal polypectomy and functional endoscopic sinus surgery (FESS) is performed following a CT scan which confirms the extent of disease and shows the important bony anatomy preoperatively. Serious complications following FESS include CSF leak and orbital problems, including orbital haematoma, and so it is important to review the level and symmetry of the anterior skull base and the integrity of the lamina papyracea on the CT scan prior to surgery. Endoscopic polypectomy is performed using a powered nasal microdebrider (Figure 46.51).

Image guidance can be used in endoscopic sinus surgery, and extended endoscopic procedures such as pituitary and anterior skull base surgery, to provide real-time feedback of instrument position in the nose based on preoperative CT or MRI scans.

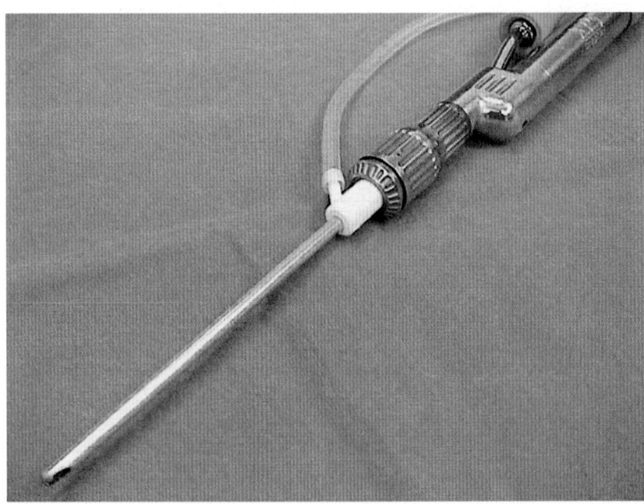

Figure 46.51 Powered nasal microdebrider.

Summary box 46.15

Nasal polyps

- Polyps are insensitive to touch and are mobile
- Inflammatory polyps are usually bilateral
- Unilateral nasal polyps should be removed for histology
- Bleeding polyps may indicate malignancy
- Meningocoele and encephalocoele must be excluded in children with polyps
- Polyps are removed using a powered microdebrider

TUMOURS OF THE NOSE AND SINUSES

Tumours arising in the nose or paranasal sinuses may present with unilateral nasal obstruction, persistent unilateral anterior rhinorrhoea, postnasal drip, epistaxis, unilateral blood-stained rhinorrhoea, facial swelling or proptosis.

Benign tumours

Simple papillomas or viral warts can grow inside the nasal vestibule. They can be confused with carcinomas and are best excised for histological diagnosis.

Osteomas of the nasal skeleton are not uncommon and are usually detected on radiology as an incidental finding (Figure 46.52). In symptomatic individuals the osteoma can be removed endoscopically or via an open procedure.

Inverted (transitional cell) papillomas can occur both in the nasal cavity and the nasal sinuses. They are inverted papillomas because histologically the hyperplastic epithelium inverts into the underlying stroma. The papillomas are covered with transitional epithelium. Calcification within the tumour may be seen on CT along with sclerosis of bone at the margins of the growth (Figure 46.53). Inverted papillomas can undergo malignant change. Full surgical resection is required and this can usually be performed endoscopically.

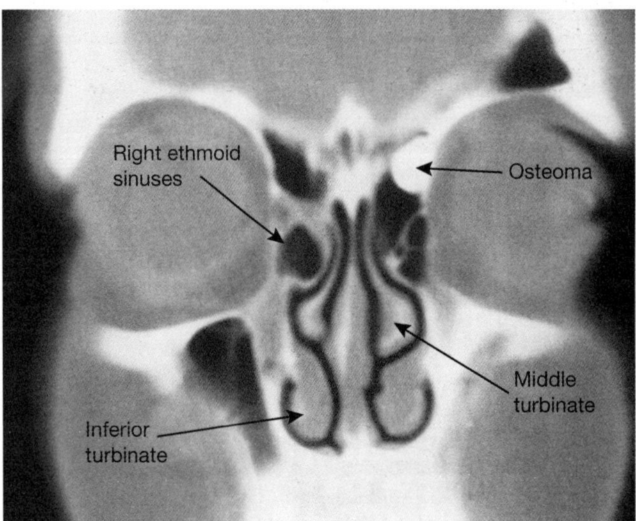

Figure 46.52 Coronal computed tomography scan showing a small osteoma in the left ethmoid sinus adjacent to the orbit.

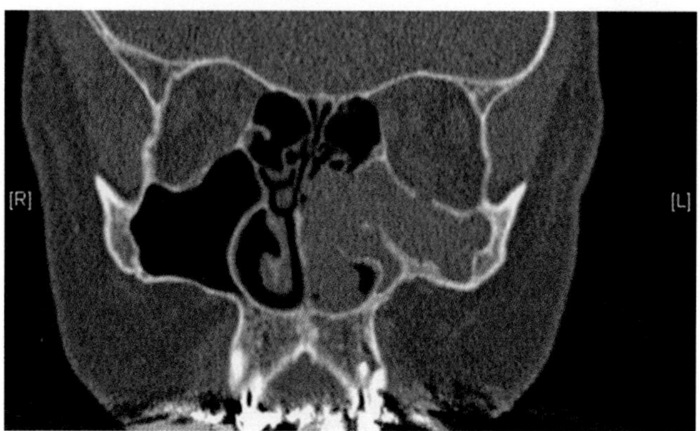

Figure 46.53 Coronal computed tomography scan showing extensive inverted papilloma involving the left maxillary antrum and ethmoid sinuses.

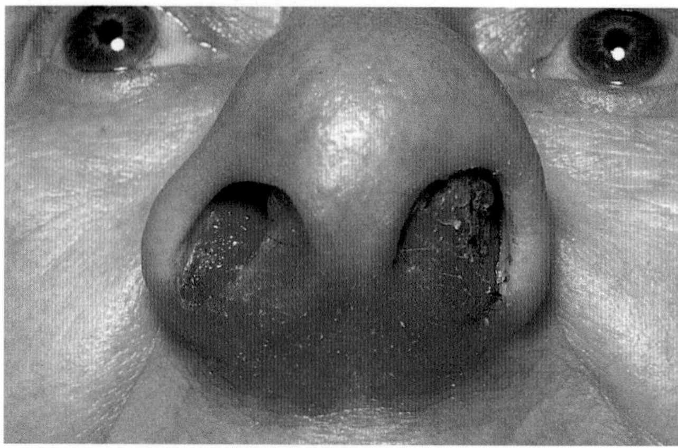

Figure 46.54 Squamous cell carcinoma of the nasal septum.

Malignant tumours

The most common malignant tumours to occur within the nasal cavity and paranasal sinuses are squamous cell carcinoma (Figure 46.54), adenoid cystic carcinoma and adenocarcinoma. Adenocarcinoma has been linked to exposure to hard wood dust in the furniture industry. Adenoid cystic carcinomas arise from minor salivary glands, which can be found in the nose. Suspicious signs of invasion of neighbouring tissues include diplopia, proptosis, loosening of the teeth (Figure 46.55), trismus, CN palsies and regional lymphadenopathy. Figure 46.56 shows invasion of a left maxillary antral carcinoma into adjacent structures, including the orbit, on an MRI scan.

Patients with sinus or intranasal malignancy are best managed in a combined clinic where the expertise of ear, nose and throat (ENT) surgeons, maxillofacial surgeons and oncologists can be employed.

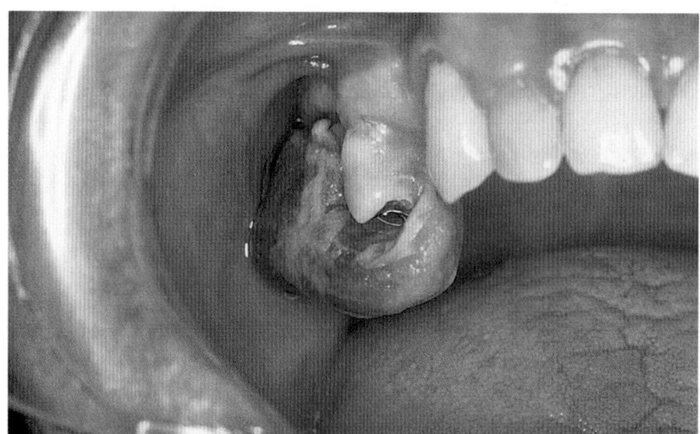

Figure 46.55 Maxillary antral carcinoma presenting through an oro-antral fistula.

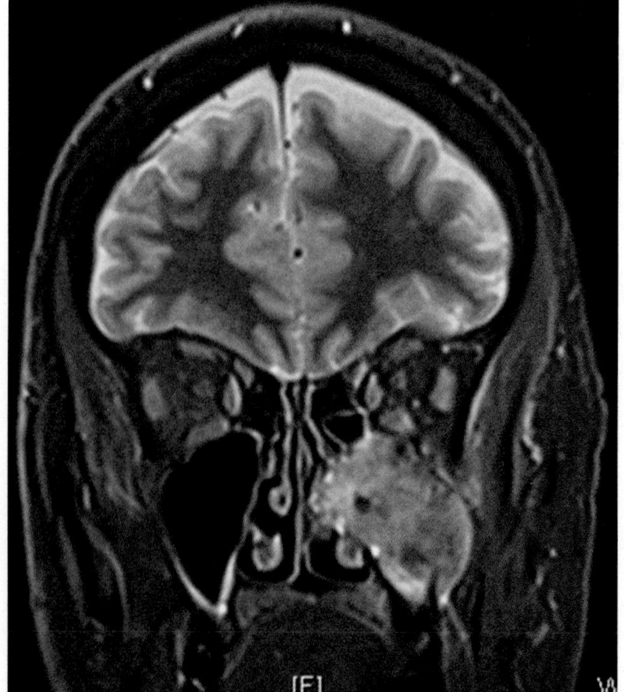

Figure 46.56 Coronal magnetic resonance imaging scan of the paranasal sinuses showing extensive left maxillary antral carcinoma invading adjacent structures.

Summary box 46.16

Tumours of the nose and sinuses

- Unilateral nasal blockage, discharge and bleeding are often presenting symptoms in nasal or sinus tumours
- Osteomas are often asymptomatic
- Inverted papilloma is a benign tumour, which presents as a unilateral polyp that can undergo malignant change
- Squamous cell carcinoma is the most common malignant tumour
- Almost 50% of sinonasal cancers arise on the lateral nasal wall and 33% in the maxillary antrum
- Multidisciplinary management of malignant sinonasal tumours requires input from Ear, Nose and Throat surgeons, maxillofacial surgeons and oncologists

FURTHER READING

Fokkens WJ, Lund VJ, Mullol J, *et al.* European position paper on rhinosinusitis and nasal polyps. *Rhinol Suppl* 2012; **23**: 1–298.

Gleeson MJ (ed). *Scott-Brown's otolaryngology: head and neck surgery*, 7th edn. London: Hodder Arnold, 2008.

Chapter 47

Pharynx, larynx and neck

Learning objectives

To understand:

- The relevant anatomy, physiology, disease processes and investigations of the pharyngolarynx and neck
- The diagnosis and emergency treatment of airway obstruction
- The aetiology, natural history, management and prevention of squamous cell carcinoma of the upper aerodigestive tract

CLINICAL ANATOMY AND PHYSIOLOGY

The pharynx

The pharynx is a fibromuscular tube forming the upper part of the respiratory and digestive passages. It extends from the base of the skull to the level of the sixth cervical vertebra at the lower border of the cricoid cartilage where it becomes continuous with the oesophagus. It is divided into three parts: the nasopharynx, oropharynx and hypopharynx (Figure 47.1).

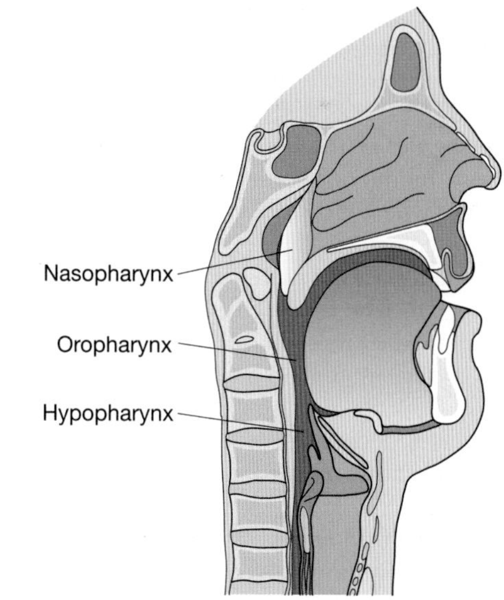

Figure 47.1 The component parts of the pharynx.

Nasopharynx

The nasopharynx lies anterior to the first cervical vertebra. The adenoids, which constitute the superior component of Waldeyer`s ring, are situated at the junction of the roof and posterior wall of the nasopharynx. Waldeyer`s ring is a ring of lymphoid tissue comprising, in addition to the adenoids, the palatine and lingual tonsils of the oropharynx. It is situated at the entry to the air and food passages and is constantly exposed to new inspired or ingested antigenic stimuli. Accordingly, it is an important part of the mucosa-associated lymphoid tissues (MALT), which process antigen and present it to T helper cells and B cells (Figure 47.2) thereby facilitating a first-line immune response mechanism, which is particularly important in childhood. The tissue of Waldeyer's ring undergoes physiological hypertrophy during early childhood as the child is exposed to increasing amounts of antigenic stimuli, and there is often a similar hypertrophy of the cervical lymph nodes.

The Eustachian tubes, leading from the middle ear cleft, open into the postero-superior aspect of the lateral wall. Dorsal and superior to the openings, bounded anteriorly by a ridge formed by the salpingopharyngeus muscle, are the fossae of Rosenmüller, a common site for the development of nasopharyngeal carcinoma.

Heinrich Wilhelm Gottfried Waldeyer-Hartz, 1836–1921, Professor of Pathological Anatomy, Berlin, Germany.
Bartolomeo Eustachio (Eustachius), ?1513–1574, appointed physician to the Pope in 1547, and Professor of Anatomy, Rome, Italy, in 1549.
Johann Christian Rosenmüller, 1771–1820, Professor of Anatomy and Surgery, Leipzig, Germany.

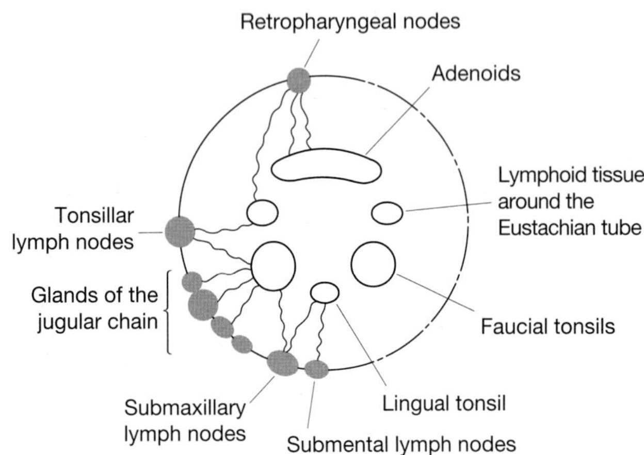

Figure 47.2 Waldeyer's ring.

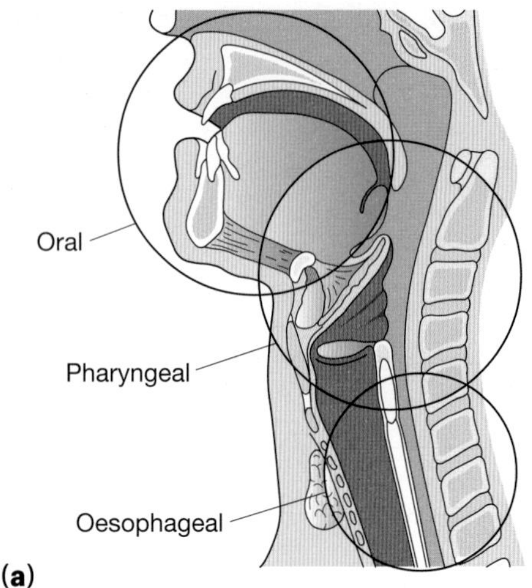

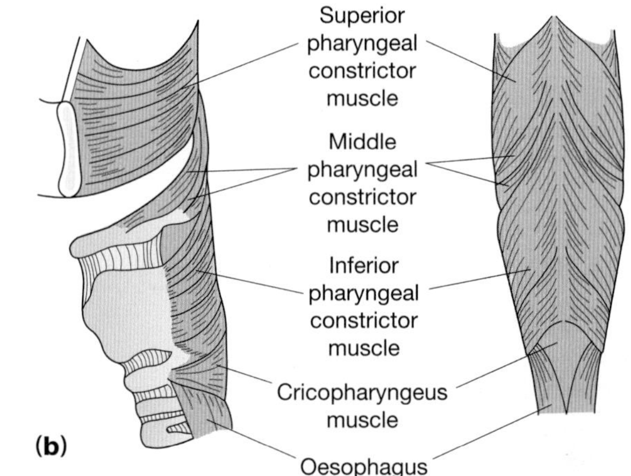

Figure 47.3 The three phases of swallowing (a) and the muscles (b).

Oropharynx

This is bounded superiorly by the soft palate, inferiorly by the upper surface of the epiglottis and anteriorly by the anterior faucial pillars and the vallate papillae of the tongue. The palatine tonsils are situated in the lateral wall between the anterior and posterior pillars of the fauces. The lateral wall, and in particular the tonsil, takes its blood supply from the facial artery, which may be closely related to the lower pole, and laterally a plexus of paratonsillar veins, which may be the source of serious venous bleeding following tonsillectomy.

Hypopharynx

The superior border of the hypopharynx is the level of the laryngeal inlet. Its inferior border is the lower border of the cricoid cartilage where it continues into the oesophagus. The hypopharynx is commonly divided into three areas: the right and left piriform fossae, the posterior pharyngeal wall and the postcricoid region. The mucosa of these areas is, however, continuous so disease processes, such as squamous cell carcinoma, often involve more than one area as a result of submucosal spread.

The multifaceted, complex process of swallowing is mediated via efferent fibres passing to the medulla oblongata through the second division of the trigeminal nerve (V), glossopharyngeal nerve (IX) and vagus nerve (X) (Figure 47.3). The afferent pathway is from the nucleus ambiguus and is mediated via the glossopharyngeal (IX), vagus (X) and hypoglossal (XII) nerves. Damage to these major cranial nerves at any point along their pathway, by trauma or disease, may cause dysphagia and/or aspiration.

Videofluoroscopy, in which the passage of a bolus of radiopaque liquid or solid from the point at which it enters the oral cavity down to its passage within the stomach is examined radiologically, is the investigation of choice when investigating swallowing (dys)function.

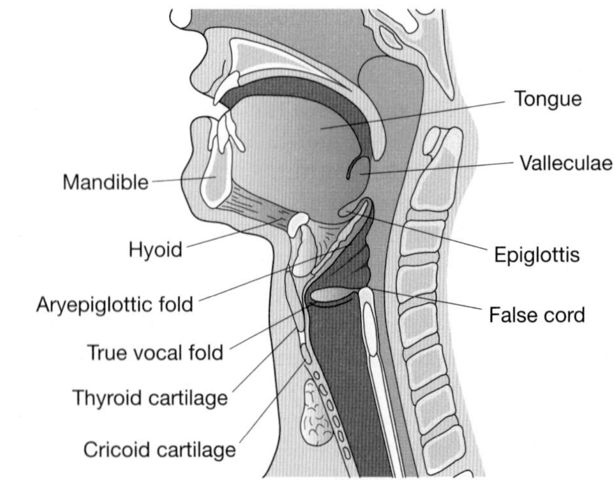

Figure 47.4 Sagittal diagram of the upper aerodigestive tract.

Anatomic relationships of the pharynx

Some of these are illustrated in Figure 47.4.

PARAPHARYNGEAL SPACE

This potential space lies lateral to the pharynx and extends from the base of the skull above to the superior mediastinum below. It is occupied by the carotid vessels, internal jugular vein, deep cervical lymph nodes, the last four cranial nerves and the cervical sympathetic trunk.

Infection and necrosis of the cervical lymph nodes in the parapharyngeal space most commonly occurs from infections of the tonsils or teeth (particularly the third lower molar tooth). As the parapharyngeal space is not anatomically divided, infection may therefore spread from the skull base cranially to the superior mediastinum caudally and consequently often presents a surgical challenge.

RETROPHARYNGEAL SPACE

This potential space lies posterior to the pharynx, bounded anteriorly by the posterior pharyngeal wall and its covering buccopharyngeal fascia and posteriorly by the prevertebral musculature and its overlying prevertebral fascia. It contains the retropharyngeal lymph nodes, which are usually paired lateral nodes but which are separated by a tough midline fibrous condensation that connects the prevertebral and buccopharyngeal fascia.

As with the lymphoid tissue of Waldeyer`s ring, these nodes are more active in infancy and young children, and it is at this age that they are most likely to be involved in inflammatory processes, which, if severe, may affect swallowing and respiration as a consequence of gross swelling and suppuration of the retropharyngeal space.

Larynx

It is important to appreciate that the main function of the larynx is not the production of voice but the protection of the tracheobronchial airway and lungs. In order to achieve this, the larynx, together with the base of the tongue, forms the protective sphincter that closes off the airway during swallowing. It is only an evolutionary by-product that, in humans and some other mammals, the larynx is responsible for the production of sound.

The larynx comprises a cartilaginous framework (that may ossify in later life), which consists of the hyoid bone above, the thyroid and cricoid cartilages and the intricate arytenoid cartilages posteriorly.

The cricoid cartilage is the only complete ring in the entire airway and bounds the subglottis, which is the narrowest point of the airway. This is the most common site for damage from an endotracheal tube used for intensive care unit ventilation in seriously ill patients.

A purely anatomical description of the larynx divides it into the supraglottis, glottis and subglottis (Figure 47.5). The true vocal folds (often incorrectly called the vocal cords) are normally white in contrast to the pink mucosa of the rest of the larynx and airway. The true vocal folds meet anteriorly at the midlevel of the thyroid cartilage, whereas posteriorly they are separate and attached to an arytenoid cartilage. This arrangement produces the 'V' shape of the glottis (Figure 47.6).

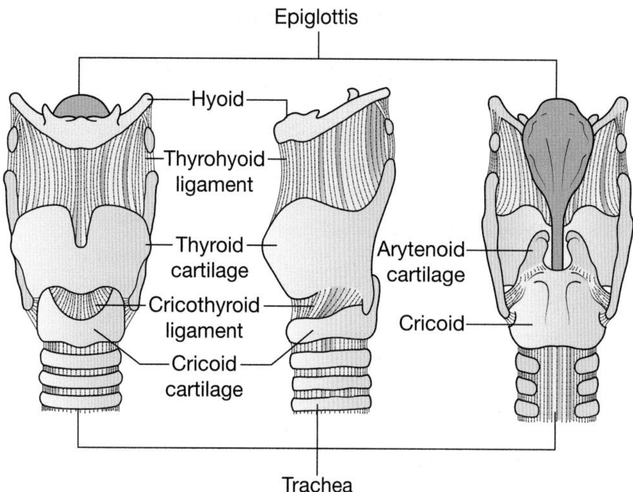

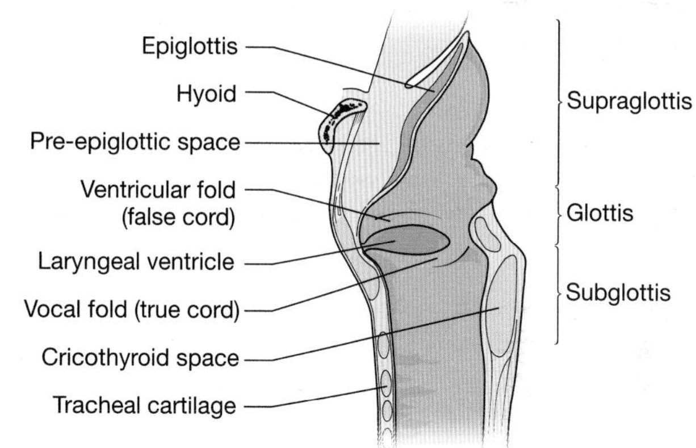

Figure 47.5 Anatomy of the larynx.

Nerve supply

The sensory nerve supply to the larynx above the vocal folds is from the superior laryngeal nerve and below the vocal folds it is from the recurrent laryngeal nerve. Both these nerves are branches of the vagus nerve (X). The motor nerve supply to the larynx is from the recurrent laryngeal nerve, which supplies all intrinsic muscles. Only one of these intrinsic muscles, the posterior cricoarytenoid, abducts the vocal folds during respiration. All other intrinsic muscles adduct the cords. As all of the intrinsic muscles of the larynx are supplied by the recurrent laryngeal nerve, damage to this nerve, or to the vagus nerve above the recurrent laryngeal nerve branch, will cause paralysis of the vocal fold on the side of the damage.

Phonation/speech

The larynx functions by closing the vocal fold against the air being exhaled from the lungs, but the rise in subglottic pressure forces the vocal folds apart slightly for an instant of time, resulting in an accompanying sinusoidal wave-like vibration of the vocal fold epithelium. The opening and closing occurs in rapid sequence to produce a vibrating column of air, which is the source of sound that can be articulated by the structure of the oral cavity to produce speech.

Paralysis or disease of the vocal folds or closely associated laryngeal structures will give rise to disturbance of the sound, producing hoarseness.

The functions of the larynx are given in *Summary box 47.1*.

Views on indirect laryngoscopy

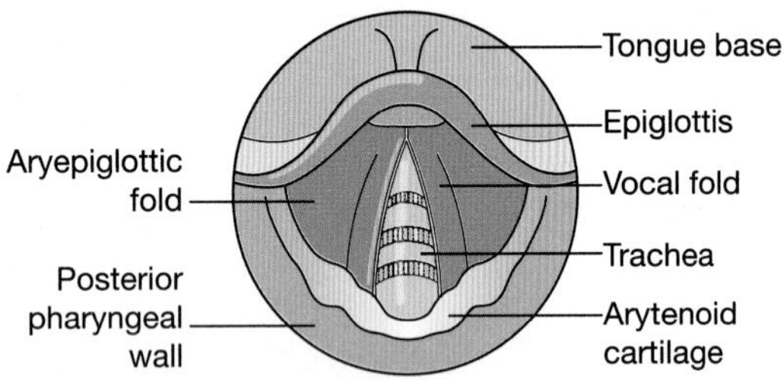

(**a**) Vocal folds abducted (open)

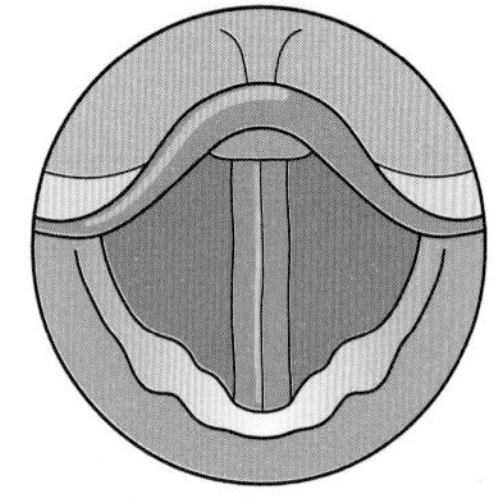

(**b**) Vocal folds adducted (closed)

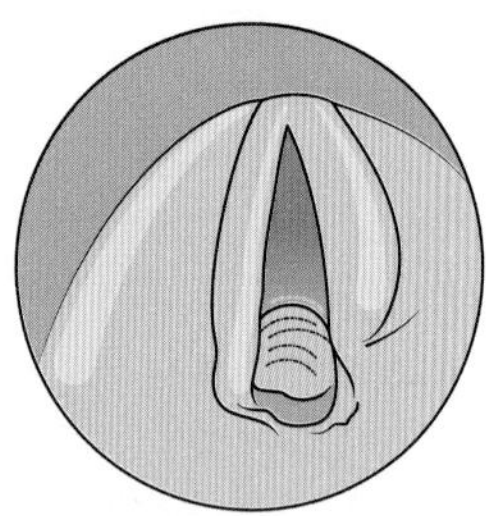

(**c**) Larynx in abduction

Figure 47.6 A view of the larynx on indirect laryngoscopy: (a) vocal folds abducted; (b) vocal folds adducted; (c) normal larynx in abduction.

Summary box 47.1

Functions of the larynx

Protection of the lower respiratory tract by

- Closure of the laryngeal inlet
- Closure of the false cords
- Closure of the glottis
- Cessation of respiration
- Cough reflex

Phonation

- Vocal folds produce sound by quasi-periodic vibration

Respiration

- Control of pressure

Fixation of chest

- Aids lifting, straining and climbing

Neck

The neck is divided into anterior and posterior triangles by the sternocleidomastoid muscle. The anterior triangle extends from the inferior border of the mandible to the sternum below, and is bounded by the midline and the sternocleidomastoid muscle. The posterior triangle extends backwards to the anterior border of the trapezius muscle and inferiorly to the clavicle. The upper part of the anterior triangle, above the hyoid bone, is commonly subdivided into the submandibular triangle above the digastric muscle and the submental triangle below. The lymphatic drainage of the head and neck is of considerable clinical importance (Figure 47.7). The most important chain of nodes are the jugular nodes (also called cervical), which run adjacent to the internal jugular vein. The other main groups are the submental, submandibular, pre- and postauricular, occipital and posterior triangle nodes.

A system of levels is used to describe the location of these neck nodes (Figure 47.8). Of particular note are

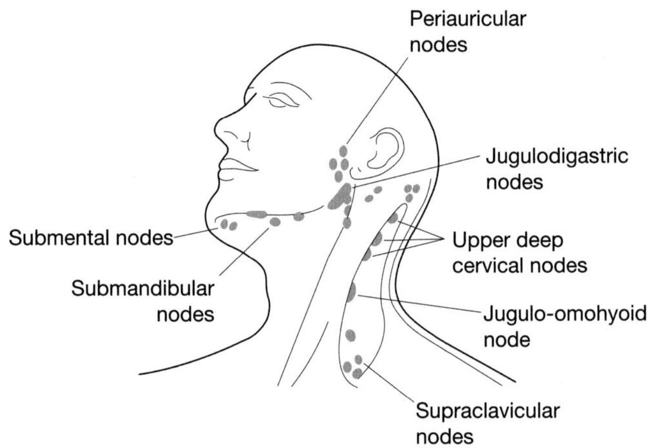

Figure 47.7 Distribution of cervical lymph nodes.

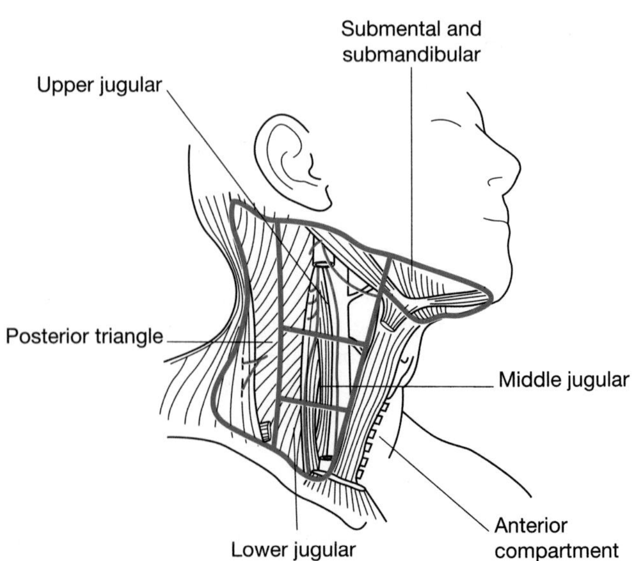

Figure 47.8 The level system for describing the location of lymph nodes in the neck. Level 1, submental and submandibular group; level II, upper jugular group; level III, middle jugular group; level IV, lower jugular group; level V, posterior triangle group; level VI, anterior compartment group.

the jugular nodal levels include levels II, III and IV, which relate to the upper, middle and inferior third of the carotid sheath, respectively. The level II nodes, which contain the large jugulodigastric node, drain the naso- and oropharynx, including the tonsils, posterolateral aspects of the oral cavity and the superior aspects of the larynx and piriform fossae. They are the most common sites of enlargement and may be palpated along the anterior border of the sternocleidomastoid muscle.

Metastatic spread of squamous cell carcinoma (80% of head and neck cancer) most commonly occurs with tumours of the nasopharynx, tongue base, tonsil, piriform fossae and supraglottic larynx. When an enlarged neck node is detected and malignant disease is suspected, these five primary sites must be carefully examined.

CLINICAL EXAMINATION

Pharynx and larynx

Before examination of the pharynx, the oral cavity should be examined with the aid of a good light and tongue depressors. Historically, a reflecting mirror on the head was used as a source of examination light. However, most practitioners in the resource-rich world now use a headband-mounted fibreoptic light source. Either option permits the use of both hands to hold instruments. Inspection should include the buccal mucosa and lips, the palate, the tongue and floor of the mouth, all surfaces of the teeth and gums, opening and closing of the mouth and dental occlusion. Patients should be asked to elevate the tongue to the roof of the mouth and protrude the tongue towards both the right and the left. Intraoral palpation may be required gently using one or two fingers to feel any swellings. Intraoral palpation may be combined with extraoral palpation of the submental and submandibular lymph nodes and salivary glands to aid the characterisation and/or localisation of any swelling detected.

Following examination of the oral cavity, the oropharynx is then inspected with the tongue depressor placed firmly onto the tongue base to depress it inferiorly. Care much be taken to, if possible, avoid provoking a gag reflex. The anterior and posterior faucial pillars, the tonsil, retromolar trigone and posterior pharyngeal wall should all be inspected for colour changes, ulceration, pus, foreign bodies and swellings. Pain and trismus as a consequence of pharyngolaryngeal or neck pathology may add to the difficulty of the examination, but are significant clinical findings in their own right.

While angled mirrors and a headlight may be used in expert hands, modern flexible fibreoptic endoscopes passed through the nose, with or without topical anaesthesia, allow high-quality examination of the entire nasopharynx, oropharynx, larynx and often the hypopharynx in almost every patient. Moreover, a camera attached to the endoscope permits the taking of high-quality photographs to record and present pertinent clinical findings. A rigid 0° fibreoptic endoscope (Hopkin`s rod) is often used in preference to inspect the nasal cavities and nasopharynx.

Neck

The patient should be examined in the sitting position with the whole neck exposed so that both clavicles are clearly seen. The neck is inspected from the front and the patient asked to swallow, preferably with the aid of a sip of water. Movements of the larynx and any swellings in the neck are noted. The patient should be asked to protrude the tongue if there is a midline neck swelling, as a thyroglossal duct cyst will move upwards with the tongue protrusion. The neck is then examined from behind with the chin flexed slightly downwards to remove any undue tension in the strap muscles, platysma and sternocleidomastoids.

On examining for a lump in the neck, it is often helpful to ask the patient to point to the lump first. Ask if the lump is tender. The neck is palpated bilaterally in a sequential manner comparing the two sides of the neck. All five palpable neck node levels (I–V) should be examined systematically.

If malignancy is suspected (hard, irregular or fixed to overlying skin or to deep structures), inspection of the nasopharynx, tonsils, tongue base, piriform fossae and supraglottic larynx is essential.

Summary box 47.2

Key points of history and examination

Mouth

- Adequate light source and two spatulas to examine the mouth
- Examine
  - Teeth, gums, gingival sulci
  - Buccal mucosa, opening of parotid duct
  - Floor of mouth
  - Hard and soft palate
  - Retromolar trigone region
  - Anterior and posterior faucial pillars, tonsils
  - Posterior pharyngeal wall
  - Tongue (observe full movements)
- Palpate
  - Salivary glands/ducts

Larynx, oropharynx and hypopharynx

- Indirect laryngoscopy
  - Mirror and headlight
- Direct flexible fibreoptic pharyngolaryngoscopy

Nasopharynx

- Rigid Hopkins' rod endoscopy
- Flexible fibreoptic nasendoscopy

Neck

- Inspection
  - Tongue protrusion
  - Observe swallowing
- Palpation
  - If a mass is palpable, evaluate for size, site, shape, consistency, superficial and deep fixation, fluctuation, transillumination, auscultation

INVESTIGATION OF THE PHARYNX, LARYNX AND NECK

Plain lateral radiographs

Plain lateral radiographs of the neck and cervical spine may show soft tissue abnormalities, although their sensitivity and specificity is low; of particular importance is the depth and outline of the prevertebral soft tissue shadow on sagittal section as an indication of retropharyngeal pathology. The outline of the laryngotracheal airway may be a useful guide to the presence of disease in the pharynx and larynx. There should be no air within the upper oesophagus. If air is seen, endoscopy is advised. Radiopaque foreign bodies may be seen impacted in the pharynx, larynx or upper oesophagus on these radiographs (Figure 47.9).

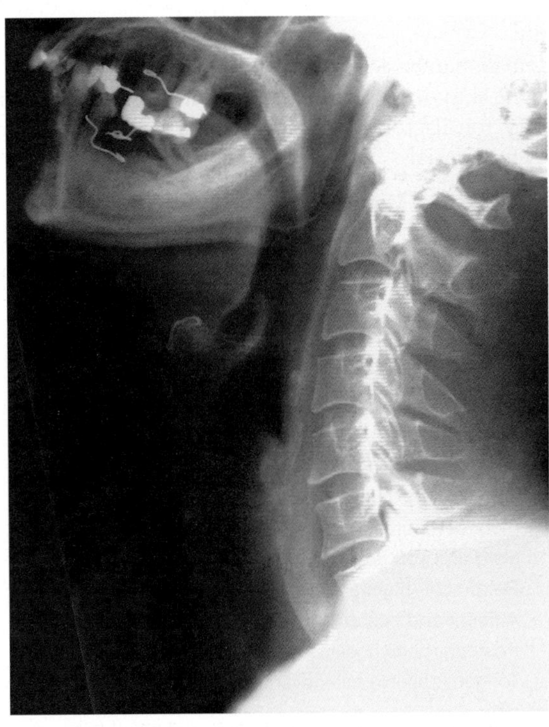

Figure 47.9 Plain lateral radiograph showing normal anatomy.

Barium swallow

Barium (or water-soluble contrast if a pharyngeal or oesophageal perforation is suspected) liquid video fluoroscopic studies record the movement of a small quantity of radiopaque liquid and allow detailed evaluation of the oral and pharyngeal phases of swallowing (Figure 47.10).

Computed tomography scanning

Computed tomography (CT) scanning provides high resolution imaging of disease in the pharynx, larynx and neck. Intravenous contrast given at the same time as the CT scan (dynamic scanning) further improves the demonstration of disease in these areas (Figure 47.11).

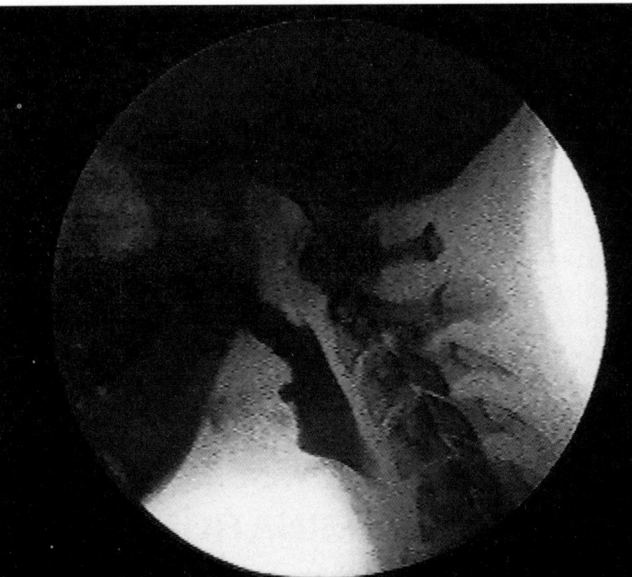

Figure 47.10 Videofluoroscopy image showing liquid barium in the upper pharynx in a normal swallow.

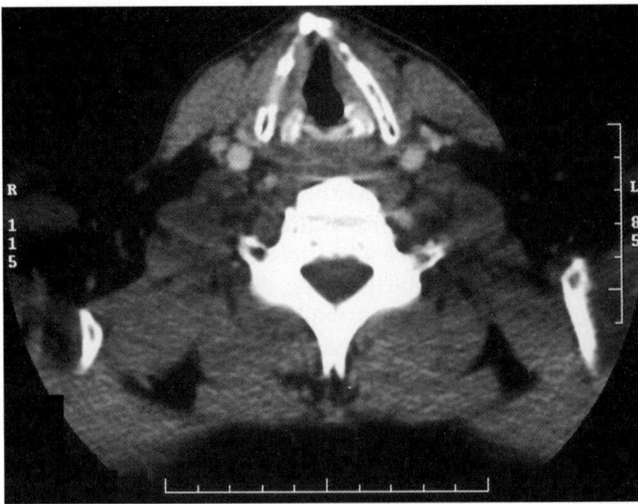

Figure 47.11 Axial computed tomography scan through the larynx at the level of the glottis.

Other imaging

Magnetic resonance imaging (MRI) may be used to give better soft tissue definition and is preferred for tumour staging in some centres. Drawbacks of this approach include a reduction in image quality due to movement artefact, poorer definition of bony and cartilaginous structures and upstaging of tumours due to oversensitivity (Figure 47.12). Ultrasound scanning can be useful in differentiating solid lesions (e.g. malignant lymph nodes from cystic lesions such as a branchial cyst) and is particularly helpful when attempting fine-needle aspiration.

If a head and neck malignancy is suspected, then CT imaging of the thorax should also be performed as the rate of synchronous primary bronchogenic tumours, while not particularly high (~5%), is significant and if detected, will change treatment options.

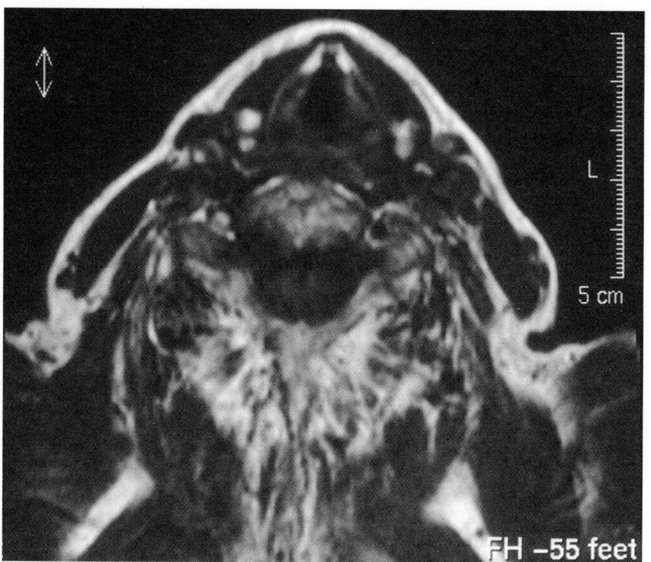

Figure 47.12 Axial magnetic resonance imaging scan at the same level as Fig. 47.11.

Fine-needle aspiration cytology

This is the investigation of choice when attempting to determine the nature of a neck or thyroid mass. Fine-needle aspiration cytology (FNAC) is considerably aided by ultrasound or CT guidance to the extent the ultrasound-guided FNAC is now routine in many units around the world. The technique is safe and well tolerated and has high diagnostic sensitivity and specificity, especially when diagnosing cervical lymph node enlargement and performed by a practitioner with a high volume practice.

Angiography or digital subtraction vascular imaging

These techniques may be indicated if a vascular lesion such as a carotid body tumour is suspected. Angiography may have a therapeutic role to play by facilitating embolisation of the lesion.

Direct pharyngoscopy and laryngoscopy

Examination of the pharynx, larynx and neck under general anaesthesia may be required if a primary head and neck malignancy is suspected or there are problems with the routine examination of patients, such as an inadequate view as a result of trismus from pain, poor patient compliance or large obstructive pharyngeal or laryngeal pathology. These examinations may be further aided by the use of an operating microscope or rigid straight and angled (30° and 70°) endoscopes (Hopkins' rods) (Figure 47.13).

The advantages and disadvantages of laryngeal examination techniques are given in *Summary box 47.3*.

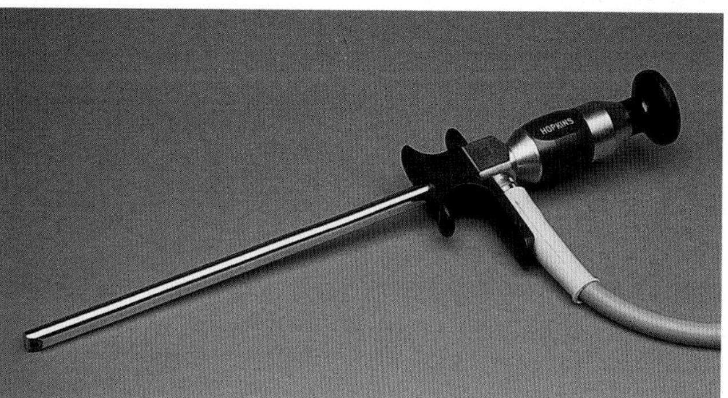

Figure 47.13 A rigid Hopkins' rod or endoscope.

Summary box 47.3

Advantages and disadvantages larynx and pharynx examination techniques

Flexible nasendoscopy
- Well tolerated examination
- Can also examine nasal passages and postnasal space
- Need fibreoptic light source

Rigid endoscopy
- Can be used with stroboscope for evaluation of voice
- High definition view
- Needs fibreoptic light source
- Bulky and difficult if prominent gag reflex present

Laryngeal mirror
- Does not need fibreoptic light source
- No record of exam, small image

Harold Horace Hopkins, 1918–1994, Professor of Applied Optics, The University of Reading, Reading, UK, invented the rigid rod endoscope (Hopkins' rod, 1954), and contributed to the development of the fibres for flexible endoscopes.

DISEASES OF THE PHARYNX

NASOPHARYNX

Enlarged adenoid

The most common cause of an enlarged adenoid (there is only one nasopharyngeal adenoid, despite the common use of the term 'adenoids') is physiological hypertrophy in childhood. The size of the adenoid alone is not an indication for removal. Of more importance is the consequences of hypertrophy (e.g. nasal obstruction). Adenoid hypertrophy is often associated with hypertrophy of the other lymphoid tissues of Waldeyer's ring. Of particular note, if excessive adenoidal hypertrophy causes blockage of the nasopharynx in association with tonsil hypertrophy, the upper airway may become compromised during sleep causing, obstructive sleep apnoea (OSA).

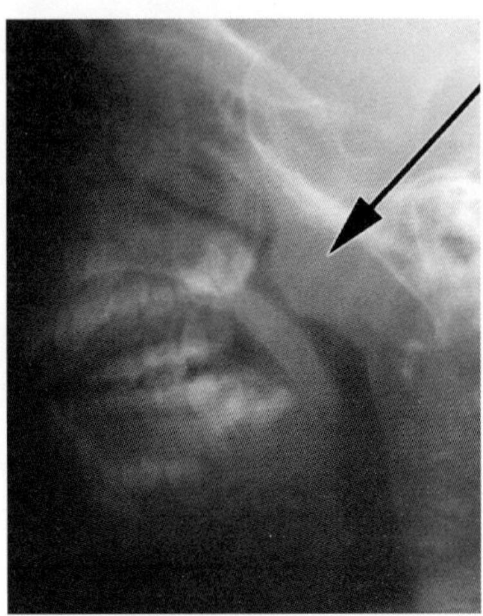

Figure 47.14 Plain lateral radiograph showing a large pad of adenoid tissue (arrow) in the postnasal space.

Obstructive sleep apnoea

This condition is becoming increasingly diagnosed in children and is important because it can cause sleep deprivation and secondary cardiac complications. It has been implicated in some cases of sudden infant death syndrome. The most common symptom is snoring, which is typically irregular, with the child actually ceasing respiration (apnoea) and then restarting with a loud inspiratory snort. The child is often restless and may take up strange sleep positions as he or she tries to improve the pharyngeal airway. Surgical removal of the tonsils and adenoid is curative, but it is important to avoid sedative premedications and opiate analgesics postoperatively because they may further depress the child's respiratory drive.

OSA may also occur in adults, where the obstruction may result from nasal deformity, a hypertrophic soft palate associated with an altered nasopharyngeal isthmus, obesity and general narrowing of the pharyngeal airway, or supraglottic laryngeal pathology. The initial investigation may include a sleep study, during which measurement of the patient's sleep pattern and arterial oxygenation are undertaken. Continuous positive airway pressure devices may ameliorate OSA by splinting the obstruction open. Surgery may also be indicated, depending on the level(s) of the obstruction.

Hypertrophy of adenoid tissue most commonly occurs between the ages of 4 and 10, but the adenoid tissue usually undergoes spontaneous atrophy during puberty, although some remnants may persist into adult life (Figure 47.14). The relationship of adenoid enlargement to recurrent secretory otitis media or recurrent acute otitis media is not entirely clear.

Adenoidectomy

Adenoid tissue can be removed alone or in conjunction with a tonsillectomy. The indications for adenoidectomy are:

- obstructive sleep apnoea associated with postnasal obstruction;
- recurrent acute otitis media or prolonged serous otitis media, usually longer than 3 months' duration;
- recurrent rhinosinusitis*;
- postnasal discharge*.

*Relative indications

Operative technique

With the patient placed in a prone position with the neck in a neutral position, the adenoid tissue is removed with a guarded curette pressed against the roof of the nasopharynx before sweeping downwards to deliver the excised adenoid into the oropharynx (Figures 47.15 and 47.16). A postnasal swab is placed into the nasopharynx until all haemorrhage

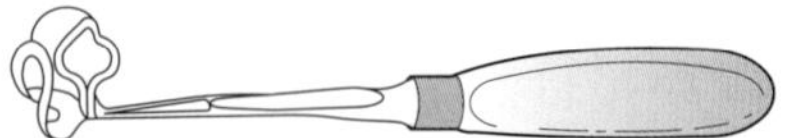

Figure 47.15 St Clair Thomson adenoid curette.

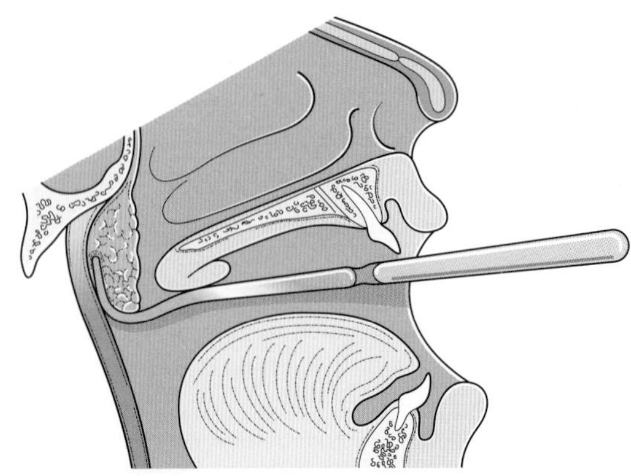

Figure 47.16 Curettage of the adenoid.

has ceased. A mirror can be used to guide the direction of the adenoid curette. Alternatively, suction monopolar diathermy may be used to remove adenoid tissue.

Reactionary or secondary haemorrhage during the recovery period may require a nasopharyngeal pack under a further anaesthetic. This can occasionally cause respiratory depression in children and adults, and strict observation is required while the pack is in place.

Tumours of the nasopharynx

Benign

There are two main types of benign tumour of the nasopharynx: the angiofibroma and the antrochoanal polyp. Both are rare.

ANGIOFIBROMA

This tumour is confined to young male patients most commonly between the ages of 8 and 20 years. It usually causes progressive nasal obstruction, recurrent severe epistaxis, purulent rhinorrhoea and occasionally loss of vision because of compression of the optic nerve by superior extension of the tumour through the skull base. Although the tumour is rare, these symptoms in a young male patient should always arouse suspicion. The tumour is more common in northern India, although the reasons for this are unknown. Clinical examination typically shows a mass in the nasal cavity or nasopharynx, but CT scanning best demonstrates the extent of the tumour and any associated bony erosion. MRI scanning defines the soft tissue extent and, with these two modern investigations, angiography is rarely indicated. Biopsy should be avoided unless clinical and radiological examinations are not diagnostic because of the risk of bleeding.

Surgical resection requires adequate exposure either through a midfacial approach or lateral rhinotomy (Figures 47.17 and 47.18). Both allow ligation of the feeding maxillary artery. More recently, endoscopic resection has been used for smaller lesions.

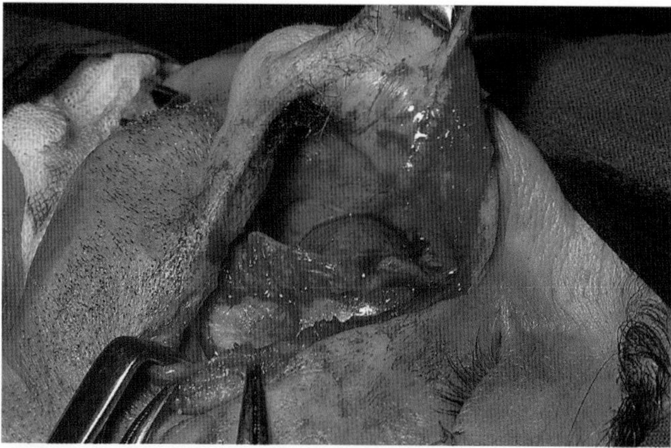

Figure 47.18 Intraoperative photograph showing an incision in lateral rhinotomy.

ANTROCHOANAL POLYP

This relatively uncommon lesion is a benign mucosal polyp that arises in the maxillary antrum and prolapses into the nasal cavity where it expands backwards into the nasopharynx and occasionally into the oropharynx (Figures 47.19 and 47.20). It may mimic an angiofibroma from which it is distinguished by its avascularity and pale colour, as well as its site of origin, which is determined on endoscopic examination and imaging. It requires complete removal via an endoscopic approach through the middle meatus of the maxillary sinus or, occasionally, via an open Caldwell–Luc approach.

Malignant

NASOPHARYNGEAL CARCINOMA

Nasopharyngeal carcinoma has a marked geographically variable incidence. In most parts of the world, the tumour

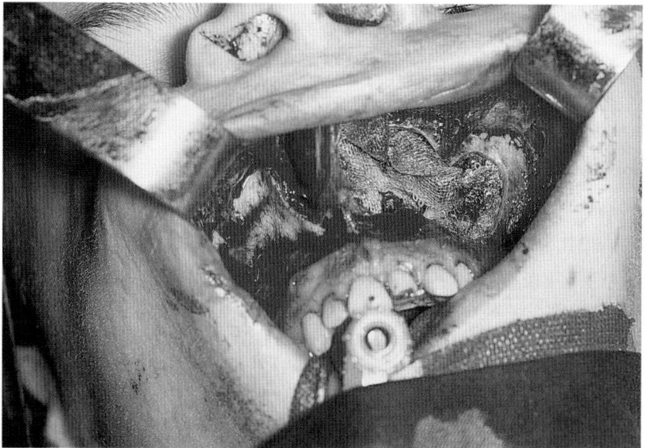

Figure 47.17 Intraoperative photograph showing exposure during a midfacial degloving approach.

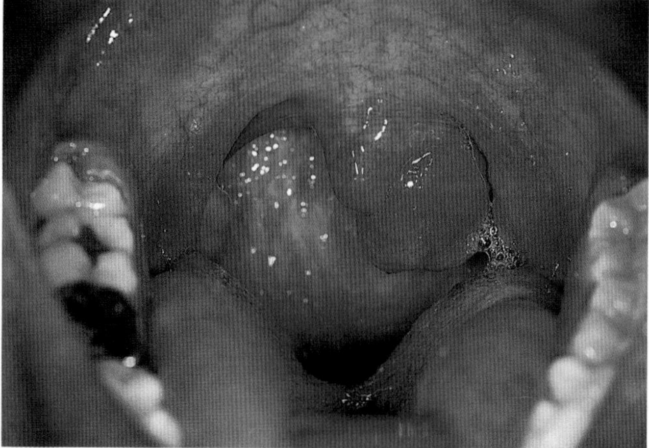

Figure 47.19 Intraoral view showing a fleshy polyp hanging in the oropharynx.

George Walter Caldwell, 1834–1918, otolaryngologist, who practised successively in New York, San Francisco, and Los Angeles, USA, devised this operation for treating suppuration in the maxillary antrum in 1893.
Henri Luc, 1855–1925, otolaryngologist, Paris, France, described his operation in 1889.

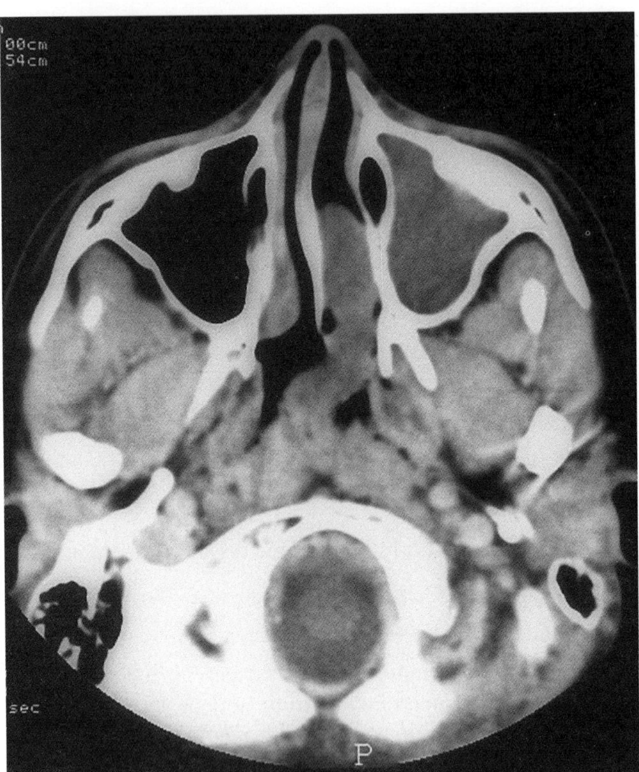

Figure 47.20 Axial computed tomogram of an antrochoanal polyp (as seen in Fig. 47.19), with opaque maxillary antrum and a mass in the nasal cavity and nasopharynx.

is rare with an annual incidence of 1 case per 100000 population; however, among southern Chinese populations the rate is 30–50 cases per 100 000 population. The aetiology of nasopharyngeal carcinoma is multifactorial. Genetic susceptibility, early infection by the Epstein–Barr virus and consumption of traditional diets, particularly salted fish, are known to contribute.

Summary box 47.4

Aetiological factors in nasopharyngeal carcinoma

- Genetic (e.g. Cantonese)
- Infective (e.g. Epstein–Barr virus)
- Environmental (e.g. salted fish)

The majority of nasopharyngeal tumours are undifferentiated with a characteristic morphology, comprising over 90% of nasopharyngeal malignancy in endemic areas. Rare epithelial tumours are adenocarcinoma and adenoid cystic carcinoma, which arise from minor salivary glands. B- and T-cell lymphomas also occur in the nasopharynx and should not be confused with the more common undifferentiated carcinoma. Nasopharyngeal carcinoma has a bimodal distribution with an increased incidence in teenagers and young adults and then again in the 50–60 age group.

Clinical features Symptoms are closely related to the position of the tumour in the nasopharynx and the degree of regional and/or distant spread. Early symptoms are often minimal and may be ignored by both patient and doctor. Approximately 50% of patients will present with a malignant node or nodes in the neck, indicating an advanced tumour. While investigation of the lymph node will involve fine-needle aspiration or a biopsy, such a clinical presentation mandates an immediate thorough examination of the nasopharynx. In about 5% of patients, the nasopharynx may look normal or minimally asymmetrical but contains submucosal nasopharyngeal carcinoma. MRI or CT of the head and neck should be performed as part of the diagnostic work-up and even if a nasopharyngeal mass is not identified clinically or radiologically, a biopsy of the nasopharynx, targeting the fossa of Rosenmüller is essential if there is suspicion of nasopharyngeal malignancy. In contrast, nasal complaints (obstruction +/- rhinorrhoea) occur in one-third of patients and aural symptoms of unilateral deafness as a consequence of Eustachian tube obstruction and secretory otitis media occur in approximately 20%. Neurological complications with cranial nerve palsies as a result of disease in the skull base occur relatively late in the disease, but are a poor prognostic sign, as is trismus resulting from tumour involvement of the medial pterygoid.

Summary box 47.5

Nasopharyngeal carcinoma: main presenting complaints

Systemic

- Cervical lymphadenopathy

Local

- Unilateral serous otitis media, otalgia
- Nasal obstruction, bloody discharge, epistaxis
- Cranial nerve palsies, especially III–VI then IX–XII
- Trismus

Investigation This is by direct inspection with a flexible or rigid nasendoscope and biopsy under topical or general anaesthesia. Serological investigation for Epstein–Barr virus-associated antigenic markers in combination with the clinical and histological examination is valuable for the early detection of disease. Highly sensitive assays for antiviral antibodies together with virus-associated serological markers are useful in early detection and in post-treatment surveillance. Immunoglobulin (Ig) A antiviral capsid antigen antibody and

Michael Anthony Epstein, born 1921, formerly Professor of Pathology, The University of Bristol, Bristol, UK.
Yvonne Barr, 1931–2016, virologist who emigrated to Australia. Epstein and Barr discovered this virus in 1964.

early antigen antibody have been evaluated in mass surveys in southern China and have been found to be an excellent screening method for early detection of nasopharyngeal carcinoma in high-risk groups.

Imaging This is essential for staging and to determine the extent of disease. The imaging of choice is MRI with gadolinium and fat suppression. This allows for assessment of brain parenchyma, cavernous sinus and the closely associated cranial foramina. CT or positron emission tomography (PET)-CT of the head, neck and chest has a major role in planning radiotherapy and assessing the response to treatment, diagnosing recurrence and detecting complications.

Treatment The primary treatment of nasopharyngeal carcinoma, depending on the stage of disease, is with external beam or intensity modulated radiotherapy +/- cisplatin-based chemotherapy, as the majority of the tumours are chemoradiosensitive, undifferentiated squamous cell carcinomas. Surgery is usually reserved for regional recurrence in the neck. For early disease, 5-year disease-free survival rates of more than 75% are common; however, in advanced disease the results are less good, with 5-year disease-free survival rates of 30–50%.

OROPHARYNX

Acute tonsillitis

This common condition is characterised by a sore throat, fever, general malaise, dysphagia, enlarged upper cervical nodes and sometimes referred otalgia. Approximately half the cases are bacterial, the most common cause being a pyogenic group A streptococcus. The remainder are viral and a wide variety of viruses have been implicated, in particular infectious mononucleosis (glandular fever), which may be mistaken for bacterial tonsillitis.

On examination, the tonsils are swollen and erythematous, and yellow or white pustules may be seen on the palatine tonsils, hence the name 'follicular tonsillitis' (Figure 47.21). A throat swab should be taken at the time of examination as well as blood for Paul–Bunnell testing to confirm or refute the diagnosis of glandular fever.

Treatment

Paracetamol or similar analgesia may be administered to relieve pain and gargles of glycerol–thymol are soothing. The condition is frequently sensitive to benzyl- or phenyoxymethylpenicillin (penicillin V) and these are given until antibiotic sensitivities are established. Ampicillin is avoided as it may precipitate a rash in patients with infectious mononucleosis. Most cases resolve in a few days.

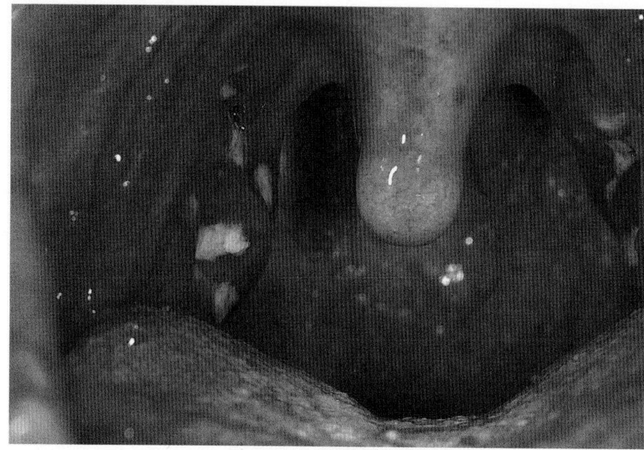

Figure 47.21 Acute follicular tonsillitis.

Quinsy

This is an abscess in the peritonsillar region that causes severe pain and trismus (Figure 47.22). The trismus caused by spasm induced in the pterygoid muscles may make examination difficult but may be overcome by instillation of local anaesthesia into the posterior nasal cavity (anaesthetising the sphenopalatine ganglion) and the oropharynx. Inspection reveals a diffuse swelling of the soft palate just superior or lateral to the involved tonsil, displacing the uvula medially. In more advanced cases, pus may be seen pointing underneath the thin mucosa.

Treatment

In the early stages, intravenous broad-spectrum antibiotics may produce resolution. However, if there is frank abscess formation, incision and drainage of the pus can be carried out under local anaesthesia. A small scalpel is best modified by winding a strip of adhesive tape around the blade so that only 1 cm of the blade projects. In teenagers and young adults, the

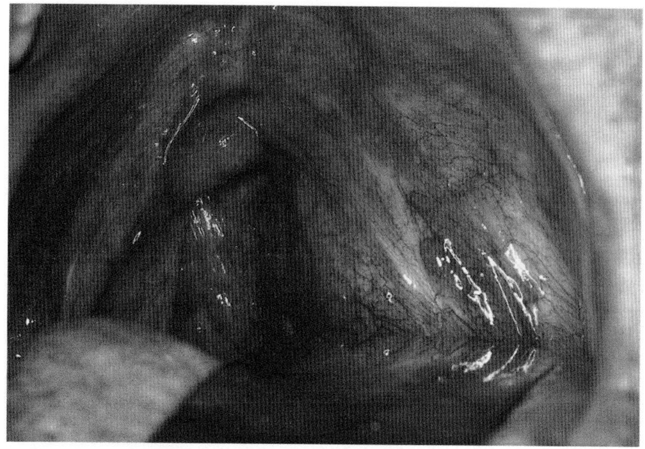

Figure 47.22 Quinsy (peritonsillar abscess).

John Rodman Paul, 1893–1971, Professor of Preventative Medicine, Yale University, New Haven, CT, USA.
Walls Willard Bunnell, 1902–1966, American physician. Paul and Bunnell described this test in 1932.

patient sits upright and an incision is made approximately midway between the base of the uvula and the third upper molar tooth (Figure 47.23). This may produce immediate release of pus, but, if not, a dressing forceps is pushed firmly through the incision and, on opening, pus may then be encountered. In small children, general anaesthesia is required.

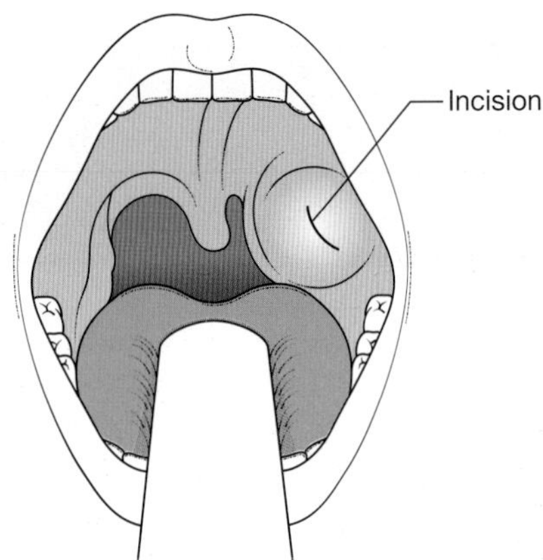

Figure 47.23 Site of incision in a peritonsillar abscess.

Chronic tonsillitis

Chronic tonsillitis usually results from repeated attacks of acute tonsillitis in which the tonsils become progressively damaged by inflammatory processes and provide a reservoir for infective organisms.

Tonsillectomy

Recurrent acute tonsillitis is the most common relative indication for tonsillectomy in children and adolescents, although it is important that these attacks are well documented, frequent and do not simply constitute a minor viral sore throat. Chronic tonsillitis more frequently affects young adults in whom it is important to establish that chronic mouth breathing secondary to nasal obstruction is not the main problem rather than the tonsils themselves. Absolute indications for tonsillectomy are when the size of the tonsils is contributing to airway obstruction or a malignancy of the tonsils is suspected (*Table 47.1*).

TABLE 47.1 Indications for tonsillectomy.

Absolute	Sleep apnoea, chronic respiratory tract obstruction, cor pulmonale
	Suspected tonsillar malignancy
Relative	Documented recurrent acute tonsillitis
	Chronic tonsillitis
	Peritonsillar abscess (quinsy)
	Tonsillar asymmetry
	Tonsillitis resulting in febrile convulsions
	Diphtheria carriers
	Systemic disease caused by β-haemolytic *Streptococcus* (nephritis, rheumatic fever)

Ideally, the procedure should be undertaken when the tonsils are not acutely infected, and it is important to discuss factors that may increase the tendency to bleed. Blood transfusion is rarely required, but it is normal practice to type and screen blood for cross-match in children under 15 kg in weight.

Dissection tonsillectomy is carried out under general anaesthesia. The mucosa of the anterior faucial pillar is incised and the tonsil capsule identified. Using blunt dissection, the tonsil is separated from its bed until only a small inferior pedicle is left (Figure 47.24). It is then separated from the lingual tonsil. A tonsil swab is placed in the tonsillar bed and pressure applied for some minutes, following which bleeding points may be controlled by ligature or by bipolar diathermy. (Coblation and laser dissection is commonly used in the resource-rich world in an attempt to reduce postoperative pain and bleeding.)

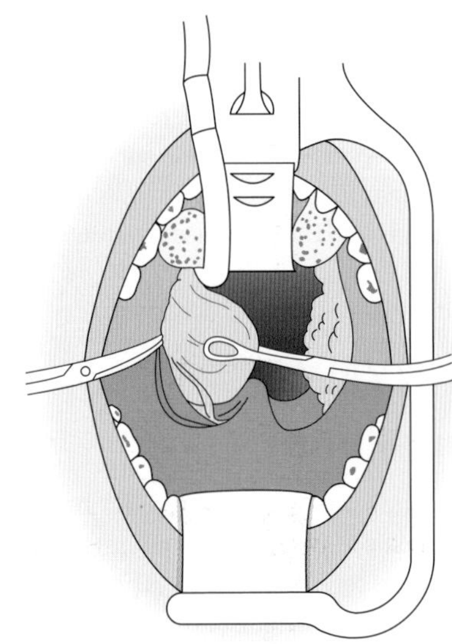

Figure 47.24 Removal of the tonsils.

Following surgery, the patient is kept under close observation for any systemic or local evidence of bleeding, with regular pulse and blood pressure measurements and observation to monitor whether the patient is swallowing excessively (Figure 47.25). Postoperatively, patients are encouraged to eat normally. Paracetamol is preferred to non-steroidal analgesics. Patients are allowed home on the same or following day and are warned that they may experience otalgia as a result of referred pain from the glossopharyngeal nerve and that secondary haemorrhage may occur up to 10 days following the surgery.

Haemorrhage is the most common complication in the immediate postoperative period. Local pressure may help in mild cases, but reactionary haemorrhage usually requires return to theatre for definitive treatment, particularly in younger patients. Under general anaesthesia, it may be possible to identify a bleeding spot, but often a more generalised ooze is observed and suturing of the tonsil bed combined with the application of haemostatic gauze and bipolar diathermy is often more successful than attempted placement of ligatures.

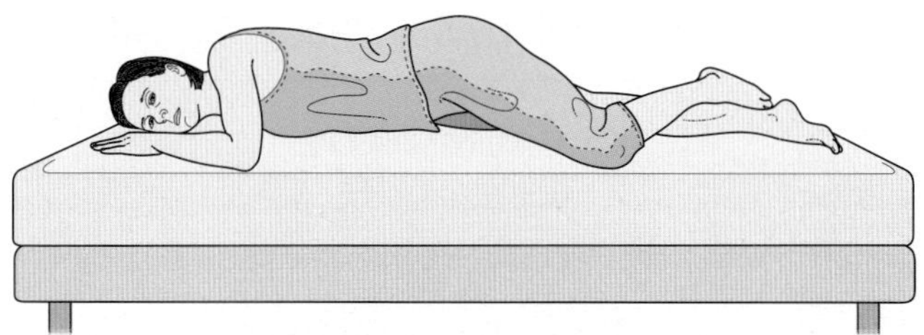

Figure 47.25 Positioning of the patient after tonsillectomy.

Late haemorrhage is sometimes secondary to infection and patients are usually started on broad-spectrum intravenous antibiotics. Any residual clot in the tonsil fossa should be removed and regular gargling with a dilute solution of hydrogen peroxide may be beneficial. Significant or persistent bleeding may require a further general anaesthetic and haemostasis, which may require diathermy and/or undersewing of the granulating, sloughy tonsil fossa. Postoperative tonsillar haemorrhage is still a serious and life-threatening complication and should not be underestimated, particularly in the younger patient.

Summary box 47.6

Complications of tonsillectomy

Anaesthetic
- Traumatic intubation
- Cardiopulmonary arrest
- Malignant hyperthermia

Surgical
- Haemorrhage (immediate or late)
- Infection
- Pain/otalgia
- Postoperative airway obstruction
- Velopharyngeal insufficiency

Parapharyngeal abscess

Parapharyngeal abscess may be confused with a peritonsillar abscess, but the maximal swelling is *behind* the posterior faucial pillar and there may be little oedema of the soft palate. The patient is usually a young child and there may be a severe general malaise and obvious neck swelling. In early cases, admission to hospital and the institution of fluid replacements coupled with intravenous antibiotics may produce resolution. In advanced cases, drainage and intravenous antibiotics are required. With an obvious abscess pointing into the oropharynx, drainage may be carried out with a blunt instrument or the glove finger, but general anaesthesia is frequently required and the expertise of a senior anaesthetist, good illumination and good suction are absolutely essential. A large parapharyngeal abscess may compromise both the airway and swallowing. MRI or CT scanning of the head and neck is often an invaluable aid to diagnosis and management as it allows assessment of the extent of the abscess and facilitates planning of the optimal surgical approach.

Acute retropharyngeal abscess

This is the result of suppuration of the retropharyngeal lymph nodes and, again, is most commonly seen in children, with most cases occurring under the age of 1 year. It is associated with infection of the upper aerodigestive tract, and is frequently accompanied by severe general malaise, neck rigidity, dysphagia, drooling, a croupy cough, an altered cry and marked dyspnoea.

Dyspnoea may be the prominent symptom and may also be accompanied by febrile convulsions and vomiting. These children should always be carefully examined by the most senior clinicians available. Inspection of the posterior wall of the pharynx may show gross swelling and an abscess pointing beneath the thinned mucosa.

In countries where diphtheria still occurs, an acute retropharyngeal abscess may be confused with this, but the presence of the greyish–green membrane aids differentiation. Occasionally, a foreign body, most commonly a fish bone which has perforated the posterior pharyngeal mucosa, will give rise to a retropharyngeal abscess in older children and young adults. Intravenous antibiotics are commenced immediately but surgical drainage of the abscess is often necessary. It requires experienced anaesthesia because, on induction, care must be taken to avoid rupturing the abscess. The airway is protected by placing the child in a head down position while a pair of dressing forceps, guided by the finger, may be thrust into an obvious abscess in the posterior wall and the contents evacuated. On other occasions, an approach anterior and medial to the carotid sheath via a cervical incision may be preferable.

Chronic retropharyngeal abscess

This condition is now rare and is most commonly the result of an extension of tuberculosis of the cervical spine, which has spread through the anterior longitudinal ligament to reach the retropharyngeal space. In addition to the retropharyngeal swelling seen intraorally, there may be fullness behind the sternocleidomastoid muscle on one side. In contrast to an acute retropharyngeal abscess, this condition occurs almost solely in adults. Radiology usually shows evidence of bone destruction and loss of the normal curvature of the cervical spine. The spine may be quite unstable and undue manipulation may precipitate a neurological event.

In contrast to an acute abscess, a chronic retropharyngeal abscess must not be opened into the mouth, as such a procedure may lead to secondary infection. Drainage of the abscess may not be necessary if suitable treatment of the underlying tuberculosis disease is instituted. If it is necessary, drainage should be carried out through a cervical incision anterior to the sternocleidomastoid muscle with an approach anterior and medial to the carotid sheath to enter the retropharyngeal space. The cavity is opened and suctioned dry after taking biopsy material. Occasionally, surgery is required to decompress or stabilise the spinal cord if there is a progressive neurological deficit.

Glandular fever (infectious mononucleosis)

This systemic condition is usually caused by the Epstein–Barr virus, but similar features can be caused by cytomegalovirus or toxoplasmosis. The tonsils are typically erythematous with a creamy grey exudate and appear almost confluent, usually symmetrical. In addition to the discomfort and dysphagia, patients may drool saliva and have respiratory difficulty, particularly on inspiration. They commonly have a high temperature and gross general malaise with marked cervical or generalised lymphadenopathy. Occasionally, an enlarged spleen or liver may be detected. The condition is most frequent in teenagers and young adults. The diagnosis can be confirmed by serological testing showing a positive Paul–Bunnell test, an absolute and relative lymphocytosis, and the presence of atypical monocytes in the peripheral blood.

Treatment

Analgesia and maintenance of fluid intake are important. A small number of patients require admission to hospital if the airway is compromised or if oral intake of fluids is not possible, and a short course of steroids may be helpful. Antibiotics are of little value and ampicillin is contraindicated because of the frequent appearance of a widespread skin rash. Rarely, if the airway is severely compromised, an elective tracheostomy under local anaesthesia is safer and less traumatic than an emergency intubation. Emergency tonsillectomy is contraindicated because of the generalised pharyngeal oedema and compromised airway.

Human immunodeficiency virus

Acquired immune deficiency syndrome (AIDS) can affect the ear, nose and throat (ENT) system at any point during the disease. The initial seroconversion may present with the symptoms of glandular fever, which is followed by an asymptomatic period of variable length. In the pre-AIDS period, before the full-blown symptoms of the AIDS-related complex, many patients have minor upper respiratory tract symptoms that are often overlooked, such as otitis externa, rhinosinusitis and a non-specific pharyngitis. As the patient moves into the full-blown AIDS-related complex, a persistent, generalised lymphadenopathy is frequently found affecting the cervical nodes, which is usually due to follicular hyperplasia. However, patients may also develop tumours such as Kaposi's sarcoma, sometimes seen in the oral cavity, and high-grade malignant B-cell lymphoma affecting the cervical lymph nodes and nasopharynx. In addition, multiple ulcers may be found in the oral cavity or pharynx associated with herpesvirus infection. Severe candida may affect the oral cavity, pharynx, oesophagus or even larynx, and a hairy leucoplakia may affect the tongue (Figure 47.26).

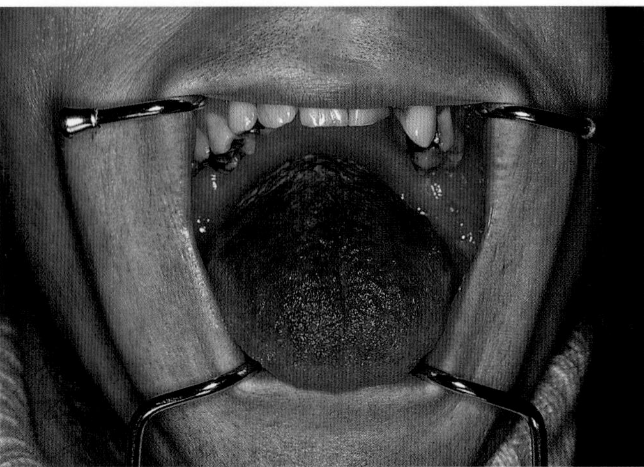

Figure 47.26 Intraoral view showing hairy tongue in a human immunodeficiency virus-positive patient.

The globus syndrome

A wide variety of patients experience the feeling of a lump in the throat (from the Latin *globus* = lump). The symptom most commonly affects adults between 30 and 60 years of age. This feeling is not true dysphagia as there is no difficulty in swallowing. Most patients notice the symptom more if they swallow their own saliva (i.e. a forced, dry swallow) rather than when they eat or drink.

The aetiology of this common symptom is unknown, but some patients may have gastro-oesophageal reflux or spasm of their cricopharyngeus muscle. Radiological and endoscopic investigation may be necessary to exclude an underlying cause and/or for patient reassurance.

Pharyngeal pouch

A pharyngeal pouch is a protrusion of mucosa though Killian's dehiscence, a weak area of the posterior pharyngeal wall between the oblique fibres of the thyropharyngeus and the transverse fibres of cricopharyngeus at the lower end of the inferior constrictor muscle (Figure 47.27). These fibres, along with the circular fibres of the upper oesophagus, form the physiological upper oesophageal sphincter mechanism. Why the pouch forms is not yet clear, even with modern videofluoroscopic and manometric studies. Many patients with pharyngeal pouches have been demonstrated to have normal relaxation of the upper oesophageal sphincter mechanism in relation to swallowing, but others have been shown to have incomplete pharyngeal relaxation, early cricopharyngeal contraction and abnormalities of the pharyngeal contraction wave. When enlarged, the pouch almost invariably deviates to the left hand side, why this is the case is also unclear.

Moritz Kaposi, 1837–1902, Professor of Dermatology, Vienna, Austria, described pigmented sarcoma of the skin in 1872.
Gustav Killian, 1860–1921, Professor of Laryngology at Freiburg, and later at Berlin, Germany.

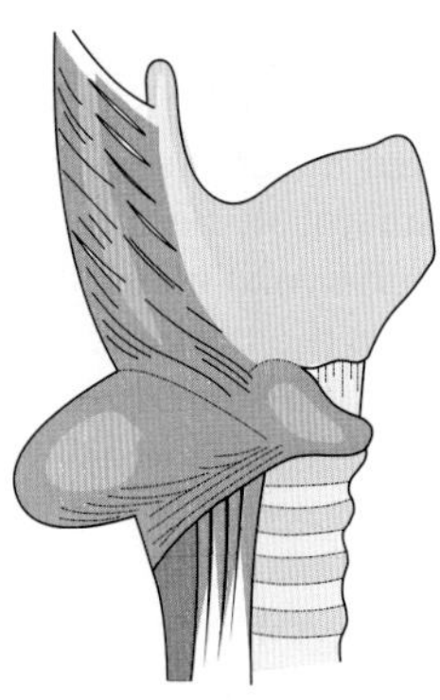

Figure 47.27 A pharyngeal pouch.

Clinical features

Patients suffering from this condition are commonly more than 60 years of age and it is more common in men than women. As the diverticulum enlarges, patients may experience regurgitation of undigested food, sometimes hours after a meal, particularly if they are bending down or turning over in bed at night. They sometimes wake at night with a feeling of tightness in the throat and a fit of coughing. Occasionally, they may present with recurrent, unexplained chest infections as a result of aspiration of the contents of the pouch. As the pouch increases in size, patients may notice gurgling noises from the neck on swallowing and the pouch may become large enough to form a visible swelling in the neck.

Radiological examination

A thin emulsion of barium is given to the patient as a barium swallow (Figure 47.28) or ideally as part of a videofluoroscopic swallowing study. Care should be exercised in patients who cough on swallowing, indicating they may have aspiration. A small volume of barium is sufficient to outline the pharynx, pouch and upper oesophagus. The videofluoroscopic study gives additional information about the pharyngeal contraction waves and the performance of the upper oesophageal sphincter.

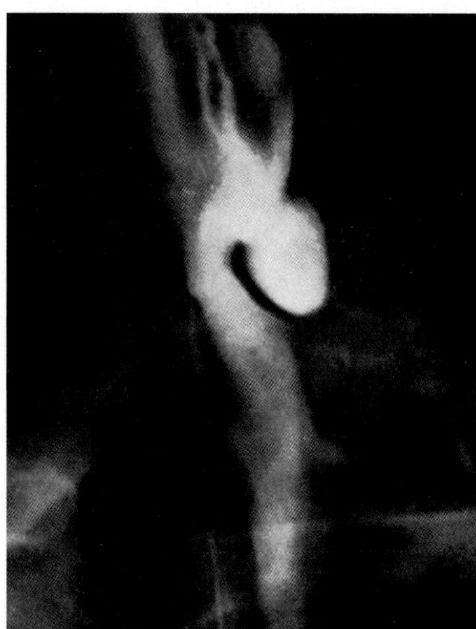

Figure 47.28 Barium swallow showing a pharyngeal pouch.

Treatment

Surgery is indicated when the pouch is associated with progressive symptoms and particularly when a prominent cricopharyngeal bar of muscle associated with abnormality of the upper oesophageal sphincter mechanism causes considerable dysphagia. In elderly patients, a decision to operate may be influenced by their general condition. However, surgical intervention is mandated in all but the most poorly patients as, in most cases, it is the pouch that is contributing significantly to the underlying debilitation. Of particular importance is the risk of recurrent pneumonia from aspiration and overspill of pouch contents, as well as increasing dysphagia as the pouch opening becomes larger than the oesophageal opening and the enlarged pouch exerts extramural pressure on the oesophagus. Accordingly, preoperative chest physiotherapy and attention to the respiratory, cardiovascular and nutritional aspects of the patient are important.

The preferred surgical technique is endoscopic stapling of the diverticular wall. A double-bladed rigid endoscope is passed, with one blade in the diverticulum and one blade positioned in the oesophagus. Opening of the bivalve scope reveals the pathonmonic 'bar' formed by the cricopharyngeus muscle and overlying mucosa, which forms the boundary between the posterior wall of the oesophagus and the anterior wall of the pouch. At this stage the pouch should be emptied of food content and the mucosa should be inspected for the rare occurrence of carcinoma in the pouch. An endoscopic linear stapler is then introduced to sit astride of the 'bar'. One jaw of the stapler is placed in the oesophagus, the other in the pouch. The stapler is fired dividing the wall separating the two. The process should be repeated until the bottom of the pouch is reached. This has the effect of opening the pouch, incorporating it as part of the oesophageal wall and dividing the cricopharyngeus muscle. If the patient is symptom free after the procedure, they may start graded per-oral intake and early discharge. Division of the 'bar' using CO_2 laser, as an alternative to stapling, is gaining popularity in some centres.

Occasionally, usually because of inadequate endoscopic access, an open excision of the pouch becomes necessary. In the classic external operation, the opening to the pouch is first identified using a pharyngoscope and a nasogastric tube placed into the oesophageal lumen for postoperative nutrition. This initial endoscopy is often difficult because the normal oesophageal opening is small compared with the lumen of the pouch, but it may be better visualised using a Dohlman's rigid endoscope. The pouch may be packed with ribbon gauze to further aid identification of its neck.

A lower neck incision along the anterior border of the left sternocleidomastoid muscle, or a transverse crease incision, is used and the muscle and carotid sheath are retracted laterally and the trachea and larynx medially. The pouch is found medially behind the lower pharynx and is carefully isolated and dissected back to its origin at Killian's dehiscence. It is then excised and the pharynx closed in two layers or, if it is small, the pouch may be invaginated into the pharyngeal lumen before closing the muscle layers. In all cases, a myotomy dividing the fibres of the cricopharyngeus muscle and the upper oesophageal circular muscle fibres must be performed. The wound is usually closed with drainage and the patient fed through a nasogastric tube for 3–7 days.

The average operating time with an endoscopic procedure is 20–30 minutes compared with 60–90 minutes with an external procedure. Inpatient stay is also decreased for patients undergoing an endoscopic procedure. The endoscopic technique is associated with a high symptomatic success rate and a low morbidity, which is particularly important in the elderly.

Complications

The classic operation has been associated with wound infection, mediastinitis, pharyngeal fistula formation, recurrent laryngeal nerve palsy and stenosis of the upper oesophagus. Endoscopic division is associated with the same risks but at much lower rates. The recurrence rates between the two procedures appears to be equal; longer-term follow up will establish this. Endoscopic stapling will also allow for safe reoperation if necessary.

In light of this risk–benefit difference, it is an option, if the main reason preventing endoscopic stapling is prominent incisors, to offer extraction of the upper incisors to facilitate access for stapling. If available, primary osseointegrated implants could be inserted at the time of stapling to allow dental restoration. This approach, despite the dental extractions, is still less risky than an open procedure.

Sideropenic dysphagia

Prolonged iron deficiency anaemia may lead to dysphagia, particularly in middle-aged women. In addition, they may have koilonychia, cheilosis and angular stomatitis together with lassitude and poor exercise tolerance. The dysphagia is caused by a postcricoid or upper oesophageal web and these patients have a higher incidence of postcricoid malignancy. The syndrome is associated with the names of Plummer and Vinson, Paterson and Brown Kelly.

Tumours of the oropharynx

Benign

Benign tumours of the oropharynx are rare, papillomas being the most common. These are usually incidental findings and are rarely of any importance.

Malignant

The most important epithelial tumour is squamous cell carcinoma, which constitutes approximately 90% of all epithelial tumours in the upper aerodigestive tract (Figures 47.29 and 47.30). In the oropharynx, the proportion is less (70%) because of the higher incidence of lymphoma (25%) and salivary gland tumours (5%). Because of the rich lymphatic drainage of the oropharynx, cervical node metastases are common. They may be the only presenting feature with an apparent occult primary tumour often being unsuspected and missed in the tonsil or tongue base.

AETIOLOGY

While it has been long established that oropharyngeal squamous cell carcinoma (OPSCC) is strongly associated with cigarette smoking and consumption of alcohol, over recent decades there has been a near epidemic increase in human papillomavirus-associated OPSCC (HPV+OPSCC) in the resource-rich world, with prevalences up to 70% being commonly reported in the USA, UK and Northern Europe. Why

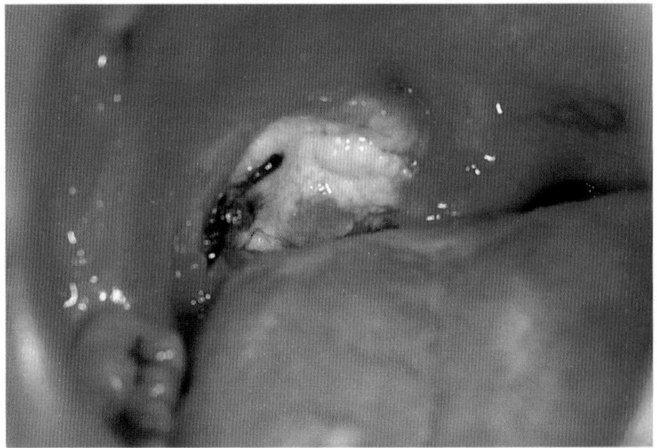

Figure 47.29 Squamous cell carcinoma of the right tonsil.

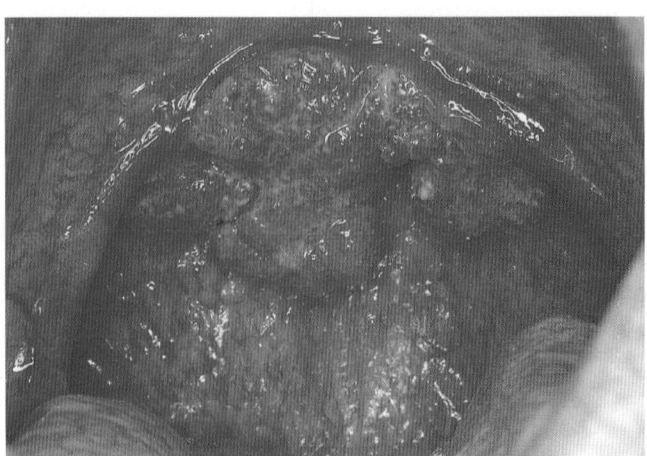

Figure 47.30 Squamous cell carcinoma of the soft palate.

Henry Stanley Plummer, 1874–1937, physician, The Mayo Clinic, Rochester, MN, USA, described this syndrome in 1912.
Porter Paisley Vinson, 1890–1959, physician, The Mayo Clinic, Rochester, MN, who later practised in Richmond, VA, USA.
Donald Rose Paterson, 1863–1939, surgeon, The Ear, Nose and Throat Department, The Royal Infirmary, Cardiff, UK.
Adam Brown Kelly, 1865–1941, surgeon, The Ear, Nose and Throat Department, The Royal Victoria Infirmary, Glasgow, UK.
Vinson, Paterson and Kelly all described this syndrome independently in 1919.

this increase has happened recently is unclear and is the subject of ongoing research. That HPV+OSCC constitutes a separate disease entity is undoubted. In contrast to patients presenting with HPV+OPSCC, those presenting with HPV-OPSCC are typically younger and fitter and smoke and drink less alcohol. Moreover, although the presenting features of HPV+OPSCC (multiple large cystic cervical lymph nodes with a high prevalence of extracapsular spread [ECS]) are usually associated with poor outcome, paradoxically, HPV+ tumours respond far better to treatment than their HPV- counterparts. Again, why this is the case is unclear and is the subject of much ongoing research.

TREATMENT

Treatment varies with facilities around the world, but early stage tumours may be cured by radiotherapy, laser excision or more conventional excision. Intermediate or late stage disease is usually managed with open surgery and reconstruction using myocutanous pedicles or free flaps, or concurrent chemoradiotherapy. Recurrent disease following radiotherapy +/- chemotherapy is a surgical challenge and usually requires open surgery and reconstruction. Neck dissection is required in most cases where surgery is the primary treatment modality and is also required for patients who have only partially responded following chemoradiotherapy. Postoperative dysphagia with aspiration as a result of interference in the complex neuromuscular control of the second phase of swallowing is a particular problem in these patients. The advent of HPV+OPSCC has created a clinical need to define novel de-intensified treatments that maintain current advantageous survival rates while reducing the late morbidity of treatment. Management of such tumours should be multidisciplinary and is best carried out in a major centre undertaking this work on a regular basis.

Lymphoma of the head and neck

Lymphomas of the head and neck may arise in nodal or extranodal sites and both Hodgkin's disease and non-Hodgkin's lymphoma commonly present as lymph node enlargement in the neck. Hodgkin's disease is rare in the oropharynx, but non-Hodgkin's lymphoma accounts for 15–20% of tumours at this site in some countries. Most are of the B-cell type and have features in common with other MALT tumours. Further evaluation with CT scanning of the thorax and abdomen and bone marrow evaluation are essential. FNAC of neck lymph nodes is now mandatory (although excision biopsy to improve tissue yield is still often required to establish a grading diagnosis) and flow cytometry of the aspirates has aided in diagnosis and classification of lymphomas.

Radiotherapy is the treatment of choice for localised non-Hodgkin's lymphoma and may give control rates as high as 75% at 5 years. For disseminated non-Hodgkin's lymphoma, systemic chemotherapy is preferred.

HYPOPHARYNX

Tumours of the hypopharynx

Benign

Benign tumours of the hypopharynx are very rare, the most common being the fibroma and the leiomyoma. They show a smooth, constant mass lying in the lumen of the hypopharynx or oesophagus.

Malignant

Malignant tumours of the hypopharynx are almost exclusively squamous cell carcinomas and typically behave aggressively. The tumours are usually classified according to their probable anatomical site of origin from the piriform fossa, postcricoid region or posterior pharyngeal wall. Marked differences in the incidence of these tumours occur globally because of factors such as iron-deficiency anaemia (see Sideropenic dysphagia, page 740). They may be associated with marked submucosal spread, which further complicates evaluation. Tumours arising from the piriform fossa and posterior pharyngeal wall may spread to upper or lower cervical nodes. Tumours arising in the postcricoid area typically metastasise to paratracheal and paraoesophageal nodes, which may not be palpable. As with other non-HPV head and neck cancers, alcohol and tobacco are two principal carcinogens. Postcricoid carcinoma, though rare, is more common in women than men.

The diagnosis of hypopharyngeal carcinoma should be considered in all patients presenting with dysphagia, hoarseness or referred otalgia, particularly if they have a history of smoking or significant alcohol consumption.

Fibreoptic endoscopic examination in the clinic may show only subtle signs such as oedema or pooling of saliva unilaterally in the piriform fossa. Note should also be made that this region is not well seen on flexible gastroscopy. The preferred investigation is with direct rigid pharyngoscopy and oesophagoscopy with biopsy under a general anaesthetic. All regions of the neck must be assessed in a systematic manner. Fine-needle aspirate is advocated for suspicious nodes.

RADIOLOGICAL EXAMINATION

As for other head and neck cancers, a suspected primary tumour requires an MRI or CT scan of the neck together with a CT scan of the thorax and upper abdomen.

TREATMENT

Squamous cell carcinoma of the hypopharynx commonly presents late and carries a poor prognosis. Early lesions may be treated with radiotherapy or transoral endoscopic carbon dioxide laser resection and a neck dissection plus postoperative radiotherapy. Non-surgical strategies for intermediate and late stage disease, designed to preserve function, rely on chemoradiotherapy. Major open excisional surgery is

---

Thomas Hodgkin, 1798–1866, Curator of the Museum and Demonstrator of Morbid Anatomy, Guy's Hospital, London, UK, described lymphadenoma in 1832.

generally used for recurrence after radiotherapy or as primary excision in advanced disease. Total laryngectomy and either partial or total pharyngectomy followed by pharyngeal reconstruction involving myocutaneous or free flap reconstruction (e.g. jejunum or anterolateral thigh) or gastric transposition is commonly required (Figure 47.31). Swallowing and voice rehabilitation are necessary to support patients after this major surgery if they are to adjust and maintain some quality of life.

Summary box 47.7

Tumours of the hypopharynx

- Variable symptoms – discomfort, pain, dysphagia, hoarseness
- Awareness increased by history of smoking and alcohol
- Expert examination with nasendoscopy
- Referral to multidisciplinary team for detailed assessment and treatment – radiotherapy +/- chemotherapy, transoral laser or extensive surgery

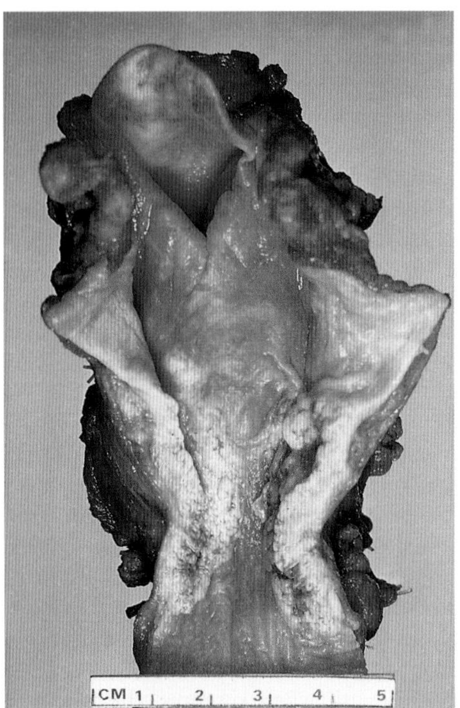

Figure 47.31 Total pharyngolaryngectomy specimen showing hypopharyngeal carcinoma (hypopharynx opened from the posterior).

DISEASES OF THE LARYNX

EMERGENCIES

Stridor

Stridor means noisy breathing. It may be inspiratory or expiratory, or occur in both phases of respiration. Inspiratory stridor is usually due to an obstruction at or above the vocal folds and is most commonly the result of an inhaled foreign body or acute infections such as epiglottitis. Expiratory stridor is usually from the lower respiratory tract and gives rise to a prolonged expiratory wheeze. It is most commonly associated with acute asthma or acute infective tracheobronchitis. Biphasic stridor is usually due to obstruction or disease of the tracheobronchial airway and distal lungs.

Summary box 47.8

Stridor

Inspiratory

- Foreign body or epiglottitis

Expiratory

- Acute asthma or infective tracheobronchitis

Biphasic

- Obstruction, disease of tracheobronchial airway or distal lungs

Stridor in children

Infants and children presenting with stridor need careful assessment with a full history and examination as appropriate. If, on presentation, a child is cyanosed and severely unwell, the airway must be secured as soon as possible, but a brief history with important pointers can often be obtained from the parents.

History

In infants in the first year of life, it is important to establish if the stridor is associated with particular activities such as swallowing, crying or movement. These may suggest congenital laryngomalacia or subglottic stenosis. If the stridor is exacerbated by feeding, particularly in the first 4 weeks of life, this suggests a vascular ring compressing the oesophagus or tracheo-oesophageal fistula. If the cry is weak or abnormal, this suggests a vocal fold palsy. If the problem only occurs in association with an upper respiratory tract infection and, in particular, is biphasic, this would suggest congenital subglottic stenosis. In a young child, inspiratory stridor and drooling suggest acute epiglottitis, whereas biphasic stridor without drooling suggests laryngotracheobronchitis or croup.

Examination

It is important when possible to observe the child carefully at rest. Once a baby starts to cry, it may be impossible to study its resting respiratory pattern for some time. Ask the mother, not a nurse or a colleague, to move a baby or young child

Summary box 47.9

Acute paediatric stridor

Congenital
- Laryngomalacia
- Laryngeal web
- Subglottic stenosis

Acquired
- Inflammatory
  Angioneurotic oedema
- Traumatic
  Impacted foreign body, laryngeal fracture
- Infective
  Epiglottis, laryngotracheobronchitis
- Neurological
  Vocal fold palsy
- Neoplasia
  Benign laryngeal papillomatosis

into different positions, such as face down and supine, and watch for changes in respiratory pattern and level of distress. Observe any drooling and, with neonates and infants, always try to watch the child being fed, listening to the trachea and chest with a stethoscope if possible. Always examine the whole child, looking for any evidence of congenital abnormalities before attempting any examination of the throat.

If a child is stridulous and drooling, do not attempt to lay it down and do not attempt to look inside the mouth. These manoeuvres are potentially life-threatening as the child may aspirate a large quantity of thick saliva contained within the oral cavity. It is particularly important in acute epiglottitis as the aspiration of thick saliva may be associated with further laryngeal spasm and a respiratory arrest. Restlessness, increasing tachycardia and cyanosis are important signs of hypoxia. If the child is not distressed and drooling, and not markedly stridulous, he/she may be cooperative enough that it is possible to look inside the mouth and check the palate, tongue and oropharynx. In stridulous children, particularly neonates and infants, a transcutaneous oximeter is invaluable. A resuscitation trolley with the necessary equipment for emergency intubation or tracheostomy should be close at hand if at all possible before commencing examination.

Investigation

Plain lateral radiographs of the neck and a chest radiograph can be obtained but only if the child's condition permits. If a child is severely stridulous, they should *not* be sent to a radiography department without access to medical staff or resuscitation equipment.

Examination under anaesthesia is essential in all children whose diagnosis remains in doubt. This requires a high level of skill and appropriate rigid laryngoscopes, bronchoscopes, endoscopic Hopkins' rods and an operating microscope should be made available if possible. Equipment should be available at all times to undertake an urgent tracheostomy to establish or maintain an airway.

Acute epiglottitis

In children acute epiglottitis is of rapid onset. It tends to occur in children of 2 years of age and over. Stridor is usually associated with drooling of saliva. The condition is caused by *Haemophilus influenzae* infection, which initially causes a severe pharyngitis that extends to involve the laryngeal inlet, causing inflammation and oedema. Further progression involves the whole of the supraglottic larynx, with severe oedema of the aryepiglottic folds and epiglottis being the most notable component, hence the commonly used term 'acute epiglottitis'.

These children frequently require intensive management with emergency intubation or tracheostomy followed by oxygenation, humidification, continuous oximetry and antibiotics such as ampicillin or chloramphenicol. There may be associated septicaemia so blood cultures should be obtained. Attempted examination with a spatula into the mouth may precipitate a respiratory arrest and should be avoided. The incidence of acute epiglottitis has plummeted where *Haemophilus influenzae* vaccination programmes are in place.

Laryngotracheobronchitis (croup)

Croup is usually of slower onset than acute epiglottitis and occurs most commonly in children under 2 years of age. It is usually viral in origin and the cases often occur in clusters. The children have biphasic stridor, and are often hoarse with a typical barking cough. Airway intervention is required less often, but admission to hospital with oxygenation and humidification, coupled with antibiotics, may be necessary if there are signs of secondary infection.

Foreign bodies

Both children and adults may inhale foreign bodies. Young children will attempt to swallow a wide variety of objects, but coins, beads and parts of toys are particularly common. In adults, the aspiration is usually food, particularly inadequately chewed bones and meat. This is more common in elderly edentulous adults. Occasionally, portions of dentures may be inhaled, particularly in association with road traffic accidents.

Clinical features

The history is paramount and a history of foreign body ingestion or inhalation in a child, even though the pain, dysphagia, coughing, etc. may have settled, should always be taken seriously.

Adults usually have a clear recall, which facilitates diagnosis. Fish bones may lodge in the tonsils or base of tongue with minimal symptoms, but small fish bones may give rise to delayed para- and retropharyngeal abscess formation.

Examination

Examination may be prevented by trismus, pain and anxiety, but the presence of a foreign body may be suspected by a salivary pool within the piriform fossa or adjacent oedema and erythema of the pharyngolaryngeal mucosa.

Radiology

Radiology may be helpful but is not critical. Fish bones are often invisible on plain radiographs and a normal plain radiograph does not exclude a foreign body within the pharynx, larynx, oesophagus or lungs.

Specialised studies may help in cases of doubt, using a CT scan or a gastrografin swallow in the case of a suspected oesophageal foreign body.

Treatment

In the case of an inhaled foreign body causing severe stridor in a neonate or infant, it may be removed either by hooking it from the pharynx with a finger or by inverting the child carefully by the ankles and slapping his/her back. In a larger child, it may be more appropriate to bend the child over your knee with the child's head hanging down and again strike the child firmly between the shoulders. In the case of adults, an impacted laryngeal foreign body may be coughed out using a Heimlich manoeuvre. This involves standing behind the patient, clasping the arms around the lower thorax, such that the knuckles of the clasped hands come into contact with the patient's xiphisternum, and then a brief, firm compression of the lower thorax may aid instant expiration of the foreign body. If none of these immediate emergency measures removes the foreign body and the patient is cyanosed and severely stridulous, an immediate cricothyroidotomy or tracheostomy may be necessary. In less urgent cases, and when a foreign body is strongly suspected, endoscopy under general anaesthesia may be indicated.

Other causes of acute pharyngolaryngeal oedema

Angioneurotic oedema, radiotherapy, laryngeal trauma associated with road traffic accidents, corrosives, scalds and smoke ingestion may all cause significant pharyngolaryngeal oedema, in addition to the acute infective conditions mentioned above. Hoarseness is the predominant symptom along with dysphagia prior to the increase in dyspnoea. If flexible laryngoscopic examination is possible, marked oedema of the supraglottis and pharynx can be seen. Humidified oxygen, adrenaline nebulisers, systemic antihistamines and steroids may be valuable. Morphine should not be given as it may cause respiratory depression and respiratory arrest. If the dyspnoea progresses, intubation or tracheostomy will be necessary.

TRACHEOSTOMY AND OTHER EMERGENCY AIRWAY MEASURES

This procedure relieves airway obstruction or protects the airway by fashioning a direct entrance into the trachea through the skin of the neck. Tracheostomy may be carried out as an emergency for acute airway obstruction when the larynx cannot be intubated, but it is not always an easy procedure, particularly in an obese patient. An easier alternative for the inexperienced is insertion of a large intravenous cannula or a small tube into the cricothyroid membrane, which lies in the midline immediately below the thyroid cartilage. *The time to do a tracheostomy is when you first think it may be necessary.*

If time allows, the following should be undertaken:

- inspection and palpation of the neck to assess the laryngotracheal anatomy in the individual patient;
- indirect or direct laryngoscopy;
- assessment of pulmonary function by auscultation.

Whenever possible, the procedure should be adequately explained to the patient beforehand, with particular emphasis on the inability to speak immediately following the operation. Ample reassurance is required that they will not have 'lost' their voice permanently. The indications for tracheostomy are shown in Summary box 47.10.

Summary box 47.10

Indications for tracheostomy

Acute upper airway obstruction

- For example, an inhaled foreign body, a large pharyngolaryngeal tumour, or acute pharyngolaryngeal infections in children

Potential upper airway obstruction

- For example, after or prior to major surgery involving the oral cavity, pharynx, larynx or neck

Protection of the lower airway

- For example, protection against aspiration of saliva in unconscious patients as a consequence of head injuries, maxillofacial injuries, comas, bulbar poliomyelitis or tetanus

Patients requiring prolonged artificial respiration

- Best performed within 10 days of ventilation

Emergency tracheostomy

If a skilled anaesthetist is unavailable, local anaesthesia is employed, but in desperate cases when the patient is unconscious, none is required. In patients who have suffered severe head and neck trauma and who may have an unstable cervical spine fracture, cricothyroidotomy may be more suitable. If it is possible, the patient should be laid supine with padding placed under the shoulders and the extended neck kept as steady as possible in the midline. This aids palpation of the thyroid and cricoid cartilage between the thumb and index finger of the free hand. The movements of the fingers of the free hand are important in this technique. The operation is more difficult in small children and thick-necked adults as the landmarks are difficult to palpate (Figures 47.32 and 47.33).

A vertical midline incision is made from the inferior aspect of the thyroid cartilage to the suprasternal notch and

Henry Jay Heimlich, 1920–2016, thoracic surgeon, Xavier University, Cincinnati, OH, USA.

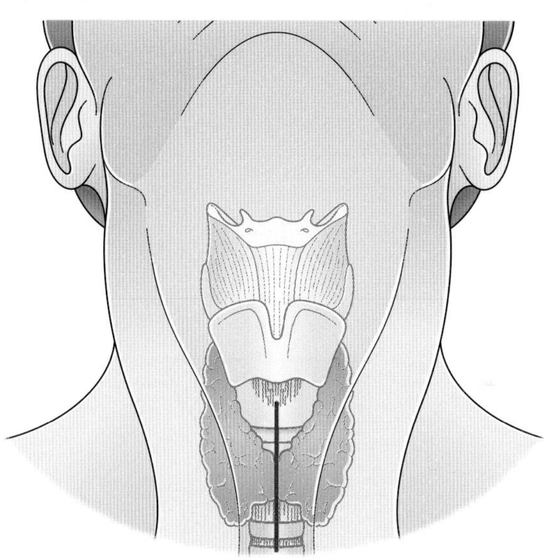

Figure 47.32 Position of the skin incision in an emergency tracheostomy.

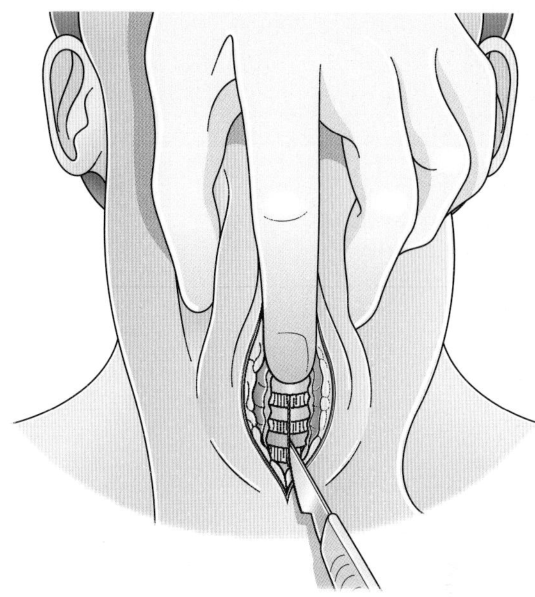

Figure 47.33 An incision in the trachea in an emergency tracheostomy.

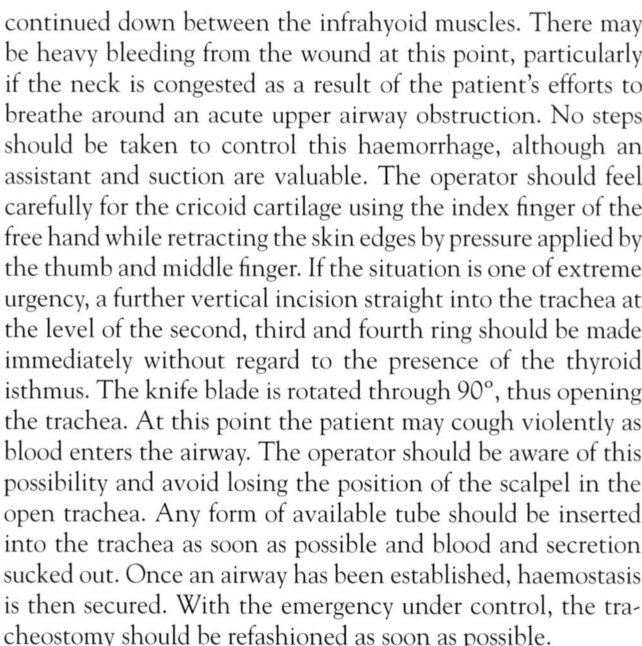

continued down between the infrahyoid muscles. There may be heavy bleeding from the wound at this point, particularly if the neck is congested as a result of the patient's efforts to breathe around an acute upper airway obstruction. No steps should be taken to control this haemorrhage, although an assistant and suction are valuable. The operator should feel carefully for the cricoid cartilage using the index finger of the free hand while retracting the skin edges by pressure applied by the thumb and middle finger. If the situation is one of extreme urgency, a further vertical incision straight into the trachea at the level of the second, third and fourth ring should be made immediately without regard to the presence of the thyroid isthmus. The knife blade is rotated through 90°, thus opening the trachea. At this point the patient may cough violently as blood enters the airway. The operator should be aware of this possibility and avoid losing the position of the scalpel in the open trachea. Any form of available tube should be inserted into the trachea as soon as possible and blood and secretion sucked out. Once an airway has been established, haemostasis is then secured. With the emergency under control, the tracheostomy should be refashioned as soon as possible.

Should additional equipment and more time be available once the cricoid cartilage has been identified, blunt finger dissection inferiorly can be used to mobilise the thyroid isthmus, which should be clipped and divided, clearing the trachea before making a vertical incision through the second to the fourth rings. A tracheal dilator is inserted through the tracheal incision and the edges of the tracheal wound are separated gently. This is likely to induce coughing and so, particularly in cases where there is a suspected infection risk, as far as possible care should be taken to minimise the risk of contaminating the operator(s). A tracheostomy tube is inserted into the trachea and the dilator removed. It is important that the surgeon keeps a finger on the tube while the assistant ties the attached tapes around the patient's neck. Return the neck to a neutral position before tying the tapes firmly.

Elective tracheostomy

The advantage of an elective surgical procedure is that there is complete airway control at all times, unhurried dissection and careful placement of an appropriate tube. Close cooperation between the surgeon, anaesthetist and scrub nurse is essential, and attention to detail will markedly reduce possible complications and morbidity from the procedure.

Following induction of general anaesthesia and endotracheal intubation, the patient is positioned with a combination of head extension and placement of an appropriate sandbag under the shoulders (Figure 47.34). There should be no rotation of the head. Children's heads should not be overextended, as it is possible to enter the trachea in the fifth and sixth rings in these circumstances. A transverse incision may be used in the elective situation (Figure 47.35). The tracheal isthmus is divided carefully and oversewn and tension sutures placed either side of the tracheal fenestration in children (Figure 47.36). A Bjork flap may be used in adults (Figures 47.37 and 47.38).

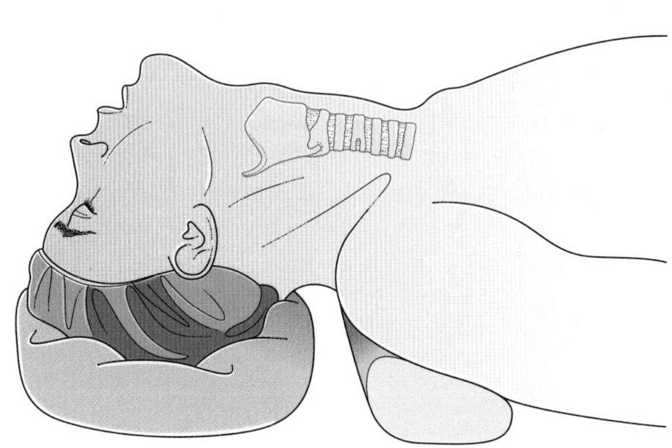

Figure 47.34 Position of the patient for elective tracheostomy.

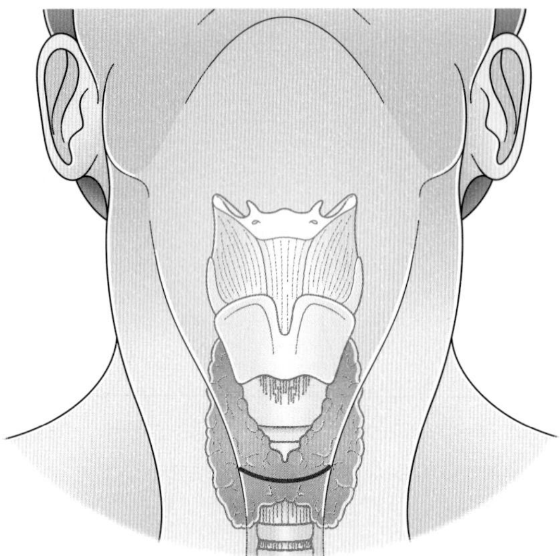
Figure 47.35 Position of the skin incision in an elective tracheostomy.

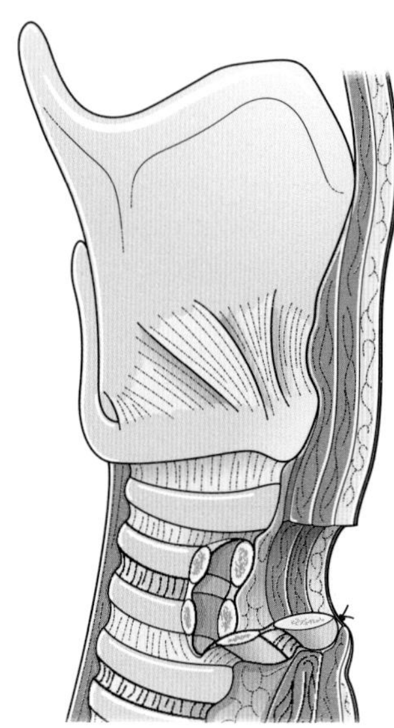
Figure 47.37 Bjork flap.

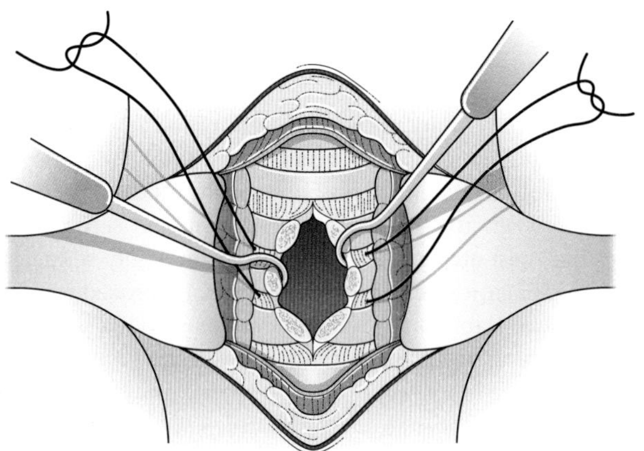
Figure 47.36 Tracheal fenestration in an elective tracheostomy.

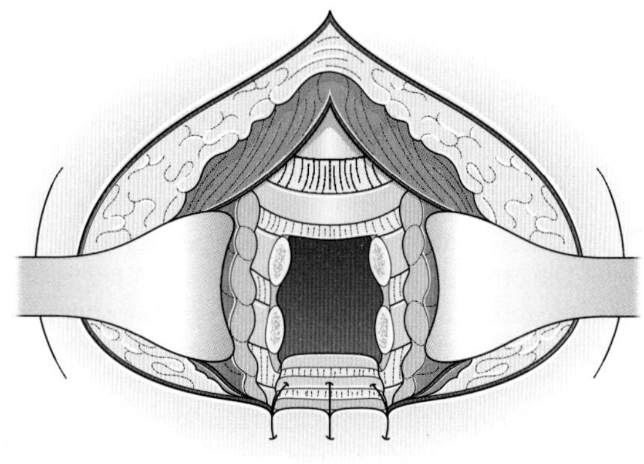
Figure 47.38 Fenestration in a Bjork flap.

The advantages of a Bjork flap outweigh the potential disadvantages, as performed correctly it is safe and allows reintroduction of a displaced tube with the minimum of difficulty, reducing the risk of replacing the displaced tube in a false track anterior to the trachea into the superior mediastinum.

The inferiorly based flap is created by starting with an incision into the trachea between the first and second or second and third tracheal rings. In order to reduce the risk of subglottic stenosis, damage to the first tracheal ring should be avoided at all costs. A stay suture is inserted around the cartilage at the free edge of the flap. Lateral incisions are made in a caudal direction extending through two tracheal rings to create the flap. One option is to leave the stay suture attached and taped to the chest wall to allow retraction of the flap to obliterate the pretracheal space when replacing a displaced tube. An alternative is to suture the free edge of the flap to the edge of the inferior transverse skin incision.

In a paediatric patient a vertical incision is made between the second and third tracheal rings. No tracheal tissue is removed. Prior to incision of the trachea, vertical stay sutures are placed lateral to the midline through the tracheal rings and left in place. These can provide traction for the trachea and allow for rapid tracheostomy tube reinsertion if accidental decannulation occurs prior to the establishment of the tract. Some surgeons will suture skin flaps to the trachea for additional safety. It is essential to stick to the midline during dissection as more lateral dissection risks a pneumothorax, as the cupula of the cervical pleura extends in to the neck on either side of the trachea.

Viking Olaf Bjork, 1918–2009, formerly cardiac surgeon, Karolinska Sjukset, Stockholm, Sweden.

Percutaneous tracheostomy

As an alternative to open tracheostomy, a percutaneous tracheostomy is commonly performed in the critical care setting. A transverse skin incision is made at the level of the first and second tracheal rings, blunt dissection of the midline is then performed. A 22-gauge needle is inserted between the second and third tracheal rings. When air is aspirated into the syringe, the guidewire is introduced. Sequentially larger dilators are then inserted over the guide wire to create a suitable sized tracheostome. Finally, the tracheotomy tube is introduced along the guidewire and dilator. The guidewire and dilator are removed, the cuff of the tracheotomy tube is inflated and the breathing circuit is connected. The endotracheal tube can then be removed.

Patients must have appropriate anatomy and no limitation of neck movement. If any doubt arises as to the suitability of a patient for percutaneous tracheostomy, a surgical approach should be adopted. Percutaneous tracheostomy is rarely performed in children.

Tracheostomy tubes

Most modern tracheostomy tubes are made of plastic (Figure 47.39). Tubes of various sizes with varying curves, angles, cuffs, inner tubes and speaking valves are available. After a newly fashioned tracheostomy is created, a cuffed tube is used initially to protect the airway from secretions or bleeding. This may be changed after 3–4 days to a non-cuffed tube. The pressure within the tube cuff should be carefully monitored and should be low enough so as not to occlude circulation in the mucosal capillaries, which promotes scar tissue formation and subglottic stenosis. When in position, the tube should retained by double tapes threaded through the flanges and passed around the patient's neck. It is important that the patient's head is flexed when the tapes are tied, otherwise they may become slack when the patient is moved from the position of extension, thereby resulting in a possible displacement of the tube if the patient coughs. Alternatively, the flanges of the plastic tube may be stitched directly to the underlying neck skin. A removable inner tube, which is easily cleaned, should always be used to prevent lumen occlusion by thickened, dried secretions from the trachea.

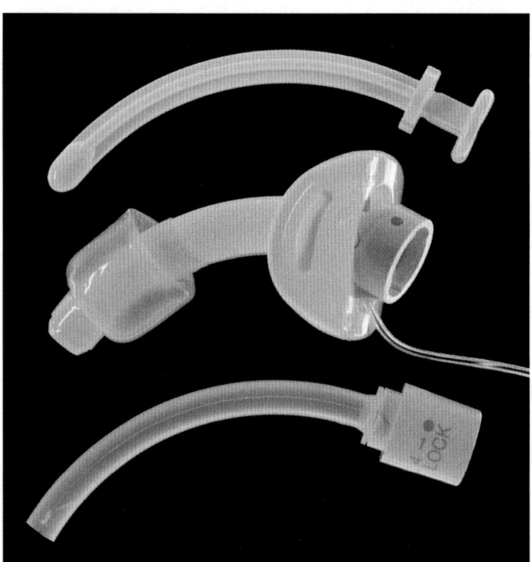

Figure 47.39 Modern plastic tracheostomy tube with introducer, low-pressure cuff and inner cannula.

All forms of tracheostomy and cricothyroidotomy bypass the upper airway and have the following advantages:

- the anatomical dead space is reduced by approximately 50%;
- the work of breathing is reduced;
- alveolar ventilation is increased;
- the level of sedation needed for patient comfort is decreased and, unlike endotracheal intubation, the patient may be able to talk and eat with a tube in place.

However, there are several disadvantages:

- loss of heat and moisture exchange in the upper respiratory tract;
- desiccation of tracheal epithelium, loss of ciliated cells and metaplasia;
- the presence of a foreign body in the trachea stimulates mucous production; where no cilia are present, the mucociliary stream is therefore impeded;
- the increased mucus is more viscid and thick crusts may form and block the tube;
- although many patients with a tracheostomy can feed satisfactorily, there is some splinting of the larynx, which may prevent normal swallowing and lead to aspiration; this aspiration may be silent.

Postoperative treatment is designed to counteract these effects and frequent suction and humidification are most important. A trolley must be placed by the bed containing a tracheal dilator, duplicate tubes and introducers, retractors and dressings. Oxygen is at hand and, in the initial period, a nurse must be in constant attendance. Humidification will render the secretions less viscid and a sucker with a catheter attached should be on hand to keep the tracheobronchial tree free from secretions.

Summary box 47.11

Tracheostomy: postoperative management

- Suction – efficient, sterile and as often as required
- Humidification (with or without oxygen)
- A warm, well-ventilated room
- Position of the tube and patient
- Spare tube, introducer, tapes, tracheal dilator
- Change of tube, inner tube, possible speaking valve
- Physiotherapy
- Initiation of local decannulation protocols where indicated

Complications of tracheostomy

The intraoperative, early and late postoperative complications of tracheostomy are listed in Table 47.2.

TABLE 47.2 Tracheostomy: complications.

Intraoperative complications	Haemorrhage
	Injury to paratracheal structures, particularly the carotid artery, recurrent laryngeal nerve and oesophagus
	Damage to the trachea
Early postoperative complications	Apnoea caused by a fall in the PCO_2
	Haemorrhage
	Subcutaneous emphysema, pneumomediastinum and pneumothorax
	Accidental extubation, anterior displacement of the tube, obstruction of the tube lumen and tip occlusion against the tracheal wall
	Infection
	Swallowing dysfunction
Late postoperative complications	Difficult decannulation
	Tracheocutaneous fistula
	Tracheo-oesophageal fistula, tracheoinnominate artery fistula with severe haemorrhage
	Tracheal stenosis

OTHER EMERGENCY AIRWAY PROCEDURES

Fibreoptic endotracheal intubation

In most emergency situations, endotracheal intubation is the most direct and satisfactory method of securing the airway. Nasotracheal 'awake' intubation in expert hands is also a well-established technique and is particularly useful if the patient has trismus, severe mandibular injuries, cervical spine rigidity or an obstructing mass within the oral cavity. This is facilitated by passing a fibreoptic endoscope through the centre of an endotracheal tube, hence guiding it into the larynx and trachea under direct vision.

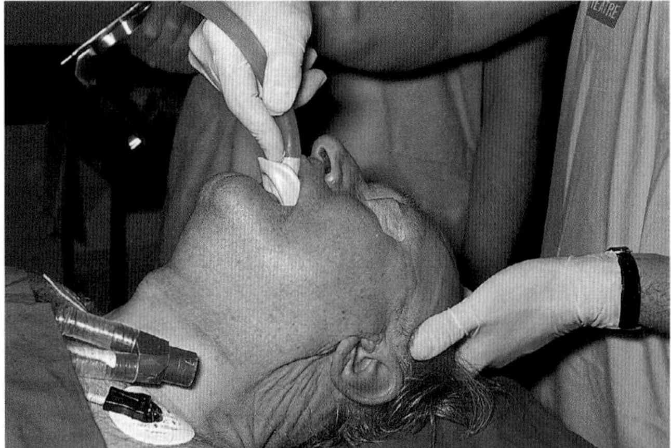

Figure 47.40 Laryngeal mask airway being inserted.

Laryngeal mask airway

The laryngeal mask airway (LMA) is a wide-bore airway with an inflatable cuff at the distal end, which forms a seal in the pharynx around the laryngeal inlet. Provided the laryngotracheal airway is clear, the LMA provides a clear and secure airway. The technique can easily be learnt by non-anaesthetists and secures an airway in most cases. It comes in a range of sizes covering infants to large adults. It is particularly useful in cases of difficult intubation where mouth opening is unimpeded (Figure 47.40).

Transtracheal ventilation

This technique is simple and effective and allows ventilation for periods in excess of 1 hour providing time to allow for more elective intubation. The cricothyroid membrane is located by palpation of the neck with the index finger, and a 14- or 16-gauge plastic sheathed intravascular needle and a 10 mL syringe containing a few millilitres of lidocaine are introduced in the midline and directed downwards and backwards into the tracheal lumen. The needle is advanced steadily and negative pressure is placed on the syringe until bubbles of air are clearly seen (Figure 47.41). The tissues of the neck may be infiltrated with the anaesthetic if desired and the tracheal mucosa likewise partly anaesthetised by the introduction of 1–2 mL after gaining the lumen. The needle is removed and the plastic sheath cannula remains in the tracheal lumen and must be carefully held and fixed in place by the operator so that it does not come out of the lumen into the soft tissues of the neck. It is attached by means of a Luer connection to the high-pressure oxygen supply. Ventilation may be undertaken in a controlled manner with a jetting device, with the chest being observed for appropriate movements.

If there is severe obstruction of the laryngopharynx by the foreign body or tumour, the exhaled outflow of gases can be

Luer was a German instrument maker who was working in Paris, France, at the end of the 19th century.

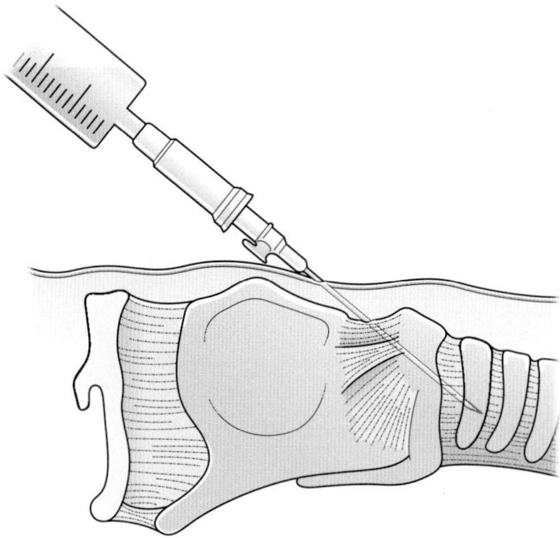

Figure 47.41 Transtracheal needle introduction.

aided by the placement of one or two further cannulas as exhalation ports. This procedure gains extremely rapid control of ventilation and requires a minimum of technical expertise. Its only notable complication is surgical emphysema of the neck tissues if the cannula dislodges from the tracheal lumen.

Cricothyroidotomy

Cricothyroidotomy has the advantages of speed and ease requiring minimal equipment and surgical expertise and has great value in the emergency setting when conditions are not optimal to perform a tracheostomy.

The patient's neck is extended and the area between the prominence of the thyroid cartilage and the cricoid cartilage below is palpated with the index finger of the free hand. In the emergency situation, a vertical skin incision is recommended with dissection rapidly carried down to the cricothyroid membrane. A 1 cm transverse incision is made through the membrane immediately above the cricoid cartilage and the scalpel twisted through a right angle to gain access to the airway. If available, an artery forceps, dilator or tracheal hook will improve the aperture and insertion of an available tube (Figures 47.42 and 47.43). As soon as practicably possible, the cricothyroidotomy should be converted to a tracheostomy. Although there is debate about the frequency of subglottic stenosis following this procedure, there is general agreement that it is much increased if any long-term ventilation is undertaken via even a modestly size tracheostomy tube through the cricothyroid membrane.

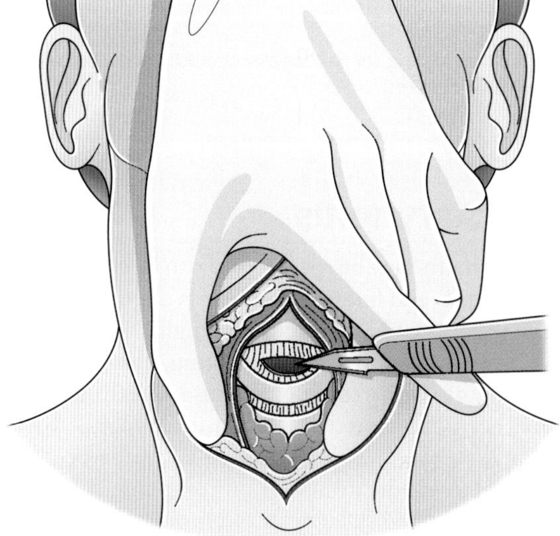

Figure 47.42 Incision in a cricothyroidotomy.

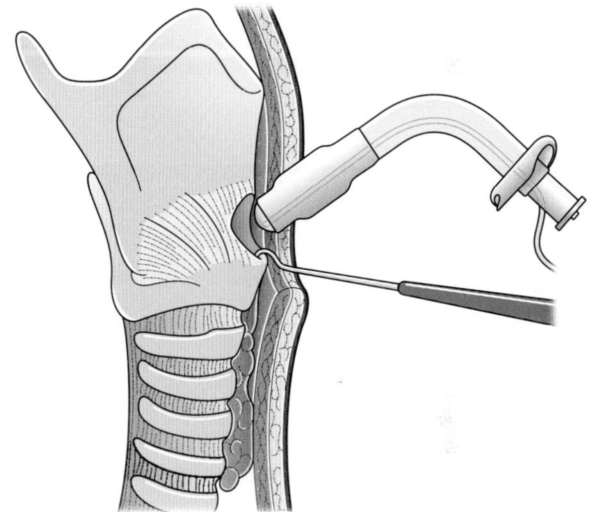

Figure 47.43 Insertion of a tube after cricothyroidotomy.

LARYNGEAL DISEASE CAUSING VOICE DISORDERS

Vocal nodules

These are fibrous thickenings of the vocal folds at the junction of the middle and anterior third (Figure 47.44) and result from vocal abuse; they are known as singers' nodules in adults and screamers' nodules in children. Speech therapy is therefore the preferred treatment and the lesions will resolve spontaneously in most cases. Occasionally, the nodules will need to be surgically removed using modern microlaryngoscopic dissection or laser techniques, but speech therapy will still be required for postoperative voice rehabilitation.

Vocal fold polyps

These are usually unilateral and may be associated with an acute infective episode, cigarette smoking or vocal abuse (Figure 47.45). Speech therapy is again indicated, but they do usually require removal by microdissection or laser surgery.

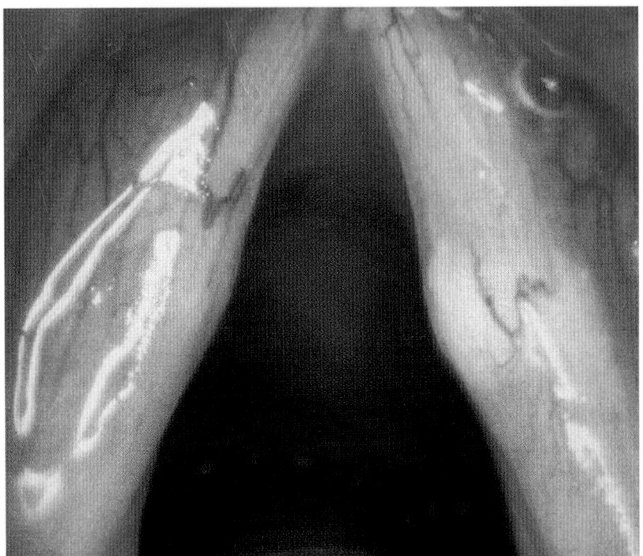

Figure 47.44 Vocal fold nodules.

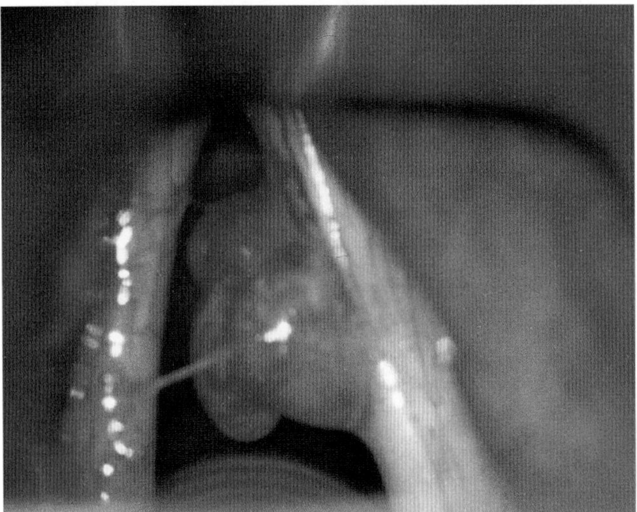

Figure 47.45 A vocal fold polyp.

Summary box 47.12

Causes of hoarseness

- Mucosal disease (e.g. vocal nodule, polyps or laryngeal papillomatosis, acute or chronic laryngitis)
- Neurological disease (e.g. vocal fold palsy)
- Neoplasia (e.g. laryngeal tumours)
- Non-specific voice disorders, functional dysphonia

Laryngeal papillomata

These are rare benign tumours occurring mainly in children, but can also present in adults. They are most commonly found on the vocal folds, but may spread throughout the larynx and tracheobronchial airway (although this is less likely in adults) (Figure 47.46). They are caused by papillomaviruses and need repeated removal by carbon dioxide laser or microsurgery to maintain a reasonable voice and airway. These patients are best managed in specialist centres, with the appropriate expertise. Antiviral treatment is of doubtful value. Papilloma vaccination is, to date, of unproven benefit.

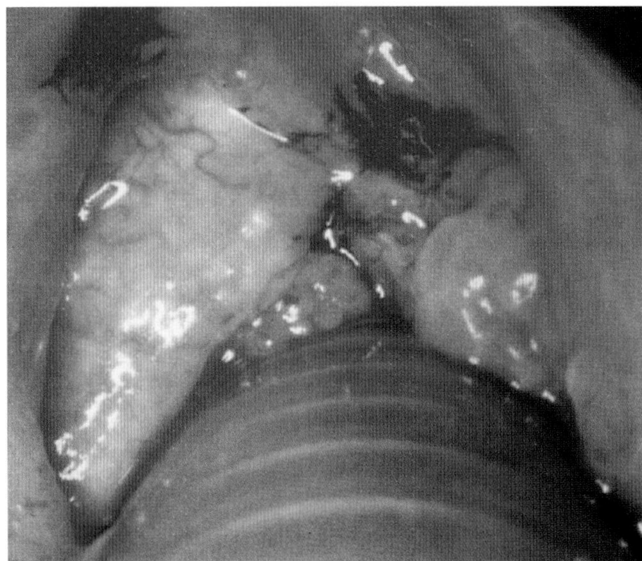

Figure 47.46 Laryngeal papillomata.

Acute laryngitis

This often occurs as part of an upper respiratory tract infection in association with a cough and pharyngitis. Usually viral, it may be localised to the larynx and it settles quickly if the voice is rested during the acute inflammation. Steam inhalations are soothing along with mild analgesia, but antibiotics are unnecessary.

Summary box 47.13

Warning

- Hoarseness lasting for 3–4 weeks should always be referred for an ENT opinion

Chronic laryngitis

Chronic laryngitis may be specific and can be caused by mycobacteria, syphilis and fungi. Treatment is directed towards the causative organism. Non-specific laryngitis is common, the main predisposing factors being smoking, chronic upper and lower respiratory sepsis and voice abuse. Gastro-oesophageal reflux has been implicated as a factor in laryngitis, vocal fold nodules and polyps, but the evidence is controversial. However, anti-reflux medication and proton pump inhibitors are commonly prescribed. Diagnosis of chronic laryngitis should not be made unless the larynx has been fully evaluated by a laryngologist.

Vocal fold palsy

This may be unilateral or bilateral (Figure 47.47). Unilateral cord palsy is most commonly idiopathic. In non-idiopathic cases, left vocal fold palsy is most common because of the long intrathoracic course of the left recurrent laryngeal nerve, which arches around the aorta and may be commonly involved in inflammatory and neoplastic conditions involving the left hilum or lung apex. Lung cancer should be considered the cause of a left vocal palsy until proved otherwise.

Tumours of the nasopharynx, larynx, thyroid gland or oesophagus may also cause vocal cord palsy. Bilateral vocal fold paralysis is uncommon and tends to occur after thyroid surgery or head injuries.

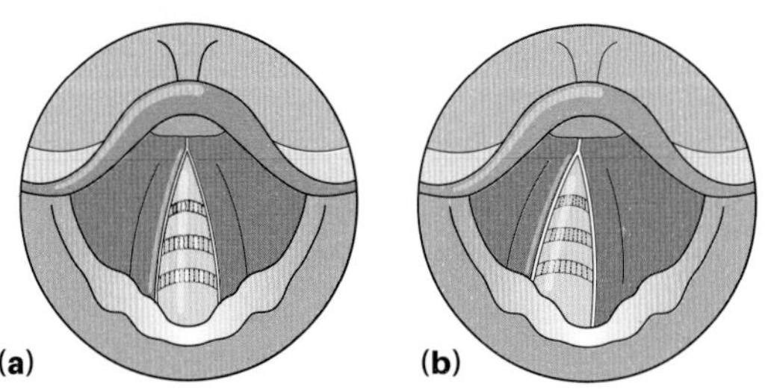

Figure 47.47 Vocal fold positions: (a) normal; (b) unilateral vocal fold palsy.

> **Summary box 47.14**
>
> Causes of vocal fold palsy
>
> **Congenital (infants)**
>
> **Acquired**
> - Traumatic
>   - Direct to neck
>   - Post-surgical (e.g. thyroidectomy)
> - Infective
>   - Viral (rare)
> - Neoplastic
>   - Carcinoma of the lung involving the left hilum
>   - Carcinoma of the nasopharynx, larynx, thyroid and oesophagus
> - Vascular
>   - Aortic aneurysm
> - Neurological
>   - Lower motor neurone disease

Clinical features

Unilateral recurrent laryngeal nerve palsy of sudden onset produces hoarseness, difficulty in swallowing liquids and a weakened cough. These symptoms may be short-lived and the voice may return to normal within a few weeks as the muscles in the opposite vocal fold compensate and move it across the midline to meet the paralysed vocal fold, which usually lies in the paramedian position. Bilateral recurrent laryngeal nerve palsy is an occasional and serious complication of total thyroidectomy. On anaesthetic reversal, acute dyspnoea occurs as a result of the paramedian position of both vocal folds, which reduce the airway to 2–3 mm and which tend to get sucked together on inspiration. In severe cases, tracheostomy or intubation is necessary immediately, otherwise death occurs from asphyxia.

Investigation of vocal fold paralysis is by a CT scan from the skull base (including posterior fossa) to the diaphragm. Approximately 20–25% of vocal fold paralysis occurs without known pathology and spontaneous recovery may occur. When compensation does not occur, a unilateral paralysed fold may be medialised by injection or external thyroplasty.

In bilateral vocal fold palsy, surgery may be carried out to remove a portion of the posterior aspect of one vocal fold or a portion of one arytenoid cartilage. These procedures are most easily performed endoscopically with a carbon dioxide laser. They increase the size of the posterior glottic airway, allowing the patient to be decannulated or even avoid an initial tracheostomy.

Tumours of the larynx

Benign tumours of the larynx are extremely rare. Squamous cell carcinoma is the most common malignant tumour, being responsible for more than 90% of tumours within the larynx. It is the second most common head and neck cancer (oral cavity is more common) and previously usually occurred in elderly male smokers. However, over the past decades, the incidence among women has risen as a consequence of increased smoking habits. The incidence of laryngeal cancer in the three compartments, supraglottis, glottis and subglottis, varies around the world. The glottis is generally the most common site for cancer in patients in the UK, followed by the supraglottis (Figure 47.48).

Clinical features

Patients typically present with voice change. If an early diagnosis can be made (i.e. confined to one vocal fold), treatment with radiotherapy or carbon dioxide laser excision is associated with a 5-year disease-free survival of approximately 90%. This rate drops dramatically once the lymphatically rich supraglottis or subglottis is involved because of spread to neck nodes. Tumour spread to just one neck gland reduces by half the overall prognosis for the patient.

Investigations

Direct laryngoscopy, preferably a microlaryngoscopy, together with angled (30° and 70°) Hopkins' rod examination, allows precise determination of the extent of the tumour and biopsy confirms the histology. CT and MRI give further details of the extent of larger tumours, demonstrating spread outside the larynx and suspicious nodal involvement within the neck, which may not be obvious clinically. The tumour–node–metastasis (TNM) classification of laryngeal cancer is given in *Table 47.3*.

Treatment

EARLY LARYNGEAL CANCER (T1 AND T2)

Early stage supraglottic and glottic tumours are optimally treated with either radiotherapy or endoscopic surgical

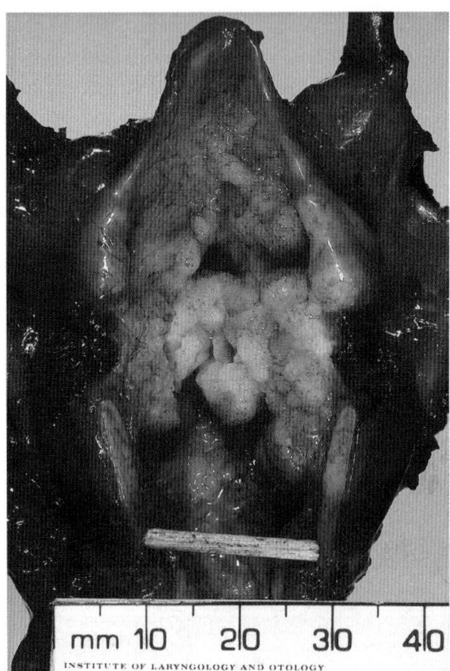

Figure 47.48 A total laryngectomy specimen with a transglottic tumour.

resection, with the aim of preservation of some function. Although both modalities are associated with similar survival rates, transoral laser resection is commonly used as it usually involves day case surgery and more therapeutic options are available for the small mumber of patients who suffer local recurrence.

ADVANCED LARYNGEAL CANCER (T3 AND T4)

Organ preservation should be a priority when treating T3 larynx cancer. The non-surgical standard of care is concurrent chemoradiotherapy, while a variety of open partial laryngectomy procedures are also available but these are best undertaken in specialist centres.

T4 disease is usually best treated with total laryngectomy and adjuvant postoperative radiotherapy or chemoradiotherapy.

After the larynx has been removed, the remaining trachea is brought out onto the lower neck as a permanent tracheal stoma and the hypopharynx, which is opened at the time of the operation, is closed to restore continuity for swallowing (Figure 47.49). Thus the upper aero- and digestive tracts are permanently disconnected. Part or all of the thyroid gland and associated parathyroid glands may also be removed, depending on the extent of the disease.

Vocal rehabilitation

The loss of the larynx as a generator of sound does not prevent patients speaking as long as an alternative source of sound can be created by vibration in the pharynx. This can be achieved in one of three ways:

1 A small one-way valve may be inserted through the back wall of the tracheal stoma into the pharynx (Figure 47.50). This allows air from the trachea to pass into

TABLE 47.3 Tumour–node–metastasis (TNM) classification of laryngeal carcinoma.

T – primary tumour

- TX Primary tumour cannot be assessed
- T0 No evidence of primary tumour
- Tis Carcinoma in situ
- Supraglottis
  - TI Tumour limited to one subsite of supraglottis, with normal vocal fold mobility
  - T2 Tumour invades more than one subsite of supraglottis, with normal vocal fold mobility
  - T3 Tumour limited to larynx with vocal fold fixation and/or invades post-cricoid area, medial wall of piriform sinus or pre-epiglottic tissues
  - T4 Tumour invades through cartilage and/or extends to other tissues beyond the larynx (e.g. to oropharynx, soft tissues of neck)
- Glottis
  - T1 Tumour limited to vocal fold(s) (may involve anterior or posterior commissures) with normal mobility
  - T1a Tumour limited to one vocal fold
  - T1b Tumour involves both vocal folds
  - T2 Tumour extends to supraglottis and/or subglottis, and/or with impaired vocal fold mobility
  - T3 Tumour limited to the larynx with vocal fold fixation
  - T4 Tumour invades through thyroid cartilage and/or extends to other tissues beyond the larynx (e.g. to oropharynx, soft tissues of the neck)
- Subglottis
  - T1 Tumour limited to the subglottis
  - T2 Tumour extends to vocal fold(s) with normal or impaired mobility
  - T3 Tumour limited to the larynx with vocal fixation
  - T4 Tumour invades through thyroid cartilage and/or extends to other tissues beyond the larynx (e.g. to oropharynx, soft tissues of the neck)

N – regional lymph nodes

- N0 No regional lymph node metastases
- N1 Metastasis in a single ipsilateral lymph node 3 cm or less in greatest diameter
- N2 Metastasis in a single ipsilateral lymph node more than 3 cm or in multiple ipsilateral nodes or in bilateral or contralateral nodes

M – distant metastasis

Stage grouping

Stage 0	Tis	N0	M0
Stage I	T1	N0	M0
Stage II	T2	N0	M0
Stage III	T1	N1	M0
	T2	N1	M0
	T3	N0, N1	M0
Stage IV	T4	N0, N1	M0
	Any T	N2, N3	M0
	Any T	Any N	M1

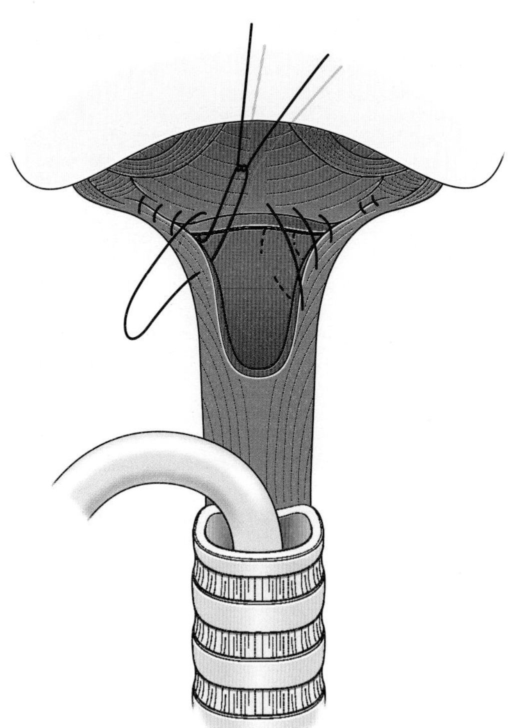

Figure 47.49 Transverse closure of the pharynx with an endotracheal tube in the end tracheostome.

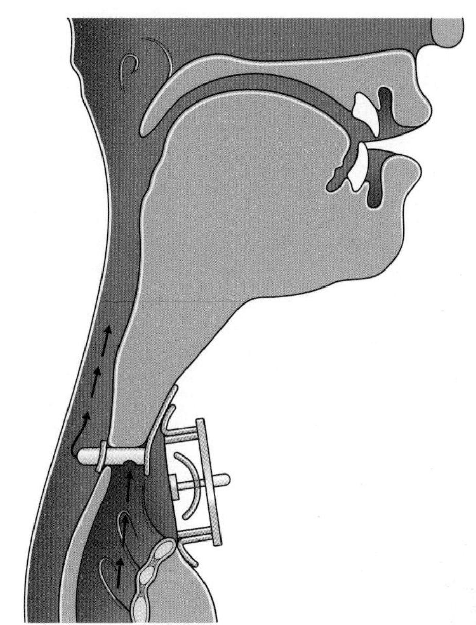

Figure 47.50 A Blom–Singer valve with a tracheo-oesophageal fistula and an outer stoma valve.

the pharynx, but does not allow food and liquid to pass into the airway. These valves must not be confused with tracheostomy tubes. Like all foreign bodies, the speaking valves are associated with minor complications, such as the formation of granulations, bleeding or leakage of pharyngeal contents, and have an ongoing financial cost due to the need for regular replacement.

2 An external battery-powered vibrating device when applied to the soft tissues of the neck produces sound, which is turned into speech by the vocal tract comprising the tongue, pharynx, oral cavity, lips, teeth and nasal sinuses.
3 Oesophageal speech when air is swallowed into the pharynx and upper oesophagus. On regurgitating the air, a segment of the pharyngo-oesophageal mucosa vibrates to produce sound, which is modified by the vocal tract into speech (Figure 47.51).

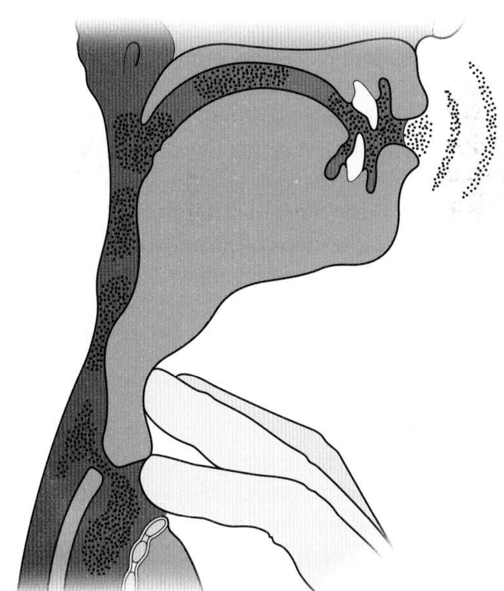

Figure 47.51 Production of oesophageal speech.

DISEASES OF THE NECK

LUMP IN THE NECK

On presentation, a careful history and examination is essential. The clinical signs of size, site, shape, consistency, fixation to skin or deep structures, pulsation, compressibility, transillumination or the presence of a bruit must be established and recorded.

Branchial cyst

A branchial cyst develops from the vestigial remnants of the second branchial cleft, is lined by squamous epithelium and contains thick, turbid fluid. The cyst usually presents in the upper neck in early or middle adulthood and is found at the junction of the upper third and middle third of the sternomastoid muscle at its anterior border. It is a fluctuant swelling that may transilluminate and is often soft in its early stages so that it may be difficult to palpate.

Summary box 47.15

Diagnosis of a lump in the neck

History

Physical signs

- Size
- Site
- Shape
- Surface
- Consistency
- Fixation: deep/superficial
- Pulsatility
- Compressibility
- Transillumination
- Bruit

If the cyst becomes infected, it becomes erythematous and tender and the differential diagnosis is broadened. Ultrasound and fine-needle aspiration both aid diagnosis and treatment is by complete excision, which is best undertaken when the lesion is quiescent. Although the anterior aspect of the cyst is easy to dissect, it may pass backwards and upwards through the bifurcation of the common carotid artery as far as the pharyngeal constrictors. It passes superficial to the hypoglossal and glossopharyngeal nerves, but deep to the posterior belly of the digastric. These structures and the spinal accessory nerve must be positively identified to avoid damage. In patients over 40 years of age, a high index of suspicion for a necrotic metastatic lymph should exists and malignancy should be excluded before excision.

Branchial fistula

A branchial fistula (Figure 47.52) may be unilateral or bilateral and is thought to represent a persistent second branchial cleft. The external orifice is nearly always situated in the lower third of the neck near the anterior border of the sternocleidomastoid, while the internal orifice is located on the anterior aspect of the posterior faucial pillar just behind the tonsil. The internal aspect of the tract may, however, end blindly at or close to the lateral pharyngeal wall, constituting a sinus rather than a fistula. The tract is lined by ciliated columnar epithelium and, as such, there may be a small amount of recurrent mucopurulent discharge onto the neck. The tract follows the same path as a branchial cyst and requires complete excision to avoid recurrence.

Cystic hygroma

Cystic hygromas (Figure 47.53) usually present in the neonate or in early infancy, and occasionally may present at birth and be so large as to obstruct labour. The cysts are filled with clear lymph and lined by a single layer of epithelium with a mosaic appearance. Swelling usually occurs in the neck and may involve the parotid, submandibular, tongue and floor of

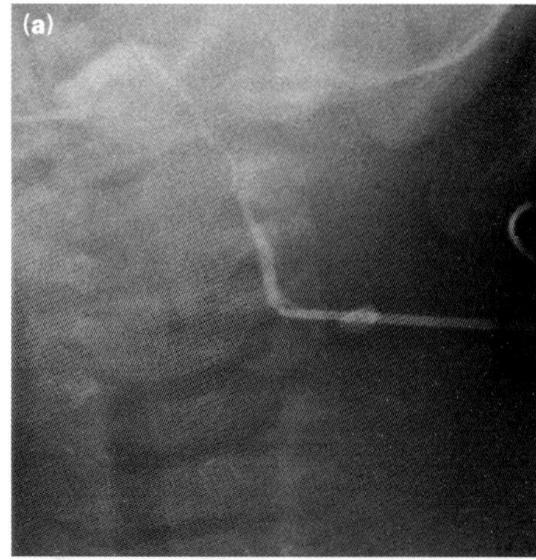

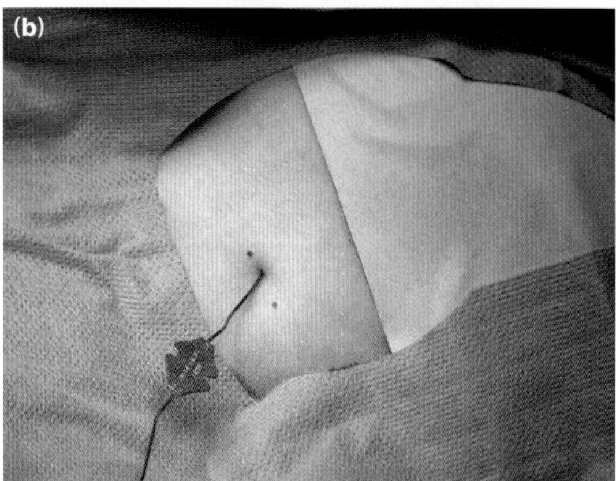

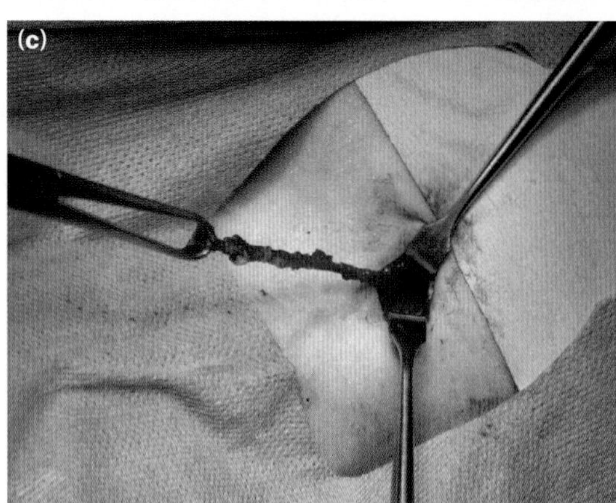

Figure 47.52 (a) Plain radiograph with radiopaque dye in the fistula tract. (b) Probing of the fistula tract. (c) Excision of the fistula tract.

mouth areas. The swelling may be bilateral and is soft and partially compressible, visibly increasing in size when the child coughs or cries. The characteristic that distinguishes it from all other neck swellings is that it is brilliantly translucent. The cheek, axilla, groin and mediastinum are other less frequent sites for a cystic hygroma.

The behaviour of cystic hygromas during infancy is unpredictable. Sometimes the cyst expands rapidly and occasionally respiratory difficulty ensues, requiring immediate aspiration and even occasionally a tracheostomy. The cyst may become infected.

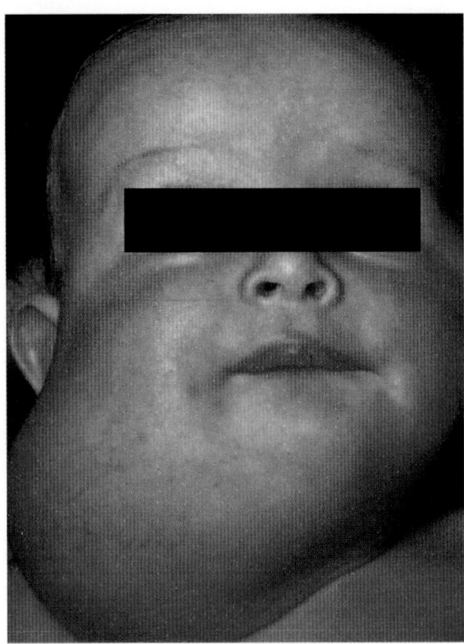

Figure 47.53 Cystic hygroma.

Definitive treatment involving complete excision of the cyst at an early stage is best if possible. Injection of a sclerosing agent is an alternative strategy and may reduce the size of the cyst; however, they are commonly multicystic and therefore complete resolution is a challenge.

Thyroglossal duct cysts

Embryology

The thyroid gland descends early in fetal life from the base of the tongue towards its position in the lower neck with the isthmus lying over the second and third tracheal rings. At the time of its descent, the hyoid bone has not been formed and the track of the descent of the thyroid gland is variable, passing in front, through or behind the eventual position of the hyoid body. Thyroglossal duct cysts represent a persistence of this track and may therefore be found anywhere in or adjacent to the midline from the tongue base to the thyroid isthmus. Rarely, a thyroglossal cyst may contain the only functioning thyroid tissue in the body.

Clinical features

The cysts almost always arise in the midline but, when they are adjacent to the thyroid cartilage, they may lie slightly to one side of the midline. Classically, the cyst moves upwards on swallowing and with tongue protrusion, but this can also occur with other midline cysts such as dermoid cysts, as it merely indicates attachment to the hyoid bone.

Thyroglossal cysts may become infected and rupture onto the skin of the neck presenting as a discharging sinus. Although they often occur in children, they may also present in adults, even as late as the sixth or seventh decade of life (Figure 47.54).

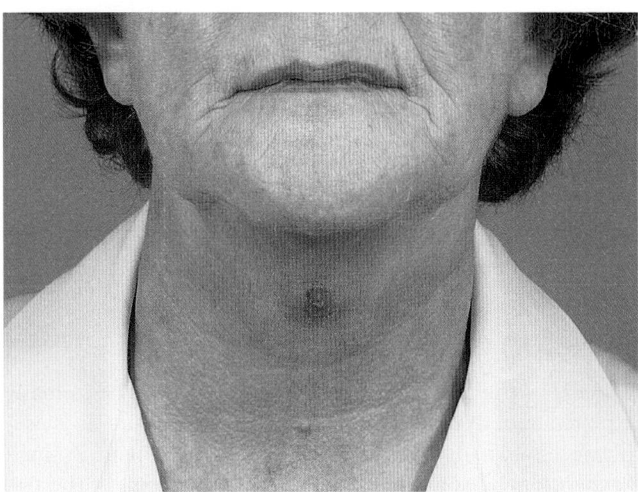

Figure 47.54 A patient with a thyroglossal fistula from a cyst in the midline of the neck.

Treatment

Treatment must include excision of the whole thyroglossal tract, which involves removal of the body of the hyoid bone and the suprahyoid tract through the tongue base to the vallecula at the site of the primitive foramen caecum, together with a core of tissue on either side. This operation is known as Sistrunk's operation and prevents recurrence, most notably from small side branches of the thyroglossal tract.

TRAUMA TO THE NECK

Wounds above the hyoid bone

The cavity of the mouth or pharynx may have been entered and the epiglottis may be divided via the pre-epiglottic space. These wounds require repair with absorbable sutures on a formal basis under a general anaesthetic. If there is any degree of associated oedema or bleeding, particularly in relation to the tongue base or laryngeal inlet, it is advisable to perform a tracheostomy to avoid any subsequent respiratory distress.

Wounds of the thyroid and cricoid cartilage

Blunt crushing injuries or severe laceration injuries to the laryngeal skeleton can cause marked haematoma formation or swelling and rapid loss of the airway. There may be significant disruption of the laryngeal skeleton. These patients should not have an endotracheal intubation for any length of time, even if this is the initial emergency way of protecting the airway. The larynx is a delicate three-tiered sphincter and the presence of a foreign body in its lumen after severe disruption gives rise to major fibrosis and loss of laryngeal function. These injuries are frequently require a low tracheostomy, following

Walter Ellis Sistrunk, Jr., 1880–1933, Professor of Clinical Surgery, Baylor University College of Medicine, Dallas, TX, USA.

which the larynx can be carefully explored, damaged cartilages repositioned and sutured or plated, and the paraglottic space drained.

An indwelling stent of soft sponge shaped to fit the laryngeal lumen and held by a nylon retaining suture through the neck may be left in place for 5–10 days to minimise webbing. This stent can be removed endoscopically after cutting the retaining suture and, as the laryngeal damage heals, the patient may then be decannulated.

Division of the trachea

Wounds of the trachea are rare. They should all be formally explored and, in order to obtain adequate exposure, it is usually necessary to divide and ligate the thyroid isthmus. A small tracheostomy below the wound followed by repair of the trachea with a limited number of submucosal sutures is appropriate. In self-inflicted wounds, the recurrent laryngeal nerves, which lie protected in the tracheo-oesophageal grooves, are rarely injured. Primary repair of the nerve is rarely possible but may be undertaken at the time of formal exploration of a major neck wound.

Neurovascular injury

Penetrating wounds of the neck may involve the common carotid or the external or internal carotid arteries. Major haemorrhagic shock may occur. Venous air embolism may occur as a result of damage to one of the major veins, most commonly the internal jugular. Compression, resuscitation and exploration under general anaesthetic, with control of vessels above and below the injury and primary repair, should be undertaken. All cervical nerves are vulnerable to injury, particularly the vagus and recurrent laryngeal nerves and cervical sympathetic chain.

Thoracic duct injury

Wounds to the thoracic duct are usually iatrogenic and usually left sided, occurring when lymph node level IV is dissected during a neck dissection. When damage to the duct is not recognised at the time of operation, chyle may subsequently leak from the wound in amounts up to 2 litres per day with profound effects on nutrition.

Treatment

Should the damage be recognised during an operation, the proximal end of the duct must be ligated. Ligation of the duct is not harmful because there are a number of anastomotic channels between the lymphatic and venous system in the lower neck. If undetected, chyle usually starts to discharge from the neck wound within 24 hours of the operation. On occasion, firm pressure by a pad to the lower neck may stop the leakage, but frequently this is unsuccessful and the wound should be re-explored and the damaged duct ligated.

INFLAMMATORY CONDITIONS OF THE NECK

Ludwig's angina

Ludwig described a clinical entity characterised by a brawny swelling of the submandibular region combined with inflammatory oedema of the mouth. These clinical features, as well as accompanying putrid halitosis define the condition.

The infection is often caused by a virulent streptococcal infection associated with anaerobic organisms. There may also be an underlying oral cavity cancer. The infection tracks deep to the mylohyoid muscle causing oedema and inflammation such that the tongue is displaced upwards and backwards, giving rise to dysphagia and subsequently to painful obstruction of the airway. Unless treated, cellulitis may extend beneath the deep fascial layers of the neck to involve the larynx, causing glottic oedema and further airway compromise.

Antibiotic therapy should be instituted as soon as possible using intravenous broad-spectrum antibiotics, with anaerobic cover. If the swelling does not subside rapidly with such treatment, or in advanced cases where pus is evident, a curved submental incision may be used to drain both submandibular triangles. The mylohyoid muscle may be incised to decompress the floor of the mouth and corrugated drains placed in the wound, which is then lightly sutured. This operation may be conducted under local anaesthetic. Rarely, a tracheostomy may be necessary.

Cervical lymphadenitis

Cervical lymphadenitis is common due to infection or inflammation in the oral and nasal cavities, pharynx, larynx, ear, scalp and face.

Acute lymphadenitis

The affected lymph nodes are enlarged and tender, and there may be varying degrees of general constitutional disturbance such as pyrexia, anorexia and general malaise. The treatment in the first instance is directed to the primary focus of infection, for example tonsillitis or a dental abscess.

Chronic lymphadenitis

Chronic, painless lymphadenopathy may be caused by tuberculosis in young children or adults, or be secondary to malignant disease, most commonly from a squamous cell carcinoma in older individuals. Lymphoma and/or HIV infection may also present in the cervical nodes.

Wilhelm Friedrich von Ludwig, 1790–1865, Professor of Surgery and Midwifery, Tubingen, Germany

Summary box 47.16

Causes of cervical lymphadenopathy

Inflammatory
- Reactive hyperplasia

Infective
- Viral
  For example, infectious mononucleosis, HIV
- Bacterial
  Streptococcus, Staphylococcus
  Actinomycosis
  Tuberculosis
  Brucellosis
- Protozoan
  Toxoplasmosis

Neoplastic
- Malignant
  Primary (e.g. lymphoma)
  Secondary (e.g. squamous cell carcinoma)
  Known primary
  Occult primary

Tuberculous adenitis

This condition most commonly affects children or young adults, but can occur at any age. The deep upper cervical nodes are most commonly affected, but there may be a widespread cervical lymphadenitis with matted nodes. In most cases, the tubercular bacilli gain entrance through the ipsilateral tonsil. In approximately 80% of patients, the tuberculous process is limited to the clinically affected group of lymph nodes, but a primary focus in the lungs must always be suspected.

As renal and pulmonary tuberculosis (TB) occasionally co-exist, the urine should be examined carefully. Rarely, the patient may develop a natural resistance to the infection and the nodes may be detected at a later date as evidenced by calcification on radiography. This can also be seen after appropriate general treatment of tuberculosis adenitis. If treatment is not instituted, the caseated node may liquefy and break down with the formation of a cold abscess in the neck. The pus is initially confined by the deep cervical fascia, but after weeks or months, this may become eroded at one point and the pus flows through the small opening into the space beneath the superficial fascia. The process has now reached the well-known stage of a 'collar-stud' abscess. The superficial abscess enlarges steadily and, unless suitably treated, a discharging sinus results.

Investigation

Fine-needle aspirate taken from neck nodes with a suspicion of TB should be tested for presence of acid-fast bacilli. Systemic investigation should not be neglected, with chest x-ray and Mantoux testing useful first line investigations. Depending on country of origin, where TB is diagnosed or suspected, the co-existence of other infectious diseases such as HIV and malaria should not be overlooked.

Treatment

The patient should be treated using appropriate chemotherapy, dependent on the sensitivities derived from the abscess contents. If an abscess fails to resolve despite appropriate chemotherapy and general measures, occasionally excision of the abscess and its surrounding fibrous capsule is necessary, together with the relevant lymph nodes. If there is active tuberculosis of another system, for example pulmonary TB, then removal of tuberculous lymph nodes in the neck is inappropriate. The matted nodes are associated with significant fibrosis making surgery difficult to the extent that the sacrifice of adjacent structures such and the internal jugular vein or sternocleidomastoid muscle may be necessary. The resected nodes should be sent for both histology and microbiology.

PRIMARY TUMOURS OF THE NECK

Neurogenic tumours

Chemodectoma (carotid body tumour)

This is a rare tumour that has a higher incidence in areas where people live at high altitudes because of chronic hypoxia leading to carotid body hyperplasia. The tumours most commonly present in the fifth decade and approximately 10% of patients have a family history. There is an association with phaeochromocytoma. The tumours arise from the chemoreceptor cells on the medial side of the carotid bulb and, at this point, the tumour is adherent to the carotid wall. The cells of the chemodectoma are not hormonally active and the tumours are usually benign with only a small number of cases producing proven metastases (Figure 47.55).

CLINICAL FEATURES

There is often a long history of a slowly enlarging, painless lump at the carotid bifurcation. About one-third of patients present with a pharyngeal mass that pushes the tonsil medially and anteriorly. The mass is firm, rubbery, pulsatile, mobile from side to side but not up and down, and can sometimes be emptied by firm pressure, after which it slowly refills in a pulsatile manner. A bruit may also be present. Swellings in the parapharyngeal space, which often displace the tonsil medially, should not be biopsied from within the mouth.

INVESTIGATIONS

When a chemodectoma is suspected, a carotid angiogram can be carried out to demonstrate the carotid bifurcation, which is usually splayed, and a blush, which outlines the tumour vessels. MRI scanning also provides excellent detail in most cases. This tumour must not be biopsied and fine-needle aspiration is also contraindicated.

TREATMENT

Because these tumours rarely metastasise and their overall rate of growth is slow, the need for surgical removal must be considered carefully as complications of surgery are potentially serious. The operation is best avoided in elderly patients. Radiotherapy has no effect. In some cases it may be possible

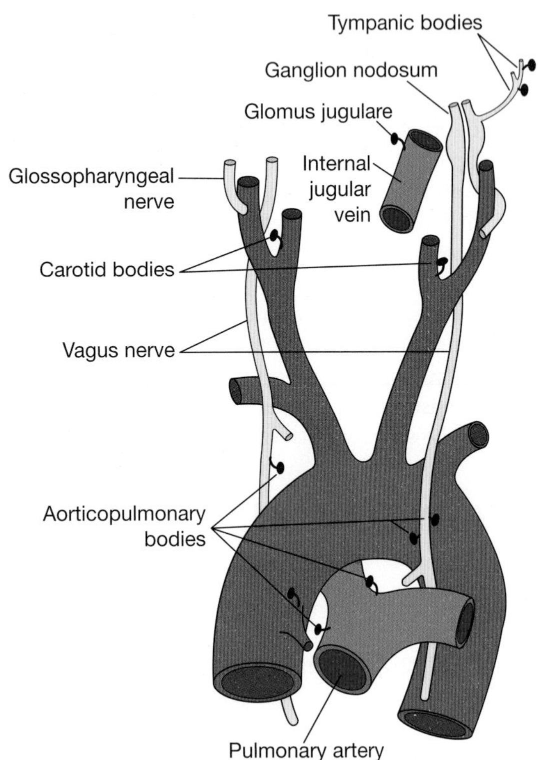

Figure 47.55 Sites for chemodectomas.

to dissect the tumour away from the carotid bifurcation but, at times, when the tumour is large, it may not be separable from the vessels and resection will be necessary, such that all appropriate facilities should be available to establish a bypass while a vein autograph is inserted to restore arterial continuity in the carotid system.

Vagal body tumours

Vagal paragangliomas arise from nests of paraganglionic tissue of the vagus nerve just below the base of the skull near the jugular foramen. They may also be found at various sites along the nerve down to the level of the carotid artery bifurcation. They also present as slowly growing and painless masses in the anterolateral aspect of the neck, and may also have a long history, commonly of 2–3 years, before diagnosis. They may spread into the cranial cavity. Diagnosis is confirmed by CT and MRI scanning and additional MR angiogram or arteriography if necessary. Treatment is surgical excision following appropriate consent of resulting hoarseness.

Peripheral nerve tumours

Schwannomas are solitary and encapsulated tumours attached to or surrounded by nerve, although paralysis of the associated nerve is unusual. The vagus nerve is the most common site. Neurofibromas also arise from the Schwann cell and may be part of von Recklinghausen's syndrome of multiple neurofibromatosis. Multiple neurofibromatosis is an autosomal dominant, hereditary disease and the neurofibromas may be present at birth and often multiple.

Diagnosis requires CT or MRI scanning to differentiate them from other parapharyngeal tumours but, on occasions, the diagnosis must wait until excision.

Secondary carcinoma

Metastatic spread of squamous cell carcinoma to the cervical lymph nodes is a common occurrence from head and neck primary cancers and may be the presenting feature of the disease. The nasopharynx, tonsil, tongue, piriform fossa and supraglottic larynx must be carefully examined by panendoscopy for the primary growth before considering biopsy or any surgery on the neck. Investigation is further assisted by ultrasound and fine needle aspirate of the neck node.

Management

The management of malignant cervical lymph nodes depends on the overall treatment regime:

- if surgery is being used to treat the primary disease and the cervical nodes are palpable and >3 cm, they may be excised with the primary lesion as part of a neck dissection;
- if radiotherapy or chemoradiotherapy is used initially with resolution of the primary tumour, but there is subsequent residual or recurrent nodal disease, then this situation will require cervical lymph node dissection.

Type of neck dissection

CLASSICAL RADICAL NECK DISSECTION (CRILE)

The classic operation involves resection of the cervical lymphatics and lymph nodes and those structures closely associated: the internal jugular vein, the accessory nerve, the submandibular gland and the sternocleidomastoid muscle. These structures are all removed *en bloc* and in continuity with the primary disease if possible. The main disability that follows the operation is weakness and drooping of the shoulder due to paralysis of the trapezius muscle as a consequence of excision of the accessory nerve.

Friedrich Theodor Schwann, 1810–1882, Professor of Anatomy and Physiology, successively at Louvain (1839–1848) and Liege (1848–1880), Belgium, described the neurilemma in 1839.
Friedrich Daniel von Recklinghausen, 1833–1910, Professor of Pathology, Strasbourg, France, described generalised neurofibromatosis in 1882.
George Washington Crile, 1864–1943, Professor of Surgery, The Western Reserve University, and one of the founders of the Cleveland Clinic, Cleveland, OH, USA.

MODIFIED RADICAL NECK DISSECTION

In selected cases, one or more of the three following structures are preserved: the accessory nerve, the sternocleidomastoid muscle or the internal jugular vein. Otherwise, all major lymph node groups and lymphatics are excised. Careful note should be made of whichever structures are preserved.

SELECTIVE NECK DISSECTION

In this type of dissection, one or more of the major lymph node groups is preserved along with the sternocleidomastoid muscle, accessory nerve and internal jugular vein. In these circumstances, the exact groups of nodes excised must be documented.

SUMMARY

The anatomical and physiological performance of the pharyngolarynx is involved in the important mechanisms of breathing, coughing, voice production and swallowing. A variety of congenital, traumatic, infectious and neoplastic conditions disturb these functions, giving rise to the common symptoms of pain, swelling, hoarseness, dyspnoea and dysphagia.

Squamous cell carcinomas are the most common malignancies, accounting for approximately 80% of all head and neck tumours. Their incidence and anatomical site vary around the world, but they are mainly caused by the preventable aetiological agents of smoking and alcohol, although nasopharyngeal and oropharyngeal squamous carcinomas have additional genetic and environmental factors. All head and neck cancers have a high morbidity and mortality, and require expert treatment.

FURTHER READING

Bull P, Clarke R. *Diseases of the ear, nose and throat*. Oxford; Blackwell, 2007.

Dhillon R, East C. *Nose and throat, head and neck surgery*, 4th edn. Amsterdam: Elsevier, 2013.

Gleeson MJ, Clarke R. (eds) *Scott Brown's otolaryngology: head and neck surgery*, 7th edn. London: Hodder & Arnold, 2008.

Lau A, Jacques T, Tandon S, Lesser T. *Evidence-based emergency ENT care*. Createspace, 2015.

Probst R, Grevers G, Iro H. *Basic otorhinolaryngology*. Stuggart: Georg Thieme, 2006.

Wackym PA, Snow JB (eds). *Ballenger's otorhinolaryngology head and neck surgery*, 18th edn. Raleigh, NC: PMPH, 2016.

Watkinson J, Gilbert RW (eds) *Stell & Maran's textbook of head and neck surgery and oncology*, 5th edn. London: Hodder & Arnold, 2012.

Chapter 48

Oral cavity malignancy

Learning objectives

To understand:

- The relationship between oral (pre)malignancy and the use of alcohol and tobacco
- The cardinal features of premalignant and malignant lesions of the oral cavity
- The investigation and treatment of these patients

INTRODUCTION

Globally, oral cancer remains a relatively uncommon disease, accounting for only 1.5% of all malignant tumours; however, there remains wide diparities in the burden of disease in specific geographic areas, such as the Indian subcontinent. Current evidence suggests that the incidence of oral cavity cancer is increasing; however, these increases are overshadowed by the rapid change in oropharyngeal cancer incidence.

EPIDEMIOLOGY

The principal aetiological agents are tobacco and alcohol. In Europe and North America this is mainly through cigarette smoking combined with alcohol abuse. Synergism between alcohol abuse and tobacco use in the development of squamous cell carcinoma (SCC) of the head and neck is well established. While the human papillomavirus (HPV; specifically HPV16) is playing a significant role in the increasing incidence of oropharyngeal cancer in resource-rich nations, its role in the oral cavity appears to be limited (<5% of incident tumours being HPV positive) and without clear relevance to outcomes. Risk factors associated with cancer of the oral cavity are outlined in *Summary box 48.1*.

In the Indian subcontinent, the use of 'pan' (a combination of betel nut, areca nut, lime and tobacco) as well as reverse smoking (smoking a cheroot with the burning end inside the mouth) are responsible for the high incidence of oral cancer. Betel quid appears to be the major carcinogen, although there is also a relationship between slaked lime and the areca nut and cancer.

Summary box 48.1

Risk factors associated with cancer of the head and neck

- Tobacco
- Alcohol
- Areca nut/pan masala

Poor nutrition

- Inherited conditions (inc. Fanconi anaemia, Li-Fraumeni syndrome)
- Human papillomavirus

INCIDENCE

The estimated age standardised ratio (ASR) for oral cavity cancer is 2.7 per 100 000 in 2012, with the proportion of incident cancers being greater in men than in women (typically 2:1). Oral cancer predominantly effects people over the age of 65. Geographic variation is incidence is profound with the highest ASRs evident in Papua New Guinea and Southern Asia countries (notably Sri Lanka, Pakistan).

ANATOMY

The oral cavity extends from the skin–vermilion border of the lips anteriorly to the junction of the hard and soft palate

Guido Fanconi, 1892–1979, Swiss paediatrician, named several conditions including Fanconi anaemia, a rare genetic disorder of DNA repair leading to bone marrow failure and the development of haematological and solid malignancies typically within early life.

Frederick Pei Li (1940–2015), Boston, MA, USA, and Joseph F Fraumeni, Jr., b.1933, NIH, MD, USA, described a familial syndrome of soft tisuue sacromas, breast cancer and other malignancies in 1969.

superiorly and the line of the circumvallate papillae on the junction of the posterior one-third third and anterior two-thirds of the tongue posteriorly. The anatomical sites that are frequently involved in mouth cancer include the floor of the mouth, the lateral border of the anterior tongue, buccal sulcus and the retromolar trigone (Figure 48.1). The retromolar trigone is defined as the attached mucosa overlying the ascending ramus of the mandible posterior to the last molar tooth and extending superiorly to the maxillary tuberosity. It is essential to appreciate the anatomical boundries of the oral cavity when defining tumour sites, particularly with respect to prognosis; the aetiological influence of HPV and its implication of improved outcomes is restricted to tumours of the oropharynx (in particular tonsillar and base of tongue subsites).

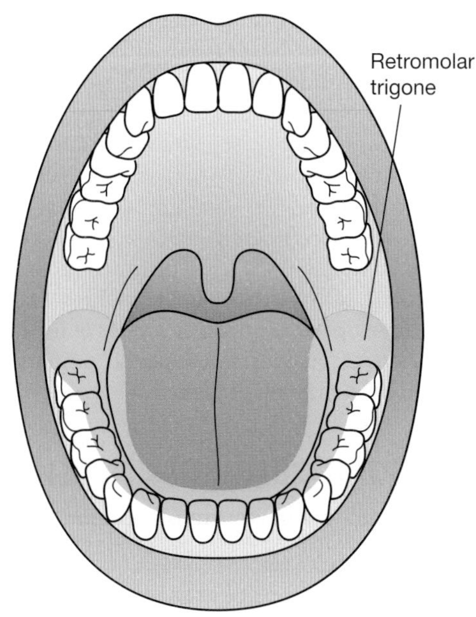

Figure 48.1 Common anatomical sites (blue) for oral squamous cell carcinoma.

PATHOLOGY

The anatomy of the oral cavity is complex and the course of the nerves, blood vessels, lymphatic pathways and fascial planes influences the spread of disease. The role that different anatomical sites play in prognosis is conflicted in the literature with both oral tongue and buccal cancer having been reported to carry worse outcomes. Whether this is a feature of anatomy or variation in biological aggression has yet to be demonstrated.

At a histological level, grade of malignancy, the presence of perineural invasion, the degree of cellular cohesion at the advancing front and angioinvasion all carry negative prognosic influence and correlate directly with regional and distant metastases. Evidence of extracapsular spread or extension (ECS or ECE) beyond the lymph node capsule in nodal metastases is a reliable predictor of poor outcome and has been included in the 8th edition of the *AJCC Cancer Staging Manual* (2017).

Histology

SCC is the predominant histology for tumours arising in the oral cavity. Tumours mainly arise from the mucosal epithelium, although malignant salivary gland tumours from the minor salivary glands are a rare but important group of lesions. Lymphomas, particularly around Waldeyer's ring (tonsils, tongue base, lingual tonsil regions, posterior one-third of the tongue), make up the last of the three principal pathological groups of oropharyngeal cancer.

Chronic exposure of the mucosal surface to carcinogenic substances (i.e. tobacco and alcohol) can produce multiple subclinical sites of carcinoma that can at any stage develop into malignant tumour. This pathological process supports the preventive measures of smoking cessation and alcohol rehabilitation in patients with both premalignant lesions and those with established head and neck cancer. This seeks to minimise the occurrence of disease progression in those with premalignant disease and, in those undergoing treatment for malignancy, it improves treatment efficacy (particulrly smoking cessation prior to radiotherapy) and to minimise synchronous and metachronous tumours development (see below).

Premalignant lesions

The majority of oral carcinomas are not preceded by or associated with clinically obvious premalignant lesions. There are, however, a group of oral pathological conditions in which an association with malignant transformation exists.

Clinical features

Leucoplakia

Leucoplakia is a clinical term used to describe any white patch or plaque that cannot be rubbed off or characterised clinically or pathologically as another disease. It is purely a descriptive term with no histological correlation. Leucoplakia varies from a small, well-circumscribed, homogenous white plaque to an extensive lesion involving large surface areas of the oral

Summary box 48.2

Conditions associated with malignant transformation

High-risk lesions

- Erythroplakia (homogenous or speckled)
- Proliferative verrucous leucoplakia
- Chronic hyperplastic candidiasis

Medium-risk lesions

- Oral submucous fibrosis
- Syphilitic glossitis

Low-risk/equivocal-risk lesions

- Oral lichen planus
- Discoid lupus erythematosus
- Discoid keratosis congenita

mucosa. It may be smooth or wrinkled, fissured and vary in white colouration depending on the thickness of the lesion. Approximately 2% of the general population have such lesions and the frequency with which dysplasia is present in the lesion varies up to approximately 20% in less homogenous lesions.

Speckled leucoplakia

This is a variation of leucoplakia arising on an erythematous base (Figure 48.2). It has the highest rate of malignant transformation.

Erythroplakia

Occurring less frequently than leucoplakia (0.02–0.5% in Asian population), erythroplakia is defined as a lesion of the oral mucosa that presents as a bright red velvety plaque that cannot be characterised clinically or pathologically as any other recognisable condition. The lesions may be irregular in outline and distinct from adjacent normal mucosa (Figure 48.3). The surfaces may be nodular or broadly atrophic in nature and frequently display contact bleeding. These lesions can coexist with leucoplakia. The risk of malignancy (or *in-situ* change) within erythroplakia is high and therefore biopsy is essential, after which surgical ablation is frequently necessary.

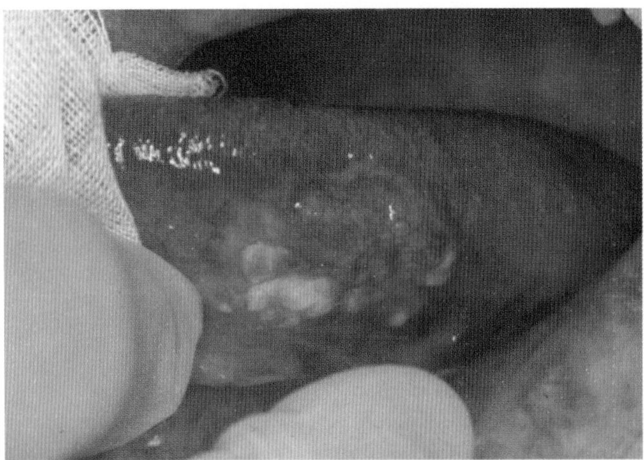

Figure 48.2 Speckled leucoplakia on the lateral border of the tongue. Histology confirmed carcinoma *in situ*.

FIELD CHANGE AND SECOND PRIMARY TUMOURS

The diffuse and chronic exposure of the mucosa of the upper aerodigestive tract to carcinogenic substances (e.g. tobacco and alcohol) causes widespread adverse changes in the mucosal epithelium. The consequence of the diffuse exposure is the development of separate tumours at different anatomical sites. These may present simultaneously, within 6 months (synchronous), or may be delayed (metachronous). Slaughter, in 1953, first proposed the concept of field change or 'cancerisation'. Separate primary tumours may not represent distinct genetic mutational events but rather the same clonal origin of cells, which migrate to separate sites in the upper aerodigestive tract. Nevertheless, minimising exposure of the mucosal surfaces to potential insults is the cornerstone of long-term management for patients with head and neck cancer.

Patients who develop a first tumour in the oral cavity and the oropharynx are more likely to develop a second primary tumour (approximately 15%, a third of which are in the head and neck). In total, 80% of these are metachronous tumours, of which 50% develop within the first 2 years of initial presentation (Figure 48.4). Synchronous second primary tumours in the head and neck are uncommon.

Potential for malignant change

The potential risk for malignant transformation includes:

- severity/grade of dysplasia;
- increases with increasing age of the patient;
- increases with increasing size of the lesion;
- may be higher in smokers (although contradictory evidence exists to suggest non-smokers are at higher risk);

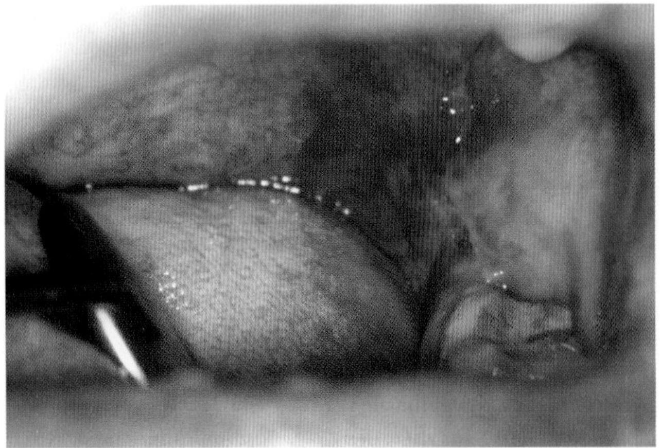

Figure 48.3 Erythroplakia of the left soft palate and lateral pharyngeal wall.

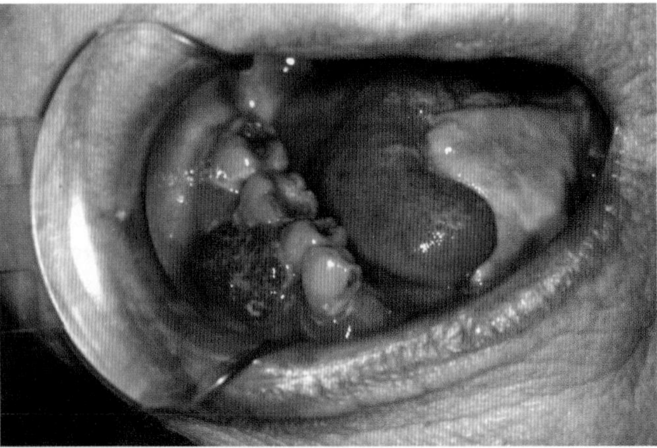

Figure 48.4 Metachronous tumour in the right mandibular alveolus after previous partial glossectomy and forearm flap reconstruction.

Danely P Slaughter, ?1911–2014, otolaryngologist, University of Illinois College of Medicine, Chicago, IL, USA.

- increases with alcohol consumption;
- depends on the anatomical site of the premalignant lesion;
- is particularly high for premalignant lesions on the lateral/ventral surface of the tongue, particularly in younger women, even in the absence of associated risk factors.

PREMALIGNANT CONDITIONS

Chronic hyperplastic candidiasis

Chronic hyperplastic candidiasis produces dense plaques of leucoplakia, particularly around the commissures of the mouth. The lesions occasionally extend on to the vermilion and even the facial skin (Figure 48.5). These lesions have a high incidence of malignant transformation, thought to be the result of invasion of the lesion by *Candida albicans*. A small percentage of patients have an associated immunological defect, which encourages the invasion of *C. albicans*, rendering the patient susceptible to malignant transformation. Specific management of chronic hyperplastic candidiasis includes prolonged (6 weeks) topical antifungal treatment or systemic antifungal treatment (2 weeks). If the lesions persist after medical therapy, particularly when dysplasia is evident on biopsy, surgical excision should be considered.

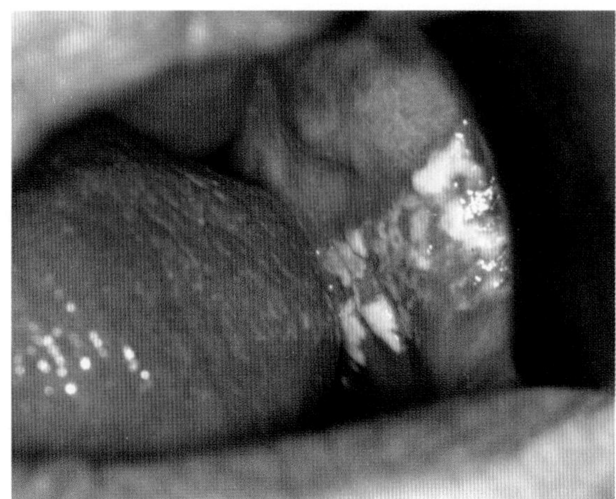

Figure 48.5 Chronic hyperplastic candidiasis of the left buccal mucosa.

Oral submucous fibrosis

Oral submucous fibrosis is a progressive disease in which fibrous bands form beneath the oral mucosa. Scarring produces contracture, resulting in limited mouth opening and restricted tongue movement. The condition is almost entirely confined to the Asian population and is characterised pathologically by epithelial fibrosis with associated atrophy and hyperplasia of the overlying epithelium (Figure 48.6). The epithelium also shows changes of epithelial dysplasia. Restricted mouth opening can be treated with intralesional steroids. Surgical excision/release and reconstruction may lead to short-term benefit only for fibrous bands to recur at the same site or progress at other sites.

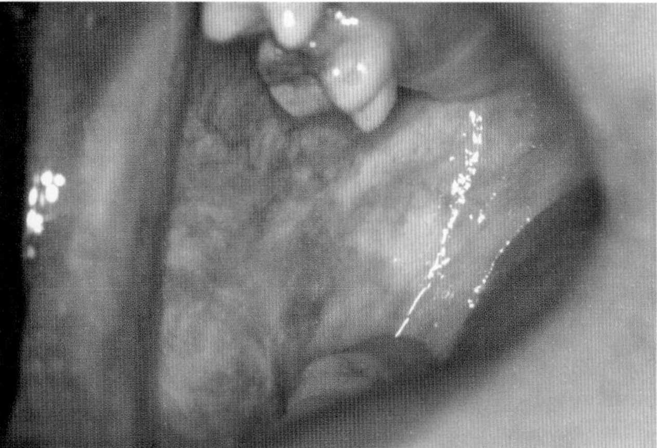

Figure 48.6 Oral submucous fibrosis of the right buccal mucosa and soft palate.

Research strongly indicates that oral submucous fibrosis is significantly associated with the use of pan masala areca nut, with or without concurrent alcohol use. Cessation of usage may halt the process but not necessarily lead to improvement. Tobacco smoking alone is not associated with oral submucous fibrosis.

Proliferative verrucous leucoplakia

Proliferative verrucous leucoplakia is a rare progressive exophytic variant of leucoplakia, which is frequently multifocal and carries a high (>50%) risk of malignant tranformation. It is a rare, yet distinct entity, frequently arising in the absence of traditional risk factors for oral premalignancy. Diagnosis is made on the basis of combined clinical and histopathological grounds. It may be localised and typically affects the gingivae or, more commonly, as a widespread varient, affects several oral mucosal sites. There is controversy as to the best approach to management; however, long-term surveillance is essential given the condition's propensity to undergo malignant transformation.

Sideropenic dysphagia (Plummer-Vinson and Paterson-Kelly syndromes)

There is a well-known relationship between sideropenia (iron deficiency in the absence of anaemia) and the development of oral cancer. Sideropenia is common in Scandinavian women and leads to epithelial atrophy, which renders the oral mucosa vulnerable to irritation from topical carcinogens. Correction of the sideropenia with iron supplements reduces the epithelial atrophy and risk of malignant transformation.

Henry S Plummer, 1874–1936 physician, Mayo Clinic, Rochester MN, USA.
Porter P Vinson, 1890–1959, surgeon, Mayo Clinic, Rochester, MN, USA.
Donald Rose Paterson, 1863–1939, surgeon, Ear, Nose and Throat Department, The Royal Infirmary, Cardiff, UK.
Adam Brown Kelly, 1865–1941, surgeon, Ear, Nose and Throat Department, The Royal Victoria Infirmary, Glasgow, UK.

CLASSIFICATION AND STAGING

TNM staging

Staging of head and neck cancer is defined by the American Joint Committee on Cancer (AJCC) and follows the TNM system. The system also takes into account the pretreatment radiological findings (either on computed tomography (CT) or magnetic resonance imaging (MRI)) of the tumour. The T classification indicates the extent of the primary tumour and the N classification relates to the extent of regional neck metastases to the cervical lymph nodes. The recent publication of the 8th edition of the *AJCC Cancer Staging Manual* (2017) has introduced profound changes, firstly on the basis of tumour aetiology (with variation on the basis of HPV status in oropharyngeal cancer) and secondly, on depth of tumour invasion as well as on greatest dimensional size. Further, as noted above, ECS or ECE is recognised as a finding worthy of upstaging of nodal stage. The introduction of these changes into clinical practice has yet to be decided in many geographic regions. The original 7th Edition of the TNM staging for oral cavity cancer is outlined in *Table 48.1*.

The M classification relates to distant metastasis. The risk of distant metastasis is related more closely to the extent of nodal disease than to the size of the primary tumour. Tumours close to the midline are at a greater risk of developing bilateral or contralateral cervical node metastasis.

TABLE 48.1 The TNM staging system.

Primary tumour (T)			
TX	Primary tumour cannot be assessed		
T0	No evidence of primary tumour		
Tis	Carcinoma in situ		
T1	Tumour <2 cm in greatest dimension		
T2	Tumour >2 but <4 cm		
T3	Tumour >4 cm but <6 cm		
T4	Tumour invades adjacent structures (e.g. mandible, skin)		
Regional lymph nodes (N)			
NX	Regional lymph nodes cannot be assessed		
N0	No regional lymph node metastasis		
N1	Metastasis in a single ipsilateral lymph node <3 cm in greatest dimension		
N2a	Metastasis in a single ipsilateral lymph node >3 cm but not more than 6 cm		
N2b	Metastasis in multiple ipsilateral lymph nodes, none >6 cm in greatest dimension		
N2c	Metastasis in bilateral or contralateral lymph nodes, none greater than 6 cm in greatest dimension		
N3	Metastasis in any lymph node >6 cm		
Distant metastasis			
M0	No evidence of distant metastasis		
M1	Evidence of distant metastasis		
Stage			
0	Tis	N0	M0
I	T1	N0	M0
II	T2	N0	M0
III	T3	N0	M0
	T1, T2, T3	N1	M0
IV	T4	N0	M0
Any T	N2	M0	
Any T	N3	M0	
Any T	Any N	M1	

Patterns of lymph node metastasis

The cervical lymph nodes are divided into five principal levels, as outlined in Figure 48.7.

The spread of tumour from the primary site has been well described. SCC in the oral cavity and lips tends to metastasise to lymph nodes at levels I, II and, to a lesser extent, level III unless higher levels are also positive. However (albeit infrequently), for SCC of the oral tongue there is a risk of skip metastasis directly to lymph node levels III or IV, without the involvement of higher-level lymph node groups. Importantly, there is also a recognised risk of contralateral neck metastasis even in well lateralised tumours of the oral tongue. Tumours arising in the oropharynx commonly metastasise to lymph node levels II, III and IV, as well as retropharyngeal and contralateral nodal groups.

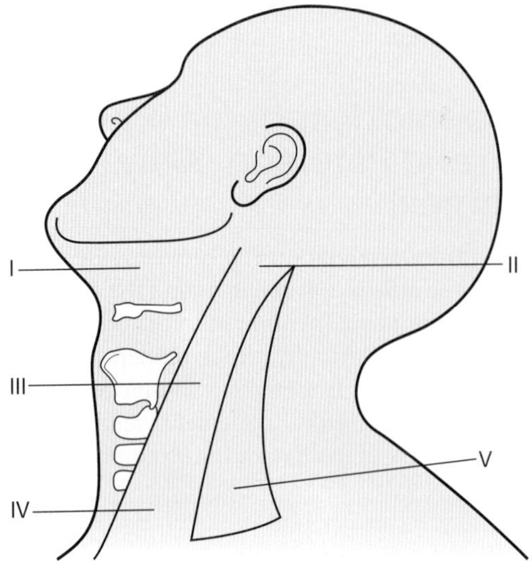

Distant metastases are relatively uncommon but sites involved include lung and, to a lesser extent, the brain, liver, bone and skin.

Figure 48.7 Cervical lymph nodes: (I) submandibular; (II) upper deep cervical; (III) mid-cervical; (IV) lower cervical; (V) posterior triangle.

CLINICAL FEATURES

Between 25% and 50% of patients with cancer of the oral cavity present late, particularly in regions of the resource-poor world and in areas of social deprevation in more affluent nations. The reasons for delay in presentation are multifactorial and not easily generalisable when considered in a global context.

Lip cancer

Lip cancer presents early as it is readily visible to the patient. It usually arises as an ulcer on the vermilion border (Figure 48.8). In total, 95% of carcinomas of the lip arise on the lower lip and 15% arise in the central one-third and commissures, reflecting the aetiological influence of UV (sunlight) radiation on the more exposed lower lip. Tumours tend to spread laterally over the mucosal surface. Lymph node metastases, usually to the submental or submandibular nodes, occur in approximately 5% of cases and reflect aggressive disease behaviour when apparent.

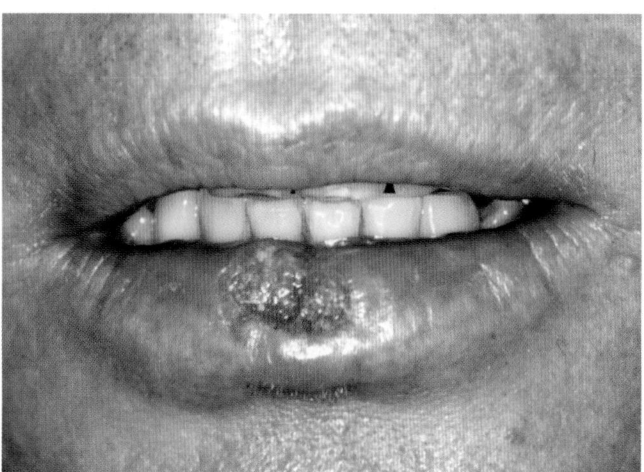

Figure 48.8 Squamous cell carcinoma of the lower lip.

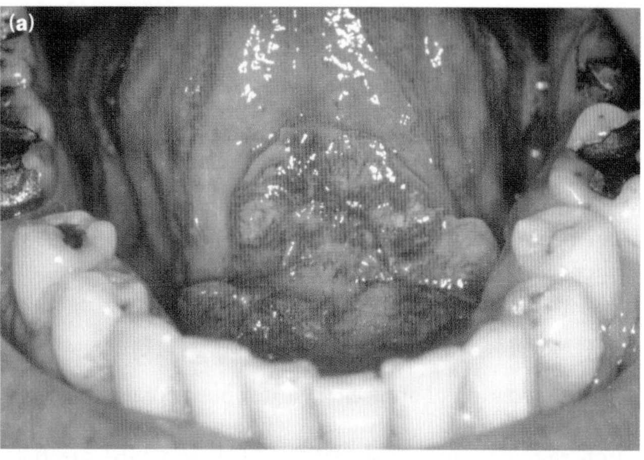

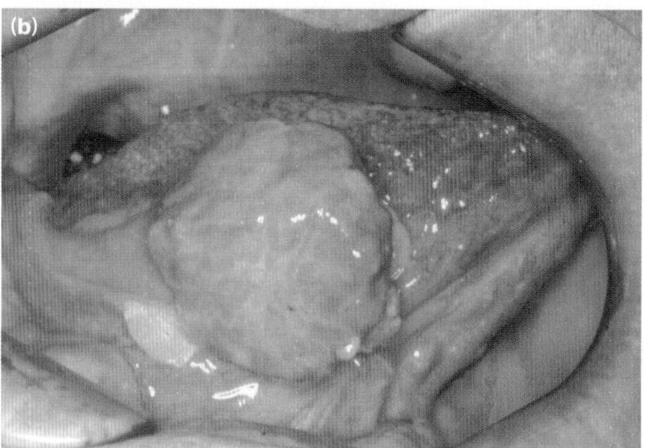

Figure 48.9 (a) Ulcerative squamous cell carcinoma of the anterior floor of the mouth. (b) Exophytic squamous cell carcinoma of the right lateral border of the tongue.

Oral cavity

Clinical presentation is markedly dependent on the anatomical site and state but classically involves mucosal ulceration with rolled margins, combinations of exophytic and endophytic neoplastic tissue, contact or spontaneous bleeding (Figure 48.9). Where involving tooth bearing areas, there may be loss of periodontal/bone support and subsequent mobility. Pain can be a feature and this may be at the site of the primary tumour or referred to adjacent structures in the case of otalgia stemming from tumours invading the lateral tongue. With advancing stage of disease comes increased risk of nutritional impairment as a result of pain and restricted oral intake. In contrast to oropharyngeal malignancy, awareness of nodal metastasis (lump in the neck) is less common in the absence of a known primary tumour.

The duration of symptoms is highly variable, from several weeks to many months.

Summary box 48.3

Clinical features of oral cancer that warrent investigation

- Persistent oral swelling for >3 weeks
- Mouth ulceration for >3 weeks
- Sore tongue
- Difficulty swallowing
- Jaw or facial swelling
- Painless neck lump
- Unexplained tooth mobility
- Trismus

INVESTIGATIONS

When a clinical diagnosis of oral cancer is suspected, a comprehensive protocol of investigations should be instituted. A tissue diagnosis, typically by way of incisional biopsy, is essential. Formal examination under anaesthetic is desirable, particularly for advanced stage disease, not only to carry out the biopsy, but also to palpate and examine the extent of the tumour, which can be exquisitely tender in the conscious patient. Under the same anaesthetic, extraction of teeth with a dubious prognosis can be performed. The biopsy should be generous and include the most suspicious area of the lesion, as well as normal adjacent tissue. Areas of necrosis or gross infection should be avoided. In circumstances where the diagnosis has already been made and where combined modality treatment proposed, consideration of insertion of a percutaneous endoscopic gastrostomy can be made at this stage.

Radiography

Plain radiography of the jaw is undertaken to facilitate adequate dental assessment rather than as a means to assessed for evidence of bone invasion.

Magnetic resonance imaging

The investigation of choice for cancer of the oral cavity, oropharynx and neck, will vary depending on institution protocol, resources and local expirtise. CT and MRI are both viable alternatives; however, MRI suffers less degredation by metallic dental restorations and provides excellent visualisation of soft-tissue infiltration of the tumour (Figure 48.10). Ideally it should be performed before diagnostic biopsy as biopsy frequently distorts the image of the primary tumour. The specificity and sensitivity of MRI in diagnosing cervical node metastasis are similar to that of CT. Patients who suffer with claustrophobia may have difficulty in tolerating the investigation. Contrast enhancement (in particular gadolinium), suppression techniques and variation in image sequence acquisition (e.g. Short Tau Inversion-Recovery; STIR) can aid interpretation. CT of the primary site and neck is an alternative favoured in some institutions.

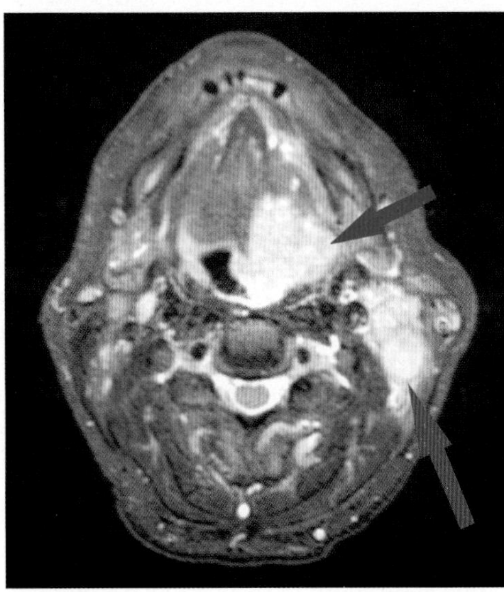

Figure 48.10 Magnetic resonance imaging of a primary tumour of the left tongue base (blue arrow) and neck node metastasis (red arrow).

Computed tomography

CT is much more widely available than MRI but its utility may be restricted by artifact degredation of images by dental restorative materials. It is useful when bony invasion is suspected. CT of the thorax is now indicated for all patients and not just those with proven cervical lymph node metastasis and large-volume disease.

Positron emmission tomography combined with CT

Positron esmission tomography combined with CT (PET-CT) of the whole body uses the anatomical capability of CT scanning in concert with radiolabelled tracers capable of localising to specific tissues. The most widely used tracer is 18 fluoro-dexoyglrucose (FDG), which is transported and trapped within hypermetabolic tissues (typically cancerous or inflammed tissues, or those that are predictably physiologically active). Evidence-based guidelines suggest targetted use of PET scanning in the work-up of patients with malignant cervical lymphadenopathy with an unknown primary. There is trial evidence for its use for surveillance following non-surgical treatment of oropharyngeal SCC and it shows promise for assessment of patients being investigated for recurrence.

Ultrasound

Ultrasound has become an integral part of head and neck services, particularly in association with one-stop clinics for the evaluation of undiagnosed neck lumps or presumed cervical metastasis. Used alongside fine-needle aspiration cytology (FNAC), ultrasound is capable of delineating and sampling cervical lymphadenopathy and both thyroid and salivary gland lesions/masses. The technique is operator dependent but benefits from exposing the patient to no ionising radiation or detrimental side-effects.

Fine-needle aspiration cytology

FNAC is useful for the assessment and pathological diagnosis of enlarged cervical lymph nodes. It involves the use of a fine-needle puncture into the mass and immediate aspiration for cytological examination. It has few complications and there is no evidence of tumour seeding along needle tracts. It requires no specialist equipment other than a 21G or 23G needle and a 10 mL syringe. Aspiration should be carried out only when the needle enters the swelling. If the specimen can be assessed immediately by an expert cytologist, then it can be sent without fixation. If there is delay in microscopic examination, then the specimen, smeared on a microscope slide, should be fixed before transfer to the laboratory. The positive yield from FNAC is dependent not only on the quality of the aspirate, but also on the skill of the cytologist.

Radionucleotide studies to assess bone invasion

A radioisotope bone scan of the facial skeleton adds little to the diagnosis and assessment of head and neck cancer, beyond that of clinical assessment, MRI and/or CT, and plain imaging. The scan is not specific and tends to show increased uptake wherever there is increased metabolic activity in bone. A false-positive diagnosis is common and 'overstaging' of the disease frequent.

TREATMENT

General principles

The management of head and neck cancer necessitates a multidisciplinary approach, integrating the combined skills and capabilities of surgeons, oncologists, radiologists, pathologists and allied health professionals to deliver an optimal treatment strategy seeking to maximise oncologic outcomes while mitigating, or restoring, loss of form and function.

Surgery remains the primary treatment modality for oral cavity cancer. Where adverse pathological features are apparent (based on resective pathology), postoperative radiotherapy or chemoradiotherapy are advocated. Given the critical normal functional demands of the oral cavity and associated structures, reconstruction of the ablated surgical defect is frequently necessary to restore (as best possible) form and function. Options for reconstruction will depend on the defect, relevant patient co-morbidities, the clinical environment/facilities and, importantly, the skill set of the treating surgeon.

In the clinically node-positive neck, a therapeutic neck dissection is normally performed at the time of pirmary resection. Management of the clinically node-negative neck in oral cavity cancer is more contentious, particularly in early stage (T1/2) disease. Recent randomised control evidence has demonstrated improved outcomes for elective neck dissection over a watch and wait policy for such patients. Sentinel lymph node biopsy as an additional staging tool in early oral cavity cancer does offer a means to avoid unnecessary elective neck dissection; however, it lacks clinical trials level evidence despite being included in some clinical guidelines.

Patient factors

Modern anaesthesia and postoperative critical care facilities have allowed major head and neck surgery to be carried out on patients with significant medical comorbidity. Advancing age is not considered to be a contraindication to major head and neck cancer surgery but may certainly influence the extent of adjuvant treatment (inclusion of chemotherapy to postoperative radiotherapy has little evidence of benefit to those over 70 years of age). Conversely, young patients should not be denied radiotherapy for fear of inducing a second malignancy (e.g. sarcoma) in later life.

Management of premalignant conditions

Elimination of associated aetiological factors is the initial basis of the management of premalignant oral mucosal lesions. Cessation of smoking, elimination of the areca nut/pan habit and reduction in alcohol consumption should be encouraged in all patients with premalignant lesions. A photographic record of the lesion is useful, particularly for long-term follow-up. All erythroplakia and speckled leucoplakia should undergo urgent incisional biopsy, as many will represent either *in-situ* or early oral cancer at presentation. Biopsy from more than one site provides a better representation of histological heterogeneity within a lesion.

Severe epithelial dysplasia and carcinoma in situ should be ablated by surgical excision where feasible. Laser vaporisation can be employed; however, it does not yeild a surgical specimen for histological examination, thus preventing assessment of resection margins and also detection of disease upstaging initially missed through sampling effects of incisional biopsies. Small lesions, particularly on the lateral border of the tongue or buccal mucosa, may be managed with surgical excision and primary closure by undermining the adjacent mucosa, or be left to granulate. Larger defects can be managed with laser excision and allowed to epithelialise spontaneously (Figure 48.11). Monitoring of less severe grades of dysplasia with elimination of causative agents is pragmatic but can be labour intensive. Use of primary care physcians/dentists can be helpful as part of a multidisciplinary follow-up regime.

Currently there are no successful chemoprevention agents; however, clinical trials are ongoing in the attractive area of clinical research with the ambition of reducing the risk of malignant transformation in high-risk oral premalignant lesions.

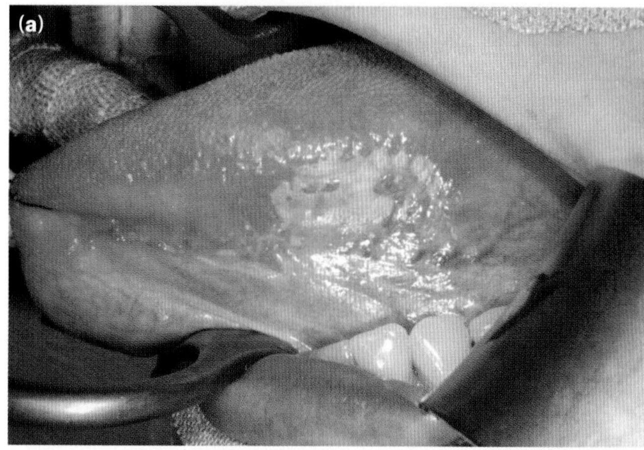

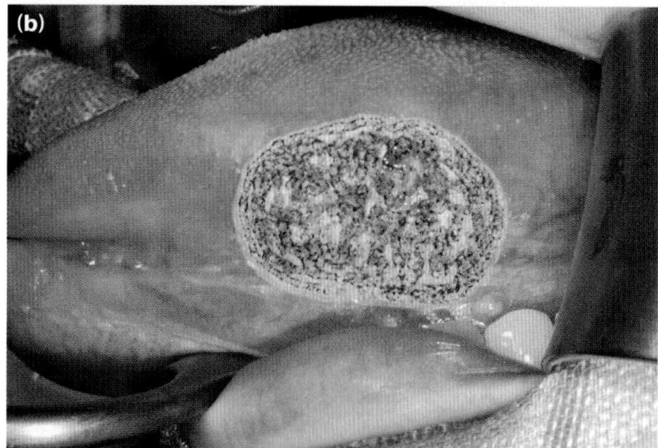

Figure 48.11 (a) Leucoplakia with severe dysplasia of the lateral border of the tongue. (b) Laser vaporisation.

LIP CANCER

Surgery and external beam radiotherapy are highly effective methods of treatment for lip cancer. The cure rate approaches 90% for either modality.

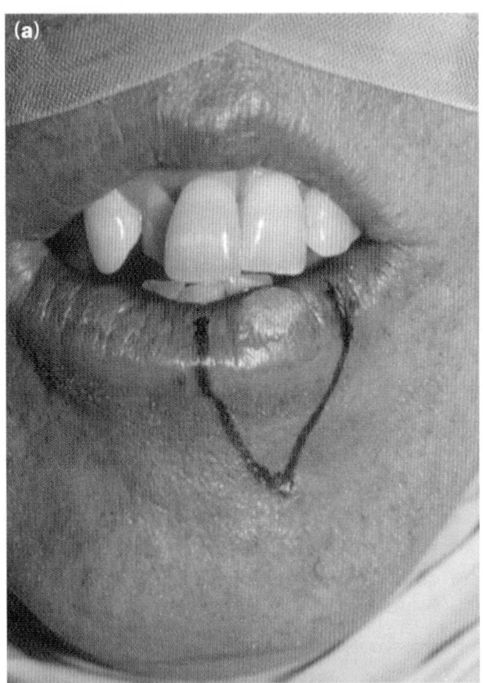

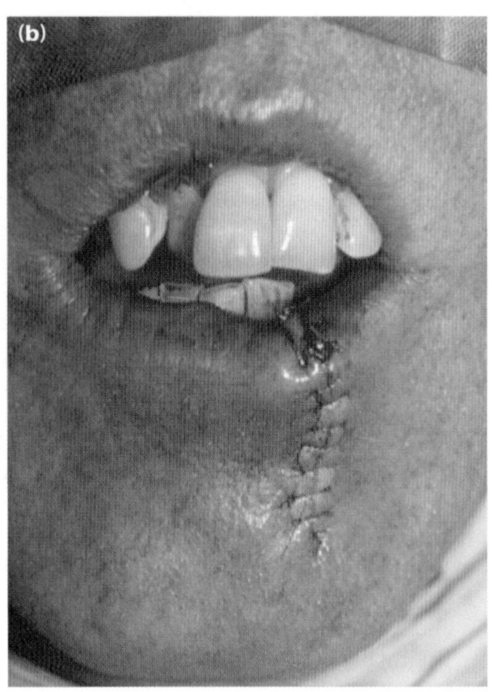

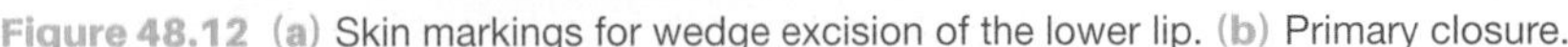

Figure 48.12 (a) Skin markings for wedge excision of the lower lip. (b) Primary closure.

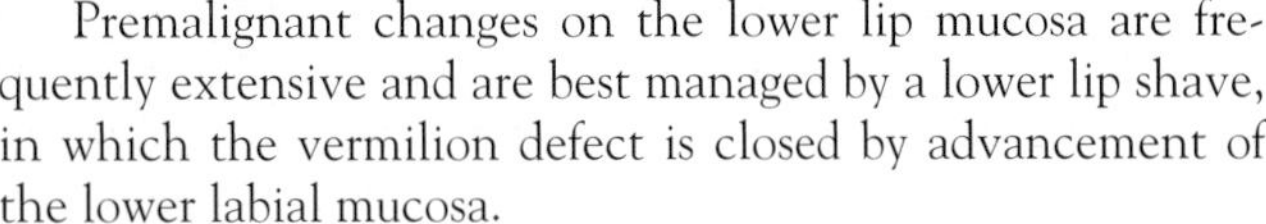

Premalignant changes on the lower lip mucosa are frequently extensive and are best managed by a lower lip shave, in which the vermilion defect is closed by advancement of the lower labial mucosa.

Small tumours

Small tumours (<2 cm) of the lip can be managed with either a V- or W-shaped excision under local or general anaesthesia. The defect, which should be no larger than one-third of the total lip size, is closed in three layers – mucosa, muscle and skin – with particular attention paid to the correct alignment of the vermilion border (Figure 48.12).

Intermediate tumours

Larger tumours, which produce defects of between one-third and two-thirds the size of the lower lip, require local flaps for reconstruction. V or W excision will result in microstomia. Large central defects can be managed using local flaps such as the Johansen step technique (Figure 48.13). This allows closure of the defect by symmetrical advancement of soft-tissue flaps, utilising the excess skin in the labiomental

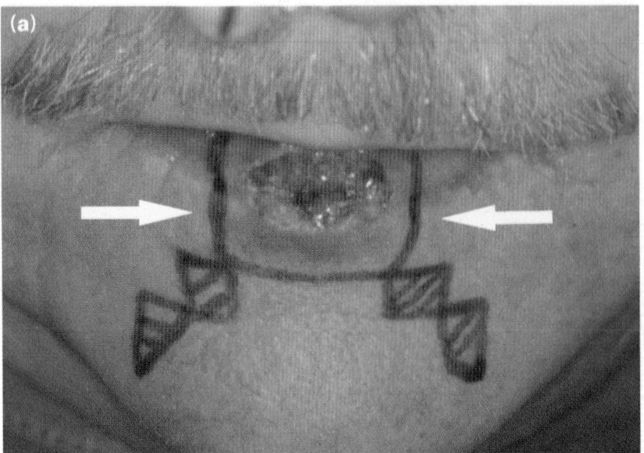

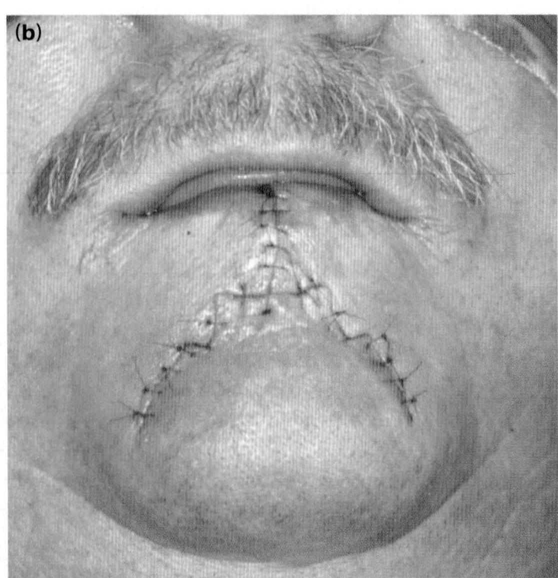

Figure 48.13 (a) Skin markings for Johansen step reconstruction. (b) Closure of lip and labiomental steps.

grooves. Alternative techniques include the Bernard or the Karapandzic advancement flaps.

Total lip reconstruction

Extensive tumours of the lower lip, which invade adjacent tissues (T4), have a high incidence of neck node metastasis. Patients with such advanced disease require surgery, which may include unilateral or bilateral selective neck dissection and total excision of the lower lip and chin, with or without adjacent mandibular resection (rim or segmental mandibulectomy). The lower lip soft-tissue defect can be reconstructed with a variety of free flaps including the radial forearm flap potentially suspended with palmaris longus tendon (Figure 48.14) or perforator flaps such as the anterolateral thigh (ALT) flap or the medial sural artery perforator (MSAP) free flap. The benefits of each vary in terms of tissue bulk, donor site morbidity and vascular pedicle length. Where segmental bony resection has been required, composite (bone including) free flaps are necessary to restore adequate mandibular continuity and soft-tissue form/function. The choice of flap will depend on the defect and the surgeons repertoire; however, the scapula free flap provides exceptional flexibility and tissue variability. Alternatives include the composite radial forearm flap, fibula free flap and perforator based osseocutaneous iliac crest free flap (DCIA; deep circumflex iliac artery free flap)

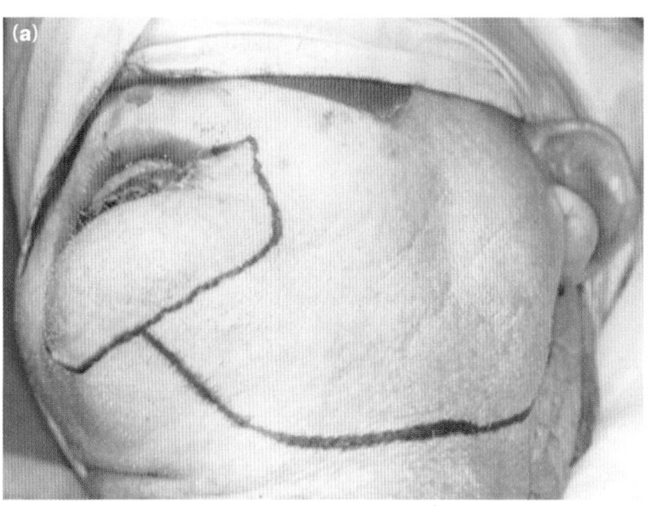

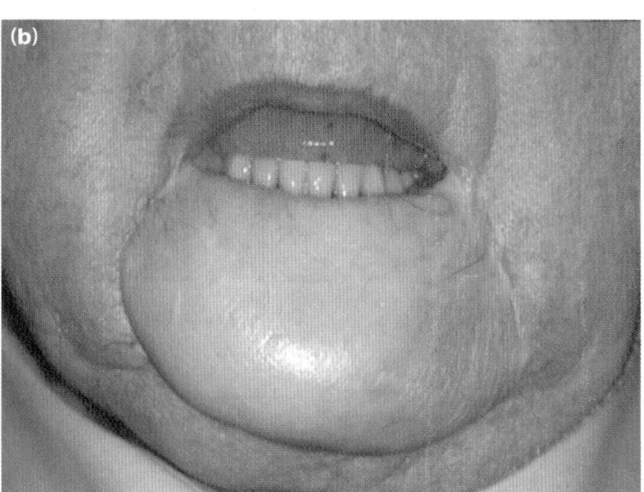

Figure 48.14 (a) Skin markings for total excision of the lower lip, chin and left selective neck dissection. (b) Postoperative view of the reconstructed lower lip using a radial artery forearm flap.

TONGUE CANCER

Management of the neck in early stage oral cavity cancer, including the oral tongue, has been discussed above; however, consideration for elective management of the node-negative neck should be made in all instances. When performing surgical excision of the primary tumour (Figure 48.15), a 1 cm margin in all planes should be attempted in seeking a complete excision with pathologically clear (>5 mm) margins. Resection resulting in partial or hemiglossectomy can be performed with either a cutting diathermy or laser if available. Advanced tumours (T3 and T4) often encroach upon the floor of the mouth and, occasionally, the mandible. In these circumstances a resection of the tongue and floor of the mouth and mandible is required. T4 tumours of the oral tongue may cross the midline, for which (sub)total glossectomy is the only option to achieve adequate tumour clearance. Decisions regarding elective neck dissections on the contralateral side will be dictated by radiological and clinical findings, in particular proximity of the tumour to the midline.

Access

Access for oral cancer is important to allow accurate assessment and clear visualisation to enable tumour clearance to be achieved. Access techniques include:

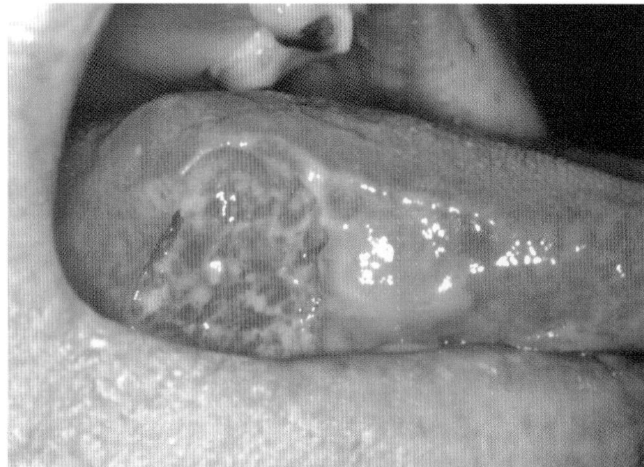

Figure 48.15 Ulcerative squamous cell carcinoma of the right lateral border of the tongue.

Camille Bernard, surgeon, presented a novel approach to the subtotal lower lip defect to the *Societé de Chirurgie de Paris* in 1852. von Burrow subsequently published his account of the flap (1855), claiming to have been using it in practice for some time. The flap is therefore referred to by some as the Bernard–von Burrow flap.
Miodrag Karapandzic, 1930–2016, maxillofacial surgeon, Professor of Plastic & Reconstructive Surgery, University of Belgrade, Yugoslavia.

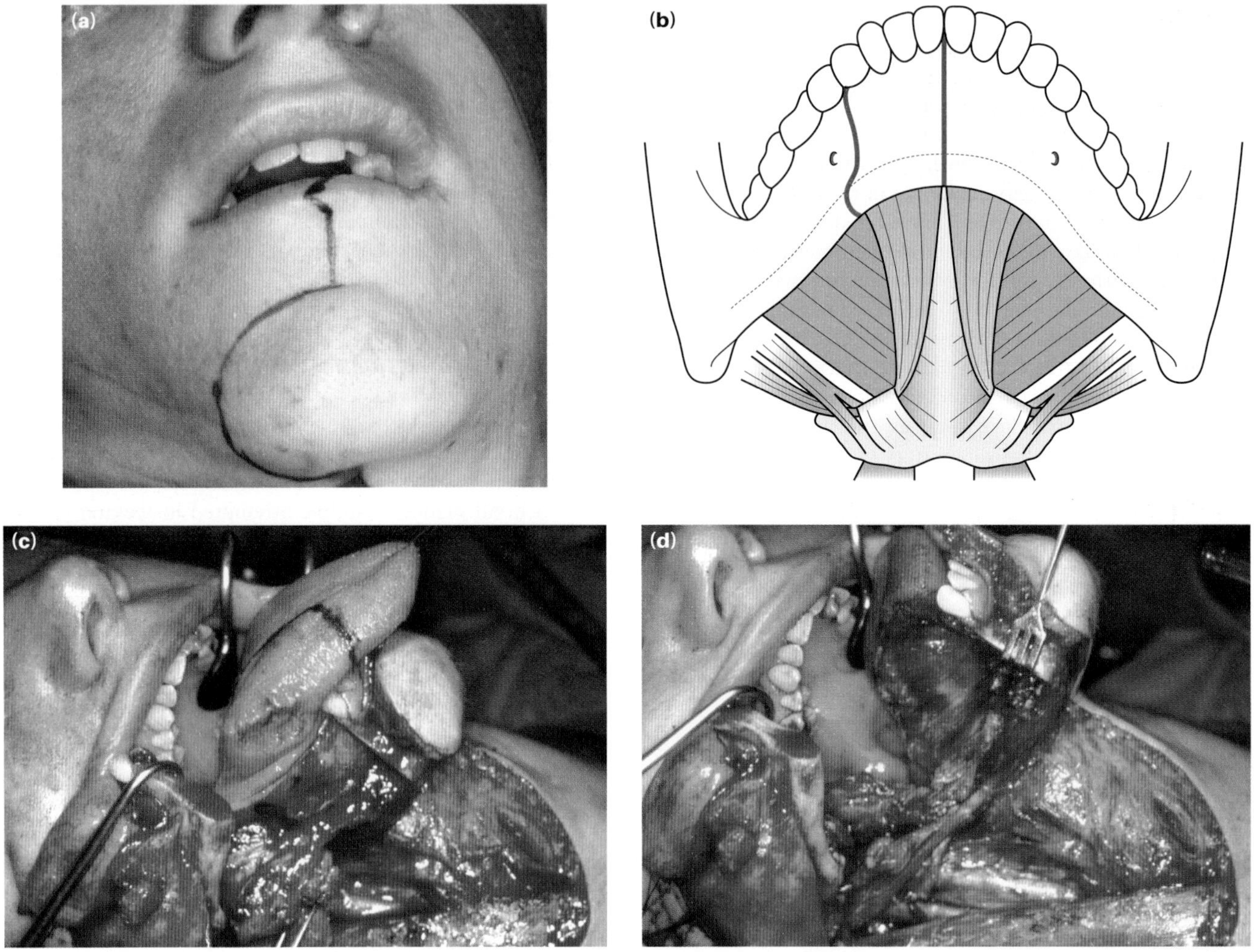

Figure 48.16 (a) Skin markings for lip split and mandibulotomy in continuity with neck dissection. (b) Paramedian and midline mandibulotomy. (c) Margins for primary tumour resection after mandibulotomy. (d) Tongue defect after right selective neck dissection, mandibulotomy and partial glossectomy.

- transoral – small –moderate sized anterior oral tumours;
- lip-split technique and paramedian or median mandibulotomy (Figure 48.16);
- visor incision (Figure 48.17) with or without drop down.

Reconstruction

Imparment of function (e.g. speech, swallowing) is related primarily to tumour size, site and reconstruction but is also influenced by patient factors (age, comorbidity, prior treatment). However, typically the more anterior the defect in the oral cavity, the greater the impact on speech, and the more posterior, the greater the detrimental impact will be on swallowing. Reconstruction of the surgical defect restores oral integrity to the neck and provides a bulk of non-dynamic tissue with an aim of restoring function benefit.

Small defects of the lateral tongue can be managed by primary closure or be allowed to heal by secondary intention

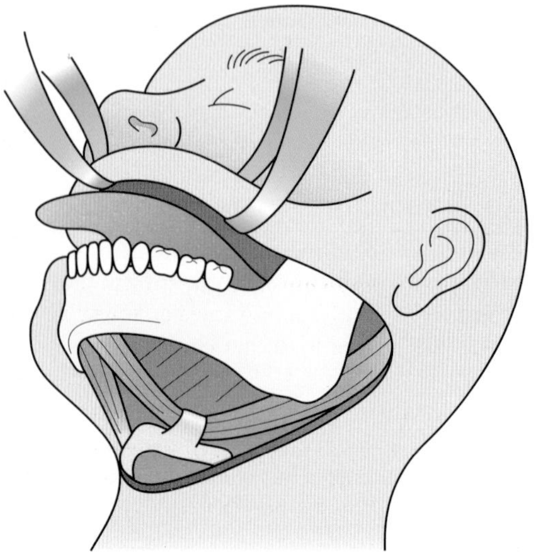

Figure 48.17 Visor approach to the anterior mandible/floor of the mouth and tongue.

with little or no functional impariment. Larger defects (e.g. T2, T3 and T4 resections) require formal reconstruction to encourage good speech and swallowing. Free tissue transfer of suitable tissue (e.g. a radial forearm flap [Figure 48.18], or ALT), utilising microvascular anastomosis in most instances, gives a good functional result. Large-volume defects, including total glossectomy, may require more bulky flaps such as the rectus abdominus free flap or ALT depending on patient body habitus. If feasible, the preservation of one or both hypoglossal nerves is useful to encourage floor of mouth function to help relearn swallowing.

The ablative surgeon should consider adequate access for the resection and consider adjunctive procedures to facilitate this where compromised (e.g. the visor procedure with drop down [see Figure 48.17]).

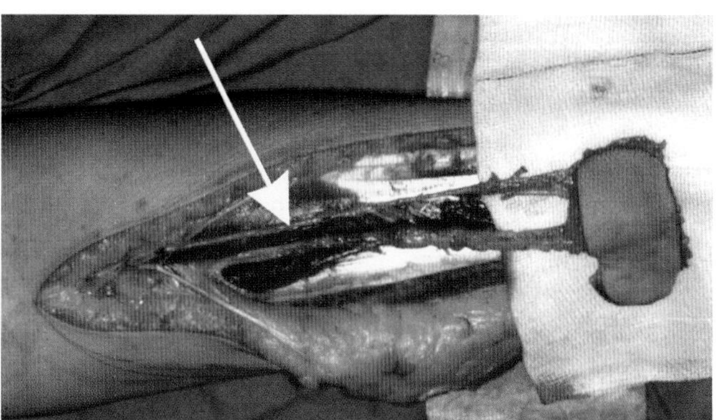

Figure 48.18 Radial artery forearm flap raised before division of a vascular pedicle and cephalic vein (arrow).

FLOOR OF MOUTH

Carcinoma of the floor of the mouth can spread to the ventral surface of the anterior tongue or encroach on the lower anterior alveolus. Surgical excision may include a partial anterior glossectomy and anterior mandibular resection. Only very small tumours of the floor of the mouth can be managed by simple excision. Management of the adjacent mandible/mandibular rim may be necessary where the tumour abuts the mandible; this may be by way of a rim resection or segmental mandibulectomy.

Reconstruction

Reconstruction will depend on the defect size (and its constituents) and ranges from healing by secondary intention to use of the thin, pilable radial forearm free flap for small defects, to ALT and composite flaps for larger resections.

Small tumours of the floor of the mouth excised with a laser frequently may avoid formal reconstruction. For larger defects, where the ventral tongue and labial mucosa are involved, reconstruction is needed to avoid severe difficulties with speech, swallowing and mastication. Smaller, simple soft-tissue defects of the anterior floor of mouth are best reconstructed with a radial artery forearm flap. If a patient is unfit for microvascular free-flap surgery or the facilities are limited, bilateral nasolabial flaps tunnelled into the mouth and interdigitated provide an acceptable alternative (Figure 48.19). Three weeks later their pedicles are divided and inset into the lateral floor of mouth defects. Large defects that involve rim resection of the anterior mandible may also be managed with soft-tissue reconstruction only. Full-thickness resection of the anterior mandible, however, requires immediate reconstruction to prevent severe functional defects or a cosmetic deformity. Vascularised bone with a soft-tissue component provides the most up-to-date method of reconstruction. A fibula flap or a vascularised iliac crest graft (DCIA) are two options in the management of anterior mandible defects with simultaneous floor of mouth defects.

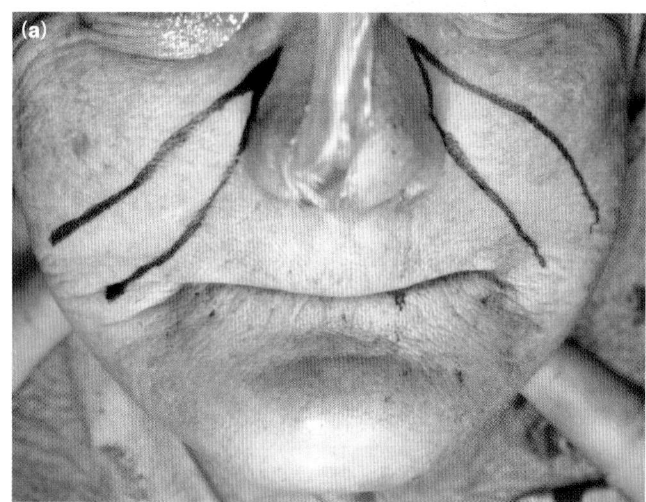

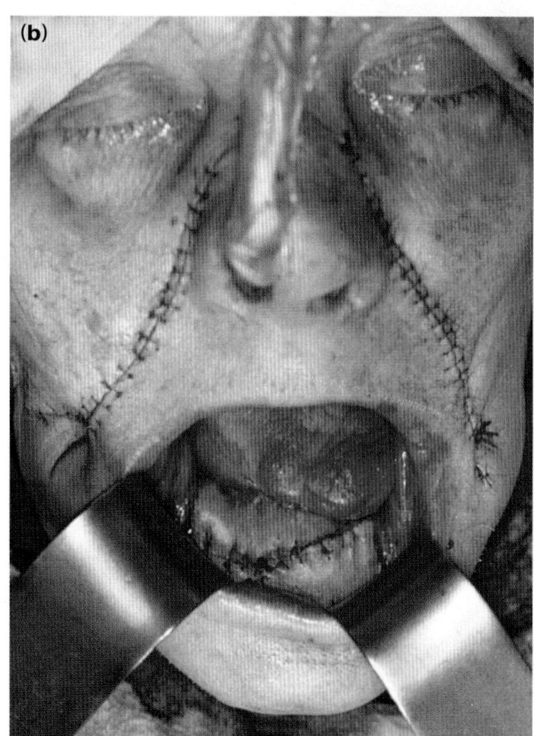

Figure 48.19 (a) Skin markings for bilateral nasolabial flaps. (b) Transposition of bilateral nasolabial flaps into the anterior floor of the mouth.

BUCCAL MUCOSA

SCC of the buccal mucosa (Figure 48.20) should be excised widely, including the underlying buccinator muscle. Larger tumours occasionally extend onto the maxillary tuberosity, tonsillar fossa or mandibular alveolus. Facial skin involvement is rare but carries a poor prognosis. Management of the clinically negative neck should be no different for tumours of the buccal mucosa and as such, a simultaneous ipsilateral selective supraomohyoid neck dissection (levels I, II, III), or sentinel lymph node biopsy, is considered good practice.

Access for buccal carcinoma can be achieved either transorally for smaller lesions (T1, T2) or using the lip-splitting technique for larger lesions (T3, T4).

Reconstruction of the buccal mucosa prevents scarring and trismus. Options include the radial artery forearm flap or a temporalis muscle flap. Raw temporalis muscle inset into the buccal mucosal defect will epithelialise spontaneously over several weeks.

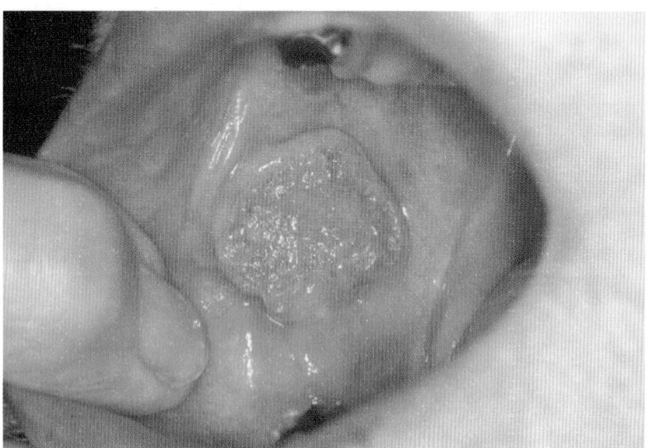

Figure 48.20 Exophytic squamous cell carcinoma of the right buccal mucosa.

LOWER ALVEOLUS

Tumours that involve the mandibular alveolus are similarly treated with surgery including (Figure 48.21a) ipsilateral selective neck dissections for lateral tumours and bilateral selective neck dissection for anterior tumours. Bone invasion (Figure 48.21b) demands segmental resection of the mandible and this may be in continuity with the neck dissection(s).

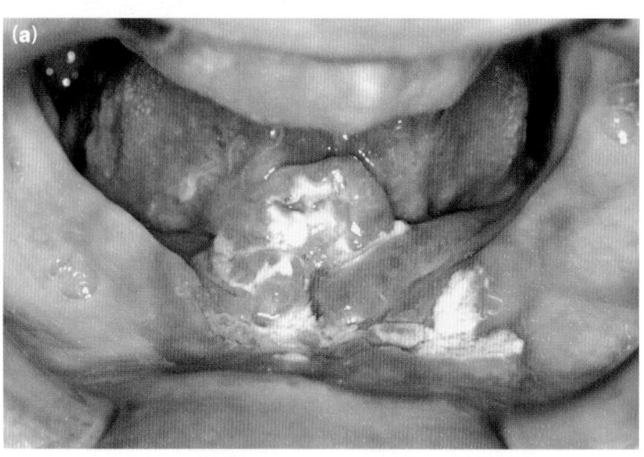

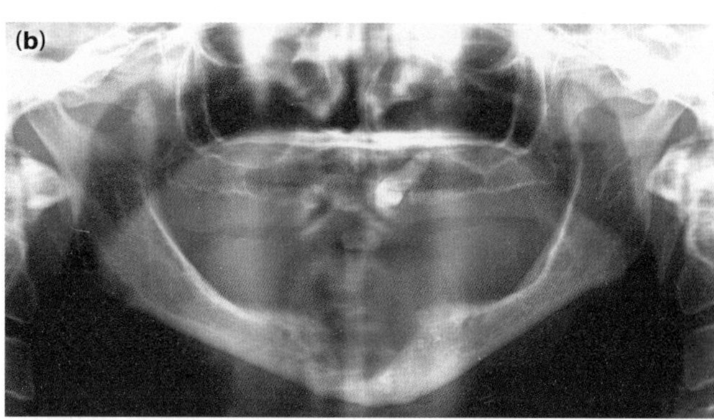

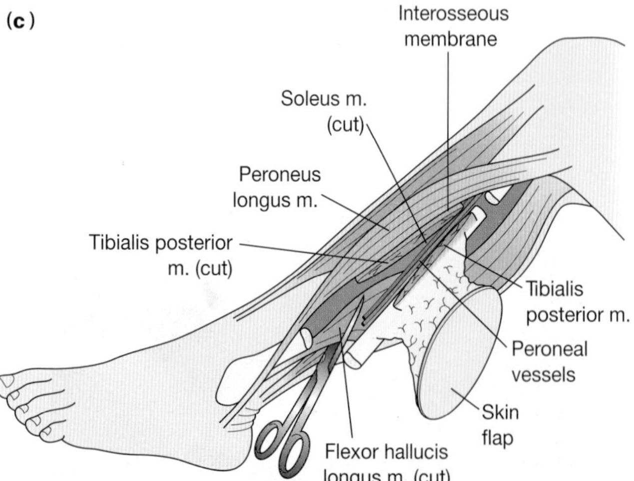

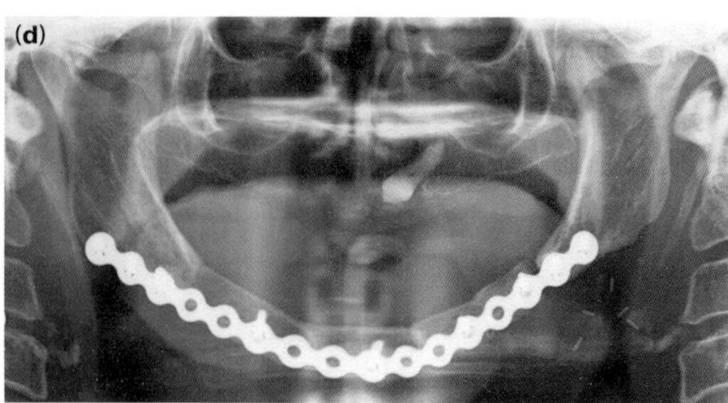

Figure 48.21 (a) Extensive squamous cell carcinoma of the anterior mandible involving the floor of the mouth. (b) Plain radiography (orthopantomogram) revealing bony destruction of the anterior mandible. (c) Osseocutaneous fibula flap. (d) Postoperative radiograph of the reconstructed mandible with fibula flap and reconstruction plate.

Primary or immediate reconstruction is preferred as the functional and cosmetic outcomes are superior to those of delayed reconstruction. Options for bony reconstruction are shown in *Table 48.2*. They include the fibula flap for the edentulous mandible (**Figures 48.21c, d**) and the iliac crest (DCIA) for patients with a dentate mandible (**Figure 48.22**). The vascularised iliac crest can be wrapped with internal oblique abdominal wall muscle, which epithelialises spontaneously. This intraoral epithelialisation provides an excellent surface for prosthetic replacement with or without osseointegrated implants.

Although non-vascularised bone grafts have been utilised for mandibular reconstruction, the long-term success is low as many patients receive postoperative radiotherapy and loss of the bone and dehiscence of the titanium tray or reconstruction plate can be expected sequelae.

TABLE 48.2 Mandibular reconstruction (reconstructive ladder).

Method	Technique
No reconstruction	Primary closure
Soft tissue only	Pectoralis major myocutaneous flap
Alloplastic material	2.4 mm reconstruction plate alone
Combination alloplastic/soft tissue	2.4 mm reconstruction plate and pectoralis major flap
Non-vascularised bone grafts	Titanium tray and cancellous chips (iliac crest)
Vascularised bone grafts	Fibula (edentulous and dentate); iliac crest (dentate); scapula (concomitant large soft-tissue defect)

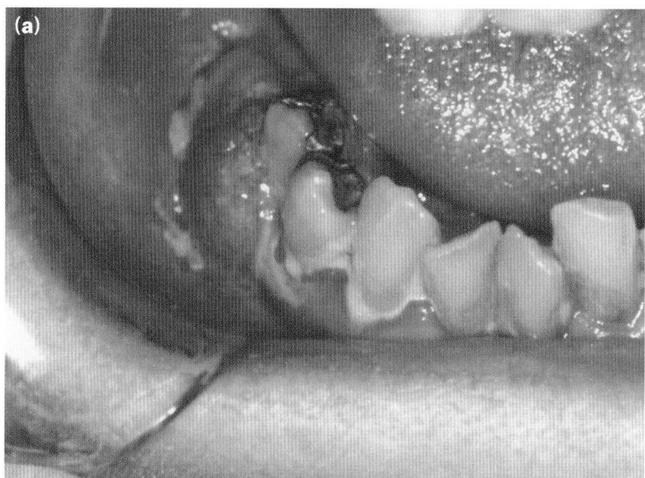
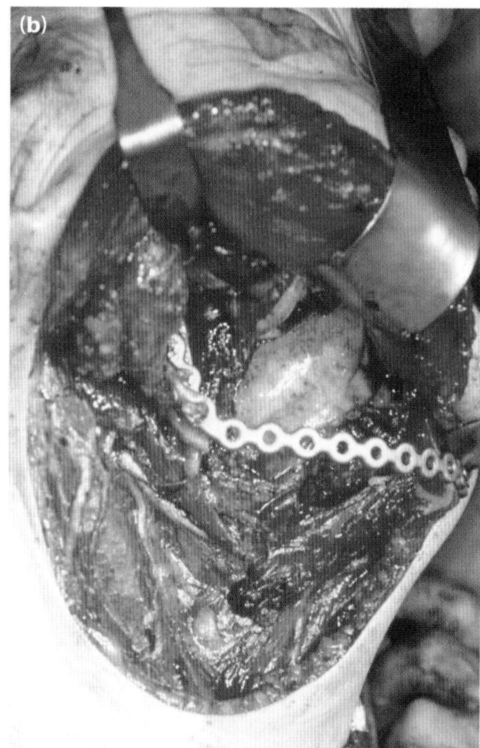
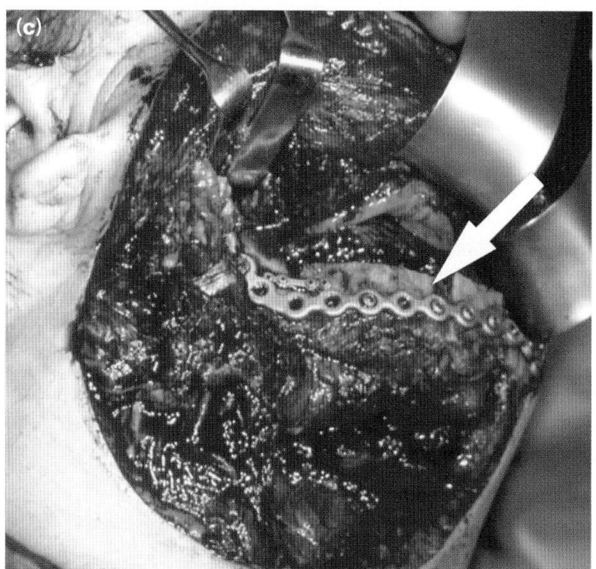
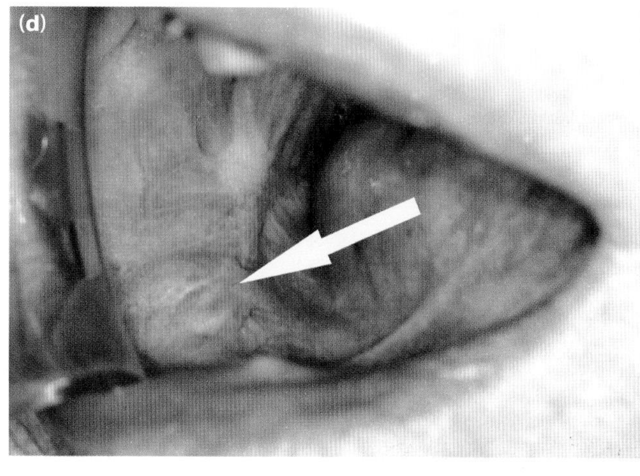
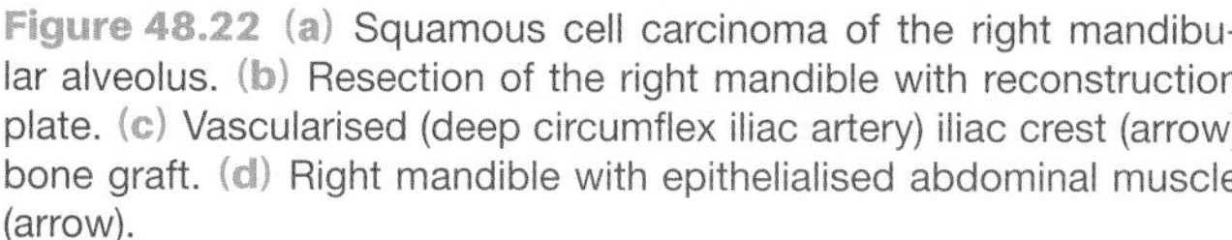

Figure 48.22 **(a)** Squamous cell carcinoma of the right mandibular alveolus. **(b)** Resection of the right mandible with reconstruction plate. **(c)** Vascularised (deep circumflex iliac artery) iliac crest (arrow) bone graft. **(d)** Right mandible with epithelialised abdominal muscle (arrow).

RETROMOLAR PAD

Tumours at this site frequently, but not always, invade the ascending ramus of the mandible. They also spread medially into the soft palate and the tonsillar fossa. Access for excision may necessitate additional access (e.g. a lip split and mandibulotomy [see Figure 48.16]). Small defects are managed ideally with a microvascular free flap, such as a radial artery forearm flap, or with a temporalis muscle flap where pedicled options are prefered. Segmental mandibular resections require vascularised bone to achieve adequate reconstruction; in such circumstances the scapula free flap provides a good source for restoration of bone continuity and abundant soft tissue capable of modification and flexible at inset, to suit larger defects.

HARD PALATE AND MAXILLARY ALVEOLUS

The maxillary alveolus and hard palate are relatively uncommon sites for SCC. A useful classification of the maxillectomy defect with suitable reconstructive options is provided by Brown *et al.* (see Further reading). A tumour arising in these areas may arise either from the oral mucosa *per se* or from the maxillary antrum penetrating the oral cavity. In the Indian subcontinent, carcinoma of the hard palate is more common and is particularly associated with reverse smoking. When they occur, malignant tumours of minor salivary glands typically present as swellings of the hard palate. Small tumours of the maxillary alveolus can be managed by transoral partial maxillectomy. More extensive tumours involving the floor of the maxillary sinus require wider access by a Weber–Fergusson incision (Figure 48.23). If the preoperative investigations demonstrate extension of the disease into the pterygoid space or the infratemporal fossa, the prognosis is poor as surgical clearance is difficult if not impossible. Tumour extending into the orbit requires simultaneous orbital exenteration or even a combined neurosurgical resection. The vascularised iliac crest graft is the method of choice for immediate maxillary reconstruction, although the fibula provides adequate bony replacement to maintain facial contour.

Microvascular free tissue transfer remains the method of choice for the management of defects in the oropharynx (*Table 48.3*). Free flaps are superior reconstructive options to pedicled or local flaps, which may be used for salvage procedures or recurrent disease. Each 'free' flap has a principal blood supply and a concomitant venous drainage. The flaps can be tailored to the defect to include skin, fascia, bone and muscle. The techniques of free tissue transfer demand specialist training and a microscope to connect blood vessels in the neck after neck dissection (e.g. facial artery to the prepared artery attached to the flap). The vascular anatomy of microvascular free flaps is summarised in *Table 48.4*.

TABLE 48.3 Primary reconstructive options in oral cancer.

Anatomical site	Primary reconstructive options	Alternative reconstruction
Floor of mouth	RFFF	Free flap – ALT, MSAP, lateral arm Pedicled/local flap – nasolabial flaps (bilateral), submental island flap
Lateral tongue	RFFF/ALT	Free flap – MSAP Pedicled/local flap – pectoralis major, platysma skin flap
Total tongue/glossectomy	ALT/rectus abdominus	Pedicled flap – pectoralis major
Buccal mucosa	RFFF	Free flap – ALT/MSAP Pedicled/local flap – pectoralis major
Mandible		
Dentate	Iliac crest (DCIA)	Free flap – fibula, composite radial, scapula or tip of scapula (angular branch of thoracodorsal A)
Edentulous	Fibula	Free flap – composite radial, scapula or tip of scapula (angular branch of thoracodorsal A) Pedicled/local flap – reconstruction plate and pectoralis major
Maxilla		
Low-level/hard palate	Obturation, RFFF/ALT	Pedicled/local flap – temporalis muscle Free flap – 'ZIP flap' - zygomatic implant retained prosthesis (perforating) RFFF/ALT
High	Iliac crest/scapula	Fibula
Soft palate/tonsil	Forearm/MSAP	Free flap – ALT for larger defects ± pharyngeal flap Pedicled/local flap – temporalis muscle, galeal flap
Tongue base	RFFF	Free flap – ALT for larger defects Pedicled/local flap – pectoralis major

ALT, anterolateral thigh; DCIA, deep circumflex iliac artery; MSAP, medial sural artery perforator; RFFF, radial forearm free flap.

Sir William Fergusson, 1808–1877, Scottish surgeon, described and published a modification of the original Weber incision to access the midface.

TABLE 48.4 Common microvascular 'free' flaps in oral cavity reconstruction.

Flap	Blood supply	Common variants
Forearm (RFFF)	Radial artery	Skin only; fascia only
Composite forearm	Radial artery	Skin and bone (radius)
Anterolateral thigh	Perforator vessels off descending (or transverse) branch of lateral circumflex femoral artery	Skin only; skin and muscle ± additional fascia (capacity for tubed reconstruction of pharynx)
Medial sural artery perforator (MSAP)	Medial sural artery	Fasciocutaneous flap
Lateral arm	Profunda brachii artery	Fasciocutaneous
Rectus abdominus	Deep inferior epigastric artery	Skin and muscle; muscle only
Fibula	Peroneal artery	Bone and skin; bone only; bone and fascia/fat
Iliac crest	Deep circumflex iliac artery	Bone only; bone and muscle; bone, muscle and skin, bone and skin as perforator flap
Scapula	Subscapular artery (+ optional angular branch of thoracodorsal artery)	Bone and skin; bone and multiple skin paddles, separate bone segments on circumflex scapula artery and angular branch of thoracodorsal artery

RFFF, radial forearm free flap.

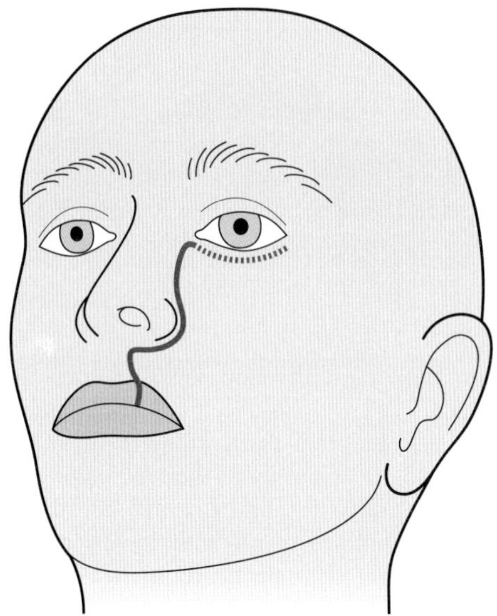

Figure 48.23 Weber–Ferguson incision for maxillectomy (lower eyelid extension may be required in extended maxillectomy).

POST-TREATMENT MANAGEMENT

As with the initial management of oral cavity cancer, the multidisciplinary team is essential for the ongoing management of oral cancer patients. For most patients, in particular those who have received combined modality treatment (surgery and (chemo)radiotherapy) medium to long-term sequelae can have a significant impact on quality of life. Speech and swallowing alteration is frequently encountered, as is the complication of osteoradionecrosis, in up to 10% of patients receiving adjuvant radiotherapy. While allied health professionals such as speech and language therapists are essential in the management of the former, surgical intervention, with its increased risks, is frequently required in the latter.

Surveillance for recurrence and, to a lesser extent, second primary tumours is necessary and development of local protocols for this can be helpful, although as a general rule recurrence reaches it peak within the first 12–24 months post treatment and therefore monitoring is most intensive in this period

FURTHER READING

Amin MB, Edge S, Greene F, Byrd DR, Brookland RK *et al.* (eds). *AJCC cancer staging manual*, 8th edn. New York: Springer International Publishing, 2017.

Brown JS, Shaw RJ. Reconstruction of the maxilla and midface: introducing a new classification. *Lancet Oncol* 2010; **11**: 1001–8.

Urken ML, Cheney ML, Sullivan M, Biller HF. *Atlas of regional and free flaps for head and neck reconstruction*. New York: Raven Press, 1995.

Wolff K-D, Hölzle F. *Raising of microvascular flaps: a systematic approach*. New York: Springer, 2011.

Chapter 49

Disorders of the salivary glands

Learning objectives

To understand:

- The surgical anatomy of the salivary glands
- The presentation, pathology and investigation of salivary gland disease
- The medical and surgical treatment of stones, infections and tumours that affect salivary glands

INTRODUCTION

There are three paired major salivary glands, two parotid glands, two submandibular glands and two sublingual glands. In addition, there are multiple minor salivary glands.

MINOR SALIVARY GLANDS

Anatomy

The mucosa of the oral cavity contains approximately 800 minor salivary glands. They are distributed in the mucosa of the lips, cheeks, palate, floor of the mouth and retromolar area. These minor salivary glands also appear in other areas of the upper aerodigestive tract including the oropharynx, larynx and trachea as well as the sinuses. They have a histological structure similar to that of mucus-secreting major salivary glands. Overall, they contribute to 10% of the total salivary volume.

Summary box 49.1

Anatomy of salivary glands

- Two parotid glands
- Two submandibular glands
- Two sublingual glands
- Approximately ~800 minor salivary glands

Common disorders of minor salivary glands

Cysts

Cysts are common and arise from trauma to the glandular parenchyma or drainage system. The minor salivary glands have the distinction that they can secrete against pressure and most cysts are of the extravasation rather than retension variety. They arise in the loose mucosa of the lower lip and the floor of mouth where saliva can easily collect. The swelling is painless and usually, but not always, translucent (Figure 49.1). Some resolve spontaneously, but most require formal surgical excision. Recurrence is rare.

Tumours

Few tumours show more diversity in histological appearance and anatomical site than those that arise from mucous glands of the upper aerodigestive tract. Tumours of minor salivary glands are histologically similar to those of major glands; however, more minor salivary gland tumours are malignant and as are almost all tumours in the sublingual glands. Tumours of minor salivary gland origin occur anywhere in the upper aerodigestive tract; however, common sites for tumour formation include the palate, upper lip and retromolar regions. Less

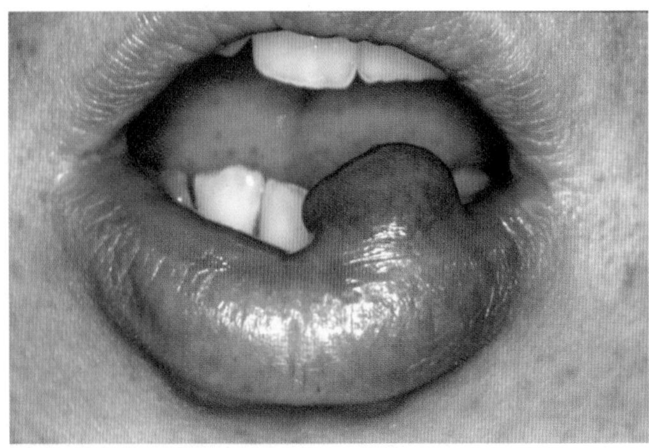

Figure 49.1 Mucous retention cyst. A translucent swelling on the lower lip is typical.

common sites for minor salivary gland tumours include the nasal and pharyngeal cavities. These tumours arise in submucosal seromucous glands that are found throughout the upper aerodigestive tract. A well-defined rubbery lump is a salivary gland tumour until proven otherwise. Benign minor salivary gland tumours present as painless, firm, slow-growing swellings. Overlying ulceration is extremely rare. Minor salivary gland tumours are managed by excision to include the overlying mucosa, with primary closure (Figure 49.2).

Benign tumours of the palate, less than 1 cm in diameter, can be managed by excisional biopsy, and the defect left to heal by secondary intention (Figure 49.3). Where the tumours are greater than 1 cm in diameter, a 3 mm punch biopsy (dermatological punch) is recommended to establish a diagnosis prior to formal excision and to avoid the embarrasment of inadvertently encountering a low-grade malignant lesion.

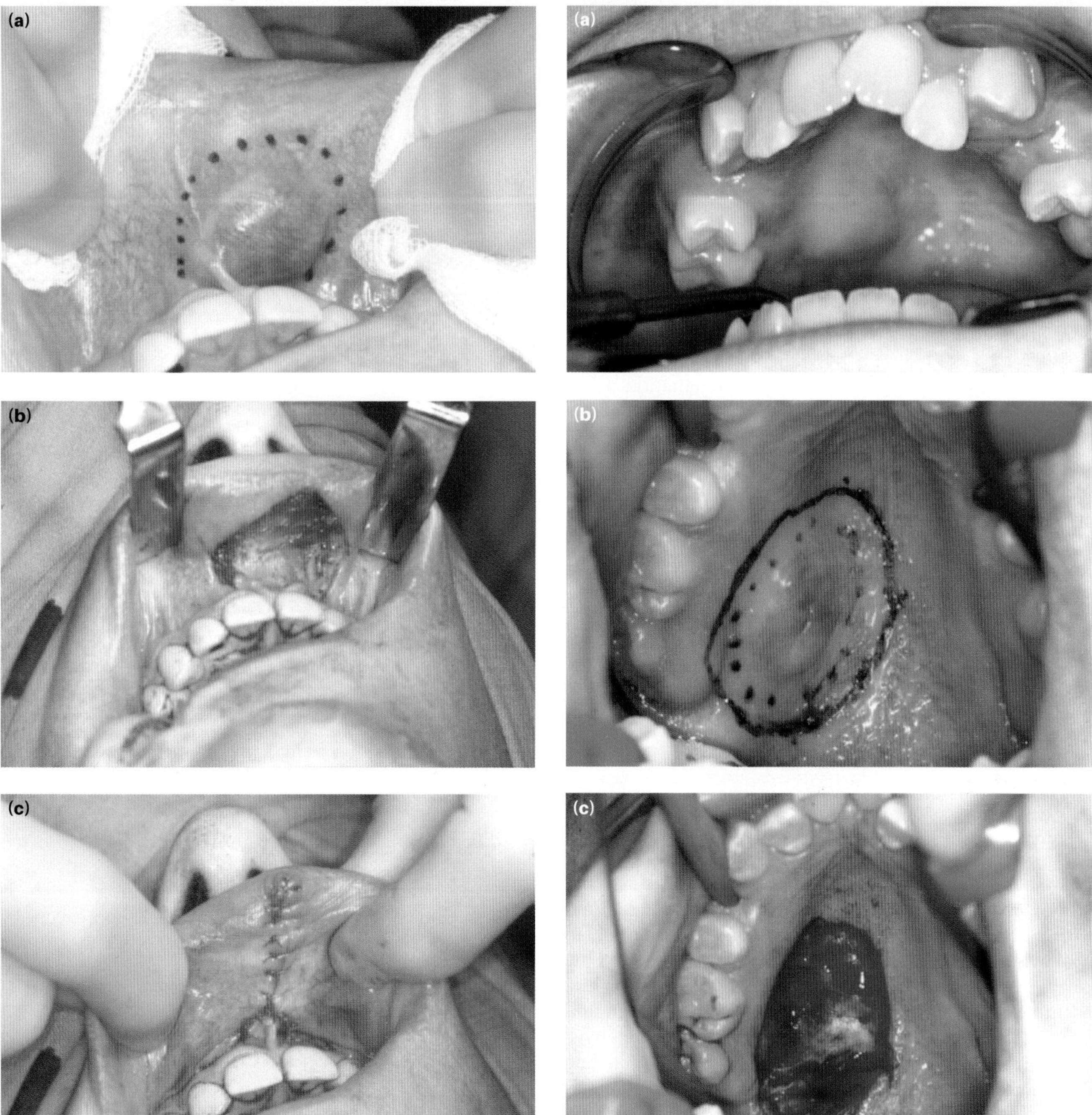

Figure 49.2 (a) Pleomorphic adenoma of the upper lip. (b) Tumour is excised with overlying mucosa. (c) Primary closure of the defect.

Figure 49.3 (a) Pleomorphic adenoma in the right palate in a 12-year-old girl. (b) Tumour is marked out with adequate margins including the overlying mucosa. (c) The subsequent defect. (d) Healing by secondary intention 3 years after surgery.

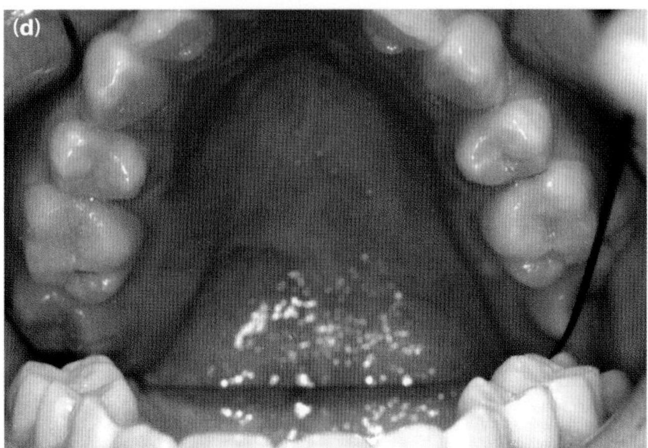

Figure 49.3 (*Continued*)

Malignant neoplasms

Malignant minor salivary gland tumours are rare (2 per million population). Most are low grade and present as apparently benign lumps. They have a firm consistency, and the overlying mucosa may have a varied discolouration from pink to blue or black (Figure 49.4). High-grade lesions usually become necrotic with ulceration as a late presentation.

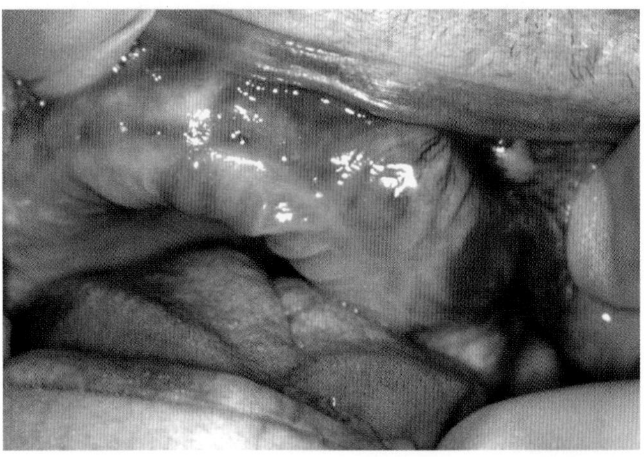

Figure 49.4 Adenoid cystic carcinoma of the left maxillary alveolus.

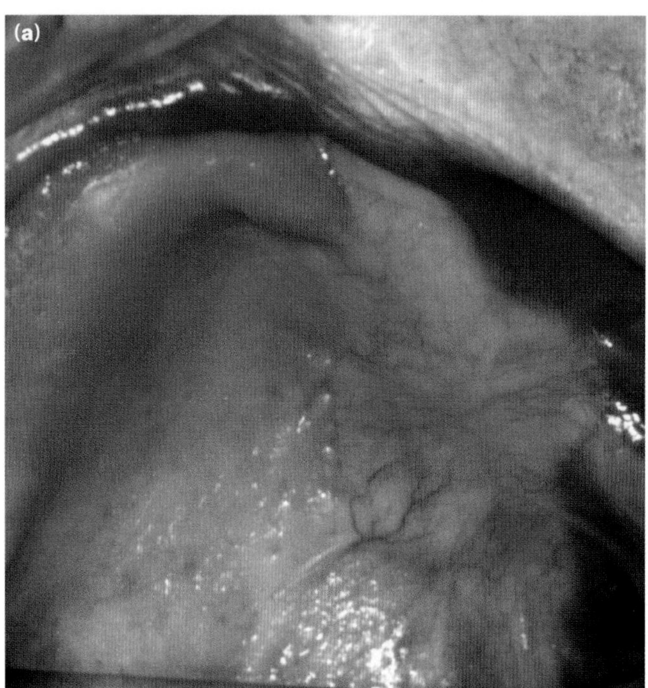

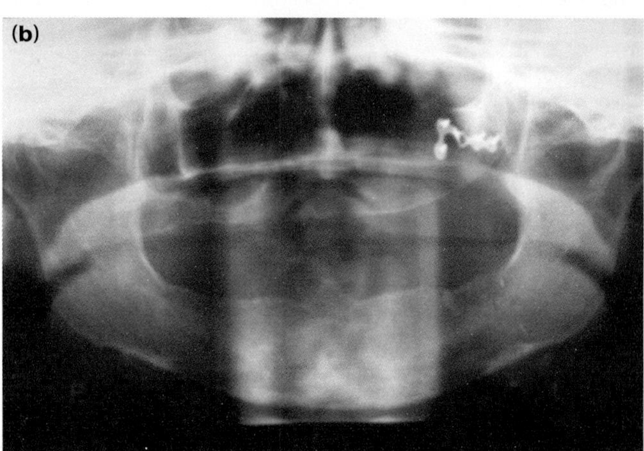

Figure 49.5 (a) Postoperative appearance following left maxillectomy and immediate reconstruction with a vascularised iliac crest graft and abdominal wall musculature (epithelialised). (b) Postoperative radiographic appearance of a reconstructed left maxilla with internal fixation.

Malignant minor salivary gland tumours of the palate that are low grade and early stage can be managed by wide excision with burring down of the underlying bone and then left to heal by secondary intention. Those that have perforated the palate may require partial or total maxillectomy. The subsequent defect can be managed by either prosthetic obturation or immediate reconstruction. Various microvascular flaps have been designed to reconstruct maxillectomy defects including radial forearm flap, fibular flap, rectus abdominus, latissimus dorsi and vascularised iliac crest graft (Figure 49.5).

Necrotising sialometaplasia

This is a well established but rare entity. Typically it occurs in the palate and mimics an aggressive cancer. It presents as a deep punched out ulcer with an indurated margin. It can not be distinguished from a neoplastic lesion except by biopsy. The diagnosis is sugested by rapid onset in a young person. The lesion resolves spontaniously with symptomatic treatment.

THE SUBLINGUAL GLANDS

Anatomy

The sublingual glands are a paired set of salivary glands lying in the anterior part of the floor of the mouth between the mucous membrane, the mylohyoid muscle and the body of the mandible close to the mental symphysis. The gland has a head portion that drains by numerous excretory ducts (Ducts of Rivinus) directly into the oral cavity and the tail that drains into the submandibular duct or directly into the mouth.

Summary box 49.2

Sublingual glands

- Problems are rare
- Minor mucous retention cysts may need surgery
- Plunging ranula is a retention cyst that tunnels deep
- Nearly all tumours are malignant

Common disorders of the sublingual glands

Cysts

The term 'ranula' is applied to a mucous extravasation cyst that arises from the sublingual gland. It produces a characteristic translucent swelling that takes on the appearance of a 'frog's belly' (ranula) (Figure 49.6). A ranula can resolve spontaneously, but many also require active treatment. The traditional and effective way is to remove the sublingual gland, but it is not an easy operation and the morbidity can be significant. New less invasive techniques are now quite effective (85% success) in resolving ranulas while preserving the gland. Incision and drainage, however tempting, usually results in recurrence.

Ranula is derived from 'rana', the Latin for frog.

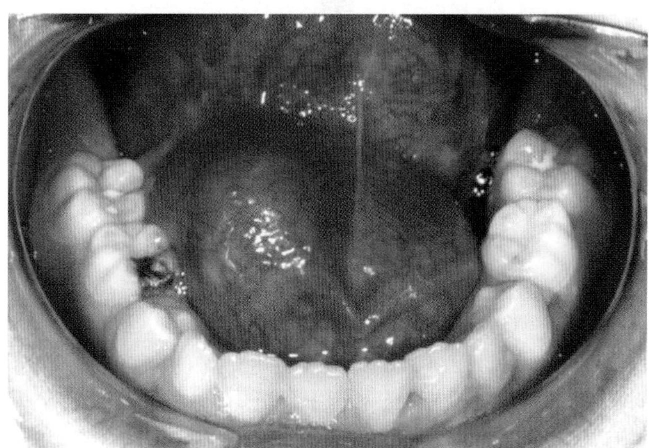

Figure 49.6 Large ranula affecting the floor of the mouth.

Plunging ranula

Plunging ranula is a rare form of mucous retention cyst that arises from the sublingual salivary glands. Mucus collects below the gland and perforates through the mylohyoid muscle diaphragm to enter the neck. Patients present with a dumb-bell-shaped swelling that is soft, fluctuant and painless in the submandibular or submental region of the neck (Figure 49.7). Diagnosis is made on ultrasound or magnetic resonance imaging (MRI) examination but clinched by aspirating thick

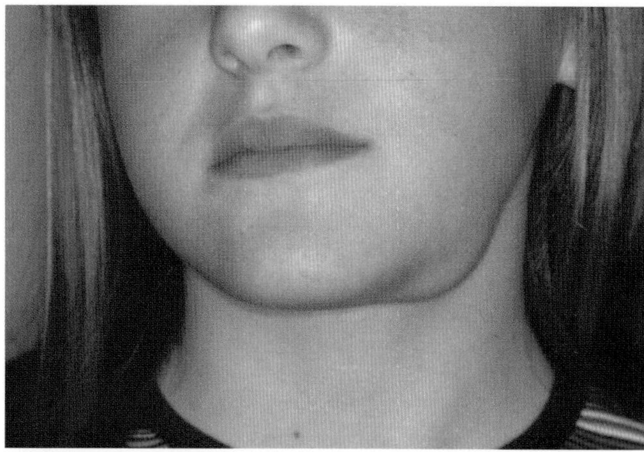

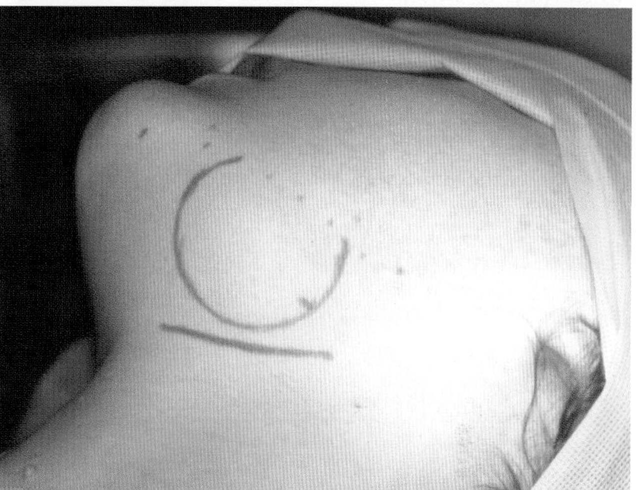

Figure 49.7 Plunging ranula in the left submandibular region.

yellow treacly fluid from the cyst. This distinguishes it from a lymphangioma. A cervical approach is now contraindicated. The cyst arises from the sublingual gland. All that is required is to remove the sublingual gland and aspirate the saliva out of the sac. The latter is formed of connective tissue not epithelium so melts away once the leak of saliva is resolved.

Tumours

Tumours involving the sublingual gland are extremely rare and are usually (90%) malignant. They present as a rubbery painless swelling in the floor of the mouth. Pain or lingual nerve paresthesia indicate a high-grade tumour. All such lumps must have a formal punch biopsy prior to formulating a treatment plan. Treatment requires *en block* wide excision involving the overlying mucosa and the adjacent periosteum with simultaneous neck dissection depending on the stage of the disease. Immediate reconstruction of the intraoral defect is recommended, especially when communication with the neck has been established. Radial artery forearm free flap or anterolateral thigh flap is usually the reconstruction of choice for fit patients, otherwise a pedicled pectoralis major flap can be used. There is normally a low threshold for adjuvant radiotherapy except for low-grade and stage lesions.

Augustus Quirinus Rivinus, 1652–1723, German physician and botanist who studied the anatomy of salivary glands and also developed ways of classifying plants.

THE SUBMANDIBULAR GLANDS

Anatomy

The submandibular glands are paired salivary glands that lie below the mandible on either side. They consist of a larger superficial and a smaller deep lobe that are continuous around the posterior border of the mylohyoid muscle. Important anatomical relations include the anterior facial vein and artery running over the surface of the gland in close association with the ramus mandibularis (marginal mandibular) of the facial nerve. The deep part of the gland lies on the hyoglossus muscle closely related to the lingual nerve and inferior to the hypoglossal nerve. The gland is surrounded by a well-defined capsule that is derived from the deep cervical fascia which splits to enclose it. The gland is drained by a single submandibular duct (Wharton's duct) that emerges from its deep surface and runs in the space between the hyoglossus and mylohyoid muscles. It drains into the anterior floor of the mouth at the sublingual papilla. There are several lymph nodes immediately adjacent and sometimes within the superficial part of the gland.

Summary box 49.3

Important anatomical relationships of the submandibular glands

- Lingual nerve
- Hypoglossal nerve
- Anterior facial vein
- Facial artery
- Marginal mandibular branch of the facial nerve

Ectopic/aberrant salivary gland tissue

The most common ectopic salivary tissue is a Stafne bone cyst, the origin of which is uncertain. It presents as an asymptomatic, clearly demarcated radiolucency of the angle of the mandible, characteristically below the inferior dental neurovascular bundle (Figure 49.8). The cavity in the lingual plate houses part of the submandibular gland or ectopic salivary tissue, but the origin of the cavity is unclear and has been attributed to the pulse pressure from the facial artery. No treatment is required.

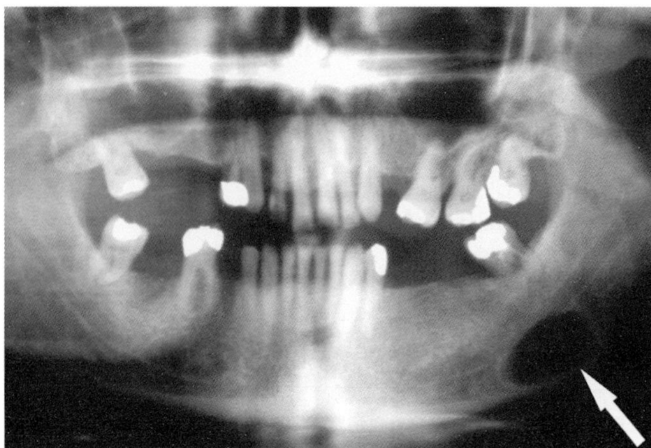

Figure 49.8 Plain radiographic appearance of a Stafne bone cyst.

Inflammatory disorders of the submandibular gland

Inflammation of the submandibular gland is termed sialadenitis. Submandibular sialadenitis may be acute, chronic or acute on chronic.

Common causes are:

- Acute submandibular sialadenitis
  - **Viral**. The paramyxovirus (mumps) is a viral illness of the salivary glands that usually produces parotitis. The submandibular glands are occasionally involved, causing painful tender swollen glands. Other viral infections of the submandibular gland are extremely rare.
  - **Bacterial**. Bacterial sialadenitis is more common than viral sialadenitis and occurs secondary to obstruction by stone. These stones can be reliably removed by minimally invasive techniques that preserve the gland.
- Chronic submandibular sialadenitis.

Obstruction and trauma

The most common cause of obstruction within the submandibular gland is stone formation (sialolithiasis) within the gland and its associated duct system. Eighty per cent of all salivary stones occur in the submandibular glands because their secretions are relatively viscous. Eighty per cent of submandibular stones are radio-opaque and can be identified on plain radiography (Figure 49.9). Stones are mainly composed of phosphate and oxalate salts.

The second most common cause of submandibular duct obstruction is stricture. The remaining 5–10% of cases are secondary to floor of mouth pathology or external pressure, particularly trauma to the floor of the mouth from an overextended flange on a lower denture that impinges on the sublingual papilla, causing inflammation and subsequent stricture.

Clinical symptoms

Patients usually present with acute painful swelling in the region of the submandibular gland, precipitated by eating (Figure 49.10). The swelling occurs rapidly and often resolves spontaneously over 1–2 hours after the meal is completed (meal-time syndrome). This classical picture occurs when the stone causes complete obstruction as it is washed forward and impacts in the lumen. The two most common sites of impaction are the hilum of the gland as the duct bends

Thomas Wharton, ?1616–1673, physician, St. Thomas's Hospital, London, UK, described the submandibular duct in 1656.
Edward C Stafne, 1894–1981, dental surgeon, The Mayo Clinic, Rochester, MN, USA, described these cysts in 1942.

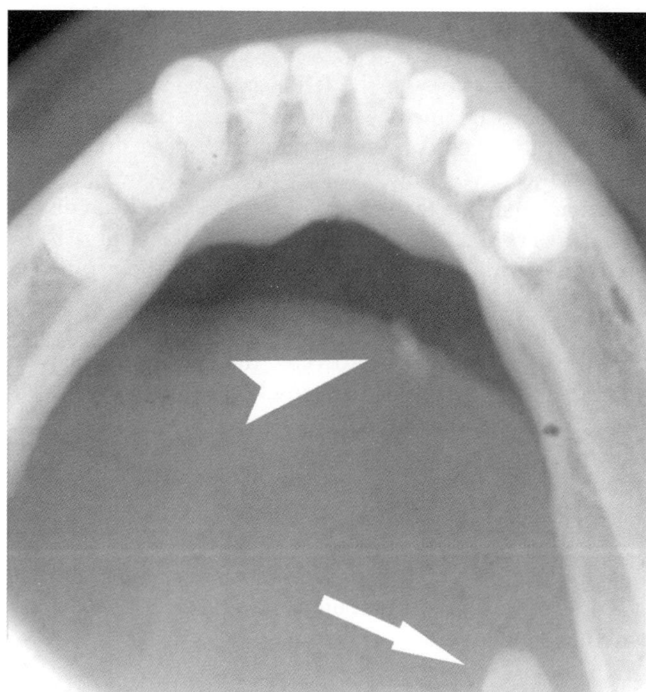

Figure 49.9 Lower occlusal X-ray highlighting a radio-opaque submandibular duct stone (arrowhead). Note the larger stone posteriorly located in the hilum of the gland (arrow).

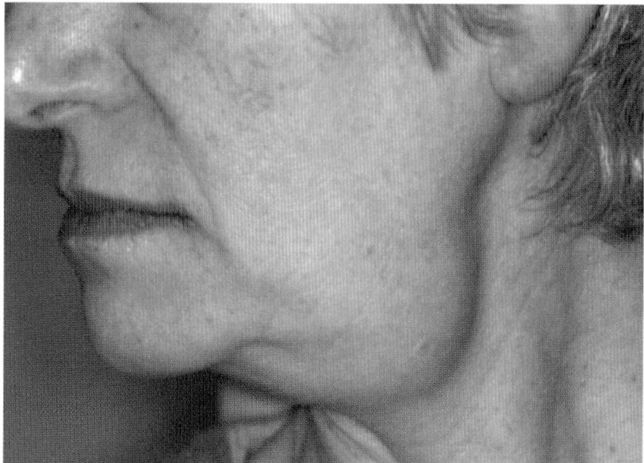

Figure 49.10 Acute left submandibular sialadenitis.

over the mylohyoid muscle and near the punctum. The symptoms are frequently intermittent as the stone can dislodge and allow the gush of saliva induced at meal times to pass. In such circumstances, symptoms are moderate with minimal discomfort and swelling. Clinical examination reveals an enlarged firm submandibular gland, tender on bimanual examination. Pus may be visible draining from the sublingual papilla or expressed by bimanual palpation of the gland (Figure 49.11).

Management

Small (less then 4 mm) mobile stones can be retrieved using a Dormia® basket. This minimally invasive procedure is usually performed under local anaestheisa either endoscopically (sialendoscopy) or under radiological control (ultrasonography). For larger stones, extracorporeal or intracorporeal lithotripsy can be employed to break the stone into smaller pieces using shock waves and the stone fragments can then removed with a basket. Recently, a pneumatic intraductal lithotripter (StoneBraker™) has been developed that can be advanced into the duct lumen under endoscopic control to fragment the stone. Results are promising, with 70% of stones being cleared in slected cases.

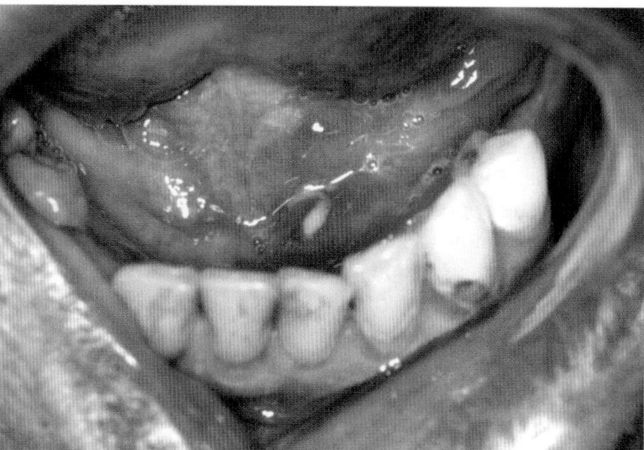

Figure 49.11 Acute suppurative submandibular sialadenitis. There is pus extruding from the left sublingual papilla.

If the stone is lying within the submandibular duct in the floor of the mouth anterior to the point at which the duct crosses the lingual nerve (second molar region), the stone can be removed under local anaesthetic but not by incising directly on to the duct. The latter runs under the sublingual gland and trauma to the head of the sublingual gland induces ranulae. Therefore, the incision has to run along the medial margin of the gland and the latter is then rotated laterally to expose the duct on its deep surface. Once the stone has been delivered via a single longitudinal incission along its surface, the duct should be closed by a resorbable suture and the incision in the floor of mouth closed.

Where the stone is proximal to the lingual nerve (i.e. at the hilum of the gland), stone retrieval via an intraoral approach can be performed quite reliably under general anaesthesia. The key is to choose cases in which the stone is palpable. This approach can be difficult and attendance on a suitable salivary course is recommended. Stone retrieval rates are excellent (95%). The risk to the lingual nerve is greatest with deep stones that are not palpable, as they lie outside the mouth below the mylohyoid. Traction injuries can occur in such circumstances. If stone retrieval fails, submandibular gland excision can be performed.

Submandibular gland excision

With the availability of more conservative techniques, submandibular gland excision is performed less frequently for benign disease as almost all benign conditions can be treated without gland removel. It is now the treatment of last rather than first resort. Submandibular gland incision is indicated for:

- sialadenitis, when minimally invasive methods have failed;
- salivary tumours.

Excision of the submandibular gland involves four distinct phases.

INCISION AND EXPOSURE OF GLAND

Surgery is usually performed under endotracheal general anaesthesia with moderate neck extension and the chin rotated to the opposite side. The incision should be marked at least 3–4 cm below the lower border of the mandible to avoid damage to the marginal mandibular branch of the facial nerve (Figure 49.12a). The incision should be sited within the nearest skin crease and should be approximately 4 cm long. Infiltration with lidocaine with adrenaline is optional. Sharp dissection is performed down to the platysma muscle, which should be clearly identified to facilitate later closure (Figure 49.12b). The muscle is incised and retracted. The underlying investing layer of deep cervical fascia is then divided, and the marginal mandibular branch of the facial nerve that normally runs on the deep surface of the platysma muscle is preserved. Posteriorly, the incision approaches the angular tract where the deep cervical fascia splits to form the investing layer around the sternomastoid muscle. Superficial veins, including the anterior facial vein, require ligation.

GLAND MOBILISATION

Deepening the incision divides the submandibular gland capsule. In inflammatory conditions, the submandibular gland is excised by intracapsular dissection, mobilising the gland by sharp dissection. For tumours of the submandibular gland it is imperative to know if the lesion is benign or malignant. This can be ascertained by Tru-Cut biopsy. This is important because if the wrong operation is undertaken on a malignant tumour, the survival rate of the patient is reduced by 20%. Malignant tumours require wide excission with neck dissection in selected cases. Benign tumours can be dealt with by extracapsular dissection and excision of the submandibular gland.

The superficial lobe of the submandibular gland is first mobilised. As dissection proceeds, the posterior belly and anterior belly of the digastric muscle are identified. Dissection posteriorly identifies the facial artery (Figure 49.13), which is divided to facilitate further mobilisation. The course of the facial artery is variable, sometimes penetrating the gland emerging on the upper border and sometimes lying in a groove on the deeper aspect of the gland. The gland is further mobilised by blunt and sharp dissection. A number of small arteries and veins are encountered, which require control with bipolar diathermy.

DISSECTION OF THE DEEP LOBE AND IDENTIFICATION OF THE LINGUAL NERVE

An important landmark in submandibular gland dissection is the posterior border of the mylohyoid muscle. Once identified, it can be retracted forwards to reveal the deep lobe of the gland. Several veins are usually encountered, which need to be controlled with diathermy. The gland is then retracted inferiorly, invariably attached to the lingual nerve through parasympathetic secretor motor fibres. In the presence of chronic infection and subsequent fibrosis, identification of the lingual nerve on the deep aspect of the gland is sometimes difficult. It is imperative that the lingual nerve is formally identified prior to division of the parasympathetic fibres. The gland is then pedicled entirely on the submandibular duct, which, once identified, is ligated. The gland is delivered and sent for histological examination. The hypoglossal nerves lie deep to the submandibular capsule and should not be damaged during intracapsular dissection (Figure 49.14).

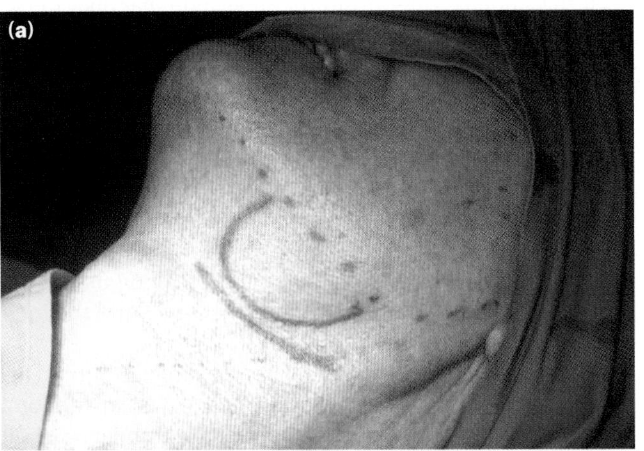

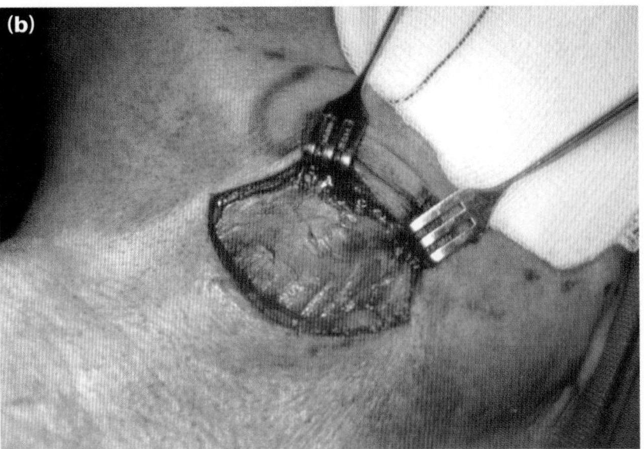

Figure 49.12 (a) Surface landmarks of submandibular gland excision. (b) Skin flaps elevated and platysma exposed.

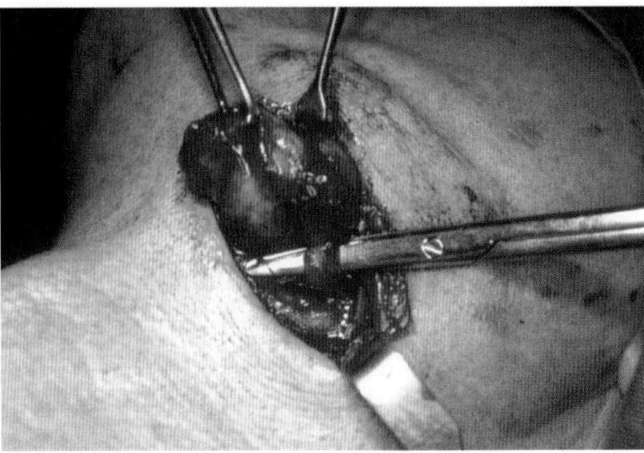

Figure 49.13 Submandibular gland mobilisation and exposure of the facial artery.

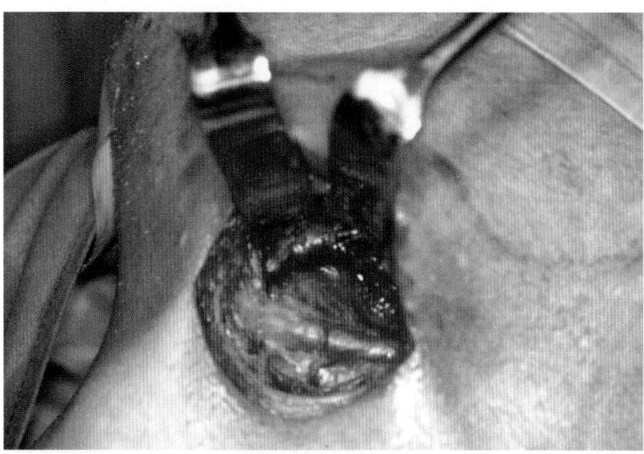

Figure 49.14 Bed of the submandibular triangle following submandibular gland removal, revealing the posterior edge of the mylohyoid muscle and the tendon of the digastric muscle.

Three cranial nerves (CNs) are at risk during removal of the submandibular gland:

1 the marginal mandibular branch of the facial nerve;
2 the lingual nerve;
3 the hypoglossal nerve.

An adequate incision coupled with meticulous haemostasis allows the surgeon to identify these important structures during surgery.

WOUND CLOSURE

Haemostasis is confirmed and a vacuum suction drain inserted. The wound is closed using a continuous resorbable suture to the platysma muscle, as the platysma muscle has a direct contribution to the depressor activity of the corner of the mouth. The skin may be closed with a subcuticular non-resorbable suture, removed 7 days after surgery. The drain remains for 24 hours.

Complications of submandibular gland excision

Complications are:

- haematoma;
- wound infection;
- marginal mandibular nerve injury;
- lingual nerve injury;
- hypoglossal nerve injury;
- transection of the nerve to the mylohyoid muscle producing submental skin anaesthesia.

Tumours of the submandibular gland

Tumours of the submandibular gland are uncommon and usually present as a slow-growing, painless swelling within the submandibular triangle (Figure 49.15). About 60–70% of submandibular gland tumours are benign, in contrast to 80–90% of parotid gland tumours (*Table 49.1*). In many circumstances, the swelling cannot, on clinical examination, be differentiated from submandibular lymphadenopathy. This can be resolved definitively by ultrasound examination. Most salivary neoplasms, even malignant tumours, are often slow-growing, painless swellings. The difficulty is to always distinguish between benign and malignant lesions prior to excision, as in up to 30% referrals of submandibular gland cancers to regional cancer centres, patients have already had surgical excison of the gland, which was subsequently found to be malignant on histological examination. Pain is not a reliable indication of malignancy; however, rapid growth, facial nerve palsy, lymph node enlargement and skin tethering are signs of a high-grade malignant lesion. The most common malignant tumour is an adenocystic carcinoma (40%), which may masquerade as a benign lump.

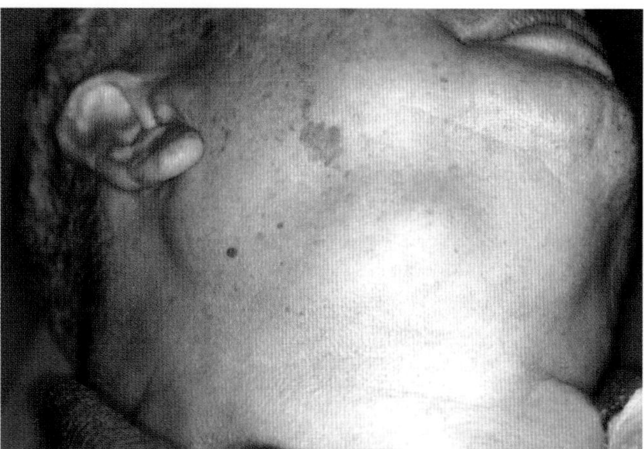

Figure 49.15 Benign tumour of the right submandibular gland.

TABLE 49.1 Salivary gland tumours – frequency and distribution.

Type	Location	Frequency	Malignant (%)
Major	Parotid Submandibular Sublingual	Common Uncommon Very rare	10–20 50 85
Minor	Upper aerodigestive tract	Rare	90

Clinical features of high-grade malignant salivary tumours

These include:

- facial nerve weakness;
- rapid enlargement of the swelling;
- induration and/or ulceration of the overlying skin;
- cervical node enlargement.

Investigation

The initial investigation of choice is ultrasound with fine-needle aspiration cytology (FNAC)/True-Cut biopsy. Once it is established that a tumour is present, computed tomography (CT) and MRI scanning are complimentary techniques for imaging tumours arising in the major salivary glands. The tumour is intrinsic to the gland. The scan will highlight the relationship of the tumour to other anatomical structures, which is helpful in planning surgery.

Open surgical biopsy is contraindicated as this may seed the tumour into surrounding tissues, making it impossible to eradicate microscopic deposits of tumour cells. Fine-needle aspiration or Tru-Cut biopsy is a safe alternative as the risk of seeding tumour is remote. The combination of careful history and examination in conjunction fine-needle aspitation cytology can identify over 95% of malignant cases. The few malignant cases that are indistinguishable from benign disease by these methods and are only identified by histology are usually indolent and act as benign tumours.

Management of submandibular gland tumours

Benign tumours of the submandibular gland can be safely removed by meticulous dissection outside the submandibular capsule. No instrument should be applied to the gland as to do so may crush it. As long as the capsule of the gland is preserved intact, the risk of recurrence is 1–1.5% at 10 years. As with all salivary gland tumours, surgical excision with a cuff of normal tissue is the goal.

The management of malignant salivary gland tumours is governed by the stage and clinical grade of the lesion. The

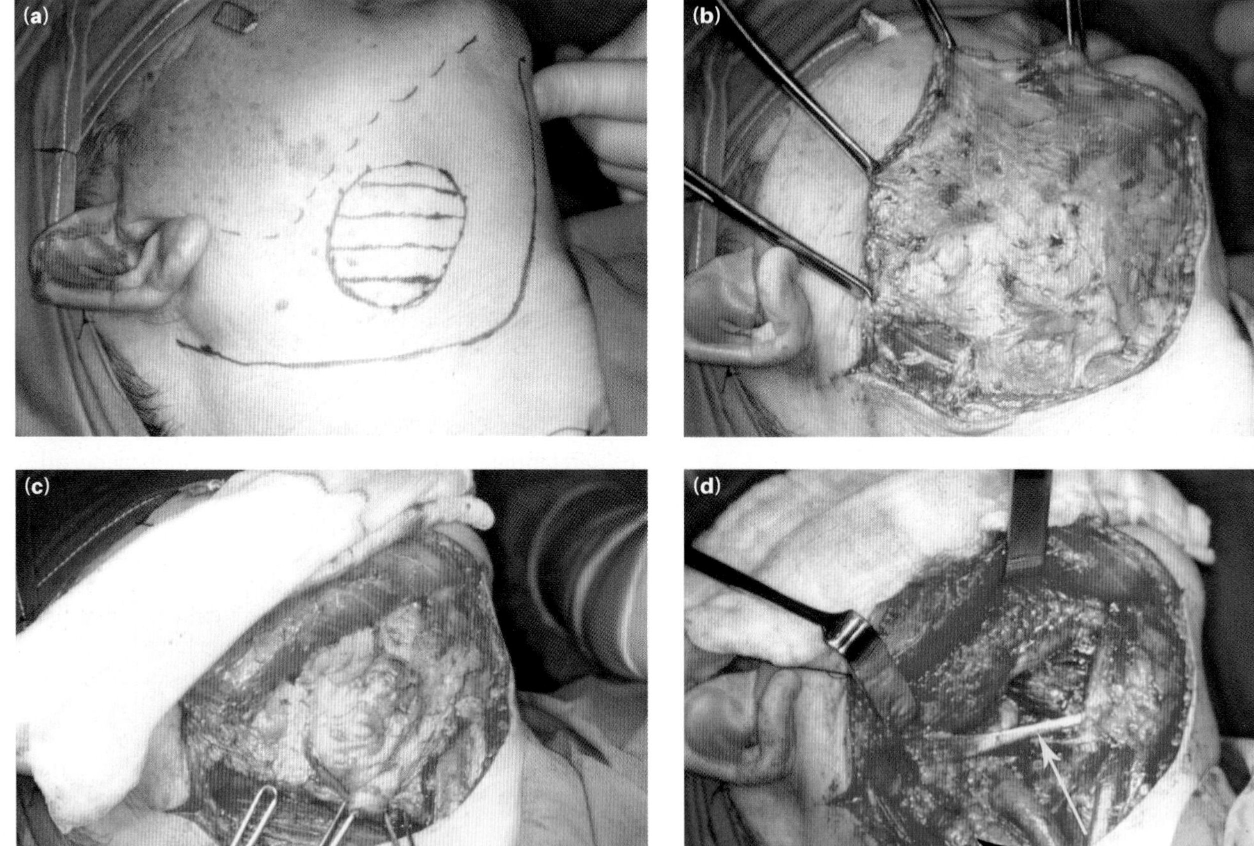

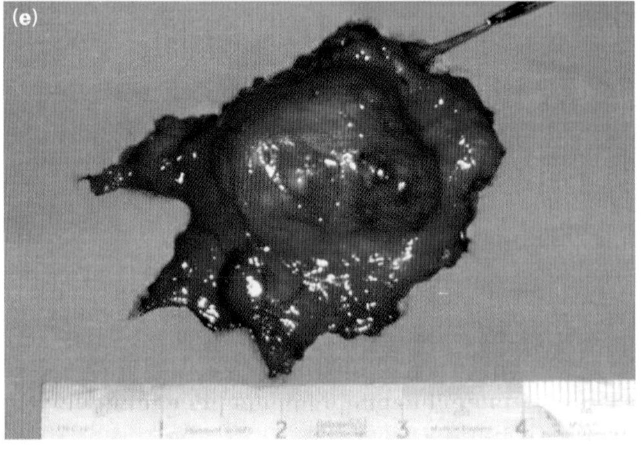

Figure 49.16 (a) Landmarks and incision for suprahyoid neck dissection to remove a large pleomorphic adenoma of the submandibular gland. (b) Skin flap raised at the subplatysmal level. (c) Mobilisation of the contents of the anterior triangle of the neck along the anterior border of the sternomastoid. (d) Suprahyoid neck dissection completed, revealing the digastric tendon (yellow arrow) and great vessels (black arrow). (e) Specimen revealing the tumour with a cuff of normal tissue with artery forceps attached to the submandibular duct.

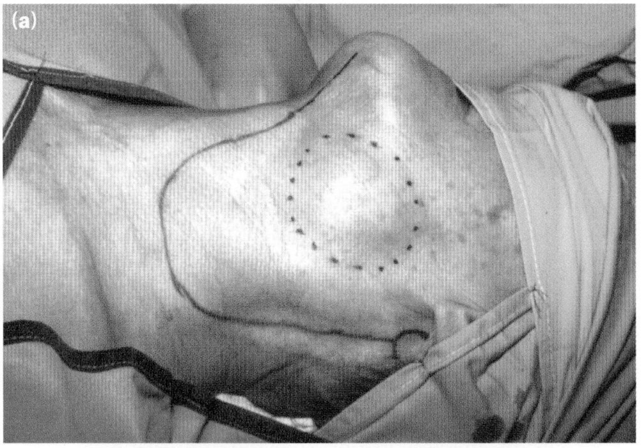
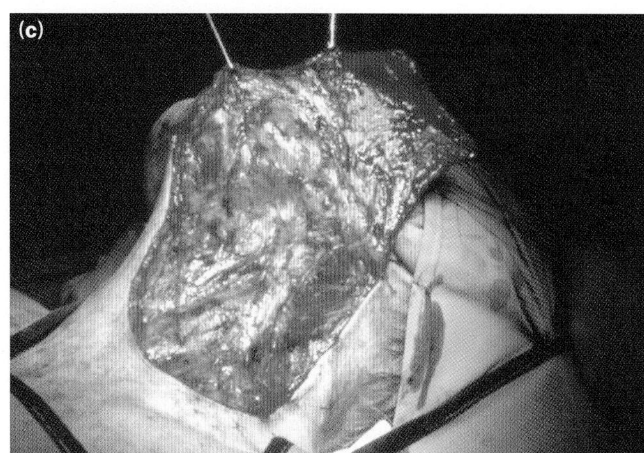
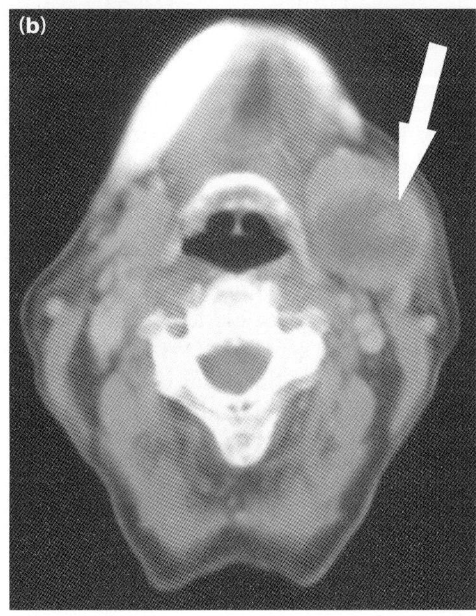
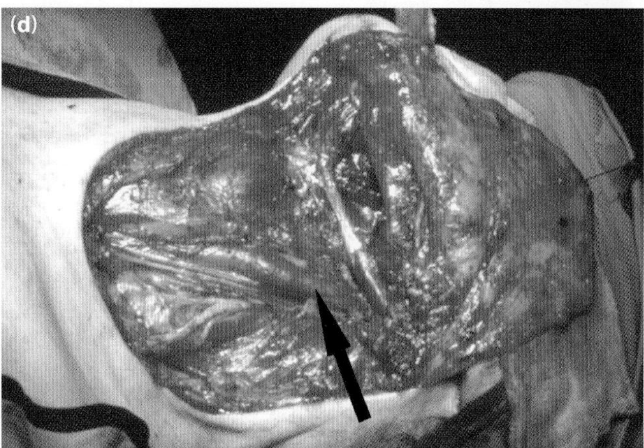

Figure 49.17 (a) Landmarks and incision for radical neck dissection for carcinoma of the left submandibular gland. (b) computed tomography scan revealing a large tumour of the left submandibular gland with central necrosis (arrow). (c) Skin flap developed for radical neck dissection. (d) Completion of radical neck dissection revealing the great vessels of the neck (arrow).

larger and more aggressive the lesion, the more radical is the surgery required. Each case has to be judged on its own merits, but wide clearance of the submandibular triangle with some form of neck dissection is normally the treatment of choice (Figure 49.16). This may neccessitate sacrifice of the lingual and hypoglossal nerves if the tumour is adherent to the deep bed of the gland (Figure 49.17). Adjuvant radiotherapy is usually dictated by pathological findings such as close margins and high-grade cancers. The prognostic cut off point for salivary cancers is 4 cm and most tumours larger than this need adjuvant therapy as will patients with adenoid cystic carcinoma if optimum results are to be achieved.

THE PAROTID GLAND

Anatomy

The parotid gland lies in a recess bounded by the ramus of the mandible, the base of the skull and the mastoid process. It lies on the carotid sheath and CNs XI and XII and extends forward over the masseter muscle. The gland is enclosed in a sheath of dense deep cervical fascia. Its upper pole extends just below the zygoma and its lower pole (tail) into the neck.

Several important structures run through the parotid gland. These include:

- the facial nerve trunk that divides into its major five branches;
- the terminal branch of the external carotid artery that divides into the maxillary artery and the superficial temporal artery;
- the retromandibular vein;
- intraparotid lymph nodes.

The gland is arbitrarily divided into deep and superficial lobes, separated by the facial nerve. Eighty per cent of the parotid gland lies superficial and 20% deep to the nerve. An accessory lobe is occasionally present lying anterior to the superficial lobe on the masseter muscle.

Developmental disorders

Developmental disorders such as agenesis, duct atresia and congenital fistula are extremely rare.

Inflammatory disorders

Viral infections

Mumps is the most common cause of acute painful parotid swelling and predominantly affects children. It is spread via airborne droplets of infected saliva. The disease starts with a prodromal period of 1–2 days, during which the patient experiences fever, nausea and headache. This is followed by pain and swelling in one or both parotid glands. Parotid pain can be very severe and exacerbated by eating and drinking. Symptoms resolve within 5–10 days. The diagnosis is based on history and clinical examination; recent contact with an infected patient with a painful parotid swelling is often sufficient to lead to a diagnosis. Atypical viral parotitis does occur and may present with predominantly unilateral swelling or even submandibular involvement. A single episode of infection confers lifelong immunity. Treatment of mumps is symptomatic with regular paracetamol and adequate oral fluid intake. Complications of orchitis, oophoritis, pancreatitis, sensorineural deafness and meningoencephalitis are rare, but are more likely to occur in adults.

Other viral agents that produce parotitis include Coxsackie A and B, parainfluenza 1 and 3, Echo and lymphocytic choriomeningitis.

Bacterial infections

Acute ascending bacterial sialadenitis is historically described in dehydrated elderly patients following major surgery. Reduced salivary flow secondary to dehydration results in ascending infection via the parotid duct into the parotid parenchyma. The more common picture today is an acute bacterial parotitis associated with a salivary calculus. The patient presents with a tender, painful parotid swelling that arises over several hours (Figure 49.18). There is generalised malaise, pyrexia and occasional cervical lymphadenopathy. The pain is exacerbated by eating or drinking. The parotid swelling may be diffuse, but often localises to the lower pole of the gland. Intraoral examination may reveal pus exuding from the parotid gland papilla. The infecting organism is usually *Staphylococcus aureus* or *Streptococcus viridans*, and treatment is with appropriate intravenous antibiotics. If the gland becomes fluctuant, ultrasound may identify abscess formation within the gland that may require aspiration with a large-bore needle or formal drainage under general anaesthesia. In the latter procedure, the skin incision should be made low to avoid damage to the lower branch of the facial nerve. Blunt dissection using sinus forceps is preferred, and the cavity is opened to facilitate drainage. A drain is inserted and left *in situ* for 24–72 hours. Sialography is contraindicated during acute infection. Chronic bacterial sialadenitis is rare in the parotid gland.

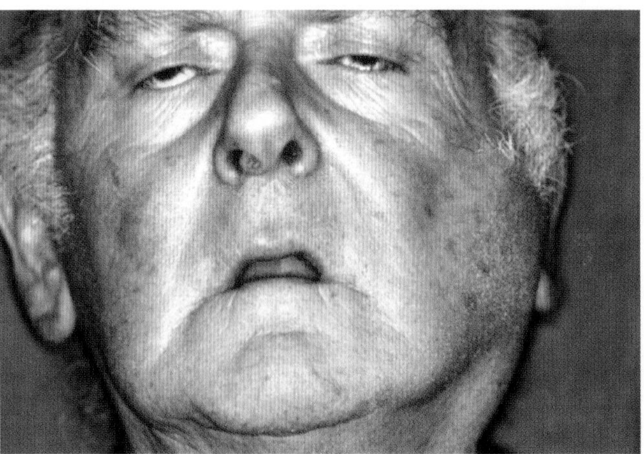

Figure 49.18 Acute left bacterial parotitis.

Recurrent parotitis of childhood

Recurrent parotitis of childhood is a distinct clinical entity of unknown aetiology and variable prognosis. It is characterised by rapid swelling of one or both parotid glands, in which the symptoms are made worse by chewing and eating. Systemic upset with fever and malaise is variable. The symptoms usually last from 3 to 7 days, and are then followed by a quiescent period of weeks to several months. Children usually present between the ages of 3 and 6 years, although symptoms have been reported in infants as young as 4 months. The diagnosis is based on the characteristic history and can be confirmed by sialography. This shows a characteristic punctate sialectasis likened to a 'snowstorm' (Figure 49.19). The condition is difficult to manage if it becomes established and so the initial treatment is important. The condition responds to regular endoscopic washouts and long courses of antibiotics. The suspicion is that in some cases the condition is caused by an incompetent punctum that leads to soiling of the parotid ducts with contaminated oral fluids.

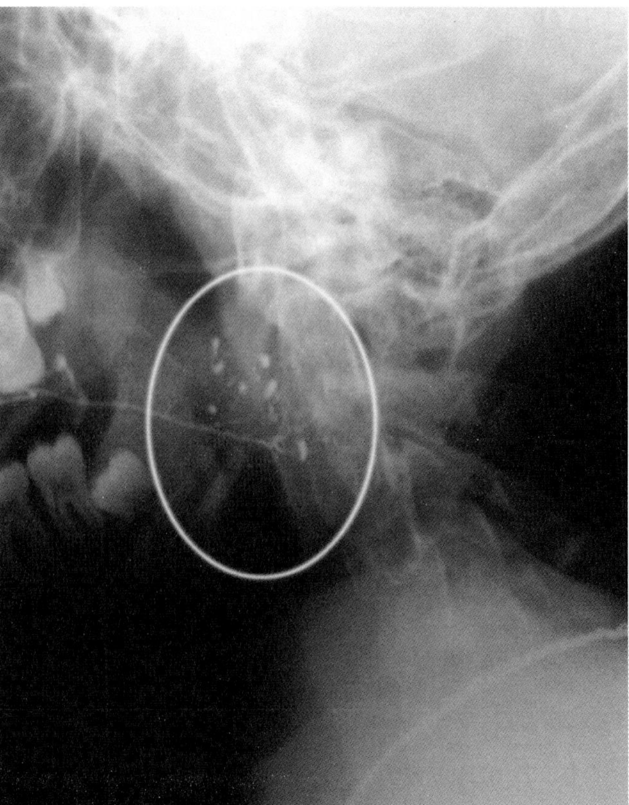

Figure 49.19 Characteristic 'snowstorm' appearance of recurrent parotitis of childhood (circled).

Human immunodeficiency virus-associated sialadenitis

Chronic parotitis in children may signify human immunodeficiency virus (HIV) infection. The presentation of HIV-associated sialadenitis is very similar to classical Sjögren's syndrome in adulthood. Although HIV-associated sialadenitis and Sjögren's syndrome are histologically similar, the former condition is usually associated with a negative autoantibody screen. Other presentations of salivary gland disease in HIV-positive patients include multiple parotid cysts, which cause gross parotid swelling and facial disfigurement. CT and MRI demonstrate the characteristic 'Swiss cheese' appearance of multiple large cystic lesions (Figure 49.20). The swollen glands are usually painless and may regress on the institution of antiviral therapy. Cysts can be aspirated.

Obstructive parotitis

There are several causes of obstructive parotitis, which produces intermittent painful swelling of the parotid gland, particularly at mealtimes.

Stone formation and strictures

Sialolithiasis is less common in the parotid gland (20%) than in the submandibular gland (80%). Parotid duct stones are usually radiolucent and rarely visible on plain radiography. They are frequently located at the confluence of the collecting ducts, at the point the duct courses over the masseter muscle or in the distal aspect of the parotid duct adjacent to the parotid papilla. The stones are easily demonstrated on ultrasound. The same rules for treatment apply to parotid stones as to submandibular duct stones. Small stones (~4 mm) can be retrieved by baskets, slightly larger stones up to 8 mm can be broken with lithotripsy and stones over 8 mm diameter should be removed by endoscopic assisted surgery while preserving the gland. Strictures are common in the parotid gland and are responsible for about 20% of obstructive cases. The symptom complex is a little different as the obstruction is due to mucus plugs. These form after periods of stagnation. Classically, the patient complains of a meal-time syndrome starting at breakfast and the saliva cannot seep past the mucus plug so the swelling persists. Massage eventually releases the plug with a gush of salty saliva. Infection is uncommon unless there is stone formation. Strictures respond to dilatation and endoscopic washouts with steroid solutions.

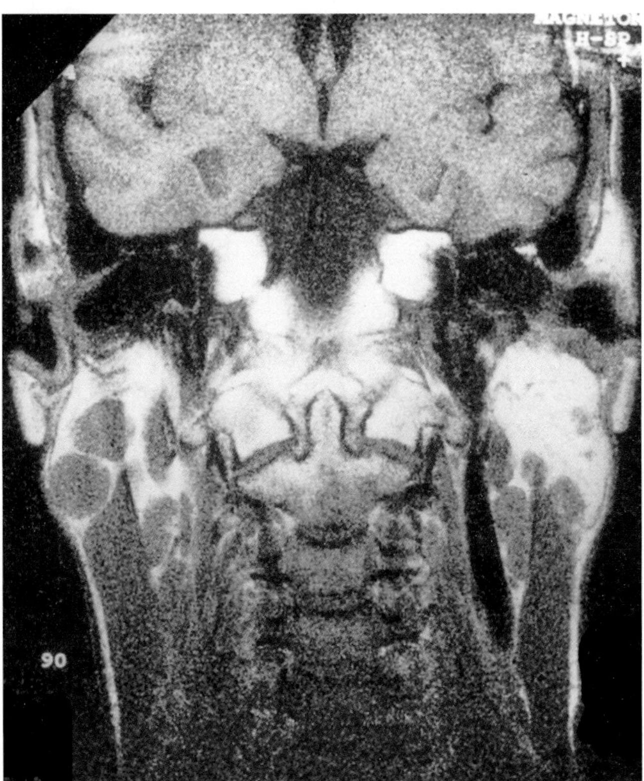

Figure 49.20 Magnetic resonance imaging scan. Giant bilateral parotid cysts in human immunodeficiency virus infection.

Papillary obstruction

Obstructive parotitis, can be caused by trauma to the parotid papilla. The subsequent inflammation and oedema obstructs salivary flow, particularly at mealtimes. This is a rare but real entity. The partial obstruction over a protracted period leads to dilation of the duct and an entity called 'mega-duct'. A large dilated duct is visible coursing over the patient's cheek. Drainage has to be re-established. This can be done by progressive dilatation of the punctum and the insertion of a stent that is kept in position for many weeks. Surgical attempts to refashion the punctum are unlikely to be successful. Papillotomy should not be performed as this often leads to stricture formation and a life time of problems. This is not the case with the submandibular gland.

Tumours of the parotid gland

The parotid gland is the most common site for salivary tumours. Most tumours arise in the superficial lobe and present as slow-growing, painless swellings below the ear (Figure 49.21a), in front of the ear (Figure 49.21b) or in the upper aspect of the neck. Less commonly, tumours may arise from the accessory lobe and present as persistent swellings within the cheek. Rarely, tumours may arise from the deep lobe of the gland and present as a parapharyngeal mass (Figures 49.21c, d). Symptoms include difficulty in swallowing and snoring. Clinical examination reveals a diffuse firm swelling in the soft palate and tonsil.

Some 80–90% of tumours of the parotid gland are benign, the most common being pleomorphic adenoma (*Table 49.2*).

Malignant salivary gland tumours are divided into two distinct sub-groups:

1 **Low-grade malignant tumours** (e.g. acinic cell carcinoma) are indistinguishable on clinical examination from benign neoplasms.

Henrik Samuel Conrad Sjögren, 1899–1986, Professor of Ophthalmology, Göthenburg, Sweden, described this condition in 1933.
A Swiss cheese is one with many holes in it.

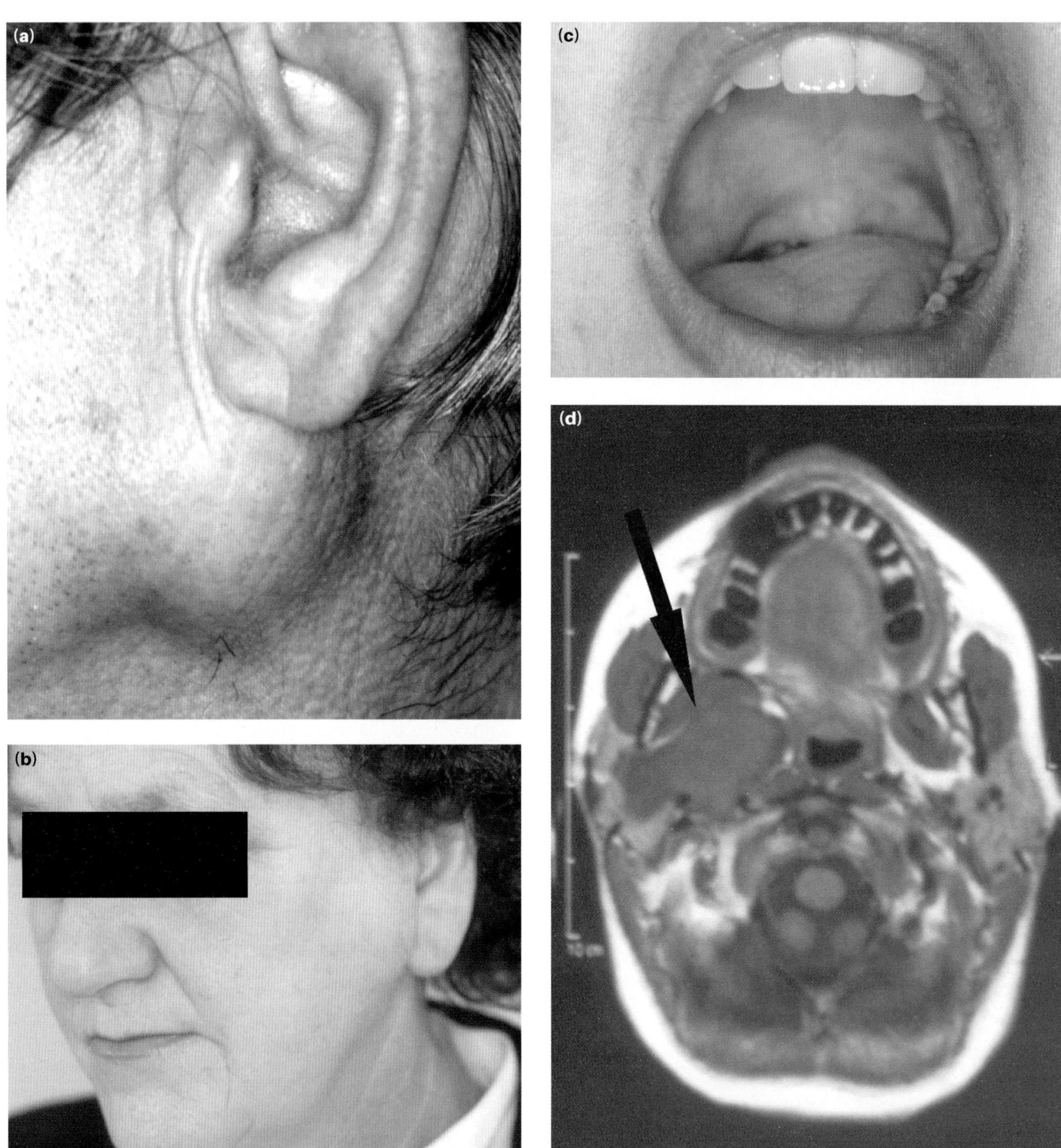

Figure 49.21 (a) Benign tumour of the left parotid gland producing characteristic deflection of the ear lobe. (b) Pleomorphic adenoma arising from the upper pole of the left parotid gland producing a preauricular swelling. (c) Deep lobe tumour of the right parotid presenting with a swelling of the right soft palate. (d) Magnetic resonance imaging scan revealing a large deep lobe tumour (arrow) of the right parotid gland, occupying the parapharyngeal space.

2 **High-grade malignant tumours** usually present as rapidly growing, often painless swellings in and around the parotid gland. The tumour presents as either a discrete mass with infiltration into the overlying skin (Figure 49.22) or a diffuse but hard swelling of the gland with no discrete mass. Presentation with advanced disease is common, and cervical lymph node metastases may be present.

Among primary parotid malignant tumours, mucoepidermoid carcinoma is the most common, followed by adenocystic carcinoma. The latter is notorious for its proclivity for perineural invasion and metastatic potential so surgery is normally supported by adjuvant radiotherapy to gain local control of the disease.

TABLE 49.2 Classification of salivary gland tumours (simplified).

Type	Subgroup	Common examples
I Adenoma	Pleomorphic Monomorphic	Pleomorphic adenoma Adenolymphoma (Warthin's tumour)
II Carcinoma	Low grade	Acinic cell carcinoma Adenoid cystic carcinoma Low-grade mucoepidermoid carcinoma
	High grade	Adenocarcinoma Squamous cell carcinoma High-grade mucoepidermoid carcinoma
III Non-epithelial tumours		Haemangioma, lymphangioma
IV Lymphomas	Primary lymphomas Secondary lymphomas	Non-Hodgkin's lymphomas Lymphomas in Sjögren's syndrome
V Secondary tumours	Local Distant	Tumours of the head and neck especially Skin and bronchus
VI Unclassified tumours		
VII Tumour-like lesions	Solid lesions	Benign lymphoepithelial lesion Adenomatoid hyperplasia
	Cystic lesions	Salivary gland cysts

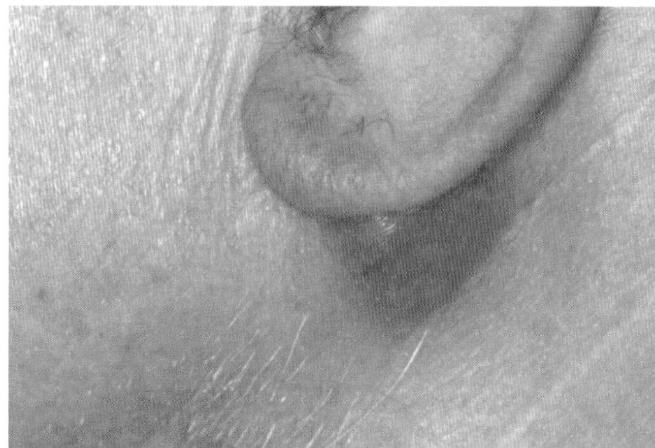

Figure 49.22 Malignant tumour of the left parotid gland with invasion of the overlying skin.

Investigations

The initial imaging modality of choice is ultrasound as it demonstrates if the lump is intrinsic to the parotid or not. It also facilitates accurate sampling of the lesion by FNAC or True-Cut biopsy. Subsequently, CT and MRI are the most useful imaging techniques (Figure 49.23). Open surgical biopsy is contraindicated unless evidence of gross malignancy is present, and preoperative histological diagnosis is required as a prelude to radical parotidectomy.

Parotidectomy

The aim of superficial parotidectomy is to remove the tumour with a cuff of normal surrounding tissue. The most important structure traversing the parotid gland in the facial nerve. Parotid tumour excision techniques are classified based on the approach onto the facial nerve. Essentially the traditional parotidectomy is in reality a dissection of the facial nerve. A parotidectomy is conservative when the nerve is spared and radical when the nerve is excised *en bloc* with the tumour. A superficial parotidectomy is when the part of the gland superficial to the facial nerve is removed. A deep lobe parotidectomy is when the part of the gland beneath the nerve is removed and total parotidectomy is when both are dissected and removed. Superficial parotidectomy can be partial in relatively small tumours that are removed with a cuff of clinically normal parenchyma without removal of the entire superficial portion of the gland.

An alternative surgical approach is to focus on the tumour itself as the principal procedure and not facial nerve dissection. Extracapsular dissection is now an established alternative to parotidectomy. It does not require formal facial nerve dissection and is a less invasive technique with reduced morbidity. Temporary facial nerve injury rates are 7% compared with 25% for superficial parotidectomy.

Superficial parotidectomy

Superficial parotidectomy is the most common procedure for parotid gland pathology. Surgery is performed under endotracheal general anaesthesia, which may or may not be accompanied by hypotensive anaesthesia to facilitate dissection, improve the visual surgical field and reduce blood loss. The operation has several distinct phases.

INCISION AND DEVELOPMENT OF A SKIN FLAP

The most commonly used incision is the 'lazy S' pre-auricular–mastoid–cervical (Figure 49.24a). The incision is marked

Aldred Scott Warthin, 1866–1931, Professor of Pathology, University of Michigan, Ann Arbor, MI, USA.
Thomas Hodgkin, 1798–1866, curator of the museum, and demonstrator of Morbid Anatomy, Guy's Hospital, London, UK, described lymphadenoma in 1832.

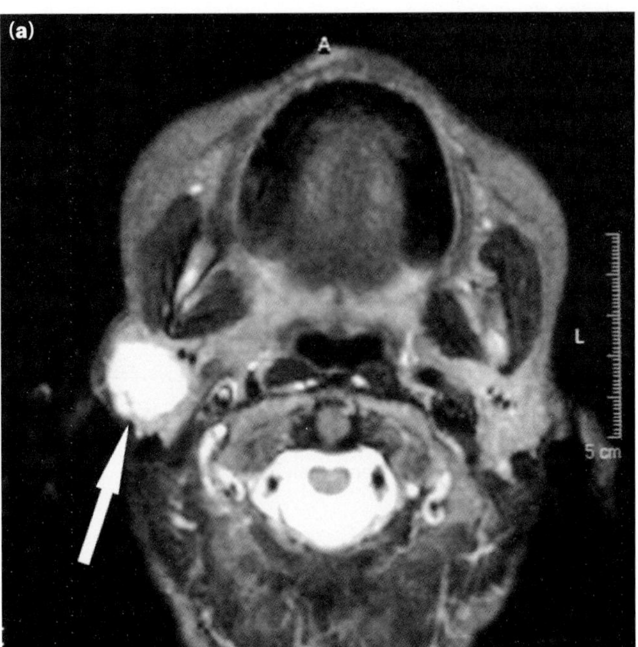

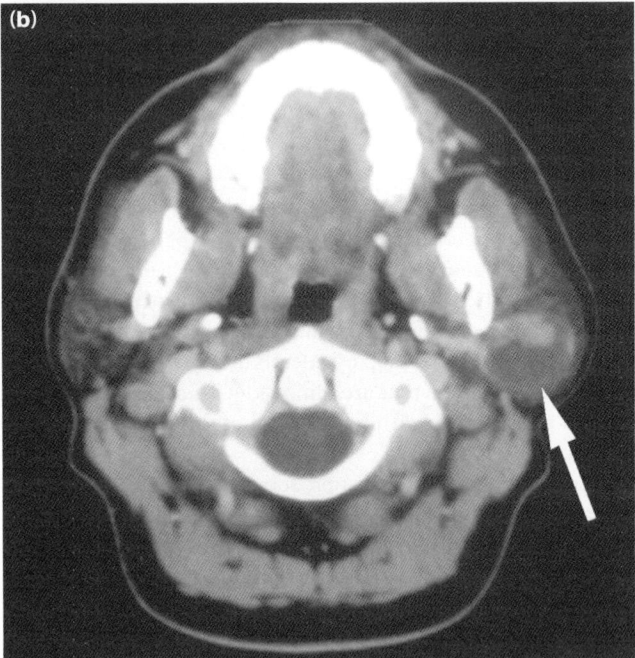

Figure 49.23 (a) Magnetic resonance imaging scan revealing a space-occupying lesion (arrow) in the right parotid gland; histology revealed pleomorphic adenoma. (b) Computed tomography scan of the left parotid gland revealing a cystic lesion (arrow). Histology revealed acinic cell carcinoma.

out and three points identified along its length to facilitate closure. Infiltration with local anaesthetic and adrenaline is optional, but does aid in the development of the skin flap, improves visibility and reduces blood loss in the initial phase. The skin flap is developed in an anterior direction by either scalpel or scissors dissection. The plane of dissection is well below the hair follicles, just above the parotid fascia. The skin flap is developed forwards to the anterior border of the gland. Posterior undermining of the incision in the cervical region facilitates access to the anterior border of the sternomastoid muscle.

MOBILISATION OF THE GLAND

This phase of the dissection aims to free the posterior margin of the gland, allowing identification of the facial nerve. Clips are applied along the fascia overlying the sternomastoid muscle, with the assistant applying traction anteriorly. By sharp dissection along the anterior border of the sternomastoid, an avascular plane is developed (Figure 49.24b), which requires elective transection of the great auricular nerve. At the lower end of the dissection, the external jugular vein is often encountered and ligated. The gland is gradually mobilised by sharp dissection up to and on to the anterior aspect of the mastoid process, identifying the posterior belly of the digastric muscle.

A second avascular plane is developed along the anterior border of the cartilaginous and bony external auditory meatus immediately anterior to the tragus. The two avascular planes are then connected by blunt and sharp dissection. By developing two broad avascular planes, identification of the facial nerve trunk is facilitated (Figure 49.24c). It is best achieved by scissors dissection in the line of the facial nerve trunk. Interoperative use of a facial nerve stimulator is recommended.

LOCATION OF THE FACIAL NERVE TRUNK

The main methods of facial nerve trunk localisation can be divided into antegrade and retrograde. The former utilises anatomical landmarks to identify the nerve trunk after its exit from the stylomastoid foramen, which is then traced distally. Landmarks commonly used are:

1. the inferior portion of the cartilaginous canal. This is termed Conley's pointer (tragal pointer) and indicates the position of the facial nerve, which lies 1 cm deep and inferior to its tip;
2. the upper border of the posterior belly of the digastric muscle. Identification of this muscle not only helps to mobilise the parotid gland, but also exposes an area immediately superior, in which the facial nerve is usually located;
3. the squamotympanic fissure;
4. the styloid process (the nerve is superficial to it);
5. the mastoid process can be drilled and the nerve identified more proximally.

Retrograde techniques rely on the identification of one of the nerve main branches (buccal in relation to the parotid duct, marginal mandibular in relation to the facial vessels, temporal branch), which is then traced proximally until the main trunk is identified. These techniques can be useful in revision cases where the anatomy is altered or postradiotherapy when significant fibrosis distorts the planes of dissection.

John J Conley, 1912–1999, otolaryngologist, St. Vincent's Hospital and Medical Center, USA, made important contributions in the treatment of head and neck cancer.

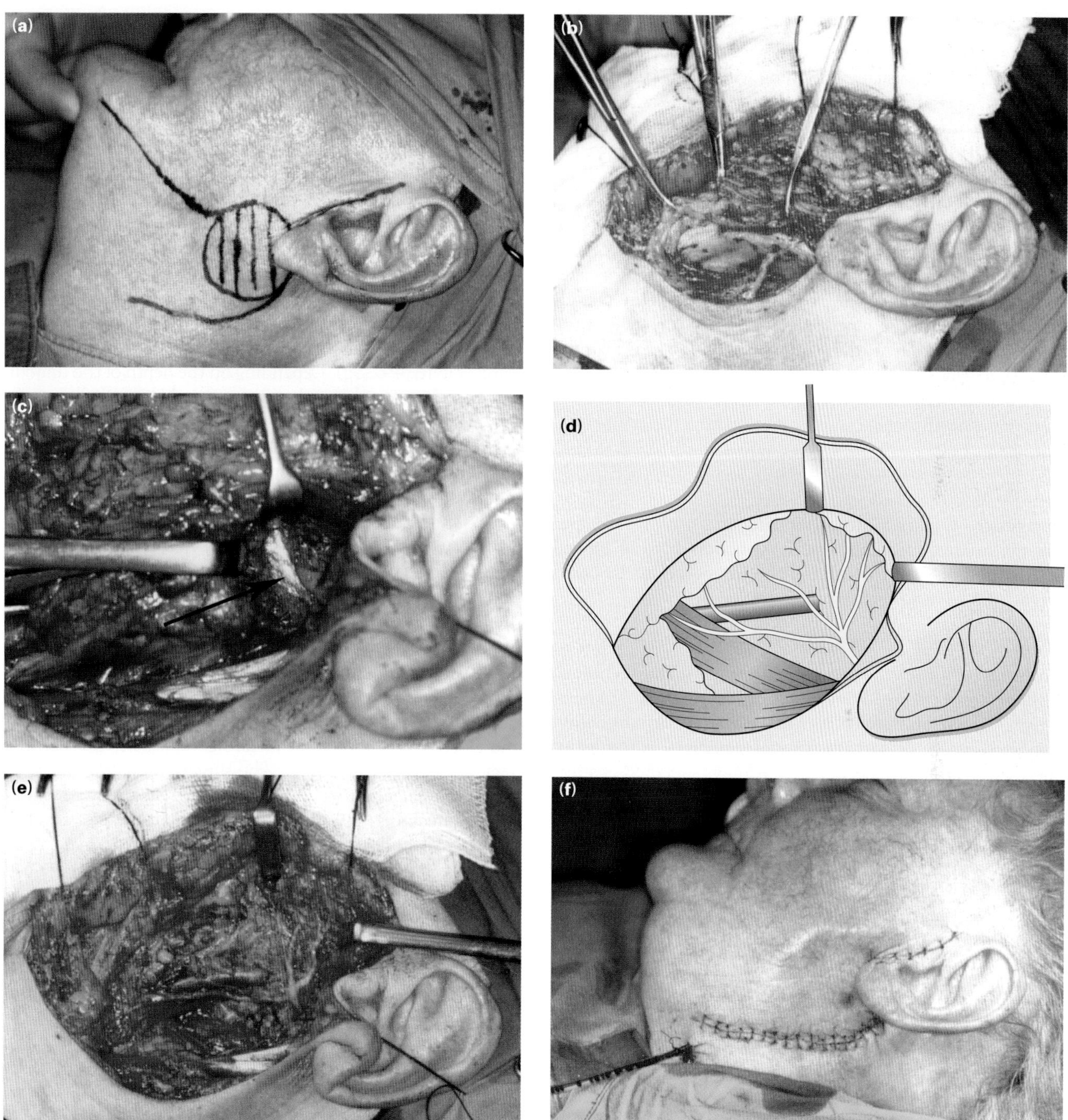

Figure 49.24 (a) Landmarks and cervical–mastoid preauricular incision for superficial parotidectomy. (b) Development of the avascular plane along the anterior border of the sternomastoid prior to sacrifice of the great auricular nerve. (c) Identification of the trunk of the facial nerve (arrow). (d) Diagram highlighting the anatomical landmarks of the parotid bed. (e) Branches of the facial nerve and retromandibular vein following delivery of the tumour. (f) Wound closure with a vacuum drain.

Once the facial nerve trunk has been identified, gentle traction anteriorly facilitates further mobilisation. Control of haemorrhage at this stage is vital as bleeding, no matter how minor, significantly impedes visibility for the surgeon. Haemostasis can be achieved with bipolar diathermy, although caution is necessary, particularly as the facial nerve is approached. Damage to the stylomastoid artery, which lies immediately lateral to the nerve, can result in troublesome bleeding immediately prior to identification. Pledget swabs soaked in adrenaline are sometimes helpful in reducing the ooze associated with this phase of the dissection.

DISSECTION OF THE GLAND OFF THE FACIAL NERVE

Once the facial nerve trunk is identified, further exposure of the branch of the facial nerve can be achieved by scissors dissection in the perineural plane immediately above the nerve.

The tunnel thus created is then laid open, and divisions and branches of the facial nerve are followed to the periphery in a sequential manner, usually beginning with the upper division. The upper division divides into a temporal and a zygomatic branch, and the lower division into mandibular and cervical branches. In this way, the superficial lobe and its associated tumour are mobilised in a superior to inferior direction (Figures 49.24d, e). The upper division of the nerve is frequently tortuous in its course and it can be damaged unless great care is taken during perineural dissection. It is often not necessary to dissect all branches of the facial nerve completely, as adequate tumour clearance can be achieved with a more conservative resection of the superficial lobe. When a branch of the facial nerve is adherent to the tumour or running through the tumour, it may require elective division. With the exception of the buccal branch, the transected nerve should be repaired immediately with a cable graft, harvested from the great auricular nerve.

CLOSURE

The patient is placed into a Trendelenburg position to identify any residual bleeding vessels. A suction drain is applied for a period of 24–48 hours and the wound closed in layers (Figure 49.24f).

Extracapsular dissection

Extracapsular dissection is an oncologically sound technique for benign parotid gland tumours. The recurrent rates of pleomorphic adenomas excision with extracapsular dissection compare favourably with traditional superficial parotidectomies (extracapsular dissection 1.3–1.5% vs superficial parotidectomy 2–2.4%) and complication rates are less (temporary facial nerve palsy 7% vs 25%: Frey's syndrome 0 vs 60%)

A preauricular incision is made, the length and position of which is adapted to the size and site of the tumour (Figure 49.25a). The dissection proceeds in the plane just immediately above the 'shining' parotid fascia (the SMAS or superficial muscular aponeurotic system layer) and continues in continuity with the platysma muscle. The skin flap should extend past the lump for at least 1 cm (Figure 49.25b).

The circumference of the tumour is marked with ink and a cruciate incision marked over the surface. The legs of the cruciate incision should extend 1 cm past the edge of the tumour. This is an essential part of the technique. Four small artery clips are then placed where the two lines bisect. The artery clips are used to tent up the parotid fascia, which is then divided along the cruciate lines (Figure 49.25c). Small rounded end scissors are then used to commence a dissection through the parotid gland. The dissection advances in a blunt fashion and only when the scissors blades are visible through the fascia may the tissue bridge be divided.

As the dissection proceeds around the tumour, the presence of a facial nerve is easy to discern (Figures 49.25d, e). It is prudent to use continuous facial monitoring during the operation, which helps alert the surgeon to the presence of a facial nerve. It is not difficult to recognise a branch of the nerve as long as the basic principle is adhered to that no parotid parenchyma is diathermised or cut unless one can see through the tissues. The key to the extracapsular dissection technique is to place traction on the artery clips, which pulls the parotid tissue away from the lump and normally reveals a plane through which the surgeon can work 2–3 mm away from the tumour. When a branch of the facial nerve is observed, it is not necessarily dissected unless in close vicinity to the tumour capsule. Retractors can be used on the normal parotid gland to improve exposure of the tumour, but direct pressure on the tumour should be avoided to minimise the risk of rupture. The tumour is removed (Figure 49.25f), leaving a parted but essentially intact parotid gland (Figure 49.25g). Depending on the depth of the tumour, a suction drain can be used at the surgeon's discretion.

The cruciate incision is re-approximated (Figure 49.25h) and the skin incision closed. It is advised that a mastoid-type pressure dressing is always applied at the end of the procedure otherwise sialoceles can occur. The pressure dressing is kept for about 48 hours.

Radical parotidectomy

Radical parotidectomy is performed for patients in whom there is clear histological evidence of a high-grade malignant tumour (e.g. squamous cell carcinoma) with invasion of facial nerve. Low-grade and low stage malignant tumours can usually be managed by standard superficial parotidectomy. Radical parotidectomy involves removal of all parotid gland tissue and elective division of the facial nerve, usually through the main trunk (Figure 49.26). The surgery inevitably removes the ipsilateral masseter muscle and may also require simultaneous neck dissection, particularly where there is clinical, radiological and cytological evidence of lymph node metastases in the ipsilateral neck. When indicated, facial nerve can be repaired using cable grafts (interpositional greater auricular or sural nerve grafts).

COMPLICATIONS OF PAROTID GLAND SURGERY

Complications of parotid gland surgery include:

- haematoma formation;
- infection;
- deformity: unsightly scar and retromandibular hollowing;
- temporary facial nerve weakness;
- transection of the facial nerve and permanent facial weakness;
- sialocele;
- facial numbness;
- permanent numbness of the ear lobe associated with great auricular nerve transection;
- Frey's syndrome.

Friedrich Trendelenburg, 1844–1924, successively Professor of Surgery at Rostock (1875–1882), Bonn (1822–1895) and Leipzig, (1895–1911), Germany. The Trendelenburg Position was first described in 1885.
Lucie Frey, 1896–1944, physician, The Neurological Clinic, Warsaw, Poland.

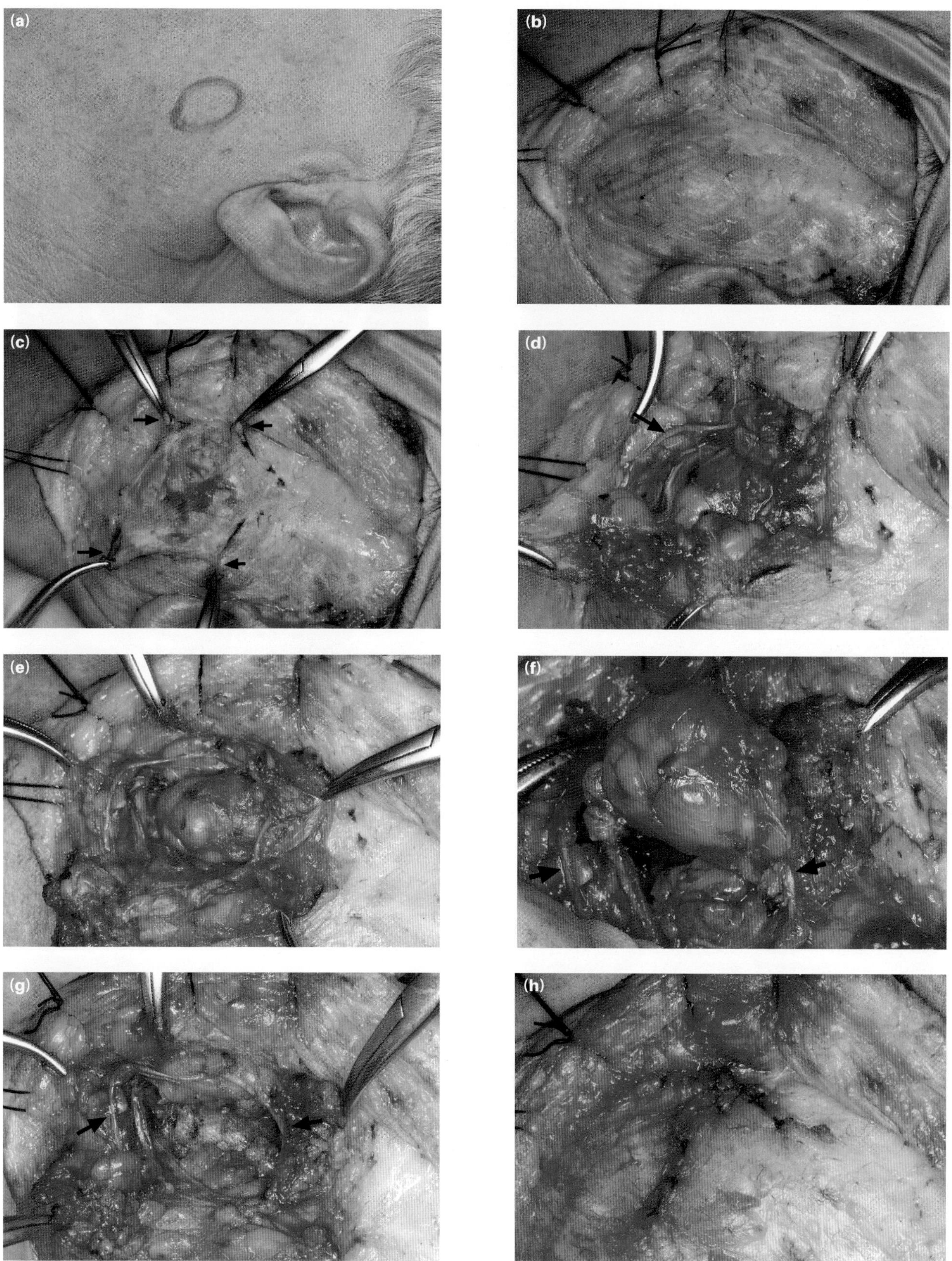

Figure 49.25 Extracapsular dissection. (a) Left parotid pleomorphic adenoma: skin marking above tumour. (b) Development of skin flap and exposure of parotid fascia. (c) Cruciate incision through parotid fascia. The leaves of parotid fascia (arrows) have been raised exposing the underlying glandular parenchyma that contains the tumour. (d) Exposure of tumour. The arrow depicts a branch of the facial nerve. (e) Gradual mobilisation of the tumour. (f) The tumour is mobilised with preservation of the facial nerve branch (arrows). (g) Excision of the tumour. The picture shows the remaining parotid bed with the facial nerve branch intact (arrows). (h) The parotid fascia leaves are replaced and sutured together in a watertight fashion. This restores the parotid capsure integrity and prevents development of Frey's syndrome.

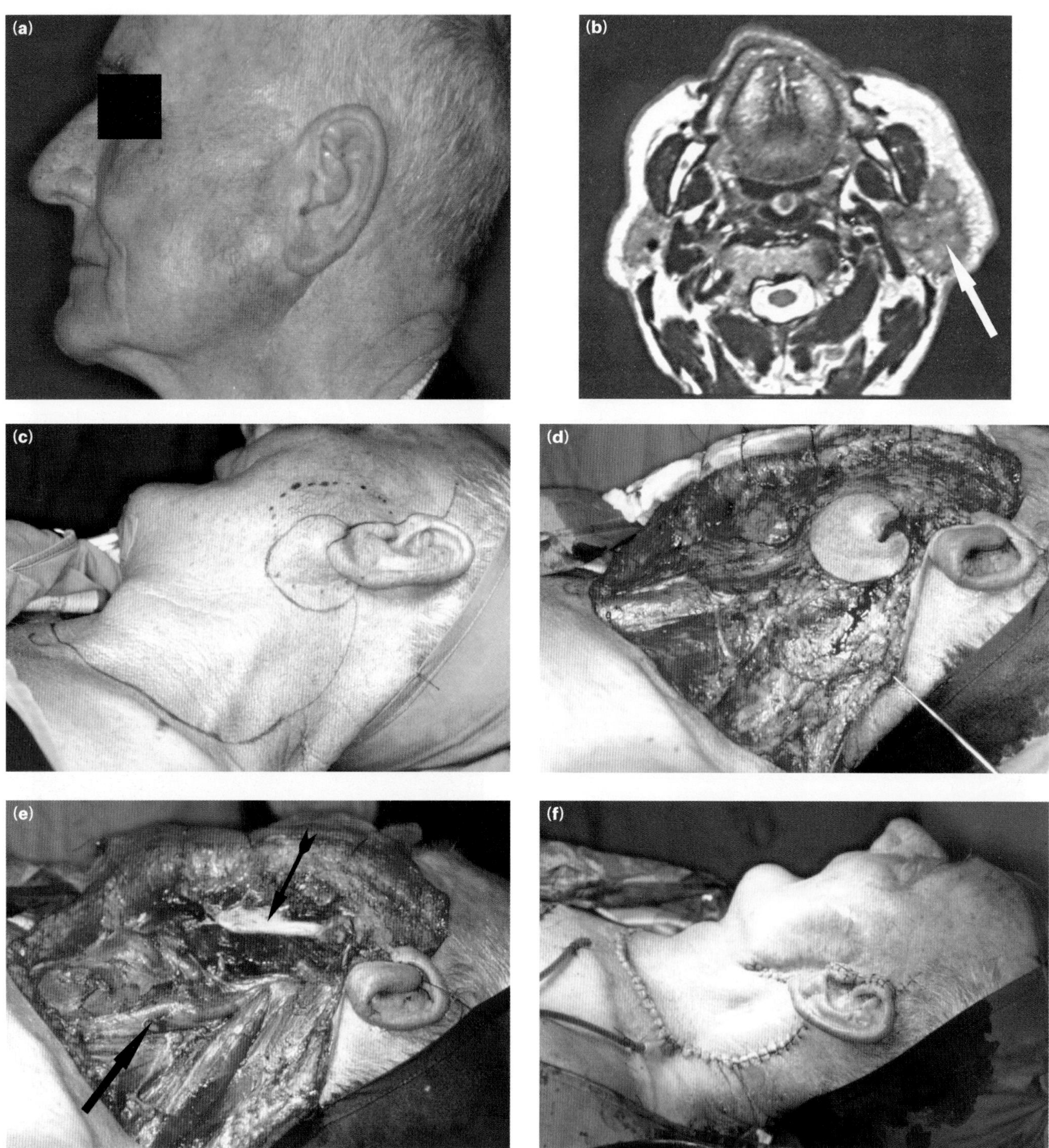

Figure 49.26 (a) High-grade malignant tumour in the left parotid gland. (b) Magnetic resonance imaging scan demonstrating a diffuse infiltrative malignant tumour of the left parotid gland (arrow). (c) Skin incision outlined for radical neck dissection and left radical parotidectomy including the removal of overlying skin. (d) Skin flap developed. (e) Appearance after left radical neck dissection and left radical parotidectomy. Posterior mandible (upper arrow) and great vessels of the neck (lower arrow) are visible. (f) Wound closure after left radical neck dissection.

Frey's syndrome

Frey's syndrome (gustatory sweating) is now considered an inevitable consequence of parotidectomy unless preventive measures are taken (see below). It results from damage to the autonomic innervation of the salivary gland with inappropriate regeneration of the postganglionic parasympathetic nerve fibres of the auriculotemporal nerve that aberrantly stimulate the sweat glands of the overlying skin. The clinical features include sweating and erythema (flushing) over the region of surgical excision of the parotid gland as a consequence of autonomic stimulation of salivation by the smellor taste of food. The symptoms are entirely variable and are clinically demonstrated by a starch iodine test. This involves painting the affected area with iodine, which is allowed to dry before applying dry starch, which turns blue on exposure to iodine in the presence of sweat. Sweating is stimulated by salivary stimulation. The management of Frey's syndrome involves the prevention as well as the management of established symptoms.

PREVENTION

The incidence of Frey's syndrome is minimal when extracapsular dissection is performed as the parotid fascia is primarily repaired and communication between denuded parotid parenchyma and subcutis sealed off.

There are a number of quite invasive techniques described to prevent Frey's syndrome following parotidectomy. These include:

- sternomastoid muscle flap;
- temporalis fascial flap;
- insertion of artificial membranes between the skin and the parotid bed.

All these methods replace the barrier between the skin and the parotid bed to minimise inappropriate regeneration of autonomic nerve fibres.

MANAGEMENT OF ESTABLISHED FREY'S SYNDROME

Methods of managing Frey's syndrome include:

- antiperspirants, usually containing aluminium chloride;
- denervation by tympanic neurectomy;
- the injection of botulinum toxin into the affected skin.

The last is the most effective and can be performed as an out-patient.

Granulomatous sialadenitis

This is a group of rare conditions that affect the salivary glands producing a variety of signs and symptoms, particularly painless swellings of the parotid and/or submandibular glands. Systemic upset is variable. These include the following:

- **Mycobacterial infection.** Tuberculosis and non-tuberculous sialadenitis typically present as a tumour-like swelling of the salivary gland. There is little pain and no fever. Preoperative investigations may be of some help, and the diagnosis is only confirmed when the swelling has been excised by either submandibular gland excision or formal parotidectomy.
- **Sarcoidosis.** Sarcoidosis can affect the salivary tissue and presents with persistent salivary gland swelling that may be associated with xerostomia. Occasionally, the patient will present with a localised tumour-like swelling in one salivary gland, more commonly the parotid – the so called sarcoid pseudotumour. In such circumstances, the diagnosis is only likely to be made following surgical excision for a presumed neoplasm. Heerfordt's syndrome is sarcoidosis that involves parotid swelling, anterior uveitis, facial palsy and fever.
- **Other.** These include cat scratch disease, toxoplasmosis, syphilis, deep mycoses and granulomatosis with polyangiitis (previously Wegener's granulomatosis), allergic sialadenitis and sialadenitis associated with radiotherapy of the head and neck.

Tumour-like lesions

There is a group of pathological conditions that affect the salivary glands and which do not fall into any particular classification or category and are often difficult to diagnose. These include such conditions as sialadenosis, adenomatoid hyperplasia and multifocal monomorphic adenomatosis.

SIALADENOSIS

Sialadenosis (sialosis) is used to describe non-inflammatory swelling particularly affecting the parotid gland. It usually occurs in association with a variety of conditions including diabetes mellitus, alcoholism, other endocrine diseases, pregnancy, drugs, bulimia and other eating disorders, and idiopathic diseases.

Most patients present between 40 and 70 years of age, and the salivary swellings are soft and often symmetrical (Figure 49.27). When the parotid glands are affected, patients may complain of a hamster-like appearance. Drug-induced sialosis

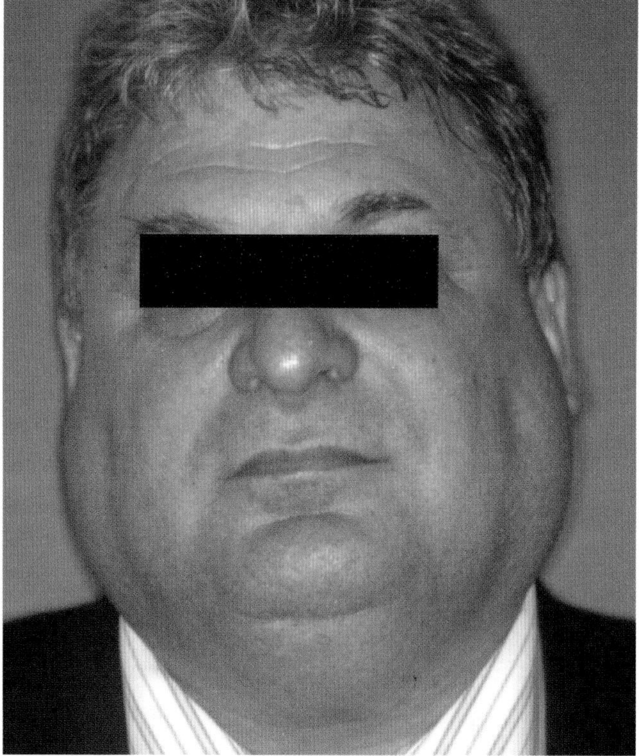

Figure 49.27 Sialosis of the parotid glands secondary to excess alcohol intake.

Christian Frederick Heerfordt, 1871–1953, Danish ophthalmologist, described this syndrome in 1909.
Friedrich Wegener, 1907–1990, Professor of Pathology, Lübeck, Germany, described this form of granulomatosis in 1939.

is particularly common with sympathomimetic drugs. In many patients, no underlying disorder can be identified. Severe and prolonged malnutrition, as seen in eating disorders, produces sialadenosis by a process of hypertrophy to compensate for swings in acid balance. The pathological mechanism of sialadenosis can be associated with a process of neuropathy, which interferes with salivary gland function and subsequent acinar cell atrophy. This may be the case in diabetes mellitus, where autonomic neuropathy is a recognised complication as well as drug-induced sialosis.

The treatment of sialosis is unsatisfactory, but treatment is aimed at correction of the underlying disorder. Drug-associated sialadenosis may regress when the drug responsible is withdrawn.

Degenerative conditions

Sjögren's syndrome

Sjögren's syndrome is an autoimmune condition causing progressive destruction of salivary and lacrimal glands. Primary Sjögren's syndrome differs from secondary Sjögren's syndrome in that xerostomia and keratoconjunctivitis sicca occur without an associated connective tissue disorder or other autoimmune condition (rhematoid arthritis, systemic lupous erythematosus, scleroderma, polymyositis, thyroiditis). However, the symptoms are often more severe, and the incidence of lymphomatous transformation (see below) in the primary group is higher than that in the secondary group (*Table 49.3*).

The incidence of Sjogren's syndrome is 0.5–2% of the population. Females are affected more than males in the ratio 10:1. Occasionally, there is enlargement of the salivary glands, more commonly the parotid rather than the submandibular glands. The glands are occasionally painful, and the patient rarely develops a bacterial sialadenitis due to ascending infection from the associated xerostomia.

The characteristic pathological feature of Sjögren's syndrome is progressive lymphocytic infiltration, acinar cell destruction and proliferation of duct epithelium in all salivary and lacrimal gland tissue. The diagnosis is based on the history as no single laboratory investigation is pathognomonic of either primary or secondary Sjögren's syndrome (Figure 49.28).

TABLE 49.3 Degenerative disorders.

Primary Sjögren's syndrome	More severe xerostomia
	Widespread exocrine gland dysfunction
	No connective tissue disorder
Secondary Sjögren's syndrome	M:F: 1:10
	Middle age
	Underlying connective tissue disorder
Benign lymphoepithelial lesion	20% develop lymphoma
	Diffuse parotid swelling 20% bilateral

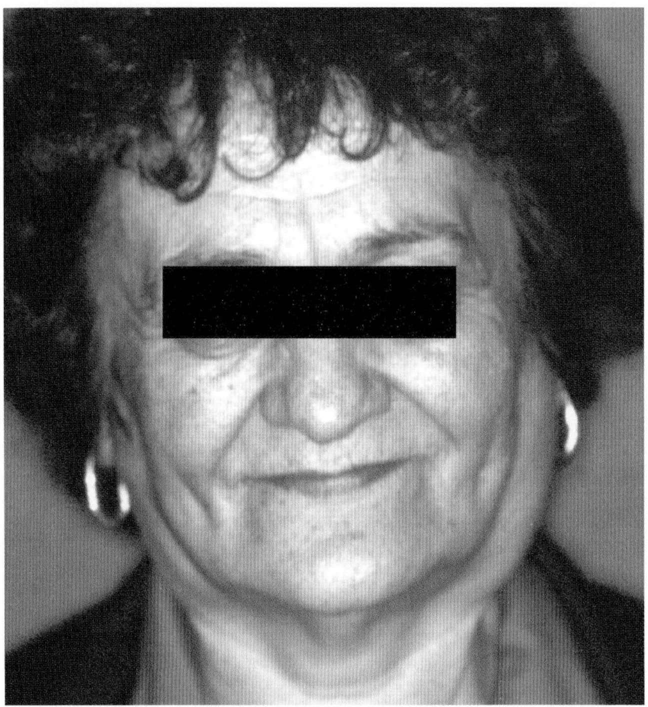

Figure 49.28 Clinical appearance of primary biliary cirrhosis associated with Sjögren's syndrome.

MANAGEMENT

Management of Sjögren's syndrome remains symptomatic. No known treatment modifies or improves the xerostomia or keratoconjunctivitis sicca. An ophthalmological assessment is important, and artificial tears are essential to preserve corneal function. For dry mouth, various artificial salivary substitutes are available, but patients often consume large volumes of water, carrying a bottle of water with them at all times. In the dentate patient, the use of salivary substitutes with fluoride is important to counter the risk of accelerating dental caries. Other oral complications include oral candidosis and accelerated periodontal disease.

COMPLICATIONS OF SJÖGREN'S SYNDROME

There is an increased incidence of developing lymphoma (most commonly non-Hodgkin's B-cell lymphoma) in patients with Sjögren's syndrome. The risk is highest within the primary group, and the onset of lymphoma is heralded by immunological change within the blood. The incidence of lymphoma in patients with Sjogren's syndrome is 4.3% (18.9 times higher than in the general population). Enlarged and painful parotid glands raise the prospect of MALT (mucosa associated lymphoid tissue) lymphoma.

Xerostomia

Xerostomia is a common symptom in many aspects of medical practice. Normal salivary flows decrease with age in both men and women, although many patients with xerostomia are postmenopausal women who also complain of a burning tongue or mouth. Common causes of xerostomia are:

1 chronic anxiety states and depression;
2 dehydration;

3 anticholinergic drugs, especially antidepressants;
4 salivary gland disorders – Sjögren's syndrome. Ascending parotitis is an occasional complication of xerostomia and is managed with antibiotics and increased fluid intake;
5 radiotherapy to the head and neck.

Sialorrhoea

Certain drugs and oral infection produce a transient increase in salivary flow rates. In healthy individuals, excess salivation is rarely symptomatic as excess saliva is swallowed spontaneously. Uncontrolled drooling is usually seen in the presence of normal salivary production in children with mental and physical handicap, most notably cerebral palsy.

MANAGEMENT

Sialorrhoea can be managed medically with antisialogogues or with intraparenchymal botulinum toxin injection.

Uncontrollable drooling is managed surgically, and many operations are available. Surgical options include:

- bilateral submandibular duct repositioning and simultaneous sublingual gland excision;
- bilateral submandibular gland excision;
- transposition of the parotid ducts and simultaneous submandibular gland excision.

Most resting salivary gland flow arises from the submandibular glands, and surgery should be focused on this gland to control uncontrolled sialorrhoea.

FURTHER READING

McGurk M, Combes J. *Controversies in the management of salivary gland disease*, 2nd edn. Oxford: Oxford University Press, 2013.

PART 8

Breast and endocrine

50	The thyroid gland	800
51	The parathyroid glands	823
52	The adrenal glands and other abdominal endocrine disorders	838
53	The breast	860

Chapter 50

The thyroid gland

Learning objectives

- To understand the development and anatomy of the thyroid gland
- To know the physiology and investigation of thyroid function
- To be able to select appropriate investigations for thyroid swellings
- To know when to operate on a thyroid swelling
- To describe thyroidectomy
- To know the risks and complications of thyroid surgery

EMBRYOLOGY

The embryology of the thyroid and parathyroid glands underlies the anatomical position, anatomical variations and congenital conditions of these structures and is therefore vital for surgery (Figure 50.1). The thyroglossal duct develops from the median bud of the pharynx. The foramen caecum at the junction of the anterior two-thirds and posterior one-third of the tongue is the vestigial remnant of the duct. This initially hollow structure migrates caudally and passes in close continuity with, and sometimes through, the developing hyoid cartilage. The parathyroid glands develop from the third and fourth pharyngeal pouches. The thymus also develops from the third pouch. As it descends, the thymus takes the associated parathyroid gland with it, which explains why the inferior parathyroid, which arises from the third pharyngeal pouch, normally lies inferior to the superior gland. However, the inferior parathyroid may be found anywhere along this line of descent (see also Chapter 51). The developing thyroid lobes amalgamate with the structures that arise in the fourth pharyngeal pouch, i.e. the superior parathyroid gland and the ultimobranchial body. Parafollicular cells (C cells) from the neural crest reach the thyroid via the ultimobranchial body.

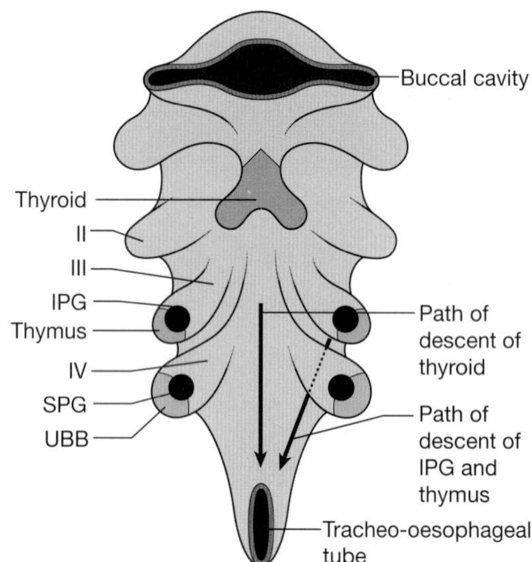

Figure 50.1 Embryology of thyroid and parathyroid. Diagram of an anterior view of the pharynx in a 4-week embryo showing the relationship of the third and fourth pharyngeal pouches to final position of the thyroid and parathyroid glands. IPG, inferior parathyroid; SPG, superior parathyroid; UBB, ultimobranchial body.

SURGICAL ANATOMY

The normal thyroid gland weighs 20–25 g. The functioning unit is the lobule supplied by a single arteriole and consists of 24–40 follicles lined with cuboidal epithelium. The follicle contains colloid in which thyroglobulin is stored (Figure 50.2). The arterial supply is rich, and extensive anastomoses occur between the main thyroid arteries and branches of the tracheal and oesophageal arteries (Figure 50.3). There is an extensive lymphatic network within and around the gland. Although some lymph channels pass directly to the deep cervical nodes, the subcapsular plexus drains principally to the central compartment juxtathyroid – 'Delphian' and paratracheal nodes

Delphi, a sacred site near the Gulf of Corinth in Greece, is the place where Phythia, the snake-woman oracle, resided. She sat on a tripod clutching the ribbons of the monolithic 'omphalos' of the world and after inhaling sulphurous fumes, would utter meaningless jargon which was interpreted equivocally by the attendent priests for those who came to consult her. Formerly the purpose of these lymph nodes was uncertain, and they were therefore called 'Delphic'.

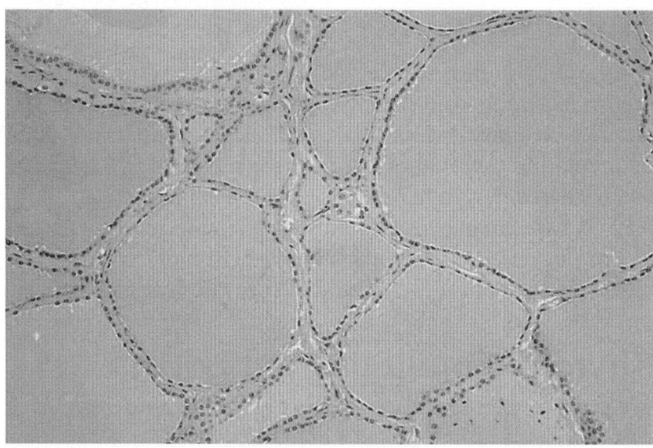

Figure 50.2 Histology of the normal thyroid.

and nodes on the superior and inferior thyroid veins (level VI), and from there to the deep cervical (levels II, III, IV and V) and mediastinal groups of nodes (level VII) (Figure 50.4).

The relationship between the recurrent laryngeal nerve (RLN) and the thyroid is of supreme importance to the operating surgeon. A branch of the vagus, the nerve recurs round the arch of the aorta on the left and the subclavian artery on the right. The clinical significance of this is that on the left the nerve has more distance in which to reach the tracheoesophageal groove and therefore runs in a medial plane. On the right, there is less distance and the nerve runs more obliquely to reach the tracheoesophageal groove. Approximately 2% of nerves on the right are non-recurrent and will enter the larynx from above.

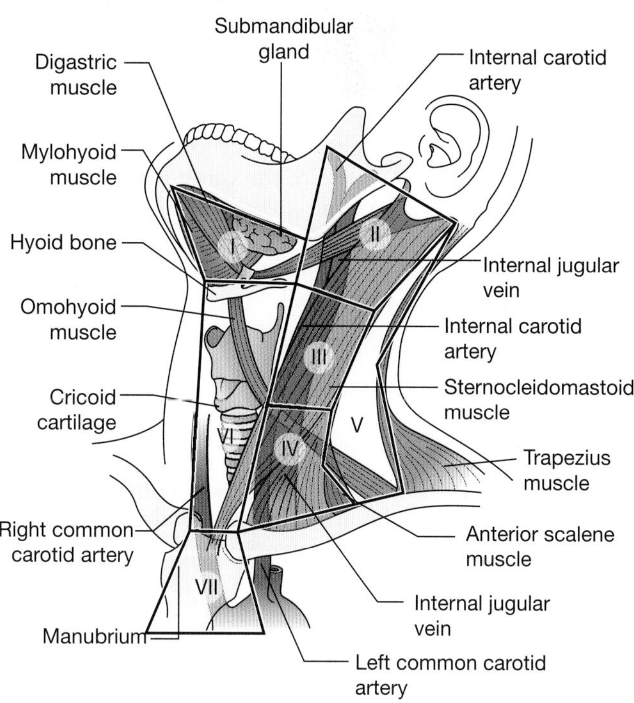

Figure 50.4 Cervical lymph node levels.

The nerve runs posterior to the thyroid and enters the larynx at the cricothyroid joint. This entry point is at

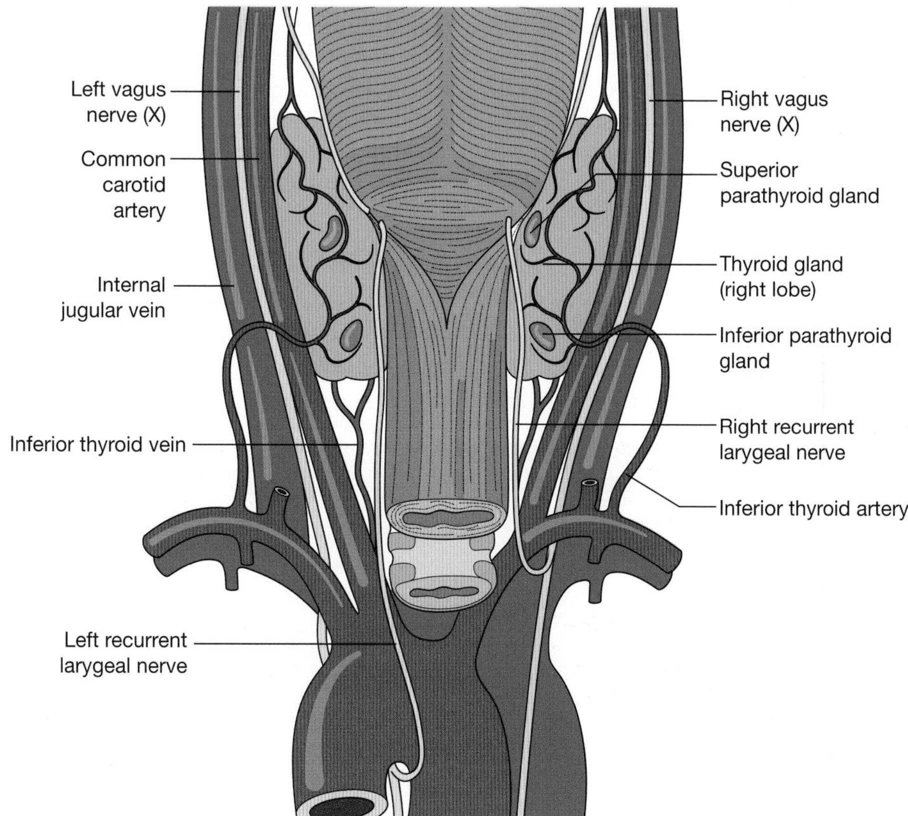

Figure 50.3 The thyroid gland from behind.

the level of Berry's ligament, a condensation of pretracheal fascia that binds the thyroid to the trachea. This is the point at which the nerve is at most risk of injury during surgery. In terms of surgical anatomy, the nerve can be located in the tracheosophageal groove where it forms one side of Beahrs' triangle (the other two sides are the carotid artery and the inferior thyroid artery) or at the cricothyroid joint. The nerve will normally be found as the thyroid lobe is mobilised laterally, lying under the most posterolateral portion of the gland called the tubercle of Zuckerkandl.

PHYSIOLOGY

Thyroxine

The hormones tri-iodothyronine (T_3) and l-thyroxine (T_4) are bound to thyroglobulin within the colloid. Synthesis within the thyroglobulin complex is controlled by several enzymes, in distinct steps:

- trapping of inorganic iodide from the blood;
- oxidation of iodide to iodine;
- binding of iodine with tyrosine to form iodotyrosine;
- coupling of monoiodotyrosines and di-iodotyrosines to form T_3 and T_4.

When hormones are required, the complex is resorbed into the cell and thyroglobulin is broken down. T_3 and T_4 are liberated and enter the blood, where they are bound to serum proteins: albumin, thyroxine-binding globulin (TBG) and thyroxine-binding prealbumin (TBPA). The small amount of hormone that remains free in the serum is biologically active.

The metabolic effects of the thyroid hormones are due to unbound free T_4 and T_3 (0.03% and 0.3% of the total circulating hormones, respectively). T_3 is the more important physiological hormone and is also produced in the periphery by conversion from T_4. T_3 is quick acting (within a few hours), whereas T_4 acts more slowly (4–14 days).

Calcitonin

The parafollicular C cells of the thyroid are of neuroendocrine origin and arrive in the thyroid via the ultimobranchial body (**Figure 50.1**). They produce calcitonin.

The pituitary-thyroid axis

Synthesis and release of thyroid hormones from the thyroid is controlled by thyroid-stimulating hormone (TSH) from the anterior pituitary. Secretion of TSH depends upon the level of circulating thyroid hormones and is modified in a negative feedback manner. In hyperthyroidism TSH production is suppressed, whereas in hypothyroidism it is stimulated. Regulation of TSH secretion also results from the action of thyrotrophin-releasing hormone (TRH) produced in the hypothalamus.

Thyroid-stimulating antibodies

A family of IgG immunoglobulins bind with TSH receptor sites (TRAbs) and activate TSH receptors on the follicular cell membrane. They have a more protracted action than TSH (16–24 versus 1.5–3 hours) and are responsible for virtually all cases of thyrotoxicosis not due to autonomous toxic nodules. Serum concentrations are very low but their measurement is not essential to make the diagnosis.

Serum thyroid hormones

Serum TSH

TSH levels can be measured accurately down to very low serum concentrations with an immunochemiluminometric assay. Interpretation of deranged TSH levels depends on knowledge of the T_3 and T_4 values. In the euthyroid state, T_3, T_4 and TSH levels will all be within the normal range. Florid thyroid failure results in depressed T_3 and T_4 levels, with gross elevation of TSH. Incipient or developing thyroid failure is characterised by low normal values of T_3 and T_4 and elevation of TSH. In toxic states, the TSH level is suppressed and undetectable (*Table 50.1*). T_3 toxicity (with a normal T_4) is a distinct entity and may only be diagnosed by measuring T_3, although a suppressed TSH in the presence of normal T_4 suggests the diagnosis.

Thyroid autoantibodies

Serum levels of antibodies against thyroid peroxidase (TPO) and thyroglobulin are useful in determining the cause of thyroid dysfunction and swellings. Autoimmune

TABLE 50.1 Results of thyroid function tests in normal and pathological states.

Thyroid functional state	TSH (0.3–3.3 mU/L)	Free T4 (10–30 nmol/L)	Free T3 (3.5–7.5 µmol/L)
Euthyroid	Normal	Normal	Normal
Thyrotoxic	Undetectable	High	High
Myxoedema	High	Low	Low
Suppressive T_4 therapy	Undetectable	High	High (often normal)
T_3 toxicity	Low/undetectable	Normal	High

Sir James Berry, 1860–1946, surgeon, Royal Free Hospital, London, UK.
Oliver H Beahrs, 1914–2006, surgeon, Mayo Clinic, MN, USA.
Emil Zuckerkandl, 1849–1901, Austro-Hungarian anatomist, brother of urologist Otto Zuckerkandl.
Myxoedema was first described in 1873 by Sir William Withey Gull, 1816–1890, physician, Guy's Hospital, London, UK.

thyroiditis may be associated with thyroid toxicity, failure or euthyroid goitre. Levels above 25 units/mL for TPO antibody and titres of greater than 1:100 for antithyroglobulin are considered significant, although a proportion of patients with histological evidence of lymphocytic (autoimmune) thyroiditis are seronegative. The presence of antithyroglobulin antibody interferes with assays of serum thyroglobulin, with implications for follow-up of thyroid cancers. TSH receptor antibodies (TSH-Rab or TRAB) are often present in Graves' disease. They are largely produced within the thyroid itself.

Summary box 50.1

Thyroid investigations

Essential

- Serum: TSH (T3 and T4 if abnormal); thyroid autoantibodies
- FNAC of palpable discrete swellings; ultrasound guidance may reduce the 'Thy1' rate

Optional

- Corrected serum calcium
- Serum calcitonin (carcinoembryonic antigen may be used as an alternative screening test for medullary cancer)
- Imaging: chest radiograph and thoracic inlet if tracheal deviation/retrosternal goitre; ultrasound, CT and MRI scan for known cancer, some reoperations and some retrosternal goitres; isotope scan if discrete swelling and toxicity coexist

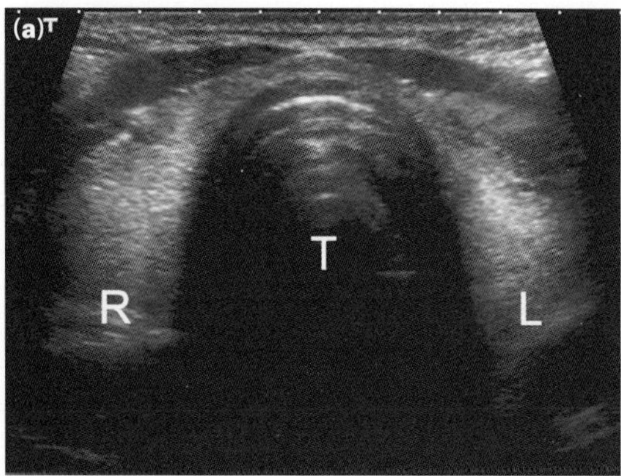

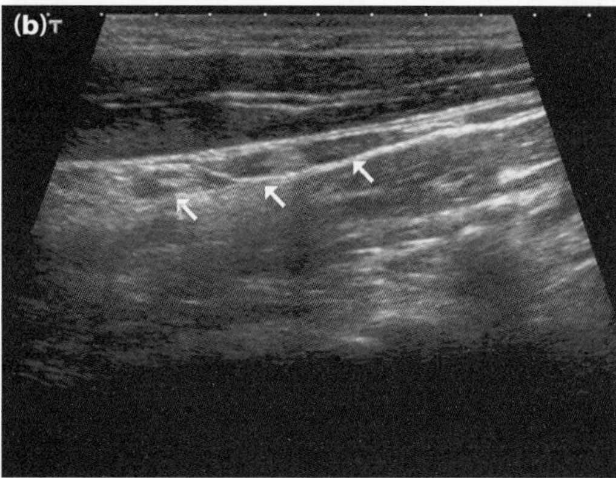

Figure 50.5 Ultrasound scanning. (a) Transverse scan of normal thyroid. R, right lobe; L, left lobe; T, trachea. (b) Longitudinal scan of normal jugular lymph nodes (white arrows).

Thyroid imaging

The workhorse investigation in thyroid disease for the surgeon is ultrasound. This modality allows assessment of the gland and the regional lymphatics. Not only can the characteristics of the gland substance be quantified, but critically the presence and features of thyroid nodules can be described. Number, size, shape, margins, vascularity and specific features such as the presence of microcalcifications can be used to predict the risk of malignancy within a specific nodule. Regional lymphatics, particularly in the lateral neck can be assessed accurately for the presence of metastatic deposits. During ultrasound, fine needle aspiration (FNA) can be performed more accurately than free-hand techniques allow.

Ultrasound has the advantages that it is not associated with ionising radiation and is non-invasive and cheap (Figure 50.5). Visualisation of the central neck nodes, in particular those behind the sternum, is however limited. For this reason, when metastatic disease is detected cross-sectional imaging is required to fully stage the disease. Retrosternal extension, which can often be predicted on plain chest x-ray (Figure 50.6), also requires more advanced techniques to determine the extent adequately prior to considering management. For most of these indications, the imaging modality of choice is computed tomography (CT). Rapid acquisition times minimise the artifact secondary to breathing and the lung fields can be accurately assessed simultaneously.

In the setting of an invasive primary thyroid cancer, both CT and magnetic resonance imaging (MRI) may have a role. Contrast enhanced CT is useful for determining the extent of airway invasion (Figure 50.7) and MRI is superior at determining the presence of prevertebral fascia invasion.

Positron emission tomography (PET) scans have limited application in thyroid disease. They may be considered in the setting of recurrent thyroid cancer. This is particularly useful when the disease does not concentrate iodine, at which point fluorodeoxyglucose (FDG) uptake increases and lesions become positive on PET scans.

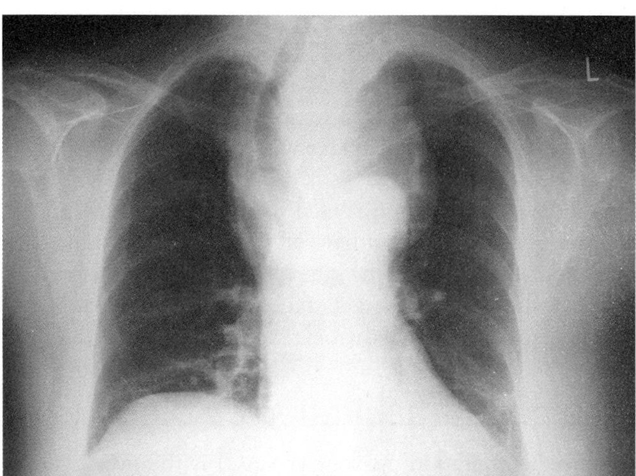

Figure 50.6 Chest radiograph showing retrosternal goitre with tracheal displacement.

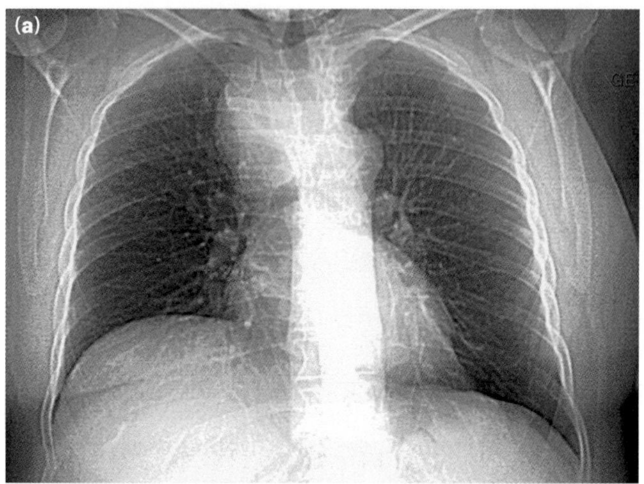

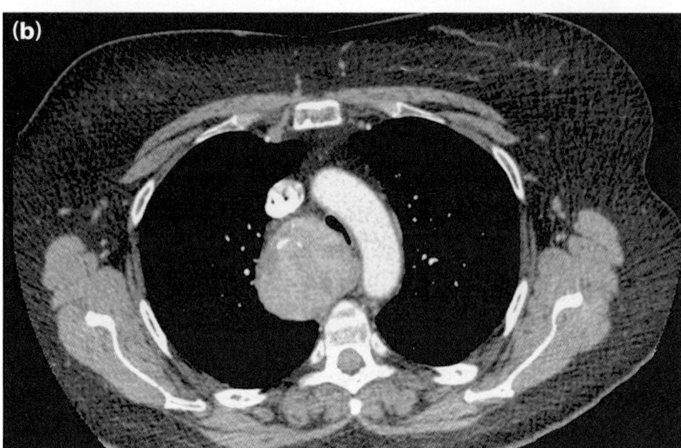

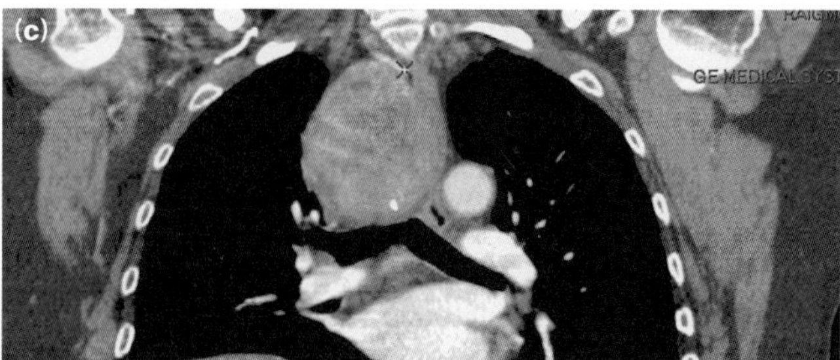

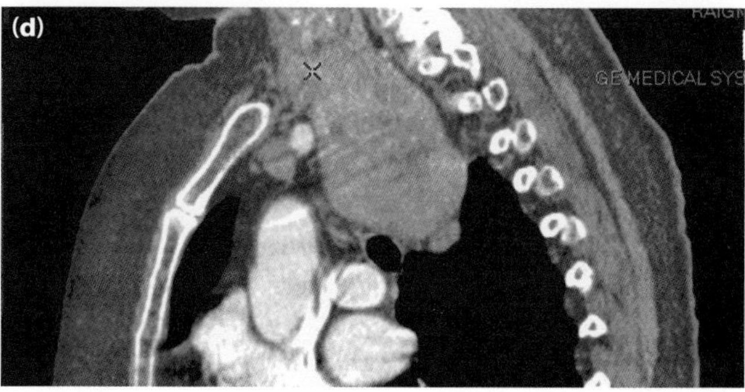

Figure 50.7 (a) Scout film showing retrosternal goitre. (b) Axial computed tomography (CT) section showing goitre extending to below the aortic arch with tracheal compression. (c) Coronal CT section showing goitre extending to the tracheal bifurcation. (d) Sagittal CT section showing goitre filling the posterior mediastinum.

Isotope scanning

The uptake by the thyroid of a low dose of either radiolabelled iodine (^{123}I) or the cheaper technetium (^{99m}Tc) will demonstrate the distribution of activity in the whole gland. Routine isotope scanning is unnecessary and inappropriate for distinguishing benign from malignant lesions because the majority (80%) of 'cold' swellings are benign and some (5%) functioning or 'warm' swellings will be malignant. Its principal value is in the toxic patient with a nodule or nodularity of the thyroid. Localisation of overactivity in the gland will differentiate between a toxic nodule with suppression of the remainder of the gland, and toxic multinodular goitre with several areas of increased uptake with important implications for therapy (Figure 50.8).

Whole-body scanning is used to demonstrate metastases. However, the patient must have all normally functioning thyroid tissue ablated either by surgery or radioiodine before the scan is performed, because metastatic thyroid cancer tissue cannot compete with normal thyroid tissue in the uptake of iodine.

Fine-needle aspiration cytology

Fine-needle aspiration cytology (FNAC) is the investigation of choice in discrete thyroid swellings. FNAC has excellent patient compliance, is simple and quick to perform in the out-patient department and is readily repeated. This technique, developed in Scandinavia 40 years ago, is now routine throughout the world. FNAC results should be reported using standard terminology (*Table 50.2*). As stated above there is a trend to

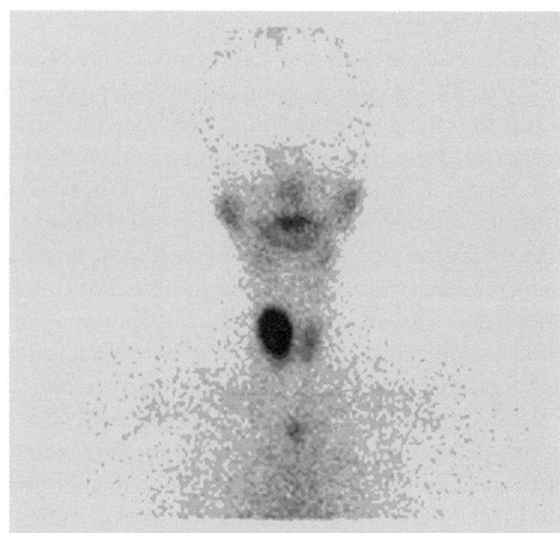

Figure 50.8 Technetium thyroid scan showing appearance of a 1-cm 'toxic' adenoma in the right thyroid lobe with suppression of uptake in the left lobe. The intense uptake gives a false impression of the size of the swelling.

TABLE 50.2 Classification of fine-needle aspiration cytology reports.	
Thy1	Non-diagnostic
Thy1c	Non-diagnostic cystic
Thy2	Non-neoplastic
Thy3	Follicular
Thy4	Suspicious of malignancy
Thy5	Malignant

use ultrasound to guide the needle to achieve more accurate sampling and reduce the rate of unsatisfactory aspirates.

THYROID ENLARGEMENT

The normal thyroid gland is impalpable. The term goitre (from the Latin guttur = the throat) is used to describe generalised enlargement of the thyroid gland. A discrete swelling (nodule) in one lobe with no palpable abnormality elsewhere is termed an isolated (or solitary) swelling. Discrete swellings with evidence of abnormality elsewhere in the gland are termed dominant.

A scheme for classifying thyroid enlargement is given in *Table 50.3*.

TABLE 50.3 Classification of thyroid swellings.		
Simple goitre (euthyroid)	Diffuse hyperplastic	Physiological Pubertal Pregnancy
	Multinodular goitre	
Toxic	Diffuse (Graves' disease)	
	Multinodular	
	Toxic adenoma	
Neoplastic	Benign	
	Malignant	
Inflammatory	Autoimmune	Chronic lymphocytic thyroiditis
		Hashimoto's disease
	Granulomatous	De Quervain's thyroiditis
	Fibrosing	Riedel's thyroiditis
	Infective	Acute (bacterial thyroiditis, viral thyroiditis, 'subacute thyroiditis')
		Chronic (tuberculous, syphilitic)
	Other	Amyloid

Summary box 50.2

Thyroid swellings

- Know how to describe thyroid swellings
- Use appropriate investigations
- Know the indications for surgery
- Select the appropriate procedure
- Describe and manage postoperative complications

Simple goitre

Aetiology

Simple goitre may develop as a result of stimulation of the thyroid gland by TSH, either as a result of inappropriate secretion from a microadenoma in the anterior pituitary (which is rare), or in response to a chronically low level of circulating thyroid hormones. The most important factor in endemic goitre is dietary deficiency of iodine (see below), but defective hormone synthesis probably accounts for many sporadic goitres (see below).

TSH is not the only stimulus to thyroid follicular cell proliferation and other growth factors, including immunoglobulins, exert an influence. The heterogeneous structural and functional response in the thyroid resulting in characteristic nodularity may be due to the presence of clones of cells particularly sensitive to growth stimulation.

IODINE DEFICIENCY

The daily requirement of iodine is about 0.1–0.15mg. In nearly all districts where simple goitre is endemic, there is a very low iodide content in the water and food. Endemic areas are in the mountainous ranges, such as the Rocky Mountains, the Alps, the Andes and the Himalayas and in the UK areas of Derbyshire and Yorkshire. Endemic goitre is also found in lowland areas where the soil lacks iodide or the water supply comes from far away mountain ranges, e.g. the Great Lakes of North America, the plains of Lombardy, the Struma valley, the Nile valley and the Congo. Calcium is also goitrogenic and goitre is common in low-iodine areas on chalk or limestone, for example Derbyshire and Southern Ireland. Although iodides in food and water may be adequate, failure of intestinal absorption may produce iodine deficiency.

DYSHORMONOGENESIS

Enzyme deficiencies of varying severity may be responsible for many sporadic goitres, i.e. in non-endemic areas (**Figure 50.9**). There is often a family history, suggesting a genetic defect. Environmental factors may compensate in areas of high iodine intake; for example, goitre is almost unknown in Iceland where the fish diet is rich in iodine. Similarly, a low intake of iodine encourages goitre formation in those with a metabolic predisposition.

Hakaru Hashimoto, 1881–1934, Director of The Hashimoto Hospital, Mie, Japan, described chronic lymphocytic thyroiditis in 1912. The link to an autoimmune basis was defined by Roitt and his co-workers.

Struma. The River Struma arises in the mountains of Bulgaria and flows into the Aegean Sea. Along its banks and those of its tributaries dwell peoples of several nationalities among whom endemic goitre has long been prevalent. Struma is a European continental term for goitre.

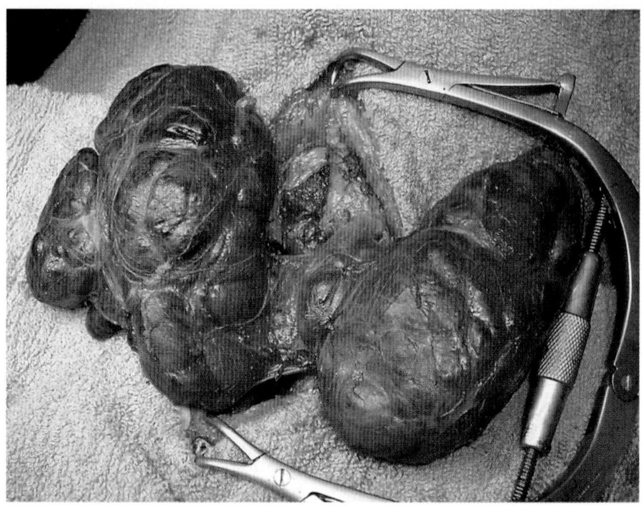
Figure 50.9 Total thyroidectomy for dyshormonogenetic goitre in a 14-year-old girl.

GOITROGENS

Well-known goitrogens are the vegetables of the brassica family (cabbage, kale and rape), which contain thiocyanate, drugs such as para-aminosalicylic acid (PAS) and the anti-thyroid drugs. Thiocyanates and perchlorates interfere with iodide trapping; carbimazole and thiouracil compounds interfere with the oxidation of iodide and the binding of iodine to tyrosine.

Surprisingly, iodides in large quantities are goitrogenic because they inhibit the organic binding of iodine and produce an iodide goitre. Excessive iodine intake may be associated with an increased incidence of autoimmune thyroid disease.

The natural history of simple goitre

Stages in goitre formation are:

- Persistent growth stimulation causes diffuse hyperplasia; all lobules are composed of active follicles and iodine uptake is uniform. This is a diffuse hyperplastic goitre, which may persist for a long time but is reversible if stimulation ceases.
- Later, as a result of fluctuating stimulation, a mixed pattern develops with areas of active lobules and areas of inactive lobules.
- Active lobules become more vascular and hyperplastic until haemorrhage occurs, causing central necrosis and leaving only a surrounding rind of active follicles.
- Necrotic lobules coalesce to form nodules filled either with iodine-free colloid or a mass of new but inactive follicles.
- Continual repetition of this process results in a nodular goitre. Most nodules are inactive, and active follicles are present only in the internodular tissue.

DIFFUSE HYPERPLASTIC GOITRE

Diffuse hyperplasia corresponds to the first stages of the natural history. The goitre appears in childhood in endemic areas but, in sporadic cases, it usually occurs at puberty when metabolic demands are high. If TSH stimulation ceases the goitre may regress, but tends to recur later at times of stress such as pregnancy. The goitre is soft, diffuse and may become large enough to cause discomfort. A colloid goitre is a late stage of diffuse hyperplasia, when TSH stimulation has fallen off and when many follicles are inactive and full of colloid (Figure 50.10).

NODULAR GOITRE

Nodules are usually multiple, forming a multinodular goitre (Figure 50.11). Occasionally, only one macroscopic nodule is found, but microscopic changes will be present throughout the gland; this is one form of a clinically solitary nodule. Nodules may be colloid or cellular, and cystic degeneration and haemorrhage are common, as is subsequent calcification. Nodules appear early in endemic goitre and later (between 20 and 30 years) in sporadic goitre, although the patient may be unaware of the goitre until his or her late 40s or 50s. All types of simple goitre are more common in the female than in the male owing to the presence of oestrogen receptors in thyroid tissue.

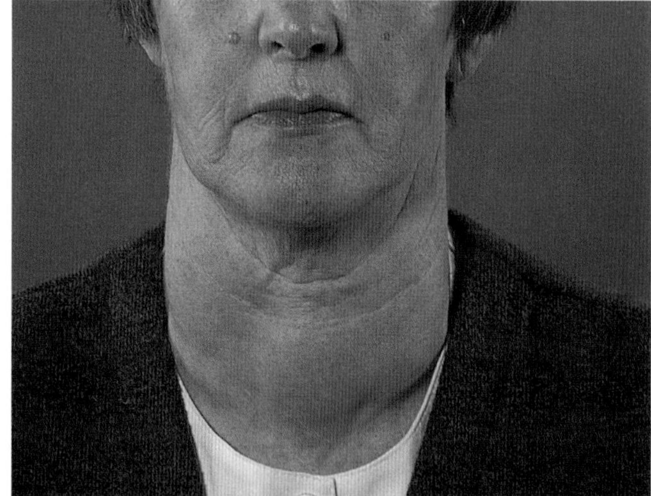
Figure 50.10 Colloid goitre.

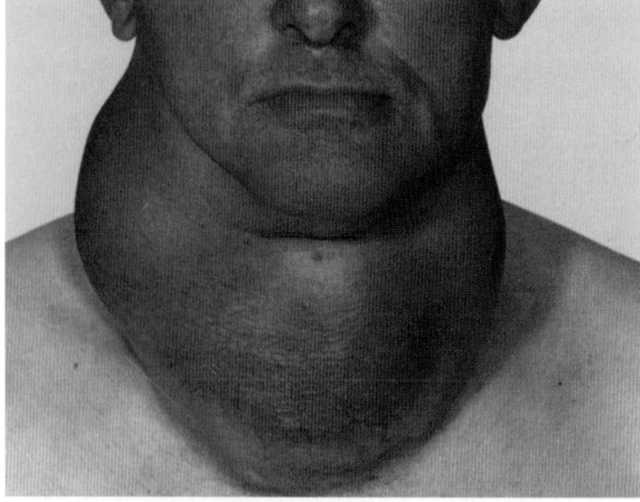
Figure 50.11 Large multinodular goitre.

Diagnosis

Diagnosis is usually straightforward. The patient is euthyroid, the nodules are palpable and often visible; they are smooth, usually firm and not hard and the goitre is painless and moves freely on swallowing. Hardness and irregularity, due to calcification, may simulate carcinoma. A painful nodule, sudden appearance or rapid enlargement of a nodule raises suspicion of carcinoma but is usually due to haemorrhage into a simple nodule. Differential diagnosis from autoimmune thyroiditis may be difficult and the two conditions frequently coexist.

Investigations

Thyroid function should be assessed to exclude mild hyperthyroidism, and the presence of circulating thyroid antibodies tested to differentiate from autoimmune thyroiditis. Ultrasound is the gold standard assessment when undertaken by a suitably trained and experienced operator. FNAC is only required for a nodule within the goitre that demonstrates ultrasonic features of concern. This may or may not be the largest 'dominant' nodule. The biopsy should be performed under ultrasonic guidance to ensure the correct nodule is sampled. If there are swallowing or breathing symptoms then a CT scan of the thoracic inlet is the best modality to assess tracheal or oesophageal compression.

Complications

Tracheal obstruction may be due to gross lateral displacement or compression in a lateral or anteroposterior plane by retrosternal extension of the goitre (Figure 50.7). Acute respiratory obstruction may follow haemorrhage into a nodule impacted in the thoracic inlet.

SECONDARY THYROTOXICOSIS

Transient episodes of mild hyperthyroidism are common, occurring in up to 30% of patients.

CARCINOMA

An increased incidence of cancer (usually follicular) has been reported from endemic areas. Dominant or rapidly growing nodules in longstanding goitres should always be subjected to aspiration cytology.

Prevention and treatment of simple goitre

In endemic areas the incidence of goitre has been strikingly reduced by the introduction of iodised salt.

In the early stages, a hyperplastic goitre may regress if thyroxine is given in a dose of 0.15–0.2 mg daily for a few months.

Although the nodular stage of simple goitre is irreversible, more than half of benign nodules will regress in size over 10 years. Most patients with multinodular goitre are asymptomatic and do not require operation. Surgery is indicated for nodular goitres with features of underlying malignancy, for swallowing symptoms if other causes have been excluded or for cosmetic reasons if the patient finds the goitre unsightly. If the goitre is causing tracheal compression then surgery should be considered. Many such patients are found incidentally and are asymptomatic and often very elderly. As these goitres often grow very slowly the risks and benefits of surgery should be considered carefully, particularly if a sternal split may be required for access.

There is a choice of surgical treatment in multinodular goitre: **total thyroidectomy** with immediate and lifelong replacement of thyroxine or some form of partial resection to conserve sufficient functioning thyroid tissue to subserve normal function while reducing the risk of hypoparathyroidism that accompanies total thyroidectomy. **Subtotal thyroidectomy** involves partial resection of each lobe removing the bulk of the gland, leaving up to 8 g of relatively normal tissue in each remnant. The technique is essentially the same as described for toxic goitre, as are the postoperative complications. More often, however, the multinodular change is asymmetrical, with one lobe more significantly involved than the other. In these circumstances, particularly in older patients, **total lobectomy** on the more affected side is the appropriate management with either subtotal resection (Dunhill procedure) or no intervention on the less affected side. In many cases, the causative factors persist and recurrence is likely.

Reoperation for recurrent nodular goitre is more difficult and hazardous and, for this reason, an increasing number of thyroid surgeons favour **total thyroidectomy** in younger patients. However, when the first operation comprised unilateral lobectomy alone for asymmetric goitre, reoperation and completion total thyroidectomy is straightforward if required for progression of nodularity in the remaining lobe. Total lobectomy and total thyroidectomy have the additional advantage of being therapeutic for incidental carcinomas (see below).

After subtotal resection, it has been customary to give thyroxine to suppress TSH secretion, with the aim of preventing recurrence. Whether this is either necessary or effective is uncertain, although the evidence of benefit in endemic areas is better than elsewhere. There is some evidence that radioactive iodine may reduce the size of recurrent nodular goitre after previous subtotal resection and, in some circumstances, this may be a safer alternative than reoperation, particularly if there has been more than one previous thyroid procedure.

Clinically discrete swellings

Discrete thyroid swellings (thyroid nodules) are common and are palpable in 3–4% of the adult population in the UK and USA. They are three to four times more frequent in women than men.

Diagnosis

A discrete swelling in an otherwise impalpable gland is termed **isolated** or **solitary**, whereas the preferred term is **dominant** for a similar swelling in a gland with clinical evidence of generalised abnormality in the form of a palpable contralateral lobe or generalised mild nodularity. About 70% of discrete thyroid swellings are clinically isolated and about 30% are dominant. The true incidence of isolated swellings is

Sir Thomas Peel Dunhill, 1876–1957, surgeon, St Bartholomew's Hospital, London, UK.

somewhat less than the clinical estimate. Clinical classification is inevitably subjective and overestimates the frequency of truly isolated swellings. When such a gland is exposed at operation or examined by ultrasonography, CT or MRI, clinically impalpable nodules are often detected. The true frequency of thyroid nodularity compared with the clinical detection rate by palpation is shown in Figure 50.12.

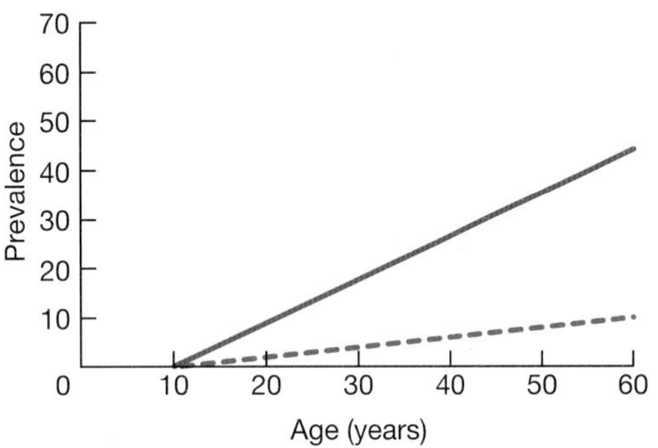

Figure 50.12 The prevalence of thyroid nodules detected on palpation (broken line) or by ultrasonography or postmortem examination (solid line) (after Mazzaferri).

Demonstrating the presence of impalpable nodules does not change the management of palpable discrete swellings and begs the question of the necessity of investigating incidentally found nodules. The importance of discrete swellings lies in the risk of neoplasia compared with other thyroid swellings. Some 15% of isolated swellings prove to be malignant and an additional 30–40% are follicular adenomas. The remainder are non-neoplastic, largely consisting of areas of colloid degeneration, thyroiditis or cysts. Although the incidence of malignancy or follicular adenoma in clinically dominant swellings is approximately half of that of truly isolated swellings, it is substantial and cannot be ignored (Figure 50.13).

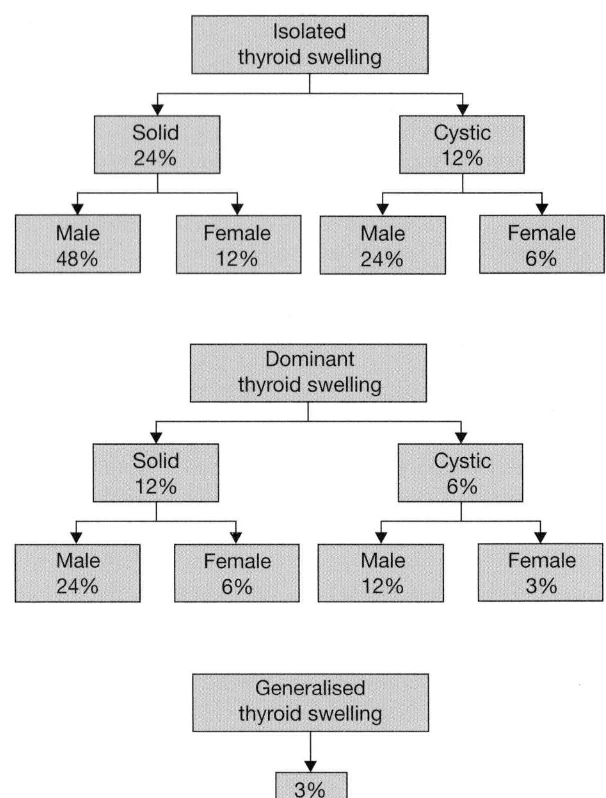

Figure 50.13 The risk of malignancy in thyroid swellings ('rule of twelve'). The risk of cancer in a thyroid swelling can be expressed as a factor of 12. The risk is greater in isolated versus dominant swellings, solid versus cystic swellings and in men versus women.

Investigation

THYROID FUNCTION

Serum TSH and thyroid hormone levels should be measured. If hyperthyroidism associated with a discrete swelling is confirmed biochemically, it indicates either a 'toxic adenoma' or a manifestation of toxic multinodular goitre. The combination of toxicity and nodularity is important and is an indication for isotope scanning to localise the area(s) of hyperfunction.

AUTOANTIBODY TITRES

The autoantibody status may determine whether a swelling is a manifestation of chronic lymphocytic thyroiditis. The presence of circulating antibodies increases the risk of thyroid failure after lobectomy.

ISOTOPE SCAN

Isotope scanning used to be the mainstay of investigation of discrete thyroid swellings but has been abandoned except when toxicity is associated with nodularity.

ULTRASONOGRAPHY

This is gold standard investigation to determine the physical characteristics of thyroid swellings. There are a number of ultrasonic features in a thyroid swelling associated with thyroid neoplasia, including microcalcification and increased vascularity, but only macroscopic capsular breach and nodal involvement are diagnostic of malignancy. Ultrasound should be used as the primary investigation of any thyroid nodule as a reassuring appearance mitigates the need for an FNAC (see below).

FINE-NEEDLE ASPIRATION CYTOLOGY

FNAC should be used, ideally under ultrasound guidance, on all nodules that do not fulfil a fully benign (U2) classification on ultrasound. FNAC is reliable in identifying papillary thyroid cancer but cannot distinguish between a benign follicular adenoma (Figure 50.14) and follicular carcinoma, as this distinction is dependent not on cytology but on histological criteria, which include capsular and vascular invasion.

FNAC is both highly specific and sensitive. Using ultrasound improves this further, particularly in part cystic, part solid nodules in which ultrasound allows targeting of the solid element for biopsy.

Ernest L Mazzaferri, 1936–2013, endocrinologist, Ohio State University School of Medicine, Columbus, OH, USA.

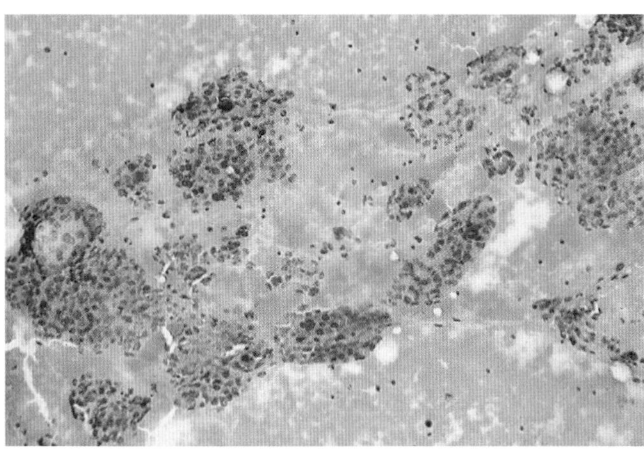

Figure 50.14 Thy3 aspiration cytology. Follicular neoplasm showing increased cellularity with a follicular pattern.

RADIOLOGY

Plain films have previously been used to assess tracheal compression and deviation, but the modality of choice now is CT scanning. CT scanning is also useful if ultrasound has identified metastatic disease in the neck as it can assist surgical planning and also assess the superior mediastinum and lungs.

LARYNGOSCOPY

Flexible laryngoscopy has rendered indirect laryngoscopy obsolete and is widely used preoperatively to determine the mobility of the vocal cords. The presence of a unilateral cord palsy coexisting with an ipsilateral thyroid nodule of concern is usually diagnostic of malignant disease.

CORE BIOPSY

Core biopsy is rarely indicated in thyroid masses due to the vascularity of the thyroid gland and the risk of postprocedure haemorrhage. It can be useful in the rapid diagnosis of widely invasive malignant disease, for example anaplastic carcinoma, or in the diagnosis of lymphadenopathy.

The main indication for operation is the risk of neoplasia, which includes follicular adenoma as well as malignant swellings. The reason for advocating the removal of all follicular neoplasms is that it is seldom possible to distinguish between a follicular adenoma and carcinoma cytologically. On this basis, some 50% of isolated swellings and 25% of dominant swellings should be removed on the grounds of neoplasia. Even when the cytology is negative, the age and sex of the patient and the size of the swelling may be relative indications for surgery, especially when a large swelling is responsible for symptoms. Some patients are happier to have a swelling removed even when cytology is negative.

There are useful clinical criteria to assist in selection for operation according to the risk of neoplasia and malignancy. Hard texture alone is not reliable as tense cystic swellings may be suspiciously hard but a hard, irregular swelling with any apparent fixity, which is unusual, is highly suspicious. Evidence of RLN paralysis, suggested by hoarseness and a non-occlusive cough and confirmed by laryngoscopy, is almost pathognomonic. Deep cervical lymphadenopathy along the internal jugular vein in association with a clinically suspicious swelling is almost diagnostic of papillary carcinoma. In most patients, however, such features are absent but there are risk factors associated with sex and age. The incidence of thyroid carcinoma in women is about three times that in men, but a discrete swelling in a male is much more likely to be malignant than in a female and it is seldom justifiable to avoid removing such a swelling in a man. The risk of carcinoma is increased at either end of the age range and a discrete swelling in a teenager of either sex must be provisionally diagnosed as carcinoma. The risk increases as age advances beyond 50 years, more so in males.

Thyroid cysts

Routine FNAC (or ultrasonography) shows that over 30% of clinically isolated swellings contain fluid and are cystic or partly cystic. Tense cysts may be hard and mimic carcinoma. Bleeding into a cyst often presents with a history of sudden painful swelling, which resolves to a variable extent over a period of weeks if untreated. Aspiration yields altered blood but reaccumulation is frequent. About 50% of cystic swellings are the result of colloid degeneration, or of uncertain aetiology because of an absence of epithelial cells in the lining. Although most of the remainder are the result of involution in follicular adenomas (Figure 50.15), some 10–15% of cystic follicular swellings are histologically malignant (30% in men and 10% in women). Papillary carcinoma is often associated with cyst formation (Figure 50.16).

Most patients with discrete swellings, however, are women, aged 20–40 years, in whom the risk of malignancy, although significant, is low and the indications for operation are not clear cut.

Ultrasound is the most useful tool for assessing cysts. If there is no discernable solid element then the cyst is almost certainly benign and does not need to be further investigated. If there is an associated solid element then consideration

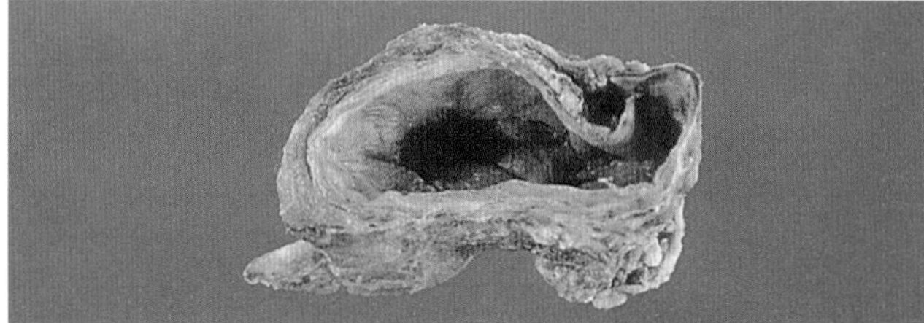

Figure 50.15 Apparently simple cystic thyroid swelling, the wall of which comprised follicular neoplastic tissue.

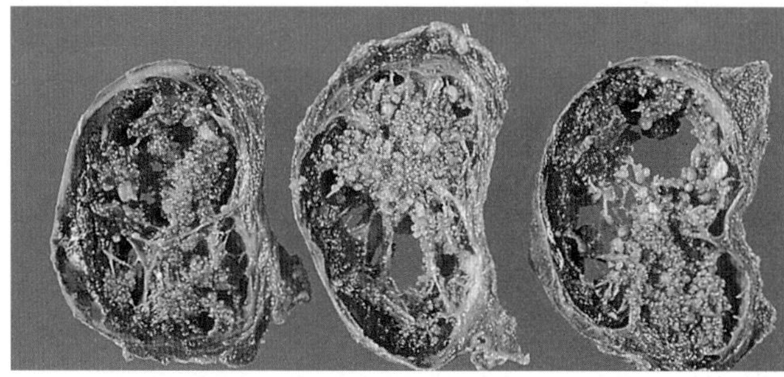

Figure 50.16 Cyst formation in a papillary carcinoma.

should be given to targeting that area with an ultrasound-guided FNAC.

The indications for operation in isolated or dominant thyroid swellings are listed in *Table 50.4*.

TABLE 50.4 Indications for operation in thyroid swellings.

Neoplasia	FNAC positive Thy3–5	
	Clinical suspicion	Age
		Male sex
		Hard texture
		Fixity
		Recurrent laryngeal nerve palsy
		Lymphadenopathy
		Recurrent cyst
Toxic adenoma		
Pressure symptoms		
Cosmesis		
Patient's wishes		

Selection of thyroid procedure

The choice of thyroid operation depends on:

- diagnosis (if known preoperatively);
- risk of thyroid failure;
- risk of RLN injury;
- risk of recurrence;
- Graves' disease;
- multinodular goitre;
- differentiated thyroid cancer;
- risk of hypoparathyroidism.

Total and near-total thyroidectomy do not conserve sufficient thyroid tissue for normal thyroid function and thyroid replacement therapy is necessary. In most patients with negative antithyroid antibodies, one thyroid lobe will maintain normal function. In subtotal thyroidectomy, the volume of thyroid tissue preserved influences the risk of thyroid failure: larger remnants have a better chance of normal function but a higher risk of recurrence in Graves' disease.

Subtotal resections for colloid goitre run the risk of later growth of the remnant and, if a second operation is required years later, this greatly increases the risk to the RLN and parathyroid glands. In young patients, total thyroidectomy should be considered. It may be preferable to leave the least affected lobe untouched to permit a straightforward lobectomy in the future if required, rather than carry out subtotal resections.

In Graves' disease, preserving large remnants increases the risk of recurrence of the toxicity and, in these cases, it is better to err on the side of removing too much thyroid tissue rather than too little (*Table 50.5*). Thyroid failure should not be regarded as a failure of treatment, but recurrent toxicity is.

The relative merits of routine total versus selective total thyroidectomy in differentiated thyroid cancer are discussed below.

Summary box 50.3

Thyroid operations

All thyroid operations can be assembled from three basic elements:

1. Total lobectomy
2. Isthmusectomy
3. Subtotal lobectomy

Total thyroidectomy = 2 × total lobectomy + isthmusectomy

Subtotal thyroidectomy = 2 subtotal lobectomy + isthmusectomy

Near-total thyroidectomy = total lobectomy + isthmusectomy + subtotal lobectomy (Dunhill procedure)

Lobectomy = total lobectomy + isthmusectomy

Retrosternal goitre

Retrosternal goitre tends to arise from the slow growth of a multinodular gland down in to the mediastinum. As the gland enlarges within the thoracic inlet, pressure may lead to dysphagia, tracheal compression and eventually airway symptoms. The vast majority of patients have minimal symptoms. Patient should be considered for surgery if there is significant airway compression, if symptoms are present or in young patients in whom symptoms are likely to develop. In elderly patients with incidentally discovered retrosternal goitres, most surgeons would observe rather than treat

TABLE 50.5 Comparison of surgical options for Graves' disease.

	Total thyroidectomy	Subtotal thyroidectomy
Control of toxicity	Immediate	Immediate
Return to euthyroid state	Immediate	Variable – up to 12 months
Risk of recurrence	None	Lifelong – up to 5%[a]
Risk of thyroid failure	100%	Lifelong – up to 100% at 30 years[a]
Risk of permanent hypoparathyroidism	5%	1%
Need for follow-up	Minimal	Lifelong

[a]The risk of recurrence and late failure are a function of the size of the remnant as a proportion of the total gland weight. Large remnants in small glands have a higher risk of recurrence and a low risk of failure, and small remnants in large glands have a higher risk of thyroid failure but a low risk of recurrence.

prophylactically. Clearly a balance between risk and benefit must be made.

If a decision is made to proceed to surgery, assessment of the extent of disease is critical. The vast majority (>95%) of retrosternal goitres can be removed transcervically. Those at most risk of requiring conversion to an open sternotomy approach include malignant or revision cases, those which extend into the posterior mediastinum and those in which the diameter of the goitre exceeds that of the thoracic inlet. In such cases a joint case with thoracic surgery should be planned.

All cases should have cross-sectional imaging. Ideally this is performed in the surgical position and when interpreting CT chest scans, the surgeon should pay attention to the arm position. If the arms are up (as for standard CT chest) a great deal of thyroid movement will be achieved when the arms are down and the neck extended.

The approach to surgery is as described below. A longer incision is required. The surgeon may mobilise the sternomastoid muscle from the strap muscles to improve access. The ligamentous tissue between the sternal heads of the clavicles may be gently divided to increase the opening for gland delivery. Blunt dissection on the capsule of the gland allows mobilisation. Gentle traction is applied to deliver the gland into the neck. If the goitre has developed from a posteriorly positioned nodule there is a risk that the RLN may be displaced anteriorly, so great care must be taken in dividing apparent fascial bands that overlie the gland. The blood supply is from the neck, reducing the risk of catastrophic bleeding from the great vessels. Nonetheless, care should be taken in the region of the major blood vessels in the neck and chest.

If the gland is fixed and immobile or too large to deliver through a cervical approach, a midline sternotomy is performed and the gland can be dissected from below to achieve a safe total thyroidectomy.

HYPERTHYROIDISM

Thyrotoxicosis

The term thyrotoxicosis is retained because hyperthyroidism, i.e. symptoms due to a raised level of circulating thyroid hormones, is not responsible for all manifestations of the disease. Clinical types are:

- diffuse toxic goitre (Graves' disease);
- toxic nodular goitre;
- toxic nodule;
- hyperthyroidism due to rarer causes.

Diffuse toxic goitre

Graves' disease, a diffuse vascular goitre appearing at the same time as hyperthyroidism, usually occurs in younger women and is frequently associated with eye signs. The syndrome is that of primary thyrotoxicosis (Figure 50.17); 50% of patients have a family history of autoimmune endocrine diseases. The whole of the functioning thyroid tissue is involved, and the hypertrophy and hyperplasia are due to abnormal TSH-RAb that bind to TSH receptor sites and produce a disproportionate and prolonged effect.

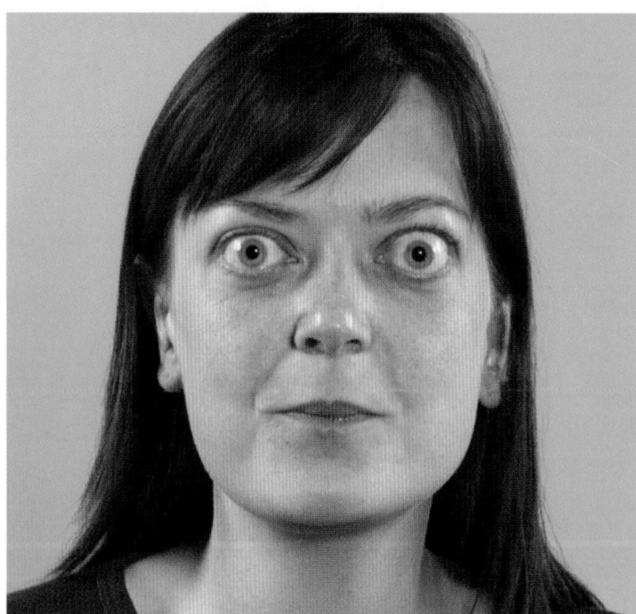

Figure 50.17 Graves' disease.

Toxic nodular goitre

A simple nodular goitre is present for a long time before the hyperthyroidism, usually in the middle-aged or elderly, and very infrequently is associated with eye signs. The syndrome is that of secondary thyrotoxicosis.

In many cases of toxic nodular goitre, the nodules are inactive, and it is the internodular thyroid tissue that is overactive. However, in some toxic nodular goitres, one or more nodules are overactive and here the hyperthyroidism is due to autonomous thyroid tissue as in a toxic adenoma.

Toxic nodule

A toxic nodule is a solitary overactive nodule, which may be part of a generalised nodularity or a true toxic adenoma. It is autonomous and its hypertrophy and hyperplasia are not due to TSH-RAb. TSH secretion is suppressed by the high level of circulating thyroid hormones and the normal thyroid tissue surrounding the nodule is itself suppressed and inactive.

HISTOLOGY

The normal thyroid gland consists of acini lined with flattened cuboidal epithelium and filled with homogeneous colloid (Figure 50.2). In hyperthyroidism (Figure 50.18), there is hyperplasia of acini, which are lined by high columnar epithelium. Many of them are empty, and others contain vacuolated colloid with a characteristic 'scalloped' pattern adjacent to the thyrocytes.

Robert James Graves, 1796–1853, physician, Meath Hospital, Dublin, Ireland, published an account of exopthalmic goitre in 1835. He was President of the Royal College of Physicians of Ireland and elected Fellow of The Royal Society of London in 1849. There is a statue of him in the Royal College of Physicians in Ireland.

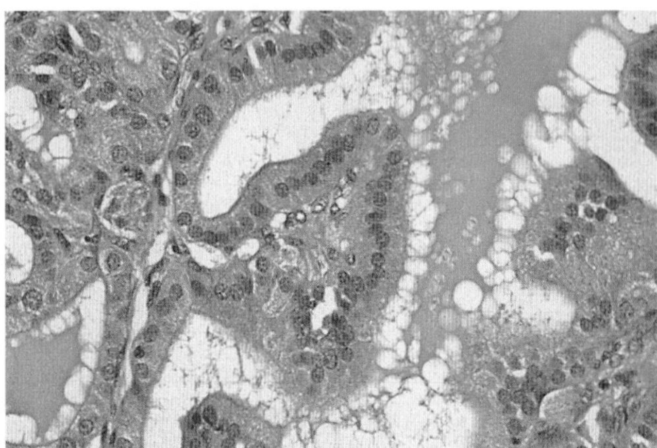

Figure 50.18 Histology of thyrotoxicosis.

Principles of treatment of thyrotoxicosis

Non-specific measures are rest and sedation and in established thyrotoxicosis should be used only in conjunction with specific measures, i.e. the use of antithyroid drugs, surgery and radioiodine.

ANTITHYROID DRUGS

Those in common use are carbimazole and propylthiouracil. Antithyroid drugs are used to restore the patient to a euthyroid state and to maintain this for a prolonged period in the hope that a permanent remission will occur, i.e. that production of thyroid-stimulating antibodies (TSH-RAb) will diminish or cease. Antithyroid drugs cannot cure a toxic nodule. The overactive thyroid tissue is autonomous and recurrence of the hyperthyroidism is certain when the drug is discontinued.

- **Advantages**. No surgery and no use of radioactive materials.
- **Disadvantages**. Treatment is prolonged and the failure rate is at least 50%. The duration of treatment may be tailored to the severity of the toxicity, with milder cases being treated for only 6 months and severe cases for 2 years before stopping therapy.

SURGERY

In diffuse toxic goitre and toxic nodular goitre with overactive internodular tissue, surgery cures by reducing the mass of overactive tissue by reducing the thyroid below a critical mass. After subtotal thyroidectomy the patient should return to a euthyroid state, albeit after a variable period of hypothyroidism. There are however, the long-term risks of recurrence and eventual thyroid failure. In contrast total/near total thyroidectomy accepts immediate thyroid failure and lifelong thyroxine replacement to eliminate the risk of recurrence and simplify follow-up. Operation may result in a reduction in TSH-RAb. In the autonomous toxic nodule, and in toxic nodular goitre with overactive autonomous toxic nodules, surgery cures by removing all the overactive thyroid tissue; this allows the suppressed normal tissue to function again.

- **Advantages**. The goitre is removed, the cure is rapid and the cure rate is high if surgery has been adequate.
- **Disadvantages**. Recurrence of thyrotoxicosis occurs in at least 5% of cases when subtotal thyroidectomy is carried out. There is a risk of permanent hypoparathyroidism and nerve injury. Young women tend to have a poorer cosmetic result from the scar.

Every operation carries a risk, but with suitable preparation and an experienced surgeon the mortality is negligible and the morbidity low.

RADIOIODINE

Radioiodine destroys thyroid cells and, as in thyroidectomy, reduces the mass of functioning thyroid tissue to below a critical level.

- **Advantages**. No surgery and no prolonged drug therapy.
- **Disadvantages**. Isotope facilities must be available. The patient must be quarantined while radiation levels are high and avoid pregnancy and close physical contact, particularly with children. Eye signs may be aggravated.

Choice of therapy

Each case must be considered individually. Below are listed guiding principles on the most satisfactory treatment for a particular toxic goitre at a particular age; these must, however, be modified according to the facilities available and the personality and wishes of the individual patient, business or family commitments and any other coexistent medical or surgical condition. Access to post-treatment care and availability of replacement thyroxine can be important considerations in resource-poor countries.

In advising treatment, compliance, influenced by social and intellectual factors, is important; many patients cannot be trusted to take drugs regularly if they feel well, and indefinite follow-up, which is essential after radioiodine or subtotal thyroidectomy is a burden for all.

DIFFUSE TOXIC GOITRE

Most patients have an initial course of antithyroid drugs with radioiodine for relapse. Exceptions are those who refuse radiation, have large goitres, progressive eye signs or are pregnant.

TOXIC NODULAR GOITRE

Toxic nodular goitre is often large and uncomfortable and enlarges still further with antithyroid drugs. A large goitre should be treated surgically because it does not respond as well or as rapidly to radioiodine or antithyroid drugs as does a diffuse toxic goitre.

TOXIC NODULE

Surgery or radioiodine treatment is appropriate. Resection is easy, certain and with a low risk of morbidity. Radioiodine is a good alternative for patients over the age of 45 years because the suppressed thyroid tissue does not take up iodine and thus there is minimal risk of delayed thyroid insufficiency.

FAILURE OF PREVIOUS TREATMENT WITH ANTITHYROID DRUGS OR RADIOIODINE

In this case, surgery or thyroid ablation with ^{123}I is appropriate.

Surgery for thyrotoxicosis

Preoperative preparation

Traditional preparation aims to make the patient biochemically euthyroid at operation. Preparation is as an out-patient and only rarely is admission to hospital necessary on account of severe symptoms at presentation, failure to control the hyperthyroidism or non-compliance with medication. Care should be coordinated with endocrinology input.

Carbimazole 30–40 mg per day is the drug of choice for preparation. When euthyroid (after 8–12 weeks), the dose may be reduced to 5 mg 8-hourly or a 'block and replace' regime used. In this case, the high dose of carbimazole is continued to inhibit T_3 and T_4 production and a maintenance dose of 0.1–0.15 mg of thyroxine is given daily. The last dose of carbimazole may be given on the evening before surgery. Iodides are not used alone because, if the patient needs preoperative treatment, a more effective drug should be given.

An alternative method of preparation is to abolish the clinical manifestations of the toxic state, using β-adrenergic blocking drugs. These act on the target organs and not on the gland itself. Propranolol also inhibits the peripheral conversion of T_4 to T_3. The appropriate dosages are propranolol 40 mg t.d.s. or the longer acting nadolol 160 mg once daily. Clinical response to β-blockade is rapid and the patient may be rendered clinically euthyroid and operation arranged in a few days rather than weeks. The dose of β-adrenergic blocking drug is increased to achieve the required clinical response and quite often larger doses (propranolol 80 mg t.d.s. or nadololol 320 mg once daily) are necessary.

β-adrenergic blocking drugs do not interfere with synthesis of thyroid hormones, and hormone levels remain high during treatment and for some days after thyroidectomy. It is, therefore, important to continue treatment for 7 days postoperatively.

Iodine may be given with carbimazole or a β-adrenergic blocking drug for 10 days before operation. Iodide alone produces a transient remission and may reduce vascularity, thereby marginally improving safety. The use of iodine preparations is not universal because of more effective alternatives. Iodine gives an additional measure of safety in case the early morning dose of β-adrenergic blocking drug is mistakenly omitted on the day of operation.

The extent of the resection depends on the size of the gland, the age of the patient, the experience of the surgeon, the need to minimise the risk of recurrent toxicity and the wish to avoid postoperative thyroid replacement (*Table 50.5*).

SURGICAL TECHNIQUE OF THYROIDECTOMY

Having made the decision to proceed to surgery, the first step is informed consent. Patients should understand the risk of scar, RLN damage, bleeding, hypocalcaemia and hypothyroidism.

Endotracheal intubation is performed, and if a nerve monitor is to be used its position should be confirmed once the patient is in the surgical position (see New technology in thyroidectomy, below).

The patient lies supine with the neck extended. Surgical preparation extends from the mandible on to the chest. A skin crease incision is placed around the level of the cricoid cartilage. Classically those patients with 'pendulous' breasts should have an incision placed more superiorly as it will tend to migrate inferiorly over years and a sternal wound is less attractive.

Subplatysmal flaps are raised to an extent that allows access to the goitre, often from thyroid notch to sternal notch. The midline is identified between the strap muscles. The plane is developed to dissect between the muscle layers, elevating sternohyoid laterally until ansa cervicalis is visualised. The sternothyroid muscle is then mobilised from the gland, taking great care with the delicate vasculature. If required, the strap muscles may be divided superiorly to afford greater exposure.

Attention is turned first to the superior pole. A plane between the larynx and superior pole is developed and the branching divisions of the superior vascular pedicle are dissected. As these insert onto the gland they are dissected, controlled with ties or bipolar diathermy and divided individually. Not only does this mobilise the superior pole, but preserves the blood supply to the superior parathyroid gland. In addition, this minimises risk to the superior laryngeal nerve, which can often be seen passing medially towards the cricothyroid muscle. Gradually the superior pole is mobilised taking care not to dissect below the cricoid cartilage, at which point the RLN is at risk.

By now, the fascia around the thyroid has been clearly identified. This plane is followed over the anterolateral aspect of the gland to the inferior pole. The tracheoesophageal groove should not be entered at this point as the RLN is yet to be identified. Inferiorly the trachea should be dissected in order to confirm the anatomical landmark.

At this point structures inferior and superior to the RLN have been identified and careful dissection toward the lateral aspect of the gland allows the gland to be rotated medially, displaying the tracheoesophageal groove. Careful dissection of this area proceeds being sure not to divide any structure that could be the nerve. The fascia from the thyroid is mobilised, being vigilant throughout. The RLN is identified and confirmed by the anatomical location, direction of travel and the nerve monitor, if in use. The nerve is then traced towards the larynx, allowing mobilisation of the lateral aspect of the gland.

During this part of the dissection the surgeon must prioritise identification of the nerve, preservation of the inferior parathyroid and its blood supply, as well as control of branches of the inferior thyroid artery. Again, these should be divided in a controlled manner as close as possible to gland in order to preserve parathyroid blood supply.

At this stage the nerve should be traced towards the cricothyroid joint as it enters the larynx. This point is the area where the nerve is most commonly damaged. The pretracheal fascia condenses into Berry's ligament at this stage. Small vessels within the ligament retract if not controlled with bipolar diathermy or ties, and the resulting bleeding can disorientate the surgeon placing the nerve at risk (**Figure 50.19**).

In order to avoid this, pre-emptive diathermy to the ligament and careful layer by layer dissection allows final mobilisation of the thyroid lobe. Some surgeons prefer to isolate the ligament and apply a careful tie to achieve haemostasis.

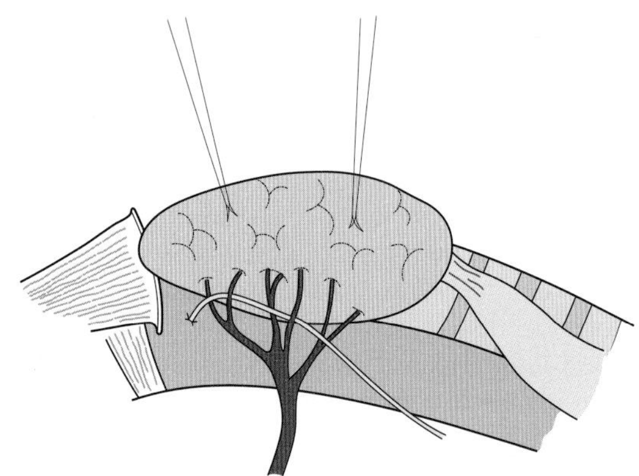

Figure 50.19 Identification of the recurrent laryngeal nerve. Note how rotating the gland medially anteriorly kinks the nerve that is normally intimately related to the terminal branches of the inferior thyroid artery.

Whichever method is preferred, great care must be taken at this point. The lobe is then mobilised medially and the nerve falls laterally.

If total thyroidectomy is indicated the procedure is repeated on the contralateral side. If, however, lobectomy alone is indicated, the isthmus should be divided between clamps and oversewn. The surgical bed is then inspected to confirm the integrity of the nerve and the state of the parathyroid glands. Consideration may be given to reimplantation of parathyroids to the sternomastoid muscle if they appear devascularised. Irrigation followed by meticulous haemostasis should follow and no bleeding is acceptable. Ideally this is performed with a Valsalva manouvre with the head down.

Following complete haemostasis the strap muscles are loosely reapproximated in order to avoid a water tight seal but to prevent adhesion between skin and trachea. The wound is then closed in layers with absorbable suture to platysma and skin closure. This may be with clips, non-absorbable sutures or subcuticular closure. It is important that those involved in postoperative care know how the wound was closed and how to perform a bedside reopening in the event of a life-threatening bleed.

The patient is then returned to the recovery room and the postoperative area for overnight monitoring. Not only is the wound regularly reviewed, but for total thyroidectomy patients postoperative calcium should be checked to identify hypocalcaemia.

NEW TECHNOLOGY IN THYROIDECTOMY

The major immediate risk following thyroidectomy is haemorrhage; conventionally, artery forceps, ligatures and sutures have been used to secure the meticulous haemostasis necessary to minimise the risk of this potentially life-threatening complication. Ultrasonic shears, enhanced bipolar diathermy and harmonic vessel sealing devices are increasingly used in thyroid surgery and may be advantageous in complex procedures.

Monitoring of the RLN and vagus nerve has become available over the last few years. By placing electrodes on the endotracheal tube between the vocal cords, movements can be detected when the nerve is stimulated. Such intermittent nerve monitoring is gaining in popularity. Advocates consider the monitor particularly useful in recurrent operations where scar tissue makes the nerve difficult to identify. In addition, some authors find operative time is reduced and that this is a valuable tool for training. There is also some support for the use of nerve monitoring during bilateral thyroid surgery, as the information provided can aid in the identification of a unilateral palsy to prevent bilateral palsy that can require tracheostomy. Those who do not support the use of the nerve monitor highlight the lack of evidence that any real difference in outcome associated with this practice. In addition, there is the expense of the base machine and the electrodes.

In contrast to intermittent nerve monitoring that allows identification of a damaged nerve, continuous nerve monitoring has now been developed. In theory, this provides the opportunity to identify a nerve when function is threatened (by excessive traction for example). This technique, although theoretically advantageous, requires an electrode placed on the vagus nerve and has not gained widespread acceptance (Figure 50.20).

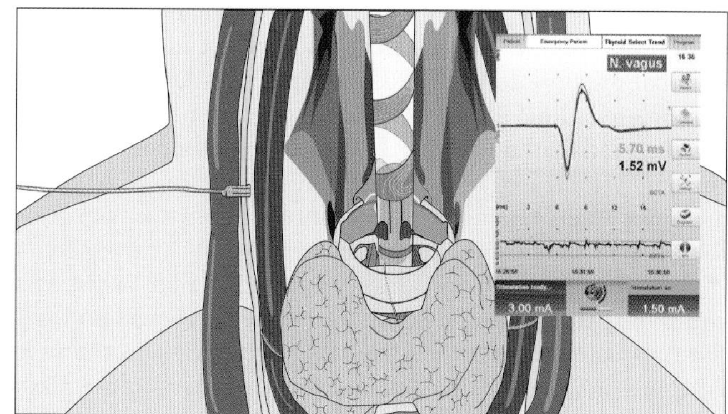

Figure 50.20 Diagram of continuous monitoring of the vagus nerve (adapted from an image provided by Inomed UK Ltd).

ALTERNATIVE SURGICAL TECHNIQUES

Over the past two decades, increasing experience has been gained in alternative approaches to thyroid surgery. Minimally invasive video assisted techniques have been developed, which allow surgeons to operate through an incision <2 cm in length. With appropriately modified dissectors, experienced operators and advanced haemostatic electrosurgical devices, such procedures offer reduced scar length. However, they are only appropriate for small volume disease and as such are not suitable for many thyroid cases.

Robots have found a role in many aspects of modern surgical practice. In the Far East, a neck scar is found to be socially unacceptable. Robotic techniques have been developed that allow access to the thyroid via an axillary incision. Such 'maximally invasive' techniques require extended dissection over the chest wall and again are most suitable for small volume disease. Experienced centres continue to expand the indications for these techniques. However, they are associated with great cost and significant time, which currently limits their application to thyroid surgical practice.

POSTOPERATIVE COMPLICATIONS

Haemorrhage Haemorrhage is the most frequent life-threatening complication of thyroidectomy. Around 1 in 50 patients will develop a haematoma, and in almost all cases this will develop in the first 24 hours. If an arterial bleed occurs, the tension in the central compartment pressure can rise until it exceeds venous pressure. Venous oedema of the larynx can then develop and cause airway obstruction leading to death. Although improvements in understanding of the blood supply to the larynx and technical developments in terms of haemostatic technologies have been made, this complication has not been eliminated. Although many surgeons worldwide practice day case thyroidectomy, bleeding is the reason that, in the UK, thyroidectomy remains an inpatient procedure.

Intraoperative attention to detail in terms of haemostasis is critical. When closing the wound, avoiding a watertight closure of the strap muscles may allow a haematoma to escape into the subcutaneous tissues. Wound drains have not been shown to have a protective effect. Close monitoring of the wound is advised postoperatively. If a haematoma develops, clinical staff should know to remove skin sutures in order to release some pressure and seek senior advice immediately. Endotracheal intubation should be used to secure the airway while the haematoma is evacuated and the bleeding point controlled.

Recurrent laryngeal nerve paralysis and voice change RLN injury may be unilateral or bilateral, transient or permanent. Early routine postoperative laryngoscopy reveals a much higher incidence of transient cord paralysis than is detectable by simple assessment of the integrity of the voice and cough. Such temporary dysfunction is not clinically important however, but voice and cord function should be assessed at first follow-up 4 weeks postoperatively. The British Association of Endocrine Surgeons audit revealed a RLN palsy rate of 1.8% at 1 month, declining to 0.5% at 3 months for first time operations. Permanent paralysis is rare if the nerve has been identified at operation.

If a RLN is injured during surgery and the transected ends are identified, they should be reanastomosed. In the event that a length of nerve is excised (due to invasion by malignancy for example), anastomosis of the ansa cervicalis may be considered. This does not return mobility of the vocal cord but maintains neurological input to the muscles of the larynx. By avoiding denervation and related muscle atrophy, the vocal quality is improved. Permanent vocal cord paralysis should be treated conservatively with speech therapy. If voice quality is unacceptable, medialisation procedures can be performed. Nerve grafting has shown promise but experience is limited.

Injury to the external branch of the superior laryngeal nerve is more common because of its proximity to the superior thyroid artery. This leads to loss of tension in the vocal cord with diminished power and range in the voice. Patients, particularly those who use their voice professionally, must be advised that any thyroid operation will result in change to the voice even in the absence of nerve trauma. Fortunately, for most patients the changes are subtle and only demonstrable on formal voice assessment.

Thyroid insufficiency Following total thyroidectomy, clearly thyroxine replacement will be required. Around one in three patients who has a lobectomy will require supplementation; rates are higher in those with thyroid autoantibodies. Subtotal thyroidectomy was at one time performed with the aim of leaving sufficient tissue to maintain thyroid function. However, this is difficult to judge and over years, the benign process that necessitated primary surgery may recur, requiring difficult revision procedures. For this reason, the practice of subtotal thyroidectomy has been more or less abandoned outside of environments where exogenous thyroxine is not available.

Parathyroid insufficiency This is due to removal of the parathyroid glands or infarction through damage to the parathyroid end arteries; often both factors occur together. Vascular injury is probably far more important than inadvertent removal. The incidence of permanent hypoparathyroidism should be less than 1% and most cases present dramatically 2–5 days after operation but, very rarely, the onset is delayed for 2–3 weeks or a patient with marked hypocalcaemia may be asymptomatic. The complication is limited to total thyroidectomy, as when lobectomy is performed the contralateral parathyroid glands are sufficient to maintain calcium levels. In particular, total thyroidectomy with central neck dissection places the parathyroid glands and their vascular supply at great risk and should only be performed when there is evidence of metastatic disease or high risk of occult disease in the regional lymph nodes.

Thyrotoxic crisis (storm) This is an acute exacerbation of hyperthyroidism. It occurs if a thyrotoxic patient has been inadequately prepared for thyroidectomy and is now extremely rare. Very rarely, a thyrotoxic patient presents in a crisis and this may follow an unrelated operation. Symptomatic and supportive treatment is for dehydration, hyperpyrexia and restlessness. This requires the administration of intravenous fluids, cooling the patient with ice packs, administration of oxygen, diuretics for cardiac failure, digoxin for uncontrolled atrial fibrillation, sedation and intravenous hydrocortisone. Specific treatment is by carbimazole 10–20 mg 6-hourly, Lugol's iodine 10 drops 8-hourly by mouth or sodium iodide 1g i.v. Propranolol intravenously (1–2 mg) or orally (40 mg 6-hourly) will block β-adrenergic effects.

Wound infection Cellulitis requiring prescription of antibiotics, often by the general practitioner, is more common than most surgeons appreciate. A significant subcutaneous or deep cervical abscess is exceptionally rare and should be drained.

Hypertrophic or keloid scar This is more likely to form if the incision overlies the sternum and in dark skinned individuals. Intradermal injections of corticosteroid should be given at once and repeated monthly if necessary. Scar revision rarely results in significant long-term improvement.

Stitch granuloma This may occur with or without sinus formation and is seen after the use of non-absorbable, particularly silk, suture material. Absorbable ligatures and sutures should be used throughout thyroid surgery. Some surgeons use a subcuticular absorbable skin suture rather than the traditional skin clips or staples.

POSTOPERATIVE CARE

Following surgery, the patient should be returned to the recovery room and nursed overnight on the ward. Wound care should include vigilance for signs of a haematoma. Following total thyroidectomy, calcium levels should be checked postoperatively. Not all patients develop immediate hypocalcaemia and they should be educated about the signs (parasthesia of the fingers and toes or round the mouth). Serial calcium monitoring should be recommended for those at highest risk. Those patients who had a total thyroidectomy require thyroxine replacement, which should start day 1 postoperatively. On clinic review, in addition to checking the histology report, the wound should be inspected and the larynx examined for vocal cord function. Biochemical assessment of thyroid function and calcium, if required, should be arranged.

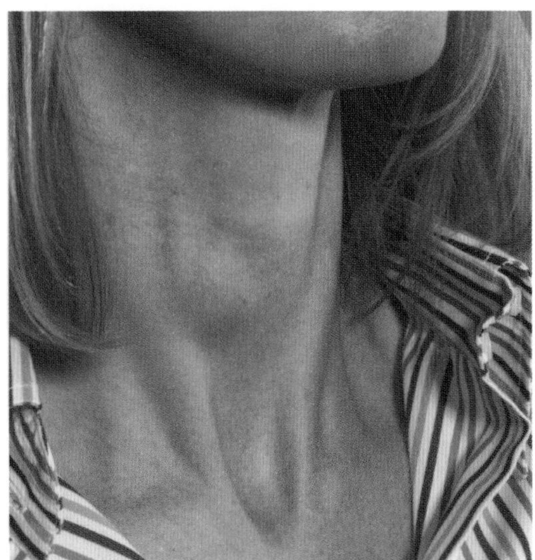

Figure 50.21 Isolated swelling in the upper pole of the right thyroid lobe.

NEOPLASMS OF THE THYROID

Classification of thyroid neoplasms is presented in *Table 50.6* and the relative incidence of malignancies in *Table 50.7*.

TABLE 50.6 Classification of thyroid neoplasms.

Benign	Follicular adenoma		
Malignant	Primary	Follicular epithelium – differentiated	Follicular Papillary
		Follicular epithelium – poorly differentiated	Anaplastic
		Parafollicular cells	Medullary
		Lymphoid cells	Lymphoma
	Secondary	Metastatic	
		Local infiltration	

TABLE 50.7 Relative incidence of primary malignant tumours of the thyroid gland.

Malignancy	Relative incidence
Papillary carcinoma	80%
Follicular carcinoma	10%
Poorly differentiated/anaplastic carcinoma	5%
Medullary carcinoma	2.5%
Lymphoma	2.5%

Benign tumours

Follicular adenomas present as clinically solitary nodules (Figure 50.21) and the distinction between a follicular carcinoma and an adenoma can only be made by histological examination; in the adenoma there is no invasion of the capsule or of pericapsular blood vessels. For this reason, FNA, which provides cytologic detail but not tissue architecture, cannot differentiate between benign and malignant follicular lesions. Diagnosis and treatment is therefore, by wide excision, i.e. total lobectomy. The remaining thyroid tissue is normal so that prolonged follow-up is unnecessary.

Malignant tumours

The vast majority of primary malignancies are carcinomas derived from the follicular cells (*Table 50.6*). Such tumors were thought of as differentiated (papillary, follicular and Hürthle cell) and undifferentiated (anaplastic). However, now an intermediate class of 'poorly differentiated carcinoma' is recognised, which is likely to represent a state of dedifferentiated, between classic differentiated and undifferentiated diseases. The parafollicular C cells can undergo malignant transformation into medullary carcinoma, and thyroid lymphoma is another primary thyroid malignancy. In addition, the thyroid can be involved by direct spread from surrounding structures (larynx and oesophagus) or metastases (most commonly from renal cell carcinoma). Lymph node and blood-borne metastases of thyroid cancer occur primarily to bone and lung and may be the mode of presentation (Figure 50.22).

Aetiology of malignant thyroid tumours

The great majority of thyroid cancers have no known aetiological factor. The most important identifiable aetiological factor in differentiated thyroid carcinoma (particularly papillary) is irradiation of the thyroid under 5 years of age. In the town of Gomel, Ukraine, the incidence of childhood thyroid cancer rose from <1 per million to 96 per million following the Chernobyl nuclear disaster.

Short latency aggressive papillary cancer is associated with the ret/PTC3 oncogene and later developing, possibly less aggressive, cancers with ret/PTC1. The incidence of follicular carcinoma is high in endemic goitrous areas, possibly due to TSH stimulation. Malignant lymphomas sometimes develop in autoimmune thyroiditis, and the lymphocytic infiltration in the autoimmune process may be an aetiological factor.

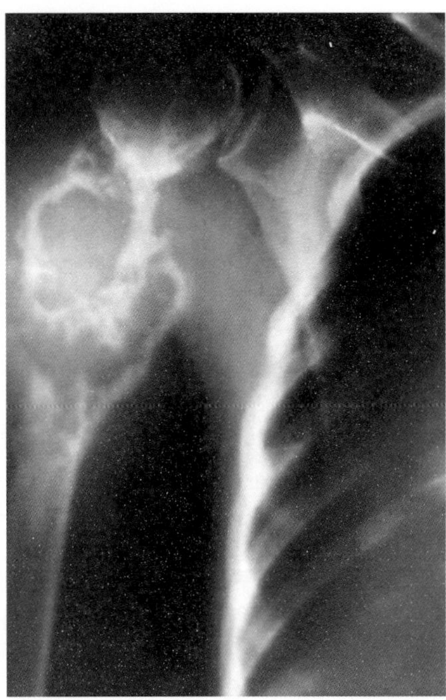

Figure 50.22 Metastasis in the humerus from thyroid carcinoma (courtesy of DS Devadatta, Vellore, India).

Clinical features of thyroid cancers

The annual incidence is about 0.6 per million of the population and the sex ratio is three females to one male. However, the incidence of papillary thyroid cancer is increasing rapidly across the world. This is mostly due to increased rates of imaging detecting previously occult disease. For that reason, although the incidence is increasing, the mortality rates remain static at over 80% 5-year survival for all groups. In particular, anaplastic carcinoma predicts poor outcome with differentiated carcinomas generally having excellent outcomes. The most common presenting symptom is a thyroid swelling (Figures 50.21 and 50.23). Enlarged cervical lymph nodes may be the presentation of papillary carcinoma (PTC). RLN paralysis is very suggestive of locally advanced disease.

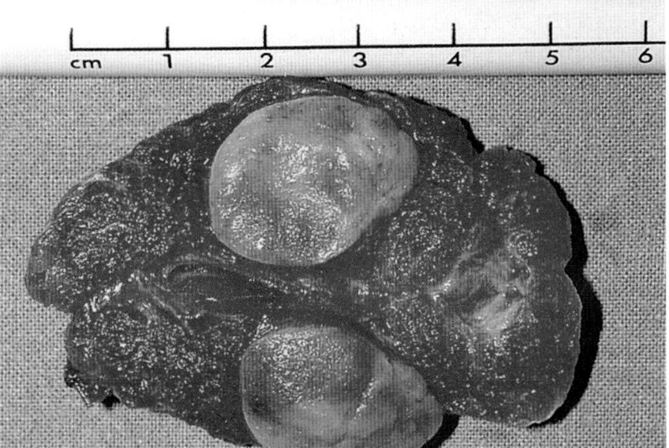

Figure 50.23 Follicular neoplasm of the thyroid presenting as an isolated swelling.

Anaplastic growths are usually hard, irregular and infiltrating. A differentiated carcinoma may be suspiciously firm and irregular, but is often indistinguishable from a benign swelling. Small papillary tumours may be impalpable, even when lymphatic metastases are present. Pain, often referred to the ear, is suggestive of nerve involvement from infiltrating tumours.

Diagnosis of thyroid neoplasms

Clinical history and examination continue to be the cornerstone of diagnosis of thyroid neoplasms. As previously mentioned, radiation exposure and family history should be discussed. Examination of the central neck and regional lymphatics should be combined with assessment of vocal cord function. Biochemical assessment of thyroid function should also be considered in this first encounter, if not already performed.

Following initial assessment, the next step is ultrasound. This non-invasive investigation is most accurate at assessing thyroid swellings. Not only can a judgement be made on the presence, size and number of thyroid nodules present, but an estimate of risk of malignancy can be made depending on these findings.

Following ultrasound, lesions can be categorised as benign, indeterminate or malignant. Benign lesions require no further assessment unless surgery is considered for compressive symptoms. Indeterminate or malignant lesions should be investigated with FNAC.

Occasionally, the surgeon will encounter a thyrotoxic patient. Such cases are one of the few indications for a radioiodine uptake scan. This allows assessment of the function of a nodule. Hot nodules are very rarely malignant. Cold nodules will require assessment as for all other thyroid neoplasms.

Following clinical, ultrasound and cytological assessment, the vast majority of lesions will be characterised as benign, malignant or indeterminate. Further treatment will be planned accordingly.

Certain situations require specific consideration. For patients with widespread nodal disease or suspicion of locally invasive disease affecting the airway, contrast enhanced imaging should be considered. This should cover the neck and chest. Not only does this allow accurate assessment of any visceral invasion, but is superior to ultrasound at defining disease in the mediastinum and thorax. Concerns over the impact of iodine-containing contrast on delays to radioactive iodine therapy have been overplayed, and it is more critical that the surgeon has an accurate assessment of disease extent prior to surgery.

Patients with a rapidly growing thyroid mass, particularly if solid and fixed, should be considered at risk of anaplastic carcinoma. However, this diagnosis can be difficult to differentiate from thyroid lymphoma or occasionally thyroiditis. Despite the difficulty, an accurate diagnosis is critical as anaplastic carcinoma is rapidly fatal and palliative measure are general recommended, whereas confounding disease processes may respond to therapy. In this setting, core or even open biopsy may be required to make a confident diagnosis.

Papillary carcinoma

Papillary carcinoma is the most common thyroid malignancy. Interestingly, up to 30% of patients who die of non-thyroid disease have deposits of PTC in autopsy studies, suggesting that many patients live with this disease undetected. Nonetheless, when papillary cancer is diagnosed most patients will be offered treatment. The disease is known for its propensity for lymph node metastases. These are more common in younger patients, in whom they do not affect the otherwise excellent survival. This finding is in contrast to most malignances, where the finding of metastatic disease confers a poor outcome. One contentious finding in patients with PTC is a high rate of occult micrometastases (as high as 40% of N0 patients in the central neck). Despite the presence of metastases, few patients progress to have clinically meaningful disease and the role of elective nodal surgery is in question. Distant metastases are uncommon in PTC.

Recently, increasing interest has focused on 'papillary microcarcinoma'. This term is used to describe PTC that is <10 mm in size. These lesions are common (detected in about 10% of benign thyroid resections) and not associated with adverse outcomes, including recurrence or non-survival. As such, management and follow-up of patients with these lesions of doubtful clinical significance is controversial. In Korea, for example, national screening has led to a significant increase in these cases. In Japan groups are opting for an observational approach without surgery. These studies have shown that at least two-thirds never progress. In the USA some groups are attempting non-surgical management with ablation techniques using ethanol or radiofrequency. In most of the world however, groups try to avoid diagnosing these small, insignificant lesions by limiting biopsies to >10 mm lesions and being conservative in the management of lesions following their diagnosis.

Follicular carcinoma

Follicular carcinoma can normally only be differentiated from follicular adenoma by the architecture on histology. For this reason, follicular lesions on FNA are unable to be diagnosed as malignant in the absence of clinical features such as metastases (Figure 50.24). Multiple foci of follicular carcinoma are seldom seen and lymph node involvement is much less common than in papillary carcinoma. Blood-borne metastases are more common and the eventual mortality rate, although still low, is twice that of papillary cancer (Figure 50.25).

Hürthle cell tumours are a rare variant of follicular neoplasm in which oxyphil (Hürthle, Askanazy) cells predominate histologically. Hürthle cell cancers are associated with a poorer prognosis.

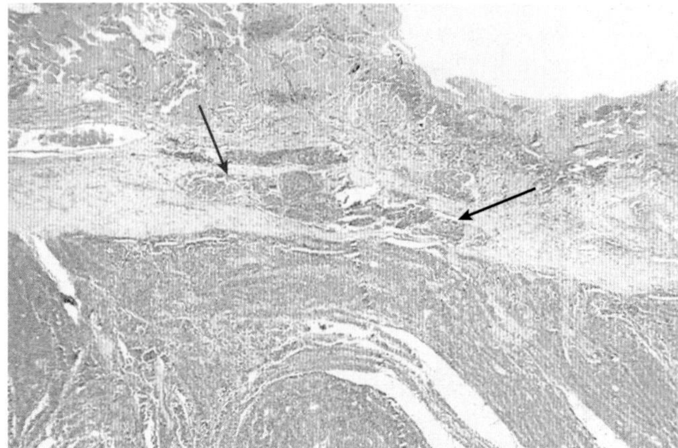

Figure 50.24 Histology of follicular thyroid carcinoma showing vascular (red arrow) and capsular (black arrow) invasion (courtesy of Dr SWB Ewen, Aberdeen, UK).

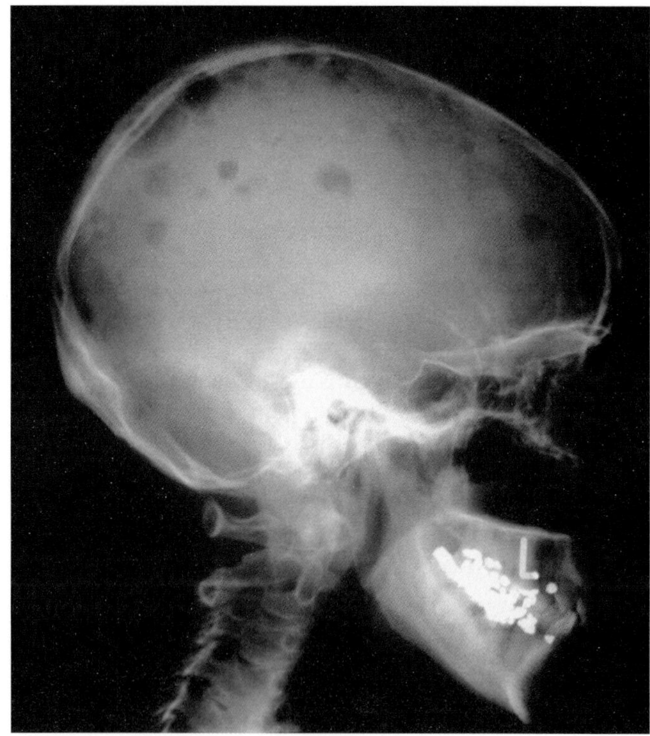

Figure 50.25 Follicular carcinoma of thyroid with skull secondaries.

Prognosis in differentiated thyroid carcinoma

The prognosis in differentiated thyroid cancers is generally excellent. In terms of survival, older patients, those with large tumors or extrathyroid extension or distant metastases have worse outcomes. A system of risk stratification can be used to predict the risk on an individual basis. In a young patient with a low-risk tumour, the risk of death following appropriate treatment is almost zero. In an older patient with a high-risk tumour (extrathyroid extension or distant metastases), the risk is as high as 50% at 5 years. Older patients with low-risk tumours and younger patients with high-risk tumours are an intermediate risk group. Nodal metastases deserve special mention. In younger patients they predict for recurrence but not for death. This is because recurrent neck disease in young

Karl Hürthle, 1866–1945, German histopathologist, first drew attention to these cells.
Max Askanazy, 1865–1940, described these cells while working at the Pathological Anatomy Institute, Tübingen, Germany.

patients can almost always be successfully salvaged. In contrast, for older patients neck metastases (particularly in the lateral neck) are a marker of distant metastases in some, and therefore carry a negative prognostic implication for both recurrence and death.

The AJCC staging system is in the process of modification. However, the current edition stages all patients <45 years as stage I unless they have distant metastases, when they are stage II. Older T1N0M0 patients are stage I and T2N0M0 are stage II. The presence of nodal disease in the central neck nodes (N1a) upstages older patients to stage III, as does T3 disease. All older patients with lateral neck disease (N1b), locally invasive primary disease (T4) or distant metastases are stage IV.

The AJCC 8th edition will raise the age cut-off to 55 years. It will also formally recognise that extrathyroid extension is less significant if identified microscopically but not evident during surgery. The extent of nodal involvement will also be included, with small numbers of low-volume nodes being considered less significant than multiple large-volume nodes.

Surgical treatment for differentiated thyroid cancer

This subject has many contentious aspects. For the vast majority of patients, outcome is excellent irrespective of the extent of surgery. The low number of recurrences and death has made prospective trials difficult and, as such, very few exist.

The aim of surgery is to rid the patient of macroscopic disease and minimise the chance of recurrence and death. An additional aim is to minimise surgical morbidity. Achieving a balance between these aims is critical. In addition, the surgeon must consider whether radioactive iodine is to be recommended. In low-risk cases this is rarely indicated, whereas in high-risk patients it is used almost universally. Risk stratification is therefore critical.

In high-risk patients with nodal or distant metastases, total thyroidectomy will be performed to eradicate disease in the thyroid and prepare the patient for radioactive iodine. For low-risk patients with a single focus of disease limited to the thyroid, a thyroid lobectomy can be offered. This has the significant advantage of protecting the contralateral RLN and parathyroid glands. This approach is now considered appropriate unless there are high-risk features of disease.

In terms of the neck, when metastatic disease is present, a therapeutic compartment-orientated neck dissection should be performed to remove disease from the central or lateral neck, depending on the site of involvement. The role of elective neck surgery, when no disease in the nodes is detected preoperatively, is far more controversial. Lateral neck dissection carries significant morbidity and despite high rates of occult metastases in papillary carcinoma, has been abandoned. The reason is that even in patients who are thought to have occult metastases, very few progress to clinically meaningful disease. In contrast, the morbidity of central neck dissection is lower, and the compartment has to be opened during a thyroidectomy. In addition, salvage surgery in the central neck carries a high risk to the RLN and parathyroid glands. For these reasons elective central neck dissection has been popular in the last few decades. However, increased recognition that performing such surgery in all patients with PTC leads to high rates of morbidity and the lack of evidence that outcomes improve due to more aggressive surgery, has led to a move away from this practice. At this point, patients who are considered at highest risk of having occult metastases in the central neck (those with extrathyroid extension for example) are considered most likely to see benefit from elective surgery and it is not recommended routinely in low-risk patients.

Many patients will only be diagnosed with their thyroid cancer following a diagnostic lobectomy. In this setting, risk assessment is again critical. If the patient is considered low risk, further surgery is unlikely to be beneficial. If, however, patient or tumour features are considered high risk, radioactive iodine may be recommended, in which case completion thyroidectomy may be required.

Given the complexity of decision making in thyroid cancer and the different groups involved (surgeons, endocrinologists, radiologists, cytologists, pathologists and nuclear medicine physicians), all cases should be discussed in a multidisciplinary setting.

Thyroxine

Following surgery, thyroid cells (both normal and malignant) can be suppressed using high doses of thyroxine. This was once considered routine for all differentiated thyroid cancers during follow-up. Again, risk stratification has modified our approach to these patients. Following surgery, patients can be considered high or low risk. For those patients at high risk from disease, thyroxine will be prescribed at levels which suppress TSH without making the patient biochemically hyperthyroid. In contrast, low-risk patients may be considered for thyroxine replacement at physiological levels. In this patient group, a balance of benefit (remember these patients have extremely low rates of recurrence or death) versus risk must be made. In particular, long-term TSH suppression can result in cardiac arrhythmia and osteoporosis. As such the treating team should consider all risks during follow-up to strike this balance.

Low-risk patients who have had lobectomy alone may require no thyroxine at all. Patients who had a total thyroidectomy will clearly require replacement and those considered high risk should be managed with suppression, in order to minimise the chance of disease recurrence.

Radioiodine

Thyroid tissue concentrates iodine. For this reason, ^{131}I can be given in order to deliver tumoricidal doses of radioactivity directly to thyroid tissue, both benign and malignant. In the setting of thyroid cancer, all normal tissue should be removed (total thyroidectomy) along with any gross neck disease (neck dissection) in order for any residual microscopic disease or distant metastases to receive an optimal dose. Radioiodine treatment is not an alternative to surgical resection for gross resectable disease.

As with many aspects of differentiated thyroid cancer management, indications for radioiodine treatment are controversial. Again, low-risk patients have little to gain and may be safely managed without adjuvant therapy. High- risk patients, however, remain candidates.

In order to effectively drive the radioiodine into cells, high levels of TSH are required. This can be achieved by rendering the patient hypothyroid (off thyroxine) or by using recombinant TSH, which is injected prior to radioiodine administration.

Following radioiodine administration, an uptake scan is performed. This demonstrates areas of iodine uptake in the whole body and can be used to identify any metastatic disease not recognised on initial imaging. This information is useful in the ongoing process of risk stratification of patients following initial therapy.

Outside the setting of primary treatment, radioiodine treatment may be considered in cases of recurrence, particularly if not used initially. Multiple doses can be used in order to treat unresectable disease, distant metastases or even a rising thyroglobulin in the absence of structural disease.

Most differentiated thyroid cancers will concentrate iodine. However, with advancing patient age and particularly if disease is multiply recurrent the tumour will lose its iodine avidity. This is called radioiodine refractory disease. Such cases may be considered for external beam radiotherapy, although this is uncommon.

Thyroglobulin

Thyroglobulin is a tumour marker produced by normal thyroid cells and most differentiated thyroid cancer. As such, this offers an extremely accurate method of following patients postoperatively. If a lobectomy has been performed the level will not be undetectable, but trends can be used to monitor for recurrence. Following total thyroidectomy, the aim is to have an undetectable thyroglobulin. Patients who achieve this point are at extremely low risk of recurrence. Serial thyroglobulin measurement (6–12 monthly) combined with ultrasound assessment of the neck can then be used to monitor patients during follow-up.

If an undetectable level is not achieved, the thyroglobulin can be followed. If it increases, imaging should be performed to look for gross recurrent disease. Resectable disease should be addressed surgically and normally further radioactive iodine (RAI) would be indicated. The role of RAI in a rising thyroglobulin without structural disease is controversial.

Undifferentiated (anaplastic) carcinoma

This is one of the most aggressive malignancies in humans. Thankfully it is rare. It may develop *de novo*, or present as dedifferentiation of a papillary or poorly differentiated carcinoma. The disease is characterised by rapid growth, visceral invasion and distant metastases. The surgeon's role in this disease is crucial. Thyroid lymphoma can be incorrectly diagnosed as anaplastic cancer and so biopsy is critical. This can be done using a core or open technique.

Management is controversial. Almost all patients will be dead within 6 months. Radiotherapy and chemotherapy have not been shown to improve survival. Occasional patients may present with disease limited to the neck, which appears resectable on imaging. Such patients seem to have a slightly better outcome if treated with aggressive surgery and postoperative adjuvant therapy (radiotherapy +/- chemotherapy). However, solid evidence is lacking and the majority of patients will not be considered for curative treatment.

Those patients who have a known diagnosis and develop airway symptoms are generally better managed without tracheostomy, despite the potentially distressing mode of death. In patients who present with airway signs and without a diagnosis, a tracheostomy may be required to buy time to confirm the diagnosis and in order to allow a few more days for patients to 'get their affairs in order'.

Medullary carcinoma

These are tumours of the parafollicular (C cells) derived from the neural crest. rather than the cells of the thyroid follicle as are other primary thyroid carcinomas. The cells are not unlike those of a carcinoid tumour and on histological analysis a characteristic amyloid stroma is seen (Figure 50.26). High levels of serum calcitonin and carcinoembryonic antigen are produced by many medullary tumours, which should be tested for in suspected cases. Calcitonin levels fall after resection and rise again with recurrence, making it a valuable tumour marker in the follow-up of patients with this disease. Diarrhoea is a feature in 30% of cases and this may be due to 5-hydroxytryptamine or prostaglandins produced by the tumour cells.

Some tumours are familial and account for 10–20% of all cases. Medullary carcinoma may occur in combination with adrenal phaeochromocytoma and hyperparathyroidism (HPT) (usually due to hyperplasia) in the syndrome known as multiple endocrine neoplasia type 2A (MEN-2A). The familial form of the disease frequently affects children and young adults, whereas the sporadic cases occur at any age with no sex predominance. When the familial form is associated with prominent mucosal neuromas involving the lips, tongue and inner aspect of the eyelids, with a Marfanoid habitus, the syndrome is referred to as MEN type 2B (see Chapter 52).

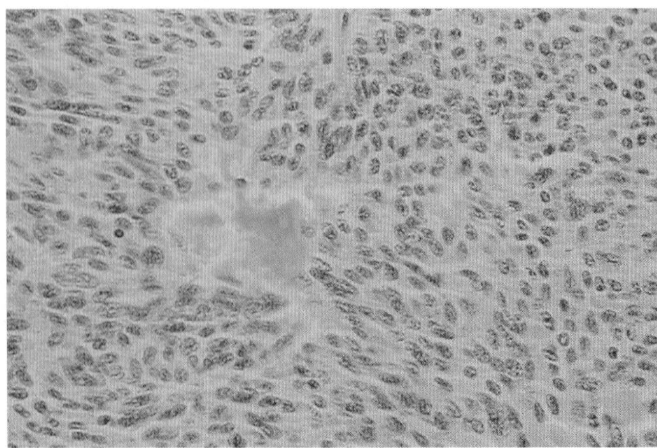

Figure 50.26 Histology of medullary carcinoma showing characteristic 'cell balls' and amyloid (courtesy of Dr SWB Ewen, Aberdeen, UK).

Involvement of lymph nodes occurs in 50–60% of cases of medullary carcinoma and blood-borne metastases are common. As would be expected, tumours are not TSH dependent and do not take up radioactive iodine. The prognosis is variable and depends on the stage at diagnosis. Any nodal involvement virtually eliminates the prospect of cure and, unfortunately, even small tumours confined to the thyroid gland may have spread by the time of diagnosis, particularly in familial cancers. In common with many endocrine tumours the progression of disease may be very slow, with a characteristically indolent course and long survival, even in the absence of cure.

In familial cases of medullary thyroid cancer, genetic screening of relatives should be recommended. This is a complex subject but individuals identified can be risk stratified dependent on the genetic abnormality. This information can be used to make recommendations concerning prophylactic thyroidectomy. Some relatives may be monitored into adulthood with serial calcitonin monitoring. In contrast, the highest-risk mutations are associated with early-onset disease and total thyroidectomy is recommended during infancy.

Treatment

When medullary carcinoma is diagnosed, staging of the neck and chest should be performed. For those patients with disease confined to the thyroid, total thyroidectomy is recommended to remove all C cells. In addition, elective dissection of the central neck nodes is also performed to optimise the chance of cure. If there is evidence of nodal metastases, cure is unlikely. In this setting, gross disease should be excised but the surgeon should be mindful of morbidity. Such patients are highly likely to recur and a pragmatic approach should be adopted.

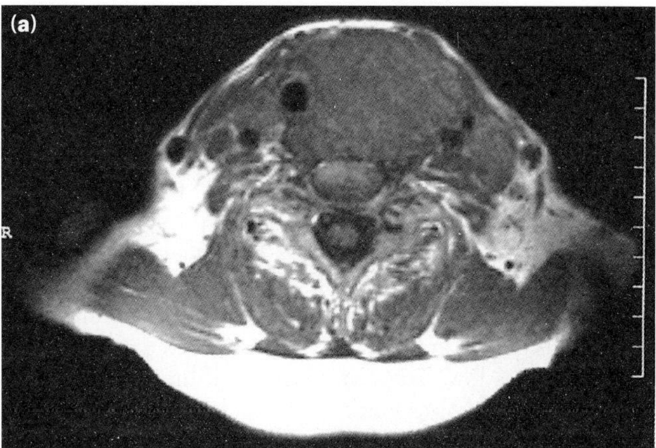

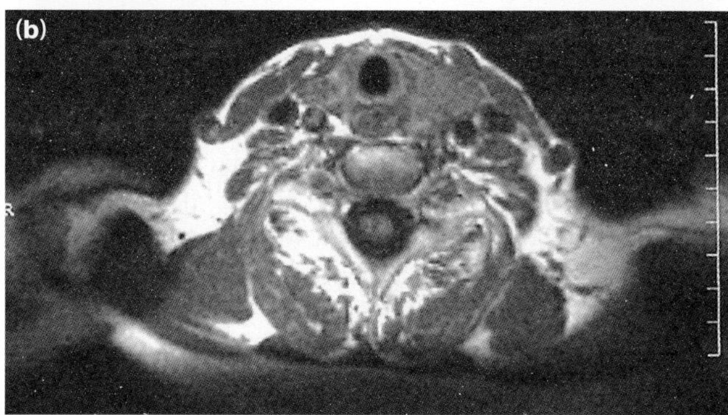

Figure 50.27 Magnetic resonance imaging scans of extensive malignant lymphoma (a) before and (b) after 7 days of external beam radiotherapy (courtesy of Dr FW Smith, Aberdeen, UK).

Malignant lymphoma

In the past, many malignant lymphomas were diagnosed as small round-cell anaplastic carcinomas. Response to irradiation is dramatic (Figure 50.27) and radical surgery is unnecessary once the diagnosis is established by biopsy. In patients with tracheal compression, isthmusectomy is the most appropriate form of biopsy although the response to therapy is so rapid that this should rarely be necessary unless there has been difficulty in making a histological diagnosis. The prognosis is good, particularly if there is no involvement of cervical lymph nodes. Rarely, the tumour is part of widespread malignant lymphoma disease and the prognosis in these cases is worse. Most lymphomas occur against a background of lymphocytic thyroiditis.

THYROIDITIS

Chronic lymphocytic (autoimmune) thyroiditis

This common condition is usually associated with raised titres of thyroid antibodies. It commonly presents as a goitre, which may be diffuse or nodular with a characteristic 'bosselated' feel or with established or subclinical thyroid failure. The diagnosis often follows investigation of a discrete swelling. Features of chronic lymphocytic (focal) thyroiditis are commonly present on histological examination in association with other thyroid disease, notably toxic goitre (Figure 50.28). Primary

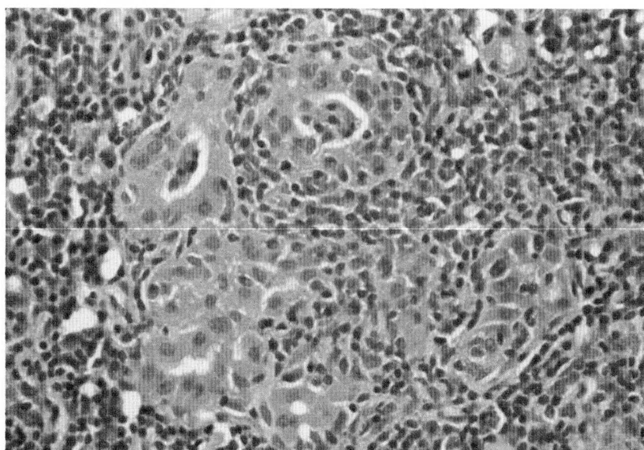

Figure 50.28 Autoimmune thyroiditis (Hashimoto's disease; struma lymphomatosa). Intense lymphocytic-plasma cell infiltration, acinar destruction and fibrosis.

Friedrich Joseph de Quervain, 1868–1940, Professor of Surgery, Berne, Switzerland, described this form of thyroiditis in 1902.

myxoedema without detectable thyroid enlargement represents the end stage of the pathological process.

Granulomatous thyroiditis (subacute thyroiditis, de Quervain's thyroiditis)

This may follow a viral infection. In a typical subacute presentation, there is pain in the neck, fever, malaise and a firm, irregular enlargement of one or both thyroid lobes. There are raised inflammatory markers, absent thyroid antibodies, the serum T_4 is high normal or slightly raised, and the ^{123}I uptake of the gland is low. The condition is self-limiting and, in a few months, the goitre subsides and there may be a period of months of hypothyroidism before eventual recovery. In 10% of cases the onset is acute, the goitre very painful and tender and there may be symptoms of hyperthyroidism. One-third of cases are asymptomatic but for the presence of the goitre. If diagnosis is in doubt, it may be confirmed by FNAC, radioactive iodine uptake and by a rapid symptomatic response to prednisone. The specific treatment for the acute case with severe pain is to give prednisone 10–20 mg daily for 7 days and the dose is then gradually reduced over the next month. If thyroid failure is prominent, treatment with thyroxine may be required until function recovers.

Riedel's thyroiditis

This is very rare, accounting for 0.5% of goitres. Thyroid tissue is replaced by cellular fibrous tissue, which infiltrates through the capsule into muscles and adjacent structures, including parathyroids, recurrent nerves and carotid sheath. It may occur in association with retroperitoneal and mediastinal fibrosis and is most probably a collagen disease. The goitre may be unilateral or bilateral and is very hard and fixed. The differential diagnosis from anaplastic carcinoma can be made with certainty only by biopsy, when a wedge of the isthmus should also be removed to free the trachea. If unilateral, the other lobe is usually involved later and subsequent hypothyroidism is common. Treatment is with high-dose steroid, tamoxifen and thyroxine replacement. Reduction in the size of the goitre and long-term improvement in symptoms are to be expected if treatment is commenced early.

FURTHER READING

Chadwick D, Kinsman R, Walton P. The British Association of Endocrine and Thyroid Surgeons Fourth National Audit Report, Dendrite Clinical Systems Ltd: Henley-on-Thames, 2012.

Chen A, Bernet V, Carty SE *et al.* American Thyroid Association statement on optimal surgical management of goiter. *Thyroid* 2014; **24**: 181–9.

Gharib H, Papini E, Valcavi R *et al.* American Association of Clinical Endocrinologists and Associazione Medici Endocrinologi medical guidelines for clinical practice for the diagnosis and management of thyroid nodules. *Endocr Pract* 2006; **12**: 63–102.

Haugen BRM, Alexander EK, Bible KC *et al.* American Thyroid Association management guidelines for adult patients with thyroid nodules and differentiated thyroid cancer. *Thyroid* 2016; **26**: 1–133.

Perros P, Boelaert K, Colley S *et al.* Guidelines for the management of thyroid cancer. *Clin Endocrinol* 2014; **81**(Suppl 1): 1–122.

Smallridge RC, Ain KB, Asa SL *et al.* American Thyroid Association guidelines for management of patients with anaplastic thyroid cancer. *Thyroid* 2012; **22**: 1104–39.

Wells SA, Jr, Asa SL, Dralle H *et al.* Revised American Thyroid Association guidelines for the management of medullary thyroid carcinoma. *Thyroid* 2015; **25**: 567–610.

Yeh MW, Bauer AJ, Bernet VA *et al.* American Thyroid Association statement on preoperative imaging for thyroid cancer surgery. *Thyroid* 2015; **25**: 3–14.

Bernhard Moritz Carl Ludwig Riedel, 1846–1916, Professor of Surgery, Jena, Germany, described this form of thyroiditis in 1896.

Chapter 51

The parathyroid glands

Learning objectives

To understand:
- The anatomy of the parathyroid glands
- The physiology of calcium regulation
- The underlying causes of hypercalcaemia and appropriate emergency management
- The aetiology, presentation, investigation and management of primary hyperparathyroidism and associated special cases
- The aetiology, presentation, investigation and management of secondary and tertiary hyperparathyroidism
- The aetiology and management of parathyroid carcinoma

INTRODUCTION

The parathyroid glands were first described by Sir Richard Owen in a neck dissection of an Indian rhinoceros at the London Zoological Gardens in 1850. Credit for recognition of the 'glandulae parathyreoidae' goes, however, to Sandström who published a monograph in 1887 on dissection of the parathyroid glands and their blood supply in animals and human cadavers. Unfortunately, Sandström committed suicide at the age of 37 and it was not until the 1890s that his work was rediscovered by Gley, who associated tetany following thyroid surgery with removal of the parathyroid glands. In 1905, MacCallum found that he could relieve postoperative tetany by the injection of parathyroid extract. While the association between parathyroid enlargement and bone disease was reported in 1907, it was not until 1925 that the first parathyroidectomy was performed by Mandl in Vienna on Albert Gahne, a tram conductor with severe primary hyperparathyroidism (PHPT) and osteitis fibrosa cystica.

ANATOMY OF THE PARATHYROID GLANDS

The developmental embryology and surgical anatomy of the parathyroid glands are intimately linked, and knowledge of both is essential for successful surgical treatment of parathyroid disease.

The parathyroid glands, of which there are four, develop from the third and fourth pharyngeal pouches between the fifth and twelfth week of gestation. They are typically described as 'Portland brick' (yellow/brown) in colour and weigh approximately 30 mg. Approximately 13% of the population have abnormal parathyroid tissue, with 5% having a true supernumerary gland. The blood supply of both the superior and inferior parathyroid glands arises from the inferior thyroidal artery. While the location of the individual glands may vary significantly, there appears to be a degree of symmetry between opposite sides that can be helpful during surgical dissection.

The inferior parathyroid gland and the thymus arise from the third pharyngeal pouch. As a result of the longer normal embryological descent, there is correspondingly more variation in their anatomical position. However, in more than 50% of cases they are located at the inferior pole of the thyroid gland, on the anterior, lateral or posterior surface. The gland itself is freely mobile within a globule of fat adjacent to the lower pole (**Figure 51.1a**).

The superior parathyroid glands arise from the dorsal portion of the fourth pharyngeal pouch. As a result of their more limited embryological descent they are more constant in

Sir Richard Owen, 1804–1892, English comparative anatomist and palaeontologist. First director of the Natural History Museum, London and Hunterian Professor at Royal College of Surgeons of England.
Ivar Viktor Sandström,1852–1889, medical student, Uppsala, Sweden.
Marcel Eugene Gley, 1857–1930, French pathologist.
William J MacCallum, 1874–1944, Professor of Pathology, Johns Hopkins Hospital, USA.
Felix Mandl, 1892–1957, Professor of Surgery, Vienna, Austria.

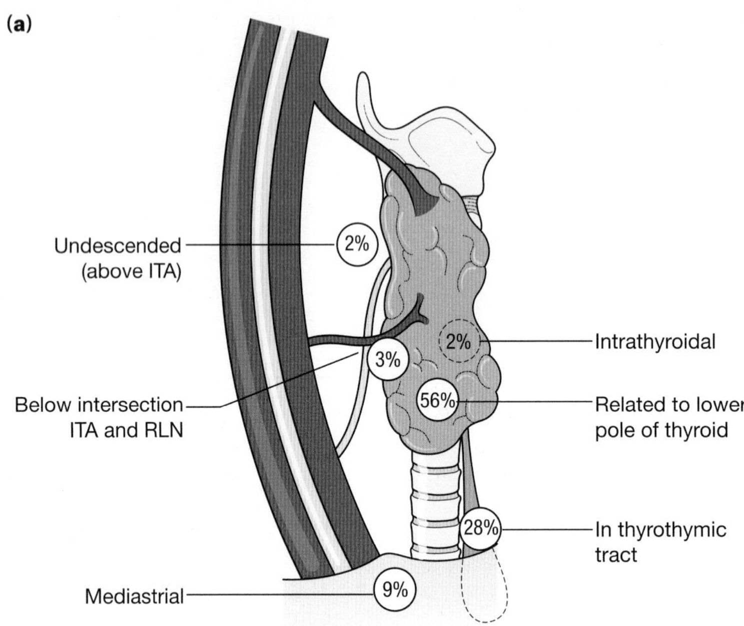

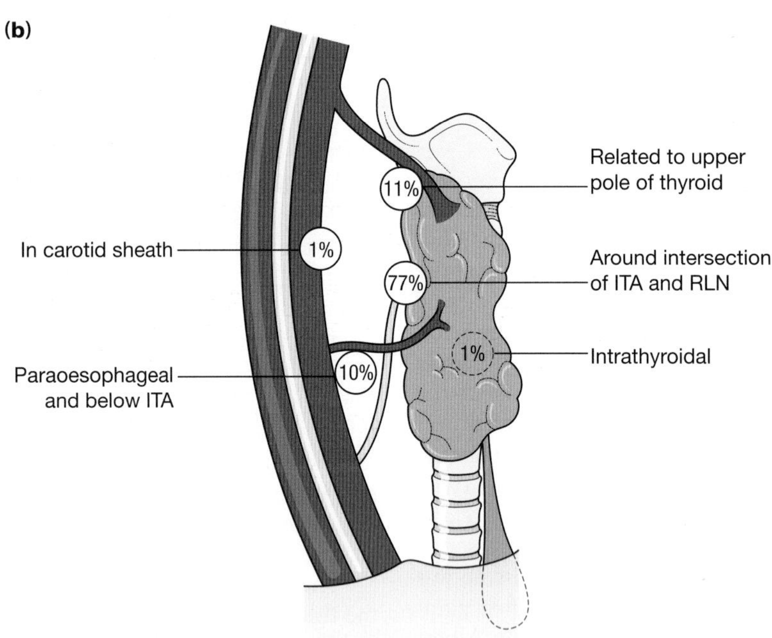

Figure 51.1 Potential locations of the inferior (a) and superior (b) parathyroid glands. ITA, inferior thyroid artery; RLN, recurrent laryngeal nerve.

position. In more than 80% of patients, the superior parathyroid glands are located at the posterior aspect of the thyroid lobe in an area 2 cm in diameter, centred 1 cm around the junction of the inferior thyroid artery and the recurrent laryngeal nerve in strict proximity to the cricothyroid junction (Figure 51.1b). The parathyroid glands are closely associated with, but contained within, a halo of fat that is freely mobile over the thyroid capsule.

CALCIUM AND PARATHYROID HORMONE REGULATION

The parathyroid glands play a central role in the regulation of serum calcium levels through the production of the active 84 amino-acid peptide, parathyroid hormone (PTH). PTH is secreted in response to low serum calcium or high serum magnesium levels. It is initially cleaved in the liver yielding an inactive C-terminal that is cleared by the kidneys. The N-terminal fragment is responsible for the biological activity of PTH on peripheral tissues. The active circulating molecule has a half life of approximately 3–5 minutes in patients with normal renal function.

PTH acts directly on the kidneys, bone and the gastrointestinal tract to activate intracellular second messengers, including cyclic AMP and calcium. In the kidneys, PTH increases serum calcium levels by increasing resorption of calcium from the renal tubules and increasing the hydroxylation of 25-hydroxyvitamin D to the biologically active 1,25-dihydroxyvitamin D. Active vitamin D increases both the resorption of phosphorus in the kidneys and the absorption of calcium from the gastrointestinal tract. In the bone, PTH acts on osteoblasts and osteoclasts to increase bone turnover, thereby increasing the amount of calcium in the extracellular space (Figure 51.2).

Calcitonin, which is synthesised by the parafollicular C cells of the thyroid gland, acts as the physiological antagonist to PTH. Calcitonin decreases serum calcium by decreasing bone turnover.

PRIMARY HYPERPARATHYROIDISM

The early descriptions of patients with PHPT were dominated by those with osteitis fibrosa cystica. Brown tumours of the long bones and associated subperiostal bone reabsorption, distal tapering of the clavicles and the classical 'salt and pepper' erosions of the skull were typical findings. Over 80% of patients had associated renal stones, significant neuromuscular dysfunction and muscle weakness. This led to the traditional mnemonic that patients with PHPT presented with 'bones, stones, abdominal groans and psychiatric overtones'. The introduction of the automated serum chemical autoanalyser in the 1970s as well as radioimmune assay to accurately measure circulating PTH levels radically improved early

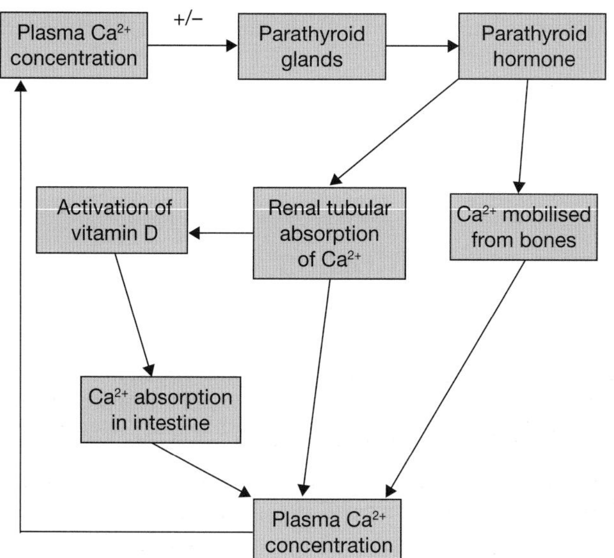

Figure 51.2 Schematic diagram of actions of parathyroid hormone.

diagnosis of PHPT, such that the majority of patients are now identified incidentally on routine biochemical investigations and are asymptomatic. The current controversies therefore, centre on the indications for intervention, either surgically or medically.

Presentation

PHPT is defined as hypercalcaemia in the presence of an unsuppressed and therefore relatively, or absolutely, elevated PTH level. Prevalence of the disease is reported to be 0.2–0.5% with approximately 100 000 new cases per year in the USA. The majority of PHPT is sporadic in nature. Familial disease can occur in multiple endocrine neoplasia (MEN) type 1 or type 2A or as a familial cluster. Patients usually present in the 5th or 6th decades and there is a female predominance with a ratio of 3:1.

Patients are typically identified incidentally with an elevated total calcium or following routine assessment of bone densitometry (DEXA scan). Most patients will, however, have some vague constitutional symptoms, such as fatigue, muscle weakness, depression or some mild memory impairment on questioning. The presence of kidney stones remains the most common clinical manifestation of symptomatic PHPT. Between 15% and 20% of patients will have nephrolithiasis and over 40% of patients will have hypercalciuria. Increasingly, postmenopausal women present with significant osteopenia or osteoporosis in the distal one-third of the radius with a minimal reduction in the lumbar spine, which prompts further investigation. This distribution arises as PTH appears to be catabolic at cortical sites (distal one-third of the radius) and anabolic at cancellous sites (lumbar spine).

PHPT may present with pancreatitis, although it is rarely seen in patients with milder forms of the disease. Common epidemiologically linked disorders, such as hypertension and peptic ulcer disease, are often encountered. Clinical examination is usually normal. Band keratopathy, pathognomonic of the disease and due to deposition of calcium phosphate crystals in the cornea, is now rarely identified.

The differential diagnosis of PHPT includes other causes of hypercalcaemia, which are usually readily distinguishable (*Table 51.1*). It is important to exclude the presence of a widespread malignancy, in which patients will typically have other symptoms. The exception to this rule is multiple myeloma, in which hypercalcaemia can be the presenting complaint. Improvements in the immuno-radiometric and immunochemiluminometric assays for PTH can help to distinguish these conditions, as in malignancy PTH levels are typically suppressed.

Hypercalcaemic crisis: presentation and management

Hypercalcaemia is documented in 0.5% of the general population and in up to 5% of hospitalised patients. The vast majority are asymptomatic with a mild to moderate elevation of serum calcium (<3 mmol/L and 3–3.5 mmol/L, respectively) and respond to treatment of the underlying aetiology with associated dietary modification. A small proportion of

TABLE 51.1 Causes of hypercalcaemia.

Endocrine	Primary hyperparathyroidism Thyrotoxicosis Phaeochromocytoma
Renal failure	Secondary hyperparathyroidism Tertiary hyperparathyroidism
Malignant disease	Skeletal metastatic disease Multiple myeloma, lymphoma, leukaemia Solid tumours (PTH-related peptide mediated): lung, renal, squamous cell carcinoma of the head and neck, oesophagus, genital tract
Nutritional	Excessive vitamin D ingestion Vitamin A intoxication Milk-alkali syndrome Aluminium intoxication
Granulomatous	Sarcoidosis Tuberculosis
Inherited disease	Hypercalciuric hypercalcaemia
Immobilisation	
Paget's disease	
Drug related	Lithium

patients will present symptomatically with a total calcium of >3.5 mmol/L. This is referred to as a hypercalcaemic crisis and requires aggressive medical management.

Although symptoms can be varied, the typical presentation is of acute confusion, abdominal pain, vomiting, dehydration and anuria. Prolongation of the P–R interval with a shortened Q–T interval can be identified on an electrocardiogram (ECG) prior to potentially lethal cardiac arrhythmias. Where the calcium is >4.5 mmol/L, coma and cardiac arrest can occur.

Treatment revolves around increasing renal excretion of calcium, reducing skeletal release of calcium and treatment of the underlying cause. Aggressive rehydration plays a pivotal role. Typically, 200–500 mL/h of normal saline is given to maintain a urine output >100 mL/h, with the caveat that this may be modified to account for associated patient comorbidities. Once intravascular volume has been adequately restored, loop diuretics, such as furosemide, can be used to enhanced the renal excretion of calcium. The majority of patients will have normalisation of their calcium with these simple measures.

In patients with advanced malignancy and a serum calcium level >3 mmol/L, agents that blunt the release of calcium from skeletal stores may be required. First-line treatment includes administration of bisphosphonates. These are pyrophosphate analogues that inhibit osteoclast activity in areas of high bone turnover. In the acute setting, these are given intravenously due to poor absorption in the gastrointestinal tract. Calcitonin can be used to both decrease osteoclastic activity and increase renal excretion of calcium. It has a short duration of action and is usually used as a bridge to reduce calcium until the sustained action of the bisphosphonates is seen. Finally, glucocorticoids (prednisolone) can be used to enhance the action of calcitonin. They increase calciuresis and decrease intestinal absorption of calcium. As a result, they may also play a role in diseases associated with vitamin D excess.

Pathology

The underlying aetiology of PHPT is usually a solitary parathyroid adenoma; however, in a small number of patients (2–4%) there are double adenomas. It may occur in a sporadic fashion or it can be familial (MEN type 1 or type 2A, hyperparathyroidism-jaw tumour syndrome (HPT-JT)) in nature. The only known risk factor for the development of PHPT is a history of prior neck irradiation. The underlying molecular basis of PHPT is heterogeneous; however, upregulation of cyclin D may lead to a clonal proliferation within the parathyroid glands. This does not alter the set point of calcium but the hyperplasic nature of the parathyroid cells themselves causes excessive secretion of PTH.

Multigland disease is less common, occurring in approximately 15% of patients. No clinical features differentiate single from multigland disease, although multigland disease is more commonly associated with familial syndromes such as MEN types 1 and 2A, as well as the chronic ingestion of lithium.

Diagnosis

PHPT is a biochemical diagnosis. Only when the disease has been confirmed biochemically should localisation studies be undertaken. Positive imaging does not confirm the diagnosis and negative findings cannot rule it out.

PHPT is defined as an elevated total, or more specifically ionised, calcium, in the presence of an inappropriately elevated or unsuppressed PTH. It is associated with a low serum phosphate in the setting of normal creatinine and vitamin D levels; 24-hour urinary excretion of calcium may be normal or elevated. It is important to perform a 24-hour urinary collection to rule out the presence of the rare familial hypocalciuric hypercalcaemia. Alkaline phosphatase may be elevated in patients in whom there is concomitant bone disease. This is important to recognise preoperatively, as the surgeon should anticipate significant postoperative hypocalcaemia due to the development of hungry bone syndrome.

Localisation studies

> "In my opinion, the only localising study required in a patient with untreated primary hyperparathyroidism is to localise an experienced parathyroid surgeon."
>
> John Doppman, 1986

Historically, preoperative localisation studies for PHPT were considered less important than identifying an experienced surgeon. However, with a shift away from the traditional four-

John L Doppman, 1928–2000, radiologist, National Institutes of Health, USA, developed the technique of selective venous sampling for parathyroid localisation.

gland (cervical neck) exploration to more minimally invasive procedures, accurate preoperative identification is critically important to guide surgical strategy.

There are a variety of both non-invasive and invasive studies commonly is use. Non-invasive radiology includes nuclear medicine-based studies, ultrasonography and 4D computed tomography (CT) scanning. Invasive imaging is largely reserved for reoperative surgery and includes ultrasound or CT-guided fine-needle aspiration with concomitant PTH assays, parathyroid angiography or selective venous sampling for the PTH gradient.

Nuclear medicine-based studies (sestamibi scanning)

The use of sestamibi (2-methoxy-2-methylpropylisonitrile (MIBI)) for parathyroid localisation was first described in 1989 and is now regarded as the most accurate and reliable method for imaging the parathyroid glands. It is safe and reproducible and while it has a sensitivity and specificity similar to ultrasound, it may image glands in ectopic positions better (Figure 51.3a).

Sestamibi accumulates in mitochondria and therefore washes out at differential rates depending on the number of mitochondria within individual tissues. Parathyroid adenomas often have a high concentration of oxyphilic cells with high mitochondrial content. These retain tracer and adenomas are therefore associated with a slow washout when compared with the thyroid gland. There are three different protocols for sestamibi scanning: single-isotope dual-phase scan, dual isotope subtraction imaging and single-photon emission computed tomography (SPECT). The sensitivity and specificity of sestamibi, regardless of the protocol used, are 79% and 90%, respectively. False positives are rare but may arise from some solid thyroid nodules, such as Hürthle cell nodules, that are associated with high oxyphilic content. These can be reduced by the addition of a thyroid-specific radioactive tracer, such as ^{99}Tc-pertechnetate and subsequent subtraction images.

Ultrasonography

Ultrasonography is a non-invasive, inexpensive method of imaging the parathyroid glands (Figure 51.3b). Parathyroid adenomas are typically oval or elongated, bi- or multilobed

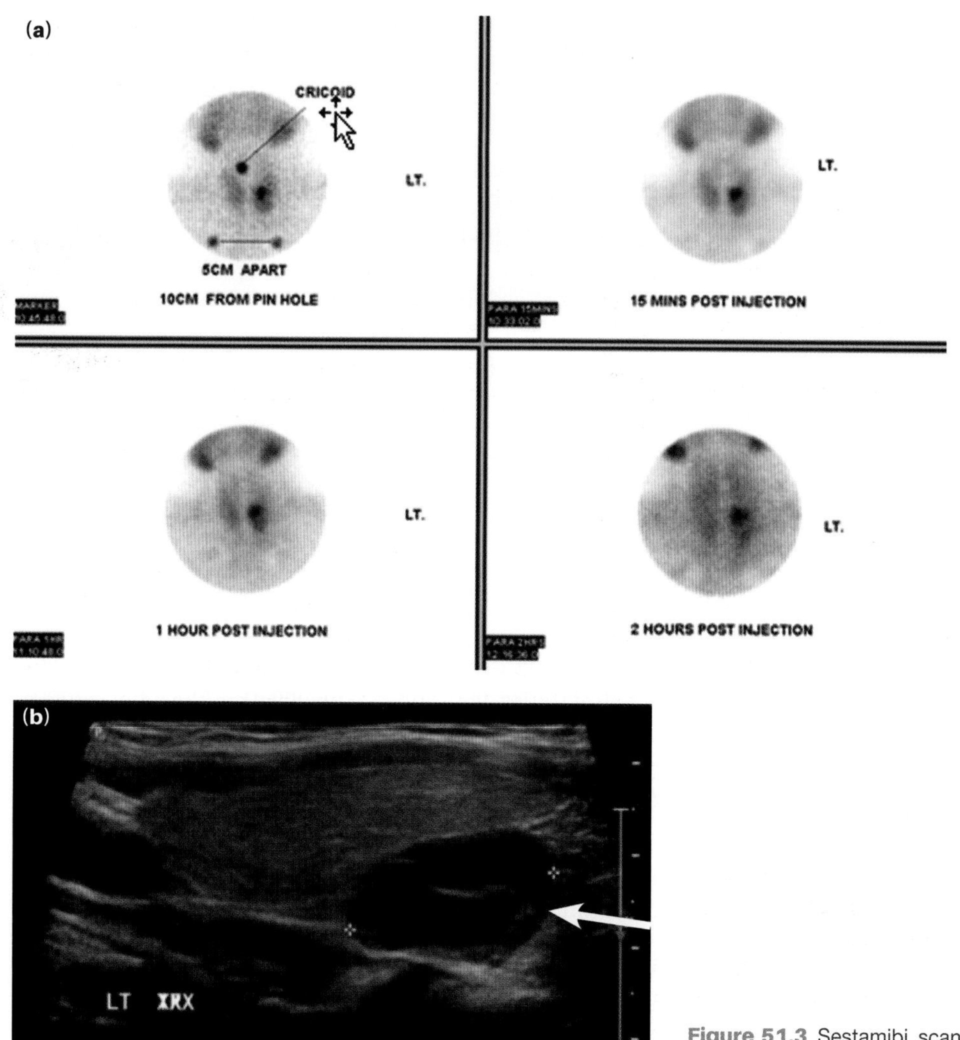

Figure 51.3 Sestamibi scan (**a**) demonstrating right inferior adenoma, with concordant ultrasound (**b**).

Karl Hürthle, 1866–1945, histopathologist, Breslau, Germany.

hypoechoic structures. Rarely, adenomas may be cystic or heterogeneous in nature. Giant adenomas are described as those over 3 cm in size. Ultrasound is not associated with any radiation exposure and has the advantage of being able to identify and facilitate biopsy of any concomitant thyroid pathology. However, ultrasonography is operator, lesion size and location dependent. Critically, ultrasound may miss adenomas located in retro-oesophageal, retrosternal or retrotracheal areas. It can also be difficult to differentiate between a small parathyroid gland and a normal appearing lymph node. A recent meta-analysis of preoperative localisation techniques in PHPT demonstrated that ultrasound and sestamibi-SPECT have comparable accuracy, with pooled sensitivities of 76.1% and 78.9% respectively, and positive predictive values (PPVs) of 93.2% and 90.7% respectively (Krakauer *et al.*, 2016).

4D Computed tomography scanning

Multiphase CT imaging (4D-CT) has become widely utilised to localise disease (Figure 51.4). It gives both anatomical as well as functional information about the parathyroid glands. Using precontrast, postcontrast and delayed images, it demonstrates not only detailed anatomic localisation but, combined with rapid uptake and wash-out, allows hyperfunctioning glands to be differentiated from lymph nodes, which demonstrate a progressive enhancement pattern. The potential disadvantage of 4D-CT scanning is the higher radiation dose when compared with traditional imaging modalities. Modification of the protocol now allows fewer phases to be obtained without compromising outcomes. The initial study in 2006 reported a sensitivity of 88% for lateralisation and 70% for localisation of parathyroid adenomas (Rodgers *et al.*, 2006). A more recent meta-analysis, although limited by the small number of studies, demonstrated a sensitivity and PPV of 89.4% and 93.5% respectively, when 4D-CT was used as the primary imaging modality. This was reduced to 71.8% and 74.9% respectively in cases of negative or inconclusive prior imaging (Cheung *et al.*, 2012).

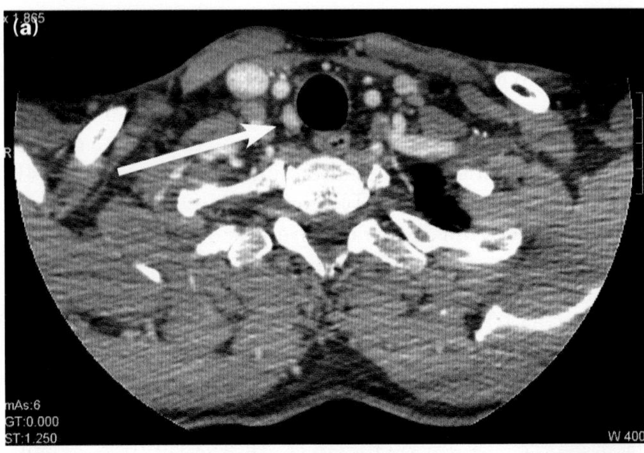

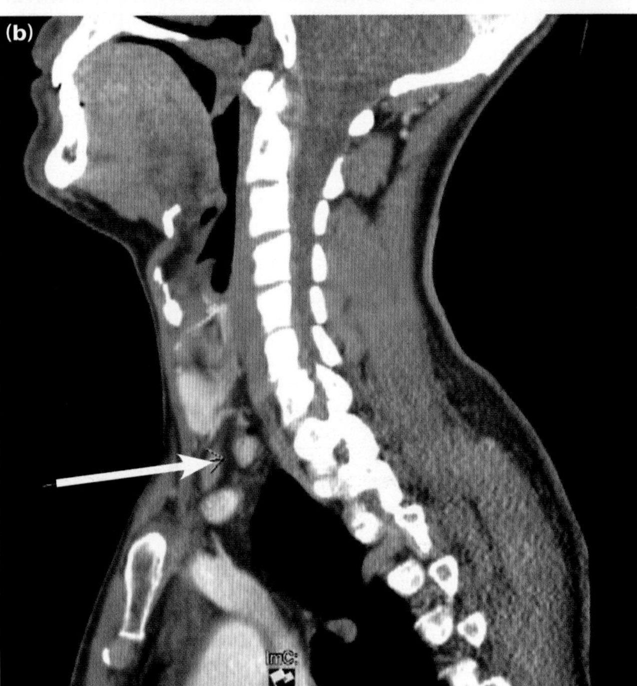

Figure 51.4 (a, b) 4D Computed tomography scanning demonstrating a right inferior parathyroid adenoma (arrows).

Magnetic resonance imaging

Magnetic resonance imaging (MRI) is not commonly used to image the parathyroid glands. However, on T2-weighted images, enlarged parathyroid glands demonstrate significantly increased intensity. In reoperative cases or where the adenoma is located in the mediastinum, MRI may be beneficial, with higher reported sensitivities (50–88%). While the sensitivity of MRI is slightly better than CT (64–88%) in primary disease, it has significant limitations. It is expensive, patients can be poorly compliant due to claustrophobia and the resolution for normal glands or adenomas <5 mm is poor. Similarly, it can be difficult to localise superior glands due to their posterior location, which allows them to be obscured by the thyroid gland.

Parathyroid angiography and venous sampling for PTH

Parathyroid angiography is reserved for reoperative cases and is now rarely required due to improvements in non-invasive imaging modalities. It involves examination of both thyrocervical trunks, both internal mammary arteries and carotids, with occasional selective superior thyroid artery catheterisation. Vascular parathyroid adenomas appear as a persistent oval or round 'stain' on angiography. Serious complications such as contrast-induced renal failure, embolisation and neurological damage have limited its utility.

Selective venous sampling for PTH can allow accurate localisation of adenomas but an experienced interventional radiologist is vital for success. The venous drainage of the lesion is established when there is a two-fold drop in the PTH between the sampled blood and the serum PTH. The sensitivity is reported to be 80% and is equally effective in localising cervical and mediastinal adenomas. However, the false-positive rate of between 6% and 18% limits its utility to reoperative cases.

Management strategies

Surgical management

The mainstay of treatment for PHPT is surgery, addressing the underlying aetiology and allowing not only resolution of biochemical abnormalities but also sustained improvements in end-organ damage. Traditionally a bilateral cervical exploration was performed with reported cure rates of 95–98%. With improvements in preoperative radiological localisation, a more minimally invasive approach has been developed and widely adopted (Figure 51.5).

All symptomatic patients should be offered surgery. An expert panel recently published recommendations on which asymptomatic patients should be considered for surgical intervention (*Table 51.2*) (Bilezikian *et al.*, 2014). When criteria have been met and where a single adenoma has been confidently identified by radiological means, a minimally invasive parathyroidectomy may be offered. Conversely, where there is discordant imaging or where imaging fails to identify any parathyroid abnormalities, then a bilateral neck exploration and three and a half-gland parathyroidectomy or a four-gland parathyroidectomy and autotransplantation should be performed.

Consent for a parathyroidectomy must include the possibility of recurrent laryngeal nerve damage (risk <1%), permanent hypoparathyroidism (requiring lifelong calcium and vitamin D supplementation, risk 0.5%), and persistent (5%) or recurrent hyperparathyroidism. Persistent disease is defined as an elevated serum calcium within 6 weeks of surgical intervention and recurrent disease is defined as an increase in calcium levels after 6 months but with an intervening period of normocalcaemia.

MINIMALLY INVASIVE (FOCUSED) PARATHYROIDECTOMY

Minimally invasive approaches are based on the principle that over 80% of individuals with PHPT have a single adenoma. Although there is no strict definition of the procedure, it commonly refers to the removal of a localised abnormal parathyroid gland through an incision less than 3 cm in length (Figure 51.6). The term encompasses open approaches (central and lateral incisions), video-assisted and radio-guided parathyroidectomies. A number of randomised studies have shown that the focused approach has similar cure rates to a cervical exploration but with reduced rates of postoperative hypocalcaemia, shorter operating times, potentially less pain and better cosmesis.

The need to convert from a focused to a cervical exploration may be guided by the use of intraoperative PTH measurements. Routine use is, however, controversial due to high false-positive and false-negative rates. The basic concept is that the half life of circulating PTH is 3–5 minutes and there should therefore be a significant drop detected in the plasma PTH following resection of a single adenoma. If no such drop is detected, then

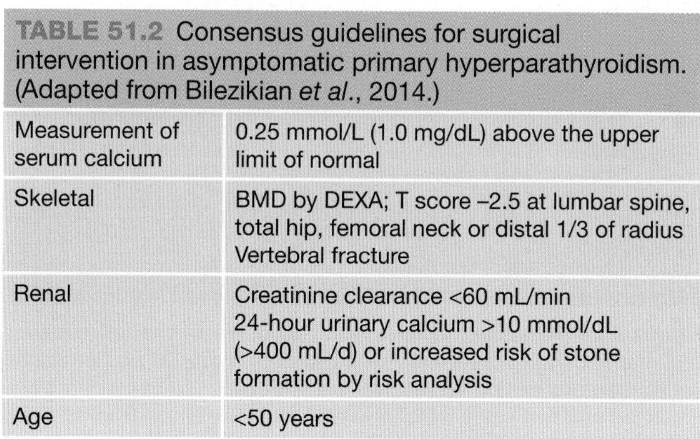

TABLE 51.2 Consensus guidelines for surgical intervention in asymptomatic primary hyperparathyroidism. (Adapted from Bilezikian *et al.*, 2014.)

Measurement of serum calcium	0.25 mmol/L (1.0 mg/dL) above the upper limit of normal
Skeletal	BMD by DEXA; T score –2.5 at lumbar spine, total hip, femoral neck or distal 1/3 of radius Vertebral fracture
Renal	Creatinine clearance <60 mL/min 24-hour urinary calcium >10 mmol/dL (>400 mL/d) or increased risk of stone formation by risk analysis
Age	<50 years

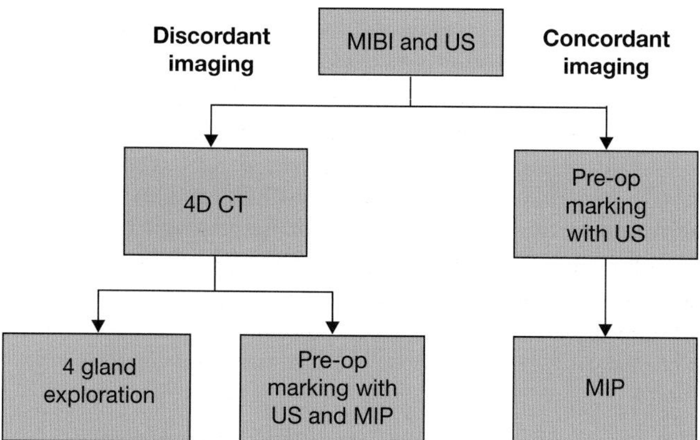

Figure 51.5 Localisation paradigm and management strategies. CT, computed tomography; MIP, minimally invasive parathyroidectomy; US, ultrasound.

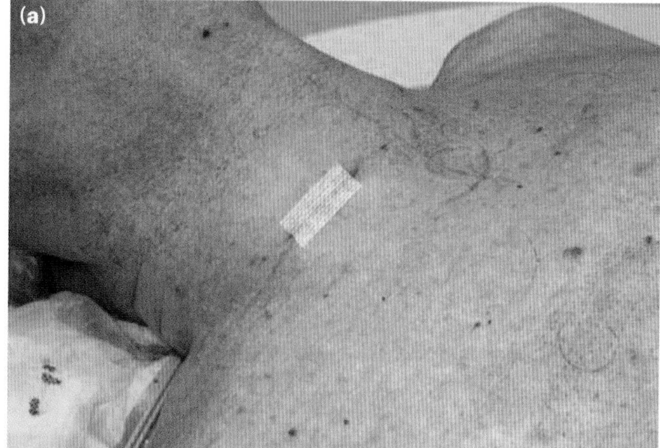

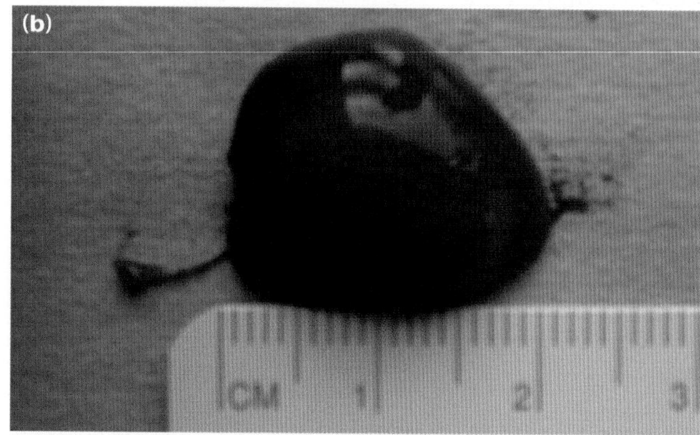

Figure 51.6 (a) Minimally invasive parathyroidectomy through a lateral approach; (b) the excised parathyroid adenoma.

multigland disease may be suspected and conversion to a bilateral neck exploration should be considered. The Miami criteria were developed to determine the extent of resection. A drop in the PTH into the normal range and to less than half the maximum preoperative PTH at 10 minutes appears to accurately predict single-gland disease (Figure 51.7).

BILATERAL NECK EXPLORATION

A traditional cervical neck exploration is required where imaging is negative or discordant, in MEN (type 1 or type 2A) or in lithium-induced PHPT. A transverse collar (Kocher's) incision is made and the subplatysmal plane developed. The deep cervical fascia is divided between the strap muscles and these are retracted. The thyroid lobes are mobilised and the middle thyroid vein may be divided when present.

Identification of the recurrent laryngeal nerve and the middle thyroid artery allows a starting point for a systematic exploration. All four glands are identified. Three and a half glands are resected, with half of a vascularised parathyroid left *in situ*. The other half of the gland should be sent for frozen section to confirm the presence of parathyroid tissue (Figure 51.8). Ideally the most normal appearing parathyroid is left *in situ*. With this caveat in mind, where possible an inferior gland should be left. It is marked with a non-absorbable suture to aid identification in the presence of recurrent disease, where resection can be achieved without increasing the risk of damage to the recurrent laryngeal nerve. Alternatively, all four glands can be resected and a forearm autotransplant created. Small pieces of parathyroid are sutured into pockets created in the brachioradialis muscle. Cure rates, persistent and recurrent disease appear to be similar, regardless of the type of procedure use. However, in recurrent disease it can be difficult to identify the location of the recurrent tissue when an autotransplant is performed.

THYMECTOMY AND RESECTION OF MEDIASTINAL ADENOMAS

The incidence of clinically significant supernumerary glands is increased in patients with multigland disease or those with hereditary syndromes. A thymectomy should be routinely undertaken for patients with MEN 1-associated PHPT or in secondary hyperparathyroidism. A cervical thymectomy is performed by dissecting close to the thymic capsule, exploring the cervical part of the gland. The mediastinal part of the gland can be removed by gentle upwards traction, with

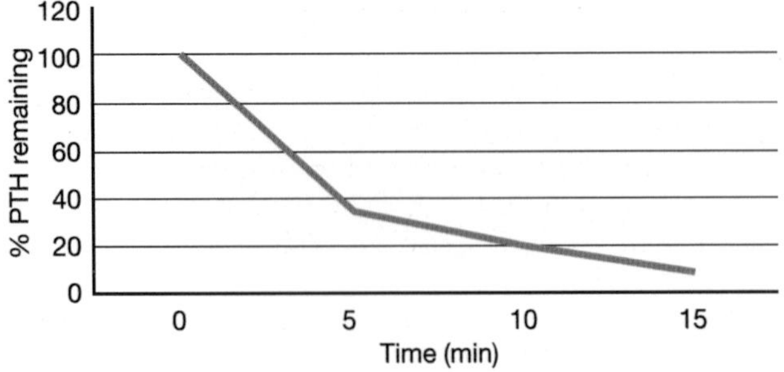

Figure 51.7 Miami criteria for intraoperative parathyroid hormone (PTH) measurement. Drop of PTH into the normal range and less than half the maximum value at 10 min postresection.

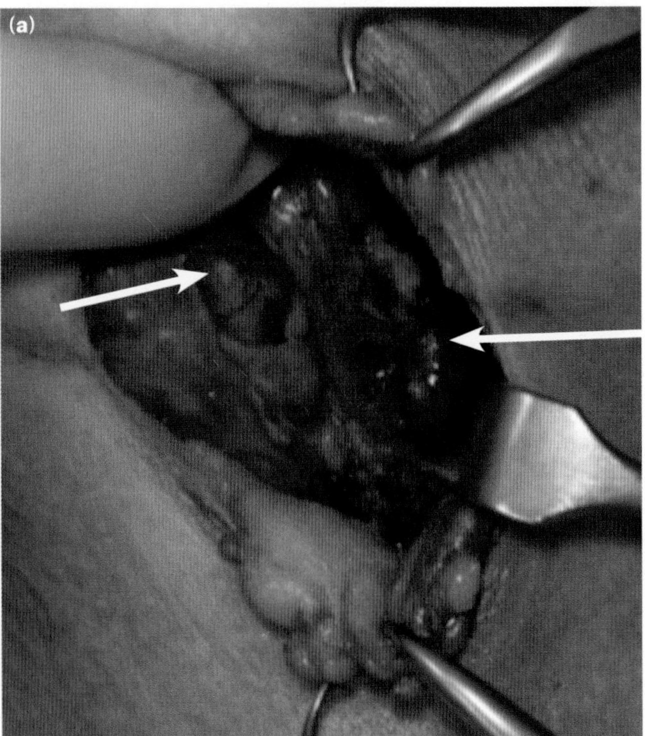

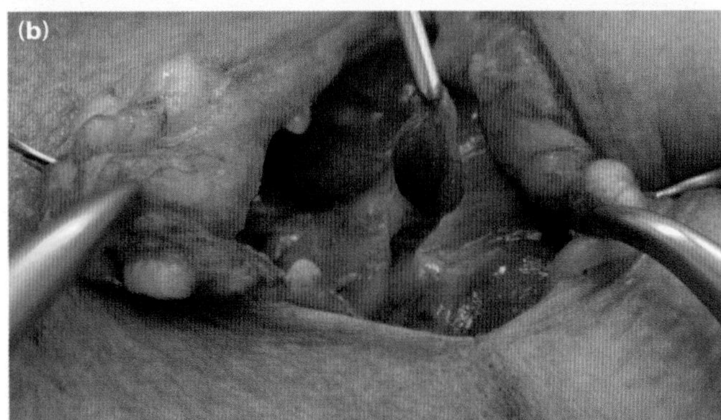

Figure 51.8 Parathyroidectomy with exposure of the left superior and inferior parathyroid glands (white arrows) *in situ* (a) and left superior gland mobilised on its vascular pedicle (b).

ligation of the veins draining into the innominate vein. The end of the gland is tapered and rarely requires formal ligation. A median sternotomy is not required where a prophylactic thymectomy is being performed.

Mediastinal adenomas are rare, accounting for less than 1% of all parathyroid adenoma. They will be typically identified on preoperative imaging. Resection can either be achieved by an open sternotomy or increasingly by a thoracoscopic approach. A minimally invasive approach can be particularly effective where the abnormal gland lies immediately deep to the mediastinal pleura. It can confer significant advantages in length of hospital stay and complication rates.

Permanent hypoparathyroidism

Permanent hypoparathyroidism is defined as the continuing need for calcium and/or vitamin D replacement at 1 year postoperatively. It is a rare complication when surgery is undertaken for PHPT (0.5%), but in secondary hyperparathyroidism it can range from 4% to 12%. Symptoms and signs relate to serum calcium levels. Symptoms include mild circumoral or digital numbness and paraesthesia, carpopedal or laryngeal spasms and cardiac arrhythmias. Chvostek's and Trousseau's signs may be elicited. Chvostek's sign refers to contraction of the ipsilateral facial muscles on percussion of the facial nerve below the zygoma. Trousseau's sign refers to the development of carpopedal spasm secondary to occlusion of the arm (usually with a blood pressure cuff).

Biochemical investigations include total and ionised calcium levels as well as serum magnesium levels. An ECG may demonstrate a prolonged QT interval or QRS complex changes. Mild hypocalcaemia can be treated with oral calcium and vitamin D supplementation. Acute symptomatic hypocalcaemia is an emergency and should be corrected with intravenous as well as oral calcium and vitamin D replacement. Traditionally, 10 mL of 10% calcium gluconate is administered slowly intravenously. Supplemental magnesium may also be required, due to the synergistic action of transporters for calcium and magnesium.

Medical management

Medical management is warranted in patients who are deemed unfit or who have contraindications to surgical intervention, in patients with failed surgical intervention or in the long-term management of parathyroid carcinoma. The aims are to prevent skeletal complications (improve bone mineral density and reduce fracture risk) and to stabilise biochemical parameters. There are only limited data on the long-term efficacy of such an approach as surgery is known to provide durable responses.

BISPHOSPHONATES

Bisphosphonates are pyrophosphate analogues that are concentrated in areas of high bone turnover. They inhibit osteoclast activity and apoptosis, thereby increasing bone mineralisation and reducing bone turnover. Studies looking at the management of PHTP utilising bisphosphonates are limited by small numbers and short follow-up. However, use does appear to stabilise bone mineral density without markedly altering the underlying serum biochemistry.

HORMONE REPLACEMENT THERAPY AND SELECTIVE OESTROGEN RECEPTOR ANTAGONISTS

Hormone replacement therapy (HRT) has been shown to improve bone mineral density and reduce the associated fracture risk in postmenopausal women by reducing bone turnover. Two non-randomised controlled trials have shown a durable and similar response to surgery for PHTP at 4 years, with improvements in bone mineral density but without any improvement in the underlying serum biochemistry. The rational for the use of selective oestrogen receptor antagonists (SERMs) is that they should confer the benefits of HRT but without the potential adverse vascular and breast effects. The effect on the bone mineral, however, appears to be less significant than that of HRT.

CALCIMIMETICS

The extracellular calcium sensing receptor (CaR) on the parathyroid cell surface negatively regulates secretion of PTH. Activation of the receptor decreases secretion of PTH, thereby decreasing bone turnover. Calcimimetics, such as cinacalcet, amplify the sensitivity of the CaR to extracellular calcium, altering the set point and thereby decreasing PTH production. The use of calcimimetics has gained widespread acceptance in secondary hyperparathyroidism, but use in PHTP is largely limited to patients unfit for surgery. Despite this, a number of small studies have shown normalisation of PTH levels and a reduction in bone remodelling, with durable results at 2 years, with the use of cinacalcet. Drug tolerance, especially gastrointestinal side effects, can be problematic and may limit the duration of usage.

SPECIAL CASES

Lithium-induced hyperparathyroidism

Lithium-induced hyperparathyroidism occurs in 10–15% of patients treated with long-term lithium. It is generally associated with a mild elevation in calcium with failure to suppress PTH. The underlying aetiology can be either gland hyperplasia, with lithium originally thought to stimulate all parathyroid tissue, or a single adenoma which has been shown to occur in 33–49% of cases. It has recently been suggested that the hyperparathyroidism may be caused by interference with the parathyroid kinase C signal transduction system and the Wnt pathway. Biochemical abnormalities may resolve with discontinuation of lithium. Surgery is indicated where ongoing treatment with lithium is required or where abnormalities persist following withdrawal of lithium. Minimally invasive surgery is relatively contraindicated in these patients due to the high incidence of multigland disease. Excision, however, should be limited to those glands that are obviously enlarged at exploration rather than a formal three and a half-gland excision.

Familial syndromes

Familial hyperparathyroidism can be part of a well-recognised endocrine disorder, but it may also occur in isolation in a non-syndromic form. PHPT occurs as a central facet in multiple MEN 1, MEN 2A, HPT-JT and familial hypocalciuric hypercalcaemia (FHH).

Familial isolated hyperparathyroidism

Isolated familial hyperparathyroidism occurs when patients have PHPT without any other associated endocrinopathies.

Frantisek Chvostek, 1835–1884, physician, The Jasefsacademie, Vienna, Austria.
Armand Trousseau, 1801–1867, physician, Hôtel Dieu, Paris, France.

The underlying genetic abnormality has yet to be fully elucidated, but the syndrome has been linked to known mutations in the *MEN 1* gene, the *HRPT2* gene as well as the calcium-sensing receptor gene. A significant proportion of patients will belong to the MEN 1 family, with documented recognised mutations but without expression of other endocrinopathies. Hyperparathyroidism should be treated with a formal bilateral neck exploration and management as per patients with MEN.

MEN 1-associated hyperparathyroidism

MEN 1 is a rare autosomal dominant syndrome consisting of tumours of the parathyroids, endocrine pancreas–duodenum and the pituitary (the three Ps). It occurs in approximately 1 per 30 000 individuals. It can also be associated with adrenal adenomas or carcinoma, foregut carcinoids and lipomas. Mutations, of which there are over 1000 identified in different families, occur in the *MEN 1* gene, which encodes the protein menin. Menin acts as a tumour suppressor. Patients typically present with young onset (20–30 years of age) of symptomatic hyperparathyroidism and over 95% of patients will have PHPT before the age of 40 years.

Surgical intervention in MEN aims to obtain and maintain normocalcaemia for the longest time possible. In general, it is associated with the presence of multigland parathyroid disease and as such has mandated a bilateral cervical exploration with at least a subtotal parathyroidectomy and cervical thymectomy. A total parathyroidectomy and forearm autotransplantation is an acceptable alternative. Half of the most normal appearing parathyroid should be left *in situ* with a marking stitch to facilitate reoperative intervention. Detailed intraoperative notes, including diagrams, should be kept. Despite meticulous and extensive surgery, the rates of both persistent and recurrent disease remain high in this group of patients (up to 62%) regardless of the type of surgery performed. Unfortunately, the rates of postoperative permanent hypocalcaemia are also high, with published rates up to 47%.

MEN 2A-associated hyperparathyroidism

MEN 2A consists of medullary thyroid carcinoma, unilateral or bilateral phaeochromocytomas and PHPT. PHPT occurs in approximately 20% of patients and is associated with mutations in codon 634 in the *RET* proto-oncogene. The majority of patients will be asymptomatic, with a mild elevation in calcium and asymmetrically enlarged parathyroid glands. It is extremely important that the presence of a phaeochromocytoma is excluded prior to surgical intervention. Surgery is usually performed for medullary thyroid carcinoma (MTC), with the parathyroid enlargement often being a coincidental intraoperative finding. In this setting, with extensive surgery for MTC, the primary aim of treatment is to avoid hypoparathyroidism. A conservative stance is adopted with resection of grossly enlarged glands, but with preservation of parathyroid tissue where possible and identification with a marking stitch in the neck.

Hyperparathyroid-jaw tumour syndrome

HPT-JT is a rare cause of PHPT. It arises due to inactivating mutations in the *HRPT2* gene on chromosome 1 q21-32, encoding parafibromin. It classically presents with early-onset PHPT (mean age of 32 years), the aetiology of which can be either single- or multiple-gland disease but is predominantly cystic in nature. It presents with severe hypercalcaemia and is associated with an increased risk of an underlying parathyroid carcinoma. Approximately 40% of patients will have the pathognomonic ossifying jaw fibromas of the maxilla or mandible. Other associated abnormalities include renal pathology (hamartomas, polycystic kidney disease and adult Wilms' tumours) and female patients may have uterine malignancies. Surgical intervention involves removal of all enlarged parathyroid glands.

Where there is concern for a parathyroid carcinoma, great care must be taken to avoid tumour spillage. Whether or not an *en bloc* resection of the enlarged suspicious parathyroid and the adjacent thyroid lobectomy is required remains controversial.

Familial hypocalciuric hypercalcaemia

FHH is not a surgical disease and therefore preoperative diagnosis is imperative for the surgeon. FHH arises as a result of heterozygous mutations in the calcium receptor gene (*CASR*) on chromosome 3. Benign familial hypocalciuric hypercalcaemia typically presents with mild hypercalcaemia in young (<10 years of age) asymptomatic patients. Patients with FHH have a normal or slightly elevated PTH level, increased serum magnesium levels and hypocalciuria. A low urinary calcium/creatinine clearance ratio is used to discriminate between FHH and mild PHPT. Patients rarely require intervention and surgical intervention is not indicated.

Summary box 51.1

Primary hyperparathyroidism

- Presentation is now typically asymptomatic rather than the classical 'bones, stones, abdominal groans and psychiatric overtones'
- The diagnosis of primary hyperparathyroidism is a biochemical one
- Presence of an elevated ionised calcium with an inappropriately elevated/not suppressed PTH level confirms the diagnosis
- Sestimibi and focused neck ultrasound are the first-line radiological investigations
- 85% of cases are due to a single adenoma
- Minimally invasive parathyroidectomy is a safe and acceptable alternative to a four-gland exploration in the presence of localised disease
- Familial syndromes and disease that is not localised require a formal four gland exploration and three and a half gland parathyroidectomy

Max Wilms, 1867–1918, Professor of Surgery, University of Heidelberg, Germany.

SECONDARY HYPERPARATHYROIDISM

Secondary hyperparathyroidism is defined as a derangement in calcium homeostasis, which leads to a compensatory increase in PTH secretion. It occurs primarily as a result of chronic kidney disease and is therefore sometimes referred to as renal hyperparathyroidism. Other underlying causes include gastrointestinal malabsorption, vitamin D deficiency, liver disease or chronic lithium usage.

The pathogenesis of secondary hyperparathyroidism is related to renal dysfunction. Abnormalities in the renal tubular absorption of phosphate lead to hyperphosphataemia. This acts directly on the parathyroid cells and stimulates PTH secretion. More recent translational research has identified a novel phosphaturia hormone, fibroblast growth factor 23 (FGF 23). This is progressively secreted from osteocytes to compensate for chronic phosphate retention that in turn leads to a reduction in 1,25-dihydroxyvitamin D, which by reducing the intestinal absorption of calcium, also acts to increase secretion of PTH. Previous studies in patients with chronic renal disease have shown that there is a reduction in the expression of the vitamin D receptor and the CaR, with associated skeletal resistance to PTH. These factors interact to form the complex pattern leading to progressive secondary hyperparathyroidism in the setting of chronic renal disease.

The pathological characteristics associated with secondary hyperparathyroidism include hyperplasia, asymmetrical glandular enlargement or nodularity. This differentiation is important, as when the parathyroid gland becomes nodular it loses expression of the vitamin D and Ca receptors. It has been proposed that nodular parathyroid glands may be resistant to calcimimetics and therefore be refractory to medical management.

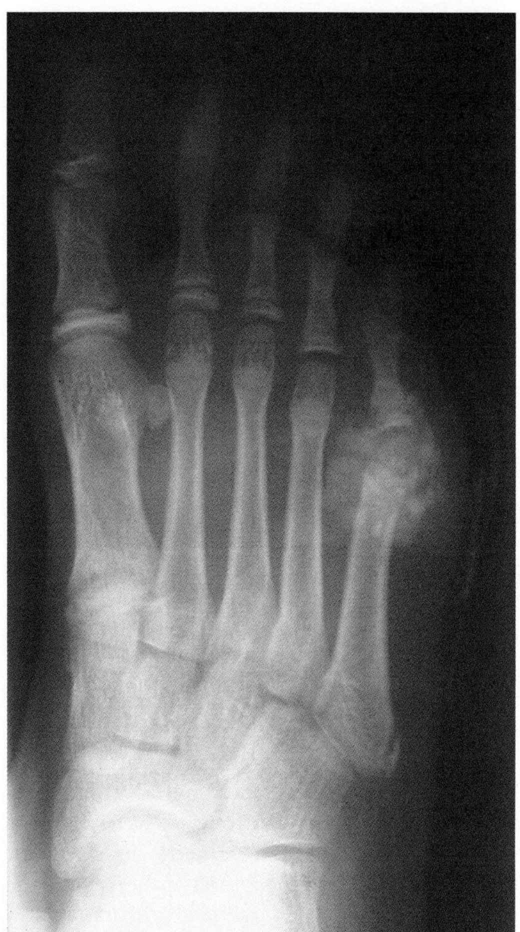

Figure 51.9 Secondary hyperparathyroidism. X-ray showing ectopic calcification.

Diagnosis

The classical symptoms associated with secondary hyperparathyroidism are seen less commonly now, with greater awareness of the disease and the resultant earlier medical intervention. However progressive bone disease, especially bone pain, can occur with associated soft tissue calcium deposits (**Figure 51.9**).

The diagnosis of secondary hyperparathyroidism is characterised by hypocalcaemia or normocalcaemia with an elevated PTH. Patients have a high serum phosphate and a low vitamin D. Traditional plain x-rays now rarely demonstrate the pathognomonic osteitis fibrosa cystica. However, bone densitometry (DEXA scan) typically demonstrates osteopenia or osteoporosis.

The diagnosis of secondary hyperparathyroidism is a biochemical one. In general, localisation studies are not undertaken as minimally invasive surgery is not indicated. However, a neck ultrasound can be performed to identify patients with nodular hyperplasia who may be refractory to medical management. Localisation studies are helpful in patients with recurrent disease, in order to identify ectopic parathyroid tissue, especially in the mediastinum. In cases of recurrent disease, when there is no evidence of active disease in the neck, and a previous allograft has been used to the forearm, then selective venous sampling for PTH in the neck and the brachial vein on the side of the graft can be useful. This is known as the Casanova test and to prove that the recurrent disease is located in the grafted arm (graft hyperplasia) the ratio must be greater than 20:1.

Calciphylaxis

Calciphylaxis (calcific uraemic arteriolopathy) is a syndrome of disseminated calcification resulting in both vascular calcification and skin necrosis. It accounts for approximately 4% of patients undergoing surgical intervention for secondary hyperparathyroidism. It presents with expanding painful cutaneous purpuritic lesions, predominantly on the extremities, although it can also be seen on the lower abdomen. The underlying tissue calcification within the arteriolar and small vascular walls leads to ischaemic necrosis and the development of gangrene, which in turn leads to overwhelming

Daniel Casanova, contemporary, University of Cantabria, Santander, Spain.

sepsis and death. The majority of these patients will have an elevated calcium × phosphate product but it is not usually associated with an extremely high PTH level. The underlying aetiology remains unclear but a number of potential factors have been postulated. A reduction in the serum levels of a calcification inhibitory protein, α-2-Heremans–Schmid glycoprotein, and abnormalities in smooth muscle cell biology in uraemic patients may play a role in the development of the syndrome. Prognosis for these patients is extremely poor, with a mortality of up to 87%. An urgent parathyroidectomy has been shown to decrease pain, improve wound healing and reduce the risk of amputation in these patients. It has also been associated with an increase in median survival.

Management

Renal transplantation remains the only definite treatment for secondary hyperparathyroidism. Other therapies are a bridge to this or aim to provide symptom relief. Standard management includes replacement of calcium and vitamin D and the reduction of phosphate levels by the use of phosphate binders. Treatment of this disease changed radically with the introduction of calcimimetic drugs, such as cinacalcet. Calcimimetics alter the set point of the CaR, thereby reducing the constant stimulation of the parathyroid glands and lowering the PTH level. This obviously does not address the underlying renal disease. It remains controversial as to which patients may benefit from the use of calcimimetics and which patients may benefit from earlier surgical intervention. Indications for pursing medical management include those patients who are deemed non-surgical candidates by reason of medical comorbidities. Similarly, where there is persistent or recurrent disease, the origin of which cannot be clearly elucidated, surgical management should be avoided. However, there are definite indications for surgical intervention in secondary hyperparathyroidism (*Table 51.3*) although these have been modified to reflect the current use, where available, of calcimimetics (*Table 51.4*).

TABLE 51.3 Indications for surgical intervention in secondary hyperparathyroidism.

Essential components
1. Persistently high serum level of intact PTH >500 pg/mL 2. Hyperphosphataemia (serum P >6 mg/dL) or hypercalcaemia (serum Ca >2.5 mmol/L or 10 mg/dL) which is refractory to medical management 3. Estimated volume of the largest gland >300–500 mm^3 or long axis >1 cm
Clinical findings
If patients have one of these symptoms, parathyroidectomy should be recommended: Severe osteitis fibrosa with associated high bone turnover Subjective symptoms (bone and joint pain, arthralgia, muscle weakness, irritability, purititis, depression) Progressive ectopic calcification Calciphylaxis Progressive reduction in bone mineral content Anaemia resistant to erythropoietin stimulating agent (ESA) Dilated cardiomyopathy/cardiac failure

TABLE 51.4 Proposed indications for surgical management of secondary hyperparathyroidism (SHPT) in the era of calcimimetics.

When SHPT is refractory to vitamin D replacement or vitamin D analogues and prolonged survival is anticipated
Severely impaired quality of life due to either SHPT or intolerance to calcimimetics
When sufficient reduction in parathyroid hormone cannot be achieved with use of calcimimetics
Thyroid surgery is also required (thyroid carcinoma)

There are a wide variety of operations that can be utilised for the management of secondary hyperparathyroidism, none of which appears significantly superior in terms of clinical outcomes (persistent or recurrent disease). These include a subtotal parathyroidectomy, a total parathyroidectomy with autograft or a total parathyroidectomy without autograft. Cryopreservation of resected tissue, where available, should be performed in case of significant postoperative hypocalcaemia. The first two procedures are most widely accepted and the type of operation performed depends upon the surgeon.

A subtotal parathyroidectomy is where three and a half parathyroid glands are excised, with the remnant being marked with a non-absorbable stitch to facilitate identification in the event of recurrent disease. A biopsy of the final gland that is to be left *in situ* is mandatory to confirm the presence of residual parathyroid tissue. Ideally an inferior gland is left *in situ* to facilitate reoperative surgery and minimise potential damage to the recurrent laryngeal nerve in that setting (**Figure 51.10**). A total parathyroidectomy with a forearm autograft involves removal of all parathyroid tissue in the neck, with reimplantation of a small amount of morcellated tissue within a pocket formed in the brachoradialis muscle. Overall, regardless of the operative approach utilised the cure rate ranges between 90% and 96%, with similar complication rates. A randomised study looking at 40 patients who either underwent a subtotal or total parathyroidectomy with autotransplant demonstrated no significant difference between the two operations in terms of efficacy and recurrence rate (Rothmund *et al.*, 1991).

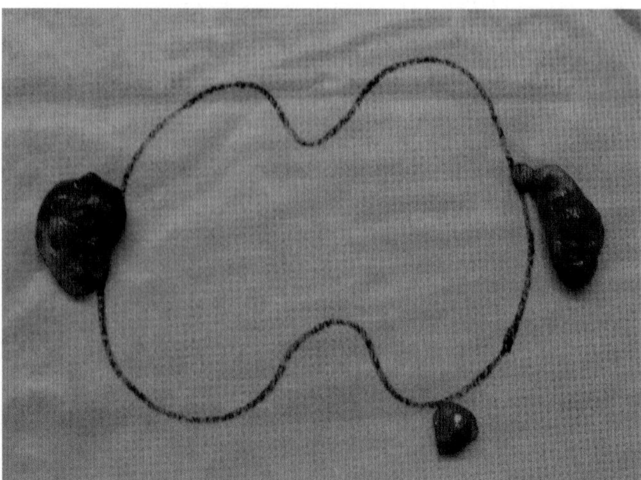

Figure 51.10 Subtotal parathyroidectomy for parathyroid hyperplasia. Right inferior gland biopsied and half left *in situ*.

The response to surgical intervention is often dramatic. The biochemical parameters may resolve almost immediately and appear to be sustained for up to 3 years postoperatively. Patients subjectively report improvements in the symptoms of secondary hyperparathyroidism including bone pain, pruritus, fatigue and depression. Finally, bone metabolism is improved with an approximate 10% increase in trabecular bone, with almost immediate suppression of bone resorption and acceleration of new bone formation.

Summary box 51.2

Secondary hyperparathyroidism

- Primarily due to underlying chronic kidney disease
- Associated with parathyroid hyperplasia
- Diagnosis is made biochemically with a low or normal calcium and an elevated PTH. High phosphate levels and low vitamin D levels are seen
- No localisation studies are required
- Mainstay of treatment is renal transplantation. Medical management with calcium and vitamin D replacements and phosphate binders is a bridge to transplantation
- Use of calcimimetics has reduced the requirement for surgical intervention
- Subtotal parathyroidectomy remains the surgical intervention of choice when indicated

TERTIARY HYPERPARATHYROIDISM

Tertiary hyperparathyroidism is a persistent autonomous hypercalcaemic hyperparathyroidism occurring after kidney transplantation. A number of proposed factors may prevent involution of the hyperplastic parathyroid glands following resolution of the underlying renal impairment. These include impaired graft function, non-suppressible PTH secretion, slow involution of enlarged glands or insufficient calcitriol conversion by the transplanted kidney.

The biochemical diagnosis is confirmed by an elevated total or ionised calcium, with an associated elevated or unsuppressed PTH and a reduced phosphate occurring at least 1-year post renal transplantation. Differentiation from PHPT can be difficult. Fewer than 1% of patients with tertiary hyperparathyroidism will require surgical intervention (*Table 51.5*). The only new evidence for intervention is the presence of nodular hyperplasia of the glands themselves. Traditionally, localisation studies or imaging of the neck was not indicated in tertiary hyperparathyroidism. However, increasing knowledge of the clonal nature of gland hyperplasia suggests that where there is a nodule within the parathyroid with a volume of tissue greater than 500 mm^3, then resolution of electrolyte abnormalities is unlikely.

TABLE 51.5 Indications for surgical intervention in tertiary hyperparathyroidism.

Subacute severe hypercalcaemia (>3 mmol/L)
Impaired graft function
Nodular hyperplasia of the parathyroid gland(s)
Progressive symptoms (>2 years following transplantation)
Worsening bone disease (pain, fractures, bone loss)
Renal stones/nephrocalcinosis
Soft tissue or vascular calcifications

The use of calcimimetics in tertiary hyperparathyroidism remains controversial and has not been approved for this indication. However, isolated reports have documented control of hypercalcaemia with minimal side effects in individual patients. Surgical intervention remains the definitive management strategy. Subtotal parathyroidectomy or total parathyroidectomy with autotransplantation are acceptable surgical options. The majority of endocrine surgeons will opt for a subtotal parathyroidectomy in this setting, leaving a gland approximately four times normal in volume to minimise postoperative complications. Total parathyroidectomy without an autograft is not a treatment option due to the postoperative and persistent difficulties in managing the associated hypocalcaemia.

Summary box 51.3

Tertiary hyperparathyroidism

- Persistent autonomous hypercalcaemic hyperparathyroidism occurring after kidney transplantation
- Diagnosis is made by demonstrating an elevated total or ionised calcium with an associated elevated or unsuppressed PTH and a reduced phosphate occurring at least 1-year post renal transplantation
- Localisation studies are not required but a focused neck ultrasound may confirm the presence of nodular enlargement
- Surgical intervention remains the mainstay of treatment and involves a subtotal parathyroidectomy

PARATHYROID CARCINOMA

Parathyroid carcinoma is a rare malignancy occurring in approximately 1% of cases of PHPT, with an estimated prevalence of 0.005% of all cancers. While the aetiology remains unclear, recent advances in molecular biology suggest that there may be an underlying genetic basis. Currently, a history of previous neck irradiation remains the only known environmental risk factor. However, given that it can arise in patients with end-stage renal disease as well as in those with MEN type 1, malignant transformation in hyperplastic glands may also occur.

A significant proportion of patients (>10%) with a parathyroid carcinoma will have HPT-JT. The underlying mutation is in the *HRPT2* gene at 1q25-32, a tumour suppressor gene that encodes the protein parafibromin. Parafibromin is involved in the regulation of cellular transcription and histone modification. *HRPT2* mutations, leading to inactivation of parafibromin, are therefore an important contributor to the pathogenesis of parathyroid carcinoma.

Parathyroid carcinoma remains difficult to diagnose preoperatively as it biochemically resembles PHPT. There are, however, a number of suggestive features. Firstly, the diagnosis is typically made a decade earlier, with an equal gender preponderance (female:male 1:1) when compared to PHPT.

Secondly, a greater proportion of these patients will be symptomatic at presentation. A palpable neck mass is found in 36–52% of patients with parathyroid carcinomas but rarely (<5%) in cases of PHPT. Finally, the biochemical abnormalities tend to be exaggerated with an average total calcium of between 3.75 and 3.97 mmol/L and a PTH level 5–10 times the normal range.

The leading cause of morbidity and mortality from parathyroid carcinoma is hypercalcaemia, due to inappropriate PTH secretion. Treatment is focused on controlling hypercalcaemia and removal of the carcinoma where possible. Surgery remains the mainstay of treatment for primary presentations and locally recurrent disease. Complete resection of the tumour avoiding spillage is vital in preventing seeding and thus recurrent disease. *En bloc* resection of the tumour, associated thyroid lobectomy and central neck dissection remains controversial. Traditionally, complete R0 resection was thought to provide the only means of a cure. However, a number of recent studies have failed to demonstrate an improvement in local recurrence rates with such comprehensive resection. Adjuvant chemotherapy has not been shown to confer a disease-free or overall survival benefit. Use of external beam radiotherapy should be considered on an individual basis. Traditionally, it has not been deemed effective, but more recent single institution case series appear to challenge this assumption. It may be considered where it is difficult to achieve a complete surgical resection or in patients with multifocal recurrent soft tissue deposits.

Histological confirmation of a parathyroid carcinoma remains difficult. The classical description included trabecular architecture, mitotic figures, thick fibrous bands and capsular and vascular invasion. However, these findings can be non-significant and new molecular markers may aid the diagnosis and stratify patients for more intensive follow-up (**Figure 51.11**). Immunohistochemical evidence of downregulation of parafibromin has a sensitivity of 67% and a specificity of 100% for detecting parathyroid carcinoma and the protein gene product 9.5 (PGP 9.5). Parafibromin immunohistochemistry may be used with immunohistochemistry for PGP 9.5. This is a protein encoded by *ubiquitin carboxyl-terminal esterase L1*. It is upregulated in parathyroid carcinoma and has a sensitivity of 78% and a specificity of 100% (**Figure 51.11**). All parafibromin-negative and PGP 9.5-positive tumours should be considered for genetic screening.

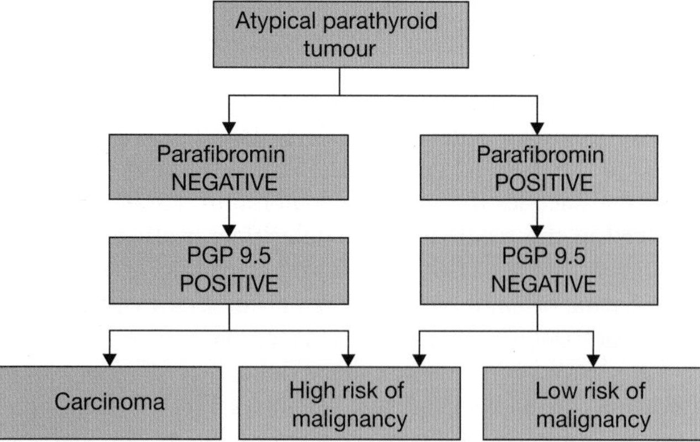

Figure 51.11 Proposed decision tree for atypical parathyroid tumours using parafibromin and PGP 9.5 immunostaining.

Parathyroid carcinoma is an indolent but progressive disease. Metastatic spread can occur to the lungs, liver and bones. Recurrence rates range from 33% to 80% and it typically occurs in the first 3 years. Overall survival is reported to be 85–90% at 5 years and 49–77% at 10 years.

Summary box 51.4

Parathyroid carcinoma

- Accounts for approximately 1% of all cases of primary hyperparathyroidism
- A history of previous neck irradiation remains the only known environmental risk factor
- The tumours remain difficult to diagnose preoperatively as they biochemically resemble primary hyperparathyroidism
- Treatment is focused on controlling hypercalcaemia and removal of the carcinoma where possible
- Surgery remains the mainstay of treatment for primary presentations and locally recurrent disease. Complete resection of the tumour avoiding spillage is vital in preventing seeding and thus recurrent disease

PERSISTENT HYPERPARATHYROIDISM

Persistent hyperparathyroidism is defined as an elevated calcium within 6 weeks of surgical intervention. For all parathyroid operations (minimally invasive parathyroidectomy (MIP) and bilateral exploration) the rate of persistent hypercalcaemia is approximately 6% in sporadic disease and between 16% and 20% in hereditary disease. It usually arises as a result of a technical error during the first operation, either due to a missed adenoma or asymmetrical disease. When this occurs all preoperative biochemistry, radiological imaging, intraoperative findings and pathology must be carefully reviewed. If reoperation is appropriate, repeat imaging of the neck and mediastinum is required (sestamibi, ultrasound and 4D-CT scanning). Surgical intervention can be straightforward where there are intact tissue planes, such as following a minimally invasive parathyroidectomy. Complications, including recurrent laryngeal nerve damage and permanent hypocalcaemia, are increased when extensive previous dissection has occurred and the patient must be consented appropriately.

RECURRENT HYPERPARATHYROIDISM

Recurrent hyperparathyroidism is defined as hypercalcaemia occurring 6 months after surgery but with an intervening period of normocalcaemia. Common causes include missed pathology at the first operation; hyperplasia in remaining or autotransplanted tissue; parathyromatosis or, very rarely, the development of a second parathyroid adenoma. Parathyromatosis refers to disseminated parathyroid tissue within the soft tissues of the neck and superior mediastinum due to rupture of the parathyroid gland during the primary surgery. A definitive indication for surgical intervention must be present prior to embarking on localisation studies. Surgical intervention will be guided by the radiological imaging. Complication rates of recurrent laryngeal nerve damage and permanent hypocalcaemia are higher in reoperative surgery.

FURTHER READING

Agarwal A, Mishra AK, Lombardi CP, Raffaelli M. Applied embryology of the thyroid and parathyroid glands. In: G.W. *Randolph surgery of the thyroid and parathyroid glands*. Philadelphia: Saunders, 2013, 15–24.

Barczyński M, Bränström R, Dionigi G, Mihai R. Sporadic multiple parathyroid gland disease – a consensus report of the European Society of Endocrine Surgeons. *Langenbecks Arch Surg* 2015; **400**(8): 887–905.

Bilezikian JP, Brandi ML, Eastell R *et al.* Guidelines for the management of asymptomatic primary hyperparathyroidism: summary statement from the Fourth International Workshop. *J Clin Endocrinol Metab* 2014; **99**: 3561–9.

Carneiro-Pla D, Pellitteri PK. Intraoperative PTH monitoring during parathyroid surgery. In: G.W. *Randolph surgery of the thyroid and parathyroid glands*. Philadelphia: Saunders, 2013, 605–12.

Certani F, Pardi E, Marcocci C. Update on parathyroid carcinoma. *J Endocrinol Invest* 2016; **39**(6): 595–606.

Cheung K, Wang TS, Farrokhyar F, Roman SA, Sosa JA. A meta-analysis of preoperative localisation techniques for patients with primary hyperparathyroidism. *Ann Surg Oncol* 2012; **19**(2): 577–83.

Howell VM, Gill A, Clarkson A *et al.* Accuracy of combined protein gene product 9.5 and parafibromin markers for immunohistochemical diagnosis of parathyroid carcinoma. *J Clin Endocrinol Metab* 2009; **94**(2): 434–41.

Iacobone M, Carnaille B, Palazzo FF, Vriens M. Hereditary hyperparathyroidism – a consensus report of the European Society of Endocrine Surgeons. *Langenbecks Arch Surg* 2015; **400**(8): 867–86.

Jeong HS, Dominguez AR. Calciphylaxis: controversies in pathogenesis, diagnosis and treatment. *Am J Med Sci* 2016; **351**(1): 217–27.

Krakauer M, Wieslander B, Myschetzky PS *et al.* A prospective comparative study of parathyroid dual-phase scintigraphy, dual-isotope subtraction scintigraphy, 4D-CT, and ultrasonography in primary hyperparathyroidism. *Clin Nucl Med* 2016; **41**(2): 93–100.

Mihai R, Simon D, Hellman P. Imaging for primary hyperparathyroidism – an evidence-based analysis. *Langenbecks Arch Surg* 2009; **394**(5): 765–84.

Pitt SC, Sipple RS, Chen H. Secondary and tertiary hyperparathyroidism: state of the art surgical management. *Surg Clin North Am* 2009; **89**(5): 1227–39.

Rodgers SE, Hunter GJ, Hamberg LM *et al.* Improved pre-operative planning for directed parathyroidectomy with 4-dimensional computed tomography. *Surgery* 2006; **140**(6): 932–40.

Rothmund M, Wagner PK, Schark C. Subtotal parathyroidectomy versus total parathyroidectomy and autotransplantation in secondary hyperparathyroidism: a randomized trial. *World J Surg* 1991; **15**(6): 745–50.

Silverberg SJ, Clarke BL, Peacock M *et al.* 2014. Current issues in the presentation of asymptomatic primary hyperparathyroidism. *Proceedings of the Fourth International Workshop* 2014; **99**: 3580–94.

Chapter 52

The adrenal glands and other abdominal endocrine disorders

Learning objectives

To understand:

- The anatomy and function of the adrenal and other abdominal endocrine glands
- The diagnosis and management of these endocrine disorders
- The role of surgery in the management of these endocrine disorders

ADRENAL GLANDS

Anatomy

The weight of a normal adrenal gland is approximately 4 g. There are two distinct components to the gland: the inner adrenal medulla and the outer adrenal cortex (**Figure 52.1**). The adrenal glands are situated near the upper poles of the kidneys, in the retroperitoneum, within Gerota's capsule. The right adrenal gland is located between the right liver lobe and the diaphragm, close to and partly behind the inferior vena cava (IVC). The left adrenal gland lies close to the upper pole of the left kidney and the renal pedicle. It is covered by the pancreatic tail and the spleen (**Figure 52.2**). The adrenal glands are well supplied by blood vessels. The arterial blood supply branches from the aorta and the diaphragmatic and renal arteries and varies considerably. A usually single large adrenal vein drains on the right side into the vena cava and on the left side into the renal vein.

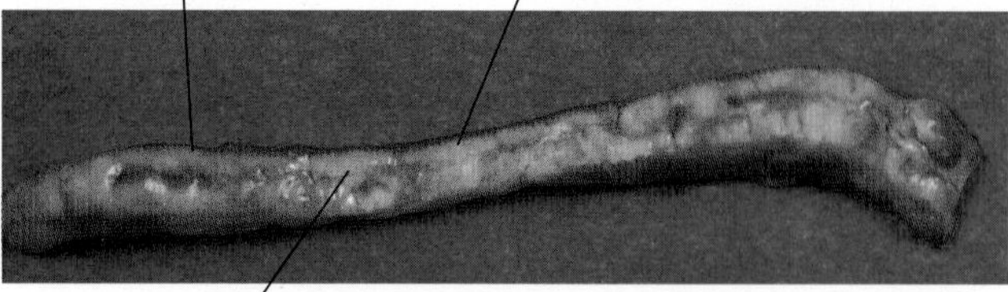

Figure 52.1 Cross-section of a normal adrenal gland. The inner, very thin layer between the two dark lines (zona reticularis) is the adrenal medulla. (DHEA, dehydroepiandrosterone; DHEAS, dehydroepiandrosterone sulphate.)

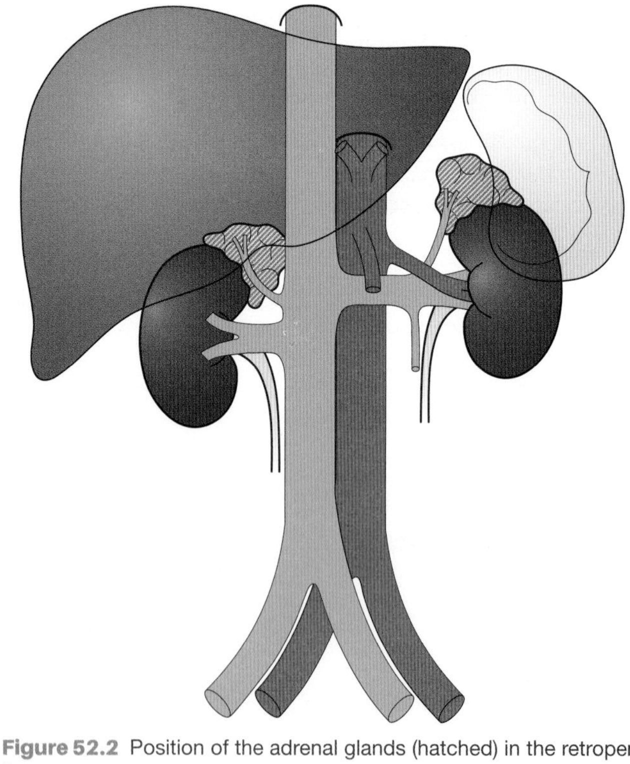

Figure 52.2 Position of the adrenal glands (hatched) in the retroperitoneum.

Dumitru Gerota, 1867–1939, Professor of Surgery, Bucharest, Romania.

Embryology

The two functional parts, the cortex and the medulla, arise from different blastodermic layers: mesodermal cells form the adrenal cortex and neuroectodermal cells migrate to the cortex from the neural crest during embryogenesis and form the adrenal medulla.

Histology

The adrenal cortex is arranged in a zonal configuration. The outer zona glomerulosa contains small, compact cells. The central zona fasciculata can be identified by larger, lipoid-rich cells, which are arranged in radial columns. Compact and pigmented cells characterise the inner zona reticularis. The adrenal medulla consists of a thin layer of large chromaffin cells, which synthesise, store and secrete catecholamine.

Function of the adrenal glands

The adrenal glands play a pivotal role in the response to stress. Catecholamines are secreted by the adrenal medulla and corticosteroids, aldosterone and cortisol are synthesised in the adrenal cortex (**Figure 52.1**). Cells of the adrenal medulla synthesise mainly adrenaline (epinephrine) but also noradrenaline (norepinephrine) and dopamine. These catecholamines act as hormones as they are secreted directly into the circulation. Their effects, which are mediated through α and β receptors on target organs, include the cardiovascular system, resulting in an increase in blood pressure and heart rate; vasoconstriction of vessels in the splanchnic system and vasodilatation of vessels in the muscles; bronchodilatation; and increased glycogenolysis in liver and muscles, all necessary for the flight/fight response. Cells of the zona glomerulosa produce aldosterone, which regulates sodium–potassium homeostasis. The target organs of aldosterone are the kidneys, the sweat and salivary glands and the intestinal mucosa. Aldosterone promotes sodium retention and potassium excretion. The most important regulators of aldosterone secretion are the renin–angiotensin system and the serum potassium concentration. Renin produced by the juxtaglomerular cells in the kidneys acts on its substrate angiotensinogen to generate angiotensin I. Angiotensin I is converted by angiotensin-converting enzyme (ACE) to the octapeptide angiotensin II, which is modified to angiotensin III. Both stimulate the secretion of aldosterone from the adrenal cortex. A decrease in renal blood flow (haemorrhage, dehydration, salt depletion, orthostasis, renal artery stenosis) or hyponatraemia increases renin secretion and leads to sodium retention, potassium excretion and an increase of plasma volume.

Cells of the zona fasciculata and zona reticularis synthesise cortisol and the adrenal androgens dehydroepiandrosterone (DHEA) and its sulphate DHEAS. DHEA and DHEAS are precursors of androgens and are converted in peripheral tissues such as fat. Cortisol secretion is regulated by adrenocorticotrophic hormone (ACTH), which is produced by the anterior pituitary gland. The hypothalamus controls ACTH secretion by secreting corticotrophin-releasing hormone (CRH). The serum cortisol level inhibits the release of CRH and ACTH via a closed-loop system (negative feedback loop).

Cortisol has numerous metabolic and immunological effects. It increases gluconeogenesis and lipolysis, decreases peripheral glucose utilisation, inhibits immunological response and, in time, reduces muscular mass. It affects fat distribution, wound healing and bone mineralisation; and alters mood (euphoria or, rarely, depression) and brain cortical activity and alertness.

DISORDERS OF THE ADRENAL CORTEX

Incidentaloma

Definition

An incidentaloma is an adrenal mass, detected incidentally by imaging studies conducted for other reasons, not known previously to have been present or causing symptoms.

Incidence

The prevalence of adrenal masses in autopsy studies ranges from 1.4% to 8.7% and increases with age. Incidentalomas may be detected on imaging studies in 1% of patients. More than 75% are non-functioning adenomas but Cushing's adenomas, phaeochromocytomas, metastases, adrenocortical carcinomas and Conn's tumours can all be found this way (*Table 52.1*).

Diagnosis

When an incidentaloma is identified, a complete history and clinical examination is required. Occasionally a previously occult endocrine disturbance will come to light. A biochemical work-up for hormone excess and sometimes additional imaging studies are also needed. The main goal is to exclude a functioning or malignant adrenal tumour.

TABLE 52.1 Prevalence of non-functioning and functioning tumours in patients with incidentalomas.

Tumour	Prevalence (%)
Non-functioning adenoma	78
Cushing's adenoma	7
Adrenocortical carcinoma	4
Phaeochromocytoma	4
Myelolipoma	2
Cyst	2
Metastases	2
Conn's adenoma	1

Harvey Williams Cushing, 1869–1939, Professor of Surgery, Harvard University Medical School, Boston, MA, USA.

Hormonal evaluation includes:

- morning and midnight plasma cortisol measurements;
- a 1-mg overnight dexamethasone suppression test;
- 24-hour urinary cortisol excretion;
- 12- or 24-hour urinary excretion of metanephrines or plasma-free metanephrines;
- serum potassium, plasma aldosterone and plasma renin activity;
- serum DHEAS, testosterone or 17-hydroxyestradiol (virilising or feminising tumour).

Cross-sectional imaging such as computed tomography (CT) or magnetic resonance imaging (MRI) should be performed in all patients with adrenal masses. The likelihood of an adrenal mass being an adrenocortical carcinoma increases with the size of the mass (25% >4 cm). Adrenal metastases are likely in patients with a history of cancer elsewhere and the sole indication for biopsy of an adrenal mass is to confirm a suspected metastasis from a distant primary site.

Summary box 52.1

Adrenal gland biopsy

- Never biopsy an adrenal mass until phaeochromocytoma has been biochemically excluded
- The indication for adrenal gland biopsy is to confirm a suspected adrenal gland metastasis

Treatment

The treatment of functional adrenal tumours is described below. Any non-functioning adrenal tumour greater than 4 cm in diameter and smaller tumours that increase in size over time should undergo surgical resection. Non-functioning tumours smaller than 4 cm should be followed-up after 6, 12 and 24 months by imaging (MRI) and hormonal evaluation. If the tumour remains non-functioning and stable in size, surveillance can be discontinued. Repeated frequent imaging using ionising radiation can lead to dangerous exposure to radiation and should be avoided.

Primary hyperaldosteronism - Conn's syndrome

Incidence

Primary hyperaldosteronism (PHA) is defined by hypertension, as a result of hypersecretion of aldosterone. In PHA, plasma renin activity is suppressed. Among patients with hypertension the incidence of PHA is approximately 2%. Recent studies have revealed that up to 12% of hypertensive patients have PHA with normal potassium levels, thus potassium levels are an inconsistent diagnostic feature of this disease, and cannot be relied on to confirm or exclude it.

Pathology

The most frequent cause of PHA with hypokalaemia is a unilateral adrenocortical adenoma (**Figure 52.3**). In 20–40% of cases, bilateral micronodular hyperplasia is present. Rare causes of PHA are bilateral macronodular hyperplasia, glucocorticoid-suppressible hyperaldosteronism or adrenocortical carcinoma. In the subset of patients with normokalaemic PHA, 70% have hyperplasia and 30% unilateral adenoma. Somatic mutations at the *KCNJ5* gene coding for the potassium channel Kir3.4 are present in aldosterone-producing adenomas and a germline *KCNJ5* mutation can cause a very rare autosomal dominant and early-onset form of PHA, characterized by bilateral adrenal hyperplasia.

Clinical features

Most patients are between 30 and 50 years of age with a female predominance. Apart from hypertension, patients complain of non-specific symptoms: headache, muscle weakness, cramps, neurological events, polyuria, polydypsia and nocturia.

Diagnosis

The key feature of the biochemical diagnosis is the assessment of the aldosterone to plasma renin activity ratio. Hypokalaemia may be present. Antihypertensive and diuretic therapy, which cause hypokalaemia and influence the renin–angiotensin–aldosterone system, have to be discontinued. Once the biochemical diagnosis is confirmed, MRI or CT should be performed to distinguish unilateral from bilateral disease. Conn's adenomas usually measure between 1 and 2 cm and are detected by CT with a sensitivity of 80–90% (**Figure 52.4**). Micronodular changes and small adenomas are often underdiagnosed. An apparent unilateral mass could be a non-functioning tumour in a patient with bilateral micronodular hyperplasia. Selective adrenal vein catheterisation can help before a decision on non-surgical or surgical treatment is

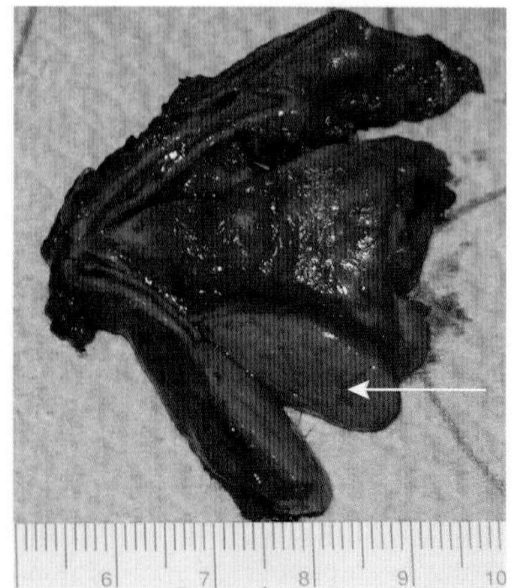

Figure 52.3 A Conn's adenoma (arrow) of the left adrenal gland; note the V-shaped normal adrenal tissue.

Jerome William Conn, 1907–1981, Professor of Internal Medicine, The University of Michigan, Michigan, MI, USA.

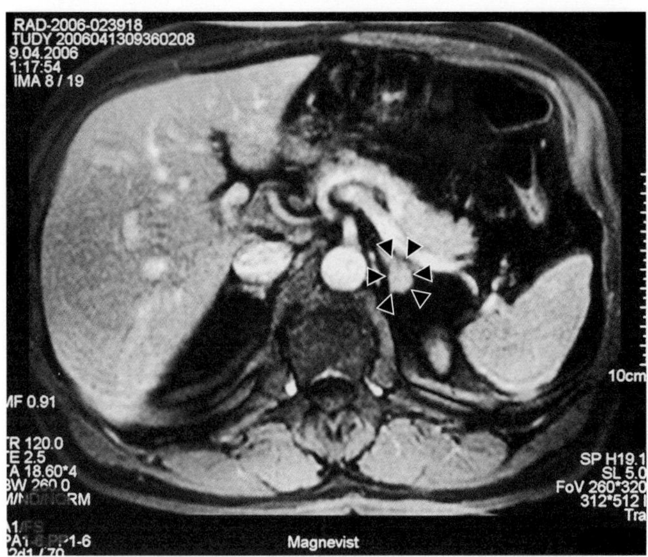

Figure 52.4 Computed tomography scan of a Conn's adenoma of the left adrenal gland (arrowheads).

made. During selective adrenal vein catheterisation, samples are obtained from the vena cava and from both adrenal veins and the aldosterone to cortisol ratio (ACR) is determined in each sample. A significant difference in the ACR ratio on one side indicates unilateral disease. In patients under age 40 with a biochemical diagnosis of Conns syndrome, a unilateral adrenal mass almost invariably represents the cause and selective adrenal vein sampling can be avoided in such cases.

Treatment

The first-line therapy for PHA with bilateral hyperplasia is medical treatment with spironolactone. In most cases supplemental antihypertensive medication is necessary to achieve satisfactory control of blood pressure.

Unilateral laparoscopic adrenalectomy is an effective therapy in patients with clear evidence of unilateral or asymmetrical bilateral disease. A subtotal adrenal resection can be considered in the case of a typical single Conn's adenoma. In 10–30% of patients who undergo an adrenalectomy, hypertension persists despite adequate diagnostic work-up and treatment, allbeit at a lower level and requiring fewer medications to control it.

Cushing's syndrome

Definition

Hypersecretion of cortisol caused by endogenous production of corticosteroids is known as Cushing's syndrome. It can be either ACTH-dependent or ACTH-independent in origin. The most common cause (85%) of ACTH-dependent Cushing's syndrome is Cushing's disease resulting from a pituitary adenoma that secretes an excessive amount of ACTH. Ectopic ACTH-producing tumours (small cell lung cancer, foregut carcinoid) and CRH-producing tumours (medullary thyroid carcinoma, neuroendocrine pancreatic tumour) are more infrequent causes of ACTH-dependent Cushing's syndrome. Excessive or prolonged administration of cortisol-like drugs will produce the same clinical picture.

In about 15% of patients, an ACTH-independent Cushing's syndrome (low ACTH levels) is caused by a unilateral adrenocortical adenoma. Adrenocortical carcinoma and bilateral macronodular or micronodular hyperplasia represent rare causes of hypercortisolism.

Clinical symptoms

The clinical features of Cushing's syndrome are shown in *Summary box 52.2*. The typical patient is characterised by a facial plethora, a buffalo hump and a moon face in combination with hypertension, diabetes and central obesity (**Figures 52.5 and 52.6**). However, clinical signs can be minimal or absent in patients with subclinical Cushing's syndrome.

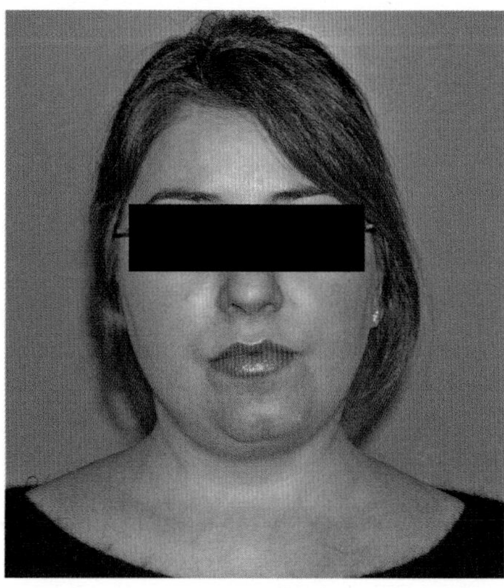

Figure 52.5 A 34-year-old patient with Cushing's syndrome whose symptoms included thickening of the face, weight gain and acne. Today patients with Cushing's syndrome rarely have the full-blown appearance as shown in older textbooks.

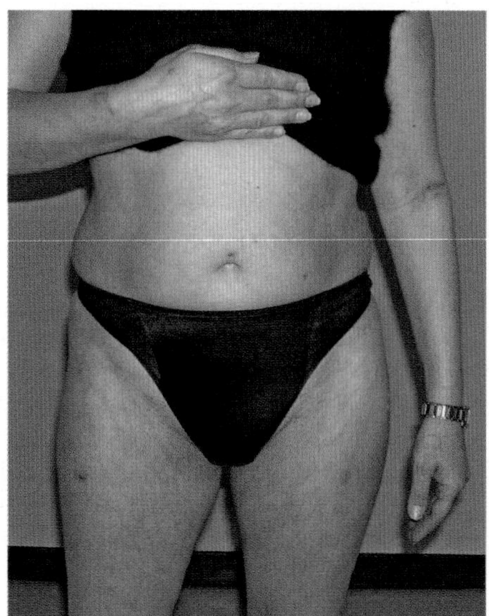

Figure 52.6 Discrete central obesity, ecchymosis and fragile skin in a patient with Cushing's syndrome.

Summary box 52.2

Clinical features of Cushing's syndrome

- Weight gain/central obesity
- Diabetes
- Hirsutism
- Hypertension
- Skin changes (abdominal striae, facial plethora, ecchymosis, acne)
- Muscle weakness
- Menstrual irregularity/impotence
- Depression/mania
- Osteoporosis
- Hypokalaemia

Diagnosis

- Morning and midnight plasma cortisol levels are elevated, usually with loss of diurnal rhythm.
- Dexamethasone fails to suppress 24-hour urinary cortisol excretion.
- Serum ACTH levels discriminate ACTH-dependent from ACTH-independent disease.

Elevated or normal ACTH levels provide evidence for an ACTH-producing pituitary tumour (85%) or ectopic ACTH production. Therefore, in patients with elevated ACTH, MRI of the pituitary gland must be performed. If MRI is negative and additional venous sampling from the inferior petrosal sinus has excluded a pituitary microadenoma, a CT scan of the chest and abdomen is warranted to detect an ectopic ACTH-producing tumour. In patients with suppressed ACTH levels, a CT or MRI scan is performed to assess the adrenal glands.

Subclinical Cushing's syndrome is diagnosed if clinical symptoms are absent in the face of abnormal cortisol secretion.

Treatment

Medical therapy with metyrapone or ketoconazole reduces steroid synthesis and secretion and can be used to prepare patients with severe hypercortisolism preoperatively or if surgery is not possible. ACTH-producing pituitary tumours are treated by trans-sphenoidal resection or radiotherapy. If an ectopic ACTH source is localised, resection will correct hypercortisolism.

A unilateral adenoma is treated by adrenalectomy. In cases of bilateral ACTH-independent disease (Figure 52.7), bilateral adrenalectomy is the primary treatment. Patients with an ectopic ACTH-dependent Cushing's syndrome and an irresectable or unlocalised primary tumour should be considered for bilateral adrenalectomy as this controls hormone excess. Subclinical Cushing's syndrome caused by unilateral adenoma can be treated by unilateral adrenalectomy.

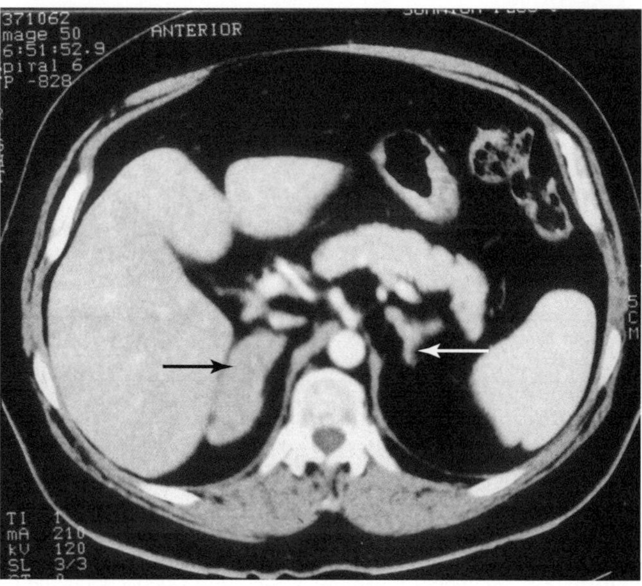

Figure 52.7 Bilateral asymmetrical hyperplasia of the adrenal glands (arrows) in a patient with Cushing's syndrome.

Preoperative management

Patients with Cushing's syndrome are at an increased risk of hospital-acquired infection, thromboembolic and myocardial complications. Therefore, prophylactic anticoagulation and the use of prophylactic antibiotics are essential. Cushing-associated diseases (diabetes, hypertension) must be controlled by medical therapy preoperatively.

Postoperative management

After unilateral adrenalectomy supplemental cortisol should be given postoperatively because the contralateral gland will be suppressed. In total, 15 mg/h is required parenterally for the first 12 hours followed by a daily dose of 100 mg for 3 days, which is gradually reduced thereafter. After unilateral adrenalectomy, the contralateral suppressed gland needs up to 1 year to recover adequate function. A synacthen test to evaluate adrenal fuction prior to stopping cortisol supplements is advised. In 10% of patients with Cushing's disease who undergo a bilateral adrenalectomy after failed pituitary surgery, the pituitary adenoma causes Nelson's syndrome due to continued ACTH secretion at high levels, causing hyperpigmentation as a result of chemical synergies between ACTH and melanocyte-stimulating hormone.

Adrenal metastases

Adrenal metastases are discovered at autopsy in one-third of patients with malignant disease (less frequently during life). In declining frequency, the most common primary tumours are breast, lung, renal, gastric, pancreatic, ovarian and colorectal cancer. In selected circumstances an adrenalectomy is appropriate, for example if it is the sole site of metastatic disease.

Don H Nelson, 1925–2010, Professor of Medicine, The University of Utah, Salt Lake City, UT, USA.

Adrenocortical carcinoma

Incidence

Adrenocortical carcinoma (ACC) is a rare malignancy with an incidence of 1–2 cases per 1 000 000 population per year and a variable but generally poor prognosis. A slight female predominance is observed (1.5:1). The age distribution is bimodal with a first peak in childhood and a second between the fourth and fifth decades.

Pathology

The differentiation between benign and malignant adrenal tumours is challenging, even in the hands of an experienced pathologist. Criteria for malignancy are tumour size, the presence of necrosis or haemorrhage and microscopic features such as capsular or vascular invasion. These should be assessed in terms of a microscopic diagnostic score. Additional information is provided by immunohistochemistry. The macroscopic features are commonly multinodularity and heterogeneous structure (**Figure 52.8**) with haemorrhage and necrosis.

Clinical presentation

Approximately 60% of patients present with evidence of cortisol excess (Cushing's syndrome). Patients with non-functioning tumours frequently complain of abdominal discomfort or back pain caused by large tumours. However, with increasing use of abdominal imaging, a growing number of adrenocortical carcinomas are detected incidentally. Adrenal tumours secreting more than one hormone in excess, or feminising/masculanising steroids are likely to be malignant.

Diagnosis

The diagnostic work-up should include measurements of DHEAS, cortisol and catecholamines to exclude a phaeochromocytoma and a dexamethasone suppression test. MRI and CT are equally effective in imaging ACC (**Figure 52.9**). MRI angiography is useful to exclude tumour thrombus in the vena cava. As distant metastases are frequently present, a preoperative staging CT scan is recommended. The World Health Organization classification of 2004 is based on the McFarlane classification and defines four stages: tumours <5 cm (stage I) or >5 cm (stage II), locally invasive tumours (III) or tumours with distant metastases (IV). Functioning tumours tend to do worse than non-functioning, but have the advantage of a serum marker that can be used for follow-up and disease monitoring.

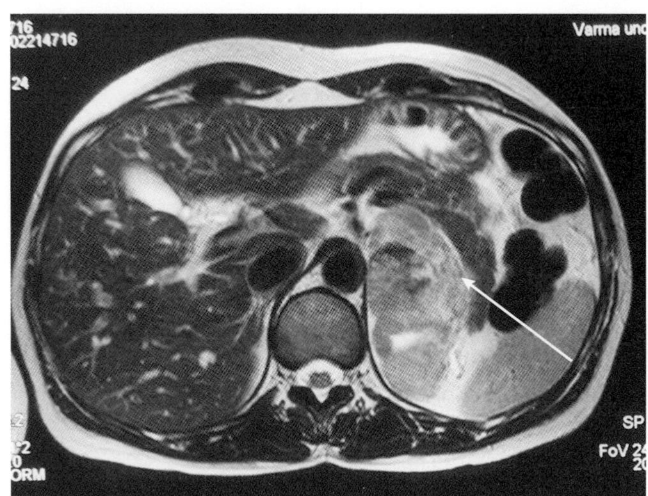

Figure 52.9 Magnetic resonance imaging of adrenocortical carcinoma (arrow) in a patient with cortisol and testosterone excess.

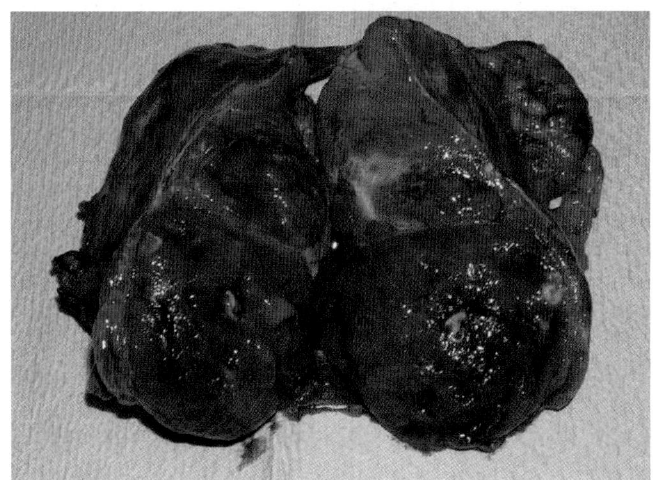

Figure 52.8 Adrenocortical carcinoma that caused Cushing's syndrome and virilisation in a female patient.

Treatment

Complete tumour resection (R0) is associated with favourable survival and should be attempted whenever possible. In order to prevent tumour spillage and implantation metastases, the capsule must not be damaged. *En bloc* resection with removal of locally involved organs is often required and in case of tumour thrombus in the vena cava, thrombectomy is needed. Laparoscopic adrenalectomy is associated with a high incidence of local recurrence and cannot be recommended. Tumour debulking plays a role in functioning tumours to control hormone excess.

Patients can be treated postoperatively with mitotane alone or in combination with etoposide, doxorubicin and cisplatin. Adjuvant radiotherapy may reduce the rate of local recurrence. After surgery, restaging every 3 months is required as the risk of tumour relapse is high. Prognosis depends on the stage of disease and complete removal of the tumour. Patients with stage I or II disease have a 5-year survival rate of 25%, whereas patients with stage III and stage IV disease have 5-year survival rates of 6% and 0% respectively. Recently, genetic sequencing of adrenocortical tumours has identified two distinct molecular subgroups that characterise aggressive and indolent ACCs and provide robust prognostic information in addition to pathological and MacFarlane staging.

---

en bloc is French for 'in a block'.

Congenital adrenal hyperplasia (adrenogenital syndrome)

Virilisation and adrenal insufficiency in children are pathognomonic of congenital adrenal hyperplasia (CAH). This is an autosomal recessive disorder caused by a variety of enzymatic defects in the synthetic pathway of cortisol and other steroids from cholesterol. The most frequent defect (95%) is the 21-hydroxylase deficiency, which has an incidence of 1 in 5000 live births. Excessive ACTH secretion is caused by the loss of cortisol and this leads to an increase in androgenic cortisol precursors and to CAH. CAH may present in girls at birth with ambiguous genitalia or as late-onset disease at puberty. Hypertension and short stature, caused by the premature epiphyseal plate closure, are common signs. Affected patients are treated by replacement of cortisol and with fludrocortisone. Large hyperplastic adrenals may need to be removed if symptomatic.

Adrenal insufficiency

Primary adrenal insufficiency is caused by the loss of function of the adrenal cortex. It was first described by Thomas Addison in 1855. An early diagnosis is a clinical challenge, even today. Symptoms are only evident when about 90% of the adrenal cortex is destroyed. Secondary adrenal insufficiency is caused by a deficiency of pituitary ACTH secretion. Tertiary adrenal deficiency is provoked by a loss of hypothalamic CRH secretion and is caused by therapeutic glucocorticoid administration, brain tumour, trauma or irradiation.

Summary box 52.3

Diseases associated with adrenal insufficiency

- Polyglandular autoimmune syndrome
- Tuberculosis
- After bilateral adrenalectomy
- Haemorrhage
- Metastases
- Systemic diseases (Boeck's disease, amyloidosis, Wilson's disease)
- Hereditary diseases (e.g. adrenoleukodystrophia, adrenogenital syndrome)
- Human immunodeficiency virus infection

Acute adrenal insufficiency

Acute adrenal insufficiency usually presents as shock in combination with fever, nausea, vomiting, abdominal pain, hypoglycaemia and electrolyte imbalance. Waterhouse–Friderichsen syndrome is a bilateral adrenal infarction associated with meningococcal sepsis and is rapidly fatal unless immediately treated. Because of intestinal symptoms and fever, the so-called Addisonian crisis is often misdiagnosed as an acute abdominal condition.

Chronic adrenal insufficiency

When symptoms develop over time, patients present with anorexia, weakness and nausea. As a result of negative feedback, ACTH and pro-opiomelanocortin (POMC) levels increase and cause hyperpigmentation of the skin and oral mucosa. Hypotension, hyponatraemia, hyperkalaemia and hypoglycaemia are commonly observed. The diagnosis of adrenal insufficiency is made using the ACTH stimulation test. Basal ACTH levels are found to be high with cortisol levels decreased. There is no rise in cortisol levels following the exogenous administration of ACTH (synacthen test).

Treatment

If a patient displays features of adrenal insufficiency, treatment must immediately be commenced, before awaiting the biochemical diagnosis. Initial blood samples can be used for later determinations of ACTH and cortisol levels. In addition to intravenous administration of hydrocortisone 100 mg every 6 hours, 3 litres of saline is given in 6 hours under careful cardiovascular monitoring. Concomitant infections, which are frequently present, require treatment.

Chronic adrenal insufficiency is treated by replacement therapy with daily oral hydrocortisone (10 mg/m^2 body surface area) and fludrocortisone (0.1 mg). Patients must be advised about the need to take lifelong glucocorticoid and mineralocorticoid replacement therapy. To prevent an Addisonian crisis, patients must be aware of the need to increase the dose in case of illness or stress. If patients with adrenal insufficiency are scheduled for surgery, appropriate steroid cover must be administrated.

DISORDERS OF THE ADRENAL MEDULLA AND NEURAL CREST-DERIVED TISSUE

Phaeochromocytoma and paraganglioma

Definition

These are tumours of the adrenal medulla and sympathetic ganglia that are derived from chromaffin cells and most commonly produce supraphysiological levels of circulating catecholamines.

Aetiology

The prevalence of phaeochromocytoma in patients with hypertension is 0.1–0.6% with an overall prevalence of 0.05% in autopsy series. In total, 4% of incidentalomas are

Thomas Addison, 1795–1860, physician, Guy's Hospital, London, England, described the effects of disease of the suprarenal capsules in 1852.
Caesar Peter Moller Boeck, 1845–1917, Professor of Medicine, The University of Oslo, Norway.
Samuel Alexander Kinnier Wilson, 1878–1936, Professor of Neurology, King's College Hospital, London, UK, described this condition in 1912.
Rupert Waterhouse, 1873–1958, physician, The Royal United Hospital, Bath, UK, described this syndrome in 1911.
Carl Friderichsen, 1886–1979, Medical Superintendent, Sundby Hospital, Copenhagen, Denmark, gave his account of the syndrome in 1918.

phaeochromocytomas. Sporadic phaeochromocytomas occur around the fourth decade, whereas patients with hereditary forms are diagnosed earlier. Phaeochromocytoma is known as the '10% tumour' as 10% of tumours are inherited, 10% are extra-adrenal, 10% are malignant, 10% are bilateral and 10% occur in children. With the recent advent of detailed genetic predisposition tests, however, the incidence of hereditary phaeochromocytomas has been shown to be higher.

Hereditary phaeochromocytomas occur in several tumour syndromes:

- **Multiple endocrine neoplasia type 2 (MEN 2)**: an autosomal dominant inherited disorder that is caused by activating germline mutations of the *RET* proto-oncogene.
- **Familial paraganglioma (PG) syndrome**: glomus tumours of the carotid body and extra-adrenal paraganglioma are characteristic in this hereditary tumour syndrome, which is caused by germline mutations within the succinate dehydrogenase complex subunit B (*SDHB*) *SDHD* and *SDHC* genes.
- **von Hippel–Lindau (VHL) syndrome**: those affected can develop early-onset bilateral kidney tumours, phaeochromocytomas, cerebellar and spinal haemangioblastomas and pancreatic tumours. Patients have a germline mutation in the *VHL* gene.
- **Neurofibromatosis (NF) type 1**: phaeochromocytomas in combination with fibromas on the skin and mucosae ('café-au-lait' skin spots) are indicative of a germline mutation in the *NF1* gene.

Pathology

Phaeochromocytomas are greyish-pink on the cut surface and are usually highly vascularised. Areas of haemorrhage or necrosis are often observed (**Figure 52.10**). Microscopically, tumour cells are polygonal but the configuration varies considerably. The differentiation between malignant and benign tumours is difficult, except when metastases are present. An increased PASS (**p**haeochromocytoma of the **a**drenal gland **s**cale **s**core), a high number of Ki-67-positive cells, vascular invasion or a breached capsule all lean more towards malignant rather than benign.

Phaeochromocytomas may also produce calcitonin, ACTH, vasoactive intestinal polypeptide (VIP) and parathyroid hormone-related protein (PTHrP). In patients with MEN 2, the onset of phaeochromocytoma is preceded by adrenomedullary hyperplasia, sometimes bilateral. Phaeochromocytoma is rarely malignant in MEN 2.

Clinical features

Symptoms and signs are caused by catecholamine excess and are typically intermittent (*Table 52.2*). In total, 90% of patients with the combination of headache, palpitations and sweating in the presence of an adrenal tumour have a phaeochromocytoma. Paroxysms may be precipitated by physical training, induction of general anaesthesia and numerous drugs and agents (contrast media, tricyclic antidepressive drugs, metoclopramide and opiates). Hypertension may occur continuously, be intermittent or absent. A subset of patients are asymptomatic. More than 25% of apparently sporadic phaeochromocytomas are caused by germline mutations in the *RET, SDHB, SDHC, SDHD* and *NF1* genes; genetic testing for these and other genes is therefore recommended, particularly in those patients aged under 50 years.

Diagnosis

The first step in the diagnosis of a phaeochromocytoma is the confirmation of excessive catecholamine levels in the patient either by the measurement of adrenaline and noradrenaline breakdown products, metanephrine and normetanephrine level, in a 12 or 24-hour urine collection, (levels that exceed the normal range by 2–40 times will be found in affected patients) or by determination of plasma-free metanephrine and normetanephrine levels. Biochemical tests should be performed at least twice. The biochemical diagnosis is then followed by localisation of the phaeochromocytoma. MRI is preferred because contrast media used for CT scans can provoke paroxysms. Classically, phaeochromocytomas show

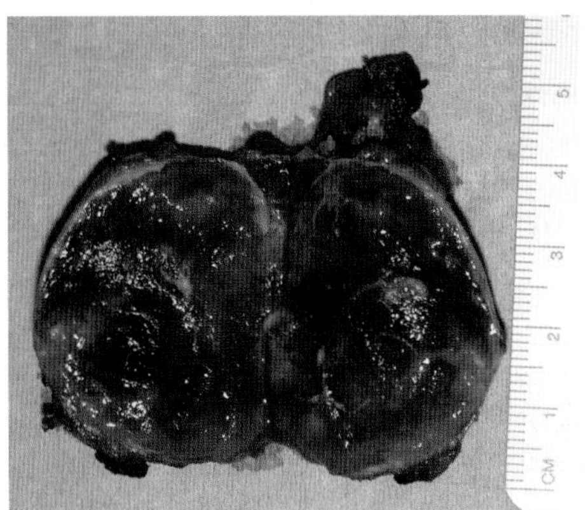

Figure 52.10 Gross appearance of a phaeochromocytoma.

TABLE 52.2 Clinical signs of phaeochromocytoma.

Symptoms	Prevalence (%)
Hypertension	80–90
Paroxysmal	50–60
Continuous	30
Headache	60–90
Sweating	50–70
Palpitation	50–70
Pallor	40–45
Weight loss	20–40
Hyperglycaemia	40
Nausea	20–40
Psychological effects	20–40

Eugen von Hippel, 1867–1939, Professor of Ophthalmology, Göttingen, Germany.
Arvid Lindau, 1892–1958, Professor of Pathology, Lund, Sweden.

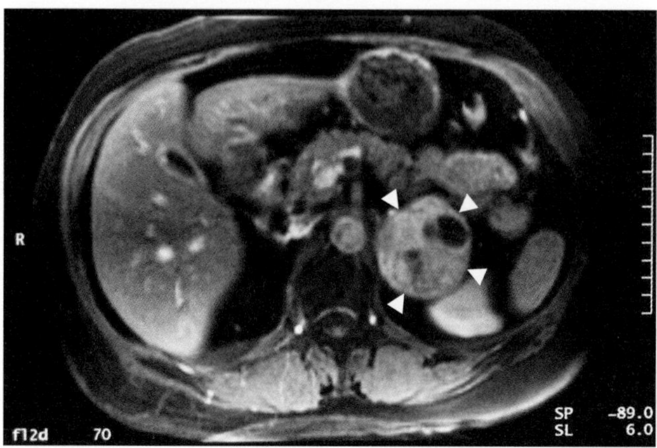

Figure 52.11 Magnetic resonance imaging of a sporadic phaeochromocytoma of the left adrenal gland (arrowheads).

a 'Swiss cheese' configuration (**Figure 52.11**). ^{123}I-MIBG (metaiodobenzylguanidine) single-photon emission computed tomography (SPECT) will identify about 90% of primary tumours and is essential for the detection of multiple extra-adrenal tumours and metastases (**Figure 52.12**). Positron emission tomography (PET) scanning using fluorodeoxyglucose (FDG) or dihydroxyphenylalanine (DOPA) is yet more sensitive in detecting metastatic foci.

Treatment

Laparoscopic resection is now routine in the treatment of phaeochromocytoma. If the tumour is larger than 8–10 cm or radiological signs of malignancy are detected, an open approach should be considered.

PREOPERATIVE

Once a phaeochromocytoma has been diagnosed, an α-adrenoreceptor blocker (phenoxybenzamine) is used to block the effects of catecholamine excess and its consequences during surgery. With adequate medical pretreatment, the perioperative mortality rate has decreased from 20–45% to less than 3%. A dose of 20 mg of phenoxybenzamine initially should be increased daily by 10 mg until a daily dose of 100–160 mg is achieved and the patient reports symptomatic postural hypotension. Additional β-blockade is required if tachycardia or arrhythmias develop; this should not be introduced until the patient is α-blocked.

With adequate α-blockade preoperatively, anaesthesia should not be more hazardous than in patients with a non-functioning adrenal tumour; however, in some patients, dramatic changes in heart rate and blood pressure may occur and require sudden administration of pressor or vasodilator agents. A central venous catheter and invasive arterial monitoring are used. Special attention is required when the adrenal vein is ligated as a sudden drop in blood pressure may occur. The infusion of large volumes of fluid or administration of noradrenaline can be necessary to correct postoperative hypotension in the presence of unopposed α-blockade.

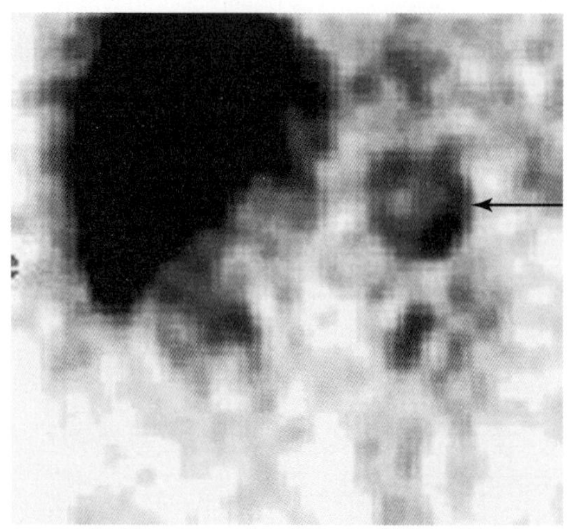

Figure 52.12 Meta-iodobenzylguanidine (MIBG) single-photon emission computed tomography scan of a phaeochromocytoma of the left adrenal gland (arrow) in the same patient as in Figure 52.11.

POSTOPERATIVE

Patients should be observed for 24 hours in the intensive care (ICU) or high dependancy unit as hypovolaemia and hypoglycaemia may occur. Lifelong yearly biochemical tests should be performed to identify recurrent, metastatic or metachronous phaeochromocytoma.

Summary box 52.4

Phaeochromocytoma

- Obtain a secure biochemical diagnosis
- Evaluate family history, refer to genetics if <50 years old
- Diagnosis confirmed, treat with α-blockers
- Plan surgical excision
- Yearly lifelong follow-up

Malignant phaeochromocytoma

Definition

Approximately 10% of phaeochromocytomas are malignant. This rate is higher in extra-adrenal tumours (paragangliomas). The diagnosis of malignancy implies metastases of chromaffin tissue, most commonly to lymph nodes, bone and liver.

Treatment

Surgical excision is the only chance for cure. Even in patients with metastatic disease, tumour debulking can be considered to reduce the tumour burden and to control the catecholamine excess. Symptomatic treatment can be obtained with α-blockers. Mitotane should be started as adjuvant or palliative treatment. Treatment with ^{131}I-MIBG or combination chemotherapy has resulted in a partial response in 30% and an improvement of symptoms in 80% of patients. The natural history is highly variable with a 5-year survival rate of less than 50%.

Phaeochromocytoma in pregnancy

Phaeochromocytomas in pregnancy may be silent and present as a hypertensive emergency, may mimic an amnion infection syndrome or pre-eclampsia. Without adequate α-blockade, mother and unborn child are threatened by hypertensive crisis during delivery. In the first and second trimesters the patient should be scheduled for laparoscopic adrenalectomy after adequate α-blockade; the risk of a miscarriage during surgery is high. In the third trimester, elective caesarean with delayed **consecutive** adrenalectomy 6 weeks later should be performed. The maternal mortality rate is 50% when a phaeochromocytoma remains undiagnosed.

Neuroblastoma

Definition

A neuroblastoma is a malignant tumour that is derived from the sympathetic nervous system in the adrenal medulla (38%) or from any site along the sympathetic chain in the paravertebral sites of the abdomen (30%), chest (20%) and, rarely, the neck or pelvis.

Pathology

Neuroblastomas have a pale and grey surface, are encapsulated and show areas with calcification. With increased tumour size, necrosis and haemorrhage may be detected. They are characterised by the presence of immature cells derived from the neuroectoderm of the sympathetic nervous system. Mature cells are found only in ganglioneuroblastomas.

Clinical features

Predominantly newborn infants and young children (<5 years of age) are affected. Symptoms are caused by tumour growth or by bone metastases. Patients present with a mass in the abdomen, neck or chest, proptosis, bone pain, painless bluish skin metastases, weakness or paralysis. Metastatic disease is present in 70% of patients at presentation.

Diagnosis

Biochemical evaluation should include urinary excretion (24-hour urine) of vanillylmandelic acid (VMA), homovanillic acid (HVA), dopamine and noradenaline, as increased levels are present in about 80% of patients. Accurate staging requires CT/MRI of the chest and abdomen, a bone scan, bone marrow aspiration and core biopsies as well as an MIBG scan. Staging is established according to the International Neuroblastoma Staging System (INSS).

Treatment

Prognosis can be predicted by the tumour stage and the age at diagnosis. Patients are classified as low, intermediate or high risk. Low-risk patients are treated by surgery alone (the addition of 6–12 weeks of chemotherapy is optional) whereas intermediate-risk patients are treated by surgery with adjuvant multiagent chemotherapy (carboplatin, cyclophosphamide, etoposide, doxorubicin). High-risk patients receive high-dose multiagent chemotherapy followed by surgical resection in responding tumours and myeloablative stem cell rescue. Patients assigned to the low-risk, intermediate-risk and high-risk groups have overall 3-year survival rates of 90%, 70–90% and 30%, respectively.

Ganglioneuroma

Definition

A ganglioneuroma is a benign neoplasm that arises from neural crest tissue. Ganglioneuromas can occur in the adrenal medulla and are characterised by mature sympathetic ganglion cells and Schwann cells in a fibrous stroma.

Clinical features

Ganglioneuroma is found in all age groups but is more common before the age of 60. Ganglioneuromas occur anywhere along the paravertebral sympathetic plexus and in the adrenal medulla (30%). Most often they are identified incidentally by CT or MRI performed for other indications.

Treatment

Treatment is by surgical excision, laparoscopic when adrenalectomy is indicated.

SURGERY OF THE ADRENAL GLANDS

Since its introduction in the 1990s, laparoscopic or retroperitoneoscopic adrenalectomy has become the ‘gold standard’ in the resection of adrenal tumours, except for tumours with signs of malignancy. The more popular approach is the laparoscopic transperitoneal approach, which offers a better view of the adrenal region than open surgery. The advantage of the retroperitoneoscopic approach is the minimal dissection required by this extra-abdominal procedure. In the case of small, bilateral tumours or in patients with hereditary tumour syndromes a subtotal resection is warranted, to avoid steroid dependence. The mortality rate ranges from 0% to 2% in specialised centres.

An open approach should be considered if radiological signs, distant metastases, large tumours (>8–10 cm) or a distinct hormonal pattern suggest malignancy.

Laparoscopic adrenalectomy

Knowledge of the anatomy of the adrenal region is essential as anatomical landmarks guide the surgeon during operation. If these landmarks are respected, injury to the vena cava or renal vein, the pancreatic tail or the spleen can be avoided. Careful haemostasis is essential as small amounts of blood can impair the surgeon’s view. To prevent tumour spillage, direct grasping of the adrenal tissue/tumour has to be avoided.

Theodor Schwann, 1810–1882, Professor of Anatomy, Louvain (1839–1848), and later at Liège (1852–1880), described the neurilemma in 1839.

Right adrenalectomy

The patient is positioned right side up, with table brake. Three ports are used to start. The dissection starts at the level of the periadrenal fat using careful coagulation and the peritoneum should be divided 2 cm below the edge of the liver from medial (IVC) to the lateral abdominal wall. This flap of peritoneum can then be used to retract the liver up and off the adrenal. A fourth port may be useful to hold the liver up. The gland is identified and mobilised gently, and the vein is secured with a clip or using one of the available energy devices; the gland is removed in a plastic catch bag (**Figure 52.13**).

Left adrenalectomy

With the patient positioned left side up, mobilisation of the spleen will displace it and the pancreatic tail medially. The incision of Gerota's fascia is followed by identification of the adrenal vein, which runs into the renal vein in the space between the medial aspect of the kidney and the posterior aspect of the pancreatic tail. The resection is completed by mobilising the adrenal gland at the level of the periadrenal fat. Remove the gland in a bag and close the 3 port sites after infiltrating each with local anaesthesia.

Retroperitoneoscopic adrenalectomy

The first port is placed at the distal end of the 12th rib with the patient in the prone position. After a digital dissection into the retroperitoneum, Gerota's fascia is displaced ventrally. The right adrenal vein is covered by the retrocaval posterior aspect of the adrenal gland. The left adrenal vein is usually located at the medial inferior pole of the adrenal gland. High inflation pressures allow bloodless dissection, effectively tamponading the veins. Being outside the abdominal cavity affords an excellent view.

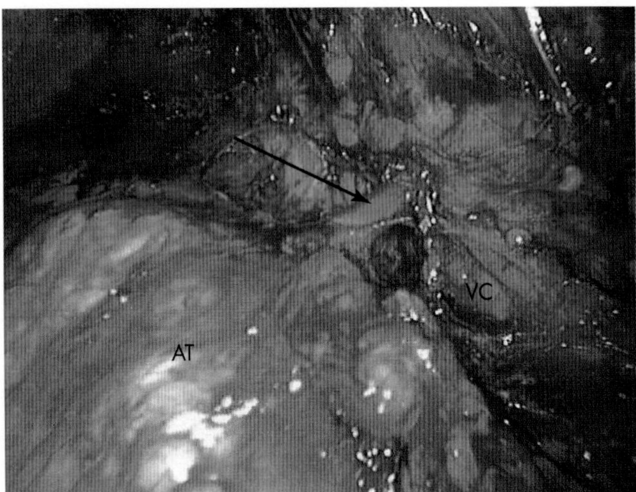

Figure 52.13 Laparoscopic view during a right adrenalectomy. Arrow indicates the adrenal vein. AT, adrenal tumour; VC, vena cava.

Open adrenalectomy

An open adrenalectomy is almost exclusively performed when a malignant adrenal tumour is suspected. On the right side the hepatic flexure of the colon is mobilised and the right liver lobe is cranially retracted to achieve an optimal exposure of the IVC and the adrenal gland. On the left side the adrenal gland can be exposed after mobilisation of the splenic flexure of the colon, through the transverse mesocolon or through the gastrocolic ligament. The remaining dissection is the same as in laparoscopic adrenalectomy. A resection of regional lymph nodes is recommended in malignant adrenal tumours and should include resection of the tissue between the renal pedicle and the diaphragm.

PANCREATIC ENDOCRINE TUMOURS

Introduction

Pancreatic endocrine tumours (PETs) represent an important subset of pancreatic neoplasms. They account for 5% of all clinically detected pancreatic tumours. They consist of single or multiple, benign or malignant neoplasms and are associated in 10–20% of cases with multiple endocrine neoplasia type 1 (MEN 1). PETs present as either functional tumours, causing specific hormonal syndromes, or non-functional tumours, with symptoms similar to those in patients with pancreatic adenocarcinoma. This section focuses on insulinomas, gastrinomas and non-functioning tumours because they represent 90% of all PETs (*Table 52.3*).

Function of the endocrine pancreas

The endocrine cells of the pancreas are grouped in the islets of Langerhans, which constitute approximately 1–2% of the mass of the pancreas (**Figure 52.14**). There are about one million islets in a healthy adult human pancreas and their combined weight is 1–1.5 g. There are four main types of cell in the islets of Langerhans, which can be classified according to their secretions:

- beta cells producing insulin (65–80% of the islet cells);
- alpha cells producing glucagon (15–20%);
- delta cells producing somatostatin (3–10%);
- pancreatic polypeptide (PP) cells containing polypeptide (1%).

Insulinoma

Definition

This is an insulin-producing tumour of the pancreas causing the clinical scenario know as Whipple's triad, i.e. symptoms of hypoglycaemia after fasting or exercise, plasma glucose levels <2.8 mmol/L and relief of symptoms on intravenous administration of glucose.

Paul Langerhans, 1847–1888, Professor of Pathological Anatomy, Freiberg, Germany.
George Hoyt Whipple, 1878–1976, Professor of Pathology, The University of Rochester, Rochester, NY, USA, described this disease in 1907. He shared the 1934 Nobel Prize for Physiology or Medicine with George Richards Minot and William Parry Murphy 'for their discoveries concerning liver therapy against anaemias'.

TABLE 52.3 Neuroendocrine tumours of the pancreas.

Tumour (syndrome)	Incidence (%)	Presentation	Malignancy (%)
Insulinoma	70–80	Weakness, sweating, tremor, tachycardia, anxiety, fatigue, dizziness, disorientation, seizures	<10
Gastrinoma	20–25	Intractable or recurrent peptic ulcer disease (haemorrhage, perforation), complications of peptic ulcer, diarrhoea	60–80
Non-functional tumours	30–50	Obstructive jaundice, pancreatitis, epigastric pain, duodenal obstruction, weight loss, fatigue	60–90
VIPoma	4	Profuse watery diarrhoea, hypotension, abdominal pain	80
Glucagonoma	4	Migratory necrolytic skin rash, glossitis, stomatitis, angular cheilitis, diabetes, severe weight loss, diarrhoea	80
Somatostatinoma	<5	Cholelithiasis, diarrhoea, neurofibromatosis	50
Carcinoid	<1	Flushing, sweating, diarrhoea, oedema	90
ACTHoma	<1	Cushing's syndrome	>90
GRFoma	<1	Acromegaly	30

ACTH, adrenocorticotrophic hormone; GRF, growth hormone-releasing factor; VIP, vasoactive intestinal polypeptide.

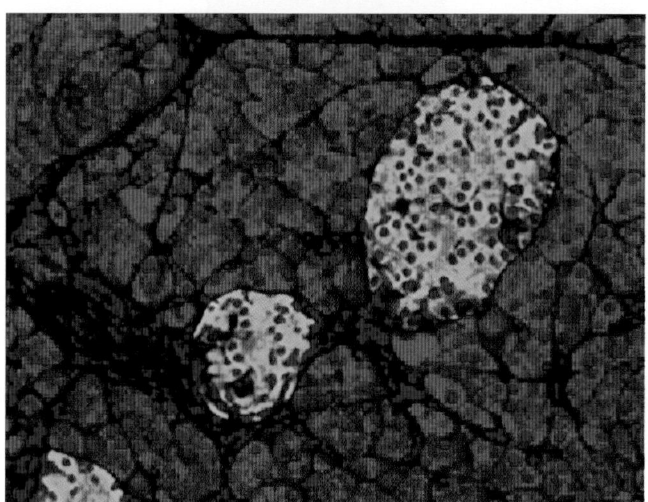

Figure 52.14 Immunofluorescent labelling of endocrine (insulin (green)) and exocrine (amylase (red)) pancreatic cells and the nuclear marker DAPI (blue) (courtesy of Dr Esni, Department of Surgery, University of Pittsburgh, USA).

Incidence

Insulinomas are the most frequent of all the functioning PETs with a reported incidence of 2–4 cases per million population per year. Insulinomas have been diagnosed in all age groups, with the highest incidence found in the fourth to the sixth decades. Women seem to be slightly more frequently affected.

Pathology

The aetiology and pathogenesis of insulinomas are unknown. No risk factors have been associated with these tumours. Virtually all insulinomas are located in the pancreas and tumours are equally distributed within the gland. Approximately 90% are solitary and about 10% are multiple and associated with MEN 1 syndrome.

Prognosis and predictive factors

No markers are available that reliably predict the biological behaviour of an insulinoma. Approximately 10% are malignant. Insulinomas of <2 cm in diameter without signs of vascular invasion or metastases are considered benign.

Clinical features

Insulinomas are characterised by fasting hypoglycaemia and neuroglycopenic symptoms. The episodic nature of the hypoglycaemic attacks is caused by intermittent insulin secretion by the tumour. This leads to central nervous system symptoms such as diplopia, blurred vision, confusion, abnormal behaviour and amnesia. Some patients develop loss of consciousness and coma. The release of catecholamines produces symptoms such as sweating, weakness, hunger, tremor, nausea, anxiety and palpitations.

Biochemical diagnosis

A fasting test that may last for up to 72 hours is regarded as the most sensitive test. Usually, insulin, proinsulin, C-peptide and blood glucose are measured in 1- to 2-hour intervals to demonstrate inappropriately high secretion of insulin in relation to blood glucose. About 80% of insulinomas are diagnosed by this test, most of them in the first 24 hours. Elevated C-peptide levels demonstrate the endogenous secretion of insulin and exclude factitious hypoglycaemia caused by insulin injection.

Differential diagnosis

The differential diagnosis of hypoglycaemia includes hormonal deficiencies, hepatic insufficiency, medication, drugs and enzyme defects. Occasionally, differentiating insulinoma from other causes of hypoglycaemia can be difficult. Nesidioblastosis is a rare disorder, mainly encountered in children, which is characterised by replacement of normal pancreatic islets by diffuse hyperplasia of islet cells.

Medical treatment of insulinoma

Medical management is reserved only for patients who are unable or unwilling to undergo surgical treatment or for unresectable metastatic disease. Diazoxide suppresses insulin secretion by direct action on the beta cells and offers reasonably good control of hypoglycaemia in approximately 50%

of patients. When surgical options to treat malignant insulinomas cannot be applied, chemotherapeutic options include doxorubicin and streptozotocin.

Surgical treatment of insulinoma

INDICATIONS FOR OPERATION

After a positive fasting test and exclusion of diffuse abdominal metastases by ultrasound or CT scan, all patients should be advised to undergo surgical excision of insulinoma.

PREOPERATIVE LOCALISATION STUDIES

Intraoperative exploration of the pancreas is the best method to use for localisation of insulinoma yet the operating surgeon will need preoperative localisation. Insulinomas are detected in about 65% of cases by endoscopic ultrasound (EUS), 33% of cases by CT scan and abdominal ultrasound and 15% of cases by magnetic resonance tomography. Intraoperative ultrasound (IOUS) of the pancreas is a vital tool after mobilisation of the gland. For preoperative localisation of an insulinoma, EUS has the highest sensitivity and should be used if laparoscopic resection is considered. If no lesion is identified and one can rely on the biochemical tests for diagnosis, laparotomy should follow, using IOUS.

BENIGN INSULINOMA

Surgical cure rates in patients with the biochemical diagnosis of insulinoma range from 90% to 100%. At open surgery an extended Kocher manoeuvre and mobilisation of the head and then the distal pancreas is performed to explore the whole gland. IOUS should then be used to confirm the presence of a tumour, to find non-palpable lesions and also to identify the relation of the tumour to the pancreatic duct (**Figure 52.15a**). Tumour enucleation is the technique of choice (**Figure 52.15b**). For superficial tumours, laparoscopic enucleation is undertaken (**Figure 52.16**). Tumours located deep in the body or tail of the pancreas and those in close proximity to the pancreatic duct require distal pancreatectomy. Postoperatively, blood sugar levels begin to rise in most patients within the first few hours after removal of the tumour. To preserve pancreatic function and reduce the risk of iatrogenic diabetes mellitus, patients in whom tumour localisation is not successful at operation should not undergo blind resection.

MALIGNANT INSULINOMA

Aggressive attempts at resection are recommended as these tumours are much less virulent than adenocarcinomas.

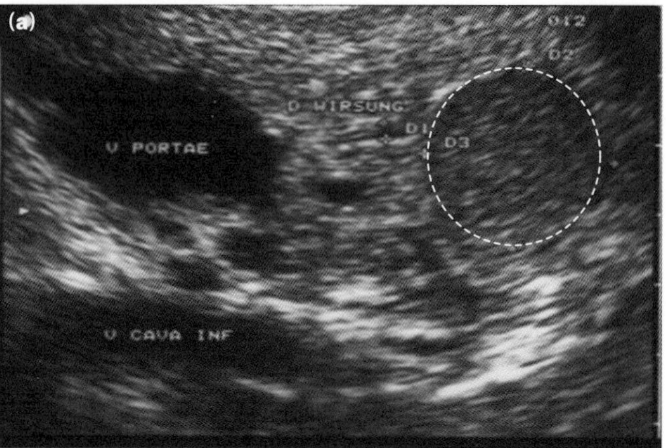

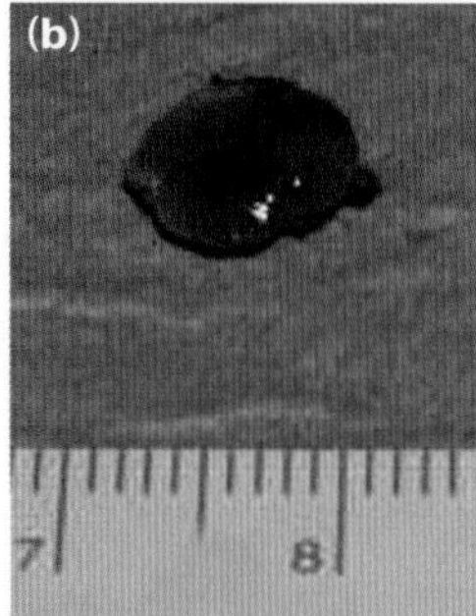

Figure 52.15 **(a)** Intraoperative ultrasound showing a typical insulinoma (dashed circle). d wirsung, pancreatic duct; v cava inf, inferior vena cava; v portae, portal vein. **(b)** Enucleated insulinoma.

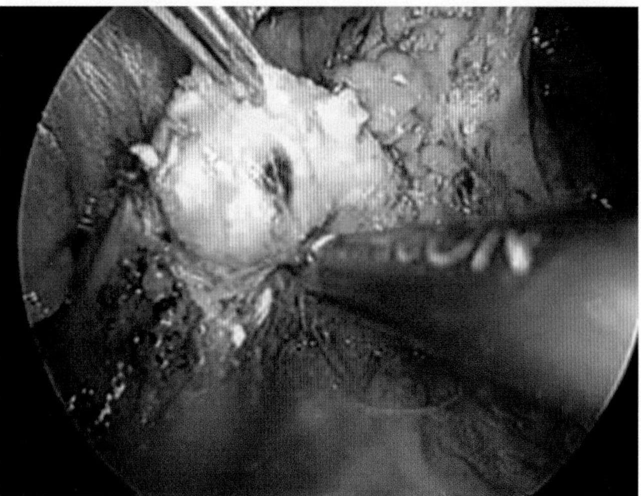

Figure 52.16 Laparoscopic enucleation of an insulinoma.

Gastrinoma (Zollinger-Ellison syndrome)

Definition

Zollinger–Ellison syndrome (ZES) is a condition that includes: (1) fulminating ulcer diathesis in the stomach, duodenum or atypical sites; (2) recurrent ulceration despite 'adequate' therapy; and (3) non-beta islet cell tumours of the pancreas (gastrinoma).

Theodor Kocher, 1841–1917, Professor of Surgery, Berne, Switzerland, awarded the Nobel Prize for Physiology or Medicine in 1909, 'for his work on the physiology, pathology, and surgery of the thyroid gland.'

Robert Milton Zollinger, 1903–1992, Professor of Surgery, The Ohio State University, Columbus, OH, USA.

Edwin Homer Ellison, 1918–1970, Professor of Surgery, Marquette University, WI, USA. Zollinger and Ellison described this condition in a joint paper in 1955 when they were both working at The Ohio State University.

Incidence

Gastrinomas account for about 20% of PET. Approximately 0.1% of patients with duodenal ulcers have evidence of ZES. The reported incidence is between 0.5 and 4 cases per million population per year. ZES is more common in males than in females. The mean age at the onset of symptoms is 38 years, and the range 7–83 years.

Pathology

The aetiology and pathogenesis of sporadic gastrinomas are unknown. At the time of diagnosis more than 60% of tumours are malignant. Pancreatic gastrinomas are mainly found in sporadic disease; most are found in the head of the pancreas. More than 70% of the gastrinomas in MEN 1 syndrome and most sporadic gastrinomas are located in the first and second part of the duodenum. Therefore, the anatomical area comprising the head of the pancreas, the superior and descending portion of the duodenum and the relevant lymph nodes has been called the 'gastrinoma triangle' because it harbours the vast majority of these tumours (Figure 52.17). All patients with gastrinomas should be tested for MEN 1 syndrome.

Prognosis and predictive factors

In general, the progression of gastrinomas is relatively slow with a 5-year survival rate of 65% and a 10-year survival rate of 51%. Patients with complete tumour resection have excellent 5- and 10-year survival rates (90–100%). Patients with pancreatic tumours have a worse prognosis than those with primary tumours in the duodenum. There is no established marker to predict the biological behaviour of gastrinoma.

Clinical and biochemical features

Over 90% of patients with gastrinomas have peptic ulcer disease, often multiple or in unusual sites. Diarrhoea is another common symptom, caused by the large volume of gastric acid secretion. Abdominal pain from either peptic ulcer disease or gastro-oesophageal reflux disease (GORD) remains the most common symptom, occurring in more than 75% of patients.

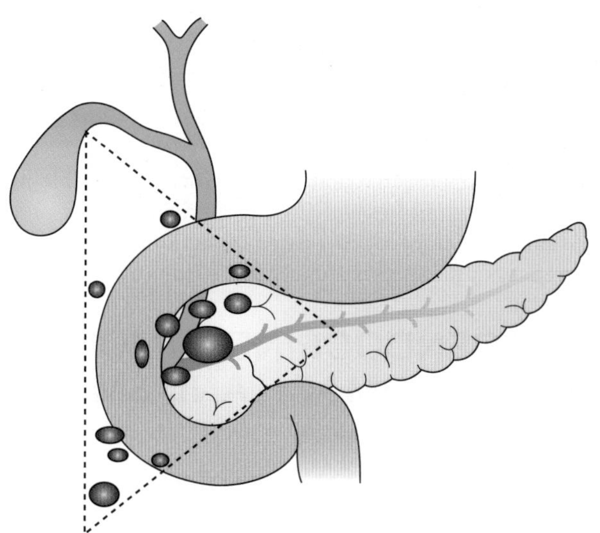

Figure 52.17 The gastrinoma triangle.

Biochemical diagnosis

If the patient presents with a gastric pH below 2.5 and a serum gastrin concentration above 1000 pg/mL (normal <100 pg/mL) then the diagnosis of ZES is confirmed. Unfortunately, the majority of patients have serum gastrin concentrations between 100 and 500 pg/mL and in these patients a secretin test should be performed. The secretin test is considered positive if an increase in serum gastrin of >200 pg/mL over the pretreatment value is obtained; this also rules out other causes of hypergastrinaemia (e.g. atrophic gastritis).

Differential diagnosis

The most common misdiagnoses are idiopathic peptic ulcer disease, chronic idiopathic diarrhoea and GORD. Other reasons for hypergastrinaemia are chronic atrophic gastritis, gastric outlet stenosis and retained antrum after gastric resection.

Medical treatment of gastrinoma

In most patients with ZES, gastric hypersecretion can be treated effectively with proton pump inhibitors. Octreotide can also help to control acid hypersecretion. Systemic chemotherapy is utilised in patients with diffuse metastatic gastrinomas. Streptozotocin in combination with 5-fluorouracil or doxorubicin is the first-line treatment.

Surgical treatment of gastrinoma

INDICATIONS FOR OPERATION

Surgical exploration should be performed in all patients without diffuse metastases, to remove known malignant gastrinomas or benign ones.

PREOPERATIVE LOCALISATION STUDIES

Pancreatic gastrinomas are often larger than 1 cm in diameter, whereas gastrinomas of the duodenum are usually smaller. Therefore, it is nearly impossible to identify duodenal gastrinomas by preoperative imaging. Pancreatic gastrinomas are detected by endoscopic ultrasound in about 80–90% of cases, by CT in 39% of cases and by MRI in 46% of cases. In approximately one-third of patients the results of conventional imaging studies are negative. On the basis of recent studies, either endoscopic ultrasound or CT and somatostatin receptor scintigraphy (SRS) scan should be performed preoperatively for staging.

PANCREATIC GASTRINOMAS

Most pancreatic gastrinomas are solitary, located in the head of the gland or uncinate process, and can be identified at operation. Enucleation with peripancreatic lymph node dissection is the procedure of choice. Rarely, tumours are situated in the body or tail and should be treated by enucleation or distal resection. Even if a tumour is found in the pancreas, duodenotomy is recommended to detect additional tumours, if the patient has MEN 1.

DUODENAL GASTRINOMAS

The duodenum should be opened with a longitudinal incision and the posterior and anterior walls palpated separately (Figure 52.18). Duodenal tumours smaller than 5 mm can

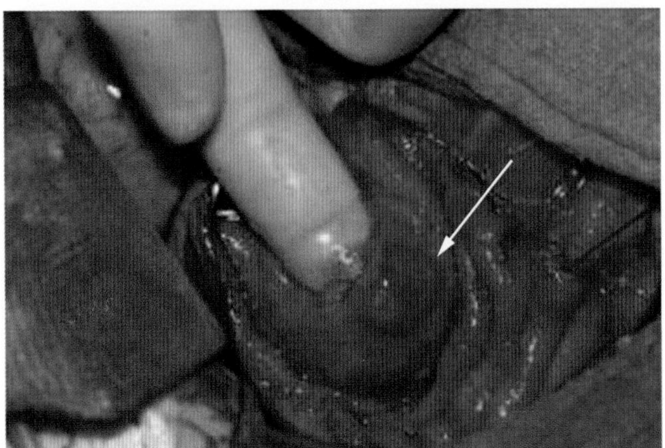

Figure 52.18 Palpation of a duodenal gastrinoma (arrow) after duodenotomy.

be enucleated with the overlying mucosa; larger tumours are excised with full-thickness excision of the duodenal wall.

Non-functional endocrine pancreatic tumours

Definition

PETs are clinically classified as non-functioning (NF-PETs) when they do not cause a clinical syndrome.

Incidence

NF-PETs account for 30–50% of all PETs. They are most often diagnosed in the fifth to sixth decades of life.

Pathology

NF-PETs cannot be differentiated from functional tumours by immunocytochemistry because they may also express hormones such as gastrin, insulin, etc. They usually stain positively for chromogranin A and synaptophysin. The tumours are usually large (>5 cm) and unifocal except in MEN 1 syndrome. They are distributed throughout the pancreas with a head to body to tail ratio of 7:1:1.5.

Prognosis and predictive factors

About 70% of all NF-PETs are malignant. Overall 5- and 10-year survival rates of 65% and 49% respectively have been described. When comparing NF-PETs with functioning PETs, the NF-PETs have a worse prognosis.

Clinical features

Patients usually present late because of the lack of a clinical/hormonal marker of tumour activity. Therefore, in contrast to functioning PETs, patients with NF-PETs present with various non-specific symptoms, including jaundice, abdominal pain, weight loss and pancreatitis. In some cases liver metastases are the first presentation.

Biochemical diagnosis

Increased levels of chromogranin A have been reported in 50–80% of NF-PETs; the level of chromogranin A sometimes correlates with the tumour burden. The combination of elevated chromogranin A and PP measurements increases the sensitivity of diagnosis from 84% to 96% in NF-PETs.

TABLE 52.4 Differences between pancreatic cancer and non-functioning endocrine pancreatic tumours (NF-PETs).

	Pancreatic cancer	NF-PETs
Tumour size	<5 cm	>5 cm
CT scan	Hypodensity	Hyperdensity
	No calcifications	Calcifications possible
Chromogranin A in blood	Negative	Positive
Somatostatin receptor scintigraphy	Negative	Positive

CT, computed tomography.

Differential diagnosis

Differentiation from the more aggressive pancreatic adenocarcinoma is extremely important (*Table 52.4*). Recognition of NF-PETs is imperative because of their resectability and excellent long-term survival compared with their exocrine counterparts.

Medical treatment of non-functioning islet cell tumours

When surgical excision is not possible, chemotherapeutic options include streptozotocin, octreotide and interferon.

Surgical treatment of non-functioning islet cell tumours

INDICATIONS FOR OPERATION

An aggressive surgical approach should be considered in malignant NF-PETs, even in the presence of distant metastases.

PREOPERATIVE LOCALISATION STUDIES

Preoperative ultrasound or CT scan are the procedures of choice as these tumours are relatively large. Also, SRS should be performed to differentiate endocrine from non-endocrine pancreatic tumours.

OPERATIVE PROCEDURES

The major goal is a potentially curative resection. This may require partial pancreaticoduodenectomy as well as the synchronous or metachronous resection of liver metastases. Using an aggressive approach, curative resections are possible in up to 62% of cases and overall 5-year survival rates of around 65% can be achieved. Repeated resections for resectable recurrences or metastases are justified to improve survival.

NEUROENDOCRINE TUMOURS OF THE STOMACH AND SMALL BOWEL

Definition and physiology

Neuroendocrine tumours (NET) of the gut and the pancreas arise from the diffuse neuroendocrine cell system, which can be found as single or clustered cells in the mucosa of the bronchi, stomach, gut, biliary tree, urogenital system and in the pancreas (see Chapters 72 and 73 for NET of the appendix and rectum respectively). This cell system was first recognised as the 'clear cell system' by Feyrter in the 1930s and is identical to the APUD (amine precursor uptake and decarboxylation) system described by Pearse in 1970. All cells of the system secrete different neuroendocrine markers, such as synaptophysin, chromogranin A and neurone-specific enolase (NSE), and produce peptide hormones that are stored in granules, e.g. serotonin, somatostatin, PP or gastrin. In clinical practice chromogranin A is utilised as a tumour marker. The main functional test for NET of the jejunum and ileum (the NET that are most often encountered) is the measurement of the serotonin metabolite 5-hydroxyindoleacetic acid (5-HIAA) in urine.

Pathology

Neuroendocrine cells can form hyperplasias or tumours. Oberndorfer coined the term 'carcinoids' for tumours arising from these cells in 1907. Although the term carcinoid continues to be used in clinical practice, these tumours do not always grow in a well-differentiated pattern reflecting the rather benign 'carcinoma-like', i.e. 'carcinoid' tumour. They can show different growth patterns, from benign tumours to high-grade undifferentiated carcinomas having a poor prognosis (neuroendocrine carcinomas). Therefore, they should always be addressed as NET, including a description of their histological pattern (benign, low- or high-grade malignant) and their anatomical site (e.g. stomach, ileum) according to the World Health Organization (WHO) classification (2000). The relative distribution of NET in different organs is given in *Table 52.5*. Another classification based on embryological principles classifies NET as foregut (lung, stomach, pancreas), midgut (small bowel and appendix) and hindgut (colon and rectum) tumours.

TABLE 52.5 Relative distribution of neuroendocrine tumours in different organs.

Site	Distribution (%)
Lung	10
Stomach	5
Duodenum	2
Small bowel	25
Appendix	40
Colon	6
Rectum	15

Neuroendocrine tumours of the stomach

These tumours are rare. They comprise about 5% of all NET of the gastrointestinal tract and have an incidence of approximately 0.2 cases per 100 000 population per year. There are four different types of gastric NET (*Table 52.6*). Types 1 and 2 are small benign tumours that arise from the enterochromaffin-like (ECL) cells in the gastric mucosa and grow in either a linear or a nodular pattern (**Figure 52.19**). Hypergastrinaemia may cause symptoms and the treatment of choice is

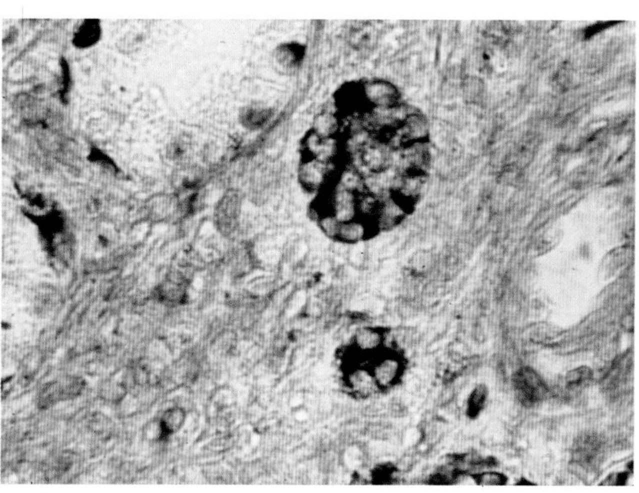

Figure 52.19 Immunostaining of chromogranin in micronodular hyperplasia of enterochromaffin-like (ECL) cells of the stomach, associated with chronic atrophic gastritis.

TABLE 52.6 Classification of gastric neuroendocrine tumours.

Type	Histological pattern	Size and location	Causative factor and prognosis
1	Benign, non-functional, well differentiated	Gastric corpus; <1 cm; mucosa/submucosa	ECLomas in chronic atrophic gastritis, hypergastrinaemia
2	Benign or low-grade malignant, differentiated	1–2 cm; angioinvasion; mucosa/submucosa	ECLomas with hypergastrinaemia as a result of gastrinoma in MEN 1
3	Low-grade malignant, differentiated	2 cm; invasion beyond submucosa	Sporadic ECLomas not related to hypergastrinaemia
4	Intermediate or small cell type, high-grade malignant (neuroendocrine carcinoma)	Different sizes	Causative factor unknown; prognosis poor

ECL, enterochromaffin-like; MEN, multiple endocrine neoplasia.

Anthony Guy Everson Pearse, 1916–2003, Professor of Histochemistry, The Royal Postgraduate Medical School, Hammersmith, London, UK.

endoscopic resection. Types 3 and 4 are almost always malignant and surgical resection should be undertaken if possible.

Pathogenesis, diagnosis and treatment

Type 1 tumours (ECLomas) are the most frequent NET of the stomach (approximately 80%); they occur mostly in elderly women. Chronic hypergastrinaemia is the result of chronic atrophic gastritis and achlorhydria, the alkaline pH being the stimulus for hypersecretion of gastrin. They do not cause symptoms and are usually detected during gastroscopy for other reasons. Endoscopic resection is the treatment of choice. Antrectomy and resection of ECLomas should be undertaken only if there is recurrent disease and multiple (more than six) tumours, with at least one measuring >1 cm and infiltration of at least one into the submucosa.

The pathogenesis, diagnosis and treatment of type 2 tumours is similar to that of type 1. The only difference is the cause of the hypergastrinaemia, which in type 2 tumours is the result of MEN 1 syndrome, with multiple gastrinomas in the duodenum or, rarely, in the pancreas.

Type 3 tumours are rare, sporadic and solitary tumours of unknown origin. Serum gastrin is normal; upper gastrointestinal bleeding is the usual symptom that leads to endoscopy. Type 3 tumours are usually larger than 2 cm and often have lymph node and liver metastases at the time of diagnosis. Gastrectomy and lymph node dissection and resection of liver metastases is the treatment of choice. Liver metastases can also be treated by chemoembolisation.

Type 4 tumours present as large ulcerating malignancies similar to adenocarcinomas and should be treated accordingly. The prognosis of types 3 and 4 is poor (*Table 52.6*).

Neuroendocrine tumours of the small bowel

Introduction

These are the tumours that are most commonly referred to as 'carcinoid' tumours, as most NET of the gastrointestinal tract are found in the small bowel. They are also called 'midgut' tumours (together with NET of the appendix and the right colon). These tumours produce serotonin and cause the 'carcinoid' syndrome, but only in patients who have a large volume of liver metastases or if there is advanced local tumour growth draining into the IVC and thereby bypassing the liver. NET of the duodenum (gastrinomas in MEN 1 syndrome, somatostatinomas and others) are very rare and are not discussed further.

Pathology

NET of the jejunum and ileum arise from a subgroup of cells of the diffuse neuroendocrine system, the enterochromaffin (EC) cells, which secrete serotonin and substance P. They are either solitary or more often multiple, are almost always malignant and metastasise early to the regional lymph nodes and the liver depending on the location of the primary tumour(s) (**Figure 52.20**).

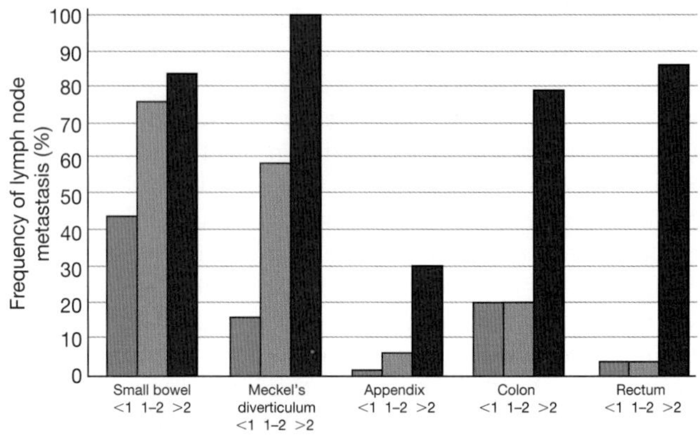

Figure 52.20 Relation of site and diameter of neuroendocrine tumours of the gut to frequency of lymph node metastasis.

Clinical symptoms

Symptoms that lead to the diagnosis are caused by either the primary tumour or its lymph node metastases. Acute or chronic, recurrent or persistent abdominal pain, ileus or, rarely, lower gastrointestinal bleeding may occur. Symptoms may be due to liver metastases, such as sudden painful reddening of the face and chest ('flushing'), diarrhoea or bronchospasm. These symptoms constitute 'carcinoid' syndrome. About 60% of patients eventually develop cardiac symptoms because of stenosis and insufficiency of the pulmonary and, more rarely, the tricuspid valve, with enlargement and thickening of the wall of the right atrium. The aetiology is unknown but local effects of serotonin and kinins may contribute.

Abdominal symptoms are caused either by obstruction of the appendix by an appendiceal NET (leading to appendectomy) or by obstruction of the mesentery or the bowel lumen by growth of lymph node metastases in the mesentery near the bowel. Pain is caused by chronic ischaemia of the bowel (**Figure 52.21**), resulting not only from mesenteric lymph

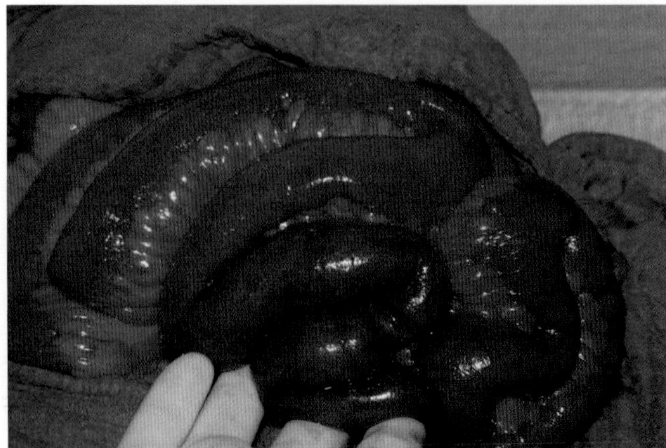

Figure 52.21 Chronic ischaemia of the small bowel caused by desmoplastic reaction and narrowing of vessels in the mesentery in a neuroendocrine tumour of the ileum.

Johann Friedrich Meckel (The Younger), 1781–1833, Professor of Anatomy and Surgery, Halle, Germany.

node metastases but also from constriction of mesenteric arteries and fibrosis of the mesentery by a so-called desmoplastic reaction.

Primary tumours in the jejunum and ileum rarely cause symptoms such as bleeding or intussusception as they usually only measure from a few millimetres up to 1 cm or at the most 2 cm in diameter (Figure 52.22). A polypoid NET of the terminal ileum may, however, cause ileocaecal intussusception.

Diagnosis

The diagnosis of NET of the small bowel is made by history, physical examination of the abdomen, imaging and an assessment of 5-HIAA in a 24-hour urine sample. It is positive in larger tumours only if metastases are present. Cross-sectional imaging, sonography, CT scan and MRI may show the primary tumour, mesenteric lymph node and liver metastases.

The best method for staging of NET is an octreotide (SRS) scan. This will show all tumour deposits provided that they are large enough and have a high somatostatin receptor density (Figure 52.23).

Surgical procedure

Surgery should be undertaken as soon as the diagnosis is made, even in the presence of liver metastases. The main goal is resection of the bowel primary tumour(s) and mesenteric lymph node metastases. This may entail resection of large amounts of bowel (100 cm or more), particularly if stage III or IV lymph node masses are found in the mesentery (Figure 52.24). In the presence of liver metastases, extrahepatic disease should be resected whenever possible. Metastatic disease in the mesenteric root will lead to long-term pain in the abdomen or back and to a poor quality of life, whereas liver metastases can be treated by chemotherapy or embolisation.

Somatostatin and its analogues provide symptomatic treatment of the 'carcinoid' syndrome caused by a large volume of liver metastases. These drugs may also have an antiproliferative effect. Surgery to remove liver metastases is possible in approximately 10% of patients. In others, embolisation, chemoembolisation, SRS using radioactively labelled octreotide, chemotherapy, biotherapy and also liver transplantation can be performed.

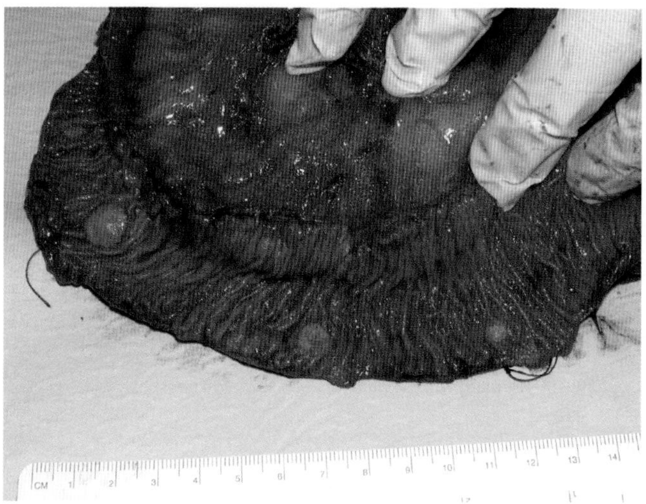

Figure 52.22 Multiple neuroendocrine tumours in the small bowel causing large lymph node metastases in the mesentery.

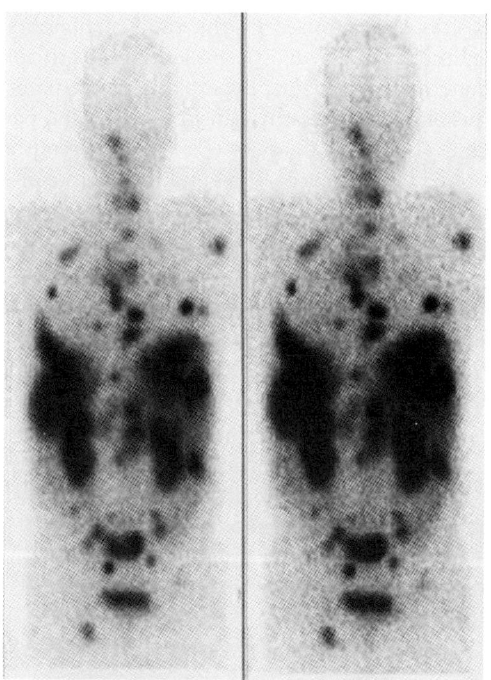

Figure 52.23 Octreotide scan of a patient with neuroendocrine tumour of the gut and diffuse metastases in different organs.

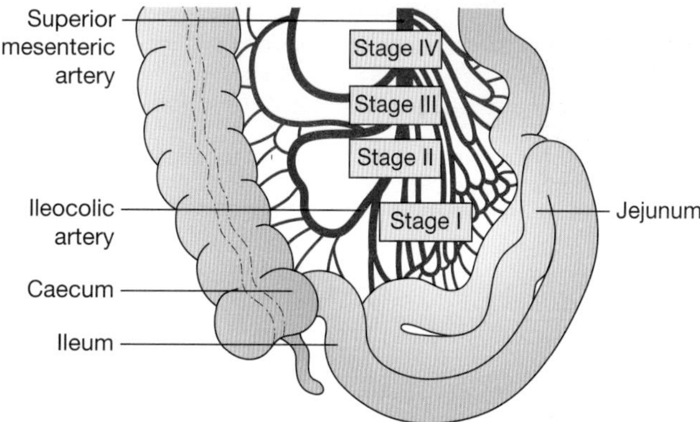

Figure 52.24 Bulky lymph node metastases can occur at different levels in the mesentery. To resect them completely, long segments of bowel must be resected, the closer to the mesenteric root the metastases are situated (adapted from Akerström G, Hellman P, Öhrvall U. Midgut and hindgut carcinoid tumours. In: Doherty GM, Skogseid B (eds.). *Surgical endocrinology*. Philadelphia, PA: Lippincott Williams & Wilkins, 2001, by kind permission.).

MULTIPLE ENDOCRINE NEOPLASIAS

Introduction

Multiple endocrine neoplasias (MEN) are inherited syndromes characterised by a combination of benign and malignant tumours in different endocrine glands. There are two main types, type 1 (MEN 1) and type 2 (MEN 2). The mode of inheritance is autosomal dominant in both.

MEN 1 is characterised by the triad of tumours in the anterior pituitary gland, mostly presenting as prolactinomas or non-functioning tumours, hyperplasia of the parathyroids causing primary hyperparathyroidism (pHPT) and pancreaticoduodenal endocrine tumours (PETs). The syndrome was first described by Wermer in 1954 and is therefore also called Wermer's syndrome. It is caused by germline mutations in the *menin* gene, located on chromosome 11.

MEN 2 is divided into three subtypes: familial medullary thyroid carcinoma (FMTC), MEN 2A and MEN 2B. Medullary thyroid carcinoma (MTC) plays the key role in all subtypes. MEN 2 is caused by germline mutations in the *RET* proto-oncogene, located on chromosome 10. MEN 2A is characterised by the combination of MTC, pHPT and mostly bilateral phaeochromocytomas. MTC combined with phaeochromocytoma alone is called Sipple's syndrome. FMTC is characterised by distinct mutations in *RET* and MTC alone as the clinical manifestation. MEN 2B comprises MTC, phaeochromocytoma and characteristic facial and oral mucosal neurinomas (**Figure 52.25**) and intestinal ganglioneuromatosis, accompanied by a Marfanoid habitus.

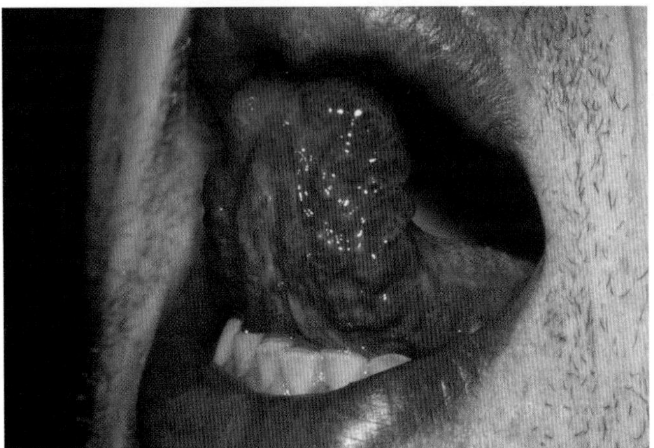

Figure 52.25 Neurinomas of the tongue in a patient with multiple endocrine neoplasia type 2B.

The most important difference between MEN 1 and MEN 2, besides the different clinical pictures, is that MEN 2 is characterised by a well-understood genotype–phenotype correlation. This means that depending on the particular mutation in the *RET* proto-oncogene, the phenotypic appearance and the onset of endocrine tumours will be different and can be predicted from the type of mutation. This is not the case in MEN 1 syndrome.

Multiple endocrine neoplasia type 1

Epidemiology

The prevalence of the syndrome is estimated to be around 0.04–0.2 cases per 1000 population per year. The penetrance is high with almost 100% of mutation carriers developing the syndrome. The disease is equally distributed between men and women.

Clinical presentation

The clinical presentation depends on the affected organs. Tumours can occur synchronously (*Table 52.7*). Most of the mutation carriers identified in screening programmes are asymptomatic.

TABLE 52.7 Affected organs in multiple endocrine neoplasia type 1.

Endocrine gland affected	Frequency (%)	Hormone	Clinical syndrome
Parathyroids	90	PTH	pHPT
Pancreas, duodenum (mostly multiple)	50–80		
Gastrinoma		Gastrin	Zollinger–Ellison syndrome
Insulinoma		Insulin	Hypoglycaemia syndrome
Non-functioning tumours		PP	–
VIPoma		VIP	Verner–Morrison syndrome
Glucagonoma		Glucagon	Glucagonoma syndrome
Anterior pituitary gland	30–60		
Prolactinoma		Prolactin	Galactorrhea
Non-functioning adenoma		–	Non-specific
Other manifestations			
Adrenals	40–50 Cortisol?	Mostly non-functioning	
NET in lung, thymus, stomach	3–10	–	–
Lipoma	5–10	–	–

NET, neuroendocrine tumours; pHPT, primary hyperparathyroidism; PP, pancreatic polypeptide; PTH, parathyroid hormone; VIP, vasoactive intestinal polypeptide.

Paul Wermer, 1898–1975, physician, The Presbyterian Hospital, New York, NY, USA, described this condition in 1954.
John H Sipple, b.1930, physician, The State University of New York, New York, NY, USA.
John V Verner, b.1927 and **Ashton B Morrison**, 1922–2008, at Duke University, USA, described the features of watery diarrhoea and hypokalaemia in 1958 and subsequently linked their observations with hyperplasia of non-beta islet cells of the pancreas in 1974.

PARATHYROIDS

In total, 90–100% of patients suffering from MEN 1 develop pHPT and it is usually the first manifestation of the disease. MEN 1 pHPT is characterised by multiglandular disease so that all four parathyroids become hyperplastic in the course of the disease. The clinical presentation of MEN 1 pHPT is similar to that of the sporadic disease. Few patients have asymptomatic disease; most common in symptomatic disease is nephrolithiasis. Diagnosis is established by determination of parathyroid hormone (PTH) and calcium in serum and urine.

ENDOCRINE PANCREAS

PETs occur in around 50–60% of MEN 1 patients. In such patients taking part in screening programmes, 70–90% are found to have non-functioning and functioning PETs. This high rate of detection of PETs is the result of the improvement in diagnostic procedures in the last decade, including EUS. MEN 1 PETs are the most common syndrome-associated cause of death. They are mostly multiple and often recur after surgery. Although most patients have multiple tumours, one hormone syndrome is usually dominant. The most common functional tumour is gastrinoma followed by insulinoma. VIPomas, glucagonomas and somatostatinomas are extremely rare. Non-functioning tumours can be asymptomatic for many years.

The diagnostic work-up is similar to that for sporadic PETs and includes hormone measurements, e.g. gastrin, insulin, PP, etc. and imaging.

ANTERIOR PITUITARY GLAND

Tumours of the anterior pituitary gland are found in 30–60% of patients with MEN 1. These are mostly microadenomas that present as prolactinomas or non-functioning tumours. Most prolactinomas can be treated with medication, thus avoiding operation.

ADRENAL TUMOURS AND OTHER ORGAN MANIFESTATIONS

Adrenal involvement is common in MEN 1 patients and affects nearly 40–50% of patients. Mostly non-functioning adenomas are found. Very rarely, adrenocortical carcinomas or phaeochromocytomas may develop.

Although very rare, manifestations of MEN 1 include NET of the lung, thymus, stomach, duodenum and small bowel. It is important to check for NETs of the thymus, as they are mostly malignant.

Genetic screening

Identification of the MEN 1 (*menin*) gene in 1997 formed the basis for direct mutational analysis of the gene and for family screening. After genetic counselling of the index patient, family members can be screened. Mutation carriers can then be included in screening programmes that make early detection of endocrine tumours possible. Screening programmes should follow the consensus guidelines published by Brandi *et al*. in 2001. In cases of apparently sporadic endocrine tumours in patients younger than 40 years, genetic testing for MEN 1 is advised.

Operative therapy

PARATHYROIDS

The indications for surgery in MEN 1 pHPT follow the same criteria as in sporadic disease but the choice of procedure is different. As multiglandular disease is present in all cases, resection follows the same rules as in secondary HPT. Therefore, the most common procedures are total parathyroidectomy, including cervical thymectomy or 31/2-gland resection, leaving approximately 50 mg of parathyroid tissue behind, and cervical thymectomy. Selective resection of enlarged glands is obsolete because of the high rates of recurrence (see Chapter 51).

ENDOCRINE PANCREAS

Indications for surgery and its extent are controversial. Most experts agree that MEN 1 gastrinoma and insulinoma have to be operated on to prevent liver metastases and to control hormonal excess, provided that diffuse liver metastases are not present. MEN 1 gastrinomas are more often located in the duodenum as multiple small tumours than in the pancreas. For gastrinomas located in the duodenum or pancreatic head (gastrinoma triangle, Figure 52.17), pylorus-preserving partial pancreaticoduodenectomy is recommended. In rare cases the gastrinoma is located in the body or tail of the pancreas. In such cases distal pancreatectomy with excision of tumours in the pancreatic head is the procedure of choice. In MEN 1 insulinoma the standard operative procedure is distal pancreatectomy with enucleation of tumours in the pancreatic head. Non-functioning PETs are operated on if they reach a size of 1 cm. Careful palpation and IOUS are essential in every pancreatic procedure for MEN 1 PETs.

ANTERIOR PITUITARY GLAND

The indications for surgery in tumours of the anterior pituitary gland are the presence of symptomatic non-functional tumours or if medical therapy of prolactinoma fails. Most procedures can be performed through a trans-sphenoidal approach.

ADRENAL TUMOURS

Functional adrenal tumours in MEN 1 are rare and have to be operated on. Non-functioning tumours should be resected if they reach a size of 4 cm. Pre- and perioperative management follow the same rules as in sporadic adrenal tumours; therefore, phaeochromocytoma has to be ruled out in every patient. In most cases a laparoscopic or retroperitoneoscopic approach can be used. If there is evidence for a malignant tumour, open surgery is preferred.

Multiple endocrine neoplasia type 2

In most patients with MEN 2A, the disease is caused by mutations of the *RET* proto-oncogene in codon 634. MTC is almost always the first manifestation of the syndrome. If phaeochromocytoma and pHPT do not occur, one must suspect the presence of the FMTC subtype. Patients with MEN 2B do not develop pHPT and in 95% of cases mutations in codon 918 of the *RET* proto-oncogene are causative (*Table 52.8*).

TABLE 52.8 Frequency of diseases in multiple endocrine neoplasia type 2 related to mutation in different codons.

Syndrome	Frequently affected codons in *RET*	MTC (%)	pHPT (%)	PCC (%)
FMTC	533, 630, 768, 844	90–100	–	–
MEN 2A	609, 634, 790, 804	90–100	20–30	10–50
MEN 2B	883, 918	100	–	10–50

FMTC, familial medullary thyroid cancer; MEN 2A, multiple endocrine neoplasia type 2A; MEN 2B, multiple endocrine neoplasia type 2B; MTC, medullary thyroid cancer; PCC, phaeochromocytoma; pHPT, primary hyperparathyroidism; *RET*, *RET* proto-oncogene (*RET* = rearranged during transfection).

Medullary thyroid carcinoma

MTC is characterised by multicentricity and is often accompanied by C-cell hyperplasia. These characteristics should lead to molecular diagnostic work-up (mutational analysis of the *RET* proto-oncogene) in patients with apparently 'sporadic' MTC. In contrast to sporadic MTC, the diagnosis in families with known mutation of the *RET* gene is mostly made much earlier, possibly as the result of mutational screening and calcitonin measurements. MTC is most aggressive in MEN 2B. It occurs in early childhood, much earlier than in MEN 2A, with lymph node metastases present in the early stages. Preventative surgery is advised around the age of 1 year.

Primary hyperparathyroidism

pHPT in MEN 2A is less common and has a milder clinical course than MEN 1 pHPT. It occurs in about 20–30% of patients with MEN 2A. Most patients are asymptomatic but all parathyroid glands can become hyperplastic, mostly metachronously. The disease develops after the third decade of life typically.

Phaeochromocytoma

The frequency of phaeochromocytoma in MEN 2 is around 10–50% and tumours can be bilateral. This can occur synchronously or metachronously. The tumours are almost always benign. Diagnostic work-up includes measurement of urinary catecholamines, abdominal CT or MRI and 131I-MIBG scintigraphy (see above).

Operative therapy

MEDULLARY THYROID CARCINOMA

Operative therapy for MEN 2 MTC in patients detected by genetic screening is a good example of efficient prophylactic surgery, as the likelihood of developing MTC is 100% for most mutations. The mutation carriers can be operated on with no evidence of tumour in the thyroid, protecting them from MTC for the rest of their lives. Different *RET* mutations are associated with early or late onset of the disease. Risk groups have been defined to determine the appropriate age for thyroidectomy (*Table 52.9*).

PHAEOCHROMOCYTOMA

The operative approach is laparoscopy or retroperitoneoscopy. Unilateral or bilateral subtotal resection may be feasible, which retains the healthy part of the gland and prevents postoperative dependence on cortisol and mineralocorticoid supplementation (see above) (**Figure 52.26**). Further phaeochromocytomas can develop in the remnants that are left, so continued surveillance is required.

PRIMARY HYPERPARATHYROIDISM

The clinical situation in MEN 2 pHPT is even more difficult than in MEN 1 pHPT because of the association with MTC in MEN 2. During neck surgery for MTC in a eucalcaemic patient, enlarged parathyroid glands should be removed. In cases in which neck surgery has already been performed for MTC, the surgical approach to MEN 2A pHPT should be more tailored to the individual patient. For example, in an older patient after thyroidectomy for MTC with mild asymptomatic hypercalcaemia, localisation procedures and a targeted approach may be appropriate.

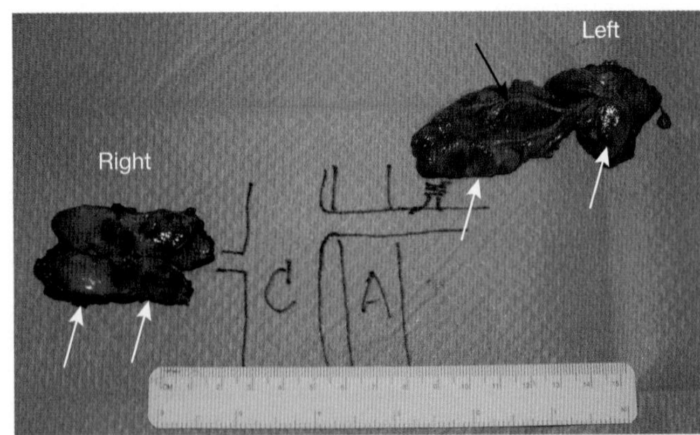

Figure 52.26 Bilateral multiple phaeochromocytomas in a patient with multiple endocrine neoplasia type 2A. A, aorta; C, vena cava; white arrows, tumours; black arrow, normal adrenal.

TABLE 52.9 Prophylactic thyroidectomy for medullary thyroid cancer depending on the site of mutation of the *RET* proto-oncogene in multiple endocrine neoplasia type 2 patients with normal calcitonin levels.

	Risk group		
	High	Medium	Low
Codon	883, 918, 922	609, 611, 618, 620, 634	768, 790, 791, 804, 891
Thyroidectomy at age (years)	<1	6	<20

FURTHER READING

Allolio B, Fassnacht M. Clinical review: adrenocortical carcinoma: clinical update. *J Clin Endocrinol Metab* 2006; **91**: 2027–37.

Assié G, Letouzé E, Fassnacht M *et al.* Integrated genomic characterization of adrenocortical carcinoma. *Nat Genet* 2014; **46**(6): 607–12.

Bartsch DK, Fendrich V, Langer P *et al.* Outcome of duodenopancreatic resections in patients with multiple endocrine neoplasia type 1. *Ann Surg* 2005; **242**: 757–64.

Brandi ML, Gagel RF, Angeli A *et al.* Guidelines for diagnosis and therapy of MEN type 1 and type 2. *J Clin Endocrinol Metab* 2001; **86**: 5658–71.

Hardy R, Lennard TWJ. Subtotal adrenalectomy. *Br J Surg* 2008; **95**: 1075–6.

Fendrich V, Langer P, Celik I *et al.* An aggressive surgical approach leads to long-term survival in patients with pancreatic endocrine tumors. *Ann Surg* 2006; **244**: 845–51.

Gaujoux S, Bonnet S, Leconte M *et al.* Risk factors for conversion and complications after unilateral laparoscopic adrenalectomy. *Br J Surg* 2011; **98**: 1392–9.

Ilias I, Pacak K. Diagnosis and management of tumors of the adrenal medulla. *Horm Metab Res* 2005; **37**: 717–21.

Madani R, Al-Hashmi M, Bliss R, Lennard TWJ. Ectopic phaeochromocytoma: does the rule of 10 apply? *World J Surg* 2007; **31**: 849–54.

Muth A, Hammarstedt L, Hellstrom M *et al.* Cohort study of patients with adrenal lesions discovered incidentally. *Br J Surg* 2011; **98**: 1383–91.

Norton JA, Fraker DL, Alexander HR *et al.* Surgery increases survival in patients with gastrinoma. *Ann Surg* 2006; **244**: 410–19.

Walz MK, Alesina PF, Wenger FA *et al.* Posterior retroperitoneoscopic adrenalectomy: results of 560 proceedures in 520 patients. *Surgery* 2006; **140**: 943–8.

Young WF Jr. Clinical practice: the incidentally discovered adrenal mass. *New Engl J Med* 2007; **356**: 601–10.

Chapter 53

The breast

Learning objectives

To understand:

- Appropriate investigation of breast disease
- Breast anomalies and the complexity of benign breast disease
- The modern management of breast cancer

COMPARATIVE AND SURGICAL ANATOMY

The protuberant part of the human breast is generally described as overlying the second to the sixth ribs and extending from the lateral border of the sternum to the anterior axillary line. Actually, a thin layer of mammary tissue extends considerably further, from the clavicle above to the seventh or eighth ribs below, and from the midline to the edge of the latissimus dorsi posteriorly. This fact is important when performing a mastectomy, the aim of which is to remove the whole breast. The anatomy of the breast is illustrated in **Figure 53.1**.

The **axillary tail** of the breast is of surgical importance. In some normal subjects it is palpable and, in a few, it can be seen premenstrually or during lactation. A well-developed axillary tail is sometimes mistaken for a mass of enlarged lymph nodes or a lipoma.

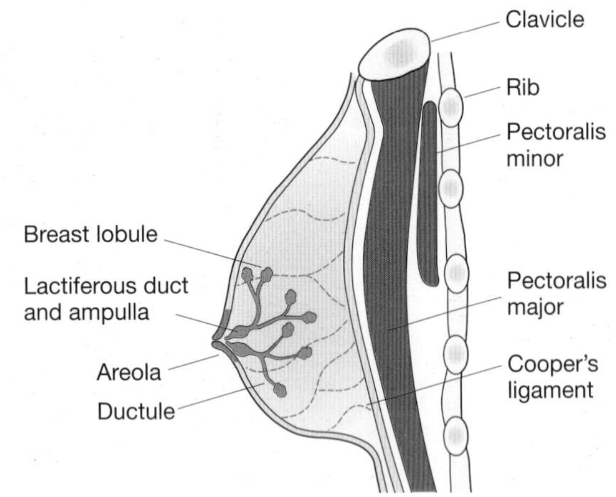

Figure 53.1 Cross-sectional anatomy of the breast.

The **lobule** is the basic structural unit of the mammary gland. The number and size of the lobules vary enormously: they are most numerous in young women. From 10 to over 100 lobules empty via ductules into a lactiferous duct, of which there are 15–20. Each lactiferous duct is lined with a spiral arrangement of contractile myoepithelial cells and is provided with a terminal ampulla, a reservoir for milk or abnormal discharges.

The **ligaments of Cooper** are hollow conical projections of fibrous tissue filled with breast tissue; the apices of the cones are attached firmly to the superficial fascia and thereby to the skin overlying the breast. These ligaments account for the dimpling of the skin overlying a carcinoma.

The **areola** contains involuntary muscle arranged in concentric rings as well as radially in the subcutaneous tissue. The areolar epithelium contains numerous sweat glands and sebaceous glands, the latter of which enlarge during pregnancy and serve to lubricate the nipple during lactation (Montgomery's tubercles).

The **nipple** is covered by thick skin with corrugations. Near its apex lie the orifices of the lactiferous ducts. The nipple contains smooth muscle fibres arranged concentrically and longitudinally; thus, it is an erectile structure, which points outwards.

The **lymphatics** of the breast drain predominantly into the axillary and internal mammary lymph nodes. The axillary nodes receive approximately 85% of the drainage and are arranged in the following groups:

- **lateral**, along the axillary vein;

Sir Astley Paston Cooper, 1768–1841, surgeon, Guy's Hospital, London, UK, described these ligaments in 1845.
William Fetherston Montgomery, 1797–1859, obstetrician, Dublin, Ireland, described these tubercles in 1837.

- **anterior**, along the lateral thoracic vessels;
- **posterior**, along the subscapular vessels;
- **central**, embedded in fat in the centre of the axilla;
- **interpectoral**, a few nodes lying between the pectoralis major and minor muscles;
- **apical**, which lie above the level of the pectoralis minor tendon in continuity with the lateral nodes and which receive the efferents of all the other groups.

The apical nodes are also in continuity with the supraclavicular nodes and drain into the subclavian lymph trunk, which enters the great veins directly or via the thoracic duct or jugular trunk. The **sentinel node** is defined as the first lymph node draining the tumour-bearing area of the breast. The importance of the sentinel node is described later.

The internal mammary nodes are fewer in number. They lie along the internal mammary vessels deep to the plane of the costal cartilages, drain the posterior third of the breast and are not routinely dissected, although they were at one time biopsied for staging.

INVESTIGATION OF BREAST SYMPTOMS

Although an accurate history and clinical examination are important methods of detecting breast disease, there are a number of investigations that can assist in the diagnosis. Examination precedes palpation and requires careful observation of the patient both with the arms at rest and also elevated to lift the breast. Small lesions may betray their presence by dimpling or minor distortions when the patient moves.

Mammography

Soft tissue radiographs are taken by placing the breast in direct contact with ultrasensitive film and exposing it to low-voltage, high-amperage x-rays (Figure 53.2). The dose of radiation is approximately 0.1 cGy and, therefore, mammography is a very safe investigation. The sensitivity of this investigation increases with age as the breast becomes less dense. In total, 5% of breast cancers are missed by population-based mammographic screening programmes; even in retrospect, such carcinomas are not apparent. Thus, a normal mammogram does not exclude the presence of carcinoma. Digital mammography is being introduced, which allows manipulation of the images and computer-aided diagnosis. Tomo-mammography is also being assessed as a more sensitive diagnostic modality.

Ultrasound

Ultrasound is particularly useful in young women with dense breasts in whom mammograms are difficult to interpret, and in distinguishing cysts from solid lesions (Figures 53.3 and 53.4). It can also be used to localise impalpable areas of breast

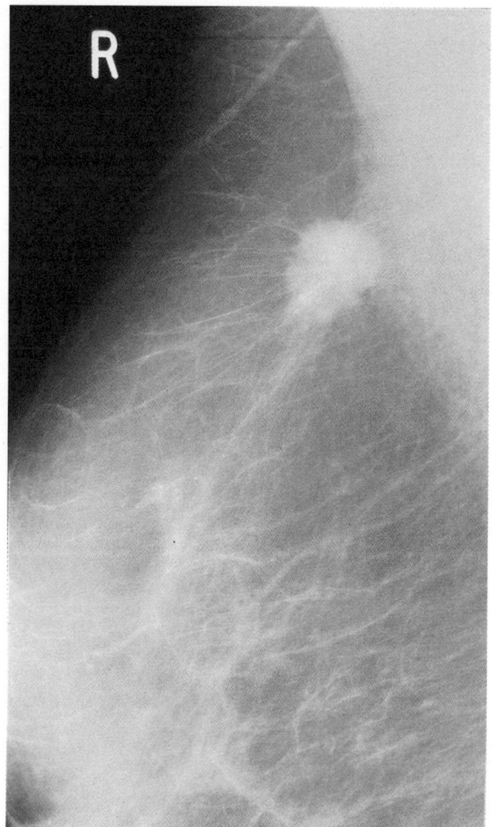

Figure 53.2 Mammogram showing a carcinoma.

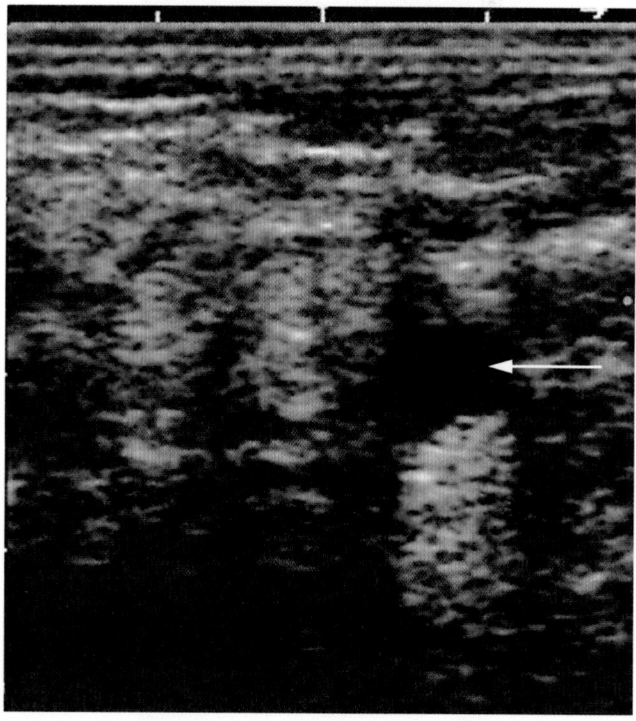

Figure 53.3 Ultrasound of the breast showing a cyst (arrow).

Gy is short for Gray, the SI unit for the absorbed dose of ionising radiation.
Louis Harold Gray, 1905–1965, Director, The British Empire Cancer Campaign Research Unit in Radiobiology, Mount Vernon Hospital, Northwood, Middlesex, UK.

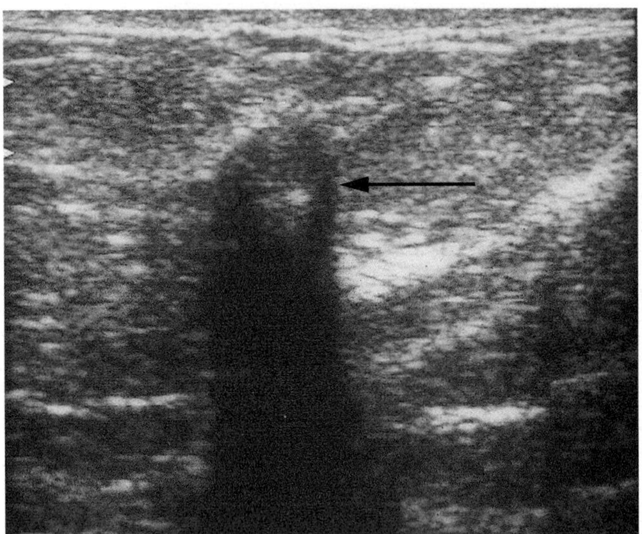

Figure 53.4 Ultrasound of the breast showing a carcinoma (arrow).

pathology. It is not useful as a screening tool and remains operator dependent. Increasingly, ultrasound of the axilla is performed when a cancer is diagnosed, with guided percutaneous biopsy of any suspicious glands.

Magnetic resonance imaging

Magnetic resonance imaging (MRI) (Figure 53.5) of the breast is useful in a number of settings:

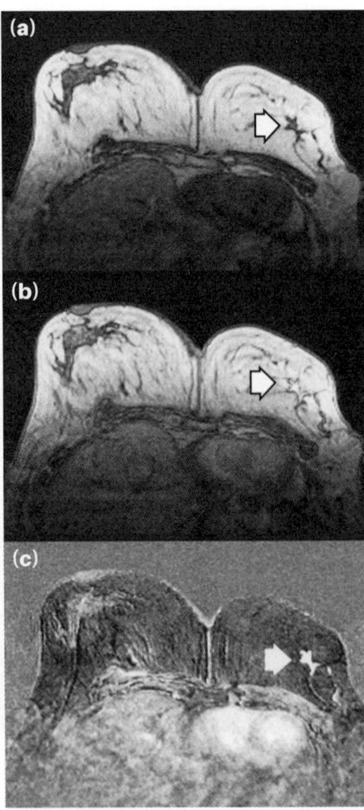

Figure 53.5 Magnetic resonance imaging scan of the breasts showing carcinoma of the left breast (arrows). (a) Precontrast; (b) postgadolinium contrast; (c) subtraction image.

- to distinguish scar from recurrence in women who have had previous breast conservation therapy for cancer (although it is less accurate within 9 months of radiotherapy because of abnormal enhancement);
- to assess multifocality and multicentricity in lobular cancer and to assess the extent of high-grade ductal carcinoma *in situ* (DCIS). It is less useful in low-grade DCIS;
- it is the best imaging modality for the breasts of women with implants;
- as a screening tool in high-risk women (because of family history).

Although biopsies can be performed with MRI guidance, this is complicated by the configuration of the imaging system. With improved ultrasound equipment, an MRI-detected lesion can often be found on a second-look ultrasound and biopsied using this modality.

Needle biopsy/cytology

Histology can be obtained under local anaesthesia using a springloaded core needle biopsy device (Figure 53.6). Cytology is obtained using a 21G or 23G needle and 10-mL syringe with multiple passes through the lump with negative pressure in the syringe. The aspirate is then smeared on to a slide, which is air dried or fixed (Figure 53.7). Fine-needle

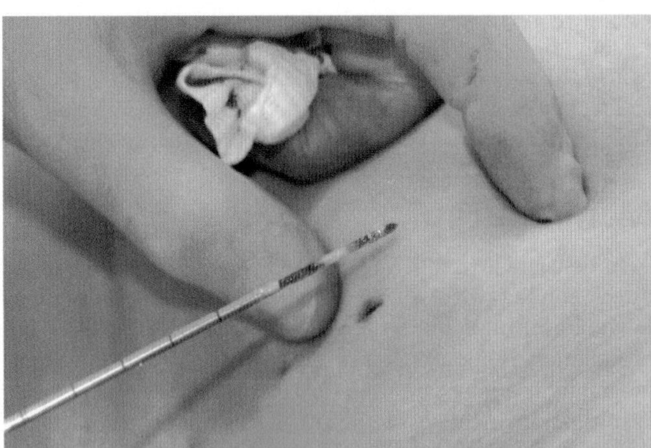

Figure 53.6 Corecut biopsy of breast.

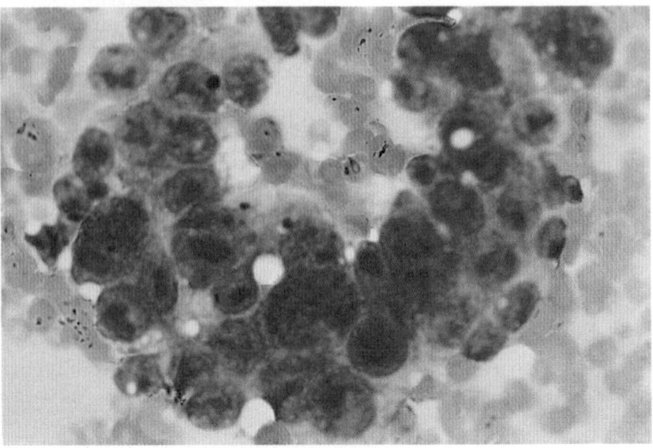

Figure 53.7 Fine-needle aspiration cytology showing grade III ductal carcinoma cells.

aspiration cytology (FNAC) is the least invasive technique of obtaining a cellular diagnosis and is rapid and very accurate if both operator and cytologist are experienced. However, false negatives do occur, mainly through sampling error, and invasive cancer cannot be distinguished from *in situ* disease. A histological specimen taken by core biopsy allows a definitive preoperative diagnosis, differentiates between DCIS and invasive disease and also allows the tumour to be stained for receptor status. This is important before commencing neoadjuvant therapy.

Large-needle biopsy with vacuum systems

The sampling error decreases as the biopsy volume increases and using 8G or 11G needles allows more extensive biopsies to be taken. This is useful in the management of microcalcifications or in the complete excision of benign lesions such as fibroadenomas.

Triple assessment

In any patient who presents with a breast lump or other symptoms suspicious of carcinoma, the diagnosis should be made by a combination of clinical assessment, radiological imaging and a tissue sample taken for either cytological or histological analysis (Figure 53.8), the so-called triple assessment. The positive predictive value (PPV) of this combination should exceed 99.9%.

THE NIPPLE

Absence of the nipple is rare and is usually associated with amazia (congenital absence of the breast).

Supernumerary nipples are not uncommon and occur along a line extending from the anterior fold of the axilla to the fold of the groin (Figure 53.9). This constitutes the milk line of lower mammals. Rarely, there is duplication of the nipple on a normal areola.

Nipple retraction

This may occur at puberty or later in life. Retraction occurring at puberty, also known as **simple nipple inversion**, is of unknown aetiology (benign horizontal inversion). In about 25% of cases it is bilateral. It may cause problems with breast-feeding and infection can occur because of retention of secretions, especially during lactation. Recent retraction of the nipple may be of considerable pathological significance. A slit-like retraction of the nipple may be caused by duct ectasia and chronic periductal mastitis (Figure 53.10a), but circumferential retraction, with or without an underlying lump, may well indicate an underlying carcinoma (Figure 53.10b).

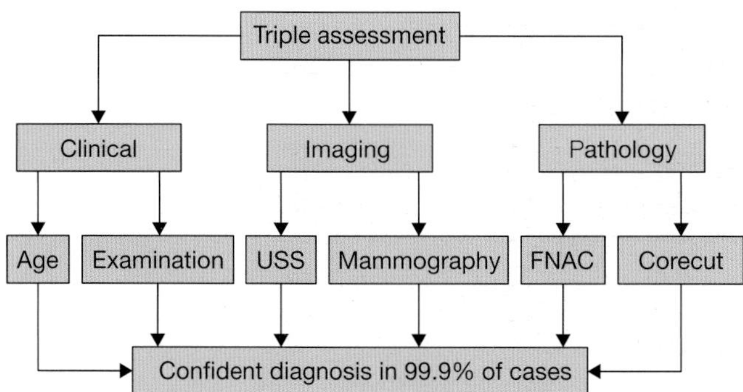

Figure 53.8 Triple assessment of breast symptoms. FNAC, fine-needle aspiration cytology; USS, ultrasound scan.

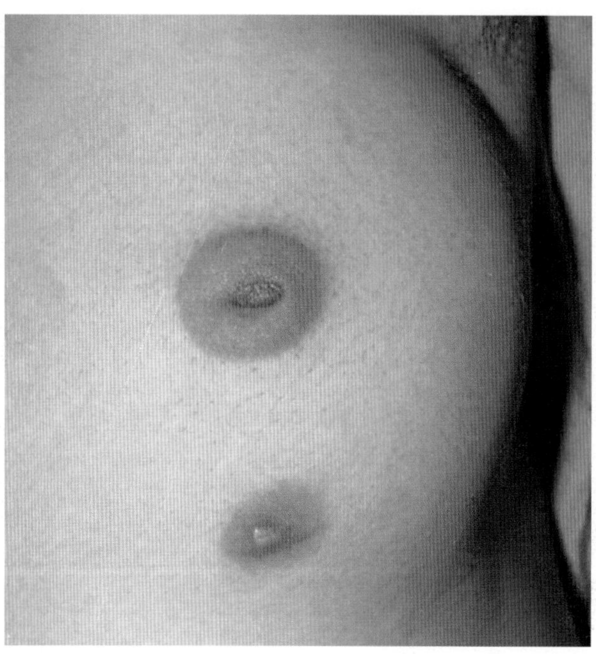

Figure 53.9 Accessory nipple with congenital retraction of the normal nipple.

Treatment

Treatment is usually unnecessary and the condition may spontaneously resolve during pregnancy or lactation.

Simple cosmetic surgery can produce an adequate correction but has the drawback of dividing the underlying ducts. Mechanical suction devices have been used to evert the nipple, with some effect.

Cracked nipple

This may occur during lactation and be the forerunner of acute infective mastitis. If the nipple becomes cracked during lactation, it should be rested for 24–48 hours and the breast should be emptied with a breast pump. Feeding should be resumed as soon as possible.

Papilloma of the nipple

Papilloma of the nipple has the same features as any cutaneous papilloma and should be excised with a tiny disc of skin. Alternatively, the base may be tied with a ligature and the papilloma will spontaneously fall off.

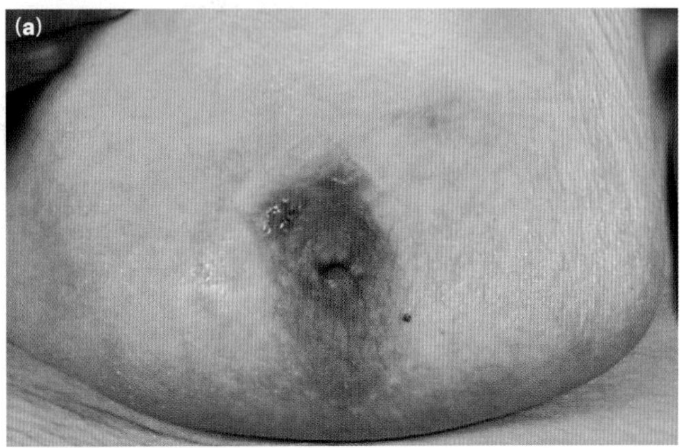

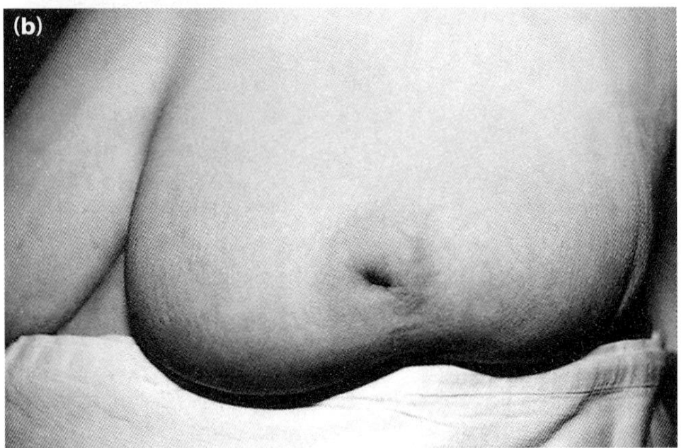

Figure 53.10 Recent nipple retraction. **(a)** Slit-like retraction of duct ectasia with mammary duct fistula. **(b)** Circumferential retraction with underlying carcinoma.

Retention cyst of a gland of Montgomery

These glands, situated in the areola, secrete sebum and if they become blocked a sebaceous cyst forms.

Eczema

Eczema of the nipples is a rare condition and is often bilateral; it is usually associated with eczema elsewhere on the body. It is treated with 0.5% hydrocortisone (not a stronger steroid preparation).

Paget's disease

Paget's disease of the nipple must be distinguished from eczema. The former is caused by malignant cells in the subdermal layer and is usually associated with a carcinoma within the breast. Eczema tends to occur in younger people who have signs of eczema elsewhere (look at the antecubital fossae).

Discharges from the nipple

Discharge can occur from one or more lactiferous ducts. Management depends on the presence of a lump (which should always be given priority in diagnosis and treatment) and the presence of blood in the discharge or discharge from a single duct. Mammography is rarely useful except to exclude an underlying impalpable mass. Cytology may reveal malignant cells but a negative result does not exclude a carcinoma or *in situ* disease.

A **clear, serous discharge** may be 'physiological' in a parous woman or may be associated with a duct papilloma or mammary dysplasia. Multiduct, multicoloured discharge is physiological and the patient may be reassured.

- A **blood-stained discharge** may be caused by duct ectasia, a duct papilloma or carcinoma. A duct papilloma is usually single and situated in one of the larger lactiferous ducts; it is sometimes associated with a cystic swelling beneath the areola.
- A **black or green discharge** is usually the result of duct ectasia and its complications.

Summary box 53.1

Discharges from the nipple (the principal causes are in bold)

Discharge from the surface
- Paget's disease
- Skin diseases (eczema, psoriasis)
- Rare causes (e.g. chancre)

Discharge from a single duct

Blood-stained:
- **Intraduct papilloma**
- **Intraduct carcinoma**
- Duct ectasia

Serous (any colour):
- **Fibrocystic disease**
- **Duct ectasia**
- Carcinoma

Discharge from more than one duct

Blood-stained:
- **Carcinoma**
- Ectasia
- Fibrocystic disease

Black or green:
- **Duct ectasia**

Purulent:
- **Infection**

Serous:
- **Fibrocystic disease**
- Duct ectasia
- Carcinoma

Milk:
- **Lactation**
- Rare causes (hypothyroidism, pituitary tumour)

Sir James Paget, 1814–1899, surgeon, St. Bartholomew's Hospital, London, UK, described this disease of the nipple in 1874.

Treatment

Treatment must firstly be to exclude a carcinoma by occult blood test and cytology. Simple reassurance may then be sufficient but, if the discharge is proving intolerable, an operation to remove the affected duct or ducts can be performed (microdochectomy).

MICRODOCHECTOMY

It is important not to express the blood before the operation as it may then be difficult to identify the duct in theatre. A lacrimal probe or length of stiff nylon suture is inserted into the duct from which the discharge is emerging. A tennis racquet incision can be made to encompass the entire duct or a periareolar incision used and the nipple flap dissected to reach the duct. The duct is then excised. A papilloma is nearly always situated within 4–5 cm of the nipple orifice.

Ductoscopy (inspection of the internal structure of the duct system) using microendoscopes is technically feasible but generally disappointing. The affected duct may not be visualised and biopsy systems are currently rudimentary.

CONE EXCISION OF THE MAJOR DUCTS (AFTER HADFIELD) (SUBAREOLAR RESECTION)

When the duct of origin of nipple bleeding is uncertain or when there is bleeding or discharge from multiple ducts, the entire major duct system can be excised for histological examination without sacrifice of the breast form. A periareolar incision is made and a cone of tissue is removed with its apex just deep to the surface of the nipple and its base on the pectoral fascia. The resulting defect may be obliterated by a series of purse-string sutures, although a temporary suction drain will reduce the chance of long-term deformity. It is vital to warn the patient that she will be unable to breast-feed after this and may experience altered nipple sensation.

BENIGN BREAST DISEASE

This is the most common cause of breast problems; up to 30% of women will suffer from a benign breast disorder requiring treatment at some time in their lives. The most common symptoms are pain, lumpiness or a lump. The aim of treatment is to exclude cancer and, once this has been done, to treat any remaining symptoms.

Congenital abnormalities

Amazia

Congenital absence of the breast may occur on one (Figure 53.11) or both sides. It is sometimes associated with absence of the sternal portion of the pectoralis major (Poland's syndrome). It is more common in males.

Polymazia

Accessory breasts (Figure 53.12) have been recorded in the axilla (the most frequent site), groin, buttock and thigh. They have been known to function during lactation.

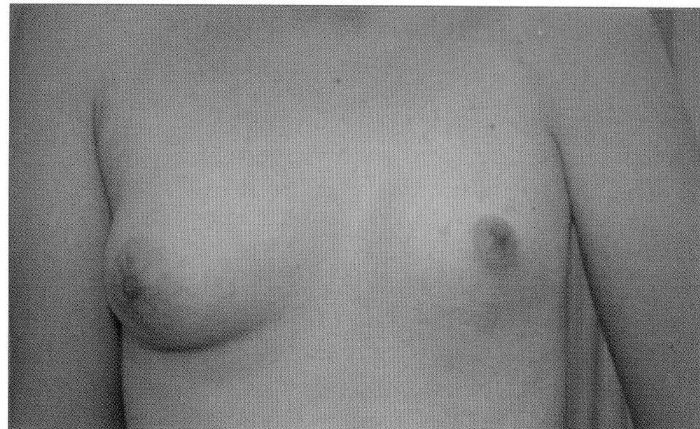

Figure 53.11 Congenital absence of the left breast.

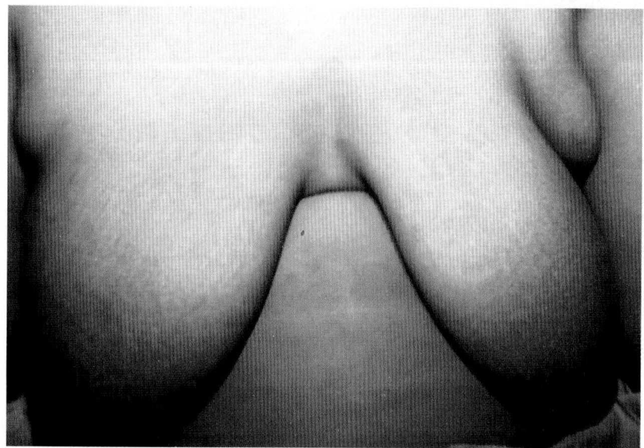

Figure 53.12 Bilateral accessory breasts.

Mastitis of infants

Mastitis of infants is at least as common in boys as in girls. On the third or fourth day of life, if the breast of an infant is pressed lightly, a drop of colourless fluid can be expressed; a few days later, there is often a slight milky secretion, which disappears during the third week. This is popularly known as 'witch's milk' and is seen only in full-term infants. It is caused by stimulation of the fetal breast by prolactin in response to the drop in maternal oestrogens and is essentially physiological. True mastitis is uncommon and is predominately caused by *Staphylococcus aureus*.

Diffuse hypertrophy

Diffuse hypertrophy of the breasts occurs sporadically in otherwise healthy girls at puberty (benign virginal hypertrophy) and, much less often, during the first pregnancy. The condition is rarely unilateral. This tremendous overgrowth is apparently caused by an alteration in the normal sensitivity of the breast to oestrogenic hormones and some success in treating it with antioestrogens has been reported. Treatment is otherwise by reduction mammoplasty.

Geoffrey John Hadfield, 1923–2006, surgeon, Stoke Mandeville Hospital, Aylesbury, Buckinghamshire, UK.
Alfred Poland, 1822–1872, surgeon, Guy's Hospital, London, UK, described this condition in 1841.

Injuries of the breast

Haematoma

Haematoma, particularly a resolving haematoma, gives rise to a lump, which, in the absence of overlying bruising, is difficult to diagnose correctly unless it is biopsied.

Traumatic fat necrosis

Traumatic fat necrosis may be acute or chronic and usually occurs in stout, middle-aged women. Following a blow, or even indirect violence (e.g. contraction of the pectoralis major), a lump, often painless, appears. This may mimic a carcinoma, even displaying skin tethering and nipple retraction, and biopsy is required for diagnosis. A history of trauma is not diagnostic as this may merely have drawn the patient's attention to a pre-existing lump. A seatbelt may transect or avulse the breast with a sudden deceleration injury, as in a road traffic accident.

Acute and subacute inflammations of the breast

Bacterial mastitis

Bacterial mastitis is the most common variety of mastitis and is associated with lactation in the majority of cases.

AETIOLOGY

Lactational mastitis is seen far less frequently than in former years. Most are caused by *S. aureus* and, if hospital acquired, are likely to be penicillin resistant. The intermediary is usually the infant; after the second day of life, 50% of infants harbour staphylococci in the nasopharynx.

Although ascending infection from a sore and cracked nipple may initiate the mastitis, in many cases the lactiferous ducts will first become blocked by epithelial debris leading to stasis; this theory is supported by the relatively high incidence of mastitis in women with a retracted nipple. Once within the ampulla of the duct, staphylococci cause clotting of milk and, within this clot, organisms multiply.

CLINICAL FEATURES

The affected breast, or more usually a segment of it, presents the classical signs of acute inflammation. Early on this is a generalised cellulitis but later an abscess will form.

TREATMENT

During the cellulitic stage, the patient should be treated with an appropriate antibiotic, such as flucloxacillin or co-amoxiclav. Feeding from the affected side may continue if the patient can manage. Support of the breast, local heat and analgesia will help to relieve pain.

If an antibiotic is used in the presence of undrained pus, an 'antibioma' may form. This is a large, sterile, brawny oedematous swelling that takes many weeks to resolve.

It used to be recommended that the breast should be incised and drained if the infection did not resolve within 48 hours or if after being emptied of milk there was an area of tense induration or other evidence of an underlying abscess. This advice has been replaced with the recommendation that repeated aspirations under antibiotic cover (if necessary using ultrasound for localisation) be performed. This often allows resolution without the need for an incision and will also allow the patient to continue breast-feeding.

The presence of pus can be confirmed with needle aspiration, and the pus should be sent for bacteriological culture. In contrast to the majority of localised infections, fluctuation is a late sign. Usually, the area of induration is sector shaped and, in early cases, about one-quarter of the breast is involved (Figure 53.13); in many late cases the area is more extensive (Figure 53.14). When in doubt, an ultrasound scan may clearly define an area suitable for drainage.

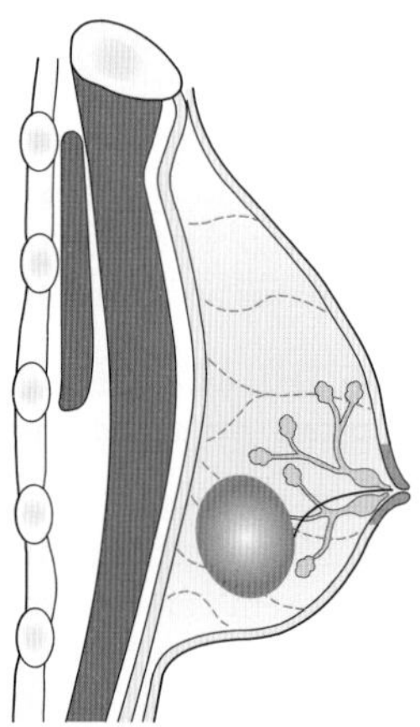

Figure 53.13 Intramammary breast abscess.

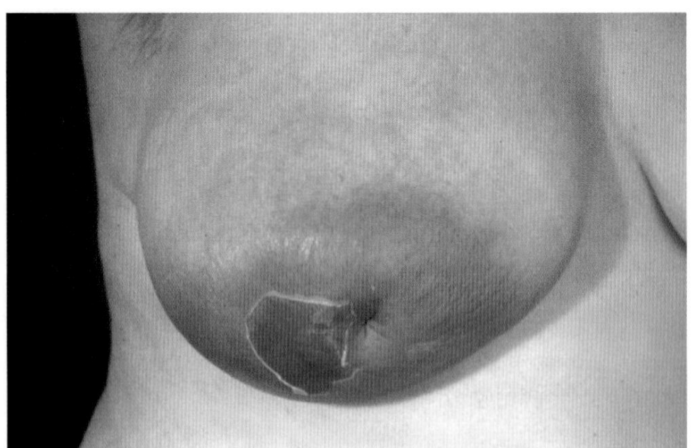

Figure 53.14 Large breast abscess.

Operative drainage of a breast abscess

This is less commonly needed as prompt commencement of antibiotics and repeated aspiration is usually successful. Incision of a lactational abscess is necessary if there is marked skin thinning and can usually be performed under local anaesthesia if an analgesic cream such as EMLA (lidocaine) is applied 30 minutes before surgery.

The usual incision is sited in a radial direction over the affected segment, although if a circumareolar incision will allow adequate access to the affected area this is preferred because it gives a better cosmetic result. The incision passes through the skin and the superficial fascia. A long artery forceps is then inserted into the abscess cavity. Every part of the abscess is palpated against the point of the artery forceps and its jaws are opened. All loculi that can be felt are entered.

Finally, the artery forceps having been withdrawn, a finger is introduced and any remaining septa are disrupted. The wound may then be lightly packed with ribbon gauze or a drain inserted to allow dependent drainage.

Chronic intramammary abscess

A chronic intramammary abscess, which may follow inadequate drainage or injudicious antibiotic treatment, is often a very difficult condition to diagnose. When encapsulated within a thick wall of fibrous tissue the condition cannot be distinguished from a carcinoma without the histological evidence from a biopsy.

Tuberculosis of the breast

Tuberculosis of the breast, which is comparatively rare, is usually associated with active pulmonary tuberculosis or tuberculous cervical adenitis.

Tuberculosis of the breast occurs more often in parous women and usually presents with multiple chronic abscesses and sinuses and a typical bluish, attenuated appearance of the surrounding skin. The diagnosis rests on bacteriological and histological examination. Treatment is with antituberculous chemotherapy. Healing is usual, although often delayed, and mastectomy should be restricted to patients with persistent residual infection.

Actinomycosis

Actinomycosis of the breast is rarer still. The lesions present the essential characteristics of faciocervical actinomycosis.

Mondor's disease

Mondor's disease is thrombophlebitis of the superficial veins of the breast and anterior chest wall, although it may also occur in the arm.

In the absence of injury or infection, the cause of thrombophlebitis (like that of spontaneous thrombophlebitis in other sites) is obscure. The pathognomonic feature is a thrombosed subcutaneous cord, usually attached to the skin. When the skin over the breast is stretched by raising the arm, a narrow, shallow, subcutaneous groove alongside the cord becomes apparent (Figure 53.15). The differential diagnosis is lymphatic permeation from an occult carcinoma of the breast. The only treatment required is to restrict arm movements. The condition usually subsides within a few months without recurrence, complications or deformity. There are case reports of Mondor's disease being associated with subsequent development of malignancy, although coincidental malignancy is more likely.

Duct ectasia/periductal mastitis

PATHOLOGY

This is a dilatation of the breast ducts, which is often associated with periductal inflammation. The pathogenesis is obscure and almost certainly not uniform in all cases, although the disease is much more common in smokers.

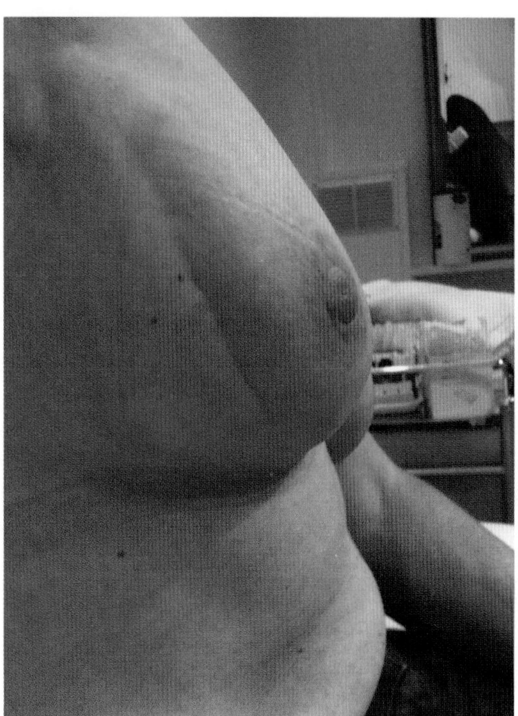

Figure 53.15 Mondor's disease evident in the lateral aspect of the right breast.

The classical description of the pathogenesis of duct ectasia asserts that the first stage in the disorder is a dilatation in one or more of the larger lactiferous ducts, which fill with a stagnant brown or green secretion. This may discharge. These fluids then set up an irritant reaction in surrounding tissue, leading to periductal mastitis or even abscess and fistula formation (Figures 53.16 and 53.17). In some cases, a chronic indurated mass forms beneath the areola, which mimics a carcinoma. Fibrosis eventually develops, which may cause slit-like nipple retraction.

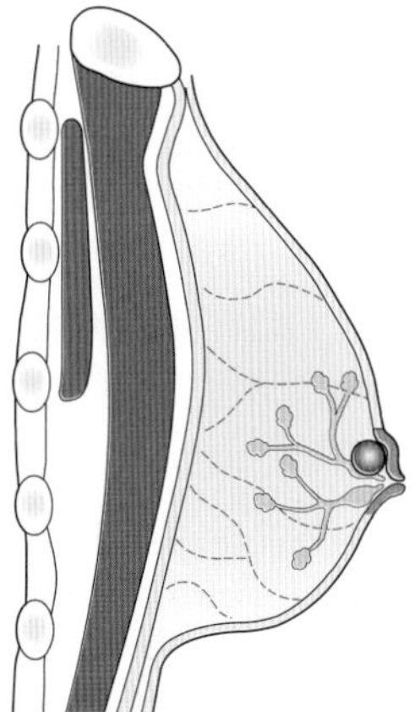

Figure 53.16 Subareolar abscess in duct ectasia.

Henri Mondor, 1885–1962, Professor of Surgery, Paris, France.

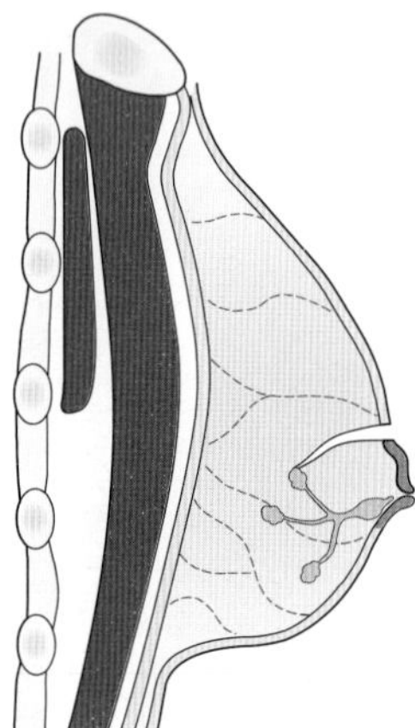

Figure 53.17 Mammary fistula originating in a chronic subareolar abscess.

An alternative theory suggests that periductal inflammation is the primary condition and, indeed, anaerobic bacterial infection is found in some cases. A marked association between recurrent periductal inflammation and smoking has been demonstrated. This was thought by some to indicate that arteriopathy is a contributing factor in its aetiology, although others believe that smoking increases the virulence of the commensal bacteria. It is certainly clear that cessation of smoking increases the chance of a long-term cure.

CLINICAL FEATURES

Nipple discharge (of any colour), a subareolar mass, abscess, mammary duct fistula and/or nipple retraction are the most common symptoms.

TREATMENT

In the case of a mass or nipple retraction, a carcinoma must be excluded by obtaining a mammogram and negative cytology or histology. If any suspicion remains the mass should be excised.

Antibiotic therapy may be tried, the most appropriate agents being co-amoxiclav or flucloxacillin and metronidazole. However, surgery is often the only option likely to bring about cure of this notoriously difficult condition; this consists of excision of all of the major ducts (Hadfield's operation). It is particularly important to shave the back of the nipple to ensure that all terminal ducts are removed. Failure to do so will lead to recurrence.

Aberrations of normal development and involution

Nomenclature

The nomenclature of benign breast disease is confusing. This is because over the last century a variety of clinicians and pathologists have chosen to describe a mixture of physiological changes and disease processes according to a variety of clinical, pathological and aetiological terminology. As well as leading to confusion, patients were often unduly alarmed or overtreated by ascribing a pathological name to a variant of physiological development. To address this confusion, a concept (Aberrations of Normal Development and Involution (ANDI)) has been developed and described by the Cardiff Breast Clinic.

Aetiology

The breast is a dynamic structure that undergoes changes throughout a woman's reproductive life and, superimposed upon this, cyclical changes throughout the menstrual cycle. (This is illustrated in Figure 53.18). The pathogenesis of ANDI involves disturbances in the breast physiology extending from a perturbation of normality to well-defined disease processes. There is often little correlation between the histological appearance of the breast tissue and the symptoms.

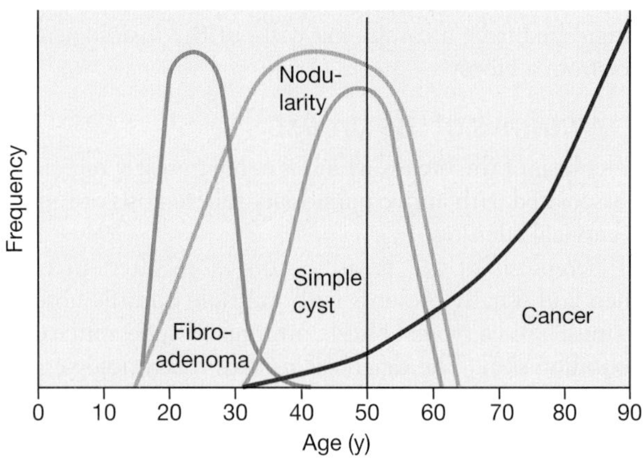

Figure 53.18 Normal breast changes throughout life. UK National Health Service Breast Screening Programme data.

Pathology

The disease consists essentially of four features that may vary in extent and degree in any one breast.

- **Cyst formation**. Cysts are almost inevitable and very variable in size.
- **Fibrosis**. Fat and elastic tissues disappear and are replaced with dense white fibrous trabeculae. The interstitial tissue is infiltrated with chronic inflammatory cells.
- **Hyperplasia** of epithelium in the lining of the ducts and acini may occur, with or without atypia.
- **Papillomatosis**. The epithelial hyperplasia may be so extensive that it results in papillomatous overgrowth within the ducts.

Clinical features

The symptoms of ANDI are many as the term is used to encompass a wide range of benign conditions, but often include an area of lumpiness (seldom discrete) and/or breast pain (mastalgia).

- A benign discrete lump in the breast is commonly a cyst or fibroadenoma. True lipomas occur rarely.
- Lumpiness may be bilateral, commonly in the upper outer quadrant or, less commonly, confined to one quadrant of one breast. The changes may be cyclical, with an increase in both lumpiness and often tenderness before a menstrual period.

- Non-cyclical mastalgia is more common in perimenopausal than postmenopausal women. It may be associated with ANDI or with periductal mastitis. It should be distinguished from referred pain, for example a musculoskeletal disorder. 'Breast' pain in postmenopausal women not taking hormonereplacement therapy (HRT) is usually derived from the chest wall, back or neck.

About 5% of breast cancers exhibit pain at presentation, but rarely as the sole presenting feature.

TREATMENT OF LUMPY BREASTS

If the clinician is confident that he or she is not dealing with a discrete abnormality (and clinical confidence is supported by mammography and/or ultrasound scanning if considered appropriate), the woman can initially be offered firm reassurance. It is perhaps worthwhile reviewing the patient at a different point in the menstrual cycle, for example 6 weeks after the initial visit as often the clinical signs will have resolved by that time. There is a tendency for women with lumpy breasts to be rendered unnecessarily anxious and to be submitted to multiple random biopsies because the clinician lacks the courage of his or her convictions. Rapid referral into the secondary health care sytem often means patients are assessed without an intervening menstrual cycle and this may lead to additional concerns.

TREATMENT OF MASTALGIA

Pronounced cyclical mastalgia may become a significant clinical problem if the pain and tenderness interfere with the woman's life, disturb her sleep and impair sexual activity. Initially, firm reassurance that the symptoms are not associated with cancer will help the majority of women. Acknowledgement that this is a real symptom, a non-dismissive attitude and an explanation of the aetiology are all helpful in managing this condition.

In the first instance, an appropriately fitting and supportive bra should be worn throughout the day and a soft bra (such as a sports bra) worn at night. Avoiding caffeine drinks is said to help, although the author remains unconvinced.

A patient symptom diary will help her to chart the pattern of pain throughout the month and thus determine whether this is cyclical mastalgia. This allows the majority of patients to adjust to the concept of a cyclical nature of their problem but, if reassurance is inadequate, then a planned escalation of treatment (*Table 53.1*) could be advised. Oil of evening primrose, in adequate doses given over 3 months, will help more than half of these women. It appears to achieve higher response rates in those over 40 years of age rather than younger women. For those with intractable symptoms, an antigonadotrophin, such as danazol, or a prolactin inhibitor, such as bromocriptine, may be tried. Very rarely it is necessary to prescribe an antioestrogen, for example tamoxifen, or a luteinising hormone-releasing hormone (LHRH) agonist to deprive the breast epithelium of oestrogenic drive.

For non-cyclical mastalgia it is important to exclude extramammary causes such as chest wall pain (Tietze syndrome). This is common in postmenopausal women who are not taking HRT, and the neck and shoulders are common sights of referred pain. It is seldom necessary these days to carry out a biopsy on a very localised tender area that might be harbouring a subclinical cancer as imaging is so much better. Treatment may be with non-steroidal analgesics or by injection with local anaesthetic on a 'trigger spot'.

Breast cysts

These occur most commonly in the last decade of reproductive life as a result of a non-integrated involution of stroma and epithelium. They are often multiple, may be bilateral and can mimic malignancy. Diagnosis can be confirmed by aspiration and/or ultrasound. They typically present suddenly and cause great alarm; prompt diagnosis and drainage provides immediate relief.

Treatment

A solitary cyst or small collection of cysts can be aspirated. If they resolve completely, and if the fluid is not blood-stained, no further treatment is required. However, 30% will recur and require reaspiration. Cytological examination of cyst fluid is no longer practised routinely. If there is a residual lump or if the fluid is blood-stained, a core biopsy or local excision for histological diagnosis is advisable, which is also the case if the cyst reforms repeatedly. This will exclude cystadenocarcinoma, which is more common in elderly women.

Galactocele

Galactocele is rare and usually presents as a solitary, subareolar cyst and always dates from lactation. It contains milk and in long-standing cases its walls tend to calcify.

TABLE 53.1 Treatment of breast pain.

Exclude cancer	
Reassure	Use pain chart if unsure if cyclical or non-cyclical. Also allows time for reassurance to become active!
Adequate support	Firm bra during the day and a softer bra at night
Exclude caffeine	Works for some although not very efficacious in author's practice
Consider medication	
Evening primrose oil (GLA)	Better effect in women over 40 years old than in younger women
Danazol, 100 mg three times a day	Start at 100 mg per day and increase (seldom used these days)
Tamoxifen	Not licensed for this indication but occasionally very helpful

Fibroadenoma

These usually arise in the fully developed breast between the ages of 15 and 25 years, although occasionally they occur in much older women. They arise from hyperplasia of a single lobule and usually grow up to 2–3 cm in size. They are surrounded by a well-marked capsule and can thus be enucleated through a cosmetically appropriate incision. A fibroadenoma does not require excision unless associated with suspicious cytology, it becomes very large or the patient expressly desires the lump to be removed. Alternatives to surgery include cryoablation, heating with high-frequency ultrasound (echotherapy) or removal with a large core vacuum biopsy system. Even if clinically obvious, a biopsy should be obtained if the patient is over 25 or there are any atypical features on ultrasound.

Giant fibroadenomas occasionally occur during puberty. They are over 5 cm in diameter and are often rapidly growing but, in other respects, are similar to smaller fibroadenomas and can be enucleated through a submammary incision. They are more common in the Afro-Caribbean population.

Phyllodes tumour

These benign tumours, previously sometimes known as serocystic disease of Brodie or cystosarcoma phyllodes, usually occur in women over the age of 40 years but can appear in younger women. They present as a large, sometimes massive, tumour with an unevenly bosselated surface (**Figure 53.19**). Occasionally, ulceration of overlying skin occurs because of pressure necrosis. Despite their size, phyllodes tumours remain mobile on the chest wall. Histologically, there is a wide variation in their appearance, with some of low malignant potential resembling a fibroadenoma and others having a higher mitotic index, which are histologically worrying. The latter may recur locally but, despite the name of cystosarcoma phyllodes, they are rarely cystic and only very rarely develop features of a sarcomatous tumour. These may metastasise via the bloodstream.

Treatment

Treatment for the benign type is enucleation in young women or wide local excision. Massive tumours, recurrent tumours and those of the malignant type will require mastectomy.

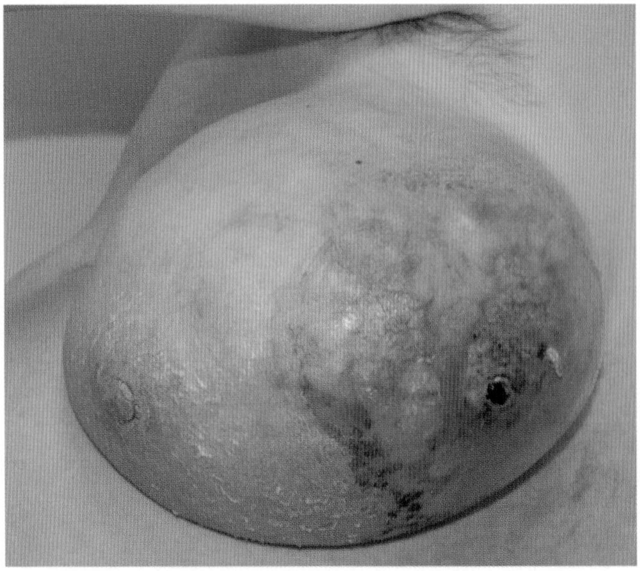

Figure 53.19 Phyllodes tumour (courtesy of Professor Mike Dixon).

Summary box 53.2

Benign breast disorder classification

Congenital disorders
- Inverted nipple
- Supernumerary breasts/nipples
- Non-breast disorders including Tietze's disease (costochondritis)
- Sebaceous cysts and other skin conditions

Injury

Inflammation/infection
- ANDI (aberations of normal differentiation and involution):
  - Cyclical nodularity and mastalgia
  - Cysts
  - Fibroadenoma
  - Duct ectasia/periductal mastitis
- Pregnancy-related:
  - Galactocele
  - Lactational abscess

When the diagnosis of carcinoma is in doubt

There will always be situations in which the clinician cannot be sure whether a particular lump in the breast is an area of mammary dysplasia, a benign tumour or an early carcinoma.

If there is doubt on clinical, cytological or radiological examination, it is essential to obtain a tissue diagnosis. This is often possible by needle biopsy. In the event of a negative result, open biopsy of the mass or large guage vacuum biopsy is necessary. Because of the possibility of reporting errors and because the histology is likely to be more difficult (if a diagnosis has not already been made), the author suggests that frozen-section reporting should be used rarely and certainly should not form the basis for a decision to undertake a mastectomy. *Table 53.2* gives an algorithm for investigating any breast lump.

Sir Benjamin Collins Brodie, 1783–1862, surgeon, St. George's Hospital, London, UK, described serocystic disease of the breast in 1840.
Alexander Tietze, 1864–1927, Professor of Surgery, Breslau, Germany (now Wroclaw, Poland), described this condition in 1921.

TABLE 53.2 Investigation of a breast lump (after imaging performed) using fine-needle aspiration cytology.

Cystic	Lump disappears; clear fluid (many colours)	Discharge patient
	Residual thickening; blood-stained fluid	Investigate – ?core biopsy
Solid	Benign	Offer excision or observe
	Atypical	Investigate – ?core biopsy
	Malignant	Treat for cancer

Risk of malignancy developing in association with benign breast pathology

The relative risks of malignancy developing according to different histological features found at biopsy are illustrated in *Table 53.3*.

These were elucidated 30 years ago but remain pertinent and a recent single-centre review reinforces the conclusion that the histological classification of the benign lesion in combination with a family history of breast cancer are important predictors of risk.

CARCINOMA OF THE BREAST

Breast cancer is the most common cause of death in middle-aged women in western countries. In England and Wales, 1 in 12 women will develop the disease during their lifetime. The incidence is expected to continue rising as the population ages, although more slowly than previously thought as the use of HRT has reduced in the USA and UK.

TABLE 53.3 Relative risk of invasive breast carcinoma based on pathological examination of benign breast tissue (American College of Pathologists Consensus Statement).[a]

No increased risk	Adenosis, sclerosing or florid
	Apocrine metaplasia
	Cysts, macro and/or micro
	Duct ectasia
	Fibroadenoma
	Fibrosis
	Hyperplasia
	Mastitis (inflammation)
	Periductal mastitis
	Squamous metaplasia
Slightly increased risk (1.5–2 times)	Hyperplasia, moderate or florid, solid or papillary
	Papilloma with a fibrovascular core
Moderately increased risk (5 times)	Atypical hyperplasia (ductal or lobular)
Insufficient data to assign a risk	Solitary papilloma of lactiferous sinus
	Radial scar lesion

After Page and Dupont (1978) by kind permission of the *Journal of the National Cancer Institute*, USA.

[a] A combination with positive family history significantly increases the risks shown above.

Aetiological factors

Geographical

Carcinoma of the breast occurs commonly in the western world, accounting for 3–5% of all deaths in women. In resource-poor countries it accounts for 1–3% of deaths.

Age

Carcinoma of the breast is extremely rare before the age of 20 years but, thereafter, the incidence steadily rises so that by the age of 90 years nearly 20% of women are affected.

Gender

Less than 0.5% of patients with breast cancer are male.

Genetic

Breast cancer occurs more commonly in women with a family history of breast cancer than in the general population. Breast cancer related to a specific mutation accounts for about 5% of breast cancers, yet has far-reaching repercussions in terms of counselling and tumour prevention in these women. This will be discussed more fully in a subsequent section.

Diet

Because breast cancer so commonly affects women in the 'developed' world, dietary factors may play a part in its causation. There is some evidence that there is a link with diets low in phytoestrogens. Alcohol consumption is associated with an increased risk.

Endocrine

Breast cancer is more common in nulliparous women and breast-feeding in particular appears to be protective. Also protective is having a first child at an early age, especially if associated with late menarche and early menopause. It is known that in postmenopausal women, breast cancer is more common in the obese. This is thought to be because of an increased conversion of steroid hormones to oestradiol in the body fat. Recent studies have clarified the role of exogenous hormones, in particular the oral contraceptive pill and HRT, in the development of breast cancer. For most women the benefits of these treatments will far outweigh the small putative risk; however, long-term exposure to the combined preparation of HRT does significantly increase the risk of developing breast cancer. The recent fall in use of HRT in USA and UK has seen a reduction in the incidence of breast cancer in the 50–60-year-old cohort.

Previous radiation

This was considered to be of historical interest, as the majority of women exposed to the atomic bombs at Hiroshima and Nagasaki have now died. It was, however, also a problem in women who had been treated with mantle radiotherapy as part of the management of Hodgkin's disease, in which significant doses of radiation to the breast were received. The risk appeared about a decade after treatment and was higher if radiotherapy occurred during breast development. A surveillance programme was organised in the UK with MRI and mammographic screening. This type of radiotherapy is now no longer used and the cohort of patients at risk is now small.

Pathology

Breast cancer may arise from the epithelium of the duct system anywhere from the nipple end of the major lactiferous ducts to the terminal duct unit, which is in the breast lobule. The disease may be entirely *in situ*, an increasingly common finding with the advent of breast cancer screening, or may be invasive cancer. The degree of differentiation of the tumour is usually described using three grades: well differentiated, moderately differentiated or poorly differentiated. Commonly, a numerical grading system based on the scoring of three individual factors (nuclear pleomorphism, tubule formation and mitotic rate) is used, with grade III cancers roughly equating to the poorly differentiated group.

Previously, descriptive terms were used to classify breast cancer ('scirrhous', meaning woody, or 'medullary', meaning brain-like). More recently, histological descriptions have been used. These have been shown to have clinical correlations in the way that the tumour behaves. However, with the increasing application of molecular markers, there is a change in the way that breast cancers are classified and it is likely that much more information about an individual tumour will be routinely reported, such as its likelihood of metastasis and to which therapeutic agents it will be susceptible. Gene array analysis of breast cancers has identified five major subtypes (luminal A and luminal B, triple negative, Her-2 receptor positive and a miscellaneous group.) Some of these correlate with known markers such as oestrogen receptor status. There are specific gene signatures that correlate with response to chemotherapy or poor prognosis. A commercial test is now available to patients with oestrogen-positive tumours to assess their risk of recurrence. This is based on analysis of 21 genes and may allow selection of patients in whom more aggressive therapy is indicated.

Current nomenclature

Ductal carcinoma is the most common variant with **lobular carcinoma** occurring in up to 15% of cases. There are subtypes of lobular cancer, including the classical type, that carry a better prognosis than the pleomorphic type. Occasionally, the picture may be mixed with both ductal and lobular features. There are different patterns of spread depending on histological type. If there is doubt whether a tumour is predominantly lobular in type, immunohistochemical analysis using the e-cadherin antibody, which reacts positively in lobular cancer, will help in diagnosis.

Rarer histological variants, usually carrying a better prognosis, include **colloid** or **mucinous carcinoma**, whose cells produce abundant mucin, **medullary carcinoma**, with solid sheets of large cells often associated with a marked lymphocytic reaction and **tubular carcinoma**. Invasive lobular carcinoma is commonly multifocal and/or bilateral, hence the increasing use of MRI for assessment. Cases detected via the screening programme are often smaller and better differentiated than those presenting to the symptomatic service and are of a special type.

Inflammatory carcinoma is a fortunately rare, highly aggressive cancer that presents as a painful, swollen breast, which is warm with cutaneous oedema. This is the result of blockage of the subdermal lymphatics with carcinoma cells. Inflammatory cancer usually involves at least one-third of the breast and may mimic a breast abscess. A biopsy will confirm the diagnosis and show undifferentiated carcinoma cells. It used to be rapidly fatal but with aggressive chemotherapy and radiotherapy and with salvage surgery the prognosis has improved considerably.

***In situ* carcinoma** is preinvasive cancer that has not breached the epithelial basement membrane. This was previously a rare, usually asymptomatic, finding in breast biopsy specimens but is becoming increasingly common because of the advent of mammographic screening; it now accounts for over 20% of cancers detected by screening in the UK. *In situ* carcinoma may be ductal (DCIS) or lobular (LCIS), the latter often being multifocal and bilateral. Both are markers for the later development of invasive cancer, which will develop in at least 20% of patients. Although mastectomy is curative, this constitutes overtreatment in many cases. The best treatment for *in situ* carcinoma is the subject of a number of on-going clinical trials. DCIS may be classified using the Van Nuys system, which combines the patient's age, type of DCIS and presence of microcalcification, extent of resection margin and size of disease. Patients with a high score benefit from radiotherapy after excision, whereas those of low grade, whose tumour is completely excised, need no further treatment.

Staining for oestrogen and progesterone receptors is now routine, as their presence will indicate the use of adjuvant hormonal therapy with tamoxifen or an aromatase inhibitor (AI) (Figure 53.20). Tumours are also stained for Her-2 or

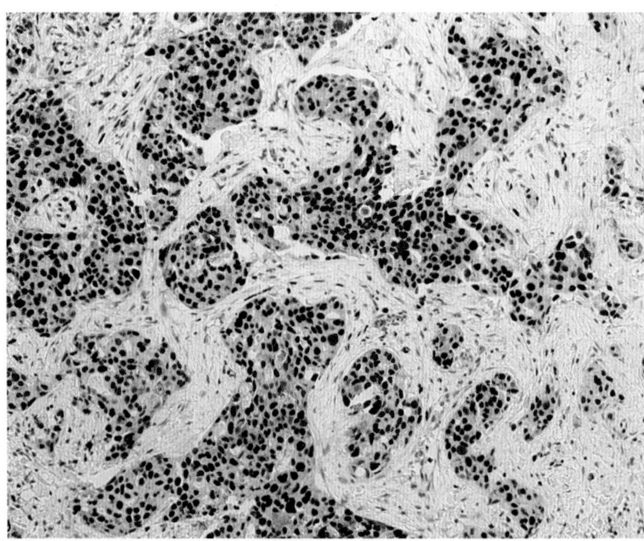

Figure 53.20 Immunohistochemical staining for oestrogen receptors.

Thomas Hodgkin, 1798–1866, Curator of the Museum, and Demonstrator of Morbid Anatomy, Guy's Hospital, London, UK.

c-erbB2 (a growth factor receptor) as patients who are positive can be treated with the monoclonal antibody trastuzumab (Herceptin®), either in the adjuvant or relapse setting.

The pathologist is an important member of the breast cancer team and will increasingly help decide which adjuvant therapies will be appropriate.

Paget's disease of the nipple

Paget's disease of the nipple (Figure 53.21) is a superficial manifestation of an underlying breast carcinoma. It presents as an eczema-like condition of the nipple and areola, which persists despite local treatment. The nipple is eroded slowly and eventually disappears. If left, the underlying carcinoma will sooner or later become clinically evident. Nipple eczema should be biopsied if there is any doubt about its cause. Microscopically, Paget's disease is characterised by the presence of large, ovoid cells with abundant, clear, pale-staining cytoplasm in the Malpighian layer of the epidermis.

The spread of breast cancer

Local spread

The tumour increases in size and invades other portions of the breast. It tends to involve the skin and to penetrate the pectoral muscles and even the chest wall if diagnosed late.

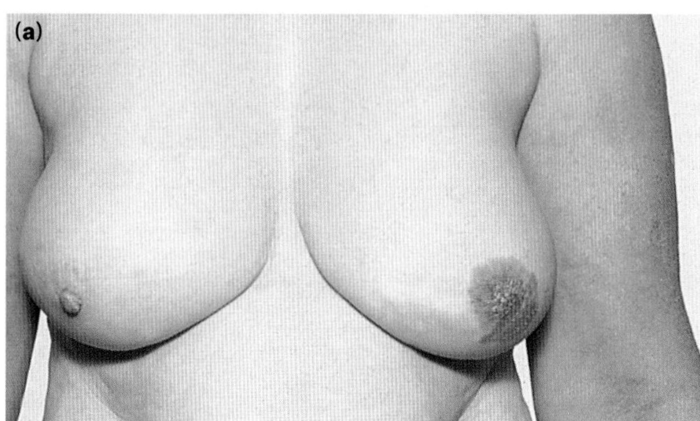

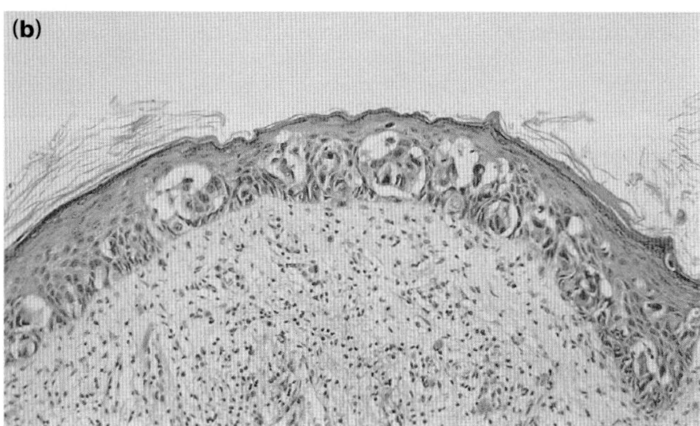

Figure 53.21 (a) Paget's disease of the nipple. (b) Histological appearance of Paget's disease.

Lymphatic metastasis

Lymphatic metastasis occurs primarily to the axillary and the internal mammary lymph nodes. Tumours in the posterior one-third of the breast are more likely to drain to the internal mammary nodes. The involvement of lymph nodes has both biological and chronological significance. It represents not only an evolutional event in the spread of the carcinoma but is also a marker for the metastatic potential of that tumour. Involvement of supraclavicular nodes and of any contralateral lymph nodes represents advanced disease.

Spread by the bloodstream

It is by this route that skeletal metastases occur, although the initial spread may be via the lymphatic system. In order of frequency the lumbar vertebrae, femur, thoracic vertebrae, rib and skull are affected and these deposits are generally osteolytic. Metastases may also commonly occur in the liver, lungs and brain and, occasionally, the adrenal glands and ovaries; they have, in fact, been described in most body sites. Analysis of peripheral blood samples for circulating tumour deoxyribonucleic acid (DNA) has shown prognostic significance and can be used to monitor response.

Clinical presentation

Although any portion of the breast, including the axillary tail, may be involved, breast cancer is found most frequently in the upper outer quadrant (Figures 53.22 and 53.23). Most breast cancers will present as a hard lump, which may be associated with indrawing of the nipple or overlying skin. As the disease advances locally there may be skin involvement with peau d'orange (Figure 53.24) or frank ulceration and fixation to the chest wall (Figure 53.25). This is described as cancer-en-cuirasse when the disease progresses around the

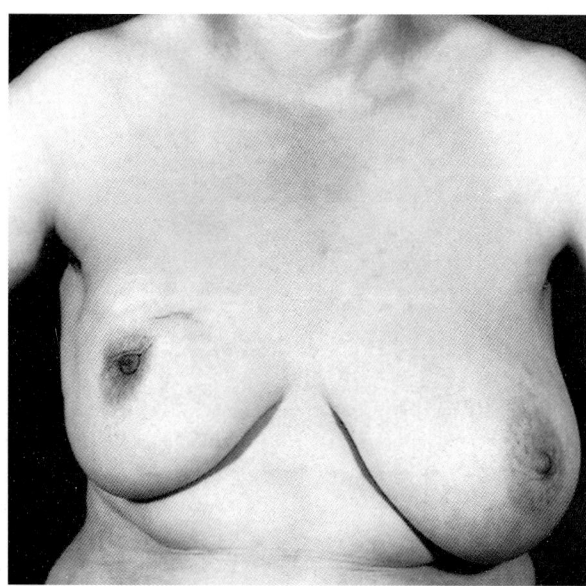

Figure 53.22 Invasive carcinoma of the right breast. Note the shrinking and elevation of the breast with nipple retraction.

Marcello Malpighi, 1628–1694, Professor of Physic successively at Bologna, Pisa and Messina, and in 1691 Physician to the Papal Court in Rome, Italy.
peau d'orange is French for 'orange skin'.

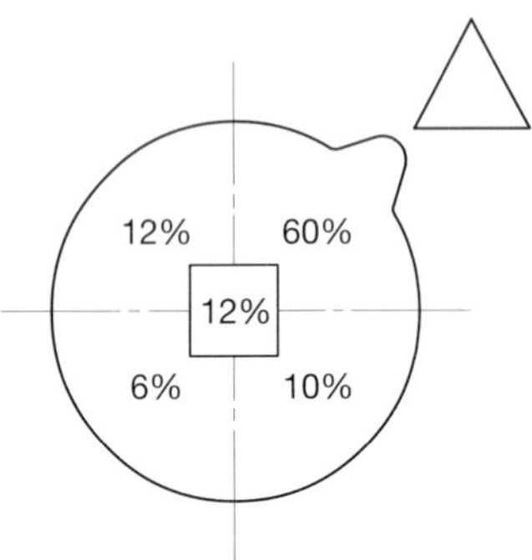

Figure 53.23 The relationship of carcinoma of the breast to the quadrants of the breast.

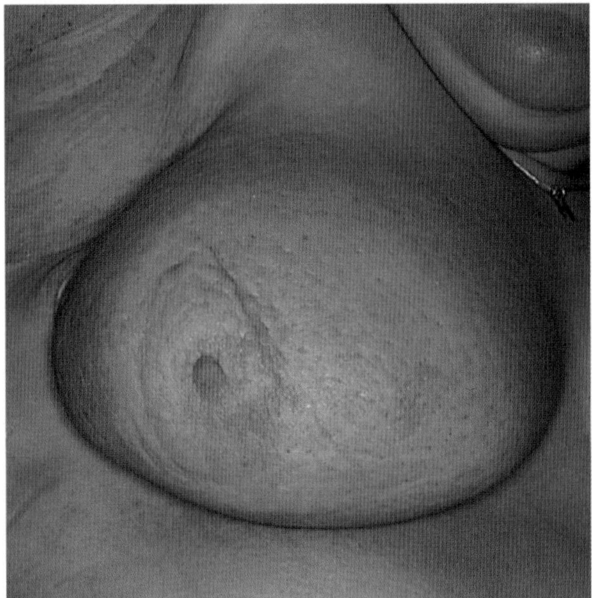

Figure 53.24 Peau d'orange of the breast.

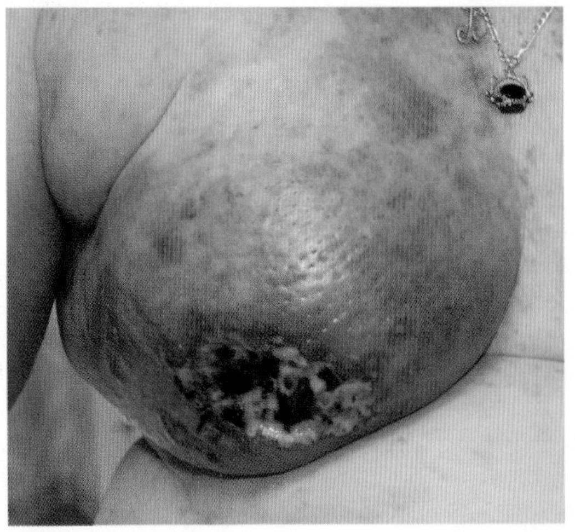

Figure 53.25 Ulcerated carcinoma of the right breast.

chest wall. About 5% of breast cancers in the UK will present with either locally advanced disease or symptoms of metastatic disease. This figure is much higher in resource-poor countries. These patients must then undergo a staging evaluation so that the full extent of their disease can be ascertained. This will include a careful clinical examination, chest radiograph, computed tomography (CT) of the chest and abdomen and a bone scan (either using isotopes or MRI) (Figure 53.26). This is important for both prognosis and treatment; a patient with widespread visceral metastases may obtain an increased length and quality of survival from systemic hormone therapy or chemotherapy, but is unlikely to benefit from surgery as she will die from her metastases before local disease becomes a problem. In contrast, patients with relatively small tumours (<2 cm in diameter) confined to the breast with negative ipsilateral lymph nodes rarely need staging beyond a good clinical examination as the pick-up rate for distant metastases is so low. Currently, there are no tests recommended for screening of patients with early-stage breast cancer.

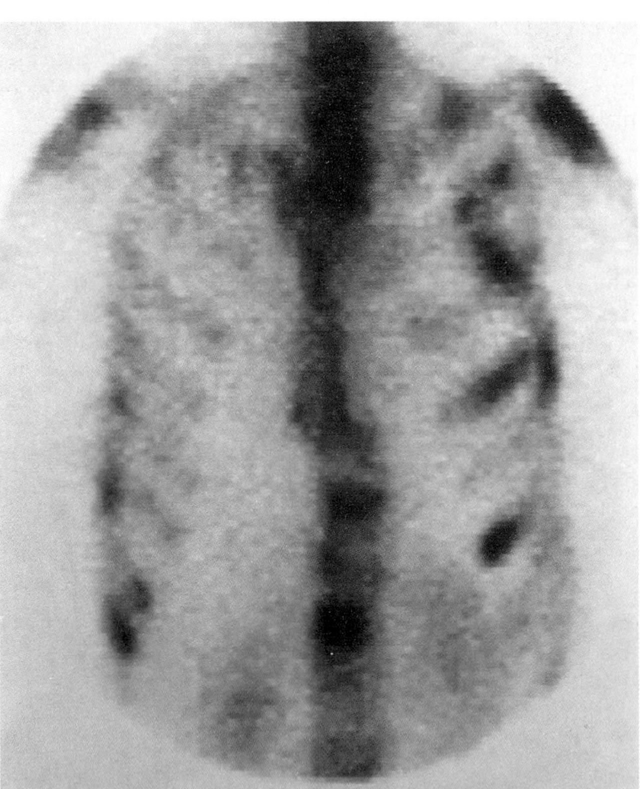

Figure 53.26 Skeletal isotope bone scan showing multiple 'hotspots' due to metastases.

Staging of breast cancer

Classical staging of breast cancer by means of the TNM (tumour–node–metastasis) or UICC (Union Internationale Contre le Cancer) criteria is used less often with increased knowledge of the biological variables that affect prognosis. It is becoming clear that these factors (discussed in more detail below) rather than anatomical mapping that influence outcome and treatment. Perhaps a more pragmatic approach would be to classify patients according to the treatment that they require (*Table 53.4*). Treatment recommendations are summarised in consensus statements such as those from the American Society of Clinical Oncology (ASCO) and the St Gallen Conference.

TABLE 53.4 A pragmatic classification of breast cancer.

Group	Approximate 5-year survival rate (%)	Example	Treatment
'Very low-risk' primary breast cancer	>90	Screen-detected DCIS, tubular or special types	Local
'Low-risk' primary breast cancer	70–90	Node negative with favourable histology	Locoregional with/without systemic
'High-risk' primary breast cancer	<70	Node positive or unfavourable histology	Locoregional with systemic
Locally advanced	<30	Large primary or inflammatory	Primary systemic
Metastatic	–	–	Primary systemic

DCIS, duct carcinoma *in situ*.

Prognosis of breast cancer

The best indicators of likely prognosis in breast cancer remain tumour size, grade and lymph node status; however, it is realised that some large tumours will remain confined to the breast for decades, whereas some very small tumours are incurable at diagnosis. Hence, the prognosis of a cancer depends not on its chronological age but on its invasive and metastatic potential. In an attempt to define which tumours will behave aggressively, and thus require early systemic treatment, a host of prognostic factors have been described. These include the histological grade of the tumour, hormone receptor status, measures of tumour proliferation such as Ki-67, growth factor analysis and oncogene or oncogene product measurements. Many others are under investigation but have proved of little practical value in patient management. Prognostic indices (such as the Nottingham prognostic index) have combined these factors to allow subdivision of patients into discrete prognostic groups. More recently, computer-aided programs (adjuvant online; www.adjuvantonline.com or in the UK Predict; www.predict.nhs.uk) have been developed, which incorporate the putative benefits of treatment allowing oncologist and patient to visualise the benefits of therapy.

Summary box 53.3

Algorithm for management of operable breast cancer

- Achieve local control
- Appropriate surgery
  - Wide local excision (clear margins) and radiotherapy, *or*
  - Mastectomy ± radiotherapy (offer reconstruction – immediate or delayed)
  - Combined with axillary procedure (see text)
  - Await final pathology and receptor measurements
  - Use risk assessment tool; stage if appropriate
- Treat risk of systemic disease
  - Offer chemotherapy if prognostic factors poor; include Herceptin if Her-2 positive
  - Radiotherapy as decided above
  - Hormone therapy if oestrogen receptor or progesterone receptor positive

Treatment of cancer of the breast

The two basic principles of treatment are to reduce the chance of local recurrence and the risk of metastatic spread. Treatment of early breast cancer will usually involve surgery with or without radiotherapy. Systemic therapy such as chemotherapy or hormone therapy is added if there are adverse prognostic factors such as lymph node involvement, indicating a high likelihood of metastatic relapse. At the other end of the spectrum, locally advanced or metastatic disease is usually treated by systemic therapy to palliate symptoms, with surgery playing a much smaller role. An algorithm for the management of breast cancer is shown in *Summary box 53.3*.

The multidisciplinary team approach

As in all branches of medicine, good doctor–patient communication plays a vital role in helping to alleviate patient anxiety. Participation of the patient in treatment decisions is of particular importance in breast cancer when there may be uncertainty as to the best therapeutic option and the desire to treat the patient within the protocol of a controlled clinical trial. As part of the preoperative and postoperative management of the patient it is often useful to employ the skills of a trained breast counsellor and also to have available advice on breast prostheses, psychological support and physiotherapy, when appropriate.

In many specialist centres the care of breast cancer patients is undertaken as a joint venture between the surgeon, medical oncologist, radiotherapist and allied health professionals such as the clinical nurse specialist. This has been shown to be good for the patient, to lead to higher trial entry and to improve the mental health of the professionals in the breast team. There are published guidelines for the optimal management of patients with breast cancer such as SIGN 84 (Scottish Intercollegiate Guidelines Network, (www.sign.ac.uk/guidelines/fulltext/84/).

Local treatment of early breast cancer

Local control is achieved through surgery and/or radiotherapy.

SURGERY

Surgery still has a central role to play in the management of breast cancer but there has been a gradual shift towards more conservative techniques, backed up by clinical trials that have

Summary box 53.4

Treatment of early breast cancer

The aims of treatment are:

- 'Cure': likely in some patients but late recurrence is possible
- Control of local disease in the breast and axilla
- Conservation of local form and function
- Prevention or delay of the occurrence of distant metastases

shown equal efficacy between mastectomy and local excision followed by radiotherapy.

It was initially hoped that avoiding mastectomy would help to alleviate the considerable psychological morbidity associated with breast cancer, but recent studies have shown that over 30% of women develop significant anxiety and depression following both radical and conservative surgery. After mastectomy women tend to worry about the effect of the operation on their appearance and relationships, whereas after conservative surgery they may remain fearful of a recurrence.

Mastectomy is indicated for large tumours (in relation to the size of the breast), central tumours beneath or involving the nipple, multifocal disease, local recurrence or patient preference. The radical Halsted mastectomy, which included excision of the breast, axillary lymph nodes and pectoralis major and minor muscles, is no longer indicated as it causes excessive morbidity with no survival benefit. The modified radical (Patey) mastectomy is more commonly performed and is thus described below. Simple mastectomy involves removal of only the breast with no dissection of the axilla, except for the region of the axillary tail of the breast, which usually has attached to it a few nodes low in the anterior group.

Patey mastectomy The breast and associated structures are dissected *en bloc* (Figure 53.27) and the excised mass is composed of:

- the whole breast;
- a large portion of skin, the centre of which overlies the tumour but which always includes the nipple;
- all of the fat, fascia and lymph nodes of the axilla.

The pectoralis minor muscle is either divided or retracted to gain access to the upper two-thirds of the axilla. The axillary vein and nerves to the serratus anterior and latissimus dorsi (the thoracodorsal trunk) should be preserved. The intercostal brachial nerves are usually divided in this operation and the patient should be warned about sensation changes postoperatively.

The wound is drained using a wide-bore suction tube. Early mobilisation of the arm is encouraged and physiotherapy helps normal function to return very quickly; most patients are able to resume light work within a few weeks.

Conservative breast cancer surgery This is aimed at removing the tumour plus a margin of normal breast tissue. This is commonly referred to as a wide local excision. The term lumpectomy should be reserved for an operation in which a benign tumour is excised and in which a large amount of normal breast tissue is not resected. A quadrantectomy involves removing the entire segment of the breast that contains the tumour. Both of these operations are usually combined with axillary surgery, usually via a separate incision in the axilla. There are various options that can be used to deal with the axilla, including sentinel node biopsy, sampling, removal of the nodes behind and lateral to the pectoralis minor (level II) or a full axillary dissection (level III). The width of the

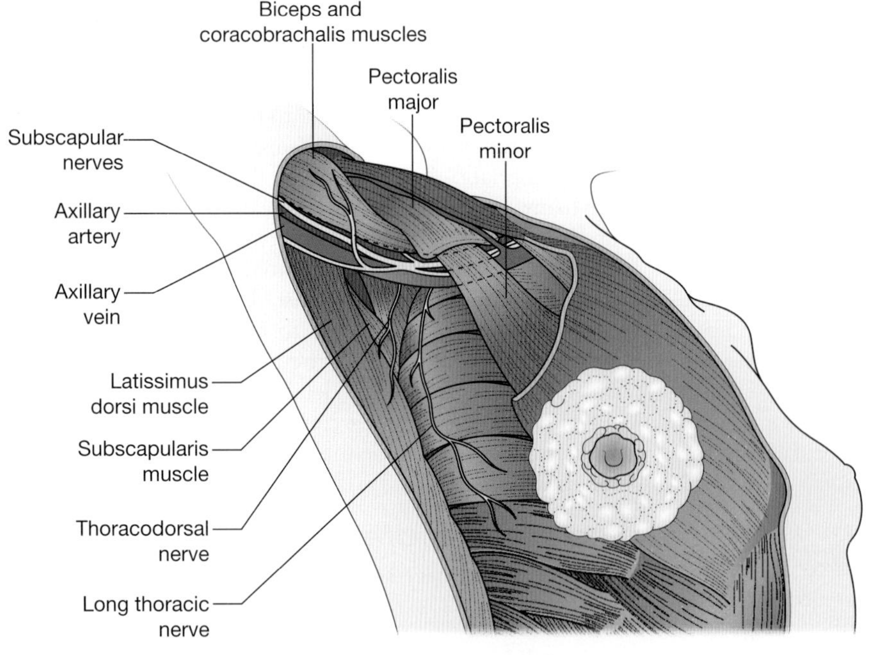

Figure 53.27 Radical mastectomy with pectoralis removed; the modified radical approach leaves the pectoralis major muscle intact.

William Stewart Halsted, 1852–1922, Professor of Surgery, Johns Hopkins Medical School, Baltimore, MD, USA.
David Howard Patey, 1899–1976, surgeon, The Middlesex Hospital, London, UK.

margin has attracted much controversy, with some units adopting a 1-cm margin and others 1 mm. A recent consensus meeting has suggested that no tumour at the inked margin is sufficient, although the trials upon which this is based have been challenged and many still regard 1 mm as a safer margin. There is no need for wider margins than this.

There is a somewhat higher rate of local recurrence following conservative surgery, even if combined with radiotherapy, but the long-term outlook in terms of survival is unaffected. Local recurrence is more common in younger women and in those with high-grade tumours and involved resection margins. Patients whose margins are involved should have a further local excision (or a mastectomy) before going on to radiotherapy. Local excision of a breast cancer without radiotherapy is associated with an unacceptably high local recurrence rate.

The role of axillary surgery is to stage the patient and to treat the axilla. The presence of metastatic disease within the axillary lymph nodes remains the best single marker for prognosis; however, treatment of the axilla does not affect long-term survival, suggesting that the axillary nodes act not as a 'reservoir' for disease but as a marker for metastatic potential. It used to be accepted that only premenopausal women should have their axilla staged by operation as there was a good case for giving chemotherapy to lymph node-positive patients; however, it is now clear that postmenopausal women also benefit from chemotherapy and so all patients require axillary staging. In postmenopausal patients, tamoxifen was once given regardless of axillary lymph node status, but it is now known that only hormone receptor-positive patients, irrespective of age, benefit from this. Axillary surgery should not be combined with radiotherapy to the axilla because of excess morbidity. Removal of the internal mammary lymph nodes is unnecessary.

Sentinel node biopsy This technique has become the standard of care in the management of the axilla in patients with clinically node-negative disease. An axillary ultrasound is now routinely performed along with the ultrasound of the breast cancer. Any suspicious nodes can be biopsied by either cytology or core biopsy The sentinel node is localised peroperatively by the injection of patent blue dye (Figure 53.28) and radioisotope-labelled albumin in the breast. The recommended site of injection is in the subdermal plexus around the nipple, although some still inject on the axillary side of the cancer. The marker passes to the primary node draining the area and is detected visually and with a hand-held gamma camera. Peropererative diagnosis allows completion axillary clearance if nodal disease is detected. This may be achieved with frozen-section analysis, touch imprint cytology (TIC) or by molecular methods. These involve homogenising the node and detection of a gene such as cytokeratin 19 or mammoglobin. In some cases there are only subcapsular micrometastases that are missed at frozen section. In patients in whom there is no tumour involvement of the sentinel node, further axillary dissection can be avoided. The utility of intraoperative diagnosis is increasingly questioned. It is time-consuming and with increasing use and experience of axillary ultrasound the rate of unexpectedly positive nodes is low. Moreover, there is increasing adoption of no further surgery even if a positive sentinel node is encountered. A nomogram outlining the chances of further axillary node positivity has been developed by the group at Memorial Sloan Kettering Hospital, New York, and is available on their website (www.mskcc.org/mskcc/html/15938.cfm). Recent trial results have called into question the utility of completion axillary clearance after a positive sentinel node has been detected but at present this remains controversial.

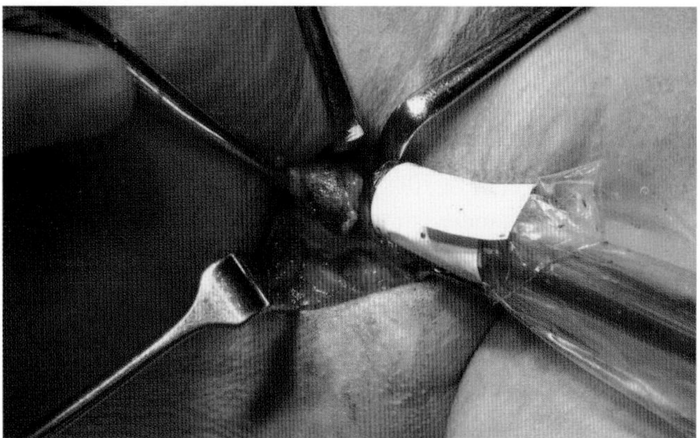

Figure 53.28 Sentinel node biopsy.

RADIOTHERAPY

Radiotherapy to the chest wall after mastectomy is indicated in selected patients in whom the risks of local recurrence are high. This includes patients with large tumours and those with large numbers of positive nodes or extensive lymphovascular invasion. There is some evidence that postoperative chest wall radiotherapy improves survival in women with node-positive breast cancer.

It is conventional to combine conservative surgery with radiotherapy to the remaining breast tissue. Recurrence rates are too high for treatment by local excision alone except in special cases (small node-negative tumours of a special type). Trials are under way to investigate whether radiotherapy can be given intraoperatively at one sitting or as an accelerated postoperative course. This would have considerable advantages in making conservative surgery available in areas where radiotherapy is not currently used. It would also relieve the burden of the current demand for radiotherapy, which accounts for up to 40% of activity in some departments.

Extrapolation from the Oxford overviews of systemic therapy (carried out every 5 years) suggests that for every four local recurrences avoided, one additional life will be spared at 15 years. This figure has recently been challenged but it does highlight the importance of getting the initial treatment right and avoiding local recurrence.

Adjuvant systemic therapy

Over the last 25 years there has been a revolution in understanding of the biological nature of carcinoma of the breast. It is now widely accepted that the outcomes of treatment are predetermined by the extent of micrometastatic disease at the time of diagnosis. Variations in the radical extent of local therapy might influence local relapse but probably do not alter long-term mortality from the disease. However, systemic therapy targeted at these putative micrometastases might be expected to delay relapse and prolong survival. As a result of many international clinical trials and recent world overview analyses it can be stated with statistical confidence that the appropriate use of adjuvant chemotherapy or hormone therapy will improve relapse-free survival by approximately 30%, which ultimately translates into an absolute improvement in survival of the order of 10% at 15 years. Bearing in mind how common breast cancer is in Northern Europe and the USA, these figures are of major public health importance.

Who to treat and with what are still questions for which absolute answers have yet to found, but the data from overviews of recent trials show that lymph node-positive and many higher-risk node-negative women should be advised to have adjuvant combined chemotherapy. Women with hormone receptor-positive tumours will obtain a worthwhile benefit from at least 5 years of endocrine therapy, either 20 mg daily of tamoxifen if premenopausal or the AIs (anastrozole, letrozole and exemestane) if postmenopausal. It is no longer appropriate to give hormone therapy to women who do not have oestrogen or progesterone receptor-positive disease. Recent trials have shown that longer durations of endocrine therapy provide a small extra benefit but with increased toxicity.

HORMONE THERAPY

Tamoxifen has been the most widely used 'hormonal' treatment in breast cancer. Its efficacy as an adjuvant therapy was first reported in 1983 and it has now been shown to reduce the annual rate of recurrence by 25%, with a 17% reduction in the annual rate of death. Beneficial effects of tamoxifen in reducing the risk of tumours in the contralateral breast have also been observed, as has its role as a preventative agent (IBIS-I and NSABP-P1 trials). Trials studying the optimal duration of treatment suggest that 5 years of treatment is preferable to 2 years.

Other hormonal agents that are also beneficial as adjuvant therapy have been developed. These include the LHRH agonists, which induce reversible ovarian suppression and thus have the same beneficial effects as surgical or radiation-induced ovarian ablation in premenopausal receptor-positive women, and the oral AIs for postmenopausal women. AIs are now licensed for treatment of all stages of disease and have been shown to be superior to tamoxifen. A large trial comparing anastrazole to tamoxifen in the adjuvant setting has shown beneficial effect for the AI in terms of relapse-free survival, although no benefit for overall survival. There is an additional reduction in contralateral disease, which makes this drug suitable for a study of prevention, and the side-effect profile is different from that of tamoxifen. AIs are more expensive than tamoxifen but are coming off patent protection and generic copies may allow more widespread use. There is an increase in bone density loss with patients taking an AI and a bone density scan is advised prior to commencement with treatment of underlying osptepaenia or osteporosis.

CHEMOTHERAPY

Chemotherapy using a first-generation regime such as a 6-monthly cycle of cyclophosphamide, methotrexate and 5-fluorouracil (CMF) will achieve a 25% reduction in the risk of relapse over a 10–15-year period. It is important to understand that this 25% reduction refers to the likelihood of an event happening. For example, a woman with a 96% chance of survival at, for example, 5 years only has a 4% chance of death over this time and the absolute benefit from chemotherapy would be an increase in survival rate of 1%, to 97%. This would not be a sufficient gain to offset the side effects of this potentially toxic therapy. However, for a woman with a 60% chance of dying (40% survival rate) a 25% reduction in risk would increase her likelihood of survival to 55% and thus treatment would be worthwhile. CMF is no longer considered adequate adjuvant chemotherapy and modern second- and third-generation regimes include an anthracycline (doxorubicin or epirubicin) and the newer agents such as the taxanes.

Chemotherapy used to be prescribed only to premenopausal women with a poor prognosis (in whom its effects are likely to be the result, in part, of a chemical castration effect) but it is now also offered to postmenopausal women with poor prognosis disease. Chemotherapy may be considered in node-negative patients if other prognostic factors, such as tumour grade, imply a high risk of recurrence. The effect of combining hormone and chemotherapy is additive, although hormone therapy is started after completion of chemotherapy to reduce side effects.

High-dose chemotherapy with stem cell rescue for patients with heavy lymph node involvement has now been shown in controlled trials to offer no advantage and has been abandoned.

Primary chemotherapy (neoadjuvant) is being used in many centres for large but operable tumours that would traditionally require a mastectomy (and almost certainly postoperative adjuvant chemotherapy). The aim of this treatment is to reduce tumour volume to enable breast-conserving surgery to be performed. This approach is successful in up to 80% of cases, but is not associated with improvements in survival compared with conventionally timed chemotherapy. Patients who achieve a complete pathological response have increased survival rates. Patients with Her-2-positive disease will receive Herceptin as part of their management and have high complete response rates. It is important that tumours have a metallic clip placed into them at the onset of therapy as otherwise there will be uncertainty about which area to resect once chemotherapy has been completed. There is debate about the safety and utility of sentinel node biopsy preinduction of chemotherapy; however, it can be safely performed after completion of chemotherapy. Neoadjuvant therapy is also used in the triple negative cohort of patients (Er, PR and Her-2 negative). In patients with breast cancer strongly positive for hormone receptors, a similar effect can be seen following 3 months of endocrine treatment.

Newer 'biological' agents will be used more frequently as molecular targets are identified – the first of these, trastuzamab (Herceptin®), is active against tumours containing the growth factor receptor c-erbB2. Other agents currently available are lapitinab, an oral combined tyrosine kinase inhibitor (TKI). Other TKIs are in development such as, pertuzumab. T-DM1 is a drug used in Her- 2-positive disease where a chemotherapy agent, emestane, is bound to an anti-Her-2 agent to allow targeted delivery of the chemotherapy to Her-2-positive cells. The antivascular growth factor bevacizumab initially showed promise but is now no longer routinely used for adjuvant therapy.

It is unclear how and when these agents will be used, whether in combination or instead of standard chemotherapy agents. They are very expensive and unaffordable in many countries. Other agents likely to be used in the next few years include CK4/CDK6 inhibitors for metastatic ER-positive cancer.

Follow-up of breast cancer

Patients with breast cancer used to be followed for life to detect recurrence and dissemination. This led to large clinics with little value for either patient or doctor. It is current practice to arrange yearly or 2-yearly mammography of the treated and contralateral breast. There is a move to return the patient early to the care of the general practitioner with fast-track access back to the breast clinic if suspicious symptoms appear. There is currently no routine role for repeated measurements of tumour markers or imaging other than mammography.

Phenomena resulting from lymphatic obstruction in advanced breast cancer

Peau d'orange

Peau d'orange is caused by cutaneous lymphatic oedema (Figure 53.24). Where the infiltrated skin is tethered by the sweat ducts it cannot swell, leading to an appearance like orange skin. Occasionally, the same phenomenon is seen over a chronic abscess.

Lymphoedema

Lymphoedema of the arm is a troublesome complication of breast cancer treatment, fortunately seen less often now that radical axillary dissection and radiotherapy are rarely combined. However, it does still occur occasionally after either mode of treatment alone and appears at any time from months to years after treatment. There is usually no precipitating cause but recurrent tumour should be excluded because neoplastic infiltration of the axilla can cause arm swelling as a result of both lymphatic and venous blockage. This neoplastic infiltration is often painful because of brachial plexus nerve involvement.

An oedematous limb is susceptible to bacterial infection following quite minor trauma and this requires vigorous antibiotic treatment. Antibiotics may need to be given for much longer than is normal and patients at risk of infection should have antibiotics readily available to enable treatment to be started promptly. Treatment of late oedema is difficult but limb elevation, elastic arm stockings and pneumatic compression devices can be useful.

Cancer-en-cuirasse

The skin of the chest is infiltrated with carcinoma and has been likened to a coat. It may be associated with a grossly swollen arm. This usually occurs in cases with local recurrence after mastectomy and is occasionally seen to follow the distribution of irradiation to the chest wall. The condition may respond to palliative systemic treatment but prognosis in terms of survival is poor.

Lymphangiosarcoma

Lymphangiosarcoma is a rare complication of lymphoedema with an onset many years after the original treatment. It takes the form of multiple subcutaneous nodules in the upper limb and must be distinguished from recurrent carcinoma of the breast. The prognosis is poor but some cases respond to cytotoxic therapy or irradiation. Interscapulothoracic (forequarter) amputation is rarely indicated.

Breast reconstruction

Despite an increasing trend towards conservative surgery, up to 40% of women still require, or want, a mastectomy. These women can now be offered immediate or delayed reconstruction of the breast. Few contraindications to breast reconstruction exist. Even those with a limited life expectancy may benefit from the improved quality of life; however, patients do require counselling before this procedure so that their expectations of cosmetic outcome are not unrealistic.

The increasing use of oncoplastic techniques such as volume displacement and volume replacement have opened up the options for increasing conservation rates. Specialist training is required and close cooperation with established plastic surgeons allows optimal selection of patients.

The easiest type of reconstruction is using a silicone gel implant under the pectoralis major muscle. The lateral portion of the implant, which was traditionally left in the subcutaneous plane, is now increasingly covered by an acellular dermal matrix (ADM). This gives a superior cosmetic result. Prior tissue expansion using an expandable saline prosthesis first (or a combined device), creates some ptosis of the new breast. If the skin at the mastectomy site is poor (e.g. following radiotherapy) or if a larger volume of tissue is required, a musculocutaneous flap can be constructed either from the latissimus dorsi muscle (an LD flap) (Figure 53.29) or using the transversus abdominis muscle (a TRAM flap as shown in Figure 53.30). The latter gives an excellent cosmetic result in experienced hands but is a lengthy procedure and requires careful patient selection. It is now usually performed as a free transfer using microvascular anastomosis, although the pedicled TRAM from the contralateral side is still used. Variations on the TRAM flap requiring less muscle harvesting, such as the DIEP flap (based on deep inferior epigastric vessels), are increasingly being used.

The timing of reconstruction may be difficult. Impediments to immediate reconstruction include insufficient theatre time and a lack of experienced reconstructive surgeons. In addition, if a patient is likely to need postoperative radiotherapy then a delayed reconstruction using a flap often gives a better result. Radiotherapy onto a prosthesis often leads to a high incidence of capsular contracture and unacceptable results.

Nipple reconstruction is a relatively simple procedure that can be performed under a local anaesthetic. Many different types of nipple reconstruction are described but the majority lose height with time. Tattooing of the reconstructed nipple is often required. Alternatively, the patient can be fitted with a prosthetic nipple. To achieve symmetry the opposite

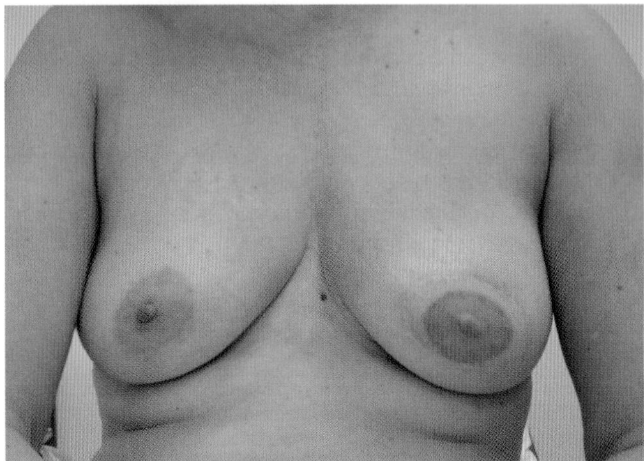

Figure 53.29 Reconstruction with latissimus dorsi flap.

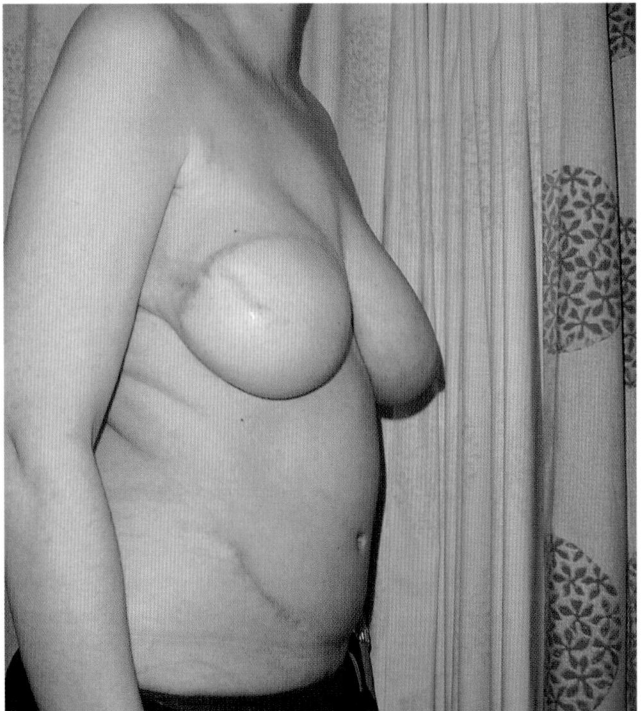

Figure 53.30 Transversus abdominus muscle flap.

breast may require a cosmetic procedure such as reduction or augmentation mammoplasty, or mastopexy. A breast reconstructive service can be offered by a suitably trained breast surgeon, a plastic surgeon or, ideally, using a combined oncoplastic approach. The patient needs to be warned that breast reconstruction is seldom, if ever, one operation.

External breast prostheses that fit within the bra are the most common method of restoring volume fill and should be available for all women who do not have an immediate reconstruction.

Screening for breast cancer

Because the prognosis of breast cancer is closely related to stage at diagnosis it would seem reasonable to hope that a population screening programme that could detect tumours before they come to the patient's notice might reduce mortality from breast cancer. Indeed, a number of studies have shown that breast screening by mammography in women over the age of 50 years will reduce cause-specific mortality by up to 30%. Following the publication in 1987 of the Forrest report, the National Health Service in the UK launched a programme of 3-yearly mammographic screening for women between the ages of 50 and 64 years (now increased to 70 years). The introduction of this programme has undoubtedly improved the quality of breast cancer services but a number of questions remain unanswered, including the value of screening women under 50 years and the ideal interval between screenings. The psychological consequences of false alarms or false reassurances still need to be addressed and self-examination programmes that have failed to show any benefit for the population in terms of earlier detection of or decreased mortality from breast cancer remain controversial. The opponents of screening rightly point out that some women will have disease detected and treated that might never harm them in their lifetime. However, this group of women cannot as yet be reliably seperated from those in whom prompt diagnosis and treatment will be benficial.

MRI is used to screen those at very high risk or where radiation might be hazardous (Li-Fraumeni syndrome). There is no place for thermography as a secreening (or diagnostic) tool.

Familial breast cancer

Recent developments in molecular genetics and the identification of a number of breast cancer predisposition genes (*BRCA1*, *BRCA2* and *p53*) have done much to stimulate interest in this area. Yet women whose breast cancer is due to an inherited genetic change actually account for less than 5% of all cases of breast cancer, that is about 1250 cases per year in the UK and 9000 cases in the USA. A much larger number of women will have a risk that is elevated above normal because of an as yet unspecified familial inheritance. These women have a risk of developing breast cancer that is 2–10 times above baseline. The risks associated with family history are summarised in *Table 53.5*. There are computer programs available to assist the clinician in assessing family history risk.

The *BRCA1* gene has been associated with an increased incidence of breast (and ovarian) cancer and is located on the long arm of chromosome 17 (17q). The gene frequency in the population is approximately 0.0006. It does, however, occur with greater frequency in certain populations such as Ashkenazi Jews, in whom there is often a common (founder) mutation. *BRCA2* is located on chromosome 13q and there is an association with male breast cancer.

Frederick Pei Li, 1940 – 2015, Dana-Farber Cancer Institute, Boston, MA USA and Joseph F Fraumeni, Jr. (b.1933), National Institutes of Health, Washington DC, USA, in 1969 identified four families with increased susceptibility to cancer. This led to the discovery of mutation in the tumour suppressor gene p53.
Sir Andrew Patrick McEwen Forrest, Regius Professor of Clinical Surgery, The University of Edinburgh, Edinburgh, UK.
Ashkenazi Jews are Jews of Eastern or Central European descent.

TABLE 53.5 Likelihood of genetic mutation with family history.

No. of family cases <50 years old	*BRCA1* (%)[a]	*BRCA2* (%)[b]
2	4	3
3	17	13
4	41	33
5	55	44

[a] *BRCA1* is also associated with ovarian and, to a lesser extent, colorectal and prostate cancer.

[b] *BRCA2* is associated with familial male breast cancer.

Women who are thought to be gene carriers may be offered breast screening (and ovarian screening in the case of *BRCA1*, which is known to impart a 50% lifetime risk of ovarian cancer), usually as part of a research programme, or genetic counselling and mutation analysis. Those who prove to be 'gene positive' have a 50–80% risk of developing breast cancer, predominantly while premenopausal. Many will opt for prophylactic mastectomy. Although this does not completely eliminate the risk, it does reduce it considerably. This work should be carried out in specialist centres.

For the great majority of women with a positive family history, who are unlikely to be carriers of a breast cancer gene, there are no currently proven breast cancer screening manoeuvres, although this is under investigation. Tamoxifen given for 5 years appears to reduce the risk of breast cancer by 30–50% as does the AI, anastrozole. Thus, these women are best served by being assessed and followed-up, preferably in a properly organised family history clinic.

Pregnancy

The effects of pregnancy on breast cancer are increasingly understood and it is thought that breast cancer presenting during pregnancy or lactation tends to be at a later stage, presumably because the symptoms are masked by the pregnancy; however, in other respects it behaves in a similar way to breast cancer in a non-pregnant young woman and should be treated accordingly. Thus, treatment is similar with some provisos: radiotherapy should be avoided during pregnancy, making mastectomy a more frequent option than breast conservation surgery; chemotherapy should be avoided during the first trimester but appears safe subsequently; most tumours are hormone receptor negative and so hormone treatment, which is potentially teratogenic, is not required. Becoming pregnant subsequent to a diagnosis of breast cancer appears not to alter the likely outcome, but women are usually advised to wait at least 2 years as it is within this time that recurrence most often occurs. The risk of developing breast cancer with oral contraceptive use is only slight, and disappears 10 years after stopping the oral contraceptive pill.

Hormone replacement therapy

HRT increases the risk of developing breast cancer if taken for prolonged periods and in certain high-risk groups. HRT may also prolong symptoms of benign breast disorders such as cysts and mastalgia and make mammographic appearances more difficult to interpret.

Patients who develop breast cancer while on HRT appear to have a more favourable prognosis. The consequences in terms of recurrence in women using HRT following breast cancer are unknown.

Treatment of advanced breast cancer

Breast cancer may occasionally present as metastatic disease without evidence of a primary tumour (that is with an occult primary). The diagnosis is made partly by exclusion of another site for the primary tumour and may be confirmed by histology with special immunohistological stains of the metastatic lesions. Management should be aimed at palliation of the symptoms and treatment of the breast cancer, usually by endocrine manipulation with or without radiotherapy.

Locally advanced inoperable breast cancer

Locally advanced inoperable breast cancer, including inflammatory breast cancer, is usually treated with systemic therapy, either chemotherapy or hormone therapy.

Occasionally, 'toilet mastectomy' or radiotherapy is required to control a fungating tumour but often incision through microscopically permeated tissues results in a worse outcome.

Metastatic carcinoma of the breast

Metastatic carcinoma of the breast will also require palliative systemic therapy to alleviate symptoms. Hormone manipulation is often the first-line treatment because of its minimal side effects. It is particularly useful for bony metastases. However, only about 30% of these tumours will be hormone responsive and, unfortunately, in time even these will become resistant to treatment. First-line hormone therapy for postmenopausal women is now anastrazole or one of the other third-generation AIs. Tamoxifen, ovarian suppression by surgery (for premenopausal women), radiotherapy and medical treatment are all in common use. When resistance to these has developed, other hormonal agents can prove useful, with about one-half of the response rate seen in the first-line therapy. The newer agents such as antiprogestins, pure antioestrogens and growth factor TKIs are all candidates for this role.

Cytotoxic therapy is used particularly in younger women or those with visceral metastases and rapidly growing tumours. A variety of regimes is available and, although none prolongs survival, contrary to expectations, quality of life and symptom control is often better with more aggressive treatments, with responses being seen in up to 70% of patients.

Local treatment may also prove useful for some metastatic disease, such as radiotherapy for painful bony deposits and internal fixation of pathological fractures.

THE MALE BREAST

Gynaecomastia

Idiopathic

Hypertrophy of the male breast may be unilateral or bilateral. The breasts enlarge at puberty and sometimes present the characteristics of female breasts.

Hormonal

Enlargement of the breasts often accompanied stilbestrol therapy for prostate cancer, now rarely used. It may also occur as a result of a teratoma of the testis, in anorchism and after castration. Rarely, it may be a feature of ectopic hormonal production in bronchial carcinoma and in adrenal and pituitary disease. Body builders may use steroids to improve their physique, which may cause gynaecomastia. Some even go so far as to take tamoxifen to mask this symptom.

Associated with leprosy

Gynaecomastia is very common in men suffering from leprosy. This is possibly because of bilateral testicular atrophy, which is a frequent accompaniment of leprosy.

Associated with liver failure

Gynaecomastia sometimes occurs in patients with cirrhosis as a result of failure of the liver to metabolise oestrogens. It is associated with drugs that interfere with the hepatic metabolism of oestrogens. It is also seen with certain drugs such as cimetidine, digitalis and spironolactone.

Associated with Klinefelter's syndrome

Gynaecomastia may occur in patients with Klinefelter's syndrome, a sex chromosome anomaly having 47XXY trisomy.

TREATMENT

Provided that the patient is healthy and comparatively young, reassurance may be sufficient. If not, mastectomy with preservation of the areola and nipple can be performed. The patient must be warned about the side effects of this procedure, which are common and a cause of many medico-legal complaints in the UK.

Carcinoma of the male breast

Carcinoma of the male breast (Figure 53.31) accounts for less than 0.5% of all cases of breast cancer. The known predisposing causes include gynaecomastia and excess endogenous or exogenous oestrogen. As in the female it tends to present as a lump and is most commonly an infiltrating ductal carcinoma.

Treatment

Stage for stage the treatment is the same as for carcinoma in the female breast and prognosis depends upon stage at presentation. Adequate local excision, because of the small size of the breast, should always be with a 'mastectomy'.

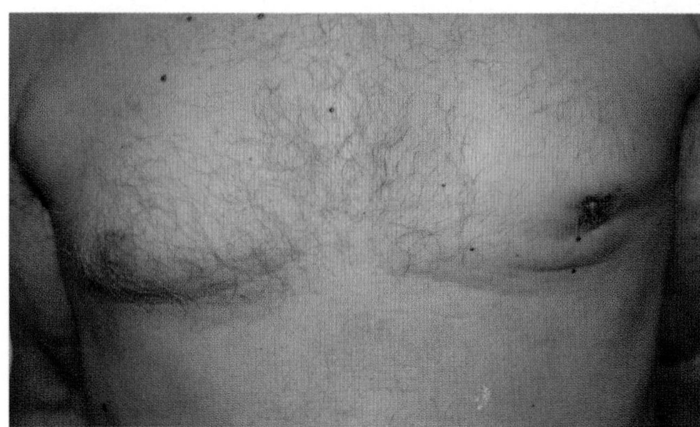

Figure 53.31 Carcinoma of the male left breast (courtesy of Professor Mike Dixon).

OTHER TUMOURS OF THE BREAST

Lipoma

A true lipoma is very rare.

Sarcoma of the breast

Sarcoma of the breast is usually of the spindle-cell variety and accounts for 0.5% of malignant tumours of the breast. Some of these growths arise in an intracanalicular fibroadenoma or may follow previous radiotherapy, e.g. for Hodgkin's lymphoma, many years previously. It may be impossible to distinguish clinically a sarcoma of the breast from a medullary carcinoma, but areas of cystic degeneration suggest a sarcoma and on incising the neoplasm it is pale and friable. Sarcoma tends to occur in younger women between the ages of 30 and 40 years. Treatment is by simple mastectomy followed by radiotherapy. The prognosis depends on the stage and histological type.

Metastases

On rare occasions cancer elsewhere may present with a metastasis in the breast. The breast is also occasionally infiltrated by Hodgkin's disease and other lymphomas.

FURTHER READING

Harris JR, Lippman M, Morrow M. Hellman S. *Diseases of the breast*. Philadelphia, PA: Lippincott, 2014.

Hughes LE, Mansel RE, Webster DJT. *Benign disorders and diseases of the breast*, 3rd edn. Edinburgh: Saunders, 2009.

Sainsbury R. Breast operations. In: Kirk R (ed). *General surgical operations*, 5th edn. Churchill Livingstone, 2006.

SIGN 84 Management of breast cancer in women. A national clinical guideline. Available online at: www.sign.ac.uk

Harry Fitch Klinefelter Jr., 1912–1990, physician of Baltimore, MD, USA, described this syndrome in 1942.

PART 9

Cardiothoracic

54 Cardiac surgery 884
55 The thorax 914

Chapter 54

Cardiac surgery

Learning objectives

To understand:

- The important role of surgery in cardiac disease
- The role of investigation in planning surgery
- The management of coronary heart disease
- The role of surgery in valvular heart disease
- The special role of surgery in congenital heart disease
- The management of aortic vascular and pericardial disease

INTRODUCTION

In 1925 Sir Henry Souttar reported the first mitral commissurotomy in the *British Medical Journal*. He wrote that the heart should be as amenable to surgery as any other organ. He saw the main problem as being maintenance of blood flow, particularly to the brain, while surgery was being performed.

The first real advances occurred in the late 1940s and early 1950s, driven by surgeons who had gained confidence and experience under the pressures and opportunities provided by war, followed by the development of cardiopulmonary bypass in the mid-1950s. Recently, the well-being and lifespan of patients with congenital, valvular and degenerative heart disease has improved drastically due to the advances in the range, complexity and technical expertise in cardiac surgery.

CARDIOPULMONARY BYPASS

Cardiopulmonary bypass (CPB) was first used successfully in 1953 by Gibbon and has since revolutionised cardiac surgery. It can be employed in any procedure in which the heart and lungs need to be stopped temporarily and their function replaced artificially. Before Gibbon's work, valve surgery under direct vision would not have been possible, nor would the precise reconstructions needed to treat extensive coronary artery disease (CAD). Much of the success of modern CPB is attributable to the development of new biomaterials and sophisticated oxygenating devices, as well as a greater understanding of the pathophysiological consequences of CPB.

Summary box 54.1

Alternative uses of cardiopulmonary bypass (CPB)

- Rewarming from profound hypothermia
- Resuscitation in severe respiratory failure
- As an adjunct in pulmonary embolectomy
- In single- and double-lung transplantation
- In cardiopulmonary trauma
- In certain non-cardiac surgical procedures (e.g. resection of highly vascular tumours and tumours invading large blood vessels)

Surgical approach to the heart

The heart is approached mainly by a median sternotomy. An incision is made from the suprasternal notch to the lower end of the xiphisternum. The sternum is divided and retracted to expose the thymus superiorly and the pericardium inferiorly. The thymus, although atrophic in adults, often remains relatively vascular. The thymus and pleurae are dissected from the pericardium and the pericardium is opened. Before cannulation for CPB, the patient is fully heparinised. Other incisions that can be used include left or right anterolateral thoracotomy for minimally invasive operations or for specific operations on the descending aorta.

Initiating cardiopulmonary bypass

Arterial cannulation

Conventionally, the great vessels are exposed and an aortic perfusion cannula is inserted into the ascending aorta, held in place by the purse-string suture. Air is excluded and the cannula connected to the bypass circuit. Alternatively, when it is inadvisable (aortic dissection), impractical (aortic root surgery) or impossible (severe adhesions) to cannulate the aorta, alternative arterial cannulation sites can be used, such as the

Sir Henry Sessions Souttar, 1875–1964, surgeon, The London Hospital, London, UK.
John Heysham Gibbon, 1903–1973, worked at Jefferson University, Philadelphia, PA, USA.

femoral artery or the axillary artery. The latter has recently been gaining more popularity, as it provides antegrade flow and can be utilised to provide selective cerebral perfusion in complex aortic operations; axillary cannulation has the theoretical advantage of reducing thromboembolic events when compared to femoral cannulation.

Venous cannulation

A purse-string suture is placed around the right atrial appendage and a single 'two-stage' venous cannula is placed to establish venous drainage. The venous pipe has end holes that sit in the inferior vena cava and side holes that sit in the right atrium (to take drainage from the superior vena cava). Alternatively, the superior and inferior vena cavae may be cannulated separately to gain better control over the venous return and to facilitate surgery within the right atrium. Venous drainage from the femoral vein can offer an alternative, particularly during thoracic aortic or minimally invasive procedures.

Cardio pulmonary bypass circuit

Once the circuit is connected (Figure 54.1) the CPB machine (the 'pump') gradually takes over the processes of circulation and ventilation. Once full flow is established (the required cardiac output depends on the body surface area of the patient), the ventilator is stopped and the heart can be isolated from the rest of the circulation. Blood is drained from the heart to the venous reservoir using the siphon effect by gravity, as it is usually placed 50–70 cm below the level of the heart and oxygenated using an oxygenator that allows gas exchange across its membrane. Blood is then pumped to the body by the bypass machine via the aortic cannula.

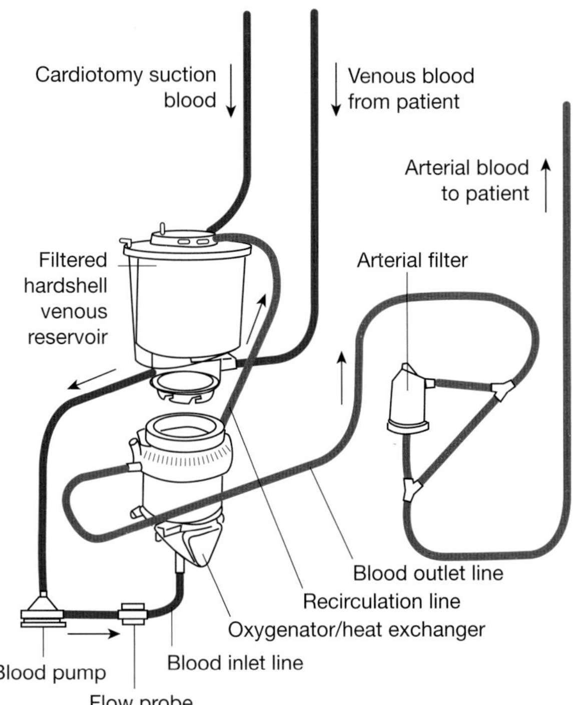

Figure 54.1 Components of the cardiopulmonary bypass (CPB) circuit. (Reproduced from Abraham JK. Cardiopulmonary bypass. *Surgery* 2000; **18**: 11, with permission from The Medical Publishing Company.)

The core systemic temperature can be lowered by passing the returning blood through a heat exchanger that can reduce the metabolic demands of the tissues. The degree of cooling is managed according to the severity and complexity of the surgical procedure, as well as the surgeon's preference.

The blood is also filtered to remove particulate emboli and returned to the systemic arterial circulation via a pump. Suction pumps can be employed to keep the area around the heart clear of blood and to decompress the heart when used as vents.

Myocardial protection

Once CPB has been established the ascending aorta is usually cross-clamped to obtain a bloodless operative field. The heart ceases to eject and becomes anoxic due to inhibition of coronary blood flow. Permanent myocardial damage can develop within 15–20 minutes, therefore most cardiac operations require some form of myocardial protection. Techniques of myocardial protection and the operative management of the myocardium have had a significant impact on the complexity of cardiac surgery. The methods of myocardial protection include intracoronary infusion of a cardioplegic solution (antegrade), infusion via the coronary sinus (retrograde), intermittent cross-clamp fibrillation and total circulatory arrest.

Cardioplegic solutions vary in terms of temperature, pH, arresting agent, osmolality and the presence of red cells and other factors. Most solutions contain potassium as the arresting agent. Potassium arrests the heart in diastole by depolarisation of the myocyte cellular membrane. Cold (4–10°C) isotonic crystalloid or blood solutions aid myocardial protection by reducing metabolic requirements through local hypothermia. Warm cardioplegic solutions, on the other hand, may facilitate better myocardial repair recovery postoperatively by aiding activation of intramyocardial enzymes.

Intermittent cross-clamp fibrillation is a technique in which intermittent ventricular fibrillation is induced by a small electrical charge. The heart does not eject and is relatively still but not bloodless. The aorta is cross-clamped to render the heart ischaemic. The heart can tolerate short periods (10–20 min) of ischaemia, provided the heart is reperfused when the cross-clamp is released and allowed to beat following cardioversion for short periods during the operation.

Total circulatory arrest becomes necessary when visibility and clarity of the operative area is crucial, as in paediatric surgery or in surgery of the ascending aorta and arch of the aorta. CPB is instituted and the core body temperature reduced to 15–18°C (profound hypothermia). The metabolic rate of all organs of the body is reduced by 50% with every 7°C drop in temperature. Using this technique, circulatory arrest can be tolerated for up to 20–30 min. Additional cerebral protection can be provided with ice packs placed around the head, pharmacological agents and cerebral perfusion techniques.

Discontinuing cardiopulmonary bypass

At the end of the procedure, air must be meticulously excluded from the cardiac chambers. Once perfusion is restored to the coronary arteries (by removing the cross-clamp) the heart may beat spontaneously. If ventricular fibrillation is present, cardioversion may be required. Epicardial pacing wires may be placed to treat postoperative bradycardia or heart block. The patient is rewarmed, acidosis and hypokalaemia are corrected and ventilation is restarted. The heart gradually takes over the circulation while the arterial flow from the CPB machine is reduced. When the blood pressure is acceptable and the surgeon is confident that the heart function is adequate, CPB is discontinued. The cannulae are removed and the anticoagulation is reversed by administering protamine.

Complications of CPB

CPB is a complex technique and requires careful interaction and communication between surgeon, anaesthetist and perfusionist to ensure that the patient remains safe. Difficulties can occur during cannulation (aortic dissection or atrial injury), at the start of CPB (oxygenator failure) and at the end of CPB (coagulopathy). Many complications can occur following blood exposure to the non-physiological surface of the CPB circuit. This leads to the activation of inflammatory cascades giving rise to a post-CPB systematic inflammatory response syndrome (SIRS) that can ultimately lead to multi-organ failure.

Recent understanding of the impact of CPB on the coagulation cascade and the patient's inflammatory response (SIRS) has resulted in the development of smaller 'mini' CPB, which has demonstrated some advantages in terms of post-CPB inflammatory responses and blood transfusion requirement. Alternative methods include surgery on beating heart 'off-pump', although despite some advantages, use remains restricted to coronory artery bypass grafting (CABG) and long-term outcomes are still a matter of debate.

CORONARY ARTERY BYPASS SURGERY

Introduction

Before the 1950s, surgical attempts to treat CAD through augmentation of non-coronary flow to the myocardium was via the creation of pericardial or omental adhesions, which had limited success. From the 1960s onwards, the importance of aortocoronary saphenous vein grafts and the value of the internal mammary (internal thoracic artery) were increasingly recognised. The outcomes of CABG surgery were carefully monitored from the beginning and by the 1970s, multiple large, prospectively randomised, multicentre trials were conducted. All these trials showed that a subset of patients had improved survival after surgery, compared with other treatments. With the advent of percutaneous coronary intervention (PCI) in the 1980s, the patient population undergoing CABG has changed, becoming progressively sicker but often with the most to gain. Over the last decade there have been major advances in PCI including the use of bare metal stents and the development of different generations of drug-eluting stents, as well as biodegradable stents, in an effort to reduce restenosis. Although the role of CABG in the treatment of ischaemic heart disease has been questioned, a recent large multicentre randomised trial carried out comparing CABG to PCI with drug-eluting stents has clearly shown that CABG is still the gold standard operation in certain groups of patients. Other more recent trials have confirmed these findings mainly in diabetic and high-risk patients.

Summary box 54.2

Potential complications of CPB

- Bleeding disorders
- Infection
- Air embolism
- Intestinal ischaemia/infarction
- Microembolisation
- Myocardial depression
- Neurological dysfunction
- Pancreatitis
- Postcardiotomy syndrome
- Pulmonary injury
- Systemic organ dysfunction
- Vascular injury

Coronary artery anatomy

The coronary arteries are branches of the ascending aorta, arising from ostia in the aortic sinuses above the aortic valve, the right from the anterior sinus and the left from the left posterior sinus (Figure 54.2).

Summary box 54.3

Coronary artery surgery

- Randomised controlled trials have confirmed improvement in survival following CABG for certain groups of patients

Left coronary artery

The left main coronary artery, which arises from the aortic root, can be the site of significant stenosis ('left main stem disease') and carries the worst prognosis in terms of survival without surgery. The artery is inaccessible at its origin and therefore grafts are anastomosed to its branches, the left anterior descending artery (LAD) or anterior interventricular artery and obtuse/marginal (OM) branches of the circumflex artery. The LAD is the most frequently diseased coronary artery and most often bypassed during CABG surgery.

Right coronary artery

The right coronary artery (RCA) passes from its origin anteriorly between the right atrial appendage and the pulmonary trunk and courses in the atrioventricular groove around the margin of the right ventricle. It usually forms an anastomosis with the circumflex artery at the junction of the right and left atria and the interventricular septum (the crux). It continues as the posterior descending artery or interventricular artery. Common sites of stenosis of the RCA are in its proximal

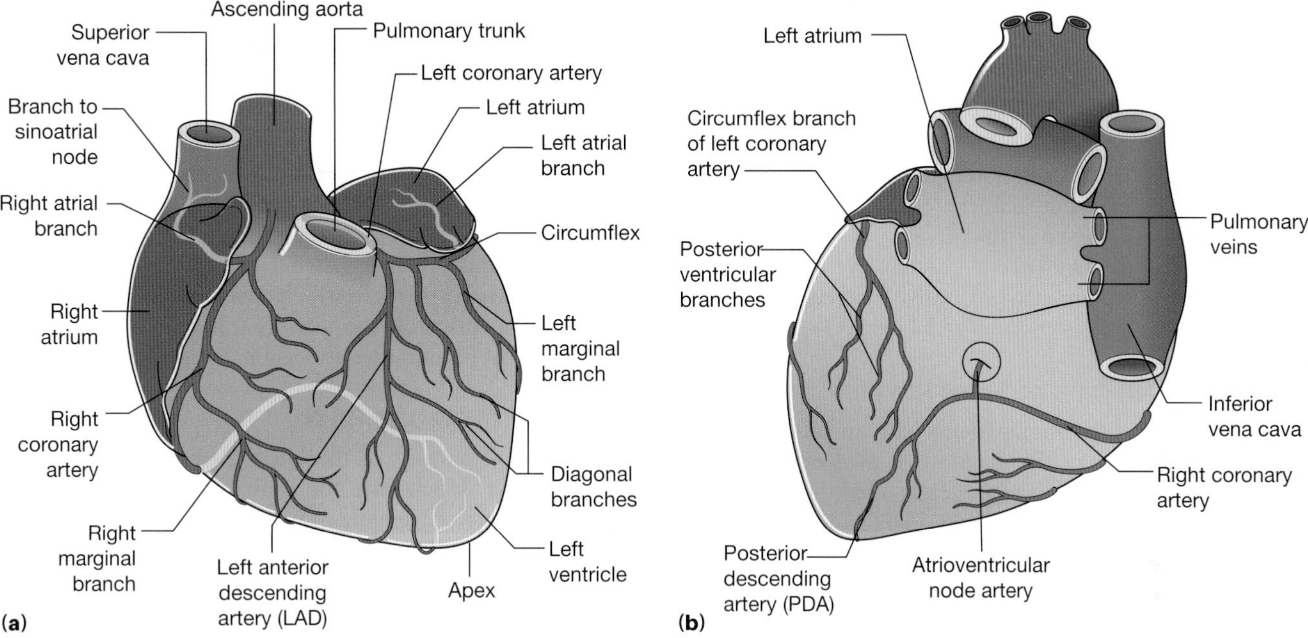

Figure 54.2 The heart, showing the distribution the of the left and right coronary arteries. (**a**) Anterior surface of the heart; (**b**) base and diaphragmatic surface of the heart.

portion or at the bifurcation or crux. In the presence of disease at the bifurcation, a graft can be placed distally to the posterior descending artery.

The question of anatomical dominance is determined by the artery that supplies the posterior descending artery. In approximately 90% of cases the posterior descending artery arises from the RCA, a pattern referred to as right dominance. The posterior descending artery can also arise from the circumflex artery, a pattern referred to as left dominance, which occurs in approximately 10% of cases. A balanced pattern is one in which two posterior descending arteries, one arising from the right coronary artery and one from the circumflex artery, can exist (**Figure 54.2**).

Ischaemic heart disease

Ischaemic heart disease (IHD) is a major cause of morbidity and mortality in resource-rich countries. The underlying pathology is mainly atherosclerosis of the coronary arteries.

Pathophysiology

Atherosclerosis is the process underlying the formation of focal obstructions or plaques in large- and medium-sized arteries. It is accepted that atherosclerosis is a chronic inflammatory process resulting from interactions between plasma lipoproteins, leukocytes (monocyte/macrophages, T lymphocytes), vascular endothelial cells and smooth muscle cells. Atherosclerotic lesions can histologically be found at different stages in blood vessels including:

- **The fatty streak**. The first evidence of atherosclerosis can be found in children 10–14 years of age. This appears as a yellow streak running along the major arteries. The streak consists of smooth muscle cells, which are filled with cholesterol, and foam cells.
- **Fibrous plaque**. A fibrous plaque consists of large numbers of smooth muscle cells, foam cells, and leukocytes. As the fibrous plaque grows, it projects into vessels leading to lumen narrowing that, in turn, can lead to ischaemia or infarction.
- **Complicated lesion**. This occurs when the fibrous plaque ruptures provoking activation of the coagulation cascade and the formation of thrombus

Clinical manifestations

The principal symptoms of IHD are chest pain or angina, breathlessness, fatigue, swelling, palpitations and syncope. Severity of symptoms and the extent to which the symptoms interfere with everyday activities form a significant part of the clinical history. An assessment of risk factors should be included. Clinical examination follows and, although often normal, any evidence of myocardial ischaemia or stigmata of associated disease, such as diabetes or peripheral vascular disease, should be noted.

Summary box 54.4

Risk factors for ischaemic heart disease (IHD)

- Advancing age
- Male gender
- Hyperlipidaemia
- Diabetes mellitus
- Hypertension
- Smoking
- Family history of IHD
- Obesity
- Reduced physical activity

Investigations

Non-invasive methods of diagnosis

RESTING ELECTROCARDIOGRAPHY

As a baseline test, a 12-lead resting electrocardiogram (ECG) often provides the first indication of ischaemic cardiac disease and is essential in the acute clinical setting. However, it is not necessarily abnormal even in the presence of severe multivessel coronary disease. Evidence of previous myocardial infarction (MI) is seen commonly, as Q waves and/or non-specific ST and T-wave changes.

TROPONIN AND CARDIAC ISOENZYMES

These are useful in assessing patients with an acute coronary syndrome (ACS) when the diagnosis is in doubt. Standard enzyme measurement such as troponin, creatine kinase MB (CKMB) and lactate dehydrogenase (LDH) can aid diagnosis, as well as having prognostic implications.

EXERCISE TOLERANCE TESTING

Exercise tolerance testing (ETT) is a valuable technique for assessing myocardial ischaemia, both for diagnostic purposes and as a prognostic tool. However, an abnormal exercise test must be interpreted in the light of the probability of CAD and the physiological response to exercise as measured by the percentage of the maximum predicted heart rate achieved. A positive test with evidence of ischaemia on the ECG (ST depression of ≤2 mm) does not always indicate IHD, and a negative test does not always exclude its presence.

ECHOCARDIOGRAPHY

Performed either through a transthoracic or transoesophageal approach, echocardiography is valuable for the evaluation of ventricular function and regional wall motion abnormalities, as well as valvular lesions.

Stress echocardiography can detect regional wall motion abnormalities brought on by exercise or the use of dobutamine or dipyridamole. It is a reliable method of identifying viable myocardium. Impaired but recoverable myocardium possesses a functional reserve that allows it to be temporarily recruited into action, whereas scar tissue does not. The development of real time 3-dimensional echocardiography (RT3DE) with the ability to carry out valve reconstruction from different aspects has recently revolutionised preoperative surgical planning in patients with complex valvular lesions.

RADIONUCLIDE STUDIES AND CARDIAC MAGNETIC RESONANCE IMAGING

The main type of radionuclide study used is myocardial perfusion scanning using specific radioiosotopes (such as thallium 201) to assess the significance of coronary disease and viability of the myocardium.

Cardiac magnetic resonance imaging (MRI) can be performed to evaluate the ischaemic burden of coronary disease (using pharmacological agents to stress the heart) and to provide details of tissue viability when using gadolinium as a contrast agent.

MRI is also very useful in assessing cardiac tumours, pericarditis and other structural heart diseases.

POSITRON EMISSION TOMOGRAPHY

Positron emission tomography (PET) provides information on myocardial perfusion, metabolism and cell membrane function. Positron-emitting isotopes are used to label physiological substances, which can measure the regional distribution of these substances. PET is valuable in the diagnosis of CAD, particularly when the more widely available imaging modalities are inconclusive. It can identify injured but viable myocardium that is potentially salvageable by revascularisation.

COMPUTED TOMOGRAPHY

With the development of the latest computed tomography (CT) scanners, which have the ability to correct for respiratory and cardiac movements, multislice high-resolution CT scanning may become an alternative to coronary angiography. It allows assessment of coronary disease, particularly proximal CAD, and gives some information about the degree of coronary artery calcification (calcium score) that is very helpful when stratifying patients to determine which ones will benefit from the more invasive coronary angiography.

Invasive methods of diagnosis

CORONARY ANGIOGRAPHY

Selective coronary angiography provides the means of accurately diagnosing the presence and extent of CAD and remains the 'gold standard' diagnostic technique (**Figure 54.3**). In spite of the availability of newer imaging techniques such as cardiac MRI, selective coronary angiography provides high image quality, demonstrating the extent, severity and location of coronary artery stenoses and the quality and size of the distal coronary arteries. Any stenosis in an artery of >70% of the diameter (90% reduction

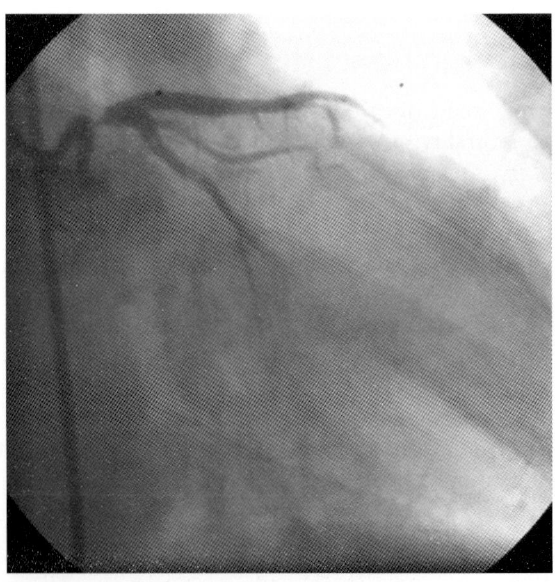

Figure 54.3 Coronary angiogram demonstrating severe stenosis in the left main stem prior to bifurcation of the left anterior descending and circumflex arteries.

of cross-sectional area) is considered 'severe'. In addition, angiography can assess ventricular function and provide the cardiac surgeon with information to determine operability, operative risk and probability of the operative result. Coronary angiography only outlines the coronary anatomy, does not demonstrate ischaemia and carries an overall complication rate of less than 1%. However, flow measurement across a stenotic area, using techniques such as fractional flow reserve (FFR), has been effective in predicting patients who are likely to benefit from revascularisation. Moreover, intravascular ultrasound (IVUS) can provide more detailed information regarding the degree of stenosis, especially in left main stem disease.

Summary box 54.5

Coronary angiography

- 'Gold standard' for imaging of anatomy
- Demonstrates extent, severity and location of stenoses
- Reduction in diameter of >70% is considered severe (90% reduction in cross-sectional area)
- Demonstrates quality and size of distal arterial tree
- Aids diagnosis of ischaemia
- Evaluates suitability for surgery
- Aids in prognostic assessment

Indications for surgery

The decision to offer CABG is based on the balance between the expected benefit and the potential risks to the patient. The two issues to be addressed when deciding if a patient is suitable to have surgery are the appropriateness of revascularisation and the relative merits of CABG versus PCI. Current best evidence shows that revascularisation can be readily justified on symptomatic grounds in patients with persistent limiting symptoms (angina or angina equivalent) despite optimal medical therapy and/or on prognostic grounds in certain anatomical patterns of disease.

Recent guidelines concerning myocardial revascularisation released by the Task Force on Myocardial Revascularization of the European Society of Cardiology (ESC) and the European Association for Cardio-Thoracic Surgery (EACTS), are useful in identifying patients with certain angiographic features who can benefit from surgery.

Summary box 54.6

Indication for surgery

- >50% stenosis of the left main stem ('critical left main stem disease')
- >50% stenosis of the proximal left anterior interventricular artery
- Two or three main coronary arteries diseased ('triple-vessel disease')
- Poor ventricular function associated with multivessel disease

Chronic stable angina

Although PCI is increasingly being used for the treatment of stable angina, CABG is still indicated in the presence of certain angiographic features. Angina can be relieved by surgical revascularisation in most patients and symptomatic improvement can be expected for over 10 years.

Acute coronary syndromes

A recently published meta-analysis showed substantial benefit with an early invasive strategy mainly in high-risk patients. An invasive strategy always starts with angiography. After defining the anatomy and its associated risk features, a decision about the type and extent of intervention can be made. The angiography in combination with ECG changes often identifies the culprit lesion and PCI, if desirable, can be recommended to treat it. Angiography should be performed urgently for diagnostic purposes in patients at high risk and in whom the differential diagnosis of other acute clinical situations is unclear. In patients stabilised after an episode of ACS, the indications for CABG are similar to those for patients with stable chronic disease.

The optimal timing of revascularisation is different for PCI and for CABG. While the benefit from PCI in patients with non-ST segment elevation acute coronary syndrome (NSTE-ACS) is related to its early performance, the benefit from CABG is greatest when patients can undergo surgery after several days of medical stabilisation.

Surgery for the complications of myocardial infarction

Myocardial infarction (MI) leads to myocyte necrosis, which may heal to form scar tissue or rupture if the ventricular wall gives way. Free rupture of the ventricle is usually fatal despite treatment. **Ventricular septal rupture** typically presents 3–7 days after infarction with pulmonary oedema, a pansystolic murmur and haemodynamic instability. The diagnosis is usually confirmed with echocardiography. Repair is with a pericardial or artificial Dacron patch. Mitral valve **papillary muscle necrosis** causes acute mitral regurgitation, a pansystolic murmur and pulmonary oedema. Diagnosis is made by echocardiography and right heart catheterisation (showing large V waves). Mitral valve replacement is usually necessary, but the mortality rate is higher than in valve replacement for non-ischaemic valvular diseases. Ventricular aneurysm occurs following partial-thickness necrosis of the ventricular wall if the free wall is replaced with noncontractile fibrous tissue. Left ventricular function is affected because the fibrous wall balloons out during systole and reduces the actual stroke volume. Repair is undertaken using CPB, and CABG is undertaken at the same time if necessary combined with valve replacement if needed.

Acute failure of percutaneous coronary angioplasty

Since the advent of intracoronary stents, the need for emergency CABG following complications of PCI is low at <1%. The mortality rate in this group is significantly higher than for elective CABG.

Preparation for surgery

Clinical assessment

Before CABG, the severity and stability of the patient's IHD, the presence of significant valvular disease and the status of left ventricular function should be properly evaluated. Any comorbid risk factors for IHD should be documented and, in particular, the state of coexisting diseases assessed. Attention is paid to the presence of carotid artery disease, peripheral vascular disease, respiratory status, preoperative diabetic control and presence of associated diabetic complications, significant renal dysfunction or coagulopathy. All medications taken by the patient are noted. Ideally, some should be stopped before surgery, in particular antiplatelet agents, including aspirin, anticoagulants and oral hypoglycaemics. Other drugs, such as diuretics and angiotensin-converting enzyme (ACE) inhibitors, are stopped at the discretion of the surgeon. However, apart from the exceptions noted, as a general rule all cardiac and antihypertensive medications should be taken preoperatively.

Risk assessment

Myocardial revascularisation is appropriate when the expected benefits, in terms of survival or health outcomes, exceed the expected negative consequences of the procedure. Therefore, risk assessment is an important aspect of contemporary clinical practice, being of value to clinicians and patients. Over the long term, it allows quality control and the assessment of health economics. Numerous different models have been developed for risk stratification in cardiac surgery including the EuroSCORE II and STS score.

EuroSCORE II is the system commonly used to predict risk for patients in the UK and can be an independent predictor of major adverse cardiac events (MACEs). Therefore, it can be used to determine the risk of revascularisation irrespective of, and even before, the selection of treatment strategy. However, it is important to acknowledge that no risk score can accurately predict events in an individual patient. Moreover, limitations exist with all databases used to build risk models, and differences in definitions and variable content can affect the performance of risk scores when they are applied across different populations. Ultimately risk stratification should be used as a guide, while clinical judgement and multidisciplinary discussion (Heart Team) remain essential.

Selection of conduit

Venous grafts

The long saphenous vein is the most common vein used as a conduit as it is straightforward to harvest, provides good length and is easy to handle. Historical studies showed limited long-term patency rate for long saphenous vein grafts (50–60% at 10 years). However, recent studies suggest that the early use of lipid-lowering agents and antiplatelet agents such as low-dose aspirin can improve vein graft long-term patency. In assessing the patient preoperatively, the legs should be checked for varicose veins. Alternative vein conduits include the short saphenous vein or upper limb veins such as the cephalic vein; however, these grafts are associated with poorer long-term patency rates.

Arterial grafts

The left internal mammary artery (LIMA), or internal thoracic artery, has become the conduit of choice for the LAD. Since the mid-1980s, long-term patency rates of >98% have been reported, with improved long-term survival and fewer reoperations. As LIMA–LAD anastomosis avoids the late complication of vein graft atherosclerosis, particular interest has focused on the use of bilateral internal mammary artery (BIMA) grafts. However, there is ongoing debate regarding the appropriateness in certain subgroups of patients, such as the obese diabetic, in whom sternal wound complications appear higher.

The use of the radial artery as a second or alternative arterial bypass graft has enjoyed a revival in recent times. This has been driven to some extent by the developing concept of total arterial revascularisation and the belief that this will help improve long-term results of coronary surgery. Different randomised controlled studies have demonstrated excellent patency rates at 1 and 5 years. In assessing a patient in whom a radial artery harvest is planned, an Allen's test should be performed. Alternative arterial bypass grafts include the gastroepiploic artery and the inferior epigastric artery.

Summary box 54.7

Allen's test

- The patient makes a tight fist while the surgeon compresses both distal and ulnar arteries digitally; this squeezes blood from the hand
- The hand is then relaxed and compression of the ulnar artery is released; the speed of returning colour to the hand is assessed
- If colour returns in 5–7 s, patency and collateral flow from the ulnar artery is confirmed

The operation

Intraoperative monitoring includes monitoring of continuous central venous pressure and blood pressure (via a central line in the internal jugular or subclavian vein and radial artery line, respectively), urine output via a urinary catheter, temperature using a nasopharyngeal probe and continuous ECG monitoring.

The operation commences with harvesting of the conduits (long saphenous vein from the leg (**Figure 54.4**), and/or radial artery) while the chest is opened via a median sternotomy and the LIMA is dissected from the chest wall (**Figure 54.5**). The patient is typically placed on CPB after heparinisation, the aorta is cross-clamped and the heart arrested with

Edgar van Nuys Allen, 1900–1961, Professor of Medicine, The Mayo Clinic, Rochester, MN, USA.

cardioplegia. The grafts are anastomosed to coronary arteries distal to the stenosis (Figure 54.6).

The aortic cross-clamp is removed and the heart is reperfused with oxygenated blood. A side-biting clamp is applied to the ascending aorta and the proximal anastomoses are completed. Occasionally, the surgeon may opt to carry out the whole operation while the cross-clamp is applied, to reduce the risks associated with aortic manipulation. The patient is warmed and weaned from CPB. The heparin is reversed and the patient is returned to the intensive care unit (ICU).

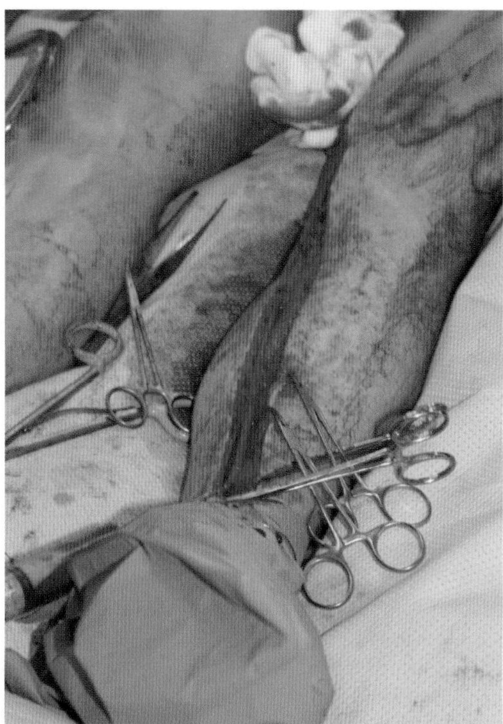

Figure 54.4 The long saphenous vein is exposed at the ankle, anterior to the medial malleolus, as far as the saphenofemoral junction (if required). The side branches are tied carefully and divided and the vein is excised. Gentle distension of the vein through a cannula at its distal end allows inspection for leaks.

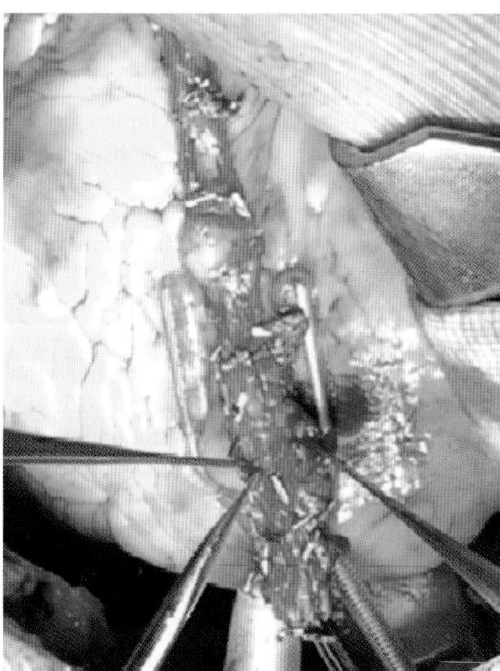

Figure 54.5 A pedicled left internal mammary artery is dissected off the chest wall and divided distally after systemic heparinisation. It is left attached to the subclavian artery proximally.

Postoperative recovery

The majority of patients are extubated a few hours after returning from surgery and remain in the ICU for 24 hours or so. In some centres, 'fast tracking' appropriate patients allows earlier transfer to a recovery area or high-dependency unit (HDU). Discharge is routinely 4–8 days after surgery.

Postoperative complications

Bleeding

Significant bleeding occurs in approximately 2–3% of patients. Rarely, acute cardiac tamponade or profound hypotension may occur in the early postoperative period and requires emergency resternotomy.

Arrhythmias

The most common postoperative arrhythmia is sinus tachycardia, closely followed by atrial fibrillation (AF). It occurs in around 30% of patients undergoing CABG and often spontaneously reverts to sinus rhythm. Treatment includes correction of potassium (>4.5 mmol/L), the use of β-blockers, amiodarone or digoxin and, if necessary, cardioversion. Bradycardia is seldom seen, but temporary pacing via epicardial pacing wires inserted intraoperatively may be required in the postoperative period.

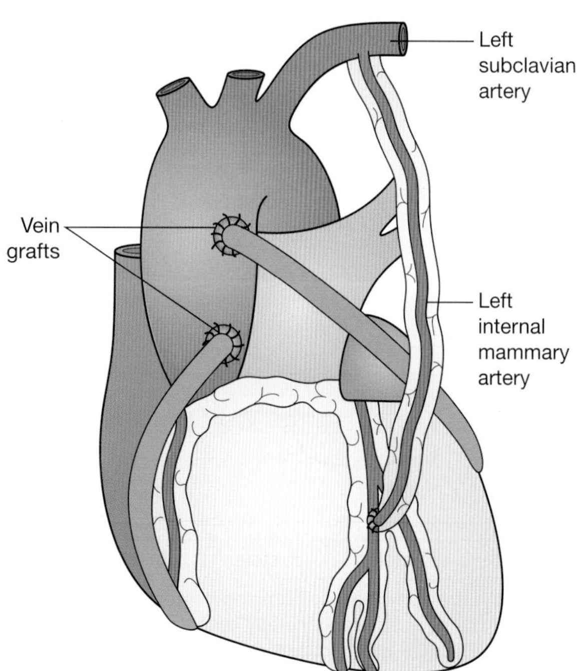

Figure 54.6 Completed coronary artery bypass grafts.

Poor cardiac output state

Myocardial function typically declines in the first few hours following cardiac surgery, presumably in response to an ischaemia/reperfusion-type injury. Inotropic agents are often required at this time to support the heart function and maintain the circulation. Occasionally, the patient develops a persistent low cardiac output state. The clinical manifestations include poor peripheral perfusion, low urine output, a developing metabolic acidosis and low blood pressure.

There are several mechanisms that account for this complication in the early postoperative period, including depressed myocardial contractility, reduced preload, increased afterload and a disturbance in heart rate or rhythm.

Treatment is aimed at the underlying cause but generally includes oxygenation, optimising preload, reducing afterload, managing any rhythm disturbances and improving contractility. If the low cardiac output state persists, the heart may require pharmacological or mechanical support.

PHARMACOLOGICAL SUPPORT

Inotropic drugs act in a variety of ways to alter the systemic vascular resistance, increase the heart rate and increase the force of myocardial contractility. Commonly used inotropes include dopamine, dobutamine, adrenaline (epinephrine) and noradrenaline (norepinephrine). These compounds are often used in conjunction with vasodilating agents that decrease the afterload.

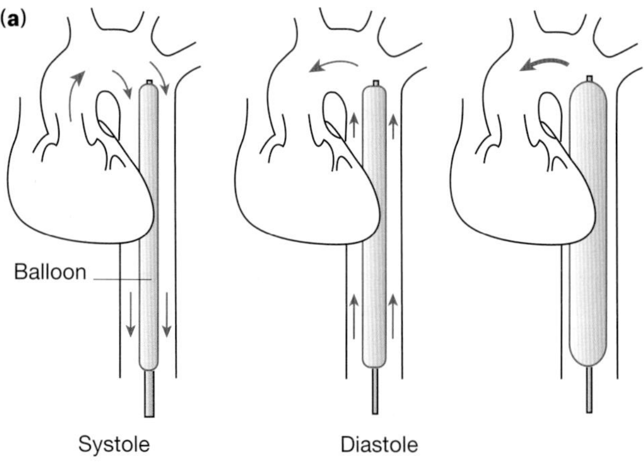

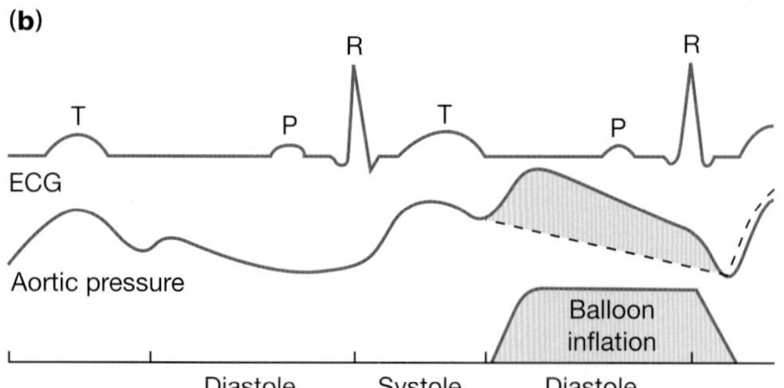

Figure 54.7 Intra-aortic balloon pump counterpulsation. (**a**) The balloon deflates during systole and thereby lowers systemic resistance. It inflates during diastole and increases coronary perfusion in addition to augmenting the systemic blood pressure. (**b**) The pressure changes and phases of the electrocardiogram (ECG) are shown.

MECHANICAL SUPPORT

If low cardiac output persists despite inotropic support, the heart may require mechanical support while it recovers its function. Mechanical support can be achieved using intra-aortic balloon pump (IABP), ventricular assist device (VAD) or extracorporeal membrane oxygenation (ECMO).

IABP is a device that is inserted, either percutaneously or under direct vision, into the common femoral artery. It is threaded into the aorta until its tip lies just distal to the arch vessels (**Figure 54.7**). The balloon is triggered by the ECG, deflating during ventricular systole (thus reducing afterload) and inflating in diastole (displacing blood that perfuses the coronary arteries retrogradely). When the heart has recovered sufficiently, the balloon is removed.

VAD is a mechanical circulatory supporting device used to replace the function of a failing heart partially or completely. It can be used as a short-term measure typically for patients recovering from heart attacks or heart surgery (bridge), or as a long-term support for patients suffering from congestive heart failure (destination). Current VAD devices are all continuous flow, based on a large trial that proved the superiority of continuous flow compared to pulsatile. Blood is exposed in these devices to a non-biological surface that can activate proinflammatory and coagulation cascades, leading to strokes and bleeding. Another important complication associated with VAD is infection.

ECMO is another circulatory support device that is similar to CPB; however ECMO can be established using venous access only (called VV-ECMO) or venous and arterial access (VA-ECMO). This mechanical support is mainly used for neonates and adults with potentially reversible respiratory failure, postcardiac surgery or as a temporary stabilisation method for patient who may need VAD (bridge therapy) as it can be easy to establish in unstable patients.

Neurological dysfunction

Stroke leading to a focal neurological deficit occurs in approximately 2% of patients following CABG. Embolisation, probably originating from the aortic arch or heart chambers, is the most common mechanism for territorial infarcts, with hypoperfusion leading to watershed infarcts. Diffuse neurological injury may occur leading to subtle cognitive abnormalities in memory, concentration and attention.

Wound infection

Significant deep wound infection resulting in sternal dehiscence and mediastinitis occurs in around 0.5–2% of patients. This can be associated with significant morbidity, with a prolonged hospital stay and further surgical interventions for debridement and/or rewiring of the sternum. It still has a significant mortality rate as high as 40%. Wound infections are more common in diabetics, dialysis patients and the obese.

Mortality

In the UK, the overall mortality rate for patients undergoing CABG is 1–3%. Multiple factors have been demonstrated to affect mortality after CABG, including age, gender, left ventricular function, use of LIMA and complete revascularisation.

Surgical outcome

Relief of symptoms

If revascularisation is complete, CABG alleviates or improves anginal symptoms in more than 90% of patients at 1 year; this falls to 80% at 5 years and 60% at 10 years. This symptomatic deterioration usually reflects progression of atherosclerotic disease in vein grafts and native coronary arteries.

Survival

Early surgical versus medical studies have reported survival rates to be >95% at 1 year, 90% at 5 years, 75% at 10 years and 60% at 15 years. Through changes in surgical practice, such as an increased use of arterial conduits and the widespread use of dual antiplatelet therapy, β-blockers and lipid-lowering agents, post-CABG survival may well improve in the future.

Summary box 54.8

Coronary artery bypass surgery outcome

Mortality
- 1–3%

Peroperative infarct
- 2–3%

Angina
- Better in >90% at 1 year
- 80% at 5 years
- 60% at 10 years

Survival
- >95% at 1 year
- 90% at 5 years
- 75% at 10 years
- 60% at 15 years

Off-pump coronary artery surgery

CABG without the use of CPB is a well-established and increasingly popular method that may be combined with a minimally invasive approach or carried out through a conventional sternotomy. It offers the advantages that it avoids the physiological stress associated with CPB and, to some extent, the aortic manipulation that can lead to neurological injury through atherosclerotic embolisation. Since the introduction of cardiac stabilising devices such as the Octopus® (Figure 54.8), off-pump coronary artery bypass (OPCAB) grafting has become widespread. One of the concerns, however, is related to the quality of anastomosis carried out on a beating heart and bloody field that can limit the surgeon's vision. The advantages of off-pump surgery over on-pump has recently been questioned, especially with the development of mini-bypass pumps, which offer a closed circuit and minimal unphysiological surface area. This reduces proinflammatory activation but at the same time allows the surgeon to operate on a still, bloodless heart. However, there is still no evidence to support the superiority of any of the above mentioned techniques and the final decision is usually based on the surgeon's skills and the required operation.

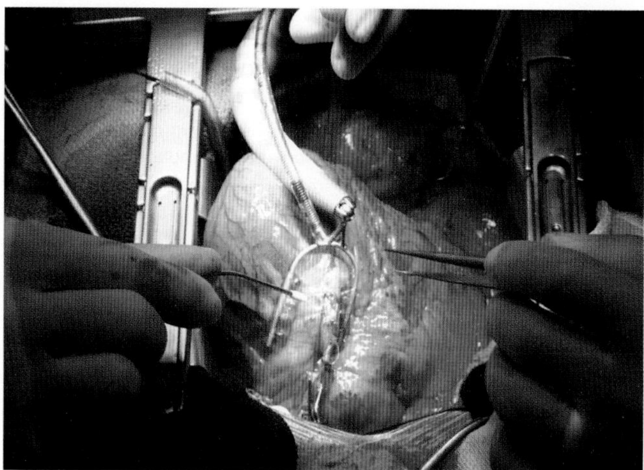

Figure 54.8 Off-pump coronary artery bypass using an Octopus® stabiliser to perform the distal anastomosis.

Minimal access surgery

Minimally invasive direct coronary artery bypass (MIDCAB) grafting is performed through a strategically placed minimal access incision and so avoids all invasive aspects of conventional CABG. Through an anterior submammary incision the LIMA can be dissected down with the aid of a thoracoscope and grafted to the LAD. More lateral MIDCAB incisions allow access to other coronary vessels, including branches of the circumflex artery. Patient selection remains, at least at present, a restriction to the ever-increasing minimally invasive methods being developed. Although not yet critically evaluated, one particular approach is to combine MIDCAB (typically LIMA to LAD) with PCI to other less accessible coronary arteries ('hybrid' coronary revascularisation).

VALVULAR HEART DISEASE

Introduction

Early surgical management of valvular heart disease concentrated on valvular repair. The heroic early procedures for valve stenosis were closed and therefore 'blind' commissurotomies. They were replaced by open procedures with full visualisation, allowing precise repair and replacement. The first prosthetic valve replacement was performed by Harken in 1960 replacing the aortic valve, followed by a mitral valve replacement by Starr a year later. Continued improvements in perioperative care, myocardial protection and, in particular,

Dwight Emary Harken, 1910–1993, formerly Chief of Thoracic Surgery, The Peter Bent Brigham Hospital, Boston, MA, USA. Innovator in heart surgery, he introduced the concept of intensive care unit and opened the first intensive care unit in 1951. Served as Chief of Thoracic Surgery at Harvard University for 22 years.
Albert Starr, b.1926, formerly Professor of Surgery, The University of Oregon, Portland, OR, USA. Medical Director, Providence Heart and Vascular Institute, Portland. Inventor of the world's first durable artificial mitral valve; winner of Lasker award in 2007 – an award given by the Lasker Foundation in the United States to a person (or persons) who has made major contributions to medical science or who has performed public service on behalf of medicine.

TABLE 54.1 Comparing options for heart valve surgery.

	Advantages	Disadvantages
Valve repair	Preservation of integral structures Improved haemodynamics Avoids long-term anticoagulation	Technical difficulties Variable failure rate
Valve replacement		
Mechanical	Readily available Extensive experience of use	Needs lifelong anticoagulation Susceptibility to infection
	Used in any age group	
	Durability, lifelong	
Biological		
Stented	Readily available	Limited lifespan
	Short period of anticoagulation	
Stentless	Readily available	Limited lifespan
	Probably better haemodynamics with less outflow tract obstruction	More difficult to insert
	Short period of anticoagulation	
Homograft	No anticoagulation Improved haemodynamics Long-term outcome uncertain	Not readily available Technical difficulties

(Adapted from Sharpe DAC, Das SR. Heart valve surgery. *Surgery* 2000; **18**: 265–9.)

the development of prosthetic heart valves have improved long-term haemodynamic results, provided symptom relief and prolonged survival. The majority of valvular operations involve surgery on the aortic or mitral valve; tricuspid and pulmonary valve surgery is rarely undertaken in isolation.

Surgical anatomy

Heart valves function to maintain pressure gradients between cardiac chambers and so ensure unidirectional flow of blood without reflux through the heart. The aortic valve is tricuspid, with semilunar leaflets attached to the aortic wall at the annulus with the aortic sinuses being above the base of each leaflet, two of which form the origin or ostium of the coronary arteries. The intrinsic shape of the aortic semilunar valve allows blood to leave the ventricle during systole and prevents regurgitation during diastole. If disease leads to disruption of the leaflets or the annulus, valve function will be affected.

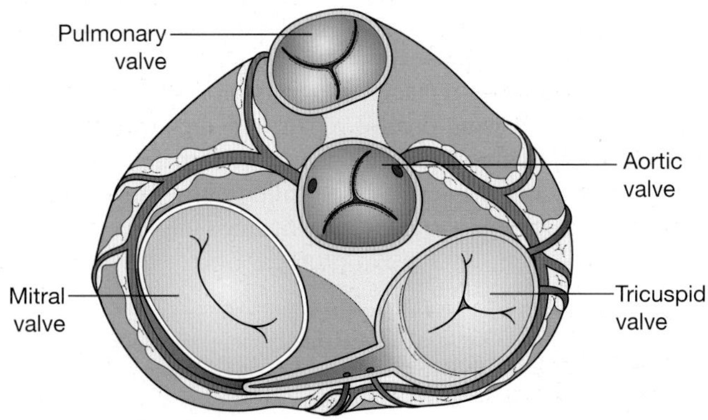

Figure 54.9 Four valves of the heart.

The mitral valve is bicuspid; the more anterior cusp is larger in area and lies between the orifices of the mitral and aortic valves. The leaflets, like those of the aortic valve, are attached to an annulus. The leaflets join at two commissures and are supported by a subvalvular apparatus, consisting of chordae tendinae and papillary muscles. The papillary muscles contract in ventricular systole, pulling the cusps towards the atrioventricular orifice and holding blood within the ventricle. The proper functioning of the mitral valve depends on the integrity of the annulus, leaflets, chordae and papillary muscles. If surgical correction is required, emphasis is on the preservation of these structures when possible (**Figure 54.9**).

Surgical options for heart valve disease

The decision of whether to repair or replace the diseased valve depends on the underlying pathology, the severity of disease and quality and/or involvement of the surrounding supporting structures. Generally, repair is increasingly favoured when possible in mitral valve disease, particularly in degenerative mitral regurgitation, in which it has been shown to have good long-term outcomes. Repair is the operation of choice in tricuspid valve disease, but aortic valve surgery generally involves replacing the diseased valve (*Table 54.1*).

Important factors in selecting the type of procedure and prosthesis include the patient's choice, age, existing comorbidities and the need for anticoagulation. Because of uncertainties about its lifespan, there is debate about when a bioprosthetic valve should be used, with most accepting its use in those over 60 years. The need for anticoagulation may have an impact on choice of valve, particularly in women of childbearing age, the elderly, the presence of congenital or acquired bleeding diathesis and when there is the need for further major surgery.

Types of prosthetic valves

Mechanical valves

Mechanical valves can be used in any age group to replace any valve (**Figure 54.10**). They are extremely durable but the components of the valve are thrombogenic and, therefore, the patient requires systemic anticoagulation, usually with warfarin. This subjects the patient to a lifetime of blood tests, medication and the constant threat of haemorrhagic (intracerebral, epistaxis, gastrointestinal bleed) or thrombotic (cerebral infarction) complications.

Biological valves

Biological valves include **homograft** (or **allograft**) valves, removed from cadavers; **autografts**, a patient's own valve; and, most commonly, **heterografts** (or **xenografts**) prepared from animal tissues. All share the basic design of three semilunar leaflets with central flow, so decreasing pressure gradients and minimising turbulence (**Figure 54.11**). Heterograft 'tissue' valves are the most commonly used valves and can be stented with a limited durability of 10–15 years, whereas stentless (or frameless) valves are expected to have less late calcific degeneration but are more technically difficult to insert.

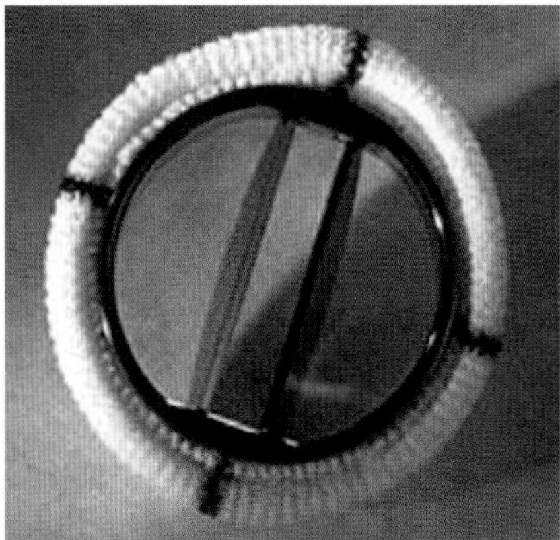

Figure 54.10 Bileaflet mechanical valve.

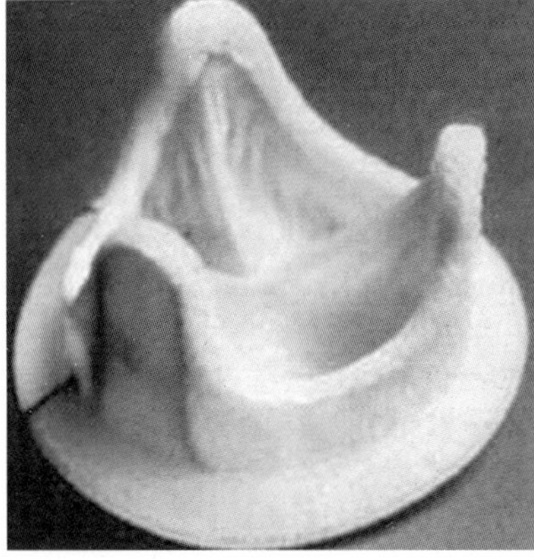

Figure 54.11 Porcine heterograft stented valve.

Prosthetic valve dysfunction and complications

Structural valve failure

Bioprosthetic valves are vulnerable to degenerative changes. Structural failure rates for biological valves, although rare in those over 70 years of age, can reach 60% after 15 years. However, newer biological valves have a reoperative rate of <10% at 20 years. Structural failure of a mechanical valve is generally uncommon.

Paravalvular leak

Early-onset paravalvular leaks usually result from technical difficulties at insertion. Late-onset leaks can occur and may be related to an episode of endocarditis or, in the presence of bioprostheses, leaflet degeneration. The leak can cause haemolytic anaemia or haemodynamic compromise and the valve may need replacement.

Thrombosis and thromboembolism

Thrombus formation on a prosthetic valve remains the most common complication of mechanical and biological valves (**Figure 54.12**). The risk of thromboembolism is greater with a valve in the mitral position (mechanical or biological) than with one in the aortic position. Improved haemodynamic function lowers the probability of thromboembolism. The incidence of thromboembolism in current mechanical valves is 0.5–3% per patient-year.

Prosthetic valve endocarditis

The incidence of prosthetic valve endocarditis (PVE) is 2–4%. The risk is lifelong and is at its greatest in the 3 months after surgery. The incidence of PVE is higher with mechanical and bioprosthetic valves and lowest with homograft and autograft valves. The diagnosis is suspected following symptoms of

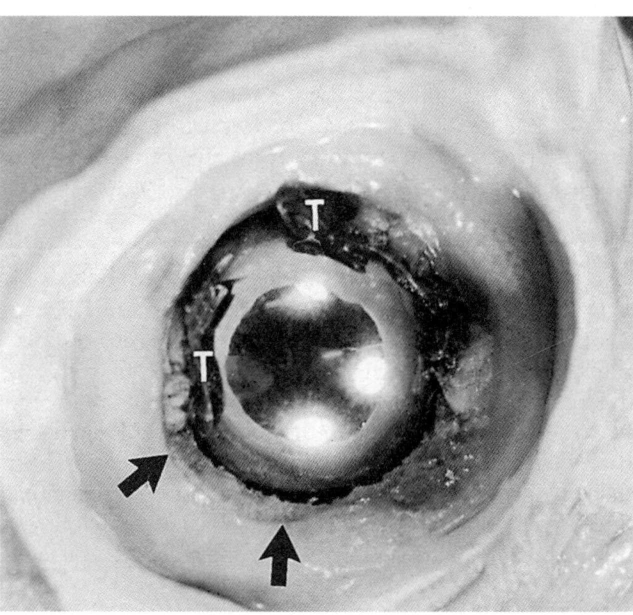

Figure 54.12 Thrombus (marked T and illustrated with the arrows) on the moving components of a ball-and-cage valve.

septicaemia, appearance of a new murmur or a septic embolus. It is confirmed with echocardiography, which may show vegetations and even abscess formation. A high index of suspicion is required and early multiple blood cultures are needed to confirm the diagnosis, identify the infective organism and choose appropriate antibiotic therapy. The most common organisms that can lead to PVE are the *Staphylococcus* species, particularly *S. epidermidis* in early PVE and *S. aureus* (at least 50% of cases); the *Streptococcus* species, usually *S. viridans* but also *S. pneumoniae*; and, less commonly, gram-negative bacilli, as well as fungal organisms.

The treatment of choice is early aggressive intravenous antibiotic therapy. Serial echocardiography to assess extent of infection into surrounding myocardial tissue, as well as functional assessment of the infected valve may help in optimising decisions on timing of surgical intervention. The prognosis of PVE remains poor, with an overall mortality rate of over 20%.

Postoperative management

Antibiotic prophylaxis

Currently; the National Institute for Health and Care Excellence (NICE) recommends that prophylactic antibiotics are not required for patients with prothetic valves undergoing dental procedures. Other leading European bodies have recently supported the above recommendation as the is no strong evidence to the contrary.

Antithrombotic therapy

All patients with mechanical valves require warfarin, usually started on the first or second postoperative day. The use of anticoagulation or antiplatelet therapy with biological valves is variable and depends on the patient's underlying rhythm postoperatively and surgeons' preference.

Mitral valve disease

Mitral regurgitation

Any pathological process affecting the mitral valve apparatus may lead to mitral regurgitation. As such, there are many causes of regurgitation and they can be broadly classified into four headings.

PATHOPHYSIOLOGY

There is an important distinction between acute and chronic mitral regurgitation. The former is usually the result of ischaemic papillary muscle rupture or following infective endocarditis, whereas the latter is the result of myxomatous degeneration or fibroelastic changes in the leaflets.

In acute mitral regurgitation, the left ventricle ejects blood back into a small, poorly compliant left atrium, imposing a sudden volume load on the left atrium during ventricular systole. This leads to an abrupt rise in left atrial pressure followed by a rise in pulmonary venous pressure and pulmonary oedema.

Summary box 54.9

Causes of mitral regurgitation and likely pathology

Degenerative

- Myxomatous degeneration of the valve and subvalvular apparatus (Barlow's disease)
- Fibroelastic deficiency (in elderly patients)
- Senile calcification: calcified annulus
- Connective tissue disorders (e.g. Marfan syndrome, Ehlers–Danlos syndrome): disruption of mitral valve apparatus

Ischaemic

- Papillary muscle rupture: following myocardial infarction
- Dynamic mitral regurgitation: as a result of transient ischaemia
- Poor left ventricular function: most common 'functional' cause secondary to myocardial ischaemia

Rheumatic

- Previous acute rheumatic fever: stiffened leaflets unable to coapt

Infective

- Endocarditis: leaflet destruction and perforation

(Adapted from Hall R. Mitral valve disease. *Medicine* 1997; **25**: 27.)

In chronic mitral regurgitation, the process is sufficiently slow to allow compensatory left ventricular dilatation and hypertrophy, and dilatation of the left atrium without any significant increase in pressure, so protecting the pulmonary circulation. As the disease advances and left atrial dilatation can no longer accomodate, left atrial pressure begins to rise, leading to a rise in pulmonary venous pressure and progressive pulmonary congestion, with eventual congestive cardiac failure.

CLINICAL FEATURES

In acute mitral regurgitation, the patient is usually unwell, presenting with clinical and radiological evidence of acute pulmonary oedema and a loud apical pansystolic murmur. Patients with mild chronic mitral regurgitation are usually asymptomatic. With progressive pulmonary congestion and left ventricular failure, the patient develops fatigue, dyspnoea on exertion and orthopnoea. The development of AF with left atrial dilatation is common. The enlarged left ventricle leads to a heaving apical impulse and a pansystolic murmur.

INVESTIGATIONS

- **ECG** may show left atrial hypertrophy (bifid P waves), left ventricular hypertrophy and atrial fibrillation.
- **Chest radiography**. There may be cardiomegaly with prominent pulmonary vasculature.
- **Echocardiography**. This is often combined with colour flow Doppler imaging, which shows the severity of the regurgitant jet of mitral regurgitation.

John Brereton Barlow, 1924–2008, South African cardiologist.
Christian Johann Doppler, 1803–1853, Professor of Experimental Physics, Vienna, Austria, enunciated the 'Doppler Principle' in 1842.

- **Coronary angiography**. In patients >40 years of age to investigate the coronary arteries.
- **Cardiac MRI**. Increasingly popular as it can give detailed information on structure and function

INDICATIONS FOR SURGERY

Indications for surgery for patients with primary mitral regurgitation include severe mitral regurgitation in symptomatic patients or severe regurgitation associated with changes in left ventricular function or dimension (such as left ventricular end-systolic diameter), as evidence suggests that any changes in ventricular function in the setting of primary mitral regurgitation is usually associated with significant mortality if not corrected (**Figure 54.13**). It is also recommended to address severe mitral disease in the same setting if a patient is undergoing cardiac surgery for a different reason.

The treatment of mitral regurgitation secondary to ischaemic heart disease remains controversial and current evidence suggests that patients with severe ischaemic regurgitation may benefit from mitral valve replacement, while patients with moderate regurgitation should usually undergo repair along with CABG if indicated.

Mitral stenosis

The most common cause of mitral stenosis worldwide remains rheumatic fever, despite the fact that the incidence of overt rheumatic fever in resource-rich countries has decreased. During the healing phase of acute rheumatic fever, the valve leaflets become adherent to each other at their free border so that the commissures become obliterated and the valve orifice narrows. Symptoms of mitral stenosis usually develop more than 10 years after the acute attack.

PATHOPHYSIOLOGY

Mitral stenosis slows ventricular filling during diastole and the pressure in the left atrium rises to maintain cardiac output. This leads to atrial hypertrophy and dilatation. Pulmonary congestion results from the rise in left atrial pressure but, with time, the lungs are protected against pulmonary oedema by constriction of the pulmonary vessels. However, this adaptive response, along with the passive 'back pressure' generated by the rise in left atrial pressure, leads to pulmonary hypertension. This leads to an increased demand on the right ventricle with eventual right heart failure and tricuspid regurgitation. The development of AF is common and can lead to a significant reduction in cardiac output. AF predisposes to thrombi forming in the left atrium, which may embolise to the systemic circulation.

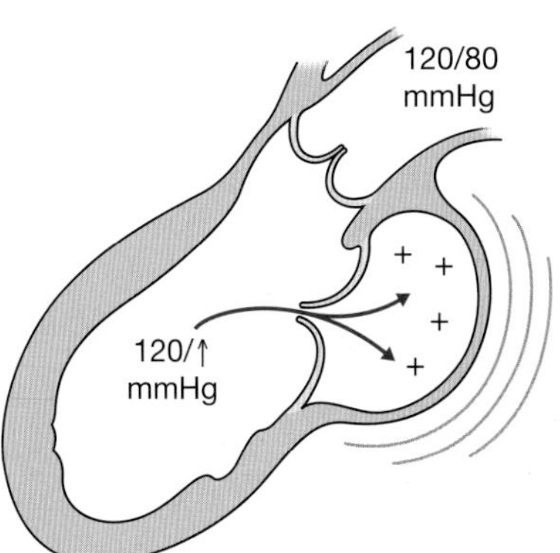

Figure 54.13 Features and pathophysiology of mitral regurgitation. There is a loud parasystolic murmur and the left atrium enlarges. The left ventricle enlarges as a consequence of volume overload.

Summary box 54.10

Causes of mitral valve disease

Stenosis
- Rheumatic heart disease (common)
- Calcification of valve or chordae
- Congenital (rare)

Regurgitation
- Rheumatic heart disease
- Valve prolapse
- Left ventricular dilatation or hypertrophy
- Ischaemia
- Bacterial endocarditis

CLINICAL FEATURES

Patients may remain asymptomatic for years and then present with symptoms when the heart is stressed by an event such as pregnancy, fever, chest infection or with the onset of AF. The common symptoms are fatigue and dyspnoea on exertion, which result from the combination of reduced forward flow and increased back pressure. The resulting pulmonary congestion adds to breathlessness and may produce a cough or haemoptysis. If mitral stenosis is advanced, there may also be a right ventricular heave due to right ventricular hypertrophy in response to pulmonary hypertension. Auscultation reveals an opening snap soon after the second heart sound, as the diseased valve is opened forcibly by the high pressure in the left atrium. The reverse happens when the valve closes and there is a loud 'tapping' first heart sound. In addition, a rumbling mid-diastolic murmur can be heard. The duration of the murmur is related to the severity of the mitral stenosis, increasing in length as the stenosis becomes more severe.

INVESTIGATIONS

- **ECG** may show left atrial enlargement (P-mitrale) or AF. Right axis deviation and other ECG signs of right ventricular hypertrophy (tall QRS complexes in the right ventricular leads V_{1-3}) may also be present.
- **Chest radiography**. There is a small aortic outline and a prominent pulmonary artery. The left atrium is enlarged (sometimes to an enormous degree) along with upper lobe diversion as a result of the raised pulmonary venous pressure. The right ventricle also appears enlarged (**Figure 54.14**).

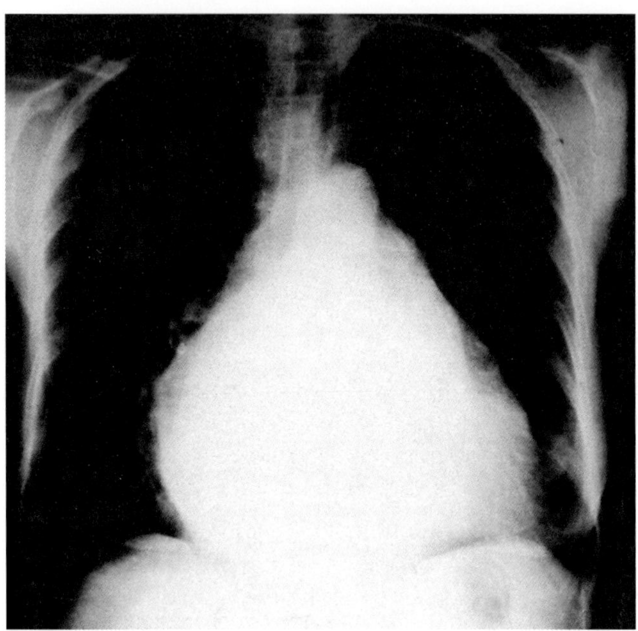

Figure 54.14 Chest radiograph of long-standing mitral stenosis, showing a massive left atrium.

- **Echocardiography**, in combination with colour flow Doppler imaging, allows assessment of the flow across the valve and, therefore, the degree of stenosis. Transoesophageal echocardiography (TOE) may be better at assessing valve morphology in detail and excluding the presence of an atrial thrombus.
- **Coronary angiography**. To investigate the coronary arteries.
- **Cardiac MRI**.
- **Right heart catheterisation**.

INDICATIONS FOR SURGERY

Medical management includes use of anticoagulation in patients with AF or left atrial enlargement. Tachyarrhythmias, including fast AF, that may lead to decompensation and cardiac failure, should be treated. Rate-controlling agents are the mainstay of treatment. Diuretics may provide some benefit. The principal invasive intervention is percutanous mitral balloon valvuloplasty (PMBV); surgery is indicated for severely symptomatic patients who have failed or who are unsuitable for PMBV. The prognosis is determined by the severity of the stenosis, the size of the atrium, the onset of AF, rising pulmonary artery pressure and the unpredictable risk of embolism from a large, fibrillating atrium (**Figure 54.15**). Surgical options include mitral valve repair or mitral valve replacement. Formerly common surgical procedures such as closed or open commissurotomy are now rarely performed.

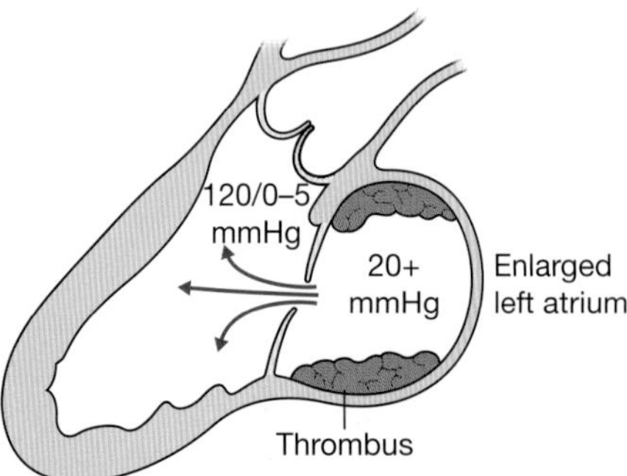

Figure 54.15 Features and pathophysiology of mitral stenosis. The aorta and left ventricle are relatively small because of chronically reduced cardiac output. The atrium is enlarged and may fibrillate, become stagnant and contain a thrombus. The ventricle fills with a turbulent jet that may be detected as a diastolic murmur or a thrill at the apex.

Mitral valve operations

Depending on the type of procedure and approach to the mitral valve, a median sternotomy or, occasionally, a right thoracotomy is performed. The mitral valve can be approached directly through the left atrium in the interatrial groove, through the right atrium and then the interatrial septum, or through the left atrial appendage.

MITRAL VALVE REPAIR

The restoration of normal valve function and preservation of the mitral apparatus is preferable to replacement in specific groups of pathology, as it can be associated with improved long-term ventricular remodelling and function. This approach reduces the bleeding complications associated with anticoagulants. The functional classification system developed by Carpentier serves as a guideline in valve reconstruction. It allows classification of any mitral insufficiency into one of three groups according to the amplitude of the leaflet motion and provides a useful framework for the mechanisms of failure of the mitral valve. As a rule, several valvular lesions or abnormalities are involved in a functional abnormality, with specific techniques developed to correct each lesion.

At surgery, the anatomy of the valvular apparatus and subvalvular structures have to be carefully inspected. In particular, the extent of annular dilatation, leaflet prolapse and chordal dysfunction are assessed. The mitral valve reconstruction is completed using various techniques, including insertion of a prosthetic ring annuloplasty (**Figure 54.16**); triangular or quadrangular resection of the leaflet; use of a sliding plasty; chordal shortening; chordal transposition and neochordea implantation.

There are many different techniques, which indicates that no one technique addresses all the issues that can occur with mitral regurgitation. Valve repair, however, offers better preservation of ventricular function and avoids the need for prolonged anticoagulation, as well as valve-related complications such as PVE or structural dysfunction. Recent advances in surgical techniques and the development of different types of rings has led to increased use of mitral valve repair with excellent results, making it the standard operation. The operative mortality is 1–3%. One of the major issues related to mitral repair is the incidence of regurgitation recurrence, which varies between series but can be up to 30% at 5 years. It seems that this is related to which leaflet is repaired and the amount of foreign material used in the repair (patch).

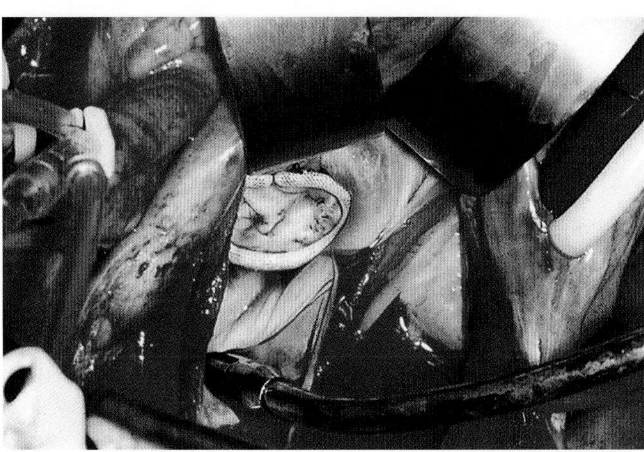

Figure 54.16 Operative view of the completed repair of a mitral valve using a Carpentier–Edwards annuloplasty ring (courtesy of A Murday, FRCS).

MITRAL VALVE REPLACEMENT

When valve repair is not feasible, mitral valve replacement is necessary. This usually involves a median sternotomy and access to the left atrium on CPB. The diseased valve is exposed, excised and a suitably sized mechanical or bioprosthetic valve is implanted. The atriotomy is closed following de-airing of the left heart. Intraoperative TOE can be used to assess adequate valve function.

The operative mortality rate for elective mitral valve replacement is approximately 5–6%. This depends largely on the state of the myocardium and the general condition (including age) of the patient. Common serious in-hospital complications include stroke (<4%) and renal failure (3%), although any complication of heart surgery is possible. The longer-term prognosis for patients following mitral valve replacement is generally good in comparison with the natural history of mitral valve disease. Indeed, more recent evidence suggests the patients with ischaemic severe mitral regurgitation can benefit more from valve replacement when compared to repair.

PERCUTANEOUS MITRAL VALVE REPAIR (MITRACLIP®)

The MitraClip® is a device used to reduce mitral valve regurgitation. The method involves suturing of the leaflets of the mitral valve together so that regurgitation into the left atrium is prevented. The valve continues to open through the sides of the suture and therefore blood continues to flow into the left ventricle. Although this method is less invasive, associated with rapid recovery and reduced in-hospital stay, it is however technically demanding and long-term durability of the results of the device is unknown.

Recent data suggest that Mitraclip® may be suitable for a small subset of high-risk patients or patients with chronic heart failure, but not for the vast majority, who are better served by surgery that leaves them with substantially less mitral regurgitation.

Aortic valve disease

Approximately two-thirds of all valve surgery performed in the UK is for aortic valve disease, which remains common despite a reduction in the incidence of rheumatic fever in resource-rich countries.

Aortic stenosis

Aortic stenosis, as opposed to aortic sclerosis, occurs when a pressure gradient can be demonstrated across the aortic valve. The difference is not absolute, as sclerosis can progress to stenosis. The common cause of aortic stenosis in adults is an acquired, degenerative, calcific process that results in immobile aortic valve cusps. Progressive fibrosis and calcification of a congenitally abnormal valve can mimic this degenerative process. The usual congenital abnormality is commissural fusion leading to a bicuspid aortic valve, which occurs in approximately 1% of the population (**Figure 54.17**).

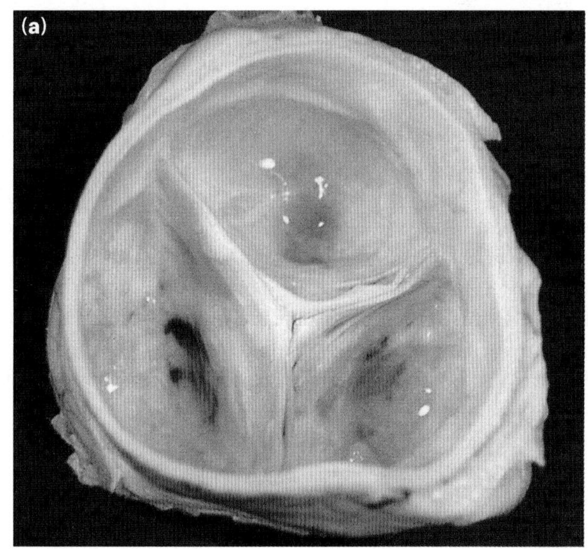

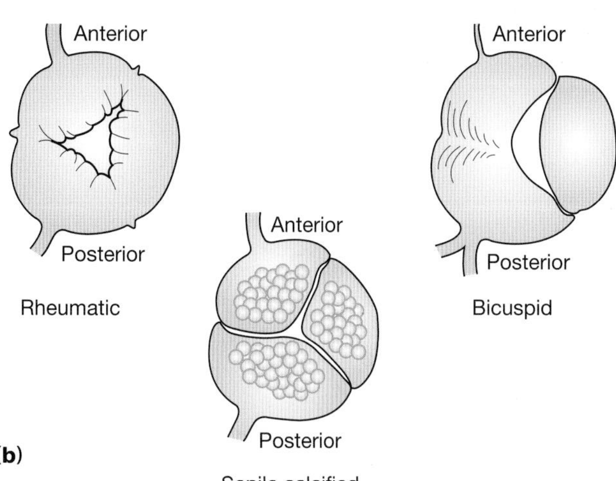

Figure 54.17 (**a**) Formaldehyde-treated aortic valve (normal tricuspid configuration). (**b**) Aortic stenosis, different pathologies.

Alain Carpentier, cardiothoracic surgeon, Hôpital European Georges Pompidou, Paris, France.

PATHOPHYSIOLOGY

A pressure gradient develops between the left ventricle and the aorta, with the left ventricle adapting to this systolic pressure overload by an increase in left ventricular wall thickness or hypertrophy. This adaptive response is an attempt to normalise left ventricular wall stress in the face of increased left ventricular systolic pressure and may maintain a normal cardiac output, prevent left ventricular dilatation and avoid significant symptoms for a number of years. Eventually, myocardial function is affected and, together with insufficient left ventricular hypertrophy to normalise wall stress (load mismatch), ventricular contractility is reduced.

When aortic stenosis is severe and cardiac output is normal, a >50 mmHg gradient between peak systolic left ventricular and aortic pressure exists. As aortic stenosis worsens, cardiac output cannot increase with exertion and eventually becomes insufficient at rest. The reduction in ventricular contractility leads to an irreversible decline in left ventricular function, with dilatation and a rise in left ventricular end-diastolic pressure, to the point of overt left heart failure.

CLINICAL FEATURES

Patients are often asymptomatic until decompensation occurs, typically presenting with dyspnoea and angina, which is due to increased oxygen needs of the hypertrophied left ventricle, reduced coronary filling and inadequate cardiac output during exertion. Patients often describe a feeling of light-headedness or 'near' syncope on effort. Cardiac arrhythmias can also occur. Auscultation of the heart demonstrates a murmur that is typically harsh, ejection in nature and best heard over the aortic area with radiation to the carotids. With critical aortic stenosis and a fall in cardiac output, the murmur may become quieter. The apex beat may be displaced in late disease along with signs of cardiac congestion (**Figure 54.18**).

INVESTIGATIONS

- **ECG**. There is left ventricular hypertrophy with tall R waves in the lateral leads and sometimes a 'strain pattern' (S–T depression with inverted T waves in the lateral leads).

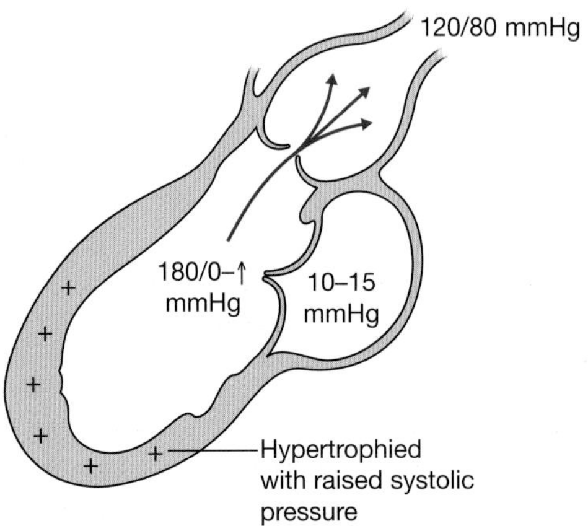

Figure 54.18 Features and pathophysiology of aortic stenosis. Haemodynamic changes in aortic stenosis. Aorta with poststenotic dilatation.

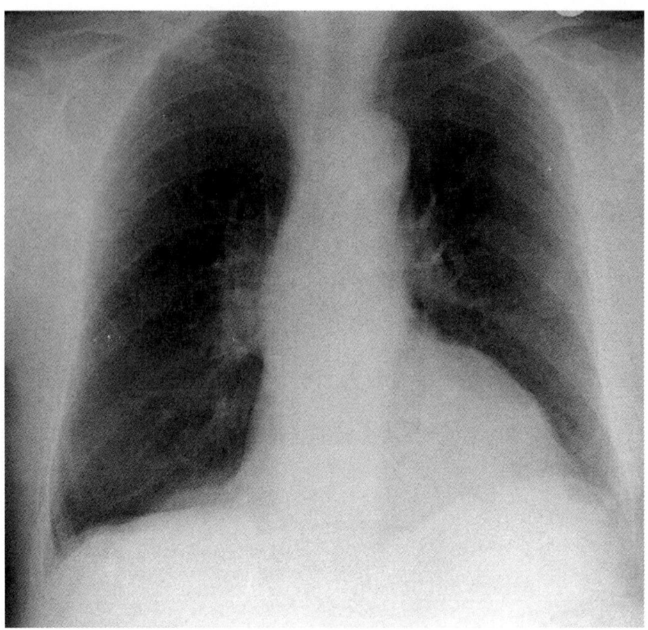

Figure 54.19 Chest radiograph in aortic stenosis.

- **Chest radiography**. May be normal. Cardiomegaly and pulmonary congestion can be seen in the presence of left ventricular failure. Poststenotic dilatation of the aorta is occasionally seen (**Figure 54.19**).
- **Echocardiography** confirms the diagnosis and, together with colour flow Doppler imaging, allows assessment of the aortic valve gradient, calculation of valve area and evaluation of left ventricular dimensions and wall thickness.
- **Coronary angiography**. To investigate the coronary arteries in patients >40 years of age.

INDICATIONS FOR SURGERY

Medical management focuses on the avoidance of systemic hypotension and arterial vasodilatation, which may reduce myocardial perfusion pressure and therefore provoke ischaemia.

The natural history of symptomatic patients with aortic stenosis is dismal, with a 10-year mortality rate of 80–90%. The patient is at risk of sudden death related to the severity of the stenosis. Severe symptomatic aortic stenosis (mean gradient >40 mmHg, velocity >4 m/s and effective orifice area <1 cm^2 are indications for surgery.

Surgery is indicated in asymptomatic patients with severe stenosis, impaired left ventricular function or when the patient is undergoing surgery for a different reason such as CABG. An abnormal blood pressure response to exercise (low blood pressure) is also a sign that there is limited reserve in asymptomatic patients.

Aortic regurgitation

The causes of aortic regurgitation can be classified according to the speed of development of the regurgitant jet (acute or chronic) or according to the anatomical location of pathology (valve leaflet or aortic wall). The causes of acute aortic regurgitation include infective endocarditis, aortic dissection and trauma. The common causes of chronic aortic regurgitation include degeneration leading to aortic root and/or annular dilatation, congenital bicuspid valve and previous rheumatic fever or endocarditis.

Summary box 54.11

Causes of aortic regurgitation according to predominant anatomical location of pathology

Valve leaflet disease

- Congenital, e.g. bicuspid valve leading to degenerative changes, occasionally with ventricular septal defect
- Rheumatic heart disease
- Infective endocarditis

Aortic wall pathology

- Inflammatory, e.g. connective tissue disorders such as ankylosing spondylitis, systemic lupus erythematosus, rheumatoid arthritis
- Systemic disease, e.g. tertiary syphilis
- Degenerative, e.g. Marfan syndrome, aortic root dissection, senile aortopathy, leading to aortic root/annular dilatation

(Adapted from Petch M. Aortic valve disease. *Medicine* 1997; 25: 31.

PATHOPHYSIOLOGY

Acute aortic regurgitation imposes a volume load on the left ventricle because of backflow. It causes a sharp rise in left ventricular end-diastolic pressure, premature closure of the mitral valve and inadequate forward left ventricular filling. The result is sudden haemodynamic deterioration and acute respiratory compromise.

In chronic aortic regurgitation, volume load and left ventricular end-diastolic pressure increase gradually, leading to compensatory left ventricular dilatation and eccentric hypertrophy to maintain adequate cardiac output. Systolic and diastolic function is abnormal, and sudden deterioration can occur.

CLINICAL FEATURES

Longstanding aortic regurgitation is usually asymptomatic until the left ventricle begins to fail, when exertional dyspnoea may be the only symptom. Angina can also develop. A wide pulse pressure due to a reduction in diastolic pressure and collapsing pulse (waterhammer pulse) are commonly seen. Other manifestations of the wide pulse pressure include visible capillary pulsation of the nail bed (Quincke's sign), pulsatile head bobbing (de Musset's sign), visible arterial pulsation in the neck (Corrigan's sign), a 'pistolshot' sound on

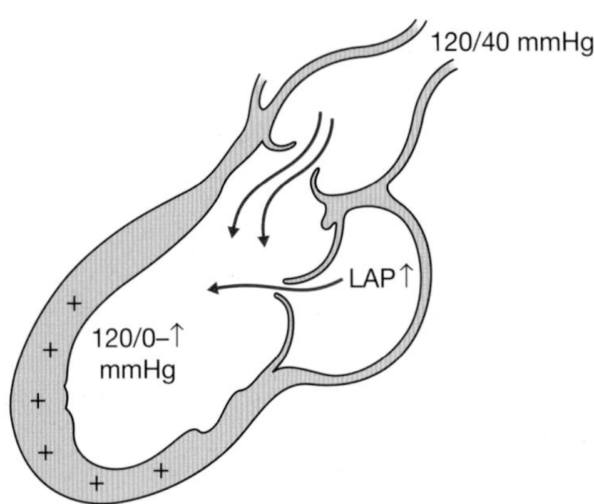

Figure 54.20 Haemodynamic consequences of aortic regurgitation. The left ventricle dilates and hypertrophies and there is a diastolic murmur. LAP, left atrial pressure.

auscultating over the femoral artery (Traube's sign) and uvular pulsation (Müller's sign). The apex is displaced laterally, often visible and hyperdynamic or 'thrusting' in nature because of the left ventricular hypertrophy. Auscultation reveals a high-pitched early diastolic murmur best heard at the left sternal edge (**Figure 54.20**).

INVESTIGATIONS

- **ECG**. There is left ventricular hypertrophy and sometimes a 'strain pattern'.
- **Chest radiography**. Cardiomegaly can be seen if the left ventricle is dilating; sometimes, the aortic shadow may also indicate dilatation.
- **Echocardiography**. This allows assessment of the underlying cause and severity of aortic regurgitation and enables the diameter of the aortic root as well as left ventricular dimensions to be determined. Colour flow Doppler imaging quantifies the size of the regurgitant jet.
- **Coronary angiography**. To investigate the coronary arteries in patients >40 years of age.

INDICATIONS FOR SURGERY

Medical therapy with vasodilator drugs for relief of dyspnoea or angina is designed to improve forward stroke volume and reduce regurgitant volume. However, symptomatic relief does not alter the need for valve surgery.

The indications for surgery include severe regurgitation in symptomatic patients. Asymptomatic patients with severe aortic regurgitation and left ventricular dysfunction should be offered surgery. Valve replacement should also be considered in asymptomatic patients with severe regurgitation if they are undergoing cardiac surgery for any other reason, or when there is evidence of progressive left ventricular dilatation

Bernard Jean Antonin Marfan, 1858–1942, physician L'Hôpital des Enfants-Malades, Paris, France, described this syndrome in 1896.
Heinrich Irenaeus Quincke, 1842–1922, Professor of Medicine, Kiel, Germany.
Louis Charles Alfred de Musset, 1810–1857, French poet and playwright in whom the sign, traditionally, was first noticed.
Sir Dominic John Corrigan, 1802–1880, physician, Jervis Street Hospital, Dublin, Ireland.
Ludwig Traube, 1818–1876, physician, The Charité, Berlin, Germany.
Friedrich von Müller, 1858–1941, physician, Munich, Germany.

Summary box 54.12

Causes of aortic valve disease

Stenosis

- Congenital
- Rheumatic heart disease
- Acquired calcification and fibrosis of valve or chordae tendineae with age

Regurgitation

- Rheumatic heart disease
- Infective endocarditis
- Congenital
- Inflammatory:
  - Systemic lupus erythematosus
  - Rheumatic ankylosing spondylitis
- Dilatation of aortic root:
  - Marfan syndrome
  - Dissection
- Systemic disease:
  - Syphilis
  - Ulcerative colitis

(left ventricular end-systolic diameter >50 mm). Aortic valve replacement is recommended if there is a decrease in systolic function.

Aortic valve surgery

Unlike mitral valve surgery, there are few occasions when the aortic valve can be repaired and usually the valve requires replacement. However, in neonates and children, aortic valve repair or valvotomy is well established. Percutaneous aortic balloon valvotomy has a role in children, but appears to only result in temporary benefit in adult aortic valve disease.

AORTIC VALVE REPLACEMENT

Aortic valve replacement (AVR) is performed through a median sternotomy on CPB. The aorta is cross-clamped and opened proximally to reveal the diseased valve. Cardioplegic solution is infused into the coronary arteries to arrest the heart in diastole. The valve is then excised leaving the annulus *in situ* but removing as much calcific debris as possible. The annulus is sized and the mechanical or biological valve is then sutured into position at the level of the native annulus and the aortotomy is closed.

The operative mortality rate for elective aortic valve surgery is 2–3%, but is higher in emergency surgery, in surgery for endocarditis and in older patients.

Major complications include stroke (2%), perioperative MI (2%) and heart block requiring a permanent pacemaker (<1%). The major determinant of late survival after aortic valve surgery is preoperative left ventricular function. The 5-year survival rate is approximately 75–85%, with the majority of late deaths related to myocardial factors.

TRANSCATHETER AORTIC VALVE IMPLANTATION

Although AVR is still the gold standard treatment, a significant number of patients affected by severe aortic stenosis requiring AVR do not undergo surgery because they are considered too old or too frail for such an invasive procedure, or because they are affected by concomitant comorbidities that noticeably increase the operative risk. In such patients transcatheter aortic valve implantation (TAVI) is an attractive alternative to standard AVR. Other indications include: heavily calcified ascending aorta ('porcelain' aorta) and the presence of a severe congenital thoracic distortion.

There are different approaches for valve implantation; the most commonly used are transapical (antegrade), and transluminal (retrograde).

- **Transapical approach**. The main advantage of performing transapical procedures is that the feasibility does not rely on the absence of a concomitant peripheral vascular disease or previous aortic surgery. This approach reduces the risk of calcium dislodgment due to the passage of a stiff transluminal device into a diseased aortic arch. In transapical TAVI, the cardiac apex is prepared through a small left anterolateral mini-thoracotomy using a purse-string or a crossing suture reinforced by pledgets and, after the procedure, a chest tube is routinely inserted into the left pleura.
- **Transluminal approach.** This can be carried out via the femoral or subclavian artery. This is a useful technique for patient with previous cardiac surgery; however, the presence of peripheral vascular disease, small vessel diameters, tortuous vessels, aortic disease or previous aortic surgery contraindicates this approach.

Whichever approach is used, a balloon catheter is advanced into the left ventricle over a guidewire and positioned at the opening of the aortic valve. The existing aortic valve is dilated in order to make room for the prosthetic valve. Rapid right ventricular pacing is used to interrupt cardiac output through the existing aortic valve and to reduce movement during implantation. The new valve, mounted on a metal stent, is manipulated into position and is either self-expanding or deployed using balloon inflation. Deployment leads to obliteration of the existing aortic valve.

Complications associated with TAVI include, mortality (5–18% at 30 days), mild-to-moderate aortic regurgitation (30–50%), stroke (3–9%), perioperative open conversion (9–12%), vascular complications (10–15%) and atrioventricular block (4–8%). A recent MI (<3 months), severe pulmonary dysfunction and the presence of an apical thrombus are contraindications for transapical TAVI. Interestingly, most recent multicentre trials have demonstrated that the role of TAVI can be expanded to include intermediate-risk patients, with satisfactory 2-year outcomes.

CONGENITAL HEART DISEASE

Introduction

Congenital heart diseases are abnormalities of cardiac structure that are present from birth. Such abnormalities in the development of the heart typically arise in the third to eighth week of gestation. The first operation for congenital heart disease was the ligation of a patent ductus arteriosus (PDA) by Gross in 1938. With the development of neonatal CPB, improved methods of myocardial protection and microsurgical techniques, an increasing number of corrective and palliative operations are possible.

Development of the heart and fetal circulation and circulatory changes at birth

By 12 weeks of fetal life the primitive vascular tube is fully developed. The fetal circulation differs from that of the adult in that the right and left ventricles pump blood in parallel rather than in series. Such an arrangement allows the heart and head to receive more highly oxygenated blood. In the fetus this is possible because of the presence of three structural shunts: the ductus venosus, the foramen ovale and the ductus arteriosus (**Figure 54.21**).

Soon after birth, pulmonary vascular resistance falls because of the action of breathing and the resulting pulmonary vasodilatation. In addition, within 30 minutes of delivery, the ductus arteriosus constricts in response to an increase in blood oxygen levels. The result is a reversal of the pulmonary–systemic pressure gradient and termination of blood flow from the pulmonary artery into the aorta.

After birth, the act of cutting and tying the umbilical cord stops venous blood flow from the placenta. This lowers the pressure in the inferior vena cava and, with the fall in pulmonary vascular resistance, right atrial pressure falls. The result is closure of the foramen ovale. The abolition of venous return from the placenta also causes the ductus venosus to close.

The closure of the fetal circulatory shunts in the few hours following birth is functional, with complete structural closure typically taking several months. In 20% of adults the structural closure of the foramen ovale remains incomplete, but is of no cardiovascular significance.

Abnormalities of cardiac structure may arise from the persistence of normal fetal channels (PDA, patent foramen ovale), failure of septation (atrial septal defect (ASD), ventricular septal defect (VSD), tetralogy of Fallot), stenosis (intracardiac–supravalvular, valvular, infravalvular or extracardiac coarctation of the aorta), atresia or abnormal connections (transposition of the great vessels (TGV), total anomalous venous drainage). Fetal echocardiography is now sufficiently sensitive to detect intracardiac lesions in the second trimester.

Incidence

Congenital heart disease is the most common congenital abnormality in the UK; the incidence of significant cardiac abnormalities is 8 cases per 1000 live births. Many spontaneous abortions or stillbirths have cardiac malformations or chromosomal abnormalities associated with structural heart defects. In neonates and children with congenital heart disease, 15% will have more than one cardiac abnormality and 15% will have another extracardiac abnormality.

Aetiology

There is often no obvious aetiology; most abnormalities appear to be multifactorial with both genetic and environmental influences. There are well-recognised associations.

Summary box 54.13

Recognised associations with congenital heart disease

Maternal (environmental) factors

- Infection: rubella
- Disease: systemic lupus erythematosus, diabetes mellitus
- Drugs/medications: alcohol abuse, warfarin, phenytoin, lithium

Genetic factors

- Single gene defects: Marfan, Noonan and Holt–Oram syndromes
- Chromosomal defects: trisomy 21 (Down syndrome), trisomy 18 (Edwards syndrome), trisomy 13 (Patau syndrome), Turner syndrome
- Deletions: DiGeorge and Williams syndromes

Diagnosis

Occasionally an antenatal diagnosis is possible, with severe congenital heart disease detected *in utero* at 16–18 weeks. If an infant is suspected of having a congenital heart disease, a diagnostic evaluation begins with an accurate history from the parents and specific questions about maternal health and drug intake during pregnancy. A detailed family history is important because some defects are familial. Clinical examination may reveal a murmur, evidence of heart failure, failure to thrive and cyanosis. In addition, congenital heart disease can present with hypertension, an arrhythmia, evidence of polycythaemia or a thromboembolic event. Investigation is much the same as for the adult patient and, with fetal echocardiography available, cardiac catheterisation is now avoided whenever possible.

Robert E Gross, 1905–1988, Surgeon-in-chief, Cardiovascular Surgery, Children's Hospital, Boston, USA.
Etienne Arthur Louis Fallot, 1850–1911, Professor of Medicine, Marseilles, France.
Jacqueline Anne Noonan, b.1921, pediatric cardiologist, The University of Kentucky College of Medicine, Lexington, KY, USA, described this condition in 1963.
Mary Clayton Holt, 1924–1993, cardiologist, The London Hospital for Women and Children, London, UK.
Samuel Oram, 1913–1991, cardiologist, King's College Hospital, London, UK. Holt and Oram described this syndrome in a joint paper in 1960.
John Hilton Edwards, 1928–2007, Professor of Genetics, The University of Oxford, Oxford, UK.
Klaus Patau, 1908–1975, German-born American geneticist, University of Wisconsin–Madison, USA.
Angelo M. DiGeorge, 1921–2009, Professor of Pediatrics, Temple University, Philadelphia, PA, USA.
John CP Williams, b.1922, New Zealand born cardiologist, described the condition in 1961.

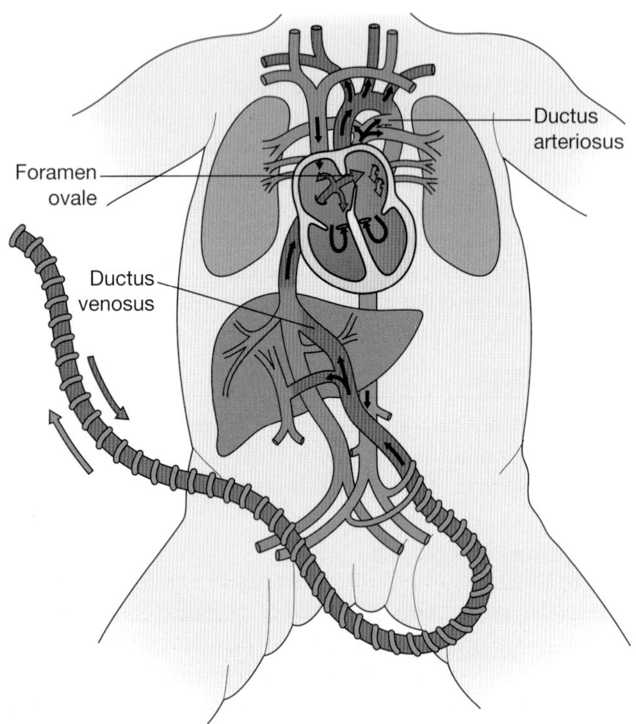

Figure 54.21 Fetal circulation.

Classification

Congenital heart disease can be broadly classified according to the presence or absence of cyanosis, although the distinction is not always clear-cut. The presence of central cyanosis, blueness of the trunk and mucous membranes, results from levels of deoxygenated haemoglobin of >3–5 g/dL in the arterial circulation.

Cyanotic congenital heart diseases make up one-third of cases and are usually more complex, although they do include simple defects. Cyanotic congenital cardiac lesions can involve:

- A right-to-left shunt resulting in decreased pulmonary blood flow. Many of these lesions consist of a septal defect in conjunction with a right-sided obstructive lesion, producing an obligatory right-to-left shunt. The most common cause of this is tetralogy of Fallot.
- Parallel systemic and pulmonary blood flow rather than in series. If there is no mixing this is incompatible with life, so typically neonates have a patent foramen ovale or VSD that allows some mixing of the two circulations at this level. The most common example of this is TGV.
- Defects in the connections of the heart in which there is mixing of the systemic and pulmonary flows. An example of such a complex lesion is total anomalous pulmonary venous drainage.

Acyanotic congenital heart diseases represent the other two-thirds of cases and are usually less complex. Such defects result in an increase in the work imposed on the heart because of either:

- A left-to-right shunt with increased pulmonary blood flow, which causes an increase in volume work of the heart. Examples include PDA, ASD and VSD.
- Obstruction of the blood flow across a heart valve on the left side of the heart, such as aortic stenosis, or in the aorta itself, as occurs with coarctation of the aorta, leading to an increase in pressure and work of the heart.

Typically, acyanotic congenital heart disease presents as heart failure in infancy because of pulmonary congestion caused by increased pulmonary blood flow, or increased pulmonary venous blood pressure resulting from an obstructive lesion. The common acyanotic cardiac defects can also present as a murmur in infancy or later.

Cyanotic congenital heart disease

Tetralogy of Fallot

This is the most common cyanotic congenital heart disease found in children surviving to 1 year and accounts for about 4–6% of all congenital heart diseases. The four intracardiac lesions originally described (**Figure 54.22**) were:

- VSD;
- overriding aorta;
- pulmonary (typically infundibular or subpulmonary) stenosis;
- right ventricular hypertrophy.

Clinically, there may be no signs initially but, as pulmonary stenosis progresses, cyanosis typically develops within the first year of life. Squatting is an adaptation by the child to hypoxic spells. This increases systemic vascular resistance and the venous return to the heart, and consequently blood is diverted into the pulmonary circulation with increased oxygenation. Lethargy and tiredness are also common. Classically

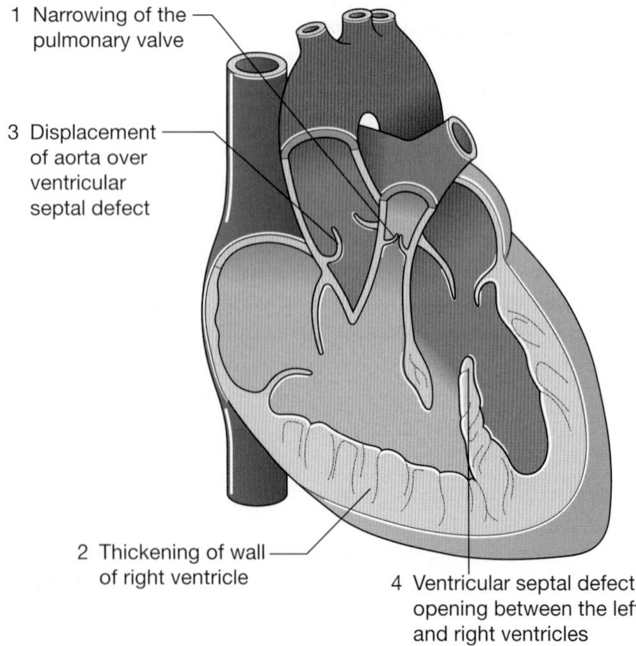

Figure 54.22 Fallot's tetralogy. Four abnormalities that result in insufficienctly oxygentated blood being pumped to the body.

the chest radiograph demonstrates a 'boot-shaped' heart with poorly developed lung vasculature. The diagnosis is confirmed with echocardiography. Surgery to correct the tetralogy is the mainstay of treatment and is usually carried out at 4–6 months of age, when possible. The repair is achieved using a patch to close the VSD and resection of the obstructing section of the infundibular septum. The results of surgery are good, with a late survival rate of 95% at 5–10 years following correction of tetralogy, an operative mortality rate for a repair of between 5% and 10%, and an incidence of reoperation following tetralogy repair of 5–10%.

Transposition of the great vessels

The condition, first described by Morgagni, is the second most common cyanotic congenital heart disease and is the most common cause of cyanosis from a congenital cardiac defect discovered in the newborn period. TGV results from abnormal development, and typically occurs when the aorta arises from the right ventricle and the pulmonary artery from the left ventricle (**Figure 54.23**). The resulting transposition causes the pulmonary and systemic circulations to run in parallel rather than in series, so that oxygenated pulmonary venous blood returns to the lungs and desaturated systemic venous blood is pumped around the body. The situation is incompatible with life and mixing of the blood must occur through associated shunts, such as a patent foramen ovale or associated VSD.

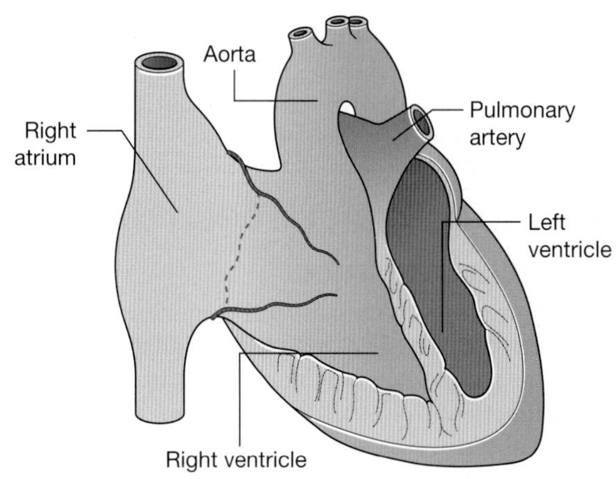

Figure 54.23 Transposition of the great vessels.

The most obvious presentation is severe central cyanosis occurring in the first 48 hours of life. However, if there is a large ASD or VSD there may be minimal cyanosis initially. Typically, progress is poor and, as pulmonary vascular resistance declines in the neonatal period, high pulmonary flow develops, with cardiac enlargement and left ventricular failure.

The chest radiograph shows pulmonary plethora, with the heart having an 'egg on its side' appearance, with a small pedicle (aorta in front of pulmonary artery). Cardiac echocardiography is sufficient to confirm the diagnosis and delineate the anatomy.

Many infants will die without treatment within 1 month of birth. Initial stabilisation can be achieved by performing percutanous balloon septostomy to increase the systemic arterial oxygen saturation. Alternatively, intravenous prostaglandins can be administered to keep the PDA open and increase systemic–pulmonary shunting. Arterial switch repair is currently the standard operation and is typically carried out within the first few weeks of birth. Long-term outcomes of the operation are excellent and many patients achieve good exercise tolerance; however, some patients will require reoperation for neopulmonary stenosis.

Total anomalous pulmonary venous drainage

Total anomalous pulmonary venous drainage (TAPVD) accounts for only 1–2% of congenital heart disease. In this condition, the pulmonary venous drainage has become disconnected from the left atrium and drains into the systemic venous circulation at some other point (inferior vena cava, superior vena cava, coronary sinus or right atrium). Typically, TAPVD presents after the first week of life with cyanosis that is mild to moderate depending on pulmonary flow. Infants with high pulmonary flow develop cardiac failure, recurrent chest infections, failure to thrive and feeding difficulties. If high pulmonary flow is associated with a large ASD, cyanosis is often minimal and the lesion is tolerated well. If there is additional venous obstruction, cyanosis presents at birth with dyspnoea and pulmonary oedema. Echocardiography and cardiac (pulmonary) angiography are necessary to confirm the diagnosis and establish the location of the anomalous drainage.

The surgical principle is to re-establish the pulmonary venous drainage into the left atrium. The exact operative technique depends on the anatomy and type of TAPVD. The long-term results for survivors of the operation are generally good. Late death following repair is uncommon but, when it occurs, it is often caused by intimal fibroplasia of the pulmonary veins away from the anastomosis.

Eisenmenger syndrome

Eisenmenger syndrome is becoming less common as corrective surgery is undertaken increasingly early and fewer patients develop a fixed increase in their pulmonary vascular resistance. It occurs following the reversal of a left-to-right shunt across a previous left-to-right shunt, such as with an ASD or VSD. These congenital anomalies cause an increase in flow and higher right-sided pressures, which lead to compensatory right ventricular hypertrophy and a subsequent rise in pulmonary artery pressure. Increasing pulmonary hypertension leads to equalisation of pressures either side of the shunt but, at some point, the right-sided pressures will exceed those on the left side, resulting in shunt reversal and desaturated blood entering the left side of the circulation. Cyanosis

Giovanni Battista Morgagni, 1682–1771, anatomist, Padua, Italy.
Victor Eisenmenger, 1864–1932, Austrian physician who described this condition in 1897, but the term 'Eisenmenger syndrome' was introduced in 1958 by an Australian cardiologist, **Paul Hamilton Wood** (1907–1962).

and dyspnoea are the most common clinical features. Closure of the shunt is contraindicated if pulmonary hypertension is irreversible because the right-to-left shunt now serves to decompress the pulmonary circulation.

Acyanotic congenital heart disease

Patent ductus arteriosus

The ductus arteriosus, a normal fetal communication, facilitates the transfer of oxygenated blood from the pulmonary artery to the aorta, shunting blood away from the lungs. Normally, functional closure of the ductus occurs within a few hours of birth; it is abnormal if it persists beyond the neonatal period. The ductus closes in response to an increase in peripheral oxygen saturation and a drop in the resistance of the pulmonary circulation as the lungs expand; this causes the ductal tissue to contract through a prostaglandin inhibition mechanism. A cyclo-oxygenase inhibitor (e.g. indomethacin) may be used therapeutically to close the ductus in the first few weeks of life. In premature babies the ductus is more likely to remain patent for longer or permanently. In the isolated case of PDA, there is a left-to-right shunt of blood, resulting in a high pulmonary blood flow. Small shunts usually cause few symptoms and signs apart from the continuous machinery murmur in the left second intercostal space. Larger ducts cause cardiac failure and can uncommonly lead to shunt reversal with cyanosis and clubbing. The diagnosis is best confirmed by echocardiography with colour flow Doppler imaging.

After 6 months of age, spontaneous closure of a PDA is rare. Most should be closed by preschool age, regardless of the absence of symptoms, if the risks of infective endocarditis, developing left ventricular failure or, rarely, Eisenmenger syndrome are to be avoided. In the adult, surgical treatment is indicated if there is a persistent left-to-right shunt, even in the presence of reversible pulmonary hypertension. In the premature infant, if medical treatment to close the ductus is unsuccessful, the PDA may be treated by interventional cardiology using an umbrella or coil duct occlusion device inserted percutaneously. If the PDA is very large or the patient very small, surgical closure via a left thoracotomy is preferred. This can be accomplished by either ligation or division of the PDA. The operative mortality rate is low and outcome generally very good.

Coarctation of the aorta

This accounts for 6–7% of congenital heart disease and is defined as a haemodynamically significant narrowing of the aorta, usually in the descending aorta just distal to the left subclavian artery, around the area of the ductus arteriosus (Figure 54.24). The coarctation typically puts a pressure load on the left ventricle, which can ultimately fail. The upper body is well perfused but the lower body, including the kidneys, is poorly perfused, leading to fluid overload, excess renin secretion and acidosis. Coarctation usually affects boys and, if it occurs in girls, is suggestive of Turner syndrome.

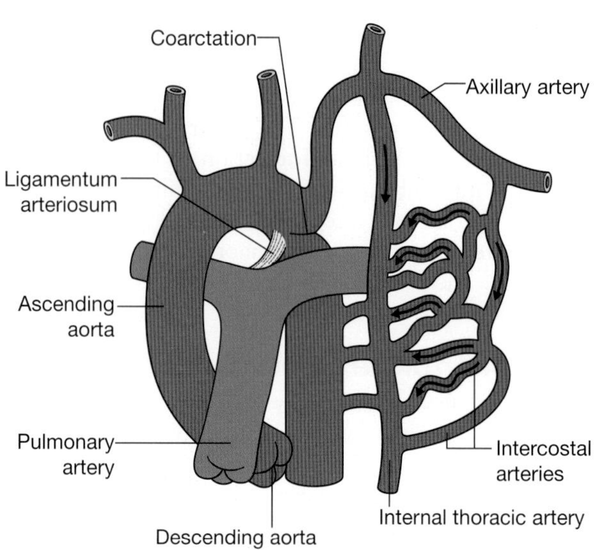

Figure 54.24 Coarctation of the aorta. Coarctation causes severe obstruction of blood flow in the descending thoracic aorta. The descending aorta and its branches are perfused by collateral channels from the axillary and internal thoracic arteries through the intercostal arteries (arrows).

In the neonatal period, coarctation, often referred to as 'infantile' or preductal coarctation, presents with symptoms of heart failure. The child may appear well in the first few days of life because the coarctation is bypassed by the ductus arteriosus and oxygenated blood reaches the entire systemic circulation. As the ductus closes, the child becomes progressively more unwell. In adult-type coarctation, which is often juxtaductal or slightly postductal, obstruction is gradual with complications developing in adolescence or early adulthood. Hypertension is a common presenting problem in older children, often upper body hypertension only with development of enormous collateral vessels that may cause rib-notching and flow murmurs over the scapula. Other symptoms include prominent pulsation in the neck, tired legs or intermittent claudication on exercise. Clinical examination of the pulses may demonstrate a radio-femoral delay and a murmur that is continuous and heard best over the thoracic spine or below the left clavicle.

The chest radiograph classically demonstrates rib-notching because of dilated posterior intercostal vessels. The heart is usually of normal size in the older child and shows a classical 'three sign' replacing the typical aortic knuckle. The upper part of the three sign is the dilated left subclavian, the middle part is the narrowing at the coarctation site and the lower part is the poststenotic dilatation of the descending aorta. Echocardiography is diagnostic. Infant coarctation typically presents with cardiac failure, often requiring vigorous medical treatment, including the administration of prostaglandin to reopen the ductus and general resuscitation, before corrective

Henry Hubert Turner, 1892–1970, Professor of Medicine, The University of Oklahoma, Oklahoma City, OK, USA.

surgery. Definitive treatment is usually surgical repair via a left thoracotomy. Coarctation presenting in the child or later typically requires surgical repair, as most patients die before the age of 40 years because of the associated complications. Percutaneous stenting is currently the standard treatment for adults with isolated coarctation. Without correction, the majority of deaths are caused by heart failure, infective endocarditis, rupture of the aorta or haemorrhagic stroke. The preoperative hypertension may not resolve despite surgical repair.

Atrial septal defects

An ASD is a defect in the septum between the left and right atria leading to a left-to-right shunt, the significance of which is determined by the size of the defect and the relative compliance of the ventricles. The development of the atrial septum is complex and abnormalities of development lead to three commonly recognised ASDs (**Figure 54.25**).

The most common type is an ostium secundum ASD. The anomaly is caused by failure of the septum primum to develop, leading to incomplete coverage of the ostium secundum. These defects are usually asymptomatic in childhood, with symptoms developing insidiously, typically presenting in middle age with congestive cardiac failure secondary to pulmonary hypertension or with atrial arrhythmias.

In ostium primum ASD, the anomaly is a form of partial atrioventricular canal defect or endocardial cushion defect. The abnormalities are confined to the atrial septum and are caused by the endocardial cushions failing to develop and so close the ostium primum part of the interatrial septum. The defect is associated with abnormalities of the mitral valve, leading to mitral regurgitation. There is a relatively high incidence of this abnormality in trisomy 21 (Down syndrome). Typically, the primum defect presents earlier than ostium secundum in childhood, with dyspnoea, recurrent chest infections and, if pulmonary hypertension develops, cyanosis.

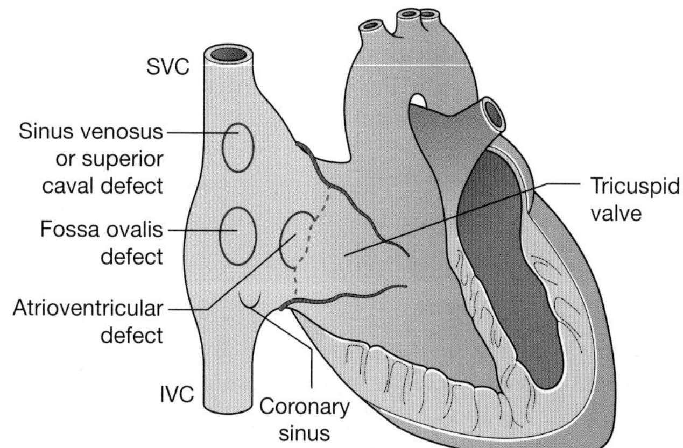

Figure 54.25 Atrial septum viewed from the right. The fossa ovalis is a useful reference point; the most common defect is in this area and is called a fossa ovalis (or ostium secundum) defect. A defect near the atrioventricular junction may be part of the spectrum of atrioventricular septal defects; if the defect is near the entry of the superior vena cava (SVC) it is commonly associated with anomalies of venous drainage into the atria. IVC, inferior vena cava.

A sinus venosus ASD is a rare defect and is the result of failure of partition of the pulmonary and systemic venous circulations. These defects are most commonly located high in the atrial septum at the junction of the superior vena cava and the right atrium. They are frequently associated with anomalous pulmonary venous drainage, with right superior pulmonary veins draining into the superior vena cava or right atrium directly.

Summary box 54.14

Atrial septal defects (ASDs)

Common defects

- Ostium secundum: fossa ovalis defect (approximately 70% of ASDs)
- Ostium primum: atrioventricular septal defect (approximately 20% of ASDs)
- Sinus venosus defect: often associated with anomalous pulmonary venous drainage (approximately 10% of ASDs)
- Patent foramen ovale: common in isolation, usually no left-to-right shunt (not strictly an ASD)

Rarer defects

- Inferior vena cava defects: a low sinus venosus defect and may allow shunting of blood into the left atrium
- Coronary sinus septal defect: also known as unroofed coronary sinus, with the left superior vena cava draining to the left atrium as part of a more complex lesion

Closure is performed during the first decade of life, even in the absence of symptoms, to avoid late-onset right ventricular failure, endocarditis and paradoxical emboli. In adults, closure is still appropriate for symptomatic improvement and avoidance of complications. The traditional method of closure involves open-heart surgery with CPB and closure of the defect, either directly with sutures, as with most secundum defects, or, if the defect is large, using a pericardial or synthetic patch. Closure of small to moderate ASDs using percutaneous catheter-delivered devices in the cardiology catheter laboratory is increasingly common. Primum atrioventricular defect repairs may require additional mitral valve repair. The operative mortality rate for isolated atrioventricular defect repairs is <1%, with an excellent prognosis. Surgical correction of complete atrioventricular canal defects, with closure of the ASD and ventricular septal components and mitral valve repair, is possible, but with a higher surgical mortality rate.

Ventricular septal defects

A VSD is a defect in the interventricular septum that allows a left-to-right shunting of blood. VSDs account for 20–30% of congenital heart disease and affect approximately 2 in 1000 live births. They may occur in isolation or as part of a more complex set of cardiac abnormalities (e.g. tetralogy of Fallot, complete atrioventricular canal defect). Four major anatomical types of VSD are described, based on the anatomical subsections of the interventricular septum (**Figure 54.26**).

John Langdon Haydon Down (sometimes given as Langdon-Down), 1828–1896, physician, The London Hospital, London, UK.

Summary box 54.15

Types of ventricular septal defects (VSD)

Perimembranous defect

- Also called conoventricular VSD; the most common defect (70–80%), usually located within the membranous septum and may extend to the tricuspid valve annulus or base of the aortic valve

Muscular defect

- Also called trabecular VSD; occurs in 10% of cases and is located within the membranous septum and often multiple

Atrioventricular defect

- Also called atrioventricular canal-type or inlet defect; occurs in 5% of cases and is located in the atrioventricular canal beneath the tricuspid valve

Subarterial defect

- Also called outlet or subarterial VSD; occurs in 5–10% of cases and lies within the conal septum immediately beneath the pulmonary valve annulus.

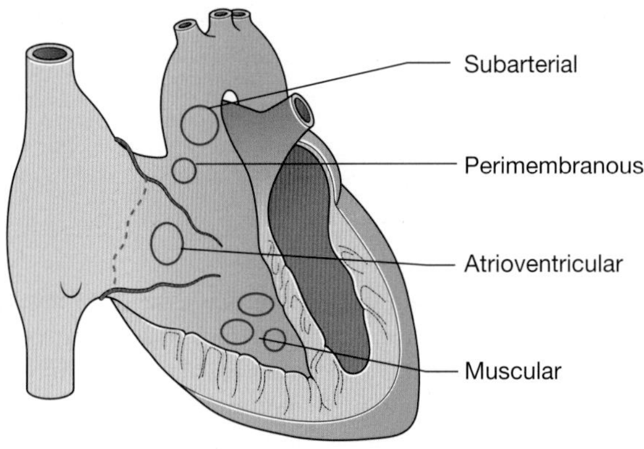

Figure 54.26 Ventricular septum viewed from the right, showing the characteristic sites of ventricular septal defects.

The VSD permits a left-to-right shunt at the ventricular level, with subsequent right ventricular volume overload and increased pulmonary blood flow. This may lead to progressive pulmonary oedema and congestive cardiac failure. Persistently elevated pulmonary blood flow and pulmonary vascular resistance also lead to irreversible pulmonary hypertension. They may eventually result in reversal of flow across the defect and Eisenmenger syndrome. The clinical presentation reflects the magnitude of the left-to-right shunt, which, in turn, depends on the size of the VSD and the pulmonary and systemic vascular resistances. Small defects may close or cause little systemic disturbance (maladie de Roger); infants are asymptomatic with normal development. In the first 5 years, up to 30–50% of VSDs close spontaneously. Clinically, a loud pansystolic murmur can be detected at the left sternal border because of high pressure flow between the ventricles. Large defects typically present with congestive cardiac failure in the first 2 months of life. Because of the size of the VSD, ventricular pressures are equalised and often only a soft systolic murmur is detected. If left untreated, pulmonary hypertensive changes start from about 1 year of age. Eisenmenger syndrome, secondary to shunt reversal in such cases, may become evident in the second decade of life.

Echocardiography confirms the diagnosis and can estimate the degree of shunting across the defect. Cardiac catheterisation can quantify the various pressures within the cardiac chambers and so assess the degree of pulmonary hypertension, as well as demonstrating a step-up in oxygen saturation between left and right ventricles. Generally, surgical closure is indicated for large defects; when there is failure to respond to medical therapy; for left-to-right shunts of >2:1; when there are signs of increasing pulmonary vascular resistance; and in the presence of complications of VSD. These include: (1) aortic regurgitation, which occurs in about 5% of defects; (2) infundibular stenosis, which tends to be progressive and leads to shunt reversal; and (3) infective endocarditis, often presenting with pneumonia or pleurisy as the infected 'emboli' in a VSD with a typical left-to-right shunt flows into the pulmonary circulation.

THE THORACIC AORTA

The most common pathologies affecting the thoracic aorta are aneurysm formation and aortic dissection.

Thoracic aortic aneurysms

A true aneurysm is a localised dilatation of a blood vessel involving all layers of the vessel, whereas a false aneurysm has compressed supporting tissue as its wall, and is usually the result of a defect in the vessel intima (from trauma, dissection or previous surgery). Aneurysms are described as fusiform when the whole circumference is affected or saccular when only part of the circumference is involved.

Aortic aneurysms can develop anywhere along its length, but thoracic aortic aneurysms, including those that extend into the upper abdomen (thoracoabdominal aneurysms) account for 25%, typically occurring in men in the fifth to seventh decade or younger in those with connective tissue disorders.

Aetiology

The most common aetiology is atherosclerosis, but connective tissue disorders account for many aneurysms in the aortic root and ascending aorta now that tertiary syphilis is rare. Marfan syndrome is associated with cystic medial degeneration involving the vessel wall and causes widening of the proximal aorta and aortic root, leading to aortic valve insufficiency. Other disorders associated with aneurysm formation and dissection include Ehlers–Danlos syndrome and osteogenesis imperfecta.

Henri Louis Roger, 1809–1891, physician, Hôpital Sainte-Eugene, Paris, France.
Edward Ehlers, 1863–1937, Professor of Clinical Dermatology, Copenhagen, Denmark.
Henri Alexandre Danlos, 1844–1912, dermatologist, Hôpital St. Louis, Paris, France, gave his account of this condition in 1908.

Trauma, typically following blunt chest injury, can lead to aneurysm formation, usually involving the descending aorta. However, these are usually false aneurysms containing haematoma from injury to the aortic vessel wall.

Clinical features

Many aneurysms are asymptomatic and are discovered incidentally on routine chest radiographs. Others present as a space occupying lesion in the thorax with pain caused by pressure on adjacent structures (vertebra), hoarseness (left recurrent laryngeal nerve), dysphagia (oesophagus) and respiratory symptoms (left main bronchus). Aortic root aneurysms may lead to dilatation of the aortic root annulus and aortic regurgitation.

Rupture can lead to cardiac tamponade or haemorrhage into the left pleural space, leading to dyspnoea and, if the tracheobronchial airway or oesophagus is involved, haemoptysis or haematemesis, respectively.

Investigations

The diagnosis is confirmed by CT or MRI. Arteriography is not necessary for diagnosis but is often required to demonstrate the relation of the arch vessels to the aneurysm.

Indications for surgery

Without treatment the aneurysm is likely to expand and ultimately rupture. Important factors to consider when planning treatment are age, comorbidity and coexisting coronary disease.

In ascending aneurysms, the presence of progressive aortic valve insufficiency is an important indication for surgery. Other indications in this group, including Marfan-related aneurysms, are a diameter of 4.5–5 cm and the presence of symptoms. In descending aneurysms, indications for surgery include symptoms, acute enlargement and a diameter of approximately 6 cm.

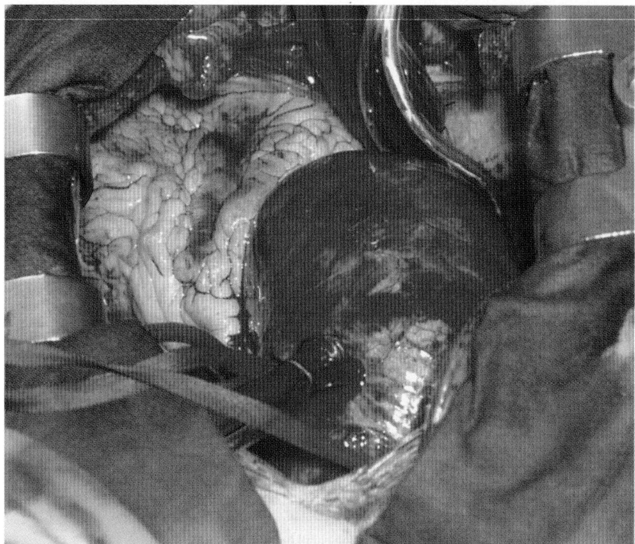

Figure 54.27 A large thoracic aortic aneurysm.

Surgical options

The approach adopted for surgical treatment depends on the location of the aneurysm, but typically involves a median sternotomy, CPB and cooling the patient to 18°C before cross-clamping the aorta above the aneurysm (**Figure 54.27**). If the aortic root is involved, the aorta, together with its annulus and valve, is resected and a composite graft is sutured to the aortic root. The circulation is arrested and, after removal of the aortic cross-clamp, the distal anastomosis is completed. The coronary ostia require reimplantation into the graft (Bentall's operation). If the ascending aorta is involved, it is resected and replaced with a tube graft. For aortic arch aneurysms, surgery on this section of the aorta is a formidable undertaking because the cerebral and subclavian vessels have to be anastomosed to the graft, either separately or *en bloc*. Typically, it involves a period of circulatory arrest and some form of cerebral protection. Excision of a descending aortic aneurysm is with graft replacement under CPB, with exposure via a left thoracotomy or with a heparin-bonded shunt. Increasingly, thoracic aneurysms at the aortic arch or more distal are repaired using a percutaneous approach via the femoral artery, with insertion of an endovascular stent under radiological guidance. The most recent guidelines support the use of endovascualr techniques over open surgical operations.

Surgical outcome

The operative mortality rate is variable depending on the location and type of repair required, but electively is between 5% and 15%. An emergency repair has a considerably higher operative mortality rate. Long-term survival depends on underlying pathology but, for ascending aneurysm repairs, the 5-year survival rate is approximately 65%. The major complications of descending aneurysm repairs include paraplegia, renal failure and ventricular dysfunction.

Aortic dissection

This occurs when a defect or flap occurs in the intima of the aorta, resulting in blood tracking into the aortic tissues splitting the medial layer and creating a false lumen. It most commonly occurs in the ascending aorta or, less often, just

Summary box 54.16

Predisposing factors for aortic dissection

- Age
- Hypertension
- Marfan syndrome
- Pregnancy
- Other connective tissue disorders, for example Ehlers–Danlos syndrome, giant cell arteritis, systemic lupus erythematosus
- Coarctation of the aorta
- Turner or Noonan syndromes
- Aortic cannulation site (iatrogenic)

Hugh Henry Bentall, 1920–2012, formerly Professor of Cardiac Surgery, The Royal Postgraduate Hospital, Hammersmith, London, UK.

distal to the left subclavian artery. It is also more common in men, typically those aged 50–70 years, and in Afro-Caribbean patients.

Aetiology

It usually occurs as a spontaneous or sporadic event, although very often a history of hypertension is noted. Other important associations include Marfan syndrome and pregnancy.

Clinical features

The presentation is often a tearing intrascapular pain not unlike the pain of myocardial ischaemia, and it may be difficult to distinguish between the two. The extent of arterial dissection may produce widespread symptoms and signs.

The dissection can extend distally down the aorta to involve:

- the renal arteries (renal pain and renal failure);
- the mesenteric arteries (abdominal pain and bowel ischaemia);
- the spinal arteries (paraplegia);
- the iliac arteries (leg pain, pallor, loss or reduced pulses and limb ischaemia).

The dissection may track proximally to involve:

- the head and neck vessels (symptoms and signs of a stroke or transient ischaemic attack);
- the coronary vessels (MI);
- the aortic root (aortic regurgitation).

The dissection may also result in aortic wall rupture into the pericardium (cardiac tamponade) or mediastinum (left haemothorax).

Classification

There are two classifications, both of which are limited in their application but widely used. The DeBakey classification is based on the pattern of dissection, whereas the Stanford classification is based on whether the ascending aorta is involved (**Figure 54.28**).

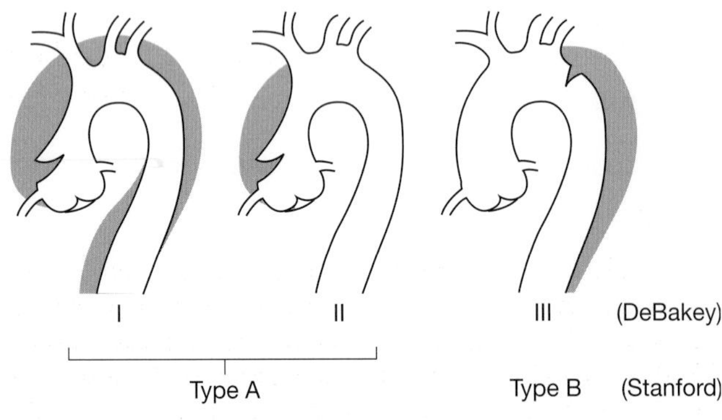

Figure 54.28 Stanford classification of aortic dissections according to whether the ascending aorta is involved (type A) or not (type B). This is simpler than the DeBakey classification (types I, II and III).

Investigations

The diagnosis is suspected based on the clinical presentation and careful history taking. Diagnosis is confirmed by CT, which is accepted as the standard method for diagnosis. Other imaging modalities such as TOE or MRI can be utilised in cases when the CT is equivocal (**Figure 54.29**).

Management

Intitial management of all types of aortic dissection includes blood pressure (which is usually high at presentation) control and strict pain management, followed by prompt referral for specialist management.

Surgical options

TYPE A (OR TYPE I AND II) DISSECTIONS

Those involving the ascending aorta usually require surgical intervention. The chest is opened through a median sternotomy and CPB is started, with core cooling down to 18°C. The aorta is cross-clamped as high as possible and opened. Cardioplegic solution is infused into the coronary ostia to arrest the heart in diastole. If the intimal tear is present and localised, the ascending aorta is excised with the tear and replaced with a synthetic graft. The distal anastomosis is performed with circulatory arrest. There has recently been attempts to carry out endovascular stenting of type A dissection with variable degrees of success.

TYPE B (OR TYPE III) DISSECTIONS

Initially, these are best managed medically with antihypertensive drugs. Intervention is indicated in complicated cases if the pain increases (signalling impending rupture) or when dissection is associated with evidence of malperfusion, such as organ, limb or neurological symptoms. The use of percutaneously placed endovascular stents is currently the standard

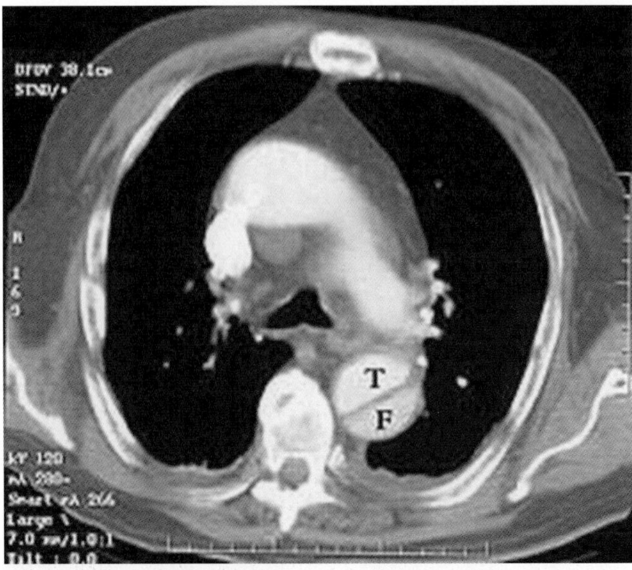

Figure 54.29 Computed tomography scan showing acute dissection of the descending thoracic aorta. F, false lumen; T, true lumen.

Michael Ellis DeBakey, 1908–2008, American cardiac surgeon, Baylor College of Medicine, Houston, Texas, USA.

intervention of choice in patients with complicated type B dissection, and surgery is only preserved for the rare cases which is not suitable for stenting.

Outcomes

If type A dissection is untreated, the mortality rate is 50% within 48 hours and 75% within 1–2 weeks, whereas patients with type B dissections have a better prognosis. The surgical mortality rate is variable but is around 20–25% for proximal aortic dissection. The overall survival rate for patients leaving hospital, regardless of the type of dissection, is around 80% at 5 years and 40% at 10 years.

PERICARDIAL DISEASES

There is a fibrous envelope covering the heart and separating it from the mediastinal structures. This fibrous structure includes a parietal layer and allows the heart to move with each beat. It is not essential for life because it can be left wide open after cardiac surgery without any ill-effects; however, there are a number of conditions affecting the pericardium that may present to the surgeon.

Pericardial effusion

There is continuous production and resorption of pericardial fluid. If a disease process disturbs this balance a pericardial effusion may develop. If the pressure exceeds the pressure in the atria, compression will occur, venous return will fall and the circulation will be compromised. This state of affairs is called 'tamponade'. A gradual build-up of fluid (e.g. malignant infiltration) may be well tolerated for a long period before tamponade occurs, and the pericardial cavity may contain 2 litres of fluid. Acute tamponade (from penetrating trauma, during coronary angiography or postoperatively) may occur in minutes with small volumes of blood. The clinical features are low blood pressure with a raised jugular venous pressure and paradoxical pulse. Kussmaul's sign is a characteristic pattern that is seen when the jugular venous pressure rises with inspiration as a result of the impaired venous return to the heart.

Emergency treatment of pericardial tamponade is aspiration of the pericardial space. A wide-bore needle is inserted under local anaesthesia to the left of the xiphisternum, between the angle of the xiphisternum and the ribcage (**Figure 54.30**). The needle is advanced towards the tip of the scapula into the pericardial space. An ECG electrode attached to the needle will indicate when the heart has been touched. This will relieve the situation temporarily until the cause of the tamponade is established. Penetrating wounds of the heart usually require exploration through a median sternotomy. Emergency room thoracotomy is rarely required. Chronic tamponade is usually a result of malignant infiltration of the pericardium (usually secondary carcinoma from breast or bronchus) or, very occasionally, uraemia or connective tissue disease. Treatment sometimes requires a pericardial window between the pericardial space and the pleural or peritoneal space.

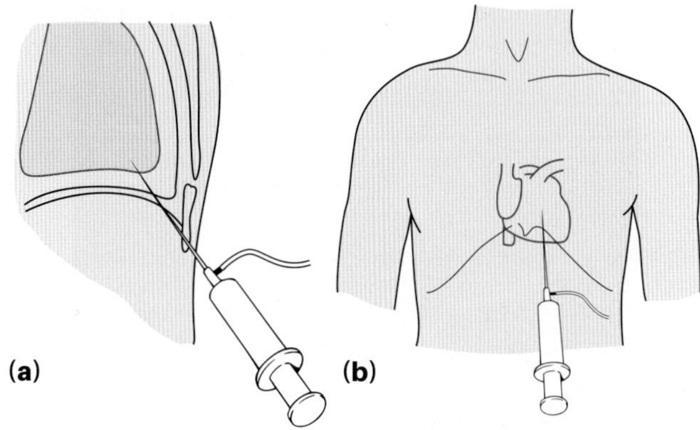

Figure 54.30 (**a**) Pericardial aspiration through the subxiphoid region. (**b**) Site of needle insertion for pericardial aspiration.

Pericarditis

Infection and inflammation may also affect the pericardium. Acute pericarditis usually occurs following a viral illness. Treatment is with non-steroidal anti-inflammatory drugs and bed rest (in case there is an underlying myocarditis). Acute purulent pericarditis is uncommon but requires urgent drainage and intravenous antibiotics, with attention to the underlying cause.

Chronic pericarditis is an uncommon condition in which the pericardium becomes thickened and non-compliant. The heart cannot move freely and the stroke volume is reduced by the constrictive process. The central venous pressure is raised and the liver becomes congested. Peripheral oedema and ascites are also a feature. Treatment is surgical and is aimed at relieving the constriction.

CARDIAC MASSES

Cardiac masses can be either thrombus (blood clots) or tumours. Thrombus can be found in patients with poor left ventricular function or long standing AF, as well as in patients with proximal pulmonary embolus, either in the ventricles or the left atrium.

Cardiac tumours can either be benign or malignant, which in turn can be secondary (from lung, esophagus, breast etc.) or primary.

Atrial myxoma

This is the most common benign cardiac mass in adult. Myxomas are neoplasm of endocardial origin and often appear as an ovid pedunculated mass most commonly seen in the left atrium (75%) or the right atrium (20%) and, rarely, in the ventricles (**Figure 54.31**). Myxomas are associated with congenital disorder (Carney complex) in 5% of cases. They usually present

---

Adolf Kussmaul, 1822–1902, successively Professor of Medicine at Heidelberg, Erlangen, Freiburg and Strasbourg, Germany.

J. Aidan Carney, b.1934, Co Roscommon, Ireland, pathologist at the Mayo Clinic, described a syndrome of myxomas, spotty pigmentation and endocrine overactivity in 1985.

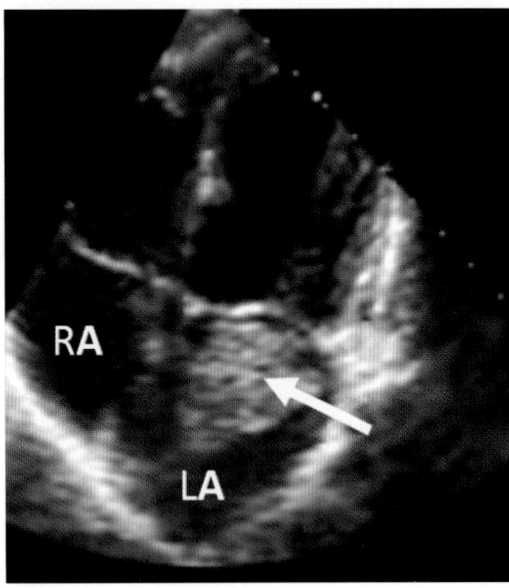

Figure 54.31 Transthoracic echocardiography view of left atrial (LA) myoma (arrow). RA, right atrium.

with symptoms related to blood flow obstruction through heart valves or systemic embolisation. Treatment is by surgical excision and recurrence rates are usually <5%.

Rhabdomyoma

This is the most common benign cardiac tumour in childern. It usually presents with symptoms related to valve dysfuction or arrhythmias. There are usually multicentric pedunculated masses in either or both ventricles. Rhabdomyoma is associated with tuberus sclerosis in >50% of the cases. Treatment is usually by surgical excision.

Primary malignant cardiac tumours

These are extremely rare and less common than secondary malignencies. They include angiosarcoma, rhabdomyosarcoma and leiomyosarcoma. Patients usually have advanced disease when they are discovered, and they are associated with poor outcomes even with multimodality treatment (surgery and chemoradiation).

MANAGEMENT OF CARDIAC ARREST AFTER CARDIAC SURGERY

Introduction

The incidence of cardiac arrest after cardiac surgery is around 0.7–2.9%, with 17–79% survival rates. Ventricular fibrillation (VF), tamponade and major bleeding account for most of arrests. Multiple variables may dictate differences in the management of cardiac arrest after cardiac surgery when compared to other situations. Therefore, EACTS published guidelines for resuscitation of cardiac arrest postcardiac surgery, which are summarised below.

Cardiac arrest with 'non-shockable' rhythm

Cardiac surgical patients who have a non-VF/ventricular tachycardia (VT) arrest may have tamponade, tension pneumothorax or severe hypovolaemia. Prompt treatment is associated with an excellent outcome. Resternotomy should be peformed promptly if connecting the pacemaker and administrating atropine fail to resolve the arrest, especially if prolonged period of CPR is needed, which will be better performed by internal massage.

Emergency resternotomy for ventricular fibrillation or pulseless ventricular tachycardia

A precordial thump may be performed if within 10 s of the onset of VF or pulseless VT; however, this should not delay cardioversion by defibrillation. In VF or pulseless VT, emergency resternotomy should be performed after three failed attempts at defibrillation.

Emergency resternotomy

After the identification of cardiac arrest, basic life support according to the Advanced Life Support (ALS) guidelines should be initiated while preparing for emergency resternotomy. Emergency resternotomy may be required in 0.8–2.7% of all patients undergoing cardiac surgery. Emergency resternotomy is a multipractitioner procedure, which should be rapidly performed with full aseptic technique.

Preparation for emergency resternotomy

- A gown and gloves should be donned in a sterile fashion.
- The thoracic drape is applied, ensuring that the whole bed is covered (if an all-in-one sterile drape is used then there is no need to prepare the skin with antiseptic).
- The scalpel is used to cut the sternotomy incision, including all sutures deeply down to the sternal wires.
- All the sternal wires are cut with the wire cutters. The sternal edges will separate a little, which may relieve tamponade.
- Suction is used to clear excessive blood or clot.
- The retractor is placed between the sternal edges and the sternum opened.
- If cardiac output is restored expert assistance should then be summoned. If there is no cardiac output, the position of any grafts should be carefully identified and internal cardiac massage and internal defibrillation performed, if required.

Internal cardiac massage

This is a potentially dangerous procedure. Risks include avulsion of a bypass graft, with the left internal mammary artery being at particular risk, and right ventricular rupture, especially if it is thin or distended. Therefore, it is important to carefully remove any clot and identify structures at risk such as grafts before placing hands around the heart.

There are several methods of internal massage; however, the two-hand technique is the safest.

TWO-HAND TECHNIQUE

The heart should be inspected to locate the internal mammary and any other grafts if present, followed by removing any blood clots. The right hand is passed over the apex of the heart and then advanced round the apex to the back of the heart, palm up and hand flat. The left hand is then placed flat onto the anterior surface of the heart and the two hands squeezed together at a rate of 100 per minute. Flat palms and straight fingers are important to avoid an unequal distribution of pressure onto the heart, thereby minimising the chance of trauma. If there is a mitral valve replacement or repair, care should be taken not to lift the apex by the right hand, as this can cause a posterior ventricular rupture.

FURTHER READING

Bojar RM. *Manual of perioperative care in cardiac surgery*, 5th edn. Oxford: Wiley-Blackwell, 2010.

Cohn LH. *Cardiac surgery in the adult*, 4th edn. New York: MaGraw Hill Professional, 2011.

Dunning J, Fabbri A, Kolh PH *et al.* Guideline for resuscitation in cardiac arrest after cardiac surgery. *Eur J Cardiothorac Surg* 2009; **36**: 3–28.

Kirklin J, Barratt-Boyce B. *Cardiac surgery*, 4th edn. Philadelphia: Elsevier Saunders, 2013.

Kolh P, Wijns W, Danchin N *et al.* Guidelines on myocardial revascularization. *Eur J Cardiothorac Surg* 2010; **38** (Suppl):S1–S52.

Mery CM, Turek JW. *TSRA Review of cardiothoracic surgery*, 2nd edn. Chicago: The Thoracic Surgery Residents Association, 2015.

Moorjani N, Viola N, Ohri S. *Key questions in cardiac surgery*. Shrewsbury: TFM publishing, 2011.

Nishimura RA, Otto CM, Bonow RO *et al.* AHA/ACC guideline for the management of patients with valvular heart disease. *J Am Coll Cardiol* 2014; **63**(22): e57–e185.

Chapter 55

The thorax

Learning objectives

To understand:

- The anatomy and physiology of the thorax
- Investigation of chest pathology
- The role of surgery in pleural disease
- The assessment of patients requiring lung surgery
- Surgical oncology as applied to chest surgery

INTRODUCTION

Anatomical development of the lungs

The lungs are derived from an outpouching of the primitive foregut during the fourth week of intrauterine life. This bud becomes a two-lobed structure, the ends of which ultimately become the lungs. The lobar arrangement is defined early and is fairly constant but anomalies of fissures and segments leading to anatomical variation in the adult are common.

The primitive lungs drain into the cardinal veins, which ultimately become the pulmonary veins draining into the left atrium. Variability in venous drainage is very common and is usually of little functional significance. At the most severe end of the spectrum is total anomalous drainage, which presents in early infant life because oxygenated blood is all directed back to the right heart.

Anatomy of the lungs

The left lung is divided by the oblique fissure, which lies nearer to the vertical than horizontal, so the upper and lower lobes could also be called anterior and posterior. On the right, the equivalent of the left upper lobe is further divided to give the middle lobe. Each lobe is composed of segments, with anatomically defined and named bronchial, pulmonary arterial and venous connections (**Figure 55.1**).

The right main bronchus (RMB) is shorter, wider and nearly vertical compared with the left main bronchus (LMB). As a consequence, inhaled foreign bodies are more likely to enter the right main bronchus than the left (**Figure 55.2**). The trachea and bronchi have a systemic arterial blood supply delivered by the bronchial arteries, which arise directly from the nearby thoracic aorta.

Lymphatic drainage tends to follow the bronchi. Lymph nodes are both named and identified by numbered 'stations'

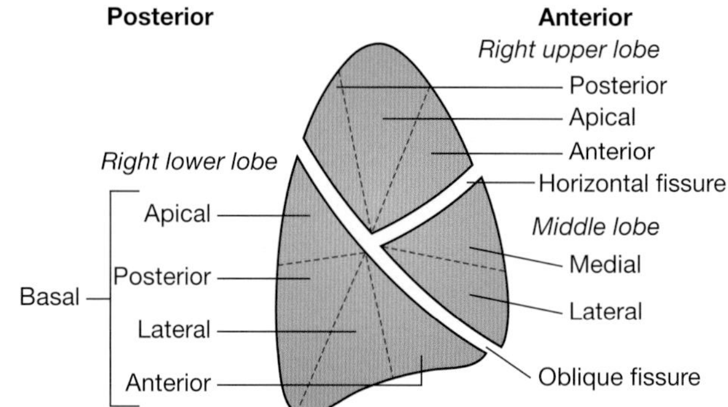

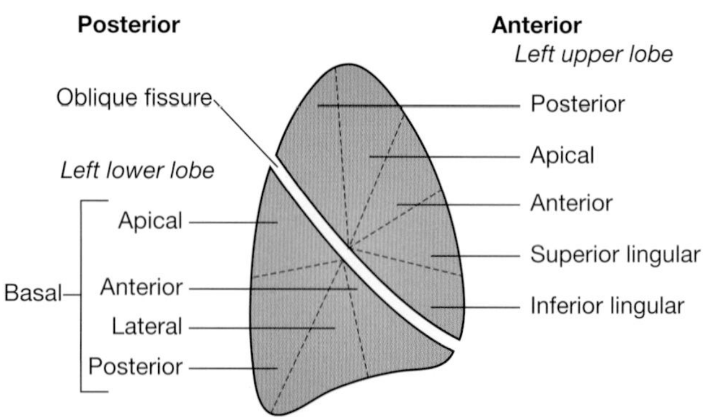

Figure 55.1 The lobar and segmental divisions of the lungs, right lung above and left lung below as if viewed from the side.

and more recently into zones, which are of importance in staging of lung cancer (**Figure 55.3**).

Mechanics of breathing

The intercostal muscles contract, causing the ribs to move upwards and outwards, thereby increasing the transverse and anteroposterior dimensions of the chest wall. The diaphragm contracts simultaneously and flattens, increasing the vertical

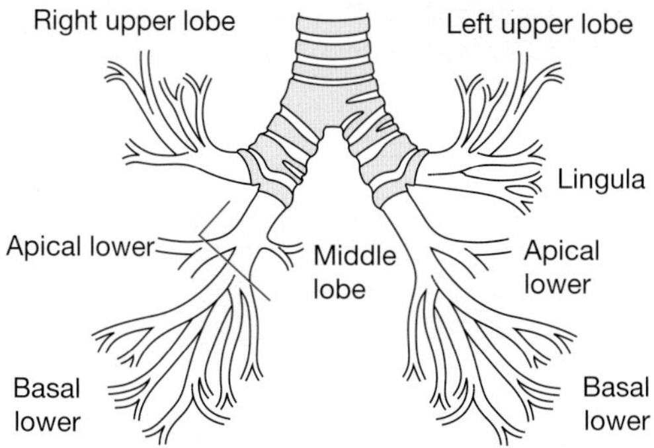

Figure 55.2 Surgical anatomy of the bronchial tree. To surgically remove the right lower lobe and conserve the middle lobe, the surgeon must be prepared to dissect and separately divide the apical bronchial segment (red line).

dimension of the chest cavity. As the volume increases, the intrathoracic pressure falls and air flows in until the alveolar pressure is the same as the atmospheric pressure. The only force used in normal expiration is the elastic recoil of the lung.

Coughing to clear sputum is an essential part of recovery from surgery. In a vigorous cough, probably the only muscle in the body that is relaxed is the diaphragm; as the abdomen and chest wall muscles contract, the limbs are braced and the sphincters are tightened. When the intrathoracic and abdominal pressure is built up, the glottis is opened and the diaphragm is forced up as a piston, or like the plunger of a syringe, to expel air at high velocity.

ASSESSMENT OF FITNESS FOR MAJOR THORACIC SURGERY

The British Thoracic Society (BTS) recommends a tripartite risk assessment model for patients undergoing lung resection, considering the risk of operative mortality, risk of perioperative myocardial events and risk of postoperative dyspnoea (Figure 55.4). (See also Chapter 17).

Risk of operative mortality

The Thoracoscore is the most widely used model to assess risk of operative mortality in thoracic patients. Risk is calculated based on nine variables – age, sex, American Society of Anesthesiologists (ASA) score, performance status, dyspnoea score, priority of surgery, extent of surgery, malignant diagnosis and composite comorbidity score. It is currently the most robust model available to estimate the risk of death when considering patients for thoracic surgery.

Risk of perioperative myocardial event

History, physical examination and resting electrocardiogram (ECG) form the basics of assessing perioperative cardiovascular risk. Patients who are found to have an active cardiac condition should be evaluated by a cardiologist and optimised (medical, revascularistion or cardiac surgery) before thoracic surgery. Surgery should be avoided within 30 days of myocardial infarction.

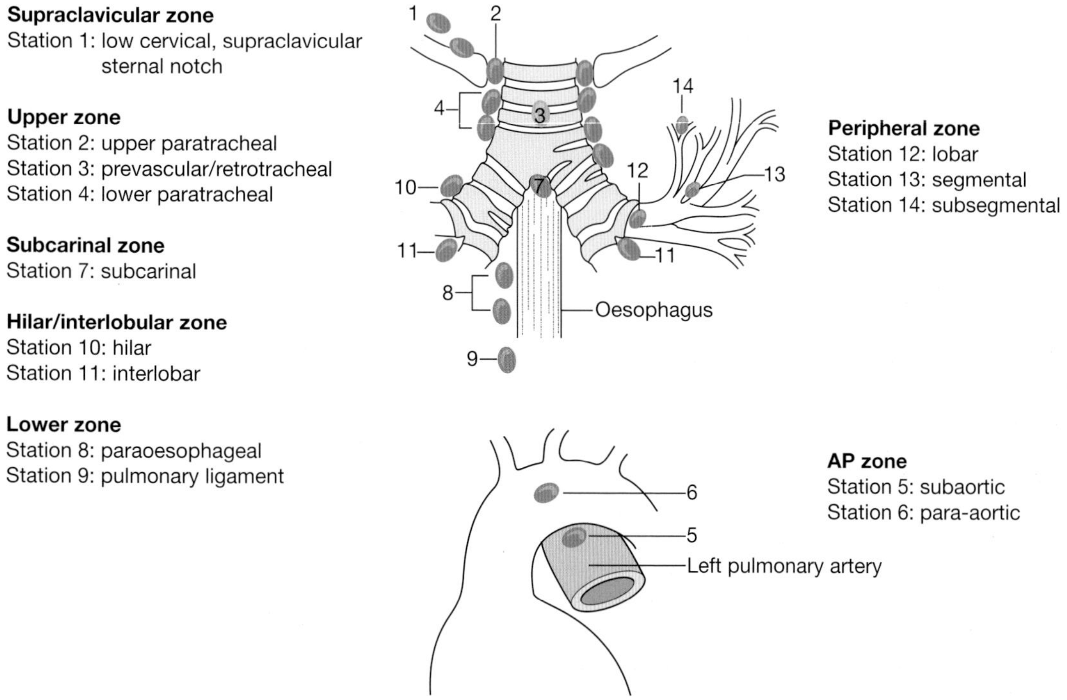

Supraclavicular zone
Station 1: low cervical, supraclavicular sternal notch

Upper zone
Station 2: upper paratracheal
Station 3: prevascular/retrotracheal
Station 4: lower paratracheal

Subcarinal zone
Station 7: subcarinal

Hilar/interlobular zone
Station 10: hilar
Station 11: interlobar

Lower zone
Station 8: paraoesophageal
Station 9: pulmonary ligament

Peripheral zone
Station 12: lobar
Station 13: segmental
Station 14: subsegmental

Oesophagus

AP zone
Station 5: subaortic
Station 6: para-aortic

Left pulmonary artery

Figure 55.3 Lymph node stations related to the bronchial tree are particularly important in the staging of lung cancer, with N1 nodes (10–14) and N2 nodes (2–9) shown.

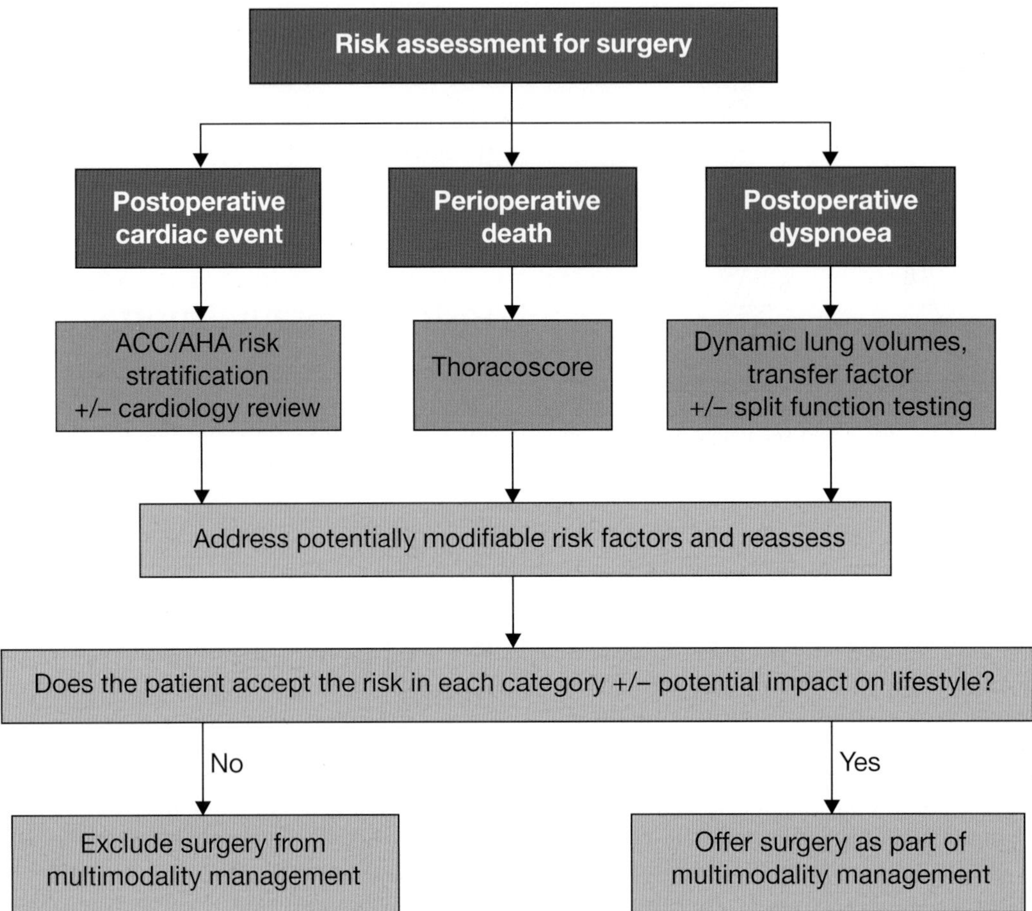

Figure 55.4 Tripartite risk assessment. ACC, American College of Cardiology; AHA, American Heart Association.

Risk of postoperative dyspnoea

Any patient undergoing general anaesthesia requires some assessment of respiratory function. This may be a clinical appraisal of fitness but more detail is necessary for patients who are undergoing lung resection.

Investigation of the respiratory system

Pulmonary function tests (PFTs) are useful in determining the functional capacity of the patient and the severity of pulmonary disease, and in predicting the response to various treatments. The tests range from simple clinic or bedside measurements to those only available in specialist centres. Spirometry is the most commonly performed PFT and measures specifically the amount (volume) and/or speed (flow rate) of air that can be inhaled or exhaled. It is reported in both absolute values and as a predicted percentage of normal. Normal values vary, depending on gender, race, age and height. The most common parameters measured in spirometry are defined below and illustrated in **Figure 55.5**.

Peak expiratory flow rate

Peak expiratory flow rate (PEFR) is measured by a Wright peak flow meter or a peak flow gauge. This is the maximum airflow velocity achieved during an expiration delivered with maximal force from the total lung capacity. It is a reliable and reproducible test but has the disadvantage of being effort dependent, and it may therefore be affected by abdominal or thoracic wound pain. PEFR measurements are often used in managing asthma, but there are many other causes of low PEFR such as a problem with large airway patency.

Forced expiratory volume in 1 second

The forced expiratory volume in 1 s (FEV_1) is the amount of air forcibly expired in 1 s. It is low in obstructive lung disease and may be normal in patients with poor gas exchange.

Basil Martin Wright, 1912–2001, member of the scientific staff of the Medical Research Council Research Centre, Northwick Park Hospital, Harrow, Middlesex, UK.

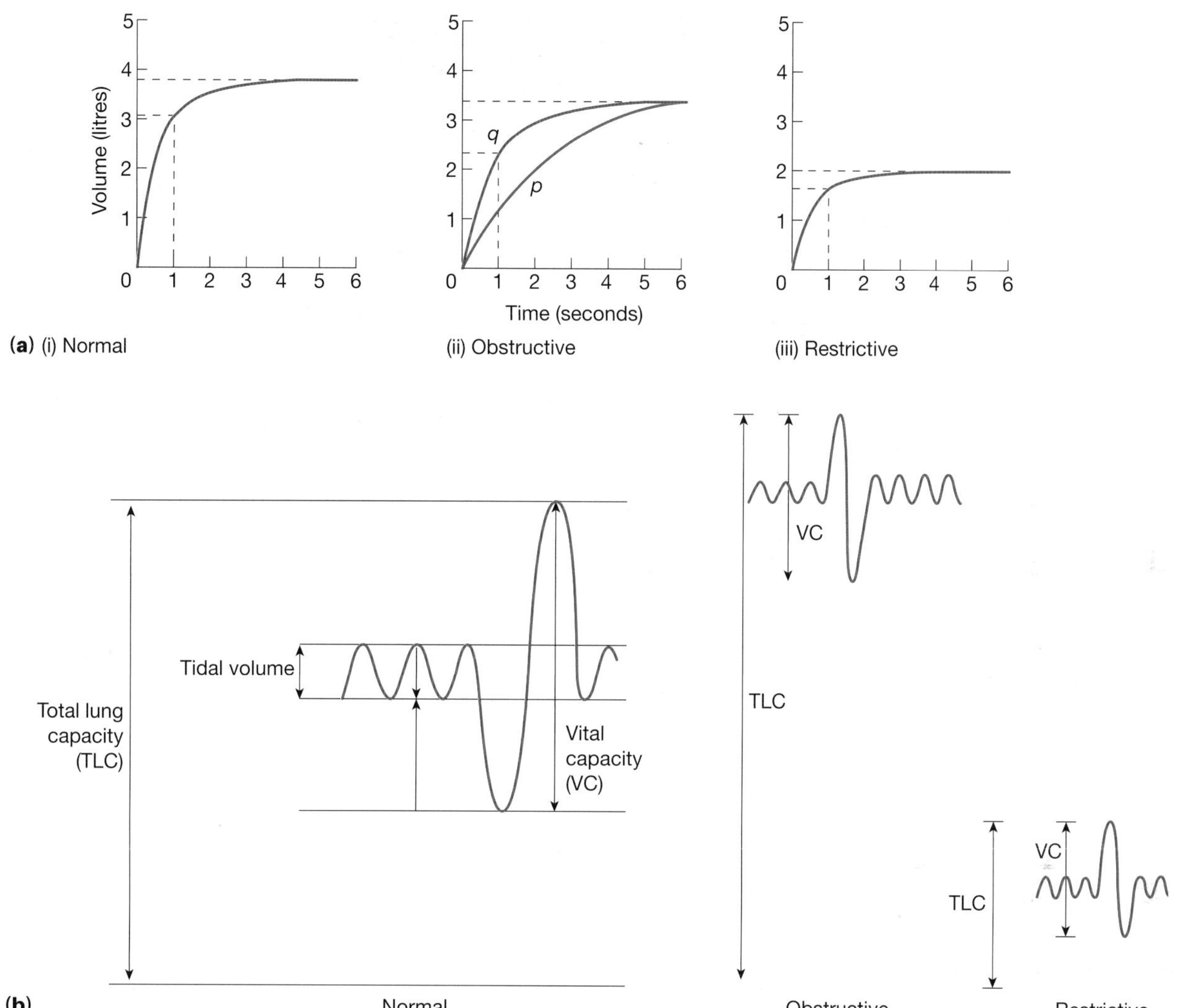

Figure 55.5 Spirometry. (**a**) Spirogram tracings obtained from a Vitallograph: (**i**) normal forced expiratory volume in 1 s (FEV_1) 3.1 litres, forced vital capacity (FVC) 3.8 litres, FEV_1/FVC 82%; (ii) obstructive defect, reversible asthma, *p* before a bronchodilator, FEV_1 1.4 litres, FVC 3.5 litres, FEV_1/FVC 40%; *q* after a bronchodilator, FEV_1 2.5 litres, FVC 3.5 litres, FEV_1/FVC 71%; (iii) restrictive defect, fibrosing alveolitis, FEV_1 1.8 litres, FVC 2.0 litres, FEV_1/FVC 90%. No change with bronchodilators. (**b**) Changes in lung volume in obstructive and restrictive lung disease. (Reproduced from Gray HH. Pulmonary embolism. *Medicine International* 1993; **21**: 477, by kind permission of the Medicine Group (Journals) Ltd.)

Forced vital capacity

The forced vital capacity (FVC) is the volume of air forcibly displaced following maximal inspiration to maximal expiration. The FEV_1 and the FVC can be measured using a Vitallograph, and a ratio (FEV_1/FVC) can be calculated (**Figure 55.5**). A low ratio indicates obstruction and the test should be repeated after bronchodilators. A normal ratio (FVC and FEV_1 reduced to the same extent) indicates a restrictive pathology.

There are two physiological categories of lung disease: obstructive and restrictive (*Table 55.1*). In obstructive conditions such as asthma or emphysema, the flow of air in and out of the lungs is impaired. In restrictive disrease, such as lung fibrosis, the lungs have lost size or elasticity, becoming 'stiff' so that they do not fill or expand properly.

TABLE 55.1 Spirometry values in obstructive and restrictive lung diseases.

	Obstructive pattern	Restrictive pattern
PEFR	↓↓	Normal or ↓
FEV_1	↓↓	Normal or ↓
FVC	Normal or ↓	↓↓
FEV_1/FVC	<70	>80

FEV_1, forced expiratory volume in 1 s; FVC, forced vital capacity; PEFR, peak expiratory flow rate.

Diffusion capacity

The diffusion capacity (DLCO) is a measurement of the lung's ability to transfer gases and is often referred to as the 'transfer factor'. It cannot be performed at the bedside, requires the patient's current haemoglobin level and is a test of the integrity of the lung's alveolar–capillary surface area for gas exchange. In lung diseases that damage the alveolar walls, such as emphysema, or that thicken the alveolar membrane, such as lung fibrosis, it may be reduced. In patients who require surgery to remove part of their lung, for example for lung cancer, measurement of DLCO is an important determitant of 'fitness' for surgery and it should be measured formally as part of a lung function test.

Oxygen saturation

Oxygen saturation (SpO_2) refers to the degree of oxygen molecules (O_2) carried in the blood attached to haemoglobin molecules (Hb). It is a measure of how much oxygen the blood is carrying as a percentage of the maximum it could carry. The common method of monitoring the oxygenation of a patient's haemoglobin is through a pulse oximeter.

Blood gases

The SpO_2 measured non-invasively with a pulse oximeter measures only oxygenation, not ventilation, and provides no information regarding a patient's carbon dioxide or bicarbonate levels, blood pH or base deficit. This requires arterial blood sampling or 'blood gases' (*Table 55.2*).

TABLE 55.2 Arterial blood gases: 'normal values'.

pH 7.35–7.45
$PaCO_2$ 4.5–6 kPa (35–50 mmHg)
PaO_2 11–14 kPa (83–105 mmHg)
Standard bicarbonate 22–28 mmol/L
Anion gap 10–16 mmol/L
Chloride 98–107 mmol/L

The FEV_1 and DLCO are often used to predict the risk of postoperative dyspnoea after lung resection. The predicted postoperative values can be calculated by considering the volume of lung, more specifically the number of bronchopulmonary segments, expected to be removed at surgery. For example if five segments of the left upper lobe are to be removed, the postoperative predicted FEV_1 in a patient with a preoperative FEV_1 of 2.5 litres (85% predicted) is $(19 - 5)/19 \times 2.5 = 1.84$ litres, and $(19 - 5)/19 \times 85\% = 62.6\%$ predicted. This assumes that all bronchopulmonary segments are functioning (e.g. not collapsed) and contribute equally to lung function. Although an optimum cut-off of postoperative predicted FEV_1 of 40% is widely cited, there are currently limited data to provide guidance on this figure to help predict an acceptable degree of postoperative dyspnoea and quality of life. Patients should still be offered surgical resection if the predicted risk of postoperative dyspnoea is moderate or high, as long as they are aware of and accept the risks of dyspnoea and associated complications.

Other functional assessments, including the shuttle walk test, 6-minute walk test, as well as cardiopulmonary exercise testing, could be considered for patients at moderate or high risk of postoperative dyspnoea.

The pleura

The key to many aspects of practical chest surgery is an understanding of the pleura and of the mechanics of breathing. Management of the essentially healthy pleural space is logical and simple and needs minimal technology. On the other hand, when pleural disease is advanced, for example when there is gross pleural sepsis surrounding a leaking and trapped lung, management is difficult and the patient may require prolonged care with repeated interventions.

The physiology of pleural fluid

The turnover of fluid in the human pleural space is about 1–2 litres in 24 hours, with only 5–10 ml of fluid present at any one time as a film, about 20 micrometres thick, between the visceral and parietal pleura.

The mechanisms and equations given are simplifications but serve to explain the clinical conditions encountered. The fluid is produced from the capillaries of the parietal pleura as a transudate, according to the Starling capillary loop pressures. However, there is a further negative force in the pleura. The elastic content of the lung causes it to recoil and collapse if not held open by the negative pressure in the pleura. This elastic recoil exerts about 4 mmHg of negative pressure and favours accumulation of fluid. The secreting forces add up to about 11 mmHg in health. Pleural fluid is mainly reabsorbed (about 90%) by the visceral pleura, whose capillaries are part of the pulmonary circulation. The principal force in absorption of pleural fluid is oncotic pressure (approximately 25 mmHg) minus the difference in mean capillary hydrostatic pressure of the pulmonary capillary (8 mmHg). Thus, the overall absorbing pressure is 25 – 8 = 17 mmHg, producing a net drying effect (17 – 11) of about 6 mmHg (**Figure 55.6**).

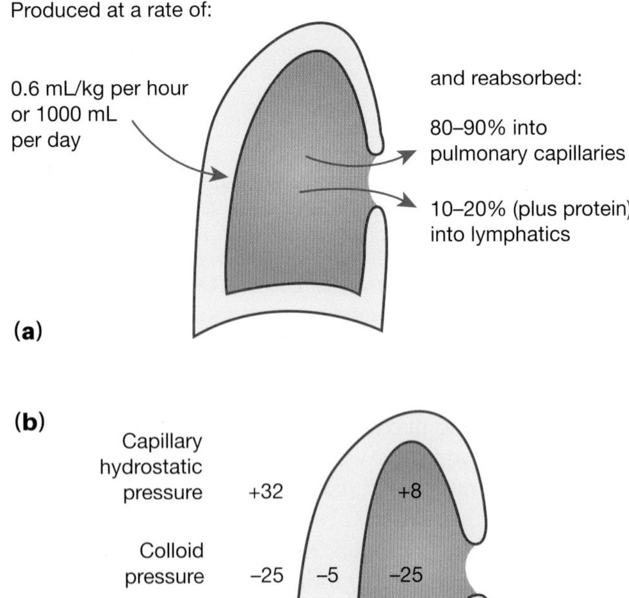

Figure 55.6 (**a**) Production and absorption of pleural fluid. (**b**) Normal pleural physiology. (See the text for an explanation of this simplistic physiological model.)

Ernest Henry Starling, 1866–1927, Professor of Physiology, University College, London, UK.

Gas in the pleural space

There is normally no free gas in the pleural space because the same physiological mechanism that absorbs air from a pneumothorax prevents any gas accumulating.

The partial pressures (water as saturated vapour pressure) of the gases in venous/end-capillary blood are:

• PO_2	40 mmHg	5.3 kPa
• PCO_2	46 mmHg	6.1 kPa
• PN_2	573 mmHg	76.4 kPa
• PH_2O	47 mmHg	6.3 kPa

These partial pressures add up to less than atmospheric pressure (760 mmHg). Free gas is therefore absorbed into the blood and lost to the atmosphere through the lungs, with the gases moving in relation to their solubility (carbon dioxide quickest and nitrogen slowest) and relative concentrations in the pleural space and the blood. This does not favour nitrogen, which constitutes about 80% of atmospheric air. Breathing oxygen accelerates nitrogen removal by reducing the content of nitrogen in the blood and increasing the gradient for its absorption. Nitrous oxide anaesthesia is dangerous in the presence of a pneumothorax; nitrous oxide is very soluble and, although not normally present in the pleural space, it will be rapidly transported into the space if the patient is given nitrous oxide to breathe.

DISORDERS OF THE PLEURA

Pneumothorax

Pneumothorax is the presence of air outside the lung, within the pleural space. It must be distinguished from bullae or air cysts within the lung. Bullae can be the cause of an air leak from the lung and can therefore coexist with pneumothorax.

Spontaneous pneumothorax occurs when the visceral pleura ruptures without an external traumatic or iatrogenic cause. Cases are divided into primary spontaneous pneumothorax (PSP) and secondary spontaneous pneumothorax (SSP). Pneumothorax can also occur following trauma or iatrogenic injury such as insertion of a central line. Tension pneumothorax is when (independent of aetiology) there is a build up of positive pressure within the hemithorax, to the extent that the lung is completely collapsed, the diaphragm is flattened, the mediastinum is distorted and, eventually, the venous return to the heart is compromised. Any pleural breach is inherently valve-like because air will find its way out through the alveoli but cannot be drawn back in because the lung tissue collapses around the hole in the pleura. Patients being mechanically ventilated following trauma are at particular risk.

Surgical emphysema is the presence of air in the tissues. It requires a breach of an air-containing viscus in communication with soft tissues, and the generation of positive pressure to push the air along tissue planes. The most serious cause is a ruptured oesophagus. Mediastinal surgical emphysema can also occur with asthma or barotrauma from positive pressure ventilation. A poorly managed chest drain with intermittent build up of pressure allows air to track into the chest wall through the point where the drain breaches the parietal pleura.

Primary spontaneous pneumothorax

This is a common condition characteristically seen in young people from their mid-teens to late 20s. About 75% of cases are in young men who tend to be tall and have a family history of the condition. It is due to leaks from small blebs, vesicles or bullae, which may become pedunculated, typically at the apex of the upper lobe or on the upper border of the lower or middle lobes.

Secondary spontaneous pneumothorax

This occurs when the visceral pleura leaks as part of an underlying lung disease; any disease that involves the pleura may cause pneumothorax, including tuberculosis, any degenerative or cavitating lung disease and necrosing tumours. As such it tends to occur in older patients, often with a history of underlying lung disease such as emphysema. The pneumothorax may be less well tolerated.

Usually, pneumothorax presents with sharp pleuritic pain and breathlessness. The pleura is exquisitely sensitive and the movement of the lung on and off the parietal pleura causes severe discomfort. As a result mild cases are more painful, whereas complete collapse is usually painless but causes more breathlessness. Bleeding and tension pneumothorax can occur. They are usually self-limiting; careful observation is wiser than too-ready resort to a chest drain. If the patient is not in respiratory distress or hypoxic there is no urgency. Tension pneumothorax should be immediately relieved by inserting a cannula into the hemithorax in as safe a position as possible (**Figure 55.7**).

The risk of recurrent pneumothorax is increased after the first episode. The best estimates of recurrence rates are:

- of patients who experience a first event, only about one-third experience recurrence;
- of those who have a second episode, about one-half go on to experience a third episode;
- those who have had three episodes will probably go on to have repeated recurrences.

Current recommendations from the BTS are that, in cases of persistent air leak following drain insertion or failure of the lung to re-expand, an early (3–5 days) thoracic surgical opinion should be sought. Other indications for thoracic surgical referral are given.

> **Summary box 55.1**
>
> Indications for surgical intervention for pneumothorax include:
>
> - Second ipsilateral pneumothorax
> - First contralateral pneumothorax
> - Bilateral spontaneous pneumothorax
> - Pneumothorax fails to settle despite chest drainage
> - Spontaneous haemothorax: professions at risk (e.g. pilots, divers)
> - Pregnancy

Current recommendations focus on the use of small bore (10–14 Fr) chest drains, usually of a Seldinger type, inserted ideally under ultrasound guidance. However, knowledge of the role of the 'surgical' chest drain and how to insert it safely is still required.

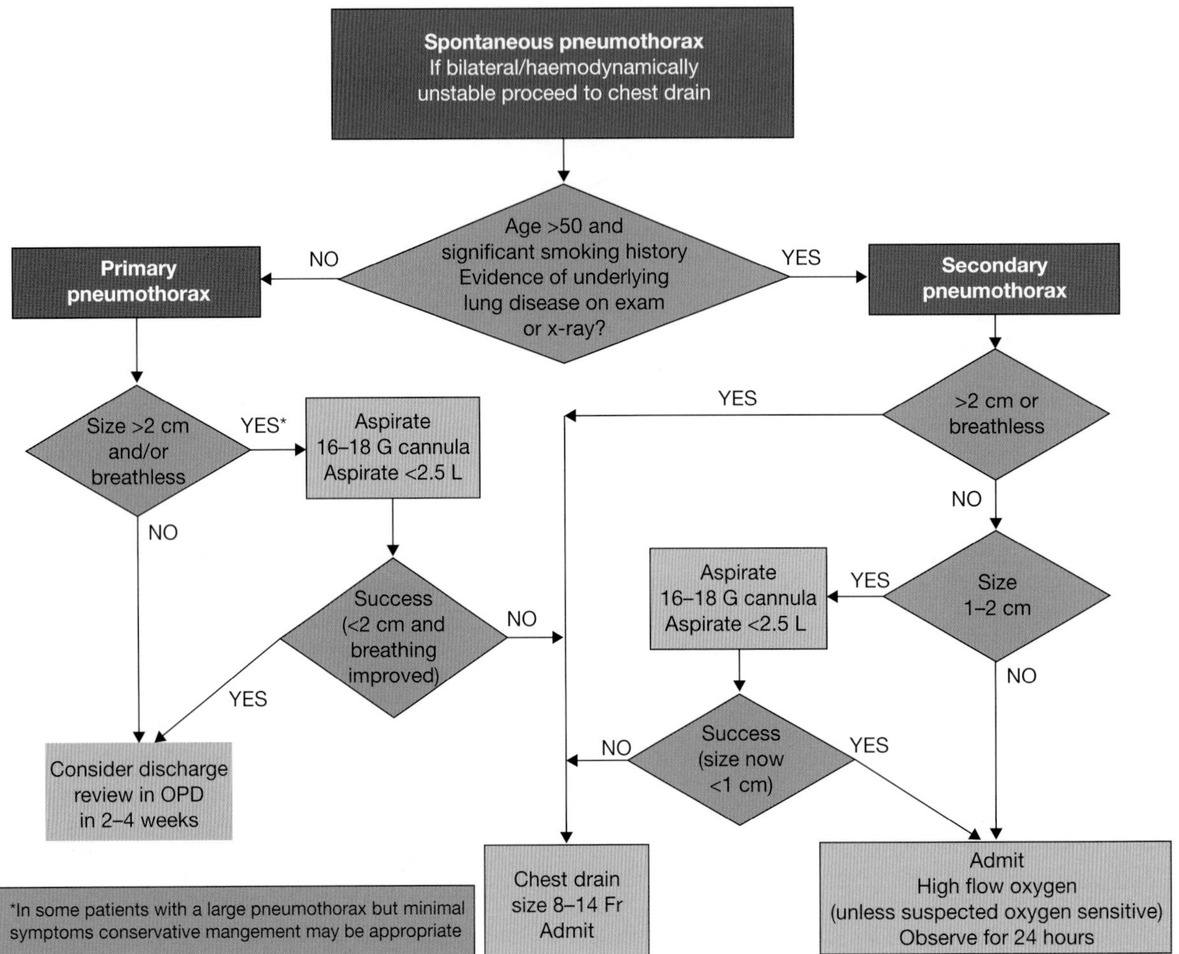

Figure 55.7 British Thoracic Society (BTS) guidelines on management of spontaneous pneumothorax (2010) (adapted from www.bts.org.uk). OPD, outpatient department.

Inserting and managing a chest drain

An intercostal tube connected to an underwater seal is central to the management of chest disease; however, the management of the pleura and of chest drains can be troublesome, even in experienced hands.

The safest site for insertion of a drain (**Figure 55.8**) is in the triangle that lies:

- anterior to the mid-axillary line;
- above the level of the nipple;
- below and lateral to the pectoralis major muscle.

This will ideally find the fifth space. The technique includes the following.

- Meticulous attention to sterility throughout.
- Adequate local anaesthesia to include the pleura.
- Sharp dissection to cut only the skin.
- Blunt dissection with artery forceps down through the muscle layers; these should only be the serratus anterior and the intercostals.
- An oblique tract, so that the skin incision and the hole in the parietal pleura do not overlie each other and the drain is in a short tunnel, which reduces the chance of entraining air.
- A drain for pneumothorax and haemothorax should aim towards the apex of the lung. A drain for pleural effusion or empyema should be nearer the base. The drain should pass over the upper edge of the rib to avoid the neurovascular bundle that lies beneath the rib.
- The retaining stitch should be secure but should not obliterate the drain.
- A vertical mattress suture is inserted for later wound closure. This is vital for pneumothorax management but should be omitted if the drain is for empyema (provided there is adherence of the pleura) because that tract should lie open.
- Connect the drain to an underwater seal device which functions as a one-way valve.
- After completion, check that the drain has achieved its objective by taking a chest radiograph.

It is preferable not to apply suction to the drain or clamp it. The danger is that the clamp may be applied for transport and forgotten. Dangers of disconnection and siphoning are small or best averted in other ways apart from clamping. A bubbling drain should (almost) never be clamped. Remove the drain when it no longer has a function.

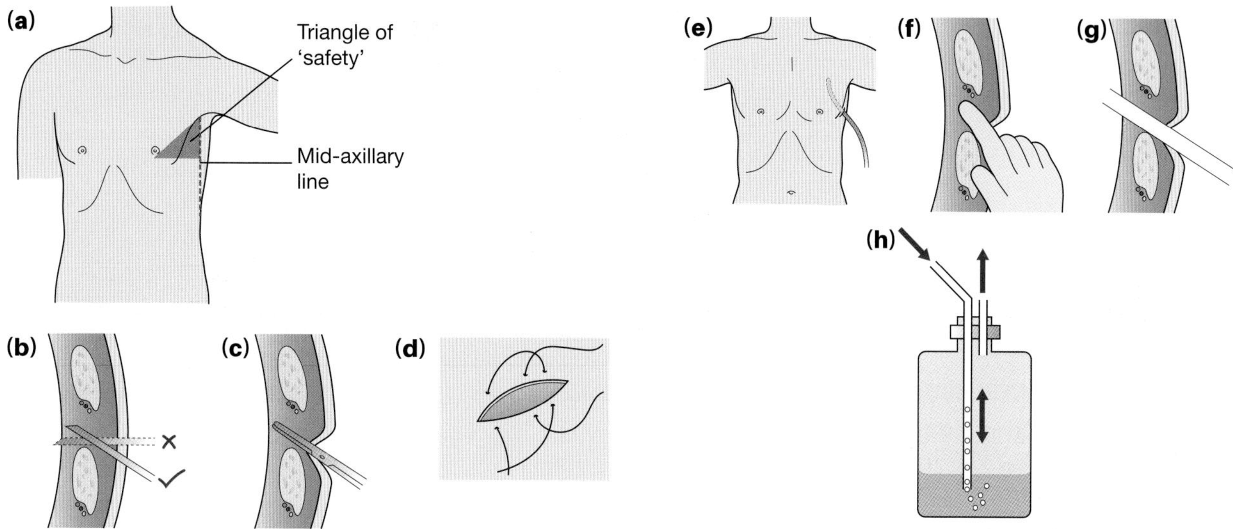

Figure 55.8 Insertion of chest drain: (**a**) triangle of safety; (**b**) penetration of the skin, muscle and pleura; (**c**) blunt dissection of the parietal pleura; (**d**) suture placement; (**e**) gauging the distance of insertion; (**f**) digital examination along the tract into the pleural space; (**g**) withdrawal of central trochar and positioning of drain; (**h**) underwater seal chest drain bottle.

Summary box 55.2

Suction on a pleural tube

- Be aware! Inserting the drain, and not the suction, is the life-saving manoeuvre
- If the lung is reluctant to expand, the suction deviates the mediastinum
- If the lung is fragile, it may worsen an air leak

Surgical management of pneumothorax

Pleurectomy and pleurodesis

Surgery for pneumothorax can be performed by video-assisted thoracoscopic surgery (VATS) or as an open procedure (thoracotomy). The object of the exercise is threefold:

- to deal with any leaks from the lung;
- to search for and obliterate any blebs and bullae;
- to make the visceral pleura adherent to the parietal pleura so that any subsequent leaks are contained and the lung cannot completely collapse.

Pleural adhesion is achieved in one of three ways:

- **Pleurectomy**: systematically stripping the parietal pleura from the chest wall.
- **Pleural abrasion**: a scourer is used to scrape off the slick surface of the parietal pleura.
- **Chemical pleurodesis**: usually talc is used and is insufflated into the chest cavity.

Pleural effusion

Pleural effusion can be readily understood with reference to the physiological mechanisms governing the flux of pleural fluid given above. Pleural effusions are divided into exudates and transudates, depending on protein content (more (exudates) or less (transudates) than 30 g/L), and characterised further according to glucose content, pH and lactate dehydrogenase content. The following are the most common ways in which the pleural fluid balance is disturbed.

- **Elevated pulmonary capillary pressure.** If left atrial pressure rises, the pulmonary capillary pressure must rise with it, as a result of either impaired cardiac performance or an overloaded circulation.
- **Reduced intravascular oncotic pressure.** If the plasma proteins fall because of renal or hepatic disease or malnutrition, the absorption mechanism fails.
- **Accumulation of pleural protein** due to obstruction of the mediastinal lymphatics secondary to lymphoma or cancers that invade the lymphatic system.
- **Excessive permeability of the capillaries** to fluid and protein as in inflammatory diseases, particularly the collagen vascular diseases. Of particular importance to the surgeon is the effusion associated with pleural infection (empyema) and malignant effusions.

Malignant pleural effusion

Pleural effusion is a common complication of cancer. This may be due to:

- lung cancer;
- pleural involvement with primary or secondary malignancy;
- mediastinal lymphatic involvement.

LUNG CANCER

There may be direct involvement of the parietal and/or visceral pleura, collapse of the lung parenchyma and spread to the mediastinal lymphatics, or a combination of these, causing pleural fluid accumulation. It is usually regarded as a feature that puts lung cancer beyond surgical cure.

PLEURAL MALIGNANCY

The only primary malignancy of the pleura seen with any regularity is malignant mesothelioma. This is a consequence of asbestos exposure, with few exceptions. The peak of asbestos importation into the UK was from 1960 to 1975 and the incidence of mesothelioma is rising and was expected to peak in 2015. Mesothelioma commonly presents with breathlessness because of pleural effusions, pain and systemic features of malignancy. Diffuse seeding of the parietal and visceral pleura is a common pattern of dissemination of cancers, particularly adenocarcinoma of any origin.

MEDIASTINAL LYMPHATIC INVOLVEMENT

In many instances, particularly in breast cancer, there is no evident disease in the pleura. The disease is in the mediastinal lymphatics, which are obstructed, and this upsets the balance of physiological forces that control pleural fluid.

SURGERY FOR PATIENTS WITH MALIGNANT PLEURAL EFFUSION

The surgeon has two roles: to make the diagnosis and to achieve effective palliation by draining the fluid and pleurodesis.

DIAGNOSIS

Pleural biopsy can be obtained by a range of techniques, with VATS being the most common. An unequivocally positive biopsy is useful but a negative biopsy may be a sampling error.

Summary box 55.3

Biopsy of the pleura

- Cytological examination of the pleural fluid (low yield)
- Abrams' needle (low yield in malignancy)
- Computed tomography (CT)-guided needle biopsy of a suspicious area
- VATS biopsy
- Open surgical biopsy

Pleural infection and empyema

Empyema is the end stage of pleural infection from any cause. It most commonly results from infection of the underlying lung, involving pneumonia or a lung abscess, but can occur as a complication of any thoracic operation. It is seen if a traumatic haemothorax becomes infected or in the course of management of pneumothorax or pleural effusions. It may be associated with pus under the diaphragm (*Table 55.3*).The pathological diagnosis requires the presence of thick pus with a thick cortex of fibrin and coagulum over the lung.

When empyema presents *de novo* it usually follows pneumonia, and three phases are described:

TABLE 55.3 Conditions that predispose to empyema formation.

Pulmonary infection	Unresolved pneumonia Bronchiectasis Tuberculosis Fungal infections Lung abscess
Aspiration of pleural effusion	Any aetiology
Trauma	Penetrating injury Surgery Oesophageal perforation
Extrapulmonary sources	Subphrenic abscess
Bone infections	Osteomyelitis of ribs or vertebrae

1. In the exudative phase, there is protein-rich (>30 g/L) effusion. If this becomes infected with the organisms from the lung (typically *Streptococcus milleri* and *Haemophilus influenzae* in children), the scene is set for empyema. At this stage antibiotics may be all that is required. Aspiration or drainage to dryness in addition is preferred.
2. Over subsequent days, the fluid thickens to what is known as the fibrinopurulent phase. Drainage at this stage is prudent as antibiotics on their own are unlikely to be curative.
3. The organising phase causes the lung to be trapped by a thick peel or 'cortex' for which surgical management may be required.

Surgical management of pleural effusions and infections

Thoracoscopy or video-assisted thoracoscopic surgery (VATS)

The direct-vision thoracoscope has been used for many years, but its use was limited mainly to performing biopsies. The instrument had a limited view and was uncomfortable to use for any length of time. All this has changed since the advent of video-assisted thoracoscopy (**Figure 55.9**); the surgeon's hands are freed because the camera is attached to the thoracoscope, which can be operated by an assistant with the image displayed on a screen. The surgeon is able to manipulate instruments with both hands to perform a variety of procedures. The number of ports required depends on the type and complexity of the surgery. The patient is usually positioned with the diseased side uppermost, having had a double lumen endotracheobronchial tube placed by the anaesthetist to allow for single-lung ventilation. The principal advantage is that a large incision is avoided, resulting in less postoperative pain and a more rapid recovery.

VATS drainage, pleural biopsy and talc pleurodesis

VATS drainage, pleural biopsy and talc pleurodesis is increasingly performed for the management of patients with an undiagnosed or malignant pleural effusion. It can be performed using a single port and allows direct visualisation of the pleural cavity for complete drainage, multiple pleural biopsies and excellent talc insufflation to achieve pleurodesis.

Leon David Abrams, 1923–2012, cardiothoracic surgeon, the United Birmingham Hospitals, Birmingham, UK.

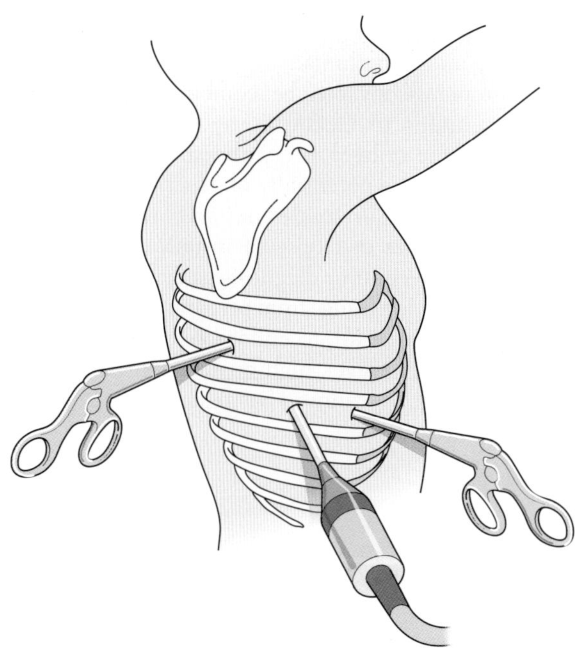

Figure 55.9 Video-assisted thoracoscopic surgery (VATS) utilises modern thoracoscopic instruments and digital technology and avoids large incisions.

VATS debridement of empyema

Pleural infection, particularly early in its evolution, requires drainage, but once the fluid component becomes fibrinopurulent and loculated it requires surgical debridement, which can often be achieved through a VATS approach. The lung is isolated through the use of a double lumen tube, the patient is positioned disease side up, and the pleural cavity is entered. The fluid and debris are vigorously debrided, freeing the lung and allowing for re-expansion. At the end of the case, carefully positioned chest drains are placed to allow for dependent drainage. The drain(s) must exit the skin anterior to the mid-axillary line otherwise the patient will have to lie on the drain(s), causing pain and possibly obstructing the tube. The drain should lie obliquely in its course through the skin and chest wall and into the pleura, or it will kink.

Following the procedure, the patient requires good analgesic control, typically using patient-controlled analgesia (PCA), and physiotherapy to help fully re-expand the lung prior to final removal of chest drains.

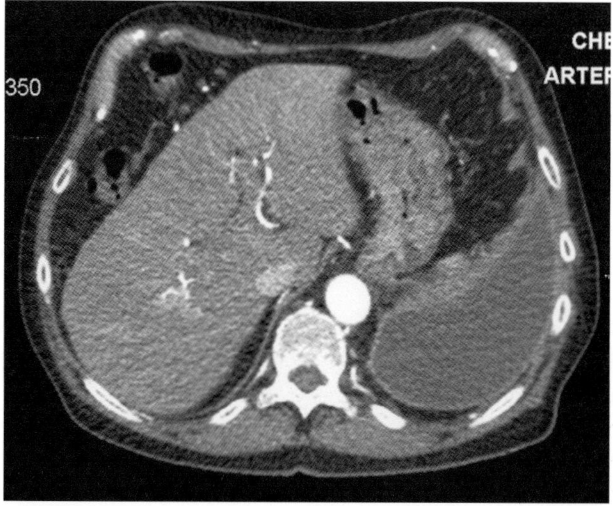

Figure 55.10 Chest computed tomography scan showing an empyema with a grossly thickened pleura.

Decortication

If the lung fails to re-expand after drainage of the empyema, the more radical operation of decortication may be required (**Figure 55.10**). The fibrous cortex or peel from the entrapped underlying lung is removed so that the lung can expand to obliterate the pleural space. This is usually performed through a posterolateral thoracotomy, though in selected cases it can be performed as a VATS procedure. It requires careful dissection to remove the parietal and visceral cortex, taking care not to damage the visceral pleura, so allowing the lung to re-expand fully.

DISORDERS OF THE AIRWAY

Haemoptysis

Diseases causing repeated haemoptysis include carcinoma, bronchiectasis, carcinoid tumours and some infections. Severe mitral stenosis is now a rare cause. Patients with repeated haemoptysis should be investigated, at the very least by chest radiography and bronchoscopy. Haemoptysis following trauma may be from a lung contusion or injury to a major airway. Treatment depends on the underlying cause.

Common associated chest symptoms include cough with or without sputum, pain, breathlessness, hoarseness and more general symptoms of systemic upset, including fatigue and loss of weight. Occasionally, chest disease may cause palpitation due to atrial fibrillation. Any of these symptoms in association with haemoptysis requires urgent investigation.

Investigation

BRONCHOSCOPY (*TABLE 55.4*)

Flexible bronchoscopy may be performed with the patient awake and the oropharynx anaesthetised with topical lignocaine (**Figure 55.11**). The bronchoscope is passed into the nose or mouth and through the vocal folds under direct vision. As the scope is flexible, its tip can be directed into the segmental bronchi with ease. Tissue and sputum samples may be obtained for diagnostic purposes. There is a greater range of movement with this instrument, but the biopsies are relatively small and suction limited.

TABLE 55.4 Uses of bronchoscopy.

Diagnostic	Confirmation of disease: carcinoma of the bronchus; inflammatory or infective processes
Investigative	Tissue biopsy
Preoperative assessment	Before lung resection Before oesophageal resection Persistent haemoptysis
Therapeutic	Removal of secretions Removal of foreign bodies Stent placement, endobronchial resection, etc.

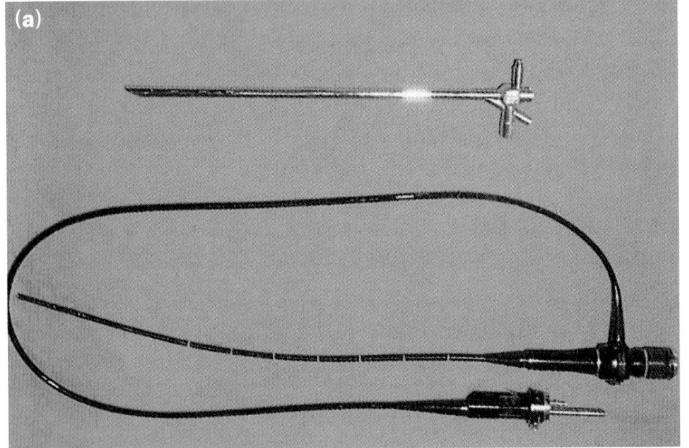

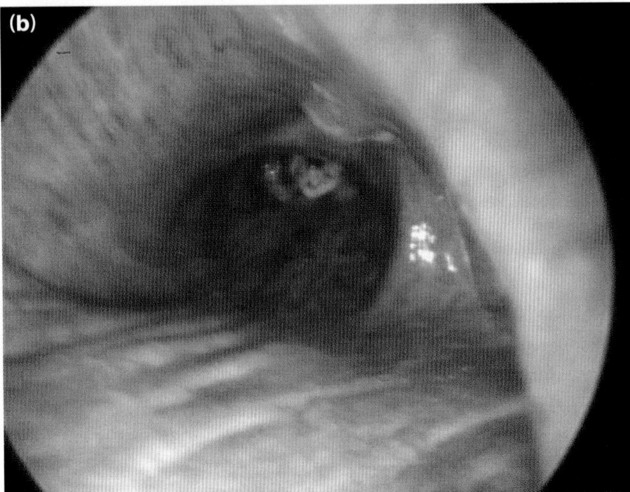

Figure 55.11 (**a**) Rigid and flexible bronchoscopes. (**b**) View past the carina into the left main bronchus with a tumour seen in the bronchial lumen.

Rigid bronchoscopy requires general anaesthesia in most instances. It is ideal for therapeutic manoeuvres, such as removal of foreign bodies, aspiration of blood and thick secretions, and intraluminal surgery (laser resection or stent placement). The surgeon and the anaesthetist share control of the airway. Continuous ECG and pulse oximetry monitoring are now essential. The technique involves the operator standing behind the patient and lifting the maxilla by the upper teeth, using the middle finger and forefinger of the left hand. The bronchoscope rests on the left thumb as it is introduced over the tongue in the midline. Care must be taken not to trap the lips or tongue between the teeth and the bronchoscope, and the fulcrum should be the left thumb and not the teeth. The bronchoscope is passed under direct vision into the oropharynx, behind the epiglottis, until the vocal folds are seen. Turning the instrument through 90° will help to negotiate the vocal folds; only then should the neck be extended.

The tracheal rings and the carina should be easily seen. Advancing the bronchoscope into the right or left main bronchus reveals the orifices of the more peripheral bronchi. Operability of an endobronchial tumour may be assessed in terms of its location (e.g. the proximity of a lesion to the carina). Complications are rare but include bleeding, pneumothorax, laryngospasm and arrhythmia.

Rigid bronchoscopy can be combined with endobronchial interventions to tackle airway tumours; these techniques include use of laser or cryotherapy, with heat or cold respectively, to excise potentially obstructing endobronchial tumours and improve airway patency and breathing.

Other techniques of biopsy of intrathoracic lesions are often necessary to confirm diagnosis, stage disease and plan treatment. The options range from percutaneous needle biopsy under radiological control, to endobronchial ultrasound and open-lung biopsy. However, high-quality, contrast-enhanced, multislice helical CT scanning has reduced the requirement for invasive assessment.

Summary box 55.4

Biopsy hazards

- Bleeding disorders
- Systemic anticoagulation
- Pulmonary hypertension

Airway obstruction

Tracheal obstruction may present acutely as a life-threatening emergency or insidiously with little in the way of symptoms until critical narrowing and stridor occur. The more common causes of airway narrowing are outlined in *Table 55.5*.

Treatment depends on the underlying cause. Tracheostomy may be required to overcome the obstruction, but there are few indications to do this as an emergency. Tracheal replacement with artificial substitutes has so far been unsuccessful, but resection of up to 6 cm of trachea is now possible. Sleeve resections of the major bronchi are also possible.

Inhaled foreign bodies

This is a fairly common occurrence in small children and is often marked by a choking incident that then apparently passes. Surprisingly large objects can be inhaled and become lodged in the wider-calibre and more vertically placed right main bronchus. There are three possible presentations:

- asymptomatic;
- wheezing (from airway narrowing) with a persistent cough and signs of obstructive emphysema;
- pyrexia with a productive cough from pulmonary suppuration.

TABLE 55.5 Causes of airway narrowing.

Intraluminal	Inhaled foreign body Neoplasm
Intramural	Congenital stenosis Fibrous stricture (post-intubation or tuberculosis)
Extramural	Neoplasm (thyroid cancer, secondary deposits) Aortic arch aneurysm

A chest radiograph is vital; even if the object is not radio-opaque there may be other changes. An experienced anaesthetist is required. Endoscopic removal may be very difficult if there is a severe inflammatory reaction to the foreign body.

NEOPLASMS OF THE LUNG

Primary lung cancer

Lung cancer is one of the most common cancers throughout the world. In the UK, there are approximately 40 000 new cases a year. From the time of diagnosis, 80% of patients are dead within 1 year and only 5% survive 5 years, making lung cancer the most common cause of cancer death.

Surgical resection has a limited role in curative treatment because at the time of presentation many cancers are locally advanced or widely disseminated and are beyond surgical cure. The proportion of lung cancers in which resection is attempted varies but in most resource-rich countries approximately 20–30% of cases are potentially surgically resectable. The thoracic surgeon working in a cancer team has a role in diagnosis, staging and palliation, in addition to resection in appropriate cases. The disease is so common that surgeons of all disciplines will encounter cases of lung cancer presenting with various manifestations.

Cigarette smoking is undoubtedly the major risk factor for developing bronchial carcinoma and accounts for 85–95% of all cases. To a lesser extent, atmospheric pollution and certain occupations (mining of radioactive ore and chromium) contribute. The risk is related to the lifetime burden of cigarette smoking, which is commonly quoted as 'pack-years' (a 'pack' being 20 cigarettes): the number of packs smoked per day multiplied by the number of years of exposure. In the UK, the mortality rate from lung cancer for individuals smoking more than 40 cigarettes per day is over 210 deaths per 100 000 population per year. This compares with a mortality rate of less than 4 deaths per 100 000 population per year in non-smokers.

Pathological types

For practical purposes, lung cancers are divided into small cell lung cancer and non-small cell lung cancer (NSCLC), which are seen in a ratio of about 1:4.

- The pattern of disease, the prognosis and the results of treatment for small cell (also known as oat cell) carcinoma differ from all other types sufficiently for these to be managed differently from the outset on the basis of the histological classification.
- Subdivisions of NSCLC according to histological characteristics are much less important, but pathological staging is critical to treatment and outcome.

Histological classification of lung cancer

Small cell lung cancers were known as oat cell cancers because of the packed nature of small dense cells. They are a type of neuroendocrine tumour (NET) and represent about 20% of all lung cancers. They tend to metastasise early to lymph nodes and by blood-borne spread. The median survival is measured in months. The tumours are very responsive to chemotherapy such that median survival may be doubled (although it is still short) but they are rarely, if ever, cured. Surgery is rarely offered unless in very limited stage disease.

Adenocarcinoma is now the most common of the NSCLC types, having overtaken squamous cancer. The increasing incidence is partly due to an increasing incidence in women and may be the result, in part, of a move towards lower-tar cigarettes that are inhaled more deeply to get the same effect.

Squamous carcinoma typically appears as a cavitating tumour.

Large cell undifferentiated is a discrete histological type of NSCLC and is included within NETs.

Bronchioalveolar carcinoma (BAC), also known as **adenocarcinoma-*in-situ***, has a distinct pattern of growth following the pre-existing pulmonary architecture and is thus much less dense; it appears as a patchy diffuse shadow ('ground glass') on radiographs rather than a solid mass and has a histological appearance to match. Recently, the pathological nomencalature for BAC, a subtype of adenocarcinoma, has changed and they are now known as 'lepidic' neoplastic lesions, which have further been classified into precursor lesions, minimal invasive lepidic adenocarcinomas and frankly malignant lepidic adenocarcinomas. After resection, the cancer can appear in another lobe or on the other side, and these are often regarded as multifocal primary tumours rather than metastatic disease. Further resection may be appropriate depending on patient fitness and extent of disease.

Neuroendocrine tumours of the lung are a group of lung cancers that incude small cell cancer and large cell undifferentiated lung cancer, but also include other less aggressive tumour types including typical carcinoid and atypical carcinoid tumours. These occur in the major (central) bronchi and 20% are found peripherally. They are characteristically slow growing and highly vascular. Most behave in a benign way; however, approximately 15% metastasise. The patient often presents with a history of recurrent pneumonia or haemoptysis, but carcinoid syndrome is rare unless there are extensive pulmonary or hepatic metastases. Surgical excision is preferred because the prognosis following complete resection is excellent (>90% 10-year survival). Segmental or wedge resection may be sufficient for a small peripheral tumour, while lobectomy or pneumonectomy may be necessary for central tumours. Where possible, a lung-sparing bronchoplastic or sleeve resection should be considered. This allows resection of proximal endobronchial lesions in an effort to preserve more distal, uninvolved lung parenchyma.

Accurate diagnosis and staging of the tumour are vital if surgery is to be considered.

Clinical features

Clinical features of lung carcinoma depend on:

- the site of the lesion;
- the invasion of neighbouring structures;
- the extent of metastases.

Common symptoms include a persistent cough, weight loss, dyspnoea and non-specific chest pain.

- Haemoptysis occurs in fewer than 50% of patients presenting for the first time.
- Cough, or a changed cough, is a common presentation but non-specific in this population.
- Severe localised pain suggests chest wall invasion with the infiltration of an intercostal nerve. Invasion of the apical area may involve the brachial plexus, leading to Pancoast's syndrome.
- Dyspnoea may come from loss of functioning lung tissue, lymphatic invasion or the development of a large pleural effusion.
- Pleural fluid is an ominous feature and the presence of blood in a pleural effusion suggests that the pleura has been directly invaded.
- Clubbing (**Figure 55.12**) and hypertrophic pulmonary osteoarthropathy accompany some lung cancers and may resolve with excision of the primary lesion.
- Invasion of the mediastinum may result in hoarseness (because of recurrent laryngeal nerve involvement), dysphagia (because of the involvement of, or extrinsic pressure on, the oesophagus) and superior vena caval obstruction.
- Small cell carcinoma is associated with the development of myopathies including the Eaton–Lambert syndrome, which is similar to myasthenia gravis.

Summary box 55.5

Symptoms of lung cancer

- Haemoptysis: <50% of patients
- Cough, new or changed pattern
- Pain
- Dyspnoea
- Clubbing
- Hoarseness
- Myopathies

Treatment of lung cancer

Careful investigation is required to determine which tumours are operable and will benefit from a major thoracic resection. The internationally agreed tumour–node–metastasis (TNM) staging system gives prognostic information on the natural history of the disease. Tumours graded up to T3, N1, M0 can be encompassed within an anatomical surgical resection and have a much improved prognosis when treated surgically so the tumour must be staged accurately before resection (*Table 55.6*). A number of non-tumour related factors, including the general fitness of the patient and the results of lung function tests, help to determine the appropriate treatment. In patients with incurable disease, treatment is palliative to maximise quality of life.

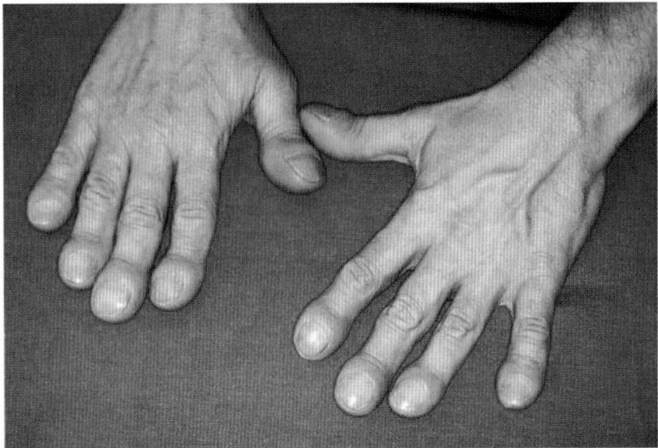

Figure 55.12 Example of finger clubbing in a patient with bronchogenic carcinoma.

Survival

Carcinoma of the bronchus generally has a low survival rate after diagnosis (*Table 55.7*). Important factors in determining prognosis are the histological type of the tumour, the spread (stage) and the general condition of the patient. Early detection and surgical resection offer the best hope for cure.

Diagnosis and staging

Increasing emphasis in recent years has been the early detection of lung cancer, with guidance on symptoms and signs of potential lung cancer that require urgent chest x-ray and referral to a lung cancer team (*Table 55.8*).

Non-invasive investigations

CHEST RADIOGRAPHY

A chest radiograph will detect most lung cancers but some, particularly early curable tumours, are hidden by other structures. Secondary effects such as pleural effusion, distal collapse and raised hemidiaphragm may be evident (**Figure 55.13**).

COMPUTED TOMOGRAPHY

Computed tomography (CT) is the first investigation in suspected lung cancer. The surgeon needs to know whether the primary is resectable (T stage) and which, if any, lymph nodes are involved (N stage). Lymph nodes more than 2 cm in diameter are likely to be involved in the disease (70%) (**Figure 55.14**) and those less than 10 mm in the shorter axis are unlikely to be involved. If the presence of cancer in the nodes is critical to management, further evidence from positron emission tomography with radiolabelled fluorodeoxyglucose (FDG-PET) or biopsy (see below) is essential. Remote metastases to the liver, adrenal glands or elsewhere may be detected.

POSITRON EMISSION TOMOGRAPHY

The patient is given radiolabelled FDG, which is taken up by all metabolising cells but more avidly by cancer cells.

Henry Khunrath Pancoast, 1875–1939, Professor of Radiology, The University of Pennsylvania, Philadelphia, PA, USA, described this condition in 1932.
Lee M. Eaton, 1905–1958, neurologist who was a professor at The Mayo Clinic, Rochester, MN, USA.
Edward H. Lambert, b.1915, Professor of Physiology, The University of Minnesota, MN, USA. Eaton and Lambert described this condition in a joint paper in 1956.

TABLE 55.6 The international tumour–node–metastasis (TNM) staging system.

T: Primary tumour	
Tx	Primary tumour cannot be assessed or tumour proven by presence of malignant cells in sputum or bronchial washings but not visualised by imaging or bronchoscopy
T0	No evidence of primary tumour
Tis	Carcinoma *in situ*
T1	Tumour ≤3 cm in greatest dimension surrounded by lung or visceral pleura without bronchoscopic evidence of invasion more proximal than the lobar bronchus (i.e. not in the main bronchus)[a]
T1a(mi)	Minimally invasive adenocarcinoma[b]
T1a	Tumour 1 cm in greatest dimension[a]
T1b	Tumour >1 cm but ≤2 cm in greatest dimension[a]
T1c	Tumour >2 cm but ≤3 cm in greatest dimension[a]
T2	Tumour >3 cm but ≤5 cm or tumour with any of the following features:[c] – involves main bronchus regardless of distance from the carina but without involvement of the carina – invades visceral pleura – associated with atelectasis or obstructive pneumonitis that extends to the hilar region, involving part or all of the lung
T2a	Tumour >3 cm but ≤4 cm in greatest dimension
T2b	Tumour >4 cm but ≤5 cm in greatest dimension
T3	Tumour >5 cm but ≤7 cm in greatest dimension or associated with separate tumour nodule(s) in the same lobe as the primary tumour or directly invades any of the following structures: chest wall (including the parietal pleura and superior sulcus tumours), phrenic nerve, parietal pericardium
T4	Tumour >7 cm in greatest dimension or associated with separate tumour nodule(s) in a different ipsilateral lobe than that of the primary tumour or invades any of the following structures: diaphragm, mediastinum, heart, great vessels, trachea, recurrent laryngeal nerve, oesophagus, vertebral body, and carina
N: Regional lymph nodes involvement	
Nx	Regional lymph nodes cannot be assessed
N0	No regional lymph node metastasis
N1	Metastasis in ipsilateral peribronchial and/or ipsilateral hilar lymph nodes and intrapulmonary nodes, including involvement by direct extension
N2	Metastasis in ipsilateral mediastinal and/or subcarinal lymph node(s)
N3	Metastasis in contralateral mediastinal, contralateral hilar, ipsilateral or contralateral scalene, or supraclavicular lymph node(s)
M: Distant metastasis	
M0	No distant metastasis
M1	Distant metastasis present
M1a	Separate tumour nodule(s) in a contralateral lobe; tumour with pleural or pericardial nodule(s) or malignant pleural or pericardial effusion[d]
M1b	Single extrathoracic metastasise
M1c	Multiple extrathoracic metastases in one or more organs

[a]The uncommon superficial spreading tumour of any size with its invasive component limited to the bronchial wall, which may proximal to the main bronchus, is also classified as T1a.
[b]Solitary adenocarcinoma, ≤3 cm with a predominately lepidic pattern and ≤5 mm invasion in any one focus.
[c]T2 tumours with these features are classified as T2a is ≤4 cm in greatest dimension or if size cannot be determined, and T2b if >4 cm but ≤5 cm in greatest dimension.
[d]Most pleural (pericardial) effusions with lung cancer are due to tumour. In a few patients, however, multiple microscopic examinations of pleural (pericardial) fluid are negative for tumour and the fluid is non-bloody and not an exudate. When these elements and clinical judgement dictate that the effusion is not related to the tumour, the effusion should be excluded as a staging descriptor.
[e]This includes involvement of a single distant (non-regional) lymph node.

The FDG enters the Kreb's cycle but cannot complete it and accumulates in proportion to the glucose avidity of the cells. High accumulation is associated with lung cancers and secondaries. Infection or other inflammation, and lymphadenopathy secondary to it, are also FDG avid (**Figure 55.15**).

SPUTUM CYTOLOGY

Sputum cytology may reveal malignant cells but the false-negative rate is high.

Invasive investigations

Once lung cancer is suspected, diagnosis and further staging are sought. The choice of investigation depends on the

Sir Hans Adolf Krebs, 1900–1981, Professor of Biochemistry, The University of Oxford, Oxford, UK.

TABLE 55.7 Survival table following operation for carcinoma of the bronchus.

	(%)
Five-year survival according to presurgical staging	
Stage I	56–67
Stage II	39–55
Stage IIIa	23
Stage IIIb	<10
Five-year survival according to cell type	
Squamous cell carcinoma	35–50
Adenocarcinoma	25–45
Adenosquamous carcinoma	20–35
Undifferentiated carcinoma	15–25
Small cell carcinoma	0–5

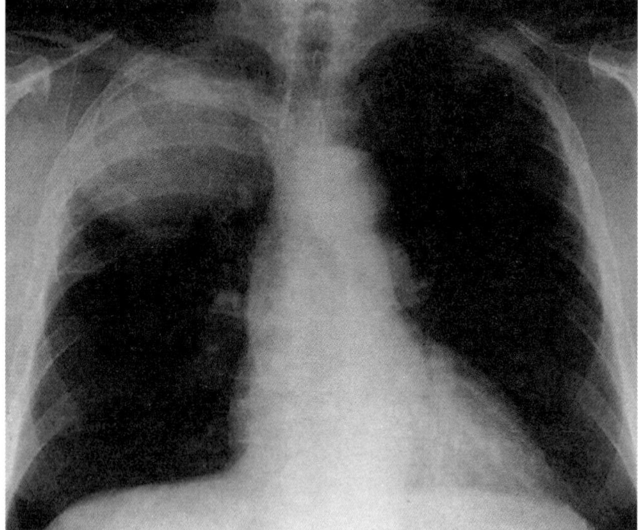

Figure 55.13 Chest x-ray of carcinoma of the lung. This patient has a large mass in the right upper lobe, causing Horner's syndrome.

position of the primary tumour in the lung (peripheral or central) and the clinical stage of the cancer (presence of enlarged lymph nodes or metastasis).

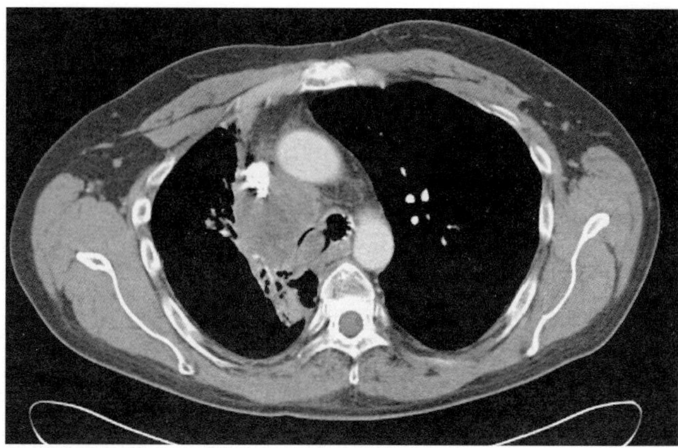

Figure 55.14 Paratracheal lymphadenopathy shown on a computed tomography scan.

BRONCHOSCOPY

Flexible bronchoscopy is usually performed under sedation, particularly in patients with more centrally placed lung cancers. It allows assessment of the segmental airway, cytological testing through brushing and washing of the concerned segmental bronchi and transbronchial needle aspiration (TBNA).

ENDOBRONCHIAL ULTRASOUND (EBUS)

EBUS allows bronchoscopic assessment of suspicious mediastinal lymph nodes with an ultrasound probe incorporated into the tip of the bronchoscope to aid TBNA (**Figure 55.16**). Endoscopic ultrasound (EUS) is a similar technique that, by passing the probe down the oesophagus, allows fine needle aspiration (FNA) of less approachable mediastinal lymph nodes.

COMPUTED TOMOGRAPHY-GUIDED BIOPSY

Percutaneous CT-guided FNA may give a good yield of cells for cytological examination. Alternatively, a core of tissue can be obtained for formal histology. These techniques are best for larger and more peripheral lesions. Pneumothorax is

TABLE 55.8 Recent National Institute for Health and Care Excellence (NICE) guidance on referral in patients with suspected lung cancer.

Symptoms and signs indicating urgent chest x-ray	Offer urgent chest x-ray to patients presenting with haemoptysis, or any of the following if unexplained or present for more than 3 weeks:	Cough Chest/shoulder pain Dyspnoea Finger clubbing Signs suggesting metastases (for example, in brain, bone, liver or skin) Weight loss Chest signs Hoarseness Cervical/supraclavicular lymphadenopathy
Symptoms and signs indicating urgent referral	Offer urgent referral to lung cancer MDT (usually the chest physician) while waiting for chest x-ray results if any of the following are present:	Persistent haemoptysis in a smoker or ex-smoker older than 40 years Signs of superior vena cava obstruction (swelling of the face and/or neck with fixed elevation of jugular venous pressure) Stridor
	Offer urgent referral to lung cancer MDT (usually the chest physician) if:	A chest x-ray or CT scan suggests lung cancer (including pleural effusion and slowly resolving consolidation) or Chest x-ray is normal, but there is a high suspicion of lung cancer

CT, computed tomography; MDT, multidisciplinary team.

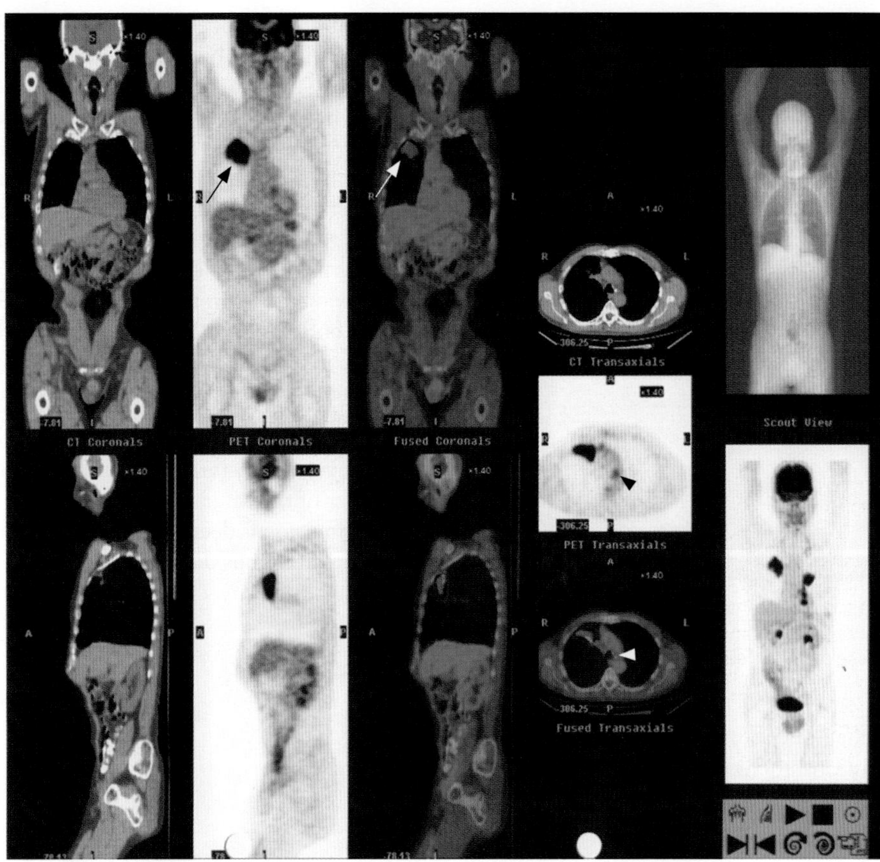

Figure 55.15 Multiple FDG-avid mediastinal lymph nodes (arrowheads) shown on a positron emission tomography/computed tomography scan (main tumour, arrows) (courtesy of Dr Sally Barrington).

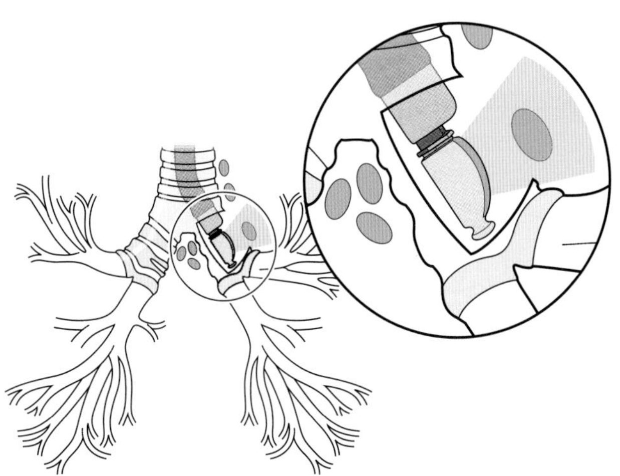

Figure 55.16 Endobronchial ultrasound (EBUS) allows accurate detection of enlarged mediastinal lymph nodes for diagnosis and staging of lung cancer.

common (30%) but rarely requires intercostal tube drainage. The contraindications include poor respiratory reserve, when even a small pneumothorax would be hazardous.

Surgical diagnosis and staging

Mediastinoscopy, mediastinotomy, VATS or thoracotomy lymph node/lung biopsy are aimed at establishing a tissue diagnosis and assessing the degree of spread (staging), which determines resectability. Histological proof of the status of mediastinal nodes may be important to avoid unnecessary thoracotomy for incurable cancers and, conversely, to avoid denying surgery to patients whose lymph nodes are enlarged but benign.

MEDIASTINOSCOPY

This procedure is performed under general anaesthesia with the patient supine and his or her neck extended (**Figure 55.17**). A transverse incision is made 2 cm above the sternal notch and deepened until the strap muscles are reached. These are retracted laterally and the thyroid isthmus is retracted superiorly to reveal the pretracheal fascia. Careful blunt dissection in this plane allows access to the paratracheal and subcarinal nodes. A mediastinoscope is introduced for direct visualisation and biopsy. Great caution should be used in the presence of superior vena caval obstruction. Complications include pneumothorax and haemorrhage.

MEDIASTINOTOMY

An incision is made through the second intercostal space to gain access to some of the mediastinal lymph nodes on the affected side. On the left, this includes lymph nodes in the para-aortic or subaortic fossa. Damage to the internal mammary artery and the phrenic nerve must be avoided. Mediastinal extension of tumour can also be assessed, for example left upper lobe tumours which invade the mediastinum around the aortic arch.

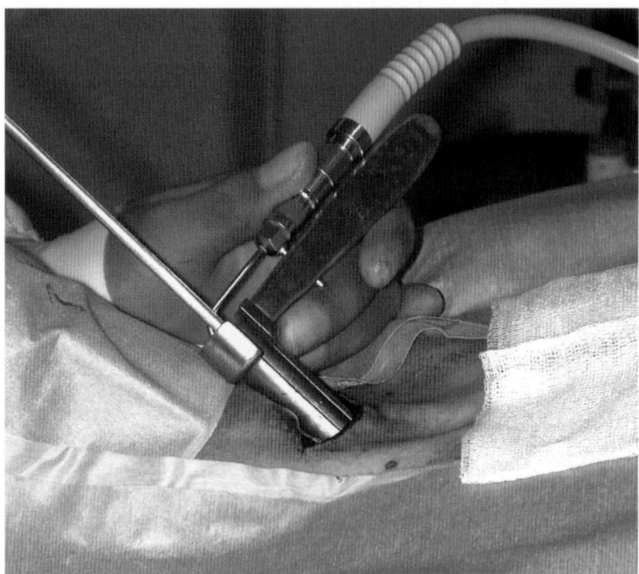

Figure 55.17 Mediastinoscopy. The mediastinoscope slides down immediately in front of the trachea, behind the aortic arch, and behind and between the great vessels of the head and neck.

These techniques may also be used in the diagnosis of other mediastinal conditions, including:

- lymphoma;
- anterior mediastinal tumours;
- thymoma;
- sarcoid, tuberculosis or any other cause of lymphadenopathy.

VATS MEDIASTINAL LYMPH NODE AND LUNG BIOPSY

For inaccessible mediastinal lymph nodes, or when diagnosis of the lung tumour has not been possible through radiological or bronchoscopic techniques, VATS performed through two or three ports allows diagnosis of the tumour, staging of the mediastinum and gives the opportunity to assess the likely operability of the lung cancer.

Surgical approach to lung cancer resection

Thoracotomy

Although the most frequent indication for thoracotomy is lung cancer, all surgeons dealing with trauma should be able to perform a thoracotomy if required. The standard route into the thoracic cavity is through a posterolateral thoracotomy. The incision is used for access to the:

- lung and major bronchi;
- pleura;
- thoracic aorta;
- oesophagus;
- posterior mediastinum.

A double-lumen endotracheal tube is used to allow ventilation of one lung while the other is collapsed, to facilitate surgery and to protect the non-operated lung and retain control of ventilation (**Figure 55.18**).

The patient is turned to the lateral position with the affected side up (**Figure 55.19**). The lower leg is flexed at the hip and the knee, with a pillow between the legs. Table supports are used to maintain the position and additional strapping is used at the hips for stability. The patient's hips are placed below the break point of the operating table to allow opening of the intercostal spaces as the table is angulated. The upper arm may be supported by a bracket in a position of 90° flexion. The lower arm is flexed and positioned near the head. It is important for both the surgeon and the anaesthetist to be completely satisfied with the position of the patient and the tube and lines at this stage.

- The incision passes 1–2 cm below the tip of the scapula, and extends posteriorly and superiorly between the medial border of the scapula and the spine.
- The incision is deepened through the subcutaneous tissues to the latissimus dorsi. This muscle is divided with coagulating diathermy, taking care over haemostasis.

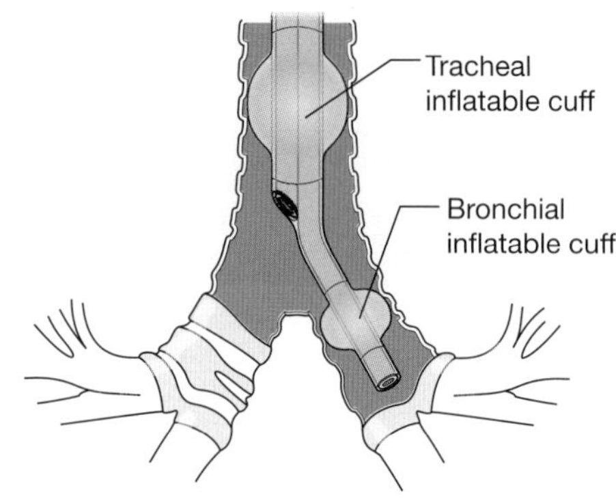

Figure 55.18 The double-lumen tube permits separate ventilation of the right and left lungs.

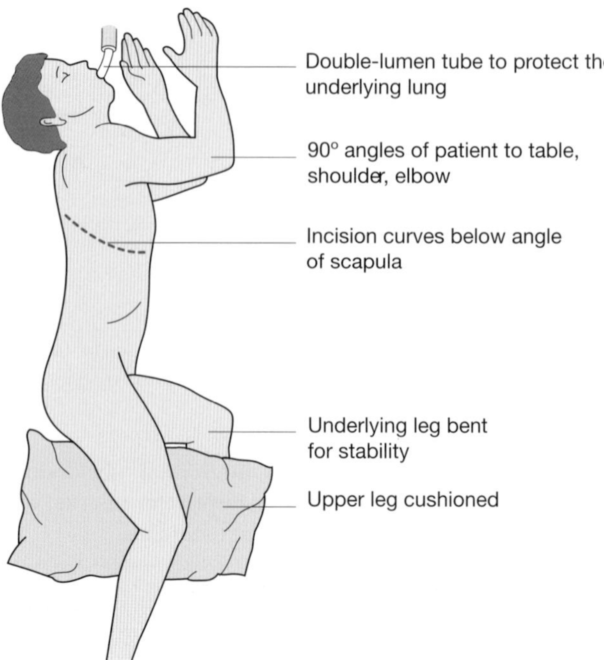

Figure 55.19 Correct positioning for thoracotomy.

- A plane of dissection is developed manually, deep to the scapula and serratus anterior. The ribs can be counted down from the highest palpable rib (which is usually the second) and the sixth rib periosteum is scored with the diathermy near its upper border. A periosteal elevator is used to lift the periosteum off the superior border of the rib or, alternatively, the intercostal muscle is cut with diathermy just above the rib (**Figure 55.20**).
- This reveals the pleura, which may be entered by blunt dissection. A rib spreader is inserted between the ribs and opened gently to prevent fracture.
- Exposure may be facilitated by dividing the rib at the costal angle or by dividing the costotransverse ligament. Resection of a rib is not usually required.
- The anaesthetist is now able to deflate the affected lung to allow a better view of the intrathoracic structures.

In an emergency thoracotomy for penetrating wounds of the heart, a more anterior approach is used and no specialised supporting equipment is required (**Figure 55.21**). The incision is taken down to the fourth or fifth rib with a scalpel, and the pleural cavity is opened using scissors. This gives rapid access to the left pleural cavity in cases of massive left hamothorax and the pericardium if cardiac tamponade is supected. A left anterior thoracotomy can be quickly converted to a clamshell or bilateral thoracotomy if necessay.

Following the operation, 24–28 Fr chest drain/s are placed, typically through the seventh or eighth intercostal space, anterior to the mid-axillary line, so that the patient does not lie on them. Even if the site to be drained is posterior, as in empyema, the drains are tunnelled to emerge more anteriorly for easier management. The thoracotomy is closed using paracostal sutures placed around the rib above and below to reapproximate the ribs or, alternatively, intercostal muscles are sutured to the intercostal muscle below the stripped rib with a continuous absorbable suture. The fascia and muscles are closed in layers using an absorbable suture. Skin closure is a matter of personal preference.

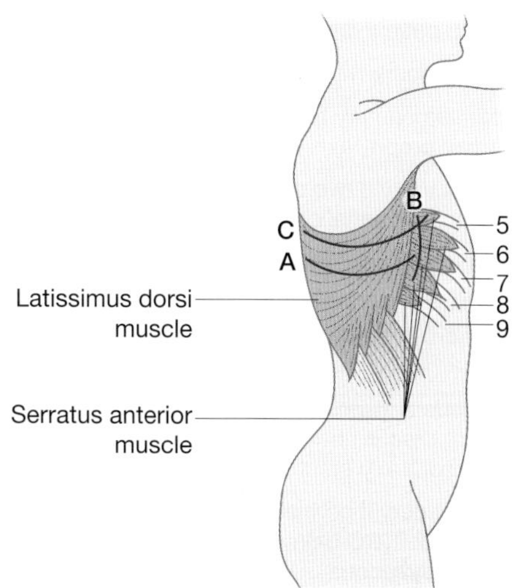

Figure 55.20 Incision and layers encountered during anterolateral thoracotomy. A, The latissimus dorsi is divided in line with the skin incision. B, If the serratus anterior is divided, it should be close to its attachment to ribs 6, 7 and 8. It can be left intact and mobilised along its inferior border. C, The intercostal muscles are stripped off the upper border of the rib.

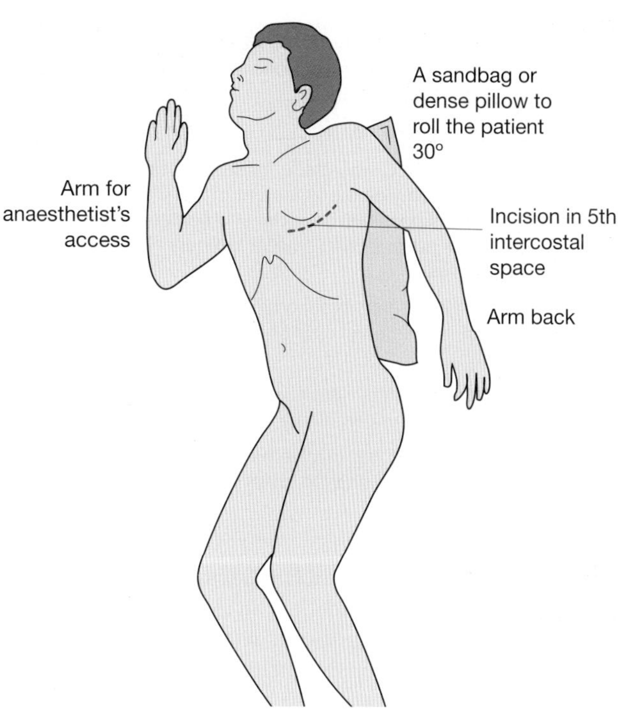

Figure 55.21 Emergency left anterior thoracotomy for access to the heart. This requires no special supports or devices.

Analgesia is an important aspect of postoperative care, and the process may be started prior to thoracotomy with an epidural catheter placed by the anaesthetist, or intraoperatively by infiltrating the intercostal nerves in the region of the incision with a long-acting local anaesthetic via a surgically sited paraveretebral catheter. Various strategies have been developed to deliver analgesics postoperatively to facilitate a normal breathing pattern.

Video assisted thoracoscopic surgery (VATS)

Various approaches utilising thoracoscopic techniques can be used to gain access to the chest cavity and facilitate lung resection. A combination of a smaller thoracotomy incision and VATS has been described, but increasingly lung resections can be performed through one to three port incisons and the dissection of hilar structures completed entirely through VATS. The technique avoids rib-spreading and appears to reduce postoperative pain and length of stay, and aids a speedier recovery.

Surgical management of lung cancer

The principle of surgery is to remove all cancer (the primary and the regional lymph nodes) but to conserve as much lung as possible. The selection of patients in terms of the stage of the lung cancer and fitness to undergo such surgery is paramount. Surgery with curative intent is offered to patients with early stage lung cancer (T1–3, N0–1) (*Table 55.9*). Assesment of a patient's fitness to undergo lung cancer resection involves considering premorbid conditions, which can be aided using

TABLE 55.9 National Institute for Health and Care Excellence (NICE) recommendations for surgery for non-small cell lung cancer (NSCLC).

Surgery with curative intent for NSCLC
Offer patients with NSCLC who are fit for surgery, open or thoracoscopic lobectomy as the treatment of first choice. If complete resection is possible, consider segmentectomy or wedge resection for patients with smaller tumours (T1a–b, N0, M0) and borderline fitness
Offer more extensive surgery (bronchoangioplastic surgery, bilobectomy, pneumonectomy) only when needed to obtain clear margins
Perform hilar and mediastinal lymph node sampling or *en bloc* resection for all patients undergoing surgery with curative intent
For T3 NSCLC with chest wall involvement, aim for complete resection by extrapleural or *en bloc* chest wall resection

risk scores such as Thorascore, Cardiovascular function and Lung function (see BTS guidelines in Assessment of Fitness for major thoracic surgery, above, and NICE guidelines in *Table 55.10*). Lung function, in particular, will aid the surgeon in selecting the type of procedure offered and the likelihood of breathlessness or dyspnoea following lung resection.

Choice of lung resection

SEGMENTECTOMY AND WEDGE RESECTION

Segmentectomy and wedge resections are performed in patients with small tumours, and with borderline fitness, through thoracotomy or VATS. Each lobe of the lung has segments, which allows anatomical dissection and ligation of the segmental pulmonary artery, vein and bronchus (segmentectomy) (see Figure 55.2), or non-anatomical excision can be performed (wedge resection) combined with removal of regional lymph nodes.

LOBECTOMY

Lobectomy remains the treatment of choice for patients with early-stage lung cancer. The surgery can be performed via thoracotomy or VATS. Following dissection of the fissure and hilar structures, the branches of the pulmonary artery and veins to the lobe are isolated and ligated. The bronchus is usually stapled but can be sewn.

At completion of the operation, the remaining lung is reinflated. Some air leak is common and usually settles within a few days. One or two intercostal drains are inserted. The patient does not routinely need intensive care and postoperative ventilation is best avoided. The 30-day mortality rate is 2–3%, with morbidity such as chest infection or cardiac arrhythmia at around 10%. The average length of stay is around 5–7 days.

PNEUMONECTOMY

Pneumonectomy is removal of a whole lung and has a higher mortality rate (5–8%). The surgeon must be satisfied that the patient is fit to tolerate this procedure from the preoperative work-up. This procedure is reserved for either centrally placed tumours involving the main bronchus or those that straddle the fissure. At thoracotomy, inspection of the lung and direct palpation of the mass will determine resectability and lymph node spread. Fixation of the tumour to the aorta, heart or oesophagus implies irresectability. Involvement of the mediastinal lymph node chain is associated with a poor prognosis. With modern preoperative imaging, resection is abandoned in only about 3% of cases.

Pneumonectomy is anatomically more straightforward than lobectomy and involves dissecting and ligating the main

TABLE 55.10 National Institute for Health and Care Excellence (NICE) recommendations for assessing fitness for treatment with curative intent (including surgery).

Perioperative mortality	Consider global risk score, such as Thoracoscore	Ensure patient is aware of risk before consenting
Cardiovascular function	Assess risk factors and cardiac functional capacity	Avoid surgery within 30 days of MI
		Optimise primary cardiac treatment and begin secondary cardiac prophylaxis as soon as possible
		Offer surgery if two or fewer risk factors and good cardiac functional capacity
		Seek cardiology review if active cardiac condition, three or more risk factors or poor cardiac functional capacity
		Consider revascularisation before surgery in stable angina
		Continue anti-ischaemic treatment in perioperative period. Discuss perioperative platelet treatment if patient has a coronary stent
Lung function	Perform spirometry, measure T_LCO if disproportionate breathlessness or other lung pathology, perform segment count and assess exercise tolerance	Offer surgery if normal FEV_1 and good exercise tolerance or FEV_1 or T_LCO below 30% and patient accepts the risks of dyspnoea
	Consider shuttle walk testing (cut-off 400 m) and cardiopulmonary exercise testing (cut-off 15 mL/kg/minute) if moderate to high risk of postoperative dyspnoea	Offer radiotherapy with curative intent if lung function poor but patient is otherwise suitable for radiotherapy with curative intent and volume of irradiated lung is small

From NICE clinical guideline 21, available from: www.nice.org.uk/nicemedia/live/13465/54208/54208.pdf. FEV_1, forced expratory volume in 1 s; MI, myocardial infarction; T_LCO, transfer factor for carbon monoxide.

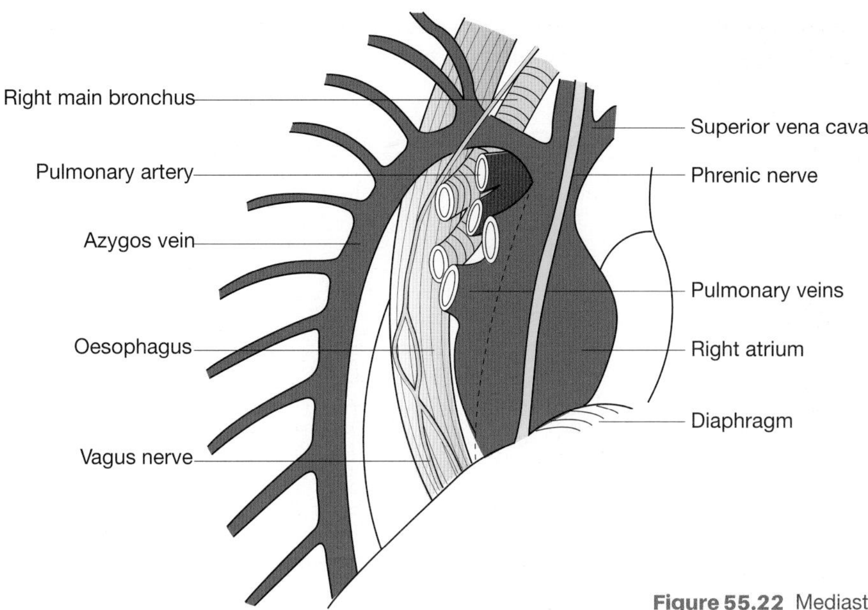

Figure 55.22 Mediastinal structures after removal of the right lung.

pulmonary artery, the superior and inferior pulmonary veins and the main bronchus, which is divided so that no blind stump remains (**Figure 55.22**). The technique of stump closure is important if a bronchopleural fistula is to be avoided. The tissues are carefully handled and the stump is usually stapled and sometimes covered using pleura, pericardium or a vascular pedicle such as an intercostal muscle. Drainage of the space is a matter of debate. Most use an underwater-seal drain and either leave it unclamped or unclamp it for 1 minute every hour until the drainage ceases; others prefer not to drain. The critical point is that no suction should be applied as there is now a sealed space with the mobile mediastinum on one side of it. The air in the pneumonectomy space is gradually absorbed and the fluid level within the space rises (**Figure 55.23**).

BRONCHOPLASTIC LUNG RESECTIONS

Increasingly, owing to the associated complications and higher mortality of a pneumonectomy, preservation of lung tissue is being considered, but without compromise of the surgical resection margins. Sleeve lung resections involve removing a central tumour that is invading a major bronchus, such as the left or right main bronchus, together with the lobe of the lung involved, with re-anastomosis of the cut major bonchus to the remaining lobar bronchus. This type of operation is particularly useful in dealing with tumours such as carcinoids that, despite low-grade malignant potential, are often found in a major bronchus.

Complications of lung resection

- **Bleeding**. Bleeding should be avoidable by the use of a careful surgical technique, but may be severe in the presence of dense adhesions.
- **Respiratory infection**. Many of these patients are ex-smokers and therefore basal collapse and hypoxaemia are common postoperatively.
- **Persistent air leak**. Chest drains are placed at the time of surgery to deal with the air leak. Rarely, the air leak persists and the remaining lung does not expand. Re-thoracotomy may then be necessary to seal the leak.
- **Bronchopleural fistula**. This is a serious complication. Following pneumonectomy the space left behind is initially filled with air. This is slowly reabsorbed and the space fills with tissue fluid. The fluid level rises until the air is finally reabsorbed. Dehiscence of the bronchial stump leads to the development of a bronchopleural fistula and the fluid in the space (which is almost inevitably infected) is expectorated in large quantities. This complication has a high morbidity and mortality rate. The patient is nursed sitting up and turned so that the affected space is dependent, to prevent infected fluid from entering the remaining lung while arrangements are made to site a pleural drain. This should be connected to an underwater seal but not suction. Bronchopleural fistulas are unlikely to resolve spontaneously and management is highly specialised.

POSTOPERATIVE CARE

Patients have limited respiratory reserve following lung resection, so infection and fluid overload are to be avoided. Once air leaks have settled, the drains are removed. Mobilisation, breathing exercises and regular physiotherapy are begun as soon as the patient's condition permits.

POSTOPERATIVE PAIN

It is important to deal with post-thoracotomy pain effectively so that a normal breathing pattern and gas exchange are achieved in the early postoperative period. Three strategies are routinely used in combination:

- patient-controlled analgesia (PCA) with intravenous boluses of opiates;
- paravertebral/extrapleural or epidural catheter-delivered local anaesthetic;
- background oral analgesia with paracetamol.

Long-term post-thoracotomy pain can be reduced by careful attention to detail during the operation. Sources of

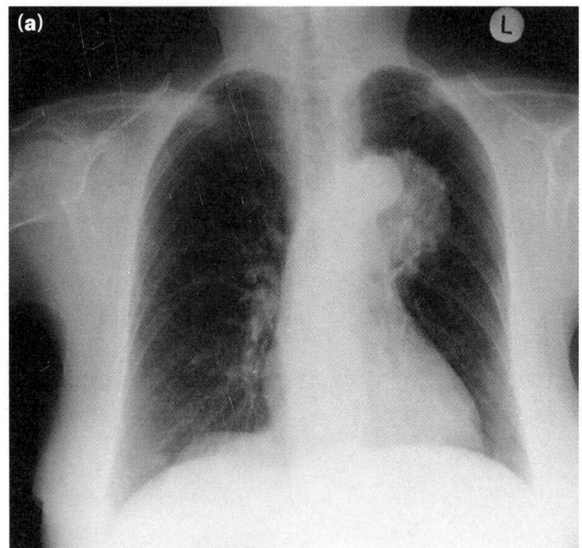

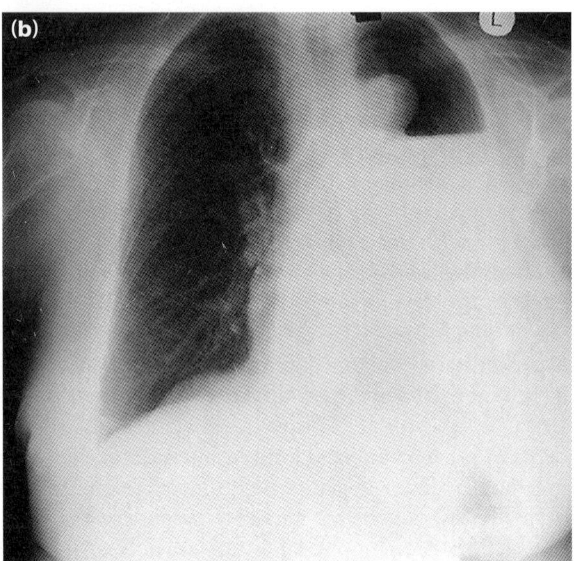

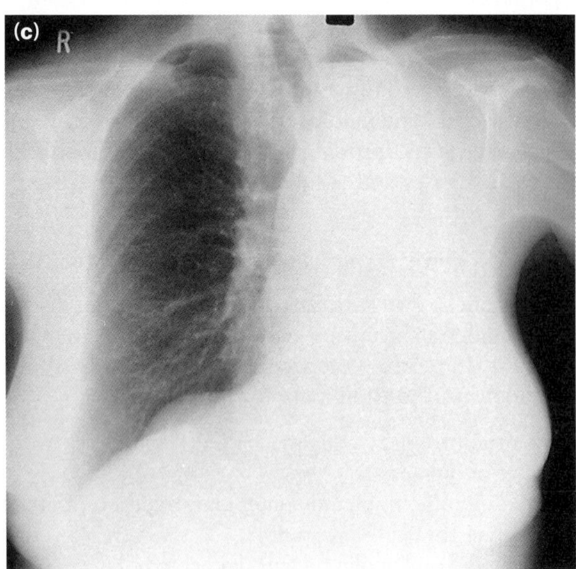

Figure 55.23 Chest radiographs (**a**) pre- and (**b**) post-pneumonectomy, with rising fluid level (**c**) in the left haemothorax.

avoidable chronic pain include rib fracture and the entrapment of intercostal nerves during wound closure.

LUNG METASTASES

For all malignancies, the lung is the most common site of metastases, that often develop through haemotogenous spread. The presence of metastases is regarded as a sign of advanced disease and few curative treatment options exist, however surgical resection of lung metastases may result in a significant survival advantage, particularly with metastases from solid tumours such as colorectal cancer. This has not yet been proven in the context of a randomised controlled trial. The selection criteria often used when considering lung metastasectomy include control of primary tumour; no evidence of metastases outside the lung; possibility of complete resection utilising lung sparing techniques; and acceptable operative risks with adequate pulmonary function.

Various approaches can be considered, though VATS is increasingly favoured over thoracotomy owing to reduced postoperative pain and length of stay, and therefore speedier recovery. The disadvantage of VATS is the inability to palpate and evaluate the lung in its entirety to locate other nodules deeper within the lung parenchyma, particularly those not identified on prior CT imaging. Median sternotomy can also be considered if there are bilateral lung metastases, located anteriorly or in the upper lobes, as this may be less painful than considering bilateral thoracotomies. The main principle when resecting lung metastases is to utilise lung-sparing techniques as much as possible, e.g. wedge resections rather than lobectomy, because it is likely that later reoperations to resect new metastases may be necessary.

Long-term outcome depends on the primary tumour type, with germ-cell tumours having the best outcome. Patients with epithelial tumours (carcinomas) generally have a 30–40% 5-year survival, as reported in several retrospective series.

BENIGN LUNG TUMOURS

Benign tumours of the lung are uncommon and account for fewer than 15% of solitary lesions seen on chest radiographs. A peripheral tumour usually causes no symptoms until it is large; a central tumour may present with haemoptysis and signs of bronchial obstruction while still small. A tumour is likely to be benign if it has not increased in size on chest radiographs for more than 2 years or it has some degree of calcification; however, a tissue diagnosis is usually pursued.

Most benign nodules are **granulomas** (tuberculosis or histoplasmosis). The most common benign tumour is a **hamartoma**, a developmental abnormality containing mesothelial and endothelial elements. Diagnosis (and definitive treatment) is achieved by excision of the lesion. Any of the mesodermal elements of the lung may form a mesodermal tumour (chondroma, lipoma, leiomyoma). Deposits of amyloid may have a similar radiographic appearance to a nodule (pseudotumour).

THE MEDIASTINUM

The mediastinum refers to the central area in the chest between the thoracic inlet and the diaphragm, between the right and left pleural surfaces, and which extends from the inner aspect of the sternum to the vertebral column. It contains the heart, great vessels, trachea and oesophagus, and is arbitrarily subdivided into compartments (superior, inferior, anterior, middle and posterior). Many of the regional lymph node chains draining the chest and its organs are also found in the mediastinum. Various surgical procedures to approach structures, and particularly lymph nodes, in the mediastinum are performed, usually as diagnostic procedures. The surgical approach when mediastinal tumours require resection depends on the antomical location of the tumour **(Figure 55.24)** and includes median sternotomy for anterior mediastinal pathology, thoracotomy or VATS for posterior mediastinal pathology and transcervical (neck incisions) for superior mediastinal pathology. The middle mediastinum can usually be approached through thoracotomy or VATS.

Primary tumours of the mediastinum

Thymoma, neurogenic tumours, germ cell tumours and lymphoma are the usual primary tumours of the mediastinum.

- **Thymoma**. This is the most common mediastinal tumour, accounting for 25% of the total, and is derived from the thymus gland **(Figure 55.25)**. Thymomas vary in behaviour from benign to aggressively invasive, as reflected in the Masoaka classification system used to stage thymomas *(Table 55.11)*. They are often related to mysthenia gravis (MG), a neuromusclar condition which can have a high associated incidence of thymomas, and interestingly may respond to excision of the thymus gland even when the gland has no associated thymoma present. The only reliable indicator of malignancy is capsular invasion. Diagnosis and treatment are best achieved by complete thymectomy, which is usually performed as a median sternotomy. However, if the thymoma is small or when the patient has MG and the thymus is being excised as a treatment, a transcervical approach with or without an additional VATS procedure can be performed.
- **Germ cell tumour**. The anterior mediastinum is the most common site of extragonadal germ cell tumours. They account for 13% of all mediastinal masses and cysts and contain elements from all three cell types (mesoderm, endoderm and ectoderm). They tend to present in young adults and 75% are benign and cystic, although they may cause compression of neighbouring structures; hence, dermoid cysts are best excised. Malignancy is suspected if elevated levels of serum alpha-fetoprotein, human chorionic gonadotrophin and carcinoembryonic antigen are detected. After initial treatment with chemotherapy, a patient with tumour marker normalisation and a persistent mass on CT may be considered for surgical resection. If tumour markers fail to normalise, further chemotherapy is usually offered.
- **Lymphoma**. Lymphoma is a common cause of a mediastinal mass lesion, particularly in the anterior mediastinum, and can lead to superior vena cava obstruction or other symptoms of local compression. The main treatment is

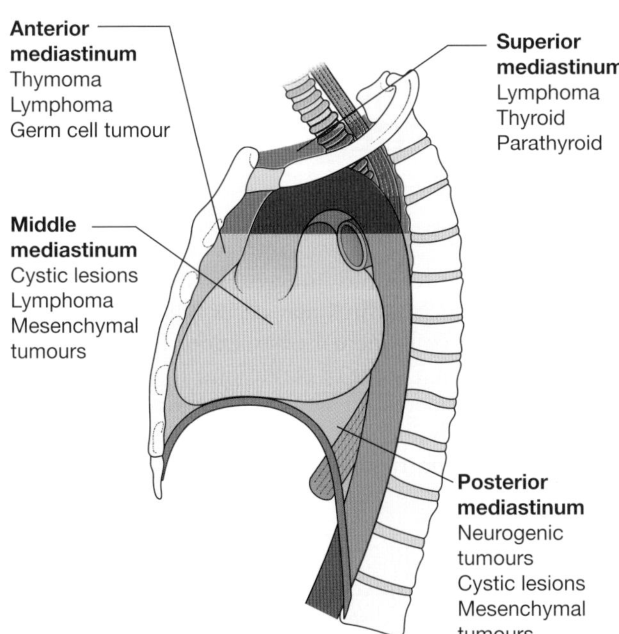

Figure 55.24 Mediastinal pathology. Subdivisions of the mediastinum with the most common mediastinal masses.

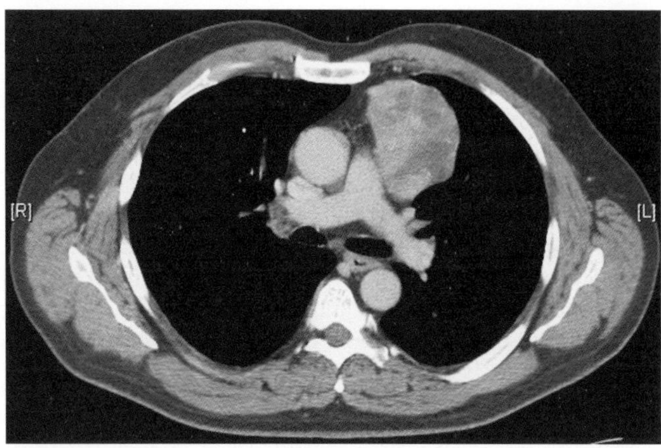

Figure 55.25 Computed tomography scan showing a thymoma presenting as a mediastinal mass.

TABLE 55.11 Masaoka thymoma staging system.

Stage	Description
I	Macroscopically completely encapsulated
	Microscopically no capsular invasion
II	Macroscopic invasion into surrounding fatty tissue or mediastinal pleura
	Microscopic invasion into the capsule
III	Macroscopic invasion into neighbouring organs (pericardium, great vessels, lungs)
IVA	Pleural or pericardial dissemination
IVB	Lymphogenous or haematogenous metastasis

After Masaoka A *et al.*, *Cancer* 1981; **48**: 2485.

chemotherapy, and surgery is rarely required apart from obtaining tissue for diagnosis.

- **Mesenchymal tumours**. Lipomas are common in the anterior mediastinum. Other mesenchymal tumours are very rare.
- **Thyroid**. Ectopic thyroid (and parathyroid) tissue may be found in the anterior mediastinum but usually the mass is an extension of a thyroid lesion (retrosternal goitre). Excision of retrosternal thyroids may be required if there is local airway compression and stridor and can be performed via a transcervical incision, but occasionally median sternotomy may be required.
- **Neurogenic tumours**. These may derive from the sympathetic nervous system or the peripheral nerves and are more prevalent in the posterior mediastinum. They may be painful but are more often discovered accidentally on routine chest radiography and can be quite large (Figure 55.26). They include neuroblastoma in childhood, and Schwannomas and neurofibromas in adults, which are usually benign. Phaeochromocytoma arises from the sympathetic chain and produces the characteristic endocrine syndrome. Excision of neurogenic tumours is generally recommended, particularly if the patient is developing symptoms. This can be performed through a thoracotomy, though for smaller tumours a VATS approach can be used (Figure 55.27).
- **Enlarged mediastinal lymph nodes** are commonly involved by metastatic tumour, mimicking a primary mediastinal lesion. Symptoms are generally secondary to compression or invasion of a structure within the mediastinum. Surgery such as mediastinoscopy is reserved for diagnosis only.

Other conditions of the mediastinum

Many of the primary tumours such as neurogenic tumours and germ cell tumours can present as cysts or have a cystic quality. In addition, the mediastinum can contain other cysts, often with an embyrological aetiology. Thymic cysts, pericardial cysts, bronchogenic and foregut cysts can all present asymptomatically or with local compression (Figure 55.28). Surgical excision is recommended if diagnosis is unclear or the patient has symptoms.

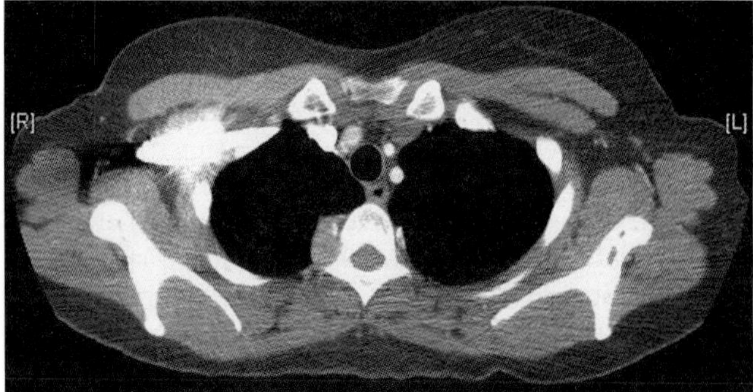

Figure 55.26 Computed tomography scan showing a right-sided paravertebral neurogenic tumour.

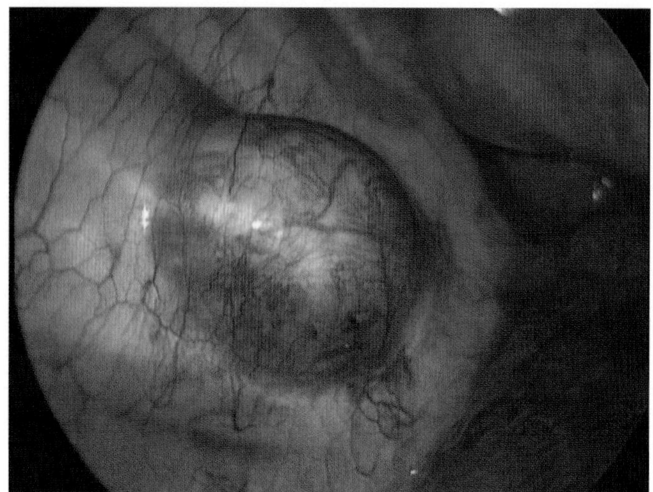

Figure 55.27 Video-assisted thoracoscopic surgery (VATS) image of a neurogenic tumour attached to the posterolateral chest wall prior to excision.

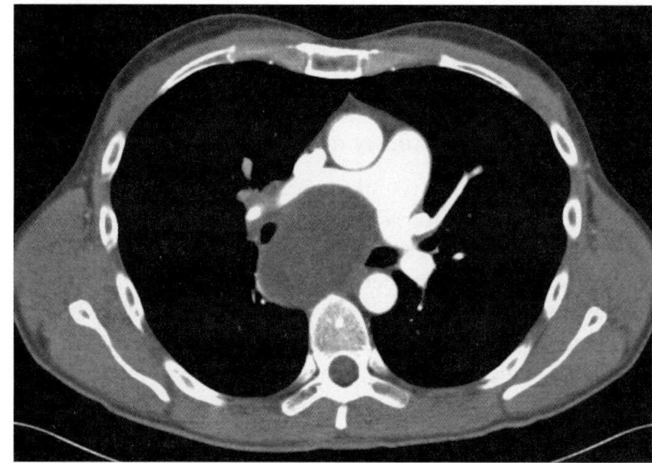

Figure 55.28 Computed tomography scan of the chest showing a bronchogenic cyst splaying the carina.

MEDICAL CONDITIONS FOR WHICH SURGERY MAY BE REQUIRED

Bronchiectasis

Bronchiechtasis is chronic irreversible dilatation of the medium-sized bronchi, which may occur following a suppurative pneumonia or bronchial obstruction. It is the pathological end stage of a range of conditions. If generalised it is almost never considered for surgical resection. Cases caused by whooping cough and measles are decreasing in frequency in resource-rich countries.

Treatment

Removal of the bronchiectatic part of the lung for symptoms of bleeding, recurrent infection or copious symptoms can be very effective when the disease is localised.

Theodor Schwann, 1810–1882, Professor of Anatomy and Physiology successively at Louvain (1839–1848) and Liege, Belgium (1849–1888).

Lung abscess

The causes of lung abscess are shown in *Table 55.12*. The chest radiograph shows a cavity with a fluid level or in myecetoma a fungal ball. Most acute abscesses resolve with appropriate antibiotic therapy and postural drainage. Surgery is avoided. Small radiologically sited drains are used sometimes in the intensive care unit.

TABLE 55.12 Causes of lung abscess.

Specific pneumonia	Streptococcal Staphylococcal Pneumococcal *Klebsiella* spp. Anaerobic
Bronchial obstruction	Carcinoma Carcinoid Foreign body Postoperative atelectasis
Chronic respiratory sepsis	Sinusitis Tonsillitis Dental infection
Septicaemia	
Penetrating lung injury	

Tuberculosis

Surgery is rarely indicated for tuberculosis in resource-rich countries but, when it is, it must be combined with adequate antitubercular chemotherapy or the benefit of surgery will be lost.

Summary box 55.6

Tuberculosis: indications for surgery

- Suspicious lesion on chest radiograph in which neoplasia cannot be excluded
- Chronic tuberculous abscess, resistant to chemotherapy
- Aspergilloma within a tuberculous cavity
- Life-threatening haemoptysis

Diagnosis

Surgical procedures may be necessary to establish the diagnosis if suspected clinically but sputum or pus cultures are persistently negative.

Complications such as an aspergilloma in a chronic cavity causing life-threatening haemoptysis may require lobectomy.

Pulmonary sequestration

This describes a section of non-functional lung separated from the normal bronchial connection with other abnormalities of development, which often include a direct systemic arterial supply from the aorta. Venous return is to the pulmomary veins in the majority of cases. The segment becomes cystic and infected, resulting in the common appearance of a solid lung mass that may be homogeneous or heterogeneous, occasionally with cystic changes on CT scan. Interlobar sequestration occurs within the lung substance. It may present with recurrent chest infections and/or haemoptysis. Patients with extralobar sequestration are usually asymptomatic because air spaces are not present, and therefore it usually presents as an incidental finding.

Lung cysts

Developmental lung cysts have a tendency to become infected. Acquired lung cysts may contain air or fluid and may be single or multiple. Pulmonary hydatid disease is a cause in endemic areas. Air cysts (bullae) may be spontaneous but may be secondary to emphysematous degeneration (**Figure 55.29**).

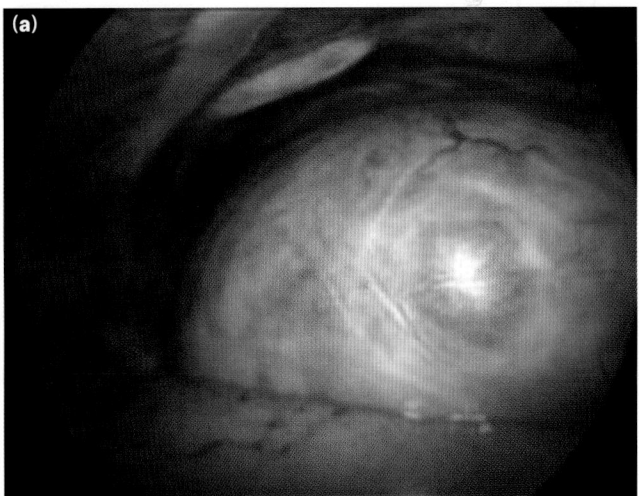

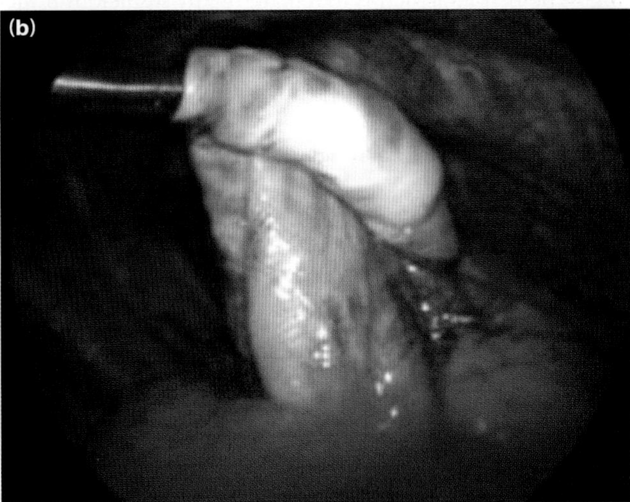

Figure 55.29 **(a)** A large solitary bulla seen on videothoracoscopy. **(b)** The bulla deflated and rolled in preparation for staple resection.

Theodor Albrecht Edwin Klebs, 1834–1913, Professor of Bacteriology successively at Prague, Czech Republic; Zurich, Switzerland; and The Rush Medical College, Chicago, IL, USA.

LUNG TRANSPLANTATION (SEE ALSO CHAPTER 82)

Lung transplantation is an established therapy for those with end-stage parenchymal or pulmonary vascular disease; it is limited by the number of donor lungs available.

CHEST TRAUMA

The approach to trauma must be methodical and exact, because the signs, particularly in the presence of other injury, may easily be missed. The general principles of resuscitation and ATLS (Advanced Trauma and Life Support) must be followed.

Thoracic trauma is responsible for over 70% of all deaths following road traffic accidents. Blunt trauma to the chest in isolation is fatal in 10% of cases, rising to 30% if other injuries are present. The indications for emergency room thoractomy in blunt chest trauma include massive haemothorax, suspected cardiac tamponade and witnessed cardiac arrest in the resuscitation area. Success rates are low. Penetrating thoracic wounds vary according to the prevalence of civil violence, with a mortality rate of 3% for simple stabbing to 15% for gunshot wounds. The indications for emergency room thoracotomy are similar to those for blunt chest trauma. The standard approach is a left anterior thoracotomy, unless the penetrating injury is in the right chest, however it may be necessary to extend the incision to bilateral thoracotomies or a clampshell incision.

Early deaths after thoracic trauma are caused by hypoxaemia, hypovolaemia and tamponade. The first steps in treating such patients should be to diagnose and treat these problems as early as possible because they may be readily corrected. Young patients have a large physiological reserve, and serious injury may be overlooked until this reserve is used up, by which time the situation is critical and may be irretrievable. The best approach is to remain highly suspicious if life-threatening conditions are to be anticipated and treated. Early consultation with a regional thoracic centre is advised in cases of doubt. In an emergency it is essential that experienced help is summoned.

Management of chest trauma is covered in detail in Chapter 27.

THE DIAPHRAGM

The diaphragm is the fibromuscular structure separating the thorax from the abdomen.

Disorders of the diaphragm

Disorders of the diaphragm can be broadly classified as disorders of innervation, leading to paralysis of the diaphragm, with elevation and reduction of thoracic volume leading to breathlessness, and disorders of anatomy, which are further categorised into congenital diaphragmatic hernias or acquired hernias, usually secondary to trauma. There are two well-recognised congenital sites where abdominal viscera can herniate into the chest (**Figures 55.30 and 55.31**).

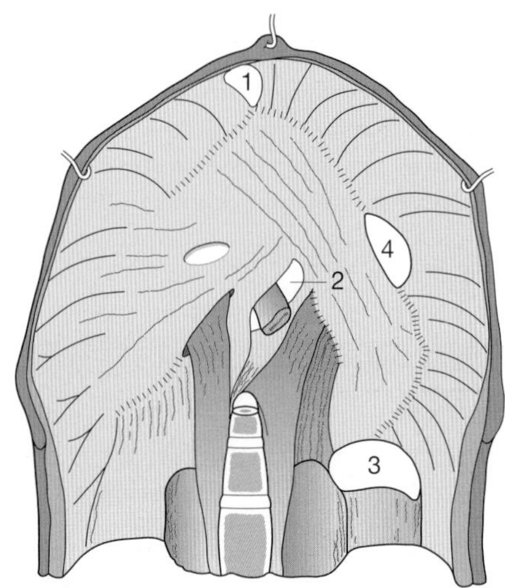

Figure 55.30 Diagram of sites of hernias. The usual sites of congenital diaphragmatic hernia: 1, foramen of Morgagni; 2, oesophageal hiatus; 3, foramen of Bochdalek (pleuroperitoneal hernia); 4, dome.

- **The foramen of Morgagni**: a hernia in the anterior part of the diaphragm with a defect between the sternal and costal attachments. The most commonly involved viscus is the transverse colon.
- **The foramen of Bochdalek**: through the dome of the diaphragm posteriorly.

Traumatic rupture of the diaphragm may occur with blunt trauma. Unless there is severe bleeding or strangulation of the viscera it is best managed after an interval. In a severely injured patient being ventilated it can wait until other injuries are dealt with and weaning from the ventilator is being considered.

When the diaphragm is breached, as in anatomical disorders, repair with either primary closure or with a mesh is usually possible via a thoracotomy. Diaphragmatic paralysis, particularly idiopathic unilateral paralysis, can be treated by plication, returning the diaphragm to a lower position and improving thoracic volume.

DISORDERS OF THE CHEST WALL

Tumours of the chest wall

These can be tumours of any component of the chest wall, i.e. bone, cartilage and soft tissue. They are treated similarly to those that occur at other sites and require specialist surgical input only if major resection and chest wall reconstruction are contemplated.

Giovanni Battista Morgagni, 1682–1771, Professor of Anatomy, Padua, Italy for 59 years, regarded as 'the founder of Morbid Anatomy'.
Victor Alexander Bochdalek, 1801–1883, Professor of Anatomy, Prague, Czech Republic.

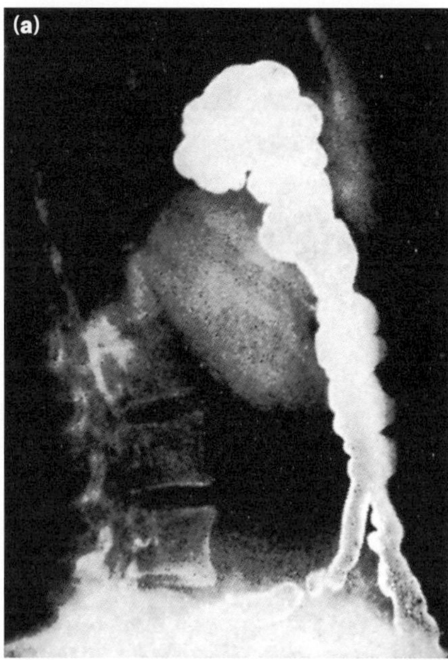

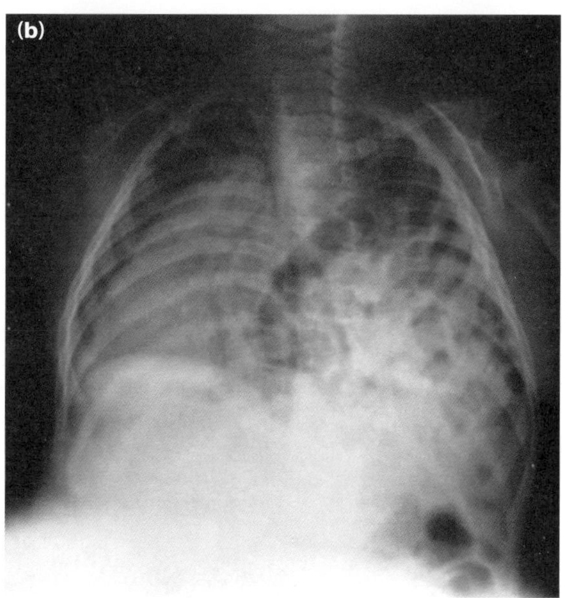

Figure 55.31 Chest x-ray of congenital diaphragmatic hernia. (**a**) Colon occupying a Morgagni hernia (courtesy of Dr Oliver Smith, Birmingham, UK). (**b**) Foramen of Bochdalek hernia on the left side in an infant. The left pleural cavity is occupied by intestine, the mediastinum is displaced to the right and the right lung is aerated very little.

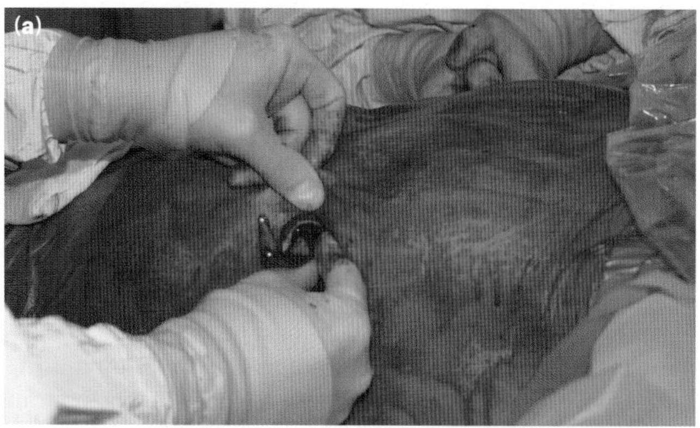

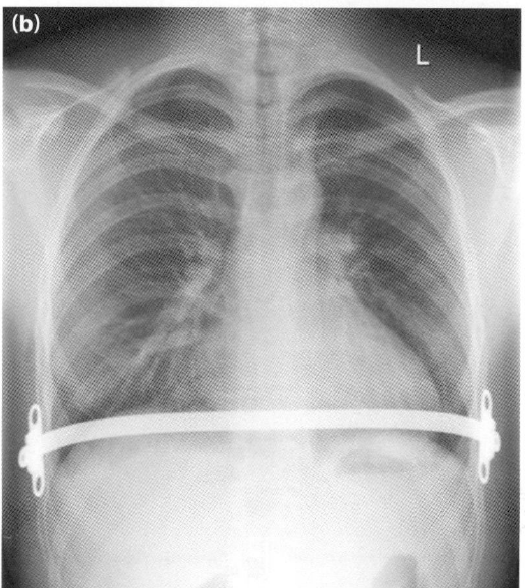

Figure 55.32 (**a**) Insertion of preformed bar placed thoracoscopically beneath the pectus excavatum. (**b**) Chest x-ray following insertion of a metal bar bracing the sternum forward (the Nuss procedure).

Other diseases of the chest wall

Congenital abnormalities are often incidental findings on chest radiography (e.g. bifid rib), but there are some important exceptions.

Cervical rib and thoracic outlet syndrome

This rib is usually represented by a fibrous band originating from the seventh cervical vertebra and inserting onto the first thoracic rib. It may be asymptomatic, but because the subclavian artery and brachial plexus course over it a variety of symptoms may occur. The lower trunk of the plexus (mainly T1) is compressed, leading to wasting of the interossei and altered sensation in the T1 distribution. Compression of the subclavian artery may result in a poststenotic dilatation with thrombus and embolus formation. The diagnosis, assessment and surgery are fraught with uncertainties and are best left to those with a well-developed interest in this problem.

Pectus excavatum

The sternum is depressed, with a dish-shaped deformity of the anterior portions of the ribs on one or both sides. It is never a cause of respiratory problems. It can be repaired to improve its cosmetic appearance either as an open procedure (the Ravitch procedure) which involves resecting the affected costal cartilages and mobilising the sternum, or as a minimally invasive technique, the Nuss procedure. A metal bar is paced behind the sternum to hold this central panel in its new position and has to be removed after a period of time (**Figure 55.32**).

Mark M Ravitch, 1910–1989, paediatric surgeon, University of Pittsburg, PA, USA.
Donald Nuss, contemporary, paediatric surgeon, Norfolk, VA, USA, described this technique in 1987.

Pectus carinatum (pigeon chest)

In this condition the sternum is elevated above the level of the ribs and treatment is offered for cosmetic reasons. The sternum is mobilised and allowed to fall back into place.

It often comes to light during the growth spurt at adolescence when, of course, the teenager is particularly sensitive about appearance. Most patients are asymptomatic and the only justification for treatment is on cosmetic grounds. Some surgeons make a very good case for this but the risk of morbidity and of a less than perfect result must be clearly spelt out to the patient and his/her parents. Surgery involves mobilising the sternum with the costal cartilages so that the sternum can be flattened to a more anatomical position. Surgery is best left until the late teens, when further growth of the chest wall is unlikely.

FURTHER READING

Baas P, Fennell D, Kerr KM *et al.* Malignant pleural mesothelioma: ESMO Clinical Practice Guidelines for diagnosis, treatment and follow-up. *Ann Oncol* 2015; **26** (Suppl 5): v31–9.

BTS Pleural Disease Guideline Group. British Thoracic Society Pleural Disease Guideline 2010. *Thorax*, 2010; **65**(Suppl 2): 1–76.

Goldstraw P, Chansky K, Crowley J *et al.* The IASLC Lung Cancer Staging Project: proposals for revision of the TNM stage groupings in the forthcoming (eighth) edition of the TNM classification for lung cancer. *J Thorac Oncol* 2016; **11**(1): 39–51.

Lim E, Baldwin D, Beckles M *et al.* Guidelines on the radical management of patients with lung cancer. *Thorax* 2010; **65**(Suppl 3): iii1–27.

NICE. *The diagnosis and treatment of lung cancer*. National Institute for Health and Clinical Excellence. NICE clinical guideline 121, 2011. Available at: guidance.nice.org.uk/cg121

Vansteenkiste J, De Ruysscher D, Eberhardt WEE *et al.* Early and locally advanced non-small-cell lung cancer (NSCLC): ESMO Clinical Practice Guidelines for diagnosis, treatment and follow-up. *Ann Oncol* 2013; **24**(Suppl 6): vi89–98.

PART 10

Vascular

56 Arterial disorders 942
57 Venous disorders 969
58 Lymphatic disorders 995

Chapter 56

Arterial disorders

Learning objectives

To understand:

- The nature and associated features of occlusive peripheral arterial disease
- The investigation and treatment options for occlusive peripheral arterial disease
- The principles of management of the severely ischaemic limb
- The nature and presentation of peripheral aneurysmal disease, particularly of the abdominal aorta
- The investigation and treatment options for peripheral aneurysmal disease
- The arteritides and vasospastic disorders

INTRODUCTION

Arterial disorders represent the most common cause of morbidity and death in Western societies. Much of this is due to the effects of atheroma on the arteries supplying the heart muscle (coronary thrombosis and myocardial infarction) and brain (stroke), although atheroma is also common at other sites. This chapter addresses diseases that are typically the province of the vascular surgeon, namely those affecting the peripheral arterial system: vascular disease that alters the normal structure and function of the aorta, its visceral branches and the arteries of the lower extremity.

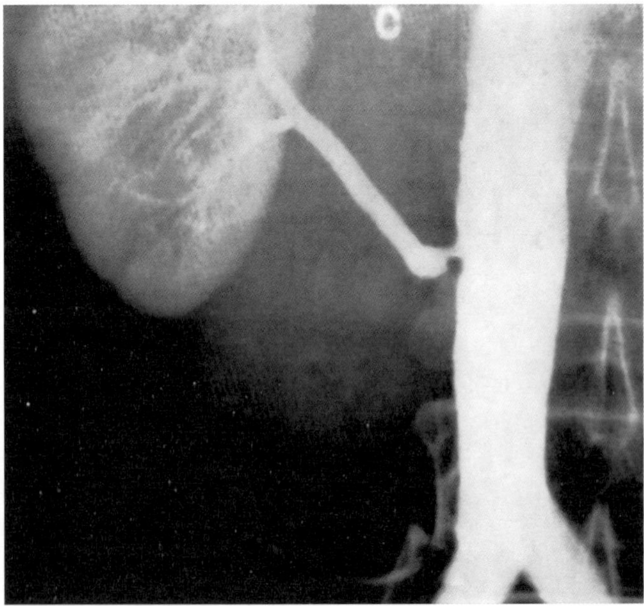

Figure 56.1 Renal artery stenosis. Angiogram by retrograde femoral catheterisation. Note the poststenotic dilatation.

ARTERIAL STENOSIS AND OCCLUSION

Cause and effect

Peripheral arterial stenosis or occlusion is predominantly caused by atherosclerosis and/or thromboembolic disease, but may also occur as a result of trauma, particularly in the younger adult. Stenosis or occlusion produces symptoms and signs that are related to the organ supplied by the artery: e.g. lower limb – claudication, rest pain and gangrene; brain – transient ischaemic attacks and stroke; myocardium – angina and myocardial infarction; kidney – hypertension and renal failure (**Figure 56.1**); intestine – abdominal pain and infarction. The severity of the symptoms is related to the size of the vessel occluded and whether the stenosis or occlusion occurs suddenly (acute) in a previously normal artery or gradually (chronic) with progressive narrowing of the artery over time. In chronic arterial narrowing, a collateral circulation may develop and provide an alternative route for blood flow that reduces symptoms until a critical stenosis or occlusion has developed (**Figure 56.2**).

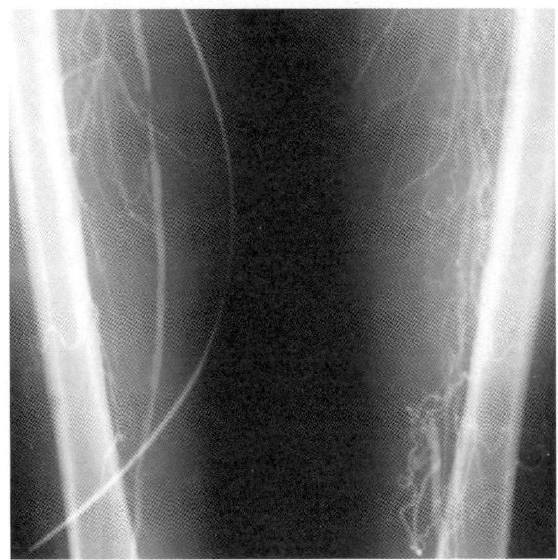

Figure 56.2 Right superficial femoral stenosis. Left superficial femoral occlusion with collateral vessels present, causing claudication.

Features of chronic arterial stenosis or occlusion in the leg

Intermittent claudication

Intermittent claudication occurs as a result of anaerobic muscle metabolism and is classically described as debilitating cramp-like pain felt in the muscles that is:

- reliably brought on by walking;
- not present on taking the first step (unlike osteoarthritis);
- reliably relieved by rest both in the standing and sitting positions; usually within 5 minutes (unlike nerve compression from a lumbar intervertebral disc prolapse or osteoarthritis of the spine or spinal stenosis, which are typically relieved only when resting in the sitting position for greater than 5 minutes).

The distance that a patient is able to walk without stopping varies (claudication distance) only slightly from day to day. It is decreased by increasing the work demands and hence oxygen requirements of the muscles affected, e.g. walking up hill, increasing the speed of walking and/or carrying heavy weights, and secondly by general health conditions that reduce the oxygen delivery capacity of the arterial system, e.g. anaemia or heart failure.

The muscle group affected by claudication is classically one anatomical level below the level of arterial disease and is usually felt in the calf because the superficial femoral artery is the most commonly affected artery (70% of cases). Aorto-iliac disease (30% of cases) may cause thigh or buttock claudication. Buttock claudication in association with sexual impotence resulting from arterial insufficiency is eponymously called Leriche's syndrome. It is very rare.

Rest pain

As disease progression occurs the claudication distance decreases and perfusion to the leg may be so severely compromised that anaerobic respiration occurs even at rest, typically affecting the foot and/or calf. The pain is exacerbated by lying down or elevation of the foot due to loss of the gravitational effects on perfusion pressure in the foot. The patient characteristically describes pain that is worse at night and may be lessened by hanging the foot out of bed or by sleeping in a chair (effects of gravity restored). Even the pressure of bedclothes on the foot may make the pain worse.

Ulceration and gangrene

Ulceration occurs with severe arterial insufficiency and may present as painful erosion between toes or as shallow, non-healing ulcers on the dorsum of the feet, on the shins and especially around the malleoli. The blackened mummified tissues of frank gangrene are unmistakable (**Figure 56.3**), and superadded infection often makes the gangrene wet. Patients with rest pain and/or ulceration/gangrene – critical limb ischaemia – should be considered to have an imminently threatened leg and require urgent vascular assessment/intervention.

Colour, temperature, sensation and movement

Unlike an acutely ischaemic foot that is often cold, white, paralysed and insensate, a chronically ischaemic limb tends to equilibrate with the temperature of its surroundings and may feel quite warm under the bedclothes. Chronic ischaemia does not produce paralysis and sensation is usually intact. Patients with critical limb ischaemia who have been waiting for a consultation with their leg in dependence may have a red swollen foot that may be mistaken for cellulitis by the unwary clinician. However, elevation of the limb reveals the severity of the ischaemia, with venous guttering and foot pallor that changes to a red/purple colour when the limb is allowed to hang down again (dependent rubor or the sunset foot sign) (**Figure 56.4**). The capillary refill time may be elicited by pressing the skin of the heel or toe causing blanching

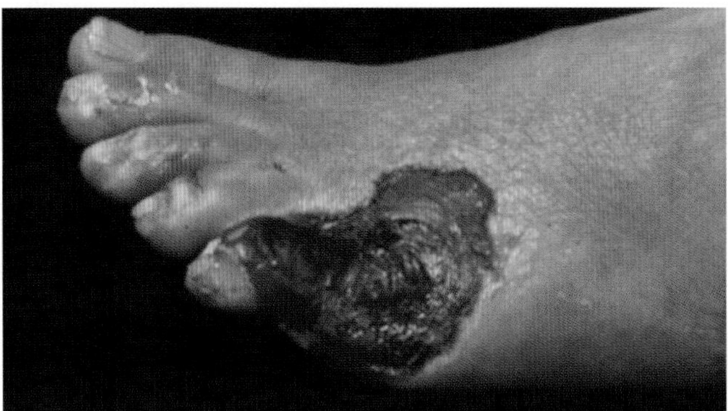

Figure 56.3 Severe chronic ischaemia with dry gangrene.

Claudication from the Latin *claudicare* – to limp. The Roman emperor Claudius (10 BC to 54 AD) walked with a limp, which was possibly due to poliomyelitis.
Rene Leriche, 1879–1955, Professor of Surgery, Strasbourg, France, described this syndrome.

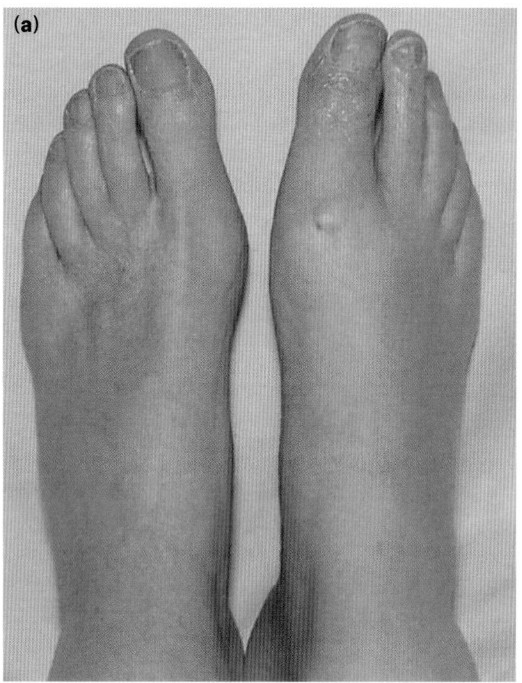
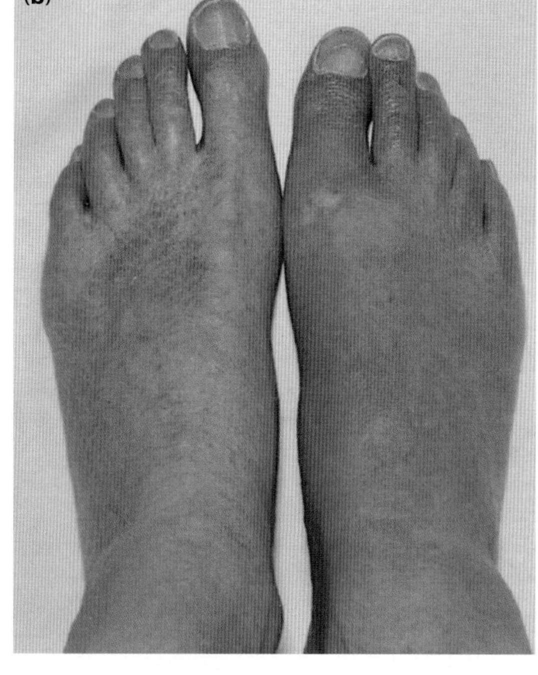

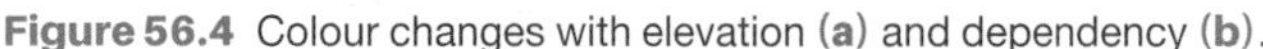
Figure 56.4 Colour changes with elevation (**a**) and dependency (**b**).

(press for 5 seconds) and then releasing to allow colour to return; normally this takes 2–3 seconds but may be prolonged to 10 seconds in severe ischaemia.

Arterial pulses

It is standard practice to examine the femoral, popliteal, posterior tibial and dorsalis pedis arteries together with the abdomen for an aortic aneurysm or renal artery bruit, which may coexist with lower limb occlusive disease. Diminution of a femoral and/or popliteal pulse can often be appreciated by comparing it with its opposite number; however, pedal pulses are either clinically palpable or absent. Popliteal pulses are often difficult to feel; a popliteal artery aneurysm should be suspected if the popliteal pulse is prominent with concomitant loss of the natural concavity of the popliteal fossa. Pulsation distal to an arterial occlusion is usually absent although the presence of a highly developed collateral circulation may allow distal pulses to be palpable – this is most likely to occur with an iliac stenosis. In this case, exercise (walking until claudication develops) usually causes the pulse to disappear as vasodilation occurs below the obstruction, causing the pulse pressure to reduce. An arterial bruit, heard on auscultation over the pulse, indicates turbulent flow and suggests a stenosis. It is an unreliable clinical sign as tight stenoses often do not have bruits. A continuous 'machinery' murmur over an artery usually indicates an arteriovenous fistula.

Relationship of clinical findings to site of disease

In most cases the site of arterial obstruction can be determined from the symptoms and signs (*Table 56.1*). Severe ischaemia (rest pain, ulceration, gangrene) is usually caused by multilevel disease, e.g. iliac and femoropopliteal disease.

Summary box 56.1

Features of chronic lower limb arterial stenosis or occlusion

- Intermittent claudication
- Rest pain
- Dependent rubor or sunset foot
- Ulceration
- Gangrene
- Arterial pulsation diminished or absent
- Arterial bruit
- Slow capillary refilling

TABLE 56.1 Relationship of clinical findings to site of disease.

Aortoiliac obstruction	Claudication in buttocks, thighs and calves
	Femoral and distal pulses absent in both limbs
	Bruit over aortoiliac region
	Impotence (Leriche)
Iliac obstruction	Unilateral claudication in the thigh and calf and sometimes the buttock
	Bruit over the iliac region
	Unilateral absence of femoral and distal pulses
Femoropopliteal obstruction	Unilateral claudication in the calf
	Femoral pulse palpable with absent unilateral distal pulses
Distal obstruction	Femoral and popliteal pulses palpable
	Ankle pulses absent
	Claudication in calf and foot

Investigation of arterial occlusive disease

Most patients with symptoms of arterial disease do not need invasive treatment, such as angioplasty or surgical reconstruction, and the decision whether or not to intervene can often be made without recourse to special investigations. When further investigation is indicated, the purpose is to confirm the presence and severity of peripheral arterial disease, identify the anatomical location of disease and assess the suitability of the patient for intervention.

General investigation

Patients with arterial disease tend to be elderly and atherosclerosis is often a multisystem disease process; the presence of arterial disease in the leg is suggestive of disease in other arterial trees, including the coronary (50%) and cerebral (25–50%). Many patients have other age-related diseases, such as chronic obstructive pulmonary disease and malignancy, that may impact on both their symptoms and suitability for intervention. Blood tests to exclude anaemia, diabetes, renal disease and lipid abnormalities should include a full blood count, blood glucose, lipid profile and serum urea and electrolytes. High blood viscosity (polycythaemia and thrombocythaemia) may be caused by smoking but may also be associated with cancer; renal impairment (raised serum creatinine and low estimated glomerular filtration rate) may be caused by drugs and may be exacerbated by intravenous contrast agents used during angiography.

Electrocardiography (ECG) may show coronary ischaemia, left ventricular hypertrophy or a cardiac dysrhythmia although a normal ECG does not rule out these conditions. More information may be gained by an echocardiogram or exercise testing. Arterial blood gases and pulmonary function test may be appropriate in patients with severe lung disease.

Doppler ultrasound blood flow detection

A hand-held Doppler ultrasound probe is very useful in the assessment of occlusive arterial disease (**Figures 56.5 and 56.6**). A continuous-wave ultrasound signal is transmitted from the probe at an artery, and a receiver within the probe itself picks up the reflected beam. The change in frequency in the reflected beam compared with that of the transmitted beam is due to the Doppler shift, resulting from the reflection of the beam by moving blood cells. The frequency change may be converted into an audio signal that is typically pulsatile. Doppler ultrasound equipment can be used in conjunction with a sphygmomanometer to assess systolic pressure in small vessels. This is possible even when the arterial pulse cannot be palpated. Both the pressure and signal quality are important; a normal artery has a triphasic signal that can be detected by a trained observer. However, although the presence of a Doppler signal indicates moving blood, it does not necessarily indicate that the blood flow is sufficient to maintain limb viability and prevent limb loss.

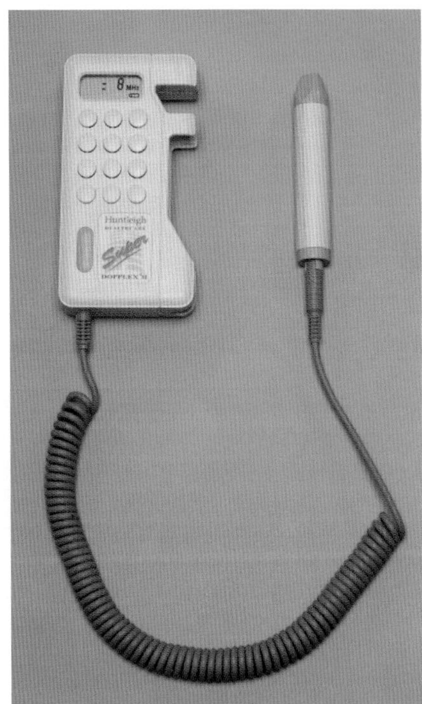

Figure 56.5 Simple hand-held Doppler ultrasound probe.

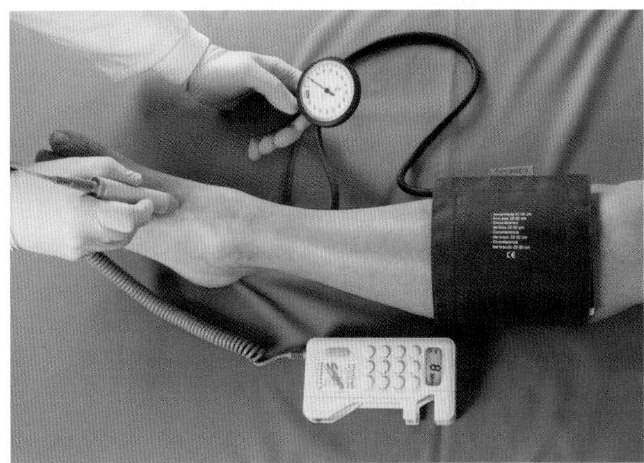

Figure 56.6 Hand-held Doppler probe and sphygmomanometer used to determine systolic pressure in the dorsalis pedis artery, as part of assessing the ankle–brachial pressure index.

Quantitative assessment can be performed at the bedside by measuring the ankle–brachial pressure index (ABPI); the ratio of systolic pressure at the ankle to that in the ipsilateral arm. The highest pressure in the dorsalis pedis, posterior tibial or peroneal artery serves as the numerator, with the highest brachial systolic pressure being the denominator. The normal resting ABPI is 0.9–1.3; values below 0.9 indicate some degree of arterial obstruction (claudication), <0.5 suggests rest pain and <0.3 indicates imminent necrosis. However, the

Christian Johann Doppler, 1803–1856, Professor of Experimental Physics, Vienna, Austria, enunciated the 'Doppler Principle' in 1842.

values are merely a guide and normal values may be present with intermittent claudication. Retesting after exercise to the onset of pain can be useful; a drop in the resting ABPI of >20% after exercise is indicative of flow-limiting arterial disease. Artificially high ABPI readings (>1.3) can be caused by calcified, incompressible arteries that are often found in diabetic patients.

Duplex scanning

This major non-invasive technique uses B-mode ultrasound to provide an image of vessels (**Figures 56.7 and 56.8**). The image is created because of the varying ability of different tissues to reflect the ultrasound beam. A second ultrasound beam is then used to insonate the imaged vessel and the Doppler shift obtained is analysed by a computer. Most scanners now have colour coding, which allows detailed visualisation of blood flow, turbulence, etc. Different colours indicate changes in direction and velocity of flow, with areas of high flow usually indicating a stenosis. In experienced hands, duplex scanning is as accurate as angiography and has the advantages of cost-effectiveness and safety. However, the aortoiliac segment can be difficult to visualise particularly in obese patients. A computed tomography (CT) angiogram can provide better imaging of this segment in these cases (see below).

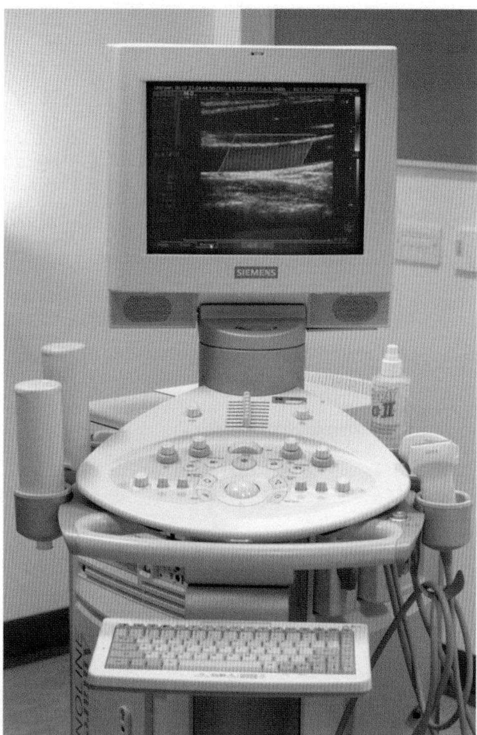

Figure 56.7 Colour duplex scanner.

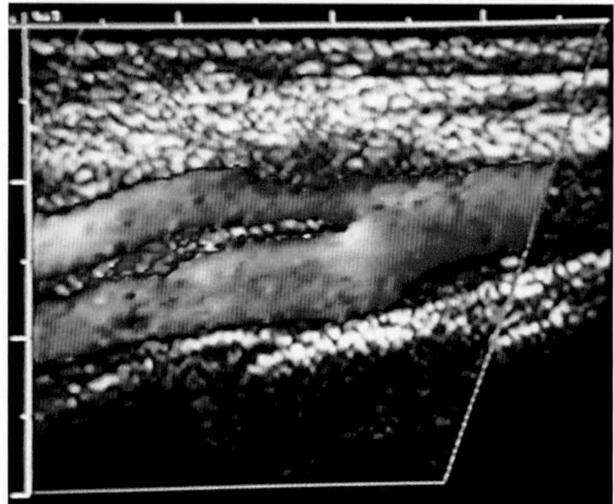

Figure 56.8 Colour duplex scan of carotid vessels in the neck showing stenosis at the common carotid bifurcation (courtesy of Dr Paul Allan, Royal Infirmary, Edinburgh, UK).

Digital subtraction percutaneous angiography

Digital subtraction percutaneous angiography (DSA) involves injection of a radio-opaque dye into the arterial tree by a percutaneous catheter method (Seldinger technique), usually involving the femoral artery (**Figures 56.9 and 56.10**). The images obtained are digitalised by computer and the extraneous background (bone, soft tissues, etc.) is removed to provide clearer images. The benefits of DSA are that it provides dynamic arterial flow information and can be combined with a definitive endovascular intervention when indicated. However, it is associated with potential complications including

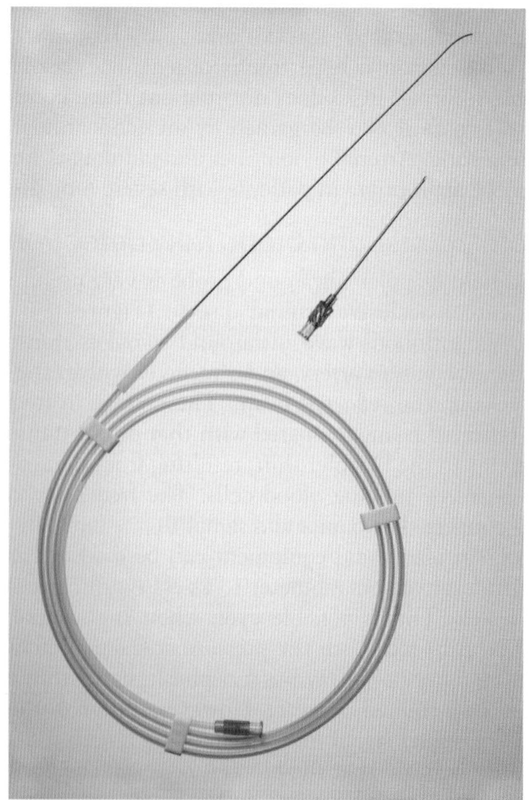

Figure 56.9 Seldinger needle and guidewire for introducing an arterial catheter.

Sven Ivar Seldinger, 1921–1998, radiologist, Karolinska Institute, Stockholm, Sweden, introduced percutaneous arterial catheterisation in 1956.

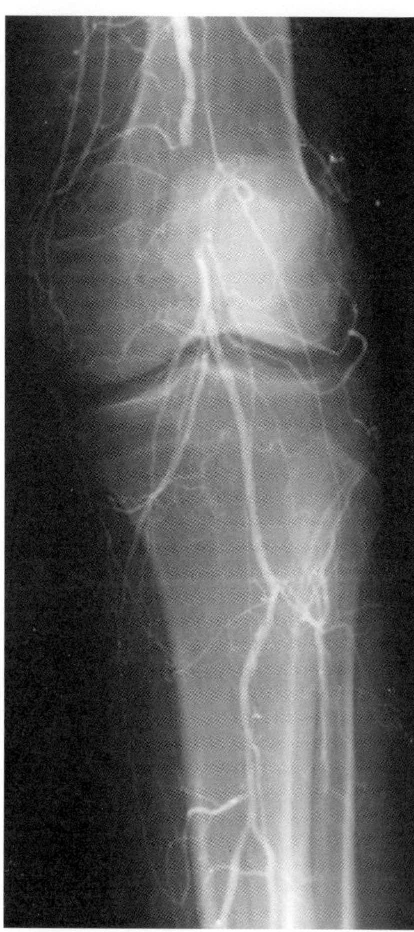

Figure 56.10 Arterial occlusion just above the knee causing claudication of the calf; good collateral circulation (a non-digital subtraction arteriogram by the Seldinger technique).

bleeding, haematoma, false aneurysm formation, thrombosis, arterial dissection, distal embolisation, renal dysfunction and allergic reaction, which may occur in up to 5% of procedures. Furthermore, it is relatively expensive compared to other investigation modalities and its usage should be limited to patients in whom a concomitant intervention is predicted.

CT angiography and magnetic resonance (MR) angiography (**Figure 56.11**) are newer techniques gaining in popularity, although the image quality is not as good as DSA. They can be useful where duplex scanning is not possible (intrathoracic arteries) or produces poor images (aortoiliac segment). MR has the added advantage of avoiding the need for ionising radiation, but may be contraindicated in patients suffering with claustrophobia or those with certain metallic implants, e.g. pacemakers.

Management of arterial stenosis or occlusion

General

Only one-quarter of patients presenting with intermittent claudication will experience symptomatic deterioration during their lifetime, but the overall risk of progression to critical leg ischaemia and amputation is small with <5% of patients requiring amputation over a 5-year period. Patients with an ABPI of <0.50 are twice as likely to deteriorate as patients with an ABPI of >0.50, and a deteriorating ABPI is predictive of future limb loss. For patients with rest pain or tissue necrosis, intervention is usually required to prevent major amputation.

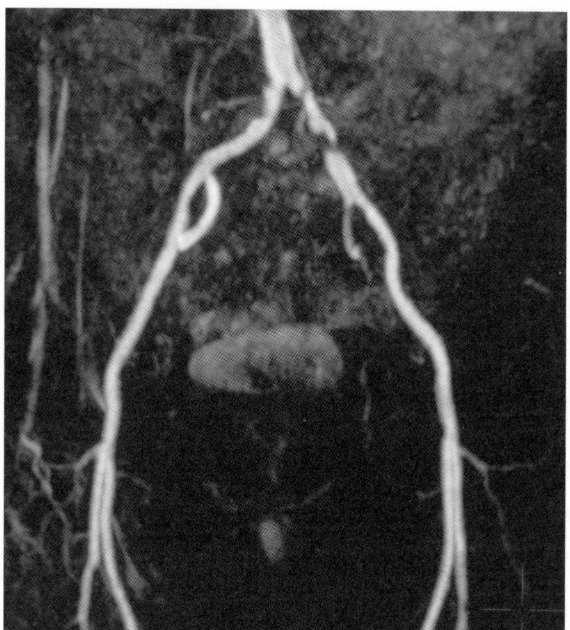

Figure 56.11 Magnetic resonance angiogram showing a tight stenosis at the midpoint of the left common iliac artery.

Claudication is often a marker of silent coronary arterial disease, whose extent correlates with the ABPI; a 0.1 decrease in ABPI below 0.9 is associated with a 10% increase in the relative risk of a major cardiovascular event. Similarly, one-quarter of patients with claudication have significant atherosclerotic disease affecting their carotid and renal arterial systems. It is thus not surprising that the risk of suffering a major cardiovascular event per year in patients with claudication is >5%, and that 50% of claudicants will die within 10 years from myocardial infarction or stroke. The common modifiable risk factors for peripheral arterial disease mirror those for coronary artery disease: smoking, diabetes mellitus, hypertension and hyperlipidaemia. Therefore, the two main aims when treating claudication are prevention of major cardiovascular morbidity through risk factor modification and symptom relief/improvement.

Non-surgical management

For many patients with claudication a structured exercise programme – at least 2 hours of exercise per week for 3 months – in combination with smoking cessation will lead to sustained improvement in claudication distance and a reduction in cardiovascular risk. Diabetes mellitus increases the risk and severity of claudication proportional to the duration of affliction. Strict control in combination with weight loss in the obese patient is vital to reduce cardiovascular risk and prevent symptom deterioration.

DRUGS

Medication may be required for diseases associated with arterial disorders, such as hypertension and diabetes; some antihypertensives (particularly β-blockers) may exacerbate claudication. Raised blood lipids require active drug treatment, but even when the lipid profile is normal a statin (HMG-CoA reductase inhibitor) should be prescribed as they may stabilise atherosclerotic plaques and protect against cardiac death independently of baseline serum lipid levels. An antiplatelet agent is also necessary: recent National Institute for Health and Care Excellence (NICE) guidelines recommend 75 mg per day of clopidogrel, or 75 mg per day of aspirin as an alternative. Other agents, such as vasodilators, are unlikely to provide either significant or sustained benefit. Drugs are now available to help with smoking cessation.

TRANSLUMINAL ANGIOPLASTY AND STENTING

Arterial occlusive disease may be treated by inserting a balloon catheter into an artery and inflating it within a narrowed or blocked area (**Figures 56.12 and 56.13**). This technique is suitable for patients with claudication, rest pain or tissue necrosis (**Figures 56.14 and 56.15**). Following percutaneous femoral artery puncture under local anaesthetic, a guidewire is inserted and negotiated through the stenosis or occlusion under fluoroscopic control. A balloon catheter is then inserted over the guidewire and positioned within the lesion. The balloon is then inflated at high pressure for approximately 30 seconds and deflated. Satisfactory dilation of the lesion is confirmed by performing an angiogram. Percutaneous transluminal angioplasty (PTA) has proved very successful in dilating the iliac and femoropopliteal segments; the results below the knee are less successful. Long occlusions may be treated by the technique of subintimal angioplasty, where the guidewire crosses the lesion in the subintimal space (in the arterial wall) and a new lumen is created by inflation of the balloon. Complications occur in about 5% of cases and include failure, haematoma, bleeding, thrombosis and distal embolisation; these may impact on the surgeons' ability to perform a subsequent open surgical revascularisation procedure.

If the vessel fails to stay adequately dilated (often caused by elastic recoil of the artery), it may be possible to hold the lumen open using a metal stent (**Figures 56.16 and 56.17**). This may be introduced on a balloon catheter and expanded by balloon inflation; or alternatively, a self-expanding stent may be used that is contained inside a plastic sheath and deployed by withdrawal of the sheath.

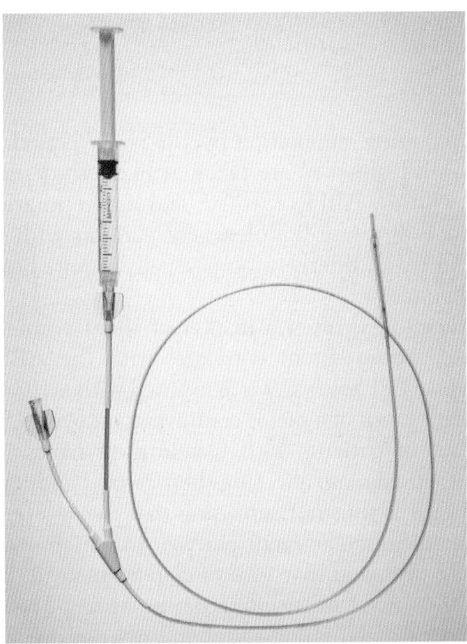

Figure 56.12 Balloon catheter for percutaneous transluminal angioplasty.

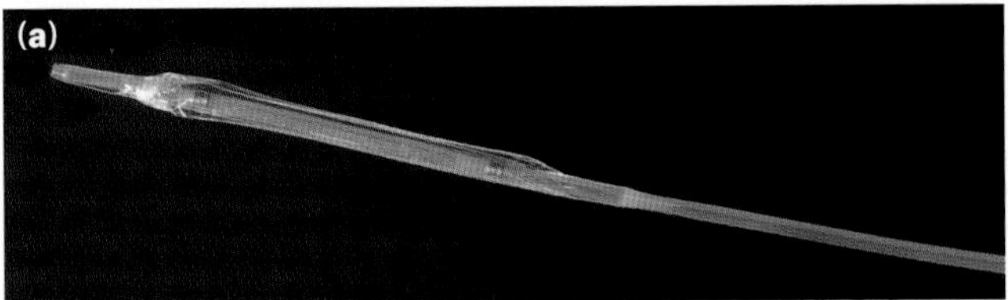

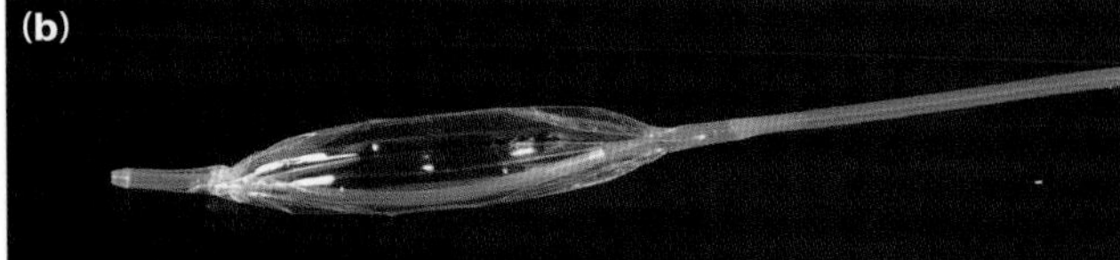

Figure 56.13 **(a)** Catheter balloon deflated; **(b)** balloon inflated.

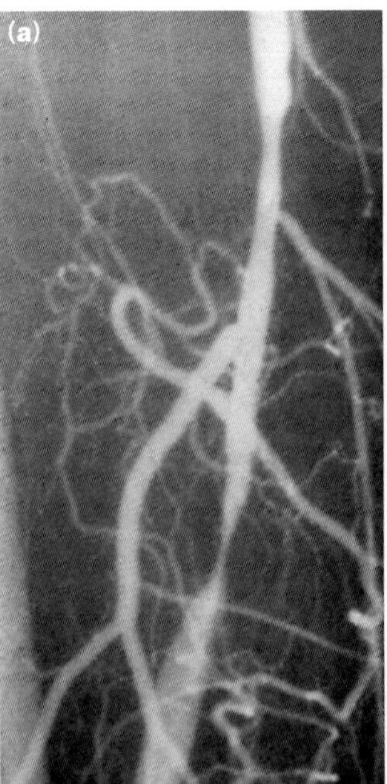

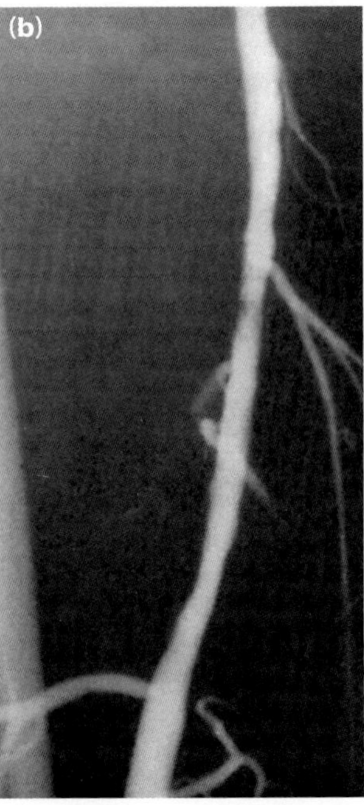

Figure 56.14 **(a, b)** Narrowed superficial femoral artery before and after transluminal angioplasty (courtesy of J McIvor, FRCR, London, UK). The advantage of this technique is that it can be carried out under local anaesthesia using the Seldinger technique of percutaneous arterial puncture, and is therefore especially useful in the treatment of patients who are medically unfit for major surgery.

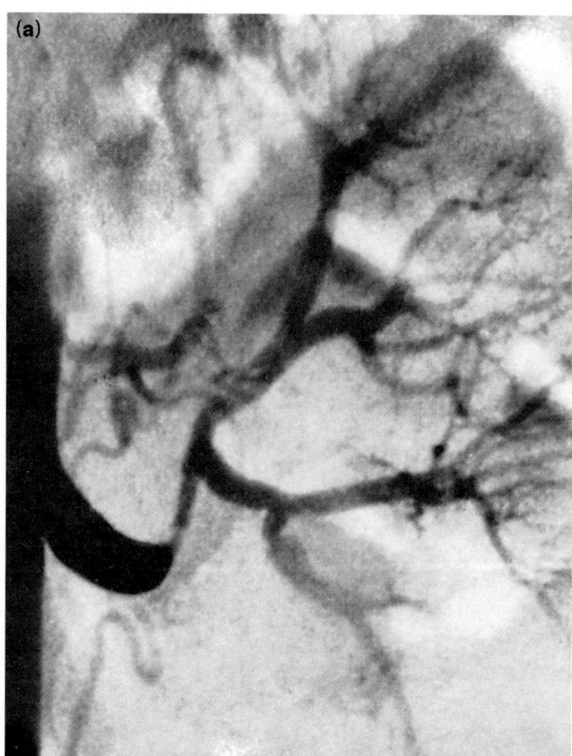
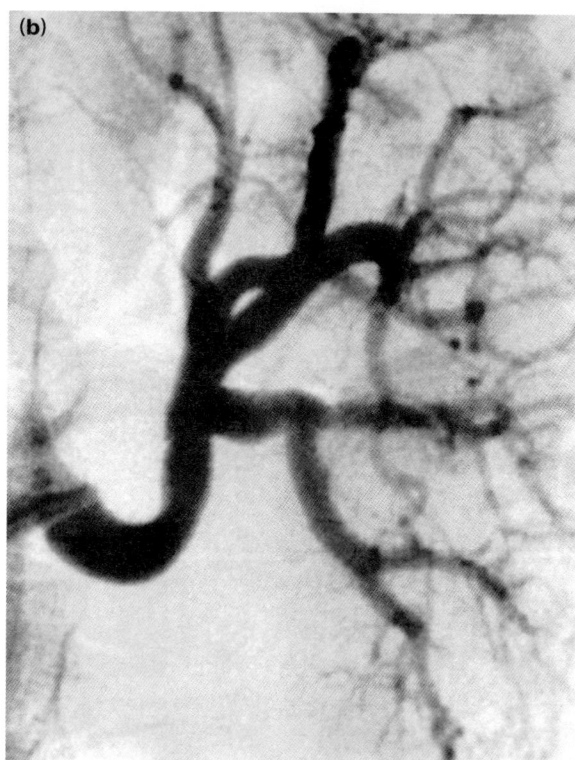

Figure 56.15 Before (**a**) and after (**b**) balloon dilatation of a severely stenosed left renal artery in a 20-year-old woman with uncontrollable hypertension. The blood pressure fell to normal after the procedure. The stenosis was probably due to fibromuscular hyperplasia, but no tissue was available for histological diagnosis.

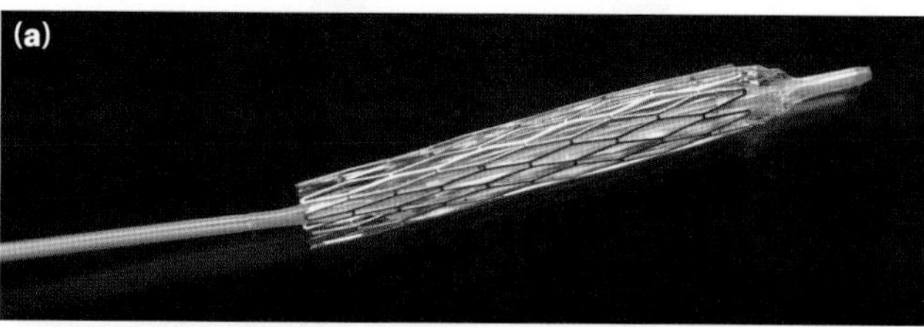
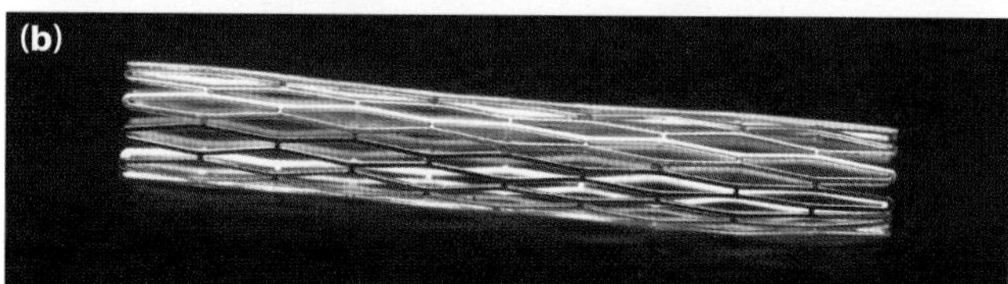

Figure 56.16 (**a**) Balloon catheter carrying stent; (**b**) expanded stent.

Operations for arterial stenosis or occlusion

Site of disease and type of operation

Surgical operations are usually reserved for patients with severe symptoms where angioplasty has failed or is not possible. Aortoiliac occlusion responds well to aortofemoral bypass (**Figure 56.18a**) using a Dacron graft (**Figure 56.19a**); although the operation carries a perioperative mortality and systemic morbidity rates of about 5% and 15%, respectively. In unfit patients, an axillofemoral bypass is an alternative, although patency rates are less. If only one iliac system is occluded, an iliofemoral or femorofemoral crossover graft may be performed.

Superficial femoral artery disease can be treated by femoropopliteal bypass (**Figure 56.18b**); long-term graft patency is determined by the quality of inflow and outflow, graft length (whether the distal anastomosis is above or below the knee) and the conduit used for the bypass. Autologous long saphenous vein (LSV) gives the best results and can be used reversed or *in situ* after valve disruption. If the LSV is not available from either leg, short saphenous or arm veins may be used. If no vein is available, a prosthetic polytetrafluoroethylene (PTFE) graft may be employed (**Figure 56.19b**) although patency rates are lower; many surgeons construct the lower anastomosis using a small collar of vein (Miller cuff) between the PTFE and the recipient artery, which may improve patency. Isolated common femoral artery or profunda disease can be treated with endarterectomy and patch (vein or prosthetic) or a short bypass in the groin.

Sometimes, in patients with critical leg ischaemia, the occlusion extends beyond the popliteal artery into the tibial vessels. Limb salvage can be attempted with a femorodistal bypass, with success even more dependent on the state of the run-off vessel and the quality of the vein conduit (minimum diameter 3 mm). The risk of early graft failure with limb loss is high and these long bypasses are only appropriate for limb salvage.

Justin H Miller, vascular surgeon, Royal Adelaide Hospital, Adelaide, SA, Australia.

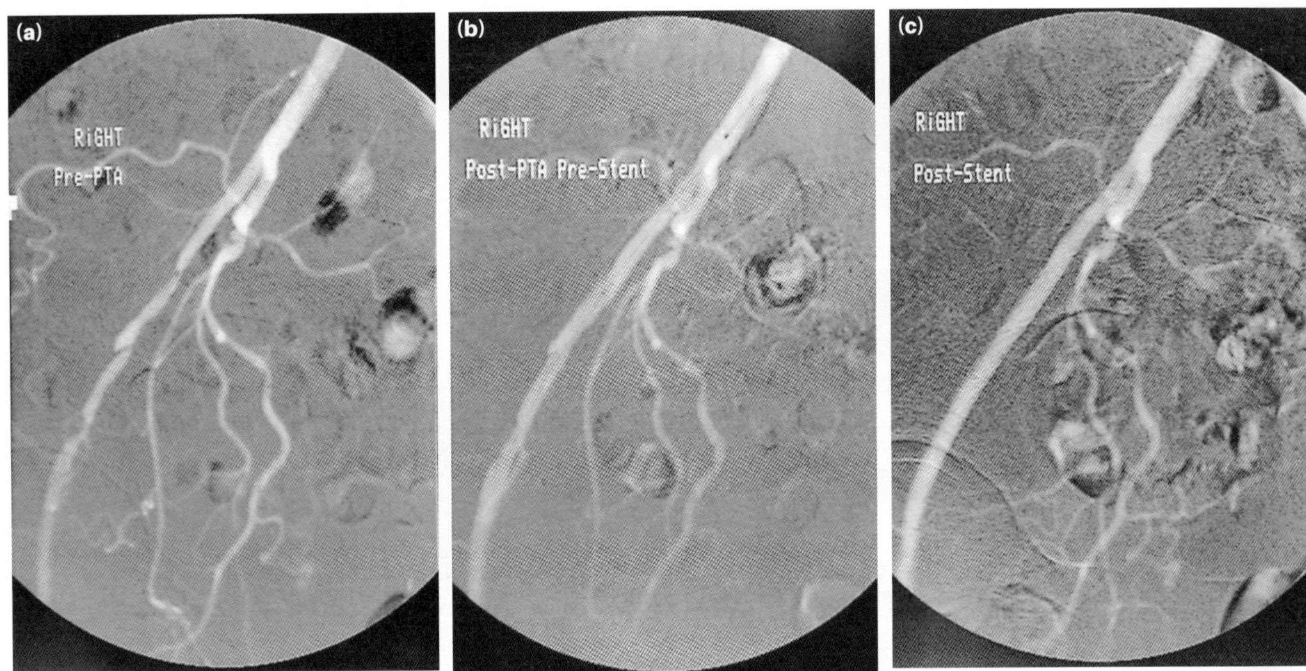

Figure 56.17 (**a**) External iliac artery stenosis before dilatation; (**b**) after dilatation by percutaneous transluminal angioplasty; and (**c**) dilated artery patency assured by stent (courtesy of Johnson and Johnson Interventional Systems, Bracknell, UK, and Dr W. Shaw, Ninewells Hospital, Dundee, UK).

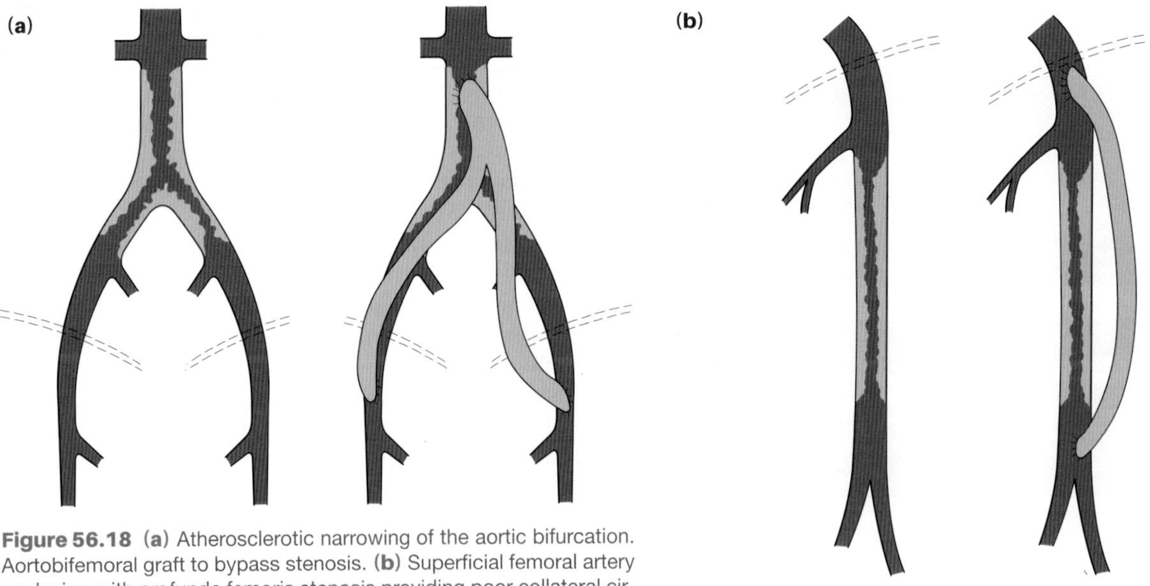

Figure 56.18 (**a**) Atherosclerotic narrowing of the aortic bifurcation. Aortobifemoral graft to bypass stenosis. (**b**) Superficial femoral artery occlusion with profunda femoris stenosis providing poor collateral circulation. Femoropopliteal graft used to bypass the occluded area into good 'run-off' below.

Technical details

For aortofemoral bypass, the aorta should be approached through a midline abdominal incision; a transverse abdominal incision divides the inferior epigastric vessels (important collateral vessel in patients with an occluded aorta) and should be avoided. The common femoral arteries and their branches are exposed through vertical groin incisions. The small bowel is retracted to the right and the posterior peritoneum opened. Retroperitoneal tunnels are made from the aorta to the groins. Heparin (5000 U) is given intravenously and the vessels clamped. A vertical incision is made in the anterior aspect of the aorta to which an obliquely cut, bifurcated Dacron® graft is sutured end-to-side with a non-absorbable suture (polypropylene). The graft limbs are then fed down to the groins where they are anastomosed end-to-side to the common femoral arteries or, if there is evidence of profunda stenosis, to an arteriotomy running from the common femoral vessel down into the profunda. The posterior

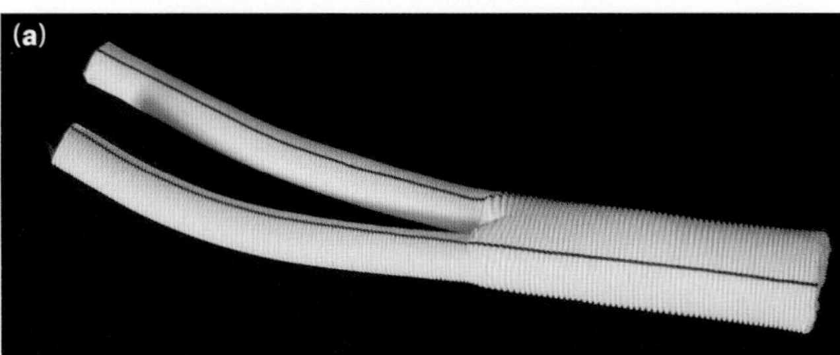

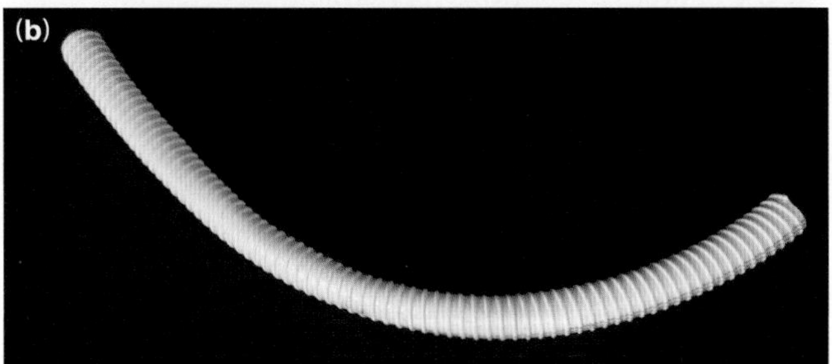

Figure 56.19 (**a**) Dacron® bifurcation graft; (**b**) polytetrafluoroethylene graft.

peritoneum is closed over the Dacron® to prevent adhesion of the graft to bowel, and the abdomen and groin wounds are closed.

For femoropopliteal bypass the popliteal artery above or below the knee is exposed through a medial incision. The common femoral artery is exposed at groin level. The LSV may be used in two different ways. First, it may be excised, its tributaries tied, and the vein used in a reversed fashion so the valves do not obstruct the flow of blood. Alternatively, it may be left in place (*in situ*) and the valves disrupted with a valvulotome. The graft is sutured to the femoral artery proximally and to the popliteal artery distally. Femorodistal bypass involves fashioning the distal anastomosis to a tibial vessel. If no suitable vein is available, prosthetic material (usually PTFE) may be used, with or without a small vein collar (Miller cuff) at its distal end (**Figures 56.20**).

A femorofemoral crossover graft involves tunnelling a prosthetic graft subcutaneously above the pubis between the groins. An axillofemoral graft is tunnelled subcutaneously between the axillary artery proximally, to reach one or both femoral arteries; the patency rate of an axillobifemoral bypass is better than that of an axillo(uni)femoral bypass.

Results of operation

Long-term results of aortoiliac reconstructive surgery are good, usually marred only by progressive infrainguinal disease. Femoropopliteal surgery is less successful. Immediate postoperative success for vein bypass exceeds 90% but the 5-year patency is around 60%. PTFE bypass yields poorer results than vein bypass, with 5-year success rates of less than 50%. Although the results of femorodistal bypass are even less satisfactory, such surgery can ensure limb salvage in patients who are generally debilitated and whose expected lifespan is limited; long-term patency is less important.

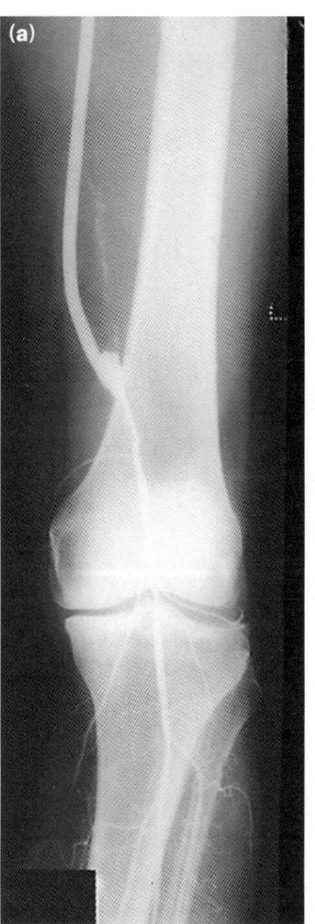

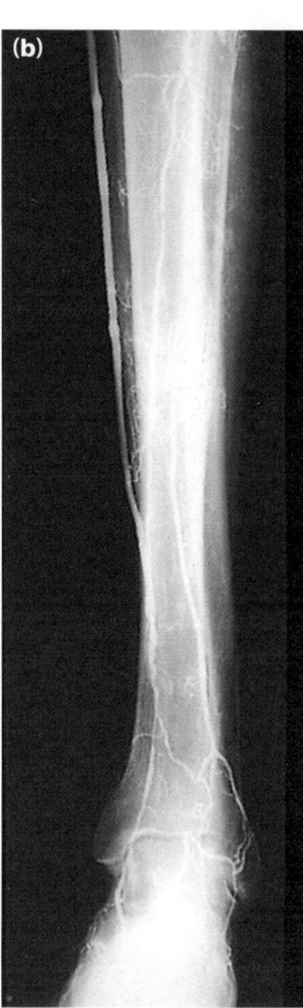

Figure 56.20 (**a**) Completion angiogram of femoropopliteal bypass graft (with Miller cuff). (**b**) Completion angiogram of femorodistal bypass graft *in situ*.

Other sites of atheromatous occlusive disease

The principles of arterial surgery outlined above can be applied at other arterial sites. Carotid stenosis (at the carotid bifurcation in the neck) may cause transient ischaemic attacks (TIAs). These short-lived mini-strokes are often recurrent and cause unilateral motor or sensory loss in the arm, leg or face, transient blindness (amaurosis fugax) or speech impairment. They are caused by distal embolisation of platelet thrombi that form on the atheromatous plaque into the cerebral circulation. They are a warning of impending major stroke. Patients should be assessed with a duplex scan. If a tight stenosis (>70%) is detected, carotid endarterectomy should be offered (**Figure 56.21**). Current guidelines for carotid endarterectomy are listed in *Summary box 56.2*. This involves clamping the vessels, an arteriotomy in the common carotid artery continued up into the internal carotid artery through the diseased segment, removal of the occlusive disease (endarterectomy) and closure of the arteriotomy, often with a patch. Many surgeons also use a temporary shunt to maintain cerebral blood flow while the carotid system is clamped.

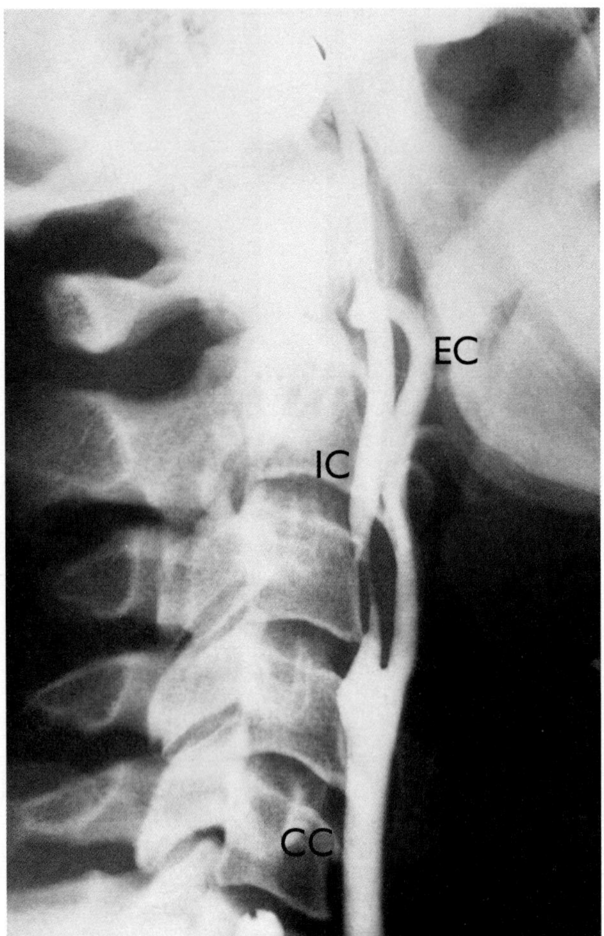

Figure 56.21 Carotid stenosis. A unilateral localised stenosis suitable for operation. CC, common carotid; EC, external carotid; IC, internal carotid.

Summary box 56.2

Indications for carotid endarterectomy in symptomatic patients

70% or greater carotid stenosis and:

- Ipsilateral amaurosis fugax or monocular blindness
- Contralateral facial paralysis or paraesthesia
- Arm/leg paralysis or paraesthesia
- Hemianopia
- Dysphasia (if dominant hemisphere)
- Sensory or visual inattention/neglect

Subclavian artery stenosis may cause claudication in the arm or digital ischaemia from distal embolisation. It may be treated by angioplasty or surgical bypass. Sometimes subclavian artery lesions are associated with neck pathology, such as a cervical rib, which should be removed during arterial repair (see Chapter 57, **Figure 57.37**). Subclavian steal syndrome may occur if the first part of the subclavian artery is occluded. Arm exercise causes syncope because of reversed flow in the vertebral artery leading to cerebral ischaemia. It can be treated by angioplasty or surgery and is rare.

Mesenteric artery occlusive disease may cause pain after eating (intestinal angina) and weight loss. In general, two of the three enteric vessels (coeliac axis, superior mesenteric artery, inferior mesenteric artery) must be occluded to produce symptoms and other intestinal disorders must be excluded before treatment with PTA, endarterectomy or bypass.

Renal artery stenosis may cause hypertension and eventual renal failure. Although it is possible to improve renal blood flow with PTA or surgery, the mainstay of treatment is the use of drugs to control hypertension, diabetes, etc.

GANGRENE

Gangrene refers to death of macroscopic portions of tissue, which turns black because of the breakdown of haemoglobin and the formation of iron sulphide. It usually affects the most distal part of a limb because of arterial obstruction (from thrombosis, embolus or arteritis). Dry gangrene occurs when the tissues are desiccated by gradual slowing of the bloodstream; it is typically the result of atheromatous occlusion of arteries. Wet gangrene occurs when superadded infection and putrefaction are present. Crepitus may be palpated as a result of infection by gas-forming organisms, commonly in diabetic foot problems, and should be considered a surgical emergency with urgent tissue debridement or amputation required.

Separation of gangrene

A zone of demarcation between the truly viable and the dead or dying tissue will eventually appear. Separation is achieved by the development of a layer of granulation tissue that forms between the dead and the living parts. In dry gangrene, if the blood supply of the proximal tissues is adequate, the final line of demarcation appears in a matter of days and separation occurs neatly and with the minimum of infection. If bone is involved, complete separation takes longer than when soft tissues alone are affected, and the stump tends to be conical as the bone has a better blood supply than its coverings. In moist gangrene, the infection and suppuration extend into the neighbouring living tissue, causing the final line of demarcation to be more proximal than in dry gangrene.

If the arterial supply to the proximal living tissue is poor, the line of final demarcation is very slow to form or does not develop at all. Unless the arterial supply can be improved, the gangrene will spread to adjacent tissues or will suddenly appear as 'skip' areas further up the limb. These skip lesions may occur on the other side of the foot, on the heel, on the dorsum of the foot or even in the calf. Infection may also cause gangrene to spread proximally into areas of extensive inflammation. To attempt local amputation in the presence of poor circulation will result in failure and gangrene will reappear in the wound or skin edges.

Treatment of gangrene

How much of a limb or digit can be salvaged depends on the blood supply proximal to the gangrene. Poor circulation can sometimes be improved by radiological or surgical intervention and this may allow a more conservative debridement or distal amputation. However, major limb amputation may be required in the presence of life-threatening sepsis, when the blood supply cannot be improved or in patients whose limb is useless because of contractures, stroke, etc.

Specific varieties of gangrene

Diabetic gangrene

Diabetic gangrene is usually caused by a combination of three factors – ischaemia secondary to macrovascular disease and microvascular dysfunction, peripheral sensorimotor neuropathy (PSN), which leads to trophic skin changes, and immunosuppression caused by excess of sugar in the tissues, which predisposes to infection (Figure 56.22). Macrovascular disease is atherosclerotic and typically affects the crural vessels with relative sparing of the pedal vessels, whereas increased microcirculatory shunting causes microvascular dysfunction. The PSN is usually sensory in the early phase, classically in a stocking distribution and renders the patients at high risk of soft tissue injury and its subsequent neglect. The PSN may extend to the joints of the foot and ankle, resulting in loss of nociceptive and proprioceptive protective reflexes and a repeated cycle of joint injury and bony destruction. Motor involvement causes an imbalance between flexors and extensor muscle groups of the foot, promoting altered foot biomechanics and abnormal pressure loading and resulting in thick callosities developing on the sole of the foot.

Ischaemia and PSN act synergistically to increase the risk of diabetic foot ulceration and reduce its subsequent healing potential. Superadded infection due to poor wound care can spread rapidly and proximally in subfascial planes leading to fulminant foot sepsis, gangrene and death.

Treatment depends on the degree of arterial involvement, which should be investigated and treated rapidly with angioplasty or surgery. The gangrene is treated by drainage of pus, liberal debridement of dead tissue and antibiotics. Unfortunately, a number of patients present with life-threatening systemic upset and should undergo primary amputation.

Bedsores

A bedsore is gangrene caused by local pressure (Figure 56.23). Bedsores are predisposed to by five factors: pressure, injury,

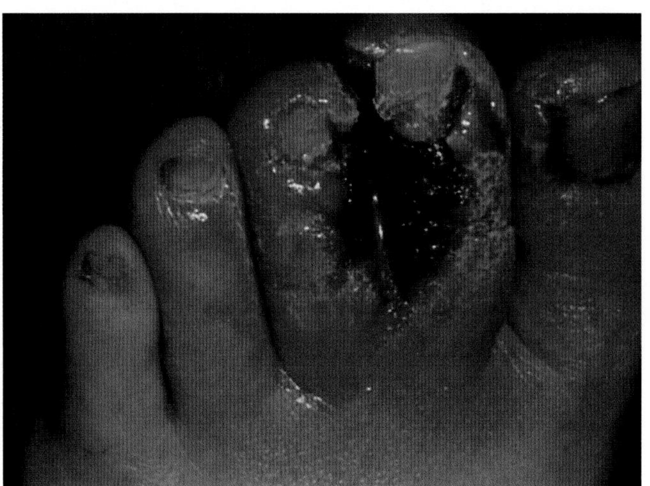

Figure 56.22 Diabetic gangrene.

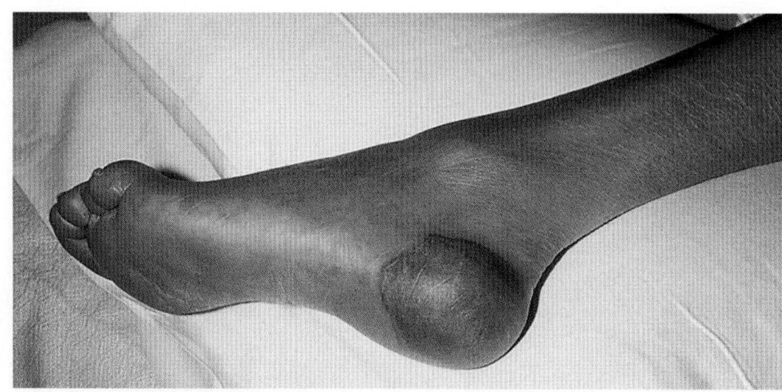

Figure 56.23 Bedsores typically appear over areas exposed to pressure, such as the sacrum and (as in this case) the heel.

anaemia, malnutrition and moisture. They can appear and extend rapidly in immobile patients and in those with debilitating illness. Prophylactic measures must be taken, including the avoidance of pressure over bony prominences by the use of foam blocks or similar, regular turning and nursing on specially designed beds that reduce the pressure to the skin. A waterbed or a ripple bed is sometimes desirable. Skilled nursing and the use of appropriate dressings must prevent maceration of the skin by sweat, urine, faeces or pus.

A bedsore can be expected if erythema appears that does not change colour on pressure. Once pressure sores develop, they are difficult to heal. They should be kept clean and debrided if necessary. Advice from a plastic surgeon should be sought for major lesions; vacuum dressings and rotation flaps can be effective.

Frostbite

Frostbite is caused by exposure to cold. It is seen both in climbers at high altitudes and in the elderly or the vagrant during cold weather (Figure 56.24). Cold injury damages the wall of the blood vessel, which causes swelling, and leakage of fluid together with severe pain. When the pain disappears, a waxy appearance remains; blistering and then gangrene follow. Treatment is gradual rewarming, analgesics and delayed conservative amputation after demarcation of devitalised tissue.

ACUTE ARTERIAL OCCLUSION

Sudden occlusion of an artery is usually caused by an embolus. It may also happen when thrombosis occurs on an atherosclerotic plaque, although the outcome is usually less dramatic because collaterals are likely to have developed in chronic arterial stenosis.

Embolic occlusion

An embolus is an object that has become lodged in a vessel causing obstruction having been carried in the bloodstream from another site. It is often a thrombus that has become detached from the heart or a more proximal vessel. Sources include the left atrium in atrial fibrillation, a left ventricular mural thrombus following myocardial infarction, vegetations on heart valves in infective endocarditis, thrombi in aneurysms and on atheroscerotic plaques. Emboli may lodge in any organ and cause ischaemic symptoms.

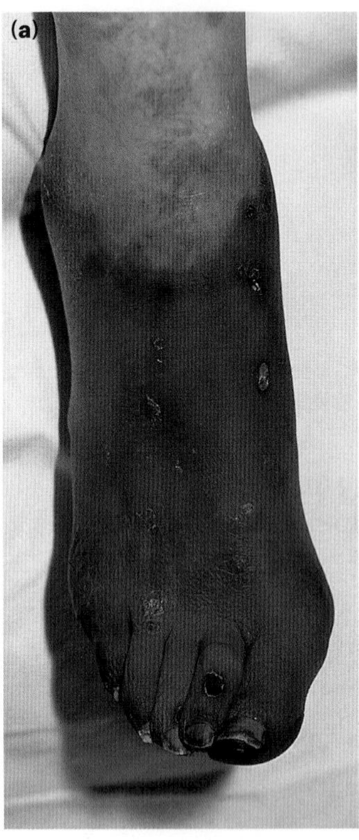

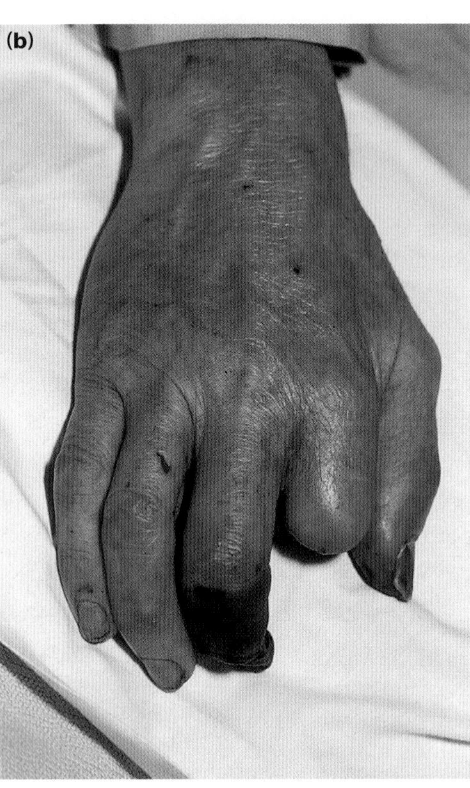

Figure 56.24 (**a**) Frostbite of the foot. Note the clear demarcation. (**b**) Frostbite of the middle finger in the same patient. The index finger was lost 2 years before, also from frostbite.

- Arm and leg – pain, pallor, paralysis, pulselessness and paraesthesia (**Figure 56.25**). Acute arterial occlusion due to an embolus differs from occlusion due to thrombosis on pre-existing atheroma; in the latter case a collateral circulation has often built up over time (**Figures 56.26 and 56.27**). It is essential to differentiate between the two, as they require different management.
- Brain – the middle cerebral artery (or its branches) is most commonly affected, resulting in major or minor (TIA) stroke.
- Retina – amaurosis fugax is fleeting blindness caused by a minute thrombus emanating from an atheromatous plaque

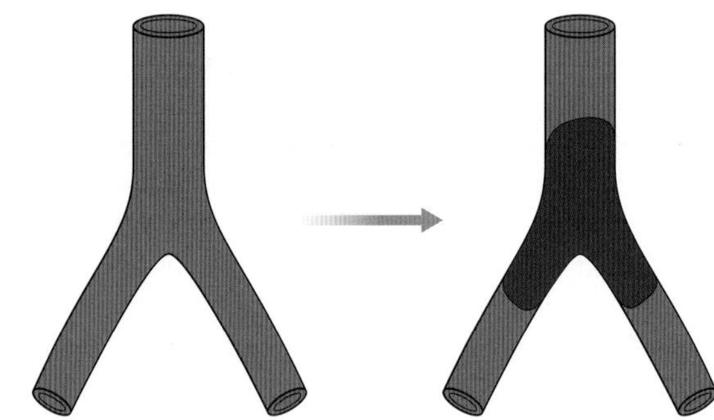

Figure 56.26 Aortic bifurcation embolus. Source of embolus is a recent myocardial infarct or atrial fibrillation. This causes severe, dramatic symptoms.

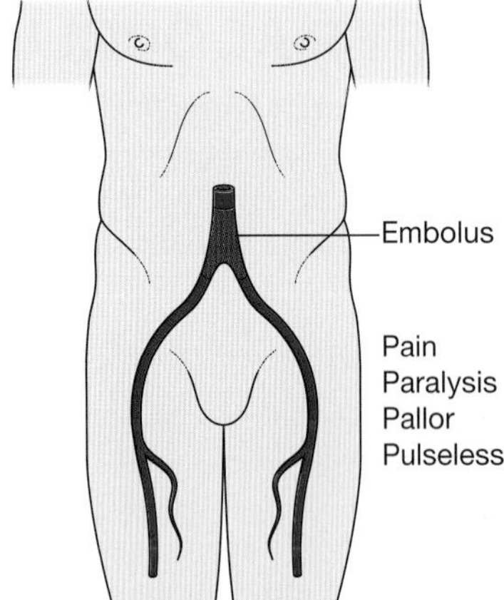

Figure 56.25 The symptoms and signs of embolism (four Ps). The fifth feature, anaesthesia, is often stated to be paraesthesia (the fifth P) but, in truth, complete loss of sensation in the toes and feet is characteristic.

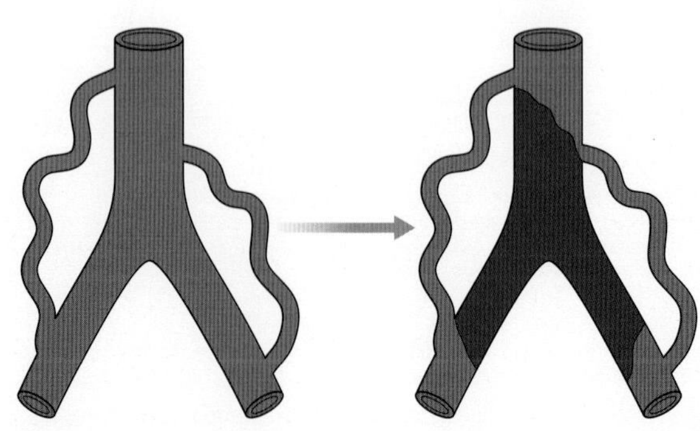

Figure 56.27 Aortic bifurcation thrombosis. No source of embolus but previous claudication worsens but there are no sudden features of distal ischaemia.

in the carotid artery passing into the central retinal artery. Lasting obstruction causes permanent blindness.

- Mesenteric vessels – possible gangrene and perforation of the corresponding loop of intestine.

Acute limb ischaemia

Clinical features

Embolic arterial occlusion is an emergency that requires immediate treatment. Ischaemia beyond 6 hours is usually irreversible and results in limb loss. The leg is often affected, with pain, pallor, paralysis, loss of pulsation and paraesthesia (or anaesthesia) **(Figure 56.25)**. The limb is cold and the toes cannot be moved, which contrasts with venous occlusion when muscle function is not affected. The diagnosis can be made clinically in a patient who has no history of claudication and has a source of emboli, who suddenly develops severe pain or numbness of the limb, which becomes cold and mottled. Movement becomes progressively more difficult and sensation is lost. Pulses are absent distally but the femoral pulse may be palpable, even thrusting, as distal occlusion results in forceful expansion of the artery with each pressure wave despite the lack of flow. A similar picture will occur in the arm with a brachial embolus.

Treatment

Because of the ensuing stasis, a thrombus can extend distally and proximally to the embolus. The immediate administration of 5000 U of heparin intravenously can reduce this extension and maintain patency of the surrounding (particularly the distal) vessels until the embolus can be treated. The relief of pain is essential because it is severe and constant. Embolectomy and thrombolysis are the treatments available for patients with limb emboli.

Embolectomy

Local or general anaesthesia may be used. The artery (usually the femoral), bulging with clot, is exposed and held in silastic vessel loops. Through a transverse incision the clot begins to extrude and is removed, together with the embolus **(Figure 56.28)**, with the help of a Fogarty balloon catheter. The catheter, with its balloon tip, is introduced both proximally and distally until it is deemed to have passed the limit of the clot. The balloon is inflated and the catheter withdrawn slowly, together with any obstructing material **(Figure 56.29)**. The procedure is repeated until bleeding occurs. An angiogram may be performed in the operating theatre at the end of the procedure to ensure that flow to the distal leg has been restored. Postoperatively, heparin therapy is continued until long-term anticoagulation with warfarin is established to reduce the chance of further embolism.

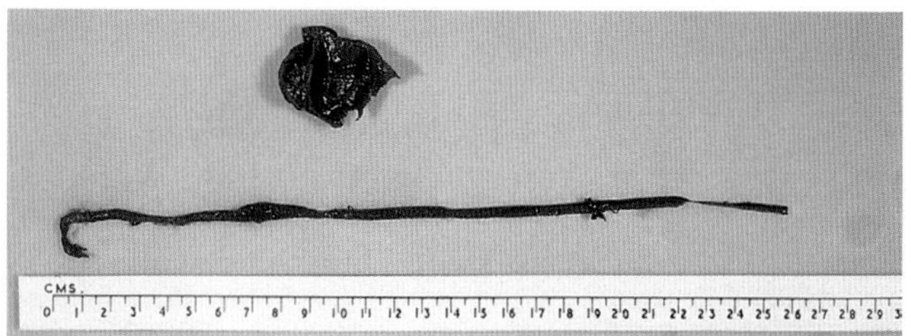

Figure 56.28 Embolic material removed from the common femoral artery, along with a long distal extension thrombus.

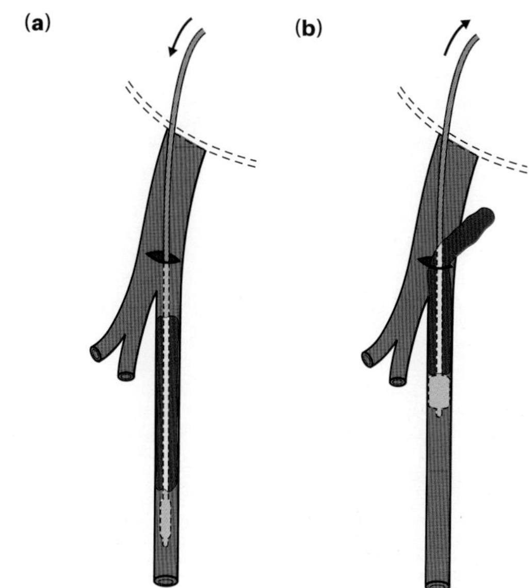

Figure 56.29 **(a)** A Fogarty catheter is inserted through an arteriotomy in the common femoral artery and fed distally down the superficial femoral artery and through the embolus. **(b)** The balloon is inflated and the catheter withdrawn, removing the embolus; the deep femoral and iliac arteries are similarly treated.

Thrombolysis

If ischaemia is not so severe that immediate operation is essential, it may be possible to treat either embolus or thrombosis by intra-arterial thrombolysis **(Figure 56.30)**. At arteriography of the ischaemic limb (usually via the common femoral artery) a narrow catheter is passed into the occluded vessel and left embedded within the clot. Tissue plasminogen activator (tPA) is infused through the catheter and regular arteriograms are carried out to check on the extent of lysis, which, in successful cases, is achieved within 24 hours. The method should be abandoned if there is no progression of dissolution of clot with time. There are several contraindications to thrombolysis, the most important of which are recent stroke, bleeding diathesis and pregnancy; results in those over 80 years old are poor.

Compartment syndrome

In limbs that have been subject to sudden ischaemia followed by revascularisation, oedema is likely. Muscles swell within confined fascial compartments and this can itself be a cause of tissue ischaemia, with both local muscle necrosis and nerve damage due to pressure, and systemic effects such as renal failure secondary to the liberation of muscle breakdown products. Liberal concomitant usage of fasciotomy following revascularisation of a prolonged ischaemic limb is advisable.

Thomas J Fogarty, b.1932, surgeon, University of Oregon Medical School, Portland, Oregon, USA.

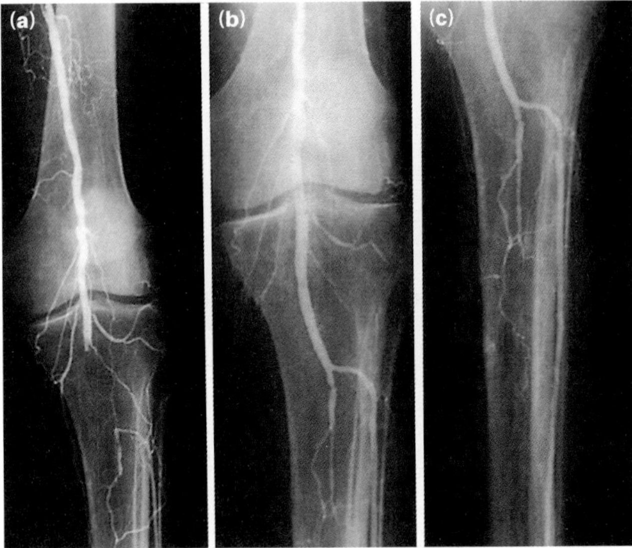

Figure 56.30 Angiogram of an occluded popliteal artery before thrombolysis (**a**), during successful lysis (**b**) and after completion of lysis (**c**).

The classical clinical picture is that of severe pain out of proportion with clinical findings that worsens with time, despite appropriate analgesia. The patient often complains of numbness/paraesthesia in the distribution of nerves running within the compartment (non-myelinated type C sensory fibres are most sensitive to hypoxia). Examination of the limb reveals a tense compartment with passive flexion and extension of muscles causing pain. The presence of palpable pulses **does not** rule out compartment syndrome.

The treatment is urgent compartment fasciotomy to release the compression. The usual site for fasciotomy is the calf (especially the anterior tibial compartment), but compartment syndrome may occasionally affect the thigh and the arm.

Acute mesenteric ischaemia

Acute mesenteric occlusion may be either thrombotic (following atheromatous narrowing) or embolic. Embolic occlusion results in sudden, severe abdominal pain, with bowel emptying (vomiting and diarrhoea) and a source of emboli present (usually cardiac). Unfortunately, the diagnosis is often only made at laparotomy with widespread infarction of the small and large bowel present; in this situation, it is often fatal. Occasionally, the degree of bowel infarction is more limited; resection of the dead bowel and embolectomy of the superior mesenteric artery or bypass surgery can reduce the otherwise high mortality rate in these patients. A 'second look' laparotomy 24 hours later to check the viability of the bowel may be indicated.

Other forms of embolism

Infective emboli of bacteria or an infected clot may cause mycotic aneurysms, septicaemia or infected infarcts. Parasitic emboli, caused by the ova of *Taenia echinococcus* and *Filaria sanguinis hominis*, may occur in some countries. Tumour cells (e.g. hypernephroma and cardiac myxoma) are rare causes of emboli. Fat embolism may follow major bony fractures. However, venous emboli to the lungs are more common.

Air embolism

Air may be accidentally injected into the venous circulation or sucked into an open vein during head and neck surgery or a cut throat. It may also occur following Fallopian tube insufflation or illegal abortion. If a large volume of air reaches the right side of the heart it may form an air lock within the pulmonary artery and cause acute right heart failure.

The treatment of air embolism is to put the patient in a head-down (Trendelenburg) position to encourage the air to enter the veins in the lower part of the body. The patient should also be placed on the left side to help the air to float to the ventricular apex, away from the ostium of the pulmonary artery. In extreme cases, air may be aspirated from the heart through a needle introduced below the left costal margin.

Therapeutic embolisation

This is used to arrest haemorrhage from the gastrointestinal, urinary (**Figure 56.31**), gynaecological and respiratory tracts, to treat arteriovenous malformations by blocking their arterial supply and to control the growth of unresectable tumours. Arterial embolisation requires accurate selective catheterisation using the Seldinger technique. A variety of materials may be used, including gelfoam sponge, plastic microspheres, balloons, ethyl alcohol, quick-setting plastics and metal coils.

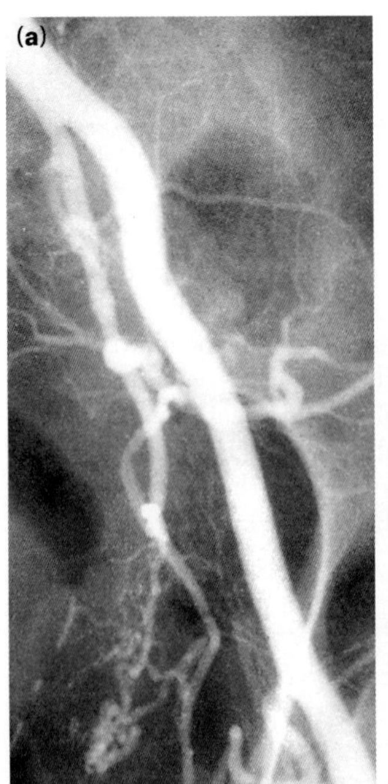

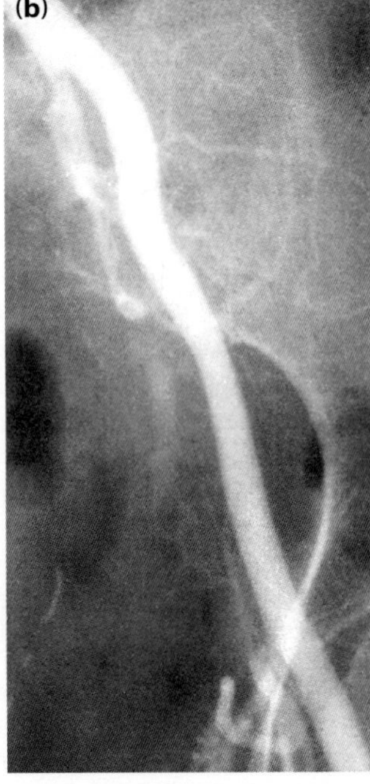

Figure 56.31 Before (**a**) and after (**b**) therapeutic embolisation of the internal iliac artery in a patient with gross haematuria from an ulcerating bladder carcinoma (courtesy of F McIvor, FRCR, London, UK).

Gabrielle Falloppio (Fallopius), 1523–1563, Professor of Anatomy, Surgery and Botany, Padua, Italy.
Friedrich Trendelenburg, 1844–1924, Professor of Surgery successively at Rostock, Bonn and Leipzig, Germany.

AMPUTATION

General

Amputation should be considered when part of a limb is dead, deadly or a dead loss. A limb is dead when arterial occlusive disease is severe enough to cause infarction of macroscopic portions of tissue, i.e. gangrene. The occlusion may be in major vessels (atherosclerotic or embolic occlusions) or in small peripheral vessels (diabetes, Buerger's disease, Raynaud's disease, inadvertent intra-arterial injection). If the obstruction cannot be reversed and the symptoms are severe, amputation is required.

A limb is deadly when the putrefaction and infection of moist gangrene spreads to surrounding viable tissues. Cellulitis and severe toxaemia are the result. Amputation is required as a life-saving operation. Antibiotic cover should be broad and massive. Other life-threatening situations for which amputation may be required include gas gangrene (as opposed to simple infection), neoplasm (such as osteogenic sarcoma) and arteriovenous fistula.

A limb may be deemed a dead loss in the following circumstances: first, when there is relentless severe rest pain without gangrene and reconstruction is not possible – amputation will improve quality of life; second, when a contracture or paralysis makes the limb impossible to use and renders it a hindrance; and third, when there is major unrecoverable traumatic damage.

Summary box 56.3

Indications for amputation

Dead limb
- Gangrene

Deadly limb
- Wet gangrene
- Spreading cellulitis
- Arteriovenous fistula
- Other (e.g. malignancy)

'Dead loss' limb
- Severe rest pain with unreconstructable critical leg ischaemia
- Paralysis
- Other (e.g. contracture, trauma)

Distal and transmetatarsal amputation

In patients with small-vessel disease, typically caused by diabetes mellitus, gangrene of the toes may occur with relatively good blood supply to the surrounding tissues. In such circumstances, local amputation of the digits can result in healing. However, if the metatarsophalangeal joint region is involved, a ray excision is required, taking part of the corresponding metatarsal bone and cutting tendons back. Most surgeons leave the wound open. Early mobility aids drainage provided that cellulitis is not present. For less extensive gangrene, if amputation is taken through a joint, healing is improved by removing the cartilage from the joint surface. A transmetatarsal amputation may be required when several toes are affected but the proximal circulation is adequate. The wound may be closed with a viable long plantar flap (**Figure 56.32**) or left open.

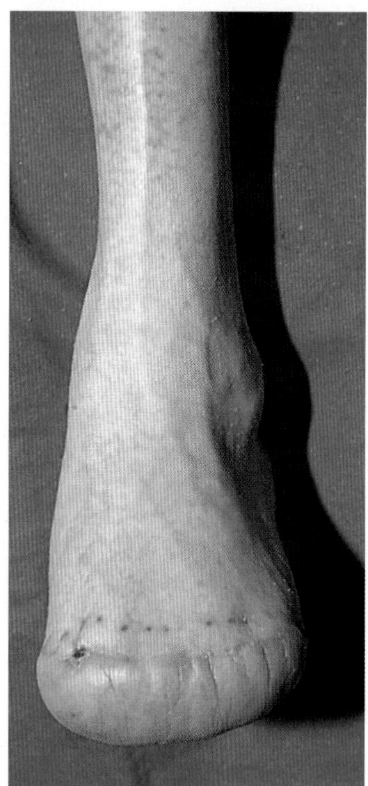

Figure 56.32 Transmetatarsal amputation for diabetic gangrene of the toes.

Major amputation

Choice of operation

The major choice is between an above- and below-knee operation. A below knee amputation preserves the knee joint and gives the best chance of walking again with a prosthesis. However, an above knee amputation is more likely to heal and may be appropriate if the patient has no prospect of walking again. If the femoral pulse is absent, the amputation should be above the knee. Unfortunately, the presence of a femoral pulse does not guarantee healing of a below-knee amputation, and sometimes a failed below-knee amputation may require revision to an above-knee procedure.

For above- or below-knee amputations with a good stump shape, it is possible to hold a prosthesis in place simply by suction, without any cumbersome and unsightly straps. The stump should be of sufficient length to give the required leverage, i.e. not less than 8 cm below the knee (preferably 10–12 cm) and not less than 20 cm above the knee.

Leo Buerger, 1879–1943, Professor of Urologic Surgery, New York Polyclinic Medical School, New York, USA, described thromboangitis obliterans in 1908.
Maurice Raynaud, 1834–1881, physician, Hospital Lariboisière, Paris, France, described this condition in 1862.

Below-knee amputation

Two types of skin flap are commonly used: long posterior flap and skew flap (described by KP Robinson). For both methods, the total length of flap must be at least one and a half times the diameter of the leg at the point of bone section.

The long posterior flap technique is the older method and remains the more popular, probably because of its relative simplicity. The proposed incision should be marked carefully: the tibial tuberosity identified and a distance 10cm measured distally and marked with a sterile marker pen; this is the anterior landmark. The circumference is measured at this landmark with a long suture tie and this length divided into two thirds. The suture is centred over the anterior landmark so that there is one-third either side. The suture ends should be pulled directly posterior; this represents the posterior limit of the transverse incision (**Figures 56.33a–c**). The transverse incision is then marked. From these posterior limits, the incision line is going to extend

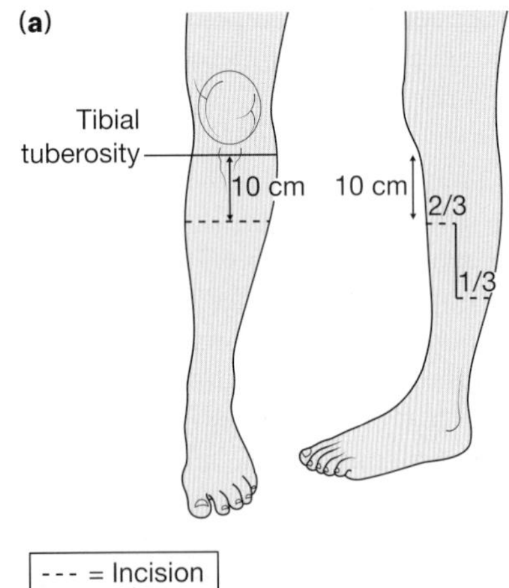

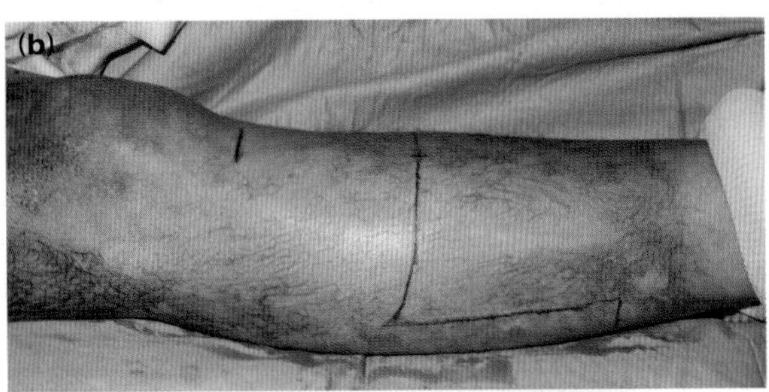

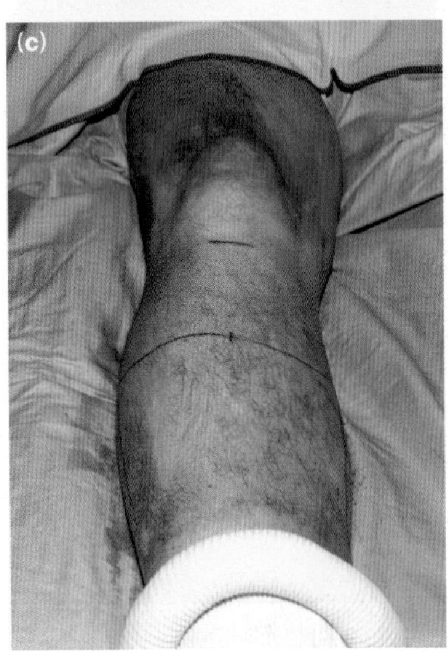

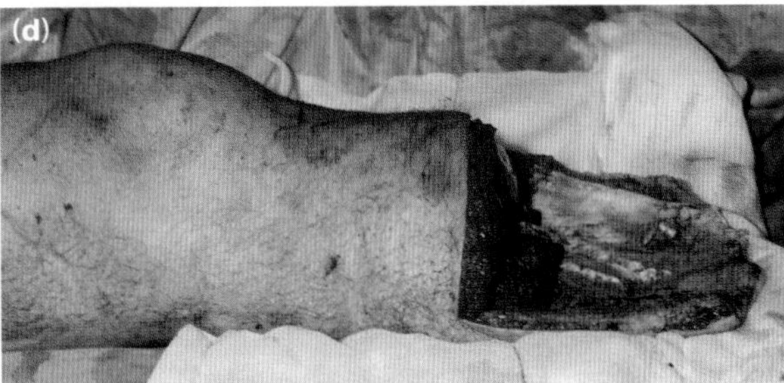

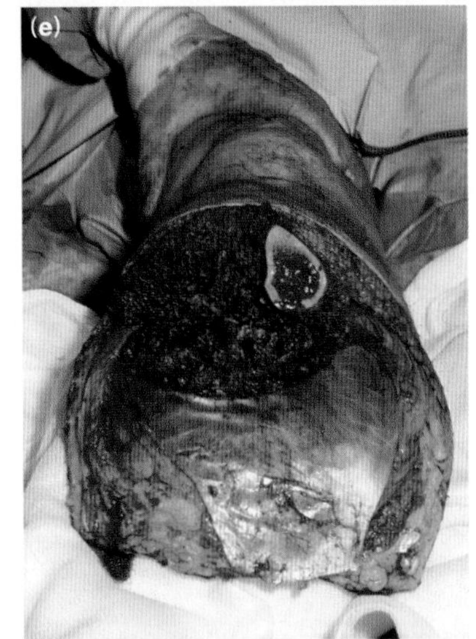

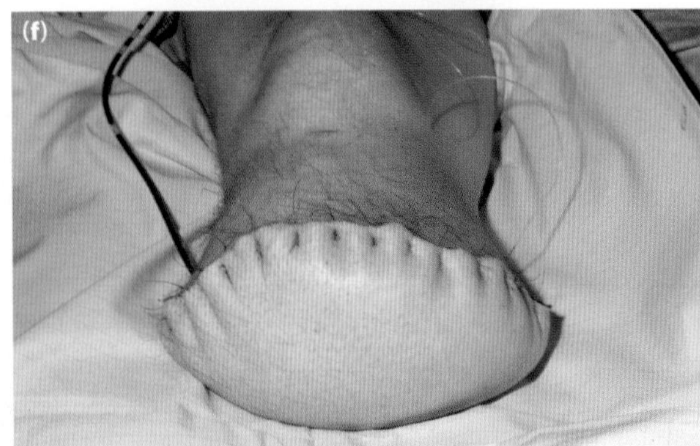

Figure 56.33 **(a)** Schematic representation of operative markings for a long posterior flap below-knee amputation. **(b)** Lateral view of operative markings. **(c)** Anterior view of operative markings. **(d)** Lateral view following removal of the leg. **(e)** Anterior view following removal of the leg. **(f)** Wound closure with suction drain and local anaesthetic infusion 'stump' catheter.

Kingsley Peter Robinson, formerly surgeon, the Westminster Hospital, London, UK.

longitudinally at least half the circumference of the leg at the level of the anterior landmark. The line of incision is now extended transversely around the back of the limb to join the distal extent of the longitudinal incisions. An incision is then made along the previously measured and marked lines through skin, subcutaneous fat and deep fascia. Anteriorly, the incision is deepened to bone and the lateral and posterior incisions are fashioned to leave the bulk of the gastrocnemius muscle attached to the flap, muscle and skin being transected together at the same level.

If bleeding is inadequate, the amputation is refashioned at a higher level. Blood vessels are identified and ligated. Nerves are not clamped but pulled down gently and sharply transected as high as possible. Vessels in nerves are ligated. The fibula is divided 2 cm proximal to the level of tibial division using bone cutters. The tibia is cleared and transected at the desired level, the anterior aspect of the bone being sawn obliquely before the cross-cut is made. This, with filing, gives a smooth anterior bevel, which prevents pressure necrosis of the flap. The long muscle/skin flap is tapered after removing the bulk of the soleus muscle (much of the gastrocnemius may be left unless it is very bulky) (**Figures 56.33d, e**). The area is washed with saline to remove bone fragments and the muscle and fascia are sutured with an absorbable material to bring the flap over the bone ends. A suction drain is placed deep to the muscle and brought out through a stab incision in the skin; a local anaesthetic infusion 'stump' catheter can be inserted for perioperative pain relief. The skin flap should lie in place with all tension taken by the deep sutures (**Figure 56.3f**). Interrupted skin sutures are inserted. Gauze, wool and crepe bandages are usually used for the stump dressing.

The skew flap amputation makes use of anatomical knowledge of the skin blood supply. Equally long fascial-cutaneous flaps are developed; they join anteriorly 2.5 cm from the tibial crest, overlying the anterior tibial compartment, and posteriorly at the exact opposite point on the circumference of the leg. After division of bone and muscle in a fashion similar to that described above, the gastrocnemius myoplastic flap is sutured over the cut bone end to the anterior tibial periosteum with absorbable sutures. Finally, drainage and skin sutures are inserted and the limb dressed as for the long posterior flap operation.

Above-knee amputation

The site is chosen as indicated above but may need to be higher if bleeding is poor on incision of the skin. Equal curved anterior and posterior skin flaps are made of sufficient total length. Skin, deep fascia and muscle are transected in the same line. Vessels are ligated. The sciatic nerve is pulled down and transected cleanly, as high as possible, and the accompanying artery ligated. Muscle and skin are retracted and the bone cleared and sawn at the point chosen. Haemostasis is achieved. The muscle ends are united over the bone by absorbable sutures incorporating the fascia. A suction drain deep to the muscle is brought out through the skin clear of the wound. The fascia and subcutaneous tissues are further brought together so that the skin can be apposed by interrupted sutures. Gauze, wool and crepe bandages form the stump dressing.

Through-knee amputation

More recently through-knee or knee disarticulation has regained popularity as an alternative to above-knee amputation if soft-tissue viability permits. This amputation preserves the full length of the femur and patella, providing a long mechanical lever that is controlled by stronger muscles as the line of muscle transection is distal and occurs through fascial tissue, as opposed to thick muscular bellies as is the case with an above-knee amputation. The bulbous nature of the amputation end, initially thought a hindrance for subsequent prosthetic fitting, is now seen as beneficial as it allows for a self-suspending prosthetic that is less likely to rotate compared to an above-knee amputation prosthetic. For the patient unlikely to mobilise with a prosthetic, e.g. elderly patients or patients with bilateral amputations, the increased length of the stump provides better counterweight to the torso, enabling better core stability.

The line of incision is marked preoperatively: equal anterior and posterior semicircular flaps are constructed, with the proximal extent of incision being the joint line laterally and medially, and the distal extent of the anterior flap being 3 cm below the tibial tuberosity and directly posterior to this level for the posterior flap. The anterior incision is carried down to the tibia and the patellar tendon insertion into the tibial tuberosity is identified and released. The patellar tendon is followed proximally to the patella, releasing it from surrounding fascial structures. The anterior knee capsule is entered and the lateral and medial capsule divided along with the collateral knee ligaments. The cruciate ligaments are released from their tibial insertions. The knee is flexed to 90° and the dense posterior capsule divided, paying attention to identify the popliteal artery and vein located immediately behind the capsule. The tibial and peroneal nerves are sharply divided. The medial head of the gastrocnemius muscle along with its vascular pedicle is transected 3 cm below the tibial plateau. The lateral head of the gastrocnemius muscle is divided at the level of the knee joint. The popliteal artery and vein are ligated distal to the medial head of gastrocnemius pedicle origin. The posterior flap incision is now carried through to join the anterior dissection and the limb is removed. The menisci do not need to be removed but can be trimmed to provide a smooth surface. With the hip flexed the patellar tendon is pulled down and sutured to the posterior cruciate ligament with polypropylene, restoring the normal position of the patellar tendon between the femoral condyles. The hamstring muscles are sutured to the posterior capsule. The residual head of gastrocnemius is retroflexed and sutured to the knee capsule, to provide a covering of the femur and reduce synovial fluid drainage. A suction drain is applied to the muscle bed and the skin flaps closed with skin clips or sutures

Postoperative care of an amputee

Opiate pain relief should be given regularly. Care of the good limb must not be forgotten, as a pressure ulcer on the remaining foot will delay mobilisation despite satisfactory healing of the stump. Exercise and mobilisation are of the greatest importance. After surgery, flexion deformity must be prevented and exercises started to build up muscle power and coordination. Mobility is progressively increased with walking between bars and the use of an inflatable artificial limb, which allows weight-bearing to be started before a pylon or temporary artificial limb is ready (**Figure 56.34**). Early assessment of the home is part of the programme; it allows time for minor alterations, such as the addition of stair rails, movement of furniture to give support near doors and provision of clearance in confined passages.

Complications

Early complications include haemorrhage, which requires return to the operating room for haemostasis; haematoma, which requires evacuation; and infection, usually in association with a haematoma. Any abscess must be drained and appropriate antibiotics given. Gas gangrene can occur in a mid-thigh stump from faecal contamination. Wound dehiscence and gangrene of the flaps are caused by ischaemia; a higher amputation may be necessary. Amputees are at risk of deep vein thrombosis and pulmonary embolism in the early postoperative period and prophylaxis with subcutaneous heparin is essential.

Later complications include pain resulting from unresolved infection (sinus, osteitis, sequestrum), a bone spur, a scar adherent to bone and an amputation neuroma. Patients frequently remark that they can feel the amputated limb (phantom limb) and sometimes remark that it is painful (phantom pain). The surgeon's attitude should be one of firm reassurance that this sensation will almost certainly disappear with time; amitriptyline or gabapentin may help. Other late complications include ulceration of the stump because of pressure effects of the prosthesis or increased ischaemia.

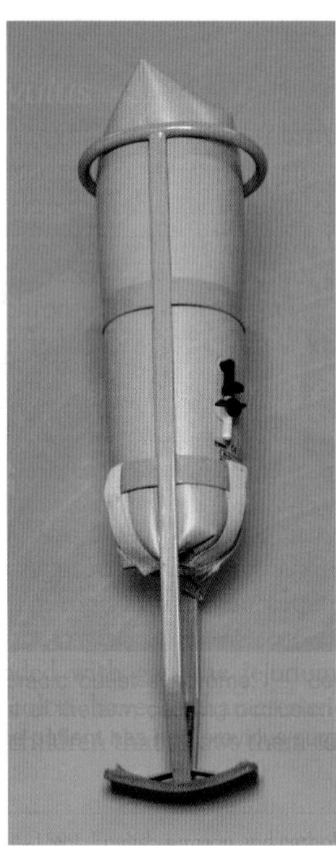

Figure 56.34 Inflatable artificial limb.

ANEURYSM

General

Dilatations of localised segments of the arterial system are called aneurysms when there is a >50% increase in the diameter of the vessel; below 50% they are termed ectactic. They can either be true aneurysms, containing the three layers of the arterial wall (intima, media, adventitia) in the aneurysm sac, or false aneurysms, having a single layer of fibrous tissue as the wall of the sac, e.g. aneurysm following trauma. Aneurysms can also be grouped according to their shape (fusiform, saccular) or their aetiology (atheromatous, traumatic, mycotic, etc.). The term mycotic is a misnomer because, although it indicates infection as the cause of the aneurysm, it is due to bacteria, not fungi. Aneurysms may occur in the aorta, iliac, femoral, popliteal, subclavian, axillary, carotid, cerebral, mesenteric, splenic and renal arteries and their branches. The majority are true fusiform atherosclerotic aneurysms.

Summary box 56.4

Classification of aneurysms

Wall

- True (three layers: intima, media, adventitia)
- False (single layer of fibrous tissue)

Morphology

- Fusiform
- Saccular

Aetiology

- Atheromatous
- Mycotic (bacterial rather than fungal)
- Collagen disease
- Traumatic

Clinical features

The majority of arterial aneurysms are asymptomatic at the time of identification and are often identified during routine health checks or investigations for other pathologies. All aneurysms can cause symptoms, but aneurysms measuring twice the size of the corresponding normal vessel are at increased risk of complications. The symptoms relate to the vessel affected and the tissues it supplies and occur as a result of compression of surrounding structures, thrombosis, rupture or the release of emboli. Many aneurysms of clinical significance can be palpated and, typically, an expansile pulsation is felt. Transmitted pulsation through a mass lesion, cyst or abscess lying adjacent to a large artery may be mistaken for aneurysmal pulsation. Before incising a swelling believed to be an abscess, it is essential to make sure that it does not pulsate. Finally, a tortuous (and often ectatic) artery, usually the innominate or carotid, may seem like an aneurysm to the inexperienced clinician.

Abdominal aortic aneurysm

Abdominal aortic aneurysm (AAA) is by far the most common type of large vessel aneurysm and is found in 2% of the population at autopsy; 95% have associated atheromatous degeneration and 95% occur below the renal arteries. Most remain asymptomatic until rupture occurs; the risk of rupture increases with increasing size (diameter) of the aneurysm. Asymptomatic aneurysms are found incidentally on physical examination, radiography or ultrasound investigation. A national screening programme for AAA has recently started in England and offers an ultrasound scan to men in their 65th year. Symptomatic aneurysms may cause minor symptoms, such as back and abdominal discomfort, before sudden, severe back and/or abdominal pain develops from expansion and rupture. Rarely, symptoms may occur as a result of erosion or compression of surrounding structures, e.g. aortoenteric fistula, ureteric obstruction.

Asymptomatic abdominal aortic aneurysm

An asymptomatic abdominal aortic aneurysm (**Figure 56.35**) in an otherwise fit patient should be considered for repair if >55 mm in diameter (measured by ultrasonography). The annual incidence of rupture rises from 1% or less in aneurysms that are <55 mm in diameter to a significant level, perhaps as high as 25%, in those that are 70 mm in diameter. Assuming open elective surgery (transabdominal) carries a 5% mortality rate, the balance is in favour of elective operation once the maximum diameter is >55 mm, provided there is no major comorbidity. Regular ultrasonographic assessment is indicated for asymptomatic aneurysms <55 mm in diameter.

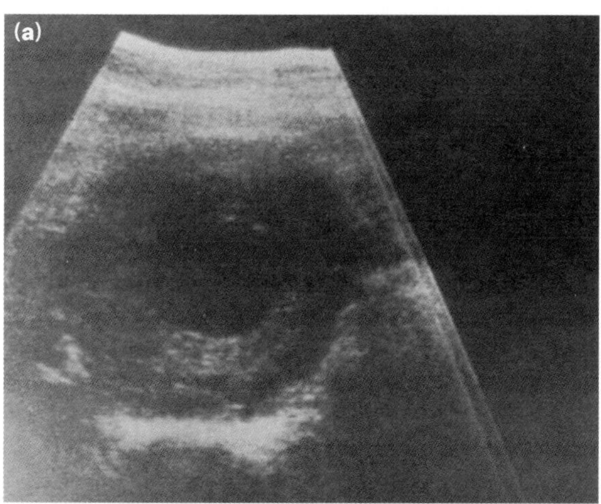

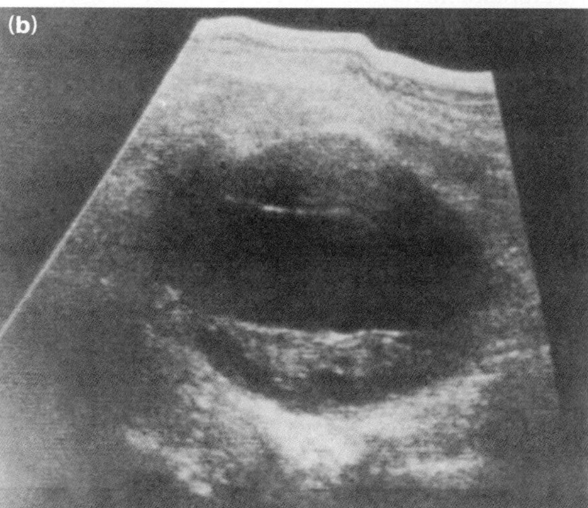

Figure 56.35 Ultrasonogram of an aortic aneurysm showing the large clot-filled sac with a small central lumen (transverse and longitudinal scans).

Investigations

Full blood count, electrolytes, liver function tests, coagulation tests and blood lipid estimation should be performed. Blood should be cross-matched a few days prior to surgery. Many patients now have an anaesthetic assessment and the need for cardiac and respiratory function tests are decided at this time. ECG and chest radiographs are essential; further assessment may include echocardiography or isotope ventriculography, cardiopulmonary exercise testing and spirometry.

The morphology of the aneurysm is best assessed by CT scan (**Figures 56.36 and 56.37**). 75% of aneurysms are suitable for endovascular (minimally invasive) repair, usually via the femoral arteries in the groin. If lower limb pulses are absent, there may be associated arterial occlusive disease that should be assessed by duplex scanning initially. Further assessment with CT, MR or DSA may be required and angioplasty may be appropriate. The aneurysm is often filled with circumferential clot (**Figure 56.38a**) that produces a falsely narrowed appearance on DSA (**Figure 56.38b**); this method should not therefore be used to assess aneurysm size.

Choice of operation – open or endovascular repair

Open aneurysm repair

Under general anaesthesia, with the patient lying supine, a full-length midline or supraumbilical transverse incision is

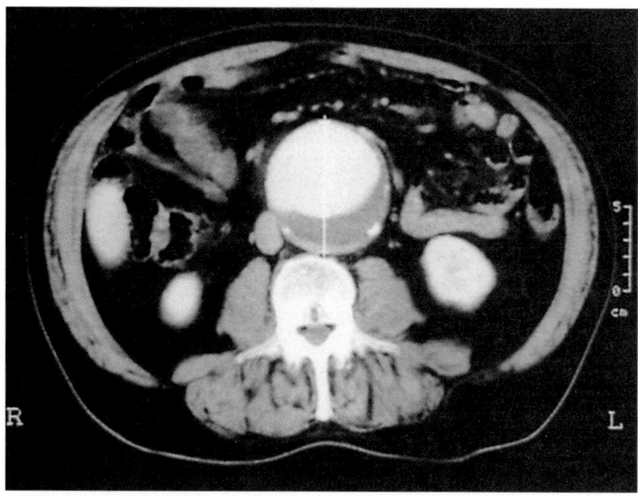

Figure 56.36 Computed tomogram of the abdomen showing an aortic aneurysm. Blood flowing through the thrombus-containing sac is enhanced with contrast agent and appears white.

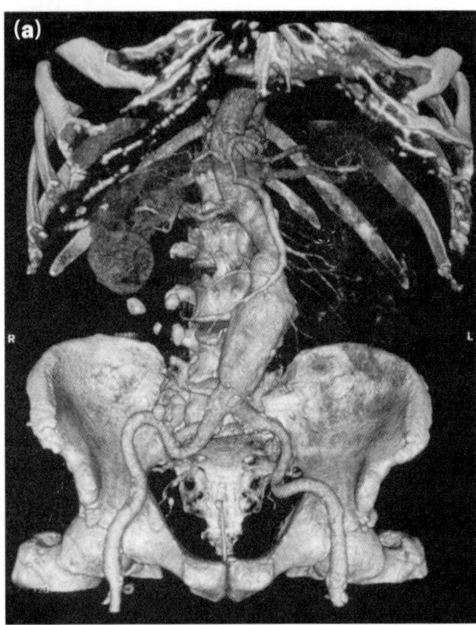

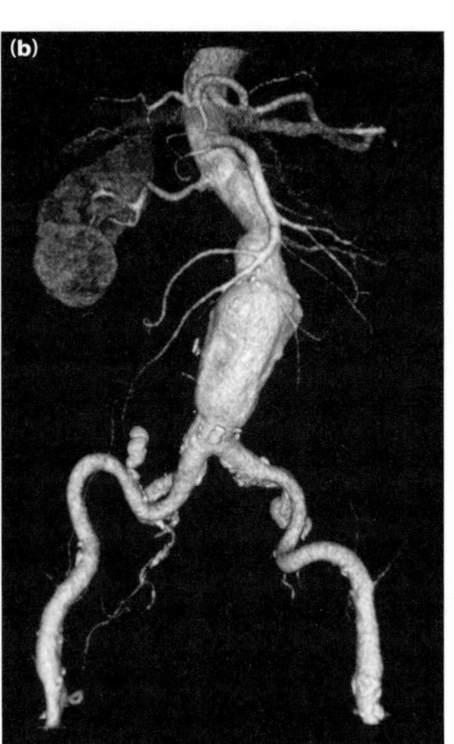

Figure 56.37 (**a**) Spiral computed tomogram showing an infrarenal abdominal aortic aneurysm; (**b**) with the bony elements subtracted.

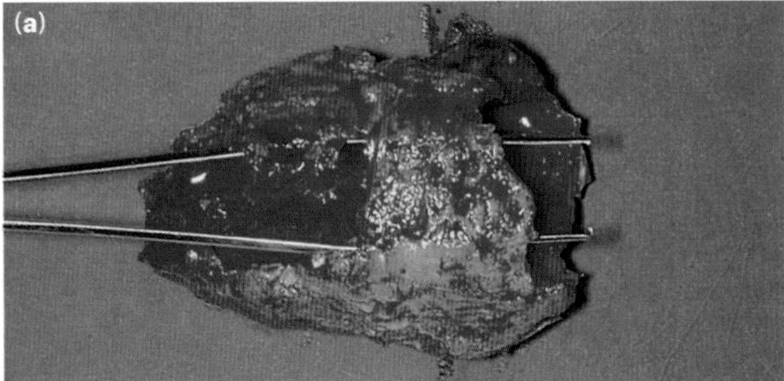

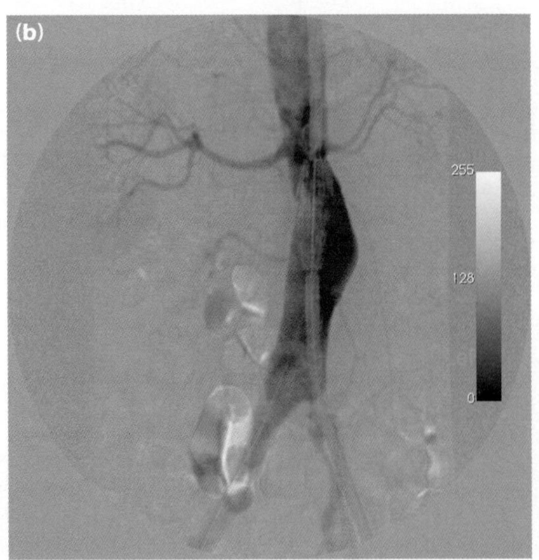

Figure 56.38 (**a**) Thrombus removed from an abdominal aortic aneurysm; this thrombus is the reason an angiogram may give a false impression of aneurysm diameter on digital subtraction angiography (**b**).

made. The small bowel is lifted to the patient's right and the aorta identified. The posterior peritoneum overlying the aorta is opened and the upper limit of the aneurysm identified. The aorta immediately above the dilatation is exposed; this is generally just inferior to the left renal vein and renal arteries (**Figure 56.39**). The common iliac arteries are then exposed and clamps applied above and below the lesion. Many surgeons give systemic heparin before clamping. The aneurysm is opened longitudinally and back-bleeding from lumbar and mesenteric vessels controlled by sutures placed from within the sac. Upper and lower aortic necks are prepared to which an aortic prosthesis is then sutured end-to-end inside the sac with a monofilament non-absorbable suture (**Figure 56.40**). Clamps are released slowly to prevent sudden hypotension. If haemostasis is satisfactory at this point, the aneurysm sac is closed around the prosthesis to exclude both it and the suture lines from the bowel, to reduce the risk of adherence and potential fistula formation. The abdomen is then closed. Occasionally, when the iliac vessels are also involved with dilatation or severe atheroma, it is necessary to construct an aortobi-iliac or aortobifemoral bypass, rather than use a simple aortoaortic tube.

Endovascular aneurysm repair

Endovascular aneurysm repair (EVAR) is now established in clinical practice and has been shown to reduce mortality compared to open repair over the first 6 years. Currently, about 75% of infrarenal aneurysms are suitable for EVAR, depending on the morphology of the aneurysm assessed by CT scan. Common causes of unsuitability include a short, flared or angulated neck and difficult iliac artery access because of

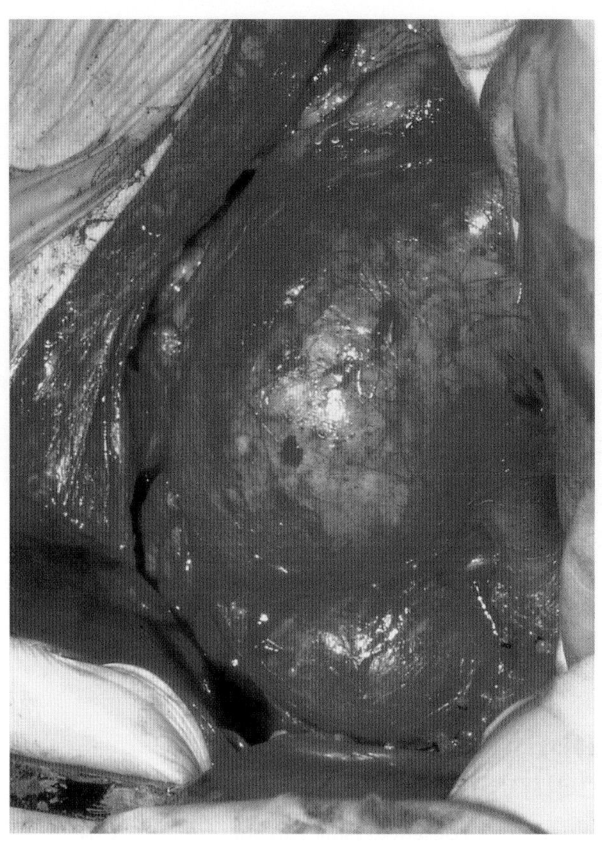

Figure 56.39 Operative appearance of a large, non-ruptured infrarenal abdominal aortic aneurysm.

narrowing or tortuosity. The usual technique is to expose both femoral arteries (under general or local anaesthetic), which allows access to the aorta. Then, under radiological control, guidewires and catheters are used to cross the aneurysm and an angiogram performed to mark the level of the renal arteries.

The endovascular prosthesis (often termed a 'stent graft') is usually made up of three separate parts – a main body (**Figure 56.41a**) and two limbs, which are enclosed in separate delivery catheters (**Figure 56.41b**). Some types have only two pieces, a main body with ipsilateral limb attached and a separate contralateral limb. The prosthesis is made from Dacron® or PTFE, with integral metallic stents for support. The delivery catheter is inserted in the aneurysm sac and the stent-graft deployed by withdrawal of the delivery system. Most systems now have hooks or barbs to anchor the prosthesis in the aortic wall and some surgeons inflate a moulding balloon catheter in the stent-graft to ensure the hooks and barbs are engaged and a good seal is obtained (**Figure 56.42**). Although the top edge of the fabric of the stent-graft has to be deployed below the renal arteries (infrarenal fixation), some systems have additional bare metal stents at the proximal end of the main body that lie across the renal arteries to give better support and fixation (suprarenal fixation). Blood flows between the metal struts of the stent into the renal arteries. Success is dependent on a good seal between the stent-graft and the proximal and distal 'landing zones' in the aorta and iliac arteries. Failure to achieve a good seal results in an endoleak, that means that the aneurysm is not excluded from the circulation and may still expand and rupture. Patients who undergo EVAR require

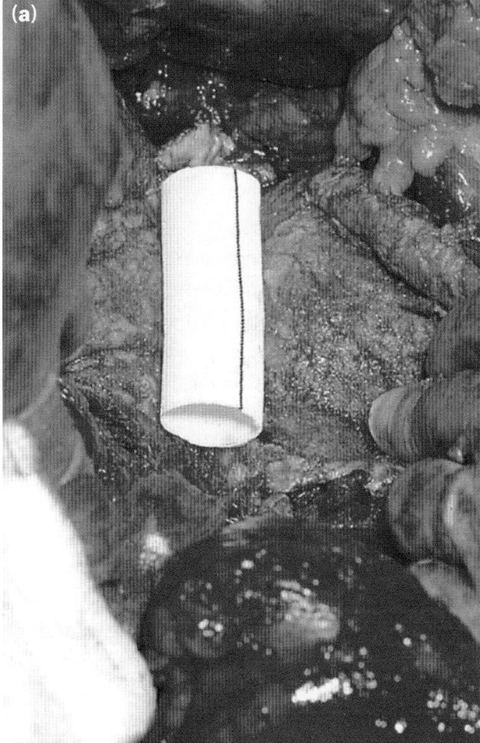

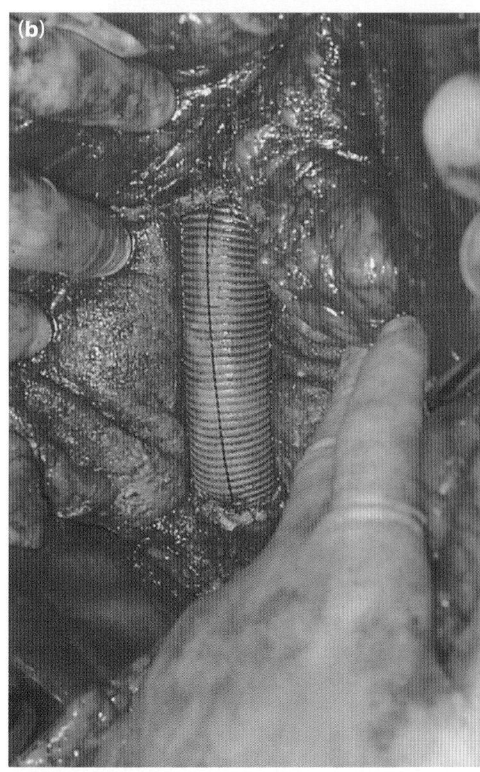

Figure 56.40 (**a**) Aneurysm sac opened. Note that the posterior wall of the aorta immediately above and below the sac is not divided. A Dacron tube graft is laid in place within the sac ready for suture. (**b**) Graft sutured in place and vascular clamps removed.

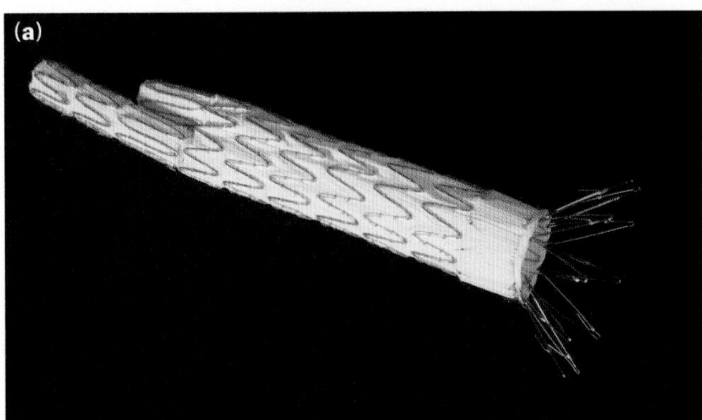

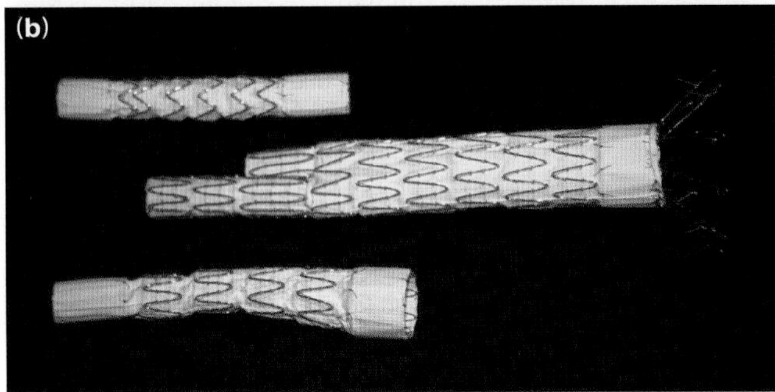

Figure 56.41 (**a**) Endovascular prosthesis main body, with separate limbs (**b**).

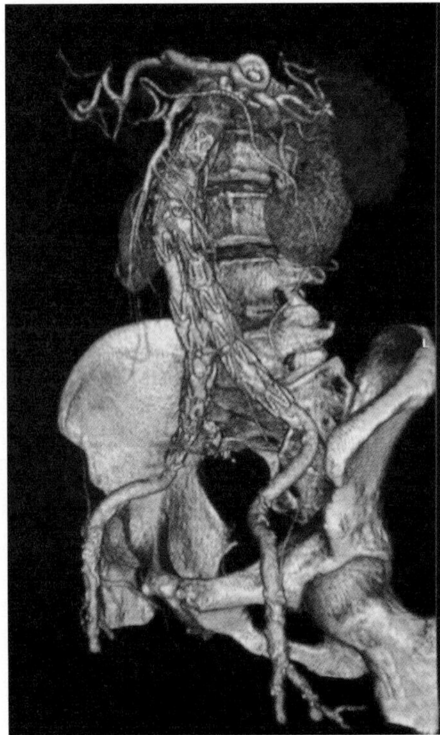

Figure 56.42 Spiral computed tomogram showing an endoluminal aortoiliac 'stent-graft'. The metallic stent structure is clearly observed.

life-long follow-up and surveillance with duplex or CT scans to detect endoleak, disconnection of the components and migration of the stent-graft, all of which predispose to late rupture (**Figure 56.43**).

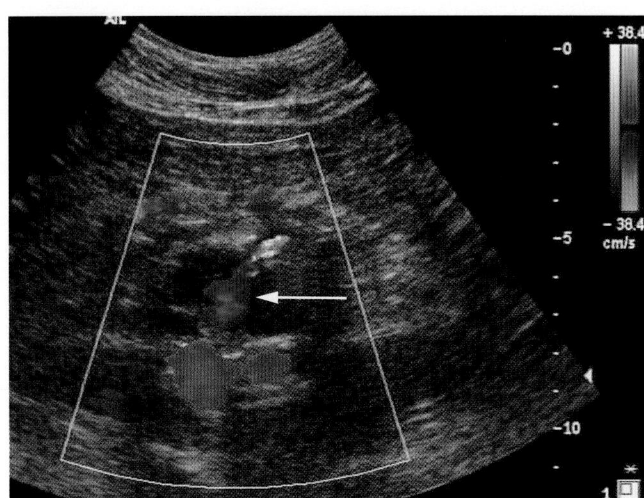

Figure 56.43 Duplex ultrasound scan post endovascular aneurysm repair (EVAR), showing the aortic sac in cross-section and two limbs of EVAR (red ovals). There is a type II endoleak from the inferior mesenteric artery, with blood flowing retrogradely into the aneurysm sac (arrow)

Ruptured abdominal aortic aneurysm

Abdominal aortic aneurysms can rupture anteriorly into the peritoneal cavity (20%) or posterolaterally into the retroperitoneal space (80%). Less than 50% of patients with rupture survive to reach hospital. Anterior rupture results in free bleeding into the peritoneal cavity; very few patients reach hospital alive. Posterior rupture, on the other hand, produces a retroperitoneal haematoma (**Figure 56.44**). Often a brief period ensues when a combination of moderate hypotension and the resistance of the retroperitoneal tissues arrests further haemorrhage and may allow transport to hospital. The patient may remain conscious but in severe pain. If no operation is performed, death is virtually inevitable. Operative mortality is around 50% and the overall combined mortality (community and hospital) is around 80–90%.

Ruptured abdominal aortic aneurysm is a surgical emergency; it should be suspected in a patient with the triad of severe abdominal and/or back pain, hypotension and a pulsatile abdominal mass. If there is doubt about the presence of an aneurysm an ultrasound scan may help, but this **cannot** diagnose rupture. CT scanning should be used to establish the diagnosis and to determine whether an endovascular repair is possible.

Good venous access is needed for infusion of saline or volume expanding fluids, but the systolic blood pressure should not be raised any more than is necessary to maintain consciousness and permit cardiac perfusion (<100 mmHg). Many surgeons now adopt a policy of permissive hypotension, where fluids are withheld if the patient is conscious (and cerebral perfusion is therefore adequate) in order to avoid provoking further uncontrolled haemorrhage. After CT scanning, the patient should be transferred immediately to an operating theatre, where a urinary catheter and arterial line are usually inserted. If the patient appears stable, surgery may be delayed

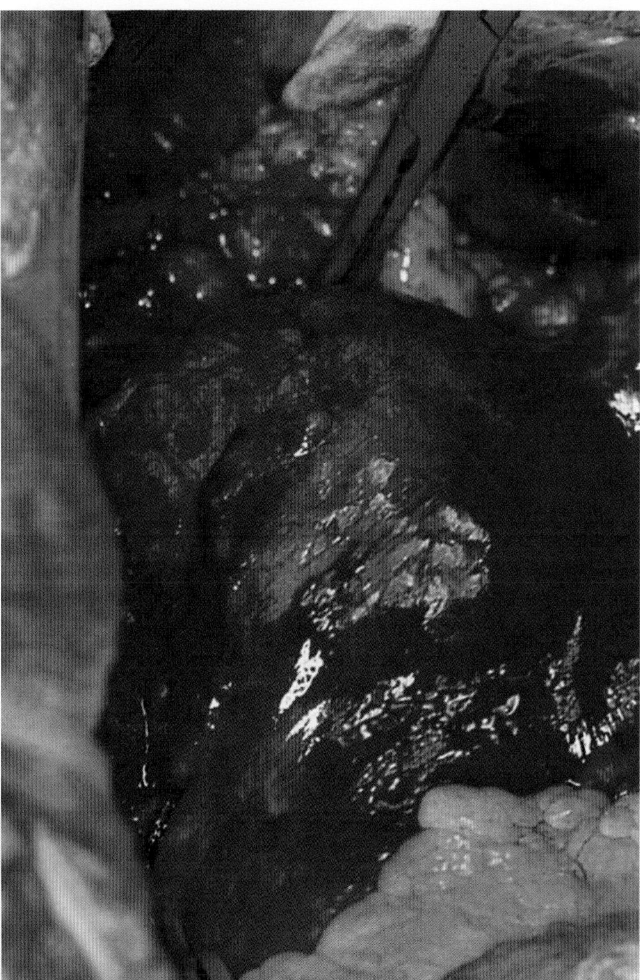

Figure 56.44 The retroperitoneal haematoma of a ruptured aortic aneurysm. The aortic pulsation is palpated through the haematoma at its upper limit and fingers are insinuated on each side of the aorta. With finger control, the upper clamp is positioned and closed on the aorta. The procedure is then as for a planned case. In this illustration, the clamp is at the proximal end of the aneurysm; the haematoma has spread from the left paracolic gutter to encircle the aneurysm and the aortic bifurcation.

until cross-matched blood is available but surgery should commence immediately if haemodynamic instability develops. The abdomen is usually prepared and draped with the patient awake. It is important to remember that the treatment of ruptured aneurysm is operation, not monitoring and resuscitation.

Summary box 56.5

Management of ruptured abdominal aortic aneurysm

- Early diagnosis (abdominal/back pain, pulsatile mass, shock)
- Immediate resuscitation (oxygen, intravenous replacement therapy, central line)
- Maintain systolic pressure, but not >100 mmHg, consider permissive hypotension
- Urinary catheter
- Cross-match 6 units of blood
- Rapid transfer to the operating room

Symptomatic abdominal aortic aneurysm

These patients most commonly present with abdominal and/or back pain but the aneurysm is not ruptured on CT scan. Pain may also occur in the thigh and groin because of nerve compression. Gastrointestinal, urinary and venous symptoms can also be caused by pressure from an abdominal aneurysm. About 3% of all aneurysms cause pain as a result of inflammation of the aneurysm itself (Figure 56.45). Finally, a few cause symptoms from distal embolisation of fragments of their intraluminal thrombus. An operation is usually indicated in patients who are otherwise reasonably fit. Pain may be a warning sign of stretching of the aneurysm sac and imminent rupture; surgery should be performed as soon as possible (usually on the next available operating list). The operative mortality of symptomatic aneurysms is usually higher than elective cases.

Postoperative complications

The most common complications after open repair are cardiac (ischaemia and infarction) and respiratory (atelectasis and lower lobe consolidation). A degree of colonic ischaemia

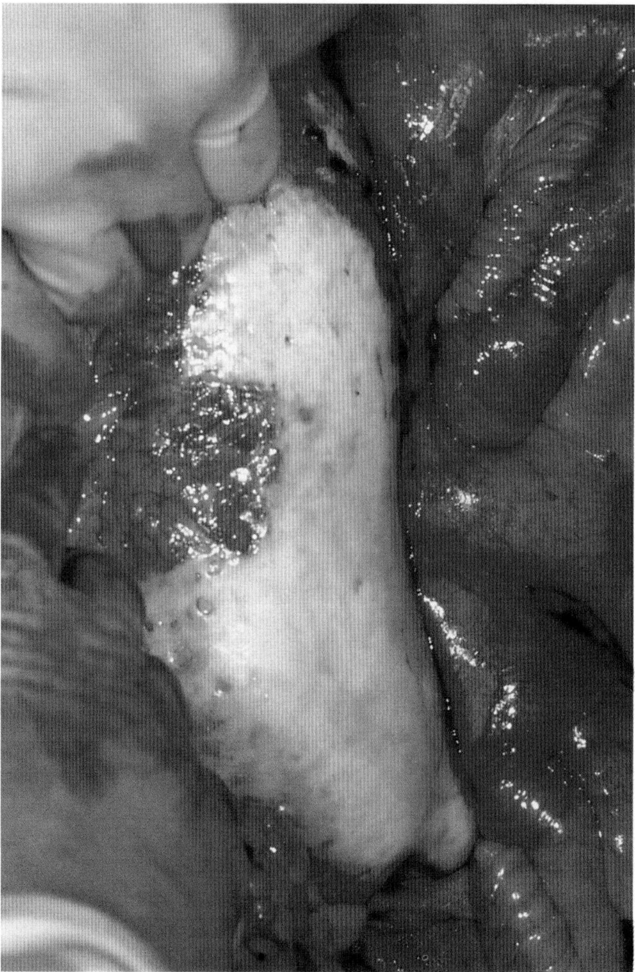

Figure 56.45 An inflammatory abdominal aortic aneurysm. Note the white 'icing' effect. Such lesions can be technically difficult to manage.

because of lack of a collateral blood supply occurs in about 10% of patients, but fortunately this usually resolves spontaneously. Renal failure is an uncommon event after elective procedures but may complicate procedures undertaken for rupture. Renal failure is more likely if there is preoperative renal impairment or considerable intraoperative blood loss. Neurological complications include sexual dysfunction and spinal cord ischaemia. An aortoduodenal fistula is an uncommon but treatable complication of abdominal aortic replacement surgery. It should be suspected whenever haematemesis or melaena occurs in the months or years after operation. Prosthetic graft infection is also uncommon; it may require explantation of the original graft and replacement with an autologous deep vein (superficial femoral vein) graft limb, or removal of the original graft with oversewing of the aortic stump and limb revascularisation by insertion of an axillobifemoral bypass. Both techniques are associated with significant risk of perioperative morbidity and mortality.

Cardiac, respiratory, renal and neurological complications are less common after endovascular repair. However, there are complications that are unique to EVAR such as endoleak, graft migration, metal strut fracture and graft limb occlusion. Life-long surveillance with duplex or CT (together with plain abdominal x-ray for strut fracture) is required to detect endoleak and migration. High-pressure endoleaks may require repeat ballooning or a proximal cuff or distal limb extension to reseal the endograft. Migration may also require extension of the graft. Overall, 10–20% of patients with EVAR will require secondary interventions to treat complications at some future date, although many of the interventions can be performed with a percutaneous approach via the femoral artery in the angiography suite.

Peripheral aneurysm

Popliteal aneurysm

Popliteal artery aneurysm accounts for 70% of all peripheral aneurysms classically diagnosed in males in their seventh decade of life; 50% are bilateral. Examination of the abdominal aorta is indicated if a popliteal aneurysm is found because one-third are accompanied by aortic dilatation.

Popliteal aneurysms present as a swelling behind the knee or with symptoms caused by complications, such as severe ischaemia following thrombosis or distal ischaemia as a result of emboli. The diagnosis is usually confirmed with duplex scanning but assessment of the distal vessels (with CT, MR or DSA) is important prior to repair if the foot pulses are diminished or absent. An asymptomatic aneurysm exceeding 20 mm in diameter should be considered for elective repair, to prevent future complications. Some surgeons would also offer elective repair for smaller diameters if the sac contains thrombus, because of a perceived increased risk of distal embolisation. All symptomatic popliteal aneurysms, including those in which single crural vessel embolisation has occurred, should be considered for repair.

Two techniques for surgical repair may be used: exclusion bypass and inlay repair. An exclusion bypass involves a medial approach to the above- and below-knee popliteal arteries, ligation of the aneurysm and restoration of flow to the foot with a bypass graft using saphenous vein. Many surgeons favour this approach because the anatomy is similar to that for a femoropopliteal bypass and therefore familiar. An inlay graft repair is performed through a posterior approach and has the benefits of allowing free ligation of feeding geniculate branches as well as aneurysmectomy in cases with neurovascular compression. However, the posterior approach limits exposure of the superficial femoral and crural arteries and should only be used when the popliteal aneurysm is confined to the popliteal fossa.

In the acute situation, the presentation is usually with a thrombosed aneurysm and an ischaemic foot; popliteal aneurysms very rarely rupture. Surgery is often unsuccessful because the distal vessels are thrombosed and difficult to clear. Attempts should be made with a Fogarty catheter and intra-arterial thrombolysis. The limb loss rate is high (50%).

Femoral aneurysm

True aneurysm of the femoral artery is uncommon. Complications occur in less than 3% so conservative treatment is generally indicated, but it is important to look for aneurysms elsewhere as over half are associated with abdominal or popliteal aneurysms. Large aneurysms should be repaired. False aneurysm of the femoral artery occurs in 2% of patients after arterial surgery at this site. Local repair may involve reanastomosis of the bypass in the groin under suitable antibiotic cover. However, if infection is the cause, the treatment may involve excision of the infected graft and insertion of a further bypass routed around the infected area. In the latter case, the failure rate is high, and limb loss may be unavoidable. For false aneurysms caused by femoral artery puncture measuring <3 cm, thrombin injection under ultrasound guidance may be successful and avoids surgery. False aneurysms measuring >3 cm are unlikely to be successfully treated by thrombin injection and require open surgical arterial repair with suturing of the puncture site.

Iliac aneurysm

This usually occurs in conjunction with aortic aneurysm and only rarely on its own. When occurring in isolation it is difficult to diagnose clinically, so about half present already ruptured. Open surgery usually involves an inlay graft but some iliac aneurysms may be suitable for EVAR.

Arteriovenous fistula

Communication between an artery and a vein (or veins) may be either a congenital malformation or the result of trauma. Arteriovenous fistulas for haemodialysis access are also created surgically. All arteriovenous communications have a structural and a physiological effect. The structural effect of arterial blood flow on the veins is characteristic; they become dilated, tortuous and thick walled (arterialised). The physiological effect, if the fistula is big enough, is an increase in cardiac output. In extreme circumstances this can cause left ventricular enlargement and even cardiac failure.

A pulsatile swelling may be present if the lesion is superficial. A thrill is detected on palpation and auscultation reveals a buzzing continuous bruit ('machinery murmur'). Dilated veins may be seen, in which there is rapid blood flow. Pressure on the artery proximal to the fistula reduces the swelling and the thrill and bruit cease.

Duplex scan and/or angiography confirms the lesion, which is noteworthy for the speed with which venous filling occurs.

Management

Treatment is by embolisation. Excision surgery can be advocated only rarely, perhaps for severe deformity or recurrent haemorrhage; the assistance of a plastic surgeon is wise. It is important to realise that ligation of a 'feeding' artery on its own is of no lasting value and is actually detrimental as it may preclude treatment by embolisation.

ARTERITIS AND VASOSPASTIC CONDITIONS

Thromboangiitis obliterans (Buerger's disease)

This is characterised by occlusive disease of small- and medium-sized arteries (plantar, tibial, radial, etc.), thrombophlebitis of the superficial or deep veins and Raynaud's syndrome; it occurs in male smokers, usually under the age of 30 years. Often, only one or two of the three manifestations are present. Histologically, there are inflammatory changes in the walls of arteries and veins, leading to thrombosis. Treatment is total abstinence from smoking, which arrests, but does not reverse, the disease. Established arterial occlusions are treated as for atheromatous disease, but amputations may eventually be required.

Other forms of arteritis

Arteritis occurs in association with many connective tissue disorders, e.g. rheumatoid arthritis, systemic lupus erythematosus and polyarteritis nodosa. This is usually the province of the specialist physician, but the surgeon may be called on to carry out minor amputations. Sympathectomy has previously been used but is usually ineffective.

Temporal arteritis is a disease in which localised infiltration with inflammatory and giant cells leads to arterial occlusion, ischaemic headache and tender, palpable, pulseless (thrombosed) arteries in the scalp. Irreversible blindness occurs if the ophthalmic artery becomes occluded. The surgeon may be required to perform a temporal artery biopsy, but this should not delay immediate steroid therapy to arrest and reverse the process before the ophthalmic artery is involved. The length of the biopsy should be at least 2.5 cm.

Takayasu's disease is an arteritis that obstructs major arteries, particularly the large vessels coming off the aortic arch. It usually pursues a relentless course.

Cystic myxomatous degeneration

This is typified by an accumulation of clear jelly (like a synovial ganglion) in the outer layers of a main artery, especially the popliteal artery. The lesion may narrow the vessel, causing claudication. Duplex scan is the investigation of choice. Decompression, by removal of the myxomatous material, is often all that is required, but the 'ganglion' may recur, necessitating excision of part of the artery with interposition vein graft repair.

Raynaud's disease

This idiopathic condition usually occurs in young women and affects the hands more than the feet. There is abnormal sensitivity in the arteriolar response to cold. These vessels constrict and the digits (usually the fingers) turn white and become incapable of fine movements. The capillaries then dilate and fill with slowly flowing deoxygenated blood, resulting in the digits becoming swollen and dusky. As the attack passes off, the arterioles relax, oxygenated blood returns into the dilated capillaries and the digits become red. Thus, the condition is recognised by the characteristic sequence of blanching, dusky cyanosis and red engorgement, often accompanied by pain. Superficial necrosis is very uncommon. This condition must be distinguished from Raynaud's syndrome, which has similar features (see below). Treatment of Raynaud's disease consists of protection from cold and avoidance of pulp and nail bed infection. Calcium antagonists, such as nifedipine, may also have a role to play and electrically heated gloves can be useful in winter. Sympathectomy has been used in the past but it is either ineffective or its effects are short-lived.

Raynaud's syndrome

Although peripheral vasospasm may be noted in atherosclerosis, thoracic outlet syndrome, carpal tunnel syndrome, etc., the term Raynaud's syndrome is most often used for a peripheral arterial manifestation of a collagen disease, such as systemic lupus erythematosus or rheumatoid arthritis. The clinical features are as for Raynaud's disease but they may be much more aggressive. Raynaud's syndrome may also follow the use of vibrating tools. In this context, it is a recognised industrial disease and is known as 'vibration white finger'.

Treatment is directed primarily at the underlying condition, although the conservative measures outlined above are often helpful. The syndrome when secondary to collagen disease leads frequently to necrosis of digits and multiple amputations. Sympathectomy yields disappointing results and is not recommended. Nifedipine, steroids and vasospastic antagonists may all have a role in treatment. Patients with vibration white finger should avoid vibrating tools.

Acrocyanosis

Acrocyanosis may be confused with Raynaud's disease but it is painless and not episodic. It tends to affect young women

Mikito Takayasu, 1860–1938, Japanese ophthalmologist, described this disease in 1908.

and the mottled cyanosis of the fingers and/or toes may be accompanied by paraesthesia and chilblains.

Cervical sympathectomy

Open cervical sympathectomy was previously performed for vasospastic conditions affecting the hands and to treat palmar (sometimes axillary) hyperhidrosis. The operation is now obsolete, having been replaced by endoscopic transthoracic sympathectomy. Furthermore, it has been increasingly recognised that the vasospastic conditions do not respond to this form of treatment, rendering the endoscopic intervention a therapy that is suitable solely for hyperhidrosis.

Lumbar sympathectomy

Lumbar sympathectomy has been used to treat chronic lower limb ischaemia in the past. Lumbar sympathectomy by open operation has, however, been obsolete for several years and even chemical sympathectomy, its minimally invasive equivalent, can now be regarded as outdated. Chemical sympathectomy requires the injection of small quantities of a sclerosant into the lumbar sympathetic chain under radiographic control.

FURTHER READING

Ascher E, Veith FJ, Gloviczki P (eds). *Haimovici's vascular surgery*, 6th edn. Oxford: Wiley-Blackwell Publishing, 2012.

Bhattacharya V, Stansby G (eds). *Postgraduate vascular surgery: the candidates' guide to the FRCS*. Cambridge: Cambridge University Press, 2011.

Cronenwett JL, Johnstone WK (eds). *Rutherford's vascular surgery*, 8th edn. Philadelphia: WB Saunders, 2014.

England T, Nasim A (eds). *ABC of arterial and venous disease*, 3rd edn. London: BMJ Books, 2014.

Moore WS (ed). *Vascular and endovascular surgery: a comprehensive review*, 8th edn. Philadelphia: WB Saunders, 2013.

Chapter 57

Venous disorders

Learning objectives

To understand:
- Venous anatomy and the physiology of venous return
- The pathophysiology of venous hypertension
- The clinical significance and management of superficial venous reflux
- The management of venous ulceration
- Venous thromboembolism

INTRODUCTION

Up to 40% of the adult population in resource-rich countries have diseases of the veins of the leg. This extraordinary prevalence along with the associated impairment in health-related quality of life make it a very important area of surgical practice. Surgical intervention has been revolutionised by the development of endovenous techniques, and level 1 evidence has demonstrated that treatment can be associated with very high clinical- and cost-effectiveness. Despite the considerable importance placed on lower limb function during the management of orthopaedic and arterial diseases, venous diseases are often forgotten or dismissed as cosmetic practice. An understanding of the nature and management of venous disease is critical to address this imbalance and improve the quality of patients' lives.

THE ANATOMY OF THE VENOUS SYSTEM OF THE LOWER LIMB

The venous system of the lower limb can be divided anatomically into the **superficial venous system**, which is located within the superficial tissues and the **deep venous system**, beneath the deep fascia of the leg, accompanying the arterial tree. The superficial veins drain into the deep system, either at junctions or via fascial perforating veins, and the deep veins then return blood to the right atrium of the heart. Venous anatomy is characteristically variable. The terminology used below is consistent with international consensus.

The deep veins of the lower limb (**Figure 57.1a**) include three pairs of venae commitantes, which accompany the three crural arteries (anterior and posterior tibial and peroneal arteries). These six veins intercommunicate and come together in the popliteal fossa to form the popliteal vein, which also receives the soleal and gastrocnemius veins. The popliteal vein passes up through the adductor hiatus to enter the subsartorial canal as the femoral vein, which receives the deep (profunda) femoral vein (or veins) in the femoral triangle before passing behind the inguinal ligament to become the external iliac vein. The internal iliac vein combines with the external iliac vein in the pelvis to form the common iliac vein. The left common iliac vein passes behind the right common iliac artery to join the right common iliac vein on the right side of the abdominal aorta to form the inferior vena cava, which goes on to the right atrium.

Far more anatomical variations exist within the superficial veins of the lower limb, but there are almost always two trunks or axes, the great and small saphenous veins (**Figures 57.1b, c**). These lie superficial to the fascia lata (deep fascia) but deep to the saphenous fascia, in the saphenous 'envelope'.

As the sole of the foot is often placed under significant pressure, the majority of the venous drainage of the foot is into the dorsal venous arch, running in the subcutaneous tissues over the metatarsal heads. The medial end of this arch drains into the first axis: the great saphenous vein (GSV). This is the longest vein in the body and the most frequently affected by superficial incompetence. The GSV passes anterior to the medial malleolus and ascends the leg accompanied by the saphenous nerve in the superficial tissues medial to the tibia, looping posteriorly at the level of the medial condyle of the femur and continuing in the medial thigh. In the groin, it unites with tributaries corresponding to the arterial branches of the common femoral artery, before piercing the cribriform fascia covering the saphenous opening (approximately 2.5 cm below and lateral to the pubic tubercle, but often somewhat higher) and terminates by draining into the common femoral vein (CFV) at the saphenofemoral junction (SFJ). Throughout its course the GSV unites variably with other superficial tributaries. The anterior (accessory) saphenous vein (ASV) is one of the most common. This is often seen originating

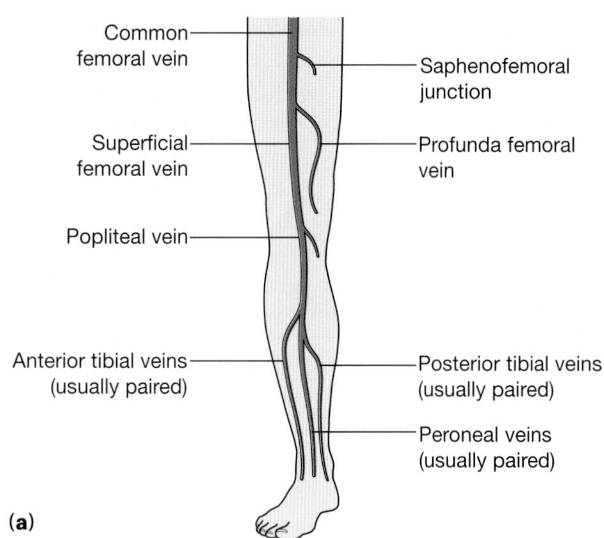

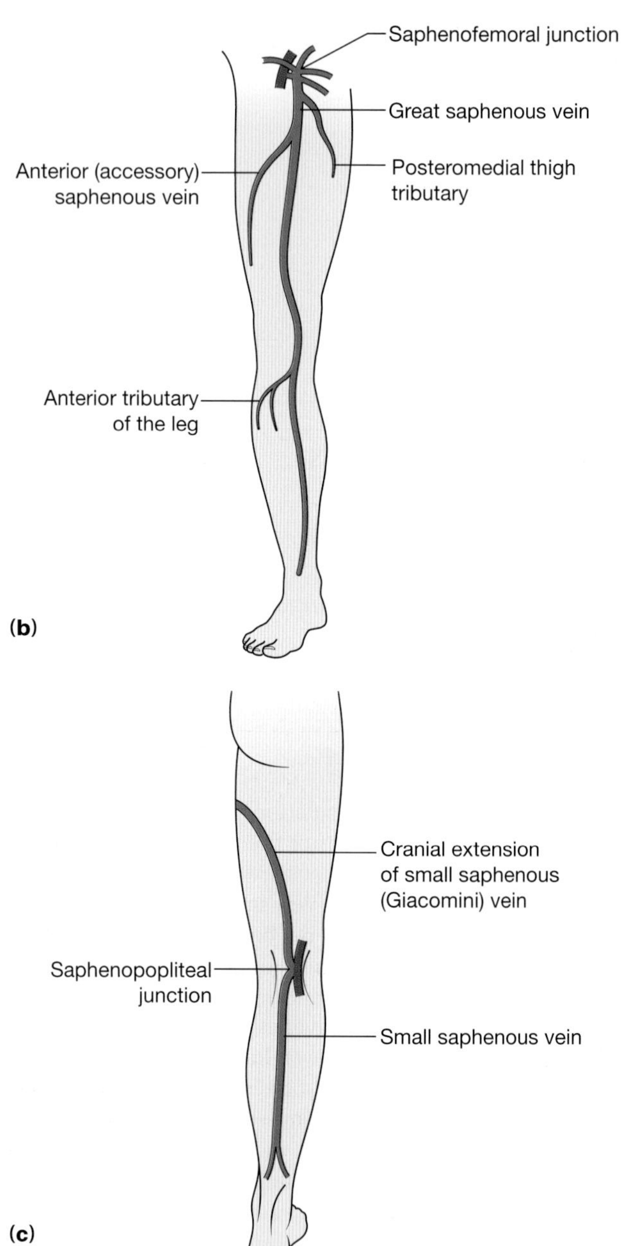

Figure 57.1 (**a**) Anatomy of the deep veins of the lower limb; (**b**) anatomy of the superficial veins of the lower limb (great saphenous axis); (**c**) anatomy of the superficial veins of the lower limb (small saphenous axis).

around the lateral border of the knee, although it sometimes originates as low as the lateral end of the dorsal venous arch. Occasionally, this vein may also course up the medial aspect of the thigh, anterolateral to the GSV following its course. In this instance, its origin is typically a confluence of small tributaries around the knee. There is usually an in-line GSV axis passing uninterrupted from the foot (in some cases this may be hypoplastic), but this pattern of ASV is commonly mistaken for the GSV itself (some surgeons will call this a duplex GSV; a true duplex GSV is rare). The ASV may drain into the GSV in the thigh, but is typically at or near the junction itself.

The small saphenous vein (SSV) originates from the lateral side of the dorsal venous arch and accompanies the sural nerve as it passes posterior to the lateral malleolus, then upwards in the posterior midline of the leg. In the proximal calf it is usually found sitting in the groove between the two muscular heads of gastrocnemius. Its termination commonly occurs by piercing the fascia of the popliteal fossa to drain into the popliteal vein at the saphenopopliteal junction (SPJ). However, this junction is highly variable and the vein may terminate as low as the mid-calf. The SSV may extend cranially beyond the SPJ, in which case it is known as either a cranial extension of the SSV, which terminates by piercing the fascia in the posterior thigh to drain into the deep system, or the Giacomini vein, which communicates with the GSV system occasionally joining the GSV at or about the SFJ. In some cases, the SSV does not terminate at or below the popliteal fossa at all, but continues on as described above.

In the calf and thigh there are a number of valved perforating (communicating) veins that join the superficial to the deep veins at inconstant sites and which allow blood to flow from the superficial to the deep venous system. The most important of these are the direct perforating veins of the medial and lateral calf and the communicating veins around the knee and in the mid-thigh.

VENOUS PATHOPHYSIOLOGY

The purpose of the venous system is primarily to return blood back to the heart so that it can be delivered into the pulmonary circulation. The venous system contains approximately 60% of the total blood volume, with an average pressure of around 5–10 mmHg. Mechanical factors, alongside the autonomic nervous and endocrine systems, control the rate

Carlo Giacomini, 1840–1898, anatomist, Turin, Italy, on his death left his skeleton to the Anatomical Museum in Turin.

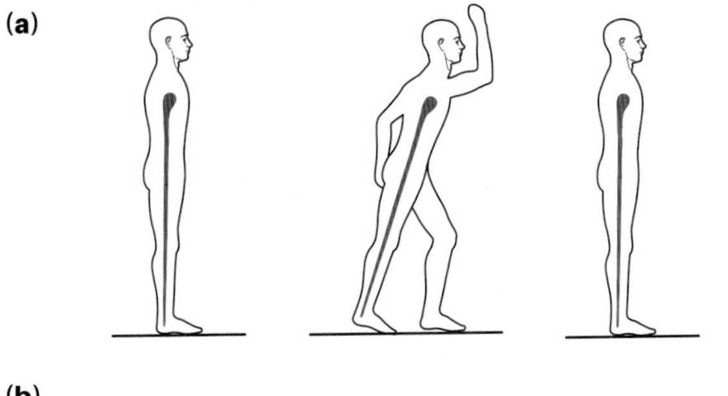

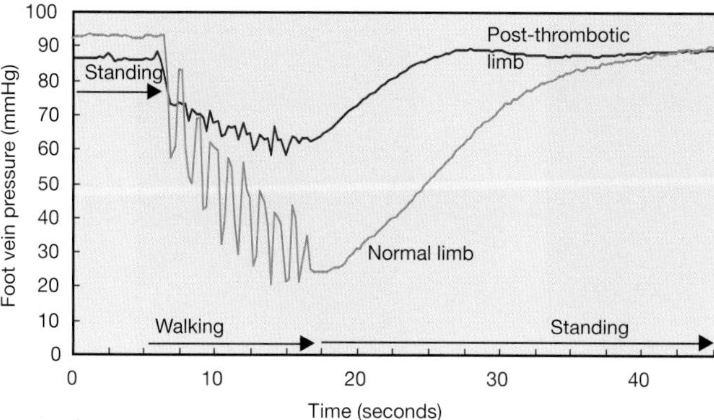

Figure 57.2 (a, b) Effect of exercise on the superficial venous pressure in health and disease.

at which blood is delivered to the right atrium. Through its effects upon myocardial contractility via the Starling mechanism, venous return is one of the factors responsible for determining cardiac output.

Blood enters the lower limb through the femoral arteries before passing through arterioles into the capillaries, which have a pressure of about 32 mmHg at their arterial ends. This pressure is reduced along the course of the capillaries and is approximately 12 mmHg at the venular end of the capillary. The pressure continues to fall in the main veins, and is as low as 5 mmHg at the upper end of the vena cava where it enters the right atrium.

The venous pressure in a foot vein on standing is equivalent to the height of a column of blood extending from the heart to the foot, e.g. approximately 100 mmHg (**Figure 57.2**). To enable blood to be returned against gravity in the standing position a pressure gradient must exist between the veins in the leg and the chest. This gradient is created in two ways. Firstly, the increase in thoracic volume during inspiration decreases intrathoracic pressure. Secondly, the pressure in the veins of the leg is increased by compression by the surrounding muscles (the 'calf muscle pump') and to a lesser extent the tone of the venous wall. The deep veins of the calf are capacious and are joined by blind-ending sacks called the soleal sinusoids, which force blood into the popliteal and crural veins during calf muscle pump contraction, e.g. walking. The foot pump also ejects blood from the plantar veins during walking. As the calf muscles contract, the veins are compressed and the valves only allow blood to pass in the direction of the heart. The pressure within the calf compartment rises to 200–300 mmHg during muscle contraction. Rapid blood flow in the deep veins at junctions and perforators draws blood from the superficial veins, driving this up the deep veins also. During muscle relaxation, the pressure falls and further blood from the superficial veins enters the deep vein. Each time this occurs the pressure falls in the superficial venous compartment until a threshold is reached, when the venous inflow keeps pace with ejection from the deep veins. This is normally around 30 mmHg, a fall of approximately two-thirds of the resting venous pressure. The net reduction in the pressure of the superficial system is dependent on the presence of a pressure gradient between the leg and the thorax and a patent and compliant venous system containing competent valves. An absence of one or more of these results in venous hypertension, which leads to further vein wall damage including loss of compliance, thickening, dilatation and valvular dysfunction. This venous damage goes on to reduce the function of the affected veins, worsening the venous hypertension in a vicious cycle. When exposed to high venous and capillary pressures chronically, the soft tissues of the leg will be damaged, causing a spectrum of damage that become irreversible. The causes of venous hypertension are listed in *Table 57.1*.

TABLE 57.1 Factors causing venous hypertension.

- Pressure gradient dysfunction:
  - Increased abdominal or thoracic pressure:
    - COPD
    - Pregnancy
    - Obesity
    - Large tumour
    - Constipation
  - Decreased calf muscle pump function:
    - Immobility
    - Ankle joint fusion
    - Paralysis
- Dysfunction of the venous system:
  - Venous structural deficit:
    - Valvular agenesis
    - Valvular incompetence
    - Venous dilatation
    - Venous tortuosity
    - Loss of vein wall compliance
    - Loss of venous tone
    - Arteriovenous fistula
  - Venous occlusion:
    - Agenesis
    - Thrombosis
    - Iatrogenic/trauma
  - Venous compression:
    - May–Thurner syndrome
    - Pelvic/abdominal tumour
    - Pelvic/abdominal radiotherapy

COPD, chronic obstructive pulmonary disease.

Ernest Henry Starling, 1866–1927, physiologist, University College, London, UK.
Rudolf Virchow, 1821–1902, pathologist Charite Hospital, Berlin, Germany, was the first to be credited with describing iliac vein compression. It was not until 1957 that May and Thurner (Innsbruck, Austria) clearly described compression of the left common iliac vein by the right common iliac artery.

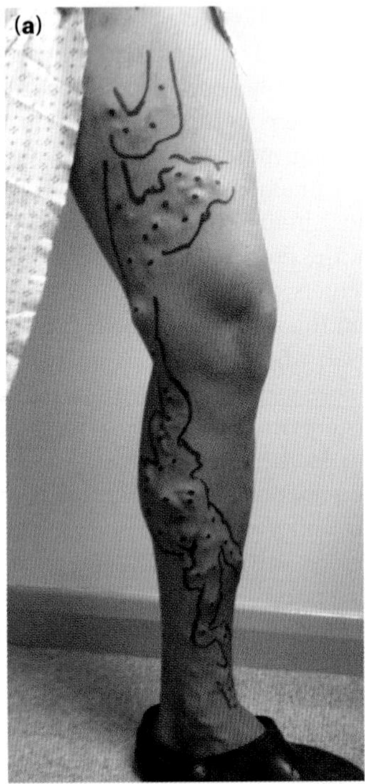

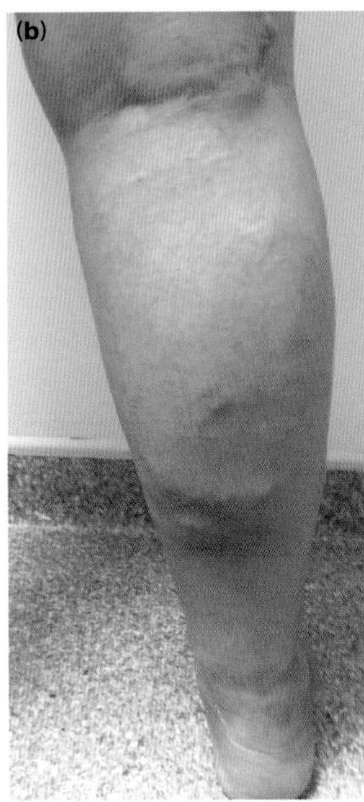

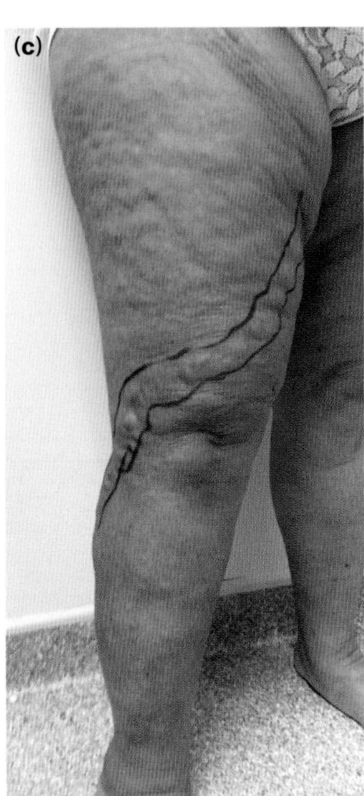

Figure 57.3 Varicose veins: (a) left leg varicose veins in the distribution of an incompetent great saphenous vein (marked for intervention); (b) right leg varicose veins in the distribution of the small saphenous system with a recent episode of phlebitis; (c) varicose veins in distribution of an isolated incompetent anterior accessory saphenous vein with associated gaiter area skin changes.

The majority of patients with venous disease have a problem primarily with the vein wall structure and in most this is confined to the superficial veins. Little is known about the mechanism of initiation of the changes in the vein wall. These changes are complex, but are typified by valvular failure allowing retrograde flow within the vein with gravity (venous incompetence). It is no longer thought that venous incompetence is caused by a primary mechanical valvular failure.

The vein wall changes include inflammatory cell infiltration and activation, dysfunctional smooth muscle cell proliferation, collagen deposition, decreased elastin content and increased matrix metalloproteinases. These effects typically lead to loss of compliance, dilatation, elongation (causing tortuosity) and secondary valvular dysfunction. This process can be initiated anywhere in the venous tree. Secondary varicose veins may develop in patients with post-thrombotic limbs and in patients with congenital abnormalities such as the Klippel–Trenaunay syndrome or multiple arteriovenous fistulae.

The extent and number of incompetent veins governs the extent of the venous hypertension and correlates to the severity of the soft tissue complications seen. Importantly however, neither the reflux burden nor the presence of skin changes, short of ulceration, correlate with the presence or degree of symptoms.

CLINICAL FEATURES OF VENOUS HYPERTENSION OF THE LEG

The following clinical features are commonly seen:

- Varicose vein: subcutaneous dilated vein 3 mm in diameter or larger. They are frequently elongated and tortuous, with intermittent 'blowouts', but are defined by the presence of reflux and may be straight and uniform tubes morphologically (Figure 57.3).
- Telangiectasia (thread veins, spider veins, and hyphen webs): represent tiny intradermal venules less than 1 mm in diameter (Figure 57.4).
- Reticular vein: small dilated 'bluish' subdermal vein 1–2.9 mm in diameter, usually tortuous, can be difficult to distinguish this from a normal subdermal vein in someone with white thin transparent skin.
- Saphena varix (Figure 57.5) is a (usually painless) groin swelling apparent on standing.
- Corona phlebectatica (malleolar flare): a fan-shaped pattern of telangiectasia on the ankle or foot. It is thought to be an early sign of advanced venous disease.
- Oedema: increased volume of fluid in the skin and soft tissues of the leg. Commonly starts distally and moves more proximally with increasing venous dysfunction. Classically this is 'pitting oedema', with firm digital pressure leaving an indentation in the soft tissues.

A gaiter is a leather or cloth covering for the lower leg and ankle. The name is derived from the French 'guetre' for the same piece of clothing.
Maurice Klippel, 1858–1942, neurologist, La Salpêtrière, Paris, France.
Paul Trenaunay, b.1875, French neurologist. Klippel and Trenaunay described this condition in a joint paper in 1900.

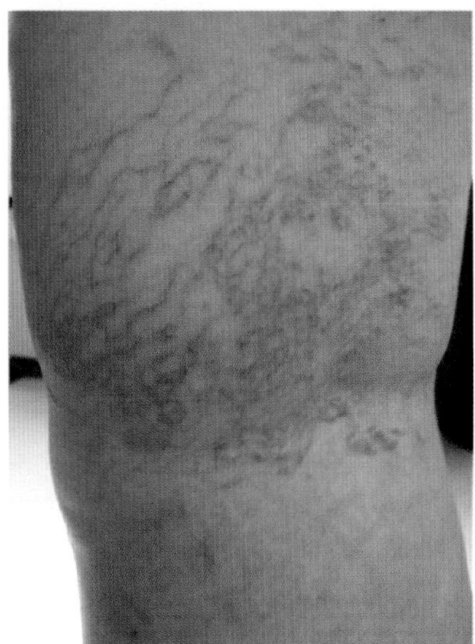

Figure 57.4 Telangiectasia and reticular veins.

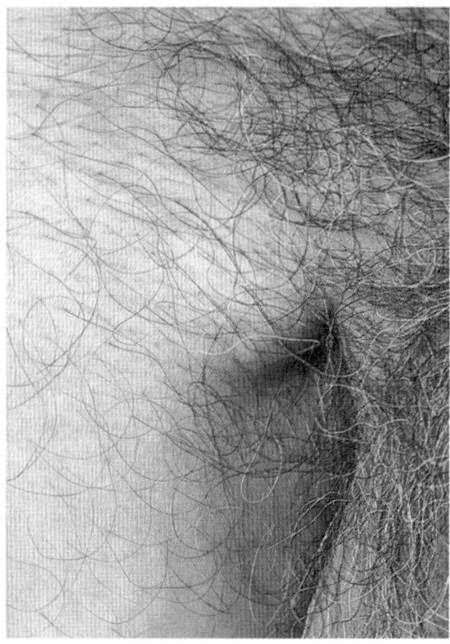

Figure 57.5 A saphena varix.

- Eczema: an erythematous dermatitis, often appears minor, although it may be associated with significant itching and discomfort. In extreme cases it may progress to blistering and weeping (Figures 57.6–57.8).
- Pigmentation (haemosiderosis): a brownish discolouration of the skin, usually permanent. It is usually seen around the ankle, but is also seen in proximity to varicose veins and incompetent perforators (Figures 57.7 and 57.9)
- Lipodermatosclerosis (LDS): chronic inflammation and fibrosis of the skin and subcutaneous tissues, resulting in a tight, contracted, 'woody' leg on examination. It occasionally results in significant contractures of the Achilles tendon. This is a sign of severe chronic venous disease (Figures 57.6 and 57.9).
- Atrophie blanche: localised areas of atrophic, white skin, often surrounded by telangiectasia and pigmentation. Some authors distinguish this from the white scarring left by ulceration, others do not. Either way, this is a sign of severe chronic venous disease (Figure 57.6).

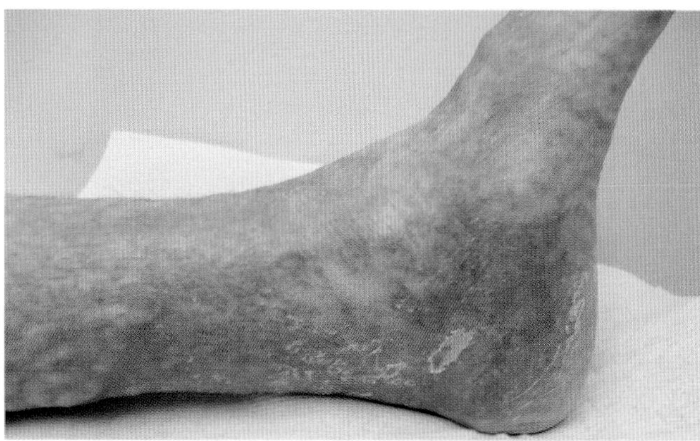

Figure 57.6 Advanced skin changes – lipodermatosclerosis, eczema and atrophie blanche.

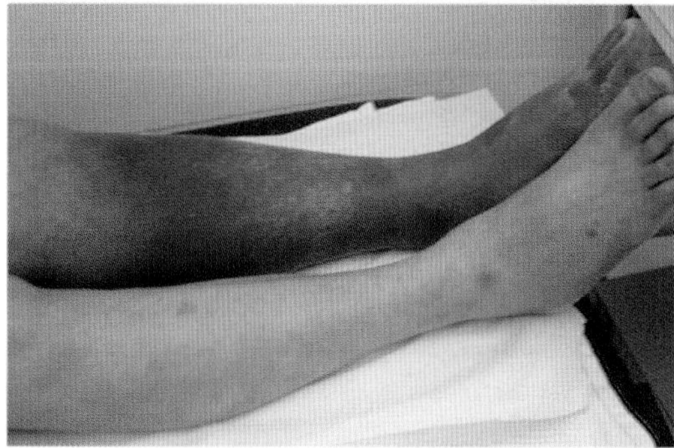

Figure 57.7 Pigmentation (haemosiderosis) and mild eczema.

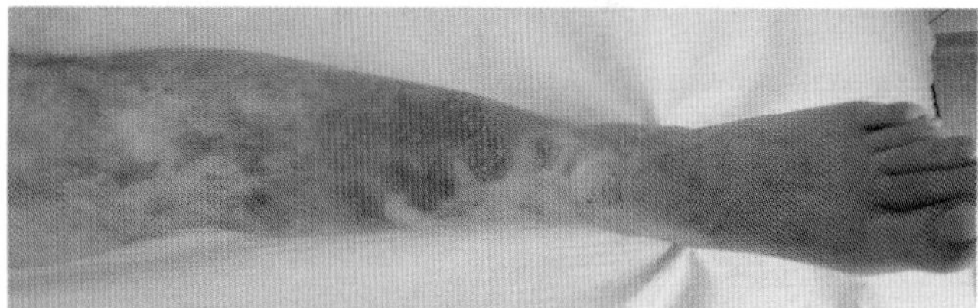

Figure 57.8 Severe eczema.

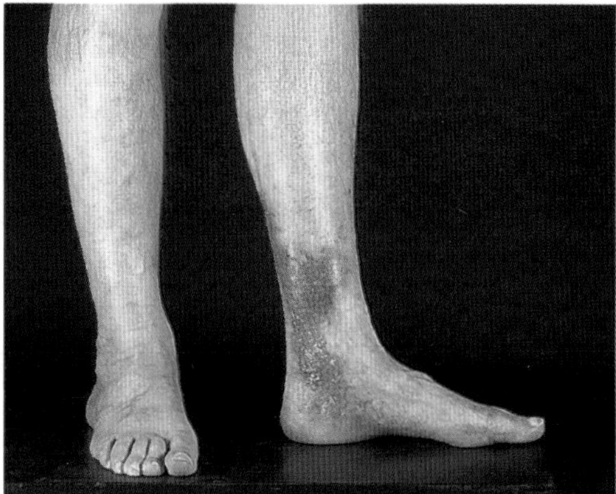

Figure 57.9 Haemosiderosis and mild lipodermatosclerosis of the calf skin.

- Venous ulcer: full-thickness skin loss, usually around the ankle, which fails to heal spontaneously and is propagated by continuing venous hypertension and the changes associated with chronic venous disease (Figure 57.10).

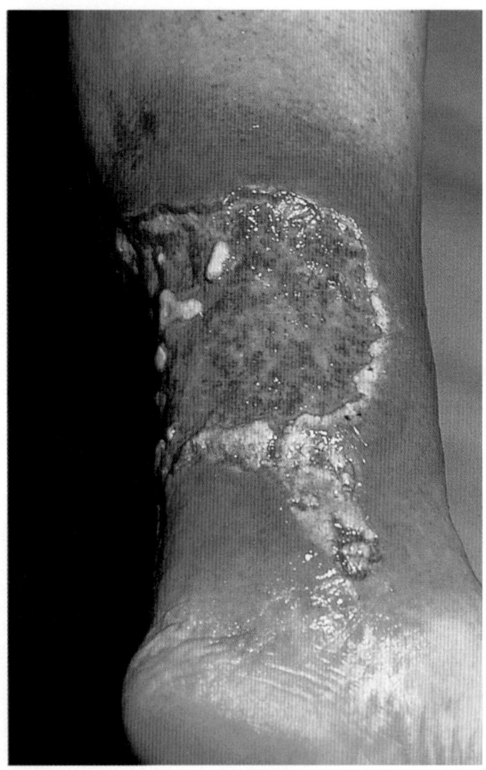

Figure 57.10 Venous ulcer.

Classification system

The descriptive CEAP (Clinical-aEtiology-Anatomy-Pathophysiology) classification for chronic venous disorders is widely utilised.

For clinical classification:

- C0: no signs of venous disease;
- C1: telangectasia or reticular veins;
- C2: varicose veins;
- C3: oedema;
- C4a: pigmentation or eczema (some include malleolar flare in this category);
- C4b: lipodermatosclerosis or atrophie blanche;
- C5: healed venous ulcer;
- C6: active venous ulcer.

Each clinical class is further characterised depending upon whether the patient is symptomatic (S) or asymptomatic (A), e.g. $C2_S$.

For aetiological classification:

- Ec: congenital;
- Ep: primary;
- Es: secondary (post-thrombotic);
- En: no venous cause identified.

For anatomical classification:

- As: superficial veins;
- Ap: perforator veins;
- Ad: deep veins;
- An: no venous location identified.

For pathophysiological classification:

- Pr: reflux;
- Po: obstruction;
- Pr,o: reflux and obstruction;
- Pn: no venous pathophysiology identifiable.

VARICOSE VEINS

In clinical practice, patients are normally categorised as having 'varicose veins' or 'venous ulcers'. Cases of varicose veins may be uncomplicated or complicated. Complications include superficial thrombophlebitis, bleeding or any of the skin changes listed above. Uncomplicated varicose veins may be asymptomatic or symptomatic.

Epidemiology

The adult prevalence of visible varicose veins is between 30% and 50%. Factors affecting prevalence include:

- Gender: the vast majority of studies report a higher prevalence in women than men, though community prevalence may differ.
- Age: the prevalence of varicose veins increases with age. In the Edinburgh Vein study, the prevalence of trunk varicosities in the age groups 18–24 years, 25–34 years, 35–44 years, 45–57 years and 55–64 years was 11.5%, 14.6%, 28.8%, 41.9% and 55.7%, respectively.
- Ethnicity: does seem to influence the prevalence of varicose veins.
- Body mass and height: increasing body mass index and height may be associated with a higher prevalence of varicose veins.
- Pregnancy: increases the risk of varicose veins.
- Family history: evidence supports familial susceptibility to varicose veins.
- Occupation and lifestyle factors: there is inconclusive evidence regarding increased prevalence of varicose veins in smokers, patients who suffer constipation and occupations that involve prolonged standing.

Symptoms

Varicose veins frequently cause symptoms. Patients describe aching, heaviness, throbbing, burning or bursting over affected areas and sometimes the whole limb. Such symptoms typically increase throughout the day or with prolonged standing, and are relieved by elevation or compression hosiery. Itching is also commonly described, though is more frequent in the presence of complications as is swelling of the ankle. Venous symptoms in the absence of complications can be vague and it may be difficult to ascertain from history alone whether they are truly venous in origin and, therefore, whether treatment will help. A trial of compression hosiery can help as venous symptoms should show some beneficial improvement.

Symptoms can be very severe and interfere with a patient's daily activities such as work, recreation and caring for children and adults. Such symptoms are independent of the degree of venous incompetence or the presence of complications, including skin changes short of ulceration. Studies have also shown that symptoms are associated with a significant deficit in health-related quality of life, and significant improvements are seen with treatment to remove or ablate the refluxing veins. The maximal benefit is seen in those with uncomplicated symptomatic varicose veins, as skin changes and a proportion of the associated morbidity are frequently irreversible.

Telangiectasia (not associated with malleolar flare) and reticular veins occur very commonly in the absence of significant reflux or obstruction and in the vast majority do not cause any physical symptoms, though cosmetic treatment is commonly sought.

Signs

The presence of tortuous dilated subcutaneous veins is usually clinically obvious. These are confined to the GSV and SSV systems in approximately 60% and 20% of cases, respectively. The distribution of varicosities may indicate which superficial axis is defective; medial thigh and calf varicosities suggest GSV incompetence (**Figure 57.3a**), posterolateral calf varicosities are suggestive of SSV incompetence (**Figure 57.3b**), whereas anterolateral thigh and calf varicosities may indicate isolated incompetence of the ASV (**Figure 57.3c**). Any of the clinical features above may be present. Large dilated veins around the SFJ may present as a (usually painless) lump, emergent when standing and disappearing when recumbent. This is a saphena varix (**Figure 57.5**). Gentle palpation over the varix during coughing may elicit a thrill, though it may be mistaken for a groin hernia.

Investigation

Tourniquet tests and the use of hand-held Doppler have now largely been abandoned. There is good evidence to support the policy of duplex ultrasound scanning for all patients with varicose veins prior to any intervention. The best clinical results come from clinicians who are personally very skilled in the use of duplex ultrasound and use it to design a bespoke treatment for each individual patient, based upon their unique anatomy.

A high-frequency linear array transducer of 7.5–13 MHz is appropriate for the majority of lower limbs in order to obtain good quality images. The B-mode settings (depth, focal zone, overall gain and dynamic gain) should be optimised to ensure the area of interest is in the centre and occupies the majority of the image, and that the lumen of the vein appears as a dark void in the subcutaneous and deep tissues. The pulsed wave spectral or colour Doppler settings should be optimised for the low-flow velocities encountered within veins. It is conventional to use blue to represent antegrade venous flow towards the heart and red for the reverse. Visible venous flow can be augmented by a calf squeeze.

The aim of the duplex scan in a patient with varicose veins is to establish:

- The presence of reflux in the deep and superficial venous system.
- The exact distribution and extent of reflux in the superficial venous system including affected junctions and perforators.
- The presence of obstruction in the deep venous system.
- The suitability of the incompetent superficial veins for the different treatments available (based upon diameter, extent, tortuosity, saphena varix).
- The presence of thrombus within the superficial veins.
- An indication of a pelvic source of reflux or obstruction.

In order to standardise measurements of venous diameter and reflux, it is recommended that examination of the superficial veins is performed with the patient standing. Superficial or crural vein reflux is defined as retrograde flow in the reverse direction to physiological flow lasting for 0.5 seconds or more. The proximal deep veins require a duration of 1 second or more to be classified as incompetent. Reflux may be elicited by release of a calf or foot squeeze for proximal or calf varicosities, respectively, manual compression over varicosity clusters, pneumatic calf cuff deflation, active foot dorsiflexion and relaxation or the Vasalva manoeuvre.

The patient should stand facing towards the examiner with the leg rotated outwards, heel on the ground and weight on the opposite limb (**Figure 57.11**). The use of a platform,

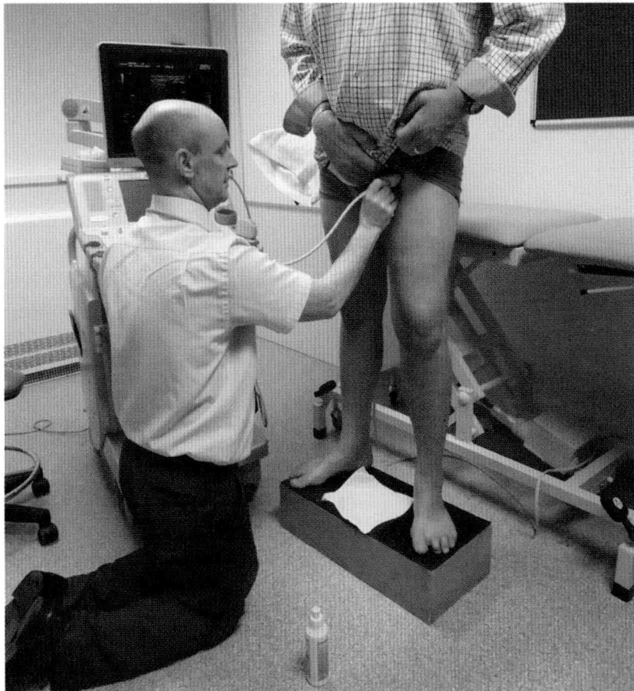

Figure 57.11 Patient position for venous duplex examination of the great saphenous system.

Christian Johann Doppler, 1803–1853, Professor of Experimental Physics, Vienna, Austria, enunciated the 'Doppler Principle' in 1842.

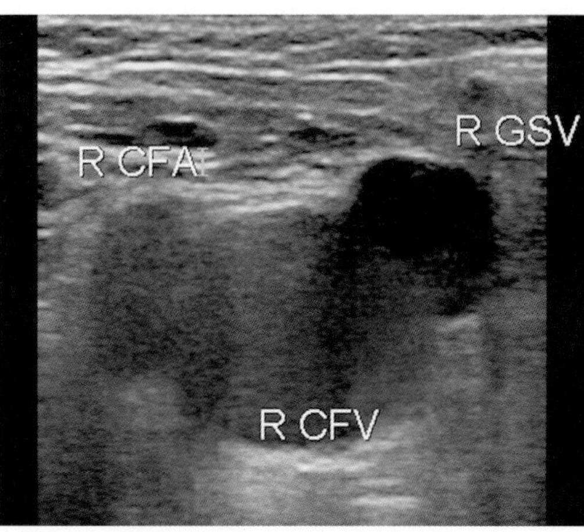

Figure 57.12 'Micky Mouse' transverse B-mode image of the right common femoral vein (CFV) and artery (CFA), great saphenous vein (GSV) and saphenofemoral junction.

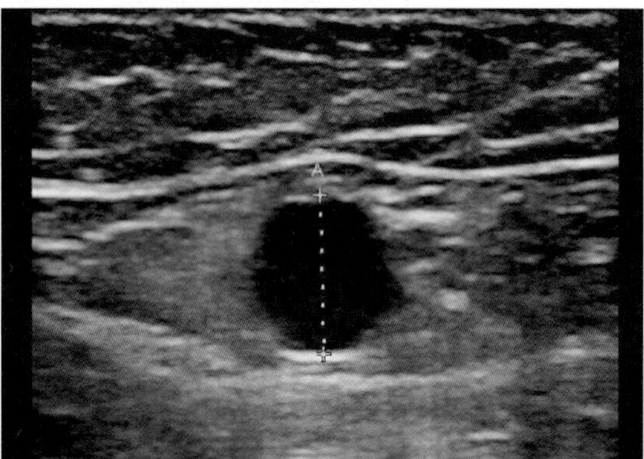

Figure 57.13 'Saphenous eye' transverse B-mode view of the great saphenous vein in fascial compartments of the thigh. The fascial line above the vein is the saphenous fascia. A true great or small saphenous vein will not cross this line, although the fascia may become discontinuous around the knee. The line deep to the vein is the fascia lata, with the muscle beneath.

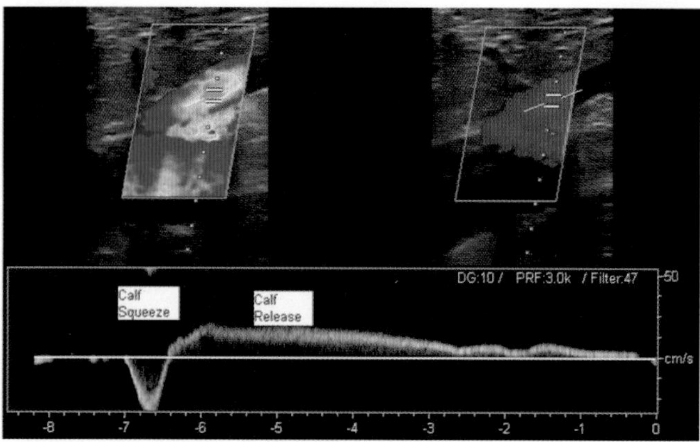

Figure 57.14 Spectral Doppler trace of the saphenofemoral junction showing antegrade and retrograde flow. The downward spike on the trace is the antegrade augmented flow and this is followed by approximately 4 seconds of retrograde flow.

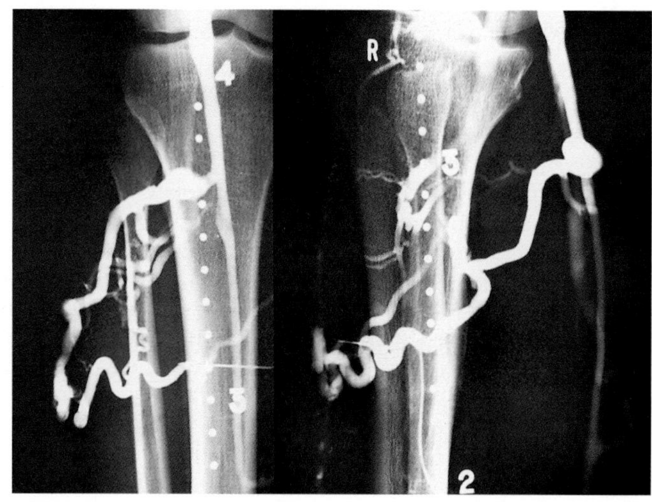

Figure 57.15 Varicogram

ideally with a handle or support bar for the patient and a stool that can drop to a low height, will improve the ergonomic comfort of both the sonographer and the patient. The scan should commence in the groin, using a transverse view to identify the GSV and CFV lying medial to the common femoral artery (the 'Micky Mouse' sign, Figure 57.12). SFJ competence is assessed in the transverse view and potential destinations for reflux, including the GSV, the ASV and other major thigh tributaries superficial to the saphenous fascia, are noted. Any indication of a pelvic source of reflux suggests the need for more proximal imaging. The full length of the GSV within its fascial compartment should be examined (Figure 57.13), and its diameter measured if required. The groin is next examined for reflux or obstruction in the CFV, superficial femoral vein, and SFJ using spectral and/or colour Doppler (Figure 57.14).

A loss of phasic flow with respiration in the CFV suggests upstream obstruction and the need for proximal imaging. The presence and competence of thigh and calf perforators should be noted and the crural veins examined for reflux or obstruction. For examination of the SSV and posterior thigh extension of the SSV (Giacomini vein), the patient is positioned facing away, knee slightly flexed, heel on the ground and the weight taken on the opposite leg. If the SPJ is incompetent, the level of the SPJ in relation to the knee crease and whether the SSV joins the popliteal vein posteriorly, medially or laterally is noted if open surgical ligation is to be entertained. In the transverse view, the SSV vein is followed distally, checking its competence and diameter in the proximal, mid and distal calf. Finally, the patency and competence of the popliteal vein is assessed.

Pelvic and iliac veins may be investigated using transabdominal or transvaginal duplex. Very occasionally investigations other than duplex are required, and these may be non-invasive, such as MR venography, or invasive such as contrast venography or intravenous ultrasound (IVUS). The use of varicography has become historical (Figure 57.15).

Management

Many patients with asymptomatic varicose veins do not progress to develop complications, although a significant proportion do, and little is known about whether treating such patients prevents the development of future complications.

There is clear evidence, however, that those with symptoms and/or complications see a significant quality of life benefit from treatment to remove or ablate refluxing superficial veins.

When interventional treatment is planned there are considerable variations in practice and treatment strategies. A detailed description of the nuances, merits and criticisms of the various options is beyond the scope of this chapter; however, a description of the basic treatment modalities available is presented below. An experienced surgeon will have his/her own preferred methods, but will frequently employ several or all methods in chosen circumstances, not infrequently in the same patient.

Compression

Compression hosiery relies on graduated external pressure to improve deep venous return and reduce venous pressures. It may be knee length or thigh length; there is no evidence which length of stocking is more effective and hence below-knee stockings are usually prescribed as they are easier to don and have much better patient acceptance. Compression hosiery are classified according to the pressure they exert: the British classification class 1 stockings exert pressure of 14–17 mmHg, class 2 exert 18–24 mmHg and class 3 exert 25–35 mmHg.

Compression hosiery significantly improves varicose vein symptoms but is not popular with patients, with compliance rates and long-term tolerance being universally poor. There is no evidence to suggest that compression hosiery prevents the occurrence or progression of varicose veins. Furthermore, incorrect application of compression hosiery can have serious consequences (pressure necrosis, tourniquet effects); thus assessment, prescription and application of compression hosiery should be limited to those with the appropriate skills and training. There are level 1 trial data to demonstrate that interventional treatment offers superior improvements in quality of life and is cost-effective. Compression is therefore to be regarded as an adjunct to assessment or treatment, unless by patient choice.

Endothermal ablation

Endothermal ablation technologies replaced surgical ligation and stripping as the gold standard treatment once randomised trials demonstrated that they were marginally safer, have extremely high technical efficacy, offer superior quality of life post procedure (with a rapid recovery) and equivalent improvements in quality of life in the longer term. The techniques are cost effective as they can be performed as an outpatient under local anaesthetic. The basic concept is that a treatment device is inserted into the incompetent axial vein percutaneously. The vein is surrounded by tumescent local anaesthetic solution. This compresses the vein onto the treatment device, emptying it of blood. It also hydro-dissects tissues such as nerves away from the zone of injury. Finally, it acts as a heat sink, mopping up excess thermal energy to prevent remote damage. The treatment device then produces thermal energy that destroys the structure of the vein, resulting in permanent occlusion. Two broad technologies exist: laser and radiofrequency ablation.

LASER ABLATION

Endovenous laser ablation (EVLA) utilises a small flexible glass fibre that is inserted into the vein. Laser energy (typically at a wavelength of 1470 nm) is transmitted down the fibre and is absorbed at the point of treatment at the end of the fibre. Absorption of this radiation results in a vigorous production of thermal energy. The tip of the fibre may be bare, focusing the energy in a very small area; divergent forward firing, spreading the energy over a larger area; or divergent side or radial firing. It is postulated that the latter two designs allow a more even distribution of energy, reducing vein wall perforations that are thought to be associated with postprocedural pain and bruising. There is no clear evidence to support one design over another. This procedure is very good for treatment of any vein that will allow the passage of a guidewire. No technique has reported a higher technical efficacy rate.

The procedure begins with ultrasound-guided marking of the truncal vein to be treated and the site of proposed cannulation. The varicosities are also marked at this stage if concomitant treatment (phlebectomy or foam sclerotherapy) is to be undertaken. The patient is then positioned on the procedure couch in the reverse Trendelenberg position. For the GSV, the patient is supine with the hip of the leg to be treated externally rotated and slightly flexed. A pillow under the contralateral hip/lower back may improve patient comfort. For the SSV the patient is positioned in the prone position. The vein is then cannulated percutaneously under ultrasound guidance, at the lowest point of reflux. Some devices allow passage of the fibre directly through a short sheath, while others use a wire first, allowing passage of a catheter that then carries the laser fibre. The former is slightly faster with fewer steps, the latter allows greater success with more tortuous veins. Accurate positioning of the fibre tip with ultrasound is crucial (Figure 57.16), but the exact location is controversial, with some surgeon positioning the tip several centimetres distal to the junction and others aiming for a flush occlusion. Proponents of the former cite that this strategy protects the deep vein from inadvertent damage and/or thrombosis. Proponents of the latter argue that neoreflux in junctional tributaries is a common pattern of recurrence

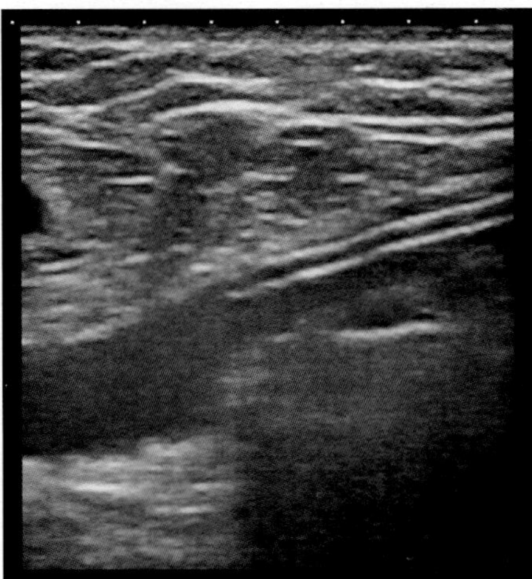

Figure 57.16 Endovenous laser ablation; B-mode image of catheter tip positioning at the saphenofemoral junction.

and that in expert hands the rate of deep vein injury is no different and the thrombosis rate may be lower (presumably as there is minimal patent stump in which to form thrombus). Following the administration of perivenous tumescent anaesthesia (**Figure 57.17**), the ablation can be performed. Practice varies as to the power of the laser and the withdrawal speed, but commonly an energy delivery of around 60 J/cm is used to achieve a durable closure. There is no clear evidence to guide the optimal power and pullback speed. Following treatment compression is applied, but there is no consensus over the method, degree or duration, and this is true of post-procedural compression with all techniques.

RADIOFREQUENCY ABLATION

Radiofrequency ablation (RFA) uses the same treatment principles, but an electromagnetic current is used to create the thermal energy. A range of different devices have been created but the most popular, which has the most supportive evidence, is the ClosureFast™ device (Medtronic) (**Figure 57.18**). This device has a wire coil on the end of a treatment catheter. The generator passes an electrical current through the coil until the surrounding temperature reaches 120°C. This is then maintained for a treatment cycle of 20 seconds. The coil is then withdrawn for a set length and another treatment cycle is commenced. Coils of 3 cm and 7 cm are produced, with the latter increasing the speed of treatment, while still being suitable for most anatomies.

There have been a range of studies comparing EVLA and RFA. The evidence is generally equivocal, with both treatments having relative advantages and disadvantages; choice often comes down to personal preference. Both are excellent treatment options and can be applied successfully to the majority of patients.

Advantages in favour of EVLA over RFA include:

- EVLA can ablate any vein that can take a guidewire successfully, with a very low rate of recanalisation. While the RFA catheter can be advanced over a 0.014 guidewire, in practice the relatively inflexible tip may not advance through very tortuous veins. Recanalisation rates may be higher for larger-diameter veins as the energy delivery and penetration are limited.
- A standard EVLA fibre may be used to treat perforators, whereas a specific additional device is required for RFA, increasing costs.

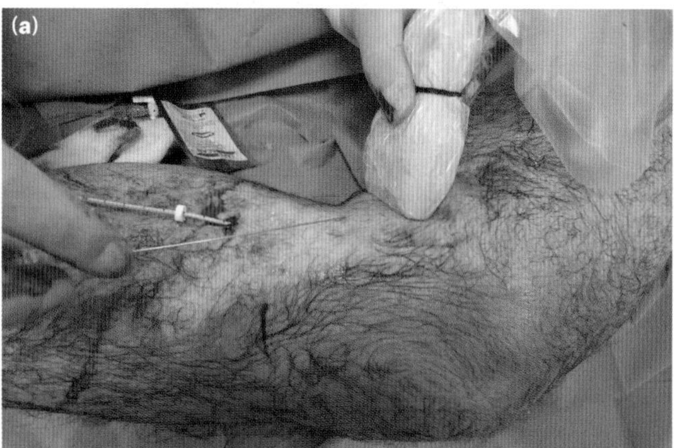

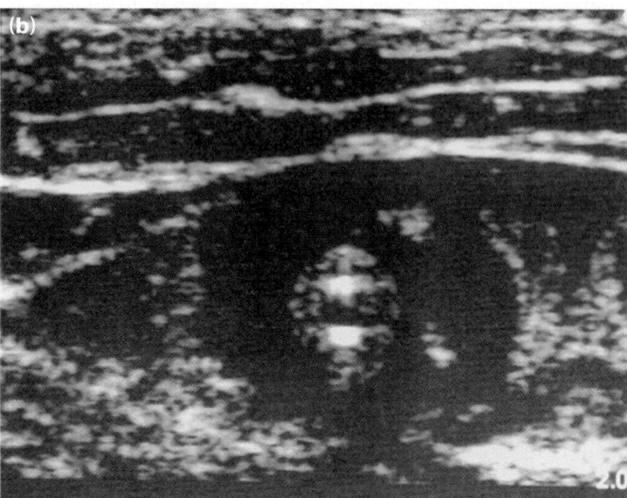

Figure 57.17 (**a**) Ultrasound-guided infiltration of perivenous tumescent anaesthetic via a long spinal needle. The anaesthetic solution is infiltrated using an electronic foot operated pump; (**b**) ultrasound image of perivenous 'halo' of anaesthetic solution around the vein and catheter in transverse section.

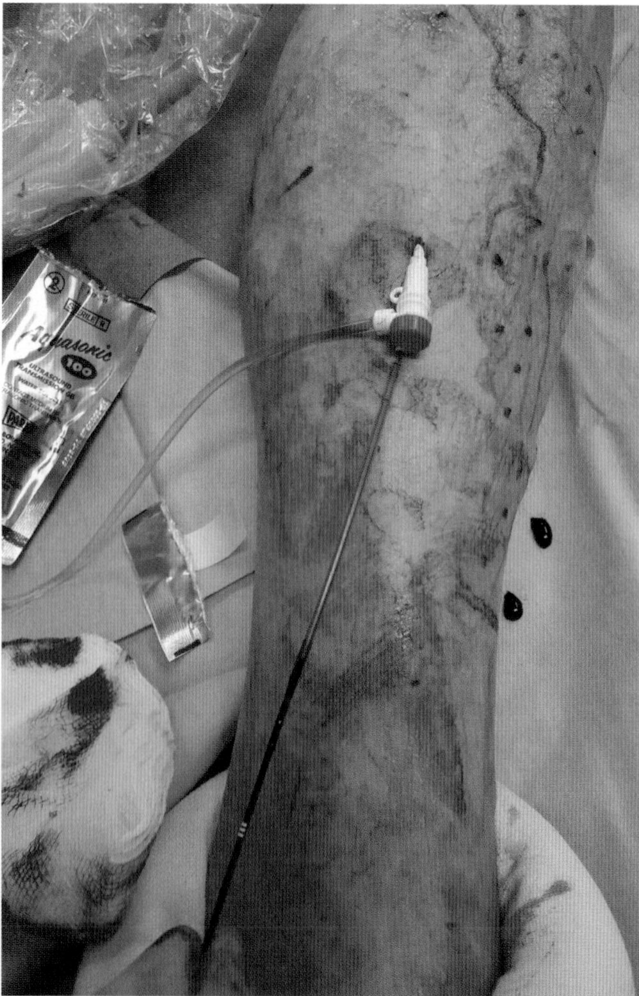

Figure 57.18 Radiofrequency ablation with ClosureFast™ introducing the treatment catheter through a sheath. The distal 7 cm of this device comprises a metal coil.

- Laser fibres are relatively inexpensive to produce, reducing the procedural costs.
- In a catheter-based system, the catheter can be used to deliver targeted foam sclerotherapy, for instance to areas of neovascularisation, prior to the actual laser fibre being inserted.

Advantages in favour of RFA over EVLA include:

- RFA has a standardised treatment protocol that is automated, minimising the uncertainty and learning curve for the ablation portion of the procedure and the possibility of a novice making a mistake with the energy delivery.
- RFA does not require a continuous pullback, again reducing the learning curve. This also frees the surgeon's focus allowing better communication with the patient and indeed, with care, concurrent treatment, e.g. infiltrating local anaesthetic into the tributaries and performing phlebectomy, reducing procedural times.
- RFA does not require laser safety precautions, reducing the administrative burden associated with setting up a service and location and allowing it to be performed in a wider range of settings with minimal adaptations.
- RFA may be associated with a marginal reduction in pain and bruising, athough this has not been shown to impact upon periprocedural quality of life or recovery.

As endothermal ablation treats only junctional and truncal incompetence, debate exists regarding the management of varicosities. These can be managed concomitantly or sequentially by either phlebectomy or sclerotherapy. Concomitant phlebectomy (**Figure 57.19**) results in a more rapid improvement in disease-specific quality of life, and allows the vast majority of patients to complete treatment in a single visit.

Non-endothermal, non-tumescent ablation

Endothermal ablation was a large step forwards in the management of superficial incompetence; however, all techniques require the injection of tumescent local anaesthetic solution and this can be uncomfortable for the patient. Other techniques that avoid injection are being developed.

ULTRASOUND-GUIDED FOAM SCLEROTHERAPY

Sclerotherapy is the original non-endothermal, non-tumescent technique and has been performed for over 100 years. It involves the injection of a sclerosing agent directly into the superficial veins. The most commonly used is sodium tetradecyl sulphate. The direct contact with detergent causes cellular death and initiates an inflammatory response, aiming to result in thrombosis, fibrosis and obliteration (sclerosis). Blood deactivates the action of the sclerosing agent and the doses administered need to be limited to avoid adverse effects, causing a trade-off between poor efficacy and safety. This led to the development of ultrasound-guided foam sclerotherapy (UGFS). The use of foam increases the effective volume of the agent, maximising endothelial contact and displacing any blood that deactivates it.

The procedure commences with the patient standing, and the sites of venous cannulation are selected and marked using ultrasound. With the patient supine, the major venous trunks and superficial varicosities to be treated are then all cannulated using ultrasound guidance prior to any injection (**Figure 57.20**). Once all injection sites are cannulated the foam can be prepared. The most widely used method is that of Tessari, which utilises two syringes connected using a three-way tap. A 1:3 or 1:4 ratio mixture of sclerosant and air is drawn into one syringe, and is then oscillated vigorously between the two syringes about 10 or 20 times (**Figure 57.21**). The foam produced in this way is stable for about 2 minutes so it should be injected as soon as it has been made. The leg is then elevated to empty the veins of blood, and injection of foam commences first with superficial varicosities and ends with injection of the GSV or SSV. Only 1 or 2 mL of foam should be injected at a time and the distribution of the foam should be monitored and massaged with the ultrasound probe. When the foam is visualised at the site of junctional incompetence no further foam should be injected. The maximum volume of foam that should be injected at a single session should not exceed 10–12 mL as the incidence of complications is directly related to the volume of foam injected. Compression is then

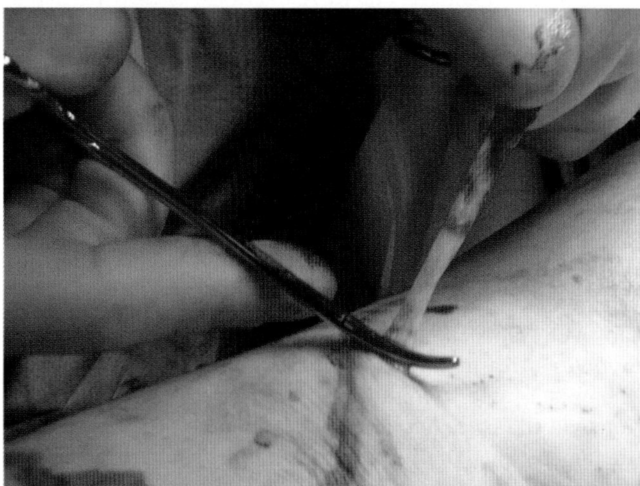

Figure 57.19 Phlebectomy performed under tumescent anaesthesia following endothermal ablation.

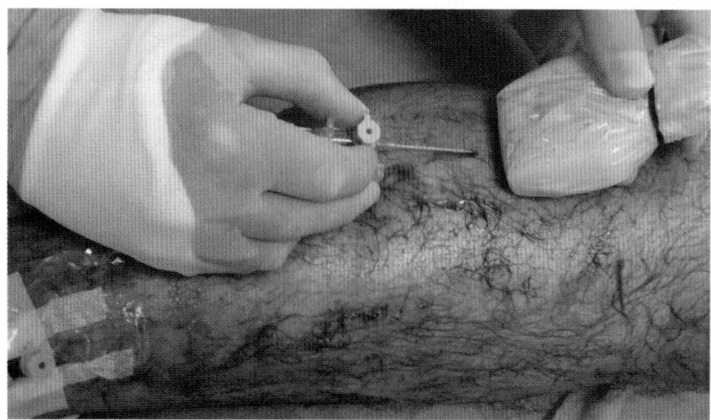

Figure 57.20 Foam sclerotherapy; cannulation of veins during ultrasound-guided foam sclerotherapy.

Lorenzo Tessari, b.1949, physician Trieste, Italy.

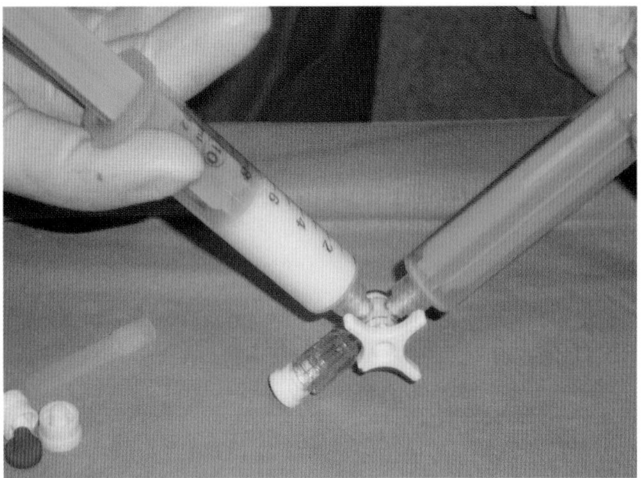

Figure 57.21 Foam sclerotherapy; Tessari method of foam sclerosant preparation.

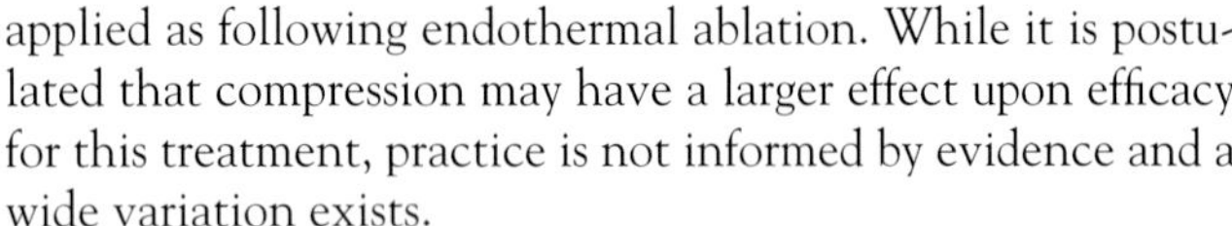

applied as following endothermal ablation. While it is postulated that compression may have a larger effect upon efficacy for this treatment, practice is not informed by evidence and a wide variation exists.

Outside of a small number of centres, the efficacy of UGFS is significantly worse than for endothermal ablation, leading to high reintervention rates, and the rates of complications such as phlebitis and pigmentation can be high. UGFS does however carry some significant advantages:

- It avoids tumescent anaesthetic and is therefore a less painful procedure (although postoperative pain is probably similar).
- No axial or tributary veins are too tortuous.
- It also allows the treatment of calf veins with overlying skin damage or ulceration without the need to pierce through damaged skin.
- Consumable treatment costs are very low.

These factors mean that many surgeons using endothermal techniques also use foam sclerotherapy as an adjunct in specific circumstances.

CATHETER-DIRECTED SCLEROTHERAPY AND MECHANICOCHEMICAL ABLATION

The efficacy of sclerotherapy relies on endothelial contact with fresh, undiluted sclerosant. Some have therefore experimented with catheter-delivered sclerotherapy rather than trying to milk the sclerosant down the vein lumen. There is no good evidence to date that this increases efficacy and the technique is not in widespread use.

A related technology that has shown more promise is mechanicochemical ablation (Figure 57.22). This involves a treatment device that deploys an angled wire from the end. This attaches to a motorised handle. The catheter is placed within the vein lumen as for endothermal ablation. The trigger on the handle is depressed, spinning the wire around and liquid sclerosant is infiltrated via the catheter simultaneously during catheter withdrawal. It is thought that the spinning wire causes physical damage to the endothelium and allows a

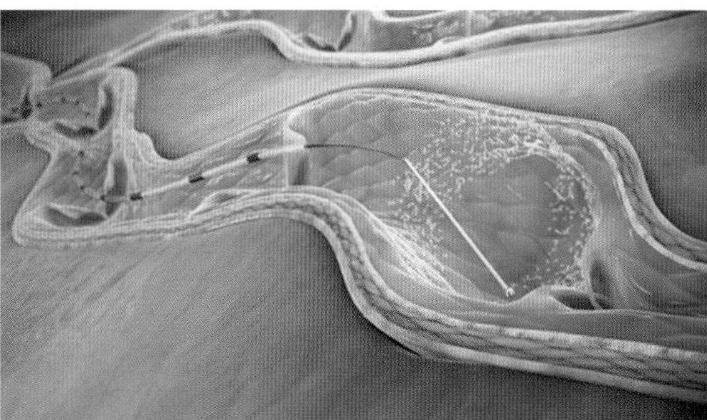

Figure 57.22 Mechanochemical ablation device (reproduced with permission of Vascular Insights).

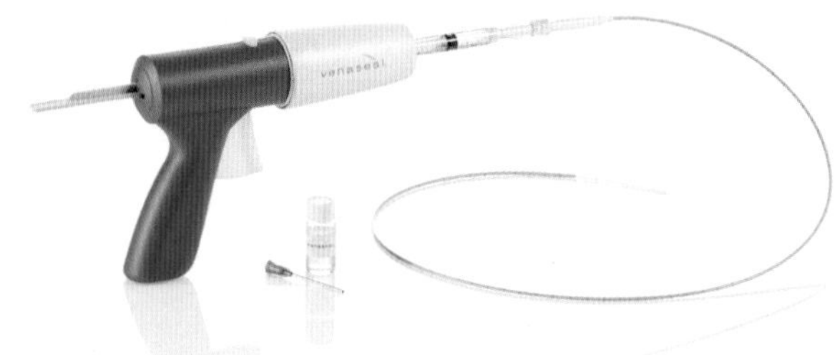

Figure 57.23 Endovenous glue device (reproduced with permission of Medtronic Inc.).

deeper penetration of the sclerosant into the vein wall. The technique is possible in most cases without tumescent anaesthesia, although a small number of patients find the procedure uncomfortable and the device can 'snag' on the vein, tearing it or rarely stripping it altogether. Early studies suggest similar early efficacy rates as for endothermal ablation, which is encouraging. The axial ablation is usually less painful than endothermal ablation, but this advantage is lost when it is combined with phlebectomy of the tributaries; therefore, it is uncertain whether it can replace endothermal ablation, unless axial ablation is to be performed in isolation. Treating longer veins can also be challenging due to limitations in catheter length and the safe dose of sclerosant. It is a good choice for a patient with needle phobia, who is happy to forgo treatment of varicose tributaries.

ENDOVENOUS GLUE

The final non-tumescent technique is the endoluminal application of cyanoacrylate adhesive (Figure 57.23). Again, this involves a treatment catheter placed within the vein lumen. A handle is used to infiltrate the adhesive in 0.1 mL applications via the catheter. The vein is then compressed, sealing the lumen closed. Early efficacy results are similarly promising and patients experience minimal intraprocedural pain. Long-term results and, similar to mechanicochemical ablation, the optimal management of tributaries are unknown. The consumable costs are currently the highest for any venous ablative technique.

Open surgery

The principles of traditional ligation and stripping are to fully dissect the point of junctional incompetence and to remove the refluxing axial vein and dilated tributaries. The operation is usually performed under general anaesthesia but loco-regional anaesthesia is used by some and the infiltration of tumescent local anaesthesia around the axial vein prior to stripping may have some advantages, but is not widely used.

The role of open surgery as a primary treatment of a refluxing superficial axis has been considerably reduced with development of the minimally invasive techniques described above, the long-term results of which are at least comparable with open surgery, but with significantly less morbidity and faster recovery. Experienced endovenous surgeons do still use open surgery in some circumstances and a venous surgeon needs to be trained and experienced in this area.

Surgical adjuncts including phlebectomy and, occasionally, perforator ligation are much more commonly used, and the former has been shown to have a significant impact upon outcome.

SAPHENOFEMORAL LIGATION AND GREAT SAPHENOUS STRIPPING

An oblique groin incision is made at the level of, and lateral to, the pubic tubercle, ideally above the groin crease. The GSV is identified and dissected to the SFJ, which should be clearly established before the vein is divided to avoid disastrous inadvertent transection of the superficial femoral vein. The anatomy is often variable but six GSV tributaries may be encountered close to the SFJ:

- Laterally:
  - superficial inferior epigastric vein;
  - superficial circumflex iliac vein;
- Medially:
  - superficial external pudendal vein;
  - deep external pudendal vein;
- Distally:
  - anterior accessory saphenous vein;
  - posteriomedial thigh vein.

Classically, these are ligated distal to their divisions. A flush SFJ ligation is then performed and the GSV retrogradely stripped to around the knee (**Figure 57.24**). Phlebectomy is performed as discussed above.

Closure of the cribriform fascia, with sutures or synthetic patches over the ligated SFJ, does not reduce groin recurrence. Stripping to the lowest point of reflux may improve results, but at a cost of increased saphenous nerve complications and is not widely performed. More recently, some surgeons argue that surgical trauma and subsequent inflammation in the groin is associated with neovascularisation, which in turn may lead to recurrence. Furthermore, others hypothesise that it is the loss of the normal groin tributaries that may be responsible for driving the process of neovascularisation. These concepts have led some to believe that ligation of the refluxing vein should be distal to the tributaries and that the junction itself should be left untouched. There is no clear clinical evidence to support these hypotheses.

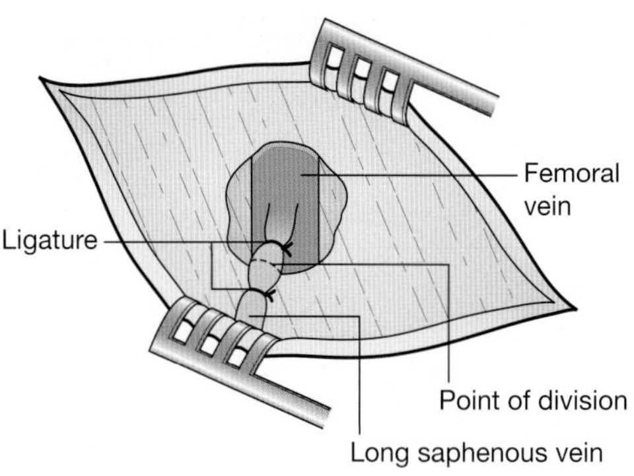

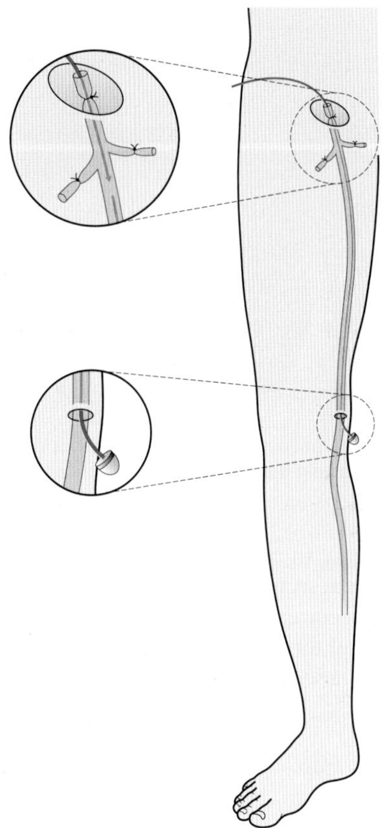

Figure 57.24 Saphenofemoral junction ligation and great saphenous vein stripping.

SAPHENOPOPLITEAL JUNCTION LIGATION AND SMALL SAPHENOUS STRIPPING

Preoperative duplex to mark the position of the SPJ is highly recommended (**Figure 57.25**). The patient is positioned in the prone position, a transverse incision is made over the premarked SPJ, the fascia is divided and the SSV is exposed. The SPJ can then be formally dissected with a flush ligation or the SSV can be gently retracted and ligated as proximally as possible. No good evidence exists to favour one technique over the other; proponents of the flush ligation would argue that it avoids leaving a stump of SSV, a common source of recurrence, while proponents of the simple SSV ligation technique argue it reduces the incidence of the most common serious complications, nerve injury and popliteal vein injury.

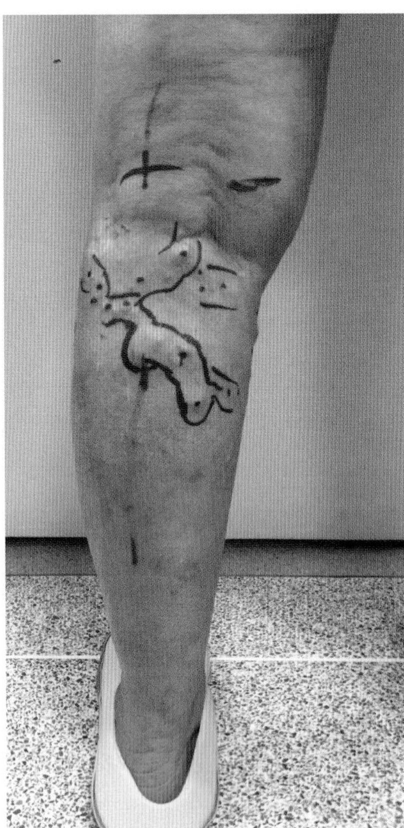

Figure 57.25 Preoperative marking of the saphenopopliteal junction and small saphenous vein mapped using duplex scanning.

The SSV can then either be stripped or the proximal section of the vein can be resected. Those who strip argue it reduces the incidence of recurrence, while opponents feel it increases the incidence of sural nerve injury. There are no randomised trials comparing these techniques. Once again, phlebectomy is then performed.

Adjunctive surgical techniques

PHLEBECTOMY

This may be performed following treatment of junctional incompetence and axial vein reflux, or as sole treatment under local anaesthetic in patients with isolated tributary incompetence, or possibly in very early axial reflux, which reverts to normal upon occlusion of the refluxing tributary on duplex ultrasound. Phlebectomy is usually performed through small stab incisions using small mosquito forceps and/or phlebectomy hooks that have been demonstrated to be superior in terms of bruising, pain and generic quality of life than transilluminated-powered phlebectomy (see Figure 57.19).

PERFORATOR LIGATION

The majority of studies assessing the role of perforator ligation have been in patients with venous ulcers, analysing the effects on ulcer healing, and even in this situation randomised data are lacking. The role of perforator ligation in patients with uncomplicated varicose veins is even less clear. In uncomplicated varicose veins, perforators may be ligated through a small, duplex-guided incision, while in patients with skin changes, subfascial endoscopic perforator ligation may be preferred, although the benefits are unproven. Perforators can also be ablated with endovenous techniques.

Complications of standard varicose vein surgery

Complications (minor and major) are reported in up to 20% of patients who undergo traditional varicose vein surgery. Wound infections, the most common complication, are reduced by prophylactic antibiotics. Nerve injury is the most common serious complication. The incidence of saphenous nerve neuralgia is up to 7% following GSV stripping to the knee (the incidence is higher with stripping to the ankle). The incidence of sural nerve neuropraxia and common peroneal nerve injury may be as high as 20% and 4%, respectively, following SSV surgery. The incidence of venous thromboembolic complications is approximately 0.5% following varicose vein surgery; however, patient risk factors must be individually assessed and appropriate prophylaxis administered according to guidelines.

Recurrent varicose veins

Approximately 10–20% of patients who present to hospital with varicose veins have had previous intervention. Prospective data on long-term results following intervention for recurrent varicose veins are sparse and the criteria for defining recurrence are variable.

Significant clinical recurrence 5–10 years following varicose vein surgery occurs in 10–35% of patients, but minor/duplex-detected recurrence is much more common, being in the order of 70%. Causes of recurrence include: neovascularisation, reflux in residual axial vein, inadequate initial surgery and new junctional reflux. Neovascularisation is the development of new veins within postsurgical tissue. These veins lack valves and over time can span the tissue between a ligated junction and nearby tributary veins. If significant in size and/or number, these may contribute to recurrent venous hypertension.

Recurrence is more common following SSV versus GSV surgery, and in patients with high body mass index, while stripping of the incompetent axial vein reduces recurrence rates. Limited data suggest recurrence rates following endovenous thermal ablation may be lower than following surgery. Recurrent varicose veins often have an atypical distribution and duplex assessment is mandatory (Figures 57.26 and 57.27). Open surgery for recurrent varicose veins is associated with a high (40%) complication rate, the most common being lymph leak and wound infection, thus endovenous interventions would seem to offer an attractive alternative, where feasible.

VENOUS LEG ULCER

Venous disease is responsible for around 85% of all chronic lower limb ulcers in resource-rich countries. Community-based prevalence is 0.1–0.3% in adults (2–4% in the elderly). Venous leg ulcer has a disproportionate cost to society, with profound impairment in health-related quality of life for

Summary box 57.1

Varicose veins

- Are one of the most common conditions causing a physical impairment in quality of life
- Interventional treatment improves quality of life and is highly cost-effective
- Anatomical and physiological assessment using duplex ultrasound is invaluable in the diagnosis and planning of treatment
- Ultrasound-guided endovenous ablation has revolutionised treatment, minimising procedural morbidity while being highly effective

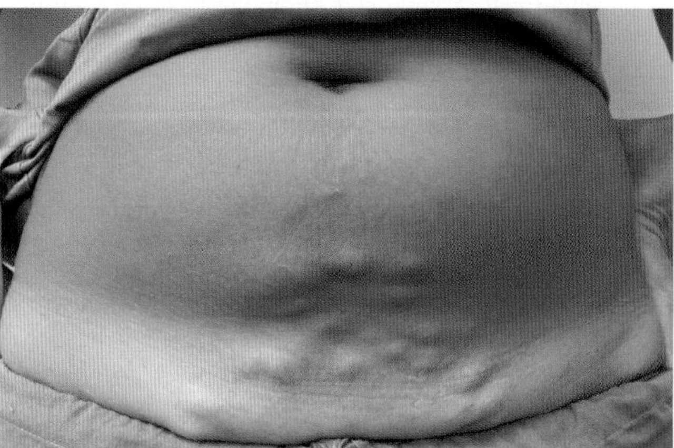

Figure 57.26 Recurrent anterior abdominal wall varicose veins following saphenofemoral junction ligation complicated by iliac deep vein thrombosis.

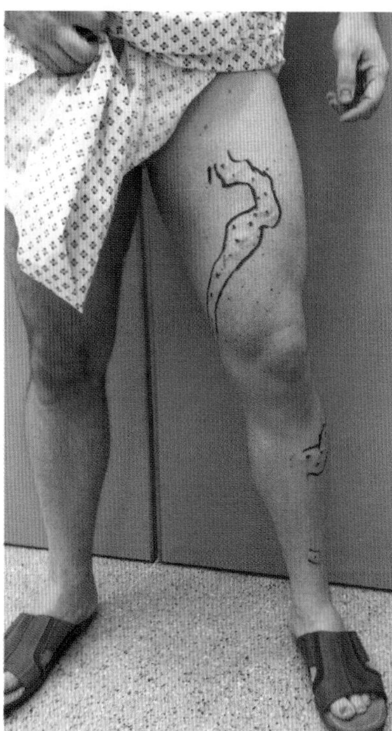

Figure 57.27 Recurrent varicose veins secondary to an incompetent thigh perforator.

both patients and their carers; the dressings alone account for 1–3% of western healthcare expenditure. Furthermore, 15–30% of patients with 'venous' leg ulcers have concomitant arterial occlusive disease. This is termed a 'mixed' ulcer. There are many other causes of leg ulcers and these must be excluded in any patient presenting with ulceration. Causes of leg ulceration include:

- venous disease: superficial incompetence, deep incompetence or obstruction;
- arterial ischaemic ulcers;
- vasculitic ulcers;
- traumatic ulcers;
- neuropathic ulcers;
- neoplastic ulcers;
- infections, especially in resource-poor countries.

Pathophysiology of ulceration

The exact pathophysiology of ulcer development has not been established. Originally, it was thought that static blood within the superficial veins led to hypoxia, which caused tissue death (stasis ulcers). This was not confirmed by investigation of venous oxygen saturation, which was found to be higher in ulcerated limbs. This led to the concept of arteriovenous fistulae, which were thought to develop in response to the high venous pressure; however, this could not be confirmed. High venous pressure was found to be associated with a pericapillary infiltrate. This includes fibrin and other proteins, which are known to lead to fibrosis. It was hypothesised that these 'cuffs' could act as an impediment to diffusion of oxygen and nutrients.

Leukocytes were found to decrease in the venous effluent coming out of dependent limbs. This decrease in leukocyte passage was shown to increase if short-term venous hypertension was induced by application of a tourniquet. This led to the concept of white cell 'trapping', which, however, has not been confirmed by further investigation. Polymorphonuclear leukocytes were not found within the tissues, but increased numbers of mast cells, monocytes and lymphocytes have been found in periulcer tissues.

Reactive oxygen species are increased in the ulcer environment and these may generate free radicals, leading to tissue damage. Proteolytic enzymes are also increased in ulcers and the fibroblasts in the ulcer surrounds are also abnormal, being in a 'senescent' state. Growth factors may be inhibited, leading to poor repair, and their absence may also lead to ulceration. It is proving difficult to show whether any of these factors is the cause of or the result of an ulcer.

At present, ambulatory venous hypertension is the only accepted underlying cause of venous ulceration. This also explains why venous ulcers are never seen in the upper limb. It is important to try to define the exact mechanism of ulcer development. Venous hypertension may be the result of primary valve incompetence of the saphenous veins, incompetence of the perforating veins or incompetence or obstruction of the deep veins.

Clinical features

The ulcer must be carefully examined. A venous ulcer usually has a gently sloping edge and the floor contains granulation tissue covered by a variable amount of slough and exudate. Any significant elevation of the ulcer edge should indicate the need for a biopsy to exclude a carcinoma (usually a squamous cell).

The venous ulcer of the leg characteristically develops in the skin of the gaiter region, the area between the muscles of the calf and the ankle. This is the region where many of the Cockett perforators join the posterior tibial vein to the surface vein, known as the posterior arch vein. The majority of ulcers develop on the medial side of the calf, but ulcers associated with SSV incompetence may develop on the lateral side of the leg. Ulcers can develop on any part of the calf skin in patients with post-thrombotic syndrome (PTS); however, venous ulcers rarely extend on to the foot or into the upper calf and, if there is ulceration at these sites, other diagnoses should be seriously considered. Ulcers often develop in response to minor trauma; many patients notice some itching, perhaps associated with mast cell degranulation, before the ulcers develop. Almost all venous ulcers have surrounding haemosiderosis (seen as pigmentation) and the more chronic ulcers develop lipodermatosclerosis with associated fibrosis of the subcutaneous tissue (see **Figure 57.10**). This is manifest as thickening, pigmentation, inflammation and induration of the calf skin. The pigmentation comes from haemosiderin and melanin and the haemosiderin itself may be an important factor in ulcer development.

A full examination of the front and back of the limbs with the patient standing should be carried out to assess the presence of varicosities and truncal incompetence of the saphenous systems (note that venous ulcers are not always accompanied by varicose veins). All patients should have their pulses palpated and, if there is any doubt, their arterial Doppler pressures should be measured. Sensation and proprioception should be assessed to exclude neuropathy, especially in diabetic patients. A careful examination of the hand and other joints may confirm the presence of rheumatoid arthritis or osteoarthritis.

Investigation

Most vascular surgeons will carry out a duplex scan when the patient with an ulcer is first seen to assess the status of the deep and superficial veins. The presence of reflux in these veins does not confirm a venous ulcer, but supports the diagnosis in the absence of another cause and helps direct treatment.

All patients presenting for the first time with a new leg ulcer should have a full blood count, blood glucose, erythrocyte sedimentation rate (ESR) or C-reactive protein (CRP) and sickle cell test if they have an appropriate racial background. Anaemia can both cause ulcers (e.g. sickle cell disease and pernicious anaemia) and be a result of ulceration (e.g. iron deficiency anaemia and the anaemia of chronic disease). Polycythaemia is a rare cause of ulceration. An antibody screen should be obtained if the ulcer appears 'atypical' or there is any suggestion of joint disease (e.g. rheumatoid arthritis). All patients presenting with a new ulcer should have their Doppler pressures measured, unless the foot pulses are easily palpable and have been confirmed as such by a vascular specialist.

Venous ulcers are characteristically difficult to heal; however, persistence may indicate that there is another or coexisting cause (e.g. malignancy, rheumatoid arthritis or arterial ischaemia). Biopsies are indicated if malignancy is suspected and it is important to remember that a Marjolin's type of ulcer (a squamous cell or basal cell carcinoma) can develop in a chronic long-standing venous ulcer (**Figure 57.28**).

Management

Compression

The very best results are seen in specialist multidisciplinary ulcer services. The cause of a venous leg ulcer is venous hypertension and the key-stone of management is to decrease this hypertension. The primary way of doing this is with the use of compression. Most patients are suitable for the classic 'four-layer bandaging system' (4LB):

- Orthopaedic wool: distributes the pressure and reduces undue pressure on sensitive areas susceptible to pressure damage. Also helps to absorb excess exudate that escapes the primary dressing.
- Cotton crepe: smooths the wool and holds it in place.

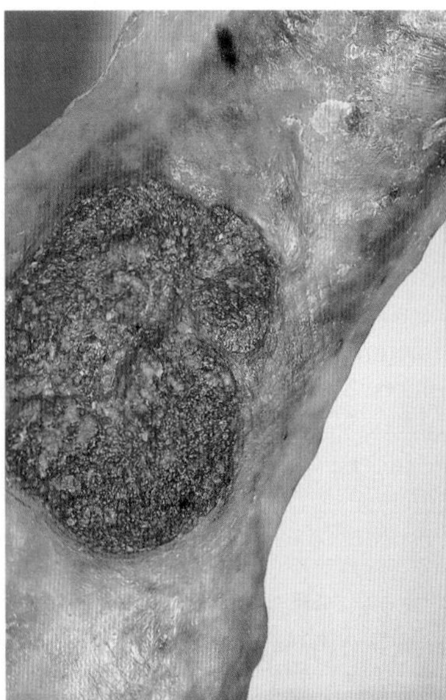

Figure 57.28 A Marjolin's ulcer (a squamous cell cancer arising in a chronic venous ulcer).

Frank Bernard Cockett, 1916–2014, surgeon, St. Thomas's Hospital, London, UK.
Jean-Nicholas Marjolin, 1780–1850, surgeon, Paris, France, described the development of malignant ulcers in scars in 1828.

- Elastic bandage: first compressive layer, contributes about one-third of the interface pressure.
- Cohesive bandage: second compressive layer, increases stiffness and adds approximately two-thirds of the interface pressure

The ideal interface pressure in pure venous ulceration is 35–40 mmHg. Skilled application of these dressings is essential for both safety and efficacy, and the best results come from specialist nursing teams either based in secondary care or in the community. Newer compression systems are being created with the aim of reducing the learning curve and variability in application, and some are designed to be applied by patients themselves. There remains little evidence that these are set to replace 4LB for the time being. The interval between bandage applications is based upon the amount of exudate and the speed of healing and best judged by an experienced nurse.

Compression in mixed ulcers is controversial, but emerging evidence suggests that it is both safe and effective when performed and monitored appropriately. With an ankle brachial pressure index (ABPI) of 0.5–0.8 modified compression with an interface pressure of 30 mmHg is safe and effective and pressures of up to 40 mmHg have been described in studies using inelastic bandages without ill effect. Contrary to conventional thinking, studies have shown an increase in perfusion in patients treated in this way, presumably by a reduction in capillary back pressure. Patients do see respectable healing rates in this group, but they remain lower than in those patients with an ABPI >0.8. It is not clear whether revascularisation followed by full compression yields better results, but this is common practice. Patients with an ABPI <0.5 or an ankle pressure <60 mmHg must undergo revascularisation prior to any compression treatment.

Superficial venous ablation or surgery

The next method of reducing venous hypertension is to treat superficial reflux. There has been only one trial of adequate power and design to answer the question of whether the abolition of superficial reflux improves ulcer healing rates. This trial has completed recruitment, but follow-up is ongoing and practice continues to vary.

Other treatments

The only drug that shows promise to date is pentoxifylline, which increases microvascular perfusion by decreasing plasma cellular viscosity and cytokine inhibition, although its exact mechanism of action is not fully understood.

A number of biological dressings have been developed, including fetal keratinocytes and collagen meshes, which have been shown to improve healing; however, they are not cost-effective for the majority of ulcers. Pinch grafts and ulcer excision with mesh grafting have been shown to provide good early healing with moderate long-term results (50% healed at 5 years).

Antibiotics do not speed ulcer healing in the absence of cellulitis and all other specific ulcer-healing drugs are of dubious validity. A large range of topical therapies and primary dressings have similarly failed to have an impact.

Prevention of recurrence

Once an ulcer has healed the patient must be re-evaluated in an attempt to prevent recurrence. If not already performed, there is level 1 evidence that patients should undergo treatment for their superficial venous incompetence, unless they have deep venous occlusion. Class II below-knee graduated compression stockings should be prescribed for all patients with residual reflux or deep venous occlusion, or those with recurrent ulceration despite not being in this group. These should be worn for life.

Prognosis

Nearly all venous ulcers can be healed but, even in those who have successful ablation or wear their stockings religiously, there is a 20–30% incidence of reulceration by 5 years. The greatest risk of reulceration is in the post-thrombotic leg.

Summary box 57.2

Venous leg ulcer

- Is associated with a profound impairment in quality of life
- Ulcers are not infrequently difficult to heal and prone to recurrence
- The treatment of these chronic wounds is associated with high costs to healthcare systems and patients
- The mainstay of treatment is the reduction in venous hypertension, with compression and increasingly superficial venous ablation

PELVIC CONGESTION SYNDROME

Pelvic congestion syndrome (PCS) is among the differential diagnoses to be considered in female patients presenting with chronic pelvic pain and may be significantly under-diagnosed. PCS sufferers are typically premenopausal, multiparous women aged 20–45 years, who present with severe dull aching pelvic pain thought to be the direct result of ovarian and pelvic varicosities. The pain is usually non-cyclical, and may be precipitated by prolonged standing. Other symptoms include dysmenorrhoea, menorrhagia, rectal discomfort or urinary frequency. Signs may include tenderness over the uterus/ovaries, vulval varicosities and haemorrhoids. There may be vulval and atypically distributed thigh varicosities. The road to a diagnosis of PCS is often a long and laborious one, usually only made following extensive investigations to exclude other more common causes of pelvic pain. Abdominal, pelvic and transvaginal duplex examination allows dynamic visualisation of pelvic blood flow and should be the initial investigation of choice, as these are rapid, readily accessible outpatient procedures that are also valuable in excluding other pathologies. Alternatives include magnetic resonance (MR) venography and diagnostic venography.

Medical treatments for PCS include psychotherapy, progestins, danazol, gonadotrophin receptor agonists (GnRH)

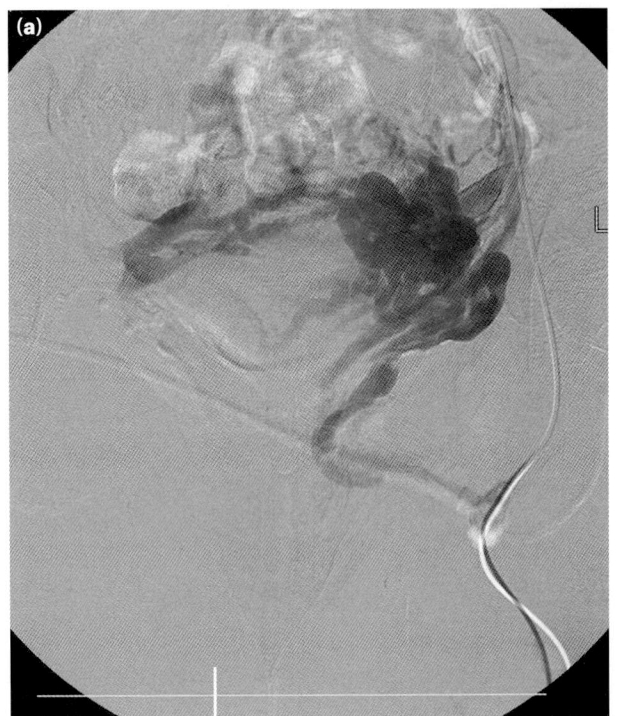

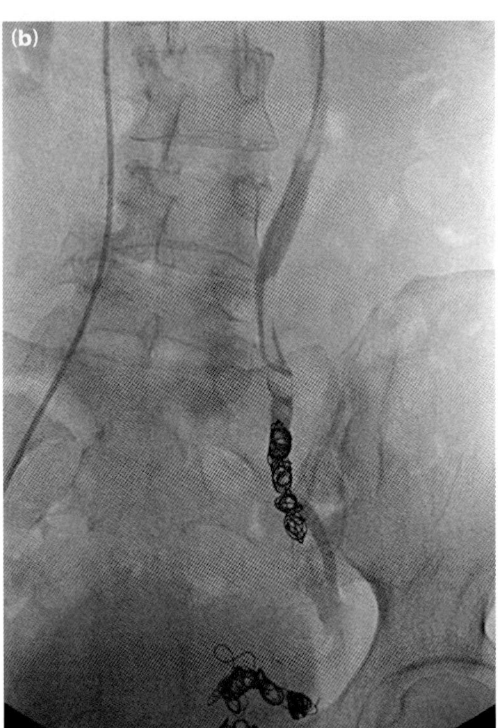

Figure 57.29 (**a, b**) Left ovarian vein incompetence supplying pelvic and pudendal varicosities: (**a**) diagnostic venogram; (**b**)therapeutic embolisation.

with hormone replacement therapy, and non-steroidal anti-inflammatory drugs. Historical open surgical procedures (extraperitoneal resection of ovarian veins) have now largely been superseded by percutaneous pelvic vein embolisation (**Figure 57.29**), reducing peri- and postprocedural morbidity while maintaining high success rates.

VENOUS THROMBOEMBOLISM

Venous thromboembolism (VTE) is an important condition within surgery, and autopsy studies suggest that it is the most common direct cause of death in surgical patients. Venous thrombosis is the formation of a semisolid coagulum within the venous system and may occur in the superficial system (usually described as superficial thrombophlebitis) or the deep system (deep venous thrombosis, DVT). Venous thrombosis of the deep veins of the leg may be complicated by the immediate risk of pulmonary embolus and sudden death. Subsequently, patients are at risk of developing PTS (**Figure 57.30**) and venous ulceration. While DVT may occur in the upper limb, it is the leg that gives rise to the vast majority of the morbidity and subsequent complications of this condition.

Aetiology

The three factors described by Virchow over a century ago are still relevant in the development of venous thrombosis. These are:

- contact of blood with an abnormal surface (e.g. endothelial damage);
- abnormal flow (e.g. stasis);
- abnormal blood (e.g. thrombophilia).

There are many predisposing causes for VTE. These are listed in *Table 57.2*. The most important factor is a hospital admission for treatment of a medical or surgical condition. Injury, especially fractures of the lower limb and pelvis, pregnancy and the oral contraceptive pill are other well-recognised predisposing factors. Endothelial damage is now known to be critically important. The interaction of the endothelium with inflammatory cells, or previous deep vein damage, renders the endothelial surface hypercoagulable and less fibrinolytic.
Stasis is a predisposing factor seen in many of the conditions described in *Table 57.2*, especially in the postoperative period, in patients with heart failure and in those with arterial ischaemia.

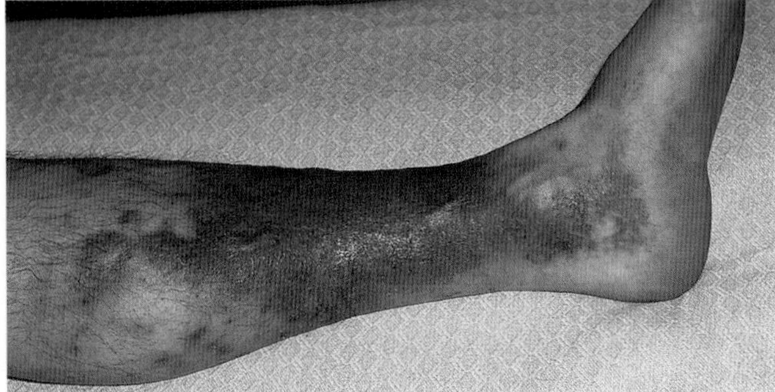

Figure 57.30 Post-thrombotic leg demonstrating features of eczema, pigmentation and mild lipodermatosclerosis.

TABLE 57.2 Risk factors for venous thromboembolism.
Patient factors
Age
Obesity
Varicose veins
Immobility
Pregnancy
Puerperium
High-dose oestrogen therapy
Previous deep vein thrombosis or pulmonary embolism
Thrombophilia (see *Table 57.3*)
Disease or surgical procedure
Trauma or surgery, especially of pelvis, hip and lower limb
Malignancy, especially pelvic, and abdominal metastatic
Heart failure
Recent myocardial infarction
Paralysis of lower limb(s)
Infection
Inflammatory bowel disease
Nephrotic syndrome
Polycythaemia
Paraproteinaemia
Paroxysmal nocturnal haemoglobinuria antibody or lupus anticoagulant
Behçet's disease
Homocystinaemia

A number of conditions are associated with increased coagulability of the blood (thrombophilia) (*Table 57.3*). Deficiencies of antithrombin, activated protein C and protein S have all been shown to predispose to venous thrombosis in young patients. Activated protein C deficiency is associated with inheritance of the factor V Leiden gene and may account for the higher incidence of venous thrombosis in Caucasian populations (being present in 6–7%). It results in a small increase in the risk of VTE, although it may act in concert with some of the other predisposing factors. A thrombophilia should be excluded in any patient presenting with an episode of VTE who gives a family history of VTE or in whom there is no other predisposing factor.

Although the development of DVT is probably multifactorial, immobility (and hence stasis) remains one of the most important factors. DVT is recognised as a complication of long-haul flights and other forms of travel.

Pathology

The thrombus commences as a platelet aggregate. Subsequently, fibrin and red cells form a mesh until the lumen of the vein wall occludes. The coralline thrombus then progresses as a propagated loose red fibrin clot containing many red cells

TABLE 57.3 Abnormalities of thrombosis and fibrinolysis (thrombophilia) that lead to an increased risk of venous thrombosis.
Congenital
Deficiency of antithrombin III, protein C or protein S
Antiphospholipid antibody or lupus anticoagulant
Factor V Leiden gene defect or activated protein C resistance
Dysfibrinogenaemias
Acquired
Antiphospholipid antibody or lupus anticoagulant

(**Figure 57.31**). This is likely to extend up to the next large venous branch and it is possible for the clot to break off and embolise to the lung as a pulmonary embolus. In this situation the embolus arising from the lower leg veins becomes detached, passes through the large veins of the limb and vena cava, through the right heart and lodges in the pulmonary arteries. This may totally occlude perfusion to all or part of one or both lungs. This results in a clinical spectrum from tachycardia and pain, through respiratory failure (despite adequate ventilation) to cardiovascular collapse and death. Moderate-sized emboli can cause pyramidal-shaped infarcts on imaging.

Diagnosis

The most common presentation of a DVT is pain and swelling, especially in the calf, usually in one leg; however, bilateral DVTs are common, occurring in up to 30%. When the

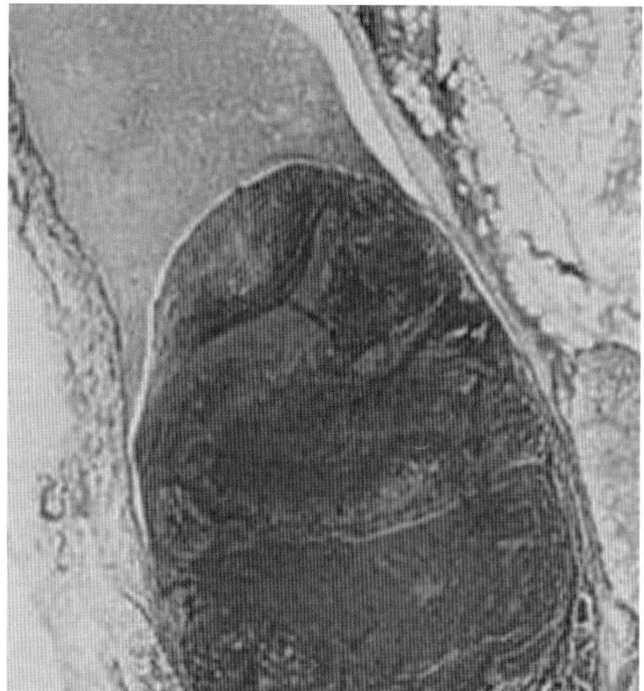

Figure 57.31 An organised thrombus.

Hulusi Behçet, 1889–1948, Turkish dermatologist described a disease of inflamed blood vessels in 1937.

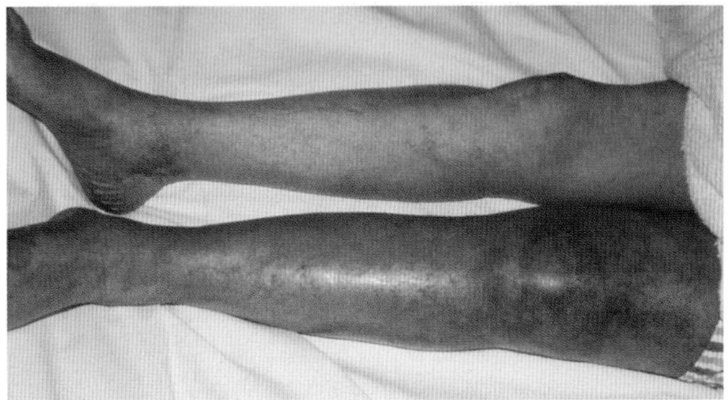

Figure 57.32 Phlegmasia cerulea dolens.

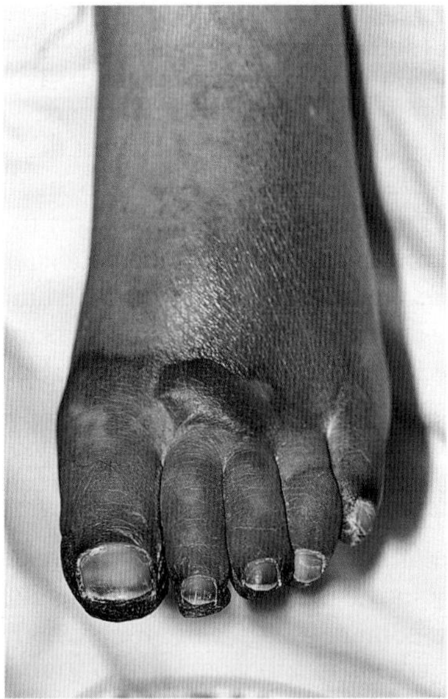

Figure 57.33 A foot with venous gangrene. The gangrene is symmetrical involving all of the toes. There is no clear-cut edge and there is marked oedema of the foot.

swelling is bilateral, DVT must be differentiated from other causes of systemic oedema, such as hypoproteinaemia, renal failure and heart failure. Some patients have no symptoms of thrombosis and may first present with signs of a pulmonary embolus, e.g. pleuritic chest pain, haemoptysis and shortness of breath. Patients may also develop shortness of breath from chronic pulmonary hypertension. Sometimes the leg appears cellulitic and very occasionally it may be white or cyanosed: phlegmasia alba dolens and phlegmasia cerulea dolens (**Figure 57.32**). This indicates venous pressures that are so high that they are impeding tissue perfusion. Patients who present with venous gangrene (**Figure 57.33**) often have an underlying neoplasm.

Clinical examination for DVT is unreliable. Physical signs may also be absent. Mild pitting oedema of the ankle, dilated surface veins, a stiff calf and tenderness over the course of the deep veins should be sought. Leg pain occurs in about 50% of patients with DVT but is nonspecific. Homans' sign – resistance (not pain) of the calf muscles to forcible dorsiflexion – is not specific and should not be elicited. Tenderness occurs in 75% of patients but is also found in 50% of patients without objectively confirmed DVT. The pain and tenderness associated with DVT does not usually correlate with the size, location or extent of the thrombus. Clinical signs and symptoms of pulmonary embolus occur in about 10% of patients with confirmed DVT.

A low-grade pyrexia may be present, especially in a patient who is having repeated pulmonary embolus. Patients may have signs of cyanosis, dyspnoea, raised neck veins, a fixed split second heart sound and a pleural rub if they have pulmonary emboli causing right heart strain, although these signs may be subtle or absent.

Investigation

The diagnosis of DVT and pulmonary embolus should be established by special investigations as the symptoms and signs are non-specific and may be absent. In addition, treatment with anticoagulation is not without risk and the diagnosis must be made with reasonable certainty.

Many centres direct investigation based upon the modified Wells score (*Table 57.4*), with further imaging dictated by these results. These scores can be unreliable though, especially in hospital inpatients, and should only be considered a guide.

Venous duplex ultrasound is commonly performed to look for evidence of thrombosis throughout the deep or superficial venous system. Ideally, this should be performed by an experienced vascular sonographer, but the volume of cases is such that compression ultrasound is frequently being performed by non-specialists. Compression ultrasound involves applying pressure with the ultrasound probe over the common femoral and popliteal veins. Under normal circumstances these veins

TABLE 57.4 Modified Wells criteria for predicting deep vein thrombosis (DVT).

Variable	Score
Lower limb trauma or surgery or immobilisation in a plaster cast	1
Bedridden for >3 days or surgery in last 4 weeks	1
Tenderness along the line of femoral or popliteal veins	1
Entire limb swollen	1
Calf >3 cm larger circumference than the other side	
10 cm below the tibial tuberosity	1
Pitting oedema	1
Dilated collateral superficial veins (not varicose veins)	1
Previous DVT	1
Malignancy (including treatment up to 6 months ago)	1
Intravenous drug abuse	3
Alternative diagnosis more likely than DVT	–2

Low probability (5%) of DVT (score –2 to 0), moderate probability (17%) of DVT (score 1–2), high probability (17–53%) of DVT (score >2).

John Homans, 1877–1957, Professor of Clinical Surgery, Harvard University Medical School, Boston, MA, USA.
Philip Wells, contemporary, physician, University of Ottawa, Canada.

will compress tightly shut. In the presence of DVT they will not fully compress. It is rapid to both learn and perform, but not ideal and most importantly misses calf vein thrombosis. Calf vein thromboses may propagate to form a more extensive thrombus, which may in turn embolise. The optimal management of calf vein thrombosis when detected is not clear, and some units use surveillance, with others anticoagulating such patients upon detection.

Ascending venography, which shows a thrombus as a filling defect, is now rarely required unless thrombolysis is being considered (**Figure 57.34**). MR venography may also be used. Pulmonary embolus is diagnosed definitively by computed tomography (CT) pulmonary angiogram, which will demonstrate the presence of filling defects in the pulmonary arteries (**Figure 57.35**). Pulmonary angiography is rarely required unless thrombolysis is being considered.

The differential diagnosis of a DVT includes a ruptured Baker's cyst, a calf muscle haematoma, a ruptured plantaris muscle, a thrombosed popliteal aneurysm and arterial ischaemia. Duplex scanning will detect many of these conditions but often patients present with non-specific pain in the calf that resolves with no firm diagnosis being made. The differential diagnosis of a pulmonary embolism includes myocardial infarction, pleurisy, pneumonia and aortic dissection.

Prophylaxis

Prophylactic methods can be divided into mechanical and pharmacological. A variety of mechanical methods have been tried, but only the use of graduated elastic compression stockings and external pneumatic compression have been shown to be worthwhile by reducing the incidence of thrombosis. Newer devices, such as electronic nerve stimulators, lack evidence of efficacy to date. Compression-based prophylactic measures should be avoided in patients with peripheral vascular disease.

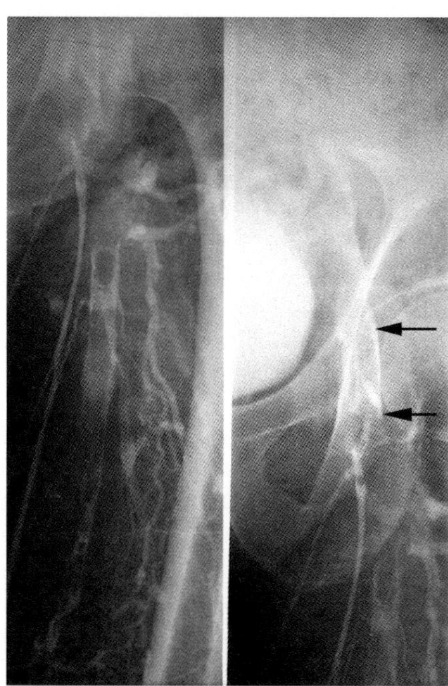

Figure 57.34 An ascending venogram of a deep vein thrombosis seen as filling defects (arrows) with contrast passing around the thrombus.

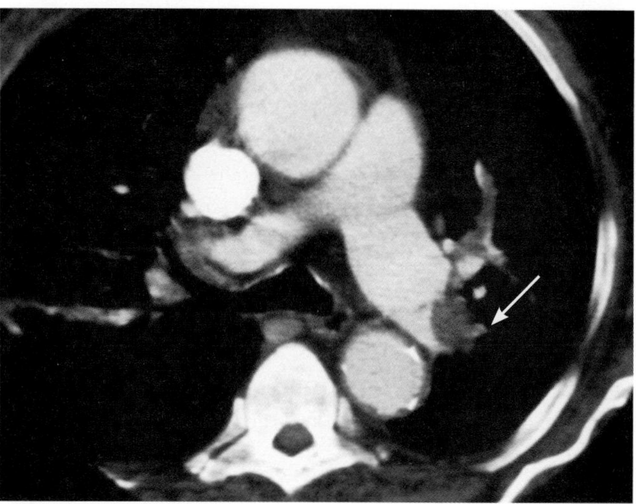

Figure 57.35 A computed tomography pulmonary angiogram showing pulmonary emboli as filling defects (arrow) in the pulmonary artery.

Pharmacological methods are more effective than mechanical methods at risk reduction, although they carry an increased risk of bleeding. In the past, low-dose unfractionated heparin was used both intravenously and subcutaneously. In the absence of renal impairment, most centres currently use low molecular weight heparin (LMWH) given subcutaneously. This is given once daily, does not require monitoring and has a lower risk of bleeding complications.

Patients who are being admitted for surgery may be graded as low, moderate or high risk for PE and VTE (*Tables 57.5* and *57.6*). Patients in the medium- or high-risk groups should be considered for pharmacological prophylaxis with an anticoagulant medication. A combination of mechanical and pharmacological treatment with heparin can be used in patients considered at high risk.

TABLE 57.5 Modified Wells criteria for predicting pulmonary embolism (PE).

Variable	Score
Clinical signs and symptoms of deep vein thrombosis (DVT) (minimum of leg swelling and pain on palpation of deep veins)	3
Alternative diagnosis less likely than PE	3
Heart rate >100 bpm	1.5
Immobilisation >3 days or surgery within past 4 weeks	1.5
Previous DVT or PE	1.5
Haemoptysis	1
Malignancy (treatment or palliation within past 6 months)	1

A score of <4 means PE is unlikely (12.4%), >4 is suggestive of PE (37.1%).

William Morrant Baker, 1839–1896, surgeon, St. Bartholomew's Hospital, London, UK, described these cysts in 1877.

TABLE 57.6 Low-, medium- and high-risk patient groups for venous thromboembolism.

LOW
Minor surgery <30 minutes; any age; no risk factors
Major surgery >30 minutes; age <40; no other risk factors
Minor trauma or medical illness
MODERATE
Major surgery; age 40+ or other risk factors
Major medical illness: heart/lung disease, cancer, inflammatory bowel disease
Major trauma/burns
Minor surgery, trauma, medical illness in patient with previous DVT, PE or thrombophilia
HIGH
Major orthopaedic surgery or fracture of pelvis, hip, lower limb
Major abdominal/pelvic surgery for cancer
Major surgery, trauma, medical illness in patient with DVT, PE or thrombophilia
Lower limb paralysis (e.g. stroke, paraplegia)
Major lower limb amputation

DVT, deep vein thrombosis; PE, pulmonary embolus.

Treatment

Deep vein thrombosis

The management of DVT has in the past been focused upon reducing the risk of pulmonary embolus. Patients who are confirmed to have a DVT on duplex imaging should be rapidly anticoagulated with a 'treatment dose' of subcutaneous LMWH. Patients with significant renal impairment should be commenced on intravenous unfractionated heparin. Patients who have a sensitivity towards heparinoids, such as those with heparin-induced thrombocytopenia, should commence on another anticoagulant, such as fondaparinux (an indirect factor Xa inhibitor) or bivalirudin (a direct thrombin inhibitor). This will achieve rapid anticoagulation and reduce the risk of embolisation. Typically, patients will then commence on warfarin for at least 3 months (or longer depending upon the persistence of risk factors or in recurrent cases). Patients who cannot be safely anticoagulated (usually due to bleeding risks) should be considered for a temporary inferior vena cava filter, until either they are safe to be anticoagulated or the risk of embolisation has subsided and the filter may be retrieved. Patients with active cancer typically remain on a LMWH. There is a range of newer or 'novel' anticoagulants (NOACs). These oral agents either directly inhibit factor Xa (rivaroxaban and apixaban) or thrombin (dabigatran). Work is ongoing to explore their place within patient management.

Alongside the risk of pulmonary embolus is the risk to the patient's leg. Two-thirds of patients will have developed a PTS within 5 years of their DVT. A PTS limb may present with any of the symptoms, signs and complications of venous hypertension discussed earlier, but are typically towards the most severe end of the spectrum and patients face a considerable deficit in their quality of life. A small number of centres are performing procedures aiming to treat this and these include venous recanalisation and stenting and sometimes venous bypass procedures. These procedures can be very challenging and although good results are possible, many patients are condemned to lifelong compression with unaddressed symptoms and complications. As the treatment of PTS is so challenging, attention is being turned towards prevention with the use of thrombolysis, endovenous thrombectomy and stenting.

During thrombolysis, an agent such as tissue plasminogen activator is administered directly into the thrombus, either via the popliteal vein or by direct puncture in the groin. New devices are being marketed that physically disrupt the thrombus at the same time as local lysis is carried out. Some thrombi can be compressed by stent grafting, allowing the venous lumen to be opened, especially in the iliac region. A meta-analysis of randomised trials has shown that these treatments result in a significant reduction in PTS at 5 years (from 67% to 39%) but at a cost of an increased risk of significant bleeding complications (from 4% to 10%). Patient selection is important. Despite such promising data, access to these treatments remains limited.

Pulmonary embolus

Most pulmonary emboli can be treated by anticoagulation and observation, but severe right heart strain and shortness of breath indicates the need for thrombolysis or radiologically guided catheter embolectomy.

Superficial thrombophlebitis

This is a superficial venous thrombosis. An abnormal endothelium is a much more common precipitating factor than in most DVTs. Common causes include external trauma (especially to varicose veins), venepunctures and infusions of hyperosmolar solutions and drugs. The presence of an intravenous cannula for longer than 24–48 hours often leads to local thrombosis. Some systemic diseases such as thromboangiitis obliterans (Buerger's disease) and malignancy, especially of the pancreas, can lead to a flitting thrombophlebitis (thrombophlebitis migrans), affecting different veins at different times. Finally, coagulation disorders such as polycythaemia, thrombocytosis and sickle cell disease are often associated, as is a concomitant DVT.

The surface vein feels solid and is tender on palpation. The overlying skin may be attached to the vein and in the early stages may be erythematous before gradually turning brown. A linear segment of vein of variable length can be easily palpated once the inflammation has died down.

A full blood count, coagulation screen and duplex scan of the deep veins should usually be obtained. Any suggestion of an associated malignancy should be investigated using

Leo Buerger, 1879–1943, Professor of Urologic Surgery, The New York Polyclinic Medical School, New York, NY, USA, described thromboangiitis obliterans in 1908.

appropriate endoscopy and imaging studies, such as an abdominal CT scan.

Most patients are treated with non-steroidal anti-inflammatory drugs and topical heparinoid preparations and the condition resolves spontaneously. Rarely, infected thrombi require incision or excision. Ligation to prevent propagation into the deep veins is almost never required, although some advocate saphenofemoral ligation when the thrombus is seen on ultrasound to be at the SFJ. Associated DVT or thrombophilia is treated by anticoagulation.

Summary box 57.3

Venous thromboembolism

- May be unprovoked, in which case an association with an inherited 'thrombophilia' should be considered
- Is much more commonly seen as a complication of illness or surgery
- Is associated with both quality of life impairment and a risk of mortality
- All healthcare professionals should actively assess the risk and consider preventative measures where this risk is increased
- Management should involve measures to reduce the risk of extension and/or embolisation, typically with systemic anticoagulation
- Consideration should be given to local thrombolysis to reduce the risk of postphlebitis limb

CONGENITAL VENOUS ANOMALIES

There are four main types of anomaly:

- aplasia;
- hypoplasia;
- duplication;
- persistence of vestigial vessels.

Aplasia is most commonly seen in the inferior vena cava and has a similar presentation to the post-thrombotic limb. Membranous occlusion of the left common iliac vein (May–Thurner syndrome) often develops where the vein passes behind the right common iliac artery (iliac vein compression syndrome). This leads to an iliac vein thrombosis, which most commonly affects the left common and external iliac veins. Membranes may also narrow the hepatic veins, which can become totally occluded, leading to a Budd–Chiari syndrome.

Hypoplasia results in a narrow vein, which frequently offers little significant venous function and amounts to a functional venous occlusion, being circumvented by enlarged collateral venous tributaries. Duplications are quite common, with double vena cava, femoral and renal veins; they often present as an incidental finding.

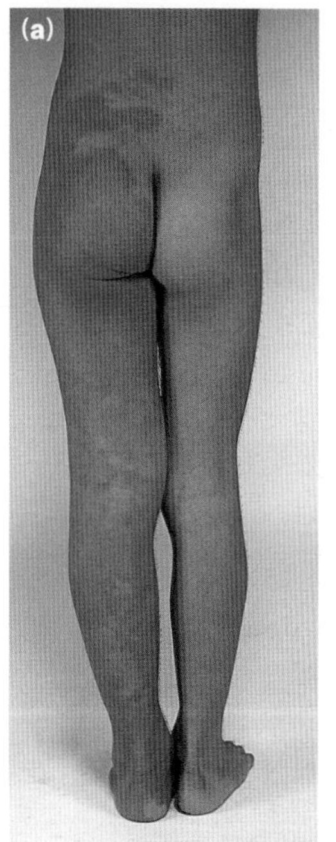

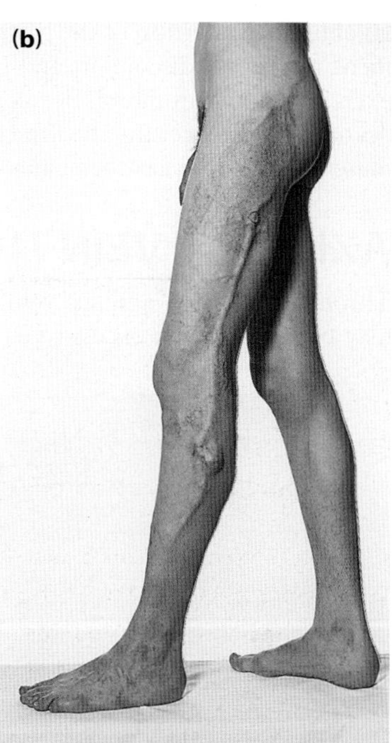

Figure 57.36 Two patients with Klippel–Trenaunay syndrome. (**a**) This patient has a longer leg and a capillary naevus; (**b**) this patient has a large lateral anomalous axial vein.

Klippel-Trenaunay syndrome

This is a combined anomaly of a cutaneous naevus, persistent vestigial veins with varicose veins and soft tissue and bone hypertrophy. The condition is a mesodermal abnormality that is not familial (**Figure 57.36**).

Segments of the deep veins are hypoplastic or aplastic and there may be an associated obstruction of the lymphatics. The condition must be distinguished from the Parkes-Weber syndrome, in which there are multiple arteriovenous fistulae causing venous hypertension, ulceration and high-output cardiac failure.

Virtually all patients with Klippel–Trenaunay syndrome should be treated conservatively with compression hosiery; however, some will benefit from laser ablation of the naevus, stapling of the bones to avoid leg length discrepancy and occasional removal of large superficial varicose veins, provided the deep veins are patent. LMWH should be given to all patients having surgery as this syndrome is associated with an increased risk of VTE.

VENOUS ENTRAPMENT SYNDROMES

The axillary vein and the popliteal vein are the two veins that are most commonly compressed. The former is compressed at the thoracic outlet between the first rib and the clavicle, where it usually presents as an axillary vein thrombosis (see below) (**Figure 57.37a**). The latter is compressed by

George Budd, 1808–1882, Professor of Medicine, King's College Hospital, London, UK, described this syndrome in 1845.
Hans Chiari, 1851–1916, Professor of Pathological Anatomy, Strasbourg, Germany (Strasbourg was returned to France after the end of World War I, in 1918), gave his account of this condition in 1898.
Frederick Parkes-Weber, 1863–1962, physician, The German Hospital, Dalston, London, UK.

an abnormal insertion of the gastrocnemius muscles. Entrapment may cause discomfort and swelling of the limb during exercise before thrombosis develops. Treatment is by surgical decompression, excising the first rib or dividing the abnormal musculature of the gastrocnemius insertion.

AXILLARY VEIN THROMBOSIS

Thrombosis of the axillary vein (Paget–Schrötter disease) may occur following excessive exercise in a patient with an anatomically abnormal thoracic outlet, but is also associated with excessive muscle bulk as found in weight lifters. The vein may be compressed by a cervical rib if this is present (**Figure 57.37b**). The arm is swollen and painful and, at an early stage, the thrombus can be disrupted by thrombolysis delivered through one of the arm veins. The vein must then be imaged to see if there is any compression on elevation of the arm. If this is confirmed, thoracic outlet decompression can be carried out by resecting the cervical rib or first rib.

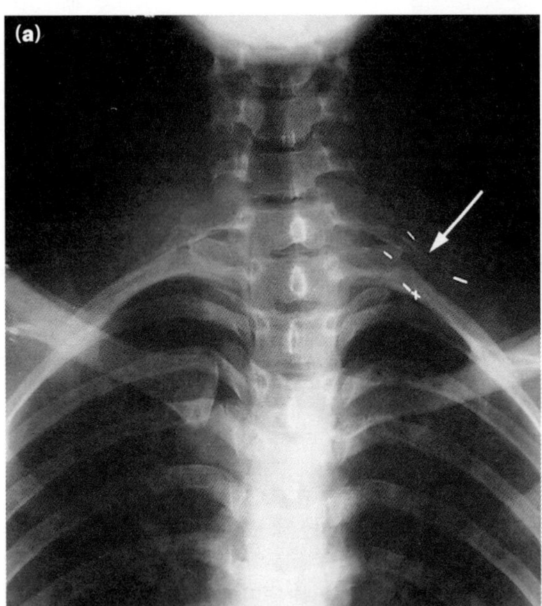

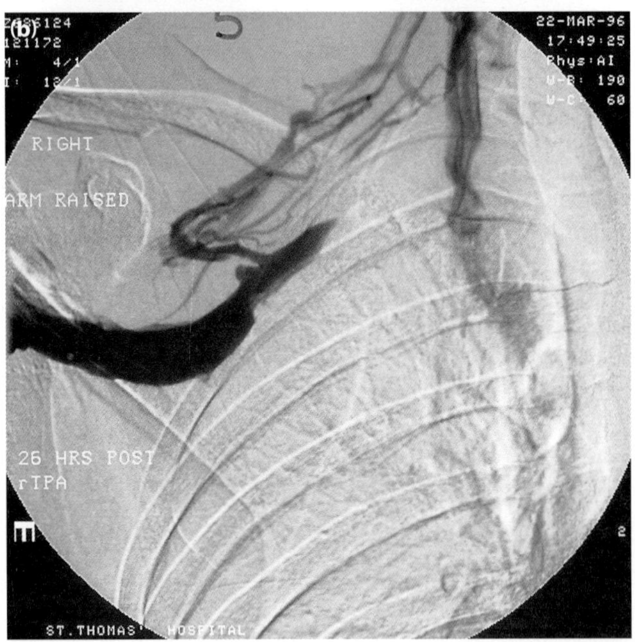

Figure 57.37 Thoracic outlet syndrome: **(a)** cervical ribs on plain x-ray; **(b)** elevation of the arm causing occlusion of the axillary vein with collaterals. The patient has had previous surgery to decompress the left side.

VENOUS INJURY

Blunt or penetrating trauma almost always damages some small- and medium-sized veins, which can be safely ignored or ligated without causing any problems. Larger axial venous channels have in the past been ligated when injured, but it is now recognised that these axial veins should be repaired whenever possible to reduce subsequent morbidity (pain and swelling in the tissues being drained) and limb loss when associated with a concomitant arterial injury. Many venous injuries remain undiagnosed at the time of injury (e.g. crural vein damage associated with a fractured tibia) and only present many years later when post-thrombotic changes become apparent. Venous injuries occur from both civilian and military trauma but the incidence of venous military injuries has been particularly well documented. In total, 40–50% of arterial injuries have concomitant venous injuries, especially in the popliteal fossa.

The mechanism may be laceration, contusion or avulsion (**Figure 57.38**). Iatrogenic injuries result from damage at the time of surgery and from punctures caused by catheter insertion. Thrombosis, haemorrhage and embolisation are all common complications and arteriovenous fistulae may develop when there is a local concomitant arterial injury.

Associated injuries to soft tissue, arteries and bones often overshadow the venous injury. Massive haemorrhage from the pelvic bones or the inferior vena cava can rapidly lead to hypovolaemic shock and death if left untreated. Haematomas are common and engorgement, cyanosis and swelling are also indicative of a major venous injury.

Management

As with all traumatic injuries, the management priorities are the assessment and management of issues affecting the airway, then breathing and then circulation. Venous injuries have the potential to threaten life through massive bleeding and patients require vascular access, circulatory support and blood products. Trauma patients with life-threatening haemorrhage are at risk of hypothermia, acidosis, functional and consumptive coagulopathy and paradoxical thrombosis, and these issues need to be prevented where possible and managed when present (see Chapter 2).

Venous pressures are low and so where there is access to the site of injury, pressure will control bleeding and in most cases offer definitive management. Intervention is required

Sir James Paget, 1814–1899, English surgeon and pathologist, best known for his description of Paget's disease of the bone.
Leopold von Schrötter, 1837–1908, Austrian physician and laryngologist, Chair of Laryngology, University of Vienna, Austria.

Chapter 58

Lymphatic disorders

Learning objectives

To understand:

- The main functions of the lymphatic system
- The development of the lymphatic system
- The various causes of limb swelling
- The aetiology, clinical features, investigations and treatment of lymphoedema

INTRODUCTION

The lymphatic system was first described by Erasistratus in Alexandria more than 2000 years ago. William Hunter, in the late eighteenth century, was the first to describe the function of the lymphatic system. Starling's pioneering work on the hydrostatic and haemodynamic forces controlling the movement of fluid across the capillary provided further insights into the function of the lymphatics. However, there is much about the lymphatic system that is not understood and debate continues over the precise aetiology of the most common abnormality of the system, namely lymphoedema.

ANATOMY AND PHYSIOLOGY OF THE LYMPHATIC SYSTEM

Functions

The principal function of the lymphatics is the return of protein-rich fluid to the circulation through the lymphaticovenous junctions in the jugular area. Thus, water, electrolytes, low molecular weight moieties (polypeptides, cytokines, growth factors) and macromolecules (fibrinogen, albumin, globulins, coagulation and fibrinolytic factors) from the interstitial fluid (ISF) return to the circulation via the lymphatics. Intestinal lymph (chyle) transports cholesterol, long-chain fatty acids, triglycerides and the fat-soluble vitamins (A, D, E and K) directly to the circulation, bypassing the liver. Lymphocytes and other immune cells also circulate within the lymphatic system.

Development and macroanatomy

In the human embryo lymph sacs develop at 6–7 weeks' gestation as four cystic spaces, one on either side of the neck and one in each groin. These cisterns enlarge and develop communications that permit lymph from the lower limbs and abdomen to drain via the cisterna chyli into the thoracic duct, which in turn drains into the left internal jugular vein at its confluence with the left subclavian vein. Lymph from the head and right arm drains via a separate lymphatic trunk, the right lymphatic duct, into the right internal jugular vein. Lymphatics accompany veins everywhere except in the cortical bony skeleton and central nervous system, although the brain and retina possess cerebrospinal fluid and aqueous humour, respectively.

The lymphatic system comprises lymphatic channels, lymphoid organs (lymph nodes, spleen, Peyer's patches, thymus, tonsils) and circulating elements (lymphocytes and other mononuclear immune cells). Lymphatic endothelial cells are derived from embryonic veins in the jugular and perimesonephric areas from where they migrate to form the primary lymph sacs and plexus. Both transcription (e.g. Prox1) and growth (e.g. vascular endothelial growth factor-C (VEGF-C)) factors are essential for these developmental events.

Microanatomy and physiology

Lymphatic capillaries

Lymphatics originate within the ISF space from specialised endothelialised capillaries (initial lymphatics) or non-endothelialised channels such as the spaces of Disse in the

Erasistratus of Chios, c.300–250BC, of the Medical School at Alexandria in Egypt is regarded by many as the first physiologist.
William Hunter, 1718–1783, anatomist and obstetrician who became the first Professor of Anatomy at the Royal Academy of Arts, London, UK. He was the elder brother of John Hunter, the anatomist and surgeon.
Ernest Henry Starling, 1866–1927, Professor of Physiology, University College, London, UK.
Josef Disse, 1852–1912, a German anatomist.

liver. Initial lymphatics are unlike arteriovenous capillaries in that:

- they are blind-ended;
- they are much larger (50 μm);
- they allow the entry of molecules of up to 1000 kDa in size because the basement membrane is fenestrated, tenuous or even absent and the endothelium itself possesses intra- and intercellular pores;
- they are anchored to interstitial matrix by filaments. In the resting state, initial lymphatics are collapsed. When ISF volume and pressure increases, initial lymphatics and their pores are held open by these filaments to facilitate increased drainage.

Terminal lymphatics

Initial lymphatics drain into terminal (collecting) lymphatics that possess bicuspid valves and endothelial cells rich in the contractile protein actin. Larger collecting lymphatics are surrounded by smooth muscle. Valves partition the lymphatics into segments (lymphangions) that contract sequentially to propel lymph into the lymph trunks.

Lymph trunks

Terminal lymphatics lead to lymph trunks, which have a structure similar to that of veins, namely a single layer of endothelial cells, lying on a basement membrane overlying a media comprising smooth muscle cells that are innervated with sympathetic, parasympathetic and sensory nerve endings. About 10% of lymph arising from a limb is transported in deep lymphatic trunks that accompany the main neurovascular bundles. The majority, however, is conducted against venous flow from deep to superficial in epifascial lymph trunks. Superficial trunks form lymph bundles of various sizes, which are located within strips of adipose tissue, and tend to follow the course of the major superficial veins.

Starling's forces

The distribution of fluid and protein between the vascular system and ISF depends on the balance of hydrostatic and oncotic pressures between the two compartments (Starling's forces), together with the relative impermeability of the blood capillary membrane to molecules over 70 kDa. In health, there is net capillary filtration, which is removed by the lymphatic system.

Transport of particles

Particles enter the initial lymphatics through interendothelial openings and vesicular transport through intraendothelial pores. Large particles are actively phagocytosed by macrophages and transported through the lymphatic system intracellularly.

Mechanisms of lymph transport

Resting ISF pressure is negative (-2 to -6 mmH$_2$O), whereas lymphatic pressures are positive, indicating that lymph flows against a small pressure gradient. It is believed that prograde lymphatic flow depends upon three mechanisms:

1. transient increases in interstitial pressure secondary to muscular contraction and external compression;
2. the sequential contraction and relaxation of lymphangions;
3. the prevention of reflux because of valves.

Lymphangions are believed to respond to increased lymph flow in much the same way as the heart responds to increased venous return, in that they increase their contractility and stroke volume. Contractility is also enhanced by noradrenaline, serotonin, certain prostaglandins and thromboxanes, and endothelin-1. Pressures of up to 30–50 mmHg have been recorded in normal lymph trunks and up to 200 mmHg in severe lymphoedema. Lymphatics may also modulate their own contractility through the production of nitric oxide and other local mediators. Transport in the thoracic and right lymph ducts also depends upon intrathoracic (respiration) and central venous (cardiac cycle) pressures. Therefore, cardiorespiratory disease may have an adverse effect on lymphatic function.

In summary, in the healthy limb, lymph flow is largely due to intrinsic lymphatic contractility, although this is augmented by exercise, limb movement and external compression. However, in lymphoedema, when the lymphatics are constantly distended with lymph, these external forces assume a much more important functional role.

ACUTE INFLAMMATION OF THE LYMPHATICS

Acute lymphangitis is an infection, often caused by *Streptococcus pyogenes* or *Staphylococcus aureus*, which spreads to the draining lymphatics and lymph nodes (lymphadenitis) where an abscess may form. Eventually this may progress to bacteraemia or septicaemia. The normal signs of infection (rubor, calor, dolor) are present and a red streak is seen in the skin along the line of the inflamed lymphatic (**Figure 58.1**). The part should be rested to reduce lymphatic drainage and elevated to reduce swelling, and the patient should be treated with intravenous antibiotics based upon actual or suspected sensitivities. Failure to improve within 48 hours suggests

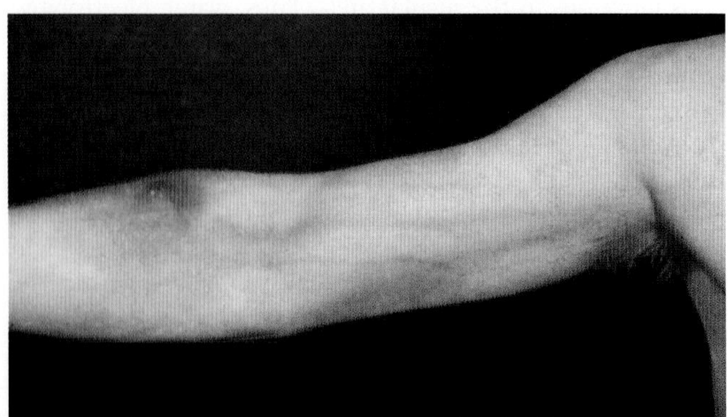

Figure 58.1 Acute lymphangitis of the arm. Erythematous streaks extend from the site of primary infection on the volar aspect of the forearm to epicondylar nodes at the elbow, and from there to enlarged and tender axillary lymph nodes.

inappropriate antibiotic therapy, the presence of undrained pus or the presence of an underlying systemic disorder (malignancy, immunodeficiency). The lymphatic damage caused by acute lymphangitis may lead to recurrent attacks of infection and lymphoedema; patients with lymphoedema are prone to so-called acute inflammatory episodes (see below).

LYMPHOEDEMA

Definition

Lymphoedema may be defined as abnormal limb swelling caused by the accumulation of increased amounts of high protein ISF secondary to defective lymphatic drainage in the presence of (near) normal net capillary filtration.

The scope of the clinical problem

At birth, 1 in 6000 people will develop lymphoedema with an overall prevalence of 0.13–2%. The condition is not only associated with significant physical symptoms and complications but is also a frequent cause of emotional and psychological distress, which can lead to difficulties with relationships, education and work.

Summary box 58.1

Symptoms frequently experienced by patients with lymphoedema

- Swelling, clothing or jewellery becoming tighter
- Constant dull ache, even severe pain
- Burning and bursting sensations
- General tiredness and debility
- Sensitivity to heat
- 'Pins and needles'
- Cramp
- Skin problems, including flakiness, weeping, excoriation and breakdown
- Immobility, leading to obesity and muscle wasting
- Backache and joint problems
- Athlete's foot
- Acute infective episodes

Despite this significant impact on quality of life, many sufferers choose not to seek medical advice because of embarrassment and a belief that nothing can be done. Patients who do come forward for help, especially those with non-cancer-related lymphoedema, often find they have limited access to appropriate expertise and treatment. Lymphoedema is often misdiagnosed and mistreated by doctors, who frequently have a poor understanding of the importance of the condition, believing it to be primarily a cosmetic problem in the early stages. However, making an early diagnosis is important because relatively simple measures can be highly effective at this stage and can prevent the development of disabling late disease, which is often very difficult to treat. It is also an opportunity for patients to make contact with patient support groups.

Summary box 58.2

What every patient with lymphoedema should receive

- An explanation of why the limb is swollen and the underlying cause
- Guidance on skin hygiene and care and the avoidance of acute infective episodes
- Antifungal prophylactic therapy to prevent athlete's foot
- Rapid access to antibiotic therapy if necessary, hospital admission for acute infective episodes
- Appropriate instructions regarding exercise therapy
- Manual lymphatic drainage (MLD)
- Multilayer lymphoedema bandaging (MLLB)
- Compression garments and, if appropriate, specialised footwear
- Advice on diet
- Access to support services and networks

The severity of unilateral limb lymphoedema can be classified as:

- mild: <20% excess limb volume;
- moderate: 20–40% excess limb volume;
- severe: >40% excess limb volume.

Pathophysiology

The ISF compartment (10–12 litres in a 70-kg man) constitutes 50% of the wet weight of the skin and subcutaneous tissues and, in order for oedema to be clinically detectable, its volume has to double. About 8 litres (protein concentration approximately 20–30 g/L, similar to ISF) of lymph is produced each day and travels in afferent lymphatics to lymph nodes. There, the volume is halved and the protein concentration doubled, resulting in 4 litres of lymph re-entering the venous circulation each day via efferent lymphatics. In one sense, all oedema is lymphoedema in that it results from an inability of the lymphatic system to clear the ISF compartment. However, in most types of oedema this is because the capillary filtration rate is pathologically high and overwhelms a normal lymphatic system, resulting in the accumulation of low-protein oedema fluid. In contrast, in true lymphoedema, when the primary problem is in the lymphatics, capillary filtration is normal and the oedema fluid is relatively high in protein. Of course, in a significant number of patients with oedema there is both abnormal capillary filtration and abnormal lymphatic drainage, as in chronic venous insufficiency (CVI) for example.

Lymphoedema results from lymphatic aplasia, hypoplasia, dysmotility (reduced contractility with or without valvular insufficiency), obliteration by inflammatory, infective or neoplastic processes, or surgical extirpation. Whatever the primary abnormality, the resultant physical and/or functional obstruction leads to lymphatic hypertension and distension, with further secondary impairment of contractility and valvular competence. Lymphostasis and lymphotension lead to the accumulation in the ISF of fluid, proteins, growth factors and other active peptide moieties, glycosaminoglycans and particulate matter, including bacteria. As a consequence, there is increased collagen production by fibroblasts, an accumulation of inflammatory cells (predominantly macrophages and lymphocytes) and activation of keratinocytes. The end result is protein-rich oedema fluid, increased deposition of ground substance, subdermal fibrosis and dermal thickening and proliferation. Lymphoedema, unlike all other types of oedema, is confined to the epifascial space. Although muscle compartments may be hypertrophied because of the increased work involved in limb movement, they are characteristically free of oedema.

Classification

Two main types of lymphoedema are recognised:

1 **Primary lymphoedema**, in which the cause is unknown (or at least uncertain and unproven); it is thought to be caused by 'congenital lymphatic dysplasia'.
2 **Secondary or acquired lymphoedema**, in which there is a clear underlying cause.

Primary lymphoedema is usually further subdivided on the basis of the presence of family history, age of onset and lymphangiographic findings (*Tables 58.1* and *58.2*).

TABLE 58.1 Aetiological classification of lymphoedema.

Primary lymphoedema	Congenital (onset <2 years old): sporadic; familial (Nonne–Milroy's disease)
	Praecox (onset 2–35 years old): sporadic; familial (Letessier–Meige's disease)
	Tarda (onset after 35 years old)
Secondary lymphoedema	Parasitic infection (filariasis)
	Fungal infection (tinea pedis)
	Exposure to foreign body material (silica particles)
	Primary lymphatic malignancy
	Metastatic spread to lymph nodes
	Radiotherapy to lymph nodes
	Surgical excision of lymph nodes
	Trauma (particularly degloving injuries)
	Superficial thrombophlebitis
	Deep venous thrombosis

TABLE 58.2 Clinical classification of lymphoedema.

Grade (Brunner)	Clinical features
Subclinical (latent)	There is excess interstitial fluid and histological abnormalities in lymphatics and lymph nodes, but no clinically apparent lymphoedema
I	Oedema pits on pressure and swelling largely or completely disappears on elevation and bed rest
II	Oedema does not pit and does not significantly reduce upon elevation, positive Stemmer's sign
III	Oedema is associated with irreversible skin changes, i.e. fibrosis, papillae

Risk factors for lymphoedema

Although the true risk factor profile for lymphoedema is not currently known, a number of factors are thought to predispose an individual to its development and predict progression, severity and outcome of the condition (*Table 58.3*).

Symptoms and signs

In most cases, the diagnosis of primary or secondary lymphoedema can be made and the condition can be differentiated from other causes of a swollen limb on the basis of history and examination without recourse to complex investigation (*Table 58.4*). Unlike other types of oedema, lymphoedema characteristically involves the foot (**Figure 58.2**). The contour of the ankle is lost through infilling of the submalleolar depressions, a 'buffalo hump' forms on the dorsum of the foot, the toes appear 'square' because of confinement of footwear and the skin on the dorsum of the toes cannot be pinched because of subcutaneous fibrosis (Stemmer's sign). Lymphoedema usually spreads proximally to knee level and less commonly affects the whole leg (**Figure 58.3**). In the early stages,

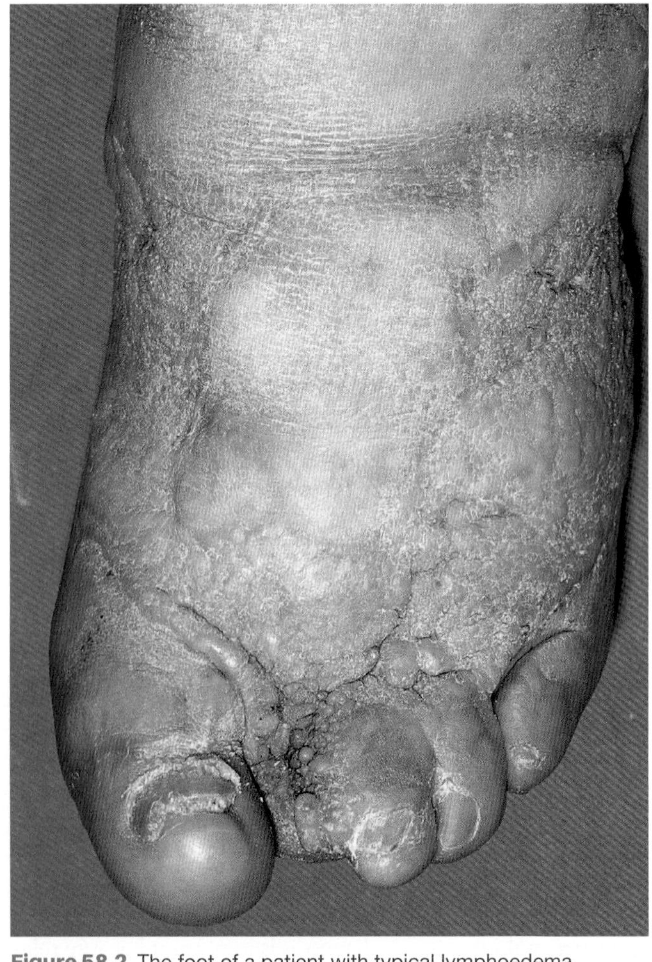

Figure 58.2 The foot of a patient with typical lymphoedema.

Robert Stemmer, 1925–2000, phlebologist, Strasbourg, France.

TABLE 58.3 Risk factors for lymphoedema.

Upper limb/trunk lymphoedema	Lower limb lymphoedema
Surgery with axillary lymph node dissection, particularly if extensive breast or lymph node surgery	Surgery with inguinal lymph node dissection
Scar formation, fibrosis and radiodermatitis from postoperative axillary radiotherapy	Postoperative pelvic radiotherapy
Radiotherapy to the breast or to the axillary, internal mammary or subclavicular lymph nodes	Recurrent soft tissue infection at the same site
Drain/wound complications or infection	Obesity
Cording (axillary web syndrome)	Varicose vein stripping and vein harvesting
Seroma formation	Genetic predisposition/family history of chronic oedema
Advanced cancer	Advanced cancer
Obesity	Intrapelvic or intra-abdominal tumours that involve or directly compress lymphatic vessels
Congenital predisposition	Orthopaedic surgery
Trauma in an 'at-risk' arm (venepuncture, blood pressure measurement, injection)	Poor nutritional status
Chronic skin disorders and inflammation	Thrombophlebitis and chronic venous insufficiency, particularly post-thrombotic syndrome
Hypertension	Any unresolved asymmetrical oedema
Taxane chemotherapy	Chronic skin disorders and inflammation
Insertion of pacemaker	Concurrent illnesses such as phlebitis, hyperthyroidism, kidney or cardiac disease
Arteriovenous shunt for dialysis	Immobilisation and prolonged limb dependency
Air travel	Air travel
Living in or visiting an area for endemic lymphatic filariasis	Living in or visiting an area for endemic lymphatic filariasis

Reproduced with permission from: Lymphoedema Framework. *Best practice management of lymphoedema*. International Consensus. London: MEP Ltd, 2006.

lymphoedema will 'pit' and the patient will report that the swelling is down in the morning. This represents a reversible component to the swelling, which can be controlled. Failure to do so allows fibrosis, dermal thickening and hyperkeratosis to occur. In general, primary lymphoedema progresses more slowly than secondary lymphoedema. Chronic eczema, fungal infection of the skin (dermatophytosis) and nails (onychomycosis), fissuring, verrucae and papillae (warts) are frequently seen in advanced disease. Ulceration is unusual, except in the presence of chronic venous insufficiency.

Lymphangiomas are dilated dermal lymphatics that 'blister' onto the skin surface. The fluid is usually clear but may be blood-stained. In the long term, lymphangiomas thrombose and fibrose, forming hard nodules that may raise concerns about malignancy. If lymphangiomas are <5 cm across, they are termed lymphangioma circumscriptum, and if they are more widespread, they are termed lymphangioma diffusum. If they form a reticulate pattern of ridges then it has been termed lymphoedema *ab igne*. Lymphangiomas frequently weep (lymphorrhoea, chylorrhoea), causing skin maceration, and they act as a portal for infection. Protein-losing diarrhoea, chylous ascites, chylothorax, chyluria and discharge from lymphangiomas suggest lymphangectasia (megalymphatics) and chylous reflux.

Ulceration, non-healing bruises and raised purple-red nodules should lead to suspicion of malignancy. Lymphangiosarcoma was originally described in postmastectomy oedema (Stewart–Treves' syndrome) and affects around 0.5% of patients at a mean onset of 10 years. However, lymphangiosarcoma can develop in any long-standing lymphoedema, but usually takes longer to manifest (20 years). It presents as single or multiple bluish/red skin and subcutaneous nodules that spread to form satellite lesions, which may then become confluent. The

Summary box 58.3

Malignancies associated with lymphoedema
- Lymphangiosarcoma (Stewart–Treves' syndrome)
- Kaposi's sarcoma (human immunodeficiency virus)
- Squamous cell carcinoma
- Liposarcoma
- Malignant melanoma
- Malignant fibrous histiocytoma
- Basal cell carcinoma
- Lymphoma

Ab igne is Latin for 'from fire'.
Fred Waldorf Stewart, 1894–1991, Chairman of Pathology, Memorial Sloan-Kettering Hospital, New York, NY, USA. An annual award was instituted in his name by the Department of Pathology called the Fred Waldorf Stewart Award.
Norman Treves, 1894–1964, American surgeon. He had a special interest in male breast cancer.
Stewart and Treves reported this condition in a joint paper in 1948.

TABLE 58.4 Differential diagnosis of the swollen limb.

Non-vascular or lymphatic	General disease states	Cardiac failure from any cause Liver failure Hypoproteinaemia due to nephrotic syndrome, malabsorption, protein-losing enteropathy Hypothyroidism (myxoedema) Allergic disorders, including angioedema and idiopathic cyclic oedema Prolonged immobility and lower limb dependency
	Local disease processes	Ruptured Baker's cyst Myositis ossificans Bony or soft-tissue tumours Arthritis Haemarthrosis Calf muscle haematoma Achilles tendon rupture
	Retroperitoneal fibrosis	May lead to arterial, venous and lymphatic abnormalities
	Gigantism	Rare All tissues are uniformly enlarged
	Drugs	Corticosteroids, oestrogens, progestagens Monoamine oxidase inhibitors, phenylbutazone, methyldopa, hydralazine, nifedipine
	Trauma	Painful swelling due to reflex sympathetic dystrophy
	Obesity	Lipodystrophy Lipoidosis
Venous	Deep venous thrombosis	There may be an obvious predisposing factor, such as recent surgery The classical signs of pain and redness may be absent
	Post-thrombotic syndrome	Swelling, usually of the whole leg, due to iliofemoral venous obstruction Venous skin changes, secondary varicose veins on the leg and collateral veins on the lower abdominal wall Venous claudication may be present
	Varicose veins	Simple primary varicose veins are rarely the cause of significant leg swelling
	Klippel–Trenaunay's syndrome and other malformations	Rare Present at birth or develops in early childhood Comprises an abnormal lateral venous complex, capillary naevus, bony abnormalities, hypo(a)plasia of deep veins and limb lengthening Lymphatic abnormalities often coexist
	External venous compression	Pelvic or abdominal tumour including the gravid uterus Retroperitoneal fibrosis
	Ischaemia–reperfusion	Following lower limb revascularisation for chronic and particularly chronic ischaemia
Arterial	Arteriovenous malformation	May be associated with local or generalised swelling
	Aneurysm	Popliteal Femoral False aneurysm following (iatrogenic) trauma

diagnosis is usually made late and confirmed by skin biopsy. Amputation offers the best chance of survival but, even then, most patients live for less than 3 years. It has been suggested that lymphoedema leads to an impairment of immune surveillance and so predisposes to other malignancies, although the causal association is not as definite as it is for lymphangiosarcoma.

William Morrant Baker, 1839–1896, surgeon, St Bartholomew's Hospital, London, UK, described these cysts in 1877.
Mauirice Klippel and Paul Trenaunay, two French physicians, described this syndrome in 1900.

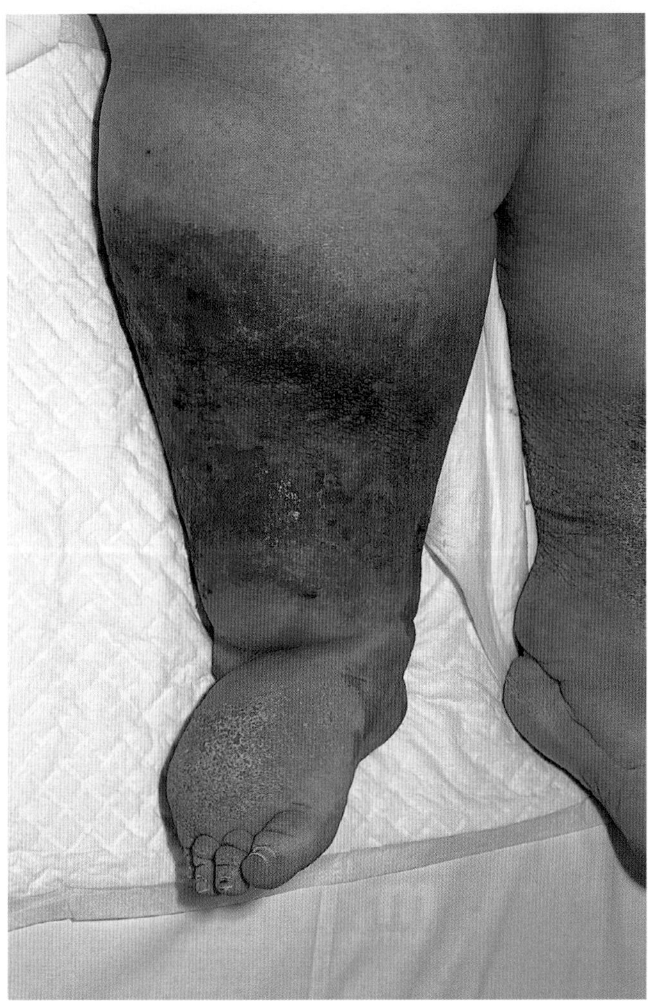

Figure 58.3 The lower leg of a patient with typical lymphoedema.

PRIMARY LYMPHOEDEMA

Aetiology

It has been proposed that all cases of primary lymphoedema are due to an inherited abnormality of the lymphatic system, sometimes termed 'congenital lymphatic dysplasia'. However, it is possible that many sporadic cases of primary lymphoedema occur in the presence of a (near-)normal lymphatic system and are actually examples of secondary lymphoedema for which the triggering events have gone unrecognised. These might include seemingly trivial (but repeated) bacterial and/or fungal infections, insect bites, barefoot walking (silica), deep venous thrombosis (DVT) or episodes of superficial thrombophlebitis. In animal models, simple excision of lymph nodes and/or trunks leads to acute lymphoedema, which resolves within a few weeks, presumably because of the development of collaterals. The human condition can only be mimicked by inducing extensive lymphatic obliteration and fibrosis. Even then, there may be considerable delay between the injury and the onset of oedema. Primary lymphoedema is much more common in the legs than the arms. This may be because of gravity and a bipedal posture, the fact that the lymphatic system of the leg is less well developed, or the increased susceptibility of the leg to trauma and/or infection. Furthermore, loss of the venoarteriolar reflex (VAR), which protects lower limb capillaries from excessive hydrostatic forces in the erect posture, with age and disease (CVI, diabetes), may be important.

Classification

Primary lymphoedema is usually classified on the basis of apparent genetic susceptibility, age of onset or lymphangiographic findings. None of these is ideal and the various classification systems in existence can appear confusing and conflicting, as various terms and eponyms are used loosely and interchangeably. This has hampered research and efforts to gain a better understanding of underlying mechanisms, the effectiveness of therapy and prognosis.

Genetic susceptibility

Primary lymphoedema can be familial or sporadic. In familial cases the genetic mutations can be inherited in an autosomal dominant, recessive or x-linked pattern. In the last few years the application of Next Generation Sequencing, which allows identification of genetic mutations, even in sporadic cases and smaller families, has increased our understanding of the genetic basis of lymphoedema.

So far, mutations in more than 20 genes have been linked to the development of primary lymphoedema. In individuals with familial mutations the penetrance of lymphoedema can often be incomplete leading to a large variability in clinical presentation. Involvement of other systems (cardiovascular, respiratory, nervous, digestive) is common and can indicate a specific mutation. Presence of isolated lower limb lymphoedema at birth, classically described as Milroy's disease, suggests mutation in FMS-like tyrosine kinase 4 (FLT4)/vascular endothelial growth factor receptor-3 (VEGFR-3) or VEGF-C. In these patients, reduced initial uptake and presence of tortuous lymphatic tracts with evidence of rerouting in lymphangiography suggests mutation in the VEGF-C gene. The unique signs and lymphangiographic features of some of the genes currently known to cause primary lymphoedema are summarised in *Table 58.5*. Lymphoedema can also be present as a minor sign in some well-recognised syndromes. Primary lymphoedema is present in less than 10% of cases of tuberous sclerosis (TSC1 and 2 gene mutations). Lymphoedema has been reported in patients with Noonan syndrome in the presence of PTPN11, SOS1 or KRAS mutations, and in patients with Turner syndrome (monosomy X) and capillary malformation-arteriovenous malformation syndrome (RAS p21 protein activator 1 (RASA1) mutation).

William Forsyth Milroy, 1855–1942, Professor of Clinical Medicine, Columbia University, New York, NY, USA, described the condition in 1892.
Jacqueline Noonan, b.1928, paediatric cardiologist, University of Kentucky, USA.
Henry Hubert Turner, 1892–1970, Professor of Medicine, The University of Oklahoma, OK, USA.

TABLE 58.5 Genes associated with primary lymphoedema.

Affected gene	Unique clinical sign(s)	Lymphoscintigraphy findings
FMS- like tyrosine kinase 4 (FLT4)	Isolated lower limb oedema present at birth (Nonne–Milroy disease)	Failure of initial lymphatic absorption (functional aplasia)
Vascular endothelial growth factor C (VEGF-C)	Milroy-like disease	Reduced initial uptake with tortuous lymphatic tracts and evidence of rerouting
Forkhead box C2 (FOXC2)	Distichiasis, cleft lip and/or palate	Hyperplastic lymphatic vessels with reflux of lymph
Gap junction protein gamma-2 (GJC2)	Lymphoedema on all four extremities (Meige syndrome)	Significant reduction in initial uptake, normal lymphatic tracts
Gap junction protein alpha – 1 (GJA1)	Oculodentodigital dysplasia	Significant reduction in initial uptake, normal lymphatic tracts
Kinesin family member 11 (KIF11)	Microcephaly, chorioretinopathy, lymphoedema and intellectual disability (MCLMR syndrome)	Failure of initial lymphatic absorption (functional aplasia)
Collagen and calcium-binding EGF domain-containing protein 1 (CCBE1)	Microcephaly, unusual face and lymphoedema affecting all four limbs (Hennekam syndrome)	Abnormal lymph drainage in all four limbs and the thoracic duct
Homolog of drosophila FAT tumor suppressor 4 (FAT4)	Microcephaly, unusual face and lymphoedema affecting all four limbs (Hennekam syndrome)	Abnormal lymph drainage in all four limbs and the thoracic duct
Gata-binding protein 2 (GATA2)	Myelodysplasia (Emberger syndrome) Warts, recurrent viral and/or bacterial infections Predisposition to several cancers	Hypoplasia of the lymphatics
Inhibitor of kappa light polypeptide gene enhancer in B-cells, kinase gamma (IKBKG)	Ectodermal dysplasia, anhidrotic, osteopetrosis and immunodeficiency (OLEDAID syndrome)	
Protein-tyrosine phosphatase non- receptor-type 14 (PTPN14)	Choanal atresia	
SRY-Box 18 (SOX18)	Hypotrichosis, lymphoedema, telangiectasia and renal defects (HLTR syndrome)	
Hepatocyte growth factor (HGF)	Lymphangectasia	
Integrin subunit alpha 9 (ITGA9)	Fetal chylothorax	

Most of the proteins encoded by these genes belong to the VEGF-C-VEGFR-3 ligand–receptor signalling complex and RAS/MAPK axis. The VEGF-C–VEGFR-3 signalling pathway is a major regulator of lymphangiogenesis. Downstream, transcription factors such as FOXC2 and ITGA9 play a major role in the development of valves in the lymphatic vessels. Mutations in the FLT4 gene that encodes VEGFR-3 protein were the first to be discovered and affect the tyrosine-kinase domain of the receptor, causing congenital primary lymphoedema. Mutations in the genes encoding the RAS/MAPK pathway cause several rare genetic conditions often called RASopathies. All RASopathies have some common clinical features such as distinct facial features and cardiac abnormalities. In addition to lymphoedema, these patients can also present with chylothorax and chylous ascites.

Age of onset

Lymphoedema congenita (onset at or within 2 years of birth) is more common in males and is more likely to be bilateral and involve the whole leg. Lymphoedema praecox (onset from 2 to 35 years) is three times more common in females, has a peak incidence shortly after menarche, is three times more likely to be unilateral than bilateral and usually only extends to the knee. Lymphoedema tarda develops, by definition, after the age of 35 years and is often associated with obesity, with lymph nodes being replaced with fibrofatty tissue. The cause is unknown. Lymphoedema developing for the first time after 50 years should prompt a thorough search for underlying (pelvic, genitalia) malignancy. It is worth noting that, in such patients, lymphoedema often commences proximally in the thigh rather than distally (**Figure 58.4**).

Max Nonne, 1861–1959, a neurologist of Hamburg, Germany, described this disease in 1891.
Raoul Hennekam, contemporary, geneticist, Amsterdam Medical Centre, the Nederlands.
Jean-Marie Emberger, contemporary, haematologist, Montpellier, France.
Henri Meige,1866-1940, physician, La Salpêtrière, Paris, France, gave his description of the disease in 1899.

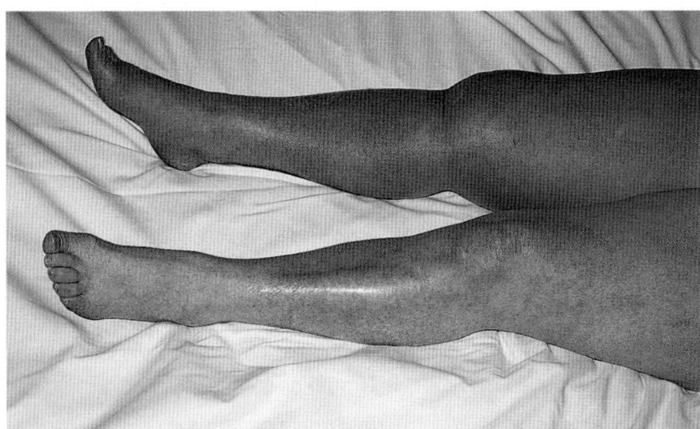

Figure 58.4 This patient, in her sixth decade, presented with rapid onset of lymphoedema of the right leg. On further investigation she was found to have locally advanced bladder carcinoma. Note that unlike most cases of lymphoedema, the swelling is greater proximally than distally.

Lymphangiographic classification

Browse has classified primary lymphoedema on the basis of lymphangiographic findings (*Table 58.6* and **Figures 58.5 and 58.6**). These findings may be related to the clinical presentations described above. Some patients with lymphatic hyperplasia possess megalymphatics in which lymph or chyle refluxes freely under the effects of gravity against the physiological direction of flow. The megalymphatics usually end in thin-walled vesicles on the skin, serous surfaces (chylous ascites, chylothorax), intestine (protein-losing enteropathy), kidney or bladder (chyluria) (**Figure 58.7**).

SECONDARY LYMPHOEDEMA

This is the most common form of lymphoedema. There are several well-recognised causes including infection, inflammation, neoplasia and trauma (*Table 58.7*).

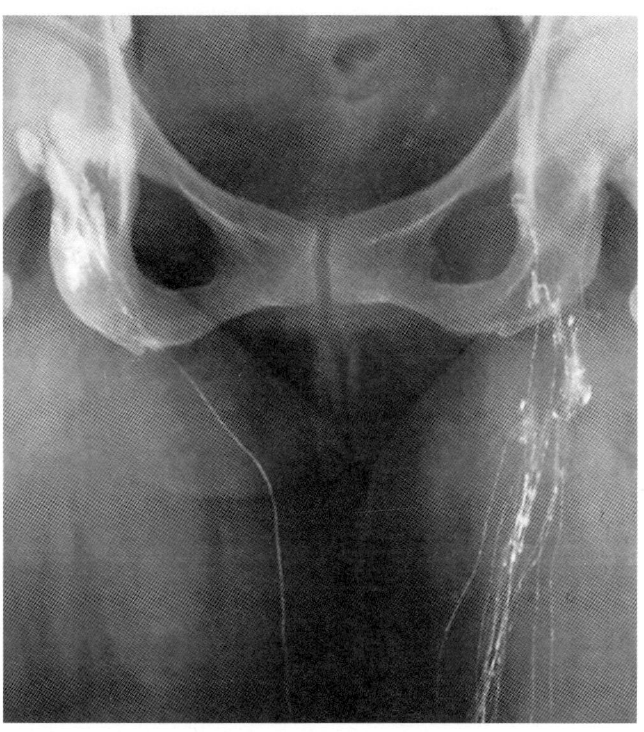

Figure 58.5 This patient presented with congenital lymphoedema of the right leg. The lymphangiogram shows lymphatic hypoplasia.

Filariasis

This is the most common cause of lymphoedema worldwide, affecting up to 100 million individuals. It is particularly prevalent in Africa, India and South America where 5–10% of the population may be affected. The viviparous nematode *Wuchereria bancrofti*, whose only host is man, is responsible for 90% of cases and is spread by the mosquito. The disease is associated with poor sanitation. The parasite enters lymphatics from the

TABLE 58.6 Lymphangiographic classification of primary lymphoedema.

	Congenital hyperplasia (10%)	Distal obliteration (80%)	Proximal obliteration (10%)
Age of onset	Congenital	Puberty (praecox)	Any age
Sex distribution	Male > female	Female > male	Male = female
Extent	Whole leg	Ankle, calf	Whole leg, thigh only
Laterality	Unilateral = bilateral	Often bilateral	Usually unilateral
Family history	Often positive	Often positive	No
Progression	Progressive	Slow	Rapid
Response to compression therapy	Variable	Good	Poor
Comments	Lymphatics are increased in number; although functionally defective, there is usually an increased number of lymph nodes. May have chylous ascites, chylothorax and protein-losing enteropathy	Absent or reduced distal superficial lymphatics. Also termed aplasia or hypoplasia	There is obstruction at the level of the aortoiliac or inguinal nodes. If associated with distal dilatation, the patient may benefit from lymphatic bypass operation. Other patients have distal obliteration as well

Sir Norman Leslie Browse, b.1931, formerly Professor of Surgery, the United Medical and Dental Schools of Guy's and St Thomas's Hospitals, London, UK; former President of the Royal College of Surgeons of England.

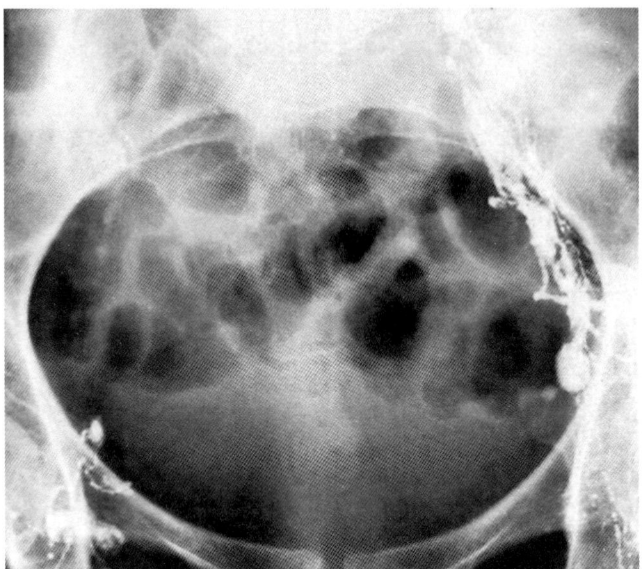

Figure 58.6 This patient presented with lymphoedema of the right leg. A bipedal lymphangiogram demonstrated normal lymphatics in the right leg up to the inguinal nodes, but no progression of contrast above the inguinal ligament – a case of proximal obstruction.

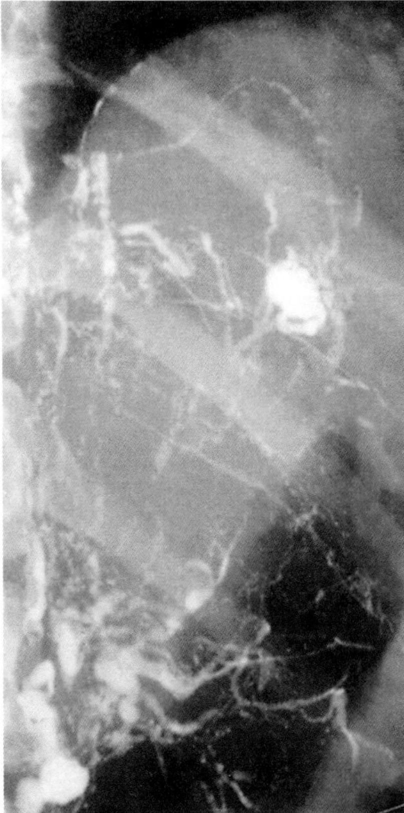

Figure 58.7 Lymphangiogram demonstrating reflux from dilated para-aortic vessels into the left kidney in a patient with filariasis who presented with chyluria.

blood and lodges in lymph nodes, where it causes fibrosis and obstruction, due partly to direct physical damage and partly to the immune response of the host. Proximal lymphatics become grossly dilated with adult parasites. The degree of

TABLE 58.7 Classification of causes of secondary lymphoedema.

Classification	Example(s)
Trauma and tissue damage	Lymph node excision
	Radiotherapy
	Burns
	Variscose vein surgery/harvesting
	Large/circumferential wounds
	Scarring
Malignant disease	Lymph node metastases
	Infiltrative carcinoma
	Lymphoma
	Pressure from large tumours
Venous disease	Chronic venous insufficiency
	Venous ulceration
	Post-thrombotic syndrome
	Intravenous drug use
Infection	Cellulitis/erysipelas
	Lymphadenitis
	Tuberculosis
	Filariasis
Inflammation	Rheumatoid arthritis
	Dermatitis
	Psoriasis
	Sarcoidosis
	Dermatosis with epidermal involvement
Endocrine disease	Pretibial myxoedema
Immobility and dependency	Dependency oedema
	Paralysis
Factitious	Self-harm

Reproduced with permission from: Lymphoedema Framework. *Best practice management of lymphoedema*. International Consensus. London: MEP Ltd, 2006.

Summary box 58.4

Features of filariasis

Acute

- Fever
- Headache
- Malaise
- Inguinal and axillary lymphadenitis
- Lymphangitis
- Cellulitis, abscess formation and ulceration
- Funiculo epididymo-orchitis

Chronic

- Lymphoedema of legs (arm, breast)
- Hydrocoele
- Abdominal lymphatic varices
  - Chyluria
  - Lymphuria

oedema is often massive, in which case it is termed elephantiasis (**Figure 58.8**). Immature parasites (microfilariae) enter the blood at night and can be identified on a blood smear, in a centrifuged specimen of urine or in lymph itself. A complement fixation test is also available and is positive in present or past infection. Eosinophilia is usually present.

Diethylcarbamazine destroys the parasites but does not reverse the lymphatic changes, although there may be some regression over time. Once the infection has been cleared, treatment is as for primary lymphoedema. Public health measures to reduce mosquito breeding, protective clothing and mosquito netting may be usefully employed to combat the condition.

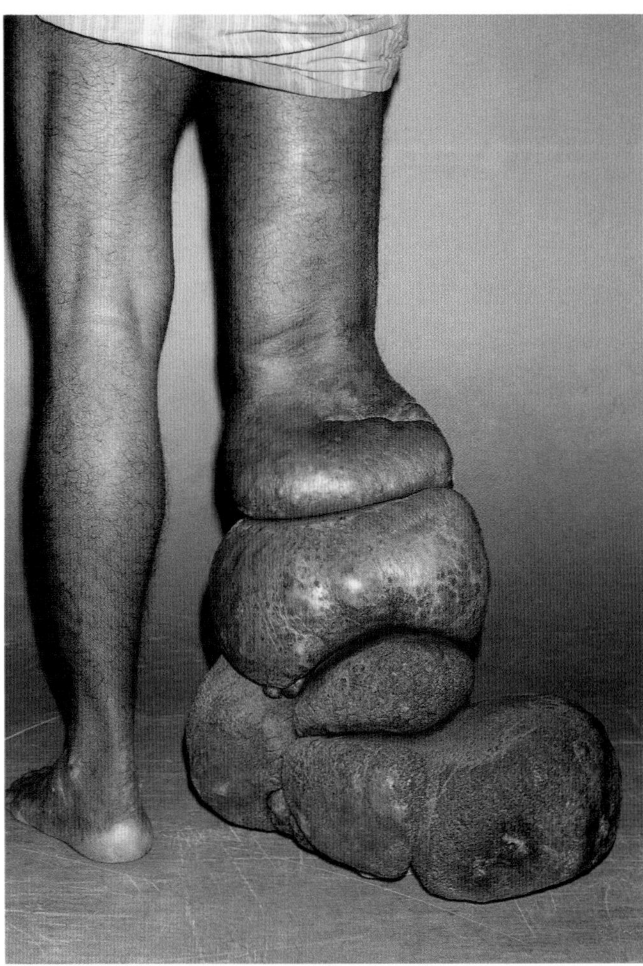

Figure 58.8 Elephantiasis due to filariasis.

Endemic elephantiasis (podoconiosis)

This is common in the tropics and affects more than 500 000 people in Africa. The barefoot cultivation of soil composed of alkaline volcanic rocks leads to destruction of the peripheral lymphatics by particles of silica, which can be seen in macrophages in draining lymph nodes. Plantar oedema develops in childhood and rapidly spreads proximally. The condition is prevented and its progression is slowed by the wearing of shoes.

Bacterial infection

Lymphangitis and lymphadenitis can cause lymphatic destruction that predisposes to lymphoedema complicated by further acute inflammatory episodes. Interestingly, in such patients, lymphangiography has revealed abnormalities in the contralateral, unaffected limb, suggesting an underlying, possibly inherited, susceptibility. Lymphatic and lymph node destruction by tuberculosis is also a well-recognised cause of lymphoedema, especially in resource-poor countries.

Malignancy and its treatment

Treatment (surgery, radiotherapy) for breast carcinoma is the most common cause of lymphoedema in resource-rich countries, but is decreasing in incidence as surgery becomes more conservative (see Chapter 53). Lymphoma may present with lymphoedema, as may malignancy of the pelvic organs and external genitalia. Kaposi's sarcoma, developing in the course of human immunodeficiency virus (HIV)-related illness, may cause lymphatic obstruction and is a growing cause of lymphoedema in certain parts of the world.

Trauma

It is not unusual for patients to develop chronic localised or generalised swelling following trauma. The aetiology is often multifactorial and includes disuse, venous thrombosis and lymphatic injury or destruction. Degloving injuries and burns are particularly likely to disrupt dermal lymphatics. Tenosynovitis can also be associated with localised subcutaneous lymphoedema, which can be a cause of troublesome persistent swelling following ankle and wrist 'sprains' and repetitive strain injury.

Lymphoedema and chronic venous insufficiency

It is important to appreciate the relationship between lymphoedema and CVI as both conditions are relatively common and so often coexist in the same patient, and it can be difficult to unravel which components of the patient's symptom complex are caused by each. There is no doubt that superficial venous thrombophlebitis (SVT) and DVT can both lead to lymphatic destruction and secondary lymphoedema, especially if recurrent. Lymphoedema is an important contributor to the swelling of the post-thrombotic syndrome. It has also been suggested that lymphoedema can predispose to DVT, and possible SVT, through immobility and acute inflammatory episodes. Certainly, tests of venous function (duplex ultrasonography, plethysmography) are frequently abnormal in patients with lymphoedema.

It is not uncommon to see patients (usually women) with lymphoedema in whom a duplex ultrasound scan has revealed superficial reflux (such reflux is present subclinically in up to one-third of the adult population). Although isolated, superficial venous reflux rarely, if ever, leads to limb swelling; such patients are frequently misdiagnosed as having venous disease

Moritz Kaposi, 1837–1902, Hungarian dermatologist, described multiple pigmented skin sarcoma in 1872.

rather than lymphoedema, and are subjected mistakenly to varicose vein surgery. Not only will such surgery invariably fail to relieve the swelling, it will usually make it worse as saphenofemoral and saphenopopliteal ligation, together with saphenous stripping, will compromise still further drainage through the subcutaneous lymph bundles (which follow the major superficial veins) and draining inguinal and popliteal lymph nodes.

Miscellaneous conditions

Rheumatoid and psoriatic arthritis (chronic inflammation and lymph node fibrosis), contact dermatitis, snake and insect bites and retroperitoneal fibrosis are all rare but well-documented causes of lymphoedema. Pretibial myxoedema is due to the obliteration of initial lymphatics by mucin.

Conditions mimicking lymphoedema

Factitious lymphoedema

This is caused by application of a tourniquet (a 'rut' and sharp cut-off is seen on examination) or 'hysterical' disuse in patients with psychological and psychiatric problems.

Immobility

Generalised or localised immobility of any cause leads to chronic limb swelling that can be misdiagnosed as lymphoedema; for example, the elderly person who spends all day (and sometimes all night) sitting in a chair (armchair legs), the hemiplegic stroke patient and the young patient with multiple sclerosis.

Lipoedema

This presents almost exclusively in women and comprises bilateral, usually symmetrical, enlargement of the legs and, sometimes, the lower half of the body because of the abnormal deposition of fat. It may or may not be associated with generalised obesity. There are a number of features that help to differentiate the condition from lymphoedema but, of course, lipoedema may coexist with other causes of limb swelling. It has been proposed that lipoedema results from, or at least is associated with, fatty obliteration of lymphatics and lymph nodes.

Summary box 58.5

Features of lipoedema that help differentiate it from lymphoedema

- Occurs almost exclusively in women
- Onset nearly always coincides with puberty
- Nearly always bilateral and symmetrical
- Involvement of trunk
- The feet are not involved, leading to an inverse shouldering effect at the malleoli
- No pitting
- No response to elevation or compression
- No skin changes of lymphoedema (negative Stemmer's sign)
- MRI shows subcutaneous fat but no fluid accumulation

INVESTIGATION OF LYMPHOEDEMA

Are investigations necessary?

It is usually possible to diagnose and manage lymphoedema purely on the basis of history and examination, especially when the swelling is mild and there are no apparent complicating features. In patients with severe, atypical and multifactorial swelling, investigations may help confirm the diagnosis, inform management and provide prognostic information.

'Routine' tests

These include a full blood count, urea and electrolytes, creatinine, liver function tests, thyroid function tests, plasma total protein and albumin, fasting glucose, C-reactive protein, urine dipstick including observation for chyluria, blood smear for microfilariae, chest radiograph and ultrasound.

Lymphangiography and isotope lymphoscintigraphy

Direct lymphangiography remains the 'gold standard' for showing structural abnormalities of larger lymphatics and nodes (**Figure 58.9**). However, it can be technically difficult, it is unpleasant for the patient, it may cause further lymphatic injury and, largely, it has become obsolete as a routine method of investigation.

Isotope lymphoscintigraphy has largely replaced lymphangiography as the primary diagnostic technique in cases of clinical uncertainty. Radioactive technetium-labelled protein or colloid particles are injected into an interdigital web space and specifically taken up by lymphatics, and serial radiographs are taken with a gamma camera. The technique provides a qualitative measure of lymphatic function rather than quantitative function or anatomical detail. Quantitative lymphoscintigraphy is performed using a dynamic (exercise) component in addition to the static test and provides information on lymphatic transport.

Computed tomography

A single, axial computed tomography (CT) slice through the mid-calf has been proposed as a useful diagnostic test for lymphoedema (coarse, non-enhancing, reticular 'honeycomb' pattern in an enlarged subcutaneous compartment), venous oedema (increased volume of the muscular compartment) and lipoedema (increased subcutaneous fat). CT can also be used to exclude pelvic or abdominal mass lesions. It can also be used to monitor response to treatment through serial measurements of cross-sectional area and tissue density.

Magnetic resonance imaging

Non-contrast magnetic resonance imaging (MRI) is also useful in identifying the classical circumferential reticular pattern (honeycomb) within the epifascial compartment.

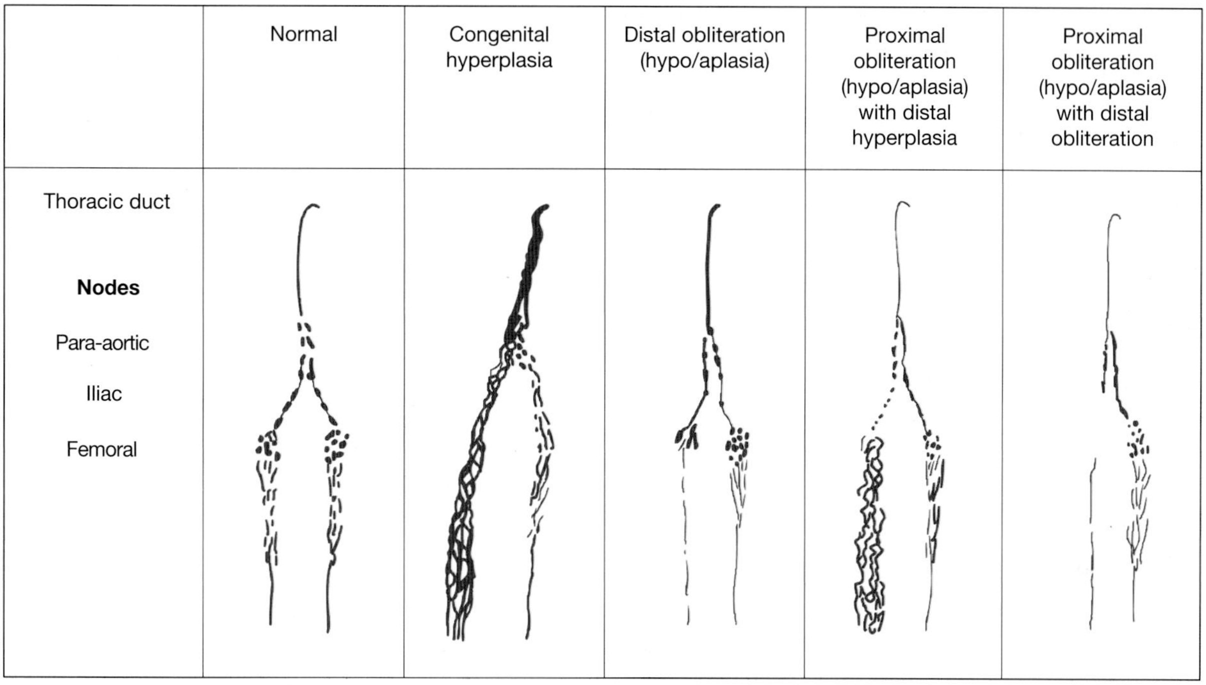

	Normal	Congenital hyperplasia	Distal obliteration (hypo/aplasia)	Proximal obliteration (hypo/aplasia) with distal hyperplasia	Proximal obliteration (hypo/aplasia) with distal obliteration
Thoracic duct **Nodes** Para-aortic Iliac Femoral					

Figure 58.9 Lymphangiographic patterns of primary lymphoedema.

Involvement of the subfascial compartment is more suggestive of venous disease. In lipoedema, there is fat deposition in the subcutaneous tissues without the typical reticular pattern and lymphatic congestion. Using the principles of spin labelling MRI, the lymphatic flow velocities can be assessed and monitored. MRI lymphography, using gadopentetate dimeglumine contrast, correlates substantially with lymphoscintigraphy and provides detailed anatomical and functional status of lymphatic vessels and lymph nodes.

Ultrasound

Ultrasound can provide useful information about venous function including DVT and venous abnormalities.

Lympho-fluoroscopies

More recently, fluorescent molecules, such as indocyanine green (ICG), are being used to image the superficial lymphatic system. When excited using appropriate light energy, these molecules emit photons with a different wavelength that can be detected using dedicated near-infrared imaging devices, providing excellent anatomic and functional details of the lymphatic system. This imaging is increasingly being used to study the lymphatic system and the effects of some therapies.

Pathological examination

In cases in which malignancy is suspected, samples of lymph nodes may be obtained by fine-needle aspiration, needle core biopsy or surgical excision. Skin biopsy will confirm the diagnosis of lymphangiosarcoma.

Limb volume measurement

While not helpful in the diagnosis of lymphoedema, limb volume measurement is a useful tool to determine severity of lymphoedema, guide management and assess response to treatment. Limb volume is typically measured at diagnosis, following intensive treatment and at follow-up. In unilateral limb swelling the affected side can be compared to the contralateral unaffected limb. In bilateral swelling the volume of both limbs is tracked with time.

Measurements are recorded in millilitres or expressed as a percentage of the normal limb. Water plethysmography (water displacement) is the 'gold standard' method, but is limited by practicalities of measurement and hygiene issues. Other options include circumferential limb measurements and perometry (infrared light beams measure the outline of the limb to calculate volume).

MANAGEMENT OF LYMPHOEDEMA

Overview

The evaluation of the lymphoedema patient needs to be 'holistic' and their care delivered by a multiprofessional team comprising physical therapists, nurses, orthotists, physicians (dermatologists, oncologists, palliative care specialists), surgeons and social service professionals. Although surgery itself has a very small role, surgeons (especially those with breast and vascular interests) are frequently asked to oversee the management of these patients. Early diagnosis and institution of management are essential because at that stage relatively simple measures can be highly effective and will prevent the development of disabling late-stage disease, which is extremely difficult to treat. There is often a latent period of several years between the precipitating event and the onset of lymphoedema. The identification, education and treatment of such 'at-risk' patients can slow down, even prevent, the onset of disease. In patients with established lymphoedema, the three goals of treatment are to relieve pain, reduce swelling and prevent the development of complications.

Summary box 58.6

Initial evaluation of the patient with lymphoedema

- History (age of onset, location, progression, exacerbating and relieving features)
- Past medical history including cancer history
- Family history
- Obesity (diet, height and weight, body mass index)
- Complications (venous, arterial, skin, joint, neurological, malignant)
- Assessment of physical, emotional and psychosocial symptoms
- Social circumstances (mobility, housing, education, work)
- Special needs (footwear, clothing, compression garments, pneumatic devices, mobility aids)
- Previous and current treatment
- Pain control
- Compliance with therapy and ability to self-care

Relief of pain

On initial presentation, 50% of patients with lymphoedema complain of significant pain. The pain is usually multifactorial and its severity and underlying cause(s) will vary depending on the aetiology of the lymphoedema. For example, following treatment for breast cancer, pain may arise from the swelling itself (radiation and surgery induced); nerve (brachial plexus and intercostobrachial nerve), bone (secondary deposits, radiation necrosis) and joint (arthritis, bursitis, capsulitis) disease; and recurrent disease. Treatment involves the considered use of non-opioid and opioid analgesics, corticosteroids, tricyclic antidepressants, muscle relaxants, antiepileptics, nerve blocks, physiotherapy and adjuvant anticancer therapies (chemo-, radio- and hormonal therapy), as well as measures to reduce swelling, if possible. In patients with non-cancer-related lymphoedema, the best way to reduce pain is to control swelling and prevent the development of complications. Whatever the cause, pain is a somatopsychic experience that is affected by mood and morale. These issues are important in patients with both cancer-related lymphoedema, who are concerned about recurrent disease and non-cancer-related disease, who often have poor self-esteem and problems with body image and perception.

Control of swelling

Physical therapy for lymphoedema, comprising bed rest, elevation, bandaging, compression garments, massage and exercises, was first described at the end of the nineteenth century, and through the twentieth century various eponymous schools developed. Although there is little doubt that physical therapy can be highly effective in reducing swelling, its general acceptance and practice has been hampered by a lack of proper research and confusing terminology. The current preferred term is decongestive lymphoedema therapy (DLT), which comprises two phases. The first is a short intensive period of therapist-led care and the second is a maintenance phase in which the patient uses a self-care regime with occasional professional intervention. The intensive phase comprises skin care, manual lymphatic drainage (MLD) and multilayer lymphoedema bandaging (MLLB), and exercises. The length of intensive treatment will depend upon the disease severity, the degree of patient compliance and the willingness and ability of the patient to take more responsibility for the maintenance phase. However, weeks rather than months should be the goal.

Skin care

The patient must be carefully educated in the principles and practice of skin care. The patient should inspect the affected skin daily, with special attention paid to skinfolds, where maceration may occur. The limb should be washed daily; the use of bath oil, e.g. Balneum, is recommended as a moisturiser and the limb must be carefully dried afterwards. A hair drier on low heat is more effective and hygienic, and less traumatic, than a towel. If the skin is in good condition daily application of a bland emollient, e.g. aqueous cream, is recommended to keep the skin hydrated. If the skin is dry and flaky then a bland ointment, e.g. 50:50 white soft paraffin/liquid paraffin (WSP/LP), should be used twice daily and, if there is marked hyperkeratosis, a keratolytic agent, such as 5% salicylic acid, should be added. Many commercially available soaps, creams and lotions contain sensitisers, e.g. lanolin in E45 cream, and are best avoided as patients with lymphoedema are highly susceptible to contact dermatitis (eczema). Apart from causing intense discomfort, eczema acts as an entry point for infection. Management comprises avoidance of the allergen (patch testing may be required) and topical corticosteroids. Fungal infections are common, difficult to eradicate and predispose to acute inflammatory episodes. Chronic application of antifungal creams leads to maceration and it is better to use powders in shoes and socks. Ointment containing 3% benzoic acid helps prevent athlete's foot and can be used safely over long periods. Painting at-risk areas with an antiseptic agent such as eosin may be helpful. Lymphorrhoea is uncommon but extremely troublesome. Management comprises emollients, elevation, compression and sometimes cautery under anaesthetic.

Apart from lymphangiosarcoma, acute inflammatory episodes are probably the most serious complications of lymphoedema and frequently lead to emergency hospital admission. About 25% of primary and 5% of secondary lymphoedema patients are affected. Acute inflammatory episodes start rapidly, often without warning or a precipitating event, with tingling, pain and redness of the limb. Patients feel 'viral'

Summary box 58.7

Skin care

- Protect hands when washing up or gardening; wear a thimble when sewing
- Never walk barefoot and wear protective footwear outside
- Use an electric razor to depilate
- Never let the skin become macerated
- Treat cuts and grazes promptly (wash, dry, apply antiseptic and a plaster)
- Use insect repellent sprays and treat bites promptly with antiseptics and antihistamines
- Seek medical attention as soon as the limb becomes hot, painful or more swollen
- Do not allow blood to be taken from, or injections to be given into, an affected arm (and avoid blood pressure measurement)
- Protect the affected skin from sun (shade, high-factor sun block)
- Consider taking antibiotics if going on holiday

and severe attacks can lead to the rapid onset of fever, rigors, headache, vomiting and delirium. Patients who have suffered previous attacks can usually predict the onset and many learn to carry antibiotics with them and self-medicate at the first hint of trouble.This may stave off a full-blown attack and prevent the further lymphatic injury that each acute inflammatory episode causes. It is rarely possible to isolate a responsible bacterium, but the majority are presumed to be caused by group A β-haemolytic streptococci and/or staphylococci. The diagnosis is usually obvious but dermatitis, thrombophlebitis and DVT are in the differential diagnosis. Oral amoxycillin is the treatment of choice with erythromycin or clarithromycin in those with penicillin allergy. Flucloxacillin should be added for those with evidence of *S. aureus* infection (folliculitis, crusted dermatitis). Oral clindamycin is a second-line agent for those with failure to respond to initial therapy. Hospital admission is required for patients with: signs of septicaemia; continuing or deteriorating systemic signs after 48 hours of antibiotic treament; unresolving or deteriorating local signs despite trials of first- and second-line antibiotics. Intravenous amoxycillin or benzyl penicillin with clindamycin in penicillin-allergic patients or as second-line therapy is most commonly recommended. Bed rest will reduce lymphatic drainage and the spread of infection, elevation will reduce the oedema and heparin prophylaxis will reduce the risk of DVT.

Analgesia is often required but non-steroidal anti-inflammatory drugs (NSAIDs) should be avoided as they have been associated with increased complications, including necrotising fasciitis. Any lymphatic massage should be ceased in the presence of active infection. Amoxycillin can be taken by patients who self-medicate. The use of long-term prophylactic antibiotics is not evidence based, but penicillin V 500 mg daily is probably reasonable in patients who suffer two or more attacks per year. However, the benefits of scrupulous compliance with physical therapy and skin care cannot be underestimated.

Manual lymphatic drainage

Several different techniques of MLD have been described and the details are beyond the scope of this chapter. However, they all aim to evacuate fluid and protein from the interstitial space and stimulate lymphangion contraction, with decongestion of impaired lymphatic pathways and development of collateral routes. The therapist should perform MLD daily; they should also train the patient (and/or carer) to perform a simpler, modified form of massage termed simple lymphatic drainage (SLD). In the intensive phase, SLD supplements MLD and, once the maintenance phase is entered, SLD will carry on as daily massage.

Multilayer lymphoedema bandaging and compression garments

Elastic bandages provide compression, produce a sustained high resting pressure and 'follow in' as limb swelling reduces. However, the sub-bandage pressure does not alter greatly in response to changes in limb circumference consequent upon muscular activity and posture. By contrast, short-stretch bandages exert support through the production of a semi-rigid casing where the resting pressure is low, but changes quite markedly in response to movement and posture. This pressure variation produces a massaging effect within the limb and stimulates lymph flow. Whether the aim is to provide support or compression, the pressure exerted must be graduated (100% ankle/foot, 70% knee, 50% mid-thigh, 40% groin).

Non-invasive assessment of the ankle–brachial pressure index (ABPI) using a hand-held Doppler ultrasound device is usually necessary prior to commencing any form of compression therapy, as it is rarely possible to feel pulses in the lymphoedematous limb. Standard MLLB and compression is used in patients with ABPI ≥0.8 and modified techniques with lower pressures in those with moderate arterial disease (ABPI 0.5–0.8). MLLB is contraindicated in severe arterial insufficiency (ABPI <0.5), uncontrolled heart failure and severe peripheral neuropathy.

It is generally believed that non-elastic MLLB is preferable (and arguably safer) in patients with severe swelling during the intensive phase of DLT, whereas compression (hosiery, sleeves) is preferable in milder cases and during the maintenance phase. MLLB is highly skilled and to be effective and safe it needs to be applied by a specially trained therapist. It is also extremely labour intensive, needing to be changed daily.

Summary box 58.8

Effects of multilayer lymphoedema bandaging

- Reduces oedema
- Restores shape to the affected area
- Reduces skin changes (hyperkeratosis, papillomatosis)
- Eliminates lymphorrhoea
- Supports inelastic skin
- Softens subcutaneous tissues

Compression garments form the mainstay of management in most clinics. The control of lymphoedema requires higher pressures (30–40 mmHg arm, 40–60 mmHg leg) than are typically used to treat CVI. These may be reduced to 15–25 mmHg in those with moderate arterial insufficiency (**Figure 58.10**). Confusingly, the British (classes I: 14–17 mmHg; II: 18–24 mmHg; III: 25–35 mmHg) and international (USA) (classes I: 20–30 mmHg; II: 30–40 mmHg; III: 40–50 mmHg; IV: 50–60 mmHg) standards are different. The patient should put the stocking on first thing in the morning before rising. It can be difficult to persuade patients to comply. Putting lymphoedema- grade stockings on and off is difficult and many patients find them intolerably uncomfortable, especially in warm climates. Furthermore, although intellectually they understand the benefits, emotionally they may find wearing them presents a greater body image problem than the swelling itself.

Enthusiasm for pneumatic compression devices has waxed and waned. Unless the device being used allows the sequential inflation of multiple chambers up to >50 mmHg, it will probably be ineffective for lymphoedema. The benefits to the patient are maximised and complications are minimised if these devices are used under the direction of a physical therapist as part of an overall package of care.

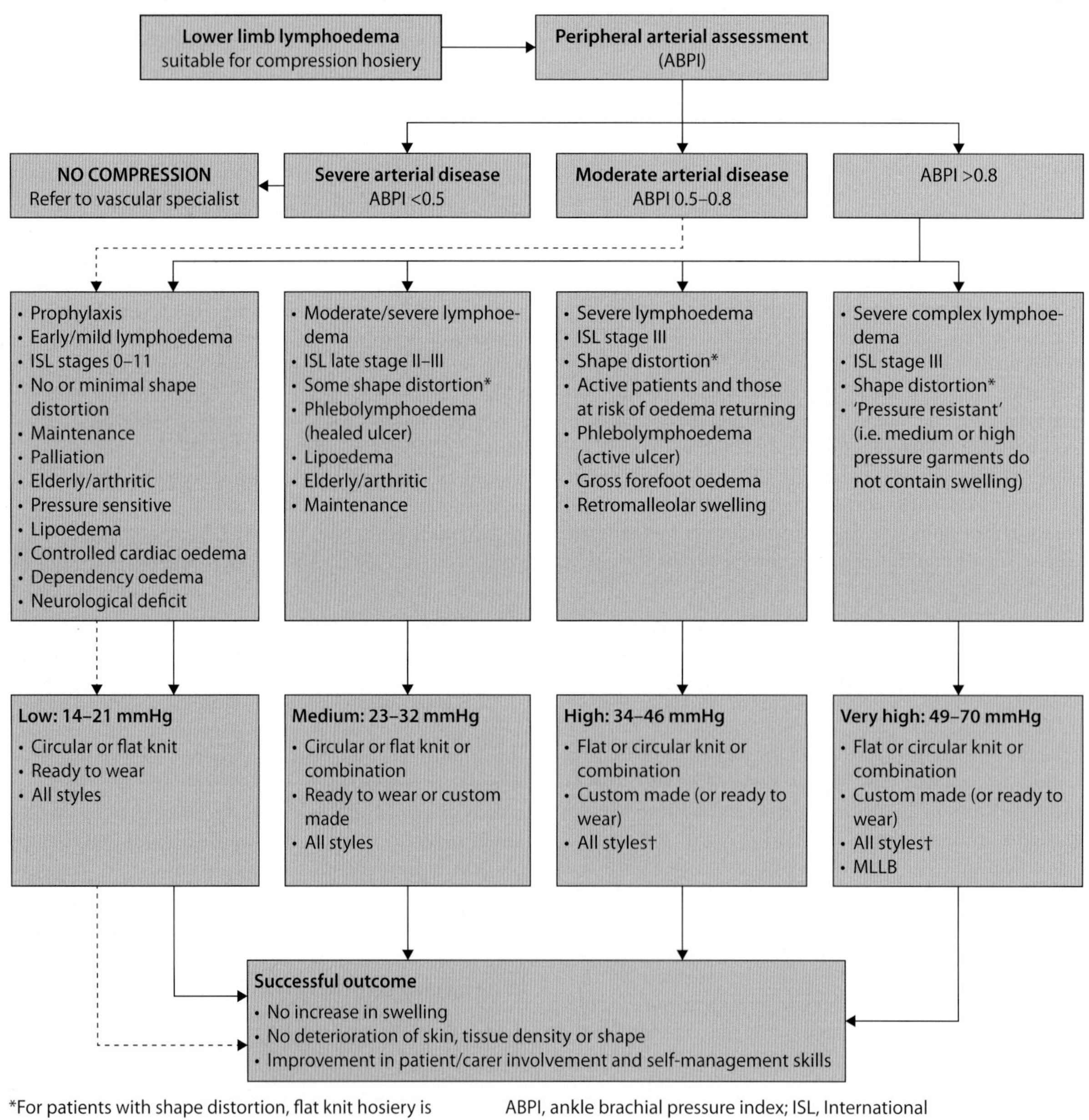

Figure 58.10 Compression garments for lower limb oedema and lymphovenous oedema. Reproduced with permission from: Lymphoedema Framework. *Best practice management of lymphoedema*. International Consensus. London: MEP Ltd, 2006. © MEP Ltd 2006.

Exercise

Lymph formation is directly proportional to arterial inflow and 40% of lymph is formed within skeletal muscle. Vigorous exercise, especially if it is anaerobic and isometric, will tend to exacerbate lymphoedema and patients should be advised to avoid prolonged static activities, for example carrying heavy shopping bags or prolonged standing. In contrast, slow, rhythmic isotonic movements (e.g. swimming) and massage will increase venous and lymphatic return through the production of movement between skin and underlying tissues (essential to the filling of initial lymphatics) and augmentation of the muscle pumps. Exercise also helps to maintain joint mobility. Patients who are unable to move their limbs benefit from passive exercises. When at rest, the lymphoedematous limb should be positioned with the foot/hand above the level of the heart. A pillow under the mattress or blocks under the bottom of the bed will encourage the swelling to go down overnight.

Drugs

There are considerable, and scientifically inexplicable, differences in the use of specific drugs for venous disease and lymphoedema between different countries. The benzpyrones are a group of several thousand naturally occurring substances, of which the flavonoids have received the most attention. Enthusiasts will argue that a number of clinical trials have shown benefit from these compounds, which are purported to reduce capillary permeability, improve microcirculatory perfusion, stimulate interstitial macrophage proteolysis, reduce erythrocyte and platelet aggregation, scavenge free radicals and exert an anti-inflammatory effect. Detractors will argue that the trials are small and poorly controlled with short follow-up and 'soft' end points, and that any benefits observed can be explained by a placebo effect. In the UK, oxerutins (Paroven®) are the only such drugs licensed for venous disease and none has a license for lymphoedema. Diuretics are of no value in pure lymphoedema. Their chronic use is associated with side effects, including electrolyte disturbance, and should be avoided.

With increasing understanding of lymphangiogenesis pathways there is hope that specific pharmacological targets or gene therapy may become available in the future, but this remains in the very early stages at present.

Surgery

Only a small minority of patients with lymphoedema benefit from surgery. Operations fall into three categories: bypass procedures, liposuction and reduction procedures.

Bypass procedures

The rare patient with proximal ilioinguinal lymphatic obstruction and normal distal lymphatic channels might benefit, at least in theory, from lymphatic bypass. A number of methods have been described, including the omental pedicle, the skin bridge (Gillies), anastomosing lymph nodes to veins (Neilubowicz) and the ileal mucosal patch (Kinmonth). More recently, direct lymphaticovenular anastomosis (LVA) has been carried out on vessels of 0.3–0.8 mm diameter using super-microsurgical techniques. The procedures are technically demanding and not without morbidity. They are more often attempted in the upper limb following lymph node resection or radiotherapy for breast cancer. The outcomes are best in patients with earlier stages of lymphoedema, for whom the majority can be controlled with best medical therapy alone. In those with later stage disease who have failed conservative management, the outcomes of LVA have generally been disappointing.

Liposuction

Liposuction has been used in the treament of chronic lymphoedema. It is usually reserved for patients who have progressed to non-pitting oedema. Case series reported thus far have shown promising results with more than 100% reduction in limb oedema volume, which can be maintained by ongoing use of compression hosiery for at least 1 year. While liposuction appears to be safe, results of long-term efficacy and effects on the incidence of future lymphoedema complications (e.g. infection) are awaited.

Limb reduction procedures

These are indicated when a limb is so swollen that it interferes with mobility and livelihood. These operations are not 'cosmetic' in the sense that they do not create a normally-shaped leg and are usually associated with significant scarring. Four operations have been described.

SISTRUNK

A wedge of skin and subcutaneous tissue is excised and the wound closed primarily. This is most commonly carried out to reduce the girth of the thigh.

HOMANS

First, skin flaps are elevated, and then subcutaneous tissue is excised from beneath the flaps, which are then trimmed to size to accommodate the reduced girth of the limb and closed primarily. This is the most satisfactory operation for the calf (**Figure 58.11**). The main complication is skin flap necrosis. There must be at least 6 months between operations on the medial and lateral sides of the limb and the flaps must not pass the midline. This procedure has also been used on the

Sir Harold Delf Gillies, 1882–1960, plastic surgeon, St Bartholomew's Hospital, London, UK. Born in New Zealand, he is widely considered the 'father of Plastic Surgery', Gillies started his craft to better the lives of the victims of the First World War. Later he became a pioneer in 'gender reassignment (sex-change) surgery'. He was joined in private practice by his cousin, the other world famous plastic surgeon, Sir Archibald McIndoe. He excelled in most sports – cricket, rowing, golf, and was an accomplished painter.

Jan Nielubowicz, 1915–2000, surgeon, Warsaw, Poland.

John Bernard Kinmonth, 1916–1982, surgeon, St Thomas's Hospital, London, UK.

Walter Ellis Sistrunk, 1880–1933, Professor of Clinical Surgery, Baylor University College of Medicine, Dallas, TX, USA.

John Homans, 1877–1957, Professor of Clinical Surgery, Harvard University Medical School, Boston, MA, USA.

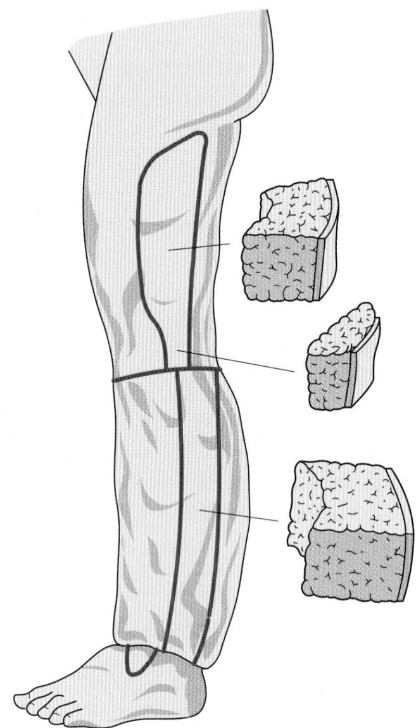

Figure 58.11 Homans' procedure involves raising skin flaps to allow the excision of a wedge of skin and a larger volume of subcutaneous tissue down to the deep fascia. Surgery to the medial and lateral aspects of the leg must be separated by at least 6 months to avoid skin flap necrosis.

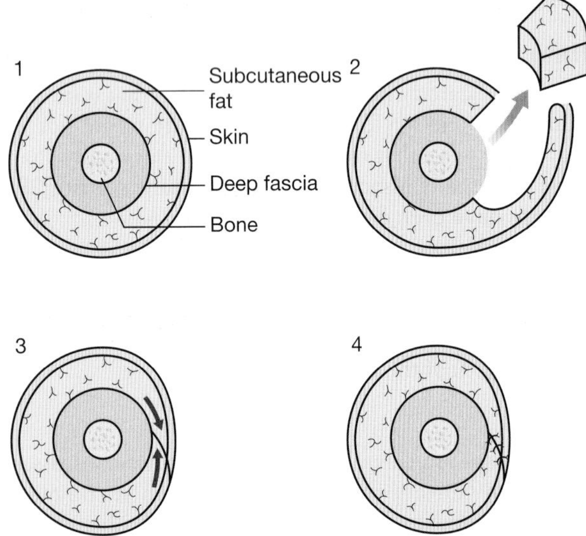

Figure 58.12 A cross-sectional representation of Thompson's reduction operation; red arrows illustrate the buried dermal flap sutured to deep fascia.

upper limb, but is contraindicated in the presence of venous obstruction or active malignancy.

THOMPSON

This is a modification of the Homans' procedure aimed to create new lymphatic connections between the superficial and deep systems. One skin flap is denuded (shaved of epidermis), sutured to the deep fascia and buried beneath the second skin flap (the so-called 'buried dermal flap') (**Figure 58.12**). This procedure has become less popular as pilonidal sinus formation is common. The cosmetic result is no better than that obtained with the Homans' procedure and there is no evidence that the buried flap establishes any new lymphatic connections.

CHARLES

This operation was initially designed for filariasis and involved excision of all of the skin and subcutaneous tissues down to the deep fascia, with coverage using split-skin grafts (**Figure 58.13**). This leaves a very unsatisfactory cosmetic result and graft failure is not uncommon. However, it does enable the surgeon to reduce greatly the girth of a massively swollen limb.

Summary box 58.9

Surgical options for lymphoedema

- Bypass procedures
  - Lymphatic bypass, e.g. omental pedicle, the skin bridge (Gillies) and the ilieal mucosal patch (Kinmonth)
  - Lymphaticovenular anastomosis (LVA)
  - Lymph nodes to vein anastomosis (Kinmonth)
- Liposuction
- Limb reduction procedures
  - Sistrunk
  - Homans
  - Thompson
  - Charles

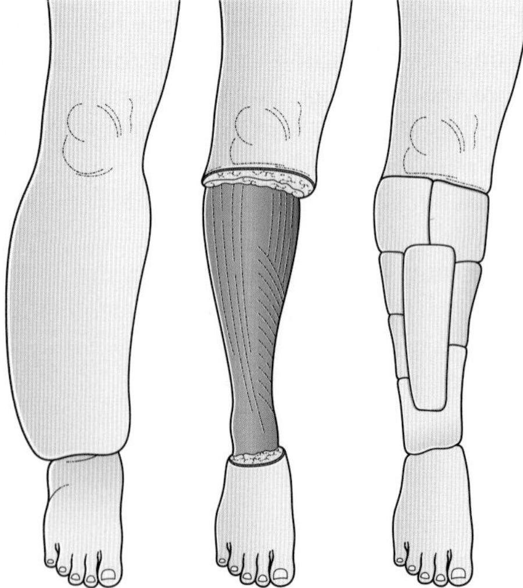

Figure 58.13 The Charles procedure involves circumferential excision of lymphoedematous tissue down to, and including, the deep fascia followed by split-skin grafting. This procedure gives a very poor cosmetic result but does allow the surgeon to remove very large amounts of tissue and is particularly useful in patients with severe skin changes.

Frederick Thompson, 1910–1975, plastic surgeon, The Middlesex Hospital, London, UK.
Major-General Sir Richard Havelock Charles, 1887–1934, surgeon in The Indian Medical Service.

Chylous ascites and chylothorax

These are associated with megalymphatics. The diagnosis may be obvious if accompanied by lymphoedema and lymphangioma. However, some patients develop chylous ascites and/or chylothorax in isolation, in which case the diagnosis can be confirmed by aspiration and the identification of chylomicrons in the aspirate. Cytology for malignant cells should also be carried out. A CT scan may show enlarged lymph nodes and CT with guided biopsy, laparoscopy or even laparotomy and biopsy may be necessary to exclude lymphoma or other malignancy. Lymphangiography may indicate the site of a lymphatic fistula that can be surgically ligated. Even if no localised lesion is identified, it may be possible to control leakage at laparotomy or even remove a segment of affected bowel. If the problem is too diffuse to be corrected surgically, a peritoneal venous shunt may be inserted, although occlusion and infection are important complications. Medical treatment comprising the avoidance of fat in the diet and the prescription of medium-chain triglycerides (which are absorbed directly into the blood rather than via the lymphatics) may reduce swelling. Chylothorax is best treated by pleurodesis, but this may lead to death from lymph-logged lungs as the excess lymph has nowhere to drain.

Chyluria

Filariasis is the most common cause, with chyluria occurring in 1–2% of cases 10–20 years after initial infestation. It usually presents as painless passage of milky white urine, particularly after a fatty meal. The chyle may clot, leading to renal colic, and hypoproteinaemia may result. Chyluria may also be caused by ascariasis, malaria, tumour and tuberculosis. Intravenous urography and/or lymphangiography will often demonstrate the lymphourinary fistula. Treatment includes a low-fat and high-protein diet, increased oral fluids to prevent clot colic, and laparotomy and ligation of the dilated lymphatics. Attempts have also been made to sclerose the lymphatics either directly or via instrumentation of the bladder, ureter and renal pelvis.

Lymphocoele

Lymphocoele is a localised collection of lymph without a distinct epithelial lining. It results from leakage of lymph into the soft tissues or body cavity secondary to surgical disruption of lymphatic vessels. They were first described as a postoperative complication after groin lymph node dissection for gynaecological tumours. Other causes include radical prostatectomy, vascular reconstructive procedures, renal transplant and body contouring surgery after massive weight loss. Clinically, lymphocoele presents as a non-tender, non-pulsatile mobile lump and can be differentiated from a seroma or a localised postoperative oedema by the presence of lymph-rich fluid. Depending upon the site and size they can deform the adjacent soft tissue structures or cause pressure symptoms. Complications include infection, chronic drainage (lymph fistula) and prolonged morbidity. In the early stages, repeated needle aspiration and compression can be attempted. However, lymphocoeles are generally refractory to these simple measures and may require insertion of drainage catheters, packing and compression or surgical excision. For a successful surgical result, combining preoperative lymphoscintigraphy with on-table isosulfan blue dye injection technique enhances the chance of accurately identifying the feeding lymphatic channels and ligation. After resecting a large lymphocoele the residual dead space may need muscle flap transposition to reduce recurrence. Other emerging concepts include performing prophylactic muscle flaps in high-risk groups and negative pressure wound therapy.

FURTHER READING

Cheng M, Chang DW, Patel KM. Principles and practice of lymphedema surgery. Amsterdam: Elsevier, 2016.

Greene AK, Slavin SA, Brorson H (eds). *Lymphedema: presentation, diagnosis and treatment.* New York: Springer, 2015.

International Lymphoedema Framework. *Best practice for the management of lymphoedema*, 2nd edn. Position document. London: ILF, 2012.

Lee B-B, Bergan J, Rockson SG. *Lymphedema: a concise compendium of theory and practice.* New York: Springer, 2011.

Lymphoedema Framework. *Best practice for the management of lymphoedema. International consensus.* London: MEP Ltd, 2006.

Szuba A, Rockson SG. Lymphedema: anatomy, physiology and pathogenesis. *Vasc Med* 1997; **2**: 321–6.

Twycross R, Jenns K, Todd J. *Lymphoedema.* Oxford: Radcliffe Medical Press, 2000.

PART 11

Abdominal

59 History and examination of the abdomen ... 1016
60 Abdominal wall, hernia and umbilicus ... 1022
61 The peritoneum, omentum, mesentery and retroperitoneal space ... 1047
62 The oesophagus ... 1067
63 Stomach and duodenum ... 1106
64 Bariatric and metabolic surgery ... 1144
65 The liver ... 1153
66 The spleen ... 1176
67 The gall bladder and bile ducts ... 1188
68 The pancreas ... 1212
69 The small intestine ... 1240
70 The large intestine ... 1258
71 Intestinal obstruction ... 1280
72 The vermiform appendix ... 1299
73 The rectum ... 1318
74 The anus and anal canal ... 1339

Chapter 59

History and examination of the abdomen

Learning objectives

To understand:

- The pathway for clinical diagnosis of a patient presenting with an abdominal complaint
- The importance of recognising the organ or system responsible for the clinical features
- The pathophysiological basis of common abdominal symptoms and signs

To identify:

- Leading questions based on the organ or system affected and reach the most likely differential diagnosis
- The relevant physical signs and come to an appropriate clinical diagnosis

INTRODUCTION

Abdominal symptoms are a frequent cause for surgical consultation. The underlying cause may be acute, presenting with the euphemistically termed 'acute abdomen', subacute, indicating an evolving disorder, or long-standing, suggesting a functional or degenerative condition. Occasionally symptoms are due to disorders outside the abdomen, in which case the term 'referred' is used, for example epigastric pain experienced as a result of a myocardial infarction.

At first presentation, a detailed clinical history and careful clinical examination are essential to establish a differential diagnosis which, in turn, leads to appropriate triage into urgent and non-urgent investigation and subsequent treatment.

GATHERING INFORMATION

The experienced clinician will recognise the acuity and severity of the patient's condition even before a history has been taken. Initial observation provides clues to the direction that the history should take: general appearance, gait, position in bed, facial expression and tone of speech all provide useful hints. In an acute presentation, it is important to realise that the patient will feel anxious and vulnerable and may well be in severe pain; therefore, the clinician should introduce him-/herself, try to comfort the patient and gain his or her confidence. This is particularly important in a busy emergency department where the patient is only one among many.

Obtaining a history

The patient's history is obtained during the initial part of the consultation. It is crucial that the patient be allowed to explain the presenting complaint without interruption, after which carefully directed questions are used to further refine the history; this will then guide subsequent clinical examination and investigation.

Presenting complaint

To establish the presenting complaint one should start with an open question inviting the patient to explain the reason for seeking medical advice. In the acute situation, pain is the most common presenting feature. The classic features of site, nature, onset, duration, radiation, and aggravating or relieving features of the pain should be established. In a non-acute presentation anorexia, weight loss, jaundice, altered bowel habit, blood loss and fatigue are all features that should be enquired about.

Once the patient has finished explaining the problem, direct questions should be used to support or exclude possible diagnoses. It should be possible to identify a likely organ or system responsible for the patient's symptoms and come to a differential diagnosis.

Past history

The past history is important because it may have a bearing on the diagnosis and management. A history of previous similar episodes or past abdominal surgery often guides the diagnosis, for example adhesive small bowel obstruction in a patient with a history of laparotomy or recurrent left iliac fossa pain in a patient with a past history of diverticulitis. Some symptoms and signs may be due to cardiac, respiratory, haematological or musculoskeletal conditions, for example abdominal pain in sickle cell crisis.

Drug history and allergies

Some drugs will have an effect on the symptoms and signs or may have to be discontinued before surgery. For example, a patient with bleeding who is taking a β-blocking drug will not have tachycardia proportionate to the blood loss, a patient taking long-term corticosteroids will need intravenous steroid supplementation to prevent an adrenal crisis in the perioperative period and a patient taking anticoagulant drugs may require reversal of the effects before surgical intervention.

Social history

The use of alcohol and illicit drugs, smoking and occupation is important. Family background will inform potential difficulties with later discharge planning.

Family history

It is important to establish a family history of similar or related conditions, particularly cancer, inflammatory bowel disease, endocrine disease (e.g. hyperparathyroidism causing hypercalcaemia or renal calculi) and genetic disorders, including adverse reactions to anaesthetics or medications.

Review of the systems

A system review should highlight any comorbid disease, such as cardiac, vascular, respiratory or endocrine problems.

Summary box 59.1

Principles of history taking

- Identify the reason for consultation – the presenting complaint
- Determine the onset, duration and evolution of the symptoms
- Deduce the most likely organ or system affected
- Refine the history with relevant direct questions
- Establish relevant past, social, family, drug and allergy history
- Complete with a thorough review of other systems
- Devise a list of differential diagnoses

CLINICAL PRESENTATION OF ABDOMINAL PROBLEMS

Pain, weight loss, anorexia or vomiting, jaundice, alteration of bowel habit, and blood loss or anaemia are the common clinical presentations of abdominal pathology. It is important to be vigilant about insidious presentations of malignancies. Classic examples are right colon cancer presenting with symptoms of anaemia, metastatic liver cancer with weight loss, gastric cancer with loss of appetite, ovarian cancer with abdominal distension, and malignant obstruction of the extrahepatic biliary tree presenting with jaundice.

Summary box 59.2

Sources of abdominal symptoms

- Abdominal pain, weight loss, anorexia or vomiting, jaundice, alteration of bowel habit, and blood loss or anaemia are the common clinical presentations of abdominal pathology
- Occult malignancies may have atypical presentation

Abdominal pain

Pain is the most common of all abdominal symptoms and may be due to inflammatory, infective, obstructive, neoplastic or ischaemic pathology. Sometimes no organic cause can be found, a situation often labelled 'functional abdominal pain' for want of a better term. Improved understanding of pain pathways and the relationship with the gastrointestinal microbiome is likely to provide a more precise diagnosis, particularly in common 'functional' disorders such as non-ulcer dyspepsia and irritable bowel syndrome (IBS).

It is essential to establish the site, nature and radiation of the pain, the rapidity of onset, and associated or relieving features. Thus biliary colic will classically result in colicky pain in the right upper quadrant of the abdomen which radiates to the angle of the scapula and is associated with food intake (which results in cholecystokinin release and gallbladder contraction). Acute pancreatitis often has an abrupt onset of severe epigastric pain radiating to the back, which may be similar to pain emanating from peptic ulcer perforation or a leaking aortic aneurysm. Intestinal colic is most frequently associated with periumbilical pain and abdominal distension: the more distal in the intestine the pathology, the greater the degree of distension. Vomiting is an early feature of proximal small bowel obstruction, whereas absolute constipation is an early feature of colonic obstruction. Renal or ureteric colic is intense, located in the flanks and radiating towards the lower midline. It is usually associated with either macroscopic or microscopic haematuria.

With regard to altered bowel habit, the onset, nature, duration, type of alteration (constipation or diarrhoea) and its relationship to abdominal pain will help to differentiate organic pathology causing obstruction or inflammation (colon cancer or inflammatory bowel disease [IBD]) from functional conditions such as IBS. When patients complain of diarrhoea, they may imply different meanings – some use the term for loose stools, others may mean frequent but normal stools. A long-standing increase in frequency of stools, with left-sided abdominal pain before defecation, that eases after defecation, is suggestive of IBS. However, if such symptoms are of recent onset or are associated with blood or mucus in the stools, colonic carcinoma or IBD is more likely. A history of progressive change in bowel habit with an acute presentation with abdominal pain, distension and absolute constipation suggests acute-on-chronic intestinal obstruction, often from a stenotic left colon cancer. Marked distension with tenderness over the caecal area suggests a closed-loop obstruction with impending caecal rupture.

Summary box 59.3

Classic presentations of abdominal pathology

- Obstructive and inflammatory pathology must be excluded in patients with abdominal pain and altered bowel habit
- Closed-loop obstruction with tenderness in the right iliac fossa is indicative of imminent caecal rupture
- Caecal cancer classically presents with anaemia
- Patients who have had previous abdominal surgery may have adhesions
- Check carefully for small incarcerated hernias, particularly femoral, in obese patients

PATHOPHYSIOLOGICAL BASIS OF COMMON ABDOMINAL SYMPTOMS AND SIGNS

The abdominal wall and parietal peritoneum are innervated by the somatic nervous system, whereas the abdominal organs and visceral peritoneum are innervated by the autonomic nervous system. Therefore pain may change in its character and distribution as the underlying pathology evolves. Visceral pain from the foregut is generally felt in the epigastrium, in the periumbilical area from the mid-gut and in the suprapubic area from the hind-gut.

The skin and the muscles of the abdominal wall are supplied by the lateral and anterior cutaneous branches of the lower six intercostal nerves, the iliohypogastric and ilioinguinal nerves (Figure 59.1). The dermatome levels of the xiphoid process, umbilicus and pubis are T7, T10 and T12, respectively. The parietal peritoneum is supplied segmentally by the same nerves that innervate the overlying muscles. The central part of the diaphragmatic peritoneum is supplied by the phrenic nerve (C4); therefore, pain arising in this region is referred to the tip of the shoulder as it has the same segmental supply. The peripheral rim of the diaphragmatic peritoneum is supplied by the intercostal nerves. The obturator nerve is the principal nerve supply of the pelvic parietal peritoneum.

Pain from the viscera is principally due to ischaemia, muscle spasm or stretching of the visceral peritoneum. Unlike somatic pain, autonomic pain is deep and poorly localised. This pain is transmitted via sympathetic fibres and so is referred to the appropriate somatic distribution of that nerve root from T1 to L2. However, when an inflamed organ touches the parietal peritoneum, the pain becomes sharp and localises to the appropriate segmental dermatome of the abdominal wall. Pain arising from the parietal peritoneum may radiate to the back or the front along the appropriate dermatome. This referral pattern is classically seen in acute cholecystitis when an inflamed gall bladder touches the parietal peritoneum. Pain then radiates round to the back along the involved dermatome. The overlying muscle and skin are supplied by the same nerve root, so, when the patient takes a deep breath, the tenderness in the right subcostal region is markedly increased, causing the patient to stop breathing; this is Murphy's sign. In children with abdominal pain, who hold their right hip in a flexed position to obtain relief from the pain, one should suspect retrocaecal appendicitis causing irritation of the psoas muscle.

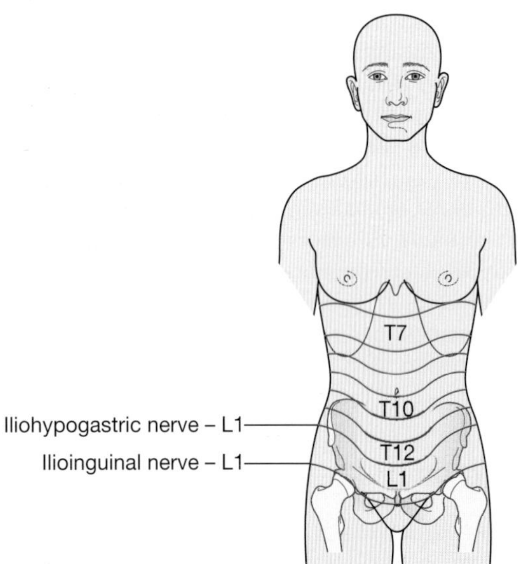

Figure 59.1 Distribution of the anterior abdominal wall dermatome and nerves.

Summary box 59.4

Nerves responsible for abdominal pain

- Abdominal wall and parietal peritoneum are supplied by the somatic nerves
- Abdominal organs and the visceral peritoneum are supplied by the autonomic nervous system
- Skin, muscles and parietal peritoneum are supplied by the iliohypogastric and ilioinguinal nerves and the lower six intercostal nerves
- Afferent pain fibres from the abdominal organs and visceral peritoneum travel with sympathetic nerves

Summary box 59.5

Specific characteristics of abdominal pain

- Visceral pain arises from ischaemia, muscle spasm or stretching of the visceral peritoneum
- Autonomic pain, deep and poorly localised, is referred to the equivalent somatic distribution of that nerve root from T1 to L2
- When an inflamed organ touches the parietal peritoneum, pain is then localised to the segmental dermatome of the abdominal wall
- The pain in the parietal peritoneum may radiate to back or front along the dermatome

Obstruction

Central colicky abdominal pain is a classic presentation of small bowel obstruction. The central distribution is because of the segmental nerve supply of the mid-gut. When the peristaltic waves hit an obstruction, the contractions increase to overcome the resistance, producing the colic. The pain reaches a crescendo and then disappears in minutes when the peristaltic wave passes. This is different from that of biliary

John Apley, 1909–1980, consultant paediatrician, Bristol, UK. The further away the chronic abdominal pain in a child is from the umbilicus, the more likely an organic cause.

John Benjamin Murphy, 1857–1916, Professor of Surgery, Northwestern University, Chicago, IL, USA, described his sign in 1903. He was the son of Irish immigrants fleeing the potato famine in Ireland, and was known as the 'Stormy Petrel' of American surgery, demonstrating the benefit of appendicectomy over conservative treatment among many things.

colic. When the gall bladder contracts against a stone, pain is relatively insidious in onset and reaches its peak in about half an hour and then eases off. A basal pain persists between the bouts of colic.

Summary box 59.6

Colicky abdominal pain

- Pain of 'small bowel colic' comes in waves and disappears completely in minutes when the peristaltic wave ceases
- Pain of biliary colic is insidious in onset, reaches the peak in half an hour or so and does not ease off completely between spasms
- Pain of ureteric colic is intense lasting one to two minutes of the ureter

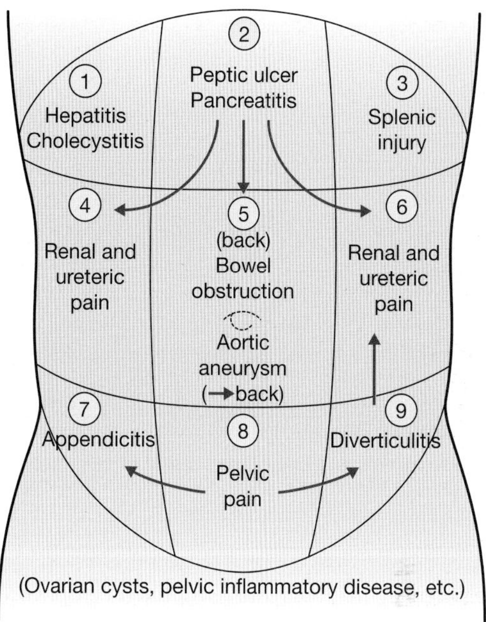

Figure 59.2 Nine sites of abdominal pain: 1, right subcostal; 2, epigastrium; 3, left subcostal; 4, right flank; 5, periumbilical; 6, left flank; 7, right iliac fossa; 8, suprapubic/hypogastrium; 9, left iliac fossa. (From Bailey and Love, 25th edn., courtesy of Mr Simon Paterson-Brown, Consultant Surgeon, Royal Infirmary of Edinburgh.)

Rupture and perforation of organs

The urinary bladder, gall bladder and gastrointestinal tract are hollow organs containing fluid. The gastrointestinal system also contains faeces, air and a high concentration of organisms. Trauma, ischaemia or tissue ulceration may cause perforation, with resulting leak of luminal contents, and peritonitis, with resulting severe abdominal pain. This may be localised to the area immediately adjacent to the perforation (for example, in a localised perforation of an appendix) or more generalised. The initial site of onset of the pain may give a clue as to the organ involved and so help with the differential diagnosis. For example, the diagnosis of a perforated peptic ulcer is supported by a past history of ulcer-type pain followed by sudden onset of upper abdominal pain.

The abdomen is divided into nine areas for ease of description (Figure 59.2). These regions are demarcated by the midclavicular lines in the vertical axis and by the transpyloric and transtubercular lines in the horizontal axis. Figure 59.2 also indicates some of the common organs and pathological processes that commonly cause pain experienced in these regions.

EXAMINATION OF THE ABDOMEN

Abdominal examination must be preceded by a detailed general examination of the patient as a whole. Physical examination should be systematic using the following sequence: inspection, palpation, percussion and auscultation.

General examination

When examining the abdomen it is essential to obtain the patient's prior consent and to ensure the presence of a chaperone if appropriate. The examination should be performed in a comfortable environment that ensures privacy. The patient must be lying flat but without causing distress (this may require provision of a pillow) and the abdomen should be adequately exposed.

The examination should be performed sequentially, beginning with general inspection looking for evidence of weight loss, dehydration, anaemia, jaundice or abnormal pigmentation. Examination of the hands may provide evidence of anaemia or chronic liver disease whereas examination of the head and neck may identify features indicative of liver disease or lymph adenopathy (particularly left supraclavicular) suggestive of intra-abdominal malignancy. The patient's vital signs (heart rate, blood pressure, respiratory rate and body temperature) should always be noted. It is wise in the elective setting also to record the patient's weight at this point.

Inspection

Scars, abdominal distension, visible peristalsis or abdominal masses, dilated veins, pulsation or abdominal wall swelling suggestive of hernia should all be carefully sought. In an abdominal emergency look for Grey Turner's sign – skin discoloration of the flanks due to retroperitoneal haemorrhage in severe acute pancreatitis and leaking abdominal aortic aneurysm. Cullen's sign – discoloration around the umbilicus – may

Vermiculation: meaning wave-like contraction similar to a worm, particularly as referring to peristalsis of the ureter (from the Latin *vermiculus* – little worm).
George Grey Turner, 1877–1951, Professor of Surgery, the University of Durham (1927–1934) and at the Royal Postgraduate Medical School, Hammersmith Hospital, London, UK (1935–1946). He had the surgical club, Grey Turner Surgical Club, named after him. It is said that he dressed shabbily so that when his friends met him they used to ask him to 'mend the clock'. He had a habit of keeping his cup of tea warm by covering it with his bowler hat!
Thomas Stephen Cullen, 1868–1953, Professor of Gynecology, the Johns Hopkins University, Baltimore, MD, USA, described the sign in ruptured ectopic pregnancy in 1916.

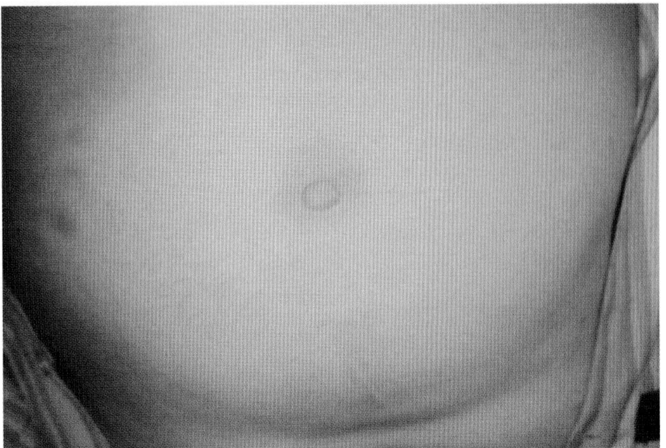

Figure 59.3 Cullen's and Grey Turner's sign of skin discoloration of flanks and around the umbilicus (courtesy of Mr Pradip Datta, Honorary Consultant Surgeon, Wick, Scotland).

indicate severe acute pancreatitis, ruptured ectopic pregnancy or trauma to the liver. In these situations, blood tracks to the umbilicus along the ligamentum teres (Figure 59.3).

In a patient with acute abdominal pain, it is important to observe if the abdominal wall moves with respiration. A thin patient with diffuse peritonitis may be unable to lie flat and the abdominal wall will have a 'scaphoid' appearance due to protective contraction of the rectus abdominis muscles. It is often appropriate to ask the patient to cough gently – this will evoke sudden discomfort in the area of underlying peritoneal irritation (equivalent to eliciting rebound tenderness, but not as distressing for the patient). A cough will also help to identify an abdominal wall hernia, if present. Visible abdominal masses, mobility on respiration and peristalsis are all best observed if the clinician kneels by the patient's bed so that the observer's eye is at the level of the patient's anterior abdominal wall. The same position is useful during palpation for abdominal masses (Figure 59.4).

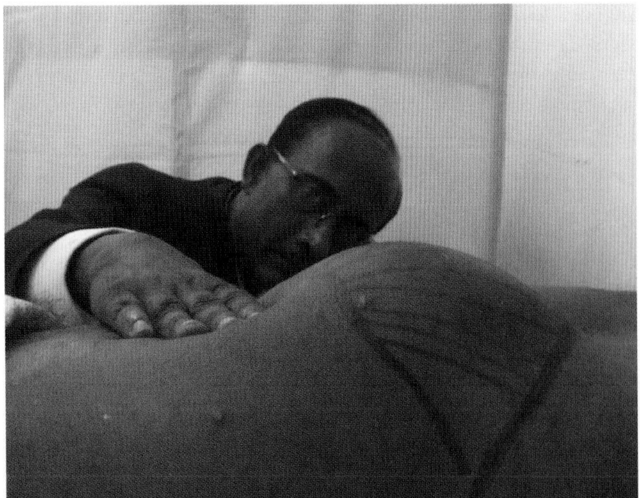

Figure 59.4 Eye at the level of patient's abdominal wall.

Palpation

Palpation should be performed in a systematic manner checking all nine regions of the abdomen (see Figure 59.2). Palpation should start in the region furthest away from the site of pain and the patient instructed to let the examiner know if tenderness is elicited. The examination should be gentle and the hands warm. The patient's facial expression will immediately reveal discomfort. Superficial palpation is followed by deep palpation if tenderness will allow. Finally, palpation during respiration is performed to identify the lower margins of the liver and spleen as they move with respiration.

Signs of parietal peritoneal irritation (tenderness, guarding, rebound tenderness, rigidity)

In the presence of abdominal pain, the degree of abdominal wall rigidity and involuntary guarding should be assessed. Guarding represents contraction of the abdominal wall muscles over the area of pain. This might occur 'voluntarily' when the patient wishes to avoid the pain from examination, or 'involuntarily' when the muscles go into spasm as the inflamed viscus touches the parietal peritoneum. This produces a reflex spasm of the overlying abdominal wall muscles. The presence of rebound tenderness indicates underlying peritoneal inflammation and is examined best using gentle percussion, although pain on coughing is also found when there is rebound tenderness. When the underlying peritoneal inflammation becomes generalised, the abdomen is 'board-like rigid' to palpation, and selective tenderness can no longer be elicited. This sign represents widespread involuntary guarding.

Abdominal masses

A mass arising from the anterior abdominal wall will usually be mobile when the patient is relaxed. On contracting the abdominal wall muscles (ask the patient to lift his or her legs with the knees extended, or perform Valsalva's manoeuvre for laterally placed swellings), lumps superficial to the abdominal wall muscles will become more obvious, and those attached to the deep fascia will become less mobile. Those arising within the muscle layer will become fixed and remain unchanged in size. Lumps arising deep to the abdominal wall (i.e. within the peritoneal cavity or behind the peritoneum) will become impalpable or less prominent on tensing the anterior abdominal wall muscles.

An intraperitoneal mass in contact with the diaphragm will move on respiration whereas retroperitoneal masses are usually fixed and do not move with respiration; an enlarged kidney is 'ballotable' and bimanually palpable. Normal aortic pulsations can be both seen and felt in a thin abdomen, but expansile pulsation is characteristic of an abdominal aortic aneurysm. This should be differentiated from transmitted pulsation of a mass sitting on the aorta (e.g. pseudocyst of the pancreas). When 'palpating during inspiration', the examining hand is placed distal to the normal site of the organ, and is held there until the edge of the organ descends

Antonio Maria Valsalva, 1666–1723, Professor of Anatomy in Bologna, of whom Morgagni wrote 'there is nobody of those times who goes ahead of him, very few who are his equals'.

and touches the examiner's fingers. Liver, spleen, gall bladder and kidneys are best palpated during inspiration. An abdominal mass in a female, the lower limit of which cannot be distinguished, is likely to arise from the pelvis. If the mass can be moved in a transverse direction, it is likely to be a uterine or ovarian mass.

Spleen

In a healthy patient the spleen is not normally palpable. An enlarged spleen descends downwards, forwards and medially. Palpation for an enlarged spleen is best performed in a supine patient. The examining hand should start in the right lower abdomen, with the tips of the fingers pointing upwards and pressed inwards. The patient is then asked to take a deep breath, and if the spleen is enlarged the lower edge with the characteristic notch will touch the fingers. If it is not palpable, then the hand is gradually moved upwards in the direction of the position of the edge of the normal-sized spleen with each breath. If the spleen is still not palpable, the patient is moved to the right lateral position and the examination repeated.

Liver

In a supine patient, the hand is placed in line with the potential enlarged liver edge lateral to the rectus muscle. The patient is then asked to take a deep breath. If the liver is enlarged sufficiently below the costal margin, then surface irregularities can also be felt.

Percussion

Percussion helps to distinguish distension due to bowel gas from solid masses and free fluid in the abdomen. Percussion is most sensitive when the examiner moves from resonant parts of the abdomen to dull areas. In patients with free fluid in the peritoneal cavity, percussion from the centre to the periphery reveals dullness of flanks. Shifting dullness is elicited if the patient is re-examined lying on his or her side. The margin of dullness is then found to shift when the patient has moved.

Percussion is a very sensitive and refined method of testing for rebound tenderness. If the patient winces with pain on abdominal percussion it denotes underlying peritonitis.

Auscultation

High-pitched bowel sounds are heard during early stages of mechanical intestinal obstruction. Aortic and iliac bruits are heard when blood flows through a stenosis. A succussion splash is a sound like 'shaking a half-filled bottle with water' and is found most often in patients with gastric stasis due to gastric outlet obstruction. In generalised peritonitis, bowel sounds will not be heard or be very few and far between.

Inspection of hernia sites, examination of genitalia, inspection of anal region and digital rectal examination

Abdominal examination is not complete until all external hernia sites and the anal area have been carefully inspected, the genitalia examined and a digital rectal examination performed. A vaginal examination may also be needed in females. The thoracic and lumbar spine and renal angles should also be examined.

VALUE OF OBSERVATION AND REVIEW

In the case of acute abdominal pain, there will be a subset of patients in whom, after full clinical assessment, the surgeon remains uncertain about the need for an urgent operation. This is probably the most difficult group to deal with compared with those in whom an urgent operation is either clearly required, or clearly not required, and undoubtedly the one in which the majority of errors occur. Further urgent investigations are obviously important in this group and these are discussed in some detail elsewhere in this book. However, while these are taking place, regular review of the patient is essential. This period of observation has now become an integral part of the early management of patients with acute abdominal pain.

FURTHER READING

Lumley JS, D'Cruz AK, Hoballah JJ, Scott-Connor CE. *Hamilton Bailey's demonstrations of physical signs in clinical surgery*, 19th edn. London: CRC Press, 2016.

Chapter 60

Abdominal wall, hernia and umbilicus

Learning objectives

To know and understand:

- Basic anatomy of the abdominal wall and its weaknesses
- Causes of abdominal hernia
- Types of hernia and classifications
- Clinical history and examination findings in hernia
- Complications of abdominal hernia
- Non-surgical and surgical management of hernia – including mesh
- Complications of hernia surgery
- Other abdominal wall conditions

THE ABDOMINAL WALL

Basic anatomy and function related to pathology

The abdominal wall is a complex structure composed primarily of muscle, bone and fascia. Its major function is to protect the enclosed organs of the gastrointestinal and urogenital tracts but a secondary role is mobility, being able to flex, extend, rotate and vary its capacity. Flexibility requires elasticity and stretch, which compromise abdominal wall strength.

The roof of the abdomen is formed by the diaphragm separating the thoracic cavity above, with negative pressure, from the abdomen below, with positive pressure. Weakness of the diaphragm can lead to much of the bowel being drawn into the chest down this pressure gradient. The bony pelvis forms the floor of the cavity but a muscular central portion, the perineum, may also weaken and allow rectum, bladder and gynaecological organs to bulge downwards, a condition called prolapse.

The overall design of the abdominal muscles is best seen on a transverse computed tomography (CT) scan through the mid-abdomen. Posteriorly the muscles are strong, further supported by the vertebral column, ribs and pelvis. Two regions called the posterior triangles represent areas of weakness which can lead to rare lumbar hernias. Laterally there are three thin muscle layers the fibres of which criss-cross for strength and flexibility. Surgeons can make use of these layers, by making releasing incisions, separating the layers and then sliding one layer over another to increase girth and allow closure of defects in the centre of the abdomen, e.g. the 'Ramirez slide' used in large incisional hernia repair (Figure 60.1).

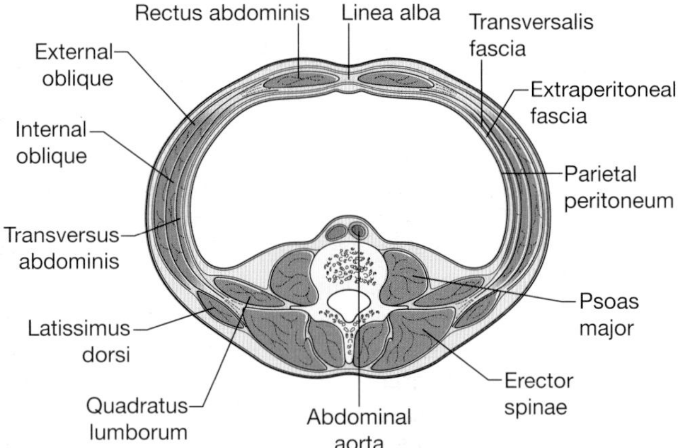

Figure 60.1 A cross-section of the midabdomen showing the muscular layout.

Anteriorly the two powerful rectus abdominis muscles extend vertically from ribs to pelvis. Herniation through these strong muscles does not occur naturally but their central join, the linea alba, is an area of weakness resulting in epigastric and paraumbilical herniation. Divarification of the recti is the condition where the linea alba stretches laterally as the two rectus muscles separate. It occurs in the upper abdomen in middle-aged, overweight men (Figure 60.2) but also as a result of birth trauma in women when it occurs below the umbilicus.

Abdominal pressure

The positive pressure within the abdomen is used by a surgeon when drains are placed to allow blood, pus, bile, bowel content and urine to flow outwards down the pressure gradient. However, this constant pressure from within can also lead to the condition of abdominal hernia where tissue, meant to be within the abdominal cavity, is forced outwards through defects in the muscular wall.

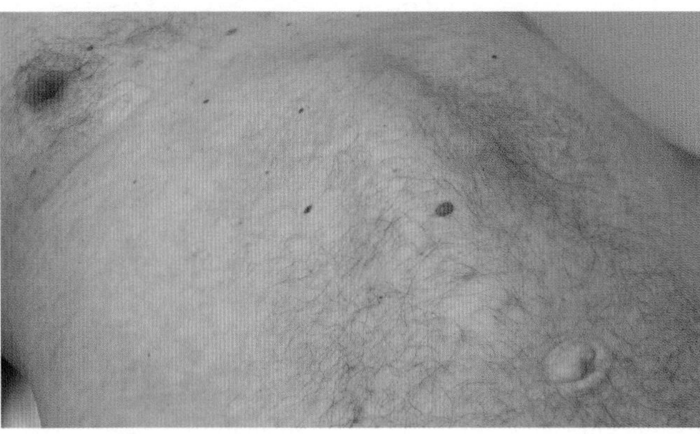

Figure 60.2 Divarification.

ABDOMINAL HERNIA

A hernia is the bulging of part of the contents of the abdominal cavity through a weakness in the abdominal wall.

Anatomical causes of abdominal wall herniation

Despite the complex design of the abdominal wall, the only natural weaknesses caused by inadequate muscular strength are the lumbar triangles and the posterior wall of the inguinal canal (Figure 60.3).

Many structures pass into and out of the abdominal cavity creating weakness which can lead to hernia formation. The most common example is the inguinal canal in males, along which the testis descends from abdomen to scrotum at the time of birth. The testicular artery, veins and vas pass though this canal (the round ligament in females). The resultant weakness leads to an indirect or lateral-type inguinal hernia. In adult surgery, 80% of all hernia repairs are for inguinal hernia. The evolutionary advantage of testicular descent must outweigh the disadvantage of a high risk of herniation. Other examples are: oesophagus → hiatus hernia, femoral vessels → femoral hernia, obturator nerve → obturator hernia, sciatic nerve → sciatic hernia.

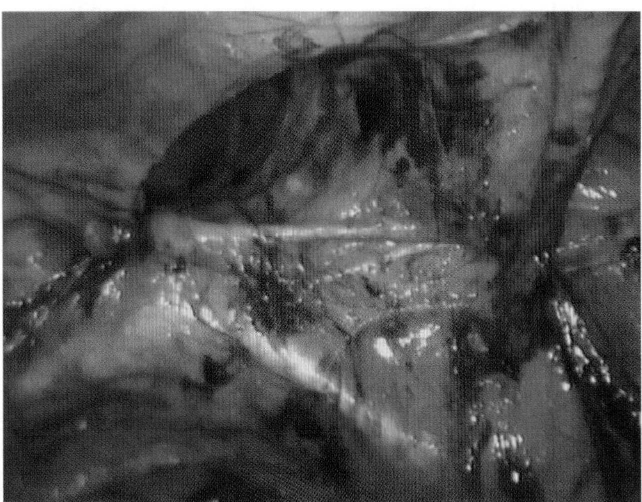

Figure 60.3 Posterior wall defect.

An inguinal hernia (indirect) also occurs through the developmental failure of the processus vaginalis to close. As the testis descends, it pulls a tube of peritoneum along with it. This tube should naturally fibrose and become obliterated but often it fails to fibrose and allows a hernia to form. Recent studies have shown that calcitonin gene-related peptide and hepatocyte growth factor influence the closure of the processus, raising the possibility of a hormonal cause of hernia development.

Failure of normal development may lead to weakness of the abdominal wall. Examples are diaphragmatic, umbilical and epigastric hernias. Muscles which should unite during development fail to form strong unions with hernia development at birth or in later life.

Herniation at the umbilicus has both components, i.e. weakness due to structures passing through the abdominal wall in fetal life and developmental failure of closure.

The risk of inguinal hernia is related to the anatomical shape of the pelvis and is higher in patients having a wider and shorter pelvis.

Weakness of abdominal muscles may be the result of sharp trauma. Most commonly, this results from abdominal surgery but also occurs after stabbing. A surgical scar, even with perfect wound healing, has only 70% of the initial muscle strength. This loss of strength can result in herniation in at least 10% of surgical incisions. Smaller laparoscopic port-site incisions have a hernia rate of 1%. Increasing use of this surgical approach should lead to a fall in the incidence of incisional hernia.

Muscle damage by blunt trauma or tearing of the abdominal muscles requires exceptional force and is rare.

The sudden presence of a mass in the rectus muscle may be a rectus sheath haematoma, occasionally due to trauma but nowadays more often due to excessive anticoagulation therapy.

Primary muscle pathology and neurological conditions can lead to muscle weakness and occasionally present to the surgeon as a 'hernia'.

Summary box 60.1

Causes of hernia

- Basic design weakness
- Weakness due to structures entering and leaving the abdomen
- Developmental failures
- Genetic weakness of collagen
- Sharp and blunt trauma
- Weakness due to ageing and pregnancy
- Primary neurological and muscle diseases
- ? Excessive intra-abdominal pressure

Pathophysiology of hernia formation

A normal abdominal wall has sufficient strength to resist high abdominal pressure and prevent herniation of content. Herniation has been attributed to high pressures from constipation, prostatic symptoms, excessive coughing in respiratory disease and obesity. However, it has been shown that hernia is no more common in Olympic weight lifters than the general population, suggesting that high pressure is not a major factor in causing a hernia. Many patients will first notice a hernia after excessive straining.

There is good evidence that hernia is a 'collagen disease' and due to an inherited imbalance in the types of collagen. This is supported by histological evidence and relationships between hernia and other diseases related to collagen, such as aortic aneurysm.

Hernia development is more common in pregnancy due to hormonally induced laxity of pelvic ligaments. It is also more common in elderly people due to degenerative weakness of muscles and fibrous tissue. A recent Swedish report has shown that inguinal hernia is less common in obese patients, with hernia risk being negatively related to body mass index (BMI), contrary to widespread belief. Hernia is more common in smokers.

Common principles in abdominal hernia

An abdominal wall hernia has two essential components, a defect in the wall and content, i.e. tissue that has been forced outwards through the defect. The weakness may be entirely in muscle, such as an incisional hernia. It may also be in fascia, similar to an epigastric hernia through the linea alba. It may have a bony component, such as a femoral hernia. The weakness in the wall is usually the narrowest part of the hernia which expands into the subcutaneous fat outside the muscle. The defect varies in size and may be very small or indeed very large. The nature of the defect is important to understanding the risk of hernia complications. A small defect with rigid walls traps the content and prevents it from freely moving in and out of the defect, increasing the risk of complications.

The content of the hernia may be tissue from the extraperitoneal space alone, such as fat within an epigastric hernia or urinary bladder in a direct inguinal hernia. However, if such a hernia enlarges then peritoneum may also be pulled into the hernia secondarily along with intraperitoneal structures such as bowel or omentum; a good example is a 'sliding type' of inguinal hernia.

More commonly, when peritoneum is lying immediately deep to the abdominal wall weakness, pressure forces the peritoneum through the defect and into the subcutaneous tissues. This 'sac' of peritoneum allows bowel and omentum to pass through the defect. In most cases, the intraperitoneal organs can move freely in and out of the hernia, a 'reducible' hernia, but if adhesions form or the defect is small, bowel can become trapped and unable to return to the main peritoneal cavity, an 'irreducible' hernia, with high risk of further complications. The narrowest part of the sac, at the abdominal wall defect, is called the 'neck of the sac'.

When tissue is trapped inside a hernia it is in a confined space. The narrow neck acts as a constriction ring impeding venous return and increasing pressure within the hernia. Resulting tension leads to pain and tenderness. If the hernia contains bowel then it may become 'obstructed', partially or totally. If the pressure rises sufficiently, arterial blood is not able to enter the hernia and the contents become ischaemic and may infarct. The hernia is then said to have 'strangulated'. The wall of the bowel perforates, releasing infected, toxic bowel content into the tissues and ultimately back into the peritoneal cavity. The risk of strangulation is highest in hernias that have a small neck of rigid tissue, leading first to irreducibility and on to strangulation. The term 'incarcerated' is not clearly defined and used to imply a hernia that is irreducible and developing towards strangulation.

Summary box 60.2

Types of hernia by complexity

- Occult – not detectable clinically; may cause severe pain
- Reducible – a swelling that appears and disappears
- Irreducible – a swelling that cannot be replaced in the abdomen, high risk of complications
- Strangulated – painful swelling with vascular compromise, requires urgent surgery
- Infarcted – when contents of the hernia have become gangrenous, high mortality

In a special circumstance (Richter's hernia) only part of the bowel wall enters the hernia. It may be small and difficult or even impossible to detect clinically. Bowel obstruction may not be present but the bowel wall may still become necrotic and perforate with life-threatening consequences. Femoral hernia may present in this way often with diagnostic delay and high risk to the patient (Figure 60.4).

An interstitial hernia occurs when the hernia extends between the layers of muscle and not directly through them. This is typical of a spigelian hernia (see below under **Spigelian hernia**).

An internal hernia is a term used when adhesions form within the peritoneal cavity. leading to abnormal pockets into which bowel can enter and become trapped. As there is no defect within the abdominal wall, the term 'hernia' is confusing.

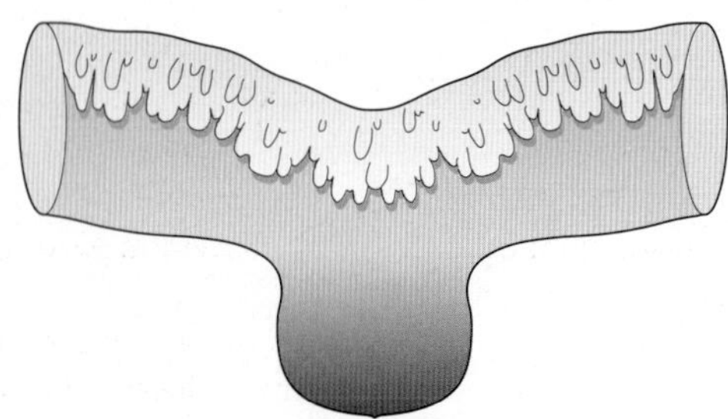

Figure 60.4 Diagrammatic representation of gangrenous Richter's hernia from a case of strangulated femoral hernia.

August Gottlieb Richter, 1742–1812, lecturer in Surgery, Göttingen, Germany described this form of hernia in 1777.

Clinical history and diagnosis in hernia cases

Patients are usually aware of a lump on the abdominal wall under the skin. Self-diagnosis is common. The hernia is usually painless but patients may complain of an aching or heavy feeling. Sharp, intermittent pains suggest pinching of tissue. Severe pain should alert the surgeon to a high risk of strangulation. One should determine whether the hernia reduces spontaneously or needs to be helped. The patient should be asked about symptoms that might suggest bowel obstruction.

It is important to know if this is a primary hernia or whether it is a recurrence after previous surgery. Recurrent hernia is more difficult to treat and may require a different surgical approach.

General questions about the cardiac and respiratory systems are necessary to assess a patient's anaesthetic risk.

In a man with a groin hernia, history of prostatic symptoms indicates a high risk of postoperative urinary retention.

Intake of anticoagulants such as warfarin is important because this impacts on future surgery. Many hernia operations can be performed as a day case or single overnight stay, so that suitability for such treatment needs to be assessed, including home support, distance from the hospital, mobility levels, etc.

Examination for hernia

The patient should be examined lying down initially and then standing as this will usually increase hernia size. In some cases no hernia will be apparent with the patient lying. The patient is asked to cough, when an occult hernia may appear. Divarification is best seen by asking a supine patient to simply lift his head off the pillow.

The overlying skin is usually of normal colour. If bruising is present this may suggest venous engorgement of the content. If there is overlying cellulitis then hernia content is strangulating and the case should be treated as an emergency.

In most cases a cough impulse is felt. Gentle pressure is applied to the lump and the patient is asked to cough. If an impulse is felt this is due to increased abdominal pressure being transmitted into the hernia. In cases where the neck is tight and the hernia irreducible there may be no cough impulse. This can lead to failure of diagnosis and is typical of femoral hernia where lack of an impulse leads the clinician to misdiagnose a lymph node. Cough impulse can also occur in a saphena varix (see Chapter 57), which may be referred to a surgeon as a suspected inguinal hernia. It is not unusual for a patient to describe an intermittent swelling but the surgeon finds nothing on examination. This is due to muscle tightening in an anxious patient.

If, on lying, the hernia does not reduce spontaneously, the surgeon asks the patient to attempt reduction because he may be well practised in this task although the surgeon might cause unnecessary discomfort. If neither the patient nor the surgeon can reduce the hernia then treatment is more urgent. An irreducible hernia may influence the decision between open and laparoscopic surgery. With the hernia reduced, the surgeon assesses the size, rigidity and number of defects. Multiple defects may be present in incisional hernia.

Summary box 60.3

Checks

- Reducibility
- Cough impulse
- Tenderness
- Overlying skin colour changes
- Multiple defects/contralateral side
- Signs of previous repair
- Scrotal content for groin hernia
- Associated pathology

Summary box 60.4

Examination

- A swelling with a cough impulse is not necessarily a hernia
- A swelling with no cough impulse may still be a hernia

Investigations for hernia

For most hernias, no specific investigation is required, the diagnosis being made on clinical examination. However, the patient may have symptoms suggesting a hernia, but no hernia is found, or have a swelling suggestive of hernia but with clinical uncertainty. It is important to be certain that any symptoms described are due to a hernia and not to coexisting pathology. There may also be a requirement for more detailed information than can be found by examination alone. A plain radiograph of the abdomen is of little value (Figure 60.5) although a hiatus hernia and diaphragmatic hernia may be seen on a chest radiograph. An ultrasound scan may be helpful in cases of irreducible hernia, where the differential diagnosis includes a mass or fluid collection, or when the nature of the hernia content is in doubt. Ultrasonography is very useful in the early postoperative period when a haematoma or seroma may develop, and be difficult to distinguish from

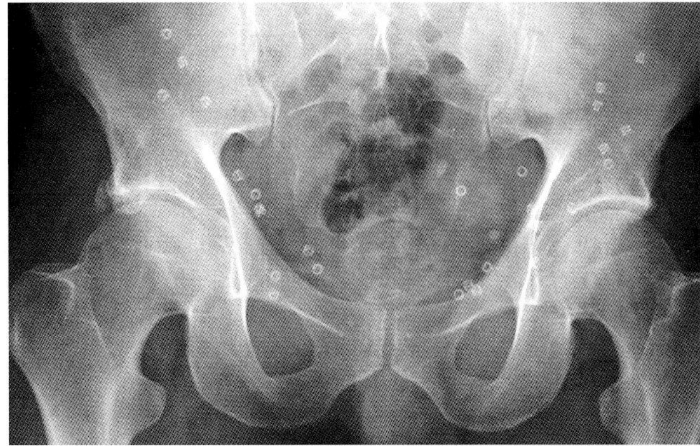

Figure 60.5 A radiograph showing spiral tacks causing chronic pain after transabdominal preperitoneal repair.

an early recurrence. Ultrasonography is non-invasive and low cost but operator dependent.

Computed tomography is helpful in complex incisional hernia, determining the number and size of muscle defects, identifying the content, giving some indication of presence of adhesions and excluding other intra-abdominal pathology such as ascites, occult malignancy and portal hypertension.

Contrast barium radiology is occasionally useful in the absence of CT. Contrast may also be injected directly into the peritoneum, a herniagram, to identify an occult sac, especially in occult inguinal hernia. Magnetic resonance imaging (MRI) can help in the diagnosis of sportsman's groin where pain is the presenting feature and the surgeon needs to distinguish an occult hernia from an orthopaedic injury.

Laparoscopy itself may be used. In incisional hernia, initial laparoscopy may determine that a laparoscopic approach is feasible or not depending on the extent of adhesions. In inguinal hernia repair by the transabdominal route, initial laparoscopy can determine the presence of an occult contralateral hernia which has been described in up to 20% of patients.

Summary box 60.5

Investigations

- Plain radiograph – of little value
- Ultrasound scan – low cost, operator dependent
- CT scan – incisional hernia
- MRI – good in sportsman's groin with pain
- Contrast radiology – especially for inguinal hernia
- Laparoscopy – useful to identify occult inguinal hernia

Management principles

An abdominal wall hernia does not necessarily require repair. A patient may request surgery for relief of symptoms of discomfort, for cosmesis or to establish the diagnosis when in doubt. The surgeon should recommend repair when complications are likely, the most worrying being strangulation with bowel obstruction and bowel infarction. All cases of femoral hernia, with high risk of strangulation, should be repaired surgically. Any case of irreducible hernia, especially where there is pain and tenderness, should be offered repair unless coexisting medical factors place the patient at very high risk from surgery or anaesthesia. Increasing difficulty in reduction and increasing size are indications for surgery. Surgery should be offered to younger adult patients as symptoms and complications are likely over time.

Summary box 60.6

Management

- Not all hernias require surgical repair
- Small hernias can be more dangerous than large
- Pain, tenderness and skin colour changes imply high risk of strangulation
- Femoral hernia should always be repaired

In reality, most patients with a hernia should be offered repair. In elderly people, if the hernia is asymptomatic, small in size, can be reduced easily and is not causing anxiety, then observation alone should be sufficient. This policy, called 'watchful waiting', has been studied in asymptomatic inguinal hernia. One study reported such a policy to be safe but a second study was abandoned when a small number of patients developed strangulation. A truss can be used to control a hernia but few surgeons would recommend this approach. Small paraumbilical hernias are often seen. They cause few symptoms and usually contain fat or omentum with a very low risk of complications.

Large incisional hernias, particularly recurrent, present a major problem. Surgical repair is a complex procedure with significant risk of complications and later recurrence. When the neck is wide, the risk of strangulation is low. In obese and elderly patients, these risks may outweigh the benefits of surgery and it is common for surgeons to adopt a conservative approach.

Any patient who presents with acute pain in a hernia, particularly if it is irreducible, should be offered surgery. Often, in a patient with an irreducible hernia, after admission to hospital and adequate analgesia, the hernia will reduce due to muscle relaxation. The likelihood of similar episodes is very high and surgery should be recommended at this admission or soon after.

Surgical approaches to hernia

All surgical repairs follow the same basic principles:

1. reduction of the hernia content into the abdominal cavity with removal of any non-viable tissue and bowel repair if necessary;
2. excision and closure of a peritoneal sac if present or replacing it deep to the muscles;
3. reapproximation of the walls of the neck of the hernia if possible;
4. permanent reinforcement of the abdominal wall defect with sutures or mesh.

Reduction of hernia content is essential for a successful repair. It is rare for a surgeon to fail to reduce the hernia but extensive dissection can lead to bowel injury, sometimes requiring bowel resection with subsequent risks of infection and bowel anastomotic complications.

Excision and closure of the peritoneal sac are ideal but not essential. During laparoscopic repair of incisional hernia, surgeons will often leave the sac *in situ* after reducing the hernia contents, and simply fix a mesh over the neck to prevent recurrence. There is risk of fluid formation within the sac (seroma). This is a common complication in all forms of hernia repair. In lateral (indirect) inguinal hernia, most surgeons excise the peritoneal sac but some leading experts recommend that it be dissected from surrounding tissue and simply pushed back through the deep inguinal ring. In laparoscopic repair of inguinal hernias, surgeons simply pull the sac back into the abdominal cavity from within and do not excise it.

Closure of the abdominal wall defect is ideal but may not be possible when the defect is large or tissues are rigid. Plastic surgical techniques have been developed to 'borrow' tissue from elsewhere in order to cover large muscle defects, but usually at the cost of leaving a weak area elsewhere. Over the past 20–30 years, surgeons have realised that simple closure of a hernia defect by sutures alone leads to a high recurrence rate.

Additional reinforcement of the defect with a non-absorbable mesh is now widely practised in most hernia repairs and evidence has shown that recurrence rates have improved but recurrence still remains a problem. There is some evidence that mesh repair delays but does not prevent recurrence. With improved surgical techniques and new meshes it is hoped that recurrence after surgery will fall further. Mesh repair has become so important in hernia surgery that some understanding of mesh technology is essential for the modern surgeon.

Mesh in hernia repair

The term 'mesh' refers to prosthetic material, either a net or a flat sheet, which is used to strengthen a hernia repair. Mesh can be used:

- to bridge a defect: the mesh is simply fixed over the defect as a tension-free patch;
- to plug a defect: a plug of mesh is pushed into the defect;
- to augment a repair: the defect is closed with sutures and the mesh added for reinforcement.

A well-placed mesh should have good overlap around all margins of the defect, at least 2 cm but up to 5 cm if possible. Suturing a mesh edge to edge into the defect (inlay), with no overlap, is not recommended. Mesh plug repairs have gained some popularity in small defects especially where overlap is hard to achieve. Plug operations are fast but plugs can form a dense 'meshoma' of plug and collagen. Other complications include migration, erosion into adjacent organs, fistula formation and chronic pain.

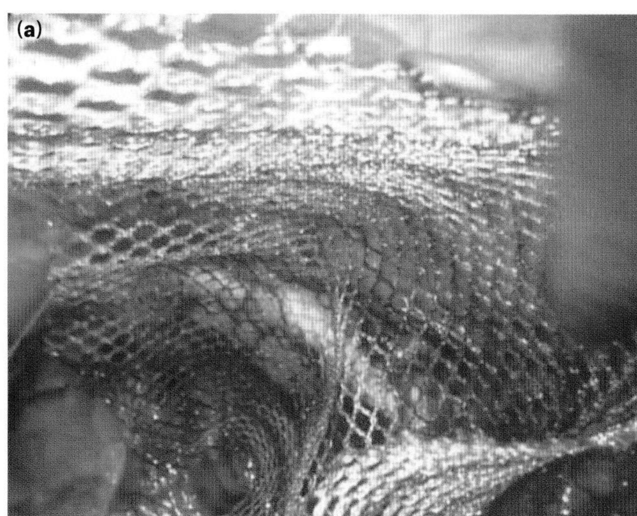

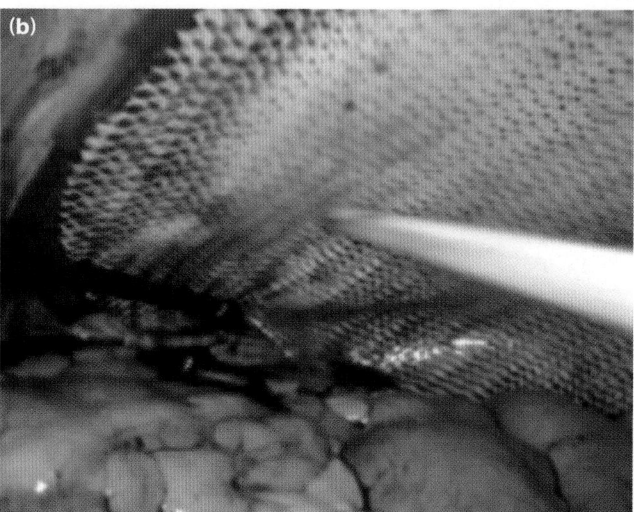

Figure 60.6 (a) Polypropylene mesh in totally extraperitoneal inguinal hernia repair and (b) polyester mesh in a paraumbilical hernia repair.

Mesh types

The wide array of meshes available can be classified as follows.

GROSS STRUCTURE

Net meshes are woven or knitted. Flat sheets are not porous but can be perforated with multiple holes. Net meshes allow fibrous tissue in growth between the strands and becoming adherent and integrated into host tissues within a few months. Initial fixation of the mesh is by glue, sutures or staples which may be absorbable. In laparoscopic inguinal hernia, no fixation is required at all as friction is sufficient to hold the mesh. 'Sheet' meshes do not allow host tissue in growth but become encapsulated by fibrous tissue. They always require strong, non-absorbable fixation to prevent mesh migration.

SYNTHETIC MESH

Most meshes used today are synthetic polymers of polypropylene, polyester or polytetrafluoroethylene (PTFE) (Figure 60.6). They are non-absorbable and provoke little tissue reaction. Polypropylene makes a strong monofilament mesh. It does not have any antibacterial properties but its hydrophobic nature and monofilament microstructure impede bacterial in-growth. Polyester is a braided filament mesh. This structure may allow infection to take hold, aided by its hydrophilic property. However, this property also allows rapid vascular and cellular infiltration within the fibrils, aiding host immune responses to infection and providing a stronger host–tissue interface. PTFE meshes are flat sheets and as a result do not allow any tissue in-growth. They are used as a non-adhesive barrier between tissue layers.

WEIGHT AND POROSITY

Synthetic meshes are very strong and early meshes were much stronger than a human abdominal wall, so they are considered as 'over-engineered'. All meshes provoke a fibrous reaction. More dense or heavyweight meshes provoke a greater reaction, leading to collagen contraction and stiffening. The term 'mesh shrinkage' is often used to describe a progressive decrease in size of a mesh over time. It is due to natural contraction of fibrous tissue embedded in the mesh, reducing the area of mesh itself. This can lead to tissue tension and pain, a common complication of mesh repair. It can also lead to hernia recurrence if the mesh no longer covers the defect. Meshes can shrink by up to 50% and, in occasional cases, even more. Meshes with thinner strands and larger spaces between them, 'lightweight, large-pore meshes', are preferred because they have better tissue integration, less shrinkage, more flexibility and improved comfort.

The terms 'light', 'medium' and 'heavy' are not precisely defined but meshes $<40\,g/m^2$ are generally referred to as light and meshes $>80\,g/m^2$ as heavy.

BIOLOGICAL MESH

There are 'biological meshes' that are sheets of sterilised, decellularised, non-immunogenic connective tissue. They derive from human or animal dermis, bovine pericardium or porcine intestinal submucosa. They provide a 'scaffold' to encourage neovascular in-growth and new collagen deposition. Host enzymes eventually break down the biological implant, which is replaced and remodelled with 'normal' host fibrous tissue. The rates of enzymatic degradation and collagen deposition vary between products and also depend on the local environment of the mesh. In the presence of infection, some biological meshes rapidly break down and weaken before remodelling can occur. Others remain strong, their labyrinthine microstructure allowing vascular in-growth to aid infection resistance. The choice of biological mesh depends on the clinical situation for which it is to be used. They are expensive.

ABSORBABLE MESHES

There are also synthetic absorbable meshes, such as those made from polyglycolic acid fibre. They are used in temporary abdominal wall closure and to buttress sutured repairs. They have no current role in hernia repair because they absorb and induce minimal collagen deposition.

TISSUE-SEPARATING MESHES

Most meshes induce fibrosis and, if placed within the peritoneal cavity, promote unwanted adhesions. New meshes have been designed for intraperitoneal use. Most of these have very different surfaces, one being sticky and one slippery. Good adherence and host–tissue in-growth is required on the parietal (muscle) side of the mesh, but the opposite (bowel) side needs to prevent adhesions to bowel. Usually one side of the mesh is coated by material that prevents adhesions (Figure 60.7), such as polycellulose, collagen, PTFE. A recent mesh made entirely of a sheet of condensed PTFE with multiple perforations can be used intraperitoneally because the peritoneum will grow in through its perforations whereas bowel will not adhere to its inside.

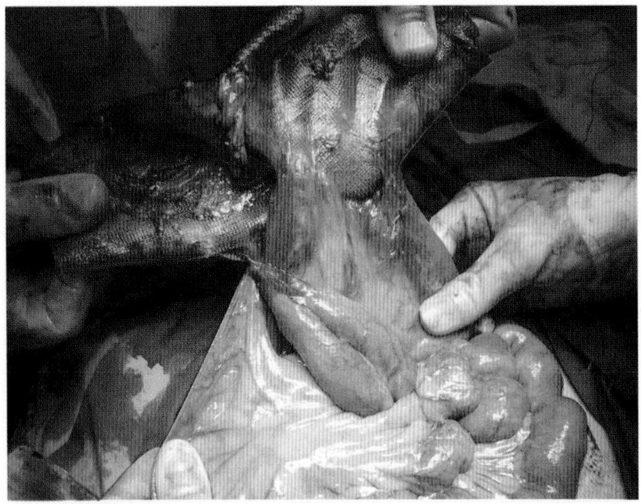
Figure 60.7 Adhesions to mesh.

Summary box 60.7

Mesh characteristics

- Woven, knitted or sheet
- Synthetic or biological – mainly synthetic
- Light, medium or heavyweight – lightweight becoming more popular
- Large pore, small pore – large pore causes less fibrosis and pain
- Intraperitoneal use or not – non-adhesive mesh on one side
- Non-absorbable or absorbable – mainly non-absorbable

Positioning the mesh

The strength of a mesh repair depends on host–tissue in-growth. Meshes should be placed on a firm, well-vascularised tissue bed with generous overlap of the defect. The mesh can be placed:

- just outside the muscle in the subcutaneous space (onlay);
- within the defect (inlay) – only applies to mesh plugs in small defects;
- between fascial layers in the abdominal wall (intraparietal or sublay);
- immediately extraperitoneally, against muscle or fascia (also sublay);
- intraperitoneally.

At open surgery all of these planes are used but laparoscopic surgeons currently use only intraperitoneal or extraperitoneal planes (Figure 60.8).

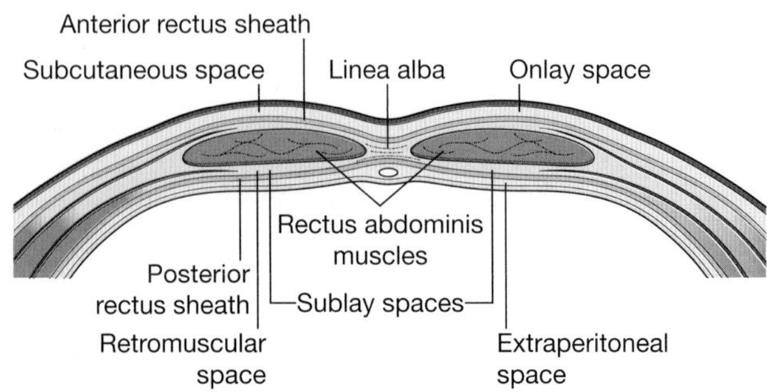

Figure 60.8 Diagrammatic representation of the various layers into which meshes are placed in ventral hernia repair.

Limitations to the use of mesh

The presence of infection limits the use of mesh, particularly heavyweight types. If a mesh becomes infected then it often needs to be removed. Some infected meshes can be salvaged using a combination of debridement of non-incorporated mesh, appropriate antibiotics and modern vacuum-assisted dressings.

Meshes are expensive, especially those for intraperitoneal use, but prices are falling and there are reports of low-cost solutions such as mosquito netting!

SPECIFIC HERNIA TYPES

Hernia sites are shown in Figure 60.9.

Inguinal hernia

The inguinal hernia, often referred to as a 'rupture' by patients, is the most common hernia in men and women but much more common in men. There are two basic types that are fundamentally different in anatomy, causation and complications. However, they are anatomically very close to each other, surgical repair techniques are very similar and ultimate reinforcement of the weakened anatomy is identical, so they are often referred to together as inguinal hernia.

Summary box 60.8

Inguinal hernia

- Types – lateral (oblique, indirect); medial (direct), sliding
- Origin – congenital or acquired
- Anatomy – inguinal canal
- Classification – latest European Hernia Society
- Diagnosis – usually clinical but radiological in special circumstances
- Surgery – open and laparoscopic

The congenital inguinal hernia is known as indirect, oblique or lateral whereas the acquired hernia is called direct or medial. There is a third 'sliding' hernia that is acquired but is lateral in position (see below).

Basic anatomy of the inguinal canal

As the testis descends from the abdominal cavity to the scrotum in males it firsts passes through a defect called the deep inguinal ring in the transversalis fascia, just deep to the abdominal muscles. This ring lies midway between the anterior superior iliac spine and the pubic tubercle, approximately 2–3 cm above the femoral artery pulse in the groin. The inferior epigastric vessels lie just medial to the deep inguinal ring, passing from the iliac vessels to rectus abdominis. Muscle fibres of the innermost two layers of the lateral abdominal wall, the transversus muscle and the internal oblique muscle, arch over the deep inguinal ring from lateral to medial before descending to become attached to the pubic tubercle. These two muscles fuse and become tendinous, hence this arch is referred to as the conjoint tendon. Below this arch there is no muscle but only transversalis fascia and external oblique aponeurosis, resulting in weakness (Figure 60.10).

The testis proceeds medially and downwards along the inguinal canal. Anterior to the canal is the aponeurosis of the external oblique muscle, the fibres of which run downwards and medially. The testis finally emerges through a V-shaped defect in the aponeurosis, the superficial inguinal ring, and descends into the scrotum. The inguinal canal is roofed by the conjoint tendon, its posterior wall is transversalis fascia, an anterior wall is the external oblique aponeurosis and a floor, which is also the external oblique, that rolls inwards at its lower margin and thickens to become the inguinal (Poupart's) ligament. The inguinal canal in males contains the testicular artery, veins, lymphatics and the vas deferens. In females, the round ligament descends through the canal to end in the vulva. Three important nerves, the ilioinguinal, the iliohypogastric and the genital branch of the genitofemoral nerve, also pass through the canal.

As the testis descends, a tube of peritoneum is pulled with the testis and wraps around it ultimately to form the tunica vaginalis. This peritoneal tube should obliterate, possibly under hormonal control, but it commonly fails to fuse either in part or totally. As a result, bowel within the peritoneal cavity is able to pass inside the tube down towards the scrotum. Inguinal hernia in neonates and young children is always of this congenital type. However, in other patients, the muscles around the deep inguinal ring can prevent a

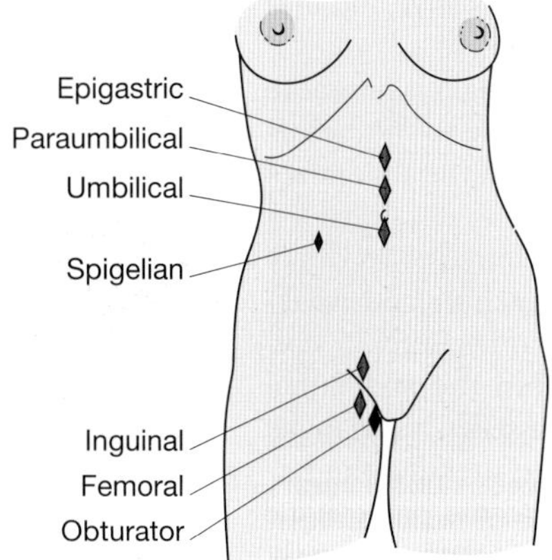

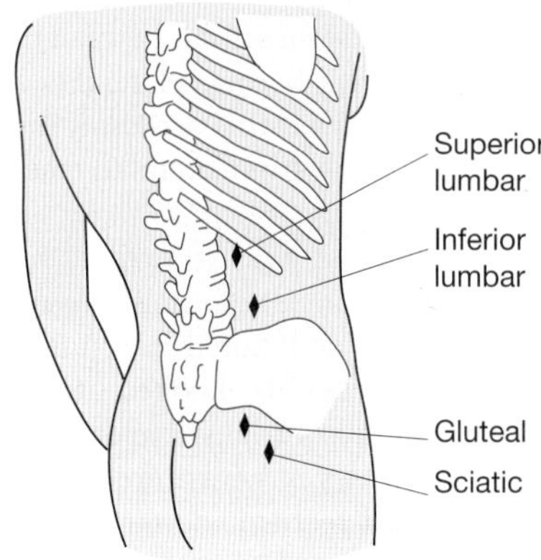

Figure 60.9 Diagram to show the sites of abdominal wall hernias, common in red and rare in black. Incisional and parastomal hernias can be found at various sites.

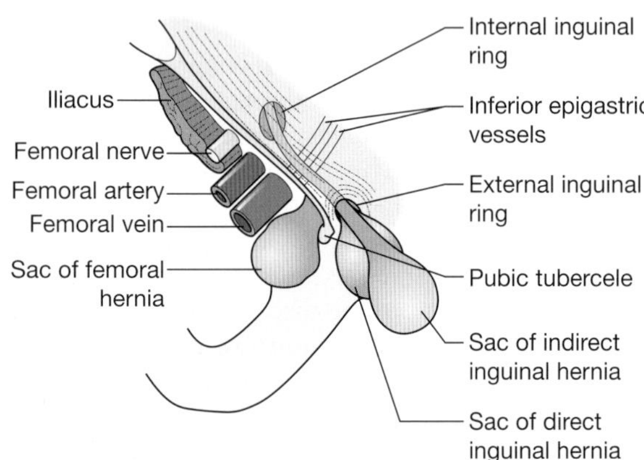

Figure 60.10 The close relationships of direct inguinal, indirect inguinal and femoral hernias.

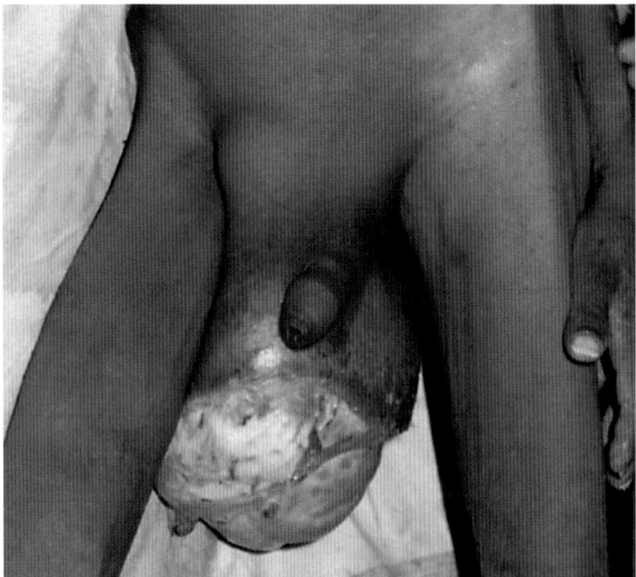

Figure 60.11 A huge scrotal hernia that has descended into the scrotum. The overlying skin has become gangrenous and sloughed away (courtesy of Dr Anupam Rai, Jabalpur, India).

hernia from developing until later in life, when, under the constant positive abdominal pressure, the deep inguinal ring and muscles are stretched and a hernia becomes apparent. As the hernia increases in size, the contents are directed down into the scrotum. These hernias can become massive and may be referred to as a scrotal hernia (Figure 60.11).

An indirect hernia is lateral because its origin is lateral to the inferior epigastric vessels. It is also oblique as the hernia passes obliquely from lateral to medial through the abdominal muscle layers.

The second type of inguinal hernia, referred to as direct or medial, is acquired. It is a result of stretching and weakening of the abdominal wall just medial to the inferior epigastric (IE) vessels. Looked at from within the abdominal cavity, there is a triangle referred to as Hasselbach's triangle, the three sides of which are the IE vessels laterally, the lateral edge of rectus abdominis medially and the pubic bone below (the iliopubic tract) (Figure 60.12). This area is weak because the abdominal wall here consists of only transversalis fascia covered by the external oblique aponeurosis. A direct, medial hernia is more likely in elderly patients. It is broadly based and therefore unlikely to strangulate. The medially placed bladder can be pulled into a direct hernia (Figure 60.13).

The third type of inguinal hernia is referred to as a sliding hernia. This is also an acquired hernia due to weakening of the abdominal wall, but occurs at the deep inguinal ring lateral to the IE vessels. Retroperitoneal fatty tissue is pushed downwards along the inguinal canal. As more tissue enters the hernia, peritoneum is pulled with it, thus creating a sac. However, the sac has formed secondarily, distinguishing it from a classic indirect hernia. On the left side, sigmoid colon may be pulled into a sliding hernia and on the right side the caecum. Surgeons need extra caution during repair because the wall of the large bowel may not be covered by peritoneum and can be damaged.

Occasionally, both lateral and medial hernias are present in the same patient (pantaloon hernia).

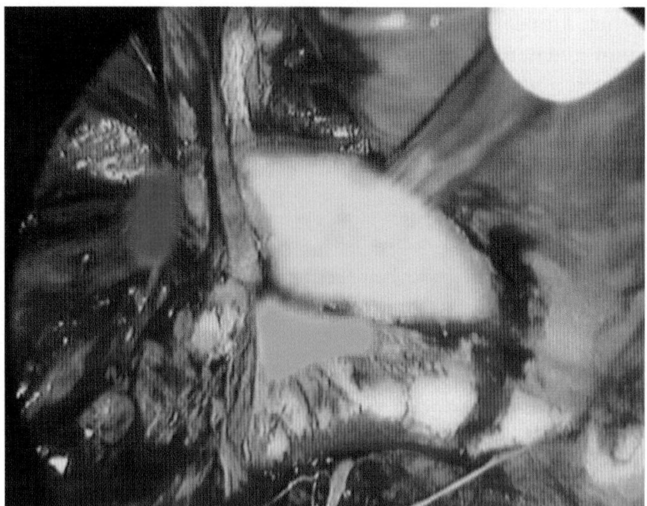

Figure 60.12 Laparoscopic view of the posterior inguinal region with hernia defects highlighted: yellow, medial inguinal; blue, lateral inguinal; green, femoral.

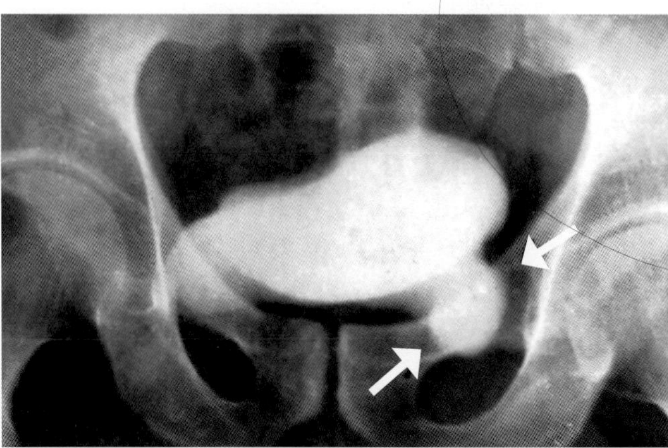

Figure 60.13 This cystogram shows the urinary bladder, part of which has descended into a left direct inguinal hernia (arrows).

Classification

Many surgeons over the past 100 years have attempted to classify inguinal (and femoral) hernias, including Casten, Halverson and McVay, Zollinger, Ponka, Gilbert and Nyhus. The European Hernia Society has recently suggested a simplified system of:

- primary or recurrent (P or R);
- lateral, medial or femoral (L, M or F);
- defect size in fingerbreadths assumed to be 1.5 cm.

A primary, indirect, inguinal hernia with a 3-cm defect size would be PL2.

Diagnosis of an inguinal hernia

In most cases, the diagnosis of an inguinal hernia is simple and patients often know their diagnosis because they are so common. Usually these hernias are reducible presenting as intermittent swellings, lying above and lateral to the pubic tubercle, with an associated cough impulse. Often the hernia will reduce on lying and reappear on standing. With the patient lying down, the patient is asked to reduce the hernia if it has not spontaneously reduced. If the patient cannot then the surgeon gently attempts to reduce the hernia. Once reduced, the surgeon identifies the bony landmarks of the anterosuperior iliac spine and pubic tubercle to landmark the deep inguinal ring at the mid-inguinal point. Gentle pressure is applied at this point and the patient asked to cough. If the hernia is controlled with pressure on the deep inguinal ring then it is likely to be indirect/lateral and if the hernia appears medial to this point then it is direct/medial. Other examination techniques have been suggested but even experienced surgeons find it difficult to distinguish lateral and medial hernias with certainty (Figure 60.14).

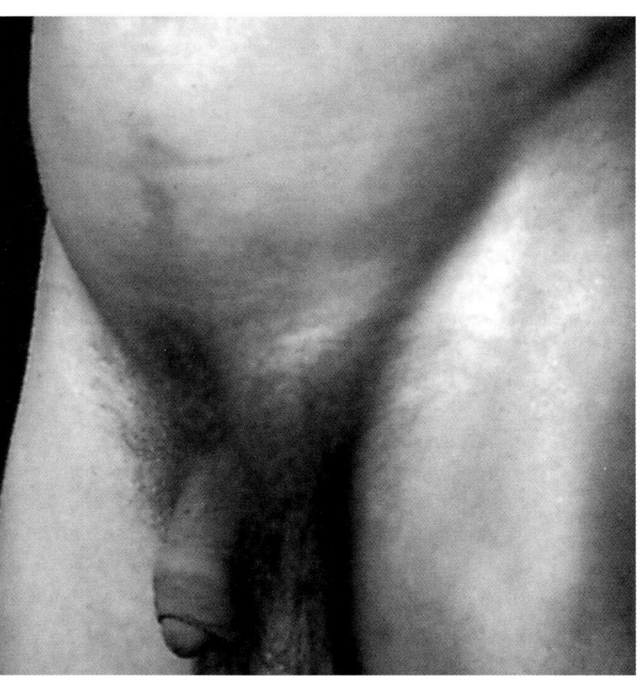

Figure 60.14 Oblique left inguinal hernia that became apparent when the patient coughed and persisted until it was reduced when he lay down.

Diagnostic difficulties

Confirmation of the diagnosis may not be possible when the patient describes an intermittent swelling but nothing is found on examination. Surgeons will often accept the diagnosis on history alone but re-examination at a later date or investigation by ultrasound scan may be requested.

If an inguinal hernia becomes irreducible and tense there may be no cough impulse. Differential diagnosis would include a lymph node groin mass or an abdominal mass (Figure 60.15). Such cases require urgent investigation by either ultrasonography or CT.

Large scrotal hernias may be misdiagnosed as a hydrocele or other testicular swelling. The surgeon should be able to identify the upper limit of a scrotal swelling but a large scrotal hernia has no upper limit because it extends back along the inguinal canal to the peritoneal cavity. In cases of doubt, ultrasonography should establish the diagnosis.

As inguinal hernia is so common, less-experienced clinicians might suggest this diagnosis when referring cases of femoral hernia or spigelian hernia. Also patients with a saphena varix may present with a swelling that increases in size on standing and with a definite cough impulse and be misdiagnosed as a hernia. The same can be true for a varicocele.

It is essential to examine the scrotal contents to exclude other pathologies and to check that the patient has two testes. It is important to examine the opposite side because contralateral hernia is common. Even if the contralateral side is weak, then bilateral repair should be recommended because the risk of contralateral recurrence is high. Of all patients 10% will present with bilateral inguinal hernias and up to 20% more will have an occult contralateral hernia on laparoscopic evaluation. A patient with a single hernia has a lifetime 33% risk of developing a hernia on the other side. Some surgeons have suggested that all patients should be offered bilateral repair, especially if laparoscopic surgery is planned, but this is not widespread practice at present.

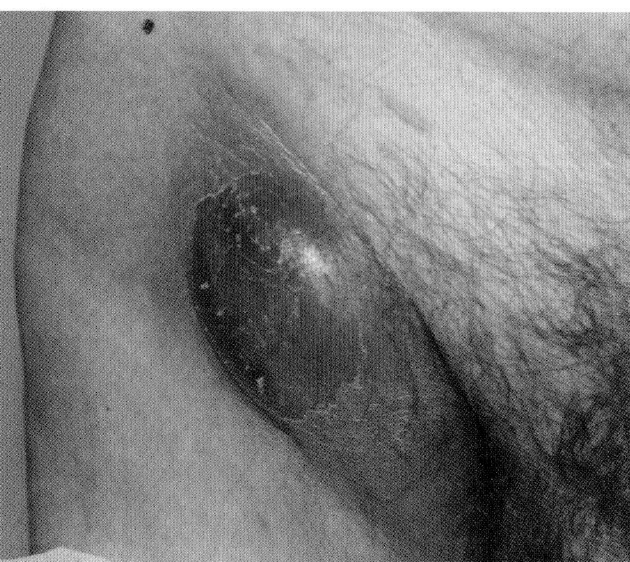

Figure 60.15 Malignant mass of nodes.

Investigations for inguinal hernia

Most cases require no diagnostic tests but ultrasonography, CT and MRI are occasionally used. A herniogram involves the injection of contrast into the peritoneal cavity followed by screening which shows the presence of a sac or asymmetrical bulging of the inguinal anatomy.

Management of inguinal hernia

It is safe to recommend no active treatment in cases of early, asymptomatic, direct hernia, particularly in elderly patients who do not wish for surgical intervention. These patients should be warned to seek early advice if the hernia increases in size or becomes symptomatic. Surgical trusses are not recommended but may be required for occasional patients who refuse any form of surgical intervention.

Elective surgery for inguinal hernia is a common and simple operation. It can be undertaken under local, regional or general anaesthesia with minimal risk, even in high-risk patients.

HERNIOTOMY

In children who have lateral hernias with a persistent processus, it is sufficient just to remove and close the sac. This is called a herniotomy. In adult surgery, herniotomy alone has a high recurrence rate and some form of muscle strengthening is added (herniorrhaphy).

OPEN SUTURE REPAIR

In 1890, Eduardo Bassini described suture repair for inguinal hernia (Figure 60.16). This was a massive leap forward and has been the basis of open repair for over 100 years. The surgeon enters the inguinal canal by opening its anterior wall, the external oblique aponeurosis. The spermatic cord is dissected free and the presence of a lateral or a medial hernia is confirmed. The sac of a lateral hernia is separated from the cord, opened and any contents reduced. The sac is then sutured closed at its neck and excess sac removed. If there is a medial hernia then it is inverted and the transversalis fascia is suture plicated. Sutures are now placed between the conjoint tendon above and the inguinal ligament below, extending from the pubic tubercle to the deep inguinal ring. The posterior wall of the inguinal canal is thus strengthened.

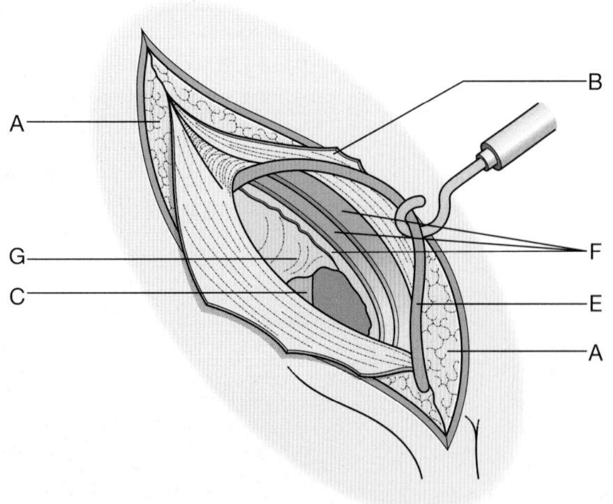

Figure 60.16 Bassini's original diagram. A, subcutaneous fat; B, external oblique; C, iliac vein; E, spermatic cord; F, nerves in inguinal canal; G, transversalis fascia.

Over 150 modifications to Bassini's operation have been described with little or no benefit except for the Shouldice modification. In this operation, the transversalis fascia is opened by a central incision from the deep inguinal ring to the pubic tubercle and then closed to create a double-thick, two-layered posterior wall (double breasting). The external oblique is closed in similar fashion. Expert centres have reported lifetime failure rates of less than 2% after Shouldice repair but it is a technically demanding operation which, in general hands, gives results identical to Bassini's repair.

Today, when a Bassini-type operation is done, most surgeons use a continuous, non-absorbable nylon or polypropylene suture which is darned between the conjoint tendon and inguinal ligament. This operation was described by Maloney, and recently published large randomised trials have reported excellent results when compared with mesh techniques. It is the most common operation performed in countries where mesh is too expensive.

Suture repair is still under development and, recently, Desarda has described an operation where a 1- to 2-cm strip of external oblique aponeurosis lying over the inguinal canal is isolated from the main muscle, but left attached both medially and laterally. It is then sutured to the conjoint tendon and inguinal ligament, reinforcing the posterior wall of the inguinal canal. As the abdominal muscles contract, this strip of aponeurosis tightens to add further physiological support to the posterior wall. This operation is currently being evaluated.

OPEN FLAT MESH REPAIR

Synthetic mesh has been used since the 1950s to reinforce hernia repair, and in the 1980s Lichtenstein described a tension-free, simple, flat, polypropylene mesh repair for inguinal hernia (Figure 60.17). The initial part of the operation is identical to Bassini's. Once the hernia sac has been removed and any medial defect closed, a piece of mesh, measuring 8 × 15 cm, is placed over the posterior wall, behind the spermatic cord, and is split to wrap around the spermatic cord at the deep inguinal ring. Loose sutures hold the mesh to the inguinal ligament and conjoint tendon. Two major advantages are claimed: lowered hernia recurrence rates and accelerated postoperative recovery. Randomised trials show that hernia recurrence within the first 2 years is lowered but acute pain scores are similar. Recent research comparing Lichtenstein's repair with laparoscopic surgery has identified chronic pain as the most common complication of open flat mesh repair with rates reported as high as 20%. Nevertheless, today, Lichtenstein's repair is the most common operation for inguinal hernia in resource-rich countries.

Eduardo Bassini, 1844–1924, Professor of Surgery, Padua, Italy, described this method of herniorraphy in 1889.

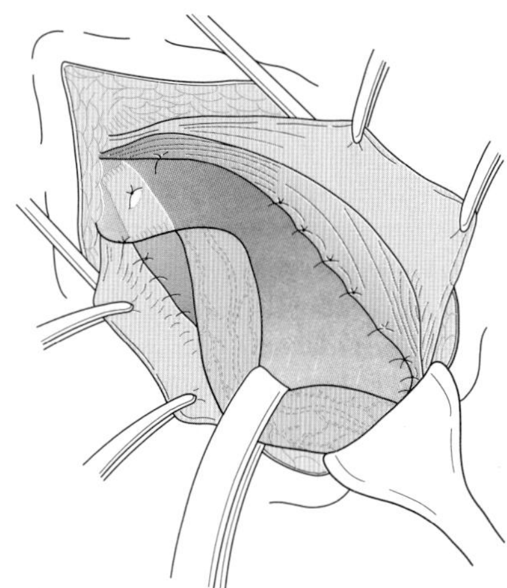

Figure 60.17 Lichtenstein's repair.

OPEN PLUG/DEVICE/COMPLEX MESH REPAIR

Surgeons and industry have been highly creative, attempting to improve on simple flat mesh repair. A surgeon in Europe has over 200 different products and techniques from which to choose. Shaped mesh plugs have gained much attention, being simple to insert into the defect and requiring little if any fixation. However, they can become solid (meshoma) and also migrate. Meshes have been designed to be placed beneath the transversalis fascia. The surgeon introduces a finger through the deep inguinal ring and bluntly (and blindly) opens the preperitoneal space deep to the inguinal canal into which a mesh is inserted. A two-layered mesh ('hernia system'), in which the inner layer is placed deep to transversalis fascia and the outer layer superficial to it, is also gaining popularity. To date, there is little evidence to show that any of these techniques is superior to Lichtenstein's operation.

OPEN PREPERITONEAL REPAIR

This approach was first described by Annandale in 1880, but was largely discarded until the 1950s when Stoppa, a French surgeon, described it with mesh reconstruction. It is useful when multiple attempts at open standard surgery have failed and the hernia(s) keeps recurring. It may now be superseded by the totally extraperitoneal laparoscopic approach, which is modelled on Stoppa's operation and first described by Ger, also French.

LAPAROSCOPIC INGUINAL HERNIA REPAIR

Two techniques are described and have been extensively studied in randomised trials. The totally extraperitoneal (TEP) approach is more widely used than the transabdominal preperitoneal (TAPP) approach. In both, the aim of surgery is to reduce the hernia and hernia sac within the abdomen, and then place a 10 × 15 cm mesh just deep to the abdominal wall, extending across the midline into the retropubic space and 5 cm lateral to the deep inguinal ring. The mesh covers Hasselbach's triangle, the deep inguinal ring and the femoral canal. In TEP, the surgeon is able to create a space just deep to the abdominal muscles without entering the peritoneal cavity whereas, in TAPP, the surgeon enters the peritoneal cavity then incises the peritoneum above the hernia defects, and reflects it away from the muscles, essentially entering the same space as in TEP. Once the hernia has been reduced, an identical mesh is inserted and the peritoneum closed over the mesh (Figures 60.18 and 60.19).

Over 60 randomised trials have compared laparoscopic surgery with Lichtenstein's repair. They show that, although the laparoscopic operation takes longer to perform, proven advantages are reduced pain both after surgery and up to 5 years later, more rapid return to full activity, and the reduced incidence of the wound complications of infection, bleeding and seroma. Laparoscopic surgery is of particular benefit in bilateral cases and in patients with hernia recurrence after open surgery. National statistics show that the proportion of cases performed laparoscopically is slowly rising, but all agree that there is a slow learning curve associated with these technically demanding operations.

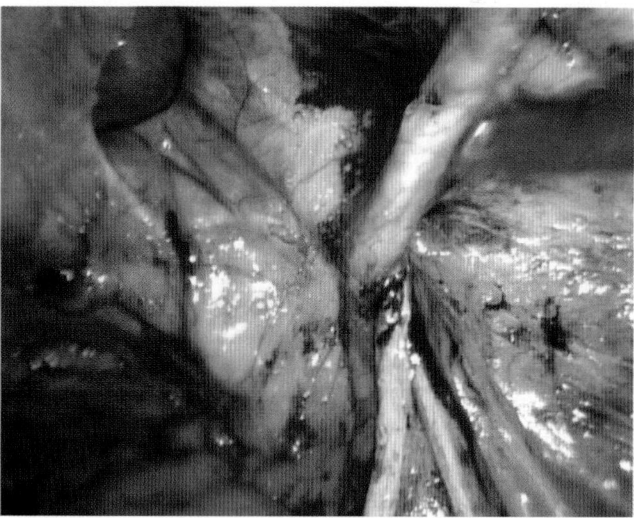

Figure 60.18 Right/medial direct hernia – laparoscopic view. Note the medial (direct) defect upper left, the inferior epigastric vessels upper right and the structures of the spermatic cord lower right.

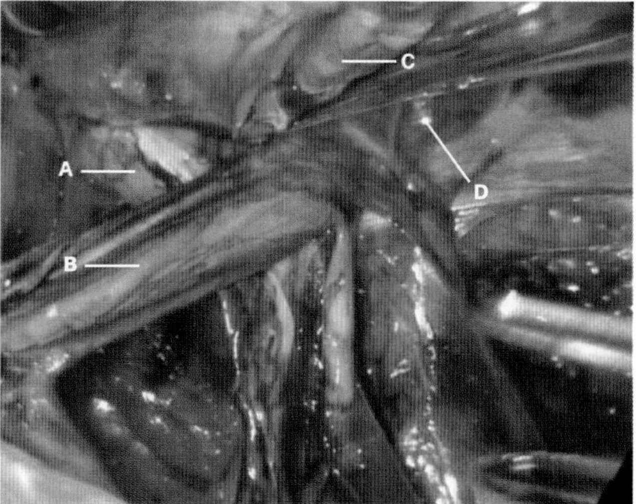

Figure 60.19 Right/lateral indirect hernia – laparoscopic view. A, arch of pubic bone; B, vas deferens and testicular vessels retracted medially; C, inferior epigastric vessels; D, deep inguinal ring (hernia defect).

Summary box 60.9

Operations for inguinal hernia

- Herniotomy
- Open suture repair
  - Bassini
  - Shouldice
  - Desarda
- Open flat mesh repair
  - Lichtenstein
- Open complex mesh repair
  - Plugs
  - Hernia systems
- Open preperitoneal repair
  - Stoppa
- Laparoscopic repair
  - TEP
  - TAPP

EMERGENCY INGUINAL HERNIA SURGERY

Of inguinal hernia patients 95% present at clinics and only 5% as an emergency with a painful irreducible hernia that may progress to strangulation and possible bowel infarction. The morbidity and mortality of emergency inguinal hernia surgery are high and surgery needs to be performed rapidly in a well-resuscitated patient with adequate postoperative high dependency or intensive care if necessary. The principles of surgery are the same as in an elective setting. Open surgery is preferred when a hernia is irreducible or if there is any risk of bowel resection. Infection may complicate these cases but most surgeons would still use a lightweight, synthetic mesh repair covered by appropriate antibiotics.

COMPLICATIONS OF INGUINAL HERNIA SURGERY

Despite this being a common procedure and technically straightforward, postoperative complications are common. Immediate complications include bleeding (which may be due to accidental damage to the inferior epigastric or iliac vessels) and urinary retention that may require catheterisation. Occasional over-enthusiastic infusion of local anaesthetic may lead to femoral nerve blockade, the patient being unable to move a leg. This usually resolves over 12 hours but is alarming.

Over the next week, seroma formation and wound infection may occur. Seroma is due to an excessive inflammatory response to sutures or mesh and cannot be prevented. In most cases the fluid resolves spontaneously but may require aspiration. After laparoscopic surgery, a seroma may be misdiagnosed as an early recurrence. Wound infection is not uncommon. Many surgeons use routine prophylactic antibiotics but recent studies suggest little benefit even when mesh is used.

In the longer term, hernia recurrence and chronic pain are the main concerns. No operation can be guaranteed to be recurrence free. Evidence shows that mesh repairs have lower recurrence rates than suture repairs, but there is no difference between the various mesh repairs and no difference between open and laparoscopic surgery. There is very strong evidence that specialist hernia surgeons will have lower recurrence rates whatever technique they use.

Chronic pain, defined as pain present 3 months after surgery, is common after all forms of surgery. It is less common and less severe after laparoscopic surgery. Different types of pain have been described but the most severe is neuralgic pain due to nerve irritation. This may be the result of nerve injury at the time of operation or chronic irritation of nerves by suture material or mesh. Careful identification and protection of all three nerves passing along the inguinal canal reduces the incidence of neuralgic pain. This type of pain is also very uncommon after laparoscopic surgery that is performed at a deeper level away from the nerves. Some contribution to chronic pain may be due to the mesh, which can become embedded in a dense collagenous reaction with shrinkage. This causes tissue tension and rigidity.

Rarely, damage to the testicular artery can lead to testicular infarction, perhaps the most serious complication of inguinal hernia surgery. There is no good evidence that hernia surgery has an effect on male fertility despite extensive study in this area.

Summary box 60.10

Complications

- Early pain, bleeding, urinary retention, anaesthetic related
- Medium seroma, wound infection
- Late chronic pain, testicular atrophy

Sportsman's hernia

This specific entity is well described and presents as severe pain in the groin area, extending into the scrotum and upper thigh. It is almost entirely restricted to young men who play contact sports such as football and rugby. The pain can be debilitating and prevent the patient from exercising. On examination there may be some tenderness in the region of the inguinal canal, over the pubic tubercle, and over the insertion of the thigh adductor muscles. Usually no hernia can be felt and only occasionally can a true inguinal hernia be found.

In most cases, the pain is due to an orthopaedic injury, such as adductor strain or pubic symphasis diastasis. However, some believe that it can be due to muscle tearing (Gilmore's groin) or stretching of the posterior wall of the inguinal canal. Other causes of pain should be excluded, such as hip, pelvic or lumbar spinal disease and bladder/prostate problems. MRI is most likely to detect an orthopaedic problem but ultrasonography, herniography or even laparoscopy may be used.

There are many anecdotal reports of successful treatment using all types of inguinal hernia surgery, suture and mesh, open and laparoscopic, but no randomised trials. Hernia surgery should be a last resort and the patient warned of a significant risk of failure to cure the pain.

Femoral hernia

Basic anatomy

The iliac artery and vein pass below the inguinal ligament to become the femoral vessels in the leg. The vein lies medially and the artery just lateral to the artery with the femoral nerve lateral to the artery. They are enclosed in a fibrous sheath. Just medial to the vein is a small space containing fat and some lymphatic tissue (node of Cloquet). It is this space which is exploited by a femoral hernia. The walls of a femoral hernia are the femoral vein laterally, the inguinal ligament anteriorly, the pelvic bone covered by the iliopectineal ligament (Astley Cooper's) posteriorly and the lacunar ligament (Gimbernat's) medially. This is a strong curved ligament with a sharp unyielding edge which impedes reduction of a femoral hernia (Figure 60.20).

The female pelvis has a different shape to the male, increasing the size of the femoral canal and the risk of hernia. In old age, the femoral defect increases and femoral hernia is commonly seen in low-weight, elderly women. There is a substantial risk of developing a femoral hernia after a sutured inguinal hernia repair (Denmark Hernia Registry).

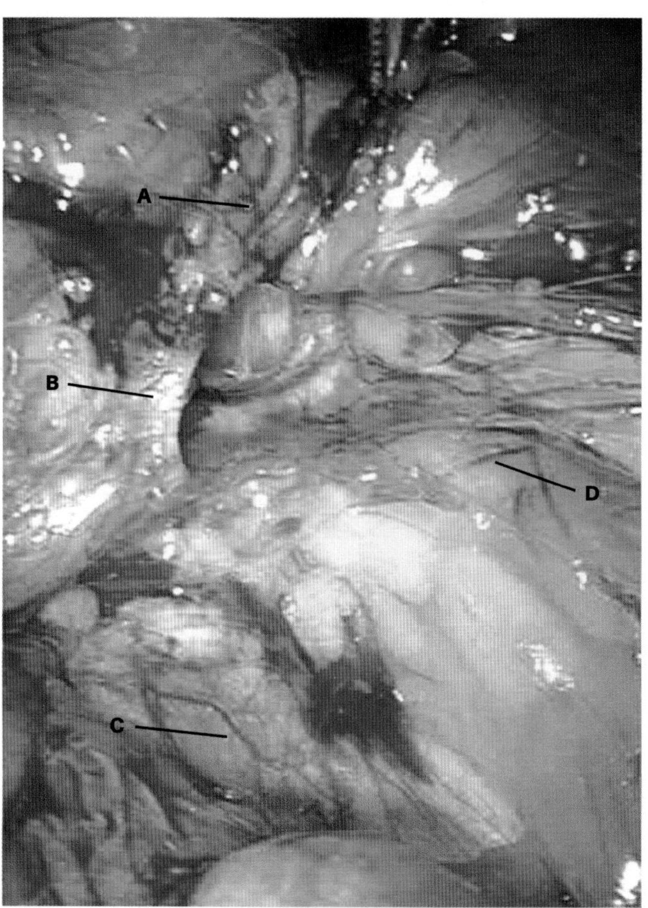

Figure 60.20 Right femoral hernia – laparoscopic view. The slightly oblique inguinal ligament can be seen superolaterally above the defect. The external iliac vein is not seen. A, Inguinal ligament; B, lacunar ligament; C, arch of pubic bone; D, fatty tissue overlying iliac vessels.

Summary box 60.11

Femoral hernia

- Less common than inguinal hernia
- It is more common in women than in men
- Easily missed on examination
- Of cases 50% present as an emergency with very high risk of strangulation

Diagnosis of femoral hernia

Diagnostic error is common and often leads to delay in diagnosis and treatment. The hernia appears below and lateral to the pubic tubercle and lies in the upper leg rather than in the lower abdomen. Inadequate exposure of this area during routine examination leads to failure to detect the hernia. The hernia often rapidly becomes irreducible and loses any cough impulse due to the tightness of the neck. It may only be 1–2 cm in size and can easily be mistaken for a lymph node. As it increases in size, it is reflected superiorly and becomes difficult to distinguish from a medial direct hernia, which arises only a few centimetres above the femoral canal. A direct inguinal hernia leaves the abdominal cavity just above the inguinal ligament and a femoral hernia just below (Figure 60.21).

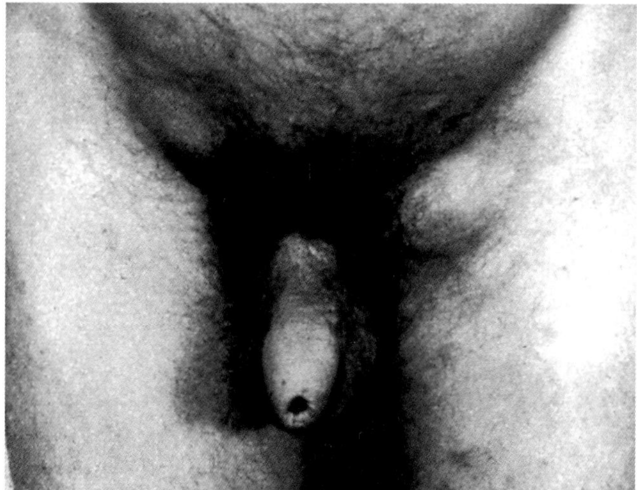

Figure 60.21 The patient has a left femoral and a right inguinal hernia.

Summary box 60.12

Differential diagnosis

- Direct inguinal hernia
- Lymph node
- Saphena varix
- Femoral artery aneurysm
- Psoas abscess
- Rupture of adductor longus with haematoma

Jules Germain Cloquet, 1790–1883, Professor of Anatomy and Surgery, Paris, France.
Sir Astley Paston Cooper, 1768–1841, surgeon, Guy's Hospital, London, UK, received a baronetcy and 1000 guineas for successfully removing an infected wen from the head of King George IV at Brighton in 1821.
Manoel Louise Antonio don Gimbernat, 1734–1816, Professor of Anatomy, Barcelona, Spain and later Director of the Royal College of Surgeons in Spain.

Investigations

In routine cases, no specific investigations are required. However, if there is uncertainly then ultrasonography or CT should be requested. In the emergency patient, bowel obstruction usually occurs and a plain radiograph is likely to show small bowel obstruction. All patients with unexplained small bowel obstruction should undergo careful examination for a femoral hernia. It is now common to perform CT scanning in cases of bowel obstruction primarily to exclude malignancy, but it can identify an obstructing femoral hernia missed by clinicians.

Surgery for femoral hernia

There is no alternative to surgery for femoral hernia and it is wise to treat such cases with some urgency. There are three open approaches and appropriate cases can be managed laparoscopically.

LOW APPROACH (LOCKWOOD)

This is the simplest operation for a femoral hernia but suitable only when there is no risk of bowel resection. It can easily be performed under local anaesthesia. A transverse incision is made over the hernia. The sac of the hernia is opened and its contents reduced. The sac is also reduced and non-absorbable sutures are placed between the inguinal ligament above and the fascia overlying the bone below. A small incision can be made in the medial lacunar ligament to aid reduction but there may be an abnormal branch of the obturator artery just deep to it, which can bleed. The femoral vein, lateral to the hernia, needs to be protected. Some surgeons place a mesh plug into the hernia defect for further reinforcement.

THE INGUINAL APPROACH (LOTHEISSEN)

The initial incision is identical to that of Bassini's or Lichtenstein's operation into the inguinal canal. The spermatic cord (or round ligament) is mobilised and the transversalis fascia opened from deep inguinal ring to the pubic tubercle. A femoral hernia lies immediately below this incision and can be reduced by a combination of pulling from above and pushing from below. If necessary, the peritoneum can be opened to help with reduction. Once reduced, the neck of the hernia is closed with sutures or a mesh plug, protecting the iliac vein throughout. The layers are closed as for inguinal hernia and the surgeon may place a mesh into the inguinal canal to protect against development of an inguinal hernia.

Some surgeons believe that exploration of the femoral canal to exclude a hernia should be a routine part of inguinal hernia surgery but most surgeons do not do this.

HIGH APPROACH (McEVEDY)

This more complex operation is ideal in the emergency situation where the risk of bowel strangulation is high. It requires regional or general anaesthesia. A horizontal incision (classically vertical) is made in the lower abdomen centred at the lateral edge of the rectus muscle. The anterior rectus sheath is incised and the rectus muscle displaced medially. The surgeon proceeds deep to the muscle in the preperitoneal space. The femoral hernia is reduced and the sac opened to allow careful inspection of the bowel, and a decision made regarding the need for bowel resection. This is performed if necessary. In dubious cases, the bowel is replaced into the peritoneal cavity for 5 minutes and then re-examined. The femoral defect is then closed with sutures, mesh or plug. This approach allows a generous incision to be made in the peritoneum, which aids inspection of the bowel and facilitates bowel resection.

LAPAROSCOPIC APPROACH

Both the TEP and TAPP approaches can be used for a femoral hernia and a standard mesh inserted. This is ideal for reducible femoral hernias presenting electively, but not for emergency cases or irreducible hernia.

VENTRAL HERNIA

This term refers to hernias of the anterior abdominal wall. Inguinal and femoral hernias are not included even though they are ventral. Lumbar hernia is included despite being dorsolateral. The European Hernia Society classification (2009) distinguished primary ventral from incisional hernia but did not include parastomal hernia. We have included parastomal hernia and traumatic hernia.

Summary box 60.13

Ventral hernias

- Umbilical–paraumbilical
- Epigastric
- Incisional
- Parastomal
- Spigelian
- Lumbar
- Traumatic

Umbilical hernia

The umbilical defect is present at birth but closes as the stump of the umbilical cord heals, usually within a week of birth. This process may be delayed, leading to the development of herniation in the neonatal period. The umbilical ring may also stretch and reopen in adult life.

Charles Barrett Lockwood, 1856–1914, surgeon, St Bartholomew's Hospital, London, UK.
George Lotheissen, 1868–1941, surgeon, the Kaiser Franz Joseph Hospital, Vienna, Austria, described this operation in 1898.
Peter George McEvedy, 1890–1951, surgeon, Ancoats Hospital, Manchester, UK.

Umbilical hernia in children

This common condition occurs in up to 10% of infants, with a higher incidence in premature babies. The hernia appears within a few weeks of birth and is often symptomless, but increases in size on crying and assumes a classic conical shape. Sexes are equally affected but the incidence in black infants is up to eight times higher than in white. Obstruction and/or strangulation is extremely uncommon below the age of 3 years.

TREATMENT

Conservative treatment is indicated under the age of 2 years when the hernia is symptomless. Parental reassurance is all that is necessary. Of hernias 95% will resolve spontaneously. If the hernia persists beyond the age of 2 years it is unlikely to resolve and surgical repair is indicated.

SURGERY

A small curved incision is made immediately below the umbilicus. The neck of the sac is defined, opened and any contents are returned to the peritoneal cavity. The sac is closed and redundant sac excised. The defect in the linea alba is closed with interrupted sutures.

Summary box 60.14

Umbilical hernia in children

- Common in infants and most resolve spontaneously
- Rarely strangulate

Umbilical hernia in adults

Conditions that cause stretching and thinning of the midline raphe (linea alba), such as pregnancy, obesity and liver disease with cirrhosis, predispose to reopening of the umbilical defect. In adults, the defect in the median raphe is immediately adjacent to (most often above) the true umbilicus, although at operation this is indistinguishable. The term 'paraumbilical hernia' is commonly used. The defect is rounded with a well-defined fibrous margin. Small umbilical hernias often contain extraperitoneal fat or omentum. Larger hernias can contain small or large bowel but, even when very large, the neck of the sac is narrow compared with the volume of its contents. As a result, in adults, umbilical hernias that include bowel are prone to become irreducible, obstructed and strangulated.

CLINICAL FEATURES

Patients are commonly overweight with a thinned and attenuated midline raphe. The bulge is typically slightly to one side of the umbilical depression, creating a crescent-shaped appearance to the umbilicus (Figure 60.22). Women are affected more than men. Most patients complain of pain due to tissue tension or symptoms of intermittent bowel obstruction. In large hernias, the overlying skin may become thinned, stretched and develop dermatitis.

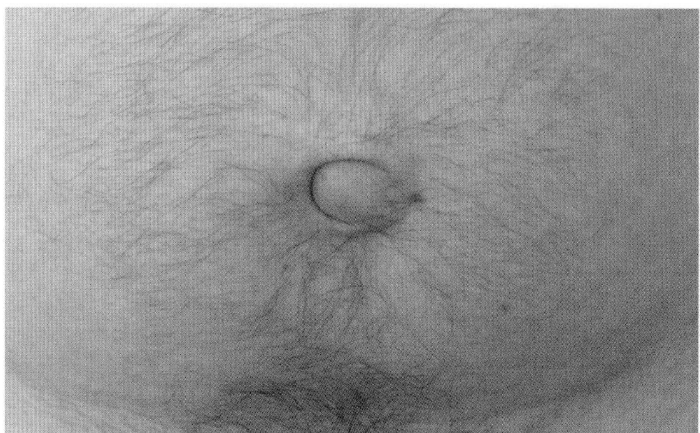

Figure 60.22 A small paraumbilical hernia.

TREATMENT

As a result of the high risk of strangulation, surgery should be advised in cases where the hernia contains bowel. Small hernias may be left alone if they are asymptomatic, but they may enlarge and require surgery at a later date. Surgery may be performed open or laparoscopically.

OPEN UMBILICAL HERNIA REPAIR

Very small defects less than 1 cm in size may be closed with a simple figure-of-eight suture, or repaired by a darn technique where a non-absorbable, monofilament suture is criss-crossed across the defect and anchored firmly to the fascia all around.

Defects up to 2 cm in diameter may be sutured primarily with minimal tension, although, the larger the defect, the more tension and the more likely it is that mesh reinforcement will be beneficial. The classic repair was described by Mayo. A transverse incision is made and the hernia sac dissected, opened and its content reduced. Any non-viable tissue is removed, sometimes involving bowel resection. The peritoneum is closed. The defect in the anterior rectus sheath is extended laterally on both sides and elevated to create an upper and lower flap. The lower flap is then inserted beneath the upper flap and sutured to it, with the upper flap being brought downwards over it so that the tissue is two layered (double breasted). Non-absorbable sutures are used. There is often a large subcutaneous space. A suction drain is placed to reduce the risk of seroma and haematoma. The skin is closed but stretched or redundant skin may need to be excised (apronectomy) to achieve a better cosmetic result. Today, with modern suture materials, surgeons simply close the anterior sheath in a single layer.

William James Mayo, 1861–1939, surgeon, the Mayo Clinic, Rochester, MN, USA, described this operation in 1901. He and his brother Charles Horace Mayo (1865–1939) joined their father's private practice in Rochester. This practice became the Mayo Clinic. Their father William Worrall Mayo was born in Manchester, UK in 1819.

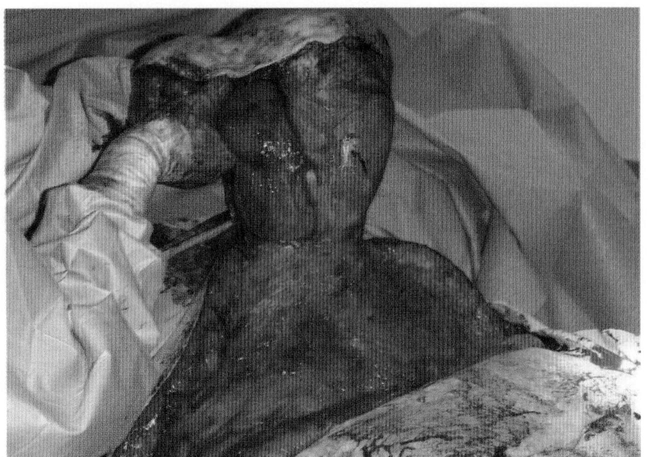
Figure 60.23 A massive paraumbilical hernia – operative view.

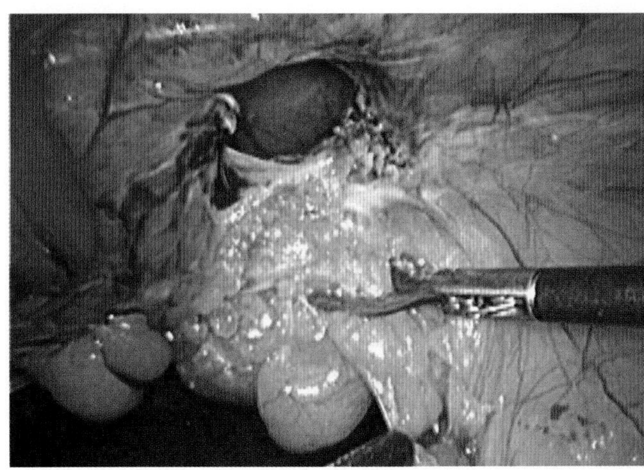
Figure 60.24 Paraumbilical defect – laparoscopic view.

For defects larger than 2 cm in diameter, mesh repair is recommended (Figure 60.23). The mesh may be placed in one of several anatomical planes:

- Within the peritoneal cavity – a tissue separating mesh is placed through the defect and spread out on the underside of the abdominal wall and fixed to it, ideally with an overlap of 5 cm in each direction. This is a quick repair but requires the use of expensive mesh.
- In the retromuscular space – the linea alba is opened vertically and both left and right posterior rectus sheaths are incised 1 cm to the side of the midline exposing the rectus muscle. The posterior sheaths are sutured together and the muscles elevated away from the sheath to develop the retromuscular space into which a sheet of mesh is placed and fixed by sutures. The mesh should overlap the midline by 5 cm laterally and the umbilicus vertically. It should therefore be a minimum diameter of 10 cm. A drain may be placed deep to the linea alba. This is a very secure repair but requires extensive dissection.
- In the extraperitoneal space – it is difficult, but possible, to develop the plane below the posterior rectus sheath, just outside the peritoneum. Care must be taken to avoid 'button-holing' the peritoneum because it is thin and fragile. Mesh can then be tucked into in this space, ensuring a good overlap as before. Ideally, the linea alba is closed over the mesh but, if this is not possible, a flap of peritoneal sac can be used to cover the mesh. This is a good repair, but, if the peritoneum is extensively damaged during the dissection, it will have to be abandoned in favour of an alternative technique.
- In the subcutaneous plane – this is the simplest technique, called an onlay mesh. The peritoneal sac and contents are dealt with as above. An attempt is made to close linea alba vertically with sutures and a disc of mesh is placed on the anterior rectus sheath and sutured to it. The mesh is lying in the subcutaneous space and is prone to infection.

LAPAROSCOPIC UMBILICAL HERNIA REPAIR

Three ports are placed laterally on the abdominal wall, usually on the left side unless adhesions from previous surgery are likely. The contents of the hernia are reduced by traction and external pressure. The falciform ligament above and the median umbilical fold below may need to be taken down if they interfere with mesh placement. A disc of non-adherent mesh, designed for intraperitoneal use, is introduced and positioned on the under surface of the abdominal wall, centred on the defect. It is then fixed to the peritoneum and posterior rectus sheaths using staples, tacks or sutures. This is a simple and secure repair, which achieves generous overlap without surgical damage to umbilicus and surrounding fascia (Figure 60.24). However, it requires specialised equipment and expensive tissue-separating mesh. Intraperitoneal meshes can cause severe pain lasting for 24–48 hours after surgery which can mimic peritonitis.

EMERGENCY REPAIR OF UMBILICAL HERNIA

Incarceration, bowel obstruction and strangulation are frequent because of the narrow neck and the fibrous edge of the defect in the midline raphe. Delay to surgery can lead to gangrene of the omentum or bowel. Large hernias are often multiloculated and there may be strangulated bowel in one component when other areas are clinically soft and a non-tender hernia.

SURGERY

In cases of simple incarceration without clinical evidence of strangulation, repair may be attempted laparoscopically but reduction of the contents can be very difficult if the hernia contains bowel. Most emergency repairs are performed by open surgery. In the presence of established strangulation it is unwise to place mesh at all because of the risk of infection, so an open sutured repair should be performed, accepting a high risk of later recurrence. Alternatively, a two-stage repair could be planned: the hernia contents being dealt with initially with little attempt made to close the defect and then subsequent definitive mesh repair once sepsis has been controlled.

Epigastric hernia

These hernias arise through the midline raphe (linea alba) any where between the xiphoid process and the umbilicus, usually midway. When close to the umbilicus they are called supraumbilical hernias. Epigastric hernias begin with a transverse split in the midline raphe so, in contrast to umbilical hernias, the defect is elliptical. It has been hypothesised that the defect occurs at the site where small blood vessels pierce the linea alba or, more likely, that it arises at weaknesses due to abnormal decussation of aponeurotic fibres related to heavy physical activity (Figure 60.25).

Epigastric hernia defects are usually less than 1 cm in maximum diameter and commonly contain only extraperitoneal fat, which gradually enlarges, spreading in the subcutaneous plane to resemble the shape of a mushroom. When very large they may contain a peritoneal sac but rarely any bowel. More than one hernia may be present. The most common cause of 'recurrence' is failure to identify a second defect at the time of original repair.

Clinical features

The patients are often fit, healthy men aged between 25 and 40 years. These hernias can be very painful even when the swelling is the size of a pea, due to the fatty contents becoming nipped sufficiently to produce partial strangulation. The pain may mimic that of a peptic ulcer but symptoms should not be ascribed to the hernia until gastrointestinal pathology has been excluded. A soft midline swelling can often be felt more easily than seen. It may be locally tender. It is unlikely to be reducible because of the narrow neck. It may resemble a lipoma. A cough impulse may or may not be felt.

Treatment

Very small epigastric hernias have been known to disappear spontaneously, probably due to infarction of the fat. Small-to-moderate-sized hernias without a peritoneal sac are not inherently dangerous and surgery should be offered only if the hernia is sufficiently symptomatic.

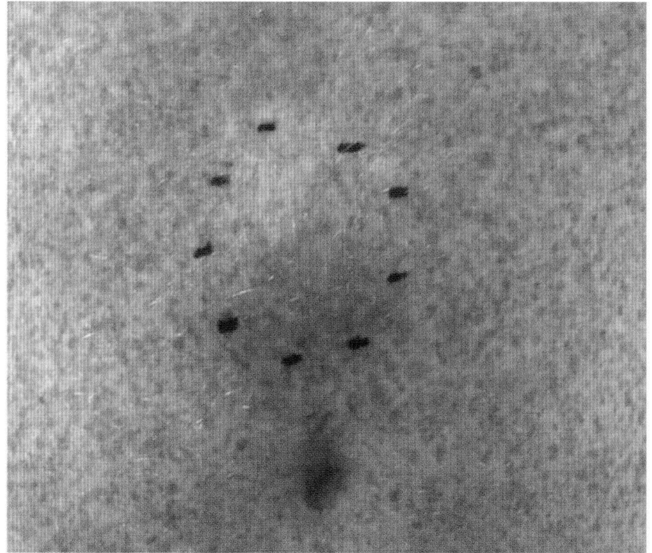

Figure 60.25 Epigastric hernia – external view.

Surgery

This may be done by open or laparoscopic surgery. At open surgery, a vertical or transverse incision is made over the swelling and down to the linea alba. Protruding extraperitoneal fat can simply be pushed back through the defect or excised. Often a small vessel is present in the hernia content that can cause troublesome bleeding. The defect in the linea alba is closed with non-absorbable sutures in adults and absorbable sutures in children. In larger hernias and when a peritoneal sac is present, the surgical approach is similar to an umbilical mesh repair.

Laparoscopic repair is very similar to that for umbilical hernia except that the defect is hidden behind the falciform ligament which must be taken down from the undersurface of the abdominal wall. The margins of the defect must be clearly exposed and the fatty contents reduced before the mesh is placed. Simply placing a mesh under the linea midline may not in fact remove the hernia when its contents are extraperitoneal fat.

Incisional hernia

These arise through a defect in the musculofascial layers of the abdominal wall in the region of a postoperative scar. Thus they may appear anywhere on the abdominal surface.

Incidence and aetiology

Incisional hernias have been reported in 10–50% of laparotomy incisions and 1–5% of laparoscopic port-site incisions. Factors predisposing to their development are patient factors (obesity, general poor healing due to malnutrition, immunosuppression or steroid therapy, chronic cough, cancer), wound factors (poor quality tissues, wound infection) and surgical factors (inappropriate suture material, incorrect suture placement).

An incisional hernia usually starts as disruption of the musculofascial layers of a wound in the early postoperative period. Often the event passes unnoticed if the overlying skin wound has healed securely. Many incisional hernias may be preventable with the use of good surgical technique. The classic sign of wound disruption is a serosanguineous discharge.

Clinical features

These hernias commonly appear as a localised swelling involving a small portion of the scar but may present as a diffuse bulging of the whole length of the incision (Figure 60.26). There may be several discrete hernias along the length of the incision and unsuspected defects are often found at surgery (Figure 60.27). Incisional hernias tend to increase steadily in size with time. The skin overlying large hernias may become thin and atrophic so that peristalsis may be seen in the underlying intestine. Vascular damage to skin may lead to dermatitis. Attacks of partial intestinal obstruction are common because there are usually coexisting internal adhesions. Strangulation is less frequent and most likely to occur when the fibrous defect is small and the sac is large. Most incisional hernias are broad-necked and carry a low risk of strangulation.

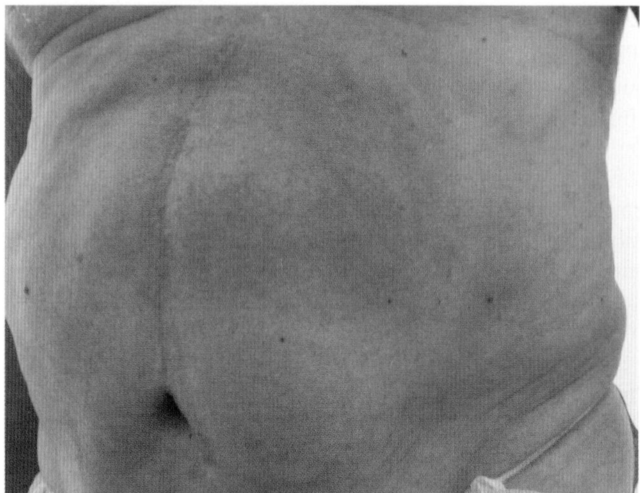

Figure 60.26 A large multilocular incisional hernia.

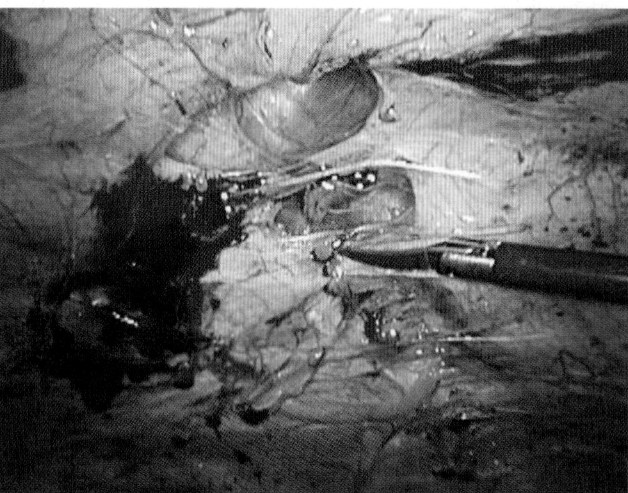

Figure 60.27 Multiple defects seen during laparoscopic operation.

Summary box 60.15

Incisional hernia

- Incidence 10–50% after surgery
- Causation due to patient, wound and surgeon factors
- Wide variation in size
- Often multiple defects within the same scar
- Obstruction is common but strangulation is rare
- Open and laparoscopic repairs possible

Treatment

Asymptomatic incisional hernias may not require treatment at all. The wearing of an abdominal binder or belt may prevent the hernia from increasing in size.

Principles of surgery

For most incisional hernias, surgery is relatively straightforward and both open and laparoscopic options are available. A number of principles apply, irrespective of the technique used.

The repair should cover the whole length of the previous incision. Approximation of the musculofascial layers should be done with minimal tension and prosthetic mesh should be used to reduce the risk of recurrence. Mesh may be contraindicated in a contaminated field, e.g. bowel injury during the dissection but, in a clean-contaminated field, such as after an elective bowel resection, mesh may be used if placed in a different anatomical plane to the contamination, such as in the extraperitoneal/retromuscular space. Appropriate systemic antibiotics should be used.

OPEN REPAIR

Simple suture techniques without the use of prosthetic mesh for reinforcement, even with layered closure such as in Mayo, 'keel' or da Silva repairs, are not recommended today because of the high risk of recurrence. However, they may be the only option in the presence of gross contamination such as peritonitis.

The previous incision is opened along its full length to reveal any clinically unsuspected defects. The hernial sac, its neck and the margins of the defect are fully exposed. The sac can be opened, contents reduced, local adhesions divided and any redundant sac excised to allow safe reclosure of the peritoneum.

Mesh can be placed in one of several planes as for umbilical hernia repair. The simplest approach is an onlay mesh but increasingly the retromuscular sublay repair is preferred by expert surgeons and is described below.

RETROMUSCULAR SUBLAY MESH REPAIR

Vertical incisions are made through the fascia surrounding the rectus abdominis muscles so that the muscle can be separated and elevated from the posterior rectus sheath below. If possible, the medial edges of the posterior rectus sheath edges are sutured together with a continuous suture. In very large defects this may not be possible and below the arcuate line where the posterior sheath is deficient, being peritoneum and transversalis fascia only. In the case of transverse incision, where the defect extends lateral to the rectus sheath, internal oblique and transversus abdominis muscles form the posterior layer. A sheet of lightweight, large-pore, prosthetic, elastic mesh is then laid between this posterior rectus sheath and belly/bellies of the rectus muscle. It is fixed to the sheath by interrupted sutures. The mesh must be large enough to ensure a 5-cm overlap of the underlying fascial defect in all directions. Careful haemostasis and meticulous asepsis are essential during this operation. The anterior rectus sheaths are then sutured together over the mesh so that, ideally, the mesh is completely covered by muscle and fascia and is not lying in the subcutaneous plane. Redundant skin may need to be excised. The risk of postoperative serous fluid collections is reduced by suction drainage.

LAPAROSCOPIC REPAIR

Incisional hernias are increasingly being repaired by laparoscopic mesh techniques. Laparoscopy and division of adhesions is initially performed. Hernia contents are reduced and the fibrous margins of the hernia defect(s) are exposed. Often the falciform ligament and median umbilical fold need to be taken down. Some surgeons prefer to suture close the muscle defects first and then reinforce with mesh. Others simply fix the mesh under the defect with adequate overlap. The use of a tissue-separating mesh is essential. Various techniques have been described to size and then position the mesh accurately. The mesh is fixed to the abdominal wall by staples or transfascial sutures which pass through all muscle layers to hold the mesh.

In the presence of dense peritoneal adhesions, the laparoscopic surgeon needs to take great care because injury to the bowel is possible and may not be recognised. Diathermy is not used. If occult bowel injury does occur it can lead to postoperative peritonitis, which is an extremely dangerous complication.

Management of the very large incisional hernia

Very large incisional hernias often require careful thought before treatment begins. If the volume of the sac is more than 25% of the volume of the abdominal cavity (and this can be calculated from CT images), then there are likely to be issues of loss of abdominal domain when the hernia is repaired. The contents of the hernia, which have been outside the abdominal cavity for a long time, will not fit back inside or, if they do, it will result in high tension. High intra-abdominal pressure can lead to visceral compression and pulmonary complications due to impaired diaphragmatic movement. A tight abdomen can lead to wound breakdown and failure of the repair.

Techniques to overcome the potential loss of abdominal domain include preoperative abdominal expansion with progressive preoperative pneumoperitoneum over several weeks, resection of the omentum and/or colon at the time of repair, the use of prosthetic mesh to span the uncloseable gap in the musculofascial layer, or the use of musculofascial advancement or transpositional flaps to achieve closure.

Even if loss of domain is not a concern, large defects can still be very difficult to close and the same special techniques may need to be used to avoid producing excessive tension in the repair. Ramirez's component separation technique, which incorporates relaxing incisions in the external oblique aponeurosis and/or the posterior sheath, is very useful because this enables either the anterior or the posterior component of the rectus sheath to be drawn together. It may then be reinforced with a mesh.

Patients with poor quality or redundant skin may benefit from a wedge excision of skin and fat (lipectomy) to improve the abdominal contour postoperatively. Repair of these very large hernias is highly specialised surgery and is best done in specialist centres.

Reducing the risk of incisional hernia

The incidence of incisional hernia may be reduced by improving the patient's general condition preoperatively where possible, e.g. weight loss for obesity or improving nutritional state for malnutrition. Closing the fascial layers with non-absorbable, or very slowly absorbable, sutures of adequate gauge is important. Traditional teaching was that sutures should be 1 cm deep and 1 cm apart. Recent work has shown that lower incisional hernia rates and reduced infection rates are gained when smaller and closer bites are used with a 2/0 suture rather than traditional heavier materials.

There is no evidence that interrupted sutures are better or worse than continuous. However, if continuous suturing is used, the tissue bites must not be too near the fascial edge or pulled too tight because they may cut out. It has also been confirmed that the optimal ratio of suture length to wound length is 4:1 (Jenkins' rule). If less length than this is used, the suture bites are too far apart or too tight and the converse applies if more length than this is used.

Drains should be brought out through separate incisions and not through the wound itself because this leads to hernia formation.

Recent reports have suggested that placement of a prophylactic mesh in patients at high risk of hernia formation will substantially reduce that risk. This has been reported in obese patients undergoing bariatric surgery and also to prevent parastomal herniation, which occurs in up to 50% of patients.

Spigelian hernia

These hernias are uncommon although are probably underdiagnosed. They affect men and women equally and can occur at any age, but are most common in elderly people. They arise through a defect in the spigelian fascia, which is the aponeurosis of transversus abdominis. Often these hernias advance through the internal oblique as well and spread out deep to the external oblique aponeurosis. The spigelian fascia extends between the transversus muscle and the lateral border of the rectus sheath from the costal margin to the groin, where it blends into the conjoint tendon. Most spigelian hernias appear below the level of the umbilicus near the edge of the rectus sheath, but they can be found anywhere along the spigelian line (Figure 60.28). There is a common

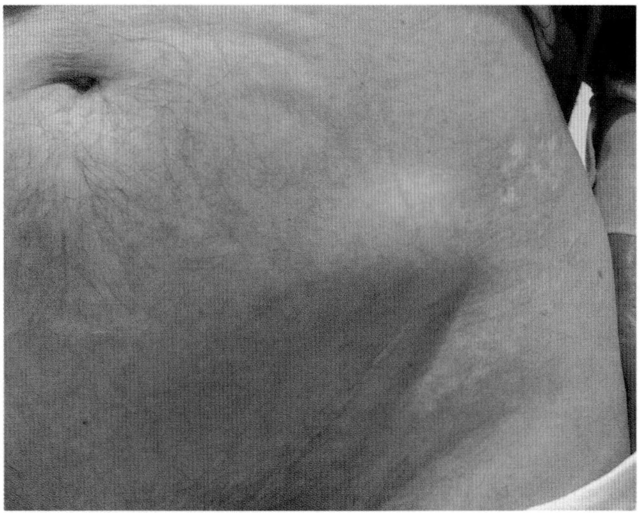

Figure 60.28 Spigelian hernia.

Adrian Van der Spieghel (Spigelius), 1578–1625, Professor of Anatomy, Padua, Italy.

misconception that they protrude below the arcuate line as a result of deficiency of the posterior rectus sheath at that level, but in fact the defect is almost always above the arcuate line. In young patients they usually contain extraperitoneal fat only but in older patients there is often a peritoneal sac and they can become very large indeed.

They have also been described in infants and may be congenital, reflecting incomplete differentiation of the mesenchymal layers within the abdominal wall.

Clinical features

Young patients usually present with intermittent pain, due to pinching of the fat, similar to an epigastric hernia. A lump may or may not be palpable because the fatty hernia is small and the overlying external oblique is intact. Older patients generally present with a reducible swelling at the edge of the rectus sheath and may have symptoms of intermittent obstruction. The diagnosis should be suspected because of the location of the symptoms and is confirmed by CT. Ultrasonography has the advantage that it can be performed in the upright patient because no defect may be visible with the patient lying down.

Treatment

Surgery is recommended because the narrow and fibrous neck predisposes to strangulation. Surgery can be open or laparoscopic. At open surgery a skin crease is made over the hernia, but no abnormality will be seen until the external oblique is opened. The sac and contents are dealt with and the small defect in the spigelian fascia is repaired by suture or mesh laid deep to the external oblique aponeurosis. The plane of the mesh can be extended medially into the posterior rectus sheath if required. The external oblique aponeurosis is closed over the mesh.

Laparoscopy is useful if no sac is palpable, but, in young patients with a hernia containing only extraperitoneal fat, no hernia will be seen from within the peritoneum. In such cases, the peritoneum can be incised and the extraperitoneal plane explored for the small defect, which can then be closed by either suture or mesh. When an intraperitoneal sac is present, laparoscopic repair can be performed using either the intraperitoneal onlay of mesh (IPOM) or TAPP technique.

Summary box 60.16

Spigelian hernia

- Rare
- Often misdiagnosed
- High risk of complications

Lumbar hernia

Most primary lumbar hernias occur through the inferior lumbar triangle of Petit bounded below by the crest of the ilium, laterally by the external oblique muscle and medially by latissimus dorsi (Figure 60.29). Less commonly, the sac comes through the superior lumbar triangle, which is bounded by the twelfth rib above, medially by sacrospinalis and laterally by the posterior border of the internal oblique muscle. Primary lumbar hernias are rare, but may be mimicked by incisional hernias arising through flank incisions for renal operations, or through incisions for bone grafts harvested from the iliac crest.

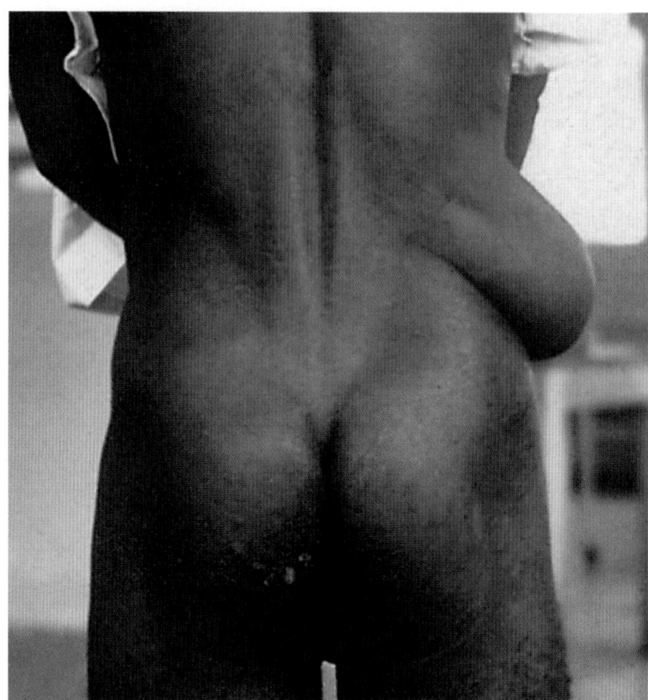

Figure 60.29 Inferior lumbar hernia, which contained caecum, appendix and small bowel. Note the filarial skin rash on the buttocks (courtesy of VJ Hartfield, formerly of south-east Nigeria).

Differential diagnosis

A lumbar hernia must be distinguished from:

- a lipoma;
- a cold (tuberculous) abscess pointing to this position;
- a pseudo-hernia due to local muscular paralysis. Lumbar pseudo-hernia can result from any interference with the nerve supply of the affected muscles, the most common cause being injury to the subcostal nerve during a kidney operation.

Treatment

The natural history is for these hernias to increase in size and surgery is recommended. Lumbar hernias can be approached by open or laparoscopic surgery. The defects can be difficult to close with sutures and mesh is recommended.

The TAPP laparoscopic approach is gaining popularity. With the patient in a semilateral position ports are inserted well away from the defect. The peritoneum is incised above the hernia and dissected back to expose the muscle defect. The content, often extraperitoneal fat, is reduced and a mesh fixed with ample overlap. The peritoneum can then be resutured or tacked back to cover the mesh.

Jean Louis Petit, 1674–1750, Director of the Academie de Chirurgie, Paris, France.

Lumbar incisional hernias can be approached in the same way but large ones, especially if there is a component of neuropathic muscle atrophy causing a diffuse bulge (pseudohernia), can be very difficult and muscle-flap double breasting with mesh reinforcement may be required.

Parastomal hernia

When surgeons create a stoma, such as a colostomy or ileostomy, they are effectively creating a hernia by bringing bowel out through the abdominal wall. The muscle defect created tends to increase in size over time and can ultimately lead to massive herniation around the stoma. The rate of parastomal hernia is over 50%. For patients, it is very difficult to manage a stoma that is lying adjacent to or atop a large hernia. Stoma appliance bags fit poorly leading to leakage.

The ideal surgical solution for the patient is to rejoin the bowel and remove the stoma altogether, but this is not always possible. The stoma may be re-sited but further recurrence is likely. Various open suture and mesh techniques have been described to repair parastomal hernia but failure rates are high. Meshes are best placed in the retromuscular space. Laparoscopic repair is also possible using a large mesh with a central hole. It can be positioned around the bowel onto the parietal peritoneum.

Recent reports (Millbourne *et al.*) have described the use of prophylactic mesh insertion at the time of formation of the stoma. A lightweight, polypropylene mesh is inserted in the retromuscular space so that the bowel passes through a hole in the mesh centre. Using this technique, parastomal hernia rates have been reduced significantly.

Traumatic hernia

These hernias arise through non-anatomical defects caused by injury. They can be classified into three types:

1. Hernias through abdominal stab wound sites. These are effectively incisional hernias.
2. Hernias protruding through splits or tears in the abdominal muscles after blunt trauma.
3. Abdominal bulging secondary to muscle atrophy that occurs as a result of nerve injury or other traumatic denervation. Akin to the lumbar pseudo-hernia seen after open nephrectomy, these can arise after a chest injury with damage to the intercostal nerves.

Clinical features

Traumatic hernias present as any other hernia. The key to the aetiology is in the history and the non-anatomical location of the hernia.

Treatment

Surgery may be justified if the hernia is sufficiently symptomatic, or if investigations suggest a narrow neck and hence a risk of obstruction or strangulation. Stab wound traumatic hernias are straightforward to repair using open or laparoscopic techniques as for other ventral hernias. Diffuse abdominal bulges are more difficult to correct and require some form of plication of the stretched musculofascial layer with mesh reinforcement to prevent further bulging in the future. Some bulging may persist, however.

Rare external hernias

Perineal hernia

This type of hernia is very rare and includes:

- postoperative hernia through a perineal scar, which may occur after excision of the rectum;
- median sliding perineal hernia, which is a complete prolapse of the rectum;
- anterolateral perineal hernia, which occurs in women and presents as a swelling of the labium majus;
- posterolateral perineal hernia, which passes through the levator ani to enter the ischiorectal fossa.

TREATMENT

A combined abdominoperineal operation is generally the most satisfactory for the last two types of hernia. The hernia is exposed by an incision directly over it. The sac is opened and its contents are reduced. The sac is cleared from surrounding structures and the wound closed. With the patient in semi-Trendelenburg position, either laparoscopically or at open surgery, the abdomen is opened and the mouth of the sac exposed. The sac is inverted, ligated and excised, and the pelvic floor repaired by muscle apposition and, if indicated, buttressing of the repair with prosthetic mesh.

Obturator hernia

Obturator hernia, which passes through the obturator canal, occurs six times more frequently in women than in men. Most patients are aged >60 years. The swelling is liable to be overlooked because it is covered by pectineus. It seldom causes a definite swelling in Scarpa's triangle, but, if the limb is flexed, abducted and rotated outwards, the hernia sometimes becomes apparent. The leg is usually kept in a semi-flexed position and movement increases the pain. In more than 50% of cases of strangulated obturator hernia, pain is referred along the obturator nerve by its geniculate branch to the knee. On vaginal or rectal examination the hernia can sometimes be felt as a tender swelling in the region of the obturator foramen.

These hernias have often undergone strangulation, frequently of the Richter type, by the time of presentation.

TREATMENT

Surgery is indicated. The diagnosis is rarely made preoperatively and so it is often approached through a laparotomy incision. The full Trendelenburg position is adopted. The constricting agent is the obturator fascia, which can be stretched by inserting the operator's index finger, or suitable forceps, through the gap in the fascia. Content is reduced. If incision

Antonio Scarpa, 1747–1832, Professor of Anatomy, Pavia, Italy.

of the fascia is required, it is made parallel to the obturator vessels and nerve. The contents of the sac are dealt with in a standard manner. The defect cannot simply be closed because one margin is bone and the obturator nerve and vessels run through it. It is best closed using a mesh plug. In the absence of mesh or in an infected field, the broad ligament can be used as a plug.

Laparoscopic TAPP repair may also be performed again using a mesh. To avoid nerve injury, glue can be used to fix a mesh over the defect.

Gluteal and sciatic hernias

Both of these hernias are very rare. A gluteal hernia passes through the greater sciatic foramen, either above or below piriformis. A sciatic hernia passes through the lesser sciatic foramen. Differential diagnosis must be made between these conditions and:

- a lipoma or other soft tissue tumour beneath gluteus maximus;
- a tuberculous abscess;
- a gluteal aneurysm.

All doubtful swellings in this situation can be characterised with CT scanning but, if in doubt, they should be explored by operation.

UMBILICAL CONDITIONS IN THE ADULT

Chronic infection

Chronic infection occurs in the umbilical area, particularly in patients with poor hygiene. It may also occur in obese people and when a paraumbilical hernia is present. It can be due to a plug of keratin causing chronic irritation. It is often encountered during elective surgery and may complicate the insertion of a laparoscope port at the umbilicus. A range of bacteria and fungi can be involved. Occasionally, a rapid-onset, superficial cellulitis occurs even after minor surgery in this region. It is normally a streptococcus and can be treated with penicillin or other appropriate antibiotic. Pre-existing infection should be treated before surgery where possible.

Chronic fistula

Patients may present with a persistent discharge from the umbilical area. This may be due to simple, superficial infection or possibly an infected epidermoid cyst within the umbilicus. However, it may also be due to a fistulous connection to deeper structures.

In normal patients, the umbilicus is connected to the liver, bladder and gynaecological organs by various ligaments. Diseases of these organs, such as infection or malignancy, can extend along these ligaments to appear at the umbilicus as a mass or fistulous discharge.

Chronic fistula may be a complication of umbilical hernia repair due to chronic infection of a mesh or around non-absorbable suture material. In most cases this problem arises soon after surgery but occasionally a chronic infection can occur months or even years after an operation. Antibiotics may help but most commonly the synthetic suture or mesh will need to be removed with a risk of recurrence of the hernia.

In fetal life the umbilicus was also connected to the gut by the vitellointestinal duct. In most patients this duct becomes totally obliterated and vanishes. The bowel end of the duct may persist as Meckel's diverticulum. More rarely, the umbilical end persists, leading to chronic discharge. If an abnormal connection between bowel and umbilicus persists, then this band can act as a cause of adhesional intestinal obstruction.

Patent urachus

A connection between the urinary bladder and umbilicus usually presents in later life. This is due to increased pressure in the bladder as a result of obstruction from conditions such as prostatic hypertrophy. The cause of obstruction should be dealt with initially, but if the problem persists then surgical excision of the patent urachus might be considered.

Malignancy at the umbilicus

Primary squamous carcinoma may occur. If tumour presents at the umbilicus it is most probably due to spread from the internal organs along internal ligaments, e.g. from the liver along the falciform ligament. A malignant mass at the umbilicus is called a Sister Joseph's nodule. It usually indicates very advanced malignant disease and surgery probably has little to offer (Figure 60.30).

GENERAL INFECTION OF THE ABDOMINAL WALL

The skin of the abdominal wall, similar to all skin, is prone to develop superficial infection that may be spontaneous, due to minor trauma or infection of skin lesions such as an epidermoid cyst. Although antibiotics will suffice in most

Johann Frederick Meckel (the Younger), 1781–1833, Professor of Anatomy and Surgery, Halle, Germany, described his diverticulum in 1809.
Alexis Littre, 1658–1726, surgeon and lecturer in anatomy, Paris, France, described Meckel's diverticulum in a hernial sac in 1700, 81 years before Meckel was born.
The neoplastic nodule sited at the umbilicus is known as Sister Joseph's nodule. Sister Mary Joseph made the observation that her patients with terminal cancer sometimes developed a red papular lesion in the umbilicus. She and William Mayo published this observation in 1928. However, it was Hamilton Bailey who coined the term 'Sister Mary Joseph's nodule' in 1949.
Sister Mary Joseph (nee Julia Dempsey), Nursing Superintendent, St Mary's Hospital, which became the Mayo Clinic, Rochester, MN, USA.

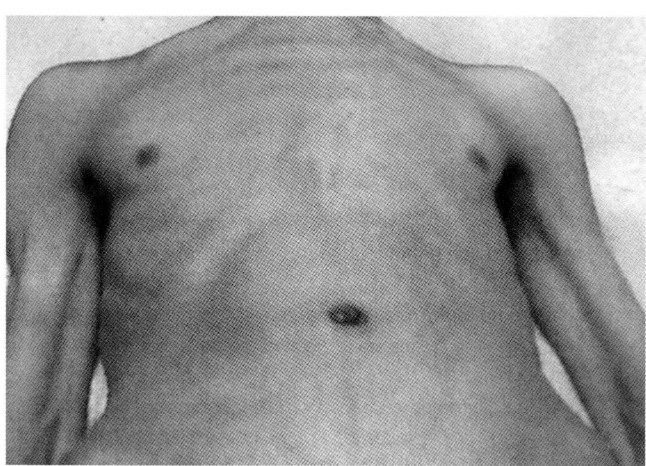

Figure 60.30 Secondary nodule at the umbilicus – Sister Joseph's nodule.

patients, if an abscess develops then surgical drainage may be required.

The close proximity of bowel and bowel organisms opens the abdominal wall to attack from a wide range of highly virulent bacteria. Most commonly, these are released during abdominal surgery such as appendicectomy and hence the need for appropriate antibiotic prophylactic cover.

Synergistic gangrene

This rare condition is due to the synergistic action of non-haemolytic streptococci and staphylococci causing rapid tissue necrosis and overwhelming systemic infection (Figure 60.31). It requires immediate administration of high-dose, broad-spectrum, powerful antibiotics in combination with early debridement of any non-viable tissue. Hyperbaric oxygen therapy has been advocated.

Other forms of severe abdominal wall infections occur, generally known as necrotising fasciitis (e.g. Fournier's gangrene). All of these conditions have a high associated morbidity and mortality. They occur in debilitated and immunocompromised patients but can occasionally occur in healthy patients. Rapid diagnosis and aggressive surgical debridement treatment are the key to success.

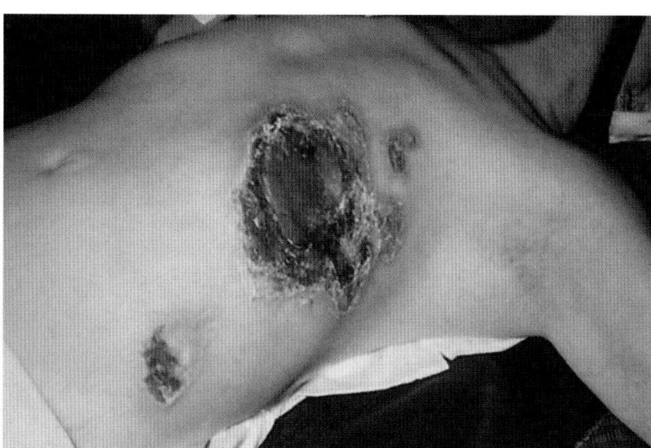

Figure 60.31 Bacterial synergistic gangrene of the chest and abdominal wall. The area has become gangrenous and looks like suede leather. Beware of amoebiasis cutis.

Cutaneous fistula

Due to the thickness of the abdominal wall, it is rare for abdominal inflammatory conditions to discharge spontaneously through the wall to the skin. Chronic intraperitoneal abscesses arising after occult bowel perforation, appendicitis, diverticulitis and cholecystitis are the most likely sources. CT will locate the internal abscess and suggest the likely origin. Treatment today is usually by CT- or ultrasound-guided drainage but the surgeon may be called on to remove the source organ, e.g. gall bladder.

Malignancy in its later stages can occasionally erode through the abdominal wall.

Crohn's disease also has a tendency to fistulate into adjacent organs and may develop an enterocutaneous fistula.

Abdominal compartment syndrome

Surgeons are increasingly aware of the harmful effect of high intra-abdominal pressures that can occur in severe intra-abdominal sepsis, such as pancreatitis and also aortic aneurysm rupture. High pressure leads to reduced blood flow and tissue ischaemia, which contributes to multiorgan failure. Although the abdominal wall has elasticity, if intra-abdominal volume increases due to fluid, gas, pus, tissue oedema, etc., then maximal capacity may be reached and pressure rises to a critical level. Tension-releasing incisions, equivalent to a fasciotomy, have been suggested, although this is not widely practised.

In some cases, after surgery for severe intraperitoneal sepsis, the surgeon cannot close the abdomen and may leave the incision wide open, covering abdominal contents with mesh or a saline-soaked dressing, planning to return at a future date to close the defect. This is called a laparostomy.

Neoplasms of the abdominal wall

As the abdominal wall is composed of muscle, fascia and bone, benign and malignant tumours can arise from each, although these are rare.

Desmoid tumour

This is usually considered by pathologists to be a hamartoma and is more common in women. Some, however, believe it to be a fibroma and possibly the result of repeated trauma. Desmoids have been reported in familial adenomatous polyposis (FAP). Histologically, they contain plasmoidal cell masses resembling giant cells. They undergo central myxomatous change. Surgical excision with a wide margin is required to prevent recurrence, which is a frequent problem.

Fibrosarcoma

These tumours can occur anywhere in the body. They are generally highly malignant and respond poorly to both radio- and chemotherapy. Wide excision will often require plastic surgical reconstruction.

FURTHER READING

Flum DR, Horvath K, Koepsell T. Have outcomes of incisional hernia repair improved with time? A population-based study. *Ann Surg* 2003; **237**: 129–35.

Kingsnorth AN, LeBlanc KA. *Management of abdominal hernias*, 4th edn. London: Edward Arnold, 2013.

Millbourn D, Cengiz Y, Israelsson LA. Effect of stitch length on wound complications after closure of midline incisions. *Arch Surg* 2009; **144**: 1056–9.

WEBSITE ADDRESSES

Classification of groin hernia: www.herniaweb.org/documents/EHS_groin_hernia_classification.pdf

Guidelines for management of groin hernia: www.herniaweb.org/documents/EHS_Guidelines.pdf

European classification of primary and incisional abdominal wall hernias: www.ncbi.nlm.nih.gov/pmc/articles/PMC2719726/

NICE guidelines for laparoscopic inguinal hernia repair: guidance.nice.org.uk/TA83

SIGN guidelines for antibiotics in surgery (including hernia): www.sign.ac.uk/pdf/sign104.pdf

Chapter 61

The peritoneum, omentum, mesentery and retroperitoneal space

Learning objectives

To recognise and understand:

- The causes and complications of localised and generalised peritonitis
- The clinical features of peritonitis and intraperitoneal abscess
- The principles of surgical management in patients with peritonitis and intraperitoneal abscess
- The causes and pathophysiology of ascites
- The pathophysiology and complications of adhesion formation
- The spectrum of mesenteric and retroperitoneal conditions

ANATOMY AND PHYSIOLOGY

Embryology

The peritoneal cavity, mesenteries and omentum have an anatomical complexity that can perhaps be truly understood only with surgical experience. Nevertheless, an understanding of the geometric alterations occurring during early gastrointestinal (GI) morphogenesis (regionalisation, elongation and coiling) of the derivatives of the endoderm (E = epithelium) and the visceral mesoderm (M = muscle and most of the rest) along with the later fusion of adjacent layers of peritoneum will give an appreciation of how the adult disposition is as it is.

Adult arrangement and functions

The peritoneal cavity is the largest cavity in the body, the surface area of its lining membrane ($2\,m^2$ in an adult) being nearly equal to that of the skin. The peritoneal membrane is composed of flattened polyhedral cells (mesothelium), one layer thick, resting on a thin layer of fibroelastic tissue. This membrane is conveniently divided into two parts – the visceral peritoneum surrounding the viscera and the parietal peritoneum lining the other surfaces of the cavity. Beneath the peritoneum, supported by a small amount of areolar tissue, lies a network of lymphatic vessels and rich plexus of capillary blood vessels from which all absorption and exudation must occur. In health, only a few millilitres of peritoneal fluid are found in the peritoneal cavity. The fluid is pale yellow, somewhat viscid, and contains lymphocytes and other leukocytes; it lubricates the viscera, allowing easy movement and peristalsis. The parietal portion is richly supplied with nerves and, when irritated, causes severe pain that is accurately localised to the affected area. The visceral peritoneum, in contrast, is poorly supplied with nerves (these being situated around blood vessels) and its irritation causes pain that is usually poorly localised to the midline.

The peritoneum has a number of functions.

Summary box 61.1

Functions of the peritoneum

In health

- Visceral lubrication
- Fluid and particulate absorption

In disease

- Pain perception (mainly parietal)
- Inflammatory and immune responses
- Fibrinolytic activity

The peritoneum has the capacity to absorb large volumes of fluid: this ability is used during peritoneal dialysis in the treatment of renal failure. However, the peritoneum can also produce large volumes of fluid (ascites) and an inflammatory exudate when injured (peritonitis). During expiration, intra-abdominal pressure is reduced and peritoneal fluid, aided by capillary attraction, travels in an upward direction towards the diaphragm. Experimental evidence shows that particulate matter and bacteria are absorbed within a few minutes into the lymphatic network through a number of 'pores' within the diaphragmatic peritoneum. The circulation of peritoneal fluids may be responsible for the occurrence of abscesses distant from primary disease. When parietal peritoneal defects are created, healing occurs not from the edges but by the development of new mesothelial cells throughout the surface of the defect. In this way, large defects heal as rapidly as small defects.

SCOPE OF DISEASE

The peritoneum, mesentery and omentum may be the site of a variety of conditions that reflect their relationship to other anatomical structures or, in some instances, their primary functions.

Summary box 61.2

Scope of disease

Intraperitoneal disease
- Peritonitis
  - Primary
  - Secondary
- Abscess
- Ascites
  - Transudate
  - Exudate
- Tumours
  - Primary
  - Secondary
- Adhesions

Omental disease
- Hernia
- Adhesions
- Torsion
- Neoplasia

Mesenteric disease
- Trauma
- Ischaemia
- Inflammation
- Cysts
- Neoplasia

Retroperitoneal disease
- Chronic inflammation/fibrosis
- Abscess
- Tumours

PERITONITIS

Peritonitis is simply defined as inflammation of the peritoneum and may be localised or generalised. Most cases of peritonitis are caused by an invasion of the peritoneal cavity by bacteria, so that, when the term 'peritonitis' is used without qualification, acute bacterial peritonitis is often implied. In this instance, free fluid spills into the peritoneal cavity and circulates, largely directed by the normal peritoneal attachments and gravity. For example, spillage from a perforated peptic ulcer may run down the right paracolic gutter, leading to presentation with pain in the right iliac fossa (Valentino's syndrome). Even in patients with non-bacterial peritonitis (e.g. acute pancreatitis, intraperitoneal rupture of the bladder or haemoperitoneum), the peritoneum often becomes infected by transmural spread of organisms from the bowel. Such translocation is a feature of the systemic inflammatory response on the bowel and it is not long (often a matter of hours) before a bacterial peritonitis develops. Most duodenal and gastric perforations are initially sterile for up to several hours before becoming secondarily infected.

Summary box 61.3

Causes of peritoneal inflammation
- Bacterial, gastrointestinal and non-gastrointestinal
- Chemical, e.g. bile, barium
- Allergic, e.g. starch peritonitis
- Traumatic, e.g. operative handling
- Ischaemia, e.g. strangulated bowel, vascular occlusion
- Miscellaneous, e.g. familial Mediterranean fever

Although acute bacterial peritonitis most commonly arises from a perforation of a viscus of the alimentary tract, other routes of infection can include the female genital tract and exogenous contamination. There are also less common forms in which the aetiology is a primary 'spontaneous' peritonitis, in which a pure infection with streptococcal, pneumococcal or haemophilus bacteria occurs.

Summary box 61.4

Paths to peritoneal infection
- Gastrointestinal perforation, e.g. perforated ulcer, appendix, diverticulum
- Transmural translocation (no perforation), e.g. pancreatitis, ischaemic bowel, **primary bacterial peritonitis**
- Exogenous contamination, e.g. drains, open surgery, trauma, **peritoneal dialysis**
- Female genital tract infection, e.g. pelvic inflammatory disease
- Haematogenous spread (rare), e.g. septicaemia

Microbiology

Bacteria from the gastrointestinal tract

The number of bacteria within the lumen of the gastrointestinal tract is normally low until the distal small bowel is reached. However, disease leading to stasis and overgrowth (e.g. obstruction, and chronic and acute motility disturbances) may increase proximal colonisation. The biliary

Rudolph Valentino, Italian actor, died during surgery for this in New York in 1926, aged 31 years.

and pancreatic tracts are also normally free from bacteria, although they may be infected in disease, e.g. gallstones. Peritoneal infection is usually caused by two or more bacterial strains. Gram-negative bacteria contain endotoxins (lipopolysaccharides) in their cell walls that have multiple toxic effects on the host, primarily by causing the release of tumour necrosis factor (TNF) from host leukocytes. Systemic absorption of endotoxin may produce endotoxic shock, with hypotension and impaired tissue perfusion. Other bacteria such as *Clostridium perfringens* produce harmful exotoxins. *Bacteroides* spp. are commonly found in peritonitis. These gram-negative, non-sporing organisms, although predominant in the lower intestine, often escape detection because they are strictly anaerobic and slow to grow on culture media unless there is an adequate carbon dioxide tension in the anaerobic apparatus (Gillespie). In many laboratories, the culture is discarded if there is no growth in 48 hours. These organisms are resistant to penicillin and streptomycin but sensitive to metronidazole, clindamycin, Augmentin (amoxicillin plus clavulanic acid) and cephalosporin compounds. Since the widespread use of metronidazole (Flagyl), bacteroides infections have greatly diminished.

Non-gastrointestinal causes of peritonitis

Pelvic infection via the fallopian tubes is responsible for a high proportion of 'non-gastrointestinal' infections. The most common offending organisms are *Chlamydia* spp. and gonococci. These organisms lead to a thinning of cervical mucus and allow bacteria from the vagina into the uterus and oviducts, causing infection and inflammation. A variant of transperitoneal spread of such organisms is perihepatitis which can cause scar tissue to form on Glisson's capsule, a thin layer of connective tissue surrounding the liver (Fitz-Hugh–Curtis syndrome). Other bacterial variants that are discussed separately include tuberculosis and other mycobacterial strains and those causing primary peritonitis (pneumococci, staphylococci and streptoccoci). Fungal peritonitis is uncommon but may complicate severely ill patients.

Summary box 61.5

Microorganisms in peritonitis

Gastrointestinal source

- *Escherichia coli*
- Streptococci
- Enterococci
- *Bacteroides* spp.
- *Clostridium* spp.
- *Klebsiella pneumoniae*

Other sources

- *Chlamydia trachomatis*
- *Neisseria gonorrhoeae*
- Haemolytic streptococci
- Staphylococci
- *Streptococcus pneumoniae*
- *Mycobacterium tuberculosis* and other species
- Fungal infections

Localised peritonitis

Anatomical and pathological factors may favour the localisation of peritonitis.

Anatomical

The greater sac of the peritoneum is divided into (1) the subphrenic spaces, (2) the pelvis and (3) the peritoneal cavity proper. The last is divided into a supracolic and an infracolic compartment by the transverse colon and transverse mesocolon, which deters the spread of infection from one to the other. When the supracolic compartment overflows, as is often the case when a peptic ulcer perforates, it does so over the colon into the infracolic compartment or by way of the right paracolic gutter to the right iliac fossa and hence to the pelvis.

Pathological

The clinical course is determined in part by the manner in which adhesions form around the affected organ. Inflamed peritoneum loses its glistening appearance and becomes reddened and velvety. Flakes of fibrin appear and cause loops of intestine to become adherent to each other and to the parietes. There is an outpouring of serous inflammatory exudate rich in leukocytes and plasma proteins that soon becomes turbid; if localisation occurs, the turbid fluid becomes frank pus. Peristalsis is retarded in affected bowel and this helps to prevent distribution of the infection. The greater omentum, by enveloping and becoming adherent to inflamed structures, often forms a substantial barrier to the spread of infection (see below).

Diffuse (generalised) peritonitis

A number of factors may favour the development of diffuse peritonitis:

- Speed of peritoneal contamination is a prime factor. If an inflamed appendix or other hollow viscus perforates before localisation has taken place, there will be an efflux of contents into the peritoneal cavity, which may spread over a large area almost instantaneously. Perforation proximal to an obstruction or from sudden anastomotic separation is associated with severe generalised peritonitis and a high mortality rate.
- Stimulation of peristalsis by the ingestion of food or even water hinders localisation. Violent peristalsis occasioned by the administration of a purgative or an enema may cause the widespread distribution of an infection that would otherwise have remained localised.
- The virulence of the infecting organism may be so great as to render the localisation of infection difficult or impossible.

William Alexander Gillespie, formerly Professor of Clinical Bacteriology, University of Bristol, Bristol, UK.
Named after the two physicians, Thomas Fitz-Hugh, Jr and Arthur Hale Curtis who first reported this condition in 1934 and 1930, respectively.

- Young children have a small omentum, which is less effective in localising infection.
- Disruption of localised collections may occur with injudicious handling, e.g. appendix mass or pericolic abscess.
- Deficient natural resistance ('immune deficiency') may result from use of drugs (e.g. steroids), disease [e.g. acquired immune deficiency syndrome (AIDS)] or old age.

With appropriate treatment, localised peritonitis usually resolves; in about 20% of cases, an abscess follows. Infrequently, localised peritonitis becomes diffuse. Conversely, in favourable circumstances, diffuse peritonitis can become localised, most frequently in the pelvis or at multiple sites within the abdominal cavity.

Clinical features

Localised peritonitis

The initial symptoms and signs of localised peritonitis are those of the underlying condition – usually visceral inflammation (hence abdominal pain, specific GI symptoms + malaise, anorexia and nausea). When the peritoneum becomes inflamed, abdominal pain will worsen and in general temperature and pulse rate will rise. The pathognomonic signs are localised guarding (involuntary abdominal wall contraction to protect the viscus from the examining hand), a positive 'release' sign (rebound tenderness) and sometimes rigidity (involuntary constant contraction of the abdominal wall over the inflamed parietes). If inflammation arises under the diaphragm, shoulder-tip ('phrenic') pain may be felt as the pain is referred to the C5 dermatome. In cases of pelvic peritonitis arising from an inflamed appendix in the pelvic position or from salpingitis, the abdominal signs are often slight; there may be deep tenderness of one or both lower quadrants alone, but a rectal or vaginal examination reveals marked tenderness of the pelvic peritoneum.

Diffuse (generalised) peritonitis

EARLY

Abdominal pain is severe and made worse by moving or breathing. It is first experienced at the site of the original lesion and spreads outwards from this point. The patient usually lies still. Tenderness and generalised guarding are found on palpation, when the peritonitis affects the anterior abdominal wall. Infrequent bowel sounds may still be heard for a few hours but they cease with the onset of paralytic ileus. Pulse and temperature rise in accord with degree of inflammation and infection.

LATE

If resolution or localisation of generalised peritonitis does not occur, the abdomen will become rigid (generalised rigidity). Distension is common and bowel sounds are absent. Circulatory failure ensues, with cold, clammy extremities, sunken eyes, dry tongue, thready (irregular) pulse, and drawn and anxious face (hippocratic facies – Figure 61.1). The patient finally lapses into unconsciousness. With early diagnosis and adequate treatment, this condition is rarely seen in modern surgical practice.

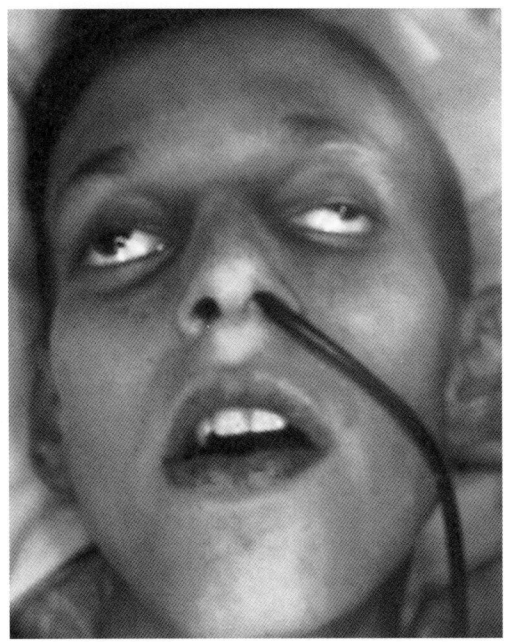

Figure 61.1 The hippocratic facies in terminal diffuse peritonitis.

Summary box 61.6

Clinical features of peritonitis

- Abdominal pain, worse on movement, coughing and deep respiration
- Constitutional upset: anorexia, malaise, fever, lassitude
- GI upset: nausea ± vomiting
- Pyrexia (may be absent)
- Raised pulse rate
- Tenderness ± guarding/rigidity/rebound of abdominal wall
- Pain/tenderness on rectal/vaginal examination (pelvic peritonitis)
- Absent or reduced bowel sounds
- 'Septic shock' (systemic inflammatory response syndrome [SIRS] and multi-organ dysfunction syndrome [MODS]) in later stages

Diagnostic aids

Investigations may elucidate a doubtful diagnosis, but the importance of a careful history and repeated examination must not be forgotten.

Bedside

- Urine dipstix for urinary tract infection.
- ECG if diagnostic doubt (as to cause of abdominal pain) or cardiac history.

Hippocrates of Kos, Greek physician and surgeon, and by common consent 'the father of medicine', was born on the island of Kos, off Turkey, about 460BC and probably died in 375BC.

Bloods

- Baseline urea and electrolytes (U&Es) for treatment.
- Full blood count for white cell count (WCC).
- Serum amylase estimation may establish the diagnosis of acute pancreatitis provided that it is remembered that moderately raised values are frequently found following other abdominal catastrophes and operations, e.g. perforated duodenal ulcer.
- Group and save may be taken as an adjunct to impending surgery.

Imaging

- Erect chest radiograph to demonstrate free subdiaphragmatic gas (Figure 61.2a).
- A supine radiograph of the abdomen may confirm the presence of dilated gas-filled loops of bowel (consistent with a paralytic ileus), and occasionally show other gas-filled structures that may aid diagnosis, e.g. biliary tree; the faecal pattern may act as a guide to colonic disease (absent in sites of significant inflammation, e.g. diverticulitis). In the patient who is too ill for an 'erect' film, a lateral decubitus film can show gas beneath the abdominal wall (if CT unavailable).
- Multiplanar computed tomography (CT) is increasingly used to identify the cause of peritonitis (Figures 61.2b and 61.3) and may also influence management decisions, e.g. surgical strategy. There is an abundance of recent published evidence to support its use in managing acute abdominal pain.
- Ultrasonography has undoubted value in certain situations such as pelvic peritonitis in women and localised right upper quadrant peritonism.

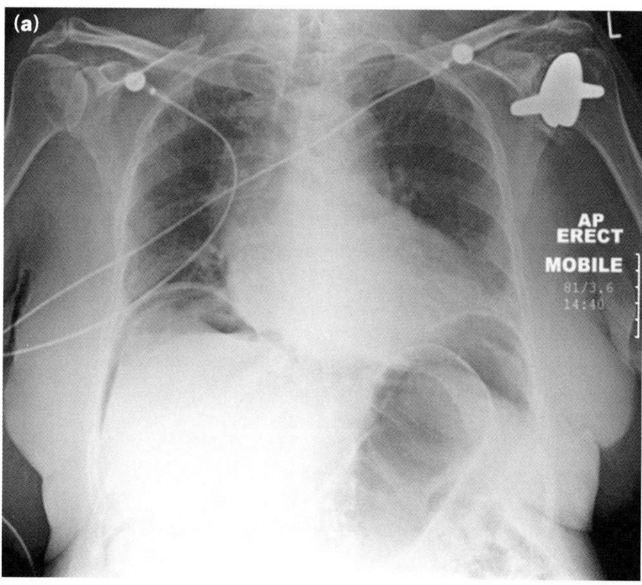

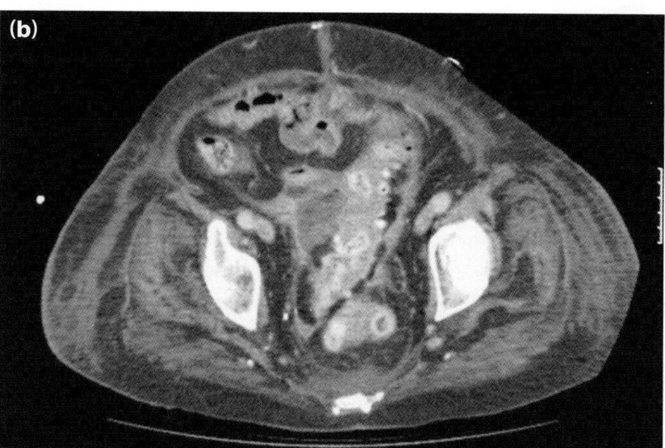

Figure 61.2 (a) Gas under the diaphragm in a patient with free perforation and peritonitis; (b) representative axial image through the pelvis of the same patient showing perforated sigmoid diverticular disease.

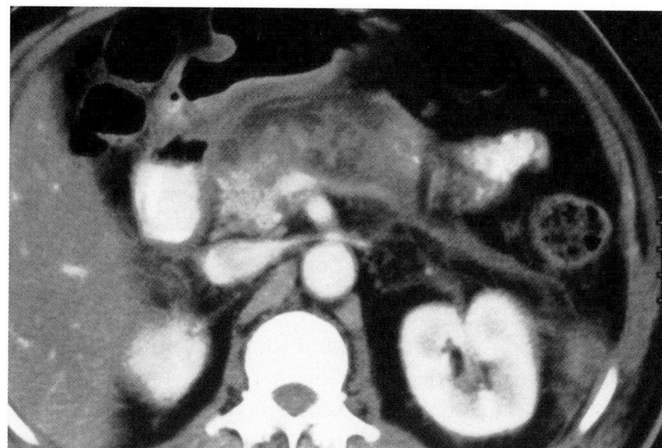

Figure 61.3 Acute pancreatitis seen on computed tomography scanning with swelling of the gland and surrounding inflammatory changes (courtesy of Dr J Healy, Chelsea and Westminster Hospital, London, UK).

Invasive

- In the era of access to high-quality CT scanning, peritoneal diagnostic aspiration has little residual value.

Management

General care of the patient

The care of critically ill surgical patients is described in detail in Chapters 2, 17 and 20. Nutritional support is covered in Chapter 19, and anaesthesia and pain relief in Chapter 18. Depending on degree (localised/generalised), duration and severity, patients will require some or all of the following.

CORRECTION OF FLUID LOSS AND CIRCULATING VOLUME

Patients are frequently hypovolaemic with electrolyte disturbances. The plasma volume must be restored and electrolyte concentrations corrected. Fluid balance should be monitored and pre-existent and ongoing losses corrected. Special measures may be needed for cardiac, pulmonary and renal support, especially if septic shock is present (see Chapter 2), including central venous pressure monitoring in patients with concurrent disease.

URINARY CATHETERISATION ± GASTROINTESTINAL DECOMPRESSION

A urinary catheter will give a guide to central perfusion and will be required if abdominal surgery is to proceed. A nasogastric tube is commonly passed to allow drainage ± aspiration until paralytic ileus has resolved.

ANTIBIOTIC THERAPY

Administration of parenteral broad-spectrum (aerobic and anaerobic) antibiotics prevents the multiplication of bacteria and the release of endotoxins.

ANALGESIA

The patient should be nursed in the sitting-up position and must be relieved of pain before and after the operation. If appropriate expertise is available, epidural infusion may provide excellent analgesia. Freedom from pain allows early mobilisation and adequate physiotherapy in the postoperative period, which helps to prevent basal pulmonary collapse, deep vein thrombosis and pulmonary embolism.

Specific treatment of the cause

Although difficult to generalise, in patients in whom specific treatment has not been guided by CT scanning, early surgical intervention is to be preferred to a 'wait and see' policy, assuming that the patient is fit for anaesthesia and that resuscitation has resulted in a satisfactory restitution of normal body physiology. This rule is particularly true for previously healthy patients and those with postoperative peritonitis. More caution is of course required in patients at high operative risk because of comorbidity or advanced age.

In those patients with a preoperative diagnosis, if the cause of peritonitis is amenable to surgery, an operation must be carried out as soon as the patient is fit. This is usually within a few hours. In peritonitis caused by pancreatitis or salpingitis, or in cases of primary peritonitis of streptococcal or pneumococcal origin, non-surgical treatment is preferred, provided that the diagnosis can be made with confidence. It is beyond the remit of this chapter to cover specific causes of peritonitis and their treatment, be it by an open or a laparoscopic approach. However, in general, surgery is directed to removing (or diverting) the cause and subsequent adequate peritoneal lavage ± drainage. In operations for generalised peritonitis it is essential that, after the cause has been dealt with, the whole peritoneal cavity be explored with the sucker and, if necessary, mopped dry until all seropurulent exudate has been removed. The use of a large volume of saline (typically 3 litres) containing dissolved antiseptic or antibiotic has been shown to be effective.

Summary box 61.7

Management of peritonitis

General care of patient

- Correction of fluid and electrolyte imbalance
- Insertion of nasogastric drainage tube and urinary catheter
- Broad-spectrum antibiotic therapy
- Analgesia
- Vital system support

Surgical treatment of cause when appropriate

- Remove or divert cause
- Peritoneal lavage ± drainage

Prognosis and complications

With modern treatment, diffuse peritonitis carries a mortality rate of about 10%, reflecting the degree and duration of peritoneal contamination, age and fitness of the patient, and the nature of the underlying cause. Paralytic ileus is covered in detail in Chapter 71, and abscess formation and adhesions are covered below.

Summary box 61.8

Systemic complications of peritonitis

- Septic shock
- Systemic inflammatory response syndrome
- Multi-organ dysfunction syndrome
- Death

Abdominal complications of peritonitis

- Paralytic ileus
- Residual or recurrent abscess/inflammatory mass
- Portal pyaemia/liver abscess
- Adhesional small bowel obstruction

SPECIAL FORMS OF PERITONITIS

Bile peritonitis

Unless there is reason to suspect that the biliary tract was damaged during surgery or the patient has proven acute cholecystitis, it is improbable that bile will be thought of as a cause of peritonitis until the abdomen has been opened.

Unless the bile has extravasated slowly and the collection becomes shut off from the general peritoneal cavity, there are symptoms (often severe pain) and signs of diffuse peritonitis. After a few hours a tinge of jaundice is not unusual. Laparotomy (or laparoscopy) should be undertaken with evacuation of the bile and peritoneal lavage. The source of bile leakage should be identified and treated accordingly. Infected bile is more lethal than sterile bile. A 'blown' duodenal stump should be drained because it is too oedematous to repair, but sometimes it can be covered by a jejunal patch. The patient is often jaundiced from absorption of peritoneal bile, but the surgeon must ensure that the abdomen is not closed until any obstruction to a major bile duct has been either excluded or relieved. Bile leaks after cholecystectomy or liver trauma may be dealt with by percutaneous (ultrasound-guided) drainage and endoscopic biliary stenting to reduce bile duct pressure. The drain is removed when dry and the stent at 4–6 weeks.

Summary box 61.9

Causes of bile peritonitis

- Perforated gall bladder secondary to inflammation or obstruction (especially empyema)
- Post-cholecystectomy:
  - Cystic duct stump leakage
  - Leakage from an accessory duct in the gall-bladder bed
  - Bile duct injury
  - T-tube drain dislodgement (or tract rupture on removal)
- Following other operations/procedures:
  - Duodenal injury
  - Leaking duodenal stump post gastrectomy
  - Leaking biliary–enteric anastomosis
  - Leakage around percutaneously placed biliary drains
- Blunt or penetrating hepatobiliary or duodenal trauma

Spontaneous bacterial peritonitis

Spontaneous bacterial peritonitis (SBP; sometimes called primary bacterial peritonitis) is an acute bacterial infection of ascitic fluid. It can occur in children and adults and can in theory occur as a complication of any disease state that produces the clinical syndrome of ascites. In practice, it is rare except in patients with cirrhosis and ascites, affecting 1.5–3.5% of outpatients and approximately 10% of inpatients.

Clinical features usually include local symptoms and/or signs of peritonitis, GI upset (secondary to ileus, e.g. nausea and vomiting), signs of systemic inflammation (hyper- or hypothermia, chills, tachycardia and tachypnoea ± signs of septic shock), worsening liver and renal function, hepatic encephalopathy and GI bleeding. It should, however, be noted that evolving infection may be asymptomatic, especially in outpatients.

The diagnosis is made by paracentesis, and this should be considered in patients with cirrhosis and ascites even when there is a low index of suspicion. Some guidelines recommend diagnostic paracentesis in all patients with cirrhosis and ascites on hospital admission. The diagnosis is made by an increased neutrophil of 250/mm^3 as determined by counting centrifuged ascitic fluid. Ascites culture is negative in as many as 60% of patients with clinical manifestations of SBP and increased ascitic neutrophil count. When culture is positive (40% of cases), the most common pathogens include gram-negative bacteria, usually *E. coli*, and gram-positive cocci (mainly streptococci and enterococci).

Empirical treatment of SBP must be initiated immediately after diagnosis before the results of culture have been received. Although the choice of antibiotic may vary internationally, a third-generation cephalosporin, e.g. cefotaxime, is the best investigated, and it avoids the renal toxicity of aminoglycosides. Alternatives are amoxicillin/clavulanic acid and quinolones such as ciprofloxacin. Complications of SBP, e.g. septic shock, GI bleeding and hypoalbuminaemia, should be managed accordingly.

When first described, the mortality rate of SBP exceeded 90%, but it has been reduced to approximately 20% with early diagnosis and treatment.

Primary pneumococcal peritonitis

This may complicate nephrotic syndrome or cirrhosis in children. Otherwise healthy children, particularly girls aged between 3 and 9 years, may also be affected, and it is likely that the route of infection is sometimes via the vagina and fallopian tubes. At other times, and always in boys, the infection is blood borne and secondary to respiratory tract or middle-ear disease. The prevalence of pneumococcal peritonitis has declined greatly and the condition is now rare. In brief, the clinical onset is sudden, with pain usually localised to the lower half of the abdomen. The temperature is raised to 39°C or more and there is usually frequent vomiting. After 24–48 hours, profuse diarrhoea is characteristic. There is usually increased frequency of micturition. The last two symptoms are caused by severe pelvic peritonitis. On examination, peritonism is usually diffuse but less prominent than in most cases of a perforated viscus, leading to peritonitis.

A leukocytosis of ≥30 000/μL, with approximately 90% polymorphs, suggests pneumococcal peritonitis rather than another cause, e.g. appendicitis. After starting antibiotic therapy and correcting dehydration and electrolyte imbalance, early surgery is required unless spontaneous infection of pre-existing ascites is strongly suspected, in which case a diagnostic peritoneal tap is useful. Laparotomy or laparoscopy may be used. Should the exudate be odourless and sticky, the diagnosis of pneumococcal peritonitis is practically certain, but it is essential to perform a careful exploration to exclude other pathology. Assuming that no other cause for the peritonitis is discovered, some of the exudate is aspirated and sent to the laboratory for microscopy, culture and sensitivity tests. Thorough peritoneal lavage is carried out and the incision closed. Antibiotics and fluid replacement therapy are continued and recovery is usual.

Other organisms are now known to cause some cases of primary peritonitis in children, including *Haemophilus* spp., group A streptococci and a few gram-negative bacteria. Underlying pathology (including an intravaginal foreign body in girls) must always be excluded before primary peritonitis can be diagnosed with certainty. Idiopathic streptococcal and staphylococcal peritonitis can also occur in adults.

Tuberculous peritonitis

Intra-abdominal tuberculosis (TB) is very common in resource-poor countries where all general surgeons are familiar with its presentation and management. The incidence is, however, also rising in resource-rich countries as a consequence of migration and immunosuppression where *Mycobacterium avium-intracellulare* is becoming increasingly prevalent with the widespread increase in human immunodeficiency virus (HIV) co-infection. The abdomen is involved in 11% of patients with extrapulmonary TB and includes intraperitoneal, GI tract and solid organ disease forms, with TB peritonitis being a common site-specific variant (ileocaecal is the most common site of involvement). Although still uncommon, TB peritonitis requires some specific mention because it is often diagnosed late in the course of the disease, resulting in undue patient morbidity and mortality.

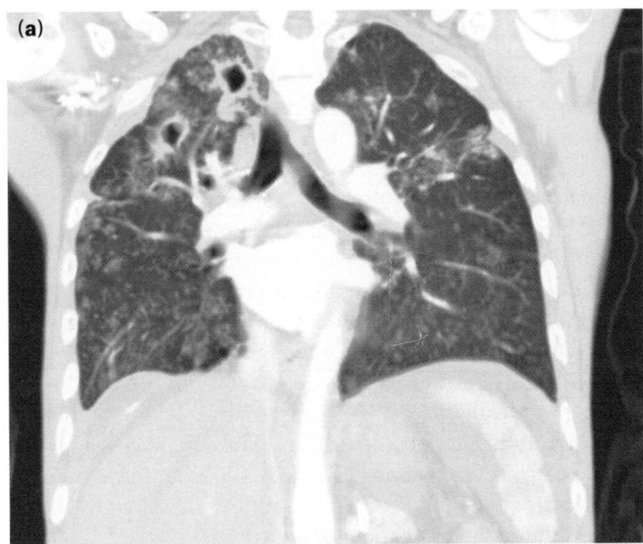

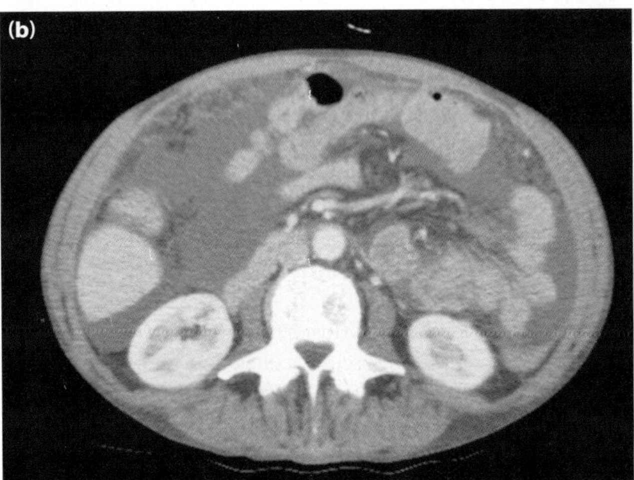

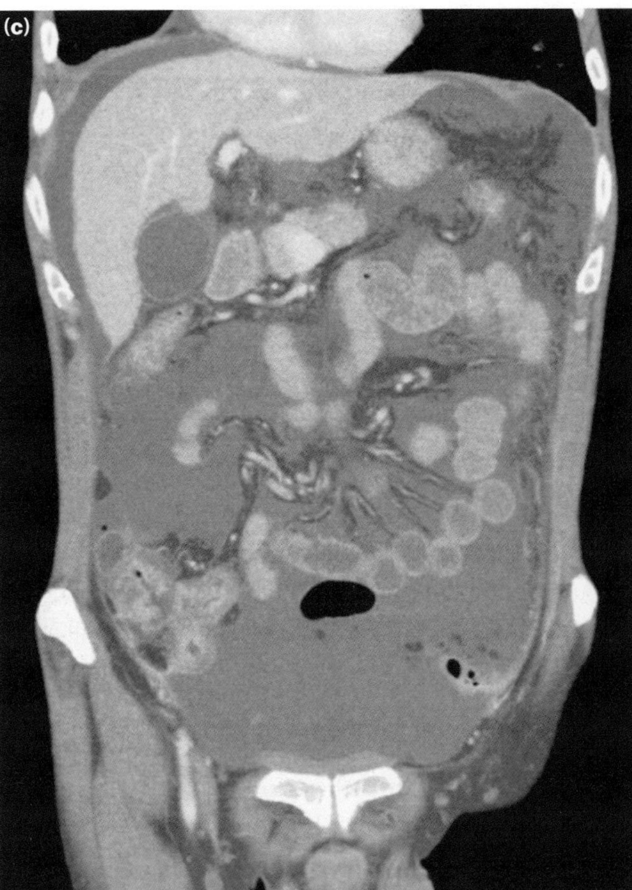

Figure 61.4 (a) Plain chest radiograph from a 55-year-old man showing miliary tuberculosis (TB); (b, c) representative computed tomography images from the same patient showing gross ascites, nodular stranding in the omentum and mesentery, as well as nodular enhancement of the peritoneum – TB peritonitis (courtesy of Dr S Burke, Homerton University Foundation Trust, London).

Tuberculosis can spread to the peritoneum through the GI tract (typically the ileocaecal region) via mesenteric lymph nodes or directly from the blood, usually from the 'miliary' (Figure 61.4a), but occasionally from the 'cavitating' form of pulmonary TB, lymph and the fallopian tubes; 50–83% of patients with abdominal TB can be expected to have peritoneal involvement. Clinical or subclinical ascites is reported in virtually all patients with TB peritonitis and is frequently a presenting feature. In the most common form of the disease, ascites may be localised or generalised throughout the peritoneal cavity. Multiple tubercle deposits appear on both layers of the peritoneum. Diagnosis is via abdominal ultrasonography or CT to detect ascites and lymphadenopathy ± diffuse thickening of the peritoneum, mesentery and/or omentum (Figure 61.4b, c). Ascitic fluid is typically a straw-coloured exudate (protein >25–30 g/L) with white cells >500 mm^3 and lymphocytes >40%. Unfortunately diagnostic smears for acid-fast bacilli are diagnostic in less than 3% of patients, and culture may take up to 4–8 weeks with no guarantee of a positive result. Laparoscopy and peritoneal biopsy may thus be helpful to couple typical appearances with histology. TB management is principally supportive (nutrition and hydration) and medical (systemic antituberculous therapy, noting that multiple-drug resistance may be higher for abdominal than for pulmonary TB), although surgery may be required for specific complications such as intestinal obstruction.

Summary box 61.10

Tuberculous peritonitis

- Acute (may be clinically indistinguishable from acute bacterial peritonitis) and chronic forms
- Abdominal pain, sweats, malaise and weight loss are frequent
- Ascites common, may be loculated
- Caseating peritoneal nodules are common – distinguish from metastatic carcinoma and fat necrosis of pancreatitis
- Intestinal obstruction may respond to anti-tuberculous treatment without surgery

Familial Mediterranean fever (periodic peritonitis)

Familial Mediterranean fever (periodic peritonitis) is characterised by abdominal pain and tenderness, mild pyrexia, polymorphonuclear leukocytosis and, occasionally, pain in the thorax and joints. The duration of an attack is 24–72 hours, when it is followed by complete remission, but exacerbations recur at regular intervals. Most of the patients have undergone appendicectomy in childhood. This disease, often familial, is limited principally to Arab, Armenian and Jewish populations; other races are occasionally affected. Mutations in the *MEFV* (Mediterranean fever) gene appear to cause the disease. This gene produces a protein called pyrin, which is expressed mostly in neutrophils; however, the exact function of pyrin is not known.

Usually, children are affected but it is not rare for the disease to make its first appearance in early adult life, with cases in women outnumbering those in men by two to one. Exceptionally, the disease becomes manifest in patients aged >40 years. At surgery, which may be necessary to exclude other causes (but should be avoided if possible), the peritoneum is inflamed, particularly in the vicinity of the spleen and the gall bladder. There is no evidence that the interior of these organs is abnormal. Colchicine therapy is used during attacks and to prevent recurrent attacks.

INTRAPERITONEAL ABSCESS

Following intraperitoneal sepsis (usually manifest first as local or diffuse peritonitis), the anatomy of the peritoneal cavity is such that with the influence of gravity (depending on patient position – sitting or supine), abscess development usually occupies one of a number of specific abdominal or pelvic sites.

In general, the symptoms and signs of a purulent collection may be vague and consist of nothing more than lassitude, anorexia and malaise, pyrexia (often low grade), mild tachycardia and localised tenderness. Certain sites have more specific clinical features. Larger abscesses will give rise to the picture of swinging pyrexia and pulse and a palpable mass. Blood tests will reveal elevated inflammatory markers.

Summary box 61.11

Clinical features of an abdominal/pelvic abscess

Symptoms

- Malaise, lethargy – failure to recover from surgery as expected
- Anorexia and weight loss
- Sweats ± rigors
- Abdominal/pelvic pain
- Symptoms from local irritation, e.g. shoulder tip/hiccoughs (subphrenic), diarrhoea and mucus (pelvic), nausea and vomiting (any upper abdominal)

Signs

- Increased temperature and pulse ± swinging pyrexia
- Localised abdominal tenderness ± mass (including on pelvic exam)

Pelvic abscess

The pelvis is the most common site of abscess formation because the vermiform appendix is often pelvic in position and the fallopian tubes are also frequent sites of infection. A pelvic abscess can also occur as a sequel to any case of diffuse peritonitis, and is common after anastomotic leakage following colorectal surgery.

Clinical features

The most characteristic symptoms are of pelvic pain, diarrhoea and the passage of mucus in the stools. Rectal examination reveals a bulging of the anterior rectal wall, which, when the abscess is ripe, becomes softly cystic.

Investigation and management

Left to nature, a proportion of these abscesses burst into the rectum, after which the patient almost always recovers rapidly. If this does not occur, the abscess should be drained deliberately. In women, vaginal drainage through the posterior fornix is often chosen. In other cases, when the abscess is definitely pointing into the rectum, rectal drainage (Figure 61.5) is employed. If any uncertainty exists, the presence of pus should be confirmed by ultrasonography or CT scanning (Figure 61.6). Laparotomy is almost never necessary and rectal drainage of a pelvic abscess is far preferable to suprapubic drainage, which risks exposing the general peritoneal cavity to infection. It is, however, increasingly common to insert drainage tubes percutaneously, e.g. via the buttock or via the vagina or rectum under CT guidance.

Abdominal abscess

Anatomy

The complicated arrangement of the peritoneum results in the formation of four intraperitoneal spaces in which pus may commonly collect (Figure 61.7).

LEFT SUBPHRENIC SPACE

This is bounded above by the diaphragm and behind by the left triangular ligament and the left lobe of the liver, the gastrohepatic omentum and the anterior surface of the stomach.

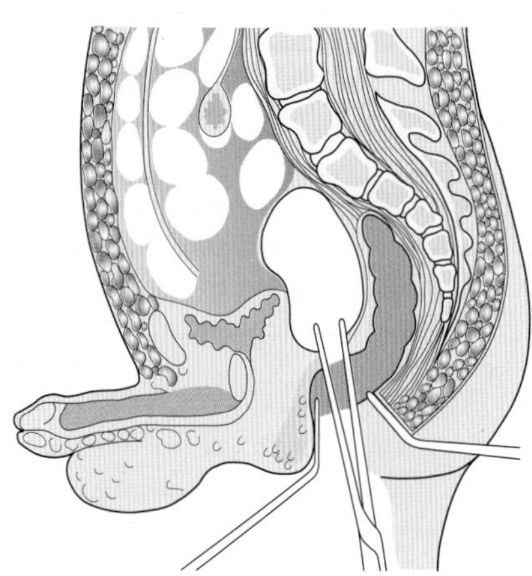

Figure 61.5 Opening a pelvic abscess into the rectum.

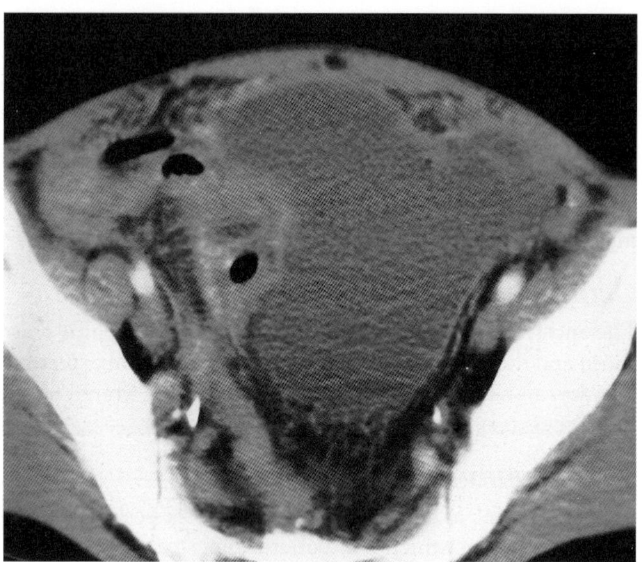

Figure 61.6 A pelvic abscess seen on CT scanning (courtesy of Dr J Healy, Chelsea and Westminster Hospital, London, UK).

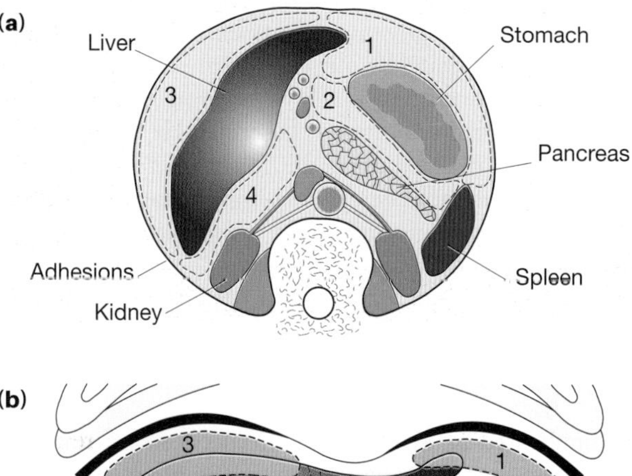

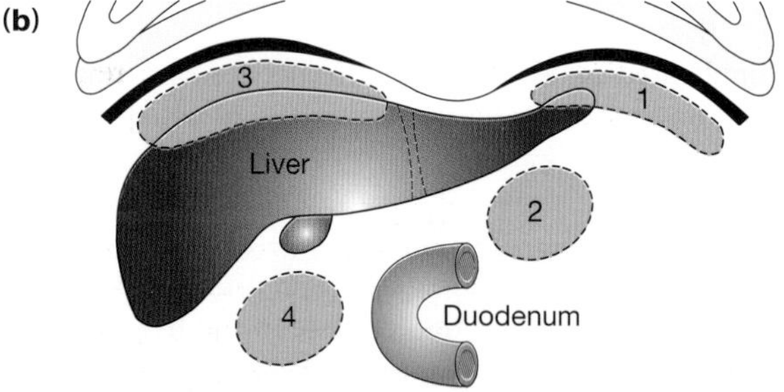

Figure 61.7 (a) Intraperitoneal abscesses on transverse section: 1, the left subphrenic space; 2, left subhepatic space/lesser sac; 3, right subphrenic space; 4, right subhepatic space. (b) Intraperitoneal abscesses on sagittal section: 1, left subphrenic; 2, left subhepatic/ lesser sac; 3, right subphrenic; 4, right subhepatic.

To the right is the falciform ligament and to the left the spleen, gastrosplenic omentum and diaphragm. The common cause of an abscess here is an operation on the stomach, the tail of the pancreas, the spleen or the splenic flexure of the colon.

LEFT SUBHEPATIC SPACE/LESSER SAC

The most common cause of infection here is complicated acute pancreatitis. In practice, a perforated gastric ulcer rarely causes a collection here because the potential space is obliterated by adhesions.

RIGHT SUBPHRENIC SPACE

This space lies between the right lobe of the liver and the diaphragm. It is limited posteriorly by the anterior layer of the coronary and the right triangular ligaments, and to the left by the falciform ligament. Common causes of abscess here are perforating cholecystitis, a perforated duodenal ulcer and a duodenal cap 'blow-out' following gastrectomy and appendicitis.

RIGHT SUBHEPATIC SPACE

This lies transversely beneath the right lobe of the liver in Rutherford Morison's pouch. It is bounded on the right by the right lobe of the liver and the diaphragm. To the left is situated the foramen of Winslow and below this lies the duodenum. In front are the liver and the gall bladder, and behind are the upper part of the right kidney and the diaphragm. The space is bounded above by the liver and below by the transverse colon and hepatic flexure. It is the deepest space of the four and the most common site of a subphrenic abscess, which usually arises from appendicitis, cholecystitis, a perforated duodenal ulcer or following upper abdominal surgery.

Clinical features

The symptoms and signs of subphrenic infection are frequently non-specific and it is well to remember the following aphorism: 'pus somewhere, pus nowhere, pus under the diaphragm'. A common history is that, when some infective focus in the abdominal cavity has been dealt with, the condition of the patient improves temporarily but, after an interval of a few days or weeks, symptoms of toxaemia reappear. The condition of the patient steadily, and often rapidly, deteriorates. Sweating, wasting and anorexia are present. There is sometimes epigastric fullness and pain, or pain in the shoulder on the affected side, because of irritation of sensory fibres in the phrenic nerve, referred along the descending branches of the cervical plexus. Persistent hiccoughs may be a presenting symptom. A swinging pyrexia is usually present. If the abscess is anterior, abdominal examination will reveal some tenderness, rigidity or even a palpable swelling. Sometimes the liver is displaced downwards but more often it is fixed by adhesions.

Investigation and management

Examination of the chest and plain radiograph are important because, in most cases, collapse of the lung or evidence of basal effusion or even an empyema is evident. The modern management of an abscess is by radiological diagnosis using ultrasound or CT guidance (Figures 61.8), followed by drainage. The same tube can be used to instil antibiotic solutions or irrigate the abscess cavity if necessary. In some instances, monitoring may be appropriate by either clinically marking out limits on the abdominal wall (if palpable) with daily examination. However, more commonly, repeat ultrasonography or CT scanning will be required. Radiolabelled white cell

James Rutherford Morison, 1853–1939, Professor of Surgery, the University of Durham, Durham, UK.
Jacob Benignus Winslow, 1669–1760, Professor of Anatomy, Physic and Surgery, Paris, France.

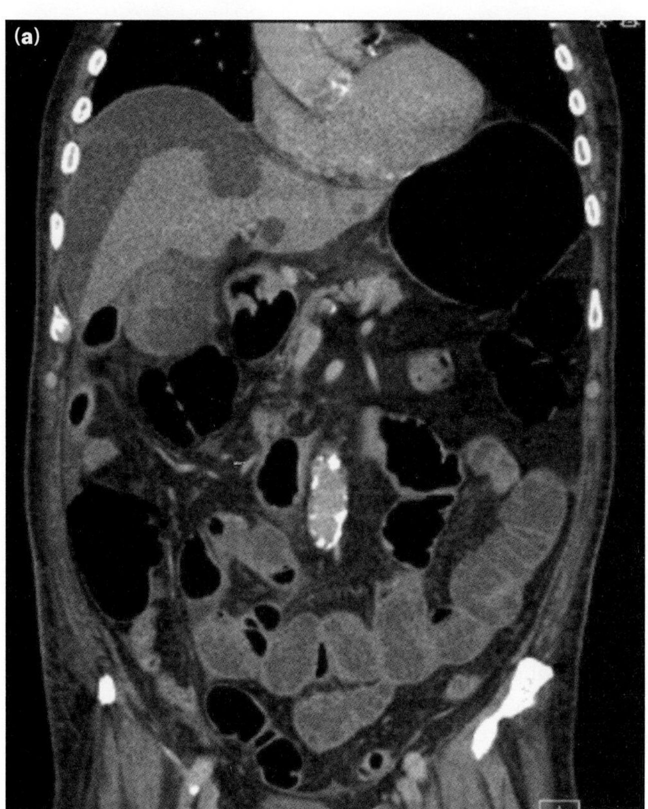

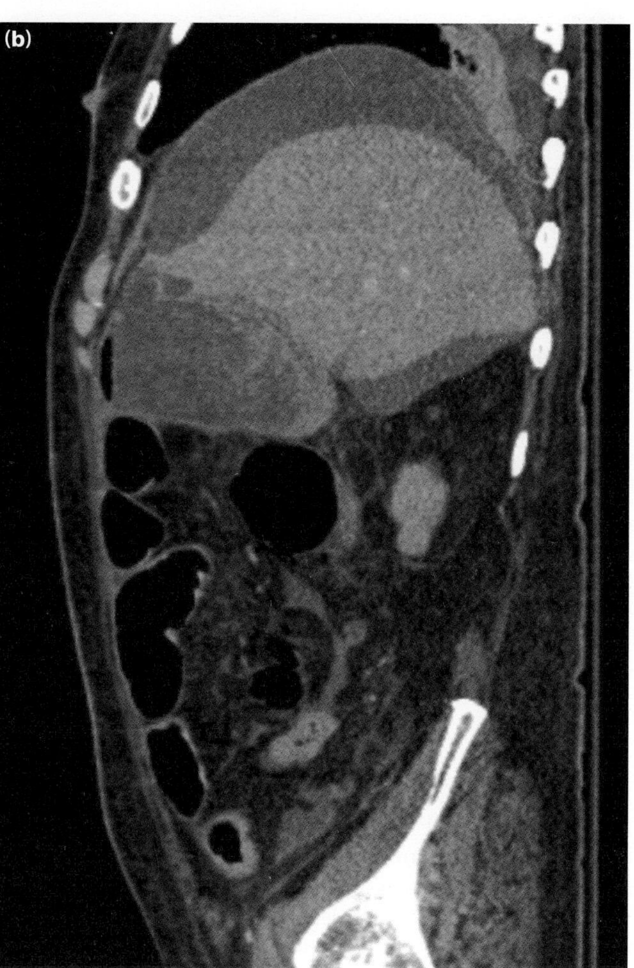

Figure 61.8 Computed tomography scans of a subphrenic abscess secondary to gallbladder empyema – (a) coronal and (b) sagittal sections (courtesy of Dr Tim Fotheringham, Consultant Interventional Radiologist, Bart's Health NHS Trust, London, UK).

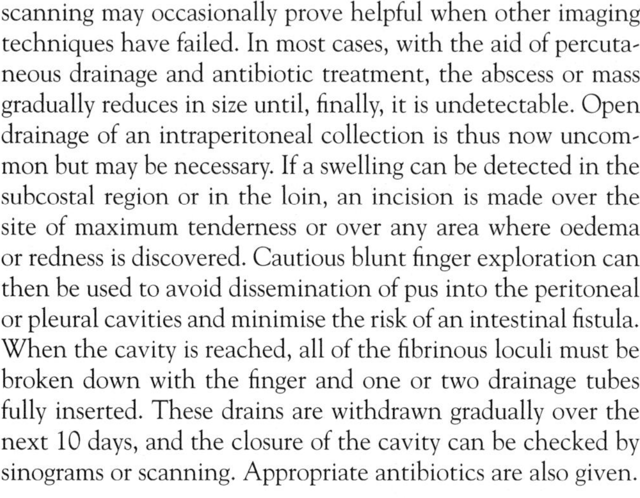

scanning may occasionally prove helpful when other imaging techniques have failed. In most cases, with the aid of percutaneous drainage and antibiotic treatment, the abscess or mass gradually reduces in size until, finally, it is undetectable. Open drainage of an intraperitoneal collection is thus now uncommon but may be necessary. If a swelling can be detected in the subcostal region or in the loin, an incision is made over the site of maximum tenderness or over any area where oedema or redness is discovered. Cautious blunt finger exploration can then be used to avoid dissemination of pus into the peritoneal or pleural cavities and minimise the risk of an intestinal fistula. When the cavity is reached, all of the fibrinous loculi must be broken down with the finger and one or two drainage tubes fully inserted. These drains are withdrawn gradually over the next 10 days, and the closure of the cavity can be checked by sinograms or scanning. Appropriate antibiotics are also given.

ASCITES

Ascites is defined as an accumulation of excess serous fluid within the peritoneal cavity.

Pathophysiology

The balanced effects of plasma and peritoneal colloid osmotic and hydrostatic pressures determine the exchange of fluid between the capillaries and the peritoneal fluid. Protein-rich fluid enters the peritoneal cavity when capillary permeability is increased, as in peritonitis and carcinomatosis peritonei. Capillary pressure may be increased because of generalised water retention, cardiac failure, constrictive pericarditis or vena cava obstruction. Capillary pressure is raised selectively in the portal venous system in the Budd–Chiari syndrome, cirrhosis of the liver or extrahepatic portal venous obstruction. Plasma colloid osmotic pressure may be lowered in patients with reduced nutritional intake, diminished intestinal absorption, abnormal protein losses or defective protein synthesis, such as occurs in cirrhosis. Peritoneal lymphatic drainage may be impaired, resulting in the accumulation of protein-rich fluid.

George Budd, 1808–1882, Professor of Medicine, King's College Hospital, London, UK, described this syndrome in 1845.
Hans Chiari, 1851–1916, Professor of Pathological Anatomy, Strasbourg, Germany (Strasbourg was returned to France in 1918 at the end of the First World War). He gave his account of this condition in 1898.

Summary box 61.12

Causes of ascites

Transudates (protein <25 g/L)

- Low plasma protein concentrations:
  - Malnutrition
  - Nephrotic syndrome
  - Protein-losing enteropathy
- High central venous pressure:
  - Congestive cardiac failure
- Portal hypertension
  - Portal vein thrombosis
  - Cirrhosis

Exudates (protein >25 g/L)

- Peritoneal malignancy
- Tuberculous peritonitis
- Budd–Chiari syndrome (hepatic vein occlusion or thrombosis)
- Pancreatic ascites
- Chylous ascites
- Meigs' syndrome

Clinical features

Ascites can usually be recognised clinically only when the amount of fluid present exceeds 1.5 L depending on body habitus: in obese individuals a greater quantity than this is necessary before there is clear evidence. The abdomen is distended evenly with fullness of the flanks, which are dull to percussion. Usually, shifting dullness is present but, when there is a very large accumulation of fluid, this sign is absent. In such cases, on flicking the abdominal wall, a characteristic fluid thrill is transmitted from one side to the other. In women, ascites must be differentiated from an enormous ovarian cyst.

Congestive heart failure results in increased venous pressure in the vena cava and consequent obstruction to the venous outflow from the liver. The ascitic fluid is light yellow and of low specific gravity, about 1.010, with a low protein concentration (<25 g/L). Patients with constrictive pericarditis (Pick's disease) have both peritoneal and pleural effusions because of engorgement of the venae cavae, consequent upon the diminished capacity of the right side of the heart. Ascites occurs with low plasma albumin concentrations, e.g. in patients with albuminuria or starvation. The ascites in this instance is caused by alterations in the osmotic pressure of the capillary blood and has a low specific gravity.

In cirrhosis, now the most common cause of ascites internationally, there is obstruction to the portal venous system, which is caused by obliterative fibrosis of the intrahepatic venous bed. In the Budd–Chiari syndrome (see Chapter 65), thrombosis or obstruction of the hepatic veins is responsible for obstruction to venous outflow from the liver. The ascites seen in patients with peritoneal metastases is caused by excessive exudation of fluid and lymphatic blockage. The fluid is dark yellow and frequently blood stained. The specific gravity, ≥1.020, and the protein content (>25 g/L) are high. Microscopic examination often reveals cancer cells, especially if large quantities of fluid are 'spun down' to produce a concentrated deposit for sampling. Rarely, ascites and pleural effusion are associated with solid fibromas of the ovary (Meigs' syndrome). The effusions disappear when the tumour is excised.

Investigation

In addition to relevant investigations to determine the underlying cause, e.g. liver function tests (LFTs), cardiac function, ultrasonography and/or CT scanning (Figure 61.9) will determine much smaller quantities of ascites than possible clinically. These will often also diagnose aetiology, e.g. carcinomatosis or liver disease. Ascitic aspiration or tap (below) is now most commonly performed under imaging guidance to minimise the risk of visceral injury. After the bladder has been emptied, puncture of the peritoneum is carried out under local anaesthetic using a moderately sized trocar and cannula. Alternatively, a peritoneal drain may be inserted. In cases where the effusion is caused by cardiac failure, the fluid must be evacuated slowly. Fluid is sent for microscopy/cytology, culture, including mycobacteria, and analysis of protein content and amylase. Unless other measures are taken the fluid soon reaccumulates, and repeated tappings remove valuable protein.

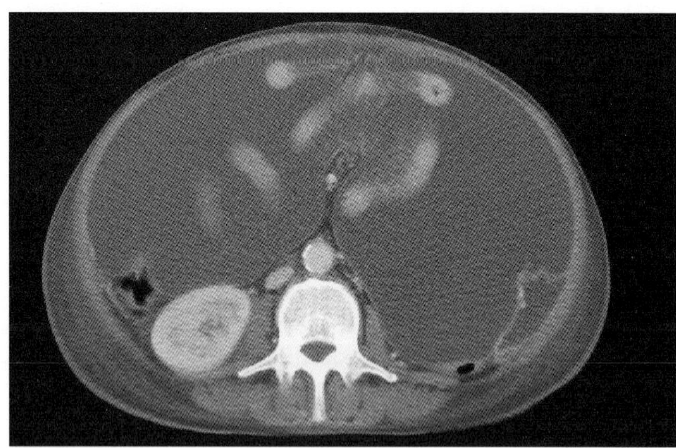

Figure 61.9 Computed tomography scan showing gross ascites.

Treatment

Treatment of the specific cause is undertaken whenever possible, e.g. if portal venous pressure is raised, it may be possible to lower it by treatment of the primary condition or by transjugular intrahepatic portosystemic shunt or transjugular intrahepatic portosystemic stent shunting (commonly abbreviated as TIPS or TIPSS). These procedures have become increasingly popular since the 1980s and are performed by interventional radiologists under fluoroscopic guidance. Access to the liver is gained via the internal jugular vein and

Joe Vincent Meigs, 1892–1963, Professor of Gynecology, Harvard University Medical School, Boston, MA, USA.
Friedel Pick, 1867–1926, physician, Prague, the former Czechoslovakia, described this disease in 1896.

a guidewire and introducer sheath facilitate cannulation of the hepatic vein. Once the catheter is in the hepatic vein, a wedge pressure is obtained to calculate the pressure gradient in the liver, and a special needle is advanced through the liver parenchyma to connect the hepatic to the portal vein. The channel for the shunt is created using an angioplasty balloon to dilate the needle tract and thence a stent placed through this track. Complications can occur, e.g. bleeding, liver injury and encephalopathy; however, in experienced hands the mortality rate is <1%. This procedure is thus, when possible, preferable to older surgical methods.

Dietary sodium restriction to 200 mg/day may be helpful, but diuretics are usually required (combination of spironolactone and furosemide). For patients failing to respond to such measures, therapeutic needle paracentesis can be performed. This is usually performed in the left of the right lower abdominal quadrant after diagnostic needle aspiration, and using a 'Z' track approach to ensure that peritoneal and skin puncture do not overlie the same point. Serial large volume paracentesis (4–6 L/day and up to 8 L in one session) can be performed safely with colloid replacement, and it can be performed in patients with cirrhosis and deranged clotting. Guidelines recommend albumin replacement after paracentesis to reduce complications. It is now also possible to leave an indwelling external drain for smaller-volume home paracentesis. In cases in which ascites accumulates rapidly after paracentesis and the patient is fit, drainage of the ascitic fluid by surgical peritoneovenous shunting (e.g. LeVeen, Denver) was previously employed; however, these procedures have been essentially abandoned due to their high rate of complications.

Special cases

Chylous ascites

In some patients the ascitic fluid appears milky because of an excess of chylomicrons (triglycerides). Most cases are associated with malignancy, usually lymphomas; other causes are cirrhosis, TB, filariasis, nephrotic syndrome, abdominal trauma (including surgery), constrictive pericarditis, sarcoidosis and congenital lymphatic abnormality. The prognosis is poor unless the underlying condition can be cured. In addition to other measures used to treat ascites, patients should be placed on a fat-free diet with medium-chain triglyceride supplements.

TUMOURS OF THE PERITONEUM

Primary tumours

Primary tumours of the peritoneum are rare and in most cases take their origin not from the serous layer but from some adjacent structure, e.g. lipoma from appendices epiploicae, fibroma from connective tissue. Mesothelioma of the peritoneum is less frequent than in the pleural cavity but equally lethal. Asbestos is a recognised cause. It has a predilection for the pelvic peritoneum. Chemocytotoxic agents are the mainstay of treatment. Desmoid tumours which have a relationship to the peritoneum are considered under familial adenomatous polyposis (see Chapter 70).

Secondary tumours

Carcinomatosis peritonei

This is a common terminal event in many cases of carcinoma of the stomach, colon, ovary or other abdominal organs, and also of the breast and bronchus. The peritoneum, both parietal and visceral, is studded with secondary growths and the peritoneal cavity becomes filled with clear, straw-coloured or blood-stained ascitic fluid.

The main forms of peritoneal metastases are:

- discrete nodules – by far the most common variety;
- plaques varying in size and colour;
- diffuse adhesions – this form occurs at a late stage of the disease and gives rise, sometimes, to a 'frozen pelvis'.

Gravity probably determines the distribution of free malignant cells within the peritoneal cavity. Cells not caught in peritoneal folds gravitate into the pelvic pouches or into a hernial sac, the enlargement of which is occasionally the first indication of the condition. Implantation occurs also on the greater omentum, the appendices epiploicae and the inferior surface of the diaphragm. The main differential diagnosis is from tuberculous peritonitis (tubercles are greyish and translucent and closely resemble the discrete nodules of peritoneal carcinomatosis). Investigation and treatment are as for underlying malignancy; however, newer treatment options such as cytoreductive surgery, intraperitoneal chemotherapy and hyperthermic intraperitoneal chemotherapy (HIPEC) are now offered in specialist centres. The last, a highly concentrated, heated (41–42°C) chemotherapy treatment is delivered directly into the abdomen for 90 minutes after cytoreductive surgery, and is progressing to a standard of care in some countries for patients without disease outside the abdomen.

Pseudomyxoma peritonei

This rare condition occurs more frequently in women. The abdomen is filled with a yellow jelly, large quantities of which are often encysted. The condition is associated with mucinous cystic tumours of the ovary and appendix. Recent studies suggest that most cases arise from a primary appendiceal tumour with secondary implantation on to one or both ovaries. It is often painless and there is frequently no impairment of general health. Pseudomyxoma peritonei does not give rise to extraperitoneal metastases but causes symptoms and complications due to tumour bulk. Although an abdomen distended with what seems to be fluid that cannot be made to shift should raise the possibility, the diagnosis is more often suggested by ultrasonography and CT scanning, or made at operation. At laparotomy, masses of jelly are scooped out. The appendix, if present, should be excised together with any ovarian tumour. More definitive treatment can be achieved by 'complete cytoreduction' (Sugarbaker technique) in which

Harry LeVeen, Professor of Surgery, the University of South Carolina, SC, USA.
Paul Sugarbaker, Director of Surgical Oncology at the Cancer Institute at Washington Hospital Center, Washington DC, USA.

the right hemicolon, spleen, gall bladder, and greater and lesser omentum are excised, along with stripping of the peritoneum from the pelvis and diaphragm, and stripping of the tumour from the surface of the liver (the uterus and ovaries are also removed in women). Intraoperative heated chemotherapy (using mitomycin C) follows and the whole procedure takes about 10 hours. There is international controversy about the effectiveness of this procedure although some large series report good 5-year survival.

Peritoneal inclusion cysts

These are usually caused by accumulation of ovarian fluid that is contained by peritoneal adhesions. The development of a peritoneal inclusion cyst thus depends on the presence of an active ovary and peritoneal adhesions. The normal peritoneum absorbs fluid easily. However, the absorptive capacity of the peritoneum is greatly diminished in the presence of mechanical injury, inflammation and peritoneal adhesions.

Peritoneal inclusion cysts occur only in premenopausal women with a history of pelvic or abdominal surgery. They range in size from several millimetres in diameter to bulky masses that may fill the entire pelvis and abdomen. Pathologically, the cyst results from non-neoplastic, reactive mesothelial proliferation.

Investigation includes the exclusion of ovarian tumour by blood tests and appropriate imaging (usually ultrasonography and magnetic resonance imaging [MRI]). Cysts may be managed expectantly or by hormonal modulation, e.g. oral contraceptives. Radiological drainage will give transient relief and may help diagnosis using cytology. Surgery can be performed to remove adhesions but the risk of recurrence is 30–50%.

Peritoneal loose bodies (peritoneal mice)

Peritoneal loose bodies (peritoneal mice) may be confused with a small tumour but almost never cause symptoms. One or more may be found in a hernial sac or in the pouch of Douglas. The loose body may come from an appendix epiploica that has undergone axial rotation followed by necrosis of its pedicle and detachment, but they are also found in those who have subacute attacks of pancreatitis. These hyaline bodies attain the size of a pea or bean and contain saponified fat surrounded by fibrin.

ADHESIONS

Pathophysiology

Adhesions are strands of fibrous tissue that form, usually as a result of surgery, between surgically injured tissues. After injury, there is bleeding and an increase in vascular permeability with extravasation of fibrinogen-rich fluid from the injured surfaces forming a temporary fibrin matrix. An inflammatory response ensues with cell migration, release of cytokines and activation of the coagulation cascade. The activation of the coagulation system results in thrombin formation, which is necessary for the conversion of fibrinogen to fibrin. In the absence of fibrinolysis, adhesions will form within 5–7 days as the matrix gradually becomes more organised with collagen secretion by fibroblasts. Fibrinolysis is therefore the key factor in determining whether an adhesion persists. This is governed by several cascades and activators that may account for interindividual differences (see Chapter 3). Of great importance to the surgeon, however, is the fact that ischaemic tissue loses its ability to break down fibrin and inhibits fibrinolysis in adjacent tissues.

Complications

The most common adhesion-related problem is small bowel obstruction (SBO). Adhesions are the most frequent cause of SBO in resource-rich countries and are responsible for 60–70% of SBOs (see Chapter 71). Adhesions are also implicated as a major cause of secondary infertility (beyond the remit of this text). The relationship of adhesions to chronic abdominal and pelvic pain is contentious. Unguided division of adhesions has not been shown to reduce chronic abdominal pain in definitive RCTs although conscious pain mapping (laparoscopy under local anaesthesia) to direct lysis may improve success rates.

Prevention

As a result of the scale of the problem there has been significant research into ways of preventing postoperative adhesion formation. Minimising the production of ischaemic tissue by careful surgical technique, including meticulous control of bleeding, remain, however, the most critical concepts. The evolution of laparoscopic bowel surgery has been shown by collective review data to result in reduced adhesion-related readmissions for a number of abdominal and pelvic procedures, e.g. cholecystectomy, hysterectomy and colectomy. It should be noted, however, that only one randomised controlled trial (after Crohn's resection) has ever shown a definitive effect, and this was not confirmed by evidence synthesis at Cochrane review.

The effect of a number of drugs including anti-inflammatory drugs such as aspirin and steroids, some hormones, anticlotting agents, antibiotics, vitamin E and even methylene blue have been investigated in adhesion prevention but have not achieved widespread use, because of either side effects or lack of consistent evidence of effectiveness. Many barrier methods of reducing adhesions have also been trialled. Adept® (4% icodextrin solution) is a solution applied inside the abdomen at the time of surgery; it has been shown to reduce the extent and severity of adhesion formation in animal models. It has also been used widely as a peritoneal dialysis solution for many years. Interceed TC7® is a mesh-like product (oxidised regenerated cellulose) which quickly forms a soft gelatinous mass around healing tissues and is absorbed within 2 weeks. It has been shown to significantly reduce the number of adhesions at the site where it is used. However, it is worth noting that a reduction in the number of adhesions in such studies does not necessarily equate to a reduction in adhesion-related problems in the future. In a review of seven randomised trials looking at a similar barrier-type product (hyaluronic acid/carboxymethyl membrane), there was a significant reduction in the incidence, extent and severity of adhesions but no reduction in the incidence of intestinal obstruction or surgical intervention. Such barriers, when placed around bowel anastomosis, also led to a significant increase in the anastomotic leaks. For these reasons barrier approaches have not gained popularity.

Special forms of intraperitoneal fibrosis

Sclerosing encapsulating peritonitis

Also known as abdominal cocoon syndrome, sclerosing encapsulating peritonitis (SEP) is described in patients as a complication of long-term peritoneal dialysis or portovenous shunting. The peritoneal cavity becomes obliterated as a result of gross subserosal thickening by fibrosis, leading to bowel obstruction and other sequelae. Surgery should be undertaken with trepidation and avoided if possible.

Diffuse fibromatosis

This is a variant of intra-abdominal fibromatosis (IAF) and is actually a rare tumour characterised by an abnormal proliferation of myofibroblasts. Although non-metastasising, and said to be benign, it can nevertheless prove widely invasive, compressing and infiltrating surrounding tissues such as the bowel and mesentery with complications thereof. IAF is very rare within the general population but has a recognised association with familial adenomatous polyposis (FAP).

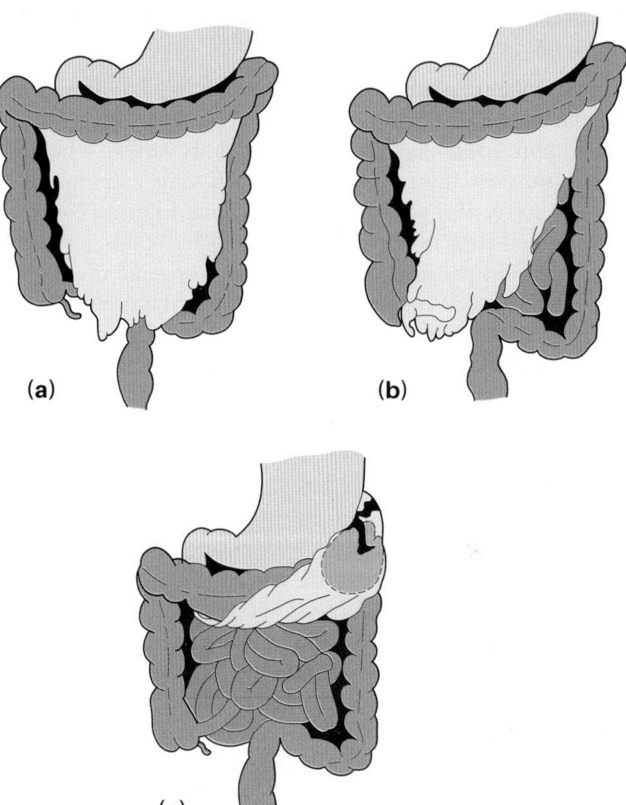

Figure 61.10 The greater omentum: (a) normal; (b) in appendicitis; (c) in a (comparatively small) laceration of the spleen.

THE OMENTUM

Rutherford Morison called the greater omentum 'the abdominal policeman'. The greater omentum attempts, often successfully, to limit intraperitoneal infective and other noxious processes (Figure 61.10). For instance, an acutely inflamed appendix is often found wrapped in omentum, and this saves many patients from developing diffuse peritonitis. Some sufferers of herniae are also greatly indebted to this structure, because it often plugs the neck of a hernial sac and prevents a coil of intestine from entering and becoming strangulated. It can of course also be a cause of obstruction (acting as a large adhesion). The omentum is usually involved in tuberculous peritonitis and carcinomatosis of the peritoneum.

Torsion of the omentum

Torsion of the omentum is a rare emergency and consequently is seldom diagnosed correctly. It is usually mistaken for appendicitis with somewhat abnormal signs. It may be primary or secondary to adhesion of the omentum to an old focus of infection or hernia. The patient is most frequently a middle-aged, obese man. A tender lump may be present in the abdomen. The blood supply having been jeopardised, the twisted mass sometimes becomes gangrenous, in which case bacterial peritonitis may follow. Treatment is surgical; the pedicle above the twist is ligated securely and the mass removed.

THE MESENTERY

Mesenteric injury

A wound of the mesentery can follow severe abdominal contusion and is a cause of haemoperitoneum. More commonly, it is injured by a torsional force, so-called seatbelt syndrome. This occurs during a vehicular collision when a seatbelt is being worn with sudden deceleration resulting in a torn mesentery. This possibility should be borne in mind, particularly as multiple injuries may distract attention from this injury (the management of abdominal trauma is covered in Chapter 27). Aside from control of any ongoing haemorrhage, associated ischaemic or ruptured gut will require resection.

Ischaemia

Torsion of the mesentery is covered under midgut volvulus and volvulus of the small intestine (see Chapter 69). Embolism and thrombosis of mesenteric vessels leading to intestinal ischaemia are also covered in Chapter 69.

Inflammation

A number of somewhat miscellaneous conditions are best described under this umbrella term.

Acute, non-specific, ileocaecal, mesenteric adenitis

Non-specific mesenteric adenitis was so named to distinguish it from specific (tuberculous) mesenteric adenitis. It is now much more common than the tuberculous variety. The aetiology often remains unknown, although some cases are associated with yersinia infection of the ileum. In other cases, an unidentified virus is blamed. In about 25% of cases, a respiratory infection precedes an attack of non-specific mesenteric adenitis. This self-limiting disease is never fatal but may be recurrent. Its significance thus mainly lies in its differential diagnosis with appendicitis in children.

DIAGNOSIS

During childhood, acute, non-specific mesenteric adenitis is a common condition. The typical history is one of short attacks of central abdominal pain lasting from 10 min to 30 min, commonly associated with vomiting. The patient seldom looks ill. In more than half the cases the temperature is elevated. Abdominal tenderness is poorly localised and, when present, shifting tenderness is a valuable sign for differentiating the condition from appendicitis. The neck, axillae and groins should be palpated for enlarged lymph nodes. There is often a leukocytosis of 10 000–12 000/μL (10–12 × 10^9/L) or more on the first day of the attack, but this falls on the second day.

TREATMENT

When the diagnosis can be made with assurance, bed rest and simple analgesia are the only treatment necessary. If, at a second examination a few hours later, acute appendicitis cannot be excluded, it is safer to perform either appendicectomy or diagnostic laparoscopy. If surgery is mistakenly undertaken, there is a small increase in the amount of peritoneal fluid. The ileocaecal mesenteric lymph nodes are enlarged, and can be seen and felt between the leaves of the mesentery. In very acute cases they are distinctly red, and many of them are the size of a walnut. The nodes nearest the attachment of the mesentery are the largest. They are not adherent to their peritoneal coats and, if a small incision is made through the overlying peritoneum, a node is extruded easily.

Tuberculosis of the mesenteric lymph nodes

Tuberculous mesenteric lymphadenitis is considerably less common than acute non-specific lymphadenitis. Tubercle bacilli, usually, but not necessarily, bovine, are ingested and enter the mesenteric lymph nodes by way of Peyer's patches. Sometimes only one lymph node is infected; usually there are several and occasionally massive involvement occurs. The presentation may be with abdominal pain (a rare differential for appendicitis) or with general constitutional symptoms (pyrexia, weight loss, etc.). Calcified lymph nodes may be demonstrated on a plain radiograph of the abdomen where they must be distinguished from other calcified lesions, e.g. renal or ureteric stones.

Misty mesentery

The term 'misty mesentery' indicates a pathological increase in mesenteric fat attenuation at CT (Figure 61.11). It is frequently observed on multidetector CT (MDCT) scans performed during daily clinical practice, and may be caused by various pathological conditions, including oedema, inflammation (especially in association with pancreatitis), haemorrhage, neoplastic infiltration (especially otherwise occult lymphoma) or sclerosing mesenteritis. In patients with acute abdominal disease, misty mesentery may be considered a feature of the underlying disease. Otherwise, it may represent an incidental finding on MDCT performed for other reasons. Follow-up scans may be required to dictate whether further investigation is required depending on progression or resolution. It should be noted that the term 'mesenteric panniculitis' is frequently used synonymously with 'misty mesentery'. Correctly this term should be reserved for the mesenteric manifestation of Weber–Christian disease; isolated lipodystrophy and mesenteric lipogranuloma. It is a very rare (200–300 cases reported worldwide) benign inflammatory or fibrotic change in the mesentery of the bowel.

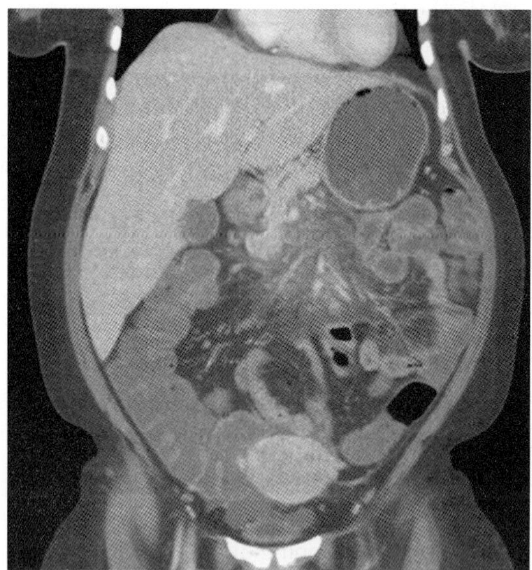

Figure 61.11 Computed tomography scan showing 'misty mesentery' in a patient with probable peritoneal inflammation secondary to acute pancreatitis (courtesy of Dr K Patel, Homerton University Foundation Trust, London).

Mesenteric cysts

Cysts may occur in the mesentery of either the small intestine (60%) or the colon (40%) and can be classified as the following:

- Chylolymphatic
- Enterogenous
- Urogenital remnant (actually retroperitoneal but project into peritoneum)
- Dermoid.

Johann Conrad Peyer, 1653–1712, Professor of Logic, Rhetoric and Medicine, Schaffhausen, Switzerland, described the lymph follicles in the intestine in 1677.

Pathology

CHYLOLYMPHATIC CYST

Although all mesenteric cysts are rare, this is the most common variety, probably arising in congenitally misplaced lymphatic tissue that has no efferent communication with the lymphatic system (most frequently in the mesentery of the ileum). The thin wall of the cyst, which is composed of connective tissue lined by flat endothelium, is filled with clear lymph or, less frequently, with chyle, varying in consistency from watered milk to cream. Occasionally, the cyst attains a great size. More often unilocular than multilocular, a chylolymphatic cyst is almost invariably solitary, although there is an extremely rare variety in which myriads of cysts are found in the various mesenteries of the abdomen. A chylolymphatic cyst has a blood supply that is independent from that of the adjacent intestine and, thus, enucleation is possible without the need for resection of gut.

ENTEROGENOUS CYSTS

These are believed to be derived either from a diverticulum of the mesenteric border of the intestine that has become sequestrated from the intestinal canal during embryonic life, or from a duplication of the intestine (see Chapter 9). An enterogenous cyst has a thicker wall than a chylolymphatic cyst and it is lined by mucous membrane, which is sometimes ciliated. The content is mucinous and either colourless or yellowish brown as a result of past haemorrhage. The muscle in the wall of an enteric duplication cyst and the bowel with which it is in contact have a common blood supply; consequently, removal of the cyst always entails resection of the related portion of intestine.

UROGENITAL REMNANT

A cyst developing in the retroperitoneal space (see below) often attains very large dimensions and has first to be distinguished from a large hydronephrosis. Even after the latter condition has been eliminated by scanning or urography, a retroperitoneal cyst can seldom be distinguished with certainty from a retroperitoneal tumour until displayed at operation. The cyst may be unilocular or multilocular. Many of these cysts are believed to be derived from a remnant of the wolffian duct, in which case they are filled with clear fluid.

Clinical features

These are shown for mesenteric cysts in general in *Summary box 61.13*.

Summary box 61.13

Mesenteric cysts: clinical features

- Cysts occur most commonly in adults with a mean age of 45 years
- Twice as common in women as in me
- Rare: incidence around 1 per 140 000
- Approximately a third of cases occur in children younger than 15 years
- The mean age of children affected is 4.9 years
- The most common presentation is of a painless abdominal swelling with characteristic physical signs
  - there is a fluctuant swelling near the umbilicus
  - the swelling moves freely in a plane at right angles to the attachment of the mesentery (Tillaux's sign) (Figure 61.12)
  - there is a zone of resonance around the cyst
- Other presentations are with recurrent attacks of abdominal pain with or without vomiting (pain resulting from recurring temporary impaction of a food bolus in a segment of bowel narrowed by the cyst or possibly from torsion of the mesentery) and acute abdominal catastrophe, due to:
  - torsion of that portion of the mesentery containing the cyst
  - rupture of the cyst, often as a result of a comparatively trivial accident
  - haemorrhage into the cyst
  - infection

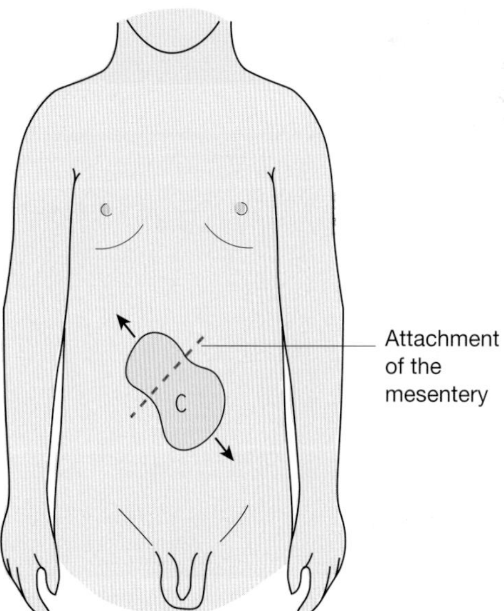

Figure 61.12 A mesenteric cyst moves freely in the direction of the arrows, i.e. at right angles to the attachment of the mesentery (Tillaux's sign).

Investigation and treatment

Ultrasonography and CT scanning will demonstrate the lesion and may allow diagnosis of cyst type (Figure 61.13a and b). There are no suitable medical therapies. The goal of surgical therapy is complete excision of the mass. The preferred treatment of mesenteric cysts is enucleation, although bowel resection is frequently required to ensure that the remaining bowel is viable. Bowel resection may be required in 50–60% of children with mesenteric cysts, whereas resection is necessary in about a third of adults (Figure 61.13c). If enucleation or resection is not possible because of either the size of the cyst or its location deep within the root of the mesentery, the third option is partial excision with marsupialisation of

Kaspar Friedrich Wolff, 1733–1794, Professor of Anatomy and Physiology, St Petersburg, Russia, described the mesonephric duct and body in 1759.
Paul Jules Tillaux, 1834–1904, surgeon, Paris, France.

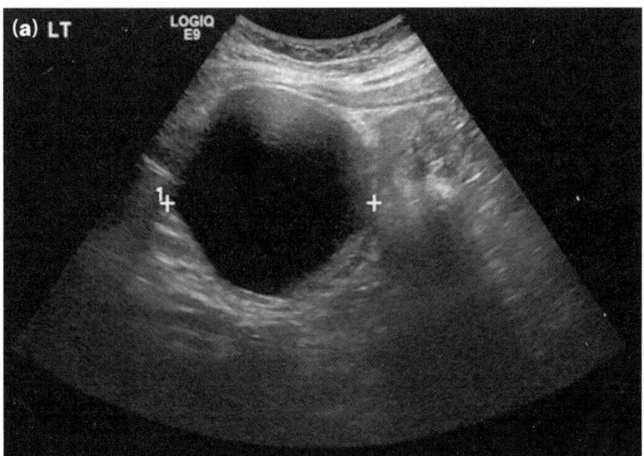

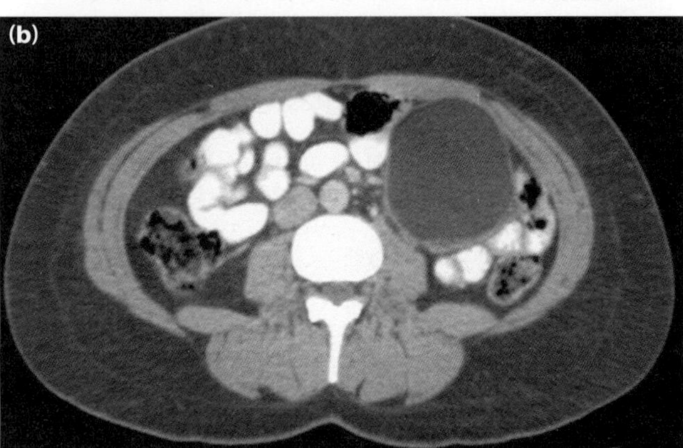

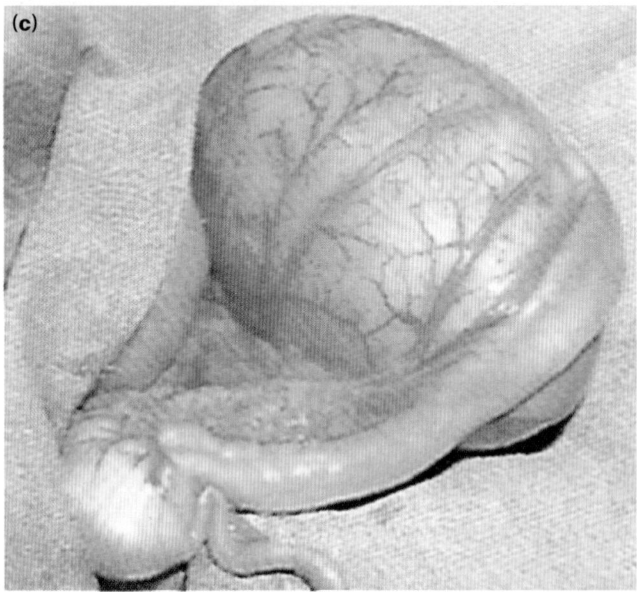

Figure 61.13 A mesenteric enterogenous cyst in a 37-year-old woman presenting with an asymptomatic palpable abdominal mass: (a) ultrasound findings; (b) computed tomography findings; and (c) intraoperative findings requiring en masse small bowel resection (courtesy of Mr F Olagbaiye, Homerton University Foundation Trust, London).

the remaining cyst into the abdominal cavity. Approximately 10% of patients require this form of therapy. If marsupialisation is performed, the cyst lining should be sclerosed with 10% glucose solution, diathermy or tincture of iodine to minimise recurrence. Recurrence rates vary from 0% to 13%.

DIFFERENTIAL DIAGNOSIS

The following, although not being mesenteric cysts in the true meaning of the term, give rise to the same physical signs:

- peritoneal inclusion cyst (see above);
- serosanguineous cyst, probably traumatic in origin although a history of an accident is seldom obtained;
- tuberculous abscess of the mesentery;
- hydatid cyst of the mesentery.

Neoplasms of the mesentery

The mesentery is necessarily affected by local lymphatic spread of carcinoma arising from the peritoneal viscera. Other benign and malignant tumours are less common.

Summary box 61.14

Mesenteric tumours

Benign
- Lipoma
- Fibroma
- Fibromyxoma

Malignant
- Lymphoma
- Secondary carcinoma

Tumours situated in the mesentery give rise to physical signs that are similar to those of a mesenteric cyst, the sole exception being that they sometimes feel solid. If indicated, a benign tumour of the mesentery is excised in the same way as an enterogenous mesenteric cyst, i.e. with resection of the adjacent intestine. A malignant tumour of the mesentery requires biopsy confirmation and specific, usually nonsurgical, treatment, e.g. chemotherapy for lymphoma.

THE RETROPERITONEAL SPACE

Retroperitoneal fibrosis

This is a relatively rare diagnosis characterised by the development of a flat grey/white plaque of tissue, which is found first in the low lumbar region but then spreads laterally and upwards to encase the common iliac vessels, ureters and aorta. Histological appearances vary from active inflammation with a high cellular content interspersed with bundles of collagen through to one of acellularity and mature fibrosis/calcification. Its aetiology is obscure in most cases (idiopathic) being allied

Summary box 61.15

Causes of retroperitoneal fibrosis

Benign

- Idiopathic (Ormond's disease)
- Chronic inflammation
- Extravasation of urine
- Retroperitoneal irritation by leakage of blood or intestinal content
- Aortic aneurysm (inflammatory type)
- Trauma
- Drugs (chemotherapeutic agents and previously methysergide)

Malignant

- Lymphoma
- Carcinoid tumours
- Secondary deposits (especially from carcinoma of stomach, colon, breast and prostate)

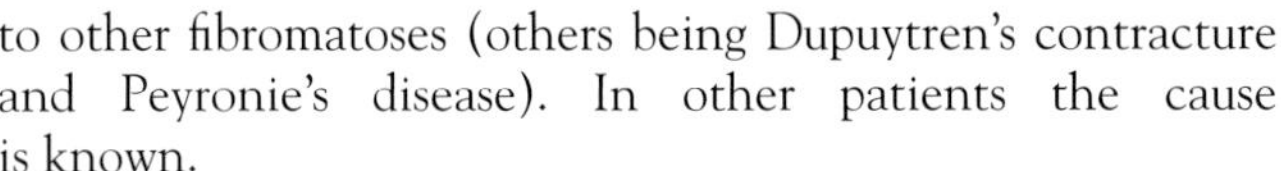

to other fibromatoses (others being Dupuytren's contracture and Peyronie's disease). In other patients the cause is known.

The clinical presentation may be one of ill-defined chronic backache or occur as a result of compromise to involved structures, e.g. lower limb or scrotal oedema secondary to venous occlusion, or chronic renal failure secondary to ureteric obstruction. Treatment will be directed to the cause, the modification of disease activity when appropriate, e.g. immunomodulation with steroids, tamoxifen and restoration of flow in affected structures, e.g. ureteric stenting.

Retroperitoneal (psoas) abscess

The retroperitoneal space can also be a site for abscess formation, which for practical purposes is almost synonymous with psoas abscess. Psoas abscess is a relatively uncommon diagnosis, the true incidence of which is not well described. At the start of the twentieth century, psoas abscess was mainly caused by TB of the spine (Pott's disease). With the decline of *M. tuberculosis* as a major pathogen in resource-rich countries, a psoas abscess was mostly found secondary to direct spread of infection from the inflamed ± perforated digestive or urinary tract. In recent years a primary psoas abscess due to haematogenous spread from an occult source is more common, especially in immunocompromised and older patients, as well as in association with intravenous drug misuse.

Clinical presentation is with back pain, lassitude and fever. A swelling may point to the groin as it tracks along iliopsoas. Pain may be elicited by passive extension of the hip or a fixed flexion of the hip evident on inspection.

Radiological investigation is via CT scanning (Figure 61.14) and treatment usually by percutaneous CT-guided drainage and appropriate antibiotic therapy.

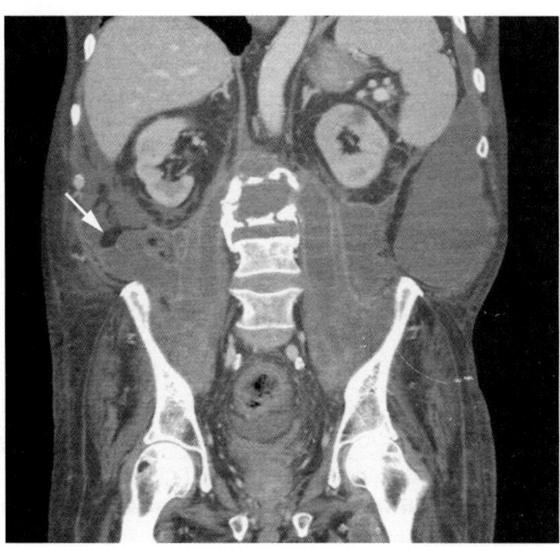

Figure 61.14 Representative sagittal computed tomography reconstruction of a right-sided psoas abscess (courtesy of Dr K Patel, Homerton University Foundation Trust, London).

Retroperitoneal tumours

Although swellings in the retroperitoneum may include abscess, haematoma, cysts (see above) and spread of malignancy from retroperitoneal organs (kidney, ureter, adrenal), the term retroperitoneal tumour is usually confined to primary tumours arising in other tissues in this region e.g. muscles, fat, lymph nodes and nerves. The management of such tumours is now frequently by referral to a specialist centre and this should be done before biopsy which may compromise subsequent surgical cure. The two commonest are briefly described.

Retroperitoneal lipoma

The patient may seek advice on account of a swelling or because of indefinite abdominal pain. Women are more often affected. These swellings sometimes reach an immense size. Diagnosis is usually by ultrasonography and CT scanning. A retroperitoneal lipoma sometimes undergoes myxomatous degeneration, a complication that does not occur in a lipoma in any other part of the body. Moreover, a retroperitoneal lipoma is often malignant (liposarcoma) (see below) and may increase rapidly in size.

Retroperitoneal sarcoma

Retroperitoneal sarcomas are rare tumours accounting for only 1–2% of all solid malignancies (10–20% of all sarcomas are retroperitoneal). The peak incidence is in the fifth decade of life, although they can occur at almost any age. The most common types of retroperitoneal soft-tissue sarcomas in adults vary from study to study. However, in most studies, the most frequently encountered cell types are:

- liposarcoma;
- leiomyosarcoma;
- malignant fibrous histiocytoma (MFH).

JK Ormond, American urologist.
Baron Guillaume Dupuytren, 1777–1835, Surgeon in Chief, Hôtel Dieu, Paris, France, described this condition in 1831.
François de la Peyronie, 1678–1747, Surgeon to King Louis XIV of France, and Founder of the Royal Academy of Surgery, Paris, France.

CLINICAL FEATURES

Patients with sarcomas present late, because these tumours arise in the large potential spaces of the retroperitoneum and can grow very large without producing symptoms. Moreover, when symptoms do occur, they are non-specific, such as abdominal pain and fullness, and are easily dismissed as being caused by other less serious processes. Retroperitoneal sarcomas are, therefore, usually very large at the time of presentation.

INVESTIGATION

Detailed multiplanar imaging (CT + MRI) with reconstructions is required not only for tumour detection, staging and surgical planning, but also for guiding percutaneous or surgical biopsy of these tumours. Such biopsies have a greater role than for other sarcomas.

TREATMENT

The definitive treatment of primary retroperitoneal sarcomas is surgical resection. Chemotherapy and radiotherapy without surgical debulking have rarely been beneficial, when used alone or in combination A multidisciplinary treatment approach with imaging review will be required when assessing operability (based on adjacency or involvement of vital structures) and approach. Up to 75% of retroperitoneal sarcoma resections involve resection of at least one adjoining intra-abdominal visceral organ (commonly large or small bowel or kidney). The most common types of vascular involvement precluding resection are involvement of the proximal superior mesenteric vessels or involvement of bilateral renal vessels.

PROGNOSIS

In the vast majority of sarcomas, cell type has no impact on treatment and long-term survival. Survival rates are in general poor, even after complete resection, being in the order of 35–50% (excluding low-grade liposarcomas, which may frequently be cured by resection).

FURTHER READING

Ahmad G, Mackie FL, Iles DA *et al.* Fluid and pharmacological agents for adhesion prevention after gynaecological surgery. *Cochrane Database Syst Rev* 2014; **9**(7): CD001298.

French FMF Consortium. A candidate gene for familial Mediterranean fever. *Nat Genet* 1997; **17**(1): 25–31.

The International FMF Consortium. Ancient missense mutations in a new member of the RoRet gene family are likely to cause familial Mediterranean fever. *Cell* 1997; **90**(4): 797–807.

Klaver CE, Musters GD, Bemelman WA *et al.* Adjuvant hyperthermic intraperitoneal chemotherapy (HIPEC) in patients with colon cancer at high risk of peritoneal carcinomatosis; the COLOPEC randomized multicentre trial. *BMC Cancer* 2015; **24**;15: 428.

Lubner MG, Hinshaw JL, Pickhardt PJ. Primary malignant tumors of peritoneal and retroperitoneal origin: clinical and imaging features. *Surg Oncol Clin N Am* 2014; 23: 821–45

Moore KP, Aithal GP. Guidelines on the management of ascites in cirrhosis. *Gut* 2006; 55(Suppl 6): vi1–12.

Rasheed S, Zinicola R, Watson D, Bajwa A, McDonald PJ. Intra-abdominal and gastrointestinal tuberculosis. *Colorectal Dis* 2007; **9**: 773–83.

Rudloff U, Langan RC, Mullinax JE *et al.* Impact of maximal cytoreductive surgery plus regional heated intraperitoneal chemotherapy (HIPEC) on outcome of patients with peritoneal carcinomatosis of gastric origin: results of the GYMSSA trial. *J Surg Oncol* 2014; **110**(3): 275–84.

Sadler TW (2010). *Langman's medical embryology* (with CD-ROM), 11th edn. Baltimore, MD: Lippincott Williams & Wilkins.

Schnüriger B, Barmparas G, Branco BC, Lustenberger T, Inaba K, Demetriades D. Prevention of postoperative peritoneal adhesions: a review of the literature. *Am J Surg* 2011; **201**: 111–21.

Sugarbaker PH, Jablonski KA. Prognostic features of 51 colorectal and 130 appendiceal cancer patients with peritoneal carcinomatosis treated by cytoreductive surgery and intraperitoneal chemotherapy. *Ann Surg* 1995; **221**(2): 124–32

Chapter 62

The oesophagus

Learning objectives

To understand:

- The anatomy and physiology of the oesophagus and their relationship to disease
- The clinical features, investigations and treatment of benign and malignant disease with particular reference to the common adult disorders

BACKGROUND

Surgical anatomy

The oesophagus is a muscular tube, approximately 25 cm long, mainly occupying the posterior mediastinum and extending from the upper oesophageal sphincter (the cricopharyngeus muscle) in the neck to the junction with the cardia of the stomach. The musculature of the upper oesophagus, including the upper sphincter, is striated. This is followed by a transitional zone of both striated and smooth muscle with the proportion of the latter progressively increasing so that, in the lower half of the oesophagus, there is only smooth muscle. It is lined throughout with squamous epithelium. The parasympathetic nerve supply is mediated by branches of the vagus nerve that has synaptic connections to the myenteric (Auerbach's) plexus. Meissner's submucosal plexus is sparse in the oesophagus.

The upper sphincter consists of powerful striated muscle. The lower sphincter is more subtle and created by the asymmetrical arrangement of muscle fibres in the distal oesophageal wall just above the oesophagogastric junction. It is helpful to remember the distances 15, 25 and 40 cm for anatomical location during endoscopy (Figure 62.1).

Physiology

The main function of the oesophagus is to transfer food from the mouth to the stomach in a coordinated fashion. The initial movement from the mouth is voluntary. The pharyngeal phase of swallowing involves sequential contraction of the oropharyngeal musculature, closure of the nasal and respiratory passages, cessation of breathing and opening of the upper oesophageal sphincter. Beyond this level, swallowing is involuntary. The body of the oesophagus propels the bolus through a relaxed lower oesophageal sphincter (LOS) into the stomach, taking air with it (Figure 62.2). This coordinated oesophageal wave which follows a conscious swallow is called primary peristalsis. It is under vagal control, although there are specific neurotransmitters that control the LOS.

The upper oesophageal sphincter is normally closed at rest and serves as a protective mechanism against regurgitation of oesophageal contents into the respiratory passages. It also serves to stop air entering the oesophagus other than the small amount that enters during swallowing.

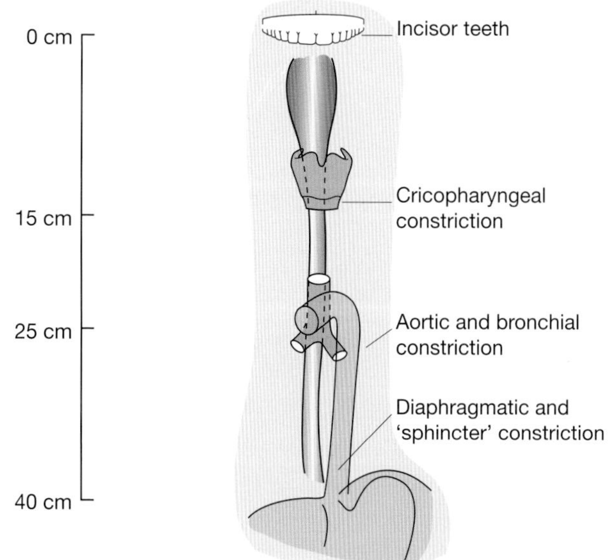

Figure 62.1 Endoscopic landmarks. Distances are given from the incisor teeth. They vary slightly with the build of the individual.

Leopold Auerbach, 1828–1897, Professor of Neuropathology, Breslau, Germany, (now Wroclaw, Poland), described the myenteric plexus in 1862.
Georg Meissner, 1829–1905, Professor of Physiology, Göttingen, Germany, described the submucosal plexus in 1852.

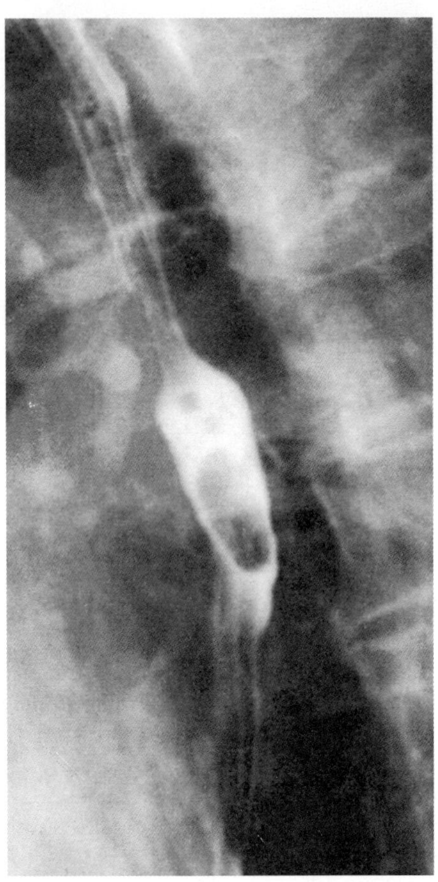

Figure 62.2 A bolus of barium or food usually takes air with it into the stomach.

The LOS is a zone of relatively high pressure that prevents gastric contents from refluxing into the lower oesophagus (Figure 62.3). In addition to opening in response to a primary peristaltic wave, the sphincter also relaxes to allow air to escape from the stomach and at the time of vomiting. A variety of factors influences sphincter tone, notably food, gastric distension, gastrointestinal (GI) hormones, drugs and smoking. The arrangement of muscle fibres, their differential responses to specific neurotransmitters and the relationship to diaphragmatic contraction all contribute to the action of the LOS. The presence of the physiological sphincter was first demonstrated by Code using manometry with small balloons. Until recently LOS pressure was measured by water-perfused tubes, but the introduction of catheters containing multiple microtransducers has meant that this approach has been superseded by high-resolution manometry. The normal LOS is 3–4 cm in length and has a pressure of 10–25 mmHg.

Manometry is also used to assess the speed and amplitude of oesophageal body contractions and ensure that peristalsis is propagated down the entire length of the oesophagus (Figure 62.4). Secondary peristalsis is the normal reflex preceded by a conscious swallow. It is worth remembering that most clearance swallows to neutralise refluxed gastric acid are, however, achieved by primary peristalsis, which carries saliva with its high bicarbonate content down to the lower oesophagus. Tertiary contractions are non-peristaltic waves that are infrequent (<10%) during laboratory-based manometry, although readily detected if manometry is undertaken while the patient eats a meal.

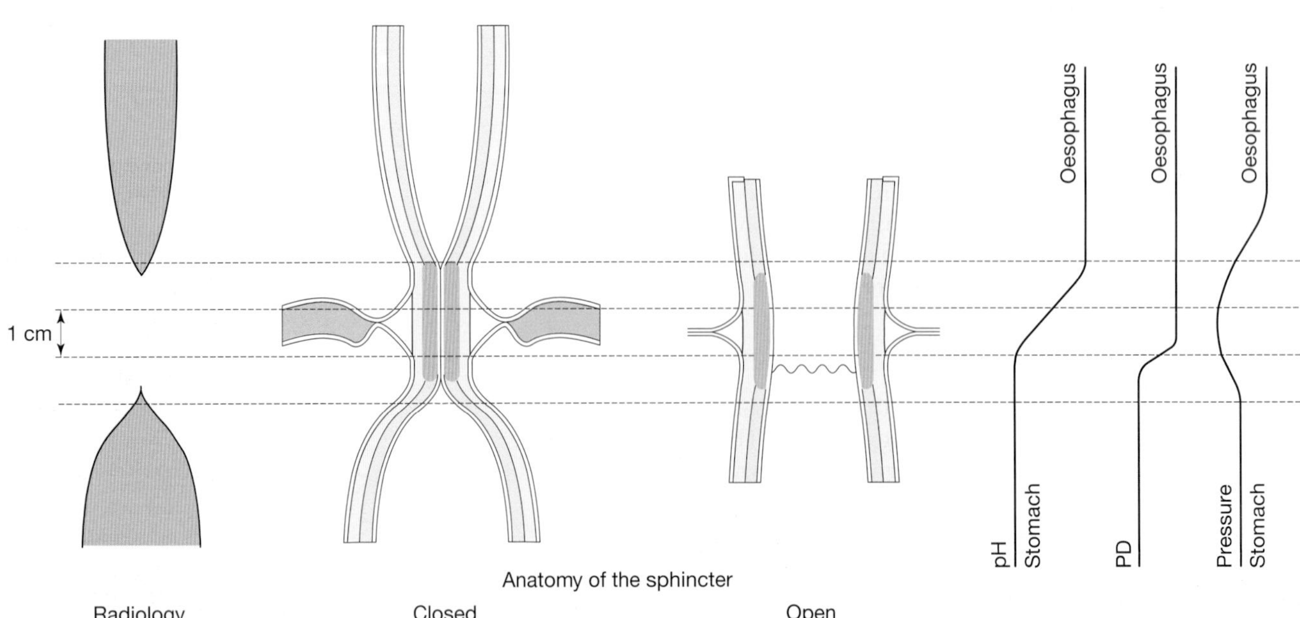

Figure 62.3 Correlation between the radiological appearances of a barium column and the lower oesophageal sphincter open and closed. The three curves on the right, set up vertically, show the pH gradient, the mucosal potential difference (PD), marking the junction of squamous and columnar epithelium, and the high-pressure zone of the sphincter.

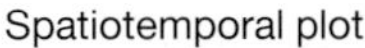

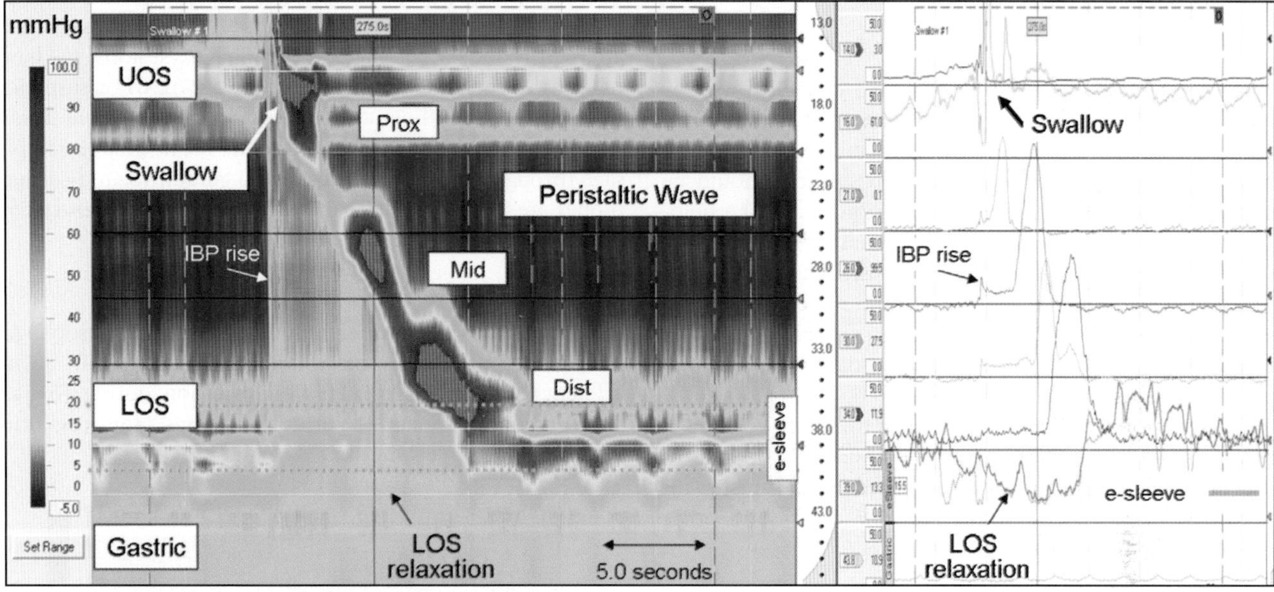

Figure 62.4 High-resolution manometry depicts oesophageal function from the pharynx to the stomach. The spatiotemporal plot presents the same information as presented in the 'conventional' line plots. Time is on the *x*-axis and distance from the nares is on the *y*-axis. Pressure is assigned a colour (legend right). The segmental anatomy of oesophagus is easy to appreciate (not seen on conventional manometry). The coordinated relaxation of the upper (UOS) and lower oesophageal sphincter (LOS) is obvious, as is the increasing pressure and duration of the peristaltic wave as it passes distally. The intrabolus pressure (IBP) between the peristaltic wave and oesophagogastric junction, and the pressure gradient across the gastro-oesophageal junction are visualized. These represent the force that drives bolus through the oesophagus and into the stomach.

Symptoms

Summary box 62.1

Symptoms of oesophageal disease

- Difficulty in swallowing described as food or fluid sticking (oesophageal dysphagia): must rule out malignancy
- Pain on swallowing (odynophagia): suggests inflammation and ulceration
- Regurgitation or reflux (heartburn): common in gastro-oesophageal reflux disease
- Chest pain: difficult to distinguish from cardiac pain

Dysphagia

Dysphagia is used to describe difficulty with swallowing. When there is a problem with swallowing in the voluntary (oral or pharyngeal) phases, patients will usually say that they cannot swallow properly, but they do not characteristically describe 'food sticking'. Instead, when they try to initiate a conscious swallow, food fails to enter the oesophagus, stays in the mouth or enters the airway, causing coughing or spluttering. Virtually all causes of this type of dysphagia are chronic neurological or muscular diseases. Oesophageal dysphagia occurs in the involuntary phase and is characterised by a sensation of food sticking. The nature of this type of dysphagia is often informative with regard to a likely diagnosis. Dysphagia may occur acutely or in a chronic fashion, can affect solids and/or fluids, and be intermittent or progressive. Although many patients point to a site of impaction, this is unreliable.

Odynophagia

Odynophagia refers to pain on swallowing. Patients with reflux oesophagitis often feel retrosternal discomfort within a few seconds of swallowing hot beverages, citrus drinks or alcohol. Odynophagia is also a feature of infective oesophagitis and may be particularly severe in chemical injury.

Regurgitation and reflux

Regurgitation and reflux are often used synonymously. It is helpful to differentiate between them, although it is not always possible. Regurgitation should strictly refer to the return of oesophageal contents from above a functional or mechanical obstruction. Reflux is the passive return of gastroduodenal contents to the mouth as part of the symptomatology of gastro-oesophageal reflux disease (GORD). Loss of weight, anaemia, cachexia, change of voice due to refluxed material irritating the vocal folds, and cough or dyspnoea due to tracheal aspiration may all accompany regurgitation and/or reflux.

Chest pain

Chest pain similar in character to angina pectoris may arise from an oesophageal cause, especially gastro-oesophageal reflux and motility disorders. Exercise-induced chest pain can be due to reflux.

Investigations

Radiography

Contrast radiography has been somewhat overshadowed by endoscopy but remains a useful investigation to demonstrate changes in oesophageal diameter, anatomical distortion or abnormal motility. An adequate barium swallow should be tailored to the problem under investigation. It may be helpful to give a solid bolus (bread or marshmallow) if a motility disorder is suspected. Video recording is useful to allow subsequent replay and detailed analysis. Barium radiology is, however, inaccurate in the diagnosis of gastro-oesophageal reflux, unless reflux is gross, and should not be used for this purpose. Plain radiographs will show some foreign bodies.

Cross-sectional imaging by computed tomography (CT) is now an essential investigation in the assessment of neoplasms of the oesophagus and can be used in place of a contrast swallow to demonstrate perforation. The role of CT and other cancer-specific tests is described later.

Endoscopy

Endoscopy is necessary for the investigation of most oesophageal conditions. It is required to view the inside of the oesophagus and the oesophagogastric junction, to obtain a biopsy or cytology specimen, for the removal of foreign bodies and to dilate strictures. Traditionally, there are two types of instrument available, the rigid oesophagoscope and the flexible video endoscope, but the rigid instrument is now virtually obsolete.

For flexible video gastroduodenoscopy, general anaesthesia is not required; most examinations can be done on an outpatient basis, and the quality of the magnified image is superb. The technology associated with video endoscopy continues to improve. Magnification is a standard feature of the modern endoscope and widely used in conjunction with agents that can be sprayed on to the mucosa, such as acetic acid to enhance mucosal detail. Novel techniques that rely on fluorescence and narrow band imaging to enhance visual contrast are becoming increasingly used for the identification of mucosal abnormalities that are not easily seen with white light, e.g. in patients with Barrett's oesophagus undergoing endoscopic surveillance.

As a matter of routine, the stomach and duodenum are examined as well as the oesophagus. If a stricture is encountered, it may be helpful to dilate it to allow a complete inspection of the upper GI tract, but this decision should be dictated by clinical circumstances and an appreciation of the perforation risk, especially if the visual appearances are thought to indicate neoplasia.

Endosonography

Endoscopic ultrasonography relies on a high-frequency (5–30 MHz) transducer located at the tip of the endoscope to provide highly detailed images of the layers of the oesophageal wall and mediastinal structures close to the oesophagus. Radial echoendoscopes have a rotating transducer that creates a circular image with the endoscope in the centre, and this type of scanner is widely used to create diagnostic transverse sectional images at right angles to the long axis of the oesophagus (Figure 62.5). Linear echoendoscopes produce a sectoral image in the line of the endoscope and are used to biopsy submucosal oesophageal lesions, mediastinal masses such as lymph nodes (Figure 62.6) or suspicious lesions that might lie outside a proposed surgical field. Radial scanners without optical components are available for passage through narrow strictures over a guidewire, and catheter probes are available that can be passed down the endoscope biopsy channel.

Oesophageal manometry

Manometry is now widely used to diagnose oesophageal motility disorders. Electronic microtransducers that are not influenced by changes in patient position during the test have gradually supplanted perfusion systems. High-resolution

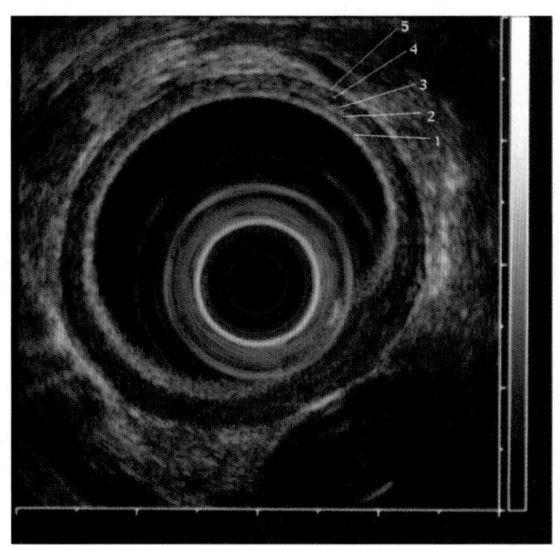

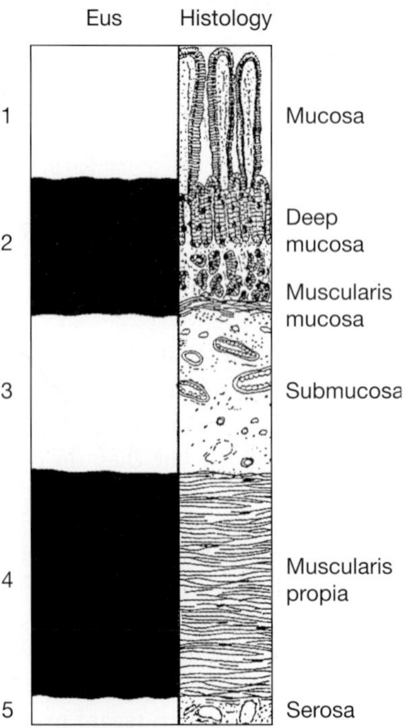

Figure 62.5 Radial endosonography indicating wall layers as alternating hyper- and hypoechoic bands.

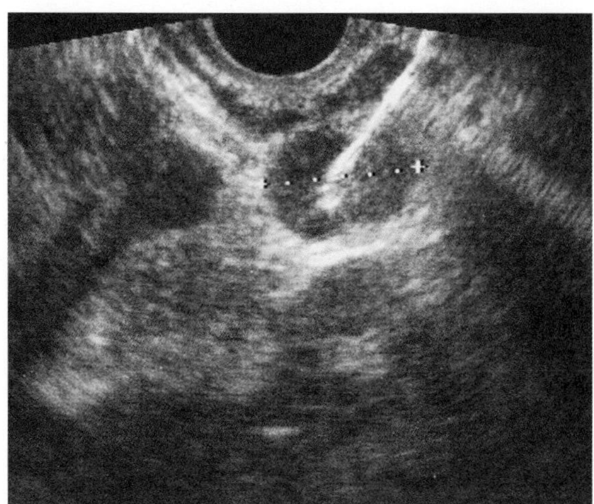

Figure 62.6 Linear endosonography with the needle traversing an ultrasound plane for guided biopsy.

manometry uses a multiple (up to 36) microtransducer catheter with the results displayed as spatiotemporal plots, and this has now largely supplanted earlier manometry systems. This system provides comprehensive information about oesophageal body function and associated behaviour of the LOS.

Twenty-four-hour pH and combined pH-impedance recording

Prolonged measurement of pH is now accepted as the most accurate method for the diagnosis of gastro-oesophageal reflux. It is particularly useful in patients with atypical reflux symptoms, those without endoscopic oesophagitis and when patients respond poorly to intensive medical therapy. A small pH probe is passed into the distal oesophagus and positioned 5 cm above the upper margin of the LOS, as defined by manometry. The probe is connected to a miniature digital recorder that is worn on a belt and allows most normal activities. Patients mark symptomatic events such as heartburn. A 24-hour recording period is usual, and the pH record is analysed by an automated computer program. An oesophageal pH <4 at the level of the pH electrode is conventionally considered the cut-off value and, in most oesophageal laboratories, the total time when pH is <4 in a 24-hour period does not exceed 4% in a healthy adult. Patterns of reflux and the correlation between symptoms and oesophageal pH <4 can be calculated. Most laboratories use a scoring system (Johnson–DeMeester) to create a numerical value, above which reflux is considered pathological. Radiotelemetry pH probes are also available that can be fixed to the oesophageal wall endoscopically without the need for a transnasal catheter. The introduction of catheter assemblies that incorporate multiple electrodes along the length of the catheter, as well as a pH probe, has resulted in combined measurement of pH and electrical impedance. Impedance measurement differentiates anterograde from retrograde bolus transit and gas from liquid, and provides a reliable measure of non-acidic or weakly acidic events that cause symptoms. This may be important in the identification of patients with non-erosive reflux disease on endoscopy.

Therapeutic procedures

Dilatation of strictures

Stricture dilatation is essentially undertaken for benign conditions and should be used with caution in the context of malignant disease. The risks associated with dilatation for malignant disease are discussed later. The advent of guidewire-directed dilatation of the oesophagus in the 1970s was a major advance over earlier blind dilatation systems. Their use is now considered standard practice. There are many different designs, but essentially they are solid dilators of increasing diameter or inflatable balloons with rigid walls. To restore normal swallowing, a stricture should be dilated to at least 16 mm in diameter, although this may need to be achieved over a series of procedures, depending on the perceived nature of the stricture. A guidewire is passed down the biopsy channel of an endoscope and through the stricture under vision. If the stricture is long or tortuous, this should be undertaken under radiological guidance to ensure that the guidewire passes easily into the stomach. The endoscope is withdrawn, leaving the guidewire in place, and graduated dilators or a balloon dilator are passed over the guidewire, sometimes with radiographic screening for safety purposes. The dilatation of reflux-induced strictures is usually straightforward. These strictures are nearly always short and at the oesophagogastric junction, so that the stomach is visible through the narrowed segment. Radiological control is rarely needed. Conversely, distal oesophageal adenocarcinomas extending into the stomach are often soft, friable and tortuous to negotiate. Caustic strictures often occur high in the thorax and may be very long.

Balloons for oesophageal use tend to have inflation diameters of 25–40 mm and may also be used for dilatation. Pneumatic dilatation is widely used to disrupt the non-relaxing LOS in achalasia.

Thermal recanalisation

Various types of laser (mainly Nd–YAG), bipolar diathermy, injection of absolute alcohol or argon-beam plasma coagulation have all been used successfully to ablate tissue in order to recanalise the oesophagus.

CONGENITAL ABNORMALITIES

See Chapter 9.

FOREIGN BODIES IN THE OESOPHAGUS

All manner of foreign bodies have become arrested in the oesophagus (Figure 62.7). Button batteries may be a troublesome problem in children. The most common impacted

Lawrence F Johnson, gastroenterologist, Birmingham, AL, USA.
Tom R DeMeester, Professor of Surgery, Los Angeles, CA, USA.

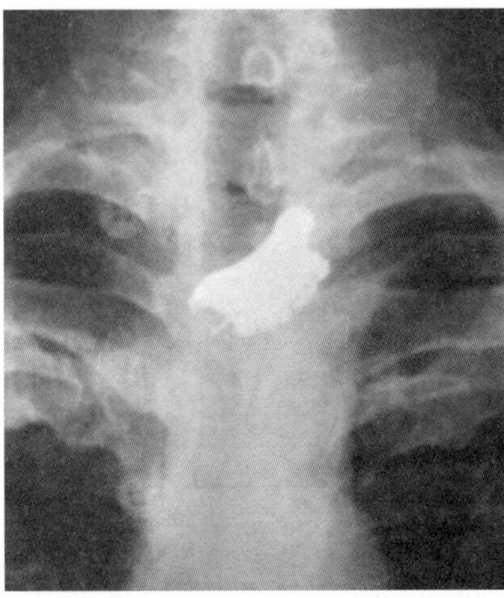

Figure 62.7 False teeth impacted in the oesophagus. (Note: modern dentures are usually radiolucent.)

material is food, and this usually occurs above a significant pathological lesion (Figure 62.8). Plain radiographs are often useful for foreign bodies, but modern denture materials are not always radiopaque. A contrast examination is not usually required and only makes endoscopy more difficult.

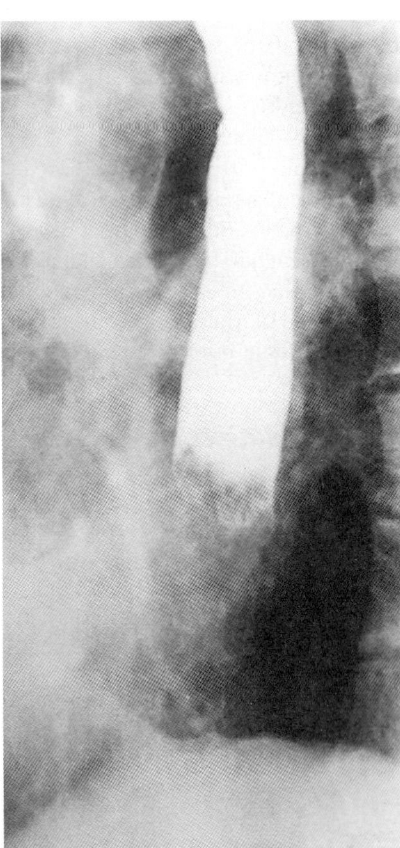

Figure 62.8 An impacted meat bolus at the lower end of the oesophagus. This may be the first presentation of a benign stricture or a malignant tumour.

Summary box 62.2

Foreign bodies

- The most common is a food bolus, which usually signifies underlying disease
- It is usually possible to remove foreign bodies by flexible endoscopy
- Beware of button batteries in the oesophagus

Foreign bodies that have become stuck in the oesophagus should be removed by flexible endoscopy using suitable grasping forceps, a snare or a basket. If the object may injure the oesophagus on withdrawal, an overtube can be used, and the endoscope and object can be withdrawn into the overtube before removal. Button batteries can be a particular worry because they are difficult to grasp, and it is tempting to push them on into the stomach. However, an exhausted battery may rapidly corrode in the GI tract and is best extracted. A multiwire basket of the type used for gallstone retrieval nearly always works. An impacted food bolus will often break up and pass on if the patient is given fizzy drinks and confined to fluids for a short time. The cause of the impaction must then be investigated. If symptoms are severe or the bolus does not pass, it can be extracted or broken up at endoscopy.

PERFORATION

Perforation of the oesophagus is usually iatrogenic (at therapeutic endoscopy) or due to 'barotrauma' (spontaneous perforation). Many instrumental perforations can be managed conservatively, but spontaneous perforation is often a life-threatening condition that regularly requires surgical intervention.

Summary box 62.3

Perforation of the oesophagus

- Potentially lethal complication due to mediastinitis and septic shock
- Numerous causes, but may be iatrogenic
- Surgical emphysema is virtually pathognomonic
- Treatment is urgent; it may be conservative or surgical, but requires specialised care

Barotrauma (spontaneous perforation, Boerhaave's syndrome)

This occurs classically when a person vomits against a closed glottis. The pressure in the oesophagus increases rapidly, and the oesophagus bursts at its weakest point in the lower third, sending a stream of material into the mediastinum and often the pleural cavity as well. The condition was first identified by Boerhaave, who reported the case of a grand admiral of

Hermann Boerhaave, 1668–1738, Professor of Medicine and Botany, the University of Leiden, the Netherlands, creator of the modern method of clinical teaching.

the Dutch fleet who was a glutton and practised autoemesis. Boerhaave's syndrome is the most serious type of perforation because of the large volume of material that is released under pressure. This causes rapid chemical irritation in the mediastinum and pleura followed by infection if untreated. Barotrauma has also been described in relation to other pressure events when the patient strains against a closed glottis (e.g. defecation, labour, weight-lifting).

Diagnosis of spontaneous perforation

The clinical history is usually of severe pain in the chest or upper abdomen after a meal or a bout of drinking. Associated shortness of breath is common. Many cases are misdiagnosed as myocardial infarction, perforated peptic ulcer or pancreatitis if the pain is confined to the upper abdomen. There may be a surprising amount of rigidity on examination of the upper abdomen, even in the absence of any peritoneal contamination.

The diagnosis can usually be suspected from the history and associated clinical features. A chest radiograph is often confirmatory with air in the mediastinum, pleura or peritoneum. Pleural effusion occurs rapidly either as a result of free communication with the pleural space or as a reaction to adjacent inflammation in the mediastinum. A contrast swallow or CT is nearly always required to guide management (Figure 62.9).

Pathological perforation

Free perforation of ulcers or tumours of the oesophagus into the pleural space is rare. Erosion into an adjacent structure with fistula formation is more common. Aerodigestive fistula is most common and usually encountered in primary malignant disease of the oesophagus or bronchus. Coughing on eating and signs of aspiration pneumonitis may allow the problem to be recognised at a time when intervention may be appropriate and feasible. Covering the communication with a self-expanding metal stent is the usual solution. Erosion into a major vascular structure is invariably fatal.

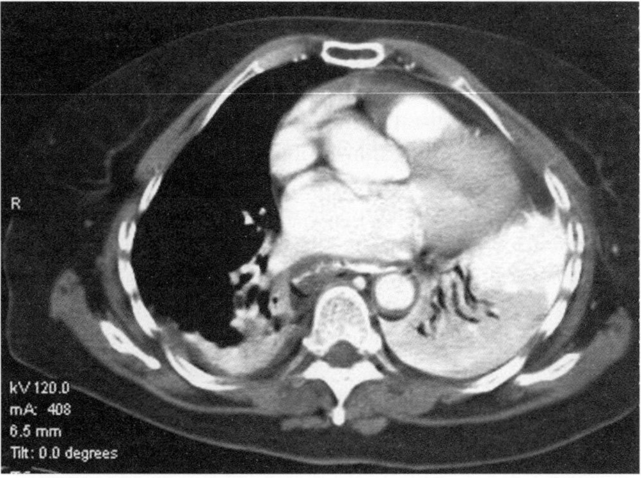

Figure 62.9 Computed tomography scan showing the site of perforation in the lower oesophagus.

Penetrating injury

Perforation by knives and bullets is uncommon, even in war, because the oesophagus is a relatively small target surrounded by other vital organs.

Foreign bodies

The oesophagus may be perforated during removal of a foreign body but, occasionally, an object that has been left in the oesophagus for several days will erode through the wall.

Instrumental perforation

Instrumentation is by far the most common cause of perforation. Modern instrumentation is remarkably safe, but perforation remains a risk that should never be forgotten.

Summary box 62.4

Instrumental perforation

- Prevention of perforation is better than cure

Perforation related to diagnostic upper GI endoscopy is unusual with an estimated frequency of about 1:4000 examinations. Perforation can occur in the pharynx or oesophagus, usually at sites of pathology or when the endoscope is passed blindly. A number of patient-related factors are associated with increased risk, including large anterior cervical osteophytes, the presence of a pharyngeal pouch and mechanical causes of obstruction. Perforation may follow biopsy of a malignant tumour.

Patients undergoing therapeutic endoscopy have a perforation risk that is at least 10 times greater than those undergoing diagnostic endoscopy. The oesophagus may be perforated by guidewires, graduated dilators or balloons, or during the placement of self-expanding stents. The risk is considerably higher in patients with malignancy.

Diagnosis of instrumental perforation

In most cases, a combination of technical difficulties and an interventional procedure should lead to a high index of suspicion. History and physical signs may be useful pointers to the site of perforation.

Cervical perforation may result in pain localised to the neck, hoarseness, painful neck movements and subcutaneous emphysema. Intrathoracic and intra-abdominal perforations, which are more common, can give rise to immediate symptoms and signs either during or at the end of the procedure, including chest pain, haemodynamic instability, oxygen desaturation or visual evidence of perforation. Within the first 24 hours, patients may additionally complain of abdominal pain or respiratory difficulties. There may be evidence of subcutaneous emphysema, pneumothorax or hydropneumothorax. In some patients, the diagnosis may be missed and recognised only at a late stage beyond 24 hours, as unexplained pyrexia, systemic sepsis or the development of a clinical fistula.

Prompt and thorough investigation is the key to management. Careful endoscopic assessment at the end of any procedure combined with a chest radiograph will identify many cases of perforation immediately. If not recognised immediately, then early and late suspected perforations should be assessed by CT. A pre-contrast scan easily demonstrates air outside the GI tract, while oral contrast localises the site of the oesophageal defect and accurately delineates specific fluid collections. Where CT is not available, a water-soluble contrast swallow should be performed although this is not always reliable in disclosing a small contained leak. If a water-soluble study is negative and clinical suspicion is high, a dilute barium swallow should be considered.

Treatment of oesophageal perforations

Perforation of the oesophagus usually leads to mediastinitis. The loose areolar tissues of the posterior mediastinum allow a rapid spread of GI contents. The aim of treatment is to limit mediastinal contamination and prevent or deal with infection. Operative repair deals with the injury directly, but imposes risks of its own; non-operative treatment aims to limit the effects of mediastinitis and provide an environment in which healing can take place.

The decision between surgical and non-surgical management rests on four factors. These are:

1. the site of the perforation (cervical vs thoracoabdominal oesophagus);
2. the event causing the perforation (spontaneous vs instrumental);
3. underlying pathology (benign or malignant);
4. the status of the oesophagus before the perforation (fasted and empty vs obstructed with a stagnant residue).

It follows that most perforations that can be managed non-surgically occur in the context of small instrumental perforations of a clean oesophagus without obstruction, where leakage is likely to be confined to the nearby mediastinum at worst (*Table 62.1*).

Instrumental perforations in the cervical oesophagus are usually small and can nearly always be managed conservatively. The development of a local abscess is an indication for cervical drainage, preventing the extension of sepsis into the mediastinum.

TABLE 62.1 Management options in perforation of the oesophagus.

Factors that favour non-surgical management	Factors that favour surgical repair
Small septic load	Large septic load
Minimal cardiovascular upset	Septic shock
Perforation confined to mediastinum	Pleura breached
Perforation by flexible endoscope	Boerhaave's syndrome
Perforation of cervical oesophagus	Perforation of abdominal oesophagus

The conservative management of an instrumental perforation in the thoracoabdominal parts of the oesophagus can be undertaken when the perforation is detected early and before oral alimentation. General guidelines for non-surgical management include:

- pain that is readily controlled with opiates;
- absence of crepitus, diffuse mediastinal gas, hydropneumothorax or pneumoperitoneum;
- mediastinal containment of the perforation with no evidence of widespread extravasation of contrast material;
- no evidence of on-going luminal obstruction or a retained foreign body.

In addition, conservative management might be appropriate in patients who have remained clinically stable despite diagnostic delay. The principles of non-interventional management involve hyperalimentation, preferably by an enteral route, nasogastric suction and broad-spectrum intravenous antibiotics.

Surgical management is required whenever patients:

- are unstable with sepsis or shock;
- have evidence of a heavily contaminated mediastinum, pleural space or peritoneum;
- have widespread intrapleural or intraperitoneal extravasation of contrast material.

Ongoing luminal obstruction (often related to malignancy) in a frail patient considered unfit for major surgery can be dealt with by placement of a covered self-expanding stent. Expanding metal stents should be used with caution in patients with benign disease because they cause significant tissue reaction and some designs are impossible to remove at a later date. Biodegradable and removable stents may be used alone or as a bridge to later definitive treatment where perforation accompanies obstruction.

For patients requiring surgery, the choice is from direct repair, the deliberate creation of an external fistula or, rarely, oesophageal resection with a view to delayed reconstruction. Direct repair is preferred by many surgeons if the perforation is recognised early (within the first 4–6 hours), and the extent of mediastinal and pleural contamination is small. After 12 hours, the tissues become swollen and friable and less suitable for direct suture. The hole in the mucosa is always bigger than the hole in the muscle, and the muscle should be incised to see the mucosal edges clearly. It is essential that there should be no obstruction distal to the repair. A variety of local tissues (gastric fundus, pericardium, intercostal muscle) have been used to buttress such repairs.

Primary repair is inadvisable with late presentation and in the presence of widespread mediastinal and pleural contamination. These patients tend to be more ill as a result of the delay, and the aim of treatment should be to achieve wide drainage with the creation of a controlled fistula and distal enteral feeding. This can usually be achieved by placing a T-tube into the oesophagus along with appropriately located drains and a feeding jejunostomy. In unusual circumstances, e.g. with extensive necrosis after corrosive ingestion, emergency oesophagectomy may be necessary. Oesophagostomy and gastrostomy should be performed with a view to delayed reconstruction.

MALLORY-WEISS SYNDROME

Forceful vomiting may produce a mucosal tear at the cardia rather than a full perforation. The mechanism of injury is different. In Boerhaave's syndrome, vomiting occurs against a closed glottis and pressure builds up in the oesophagus. In Mallory–Weiss syndrome, vigorous vomiting produces a vertical split in the gastric mucosa, immediately below the squamocolumnar junction at the cardia in 90% of cases. In only 10% is the tear in the oesophagus (Figure 62.10). The condition presents with haematemesis. Usually, the bleeding is not severe, but endoscopic injection therapy may be required for the occasional, severe case. Surgery is rarely required. There are two other injuries to the oesophagus that lie within the spectrum of the mucosal tear of Mallory–Weiss and the full-thickness tear of Boerhaave. Intramural rupture produces a dissection within the oesophageal wall that causes severe chest pain, often with odynophagia. It is best diagnosed by contrast radiology. Intramural haematoma is seen most often in elderly patients on anticoagulants or patients with coagulation disorders, and usually follows an episode of vomiting. Large haematomas causing dysphagia can occur, extending from the cardia up to the carina. The diagnosis is readily made on endoscopy. Both intramural rupture and intramural haematoma can be managed conservatively. Symptoms usually resolve in 7–14 days, and oral intake can be reinstituted as soon as symptoms allow.

CORROSIVE INJURY

Corrosives such as sodium hydroxide (lye, caustic soda) or sulphuric acid may be taken in an attempted suicide. Accidental ingestion occurs in children and when corrosives are stored in bottles labelled as beverages. All can cause severe damage to the mouth, pharynx, larynx, oesophagus and stomach. The type of agent, its concentration and the volume ingested largely determine the extent of damage. In general, alkalis are relatively odourless and tasteless, making them more likely to be ingested in large volume. Alkalis cause liquefaction, saponification of fats, dehydration and thrombosis of blood vessels which usually leads to fibrous scarring. Acids cause coagulative necrosis with eschar formation, and this coagulant may limit penetration to deeper layers of the oesophageal wall. Acids also cause more gastric damage than alkalis because of the induction of intense pylorospasm with pooling in the antrum.

Symptoms and signs are notoriously unreliable in predicting the severity of injury. The key to management is early endoscopy by an experienced endoscopist to inspect the whole of the oesophagus and stomach (Figure 62.11). Deep ulcers and the recognition of a grey or black eschar signify the most severe lesions with the greatest risk of perforation. Minor injuries with only oedema of the mucosa resolve rapidly with no late sequelae. These patients can safely be fed. With more severe injuries, a feeding jejunostomy may be appropriate until the patient can swallow saliva satisfactorily. The widespread use of broad-spectrum antibiotics and steroids is not supported by evidence.

Regular endoscopic examinations are the best way to assess stricture development (Figure 62.12). Significant stricture formation occurs in about 50% of patients with extensive mucosal damage (Figure 62.13). The role and timing of repeat endoscopies with or without dilatation in such patients

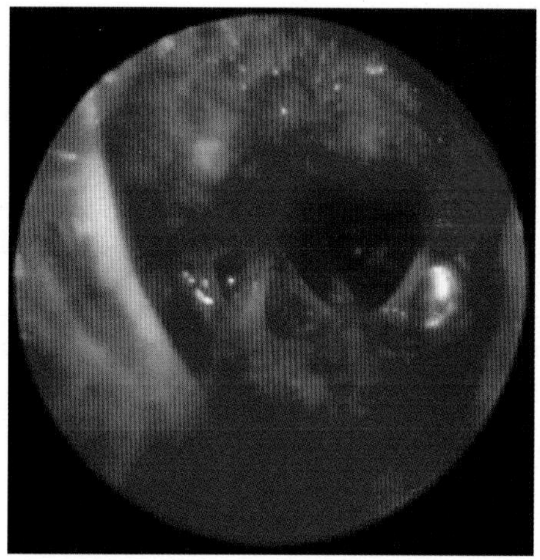

Figure 62.11 Acute caustic burn in the haemorrhagic phase.

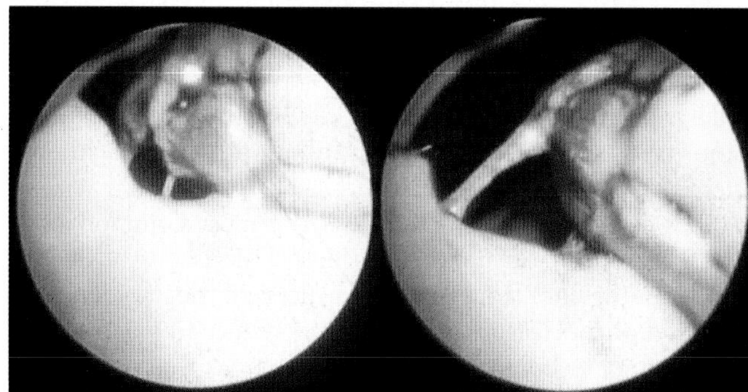

Figure 62.10 The endoscopic appearance of a mucosal tear at the cardia (Mallory–Weiss).

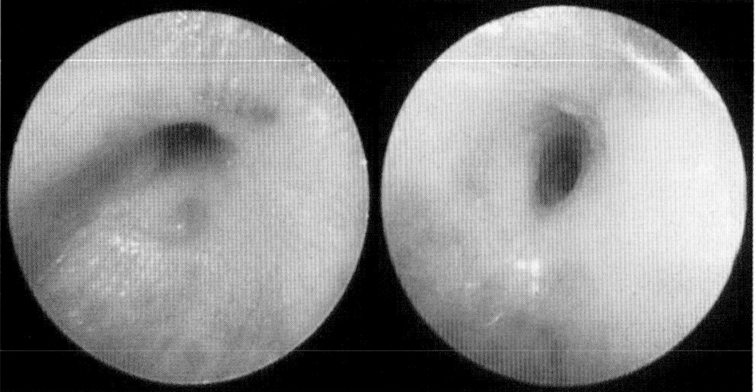

Figure 62.12 The late result of a caustic alkali burn with a high oesophageal stricture.

George Kenneth Mallory, b.1926, Professor of Pathology, Boston University, Boston, MA, USA.
Soma Weiss, 1898–1942, Professor of Medicine, Harvard University Medical School, Boston, MA, USA.

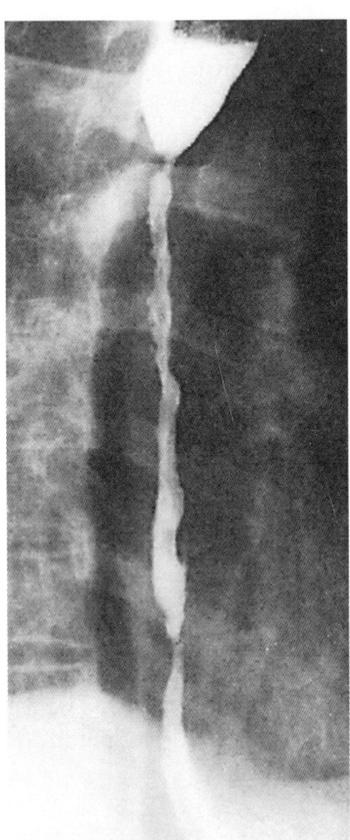

Figure 62.13 Caustic or lye stricture with marked stenosis high in the body of the oesophagus. The strictures are frequently multiple and difficult to dilate unless treated energetically at an early stage.

remain controversial. Other than the need for emergency surgery for bleeding or perforation, elective oesophageal resection should be deferred for at least 3 months until the fibrotic phase has been established. Oesophageal replacement is usually required for very long or multiple strictures. Resection can be difficult because of perioesophageal inflammation in these patients. Because of associated gastric damage, colon may have to be used as the replacement conduit.

There is also controversy with regard to the risk of developing carcinoma in the damaged oesophagus and stomach and how this might influence management. The lifetime risk is certainly less than 5%. Some surgeons advocate resection and replacement, whereas others believe that oesophageal bypass and endoscopic surveillance are preferable, because removal of the badly damaged oesophagus from a scarred mediastinum can be hazardous.

Summary box 62.5

Corrosive injury

- Skilled early endoscopy is mandatory

DRUG-INDUCED INJURY

Many medications, such as antibiotics and potassium preparations, are potentially damaging to the oesophagus, because tablets may remain for a long time, especially if taken without an adequate drink. Acute injury presents with dysphagia and odynophagia, which may be severe. The inflammation usually resolves within 2–3 weeks, and no specific treatment is required apart from appropriate nutritional support. A stricture may follow.

GASTRO-OESOPHAGEAL REFLUX DISEASE

Aetiology

Normal competence of the gastro-oesophageal junction is maintained by the LOS. This is influenced by both its physiological function and its anatomical location relative to the diaphragm and the oesophageal hiatus. In normal circumstances, the LOS transiently relaxes as a coordinated part of swallowing, as a means of allowing vomiting to occur and in response to stretching of the gastric fundus, particularly after a meal to allow swallowed air to be vented. Most episodes of physiological reflux occur during postprandial transient LOS relaxations (TLOSRs). In the early stages of GORD, most pathological reflux occurs as a result of an increased number of TLOSRs rather than a persistent fall in overall sphincter pressure. In more severe GORD, LOS pressure tends to be generally low, and this loss of sphincter function seems to be made worse if there is loss of an adequate length of intra-abdominal oesophagus.

The absence of an intra-abdominal length of oesophagus results in a sliding hiatus hernia. The normal condensation of peritoneal fascia over the lower oesophagus (the phreno-oesophageal ligament) is weak, and the crural opening widens, allowing the upper stomach to slide up through the hiatus. The loss of the normal anatomical configuration exacerbates reflux, although sliding hiatus hernia alone should not be viewed as the cause of reflux. Sliding hiatus hernia is associated with GORD and may make it worse but, as long as the LOS remains competent, pathological GORD does not occur. Many GORD sufferers do not have a hernia, and many of those with a hernia do not have GORD. It should be noted that rolling or paraoesophageal hiatus hernia is a quite different and potentially dangerous condition (see below). A proportion of patients have a rolling hernia and symptomatic GORD or a mixed hernia with both sliding and rolling components. Reflux oesophagitis that is visible endoscopically is a complication of GORD and occurs in a minority of sufferers overall, but in around 40% of patients referred to hospital.

In western societies, GORD is the most common condition affecting the upper GI tract. This is partly due to the declining incidence of peptic ulcer as the incidence of infection with *Helicobacter pylori* has reduced as a result of improved socioeconomic conditions, along with a rising incidence of GORD in the last 30 years. The cause of the increase is unclear, but may be due in part to increasing obesity. The strong association between GORD, obesity and the parallel rise in the incidence of adenocarcinoma of the oesophagus represents a major health challenge for most western countries.

Clinical features

The classic triad of symptoms is retrosternal burning pain (heartburn), epigastric pain (sometimes radiating through to the back) and regurgitation. Most patients do not experience all three. Symptoms are often provoked by food, particularly those that delay gastric emptying (e.g. fats, spicy foods). As the condition becomes more severe, gastric juice may reflux to the mouth and produce an unpleasant taste, often described as 'acid' or 'bitter'. Heartburn and regurgitation can be brought on by stooping or exercise. A proportion of patients have odynophagia with hot beverages, citrus drinks or alcohol. Patients with nocturnal reflux and those who reflux food to the mouth nearly always have severe GORD. Some patients present with less typical symptoms such as angina-like chest pain, pulmonary or laryngeal symptoms. Dysphagia is usually a sign that a stricture has occurred, but may be caused by an associated motility disorder.

As GORD is such a common disorder, it should always be the first thought when a patient presents with oesophageal symptoms that are unusual or that defy diagnosis after a series of investigations.

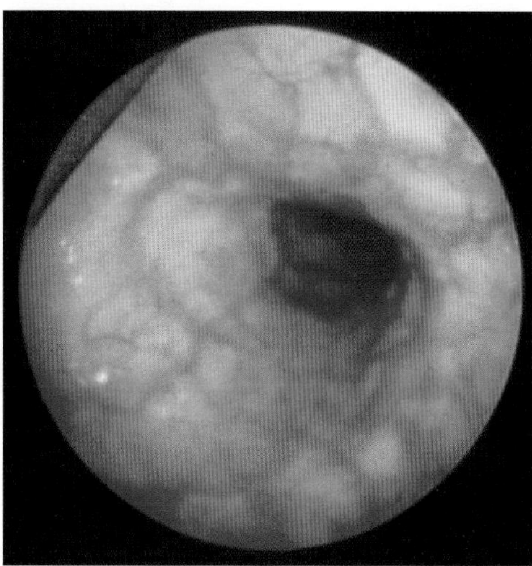

Figure 62.14 The endoscopic appearance of the normal squamous mucosa in the body of the oesophagus.

Diagnosis

In most cases, the diagnosis is assumed rather than proven, and treatment is empirical. Investigation is required only when the diagnosis is in doubt, when the patient does not respond to a proton pump inhibitor (PPI) or if dysphagia is present. The most appropriate examination is endoscopy with biopsy. If the typical appearance of reflux oesophagitis, peptic stricture or Barrett's oesophagus is seen, the diagnosis is clinched, but visible oesophagitis is not always present, even in patients selected as above. This is compounded in clinical practice by the widespread use of PPIs, which cause rapid healing of early mucosal lesions. Many patients will have received such treatment before referral. The endoscopic appearances of the normal oesophagus, hiatus hernia, oesophagitis and stricture are shown in Figures 62.14–62.20. It is worth remembering that the correlation between symptoms and endoscopic appearances is poor. On the other hand, there is a strong correlation between worsening endoscopic appearances and the duration of oesophageal acidification on pH testing.

In patients with atypical or persistent symptoms despite therapy, oesophageal manometry and 24-hour oesophageal pH recording (ideally with impedance measurement) may be justified to establish the diagnosis and guide management.

Summary box 62.6

Diagnostic measurement in GORD

- 24-hour pH recording is the 'gold standard' for diagnosis of GORD
- Length and pressure of the LOS are important

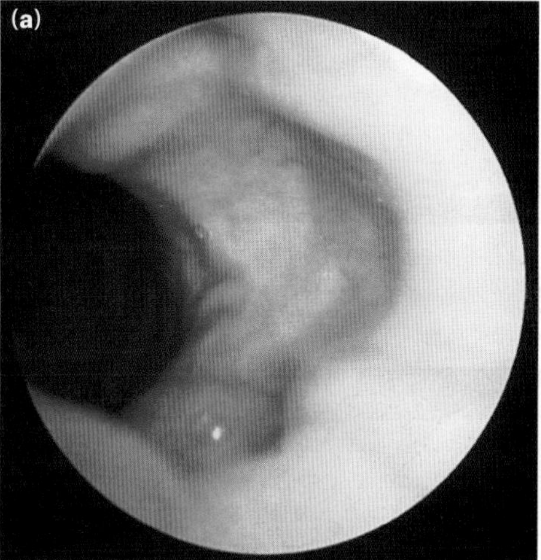

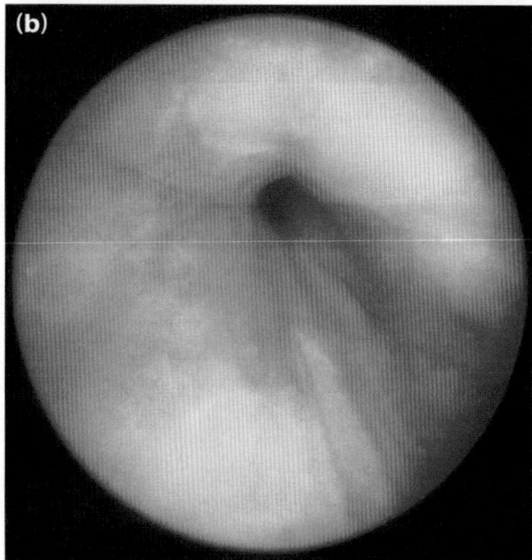

Figure 62.15 The normal lower oesophageal sphincter: (a) open; (b) closed.

Norman Rupert Barrett, 1903–1979, surgeon, St Thomas' Hospital, London, UK.

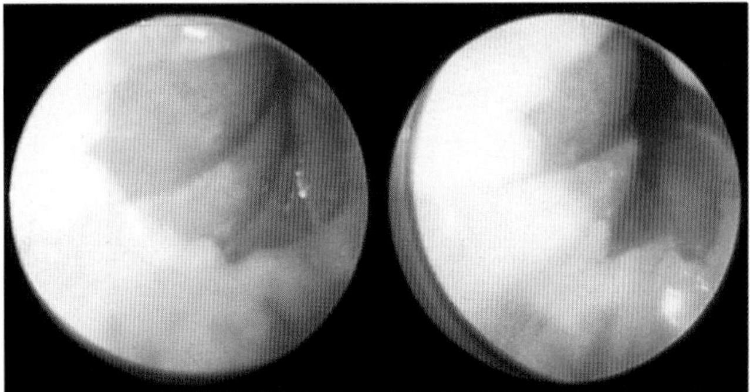

Figure 62.16 The squamocolumnar junction is clearly seen in the lower oesophagus with a normal sharp demarcation.

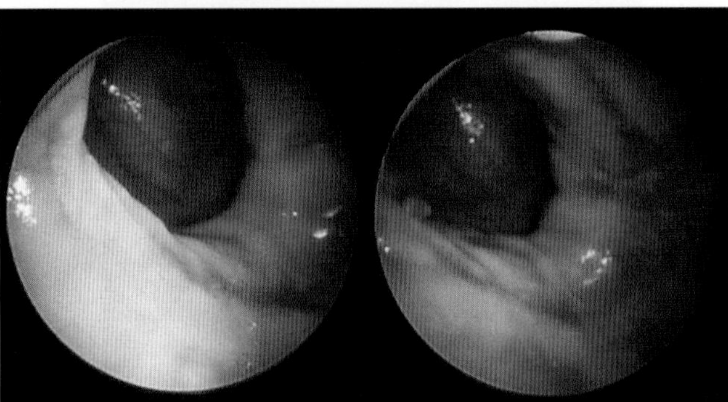

Figure 62.17 Sliding hiatus hernia. The diaphragm can be seen constricting the upper stomach.

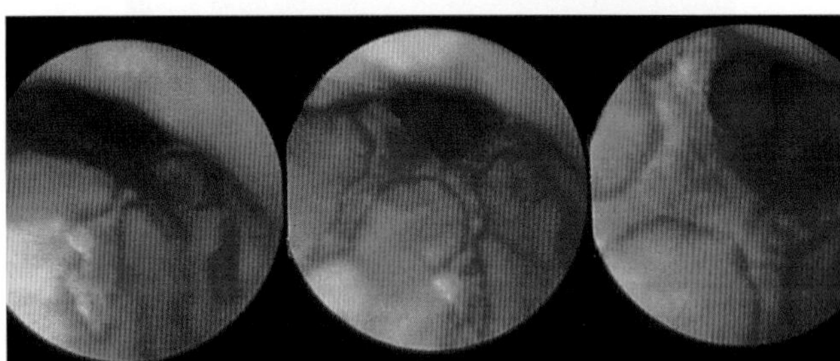

Figure 62.18 Reflux oesophagitis.

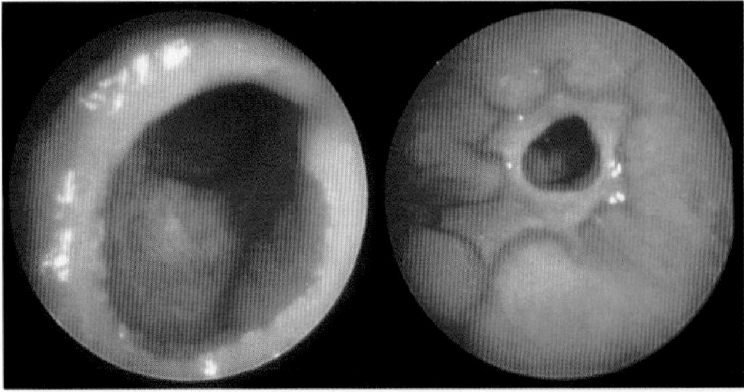

Figure 62.19 Benign stricture with active oesophagitis (left) and healed with columnar epithelium (right).

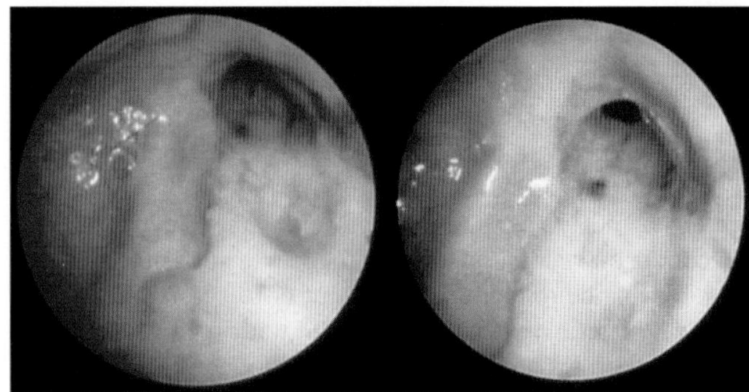

Figure 62.20 Ulceration associated with a benign peptic stricture.

As a matter of routine, proton pump inhibitors (PPIs) are stopped 1 week before oesophageal pH recording, but acid secretion is sometimes reduced for 2 weeks or more, and this can necessitate repeat examination after a prolonged interval without a PPI. Manometry and pH recording are essential in patients being considered for antireflux surgery. Although the main purpose of the test is objectively to quantify the extent of reflux disease, it is also used to rule out a diagnosis of achalasia. In the early stages of achalasia, chest pain can dominate the clinical picture and, when associated with intermittent swallowing problems and non-specific symptoms, it is easy to see how a clinical diagnosis of GORD might be made. Patients with achalasia can also have an abnormal pH study as a result of fermentation of food residue in a dilated oesophagus. Usually, the form of the pH trace is different from that of GORD, with slow undulations of pH rather than rapid bursts of reflux, but the complete absence of peristalsis on manometry is pathognomonic of achalasia.

A CT scan gives the best appreciation of gastro-oesophageal anatomy. This may be important in the context of surgery for rolling or mixed hiatus hernias, but it is unimportant in most patients with GORD.

Management of uncomplicated GORD

Medical management

Most sufferers from GORD do not consult a doctor and do not need to do so. They self-medicate with over-the-counter medicines such as simple antacids, antacid–alginate preparations, H_2-receptor antagonists or PPIs. Consultation is more likely when symptoms are severe, prolonged and unresponsive to the above treatments. Simple measures that are often neglected include advice about weight loss, smoking, excessive consumption of alcohol, tea or coffee, the avoidance of large meals late at night and a modest degree of head-up tilt of the bed. Tilting the bed has been shown to have an effect that is similar to taking an H_2-receptor antagonist. The common practice of using additional pillows has no significant effect.

PPIs are the most effective drug treatment for GORD. Indeed, they are so effective that, once started, patients are very reluctant to stop taking them. Given an adequate dose for 8 weeks, most patients have a rapid improvement in symptoms (within a few days), and more than 90% can expect full mucosal healing at the end of this time. For this reason, a policy of 'step-down' medical treatment is advocated based on the general advice outlined above and a standard dose of a PPI given for 8 weeks. At the end of that time, the dose of PPI is reduced to that which keeps the patient free of symptoms, and this might even mean the cessation of PPI treatment. As most patients do not make major lifestyle changes and as PPIs are so effective, many remain on long-term treatment. For the minority who do not respond adequately to a standard dose, a trial at an increased dose or the addition of an H_2-receptor antagonist is recommended. If unsuccessful, these patients should be formally investigated.

PPI therapy is also important in patients with reflux-induced strictures, resulting in significant prolongation of the intervals between endoscopic dilatation. As yet, fears that chronic acid suppression might have serious long-term side effects including the risk of gastric cancer seem unwarranted.

Surgery

Strictly speaking, the need for surgery should have been reduced as medication has improved so much. Paradoxically, the number of antireflux operations has remained relatively constant and may even be increasing. This is probably due partly to increased patient expectations and partly to the advent of minimal access surgery, which has improved the acceptability of procedures.

Endoscopic treatments

A number of endoscopic treatments have been tried in the last 10 years that attempt to augment a failing LOS. These involve endoscopic suturing devices that plicate gastric mucosa just below the cardia to accentuate the angle of His, radiofrequency ablation (RFA) to the level of the sphincter and the injection of submucosal polymers into the lower oesophagus. The procedures have generally been applied to patients with only small hiatus hernias or none at all, so only a small proportion of patients who present to hospitals are suitable. Although most methods produce some temporary improvement in symptoms and objective assessments of reflux, failure rates at 1 year are high and can be over 50%. There are few large series that have reported long-term outcomes. Only RFA has been shown to be effective for as long as 10 years when around two-thirds patients remain off PPI medication.

Surgical treatments

The indication for surgery in uncomplicated GORD is essentially patient choice. The risks and possible benefits need to be discussed in detail. Risks include a small mortality rate (0.1–0.5%, depending on patient selection), failed operation (5–10%) and side effects such as dysphagia, gas bloat or abdominal discomfort (10%). With current surgical techniques, 85–90% of patients should be satisfied with the result of an antireflux operation. Patients who are asymptomatic on a PPI need a careful discussion of the risk side of the equation. Those who are symptomatic on a PPI need a careful clinical review to make sure that they will benefit from an operation. Reasons for failure on a PPI include 'volume' reflux (a good indication for surgery), a 'hermit' lifestyle in which the least deviation from lifestyle rules leads to symptoms (a good indication), psychological distress with intolerance of minor symptoms (a poor indication; these patients are likely to be dissatisfied with surgery), poor compliance (a good indication if the reason for poor compliance is the side effects of treatment, otherwise a bad indication) and misdiagnosis of GORD.

WHICH SURGERY?

There are many operations for GORD, but they are virtually all based on the creation of an intra-abdominal segment of oesophagus, crural repair and some form of wrap of the upper stomach (fundoplication) around the intra-abdominal oesophagus. The contribution of each component to operative success is widely debated, but it is clear that operations that fail to address all three components have inferior success rates. The major types of anti-reflux operation were all developed in the 1950s (Figure 62.21). When performed correctly, nearly all are effective. Most randomised trials do not show a clear advantage for any one operation over the

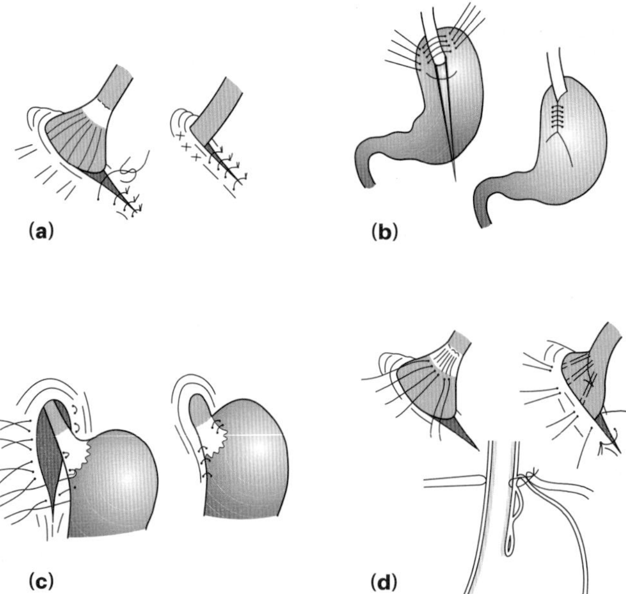

Figure 62.21 Various operations for the surgical correction of gastro-oesophageal reflux disease. (a) The original Allison repair of hiatus hernia (this is ineffective and is no longer done); (b) Nissen fundoplication; (c) Hill procedure; (d) Belsey mark IV operation.

Philip Rowland Allison, 1907–1974, Professor of Surgery, Oxford University, Oxford, UK.
Rudolph Nissen, 1896–1981, Professor of Surgery, Istanbul, Turkey, and later at Basle, Switzerland.
Lucius Davis Hill, surgeon, the Mason Clinic, Seattle, MN, USA.
Ronald Herbert Robert Belsey, d.2007, thoracic surgeon, Frenchay Hospital, Bristol, UK.

others, although one meta-analysis has come down in favour of posterior partial fundoplication over total fundoplication when performed laparoscopically.

Total fundoplication (Nissen) tends to be associated with slightly more short-term dysphagia but is the most durable repair in terms of long-term reflux control. Partial fundoplication, whether performed posteriorly (Toupet) or anteriorly (Dor, Watson), has fewer short-term side effects, although this is sometimes at the expense of a slightly higher long-term failure rate. One disadvantage of total fundoplication is the creation of an overcompetent cardia, resulting in the 'gas bloat' syndrome in which belching is impossible. The stomach fills with air, the patient feels very full after small meals and passes excessive flatus. This does not seem to occur with partial fundoplication. The problem has been largely overcome by the 'floppy' Nissen technique in which the fundoplication is loose around the oesophagus and is kept short in length. Although the other short-term side effects of fundoplication usually resolve within 3 months of surgery, this is rarely the case for gas bloat. The problem is best remedied by conversion to a partial fundoplication.

As with primary surgery, various revisional procedures have been described, usually for recurrent reflux or persistent dysphagia. For most patients, recurrent reflux relates to anatomical failure, so the solution is a revisional fundoplication. The results of surgery for recurrent reflux tend to be better than those for dysphagia, because the latter problem has many causes (too tight a wrap, slipping of the wrap, hiatal fibrosis) A very small proportion of patients may undergo more than two operations to correct recurrent reflux or unacceptable side effects. Revisional surgery carries a lower chance of success and, in some patients, local revision becomes technically impossible. The final resort is antrectomy with a Roux-en-Y reconstruction. This reduces gastric acid secretion and diverts bile and pancreatic secretions away from the stomach. Thus, the volume of potential refluxate in the stomach is reduced and, because of its changed composition, it is less damaging to the oesophagus.

For many years, the relative merits of thoracic and abdominal approaches were hotly debated. The introduction of minimal access surgery has made this debate obsolete. Most antireflux operations are now done with a laparoscopic approach.

LAPAROSCOPIC FUNDOPLICATION

Five cannulae are inserted in the upper abdomen (Figure 62.22). The cardia and lower oesophagus are separated from the diaphragmatic hiatus. An appropriate length of oesophagus is mobilised in the mediastinum. The fundus may be mobilised by dividing the short gastric vessels that tether the fundus to the spleen, although some surgeons feel that this is unnecessary. The hiatus is narrowed by sutures placed behind the oesophagus. In total (Nissen) fundoplication, the fundus is drawn behind the oesophagus and then sutured to itself in front of the oesophagus (Figure 62.23a). In partial fundoplication, the fundus is drawn either behind or in front of the oesophagus and sutured to it on each side, leaving a strip of exposed oesophagus either at the front (Figure 62.23b) or at the back. Robotic fundoplication has been described but comparisons with laparoscopic surgery do not indicate any clear clinical benefits.

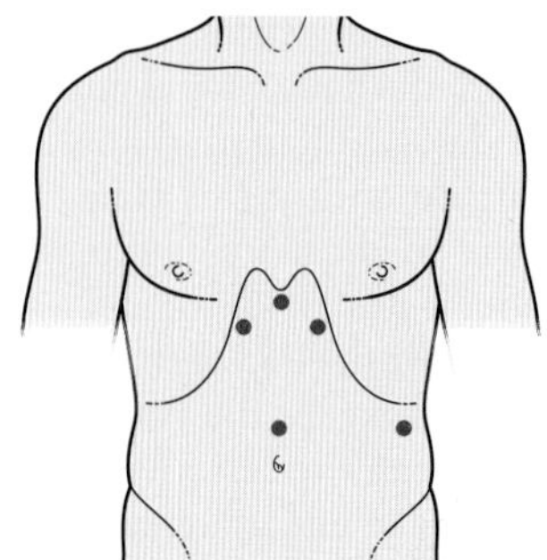

Figure 62.22 Laparoscope cannula sites for laparoscopic fundoplication.

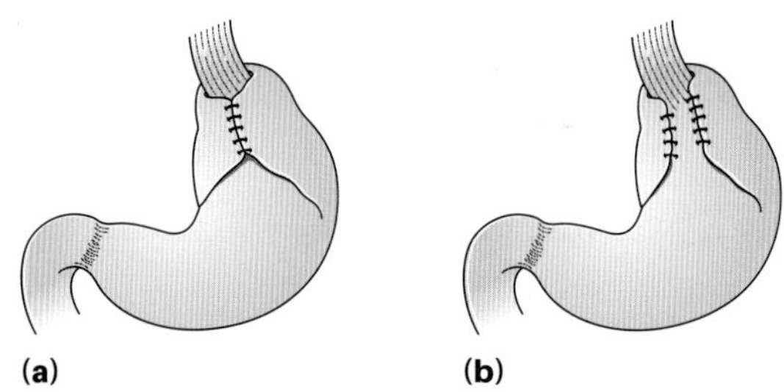

Figure 62.23 (a) Total (Nissen) fundoplication; (b) partial fundoplication (Toupet).

Complications of GORD

Stricture

Reflux-induced strictures (see Figure 62.20) occur mainly in late middle-aged and elderly people, but they may present in children. It is important to distinguish a benign reflux-induced stricture from a carcinoma. This is not usually difficult on the basis of location (immediately above the oesophagogastric junction), length (only about 1–2 cm) and smooth mucosa, but sometimes a cancer spreads under the oesophageal mucosa at its upper margin, producing a benign-looking stricture.

Peptic strictures generally respond well to dilatation and long-term treatment with a PPI. As most patients are elderly, antireflux surgery is not usually considered. However, it is an alternative to long-term PPI treatment, just as in uncomplicated GORD in younger and fitter patients. Most patients do not require anything other than a standard operation.

Summary box 62.7

Peptic stricture

- Day-case dilatation and PPI for peptic stricture

AM Toupet, French surgeon.
Cesar Roux, 1857–1934, Professor of Surgery and Gynaecology, Lausanne, Switzerland, described this method of forming a jejunal conduit in 1908.

Oesophageal shortening

The issue of oesophageal shortening continues to provoke debate. There can be no doubt that, in the presence of a large sliding hiatus hernia, the oesophagus is short, but this does not necessarily mean that, with mobilisation from the mediastinum, it cannot easily be restored to its normal length. The extent to which severe inflammation in the wall of the oesophagus causes fibrosis and real shortening is less clear. If a good segment of intra-abdominal oesophagus cannot be restored without tension, a Collis gastroplasty should be performed (Figure 62.24). This produces a neo-oesophagus around which a fundoplication can be done (Collis–Nissen operation).

Summary box 62.8

GORD

- Is due to loss of competence of the LOS and is extremely common
- May be associated with a hiatus hernia, which may be sliding or, less commonly, rolling (paraoesophageal)
- The most common symptoms are heartburn, epigastric discomfort and regurgitation, often made worse by stooping and lying
- Achalasia and GORD are diagnostically easily confused
  - Dysphagia may occur, but a neoplasm must be excluded
  - Diagnosis and treatment can be instituted on clinical grounds
- Endoscopy may be required and 24-hour pH is the 'gold standard'
  - Management is primarily medical (PPIs being the most effective), but surgery may be required; laparoscopic fundoplication is the most popular technique
  - Stricture may develop in time

Barrett's oesophagus (columnar-lined lower oesophagus)

Barrett's oesophagus is a metaplastic change in the lining mucosa of the oesophagus in response to chronic gastro-oesophageal reflux (Figure 62.25). Many of these patients do not have particularly severe symptoms, although they do have the most abnormal pH profiles. This adaptive response involves a mosaic of cell types, probably beginning as a simple columnar epithelium which becomes 'specialised' with time. The hallmark of 'specialised' Barrett's epithelium is the presence of mucus-secreting goblet cells (intestinal metaplasia). One of the great mysteries of GORD is why some people develop oesophagitis and others develop Barrett's oesophagus, often without significant oesophagitis. In Barrett's oesophagus, the junction between squamous oesophageal mucosa and gastric mucosa moves proximally. It may be difficult to distinguish a Barrett's oesophagus from a tubular, sliding hiatus hernia during endoscopy, as the two often coexist (Figure 62.26) or where the visible Barrett's segment is very short. The key

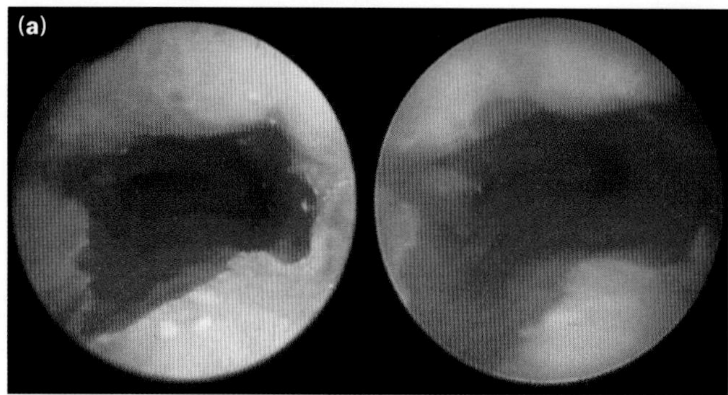

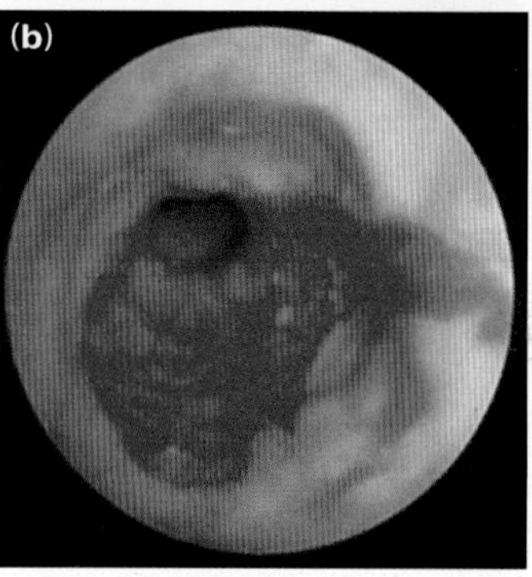

Figure 62.25 Barrett's oesophagus with (a) proximal migration of the squamocolumnar junction and (b) a view of the distal oesophagus.

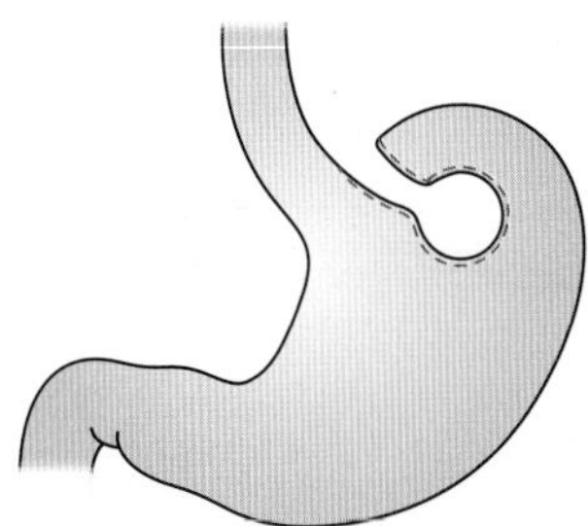

Figure 62.24 Collis gastroplasty to produce a neo-oesophagus around which a Nissen fundoplication is done. The operation may be performed by a laparoscopic as well as an open approach, using circular and linear staplers.

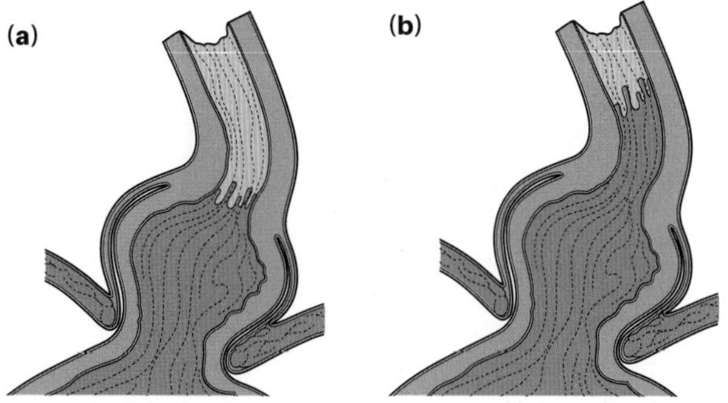

Figure 62.26 (a) The interrelationship of the lower oesophageal sphincter, the squamocolumnar junction and the diaphragm in sliding hiatus hernia. (b) Barrett's oesophagus and sliding hernia.

John Leigh Collis, 1911–2003, Professor of Thoracic Surgery, the University of Birmingham, Birmingham, UK.

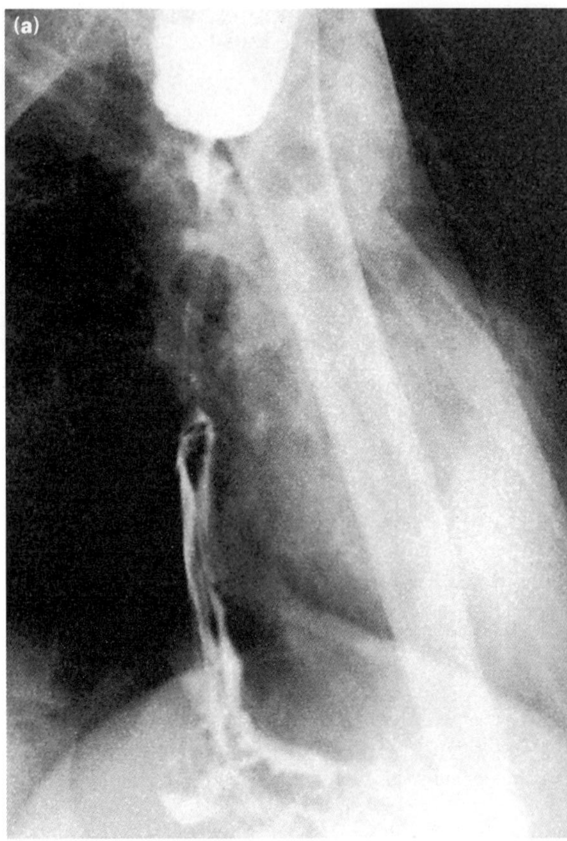

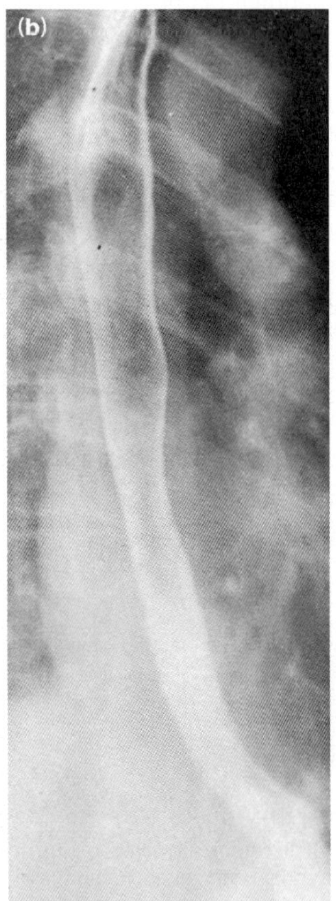

Figure 62.27 The radiological appearance of a midoesophageal stricture in (a), a patient with Barrett's oesophagus and in (b) a normal lumen after dilatation.

is where the gastric mucosal folds end along with recognition of the mucosal vascular pattern. The mucosa in the body of the stomach has longitudinal folds; the columnar lining of Barrett's oesophagus is smooth. The lower oesophagus is characterised by palisade vessels that run longitudinally and are easily seen through the lower oesophageal mucosa. Strictures can occur in Barrett's oesophagus and nearly always appear at the new squamocolumnar junction (Figure 62.27). Rarely, a stricture may occur in the columnar segment after healing of a Barrett's ulcer (Figure 62.28). Although intestinal metaplasia and length of the Barrett's segment are important risk factors for the development of carcinoma, neither represents an essential feature for cancer development. The risk of transformation to cancer is probably no more than 0.5% per patient per year, which is about 25 times that of the general population (Figures 62.29 and 62.30).

Summary box 62.9

Barrett's oesophagus

- Intestinal metaplasia is a risk factor for the development of adenocarcinoma
- Do not confuse Barrett's ulcer with oesophagitis

Patients who are found to have Barrett's oesophagus may be submitted to regular surveillance endoscopy with multiple biopsies in the hope of finding dysplasia or in situ cancer, rather than allowing invasive cancer to develop and cause symptoms. There is no general agreement about the benefits of surveillance endoscopy, or its ideal frequency. Endoscopy at 2-year intervals is probably adequate, provided that no dysplasia has been detected. A significant problem is that the incidence of Barrett's oesophagus in the community is

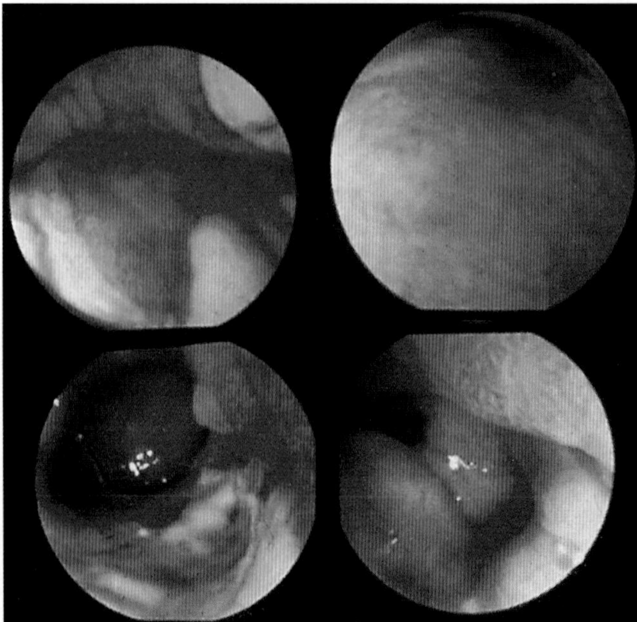

Figure 62.28 Barrett's ulcer in the columnar cell-lined oesophagus.

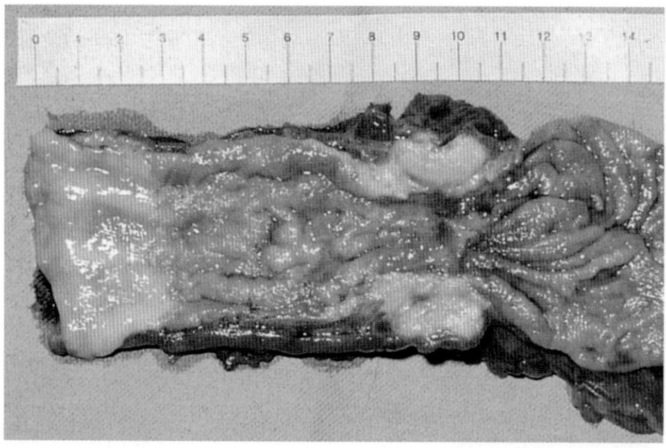
Figure 62.29 The macroscopic appearances of an adenocarcinoma in Barrett's oesophagus.

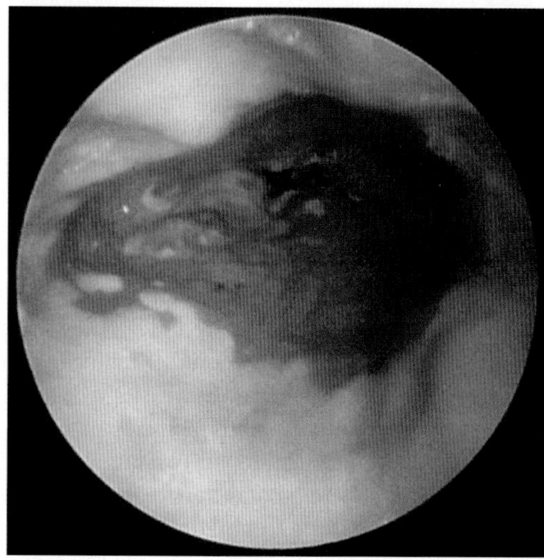
Figure 62.30 Endoscopic view of carcinoma in Barrett's oesophagus.

estimated to be at least 10 times the incidence discovered in dyspeptic patients referred for endoscopy. Thus, adenocarcinoma in Barrett's oesophagus often presents with invasive cancer without any preceding reflux symptoms.

Until recently, Barrett's oesophagus was not diagnosed until there was at least 3 cm of columnar epithelium in the distal oesophagus. With the better appreciation of the importance of intestinal metaplasia, Barrett's oesophagus may be diagnosed if there is any intestinal metaplasia in the oesophagus. The relative risk of cancer rises with increasing length of abnormal mucosa. The following terms are widely used:

- classic Barrett's (≥3 cm columnar epithelium);
- short-segment Barrett's (<3 cm of columnar epithelium);
- cardia metaplasia (intestinal metaplasia at the oesophagogastric junction without any macroscopic change at endoscopy).

When Barrett's oesophagus is discovered, the treatment is that of the underlying GORD. There has been considerable interest in recent years in endoscopic methods of treating Barrett's mucosa in the hope of eliminating the risk of cancer development. Laser, photodynamic therapy, argon-beam plasma coagulation, RFA and endoscopic mucosal resection (EMR) have all been used. Until recently, it was felt that intervention should only be offered in patients with high-grade dysplasia, but recent evidence suggests that patients with low-grade dysplasia also have a substantial risk of progressing to high-grade dysplasia of around 9% per year. For this reason endoscopic treatment is considered appropriate for patients with low-grade dysplasia when confirmed by a second independent histopathologist. EMR of dysplastic areas followed by RFA seems to be the most popular approach and, together with PPI treatment, these endoscopic methods can result in a neosquamous lining. Fears of buried glands that might give rise to cancer seem unfounded.

PARAOESOPHAGEAL ('ROLLING') HIATUS HERNIA

True paraoesophageal hernias in which the cardia remains in its normal anatomical position are rare. The vast majority of rolling hernias are mixed hernias in which the cardia is displaced into the chest and the greater curve of the stomach rolls into the mediastinum (Figure 62.31). Sometimes, the whole of the stomach lies in the chest (Figure 62.32). Colon or small intestine may sometimes lie in the hernia sac. The hernia is most common in elderly people, but may occur in young fit people. As the stomach rolls up into the chest, there is always an element of rotation (volvulus).

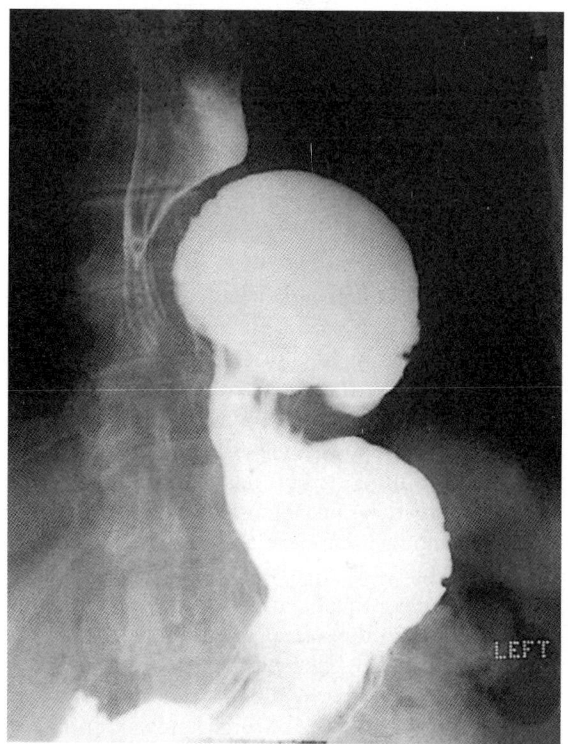

Figure 62.31 A paraoesophageal hernia showing the gastro-oesophageal junction just above the diaphragm and the fundus alongside the oesophagus, compressing the lumen.

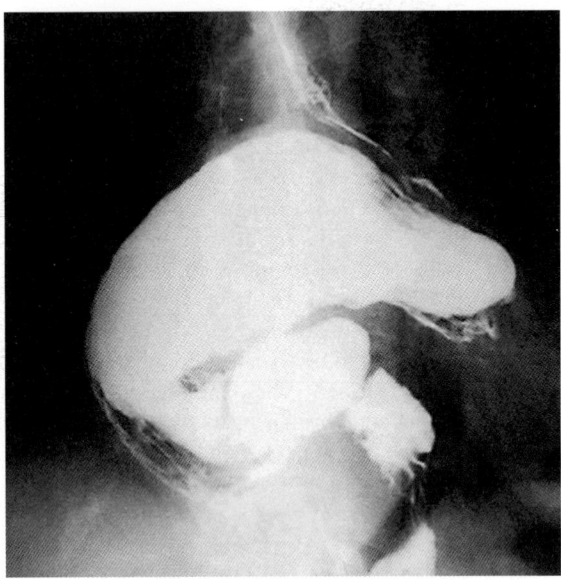

Figure 62.32 A huge paraoesophageal hernia with an upside-down stomach and the pylorus just below the hiatus.

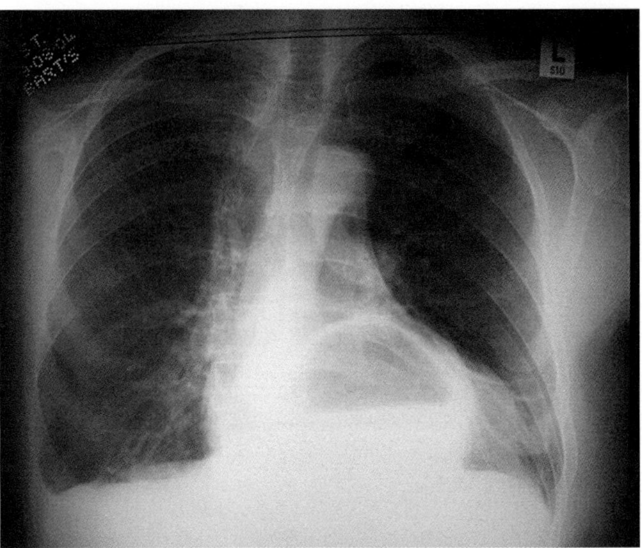

Figure 62.33 A gas bubble seen on a plain chest radiograph, showing the fundus of the stomach in the chest (courtesy of Dr Stephen Ellis, Bart's and the London NHS Trust).

Summary box 62.10

'Rolling' hiatus hernia

- Potentially dangerous, because of volvulus

The symptoms of rolling hernia are mostly due to twisting and distortion of the oesophagus and stomach. Dysphagia is common. Chest pain may occur from distension of an obstructed stomach. Classically, the pain is relieved by a loud belch. Symptoms of GORD are variable. Strangulation, gastric perforation and gangrene can occur. Emergency presentation with any of these complications carries high mortality on account of a combination of late diagnosis, generally elderly patients with comorbid diseases and the complexity of surgery involved.

The hernia may be visible on a plain radiograph of the chest as a gas bubble, often with a fluid level behind the heart (Figure 62.33). A CT scan with oral contrast is the best method of diagnosis, highlighting the gastric anatomy but also identifying other structures involved in the hernia. The endoscopic appearances may be confusing, especially in large hernias when it is easy to become disoriented.

Symptomatic rolling hernias nearly always require surgical repair because they are potentially dangerous. The risk of an asymptomatic patient developing a significant problem when a rolling hiatus hernia is discovered incidentally has probably been underestimated in the past. The annual risk is probably greater than the historical estimate of 1%. Patients who present as an emergency with acute chest pain may be treated initially by nasogastric tube, to relieve the distension that causes the pain, followed by surgical repair. Endoscopy is useful if nasogastric intubation is unsuccessful. If the pain is not relieved or perforation is suspected, immediate operation is mandatory.

Emergency surgery needs to be tailored to the problem encountered and the fitness of the patient. Elective surgery involves reduction of the hernia, excision of the sac, reduction of the crural defect and some form of retention of the stomach in the abdomen. Some surgeons perform a fundoplication, arguing that this is a very effective means of maintaining reduction and that it deals with the associated GORD. Others argue that fundoplication should be done only if reflux can be conclusively demonstrated beforehand. Surprisingly, both philosophies achieve good results. Laparoscopic repair has recently become popular. Full anatomical repair of a large rolling hernia can be difficult using this approach and requires considerable expertise. Secure closure of the hiatal defect can be a problem, and some surgeons advocate mesh to reinforce the repair.

NEOPLASMS OF THE OESOPHAGUS

Benign tumours

Benign tumours of the oesophagus are relatively rare. True papillomas, adenomas and hyperplastic polyps do occur, but most 'benign' tumours are not epithelial in origin and arise from other layers of the oesophageal wall (GI stromal tumour [GIST], lipoma, granular cell tumour). Most benign oesophageal tumours are small and asymptomatic, and even a large benign tumour may cause only mild symptoms (Figure 62.34). The most important point in their management is usually to carry out an adequate number of biopsies to prove beyond reasonable doubt that the lesion is not malignant (Figure 62.35).

Malignant tumours

Non-epithelial primary malignancies are also rare, as is malignant melanoma. Secondary malignancies rarely involve the oesophagus, with the exception of bronchogenic carcinoma

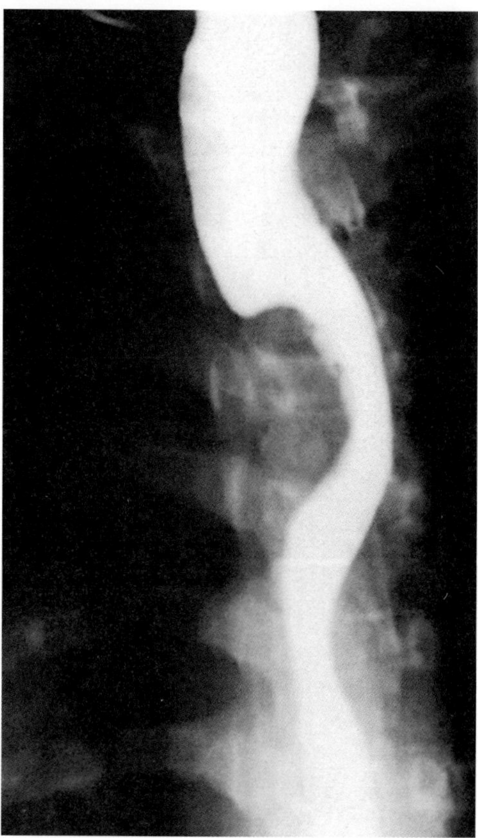

Figure 62.34 Classic appearance of a large oesophageal gastrointestinal stromal tumour on barium swallow.

by direct invasion of either the primary and/or contiguous lymph nodes.

Carcinoma of the oesophagus

Cancer of the oesophagus is the sixth most common cancer in the world. In general, it is a disease of mid to late adulthood, with a poor survival rate. Only 5–10% of those diagnosed will survive for 5 years.

Summary box 62.11

Carcinoma of the oesophagus

- Squamous cell usually affects the upper two-thirds; adenocarcinoma usually affects the lower third
- Common aetiological factors are tobacco and alcohol (squamous cell), GORD and obesity (adenocarcinoma)
- The incidence of adenocarcinoma is increasing
- Lymph node involvement is a bad prognostic factor
- Dysphagia is the most common presenting symptom, but is a late feature
- Accurate pretreatment staging is essential in patients thought to be fit to undergo 'curative' treatment

Pathology and aetiology

Squamous cell cancer (Figures 62.36 and 62.37) and adenocarcinoma (Figures 62.38 and 62.39) are the most common types. Squamous cell carcinoma generally affects the upper

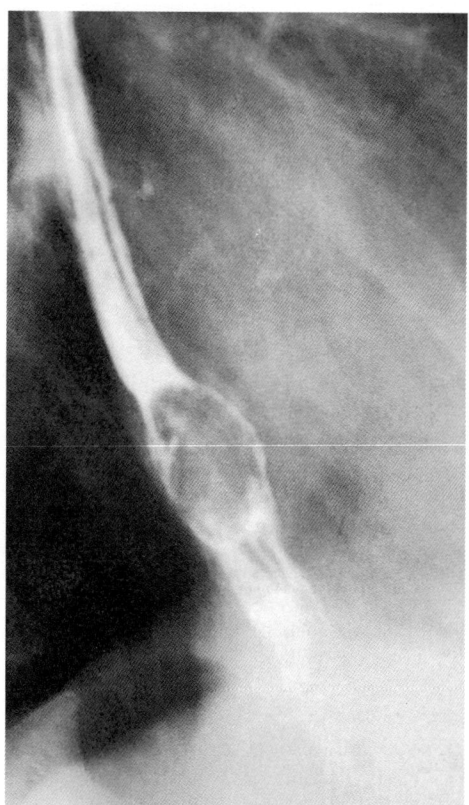

Figure 62.35 An intraluminal polyp that proved to be a leiomyosarcoma.

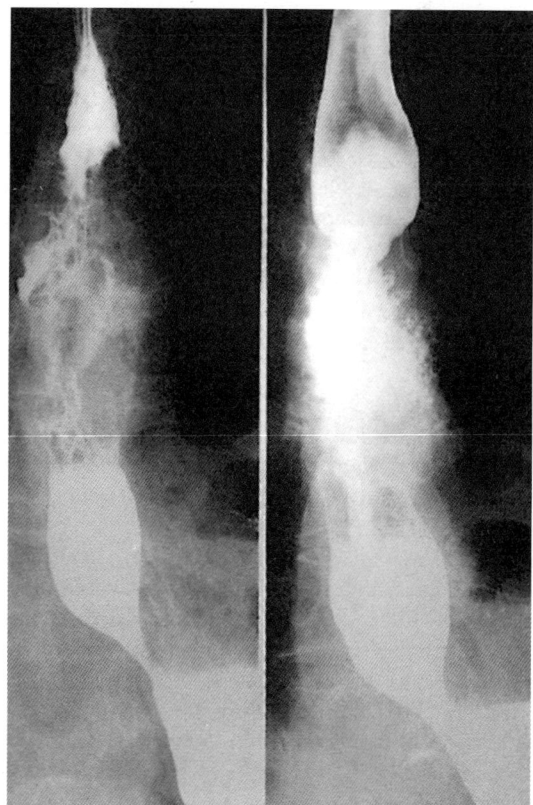

Figure 62.36 The classic appearances of a midoesophageal proliferative squamous cell carcinoma.

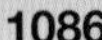

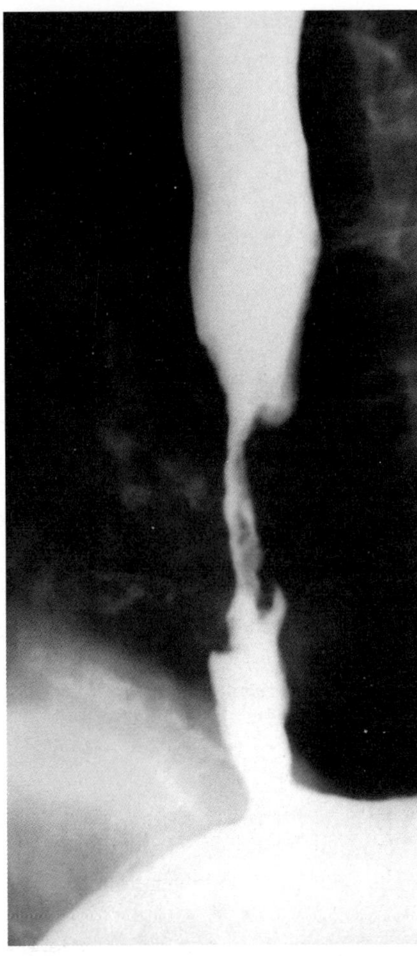

Figure 62.37 Squamous cell carcinoma of the oesophagus producing an irregular stricture with shouldered margins.

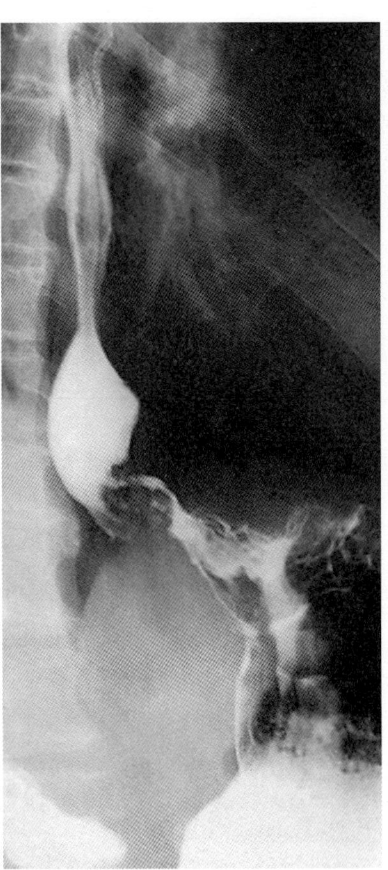

Figure 62.38 Adenocarcinoma of the lower oesophagus, spreading upwards from the cardia.

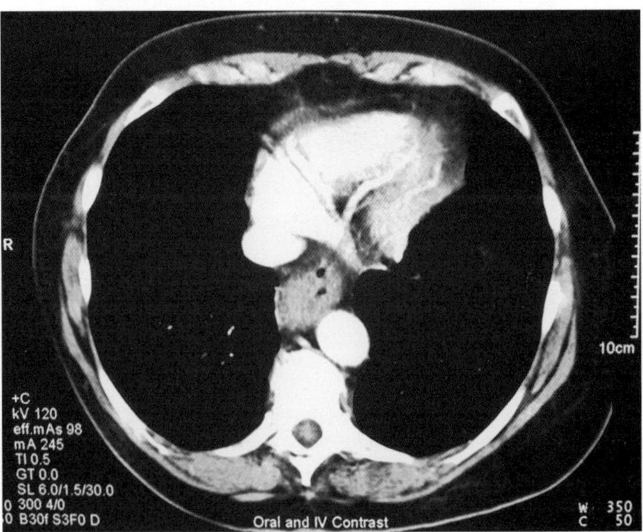

Figure 62.39 Computed tomography scan showing a primary tumour of the lower oesophagus.

two-thirds of the oesophagus and adenocarcinoma the lower third. Worldwide, squamous cell cancer is most common, but adenocarcinoma predominates in the west and is increasing in incidence.

Geographical variation in oesophageal cancer

The incidence of oesophageal cancer varies more than that of any other cancer. Squamous cell cancer is endemic in the Transkei region of South Africa and in the Asian 'cancer belt', which extends across the middle of Asia from the shores of the Caspian Sea (in northern Iran) to China. The highest incidence in the world is in Linxian in Henan province in China, where it is the most common single cause of death, with more than 100 cases per 100 000 population per annum. The cause of the disease in the endemic areas is not known. Although there is evidence of genetic susceptibility across much of central Asia, a variety of environmental factors along with nutritional deficiencies are probably involved. In Linxian, supplementation of the diet with β-carotene, vitamin E and selenium has been shown to reduce the incidence.

Away from the endemic areas, tobacco and alcohol are major factors in the occurrence of squamous cancer. Incidence rates vary from less than 5:100 000 in white people in the USA to 26.5:100 000 in some regions of France.

In many western countries, the incidence of squamous cell cancer has fallen or remained static, but the incidence of adenocarcinoma of the oesophagus has increased dramatically since the mid-1970s at a rate of 5–10% per annum.

The change is greater than that of any other neoplasm in this time. Adenocarcinoma now accounts for 60–75% of all oesophageal cancers in several countries. The reason for this change is not understood. A similar rate of increase in GORD over the same period, which mirrors an increase in obesity in the west, is likely to be an important factor, particularly through the link to Barrett's oesophagus. Obese, white men in their 60s represent the highest-risk group. There has also been an increase in the incidence of carcinoma of the cardia of the stomach, which suggests that cancer of the cardia and adenocarcinoma of the oesophagus may share common aetiological factors. With a falling incidence of cancer in the rest of the stomach, more than 60% of all upper GI cancers in the west involve the cardia or distal oesophagus.

Both adenocarcinomas and squamous cell carcinomas tend to disseminate early. Sadly, the classic presenting symptoms of dysphagia, regurgitation and weight loss are often absent until the primary tumour has become advanced, and so the tumour is often well established before the diagnosis is made. Tumours can spread in three ways: invasion directly through the oesophageal wall, via the lymphatics or in the bloodstream. Direct spread occurs both laterally, through the component layers of the oesophageal wall, and longitudinally within the oesophageal wall. Longitudinal spread is mainly via the submucosal lymphatic channels of the oesophagus. The pattern of lymphatic drainage is therefore not segmental, as in other parts of the GI tract. Consequently, the length of oesophagus involved by tumour is frequently much longer than the macroscopic length of the malignancy at the epithelial surface. Lymph node spread occurs commonly. Although the direction of spread to regional lymphatics is predominantly caudal, the involvement of lymph nodes is potentially widespread and can also occur in a cranial direction. Any regional lymph node from the superior mediastinum to the coeliac axis and lesser curve of the stomach may be involved, regardless of the location of the primary lesion within the oesophagus. Haematogenous spread may involve a variety of different organs including the liver, lungs, brain and bones. Tumours arising from the intra-abdominal portion of the oesophagus may also disseminate transperitoneally.

Clinical features

Most oesophageal neoplasms present with mechanical symptoms, principally dysphagia, but sometimes also regurgitation, vomiting, odynophagia and weight loss. Clinical findings suggestive of advanced malignancy include recurrent laryngeal nerve palsy, Horner's syndrome, chronic spinal pain and diaphragmatic paralysis. Other factors making surgical cure unlikely include weight loss of more than 20% and loss of appetite. Cutaneous tumour metastases or enlarged supraclavicular lymph nodes may be seen on clinical examination and indicate disseminated disease. Hoarseness due to recurrent laryngeal nerve palsy is a sign of advanced and incurable disease. Palpable lymphadenopathy in the neck is likewise a sign of advanced disease.

Patients with early disease may have non-specific dyspeptic symptoms or a vague feeling of 'something that is not quite right' during swallowing. Some are diagnosed during endoscopic surveillance of patients with Barrett's oesophagus and, although this does identify patients with the earliest stages of disease, such programmes have little overall impact, because most patients with Barrett's oesophagus are unknown to the medical profession and make their first presentation with a symptomatic, and therefore usually locally advanced, oesophageal cancer. The widespread use of endoscopy as a diagnostic tool does, nevertheless, provide an opportunity for early diagnosis (Figure 62.40). Biopsies should be taken of all lesions in the oesophagus (Figures 62.41 and 62.42), no matter how trivial they appear and irrespective of the indication for the examination.

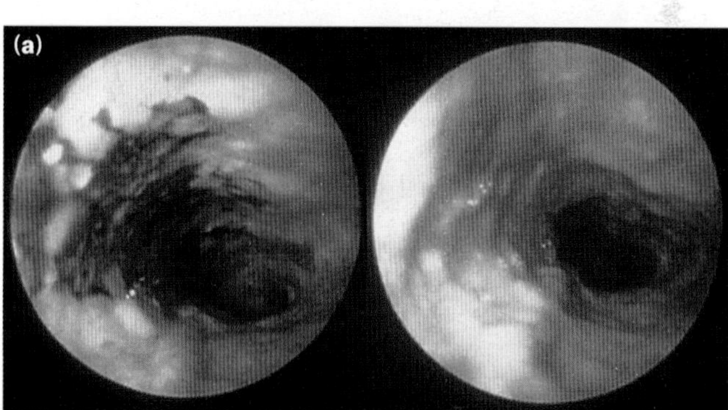

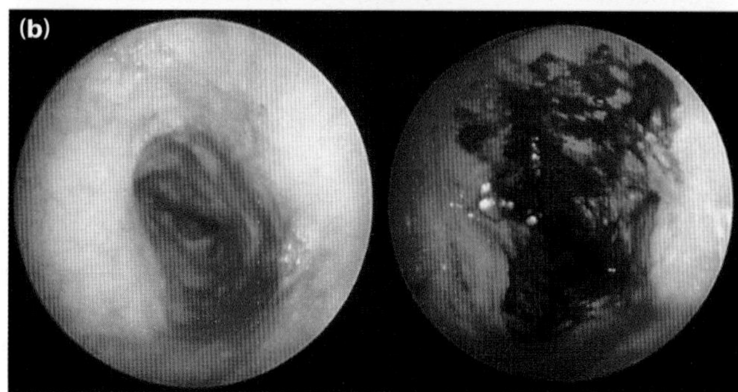

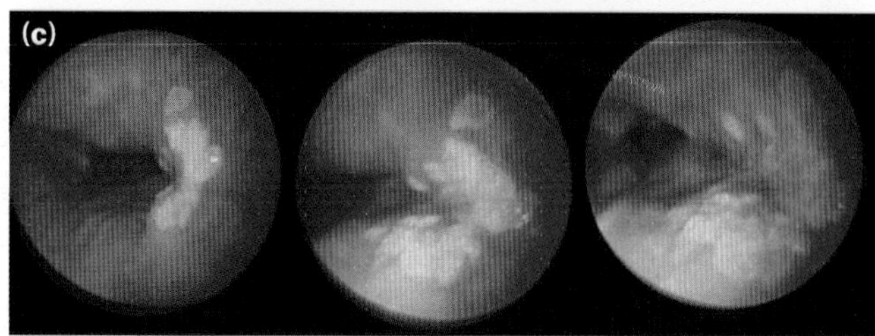

Figure 62.40 Carcinoma *in situ* showing the varied presentations: (a) occult form; (b) erythroplakia; (c) leukoplakia. The right-hand pictures in (a) and (b) demonstrate the use of vital staining with methylene blue.

Johann Friedrich Horner, 1831–1886, Professor of Ophthalmology, Zurich, Switzerland, described this syndrome in 1869.

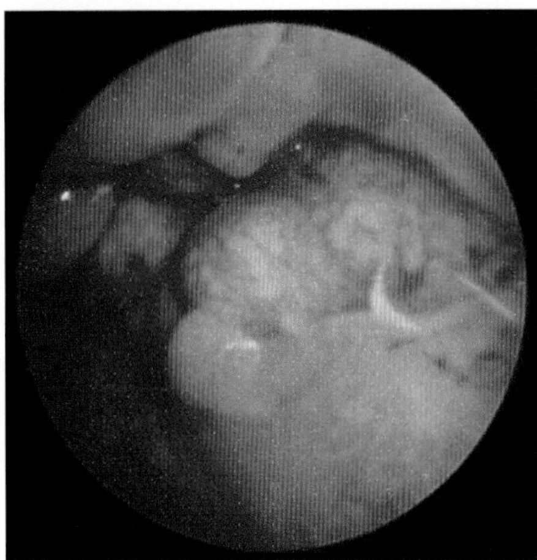

Figure 62.41 Endoscopic appearances of a midoesophageal squamous cell carcinoma.

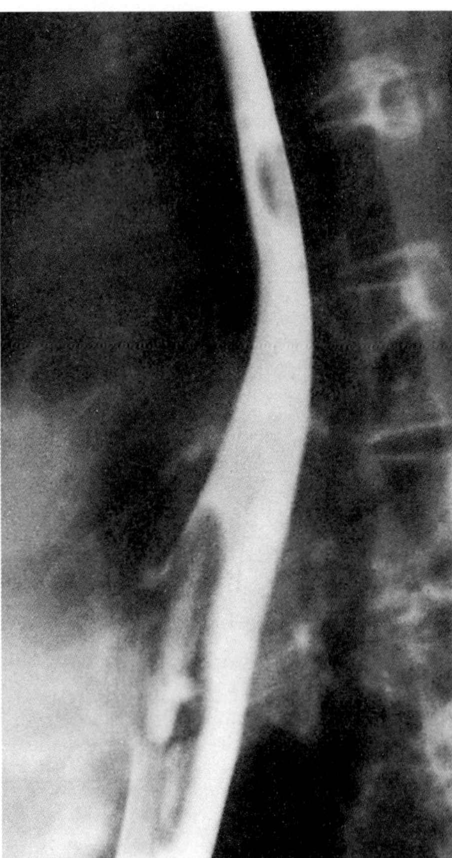

Figure 62.42 Beware the differential diagnosis of infection, for what appears to be a tumour. This midoesophageal mass was actually tuberculosis.

Investigation

Endoscopy is the first-line investigation for most patients. It provides an unrivalled direct view of the oesophageal mucosa and any lesion allowing its site and size to be documented. Cytology and/or histology specimens taken via the endoscope are crucial for accurate diagnosis. The combination of histology and cytology increases the diagnostic accuracy to more than 95%. The chief limitation of conventional endoscopy is that only the mucosal surface can be studied and biopsied. Other investigations are therefore usually required to define the extent of local or distant spread. The improved image resolution of modern endoscopes and novel techniques involving magnification and the use of dyes to enhance surface detail may lead to more early lesions being recognised.

GENERAL ASSESSMENT AND STAGING

Once the initial diagnosis of a malignant oesophageal neoplasm has been made, patients should be assessed first in terms of their general health and fitness for potential therapies. Their preferences should also be considered. Most potentially curative therapies include radical surgery, although definitive chemoradiotherapy is an alternative in squamous cell carcinoma. Patients who are unfit for, or who do not wish to contemplate, radical treatments should not be investigated further, but should be diverted to appropriate palliative therapies, depending on the symptoms and current quality of life. Only those patients suitable for potentially curative therapies should proceed to staging investigations to rule out haematogenous spread (CT scan) and then to assess locoregional stage (endoscopic ultrasonography [EUS] ± laparoscopy). This will distinguish between early (T1/T2, N0) and advanced lesions (T3/T4, N1) and indicate whether surgery alone or multimodal therapy is most appropriate. Where attempted cure is deemed possible, the aim should be to provide the best chance of cure while minimising procedural risks. In general, surgery alone should be reserved for patients with early disease, and multimodal therapy should be used in patients with locally advanced disease, in whom the chance of cure by surgery alone is small (generally <20%).

The most widely used pathological staging system is that of the World Health Organization (tumour–nodes–metastasis TNM).

Table 62.2 shows the TNM system for oesophageal cancer. Similar to all pathological systems, it relies on the nature and extent of the surgery performed, e.g. performing more

TABLE 62.2 TNM staging scheme for oesophageal cancer.

Tis	High-grade dysplasia
T1	Tumour invading lamina propria or submucosa
T2	Tumour invading muscularis propria
T3	Tumour invading beyond muscularis propria
T4a	Tumour invading adjacent structures (pleura, pericardium, diaphragm)
T4b	Tumour invading adjacent structures (trachea, bone, aorta)
N0	No lymph node metastases
N1	Lymph node metastases in 1–2 nodes
N2	Lymph nodes metastases in 3–6 nodes
N3	Lymph node metastases in 7 or more lymph nodes
M0	No distant metastases
M1	All other distant metastases
Stage	1A: T1N0M0; 1B: T2N0M0; 2A: T3N0M0; 2B: T1/2N0M0; 3A: T4aN0M0, T3N1M0, T1/2N2M0
Stage	3B: T3N2M0; 3C: T4aN1/2M0, T4bN0–3M0, T1–4N3M0; 4T:1–4N1–3M1

extensive radical surgical lymphadenectomy provides a more accurate assessment of the 'N' stage. There is evidence that many patients described as N0 in the past were probably N1, a phenomenon described as stage migration.

Staging information may be gathered before the commencement of therapy, during therapy (e.g. at open operation) or following treatment (histology or postmortem examination). The techniques commonly used to provide preoperative staging data are described in Figure 62.43, along with a suggested algorithm.

BLOOD TESTS

These are of limited value. Blood tests reveal nothing about local invasion or regional lymph node spread and, to date, no reliable tumour marker for oesophageal cancer has been isolated from peripheral blood. The presence of abnormal liver function tests (LFTs) may suggest the presence of liver metastases, but this is generally too insensitive to be diagnostic. Many patients with known liver metastases have normal LFTs. At best, abnormal LFTs only reinforce the clinical suspicion of spread to the liver, and further imaging is usually required to confirm the diagnosis.

TRANSCUTANEOUS ULTRASONOGRAPHY

It is difficult to visualise mediastinal structures with transcutaneous ultrasonography. With the relatively low-frequency sound waves used, good depth of tissue penetration is achieved at the expense of poor image resolution. In addition, the mediastinal organs are surrounded by bone and air, which renders them largely inaccessible to external ultrasound. The technique is therefore used mainly to assess spread to the liver, the whole of which can be clearly visualised by standard transcutaneous ultrasonography. Haematogenous spread can be more fully assessed by combining ultrasonography with chest radiography, although this combination is less accurate than CT scanning.

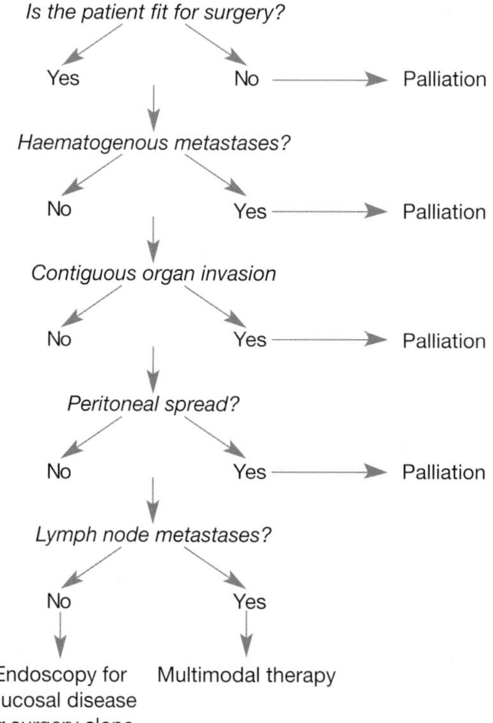

Figure 62.43 Algorithm for the management of oesophageal cancer.

BRONCHOSCOPY

Many middle- and upper-third oesophageal carcinomas (and therefore usually squamous carcinomas) are sufficiently advanced at the time of diagnosis that the trachea or bronchi are already involved (Figure 62.44). Bronchoscopy may reveal either impingement or invasion of the main airways in over 30% of new patients with cancers in the upper third of the oesophagus. In some cases, therefore, bronchoscopy alone can confirm that the tumour is locally unresectable.

LAPAROSCOPY

This is a useful technique for the diagnosis of intra-abdominal and hepatic metastases. It has the advantage of enabling tissue samples or peritoneal cytology to be obtained and is the only modality reliably able to detect peritoneal tumour seedlings (Figure 62.45). This is particularly important for tumours arising from the intra-abdominal portion of the oesophagus,

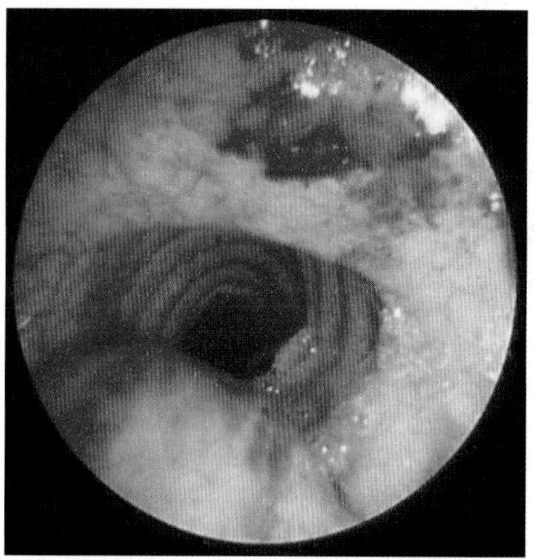

Figure 62.44 Invasion into the posterior wall of the trachea from an oesophageal carcinoma.

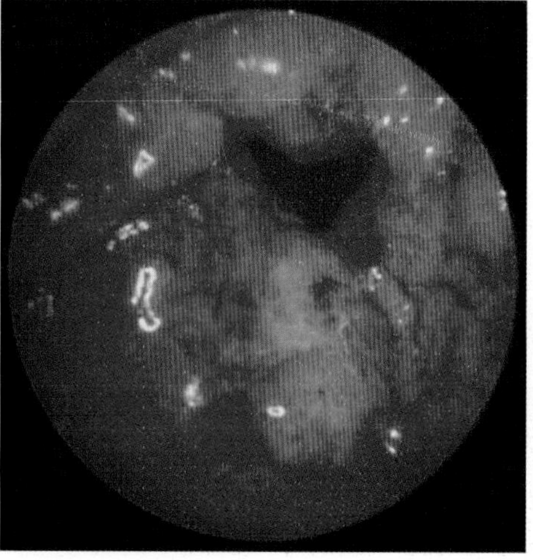

Figure 62.45 Adenocarcinoma of the cardia. Transcoelomic spread may occur with this type of lesion.

cardia and where there is a potential communication between a full-thickness tumour and the peritoneal cavity, for instance where there is a hiatus hernia.

COMPUTED TOMOGRAPHY

Computed tomography (CT) from the neck to the pelvis with intravenous contrast is the modality most used to identify haematogenous metastases (Figure 62.46). Distant organs are easily seen and metastases within them visualised with high accuracy (94–100%). The normal thoracic oesophagus is easily demonstrated by CT scanning. The mediastinal fat planes are usually clearly imaged in healthy individuals, and any blurring or distortion of these images is a fairly reliable indicator of abnormality. In cachectic patients with dysphagia and malnutrition, the mediastinal fat plane may be virtually absent, making local invasion difficult to assess. Thin-slice CT permits structures such as lymph nodes to be adequately imaged, down to a minimum diameter of about 5 mm. Smaller nodes cannot be reliably visualised, and it is not possible to distinguish between enlarged lymph nodes that have reactive changes only and metastatic nodes. Similarly, micrometastases within normal-sized nodes cannot be detected.

MAGNETIC RESONANCE IMAGING

Magnetic resonance imaging (MRI) does not expose the patient to ionising radiation and needs no intravascular contrast medium, although intraoesophageal air or contrast media may help to assess wall thickness. Distant metastases to organs such as the liver are usually reliably identified by MRI but, at the moment, there do not seem to be additional benefits over CT.

ENDOSCOPIC ULTRASONOGRAPHY

After haematogenous spread, the two principal prognostic factors for oesophageal cancer are the depth of tumour penetration through the oesophageal wall and regional lymph node spread. Although CT will detect distant metastasis, its limited axial resolution precludes a reliable assessment of both the depth of wall penetration and lymph node involvement. Endoscopic ultrasonography (EUS) can determine the depth of spread of a malignant tumour through the oesophageal wall (T1–3), the invasion of adjacent organs (T4) and metastasis to lymph nodes (N0 or N1) (Figures 62.47–62.49). It can also detect contiguous spread downward into the cardia and more distant metastases to the left lobe of the liver.

EUS visualises the oesophageal wall as a multilayered structure. The layers represent ultrasound interfaces rather than true anatomical layers, but there is close enough correlation to allow accurate assessment of the depth of invasion through the oesophageal wall. Structures smaller than 5 mm can be clearly seen, enabling very small nodes to be imaged. The EUS image morphology of such structures provides an additional means of distinguishing malignant from reactive or benign lymph nodes. For submucosal lesions, EUS can demonstrate the wall layer of origin of a lesion, suggesting the likely histological type.

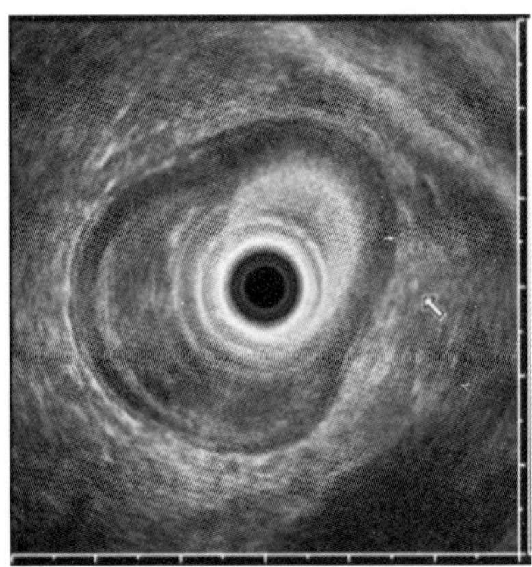

Figure 62.47 Endosonography demonstrating an 'early' tumour. Note the preservation of the outer dark wall layer that represents the muscle coat.

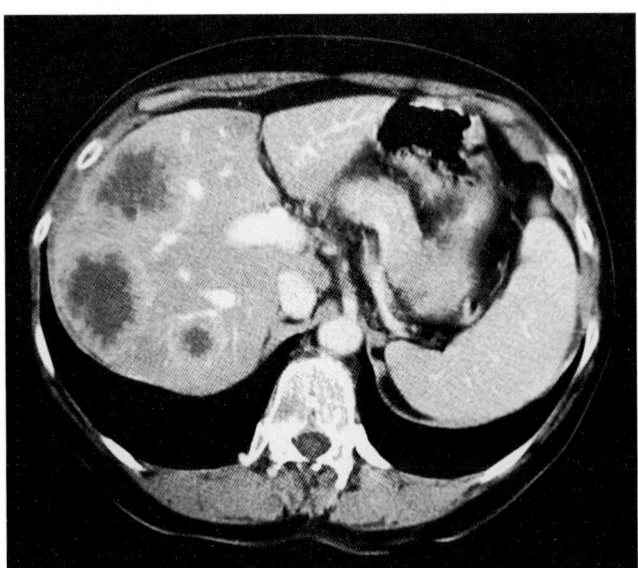

Figure 62.46 Computed tomography scan demonstrating liver metastases.

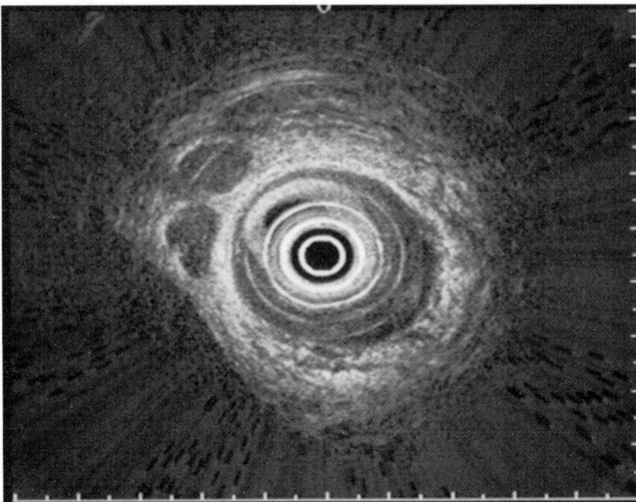

Figure 62.48 Endosonography demonstrating an 'advanced' local tumour. Note the breach of the outer white line that represents the interface between the oesophageal wall and the mediastinum.

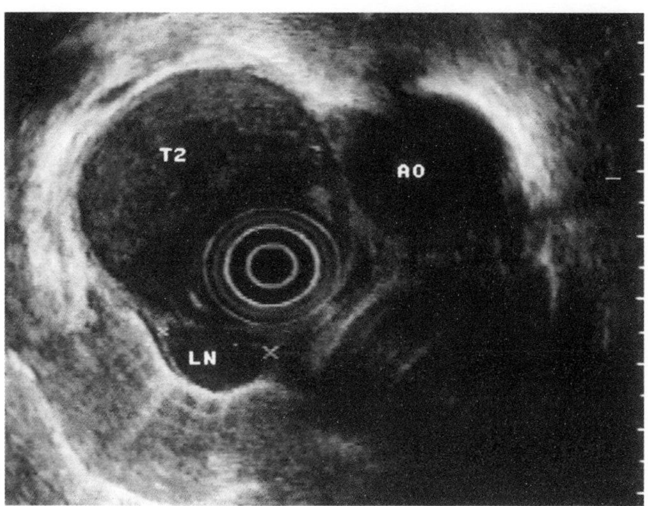

Figure 62.49 Endosonography demonstrating malignant nodes. These are usually large, hypoechoic and round compared with normal nodes.

Narrow EUS instruments are available for insertion over a guidewire to minimise the risk of technical failure, and linear array echoendoscopes can be used to biopsy lesions that might signify incurability outside the wall of the GI tract which might be considered to lie outside the proposed field of resection (usually lymph nodes outside a standard field).

Positron emission tomography with CT

Positron emission tomography (PET) with CT (PET-CT) in the context of cancer staging relies on the generally high metabolic activity (particularly in the glycolytic pathway) of tumours compared with normal tissues. The patient is given a small dose of the radiopharmaceutical agent [^{18}F]fluorodeoxyglucose (FDG). This enters cells and is phosphorylated. FDG 6-phosphate cannot be metabolised further and, as it is a highly polar molecule, it cannot easily diffuse back out of the cell. After intravenous injection of FDG, it continuously accumulates in metabolically active cells. Primary oesophageal cancers are usually sufficiently active to be easily visible, and spatial resolution of positive PET areas occurs down to about 5–8 mm. When used in isolation, there are problems with the anatomical location of these areas. This has been significantly improved by combining PET with CT (Figure 62.50), which covers the whole body. The main value of PET-CT is the identification of distant metastatic disease not seen on CT alone. Although there are wide variations between centres, a change in stage is frequently reported in around 15% of patients, but the timing of the scan in relation to the last date of treatment is important and probably accounts for differences in perceived effect. It has also been suggested that a reduction in PET activity after chemotherapy might be a way of predicting 'responders' to this approach, although the persistence of PET activity after a neoadjuvant treatment seems to be a poor prognostic sign.

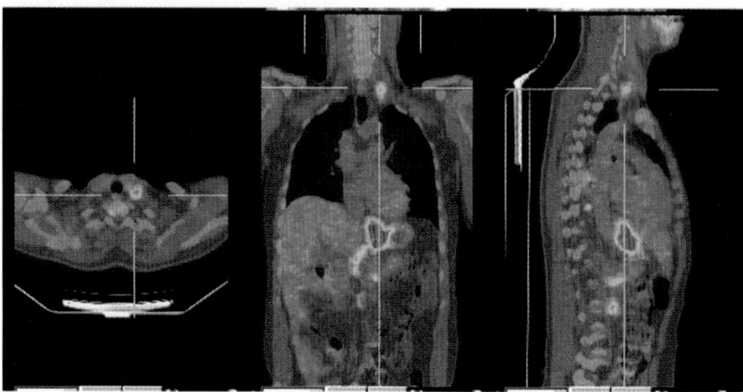

Figure 62.50 Positron emission tomography/computed tomography demonstrating a primary tumour and a distant metastatic node.

Treatment of malignant tumours

PRINCIPLES

At the time of diagnosis, around two-thirds of all patients with oesophageal cancer will already have incurable disease. The aim of palliative treatment is to overcome debilitating or distressing symptoms while maintaining the best quality of life possible for the patient. Some patients do not require specific therapeutic interventions, but do need supportive care and appropriate liaison with community nursing and hospice care services.

As dysphagia is the predominant symptom in advanced oesophageal cancer, the principal aim of palliation is to restore adequate swallowing. A variety of methods is available and, given the short life expectancy of most patients, it is important that the choice of treatment should be tailored to each individual. Tumour location and endoscopic appearance are important in this regard, as is the general condition of the patient.

Once oesophageal neoplasms reach the submucosal layer of the oesophagus, the tumour has access to the lymphatic system, meaning that, even at this early local stage, there is an incidence of nodal positivity for both squamous cell carcinoma and adenocarcinomas of about 20%. The principle of oesophagectomy is to deal adequately with the local tumour in order to minimise the risk of local recurrence and achieve an adequate lymphadenectomy to reduce the risk of staging error. Although studies in Japan would indicate that more extensive lymphadenectomy is associated with better survival, this may simply reflect more accurate staging. A number of studies support the view that the proximal extent of resection should ideally be 10 cm above the macroscopic tumour and 5 cm distal. When such a margin cannot be achieved proximally, particularly with squamous cell carcinoma, there is evidence that postoperative radiotherapy can minimise local recurrence, although this does not improve survival.

Adenocarcinoma commonly involves the gastric cardia and may therefore extend into the fundus or down the lesser curve. Some degree of gastric excision is essential in order to achieve adequate local clearance and accomplish an appropriate lymphadenectomy. Excision of contiguous structures, such as the crura, diaphragm and mediastinal pleura, needs to be considered as a method of creating negative resection margins.

The rarity of intramucosal cancer in symptomatic patients means that there are no randomised studies to compare different approaches to this type of very early disease. EMR for these apparently early (T1a) lesions has become increasingly popular, providing either a cure or at least sufficient histological information on which to base a further management strategy.

Surgery alone is best suited to patients with disease confined to the oesophagus (T1b, T2) without nodal metastasis (N0). The problem here is ensuring that patients are truly node negative. Despite careful preoperative investigation, these patients are not easily identified and so there is an argument for neoadjuvant therapy followed by surgery. A cure rate for the patient who is truly node negative having surgery alone of between 50% and 80% needs to be balanced against adverse events related to neoadjuvant therapy, the likelihood of response and the potential impact on survival. Patients with more advanced stages of disease require either multimodal approaches or entry into appropriate trials.

It is essential that oesophagectomy should be performed with a low hospital mortality and complication rate. Patient selection, volume and experience of the surgical team are all important. Preoperative risk analysis has shown that this can play a major part in reducing hospital mortality. There are really no circumstances in the western world in which surgery should be undertaken if it is not part of an overall treatment plan aimed at cure.

Summary box 62.12

Treatment of carcinoma of the oesophagus

- Radical oesophagectomy is the most important aspect of curative treatment
- Neoadjuvant treatments before surgery may improve survival in a proportion of patients
- Chemoradiotherapy alone may cure selected patients, particularly those with squamous cell cancers
- Useful palliation may be achieved by chemo-/radiotherapy or endoscopic treatments

Treatments with curative intent

SURGERY

Histological tumour type, location and the extent of the proposed lymphadenectomy all influence the surgical approach. This is largely an issue of surgical preference, although it should be recognised that a left thoracoabdominal approach is limited proximally by the aortic arch and should be avoided when the primary tumour is at or above this level. Similarly, transhiatal oesophagectomy is unsuitable for most patients with squamous cell carcinoma because a complete mediastinal lymphadenectomy is not easily achieved by this approach. The most widely practised approach in the west is the two-phase Ivor Lewis (sometimes called Lewis–Tanner) operation (Figure 62.51), with an initial laparotomy and construction of a gastric tube, followed by a right thoracotomy to excise the tumour and create an oesophagogastric anastomosis. The closer this is placed to the apex of the thoracic cavity, the fewer problems there are with reflux disease. Three-phase oesophagectomy (McKeown) may be more appropriate for more proximal tumours in order to achieve better longitudinal clearance, although the additional distance gained is less than many surgeons believe. A third cervical incision also permits lymphadenectomy in this region.

The extent of lymphadenectomy is highly controversial. For squamous cell carcinoma, because a higher proportion of patients will have middle- and upper-third tumours in the thoracic oesophagus, the rationale behind a three-phase operation with three-field lymphadenectomy is more understandable, even though this approach has not been widely adopted in the west. For adenocarcinoma, the incidence of metastases in the neck is relatively low in the context of patients who would otherwise be curable. For this reason, two-phase operations with two-field lymphadenectomy seem the most logical operations. Although two-field lymphadenectomy does not substantially increase surgical morbidity or mortality, the same cannot be said for more extended operations.

Minimal access techniques, pioneered in Australia by Gotley and Smithers and in North America by Luketich, have enjoyed increasing popularity, often combined with enhanced recovery programmes after surgery (ERAS). Hybrid (where at least one phase is performed as open surgery), total minimally invasive and robotic oesophagectomy all have their advocates, although there are no high-quality comparative studies and little evidence to indicate clear superiority of one approach

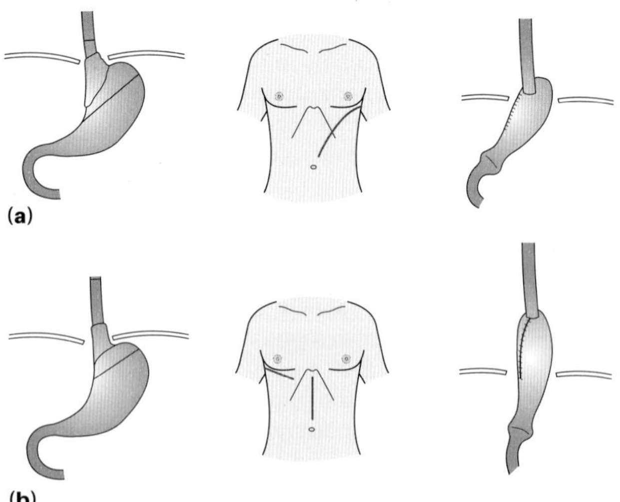

Figure 62.51 The two usual approaches for surgery of the oesophagus are (a) the thoracoabdominal, which opens the abdominal and thoracic cavities together, and (b) the two-stage Ivor Lewis approach, in which the abdomen is opened first, closed and then the thoracotomy is performed. In the McKeown operation, a third incision in the neck is made to complete the cervical anastomosis.

Ivor Lewis, 1895–1982, surgeon, the North Middlesex Hospital, London, UK, and later at Rhyl, North Wales, UK.
Norman Cecil Tanner, 1906–1982, surgeon, Charing Cross Hospital, London, UK.
Kenneth Charles McKeown, 1912–1995, surgeon, Darlington Memorial Hospital, Darlington, County Durham, UK.

over the others. In experienced hands, the open operation can be reproduced by less invasive approaches, without significant compromise. Many groups have reported similar lymph node yields and rates of resection margin positivity with open and minimal access approaches. As yet, benefits seem to be confined to reduced wound pain and the absence of specific complications associated with long incisions.

Although many centres have reduced hospital mortality to low single figures after oesophagectomy, the complication rate remains high. At least a third of all patients will develop some significant complication after surgery. The most common of these is respiratory, followed by anastomotic leakage, chylothorax and injury to the recurrent laryngeal nerves. The most common late problem is benign anastomotic stricture, which seems to be higher with cervical rather than with intrathoracic anastomoses, although the problem is usually easily dealt with by endoscopic dilatation.

Lesions of the cardia that do not involve the oesophagus to any significant extent may be dealt with by extended total gastrectomy to include the distal oesophagus, or by proximal gastrectomy and distal oesophagectomy.

Summary box 62.13

Oesophagogastric surgery

- Beware of satellite nodules proximal to the primary lesion
- Carefully preserve the blood supply of the stomach, both venous and arterial
- Right thoracic approach gives easy access to the oesophagus

TWO-PHASE OESOPHAGECTOMY (ABDOMEN AND RIGHT CHEST, IVOR LEWIS)

Mobilisation of the stomach must be done with care because it is essential to have a tension-free, well-vascularised stomach for transposition. The left gastric, short gastric and left gastroepiploic arteries are all divided. The viability of the transposed stomach mainly depends on the right gastroepiploic and, to a lesser extent, the right gastric vessels. It should be noted that venous drainage is as important as arterial supply, and it is essential to perform an accurate anatomical dissection that preserves the right gastroepiploic vein as well as the artery. The stomach is divided to remove the cardia and the upper part of the lesser curve, including the whole of the left gastric artery and its associated lymph nodes.

The approach to the oesophagus through the right chest is straightforward, providing excellent access to the mediastinum, the thoracic inlet and the hiatus. The azygos vein is divided, and the whole of the intrathoracic oesophagus can be mobilised along with the thoracic duct (which is ligated by most surgeons) and the mediastinal lymph nodes. The oesophagus is divided just below the thoracic inlet. As most lesions are in the lower or middle third, this usually gives adequate proximal clearance of at least 5 cm. Carcinomas of the upper thoracic oesophagus are almost always incurable at the time of diagnosis, and invasion of the trachea is common. If one of these lesions is resectable, it is essential to use an incision in the neck (McKeown or three-phase operation) and to resect more of the oesophagus than is customary in the operation of subtotal oesophagectomy.

Oesophagogastric anastomosis may be performed equally well by hand or stapler. Both methods require attention to detail. In experienced hands, clinical anastomotic leakage should be less than 10%. Most surgeons still prefer to keep patients nil by mouth for 5–7 days. Most centres have abandoned the use of routine contrast swallows in patients who are clinically well. Conversely, aggressive investigation of a suspected leak is mandatory for any unexplained fever or clinical event. This should involve early endoscopy, which has been shown to be safe and is the most reliable method for identifying necrosis in any part of the replacement conduit and/or CT scan to resolve the situation adequately.

Postoperative nutritional support remains controversial. There is general agreement that parenteral feeding is associated with more nosocomial infection, including pneumonia, than enteral feeding. It is also expensive. The simplicity of placing a modern feeding jejunostomy device at the time of resection means that this is in routine use in many centres.

TRANSHIATAL OESOPHAGECTOMY (WITHOUT THORACOTOMY)

This approach was popularised for cancer by Orringer, adapting a technique developed in Brazil by Pinotti for the removal of chagasic megaoesophagus (see the section on achalasia, p. 1095). The stomach is mobilised through a midline abdominal incision or by laparoscopy, and the cervical oesophagus is mobilised through an incision in the neck. The diaphragm is then opened from the abdomen, and the posterior mediastinum is entered. The lower oesophagus and the tumour are mobilised under direct vision, and the upper oesophagus is mobilised by blunt dissection. This approach can provide an adequate removal of the tumour and lymph nodes in the lower mediastinum, but it is not possible to remove the nodes in the middle or upper mediastinum. It may be a useful procedure for lesions of the lower oesophagus, but is hazardous for a middle third lesion that may be adherent to the bronchus or to the azygos vein.

NEOADJUVANT TREATMENTS WITH SURGERY

Apart from the earliest stages of disease, surgery alone produces relatively few cures in either squamous cell carcinoma or adenocarcinoma patients. This led to a number of trials throughout the 1980s and 1990s to investigate the value of chemotherapy and surgery or chemoradiotherapy and surgery compared with surgery alone. Some studies relate only to squamous cell cancer, and many are open to criticism on the grounds of trial design or patient numbers. Nevertheless,

Mark Burton Orringer, surgeon, Ann Arbor, MI, USA.
Walter Pinotti, Professor of Surgery, Sao Paulo, Brazil.
Carlos Justiniano Ribeiro Chagas, 1879–1934, Director of the Oswaldo Cruz Institute and Professor of Tropical Medicine, the University of Rio de Janeiro, Brazil.

positive results in favour of neoadjuvant therapy for adenocarcinoma in two large studies as well as a limited meta-analysis indicated that it was no longer appropriate to consider surgery alone as the 'gold standard' treatment for most patients who are surgical candidates with adenocarcinoma. The Dutch trial (CROSS) that compared chemoradiotherapy and surgery versus surgery alone has provided the most convincing evidence so far of survival benefit for squamous cell carcinoma. The same study was initially unable to show a survival benefit for adenocarcinomas, although subsequent analyses again suggested survival benefit of similar magnitude to that seen with chemotherapy and surgery.

GASTRO-OESOPHAGEAL REFLUX FOLLOWING OESOPHAGOGASTRIC RESECTION

Gastro-oesophageal reflux may be a major problem after any operation that involves resecting the cardia. Reflux may present with the typical symptoms of GORD or with a peptic stricture at the site of the anastomosis. However, the presentation may be different with a miserable patient who fails to thrive after the operation and who is then suspected of having recurrent cancer. This atypical presentation is particularly common after total gastrectomy with an inadequate reconstruction that allows bile reflux.

Summary box 62.14

Postoesophagectomy

- Reflux may be a problem after resection
- Symptoms may be atypical
- Reflux may be limited or avoided by subtotal oesophagectomy and gastric transposition high in the chest

Non-surgical treatments

Radiotherapy alone was widely used as a single-modality treatment for squamous cell carcinoma of the oesophagus until the late 1970s. The 5-year survival overall rate was 6%. As a result, multimodal approaches were adopted throughout the 1980s, initial trials indicating that similar long-term survival rates could be obtained with surgery. Subsequent randomised studies, essentially confined to patients with squamous cell carcinoma, have indicated significant survival advantages with chemoradiotherapy over radiotherapy alone. Although it is clear that chemoradiotherapy does offer a prospect of cure for patients who may not be fit for surgery, particularly in squamous cell carcinoma, the high rate of locoregional failure has meant that surgery remains the mainstay of attempted curative treatments for both adenocarcinoma and squamous cell carcinoma in patients who have potentially resectable disease and are fit for oesophagectomy. In most western series, this represents about a third of patients with adenocarcinoma and a slightly lower percentage of patients with squamous cell carcinoma. There has been no high-quality randomised comparison of the results of definitive radiotherapy versus chemoradiotherapy and surgical resection, and it is therefore impossible to make dogmatic statements about the relative merits of each form of treatment.

Summary box 62.15

Alternative therapeutic approaches

- Chemoradiotherapy may be a useful alternative to surgery, especially in unfit patients

Palliative treatment

Surgical resection and external beam radiotherapy may be used for palliation, but are not suitable when the expected survival is short, because most of the remainder of life will be spent recovering from the 'treatment'. Surgical bypass is likewise too major a procedure for use in a patient with limited life expectancy. A variety of relatively simple methods of palliation is now available that will produce worthwhile relief of dysphagia with minimal disturbance to the patient.

Summary box 62.16

Palliation

- Palliation should be simple and effective

Intubation has been used for many years after the invention of the Souttar tube, which was made of coiled silver wire. A variety of rigid plastic or rubber tubes had been developed for placement under endoscopic and/or radiological control. The technology of intubation has now moved on with the development of various types of expanding metal stent (Figure 62.52). These are also inserted under radiographic or endoscopic control. The stent is collapsed during insertion and released when it is in the correct position. Expanding stents produce a wider lumen for swallowing than rigid tubes. More importantly, it is not necessary to dilate the oesophagus to beyond 8 mm to insert the unexpanded stent through the tumour, so there is a lower risk of injury to the oesophagus.

Endoscopic laser treatment may be used to core a channel through the tumour. It is based on thermal tumour destruction. It produces a worthwhile improvement in swallowing, but has the disadvantage that it has to be repeated every few weeks. Lasers may also be used to unblock a stent that has become occluded by tumour overgrowth. Other endoscopic

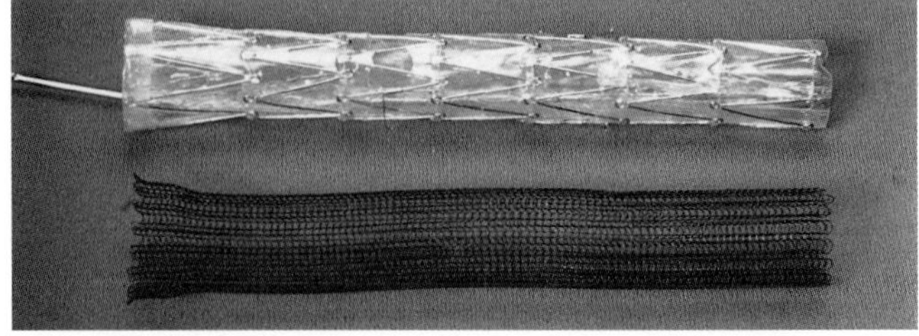

Figure 62.52 Expanding metal stents, covered and uncovered.

Sir Henry Sessions Souttar, 1875–1964, surgeon, the London Hospital, London, UK.

methods include bipolar diathermy, argon-beam plasma coagulation and alcohol injection.

Brachytherapy is a method of delivering intraluminal radiation with a short penetration distance (hence the prefix 'brachy') to a tumour. An introduction system is inserted through the tumour, and the treatment is then delivered in a single session lasting approximately 20 minutes. The equipment is expensive to purchase, but running costs are low.

Although the above methods are suitable for patients with very advanced disease, elderly people and those with significant comorbidities that would make more aggressive strategies inappropriate, an increasing proportion of patients (particularly with adenocarcinoma) are being treated with platinum-based chemotherapy. In general, this leads to only a modest prolongation of survival but a better quality of life than in those receiving an endoscopic treatment alone.

Malignant tracheo-oesophageal fistula

Malignant tracheo-oesophageal fistula is a sign of incurable disease. Some have advocated surgical bypass and oesophageal exclusion, but this is a major procedure. An expanding metal stent is probably the best treatment.

Post-cricoid carcinoma

Post-cricoid carcinoma is considered in Chapter 47.

MOTILITY DISORDERS AND DIVERTICULA

Oesophageal motility disorders

A motility disorder can be readily understood when a patient has dysphagia in the absence of a stricture, and a barium-impregnated food bolus is seen to stick in the oesophagus. If this can be correlated with a specific abnormality on oesophageal manometry, accepting that this is the cause of the patient's symptoms may be straightforward. Unfortunately, this is often not the case. Pain, with or without a swallowing problem, is frequently the dominant symptom, and patients often undergo extensive hospital investigation before the oesophagus is considered as a source of symptoms. Symptoms are often intermittent, and the correlation between symptoms and test 'abnormalities' is poor. Confirmation of a specific motility disturbance is made by high-resolution manometry. Much harm may be done by inappropriate enthusiastic surgery for ill-defined conditions. It should also be remembered that oesophageal dysmotility may be only a feature of a general disturbance in GI function.

Summary box 62.17

Oesophageal motility disorders

- May be part of a more diffuse GI motility problem
- May be associated with GORD

Oesophageal motility disorders are currently best classified by incorporation of the Chicago classification developed for use with high-resolution manometry as shown in *Tables 62.3 and 62.4*.

Functional pain and the oesophagus

Pain that is assumed to arise from dysfunction of the GI tract may reflect abnormal motor activity, abnormal perception or a combination of the two. There is evidence that all three exist. Very high-pressure uncoordinated contractions ('spasm') have been shown to correlate with pain. Distension of a balloon in the oesophagus indicates that some patients have a low threshold for the sensation of pain (visceral hypersensitivity), and this itself may reflect local or central neuronal dysfunction. In practice, the difficulty is in understanding the relative contributions of these elements, so that a logical treatment might follow.

Achalasia

Pathology and aetiology

Achalasia (Greek 'failure to relax') is uncommon, but merits prominence because it is reasonably understood and responds to treatment. It is due to loss of the ganglion cells in the myenteric (Auerbach's) plexus, the cause of which is unknown. In South America, chronic infection with the parasite *Trypanosoma cruzi* causes Chagas' disease, which has marked clinical similarities to achalasia. Achalasia differs

TABLE 62.3 General classification of oesophageal motility disorders.

Disorders of the pharyngo-oesophageal junction
Neurological – stroke, motor neuron disease, multiple sclerosis, Parkinson's disease
Myogenic – myasthenia, muscular dystrophy
Pharyngo-oesophageal (Zenker's) diverticulum
Disorders of the body of the oesophagus
Diffuse oesophageal spasm
Nutcracker oesophagus
Autoimmune disorders – especially systemic sclerosis (CREST)
Reflux associated
Idiopathic
Allergic
Eosinophilic oesophagitis
Non-specific oesophageal dysmotility
Disorders of the lower oesophageal sphincter
Achalasia
Incompetent lower sphincter (i.e. GORD)

CREST, calcinosis, Raynaud's syndrome, (o)esophageal motility disorders, sclerodactyly and telangiectasia.
GORD, gastro-oesophageal reflux disease.

TABLE 62.4 The Chicago Classification of oesophageal motility v3.0.

Achalasia and EGJ outflow obstruction	Criteria
Type I achalasia (classic achalasia)	Elevated median IRP (>15 mmHg), 100% failed peristalsis (DCI <100 mmHg·s·cm) *Premature contractions with DCI values* <450 mmHg·s·cm *satisfy criteria for failed peristalsis*
Type II achalasia (with oesophageal compression)	Elevated median IRP (>15 mmHg), 100% failed peristalsis, panoesophageal pressurisation with ≥20% of swallows *Contractions may be masked by oesophageal pressurisation and DCI should not be calculated*
Type III achalasia (spastic achalasia)	Elevated median IRP (>15 mmHg), no normal peristalsis, premature (spastic) contractions with DCI >450 mmHg·s·cm with ≥20% of swallows *May be mixed with panoesophageal pressurisation*
EGJ outflow obstruction	Elevated median IRP (>15 mmHg), sufficient evidence of peristalsis such that criteria for types I–III achalasia are not met
Major disorders of peristalsis	(Not encountered in normal individuals)
Absent contractility	Normal median IRP, 100% failed peristalsis *Achalasia should be considered when IRP values are borderline and when there is evidence of oesophageal pressurisation* *Premature contractions with DCI values* <450 mmHg·s·cm *meet criteria for failed peristalsis*
Distal oesophageal spasm	Normal median IRP, ≥20% premature contractions with DCI >450 mmHg·s·cm. Some normal peristalsis may be present
Hypercontractile oesophagus (jackhammer)	At least two swallows with DCI >8000 mmHg·s·cm *Hypercontractility may involve, or even be localised to, the LES*
Minor disorders of peristalsis	(Characterised by contractile vigour and contraction pattern)
Ineffective oesophageal motility (IEM)	≥50% ineffective swallows *Ineffective swallows can be failed or weak (DCI <450 mmHg·s·cm)* *Multiple repetitive swallow assessment may be helpful in determining peristaltic reserve*
Fragmented peristalsis	≥50% fragmented contractions with DCI >450 mmHg·s·cm
Normal oesophageal motility	Not fulfilling any of the above classifications

DCI, distal contractile integral (mmHg·s·cm); EGJ, o(e)sophaogastric junction; IRP, integrated relaxation pressure (mmHg); LES, lower o(e)sophageal sphincter. (From Kahrilas PJ *et al*. The Chicago Classification of esophageal motility disorders v3.0. *Neurogastroenterology and Motility* 2015; **27**(2): 160–74, with kind permission, John Wiley & Sons.)

from Hirschsprung's disease of the colon because the dilated oesophagus usually contains few ganglion cells, whereas the dilated colon contains normal ganglion cells proximal to a constricted, aganglionic segment. Histology of muscle specimens generally shows a reduction in the number of ganglion cells (and mainly inhibitory neurons) with a variable degree of chronic inflammation. When powerful non-peristaltic contractions are still present, perhaps representing an early stage of the disease, inflammation and neural fibrosis may be seen with normal numbers of ganglion cells.

Summary box 62.18

Achalasia

- Is uncommon
- Is due to selective loss of inhibitory neurons in the lower oesophagus
- The causes dysphagia and carcinoma must be excluded
- Treatment is by either endoscopic dilatation, or endoscopic or surgical myotomy

The classic physiological abnormalities are a non-relaxing LOS and absent peristalsis in the body of the oesophagus. The Chicago classification identifies three variants. Although most patients have almost no recognisable contractions (type I), some patients continue to exhibit pressurisation throughout the oesophagus (type 2), whereas in others the oesophagus is of normal calibre and exhibits high-pressure contractile (although non-peristaltic) activity (spastic oesophagus, vigorous achalasia). In some patients, these uncoordinated contractions result in pain as much as a sense of food sticking. High-resolution manometry recognises these contraction patterns, which may be important in predicting the outcome of treatment. With time, the oesophagus dilates and contractions disappear, so that the oesophagus empties mainly by the hydrostatic pressure of its contents. This is nearly always incomplete, leaving residual food and fluid. The gas bubble in the stomach is frequently absent, as no bolus with its accompanying normal gas passes through the sphincter. The 'megaoesophagus' becomes tortuous with a persistent retention oesophagitis due to fermentation of food residues (Figure 62.53), and this may account for the increased incidence of carcinoma of the oesophagus

Harald Hirschsprung, 1831–1916, physician, the Queen Louise Hospital for Children, and Professor of Paediatrics, Copenhagen, Denmark, described congenital megacolon in 1888.

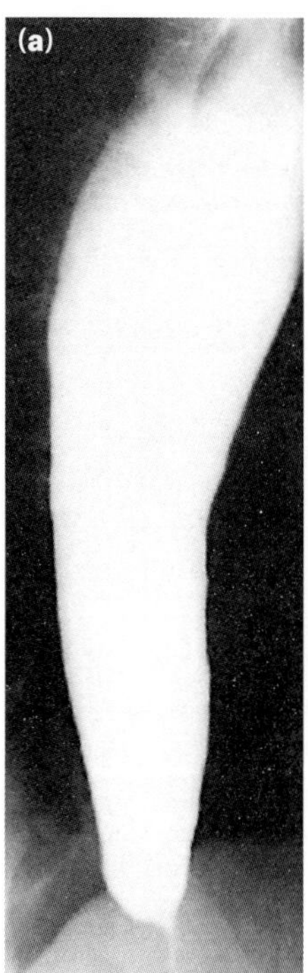

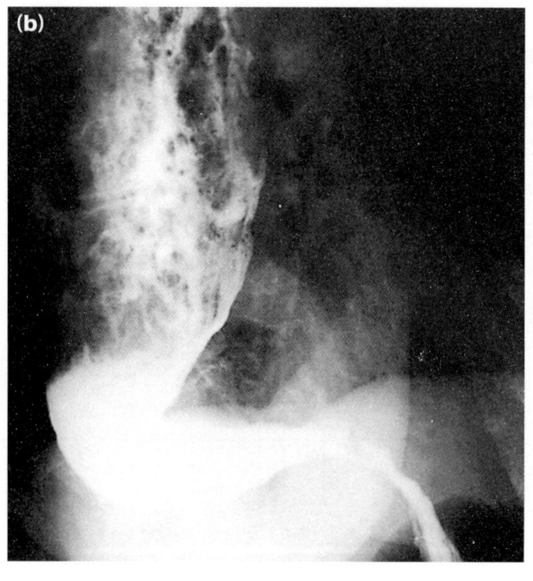

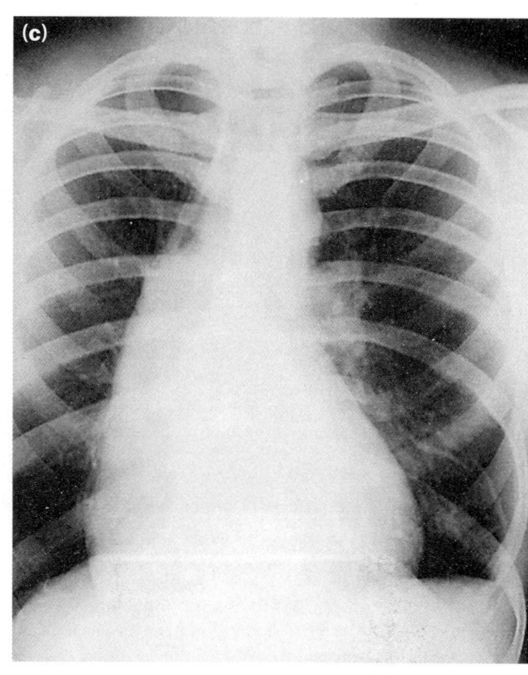

Figure 62.53 Achalasia of the oesophagus. (a) Barium swallow showing the smooth outline of the stricture, which narrows to a point at its lower end. (b) Tortuosity and sigmoid appearance of the lower oesophagus. (c) Mediastinal shadow due to a large, fluid-filled oesophagus.

Summary box 62.19

Lower oesophageal stricture

- Beware pseudoachalasia; look for tumour

Pseudoachalasia is an achalasia-like disorder that is usually produced by adenocarcinoma of the cardia (Figure 62.54), but has also been described in relation to benign tumours at this level. It has been presumed that the inability of the sphincter to relax is linked to the loss of body peristalsis, although other cancers outside the oesophagus (bronchus, pancreas) have also been associated with pseudoachalasia.

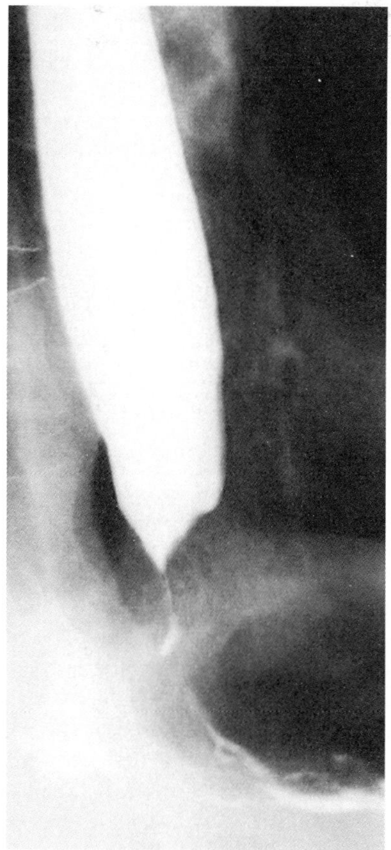

Figure 62.54 Almost achalasia, but note the irregularity of the taper, which indicates carcinoma of the cardia.

Clinical features

The disease is most common in middle life, but can occur at any age. It typically presents with dysphagia, although pain (often mistaken for reflux) is common in the early stages. Patients often present late and, having had relatively mild symptoms, remain untreated for many years. Regurgitation is frequent, and there may be overspill into the trachea, especially at night.

Diagnosis

Achalasia may be suspected at endoscopy by finding a tight cardia and food residue in the oesophagus. Barium radiology may show hold-up in the distal oesophagus, abnormal contractions in the oesophageal body and a tapering stricture in the distal oesophagus, often described as a 'bird's beak' (see

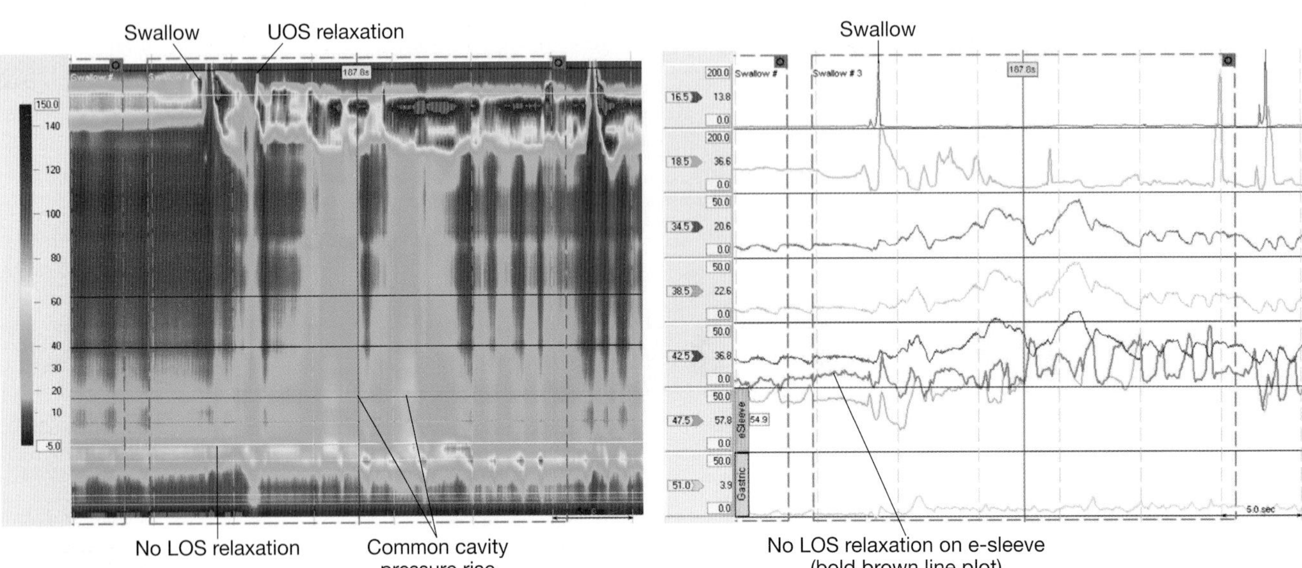

Figure 62.55 High-resolution oesophageal manometry from a patient presenting with dysphagia and regurgitation. The swallow is followed by a common cavity rise in oesophageal pressure indicating filling. Lower oesophageal sphincter (LOS) relaxation is absent and there is a positive oesophagogastric pressure gradient. Upper oesophageal sphincter (UOS) relaxation shortly after the swallow was related to regurgitation of oesophageal contents.

Figure 62.53). The gastric gas bubble is usually absent. These typical features of well-developed achalasia are often absent, and endoscopy and radiology can be normal. A firm diagnosis is established by high-resolution oesophageal manometry. Classically, the LOS does not relax completely on swallowing, there is no peristalsis and there is a raised resting pressure in the oesophagus (Figure 62.55). The LOS pressure may be elevated, but is often normal.

Treatment

Alone among motility disorders, achalasia responds well to treatment. The two main methods are forceful dilatation of the cardia and laparoscopic cardiomyotomy (conventionally performed together with a partial fundoplication), although in recent years there has been growing interest in the use of peroral endoscopic myotomy (POEM). Comparative studies between pneumatic dilatation and surgical myotomy suggest equivalence in terms of safety, effectiveness and cost when considered over a number of years.

PNEUMATIC DILATATION

This involves stretching the cardia with a balloon to disrupt the muscle and render it less competent. The treatment was first described by Plummer. Many varieties of balloon have been used but, nowadays, plastic balloons with a precisely controlled external diameter are used. If the pressure in the balloon is too high, the balloon is designed to split along its length rather than expanding further. Balloons of 30–40 mm in diameter are available and are inserted over a guidewire (Figure 62.56). Perforation is the major complication. With a 30-mm balloon, the incidence of perforation should be less than 0.5%. The risk of perforation increases with bigger balloons, and they should be used cautiously for progressive dilatation over a period of weeks. Forceful dilatation is curative in 75–85% of cases. The results are best in patients aged over 45 years.

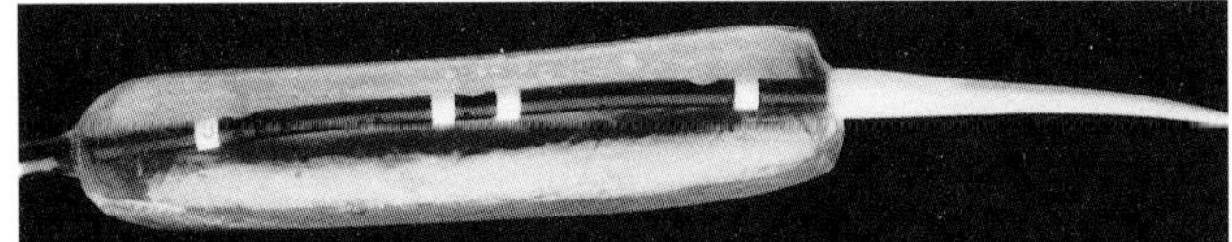

Figure 62.56 Balloon dilator for the treatment of achalasia by forceful dilatation.

Summary box 62.20

Achalasia

- Beware perforation due to dilatation of achalasia
- Beware postoperative reflux

HELLER'S MYOTOMY

This involves cutting the muscle of the lower oesophagus and cardia (Figure 62.57). The major complication is

Henry Stanley Plummer, 1874–1937, physician, the Mayo Clinic, Rochester, MN, USA.
Ernst Heller, 1877–1964, surgeon, St George's Krankenhaus, Leipzig, Germany.

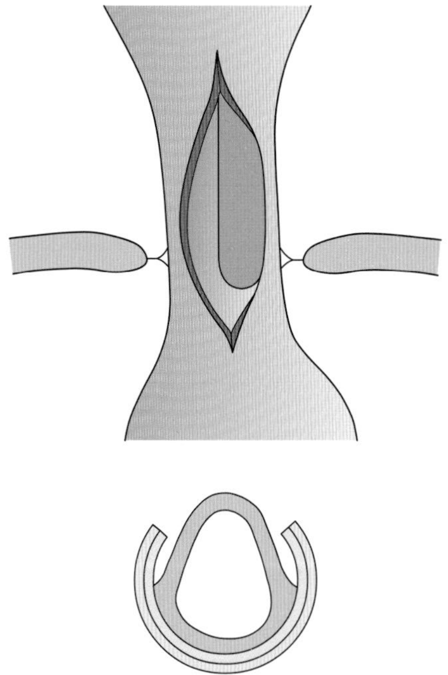

Figure 62.57 Heller's myotomy: the incision should not go too far on to the stomach. The lateral extent must enable the mucosa to pout out, to prevent the edges healing together.

gastro-oesophageal reflux, and most surgeons therefore add a partial anterior fundoplication (Heller–Dor operation). The procedure is ideally suited to a minimal access laparoscopic approach, and most surgeons use intraoperative endoscopy to judge the extent of the myotomy and to ensure that the narrow segment is abolished.

It is successful in more than 90% of cases and may be used after failed dilatation.

ENDOSCOPIC MYOTOMY

This was introduced in Japan in 2009. It involves the creation of a submucosal tunnel in the midoesophagus that can be developed distally, allowing a long myotomy to be performed. The oesophageal mucosal defect is clipped shut at the end. Many cohort studies indicate that the procedure can be performed safely and early clinical results imply equivalence to other approaches.

BOTULINUM TOXIN

This is done by endoscopic injection into the LOS. It acts by interfering with cholinergic excitatory neural activity at the LOS. The effect is not permanent, and the injection usually has to be repeated after a few months. For this reason, its use is restricted to elderly patients with other comorbidities.

DRUGS

Drugs such as calcium channel antagonists have been used but are ineffective for long-term use. However, sublingual nifedipine may be useful for transient relief of symptoms if definitive treatment is postponed.

Other oesophageal motility disorders

Disorders of the pharyngo-oesophageal junction

With the exception of Zenker's diverticulum (see below), most patients with oropharyngeal dysphagia have generalised neurological or muscular disorders with pharyngeal involvement. A small number of patients who have sustained a cerebrovascular accident benefit from myotomy of cricopharyngeus to alleviate pooling of saliva and nocturnal aspiration, but they should have good deglutition and phonation before this is performed. The operation is also effective in patients with oculopharyngeal muscular dystrophy.

Disorders of the body of the oesophagus

The older terms, 'diffuse oesophageal spasm' and 'jackhammer (nutcracker) oesophagus', have been replaced in the Chicago classification. There are, nevertheless, patients with incoordinate contractions of the oesophagus who experience dysphagia and/or chest pain. The condition may be dramatic, with spastic pressures on manometry of 400–500 mmHg, marked hypertrophy of the circular muscle and a corkscrew oesophagus on barium swallow (Figure 62.58). These abnormal contractions are more common in the distal two-thirds of the oesophageal body (Figure 62.59) and this may have some relevance to treatment. Making the diagnosis when chest pain is the only symptom may be difficult. Prolonged oesophageal manometry that correlates episodes of chest pain with manometric abnormalities may establish the diagnosis.

There is no proven pharmacological or endoscopic treatment. Calcium channel antagonists, vasodilators and endoscopic dilatation have only transient effects. Although the severity and frequency of symptoms may be tolerated by most

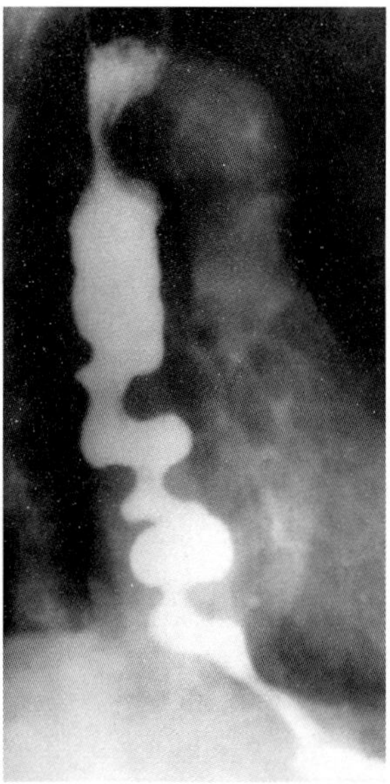

Figure 62.58 Corkscrew oesophagus in diffuse oesophageal spasm.

Friedrich Albert Zenker, 1825–1898, Professor of Pathology, Dresden, Germany.

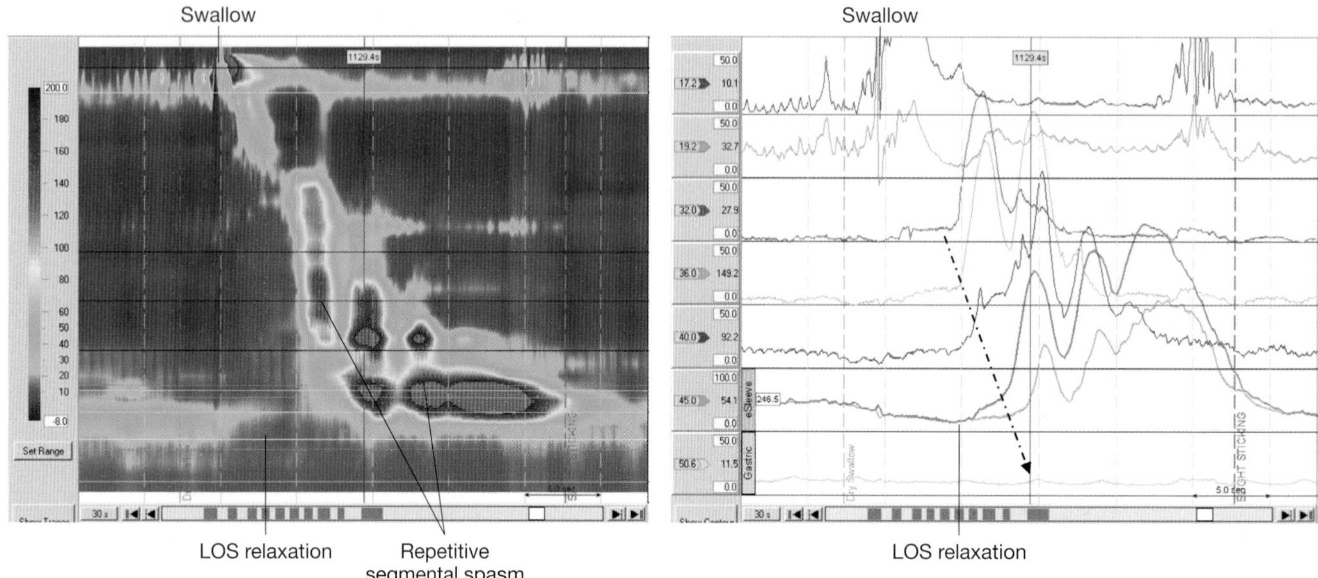

Figure 62.59 High-resolution oesophageal manometry from a patient presenting with dysphagia and chest pain. The swallow is followed by simultaneous, repetitive contractions in the mid-distal smooth muscle oesophagus. Lower oesophageal sphincter (LOS) relaxation is preserved. Note the sequential simultaneous contractions first in the mid- and distal segments of the oesophagus and then in the LOS make it appear as if there is progressive peristalsis on the conventional line plots (dotted arrow). Repetitive contractions are seen clearly on both.

patients, sometimes the combination of chest pain and dysphagia is sufficiently severe that malnutrition begins. In these patients, extended oesophageal myotomy up to the aortic arch may be required. Surgical treatment is more successful in improving dysphagia than chest pain, and caution should be exercised in patients in whom chest pain is the only symptom.

Jackhammer or nutcracker oesophagus is a condition with characteristic high-pressure manometric features (see Table 62.4). The correlation of manometric abnormalities with symptoms remains poor.

OESOPHAGEAL INVOLVEMENT IN AUTOIMMUNE DISEASE

Oesophageal involvement is mainly seen in systemic sclerosis, but may be a feature of polymyositis, dermatomyositis, systemic lupus erythematosus, polyarteritis nodosa and rheumatoid disease. Although most involve weak peristalsis, swallowing difficulties may be compounded by pharyngeal problems in the disorders that primarily affect skeletal muscle (e.g. polymyositis) or extraoesophageal problems such as involvement of the cricoarytenoid joint in rheumatoid disease or dry mouth in Sjögren's syndrome. In systemic sclerosis, smooth muscle atrophy causes hypoperistalsis (Figure 62.60). The LOS is involved, leading to a loss of the antireflux barrier. A wide range of symptoms can follow from mild to severe dysphagia accompanied by regurgitation and aspiration. Reflux can be severe and is exacerbated by weak acid clearance so that strictures can occur. There are no drugs that specifically correct the motor disorder, and medical treatment is mainly directed at minimising reflux-induced damage with PPIs. A small number of patients may require anti-reflux surgery.

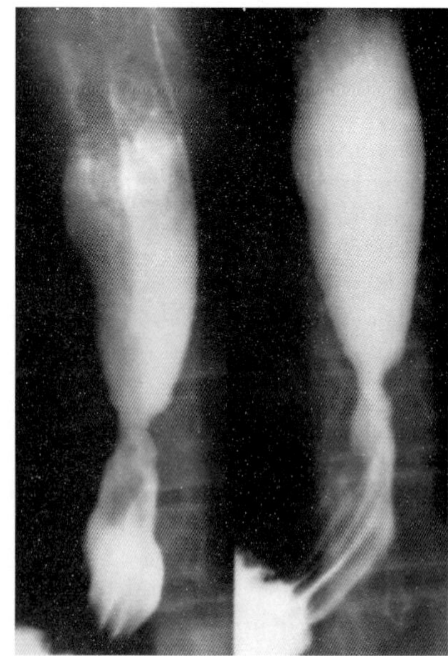

Figure 62.60 Advanced scleroderma of the oesophagus. The oesophagus dilates, and the lower oesophageal sphincter is widely incompetent.

Eosinophilic oesophagitis is a disorder that occurs in children and adults either alone or as a manifestation of

Henrik Samuel Conrad Sjögren, 1899–1986, Professor of Ophthalmology, Gothenburg, Sweden.

eosinophilic gastroenteritis. It is characterised by eosinophilic infiltration of the oesophageal wall, presumably of allergic or idiopathic origin. The most common presenting symptom is dysphagia, and more than half have some history of atopy. The oesophagus often seems narrow and friable on endoscopy and may include mucosal rings. The most important feature is the development of deep ulcers, leading to stricture development, especially in the proximal oesophagus. The diagnosis is established by endoscopic biopsy.

Elimination diets, and topical and systemic steroids all seem to be helpful in the short term, but there is scant information on the long-term impact of any particular approach. Immunotherapy directed against interleukin (IL)-5, which has a major role in eosinophil recruitment, seems to be a promising innovative approach. Although endoscopic dilatation has been recommended, this can create deep ulcers and further scarring, so should be used with caution and only when the above therapies fail.

Pharyngeal and oesophageal diverticula

Most oesophageal diverticula are **pulsion** diverticula that develop at a site of weakness as a result of chronic pressure against an obstruction. Symptoms are mostly caused by the underlying disorder unless the diverticulum is particularly large. Traction diverticula (Figure 62.61) are much less common. They are mostly a consequence of chronic granulomatous disease affecting the tracheobronchial lymph nodes due to tuberculosis, atypical mycobacteria or histoplasmosis. Fibrotic healing of the lymph nodes exerts traction on the oesophageal wall and produces a focal outpouching which is usually small and has a conical shape. There may be associated broncholithiasis, and additional complications may occur, such as aerodigestive fistulation (Figure 62.62) and bleeding.

Zenker's diverticulum (pharyngeal pouch) is not really an oesophageal diverticulum as it protrudes posteriorly above the cricopharyngeal sphincter through the natural weak point (the dehiscence of Killian) between the oblique and horizontal (cricopharyngeus) fibres of the inferior pharyngeal constrictor (Figures 62.63 and 62.64). The exact mechanism that leads to its formation is unknown, but it involves loss of the coordination between pharyngeal contraction and opening of the upper sphincter. When the diverticulum is small, symptoms largely reflect this incoordination with predominantly pharyngeal dysphagia. As the pouch enlarges, it tends to fill with food on eating, and the fundus descends into the mediastinum. This leads to halitosis and oesophageal dysphagia. Treatment can be undertaken endoscopically with a linear cutting stapler to divide the septum between the diverticulum and the upper oesophagus, producing a

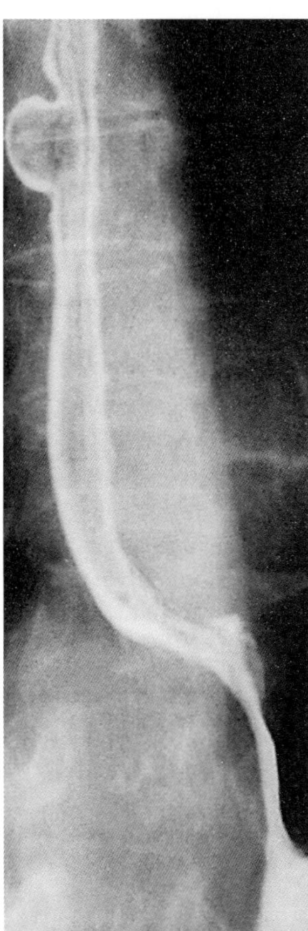

Figure 62.61 Midoesophageal traction diverticulum with the mouth facing downwards.

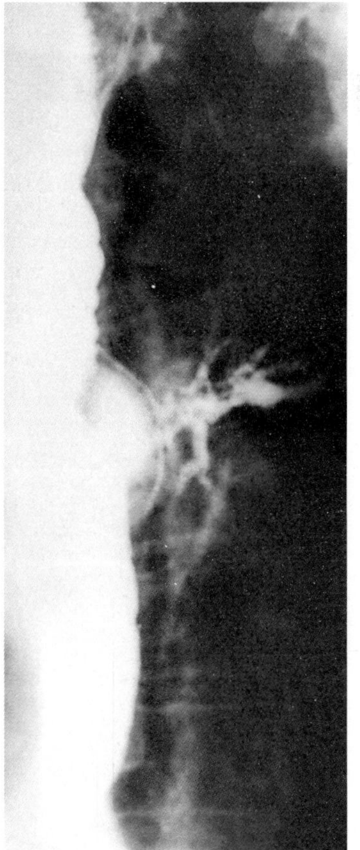

Figure 62.62 Midoesophageal diverticulum with a trachea-oesophageal fistula.

Gustav Killian, 1860–1921, Professor of Laryngology at Freiburg, and later at Berlin, Germany.

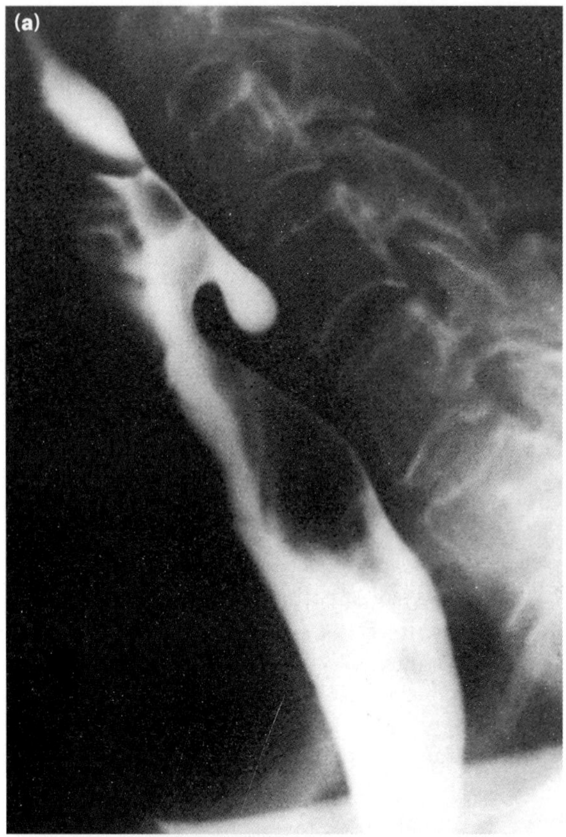

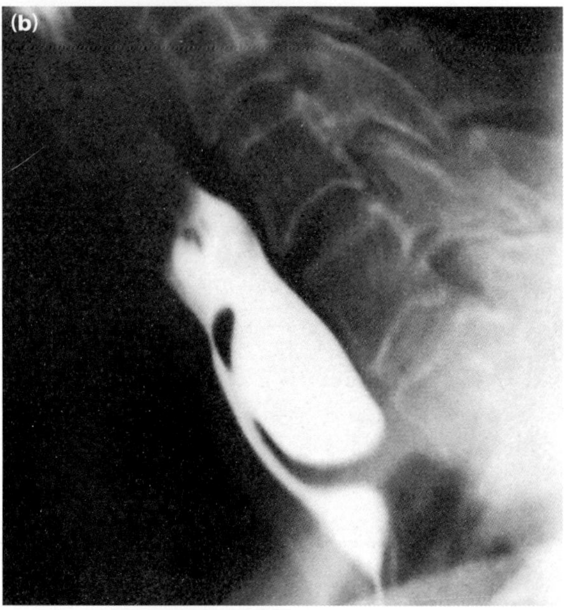

Figure 62.63 The typical appearances of: (a) a small pharyngeal pouch with a prominent cricopharyngeal impression and 'streaming' of barium, indicating partial obstruction; and (b) a large pouch extending behind the oesophagus towards the thoracic inlet.

diverticulo-oesophagostomy, or can be done by open surgery involving pouch excision, pouch suspension (diverticulopexy) and/or myotomy of cricopharyngeus. All techniques have good results.

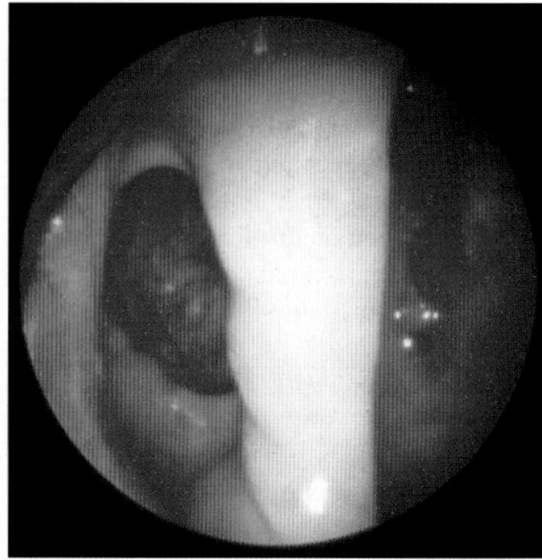

Figure 62.64 The endoscopic appearance of the mouth of a pharyngeal pouch posterior to the normal opening (left) of the oesophagus.

Midoesophageal diverticula are usually small pulsion diverticula of no particular consequence. The underlying motility disorder does not usually require treatment. Some pulsion diverticula may fistulate into the trachea (see Figure 62.62), but this is more common with traction diverticula in granulomatous disease.

Epiphrenic diverticula are pulsion diverticula situated in the lower oesophagus above the diaphragm (Figure 62.65). They may be quite large, but cause surprisingly few symptoms. They again probably reflect some loss of coordination between an incoming pressure wave and appropriate relaxation of the LOS. This needs to be acknowledged in the surgical management of the patient. The diverticulum, in isolation, should not be assumed to account for a patient's illness just because it looks dramatic on a radiograph. Large diverticula may be excised, and this should be combined with a myotomy from the site of the diverticulum down to the cardia to relieve functional obstruction.

Summary box 62.21

Oesophageal diverticula

- Diverticula are indicators of a motor disorder and not necessarily the cause of symptoms

Diffuse intramural pseudodiverticulosis is a rare condition in which there are multiple tiny outpouchings from the lumen of the oesophagus. The pseudodiverticula are dilated excretory ducts of oesophageal sebaceous glands. It is questionable whether the condition produces any symptoms in its own right.

OTHER NON-NEOPLASTIC CONDITIONS

Schatzki's ring

Schatzki's ring is a circular ring in the distal oesophagus (Figure 62.66), usually at the squamocolumnar junction. The

Richard Schatzki, 1901–1992, American radiologist.

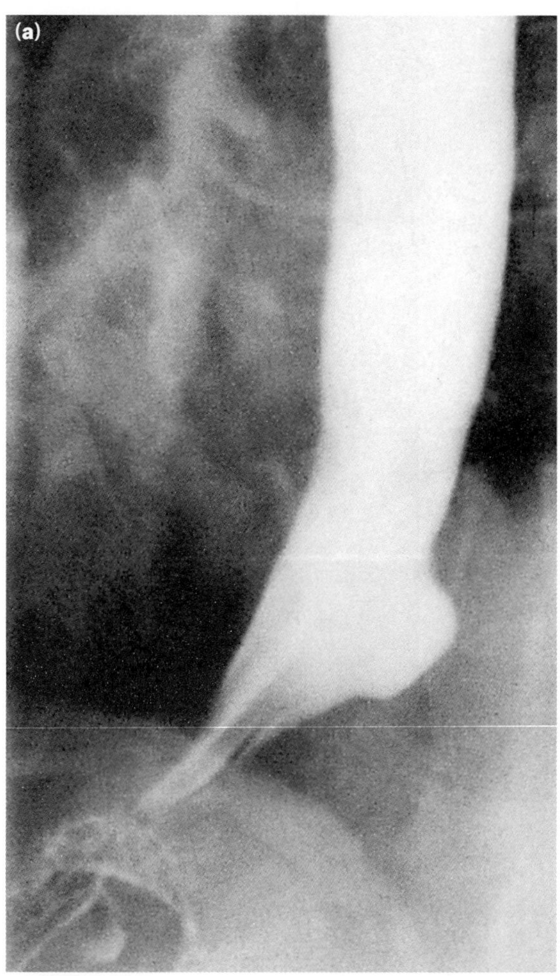

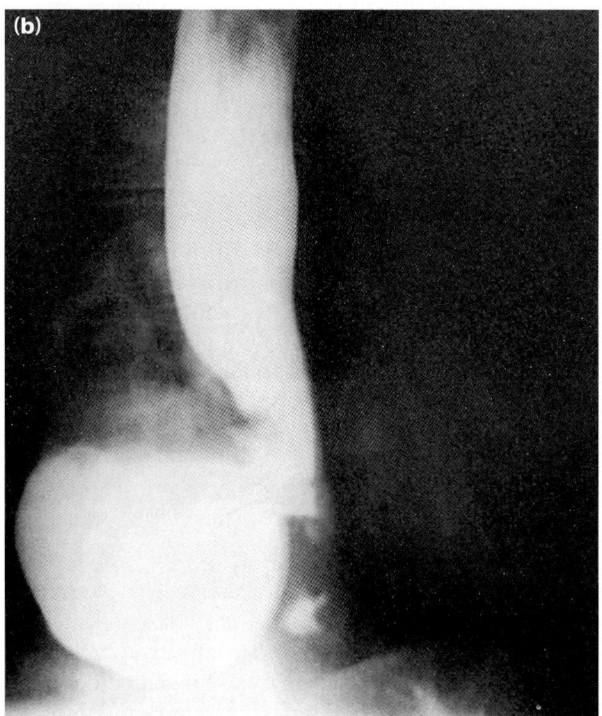

Figure 62.65 Epiphrenic diverticulum proximal to the gastro-oesophageal sphincter. (a) Small and asymptomatic; (b) large, symptomatic and appearing as a gas-filled bubble on the chest radiograph.

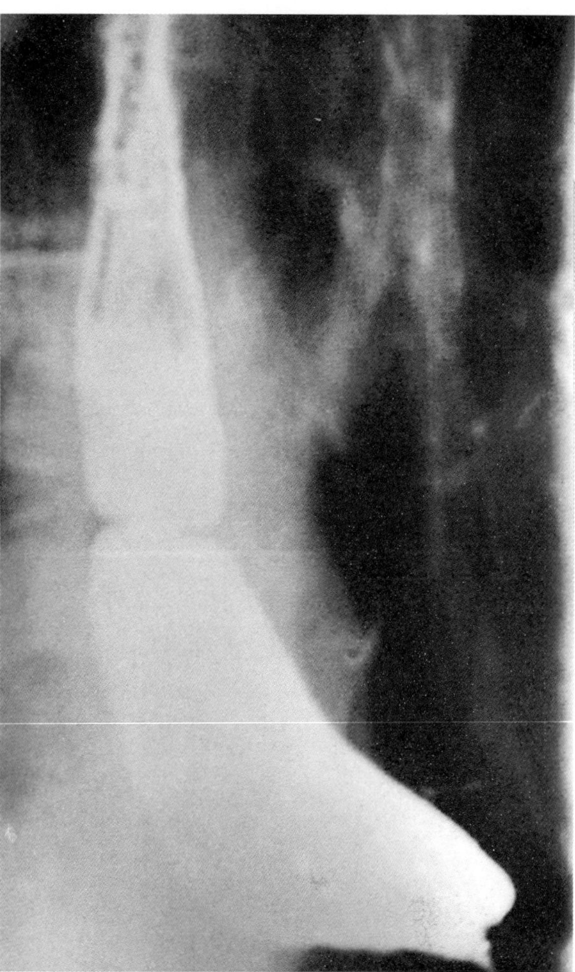

Figure 62.66 Schatzki's ring, a thin submucosal web completely encircling the whole of the lumen, usually situated at the squamo-columnar junction.

cause is obscure, but there is a strong association with reflux disease. The core of the ring consists of variable amounts of fibrous tissue and cellular infiltrate. Most rings are incidental findings. Some are associated with dysphagia and respond to dilatation in conjunction with medical antireflux therapy.

Oesophageal infections

Bacterial infection of the oesophagus is rare, but fungal and viral infections do occur. They are particularly important in immunocompromised patients.

Oesophagitis due to *Candida albicans* is relatively common in patients taking steroids (especially transplant recipients) or those undergoing cancer chemotherapy. It may present with dysphagia or odynophagia. There may be visible thrush in the throat. Endoscopy shows numerous white plaques that cannot be moved, unlike food residues (Figure 62.67). Biopsies are diagnostic. In severe cases, a barium swallow may show dramatic mucosal ulceration and irregularity that is surprisingly similar to the appearance of oesophageal varices (Figures 62.68 and 62.69). Treatment is with a topical antifungal agent.

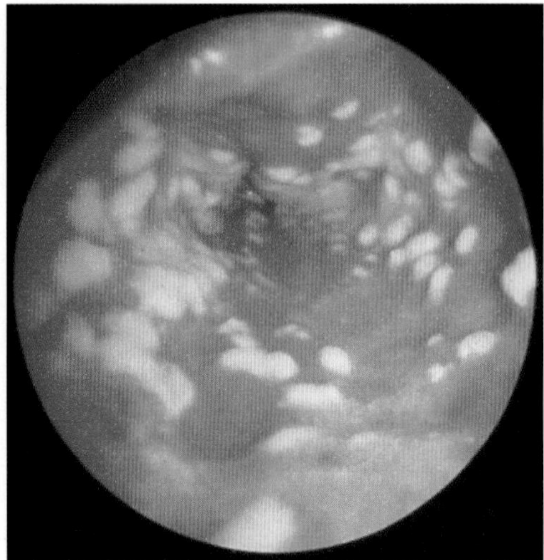

Figure 62.67 Endoscopic appearance of oesophageal candidiasis.

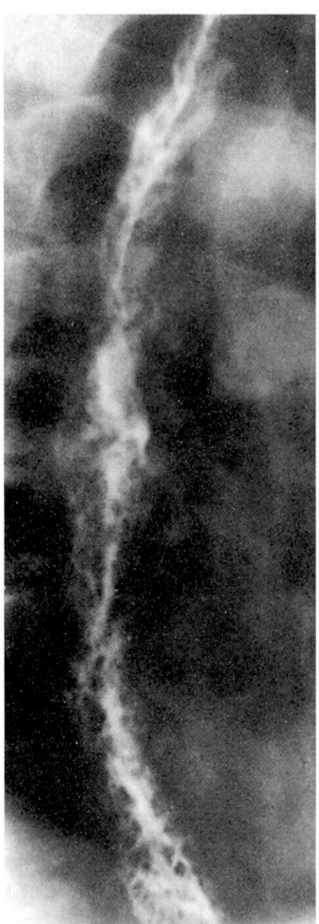

Figure 62.68 Oesophageal candidiasis with shaggy appearance of mucosal defects.

Dysphagia and odynophagia can also be caused by herpes simplex virus and cytomegalovirus (CMV). With the former, there may be a history of a herpetic lesion on the lip some days earlier, and endoscopy may reveal vesicles or small ulcers with raised margins, usually in the upper half of the oesophagus. CMV infection may be apparent in graft-versus-host disease following bone marrow transplantation. It has a characteristic endoscopic appearance with a geographical, serpiginous border. In both cases, endoscopic biopsy is diagnostic.

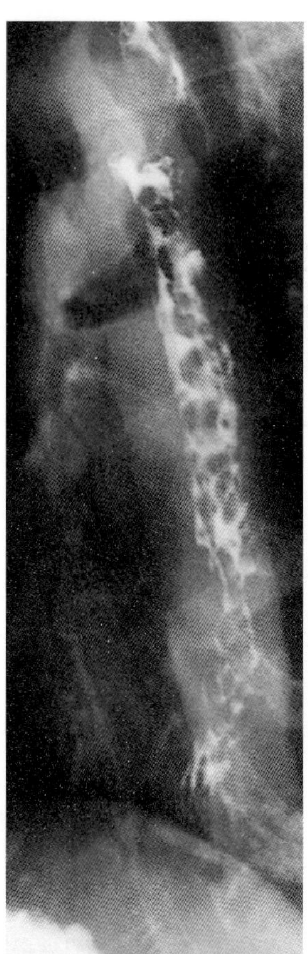

Figure 62.69 Oesophageal varices with smooth outline of the filling defects.

Chagas' disease

This condition is confined to South American countries, but is of interest because oesophageal symptoms occur that are similar to severe achalasia. It is caused by a protozoan, Trypanosoma cruzi, transmitted by an insect vector. Parasites reach the bloodstream and, after a long latent period, there is damage particularly to cardiac and smooth muscle. Destruction of both Auerbach's and Meissner's plexus leads to acquired megaoesophagus.

Crohn's disease

The oesophagus is not commonly affected by symptomatic Crohn's disease. However, pathological studies indicate that it may be present in 20% of patients without symptoms. Symptoms are often severe, and a diagnosis of reflux oesophagitis is usually made on the basis of retrosternal pain and dysphagia.

Burrill Bernard Crohn, 1884–1983, gastroenterologist, Mount Sinai Hospital, New York, NY, USA, described regional ileitis in 1932.

Endoscopy shows extensive oesophagitis that extends much further proximally than reflux oesophagitis. Biopsies may be diagnostic, but may show only non-specific inflammation. In severe cases, deep sinuses occur, and fistulation has been described. Crohn's oesophagitis is said to respond poorly to medical treatment and, although balloon dilatation of strictures and surgical resection for multiple internal fistulae have both been described, these interventions should be used with great caution.

Plummer-Vinson syndrome

This is also called the Paterson–Kelly (or Paterson–Brown Kelly) syndrome or sideropenic dysphagia. The original descriptions are vague and poorly supported by evidence of a coherent syndrome. Dysphagia is said to occur because of the presence of a postcricoid web that is associated with iron deficiency anaemia, glossitis and koilonychia. The classic syndrome is rarely complete. Some patients may have oropharyngeal leukoplakia, and this may account for an alleged increased risk of developing hypopharyngeal cancer.

Webs certainly occur in the upper and middle oesophagus, usually without any kind of associated syndrome. They are nearly always thin diaphanous membranes identified coincidentally by contrast radiology. Even symptomatic webs that cause a degree of obstruction may be inadvertently ruptured at endoscopy. Few require formal endoscopic dilatation.

Vascular abnormalities affecting the oesophagus

Several congenital vascular anomalies may produce dysphagia by compression of the oesophagus. Classically, this results from an aberrant right subclavian artery (arteria lusoria). However, the oesophagus is more commonly compressed by vascular rings, such as a double aortic arch. Dysphagia occurs in only a minority of cases and usually presents early in childhood, although it can occur in the late teens. Treatment is usually by division of the non-dominant component of the ring.

In adults, acquired causes include aneurysm of the aorta, diffuse cardiac enlargement and pressure from the left common carotid or vertebral arteries. It is rare that symptom severity justifies surgical intervention.

Mediastinal fibrosis

This rare condition can occur alone or together with retroperitoneal fibrosis. The cause is unknown and, although the major consequences are usually cardiovascular as a result of caval compression, dysphagia can occur. The existence of irreparable cardiovascular problems usually precludes surgical intervention on the oesophagus.

FURTHER READING

Castell DO, Richter JE. *The esophagus*, 5th edn. Oxford: Wiley-Blackwell, 2011.

Griffin SM, Raimes SA, Shenfine J. *Oesophago-gastric surgery*, 5th edn. Philadelphia, PA: Saunders Ltd, 2013.

Luketich JD. *Master techniques in surgery: esophageal surgery*. Philadelphia, PA: Wolters Kluwer, 2014.

Pleskow D, Erim T. *Barrett's esophagus: emerging evidence for improved clinical practice*. Cambridge, MA: Academic Press, 2016.

Sharma P, Sampliner RE, Ilson D. *Esophageal cancer and Barrett's oesophagus*, 3rd edn. Hoboken, NJ: John Wiley & Sons, 2015.

Takubo K. *Pathology of the esophagus*. New York: Springer, 2010.

Henry Stanley Plummer, 1874–1936, American internist and endocrinologist.
Porter Paisley Vinson, 1890–1959, Physician, the Mayo Clinic, Rochester, MN, who later practised in Richmond, VA, USA.
Adam Brown Kelly, 1865–1941, surgeon, Ear, Nose and Throat Department, the Royal Victoria Infirmary, Glasgow, UK.
Donald Rose Paterson, 1863–1939, surgeon, Ear, Nose and Throat Department, the Royal Infirmary, Cardiff, UK.
Vinson, Kelly and Paterson all described this syndrome independently in 1919.

Chapter 63

Stomach and duodenum

Learning objectives

- To understand the gross and microscopic anatomy and pathophysiology of the stomach in relation to disease
- To be able to decide on the most appropriate techniques to use in the investigation of patients with complaints relating to the stomach and duodenum
- To understand the critical importance of gastritis and *Helicobacter pylori* in upper gastrointestinal disease
- To be able to investigate and treat peptic ulcer disease and its complications
- To be able to recognise the presentation of gastric cancer and understand the principles involved in its treatment
- To know about the causes of duodenal obstruction and the presentation of duodenal tumours

INTRODUCTION

The function of the stomach is to act as a reservoir for ingested food. It also serves to break down foodstuffs mechanically and commence the processes of digestion before these products are passed on into the duodenum.

GROSS ANATOMY OF THE STOMACH AND DUODENUM

Blood supply

Arteries

The stomach has an arterial supply on both lesser and greater curves (Figure 63.1). On the lesser curve, the left gastric artery, a branch of the coeliac axis, forms an anastomotic arcade with the right gastric artery, which arises from the common hepatic artery. Branches of the left gastric artery pass up towards the cardia. The gastroduodenal artery, which is also a branch of the hepatic artery, passes behind the first part of the duodenum, highly relevant with respect to the bleeding duodenal ulcer. Here it divides into the superior pancreaticoduodenal artery and the right gastroepiploic artery. The superior pancreaticoduodenal artery supplies the duodenum and pancreatic head, and forms an anastomosis with the inferior pancreaticoduodenal artery, a branch of the superior mesenteric artery. The right gastroepiploic artery runs along the greater curvature of the stomach, eventually forming an anastomosis with the left gastroepiploic artery, a branch of the splenic artery. This vascular arcade, important for the construction of the gastric conduit in oesophageal resection, is often variably incomplete. The fundus of the stomach is supplied by the vasa brevia (or short gastric arteries), which arise from near the termination of the splenic artery.

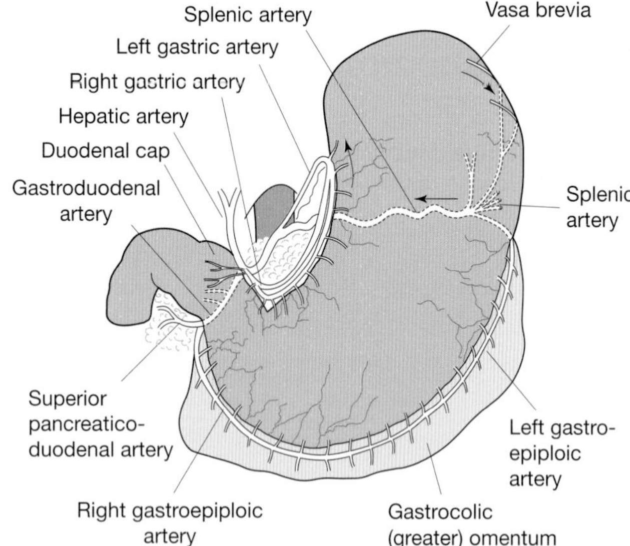

Figure 63.1 The arterial blood supply of the stomach.

Veins

In general, the veins are equivalent to the arteries, those along the lesser curve ending in the portal vein and those on the greater curve joining via the splenic vein. On the lesser curve, the coronary vein is particularly important. It runs up the lesser curve towards the oesophagus and then passes left to right to join the portal vein. This vein becomes markedly dilated in portal hypertension.

Lymphatics

The lymphatics of the stomach are of considerable importance in the surgery of gastric cancer and are therefore described in detail in that section.

Nerves

As with the entire gastrointestinal tract, the stomach and duodenum possess both intrinsic and extrinsic nerve supplies. The intrinsic nerves exist principally in two plexuses, the myenteric plexus of Auerbach and the submucosal plexus of Meissner. Compared with the rest of the gut, the submucosal plexus of the stomach contains relatively few ganglionic cells, as does the myenteric plexus in the fundus. However, in the antrum the ganglia of the myenteric plexus are well developed. The extrinsic supply is derived mainly from the vagus nerves (CN XI), fibres of which originate in the brainstem. The vagal plexus around the oesophagus condenses into bundles that pass through the oesophageal hiatus (Figure 63.2), the posterior bundle being usually identifiable as a large nerve trunk. Vagal fibres are both afferent (sensory) and efferent. The efferent fibres are involved in the receptive relaxation of the stomach and the stimulation of gastric motility, as well as having the well-known secretory function. The sympathetic supply is derived mainly from the coeliac ganglia.

MICROSCOPIC ANATOMY OF THE STOMACH AND DUODENUM

The gastric epithelial cells are mucus producing and are turned over rapidly. In the pyloric part of the stomach, and also the duodenum, mucus-secreting glands are found. Most of the specialised cells of the stomach (parietal and chief cells) are found in the gastric crypts (Figure 63.3). The stomach also has numerous endocrine cells.

Parietal cells

These are in the body (acid-secreting portion) of the stomach and line the gastric crypts, being more abundant distally. They are responsible for the production of hydrogen ions to form hydrochloric acid. The hydrogen ions are actively secreted by the proton pump, a hydrogen–potassium-ATPase (Sachs), which exchanges intraluminal potassium for hydrogen ions. The potassium ions enter the lumen of the crypts passively, but the hydrogen ions are pumped against an immense concentration gradient (1 000 000:1).

Chief cells

These lie principally proximally in the gastric crypts and produce pepsinogen. Two forms of pepsinogen are described: pepsinogen I and pepsinogen II. Both are produced by the chief cell, but pepsinogen I is produced only in the stomach. The ratio between pepsinogens I and II in the serum decreases with gastric atrophy. Pepsinogen is activated in the stomach to produce the digestive protease, pepsin.

Endocrine cells

The stomach has numerous endocrine cells, which are critical to its function. In the gastric antrum, the mucosa contains G cells, which produce gastrin. Throughout the body of the stomach, enterochromaffin-like (ECL) cells are abundant and produce histamine, a key factor in driving gastric acid secretion. In addition, there are large numbers of somatostatin-

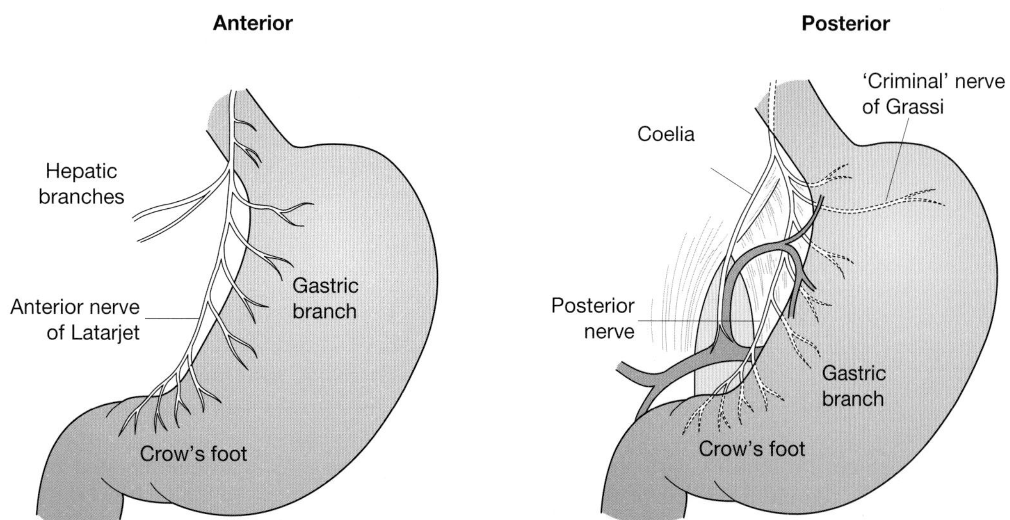

Figure 63.2 The anatomy of the anterior and posterior vagus nerves in relation to the stomach.

Leopold Auerbach, 1828–1897, Professor of Neuropathology, Breslau, Germany (now Wroclaw, Poland), described the myenteric plexus in 1862.
George Meissner, 1829–1905, Professor of Physiology, Gottingen, Germany.
George Sachs, Professor of Medicine, CURE, Los Angeles, CA, USA, discoverer of the proton pump.

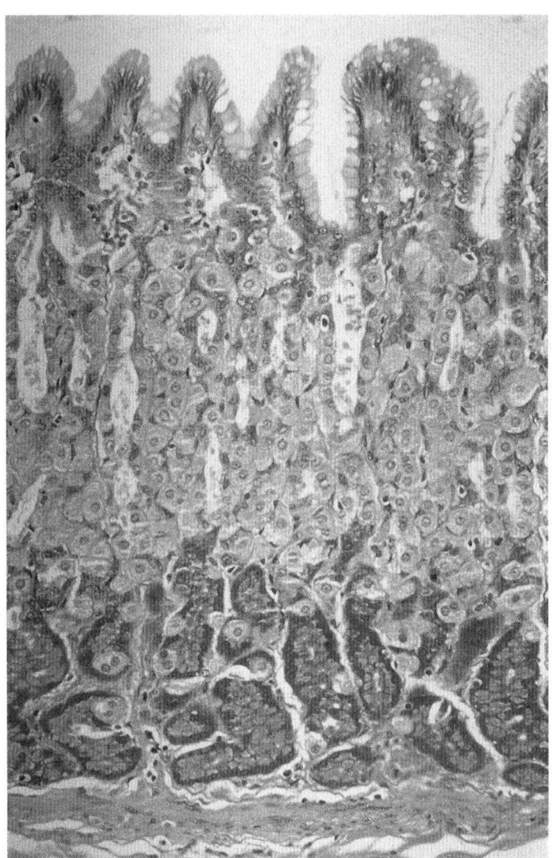

Figure 63.3 The histological appearance of a gastric gland. The mucus-secreting cells are seen at the mucosal surface, the eosinophilic parietal cells superficially in the glands and the basophilic chief cells in the deepest layer.

producing D cells throughout the stomach, and somatostatin has a negative regulatory role. The peptides and neuropeptides produced in the stomach are discussed later.

Duodenum

The duodenum is lined by a mucus-secreting columnar epithelium. In addition, Brunner's glands lie beneath the mucosa and are similar to the pyloric glands in the pyloric part of the stomach. Endocrine cells in the duodenum produce cholecystokinin and secretin.

PHYSIOLOGY OF THE STOMACH AND DUODENUM

The stomach mechanically breaks up ingested food and, together with the actions of acid and pepsin, forms chyme that passes into the duodenum. In contrast with the acidic environment of the stomach, the environment of the duodenum is alkaline, due to the secretion of bicarbonate ions from both the pancreas and the duodenum. This neutralises the acid chyme and adjusts the luminal osmolarity to approximately that of plasma. Endocrine cells in the duodenum produce cholecystokinin, which stimulates the pancreas to produce trypsin and the gall bladder to contract. Secretin is also produced by the endocrine cells of the duodenum. This hormone inhibits gastric acid secretion and promotes production of bicarbonate by the pancreas.

Summary box 63.1

The anatomy and physiology of the stomach

- The stomach acts as a reservoir for food and commences the process of digestion
- Gastric acid is produced by a proton pump in the parietal cells, which in turn is controlled by histamine acting on the H_2-receptors
- The histamine is produced by the endocrine gastric ECL cells in response to a number of factors, particularly gastrin and the vagus
- Proton pump inhibitors abolish gastric acid production, whereas H_2-receptor antagonists only markedly reduce it
- The gastric mucous layer is essential to the integrity of the gastric mucosa

Gastric acid secretion

The secretion of gastric acid and pepsin tends to run in parallel, although the understanding of the mechanisms of gastric acid secretion is considerably greater than that of pepsin. Numerous factors are involved to some degree in the production of gastric acid. These include neurotransmitters, neuropeptides and peptide hormones. This complexity need not detract from the fact that there are basic principles that are relatively easily understood (Figure 63.4). Hydrogen ions are produced by the parietal cell by the proton pump. Although numerous factors can act on the parietal cell, the most important of these is histamine, which acts via the H_2-receptor. Histamine is produced, in turn, by the ECL cells of the stomach and acts in a paracrine (local) fashion on the parietal cells. These relationships explain why proton pump inhibitors can abolish gastric acid secretion, as they act on the final common pathway – hydrogen ion secretion. H_2-receptor antagonists have profound effects on gastric acid secretion, but this is not insurmountable (Figure 63.4). The ECL cell produces histamine in response to a number of stimuli that include the vagus nerve and gastrin. Gastrin is released by the G cells in response to the presence of the food in the stomach. The production of gastrin is inhibited by acid, creating a negative feedback loop. Various other peptides, including secretin, inhibit gastric acid secretion.

Classically, three phases of gastric secretion are described. The cephalic phase is mediated by vagal activity, secondary to sensory arousal as first demonstrated by Pavlov. The gastric phase is a response to food within the stomach, which is mediated principally, but not exclusively, by gastrin. In the intestinal phase, the presence of chyme in the duodenum and small bowel inhibits gastric emptying, and the acidification

Johann Conrad Brunner, 1653–1729, Professor of Anatomy, Heidelberg, Germany, and later at Strasbourg, France.
Ivan Petrovich Pavlov, 1849–1936, Professor of Physiology, The Medico-Chirurgical Academy, St Petersburg, Russia.

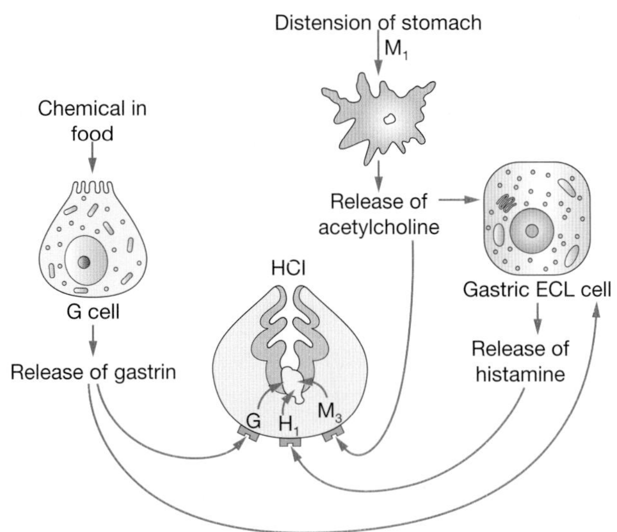

Figure 63.4 The parietal cell in relation to the mechanism of gastric acid secretion. ECL, enterochromaffin-like; G, gastrin receptor; H, histamine receptor; HCl, hydrochloric acid; M, muscarinic receptor.

of the duodenum leads to the production of secretin, which inhibits gastric acid secretion, along with numerous other peptides originating from the gut. The stomach also possesses somatostatin-containing D cells. Somatostatin is released in response to a number of factors including acidification. This peptide acts probably on the G cell, the ECL cell and the parietal cell itself to inhibit the production of acid.

Gastric mucus and the gastric mucosal barrier

The gastric mucous layer is essential to the integrity of the gastric mucosa. It is a viscid layer of mucopolysaccharides produced by the mucus-producing cells of the stomach and the pyloric glands. Gastric mucus is an important physiological barrier to protect the gastric mucosa from mechanical damage, and also the effects of acid and pepsin. Its considerable buffering capacity is enhanced by the presence of bicarbonate ions within the mucus. Many factors can lead to the breakdown of this gastric mucous barrier. These include bile, non-steroidal anti-inflammatory drugs (NSAIDs), alcohol, trauma and shock. Tonometry studies have shown that, of the entire gastrointestinal tract, the stomach is the most sensitive to ischaemia following a hypovolaemic insult and also the slowest to recover. This may explain the high incidence of stress ulceration in the stomach.

Peptides and neuropeptides in the stomach and duodenum

As with most of the gastrointestinal tract, the endocrine cells of the stomach produce peptide hormones and neurotransmitters. Previously, nerves and endocrine cells were considered distinct in terms of their products. However, it is increasingly realised that there is enormous overlap within these systems. Many peptides recognised as hormones may also be produced by neurones, hence the term neuropeptides. The term 'messenger' can be used to describe all such products. There are three conventional modes of action that overlap.

1 **Endocrine**. The messenger is secreted into the circulation, where it affects tissues that may be remote from the site of origin (Bayliss and Starling).
2 **Paracrine**. Messengers are produced locally and have local effects on tissues. Neurones and endocrine cells both act in this way.
3 **Neurocrine** (classical neurotransmitter). Messengers are produced by the neurone via the synaptic knob and pass across the synaptic cleft to the target.

Many peptide hormones act on the intrinsic nerve plexus of the gut (see later) and influence motility. Similarly, neuropeptides may influence the structure and function of the mucosa. Some of these peptides, neuropeptides and neurotransmitters are shown in *Table 63.1*. The stomach is vital in the regulation of appetite and weight control via a combination of mechanical and hormonal mechanisms; these are discussed further in following chapters.

Gastroduodenal motor activity

The motility of the entire gastrointestinal tract is modulated to a large degree by its intrinsic nervous system. Critical in this process is the migrating motor complex (MMC). In the fasted state, and after food has cleared, in the small bowel there is a period of quiescence lasting in the region of 40 minutes (phase I). There follows a series of waves of electrical and motor activity, also lasting for about 40 minutes, propagated from the fundus of the stomach in a caudal direction at a rate of about three per minute (phase II). These pass as far the pylorus, but not beyond. Duodenal slow waves are generated in the duodenum at a rate of about 10 per minute, which carry down the small bowel. The amplitude of these contractions increases to a maximum in phase III, which lasts for about 10 minutes. This 90-minute cycle of activity is then repeated. From the duodenum, the MMC moves distally at 5–10 cm/min, reaching the terminal ileum after 1.5 hours.

Following a meal, the stomach exhibits receptive relaxation, which lasts for a few seconds. Following this, adaptive relaxation occurs, which allows the proximal stomach to act as a reservoir. Most of the peristaltic activity is found in the distal stomach (the antral mill) and the proximal stomach demonstrates only tonic activity. The pylorus, which is most commonly open, contracts with the peristaltic wave and allows only a few millilitres of chyme through at a time. The antral contraction against the closed sphincter is important in the milling activity of the stomach. Although the duodenum is capable of generating 10 waves per minute, after a meal it only contracts after an antral wave reaches the pylorus. The coordination of the motility of the antrum, pylorus and duodenum

Sir William Maddock Bayliss, 1860–1924, physiologist, University College, London, UK.
Ernest Henry Starling, 1866–1927, physiologist, University College, London, UK.

TABLE 63.1 Function and source of peptides and neuropeptides in the stomach.

Function	Source
Stimulate secretion	
Gastrin	G cells
Histamine	ECL cells
Acetylcholine	Neurones
Gastrin-releasing peptide	Neurones and mucosa
Cholecystokinin (CCK)	Duodenal endocrine cells
Inhibit secretion	
Somatostatin	D cells and neurones
Secretin	Duodenal endocrine cells
Enteroglucagon	Small intestinal endocrine cells
Prostaglandins	Mucosa
Neurotensin	Neurones
GIP	Duodenal and jejunal endocrine cells
PYY	Small intestinal endocrine cells
Stimulate motility	
Acetylcholine	Neurones
5-HT	Neurones
Histamine	ECL cell
Substance P	Neurones
Substance K	Neurones
Motilin	Neurones
Gastrin	G cells
Angiotensin	
Inhibit motility	
Somatostatin	D cells and neurones
VIP	Neurones
Nitric oxide	Neurones and smooth muscle
Noradrenaline	Neurones
Encephalin	Neurones
Dopamine	Neurones

ECL, enterochromaffin-like cells; GIP, gastric inhibitory polypeptide; PYY, peptide YY; VIP, vasoactive intestinal peptide.

means that only small quantities of food reach the small bowel at a time. It is important to consider that this control of gastric emptying can be abolished after gastric surgery leading to significant symptoms (discussed in later sections). Motility is influenced by numerous factors, including mechanical stimulation and neuronal and endocrine influences (*Table 63.1*).

INVESTIGATION OF THE STOMACH AND DUODENUM

Flexible endoscopy

Flexible endoscopy is the 'gold standard' investigation of the upper gastrointestinal tract. The original flexible endoscopes were fibreoptic (Hirschowitz), but now most use a solid-state camera mounted at the instrument's tip (Figures 63.5 and 63.6). Other members of the endoscopy team see the image and this is useful when taking biopsies or performing interventional techniques, and it also facilitates teaching and training.

(a)
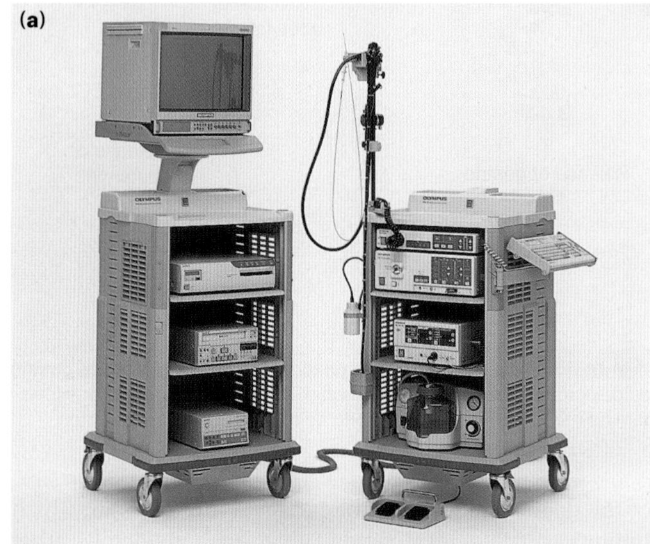

(b)
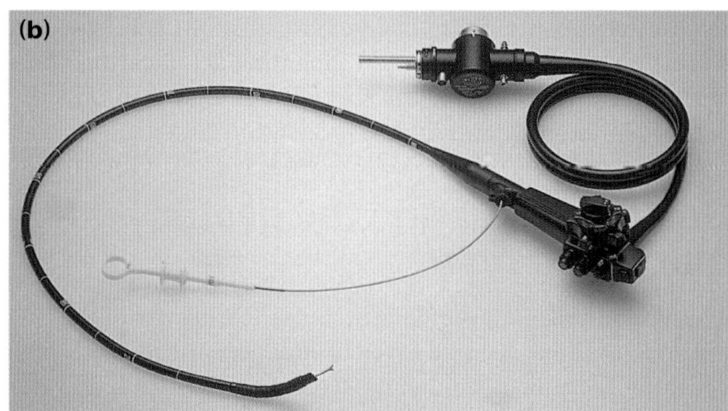

Figure 63.5 A video-gastroscope (courtesy of Keymed (Medical and Industrial Equipment Ltd)). (a) The camera stack; (b) the gastroscope and biopsy forceps in the working channel.

Summary box 63.2

The investigation of gastric disorders

- Flexible endoscopy is the most commonly used and sensitive technique for investigating the stomach and duodenum
- Great care needs to be exercised in performing endoscopy to avoid complications and missing important pathology
- Axial imaging, particularly multislice CT, is useful in the staging of gastric cancer, although it may be less sensitive in the detection of liver metastases than other modalities
- Endoscopic ultrasound is the most sensitive technique in the evaluation of the 'T' stage of gastric cancer and in the assessment of duodenal tumours
- Laparoscopy is very sensitive in detecting peritoneal metastases, and laparoscopic ultrasound provides an accurate evaluation of lymph node and liver metastases

Basil I Hirschowitz, Professor of Medicine, Birmingham, AL, USA.

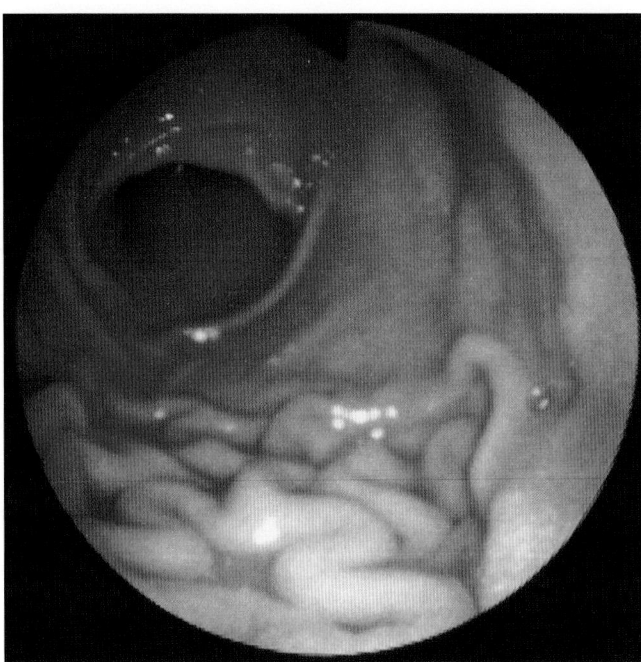

Figure 63.6 A view of the normal stomach during endoscopy (courtesy of GNJ Tytgat, Amsterdam, The Netherlands).

Flexible endoscopy is more sensitive than conventional radiology in the assessment of the majority of gastroduodenal conditions. This is particularly the case for peptic ulceration, gastritis and duodenitis. In upper gastrointestinal bleeding, endoscopy is far superior to any other investigation and offers the possibility of endoscopic therapy. In most circumstances it is the only investigation required.

Fibreoptic endoscopy is generally a safe investigation, but it is important that all personnel undertaking these procedures are adequately trained. Careless and rough handling of the endoscope during intubation of a patient may result in perforations of the pharynx and oesophagus. Any other part of the upper gastrointestinal tract may also be perforated. An inadequately performed endoscopy is also dangerous as a serious condition may be overlooked. This is particularly the case in respect of early and curable gastric cancer, the appearances of which may often be extremely subtle and may be missed by inexperienced endoscopists. A more experienced endoscopist will have a higher index of suspicion for any mucosal abnormalities and will take more biopsies. Spraying the mucosa with dye endoscopically may allow better discrimination between normal and abnormal mucosa, so allowing a small cancer to be more easily seen. In the future, advances in technology may allow 'optical biopsy' to determine the nature of mucosal abnormalities in real time.

Upper gastrointestinal endoscopy can be performed without sedation, but when sedation is required incremental doses of a benzodiazepine are usually administered. Sedation is of particular concern in the case of gastrointestinal bleeding as it may have a more profound effect on the patient's cardiovascular stability. It has now become the standard to use pulse oximetry to monitor patients during upper gastrointestinal endoscopy, and nasal oxygen is often also administered. Buscopan is useful to abolish duodenal motility for examinations of the second and third parts of the duodenum. Examinations of this type are best carried out using a side-viewing endoscope such as is used for endoscopic retrograde cholangiopancreatography (ERCP).

Some patients are relatively resistant to sedation with benzodiazepines, particularly those who are accustomed to drinking alcohol. Increasing the dose of benzodiazepines in these patients may not result in any useful sedation, but merely make the patient more restless and confused. Such patients are sometimes better endoscoped fully awake using a local anaesthetic throat spray and a narrow-gauge endoscope. Whatever the circumstances, it is important that resuscitation facilities are available including agents that reverse the effects of benzodiazepines, such as flumazenil.

The technology associated with upper gastrointestinal endoscopy is continuing to advance. Instruments which allow both endoscopy and endoluminal ultrasound to be performed simultaneously (see later) are used routinely. Bleeding from the stomach and duodenum can be treated with a number of haemostatic measures. These include injection with various substances, diathermy, heater probes, lasers and clips. These approaches appear to be useful in the treatment of bleeding ulcers, although there are few good controlled trials in this area. There is no good evidence that such interventional procedures at the moment work in patients who are bleeding from very large vessels, such as the gastroduodenal artery or splenic artery, although technology may overcome this problem in the future.

Contrast radiology

Upper gastrointestinal radiology is not used as much as in previous years, as endoscopy is a more sensitive investigation for most gastric problems. Computed tomography (CT) imaging with oral contrast has also replaced contrast radiology in many of the areas where anatomical information is sought, eg large hiatus hernias of the rolling type and chronic gastric volvulus. In these conditions it may be difficult for the endoscopist to determine exactly the anatomy or, indeed, negotiate the deformity to see the distal stomach.

Ultrasonography

Standard ultrasound imaging can be used to investigate the stomach, but used conventionally it is less sensitive than other modalities. In contrast, endoluminal ultrasound and laparoscopic ultrasound are probably the most sensitive techniques available in the preoperative local staging of gastric cancer. In endoluminal ultrasound, the transducer is usually attached to the distal tip of the instrument. However, devices have been developed which may be passed down the biopsy channel, albeit with poorer image quality. Five layers (Figure 63.7) of the gastric wall may be identified on endoluminal ultrasound and the depth of invasion of a tumour can be assessed with exquisite accuracy (90% accuracy for the 'T' component of the staging). Enlarged lymph nodes can also be identified and the technique's accuracy in this situation is about 80%.

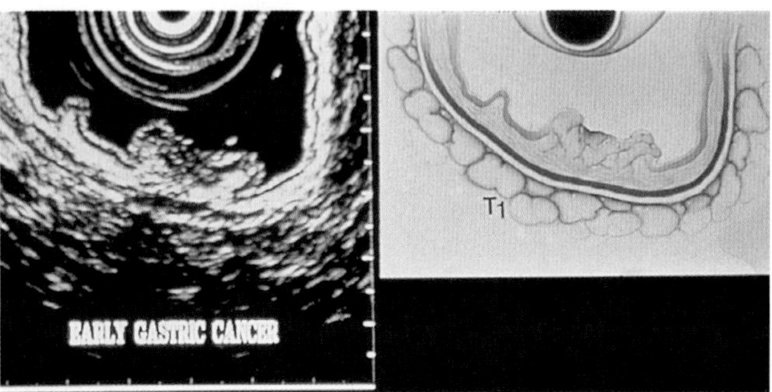

Figure 63.7 Endoscopic ultrasound of the stomach. Five layers can be identified in the normal stomach. A gastric cancer is shown invading the muscle of the gastric wall (courtesy of KeyMed (Medical and Industrial Equipment Ltd)).

Finally, it may be possible to identify liver metastases not seen on axial imaging. Laparoscopic ultrasound is also a very sensitive imaging modality to a large measure because of the laparoscopy itself (see below). It is one of the most sensitive methods of detecting liver metastases from gastric cancer.

An additional use of ultrasound is in the assessment of gastric emptying. Swallowed contrast is utilised, which is designed to be easily seen using an ultrasound transducer. The emptying of this contrast is then followed directly. The accuracy of the technique is similar to that of radioisotope gastric emptying studies (see below).

CT scanning and magnetic resonance imaging

The resolution of CT scanners is continuing to improve, and multislice CT is of increasing value in the investigation of the stomach, especially gastric malignancies (Figure 63.8). The presence of gastric wall thickening associated with a carcinoma of any reasonable size can be easily detected by CT, but the investigation lacks sensitivity in detecting smaller lesions. It is much less accurate in 'T' staging than endoluminal ultrasound. Lymph node enlargement can be detected and, based on the size and shape of the nodes, it is possible to be reasonably accurate in detecting nodal involvement with tumour. However, as with all imaging techniques, it is limited. Microscopic tumour deposits in lymph nodes cannot be detected when the node is not enlarged and, in contrast, lymph nodes may undergo reactive enlargement but not contain tumour. These problems apply to all imaging techniques.

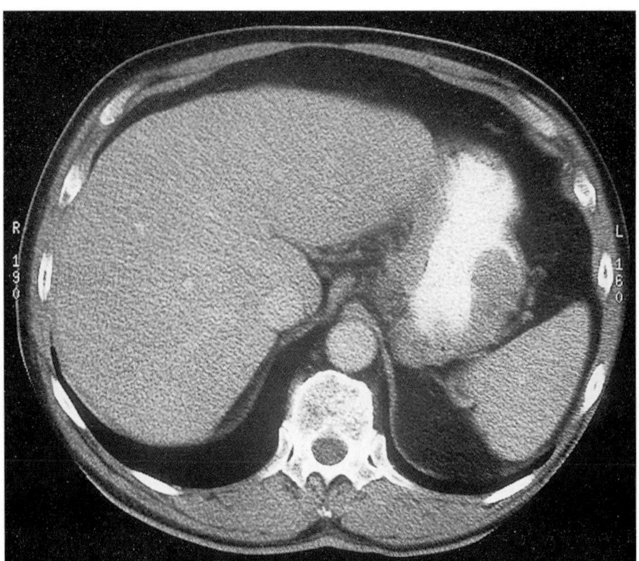

Figure 63.8 A computed tomography scan of the abdomen, showing a gastric cancer arising in the body of the stomach.

The detection of small liver metastases is improving, although in general terms metastases from gastric cancer are less easy to detect using CT than those, for instance, from colorectal cancer. This is because metastases from gastric cancer may be of the same density as liver and may not handle the intravenous contrast any differently. At present, magnetic resonance imaging (MRI) scanning does not offer any specific advantage in assessing the stomach, although it has a higher sensitivity for the detection of gastric cancer liver metastases than conventional CT imaging.

CT/positron emission tomography

Positron emission tomography (PET) is a functional imaging technique which relies on the uptake of a tracer in most cases by metabolically active tumour tissue. Fluorodeoxyglucose (FDG) is the most commonly used tracer. This tracer has a short half-life hence manufacture and use have to be carefully coordinated. To be of value, anatomical and functional information need to be linked, hence PET/CT is now used universally. It is increasingly being used in the preoperative staging of gastro-oesophageal cancer as it will demonstrate occult spread which renders the patient surgically incurable in up to 10% of patients who would otherwise have undergone major resections (Figure 63.9). PET/CT may also be used to determine the response to neoadjuvant chemotherapy in oesophagogastric malignancies although this is the subject of ongoing studies.

Laparoscopy

This technique is routine in the assessment of patients with gastric cancer. Its particular value is in the detection of peritoneal disease, which is difficult by any other technique, unless the patient has ascites or bulky intraperitoneal deposits. Its main limitation is in the evaluation of posterior extension but other techniques are available to evaluate posterior invasion, especially CT and endoluminal ultrasound. Usually laparoscopy is combined with peritoneal cytology unless laparotomy follows immediately.

Gastric emptying studies

These are useful in the study of gastric dysmotility problems, particularly those that follow gastric surgery. The principle of the examination is that radioisotope-labelled liquid and solid meals are ingested by the patient and the emptying of the stomach is followed on a gamma camera. This allows the

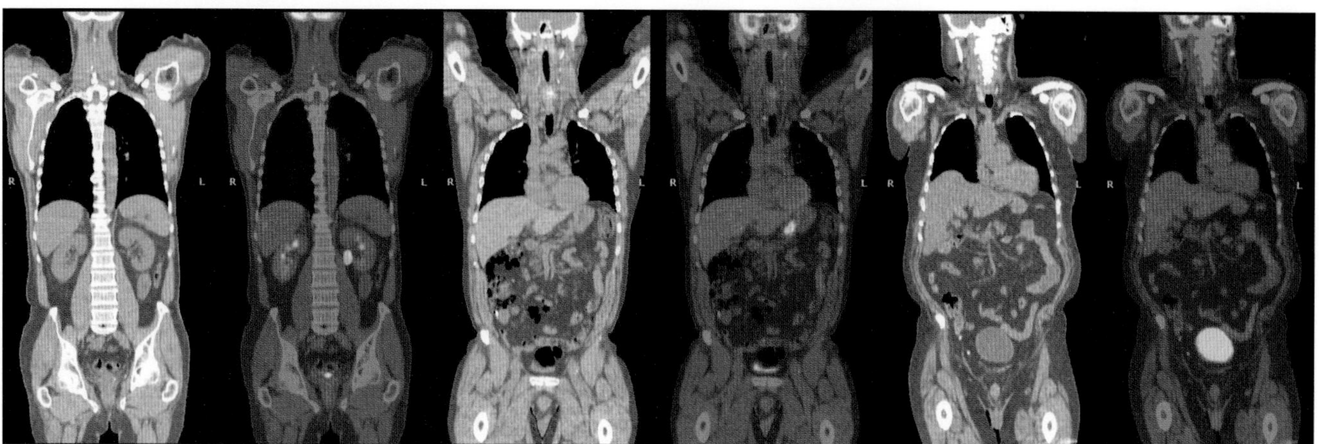

Figure 63.9 Computed tomography/positron emission tomography of a patient with gastric cancer. The middle pair of images shows the primary tumour. The two images on the left show unsuspected liver metastases, whereas the two on the right show a left cervical node positive for metastases.

proportion of activity in the remaining stomach to be assessed numerically, and it is possible to follow liquid and solid gastric emptying independently (Figure 63.10).

Angiography

Angiography is used most commonly in the investigation of upper gastrointestinal bleeding that is not identified using endoscopy. Therapeutic embolisation may also be of value in the treatment of bleeding in patients in whom surgery is difficult or inadvisable. In expert centres embolisation now replaces surgery in the majority of cases.

HELICOBACTER PYLORI

Over the last 30 years, this organism has proved to be of overwhelming importance in the aetiology of a number of common gastroduodenal diseases such as chronic gastritis, peptic ulceration and gastric cancer. The organism had unquestionably been observed by a number of workers since Bircher's first description in 1874, but it was not until 1980 that Warren and Marshall, with enthusiasm but perhaps a lack of caution, ingested the organism to confirm that Koch's postulates could be fulfilled with respect to the gastritis that they succeeded in causing in themselves. Eradication therapy was then employed with mixed success, but both received the Nobel

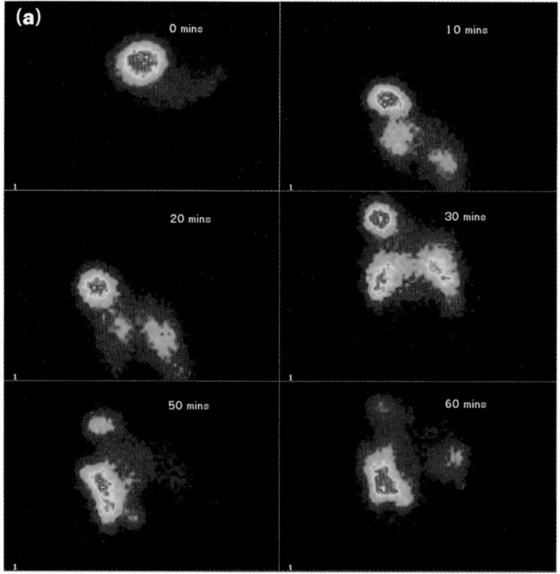

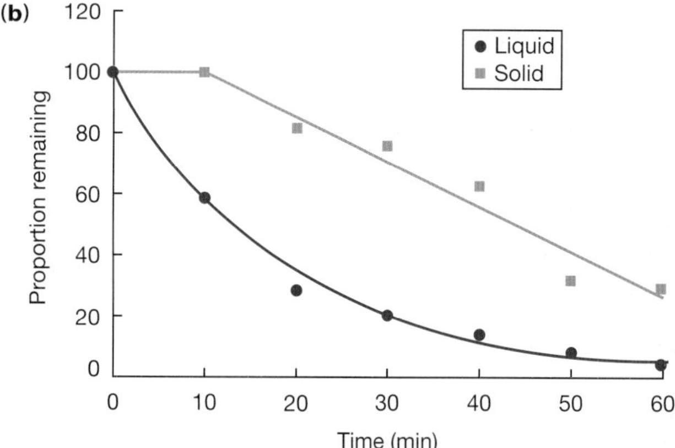

Figure 63.10 Dual-phase solid and liquid gastric emptying. The use of two isotopic labels allows the liquid and solid phases of the emptying to be followed separately. (a) Image acquisition. (b) Gastric emptying curves in a normal individual showing typical lag period in the solid phase before linear emptying (courtesy of Dr V Lewington, Southampton, UK).

C.S. Warren, Perth, Australia, now Chicago, IL, USA, credited with awakening the current interest in *Helicobacter*.

Barry Marshall, Perth, Australia, now Charlottesville, VA, USA, credited with awakening the current interest in *Helicobacter*.

Robert Koch, 1843–1910, Professor of Hygiene and Bacteriology, Berlin, Germany. Stated his 'postulates' in 1882. The postulates define the conditions that must be met before an organism can be shown to be the causal agent for a particular disease.

Prize for Medicine and Physiology in 2005. The organism is spiral shaped and is fastidious in its requirements, being difficult to culture outside the mucous layer of the stomach.

One of the characteristics of the organism is its ability to hydrolyse urea, resulting in the production of ammonia, a strong alkali. The effect of ammonia on the antral G cells is to cause the release of gastrin via the previously described negative-feedback loop. This is probably responsible for the modest, but inappropriate, hypergastrinaemia in patients with peptic ulcer disease, which, in turn, may result in gastric acid hypersecretion. The organism's obligate urease activity is utilised by various tests used to detect the presence of the organism, including the ^{13}C and ^{14}C breath tests and the CLO test (a commercially available urease test kit), which is performed on gastric biopsies. The organism can also be detected histologically (Figure 63.11), using the Giemsa or the Warthin–Starry stains, and cultured using appropriate media. Previous or current infection with the organism may also be detected serologically. Breath tests or faecal antigen tests are recommended for the pre-treatment diagnosis of *H. pylori* infection in the community. Less accurate, hospital-based serology tests have a place within the non-invasive test-and-treat strategy.

Infection with *H. pylori* leads to the disruption of the gastric mucous barrier by the enzymes produced by the organism, and the inflammation induced in the gastric epithelium is the basis of many of the associated disease processes. The association of the organism with chronic (type B) gastritis is not in doubt. Some strains of *H. pylori* produce cytotoxins, notably the *Cag A* and *Vac A* products, and the production of cytotoxins seems to be associated with the ability of the organism to cause gastritis, peptic ulceration and cancer. The effect of the organism on the gastric epithelium is to incite a classical inflammatory response that involves the migration and degranulation of acute inflammatory cells, such as neutrophils, and also the accumulation of chronic inflammatory cells, such as macrophages and lymphocytes.

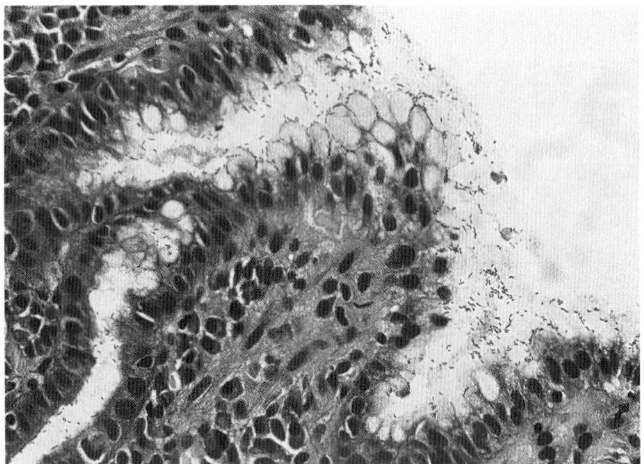

Figure 63.11 Antral mucosa showing colonisation with *Helicobacter pylori* (modified Giemsa stain).

It is evident how *H. pylori* infection results in chronic gastritis and also how this may progress to gastric ulceration, but for a while it remained an enigma as to how the organism could be involved in duodenal ulceration, as the normal duodenum is not colonised. As mentioned above, the production of ammonia does increase the level of circulating gastrin and it has been shown subsequently that eradication of the organism in patients with duodenal ulcer disease will reduce the acid levels to normal. However, the overlap in gastric acid secretion between normal subjects and those with duodenal ulcers is considerable and the modestly increased acid levels in patients with *Helicobacter*-associated antral gastritis are insufficient to explain the aetiology of duodenal ulceration.

The explanation can probably be found in the phenomenon of duodenal gastric metaplasia. Gastric metaplasia is the normal response of the duodenal mucosa to excess acidity. It can be thought of in the same way as any other metaplasia in the gastrointestinal tract: an attempt by the mucosa to resist an injurious stimulus. Although normal duodenal mucosa cannot be infected with *H. pylori*, gastric metaplasia in the duodenum is commonly infected and this infection results in the same inflammatory process that is observed in the gastric mucosa. The result is duodenitis, which is almost certainly the precursor of duodenal ulceration.

Infection with *H. pylori* may be the most common human infection. The incidence of infection within a population increases with age, and in many populations infection rates of 80–90% are not unusual. Up to 50% of the world's population may be infected with *Helicobacter*. It appears that most infection is acquired in childhood and the possibility of infection is inversely related to socioeconomic group. The means of spread has not been identified, but the organism can occur in the faeces and faecal–oral spread seems most likely. The organism is not normally found in saliva or dental plaque. There is evidence in different environments and in different population groups that the manifestations of the infection may be different. Predominantly antral gastritis, which is commonly seen in resource-rich countries, results initially in increased levels of acid production and peptic ulcer disease, whereas gastritis affecting the body, common in resource-poor countries, may lead to hypochlorhydria and gastric neoplasia.

It has been known since 1984 that *Helicobacter* infection is amenable to treatment with antibiotics. The profound hypochlorhydria produced by proton pump inhibitors combined with antibiotics is also effective in eradicating the organism. Commonly used eradication regimes include a proton pump inhibitor and two antibiotics, such as metronidazole and amoxycillin. Very high eradication rates, in the region of 90%, can be achieved with combinations that include the antibiotic clarithromycin, although it may be that in the future antibiotic resistance will become a problem. Reinfection following successful eradication appears rare (<0.5%) but incomplete eradication is a more important clinical problem.

Gustav Giemsa, 1867–1948, bacteriologist who became Privatdozent in Chemotherapy at the University of Hamburg, Hamburg, Germany.
Aldred Scott Warthin, 1866–1931, pathologist, the University of Michigan, USA.
Allen Chronister Starry, 1890–1973, pathologist, the University of Michigan, USA.

At present, eradication therapy is recommended for patients with duodenal ulcer disease, but not for patients with non-ulcer dyspepsia or in asymptomatic patients who are infected. However, recent data show that a proportion of patients with non-ulcer dyspepsia do respond to treatment. *H. pylori* is now classed by the World Health Organisation as a class 1 carcinogen and it may be that further epidemiological studies on the risk of gastric cancer change the current advice on treatment.

GASTRITIS

The great variety of names and classification systems used in gastritis is confusing. Thankfully, the understanding of gastritis has increased markedly following elucidation of the role of *H. pylori* in chronic gastritis and there is broad agreement that gastritis should be classified according to the underlying aetiology. Gastritis describes any histologically confirmed inflammation of the gastric mucosa. In most modern classification systems the amount of inflammatory infiltrate and the degree of gastric atrophy will be included.

Summary box 63.3

Gastritis

- The spiral bacterium *Helicobacter pylori* is critical in the development of gastritis, peptic ulceration and gastric cancer
- Infection appears to be acquired mainly in childhood and the infection rate is inversely associated with socioeconomic status
- Eradication, recommended specifically in patients with peptic ulcer disease, can be achieved in up to 90% of patients with a combination of a proton pump inhibitor and antibiotics, and reinfection is uncommon (<0.5%)
- Erosive gastritis is usually related to the use of NSAIDs
- Autoimmune gastritis is associated with the development of pernicious anaemia and gastric cancer

Autoimmune gastritis

This is an autoimmune condition in which there are circulating antibodies to the parietal cell. This results in the atrophy of the parietal cell mass, hence hypochlorhydria and ultimately achlorhydria. As intrinsic factor is also produced by the parietal cell there is malabsorption of vitamin B12, which, if untreated, may result in pernicious anaemia. The antrum is not affected and the hypochlorhydria leads to the production of high levels of gastrin from the antral G cells. This results in chronic hypergastrinaemia. This, in turn, results in hypertrophy of the ECL cells in the body of the stomach, which are not affected by the autoimmune damage. Over time it is apparent that microadenomas develop in the ECL cells of the stomach, sometimes becoming identifiable tumour nodules. Very rarely, these tumours can become malignant. Patients with autoimmune gastritis are predisposed to the development of gastric cancer, and screening such patients endoscopically may be appropriate.

H. pylori gastritis

Previously described as type B gastritis, this affects the antrum, and it is these patients who are prone to peptic ulcer disease. *Helicobacter*-associated pangastritis is also a very common manifestation of infection, but gastritis affecting the corpus alone does not seem to be associated. However, there are some data to suggest that *Helicobacter* may be involved in the initiation of the process. Patients with pangastritis seem to be most prone to the development of gastric cancer.

Intestinal metaplasia is associated with chronic pangastritis with atrophy. Although intestinal metaplasia per se is common, intestinal metaplasia associated with dysplasia has significant malignant potential and, if this condition is identified, endoscopic screening may be appropriate.

Reflux gastritis

This is caused by enterogastric reflux and is particularly common after gastric surgery. Its histological features are distinct from other types of gastritis. Although commonly seen after gastric surgery, it is occasionally found in patients with no previous surgical intervention or who have had a cholecystectomy. Bile chelating or prokinetic agents may be useful in treatment and as a temporising measure to avoid consideration of revisional surgery. Operation for the condition should be reserved for the most severe cases.

Erosive gastritis

This is caused by agents that disturb the gastric mucosal barrier; NSAIDs and alcohol are common causes. The NSAID-induced gastric lesion is associated with inhibition of the cyclo-oxygenase type 1 (COX-1) receptor enzyme, hence reducing the production of cytoprotective prostaglandins in the stomach. Many of the beneficial anti-inflammatory activities of NSAIDs are mediated by COX-2, and the use of specific COX-2 inhibitors reduces the incidence of these side effects. However, taken in the long term COX-2 inhibitors are associated with cardiovascular complications in common with many NSAIDs.

Stress gastritis

This is a common sequel of serious illness or injury and is characterised by a reduction in the blood supply to superficial mucosa of the stomach. Although common, this is not usually recognised unless stress ulceration and bleeding supervene, in which case treatment can be extremely difficult. The condition also sometimes follows cardiopulmonary bypass. Prevention of the stress bleeding from the stomach is much easier than treating it, and hence the routine use of H_2 antagonists with or without barrier agents, such as sucralfate, in patients who are on intensive care. These measures have been shown to reduce the incidence of bleeding from stress ulceration.

Ménétrier's disease

This is an unusual condition characterised by gross hypertrophy of the gastric mucosal folds, mucus production and hypochlorhydria. The condition is premalignant and may present with hypoproteinaemia and anaemia. There is no treatment other than a gastrectomy. The disease seems to be caused by overexpression of transforming growth factor alpha (TGF-α). Like epidermal growth factor (EGF), this peptide also binds to the EGF receptor. The histological features of Ménétrier's disease may be reproduced in transgenic mice overexpressing TGF-α.

Lymphocytic gastritis

This type of gastritis is seen rarely. It is characterised by the infiltration of the gastric mucosa by T cells and is probably associated with *H. pylori* infection. The pattern of inflammation resembles that seen in coeliac disease or lymphocytic colitis.

Summary box 63.4

Peptic ulceration

- Most peptic ulcers are caused by *H. pylori* or NSAIDs and changes in epidemiology mirror changes in these principal aetiological factors
- Duodenal ulcers are more common than gastric ulcers, but the symptoms are indistinguishable
- Gastric ulcers may become malignant and an ulcerated gastric cancer may mimic a benign ulcer
- Gastric antisecretory agents and *H. pylori* eradication therapy are the mainstay of treatment, and elective surgery is very rarely performed
- The long-term complications of peptic ulcer surgery may be difficult to treat
- The common complications of peptic ulcers are perforation, bleeding and stenosis
- The treatment of the perforated peptic ulcer is primarily surgical, although some patients may be managed conservatively

Other forms of gastritis

Eosinophilic gastritis appears to have an allergic basis, and is treated with steroids and cromoglycate. Granulomatous gastritis is seen rarely in Crohn's disease and also may be associated with tuberculosis. Acquired immunodeficiency syndrome (AIDS) gastritis is secondary to infection with cryptospiridiosis. Phlegmonous gastritis is a rare bacterial infection of the stomach found in patients with severe intercurrent illness. It is usually an agonal event.

PEPTIC ULCER

Although the name 'peptic' ulcer suggests an association with pepsin, this is essentially unimportant as in the absence of acid, peptic ulcers do not occur. Nearly all peptic ulcers can be healed by using proton pump inhibitors, which can render a patient virtually achlorhydric.

Common sites for peptic ulcers are the first part of the duodenum and the lesser curve of the stomach, but they also occur on the stoma following gastric surgery, the oesophagus and even in a Meckel's diverticulum, which contains ectopic gastric epithelium. In general, the ulcer occurs at a junction between different types of epithelia, the ulcer occurring in the epithelium least resistant to acid damage.

In the past, much distinction has been made between acute and chronic peptic ulcers, but this difference can sometimes be difficult to determine clinically. It is probably best to consider that there is a spectrum of disease from the superficial gastric and duodenal ulceration, frequently seen at endoscopy, to deep chronic penetrating ulcers. This does not minimise the importance of acute stress ulceration. These ulcers can both perforate and bleed.

For many years, the cause of peptic ulceration remained an enigma. When comparing groups of patients with duodenal and pre-pyloric peptic ulcers with normal subjects, gastric acid levels are higher, but the overlap is very considerable. Patients with gastric ulceration have relatively normal levels of gastric acid secretion. As peptic ulceration will occur in the presence of very high acid levels, such as those found in patients with a gastrinoma (Zollinger–Ellison syndrome), and as all ulcers can be healed in the absence of acid, it is clear that acid is important. In patients with a gastrinoma it may be the only aetiological factor, but this is not the case in the majority of patients. As with many diseases, genetic factors may be involved to a limited degree and social stress has also been falsely implicated (Asher).

It is now widely accepted that infection with *H. pylori* and the consumption of NSAIDs are the most important factors in the development of peptic ulceration. In combination *H. pylori* and NSAIDs act synergistically to promote ulcer development and ulcer bleeding. Cigarette smoking predisposes to peptic ulceration and increases the relapse rate after treatment, with either gastric antisecretory agents or, in the past, elective surgery. Multiple other factors may be involved in transition between the superficial and the deep penetrating chronic ulcer, but they are of lesser importance.

Pierre Ménétrier, 1859–1935, French physician.

Burrill Bernard Crohn, 1884–1956, gastroenterologist, Mount Sinai Hospital, New York, NY, USA. Described regional ileitis in 1932.

Johann Friedrich Meckel (The Younger), 1781–1833, Professor of Anatomy and Surgery, Halle, Germany. Described the diverticulum in 1809.

Robert Milton Zollinger, 1903–1992, Professor of Surgery, Ohio State University, Columbus, OH, USA.

Edwin Homer Ellison, 1918–1970, Professor of Surgery, Marquette University, Milwaukee, WI, USA. Zollinger and Ellison described this condition in a joint paper in 1955 when they were both working at the Ohio State University.

Richard Asher, 1912–1969, physician, the Central Middlesex Hospital, London, UK. Ridiculed the concept that the stress of modern living caused peptic ulceration by pointing out that the same claim was made for syphilis! It is an interesting coincidence that both diseases have strong aetiological associations with spiral organisms.

Duodenal ulceration

Incidence

There have been marked changes in the last two decades in the demography of patients presenting with duodenal ulceration in resource-rich countries. First, even before the introduction of H_2-receptor antagonists, the incidence of duodenal ulceration and the frequency of elective surgery for the condition were falling. This trend has continued and now, dyspeptic patients presenting with a duodenal ulcer at gastroscopy are uncommon. In part, this may relate to the widespread use of gastric antisecretory agents and *H. pylori* eradication therapy for patients with dyspepsia. Second, the peak incidence is now in a much older age group than previously and, although it is still more common in men, the difference is less marked. These changes mirror the changes, at least in part, in the epidemiology of *H. pylori* infection. In Eastern Europe, the disease remains common and, from having been uncommon in some resource-poor nations, it is now observed more frequently. Again, the relationship with *H. pylori* appears convincing.

Pathology

Most occur in the first part of the duodenum (Figures 63.12 and 63.13). A chronic ulcer penetrates the mucosa and into the muscle coat, leading to fibrosis. The fibrosis causes deformities such as pyloric stenosis. When an ulcer heals, a scar can be observed in the mucosa. Sometimes there may be more than one duodenal ulcer. The situation in which there is both a posterior and an anterior duodenal ulcer is referred to as 'kissing ulcers'. Anteriorly placed ulcers tend to perforate and, in contrast, posterior duodenal ulcers tend to bleed, sometimes by eroding into the gastroduodenal artery. Occasionally, the ulceration may be so extensive that the entire duodenal cap is ulcerated and devoid of mucosa. With respect to the giant duodenal ulcer, malignancy in this region is so uncommon that under normal circumstances surgeons can be confident that they are dealing with benign disease, even though from external palpation it may not appear so. In the stomach the situation is different.

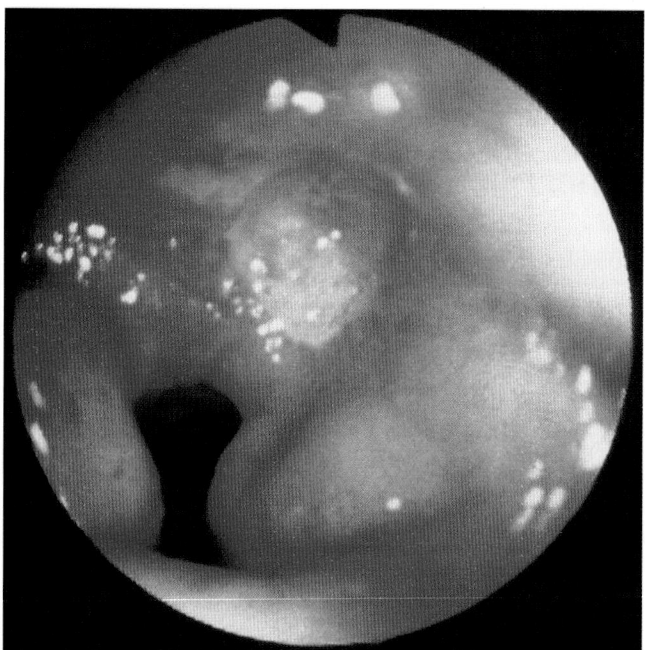

Figure 63.12 Duodenal ulcer at gastroduodenoscopy (courtesy of Dr GNJ Tytgat, Amsterdam, The Netherlands).

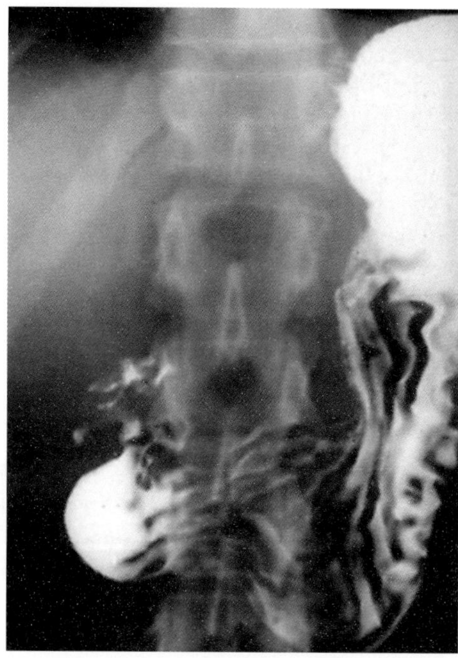

Figure 63.13 Duodenal ulcer shown by barium meal.

Histopathology

Microscopically, destruction of the muscular coat is observed and the base of the ulcer is covered with granulation tissue, the arteries in this region showing the typical changes of endarteritis obliterans. Sometimes the terminations of nerves can be seen among the fibrosis. The pathological appearances of the healing ulcer must be carefully interpreted as some of the epithelial downgrowths can be misinterpreted as invasion. This is unlikely to be important in duodenal ulcers when malignancy rarely, if ever, occurs, but it is much more important with gastric ulcers.

Gastric ulcers

Incidence

As with duodenal ulceration, *H. pylori* and NSAIDs are the important aetiological factors. Gastric ulceration is also associated with smoking; other factors are of lesser importance.

There are marked differences between the populations afflicted by chronic gastric ulceration compared with duodenal ulceration. First, gastric ulceration is substantially less common than duodenal ulceration. The sex incidence is equal and the population with gastric ulcers tends to be older. It is more prevalent in low socioeconomic groups and is considerably more common in resource-poor countries than in richer ones.

Pathology

This is essentially similar to that of a duodenal ulcer, except that gastric ulcers tend to be larger. Fibrosis, when it occurs, may result in the now rarely seen hourglass contraction of the stomach. Large chronic ulcers may erode posteriorly into the pancreas and, on other occasions, into major vessels such as the splenic artery. Less commonly, they may erode into other organs such as the transverse colon. Chronic gastric ulcers are much more common on the lesser curve (especially at the incisura angularis; Figures 63.14 and 63.15) than on the greater curve and, even when high on the lesser curve, they tend to be at the boundary between the acid-secreting and the non-acid-secreting epithelia. With atrophy of parietal cell mass, non-acid-secreting epithelium migrates up the lesser curvature.

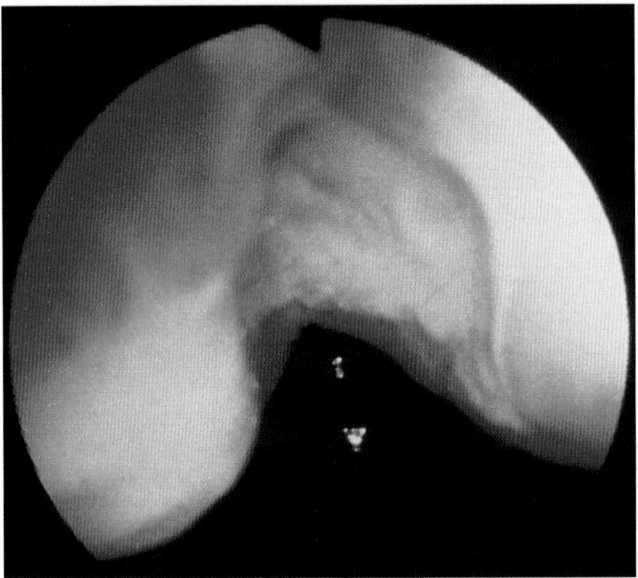

Figure 63.14 Benign incisural gastric ulcer shown at gastroscopy (courtesy of Dr GNJ Tytgat, Amsterdam, The Netherlands).

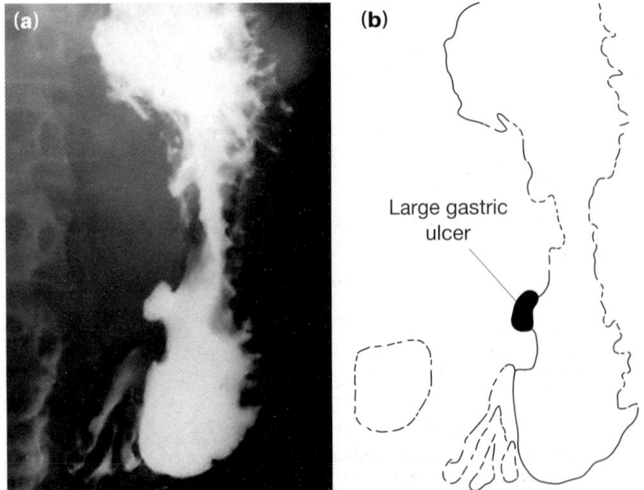

Figure 63.15 Benign gastric ulcer shown on barium meal. (a) Radiograph; (b) diagrammatic outline.

Malignancy in gastric ulcers

Chronic duodenal ulcers are not associated with malignancy and, in contrast, gastric ulcers are. Widely varying estimates are made of the incidence of gastric malignancy in gastric ulcers. The reason for this is that the authors reporting such diverse incidences are describing different clinical situations. Two clinical extremes must be distinguished to understand this problem properly. First, there is the situation in which a benign chronic gastric ulcer undergoes malignant transformation. This is known to happen, albeit rarely. The contrasting clinical extreme is the patient identified as having an ulcer in the stomach, either endoscopically or on contrast radiology, which is assessed as benign but biopsies reveal malignancy. In this situation the patient does not have, and probably never has had, chronic peptic ulceration in the stomach but has presented with an ulcerated cancer. This situation is common, although whether a lesion found in the stomach is described as being benign or malignant on clinical grounds depends very much on the skill and experience of the endoscopist or radiologist.

It is fundamental that any gastric ulcer should be regarded as being malignant, no matter how classical the features of a benign gastric ulcer. Multiple biopsies should always be taken, perhaps as many as 10 well-targeted biopsies, before an ulcer can be tentatively accepted as being benign. Even then it is important that further biopsies are taken while the ulcer is healing and when healed. Modern antisecretory agents can frequently heal the ulceration associated with gastric cancer but, clearly, are ineffective in treating the malignancy itself. At operation, even experienced surgeons may have difficulty distinguishing between the gastric cancer and a benign ulcer. Operative strategies differ so radically that it is essential, if at all possible, that a confident diagnosis is made before operation. If, at operation for perforation, it is determined that the ulcer is probably benign it should, nonetheless, be excised, in totality if possible, and submitted for histological examination. It is not known whether a patient's survival is compromised by this approach if the ulcer turns out to be malignant on biopsy, as convincing data are not available.

Other peptic ulcers

The pre-pyloric gastric ulcer was in the past difficult to treat, a problem overcome with the introduction of proton pump inhibitors. Pyloric channel ulcers are similar to duodenal ulcers. Both pre-pyloric and pyloric ulcers may be malignant, and biopsy is essential. Stomal ulcers occur after a gastroenterostomy (now most commonly after bariatric surgery; see later) or a gastrectomy of the Billroth II type. The ulcer is usually found on the jejunal side of the stoma.

Clinical features of peptic ulcers

Although many textbooks try to create differences in the clinical feature of gastric and duodenal ulceration, detailed analysis has shown that they cannot be differentiated on the

Christian Albert Theodor Billroth, 1829–1894, Professor of Surgery, Vienna, Austria.

basis of symptoms. The demographic characteristics of groups of patients with gastric and duodenal ulceration do differ but this does not allow discrimination.

Pain

The pain is epigastric, often described as gnawing and may radiate to the back. Eating may sometimes relieve the discomfort. The pain is normally intermittent rather than intractable.

Periodicity

One of the classical features of untreated peptic ulceration is periodicity. Symptoms may disappear for weeks or months to return again. This periodicity may be related to the spontaneous healing of the ulcer.

Vomiting

While this occurs, it is not a notable feature unless stenosis has occurred.

Alteration in weight

Weight loss or, sometimes, weight gain may occur. Patients with gastric ulceration are often underweight but this may precede the occurrence of the ulcer.

Bleeding

All peptic ulcers may bleed. The bleeding may be chronic and presentation with microcytic anaemia is not uncommon. All such patients should be investigated with endoscopy. Acute presentation with haematemesis and melaena is discussed later.

Clinical examination

Examination of the patient may reveal epigastric tenderness but, except in extreme cases (for instance, gastric outlet obstruction), there is unlikely to be much else to find.

Investigation of the patient with suspected peptic ulcer

Gastroduodenoscopy

This is the investigation of choice in the management of suspected peptic ulceration and in the hands of a well-trained operator is highly sensitive and specific.

In the stomach, any abnormal lesion should be multiply biopsied, and in the case of a suspected benign gastric ulcer numerous biopsies must be taken in order to exclude, as far as possible, the presence of a malignancy. Commonly, biopsies of the antrum will be taken to see whether there is histological evidence of gastritis and a CLO test performed to determine the presence of *H. pylori*. A 'U' manoeuvre should be performed to exclude ulcers around the gastro-oesophageal junction. This is important as the increasing incidence of cancer at the gastro-oesophageal junction requires that all mucosal abnormalities in this region should undergo multiple biopsy. Similarly, if a stoma is present, for instance after gastroenterostomy or Billroth II gastrectomy, it is important to enter both afferent and efferent loops. Almost all stomal ulcers will be very close to the junction between the jejunal and gastric mucosa. Attention should be given to the pylorus to note whether there is any pre-pyloric or pyloric channel ulceration, and also whether it is deformed, which is often the case with chronic duodenal ulceration. In the duodenum, care must be taken to view all of the first part. It is not infrequent for an ulcer to be just beyond the pylorus and easily overlooked.

Treatment of peptic ulceration

The vast majority of uncomplicated peptic ulcers are treated medically. Surgical treatment of uncomplicated peptic ulceration has decreased markedly since the 1960s and is now seldom performed in resource-rich countries. Surgical treatment was aimed principally at reducing gastric acid secretion and, in the case of gastric ulceration, removing the diseased mucosa. When originally devised, medical treatment also aimed to reduce gastric acid secretion, initially using the highly successful H_2-receptor antagonist and, subsequently, proton pump inhibitors. This has now largely given way to eradication therapy.

Medical treatment

It is reasonable that a doctor managing a patient with an uncomplicated peptic ulcer should suggest modifications to the patient's lifestyle, particularly the cessation of cigarette smoking. This advice is rarely followed and pharmacological measures form the mainstay of treatment.

H_2-receptor antagonists and proton pump inhibitors

H_2-antagonists (Black) revolutionised the management of peptic ulceration. Most duodenal ulcers and gastric ulcers can be healed by a few weeks of treatment with these drugs provided that they are taken and absorbed. There remained, however, a group of patients who were relatively refractory to conventional doses of H_2-receptor antagonists. This is largely now irrelevant as proton pump inhibitors can effectively render a patient achlorhydric and all benign ulcers will heal using these drugs, the majority within 2 weeks. Symptom relief is impressively rapid, most patients being asymptomatic within a few days. Like H_2-antagonists, proton pump inhibitors are safe and relatively devoid of serious side effects. The problem with all gastric antisecretory agents is that following cessation of therapy relapse is almost universal.

Eradication therapy

Eradication therapy is now routinely given to patients with peptic ulceration, and this is described earlier in this chapter. Evidence suggests that if a patient has a peptic ulcer and *H. pylori* is the principal aetiological factor (essentially the patient not taking NSAIDs) then complete eradication of the organism will cure the disease and reinfection as an adult is

Sir James Black, 1924–2002, Professor of Pharmacology, King's College Hospital Medical School, London, UK, introduced beta-blockers and H_2-receptor antagonists. He received the Nobel Prize for Physiology or Medicine in 1988.

uncommon. Eradication therapy is therefore the mainstay of treatment for peptic ulceration. It is extremely economical by comparison with prolonged courses of antisecretory agents or surgery. It is also considerably safer than surgical treatment.

There are some patients with peptic ulcers in whom eradication therapy may not be appropriate and this includes patients with NSAID-associated ulcers. Such patients should avoid these drugs if possible and, if not, they should be co-prescribed with a potent antisecretory agent. Similarly, patients with stomal ulceration are not effectively treated with eradication therapy and require prolonged prescription of antisecretory agents. Patients with Zollinger–Ellison syndrome should be treated in the long term with proton pump inhibitors unless the tumour can be adequately managed by surgery.

Ulcers that fail to heal

The introduction of antisecretory agents and effective treatments for *H. pylori* have revolutionised the management of peptic ulcers. Despite these advances peptic ulceration fails to heal in a small minority of patients. Endoscopic re-evaluation should be regarded as mandatory to confirm healing of all gastric ulcers. Furthermore, endoscopy permits the differentiation between a refractory ulcer and persistent symptoms despite ulcer healing. The most common cause of failed healing is persistent *H. pylori* infection. Biopsies should be repeated at the time of endoscopy as false-negative results with breath tests may be expected soon after eradication therapy and serum antibody titres may not fall for 6 months after successful eradication. Failure of eradication is usually due to poor compliance or bacterial resistance and bacteriological culture will guide further attempts at *H. pylori* eradication. The ingestion of NSAIDs should once again be addressed. A diagnosis of Zollinger-Ellison syndrome (described in detail later) should be suspected in *H. pylori* negative, non-NSAID-related peptic ulceration and serum gastrin levels should be measured. Very rarely, a recently described autoimmune IgG4-related phenomenon is the cause of resistant and recurrent gastric ulceration.

Surgical treatment of uncomplicated peptic ulceration

From its peak in the 1960s, the incidence of surgery for uncomplicated peptic ulceration has fallen markedly, to the extent that peptic ulcer surgery is now of little more than historical interest. A description of operations used in the treatment of peptic ulcers is still necessary because surgery is occasionally employed for the complicated ulcer and, in addition, many patients are left suffering from the consequences of the more destructive operations.

Operations for duodenal ulceration

Duodenal ulcer surgery (rationale)

Procedures devised for the treatment of duodenal ulcers have the common aim of excluding the damaging effects of acid from the duodenum. This has been achieved by diversion of the acid away from the duodenum, reducing the secretory potential of the stomach, or both. All of the operations devised achieved their aim to some extent, but with varying degrees of morbidity, mortality and postoperative side effects. There is now no role for acid-reducing operations in the routine management of peptic ulcer disease but occasionally operations which involve gastrectomy have to be performed in the emergency situation. In addition many patients have had such operations performed and suffer from the sequelae. Hence it is important for the clinician to understand the anatomical and physiological consequences of surgery. The operations are described in historical sequence.

Billroth II gastrectomy

The first successful gastrectomy was performed by Billroth in January 1881, and Wolfler performed the first gastroenterostomy in the same year. The original Billroth operations consisted of a gastric resection with gastroduodenal anastomosis (Billroth I technique) (Figure 63.16). The Billroth II operation was devised more by accident than design (Figure 63.17). A gastroenterostomy (Figure 63.18) was performed on a gravely ill patient with a pyloric cancer, who was not expected to survive. Contrary to expectations, the patient improved and the stomach distal to the anastomosis was resected. It soon became evident that the use of gastrojejunal anastomosis after gastric resection could be safer and easier than the Billroth I procedure, and it became popular and effective in the surgical treatment of duodenal ulcer. Because of its disadvantages, such as higher operative mortality and morbidity, it has not been used for many years in the patient with an uncomplicated ulcer, but it is still used occasionally

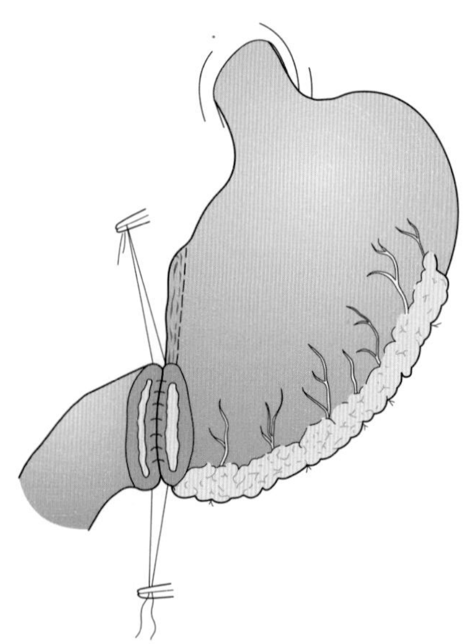

Figure 63.16 Billroth I gastrectomy. The lower half of the stomach is removed and the cut stomach anastomosed to the first part of the duodenum.

Anton Wolfler, 1850–1917, Professor of Surgery, Prague, Czechoslovakia.

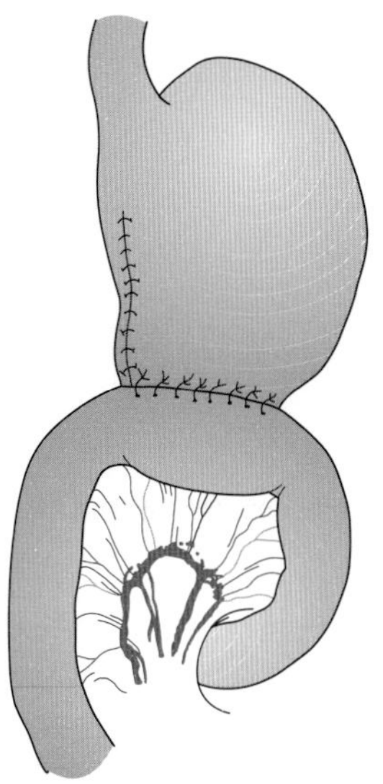

Figure 63.17 Billroth II. Two-thirds of the stomach is removed, the duodenal stump is closed and the stomach anastomosed to the jejunum.

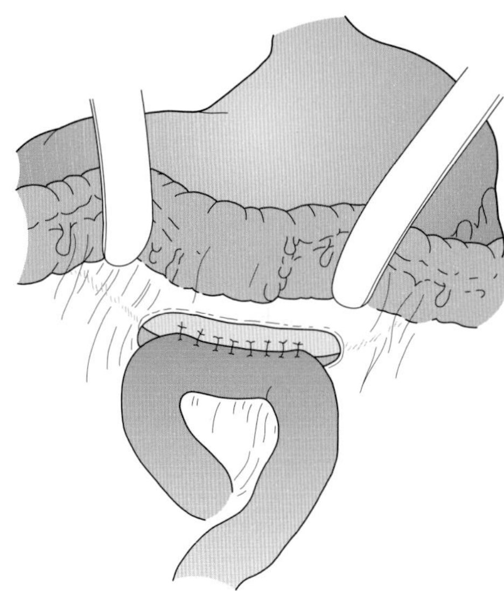

Figure 63.18 Gastroenterostomy. The jejunum is anastomosed to the posterior, dependent, wall of the stomach.

in the treatment of a complicated ulcer with a 'difficult' duodenum. In Billroth II gastrectomy, or its close relation Pólya gastrectomy, the antrum and distal body of the stomach are mobilised by opening the greater and lesser omentum and dividing the gastroepiploic arteries, right gastric artery and the left gastric artery arcade at the limit of the resection. The duodenum is closed off either by suture or using staples, sometimes with difficulty in patients with a very deformed duodenum. Various techniques are available to close the difficult duodenum and, in extremis, a catheter may be placed in the duodenal stump, the duodenum closed around it and a catheter brought out through the abdominal wall. Following resection, the distal end of the stomach is narrowed by the closure of the lesser curve aspect of the remnant. The greater curve aspect is then anastomosed, usually in a retrocolic fashion, to the jejunum, leaving as short an afferent loop as feasible (Figure 63.17). Even when well performed, this procedure has an operative mortality rate of a few per cent and morbidity is not unusual. A common cause of morbidity is leakage from the duodenal stump, which is particularly associated with kinking of the afferent loop. Leakage from the gastrojejunal anastomosis is unusual unless it is under tension or the stomach has been devascularised during the mobilisation. The incidence of side effects following gastrectomy is considerable, as shown in *Table 63.2*. Recurrence of the ulcer at the stoma is uncommon but can occur, especially as this procedure is traditionally not combined with the vagotomy. In the majority of expert centres a Roux-en-Y reconstruction rather than the Billroth II procedure is performed because postoperative function is better.

TABLE 63.2 Operative mortality, side effects and incidence of recurrence following duodenal ulcer operations.

Operation	Operative mortality (%)	Significant side effects (%)	Recurrent ulceration (%)
Gastrectomy	<1–2	<20–40	1–4
Gastroenterostomy alone	<1	<10–20	50
Truncal vagotomy and drainage	<1	<10–20	2–7
Selective vagotomy and drainage	<1	<10–20	5–10
Highly selective vagotomy	<0.2	<5	2–10
Truncal vagotomy and antrectomy	<1	<10–20	1

Gastrojejunostomy

Because of the potential for mortality after gastrectomy, the use of gastrojejunostomy alone in the treatment of duodenal ulceration was developed (Figure 63.18). Reflux of alkali from the small bowel into the stomach reduced duodenal acid exposure and was often successful in healing the ulcer. However, because the jejunal loop was exposed directly to gastric acid, stomal ulceration was extremely common, hence the procedure in isolation was ineffective.

Truncal vagotomy and drainage

Truncal vagotomy was first introduced in 1943 by Dragstedt and, for many years, combined with drainage, was the mainstay of treatment of duodenal ulceration (Figure 63.19). The principle of the operation is that section of the vagus nerves, which are critically involved in the secretion of gastric acid,

Eugen (Jeno) Alexander Pólya, 1876–1944, surgeon, St Stephen's Hospital, Budapest, Hungary.
César Roux, 1857–1934, Professor of Surgery and Gynaecology, Lausanne, Switzerland. Described this method of forming a jejunal conduit in 1908.
Lester Reynold Dragstedt, 1893–1975, Professor of Surgery, Chicago, IL, USA.

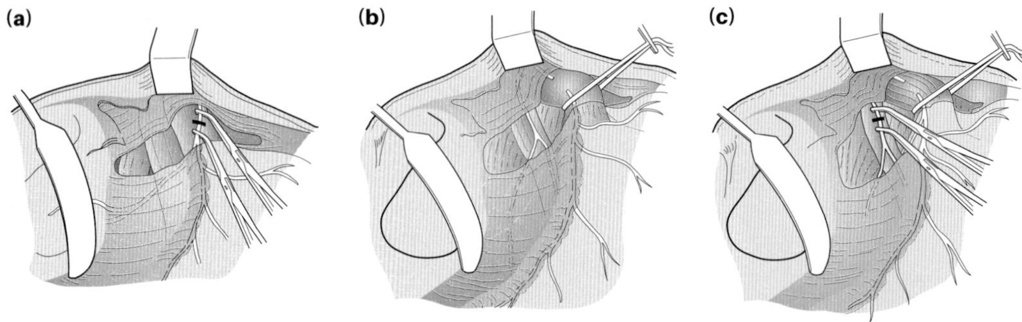

Figure 63.19 Truncal vagotomy: (a) division of the anterior vagus; (b) mobilisation of the oesophagus; (c) division of the posterior vagus.

reduces the maximal acid output by approximately 50%. Because the vagal nerves are motor to the stomach, denervation of the antropyloroduodenal segment results in gastric stasis in a substantial proportion of patients on whom truncal vagotomy alone is performed. This was first noted by Dragstedt, who did not perform a drainage procedure when he first introduced the operation. The most popular drainage procedure is the Heineke–Mikulicz pyloroplasty (Figure 63.20). It is simple to perform and involves the longitudinal section of the pyloric ring. The incision is closed transversely. Gastrojejunostomy (Figure 63.18) was the alternative drainage procedure to pyloroplasty. This is performed through opening the lesser sac and performing an anastomosis between the most dependent part of the antrum and the first jejunal loop. An isoperistaltic anastomosis was most commonly performed. The operation of truncal vagotomy and drainage is substantially safer than gastrectomy (*Table 63.2*). However, the side effects of surgery are, in fact, little different from those that follow gastrectomy.

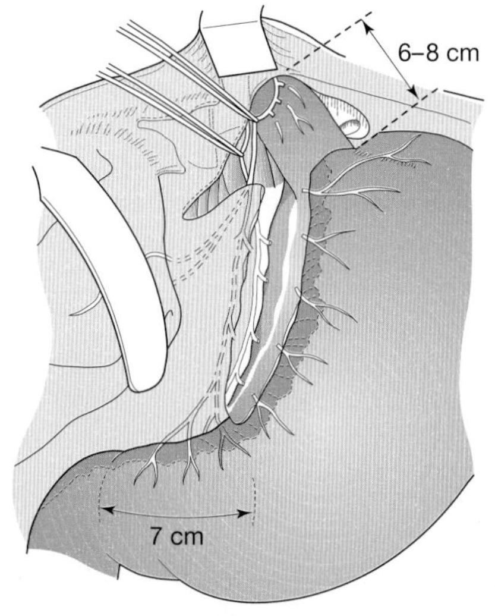

Highly selective vagotomy

In 1968 Johnston and Amdrup independently devised the operation of highly selective vagotomy in which only the parietal cell mass of the stomach was denervated (Figure 63.21). This proved to be the most satisfactory operation for duodenal ulceration, with a low incidence of side effects and acceptable recurrence rates when performed to a high technical standard. This operation became the gold standard for operations on duodenal ulceration in the 1970s. The operative mortality was lower than any other definitive operation for duodenal ulceration, in all probability because the gastrointestinal tract was not opened during this procedure. The unpleasant effects of peptic ulcer surgery were largely avoided, although loss of receptive relaxation of the stomach did occur, leading to epigastric fullness and sometimes mild dumping. However, the severe symptoms that occur after other more destructive gastric operations did not occur. It is often said that recurrent ulceration is the Achilles' heel of this operation although, when performed well, recurrence was no more common than after truncal vagotomy. The operation disappeared from routine use with the advent of antisecretory agents and eradication therapy.

Figure 63.21 Highly selective vagotomy. The anterior and posterior vagus nerves are preserved but all branches to the fundus and body of the stomach are divided.

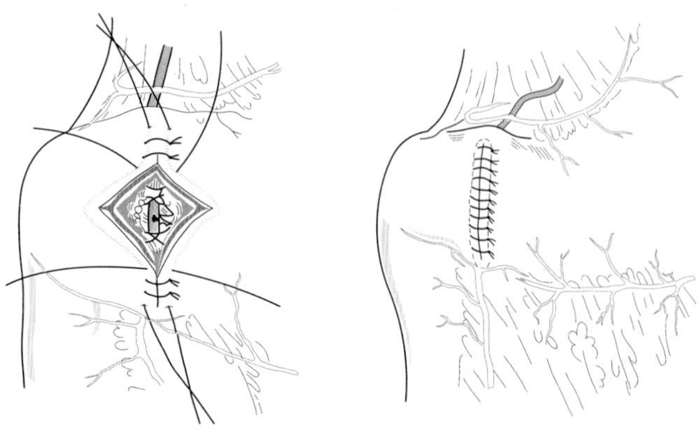

Figure 63.20 Pyroplasty.

Walther Hermann Heineke, 1834–1901, surgeon, Erlangen, Germany.
Johann von Mikulicz-Radecki, 1850–1905, Professor of Surgery, Breslau, Germany (now Wroclaw, Poland).
David Johnston, contemporary, Professor of Surgery, University of Leeds, Leeds, UK.
Eric Amdrup, 1923–1998, Professor of Surgery, Aarhus, Denmark.

Truncal vagotomy and antrectomy

For completeness, this operation should be mentioned as at one stage it was popular in the USA. In addition to a truncal vagotomy, the antrum of the stomach is removed, thus removing the source of gastrin, and the gastric remnant is joined to the duodenum. The recurrence rates after this procedure are exceedingly low. However, the operative mortality is higher than after vagotomy and drainage (*Table 63.2*) and the incidence of unpleasant side effects is similar.

Operations for gastric ulcer

In contrast with duodenal ulcer surgery, when the principal objective was to reduce duodenal acid exposure, in gastric ulceration the diseased tissue is usually removed as well. This has the advantage that malignancy can then be confidently excluded. As with duodenal ulceration such surgery is not now performed except for complications of gastric ulcer.

Billroth I gastrectomy

This was the standard operation (Figure 63.16) for gastric ulceration until medical treatments became prevalent. The distal stomach is mobilised and resected in the same way as in the Billroth II gastrectomy. This resection should include the ulcer that is usually situated on the lesser curve. The cut edge of the remnant is then partially closed from the lesser curve aspect, leaving a stoma at the greater curve aspect, which should be similar in size to the duodenum. Reconstruction may be facilitated by mobilising the duodenum using Kocher's manoeuvre. The incidence of recurrent ulceration after this operation is low, but it carries with it the morbidity and mortality associated with any gastric resection. This operation is virtually never performed now.

Sequelae of peptic ulcer surgery

There are a number of sequelae of peptic ulcer surgery, which include recurrent ulceration, small stomach syndrome, bilious vomiting, early and late dumping, diarrhoea and malignant transformation. These sequelae principally follow from the more destructive operations that are now seldom performed. However, a substantial number of patients suffer from side effects from operations undertaken in the past. Approximately 30% of patients can expect to suffer a degree of dysfunction following peptic ulcer surgery (*Table 63.2*) and, in about 5% of such patients, the symptoms will be intractable.

Recurrent ulceration

Although mentioned first, this is by far the easiest problem to treat. Just as all peptic ulcers will heal with potent antisecretory agents, so will ulcers that are recurrent after ulcer surgery.

As with other peptic ulcers, recurrent ulcers may present with complications, particularly bleeding and perforation. In this respect, the complication of gastrojejunal colic fistula requires a particular mention. In this rare condition, the anastomotic ulcer penetrates into the transverse colon. Patients suffer from diarrhoea that is severe and follows every meal. They have foul breath and may vomit formed faeces. Severe weight loss and dehydration are rapid in onset, and for this reason the condition may be mistaken for malignancy. The major factor producing the nutritional disturbance is the severe contamination of the jejunum with colonic bacteria. A number of imaging techniques can be used to detect the fistula, most commonly CT with oral contrast or indeed a barium enema. Endoscopy may not convincingly demonstrate the fistula and, in about one-half of such cases, the barium meal will not reveal the problem. The treatment of gastrocolic fistula consists of first correcting the dehydration and malnutrition and then performing revisional surgery.

Small stomach syndrome

Early satiety follows most ulcer operations to some degree, including highly selective vagotomy. In this latter circumstance, although there is no anatomical disturbance of the stomach there is loss of receptive relaxation. Fortunately, this problem does tend to get better with time and revisional surgery is not necessary.

Bile vomiting

Bile vomiting can occur after any form of vagotomy with drainage or gastrectomy. Commonly, the patient presents with vomiting a mixture of food and bile or sometimes some bile alone after a meal. Often eating will precipitate abdominal pain and reflux symptoms are common. Bile chelating agents can be tried but are usually ineffective. In intractable cases, revisional surgery may be indicated. The nature of that revisional surgery depends very much on the original operation. Following gastrectomy, Roux-en-Y diversion is probably the best treatment. In patients with a gastroenterostomy, this can be taken down and, in most circumstances a small pyloroplasty can be performed. In patients with a pyloroplasty, reconstruction of the pylorus has been attempted but, in general terms, the results of this operation have been rather poor. Antrectomy and Roux-en-Y reconstruction may be the better option.

Early and late dumping

Although considered together because the symptoms are similar, early and late dumping have different aetiologies. A common feature, however, is early rapid gastric emptying. Many patients have both early and late dumping.

EARLY DUMPING

Early dumping consists of abdominal and vasomotor symptoms that are found in about 10% of patients following gastrectomy or vagotomy and drainage. It also affects a small percentage of patients following highly selective vagotomy due to the loss of receptive relaxation of the stomach. The small bowel is filled with foodstuffs from the stomach, which have a high osmotic load, and this leads to the sequestration of fluid from the circulation into the gastrointestinal tract. This can be observed by the rise in the packed cell volume

Emil Theodor Kocher, 1841–1917, Professor of Surgery, Berne, Switzerland.

while the symptoms are present. All of the symptoms shown in Table 63.3 can be related to this effect on the gut and the circulation.

The principal treatment is dietary manipulation. Small, regular meals based on fat and protein are best, and avoiding fluids with a high carbohydrate content also helps. Fortunately, following operation, the syndrome tends to improve with time. For some reason, however, there is a group of patients who suffer intractable dumping regardless of any of these measures. The somatostatin analogue octreotide given before meals has been shown to be useful in some individuals and the long-acting preparation may also be useful. However, this treatment can lead to the development of gallstones and it does not help the diarrhoea from which many patients with dumping also suffer.

Revisional surgery may be occasionally required. In patients with a gastroenterostomy, the drainage may be taken down or, in the case of a pyloroplasty, repaired. Alternatively, antrectomy with Roux-en-Y reconstruction is often effective, although the procedure is of greater magnitude; following gastrectomy, it is the revisional procedure of choice.

TABLE 63.3 Features of early and late dumping.

	Early	Late
Incidence	5–10%	5%
Relation to meals	Almost immediate	Second hour after meal
Durations of attack	30–40 minutes	30–40 minutes
Relief	Lying down	Food
Aggravated by	More food	Exercise
Precipitating factor	Food, especially carbohydrate-rich and wet	As early dumping
Major symptoms	Epigastric fullness, sweating, light-headedness, tachycardia, colic, sometimes diarrhoea	Tremor, faintness, prostration

LATE DUMPING

This is reactive hypoglycaemia. The carbohydrate load in the small bowel causes a rise in the plasma glucose, which, in turn, causes insulin levels to rise, causing a secondary hypoglycaemia. This can be easily demonstrated by serial measurements of blood glucose in a patient following a test meal. The treatment is essentially the same as for early dumping. Octreotide is very effective in dealing with this problem.

Post-vagotomy diarrhoea

This can be the most devastating symptom to afflict patients having peptic ulcer surgery. Most patients will suffer some looseness of bowel action to some degree (with the exception of highly selective vagotomy) but, in about 5%, it may be intractable. Despite much investigation, the precise aetiology of the problem is uncertain. It is related, to some degree, to rapid gastric emptying. In all probability, the denervation of the upper gastrointestinal tract as a result of the vagotomy is also important. Exaggerated gastrointestinal peptide responses may also aggravate the condition.

The diarrhoea in post-vagotomy patients may take several forms. It may be severe and explosive, the patient experiencing a considerable degree of urgency. The patients sometimes describe the diarrhoea as feeling like passing boiling water. At the other extreme, some patients only have minor episodes of diarrhoea, which are not as directly related to food.

Many authors regard diarrhoea and dumping as being essentially the same problem. However, many patients with severe diarrhoea do not have any of the other symptoms of dumping and likewise some patients with dumping do not experience any significant diarrhoea.

The condition is difficult to treat. The patient should be managed as for early dumping and antidiarrhoeal preparations may be of some value. Octreotide is not effective in this condition and the results of revisional surgery are too unpredictable to make this an attractive treatment option.

Malignant transformation

Many large studies now confirm that operations such as gastrectomy or vagotomy and drainage are independent risk factors for the development of gastric cancer. The increased risk appears to be approximately four times that of the control population.

It is not difficult to understand the increased incidence of gastric cancer, as bile reflux gastritis, intestinal metaplasia and gastric cancer are linked. The lag phase between operation and the development of malignancy is at least 10 years. Highly selective vagotomy does not seem to be associated with an increased incidence of gastric cancer in the long term.

Nutritional consequences

Nutritional disorders are more common after gastrectomy than after vagotomy and drainage. Weight loss is common after gastrectomy and the patient may, in fact, never return to their original weight. Nutritional advice advising the taking of small meals is often more useful. Anaemia may be due to either iron or vitamin B12 deficiency.

Iron-deficiency anaemia occurs after both gastrectomy and vagotomy and drainage and is probably multifactorial in origin. Reduced iron absorption is probably the most important factor, although the loss of blood from the gastric mucosa may also be important. Vitamin B12 deficiency is prone to occur after total gastrectomy. However, because of the very large vitamin B12 stores that most patients have, this may be very late in occurring. Vitamin B12 supplementation after total gastrectomy is essential. Rarely, vitamin B12 deficiency may occur after lesser forms of gastrectomy. In such patients the cause is probably a combination of reduced intrinsic factor production and also the fact that some patients have bacterial colonisation, which results in the destruction of the vitamin B12 in the gut.

Bone disease is seen principally after gastrectomy and mainly in women. The condition is essentially indistinguishable from the osteoporosis commonly seen in post-menopausal women. It is only the frequency and magnitude of the disorder that distinguish it. Treatment is with dietary supplementation, calcium and vitamin D, and exercise.

Gallstones

The development of gallstones is strongly associated with truncal vagotomy. Following truncal vagotomy, the biliary tree, as well as the stomach, is denervated, leading to stasis and hence stone formation. Patients developing symptomatic gallstones will require cholecystectomy. However, this may induce or worsen other postpeptic ulcer surgery syndromes such as bilious vomiting and postvagotomy diarrhoea.

The complications of peptic ulceration

The common complications of peptic ulcer are perforation, bleeding and stenosis. Bleeding and stenosis are considered below in the relevant sections.

Perforated peptic ulcer

EPIDEMIOLOGY

Despite the widespread use of gastric antisecretory agents and eradication therapy, the incidence of perforated peptic ulcer has changed little. However, there has been a considerable change in the epidemiology of perforated peptic ulcer in resource-rich countries over the last two decades. Previously, most patients were middle aged, with a ratio of 2:1 of male:female. With time there has been a steady increase in the age of the patients suffering this complication and an increase in the numbers of females, such that perforations now occur most commonly in elderly female patients. NSAIDs appear to be responsible for most of these perforations.

CLINICAL FEATURES

The classical presentation of perforated duodenal ulcer is instantly recognisable (Figure 63.22). The patient, who may have a history of peptic ulceration, develops sudden-onset severe generalised abdominal pain due to the irritant effect of gastric acid on the peritoneum. Although the contents of an acid-producing stomach are relatively low in bacterial load, bacterial peritonitis supervenes over a few hours, usually accompanied by a deterioration in the patient's condition. Initially, the patient may be shocked with a tachycardia but a pyrexia is not usually observed until some hours after the event. The abdomen exhibits a board-like rigidity and the patient is disinclined to move because of the pain. The abdomen does not move with respiration. Patients with this form of presentation need an operation, without which the patient will deteriorate with a septic peritonitis.

This classical presentation of the perforated peptic ulcer is observed less commonly than in the past. Very frequently the elderly patient who is taking NSAIDs will have a less dramatic presentation, perhaps because of the use of potent anti-inflammatory drugs (steroids). The board-like rigidity seen in the abdomen of younger patients may also not be observed and a higher index of suspicion is necessary to make the correct diagnosis. In other patients, the leak from the ulcer may not be massive. They may present only with pain in the epigastrium and right iliac fossa as the fluid may track down the right paracolic gutter. Sometimes perforations will seal owing to the inflammatory response and adhesion within the abdominal cavity, and so the perforation may be self-limiting. All of these factors may combine to make the diagnosis of perforated peptic ulcer difficult.

By far the most common site of perforation is the anterior aspect of the duodenum. However, the anterior or incisural gastric ulcer may perforate and, in addition, gastric ulcers may perforate into the lesser sac, which can be particularly difficult to diagnose. These patients may not have obvious peritonitis.

INVESTIGATIONS

An erect plain chest radiograph will reveal free gas under the diaphragm in excess of 50% of cases with perforated peptic ulcer (Figure 63.23) but CT imaging is more accurate (see below). All patients should have serum amylase performed, as distinguishing between peptic ulcer, perforation and pancreatitis can be difficult. Measuring the serum amylase, however, may not remove the diagnostic difficulty. It can be elevated following perforation of a peptic ulcer although, fortunately, the levels are not usually as high as the levels commonly seen

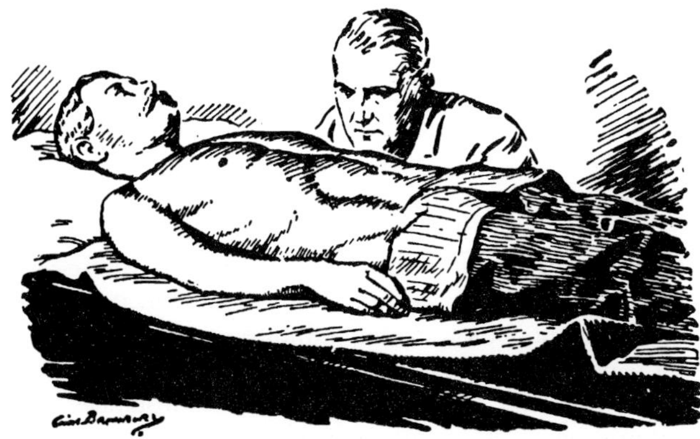

Figure 63.22 A sketch of Mr Hamilton Bailey watching for abdominal movement on respiration. In the case of a classically presenting perforated ulcer, the abdominal movement is restricted or absent.

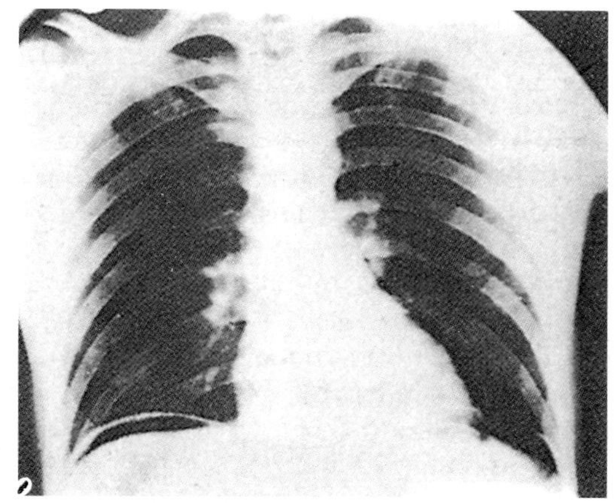

Figure 63.23 Plain abdominal radiograph of a perforated ulcer, showing air under the diaphragm.

Henry Hamilton Bailey, 1894–1961, surgeon, The Royal Northern Hospital, London, UK.

in acute pancreatitis. Several other investigations are useful if doubt remains. A CT scan will normally be diagnostic in both conditions.

TREATMENT

The initial priorities are resuscitation and analgesia. Analgesia should not be withheld for fear of removing the signs of an intra-abdominal catastrophe. In fact, adequate analgesia makes the clinical signs more obvious. It is important, however, to titrate the analgesic dose. Following resuscitation, the treatment is principally surgical. Laparotomy is performed, usually through an upper midline incision if the diagnosis of perforated peptic ulcer can be made with confidence. This is not always possible and hence it may be better to place a small incision around the umbilicus to localise the perforation with more certainty. Alternatively, laparoscopy may be used. The most important component of the operation is a thorough peritoneal toilet to remove all of the fluid and food debris. If the perforation is in the duodenum it can usually be closed by several well-placed sutures, closing the ulcer in a transverse direction as with a pyloroplasty. It is important that sufficient tissue is taken in the suture to allow the edges to be approximated, and the sutures should not be tied so tight that they tear out. It is common to place an omental patch over the perforation in the hope of enhancing the chances of the leak sealing. If the perforation is difficult to close primarily it is frequently possible to seal the leak with an omental patch alone, and many surgeons now employ this strategy for all perforations. When securing the omental patch it is important not to tie the sutures too tight so as to obliterate the omental blood supply. Gastric ulcers should, if possible, be excised and closed, so that malignancy can be excluded. Occasionally a patient is seen who has a massive duodenal or gastric perforation such that simple closure is impossible; in these patients a distal gastrectomy with Roux-en-Y reconstruction is the procedure of choice.

All patients should be treated with systemic antibiotics in addition to a thorough peritoneal lavage. In the past, many surgeons performed definitive procedures such as either truncal vagotomy and pyloroplasty or, more recently and probably more successfully, highly selective vagotomy during the course of an operation for a perforation. Studies show that in well-selected patients and in expert hands this is a very safe strategy. However, nowadays, surgery is confined to first-aid measures most commonly, and the peptic ulcer is treated medically as described earlier in this chapter. Following operation, gastric antisecretory agents should be started immediately. *H. pylori* eradication is mandatory.

Perforated peptic ulcers can often be managed by minimally invasive techniques if the expertise is available. The principles of operation are, however, the same; thorough peritoneal toilet is performed and the perforation is closed by intracorporeal suturing. Whatever technique is used, it is important that the stomach is kept empty postoperatively by nasogastric suction, and that gastric antisecretory agents are commenced to promote healing in the residual ulcer.

A great deal has been written about the conservative management of perforated ulcer. Some writers say that virtually all patients can be managed conservatively, whereas most surgeons have difficulty in understanding how a patient who is ill with widespread peritonitis and who has food debris widely distributed through the abdominal cavity will improve without an operation. However, undoubtedly, there are patients who have small leaks from a perforated peptic ulcer and relatively mild peritoneal contamination, who may be managed with intravenous fluids, nasogastric suction and antibiotics. These patients are in the minority. A number of factors have been associated with poor outcome after perforated peptic ulcer, including:

- delay in diagnosis (>24 hours);
- medical comorbidities;
- shock;
- increasing age (>75).

There is little evidence to advocate the conservative management of patients who exhibit any of these characteristics.

Patients who have suffered one perforation may suffer another one. Therefore, they should be managed aggressively to ensure that this does not happen. Lifelong treatment with proton pump inhibitors is a reasonable option especially in those who have to continue with NSAID treatment.

HAEMATEMESIS AND MELAENA

Upper gastrointestinal haemorrhage remains a major medical problem with an incidence over 100/100 000 per year in western practice that increases with increasing age. Haemorrhage is strongly associated with NSAID use. Despite improvements in diagnosis and the proliferation in treatment modalities over the last few decades, an in-hospital mortality of 5–10% can be expected. This rises to 33% when bleeding is first observed in patients who are hospitalised for other reasons. In patients in whom the cause of bleeding can be found, the most common causes are peptic ulcer, erosions, Mallory–Weiss tear and bleeding oesophageal varices (Table 63.4).

Whatever the cause, the principles of management are identical. First, the patient should be adequately resuscitated and, following this, the patient should be investigated urgently to determine the cause of the bleeding. Only then should treatment of a definitive nature be instituted. For any significant gastrointestinal bleed, intravenous access should be established and, for those with severe bleeding, central venous pressure monitoring should be set up and bladder catheterisation performed. Blood should be cross-matched and the patient transfused as clinically indicated, usually when >30% of blood volume has been lost. There is no evidence for the use of intravenous proton pump inhibitors prior to endoscopy. As a general rule, most gastrointestinal bleeding will stop, albeit temporarily, but there are sometimes instances when this is not the case. In these circumstances, resuscitation, diagnosis and treatment should be carried out simultaneously. There are occasions when life-saving manoeuvres have to

George Kenneth Mallory, b.1926, Professor of Pathology, Boston, MA, USA.
Soma Weiss, 1899–1942, Professor of Medicine, Boston, MA, USA.

TABLE 63.4 Causes of upper gastrointestinal bleeding.

Condition	%
Ulcers	60
Oesophageal	6
Gastric	21
Duodenal	33
Erosions	26
Oesophageal	13
Gastric	9
Duodenal	4
Mallory–Weiss tear	4
Oesophageal varices	4
Tumour	0.5
Vascular lesions, e.g. Dieulafoy's disease	0.5
Others	5

be undertaken without the benefit of an absolute diagnosis. For instance, in patients with known oesophageal varices and uncontrollable bleeding, a Sengstaken–Blakemore tube may be inserted before an endoscopy has been carried out. This practice is not to be encouraged, except in extremis. In some patients, bleeding is secondary to a coagulopathy. The most important current causes of this are liver disease and inadequately controlled warfarin therapy. In these circumstances the coagulopathy should be corrected, if possible, with fresh-frozen plasma or concentrated clotting factors.

Upper gastrointestinal endoscopy should be carried out by an experienced operator as soon as practicable after the patient has been stabilised. In patients in whom the bleeding is relatively mild, endoscopy may be carried out on the morning after admission; this is usually guided by local policy. In all cases of severe bleeding it should be carried out immediately. A number of scoring systems have been advocated for the assessment of rebleeding and death after upper gastrointestinal haemorrhage. Perhaps the most useful of these is the Rockall score. This can be used in a pre-endoscopy format to stratify patients to safe early discharge and postendoscopy it can relatively accurately predict rebleeding and death.

Bleeding peptic ulcers

The epidemiology of bleeding peptic ulcers exactly mirrors that of perforated ulcers. In recent years, the population affected has become much older and the bleeding is commonly associated with the ingestion of NSAIDs. Diagnosis can normally be made endoscopically, although occasionally the nature of the blood loss precludes accurately identifying the lesion. However, the more experienced the endoscopist, the less likely this is to be a problem.

Medical and minimally interventional treatments

Medical treatment has limited efficacy. All patients are commonly started on either an H_2-antagonist or a proton pump antagonist, and recent evidence confirms the benefit of proton pump inhibitor administration to prevent rebleeding after endoscopy. Furthermore, meta-analysis of studies suggests that tranexamic acid, an inhibitor of fibrinolysis, may reduce overall mortality.

Therapeutic endoscopy can achieve haemostasis in approximately 70% of cases, with the best evidence supporting a combination of adrenaline injection with heater probe and/or clips. Therapeutic endoscopy will probably never be effective in patients who are bleeding from large vessels and with which the majority of the mortality is associated.

In patients where the source of bleeding cannot be identified or in those who rebleed after endoscopy, angiography with transcatheter embolisation may offer a valuable alternative to surgery in expert centres. The risk of significant ischaemia following embolisation is low because of the rich collateral blood supply of the stomach and duodenum. The surgeon should be mindful that rescue surgery after failed embolisation is associated with poor outcome and it may be advantageous to proceed directly to surgery.

Surgical treatment

Criteria for surgery are well worked out. A patient who continues to bleed requires surgical treatment. The same applies to a significant rebleed. The only exception applies in expert centres with 24-hour interventional radiology and experience of angiographic embolisation where attempts may be made to arrest bleeding and avoid surgery. The surgical team should care for these patients and an operation should not be delayed if any concerns remain. Patients with a visible vessel in the ulcer base, a spurting vessel or an ulcer with a clot in the base are statistically likely to require surgical treatment to stop the bleeding. Elderly and unfit patients are more likely to die as a result of bleeding than younger patients. Ironically, they should have early surgery. A patient who has required more than six units of blood in general needs surgical treatment.

The aim of the operation is to stop the bleeding. The advent of endoscopy has greatly helped in the management of upper gastrointestinal bleeding as a surgeon can usually be confident about the site of bleeding prior to operation. The most common site of bleeding from a peptic ulcer is the duodenum. In tackling this, it is essential that the duodenum is fully mobilised. This should be done before the duodenum is opened as it makes the ulcer much more accessible and also allows the surgeon's hand to be placed behind the gastroduodenal artery, which is commonly the source of major bleeding. Following mobilisation, the duodenum, and usually the pylorus, is opened longitudinally as in a

Robert William Sengstaken, b.1923, surgeon, Garden City, NY, USA.
Arthur Hendley Blakemore, 1897–1970, Associate Professor of Surgery, the Columbia College of Physicians and Surgeons, New York, NY, USA. Sengstaken and Blakemore originally described the tube in 1950.
Timothy A Rockall, contemporary, Professor of Surgery, University of Surrey, UK.

pyloroplasty. This allows good access to the ulcer, which is usually found posteriorly or superiorly. Accurate haemostasis is important and can be achieved initially by direct pressure. It is the vessel within the ulcer that is bleeding and this should be controlled using well-placed sutures on a small round-bodied needle that under-run the vessel. The placing of more and more inaccurately positioned sutures is counter-productive. Following under-running, it is often possible to close the mucosa over the ulcer. The pyloroplasty is then closed with interrupted sutures in a transverse direction as in the usual fashion. In a giant ulcer the first part of the duodenum may be destroyed making primary closure impossible. In this circumstance one should proceed to distal gastrectomy with Roux-en-Y reconstruction. The duodenal stump may then be closed using the Nissen technique with T-tube drainage.

The principles of management of bleeding gastric ulcers are essentially the same. The stomach is opened at an appropriate position anteriorly and the vessel in the ulcer under-run. If the ulcer is not excised then a biopsy of the edge needs to be taken to exclude malignant transformation. Sometimes the bleeding is from the splenic artery and if there is a lot of fibrosis present then the operation may be challenging. However, most patients can be managed by conservative surgery. Gastrectomy for bleeding has been widely practised in the past, but is associated with a high perioperative mortality even if the incidence of recurrent bleeding is less.

Bearing in mind that most patients nowadays are elderly and unfit, the minimum surgery that stops the bleeding is probably optimal (damage control surgery). Acid can be inhibited by pharmacological means and appropriate eradication therapy will prevent ulcer recurrence. Definitive acid-lowering surgery is not now required. Patients on long-term NSAIDs can be managed as outlined earlier.

Stress ulceration

This commonly occurs in patients with major injury or illness, who have undergone major surgery or who have major comorbidity. Many such patients are found in intensive care units. There seems little doubt that the incidence of this problem has reduced in recent years due to the widespread use of prophylaxis. Acid inhibition and the nasogastric or oral administration of sucralfate has been shown to reduce the incidence of stress ulceration. There is no doubt that it is far better to prevent this condition than to try to treat it once it occurs. Endoscopic means of treating stress ulceration may be ineffective and operation may be required. The principles of management are the same as for the chronic ulcer.

Gastric erosions

Erosive gastritis has a variety of causes, especially NSAIDs. Fortunately, most such bleeding settles spontaneously, but when it does not it can be a major problem to treat. In general terms, although there is a diffuse erosive gastritis, there is one (or more) specific lesion that has a significant-sized vessel within it. This should be dealt with appropriately, preferably endoscopically, but sometimes surgery is necessary.

Mallory-Weiss tear

This is a longitudinal tear at the gastro-oesophageal junction, which is induced by repetitive and strenuous vomiting. Doubtless, many such lesions occur and do not cause bleeding. When it is a cause of haematemesis, the lesion may often be missed as it can be difficult to see as it is just below the gastro-oesophageal junction, a position that can be difficult for the inexperienced endoscopist. Occasionally these lesions continue to bleed and require surgical treatment. Often the situation arises in which the surgeon does not have guidance from the endoscopists as regards the site of bleeding, and a high index of suspicion in such circumstances is important. The experienced surgeon will perform on-table endoscopy prior to embarking on surgery. The stomach is opened by longitudinal gastrotomy and the upper section is carefully inspected. It is normally possible to palpate the longitudinal mucosal tear with a little induration at the edges, which gives a clue to the lesion's location. Under-running is all that is required.

Dieulafoy's disease

This is essentially a gastric arterial venous malformation that has a characteristic histological appearance. Bleeding due to this malformation is one of the most difficult causes of upper gastrointestinal bleeding to treat. The lesion itself is covered by normal mucosa and, when not bleeding, it may be invisible. If it can be seen while bleeding, all that may be visible is profuse bleeding coming from an area of apparently normal mucosa. If this occurs, the cause is instantly recognisable. If the lesion can be identified endoscopically there are various means of dealing with it, including injection of sclerosant and endoscopic clips. If it is identified at operation then only a local excision is necessary. Occasionally, a lesion is only recognised after gastrectomy and sometimes not even then. The pathologist, as well as the endoscopist, may have difficulty in finding it.

Tumours

All of the gastric tumours described below may present with chronic or acute upper gastrointestinal bleeding. Bleeding is not normally torrential but can be unremitting. Gastric stromal tumours commonly present with bleeding and have a characteristic appearance, as the mucosa breaks down over the tumour in the gastric wall (Figure 63.24). Whatever the nature, the tumours should be dealt with as appropriate.

Rudolph Nissen, 1896–1981, Professor of Surgery, Istanbul, Turkey, and later at Basle, Switzerland.
Georges Dieulafoy, 1839–1911, physician, Paris, France.

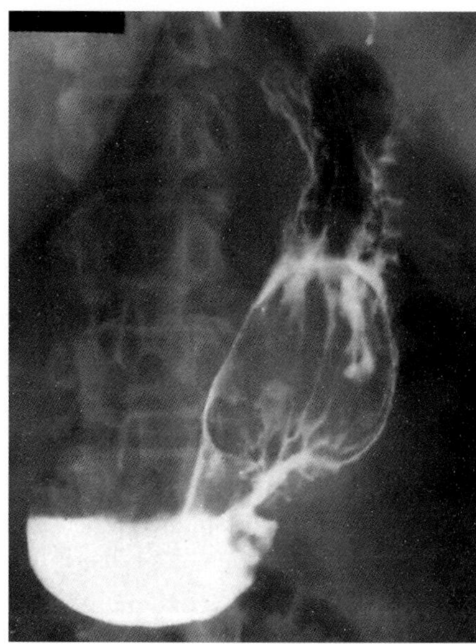

Figure 63.24 Smooth muscle tumour of the stomach, with ulceration.

Portal hypertension and portal gastropathy

The management of bleeding gastric varices is very challenging. Fortunately, most bleeding from varices is oesophageal and this is much more amenable to sclerotherapy, banding and balloon tamponade. Gastric varices may also be injected, although this is technically more difficult. Banding can also be used, again with difficulty. The gastric balloon of the Sengstaken–Blakemore tube can be used to arrest the haemorrhage if it is occurring from the fundus of the stomach or gastro-oesophageal junction. Octreotide is a somatostatin analogue that reduces portal pressure in patients with varices, and trials suggest that it is of value in arresting haemorrhage in these patients, although its overall effect on mortality remains in doubt. Glypressin is also said to be of use.

Most surgeons prefer to avoid acute surgery on bleeding varices as, in contrast with elective operations for portal hypertension, acute shunts are attended by considerable operative mortality. For this reason the acute TIPSS procedure (transjugular intrahepatic portosystemic shunt), which is described in Chapter 65, can be an extremely useful, although technically demanding, procedure.

Portal gastropathy

Portal gastropathy is essentially the same disease process as described above. The mucosa is affected by the increased portal pressure and may exude blood, even in the absence of well-developed visible varices. The treatment is as above.

Aortic enteric fistula

This diagnosis should be considered in any patient with haematemesis and melaena that cannot be otherwise explained. Contrary to expectation, the bleeding from such patients is not always massive, although it can be. Very often there is nothing much to distinguish between the bleeding from the aortic enteric fistula and any other recurrent upper gastrointestinal bleeding. The vast majority of patients will have had an aortic graft and, in the absence of this, the diagnosis is unlikely. However, it is occasionally seen in patients with an untreated aortic aneurysm. A well-performed CT scan will commonly allow the diagnosis to be made with certainty. The condition should be managed by an expert vascular surgeon as, whether secondary or primary, the morbidity and mortality are high.

GASTRIC OUTLET OBSTRUCTION

The two common causes of gastric outlet obstruction are gastric cancer (see below) and pyloric stenosis secondary to peptic ulceration. Previously, the latter was more common. Now, with the decrease in the incidence of peptic ulceration and the advent of potent medical treatments, gastric outlet obstruction should be considered malignant until proven otherwise, at least in resource-rich countries.

The term 'pyloric stenosis' is normally a misnomer. The stenosis is seldom at the pylorus. Commonly, when the condition is due to underlying peptic ulcer disease, the stenosis is found in the first part of the duodenum, the most common site for a peptic ulcer. True pyloric stenosis can occur due to fibrosis around a pyloric channel ulcer. However, in recent years the most common cause of gastric outlet obstruction has been gastric cancer. In this circumstance the metabolic consequences may be somewhat different from those of benign pyloric stenosis because of the relative hypochlorhydria found in patients with gastric cancer.

Summary box 63.5

Gastric outlet obstruction

- Gastric outlet obstruction is most commonly associated with longstanding peptic ulcer disease and gastric cancer
- The metabolic abnormality of hypochloraemic alkalosis is usually only seen with peptic ulcer disease and should be treated with isotonic saline with potassium
- Endoscopic biopsy is essential to determine whether the cause of the problem is malignancy
- Aggressive medical therapy for peptic ulcer disease often leads to resolution
- Endoscopic dilatation of the gastric outlet may be effective in less severe cases of benign stenosis
- Operation is frequently required, with a drainage procedure being performed for benign disease and appropriate resectional surgery if malignant

Clinical features

In benign gastric outlet obstruction there is usually a long history of peptic ulcer disease. Nowadays, as most patients with peptic ulcer symptoms are treated medically, it is easy to understand why the condition is becoming much less common. In some patients the pain may become unremitting and in other cases it may largely disappear. The vomitus is characteristically unpleasant in nature and is totally lacking in bile. Very often it is possible to recognise foodstuff taken several days previously. The patient commonly complains of losing weight, and appears unwell and dehydrated. When examining the patient, it may be possible to see the distended stomach and a succussion splash may be audible on shaking the patient's abdomen.

Metabolic effects

These are most interesting, as the metabolic consequences of benign pyloric stenosis are unique. The vomiting of hydrochloric acid results in hypochloraemic alkalosis. Initially the sodium and potassium may be relatively normal. However, as dehydration progresses, more profound metabolic abnormalities arise, partly related to renal dysfunction. Initially, the urine has a low chloride and high bicarbonate content, reflecting the primary metabolic abnormality. This bicarbonate is excreted along with sodium, and so with time the patient becomes progressively hyponatraemic and more profoundly dehydrated. Because of the dehydration, a phase of sodium retention follows and potassium and hydrogen are excreted in preference. This results in the urine becoming paradoxically acidic and hypokalaemia ensues. Alkalosis leads to a lowering in the circulating ionised calcium, and tetany can occur.

Management

Treating the patient involves correcting the metabolic abnormality and dealing with the mechanical problem. The patient should be rehydrated with intravenous isotonic saline with potassium supplementation. Replacing the sodium chloride and water allows the kidney to correct the acid–base abnormality. Following rehydration, it may become obvious that the patient is also anaemic, the haemoglobin being spuriously high on presentation.

It is notable that the metabolic abnormalities may be less if the obstruction is due to malignancy, as the acid–base disturbance is less pronounced.

The stomach should be emptied using a wide-bore gastric tube. A large nasogastric tube may not be sufficiently large to deal with the contents of the stomach, and it may be necessary to pass an orogastric tube and lavage the stomach until it is completely emptied. This then allows investigation of the patient with endoscopy and contrast radiology. Biopsy of the area around the pylorus is essential to exclude malignancy. The patient should also have a gastric antisecretory agent, initially given intravenously to ensure absorption.

Early cases may settle with conservative treatment, presumably as the oedema around the ulcer diminishes as the ulcer is healed. Traditionally, severe cases are treated surgically, usually with a gastroenterostomy rather than a pyloroplasty. Endoscopic treatment with balloon dilatation has been practised and may be most useful in early cases. However, this treatment is not devoid of problems. Dilating the duodenal stenosis may result in perforation. The dilatation may have to be performed several times and may not be successful in the long term. Occasionally duodenal stent insertion will be considered in specialist centres.

Other causes of gastric outlet obstruction

Adult pyloric stenosis

This is a rare condition and its relationship to the childhood condition is unclear, although some patients have a long history of problems with gastric emptying. It is commonly treated by pyloroplasty rather than pyloromyotomy.

Pyloric mucosal diaphragm

The origin of this rare condition is unknown. It usually does not become apparent until middle life. When found, simple excision of the mucosal diaphragm is all that is required.

GASTRIC POLYPS

A number of conditions manifest as gastric polyps. Their main importance is that they may actually represent early gastric cancer. Biopsy is essential.

The most common type of gastric polyp is metaplastic. These are associated with *H. pylori* infection and regress following eradication therapy. Inflammatory polyps are also common. Fundic gland polyps deserve particular attention. They seem to be associated with the use of proton pump inhibitors and are also found in patients with familial polyposis. None of the above polypoid lesions has proven malignant potential. True adenomas have malignant potential and should be removed, but they account for only 10% of polypoid lesions. Gastric carcinoids arising from the ECL cells are seen in patients with pernicious anaemia and usually appear as small polyps.

GASTRIC CANCER

Carcinoma of the stomach is a major cause of cancer mortality worldwide. Its prognosis tends to be poor, with cure rates little better than 5–10%, although better results are obtained in Japan, where the disease is common. Gastric cancer is actually an eminently curable disease provided that it is detected at an appropriate stage and treated adequately. It rarely disseminates widely before it has involved the lymph nodes and, therefore, there is an opportunity to cure the disease prior to dissemination. Early diagnosis is therefore the key to success with this disease. Unfortunately, the late presentation of many cases is the cause of the poor overall survival figures. The only treatment modality able to cure the disease is resectional surgery.

Incidence

There are marked variations in the incidence of gastric cancer worldwide. In the UK it is approximately 15 per 100 000 per year, in the USA 10 per 100 000 per year and in Eastern Europe 40 per 100 000 per year. In Japan, the disease is much more common, with an incidence of approximately 70 per

Summary box 63.6

Gastric cancer

- Gastric cancer is one of the most common causes of cancer death in the world
- The outlook is generally poor, owing to the advanced stage of the tumour at presentation
- Better results are obtained in Japan, which has a high population incidence, screening programmes and a high-quality surgical treatment
- The aetiology of gastric cancer is multifactorial, but *H. pylori* is an important factor for distal but not proximal gastric cancer
- Early gastric cancer is associated with very high cure rates
- Gastric cancer can be classified into intestinal and diffuse types, the latter having a worse prognosis
- In western resource-rich countries, proximal gastric cancer is now more common than distal cancer and is usually of the diffuse type
- Spread may be by lymphatics, blood, transcoelomic or direct, but distant metastases are uncommon in the absence of lymph node involvement
- The treatment of curable cases is by radical surgery and removal of the second tier of nodes (around the principal arterial trunks) may be advantageous
- Gastric cancer is chemosensitive and chemotherapy improves survival in patients having surgery for the condition and in advanced disease

100 000 per year, and there are small geographical areas in China where the incidence is double that in Japan. These underlying epidemiological data make it clear that this is an environmental disease. In general, men are more affected by the disease than women and, as with most solid organ malignancies, the incidence increases with age.

At present, marked changes are being observed in resource-rich countries in terms of the incidence and site of gastric cancer and the population affected, changes that to date have not been observed in Japan. First, the incidence of gastric cancer is continuing to fall at about 1% per year. This reduction exclusively affects carcinoma arising in the body and distal stomach. In contrast, there appears to be an increase in the incidence of carcinoma in the proximal stomach, particularly the oesophagogastric junction. Carcinoma of the distal stomach and body of the stomach is most common in low socioeconomic groups, whereas the increase in proximal gastric cancer seems to affect principally higher socioeconomic groups. Proximal gastric cancer does not seem to be associated with *H. pylori* infection, in contrast with carcinoma of the body and distal stomach.

Aetiology

Gastric cancer is a multifactorial disease (Correa). Epidemiological studies point to a role for *H. pylori*, although there is argument about how important this factor is. Studies reveal a correlation between the incidence of gastric cancer in various populations and the prevalence of *H. pylori* infection, but other factors are also important. There is insufficient evidence at the moment to support eradication programmes in asymptomatic patients who are infected with *Helicobacter*, with a view to reducing the population incidence of gastric cancer. However, clinical trials may subsequently change this view. As mentioned above, *Helicobacter* seems to be principally associated with carcinoma of the body, stomach and distal stomach rather than the proximal stomach. As *Helicobacter* is associated with gastritis, gastric atrophy and intestinal metaplasia, the association with malignancy is perhaps not surprising.

Several other risk factors have been identified as being important in the aetiology of gastric cancer. Patients with pernicious anaemia and gastric atrophy are at increased risk, as are those with gastric polyps. Patients who have had peptic ulcer surgery, particularly those who have had drainage procedures such as Billroth II or Polya gastrectomy, gastroenterostomy or pyloroplasty, are at approximately four times the average risk. Presumably duodenogastric reflux and reflux gastritis are related to the increased risk of malignancy in these patients. Intestinal metaplasia is a risk factor. Carcinoma is associated with cigarette smoking and dust ingestion from a variety of industrial processes. Diet appears to be important, as illustrated by the often quoted example of the change in the incidence of gastric cancer in Japanese families living in the USA. The high incidence of gastric cancer in some pockets in China is probably environmental and probably diet related. The ingestion of substances such as spirits may induce gastritis and, in the long term, cancer. Excessive salt intake, deficiency of antioxidants and exposure to *N*-nitroso compounds are also related. The aetiology of proximal gastric cancer remains an enigma. It is not associated with *Helicobacter* but is associated with obesity and higher socioeconomic status. Genetic factors are also important but imperfectly elucidated (see below).

Clinical features

The features of advanced gastric cancer are usually obvious. However, curable gastric cancer has no specific features to distinguish it symptomatically from benign dyspepsia. The key to improving the outcome of gastric cancer is early diagnosis and, although in Japan there is a screening programme, most curable cases are picked up by the liberal use of gastroscopy in patients with dyspepsia. In western resource-rich countries it is much more difficult as the population incidence is much lower. Hence the cost effectiveness of performing gastroscopy for mild dyspeptic symptoms is low. However a high index of suspicion is necessary as only endoscoping patients with symptoms of advanced cancer is unlikely to be beneficial as such patients are not surgically curable. It is important to note that gastric antisecretory agents will improve the symptoms of gastric cancer so the disease should be excluded, preferably before therapy is started.

P. Correa, contemporary, pathologist, New Orleans, LA, USA. Produced a cogent hypothesis to explain the development of the intestinal type of gastric cancer.

In advanced cancer, early satiety, bloating, distension and vomiting may occur. The tumour frequently bleeds, resulting in iron deficiency anaemia. Obstruction leads to dysphagia, epigastric fullness or vomiting. Weight loss can be profound. With pyloric involvement the presentation may be of gastric outlet obstruction, although the alkalosis is usually less pronounced or absent compared with when duodenal ulceration leads to obstruction. In recent years, gastric outlet obstruction is more commonly associated with malignancy than benign disease. Non-metastatic effects of malignancy are seen, particularly thrombophlebitis (Trousseau's sign) and deep venous thrombosis. These features result from the effects of the tumour on thrombotic and haemostatic mechanisms.

Site

The proximal stomach is now the most common site for gastric cancer in resource-rich western countries. Because so many malignancies occur at the oesophageal–gastric junction, and because the lower oesophagus is also a very common site of adenocarcinoma, it is artificial to separate the stomach from the oesophagus. Therefore, it is best to consider the whole of the upper gastrointestinal tract from the cricopharyngeus to the pylorus. The incidence of cancer at these various sites is shown in Figure 63.25. It can be seen that just under 60% of all of the malignancies occurring in the oesophagus and stomach occur in proximity to the oesophagogastric junction. Adenocarcinoma at this site has doubled in incidence in the UK over the last 30 years. This high prevalence of proximal gastric cancer is not seen in Japan, where distal cancer still predominates, as it does in most of the rest of the world.

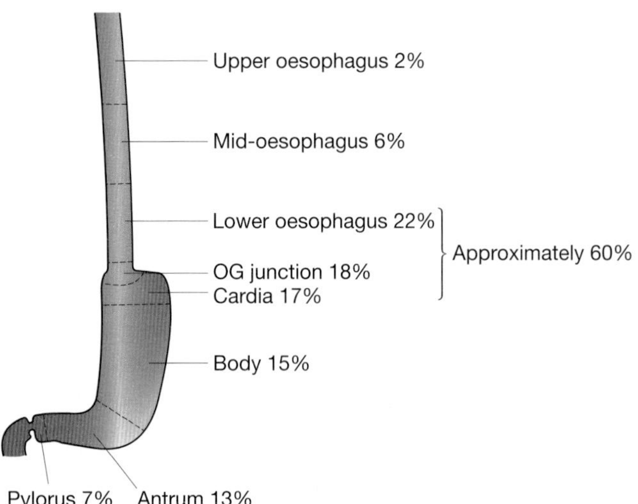

Figure 63.25 The incidence of cancer in the various parts of the upper gastrointestinal tract in the UK. OG, oesophagogastric.

Pathology

The most useful clinicopathological classification of gastric cancer is the Lauren classification. In this system there are principally two forms of gastric cancer: intestinal gastric cancer and diffuse gastric cancer (often with signet ring cells). In intestinal gastric cancer, the tumour resembles a carcinoma elsewhere in the tubular gastrointestinal tract and forms polypoid tumours or ulcers. It probably arises in areas of intestinal metaplasia. In contrast, diffuse gastric cancer infiltrates deeply into the stomach without forming obvious mass lesions, but spreads widely in the gastric wall. Not surprisingly, this has a much worse prognosis. A small proportion of gastric cancers are of mixed morphology.

Gastric cancer can be divided into early gastric cancer and advanced gastric cancer. Early gastric cancer is defined as cancer limited to the mucosa and submucosa with or without lymph node involvement (T1, any N). The classification is shown in Figures 63.26 and 63.27. This can be either protruding, superficial or excavated in the Japanese classification. This type of cancer is eminently curable, and even early gastric cancers associated with lymph node involvement have 5-year survival rates in the region of 90%. In Japan, approximately one-third of gastric cancers diagnosed are in this stage. However, in the UK it is uncommon to detect gastric cancers at this stage. A number of reasons probably still account for this. First, because gastric cancer is less common in the UK, dyspeptic patients are not always referred for endoscopy at an appropriate stage. Second, endoscopists are unfamiliar with the appearances of early gastric cancer and in all probability many such cases are missed.

Advanced gastric cancer involves the muscularis. Its macroscopic appearances have been classified by Bormann into four types (Figures 63.28 and 63.29). Types III and IV are commonly incurable.

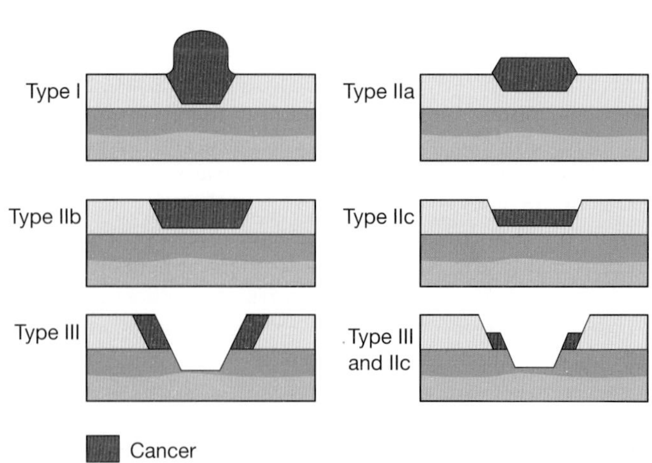

Figure 63.26 Early gastric cancer, Japanese classification.

Armand Trousseau, 1801–1867, physician, Hôtel Dieu, Paris, France. This sign led him to suspect himself of having gastric cancer. He actually had pancreatic cancer, which was diagnosed at postmortem.
Pekka A. Lauren, contemporary, pathologist, University of Turku, Finland.

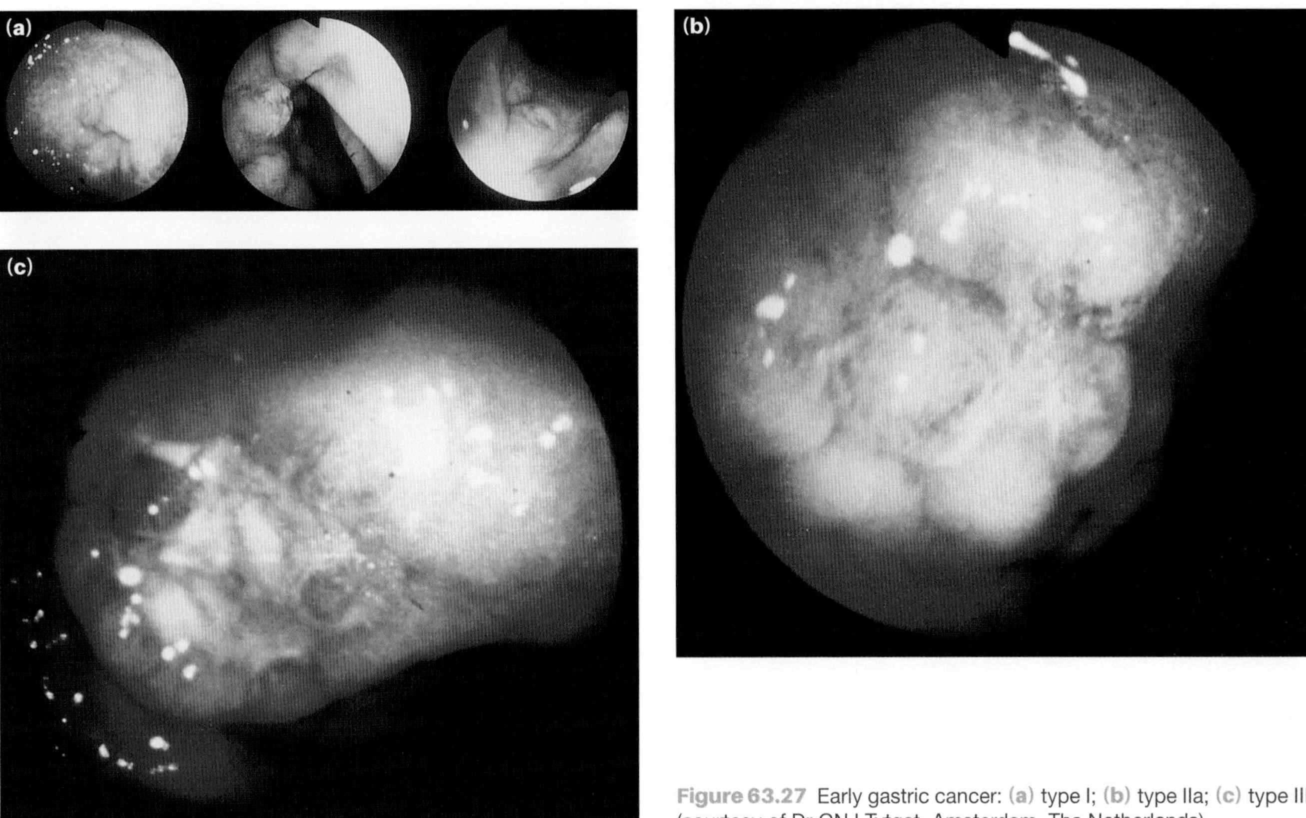

Figure 63.27 Early gastric cancer: (a) type I; (b) type IIa; (c) type III (courtesy of Dr GNJ Tytgat, Amsterdam, The Netherlands).

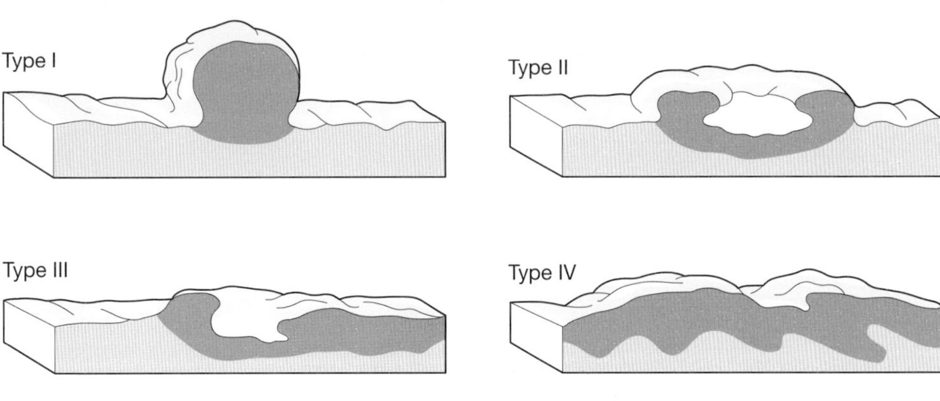

Figure 63.28 Bormann classification of advanced gastric cancer.

The molecular pathology of gastric cancer

Our understanding of the molecular pathology of gastric cancer has been revolutionised by the application of next-generation sequencing platforms to the disease. In a recent landmark paper The Cancer Genome Atlas (TCGA) group described four molecular subtypes of gastric cancer: Epstein–Barr virus positive, microsatellite instable, genomically stable and chromosomal instability. Recognition of these sub-groups and their underlying common gene mutations and driver events is leading to the development of targeted therapies including immunotherapies. Similar genetic classifications are now available for other tumours of the gastrointestinal tract meaning that novel treatments can be applied across tumour types. A range of mutations in genes related to genome integrity (e.g. *BRCA2*, *TP53*, *ARID1A*), chromatin remodelling (e.g. *SMARCA1*, *CHD3&4*) and cell–cell adhesion and

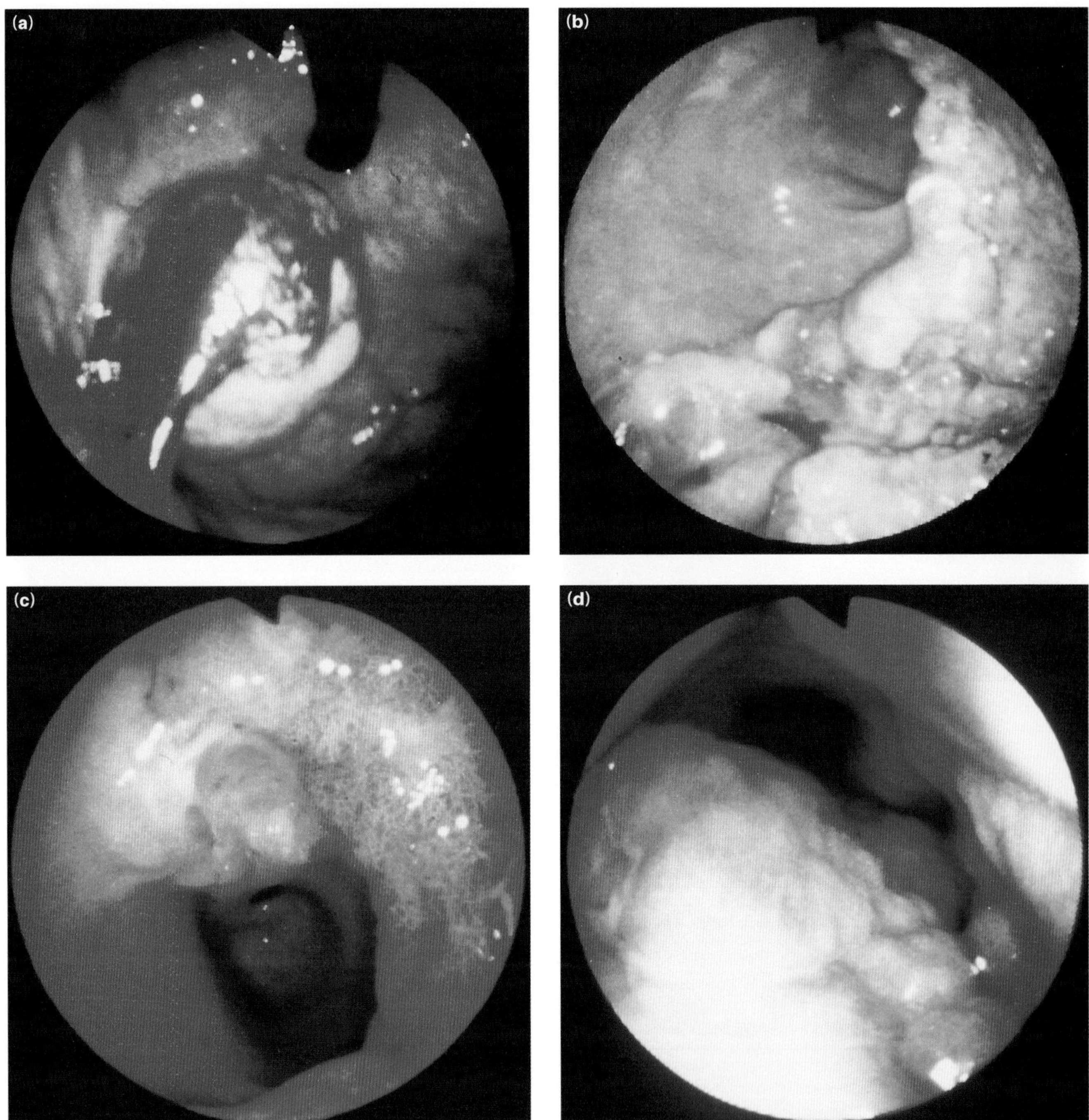

Figure 63.29 Advanced gastric cancer: (a) type I; (b) type II; (c) type III; (d) type IV (linitus plastica) (courtesy of Dr GNJ Tytgat, Amsterdam, The Netherlands).

motility (e.g. *RHOA*, *CDH1*) have been described in gastric cancer. In addition, cell signalling pathways commonly mutated in other solid organ tumours are commonly found perturbed in gastric cancer. For example, the Wnt pathway may be amenable to specific small molecule inhibitors. Unsurprisingly, gastric cancer exhibits a range of mutations in receptor tyrosine kinases and PI3K/MAPK signalling.

The rapid development of sequencing technologies, including single-cell platforms and the development of real-time sequencing, offers the promise of precision therapy for gastric cancer in the future, but currently treatment is still based on surgery with or without conventional chemo/radiotherapy.

Staging

The International Union Against Cancer (UICC) staging system is shown in Table 63.5. Important changes have been made in the seventh edition of the TNM staging system that are worthy of discussion. In an attempt to reflect the current

TABLE 63.5 UICC staging of gastric cancer.

T1	Tumour involves lamina propria, submucosa		
	T1a lamina propria		
	T1b submucosa		
T2	Tumour invades muscularis propria		
T3	Tumour involves subserosa		
T4a	Tumour perforates serosa		
T4b	Tumour invades adjacent organs		
N0	No lymph nodes		
N1	Metastasis in 1–2 regional nodes		
N2	Metastasis in 3-6 regional nodes		
N3a	Metastasis in 7–15 regional nodes		
N3b	Metastasis in more than 15 regional nodes		
M0	No distant metastasis		
M1	Distant metastasis (this includes peritoneum and distant lymph nodes)		
Staging			
IA	T1	N0	M0
IB	T1	N1	M0
T2	N0	M0	
IIA	T1	N2	M0
T2	N1	M0	
T3	N0	M0	
IIB	T1	N3	M0
T2	N2	M0	
T3	N1	M0	
T4a	N0	M0	
IIIA	T2	N3	M0
T3	N2	M0	
T4a	N1	M0	
IIIB	T3	N3	M0
T4a	N2	M0	
T4b	N0-1	M0	
IIIC	T4a	N3	M0
T4b	N2-3	M0	
IV	Any T	Any N	M1

evidence base and to improve outcome prediction for individual patients, all gastric tumours whose epicentre is within 5 cm of the gastro-oesophageal junction and which extend into the oesophagus are now classified according to the oesophageal system. Tumours whose epicentre is within 5 cm of the gastro-oesophageal junction but which do not extend into the oesophagus, and all other gastric cancers, are staged using the revised gastric staging system. In addition, any tumour that perforates the serosa is now classified as T4 disease.

Spread of carcinoma of the stomach

No better example of the various modes by which carcinoma spreads can be given than the case of stomach cancer. It is important to note that this distant spread is unusual before the disease spreads locally, and distant metastases are uncommon in the absence of lymph node metastases. The intestinal and diffuse types of gastric cancer spread differently. The diffuse type spreads via the submucosal and subserosal lymphatic plexus and it penetrates the gastric wall at an early stage.

Direct spread

The tumour penetrates the muscularis, serosa and ultimately adjacent organs such as the pancreas, colon and liver.

Lymphatic spread

This is by both permeation and emboli to the affected tiers (see below) of nodes. This may be extensive, the tumour even appearing in the supraclavicular nodes (Troisier's sign). Unlike malignancies such as breast cancer, nodal involvement does not imply systemic dissemination.

Blood-borne metastases

These occur first to the liver and subsequently to other organs, including lung and bone. This is uncommon in the absence of nodal disease.

Transperitoneal spread

This is a common mode of spread once the tumour has reached the serosa of the stomach and indicates incurability. Tumours can manifest anywhere in the peritoneal cavity and commonly give rise to ascites. Advanced peritoneal disease may be palpated either abdominally or rectally as a tumour 'shelf'. The ovaries may sometimes be the sole site of transcoelomic spread (Krukenberg's tumours). Tumour may spread via the abdominal cavity to the umbilicus (Sister Joseph's nodule). Transperitoneal spread of gastric cancer can be detected most effectively by laparoscopy and cytology.

Lymphatic drainage of the stomach

Understanding the lymphatic drainage of the stomach is the key to comprehending the radical surgery of gastric cancer. The lymphatics of the antrum drain into the right gastric lymph node superiorly, and right gastroepiploic and subpyloric lymph nodes inferiorly. The lymphatics of the pylorus drain into the right gastric suprapyloric nodes superiorly and the subpyloric lymph nodes situated around the gastroduodenal artery inferiorly. The efferent lymphatics from suprapyloric lymph nodes converge on the para-aortic nodes around the coeliac axis, whereas the efferent lymphatics from the subpyloric lymph nodes pass up to the main superior mesenteric lymph nodes situated around the origin of the superior mesenteric artery. The lymphatic vessels related to the cardiac

Charles Emile Troisier, 1844–1919, Professor of Pathology, Paris, France.
Friedrich Ernst Krukenberg, 1870–1946, ophthalmologist, Halle, Germany, wrote a classic paper on malignant tumours of the ovary in 1896.
Sister Mary Joseph (Julia Dempsey), 1856–1939, Nursing Superintendent, St Mary's Hospital, Rochester, MN, USA, noted the presence of an umbilical nodule in many patients who proved to have advanced gastric cancer and pointed this out to William Mayo while she was working as theatre sister at the Mayo Clinic.

orifice of the stomach communicate freely with those of the oesophagus.

The prognosis of operable cases of carcinoma of the stomach depends on whether or not there is histological evidence of regional lymph node involvement. Retrograde (downwards) spread may occur if the upper lymphatics are blocked. In Japan, the lymph node dissection is highly advanced and the Japanese Research Society for Gastric Cancer has assigned a number to each lymph node station to aid the pathological staging (Figure 63.30). Many centres in resource-rich countries now perform surgery that involves a radical lymphadenectomy but, in other centres, both the staging and surgery are less developed.

Operability

It is important that patients with incurable disease are not subjected to radical surgery that cannot help them, hence the value of CT/PET and preoperative laparoscopy. Unequivocal evidence of incurability is haematogenous metastases, involvement of the distant peritoneum, N4 nodal disease and disease beyond the N4 nodes, and fixation to structures that cannot be removed. It is important to note that involvement of another organ per se does not imply incurability, provided that it can be removed. Controversies with respect to operability include N3 nodal involvement and involvement of the adjacent peritoneum, performed in Japan but seldom elsewhere. Curative resection should be considered on the remaining patients.

Most operable patients should have neoadjuvant chemotherapy as described below as this improves survival.

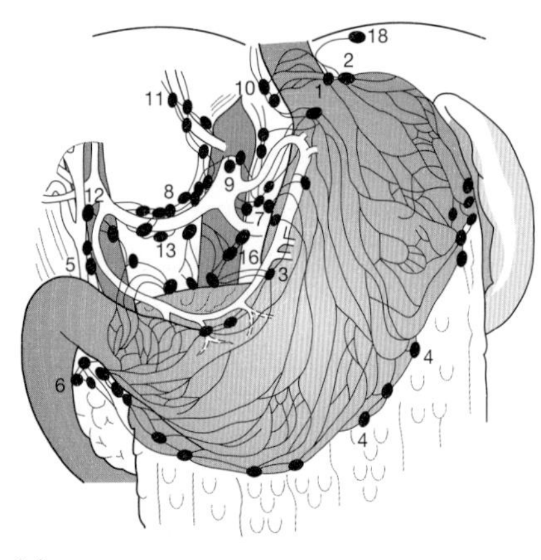

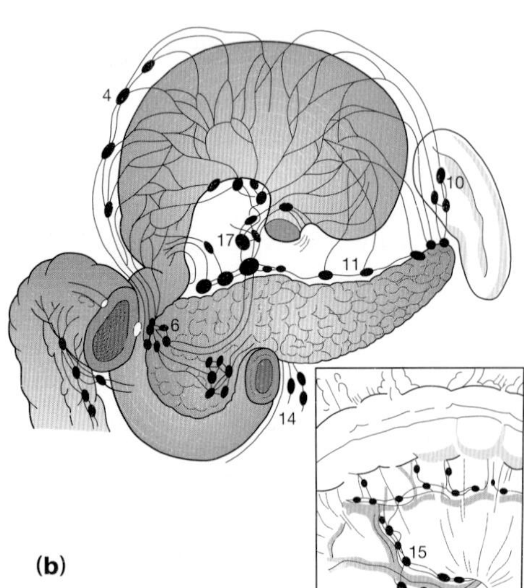

Figure 63.30 Lymphatic drainage of the stomach and nodal stations by the Japanese classification: (a) the anterior view of the stomach; (b) the posterior view.

Total gastrectomy

This is best performed through a long upper midline incision. The stomach is removed en bloc, including the tissues of the entire greater omentum and lesser omentum (Figure 63.31). In commencing the operation, the transverse colon is completely separated from the greater omentum. The dissection may then be commenced proximally or, more usually, distally. The subpyloric nodes are dissected and the first part of the duodenum is divided, usually with a surgical stapler. The hepatic nodes are dissected down to clear the hepatic artery; this dissection also includes the suprapyloric nodes. The right gastric artery is taken on the hepatic artery. The lymph node dissection is continued to the origin of the left gastric artery, which is divided flush with its origin. The dissection is continued along the splenic artery, taking all of the nodes at the superior aspect of the pancreas and accessible nodes in the splenic hilum. Separation of the stomach from the spleen, if this organ is not going to be removed, is carried out and this then allows access to the nodal tissues around the upper stomach and oesophagogastric junction. The oesophagus can then be divided at an appropriate point using a combination of stay sutures and a soft non-crushing clamp, usually of the right-angled variety. It is important that the resection margins are well clear of the tumour (>5 cm). Involvement of either proximal or distal resection margin carries an appalling prognosis and, if in doubt, frozen section should be performed. There is some controversy regarding the management of the spleen and distal pancreas in this procedure and this is discussed below.

Gastrointestinal continuity is reconstituted by means of a Roux loop. Other methods of reconstruction should be discouraged because of poor functional results. The alimentary limb of the Roux loop should be at least 50 cm long to avoid bile reflux oesophagitis. The simplest means of effecting the oesophagojejunostomy is to place a purse string in the cut end of the oesophagus and, using a circular stapler introduced through the blind end of the Roux loop, staple the end of the oesophagus onto the side of the Roux loop. The blind open end of the Roux loop may then be closed either with sutures or, alternatively, with a linear stapler. The anastomosis can also be fashioned end to end. The Roux loop may be placed in either an anticolic or retrocolic position. The jejunojejunostomy is undertaken at a convenient point in the usual fashion (end to side, Figure 63.32).

There remains some controversy about the extent of the lymphadenectomy required for the optimal treatment of curable gastric cancer. In Japan, at least a D2 gastrectomy (removal of the second tier of nodes) is performed on all

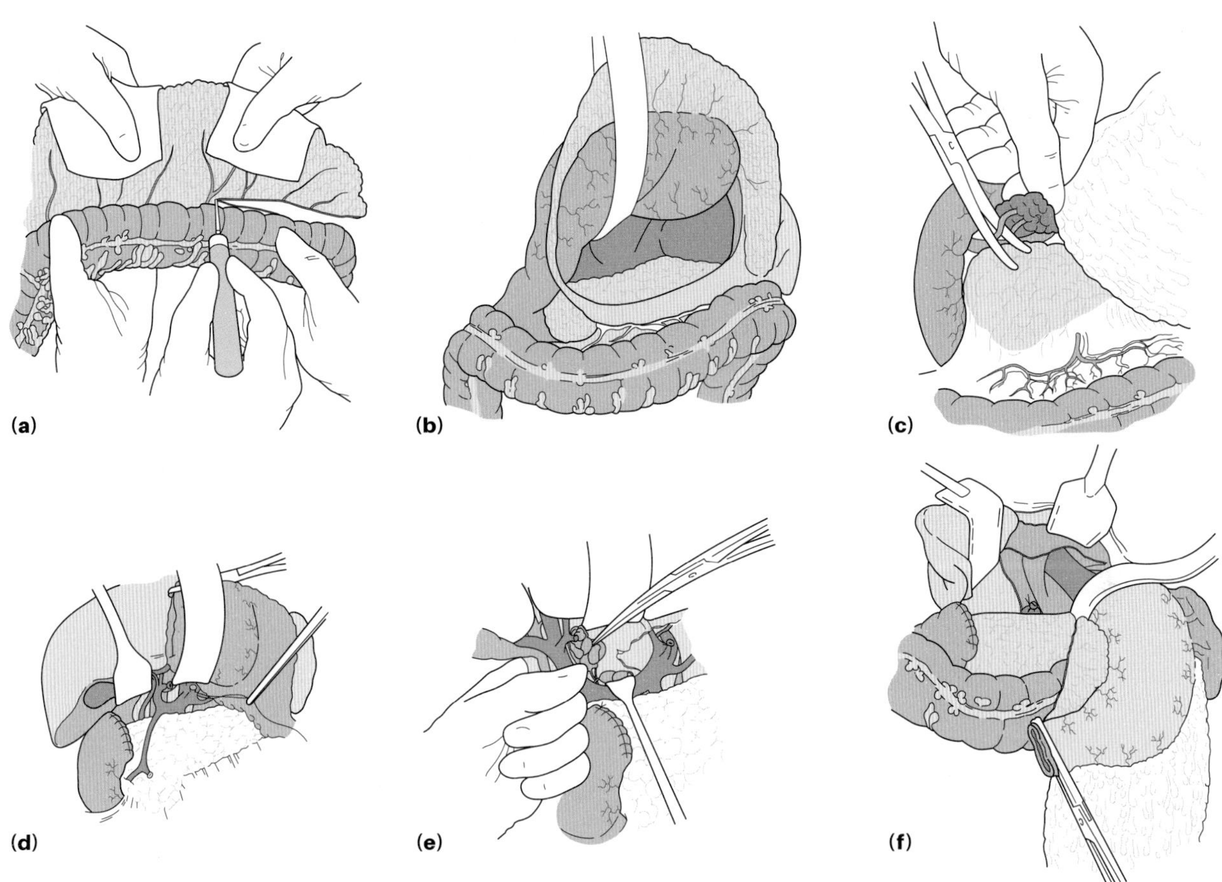

Figure 63.31 Radical total gastrectomy: (a) dissection of omentum off the transverse colon; (b) exposure of the lesser sac; (c) splenectomy; (d) division and oversewing of the duodenum; (e) dissection of the left gastric artery nodes (group 17); (f) mobilisation of the oesophagus.

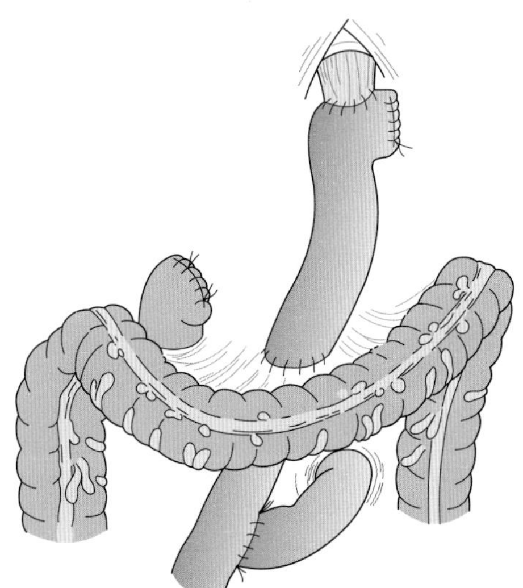

Figure 63.32 Oesophagojejunostomy Roux-en-Y.

operable gastric cancer and some centres are practicing more radical surgery (D3 and even D4 resections). Certainly, the results of surgical treatment stage for stage in Japan are much better than commonly reported in western resource-rich countries, and the Japanese contention is that the difference is principally related to the staging and the quality of the surgery. It is observed that the physical proportions of the average Japanese patient favour the performance of more radical procedures compared with the average patient in western countries. However, radical lymphadenectomies above D2 have not been subjected to any randomised controlled trials. In the UK and Europe, randomised trials have been set up to compare D1 and D2 gastrectomy, but the results are difficult to interpret. One of the problems relates to standardisation of the operation. Overall, it seems that the oncological outcome may be better following a D2 gastrectomy, but this operation is associated with higher levels of morbidity and perioperative mortality. It is clear that most of this morbidity and mortality relates to the removal of the spleen with or without the distal pancreas. The traditional radical gastrectomy removes the spleen and distal pancreas en bloc with the stomach and, although this is indeed an adequate means of performing clearance of the lymph nodes around the splenic artery, there now seems little doubt that adding this substantially increases the complication rate. The Japanese D2 gastrectomy will commonly preserve spleen and pancreas and this practice has been widely adopted by specialist centres in western countries.

The differentiation between a D1 and a D2 operation depends upon the tiers of nodes removed. Different tiers need to be removed depending on the positions of primary tumour and this is outlined in Table 63.6. In general, a D1 resection involves the removal of the perigastric nodes and a D2

TABLE 63.6 The lymph node stations (see Figure 63.30) that need to be removed in a D1 (N1 nodes removed) or a D2 (N2 nodes removed) resection.

LN number		Site of cancer			
		Antrum	Middle	Cardia	Cardia and oesophagus
1	Right cardia	N2	N1	N1	N1
2	Left cardial		N1	N1	N1
3	Lesser curve	N1	N1	N1	N1
4sa	Short gastric	N1	N1	N1	N1
4sb	Left gastroepiploic	N1	N1	N1	N1
4d	Right gastroepiploic	N1	N1	N2	N2
5	Suprapyloric	N1	N1	N2	N2
6	Infrapyloric	N1	N1	N2	N2
7	Left gastric artery	N2	N2	N2	N2
8a	Anterior hepatic artery	N2	N2	N2	N2
9	Coeliac artery	N2	N2	N2	N2
10	Splenic hilum		N2	N2	N2
11	Splenic artery		N2	N2	N2
19	Infradiaphragmatic				N2
20	Oesophageal hiatus			N2	N1
110	Lower oesophagus				N2
111	Supradiaphragmatic				N2

The nodes in stations 12–18 are not routinely removed in a D1 or D2 gastrectomy.

resection involves the clearance of the major arterial trunks. In practice the majority of specialist centres will perform a radical total gastrectomy, conserving the spleen and pancreas, with D2 lymphadenectomy sparing station 10 lymph nodes.

Subtotal gastrectomy

For tumours distally placed in the stomach, it appears unnecessary to remove the whole stomach. However, the operation is very similar to that of a total gastrectomy except that the proximal stomach is preserved, the blood supply being derived from the short gastric arteries. Following the resection, the simplest form of reconstruction is to close the stomach from the lesser curve, near the oesophagogastric junction, with either sutures or staples and then perform an anastomosis of the greater curve to the jejunum. Although this can be performed as in a Billroth II/Polya-type gastrectomy, this reconstruction may result in quite marked enterogastric reflux and bile reflux oesophagitis, and the preferred method is to perform the reconstruction using a Roux loop.

Palliative surgery

In patients suffering from significant symptoms of either obstruction or bleeding, palliative resection is appropriate. A palliative gastrectomy need not be radical and it is sufficient to remove the tumour and reconstruct the gastrointestinal tract. Sometimes it is impossible to resect an obstructing tumour in the distal stomach and other palliative procedures need to be considered, although the prognosis in such patients, even in the short term, is poor. A high gastroenterostomy is a poor operation that very frequently does not allow the stomach to empty adequately, but may produce the additional problem of bile reflux. A Roux loop with a wide anastomosis between the stomach and jejunum may be a better option, although even this may not allow the stomach to empty particularly well. Gastric exclusion and oesophagojejunostomy is practised by some surgeons. For inoperable tumours situated in the cardia, either palliative intubation, stenting or another form of recanalisation can be used (Chapter 62). Recanalisation appears to offer better functional results.

Postoperative complications of gastrectomy

Radical gastrectomy is complex major surgery and predictably there are a large number of potential complications of the operation. Leakage of the oesophagojejunostomy should be uncommon in experienced hands. When it occurs it can often be managed conservatively as the Roux-en-Y reconstruction means that it is mainly saliva and ingested food that leaks. Some patients may establish a fistula from the wound or drain site and others may need radiological or surgically placed drains. It is unclear whether a nasoenteric tube should be used routinely. Many surgeons use such tubes routinely, but this is not supported by any evidence base. It is unusual to detect a major anastomotic leak in the absence of clinical signs and the use of postoperative water-soluble contrast swallows is not now routine in expert centres. Physiological scoring systems to predict those patients likely to experience significant complications offer potential in this area.

As with any gastrectomy, leakage from the duodenal stump can occur. This is usually due to a degree of distal obstruction and care must be taken when performing the Roux-en-Y anastomosis that there is no kinking. Paraduodenal collections can be drained radiologically, which will often convert the collection into an external fistula. Biliary peritonitis requires a laparotomy and peritoneal toilet, and in this circumstance it is best to leave a Foley catheter in the duodenum to establish a controlled duodenal fistula. If it is established that there is no distal obstruction, or if any such obstruction is managed, then with time the fistula will close.

The presence of septic collections along with a very radical vascular dissection may lead to catastrophic secondary haemorrhage from the exposed or divided blood vessels. This situation may be very difficult to manage, whether or not reoperation or interventional radiology is employed.

Long-term complications of surgery

It is surprising that, considering the radical nature of the total gastrectomy, many patients, particularly the younger ones, have good functional results. However, most patients will have a reduced capacity, particularly in the short term. They need to be given detailed nutritional advice, the substance of which is to eat small meals and often, while the jejunum or small gastric remnant adapts. In fact, there is very little functional difference between patients who have a total gastrectomy and those who have a subtotal gastrectomy. Various attempts have been made to try to improve the short-term functional results by a forming a jejunal pouch and attaching this to the oesophagus. Most surgeons do not perform this as in the long term there seems little functional advantage. It is surprising that these patients only infrequently suffer from the complications of gastric surgery, such as dumping and diarrhoea. Nutritional deficiencies may occur and the patient should be monitored with this in view. The loss of the parietal mass leads to vitamin B12 deficiency and replacement should be given routinely.

Outlook after surgical treatment

The outlook after surgical treatment varies considerably between western countries and Japan. In Japan, approximately 75% of patients will have a curative resection and, of these, the overall 5-year survival rate will be in the region of 50–70%. In contrast, in western countries most series show that only 25–50% of patients undergoing surgery will have a curative operation and the 5-year survival rate in such patients is only about 25–30%, although in some series it approaches Japanese levels. A combination of differences in staging and a higher standard of surgery in Japan probably accounts for the differences. Staging is clearly crucial when survival figures are being compared. The more thorough the staging, the higher the stage is likely to be and, therefore, stage for stage the outcome seems better in patients who are adequately staged pathologically. This phenomenon is termed 'stage migration'.

Other treatment modalities

Because of the failure of radical surgery to cure advanced gastric cancer, there has been an interest in the use of radiotherapy and chemotherapy.

Radiotherapy

The routine use of radiotherapy is controversial as the results of clinical trials are inconclusive. There are a number of radiosensitive tissues in the region of the gastric bed, which limits the dose that can be given. Radiotherapy has a role in the palliative treatment of painful bony metastases.

Chemotherapy

Gastric cancer may respond well to combination cytotoxic chemotherapy and neoadjuvant chemotherapy improves the outcome following surgery. Most patients therefore should have prior chemotherapy. There are a number of well-investigated regimes, but the best results are currently obtained using a combination of epirubacin, *cis*-platinum and infusional 5-FU or an oral analogue such as capecitabine. The same regimen is used as first line for patients with inoperable disease although oxaliplatin is being substituted for *cis*-platinum as it has fewer side effects. Second-line treatment using combinations which include taxotere are increasingly being used. Chemotherapy for advanced disease is palliative. Newer biological agents such as trastuzumab (Herceptin) offer potential advantages to survival in the minority of patients (<20%) with *HER2*-positive gastric cancer. However the absolute survival advantages are small (~4 months) and the cost of treatment is high. Nevertheless, trastuzumab has been approved for use in metastatic *HER2*-positive gastric cancer in the UK and the European Union.

Pattern of relapse following surgical treatment

As might be expected, the most common site of relapse following radical gastrectomy is the gastric bed, representing inadequate extirpation of the primary tumour. Widespread nodal intraperitoneal metastases, distant nodal metastases and liver metastases are all common. Dissemination to the lung and bones usually only occurs after liver metastases are already established.

GASTROINTESTINAL STROMAL TUMOURS

Gastrointestinal stromal tumours (GISTs) may arise in any part of the gastrointestinal tract but 50% will be found in the stomach. Previously named leiomyoma and leiomyosarcoma, the term GIST is now used, recognising their particular

Frederic Eugene Basil Foley, 1891–1966, urologist, Ankher Hospital, St Paul, MN, USA.

distinct phenotype. They are tumours of mesenchymal origin and are observed equally commonly in males and females. The tumours are universally associated with a mutation in the tyrosine kinase *c-kit* oncogene. These tumours are sensitive to the tyrosine kinase antagonist imatinib, and an 80% objective response rate can be observed. Tumours with mutations in exon 11 of *c-kit* are particularly sensitive to this drug. The biological behaviour of these tumours is unpredictable but size and mitotic index are the best predictors of metastasis. Peritoneal and liver metastases are most common but spread to lymph nodes is extremely rare.

The incidence of the condition is unclear as small stromal tumours of the stomach are probably quite common and remain unnoticed. Clinically obvious tumours are considerably less common than gastric cancer. GISTs comprise 1–3% of all gastrointestinal neoplasia.

The only ways that many stromal tumours are recognised are either that the mucosa overlying the tumour ulcerates (see Figure 63.24), leading to bleeding, or that they are noticed incidentally at endoscopy. Because the mucosa overlying the tumour is normal, endoscopic biopsy can be uninformative unless the tumour has ulcerated. Targeted biopsy by endoscopic ultrasound is more helpful. Larger tumours present with non-specific gastric symptoms and, in many instances, they may be thought to be gastric cancer initially (Figure 63.33).

As the biological behaviour is difficult to predict, the best guide is to consider the size of the tumour. Tumours over 5 cm in diameter should be considered to have metastatic potential. If easily resectable, surgery is the primary mode of treatment. Smaller tumours can be treated by wedge excision although the appropriate management of asymptomatic diminutive tumours found incidentally at endoscopy is unclear. Larger tumours may require a gastrectomy or duodenectomy (see Chapter 68) but lymphadenectomy is not required. Larger tumours which require multivisceral resection may be better treated with 3–6 months of imatinib prior to operation as this will usually radically reduce the size and vascularity of the tumours. Adjuvant imatinib for large resected tumours of high malignant potential should probably be continued indefinitely.

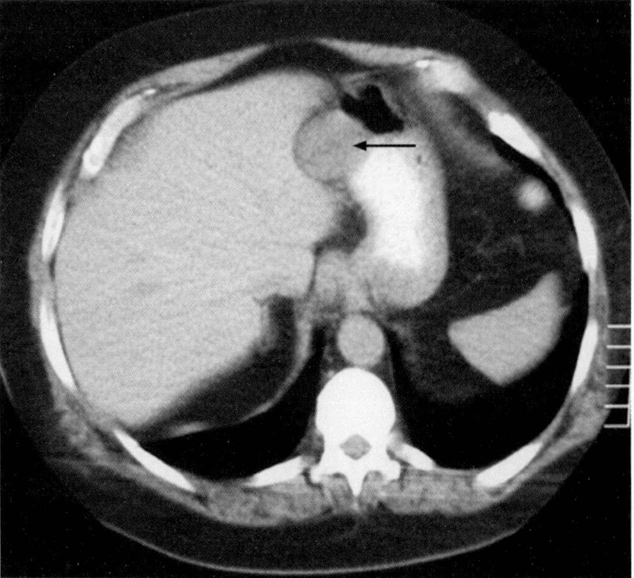

Figure 63.33 Computed tomography scan of the upper abdomen showing a 3.5 cm gastrointestinal stromal tumour arising from the gastric wall.

The prognosis of advanced metastatic GISTs has been dramatically improved with imatinib chemotherapy but resection of metastases, especially from the liver, still has an important role.

GASTRIC LYMPHOMA

Gastric lymphoma is an interesting disease and some aspects of its management are controversial. It is first important to distinguish primary gastric lymphoma from involvement of the stomach in a generalised lymphomatous process. This latter situation is more common than the former. Unlike gastric carcinoma, the incidence of lymphoma seems to be increasing. Primary gastric lymphoma accounts for approximately 5% of all gastric neoplasms.

Gastric lymphoma is most common in the sixth decade and the presentation is no different from gastric cancer, the common symptoms being pain, weight loss and bleeding. Acute presentations of gastric lymphoma such as haematemesis, perforation or obstruction are not common. Primary gastric lymphomas are B-cell derived, the tumour arising from the mucosa-associated lymphoid tissue (MALT). Primary gastric lymphoma remains in the stomach for a prolonged period before involving the lymph nodes. At an early stage, the disease takes the form of a diffuse mucosal thickening, which may ulcerate. Diagnosis is made as a result of the endoscopic biopsy and seldom on the basis of the endoscopic features alone, which are not specific.

Following diagnosis, adequate staging is necessary, primarily to establish whether the lesion is a primary gastric lymphoma or part of a more generalised process. CT scans of the chest and abdomen and bone marrow aspirate are required, as well as a full blood count.

Although the treatment of primary gastric lymphoma is somewhat controversial, it seems most appropriate to use surgery alone for the localised disease process. No benefit has been shown from adjuvant chemotherapy, although some oncologists contend that primary gastric lymphoma can be treated by chemotherapy alone. Chemotherapy alone is appropriate for patients with systemic disease.

Some of the more controversial aspects of gastric lymphoma concern the role of *H. pylori*. Lymphocytes are not found to any degree in normal gastric mucosa, but are found in association with *Helicobacter* infection. It has also been shown that early gastric lymphomas may regress and disappear when the *Helicobacter* infection is treated (Isaacson).

Peter Gersohn Isaacson, contemporary, Professor of Morbid Anatomy, University College, London, UK.

Gastric involvement with diffuse lymphoma

These patients are treated with chemotherapy, sometimes with dramatic and rapid responses. Surgeons are frequently asked to deal with the complications of gastric involvement. The two common complications are bleeding and perforation. Both may occur at presentation, but more usually may follow the chemotherapy when there is rapid regression and necrosis of the tumour. These operations can be technically very challenging and normally require gastrectomy.

DUODENAL TUMOURS

Benign duodenal tumours

Duodenal villous adenomas occur principally in the periampullary region. Although generally uncommon, they are often found in patients with familial adenomatous polyposis. The appearances are similar to those adenomas arising in the colon and, as they have malignant potential, they should be locally excised with histologically clear margins.

Summary box 63.7

Duodenal tumours

- Duodenal villous adenomas are commonly found around the ampulla of Vater and are premalignant
- Duodenal carcinoma is uncommon, but the commonest site for adenocarcinoma is in the small intestine
- Both adenoma and carcinoma occur commonly in patients with familial polyposis and screening these patients is advised
- Pancreatic cancer is the most common cause of duodenal obstruction

Duodenal adenocarcinoma

Although uncommon, this is the most common site for adenocarcinoma arising in the small bowel. Most tumours originate in the periampullary region and commonly arise in pre-existing villous adenomas. Patients present with anaemia due to ulceration of the tumour or obstruction as the polypoid neoplasm begins to obstruct the duodenum. Direct involvement in the ampulla leads to obstructive jaundice. Histologically, the lesion is a typical adenocarcinoma and the metastases are commonly to regional lymph nodes and the liver. At presentation, about 70% of the patients have resectable disease and for those who survive operation the 5-year survival rate is in the region of 20%, this approximately equating to cure. Poor prognostic features in the resected specimen include regional lymph node metastases, transmural involvement and perineural invasion. Curative surgical treatment will normally involve a pancreaticoduodenectomy (Whipple's procedure). Patients with familial polyposis, which is due to a mutation in the *APC* gene on chromosome 5, are predisposed to periampullary cancer, which is one of the most common causes of death in patients who have had their colon removed. Other duodenal malignancies include GISTs (see above) and neuroendocrine tumours.

Neuroendocrine tumours

A number of neuroendocrine neoplasms occur in the duodenum. It is a common site for primary gastrinoma (Zollinger–Ellison syndrome). Non-functioning neuroendocrine tumours (usually called carcinoid tumours) also occur but uncommonly in comparison to the ileum.

Zollinger-Ellison syndrome

This syndrome is mentioned here because the gastrin-producing endocrine tumour is often found in the duodenal loop, although it also occurs in the pancreas, especially the head. It is a cause of persistent peptic ulceration. Before the development of potent gastric antisecretory agents, the condition was recognised by the sometimes fulminant peptic ulceration which did not respond to gastric surgery short of total gastrectomy. It was also recognisable from gastric secretory studies in which the patient had a very high basal acid output but no marked response to pentagastrin, as the parietal cell mass was already nearly maximally stimulated by pathological levels of gastrin. The advent of proton pump inhibitors such as omeprazole has rendered this extreme endocrine condition fully controllable, but also less easily recognised.

Gastrinomas may be either sporadic or associated with the autosomal dominantly inherited multiple endocrine neoplasia (MEN) type I (in which a parathyroid adenoma is almost invariable). The tumours are most commonly found in the 'gastrinoma triangle' (Passaro) defined by the junction of the cystic duct and common bile duct superiorly, the junction of the second and third parts of the duodenum inferiorly, and the junction of the neck and body of the pancreas medially (essentially the superior mesenteric artery). Many are found in the duodenal loop, presumably arising in the G cells found in Brunner's glands. It is extremely important that the duodenal wall is very carefully inspected endoscopically and also at operation. Very often all that can be detected is a small nodule that projects into the medial wall of the duodenum.

Even malignant sporadic gastrinomas may have a very indolent course. The palliative resection of liver metastases may be beneficial and liver transplantation is practised in some centres, as for other gut endocrine tumours, with reasonable long-term results. However, the minority of tumours found to the left of the superior mesenteric artery (outside the 'triangle') seem to have a worse prognosis, more having liver metastases at presentation. In MEN type I, the tumours may be multiple and the condition is incurable. Even in this situation,

Abraham Vater, 1684–1751, Professor of Anatomy and Biology, Wittenburg, Germany.
Allen Oldfather Whipple, 1881–1963, Valentine Mott Professor of Surgery, The College of Physicians and Surgeons, Columbia University, New York, NY, USA.
Edward Passaro, Emeritus Professor of Surgery 1974–1997, Los Angeles, CA, USA.

as with sporadic gastrinoma, surgical treatment should be employed to remove any obvious tumours and associated lymphatic metastases, as the palliation achieved may be good.

DUODENAL OBSTRUCTION

Duodenal obstruction in the adult is usually due to malignancy, and cancer of the pancreas is the most common cause. About one-fifth of patients with pancreatic cancer treated with endoscopic stenting will develop obstruction. Treatment is usually by gastroenterostomy but duodenal stenting is increasingly being used. In patients having a surgical biliary bypass for pancreatic cancer, gastric drainage may be necessary.

A variety of other malignancies can cause duodenal obstruction, including metastases from colorectal and gastric cancer. Primary duodenal cancer is much less common as a cause of obstruction than these other malignancies.

Annular pancreas may rarely cause duodenal obstruction. Obstruction usually follows an attack of pancreatitis and, on occasions, the obstruction may be mistaken for malignancy.

Arteriomesenteric compression is an ill-defined condition in which it is proposed that the fourth part of the duodenum is compressed between the superior mesenteric artery and the vertebral column; when it is convincingly demonstrated and causing weight loss, duodenojejunostomy may be performed.

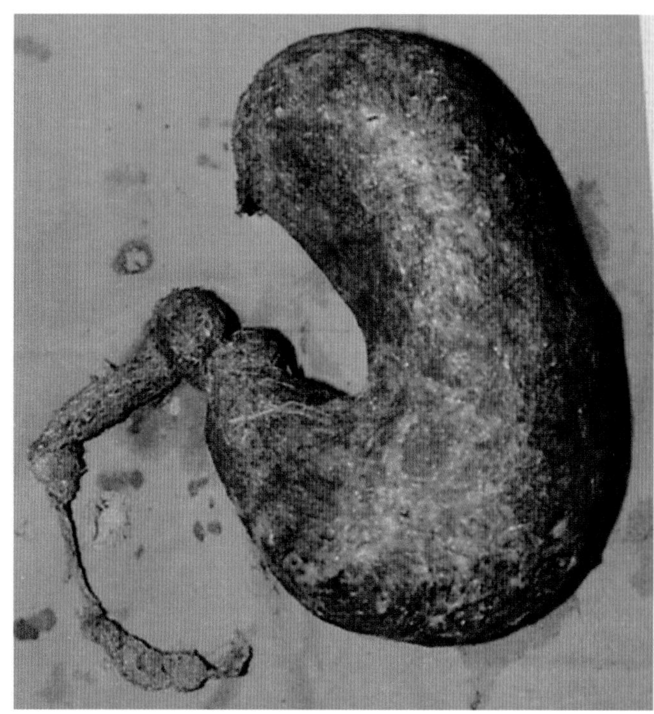

Figure 63.34 Trichobezoar of the stomach in a girl aged 15 years.

OTHER GASTRIC CONDITIONS

Acute gastric dilatation

This condition usually occurs in association with pyloroduodenal disorders or postsurgery without nasogastric suction. The stomach, which may also be atonic, dilates enormously. Often the patient is also dehydrated and has electrolyte disturbances. Failure to treat this condition can result in a sudden massive vomit with aspiration into the lungs. The treatment is nasogastric suction, with a large-bore tube, fluid replacement and treatment of the underlying condition.

Trichobezoar and phytobezoar

Trichobezoar (hair balls) (Figure 63.34) are unusual and are virtually exclusively found in female psychiatric patients, often young. It is caused by the pathological ingestion of hair, which remains undigested in the stomach. The hair ball can lead to ulceration and gastrointestinal bleeding, perforation or obstruction. The diagnosis is made easily at endoscopy or, indeed, from a plain radiograph. Treatment consists of removal of the bezoar, which may require open surgical treatment. Phytobezoars are made of vegetable matter and found principally in patients who have gastric stasis. Often this follows gastric surgery.

Foreign bodies in the stomach

A variety of ingested foreign bodies reach the stomach, and very often these can be seen on a plain radiograph. If possible, they should be removed endoscopically but, if not, most can be left to pass normally. Even objects such as needles, with which there is understandable anxiety, will seldom cause harm. In general, an object which leaves the stomach will pass spontaneously. In contrast, attempted removal at laparotomy can be very difficult as the object may be much more difficult to find than might be expected. Most adults who swallow foreign bodies have ill-defined psychiatric problems and may appear to relish the attention associated with serial laparotomies. The treatment should therefore be expectant and intervention reserved for patients with symptoms in whom the foreign body is failing to progress.

Volvulus of the stomach

Rotation of the stomach usually occurs around the axis and between its two fixed points, i.e. the cardia and the pylorus. In theory, rotation can occur in the horizontal (organoaxial) or vertical (mesenteroaxial) direction but, commonly, it is the former which occurs. This condition is usually associated with a large diaphragmatic defect around the oesophagus (paraoesophageal herniation) (Figure 63.35). What commonly happens is that the transverse colon moves upwards to lie under the left diaphragm, thus taking the stomach with it, and the stomach and colon may both enter the chest through the eventration of the diaphragm. The condition is commonly chronic, the patient presenting with difficulty in eating. An acute presentation with ischaemia may occur. Endoscopically, it can be extremely difficult to sort out the anatomy, and this is one situation in which the contrast radiograph is superior.

Treatment

If the problem is causing symptoms then surgical treatment is the only satisfactory approach. Traditionally, open surgery

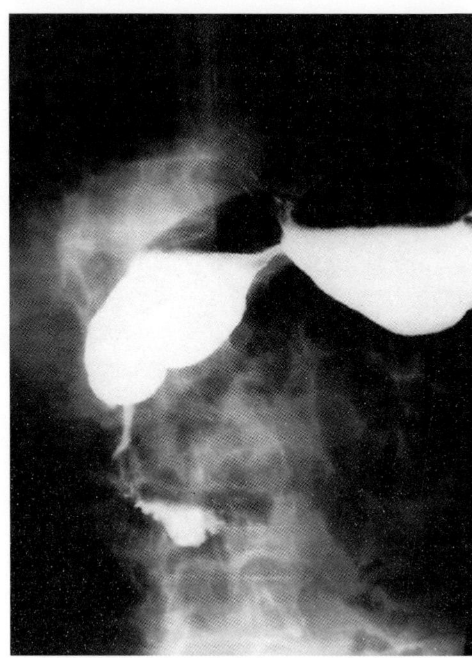

Figure 63.35 Barium meal showing organoaxial volvulus of the stomach associated with eventration of the diaphragm.

has been employed but this problem is suitable for laparoscopic treatment if appropriate skill is available. If there is a hernia, the sac and its contents (usually the stomach) should be reduced. The defect in the diaphragm should be closed, if necessary, with a mesh. It is advisable to separate the stomach from the transverse colon and then perform an anterior gastropexy to fix the stomach to the anterior abdominal wall. The results from this treatment are good.

FURTHER READING

Best LM, Mughal M, Gurusamy KS. Laparoscopic versus open gastrectomy for gastric cancer. *Cochrane Database Syst Rev*. 2016; Mar 31;3:CD011389.

Cancer Genome Atlas Research Network. Comprehensive molecular characterisation of gastric adenocarcinoma. *Nature* 2014; **513**(7517):202–9.

Gurusamy KS, Pallari E. Medical versus surgical treatment for refractory or recurrent peptic ulcer. *Cochrane Database Syst Rev*. 2016; Mar 29;3:CD011523.

Pelletier JS, Gill RS, Gazala S, Karmali S. A systematic review and meta-analysis of open vs. laparoscopic resection of gastric gastrointestinal stromal tumours. *J. Clin. Med. Res*. 2015; **7**(5): 289–96.

Sano T, Aiko T. New Japanese classifications and treatment guidelines for gastric cancer: revision concepts and major revised points. *Gastric Cancer* 2011; **14**: 97–100.

Sobin LH, Gospodarowicz MK, Wittekind C (eds). *UICC TNM classification of malignant tumours*, 7th edn. New York: Wiley, 2009.

Chapter 64

Bariatric and metabolic surgery

Learning objectives

To know and understand:

- What severe and complex obesity is
- Rationale for surgery and the concept of metabolic surgery
- Eligibility and NICE guidelines
- Multidisciplinary assessment
- The common operations and how they work
- How to assess and treat perioperative complications
- Follow-up, nutritional supplements and biochemical monitoring

INTRODUCTION

Obesity is becoming the plague of the 21st century. With overweight becoming the norm in most western countries and newly resource-rich countries, two-thirds of adults are overweight or obese (*Table 64.1*). Every clinician faces the condition and its associated diseases, such as type 2 diabetes, as part of their practice. Obesity and lack of physical activity have the second largest public health impact after smoking. Severe obesity increases the risk of cancer, is associated with multiple other diseases, affects quality of life and reduces life expectancy by 5–20 years. Obese people will more often be of lower social class, unemployed and/or on state benefits. Obesity runs in families and social networks and very few obese people have an identifiable genetic, hormonal basis such as Prader–Willi syndrome. Surgeons encounter the problem of obesity on a daily basis as it affects the treatment of nearly every abdominal pathology in terms of approach and outcomes.

Dieting, increasing energy expenditure through exercise, and intensive lifestyle intervention, are successful for most obese people in helping them lose 6–8% body weight in the short term, up to 1–3 years. Reaching a plateau and cyclical rebound weight regain is, however, expected with all diets. Currently there is no available pharmacotherapy that is safe and clinically or cost-effective in the long term, and there is none on the horizon remotely as effective as bariatric surgery.

Bariatric surgery is the branch of surgery involving manipulation of the stomach and/or small bowel to aid weight loss. Severe and complex obesity is a phrase commonly used for patients with body mass index (BMI) ≥35 and obesity-related disease, or BMI ≥40 by itself (*Table 64.2*).

TABLE 64.1 Definitions of overweight and obesity*.

Adult weight status	BMI (kg/m^2)
Normal	18.5–24.9
Overweight	25–29.9
Class 1 obesity	30–34.9
Class 2 obesity	35–39.9
Class 3 obesity	≥40
Body mass index (BMI) = weight (kg)/height (m)^2.	

* Obesity for children is defined as BMI at or above the 95th centile.

TABLE 64.2 Conditions that are associated with severe and complex obesity.
Type 2 diabetes
Hypertension
Dyslipidaemia
Obstructive sleep apnoea (OSA)
Arthritis and functional impairment
Gastro-oesophageal reflux disease
Non-alcoholic fatty liver disease/non-alcoholic steatohepatosis
Polycystic ovary syndrome
Clinical depression
Functional impairment

Bariatric surgery comes from the Greek *baros*: weight/pressure, and -iatric: the medicine or surgery thereof.
Andrea Prader, 1919–2001, paediatric endocrinologist, Zurich, Switzerland.
Heinrich Willi, 1900–1971, paediatrician, Zurich, Switzerland.

RATIONALE

Bariatric surgery leads to weight loss of 25–35% of body weight (usually at least 15 kg) after 1 year, and this is sustained at 15–25% after 20 years. Additional benefits are that most or all of the obesity-related diseases improve as weight is lost. Quality of life improves. A number of randomised controlled trials (RCTs) have reported on the outcomes of bariatric surgery versus intensive lifestyle interventions, and all favour surgery. The longest follow-up in an RCT is 5 years. However, the non-randomised Swedish Obese Subjects (SOS) study has now shown sustained weight loss and improvement in obesity-related disease up to 20 years after surgery. In this study 2010 patients who chose to have surgery were compared to 2037 controls who did not. All had best medical care throughout and follow-up was better than 99%.

The SOS study was among the first to demonstrate that bariatric surgery also leads to survival benefit. The primary end point was overall mortality and a significant difference was found at mean follow-up of 10 years. Several other studies have found similarly, including one of nearly 8000 operated patients from Utah, USA.

The SOS study also reported a lower incidence of both microvascular and macrovascular complications at 15 years' follow-up in the surgical group. Although there are no RCT data available for this potential outcome, the Swedish registry (SOREG) data indicate lower mortality within only 3–4 years after surgery in diabetic patients. Both the SOS and Utah studies have shown that bariatric surgery also effectively reduces cancer risk in large series of patients.

Summary box 64.1

Rationale for surgery

- Due to the tendency for basal metabolic rate to decrease with dieting, most people will regain all their weight, returning to the previous homeostatic set point
- Bariatric surgery appears to alter this mechanism and 'reset' this point, with 15–25% weight loss maintenance up to 20 years
- Bariatric surgery leads to long-term survival benefit and improves obesity-related disease and quality of life

METABOLIC SURGERY

'Metabolic' or 'diabetes' surgery is increasingly being used in conjunction with, or instead of, 'bariatric surgery' due to the highly effective way surgery improves the metabolic syndrome, with weight loss being a welcomed additional effect. Type 2 diabetes is part of the 'metabolic syndrome' that includes high blood pressure, dyslipidaemia and polycystic ovary syndrome.

It has been known for more than 20 years that control of type 2 diabetes improves with weight loss. Remarkably, after several types of bariatric surgery diabetes control appears to improve **before** significant weight loss occurs. Some of the effects on glucose metabolism can be attributed to the caloric restriction, but changes in gut hormone levels, particularly glucagon-like-peptide 1 (GLP-1), have provoked much interest. GLP-1 is an incretin, which stimulates the beta cells in the pancreas to restore the normal first phase insulin response after eating. Bile acids are also involved.

Although type 2 diabetes is a chronic disease, surgeons initially claimed to 'cure' it. The emphasis has now changed to improving glycaemic control by lowering HbA1c and improving insulin resistance. Patients with the shortest duration of type 2 diabetes have a higher rate of remission or improvement. Even so, patients with depleted pancreatic beta cell reserve, associated with longer disease duration and being on insulin, still benefit from the improved glycaemic control. As they are usually able to reduce or stop their diabetes medications as well, including insulin, it adds to the cost effectiveness. Diabetes 'remission' is defined as patients being off all medication with normal glucose homeostasis. In the SOS study, diabetic patients not only went into remission after surgery, but there was a decreased incidence of patients becoming diabetic.

Many surgical societies have added the word 'metabolic' to their titles, e.g. American Society for Metabolic and Bariatric Surgery (ASMBS), and British Obesity and Metabolic Surgery Society (BOMSS), to emphasise the goal of surgery as an accepted treatment option for metabolic syndrome, rather than just for weight loss. It is hoped that this approach will improve the acceptability in public funded healthcare systems of bariatric/metabolic surgery.

Summary box 64.2

Metabolic surgery

- The term refers to the marked effects of some operations on diabetes and the metabolic syndrome, which may have an impact more important than weight loss itself
- The improvement in type 2 diabetes may be additional to the weight loss
- Surgery is very cost effective since medications reduce or stop as glycaemic control improves

In the wrong place at the wrong time. The Utah paper was the first large study to show improved survival after gastric bypass surgery compared to matched population controls. One of the operated patients was staying in a hotel and killed by a stray bullet fired from the next room by a complete stranger. The mortality still had to be included as a death after surgery (source Dr Ted Adams, author of the Utah study).

COST EFFECTIVENESS

The cost effectiveness of bariatric surgery has been shown in studies from several different countries. A 2009 Health Technology Assessment report in the UK showed bariatric surgery to be cost effective compared to non-surgical options. The

When the SOS study was conceived in 1987, all surgery was done by laparotomy and it was considered unethical to attempt to randomise patients between best medical therapy and bariatric surgery as the latter was considered too risky.

incremental cost-effectiveness ratio (ICER) compared to no surgery was between £2000 and £4000 per Quality Adjusted Life Year (QALY) gained for patients with BMI ≥40 kg/m^2 over 20 years. For patients with BMI 30–40 kg/m^2 the ICER was £1367 per QALY gained. Regarding maximum willingness to pay, compared with non-surgical interventions, if a decision-maker is willing to pay £20 000 for an additional QALY, then the probability of surgery being cost effective over a 20-year time horizon was reported as 100%. The ICERs are similar to the cost effectiveness of stopping smoking and routine statin therapy for the primary prevention of cardiovascular disease. In practice it means that the cost of the operation is recouped within 1–2 years after surgery from reduced medication costs. All the cost-effectiveness studies assess direct or indirect healthcare costs, but not additional benefits of surgery. Thus, return to paid work, coming off state benefits, improved functional capacity and quality of life are 'add-ons' that incur no cost.

ELIGIBILITY

Eligibility criteria were first proposed by the United States' National Institutes of Health in 1991, when the obesity epidemic was just starting. All bariatric surgery was done by laparotomy, and the safety profile was very different. The National Institute of Health and Care Excellence (NICE) in the UK recommends consideration of bariatric surgery for people with severe obesity in whom all non-surgical measures have been tried with no adequate weight loss achieved or maintained. Commitment to long-term follow-up and behaviour change are also advised. After a review of recent RCTs NICE updated its guidance and lowered the BMI threshold to 30 kg/m^2 for recent-onset type 2 diabetes (*Table 64.3*).

NICE estimated that about 80% of people fulfilling the eligibility criteria would have no medical or psychological reason why they would not be fit for surgery. An estimate is that perhaps 10% of these might want it.

TABLE 64.3 Summary of 2014 updated NICE guidance on bariatric surgery (CG 189).

Bariatric surgery is a treatment option for anyone with a BMI ≥40
Offer an expedited assessment for people with a BMI ≥35 with onset of type 2 diabetes in the past 10 years
Consider an assessment for people with a BMI of 30–34.9 with onset of type 2 diabetes within 10 years
Consider an assessment for people of Asian origin with onset of type 2 diabetes at a lower BMI than other populations
Bariatric surgery is the option of choice for adults with BMI >50 when other interventions have not been effective
People fitting the above criteria are also required to be receiving, or to receive, assessment in a specialist weight-management service before referral to a surgical team

There is far more accumulated evidence now that surgery is an effective treatment option for severe and complex obesity than there was historically for the first effective therapies for human immunodeficiency virus infection, which were universally taken up in western countries. The uptake of bariatric surgery worldwide is much less than 1% of those who could benefit.

PRINCIPLES OF SETTING UP A BARIATRIC/METABOLIC SURGERY SERVICE

As for gastrointestinal cancer surgery where oncologists and surgeons routinely work together, it is now agreed that 'bariatric physicians/internists' should be part of the team assessing and managing long-term care after bariatric surgery (*Table 64.4*). Very obese sick patients with, for instance, sleep apnoea with complications need careful multidisciplinary team (MDT) work-up. Using risk scores such as the Edmonton Obesity Staging System (EOSS) and Obesity Surgery-Mortality Risk Score (OS-MRS) can help the team discuss with patients the likely prognosis without surgery, and the risk of complications. The OS-MRS scores one point for each of: age ≥45, BMI ≥50, male gender (due to central obesity), hypertension (due to central obesity), increased deep vein thrombosis (DVT)/pulmonary embolus (PE) risk. The more points that are present the greater is the risk. Swedish registry data indicate that obstructive sleep apnoea (OSA) is a risk factor for anastomotic leak. Therefore, OSA should be actively investigated, as treatment with continuous positive airway pressure might reduce risk. Uncontrolled diabetes must also be considered a risk factor, as it is for all other operations.

Better surgical results are likely in high-volume surgical units. The International Federation for Surgery of Obesity (IFSO) and the ASMBS recommended 100–125 cases per year, and there should be at least two surgeons each performing 50 or more cases. Surgeons early in the learning curve (about 100 for gastric bypass) need to be mentored before independent practice. Irrespective of the technical expertise of each surgeon, higher volumes usually mean that there are sufficient MDT members available to provide support and follow-up. Each unit should have expertise in a variety of surgical procedures including revisions.

It is routine to put patients on a 'liver shrinkage diet' for at least 2 weeks before surgery, especially when there is central obesity, as this is associated with large livers that can make surgery impossible. If a patient cannot lose weight or comply with the liver diet it implies there may be important psychological blocks that need addressing. Male patients especially, with

TABLE 64.4 NICE-accredited guidance on the make-up of the medical and surgical bariatric multidisciplinary team.

Bariatric physician in primary (can be the general practitioner) or secondary care (usually a diabetologist)
Dietitian
Specialist nurse
Appropriately trained mental health professional
Bariatric surgeon
Anaesthetist
Radiologist
± Exercise therapists
Other secondary care specialities, e.g. respiratory/sleep medicine, cardiology

central obesity, a very dense/hard abdomen, OSA/diabetes and a BMI >50 may need more, supervised, mandatory weight loss to make surgery safe.

Although not stipulated in any national guidance, every successful bariatric unit depends on active patient support groups and preoperative education sessions, best run by bariatric nurses and dietitians. These are invaluable in preparing patients for surgery and it is difficult to conceive how a programme can run without them. Also, the ward and outpatient environment must be suitably equipped for severely obese patients, to include scales that can measure up to 250 kg.

Summary box 64.3

Multidisciplinary assessment

Every patient should be assessed and managed by a coherent and well-functioning team of healthcare professionals with a varied background and expertise

Improved outcomes are usually achieved in high-volume, specialised units

Data collection and submission to national registries are recommended to provide quality assurance and long-term outcome data

Laparoscopic surgery and enhanced recovery

Bariatric surgery has been transformed by its amenability to laparoscopic techniques, including intracorporeal suturing and modern laparoscopic stapling devices. Probably equally important is enhanced recovery with the avoidance of catheters, central venous and arterial lines. Free access to fluids is routine immediately after surgery, and due to the relative lack of pain patients can mobilise straightaway. It is usual for gastric bypass and sleeve gastrectomy patients to go home on postoperative day 2 or 3. Gastric banding patients go home as day cases or within 24 hours. The main cause of death after surgery is now DVT/PE, rather than anastomotic leakage or bleeding, and appropriate prophylaxis is usually used for at least 1 week.

Randomised controlled trial evidence for the different types of surgery

Bariatric surgery needs more RCTs comparing different procedures, with long-term follow-up. One of the challenges is keeping the research question relevant, given the rapidity with which surgeons adopt different techniques. Long-term, large scale, pragmatic RCTs with good follow-up are needed to inform practice. The By-Band-Sleeve study is an ongoing pragmatic, multicentre, 3-arm RCT in the UK assessing weight loss and quality of life at 3 years between gastric banding, gastric bypass and sleeve gastrectomy in 1341 patients.

In the 1970s a hospital in the USA designed lavatories to be wall-mounted to make cleaning the floor easier. A bariatric patient broke the lavatory, resulting in a 20-storey waterfall (source Dr Neil Hutcher, past-president ASBS).

Summary box 64.4

Evidence for the different operations

Usually the operation choice is guided by patient, surgeon and unit preference

Well-conducted RCTs comparing the the different operations, with comprehensive follow-up, are needed

The common operations

An international survey by IFSO in 2013 indicated that there were nearly 500 000 procedures done annually. Gastric bypass comprised 45%, sleeve gastrectomy 37%, gastric banding 10% and biliopancreatic diversion/duodenal switch (BPD/DS) 1.5%. The variety of procedures usually reflects surgeon expertise and surgeon and patient preferences, as there are no RCTs beyond 5 years comparing different operations. Sleeve gastrectomy is rapidly gaining popularity at the expense of gastric banding and to a lesser extent gastric bypass. Some clinical outcomes are shown in *Table 64.5*). The mechanism of action of most weight-loss procedures remains incompletely understood. Reduced appetite and early satiety are common features that are potentially explained by changes in levels of gut hormones, such as PYY and GLP-1, and how these interact with the brain.

TABLE 64.5 Malabsorption, percent excess weight loss (EWL)* and diabetes remission after bariatric surgery.

	Protein/calorie malabsorption	3-year % EWL	3-year % diabetes remission
Gastric band	No	40–50%	20%
Gastric bypass	No	50–60%	50%
Sleeve gastrectomy	No	50–60%	50%
BPD/DS	Yes	70–80%	80%

BPD, biliopancreatic diversion; DS, duodenal switch.
* % EWL refers to the excess weight lost above a notional upper normal BMI of 25. Percent weight loss is another way of measuring weight change, preferred by physicians.

Gastric banding

Although adjustable gastric banding is declining in the UK and elsewhere, it did boost the popularity of bariatric surgery due to the perioperative safety, the lack of nutritional complications and its relative ease and availability. The pars flaccida technique (through the window of the lesser omentum) is now standard practice with a band placed just below the oesophagogastric junction, making a small 'virtual' gastric pouch (**Figure 64.1**). The band is sutured into place anteriorly with gastrogastric tunneling sutures to reduce slippage.

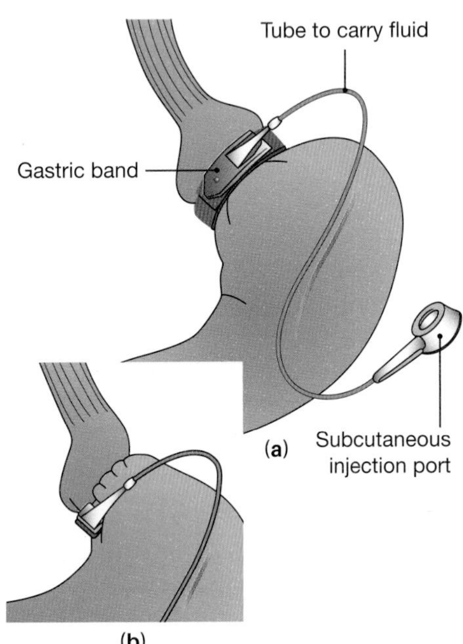

Figure 64.1 Adjustable gastric band. Gastric band surgery showing (a) a small 'virtual' pouch of stomach below the gastro-oesophageal junction and (b) gastrogastric tunnelling sutures. (Reproduced from Griffin SM, Raimes SA, Shenfine J. *Oesophagogastric surgery*, 5th edn. Saunders Elsevier, 2013.)

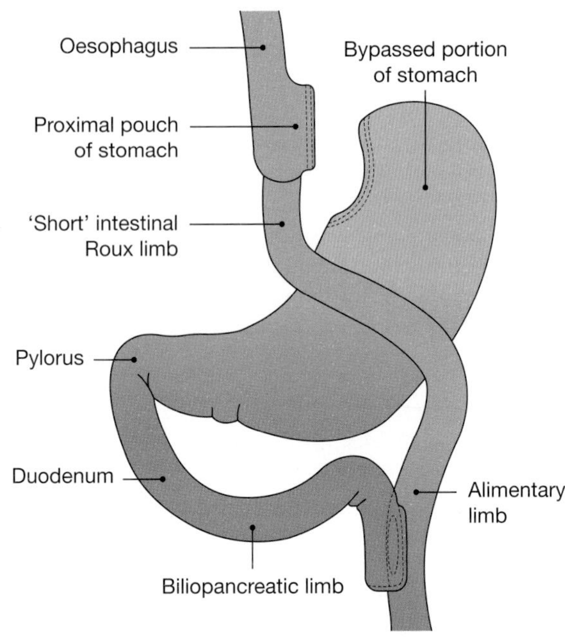

Figure 64.2 Gastric bypass showing a short vertical lesser curve-based gastric pouch with Roux-en-Y jejunojejunostomy reconstruction. (Reproduced from Griffin SM, Raimes SA, Shenfine J. *Oesophagogastric surgery*, 5th edn. Saunders Elsevier, 2013.)

The access port is routinely sutured to the rectus sheath in the upper abdomen for ease of access by a non-coring, Huber needle for band adjustments.

The operation appears to work by reducing hunger, probably vagally mediated. The initial surgical placement is only the beginning of the treatment. Specialist nurses, physicians and surgeons do 'band consultations' to assess eating habits and then perform an adjustment with injection or aspiration of saline if indicated. The objective is to reach the so-called 'sweet spot' of optimal appetite control. Follow-up should be monthly to begin with as needed during the first year, with full MDT support to help patients get the best use out of their bands. Lack of appropriate follow-up accounts for why some of the results in the literature vary so much, with a consequent high band removal rate.

Roux-en-Y gastric bypass

Despite the variety in laparoscopic techniques described and the lack of standardisation, most agree that Roux-en-Y gastric bypass includes a short vertical lesser curvature-based gastric pouch. The available techniques of pouch-jejunostomy are linear stapler with suture closure of the defect, circular stapler and entirely hand sewn. It is routine to perform a leak test. The Roux limb can be retro- or antecolic. Again, there is no standard length of the biliary and Roux limbs; however, the biliary limb is usually kept short with the objective to reduce vitamin and mineral deficiencies and the Roux limb length is varied between 100 and 150 cm (Figure 64.2). There are no consistent data regarding the effect of different limb lengths on weight loss. Bowel continuity is restored by a 'Y' jejunojejunostomy, which is either stapled with suture closure of the defect, or stapled in its entirety.

Despite the widespread belief that the mechanism of action is a combination of restriction and malabsorption of calories, there is no evidence to suggest this. Patients lose weight, at least in part, because they eat less, due to a change in appetite, facilitated by a change in satiety gut hormones. Other mechanisms such as changes in energy expenditure and change in food preferences, may also play a role.

Sleeve gastrectomy

This operation is less challenging to perform than gastric bypass. It evolved from the Magenstrasse and Mill operation, where the divided fundus (the 'mill') was left in continuity with the lesser curve-based tube (the 'main street'). At the same time, it was acting as the first step of the DS operation and proving to be effective on its own.

The lesser curve-based gastric tube is constructed over a size 32–36 Fr bougie, although some advocate that even larger sizes reduce the risk of staple line leakage (Figure 64.3). Linear stapling devices are used and again there is variation in the different techniques between how wide the staplers should be and whether reinforcement strips should be used. The 'Achilles heel' of the sleeve is the risk of staple line leaks at the angle of His, which can take months to heal due to the high-pressure system in the stomach with an intact pylorus. There is no consensus on how these should be treated and many patients become severely catabolic, having multiple procedures with long hospital stays. However, the sleeve is considered to be associated with lower perioperative risk and similar weight-loss outcomes to gastric bypass up to 3 or more years. Long-terms results are still awaited. A proportion of patients will need revisional surgery in future for weight regain.

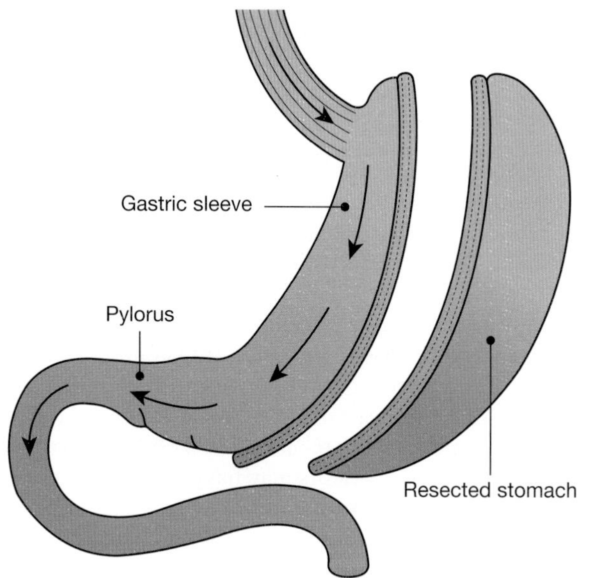

Figure 64.3 Sleeve gastrectomy. (Reproduced from Griffin SM, Raimes SA, Shenfine J. *Oesophagogastric surgery*, 5th edn. Saunders Elsevier, 2013.)

The mechanism of action is still being investigated. The initial thought that this is a restrictive procedure has been challenged with studies suggesting that gastric emptying is accelerated rather than delayed after sleeve gastrectomy. A change in satiety gut hormones and bile salt metabolism, similar to those described after gastric bypass, may explain some of the phenomena observed.

Biliopancreatic diversion/duodenal switch

BPD, described by Scopinaro in Naples, produces greater weight loss than other procedures, but is associated with a higher nutritional complication rate. The mechanism of action appears to be mainly malabsorption of calories. The DS is a variant of the BPD (Figure 64.4). A sleeve gastrectomy is followed by division of the duodenum just distally to the pylorus. The ileum is divided with a linear stapler, followed by a duodenoileostomy and ileoileostomy with the objective to create a common channel of 75–125 cm and an alimentary channel of 100–250 cm. The long remaining biliary limb is not measured.

DS is increasingly seen as a definitive procedure, particularly after significant weight regain following sleeve gastrectomy. A high protein diet and regular vitamin and mineral supplements with life-long monitoring and patient commitment, to avoid malnutrition, are essential postoperatively. Only a few centres offer these procedures.

Banded Roux-en-Y gastric bypass

Less common procedures include the banded bypass of Fobi and Capella, where a silicone ring is placed around the gastric pouch above the gastrojejunostomy with the objective to reduce weight regain. The design is not supported by our current understanding of the mechanism of action of gastric bypass and no benefit has been demonstrated by RCT.

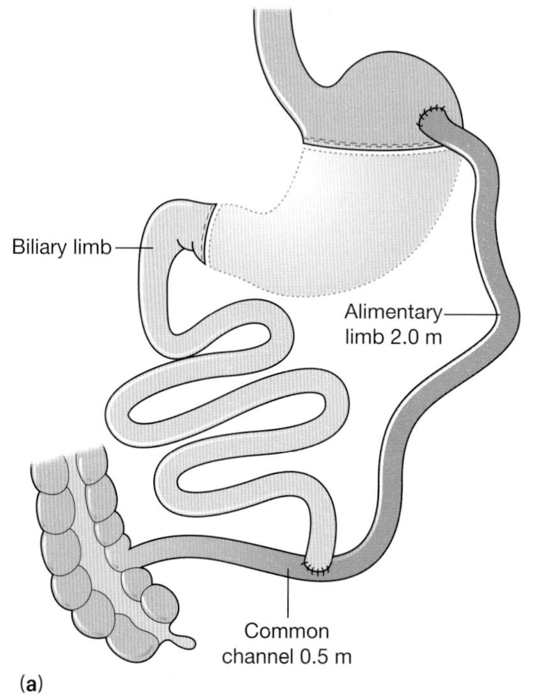

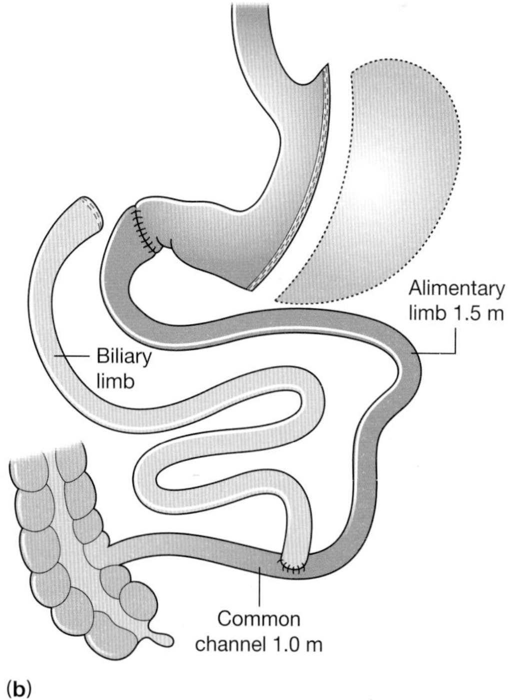

Figure 64.4 (a) Biliopancreatic diversion (BPD); (b) BPD with duodenal switch variant (BPD/DS).

Nicola Scopinaro, contemporary, Professor of Surgery, University of Genoa, Italy.
Mathias Fobi, contemporary, surgeon, California, USA.
Rafael Capella, contemporary, Assistant Professor of Surgery, New Jersey Medical School of Newark, NJ, USA.

One anastomosis gastric bypass

One anastomosis gastric bypass, also known as mini-gastric bypass, was first described by Rutledge. The objective was to develop a technique that is technically less demanding, with only one anastomosis (antecolic loop gastrojejunostomy without a Roux-en-Y configuration) and a longer gastric pouch than for standard gastric bypass. Similar weight-loss outcomes have been reported, but there is concern regarding symptomatic biliary reflux causing gastritis or oesophagitis, marginal ulcers and the management of anastomotic leaks due to a potentially high volume of biliary and pancreatic secretions. With the Roux-en-Y historically the standard in surgery of the stomach for ulcer disease and cancer, there is further concern due to possibly increased risk of Barrett's oesophagus and gastric or oesophageal cancer associated with biliary reflux. These outcomes will need long-term investigation.

Single anastomosis duodenoileal bypass with sleeve gastrectomy

Single anastomosis duodenoileal bypass with sleeve gastrectomy (SADI-S) is a novel procedure based on the BPD-DS. A sleeve gastrectomy is followed by an end-to-side duodenoileal anastomosis. The length of the common channel–alimentary limb is 200 cm. Potential advantages include the preservation of the pylorus, elimination of one anastomosis compared to the DS, reduced operating time and reduced risk of perioperative complications.

Sleeve gastrectomy and ileal transposition

Addition to the sleeve gastrectomy of an ileal transposition has also been suggested as an alternative option. In this operation, a large part of the ileum is transposed to the jejunum, in continuity. The lack of a bypass component with the potential benefits on glucose homeostasis should be balanced against the addition of three anastomoses and the creation of mesenteric defects at risk of internal herniation. This technique remains experimental and comparative studies are needed to establish the role of this procedure.

Complications

The common complications are shown in Table 64.6. Very few gastric banding patients develop early intra-abdominal complications. Unfortunately, a large number of patients have their bands removed later on if there is inadequate follow-up or a late complication.

Anastomotic leakage, bleeding and closed loop obstruction after gastric bypass can be life-threatening. If a bypass patient is not well after 24 hours, urgent consideration should be given to oral contrast x-ray swallow or computed tomography (CT) scanning and/or relaparoscopy. Other than a feeling of 'impending doom' patients may have few overt features of sepsis and abdominal examination can be very misleading. Deterioration after an anastomotic leak can be very rapid and there is no time for delay.

In sleeve gastrectomy, a staple line leak at the angle of His usually presents any time **after** discharge up to 30 days, and patients can also deteriorate rapidly with sepsis. Urgent CT scanning and relaparoscopy are indicated, with source control by drainage the major goal. Patients are typically in hospital for months and need multiple reinterventions, including any of stenting, making a controlled fistula, conversion to gastric bypass and fistula enterostomy. Long-term nutritional support is needed as patients are severely catabolic after complications from both bypass and sleeve surgery.

A 7-month pregnant patient presented with 48 hours of colicky abdominal pain and vomiting 5 years after a gastric bypass. At laparoscopy/laparotomy there was an internal hernia at the jejunojejunostomy. The patient lost two-thirds of her small bowel and the pregnancy. A Swedish RCT has now shown that closure of hernia defects at the time of surgery reduces the incidence of symptomatic internal hernias.

TABLE 64.6 Estimated early surgical complication rates, operative mortality after gastric banding, gastric bypass and sleeve gastrectomy and late complications.

	Early	Mortality	Late
Gastric band	Access port infection (1%) DVT/PE (<0.1%)	0.05–0.1%	Band infection Tubing leak Slippage Erosion into stomach Band intolerance Failure to lose weight/weight regain
Gastric bypass	Anastomotic leak (<1%) Intra-abdominal bleed (2–3%) Unspecified obstruction (1–2%) DVT/PE (<1%)	0.1–0.2%	Internal hernia Chronic abdominal pain Malnutrition if long limb bypass Anastomotic ulcer/stricture Weight regain
Sleeve gastrectomy	Leak at angle of His (2–3%) Intra-abdominal bleed (2–3%) DVT/PE (<1%)	0.1–0.2%	Gastro-oesophageal reflux Weight regain

DVT, deep vein thrombosis; PE, pulmonary embolus.

Robert Rutledge, contemporary, surgeon, Las Vegas USA.

Summary box 64.5

Acute complications

Anastomotic leak and staple line dehiscence can be rapidly fatal and require emergency laparoscopy

Internal hernias developing after surgery, e.g. gastric bypass, are very difficult to diagnose other than by prompt laparoscopy, and require a high index of suspicion

The incidence of late complications is difficult to estimate, as so many patients are lost to follow-up. Internal hernias develop as weight is lost and hernia spaces open up after gastric bypass. CT scanning has a high rate of false negatives for internal hernia, so anyone presenting with severe, cramping abdominal pain 2–3 years after surgery needs to be high priority for investigation by laparoscopy.

Outcomes reported

There is wide variation in how surgeons report the results of surgery, which means that it is often difficult to compare studies. There is a need to standardise clinician reported outcomes and patient reported outcome measures (PROMs) into an agreed core outcome set that includes risk stratification. Obvious PROMs include quality of life.

Follow-up and a shared-care model of chronic disease

Shared-care arrangements with surgeons/physicians and primary care need to be in place so that diabetes and hypertension medications and dosage can be appropriately reduced as weight is lost. Every diabetic needs at least an annual review. Although gastric banding, gastric bypass and sleeve gastrectomy do not cause protein–calorie malabsorption, bariatric surgery can cause severe vitamin and mineral deficiencies, amplifying pre-existing deficiencies caused by being obese.

TABLE 64.7 Summary of British Obesity and Metabolic Surgery Society (BOMSS) biochemical guidance after bariatric surgery.

Blood tests all patients should have at baseline:
Full blood count, urea and electrolytes, liver function tests, thyroid function tests, ferritin, folate, vitamin D, Ca^{++}, parathyroid hormone plus HbA1c, fasting glucose, lipid profile if diabetic
After gastric banding:
Annual full blood count, urea and electrolytes, HbA1c, fasting glucose, lipids as appropriate
After gastric bypass, sleeve gastrectomy, BPD/DS:
As for bands + liver function tests, ferritin, folate, vitamin D, Ca^{++}, parathyroid hormone at 3, 6, 12 months then annually; vitamin B12 at 6, 12 months then annually; zinc, copper annual; vitamin A, E, K, selenium if concern (e.g. steatorrhoea, night blindness, unexplained fatigue, anaemia, metabolic bone disease, chronic diarrhoea, heart failure)

BPD, biliopancreatic diversion; DS, duodenal switch.

TABLE 64.8 Summary of British Obesity and Metabolic Surgery Society (BOMSS) nutritional and micronutrient guidance after bariatric surgery.

After gastric banding:
Multivitamin and mineral supplement, thiamine if vomiting, vitamin D, iron
After gastric bypass, sleeve gastrectomy, BPD/DS:
As for banding + selenium, copper, zinc, folic acid, vitamins B12, A, E, K (BPD/DS may require higher doses)

BPD, biliopancreatic diversion; DS, duodenal switch.

All patients should have routine metabolic and nutritional monitoring lifelong (*Table 64.7*). Patients need regular multivitamins/trace element supplements (*Table 64.8*). The minimum frequency of assessment is 3–6 monthly in the first postoperative year, 6–12 monthly in the second year and at least annually thereafter. Folic acid supplementation should be considered in all sexually active women of child-bearing age, due to the risk of neural tube defects. This is especially important as fertility often improves after surgery. The MDT also needs to support the small number of patients who develop severe mental health issues after surgery, as there is a slightly increased risk of suicide after gastric bypass.

A female patient travelled abroad to have a self-funded laparoscopic Roux-en-Y gastric bypass. Three months after returning she came to the clinic in a wheelchair, unable to stand, with polyneuropathy and severe paraesthesia up to her chest ('bariatric beriberi'). She had not received multidisciplinary care or been advised to take multivitamins and have nutritional monitoring. After prompt thiamine injections and multivitamin support, she made a partial recovery.

Summary box 64.6

Shared-care model of chronic disease

Close collaboration between surgeons, physicians and primary care clinicians is needed to enable seamless follow-up before and after surgery, with a focus on long-term care of patients

Patients should be committed to lifelong vitamin and micronutrient monitoring and replacement

FUTURE CHALLENGES

Patients with obesity suffer from widespread prejudice. Understanding that the obesity epidemic currently experienced in different parts of the world is driven by a change in the environment towards becoming 'obesogenic', and not lack of willpower, would be the first step in removing the barriers to more surgery.

All surgeons should contribute their results to national registries so that safety can be monitored and operation trends established. Ideally, registries should also link to other national healthcare records, e.g. diabetes databases, so that long-term outcomes data can be collected outside of funded RCTs.

FURTHER READING

Adams TD, Gress RE, Smith SC *et al.* Long-term mortality after gastric bypass surgery. *NEJM* 2007; **357**: 753–61.

BOMSS Guidelines on perioperative and postoperative biochemical monitoring and micronutrient replacement for patients undergoing bariatric surgery. 2014. http://www.bomss.org.uk/wp-content/uploads/2014/09/BOMSS-guidelines-Final-version1Oct14.pdf.

Mingrone G, Panunzi S, De Gaetano A *et al.* Bariatric–metabolic surgery versus conventional medical treatment in obese patients with type 2 diabetes: 5-year follow-up of an open-label, single-centre, randomised controlled trial. *Lancet* 2015; **386**: 964–73.

NICE. Obesity: identification, assessment and management. NICE guidelines (CG189) 2014. https://www.nice.org.uk/guidance/cg189.

Sjöström L. Review of the key results from the Swedish Obese Subjects (SOS) trial – a prospective controlled intervention study of bariatric surgery. *J Int Med* 2013; **273**: 219–34.

Welbourn R, Dixon J, Barth JH *et al.* NICE-accredited commissioning guidance for weight assessment and management clinics: a model for a specialist multidisciplinary team approach for people with severe obesity. *Obes Surg* 2016; **26**: 649–59.

Welbourn R, le Roux CW, Owen-Smith A *et al.* Why the NHS should be doing more bariatric surgery; how much should we do? *BMJ* 2016; **353**: i1472.

Chapter 65

The liver

Learning objectives

To understand:

- The anatomy of the liver
- The signs of acute and chronic liver disease
- The investigation of liver disease
- The management of liver trauma
- The management of liver infections
- The management of colorectal liver metastases
- The management of hepatocellular carcinoma

INTRODUCTION

The liver is the largest organ in the body, weighing 1.7 kg in the average 80-kg man. It sits in the right upper quadrant beneath the diaphragm, and is protected by the rib cage. The liver parenchyma is entirely covered by a thin capsule (Glisson's capsule) and by visceral peritoneum on all but the posterior surface of the liver, termed the 'bare area'. The liver is divided into a large right lobe, which constitutes three-quarters of the liver volume, and a smaller left lobe.

ANATOMY OF THE LIVER

Ligaments and peritoneal reflections

The liver is fixed in the right upper quadrant by peritoneal reflections that form ligaments. On the superior surface of the left lobe is the left triangular ligament. Dividing the anterior and posterior folds of this ligament allows the left lobe to be mobilised from the diaphragm and the left lateral wall of the inferior vena cava (IVC) to be exposed. The right triangular ligament fixes the entire right lobe of the liver to the undersurface of the right hemidiaphragm. Division of this ligament allows the liver to be mobilised from under the diaphragm and rotated to the left. Another major supporting structure is the falciform ligament (remnant of the umbilical vein), which runs from the umbilicus to the liver between the right and left lobes, passing into the interlobar fissure. From the fissure, it passes anteriorly on the surface of the liver, attaching it to the posterior aspect of the anterior abdominal wall. Division of the superior leaves of the falciform ligament allows exposure of the suprahepatic IVC, lying within a thin sheath of fibrous tissue. The final peritoneal reflection is between the stomach and the liver. This lesser omentum is often thin and fragile, but contains the hilar structures in its free edge.

Liver blood supply

The blood supply to the liver is unique, 80% being derived from the portal vein and 20% from the hepatic artery. The arterial blood supply in most individuals is derived from the coeliac trunk of the aorta, where the hepatic artery arises along with the splenic and left gastric artery. After supplying the gastroduodenal artery, the hepatic artery branches at a very variable level to produce the right and left hepatic arteries. The right artery supplies the majority of the liver parenchyma and is, therefore, the larger of the two arteries. There are many anatomical variations, knowledge of which is essential for safe surgery on the liver. The blood supply to the right lobe of the liver may be partly or completely supplied by a right hepatic artery arising directly from the superior mesenteric artery, rather than the coeliac trunk. This vessel passes posterior to the uncinate process and head of the pancreas, and runs to the liver on the posterior wall of the bile duct. Similarly, the arterial blood supply to the left lobe of the liver may be derived from a branch of the left gastric artery. This vessel runs between the lesser curve of the stomach and the left lobe of the liver in the lesser omentum.

Structures in the hilum of the liver

The porta hepatis, a transverse fissure on the visceral surface of the liver, is the hilum of the liver. The hepatic artery, portal vein and bile duct are present within the free edge of the lesser omentum (the hepatoduodenal ligament) and together with nerves and lymphatics enter the liver at the porta hepatis.

Francis Glisson, 1597–1677, Regius Professor of Physic, Cambridge, UK, described the capsule of the liver and its blood supply in his book *Anatomia hepatis* (1654).

The usual anatomical relationship of these structures is for the bile duct to be within the free edge, the hepatic artery to be above and medial, and the portal vein to lie posteriorly. Within this ligament, the common hepatic duct is joined by the cystic duct (draining the gallbladder) at a varying level to form the common bile duct (CBD). The common hepatic artery branches at a variable level within the ligament, with the right hepatic artery crossing the bile duct either anteriorly or posteriorly before giving rise to the cystic artery. Multiple small hepatic arterial branches provide blood to the bile duct, predominantly from the right hepatic artery. The portal vein arises from the confluence of the splenic vein and the superior mesenteric vein behind the neck of the pancreas. It has some important tributaries, including the left gastric vein, which joins just above the pancreas.

Division of structures at the hilum

At the hilum, the major structures divide into right and left branches. The right and left hepatic ducts arise from the hepatic parenchyma and join to form the common hepatic duct. The left duct has a longer extrahepatic course of approximately 2 cm. Once within the liver parenchyma, the duct accompanies the branches of the hepatic artery and portal vein within a fibrous sheath. The portal vein often gives off two large branches to the right lobe, which are usually outside the liver for a short length, before giving a left portal vein branch that runs behind the left hepatic duct.

Venous drainage of the liver

The venous drainage of the liver is via the hepatic veins into the IVC. The vena cava lies within a groove in the posterior wall of the liver. Above the liver, it immediately penetrates the diaphragm to join the right atrium, whereas below the liver parenchyma, there is a short length of vessel before the insertion of the renal veins. The inferior hepatic veins are short vessels that pass directly between the liver parenchyma and the anterior wall of the IVC. The major venous drainage is through three large veins that join the IVC immediately below the diaphragm. Outside the liver, these vessels are surrounded by a thin fibrous layer. The right hepatic vein can be exposed fully outside the liver, but the middle and left veins usually join within the liver parenchyma. The right kidney and adrenal gland lie immediately adjacent to the retrohepatic IVC. The right adrenal vein drains into the IVC at this level, usually via one main branch. The IVC can be mobilised fully from the retroperitoneal tissues and, in the healthy state, there are no large vessels in this tissue plane.

Segmental anatomy of the liver

Understanding the internal anatomy of the liver has greatly facilitated safe liver surgery. Couinaud, a French surgeon,

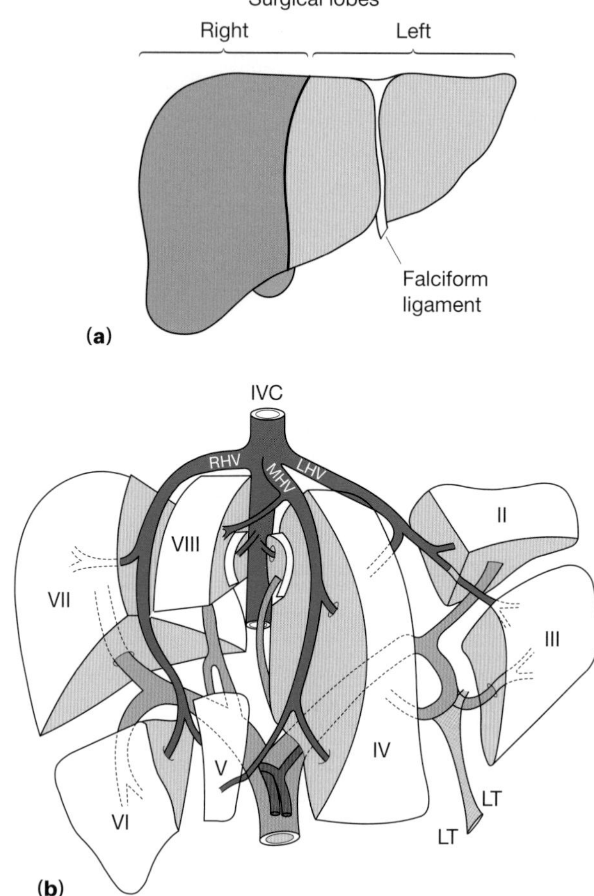

Figure 65.1 (a) The 'surgical' labels of the liver compared with the usual anatomical division into right and left lobes by the falciform ligament. (b) Segments of the liver (after Couinaud). IVC, inferior vena cava; LHV, left hepatic vein; LT, ligamentum teres; MHV, middle hepatic vein; RHV, right hepatic vein.

described the liver as being divided into eight segments (Figure 65.1). Each of these segments can be considered as a functional unit, with a branch of the hepatic artery, portal vein and bile duct, and drained by a branch of the hepatic vein. It is the concept of these segments as distinct functional units that guides 'anatomical' liver resection. The overall anatomy of the liver is divided into a functional right and left 'unit'

Summary box 65.1

Liver anatomy

- There are two anatomical lobes with separate blood supply, bile duct and venous drainage
- Dual blood supply (20% hepatic artery and 80% portal vein)
- The liver regenerates fully after partial resection
- Resection is based on anatomical lines to preserve maximal functioning liver

Claude Couinaud, 1922–2008, French surgeon and anatomist, described the segmental anatomy of the liver in his seminal book *Le Foie: Études anatomiques et chirurgicales*.
Sir James Cantlie, 1851–1926, Scottish born physician who cofounded the Hong Kong College of Medicine for Chinese (now Hong Kong University School of Medicine).

along the line between the gallbladder fossa and the middle hepatic vein (Cantlie's line). Liver segments (V–VIII) to the right of this line are supplied by the right hepatic artery and the right branch of the portal vein, and drain bile via the right hepatic duct. To the left of this line (segments I–IV), functionally, is the left liver, which is supplied by the left branch of the hepatic artery and the left portal vein branch, and drains bile via the left hepatic duct. Resections can be performed of individual segments or of the whole of the left or right hemiliver.

The hepatic lobules

The functional units within the liver segments are the liver lobules. These comprise plates of liver cells separated by the hepatic sinusoids, large, thin-walled venous channels that carry blood to the central vein, a tributary of the hepatic vein, from the portal tracts, which contain branches of the hepatic artery and portal vein. During passage through the sinusoids, the many functions of the liver take place, including bile formation, which is channelled in an opposite direction to the blood flow to drain via the bile duct tributaries within the portal tracts.

Embryology

The liver is a foregut structure and forms as a small endodermal bud early in gestation. The cell population is bipotential, and cells may develop into hepatocytes or intrahepatic ductal cells. The liver endothelium is derived from the vitelline and umbilical veins, which merge with the endodermal bud to form the liver sinusoids. The supporting connective tissue, haemopoietic cells, and Kupffer cells are derived from the mesoderm of the septum transversum, which is a mass of mesenchymal connective tissue.

ACUTE AND CHRONIC LIVER DISEASE

Liver function and tests

Adequate liver function is essential to survival; humans will survive for only 24–48 hours in the anhepatic state despite full supportive therapy. The liver is central to many key metabolic pathways.

Summary box 65.2

Main functions of the liver

- Maintaining core body temperature
- pH balance and correction of lactic acidosis
- Synthesis of clotting factors
- Glucose metabolism, glycolysis and gluconeogenesis
- Urea formation from protein catabolism
- Bilirubin formation from haemoglobin degradation
- Drug and hormone metabolism and excretion
- Removal of gut endotoxins and foreign antigens

TABLE 65.1 Routinely available tests of liver function.

Test	Normal range
Bilirubin	5–17 μmol/L
Alkaline phosphatase (ALP)	35–130 IU/L
Aspartate transaminase (AST)	5–40 IU/L
Alanine transaminase (ALT)	5–40 IU/L
Gamma-glutamyl transpeptidase (GGT)	10–48 IU/L
Albumin	35–50 g/L
Prothrombin time (PT)	12–16 s

An awareness of the currently available liver function tests and their significance is essential (*Table 65.1*).

Bilirubin is synthesised in the liver and excreted in bile. Increased levels may be associated with increased haemoglobin breakdown, hepatocellular dysfunction resulting in impaired bilirubin transport and excretion or biliary obstruction. In patients with known parenchymal liver disease, progressive elevation of bilirubin in the absence of a secondary complication suggests deterioration in liver function. The serum alkaline phosphatase (ALP) is particularly elevated with cholestatic liver disease or biliary obstruction. It is important to note that routine laboratory analysis of ALP is not isoform-specific and so alkaline phosphatase from a skeletal source may also lead to elevation. The transaminase levels (aspartate transaminase (AST) and alanine transaminase (ALT)) reflect acute hepatocellular damage, as does the gamma-glutamyl transpeptidase (GGT) level, which may be used to detect the liver injury associated with acute alcohol ingestion. However, marked liver injury can occur in the presence of normal liver function tests. The synthetic functions of the liver are reflected in the ability to synthesise proteins (albumin level) and clotting factors (prothrombin time). The standard method of monitoring liver function in patients with chronic liver disease is therefore serial measurement of bilirubin, albumin and prothrombin time.

Clinical signs of impaired liver function

These signs depend on the severity of dysfunction and whether it is acute or chronic.

Acute liver failure

Causes of acute liver failure

In the early stages, there may be no objective signs, but with severe dysfunction the onset of clinical jaundice may be associated with neurological signs of liver failure (hepatic encephalopathy), consisting of a liver flap, drowsiness, confusion and, eventually, coma.

Karl Wilhelm von Kupffer, 1829–1902, Professor of Anatomy at Kiel (1867), Königsberg (1875) and Munich, Germany (1880), described these 'stellate cells' in 1880.

rarely seen throughout their entire course. The advent of contrast enhanced ultrasound scanning (CEUS), which employs transient intravascular bubbles to delineate normal liver parenchyma from solid tumours, has significantly increased the sensitivity and specificity of ultrasound scanning. CEUS assesses real-time lesion vascularity with a temporal resolution superior to that of other imaging modalities.

Computed tomography

Modern spiral computed tomography (CT) technology has increased the accuracy of diagnosis and staging of liver lesions, and contrast-enhanced CT is currently the most widely used and best validated modality for liver imaging. It provides fine detail of liver lesions down to less than 1 cm in diameter and gives information on their nature (Figure 65.3). Oral contrast enhancement allows visualisation of the stomach and duodenum in relation to the liver hilum. The early arterial phase of the intravenous contrast vascular enhancement is particularly useful for detecting small primary liver cancers, owing to their preferential arterial blood supply. The venous phase maps the branches of the portal vein within the liver and the drainage via the hepatic veins. Inflammatory liver lesions often exhibit rim enhancement with intravenous contrast, whereas commonly found haemangiomas characteristically show late venous enhancement. The density of any liver lesion can be measured, which is useful in establishing the presence of a cystic lesion. CT has high accuracy in determining the stage, and high sensitivity and specificity in determining resectability, of liver tumours. Local and distant metastases can also be detected, although peritoneal metastases are often missed on CT.

Magnetic resonance imaging

Magnetic resonance (MR) of the liver is superior to CT in characterising liver lesions and detecting small liver metastases (Figure 65.4). The advent of liver-specific contrast

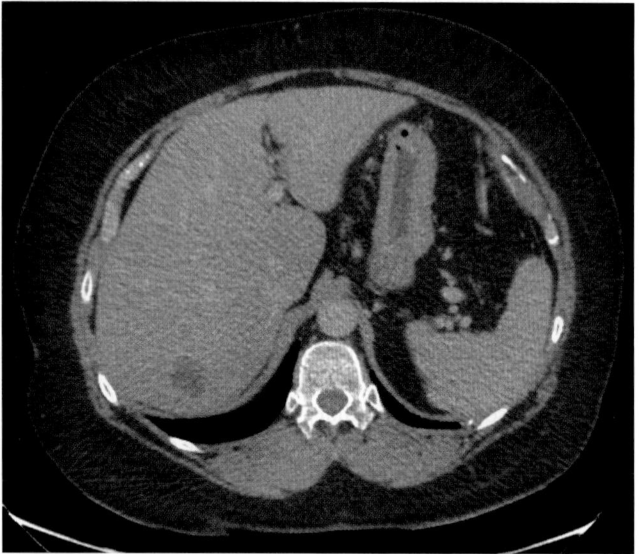

Figure 65.3 Computed tomography scan of a patient with a liver tumour in the right lobe of the liver, using intravenous contrast enhancement.

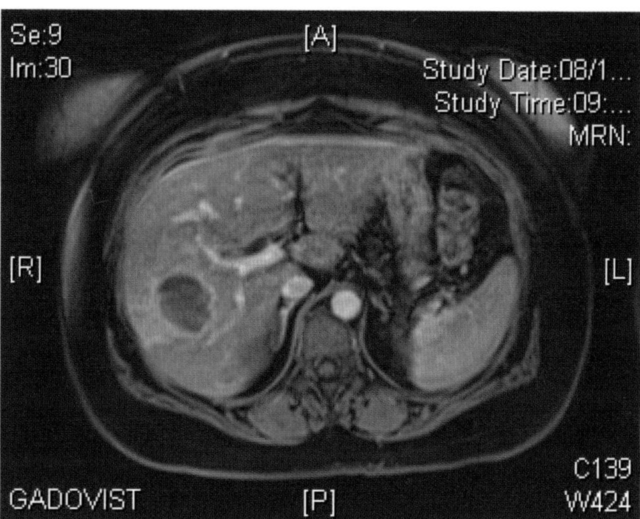

Figure 65.4 Magnetic resonance imaging (MRI) is increasingly used for the diagnosis and staging of liver cancers. This figure shows a colorectal liver metastasis as seen on contrast MRI.

agents has significantly improved lesion characterisation and detection, particularly in differentiating small hepatocellular carcinoma (HCC) from regenerative nodules. These contrast agents are taken up by normally functioning hepatocytes. A lesion not containing hepatocytes will not take up contrast, and will appear dark against an enhancing background liver. These contrast agents are now being used more frequently due to the increased detection of lesions on liver-specific phase CT scans. This observation is particularly important for colorectal liver metastases prior to consideration of liver resection. In addition to standard MR scanning, magnetic resonance cholangiopancreatography (MRCP) provides excellent quality non-invasive imaging of the biliary tract, the accuracy of which is comparable to direct cholangiography by endoscopic retrograde cholangiopancreatography (ERCP) or percutaneous transhepatic cholangiography (PTC).

Endoscopic retrograde cholangiopancreatography

ERCP (Figure 65.5) is performed in patients with obstructive jaundice when an endoscopic intervention is anticipated based on prior imaging (endoscopic removal of CBD stones, biliary drainage in septic patient or insertion of a biliary tract stent). Preoperative assessment of coagulation is essential, and if abnormal it is appropriately corrected, along with prophylactic antibiotics and an explanation of the main complications, which include pancreatitis, cholangitis and bleeding or perforation of the duodenum related to sphincterotomy.

Direct endoscopic cholangioscopy

Cholangioscopy enables direct visualisation of the bile ducts, either operatively or endoscopically. Originally, 'mother and baby' ERCP cholangioscopy only visualised the biliary mucosa of the common duct, and required two endoscopists to operate. This has changed with the development of the

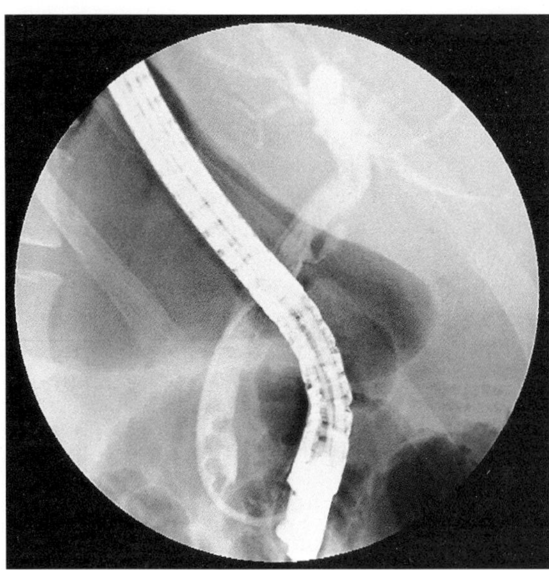

Figure 65.5 Endoscopic retrograde cholangiopancreatography demonstrating the biliary tract with multiple stones in the distal common bile duct.

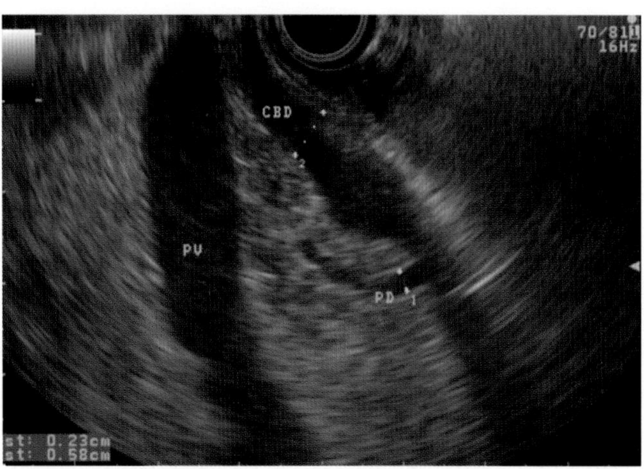

Figure 65.6 Endoscopic ultrasound gives excellent views of the head of pancreas and distal biliary tree, and is a sensitive method of detecting microcalculi not seen on standard transabdominal ultrasonography. This figure demonstrates the common bile duct (CBD) and confluence with the pancreatic duct (PD), with the portal vein lying deep to this (PV).

new SpyGlass™ (Boston Scientific) cholangioscope. SpyGlass™ cholangioscopy enables a single operator to visualise the biliary mucosa to at least second- and third-order ducts, with the benefit of a working channel to allow directly visualised biopsies and application of targeted therapy. Directly targeted biopsies improve the diagnostic yield to >80% in patients with indeterminate biliary strictures.

Endoscopic ultrasound

EUS evaluates the extrahepatic biliary tree, including indeterminate lymphadenopathy at the porta hepatis and para-aortic regions. EUS provides detailed views of the bile ducts, ampulla, pancreas and liver hilum, but does not carry the associated risks of ERCP. Radial EUS provides a 360° image, whereas linear EUS provides a view in the plane of the scope and allows for the sampling of tissue via biopsy or fine-needle aspiration (FNA). EUS is also the most sensitive tool for diagnosing small bile duct calculi (Figure 65.6).

Percutaneous transhepatic cholangiography

PTC is indicated where endoscopic cholangiography has failed or is impossible, e.g. in patients with previous pancreatoduodenectomy or gastrectomy. It is often required in patients with hilar bile duct tumours to guide external drainage of the obstructed bile ducts to relieve jaundice, evaluate resectability and to direct stent insertion (Figure 65.7).

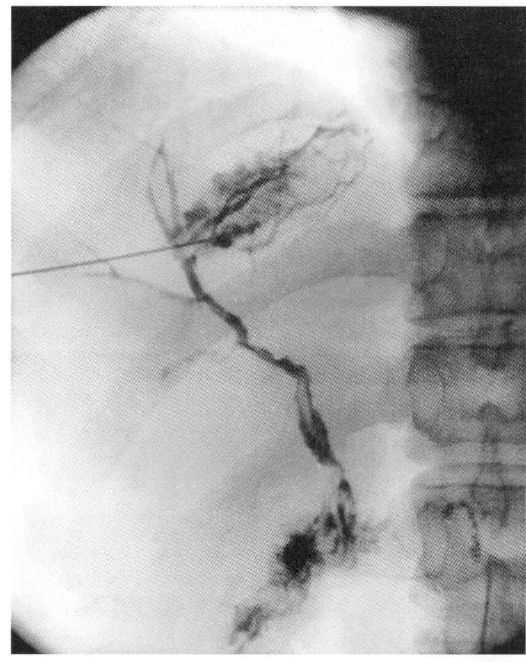

Figure 65.7 Percutaneous transhepatic cholangiography. Some contrast has extravasated at the site of hepatic puncture of the percutaneously placed needle, but the biliary tract is clearly demonstrated and shows the multiple strictures typical of primary sclerosing cholangitis.

Angiography

Angiography is generally employed only for direct therapeutic intervention. Therapeutic interventions include the occlusion of arteriovenous malformations, the embolisation of bleeding sites in the liver and the treatment of liver tumours (transarterial chemoembolisation, TACE).

Positron emission tomography

18F-2-fluoro-2-deoxy-D-glucose positron emission tomography (FDG–PET) depends on the avid uptake of glucose by cancerous tissue in comparison with benign or inflammatory tissue. Deoxyglucose is labelled with the positron emitter fluorine-18 (18FDG), and this is administered to the patient prior to imaging by PET. A three-dimensional image of the whole body is obtained, highlighting areas of increased glucose metabolism (Figure 65.8). PET or integrated PET-CT can be useful in the diagnosis of regional lymph node metastases and distant metastases.

Laparoscopy

Laparoscopy is useful for the staging of primary hepatopancreatobiliary cancers. Lesions overlooked by conventional imaging are mainly peritoneal metastases and superficial liver tumours. These lesions can be detected at laparoscopy thus avoiding an unnecessary laparotomy. A liver biopsy to confirm or exclude chronic liver disease can also be performed during laparoscopy, but routine biopsy of resectable lesions should be avoided because of the risk of tumour seeding. There is no role for routine laparoscopy in patients with colorectal liver metastases.

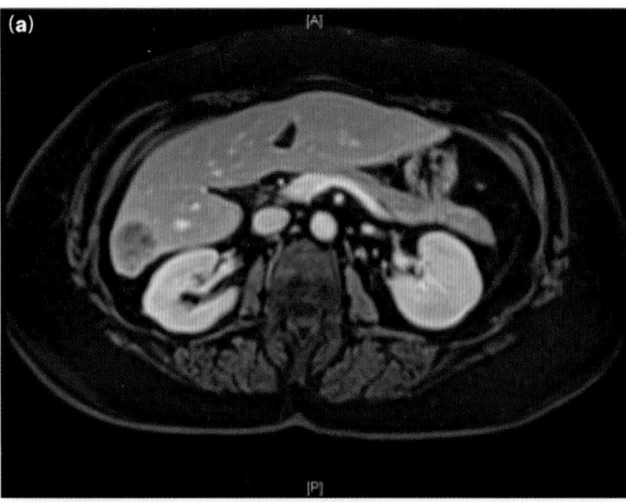

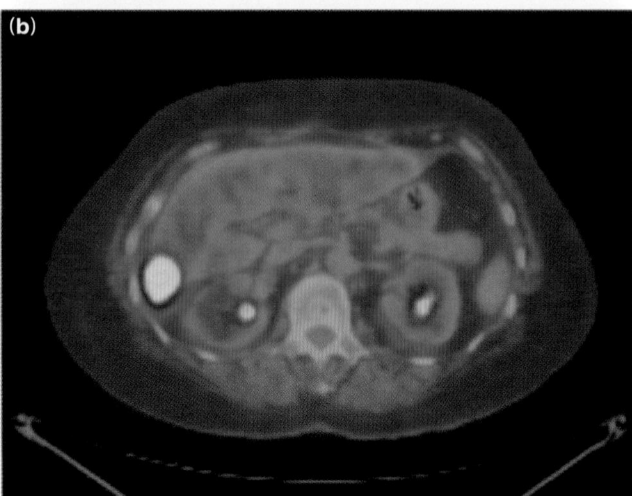

Figure 65.8 Patient with colorectal liver metastasis seen on (a) an MRI liver and (b) 18F-2-fluoro-2- deoxy-D-glucose uptake on a combined PET-CT scan. Similar uptake outside the liver usually precludes curative intent surgery as it indicates distant metastases. As seen in these images, some background renal activity is expected.

LIVER TRAUMA

General

The liver is the second most common organ injured in abdominal trauma after the spleen.

Liver trauma can be divided into blunt and penetrating injuries. Blunt injury produces contusion, laceration and avulsion injuries to the liver, often in association with splenic, mesenteric or renal injury. Penetrating injuries, such as stab and gunshot wounds, are often associated with chest or pericardial involvement. Blunt injuries are more common and have a higher mortality than penetrating injuries.

Summary box 65.7

Management of liver trauma

- Remember associated injuries
- At-risk groups
  - Stabbing/gunshot in lower chest or upper abdomen
  - Crush injury with multiple rib fractures
- Resuscitate
  - Airway
  - Breathing
  - Circulation
- Assessment of injury
  - CT chest and abdomen with contrast
  - Laparotomy if haemodynamically unstable
- Treatment
  - Correct coagulopathy
  - Suture lacerations
  - Resect if major vascular injury
  - Packing if diffuse parenchymal injury

Diagnosis of liver injury

The liver is an extremely well-vascularised organ, and blood loss is therefore the major early complication of liver injuries. Clinical suspicion of a possible liver injury is essential, as a laparotomy by an inexperienced surgeon with inadequate preoperative preparation is doomed to failure. All lower chest and upper abdominal stab wounds should be suspect, especially if considerable blood volume replacement has been required. Similarly, severe crushing injuries to the lower chest or upper abdomen often combine rib fractures, haemothorax and damage to the spleen and/or liver. Focused assessment sonography in trauma (FAST) performed in the emergency room by an experienced operator can reliably diagnose free intraperitoneal fluid. Patients with free intraperitoneal fluid on FAST and haemodynamic instability, and patients with a penetrating wound, will require a laparotomy and/or thoracotomy once active resuscitation is under way. Owing to the opportunity for massive ongoing blood loss and the rapid development of a coagulopathy, the patient should be directly transferred to the operating theatre while blood products are obtained and volume replacement is taking place. Patients who are haemodynamically stable should have a contrast-enhanced CT scan of the chest and abdomen as the next step. This scan will demonstrate evidence of parenchymal damage to the liver or spleen, as well as associated traumatic injuries to their feeding vessels. Free fluid can also be clearly established. The chest scan will help to exclude injuries to the great vessels and demonstrate damage to the lung parenchyma.

Initial management of liver injuries

Penetrating

The initial management is maintenance of airway patency, breathing and circulation (ABC) following the principles of advanced trauma life support (ATLS). Peripheral venous access is gained with two large-bore cannulae and blood sent for cross-match of 10 units of blood, full blood count, urea and electrolytes, liver function tests, clotting screen, glucose and amylase. Initial volume replacement should be with blood. Arterial blood gases should be obtained and the patient intubated and ventilated if the gas exchange is inadequate. Intercostal chest drains should be inserted if associated pneumothorax or haemothorax is suspected. Once initial resuscitation has commenced, the patient should be transferred to the operating theatre, with further resuscitation performed on the operating table. The necessity for fresh frozen plasma and cryoprecipitate should be discussed with the blood transfusion service immediately the patient arrives in the hospital (often by activation of a major transfusion protocol), as these patients rapidly develop irreversible coagulopathies due to a lack of fibrinogen and clotting factors. Standard coagulation profiles are inadequate to evaluate this acute loss of clotting factors, and factors should be given empirically, aided by the results of thromboelastography (TEG), if available (Figure 65.9). A contrast CT prior to laparotomy should be considered if the patient is haemodynamically stable.

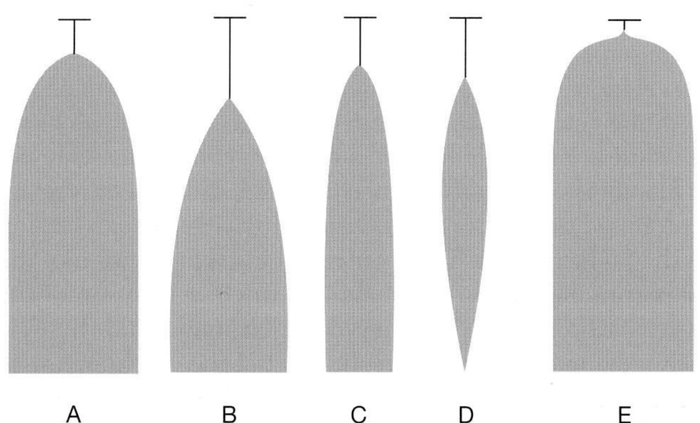

Figure 65.9 Thromboelastography (TEG). This dynamic form of assessing the coagulation status is being used increasingly for intraoperative monitoring. The shape of the TEG trace defines the nature of the underlying coagulation deficiency as shown. A, normal; B, delayed clot formation; C, reduced clot strength; D, clot lysis; E, hypercoagulable.

Blunt trauma

With blunt injuries, the initial plan for resuscitation and management is as outlined above for penetrating injuries. Patients who are haemodynamically unstable will require an immediate laparotomy. For the patient who is haemodynamically stable, imaging by CT should be performed to further evaluate the nature of the injury. Most patients with blunt liver injury who are haemodynamically stable can be managed conservatively. The indication for discontinuing conservative treatment is the development of haemodynamic instability, evidence of ongoing blood loss despite correction of any underlying coagulopathy and the development of signs of generalised peritonitis. Interventional radiology has an important role in management of liver trauma and embolisation to control hepatic artery bleeding is safe and effective in a stable patient with no evidence of hollow viscus perforation.

The surgical approach to liver trauma

Good access is vital. A 'rooftop' incision with midline extension to the xiphisternum and retraction of the costal margins gives excellent access to the liver and spleen. If the laparotomy has been started through a midline incision, a transverse lateral extension to the right can be added to improve access to the liver. Compression of the liver with packs and correction of coagulopathy, if present, will control most of the active bleeding. If bleeding persists, further control can be acheived by vascular inflow occlusion by placing an atraumatic clamp across the foramen of Winslow (the Pringle manoeuvre). A stab incision in the liver can be sutured with a fine absorbable monofilament suture. Lacerations to the hepatic artery should be identified and repaired with 6/0 Prolene suture. If unavoidable, the hepatic artery may be ligated, although parenchymal necrosis and abscess formation will result in some individuals. Portal vein injuries should be repaired with 5/0 Prolene. Inflow occlusion facilitates suturing of lacerations and vessels.

If bleeding persists despite inflow occlusion, consider major hepatic vein or IVC injuries, and also look for abberant arteries to the liver. Deceleration injuries often produce lacerations of the liver parenchyma adjacent to the anchoring ligaments of the liver. These may be amenable to suture with an absorbable monofilament suture. Again, inflow occlusion may facilitate this suturing and, if necessary, the sutures can be buttressed to prevent them cutting through the liver parenchyma. With more severe deceleration injuries, a portion of the liver may be avulsed. These injuries are more complex as they are associated with a devitalised portion of the liver and, often, major injuries to the hepatic veins and IVC. Diffuse parenchymal injuries should be treated by packing the liver to achieve haemostasis (Figure 65.10). This is effective for the majority of liver injuries if the liver is packed against the natural contour of the diaphragm by packing from below. Large

Jacob Benignus Winslow, 1669–1760, Professor of Anatomy, Physic and Surgery, Paris, France.

James Hogarth Pringle, 1863–1941, surgeon, The Royal Infirmary, Glasgow, UK. Born in Australia and trained in Edinburgh, he was a strong supporter of women in medicine; he performed the first successful autologous vein graft in the UK and the first excision and block dissection for malignant melanoma. He and his father, George Hogarth Pringle (1830 –1872, who practised in Australia), formed a famous team of surgical innovators.

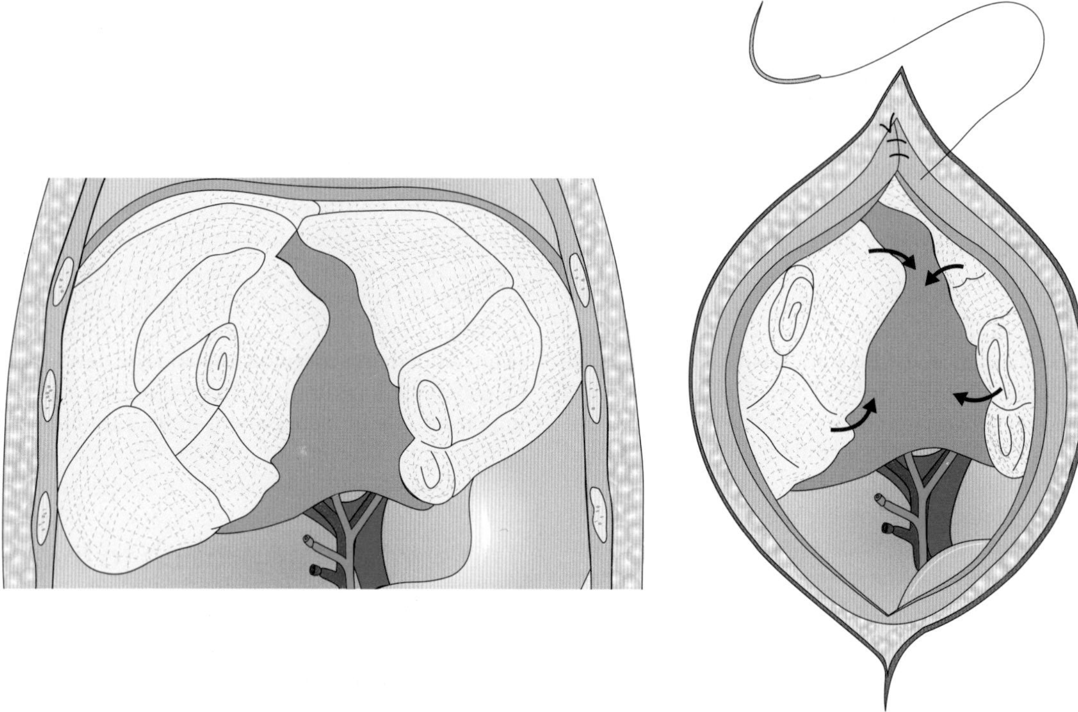

Figure 65.10 Packing the liver to achieve haemostasis. The abdomen can then be closed and the patient transferred to critical care for stabilisation prior to relook laparotomy 24–48 hours later. (Adapted from Poston, D'Angelica, Adam (eds). *Surgical management of hepatobiliary and pancreatic disorders*. Boca Raton: CRC Press, 2010.)

abdominal packs should be used to ease their removal, and the abdomen closed to facilitate compression of the parenchyma. Care should be taken to avoid overzealous packing, as this may produce pressure necrosis of the liver parenchyma or abdominal compartment syndrome.

Crush injuries to the liver often result in large parenchymal haematomas and diffuse capsular lacerations (Figure 65.11). Suturing is usually ineffective, and perihepatic packing, which involves placing packs above, behind and below the liver, is the most useful method of providing haemostasis. Necrotic tissue should be removed, but poorly perfused, though viable, liver left *in situ*. If packing is necessary, the patient should have the packs removed after 48 hours, and usually no further surgical intervention is required. Antibiotic cover is advisable, and full reversal of any coagulopathy is essential. If a major liver vascular injury (hepatic vein or vena cava, grade V or VI) is suspected at the time of the initial laparotomy, then packing and referral to a specialist centre should be considered. A common surgical approach in these circumstances would be to place the patient on venovenous bypass, using cannulae in the femoral vein via a long saphenous cut-down, with the blood returned using a roller pump to the superior vena cava (SVC) via an internal jugular line. Venovenous bypass allows the IVC to be safely clamped to facilitate caval or hepatic vein repair. A rapid infuser blood transfusion machine facilitates the delivery of large volumes of blood instantaneously. Once prepared, the patient is relaparotomised via the rooftop incision with a midline extension to the xiphisternum. The liver is mobilised by division of the supporting ligaments, and complete vascular isolation of the liver is achieved by occluding the hilar inflow and the IVC above the renal veins and at the level of the diaphragm with atraumatic vascular clamps. Venous return is provided by the venovenous bypass. Warm ischaemia of the liver is tolerated for up to 45 minutes, allowing sufficient time in a blood-free field for repair of injuries to the IVC or hepatic veins.

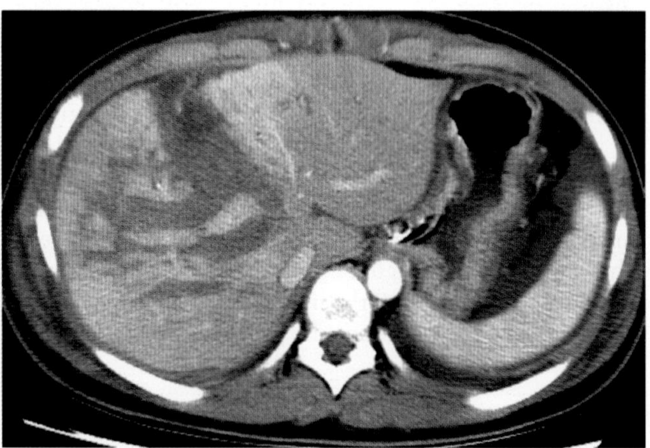

Figure 65.11 Computed tomography scan demonstrating grade IV liver injury.

Other complications of liver trauma

A subcapsular or intrahepatic haematoma requires no specific intervention and should be allowed to resolve spontaneously. Abscesses may form as a result of secondary infection of an area of parenchymal ischaemia, especially after penetrating trauma. Treatment is with systemic antibiotics and aspiration under ultrasound guidance once the necrotic tissue has liquefied. Bile collections require aspiration under ultrasound guidance or percutaneous insertion of a pigtail drain. The site of origin of a biliary fistula should be determined by endoscopic or percutaneous cholangiography, and biliary decompression achieved by nasobiliary or percutaneous transhepatic drainage or stent insertion. If this fails to control the fistula, the affected portion of the liver may require resection. Late vascular complications include hepatic artery aneurysm and arteriovenous (precipitating acute heart failure if between the hepatic artery and hepatic vein and acute portal hypertension if arterioportal) or arteriobiliary fistulae (resulting in often painful haemobilia) (Figure 65.12). These are best treated non-surgically by a specialist hepatobiliary interventional radiologist. The feeding vessel can be embolised transarterially.

Hepatic failure may occur following extensive liver trauma. This will usually reverse with conservative supportive treatment if the blood supply and biliary drainage of the liver are intact.

Summary box 65.8

Complications of liver trauma

- Intrahepatic haematoma
- Liver abscess
- Bile collection
- Biliary fistula
- Hepatic artery aneurysm
- Arteriovenous fistula
- Arteriobiliary fistula
- Liver failure

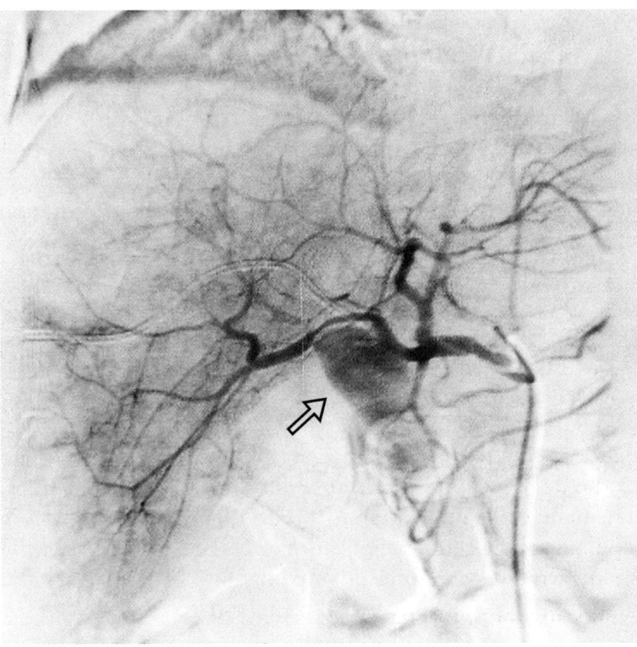

Figure 65.12 Hepatic aneurysm following liver trauma. An aneurysm arising from the right hepatic artery (arrow), which can be optimally treated by the interventional radiologist using transarterial embolisation.

Long-term outcome of liver trauma

The capacity of the liver to recover from extensive trauma is remarkable, and parenchymal regeneration occurs rapidly. Late complications are rare, but the development of biliary strictures many years after recovery from liver trauma has been reported. The treatment depends on the mode of presentation and the extent and site of stricturing. A segmental or lobar stricture, associated with atrophy of the corresponding area of liver parenchyma and compensatory hypertrophy of the other liver lobe, may be treated expectantly. A dominant extrahepatic bile duct stricture associated with obstructive jaundice may be treated initially with endobiliary balloon dilatation or stenting, but will usually require surgical correction using a Roux-en-Y hepatodochojejunostomy.

PORTAL HYPERTENSION

An elevation in portal pressure is most commonly found in the presence of liver cirrhosis, although it may be present in patients with extrahepatic portal vein occlusion, intrahepatic veno-occlusive disease or occlusion of the main hepatic veins (Budd–Chiari syndrome (BCS)). As portal hypertension *per se* produces no symptoms, it is usually diagnosed following presentation with decompensated chronic liver disease and encephalopathy, ascites or variceal bleeding.

Management of bleeding varices

General resuscitation

Varices usually present with the acute onset of a large-volume haematemesis, the lower oesophagus being the most common site for variceal bleeding. The diagnosis may be suspected if the patient is known to have liver cirrhosis, but it needs to be confirmed following initial resuscitation of the patient. Variceal haemorrhage is a medical emergency. Patients with massive hemorrhage should be admitted to the intensive care unit. Venous access should be obtained through two large-bore peripheral cannulae. Resuscitation should be commenced, ideally with blood. Liver function tests will reveal underlying liver disease, and a coagulation profile will reveal any underlying coagulopathy. Hypervolaemia should be avoided since this may increase portal pressure and exacerbate the bleeding. Vitamin K is administered (10 mg intravenously (i.v.)) as well as tranexamic acid (1 g i.v.), but correction of a coagulopathy will require the administration of fresh frozen plasma (FFP). A major transfusion protocol should be activated. An associated thrombocytopenia is usually secondary to hypersplenism due to cirrhosis and is treated if the platelet count falls below 50×10^9/L. Treatment with a splanchnic vasoconstrictor (such as terlipressin) should be started. Administration of a prophylactic antibiotic is recommended to prevent or treat associated bacterial infection. As soon as the patient is haemodynamically stabilised, an upper gastrointestinal endoscopy should be performed to establish the diagnosis because 50% of patients with portal hypertension will have a non-variceal source of bleeding. Variceal bleeding is often associated with hepatic encephalopathy and, in these circumstances and when bleeding is severe, endotracheal intubation will be required to provide definitive airway protection prior to endoscopy. Bronchial aspiration is a frequent complication of variceal bleeding.

Summary box 65.9

Management of bleeding oesophageal varices

- Blood transfusion
- Correct coagulopathy
- Oesophageal balloon tamponade (Sengstaken–Blakemore tube)
- Drug therapy (terlipressin)
- Endoscopic sclerotherapy or banding
- Assess portal vein patency (Doppler ultrasound or CT)
- Transjugular intrahepatic portosystemic stent shunts (TIPSS)
- Surgery
    - Portosystemic shunts
    - Splenectomy and gastric devascularisation

If the rate of blood loss prohibits endoscopic evaluation, a Sengstaken–Blakemore tube may be inserted to provide temporary haemostasis (Figure 65.13). Once inserted, the gastric balloon is inflated with 300 mL of air and retracted to the gastric fundus, where the varices at the oesophagogastric junction are tamponaded by the subsequent inflation of the oesophageal balloon to a pressure of 40 mmHg. The two remaining channels allow gastric and oesophageal aspiration. The position of the tube is confirmed radiologically. The balloons should be temporarily deflated after 12 hours to prevent pressure necrosis of the oesophagus. Aspiration pneumonia and oesophageal ulceration are other complications. Balloon tamponade is very effective in stopping bleeding and once the patient is stabilised, a more definitive treatment can be carried out.

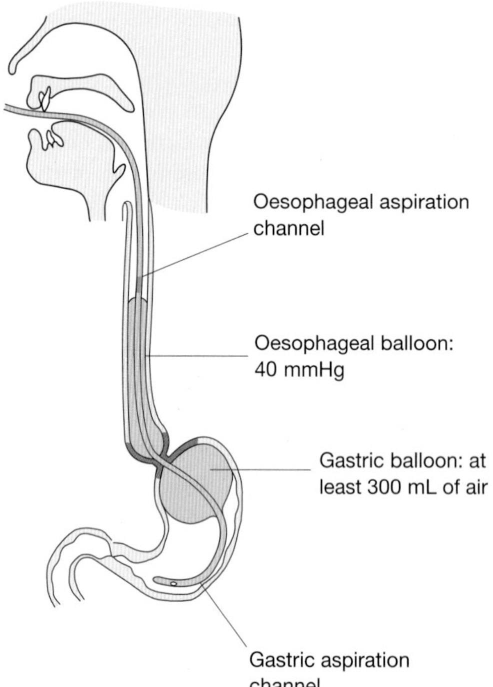

Figure 65.13 Oesophageal balloon tamponade with a Sengstaken–Blakemore tube. The tube should be decompressed every 12 hours to prevent necrosis.

Endoscopic treatment of varices

Treatment with a vasoconstrictor combined with endoscopic therapy is the standard medical treatment for acute variceal bleeding. The two most commonly used endoscopic techniques are endoscopic band ligation, which involves placing a constricting rubber band at the base of the varix, and endoscopic sclerotherapy, which involves injection of a sclerosant into or around the varix. Although both are effective in controlling the bleed, banding is signficantly better in preventing rebleeding and is the preferred option. The majority of variceal bleeds will respond to a single course of endoscopic treatment.

Transjugular intrahepatic portosystemic stent shunts

The emergency management of variceal haemorrhage has been revolutionised by the introduction of transjugular intrahepatic portosystemic stent shunts (TIPSS). Over a short period, this has become the main treatment of variceal haemorrhage that has not responded to drug treatment and endoscopic therapy. The shunts are inserted under local anaesthetic, analgesia and sedation, using fluoroscopic guidance and ultrasonography. Via the internal jugular vein and SVC, a guidewire is inserted into a hepatic vein and through the hepatic parenchyma into a branch of the portal vein. The track through the parenchyma is then dilated with a balloon catheter to allow insertion of a metallic stent, which is expanded once a satisfactory position is achieved (Figure 65.14) to form a channel between systemic and portal venous systems. A satisfactory drop in portal venous pressure is usually associated with good control of the variceal haemorrhage. The main early complication of this technique is perforation of the liver capsule, which can be associated with fatal intraperitoneal haemorrhage. TIPSS occlusion may result in further variceal haemorrhage and occurs more commonly in patients with well-compensated liver disease and good synthetic function. Post-shunt encephalopathy is a confusional state caused by the portal blood bypassing the detoxification of the liver. It occurs in about 40% of patients, a similar incidence to that found after surgical shunts. If severe, the lumen of the TIPSS can be reduced by insertion of a smaller stent. The main contraindication to TIPSS is portal vein occlusion. The main long-term complication of TIPSS is stenosis of the shunt, which is common (approximately 50% at 1 year) and may present as further variceal haemorrhage.

Robert William Sengstaken Sr., 1923–1978, neurosurgeon, Garden City, New York, NY, USA.
Arthur Blakemore, 1897–1970, surgeon, The Columbia College of Physicians and Surgeons, New York, NY, USA.

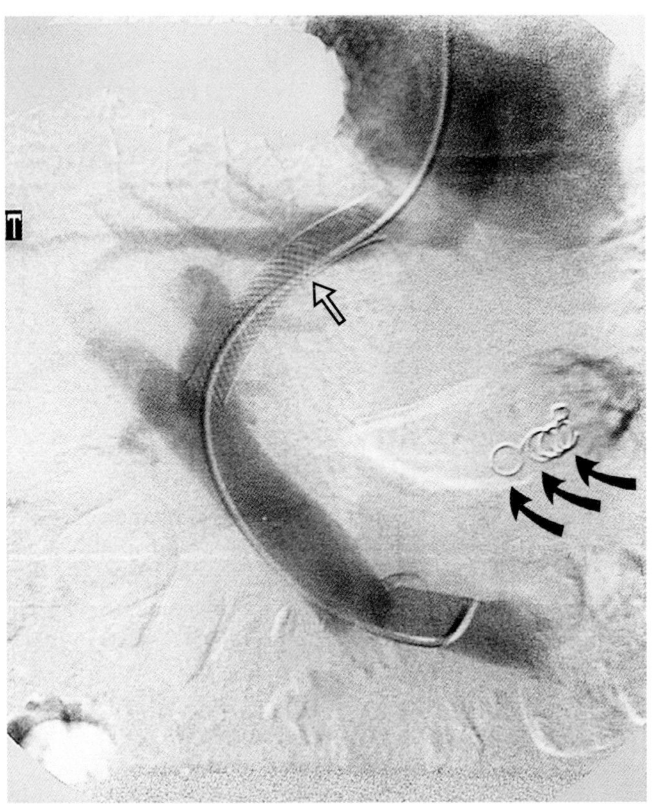

Figure 65.14 A check angiogram following insertion of a TIPSS (transjugular intrahepatic portosystemic stent shunt) (open arrow). Injection of contrast into the portal vein flows through the metallic stent and outlines the right hepatic vein. Pressure measurements are taken from within the portal vein before and after insertion. Solid arrows indicate coils placed at the site of previous embolisation.

Surgical shunts for variceal haemorrhage

The increasing availability of liver transplantation and TIPSS has greatly reduced the indications for surgical shunts. It is rarely considered for the acute management of variceal haemorrhage, as the morbidity and mortality in these circumstances are high. The main current indication for a surgical shunt is a patient with CTP grade A cirrhosis, in whom the initial bleed has been controlled by sclerotherapy. Long-term β-blocker therapy and chronic sclerotherapy or banding are the main alternatives. β-blockers lower portal pressure by a combination of vasodilation and decreasing cardiac output, reducing the risk of subsequent rebleeds.

Surgical shunts are an effective method of preventing rebleeding from oesophageal or gastric varices, as they reduce the pressure in the portal circulation by diverting the blood into the low-pressure systemic circulation. Shunts may be divided into selective (e.g. splenorenal) and non-selective (e.g. portocaval), the former attempting to preserve blood flow to the liver while decompressing the left side of the portal circulation responsible for giving rise to the oesophageal and gastric varices (Figure 65.15). Selective shunts are associated with a lower incidence of portal systemic encephalopathy (PSE), a confusional state commonly found in patients with chronic liver disease who have undergone radiological or surgical portosystemic shunts. There is no evidence that prophylactic shunting is beneficial in patients with varices that have not bled.

Management of recurrent variceal bleeds secondary to splenic or portal vein thrombosis

Treatment is by splenectomy and gastro-oesophageal devascularisation, in which the blood supply to the greater and lesser curve of the stomach and lower oesophagus is divided. Splenic vein thrombosis may be seen secondary to chronic

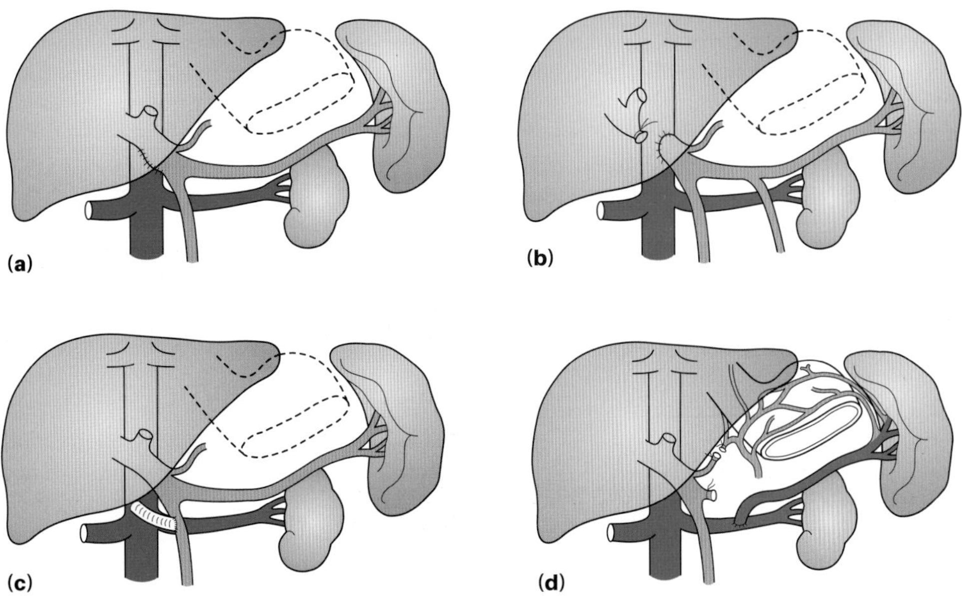

Figure 65.15 (a-d) Surgical shunts. Surgical shunts for portal hypertension involve shunting portal blood into the systemic veins. This commonly involves a side-to-side portocaval anastomosis (a) or end-to-side portocaval (b), mesocaval (c) or splenorenal (d) anastomoses.

pancreatitis, and portal vein thrombosis is a common late complication of liver cirrhosis.

Variceal bleeding and orthotopic liver transplantation

Liver transplantation is the only therapy that will treat both portal hypertension and the underlying liver disease. The management of variceal bleeding should always take into account the possibility of liver transplantation when this is available. Previous surgical shunts greatly increase the morbidity associated with orthotopic liver transplantation. TIPSS would be the preferred management for bleeds resistant to sclerotherapy, as long as placement is optimal.

Ascites

The accumulation of ascites is a common feature of advanced liver disease independent of the aetiology. The fluid accumulation is usually associated with abdominal discomfort and a dragging sensation. Development is usually insidious. The aetiology of the ascites must be established.

Summary box 65.10

Determining the cause of ascites

- Imaging (ultrasound or CT)
    - Irregular cirrhotic liver
    - Portal vein patency
    - Splenomegaly of cirrhosis
- Aspiration
    - Culture and microscopy
    - Protein content
    - Cytology
    - Amylase level

Imaging by CT will confirm the ascites and demonstrate the irregular and shrunken nature of a cirrhotic liver and associated portal hypertension and splenomegaly. Intravenous contrast enhancement will allow abdominal varices to be demonstrated and assess patency of the portal vein, as portal vein thrombosis is a common predisposing factor to the development of ascites in chronic liver disease. In patients without evidence of liver disease, malignancy is a common cause, and the primary site may also be established on CT. Aspiration of the peritoneal fluid allows the measurement of protein content to determine whether the fluid is an exudate or transudate, and an amylase estimation to exclude pancreatic ascites. Cytology will determine the presence of malignant cells, and both microscopy and culture will exclude primary bacterial and tuberculous peritonitis.

Treatment of ascites in chronic liver disease

The initial treatment is to restrict additional salt intake and commence diuretics using either spironolactone or furosemide. This should be combined with advice on avoiding any precipitating factors for impaired liver function, such as alcohol intake in patients with alcoholic cirrhosis. Patients on diuretics should be monitored for the development of hyponatraemia and hypokalaemia.

Summary box 65.11

Treatment of ascites in chronic liver disease

- Salt restriction
- Diuretics
- Abdominal paracentesis
- TIPSS
- Liver transplantation

Abdominal paracentesis

Patients who fail to respond to diuretic treatment may require repeated percutaneous aspiration of large volumes of the ascites (abdominal paracentesis), combined with volume replacement using salt-poor or standard human albumin solution, dependent on the serum sodium level. Paracentesis provides only short-term symptomatic relief.

TIPSS for ascites

The use of TIPSS for ascites is for symptomatic relief. In patients with intractable ascites, TIPSS is a good alternative to repeated paracentesis but post-stent encephalopathy is common (about 40%), and the majority of stents will stenose or thrombose on follow-up (approximately 50% by 1 year).

Liver transplantation for ascites

Diuretic-resistant ascites is an indication for liver transplantation if associated with deterioration in liver function (rising bilirubin, dropping albumin, prolonged prothrombin time). The patient's age, underlying aetiology of liver disease and associated medical problems will be the major factors determining suitability for liver transplantation. In those considered inappropriate for liver transplantation, management is aimed at symptomatic control of ascites.

CHRONIC LIVER CONDITIONS

There are several chronic liver conditions, which, although rare, are important to recognise because they require a specific plan for investigation and treatment, and may present mimicking a more common clinical condition (*Table 65.4*).

Budd-Chiari syndrome

Budd–Chiari syndrome (BCS) is a condition principally affecting young females, in which the venous drainage of the liver is occluded by hepatic venous thrombosis or obstruction from a venous web. As a result of venous outflow obstruction, the liver becomes acutely congested, with the development of impaired liver function and, subsequently, portal hypertension, ascites and oesophageal varices. In an acute thrombosis, the patient may rapidly progress to fulminant liver failure but,

TABLE 65.4 Important chronic liver conditions.

Condition	Common presentations
Budd–Chiari syndrome	Ascites
Primary sclerosing cholangitis	Abnormal LFTs or jaundice
Primary biliary cirrhosis	Malaise, lethargy, itching, abnormal LFTs
Caroli's disease	Abdominal pain, sepsis
Simple liver cysts	Coincidental finding, pain
Polycystic liver disease	Hepatomegaly, pain

LFTs, liver function tests.

in the majority of cases, abdominal discomfort and ascites are the main presenting features. If chronic, the liver progresses to established cirrhosis. The cause of the venous thrombosis needs to be established, and an underlying myeloproliferative disorder or procoagulant state is commonly found, such as antithrombin 3, protein C or protein S deficiency. The diagnosis is commonly suspected in a patient presenting with ascites, in whom a CT scan shows a large congested liver or a small cirrhotic liver in which there is gross enlargement of segment I (the caudate lobe); this feature results from preservation and hypertrophy of the segment with direct venous drainage to the IVC in the face of atrophy of the rest of the liver due to venous obstruction. IVC compression or occlusion from the segment I hypertrophy is also a common feature, as is portal vein thrombosis.

Treatment of BCS must be tailored to the individual patient and, in particular, to the stage of disease at presentation. Patients presenting in fulminant liver failure should be considered for liver transplantation, as should those with established cirrhosis and the complications of portal hypertension. Those in whom cirrhosis is not established may be considered for portosystemic shunting by TIPSS. IVC compression may be relieved by the insertion of a retrohepatic expandable metallic stent. If the BCS is treated satisfactorily, the prognosis of this patient group is largely dependent on the underlying aetiology and whether this is amenable to treatment. Patients are usually left on lifelong anticoagulation.

Primary sclerosing cholangitis

This condition often presents in young adults with mild non-specific symptoms, and biliary disease is suggested by the finding of abnormal liver function tests. Rarely, the first presentation is with jaundice due to biliary obstruction. The disease process results in progressive fibrous stricturing and obliteration of both the intrahepatic and the extrahepatic bile ducts. Although the aetiology is unknown, a genetic predisposition is likely, owing to its association with ulcerative colitis (UC). In patients with primary sclerosing cholangitis (PSC) and UC, the condition usually progresses even if the diseased colon is removed. The diagnosis is principally based on the findings at cholangiography, in which irregular, narrowed bile ducts are demonstrated in both the intrahepatic and the extrahepatic biliary tree (Figure 65.16). If the radiological appearances are equivocal, a liver biopsy is required to demonstrate the fibrous obliteration of the biliary tracts. There is no specific treatment that can reverse the ductal changes, and the patients usually slowly progress to progressive cholestasis and death from liver failure. There is a strong predisposition to cholangiocarcinoma (CCA) and gallbladder cancer, and this should be considered in any patient with PSC in whom a new or dominant stricture is demonstrated on cholangiography, or in whom gallbladder polyps are identified.

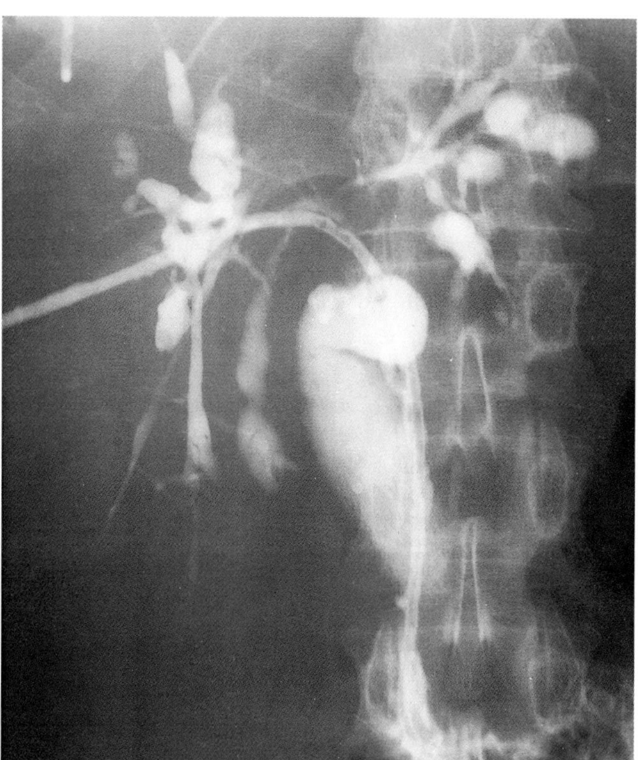

Figure 65.16 Primary sclerosing cholangitis (PSC). Percutaneous cholangiography showing the characteristic extensive bile duct strictures and dilatations associated with PSC.

Diagnosis of CCA in PSC is greatly facilitated by biliary brush cytology and direct endoscopic inspection (Spyglass, see above), as imaging rarely shows evidence of a mass lesion even in patients with advanced CCA. Further, imaging cannot reliably differentiate between inflammatory and malignant biliary strictures. Serum CA 19-9 level may be increased but the sensitivity of CA 19-9 in detecting CCA in PSC is only 60%. Patients with good liver function, no dominant strictures and negative biliary cytology may simply be monitored for disease progression. The only useful treatment modality is liver transplantation, which is associated with excellent results if carried out before bile duct cancer has developed. Temporary relief of obstructive jaundice due to a dominant bile duct stricture can be achieved by biliary stenting, although there is considerable risk of cholangitis from the introduction of bacteria to the biliary tract.

Primary biliary cirrhosis

As with PSC, the presentation of patients with primary biliary cirrhosis (PBC) is often hidden, with general malaise, lethargy and pruritus prior to the development of clinical jaundice or the finding of abnormal liver function tests. The condition is largely confined to females. Diagnosis is suggested by the finding of circulating antismooth muscle antibodies and, if necessary, is confirmed by liver biopsy. The condition is slowly progressive, with deterioration in liver function resulting in lethargy and malaise. It may be complicated by the development of portal hypertension and the secondary complications of ascites and variceal bleeding. The mainstay of treatment is liver transplantation, which should be considered when the patient's general condition starts to deteriorate with inability to lead a normal lifestyle.

Caroli's disease

This is congenital dilatation of the intrahepatic biliary tree, which is often complicated by the presence of intrahepatic stone formation. Presentation may be with abdominal pain or sepsis. Imaging is usually diagnostic, with the finding on ultrasound or CT of intrahepatic biliary lakes containing stones. Biliary stasis and stone formation combine to predispose to biliary sepsis, which may be life-threatening. No specific treatment is available. Acute infective episodes are treated with antibiotics. Obstructed and septic bile ducts may be drained either radiologically or surgically. Malignant change within the ductal system results in cholangiocarcinoma, which may be amenable to resection. Segmental involvement of the liver by Caroli's disease may be treated by resection of the affected part, although the ductal dilatation is usually diffuse. Liver transplantation is a radical but definitive treatment.

Simple cystic disease

Simple cysts are generally solitary, and occur more frequently in women. Most are incidental findings, and have a characteristic blue hue when seen at laparoscopy. Indications for surgical intervention include symptoms, rupture, haemorrhage, infection or indeterminate diagnosis. Surgical resection typically involves laparoscopic deroofing, with oversewing of the cyst wall. Polycystic liver disease is less common. It is an autosomal dominant condition, more commonly seen in women, and around half of patients will also have polycystic kidneys. Indications for surgical intervention are broadly similar to those for simple cysts, although the large number of lesions means that deroofing a single cyst is unlikely to relieve symptoms.

LIVER INFECTIONS

Ascending cholangitis

Ascending bacterial infection of the biliary tract is usually associated with obstruction and presents with clinical jaundice, rigors and a tender right upper quadrant (Charcot's triad). The diagnosis is confirmed by the finding of dilated bile ducts on ultrasound, an obstructive picture of liver function tests and the isolation of an organism from the blood on culture. The condition is a medical emergency, and delay in appropriate treatment results in multiorgan failure secondary to septicaemia. Once the diagnosis has been confirmed, the patient should be commenced on a first-line broad spectrum antibiotic and rehydrated, and arrangements should be made for urgent endoscopic or percutaneous transhepatic drainage of the biliary tree. Biliary stone disease is a common predisposing factor, and the causative ductal stones may be removed at the time of endoscopic cholangiography by endoscopic sphincterotomy.

Pyogenic liver abscess

The aetiology of a pyogenic liver abscess is unexplained in the majority of patients. Common causes include biliary stone disease and other causes of intra-abdominal sepsis, including appendicitis and diverticular disease. It has an increased incidence in the elderly, diabetics and the immunosuppressed, who usually present with anorexia, fevers and malaise, accompanied by right upper quadrant discomfort. The diagnosis is suggested by the finding of a multiloculated cystic mass on ultrasound or CT scan (Figure 65.17) and is confirmed by aspiration for culture and sensitivity. The most common organisms are *Streptococcus milleri* and *Escherichia coli*, but other enteric organisms such as *Streptococcus faecalis*, *Klebsiella* and *Proteus vulgaris* also occur, and mixed growths are common. Opportunistic pathogens include staphylococci. Treatment is with antibiotics and ultrasound-guided aspiration. First-line antibiotics to be used are a penicillin, aminoglycoside and metronidazole or a cephalosporin and metronidazole. Often repeated aspirations may be necessary. Percutaneous drainage without ultrasound guidance should be performed with caution as an empyema may follow drainage through the pleural space. A source for the liver abscess should be sought,

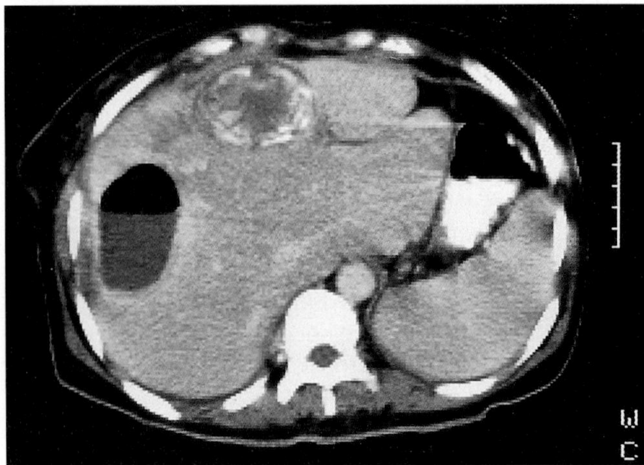

Figure 65.17 Liver abscess. Computed tomography scan showing an air–fluid level and rim enhancement with intravenous contrast typical of a liver abscess. In the adjacent liver is a calcified hydatid cyst.

Jacques Caroli, 1902–1979, Professor of Medicine, St Antoine Hospital, Paris, France, described the disease in 1958.
Jean-Martin Charcot, 1825–1893, French neurologist and Professor of Pathology at Pitié-Salpêtrière Hospital, Paris, France.

particularly from the colon. Atypical clinical or radiological findings should raise the possibility of a necrotic neoplasm.

Amoebic liver abscess

Entamoeba histolytica is endemic in many parts of the world. It exists in vegetative form outside the body and is spread by the faecal–oral route. The most common presentation is with dysentery, but it may also present with an amoebic abscess, the common sites being paracaecal and in the liver. The amoebic cyst is ingested and develops into the trophozoite form in the colon, and then passes through the bowel wall and to the liver via the portal blood. Diagnosis is by isolation of the parasite from the liver lesion or the stool and confirming its nature by microscopy. Often patients with clinical signs of an amoebic abscess will be treated empirically with metronidazole (400–800 mg t.d.s. for 7–10 days) and investigated further only if they do not respond. Resolution of the abscess can be monitored using ultrasound.

Hydatid liver disease

This is a very common condition in countries around the Mediterranean and Middle East. The causative tapeworm, *Echinococcus granulosus*, is present in the dog intestine, and ova are ingested by humans and pass in the portal blood to the liver. Liver abscesses are often large by the time of presentation with upper abdominal discomfort or may present after minor abdominal trauma as an acute abdomen due to rupture of the cyst into the peritoneal cavity. Diagnosis is suggested by the finding of a multiloculated cyst on ultrasound and is further supported by the finding of a floating membrane within the cysts on CT scan (Figure 65.18). Active cysts contain a large number of smaller daughter cysts (Figure 65.19), and rupture can result in these implanting and growing within the peritoneal cavity. Liver cysts can also rupture through the diaphragm producing an empyema, into the biliary tract producing obstructive jaundice, or into the stomach. Clinical and radiological diagnosis can be supported by serology

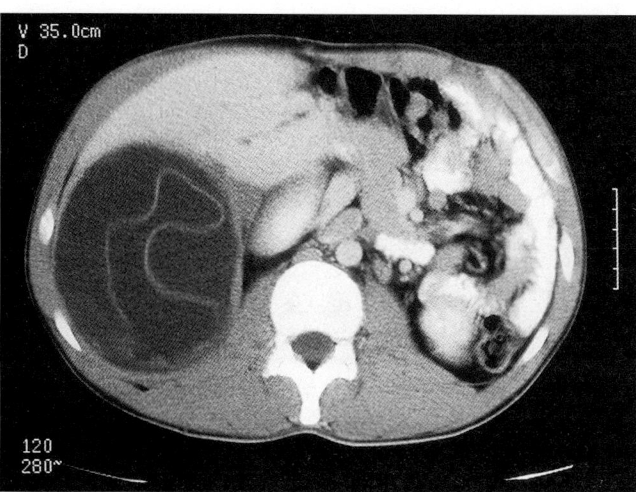

Figure 65.18 Hydatid liver cyst. Active hydatid disease usually produces a non-calcified liver cyst and, within the cyst, floating layers of the germinal membrane can be seen.

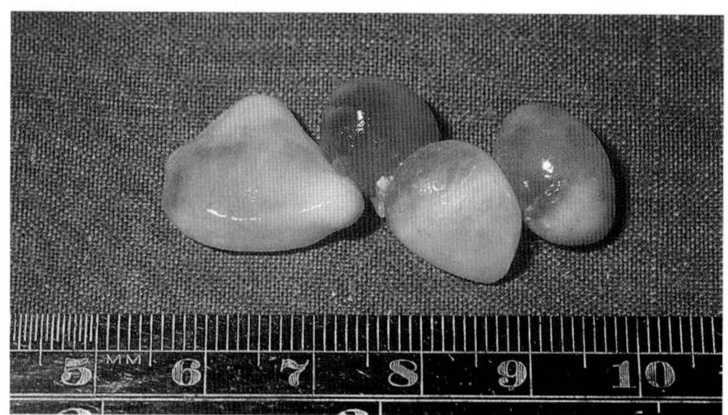

Figure 65.19 Hydatid 'daughter' cysts. These were removed from the bile duct of a patient presenting with obstructive jaundice due to a hydatid liver cyst communicating with the bile duct. Endoscopic removal should also be considered.

for antibodies to hydatid antigen, in the form of an enzyme-linked immunosorbent assay (ELISA). Treatment is indicated to prevent progressive enlargement and rupture of the cysts. In the first instance, a course of albendazole or mebendazole may be tried. There are many reports that percutaneous treatment of hydatid cysts is safe and effective. Percutaneous treatment (PAIR) constitutes of an intial course of albendazole followed by puncture of the cyst under image guidance, aspiration of the cyst's contents, instillation of hypertonic saline in the cyst cavity and reaspiration. PAIR should only be attempted if there is no communication with the biliary tree. Failure to respond to medical treatment or percutaneous treatment usually requires surgical intervention. The surgical options range from liver resection or local excision of the cysts to deroofing with evacuation of the contents. Contamination of the peritoneal cavity at the time of surgery with active hydatid daughters should be avoided by continuing drug therapy with albendazole and adding peroperative praziquantel. This should be combined with packing of the peritoneal cavity with 20% hypertonic saline-soaked packs and instilling 20% hypertonic saline into the cyst before it is opened. A biliary communication should be actively sought and sutured. The residual cavity may become infected, and this may be reduced, as may bile leakage, by packing the space with pedicled greater omentum (an omentoplasty). Calcified cysts may well be dead. If doubt exists as to whether a suspected cyst is active, it can be followed on ultrasound, as active cysts gradually become larger and more superficial in the liver. Rupture of daughter hydatids into the biliary tract may result in obstructive jaundice or acute cholangitis. This may be treated by endoscopic clearance of the daughter cysts prior to cyst removal from the liver.

LIVER TUMOURS

Surgical approaches to resection of liver tumours

Adequate exposure of the liver is an absolute prerequisite to safe liver surgery. A transverse abdominal incision in the right upper quadrant with a vertical midline extension to the xiphoid provides excellent access to the liver if adequate retraction of the costal margin is employed, using a costal margin retractor. If necessary the incision can be extended across the midline transversely in the left upper quadrant. Thoracoabdominal incisions are very rarely required. The procedure for complete mobilisation of the liver is described, although this will not be necessary in all cases. There are many variations in surgical technique.

Mobilisation of the liver

The falciform ligament is first divided and followed along the anterosuperior surface of the liver towards the suprahepatic IVC. The left triangular ligament is divided, facilitated by placing a swab in front of the oesophagogastric junction. The right triangular ligament is then divided by retraction of the diaphragm away from the right lobe. On exposure of the bare area of the liver, the IVC can be seen as it passes behind the liver, and this can be slung above the renal veins below the liver and at the level of the main hepatic veins. Mobilisation of the liver is completed by division of the lesser omentum. Separating the liver from the IVC is achieved by lifting the liver anteriorly, to expose the multiple small veins (inferior hepatic veins) passing between the liver parenchyma and the IVC. These should be suture ligated to ensure haemostasis. This proceeds from above the renal veins until the main named hepatic veins are reached below the diaphragm.

Dissection of the hilum

The peritoneum overlying the hilum is divided. The CBD is then exposed on the free edge of the lesser omentum, mobilisation being facilitated by ligation and division of the cystic duct and artery followed by removal of the gallbladder. Slinging the CBD with an elastic sling allows exposure of the common hepatic artery and dissection of the main right and left branches. These again may be slung to allow the remaining lymphatic tissue surrounding the portal vein to be ligated and divided. The possibility of a replaced right hepatic artery should be sought arising from the superior mesenteric artery and lying posterior to the bile duct (25% of people), and an accessory left hepatic artery from the left gastric artery in the lesser omentum (25% of people). Dissection of the hilar bile ducts requires careful retraction on segment IV of the liver, and division of the small vessels and bile duct branches passing between segment IV and the confluence of the right and left hepatic ducts.

Division of the parenchyma: hemihepatectomy

Once the liver has been adequately mobilised and the hilar vessels have been exposed, the main inflow vessels and bile duct to the liver to be resected can be divided. The arterial branch, bile duct and portal vein branch are all suture ligated. For a hemihepatectomy, division of the inflow vessels in the portal pedicle produces a line of demarcation between the right and left liver, passing to the right of, and parallel with, the falciform ligament. The parenchyma is divided along this plane of demarcation, commencing by diathermy of the liver capsule. The ultrasound dissector (CUSA®, Cavitron ultrasonic surgical aspirator) is the most common method used for division of the parenchyma, but alternative methods including stapling, Kelly-clasia crushing and Aquaseal have all been used. Prospective evidence suggests there is no difference in speed of transection or blood loss between these methods. As the parenchyma is divided, vessels and bile duct branches are diathermised or ligated depending on their size. Dissection continues on until the hepatic vein branches are approached from within the liver parenchyma, when they are ligated or stapled then divided. Alternatively, the hepatic veins can be divided outside the liver at the time of mobilisation (Figure 65.20).

Segmental and local resections

Traditionally, surgical strategy has involved removal of the entire liver segment or hemiliver containing disease, with a view to providing the largest possible negative margin. Although anatomical resection remains the treatment of choice for patients with HCC (Figure 65.21), for those with colorectal liver metastasis a parenchymal-sparing non-anatomical approach involving multiple metastectomies is now considered the standard of care (Figure 65.22). This approach has no impact on long-term oncological outcome, and preserves liver remnants, so allowing the opportunity for further resection in the case of recurrent disease.

Laparoscopic liver resections

Laparoscopic liver surgery aims to provide curative resection while minimising postoperative time to recovery. There are

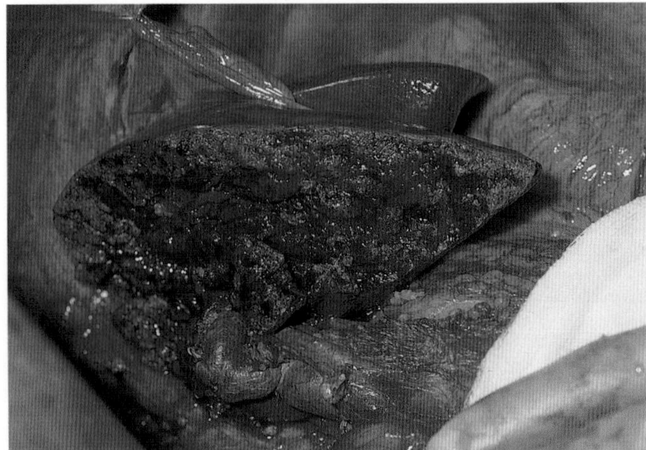

Figure 65.20 Hepatectomy post resection. Cut surface of the residual liver following a right hepatectomy in which segments V–VIII have been removed. On the lower edge, the portal vein and bile duct can be visualised.

Howard A Kelly, 1858–1943, American gynaecologist, who together with William Osler, William Halstead and William Welsh, was one of the founding professors of Johns Hopkins Hospital in Baltimore, MD, USA.

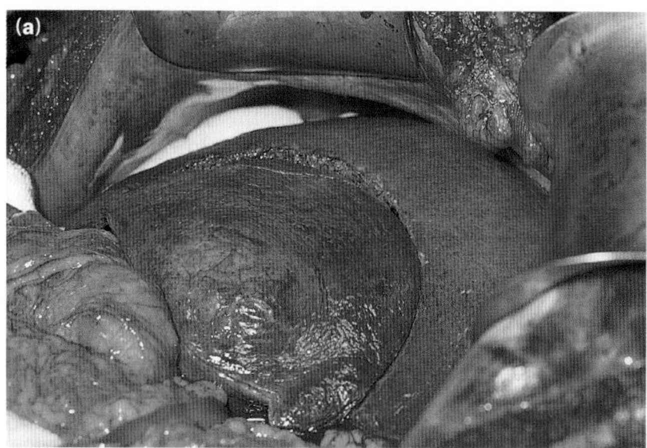

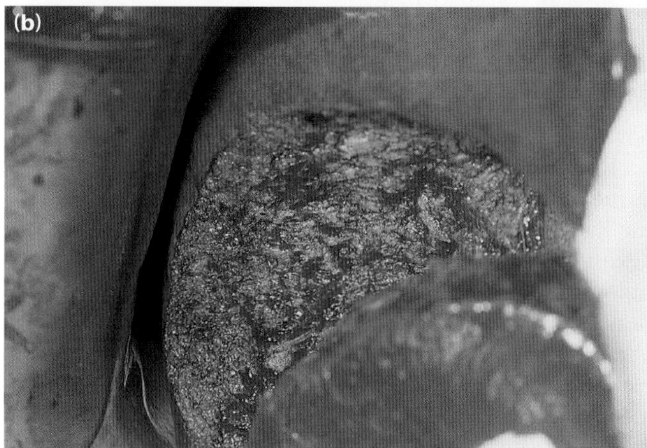

Figure 65.21 (a, b) Segmental resection. Removal of a primary liver tumour by resection of liver segment VI in a patient with well-compensated liver cirrhosis.

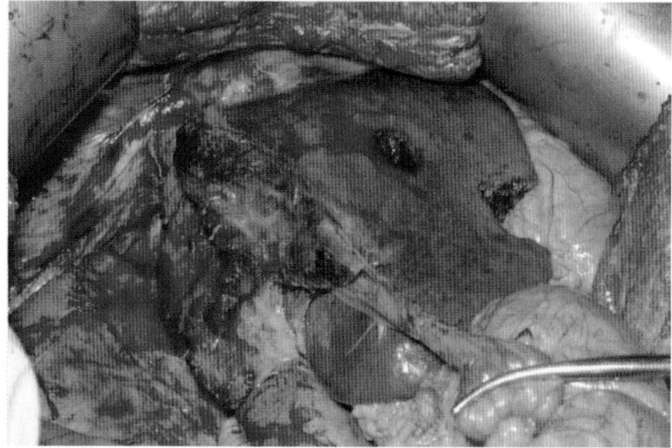

Figure 65.22 Combined anatomical and non-anatomical resection with formal right hemihepatectomy and multiple metastectomies. Sparing the maximal amount of parenchyma is critical for patients with colorectal liver metastases, as it maximises the chance of further resection in the event of disease recurrence.

no randomised controlled trials comparing laparoscopic and open surgery, and so the evidence is based on retrospective series. Meta-analysis suggests that blood loss and duration of hospital stay are significantly reduced after laparoscopic surgery, with no impact on oncological clearance. Prospective studies are underway to validate these findings.

Blood loss and transfusion

The reduction of blood loss during liver surgery has been one of the major achievements in the last 20 years, and resection is often possible without blood transfusion. Better understanding of the segmental anatomy of the liver, better patient selection for surgery and low central venous pressure anaesthesia (<10 mmHg) have all helped to reduce the need for blood transfusions. Better control of the coagulation cascade has been achieved using TEG, and the antifibrinolytic drug aprotinin has significantly reduced bleeding in patients with liver disease and an underlying coagulopathy. Oozing from the resected surface of the remnant liver can be reduced by the topical application of fibrin glue or fibrin-impregnated collagen fleece. The main alternative is use of an argon-beam coagulator. Intermittant temporary clamping of the portal vein and hepatic artery in the hepatoduodenal ligament (Pringle manoeuvre) can reduce blood loss during parenchymal transection. The optimal duration of the Pringle manoeuvre is unknown, but it can be applied intermittently, e.g. cycles of 15 minutes inflow occlusion followed by 5 minutes of reperfusion, until parenchymal transection is complete.

Ablation for liver tumours

Ablative therapies aim to destroy tumour by the direct application of energy to discrete lesions and can be perfomed percutaneously, laparoscopically or at open surgery. There is wide variation in overall survival and local recurrence rates after ablation, so surgery remains the gold standard treatment for resectable disease. Despite these concerns, ablation still has a role as an adjunct to resection. Patients with small volume resectable lesions who are not sufficiently fit to undergo liver resection should be considered for ablation, as should those with limited liver metastases who have insufficient liver volume to undergo resection. In addition, a combined resection/ablation approach has also been advocated.

Radiofrequency ablation (RFA) is the most widely used ablative technique and relies on direct current transmission through tissue to generate heat and ablation of the tumour. Increasing lesion size leads to exponential increases in resistance to current, limiting the size of the effective ablation zone and explaining the increased risk of local recurrence and diminished survival with lesions >3 cm. Microwave ablation has been designed to overcome some of the limitations of RFA and offers higher intratumoural temperatures, larger tumour ablation volumes and faster ablation times. Despite this, local recurrence after microwave ablation has been reported at between 5% and 13%.

Benign liver tumours

Haemangiomas

These are the most common liver lesions, and the reported incidence has increased with the widespread availability of diagnostic ultrasound. They consist of an abnormal plexus of vessels, and their nature is usually apparent on ultrasound. If diagnostic uncertainty exists, CT scanning with delayed contrast enhancement shows the characteristic appearance of slow contrast enhancement due to small vessel uptake in the haemangioma. Often, haemangiomas are multiple. Lesions found incidentally require radiological confirmation of their nature and no further treatment. The management of 'giant' haemangiomas is more controversial. Occasional reports of rupture of haemangiomas have led some to consider resection for large lesions, especially if they appear to be symptomatic. Diagnosis is usually incidental, and surgical resection only recommended if patients are significantly symptomatic or significant diagnostic uncertainty remains after multimodal imaging.

Hepatic adenoma

Adenomas are benign liver tumours seen almost exclusively in women aged between 25 and 50 years. These well-defined and vascular lesions are classically associated with use of the oral contraceptive pill, and are generally solitary. The majority are found incidentally on imaging, although up to one-third may present with pain because of rupture or bleeding. Adenomas are recognised as having malignant potential, with up to 10% developing into hepatocellular carcinoma. The risk of rupture and malignancy means that surgical excision is generally recommended if >5 cm in size, although some lesions may regress after discontinuation of the oral contraceptive pill.

Focal nodular hyperplasia

Focal nodular hyperplasia (FNH) is an unusual but not uncommon benign condition of unknown aetiology, in which there is a focal overgrowth of functioning liver tissue supported by fibrous stroma. Patients are usually middle-aged females, and there is no association with underlying liver disease. Ultrasound shows a solid tumour mass. Contrast CT or MRI may show central scarring and a hypervascular lesion. FNH contains both hepatocytes and Kupffer cells. MRI using liver-specific contrast agents, such as gadoxetic acid, which is taken up by hepatocytes and excreted in bile, or superparamagnetic iron oxide, which is taken up by Kupffer cells, may be useful in determining the hepatocellular origin of FNH and allowing differentiation of FNH from metastatic cancer. FNH does not have any malignant potential and once the diagnosis is confirmed, does not require any treatment or follow-up.

Colorectal liver metastases

Twenty years ago, a diagnosis of stage IV (metastatic) colorectal cancer was associated with a survival of less than 3% at 5 years. A small minority of patients with liver-only metastatic disease were offered surgical resection and these patients had a 50% chance of being alive after 5 years. These excellent long-term outcomes highlighted the potential survival benefits of resection in appropriate cases, and lead to a revolution in the approach to metastatic colorectal disease. Instead of a terminal diagnosis, it was recognised that in certain situations resection could offer a cure.

Around 30% of patients with colorectal cancer will have metastatic disease at the time of presentation, and a further 20% will develop liver disease after the primary colorectal malignancy has been resected. In 2016, 20% of these patients will be candidates for upfront curative liver surgery and a further 20–30% of patients with initially unresectable liver disease may achieve a response to systemic therapy of sufficient magnitude to render the liver disease resectable (see below).

Defining resectability for colorectal liver metastases

Previously, patients with synchronous disease, rectal primary, multiple diffuse metastases, metastases larger than 5 cm, disease-free interval of less than 1 year from the diagnosis of primary disease or a high serum carcinoembryonic antigen (CEA) were considered irresectable and suitable only for palliative treatment. Modern surgical techniques and chemotherapeutic regimes mean none of these contraindications now hold true.

Resectability with curative intent is now loosely defined as the ability to successfully remove all residual disease from the liver with clear surgical margins, while leaving adequate disease-free viable liver tissue to sustain life. Technical contraindications to resection are related to the anatomical location of metastases, mainly due to close proximity to major vascular or biliary drainage structures. The boundaries of technical resectability have been extended by the development of techniques such as total vascular exclusion, which offer hope for certain patients with involvement of major vessels. Resection with a negative surgical margin of 1 cm (R0) has always been considered the gold standard, but in an era of effective modern chemotherapy, patients with R1 (microscopically negative) resection have similar survival to those with R0 resections. A future liver remnant (FLR) of 25% preoperative volume is considered sufficient to prevent postoperative hepatic failure, although patients with impaired hepatic function, including those with chemotherapy-induced liver damage, may require a larger FLR. The regenerative nature of liver parenchyma means that significant regrowth takes place after resection, and this unique feature means that two-stage procedures are feasible, with parenchymal regeneration between resections ensuring adequate FLR. This regenerative capacity can be further manipulated further using preoperative portal vein embolisation (PVE) to cause reactive hypertrophy in the proposed FLR.

The ALPPS procedure (associating liver partition and portal vein ligation for staged hepatectomy) combines both these procedures, maximising hypertrophy of the FLR, but is associated with significant operative mortality (10%) and morbidity (>50%). For some patients, a combination of resection and thermal ablation may also offer long-term benefits.

Oncological contraindications to hepatic resection include unresectable extrahepatic malignancy. Twenty years ago, any extrahepatic metastatic disease was considered a contraindication to liver resection. However, long-term survival is now possible in selected groups of patients with resected extrahepatic disease. Survival after lung resection for colorectal metastases is similar to that seen after liver resection, with most series quoting a 5-year survival in the order of 40–50%, with low operative morbidity and mortality.

Staging and selection of patients for liver surgery

Patients with colorectal liver metastases must be fully staged prior to any treatment plan and this should be coordinated by a specialist multidisciplinary team. Routine staging commonly involves triple phase CT chest/abdomen/pelvis (Figure 65.23), contrast MRI scan of the liver and whole body PET-CT to identify metastatic disease.

Chemotherapy for colorectal liver metastases

The precise role of adjuvant and neoadjuvant chemotherapy in the management of resectable disease remains controversial. Current consensus is that the majority of patients with colorectal liver metastases should receive perioperative chemotherapy irrespective of their initial resectability, with the rationale that this will result in the destruction of occult disease, and allow a test of biology where progression despite chemotherapy signifies poorer prognosis, as well as reducing lesion size and so improving resectability.

A major development in the chemotherapeutic management of advanced disease over the last 20 years has been the recognition that there is a subgroup of patients who may not be resectable at presentation, but become resectable after systemic chemotherapy as lesions decrease in size and move away from critical vascular and biliary structures. Resectability rates after chemotherapy for initially irresectable disease vary widely from 6% to 60%. Attempting to convert irresectable disease into resectable is a worthwhile aim, with 5-year survival around 35–50% if liver resection becomes feasible, similar to those patients who are able undergo resection at the time of presentation. Chemotherapy with 5-fluorouracil (5FU) and folinic acid produces a response rate of approximately 30% but, when combined with oxaliplatin, the response rate increases to 50–60%, often with a dramatic size reduction of the lesions. The combination of chemotherapy with monoclonal antibodies (mAbs) that recognise vascular endothelial growth factor receptor (VEGFR) or the epidermal growth factor receptor (EGFR) may provide additional benefit.

Hepatocellular carcinoma

HCC comprises the overwhelming majority of primary liver cancers, with a steadily rising global burden. There is wide variation in the geographical incidence of HCC, with >80% of cases occurring in Asia and sub-Saharan Africa, with an incidence of 99 per 100 000. By contrast, the incidence in Europe is considerably lower (approximately 5 per 100000). The wide variations in distribution reflect the varying incidence of aetiological factors known to be integral to the development of hepatocellular carcinogenesis (*Table 65.5*). Chronic hepatitis B virus (HBV) infection accounts for >50% of cases of HCC worldwide. HBV as a risk factor for HCC is supported by strong evidence that HBV vaccination programmes have led to falls in the incidence of HCC in high-risk areas such as Hong Kong. Hepatitis C virus (HCV) increases the risk of HCC by 17 times, primarily by promoting end-stage liver disease. There is clear evidence that lifetime alcohol exposure correlates with the incidence of HCC. Hepatic metabolism of alcohol is thought to lead to the production of free radicals, causing intracellular oxidative stress eventually leading to a chronic inflammatory state. Because of the critical role of the liver in glucose metabolism, it is not surprising that obesity and diabetes mellitus (both of which involve impaired glucose handling) are significant independent risk factors for the development of HCC, and the global rise in obesity and diabetes is likely to lead to a significant increase in HCC developing on a background of hepatic non-alcoholic fatty liver disease (NAFLD).

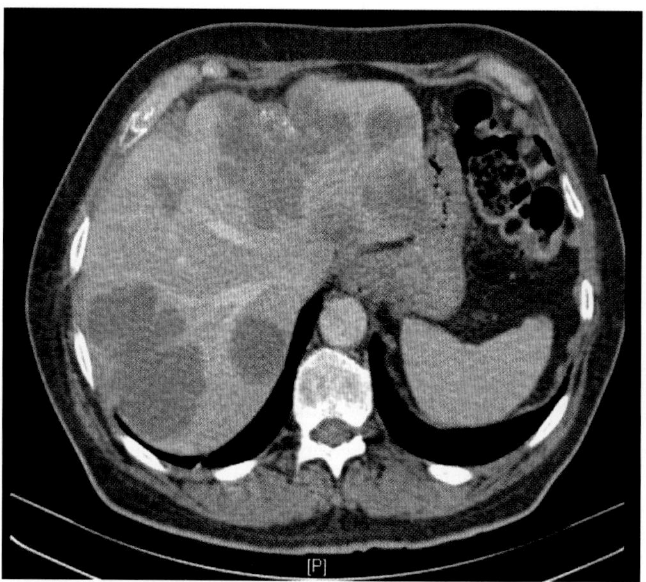

Figure 65.23 Colorectal liver metastases on a computed tomography scan.

TABLE 65.5 Liver infections and their treatment.

Condition	Causative agent	Treatment
Viral hepatitis	Hepatitis A, B, C	Supportive, antiviral agents (lamivudine, interferon, ribavirin)
		Liver transplant for cirrhosis
Ascending cholangitis	Enteric bacteria	Antibiotics (cephalosporin)
		Relieve obstruction
Pyogenic liver abscess	*Streptococcus milleri*	Antibiotics
	Escherichia coli	Aspiration
	Streptococcus faecalis	Drainage
Amoebic liver abscess	Entamoeba	Metronidazole
Hydatid liver disease	Echinococcus	Mebendazole, Resection/omentoplasty

Cohort studies have suggested that 60% of patients with HCC die of cancer-related causes, with the remaining 40% succumbing to underlying parenchymal liver disease. It is therefore critical that treatments for patients with HCC are considered in the context of both the cancer and the underlying parenchymal disease.

Staging of hepatocellular carcinoma

Clinical staging systems for HCC are often designed to guide choice of therapy, the most commonly used being the Barcelona Clinic Liver Group (BCLC) staging system, which was initially designed to define both prognosis and optimal treatment for patients with HCC (Figure 65.24). As patients with HCC usually have underlying liver disease as well as cancer (both of which have a marked impact on prognosis), the BCLC system was designed to reflect underlying liver function and patient performance status as well as characteristics of the tumour. Underlying liver function is assessed using the CTP system (see *Table 65.2*).

Surgical resection for HCC

Only 20–40% of patients with HCC are considered candidates for surgical resection. However, with the introduction of surveillance programmes for those patients identified to be at risk, improved imaging and better perioperative management, surgical resection is increasingly considered the mainstay of treatment for patients with preserved hepatic function.

Considerable controversy remains over which patients should be considered surgical candidates. Although tumour size, vascular invasion and multifocal disease are recognised as poor prognostic indicators, none is considered an absolute contraindication to surgical intervention. Multinodular lesions present a particular management challenge. These may represent multiple discrete lesions occurring independently against a background of procarcinogenic parenchymal damage, or may represent aggressive tumour biology with intrahepatic metastases.

In general, oncological contraindications to resection now include: (1) extrahepatic metastasis; (2) multiple and

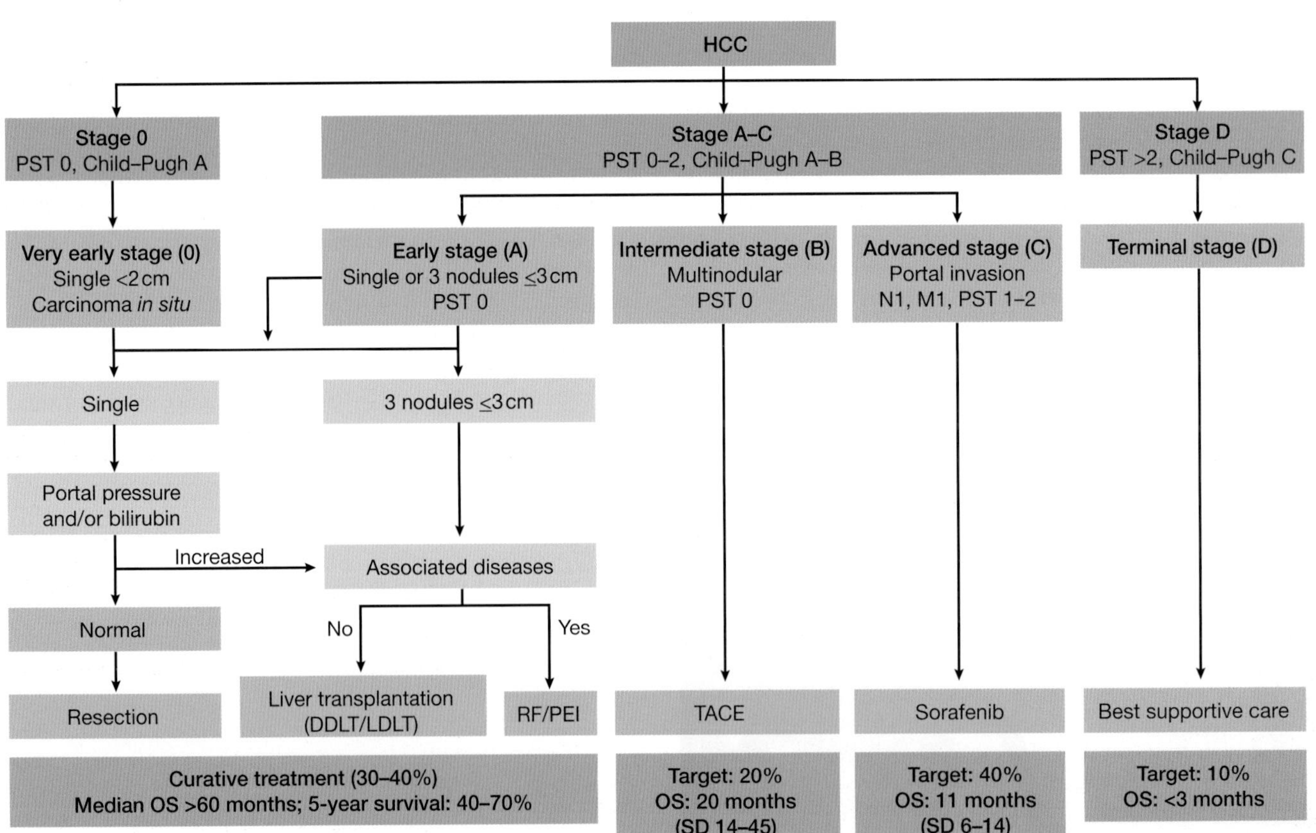

Figure 65.24 The Barcelona Clinic Liver Group staging system for the management of hepatocellular carcinoma (HCC). Patients with asymptomatic early tumours (stage 0–A) are candidates for curative therapies (resection, transplantation or local ablation). Asymptomatic patients with multinodular HCC (stage B) are suitable for chemoembolisation (TACE), whereas patients with advanced symptomatic tumours and/or an invasive tumoural pattern (stage C) are candidates for sorafenib. End-stage disease (stage D) includes patients with grim prognosis who should be treated by best supportive care. DDLT, deceased donor liver transplantation; LDLT, living donor liver transplantation; OS, overall survival; PEI, percutaneous ethanol injection; PST, ECOG performance status; RF, radiofrequency ablation; SD, standard deviation; TACE, transcatheter arterial chemoembolisation. (Reproduced with permission from Villanueva A. Medical therapies for hepatocellular carcinoma: a critical view of the evidence. *Nature Rev Gastroenterolol Hepatol* 2013; **10**: 34–42).

bilobar tumours; (3) involvement of the main bile duct; and (4) presence of tumour thrombus in the main portal vein/vena cava. However, reasonable long-term outcomes from highly selected patients outside these contraindications have also been reported.

Preoperative evaluation of patients with HCC

Ensuring good outcome for patients undergoing surgical resection for HCC relies on an accurate assessment of tumour stage, patient fitness and underlying liver function. This is particularly important when considering patients for larger resections, where the function of the FLR becomes critical. Postoperative morbidity and mortality are known to increase with a higher CTP score, and major liver resection is generally only considered feasible in patients with CTPA disease. Minor liver resection may be considered in CTP grade B, but remains a high-risk procedure. CTP grade C score patients are not candidates for liver resection. For some patients, inadequate FLR may the only contraindication to surgical resection. For this group, preoperative radiological portal vein embolisation can be performed to induce hypertrophy in the proposed remnant liver, increasing the FLR.

Preoperative imaging for HCC

Imaging is a critical part of the pretreatment assessment of HCC. Accurate tumour staging and anatomical assessment is essential, to determine both technical and oncological resectability, as well as to exclude distant metastatic spread. Triple phase CT chest/abdomen/pelvis and MRI of the liver is considered standard of care in most units. However, both MRI and CT have limited sensitivity and specificity for detection of lesions <1 cm, although this is improved with the use of liver-specific contrast agents. There is also growing interest in the assessment of background liver fibrosis and cirrhosis with functional imaging techniques that use hepatospecific contrast medium. The use of FDG-PET to exclude extrahepatic involvement has been investigated, but it remains unclear whether this offers any benefit over standard CT chest/abdomen/pelvis.

Surgical principles for HCC

The objectives of surgical resection for HCC can appear contradictory: (1) resection of all malignant and as much preneoplastic tissue as possible; and (2) preserving enough functional hepatic parenchyma to reduce the risk of postoperative liver failure. HCC spreads within the liver by direct invasion of both the portal and hepatic venous systems, and anatomical resection that includes removal of the entire venous drainage of a HCC is therefore considered the optimal approach to increase the removal of occult micrometastases. There is a clear long-term survival advantage to anatomical versus non-anatomical resection, and this approach is now considered standard of care where underlying liver function allows. Improvements in patient selection and surgical technique have led to a reduction in mortality, with 30-day postoperative death rates consistently quoted as <5%, including patients with underlying cirrhosis.

Disease recurrence after resection

Intrahepatic recurrence occurs in around 80% of cases within 5 years of resection. There are no effective neoadjuvant or adjuvant treatment options to reduce the risk of recurrence after resection. Intrahepatic recurrence after surgery is thought to consist of two discrete groups: patients who had missed micrometastases at initial staging, and those who developed lesions *de novo* in diseased background liver. The most effective approach to reducing intrahepatic recurrence of HCC is to remove both of these possibilities by performing liver transplantation.

Liver transplantation

Liver transplantation for HCC offers the advantage of not only definitively treating the tumour but also removing the diseased hepatic parenchyma, so reducing the potential for intrahepatic recurrence. The concept of organ transplantation for primary liver cancer was first described by Mazzaferro in 1996, who performed liver transplantation for patients with one hepatocellular carcinoma of ≤5 cm, or up to three nodules of ≤3 cm, and reported a 4-year overall survival of 75% and recurrence-free survival of 83%. Other groups have since replicated these results, and these inclusion criteria (Milan criteria) are now considered the benchmark indications for transplantation for HCC. Patients outside these criteria can also be successfully downstaged using locoregional therapies (such as ablation), and following a period of observation with adequate disease control may be considered suitable candidates for transplantation.

FURTHER READING

Belghiti J, Clavien PA, Gadzijev E *et al.* The Brisbane 2000 terminology of liver anatomy and resections terminology committee of the international hepato-pancreato-biliary association: Chairman, SM Strasberg (USA). *HPB* 2000; **2**(3): 333–9.

Clavien PA. Recommendations for liver transplantation for hepatocellular carcinoma: an international consensus statement. *Lancet Oncol* 2012; **13**(1): 11–22.

Forner A, Llovet JM, Bruix J. Hepatocellular carcinoma. *Lancet* 2012; **379**(9822): 1245–55.

Franklin JM, Sharma RA, Harris AL, Gleeson FV. Imaging oligometastatic cancer before local treatment. *Lancet Oncol* 2016; **17**(9): 406–14.

Jarnagin W. Surgical treatment of hepatocellular carcinoma: expert consensus statement. *HPB* 2010; **12**(5):302–10.

Jones RP, Brudvik KW, Franklin JM, Poston GJ. Precision surgery for colorectal liver metastases: opportunities and challenges of omics-based decision making. *Eur Journ Surg Oncol* 2017; **43**(5): 875–83.

Jones RP, Poston GJ. Resection of liver metastases in colorectal cancer in the era of expanding systemic therapy. *Ann Rev Med* 2017; **68**: 183–96.

Vincenzo Mazzaferro, contemporary surgeon, Milan, Italy.

Chapter 66

The spleen

Learning objectives

To understand:

- The function of the spleen
- The common pathologies involving the spleen
- The principles and potential complications of splenectomy
- The potential advantages of laparoscopic splenectomy
- The benefits of splenic conservation
- The importance of prophylaxis against infection following splenectomy

EMBRYOLOGY, ANATOMY AND PHYSIOLOGY

Embryology

Fetal splenic tissue develops from condensations of mesoderm in the dorsal mesogastrium. This peritoneal fold attaches the dorsal body wall to the fusiform swelling in the foregut that develops into the stomach. This condensation divides the mesogastrium into two parts, one between the fetal splenic tissue and the stomach to form the gastrosplenic ligament and the other between it and the left kidney to form the lienorenal ligament.

Anatomy

The weight of the normal adult spleen is 75–250 g and it measures up to 10 × 7 × 3 cm. It lies in the left hypochondrium between the gastric fundus and the left hemidiaphragm, with its long axis lying along the 10th rib. The hilum sits in the angle between the stomach and the kidney and is in contact with the tail of the pancreas. The concave visceral surface lies in contact with these structures, and the lower pole extends no further than the mid-axillary line. There is a notch on the inferolateral border, and this may be palpated when the spleen is enlarged. The tortuous splenic artery arises from the coeliac axis, usually from a common stem with a hepatic artery, and runs along the upper border of the body and tail of the pancreas, to which it gives small branches. The short gastric and left gastroepiploic branches pass between the layers of the gastrosplenic ligament. The main splenic artery generally divides into superior and inferior branches, which, in turn, subdivide into several segmental branches (Figure 66.1).

The splenic vein is formed from several tributaries that drain the hilum. The vein runs behind the pancreas, receiving several small tributaries from the pancreas before joining the superior mesenteric vein at the neck of the pancreas to form the portal vein.

The splenic pulp is invested by an external serous and internal fibroelastic coat which is reflected inwards at the hilum onto the vessels to form vascular sheaths. The lymphatic drainage comprises efferent vessels in the white pulp that run with the arterioles and emerge from nodes at the hilum. These nodes and lymphatics drain via retropancreatic nodes to the coeliac nodes.

Sympathetic nerve fibres run from the coeliac plexus and innervate splenic arterial branches.

Physiology

The splenic parenchyma consists of white and red pulp that is surrounded by serosa and a collagenous capsule with smooth muscle fibres. These penetrate the parenchyma as trabeculae of dense connective tissue fibres rich in collagen and elastic tissue. These, with the reticular framework, support the cells of the spleen and surround the vessels in the splenic pulp. The white pulp comprises a central trabecular artery surrounded by nodules with germinal centres and periarterial lymphatic sheaths that provide a framework filled with lymphocytes and macrophages. Arteries from the central artery and the peripheral 'penicillar' arteries pass into the marginal zone that lies at the edge of the white pulp. Plasma-rich blood that has passed through the central lymphatic nodules is filtered as it passes through the sinuses within the marginal zone, and particles are phagocytosed.

Immunoglobulins produced in the lymphatic nodules enter the circulation through the sinuses in the marginal

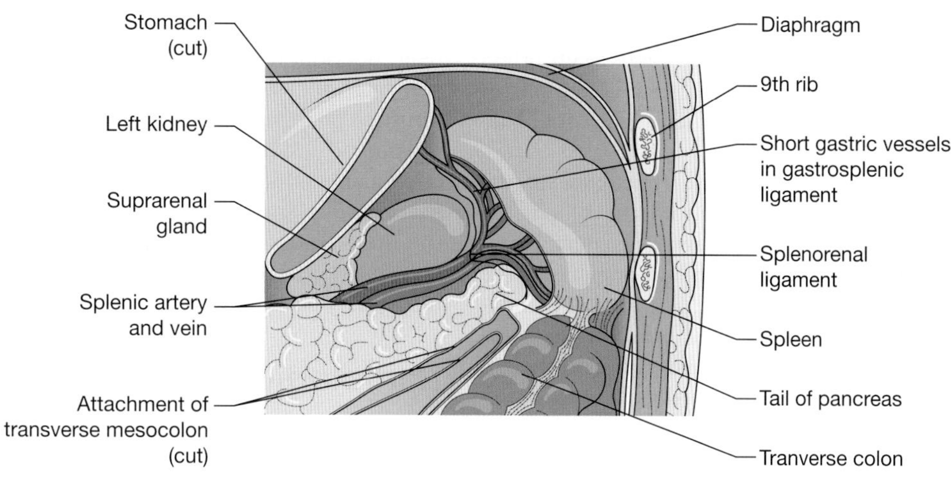

Figure 66.1 Anatomy of the spleen.

zone, beyond which lies the red pulp, which consists of cords and sinuses. Cell-concentrated blood passes in the trabecular artery through the centre of the white pulp to the red pulp cords. Red cells must elongate and become thinner to pass from the cords to the sinuses, a process that removes abnormally shaped cells from the circulation (Figure 66.2). As 90% of the blood passing through the spleen moves through an open circulation in which blood flows from arteries to cords, and thence sinuses, splenic pulp pressure reflects the pressure throughout the portal system. The remaining 10% of the blood flow through the spleen bypasses the cords and sinuses by direct arteriovenous communications. The overall flow rate of blood is about 300 mL/min.

FUNCTIONS OF THE SPLEEN

Although the spleen was previously thought to be dispensable, increasing knowledge of its function has led to a conservative approach in the management of conditions involving the spleen. It is now recognised that an incidental splenectomy during the course of another operative procedure increases the risk of complication and death. The surgeon should therefore normally endeavour to preserve the spleen to maintain the following functions:

- **Immune function**. The spleen contains 66.5% and 10–15% of the body's total T and B lymphocyte population, respectively. It processes foreign antigens and is the

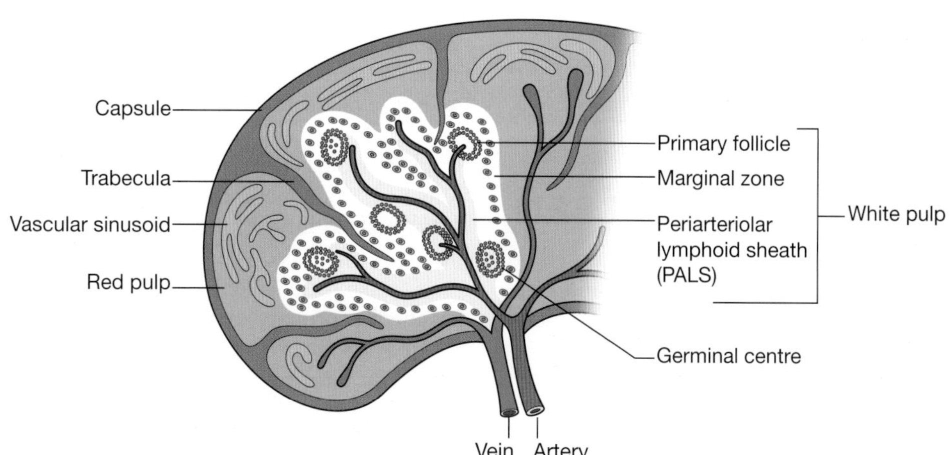

Figure 66.2 Functional anatomy of the spleen. Blood from a central trabecular artery passes through the white pulp into the surrounding red pulp and hence to the vascular cords and sinuses that drain into the trabecular vein.

major site of specific immunoglobulin M (IgM) production. The non-specific opsonins, properdin and tuftsin, are synthesised. These antibodies are of B- and T-cell origin and bind to the specific receptors on the surface of macrophages and leukocytes, stimulating their phagocytic, bactericidal and tumoricidal activity.

- **Filter function**. Macrophages in the reticulum capture cellular and non-cellular material from the blood and plasma. This will include the removal of effete platelets and red blood cells. This process takes place in the sinuses and the splenic cords by the action of the endothelial macrophages. Iron is removed from the degraded haemoglobin during red cell breakdown and is returned to plasma. Removed non-cellular material may include bacteria and, in particular, pneumococci.
- **Pitting**. Particulate inclusions from red cells are removed, and the repaired red cells are returned to the circulation. These include Howell–Jolly and Heinz bodies, which represent nuclear remnants and precipitated haemoglobin or globin subunits, respectively.
- **Reservoir function**. This function in humans is less marked than in other species, but the spleen does contain approximately 8% of the red cell mass. An enlarged spleen may contain a much larger proportion of the blood volume.
- **Cytopoiesis**. From the fourth month of intrauterine life, some degree of haemopoiesis occurs in the fetal spleen. Stimulation of the white pulp may occur following antigenic challenge, resulting in the proliferation of T and B cells and macrophages. This may also occur in myeloproliferative disorders, thalassaemias and chronic haemolytic anaemias.

Summary box 66.1

Functions of the spleen

- Immune
- Filter function
- Pitting
- Reservoir
- Cytopoiesis

INVESTIGATION OF THE SPLEEN

Conditions that result in splenomegaly can be diagnosed on the basis of the history and examination findings and from laboratory examination. In haemolytic anaemia, a full blood count, reticulocyte count and tests for haemolysis will determine the cause of the anaemia. Splenomegaly associated with portal hypertension caused by cirrhosis is diagnosed on the history, physical signs of liver dysfunction, abnormal tests of liver function, often anaemia, leukopenia and thrombocytopenia, as well as endoscopic evidence of oesophageal varices. Sinistral or segmental portal hypertension may result from isolated occlusion of the splenic vein by thrombosis, pancreatic inflammation or tumour infiltration. As many conditions that cause splenomegaly are associated with lymphadenopathy, investigation should be directed at those disease processes known to be associated with both physical signs. Lymph node biopsy may be required.

Radiological imaging

Plain radiology is rarely used in investigation, but the incidental finding of calcification of the splenic artery or spleen may raise the possible diagnosis of a splenic artery aneurysm, an old infarct, a benign cyst or hydatid disease. Multiple areas of calcification may suggest splenic tuberculosis. Ultrasonography can determine the size and consistency of the spleen, and whether a cyst is present. However, computed tomography (CT) with contrast enhancement is more commonly undertaken to better characterise the nature of the suspected splenic pathology and to exclude other intra-abdominal pathology. Magnetic resonance imaging (MRI) may be similarly useful. Radioisotope scanning is used occasionally to provide information about the spleen. The use of technetium-99m (^{99m}Tc)-labelled colloid is normally restricted to determining whether the spleen is a significant site of destruction of red blood cells.

CONGENITAL ABNORMALITIES OF THE SPLEEN

Splenic agenesis is rare but is present in 5% of children with congenital heart disease. Polysplenia is a rare condition resulting from failure of splenic fusion.

Splenunculi are single or multiple accessory spleens that are found in approximately 10–30% of the population. They are located near the hilum of the spleen in 50% of cases and are related to the splenic vessels, or behind the tail of the pancreas in 30%. The remainder are located in the mesocolon, greater omentum or the splenic ligaments. Their significance lies in the fact that failure to identify and remove these at the time of splenectomy may give rise to persistent disease.

Hamartomas are rarely found in life and vary in size from 1 cm in diameter to masses large enough to produce an abdominal swelling. One form is mainly lymphoid and resembles the white pulp, whereas the other resembles the red pulp.

Non-parasitic **splenic cysts** are rare. Splenic cysts are classified as primary cysts (true) or pseudocysts (secondary) on the basis of the presence or absence of lining epithelium. True cysts form from embryonal rests and include dermoid

William Henry Howell, 1860–1945, Professor of Physiology, Johns Hopkins University, Baltimore, MD, USA.
Justin Marie Jules Jolly, 1870–1953, Professor of Histopathology, College de France, Paris, France.
Robert Heinz, 1865–1962, Professor of Pharmacology and Toxicology, Erlangen, Germany.

and mesenchymal inclusion cysts (Figure 66.3). True cysts of the spleen are very rare, and are frequently classified as cystic haemangiomas, cystic lymphangiomas, and epidermoid and dermoid cysts. Epidermoid cysts are thought to be of congenital origin and represent 10% of splenic cysts. They are lined by flattened squamous epithelium and more frequent in children and young patients. Splenectomy or partial splenectomy is usually considered for cysts larger than 5 cm in diameter. These should be differentiated from false or secondary cysts that may result from trauma and contain serous or haemorrhagic fluid. The walls of such degenerative cysts may be calcified and therefore resemble the radiological appearances of a hydatid cyst. The spleen is also a common site for pseudocyst development following a severe attack of pancreatitis (Figure 66.4). Pseudocysts can easily be diagnosed on scanning, and intervention is normally required for symptomatic lesions that persist following a period of observation.

SPLENIC ARTERY ANEURYSM, INFARCT AND RUPTURE

Splenic artery aneurysm

Aneurysms involving the splenic artery are estimated to be identified at 0.04–1% of postmortem examinations. They are twice as common in women and are usually situated in the main arterial trunk. Although these are generally single, more than one aneurysm is found in one-quarter of cases. These may be a consequence of intra-abdominal sepsis and pancreatic necrosis, in particular. They are more likely to be associated with arteriosclerosis in elderly patients.

The aneurysm is symptomless unless it ruptures and is more likely to be detected on a plain abdominal radiograph or scan. It is unlikely to be palpable, although a bruit may be present. Rupture is unsuspected in the majority of cases and, as it will generally rupture into the peritoneal cavity, the symptoms mimic those of splenic rupture. Almost half the cases of rupture occur in patients younger than 45 years of age, and one-quarter are in pregnant women, usually in the third trimester of pregnancy or at labour. Aneurysmal rupture carries a high mortality rate and this increases disproportionately in pregnant women, with almost inevitable fetal death.

The treatment of choice previously consisted of splenectomy and removal of the diseased artery. Some surgeons advocate ligation of the proximal and distal ends of the sac to allow thrombosis of the aneurysm and partial or complete splenectomy, if necessary. The procedure has been performed laparoscopically with success. Embolisation or endovascular stenting following selective splenic artery angiography can be considered, and is now more commonly undertaken. In the younger patient with an asymptomatic splenic artery aneurysm, surgery or interventional radiology is indicated depending on local expertise after CT scan, MRI or selective coeliac angiography has confirmed the diagnosis (Figure 66.5). In the elderly patient with a calcified aneurysm, there is less risk of rupture, and observation may be preferred. In patients with pancreatic necrosis, the treatment will include drainage of the septic focus.

Splenic infarction

This condition commonly occurs in patients with a massively enlarged spleen from myeloproliferative syndrome, portal hypertension or vascular occlusion produced by previous surgical intervention (such as spleen-preserving distal pancreatectomy), pancreatic disease, splenic vein thrombosis or sickle cell disease. The infarct may be asymptomatic or give rise to left upper quadrant and left shoulder tip pain. Contrast-enhanced CT will show the characteristic perfusion defect in the enlarged spleen (Figure 66.6). Treatment is conservative, and splenectomy should be considered only when a septic infarct causes an abscess.

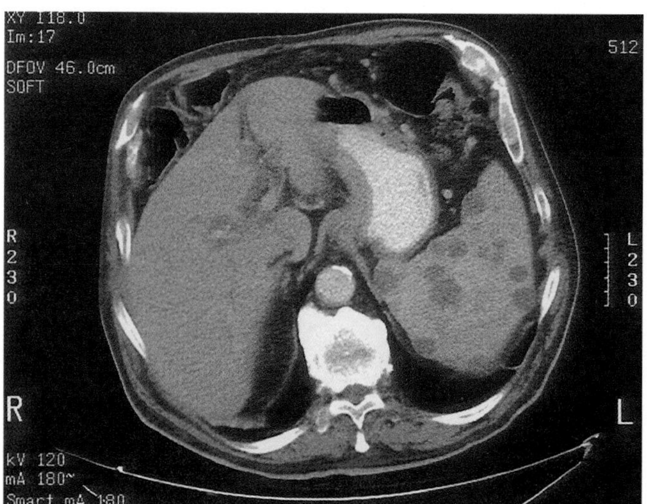

Figure 66.3 Computed tomography scan showing multiple low-density areas in the spleen consistent with multiple benign splenic cysts.

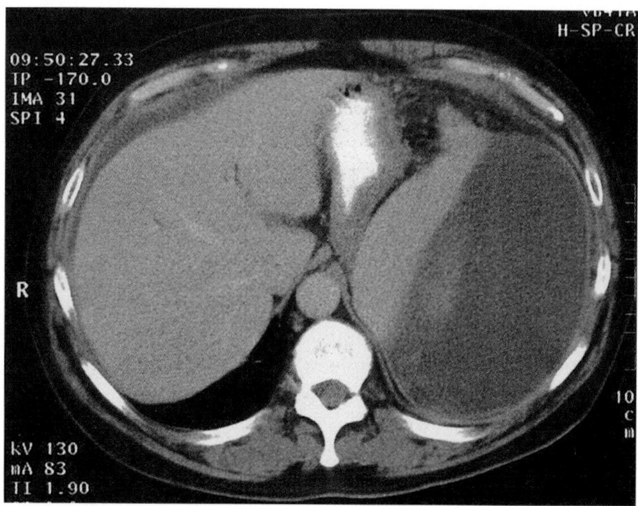

Figure 66.4 Computed tomography scan showing a large pseudocyst involving the spleen. There is displacement of the stomach medially, and a trace of ascitic fluid is present above the liver.

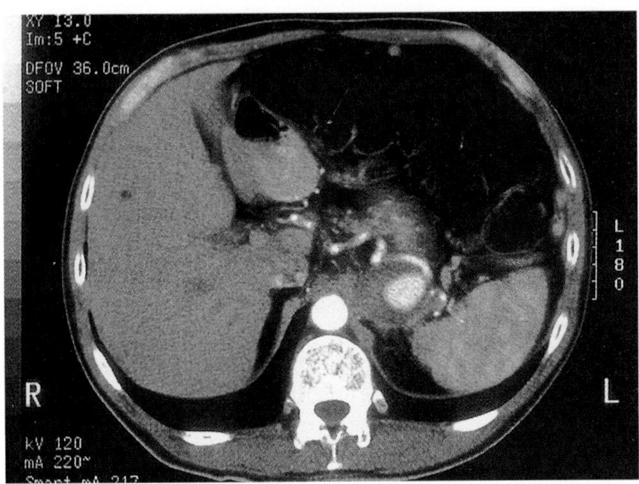

Figure 66.5 Computed tomography scan showing a pool of contrast in a pseudoaneurysm situated in the tail of the pancreas adjacent to the spleen.

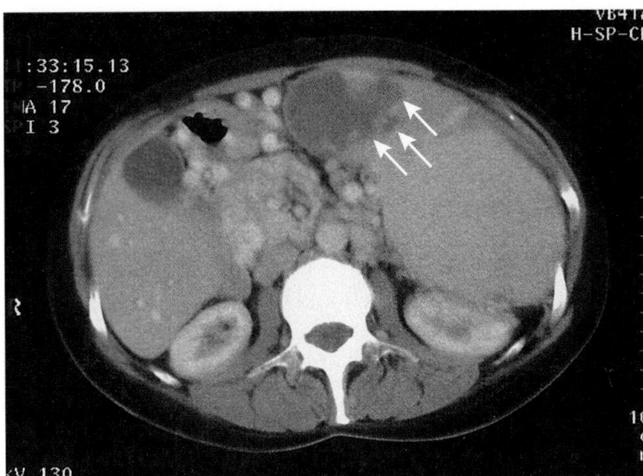

Figure 66.6 Computed tomography scan showing a splenic infarct (arrows) in a patient with splenomegaly and hypersplenism secondary to portal hypertension and portal vein thrombosis. The varices are evident at the hilus and at the greater curvature of the stomach.

Splenic rupture

Splenic rupture should be considered in any case of blunt abdominal trauma, particularly when the injury occurs to the left upper quadrant of the abdomen. Iatrogenic injury to the spleen remains a frequent complication of any surgical procedure, particularly those in the left upper quadrant when adhesions are present.

Rupture of a malarial spleen

In tropical countries, rupture of a spleen enlarged due to malaria is not uncommon (see Tropical spleen, below). Delayed presentation following a 'trivial' injury is not infrequent. In such patients, radiological embolisation may be performed if available, and splenectomy should be considered before a perisplenic haematoma ruptures, a complication that is associated with a worse prognosis.

Surgery in such patients is challenging, and early ligation of the splenic vessels along the superior border of the pancreatic body should be considered before disturbing the haematoma.

SPLENOMEGALY AND HYPERSPLENISM

Splenomegaly is a common feature of many disease processes, although the spleen has to enlarge three times before it is palpable (*Table 66.1*). It should be borne in mind that many conditions affecting the spleen, such as idiopathic thrombocytopenic purpura, may be associated with enlargement, but the gland is seldom palpable. Few conditions that cause splenomegaly will require splenectomy as part of treatment. **Hypersplenism** is an indefinite clinical syndrome that is characterised by splenic enlargement, any combination of anaemia, leucopenia or thrombocytopenia, compensatory bone marrow hyperplasia and improvement after splenectomy. Careful clinical judgement is required to balance the long- and short-term risks of splenectomy against continued conservative management.

Splenic abscess

Splenic abscess may arise from an infected splenic embolus or in association with typhoid and paratyphoid fever, osteomyelitis, otitis media and puerperal sepsis. In general surgical practice, it may be associated with pancreatic necrosis or other intra-abdominal infection (Figure 66.7). An abscess may rupture and form a left subphrenic abscess, or result in diffuse peritonitis. Treatment involves that of the underlying cause; percutaneous drainage of the splenic abscess under radiological guidance is normally required, with splenectomy being reserved when interventional radiology is not available.

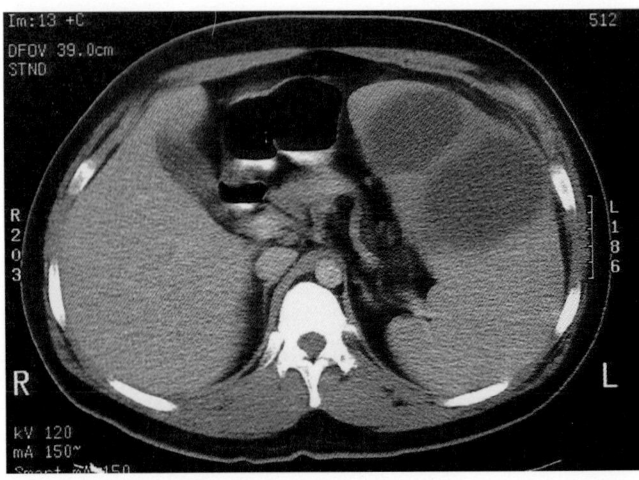

Figure 66.7 Computed tomography scan showing a multiloculated abscess in the enlarged spleen. This was managed successfully by percutaneous drainage under ultrasound guidance.

TABLE 66.1 Causes of splenic enlargement.

Infective	Bacterial	Typhoid and paratyphoid
		Typhus
		Tuberculosis[a]
		Psittacosis
		Septicaemia
		Splenic abscess[b]
	Spirochaetal	Weil's disease
		Syphilis
	Viral	Infectious mononucleosis
		HIV-related thrombocytopenia[b]
	Protozoal and parasitic	Malaria
		Schistosomiasis[a]
		Trypanosomiasis
		Kala-azar
		Hydatid cyst[c]
		Tropical splenomegaly[a]
Blood disease	Acute leukaemia	Idiopathic thrombocytopenic purpura[c]
	Chronic leukaemia	Hereditary spherocytosis[a]
	Pernicious anaemia	Autoimmune haemolytic anaemia[a]
	Polycythaemia vera	Thalassaemia[a]
	Erythroblastosis fetalis	Sickle cell disease[a]
Metabolic	Rickets	
	Amyloid	
	Porphyria	
	Gaucher's disease[b]	
Circulatory	Infarct	
	Portal hypertension	
	Segmental portal hypertension[b]	(Pancreatic carcinoma, splenic vein thrombosis)
Collagen disease	Still's disease	
	Felty's syndrome[a]	
Non-parasitic cysts	Congenital	
	Acquired	
Neoplastic	Angioma	
	Primary fibrosarcoma	
	Hodgkin's lymphoma[b]	
	Other lymphomas	
	Myelofibrosis[b]	

HIV, human immunodeficiency virus.
[a] Often benefited by splenectomy.
[b] Splenectomy may be indicated.
[c] Benefited by splenectomy.

Adolph Weil, 1848–1916, physician, Dorpat (now Tartu), Estonia, described leptospirosis icterohaemorrhagica in 1886.
Sir George Frederic Still, 1868–1941, Professor of Diseases of Children, King's College Hospital, London, UK, described chronic articular rheumatism in children in 1896.
Augustus Roy Felty, 1895–1964, physician Hartford CT, USA, described the combination of arthritis, splenomegally and leukopenia in 1924, while still a medical student at Johns Hopkins School of Medicine, Baltimore, ML, USA.

Tuberculosis

The diagnosis of tuberculosis should be considered in young adults with splenomegaly presenting with asthenia, loss of weight and fever. Tuberculosis of the spleen may produce portal hypertension or, rarely, cold abscess. Treatment with antituberculous drugs will normally produce improvement. Splenectomy is not normally required and is made difficult by the inflammatory adhesions.

Tropical splenomegaly

Massive splenic enlargement frequently occurs in the tropics from malaria, kala-azar and schistosomiasis. Occasionally, splenomegaly cannot be fully attributed to these diseases. It may result from occult infection or be related to malnutrition. The massive splenomegaly observed in this condition may require removal in those patients disabled by anaemia or local symptoms. Lifelong antimalarial therapy is indicated in malaria endemic areas.

Schistosomiasis

This condition is prevalent in Africa, Asia and South America. It is caused by infection with *Schistosoma mansoni* in 75% of cases and by *S. haematobium* in the remainder. The splenic enlargement may result from portal hypertension associated with hepatic fibrosis, but can also result from hyperplasia induced by the phagocytosis of disintegrated worms, ova and toxin. Splenomegaly can occur at any age. The diagnosis is based on examination of the urine and faeces for ova, abnormal liver function tests and the presence of hypochromic anaemia.

Successful medical treatment of established cases does not result in regression of splenomegaly, and removal of the painful and bulky spleen is indicated where there is no evidence of hepatic or renal insufficiency. Splenectomy may be required as part of a devascularisation procedure in patients with portal hypertension associated with schistosomiasis.

Leukaemia

Leukaemia should be considered in the differential diagnosis of splenomegaly and the diagnosis is made by examining blood or marrow film. Splenectomy is reserved for hypersplenism that occurs during the chronic phase of chronic granulocytic leukaemia.

Idiopathic thrombocytopenic purpura

In most cases of idiopathic thrombocytopenic purpura (ITP), the low platelet count results from the development of antibodies to specific platelet membrane glycoproteins (antiplatelet IgG autoantibodies) that damage the patient's own platelets. It is also known as immune and autoimmune thrombocytopenic purpura. It is defined as isolated thrombocytopenia with normal bone marrow and the absence of other causes of thrombocytopenia. Two distinct clinical types are evident: the acute condition in children and a chronic condition in adults. Acute ITP often follows an acute infection and has a spontaneous resolution within 2 months. Chronic ITP persists longer than 6 months without a specific cause being identified. Approximately 50–75 cases per million arise each year in adults compared with 50 cases per million each year in children.

Clinical features

The adult form normally affects females between the ages of 15 and 50 years, although it can be associated with other conditions, including systemic lupus erythematosus, chronic lymphatic leukaemia and Hodgkin's disease. The childhood form is distributed equally between males and females and commonly presents before the age of 5 years. Purpuric patches (ecchymoses) occur on the skin and mucous membranes. Following trauma or pressure, examination often reveals numbers of petechial haemorrhages in the skin. There is a tendency to spontaneous bleeding from mucous membranes (e.g. epistaxis); in women, menorrhagia and the prolonged bleeding of minor wounds are common. Haemorrhage from the urinary and gastrointestinal tracts and haemarthrosis are rare. Although intracranial haemorrhage is also uncommon, it is the most frequent cause of death. The diagnosis is made based upon the presence of cutaneous ecchymoses and a positive tourniquet test. The spleen is palpable in fewer than 10% of patients, and the presence of gross splenic enlargement should raise the suspicion of an alternative diagnosis.

Investigations

Coagulation studies are normal, and a bleeding time is not helpful in diagnosis. Platelet count in the peripheral blood film is reduced (usually $<60 \times 10^9$/L). Bone marrow aspiration reveals a plentiful supply of platelet-producing megakaryocytes.

Treatment

The course of the disease differs in children and adults. The disease regresses spontaneously in 75% of paediatric cases following the initial attack. Short courses of corticosteroids in both adult and child are usually followed by recovery. Prolonged steroid therapy should not be continued if this does not produce remission. Splenectomy is usually recommended if a patient has two relapses on steroid therapy, or if the platelet count remains low. Generally, this is indicated where the ITP has persisted for more than 6–9 months.

Up to two-thirds of patients will be cured by surgical intervention, and 15% will be improved, but no benefit will be

Sir Patrick Manson, 1844–1922, practised in Formosa (now Taiwan) and Hong Kong before becoming physician to the Dreadnought Hospital, Greenwich, London, UK. He is regarded as 'the father of tropical medicine'.
Thomas Hodgkin, 1798–1866, lecturer in morbid anatomy and curator of the Museum, Guy's Hospital, London, UK, described lymphadenoma in 1836.

derived in the remainder. The response to steroids predicts a good response to splenectomy. In the acute setting, if severe bleeding has not been controlled by steroid therapy, fresh blood transfusion or transfusion with platelet concentrates before operation is necessary, although these are generally withheld until the splenic vessels have been controlled at operation.

Haemolytic anaemias

There are four causes of haemolytic anaemia that are generally amenable to splenectomy.

Hereditary spherocytosis

Hereditary spherocytosis is an autosomal dominant hereditary disorder characterised by the presence of spherocytic red cells, caused by various molecular defects in the genes that code for alpha- and beta-spectrin, ankyrin, band 3 protein, protein 4.2 and other erythrocyte membrane proteins. These proteins are necessary to maintain the normal biconcave shape of the erythrocyte. Spherocytosis arises essentially from an increase in permeability of the red cell membranes to sodium. As this ion leaks into the cell, the osmotic pressure rises, resulting in swelling and increased fragility of the spherocyte. As the sodium pump has to work harder to rid the cells of sodium, there is greater loss of membrane phospholipid, resulting in an increased fragility of the membrane, and the energy and oxygen requirements increase. A large number of red cells are destroyed in the spleen, where there is a relative deficiency of both glucose and oxygen.

The clinical presentation is generally in childhood, but may be delayed until later life. Mild intermittent jaundice is associated with mild anaemia, splenomegaly and gallstones. Circulating bilirubin is not conjugated with glucuronic acid, and is not therefore excreted in the urine as it is bound to albumin. Excretion of the resulting bilirubin complex by the liver favours the formation of pigment gallstones. Once the disease manifests itself, spontaneous remissions are uncommon; the patient is often pale and jaundiced at presentation and, in established cases, lassitude and undue fatigue are present.

In some families, the disease is characterised by a severe crisis of red blood cell destruction, during which the erythrocyte count may fall from 4.5×10^6/mL to 1.5×10^6/mL within 1 week. Such crises are characterised by the onset of pyrexia, abdominal pain, nausea, vomiting and extreme pallor, followed by increased jaundice. These episodes may be precipitated by acute infection. Any child with gallstone disease should be investigated for hereditary spherocytosis and a family history sought.

Examination reveals splenomegaly, and the liver may also be palpable. Chronic leg ulcers may arise in adults with the disease.

Haematological investigations include the fragility test. Erythrocytes begin to haemolyse in 0.47% saline solution but, in this condition, haemolysis may occur in 0.6% or even stronger solutions. Immature red blood cells (reticulocytes), which differ from adult cells by possessing a reticulum, are discharged into the circulation by the bone marrow to compensate for the loss of erythrocytes by haemolysis.

Faecal urobilinogen is increased as this route excretes most of the urinobilinogen.

Radioactive chromium (^{51}Cr) labelling of the patient's own red cells will demonstrate the severity of red cell destruction. Daily scanning over the spleen will show the degree of red cell sequestration by the spleen. The presence of high levels of splenic radioactivity generally predicts a good response to splenectomy, but this test is used less commonly.

All patients with hereditary spherocytosis should be treated by splenectomy but, in juvenile cases, this is generally delayed until 6 years of age to minimise the risk of postsplenectomy infection, but before gallstones have had time to form. Ultrasonography should be performed preoperatively to determine the presence or absence of gallstones.

Acquired autoimmune haemolytic anaemia

This condition is divided into immune- and non-immune-mediated forms. It may arise following exposure to agents such as chemicals, infection or drugs, e.g. alpha-methyldopa, or be associated with another disease (e.g. systemic lupus erythematosus). In most instances, the cause is unknown, and red cell survival is reduced because of an immune reaction triggered by immunoglobulin or complement on the red cell surface. This condition is more common in women after the age of 50 years. In half the patients, the spleen is enlarged and, in 20% of cases, pigment gallstones are present.

Anaemia is invariably present and may be associated with spherocytosis because of red cell membrane damage. In the immune type, antibody, which coats the red cells, can be detected by agglutination when antihuman globulin is added to a suspension of the patient's erythrocytes (Coombs' test positive). The disease runs an acute self-limiting course, and no treatment is necessary. Splenectomy should, however, be considered if corticosteroids are ineffective, when the patient is developing complications from long-term steroid treatment or if corticosteroids are contraindicated; 80% of patients respond to splenectomy.

Thalassaemia (synonyms: Cooley's anaemia, Mediterranean anaemia)

This condition results from a defect in haemoglobin peptide chain synthesis and is transmitted most commonly as a recessive trait. The disease is really a group of related diseases, alpha, beta and gamma, depending upon which haemoglobin peptide chain's rate of synthesis is reduced. Most patients suffer from beta-thalassaemia, in which a reduction in the rate of beta-chain synthesis results in a decrease in haemoglobin A. Intracellular precipitates (Heinz bodies) contribute to premature red cell destruction.

Robin Royston Amos Coombs, 1921–2006, Quick Professor of Biology, University of Cambridge, Cambridge, UK, described this test in 1945.
Thomas Benton Cooley, 1871–1945, Professor of Pediatrics, Wayne University, Detroit, MI, USA, described this type of anaemia in 1927.

Graduations of the disease range from heterozygous thalassaemia minor to homozygous thalassaemia major, which is associated with chronic anaemia, jaundice and splenomegaly. Patients with homozygous thalassaemia major frequently develop clinical signs in the first year of life, and these include retarded growth, enlarged head with slanting eyes and depressed nose, leg ulcers, jaundice and abdominal distension secondary to splenomegaly.

Red cells are small, thin and misshapen and have a characteristic resistance to osmotic lysis. In the more severe forms, nucleated red cells and other immature blood cells are seen. The final diagnosis is by haemoglobin electrophoresis.

Blood transfusion may be required to correct profound anaemia, but the patient may become transfusion dependent because of the development of hypersplenism. Splenectomy is therefore of benefit in patients who require frequent blood transfusion, and if haemolytic antibodies have developed as a result.

Sickle cell disease

Sickle cell disease is a hereditary, autosomal recessive haemolytic anaemia occurring mainly among those of African origin, in whom the normal haemoglobin A is replaced by haemoglobin S (HbS). The HbS molecule crystallises when the blood oxygen tension is reduced, thus distorting and elongating the red cell. The resulting increased blood viscosity may obstruct the flow of blood in the spleen. Splenic microinfarcts are therefore common.

The sickle cell trait can be detected in 9% of those of African origin, but most are asymptomatic; sickle cell disease occurs in about 1% of Africans. Depending upon the vessels affected by vascular occlusion, patients may complain of bone or joint pain, priapism, neurological abnormalities, skin ulcers or abdominal pain due to visceral blood stasis. The diagnosis is made by the finding of characteristic sickle-shaped cells on blood film, although this investigation has largely been replaced by haemoglobin electrophoresis.

Hypoxia that provokes a sickling crisis should be avoided and is particularly relevant in patients undergoing general anaesthesia. Adequate hydration and partial exchange transfusion may help in a crisis. Splenectomy is of benefit in a few patients in whom excessive splenic sequestration of red cells aggravates the anaemia. Chronic hypersplenism usually occurs in late childhood or adolescence, although *Streptococcus pneumoniae* infection may precipitate an acute form in the first 5 years of life.

Porphyria

Porphyria is a hereditary error of haemoglobin catabolism in which porphyrinuria occurs. Abdominal crises, characterised by severe intestinal colic and constipation, can be precipitated by the administration of barbiturates. The patient is anaemic and may suffer from photosensitivity; in advanced forms of the disease, neurological and mental symptoms are present. The splenomegaly associated with this condition may be overlooked. The urine may be orange and develops a port-wine colour after a few hours of exposure to the air. Splenectomy has little role to play in the management of this condition.

Gaucher's disease

This lipid storage disease is characterised by storage of glucocerebroside in the reticuloendothelial system and in the spleen. Enormous splenic enlargement may be associated with yellowish brown discolouration of the skin on the hands and face, anaemia and conjunctival thickening (pinguecula). Slavonic and Jewish races are more prone to the disease, and the detection of Gaucher cells in the bone marrow confirms the diagnosis. Splenectomy is indicated only for severe symptoms related to the splenomegaly.

Hypersplenism due to portal hypertension

Splenomegaly is an invariable feature of portal hypertension (Figure 66.8) and results in the thrombocytopenia and granulocytopenia observed in these patients. These may be improved if the portal hypertension is relieved by shunt surgery or liver transplantation. Splenectomy would normally be required only in those patients whose segmental portal hypertension has resulted in symptomatic oesophagogastric varices.

Felty's syndrome

Patients with rheumatoid arthritis may develop leukopenia. This is referred to as Felty's syndrome if it is extreme and associated with splenomegaly. There is no definite relationship between the severity of the arthritic changes and the leukopenia and splenomegaly. Splenectomy produces only a transient

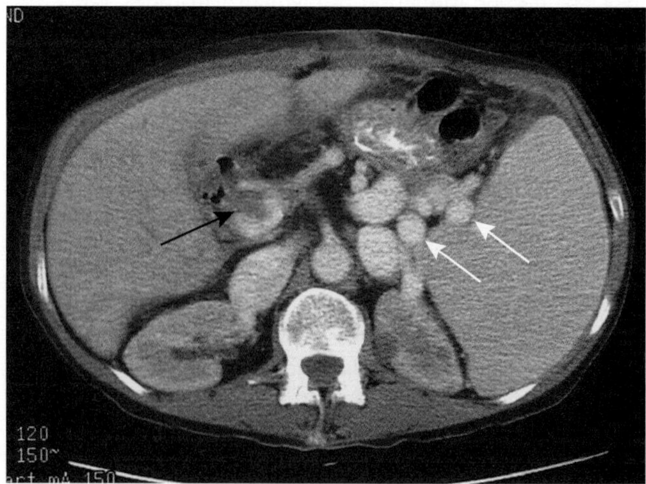

Figure 66.8 Computed tomography scan showing an enlarged spleen in a patient with portal hypertension secondary to portal vein thrombosis. Clot is evident within the lumen of the portal vein (black arrow), and large varices (white arrows) are present at the splenic hilus.

Philippe Charles Ernest Gaucher, 1854–1918, physician, Hôpital St Louis, Paris, France, described familial splenic anaemia in 1882.

improvement in the blood picture, but rheumatoid arthritis may respond to steroid therapy to which it had previously become resistant.

NEOPLASMS

Haemangioma is the most common benign tumour of the spleen and may rarely develop into a haemangiosarcoma that is managed by splenectomy. The spleen is rarely the site of metastatic disease. Lymphoma is the most common cause of neoplastic enlargement, and splenectomy may play a part in its management. Splenectomy may be required to achieve a diagnosis in the absence of palpable lymph nodes or to relieve the symptoms of gross splenomegaly. However, the need for staging laparoscopy has largely receded with the advent of CT. Its use has been restricted to those patients in whom a definite histological diagnosis of intra-abdominal disease will affect management. Thus, selected patients with stage IA or IIA Hodgkin's disease may be candidates for staging laparotomy or laparoscopy, although percutaneous biopsy under ultrasound or CT guidance is more commonly performed. In the absence of obvious liver or intra-abdominal nodal disease, splenectomy is an integral part of the staging procedure to exclude splenic involvement, which would alter the method of treatment.

Myelofibrosis results from an abnormal proliferation of mesenchymal elements in the bone marrow, spleen, liver and lymph nodes. Most patients present over the age of 50 years, and the spleen may produce pain, owing to its gross enlargement (Figure 66.9) or from splenic infarcts. Splenectomy reduces the need for transfusion and may relieve the discomfort resulting from the splenomegaly.

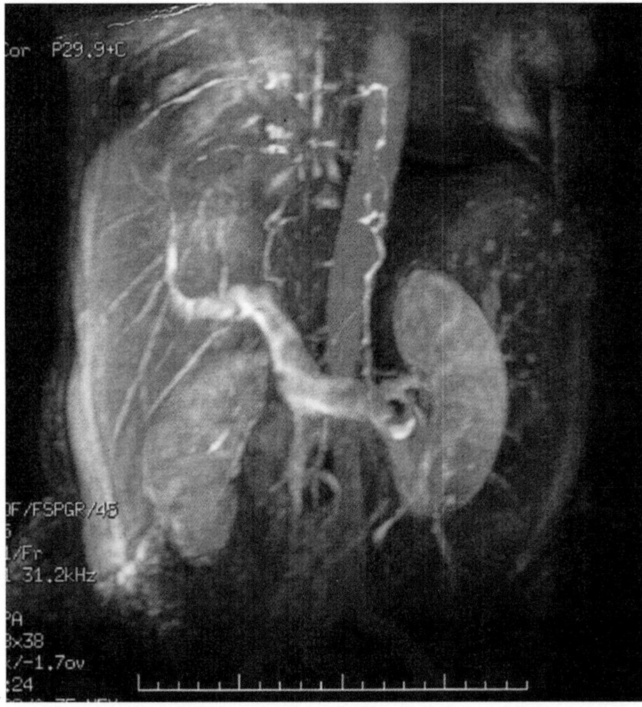

Figure 66.9 Magnetic resonance imaging scan showing massive hepatosplenomegaly secondary to myelofibrosis. Note the prominent portal system and the left kidney, which is superimposed over the grossly enlarged spleen.

SPLENECTOMY

The common indications for splenectomy are:

- trauma resulting from an accident or during a surgical procedure, as for example during mobilisation of the oesophagus, stomach, distal pancreas or splenic flexure of the colon;
- removal *en bloc* with the stomach as part of a radical gastrectomy, or with the pancreas as part of a distal or total pancreatectomy;
- to reduce anaemia or thrombocytopenia in spherocytosis, idiopathic thrombocytopenic purpura or hypersplenism;
- in association with shunt or variceal surgery for portal hypertension.

Summary box 66.2

Indications for splenectomy

Trauma
- Accidental
- Operative

Oncological
- Part of *en bloc* resection
- Diagnostic
- Therapeutic

Haematological
- Spherocytosis
- Purpura (ITP)
- Hypersplenism

Portal hypertension
- Variceal surgery

Preoperative preparation

In the presence of a bleeding tendency, transfusion of blood, fresh-frozen plasma, cryoprecipitate or platelets may be required. Coagulation profiles should be as near normal as possible at operation, and platelets should be available for patients with thrombocytopenia at operation and in the early postoperative period.

Antibiotic prophylaxis appropriate to the operative procedure should be given, and consideration should be given to the risk of postsplenectomy sepsis (see below).

Technique of open splenectomy

Most surgeons use a midline or transverse left subcostal incision for open splenectomy with the patient in the supine position. Rarely, a thoracoabdominal incision may be necessary for a massive spleen that is adherent to the diaphragm. Passage of a nasogastric tube following induction of the anaesthetic enables the stomach to be emptied.

In elective splenectomy, the gastrosplenic ligament is opened up, and the short gastric vessels are divided. The splenic vessels at the superior border of the pancreas are suture-ligated. The posterior surface of the spleen is exposed, the posterior leaf of the lienorenal ligament divided with long curved scissors, and the spleen rotated medially along with the tail and body of the pancreas (Figure 66.10). The pancreas is separated from the hilar vessels, which are normally doubly ligated separately and divided. Accessory splenic tissue in the splenic hilum or omentum should be excluded by a careful search at operation. There is no need to drain the wound if haemostasis is adequate.

The segmental vasculature of the spleen does make it possible to undertake limited resection of the parenchyma. Haemostasis can be achieved by ligation of, or application of metal clips to, intrasplenic vessels, and by careful application of topical haemostatic agents such as fibrin pad (EVARREST®). Conservative splenic surgery is therefore possible in some cases of splenic trauma and other pathology such as splenic cysts.

Technique of laparoscopic splenectomy

The patient is placed on the right side with the space between the left ilium and costal margin exposed. Placement of access ports is often determined by the size of the patient and the spleen. Insufflation of the abdomen can be performed once access is obtained through an incision 1 cm from the costal margin at the left mid-clavicular line. A further trocar is inserted close to the costal margin below the xiphoid. A 12-mm trocar is inserted at a similar distance from the costal margin at the posterior axillary line. The splenocolic ligament is divided to give access to the lower splenic pole. The spleen is separated from the kidney and diaphragm before the gap between the splenic hilum and the tail of the pancreas is enlarged. The spleen is elevated to expose the splenic hilum, which is secured and divided with an endoscopic vascular stapler (Figure 66.11). Two or three applications of the instrument may be required to secure the hilum and the short gastric vessels. Any remaining attachments to the diaphragm are divided before a self-retaining opening bag is introduced through the incision of the open laparoscopy, after removal of the 12-mm port. The spleen is placed in the bag, the mouth of which is pulled out of the abdominal opening before the spleen is crushed and retrieved with an instrument. The operation may be undertaken as a hand-assisted procedure, particularly when the spleen is grossly enlarged.

Postoperative complications

Immediate complications specific to splenectomy include haemorrhage resulting from a slipped ligature. Haematemesis from gastric mucosal damage and gastric dilatation is uncommon. Left basal atelectasis is common, and a pleural effusion may be present. Adjacent structures at risk during the procedure include the stomach and pancreas. A fistula may result from damage to the greater curvature of the stomach during ligation of the short gastric vessels. Damage to the tail of the pancreas may result in pancreatitis, a localised abscess or a pancreatic fistula.

Postoperative thrombocytosis may arise and, if the blood platelet count exceeds 1×10^6/mL, prophylactic aspirin is recommended. Long-term surveillance programmes have emphasised an increased risk of deep vein thrombosis and pulmonary embolism. The relative risk and benefit of thromboprophylaxis in this setting has not been assessed adequately.

Postsplenectomy septicaemia may result from *Streptococcus pneumoniae*, *Neisseria meningitides*, *Haemophilus influenzae* and *Escherichia coli*. Long-term surveillance programmes have

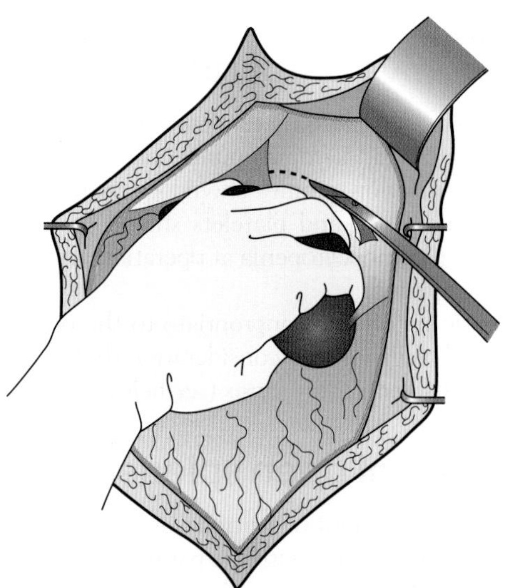

Figure 66.10 Diagrammatic view of the approach required to divide the short gastric vessels anteriorly and the lienorenal ligament posteriorly.

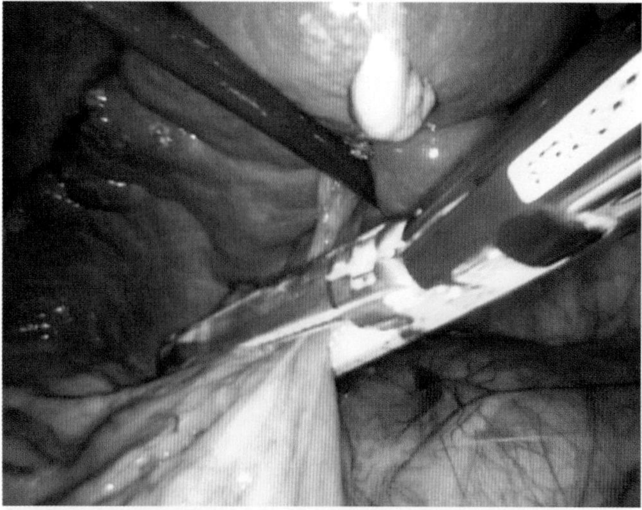

Figure 66.11 Photograph showing a stapling device across the splenic hilus for division of the splenic vessels during laparoscopic splenectomy.

Albert Ludwig Siegmund Neisser, 1855–1916, Director of the Dermatological Institute, Breslau, Germany (now Wroclaw, Poland).
Theodor Escherich, 1857–1911, Professor of Paediatrics, Vienna, Austria.

suggested that the risk of pneumonia, meningitis and major sepsis following splenectomy is increased three-fold. However, the risk is greater in the young patient, in splenectomised patients treated with chemoradiotherapy and in patients who have undergone splenectomy for thalassaemia, sickle cell disease and autoimmune anaemia or thrombocytopenia.

Opportunist postsplenectomy infection (OPSI) is a major concern. Published guidelines emphasise that most infections after splenectomy could be avoided through measures that include offering patients appropriate and timely immunisation, antibiotic prophylaxis, education and prompt treatment of infection. The benefit of prophylactic antibiotics in this setting remains controversial. It is thought that children who have undergone splenectomy before the age of 5 years should be treated with a daily dose of penicillin until the age of 10 years. Prophylaxis in older children should be continued at least until the age of 16 years, but its use is less well defined in adults. Furthermore, compliance is problematic in the long term but, as the risk of overwhelming sepsis is greatest within the first 2–3 years after splenectomy, it seems reasonable to give prophylaxis during this time. However, all patients with compromised immune function should receive prophylaxis. Satisfactory oral prophylaxis can be obtained with penicillin, erythromycin, amoxicillin or co-amoxiclav. Suspected infection can be treated intravenously with these same antibiotics and cefotaxime or ceftriaxone, or chloramphenicol in patients allergic to penicillin and cephalosporins.

If elective splenectomy is planned, consideration should be given to vaccinating against pneumococcus, meningococcus C (both repeated every 5 years) and *H. influenzae* type B (Hib) (repeated every 10 years). The latter two vaccines are commonly delivered as a combined preparation. Yearly influenza vaccination has been recommended, as there is some evidence that it may reduce the risk of secondary bacterial infection. Such vaccinations should be administered at least 2 weeks before elective surgery or as soon as possible after recovery from surgery but before discharge from hospital. Pneumococcal vaccination is recommended in those patients aged over 2 years. *Haemophilus influenzae* type b vaccination is recommended irrespective of age. Asplenic patients should carry a medical alert and an up-to-date vaccination card. They require specific advice regarding travel and animal handling. Patients who have undergone splenectomy and are travelling to countries where malaria is present are strongly advised to use all physical antimosquito barriers as well as antimalarial therapy since they are at increased risk of severe malaria. Overwhelming postsplectomy sepsis due to *Capnocytophaga canimorsus* may result from dog, cat or other animal bites.

In the trauma victim, vaccination can be given in the postoperative period, and the resulting antibody levels will be protective in the majority of cases. Antibody levels are, however, less than 50% of those achieved if vaccination is given in the presence of an intact spleen. Protection following vaccination is not always guaranteed.

Summary box 66.3

Splenectomy

- Remember preoperative immunisation
- Prophylactic antibiotics in the long term
- Opportunistic postsplenectomy infection is a real clinical danger
- Splenic conservation should be considered

FURTHER READING

Boyle S, White RH, Brunson A, Wun T. Splenectomy and the incidence of venous thromboembolism and sepsis in patients with immune thrombocytopenia. *Blood* 2013; **121**: 4782–90.

Di Sabatino A, Carsetti R, Corazza GR. Postsplenectomy and hyposplenic states. *Lancet* 2011; **378**: 86–97.

Easow MM, Sharma A, Aravindakshan R. Splenectomy for people with thalassaemia major or intermedia. *Cochrane Database Syst Rev* 2014; **6**: CDO10517.

Edgren G, Almqvist R, Hartman M, Utter GH. Splenectomy and the risk of sepsis: a population-based cohort study. *Ann Surg* 2014; **260**: 1081–7.

Glasgow RE, Mulvihill SJ Laparoscopic splenectomy. *World J Surg* 1999; **23**: 384–8.

Mourtzoukou EG, Mikhael J, Northridge K *et al.* Short-term and long-term failure of laparoscopic splenectomy in adult immune thrombocytopenic purpura patients: a systematic review. *Am J Hematol* 2009; **84**(11): 743–8.

Pappas G, Peppas G, Falagas ME. Vaccination of asplenic or hyposplenic adults. *Br J Surg* 2008; **95**(3): 273–80.

Weatherall DJ. The hereditary anaemias. *Br Med J* 1997; **314**: 492–6.

Chapter 67

The gallbladder and bile ducts

Learning objectives

- To understand the anatomy and physiology of the gallbladder and bile ducts
- To be familiar with the pathophysiology and management of gallstones
- To be aware of unusual disorders of the biliary tree
- To be aware of malignant disease of the gallbladder and bile ducts

SURGICAL ANATOMY AND PHYSIOLOGY

The gallbladder lies on the underside of the liver in the main liver scissura at the junction of the right and left lobes of the liver. The relationship of the gallbladder to the liver varies between being embedded within the liver substance to being suspended by a mesentry. It is a pear-shaped structure, 7.5–12 cm long, with a normal capacity of about 25–30 mL. The anatomical divisions are a fundus, a body and a neck that terminates in a narrow infundibulum. The muscle fibres in the wall of the gallbladder are arranged in a criss-cross manner, being particularly well developed in its neck. The mucous membrane contains indentations of the mucosa that sink into the muscle coat; these are the crypts of Luschka.

The cystic duct is about 3 cm in length but the length is variable. The lumen is usually 1–3 mm in diameter. The mucosa of the cystic duct is arranged in spiral folds known as the valves of Heister and the wall is surrounded by a sphincteric structure called the sphincter of Lütkens. The cystic duct joins the supraduodenal segment of the common hepatic duct in 80% of cases, however the anatomy may vary and the junction may be much lower in the retroduodenal or even retropancreatic part of the bile duct. Occasionally, the cystic duct may join the right hepatic duct or even a right hepatic sectorial duct (see below).

The common hepatic duct is usually less than 2.5 cm long and is formed by the union of the right and left hepatic ducts. The common bile duct is about 7.5 cm long and formed by the junction of the cystic and common hepatic ducts. It is divided into four parts:

- the supraduodenal portion, about 2.5 cm long, runs in the free edge of the lesser omentum;
- the retroduodenal portion;
- the infraduodenal portion lies in a groove, but at times in a tunnel, on the posterior surface of the pancreas;
- the intraduodenal portion passes obliquely through the wall of the second part of the duodenum, where it is surrounded by the sphincter of Oddi, and terminates by opening on the summit of the ampulla of Vater.

The cystic artery, a branch of the right hepatic artery, usually arises behind the common hepatic duct (Figure 67.1). Occasionally, an accessory cystic artery arises from the gastroduodenal artery. In 15% of cases the right hepatic artery and/or the cystic artery crosses in front of the common hepatic duct and the cystic duct.

Calot's triangle, or the hepatobiliary triangle, was initially described by Calot as the space bordered by the cystic duct inferiorly, the common hepatic duct medially and the superior border of the cystic artery. This has been modified in contemporary literature to be the area bound superiorly by the inferior surface of the liver, laterally by the cystic duct and the medial border of the gallbladder and medially by the common hepatic duct. It is an important surgical landmark as the cystic artery usually can be found within its boundaries and should be identified by surgeons performing a cholecystectomy to avoid damage to the extrahepatic biliary system (Figure 67.2a).

The most dangerous anomalies are where the hepatic artery takes a tortuous course on the front of the origin of the cystic duct (Figure 67.2b), or the right hepatic artery

Hubert Luschka, 1820–1875, Professor of Anatomy, Tübingen, Germany.
Ulrich Lütkens, b.1894, surgeon at the University Clinic, Berlin, Germany, published a monograph on the structure and function of the extrahepatic biliary tract in 1926.
Lorenz Heister, 1683–1758, Professor of Surgery and Botany, Helmstädt, Germany.
Ruggero Oddi, 1845–1906, physiologist, Perugia, Italy.
Abraham Vater, 1684–1751, Professor of Anatomy and Botany, Wittenberg, Germany.

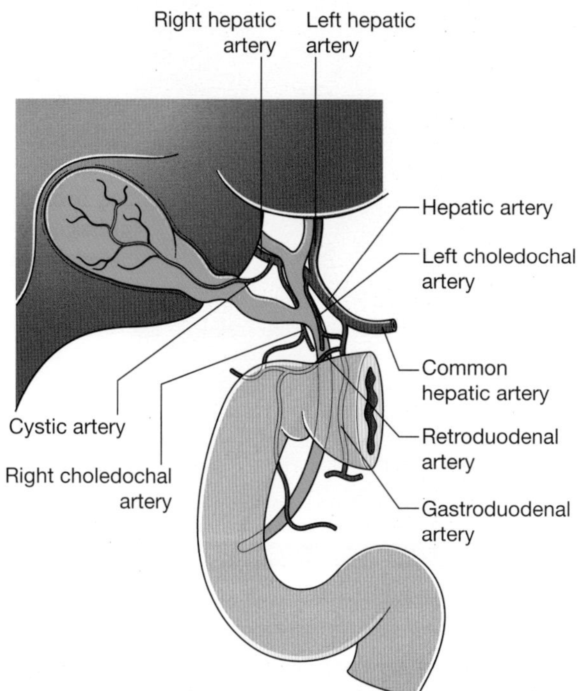

Figure 67.1 The anatomy of the gallbladder and bile ducts. Note the arrangement of the arterial tree.

is tortuous and the cystic artery short (**Figure 67.2c**). The tortuosity is known as the 'caterpillar turn' or 'Moynihan's hump'. This variation is the cause of many problems during a difficult cholecystectomy with inflammation in the region of the cystic duct.

Lymphatics

The lymphatic vessels of the gallbladder (subserosal and submucosal) drain into the cystic lymph node of Lund (the sentinel lymph node), which lies in the fork created by the junction of the cystic and common hepatic ducts. Efferent vessels from this lymph node go to the hilum of the liver, and to the coeliac lymph nodes. The subserosal lymphatic vessels of the gallbladder also connect with the subcapsular lymph channels of the liver, and this accounts for the frequent spread of carcinoma of the gallbladder to the liver.

Surgical physiology

Bile is produced by the liver and stored in the gallbladder, from which it is released into the duodenum. As it leaves the liver it is composed of 97% water, bile salts (cholic and chenodeoxycholic acids, deoxycholic and lithocholic acids), phospholipids, cholesterol and bilirubin. The liver excretes bile at a rate estimated to be approximately 40 mL/hour. About 95% of bile salts are reabsorbed in the terminal ileum (enterohepatic circulation).

Functions of the gallbladder

The gallbladder is a reservoir for bile. During fasting, resistance to flow through the sphincter of Oddi is high, and bile excreted by the liver is diverted to the gallbladder. After feeding, the resistance to flow through the sphincter is reduced, the gallbladder contracts and the bile enters the duodenum. These motor responses of the biliary tract are in part affected by the hormone cholecystokinin.

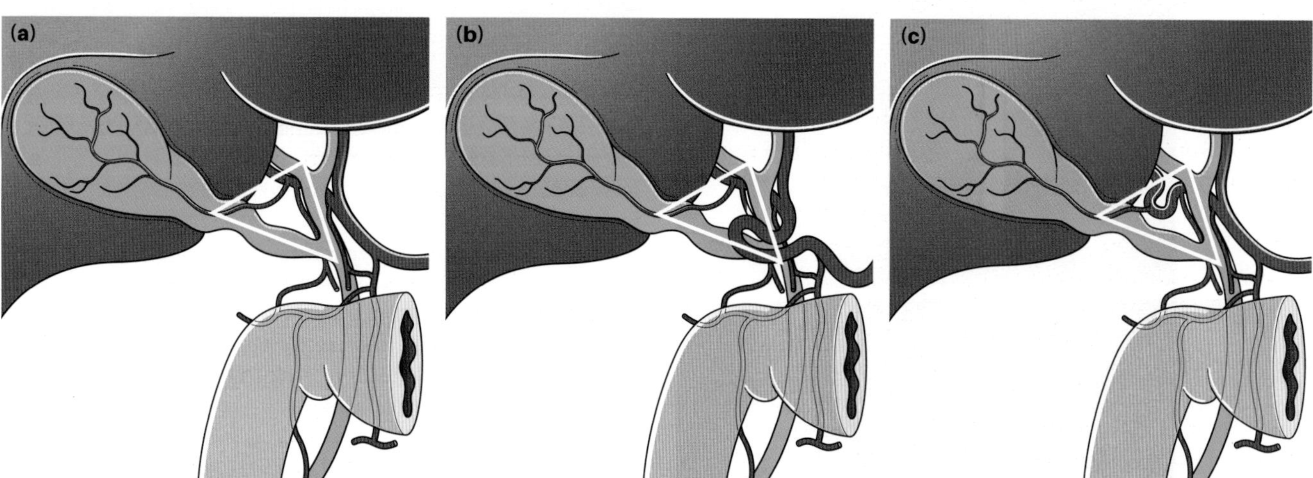

Figure 67.2 **(a)** Usual anatomy of Calot's triangle; **(b)** tortuous common hepatic artery; **(c)** tortuous right hepatic artery with short cystic artery; **(b)** and **(c)** are examples of so-called 'caterpillar turn' or 'Moynihan's hump', which if not recognised can lead to inadvertent arterial injury or bleeding during cholecystectomy.

Berkeley George Andrew Moynihan (Lord Moynihan), 1865–1936, Professor of Clinical Surgery, Leeds, UK.
Jean François Calot, 1861–1944, surgeon, Paris, France.
Fred Bates Lund, 1865–1950, surgeon, Boston City Hospital, Boston, MA, USA.

The second function of the gallbladder is concentration of bile by active absorption of water, sodium chloride and bicarbonate via the mucous membrane of the gallbladder. The hepatic bile which enters the gallbladder becomes concentrated 5–10 times, with a corresponding increase in the proportion of bile salts, bile pigments, cholesterol and calcium.

The third function of the gallbladder is the secretion of mucus – approximately 20 mL is produced per day. With complete obstruction of the cystic duct in an otherwise healthy gallbladder, a mucocoele may develop as a result of ongoing mucus secretion by the gallbladder mucosa.

RADIOLOGICAL INVESTIGATION OF THE BILIARY TRACT

Plain radiographs

The skillfully taken plain radiograph of the gallbladder will show radiopaque gallstones in 10% of patients (Figure 67.3). Rarely, the centre of a stone may contain radiolucent gas in a triradiate or biradiate fissure and this gives rise to characteristic dark shapes on a radiograph: the 'Mercedes–Benz' or 'seagull' sign.

A plain x-ray may also show the rare cases of calcification of the gallbladder, a so-called 'porcelain' gallbladder (Figure 67.4). This is more commonly seen on computed tomography (CT) (Figure 67.5). Traditionally, this has been considered an indication for cholecystectomy as it was associated with a high incidence of gallbladder carcinoma. However, contemporary data suggest that this may not be the case, with the true incidence of cancer being less than 5%. Therefore, decisions on whether or not a cholecystectomy should be performed should be individualised depending on the age of the patient, comorbidities and presence or absence of symptoms.

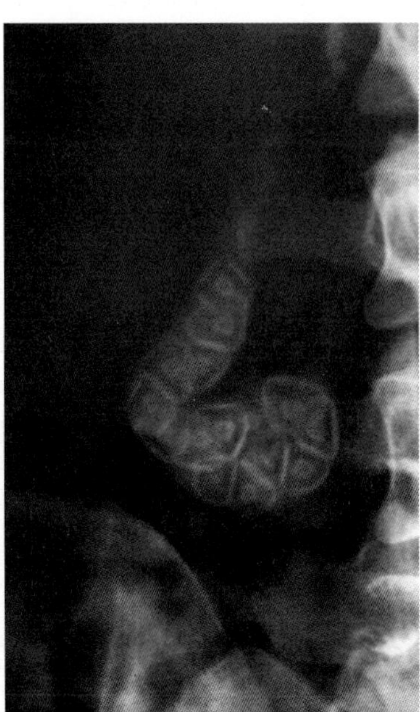

Figure 67.3 Plain radiograph showing radiopaque stones in the gallbladder. Radiopaque stones are rare (10%).

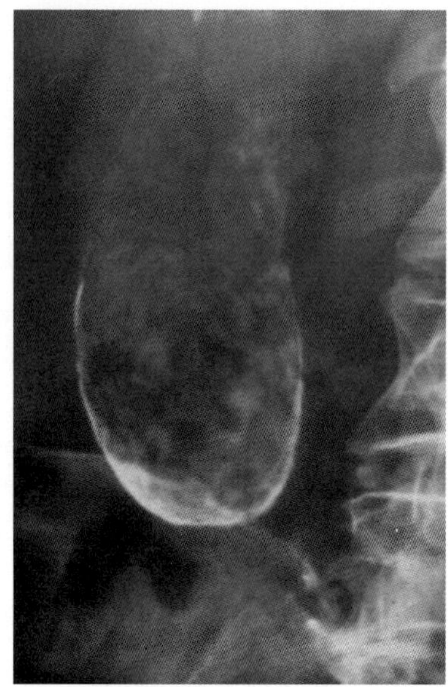

Figure 67.4 Porcelain gallbladder.

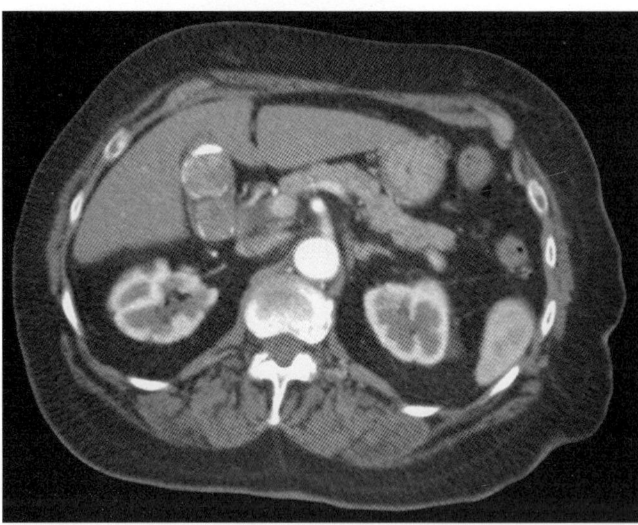

Figure 67.5 Computed tomography scan demonstrating calicification in the gallbladder wall ('porcelain gallbladder').

Gas may be seen in the wall of the gallbladder (emphysematous cholecystitis) (Figure 67.6). Gas in the biliary tree may also be seen normally after endoscopic sphincterotomy or following a surgical anastomosis

Oral cholecystography and intravenous cholangiography

Oral and intravenous cholecystography are of interest for historical purposes only as they have been replaced by more accurate imaging modalities.

The Mercedes–Benz sign takes its name from the insignia displayed on the bonnet of a Mercedes–Benz car.

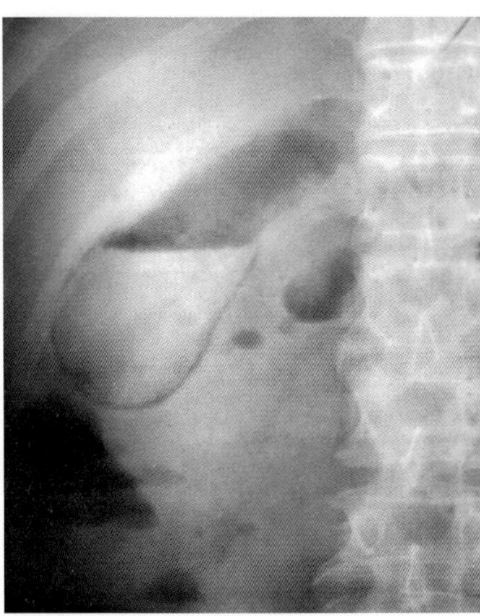

Figure 67.6 Gas in the gallbladder and gallbladder wall (*Clostridium perfringens*). Emergency surgery is indicated.

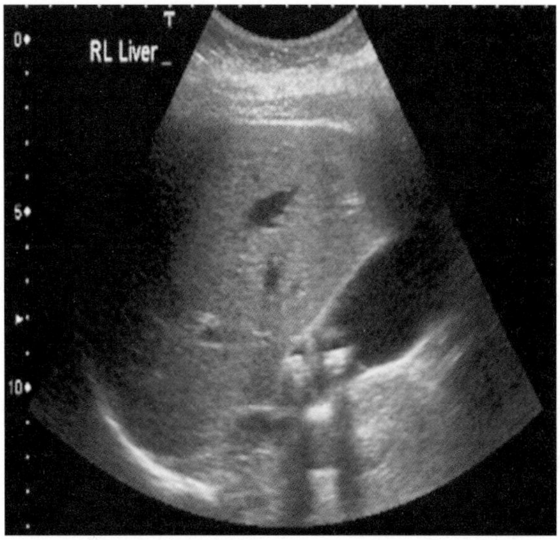

Figure 67.8 Ultrasound examination. Gallstones noted at the neck of the gallbladder with associated acoustic shadowing.

Ultrasonography

Transabdominal ultrasonography (US) (Figures 67.7 and 67.8) is the initial imaging modality of choice as it is accurate, readily available, inexpensive and quick to perform. However, it is operator dependent and may be compromised by excessive body fat and intraluminal bowel gas. The size of the gallbladder can be seen, the presence of stones or polyps determined and the thickness of the wall measured. Additionally, the presence of inflammation around the gallbladder, the size of the common bile duct and, occasionally, the presence of stones within the extrahepatic biliary tree can be determined.

For the patient who presents with obstructive jaundice, ultrasonography is particularly helpful because it can identify intra- and extrahepatic biliary dilatation and often the level of obstruction. In addition, the cause of the obstruction may also be determined, such as gallstones in the gallbladder, common hepatic or common bile duct stones, lesions within the wall of the common bile duct suggestive of a cholangiocarcinoma or enlargement of the pancreatic head indicative of a pancreatic carcinoma.

Endoscopic ultrasonography (EUS) utilises a specially designed endoscope with an ultrasound transducer at its tip which allows the gastroenterologist to visualise the liver and biliary tree from within the stomach and duodenum (Figure 67.9). It is accurate in imaging the bile duct and detecting the presence of choledocholithiasis. In addition, it has been shown to be useful in diagnosing and staging both pancreatic and periampullary cancers. Biopsies can be taken from suspicious areas for either cytological or histopathological analysis.

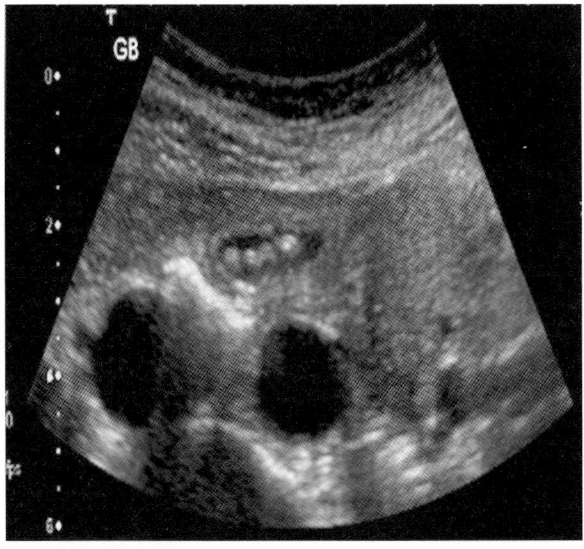

Figure 67.7 Ultrasound examination. Multiple gallstones noted within the gallbladder.

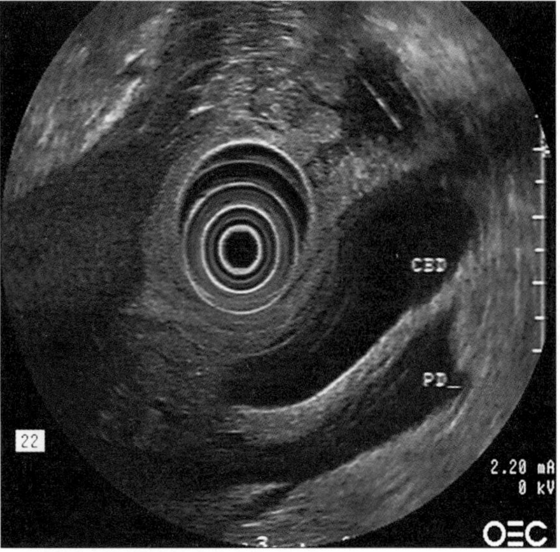

Figure 67.9 Endoscopic ultrasonography. CBD, common bile duct; PD, pancreatic duct.

Cholescintigraphy

Technetium-99m (^{99m}Tc)-labelled derivatives of iminodiacetic acid (HIDA, IODIDA) when injected intravenously are selectively taken up by the retroendothelial cells of the liver and excreted into the bile. This allows visualisation of the biliary tree and gallbladder. In 90% of normal individuals the gallbladder is visualised within 30 minutes following injection, with 100% being seen within 1 hour (Figure 67.10). The bowel is seen, usually within 1 hour, in the majority of patients.

Non-visualisation of the gallbladder is suggestive of acute cholecystitis. If the patient has a contracted gallbladder, as often seen in chronic cholecystitis, the gallbladder visualisation may be reduced or delayed.

An abnormally low gallbladder ejection fraction may be suggestive of gallbladder dyskinesia; however, the diagnosis and interpretation of cholescintigraphy in this context are controversial.

Biliary scintigraphy may also be helpful in diagnosing bile leaks and iatrogenic biliary obstruction.

Computed tomography (CT)

Unlike ultrasonography, CT is less affected by body habitus and is not operator dependent. It allows visualisation of the liver, bile ducts, gallbladder and pancreas (Figure 67.11). It is particularly useful in detecting hepatic and pancreatic lesions and is the modality of choice in the staging of cancers of the liver, gallbladder, bile ducts and pancreas. It can identify the extent of the primary tumour and define the relationship of the tumour to other organs and blood vessels (Figure 67.12). In addition, the presence of enlarged lymph nodes or metastatic disease may be seen. However, as only 75% of gallstones are identified by CT, it is not used as a screening modality for uncomplicated gallstones.

Magnetic resonance cholangiopancreatography (MRCP)

Magnetic resonance cholangiopancreatography is a non-invasive modality that provides excellent imaging of the gallbladder and biliary system (Figures 67.13 and 67.14). Images can be obtained of the biliary tree demonstrating ductal obstruction, strictures or other intraductal abnormalities. Images comparable to those obtained using ERCP or PTC (see below) can be achieved non-invasively without the potential complications of either technique.

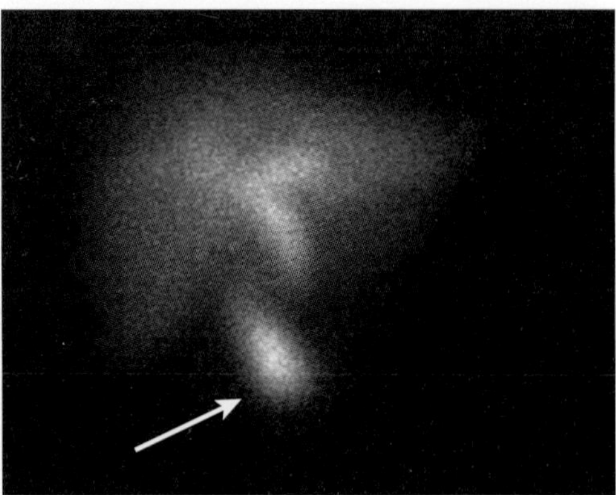

Figure 67.10 Dimethyl iminodiacetic acid (HIDA) scan (arrow indicates the gallbladder).

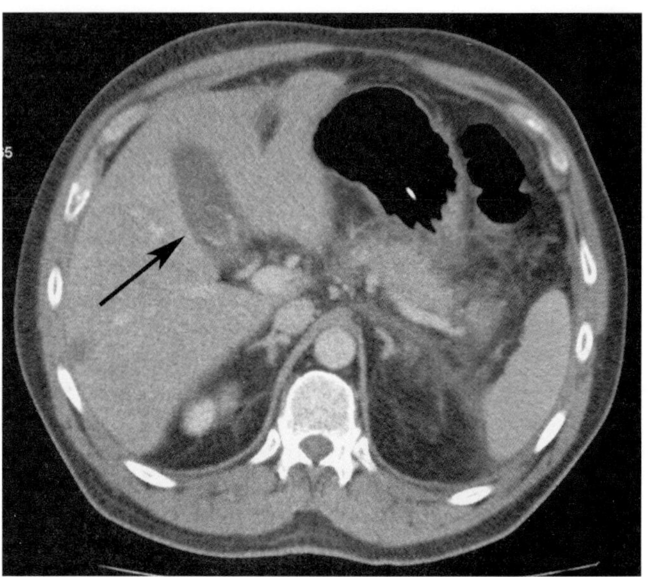

Figure 67.11 Computed tomography scan demonstrating a gallstone within the gallbladder (arrow).

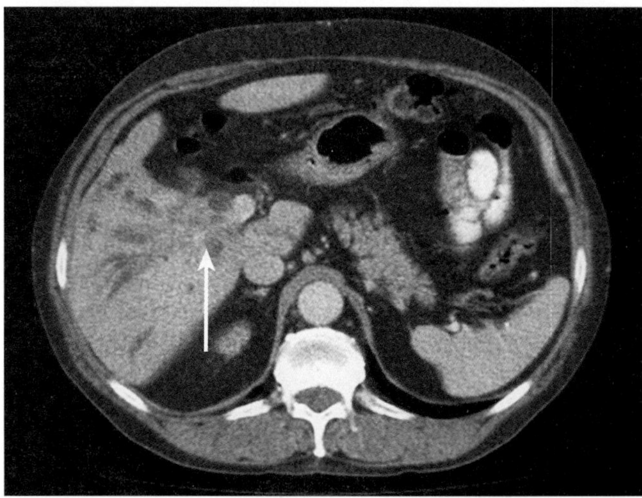

Figure 67.12 Computed tomography scan demonstrating a hilar mass (arrow).

Endoscopic retrograde cholangiopancreatography (ERCP)

This technique remains widely used as both a diagnostic and a therapeutic modality. Using a side-viewing endoscope the ampulla of Vater can be identified and cannulated. Injection of water-soluble contrast directly into the bile duct provides excellent images of the ductal anatomy (Figure 67.15) and can identify causes of obstruction such as calculi (Figure 67.16) or malignant strictures (Figure 67.17). While the widespread availability of ultrasound and MRCP has reduced

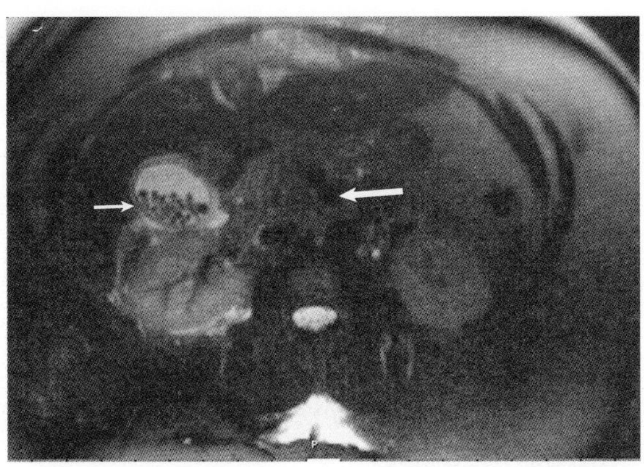

Figure 67.13 Magnetic resonance cholangiopancreatography: cross-sectional image demonstrating a hilar mass (thick arrow) and gallstones (thin arrow).

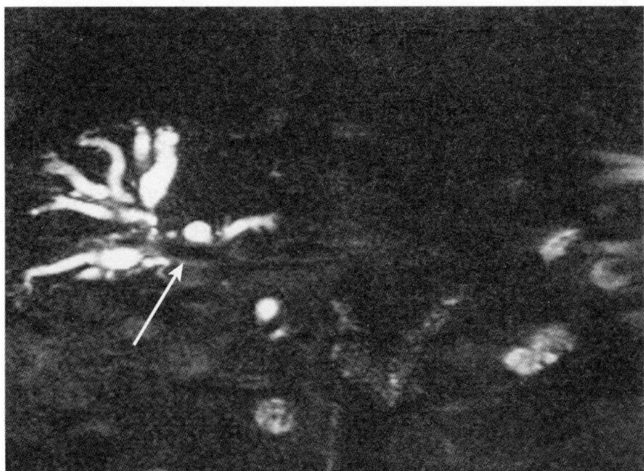

Figure 67.14 Magnetic resonance cholangiopancreatography: projectional images demonstrating stones and hilar obstruction (arrow).

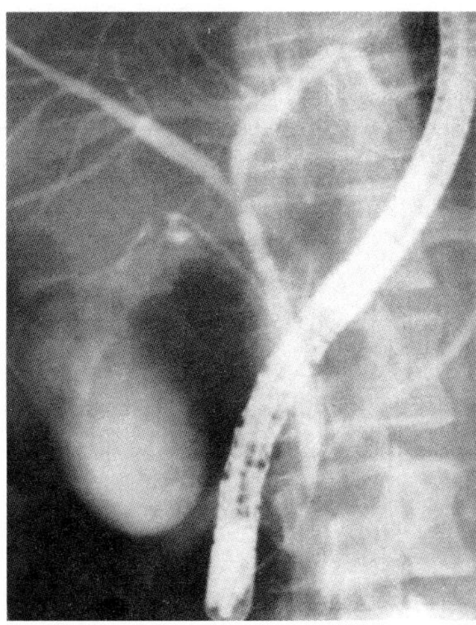

Figure 67.15 Endoscopic retrograde cholangiopancreatography: normal cholangiogram.

its diagnostic use, ERCP still has an important role in the assessment of the patient with obstructive jaundice. In this group of patients it is especially useful in determining the cause and level of obstruction.

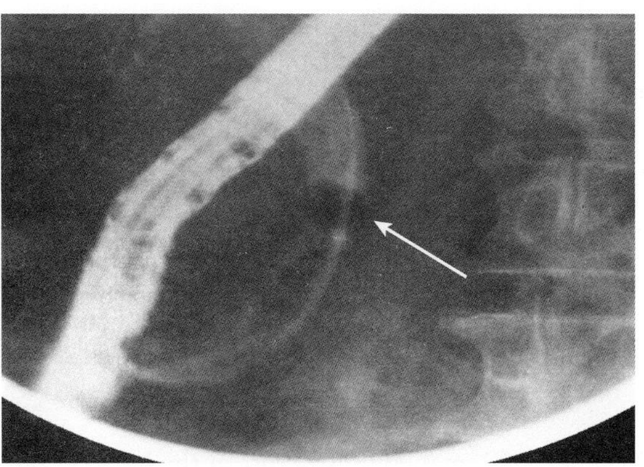

Figure 67.16 Endoscopic retrograde cholangiopancreatography: common duct obstruction (arrow).

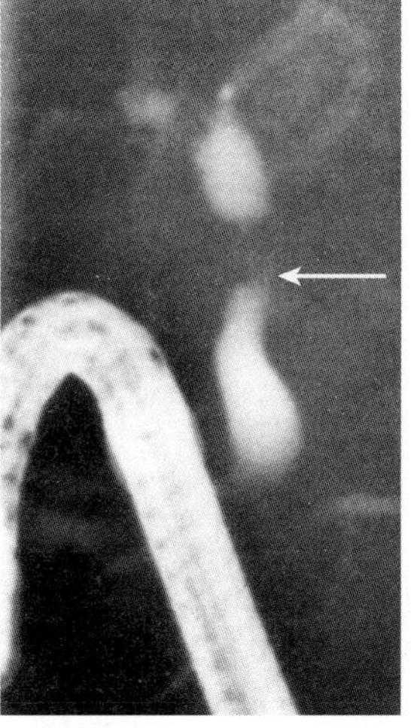

Figure 67.17 Endoscopic retrograde cholangiopancreatography: partial occlusion of the bile duct by a malignant stricture (arrow).

During ERCP, bile aspirates can be sent for cytological and microbiological examination, and endoluminal brushings can be taken from strictures for cytological studies. Therapeutic interventions such as stone removal or stent placement to relieve the obstruction can be performed. Thus, ERCP has evolved into a mainly therapeutic rather than a diagnostic technique.

Percutaneous transhepatic cholangiography (PTC)

This is an invasive technique in which the bile ducts are cannulated percutaneously. It is only undertaken once a bleeding tendency has been excluded and if the patient's prothrombin time is normal. Antibiotics should be given prior to the procedure. Usually, under fluoroscopic control, a needle (the Chiba or Okuda needle) is introduced percutaneously into the liver substance. Under radiological control (either ultrasound or CT) a bile duct is cannulated. Successful entry is confirmed

Evarts Ambrose Graham, 1883–1957, Bixby Professor of Surgery, Washington University, St Louis, MO, USA.
Warren Henry Cole, 1898–1990, Emeritus Professor of Surgery, University of Illinois, Chicago, IL, USA, introduced cholecystography in 1924.
Kunio Okuda, 1921–2003, Professor of Medicine, Chiba University, Japan.

by contrast injection or aspiration of bile. Water-soluble contrast medium is injected to visualise the biliary system. Multiple images can be taken demonstrating areas of strictures or obstruction (Figure 67.18). Bile can be sent for cytology. In addition, this technique enables placement of a catheter into the bile ducts to provide external biliary drainage or the insertion of indwelling stents. The scope of this procedure can be further extended by leaving the drainage catheter *in situ* for a number of days and then dilating the track sufficiently for a fine flexible choledochoscope to be passed into the intrahepatic biliary tree in order to diagnose strictures, take biopsies and remove stones.

In general, if a malignant stricture at the level of the confluence of the right and left hepatic ducts or higher is suspected in a jaundiced patient, a PTC is preferred to ERCP because successful drainage is more likely.

Summary box 67.1

Radiological investigation of the biliary tree

- Plain radiograph: calcification, air within biliary system
- Ultrasound: stones and biliary dilatation
- MRCP: anatomy and stones
- CT scan: anatomy, liver, gallbladder and pancreatic cancer
- Radioisotope scanning (HIDA scan): function
- ERCP: anatomy, stones and biliary strictures
- PTC: anatomy and biliary strictures
- EUS: anatomy, stones

Intraoperative imaging techniques

Peroperative cholangiography

During open or laparoscopic cholecystectomy a catheter can be placed in the cystic duct and contrast injected directly into the biliary tree. The technique defines the anatomy and is used mainly to exclude the presence of stones within the bile ducts (Figures 67.19–67.21). A single x-ray plate or image intensifier can be used to obtain and review the images intraoperatively. Irrespective of the technique used the operating table should be tilted head down by approximately 20° to facilitate filling of the intrahepatic ducts. In addition, care should be taken when injecting contrast not to introduce air bubbles into the system as these may give the appearance of stones and lead to a false-positive result.

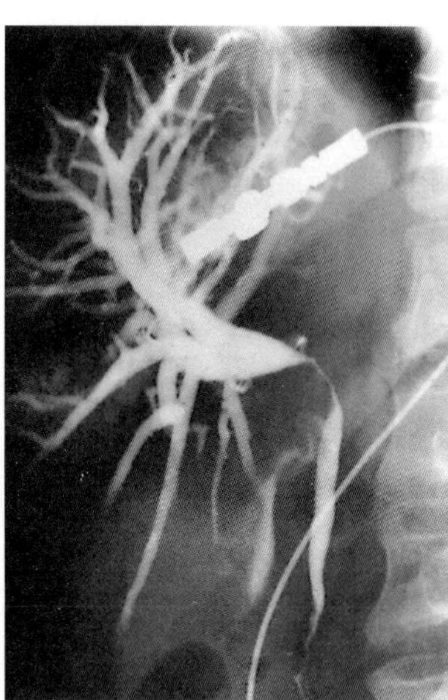

Figure 67.18 Transhepatic cholangiogram showing a stricture of the common hepatic duct (courtesy of Miss Phyllis George, FRCS, London, UK).

Operative biliary endoscopy (choledochoscopy)

At operation, a flexible fibreoptic endoscope can be passed either via the cystic duct or directly via a choledochotomy into the common bile duct, enabling stone identification and removal under direct vision. After exploration of the bile duct, a tube can be left in the cystic duct remnant or in the common bile duct (a T-tube) and drainage of the biliary tree established. After 7–10 days, a track will be established. This track can be used subsequently for the passage of a choledochoscope to remove residual stones in the awake patient in an endoscopy suite.

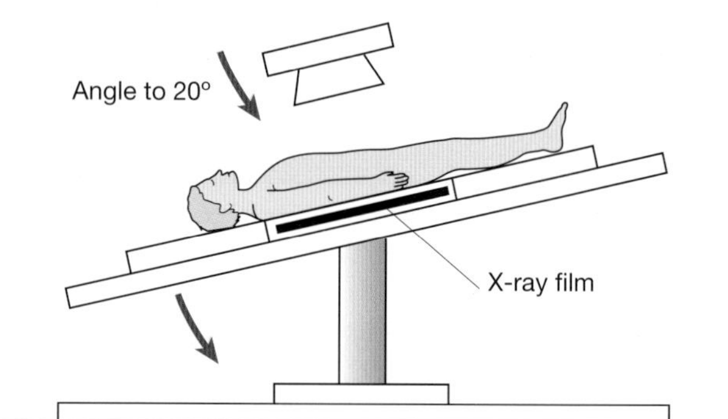

Figure 67.19 Peroperative cholangiography using a radiolucent table-top.

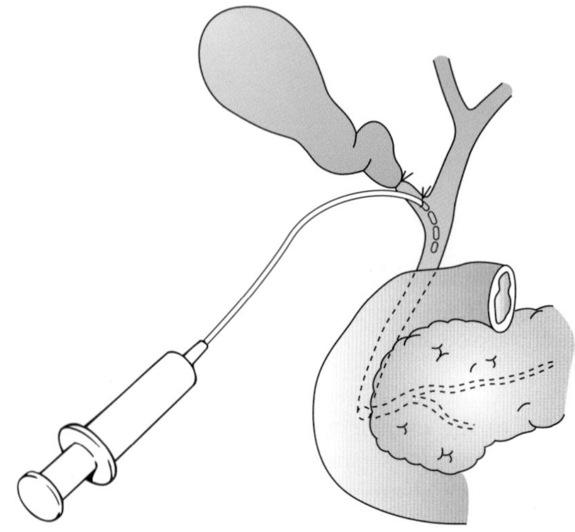

Figure 67.20 Peroperative cholangiography. Technique of introducing contrast.

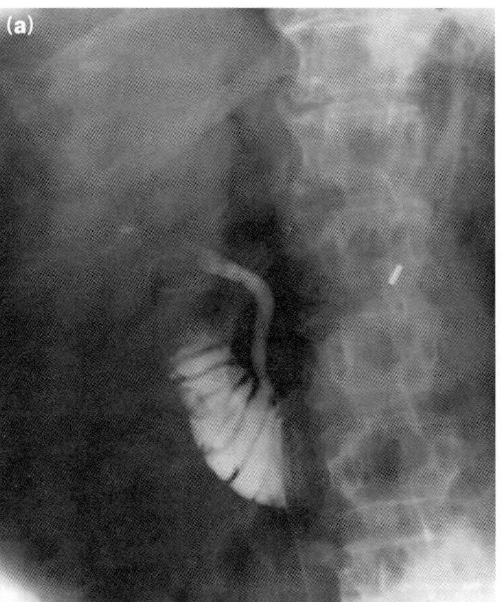

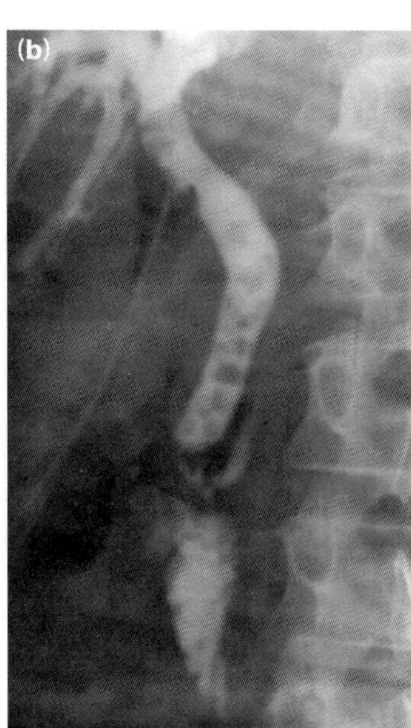

Figure 67.21 Peroperative cholangiography. (a) Gentle infusion of contrast, passing without hindrance into the duodenum. A normal duct with no problems. (b) The duct is dilated and contains multiple stones. There is hold-up of contrast passing into the duodenum. A sphincterotomy was performed.

Laparoscopic ultrasonography

At laparoscopy, the use of a laparoscopic ultrasound probe can be used to image the extrahepatic biliary system. It is a useful technique in biliary and pancreatic tumour staging as it can identify the primary tumour and determine its relationship to major vessels such as the hepatic artery, superior mesenteric artery, portal vein and superior mesenteric vein.

CONGENITAL ABNORMALITIES OF THE GALLBLADDER AND BILE DUCTS

Embryology

The hepatic diverticulum arises from the ventral wall of the foregut and elongates into a stalk to form the choledochus. A lateral bud is given off, which is destined to become the gallbladder and cystic duct. The embryonic hepatic duct sends out many branches which join up the canaliculi between the liver cells. As is usual with embryonic tubular structures, hyperplasia obliterates the lumina of this ductal system; normally recanalisation subsequently occurs and bile begins to flow. During early fetal life the gallbladder is entirely intrahepatic.

Absence of the gallbladder

Occasionally, the gallbladder is absent. Failure to visualise the gallbladder does not necessarily indicate a pathological problem.

The Phrygian cap

The Phrygian cap (Figure 67.22) is present in 5% of cases and may be mistaken for a pathological deformity of the organ. ‘Phrygian cap’ refers to hats worn by the people of Phrygia, an ancient country of Asia Minor; it was rather like a liberté cap of the French Revolution.

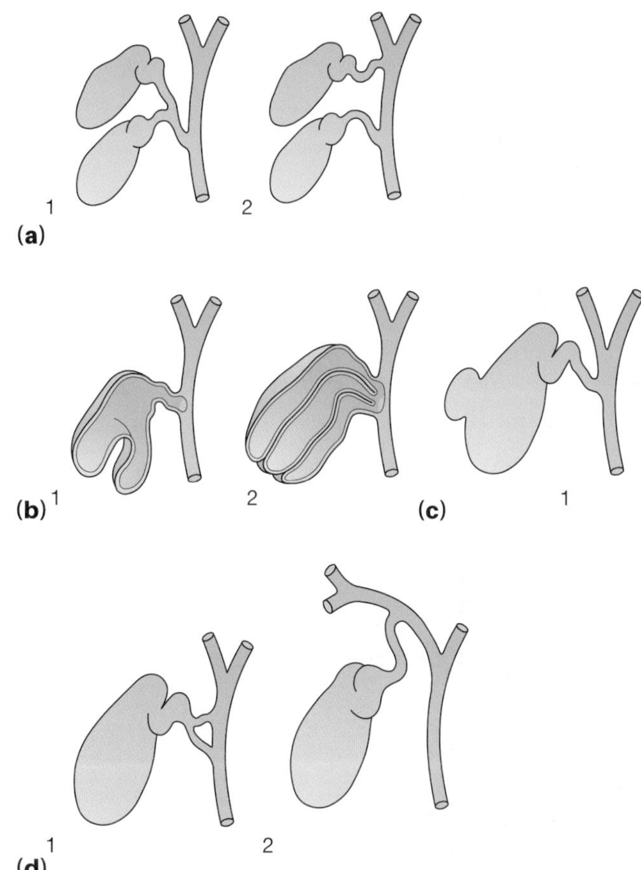

Figure 67.22 The main variations in gallbladder and cystic duct anatomy. (a) Double gallbladder. (b) Septum of the gallbladder: 1 is the most common, the so-called ‘Phrygian cap’. (c) Diverticulum of the gallbladder. (d) Variations in cystic duct insertion.

Floating gallbladder

The gallbladder may hang on a mesentery, which makes it liable to undergo torsion.

Absence of the cystic duct

This is usually a pathological, as opposed to an anatomical, anomaly and indicates the recent passage of a stone or the presence of a stone at the lower end of the cystic duct, which is ulcerating into the common bile duct. The main danger at surgery is damage to the bile duct, and particular care to identify the correct anatomy is essential before division of any duct.

Low insertion of the cystic duct

The cystic duct opens into the common bile duct near the ampulla. Variations of this anomaly can occur (Figure 67.23). It is important that the operating surgeon correctly identifies the anatomy to avoid inadvertent damage to the common hepatic or common bile duct. Complete dissection of a cystic duct which is inserted low into the bile duct (Figure 67.24) should be avoided because there is a potential to devascularise the common bile duct, which could result in stricture formation.

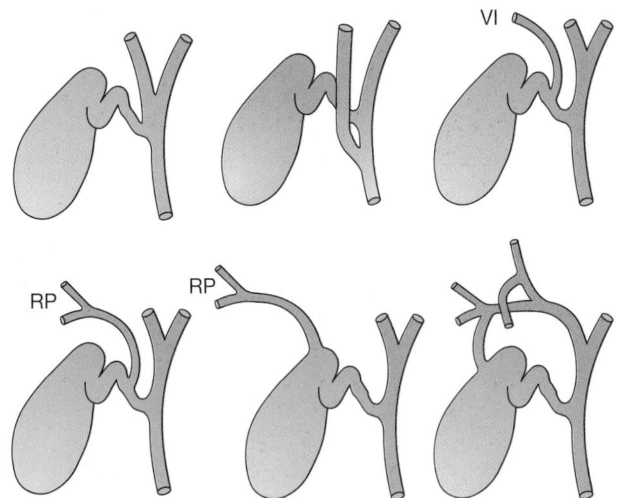

Figure 67.23 Patterns of cystic duct anatomy – note segment VI drainage into the cystic duct and the drainage of the right posterior sectorial duct (RP) into the neck of the gallbladder, or an accessory duct, the so-called duct of Luschka.

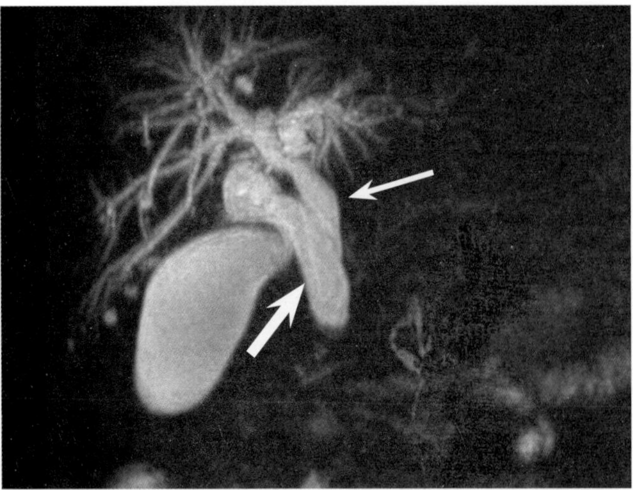

Figure 67.24 Magnetic resonance cholangiopancreatography demonstrating low insertion of the cystic duct (thick arrow) into the common bile duct (thin arrow).

An accessory cholecystohepatic duct

Ducts passing directly into the gallbladder from the liver are not uncommon. Larger ducts should be closed, but before doing so the precise anatomy should be carefully ascertained to ensure that a right hepatic duct is not being ligated (Figure 67.23).

EXTRAHEPATIC BILIARY ATRESIA

Aetiology and physiology

Atresia is present in approximately 1 per 12 000 live births, and affects males and females equally. The extrahepatic bile ducts are progressively destroyed by an inflammatory process which starts around the time of birth. The aetiology is unclear. Intrahepatic changes also occur and eventually result in biliary cirrhosis and portal hypertension. Untreated, death from the consequences of liver failure occurs before the age of 3 years.

The inflammatory destruction of the bile ducts has been classified into three main types (Figure 67.25):

- type I: atresia restricted to the common bile duct;
- type II: atresia of the common hepatic duct;
- type III: atresia of the right and left hepatic ducts.

Associated anomalies occur in about 20% of cases and include cardiac lesions, polysplenia, situs inversus, absent vena cava and a preduodenal portal vein.

Clinical features

About one-third of patients are jaundiced at birth. In all, however, jaundice is present by the end of the first week and deepens progressively. Liver function tests show an obstructive pattern with elevated bilirubin and alkaline phosphatase. The meconium may be a little bile stained, but later the stools are pale and the urine is dark. Prolonged steatorrhoea gives rise to osteomalacia (biliary rickets). Pruritus is severe. Clubbing and skin xanthomas, probably related to raised serum cholesterol, may be present.

Differential diagnosis

This includes any form of jaundice in a neonate giving a cholestatic picture. Examples are α_1-antitrypsin deficiency, cholestasis associated with intravenous feeding, choledochal cyst and inspissated bile syndrome. Neonatal hepatitis is the most difficult to differentiate. Both extrahepatic biliary atresia and neonatal hepatitis are associated with giant cell transformation of the hepatocytes. Liver biopsy and radionuclide excretion scans are essential.

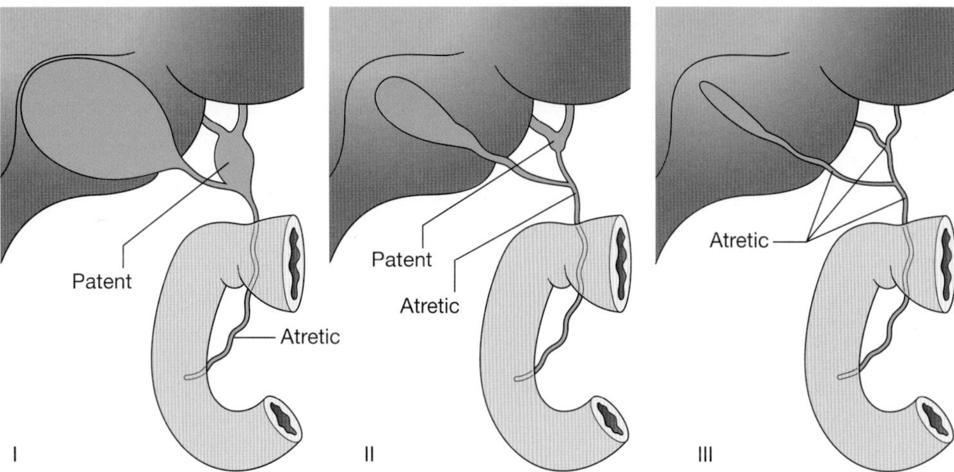

Figure 67.25 Classification of biliary atresia. Gallbladder filling provides a clue to the type of atresia.

Treatment

Patent segments of proximal bile duct are found in 10% of type I lesions. A direct Roux-en-Y hepaticojejunostomy will achieve bile flow in 75%, but progressive fibrosis results in disappointing long-term results. A simple biliary–enteric anatomosis is not possible in the majority of cases in which the proximal hepatic ducts are either very small (type II) or atretic (type III). These are treated by the Kasai procedure, in which radical excision of all bile duct tissue up to the liver capsule is performed. A Roux-en-Y loop of jejunum is anastomosed to the exposed area of liver capsule above the bifurcation of the portal vein, creating a portoenterostomy. The chances of achieving effective bile drainage after portoenterostomy are maximal when the operation is performed before the age of 8 weeks, and approximately 90% of children whose bilirubin falls to within the normal range can be expected to survive for 10 years or more. Early referral for surgery is critical.

Postoperative complications include bacterial cholangitis, which occurs in 40% of patients. Repeated attacks lead to hepatic fibrosis, and 50% of long-term survivors develop portal hypertension, with one-third having variceal bleeding.

Liver transplantation should be considered in children in whom a portoenterostomy is unsuccessful. Results are improving, with 70–80% alive 2–5 years following transplant.

CONGENITAL DILATATION OF THE INTRAHEPATIC DUCTS (CAROLI'S DISEASE)

This rare congenital condition is characterised by multiple irregular saccular dilatations of the intrahepatic ducts, separated by segments of normal or stenotic ducts, with a normal extrahepatic biliary system. In Caroli's syndrome, the biliary dilatation is associated with congenital hepatic fibrosis. The presentation is varied, with many patients presenting with abdominal pain, cholangitis or end-stage liver disease. The majority of patients present before the age of 30. Sex distribution is equal. Management is multidisciplinary: cholangitis or jaundice are treated with appropriate antibiotic therapy and endoscopic or interventional stenting. Malignancy is a complication of long-standing disease. Hepatic resection is indicated for patients with limited disease. Patients with diffuse disease and concomitant hepatic fibrosis are candidates for liver transplantation. Recurrence is common, particularly after resection, and long-term surveillance is required.

CHOLEDOCHAL CYST

Cystic disease of the biliary system is rare. Choledochal cysts are congenital dilations of the intra and/or extrahepatic biliary system. The pathogenesis is unclear. Anomalous junctions of the biliary pancreatic junction are frequently observed, but whether or not these play a role in the pathogenesis of the condition is unclear. Todani and colleagues proposed a classification of cystic disease of the biliary tract (Figure 67.26). Type I cysts are the most common and account for approximately 75% of patients.

Patients may present at any age with jaundice, fever, abdominal pain and a right upper quadrant mass on examination; however, 60% of cases are diagnosed before the age of 10 years. Pancreatitis is not an infrequent presentation in adults. Patients with choledochal cysts have an increased risk of developing cholangiocarcinoma with the risk varying directly with the age at diagnosis.

Ultrasonography will confirm the presence of an abnormal cyst and magnetic resonance imaging (MRI/MRCP) will reveal the anatomy, in particular the relationship between the lower end of the bile duct and the pancreatic duct. CT is also useful for delineating the extent of the intra- or extrahepatic dilatation.

César Roux, 1857–1934, Professor of Surgery and Gynaecology, Lausanne, Switzerland. Described the Roux-en-Y loop in 1908.
Morio Kasai, 1922–2008, Professor of Surgery, Tokyo University, Japan.
Jacques Caroli, 1902–1979, gastrogenterologist, Hôpital St Antoine, Paris, described cavernous ectasia in the biliary tree in 1958.
Takuji Todani, b.1931, Department of Surgery, Okayama University Medical School, Japan, modified Alonso-Lej's classification of choledochal cysts in 1977.

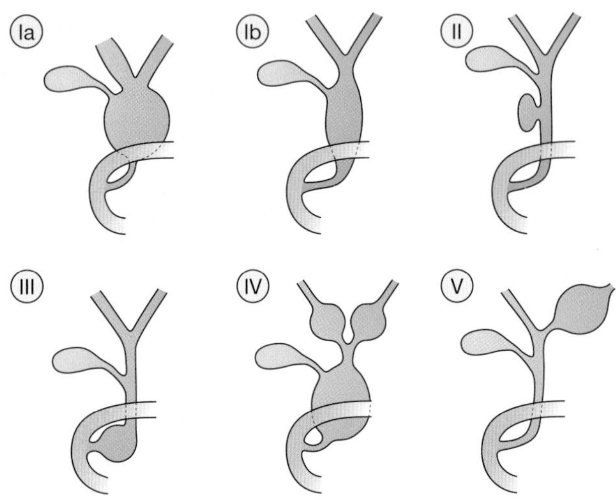

Figure 67.26 Classification of types of choledochal cyst. Type Ia and b: diffuse cystic. Note extension into pancreas of type Ib. Type II: diverticulum of common bile duct. Type III: diverticulum within pancreas. Type IV: extension into the liver. Type V: cystic dilatation only of the intrahepatic ducts.

Radical excision of the cyst is the treatment of choice, with reconstruction of the biliary tract using a Roux-en-Y loop of jejunum. Complete resection of the cyst is important because of the association with the development of cholangiocarcinoma. Resection and roux-en-Y reconstruction are also associated with a reduced incidence of stricture formation and recurrent cholangitis.

TRAUMA

Injuries to the gallbladder and extrahepatic biliary tree are rare. They occur as a result of blunt or penetrating abdominal trauma. Iatrogenic injury is perhaps more frequent than external trauma. The physical signs are those of an acute abdomen. Management depends on the location and extent of the biliary and associated injury. In the stable patient a transected bile duct is best repaired by a Roux-en-Y choledochojejunostomy. Injuries to the gallbladder can be dealt with by cholecystectomy.

TORSION OF THE GALLBLADDER

This is very rare and requires a long mesentery, and therefore often occurs in an older patient with a large mucocoele of the gallbladder. The patient presents with extreme pain and an acute abdomen. Immediate exploration is indicated, with cholecystectomy as the only treatment.

GALLSTONES (CHOLELITHIASIS)

Gallstones are the most common biliary pathology. It is estimated that gallstones affect 10–15% of the population in Western societies. They are asymptomatic in the majority of cases (>80%). In the UK, the prevalence of gallstones at the time of death is estimated to be 17% and may be increasing. Approximately 1–2% of asymptomatic patients will develop symptoms requiring surgery per year, making cholecystectomy one of the most common operations performed by general surgeons.

Causal factors in gallstone formation

Gallstones can be divided into three main types: cholesterol, pigment (brown/black) or mixed stones. In the USA and Europe 80% are cholesterol or mixed stones, whereas in Asia 80% are pigment stones. Cholesterol or mixed stones contain 51–99% pure cholesterol plus an admixture of calcium salts, bile acids, bile pigments and phospholipids.

Cholesterol, which is insoluble in water, is secreted from the canalicular membrane in phospholipid vesicles. Whether cholesterol remains in solution depends on the concentration of phospholipids and bile acids in the bile, and on the type of phospholipid and bile acid. Micelles formed by the phospholipid hold cholesterol in a stable thermodynamic state. When bile is supersaturated with cholesterol or bile acid concentrations are low, unstable unilamellar phospholipid vesicles form, from which cholesterol crystals may nucleate, and stones may form. The process of gallstone formation is complex (Figure 67.27), and many areas remain unclear. Obesity, high-caloric diets and certain medications (e.g. oral contraceptives) can increase secretion of cholesterol and supersaturate the bile, increasing the lithogenicity of bile. Resection of the terminal ileum, which diminishes the enterohepatic circulation, will deplete the bile acid pool and result in cholesterol supersaturation. Nucleation of cholesterol monohydrate crystals from multilamellar vesicles is a crucial step in gallstone formation. Abnormal emptying of the gallbladder may aid the aggregation of nucleated cholesterol crystals; hence, removing gallstones without removing the gallbladder inevitability leads to gallstone recurrence.

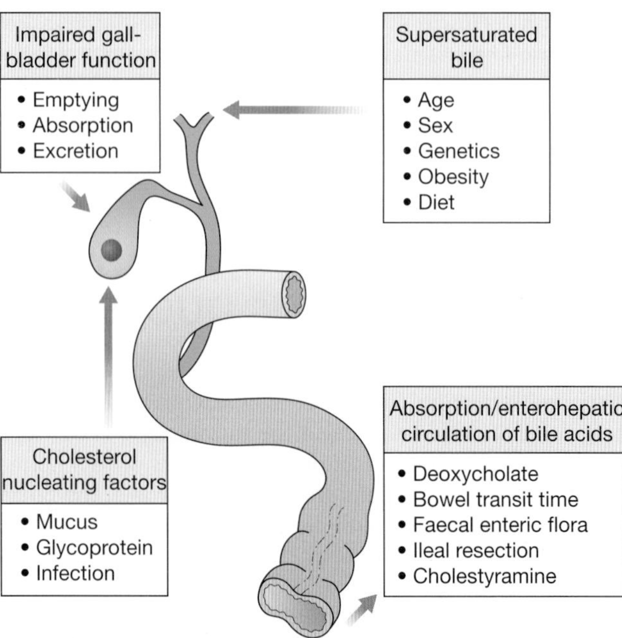

Figure 67.27 Factors associated with gallstone formation.

Pigment stone is the name used for stones containing <30% cholesterol. There are two types: black and brown. Black stones are largely composed of an insoluble bilirubin pigment polymer mixed with calcium phosphate and calcium bicarbonate. Overall, 20–30% of stones are black. The incidence rises with age. Black stones are associated with haemolysis, usually hereditary spherocytosis or sickle cell disease. For reasons that are unclear, patients with cirrhosis have a higher instance of pigmented stones.

Brown pigment stones contain calcium bilirubinate, calcium palmitate and calcium stearate, as well as cholesterol. Brown stones are rare in the gallbladder. They form in the bile duct and are related to bile stasis and infected bile. Stone formation is related to the deconjugation of bilirubin deglucuronide by bacterial β-glucuronidase. Insoluble unconjugated bilirubinate precipitates. Brown pigment stones are also associated with the presence of foreign bodies within the bile ducts such as endoprostheses (stents) or parasites such as *Clonorchis sinensis* and *Ascaris lumbricoides*.

Clinical presentation

Gallstones may remain asymptomatic, being detected incidentally as imaging is performed for other symptoms. If symptoms occur, patients typically complain of right upper quadrant or epigastric pain, which may radiate to the back. This may be described as colicky but more often is dull and constant. Other symptoms include dyspepsia, flatulence, food intolerance particularly to fats and some alteration in bowel frequency. Biliary colic is typically present in 10–25% of patients. This is described as a severe right upper quadrant pain which ebbs and flows, associated with nausea and vomiting. Pain may radiate to the chest. The pain is usually severe and may last for minutes or even several hours. Frequently, the pain starts during the night and wakes the patient. Minor episodes of the same discomfort may occur intermittently during the day. Dyspeptic symptoms may coexist and be worse after such an attack. As the pain resolves the patient improves and is able to eat and drink again, often only to suffer further episodes. It is of interest that a patient may have several episodes of this nature over a period of a few weeks and then no more trouble for some months. Jaundice may result if the stone migrates from the gallbladder and obstructs the common bile duct. Rarely, a gallstone can lead to bowel obstruction (gallstone ileus).

When the symptoms do not resolve but progress to continued pain with fever and leukocytosis, the diagnosis of acute cholecystitis should be considered. The differential diagnosis is given in *Summary box 67.3*.

Summary box 67.2

Effects and complications of gallstones

- Biliary colic
- Acute cholecystitis
- Chronic cholecystitis
- Empyema of the gallbladder
- Mucocoele
- Perforation
- Biliary obstruction
- Acute cholangitis
- Acute pancreatitis
- Intestinal obstruction (gallstone ileus)

Summary box 67.3

Differential diagnosis of acute cholecystitis

Common

- Appendicitis
- Perforated peptic ulcer
- Acute pancreatitis

Rare

- Acute pyelonephritis
- Myocardial infarction
- Pneumonia – right lower lobe

Diagnosis

A diagnosis of gallstone disease is based on the history and physical examination with confirmatory radiological studies such as transabdominal ultrasonography and radionuclide scans (see above). In the acute phase the patient may have right upper quadrant tenderness that is exacerbated during inspiration by the examiner's right subcostal palpation (Murphy's sign). A positive Murphy's sign suggests acute inflammation and may be associated with a leukocytosis and moderately elevated liver function tests. A mass may be palpable as the omentum walls off an inflamed gallbladder. While the presentation and examination may suggest acute cholecystitis, a definitive diagnosis can only be made following appropriate imaging studies (US or CT). Fortunately, in the majority of cases the process is limited by the stone slipping back into the body of the gallbladder and the contents of the gallbladder escaping by way of the cystic duct. This achieves adequate drainage of the gallbladder and enables the inflammation to resolve.

If resolution does not occur, an empyema of the gallbladder may result. The wall may become necrotic and perforate, with development of localised peritonitis. The abscess may then perforate into the peritoneal cavity with a septic peritonitis; however, this is uncommon, because the inflamed gallbladder is usually localised by omentum which contains the perforation.

A palpable, non-tender gallbladder (Courvoisier's sign) portends a more sinister diagnosis. This usually results from a distal common duct obstruction secondary to a peripancreatic

John Benjamin Murphy, 1857–1916, surgeon, Mercy Hospital Chicago, IL, USA.
Ludwig Courvoisier, 1843–1918, Professor of Surgery, Basle, Switzerland.

malignancy. Rarely, a non-tender, palpable gallbladder results from complete obstruction of the cystic duct with reabsorption of the intraluminal bile salts and secretion of uninfected mucus by the gallbladder epithelium, leading to a mucocoele of the gallbladder.

Treatment

Most consider that it is safe to observe patients with asymptomatic gallstones, with cholecystectomy reserved for patients who develop symptoms or complications. However, prophylactic cholecystectomy may be considered for diabetic patients, those with congenital haemolytic anaemia and those patients who are undergoing bariatric surgery for morbid obesity because it has been found in these groups that the risk of developing symptoms is increased. For patients with symptomatic gallstones, cholecystectomy is the treatment of choice if there are no medical contraindications.

Experience shows that, in more than 90% of cases, the symptoms of acute cholecystitis subside with conservative measures. Non-operative treatment is based on four principles:

- Nil per mouth (NPO) and intravenous fluid administration until the pain resolves.
- Administration of analgesics.
- Administration of antibiotics. As the cystic duct is blocked in most instances, the concentration of antibiotic in the serum is more important than its concentration in bile. A broad-spectrum antibiotic effective against gram-negative aerobes is most appropriate (e.g. cefazolin, cefuroxime or ciprofloxacillin).
- Subsequent management. When the temperature, pulse and other physical signs show that the inflammation is subsiding, oral fluids are reinstated, followed by a regular diet. Ultrasonography is performed to confirm the diagnosis. If jaundice is present MRCP is performed to exclude choledocholithiasis. If there is any concern regarding the diagnosis or presence of complications such as perforation CT should be performed. Cholecystectomy may be performed on the next available list, or the patient may be allowed home to return later when the inflammation has completely resolved.

The 2013 Toyko guidelines allow assessment of severity to be made (*Table 67.1*). In patients with grade III disease depending on the status of the patient either operative intervention and cholecystectomy should be performed or if the patient has comorbid conditions, a percutaneous cholecystostomy can be performed by a radiologist under ultrasound control. This will usually rapidly relieve symptoms, however an interval cholecystectomy will be required once the patient's condition has stablised.

The timing of surgery in acute cholecystitis remains controversial, with many units favouring an early intervention within the first week whereas others suggest that a delayed approach is preferable. Early cholecystectomy during acute cholecystitis appears to be safe and shortens the total hospital stay.

Provided that the operation is undertaken within 5–7 days of the onset of the attack, the surgeon is experienced and excellent operating facilities are available, good results are achieved. Nevertheless, the conversion rate in laparoscopic cholecystectomy is higher in acute than in elective surgery. If an early operation is not indicated one should wait approximately 6 weeks for the inflammation to subside before operating.

TABLE 67.1 Tokyo Consensus Guidelines for severity grading of acute cholecystitis. Reproduced with permission from Yokoe *et al. J Hepatobiliary Pancreat Sci* 2013; **30**: 35–46.

Grade III (severe) acute cholecystitis	
Associated with dysfunction of any one of the following organs/systems:	
1 Cardiovascular dysfunction	Hypertension requiring treatment with dopamine ≤5 µg/kg/min, or any dose of norepinephrine (noradrenaline)
2 Neurological dysfunction	Decreased level of consciousness
3 Respiratory dysfunction	P_aO_2/FiO_2 ratio <300
4 Renal dysfunction	Oliguria; creatinine >2.0 mg/dL
5 Hepatic dysfunction	Prothrombin time (PT-INR) >1.5
6 Haematological dysfunction	Platelet count <100 000/mm^3
Grade II (moderate) acute cholecystitis	
Associated with any one of the following conditions: 1 Elevated white cell count (>18 000/mm^3) 2 Palpable tender mass in the right upper abdominal quadrant 3 Duration of complaints >72 hours 4 Marked local inflammation (gangrenous cholecystitis, pericholecystic abscess, hepatic abscess, biliary peritonitis, emphysematous cholecystitis)	
Grade I (mild) acute cholecystitis	
Does not meet the criteria of grade II or grade III acute cholecystitis. Grade I can also be defined as acute cholecystitis in a healthy person with no organ dysfunction and mild inflammatory changes in the gallbladder, making cholecystectomy a safe and low-risk operative procedure	

EMPYEMA OF THE GALLBLADDER

Empyema may be a sequel to acute cholecystitis or the result of a mucocoele becoming infected. The gallbladder is distended with pus. The optimal treatment is drainage (cholecystostomy, see above) and, later, cholecystectomy.

Acalculous cholecystitis

Acute and chronic inflammation of the gallbladder can occur in the absence of stones and give rise to a clinical picture similar to that of calculous cholecystitis. Some patients have non-specific inflammation of the gallbladder, whereas others have one of the cholecystoses (see below). Acute acalculous cholecystitis is particularly seen in critically ill patients and those recovering from major surgery, trauma and burns. The diagnosis is often missed and the mortality rate is high.

THE CHOLECYSTOSES (CHOLESTEROSIS, POLYPOSIS, ADENOMYOMATOSIS AND CHOLECYSTITIS GLANDULARIS PROLIFERANS)

This is a relatively uncommon group of conditions affecting the gallbladder, in which there are chronic inflammatory changes with hyperplasia of all tissue elements.

Cholesterosis ('strawberry gallbladder')

In the fresh state, the interior of the gallbladder looks something like a strawberry in patients with this condition; the yellow specks (submucous aggregations of cholesterol crystals and cholesterol esters) correspond to the seeds (Figure 67.28). It may be associated with cholesterol stones.

Cholesterol polyposis of the gallbladder

Ultrasound may show a non-mobile defect in the gallbladder lumen which does not exhibit an associated acoustic shadow. The differential is an adenomatous polyp, and interval follow-up is indicated to ensure stability. Surgery is only advised if there is a diagnostic dilemma.

Cholecystitis glandularis proliferans (polyp, adenomyomatosis and intramural diverticulosis)

Figure 67.29 summarises the varieties of this condition. A polyp of the mucous membrane is fleshy and granulomatous.

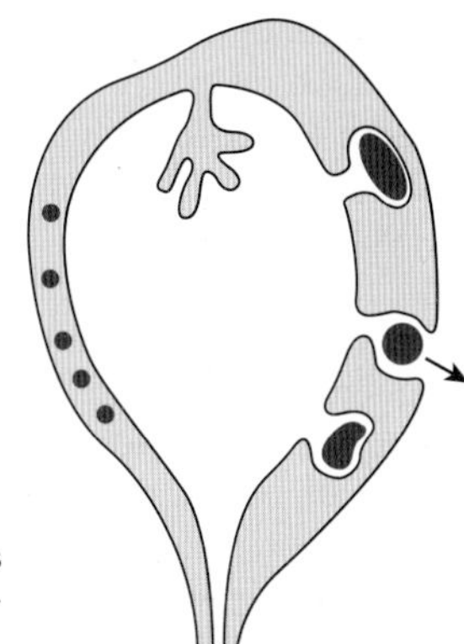

Figure 67.29 Types of cholecystitis glandularis proliferans (polypus, intramural or diverticular stones and fistula).

All layers of the gallbladder wall may be thickened, but sometimes an incomplete septum forms that separates the hyperplastic from the normal. Intraparietal 'mixed' calculi may be present. These can be complicated by an intramural, and later extramural, abscess and potentially fistula formation. If symptomatic, the patient is treated by cholecystectomy.

Diverticulosis of the gallbladder

Diverticulosis of the gallbladder is usually manifest as black pigment stones impacted in the outpouchings of the lacunae of Luschka. Diverticulosis of the gallbladder may be demonstrated by cholecystography, especially when the gallbladder contracts after a fatty meal. There are small dots of contrast medium just within and outside the gallbladder (Figure 67.30). A septum may also be present, to be distinguished from the Phrygian cap. The treatment is cholecystectomy.

Typhoid infection of the gallbladder

Salmonella typhi or *Salmonella typhimurium* can infect the gallbladder. Acute cholecystitis can occur. More frequently,

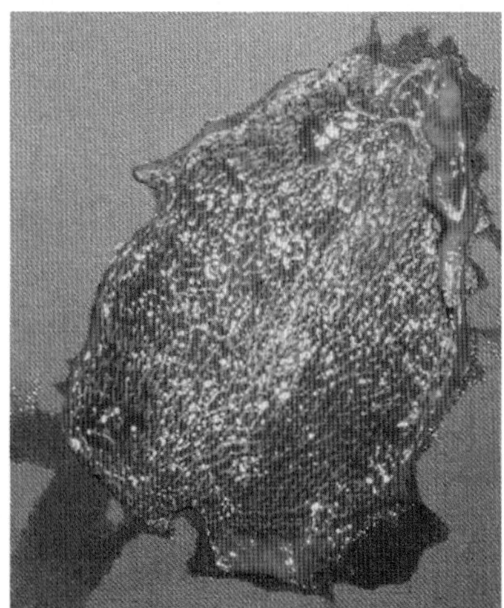

Figure 67.28 The interior of a strawberry gallbladder (cholesterosis) (courtesy of Dr Sanjay P Thakur, Patna, India).

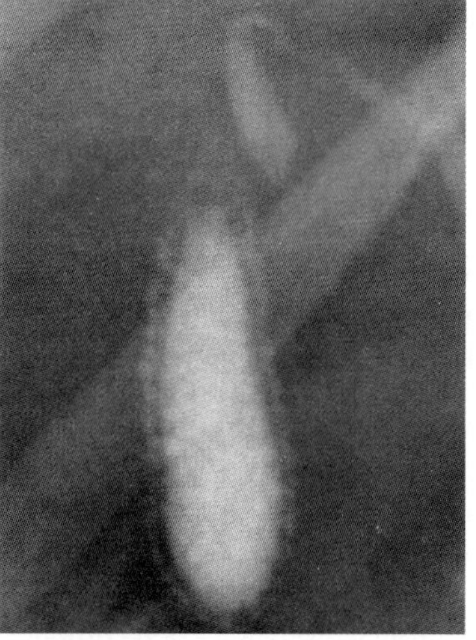

Figure 67.30 Cholecystogram showing diverticulosis with dots of contrast medium in the gallbladder wall.

Daniel Elmer Salmon, 1850–1914, veterinary pathologist, Chief of the Bureau of Animal Industry, Washington, DC, USA.

chronic cholecystitis occurs, the patient becoming a typhoid carrier excreting the bacteria in the bile. Gallstones may be present (surgeons should not give patients their stones after their operation if there is any suspicion of typhoid!). It is debatable whether the stones are secondary to the *Salmonella* cholecystitis or whether pre-existing stones predispose the gallbladder to chronic infection. Salmonellae can, however, frequently be cultured from these stones. Treatment with ampicillin and cholecystectomy are indicated. In cases of penicillin allergy a quinolone antibiotic can be used.

CHOLECYSTECTOMY

Preparation for operation

After appropriate history taking and assessment of the patient's fitness for the procedure, a full blood count and biochemical profile should be performed to exclude anaemia and to identify abnormal liver function. A blood coagulation screen should be checked if there is a history of jaundice or liver function is abnormal. Prophylactic antibiotics should be administered either with the premedication or at the time of induction of anaesthesia. A second-generation cephalosporin is appropriate. Subcutaneous heparin or antiembolic stockings should be prescribed. The patient must sign a consent form to indicate that he or she is fully aware of the procedure being undertaken, alternative options and the risks involved and complications that may occur.

Summary box 67.4

Preparation for cholecystectomy

- Full blood count
- Renal profile and liver function tests
- Prothrombin time
- Chest x-ray and electrocardiogram (if over 45 years or medically indicated)
- Antibiotic prophylaxis
- Deep vein thrombosis prophylaxis
- Informed consent

Laparoscopic cholecystectomy

The preparation and indications for cholecystectomy are the same whether it is performed by laparoscopy or by open techniques. Laparoscopic cholecystectomy is the procedure of choice for the majority of patients with gallbladder disease. The key, as in open surgery, is the identification and safe dissection of Calot's triangle (Figure 67.31).

The patient is placed supine on the operating table. Following induction and maintenance of general anaesthesia, the abdomen is prepared in a standard fashion. Pneumoperitoneum is established. A number of techniques are described. The author's preference is to use an open subumbilical cutdown with direct visualisation of the peritoneum, to place the initial port. This port will function as the camera port. An angled telescope (30°) is preferred. Many surgeons perfer a 'closed' technique using a Verres needle to establish pneumoperitoneum prior to placing the initial trocar. Recently, single-port laparoscopic cholecystectomy has been described. Proponents report decreased postoperative pain and improved cosmesis. However, recent systematic reviews have reported a higher failure rate, longer operative time and increased blood loss without any substantive benefits for the technique.

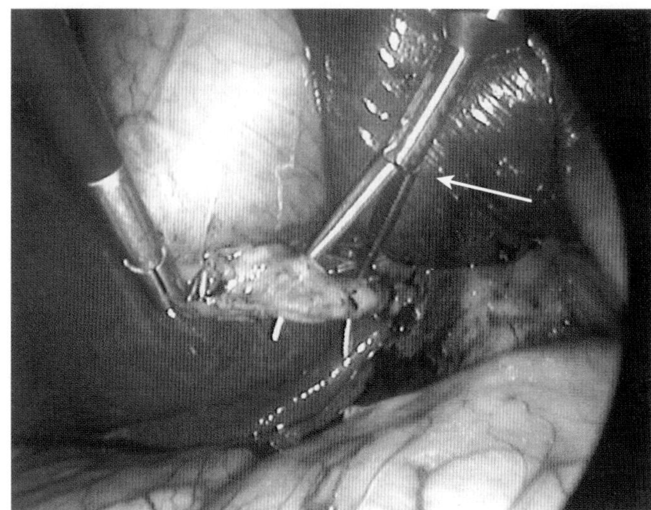

Figure 67.31 Operative image of a laparoscopic cholecystectomy. Laparoscopic forceps (arrow) are used to dissect Calot's triangle.

Additional operating ports are inserted in the subxiphoid area and in the right subcostal area. The patient is placed in a reverse Trendelberg position slightly rotated to the left. This exposes the fundus of the gallbladder which is retracted towards the diaphragm. The neck of the gallbladder is then retracted towards the right iliac fossa, exposing Calot's triangle. This area is laid wide open by dividing the peritoneum on the posterior and on the anterior aspect. The cystic duct is carefully defined, as is the cystic artery. The gallbladder is separated from the liver bed for about 2 cm to allow confirmation of the anatomy. Unless there are specific indications (see below) a routine cholangiogram is not performed. However, if doubt exists regarding the anatomy a cholangiogram is warranted. Once the anatomy is clearly defined and the triangle of Calot has been laid wide open, the cystic duct and artery are clipped and divided. The gallbladder is then removed from the gallbladder bed by sharp or cautery dissection and, once free, removed via the umbilicus.

Open cholecystectomy

For patients in whom a laparoscopic approach is not indicated or in whom conversion from a laparoscopic approach is required an open cholecystectomy is performed.

Either an upper midline or a short right upper transverse incision is made, centred over the lateral border of the rectus muscle. The gallbladder is appropriately exposed and packs are placed on the hepatic flexure of the colon, the duodenum and the lesser omentum to ensure a clear view of the anatomy of the porta hepatis. These packs may be retracted by the assistant's hand ('It is the left hand of the assistant that does all the work' – Moynihan). Alternatively, a stabilised ring retractor is used to keep the packs in position.

An artery or Duval forceps is placed on the infundibulum of the gallbladder and the peritoneum overlying Calot's triangle is placed on a stretch. The peritoneum is then divided close to the wall of the gallbladder and the fat in the triangle of Calot carefully dissected away to expose the cystic artery and the cystic duct. The cystic duct is cleaned down to the common bile duct, whose position is clearly ascertained. The cystic artery is tied and divided. The whole of the triangle of Calot is displayed to ensure that the anatomy of the ducts is clear and the cystic duct is then divided between ligatures (Figure 67.32). The gallbladder is then dissected away from the gallbladder bed.

Some golden rules to observe in case of difficulty:

- When the anatomy of the triangle of Calot is unclear, blind dissection should stop.
- Bleeding adjacent to the triangle of Calot should be controlled by pressure and not by blind clipping or clamping.
- When there is doubt about the anatomy, a retrograde or 'fundus-first' cholecystectomy dissection on the gallbladder wall from the fundus to the cystic duct can be helpful.
- If the cystic duct is densely adherent to the common bile duct and there is the possibility of a Mirizzi syndrome (a stone ulcerating through the neck of the gallbladder into the common hepatic duct), the infundibulum of the gallbladder should be opened, the stone removed and the infundibulum oversewn. Attempts to dissect out the cystic duct completely will only lead to injury to the common hepatic or common bile duct.
- A cholecystostomy is rarely indicated but, if required, as many stones as possible should be extracted and a large Foley catheter (14 Fr) placed in the fundus of the gallbladder with a direct track externally. By so doing, stones retained in the gallbladder can be subsequently extracted with a choledochoscope.

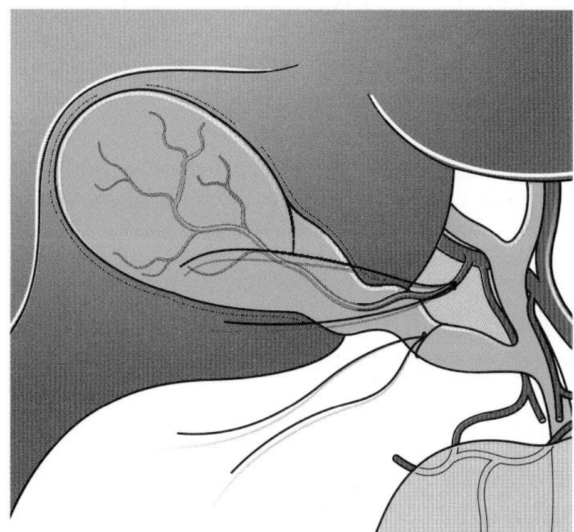

Figure 67.32 Ligatures are passed and tied around the cystic artery and cystic duct. The grey shaded area represents Calot's triangle.

Indications for choledochotomy

In an environment in which neither the modern diagnostic armamentarium described at the beginning of this chapter nor peroperative cholangiography is available, it is well to remember the traditional indications for choledochotomy, which are:

- palpable duct stones;
- jaundice or a history of jaundice or cholangitis;
- a dilated common bile duct;
- abnormal liver function tests, in particular a raised alkaline phosphatase.

Unless the expertise is available, it is probably inadvisable to perform a choledochotomy laparoscopically; rather, one should rely on endoscopic techniques or convert to an open operation. The incidence of symptomatic stones in the bile duct varies from 5% to 8%. These can, in the main, be dealt with endoscopically without resort to opening the duct. However, current trials suggest that in experienced hands the morbidity associated with the two techniques is identical.

Complications of cholecystectomy

Recovery after laparoscopic cholecystectomy is associated with less pain and faster return to normal activity than after open cholecystectomy. The majority of patients undergoing an elective laparoscopic cholecystectomy can have this performed as a day case, avoiding hospital admission. Any untoward symptoms in the postoperative period such as fevers, chills or abdominal pain require immediate investigation.

The operative mortality for cholecystectomy is less than 1%. Factors increasing the risk for postoperative mortality include advanced age, comorbid conditions and acute presentation. Complications can occur in 10–15% of cases. Serious complications of laparoscopic cholecystectomy fall into two major areas: access complications and bile duct injuries. The latter are rare, occurring in approximately 0.5% of cases. In the main, biliary injury results from poor dissection and failure to define the surgical anatomy adequately. Controversy exists as to whether or not the use of operative cholangiography reduces the incidence of bile duct injury. The majority of surgeons use cholangiography only in selected cases.

Patients who develop jaundice in the postoperative period require urgent investigation. This is especially true if the jaundice is associated with infection, a condition called cholangitis.

The first step in management following resuscitation and administration of appropriate antibiotics is to undertake an urgent ultrasound scan. This will demonstrate whether there is intra- or extrahepatic ductal dilatation. The anatomy needs to be defined by either an ERCP or a MRCP. The former will also allow therapeutic manoeuvres such as removal

Pierre Alfred Duval, 1874–1941, French surgeon.
Pablo Luis Mirizzi, 1893–1964, Argentinian surgeon, described this condition in 1932.
Frederic Eugene Basil Foley, 1891–1965, urologist, The Miller and Anker Hospitals, St Paul, MN, USA.

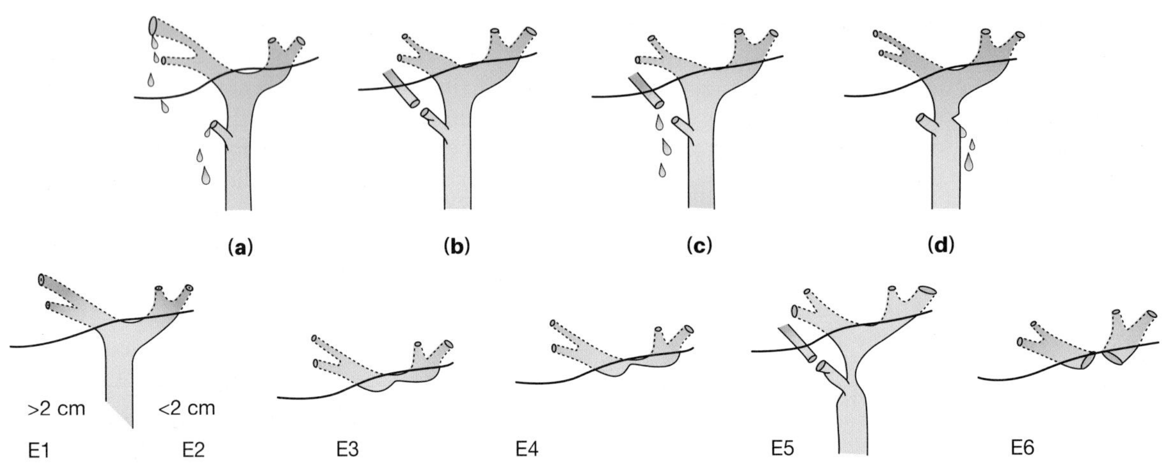

Figure 67.33 Schematic representation of the Strasberg classification of bile duct injuries. (a) Bile leak from cystic duct stump or a minor biliary radical in gallbladder fossa. (b) Occluded right posterior sectoral duct. (c) Bile leak from divided right posterior sectoral duct. (d) Bile leak from main bile duct without major tissue loss. E1: Transected main bile duct with a stricture more than 2 cm from the hilus. E2: Transected main bile duct with a stricture less than 2 cm from the hilus. E3: Stricture of the hilus with right and left ducts in communication. E4: Stricture of the hilus with separation of right and left hepatic ducts. E5: Stricture of the main bile duct and the right posterior sectoral duct. E6: Complete excision of the extrahepatic ducts involving the confluence (this injury is not described in Strasberg's classification). (After Connor S, Garden OJ, *Br J Surg* 2006; **93**: 158–168.)

of an obstructing stone or insertion of a stent across a biliary leak. If a fluid collection is present in the subhepatic space, drainage catheters may be required. These can be inserted under radiological control or, if this expertise is not available, at open operation. Small biliary leaks will usually resolve spontaneously, especially if there is no distal obstruction. Should the common bile duct be damaged, the patient should be referred to an appropriate expert for reconstruction of the duct.

About 15% of injuries to the bile ducts are recognised at the time of operation; in the remaining 85% of cases, the injury declares itself postoperatively by either a profuse and persistent leakage of bile, if drainage has been provided, bile peritonitis if such drainage has not been provided, or deepening obstructive jaundice. When the obstruction is incomplete, jaundice is delayed until subsequent fibrosis renders the lumen of the duct inadequate.

Any postoperative elevation in serum bilirubin or suggestion of duct damage requires investigation and the nature of the bile duct injury clarified.

HIDA scanning may be helpful as it can confirm the presence of a leak or biliary obstruction. It can be used to identify and quantitate the leak. If available, ERCP should be considered because this is both diagnostic and potentially therapeutic. The most common bile leak following cholecystectomy is from the cystic duct. This can be treated by a gastroenterologist placing a biliary endoprosthesis (stent) in the common bile duct across the origin of the cystic duct. MRCP is also helpful in determining the level and degree of injury.

The surgical repair and subsequent outcome are related to the level and degree of injury, in conjunction with the presence or absence of concomitant vascular injury. A number of classification systems have been proposed, with the Strasberg classification being commonly utilised (Figure 67.33).

In a debilitated patient, temporary external biliary drainage may be achieved by passing a catheter percutaneously into an intrahepatic duct. Also, stents may be passed through strictures at the time of ERCP and left to drain into the duodenum. When the general condition of the patient has improved, definitive surgery can be undertaken. The principles of surgical repair are maintenance of duct length and restoration of biliary drainage. For benign stricture or duct transection, the preferred treatment is Roux-en-Y choledochojejunostomy performed by an experienced hepatobiliary surgeon. For a stricture of recent onset through which a guidewire can be passed, balloon dilatation with insertion of a stent is an acceptable alternative, provided that the services of an experienced endoscopist are available. The outcome of such surgery is good, with 90% of patients having no further cholangitis or stricture formation.

Late symptoms after cholecystectomy

In up to 15% of patients, cholecystectomy fails to relieve the symptoms for which the operation was performed. Such patients may be considered to have a 'post-cholecystectomy' syndrome. However, such problems are usually related to the preoperative symptoms and are merely a continuation of those symptoms. Full investigation should be undertaken to confirm the diagnosis and exclude the presence of a stone in the bile duct, a stone in the cystic duct stump or operative damage to the biliary tree. This is best performed by MRCP or ERCP, the latter of which has the added advantage that if a stone is in the common bile duct it can be removed.

Post-cholecystectomy choledocholithiasis

Duct stones may occur many years after a cholecystectomy or be related to the development of new pathology, such as infection of the biliary tree or infestation by *Ascaris lumbricoides* or *Clinorchis sinensis*. Any obstruction to the flow of bile can give rise to stasis with the formation of stones within the duct. The consequence of duct stones is either obstruction to bile flow or infection. Stones in the bile ducts are more often associated with infected bile (80%) than are stones in the gallbladder.

Symptoms

The patient may be asymptomatic but usually has bouts of pain, jaundice and fever. The patient is often ill and feels unwell. The term 'cholangitis' is given to the triad of pain, jaundice and fevers sometimes known as 'Charcot's triad'.

Signs

Tenderness may be elicited in the epigastrium and the right hypochondrium. In the jaundiced patient it is useful to remember Courvoisier's law: 'in obstruction of the common bile duct due to a stone, distension of the gallbladder seldom occurs; the organ usually is already shrivelled'. In obstruction from other causes, distension is common, by comparison. However, if there is no disease in the gallbladder and the obstruction is due to a cancer of the ampulla, pancreas or bile duct, then the gallbladder may well be distended.

Management

It is essential to determine whether the jaundice is due to liver disease, disease within the duct, such as sclerosing cholangitis, or obstruction. Ultrasound scanning, liver function tests, liver biopsy if the ducts are not dilated, and MRI or ERCP will identify the nature of the obstruction.

The patient may be ill. Pus may be present within the biliary tree and liver abscesses may develop. Full supportive measures are required with rehydration, attention to clotting, exclusion of diabetes and administration of appropriate broad-spectrum antibiotics. As soon as resuscitation has taken place, relief of the biliary obstruction is essential. Endoscopic papillotomy is the preferred first technique, by means of a sphincterotomy, removal of the stones using a Dormia basket or placement of a stent if stone removal is not possible (Figures 67.34 and 67.35). If this technique fails, percutaneous transhepatic cholangiography can be performed to provide drainage and subsequent percutaneous choledochoscopy. Surgery, in the form of choledochotomy, is now rarely used for this situation as most patients can be managed by minimally invasive techniques.

Choledochotomy

When faced with a sick patient whose investigations show that the cause of the cholangitis is stones in the common bile duct and minimally invasive techniques for stone extraction are not available, the surgeon has no alternative but to undertake a laparotomy. The aim of this surgery is to drain the common bile duct and remove the stones through a longitudinal incision in the duct. When the duct is clear of stones, a T-tube is inserted and the duct closed around it; the long limb is brought out on the right side and the bile allowed to drain externally. When the bile has become clear and the patient has recovered, a cholangiogram is performed. If residual stones are found, the tube is left in place for 6 weeks so that the track is 'mature'. The radiologist can then use the tract for percutaneous removal of the stones (Figure 67.36). Once the radiologist has removed the tube, the track will close and the patient will make a rapid recovery.

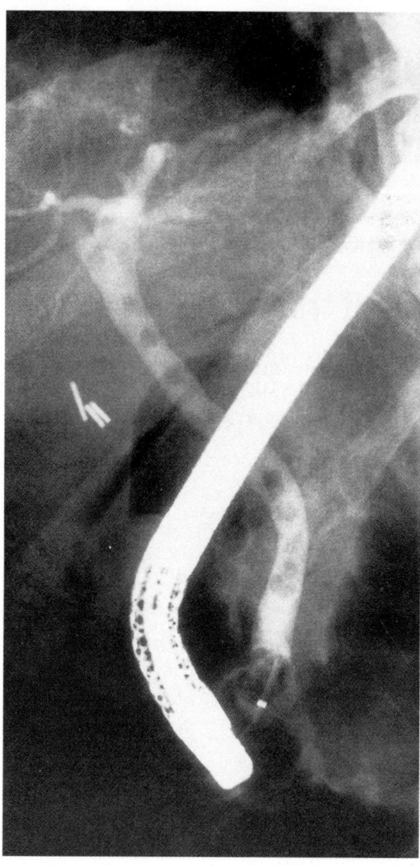

Figure 67.34 This patient presented with jaundice 4 days after a laparoscopic cholecystectomy. The duct contained multiple stones.

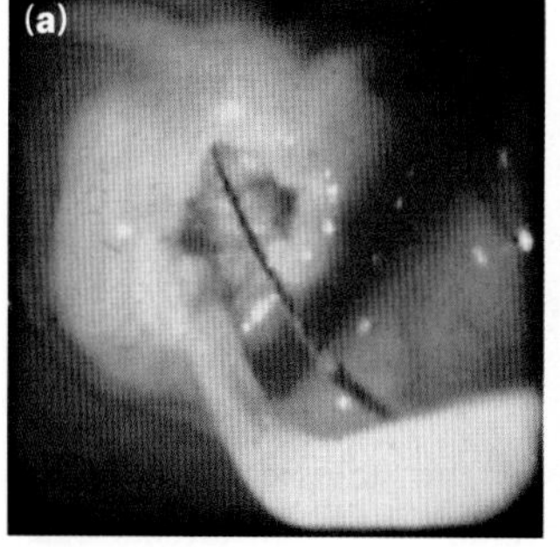

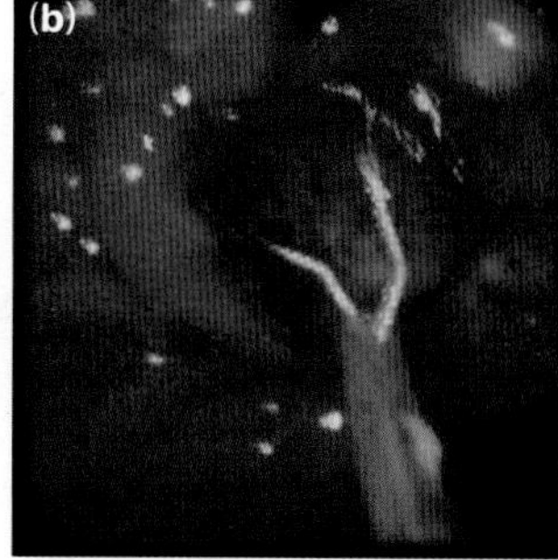

Figure 67.35 **(a)** Endoscopic sphincterotomy; **(b)** extraction of a stone from the bile duct through the ampulla.

Jean Martin Charcot, 1825–1893, physician, La Salpêtrière, Paris, France.

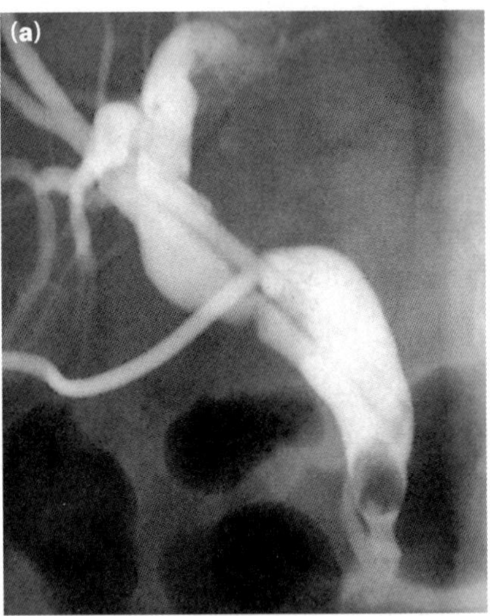
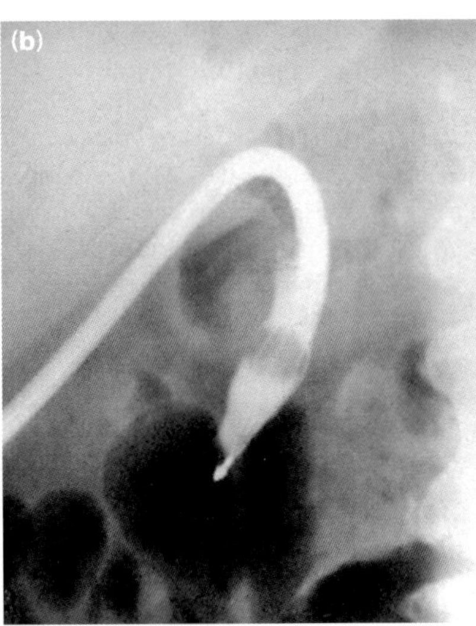
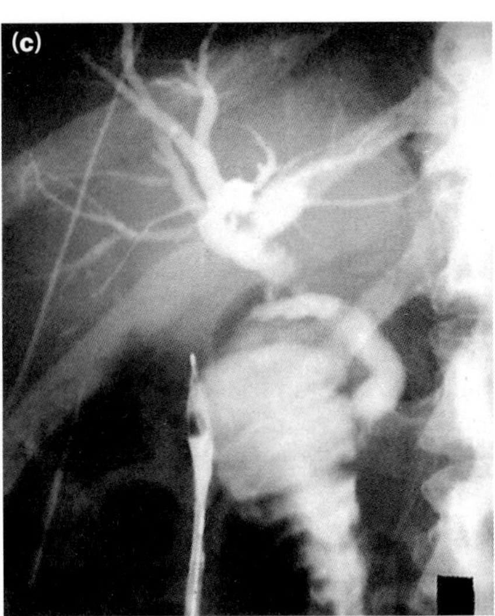

Figure 67.36 Extraction of a stone from the common bile duct by the Burhenne technique. (a) A T-tube in situ with a stone in the duct. (b) A steerable catheter has been manipulated into the duct and a basket placed around the stone. (c) The stone being extracted from the bile duct along the T-tube track.

Stricture of the bile duct

The causes of benign biliary stricture are given in *Summary box 67.5*. Bile duct strictures may be investigated radiologically as described in *Summary box 67.6*.

Summary box 67.5

Causes of benign biliary stricture

Congenital
- Biliary atresia

Bile duct injury at surgery
- Cholecystectomy
- Choledochotomy
- Gastrectomy
- Hepatic resection
- Transplantation

Inflammatory
- Stones
- Cholangitis
- Parasitic
- Pancreatitis
- Sclerosing cholangitis
- Radiotherapy

Trauma

Idiopathic

Summary box 67.6

Radiological investigation of biliary strictures
- Ultrasonography
- Cholangiography via T-tube, if present
- ERCP
- MRCP
- Percutaneous transhepatic cholangiography
- CT scan

PRIMARY SCLEROSING CHOLANGITIS

Primary sclerosing cholangitis is an idiopathic fibrosing inflammatory condition of the biliary tree that affects both intrahepatic and extrahepatic ducts. It is of unknown origin but the association of hypergammaglobulinaemia and elevated markers such as smooth muscle antibodies and antinuclear factor suggest an immunological basis. The majority of patients are between 30 and 60 years of age. There appears to be a male predominance and a strong association with inflammatory bowel disease, especially ulcerative colitis.

Common symptoms include right upper quadrant discomfort, jaundice, pruritus, fever, fatigue and weight loss. Investigation reveals a cholestatic pattern to the liver function tests with elevation of the serum alkaline phosphatase and γ-glutamyl transferase and smaller rises in the aminotransferases. Bilirubin values can be variable and may fluctuate. Imaging studies such as MRCP or ERCP may demonstrate stricturing and beading of the bile ducts (Figure 67.37). A liver biopsy is helpful to confirm the diagnosis and may help guide therapy by excluding cirrhosis. The important differential diagnoses are secondary sclerosing cholangitis and cholangiocarcinoma. The latter may be very difficult to diagnose and a high index of suspicion is required especially in the setting of unexplained clinical deterioration.

Medical management with antibiotics, vitamin K, cholestyramine, steroids and immunosuppressant drugs such as azathioprine is generally unsuccessful. Endoscopic stenting of dominant strictures and, in selected patients with predominantly extrahepatic disease, operative resection may be worthwhile. For patients with cirrhosis, liver transplantation is the best option. Five-year survival following transplantation in high-volume centres is in excess of 80%.

Joachim Burhenne, 1926–1996, radiologist, Vancouver, Canada. His technique transformed stone management in the 1970s.

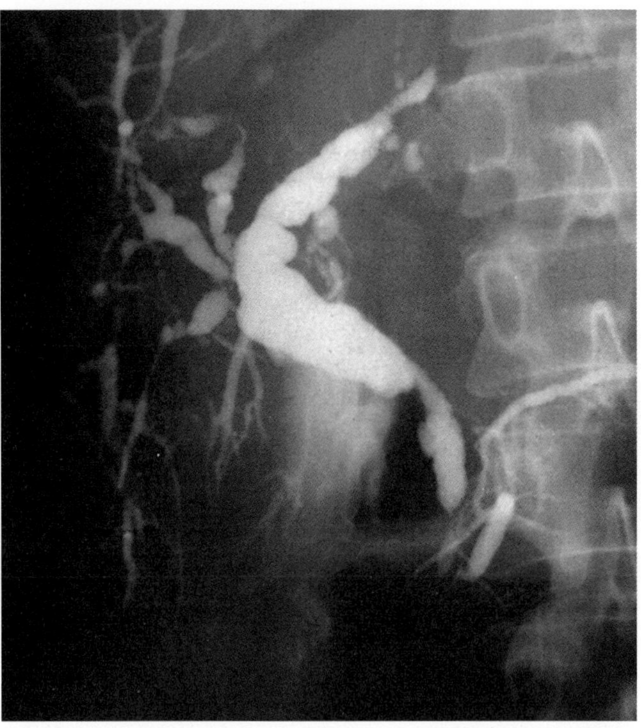

Figure 67.37 Sclerosing cholangitis in a patient with ulcerative colitis, visualised by endoscopic retrograde cholangiopancreatography.

Immunoglobulin (Ig) G_4-related cholangitis

This recently recognised entity presents with diffuse or segmental narrowing of the intra- or extrahepatic bile ducts. Its features may make differentiation from primary sclerosing cholangitis (PSC), cholangiocarcinoma or pancreatic cancer difficult. However, patients often have elevated serum IgG_4 levels and concomitant autoimmune pancreatitis, IgG_4-related sialadenitis or retroperitoneal fibrosis. Biliary biopsies show lymphoplasmacytic sclerosing cholangitis. Treatment is with systemic steroids. Failure to respond to steroid therapy should make one reconsider the diagnosis and exclude an underlying malignancy.

PARASITIC INFESTATION OF THE BILIARY TRACT

Biliary ascariasis

The roundworm *Ascaris lumbricoides* commonly infests the intestines of inhabitants of Asia, Africa and Central America. It may enter the biliary tree through the ampulla of Vater and cause biliary pain. Complications include strictures, suppurative cholangitis, liver abscesses and empyema of the gallbladder. In the uncomplicated case, antispasmodics can be given to relax the sphincter of Oddi and the worms will return to the small intestine to be dealt with by anthelminthic drugs. Operation may be necessary to remove the worms or deal with complications. Worms can be extracted via the ampulla of Vater by ERCP.

Clonorchiasis (Asiatic cholangiohepatis)

This disease is endemic in the Far East. The fluke, up to 25 mm long and 5 mm wide, inhabits the bile ducts, including the intrahepatic ducts. Fibrous thickening of the duct walls occurs. Many cases are asymptomatic. Complications include biliary pain, stones, cholangitis, cirrhosis and bile duct carcinoma. Choledochotomy and T-tube drainage and, in some cases, choledochoduodenostomy are required. Because a process of recurrent stone formation is set up, a choledochojejunostomy with a Roux loop fixed to the adjacent abdominal wall is performed in some centres to allow easy subsequent access to the duct system.

Hydatid disease

A large hydatid cyst may obstruct the hepatic ducts. Sometimes, a cyst will rupture into the biliary tree and its contents cause obstructive jaundice or cholangitis, requiring appropriate surgery (see Chapter 6).

TUMOURS OF THE BILE DUCT

Benign tumours of the bile duct

These are uncommon and may be an incidental finding. For symptomatic patients, the duration of symptoms may vary from a few days to months and their clinical presentation may in fact mimic conditions such as cholecystitis, choledocholithiasis, cholangiocarcinoma or pancreatic cancer.

Benign neoplasms causing biliary obstruction may be classified as follows:

- papilloma and adenoma;
- multiple biliary papillomatosis;
- granular cell myoblastoma;
- neural tumours;
- leiomyoma;
- endocrine tumours.

Papilloma and adenoma

The most common benign neoplasms arise from the glandular epithelium lining the bile ducts. They can occur throughout the biliary system but are more frequent in the periampullary area. Lesions in this area may protrude through the ampulla of Vater and be visible at endoscopy. Jaundice is the most common symptom, occurring in >90% of cases. Coexisting gallstones are uncommon.

Treatment depends on the age, the general status of the patient and site of the disease but in general should consist of total resection of the lesion. In some cases a wide local resection can be performed.

Papillomatosis

This rare condition is characterised by the presence of multiple mucus-secreting tumours of the biliary epithelium. Patients present with obstructive jaundice, which may be intermittent, often complicated by cholangitis. These tumours have malignant potential and should be resected. This may involve liver resection if the disease is confined to a hepatic lobe. If both lobes are affected then liver transplantation may be required.

Granular cell myoblastoma, neural tumours, leiomyoma and endocrine tumours are extremely uncommon. In general, if biliary obstruction occurs it should be relieved by biliary resection, bypass or endoscopic stenting.

Malignant tumours of the biliary tract

Malignant tumours of the gallbladder and extrahepatic biliary tree are uncommon. Gallbladder cancer is the predominant type, accounting for 60–70% of cases with the remainder distributed between the intra- and extrahepatic biliary trees.

Unfortunately, owing to advanced stage at presentation, surgical resection, which offers the best survival, is only possible for a minority of patients. Thus, for most patients treatment is generally palliative in nature and survival is limited.

Summary box 67.7

Bile duct cancer (cholangiocarcinoma)

- Rare, but incidence increasing
- Most patients present with abnormal liver function tests or frank jaundice
- Diagnosis by ultrasound, CT or MRCP scanning
- The majority of patients receive palliative care only
- Complete surgical excision possible in <10%
- Prognosis poor: 90% die within 1 year, from liver failure or biliary sepsis
- Adjuvant chemoradiation therapy has a limited role

Incidence

Cholangicarcinoma is a rare malignancy. The overall annual incidence is 1–1.5 per 100 000 with the peak incidence in the 8th decade. The male:female ratio is approximately 1.5:1.

Anatomically, tumours involving the biliary confluence (hilar cholangiocarcinoma or Klatskin tumours) account for 60% of cases, with the remainder involving the distal bile duct (20–30%) or intrahepatic ducts (10–20%).

Risk factors

A minority of patients presenting with cholangiocarcinoma have a known risk factor. The major risk factor in Western practice is primary sclerosing cholangitis (PSC). It is estimated that a long-standing history of PSC increases the risk of developing biliary tract cancer by 20-fold compared to the normal population. It appears that patients with PSC and concomitant inflammatory bowel disease are at significantly higher risk of developing cancer compared to those without the disease. Cholangiocarcinoma appears to occur at an earlier age in patients with PSC (30–50 years of age) compared to the general population. In addition, disease is usually multifocal and detected at advanced stage with resultant poor prognosis.

Congenital cystic disease (Caroli's disease, choledochal cysts), hepatolithiasis, oriental cholangiohepatitis, hepatitis C viral infection and infestation with liver flukes have also been associated with an increased risk of cholangiocarcinoma. Liver fluke infestations are particularly important in South-East Asia. *Opisthorchis viverrini* and *Clonorchis sinensis* infestations are important in Thailand, Laos and western Malaysia. While the pathophysiology is unclear, it is thought that these parasites cause chronic inflammation that leads to DNA mutations through production of carcinogens and free radicals, which stimulate cellular proliferation in the intrahepatic bile ducts and ultimately can lead to invasive cancer.

Other risk factors suggested include chemical carcinogens such as thorium dioxide, vinyl chloride, dioxin and asbestos.

Summary box 67.8

Risk factors for cholangiocarcinoma

Chronic inflammatory conditions
- Primary sclerosing cholangitis (PSC)
- Oriental cholangiohepatitis
- Hepatitis C infection

Parasitic infections
- *Opisthorchis viverrini*
- *Clonorchis sinensis*

Congenital
- Choledochal cysts
- Caroli's disease

Chemical agents
- Thorium dioxide (Thorotrast)
- Vinyl chloride
- Dioxin
- Asbestos

Post surgical
- Biliary–enteric anastomosis

Clinical features

Early symptoms of cholangiocarcinoma are often non-specific, with abdominal pain, early satiety, anorexia and weight loss commonly seen. Symptoms associated with biliary obstruction (puritus and jaundice) may be present in a minority of patients. In these patients, examination often demonstrates clinical signs of jaundice, cachexia is often noticeable and a palpable gallbladder present if the obstruction is in the distal common bile duct (Courvoisier's sign).

Investigations

Biochemical investigations will confirm the presence of obstructive jaundice (elevated bilirubin, alkaline phosphatase and γ-glutamyltransferase). The tumour-marker CA 19-9 may also be elevated. Imaging studies such as ultrasound, MDR-CT and MRI/MRCP are essential for diagnosis and staging. These studies allow the level of biliary obstruction to be defined and determine the locoregional extent of disease and the presence of metastases (Figure 67.38).

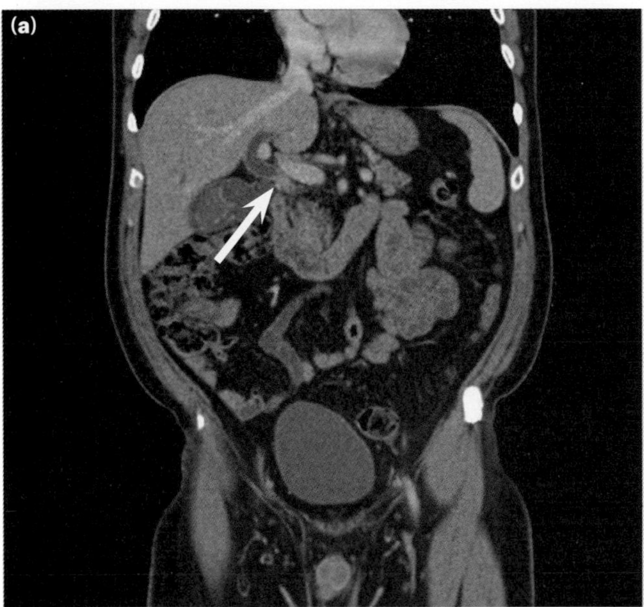

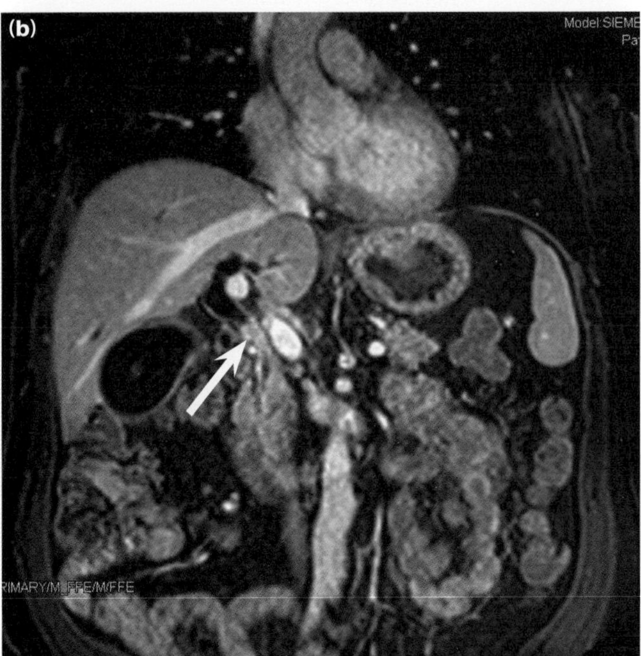

Figure 67.38 (a) A computed tomography scan demonstrating a cholangiocarcinoma obstructing the common hepatic duct (arrow). (b) Magnetic resonance cholangiopancreatography showing the level of obstruction (arrow).

Direct cholangiography using ERCP or PTC is also used following non-invasive studies. Both can define the level of obstruction and allow access to the biliary system for biopsy and placement of endobiliary stents for biliary drainage. The choice between the modalities depends on local availability and the anatomical site of the tumour, with PTC preferred for more proximal lesions and ERCP favoured for distal tumours. Cytology can be obtained from either procedure but it is often non-diagnostic.

Positron emission tomography (PET) is useful in detecting lymph node and distant metastases but has limited value in assessment of local resectability.

The anatomical extent of the disease is classified according to either the Bismuth–Corette or Memorial Sloan–Kettering Cancer Centre Classification (Figure 67.39).

Treatment

A multidisciplinary approach is required in all cases. The choice of treatment depends on the site and extent of the disease. Unfortunately, the majority of patients present with advanced disease. However, 10–15% are suitable for surgical resection, which offers the only hope for long-term survival. The aim of surgical resection is to achieve a complete resection with negative pathological margins (R0 resection) and safely restore biliary–enteric continuity.

Whether or not the disease is resectable depends on patient factors (comorbidities, presence or absence of chronic liver disease), and tumour factors (extent of disease within the biliary tree, vascular involvement, presence or absence of metastatic disease). Depending on the site of disease, surgery may involve either a standard or extended hepatic resection with *en bloc* lymphadenectomy and reconstruction of the biliary tree. Distal common duct tumours may require a pancreaticoduodenectomy (Whipple procedure). Local resection should be avoided.

In selected patients, liver transplantation has been recommended for those with locally unresectable disease without evidence of distant metastases. Transplantation is often combined with neoadjuvant chemoradiation therapy. While emerging data are encouraging, this aggressive approach remains controversial and is reserved for selected patients in specialised centres.

Following resection, disease-specific survival is related to the T-stage, nodal and margin status. Approximately 35% of patients will survive 5 years after surgery. Adjuvant chemotherapy and radiotherapy have a limited role to play and have not been demonstrated to add survival benefit following surgical resection. However, patients at high risk for recurrence (positive surgical margins or node positive) may benefit from adjuvant therapy and should be referred for a medical or radiation oncology opinion.

The majority of patients who present with unresectable disease are candidates for palliative therapy. The aim is to maintain or improve quality of life by relieving symptoms and preventing cholestatic liver failure. Biliary obstruction can be relieved by either endoscopic (ERCP) or percutaneous (PTC) methods. Surgical bypass rarely has a role apart from in patients who present with a distal bile duct lesion and are found to have unresectable disease at operation.

Cancer of the gallbladder

Incidence

Carcinoma of the gallbladder is a rare disease, but extremely variable by geographical region and racial–ethnic groups. The

Herni Bismuth, contemporary, hepatobiliary surgeon, Hôpital Paul Bruce, Villejif, France, with Dr Marvin Corlette described the classification of cholangiocarcinoma in 1975.

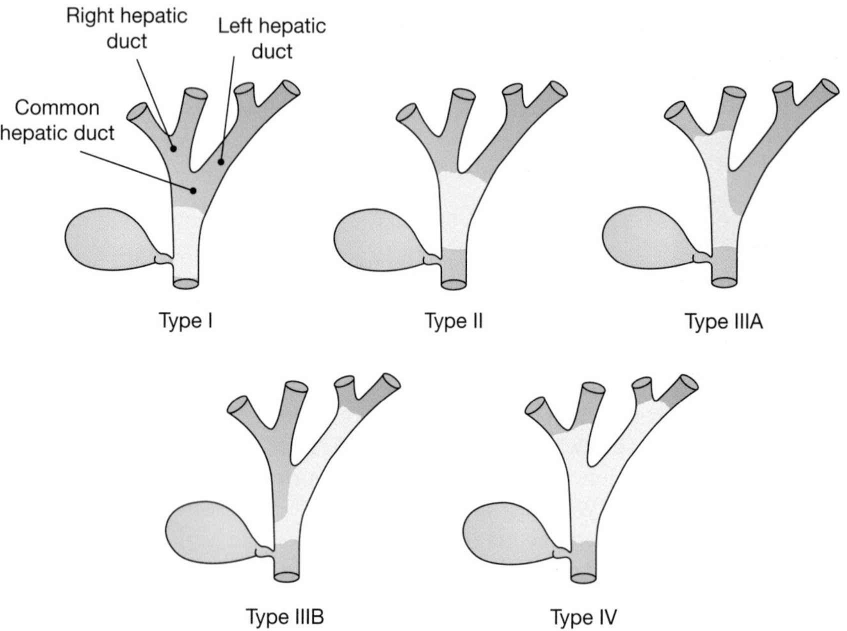

Figure 67.39 Bismuth-Corlette Classification for cholangiocarcinoma.

highest incidence is among Chileans, American Indians and residents in parts of northern India, where it accounts for as much as 9% of all biliary tract disease. Women appear to have a higher incidence across all geographical areas. In Western practice, gallbladder cancer accounts for less than 1% of new cancer diagnoses. The disease usually presents in the 7th or 8th decade. The aetiology is unclear but there appears to be an association with pre-existing gallstone disease, suggesting that chronic inflammation may play a role in a manner similar to tumours of the common bile duct. Calcification of the gallbladder wall, presumably due to chronic inflammation (porcelain gallbladder), is also associated with a small increased risk of cancer (see Figure 67.4). Chronic infection may also promote development of gallbladder cancer and the risk in typhoid carriers is significantly increased over the general population.

Gallbladder polyps may be found in approximately 5% of patients who undergo ultrasonography (Figure 67.40). The majority are either adenomyomatosis or cholesterol polyps and have no malignant potential. True adenomatous polyps occur in 0.3–0.5% of the population. The risk of malignant transformation increases with increasing size of the polyp.

Summary box 67.9

Gallbladder cancer

- Very rare
- Similar presentation to benign biliary disease i.e., gallstones
- Diagnosis by ultrasound, CT, MRI/MRCP
- Most patients present with advanced disease
- Surgical resection in less than 10% – remainder receive palliative treatment
- Prognosis is poor – median survival approximately 6 months

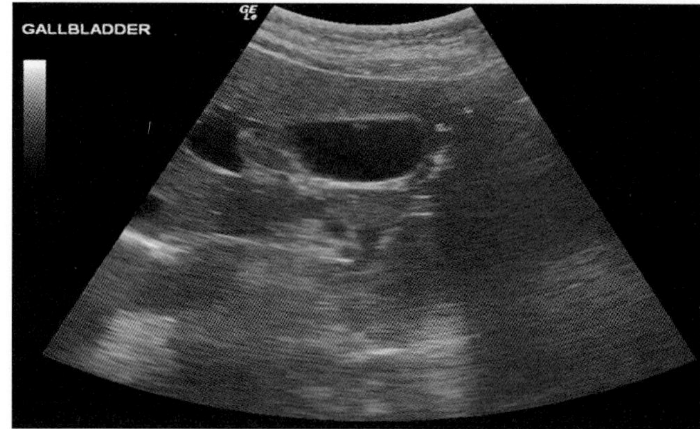

Figure 67.40 Ultrasound demonstrating a gallbladder polyp. Note the lack of the acoustic shadow.

Pathology

The majority (90%) of tumours are adenocarcinomas. Squamous carcinomas also occur and are believed to arise from areas of mucosal squamous metaplasia.

At operation, localised carcinomas are difficult to differentiate from chronic cholecystitis; the tumour most commonly is nodular and infiltrative, with thickening of the gallbladder wall, often extending to the whole gallbladder. The tumour spreads by direct extension into the liver, seeding of the peritoneal cavity and involvement of the perihilar lymphatics and neural plexuses. At the time of presentation the majority of tumours are advanced.

Clinical features

Patients may be asymptomatic at the time of diagnosis. Symptoms, if present, are usually indistinguishable from those of benign gallbladder disease such as biliary colic or cholecystitis, particularly in older patients. Jaundice and anorexia are late features. A palpable mass is a late sign.

Investigation

Laboratory findings are generally non-specific but may be consistent with biliary obstruction. Non-specific findings such as anaemia, leukocytosis, mild elevation in transaminases and increased inflammatory markers such as ESR or C-reactive protein may be present. Serum CA19-9 is elevated in approximately 80% of patients.

The preoperative diagnosis is often made on ultrasonography, and confirmed by a CT scan or MRI/MRCP. Preoperative staging should aim to determine the local extent of disease and exclude the presence of distant metastases. A percutaneous biopsy under radiological guidance is often done to obtain tissue for pathological examination. In selected cases, laparoscopic examination is useful in staging the disease. Laparoscopy can detect peritoneal or liver metastases which would preclude further surgical resection (Figure 67.41).

PET scanning also has a role in detecting metastatic disease.

Summary box 67.10

Aims of staging gallbladder cancer

- Assessment of local disease
- Detection of metastatic disease:
  - Liver
  - Peritoneal
  - Lymphatic
  - Extra-abdominal disease

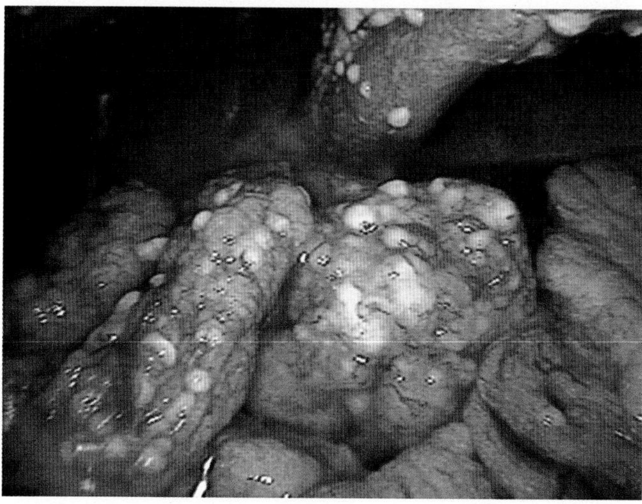

Figure 67.41 Laparoscopic staging in a patient with gallbladder carcinoma demonstrating gross peritoneal metastases.

Treatment and prognosis

The majority of patients have advanced disease at presentation, and are not candidates for surgical therapy. Surgery is indicated in only very selected cases.

Cholecystectomy should be performed for all gallbladder polyps greater than 1 cm. Polyps less than 1 cm can be followed with serial ultrasonography to detect any change in size or character as the incidence of malignancy in polyps less than 1 cm is extremely low.

Radical *en bloc* resection that may include segmental or extended hepatectomy, bile duct resection and regional lymphadenectomy should be considered in selected patients. The aim is to remove the tumour entirely and achieve negative histopathological margins.

Patients can have the disease diagnosed following histopathological examination of the gallbladder removed for presumed benign disease. In these cases, the need for further surgery is determined by the stage of disease. For early-stage disease, confined to the mucosa or muscle of the gallbladder, no further treatment is indicated. However, for transmural disease, a radical *en bloc* resection of the gallbladder fossa and surrounding liver along with the regional lymph nodes should be performed. If the initial procedure was performed laparoscopically, the surgeon should examine the laparoscopic port sites. Routine resection of port sites is no longer recommended. However, it is recognised that the finding of disease at the port sites is a sign of generalised peritoneal disease and carries a very poor prognosis.

For the majority of patients a non-operative approach to palliation is best. Obstructive jaundice can be relieved by endoscopic and/or percutaneous methods. The value of adjuvant therapy is unproven.

Gallbladder cancer for most patients is a lethal disease with a grim prognosis. The median survival is less than 6 months and a 5-year survival figure of 5% has been reported.

FURTHER READING

Carter DC, Russell RCG, Pitt HA, Bismuth H (eds). *Rob and Smith's operative surgery: hepatobiliary and pancreatic surgery*. London: Chapman & Hall, 1996.

Dooley JS, Lok A, Burroughs A, Heathcoate J (eds). *Sherlock's diseases of the liver and biliary system*, 12th edn. Oxford: Wiley-Blackwell, 2011.

Garden OJ, Parks RW. *Hepatobiliary and pancreatic surgery: a companion to specialist practice*, 5th edn. New York: Saunders Elsevier, 2013.

Jarnagin W. *Blumgart's surgery of the liver, pancreas and biliary tract*, 5th edn. New York: Elsevier, 2012.

Chapter 68

The pancreas

Learning objectives

To understand:

- The anatomy and physiology of the pancreas
- Investigations of the pancreas
- Congenital abnormalities of the pancreas
- Assessment and management of pancreatitis
- Diagnosis and treatment of pancreatic cancer

ANATOMY AND PHYSIOLOGY

Anatomy

The name 'pancreas' is derived from the Greek '*pan*' (all) and '*kreas*' (flesh). For a long time, its glandular function was not understood, and it was thought to act as a cushion for the stomach. The pancreas is situated in the retroperitoneum. It is divided into a head, which occupies 30% of the gland by mass, and a body and tail, which together constitute 70%. The head lies within the curve of the duodenum, overlying the body of the second lumbar vertebra and the vena cava. The aorta and the superior mesenteric vessels lie behind the neck of the gland. Coming off the side of the pancreatic head and passing to the left and behind the superior mesenteric vein is the uncinate process of the pancreas. Behind the neck of the pancreas, near its upper border, the superior mesenteric vein joins the splenic vein to form the portal vein (Figures 68.1 and 68.2). The tip of the pancreatic tail extends up to the splenic hilum.

The pancreas weighs approximately 80 g. Of this, 80–90% is composed of exocrine acinar tissue, which is organised into lobules. The main pancreatic duct branches into interlobular and intralobular ducts, ductules and, finally, acini. The main duct is lined by columnar epithelium, which becomes cuboidal in the ductules. Acinar cells are clumped around a central lumen, which communicates with the duct system. Clusters of endocrine cells, known as islets of Langerhans, are distributed throughout the pancreas. Islets consist of different cell types: 75% are B cells (producing insulin); 20% are A cells (producing glucagon); and the remainder are D cells (producing somatostatin) and a small number of pancreatic polypeptide cells. Within an islet, the B cells form an inner core surrounded by the other cells. Capillaries draining the islet cells drain into the portal vein, forming a pancreatic portal system.

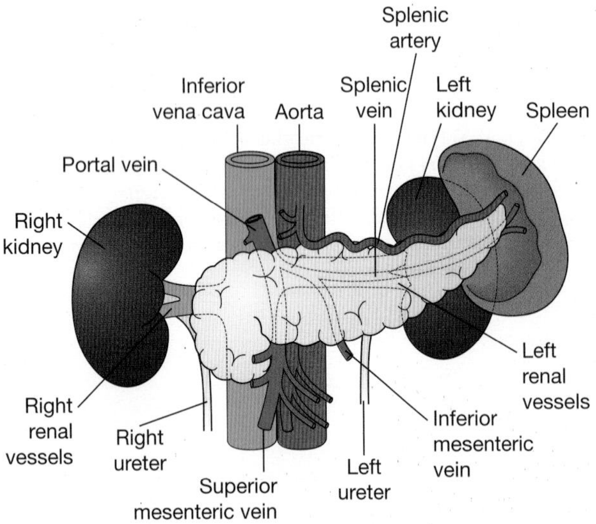

Figure 68.1 The posterior relations of the pancreas.

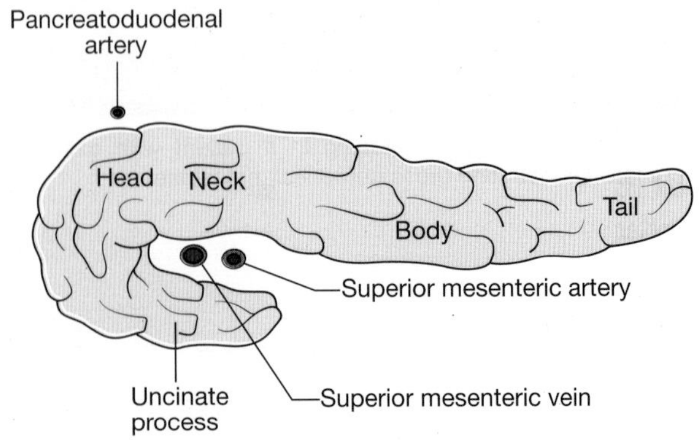

Figure 68.2 Transverse section of the pancreas. Note the position of the uncinate process behind the vessels.

Paul Langerhans, 1847–1888, Professor of Pathological Anatomy, Freiberg, Germany, described the islets in 1869, in his doctoral thesis. He later contracted tuberculosis, resigned and moved to warmer climes in Madeira, where he also studied marine worms.

There are nine key processes that occur during pancreatic embryogenesis (*Table 68.1*). Malrotation of the ventral bud in the fifth week results in an annular pancreas, while the mode of ductule fusion in the seventh week produces the various possible ductular patterns. Between the 12th and 40th weeks of fetal life, the pancreas differentiates into exocrine and endocrine elements. The primitive ducts and their ductules are responsible for the lobular arrangement of the pancreas. Congenital anomalies of the pancreas are varied and arise during the early phase of development. The anatomy of the pancreatic duct is variable as a result of the primordial bud development. The dorsal duct is expressed in a variable manner in the adult, as outlined in Figure 68.3. Approximately 10% of patients will have a significant flow from the main duct through the accessory papilla. The anatomy of the main duodenal papilla, also known as the ampulla of Vater, is also variable (Figure 68.4).

TABLE 68.1 Steps in the development of the pancreas.

1	Day 26	Dorsal pancreatic duct arises from the dorsal side of the duodenum
2	Day 32	Ventral bud arises from the base of the hepatic diverticulum
3	Day 37	Contact occurs between the two buds. Fusion by the end of week 6
4	Week 6	Ventral bud produces the head and uncinate process
5	Week 6	Ducts fuse
6	Week 6	Ventral duct and distal portion of the dorsal duct form the main duct (duct of Wirsung)
7	Week 6	Proximal dorsal duct forms the duct of Santorini
8	Month 3	Acini appear
9	Months 3–4	Islets of Langerhans appear and become biologically active

Summary box 68.1

Anomalies of the pancreas

- Aplasia
- Hypoplasia
- Hyperplasia
- Hypertrophy
- Dysplasia
- Variations and anomalies of the ducts[a]
  - Pancreas divisum
  - Rotational anomalies
- Annular pancreas[a]
- Pancreatic gall bladder
- Polycystic disease[a]
- Congenital pancreatic cysts
  - Cystic fibrosis[a]
  - von Hippel–Lindau syndrome
- Ectopic pancreatic tissue, accessory pancreas[a]
- Vascular anomalies
- Choledochal cysts[a]
- Horseshoe pancreas

[a]The more frequent anomalies encountered in surgical practice.

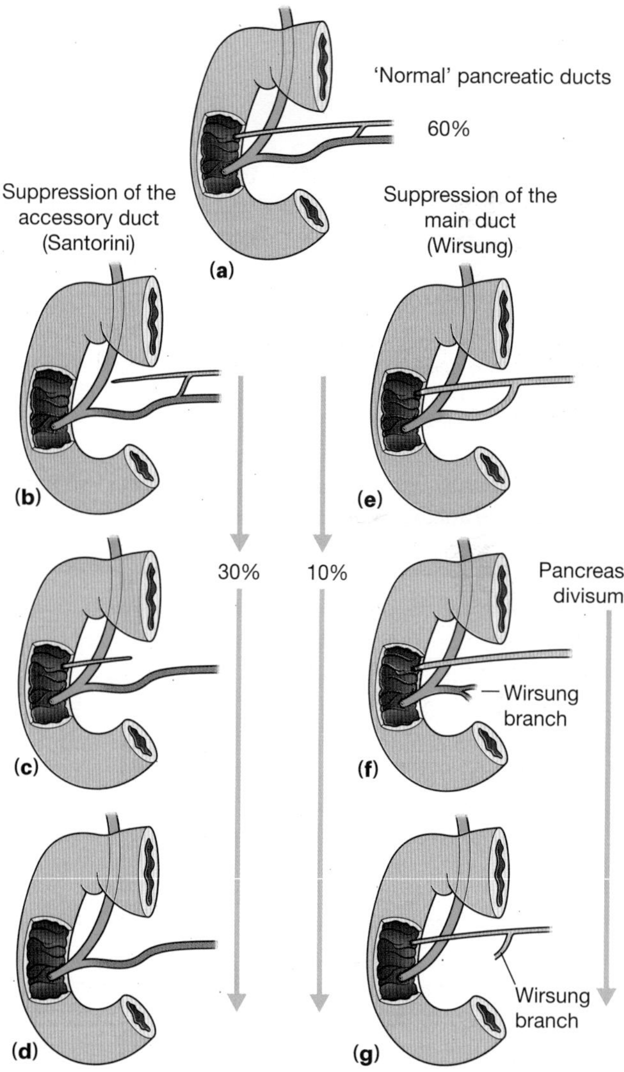

Figure 68.3 Variations in the pancreatic ducts. (a) Normal. (b-d) Progressive suppression of the accessory duct (30%). (e-g) Progressive suppression of the main duct (10%). (f, g) Pancreas divisum.

Giovanni Domenico Santorini, 1681–1737, Professor of Anatomy and Medicine, Venice, Italy. His drawings of the accessory pancreatic duct were published after his death.

Johann Georg Wirsung, 1589–1643, Professor of Anatomy, Padua, Italy, described the pancreatic duct in 1642, when dissecting the cadaver of a man hanged for murder. He died a year later from an assassin's bullet, on his doorstep.

Eugen von Hippel, 1866–1939, Professor of Ophthalmology, Göttingen, Germany.

Arvid Lindau, 1892–1958, pathologist, Lund, Sweden, established the link between the retinal angiomatosis described by von Hippel and the cerebellar and visceral components of the syndrome.

Abraham Vater, 1684–1751, Professor of Anatomy and Botany, and later of Pathology and Therapeutics, Wittenberg, Germany.

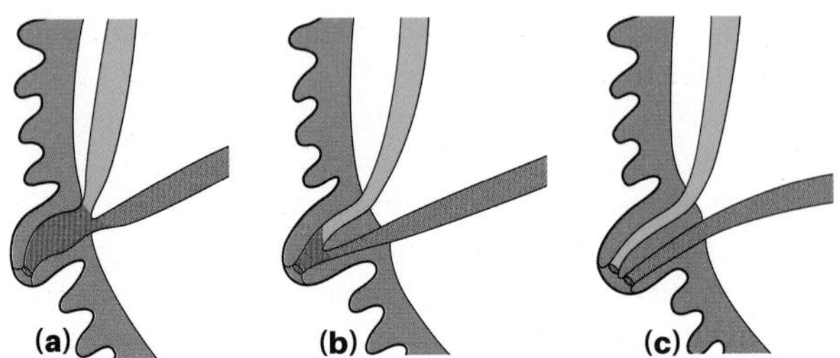

Figure 68.4 Variations in the relation of the common bile duct and main pancreatic duct at the main duodenal papilla. In (a), there is a common channel with no sphincter mechanism protecting flow between the ducts. In (b), there is a partial common channel, while in (c), there is separation of the two channels. Gallstone pancreatitis is more likely with (a) and (b).

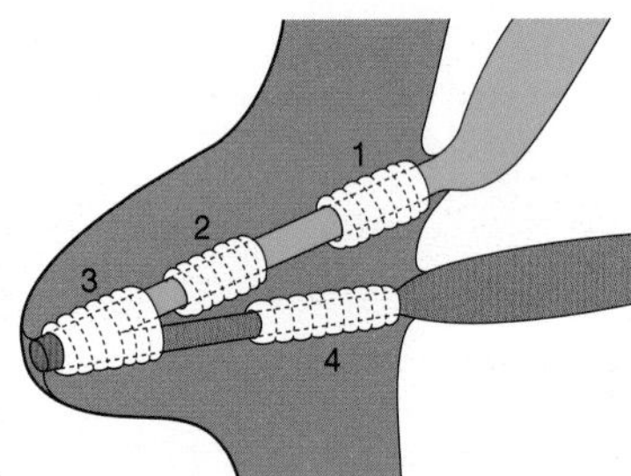

Figure 68.5 The complexity of the sphincter of Oddi. (1) Superior choledochal sphincter; (2) inferior choledochal sphincter; (3) ampullary sphincter; (4) pancreatic sphincter.

The outlet of each duct is protected by a complex sphincter mechanism (sphincter of Oddi) (Figure 68.5).

Physiology

In response to a meal, the pancreas secretes digestive enzymes in an alkaline (pH 8.4) bicarbonate-rich fluid. Spontaneous secretion is minimal; the hormone secretin, which is released from the duodenal mucosa, evokes a bicarbonate-rich fluid. Cholecystokinin (CCK) (synonym: pancreozymin) is released from the duodenal mucosa in response to food. CCK is responsible for enzyme release. Vagal stimulation increases the volume of secretion. Protein is synthesised at a greater rate (per gram of tissue) in the pancreas than in any other tissue, with the possible exception of the lactating mammary gland. About 90% of this protein is exported from the acinar cells as a variety of digestive enzymes. Approximately 6–20 g of digestive enzymes enters the duodenum each day. Nascent proteins are synthesised as preproteins and undergo modification in a sequence of steps. The proteins move from the rough endothelial endoplasmic reticulum to the Golgi complex, where lysosomes and mature zymogen storage granules containing proteases are stored, and then to the ductal surface of the cell, from which they are extruded by exocytosis. During this phase, the proteolytic enzymes are in an inactive form, the maintenance of which is important in preventing pancreatitis.

INVESTIGATIONS (*TABLE 68.2*)

Estimation of pancreatic enzymes in body fluids

When the pancreas is damaged, enzymes such as amylase, lipase, trypsin, elastase and chymotrypsin are released into the serum. Measurement of serum amylase is the most widely used test of pancreatic damage (serum lipase is more sensitive and specific, but is not widely available). The serum amylase rises within a few hours of pancreatic damage and declines over the next 4–8 days. A markedly elevated serum level is highly suspicious but not diagnostic of acute pancreatitis. Urinary amylase and amylase–creatinine clearance ratios add little to diagnostic accuracy. If confirmation of the diagnosis is required, computed tomography (CT) of the pancreas is of greater value.

TABLE 68.2 Investigation of the pancreas.
Serum enzyme levels
Pancreatic function tests
Morphology
Ultrasound scan
Computed tomography
Magnetic resonance imaging
Endoscopic retrograde cholangiopancreatography
Endoscopic ultrasound
Plain radiography
Chest
Upper abdomen

Summary box 68.2

Causes of raised serum amylase level other than acute pancreatitis

- Upper gastrointestinal tract perforation
- Mesenteric infarction
- Torsion of an intra-abdominal viscus
- Retroperitoneal haematoma
- Ectopic pregnancy
- Macroamylasaemia
- Renal failure
- Salivary gland inflammation

Pancreatic function tests

Pancreatic exocrine function can be assessed by directly measuring pancreatic secretion in response to a standardised stimulus. The stimulus to secretion can be physiological, e.g. ingestion of a test meal, as in the Lundh test, or pharmacological, e.g.

Ruggero Oddi, 1866–1913, anatomist and physiologist, Perugia, Italy, wrote about the structure and function of the ampullary sphincter in 1887, when still a student. He struggled in later life with drug addiction.

Camillo Golgi, 1844–1926, Professor of Anatomy and Histology at Pavia, and later at Siena, Italy, developed silver staining of neural tissue and received the Nobel Prize in 1906 (with Ramon y Cajal) for his studies in neuroanatomy.

Göran Lundh, 1926–1999, surgeon, Södersjukhuset, Stockholm, Sweden. Working with Bengt Borgstrom, a biochemist at Lund University, he described this test of pancreatic function in 1962. The test has largely been superseded by measurement of faecal elastase.

intravenous injection of a hormone such as secretin or CCK. Duodenal intubation has to be performed with a triple-lumen tube so that the gastric and duodenal juices can be aspirated, and a non-absorbable marker such as polyethylene glycol is used to assess the completeness of the aspiration. The nitroblue tetrazolium–*para*-aminobenzoic acid (NBT–PABA) test provides an indirect measure of pancreatic function. The substance is administered orally and degraded in the gut by a pancreatic enzyme, and the breakdown product (PABA) is absorbed by the intestine and excreted in the urine; its urinary level is measured. The pancreolauryl test works on a similar principle. These tests are cheap and easy to perform, but are non-specific, especially following gastrectomy and in conditions that may alter gastrointestinal transit and intestinal absorptive capacity. Measurement of the enzyme elastase in stool is simple, specific and now used widely. A low level of faecal elastase indicates exocrine insufficiency.

Imaging investigations

Ultrasonography

Ultrasonography is the initial investigation of choice in patients with jaundice to determine whether or not the bile duct is dilated, the coexistence of gallstones or gross disease within the liver such as metastases. It may also define the presence or absence of a mass in the pancreas (Figure 68.6). However, obesity and overlying bowel gas often make interpretation of the pancreas itself unsatisfactory.

Computed tomography

Most significant pathologies within the pancreas can be diagnosed on high-quality CT scans, with three-dimensional reconstruction if necessary. A specific pancreatic protocol should be followed. An initial unenhanced CT scan is essential to determine the presence of calcification within the pancreas and gall bladder (Figure 68.7). Then, following rapid injection of intravenous contrast, scanning is performed in the arterial and venous phases. The stomach and duodenum should be outlined with water and distended to define the duodenal loop. Pancreatic carcinomas of 1–2 cm in size can usually be demonstrated (Figure 68.8). Endocrine tumours are also well imaged on CT (Figure 68.9). In patients with pancreatitis, necrotic areas within the gland can be identified by the absence of contrast enhancement on CT. Inflammatory collections and pseudocysts can be seen (Figure 68.10). CT-guided drainage is helpful in the treatment of pancreatic collections, cysts and pseudocysts, and facilitates percutaneous fine-needle or Trucut biopsy.

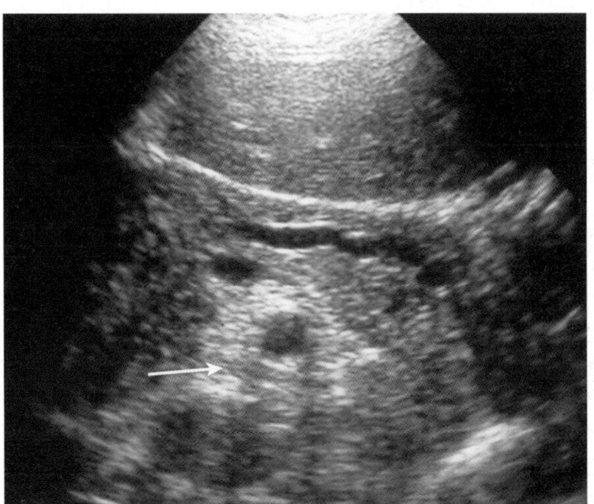

Figure 68.6 Ultrasound scan showing a mass in the head of the pancreas (marked by an arrow) and a dilated pancreatic duct in the body of the gland (courtesy of Dr Alison McLean).

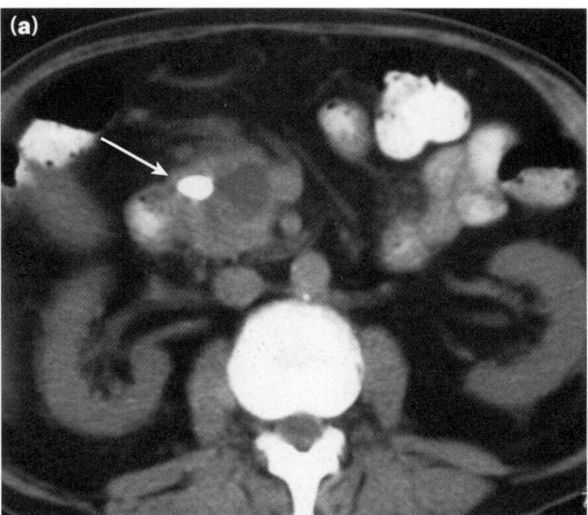

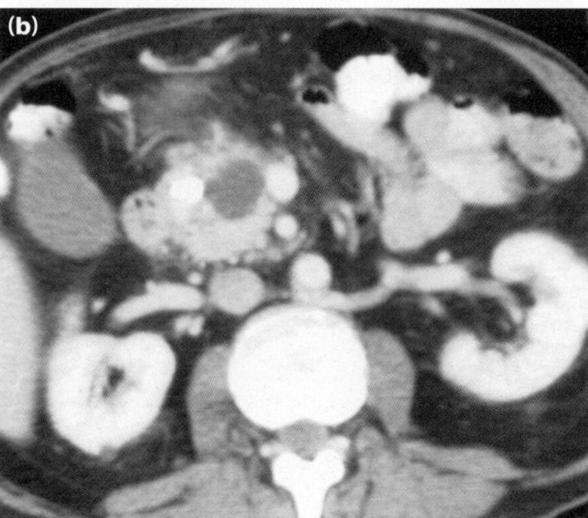

Figure 68.7 (a) Unenhanced computed tomography scan of a man with chronic pancreatitis, showing a focus of calcification (marked by an arrow) in the head of the pancreas and a cyst adjacent to that. Oral contrast has been administered. (b) The same area after injection of intravenous contrast.

Magnetic resonance imaging

With magnetic resonance imaging (MRI), the pancreas can be clearly identified, and the anatomy of the bile duct and the pancreatic duct, together with fluid collections, can be defined. Magnetic resonance cholangiography and pancreatography (MRCP) may well replace *diagnostic* endoscopic cholangiography and pancreatography (ERCP) as it is non-invasive and less expensive (Figure 68.11). Using the technique in conjunction with intravenous injection of secretin, emptying of the pancreatic duct can be demonstrated to show the absence or presence of obstruction.

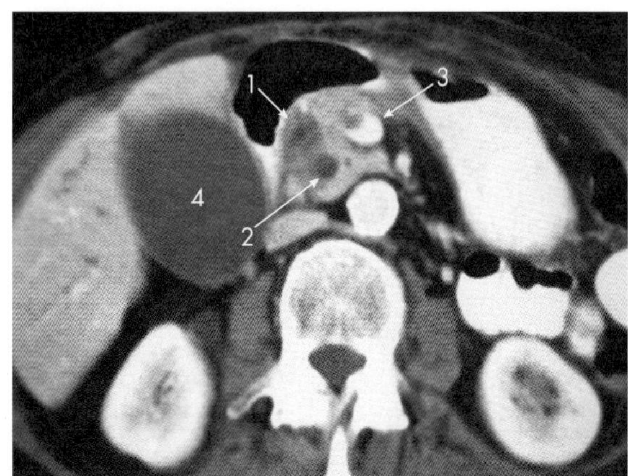

Figure 68.8 Contrast-enhanced computed tomography scan of a patient with a carcinoma of the pancreatic head. The main bulk of the tumour lies inferior to the section shown here. The dilated bile duct (1) and main pancreatic duct (2) can be seen, with tumour infiltration around them. There is a thrombus in the superior mesenteric vein (3). The gall bladder is distended (4).

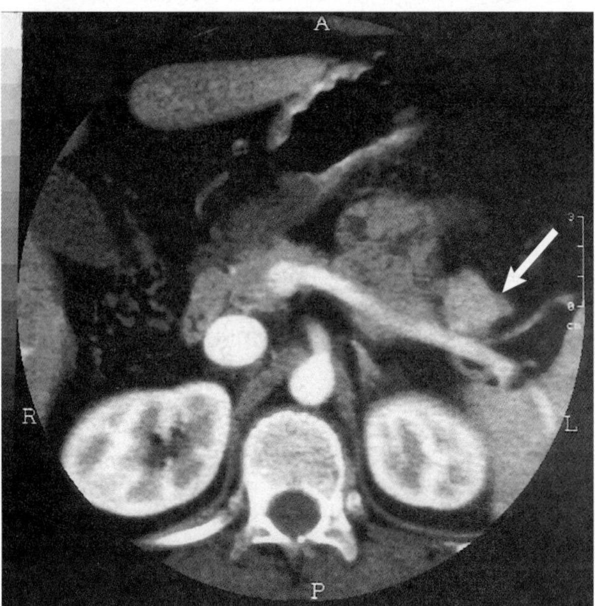

Figure 68.9 Computed tomography scan showing a hypervascular insulinoma (arrow) adjacent to the splenic vein. Local excision of the tumour resulted in normoglycaemia.

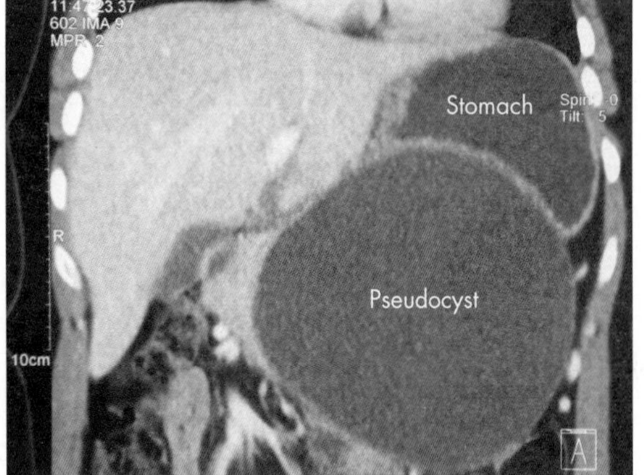

Figure 68.10 Computed tomography scan of a large pseudocyst in relation to the body and tail of the pancreas.

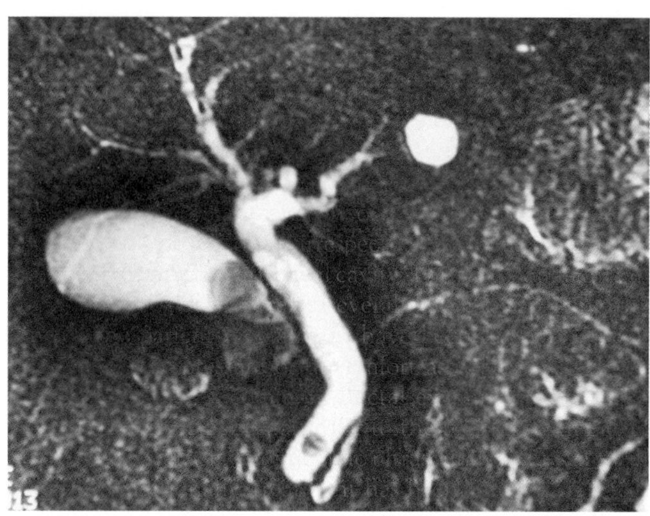

Figure 68.11 Magnetic resonance cholangiopancreatography in a patient with obstructive jaundice. A dilated common bile duct was seen on ultrasound, but no pancreatic mass lesion was visible on computed tomography. The bile duct and the main pancreatic duct are seen very well, with a stone visible in the lower part of the bile duct and another in the neck of the gall bladder.

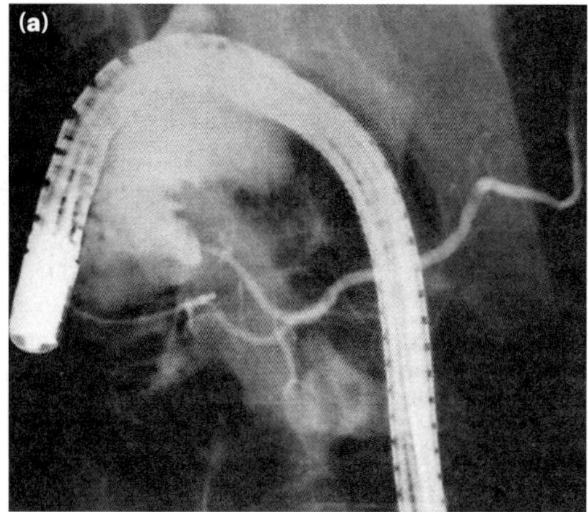

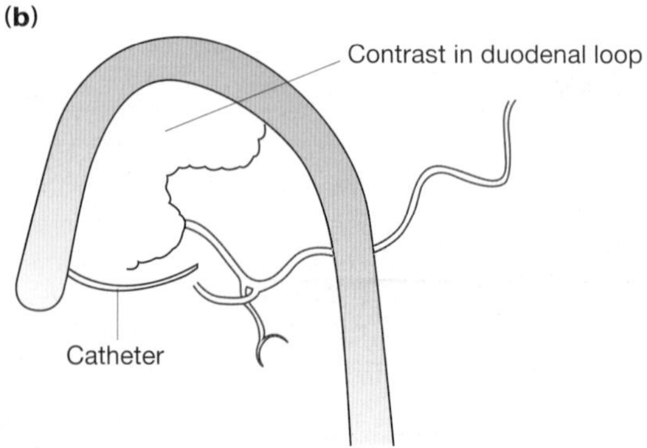

Figure 68.12 Endoscopic retrograde cholangiopancreatography. (a) Normal pancreatic duct with filling of the duct of Santorini from the duct of Wirsung. (b) Diagrammatic outline of (a).

Endoscopic retrograde cholangiopancreatography

ERCP is performed using a side-viewing fibreoptic duodenoscope. The ampulla of Vater is intubated, and contrast is injected into the biliary and pancreatic ducts to display the anatomy radiologically (Figure 68.12). In pancreatic carcinoma, the main pancreatic duct may be narrowed or completely obstructed at the site of the tumour (Figure 68.13), or the distal bile duct may be narrowed. Concurrent narrowing of both ducts results in the so-called double duct sign (Figure 68.14). Changes seen in chronic pancreatitis include the presence of pancreatic duct strictures, dilatation of the main pancreatic duct with stones, abnormalities of pancreatic duct side branches, communication of the pancreatic duct with cysts, and bile duct strictures (Figures 68.15–68.17). A plain radiograph before contrast studies is essential to delineate calcification (Figure 68.18). In addition to imaging, bile or pancreatic fluid and brushings from duct strictures can yield cells that confirm the suspected diagnosis of carcinoma (Figure 68.19). Brush cytology taken from malignant strictures at the time of ERCP yields a positive diagnosis in 40–50% of patients. ERCP also allows the placement of biliary and pancreatic stents.

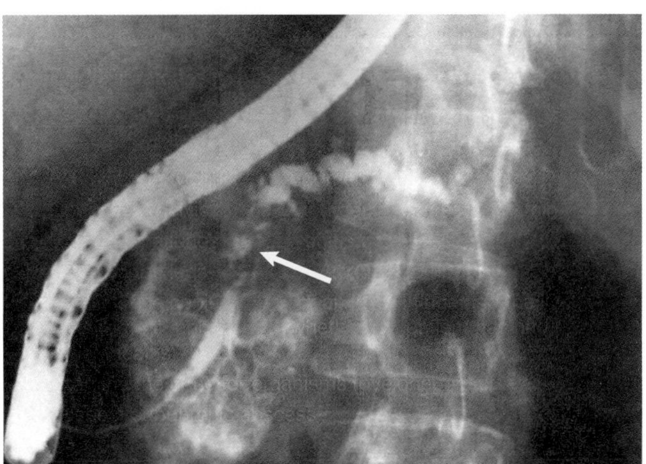

Figure 68.13 Endoscopic retrograde cholangiopancreatography: pancreatic carcinoma. Irregular stricture of the main pancreatic duct (arrow) with dilatation distal to the obstruction.

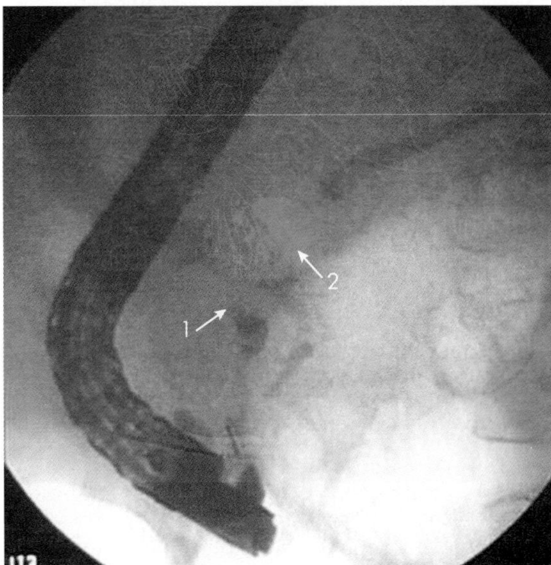

Figure 68.14 Endoscopic retrograde cholangiopancreatography depicting a malignant stricture in the lower part of the common bile duct (1) and in the main pancreatic duct (2), an appearance referred to as the double duct sign (courtesy of Dr George Webster).

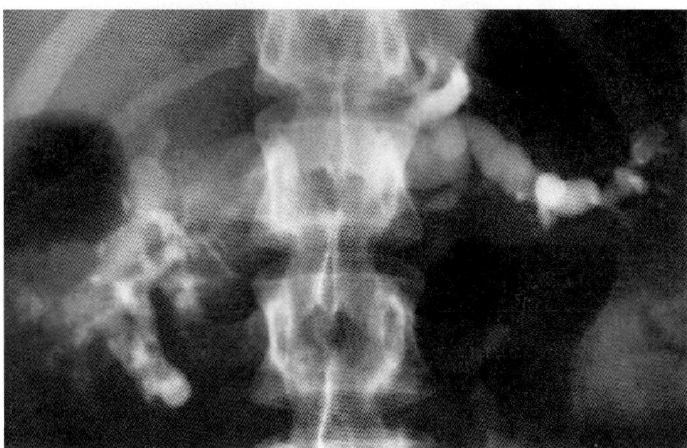

Figure 68.15 Endoscopic retrograde cholangiopancreatography: chronic pancreatitis. Most of the opacities lie within the duct system and are stones. Gross dilatation of ducts in the body and tail are due to obstruction by stones in the head of the pancreas.

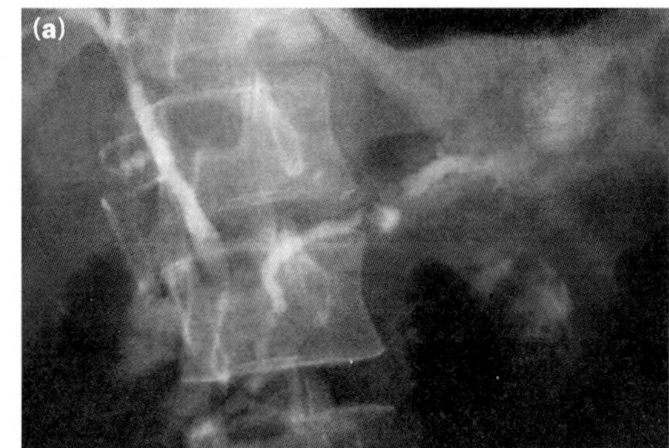

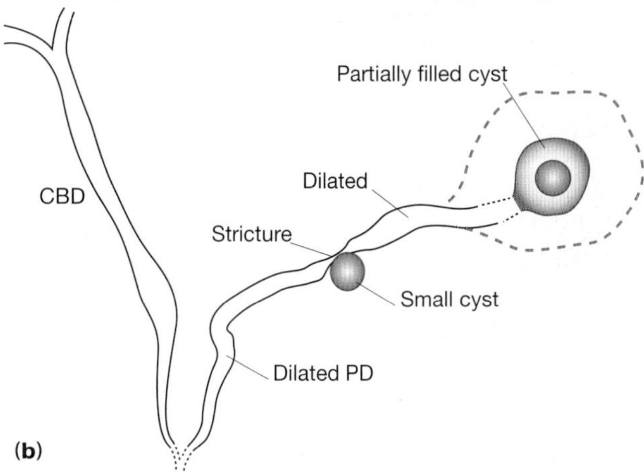

Figure 68.16 (a) Endoscopic retrograde cholangiopancreatography: relapsing acute pancreatitis. Normal biliary tree. Pancreatogram shows stricture of the main duct in the body with distal dilatation and cyst formation. (b) Diagrammatic outline of (a). CBD, common bile duct; PD, pancreatic duct.

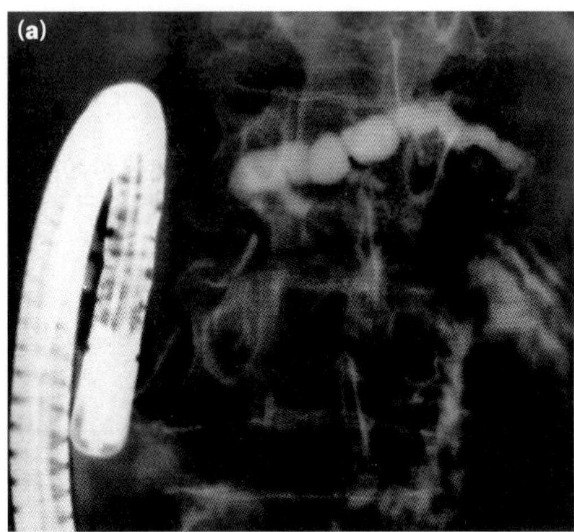

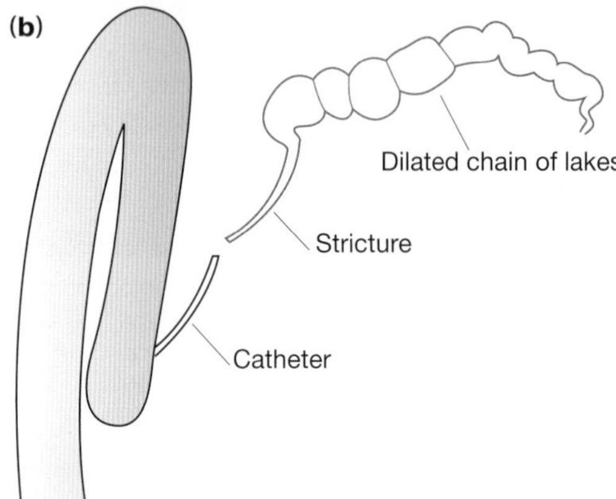

Figure 68.17 (a) Endoscopic retrograde cholangiopancreatography: chronic pancreatitis. Long stricture of the pancreatic duct in the head; distal pancreatic duct shows sacculation with intervening short strictures, 'chain of lakes'. (b) Diagrammatic outline of (a).

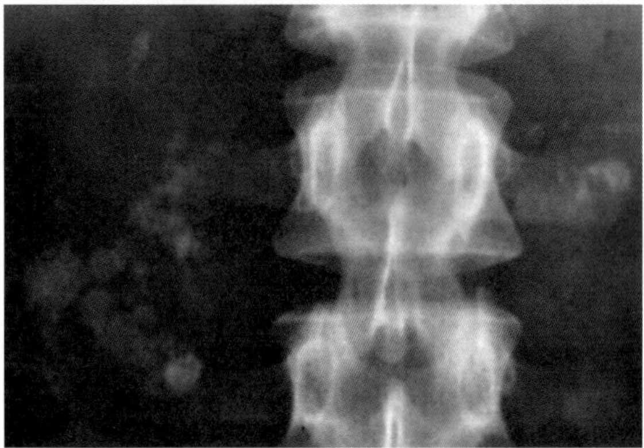

Figure 68.18 Plain abdominal radiograph: chronic pancreatitis. Multiple opacities can be seen in the region of the head and tail of the pancreas.

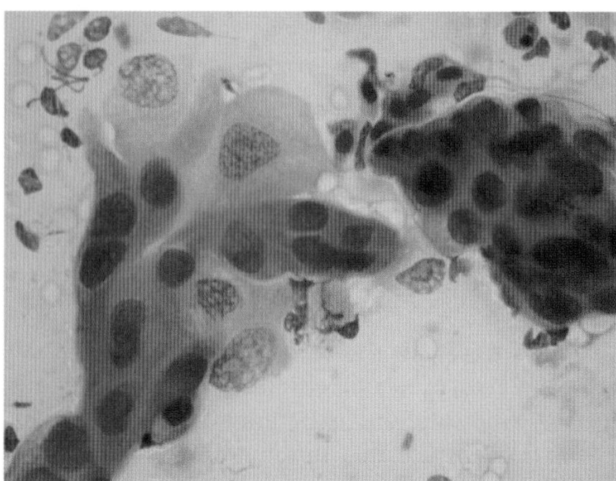

Figure 68.19 A group of adenocarcinoma cells identified in pancreatic juice collected at the time of endoscopic retrograde cholangiopancreatography (courtesy of Professor Roger Feakins).

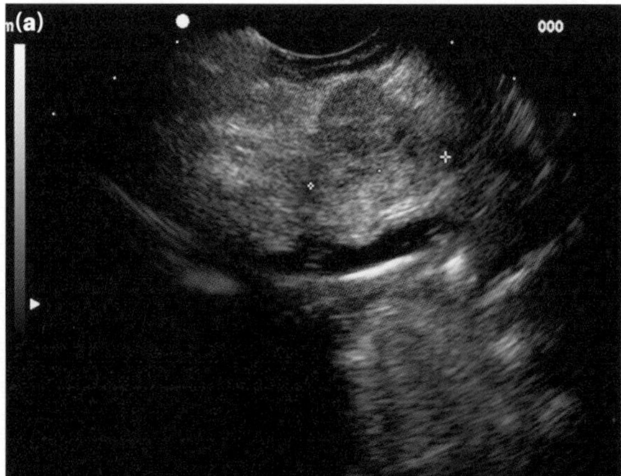

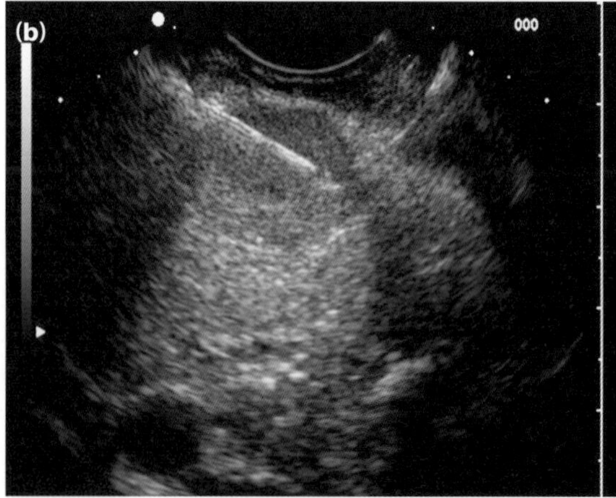

Figure 68.20 (a) Carcinoma of the pancreatic head as seen on endoscopic ultrasound (EUS). (b) Aspiration biopsy carried out under EUS guidance: needle seen entering the tumour (courtesy of Dr Peter Fairclough).

Endoscopic ultrasound

Endoscopic ultrasound (EUS) is performed using a special endoscope that has a high-frequency ultrasonic transducer at its tip. When the endoscope is in the lumen of the stomach or duodenum, the pancreas and its surrounding vasculature and lymph nodes can be assessed (Figure 68.20). This is particularly useful in identifying small tumours that may not show up well on CT or MRI, and in demonstrating the relationship of a pancreatic tumour to major vessels nearby. EUS can clarify the relationship of a neuroendocrine tumour to the main pancreatic duct (important if enucleation is being considered).

It helps to distinguish cystic tumours from pseudocysts. Transduodenal or transgastric fine needle aspiration (FNA) or Trucut biopsy performed under EUS guidance avoids spillage of tumour cells into the peritoneal cavity.

CONGENITAL ABNORMALITIES

Cystic fibrosis

This is inherited as an autosomal recessive condition. It occurs most frequently among Caucasians, in whom it is the most common inherited disorder (incidence of 1:2000 live births in the UK). Cystic fibrosis (CF) develops when there is a mutation in the *CFTR* (cystic fibrosis transmembrane conductance regulator) gene on chromosome 7. This gene creates a cell membrane protein that helps to control the movement of chloride across the cell membrane.

CF is a multisystem disorder of exocrine glands that affects the lungs, intestines, pancreas and liver, and is characterised by elevated sodium and chloride ion concentrations in sweat. The mother may notice that the child is salty when kissed.

Most of the organ damage is due to blockage of narrow passages by thickened secretions. Chronic pulmonary disease arises from plugging of bronchi and bronchioles. CF is the most common cause of chronic lung disease among children in resource-rich countries. Cor pulmonale may develop later. At birth, the meconium may set in a sticky mass and produce intestinal obstruction (meconium ileus) (see Chapter 9). Secretions precipitate in the lumen of the pancreatic duct causing blockage, which results in duct ectasia and fatty replacement of exocrine acinar tissue. Pancreatic exocrine insufficiency leads to fat malabsorption. Steatorrhoea is usually present from birth, resulting in stools that are bulky, oily and offensive. The islets of Langerhans usually appear normal, but diabetes mellitus can occur in older patients. The liver may become cirrhotic as a result of bile duct plugging, and signs of portal hypertension may appear. Infertility is common, due to the absence of the vas deferens in men and thick cervical mucus in women.

Outside the newborn period, the earliest clinical signs of CF are poor growth, poor appetite, rancid greasy stools, abdominal distension, chronic respiratory disease and finger clubbing. The appearance of secondary sexual characteristics may be delayed. The diagnosis can be made by genetic testing (which may be part of prenatal or newborn screening) and by the sweat test. Levels of sodium and chloride ions in the sweat above 90 mmol/L confirm the diagnosis.

Treatment is aimed at control of the secondary consequences of the disease. Pulmonary function is preserved with aggressive physiotherapy and antibiotics. Malabsorption is treated by administration of oral pancreatic enzyme preparations. The diet should be low in fat but contain added salt to replace the high losses in the sweat. With early diagnosis and optimal treatment, patients in resource-rich countries can now expect to survive to their mid-thirties. Those with end-stage lung disease may be considered for lung transplantation. Heterozygous carriers of the various gene mutations are asymptomatic but can be identified by DNA analysis. There is a suggestion that such patients may develop pancreatitis later in life.

Pancreas divisum

Pancreas divisum occurs when the embryological ventral and dorsal parts of the pancreas fail to fuse (Figure 68.3). The dorsal pancreatic duct becomes the main pancreatic duct and drains most of the pancreas through the minor or accessory papilla. The incidence of pancreas divisum ranges from 5% in autopsy series to 10% in some ERCP and MRCP series. Pancreas divisum found incidentally in an asymptomatic person does not warrant any intervention. But the incidence of pancreas divisum ranges from 25–50% in patients with recurrent acute pancreatitis, chronic pancreatitis and pancreatic pain. The minor papilla is substantially smaller than the major papilla (and many of these patients probably have papillary stenosis). A large volume of secretions flowing through a narrow papilla probably leads to incomplete drainage, which may then cause obstructive pain or pancreatitis. Certainly in patients with idiopathic recurrent pancreatitis, pancreas divisum should be excluded. The diagnosis can be arrived at by MRCP, EUS or ERCP, augmented by injection of secretin if necessary. There may be changes indicative of obstruction or chronic inflammation in the dorsal duct system. Endoscopic sphincterotomy and stenting of the minor papilla may relieve the symptoms. Surgical intervention can take the form of sphincteroplasty, pancreatojejunostomy or even resection of the pancreatic head.

Annular pancreas

This is the result of failure of complete rotation of the ventral pancreatic bud during development, so that a ring of pancreatic tissue surrounds the second or third part of the duodenum. It is most often seen in association with congenital duodenal stenosis or atresia and is therefore more prevalent in children with Down syndrome. Duodenal obstruction typically causes vomiting in the neonate (see Chapter 9). The usual treatment is bypass (duodenoduodenostomy). The disease may occur in later life as one of the causes of pancreatitis, in which case resection of the head of the pancreas is preferable to lesser procedures.

Ectopic pancreas

Islands of ectopic pancreatic tissue can be found in the submucosa in parts of the stomach, duodenum or small intestine (including Meckel's diverticulum), the gall bladder, adjoining the pancreas, in the hilum of the spleen and within the liver. Ectopic pancreas may also be found in the wall of an alimentary tract duplication cyst.

John Langdon Haydon Down, (sometimes given as Haydon-Down), 1828–1896, physician, The London Hospital, London, and Superintendent, Earlswood Asylum for Idiots, Surrey, UK, described this syndrome in 1866.
Johann Friedrich Meckel (The Younger), 1781–1833, Professor of Anatomy and Surgery, Halle, Germany, described the embryological origin of the eponymous diverticulum in 1809.

Congenital cystic disease of the pancreas

This sometimes accompanies congenital disease of the kidneys and liver, and occurs as part of the von Hippel–Lindau syndrome.

INJURIES TO THE PANCREAS

External injury

Presentation and management

The pancreas, thanks to its somewhat protected location in the retroperitoneum, is not frequently damaged in blunt abdominal trauma. If there is damage to the pancreas, it is often concomitant with injuries to other viscera, especially the liver, the spleen and the duodenum. Occasionally, a forceful blow to the epigastrium (such as a kick from a human or a horse, or pressure from the steering wheel in a car accident) may crush the body of the pancreas against the vertebral column. Penetrating trauma to the upper abdomen or the back carries a higher chance of pancreatic injury. Pancreatic injuries may range from a contusion or laceration of the parenchyma *without* duct disruption to major parenchymal destruction *with* duct disruption (sometimes complete transection) and, rarely, massive destruction of the pancreatic head. The most important factor that determines treatment is whether the pancreatic duct has been disrupted.

Blunt pancreatic trauma usually presents with epigastric pain, which may be minor at first, with the progressive development of more severe pain due to the sequelae of leakage of pancreatic fluid into the surrounding tissues. The clinical presentation can be quite deceptive; careful serial assessments and a high index of suspicion are required. A rise in serum amylase occurs in most cases. A CT scan of the pancreas will delineate the damage that has occurred to the pancreas (Figure 68.21). If there is doubt about duct disruption, an urgent ERCP should be sought. MRCP may also provide the answer, but the images can be difficult to interpret. Support with intravenous fluids and a 'nil by mouth' regimen should be instituted while these investigations are performed. There is no need to rush to a laparotomy if the patient is haemodynamically stable, without peritonitis. It is preferable to manage conservatively at first, investigate and, once the extent of the damage has been ascertained, undertake appropriate action. Operation is indicated if there is disruption of the main pancreatic duct; in almost all other cases, the patient will recover with conservative management.

In penetrating injuries, especially if other organs are injured and the patient's condition is unstable, there is a greater need to perform an urgent surgical exploration. Assessment of pancreatic damage and duct disruption at the time of surgery can be difficult, because the bruising associated with the retroperitoneal damage prevents clear visualisation of the pancreas. A patient and thorough examination of the gland should be carried out. Haemostasis and closed drainage is adequate for minor parenchymal injuries. If the gland is transected in the body or tail, a distal pancreatectomy should be performed, with or without splenectomy. If damage is purely confined to the head of the pancreas, haemostasis and external drainage is normally effective. In the emergency setting, in an unstable patient with concomitant injuries, a surgeon unaccustomed to pancreatic surgery should refrain from trying to ascertain whether the duct in the pancreatic head is intact or embarking on a major resection. However, if there is severe injury to the pancreatic head and duodenum, then a pancreatoduodenectomy may be necessary.

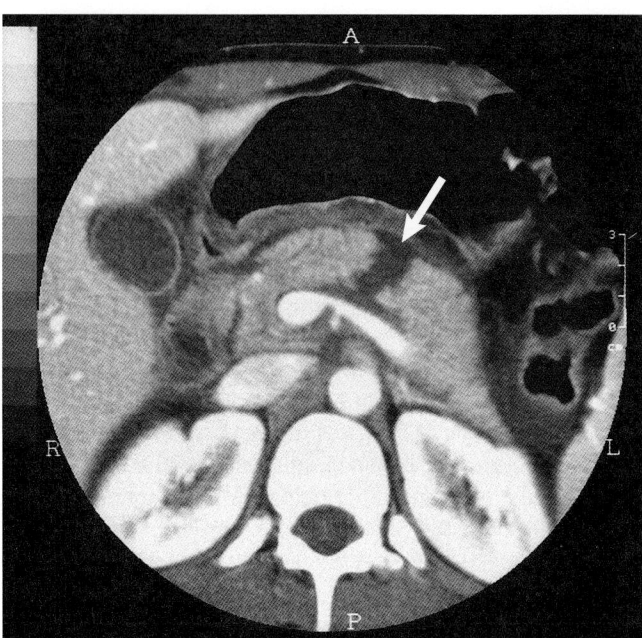

Figure 68.21 Computed tomography scan showing a pancreatic transection due to a bicycle handlebar injury. A distal pancreatectomy was performed.

Summary box 68.3

External injury to the pancreas

- Other organs are likely to be injured
- It is important to ascertain if the pancreatic duct has been disrupted
- CT and ERCP are the most useful tests
- Surgery is indicated if the main pancreatic duct is disrupted

Prognosis

The most common cause of death in the immediate period is bleeding, usually from associated injuries. Once the acute phase has passed, the mortality and morbidity related to the pancreatic injury itself are treatable, with a complete return to normal activity the usual outcome.

Persistent drain output occurs in up to a third of patients (see the section on pancreatic fistulae below). Sometimes, in the aftermath of trauma that has been treated conservatively, duct stricturing develops, leading to recurrent episodes of pancreatitis. The appropriate treatment in such cases is resection of the tail of the pancreas distal to the site of duct disruption.

Also, a pancreatic pseudocyst may develop. If the main duct is intact, the cyst can be aspirated percutaneously in the first instance; it may not be necessary to undertake a cystgastrostomy. If the cyst develops in the presence of complete disruption of the pancreas, there is no alternative but to undertake a distal resection or, occasionally, a pancreatojejunostomy with a Roux-en-Y loop. In a patient who presents with a peripancreatic cyst and a history of previous blunt abdominal trauma, do not assume that it is a post-traumatic pseudocyst. The possibility of a cystic neoplasm should be considered and excluded.

Iatrogenic injury

This can occur in several ways:

- Injury to the tail of the pancreas during splenectomy, resulting in a pancreatic fistula.
- Injury to the pancreatic head and the accessory pancreatic duct (Santorini), which is the main duct in 7% of patients, during Billroth II gastrectomy. A pancreatogram performed by cannulating the duct at the time of discovery of such an injury will demonstrate whether it is safe to ligate and divide the duct. If no alternative drainage duct can be demonstrated, then the duct should be reanastomosed to the duodenum or alternatively resection of the pancreatic head should be considered.
- Enucleation of islet cell tumours of the pancreas can result in fistulae.
- Duodenal or ampullary bleeding following sphincterotomy. This injury may require duodenotomy to control the bleeding.

Pancreatic fistula

Pancreatic fistula usually follows operative trauma to the gland or occurs as a complication of acute or chronic pancreatitis. It is important to define the site of the fistula and the epithelial structure with which it communicates (e.g. externally to skin, or internally to bowel). If there is uncertainty about whether the fluid issuing from a drain site or a wound is pancreatic juice, measurement of the amylase content will be diagnostic.

Management includes correction of metabolic and electrolyte disturbances and adequate drainage of the fistula into a stoma bag with protection of the skin. Investigation of the cause of the fistula is required as the underlying cause must be treated before the fistula will close. Frequently, the cause is related to obstruction within the pancreatic duct, which can be overcome by the insertion of a stent or catheter endoscopically into the pancreatic duct. While waiting for closure of the fistula, the patient should be given parenteral or nasojejunal nutritional support (as opposed to nasogastric or oral feeding; the rationale is that parenteral or nasojejunal feeding reduces the volume of pancreatic secretion). The use of octreotide will also suppress pancreatic secretion.

Summary box 68.4

Management of pancreatic fistulae

Tests

- Measure amylase level in fluid
- Determine the anatomy of the fistula
- Check if the main pancreatic duct is blocked or disrupted

Measures

- Correct fluid and electrolyte imbalances
- Protect the skin
- Drain adequately
- Parenteral or nasojejunal feeding
- Octreotide to suppress secretion
- Relieve pancreatic duct obstruction if possible (ERCP and stent)
- Treat underlying cause

PANCREATITIS

Pancreatitis is inflammation of the pancreatic parenchyma. For clinical purposes, it is useful to divide pancreatitis into acute, which presents as an emergency, and chronic, which is a prolonged and frequently lifelong disorder resulting from the development of fibrosis within the pancreas. It is possible that acute and chronic pancreatitis are different phases of the same process.

Acute pancreatitis is defined as an acute condition presenting with abdominal pain, a threefold or greater rise in the serum levels of the pancreatic enzymes amylase or lipase, and/or characteristic findings of pancreatic inflammation on contrast-enhanced CT. Acute pancreatitis may recur.

The underlying mechanism of injury in pancreatitis is thought to be premature activation of pancreatic enzymes within the pancreas, leading to a process of autodigestion. Anything that injures the acinar cell and impairs the secretion of zymogen granules, or damages the duct epithelium and thus delays enzymatic secretion, can trigger acute pancreatitis. Once cellular injury has been initiated, the inflammatory process can lead to pancreatic oedema, haemorrhage and, eventually, necrosis. As inflammatory mediators are released into the circulation, systemic complications can arise, such as haemodynamic instability, bacteraemia (due to translocation of gut flora), acute respiratory distress syndrome and pleural effusions, gastrointestinal haemorrhage, renal failure and disseminated intravascular coagulation (DIC).

Acute pancreatitis may be categorised as mild (*interstitial oedematous pancreatitis*) or severe (*necrotising pancreatitis*). The former is characterised by interstitial oedema of the gland and minimal organ dysfunction. The majority of patients will have a mild attack of pancreatitis, the mortality from which is around 1%. Severe acute pancreatitis is seen in 5–10% of patients, and is characterised by pancreatic necrosis, a severe systemic inflammatory response and often multi-organ failure.

Cesar Roux, 1857–1934, Professor of Surgery and Gynaecology, Lausanne, Switzerland, described this method of forming a jejunal conduit in 1908.
Christian Albert Theodor Billroth, 1829–1894, Professor of Surgery, Vienna, Austria. A hugely influential surgical teacher and an early proponent of surgical audit, Billroth performed the first oesophagectomy, first laryngectomy and first successful gastrectomy.

In those who have a severe attack of pancreatitis, the mortality varies from 20 to 50%.

Acute pancreatitis has an *early phase* that usually lasts a week. It is characterised by a systemic inflammatory response syndrome (SIRS) which – if severe – can lead to transient or persistent organ failure (deemed persistent if it lasts for over 48 hours). About one-third of deaths occur in the early phase of the attack, from multiple organ failure. The *late* phase is seen typically in those who suffer a severe attack, and can run from weeks to months. It is characterised by persistent systemic signs of inflammation, and/or local complications, particularly fluid collections and peripancreatic sepsis. Deaths occurring after the first week of onset are often due to septic complications.

Chronic pancreatitis is defined as a continuing inflammatory disease of the pancreas characterised by irreversible morphological change typically causing pain and/or permanent loss of function. Many patients with chronic pancreatitis have painful exacerbations, but the condition may be completely painless.

Acute pancreatitis

Incidence

Acute pancreatitis accounts for 3% of all cases of abdominal pain among patients admitted to hospital in the UK. The hospital admission rate for acute pancreatitis is 9.8 per year per 100 000 population in the UK, although worldwide, the annual incidence may range from 5 to 50 per 100 000. The disease may occur at any age, with a peak in young men and older women.

Aetiology

The two major causes of acute pancreatitis are biliary calculi, which occur in 50–70% of patients, and alcohol abuse, which accounts for 25% of cases. Gallstone pancreatitis is thought to be triggered by the passage of gallstones down the common bile duct. If the biliary and pancreatic ducts join to share a common channel before ending at the ampulla, then obstruction of this passage may lead to reflux of bile or activated pancreatic enzymes into the pancreatic duct. Patients who have small gallstones and a wide cystic duct may be at a higher risk of passing stones. The proposed mechanisms for alcoholic pancreatitis include the effects of diet, malnutrition, direct toxicity of alcohol, concomitant tobacco smoking, hypersecretion, duct obstruction or reflux, and hyperlipidaemia. The remaining cases may be due to rare causes or be idiopathic.

Among patients who undergo ERCP, 1–3% develop pancreatitis, probably as a consequence of duct disruption and enzyme extravasation. Patients with sphincter of Oddi dysfunction or a history of recurrent pancreatitis, and those who undergo sphincterotomy or balloon dilatation of the sphincter, carry a higher risk of developing post-ERCP pancreatitis. Patients who have undergone upper abdominal or cardiothoracic surgery may develop acute pancreatitis in the postoperative phase, as may those who have suffered blunt abdominal trauma.

Hereditary pancreatitis is a rare familial condition associated with mutations of the cationic trypsinogen gene. Patients have a tendency to suffer acute pancreatitis while in their teens, progress to chronic pancreatitis in the next two decades and have a high risk (possibly up to 40%) of developing pancreatic cancer by the age of 70 years.

Occasionally, tumours at the ampulla of Vater may cause acute pancreatitis. It is important to check the serum calcium level, a fasting lipid profile, autoimmune markers and viral titres in patients with so called idiopathic acute pancreatitis. It is equally important to take a detailed drug history and remember the association of corticosteroids, azathioprine, asparaginase and valproic acid with acute pancreatitis. Statins (taken over a long time) and gliptins have been linked with pancreatitis, but the evidence is slim. It is essential to exclude tiny gallstones. A careful search for the aetiology must be made in all cases, and no more than 20% of cases should fall into the idiopathic category.

Summary box 68.5

Possible causes of acute pancreatitis

- Gallstones
- Alcoholism
- Post ERCP
- Abdominal trauma
- Following biliary, upper gastrointestinal or cardiothoracic surgery
- Ampullary tumour
- Drugs (corticosteroids, azathioprine, asparaginase, valproic acid, thiazides, oestrogens)
- Hyperparathyroidism
- Hypercalcaemia
- Pancreas divisum
- Autoimmune pancreatitis
- Hereditary pancreatitis
- Viral infections (mumps, coxsackie B)
- Malnutrition
- Scorpion bite
- Idiopathic

Summary box 68.6

Aetiology of acute pancreatitis

- It is essential to establish the aetiology
- Investigate thoroughly before labelling it as 'idiopathic'
- After the acute episode resolves, remember further management of the underlying aetiology
- If the aetiology is gallstones, cholecystectomy is desirable during the same admission

Clinical presentation

Pain is the cardinal symptom. It characteristically develops quickly, reaching maximum intensity within minutes rather than hours and persists for hours or even days. The pain is frequently severe, constant and refractory to the usual doses of analgesics. Pain is usually experienced first in the epigastrium but may be localised to either upper quadrant or felt diffusely throughout the abdomen. There is radiation to the back in about 50% of patients, and some patients may gain relief by sitting or leaning forwards. The suddenness of onset may simulate a perforated peptic ulcer, while biliary colic or acute cholecystitis can be mimicked if the pain is maximal in the right upper quadrant. Radiation to the chest can simulate myocardial infarction, pneumonia or pleuritic pain. In fact, acute pancreatitis can mimic most causes of the acute abdomen and should seldom be discounted in differential diagnosis.

Nausea, repeated vomiting and retching are usually marked accompaniments. The retching may persist despite the stomach being kept empty by nasogastric aspiration. Hiccoughs can be troublesome and may be due to gastric distension or irritation of the diaphragm.

On examination, the appearance may be that of a patient who is well or, at the other extreme, one who is gravely ill with profound shock, toxicity and confusion. Tachypnoea is common, tachycardia is usual, and hypotension may be present. The body temperature is often normal or even subnormal, but frequently rises as inflammation develops. It is useful to reiterate here that SIRS is defined by the presence of two or more of the following criteria: heart rate >90/min, core temperature <36° C or >38° C, respirations >20/min or pCO_2 <32 mmHg, and white blood cell count <4000 or >12 000/mm^3. Mild icterus can be caused by biliary obstruction in gallstone pancreatitis, and an acute swinging pyrexia suggests cholangitis. Bleeding into the fascial planes can produce bluish discolouration of the flanks (Grey Turner's sign) or umbilicus (Cullen's sign). Neither sign is pathognomonic of acute pancreatitis; Cullen's sign was first described in association with rupture of an ectopic pregnancy. Subcutaneous fat necrosis may produce small, red, tender nodules on the skin of the legs.

Abdominal examination may reveal distension due to ileus or, more rarely, ascites with shifting dullness. A mass can develop in the epigastrium due to inflammation. There is usually muscle guarding in the upper abdomen, although marked rigidity is unusual. A pleural effusion is present in 10–20% of patients. Pulmonary oedema and pneumonitis are also described and may give rise to the differential diagnosis of pneumonia or myocardial infarction. The patient may be confused and exhibit the signs of metabolic derangement together with hypoxaemia.

Investigations

Typically, the diagnosis is made on the basis of the clinical presentation and an elevated serum amylase level. A serum amylase level three times above normal is indicative of the disease. A normal serum amylase level does not exclude acute pancreatitis, particularly if the patient has presented a few days later. If the serum lipase level can be checked, it provides a slightly more sensitive and specific test than amylase. If there is doubt, and other causes of acute abdomen have to be excluded, contrast-enhanced CT is probably the best single imaging investigation (see below).

Summary box 68.7

Investigations in acute pancreatitis should be aimed at answering three questions:

- Is a diagnosis of acute pancreatitis correct?
- How severe is the attack?
- What is the aetiology?

ASSESSMENT OF SEVERITY

It is important to define that group of patients who will develop severe pancreatitis, as they are the ones with poorer outcomes and therefore they require aggressive early management and possibly transfer to a specialist unit. A severe attack may be heralded by an initial clinical impression of a very ill patient and a worsening physiological state at 24–48 hours. Various prognostic scoring systems have been used, all aimed at predicting persistent organ failure, particularly respiratory, cardiac and renal. Severity stratification assessments should be performed in patients at 24 hours, 48 hours and 7 days after admission. The Ranson and Glasgow scoring systems are specific for acute pancreatitis, and a score of 3 or more at 48 hours indicates a severe attack (*Table 68.3*). Several other systems that are used in intensive care units can also be applied. These include the APACHE, SAPS, SOFA, MODS and modified Marshall scoring systems (the latter has the advantage of simplicity). Regardless of the system used, persisting organ failure indicates a severe attack. A serum C-reactive protein level >150 mg/L at 48 hours after the onset of symptoms is also an indicator of severity. Patients with a body mass index over 30 are at higher risk of developing complications. A revision in 2013 of the Atlanta classification of acute pancreatitis (1992) recommends that patients with acute pancreatitis be stratified into 3 groups:

- Mild acute pancreatitis:
  - no organ failure;
  - no local or systemic complications.
- Moderately severe acute pancreatitis:
  - organ failure that resolves within 48 hours (transient organ failure); and/or
  - local or systemic complications without persistent organ failure.

George Grey Turner, 1877–1951, Professor of Surgery, The University of Durham, Durham (1927–1934), and at the Postgraduate Medical School, Hammersmith, London, UK (1934–1945).
Thomas Stephen Cullen, 1868–1953, Professor of Gynecology, The Johns Hopkins University, Baltimore, MD, USA. Described bluish discoloration of the peri-umbilical skin as a sign of ruptured ectopic pregnancy.
John HC Ranson, 1938–95, Professor of Surgery, The New York University School of Medicine, New York, NY, USA. Published his scoring criteria for severe acute pancreatitis in 1974.
John C Marshall, contemporary, trauma surgeon and intensivist, St Michael's Hospital, Toronto, Canada.

TABLE 68.3 The Ranson and Glasgow scoring systems to predict the severity of acute pancreatitis: in both systems, disease is classified as severe when three or more factors are present.

Ranson score	Glasgow score
On admission	**Within 48 hours**
Age >55 years	Age >55 years
White blood cell count >16 × 10^9/L	White blood cell count >15 × 10^9/L
Blood glucose >1.1 mmol/L (>200 mg/dL)	Blood glucose >10 mmol/L (no history of diabetes)
LDH >350 units/L	LDH > 600 units/L
AST >250 units/L	Serum urea >16 mmol/L (no response to intravenous fluids)
Within 48 hours	Arterial oxygen saturation (PaO_2) <8 kPa (60 mmHg)
Haematocrit fall of 10% or greater	Serum calcium <2.0 mmol/L
Blood urea nitrogen rise >5 mg/dL (1.8 mmol/L) despite fluids	Serum albumin <32 g/L
Arterial oxygen saturation (PaO_2) <8 kPa (60 mmHg)	
Serum calcium <2.0 mmol/L	
Base deficit >4 mmol/L	
Fluid sequestration >6 litres	

AST, aspartate aminotransferase; LDH, lactate dehydrogenase; PaO_2, arterial oxygen tension.

- Severe acute pancreatitis:
  - persistent organ failure (>48 hours);
  - single organ failure;
  - multiple organ failure.

IMAGING

Plain erect chest and abdominal radiographs are not diagnostic of acute pancreatitis, but are useful in the differential diagnosis. Non-specific findings in pancreatitis include a generalised or local ileus (sentinel loop), a colon cut-off sign and a renal halo sign. Occasionally, calcified gallstones or pancreatic calcification may be seen. A chest radiograph may show a pleural effusion and, in severe cases, a diffuse alveolar interstitial shadowing may suggest acute respiratory distress syndrome.

Ultrasound does not establish a diagnosis of acute pancreatitis. The swollen pancreas may be seen, but ultrasonography should be performed within 24 hours in *all* patients to detect gallstones as a potential cause, rule out acute cholecystitis as a differential diagnosis and determine whether the common bile duct is dilated.

CT is not necessary for all patients, particularly those deemed to have a mild attack on prognostic criteria. But a contrast-enhanced CT is indicated in the following situations:

- If there is diagnostic uncertainty.
- In patients with severe acute pancreatitis, to distinguish interstitial from necrotising pancreatitis (Figure 68.22). In the first 72 hours, CT may underestimate the extent of necrosis. The severity of pancreatitis detected on CT may be staged according to the Balthazar criteria.
- In patients with organ failure, signs of sepsis or progressive clinical deterioration.
- When a localised complication is suspected, such as fluid collection, pseudocyst or a pseudoaneurysm.

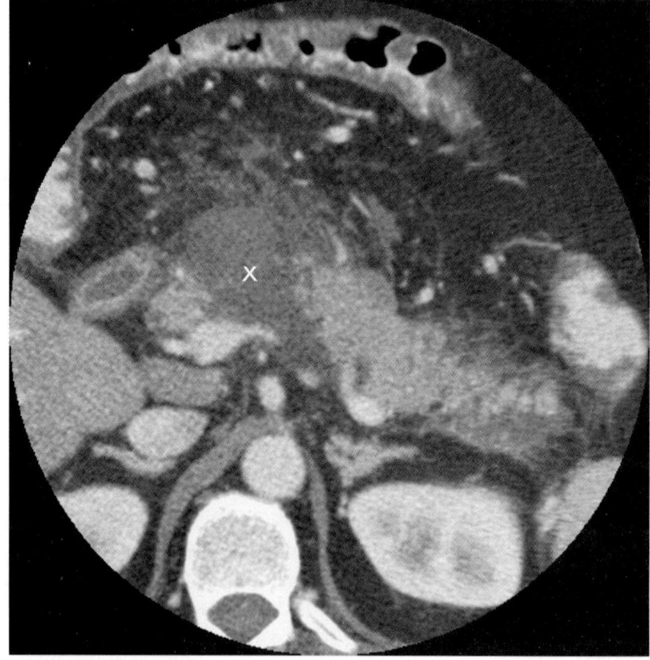

Figure 68.22 Contrast-enhanced computed tomography scan showing acute necrotising pancreatitis. Note the area of reduced enhancement in the pancreas (marked X), the peripancreatic oedema and stranding of the fatty tissues (courtesy of Dr Niall Power).

Cross-sectional MRI can yield similar information to that obtained by CT. EUS and MRCP can help in detecting stones in the common bile duct and directly assessing the pancreatic parenchyma, but are not widely available. ERCP allows the identification and removal of stones in the common bile duct in gallstone pancreatitis. In patients with severe acute gallstone pancreatitis and signs of ongoing biliary obstruction and cholangitis, an urgent ERCP should be sought (see below).

Emil J Balthazar, contemporary, Professor Emeritus, The Department of Radiology, The New York University, New York, NY, USA.

The presentation is so variable that sometimes even an experienced clinician can be mistaken. While this is not desirable, occasionally the diagnosis is only made at laparotomy. The appearances at laparotomy are characteristic (Figure 68.23).

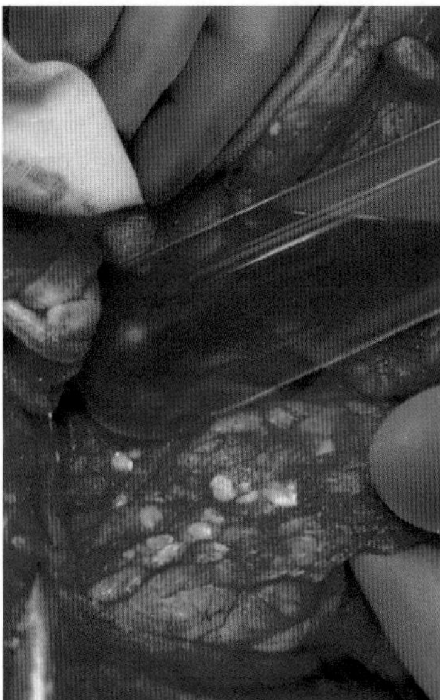

Figure 68.23 Widespread fat necrosis of the omentum. A test tube has been filled with blood-stained peritoneal fluid. This specimen was rich in amylase. Fat necroses are dull, opaque, yellow-white areas suggestive of drops of wax. They are most abundant in the vicinity of the pancreas, but are widespread in the greater omentum and the mesentery. At necropsy, they can sometimes be demonstrated beneath the pleura and pericardium, and even in the subsynovial fat of the knee joint. Fat necroses consist of small islands of saponification caused by the liberation of lipase, which splits into glycerol and fatty acids. Free fatty acids combine with calcium to form soaps (fatty necrosis) (courtesy of Dr GD Adhia, Mumbai, India).

Management

If after initial assessment a patient is considered to have a mild attack of pancreatitis, a conservative approach is indicated with intravenous fluid administration and frequent, but non-invasive, observation. A brief period of fasting may be sensible in a patient who is nauseated and in pain, but there is little physiological justification for keeping patients on a prolonged 'nil by mouth' regimen. Antibiotics are not indicated. Apart from analgesics and anti-emetics, no drugs or interventions are warranted, and CT scanning is unnecessary unless there is evidence of deterioration. However, if a stable patient meets the prognostic criteria for a severe attack of pancreatitis, then a more aggressive approach is required, with the patient being admitted to a high-dependency or an intensive care unit and monitored invasively.

Patients with a severe attack should be admitted to an intensive care or high-dependency unit (*Table 68.4*). Adequate analgesia should be administered. Aggressive fluid resuscitation is important, guided by frequent measurement of vital signs, urine output and central venous pressure. Supplemental oxygen should be administered and serial arterial blood gas analysis performed. The haematocrit, clotting profile, blood glucose and serum levels of calcium and magnesium should be closely monitored.

TABLE 68.4 Early management of severe acute pancreatitis.
Admission to HDU/ICU
Analgesia
Aggressive fluid rehydration
Supplemental oxygen
Invasive monitoring of vital signs, central venous pressure, urine output, blood gases
Frequent monitoring of haematological and biochemical parameters (including liver and renal function, clotting, serum calcium, blood glucose)
Nasogastric drainage (only initially)
Antibiotics if cholangitis suspected; prophylactic antibiotics can be considered
CT scan essential if organ failure, clinical deterioration or signs of sepsis develop
ERCP within 72 hours for severe gallstone pancreatitis or signs of cholangitis
Supportive therapy for organ failure if it develops (inotropes, ventilatory support, haemofiltration, etc.)
If nutritional support is required, consider enteral (nasogastric) feeding

CT, computed tomography; ERCP, endoscopic retrograde cholangiopancreatography; HDU, high-dependency unit; ICU, intensive care unit.

A nasogastric tube is not essential but may be of value in patients with vomiting. Specific treatments such as aprotinin, somatostatin analogues, platelet-activating factor inhibitors and selective gut decontamination have failed to improve outcome in numerous clinical trials and should not be given. There are no data to support a practice of 'resting' the pancreas and feeding only by the parenteral or nasojejunal routes. If nutritional support is felt to be necessary, enteral nutrition (e.g. feeding via a nasogastric tube) should be used.

There is some evidence to support the use of prophylactic antibiotics in patients with severe acute pancreatitis but there is no consensus. The rationale is to prevent local and other septic complications. The regimens used include intravenous cefuroxime, or imipenem, or ciprofloxacin plus metronidazole. The duration of antibiotic prophylaxis should not exceed 14 days. Additional antibiotic use should be guided by microbiological cultures. If however there is evidence of cholangitis, or concomitant respiratory or urinary infection, then antibiotics should be given promptly.

If gallstones are the cause of an attack of predicted or proven severe pancreatitis, or if the patient has jaundice, cholangitis or a dilated common bile duct, urgent ERCP should be carried out within 72 hours of the onset of symptoms. There is evidence that sphincterotomy and clearance of the bile duct can reduce the incidence of infective complications in these patients. In patients with cholangitis, sphincterotomy should be carried out or a biliary stent placed to drain the duct. ERCP is an invasive procedure and carries a small risk of worsening the pancreatitis.

Systemic complications

Pancreatitis may involve all organ systems (Table 68.5) and place demands on the surgeon beyond his or her skills. Patients with systemic complications should be managed by a multidisciplinary team that includes intensive care specialists. When there is organ failure, appropriate supportive therapies may include inotropic support for haemodynamic instability, haemofiltration in the event of renal failure, ventilatory support for respiratory failure and correction of coagulopathies (including DIC). There is no role for surgery during the initial period of resuscitation and stabilisation; surgical intervention is contemplated only in the patient who deteriorates as a result of local complications following successful stabilisation.

Local complications and their management

Once the acute phase has been survived, usually by the end of the first week, and major organ failure is under control, then local complications become pre-eminent in the management of these patients. The course of the patient should be followed carefully. If pain persists or recurs, clinical resolution does not progress as expected, signs of sepsis develop, organ dysfunction worsens, or there is a further spike in the serum amylase level, a CT scan should be performed. Local complications in pancreatic disease are serious and carry a significant mortality. The management approach is conservative on the whole, with surgery restricted to situations in which conservative management has failed. It is important to be clear about the definitions. Certain terms are confusing, such as 'phlegmon', which may refer to an abscess or to an inflammatory mass in the pancreas, and are best avoided.

TABLE 68.5 Complications of acute pancreatitis.

Systemic	Local
(More common in the first week)	*(Usually develop after the first week)*
Cardiovascular	Acute fluid collection
Shock	Sterile pancreatic necrosis
Arrhythmias	Infected pancreatic necrosis
Pulmonary	Pancreatic abscess
ARDS	Pseudocyst
Renal failure	Pancreatic ascites
Haematological	Pleural effusion
DIC	Portal/splenic vein thrombosis
Metabolic	Pseudoaneurysm
Hypocalcaemia	
Hyperglycaemia	
Hyperlipidaemia	
Gastrointestinal	
Ileus	
Neurological	
Visual disturbances	
Confusion, irritability	
Encephalopathy	
Miscellaneous	
Subcutaneous fat necrosis	
Arthralgia	

ARDS, acute respiratory distress syndrome; DIC, disseminated intravascular coagulation.

ACUTE PERIPANCREATIC FLUID COLLECTION (APFC)

This occurs early in the course of mild pancreatitis without necrosis, and is located adjacent to the pancreas. It has no encapsulating wall and is confined within normal fascial planes. The fluid is sterile, and most such collections resolve. No intervention is necessary unless a large collection causes symptoms or pressure effects, in which case it can be percutaneously aspirated under ultrasound or CT guidance. Transgastric drainage under EUS guidance is another option.

STERILE AND INFECTED PANCREATIC NECROSIS

The term 'pancreatic necrosis' refers to a diffuse or focal area of non-viable parenchyma. This can be identified by an absence of parenchymal enhancement on CT with intravenous contrast. Pancreatic necrosis is typically associated with lysis of peripancreatic fat. This may lead to what is described as an *acute necrotic collection* (ANC). This is typically an intra- or extrapancreatic collection containing fluid and necrotic material, with no definable wall. Gradually, over a period of over 4 weeks, this may develop a well-defined inflammatory capsule, and evolve into what is termed *walled-off necrosis* (WON). Collections associated with necrotising pancreatitis are sterile to begin with but often become subsequently infected, probably due to translocation of gut bacteria. Infected necrosis is associated with a mortality rate of up to 50%. Sterile necrotic material should not be drained or interfered with. But if the patient shows signs of sepsis, then one should determine whether the collection is infected (Figure 68.24). A CT scan should be performed and a needle passed into the area under CT guidance, choosing a path that does

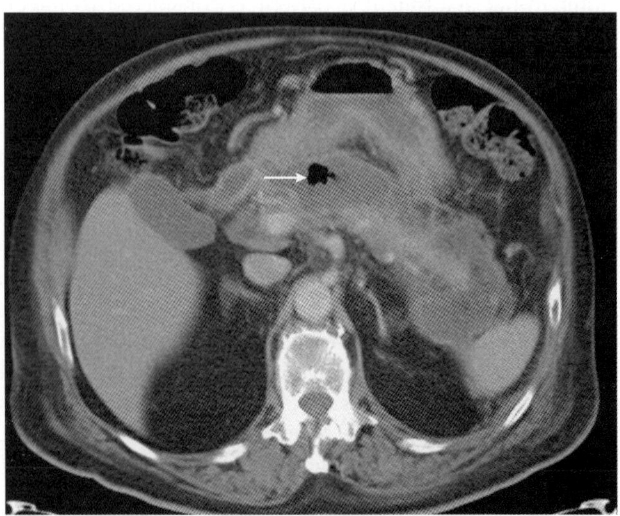

Figure 68.24 Infected pancreatic necrosis in an elderly patient. Note the areas of reduced enhancement in the pancreas and the peripancreatic fluid collection with pockets of gas within it (arrow). This resolved after percutaneous drainage and antibiotic therapy.

not traverse hollow viscera. This may be done under ultrasonographic guidance as well. If the aspirate is purulent, percutaneous drainage of the infected fluid should be carried out. The tube drain inserted should have the *widest* bore possible. The aspirate should be sent for microbiological assessment, and appropriate antibiotic therapy should be commenced as per the sensitivity report. The fluid can be quite viscous with particulate matter, and the drain may need regular flushing with full aseptic precautions. Often, repeated imaging and repeated insertion of progressively wider drains is necessary.

If the sepsis worsens despite this, then a pancreatic necrosectomy should be considered. This is a challenging operation that carries a high morbidity and mortality, and is best carried out in a specialist unit. The overwhelming majority of patients with peripancreatic sepsis can be successfully treated by conservative means, and necrosectomy should be necessary in a very small proportion of patients. The surgical approach may be through a mid-line laparotomy, especially if the area involved is around the head of the gland. The duodenocolic and gastrocolic ligaments should be divided and the lesser sac opened. Thorough debridement of the dead tissue around the pancreas should be carried out. If the body and tail of the gland are primarily involved (Figure 68.25), a retroperitoneal approach through a left flank incision may be more appropriate. The tissues are inevitably friable, and one should be careful not to precipitate excessive bleeding or inadvertently breach the bowel wall. Blunt dissection is preferable to sharp dissection. A feeding jejunostomy may be a useful adjunct to the procedure. If gallstones are the precipitating factor of the pancreatitis, a cholecystectomy should be included. Some prefer a minimally invasive approach to a formal laparotomy. A rigid laparoscope is inserted into the peripancreatic area through a retroperitoneal approach, and vigorous irrigation and suction is combined with a gradual nibbling away of the necrotic debris.

Once a necrosectomy has been completed, further necrotic tissue may form. There are several possible ways of dealing with this (listed below), none of which has been proved to be more effective than the others. The last two approaches make greater logistic demands as one is committed to a re-exploration every 48–72 hours.

- **Closed continuous lavage.** Tube drains are left in and the raw area flushed (Beger) (Figure 68.26).
- **Closed drainage.** The incision is closed, but the cavity is packed with gauze-filled Penrose drains and closed suction drains. The Penrose drains are brought out through the flank and slowly pulled out and removed after 7 days.
- **Open packing.** The incision is left open, and the cavity is packed with the intention of returning to the operating room at regular intervals and repacking until there is a clean granulating cavity.
- **Closure and relaparotomy.** The incision is closed with drains with the intention of performing a series of planned relaparotomies every 48–72 hours until the raw area granulates (Bradley).

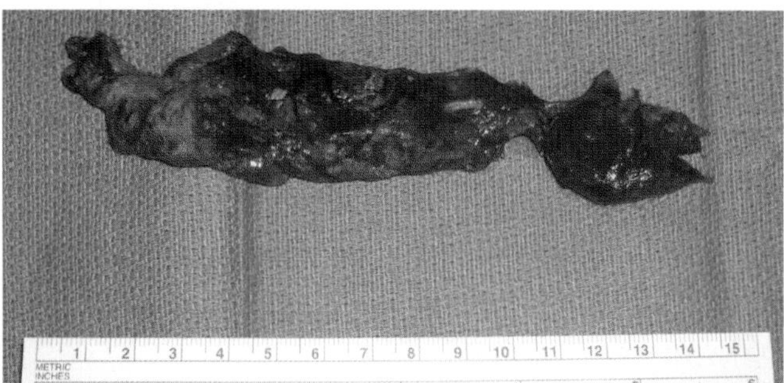

Figure 68.25 Necrotic body and tail of the pancreas removed as an intact specimen rather than piecemeal. The patient had suffered severe necrotising gallstone pancreatitis complicated by persistent pancreatic sepsis. Necrosectomy was carried out through a left flank retroperitoneal approach.

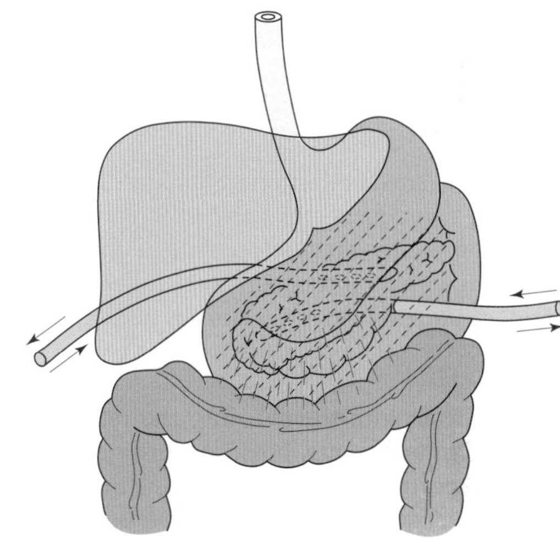

Figure 68.26 Continuous postoperative closed lavage of the lesser sac as advised by Beger. Lavage is carried out through several double-lumen and single-lumen catheters. Each time, 1 litre of saline is infused through and then drained over a period of hours, and the process is repeated.

There is a subgroup of patients who respond initially to percutaneous treatment but then develop recurrent sepsis that requires repeated insertion of drains, and fail to thrive. Necrosectomy should be considered in these patients, but it can be a difficult judgement call.

Patients with peripancreatic sepsis are ill for long periods of time, and may require management in an intensive care unit. Nutritional support is essential. The parenteral and nasojejunal approaches are more popular (on the assumption that they rest the pancreas), although there is little evidence to show that nasogastric feeding, if tolerated, is harmful in any way.

PANCREATIC ABSCESS

This is a circumscribed intra-abdominal collection of pus, usually in proximity to the pancreas. It may be an ANC or a WON that has become infected. The principles of diagnosis

Hans Beger, contemporary, Emeritus Professor of Surgery, Ulm, Germany.
Charles Bingham Penrose, 1862–1925, Professor of Gynecology, The University of Pennsylvania, Philadelphia, PA, USA.
Edward Bradley III, contemporary, Professor, The Department of Clinical Sciences, Florida State University College of Medicine, FL, USA.

and management are as outlined above for infected pancreatic necrosis. Percutaneous drainage with the widest possible drains placed under imaging guidance is the treatment, along with appropriate antibiotics and supportive care. Repeated scans may be required depending on the progress of the patient, and drains may need to be flushed, repositioned or re-inserted. Very occasionally, open drainage of the abscess may be necessary.

PANCREATIC ASCITES

This is a chronic, generalised, peritoneal, enzyme-rich effusion usually associated with pancreatic duct disruption. Paracentesis will reveal turbid fluid with a high amylase level. Adequate drainage with wide-bore drains placed under imaging guidance is essential. Measures that can be taken to suppress pancreatic secretion include parenteral or nasojejunal feeding and administration of octreotide. An ERCP may allow demonstration of the duct disruption and placement of a pancreatic stent.

PANCREATIC EFFUSION

This is an encapsulated collection of fluid in the pleural cavity, arising as a consequence of acute pancreatitis. Concomitant pancreatic ascites may be present, or there may be a communication with an intra-abdominal collection. Percutaneous drainage under imaging guidance is necessary.

HAEMORRHAGE

Bleeding may occur into the gut, into the retroperitoneum or into the peritoneal cavity. Possible causes include bleeding into a pseudocyst cavity, diffuse bleeding from a large raw surface, or a pseudoaneurysm. The last is a false aneurysm of a major peripancreatic vessel confined as a clot by the surrounding tissues and often associated with infection. Recurrent bleeding is common, often culminating in fatal haemorrhage. CT, angiography or MR angiography helps to make the diagnosis. Treatment involves embolisation or surgery.

PORTAL OR SPLENIC VEIN THROMBOSIS

This may often develop silently and is identified on a CT scan. A marked rise in the platelet count should raise suspicions. In the context of acute pancreatitis, treatment is usually conservative. The patient should be screened for pro-coagulant tendencies. If varices or other manifestations of portal hypertension develop, they will require treatment, such as endoscopic injection or banding, β-blockade, etc. Thrombocytosis may mandate the use of aspirin or other antiplatelet drugs for a period. Systemic anticoagulation, if instituted early in the process, may achieve recanalisation of the vein, but it is not routinely used as it carries considerable risks in a patient with ongoing pancreatitis.

PSEUDOCYST

A pseudocyst is a collection of amylase-rich fluid enclosed in a well-defined wall of fibrous or granulation tissue. Pseudocysts typically arise following an attack of mild acute pancreatitis, lie outside the pancreas, and represent an APFC that has not resolved and matured. Formation of a pseudocyst requires 4 weeks or more from the onset of acute pancreatitis. The term 'pseudocyst' is often used more loosely, to include sterile WON that has failed to resolve, or a collection that has developed in the context of chronic pancreatitis or after pancreatic trauma. (Figure 68.27; see also Figure 68.10). If carefully investigated, more than half of these will be found to have a communication with the main pancreatic duct. Pseudocysts are often single but, occasionally, patients will develop multiple pseudocysts.

A pseudocyst is usually identified on ultrasound or a CT scan. It is important to differentiate a pseudocyst from an APFC; the clinical scenario and the radiological appearances should allow that distinction to be made. Occasionally, a cystic neoplasm may be confused with a chronic pseudocyst. EUS and aspiration of the cyst fluid is very useful in such a situation. The fluid should be sent for measurement of carcinoembryonic antigen (CEA) levels, amylase levels and cytology. Fluid from a pseudocyst typically has a low CEA level, and levels above 400 ng/mL are suggestive of a mucinous neoplasm. Pseudocyst fluid usually has a high amylase level, but that is not diagnostic, as a tumour that communicates with the duct system may yield similar findings. Cytology typically reveals inflammatory cells in pseudocyst fluid. If there is no access to EUS, then percutaneous FNA is acceptable (just aspiration, *not* percutaneous insertion of a drain). ERCP and MRCP may demonstrate communication of the cyst with the pancreatic duct system, demonstrate ductal anomalies, or diagnose chronic pancreatitis and thus help in planning treatment.

Pseudocysts will resolve spontaneously in most instances, but complications can develop (*Table* 68.6). Pseudocysts that are thick-walled or large (over 6 cm in diameter), have lasted for a long time (over 12 weeks), or have arisen in the context of chronic pancreatitis are less likely to resolve spontaneously,

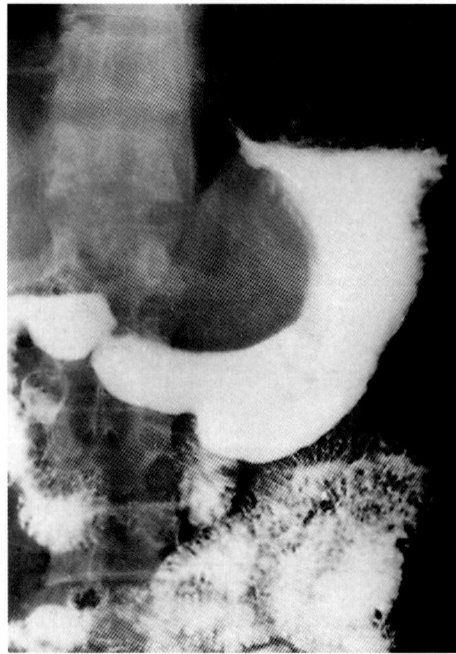

Figure 68.27 Barium meal. Pseudocyst displacing the stomach (courtesy of Professor VK Kapoor, Lucknow, India).

TABLE 68.6 Possible complications of a pancreatic pseudocyst.

Process	Outcomes
Infection	Abscess
	Systemic sepsis
Rupture	
Into the gut	Gastrointestinal bleeding
	Internal fistula
Into the peritoneum	Peritonitis
Enlargement	
Pressure effects	Obstructive jaundice from biliary compression
	Bowel obstruction
Pain	
Erosion into a vessel	Haemorrhage into the cyst
	Haemoperitoneum

but these factors are not specific indications for intervention. Therapeutic interventions are advised only if the pseudocyst causes symptoms, if complications develop, or if a distinction has to be made between a pseudocyst and a tumour.

There are three possible approaches to draining a pseudocyst: percutaneous, endoscopic and surgical. Percutaneous drainage to the exterior under radiological guidance should be avoided. It carries a very high likelihood of recurrence. Moreover, it is not advisable unless one is absolutely certain that the cyst is not neoplastic and that it has no communication with the pancreatic duct (or else a pancreaticocutaneous fistula will develop). A percutaneous transgastric cystgastrostomy can be done under imaging guidance, and a double-pigtail drain placed with one end in the cyst cavity and the other end in the gastric lumen. This requires specialist expertise but, in experienced hands, the recurrence rates are no more than 15%. Endoscopic drainage usually involves puncture of the cyst through the stomach or duodenal wall under EUS guidance, and placement of a tube drain with one end in the cyst cavity and the other end in the gastric lumen. The success rates depend on operator expertise. Occasionally, ERCP and placement of a pancreatic stent across the ampulla may help to drain a pseudocyst that is in communication with the duct. Surgical drainage involves internally draining the cyst into the gastric or jejunal lumen (Figure 68.28). Recurrence rates should be no more than 5%, and this still remains the standard against which the evolving radiological and endoscopic approaches are measured. The approach is conventionally through an open incision, but laparoscopic cystgastrostomy is also feasible. Pseudocysts that have developed complications are best managed surgically.

There is a small group of patients who, having suffered an attack of necrotising pancreatitis with duct disruption, go on to suffer repeated complications in the form of recurrent fluid collections, pseudocysts, pleural effusions or pancreatic ascites. Very often disruption of the main pancreatic duct in the neck, body or tail is compounded by a stricture or a stone in the head that cannot be treated endoscopically. In such patients, some form of surgical resection and/or a drainage procedure – even though it may be technically challenging – may be the only way to achieve lasting resolution.

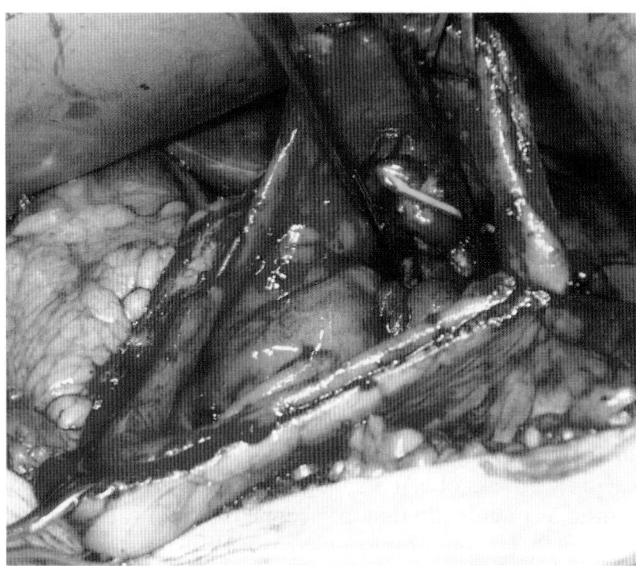

Figure 68.28 Cystgastrostomy for the pancreatic pseudocyst shown in Figure 68.10. The anterior wall of the stomach has been opened and the edges drawn back, held by Babcock's forceps. An opening has been made through the posterior wall of the stomach into the pseudocyst, and the tips of the dissecting forceps are in the cavity of the pseudocyst, which is lined by slough and granulation tissue. The tip of a nasogastric tube is visible. A running stitch will next be placed along the edges of this opening, suturing the full thickness of the posterior gastric wall to the capsule of the pseudocyst.

Summary box 68.8

Distinguishing a pseudocyst from a cystic neoplasm

- History
- Appearance on computed tomography and ultrasound (US)
- Fine needle aspiration of fluid, preferably under endoscopic US guidance:
  - Carcinoembryonic antigen (high level in mucinous tumours)
  - Amylase (level usually high in pseudocysts but occasionally in tumours)
  - Cytology

Outcomes and follow-up of acute pancreatitis

The overall mortality from acute pancreatitis has remained at 10–15% over the past 20 years. There is a clear responsibility before the patient is discharged to determine the aetiology of the attack of pancreatitis, and the causes listed in *Summary box* 68.5 must be looked for and excluded. Failure to remove a predisposing factor could lead to a second attack of pancreatitis,

William Wayne Babcock, 1872–1963, surgeon, Philadelphia, PA, USA.

which could be fatal. A proportion of patients in the idiopathic group who suffer repeated attacks may prove to have biliary microlithiasis, which can be identified only by bile sampling at ERCP or by endoscopic ultrasound. In a patient who has gallstone pancreatitis, the gallbladder and gallstones should be removed as soon as the patient is fit to undergo surgery and, preferably, before discharge from hospital.

Chronic pancreatitis

Chronic pancreatitis is a progressive inflammatory disease in which there is irreversible destruction of pancreatic tissue. Its clinical course is characterised by severe pain and, in the later stages, exocrine and endocrine pancreatic insufficiency. In the early stages of its evolution, it is frequently complicated by attacks of acute pancreatitis, which are responsible for the recurrent pain that may be the only clinical symptom. The incidence of chronic pancreatitis in several European, North American and Japanese studies ranges from 2 to 10 new cases per 100 000 population per year, with a prevalence of around 13 cases per 100 000, although there are suspicions that the prevalence is actually higher. In certain parts of the world, such as southern India, the prevalence is much higher (100–200 per 100 000). The disease occurs more frequently in men (male:female ratio of 4:1), and the mean age of onset is about 40 years.

Aetiology and pathology

High alcohol consumption is the most frequent cause of chronic pancreatitis, accounting for 60–70% of cases, but only 5–10% of people with alcoholism develop chronic pancreatitis. The exact mechanism of how alcohol causes chronic inflammation in these patients is unclear; genetic and metabolic factors may be at play.

Other causes include pancreatic duct obstruction resulting from stricture formation after trauma, after acute pancreatitis, or even occlusion of the duct by pancreatic cancer. Congenital abnormalities, such as pancreas divisum and annular pancreas, if associated with papillary stenosis, are rare causes of chronic pancreatitis.

Hereditary pancreatitis, CF, infantile malnutrition and a large unexplained idiopathic group make up the remainder. Normally, if trypsinogen does become prematurely activated within the pancreas, it is inhibited by *SPINK1* and then gets destroyed. Hereditary pancreatitis is an autosomal dominant disorder with an 80% penetrance, associated with a gain-of-function mutation in the cationic trypsinogen gene (*PRSS1*) on chromosome 7, which leads to production of a degradation-resistant form of trypsin. A loss-of-function mutation in *SPINK1* also predisposes to idiopathic pancreatitis. Some patients with idiopathic chronic pancreatitis have mutations in the *CFTR* gene. Idiopathic chronic pancreatitis accounts for approximately 30% of cases and has been subdivided into early-onset and late-onset forms.

The importance of hereditary pancreatitis and pancreatitis occurring at a young age is that there is a markedly increased risk of developing pancreatic cancer, particularly if the patient smokes tobacco. Hyperlipidaemia and hypercalcaemia can lead to chronic pancreatitis.

Tropical pancreatitis is a form of idiopathic pancreatitis that begins at a young age and is associated with a high incidence of diabetes mellitus and stone formation. This has been described in Kerala, in southern India, as well as in resource-poor countries in Asia, Africa and central America. Malnutrition, ingestion of cyanogenic glycosides in cassava, and exposure to hydrocarbons released by kerosene or paraffin lamps have been proposed as possible mechanisms for tropical pancreatitis.

Autoimmune pancreatitis has been described relatively recently. Features include diffuse enlargement of the pancreas, and diffuse and irregular narrowing of the main pancreatic duct. It may occur in association with other autoimmune diseases, as a multisystem disorder, or may affect the pancreas alone. There may be changes in the biliary tree (autoimmune cholangiopathy) as well. The changes may be confused with neoplasia. Autoantibodies may be present, and levels of the immunoglobulin subtype IgG4 are elevated.

At the onset of the disease when symptoms have developed, the pancreas may appear normal. Later, the pancreas enlarges and becomes hard as a result of fibrosis. The ducts become distorted and dilated with areas of both stricture formation and ectasia. Calcified stones weighing from a few milligrams to 200 mg may form within the ducts. The ducts may become occluded with a gelatinous proteinaceous fluid and debris, and inflammatory cysts may form. Histologically, the lesions affect the lobules, producing ductular metaplasia and atrophy of acini, hyperplasia of duct epithelium and interlobular fibrosis.

Clinical features

Pain is the outstanding symptom in the majority of patients. The site of pain depends to some extent on the main focus of the disease. If the disease is mainly in the head of the pancreas, then epigastric and right subcostal pain is common, whereas if it is limited to the left side of the pancreas, left subcostal and back pain are the presenting symptoms. In some patients, the pain is more diffuse. Radiation to the shoulder can occur. Nausea is common during attacks, and vomiting may occur. The pain is often dull and gnawing. Severe flare-ups of pain may be superimposed on background discomfort. All the complications of acute pancreatitis can occur with chronic pancreatitis. Weight loss is common, because the patient does not feel like eating. The pain prevents sleep and time off work is frequent. The number of hospital admissions for acute exacerbations is a pointer towards the severity of the disease. Analgesic use and abuse is frequent. This, too, gives an indication of the severity of the disability. The patient's lifestyle is gradually destroyed by pain, analgesic dependence, weight loss and inability to work. Loss of exocrine function leads to steatorrhoea in more than 30% of patients with chronic pancreatitis. Loss of endocrine function and the development of diabetes are not uncommon, and the incidence increases as the disease progresses. Complications frequently bring the patient to the attention of the surgeon. Infection is not infrequent, possibly related to the diabetes mellitus.

Investigations

Only in the early stages of the disease will there be a rise in serum amylase. Tests of pancreatic function merely confirm the presence of pancreatic insufficiency or that more than 70% of the gland has been destroyed.

Pancreatic calcifications may be seen on abdominal X-ray (see Figure 68.18). CT or MRI scan will show the outline of the gland, the main area of damage and the possibilities for surgical correction (Figure 68.29; see also Figure 68.7). Calcification is seen very well on CT but not on MRI. An MRCP will identify the presence of biliary obstruction and the state of the pancreatic duct (Figure 68.30). The use of intravenous secretin during the study may demonstrate a pancreatic duct stricture that is not apparent on a standard MRCP, but a normal-looking pancreas on CT or MRI does not rule out chronic pancreatitis. ERCP is the most accurate way of elucidating the anatomy of the duct and, in conjunction with the whole organ morphology, can help to determine the type of operation required, if operative intervention is indicated (Figures 68.15 and 68.17). Histologically proven chronic pancreatitis can, however, occur in the setting of normal findings on pancreatography. EUS can also be very useful. Sonographic findings characteristic of chronic pancreatitis include the presence of stones, visible side branches, cysts, lobularity, an irregular main pancreatic duct, hyperechoic foci and strands, dilatation of the main pancreatic duct and hyperechoic margins of the main pancreatic duct. The presence of four or more of these features is highly suggestive of chronic pancreatitis.

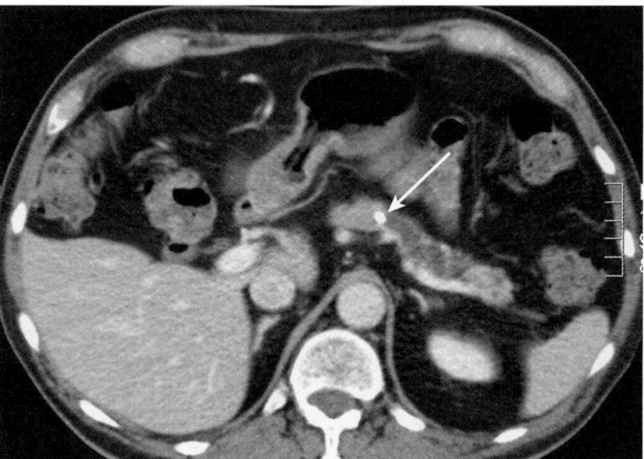

Figure 68.29 Computed tomography scan in a patient with chronic pancreatitis. A stone (arrow) is obstructing the main pancreatic duct in the body of the gland. The duct is markedly dilated upstream of the obstruction.

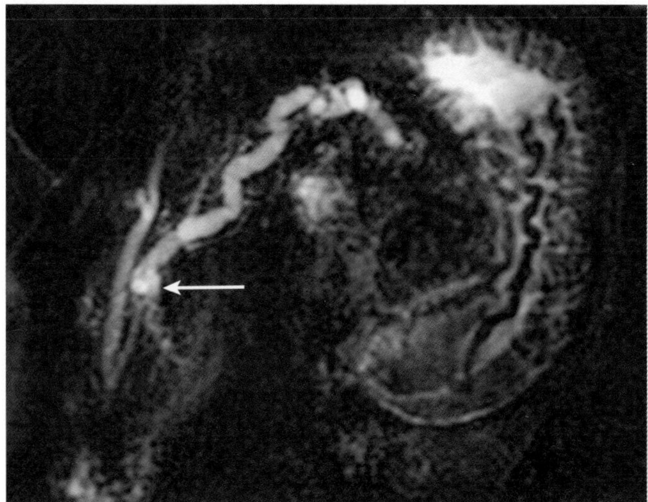

Figure 68.30 Magnetic resonance cholangiopancreatography in a patient with chronic pancreatitis, showing a stricture of the pancreatic duct in the body of the gland (arrow), with dilatation upstream.

Treatment

Most patients can be managed with medical measures. There is no single therapeutic agent that has been shown to relieve symptoms (*Summary box 68.9*).

Summary box 68.9

Medical treatment of chronic pancreatitis

Treat the addiction

- Help the patient to stop alcohol consumption and tobacco smoking
- Involve a dependency counsellor or a psychologist

Alleviate abdominal pain

- Eliminate obstructive factors (duodenum, bile duct, pancreatic duct)
- Escalate analgesia in a stepwise fashion
- Refer to a pain management specialist
- For intractable pain, consider CT/EUS-guided coeliac axis block

Nutritional and pharmacological measures

- Diet: low in fat and high in protein and carbohydrates
- Pancreatic enzyme supplementation with meals
- Correct malabsorption of the fat-soluble vitamins and vitamin B12
- Micronutrient therapy with methionine, vitamins C & E, selenium (may reduce pain and slow disease progression)
- Steroids (only in autoimmune pancreatitis, for relief of symptoms)
- Medium-chain triglycerides in patients with severe fat malabsorption (they are directly absorbed by the small intestine without the need for digestion)
- Reducing gastric secretions may help

Treat diabetes mellitus

Endoscopic, radiological or surgical interventions are indicated mainly to relieve obstruction of the pancreatic duct, bile duct or the duodenum, or in dealing with complications (e.g. pseudocyst, abscess, fistula, ascites or variceal haemorrhage). Decompressing an obstructed pancreatic duct can provide pain relief in some patients (the assumption is that ductal hypertension causes the pain).

Endoscopic pancreatic sphincterotomy might be beneficial in patients with papillary stenosis and a high sphincter pressure and pancreatic ductal pressure. Patients with a dominant pancreatic duct stricture and upstream dilatation may benefit by placement of a stent across the stricture. The stent should be left in for no more than 4–6 weeks as it will block. The complication rate is high, and less than two-thirds of patients experience pain relief, but those who do get relief may benefit from a surgical bypass. Pancreatic duct stones may be extracted at ERCP, and this may sometimes be combined with extracorporeal shock wave lithotripsy. Pseudocysts may be drained internally under EUS guidance. Percutaneous or transgastric drainage of pseudocysts under ultrasound or CT guidance may be performed.

The role of surgery is to overcome obstruction and remove mass lesions. Some patients have a mass in the head of the pancreas, for which either a pancreatoduodenectomy or a Beger procedure (duodenum-preserving resection of the pancreatic head) is appropriate. If the duct is markedly dilated, then a longitudinal pancreatojejunostomy or Frey procedure can be of value (Figure 68.31). The natural evolution of the disease may not be altered significantly, but around half the patients get long-term pain relief. The rare patient with disease limited to the tail will be cured by a distal pancreatectomy. Patients with intractable pain and diffuse disease may plead for a total pancreatectomy in the expectation that removing the offending organ will relieve their pain. However, one should keep in mind that pancreatic function and quality of life are significantly impaired after this procedure, and the operative mortality rate is not trivial. Moreover, there is no guarantee of pain relief (approximately a third of patients get resolution, a third show some benefit, and a third see no benefit at all). Total pancreatectomy and islet autotransplantation has been reported in selected patients, but it is difficult to demonstrate any overall benefit.

Prognosis

Chronic pancreatitis is a difficult condition to manage. Patients often suffer a gradual decline in their professional, social and personal lives. The pain may abate after a surgical or percutaneous intervention, but tends to return over a period of time. In a proportion of patients, the inflammation may gradually burn out over a period of years, with disappearance of the pain, leaving only the exocrine and endocrine insufficiencies. Development of pancreatic cancer is a risk in those who have had the disease for more than 20 years. New symptoms or a change in the pattern of symptoms should be investigated and malignancy excluded.

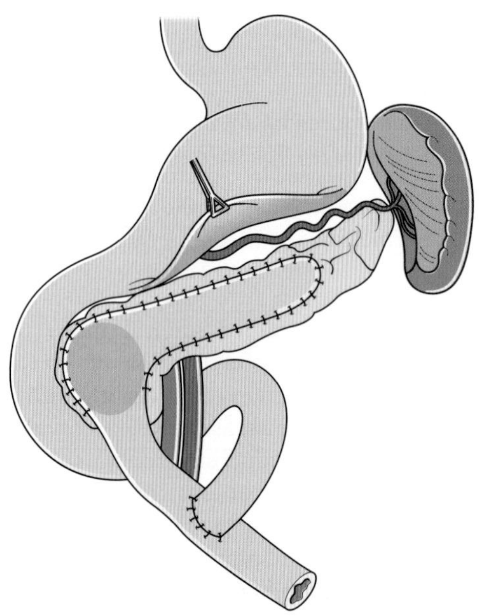

Figure 68.31 Pancreatojejunostomy. The pancreatic duct is opened longitudinally, and a loop of jejunum is sutured to the duct. In the Frey procedure, the superficial part of the head of the pancreas is removed to achieve drainage.

Sphincter of Oddi dysfunction

Separate mention is warranted of this condition, which should be considered in the differential diagnosis of chronic biliary or pancreatic pain. The sphincter of Oddi is 6–10 mm long and lies within the duodenal wall. A part of it encircles the common channel, and then there are separate biliary and pancreatic components (see Figure 68.5). In most mammals the bile duct and pancreatic duct have separate openings into the duodenum. The one other animal that has a sphincter anatomy very similar to that of humans is the Australian possum. Sphincter of Oddi dyskinesia or dysfunction (SOD) is a clinical syndrome in which pain, biochemical abnormalities and dilatation of the bile duct and/or pancreatic duct are attributed to abnormal function of the sphincter of Oddi. The true incidence of SOD is unknown. Females are more commonly affected than males. SOD may result from stenosis of the sphincter, or from dysmotility. Scarring or stenosis of the sphincter can result from passage of stones, pancreatitis or prior endoscopic sphincterotomies.

There are two clinical types of SOD. Biliary-type SOD is characterised by biliary pain, which may be accompanied by abnormally raised liver enzymes and/or dilation of the bile duct and/or evidence of delayed emptying on biliary scintigraphy. It may be a cause of persistent post-cholecystectomy symptoms. A predominance of pancreatic problems, especially recurrent episodes of acute pancreatitis, is known as pancreatic-type SOD. Each type of SOD is further divided into types I, II and III (*Table 68.7*). This classification helps to predict the underlying pathology and the likelihood of successful treatment. Type I disease is thought to result from a fixed stenosis and responds best to therapy. An episodic dysmotility is the presumed underlying abnormality in the other types and often does not respond as well to treatment.

Biliary type SOD should be considered and excluded in patients with the post-cholecystectomy syndrome. Pancreatic type SOD should be excluded in patients with recurrent acute pancreatitis of unexplained aetiology. The role of SOD in chronic pancreatitis is unclear. A careful history is essential. CT and MRCP can demonstrate dilatation of the biliary and pancreatic ducts. MRCP with intravenous secretin injection can particularly demonstrate pancreatic duct dilatation due to raised sphincter pressures. EUS may achieve the same end. Quantitative cholescintigraphy (HIDA scan) may demonstrate delayed biliary transit. The gold standard for diagnosing SOD is ERCP with manometry of the biliary and pancreatic sphincters, though many would say that this is not essential for diagnosis of type I SOD. ERCP with manometry

Charles Frederick Frey, b.1929, Professor of Surgery, The University of California, Davids, CA, USA.

TABLE 68.7 Milwaukee classification of sphincter of Oddi (SOD) dysfunction.
1. Biliary type SOD:
Type I: Typical biliary type pain Liver enzymes (AST, ALT or ALP) >2 times normal limit documented on at least 2 occasions during episodes of pain Dilated CBD >12 mm in diameter Prolonged biliary drainage time (>45 min)*
Type II: Biliary type pain, and One or two of the above criteria
Type III: Biliary type pain only
2. Pancreatic type SOD:
Type I: Pancreatic type pain Amylase and/or lipase >2 times upper normal limit on at least 2 occasions during episodes of pain Dilated pancreatic duct (head >6 mm, body >5 mm) Prolonged pancreatic drainage time (>9 min)*
Type II: Pancreatic type pain, and One or two of the above criteria
Type III: Pancreatic type pain only

* difficult to measure and often eschewed in clinical practice

is indicated if the pain disabling, noninvasive investigations have not shown structural abnormalities and conservative therapy has not helped. The variables customarily assessed at manometry are basal pressure and amplitude, duration, frequency, and propagation pattern of the phasic waves. Basal sphincter pressure higher than 40 mm Hg is the manometric criterion used to diagnose SOD.

Endoscopic sphincterotomy is the treatment of choice for type I SOD. The question of whether dual sphincterotomies (biliary and pancreatic) should be carried out remains unanswered. There is however a particularly high risk of post-ERCP pancreatitis (30% or more), though placement of a pancreatic stent at the time of the procedure appears to reduce this risk. Such treatments are best carried out in tertiary units by expert gastroenterologists. For patients with type II SOD, manometry should be done before considering sphincterotomy, and the results of sphincterotomy are less consistent. Patients with type III SOD are even more difficult, with response rates to sphincterotomy ranging from 8% to 65%. Medical therapy should be tried before proceeding to manometry. Proton pump inhibitors, spasmolytic drugs, calcium blockers (nifedipine), and psychotropic agents have all been tried with varying degrees of success. Injection of botulinum toxin (which can cause a chemical sphincterotomy for up to 3 months) or placement of a pancreatic stent (these are usually removed after 6 weeks) do not provide lasting relief, but can be used to identify patients who may benefit from a sphincterotomy.

A recent study in patients with abdominal pain after cholecystectomy and suspected SOD casts doubt on the efficacy of endoscopic sphincterotomy. In patients undergoing ERCP with manometry, sphincterotomy versus sham did not reduce disability due to pain. Manometry results were not associated with the outcome. No clinical subgroups appeared to benefit from sphincterotomy more than others.

In a small subgroup of patients who have experienced significant but short-lived relief with sphincterotomy or stenting, surgical transduodenal sphincteroplasty may be considered. But the long-term results of surgical sphincteroplasty are often poor. In exceptional circumstances, where the pancreatic head is badly scarred and sphincteroplasty has failed or is unlikely to succeed, there may be grounds for surgical resection of the pancreatic head.

CARCINOMA OF THE PANCREAS

Pancreatic cancer is the sixth leading cause of cancer death in the UK, and the incidence is 10 cases per 100 000 population per year. Worldwide, it constitutes 2–3% of all cancers and, in the USA, is the fourth highest cause of cancer death. The incidence has declined slightly over the last 25 years. There is no simple screening test; however, patients with an increased inherited risk of pancreatic cancer (*Table 68.8*) should be referred to specialist units for screening and counselling.

TABLE 68.8 Risk factors for the development of pancreatic cancer.
Demographic factors
Age (peak incidence 65–75 years)
Male gender
Black ethnicity
Environment/lifestyle
Cigarette smoking
Genetic factors and medical conditions
Family history
Two first-degree relatives with pancreas cancer: relative risk increases 18- to 57-fold
Germline BRCA2 mutations in some rare high-risk families
Hereditary pancreatitis (50- to 70-fold increased risk)
Chronic pancreatitis (5- to 15-fold increased risk)
Lynch syndrome (HNPCC)
Ataxia telangiectasia
Peutz–Jeghers syndrome
Familial breast–ovarian cancer syndrome
Familial atypical multiple mole melanoma
Familial adenomatous polyposis – risk of ampullary/duodenal carcinoma
Diabetes mellitus

HNPCC, hereditary non-polyposis colorectal cancer.

Henry T Lynch, b.1928, Professor of Preventative Medicine, Creighton University, Omaha, NE, USA.
John Law Augustine Peutz, 1886–1968, Chief Specialist for Internal Medicine, St. John's Hospital, The Hague, The Netherlands.
Harold Joseph Jeghers, 1904–1990, Professor of Internal Medicine, The New Jersey College of Medicine and Dentistry, Jersey City, NJ, USA.

Pathology

More than 85% of pancreatic cancers are ductal adenocarcinomas. The remaining tumours constitute a variety of pathologies with individual characteristics. Endocrine tumours of the pancreas are rare. These are covered in Chapter 52.

Ductal adenocarcinomas arise most commonly in the head of the gland. They are solid, scirrhous tumours, characterised by neoplastic tubular glands within a markedly desmoplastic fibrous stroma. Fibrosis is also a characteristic of chronic pancreatitis, and histological differentiation between tumour and pancreatitis can cause diagnostic difficulties. Ductal adenocarcinomas infiltrate locally, typically along nerve sheaths, along lymphatics and into blood vessels. Liver and peritoneal metastases are common. Proliferative lesions in the pancreatic ducts can precede invasive ductal adenocarcinoma. These are termed pancreatic intraepithelial neoplasia or PanIN, and can demonstrate a range of structural complexity and cellular atypia.

Cystic tumours of the pancreas may be serous or mucinous. Serous cystadenomas are typically found in older women, and are large aggregations of multiple small cysts, almost like bubblewrap. They are benign. Mucinous tumours, on the other hand, have the potential for malignant transformation. They include mucinous cystic neoplasms (MCNs) and intraductal papillary mucinous neoplasms (IPMNs). MCNs are seen in perimenopausal women, show up as multilocular thick-walled cysts in the pancreatic body or tail, and, histologically, contain an ovarian-type stroma. IPMNs are more common in the pancreatic head and in older men, but an IPMN arising from a branch duct can be difficult to distinguish from an MCN. IPMNs arising within the main duct are often multifocal and have a greater tendency to prove malignant. Thick mucus seen extruding from the ampulla at ERCP is diagnostic of a main duct IPMN. Mucinous tumours can be confused with pseudocysts (see *Summary box* 68.8). Occasionally, lymphoepithelial cysts, lymphangiomas, dermoid cysts and intestinal duplication cysts can show up in the pancreas. Solid pseudopapillary tumour is a rare, slowly progressive but malignant tumour, seen in women of childbearing age, and manifests as a large, part-solid, part-cystic tumour.

Tumours arising from the ampulla or from the distal common bile duct can present as a mass in the head of the pancreas, and constitute around a third of all tumours in that area. Adenomas of the ampulla of Vater are diagnosed at endoscopy as polypoid submucosal masses covered by a smooth epithelium. They can harbour foci of invasive carcinoma; the larger the adenoma, the greater the risk. Biopsies taken at endoscopy may not always include the malignant focus. Endoscopic surveillance, endoscopic resection or even surgical transduodenal ampullary excision should be considered (Figure 68.32). Patients with familial adenomatous polyposis (FAP) can present with multiple duodenal polyps. Malignant transformation in a duodenal polyp is a significant cause of mortality in these patients, mandating endoscopic follow-up and pancreatoduodenectomy in selected patients with high-grade dysplasia within the polyp.

Ampullary adenocarcinomas often present early with biliary obstruction. Their natural history is distinctly more favourable compared with pancreatic ductal adenocarcinoma. Ampullary carcinomas are relatively small when diagnosed, which may account for their better prognosis. Occasionally, other malignant neoplasms can arise at the ampulla, such as carcinoid tumours and high-grade neuroendocrine carcinomas.

Clinical features

Jaundice secondary to obstruction of the distal bile duct is the most common symptom that draws attention to ampullary and pancreatic head tumours. It is characteristically painless jaundice but may be associated with nausea and epigastric discomfort. Pruritus, dark urine and pale stools with steatorrhoea are common accompaniments of jaundice. In the absence of jaundice, symptoms are often non-specific, namely vague discomfort, anorexia and weight loss, and are frequently dismissed by both patient and doctor. Upper abdominal symptoms in a recently diagnosed diabetic, especially in one above 50 years of age, with no family history or obesity, should raise suspicion. Occasionally, a patient will present with an unexplained attack of pancreatitis; all such patients should have follow-up imaging of the pancreas. Tumours of the body and tail of the gland often grow silently, and present at an advanced unresectable stage. Back pain is a worrying symptom, raising the possibility of retroperitoneal infiltration.

On examination, there may be evidence of jaundice, weight loss, a palpable liver and a palpable gall bladder. Courvoisier first drew attention to the association of an enlarged

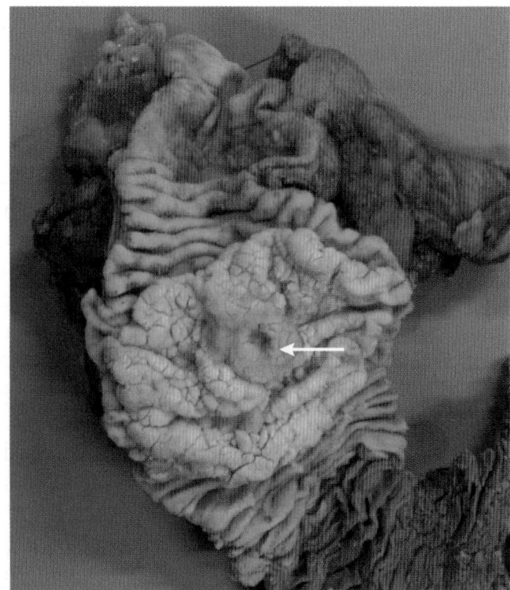

Figure 68.32 A large ampullary adenoma that turned into an adenocarcinoma; the arrow indicates the ampulla. Photograph taken after resection in the form of a pancreatoduodenectomy (courtesy of Dr Joanne Chin-Aleong).

Ludwig Courvoisier, 1843–1918, surgeon, Basel, Switzerland, was one of the first surgeons to remove stones from the common bile duct.

gall bladder and a pancreatic tumour in 1890, when he noted that, when the common duct is obstructed by a stone, distension of the gall bladder (which is likely to be chronically inflamed) is rare; when the duct is obstructed in some other way, such as a neoplasm, distension of the normal gall bladder is common. Other signs of intra-abdominal malignancy should be looked for with care, such as a palpable mass, ascites, supraclavicular nodes and tumour deposits in the pelvis; when present, they indicate a grim prognosis.

Investigation

In a jaundiced patient, the usual blood tests and ultrasound scan should be performed. Ultrasound will determine if the bile duct is dilated. If it is, and there is a genuine suspicion of a tumour in the head of the pancreas, the preferred test is a contrast-enhanced CT scan (see Figure 68.8). In the majority of instances, this should establish if there is a tumour in the pancreas and if it is resectable. The presence of hepatic or peritoneal metastases, lymph node metastases distant from the pancreatic head, or encasement of the superior mesenteric, hepatic or coeliac artery by tumour are clear contraindications to surgical resection. Tumour size, continuous invasion of the duodenum, stomach or colon, and lymph node metastases within the operative field are not contraindications. If the tumour abuts or minimally invades the portal or superior mesenteric vein, this is not a contraindication to surgery (as part of the vein can be resected if necessary), but complete encasement and occlusion of the vein is. MRI and MR angiography can provide information comparable to CT.

ERCP and biliary stenting should be carried out if there is any suggestion of cholangitis, if there is diagnostic doubt (small ampullary lesions may not be seen on CT, and ERCP is the best way to identify them) or if there is likely to be a delay between diagnosis and surgery and the patient is deeply jaundiced with distressing pruritus. It relieves the jaundice and can also provide a brush cytology or biopsy specimen to confirm the diagnosis (see Figures 68.13, 68.14 and 68.19). Otherwise, however, preoperative ERCP and biliary stenting is not mandatory in patients with resectable disease; there is evidence to suggest that it is associated with a slightly higher incidence of infective complications after surgery. The prothrombin time should be checked, and clotting abnormalities should be corrected with vitamin K or fresh-frozen plasma prior to ERCP. If a stent is placed in a patient who may undergo resection, it should be a plastic stent or a covered metal stent, as these can be easily pulled out during surgery. If a naked metal self-expanding stent is placed (that will get embedded in its position), it should be a relatively short one that does not extend too high up the bile duct towards the biliary confluence.

EUS is useful if CT fails to demonstrate a tumour, if tissue diagnosis is required prior to surgery (e.g. a mass has developed on a background of chronic pancreatitis and a distinction needs to be made between inflammation and neoplasia), if vascular invasion needs to be confirmed, or in separating cystic tumours from pseudocysts (Figure 68.33; see also Figure 68.20). Transduodenal or transgastric FNA or Trucut biopsy performed under EUS guidance avoids spillage of tumour cells into the peritoneal cavity. Percutaneous transperitoneal biopsy of potentially resectable pancreatic tumours should be avoided as far as possible. Histological confirmation of malignancy is desirable but not essential, particularly if the imaging clearly demonstrates a resectable tumour. The lack of a tissue diagnosis should not delay appropriate surgical therapy. In patients judged to have unresectable disease, tissue diagnosis should be obtained prior to starting palliative therapy.

Diagnostic laparoscopy prior to an attempt at resection can spare a proportion of patients an unnecessary laparotomy by identifying small peritoneal and liver metastases. It can be combined with laparoscopic ultrasonography. The tumour marker CA19-9 is not highly specific or sensitive, but a baseline level should be established; if it is initially raised, it can be useful later in identifying recurrence.

Management

At the time of presentation, more than 85% of patients with ductal adenocarcinoma are unsuitable for resection because the disease is too advanced. If imaging shows that the tumour is potentially resectable, the patient should be considered

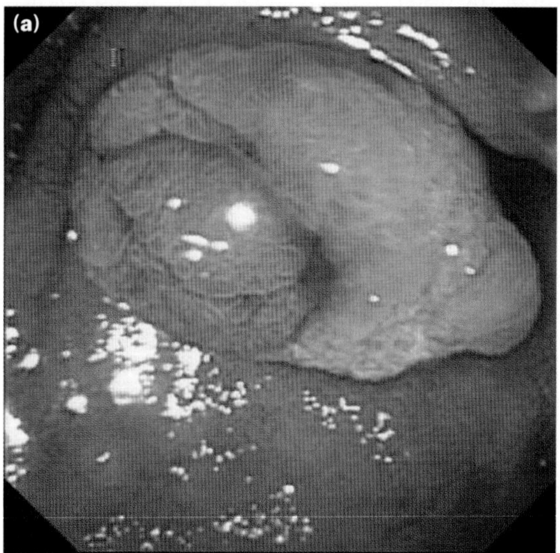

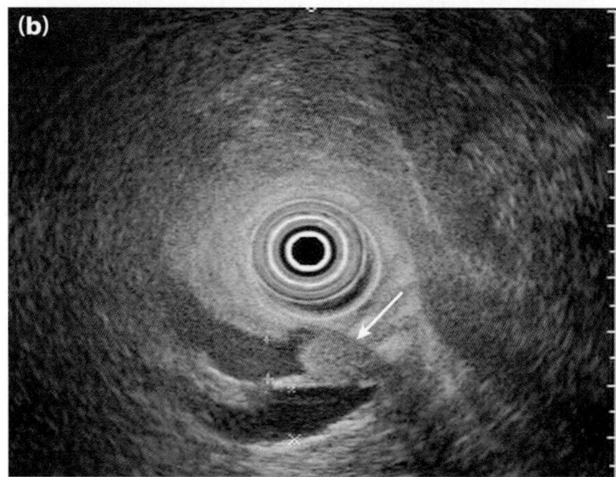

Figure 68.33 (a) Carcinoma of the ampulla as seen at endoscopy. (b) Appearance of the same tumour (arrow) on endoscopic ultrasound (courtesy of Dr Peter Fairclough).

for surgical resection, as that offers the only (albeit small) chance of a cure. Comorbidities should be taken carefully into account. Biological rather than chronological age should be the consideration. If a cystic tumour is encountered, no matter how large, surgical resection should be considered, as it carries a reasonable chance of cure. Tumours of the ampulla have a good prognosis and should, if at all possible, be resected. Some of the rare tumours and the neuroendocrine lesions should also be resected if at all possible. For those patients who have inoperable disease, palliative treatment should be offered.

Surgical resection

The standard resection for a tumour of the pancreatic head or the ampulla is a pylorus-preserving pancreatoduodenectomy (PPPD). This involves removal of the duodenum and the pancreatic head, including the distal part of the bile duct. The original pancreatoduodenectomy as proposed by Whipple included resection of the gastric antrum. Preserving the antrum and the pylorus is thought to result in a more physiological outcome with no difference in survival or recurrence rates. The Whipple procedure is now reserved for situations in which the entire duodenum has to be removed (e.g. in FAP) or where the tumour encroaches on the first part of the duodenum or the distal stomach and a PPPD would not achieve a clear resection margin. Total pancreatectomy is warranted only in situations where one is dealing with a multifocal tumour (e.g. a main duct IPMN), or the body and tail of the gland are too inflamed or too friable to achieve a safe anastomosis with the bowel. The PPPD procedure includes a local lymphadenectomy. Extended lymphadenectomy has not been shown to be beneficial in improving survival and is associated with increased morbidity. If the tumour is adherent to the portal or superior mesenteric vein, but can still be removed by including a patch or a short segment of vein in the resection, with an appropriate reconstruction of the vessel, then that should be done. This is not associated with an increase in the morbidity or mortality of the procedure, and the outcomes are similar.

For tumours of the body and tail, distal pancreatectomy with splenectomy is the standard. Infiltration of the splenic artery or vein by the tumour is not a contraindication to resection. When resecting the pancreatic tail for a benign lesion, one may attempt to preserve the spleen if possible. When removing the spleen, prior vaccinations against pneumococci, meningococci and *Haemophilus influenzae* B should be administered, and subsequent antibiotic prophylaxis given (see Chapter 66).

While the majority of pancreatic resections continue to be performed via the open approach, there is evidence that the laparoscopic and robotic approaches are also feasible and may yield comparable results. Laparoscopic pancreatic resections are technically challenging, pose additional demands on operating room time and equipment, and involve a significant learning curve for the surgeon and the entire team. Distal pancreatectomy, especially for smaller tumours, lends itself more easily to the laparoscopic approach than a pancreatic head resection.

PANCREATODUODENECTOMY

The patient's coagulation screen should be checked preoperatively and adequate hydration ensured. The patient should be aware of the diagnosis, the gravity of the operation and the risks involved. The operation has three distinct phases:

- exploration and assessment;
- resection;
- reconstruction.

A cholecystectomy is performed. The bile duct and hepatic artery are exposed, removing the lymphatic tissue in this area. Exposure of the hepatic artery enables division of the gastroduodenal artery and visualisation of the portal vein. The distal part of the gastric antrum is mobilised. The duodenum and right colon are mobilised from the retroperitoneal tissues. The superior mesenteric vein is exposed inferior to the pancreatic neck. Careful dissection into the plane between the vein and the pancreatic substance (see Figure 68.2) will reveal whether the tumour is adherent to the vein. At this juncture, a decision has to be made whether to proceed to the next phase of resection or not. If resection is to be performed, the fourth part of the duodenum is dissected and freed from the ligament of Treitz so that the upper jejunum can be brought into the supracolic compartment. The jejunum is divided 20–30 cm downstream from the duodenojejunal flexure, and the mesentery of the proximal jejunum is detached. The first part of the duodenum is divided. The neck of the pancreas is divided, and then the uncinate process is separated from the superior mesenteric vein and artery working up towards the upper bile duct, which is divided, releasing the specimen (Figure 68.34). Retroperitoneal lymph nodes within the operative field are completely removed with the specimen. Reconstruction is carried out as in Figure 68.35. The pancreatic stump, the divided bile duct and the duodenal stump are anastomosed on to the jejunum, in that order. Some surgeons prefer to anastomose the pancreas to the posterior wall of the stomach instead; others prefer to create a separate Roux loop of the jejunum and anastomose the pancreas to that. The operation should take between 3 and 6 hours. Blood loss should be low, and transfusion is often not necessary. The patients are usually nursed in a high-dependency area for the first 24–48 hours after surgery. Prolonged nasogastric drainage is unnecessary, and early feeding can be commenced.

Resection for pancreatic cancer should be carried out in specialist units. There is a clear correlation between higher caseload volume and lower hospital mortality and morbidity.

Allen Oldfather Whipple, 1881–1963, Director of Surgical Services, The Presbyterian Hospital, and Professor of Surgery, Columbia University, New York, NY, USA, began to perform two-stage pancreatoduodenectomies in 1934 and shortened the procedure into a one-stage process in 1940. Alessandro Codivilla (1861–1912) and Walter Kausch (1867–1928) had performed the operation before him, but Whipple was the surgeon who established pancreatoduodenectomy as an operation.

Wenzel Treitz, 1819–1872, Professor of Anatomy and Pathology, at Krakow, Poland, and later at Prague, The Czech Republic. He was involved in the struggle for Czech nationalism and at 52 committed suicide by taking potassium cyanide.

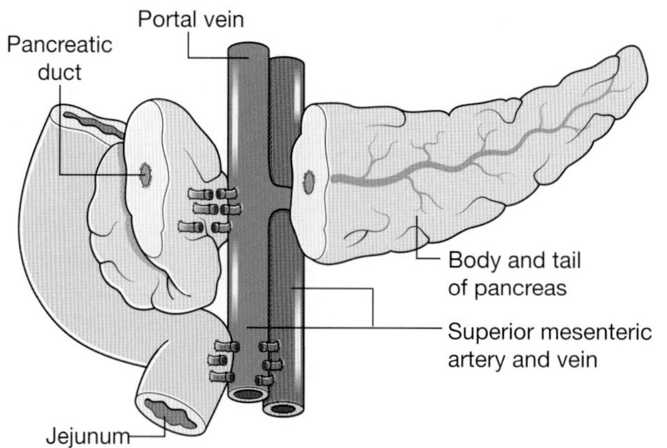

Figure 68.34 Resection of the head of the pancreas in a pylorus-preserving pancreatoduodenectomy.

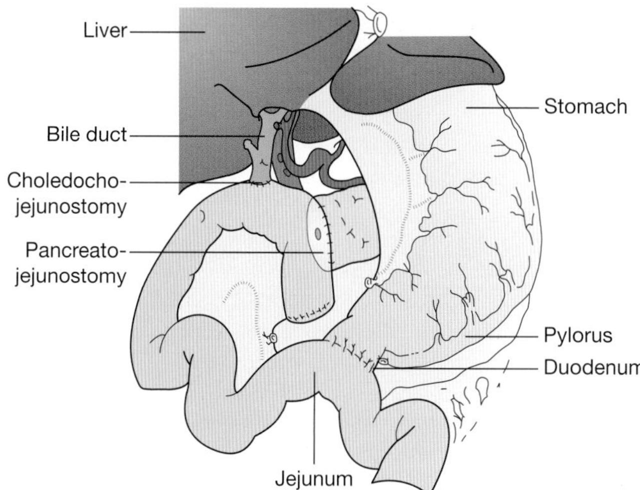

Figure 68.35 Reconstruction after a pylorus-preserving pancreatoduodenectomy.

PPPD should carry a mortality of no more than 3–5%. The morbidity remains high, with some 30–40% of patients developing a complication in the postoperative period. These complications are usually infective, but a leak from the anastomosis between the pancreas and the bowel is known to occur in at least 10% of patients, and this may give rise to major complications. Octreotide may be administered in the perioperative period to suppress secretion and reduce the likelihood of a leak, but the evidence for its efficacy is still debatable. Following surgical resection, the pathological tumour–node–metastasis stage should be documented.

ADJUVANT THERAPY

At the beginning of this century, the reported 5-year survival following resection of a pancreatic adenocarcinoma ranged from 7% to 25% (around 10% for most centres). The median survival was 11–20 months. Considering that, at best, 15% of patients had resectable disease to begin with, this meant only two or three out of 100 patients with this disease could expect to survive to 5 years. Moreover, recurrences could and did show up even beyond the 5-year cut-off. The high recurrence rate following resection inevitably led to the consideration of adjuvant treatments to improve outcome. In a large multicentre European study (ESPAC-1) reported in 2004, adjuvant radiotherapy or chemoradiotherapy was shown to confer no advantage, but chemotherapy with 5-fluorouracil (5-FU) provided an overall benefit; median survival with chemotherapy was 20 months compared with 16 months without. Another trial (ESPAC-3) showed that gemcitabine works equally well. A further trial (ESPAC-4), of gemcitabine alone versus gemcitabine with capecitabine (a fluorouracil that can be taken orally) has indicated that the latter regimen can push the median survival above 2 years and the 5-year survival close to 30%. Most patients with resected ductal adenocarcinoma are now offered 6 months of adjuvant chemotherapy with gemcitabine and/or 5-FU. Some centres continue to offer chemoradiotherapy, particularly in patients with involved (R1) resection margins, and further trials of adjuvant chemoradiation are in progress.

It should be emphasised, however, that these depressing statistics apply to ductal adenocarcinomas. Patients with resected ampullary tumours have a 5-year survival of 40%, and cystic tumours and neuroendocrine tumours can often be cured by surgical resection.

Palliation

The median survival of patients with unresectable, locally advanced, non-metastatic pancreatic cancer is 6–10 months and, in patients with metastatic disease, it is 2–6 months.

If unresectable disease is found in the course of a laparotomy that was commenced with the intent to resect, a choledochoenterostomy and a gastroenterostomy should be carried out to relieve (or pre-empt) jaundice and duodenal obstruction. The bile duct may be anastomosed to the duodenum, or to a loop of jejunum. It is preferable to use the bile duct rather than the gall bladder. Cholecystojejunostomy is easier to perform, but the bile must then drain through the cystic duct, which is narrow and, if inserted low into the bile duct, is vulnerable to occlusion by tumour growth. A coeliac plexus block can also be administered. A transduodenal Tru-cut biopsy of the tumour should be obtained.

In patients found to have unresectable disease on imaging, jaundice is relieved by stenting at ERCP (Figure 68.36a). Stents may be made of plastic or self-expanding metal mesh. Plastic stents are cheaper but tend to occlude faster and, if the patient is likely to have a longer life expectancy, a metal stent can be used. If the patient is not a suitable candidate for endoscopic biliary stenting, a percutaneous transhepatic stent can be placed (Figure 68.36b). Obstruction of the duodenum occurs in approximately 15% of cases. If this occurs early in the course of the disease, surgical bypass by gastrojejunostomy is appropriate but, if it is late in the course of the disease, then the use of expanding metal stents inserted endoscopically is preferable, as many of these patients have prolonged delayed gastric emptying following surgery (Figure 68.36c). If both biliary and duodenal metal stents are to be placed endoscopically, the biliary one should be placed first.

If no operative procedure is undertaken, an EUS-guided or percutaneous biopsy of the tumour should be performed before consideration of chemotherapy or chemoradiation.

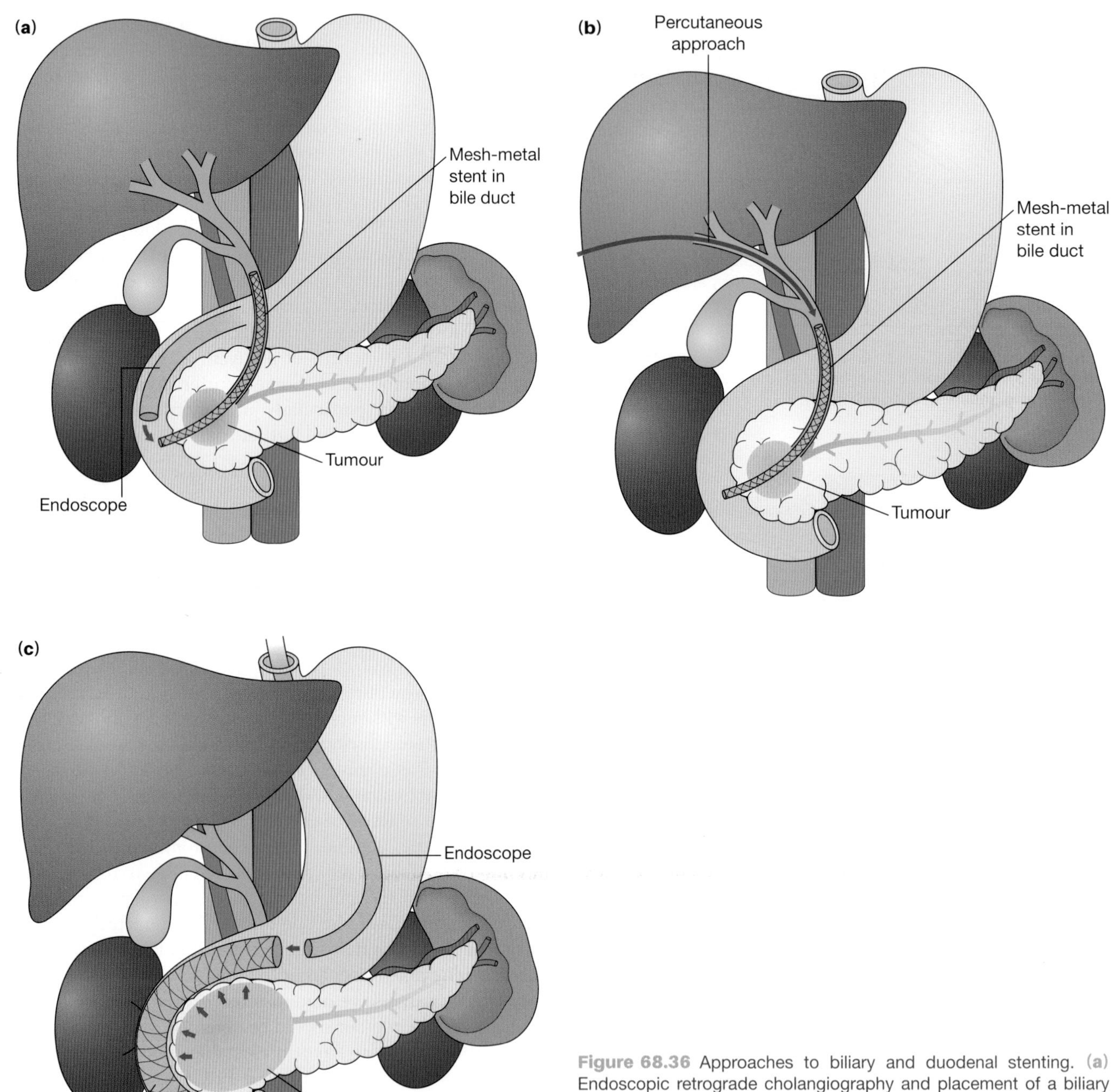

Figure 68.36 Approaches to biliary and duodenal stenting. (a) Endoscopic retrograde cholangiography and placement of a biliary stent; (b) percutaneous transhepatic cholangiography followed by cannulation of the biliary system and percutaneous placement of a biliary stent (mesh metal in this instance); (c) endoscopic placement of a duodenal stent (mesh metal).

Lymphomas of the pancreas are rare and constitute less than 3% of all pancreatic cancers. These respond to chemoradiotherapy and surgical resection is not indicated. For patients with ductal adenocarcinoma, 5-FU or gemcitabine will produce a remission in 15–25%, while the remainder will receive no benefit from the therapy. Better tumour responses are now being achieved with multiagent chemotherapy regimens such as the combination of fluorouracil, irinotecan, oxaliplatin, and leucovorin (FOLFIRINOX) and gemcitabine plus albumin-bound paclitaxel particles (nab-paclitaxel). However the 2–5 months' increase in median survival with these regimens has to be offset against the higher toxicity and cost. No long-term cures have been described with chemotherapy or radiotherapy.

Attempts to downstage unresectable disease with chemotherapy or chemoradiation and render it resectable are rarely successful. In a very small proportion of patients who have been deemed unresectable due to major vascular involvement and do not have metastatic disease, attempts have been made to downstage the tumour with one of the newer combination chemotherapy regimens, sometimes with chemoradiation thrown in, to try to render them resectable. Such neoadjuvant therapies should ideally be considered within a clinical trial.

Steatorrhoea is treated with enzyme supplementation. Diabetes mellitus, if it develops, is treated with oral hypoglycaemics or insulin as appropriate, and pain with either analgesics or an appropriate nerve block.

Summary box 68.10

Palliation of pancreatic cancer

Relieve jaundice and treat biliary sepsis

- Surgical biliary bypass
- Stent placed at ERCP or percutaneous transhepatic cholangiography

Improve gastric emptying

- Surgical gastroenterostomy
- Duodenal stent

Pain relief

- Stepwise escalation of analgesia
- Coeliac plexus block
- Transthoracic splanchnicectomy

Symptom relief and quality of life

- Encourage normal activities
- Enzyme replacement for steatorrhoea
- Treat diabetes

Consider chemotherapy

FURTHER READING

Ayub K, Imada R, Slavin J. Endoscopic retrograde cholangiopancreatography in gallstone-associated acute pancreatitis. *Cochrane Reviews* 2004; **(2)**: CD003630.

Banks PA, Bollen TL, Dervenis C *et al.* Acute Pancreatitis Classification Working Group Classification of acute pancreatitis 2012: revision of the Atlanta classification and definitions by international consensus. *Gut* 2013; **62**:102–111.

Braganza JM, Lee SH, McCloy RF, McMahon MJ. Chronic pancreatitis. *Lancet* 2011; **377**: 1184–97.

Jarnagin W. *Blumgart's Surgery of the liver, biliary tract and pancreas*, 5th edn. Elsevier, 2012.

Moss AC, Morris E, MacMathuna P. Palliative biliary stents for obstructing pancreatic carcinoma. *Cochrane Reviews* 2006; **(2)**:CD004200.

Pancreatic Section, British Society of Gastroenterology; Pancreatic Society of Great Britain and Ireland; Association of Upper Gastrointestinal Surgeons of Great Britain and Ireland; Royal College of Pathologists; Special Interest Group for Gastro-Intestinal Radiology. Guidelines for the management of patients with pancreatic cancer, periampullary and ampullary carcinomas. *Gut* 2005; **54** (Suppl V):1–16.

Ryan DP, Hong TS, Bardeesy N. Pancreatic adenocarcinoma. *N Engl J Med* 2014; **371**:1039-1049.

van der Gaag NA, Rauws EAJ, van Eijck CSJ *et al.* Preoperative biliary drainage for cancer of the head of the pancreas. *N Engl J Med* 2010; **362**:129–137.

Working Party of the British Society of Gastroenterology; Association of Surgeons of Great Britain and Ireland, Pancreatic Society of Great Britain and Ireland; Association of Upper GI Surgeons of Great Britain and Ireland. UK guidelines for the management of acute pancreatitis. *Gut* 2005; **54** (Suppl III):1–9.

Chapter 69

The small intestine

Learning objectives

To appreciate:

- The basic anatomy and physiology of the small intestine
- The range of conditions that may affect the small intestine

To understand:

- The aetiology and pathology of common small intestinal conditions
- The principles of investigation of small intestinal symptoms
- The importance of non-surgical management of small intestinal problems
- The principles of small intestinal surgery
- That complex intestinal problems are best managed by a multidisciplinary team
- The management of acute surgical problems of the intestines

ANATOMY OF THE SMALL INTESTINE

Although the duodenum is anatomically indistinguishable from the small intestine, it is subject to some specific pathologies and surgical therapies; therefore, in purely surgical terms it may be regarded as a distinct entity and is covered in Chapter 63. The length of the small bowel varies from 300 to 850cm between the duodenojejunal (DJ) flexure to the ileocaecal valve (Figure 69.1). It is notoriously difficult to establish the length of the small intestine, and estimates gathered at surgery, at postmortem and during radiological investigations may vary widely, even in the same individual. In addition, there is considerable inter-individual variability and the small intestine has been said to be longer in men.

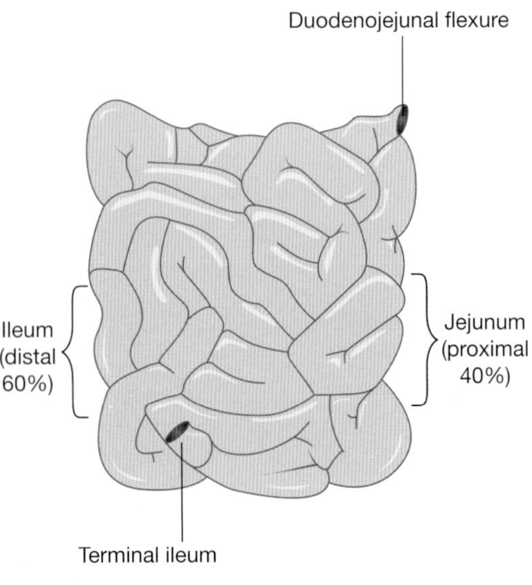

Figure 69.1 Portions of the small bowel and their relations to the colon.

The proximal 40% of the small intestine is referred to as the jejunum; the remainder is the ileum. There is no clear demarcation between jejunum and ileum, but the small bowel does change gradually in character from proximal to distal. The jejunum tends to have a wider diameter and a thicker wall, with more prominent mucosal folds (valvulae conniventes), while the ileum has a thicker, more fatty mesentery with more complex arterial arcades. The ileum also contains larger aggregates of lymph nodes (Peyer's patches), which can occasionally become lead points in intussusception in childhood.

The small intestine has a very rich blood supply, derived from the superior mesenteric artery, while venous drainage is via the portal venous system, into which the superior mesenteric vein drains blood rich in nutrients after a meal. This arrangement facilitates processing of the nutrients by the liver, into which the portal vein drains in turn. The lymphatic drainage of the small intestine follows the arterial supply.

The small intestine has a rich autonomic innervation arising from the splanchnic nerves, which contribute a dense network of sympathetic fibres around the superior mesenteric artery and its branches. Referred pain from the small intestine is usually felt in the periumbilical region (T10). The blood and nerve supply to the small intestine runs in the attached mesentery, which originates on the posterior abdominal wall and runs obliquely downwards to the right between the duodenojejunal flexure to the left of the second lumbar vertebra and the right sacroiliac joint.

Summary box 69.1

Important features of small bowel anatomy

- Comprises jejunum and ileum
- Has valvulae conniventes
- Blood supply from superior mesenteric artery

PHYSIOLOGY OF THE SMALL INTESTINE

The principal function of the small intestine is the digestion of food and the absorption of nutrients, water and electrolytes. Carbohydrates and proteins are broken down in the intestinal lumen by pancreatic enzymes, but the final hydrolysis takes place at the brush border of the jejunum, after which they are absorbed. Fats are digested chiefly by the actions of pancreatic lipase and bile salts. The products of fat digestion, fatty acids and monoglycerides, separate from bile salts in the jejunum and are absorbed for further processing. The jejunum is the principal site for digestion and absorption of fluid, electrolytes, iron, folate, fat, protein and carbohydrate, but the absorption of bile salts and vitamin B12 only occurs in the terminal ileum, where there are specific transporters. If the jejunum is resected, the ileum can assume all the required absorptive functions, but resection of the terminal ileum will result in a diminished bile salt pool, B12 deficiency and may lead to deficiency of the fat-soluble vitamins A, D, E and K.

The small intestine plays an important role in the metabolism of plasma lipoproteins, as it is the main site of synthesis of high-density, low-density and very low-density lipoproteins (HDL, LDL, VLDL). These particles transport most of the absorbed dietary fat to the systemic circulation via the lymph. The small bowel also synthesises intestinal hormones such as glucagon-like peptides GLP-1 and 2, peptide YY and motilin, which interact with the enteric nervous system to modulate intestinal function, growth and differentiation.

INFLAMMATORY BOWEL DISEASE

By definition, the term 'inflammatory bowel disease' is reserved for conditions characterised by the presence of idiopathic intestinal inflammation, while conditions such as infective or ischaemic enteritis are excluded. Crohn's disease (CD) is the only known 'inflammatory bowel disease' affecting the small intestine.

Crohn's disease (regional enteritis)

The label 'Crohn's disease' (CD) became attached to a chronic inflammatory disease of the ileum following a key publication by Crohn and colleagues in 1932. CD is characterised by a chronic full-thickness inflammatory process that can affect any part of the gastrointestinal tract from the lips to the anal margin. It is most common in North America and Northern Europe with an annual incidence of 8 per 100000. Prevalence rates of around 145 per 100000 have been reported in the UK. Over the last four decades, the incidence appears to have increased three-fold, thought to possibly be a consequence of environmental factors, improved diagnostic modalities, or both. It is slightly more common in women than in men, and is most commonly diagnosed between the ages of 25 and 40 years. There is a second peak of incidence around the age of 70 years. In those countries with high prevalence of CD, the groups with the highest prevalence seem to be Caucasian, notably American Whites and Northern Europeans, whereas it is less common, even in high prevalence countries, in those originating from Central Europe and less prevalent still in those originating from South America, Asia and Africa. CD seems to be especially prevalent (three- to five-fold higher) in the Ashkenazi Jewish population, although interestingly, the prevalence of CD in the Jewish population in Israel is lower than that in Europe or the United States, suggesting that environmental factors are also important.

Aetiology

The aetiology of CD is incompletely understood but is thought to involve a complex interplay of genetic and environmental factors. Although CD shares some features with chronic

Valvulae conniventes describes a fold of mucous membrane that passes across two-thirds of the bowel circumference.
Johann Conrad Peyer, 1653–1712, Professor of Logis, Rhetoric and Medicine, Schaffausen, Switzerland, described the lymph follicles in the intestine in 1677.

infection, no causative organism has ever been demonstrated. An intriguing similarity to Johne's disease of cattle, a chronic inflammatory enteropathy resulting from infection with *Mycobacterium paratuberculosis*, suggests that CD in man may share a similar aetiology. Some studies of tissue affected by CD have identified mycobacterial DNA more frequently in patients with CD than in controls, but others have been less conclusive and, importantly, randomised controlled trials have failed to show a significant therapeutic benefit of treating CD with antituberculous drugs.

A wide variety of foods have been implicated, in particular a diet high in refined foodstuffs, but none conclusively. An association with high levels of sanitation in childhood has been suggested. Smoking increases the relative risk of CD three-fold and is certainly an exacerbating factor after diagnosis, contrary to the protective effect seen in ulcerative colitis (UC). Smoking cessation has a beneficial effect on disease activity that is comparable to that of very strong medical therapies, such as the antitumour necrosis factor drugs, and is therefore an essential component in the management of CD.

Genetic factors are also clearly extremely important. Approximately 10% of patients have a first-degree relative with the disease, and concordance has been shown to approach 50% in monozygotic twins. Inheritance is thought to involve multiple genes with low penetrance. The *NOD2/CARD15* gene has excited particular interest as variants of this gene have been shown to have strong associations with CD. Genetic manipulation of these genes in mice seems to induce the development of a disease resembling CD and abnormalities of these genes have been shown to be present in some members of families with a particularly high incidence of CD. It should be noted, however, that the vast majority of individuals with CD have no abnormalities of these genes. Since these genes are involved in intracellular recognition of bacteria, their discovery provides potentially valuable insight into the pathogenesis of CD, as a disease in which the relationship between the gut mucosa and the normal gut bacteria becomes deranged, resulting in uncontrolled intestinal inflammation.

Pathogenesis

As in UC, increased gut mucosal permeability appears to develop at a relatively early stage of the disease. This may lead to increased passage of luminal antigens, which then induce a cell-mediated inflammatory response. This results in the release of proinflammatory cytokines, such as interleukin-2 and tumour necrosis factor, which coordinate local and systemic inflammatory responses. It has been suggested that CD is associated with a defect in suppressor T-cells, which usually act to prevent escalation of the inflammatory process. As in UC, however, it remains unclear whether the proposed increase in intestinal permeability is a cause or consequence of the disease process. Studies of intestinal permeability in healthy and apparently unaffected first-degree relatives of patients with CD have also, however, suggested that gut permeability is increased, suggesting that a global, and potentially genetically determined increase in gut permeability, combined perhaps with an abnormal immune-mediated response to colonisation of the gut with some subspecies of the normal enteric microflora, may initiate the disease.

Pathology

The terminal ileum is most commonly involved (65%), either in isolation or in combination with colonic disease. Colitis alone occurs in up to a one-third of cases and the remainder are patients with more proximal small bowel involvement. The stomach and duodenum are affected in around 5%, but perianal lesions are common, affecting up to 50–75% of patients. Perianal disease occurs in 25% per cent of patients with small bowel disease, but in 75% of patients with Crohn's colitis.

Macroscopically, resection specimens show fibrotic thickening of the intestinal wall with narrowing of the lumen and fat wrapping (encroachment of mesenteric fat around the bowel, Figure 69.2). There is usually dilated bowel just proximal to the stricture and deep mucosal ulcerations with linear or snake-like patterns in the strictured area itself. Oedema in between the ulcers gives rise to a cobblestone appearance of the mucosa. The transmural inflammation (which is a characteristic feature of CD) may lead to segments of bowel becoming adherent to each other and to surrounding structures, inflammatory masses with mesenteric abscesses and fistulae into adjacent organs. The serosa is usually opaque, with thickening of the mesentery and enlarged mesenteric lymph nodes. CD is characteristically discontinuous, with inflamed areas separated by normal intestine, so-called 'skip' lesions.

Microscopically, there are focal areas of chronic inflammation involving all layers of the intestinal wall with lymphoid aggregates. Non-caseating giant cell granulomas are found in 60% of patients and when present clearly allow a confident diagnosis of CD. They are most common in anorectal disease.

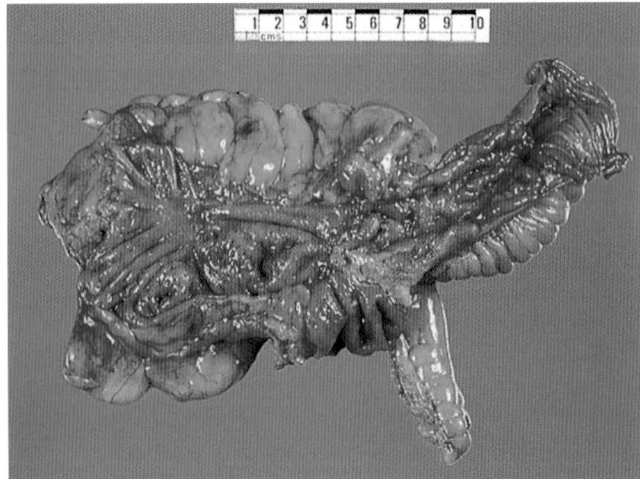

Figure 69.2 Crohn's disease of the ileocaecal region showing typical thickening of the wall of the terminal ileum with narrowing of the lumen (courtesy of Dr B Warren, John Radcliffe Hospital, Oxford, UK).

A first-degree relative, defined as the individual's parents, siblings or children.

Burrill Bernard Crohn, 1884–1983, gastroenterologist, Mount Sinai Hospital, New York, NY, USA, along with Leon Ginzburg and Gordon Oppenheimer, described regional ileitis in 1932.

Multifocal arterial occlusions are found in the muscularis propria, which is thickened. There may be nerve cell hyperplasia and there is deep, fissuring ulceration within affected areas. Characteristically, and unlike in UC, there may be completely normal areas immediately next to areas of severe inflammation.

Clinical features

Presentation depends on the pattern of disease. Occasionally, CD presents acutely with ileal inflammation and symptoms and signs resembling those of acute appendicitis, or even with free perforation of the small intestine, resulting in a local or diffuse peritonitis. CD may present with fulminant colitis but this is considerably less common than in UC.

Summary box 69.2

Differences between ulcerative colitis (UC) and Crohn's disease (CD)

- UC affects the colon; CD can affect any part of the gastrointestinal tract, but particularly the small and large bowel
- UC is a mucosal disease, whereas CD affects the full thickness of the bowel wall
- UC produces confluent disease in the colon and rectum, whereas CD is characterised by skip lesions
- CD more commonly causes stricturing and fistulation
- Granulomas may be found on histology in CD, but not in UC
- CD is often associated with perianal disease, whereas this is unusual in UC
- CD affecting the terminal ileum may produce symptoms mimicking appendicitis, but this does not occur in UC
- Resection of the colon and rectum cures the patient with UC, whereas recurrence is common after resection in CD

CD more commonly presents with features of chronicity. Small bowel CD is often characterised by abdominal colicky pain, which may be postprandial, and mild diarrhoea extending over many months occurring in bouts. A tender mass may be palpable in the right iliac fossa. Intermittent fevers, secondary anaemia and weight loss are common. After months of repeated attacks characterised by acute inflammation, the affected area of intestine begins to narrow with fibrosis, causing more chronic obstructive symptoms. Children developing the illness before puberty may have retarded growth and sexual development. With progression of the disease, adhesions and transmural fissuring, intra-abdominal abscesses and fistulae may develop.

Fistulation may occur into adjacent loops of bowel (enteroenteric or interloop fistulae). Occasionally, the (healthy) sigmoid loop may become adherent to the affected terminal ileum, resulting in ileosigmoid fistulation. The fistula tracks in such cases are usually small and the profuse diarrhoea that results from ileosigmoid fistulation is due primarily to bacterial overgrowth (attributable to colonisation of the small bowel with colonic flora) rather than passage of small bowel content into the colon. Fistulation may also occur into the bladder (ileovesical) or the female genital tract and, less commonly, the duodenum. Fistulation into the abdominal wall (enterocutaneous fistulation) may also develop spontaneously, but it far more commonly occurs as a complication of abdominal surgery (see below).

Colonic CD presents with symptoms of colitis and proctitis as described for UC (Chapter 70), although toxic megacolon is much less common.

Many patients with CD present with perianal problems. In the presence of active disease, the perianal skin appears bluish. Superficial ulcers with undermined edges are relatively painless and can heal with bridging of epithelium. Deep cavitating ulcers are usually found in the upper anal canal; they can be painful and cause perianal abscesses and fistulae, discharging around the anus and sometimes forwards into the genitalia. Fistulation through the posterior wall of the vagina may lead to rectovaginal fistula and continuous leakage of gas and/or faeces per vaginam.

The rectal mucosa is often spared in CD and may feel normal on rectal examination. If it is involved, however, it will feel thickened, nodular and irregular. Perianal disease is frequently associated with dense, fibrous stricturing at the anorectal junction. Incontinence may develop as a result of destruction of the anal sphincter musculature because of inflammation, abscess formation, fibrotic change and repeated episodes of surgical drainage. In severe cases, the perineum may become densely fibrotic, rigid and covered with multiple discharging openings (watering-can perineum).

Each patient with CD should have their disease phenotype (manifestations) classified according to the Montreal classification. This is important as it allows an overview of disease progression in the individual patient over time, and it enables group comparisons and evaluations. The Montreal classification specifies age of onset, location and behaviour. As discussed above, the behaviour of CD can be dominated by inflammation without stricturing or penetration, stricturing or penetration (causing phlegmons, abscesses and fistulae).

EXTRAINTESTINAL MANIFESTATIONS

The extraintestinal manifestations of CD are similar to those that occur in UC and are outlined in Summary box 69.3. Primary sclerosing cholangitis is relatively rare in CD, compared with UC. Gallstones are common, as an inflamed or excised terminal ileum leads to reduced absorption of bile salts. Amyloidosis is common at postmortem examination, but is rarely symptomatic. 'Metastatic' CD can occur in the vagina and/or skin with nodular ulcers, which demonstrate non-caseating granulomas when biopsied. Such 'cutaneous' CD can be virtually indistinguishable macroscopically from hidradenitis suppurativa.

Investigations

LABORATORY

A full blood count should be performed, as anaemia is common and usually multifactorial. It may result from the anaemia of chronic disease, or from iron deficiency as a result of blood loss or malabsorption. Vitamin B12 deficiency may occur as a consequence of terminal ileal disease or resection. Folate deficiency may also result from diffuse small bowel disease or

Summary box 69.3

Extraintestinal manifestations of Crohn's disease

- Related to disease activity
  - Erythema nodosum
  - Pyoderma gangrenosum
  - Arthropathy
  - Eye complications (iritis/uveitis)
  - Aphthous ulceration
  - Amyloidosis
- Unrelated to disease activity
  - Gallstones
  - Renal calculi
  - Primary sclerosing cholangitis
  - Chronic active hepatitis
  - Sacroiliitis

resection. Active inflammatory disease is usually associated with a fall in serum albumin, magnesium, zinc and selenium. Acute phase protein measurements (C-reactive protein and orosomucoid) and the erythrocyte sedimentation rate may correlate with disease activity.

Finding an elevated concentration in the stools of calprotectin, a specific marker of inflammation, may support a diagnosis of CD in patients with new onset of persistent gastrointestinal symptoms. It can also be used to monitor disease activity in the long-term management of established CD.

ENDOSCOPY

Colonoscopic examination may be normal or show patchy inflammation. Characteristically, there are areas of normal mucosa in between areas of inflammation that are irregular and ulcerated, with a mucopurulent exudate. The earliest findings are of aphthous ulcers surrounded by a rim of erythematous mucosa. These become larger and deeper with increasing severity of disease. There may be stricturing, and it is important to exclude malignancy at these sites by multiple and often repeated mucosal biopsies. An irregular Crohn's stricture with polypoid mucosa may be almost macroscopically indistinguishable from malignancy. The terminal ileum may be ulcerated and strictured. In patients who have had previous ileocaecal resection and anastomosis, recurrent disease usually presents first with aphthous ulceration just proximal to the anastomosis. Interval colonoscopy is therefore important in the follow-up after surgery for CD.

Upper gastrointestinal symptoms may require upper gastrointestinal endoscopy, which may reveal deep longitudinal ulcers and cobblestoning of mucosa in the duodenum, stomach or, rarely, in the oesophagus.

Enteroscopy may reveal jejunal ulceration and stricturing. Capsule endoscopy should not be undertaken where there is a suspicion of stricture, because of the possibility of the capsule becoming stuck in the narrow segment. A biodegradable test capsule can be used if this is a source of concern. Capsule endoscopy has a useful role in those patients with evidence of chronic gastrointestinal symptoms or blood loss where no evidence of ulceration can be found with more conventional endoscopic assessment.

IMAGING

High-resolution ultrasound in expert hands can demonstrate inflamed and thickened bowel loops, as well as fluid collections and abscesses. The small intestine is traditionally imaged by a small bowel enema (Figure 69.3). This is performed by instilling contrast into the small bowel via a nasoduodenal tube, and will show up areas of stricturing and prestenotic dilatation. The involved areas tend to be narrowed, irregular and, sometimes, when a length of terminal ileum is involved, there may be the 'string sign' of Kantor (Figure 69.3).

Computed tomography (CT) scans with oral contrast are widely used in the investigation of abdominal symptoms and can demonstrate fistulae, intra-abdominal abscesses and bowel thickening or dilatation. Magnetic resonance imaging (MRI) is useful in assessing complex perianal disease and, more recently, has been shown to be an excellent method for investigating the small bowel. MR enterography (oral contrast) or enteroclysis (contrast administered via nasoduodenal tube) is particularly effective at demonstrating small bowel stricturing and avoids the need for repeated exposure to large

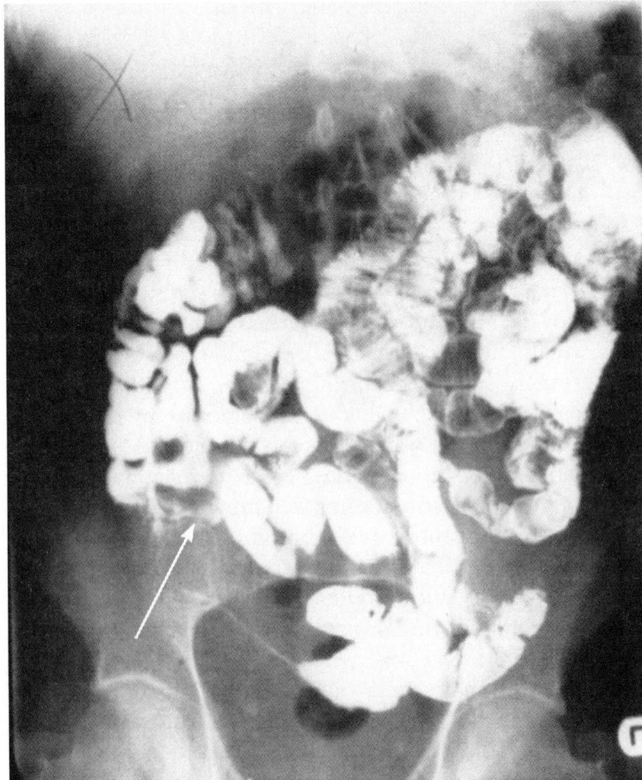

Figure 69.3 Small bowel enema examination showing a narrowed terminal ileum involved with Crohn's disease (arrow) – the 'string' sign of Kantor (courtesy of Pradip K Datta, Caithness General Hospital, Wick, UK).

John Leonard Kantor, 1890–1947, gastroenterologist, the Presbyterian Hospital, New York, NY, USA, described his 'string sign' in 1934.

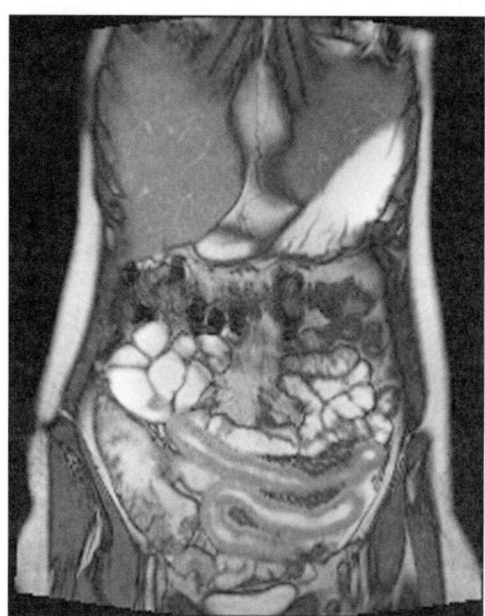

Figure 69.4 Magnetic resonance enteroclysis demonstrating small bowel inflammation (courtesy of Dr D Kasir, Hope Hospital, Salford, UK).

doses of ionising radiation in young patients (Figure 69.4). A labelled white cell scan is occasionally of value to determine whether or not a segment of bowel is actively inflamed and guide decisions on medical treatment.

In patients with enterocutaneous fistulae, fistulography will be required to demonstrate the anatomy and complexity of the fistulae and allow adequate planning for future surgery.

Treatment

MEDICAL TREATMENT

Steroids Steroids are the traditional method for inducing remission in CD, and remain important when rapid remission is required. They induce remission in 70–80% of cases with moderate to severe disease. They should be used in short courses only and tapered when a response has been achieved. They reduce inflammation and are therefore ineffective in fibrostenotic disease, where the symptoms relate mainly to obstruction. Steroids can also be used as topical agents in the rectum where the benefits include reduced systemic bioavailability, but long-term use can still cause adrenal suppression. More recently, oral steroid formulations such as budesonide have been devised, to ensure that the steroid moiety is removed in the portal circulation, reducing systemic side effects. Steroids should not be used for maintenance therapy for CD and are usually replaced with immunomodulatory agents (see below) in order to minimise the risk of side effects associated with long-term steroid use.

Aminosalicylates Colonic symptoms can be treated by 5-ASA agents in a similar manner to that in UC. These agents have limited efficacy in small bowel CD.

Antibiotics Metronidazole and ciprofloxacin may be used, particularly for periods of a few weeks at a time, especially in perianal disease. Long-term use of metronidazole is to be especially avoided, as there is a risk of peripheral neuropathy. Ciprofloxacin also has significant side effects when used in the long term, such as Achilles tendinitis and tendon rupture. Antibiotics may also be used to decrease systemic symptoms resulting from an inflammatory mass or an abscess. In general, however, a confirmed abscess should be treated by percutaneous drainage and/or surgery as antibiotics alone will not treat a Crohn's mass effectively.

Immunomodulatory agents Azathioprine is used for its additive and steroid-sparing effects and currently represents standard maintenance therapy. It is a purine analogue, which is metabolised to 6-mercaptopurine (6-MP) and works by inhibiting cell-mediated immune responses. 6-MP may be given directly for the same effects. Approximately 10% of people have deficient thiopurine methyltransferase (TPMT) and 1 in 300 people have no enzyme activity, causing inefficient metabolism of 6-MP. The resulting supra-pharmacological concentrations may cause severe adverse effects such as myelosuppression. Testing TPMT activity is usually undertaken before commencing treatment.

Cyclosporin also acts by inhibiting cell-mediated immunity. Short-course intravenous cyclosporin treatment is associated with 80% remission; however, there is relapse after completion of treatment in many cases.

Monoclonal antibody therapy Several commercially available agents have been developed based on monoclonal antibodies targeting tumour necrosis factor alpha and other key pro-inflammatory mediators.

Infliximab, a murine chimeric monoclonal antibody, was the first available monoclonal antibody for the treatment of CD. This needs to be administered as an intravenous infusion and is typically given every 8 weeks for maintenance of remission.

Adalimumab, an entirely human monoclonal antibody, is an alternative to infliximab. This is administered subcutaneously every 1–2 weeks, depending on response, and most patients can self-administer this agent.

Third-generation monoclonal antibody therapies include integrin antibodies vedulizumab and etrolizumab. Both prevent leucocyte migration preferentially in the gastrointestinal tract and may therefore have fewer side effects than the earlier monoclonal antibodies, although they are both currently in limited use.

The roles of monoclonal antibodies have expanded from initially being used exclusively in the most severe cases of CD when other therapies failed, to having a more central role in the management of moderate to severe CD. They are currently widely used for induction and maintenance of remission. Furthermore, there is evidence that early and aggressive use of these agents in patients at high risk for early recrudescent disease after surgery (for example, penetrating phenotype, early mucosal inflammation or aphthous ulceration at follow-up colonoscopy) may reduce the need for subsequent surgery.

These agents also appear to be effective treatments for perianal disease. Recent studies have suggested, however, that while they may reduce the inflammation associated with the process of fistulation and can achieve healing of fistula openings, the fistula tracks may remain patent and cessation of therapy is usually associated with a high risk of reactivation of the fistulae.

Overall, monoclonal antibodies are expensive forms of treatment that are associated with a small but definable risk of overwhelming bacterial infection and specific malignancies over the long term. Active infection, tuberculosis and a past history of malignancy are specific contraindications.

Nutritional support It is essential that nutritional status is evaluated in all patients with CD. Nutritional support is frequently required. Patients with moderate nutritional impairment will require nutritional supplementation and severely malnourished patients may require enteral tube or even intravenous feeding. Anaemia, hypoproteinaemia and electrolyte, vitamin and metabolic bone problems must all be addressed. Elemental diet or parenteral nutrition can induce remission in up to 80% of patients, an effect comparable to steroids. However, almost all patients relapse rapidly after cessation of therapy.

Summary box 69.4

Principles of management of Crohn's disease (CD)

- Close liaison between physician and surgeon is crucial
- Medical therapy should always be considered as an alternative to surgery, although surgery should not be delayed when a clear indication for surgery exists
- Patients must be optimised as far as possible prior to surgery, and this may require preoperative total parenteral nutrition
- CD is a chronic relapsing disease with a high likelihood of reoperation; the surgeon must take every reasonable effort to preserve bowel length and sphincter function

ENDOSCOPIC DILATATION IN CROHN'S DISEASE

Although penetrating disease will often require surgical resection (see below under Surgery), stricturing may be amenable to endoscopic treatment, provided the strictures can be reached with an endoscope and negotiated with a guidewire. This may be accomplished by enteroscopy or colonoscopy, depending on the site of the stricture. Dilatation of an inflamed or ulcerated stricture is contraindicated because of the risks of perforation, but balloon dilatation of fibrostenotic disease may result in substantial symptomatic improvement and obviate the need for surgery in selected cases.

INDICATIONS FOR SURGERY

Surgical resection will not cure CD. Surgery therefore focuses on managing the complications of the disease. As many of these indications for surgery may be relative, joint management by an aggressive physician and a conservative surgeon is ideal (see Summary box 69.4). CD is a complicated condition and decisions regarding management are best made jointly by members of a multidisciplinary team.

Complications or manifestations of CD for which surgery is usually appropriate include the following:

- recurrent intestinal obstruction;
- persistent or, less commonly, massive acute bleeding;
- free perforation of the bowel;
- failure of medical therapy;
- steroid dependent disease;
- intestinal fistula;
- perianal disease (abscess, fistula, stenosis);
- malignant change (notably in the colon and less commonly as a complication of small bowel disease).

TOP-DOWN APPROACH TO MANAGEMENT OF CROHN'S DISEASE

Traditionally, active Crohn's disease is treated in a 'step-up' approach where newer, more aggressive therapies are added only when more established and less toxic therapies have failed. Thus, active ileocolic CD may be treated initially with a thiopurine, adding steroids and then a monoclonal antibody only if and when required. Some centres instead advocate a top-down approach, where rapid remission is obtained by initiating therapy with a monoclonal antibody agent (unless contraindicated), often in combination with a thiopurine. Studies suggest advantages mainly in the form of rapid remission, steroid sparing and increased rates of mucosal healing.

Whether surgical resection should be part of a top-down approach is currently being debated. While surgery carries perioperative risks, these have been reduced during the past decades with the development of perioperative enhanced-recovery protocols and laparoscopic surgery. It has been suggested that the balance of risk and benefit between surgical resection and non-operative treatment, typically involving long-term medical therapy, is finely balanced and requires more detailed evaluation.

SURGERY FOR CROHN'S DISEASE

Population-based studies show that roughly 70% of patients with CD will require a bowel resection in the first decade after diagnosis, and 40% will require a further resection in the decade following their index resection. Recent population-based data in the era of monoclonal antibodies suggest that the incidence of surgery may be falling, but nevertheless still remains substantial.

Since surgery does not cure CD, the fundamental principle is to preserve healthy gut and to maintain adequate function. The whole of the gastrointestinal tract should be examined carefully at surgery and intestinal resection kept to the minimum required to treat the local consequences of disease. In laparoscopic surgery, it may be difficult to fully assess the full length of the small intestine. Up-to-date and accurate preoperative small bowel imaging is therefore paramount, particularly in laparoscopic surgery for CD.

Occasionally, unsuspected ileitis is diagnosed during the course of an operation for suspected appendicitis. Determining whether to resect the ileum in this situation is a complex clinical decision that should be made by a senior surgeon. This decision involves an assessment of the likelihood that the ileitis is an expression of CD rather than of another aetiology such as *Yersinia* infection; an assessment of the likelihood of remission with medical therapy rather than surgery; and an assessment of the rest of the small bowel for presence of additional sites of inflammation. Thus, it would be advisable to surgically resect a mass caused by penetrating CD of the terminal ileum, as such complex disease is unlikely to resolve with medical therapy. On the other hand, it would be controversial in the current era of monoclonal therapy to resect uncomplicated terminal ileitis found during an emergency procedure for suspected appendicitis, as uncomplicated Crohn's ileitis is likely to respond to medical therapy. Many cases fall in between these two extremes, requiring a considered decision.

A further consideration is whether to perform an appendicectomy when terminal ileitis is found. There is a risk of fistulation in the setting of CD, so unless the appendix itself is grossly inflamed with a healthy base, isolated appendicectomy should be avoided in this setting.

The course of CD after surgery is unpredictable, but recrudescence (a better term than 'recurrence', as surgery never cures CD) is common. Symptomatic recrudescence does not seem to be related to the presence of disease at the resection line. The cumulative probability of recrudescence requiring surgery for ileal disease is approximately 20, 40, 60 and 80% at 5, 10, 15 and 20 years, respectively, after a previous resection.

Surgery for CD is technically demanding as the involved mesentery is thickened and oedematous and healing may be impaired. The patient may be malnourished, immunosuppressed or suffer from sepsis (and potentially all three). Decision-making regarding the timing and nature of surgery to be undertaken is the key to satisfactory outcome of surgical treatment, and frequently requires experience and considerable discussion with other health professional and, most importantly, the patient. A key decision has to be made whether to anastomose the apparently healthy bowel ends after macroscopically apparent disease has been resected, as anastomotic leaks and fistulation represent a considerable problem after surgery for CD. Intra-abdominal septic complications are more common if one or more of the following risk factors are present:

- current high-dose steroid therapy (≥10 mg prednisolone for ≥4 weeks before surgery);
- current preoperative monoclonal antibody therapy;
- preoperative significant weight loss (>10% premorbid weight);
- pre-existing abdominal sepsis (notably abscess or fistula);
- serum albumin <32 g/L.

If any these risk factors are present (and particularly if more than one risk factor is present as the risks appear to be additive), one should consider exteriorising the bowel and planning a delayed anastomosis when the risk factor has been corrected.

Ileocaecal or colonic resections can be undertaken laparoscopically, with the potential advantage of smaller incisions and potentially shorter recovery time. Reoperative surgery is technically demanding and studies suggest that ileosigmoid or ileoduodenal adhesions and fistulae can be difficult to safely dissect laparoscopically and conversion to laparotomy may be advisable in this setting.

A range of operations is performed for CD, depending on the pattern of disease – the most common are outlined below:

- Ileocaecal resection is the usual procedure for terminal ileal disease, with a primary anastomosis between the ileum and the ascending or transverse colon, depending on the extent of the disease.
- Segmental resection of short segments of small or large bowel strictures can be performed.
- Colectomy and ileorectal anastomosis may be undertaken for colonic CD with rectal sparing and a normal anus.
- Subtotal colectomy and ileostomy for Crohn's colitis accounts for 8% of such procedures for acute colonic disease. The indications are similar to those for UC.
- Temporary loop ileostomy. This can be used either in patients with acute distal CD, allowing remission and later restoration of continuity, or in patients with severe perianal or rectal disease.
- Proctectomy and proctocolectomy. Many patients with severe anal disease failing to respond to medical treatment will eventually require a permanent colostomy. When this occurs in a setting of severe colonic disease, proctocolectomy and permanent ileostomy may be required.
- Strictureplasty. Strictured areas of CD (Figure 69.5) can be treated by strictureplasty, a local widening procedure, to avoid small bowel resection and is thus an important bowel sparing technique (Figure 69.6). Strictureplasty is particularly useful for the treatment of fibrostenotic disease, when there is little or no active inflammation in the involved segment. Multiple strictureplasties can be performed and strictureplasty can be combined with resection.

Anal disease should be treated conservatively by simple drainage of abscesses and the use of setons through fistulae to avoid sphincter injury. Infliximab or adalimumab therapy may be combined with seton insertion in the early phase of management of perianal fistulae. Once the fistula has dried up, typically after 2–3 doses, the seton can be removed. Laying open of fistulae (fistulotomy), commonly performed for fistulae resulting from the common cryptoglandular perianal

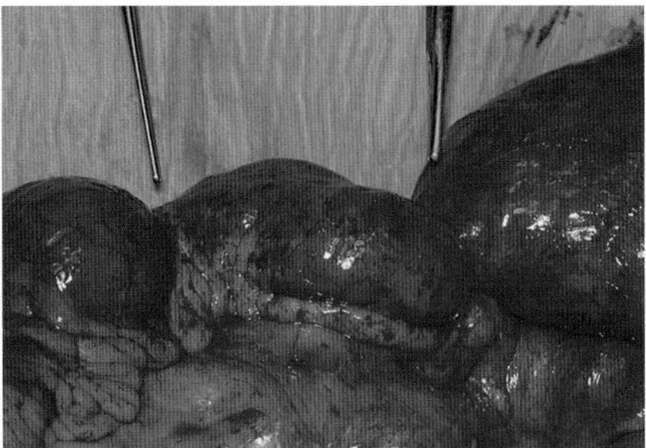

Figure 69.5 Small bowel strictures in Crohn's disease with dilatation between strictures.

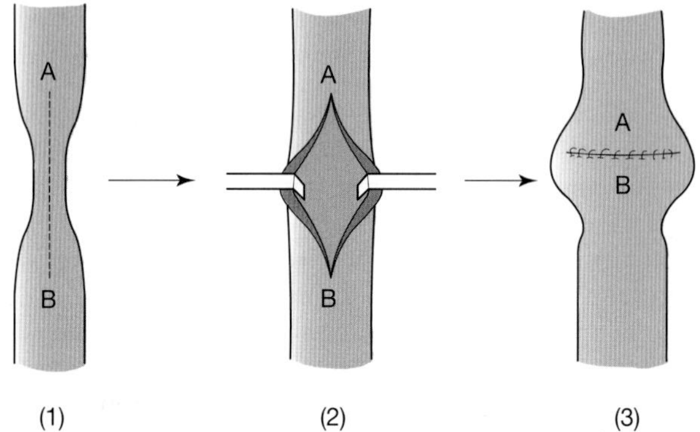

Figure 69.6 Heineke–Mikulicz strictureplasty. (1) A strictured length of intestine is incised along its length. (2) The bowel is opened and the walls are retracted as shown. (3) The bowel is resutured transversely to widen the narrowed segment. Other types of strictureplasty are also used.

abscess, should be avoided in CD as the wound edges heal very slowly or not at all.

INFECTIVE ENTERITIS

Campylobacteriosis

Infection with *Campylobacter jejuni* (a gram-negative rod with a distinctive spiral shape) is the most common form of bacterial gastroenteritis in the UK, typically acquired from eating infected poultry. It causes diarrhoea and abdominal pain and may mimic an acute abdomen. Severe cases may resemble UC, with rectal bleeding and colorectal ulceration, causing diagnostic difficulty. The organism is very sensitive and may take several days to isolate on stool culture. Toxic dilatation and even disintegrative colitis have rarely been reported to occur. Treatment is generally supportive as the condition usually resolves without antibiotics. It is a notifiable disease.

Yersiniosis

Yersinia enterocolitica is a gram-negative rod that can infect the terminal ileum, appendix, ascending colon and mesenteric lymph nodes, and can cause a granulomatous inflammatory process that mimics CD. *Yersinia* typically causes a fever and gastroenteritis, but may persist and cause a terminal ileitis, which, on occasion, may perforate. The diagnosis may be made on stool culture, but is more often confirmed serologically. If discovered at laparotomy, the terminal ileum and mesenteric nodes will look thickened and inflamed and a lymph node biopsy can be taken for diagnostic purposes. The disease is normally self-limiting, but responds to treatment with cotrimoxazole or chloramphenicol.

Salmonellosis, typhoid and paratyphoid

Salmonella are a family of gram-negative rods that can cause a range of enteric infections. *Salmonella* gastroenteritis is typically caused by *S. enteritidis* from poultry, and is most often a self-limiting illness comprising headache, fever and watery diarrhoea. When severe, antibiotics and hospitalisation and intravenous fluids may be needed. The diagnosis is based on stool culture. *Shigella* and enteropathogenic strains of *E. coli* may cause similar diarrhoeal illnesses.

Typhoid fever is caused by *S. typhi* and presents with fever and abdominal pain after an incubation period of 10–20 days. Over the next week, the patient can develop distension, diarrhoea, splenomegaly and characteristic 'rose spots' on the abdomen caused by a vasculitis. Typhoid is a systemic infection and diagnosis of typhoid is confirmed by culture of blood or stool. Treatment is by antibiotics, usually chloramphenicol. A number of surgical complications can result, including paralytic ileus, intestinal haemorrhage, free ileal perforation and cholecystitis.

In addition, invasion of the systemic circulation, which is a characteristic feature of salmonellosis, may cause severe gram-negative sepsis, resulting in septic shock. Some patients develop metastatic sepsis, including septic arthritis and osteomyelitis, meningitis, encephalitis, disseminated intravascular coagulation and pancreatitis.

Perforation of a typhoid ulcer characteristically occurs during the third week of the illness, although it is sometimes the first clinical sign of the disease. The ulcer is parallel to the long axis of the gut and is usually situated in the distal ileum. Perforation requires surgery to wash out and close the ulcer and intestinal resection is usually avoided. In unstable patients, notably with evidence of septic shock, the bowel should be exteriorised and the perforation closed after recovery. Paratyphoid infection (with *S. paratyphi*) resembles typhoid fever and is treated in a similar manner.

Tuberculosis of the intestine

Tuberculosis, like CD, can affect any part of the gastrointestinal tract from the mouth to the anus. The sites affected most often are the ileum, proximal colon and peritoneum. There are two principal disease presentations.

Ulcerative tuberculosis

Ulcerative tuberculosis develops secondary to pulmonary tuberculosis and arises as a result of swallowing tubercle bacilli. Multiple ulcers, lying transversely, develop in the terminal ileum and the overlying serosa is thickened, reddened and covered in tubercles. Patients typically present with diarrhoea and weight loss, although subacute obstruction and even local perforation and fistula formation can occur. A barium follow-through or CT examination fails to show filling of the lower ileum, caecum and the ascending colon as a result of narrowing of the ulcerated segment (Figure 69.7).

A course of antituberculous chemotherapy usually leads to cure, provided the pulmonary tuberculosis is adequately treated. Surgery is usually undertaken only in the rare event of a perforation or complete intestinal obstruction.

Hyperplastic tuberculosis

This is caused by the ingestion of *Mycobacterium tuberculosis* by patients with a high resistance to the organism. The infection usually occurs in the ileocaecal region, although solitary and multiple lesions in the lower ileum are also sometimes

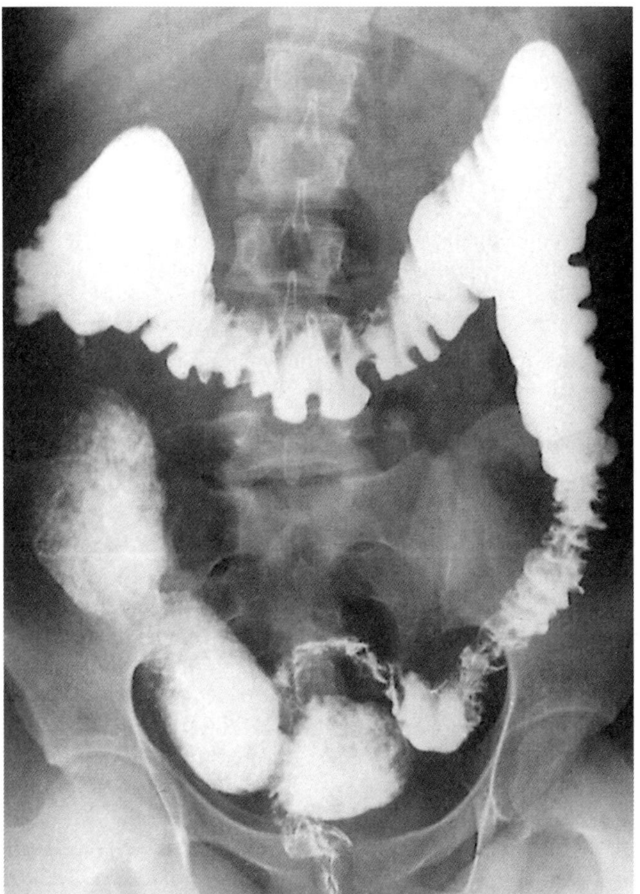

Figure 69.7 Ileocaecal tuberculosis. Absent ascending colon and caecum with dilatation of terminal ileum (courtesy of Dr VK Kapoor, Delhi, India).

seen. The infection establishes itself in lymphoid follicles, and the resulting chronic inflammation causes thickening of the intestinal wall and narrowing of the lumen. There is early involvement of the regional lymph nodes, which may caseate. Unlike in CD, abscess and fistula formation are rare.

Patients usually present with attacks of abdominal pain and intermittent diarrhoea. There is incomplete ileal obstruction, leading to stasis and bacterial overgrowth. This in turn causes steatorrhoea, anaemia and loss of weight. Patients may present with a mass in the right iliac fossa and vague ill health. The differential diagnosis is that of an appendix mass, lymphoma, carcinoma of the caecum, CD, tuberculosis or actinomycosis. A barium follow-through or small bowel enema will show a long narrow filling defect in the terminal ileum (which may result in a differential diagnosis of CD). CT will also demonstrate the narrowed segment with proximal distension and the associated lymphadenopathy. When the diagnosis is clear and the patient has not yet developed obstructive symptoms, treatment with chemotherapy is advised and may be curative. Where obstruction is present, or the possibility of CD or lymphoma require clarification, ileocaecal resection is often required.

Actinomycosis

Abdominal actinomycosis is rare. It is caused by infection with *Actinomyces israelii* and infection usually develops several weeks after an apparently straightforward perforated appendicitis. An abscess develops and spreads to the retroperitoneal tissues and the adjacent abdominal wall, eventually becoming the seat of multiple indurated discharging sinuses. At first, the discharge from the sinuses is thin, watery and inoffensive, but it may later become thicker and malodorous. Secondary fistulation may occur and the tissues may become extensively indurated and woody. In contrast to tuberculosis, however, mesenteric lymph nodes are not involved and the lumen of the intestine is not narrowed. Haematogenous spread via the portal vein may lead to multiple liver abscesses.

Pus should be sent for bacteriological examination, which will reveal the characteristic sulphur granules. Penicillin or cotrimoxazole treatment is required and should be prolonged and in high dosage.

Human immunodeficiency virus

Human immunodeficiency virus (HIV) infection is associated with a number of proctological problems, as discussed in Chapter 73. Intestinal complications are common after the development of AIDS when opportunistic organisms can cause gastroenteritis (see Summary box 69.5.). HIV1 may also cause a specific enteropathy. Treatment is directed towards the relevant organism and surgery should be avoided if possible.

Summary box 69.5

Opportunistic intestinal infections in patients with AIDS

- Bacteria
  - Salmonella
  - Shigella
  - Yersinia
  - Campylobacter
  - *Mycobacterium avium intracellulare* (MAI)
- Viral
  - Cytomegalovirus
- Protozoa
  - Cryptosporidium
  - Giardia
- Fungal
  - *Candida albicans*

TUMOURS OF THE SMALL INTESTINE

Small bowel tumours are rare and in total account for less than 10% of gastrointestinal neoplasia.

James Israel, 1848–1926, first found sulphur granules in pus from a discharging sinus in a man's neck. Later, he became a famous Berlin urologist.

Benign

The majority of small bowel neoplasms are benign, comprising adenomas, lipomas, haemangiomas and neurogenic tumours. They are frequently asymptomatic and identified incidentally, but can present with intussusception, small bowel obstruction and bleeding that may cause anaemia or may even be overt. Where these lesions do cause anaemia, the cause can be difficult to diagnose, as CT or small bowel contrast studies do not show them easily. Capsule endoscopy or small bowel endoscopy has been used successfully where the facilities exist. Symptomatic lesions can be treated by small bowel resection and anastomosis.

Peutz-Jeghers syndrome

This is an autosomal dominant disease characterised by melanosis of the mouth and lips, with multiple hamartomatous (benign tumour-like malformation resulting from faulty development in an organ) polyps in the small bowel and colon (Figure 69.8). Melanin spots can also occur on the digits and perianal skin. The gene *STK11* on chromosome 19 has been found in a proportion of patients with this condition. Long-term follow-up of the original family described by Peutz has shown reduced survival as a consequence of complications of bowel obstruction and the development of a range of cancers. It is logical to perform regular colonic surveillance and encourage female patients to attend breast and cervical screening. Despite the increased risk of malignancy in general, malignant change in the polyps themselves rarely occurs and the polyps can be left alone unless they are the cause of symptoms. Resection may be indicated, however, for heavy and persistent or recurrent bleeding or intussusception. Polyps may be removed by enterotomy or, at laparotomy, snared via a colonoscope introduced via an enterotomy. Heavily involved segments of small intestine may occasionally be resected.

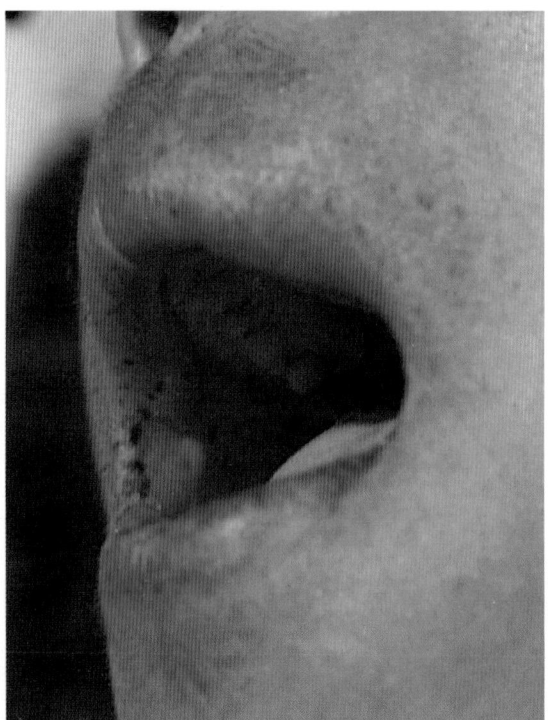

Figure 69.8 Melanin spots on the lips of a patient afflicted with Peutz–Jeghers syndrome (courtesy of Major PCM Manta, Indian Medical Service).

Malignant

Small bowel malignancy is rare and classically presents late, most often diagnosed after surgery for small bowel obstruction. Four types will be considered, which account for over 99% of small bowel malignancies: adenocarcinoma, carcinoid tumours, lymphomas and mesenchymal tumours (gastrointestinal stromal tumours [GIST]).

Adenocarcinoma

Small bowel adenocarcinoma is more often found in the jejunum than the ileum and although the aetiology is unknown, it is more common in patients with CD, coeliac disease, familial adenomatous polyposis, hereditary non-polyposis colon cancer and Peutz–Jeghers syndrome. The tumours present with anaemia, overt gastrointestinal bleeding, intussusception or obstruction. Prognosis is poor, particularly in patients with CD, in whom these tumours often present late, because the symptoms are commonly mistaken for those of CD and treated conservatively. When suspected, the advised surgical treatment is a resection of 5 cm of non-involved bowel either side of the lesion and the affected mesentery (Figure 69.9). A right hemicolectomy is likely to be required for tumours of the distal ileum.

Carcinoid tumours

These neuroendocrine tumours occur throughout the gastrointestinal tract, most commonly in the appendix, ileum and rectum in decreasing order of frequency. Appendicular carcinoid tumours are commonly noted as an incidental finding at appendicectomy, and are said to occur in approximately 2% of appendices removed surgically. The tumour arises from Kulchitsky cells at the base of intestinal crypts (of Lieberkuhn). The primary is usually small, although significant lymph node metastases can occur. In up to one-third of cases of small bowel carcinoids, the tumours are multiple. They

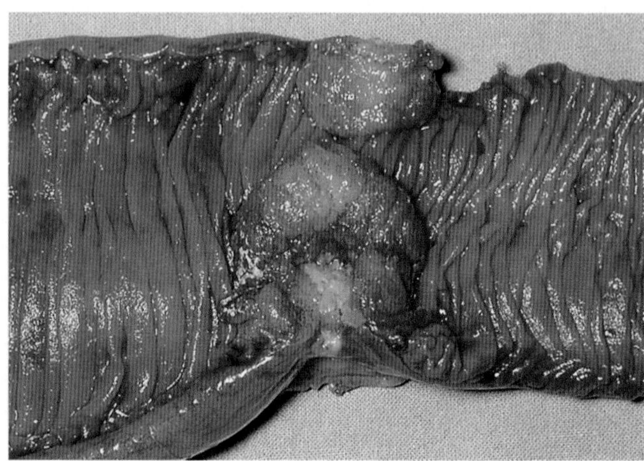

Figure 69.9 Small bowel adenocarcinoma.

may produce dense fibrosis in the surrounding tissues, resulting in distortion and scarring of the bowel and associated mesentery, giving them a characteristic radiological appearance. Carcinoid tumours can produce a number of vasoactive peptides, most commonly 5-hydroxytryptamine (serotonin), but also histamine, prostaglandins and kallikrein. When they metastasise to the liver, the 'carcinoid syndrome' can become evident, because the vasoactive substances escape the filtering actions of the liver. The clinical syndrome itself consists of reddish-blue cyanosis, flushing attacks, diarrhoea, borborygmi, asthmatic attacks and, eventually, pulmonary and tricuspid stenosis (see *Summary box* 69.6). Classically, the flushing attacks are induced by alcohol.

Summary box 69.6

Carcinoid syndrome
- Diarrhoea
- Bronchospasm
- Facial/upper chest flushing
- Palpitations
- Tricuspid regurgitation

Surgical resection is usually sufficient for patients with primary disease, but the incidence of recurrence is significant. The extent of disease can be assessed preoperatively using octreotide scanning, which may detect otherwise clinically unapparent primary and secondary tumours. Plasma markers of tumour bulk, such as chromogranin A concentrations, may be useful markers of disease recurrence, as well as of prognostic value.

Hepatic resection can be carried out in patients with metastatic disease. The treatment has been transformed by the use of octreotide (a somatostatin analogue), which reduces both flushing and diarrhoea, and octreotide cover is usually used in patients with a carcinoid syndrome who have surgery to prevent a carcinoid crisis resulting from liberation of vasoactive substances following handling of the tumour. Carcinoid tumours generally grow more slowly than most metastatic malignancies and patients may live with the syndrome of metastatic disease for many years. They are not usually sensitive to chemo- or radiotherapy.

Lymphoma

Small bowel lymphoma may be primary or, more commonly, secondary to systemic lymphoma. The incidence of small bowel lymphoma is increased in patients with CD and immunodeficiency syndromes. The classification of lymphoma is beyond the scope of this chapter but a number of points are worth noting briefly. It is rare for Hodgkin's lymphoma to affect the small bowel and most western-type lymphomas are non-Hodgkin's B-cell lymphomas. They usually present with anaemia, bleeding, perforation, anorexia and weight loss.

T-cell lymphoma develops in patients with coeliac disease. It usually presents with worsening of the patient's diarrhoea, pyrexia of unknown origin and local obstructive symptoms. Mediterranean lymphoma is found mostly in North Africa and the Middle East and is often widespread at diagnosis. Burkitt's lymphoma can aggressively affect the ileocaecal region, particularly in children. The mainstay of treatment for these conditions is chemotherapy; however, surgery may be required for obstruction, perforation or bleeding.

Gastrointestinal stromal tumours

Gastrointestinal stromal tumours (GISTs) are mesenchymal tumours and the distinction between benign or malignant types is difficult even on histological examination. Increased size and high levels of c-kit (CD117) staining are associated with malignant potential. GISTs are found most commonly in the stomach, but can be found in other parts of the gut. They occur most commonly in the 50- to 70-year age group. Although the cause is unknown, patients with neurofibromatosis have an increased risk of developing these types of tumour. Patients may be asymptomatic and the tumour may present as an incidental mass on a CT scan. Symptoms include lethargy, pain, nausea, haematemesis or melaena. Surgery is the most effective way of treating GISTs, as the tumour is radioresistant and is not sensitive to conventional chemotherapy. Glivec® (imatinib) is a tyrosine kinase inhibitor that has been shown to be effective in advanced cases and may also have a role in adjuvant treatment.

CONNECTIVE TISSUE DISORDERS

Intestinal diverticulae

Diverticulae (hollow out-pouchings) are a common structural abnormality that can occur from the oesophagus to the rectosigmoid junction (but not usually in the rectum). Small bowel diverticulae may be congenital or acquired. In congenital diverticulae, all three coats of the bowel are present in the wall of the diverticulum (e.g. Meckel's diverticulum).

Acquired diverticulae

These invariably develop in the jejunum and arise from the mesenteric side of the bowel as a result of mucosal herniation at the point of entry of the blood vessels. There is thus no muscularis layer present in the wall. Jejunal diverticulae can vary in size and are frequently multiple. They are commonly asymptomatic and present as an incidental finding at surgery or on radiological imaging (Figure 69.10). However, they can result in malabsorption, as a result of bacterial stasis, or present as an acute abdominal emergency if they become inflamed or perforate. Bleeding from a jejunal diverticulum is a rare complication (compared with sigmoid diverticular disease). Elective resection of an affected small bowel segment that is causing malabsorption can be effective, provided there

Thomas Hodgkin, 1798–1866, lecturer in morbid anatomy and curator of the museum, Guy's Hospital, London, UK, described lymphadenoma in 1832.
Johann Friedrich Meckel (the younger), 1781–1833, Professor of Anatomy and Surgery, Halle, Germany, described the diverticulum in 1809.

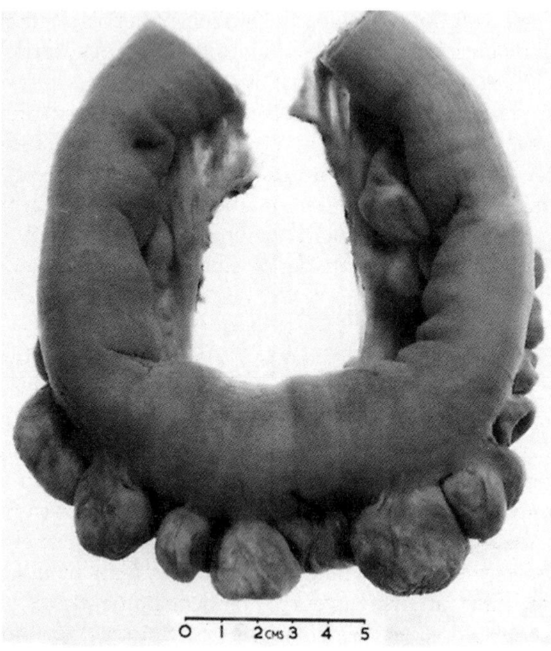

Figure 69.10 Jejunal diverticula.

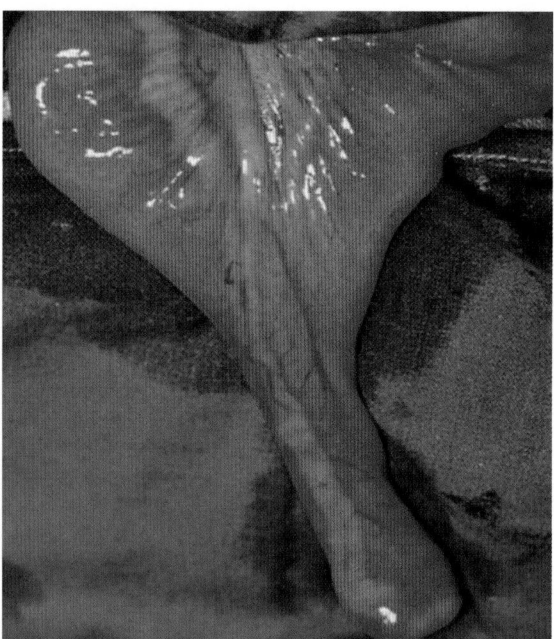

Figure 69.11 Meckel's diverticulum.

is only a limited amount of jejunum affected by the condition. If perforated jejunal diverticulitis is found at emergency laparotomy, a small bowel resection should be performed and a decision made between anastomosis and stoma formation. This will depend on the degree of contamination, physiological stability and local resources for managing a patient with a high output jejunostomy.

Complications resulting from extensive jejunal diverticulosis can be extremely difficult to treat. In severe cases, much of the proximal small intestine may be involved, effectively precluding resection. Prolonged antibiotic therapy for bacterial overgrowth may be preferable, and antibiotics (metronidazole, ciprofloxacin, rifaximin) are frequently rotated in an attempt to avoid the development of antibiotic resistance. Limited resection, leaving remaining segments of affected jejunum, may be feasible, but may also fail to deal adequately with bacterial overgrowth, recurrent attacks of inflammation or bleeding.

Meckel's diverticulum

A Meckel's diverticulum is a persistent remnant of the vitellointestinal duct and is present in about 2% of the population. It is found on the antimesenteric side of the ileum, commonly approximately 60 cm from the ileocaecal valve and is classically 5 cm long (Figure 69.11). A Meckel's diverticulum is a congenital diverticulum. It contains all three coats of the bowel wall and has its own blood supply. It may be vulnerable to obstruction and inflammation in the same way as the appendix; indeed, when a normal appendix is found at surgery for suspected appendicitis, a Meckel's diverticulum should be looked for by examining the small bowel, particularly if free fluid or pus is found. In approximately 20% of cases, the mucosa of a Meckel's diverticulum contains heterotopic epithelium of gastric, colonic or pancreatic type. The presence of heterotopic mucosa may predispose to the development of complications. The vast majority of Meckel's diverticulae are asymptomatic and Meckel's diverticulum is notoriously difficult to see with contrast radiology. Meckel's diverticulum may, however, present clinically in the following ways:

- Haemorrhage. If gastric mucosa is present, peptic ulceration can occur and present as painless dark rectal bleeding or melaena. If the stomach, duodenum and colon are excluded as a source of bleeding by endoscopy, radioisotope scanning with technetium-99m may demonstrate a Meckel's diverticulum.
- Diverticulitis. Meckel's diverticulitis presents like appendicitis, although if perforation occurs the presentation may resemble a perforated duodenal ulcer.
- Intussusception. A Meckel's diverticulum can be the lead point for ileoileal or ileocolic intussusception.
- Chronic ulceration. Pain is felt around the umbilicus, as the site of the diverticulum is midgut in origin.
- Intestinal obstruction. A band between the apex of the diverticulum and the umbilicus (also part of the vitellointestinal duct) may cause obstruction directly, or by predisposing to the development of a volvulus around it.
- Perforation. (Figure 69.12).

When found in the course of abdominal surgery, a Meckel's diverticulum can safely be left alone, provided it has a wide mouth and is not thickened. When there is doubt, it can be resected. The finding of a Meckel's diverticulum in an inguinal or femoral hernia has been described as 'Littre's hernia'.

Alexis Littre, 1658–1726, surgeon and lecturer in Anatomy, Paris, France, described Meckel's diverticulum in a hernial sac in 1700, 81 years before Meckel was born.

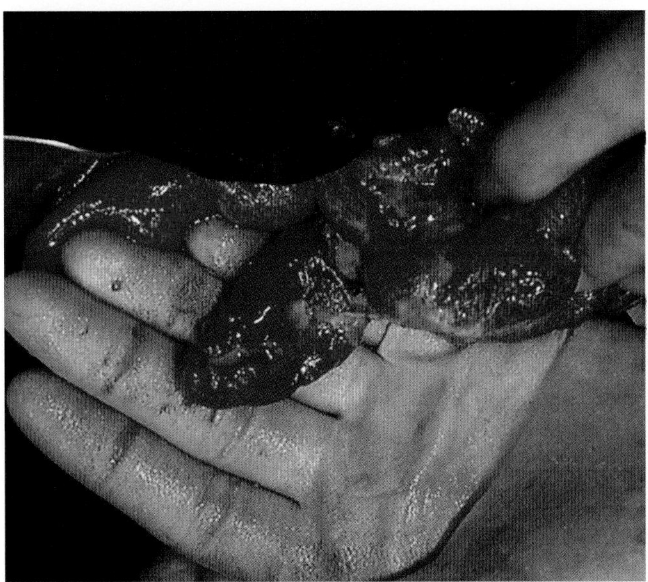

Figure 69.12 Gangrenous Meckel's diverticulitis.

Summary box 69.7

Features of Meckel's diverticulum

- Remnant of vitellointestinal duct
- Occurs in 2% of patients, 2 inches (5 cm) long, 2 feet (60 cm) from the ileocaecal valve, 20% heterotopic epithelium
- Should be looked for when a normal appendix is found at surgery for suspected appendicitis
- If a Meckel's is found incidentally at surgery, it can be left provided it has a wide mouth and is not thickened
- Can be source of gastrointestinal bleeding if it contains ectopic gastric mucosa

Meckel's diverticulectomy

A broad-based Meckel's diverticulum should not be amputated at its base and invaginated (as for an appendix), as there is the risk of stricture and of leaving heterotopic epithelium behind. It is safer simply to excise the diverticulum, either by resecting it and suturing the defect at its base, or with a linear stapler-cutter. If the base of the diverticulum is indurated, it is on balance more logical to perform a limited small bowel resection of the involved segment followed by an anastomosis.

VASCULAR ANOMALIES OF THE INTESTINE

Mesenteric ischaemia

Mesenteric vascular disease may be classified as acute intestinal ischaemia – with or without occlusion – venous, chronic arterial, central or peripheral. The superior mesenteric vessels are the visceral vessels most likely to be affected by embolisation or thrombosis, with the former being most common. Occlusion at the origin of the superior mesenteric artery (SMA) is almost invariably the result of thrombosis, whereas emboli tend to lodge at the origin of the middle colic artery. Inferior mesenteric involvement is usually clinically silent because the collateral circulation is better.

Possible sources for embolisation of the SMA include the left atrium in atrial fibrillation, the left ventricle after mural myocardial infarction, vegetations on mitral and aortic valves associated with endocarditis and an atheromatous plaque from an aortic aneurysm. Primary thrombosis is associated with atherosclerosis and vasculitides, including conditions such as thromboangitis obliterans and polyarteritis nodosa. Primary thrombosis of the superior mesenteric veins may occur in association with factor V Leiden, portal hypertension, portal pyaemia and sickle cell disease and in women taking the oral contraceptive pill. A specific form of 'non-occlusive mesenteric ischaemia' may complicate critical illness, possibly due to alterations in splanchnic blood flow.

Irrespective of whether the occlusion is arterial or venous, haemorrhagic infarction occurs. The mucosa is especially sensitive to ischaemic injury because of its high metabolic activity. The intestine and its mesentery become swollen and oedematous, especially with venous occlusion. Blood-stained fluid exudes into the peritoneal cavity and bowel lumen. The changes develop rapidly and irreversible injury, ranging in severity from mucosal necrosis and sloughing, to full-thickness infarction usually occurs within a few hours at most. If the main trunk of the SMA is involved, the infarction usually covers an area from just distal to the DJ flexure to the splenic flexure. Usually, a branch of the main trunk is implicated and the area of infarction is less.

Clinical features

The most important clue to an early diagnosis of acute mesenteric ischaemia is the sudden onset of severe abdominal pain in a patient with atrial fibrillation or atherosclerosis. The pain is typically in the central abdomen and out of all proportion to the physical findings. Persistent vomiting and defaecation occur early, with the subsequent passage of altered blood. Abdominal tenderness may be mild initially, with rigidity being a late feature. Shock, with features of both hypovolaemia and sepsis, rapidly ensues.

Investigation

Investigation will usually reveal a profound neutrophil leucocytosis with an absence of gas in the lumen of the thickened small intestine on abdominal radiographs and CT scans. Gas may be present within the intestinal wall and occasionally in the mesenteric and portal veins.

Treatment

Treatment should be tailored to the individual. In conjunction with full resuscitation, laparotomy with embolectomy via the ileocolic artery or revascularisation of the SMA by vascular bypass may be considered in early cases. Anticoagulation should be implemented early in the postoperative period. However, the condition is usually diagnosed late in the disease process and the mortality rate is extremely high. In the young, all affected bowel should be resected, whereas in the elderly or infirm the situation may be deemed incurable.

After extensive enterectomy, it is usual for patients to require intravenous alimentation. The young, however, may sometimes develop sufficient intestinal digestive and absorptive function to lead relatively normal lives. In selected cases, consideration may be given to small bowel transplantation.

Chronic small intestinal ischaemia

Chronic small intestinal ischaemia almost invariably results from atherosclerosis and affects the proximal superior mesenteric and coeliac vessels. Patients classically present with symptoms of severe central abdominal pain that comes on within 30–60 minutes of eating (mesenteric angina). Weight loss and diarrhoea due to malabsorption may also occur. The condition may be difficult to diagnose and is often overlooked initially, the symptoms being mistaken for those of peptic ulcer disease or irritable bowel syndrome. The presence of significant vascular disease on visceral angiography is common in elderly patients and in those with severe vascular disease, and should not necessarily be assumed to indicate that abdominal symptoms are attributable to chronic ischaemia. Treatment is usually by selective visceral angiography, with stenting/angioplasty and, where this is not possible, bypass surgery. Smoking cessation in imperative and patients are usually anticoagulated.

STOMAS

A colostomy (or ileostomy) stoma is an artificial opening made in the colon (or small intestine) to divert faeces and flatus out-side the abdomen where they can be collected in an external appliance. Depending on the purpose for which the diversion has been necessary, a stoma may be temporary or permanent.

Summary box 69.8

Stomas

- May be colostomy or ileostomy
- May be temporary or permanent
- Temporary or defunctioning stomas are usually fashioned as loop stomas
- An ileostomy is spouted; a colostomy is flush
- Ileostomy effluent is usually liquid, whereas colostomy effluent is usually solid
- Ileostomy patients are more likely to develop fluid and electrolyte problems
- An ileostomy is usually sited in the right iliac fossa
- End-colostomy is usually sited in the left iliac fossa
- Whenever possible, patients should be counselled and sited by a stoma care nurse before operation

Loop ileostomy

A loop ileostomy is often used for defunctioning a low rectal anastomosis or an ileal pouch. A knuckle of ileum is exteriorised through a skin trephine in the right iliac fossa. An incision is made in the distal part of the knuckle, and this is then pulled over the top of the more proximal part to create a spout on the proximal side of the loop with a flush distal side still in continuity. This allows near perfect defunctioning, but also the possibility of restoration of continuity, by taking down the spout and reanastomosing the partially divided ileum.

The advantages of a loop ileostomy over a loop colostomy are the ease with which the bowel can be brought to the surface and the relative absence of odour. Care is needed when the ileostomy is closed, so that suture line obstruction does not occur. Closure of a loop ileostomy can be a technically challenging procedure, particularly if there are dense adhesions resulting from previous surgery.

End ileostomy

An end ileostomy is formed after a subtotal colectomy without anastomosis, when it may later be reversed, or may be permanent after a panproctocolectomy. The ileum is normally brought through the rectus abdominis muscle. Careful attention to the terminal ileal mesentery should be taken to ensure that it is not too bulky. The use of a spout was originally described by Bryan Brooke; this should project some 2–4 cm from the skin surface (Figure 69.13). A disposable appliance is placed over the ileostomy so that it is a snug fit at skin level.

There may be an 'ileostomy flux' while the ileum adapts to the loss of the colon. While ileostomy output can amount to 4 or 5 litres per day, losses of 1–2 litres are more common. A consistent ileostomy output in excess of 1.5 litres is usually associated with dehydration and sodium depletion in the absence of intravenous therapy. The stools thicken in a few weeks and are semisolid in a few months. The help, skill and advice of the stoma care nurse specialist are essential. Modern appliances have transformed stoma care, and skin problems are unusual (Figure 69.14). Complications of an ileostomy include prolapse, retraction, stenosis, bleeding, fistula and parastomal hernia.

Stoma bags and appliances

Stoma output is collected in disposable adhesive bags. Ileostomy appliances tend to be drainable bags, which are left

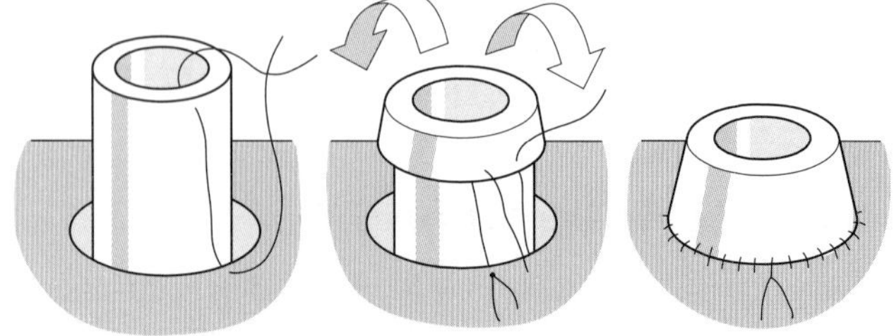

Figure 69.13 Ileostomy formation. Suturing the free extremity of the proximal ileum to the skin edges after eversion to form a spout (after Brooke).

Bryan Nicholas Brooke, 1915–1998, Professor of Surgery, St George's Hospital, London, UK.

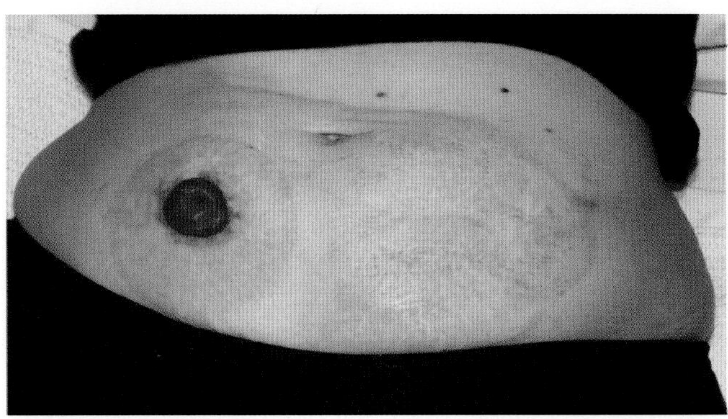

Figure 69.14 Spouted ileostomy in the right iliac fossa.

in place for 48 hours, while colostomy appliances are simply changed two or three times each day. A wide range of such bags is currently available. Many now incorporate an adhesive backing, which can be left in place for several days. In most hospitals, a stoma care service is available to offer advice to patients, to acquaint them with the latest appliances and to provide the appropriate psychological and practical help.

Complications of stomas

Stoma complications are underestimated and common. On occasion, these complications require surgical revision. Sometimes, this can be achieved with an incision immediately around the stoma, but on occasion reopening the abdomen and freeing up the stoma may be necessary. Repair of parastomal hernias is particularly technically challenging and the recurrence rate is high. Simple suture of the parastomal hernia is associated with an almost 100% risk of recurrence and transfer to the opposite side of the abdomen, or insertion of a piece of prosthetic material within the abdominal wall around the stoma may be necessary.

Summary box 69.9

Stoma complications

- Skin irritation
- Prolapse
- Retraction
- Ischaemia
- Stenosis
- Parastomal hernia
- Bleeding
- Fistulation

CONDITIONS CAUSING MALABSORPTION

Coeliac disease

Coeliac disease is the most common cause of malabsorption in the UK with a stated prevalence of 1:1800, although this may be an underestimate. It is characterised by a hypertrophic small bowel mucosa with atrophic villi and deep crypts. It is thought that the loss of surface area and brush border enzymes results in malabsorption.

Coeliac disease is caused by an abnormal immune response to gluten, a cereal protein, although the exact mechanism remains unclear. There is a genetic component, as the disease is more common in first-degree relatives and has an association with HLA B8. In children, coeliac disease presents with steatorrhoea and growth retardation. In adults, it may result in diarrhoea and weight loss but many patients simply present with an iron deficiency anaemia. Some patients develop a characteristic skin rash (dermatitis herpetiformis)

The diagnosis is usually made after an endoscopic duodenal biopsy allows pathological examination of mucosa. The antiendomysial antibody tests have a very high sensitivity and specificity for coeliac disease, but a duodenal biopsy is usually indicated to confirm the diagnosis. The biopsy usually shows flattening of the mucosa, marked inflammatory changes and characteristic findings of intraepithelial lymphocytes.

Patients with coeliac disease may develop an acute inflammatory condition of the small intestine (ulcerative jejunoileitis) and have an increased risk of small bowel lymphoma and adenocarcinoma.

The main treatment for coeliac disease is the withdrawal of gluten from the diet by avoiding wheat, rye and barley. Surgery does not usually play a role in the management of coeliac disease and is primarily reserved for resection of malignancy.

Bacterial overgrowth

The small intestine can become colonised with bacteria normally confined to the colon if there is stasis resulting in delayed bacterial clearance (blind loop syndrome, Figure 69.15). Similar complications may result from chronic small bowel obstruction, jejunal diverticulosis and ileosigmoid fistulation

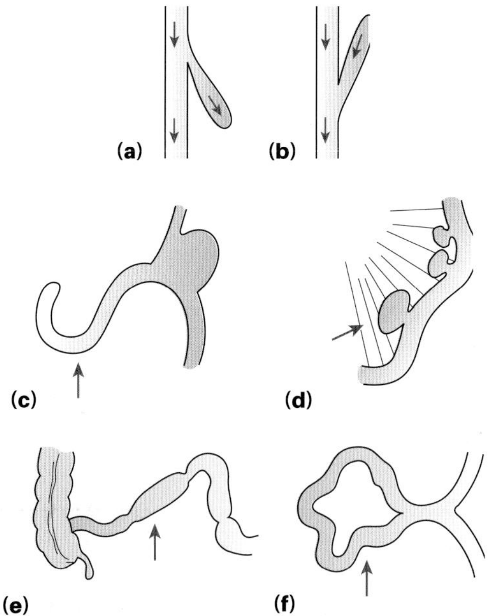

Figure 69.15 Common types of blind loop: (a) self-filling: deficiency occurs; (b) self-emptying: no deficiency occurs; (c) long afferent loop stasis in Pólya gastrectomy; (d) jejunal diverticula; (e) intestinal stricture causing stasis; (f) 'stenosis–anastomosis loop' syndrome.

(see above). If overgrowth occurs in the upper small intestine, the defect is chiefly of fat absorption; if in the lower intestine, there is vitamin B12 deficiency. There is usually relatively little effect on carbohydrate or protein metabolism. Stasis results in an abnormal bacterial flora, which prevents adequate breakdown of fat. Sometimes, the only manifestation is anaemia, resulting from vitamin B12 deficiency but, if steatorrhoea occurs, other serious malabsorption features may follow, including glossitis, osteomalacia, paraesthesia and peripheral neuropathy.

Improvement normally follows after intermittent therapy with oral antibiotics; metronidazole, ciprofloxacin, tetracycline and rifaximin are commonly used. Definitive treatment is surgical when the anatomical abnormality can be corrected, but this is not always possible.

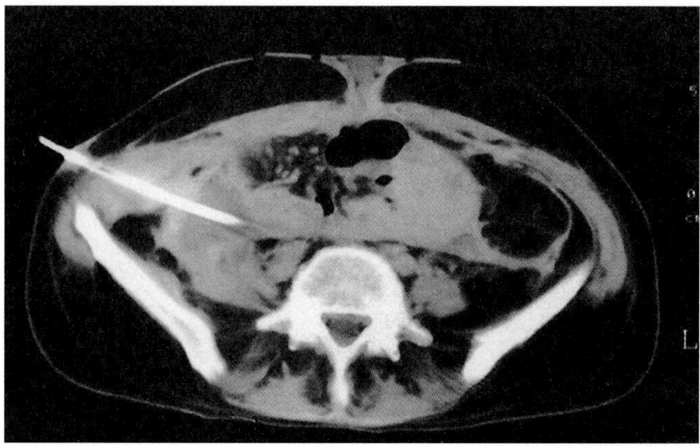

Figure 69.16 Computed tomography (CT) scan in a patient with a complex enterocutaneous fistula and an intra-abdominal abscess being drained with a CT-guided catheter.

ENTEROCUTANEOUS FISTULA

An abnormal connection between the small intestine and the skin can occur as a result of fistulating CD, radiotherapy or abdominal trauma, but the condition most commonly follows a surgical complication – either a leak from an anastomosis or an inadvertent enterotomy during dissection. At least 50% of small bowel enterocutaneous fistulae develop after surgery in which no small bowel has been resected, as a result of injury to the intestine following division of adhesions. The frequency of this complication has been shown to increase with the number of previous laparotomies. Management of patients with enterocutaneous fistulae can be very challenging, especially when the fistula output is high (usually defined as >500 mL of effluent/day). The majority of fistulae can be expected to heal spontaneously, provided there is no distal obstruction or disease at the fistula site. Reasons for failure of spontaneous healing also include epithelial continuity between the gut and the skin and an associated complex abscess.

The management of fistulas is based on well-established principles ('SNAP', see Summary box 69.10). An early return to theatre to try and treat the problem definitively in a septic, malnourished patient is doomed to failure.

Infected collections are best identified at CT (Figure 69.16) and can be drained percutaneously. Skin protection is important, as small bowel effluent is caustic. Nutritional support must include fluid and electrolytes, which can be lost in high quantities from a proximal fistula, as well as carbohydrates, protein, fat and vitamins. Judgements have to be made between enteral and parenteral feeding – enteral feeding has advantages but if the fistula is proximal or high output, total parenteral nutrition will be required. Defining anatomy is best done after careful discussion with the radiologist – a sequence of contrast studies (follow-through, fistulogram and enema) may well be required to define bowel length and plan a surgical strategy. Surgery can be extremely technically demanding, and an anastomosis should not be fashioned in the presence of continuing intra-abdominal sepsis or when the patient is hypoalbuminaemic (<32 g/dL).

Summary box 69.10

Principles of management of enterocutaneous fistulae (SNAP)

- **S**, elimination of Sepsis and skin protection
- **N**, Nutrition – a period of parenteral nutrition may well be required
- **A**, Anatomical assessment
- **P**, definitive **P**lanned surgery

SHORT BOWEL SYNDROME

Intractable diarrhoea with impaired absorption of nutrients following resection or bypass of the small intestine, ultimately leading to progressive malnutrition, is referred to as 'short bowel syndrome'. The most common causes of short bowel syndrome are resection resulting from the management of CD and its complications (which accounts for almost half of cases), mesenteric vascular thrombosis, radiation enteritis and tumours. Although features of short bowel syndrome usually appear when there is less than 200 cm of small bowel, the length and nature of the remaining intestine are also important. In general, diseases which result in short bowel syndrome tend to preferentially affect the distal small intestine, and there is some evidence that the ileum, with its tighter intercellular junctions and consequently better fluid absorptive capacity, can assume the functions of a missing jejunum, but not *vice versa*. While the ileocaecal valve used to be considered important with regard to preservation of absorptive function, it is more likely that this is a reflection of the associated preservation of the distal ileum and right colon than the valve itself.

Patients with an intact colon are relatively protected from the effects of massive small bowel resection because of the ability of the colon to absorb not only fluid and electrolytes, but a modest amount of nutrient energy. Patients with as little as 100–200 cm of jejunum anastomosed to an intact colon may therefore be able to maintain satisfactory macronutrient, fluid and electrolyte status, although they will, of course, be at risk of fat-soluble and B12 vitamin deficiencies and will also generally need oral nutritional supplements of trace elements, vitamins and minerals. Some (but not all) patients with

50–100 cm of small intestine and an intact colon will need long-term parenteral nutrition, as will almost all patients with 50 cm or less of jejunum anastomosed to an intact colon. In contrast, most patients with less than 200 cm of small intestine ending in a jejunostomy will require regular infusions of parenteral fluid and electrolytes, and almost all of those with less than 100 cm of small bowel ending in a jejunostomy will require long-term parenteral nutrition.

Medical management of patients with short bowel syndrome relies on the use of antidiarrhoeal agents (loperamide and codeine phosphate), drugs to reduce diarrhoea related to bile-salt malabsorption (colestyramine) and enteral and parenteral vitamin and trace element supplements. Although there has also been interest in the use of drugs to promote intestinal adaptation, such as growth hormone, glutamine and, most recently, glucagon-like peptide 2 agonists, the mainstay of treatment for short bowel syndrome remains home parenteral nutrition (HPN). The development of this treatment in the late 1960s enabled the majority of patients with short bowel syndrome to enjoy a reasonably good quality of life, with long-term survival related principally to the underlying disease. HPN is, however, expensive and demanding and patients with short bowel syndrome receiving HPN are at risk from catheter-related complications (notably catheter-related sepsis and occlusion), as well as metabolic complications (fibrotic liver disease, gallstones, metabolic bone disease and kidney stones).

Surgical procedures designed to improve the surface area or reduce the speed of transit of the remaining small intestine (and thus improve absorptive capacity) have shown some promise in children, but their place in managing adults with established short bowel syndrome is currently unclear. In some patients, the loss of venous access resulting from the complications of long-term intravenous feeding or the development of progressive liver dysfunction may represent indications for small bowel transplantation. The results of small bowel transplantation have progressively improved and 5-year patient survival now exceeds 80% in some centres.

FURTHER READING

Bland KI, Sarr MG, Büchler MW, Csendes A, Garden OJ, Wong J (eds). *Surgery of the small bowel. Handbooks in general surgery*. London: Springer-Verlag, 2011.

Gionchetti P, Dignass A, Danese S *et al*. *3rd European Evidence-based Consensus on the Diagnosis and Management of Crohn's Disease 2016: Part 2: Surgical Management and Special Situations*. ECCO Guideline/Consensus Paper. Oxford: Oxford University Press, 2016.

Keighley MRB, Williams NS. *Surgery of the anus rectum and colon*. 3rd edn. Philadelphia: Elsevier Saunders, 2008.

Mowat C, Cole A, Windsor A *et al*. Guidelines for the management of inflammatory bowel disease in adults. *Gut* 2011; **60**: 571–607.

Slade DAJ, Carlson GL. Takedown of enterocutaneous fistula and complex abdominal wall reconstruction. *Surg Clin N Am* 2013; **93**: 1163–83.

Chapter 70

The large intestine

Learning objectives

To appreciate:
- The basic anatomy and physiology of the large intestine
- The range of conditions that may affect the large intestine

To understand:
- The aetiology and pathology of common large intestinal conditions
- The principles of investigation of large intestinal symptoms
- The importance of non-surgical management of large intestinal problems
- The principles of colonic surgery
- That complex intestinal problems are best managed by a multidisciplinary team
- The management of acute surgical problems of the intestines

ANATOMY OF THE LARGE INTESTINE

The large intestine begins at the ileocaecal valve and extends to the anus. It is divided into the caecum, ascending colon, hepatic flexure, transverse colon with attached greater omentum, splenic flexure, descending colon, sigmoid and rectum. The large intestine is approximately 1.5 m long, but can be straightened at endoscopy so the caecum can be reached with 70 cm of colonoscope.

The colon is distinguished from the small bowel by having fat-filled peritoneal tags known as appendices epiploicae and the taenia coli. These are three flat bands of longitudinal muscle that run from the appendix base to the rectosigmoid junction. They act to pull the colon into its sacculated state, producing a series of haustrations. Distended small and large intestine can be distinguished on an abdominal radiograph as the small bowel has complete transverse markings caused by the valvulae conniventes, while the colon has incomplete lines from the sacculation caused by the taeniae. The important posterior relations of the caecum and ascending colon are the right ureter, right gonadal vessels and duodenum and these must be protected at surgery. The left ureter, left gonadal vessels and tail of the pancreas must be protected when operating on the left colon.

The blood supply of the large intestine is derived from branches of the superior mesenteric artery from the caecum to the distal transverse colon and the inferior mesenteric artery and its branches more distally. Adjacent branches anastomose so there is usually a complete vascular supply along the colon, named the marginal artery of Drummond. This vessel is often the key blood supply to the vascular arcades, ensuring adequate perfusion of a colonic anastomosis, but blood flow in the 'watershed' area of the splenic flexure representing the junction between the superior and inferior mesenteric supply may be tenuous. Sudden occlusion of the inferior mesenteric artery may leave the area of the splenic flexure poorly perfused, leading to an ischaemic colitis. Venous and lymphatic drainage of the colon follows the arterial supply and venous drainage is into the portal system. High ligation of the artery supplying a segment of colon will therefore also remove the draining lymph nodes, a key technical point in cancer surgery. The nerve supply to the large intestine is derived from the splanchnic nerves via a dense sympathetic plexus surrounding the superior and inferior mesenteric arteries. Visceral pain from the part of the colon supplied by the superior mesenteric artery is thus felt, like that of the small intestine, in the periumbilical region, while pain from the colon distal to that point is felt suprapubically.

Valvulae conniventes describes a fold of mucous membrane that passes across two-thirds of the bowel circumference.
David Drummond, 1852–1932, English physician.

PHYSIOLOGY OF THE LARGE INTESTINE

The principle function of the colon is absorption of water; 1000 mL of ileal content enters the caecum every 24 hours, of which only approximately 200 mL is excreted as faeces. Sodium absorption is efficiently accomplished by an active transport system, while chloride and water are absorbed passively. Fermentation of dietary fibre in the colon by the normal colonic microflora leads to the generation of short chain fatty acids, which are an important metabolic fuel for the colonic mucosa. Diversion of the faecal stream may lead to inflammatory changes in the colon downstream (diversion colitis). Absorption of nutrients including glucose, fatty acids, amino acids and vitamins can also take place in the colon.

Colonic motility is variable. In general, faecal residue reaches the caecum 4 hours after a meal and the rectum after 24 hours. Passage of stool is not orderly because of mixing within the colon, so it is not uncommon for residue from a single meal to still be passed 4 days later.

TUMOURS OF THE LARGE INTESTINE

Benign

The term 'polyp' is a clinical description of any protrusion of the mucosa. It encompasses a variety of histologically different tumours (*Table 70.1*). Polyps can occur singly, synchronously in small numbers or as part of a polyposis syndrome.

Adenomatous polyps

Adenomatous polyps vary from a tubular adenoma (Figure 70.1), rather like a berry on a stalk, to the villous adenoma, a flat spreading lesion. Villous tumours can cause diarrhoea, mucus discharge and, occasionally hypokalaemia and hypoalbuminaemia. The risk of malignancy developing in an adenoma increases with size; there is a 10% risk of cancer in a 1-cm diameter tubular adenoma, whereas almost one-third of large (>3 cm) colonic adenomas will have an area of invasive malignancy within them. Adenomas larger than 5 mm in diameter are usually excised because of their malignant potential. Snare polypectomy is usually possible for colonic polyps but larger sessile polyps may require endoscopic mucosal resection after infiltration of a solution containing dilute adrenaline. Larger rectal adenomas may require transanal resection or, where the adenoma is too high, transanal endoscopic microsurgery or resection via transanal placement of laparoscopic instruments. Extensive villous lesions of the rectum may require argon beam ablation when the patient is frail but symptomatic.

TABLE 70.1 Classification of intestinal polyps.

Inflammatory	Inflammatory polyps (pseudopolyps in UC)	
Metaplastic	Metaplastic or hyperplastic polyps	
Hamartomatous	Peutz–Jeghers polyp	
	Juvenile polyp	
Neoplastic	Adenoma	Tubular
		Tubulovillous
		Villous
	Adenocarcinoma	
	Carcinoid tumour	

UC, ulcerative colitis.

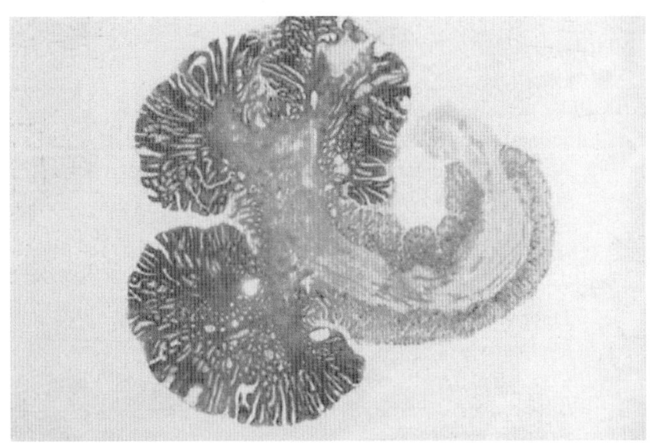

Figure 70.1 Pedunculated adenomatous polyp of the large intestine, longitudinal section (courtesy of Dr P Millard, John Radcliffe Hospital, Oxford, UK).

Familial adenomatous polyposis

Familial adenomatous polyposis (FAP) is defined clinically by the presence of more than 100 colorectal adenomas, but is also characterised by duodenal adenomas and multiple extraintestinal manifestations (*Summary box 70.1*). Over 80% of cases come from patients with a positive family history. The remainder arise as a result of new mutations in the adenomatous polyposis coli (APC) gene on the short arm of chromosome 5. FAP is inherited as an autosomal dominant condition and is consequently equally likely in men and women. The lifetime risk of colorectal cancer is 100% in patients with FAP. FAP can also be associated with benign mesodermal tumours such as desmoid tumours and osteomas. Epidermoid cysts can also occur (Gardner's syndrome); desmoid tumours in the abdomen spread locally to involve the intestinal mesentery and, although non-metastasising, they may become unresectable. Up to 50% of patients with FAP have congenital hypertrophy of the retinal pigment epithelium (CHRPE), which can be used to screen affected families if genetic testing is unavailable.

CLINICAL FEATURES

Polyps are usually visible on sigmoidoscopy by the age of 15 years and will almost always be visible by the age of 30 years. Carcinoma of the large bowel develops 10–20 years after the onset of the polyposis. If there are no adenomas by the age of 30 years, FAP is unlikely. If the diagnosis is made during

Eldon John Gardner, 1909–1989, geneticist, The University of Utah, Salt Lake City, UT, USA, described this syndrome in 1950.

Summary box 70.1

Extracolonic manifestations of FAP

- Endodermal derivatives
  - Adenomas and carcinomas of the duodenum, stomach, small intestine, thyroid and biliary tree
  - Fundic gland polyps
  - Hepatoblastoma
- Ectodermal derivatives
  - Epidermoid cysts
  - Pilomatrixoma
  - Congenital hypertrophy of the retinal pigment epithelium (CHRPE)
  - Brain tumours
- Mesodermal derivatives
  - Desmoid tumours
  - Osteomas
  - Dental problems

adolescence, surgery is usually deferred to the age of 17 or 18 years unless symptoms develop. Malignant change is rare before the age of 20 years. Examination of blood relatives, including cousins, nephews and nieces, is essential; a family tree should be constructed and a register of affected families maintained. Referral to a medical geneticist is essential. If over 100 adenomas are present at colonoscopy, the diagnosis can be made confidently (Figure 70.2).

Summary box 70.2

Features of FAP

- Autosomal dominant inherited disease due to mutation of the *APC* gene
- More than 100 colonic adenomas are diagnostic
- Prophylactic surgery is indicated to preventing colorectal cancer
- Polyps and malignant tumours can develop in the duodenum and small bowel

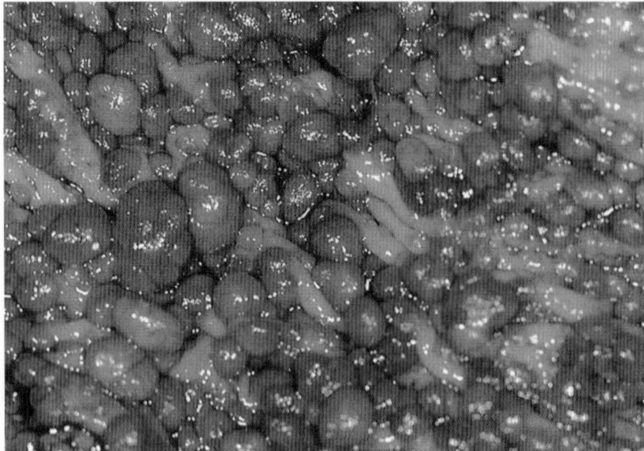

Figure 70.2 Familial adenomatous polyposis.

TREATMENT

The aim of surgery in FAP is to prevent the development of colorectal cancer. The surgical options are:

1. colectomy with ileorectal anastomosis (IRA);
2. restorative proctocolectomy with an ileal pouch–anal anastomosis (RPC);
3. total proctectomy and end ileostomy.

The patient is almost always young and likely to prefer to avoid a permanent stoma and so the choice is normally between the first two options. The advantage of an IRA is that it avoids the temporary stoma frequently required for an RPC and avoids the potential compromise to sexual function accompanying proctectomy. It is also has a lower morbidity and mortality. However, the rectum requires regular surveillance. Even with optimal surveillance of the rectal remnant, up to 10% of patients will develop invasive malignancy within a 30-year follow up period. Restorative proctocolectomy has the advantage of removing the whole colon and rectum. However, there is a pouch failure rate of approximately 10%. In addition, and particularly where a stapled anastomosis has been created, there remains a small but definite incidence of cancer developing in the small strip of rectal mucosa between the pouch and the dentate line. Some advocate complete mucosectomy of the residual cuff and a transanal anastomosis, although this may result in worse function. In experienced hands a laparoscopic approach to these operations can be successful, with swifter recovery and improved cosmesis.

POSTOPERATIVE SURVEILLANCE

Because of the risk of further tumour formation, follow-up is important and takes the form of rectal/pouch surveillance, with biopsy of the cuff recommended yearly. Gastroscopies are also carried out to detect upper gastrointestinal tumours (notably duodenal adenomas). Despite this, lifespan is reduced because of the development of duodenal and ampullary cancers and complications of desmoid tumours.

Hereditary non-polyposis colorectal cancer (Lynch syndrome)

Hereditary non-polyposis colorectal cancer (HNPCC) is characterised by an increased risk of colorectal cancer and also cancers of the endometrium, ovary, stomach and small intestine. It is an autosomal dominant condition caused by a mutation in one of the DNA mismatch repair genes. The most commonly affected genes are *MLH1* and *MSH2*. The lifetime risk of developing colorectal cancer is 80%, and the mean age of diagnosis is 45 years. Most cancers develop in the proximal colon. Females have a 30–50% lifetime risk of developing endometrial cancer.

DIAGNOSIS

HNPCC can be diagnosed by genetic testing or by the Amsterdam II criteria:

- three or more family members with an HNPCC-related cancer (colorectal, endometrial, small bowel, ureter, renal

pelvis), one of whom is a first-degree relative of the other two;
- two successive affected generations;
- at least one colorectal cancer diagnosed before the age of 50 years;
- FAP excluded;
- tumours verified by pathological examination.

Patients with HNPCC are offered regular endoscopic surveillance. The small intestine may also be radiologically assessed but this is of unproven benefit.

Malignant - colorectal cancer

Epidemiology

In the UK, colorectal cancer is the second most common cause of cancer death. Approximately 35 000 patients are diagnosed with colorectal cancer every year in the UK. Approximately one-third of these tumours are in the rectum and two-thirds in the colon. The burden of disease is similar in men and women. Colorectal cancer occurs less frequently in the resource-poor world than in resource-rich countries.

Aetiology

The accepted model of colorectal cancer development is that it arises from adenomatous polyps after a sequence of genetic mutations influenced by environmental factors. This adenoma–carcinoma sequence is based on strong observational evidence as outlined in *Summary box 70.3*. The adenoma–carcinoma sequence is not a simple stepwise progression of mutations but a complicated array of multiple genetic alterations, ultimately resulting in an invasive tumour. Mutations of the adenomatous polyposis coli (APC) gene occur in two-thirds of colonic adenomas and are thought to develop early in the carcinogenesis pathway. K-ras mutations result in activation of cell signalling pathways and are more common in larger lesions, suggesting that that they are later events in mutagenesis. The p53 gene is frequently mutated in carcinomas but not in adenomas and therefore thought to be a marker of invasion.

Summary box 70.3

Evidence for adenoma-carcinoma sequence

- The prevalence of adenomas and carcinomas is very similar – carcinoma patients are about 5 years older
- The distribution of adenomas in the colon is the same as that of cancers (70% left sided)
- When small cancers are studied they almost always have adjacent adenomatous tissue
- Adenomas are found in one-third of specimens resected for colorectal cancer
- Sporadic adenomas are identical to the adenomas of FAP, which is associated with a 100% chance of colorectal adenocarcinoma unless treated
- Larger adenomas are more likely to be dysplastic and to have higher grades of dysplasia than small adenomas
- Incidence of colorectal cancer falls within a screening programme that involves colonoscopy and polypectomy

There has been much interest in the association between diet and colon cancer. Worldwide, the prevalence of colorectal cancer is closely associated with intake of red meat and particularly processed meat products (haem and N-nitroso compounds). These adversely affect DNA in the colorectal mucosa. A protective effect of dietary fibre is also suggested by epidemiological studies. The hypothesis is that increased roughage is associated with reduced colonic transit times, and this in turn reduces the exposure of the mucosa to dietary carcinogens. Increased risk for colorectal cancer has also been associated with dietary animal fat, smoking and alcohol. Cholecystectomy may marginally increase the risk of right-sided colon cancer and inflammatory bowel disease is a well-recognized risk factor (see below).

Pathology

Macroscopically, the tumour may take one of four forms (Figure 70.3). The annular variety tends to give rise to obstructive symptoms, whereas the others present more commonly with bleeding. Most large bowel cancers arise from the left colon, notably the rectum (38%), sigmoid (21%), and descending colon (4%). Cancer of the caecum (12%) and ascending colon (5%) are less common, but may be gradually increasing in incidence. Cancer of the transverse colon (5.5%), flexures (2–3%) and appendix (0.5%) are relatively uncommon. Microscopically, the neoplasm is a columnar cell adenocarcinoma. Origin from a benign polyp may be evident in early cases, before the benign architecture is destroyed by malignant infiltration.

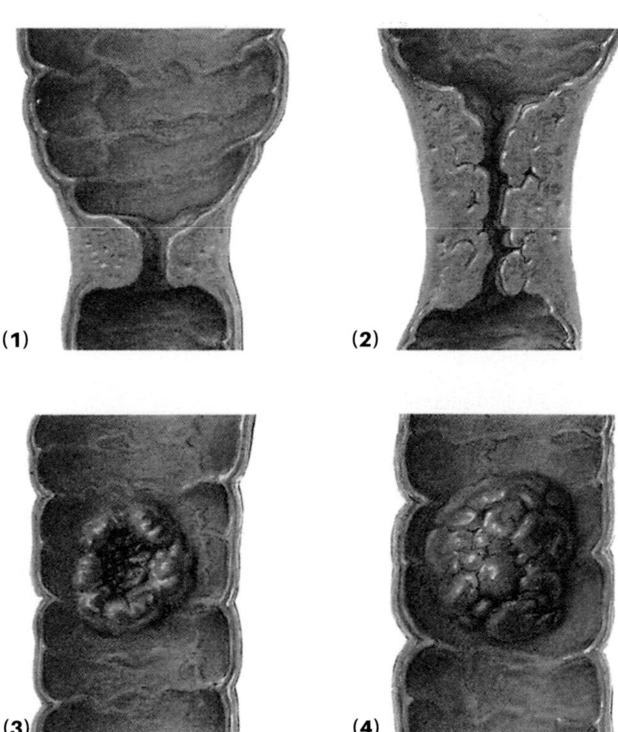

Figure 70.3 The four common macroscopic varieties of carcinoma of the colon: (1) annular; (2) tubular; (3) ulcer; (4) cauliflower.

Spread

Colonic cancer can spread locally or via the lymphatics, bloodstream or transcoelomically across the peritoneal cavity. Direct spread may be longitudinal or radial. Radial spread may be retroperitoneal into the ureter, duodenum and posterior abdominal wall muscles or intraperitoneal into adjacent organs or the anterior abdominal wall.

In general, involvement of the lymph nodes by the tumour progresses from those closest to the bowel along the course of lymphatics to central nodes. However, this orderly process does not always occur. Haematogenous spread is most commonly to the liver via the portal vein. One-third of patients will have liver metastases at the time of diagnosis and 50% will develop them at some point, accounting for the majority of deaths. The lung is the next most common site; metastasis to ovary, brain, kidney and bone is less common. Colorectal cancer can spread from the serosa of the bowel or via subperitoneal lymphatics to other structures within the peritoneal cavity, including peritoneum, ovary and omentum.

Staging colon cancer

A variety of staging systems are described for colorectal cancer based on pathological reporting to predict prognosis and guide adjuvant treatment. Dukes' classification was originally described for rectal tumours but has been adopted for histopathological reporting of colon cancer. Although it is simple and widely recognised (*Summary box 70.4*) the more detailed TNM system is regarded as the international standard (*Summary box 70.5*).

Summary box 70.4

Dukes' staging for colorectal cancer

- A: invasion of but not breaching the muscularis propria
- B: breaching the muscularis propria but not involving lymph nodes
- C: lymph nodes involved.

Dukes himself never described a stage D, but this is often used to describe metastatic disease

Summary box 70.5

TNM classification for colonic cancer

- T Tumour stage
  - T1 Into submucosa
  - T2 Into muscularis propria
  - T3 Into pericolic fat or subserosa but not breaching serosa
  - T4 Breaches serosa or directly involving another organ
- N Nodal stage
  - N0 No nodes involved
  - N1 1-3 nodes involved
  - N2 Four or more nodes involved
- M Metastases
  - M0 No metastases
  - M1 Metastases

Clinical features

Carcinoma of the colon typically occurs in patients over 50 years of age and is most common in the 8th decade of life. Emergency presentation occurs in 20% of cases and is associated with a considerably worse prognosis, even when matched for disease stage. A careful family history should be taken. Those with first-degree relatives who have developed colorectal cancer before the age of 45 years may be part of one of the colorectal cancer familial syndromes. Tumours of the left side of the colon usually present with a change in bowel habit or rectal bleeding, while proximal lesions typically present later, with iron deficiency anaemia or a mass (Figure 70.4). Patients commonly present with metastatic disease. Lesions of the flexures may present with vague upper abdominal symptoms for many months before symptoms suggestive of colonic disease appear.

Investigation of colon cancer

SCREENING

Colon cancer is suited to screening as prognosis is better for early stage disease and polypectomy allows the prevention of cancer development. In the UK, a screening programme has been introduced based on faecal occult blood testing of people aged 60–69 years, followed by colonoscopy in those who test positive. A guaiac-based test is used, which detects peroxidase-like activity of faecal haematin. Studies have suggested a 15–20% reduction in colorectal cancer specific mortality in the screened population. Flexible sigmoidoscopy can also be used as the initial screening tool, with a similar reduction in colorectal cancer specific mortality.

ENDOSCOPY

The 60-cm, fibreoptic, flexible sigmoidoscope is increasingly being used in 'one-stop' rectal bleeding clinics. The patient is prepared with an enema and sedation is not usually necessary. It is usually possible to assess the bowel up to the splenic flexure, which will detect up to 70% of cancers and almost all that cause fresh rectal bleeding (Figure 70.5). Colonoscopy is the investigation of choice if colorectal cancer is suspected,

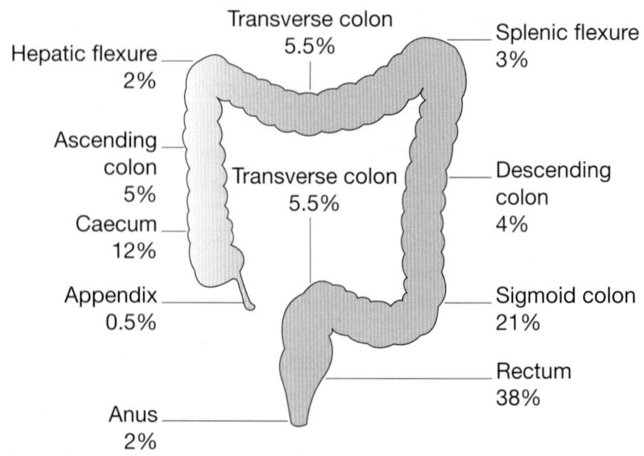

Figure 70.4 Distribution of colorectal cancer by site.

Cuthbert Esquire Dukes, 1890–1977, pathologist, St Mark's Hospital, London, UK. The original Dukes' classification in 1932 gave three stages, A–C.

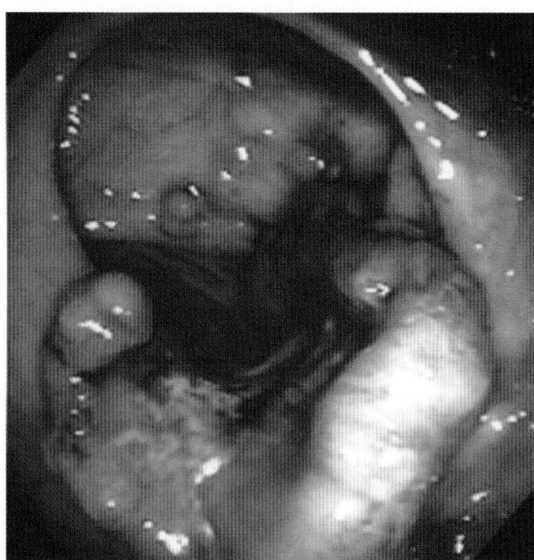

Figure 70.5 A cancer seen at colonoscopy.

provided the patient is fit enough to undergo the mechanical bowel preparation required. It has the advantage of not only picking up a primary cancer but also having the ability to detect synchronous polyps or other carcinomas, which occur in 3–5% of cases. There is a small risk of perforation (1:1000).

RADIOLOGY

Double-contrast barium enema has traditionally been used and shows a cancer of the colon as a constant irregular filling defect, often described as looking like an apple-core (Figure 70.6). False positives occur in 1–2% of cases and false negatives in 7–9% of cases. It has now been largely replaced by computed tomography (CT) virtual colonoscopy, which is extremely sensitive in picking up polyps down to a size of 6 mm (Figure 70.7). It has the advantage of being less invasive than colonoscopy but if a biopsy is required, an endoscopy will still be needed. CT is used as a diagnostic tool in patients with palpable abdominal masses. Spiral CT of the chest, abdomen and pelvis now represents the standard means of staging colorectal cancer, although chest x-ray and liver ultrasound are alternatives if CT is not readily available. Rectal cancer usually requires additional staging for local spread, using magnetic resonance imaging.

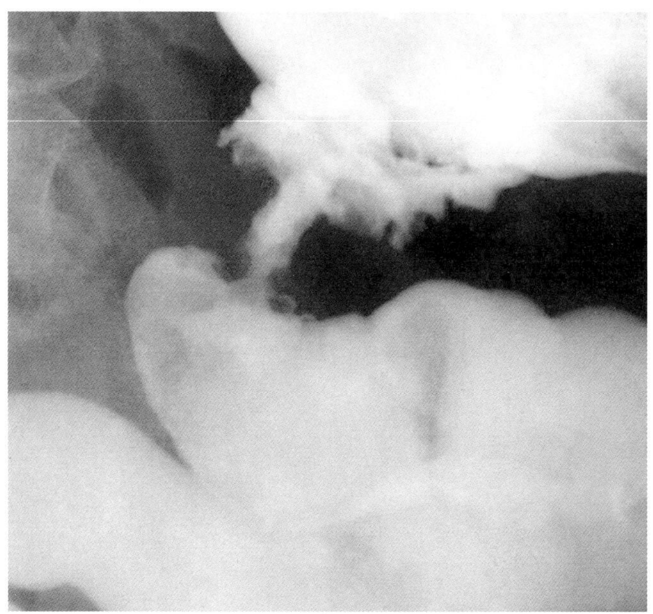

Figure 70.6 Barium enema showing a carcinoma of the sigmoid colon. It may have an 'apple core' appearance (i.e. a short, irregular stenosis with sharp shoulders at each end).

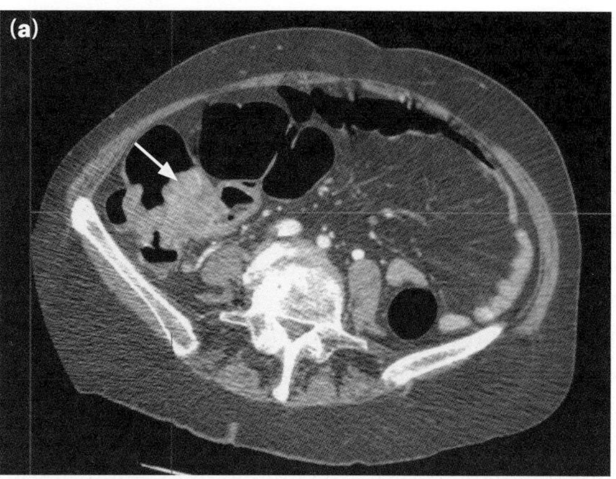

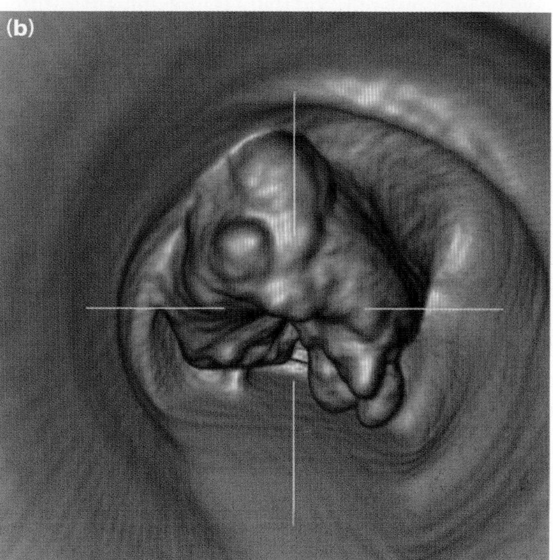

Figure 70.7 Virtual colonoscopy of the right colon. (a) Computed tomography scan of the abdomen showing a caecal tumour (arrow). (b) Formatted 'virtual' image of the same lesion as in (a) (courtesy of Dr A Slater, John Radcliffe Hospital, Oxford, UK).

Surgical treatment

PREOPERATIVE PREPARATION

Mechanical bowel preparation has fallen out of favour in surgery for colon cancer, with little evidence of benefit and some of an increased rate of wound infection. It currently remains in use largely for low rectal resection, where unprepared bowel may be associated with a higher infection rate. Anti-embolism stockings should be fitted and the patient started on prophylactic subcutaneous low molecular weight heparin. If available, manual compression boots are used perioperatively. Intravenous prophylactic antibiotics are given immediately before the start of surgery, to reduce the risk of surgical site infection. A single dose of antibiotics covering bowel organisms is as effective as multiple doses. In all cases where a stoma seems likely, careful preoperative counselling and marking of an appropriate site by an enterostomal therapist is essential.

OPERATIONS

The operations described are designed to remove the primary tumour and its draining locoregional lymph nodes. It is unusual to find unsuspected metastases at laparotomy (or laparoscopy) after CT staging, but the presence of peritoneal metastases may predicate a palliative strategy with a segmental resection and less aggressive lymphadenectomy. The use of stapling and hand-suturing techniques for colonic anastomoses have been compared, and there is probably little difference in leak rate. It is more important that healthy bowel, free of tension or distal obstruction, is used to construct an anastomosis and that patients are adequately nourished and free from active infection if anastomotic leakage is to be avoided.

Right hemicolectomy Carcinoma of the caecum or ascending colon (Figure 70.8) is treated by right hemicolectomy (Figure 70.9). At open surgery the peritoneum lateral to the ascending colon is incised, and the incision is carried around the hepatic flexure. The right colon and mesentery are elevated, taking care not to injure the ureter, gonadal vessels or the duodenum. The ileocolic artery is ligated close to its origin from the superior mesenteric artery ('high-tie') and divided. Where the right colic artery has a separate origin from the superior mesenteric artery (around 10% of patients) this is separately ligated. The mesentery of the distal 20 cm of ileum and the mesocolon as far as the proximal third of the transverse colon is divided. The greater omentum is divided up to the point of intended division of the transverse colon. When it is clear that there is an adequate blood supply at the resection margins, the right colon is resected, and an anastomosis is fashioned between the ileum and the transverse colon. If the tumour is at the hepatic flexure the resection must be extended further along the transverse colon and will involve dividing the right branch of the middle colic artery.

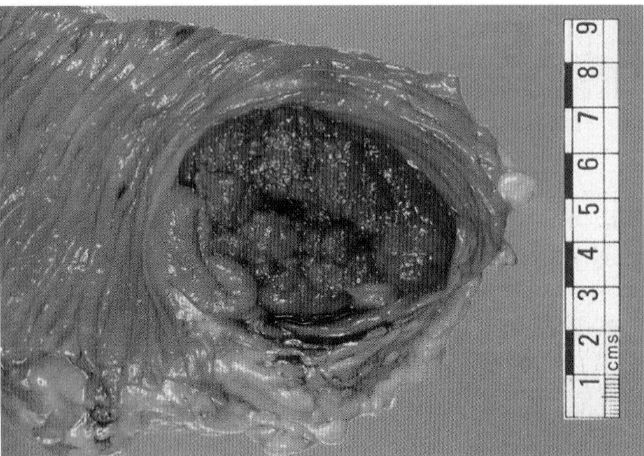

Figure 70.8 Large villous tumour of the caecum with malignant change.

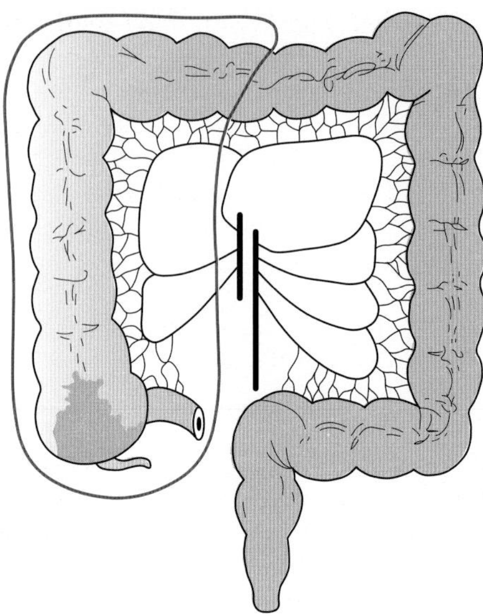

Figure 70.9 Schematic showing right hemicolectomy.

Extended right hemicolectomy Carcinomas of the transverse colon and splenic flexure are most commonly treated by an extended right hemicolectomy. The extent of the resection is from the right colon to the descending colon. The mobilisation is as for a right hemicolectomy but dissection continues to take down the splenic flexure and the whole transverse mesocolon is ligated. Some surgeons prefer to perform a left hemicolectomy for a splenic flexure cancer.

Left hemicolectomy This is the operation of choice for descending colon and sigmoid cancers (Figure 70.10). The left half of the colon is mobilised completely along the 'white line' that marks the lateral attachment of the mesocolon. As the sigmoid mesentery is mobilised, the left ureter and gonadal vessels must be identified and protected. The splenic flexure may be mobilised by extending the lateral dissection

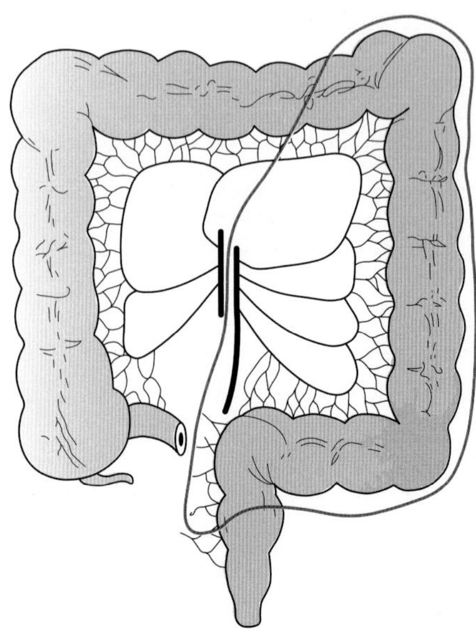

Figure 70.10 Schematic showing left hemicolectomy.

from below and completed by entering the lesser sac. The inferior mesenteric artery below its left colic branch, together with the related paracolic lymph nodes, is included in the resection by ligating the inferior mesenteric artery close to its origin ('high-tie'). For full mobility the inferior mesenteric vein is also ligated and divided at the lower border of the pancreas. The bowel and mesentery can then be resected to allow a tension-free anastomosis. A temporary diverting stoma may be fashioned upstream, usually by formation of a loop ileostomy. This is usually undertaken if the anastomosis is below the peritoneal reflection of the rectum, because healing is more likely to be impaired distally.

Laparoscopic surgery Laparoscopic surgery for colon cancer has been shown to have equivalent overall and cancer-related outcomes to open surgery. Lymph node harvests are equivalent to open surgery and initial concerns about reports of port site recurrence have been dispelled as the world experience has grown. In the UK, the National Institute for Health and Care Excellence has stated that laparoscopic colorectal surgery should be offered to suitable patients. Operation times are longer but wound infection rates, blood loss and postoperative pain scores are lower than for open surgery. The costs of laparoscopic surgery are, however, generally higher and this may particularly relevant where funds are limited.

It is not possible to palpate lesions, so if laparoscopic surgery is planned it is useful to tattoo the lesion at prior colonoscopy. The laparoscopic operation has particular advantages if performed in a medial to lateral manner – that is starting the dissection by controlling and dividing the major vascular pedicles and only taking the lateral peritoneal reflection once the mesocolon is completely free. Specimen retrieval and bowel anastomosis can then be performed via small incisions. Dedicated training in laparoscopic colorectal surgery is important, as there is a relatively long learning curve.

Emergency surgery

In the UK, 20% of patients with colonic cancer will present as an emergency, the majority with obstruction, but occasionally with haemorrhage or perforation. If the lesion is right sided, it is usually possible to perform a right hemicolectomy and anastomosis in the usual manner. If there has been perforation with substantial contamination or if the patient is unstable, it may be advisable to bring out an ileocolostomy rather than forming an anastomosis. For a left-sided lesion the decision lies between a Hartmann's procedure or resection and anastomosis. Where endoscopic and radiological facilities are present an obstructing left-sided lesion can be treated with an expanding metal stent (Figure 70.11). This has the advantage of converting an emergency operation with a high chance of a stoma to a situation that can be managed semi-electively by resection and anastomosis. Although early studies cast doubt on the benefits of colorectal stenting, more recently evidence has emerged that stenting leads to a reduction in stoma rates.

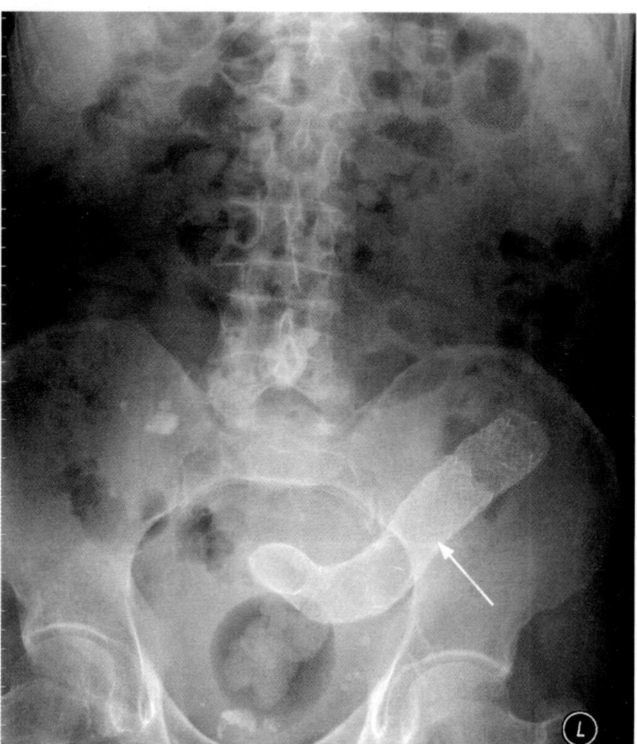

Figure 70.11 Abdominal radiograph demonstrating a colonic stent in position ((arrow) courtesy of Dr D Kasir, Hope Hospital, Salford, UK)

Postoperative care

After colonic surgery patients should be closely monitored, as there is a small incidence of postoperative bleeding. Antithrombosis measures should be continued as discussed in the preoperative section and are currently recommended for 28 days postoperatively. There is no advantage to placing intra-abdominal drains after colonic surgery. Wound infections are relatively common after colonic surgery and may well be more frequent than the 10% usually quoted. Anastomotic leaks occur in 4–8% of ileocolic or colocolic anastomoses. The possibility should be borne in mind in any patient not progressing as expected or with unexplained cardiac abnormalities, fever or worsening abdominal pain. Early investigation with contrast enhanced CT scan is appropriate. In the presence of sepsis or peritonitis, early return to theatre and taking down the leaking anastomosis with the formation of stomas is usually advised.

Prolonged nasogastric drainage, intravenous fluid therapy and cautious introduction of oral fluid and diet represented traditional postoperative practice. Enhanced recovery programmes have been shown to reduce length of hospital stay from 10–14 days to as little as 2–3 days, by modulating the surgical stress response and reducing post-operative ileus. It is important to appreciate that these programmes require multiple interventions to be instituted and considerable time, effort and education from the surgical, anaesthetic and ward teams.

Henri Albert Antoine Hartmann, 1860–1952, Professor of Clinical Surgery in the Faculty of Medicine, University of Paris, France.

Summary box 70.6

Key elements of an enhanced recovery programme

- Preadmission counselling
- Avoidance of mechanical bowel preparation
- Preoperative carbohydrate loading
- Avoidance of preoperative dehydration
- No nasogastric tubes
- Short, transverse incisions (or laparoscopic procedure)
- Short-acting anaesthetic drugs
- Avoidance of perioperative fluid/salt overload
- Thoracic epidurals
- Avoidance of opiate analgesia
- Maintenance of perioperative temperature
- Prevention of postoperative nausea and vomiting
- Early mobilisation
- Early introduction of oral fluids/diets/supplements
- Early removal of urinary catheters
- Continual audit of outcomes

Adjuvant therapy

In most patients with colon cancer there is little clear benefit of preoperative chemotherapy, although trials in selected patient groups with locally advanced disease are ongoing. There is evidence that adjuvant chemotherapy improves outcome after surgery in patients with node-positive disease (Dukes C).

Metastatic disease

Hepatic metastases can be resected and series have demonstrated 5-year survival of over 30% in resectable disease. Liver surgeons are increasingly aggressive in treatment and the only absolute limitation on what can be resected relates to leaving behind sufficient functioning liver, although this clearly has to be moderated by patient factors. It is important not to biopsy potentially resectable hepatic metastases as this may cause tumour dissemination. Imaging will usually correctly identify colorectal metastases and assess patients suitable for liver resection (Figure 70.12). The role of chemotherapy and the timing of colonic and hepatic surgery in synchronous metastases is still a matter of debate and such cases should be carefully discussed by a multidisciplinary team. Isolated lung metastases may occasionally be suitable for resection but they are more commonly accompanied by metastases elsewhere. In patients with widespread disease, palliative chemotherapy is offered alongside symptomatic treatment and support by a palliative care team.

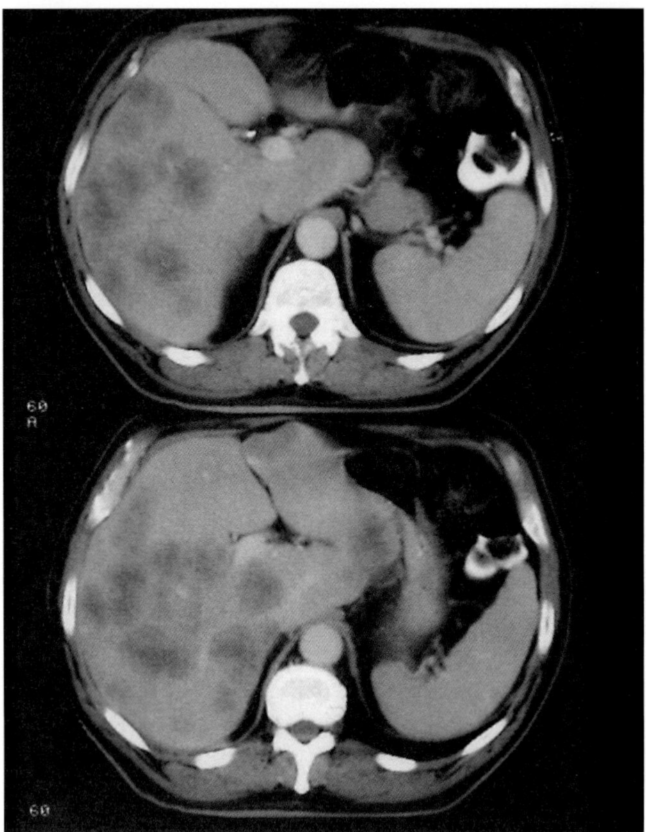

Figure 70.12 Computed tomography scan of the liver showing multiple metastases from carcinoma of the colon.

Prognosis

Overall 5-year survival for colorectal cancer is approximately 50%. The most important determinant of prognosis is tumour stage and, in particular, lymph node status. Patients with disease confined to the bowel wall (Dukes stage A) will usually have cure by surgical resection alone and over 90% will have disease-free survival at 5 years. Spread beyond the bowel wall (Dukes B) reduces 5-year survival to approximately 60–70%. Patients with lymph node metastases (Dukes C) have a 5-year survival of 30%, while fewer than 10% of patients presenting with metastatic disease at the outset will be alive 5 years later.

Colorectal cancer follow-up

Since the advent of safe liver resection for metastases the outcome benefit of follow-up has been clearly demonstrated. Follow-up aims to identify synchronous bowel tumours (present in 3%) that were not picked up at the time of original diagnosis due to emergency presentation or incomplete assessment. Similarly, 3% of patients will develop a metachronous (at a different time) colonic cancer and surveillance colonoscopy is designed to diagnose these. Up to a half of all patients with colorectal cancer will develop liver metastases at some point and regular imaging of the liver (by ultrasound and CT scan) and measurement of carcinoembryonic antigen (CEA) is designed to diagnose this early, in order to allow curative metastectomy. Trials of the optimum follow-up pathway have suggested that CEA measurement alone can be as effective as regular imaging.

INFLAMMATORY BOWEL DISEASE

The term 'inflammatory bowel disease' is reserved for conditions characterised by the presence of idiopathic intestinal inflammation (i.e. ulcerative colitis [UC] and Crohn's disease [CD]. Although the availability of population genetics and molecular biology has contributed to our understanding of the pathogenesis of inflammatory bowel disease, the aetiology remains unclear.

Ulcerative colitis

UC is a disease of the rectum and colon with extraintestinal manifestations. The incidence is 10 per 100000 per year in the UK with a prevalence of 160 per 100000 population. UC affects men and women equally in early life, although it is said to be more common in males in later life. It is most commonly diagnosed between the ages of 20 and 40. UC is far more common in the USA and Western Europe but relatively rare in the Far East and tropics. Asians who spent their childhood before the age of 14 in Asia have a much lower incidence of UC than Asians born and raised in the UK, suggesting an important effect of environmental exposure in childhood.

Aetiology

The cause of UC is unknown. There is clearly a genetic contribution, as 10–20% of patients have a first-degree relative with inflammatory bowel disease. Patients with severe colitis have a reduction in the number of anaerobic bacteria and in the variability of bacterial strains in the colon, but no causative link with any specific organism has been identified. Unlike CD, smoking seems to have a protective effect in UC and has even been the basis of therapeutic trials of nicotine. Relapses are occasionally said to be associated with periods of stress, but personality and psychiatric profiles in patients with UC are the same as those of the normal population.

Pathology

In virtually all cases the disease starts in the rectum and extends proximally in continuity. Colonic inflammation is diffuse, confluent and superficial, primarily affecting the mucosa and superficial submucosa. 'Pseudopolyposis' occurs in almost one-quarter of cases. Stricturing in UC is very unusual (unlike CD) and should prompt urgent assessment because of the possibility of coexisting carcinoma. A small proportion of patients develop irregular mucosal swellings (dysplasia-associated lesions or mass [DALMs]), which are highly predictive of coexisting carcinoma.

Histological examination reveals an increase in inflammatory cells in the lamina propria and the crypts of Lieberkuhn and there are 'crypt abscesses'. There is depletion of goblet cell mucin. With time, precancerous changes can develop (dysplasia). High-grade dysplasia is regarded as an indication for surgery as 40% of colectomy specimens in which high-grade dysplasia was detected will have evidence of a colorectal cancer. In contrast, optimum management of low-grade dysplasia is currently controversial. Ten to twenty per cent of patients with low-grade dysplasia will have a cancer at colectomy. The progression rate of low-grade dysplasia to invasive cancer is unclear and many cancers in patients with low-grade dysplasia probably develop without high-grade dysplasia.

Symptoms

Clinical presentation depends in large part on the extent of disease. If confined to the rectum (proctitis), there is usually no systemic upset and extra-alimentary manifestations are rare. The main symptoms are rectal bleeding, tenesmus and mucous discharge. The disease remains confined to the rectum in 90% of cases but proctitis may extend proximally. Colitis is almost always associated with bloody diarrhoea and urgency. Severe and/or extensive colitis may result in anaemia, hypoproteinaemia and electrolyte disturbances. Pain is unusual. Children with poorly controlled colitis may have impaired growth. The more extensive the disease the more likely extraintestinal manifestations are to occur. Extensive colitis is also associated with systemic illness, characterised by malaise, loss of appetite, and fever.

Classification of colitis severity

The assessment of severity of UC is determined by frequency of bowel action and the presence of systemic signs of illness:

- Mild disease is characterized by fewer than four stools daily, with or without bleeding. There are no systemic signs of toxicity.
- Moderate disease corresponds to more than four stools daily, but with few signs of systemic illness. There may be mild anaemia. Abdominal pain may occur. Inflammatory markers, including erythrocyte sedimentation rate and C-reactive protein, are often raised.
- Severe disease corresponds to more than six bloody stools a day and evidence of systemic illness, with fever, tachycardia, anaemia and raised inflammatory markers. Hypoalbuminaemia is common and an ominous finding.
- Fulminant disease is associated with more than 10 bowel movements daily, fever, tachycardia, continuous bleeding, anaemia, hypoalbuminaemia, abdominal tenderness and distension, the need for blood transfusion and, in the most severe cases, progressive colonic dilation ('toxic megacolon'). This is a very significant finding, suggestive of disintegrative colitis, and an indication for emergency surgery if colonic perforation is to be avoided.

Extraintestinal manifestations

Arthritis occurs in around 15% of patients and is typically a large joint polyarthropathy, affecting knees, ankles, elbows and wrists. Sacroiliitis and ankylosing spondylitis are 20 times more common in patients with UC than the general population and are associated with the HLA-B27 genotype. Sclerosing cholangitis is associated with UC and can progress to cirrhosis and hepatocellular failure. Patients with UC and sclerosing cholangitis are also at a significantly greater risk of development of large bowel cancer. Cholangiocarcinoma is an extremely rare association and its frequency is not influenced by colectomy. The skin lesions erythema nodosum and pyoderma gangrenosum are associated with UC and both normally resolve with good colitis control. The eyes can also be affected by uveitis and episcleritis.

Acute colitis

Approximately 5% of patients present with severe acute (fulminant) colitis. Intensive medical treatment leads to remission in 70% but the remainder require urgent surgery. Toxic dilatation should be suspected in patients who develop severe abdominal pain and confirmed by the presence on a plain abdominal radiograph of a colon with a diameter of more than 6 cm (Figure 70.13). A reduction in stool frequency is not always a sign of improvement in patients with severe UC, and a falling stool frequency, abdominal distension and abdominal pain (resulting from progression of the inflammatory process through the colonic wall) are strongly suggestive of disintegrative colitis and impending perforation. Plain abdominal radiographs should be obtained daily in patients with severe colitis, and a progressive increase in colon diameter despite medical therapy is an indication for urgent surgery. Colonic perforation is a grave complication with a mortality rate of 40%. Steroids may mask the physical signs. Severe haemorrhage is uncommon (1–2%) but may occasionally require urgent surgical intervention.

Cancer risk in colitis

The risk of cancer in ulcerative colitis increases with duration of disease. At 10 years from diagnosis it is approximately 1%, increasing to 10–15% at 20 years and 20% at 30 years. Patients with pancolitis (defined as the presence of inflammation proximal to the splenic flexure) of more than ten years duration should be entered into screening programmes in order to detect clinically silent dysplasia, which is predictive of increased cancer risk. The value of screening programmes remains somewhat controversial, however, with most UC patients who develop cancer (approximately 3.5% of all patients) presenting with their tumours in-between attendances for screening colonoscopy. Carcinoma is more likely to occur if the whole colon is involved (Figure 70.14) or if the disease started early in life. Malignant change, often atypical and high grade, may occur at many sites at once. Colonoscopic surveillance with dye-spray (chromo-endoscopy) or multiple biopsies every 10 cm is undertaken to look for subtle mucosal abnormalities, which can occur in flat mucosa, or a DALM.

Investigations

ENDOSCOPY AND BIOPSY

Rigid/flexible sigmoidoscopy can detect proctitis in the clinic; the mucosa is hyperaemic and bleeds on touch, and there may be a purulent exudate. Where there has been remission and relapse, there may be regenerative mucosal nodules or pseudopolyps. Later, tiny ulcers may be seen that appear to coalesce. Colonoscopy and biopsy has a key role in diagnosis and management:

1 to establish the extent of inflammation, although colonoscopy is contraindicated in severe acute colitis because of the risk of colonic perforation;
2 to distinguish between UC and Crohn's colitis (although this can be exceptionally difficult, *Table 70.2*);
3 to monitor the response to treatment;
4 to assess longstanding cases for malignant change.

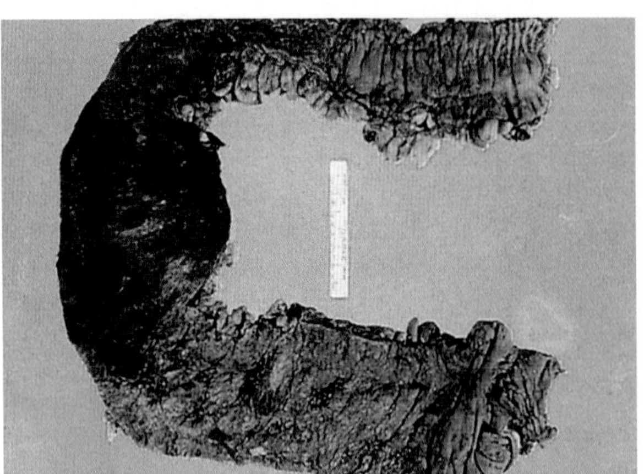

Figure 70.13 Fulminating ulcerative colitis with toxic dilatation of the transverse colon.

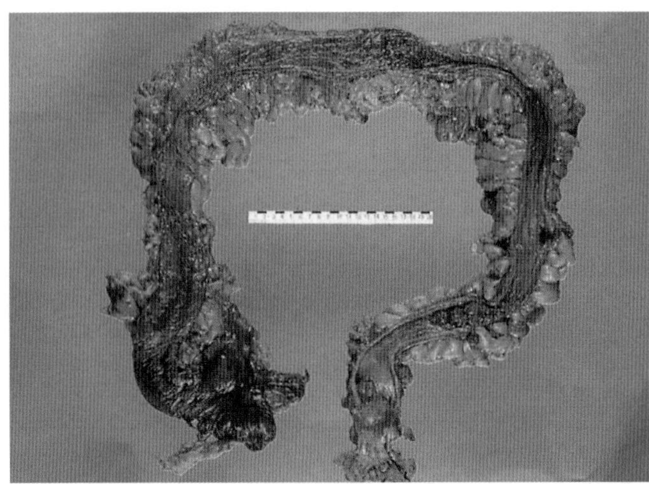

Figure 70.14 Resection specimen from a patient with long-standing ulcerative colitis showing a narrow tubular colon with areas of cancerous change in the rectum and sigmoid (courtesy of Dr B Warren, John Radcliffe Hospital, Oxford, UK).

RADIOLOGY

A plain abdominal film may indicate the severity of disease in the acute setting and is particularly valuable in demonstrating the development of toxic megacolon. Barium enema has largely been replaced by CT, although a contrast study will

TABLE 70.2 Distinguishing ulcerative colitis (UC) and Crohn's disease (CD).

	UC	CD
Macroscopic		
Distribution	Colon/rectum	Anywhere in the gastrointestinal tract
Rectum	Always involved	Often spared
Perianal disease	Rare	Common
Fistula formation	Rare	Common
Stricture	Rare	Common
Microscopic		
Layers involved	Mucosa/submucosa	Full thickness
Granulomas	No	Common
Fissuring	No	Common
Crypt abscesses	Common	Rare

show a featureless colon. CT findings in pancolitis may show significant thickening of the colonic wall, as well as inflammatory stranding in the colonic mesentery (Figure 70.15).

BACTERIOLOGY

A stool specimen should be sent for microbiological analysis when UC is suspected, in order to exclude infective colitides, notably *Campylobacter*, which may be very difficult to distinguish from acute severe UC. *Clostridium difficile* colitis may need to be considered in populations at risk of this disease (see below).

Treatment

Effective treatment of UC requires a multidisciplinary approach to management. This involves the gastroenterologist, nurses, nutritionist, enterostomal therapists and, occasionally, clinical psychologists and social workers as well as the surgeon.

Summary box 70.7

Principles of management of ulcerative colitis

- Many patients can be adequately maintained for years on medical therapy
- Toxic dilatation must be suspected in any colitic patient who develops severe abdominal pain; missed colonic perforation is associated with a high mortality
- Colitic patients are at increased risk of developing cancer; those with pancolitis of long duration are most at risk

MEDICAL TREATMENT

Medical therapy is based on anti-inflammatory agents. The 5-aminosalicylic acid (5-ASA) derivatives can be given topically (per rectum) or systemically. They act as inhibitors of the cyclo-oxygenase enzyme system and are formulated to protect the aspirin-related drug from degradation before reaching the colon. They can be used long term as maintenance therapy.

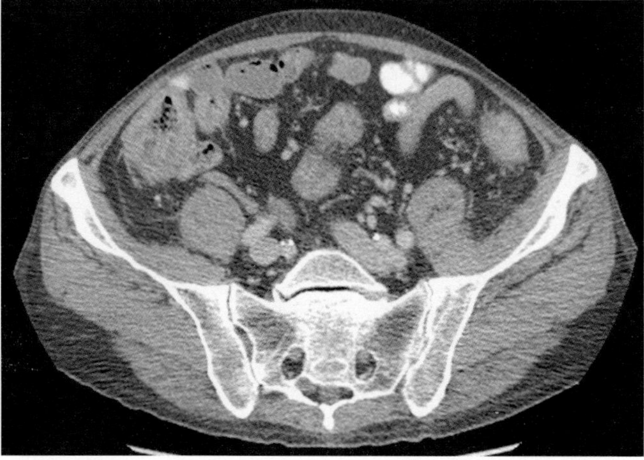

Figure 70.15 Computed tomography scan demonstrating colitis with thickened colonic wall and inflammatory stranding in the mesentery (courtesy of Dr D Kasir, Hope Hospital, Salford, UK).

Corticosteroids are the mainstay of treatment for 'flare-ups', either topically or systemically, and have a widespread anti-inflammatory action. The immunosuppressive drugs azathioprine and cyclosporin can be used to maintain remission and as 'steroid-sparing' agents. The monoclonal antibodies infliximab and adalimumab both act against antitumour necrosis factor alpha, which has a central role in inflammatory cascades. Most recently, vedolizumab, which blocks integrins, has been used as 'rescue therapy' for severe colitis, to try and avoid emergency colectomy.

ACUTE COLITIS

Patients with a mild attack usually respond to a course of oral prednisolone. A moderate attack often responds to oral prednisolone, twice-daily steroid enemas and 5-ASA. Failure to achieve remission as an outpatient is an indication for admission. Severe attacks of UC occur in up to 10% of patients and are emergencies, requiring hospital admission. Regular assessment of vital signs, weight and the abdomen is required. A stool chart should be kept and a plain abdominal radiograph is taken daily and inspected for dilatation of the transverse colon. The presence of mucosal islands or intramural gas on plain radiographs, increasing colonic diameter or a sudden increase in pulse and temperature may indicate a colonic perforation. Fluid and electrolyte balance is maintained, anaemia corrected and adequate nutrition is provided, sometimes intravenously in severe cases. The patient is treated with intravenous hydrocortisone four times daily, as well as rectal steroids. If there is failure to gain an improvement within 48 hours of commencing high-dose intravenous steroids, then surgery should be considered and it is certainly advisable if there has been no improvement within 3–5 days. Regular and joint review by gastroenterologist and surgeon is essential to identify patients who are failing to make anticipated progress and to ensure that surgery is neither inappropriately delayed nor undertaken. Gastroenterologists will use azathioprine, cyclosporin or infliximab in severe acute attacks to attempt to induce remission.

INDICATIONS FOR SURGERY

The greatest likelihood of a patient with UC requiring surgery is during the first year after diagnosis. The overall risk of colectomy is 20%. Indications for surgery in UC are:

- severe or fulminating disease failing to respond to medical therapy;
- chronic disease with anaemia, frequent stools, urgency and tenesmus;
- steroid-dependent disease – here, the disease is not severe but remission cannot be maintained without substantial doses of steroids;
- inability of the patient to tolerate medical therapy required to control the disease (steroid psychosis or other side effects, azathioprine-induced pancreatitis), such that remission cannot be maintained;
- neoplastic change: patients who have severe dysplasia or carcinoma on review colonoscopy;
- extraintestinal manifestations;
- rarely, severe haemorrhage or stenosis causing obstruction.

OPERATIVE TREATMENT FOR UC

Emergency In the emergency situation, (or for a patient who is malnourished or on steroids), the 'first aid' procedure is a subtotal colectomy and end ileostomy. The rectosigmoid stump is left long and can either be brought out as a mucous fistula or closed just beneath the skin. This operation has the advantages that the patient avoids a pelvic operation while unwell, that colonic histology can be assessed and restorative surgery can be contemplated at a later date when the patient is no longer on steroids and has fully recovered. The mesentery is divided close to the bowel and the omentum should be preserved if possible. Dissection of the left colon is continued to divide the sigmoid at a level that will comfortably reach the skin as a mucous fistula. The temptation to close the rectal stump and leave it stapled off in the pelvis should be avoided if at all possible. The diseased rectum may disintegrate, causing a pelvic abscess and severe sepsis, with potentially fatal consequences. Allowing the rectal remnant to discharge through the mucous fistula not only minimises the risk of this serious complication but may also allow the delivery of a high-dose topical steroid or 5-ASA compound, via the mucous fistula, into the isolated rectum. An emergency subtotal colectomy can be performed laparoscopically, provided the surgeon and theatre team has adequate experience.

Elective surgery The indications for elective surgery include:

1 failure of medical therapy/steroid dependence;
2 growth retardation in the young;
3 extraintestinal disease (polyarthropathy and pyoderma gangrenosum respond to colectomy);
4 malignant change.

In the elective setting four operations are available – all of these can be successfully performed laparoscopically in experienced hands:

1 subtotal colectomy and ileostomy (as in an emergency);
2 proctocolectomy and permanent end ileostomy;
3 restorative proctocolectomy with ileoanal pouch;
4 subtotal colectomy and ileorectal anastomosis.

Segmental resections are not recommended as even when the right side is not obviously involved there is a high recurrence rate in the remaining colon. Subtotal colectomy with ileostomy is performed electively for a frail patient, a patient who cannot be weaned from steroids and when there is doubt as to whether the colitis may represent CD. A pouch, a completion proctectomy and even an ileorectal anastomosis can be considered at a future date.

Proctocolectomy and ileostomy This operation removes all the colon and rectum, removing any risk of colorectal neoplasia or colitic symptoms, but it leaves a permanent stoma. It has a lower complication rate compared with a pouch procedure, although the perineal wound can be problematic (10% fail to heal) and stoma problems are common. It is indicated for patients who are not candidates for restorative surgery due to sphincter problems or patient preference. The colectomy is performed as above. Provided there is no concern regarding rectal cancer, a close rectal dissection may be performed to minimise damage to the pelvic nerves, avoiding erectile and bladder dysfunction. An intersphincteric excision of the anus is undertaken, which results in a smaller perineal wound and fewer healing problems. A permanent end ileostomy is formed. The position of the ileostomy should be carefully chosen by the patient with the help of a stoma care nurse specialist.

Restorative proctocolectomy with an ileoanal pouch (Parks) In this operation, a pouch is made out of ileum (Figure 70.16) as a substitute for the rectum and sewn or stapled to the anal canal. This avoids a permanent stoma. It is reserved for patients with adequate anal sphincters and

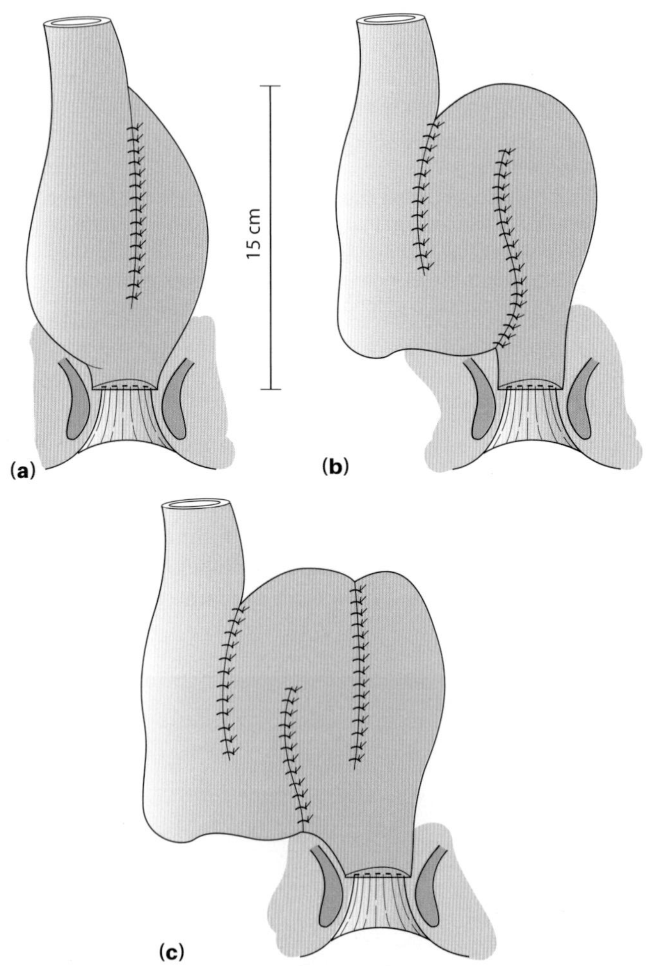

Figure 70.16 Ileoanal anastomosis with pouch. A substitute rectum is made from joined folds of ileum to form an expanded pouch of small intestine. The pouch is then joined directly to the anus at the level of the dentate line, all other rectal mucosa having been removed. Three ways of forming a pouch are illustrated: (a) a simple reversed 'J'; (b) an 'S' pouch; (c) a 'W' pouch.

Sir Alan Guyatt Parks, 1920–1982, surgeon, St Mark's Hospital and the London Hospital, London, UK, former President of the Royal College of Surgeons of England.

should be avoided if CD is a possibility. Various pouch designs have been described, but the 'J' is the most popular and the most easily made using staplers (Figure 70.17). There is some controversy over the correct technique for ileoanal anastomosis. In the earliest operations, the mucosa from the dentate line up to mid-rectum was stripped off the underlying muscle, but it is now known that a long muscle cuff is not needed. Although mucosectomy of the upper anal canal with an anastomosis at the dentate line is claimed to remove all of the at-risk mucosa and any problem of subsequent cancer, it may also increase the risk of incontinence with nocturnal seepage. The alternative is an anastomosis double-stapled to the top of the anal canal, preserving the upper anal mucosa. Continence appears to be better, but there is a theoretical risk of leaving inflamed mucosa behind. The procedure can be carried out in stages and a covering loop ileostomy is virtually always used.

Complications include pelvic infection (usually resulting from a leak at the ileoanal anastomosis or, in a J pouch, from the top of the 'J'), postoperative small bowel obstruction (which may occur in as many as 10–15% of patients) and pouch vaginal fistula. Frequency of evacuation is determined by pouch volume, completeness of emptying, reservoir inflammation and intrinsic small bowel motility, but is typically between three and eight evacuations in each 24-hour period. Increased frequency, urgency and faecal incontinence are common (20%, 5% and 5%, respectively), but usually reduce with time. Approximately 50% of patients with ileoanal pouches have a very good quality of life, whereas 35% of patients are less satisfied but choose to retain their pouches. Pouch function is so poor in 15% that the pouch is removed. The main reasons for failure are pelvic infection (50%), poor function (30%) and pouchitis or inflammation of the pouch (10%). It is also important for women of reproductive age to be advised that they may suffer from reduced fertility, as well as vaginal dryness, due to denervation of the secretory glands of the vaginal mucosa. Women who have not completed their families may elect for a colectomy with ileostomy and a pouch later.

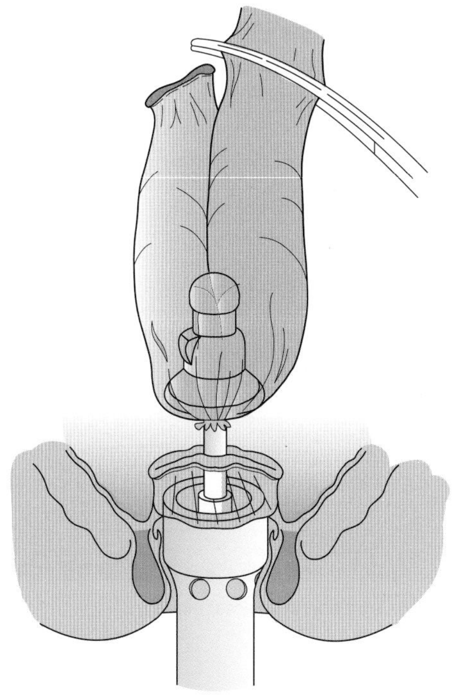
Figure 70.17 Stapled 'J' pouch with stapler creating a pouch–anus anastomosis.

Pouchitis describes an inflammatory condition, which may affect 30% of patients with an ileoanal pouch for colitis. It is characterised not only by the presence of inflammation in the pouch (which is common and frequently asymptomatic) but also by symptoms of pouch dysfunction (increased frequency, tenesmus, bleeding, purulent discharge) and systemic illness (malaise, fever, raised inflammatory markers). The cause of pouchitis is unknown but it appears to relate to inflammatory bowel disease (pouchitis does not usually occur in pouches created for other indications). Alterations in bacteria flora may be relevant as pouchitis usually responds to a short course of antibiotic therapy, notably with metronidazole or ciprofloxacin and can be followed by maintenance with probiotics.

Colectomy and ileorectal anastomosis This procedure is occasionally performed in UC if there is minimal rectal inflammation. A very considerable percentage (at least 50%) of patients with a quiescent rectum after total colectomy will develop significant mucosal inflammation in the rectum once the faecal stream has been re-established. Although rectal inflammation can be controlled with medical treatment, functional results may be disappointing. If the rectum is preserved, then annual rectal inspection is advocated. Although this procedure has the advantage of avoiding a stoma and the risk to sexual function associated with rectal dissection, it has largely fallen out of favour due to the ongoing risk of persisting inflammation and malignancy in the retained rectum.

Indeterminate colitis

Ten percent of patients with colitis present with histological features that make their disease difficult to characterise. Such patients may be said to have an 'indeterminate colitis'. Indeterminate colitis is, therefore, an indication by a pathologist that the nature of the underlying colitis (and therefore the likely course of the illness) is unclear. While the clinical history may suggest the diagnosis in some cases (for example, a history of recurrent perianal sepsis and fistulation would make a diagnosis of CD more likely), in others it may remain unclear whether a patient has UC or CD. In such cases, it may still be appropriate to offer a pouch after detailed informed consent, but the risks of pouch failure appear to be significantly higher (up to 25–30%) and patients should be advised accordingly.

Crohn's disease of the colon

CD affecting the small bowel is discussed in Chapter 69. Colonic involvement is found in 30% of patients with CD, frequently in association with perianal disease and it may coexist with small bowel pathology. Colonic CD presents

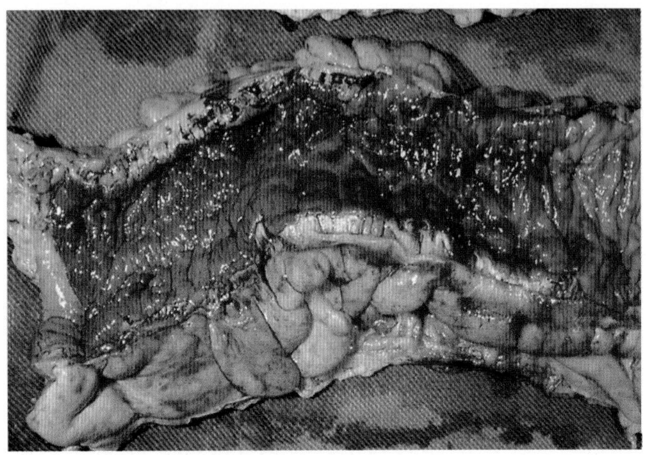

Figure 70.18 Colonic Crohn's disease. Note the normal mucosa on either side of the inflammatory stricture (courtesy of Dr B Warren, John Radcliffe Hospital, Oxford, UK).

with symptoms of colitis and proctitis as described for UC, although toxic megacolon is much less common (Figure 70.18). Colonic strictures may form just as are seen in small bowel CD. Endoscopic dilatation may be performed in expert hands as an alternative to surgical resection. Distinguishing between CD and UC is often difficult and requires clinical and pathological patterns to be combined. The presence of skip lesions, rectal sparing, non-caseating granulomas or perianal disease will point to CD.

Colonoscopic examination may be normal or show patchy inflammation. There will be areas of normal colon or rectum in between areas of inflamed mucosa that are irregular and ulcerated, with a mucopurulent exudate. The earliest appearances are aphthous ulcers surrounded by a rim of erythematous mucosa. These become larger and deeper with increasing severity of disease. There may be stricturing, and it is important to exclude malignancy in these sites. An irregular Crohn's stricture with polypoid mucosa may be almost indistinguishable from malignancy.

Treatment

There is great overlap in the treatment of Crohn's colitis and UC. Disease activity can be controlled with 5-ASA compounds and flare-ups treated with steroids. Rectal agents can be particularly effective if the disease activity is localised to the rectum. Immunomodulatory agents are frequently used, particularly if there is evidence of CD activity in large and small bowel.

Although CD is usually regarded as a contraindication to pouch surgery, the other options (panproctocolectomy or total colectomy with ileorectal anastomosis) are frequently appropriate and there may be considerable rectal sparing in CD, justifying the latter. Where the diagnosis of CD is firmly established, segmental rather than total colectomy may be appropriate.

INFECTIONS OF THE LARGE INTESTINE

Campylobacter

Infection with *Campylobacter jejuni* (a gram-negative rod with a distinctive spiral shape) is the commonest form of gastroenteritis in the UK, typically acquired from eating infected poultry. It causes diarrhoea and abdominal pain. Severe cases may resemble UC. The organism may take several days to isolate on stool culture. Treatment is supportive as it usually resolves without antibiotics, but severe colitis and even perforation may occur. It is a notifiable disease.

Intestinal amoebiasis

Entamoeba histolytica has a worldwide distribution and is transmitted mainly in contaminated drinking water. It can cause colonic ulcers, which are described as 'bottlenecked' because they have considerably undermined edges. The ulcers typically also have a yellow necrotic floor, from which blood and pus exude. In the majority of cases they are confined to the distal sigmoid colon and the rectum. Clinically amoebiasis can mimic UC, most commonly causing bloody diarrhoea, but more severe colonic complications can occur, including severe haemorrhage, stricture formation or perforation. A pericolitis is not uncommon and results in adhesions and may cause intestinal obstruction. Amoebiasis may cause liver abscesses or an amoebic mass ('amoeboma') of the caecum or sigmoid which is difficult to distinguish from a carcinoma. Surgery is fraught with danger as the bowel is extremely friable.

Endoscopic biopsies or fresh hot stools are examined to look for the presence of amoebae (Figure 70.19). It is important to emphasise, however, that the presence of the parasite does not indicate that it is pathogenic. It is especially important to exclude amoebic infection in patients suspected of having UC. Treatment is by metronidazole in the acute setting,

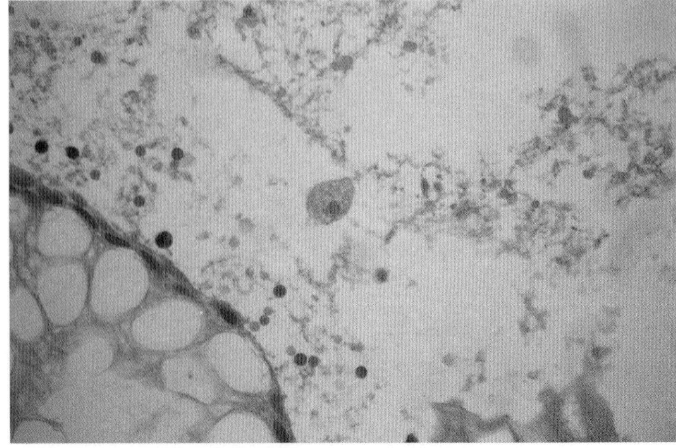

Figure 70.19 An amoeba in a rectal biopsy.

Burrill Bernard Crohn, 1884–1983, gastroenterologist, Mount Sinai Hospital, New York, NY, USA, along with Leon Ginzburg and Gordon Oppenheimer described regional ileitis in 1932.

three times daily for 7–10 days. Diloxanide furoate is effective against chronic infections associated with the passage of cysts in stools.

Salmonellosis, typhoid and paratyphoid

Salmonella are a family of gram-negative rods that can cause a range of enteric infections. Salmonella gastroenteritis is typically caused by *S. enteritidis* from poultry, and is most often a self-limiting illness comprising headache, fever and watery diarrhoea. When severe, antibiotics and indeed hospitalisation and intravenous fluids may be needed. The diagnosis is based on stool culture. *Shigella* and enteropathogenic strains of *E. coli* may cause similar diarrhoeal illnesses.

Typhoid fever is caused by *S. typhi* and presents with fever and abdominal pain after a 10–20-day incubation period. Over the next week, the patient can develop distension, diarrhoea, splenomegaly and characteristic 'rose spots' on the abdomen caused by a vasculitis. A number of surgical complications can result:

- paralytic ileus;
- intestinal haemorrhage;
- perforation;
- cholecystitis.

In addition, invasion of the systemic circulation, which is a characteristic feature of salmonellosis, may cause severe gram-negative sepsis and septic shock may develop. Some patients may develop metastatic sepsis, including septic arthritis and osteomyelitis, meningitis, encephalitis and pancreatitis.

Human immunodeficiency virus (HIV)

Intestinal complications are common after the development of AIDS when opportunistic organisms can cause gastroenteritis (*Summary box 70.8*). HIV1 may also cause a specific enteropathy. Treatment is directed towards the responsible organism and surgery should be avoided.

Clostridium difficile

Clostridium difficile is a toxin-producing gram-positive bacillus that is an increasing concern in many hospitals. Although normally present in around 2% of the population, it proliferates after antibiotic treatment (especially cephalosporins). Clinically, *C. difficile* infection presents with diarrhoea, abdominal pain and fever. Infection may progress to pseudomembranous colitis, so called because on visualisation of the bowel, plaques of inflammatory exudate between oedematous mucosa are seen. Diagnosis is usually made by detection of the toxin in stool samples, rather than by culture. Treatment is by metronidazole or vancomycin alongside supportive care.

Summary box 70.8

Opportunistic intestinal infections in patients with AIDS

- Bacteria
  - Salmonella
  - Shigella
  - Yersinia
  - Campylobacter
  - *Mycobacterium avium intracellulare* (MAI)
- Viral
  - Cytomegalovirus
- Protozoa
  - Cryptosporidium
  - Giardia
- Fungal
  - *Candida albicans*

If the colitis does not settle, an emergency subtotal colectomy and ileostomy may be necessary.

Colonic diverticula

Diverticula (hollow out-pouchings) are a common structural abnormality. They can be classified as:

1. Congenital. All three coats of the bowel are present in the wall of the diverticulum (e.g. Meckel's diverticulum).
2. Acquired. There is no muscularis layer present in the diverticulum (e.g. sigmoid diverticular disease).

Diverticula are found in the left colon in around 75% of over 70 year olds in the Western world. The condition is overwhelmingly found in the sigmoid but can affect the whole colon. Interestingly, in South-East Asia right-sided diverticular disease is more common. Diverticula are most often asymptomatic (diverticulosis) and found incidentally, but they can present clinically with sepsis or haemorrhage.

Aetiology

Epidemiological studies indicate that diverticular disease is a consequence of a refined Western diet, deficient in dietary fibre. The combination of altered collagen structure with ageing, disordered motility and increased intraluminal pressure, most notably in the narrow sigmoid colon, results in herniation of mucosa through the circular muscle at the points where blood vessels penetrate the bowel wall. The rectum has a complete muscular coat and a wider lumen and is thus very rarely affected. Diverticular disease is rare in Africa and Asia where the diet is high in natural fibre.

Complications of diverticular disease

The majority of patients with diverticula are asymptomatic but historical studies suggest that somewhere between 10 and 30% will have symptomatic complications (*Summary box 70.9*). These complications are:

Johann Friedrich Meckel (the younger), 1781–1833, Professor of Anatomy and Surgery, Halle, Germany, described the diverticulum in 1809.

1. Pain and inflammation (diverticulitis).
2. Perforation: most often contained leading to pericolic abscess formation but occasionally leading to generalised peritonitis.
3. Intestinal obstruction: progressive fibrosis can cause stenosis of the sigmoid and large bowel obstruction or loops of small intestine can adhere to an inflamed sigmoid, resulting in small bowel obstruction.
4. Haemorrhage: diverticular disease may present with profuse and recurrent) colonic haemorrhage due to erosion of vessels adjacent to a diverticulum.
5. Fistula formation (colovesical, colovaginal, enterocolic, colocutaneous): occurs in 5% of cases, colovesical fistulation is most commonly seen.

Summary box 70.9

Complications of diverticular disease

- Diverticulitis
- Abscess
- Peritonitis
- Intestinal obstruction
- Haemorrhage
- Fistula formation

Clinical features

In mild cases, symptoms such as distension, flatulence and a sensation of heaviness in the lower abdomen may be indistinguishable from those of irritable bowel syndrome. These symptoms are thought to result from a combination of increased luminal pressure affecting wall tension and increased visceral hypersensitivity. Surgical treatment is rarely, if ever appropriate for diverticular disease in the absence of complications.

Diverticulitis typically presents as persistent lower abdominal pain, usually in the left iliac fossa. There may be accompanying diarrhoea or constipation. The lower abdomen is tender, especially on the left, but occasionally also in the right iliac fossa if the sigmoid loop lies across the midline. The sigmoid colon may be tender and thickened on palpation and rectal examination may reveal a tender mass if an abscess has formed. Distinguishing between diverticulitis and abscess formation is difficult on clinical grounds alone and radiological imaging is essential. Generalised peritonitis as a result of free perforation presents in the typical manner with systemic upset and generalised tenderness and guarding.

Haemorrhage from colonic diverticula is typically painless and profuse. Bleeding from the sigmoid will be bright red with clots, whereas right-sided bleeding will be darker. Torrential bleeding is fortunately rare and, in fact, more commonly due to angiodysplasia, but diverticular bleeding may persist or recur requiring transfusion and resection. The presentation of a fistula resulting from diverticular disease depends on the site. The most common colovesical fistula results in recurrent urinary tract infections and pneumaturia (flatus in the urine) or even faeces in the urine. Colovaginal fistulae are more common after hysterectomy. Colocutaneous fistulation is rare in the absence of prior intervention (e.g. radiological drainage). Rarely, diverticular disease may perforate into the retroperitoneum, leading to a psoas abscess, and even groin fistulation.

Classification of contamination

The degree of infection has a major impact on outcome in acute diverticulitis. Patients with inflammatory masses have a lower mortality than those with perforation (3% versus. 33%). Classification systems have been developed for acute diverticulitis to try and rationalise the literature, the most commonly used being the Hinchey classification (*Table 70.3*).

Radiology

Plain radiographs can demonstrate a pneumoperitoneum. Spiral CT has excellent sensitivity and specificity for identifying bowel wall thickening, abscess formation and extraluminal disease and has revolutionised the assessment of complicated diverticular disease (Figure 70.20). On identification of abscesses in stable patients, drainage may be carried out percutaneously, avoiding the need for laparotomy/laparoscopy. Contrast studies and endoscopy are usually avoided for 6 weeks after an acute attack for fear of causing perforation. They are used subsequently, however, to exclude a coexisting carcinoma and assess the extent of diverticular disease. Contrast examination or CT can demonstrate a fistula.

Colonoscopy

Endoscopic assessment may demonstrate the necks of diverticula within the bowel lumen (Figure 70.21). A narrowed

TABLE 70.3 Hinchey classification of complicated diverticulitis.

Grade I	Mesenteric or pericolic abscess
Grade II	Pelvic abscess
Grade III	Purulent peritonitis
Grade IV	Faecal peritonitis

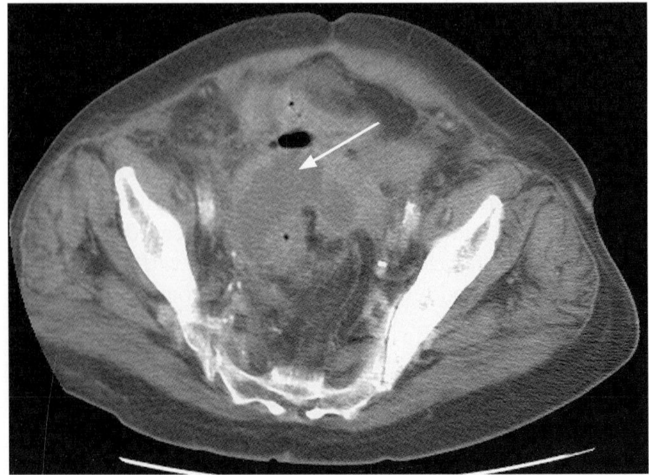

Figure 70.20 Computed tomography scan demonstrating an abscess associated with diverticulitis (arrow) (courtesy of Dr D Kasir, Hope Hospital, Salford, UK)

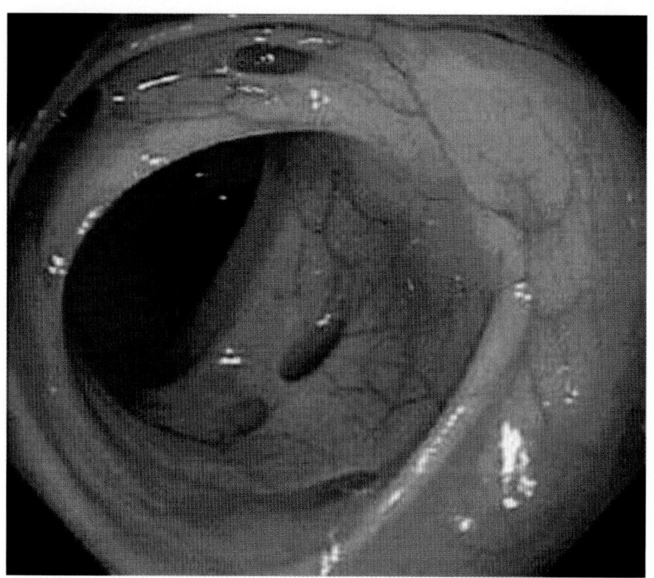

Figure 70.21 Colonoscopic view of sigmoid diverticula. Note the mouths of diverticula between the hypertrophied colonic walls.

area of diverticular disease may be impassable because of the severity of disease and there is a significant risk of endoscopic perforation. Colonoscopy in these circumstances requires judgement and experience. Biopsies may be taken if possible and corroboration with barium enema or CT virtual colonoscopy is required. Excluding a carcinoma may not always be possible and may represent an indication for resection.

Management

Patients are frequently recommended to take a high-fibre diet and bulk-forming laxatives, although the evidence for their effectiveness in diverticulosis or after an attack of diverticulitis is limited. Antispasmodics may have a role if recurrent pain is a problem. Acute diverticulitis is treated by intravenous antibiotics (to cover gram-negative bacilli and anaerobes) alongside appropriate resuscitation and analgesia. Nil by mouth to 'rest the bowel' and catheterisation to reduce the risk of colovesical fistulation are often advocated, but there is little evidence to support these practices. A CT scan can confirm the diagnosis and assess for complications. After the acute attack has subsided the bowel should be investigated by endoscopy, barium enema or CT virtual colonoscopy. Some pericolic abscesses can be drained percutaneously. A diameter of 5 cm is frequently regarded as the cut off between an abscess likely to settle with antibiotics and one likely to require intervention.

Operative procedures for diverticular disease

The aim of emergency surgery is to control peritoneal infection; indications are generalised peritonitis and failure to respond to optimum medical management. Laparotomy for diverticular disease in the acute setting has considerable risk with mortality in most series of 15% and, in the case of faecal peritonitis, mortality approaches 50%. Alongside operative technique, resuscitation, anaesthesia and postoperative management should be optimised.

Laparotomy and thorough washout of contamination are performed and then a choice has to be made between a Hartmann's procedure (sigmoid resection with formation of left iliac fossa colostomy and closure of the rectal stump) and resection with colonic washout and anastomosis (with consideration of a defunctioning loop ileostomy). Primary anastomosis should be used selectively but is appealing in a young fit patient without gross contamination or overwhelming sepsis. However, this is a relatively rare scenario and the majority of emergency operations for perforated diverticular disease are Hartmann's procedures (Figure 70.22). There is good evidence that simple defunctioning with a proximal stoma is associated with higher mortality than a resection. There may be a role for emergency laparoscopy in diverticular disease with washout if there is no faecal contamination (i.e. Hinchey grade III or less), allowing sigmoid resection to be avoided, but this remains somewhat controversial as some trials have suggested a higher mortality.

Elective surgery is usually undertaken for management of complications. Diverticular fistulae can only be cured by resecting the affected bowel, although a defunctioning stoma can ameliorate symptoms. In colovesical fistula the sigmoid can often be pinched off the bladder and the sigmoid resected. If an anastomosis is performed, it is wise to place an omental pedicle between the bowel and bladder to prevent recurrent

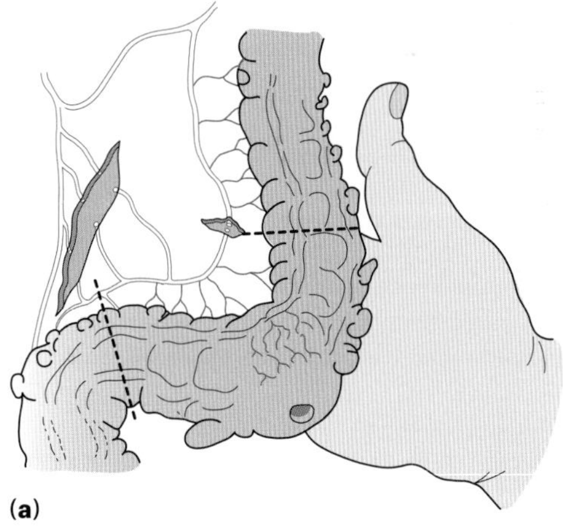

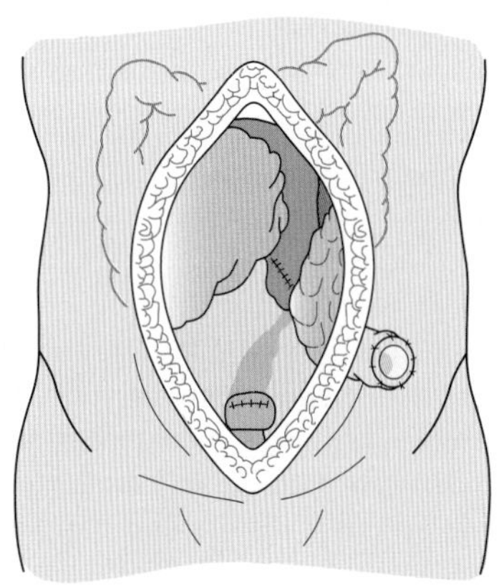

Figure 70.22 (a) Perforated sigmoid diverticular disease. (b) The Hartmann procedure – oversewn rectal stump and left iliac fossa colostomy.

fistulation. These procedures can be technically challenging and ureteric stents are commonly required to reduce the risk of ureteric injury. Partial cystectomy may be required and assistance from a urological surgeon is often very helpful

Haemorrhage from diverticular disease should be distinguished from angiodysplasia. It usually responds to conservative management and only occasionally requires resection. Where available, angiography is helpful to localise bleeding points. On-table lavage and colonoscopy may be necessary to localise the bleeding site. If the source cannot be located, then subtotal colectomy and ileostomy may be the safest option.

Indications for surgery in an elective setting, in the absence of complications of the disease, are controversial. There are undoubtedly a small number of patients with recurrent attacks who should be offered an elective sigmoid colectomy (with anastomosis). This could be performed laparoscopically in experienced hands with a likely swifter recovery as well as improved cosmesis. Cohort studies suggest that in patients under 50 years old admitted with diverticulitis, 25% will have a further episode. This may be used as an argument for offering elective resection but equally suggests that 75% will not get another severe attack. Many surgeons would discuss the pros and cons of elective surgery after two emergency admissions, although general health must be carefully considered. There has been an increasing tendency, in recent years, to treat even patients with recurrent attacks of diverticulitis conservatively in the absence of complications.

Summary box 70.10

Principles of surgical management of diverticular disease

- Hartmann's procedure is the safest option in emergency surgery
- Primary anastomosis can be considered in selected patients
- Elective resection may be offered for recurrent attacks
- Definitive treatment of colovesical fistula will require resection

VASCULAR ANOMALIES OF THE INTESTINE

Angiodysplasia

Angiodysplasia is a vascular malformation that commonly causes haemorrhage from the colon in patients over the age of 60. The malformations consist of dilated tortuous submucosal veins.

Clinical features

In the majority of cases, the symptoms are subtle and patients can present with anaemia. About 10–15% have brisk bleeds, which may present as melaena or significant rectal bleeding. Many patients in whom rectal bleeding has been attributed to diverticular disease have probably bled from angiodysplasia. There is an association with aortic stenosis (Heyde's syndrome).

Investigation

Colonoscopy may show the characteristic lesion in the right colon. The lesions are only a few millimetres in size and appear as reddish, raised areas at endoscopy. Selective superior and inferior mesenteric angiography shows the site and extent of the lesion by a 'blush' of contrast, provided bleeding is above 1 mL/minute. If this fails, a technetium-99m (99mTc)-labelled red cell scan may confirm and localise the source of haemorrhage.

Treatment

The first principle is to stabilise the patient. Following this, the bleeding needs to be localised. Colonoscopy may allow cauterisation to be carried out and an argon laser can be helpful. In severe uncontrolled bleeding, surgery becomes necessary. On-table colonoscopy is carried out to confirm the site of bleeding. Angiodysplastic lesions are sometimes demonstrated by transillumination through the caecum (Figure 70.23). If it is still not clear exactly which segment of the colon is involved, then a subtotal colectomy may be necessary.

Ischaemic colitis

Ischaemia of the colon typically results from thrombosis or embolism. Sudden embolic events present with severe pain out of proportion to the degree of peritonism, bloody diarrhoea, haemodynamic instability and shock. Resuscitation and laparotomy are required with resection of gangrenous

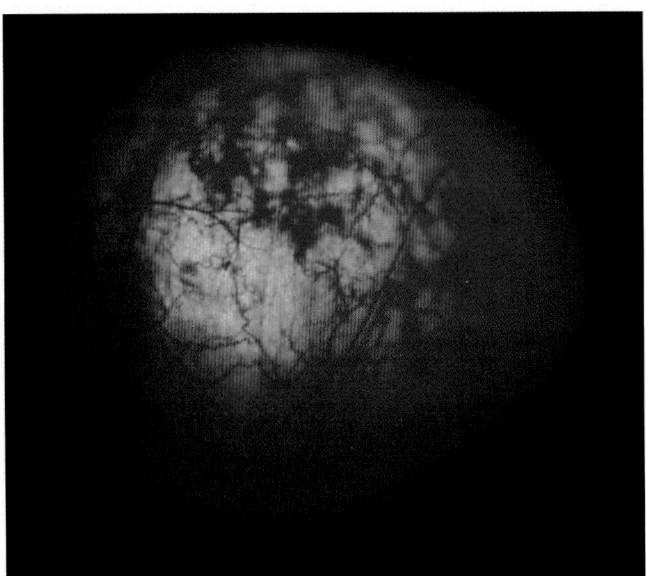

Figure 70.23 Angiodysplasia of the caecum demonstrated by transillumination with a colonoscope intraoperatively.

Edward Heyde, American internist, published his findings on the association between aortic valve stenosis and angiodysplasia in a letter to the *New England Journal of Medicine* in 1958.

bowel and exteriorisation of viable bowel ends. Mortality is extremely high. Thrombotic occlusion usually occurs in the context of global atherosclerosis and the presentation tends to be less dramatic with abdominal pain and rectal bleeding. A plain abdominal radiograph may show 'thumb-printing' and endoscopy may demonstrate haemorrhagic oedema. The left colon and, in particular, the splenic flexure are usually the worst affected. Symptoms usually settle spontaneously. In some cases, ulceration at the splenic flexure associated with ischaemic colitis may heal with stricturing and present with subsequent large bowel obstruction.

COLOSTOMIES

A colostomy (or ileostomy) stoma is a planned opening made in the colon (or small intestine) to divert faeces and flatus to the abdominal wall where they can be collected in an external appliance. Depending on the purpose for which the diversion has been necessary, a stoma may be temporary or permanent.

Loop colostomy

A transverse loop colostomy has in the past been used to defunction an anastomosis after an anterior resection. It is now less commonly employed, as it is difficult to manage and potentially disrupts the marginal arterial supply to the anastomosis. Loop transverse colostomies are also particularly prone to prolapse. A loop ileostomy is now more commonly used.

A loop left iliac fossa colostomy is still sometimes used to prevent faecal peritonitis developing following traumatic injury to the rectum, to facilitate the operative treatment of a high anal fistula, for incontinence and to defunction an obstructing low rectal cancer prior to long course chemoradiotherapy.

A temporary loop colostomy is made by bringing a mobilised loop of colon to the surface, where it is held in place by a plastic bridge passed through a mesenteric window. Once the abdomen has been closed, the colostomy is opened, and the edges of the colonic incision are sutured to the adjacent skin margin (Figure 70.24). When firm adhesion of the colostomy to the abdominal wall has taken place, the bridge can be removed.

Following healing of the distal lesion for which the temporary stoma was constructed, the colostomy can be closed. It is usual to perform a contrast examination (proctogram) to check that there is no distal obstruction or continuing problem at the site of previous surgery. Colostomy closure is most easily and safely accomplished if the stoma is mature, typically after the colostomy has been established for at least 2 months. Closure is usually possible with a circumstomal incision, which avoids a full laparotomy, but it is important for patient and surgeon to consider the risks of closure carefully as it does involve a bowel anastomosis. In some cases, a full laparotomy may be required for safe closure of the stoma.

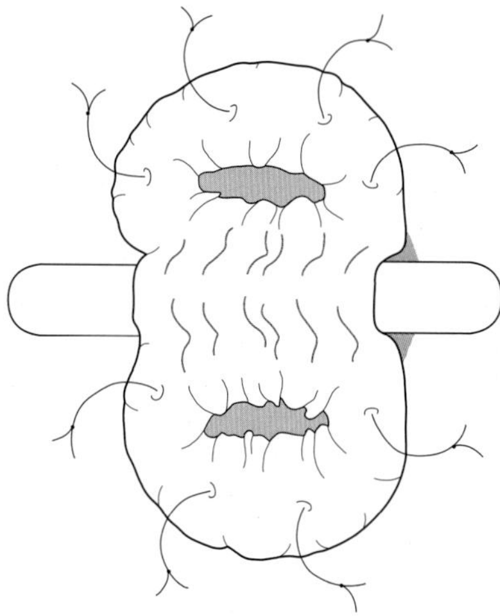

Figure 70.24 Temporary (loop) colostomy opened over a rod, and immediate suture of the colon wall to surrounding skin (alternatively, a skin bridge is used).

End colostomy

This is formed after an abdominoperineal excision of the rectum or as part of a Hartmann's procedure, bringing the divided colon through a left iliac fossa trephine in rectus abdominis and skin. The colonic margin is then sutured to the adjoining skin.

The point at which the colon is brought to the surface must be carefully selected to allow a colostomy bag to be applied without impinging on the anterior-superior iliac spine. The best site is usually through the lateral edge of the rectus sheath (Figure 70.25).

Stoma bags and appliances

Stoma output is collected in disposable adhesive bags. Colostomy appliances are simply changed two or three times each day. A wide range of such bags is currently available. In most hospitals, a stoma care service is available to offer advice to patients, to acquaint them with the latest appliances and to provide the appropriate psychological and practical help.

Summary box 70.11

Stomas

- May be colostomy or ileostomy
- May be temporary or permanent
- Temporary or defunctioning stomas are usually fashioned as loop stomas
- An ileostomy is spouted; a colostomy is flush
- Ileostomy effluent is usually liquid whereas colostomy effluent is usually solid
- Ileostomy patients are more likely to develop fluid and electrolyte problems
- An ileostomy is usually sited in the right iliac fossa
- End-colostomy is usually sited in the left iliac fossa
- Whenever possible patients should be counselled and sited by a stoma care nurse before operation

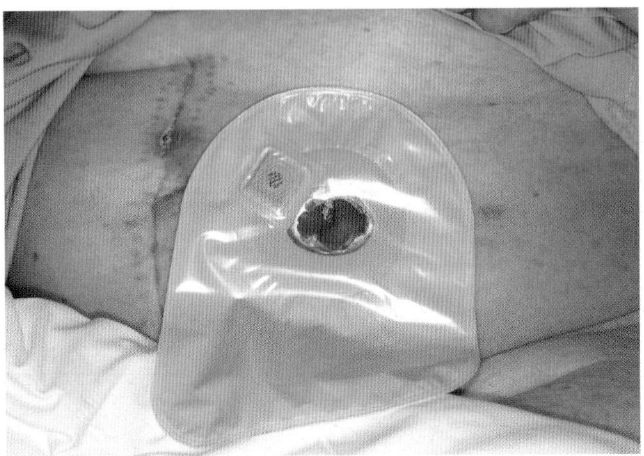

Figure 70.25 A colostomy in the left iliac fossa.

Complications of stomas

Stoma complications are underestimated and common (*Summary box 70.12*). On occasion these complications may require surgical treatment. Sometimes, this can be achieved with an incision immediately around the stoma but on occasion reopening the abdomen and freeing up the stoma may be necessary. Repair of parastomal hernias is particularly technically challenging and the recurrence rate is high. Simple suture is associated with an almost 100% risk of recurrence and transfer to the opposite side of the abdomen, or insertion of a piece of prosthetic material within the abdominal wall around the stoma may be necessary. There is some evidence that stoma trephine reinforcement with mesh at the time of initial stoma formation may reduce the incidence of parastomal herniation, which may be as high as 50% over the long term.

Summary box 70.12

Stoma complications
- Skin irritation
- Prolapse
- Retraction
- Ischaemia
- Stenosis
- Parastomal hernia
- Bleeding
- Fistulation

FUNCTIONAL ABNORMALITIES

Constipation

There is no single definition of constipation; however, a bowel frequency of less than one every 3 days is commonly considered to be abnormal. Constipation is an extremely prevalent complaint in western society and some patients are greatly disabled by abdominal pain, distension, reliance on laxatives and difficulty with defaecation.

Drugs and a range of illnesses can result in constipation (*Summary boxes 70.13, 70.14*). Altering medication or addition of laxatives can be helpful for drug-related constipation and correction of underlying illness is clearly ideal where possible.

Summary box 70.13

Drugs that can cause constipation
- Benzodiazepines
- Carbamazepine
- Chlorpromazine
- Cholestyramine
- Iron
- Opiates, particularly codeine and morphine
- Tricyclic antidepressants
- Statins

Summary box 70.14

Illnesses associated with constipation
- Neurological conditions
- Parkinson's disease
- Multiple sclerosis
- Diabetic nephropathy
- Spinal cord lesion
- Endocrine conditions
- Hypothyroidism
- Hypercalcaemia

There remains a group of patients with constipation who do not have any structural, pharmacological or other pathology to explain their symptoms. Some will have obstructed defaecation (a syndrome of impaired rectal emptying associated with pelvic floor dysfunction). Others will have slow colonic transit, a disorder usually seen in women, which may have been present since childhood or may suddenly follow abdominal or pelvic surgery. Some patients have a combination of both conditions.

Investigation

It is important to exclude a structural abnormality (notably large bowel obstruction) by conventional investigation (colonoscopy, CT virtual colonoscopy or barium enema) before diagnosing a functional bowel disorder.

Whole-gut transit time can be measured by asking the patient to stop all laxatives and take a capsule containing radiopaque markers (Figure 70.26). Retention of more than 80% of the shapes, 120 hours after ingestion, is abnormal.

Defaecating proctography may demonstrate impaired pelvic floor relaxation, rectal intussusception and/or rectocoele if they are causing obstructed defaecation. Anorectal manometry may confirm an abnormal pattern of straining in patients with obstructed defaecation, with failure to reduce (or even inappropriately increase) anal canal pressures on bearing down.

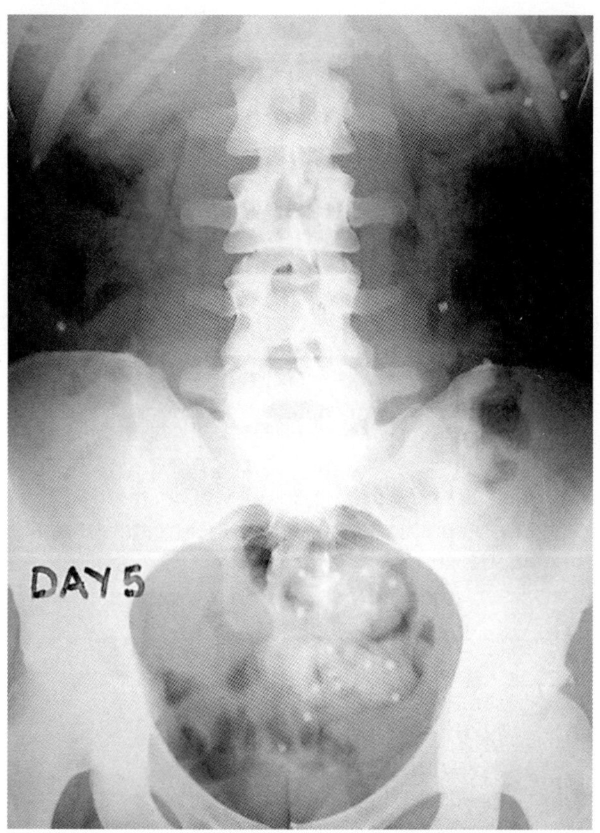

Figure 70.26 Whole-gut transit studied using radiopaque markers. More than 80% should have passed by day 5, demonstrating delayed transit here (courtesy of Dr D Nolan, John Radcliffe Hospital, Oxford, UK).

Treatment of slow colonic transit and obstructed defaecation

Dietary fibre This is the first-line treatment for mild constipation. Constipation only resolves after several weeks of therapy, which usually needs to be continued in the long term.

Laxatives It is important that patients do not fall into a cycle of laxative abuse. A number of types are available including bulk, osmotic and stimulant agents.

New agents Newer agents such as prucalopride, which selectively activates serotonin (5HT-4) receptors, may have a role in chronic constipation.

Rectal irrigation Rectal irrigation may improve quality of life in some patients, who can be trained to do this for themselves using commercially available kits.

Biofeedback This involves training in pelvic floor function. It has been shown to be effective in up to 50% of patients with obstructed defaecation.

Sacral nerve stimulation Although primarily used for the treatment of faecal incontinence, sacral neuromodulation has recently been suggested to be of value in the treatment of obstructed defaecation.

Surgery The results of surgery are relatively poor. Surgery is justified only after careful evaluation and when appropriate medical options have been exhausted. Total colectomy and ileorectal anastomosis is the preferred procedure for slow transit constipation but the results are unpredictable.

Complications include intermittent small bowel obstruction (60%), further surgery (30%), constipation (25%), diarrhoea (25%) and incontinence (10%). Patients need to be carefully selected for surgery and psychological evaluation may be of benefit. An ileostomy may be required in some cases.

Obstructed defaecation may be amenable to surgical treatment if there is evidence of rectal intussusception or a sizeable rectocele. These can be corrected by a ventral mesh rectopexy and repair (transrectal or transvaginal), respectively. If there is coexisting evidence of impaired pelvic floor relaxation, the results of surgical treatment tend to be disappointing.

Irritable bowel syndrome

The term irritable bowel syndrome (IBS) covers a range of symptoms with a functional basis. Clinical features are variable but abdominal discomfort, bloating, irregularity of bowel habit and passage of mucus are common. By definition, the symptoms of pain have to have been present for at least 3 days per month for at least the 3 previous months in the 6-month period prior to diagnosis (Rome criteria). IBS is common and symptoms have been said to occur in up to 20% of the population.

Colonic investigations are typically performed to rule out organic disease (colonoscopy, barium enema or CT virtual colonoscopy) but are, by definition, normal.

Treatment of IBS is difficult. Many patients benefit from reassurance and symptomatic treatment; dietary modifications, including fibre for constipation and avoidance of fermentable carbohydrates, reduction of caffeine and nicotine intake, may be of value. Antidiarrhoeals and antispasmodic agents are commonly prescribed, but the evidence of benefit is poor. There is some evidence of benefit for low-dose tricyclic antidepressants but patients are often reluctant to use them. Psychological treatments, including hypnotherapy and cognitive behavioural therapy, may be beneficial. Surgery is contraindicated.

FURTHER READING

Herold A, Lehur P-A, Matzel KE, O'Connell PR (eds). *European manual of medicine: coloproctology*, 2nd edn. New York: Springer, 2017.

Phillips RKS, Clark S *Colorectal surgery: a companion to specialist surgical practice*, 4th edn. Philadelphia: Elsevier Saunders, 2013.

Chapter 71

Intestinal obstruction

Learning objectives

To understand:

- The pathophysiology of dynamic and adynamic intestinal obstruction
- The cardinal features on history and examination
- The causes of small and large bowel obstruction
- The indications for surgery and other treatment options in bowel obstruction

CLASSIFICATION

Intestinal obstruction may be classified into two types:

- **Dynamic**, in which peristalsis is working against a mechanical obstruction. It may occur in an acute or a chronic form (Figure 71.1).
- **Adynamic**, in which there is no mechanical obstruction; peristalsis is absent or inadequate (e.g. paralytic ileus or pseudo-obstruction).

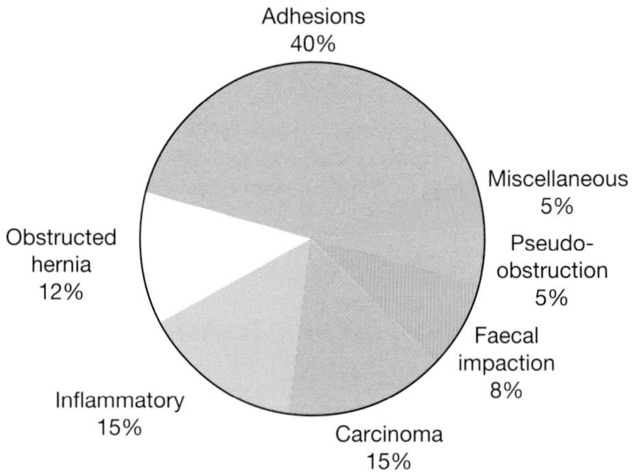

Summary box 71.1

Causes of intestinal obstruction

Dynamic

- Intraluminal
  - Faecal impaction
  - Foreign bodies
  - Bezoars
  - Gallstones
- Intramural
  - Stricture
  - Malignancy
  - Intussusception
  - Volvulus
- Extramural
  - Bands/adhesions
  - Hernia

Adynamic

- Paralytic ileus
- Pseudo-obstruction

Figure 71.1 Pie chart showing the common causes of intestinal obstruction and their relative frequencies.

PATHOPHYSIOLOGY

Irrespective of aetiology or acuteness of onset, in dynamic (mechanical) obstruction the bowel proximal to the obstruction dilates and the bowel below the obstruction exhibits normal peristalsis and absorption until it becomes empty and collapses. Initially, proximal peristalsis is increased in an attempt to overcome the obstruction. If the obstruction is not relieved, the bowel continues to dilate; ultimately there is a reduction in peristaltic strength, resulting in flaccidity and paralysis.

The distension proximal to an obstruction is caused by two factors:

- **Gas**: there is a significant overgrowth of both aerobic and anaerobic organisms, resulting in considerable gas production. Following the reabsorption of oxygen and carbon dioxide, the majority is made up of nitrogen (90%) and hydrogen sulphide.

- **Fluid**: this is made up of the various digestive juices. (saliva 500 mL, bile 500 mL, pancreatic secretions 500 mL, gastric secretions 1 litre – all per 24 hours). This accumulates in the gut lumen as absorption by the obstucted gut is retarded. Dehydration and electrolyte loss are therefore due to:
  - reduced oral intake;
  - defective intestinal absorption;
  - losses as a result of vomiting;
  - sequestration in the bowel lumen;
  - transudation of fluid into the peritoneal cavity.

STRANGULATION

It is important to appreciate that the consequences of intestinal obstruction are not immediately life-threatening unless there is superimposed strangulation. When strangulation occurs, the blood supply is compromised and the bowel becomes ischaemic.

Summary box 71.2

Causes of strangulation

Direct pressure on the bowel wall
- Hernial orifices
- Adhesions/bands

Interrupted mesenteric blood flow
- Volvulus
- Intussusception

Increased intraluminal pressure
- Closed-loop obstruction

Ischaemia from direct pressure on the bowel wall from a constricting band such as a hernial orifice is easy to understand.

Distension of the obstructed segment of bowel results in high pressure within the bowel wall. This can happen when only part of the bowel wall is obstructed as seen in Richter's hernias. Venous return is compromised before the arterial supply. The resultant increase in capillary pressure leads to impaired local perfusion and once the arterial supply is impaired, haemorrhagic infarction occurs. As the viability of the bowel is compromised, translocation and systemic exposure to anaerobic organisms and endotoxin occurs.

The morbidity and mortality associated with strangulation are largely dependent on the duration of the ischaemia and its extent. Elderly patients and those with comorbidities are more vulnerable to its effects. Although in strangulated external hernias the segment involved is often short, any length of ischaemic bowel can cause significant systemic effects secondary to sepsis and obstruction proximal to the obstruction can result in significant dehydration. When bowel involvement is extensive circulatory failure is common.

Closed-loop obstruction

This occurs when the bowel is obstructed at both the proximal and distal points (Figure 71.2). The distension is principally confined to the closed loop; distension proximal to the obstructed segment is not typically marked.

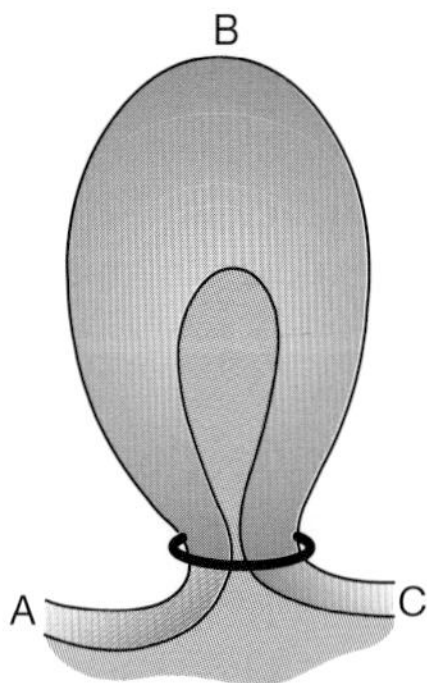

Figure 71.2 Distension. Closed-loop obstruction with no proximal (A) or distal (C) distension and impending strangulation (B).

A classic form of closed-loop obstruction is seen in the presence of a malignant stricture of the colon with a competent ileocaecal valve (present in up to one-third of individuals). This can occur with lesions as far distally as the rectum. The inability of the distended colon to decompress itself into the small bowel results in an increase in luminal pressure, which is greatest at the caecum, with subsequent impairment of blood flow in the wall. Unrelieved, this results in necrosis and perforation (Figure 71.3).

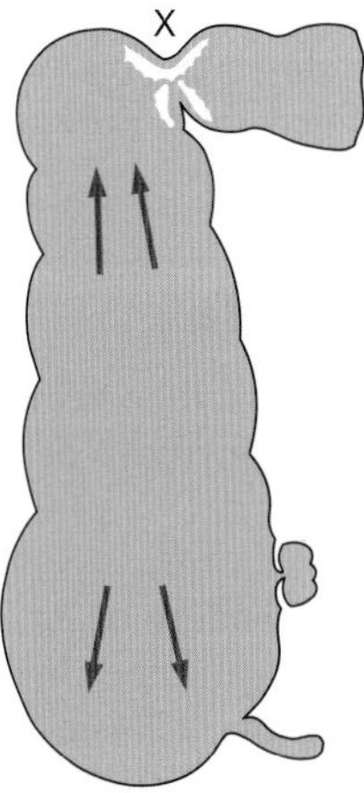

Figure 71.3 Carcinomatous stricture (X) of the hepatic flexure: closed-loop obstruction.

August Gottlieb Richter, 1742–1812, lecturer in surgery, Göttingen, Germany, described this form of hernia in 1777.

SPECIAL TYPES OF MECHANICAL INTESTINAL OBSTRUCTION

Internal hernia

Internal herniation occurs when a portion of the small intestine becomes entrapped in one of the retroperitoneal fossae or in a congenital mesenteric defect.

The following are potential sites of internal herniation (all are rare):

- the foramen of Winslow;
- a defect in the mesentery;
- a defect in the transverse mesocolon;
- defects in the broad ligament;
- congenital or acquired diaphragmatic hernia;
- duodenal retroperitoneal fossae – left paraduodenal and right duodenojejunal;
- caecal/appendiceal retroperitoneal fossae – superior, inferior and retrocaecal;
- intersigmoid fossa.

Internal herniation in the absence of adhesions is rare and a preoperative diagnosis is unusual. The standard treatment of an obstructed hernia is to release the constricting agent by division. This should not be undertaken in cases of herniation involving the foramen of Winslow, mesenteric defects and the paraduodenal/duodenojejunal fossae as major blood vessels run in the edge of the constriction ring. The distended loop in such circumstances must first be decompressed (minimising contamination) and then reduced.

Obstruction from enteric strictures

Small bowel strictures usually occur secondary to tuberculosis or Crohn's disease. Malignant strictures associated with lymphoma are uncommon, whereas carcinoma and sarcoma are rare. Presentation is usually subacute or chronic. Standard surgical management consists of resection and anastomosis. Resection is important to establish a histological diagnosis as this can be uncertain clinically. In Crohn's disease, strictureplasty may be considered in the presence of short multiple strictures without active sepsis.

Bolus obstruction

Bolus obstruction in the small bowel may be caused by gallstones, food, trichobezoar, phytobezoar, stercoliths and worms.

Gallstones

This type of obstruction tends to occur in the elderly secondary to erosion of a large gallstone directly through the gall bladder into the duodenum. Classically, there is impaction about 60 cm proximal to the ileocaecal valve. The patient may have recurrent attacks as the obstruction is frequently incomplete or relapsing as a result of a ball-valve effect. The characteristic radiological sign of gallstone ileus is Rigler's triad, comprising: small bowel obstruction, pneumobilia and an atypical mineral shadow on radiographs of the abdomen. The presence of two of these radiological signs has been considered pathognomic of gallstone ileus and is encountered in 40–50% of the cases (note than pneumobilia is common following endoscopic retrograde cholangiopancreatography (ERCP) with sphincterotomy). At laparotomy, the stone is milked proximally away from the site of impaction. It may be possible to crush the stone within the bowel lumen; if not, the intestine is opened at this point and the gallstone removed. If the gallstone is faceted, a careful check for other enteric stones should be made. The region of the gall bladder should not be explored.

Food

Bolus obstruction may occur after partial or total gastrectomy when unchewed articles can pass directly into the small bowel. Fruit and vegetables are particularly liable to cause obstruction. The management is similar to that for gallstone, with intraluminal crushing usually being successful.

Trychobezoars and phytobezoars

These are firm masses of undigested hair ball and fruit/vegetable fibre respectively. The former is due to persistent hair chewing or sucking, and may be associated with an underlying psychiatric abnormality. Predisposition to phytobezoars results from a high fibre intake, inadequate chewing, previous gastric surgery, hypochlorhydria and loss of the gastric pump mechanism. When possible, the lesion may be kneaded into the caecum; otherwise open removal is required. A preoperative diagnosis is difficult even with high-resolution computed tomography (CT) scanning.

Stercoliths

These are usually found in the small bowel in association with a jejunal diverticulum or ileal stricture. Presentation and management are identical to that of gallstones.

Worms

Ascaris lumbricoides may cause low small bowel obstruction, particularly in children, the institutionalised and those near the tropics (Figure 71.4). An attack may follow the initiation of antihelminthic therapy. Debility is frequently out of proportion to that produced by the obstruction. If worms are not seen in the stool or vomitus the diagnosis may be indicated by eosinophilia or the sight of worms within gas-filled small bowel loops on a plain radiograph (Naik). At laparotomy it may be possible to knead the tangled mass into the caecum; if not it should be removed. Occasionally, worms may cause

Jacob Benignus Winslow, 1669–1760, Professor of Anatomy, Physic and Surgery, Paris, France.
Burrill Bernard Crohn, 1884–1983, gastroenterologist, Mount Sinai Hospital, New York, NY, USA, described regional ileitis in 1932.
Leo George Rigler, 1896–1979, Professor of Radiology, University of California, Los Angeles, CA, USA.
Vinod C Naik, a doctor from Nansari, India.

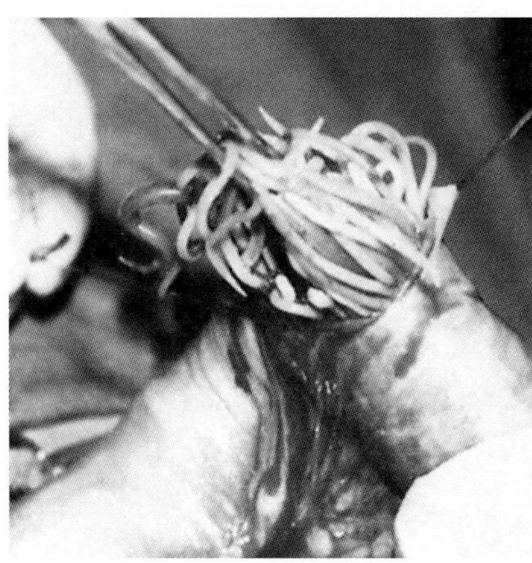

Figure 71.4 Obstruction of the small intestine due to *Ascaris lumbricoides* (courtesy of Asal Y Izzidien, Nenavah, Iraq).

a perforation and peritonitis, especially if the enteric wall is weakened by such conditions as ameobiasis.

Obstruction by adhesions and bands

Adhesions

In Western countries where abdominal operations are common, adhesions and bands are the most common cause of intestinal obstruction. The lifetime risk of requiring an admission to hospital for adhesional small bowel obstruction susequent to abdominal surgery is around 4% and the risk of requiring a laparotomy around 2%. Adhesions start to form within hours of abdominal surgery. In the early postoperative period, the onset of such a mechanical obstruction may be difficult to differentiate from paralytic ileus.

The causes of intraperitoneal adhesions are shown in *Table 71.1*. Any source of peritoneal irritation results in local fibrin production, which produces adhesions between apposed surfaces. Early fibrinous adhesions may disappear when the cause is removed or they may become vascularised and be replaced by mature fibrous tissue.

There are several factors that may limit adhesion formation.

TABLE 71.1 The common causes of intra-abdominal adhesions.

Acute inflammation	Sites of anastomoses, reperitonealisation of raw areas, trauma, ischaemia
Foreign material	Talc, starch, gauze, silk
Infection	Peritonitis, tuberculosis
Chronic inflammatory conditions	Crohn's disease
Radiation enteritis	

Summary box 71.3

Prevention of adhesions

Factors that may limit adhesion formation include:

- Good surgical technique
- Washing of the peritoneal cavity with saline to remove clots
- Minimising contact with gauze
- Covering anastomosis and raw peritoneal surfaces

Laparoscopic technique

Numerous substances have been instilled in the peritoneal cavity to prevent adhesion formation, including hyaluronidase, hydrocortisone, silicone, dextran, polyvinylpropylene (PVP), chondroitin and streptomycin, anticoagulants, antihistamines, non-steroidal anti-inflammatory drugs and streptokinase. Currently, no single agent or combination of agents has been convincingly shown to be effective.It is hoped that with the more widespread use of laparoscopic surgery the incidence of intra-abdominal adhesions will reduce.

Adhesions may be classified into various types by virtue of whether they are early (fibrinous) or late (fibrous) or by underlying aetiology. From a practical perspective there are only two types – 'easy' flimsy ones and 'difficult' dense ones.

Postoperative adhesions giving rise to intestinal obstruction usually involve the lower small bowel and almost never involve the large bowel.

Bands

Usually only one band is culpable. This may be:

- congenital, e.g. obliterated vitellointestinal duct;
- a string band following previous bacterial peritonitis;
- a portion of greater omentum, usually adherent to the parietes.

Acute intussusception

This occurs when one portion of the gut invaginates into an immediately adjacent segment; almost invariably, it is the proximal into the distal.

The condition is encountered most commonly in children, with a peak incidence between 5 and 10 months of age. About 90% of cases are idiopathic but an associated upper respiratory tract infection or gastroenteritis may precede the condition. It is believed that hyperplasia of Peyer's patches in the terminal ileum may be the initiating event. Weaning, loss of passively acquired maternal immunity and common viral pathogens have all been implicated in the pathogenesis of intussusception in infancy.

Children with intussusception associated with a pathological lead point such as Meckel's diverticulum, polyp, duplication, Henoch–Schönlein purpura or appendix are usually older than those with idiopathic disease. After the age of

Johann Conrad Peyer, 1653–1712, Professor of Logic, Rhetoric and Medicine, Schaffhausen, Switzerland, described the lymph follicles in the intestine in 1677.
Johann Friedrich Meckel, (The Younger), 1781–1833, Professor of Anatomy and Surgery, Halle, Germany, described the diverticulum in 1809.
Eduard Heinrich Henoch, 1820–1910, Professor of Diseases of Children, Berlin, Germany, described this form of purpura in 1868.
Johann Lucas Schönlein, 1793–1864, Professor of Medicine, Berlin, Germany, gave his account of this disease in 1837.

2 years, a pathological lead point is found in at least one-third of affected children. Adult cases are invariably associated with a lead point, which is usually a polyp (e.g. Peutz–Jeghers syndrome), a submucosal lipoma or other tumour.

Pathology

An intussusception is composed of three parts (Figure 71.5):

- the entering or inner tube (intussusceptum);
- the returning or middle tube;
- the sheath or outer tube (intussuscipiens).

The part that advances is the apex, the mass is the intussusception and the neck is the junction of the entering layer with the mass.

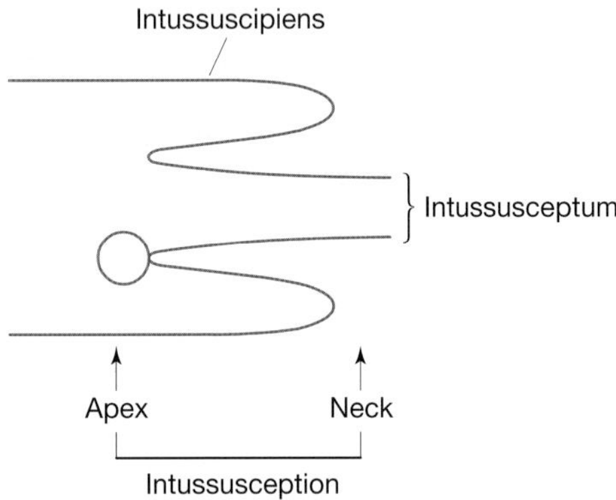

Figure 71.5 Mechanism and nomenclature of intussusception.

Intussusception may be anatomically defined according to the site and extent of invagination (*Table 71.2*). In most children, the intussusception is ileocolic. In adults, colocolic intussusception is more common. The degree of ischaemia is dependent on the tightness of the invagination, which is usually greatest as it passes through the ileocaecal valve. On CT scanning the target sign may be evident and if present is pathognomonic. It is worth noting that, rarely, intussuception has been noted on CT scanning in asymptomatic adults.

TABLE 71.2 Types of intussusception in children (after RE Gross) (n = 702).

	Percentage of series
Ileoileal	5
Ileocolic	77
Ileoileocolic	12
Colocolic	2
Multiple	1
Retrograde	0.2
Others	2.8

Summary box 71.4

Intussusception

- Most common in children
- Adult cases are secondary to intestinal pathology, e.g. polyp, Meckel's diverticulum
- Ileocolic is the commonest variety
- Can lead to an ischaemic segment
- Radiological reduction is indicated in most paediatric cases
- Adults require surgery

Volvulus

A volvulus is a twisting or axial rotation of a portion of bowel about its mesentery. The rotation causes obstruction to the lumen (>180° torsion) and if tight enough also causes vascular occlusion in the mesentery (>360° torsion). Bacterial fermentation adds to the distension and increasing intraluminal pressure impairs capillary perfusion. Mesenteric veins become obstructed as a result of the mechanical twisting and thrombosis results and contributes to the ischaemia.

Volvuli may be primary or secondary. The primary form occurs secondary to congenital malrotation of the gut, abnormal mesenteric attachments or congenital bands. Examples include volvulus neonatorum, caecal volvulus and sigmoid volvulus. A secondary volvulus, which is the more common variety, is due to rotation of a segment of bowel around an acquired adhesion or stoma.

Summary box 71.5

Volvulus

- May involve the small intestine, caecum or sigmoid colon; neonatal midgut volvulus secondary to midgut malrotation is life-threatening
- The commonest spontaneous type in adults is sigmoid
- Sigmoid volvulus can be relieved by decompression per anum
- Surgery is required to prevent or relieve ischaemia

Volvulus neonatorum

This occurs secondary to intestinal malrotation (see Chapter 9) and is potentially catastrophic.

Sigmoid volvulus

This is uncommon in Europe and the USA but more common in Eastern Europe and Africa. Indeed, it is the most common cause of large bowel obstruction in the indigenous black African population. Rotation nearly always occurs in the anticlockwise direction. The predisposing clinical features are summarised in Figure 71.6. Other predisposing factors include a high-residue diet and constipation. In

John Law Augustine Peutz, 1886–1968, Chief Specialist for Internal Medicine, St. John's Hospital, The Hague, The Netherlands.
Harold Joseph Jeghers, 1904–1990, Professor of Internal Medicine, New Jersey College of Medicine and Dentistry, Jersey City, NJ, USA.

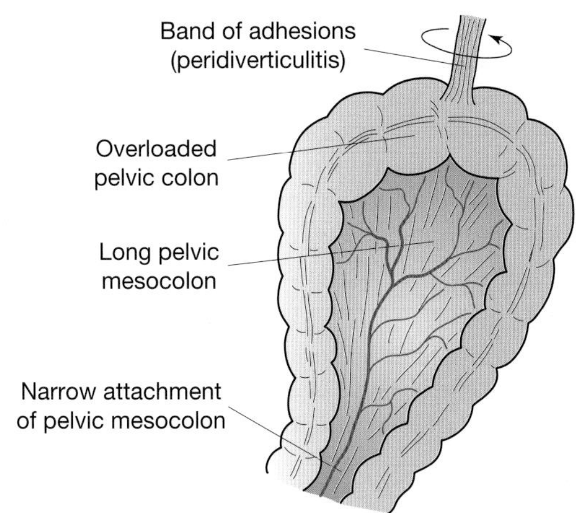

Figure 71.6 Causes predisposing to volvulus of the sigmoid colon. Idiopathic megacolon usually precedes the volvulus in African people.

western populations, the condition is seen most often in elderly patients with chronic constipation; comorbidities are common and chronic psychotropic drug use is associated with this condition. Younger patients present earlier and the prognosis is inversely related to the duration of symptoms. Presentation can be classified as:

- **Fulminant**: sudden onset, severe pain, early vomiting, rapidly deteriorating clinical course;
- **Indolent**: insidious onset, slow progressive course, less pain, late vomiting.

Compound volvulus

This is a rare condition also known as ileosigmoid knotting. The long pelvic mesocolon allows the ileum to twist around the sigmoid colon, resulting in gangrene of either or both segments of bowel. The patient presents with acute intestinal obstruction, but distension is comparatively mild. Plain radiography reveals distended ileal loops in a distended sigmoid colon. At operation, decompression, resection and anastomosis are required.

CLINICAL FEATURES OF INTESTINAL OBSTRUCTION

Dynamic obstruction

The diagnosis of dynamic intestinal obstruction is based on the classic quartet of pain, distension, vomiting and absolute constipation. Obstruction may be classified clinically into two types:

- small bowel obstruction – high or low;
- large bowel obstruction.

The nature of the presentation will also be influenced by whether the obstruction is:

- complete;
- incomplete.

A complete small bowel obstruction has all the cardinal features. In cases of complete large bowel obstruction there is often a surprising lack of preceeding symptoms. Both small and large bowel obstruction can present with more chronic symptoms in which the symptoms are intermittent or the obstruction is incomplete. Incomplete obstruction is also referred to as partial or subacute.

Summary box 71.6

Features of obstruction

- In **high small bowel obstruction**, vomiting occurs early, is profuse and causes rapid dehydration. Distension is minimal with little evidence of dilated small bowel loops on abdominal radiography
- In **low small bowel obstruction**, pain is predominant with central distension. Vomiting is delayed. Multiple dilated small bowel loops are seen on radiography
- In **large bowel obstruction**, distension is early and pronounced. Pain is less severe and vomiting and dehydration are later features. The colon proximal to the obstruction is distended on abdominal radiography. The small bowel will be dilated if the ileocaecal valve is incompetent.

Summary box 71.7

Cardinal clinical features of acute obstruction

- Abdominal pain
- Distension
- Vomiting
- Absolute constipation

Presentation will be further influenced by whether the obstruction is:

- simple – in which the blood supply is intact;
- strangulating/strangulated – in which there is interference to blood flow.

The common causes of intestinal obstruction in Western countries and their relative frequencies are shown in Figure 71.1. The underlying mechanisms are shown in *Summary box 71.2*.

The clinical features vary according to:

- the location of the obstruction;
- the duration of the obstruction;
- the underlying pathology;
- the presence or absence of intestinal ischaemia.

Late manifestations of intestinal obstruction that may be encountered include dehydration, oliguria, hypovolaemic shock, pyrexia, septicaemia, respiratory embarrassment and peritonism. In all cases of suspected intestinal obstruction, the hernial orifices must be examined.

Pain

Pain is the first symptom encountered; it occurs suddenly and is usually severe. It is colicky in nature and usually centred on the umbilicus (small bowel) or lower abdomen (large bowel).

The pain coincides with increased peristaltic activity. With increasing distension, the colicky pain is replaced by a mild and more constant diffuse pain. If there is no ischaemia and the obstruction persists over several days, pain reduces and can disappear.

The development of severe pain is suggestive of the presence of strangulation, especially if that severe pain is continuous. Beware the patient whose pain is not controlled with intravenous opiates. Colicky pain may not be a significant feature in postoperative simple mechanical obstruction and pain does not usually occur in paralytic ileus.

Vomiting

The more distal the obstruction, the longer the interval between the onset of symptoms and the appearance of nausea and vomiting. As obstruction progresses the character of the vomitus alters from digested food to faeculent material, as a result of the presence of enteric bacterial overgrowth.

Distension

In the small bowel the degree of distension is dependent on the site of the obstruction and is greater the more distal the lesion. Visible peristalsis may be present (Figure 71.7). This can sometimes be provoked by 'flicking' the abdominal wall. Distension is a later feature in colonic obstruction and may be minimal or absent in the presence of mesenteric vascular occlusion.

Constipation

This may be classified as absolute (i.e. neither faeces nor flatus is passed) or relative (where only flatus is passed). Absolute constipation is a cardinal feature of complete intestinal obstruction. Some patients may pass flatus or faeces after the onset of obstruction as a result of the evacuation of the distal bowel contents. The administration of enemas should be avoided in cases of suspected obstruction. This merely stimulates evacuation of bowel contents distal to the obstruction and confuses the clinical picture.

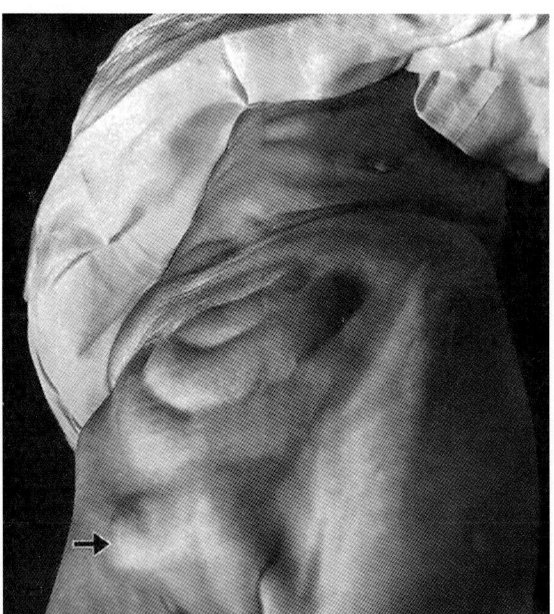

Figure 71.7 Visible peristalsis. Intestinal obstruction due to a strangulated right femoral hernia, to which the arrow points.

The rule that absolute constipation is present in intestinal obstruction does not apply in:

- Richter's hernia;
- gallstone ileus;
- mesenteric vascular occlusion;
- functional obstruction associated with pelvic abscess;
- all cases of partial obstruction (in which diarrhoea may occur).

Other manifestations

Dehydration

Dehydration is seen most commonly in small bowel obstruction because of repeated vomiting and fluid sequestration. It results in dry skin and tongue, poor venous filling and sunken eyes with oliguria. The blood urea level and haematocrit rise, giving a secondary polycythaemia.

Hypokalaemia

Hypokalaemia is not a common feature in simple mechanical obstruction. An increase in serum potassium, amylase or lactate dehydrogenase may be associated with the presence of strangulation, as may leucocytosis or leucopenia.

Pyrexia

Pyrexia in the presence of obstruction is rare and may indicate:

- the onset of ischaemia;
- intestinal perforation;
- inflammation or abscess associated with the obstructing disease.

Hypothermia indicates septicaemic shock or neglected cases of long duration.

Abdominal tenderness

Localised tenderness indicates impending or established ischaemia. The development of peritonism or peritonitis indicates overt infarction and/or perforation. In cases of large bowel obstruction, it is important to elicit these findings in the right iliac fossa as the caecum is most vulnerable to ischaemia.

Bowel sounds

High-pitched bowel sounds are present in the vast majority of patients with intestinal obstruction. Normal bowel sounds are of negative predictive value. Bowel sounds may be scanty or absent if the obstruction is longstanding and the small bowel has become inactive.

Clinical features of strangulation

It is vital to distinguish strangulating from non-strangulating intestinal obstruction because the former is a surgical emergency. The diagnosis is almost entirely clinical.

Summary box 71.8

Clinical features of strangulation

- Constant pain, severe pain
- Tenderness with rigidity and peritonism
- Shock

In addition to the features above, it should be noted that:

- The presence of shock suggests underlying ischaemia, especially if the shock is resistant to simple fluid resuscitation.
- In impending or established strangulation, pain is never completely absent.
- The presence and character of any local tenderness are of great significance and, however mild, tenderness requires frequent reassessment.
- Generalised tenderness and the presence of rigidity indicate the need for early laparotomy.
- In cases of intestinal obstruction in which pain persists despite conservative management, even in the absence of the above signs, strangulation should be presumed.
- When strangulation occurs in an external hernia, the lump is tense, tender and irreducible and there is no expansile cough impulse. Skin changes with erythema or purplish discolouration are associated with underlying ischaemia (Figures 71.8 and 71.9).

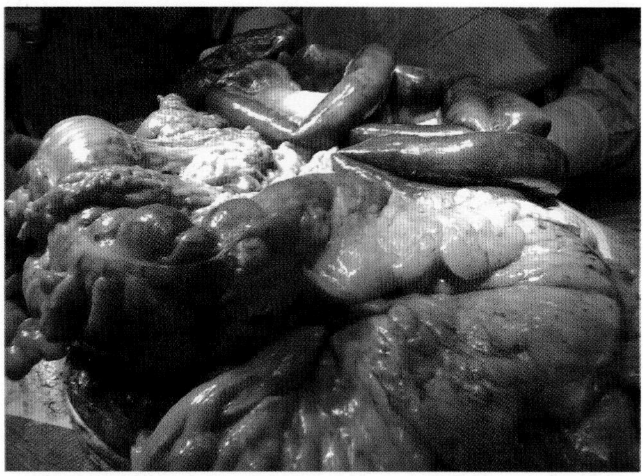

Figure 71.9 Ischaemic small and large bowel in a strangulated incisional hernia.

Clinical features of intussusception

The classical presentation of intussusception is with episodes of screaming and drawing up of the legs in a previously well male infant. The attacks last for a few minutes and recur repeatedly. During attacks the child appears pale; between episodes he may be listless. Vomiting may or may not occur at the outset but becomes conspicuous and bile-stained with time. Initially, the passage of stool may be normal, whereas, later, blood and mucus are evacuated – the 'redcurrant jelly' stool.

Whenever possible, examination should be undertaken between episodes of colic, without disturbing the child. Classically, the abdomen is not initially distended; a lump that hardens on palpation may be discerned but this is present in only 60% of cases (Figure 71.10). There may be an associated feeling of emptiness in the right iliac fossa (the sign of Dance). On rectal examination, blood-stained mucus may be found on the finger. Occasionally, in extensive ileocolic or colocolic intussusception, the apex may be palpable or even protrude from the anus.

Unrelieved, progressive dehydration and abdominal distension from small bowel obstruction will occur, followed by peritonitis secondary to gangrene. Rarely, natural cure may occur as a result of sloughing of the intussusception.

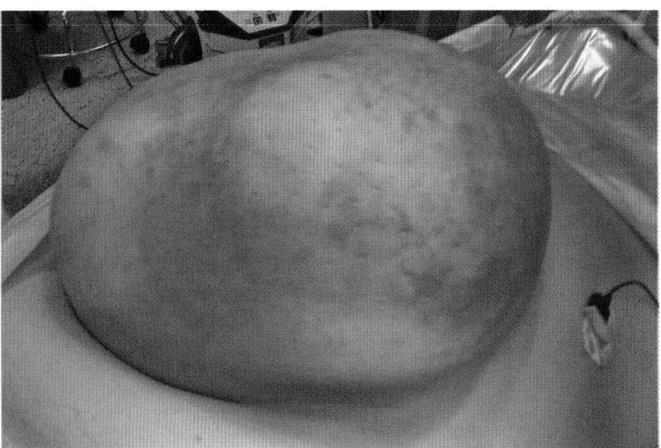

Figure 71.8 Skin discolouration over a strangulated incisional hernia.

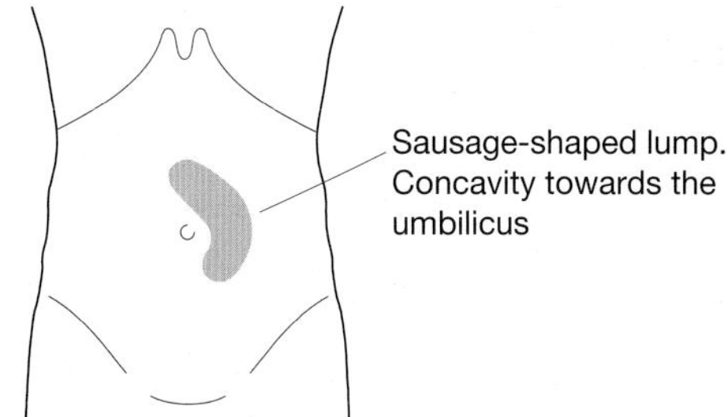

Figure 71.10 The physical signs as recorded by Hamilton Bailey in a typical case of intussusception in an infant.

Differential diagnosis

ACUTE GASTROENTERITIS

Although abdominal pain and vomiting are common in acute gastroenteritis, with occasional blood and mucus in the stool,

Henry Hamilton Bailey, 1894–1961, surgeon, The Royal Northern Hospital, London, UK.
Jean Baptiste Hippolyte Dance, 1797–1832, physician, Hôpital Cochin, Paris, France.

diarrhoea is a leading symptom and faecal matter or bile is always present in the stool.

HENOCH-SCHÖNLEIN PURPURA

Henoch–Schönlein purpura is associated with a characteristic rash and abdominal pain; intussusception may occur.

RECTAL PROLAPSE

This may be easily differentiated by the fact that the projecting mucosa can be felt in continuity with the perianal skin whereas in intussusception the finger may pass indefinitely into the depths of a sulcus.

Clinical features of volvulus

Volvulus of the small intestine

This may be primary or secondary and usually occurs in the lower ileum. It may occur spontaneously in African people, particularly following the consumption of a large volume of vegetable matter, whereas in western countries it is usually secondary to adhesions passing to the parietes or female pelvic organs.

Caecal volvulus

This may occur as part of volvulus neonatorum or *de novo* and is usually a clockwise twist. It is more common in females in the 4th and 5th decades and usually presents acutely with the classic features of obstruction. Ischaemia is common. At first the obstruction may be partial, with the passage of flatus and faeces. In 25% of cases, examination may reveal a palpable tympanic swelling in the midline or left side of the abdomen. The volvulus typically results in the caecum lying in the left upper quadrant. The diagnosis is not usually made preoperatively.

Sigmoid volvulus

The symptoms are of large bowel obstruction. Presentation varies in severity and acuteness, with younger patients appearing to develop the more acute form. Abdominal distension is an early and progressive sign, which may be associated with hiccough and retching. Constipation is absolute. In the elderly, a more chronic form may be seen. In some patients the grossly distended torted left colon is visible through the abdominal wall

IMAGING

Erect abdominal films are no longer routinely obtained and the radiological diagnosis is based on a supine abdominal film (Figure 71.11). An erect film may subsequently be requested when further doubt exists.

When distended with gas, the jejunum, ileum, caecum and remaining colon have a characteristic appearance in adults and older children that allows them to be distinguished radiologically.

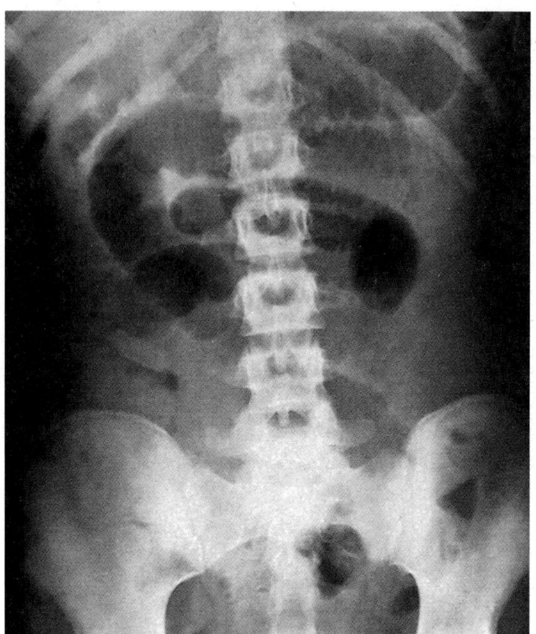

Figure 71.11 Gas-filled small bowel loop; patient supine.

> **Summary box 71.9**
>
> **Radiological features of obstruction (on plain x-ray)**
>
> - The obstructed small bowel is characterised by straight segments that are generally central and lie transversely. No/minimal gas is seen in the colon
> - The jejunum is characterised by its valvulae conniventes, which completely pass across the width of the bowel and are regularly spaced, giving a 'concertina' or ladder effect
> - Ileum – the distal ileum has been piquantly described by Wangensteen as featureless
> - Caecum – a distended caecum is shown by a rounded gas shadow in the right iliac fossa
> - Large bowel, except for the caecum, shows haustral folds, which, unlike valvulae conniventes, are spaced irregularly, do not cross the whole diameter of the bowel and do not have indentations placed opposite one another

In intestinal obstruction, fluid levels appear later than gas shadows as it takes time for gas and fluid to separate (Figure 71.12). These are most prominent on an erect film. In adults, two inconstant fluid levels – one at the duodenal cap and the other in the terminal ileum – may be regarded as normal. In infants (less than 1 year old), a few fluid levels in the small bowel may be physiological. In this age group it is difficult to distinguish large from small bowel in the presence of obstruction, because the characteristic features seen in adults are not present or are unreliable.

During the obstructive process, fluid levels become more conspicuous and more numerous when paralysis has occurred. When fluid levels are pronounced, the obstruction is advanced. In the small bowel, the number of fluid levels is directly proportional to the degree of obstruction and to its site, the number increasing the more distal the lesion.

Owen Harding Wangensteen, 1898–1981, Professor of Surgery, The University of Minnesota, Minneapolis, MN, USA.

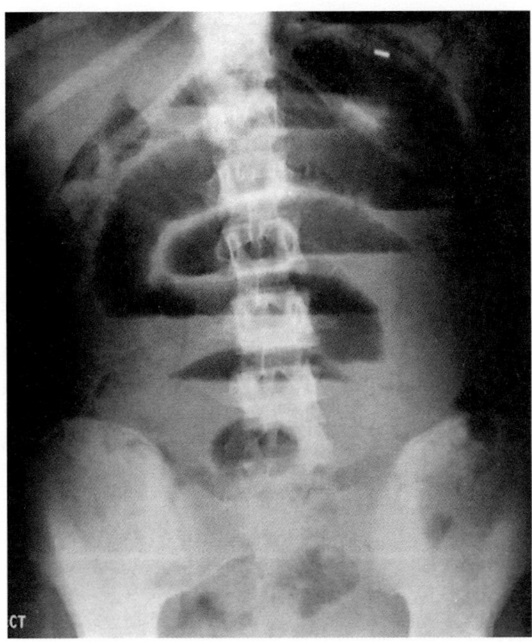

Figure 71.12 Fluid levels with gas above; 'stepladder pattern'. Ileal obstruction by adhesions; patient erect.

In patients without evidence of strangulation there is a role for other imaging modalities. A recent systematic review and meta-analysis of the diagnostic and therapeutic role of 50–100mL water-soluble contrast agent in adhesive small bowel obstruction included 14 prospective studies. The appearance of contrast in the colon 4–24 hours after administration had a sensitivity of 96% and a specificity of 98% in predicting resolution of small bowel obstruction. If contrast does not reach the colon, sugery is required in about 90% of patients. Administration of a water-soluble agent was also effective in reducing the need for surgey (OR 0.62; $p = 0.007$) and shortening hospital stay.

In contrast, low colonic obstruction does not commonly give rise to small bowel fluid levels unless advanced, whereas high colonic obstruction may do so in the presence of an incompetent ileocaecal valve. Colonic obstruction is usually associated with a large amount of gas in the caecum. A limited water-soluble enema should be undertaken to differentiate large bowel obstruction from pseudo-obstruction. A barium follow-through is contraindicated in the presence of acute obstruction and may be life-threatening.

The CT scan is now used very widely to investigate all forms of intestinal obstruction. It is highly accurate and its only limitations are in diagnosing ischaemia. Two CT scan findings may be used in clinical practice when looking for intestinal ischaemia: reduced enhanced bowel wall is highly predictive of ischaemia and absence of mesenteric fluid is a reliable finding to rule out strangulation. It is important to remember that even with the best imaging techniques, the diagnosis of strangulation remains a clinical one.

Key points:

- Reduced bowel wall enhancement on CT increases the probability of strangulation 11-fold.
- Absence of mesenteric fluid on CT decreases the probability of strangulation 6-fold.
- The clinical reliability of other CT signs is doubtful for predicting strangulation.

Impacted foreign bodies may be seen on abdominal radiographs. It is noteworthy that gas-filled loops and fluid levels in the small and large bowel can also be seen in established paralytic ileus and pseudo-obstruction. The former can, however, normally be distinguished on clinical grounds whereas the latter can be confirmed radiologically. Fluid levels may also be seen in nonobstructing conditions such as gastroenteritis, acute pancreatitis and intra-abdominal sepsis.

Imaging in intussusception

A plain abdominal field usually reveals evidence of small or large bowel obstruction with an absent caecal gas shadow in ileocolic cases. A soft tissue opacity is often visible in children. A barium enema may be used to diagnose the presence of an ileocolic intussusception (the claw sign) (Figure 71.13) but does not demonstrate small bowel intussusception. An abdominal ultrasound scan has a high diagnostic sensitivity in children, demonstrating the typical doughnut appearance of concentric rings in transverse section. CT scanning is currently considered the most sensitive radiological method to confirm intussusception, with a reported diagnostic accuracy of 58–100%. The characteristic features of CT scan include a 'target'- or 'sausage'- shaped soft-tissue mass with a layering effect; mesenteric vessels within the bowel lumen are also typical.

Imaging in volvulus

- In **caecal volvulus**, radiological abnormalities are identifiable in nearly all patients, but are often nonspecific, with caecal dilatation (98–100%), single air-fluid level

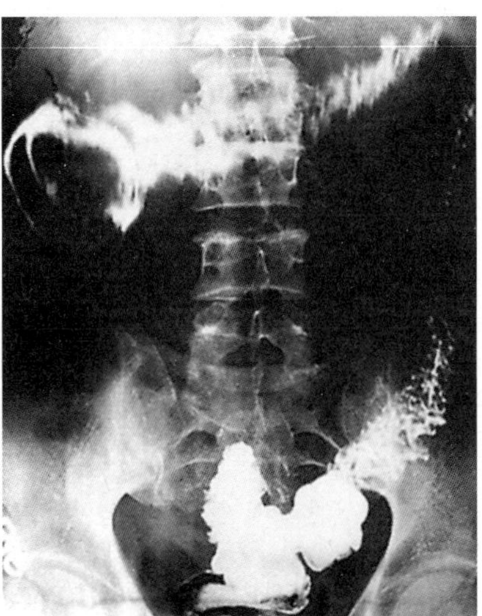

Figure 71.13 'Claw' sign of iliac intussusception. The barium in the intussusception is seen as a claw around a negative shadow of the intussusception (courtesy of RS Naik, Durg, India).

(72–88%), small bowel dilatation (42–55%) and absence of gas in distal colon (82–91%) reported as the most common abnormalities. A barium enema may be used to confirm the diagnosis if there are no concerns about ischaemia, with an absence of barium in the caecum and a bird beak deformity. CT scanning is replacing barium enema as the imaging of choice in these less urgent cases.
- In **sigmoid volvulus**, a plain radiograph shows massive colonic distension. The classic appearance is of a dilated loop of bowel; the two limbs are seen running diagonally across the abdomen from right to left, with two fluid levels seen, one within each loop of bowel (if an erect film is taken).
- In **volvulus neonatorium**, the abdominal radiograph shows a variable appearance. Initially, it may appear normal or show evidence of duodenal obstruction but, as the intestinal strangulation progresses, the abdomen becomes relatively gasless.

TREATMENT OF ACUTE INTESTINAL OBSTRUCTION

There are three main measures used to treat acute intestinal obstruction.

Summary box 71.10

Treatment of acute intestinal obstruction

- Gastrointestinal drainage via a nasogastric tube
- Fluid and electrolyte replacement
- Relief of obstruction
- Surgical treatment is necessary for most cases of intestinal obstruction but should be delayed until resuscitation is complete, provided there is no sign of strangulation or evidence of closed-loop obstruction

The first two steps are always necessary before attempting the surgical relief of obstruction and are the mainstay of postoperative management.

Summary box 71.11

Principles of surgical intervention for obstruction

Management of:

- The segment at the site of obstruction
- The distended proximal bowel
- The underlying cause of obstruction

Supportive management

Nasogastric decompression is achieved by the passage of a nonvented (Ryle) or vented (Salem) tube. The tubes are normally placed on free drainage with 4-hourly aspiration but may be placed on continuous or intermittent suction. As well as facilitating decompression proximal to the obstruction, they are essential to reduce the risk of subsequent aspiration during induction of anaesthesia and post-extubation.

The basic biochemical abnormality in intestinal obstruction is sodium and water loss, and therefore the appropriate replacement is Hartmann's solution or normal saline. The volume required varies and should be determined by clinical haematological and biochemical criteria.

Antibiotics are not mandatory but many clinicians initiate broad-spectrum antibiotics early in therapy because of bacterial overgrowth. Antibiotic therapy is mandatory for all patients undergoing surgery for intestinal obstruction.

Surgical treatment

The timing of surgical intervention is dependent on the clinical picture. There are several indications for early surgical intervention.

Summary box 71.12

Indications for early surgical intervention

- Obstructed external hernia
- Clinical features suspicious of intestinal strangulation
- Obstruction in a 'virgin' abdomen

The classic clinical advice that 'the sun should not both rise and set' on a case of unrelieved acute intestinal obstruction was based on the concern that intestinal ischaemia would develop while the patient was waiting for surgery. If there is complete obstruction, but no evidence of intestinal ischaemia, it is reasonable to defer surgery until the patient has been adequately resuscitated. Where obstruction is likely to be secondary to adhesions, conservative management may be continued for up to 72 hours in the hope of spontaneous resolution.

If the site of obstruction is unknown, adequate exposure is best achieved by a midline incision. Assessment is directed to:

- the site of the obstruction;
- the nature of the obstruction;
- the viability of the gut.

In cases of small bowel obstruction, the first manoeuvre is to deliver the distended small bowel into the wound. This

John Alfred Ryle, 1889–1950, Regius Professor of Physic, The University of Cambridge, and later Professor of Social Medicine, The University of Oxford, UK, introduced the Ryle's tube in 1921.
Henri Albert Charles Antoine Hartmann, 1860–1952, Professor of Clinical Surgery, The Faculty of Medicine, The University of Paris, France.

permits access to the site of obstruction. The small bowel should be covered with moist swabs and the weight of the fluid-filled bowel supported such that the blood supply to the mesentery is not impaired.

Operative decompression should be performed whenever possible. This reduces pressure on the abdominal wound, reducing pain and improving diaphragmatic movement. The simplest and safest method is to insert a large-bore orogastric tube and to milk the small bowel contents in a retrograde manner to the stomach for aspiration. All volumes of fluid removed should be accurately measured and appropriately replaced. It is important to ensure that the stomach is empty at the end of the procedure to prevent postoperative aspiration.

Rarely, decompression using Savage's decompressor within a seromuscular purse-string suture may be required. Its benefits should be balanced against the potential risk of septic complications from spillage and the risk of leakage from the suture line postoperatively. The type of surgical procedure required will depend upon the cause of obstruction – division of adhesions (enterolysis), excision, bypass or proximal decompression.

Following relief of obstruction, the viability of the involved bowel should be carefully assessed (*Table 71.3*). Although frankly infarcted bowel is obvious, the viability status in many cases may be difficult to discern. If in doubt, the bowel should be wrapped in hot packs for 10 minutes with increased oxygenation and then reassessed. The state of the mesenteric vessels and pulsation in adjacent arcades should be sought. Viability is also confirmed by colour, sheen and peristalsis. If, at the end of this period, there is still uncertainty about gut viability, the gut should be resected if this does not result in short bowel syndrome. If the patient is septic such that they require inotropic therapy or would require postoperative level 3 intensive care treatment following resection, consideration should be given to raising both ends of the bowel as stomas. This is not only safe but also allows regular assessment of the bowel.

Intestinal ischaemia/reperfusion injury has been described following reperfusion of ischaemic bowel with remote lung injury resulting from the release of inflammatory mediators. This should be borne in mind when dealing with ischaemic bowel. For example if there is a volvulus with established infarction, detorsion should be avoided until the affected mesentery has been clamped and thus reperfusion injury prevented. When no resection has been undertaken or there are multiple ischaemic areas (mesenteric vascular occlusion), a second-look laparotomy at 24–48 hours may be required.

Special attention should always be paid to the sites of constriction at each end of an obstructed segment. If of doubtful viability they should be infolded by the use of a seromuscular suture and can also be covered with omentum (**Figures 71.14 and 71.15**).

The surgical management of massive infarction is dependent on the patient's overall prognostic criteria. In the elderly, infarction of the small bowel from the duodenojejunal flexure to the right colon may be considered incurable, whereas in the young, with the potential for long-term intravenous alimentation and small bowel transplantation, a policy of excision may be justified.

Whenever the small bowel is resected, the exact site of resection, the length of the resected segment and that of the residual bowel should be recorded.

As laparoscopic surgery is now so common, it is important to note that small bowel obstruction and strangulation occur in relation to port site hernias. The risk of port site herniation is related to older age, higher body mass, trocar diameter and extension of the port site for tissue extraction. For laparoscopic cholecystectomy, the hernia rate is reported to be around 2%. Obstruction and strangulation have even been reported through 5-mm port sites. Complications from these hernias may present in the early postoperative period and as a Richter's hernia. They can be easily overlooked and careful examination of port sites in patients with small bowel obstruction is essential.

TABLE 71.3 Differentiation between viable and non-viable intestine.

	Viable	Non-viable
Circulation	Dark colour becomes lighter Visible pulsation in mesenteric arteries	Dark colour remains No detectable pulsation
General appearance	Shiny	Dull and lustreless
Intestinal musculature	Firm	Flabby, thin and friable
	Peristalsis may be observed	No peristalsis

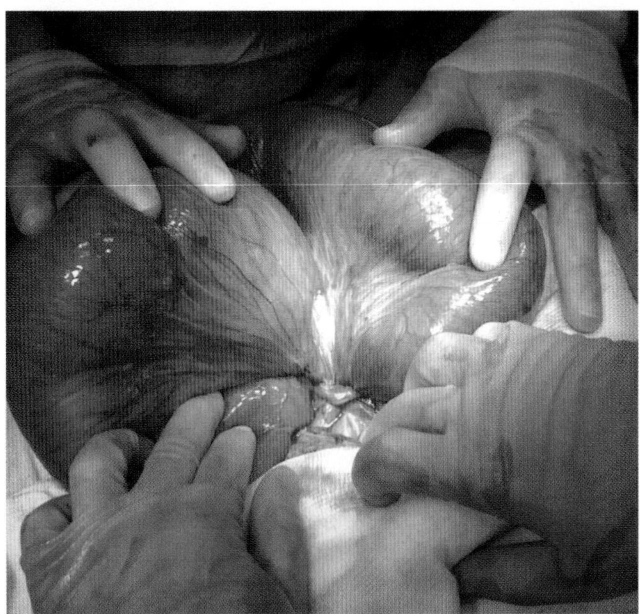

Figure 71.14 Band adhesion causing closed-loop obstruction.

Paul Thwaites Savage, formerly surgeon, The Whittington Hospital, London, UK.

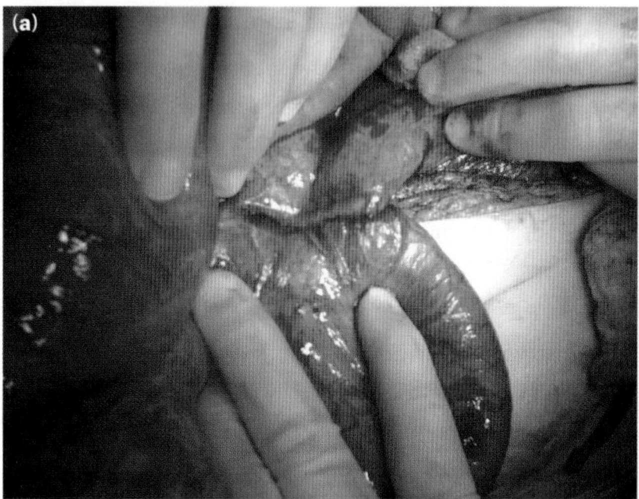

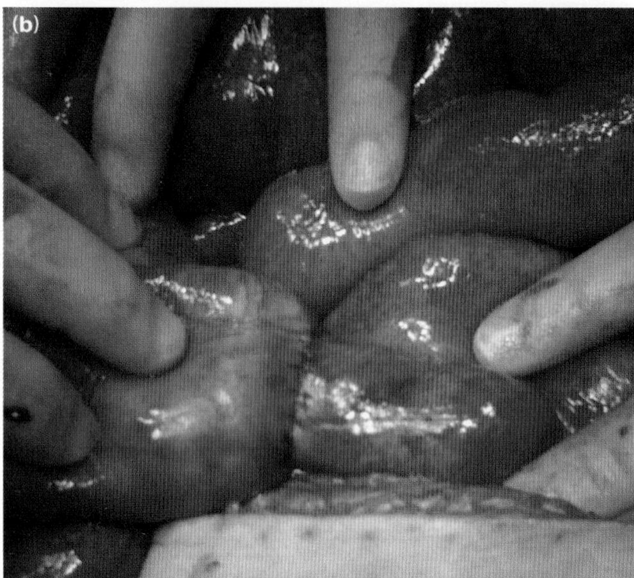

Figure 71.15 (a, b) Wall injury resulting from band compression, oversewn with an absorbable seromuscular suture.

Treatment of adhesions

Initial management is based on intravenous rehydration and nasogastric decompression; occasionally, this treatment is curative. Although an initial conservative regimen is considered appropriate, regular assessment is mandatory to ensure that strangulation does not occur. Conservative treatment should not usually be prolonged beyond 72 hours.

When laparotomy is required, although multiple adhesions may be found, only one may be causative. If there is absolute certainty that this is the cause of the obstruction, this should be divided and the remaining adhesions can be left *in situ* unless severe angulation is present. Division of these adhesions will only cause further adhesion formation.

When obstruction is caused by an area of multiple adhesions, the adhesions should be freed by sharp dissection from the duodenojejunal junction to the caecum. Following the release of band obstruction, the constriction sites that have suffered direct compression should be carefully assessed and, if they show residual colour changes, invaginated with a seromuscular suture (Figure 71.15).

Laparoscopic adhesiolysis may be considered in highly selected cases of small bowel obstruction. This is classed as an advanced laparoscopic procedure and should only be undertaken by surgeons with advanced laparoscopic skills.

Summary box 71.13

Treatment of adhesive obstruction

- Initially treat conservatively provided there are no signs of strangulation; should rarely continue conservative treatment for longer than 72 hours
- At operation, divide only the causative adhesion(s) and limit dissection
- Repair serosal tears; invaginate (or resect) areas of doubtful viability
- Laparoscopic adhesiolysis in the hands of advanced laparoscopic practitioners

Treatment of recurrent intestinal obstruction caused by adhesions

Several procedures may be considered in the presence of recurrent obstruction including:

- repeat adhesiolysis (enterolysis) alone;
- Noble's plication operation;
- Child–Phillips transmesenteric plication;
- intestinal intubation.

The latter three operations are now very rarely performed and can probably be consigned to the history books (they have never been required by the author).

Postoperative intestinal obstruction

Differentiation between persistent paralytic ileus and early mechanical obstruction may be difficult in the early postoperative period. Mechanical obstruction is more likely if the patient has regained bowel function postoperatively which subsequently stops. Obstruction is usually incomplete and the majority settle with continued conservative management. Postoperative intra-abdominal sepsis is a potent cause of postoperative obstruction; CT scanning with oral contrast is of particular value in the assessment of the postoperative abdomen. Instant gastrografin enemas are also of value.

Thomas Benjamin Noble, 1895–1965, surgeon, The Community Hospital, Indianapolis, IN, USA.
Richard V Phillips, surgeon, Albuquerque, NM, USA.

Treatment of intussusception

In the infant with ileocolic intussusception, after resuscitation with intravenous fluids, broad-spectrum antibiotics and nasogastric drainage, non-operative reduction can be attempted using an air or barium enema. Successful reduction can only be accepted if there is free reflux of air or barium into the small bowel, together with resolution of symptoms and signs in the patient. Non-operative reduction is contraindicated if there are signs of peritonitis or perforation, there is a known pathological lead point or in the presence of profound shock. In experienced units, more than 70% of intussusceptions can be reduced non-operatively. Strangulated bowel and pathological lead points are unlikely to reduce. Perforation of the colon during pneumatic or hydrostatic reduction is a recognised hazard but is rare. Recurrent intussusception occurs in up to 10% of patients after non-operative reduction.

Surgery is required when radiological reduction has failed or is contraindicated. After resuscitation, a transverse right-sided abdominal incision provides good access. Reduction is achieved by gently compressing the most distal part of the intussusception toward its origin (Figure 71.16), making sure not to pull. The last part of the reduction is the most difficult (Figure 71.17). After reduction, the terminal part of the small bowel and the appendix will be seen to be bruised and oedematous. The viability of the whole bowel should be checked carefully. An irreducible intussusception or one complicated by infarction or a pathological lead point requires resection and primary anastomosis.

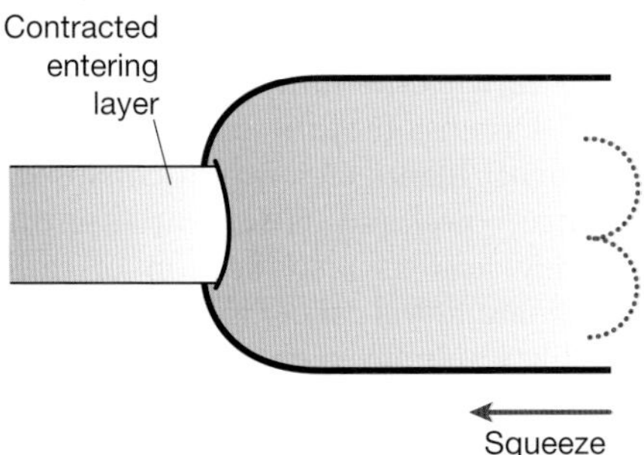

Figure 71.16 Diagram showing the method used to reduce an intussusception.

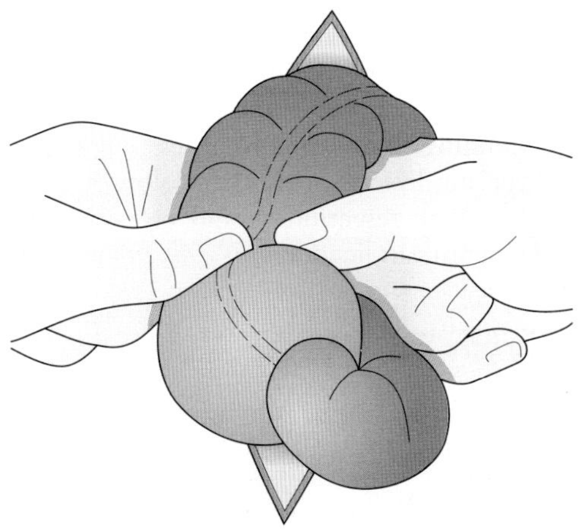

Figure 71.17 Reducing the terminal part of the intussusception (after RE Gross).

Acute intestinal obstruction of the newborn

Neonatal intestinal obstruction has many potential causes. Congenital atresia and stenosis are the most common. Intestinal malrotation with midgut volvulus, meconium ileus, Hirschprung's disease, imperforate anus, necrotising enterocolitis and an incarcerated inguinal hernia may also be responsible. Many of these conditions are discussed in Chapter 9.

Intestinal atresia

Duodenal atresia and stenosis are the commonest forms of intestinal obstruction in the newborn (see Chapter 9). Jejunal or ileal atresias are next in frequency whereas colonic atresia is rare. The possibility of multiple atresias makes intraoperative assessment of the whole small and large bowel mandatory. As with all congenital anomalies, associated malformations are common and should be excluded.

There are four main types of jejunal/ileal atresia, ranging from an obstructing membrane with continuity of the bowel wall, through blind-ended segments of bowel separated by a fibrous cord or V-shaped mesenteric defect (including the so called apple-peel atresia) (Figure 71.18), to multiple atresias ('string of sausages'). The obstructed proximal bowel is at risk of perforation, which may happen prenatally causing meconium peritonitis in the fetus.

Small bowel atresias present with intestinal obstruction soon after birth. Bilious vomiting is the dominant feature in jejunal atresia whereas abdominal distension is more

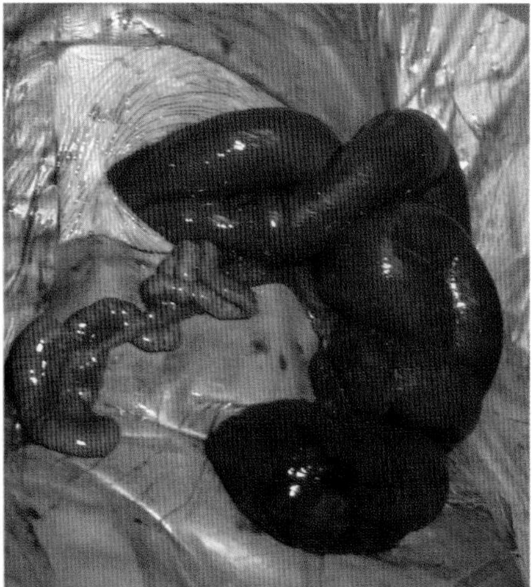

Figure 71.18 Apple-peel jejunal bowel atresia with obstructed proximal jejunum and collapsed distal ileum coiled round a remnant ileocolic artery (courtesy of MD Stringer, Leeds, UK).

Harald Hirschsprung, 1830–1916, physician, The Queen Louise Hospital for Children, Copenhagen, Denmark, described congenital megacolon in 1887.

prominent with ileal atresia. A small amount of pale meconium may be passed despite the atresia.

Plain abdominal radiographs show a variable number of dilated loops of bowel and fluid levels according to the level of obstruction. In a stable infant, a contrast enema may be required to clarify the cause of a distal bowel obstruction.

SURGERY

Duodenal atresia is corrected by a duodenoduodenostomy. In most cases of jejunal/ileal atresia, the distal end of the dilated proximal small bowel is resected and a primary end-to-end anastomosis is possible. If the proximal bowel is extremely dilated it may need to be tapered to the distal bowel before anastomosis. Occasionally, a temporary stoma is required before definitive repair.

Meconium ileus

Cystic fibrosis is almost always the underlying cause of this condition. Meconium is normally kept fluid by the action of pancreatic enzymes. In meconium ileus the terminal ileum becomes filled with thick viscid meconium, resulting in progressive intestinal obstruction. A sterile meconium peritonitis may have occurred *in utero*.

Visibly dilated loops of bowel are often palpable in the newborn with meconium ileus. An abdominal radiograph may show a dilated small intestine with mottling. Fluid levels are generally not seen. Unlike ileal atresia there is no abrupt termination of the gas-filled intestine. A contrast enema shows an unused microcolon. As the condition is caused by an autosomal recessive genetic defect, a family history may be present. Further assessment includes gene mutation analysis and, beyond the neonatal period, a sweat test, which shows elevated sodium and chloride levels (>70 mmol/L).

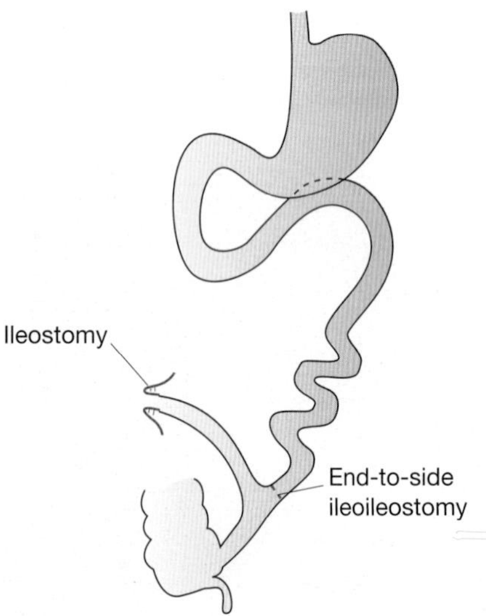

Figure 71.19 Bishop–Koop operation. This shows the completed procedure after a grossly distended ileum has been resected. Because intestinal continuity is preserved, early closure of the ileostomy is not essential.

Uncomplicated meconium ileus may respond to treatment with a hyperosmolar gastrografin enema; this draws fluid into the gut lumen and also has detergent properties, which help to liquefy the meconium. Infants treated in this way need extra intravenous fluids to compensate for fluid shifts. Meconium ileus complicated by intestinal perforation, volvulus or atresia, or unresponsive to enemas, demands surgery. Various surgical procedures are used including intestinal resection and temporary stoma formation, resection and primary anastomosis, and, in uncomplicated cases, enterotomy and irrigation of the bowel. The Bishop–Koop operation (Figure 71.19) with its irrigating stoma is now only rarely used.

TREATMENT OF ACUTE LARGE BOWEL OBSTRUCTION

Large bowel obstruction is usually caused by an underlying carcinoma or occasionally diverticular disease, and presents in an acute or chronic form. The condition of pseudo-obstruction should always be considered and excluded by a limited contrast study or CT scan to confirm organic obstruction.

After full resuscitation, the abdomen should be opened through a midline incision. Care should be taken to ensure that the loss of tamponade of the abdominal wall does not lead to increased caecal distension and rupture (this starts with splitting along the line of the taenia coli on the antimesenteric border). Distension of the caecum will confirm large bowel involvement. Identification of a collapsed distal segment of the large bowel and its sequential proximal assessment will readily lead to identification of the cause. As surgery for malignant bowel cancer is technically challenging, wherever possible a suitably trained surgeon should perform the procedure. When a removable lesion is found in the caecum, ascending colon, hepatic flexure or proximal transverse colon, an emergency right hemicolectomy should be performed. A primary anastomosis is safe if the patient's general condition is reasonable. If the lesion is irremovable (this is rarely the case) a proximal stoma (colostomy or ileosotomy if the ileocaecal valve is incompetent) or ileotransverse bypass should be considered. Obstructing lesions at the splenic flexure should be treated by an extended right hemicolectomy with ileodescending colonic anastomosis.

For obstructing lesions of the left colon or rectosigmoid junction, immediate resection should be considered unless there are clear contraindications.

Summary box 71.14

Management of left-sided large bowel obstruction

Contraindications to immediate resection include:

- Inexperienced surgeon
- Moribund patient
- Advanced disease

Harry C Bishop, 1921–2009, Professor of Surgery, University of Philadelphia, PA, USA.
Charles Everett Koop, 1916–2013, paediatric surgeon and public health administrator, served as the 13th Surgeon General of the United States (1982–1989).

In rare instances, or when caecal perforation is imminent, additional time to improve the patient's clinical condition can be bought by performing an emergency caecostomy (or ileostomy in the presence of an incompetent ileocaecal valve).

In the absence of senior clinical staff it is safest to bring the proximal colon to the surface as a colostomy. When possible the distal bowel should be brought out at the same time (Paul–Mikulicz procedure) to facilitate subsequent closure. In the majority of cases, the distal bowel will not reach and is closed and returned to the abdomen (Hartmann's procedure). A second-stage colorectal anastomosis can be planned when the patient is fit.

If an anastomosis is to be considered using the proximal colon, in the presence of obstruction, it must be decompressed and cleaned by an on-table colonic lavage.

In the palliative situation, where there is advanced incurable disease, the patient is unfit for major surgery or a combination of the two, insertion of a self-expanding metal stent (SEMS) has been demonstrated to be preferable to surgery; there is now good evidence of reduced mortality and morbidity and stoma formation. Technical and clinical success rates for stenting are of the order of 80–90%.

For patients with potentially curative disease, stenting as a bridge to surgery (usually performed 1–4 weeks poststenting) has been shown to reduce stoma formation but not to reduce postoperative mortality, and the long-term oncological effects of stenting are still uncertain. The current recommendation is that stenting as a bridge to surgery in patients with potentially curative disease should only be used in patients with a high risk of postoperative morbidity and mortality (Figure 71.20).

Treatment of caecal volvulus

At operation the volvulus is usually found to be ischaemic and needs resection. If viable, the volvulus should be reduced. Sometimes, this can only be achieved after decompression of the caecum using a needle. Further management consists of fixation of the caecum to the right iliac fossa (caecopexy) and/or a caecostomy. Recurrence of volvulus after caecopexy has been reported in up to 40% of cases.

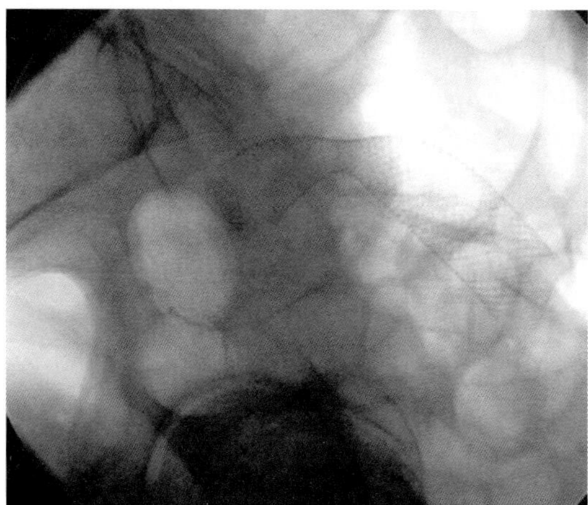

Figure 71.20 X-ray of a stent inserted for malignant colonic obstruction.

Treatment of sigmoid volvulus

Flexible sigmoidoscopy or rigid sigmoidoscopy and insertion of a flatus tube should be carried out to allow deflation of the gut. The tube should be secured in place with tape for 24 hours and a repeat x-ray taken to ensure that decompression has occurred. Success, as long as ischaemic bowel is excluded, will resolve the acute problem.

In young patients, an elective sigmoid colectomy is required. It is reasonable not to offer any further treatment following successful endoscopic decompression in the elderly as there is a high death rate (~80% at two years) from causes other than recurrent volvulus. In elderly patients with co-morbidities and recurrent episodes of volvulus, the options are resection or two-point fixation with combined endoscopic/percutaneous tube insertion (gastrostomy tubes are frequently used for this purpose). Failure results in an early laparotomy, with untwisting of the loop and per anum decompression (Figure 71.21).

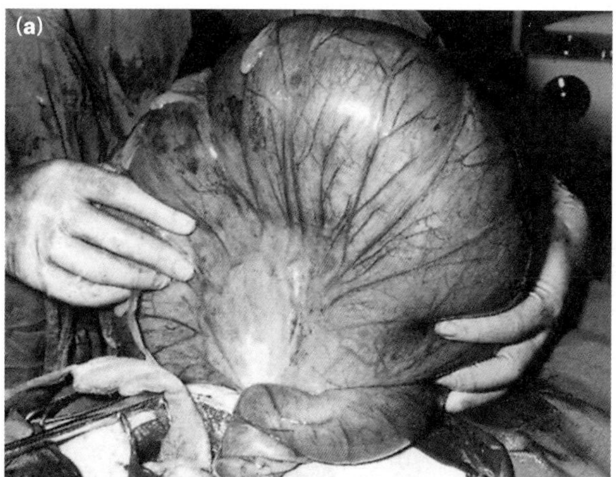

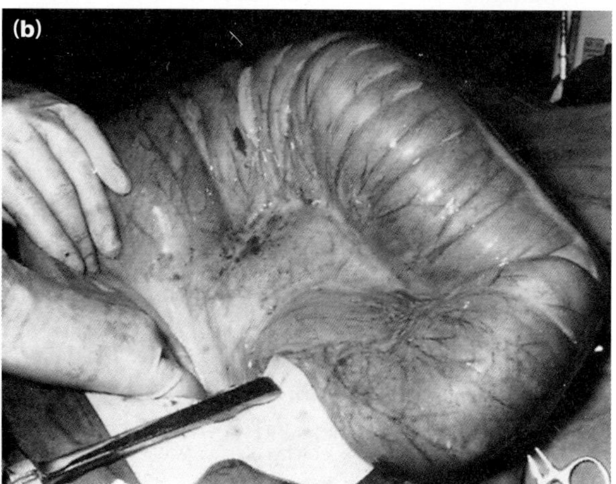

Figure 71.21 Volvulus of the sigmoid colon (a) before and (b) after untwisting (courtesy of SU Rahman, Manchester, UK).

Frank Thomas Paul, 1851–1941, surgeon, The Royal Infirmary, Liverpool, UK.
Johann von Mikulicz-Radecki, 1850–1905, Professor of Surgery, Breslau, Germany, (now Wroclaw, Poland).

When the bowel is viable, fixation of the sigmoid colon to the posterior abdominal wall may be a safer manoeuvre in inexperienced hands. Resection is preferable if it can be achieved safely. A Paul–Mikulicz procedure is useful, particularly if there is suspicion of impending gangrene (Figure 71.22); an alternative procedure is a sigmoid colectomy and, when anastomosis is considered unwise, a Hartmann's procedure with subsequent reanastomosis can be carried out.

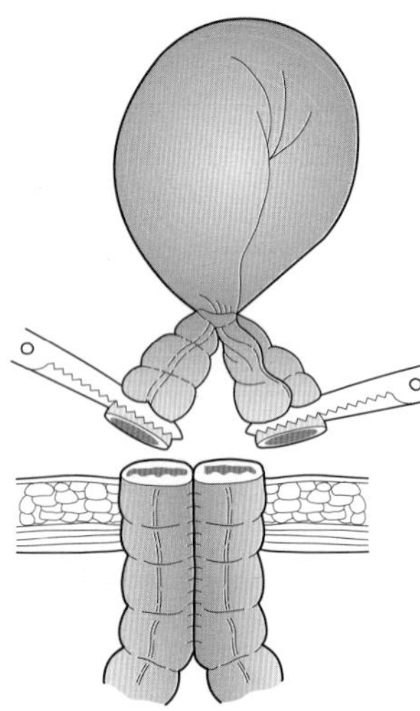

Figure 71.22 The Paul–Mikulicz operation applied to volvulus of the pelvic colon.

CHRONIC LARGE BOWEL OBSTRUCTION

The symptoms of chronic intestinal obstruction may arise from two sources – the cause and the subsequent obstruction.

The causes of obstruction may be organic:

- intraluminal (rare) – faecal impaction;
- intrinsic intramural – strictures (Crohn's disease, ischaemia, diverticular), anastomotic stenosis;
- extrinsic intramural (rare) – metastatic deposits (ovarian), endometriosis, stomal stenosis;

or functional:

- Hirschsprung's disease, idiopathic megacolon, pseudo-obstruction.

The symptoms of chronic obstruction differ in their predominance, timing and degree from acute obstruction. In functional cases, the symptoms may have been present for months or years. Constipation appears first. It is initially relative and then absolute, associated with distension. In the presence of large bowel disease, the point of greatest distension is in the caecum, and this is heralded by the onset of pain. Vomiting is a late feature and therefore dehydration is less severe. Examination is unremarkable, save for confirmation of distension, which can be profound (Figure 71.23) and the onset of peritonism in late cases. Rectal examination may confirm the presence of faecal impaction or a tumour.

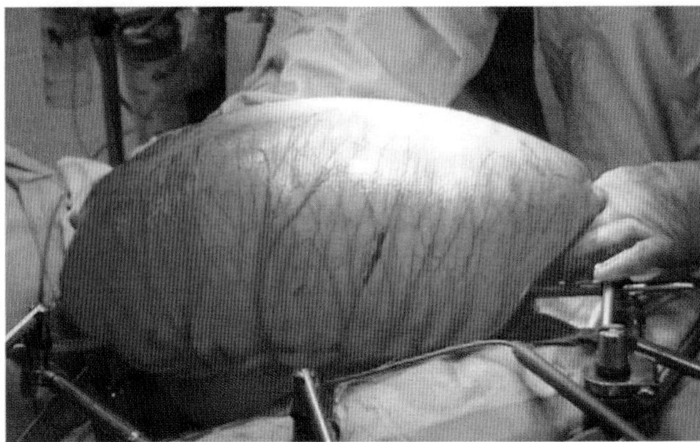

Figure 71.23 Gross functional distension.

Investigation

Plain abdominal radiography confirms the presence of large bowel distension. All such cases should be investigated by a subsequent single-contrast water-soluble enema study, CT scan or endoscopic assessment to rule out functional disease.

Organic disease requires decompression with either a laparotomy or stent. Stomal stenosis can usually be managed at the abdominal wall level (Figure 71.24). Surgical management after resuscitation depends on the underlying cause and the relevant chapters in this book should be consulted.

Functional disease requires colonoscopic decompression in the first instance and conservative management. Intestinal perforation can occur in patients with functional obstruction. Those at risk have such gross distension that the abomen is rigid on palpation.

Summary box 71.15

Principles of investigation of possible large bowel obstruction

- In the presence of large bowel obstruction, a single-contrast water-soluble enema or CT should be undertaken to exclude a functional cause

ADYNAMIC OBSTRUCTION

Paralytic ileus

This may be defined as a state in which there is failure of transmission of peristaltic waves secondary to neuromuscular failure (i.e. in the myenteric (Auerbach's) and submucous

Leopold Auerbach, 1828–1897, Professor of Neuropathology, Breslau, Germany, (now Wroclaw, Poland), described the myenteric plexus in 1862.

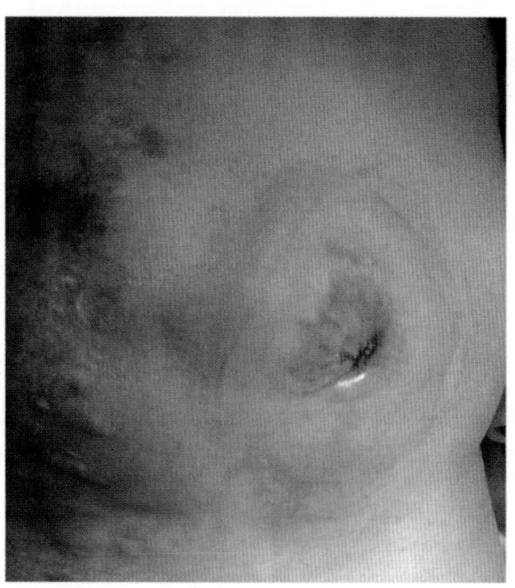

Figure 71.24 Stomal stenosis causing large bowel obstruction.

(Meissner's) plexuses). The resultant stasis leads to accumulation of fluid and gas within the bowel, with associated distension, vomiting, absence of bowel sounds and absolute constipation.

Varieties

The following varieties are recognised:

- **Postoperative**: a degree of ileus usually occurs after any abdominal procedure and is self-limiting, with a variable duration of 24–72 hours. Postoperative ileus may be prolonged in the presence of hypoproteinaemia or metabolic abnormality (see below).
- **Infection**: intra-abdominal sepsis may give rise to localised or generalised ileus.
- **Reflex ileus**: this may occur following fractures of the spine or ribs, retroperitoneal haemorrhage or even the application of a plaster jacket.
- **Metabolic**: uraemia and hypokalaemia are the most common contributory factors.

Clinical features

Paralytic ileus takes on a clinical significance if, 72 hours after laparotomy:

- there has been no return of bowel sounds on auscultation;
- there has been no passage of flatus.

Abdominal distension becomes more marked and tympanitic. Colicky pain is not a feature. Distension increases pain from the abdominal wound. In the absence of gastric aspiration, effortless vomiting may occur. Radiologically, the abdomen shows gas-filled loops of intestine with multiple fluid levels (if an erect film is felt necessary).

Management

Nasogastric tubes are not required routinely after elective intra-abdominal surgery. Paralytic ileus is managed with the use of nasogastric suction and restriction of oral intake until bowel sounds and the passage of flatus return. Electrolyte balance must be maintained. The use of an enhanced recovery programme with early introduction of fluids and solids is, however, becoming increasingly popular.

Specific treatment is directed towards the cause, but the following general principles apply:

- If a primary cause is identified this must be treated.
- Gastrointestinal distension must be relieved by decompression.
- Close attention to fluid and electrolyte balance is essential.
- There is no convincing evidence for the use of prokinetic drugs to treat postoperative adynamic ileus.
- If paralytic ileus is prolonged CT scanning is the most effective investigation; it will demonstrate any intra-abdominal sepsis or mechanical obstruction and therefore guide any requirement for laparotomy. Otherwise the decision to take a patient back to theatre in these circumstances is always difficult. The need for a laparotomy becomes increasingly likely the longer the bowel inactivity persists, particularly if it lasts for more than seven days or if bowel activity recommences following surgery and then stops again.

Pseudo-obstruction

This condition describes an obstruction, usually of the colon, that occurs in the absence of a mechanical cause or acute intra-abdominal disease. It is associated with a variety of syndromes in which there is an underlying neuropathy and/or myopathy and a range of other factors.

Small intestinal pseudo-obstruction

This condition may be primary (i.e. idiopathic or associated with familial visceral myopathy) or secondary. The clinical picture consists of recurrent subacute obstruction. The diagnosis is made by the exclusion of a mechanical cause. Treatment consists of initial correction of any underlying disorder. Metoclopramide and erythromycin may be of use.

Colonic pseudo-obstruction

This may occur in an acute or a chronic form. The former, also known as Ogilvie's syndrome, presents as acute large bowel obstruction. Abdominal radiographs show evidence of colonic obstruction, with marked caecal distension being a common feature. Indeed, caecal perforation is a well-recognised complication. The absence of a mechanical cause requires urgent confirmation by colonoscopy or a single-contrast water-soluble barium enema or CT. Once confirmed, pseudo-obstruction requires treatment of any identifiable cause. If this is ineffective, intravenous neostigmine should be given (1 mg intravenously), with a further 1 mg given intravenously within a few minutes if the first dose is ineffective. During this procedure, it is best to sit the patient on a

Georg Meissner, 1829–1905, Professor of Physiology, Gottingen, Germany, described the submucous plexus of the alimentary tract in 1852.
Sir William Heneage Ogilvie, 1887–1971, surgeon, Guy's Hospital, London, UK.

Summary box 71.16

Factors associated with pseudo-obstruction

- Metabolic
  - Diabetes
  - Hypokalaemia
  - Uraemia
  - Myxodoema
  - Intermittent porphyria
- Severe trauma (especially to the lumbar spine and pelvis)
- Shock
  - Burns
  - Myocardial infarction
  - Stroke
- Idiopathic
- Septicaemia
- Postoperative (for example fractured neck of femur)
- Retroperitoneal irritation
  - Blood
  - Urine
  - Enzymes (pancreatitis)
  - Tumour
- Drugs
  - Tricyclic antidepressants
  - Phenothiazines
  - Laxatives
- Secondary gastrointestinal involvement
  - Scleroderma
  - Chagas' disease

commode. Electrocardiograph (ECG) monitoring is required and atropine should be available. If neostigmine is not effective, colonoscopic decompression should be peformed. Caecal perforation can occur in pseudo-obstruction. Abdominal examination should pay attention to tenderness and peritonism over the caecum and as with mechanical obstruction, caecal perforation is more likely if the caecal diameter is 14 cm or greater. Surgery is associated with high morbidity and mortality and should be reserved for those with impending perforation when other treatments have failed or perforation has occurred.

Rarely, an endoscopically placed tube colostomy is used as a vent for patients with a chronic unremitting condition.

FURTHER READING

Becker JM, Stucchi AF. Intra-abdominal adhesion prevention: are we getting any closer? *Ann Surg* 2004: **240**: 202–4.

Bickell NA, Federman AD, Aufses AH. Influence of time on risk of bowel resection in complete small bowel obstruction. *J Am Coll Surg* 2005; **201**: 847–54.

Branco BC, Barmparas G, Schnuriger B *et al.* Systematic review and meta-analyis of the diagnostic and therapeutic role of water-soluble contrast agent in adhesive small bowel obstruction. *Br J Surg* 2010; **97**:470–8.

ten Broek RP, Stommel MW, Strik C, van Laarhoven CJ, Keus F, van Goor H. Benefits and harms of adhesion barriers for abdominal surgery: a systematic review and meta-analysis. *Lancet* 2014; **383**(9911):48–59.

Ceresoli M, Coccolini F, Catena F, Montori G, Di Saverio S, Sartelli M, Ansaloni L. Water-soluble contrast agent in adhesive small bowel obstruction: a systematic review and meta-analysis of diagnostic and therapeutic value. *Am J Surg* 2016; **211**(6):1114–25.

Fazio VW, Cohen Z, Fleshman JW *et al.* Reduction in adhesive small-bowel obstruction by Seprafilm® stop adhesion barrier after intestinal resection. *Dis Colon Rectum* 2006; **49**: 1–11.

Fevang BT, Fevang J, Lie S, Soreide O, Svanes K, Viste A. Long-term prognosis after operation for adhesive small bowel obstruction. *Ann Surg* 2004; **240**: 193–201.

Ha GW, Lee MR, Kim JH. Adhesive small bowel obstruction after laparoscopic and open colorectal surgery: a systematic review and meta-analysis. *Am J Surg* 2016; **212**(3):527–36.

Raveenthiran V, Madiba TE, Atamanalp SS. Volvulus of the sigmoid colon. *Colorectal Dis* 2010;**12**:1–17.

Sajja SB, Schein M. Early postoperative small bowel obstruction. *Br J Surg* 2004; **91**: 683–91.

Stenberg E, Szabo E, Ågren G *et al.* Closure of mesenteric defects in laparoscopic gastric bypass: a multicentre, randomised, parallel, open-label trial. *Lancet* 2016; **387**(10026):1397–404.

Williams SB, Greenspon J, Young HA, Orkin BA. Small bowel obstruction: conservative vs. surgical management. *Dis Colon Rectum* 2005; **48**: 1140–6.

Wolthuis AM, Bislenghi G, Fieuws S *et al.* (2016) Incidence of prolonged postoperative ileus after colorectal surgery: a systematic review and meta-analysis. *Colorectal Dis* 2016; **18**(1):O1-9.

Carlos Justiniano Ribeiro Chagas, 1879–1934, Director of The Oswald Cruz Institute, and Professor of Tropical Medicine, The University of Rio de Janeiro, Brazil.

The vermiform appendix

Learning objectives

To understand:

- The aetiology and surgical anatomy of acute appendicitis
- The clinical signs and differential diagnoses of appendicitis
- The investigation of suspected appendicitis
- Evolving concepts in management of acute appendicitis
- Basic surgical techniques, both open and laparoscopic
- The management of postoperative problems
- Tumours of the appendix and pseudomyxoma peritonei

INTRODUCTION

The importance of the vermiform appendix in surgery results primarily from its propensity for inflammation, which results in the clinical syndrome known as acute appendicitis. Acute appendicitis is the most common cause of an 'acute abdomen' in young adults and, as such, the associated symptoms and signs have become a paradigm for clinical teaching. Appendicitis is sufficiently common that appendicectomy (termed appendectomy in North America) is the most frequently performed urgent abdominal operation and is often the first major procedure performed by a surgeon in training. Advances in modern radiographic imaging have improved diagnostic accuracy; however, the diagnosis of appendicitis remains essentially clinical, requiring a mixture of observation, clinical acumen and surgical science and as such it remains an enigmatic challenge and a reminder of the art of surgical diagnosis. Although much more uncommon, the appendix also has a propensity to the formation of tumours which, despite humble and innocuous beginnings, may disseminate widely with dramatic clinical consequences.

Aside from its tendancy to cause surgical pathology the appendix, long thought to be a vistigial organ, may also have important roles in both immune function and maintaining the gut microbiota. The putative role of the appendix in the pathogenesis of ulcerative colitis (appendicectomy seems to be protective) for example, may be explained by its interaction with the intestinal flora and gut immune function.

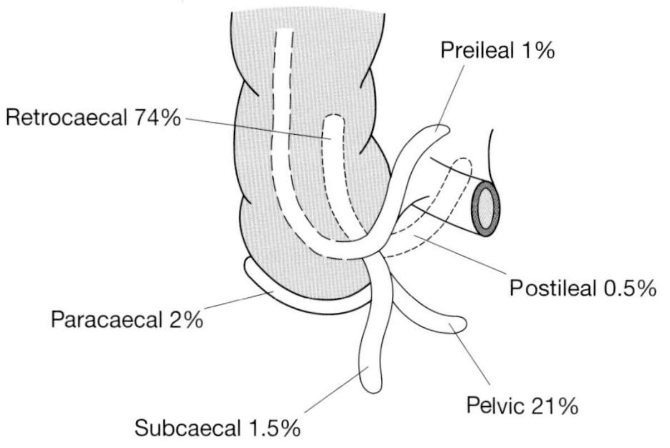

Figure 72.1 The various positions of the appendix (after Sir C Wakeley, London, formerly PRCS).

ANATOMY

The vermiform appendix is present only in humans, certain anthropoid apes and the wombat. It is a blind muscular tube with mucosal, submucosal, muscular and serosal layers. Morphologically, it is the undeveloped distal end of the large caecum found in many lower animals. At birth, the appendix is short and broad at its junction with the caecum, but differential growth of the caecum produces the typical tubular structure by about the age of 2 years (Condon). During childhood, continued growth of the caecum commonly rotates the appendix into a retrocaecal but intraperitoneal position (Figure 72.1). In approximately one-quarter of cases, rotation of the appendix does not occur, resulting in a pelvic, subcaecal or paracaecal position. Occasionally, the tip of the appendix becomes extraperitoneal, lying behind the caecum or ascending colon. Rarely, the caecum does not migrate

A wombat is a nocturnal, burrowing Australian marsupial.
Robert E Condon, 1929–2015, Emeritus Professor of Surgery, The Medical College of Wisconsin, WI, USA.

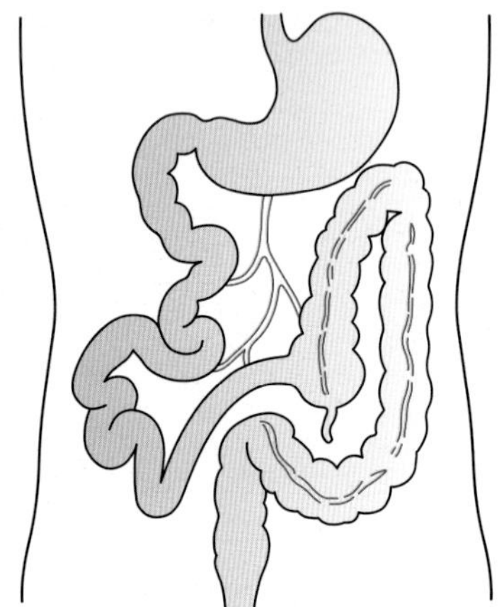

Figure 72.2 Left-sided caecum and appendix due to intestinal malrotation (after Findley and Humphreys).

during development to its normal position in the right lower quadrant of the abdomen. In these circumstances, the appendix can be found near the gall bladder or, in the case of intestinal malrotation, in the left iliac fossa, causing diagnostic difficulty if appendicitis develops (Figure 72.2).

The position of the base of the appendix is constant, being found at the confluence of the three taeniae coli of the caecum, which fuse to form the outer longitudinal muscle coat of the appendix. At operation, use can be made of this to find an elusive appendix, as gentle traction on the taeniae coli, particularly the anterior taenia, will lead the operator to the base of the appendix.

The mesentery of the appendix or mesoappendix arises from the lower surface of the mesentery or the terminal ileum and is itself subject to great variation. Sometimes, as much as the distal one-third of the appendix is bereft of mesoappendix. Especially in childhood, the mesoappendix is so transparent that the contained blood vessels can be seen (Figure 72.3). In many adults, it becomes laden with fat, which obscures these vessels. The appendicular artery, a branch of the lower division of the ileocolic artery, passes behind the terminal ileum to enter the mesoappendix a short distance from the base of the appendix. It then comes to lie in the free border of the mesoappendix. An accessory appendicular artery may be present but, in most people, the appendicular artery is an 'end-artery', thrombosis of which results in necrosis of the appendix (synonym: gangrenous appendicitis). Four, six or more lymphatic channels traverse the mesoappendix to empty into the ileocaecal lymph nodes.

Microscopic anatomy

The appendix varies considerably in length and circumference. The average length is between 7.5 and 10 cm. The lumen is irregular, being encroached on by multiple longitudinal folds of mucous membrane lined by columnar cell intestinal mucosa of colonic type (Figure 72.4). Crypts are present but are not numerous. In the base of the crypts lie argentaffin cells (Kulchitsky cells), which may give rise to carcinoid tumours (see below). The appendix is the most frequent site for carcinoid tumours, which may present with appendicitis due to occlusion of the appendiceal lumen. The submucosa contains numerous lymphatic aggregations or follicles. While no discernible change in immune function results from appendicectomy, the prominence of lymphatic tissue in the appendix of young adults seems to be important in the aetiology of appendicitis (see below).

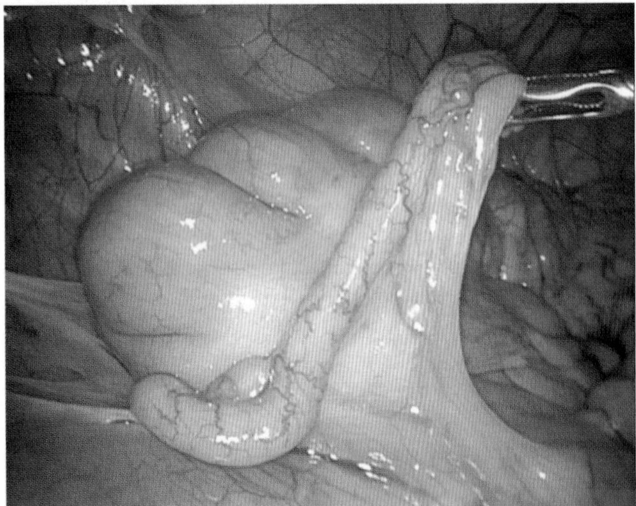

Figure 72.3 Laparoscopic view of a normal appendix with mesoappendix displaying the appendicular artery.

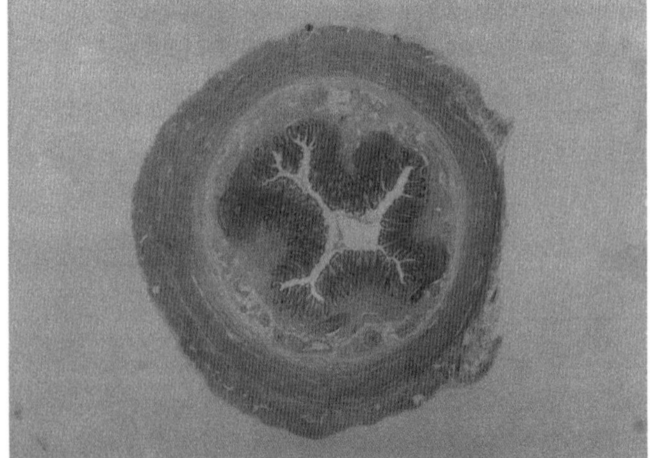

Figure 72.4 Normal vermiform appendix. The narrow lumen is bounded by mucosa, which may be arranged in folds. There is usually abundant lymphoid tissue in the mucosa, especially in younger individuals. This may encroach on and further narrow the lumen. The mucosa is bounded by a relatively thin muscularis mucosa (courtesy of Dr P Kelly, FRCPath, Dublin, Ireland).

Nikolai Kulchitsky, 1856–1925, Professor of Histology, Kharkov, Ukraine, who left Russia after the Revolution of 1917 and later worked at University College, London, UK. He described these cells in 1897.

ACUTE APPENDICITIS

While there are isolated reports of perityphlitis (fatal inflammation of the caecal region) from the late 1500s, recognition of acute appendicitis as a clinical entity is attributed to Reginald Fitz, who presented a paper to the first meeting of the Association of American Physicians in 1886 entitled 'Perforating inflammation of the vermiform appendix'. Soon afterwards, Charles McBurney described the clinical manifestations of acute appendicitis including the point of maximum tenderness in the right iliac fossa that now bears his name.

The incidence of appendicitis seems to have risen greatly in the first half of this century, particularly in Europe, America and Australasia, with up to 16% of the population undergoing appendicectomy. In the past 30 years, the incidence has fallen dramatically in these countries, such that the individual lifetime risk of appendicectomy is 8.6% and 6.7% among males and females, respectively.

Acute appendicitis is relatively rare in infants and becomes increasingly common in childhood and early adult life, reaching a peak incidence in the teens and early 20s. After middle age, the risk of developing appendicitis is quite small. The incidence of appendicitis is equal among males and females before puberty. In teenagers and young adults, the male–female ratio increases to 3:2 at age 25; thereafter, the greater incidence in males declines.

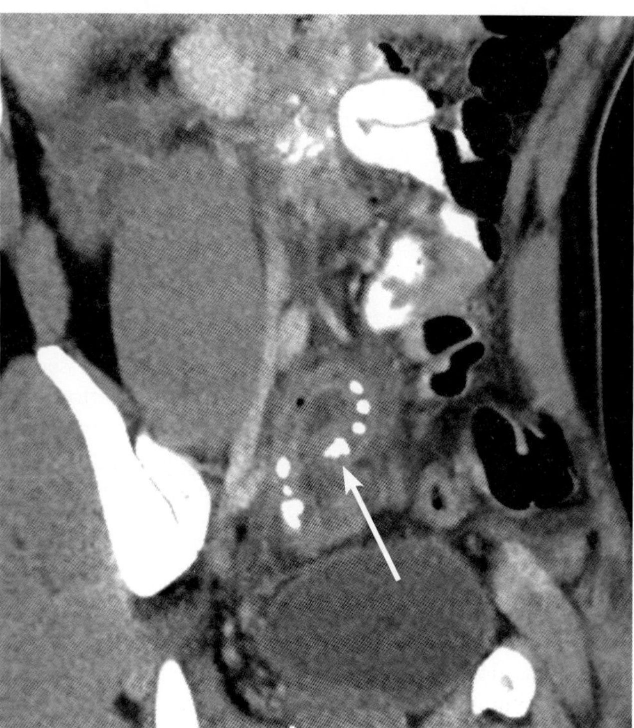

Figure 72.5 Coronal reformat of a computed tomography scan of the abdomen obtained with oral and intravenous contrast, demonstrating an inflamed, enhancing and enlarged appendix that is curled in the midline extending towards the pelvis (arrow). It contains multiple radiopaque appendicoliths. There is extensive periappendiceal fat stranding (courtesy of Dr P MacMahon, FRCR, Dublin, Ireland).

Aetiology

There is no unifying hypothesis regarding the aetiology of acute appendicitis. Decreased dietary fibre and increased consumption of refined carbohydrates may be important. As with colonic diverticulitis, the incidence of appendicitis is lowest in societies with a high dietary fibre intake. In resource-poor countries that are adopting a more refined western-type diet, the incidence continues to rise. This is in contrast to the dramatic decrease in the incidence of appendicitis in western countries observed in the past 30 years. No reason has been established for these paradoxical changes; however, improved hygiene and a change in the pattern of childhood gastrointestinal infection related to the increased use of antibiotics may be responsible.

While appendicitis is clearly associated with bacterial proliferation within the appendix, no single organism is responsible. A mixed growth of aerobic and anaerobic organisms is usual. The initiating event causing bacterial proliferation is controversial. Obstruction of the appendix lumen has been widely held to be important, and some form of luminal obstruction, either by a faecolith (Figure 72.5) or a stricture, is found in the majority of cases.

A faecolith (sometimes refered to as an appendicolith) is composed of inspissated faecal material, calcium phosphates, bacteria and epithelial debris (Figure 72.6). Rarely, a foreign body is incorporated into the mass. The incidental finding of a faecolith is a relative indication for prophylactic

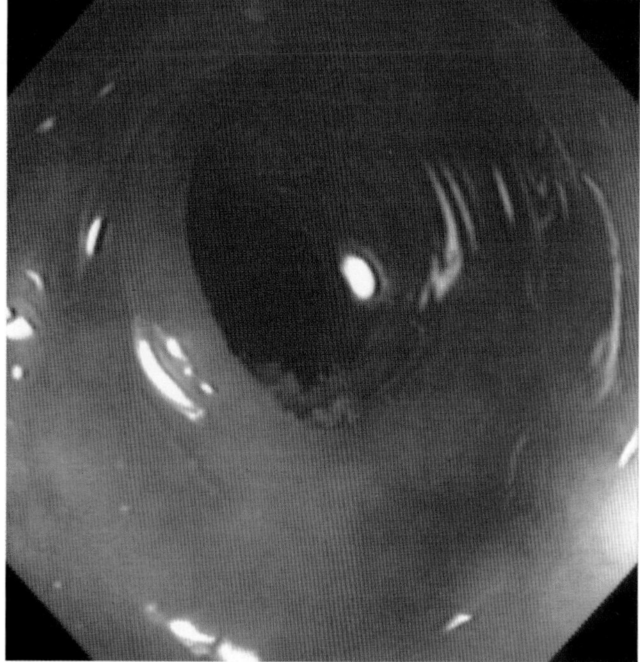

Figure 72.6 Colonoscopic view of the lumen of the appendix showing intraluminal debris (courtesy of Professor D Winter, FRCSI, Dublin, Ireland).

Reginald Heber Fitz, 1843–1913, Professor of Medicine, Harvard University, Boston, MA, USA.
Charles McBurney, 1854–1913, Professor of Surgery, Columbia College of Physicians and Surgeons, New York, NY, USA. In 1889 McBurney published a paper on appendicitis in which he stated 'I believe that in every case the seat of greatest pain "determined by the pressure of one finger" has been very exactly between an inch and a half and two inches from the anterior spirious process of the ilium on a straight line drawn from that process to the umbilicus.'

appendicectomy or an interval appendicetomy in a patient treated conservatively. A fibrotic stricture of the appendix usually indicates previous appendicitis that resolved without surgical intervention. Obstruction of the appendiceal orifice by tumour, particularly carcinoma of the caecum, is an occasional cause of acute appendicitis in middle-aged and elderly patients. Intestinal parasites, particularly *Oxyuris vermicularis* (pinworm), can proliferate in the appendix and occlude the lumen.

Pathology

Obstruction of the appendiceal lumen seems to be essential for the development of appendiceal gangrene and perforation. However, in many cases of early appendicitis, the appendix lumen is patent despite the presence of mucosal inflammation and lymphoid hyperplasia. Occasional clustering of cases among children and young adults suggests an infective agent, possibly viral, which initiates an inflammatory response. Seasonal variation in the incidence is also observed, with more cases occurring between May and August in northern Europe than at other times of the year.

Lymphoid hyperplasia narrows the lumen of the appendix, leading to luminal obstruction. Once obstruction occurs, continued mucus secretion and inflammatory exudation increase intraluminal pressure, obstructing lymphatic drainage. Oedema and mucosal ulceration develop with bacterial translocation to the submucosa. Resolution may occur at this point either spontaneously or in response to antibiotic therapy. If the condition progresses, further distension of the appendix may cause venous obstruction and ischaemia of the appendix wall. With ischaemia, bacterial invasion occurs through the muscularis propria and submucosa, producing acute appendicitis (**Figure 72.7**). Finally, ischaemic necrosis of the appendix wall produces gangrenous appendicitis, with free bacterial contamination of the peritoneal cavity. Alternatively, the greater omentum and loops of small bowel become adherent to the inflamed appendix, walling off the spread of peritoneal contamination and resulting in a phlegmonous mass or paracaecal abscess. Rarely, appendiceal inflammation resolves, leaving a distended mucus-filled organ termed a mucocele of the appendix.

It is the potential for diffuse peritonitis that is the great threat of acute appendicitis. Peritonitis occurs as a result of free migration of bacteria through an ischaemic appendicular wall, frank perforation of a gangrenous appendix or delayed perforation of an appendix abscess. Factors that promote this process include extremes of age, immunosuppression, diabetes mellitus and faecolith obstruction of the appendix lumen, a free-lying pelvic appendix and previous abdominal surgery that limits the ability of the greater omentum to wall off the spread of peritoneal contamination. In these situations, a rapidly deteriorating clinical course is accompanied by signs of diffuse peritonitis and systemic sepsis syndrome.

Summary box 72.1

Risk factors for perforation of the appendix

- Extremes of age
- Immunosuppression
- Diabetes mellitus
- Faecolith obstruction
- Pelvic appendix
- Previous abdominal surgery

Clinical diagnosis

History

The classical features of acute appendicitis begin with poorly localised colicky abdominal pain. This is due to mid-gut visceral discomfort in response to appendiceal inflammation and obstruction. The pain is frequently first noticed in the periumbilical region and is similar to, but less intense than,

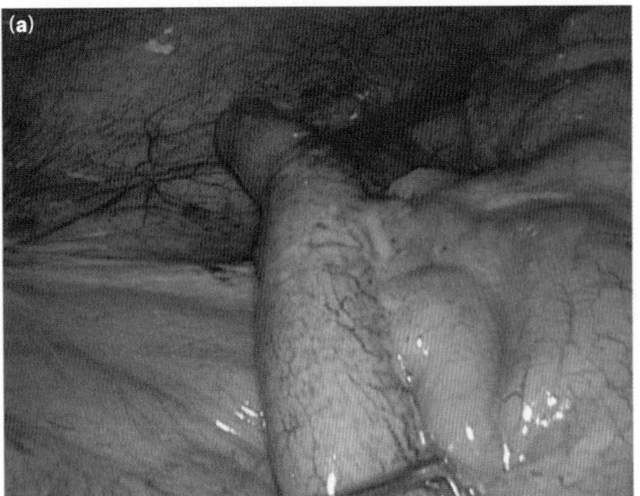

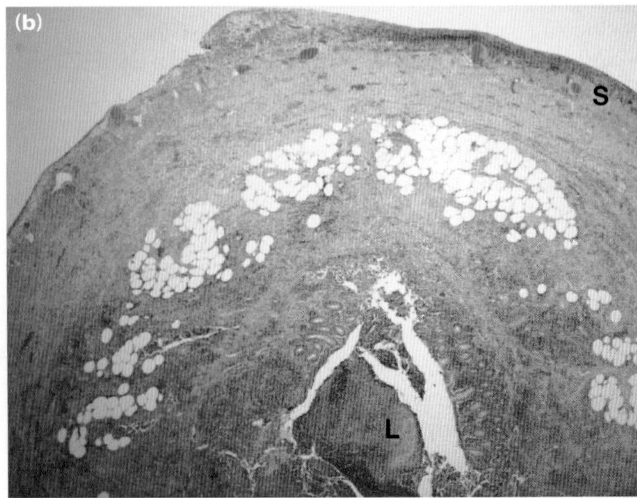

Figure 72.7 Acutely inflammed appendix with purulent exudate extending to the mesoappendix in a 28-year-old male as seen at laparoscopy (a) and a photomicrograph (original magnification ×20) from the same patient showing the appendix with pus-filled lumen (L) and inflammation extending to inflamed serosa (S) (courtesy of Professor C O'Keane, FFPath, FRCPI, Dublin, Ireland).

the colic of small bowel obstruction. Central abdominal pain is associated with anorexia, nausea and usually one or two episodes of vomiting that follow the onset of pain (Murphy). Anorexia is a useful and constant clinical feature, particularly in children. The patient often gives a history of similar discomfort that settled spontaneously. A family history is also useful as up to one-third of children with appendicitis have a first-degree relative with a similar history.

Summary box 72.2

Symptoms of appendicitis

- Periumbilical colic
- Pain shifting to the right iliac fossa
- Anorexia
- Nausea

With progressive inflammation of the appendix, the parietal peritoneum in the right iliac fossa becomes irritated, producing more intense, constant and localised somatic pain that begins to predominate. Patients often report this as an abdominal pain that has shifted and changed in character. Typically, coughing or sudden movement exacerbates the right iliac fossa pain.

The classic visceral–somatic sequence of pain is present in only about half of those patients subsequently proven to have acute appendicitis. Atypical presentations include pain that is predominantly somatic or visceral and poorly localised. Atypical pain is more common in the elderly, in whom localisation to the right iliac fossa is unusual. An inflamed appendix in the pelvis may never produce somatic pain involving the anterior abdominal wall, but may instead cause suprapubic discomfort and tenesmus. In this circumstance, tenderness may be elicited only on rectal examination and is the basis for the recommendation that a rectal examination should be performed on every patient who presents with acute lower abdominal pain.

During the first 6 hours, there is rarely any alteration in temperature or pulse rate. After that time, slight pyrexia (37.2–37.7°C) with a corresponding increase in the pulse rate to 80 or 90 is usual. However, in 20% of patients there is no pyrexia or tachycardia in the early stages. In children, a temperature greater than 38.5°C suggests other causes (e.g. mesenteric adenitis [see below]).

Typically, two clinical syndromes of acute appendicitis can be discerned, *acute catarrhal* (*non-obstructive*) appendicitis and *acute obstructive* appendicitis, the latter characterised by a more acute course. The onset of symptoms is abrupt and there may be generalised abdominal pain from the start. The temperature may be normal and vomiting is common, so the clinical picture may mimic acute intestinal obstruction.

Signs

The diagnosis of appendicitis rests more on thorough clinical examination of the abdomen than on any aspect of the history or laboratory investigation. The cardinal features are those of an unwell patient with low-grade pyrexia, localised abdominal tenderness, muscle guarding and rebound tenderness. Inspection of the abdomen may show limitation of respiratory movement in the lower abdomen. The patient is then asked to point to where the pain began and where it moved (the pointing sign). Gentle superficial palpation of the abdomen, beginning in the left iliac fossa and moving anticlockwise to the right iliac fossa, will detect muscle guarding over the point of maximum tenderness, classically McBurney's point. Asking the patient to cough or gentle percussion over the site of maximum tenderness will elicit rebound tenderness.

Summary box 72.3

Clinical signs in appendicitis

- Pyrexia
- Localised tenderness in the right iliac fossa
- Muscle guarding
- Rebound tenderness

Deep palpation of the left iliac fossa may cause pain in the right iliac fossa, Rovsing's sign, which is helpful in supporting a clinical diagnosis of appendicitis. Occasionally, an inflamed appendix lies on the psoas muscle, and the patient, often a young adult, will lie with the right hip flexed for pain relief (the psoas sign). Spasm of the obturator internus is sometimes demonstrable when the hip is flexed and internally rotated. If an inflamed appendix is in contact with the obturator internus, this manoeuvre will cause pain in the hypogastrium (the obturator test; Zachary Cope). Cutaneous hyperaesthesia may be demonstrable in the right iliac fossa, but is rarely of diagnostic value.

Summary box 72.4

Signs to elicit in appendicitis

- Pointing sign
- Rovsing's sign
- Psoas sign
- Obturator sign

John Benjamin Murphy, 1857–1916, Professor of Surgery, Northwestern University, Chicago, IL, USA.
Neils Thorkild Rovsing, 1862–1937, Professor of Surgery, Copenhagen, Denmark.
Sir Vincent Zachary Cope, 1881–1975, surgeon, St. Mary's Hospital, London, UK.

Special features, according to position of the appendix

Retrocaecal

Rigidity is often absent, and even application of deep pressure may fail to elicit tenderness (silent appendix), the reason being that the caecum, distended with gas, prevents the pressure exerted by the hand from reaching the inflamed structure. However, deep tenderness is often present in the loin, and rigidity of the quadratus lumborum may be in evidence. Psoas spasm, due to the inflamed appendix being in contact with that muscle, may be sufficient to cause flexion of the hip joint. Hyperextension of the hip joint may induce abdominal pain when the degree of psoas spasm is insufficient to cause flexion of the hip.

Pelvic

Occasionally, early diarrhoea results from an inflamed appendix being in contact with the rectum. When the appendix lies entirely within the pelvis, there is usually complete absence of abdominal rigidity, and often tenderness over McBurney's point is also lacking. In some instances, deep tenderness can be made out just above and to the right of the symphysis pubis. In either event, a rectal examination reveals tenderness in the rectovesical pouch or the pouch of Douglas, especially on the right side. Spasm of the psoas and obturator internus muscles may be present when the appendix is in this position. An inflamed appendix in contact with the bladder may cause frequency of micturition. This is more common in children.

Postileal

In this case, the inflamed appendix lies behind the terminal ileum. It presents the greatest difficulty in diagnosis because the pain may not shift, diarrhoea is a feature and marked retching may occur. Tenderness, if any, is ill defined, although it may be present immediately to the right of the umbilicus.

Special features, according to age

Infants

Appendicitis is relatively rare in infants under 36 months of age and, for obvious reasons, the patient is unable to give a history. Because of this, diagnosis is often delayed, and thus the incidence of perforation and postoperative morbidity is considerably higher than in older children. Diffuse peritonitis can develop rapidly because of the underdeveloped greater omentum, which is unable to give much assistance in localising the infection.

Children

It is rare to find a child with appendicitis who has not vomited. Children with appendicitis usually have complete aversion to food.

The elderly

Gangrene and perforation occur much more frequently in elderly patients. Elderly patients with a lax abdominal wall or obesity may harbour a gangrenous appendix with little evidence of it, and the clinical picture may simulate subacute intestinal obstruction. These features, coupled with coincident medical conditions, produce a much higher mortality for acute appendicitis in the elderly.

The obese

Obesity can obscure and diminish all the local signs of acute appendicitis and the clinician may have to rely on imaging to establish the diagnosis. Laparoscopy is particularly useful in the obese patient as it may obviate the need for a large abdominal incision.

Pregnancy

Appendicitis is the most common extrauterine acute abdominal condition in pregnancy, with a frequency of 1:1500–2000 pregnancies. Diagnosis is complicated by delay in presentation as early non-specific symptoms are often attributed to the pregnancy. Obstetric teaching has been that the caecum and appendix are progressively pushed to the right upper quadrant of the abdomen as pregnancy develops during the second and third trimesters. However, pain in the right lower quadrant of the abdomen remains the cardinal feature of appendicitis in pregnancy. Fetal loss occurs in 3–5% of cases, increasing to 20% if perforation is found at operation.

Differential diagnosis

Although acute appendicitis is the most common abdominal surgical emergency, the diagnosis can be extremely difficult at times. There are a number of common conditions that it is wise to consider carefully and, if possible, exclude. The differential diagnosis differs in patients of different ages; in women, additional differential diagnoses are diseases of the female genital tract (*Table 72.1*).

Children

The diseases most commonly mistaken for acute appendicitis are acute gastroenteritis and mesenteric lymphadenitis. In mesenteric lymphadenitis, the pain is colicky in nature and cervical lymph nodes may be enlarged. It may be impossible to clinically distinguish Meckel's diverticulitis from acute appendicitis. The pain is similar; however, signs may be central or left sided. Occasionally, there is a history of antecedent abdominal pain or intermittent lower gastrointestinal bleeding.

It is important to distinguish between acute appendicitis and intussusception. Appendicitis is uncommon before the age of 2 years, whereas the median age for intussusception is 18 months. A mass may be palpable in the right lower quadrant, and the preferred treatment of intussusception is reduction by careful barium enema.

James Douglas, 1715–1742, anatomist and midwife who practised in London, UK, described this pouch in 1730.
Johann Friedrich Meckel, 1781–1883, Professor of Anatomy and Surgery, Halle, Germany.

TABLE 72.1 Differential diagnosis of acute appendicitis.

Children	Adult	Adult female	Elderly
Gastroenteritis	Regional enteritis	Mittelschmerz	Diverticulitis
Mesenteric adenitis	Ureteric colic	Pelvic inflammatory disease	Intestinal obstruction
Meckel's diverticulitis	Perforated peptic ulcer	Pyelonephritis	Colonic carcinoma
Intussusception	Torsion of testis	Ectopic pregnancy	Torsion appendix epiploicae
Henoch–Schönlein purpura	Pancreatitis	Torsion/rupture of ovarian cyst	Mesenteric infarction
Lobar pneumonia	Rectus sheath haematoma	Endometriosis	Leaking aortic aneurysm

Henoch–Schönlein purpura is often preceded by a sore throat or respiratory infection. Abdominal pain can be severe and can be confused with intussusception or appendicitis. There is nearly always an ecchymotic rash, typically affecting the extensor surfaces of the limbs and on the buttocks. The face is usually spared. The platelet count and bleeding time are within normal limits. Microscopic haematuria is common.

Lobar pneumonia and pleurisy, especially at the right base, may give rise to right-sided abdominal pain and mimic appendicitis. Abdominal tenderness is minimal, pyrexia is marked and chest examination may reveal a pleural friction rub or altered breath sounds on auscultation. A chest radiograph is diagnostic.

Adults

Terminal ileitis in its acute form may be clinically indistinguishable from acute appendicitis unless a doughy mass of inflamed ileum can be felt. An antecedent history of abdominal cramping, weight loss and diarrhoea suggests regional ileitis rather than appendicitis. The ileitis may be non-specific, due to Crohn's disease (Figure 72.8) or *Yersinia* infection. *Yersinia enterocolitica* causes inflammation of the terminal ileum, appendix and caecum with mesenteric adenopathy. If suspected, serum antibody titres are diagnostic, and treatment with intravenous tetracycline is appropriate. If *Yersinia* infection is suspected at operation, a mesenteric lymph node should be excised and divided, with half submitted for microbiological culture (including tuberculosis) and half for histological examination.

Ureteric colic does not commonly cause diagnostic difficulty, as the character and radiation of pain differs from that of appendicitis. Urinalysis should always be performed, and the presence of red cells should prompt a supine abdominal radiograph. Renal ultrasound or intravenous urogram is diagnostic.

Right-sided acute pyelonephritis is accompanied and often preceded by increased frequency of micturition. It may cause difficulty in diagnosis, especially in women. The leading features are tenderness confined to the loin, fever (temperature 39°C) and possibly rigors and pyuria.

In perforated peptic ulcer, the duodenal contents pass along the paracolic gutter to the right iliac fossa. As a rule, there is a history of dyspepsia and a very sudden onset of pain that starts in the epigastrium and passes down the right paracolic gutter. In appendicitis, the pain starts classically in the umbilical region. Rigidity and tenderness in the right iliac fossa are present in both conditions but, in perforated duodenal ulcer, the rigidity is usually greater in the right hypochondrium. An erect chest radiograph will show gas under the diaphragm in 70% of patients. An abdominal computed tomography (CT) examination is valuable when there is diagnostic difficulty.

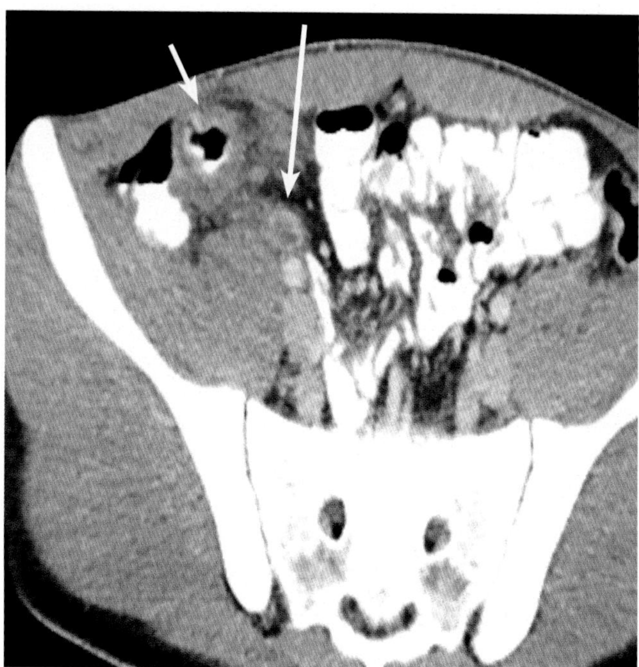

Figure 72.8 First presentation in a 19-year-old male with terminal ileitis, later confirmed to be Crohn's disease. Short arrow demonstrates abnormally thickened and inflamed terminal ileum. Long arrow indicates wall enhancement and enlargement of the appendix, indicating secondary acute appendicitis (courtesy of Dr P MacMahon, FRCR, Dublin, Ireland).

Eduard Heinrich Henoch, 1820–1910, Professor of Diseases of Children, Berlin, Germany, described this form of purpura in 1868.
Johann Lucas Schönlein, 1793–1864, Professor of Medicine, Berlin, Germany, described this form of purpura in 1837.
Burrill Bernard Crohn, 1884–1983, gastroenterologist, Mount Sinai Hospital, New York, NY, USA, described regional ileitis in 1932.
Alexandre Emile Yersin, 1863–1943, bacteriologist, Paris, France.

Testicular torsion in a teenage or young adult male is easily missed. Pain can be referred to the right iliac fossa, and shyness on the part of the patient may lead the unwary to suspect appendicitis unless the scrotum is examined in all cases.

Acute pancreatitis should be considered in the differential diagnosis of all adults suspected of having acute appendicitis and, when appropriate, should be excluded by serum or urinary amylase measurement.

Rectus sheath haematoma is a relatively rare but easily missed differential diagnosis. It usually presents with acute pain and localised tenderness in the right iliac fossa, often after an episode of strenuous physical exercise. Localised pain without gastrointestinal upset is the rule. Occasionally, in an elderly patient, particularly one taking anticoagulant therapy, a rectus sheath haematoma may present as a mass and tenderness in the right iliac fossa after minor trauma.

Adult female

It is in women of childbearing age that pelvic disease most often mimics acute appendicitis. A careful gynaecological history should be taken in all women with suspected appendicitis, concentrating on menstrual cycle, vaginal discharge and possible pregnancy. The most common diagnostic mimics are pelvic inflammatory disease (PID), Mittelschmerz, torsion or haemorrhage of an ovarian cyst and ectopic pregnancy.

PELVIC INFLAMMATORY DISEASE

PID comprises a spectrum of diseases that include salpingitis, endometritis and tubo-ovarian sepsis. The incidence of these conditions is increasing, and the diagnosis should be considered in every young adult female. Typically, the pain is lower than in appendicitis and is bilateral. A history of vaginal discharge, dysmenorrhoea and burning pain on micturition is a helpful differential diagnostic point. The physical findings include adenexal and cervical tenderness on vaginal examination. When suspected, a high vaginal swab should be taken for *Chlamydia trachomatis* and *Neisseria gonorrhoeae* culture, and the opinion of a gynaecologist should be obtained. Treatment is usually a combination of ofloxacin and metronidazole for 14 days. Transvaginal ultrasound can be particularly helpful in establishing the diagnosis. When serious diagnostic uncertainty persists, diagnostic laparoscopy should be undertaken.

MITTELSCHMERZ

Midcycle rupture of a follicular cyst with bleeding produces lower abdominal and pelvic pain, typically midcycle. Systemic upset is rare, a pregnancy test is negative and symptoms usually subside within hours. Occasionally, diagnostic laparoscopy is required. Retrograde menstruation may cause similar symptoms.

TORSION/HAEMORRHAGE OF AN OVARIAN CYST

This can prove a difficult differential diagnosis. When suspected, pelvic ultrasound and a gynaecological opinion should be sought. If encountered at operation, untwisting of the involved adnexa and ovarian cystectomy should be performed, if necessary, in women of childbearing years. Documented visualisation of the contralateral ovary is an essential medico-legal precaution prior to oophorectomy for any reason.

ECTOPIC PREGNANCY

It is unlikely that a ruptured ectopic pregnancy, with its well-defined signs of haemoperitoneum, will be mistaken for acute appendicitis, but the same cannot be said for a right-sided tubal abortion or, still more, for a right-sided unruptured tubal pregnancy. In the latter, the signs are very similar to those of acute appendicitis except that the pain commences on the right side and stays there. The pain is severe and continues unabated until operation. Usually, there is a history of a missed menstrual period, and a urinary pregnancy test may be positive. Severe pain is felt when the cervix is moved on vaginal examination. Signs of intraperitoneal bleeding usually become apparent, and the patient should be questioned specifically regarding referred pain in the shoulder. Pelvic ultrasonography should be carried out in all cases in which an ectopic pregnancy is a possible diagnosis.

Elderly

DIVERTICULITIS

In some patients with a long sigmoid loop, the colon lies to the right of the midline and it may be impossible to differentiate between diverticulitis and appendicitis. Abdominal CT scanning is particularly useful in this setting and should be considered in the management of all patients over the age of 60 years. A trial of conservative management with intravenous fluids and antibiotics is often appropriate, with a low threshold for laparoscopy or exploratory laparotomy in the face of deterioration or lack of clinical response. Right-sided diverticulitis is unusual and may be clinically indistinguishable from appendicitis. Abdominal CT scanning is particularly useful in making the distinction. As with left-sided diverticulatis, treament should be conservative with intravenous antibiotics with recourse to laparoscopy or laparotomy in the face of clinical deterioration

INTESTINAL OBSTRUCTION

The diagnosis of intestinal obstruction is usually clear; the subtlety lies in recognising acute appendicitis as the occasional cause in the elderly. As with diverticulitis, intravenous fluids, antibiotics and nasogastric decompression should be instigated, with early resort to laparotomy.

CARCINOMA OF THE CAECUM

When obstructed or locally perforated, carcinoma of the caecum may mimic or cause obstructive appendicitis in adults. A history of antecedent discomfort, altered bowel habit or unexplained anaemia should raise suspicion. A mass may be palpable (see below) and an abdominal CT scan diagnostic.

Rare differential diagnoses

Preherpetic pain of the right 10th and 11th dorsal nerves is localised over the same area as that of appendicitis. It does not shift and is associated with marked hyperaesthesia. There is no intestinal upset or rigidity. The herpetic eruption may be delayed for 3–8 hours.

Tabetic crises are now rare. Severe abdominal pain and vomiting usher in the crisis. Other signs of tabes confirm the diagnosis.

Spinal conditions are sometimes associated with acute abdominal pain, especially in children and the elderly. These may include tuberculosis of the spine, metastatic carcinoma, osteoporotic vertebral collapse and multiple myeloma. The pain is due to compression of nerve roots and may be aggravated by movement. There is rigidity of the lumbar spine and intestinal symptoms are absent.

The abdominal crises of porphyria and diabetes mellitus need to be remembered. A urinalysis should be undertaken in every abdominal emergency. In cyclical vomiting of infants or young children, there is a history of previous similar attacks and abdominal rigidity is absent. Acetone is found in the urine but is not diagnostic as it may accompany starvation.

Typhlitis or leukaemic ileocaecal syndrome is a rare but potentially fatal enterocolitis occurring in immunosuppressed patients. Gram-negative or clostridial (especially *Clostridium septicum*) septicaemia can be rapidly progressive. Treatment is with appropriate antibiotics and haematopoietic factors. Surgical intervention is rarely indicated.

Investigation

The diagnosis of acute appendicitis is essentially clinical; however, a decision to operate based on clinical suspicion alone can lead to the removal of a normal appendix in 15–30% of cases. The premise that it is better to remove a normal appendix than to delay diagnosis does not stand up to close scrutiny, particularly in the elderly. A number of clinical and laboratory-based scoring systems have been devised to assist diagnosis. The most widely used is the Alvarado score (*Table 72.2*). A score of 7 or more is strongly predictive of acute appendicitis.

In patients with an equivocal score (5–6), abdominal ultrasound or contrast-enhanced CT examination further reduces the rate of negative appendicectomy. Abdominal ultrasound examination is more useful in children and thin adults, particularly if gynaecological pathology is suspected, with a diagnostic accuracy in excess of 90% (**Figure 72.9**). Modern CT is both sensitive and specific (approximately 95%) in the diagnosis of acute appendicitis (**Figure 72.10**) and worldwide there has been a steady increase in its use for this purpose. In the United States, for example, the majority of patients will undergo CT prior to surgery. CT has been shown to reduce the rate of negative appendicectomy without an associated increased perforation rate (due to delay in diagnosis) and may be cost-effective due to shorter hospital stay. While the diagnostic accuracy of modern CT scanning for appendicitis is well established, radiation exposure and the theoretical carcinogenic effect are a concern. Low-dose protocols, which reduce the radiation dose to the patient by up to 80%, can be as reliable as standard dose scanning and may be more appropriately applied when considering a diagnosis of acute appendicitis, particularly in the younger adult (Kim).

Contrast-enhanced standard dose CT is especially useful in patients in whom there is diagnostic uncertainty, particularly older patients, where acute diverticulitis, intestinal obstruction and neoplasm are likely differential diagnoses.

Summary box 72.5

Preoperative investigations in appendicitis

- Routine
  - Full blood count
  - Urinalysis
- Selective
  - Pregnancy test
  - Urea and electrolytes
  - Supine abdominal radiograph
  - Ultrasound of the abdomen/pelvis
  - Contrast-enhanced abdomen and pelvic computed tomography scan
  - Consider low-dose protocol in young adults

TABLE 72.2 The Alvarado (MANTRELS) score.

	Score
Symptoms **M**igratory RIF pain	1
Anorexia	1
Nausea and vomiting	1
Signs	
Tenderness (RIF)	2
Rebound tenderness	1
Elevated temperature	1
Laboratory	
Leucocytosis	2
Shift to left	1
Total	10

RIF, right iliac fossa; MANTRELS, Migration of pain, Anorexia, Nausea or vomiting, Tenderness, Rebound pain, Elevation of temperature, Leucocytosis, Shift to left (segmented neutrophils).

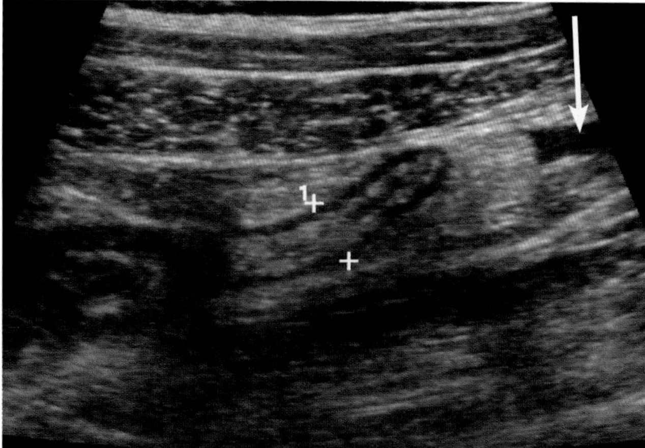

Figure 72.9 Ultrasound image of the right iliac fossa (RIF) demonstrating a mildly enlarged appendix, measuring 8 mm in diameter, consistent with acute appendicitis in a 40-year-old male. Arrow indicates small pocket of free fluid more inferiorly in the RIF (courtesy of Dr D Byrne, MB, Dublin, Ireland).

Alfredo Alvarado, contemporary, surgeon, Plantation, FL, USA.

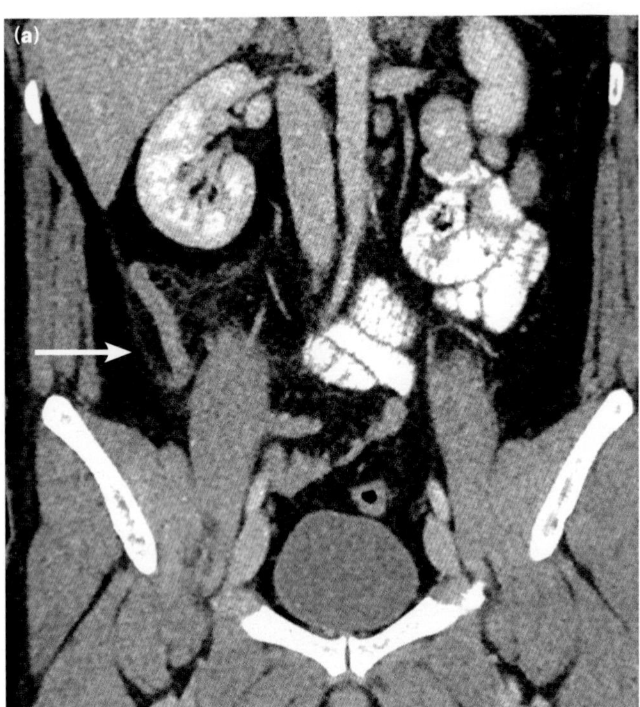

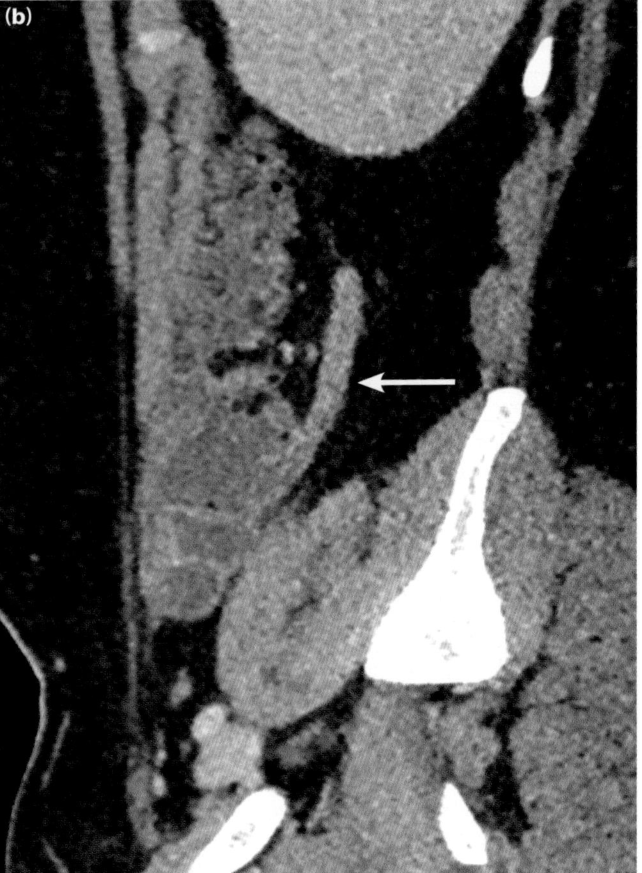

Figure 72.10 Coronal (a) and sagittal (b) reformat of a computed tomography scan of the abdomen obtained with oral and intravenous contrast, demonstrating an enlarged (10 mm), enhancing retrocaecal appendix with periappendiceal fat stranding. No evidence of necrosis, perforation or collection. No radiopaque appendicolith seen. Images in Figure 72.7 refer to the same patient (courtesy of Dr P MacMahon, FRCR, Dublin, Ireland).

Treatment

Non-operative management

While surgery remains the standard teaching, there is an emerging body of literature to support a trial of conservative mangement in patients with uncomplicated (absence of appendicolith, perforation or abscess) appendicitis. Treatment is bowel rest and intravenous antibiotics, often metronidazole and 3rd generation cephalosprin. More recently, ertapenem has been used in this setting and has the benefit of broad antimicrobial cover administered as a single daily dose. The available data indicate initial successful outcomes in more than 90% of patients with CT confirmed appendicitis; however, approximately one-quarter of patients initially treated conservatively will require surgery within 1 year for recurrent appendicitis (Salminen). Subsequent surgery, if needed, tends to be uncomplicated. This approach may be considered in the well patient with limited signs or those with high operative risk (multiple co-morbidities). As with conservative treatment of an appendix mass, patients over the age of 40 should be followed up to ensure there is no underlying malignancy (see below).

Operative management

The traditional treatment for acute appendicitis is appendicectomy. While there should be no unnecessary delay, all patients, particularly those most at risk of serious morbidity, benefit by a short period of intensive preoperative preparation. Intravenous fluids, sufficient to establish adequate urine output (catheterisation is needed only in the very ill), and appropriate antibiotics should be given. There is ample evidence that in the absence of purulent peritonitis, a single peroperative dose of antibiotics reduces the incidence of postoperative wound infection. When peritonitis is suspected, therapeutic intravenous antibiotics to cover gram-negative bacilli as well as anaerobic cocci should be given. Hyperpyrexia in children should be treated with salicylates in addition to antibiotics and intravenous fluids. With appropriate use of intravenous fluids and parenteral antibiotics, a policy of deferring appendicectomy after midnight to the first case on the following morning does not increase morbidity. However, when acute obstructive appendicitis is recognised, operation should not be deferred longer than it takes to optimise the patient's condition.

Appendicectomy

Claudius Amyand successfully removed an acutely inflamed appendix from the hernial sac of a boy in 1736. The first surgeon to perform deliberate appendicectomy for acute appendicitis was Lawson Tait in May 1880. The patient recovered; however, the case was not reported until 1890. Meanwhile,

Claudius Amyand, 1685–1740, surgeon, St. George's Hospital, London, UK.
Robert Lawson Tait, 1845–1899, surgeon, The Hospital for Diseases of Women, Birmingham, UK.

Thomas Morton was the first to diagnose appendicitis, drain the abscess and remove the appendix with recovery, publishing his findings in 1887.

Appendicectomy should be performed under general anaesthetic with the patient supine on the operating table and may be undertaken using either an open or laparoscopic approach. When the appropriate equipment and expertise are available and cost allows, the laparoscopic approach is advantageous. The initial laparoscopy allows the diagnosis to be established and may reduce the negative appendicectomy rate. Furthermore, the patient may benefit from the quicker recovery afforded by a minimally invasive approach, the rate of wound infection is lower (when compared with open surgery) and, contrary to initial concerns, the incidence of postoperative pelvic collection does not appear to be increased (van Rossem). There remains much variability in the operative approach to appendicitis. In the United Kingdom, for example, despite the widespread familiarity with and availability of laparoscopy, an initial laparoscopic approach is performed in only two-thirds of patients and the negative appendicectomy rate remains high (20%).

When a laparoscopic technique is used, the bladder must be empty (ensure that the patient has voided before leaving the ward). Prior to preparing the entire abdomen with an appropriate antiseptic solution, the right iliac fossa should be palpated for a mass. If a mass is felt, it may, on occasion, be preferable to adopt a conservative approach (see below). Draping of the abdomen is in accordance with the planned operative technique, taking account of any requirement to extend the incision or convert a laparoscopic technique to an open operation.

CONVENTIONAL APPENDICECTOMY

When the preoperative diagnosis is considered reasonably certain, the incision that is widely used for appendicectomy is the so-called gridiron incision (gridiron: a frame of crossbeams to support a ship during repairs). The gridiron incision (described first by McArthur) is made at right angles to a line joining the anterior superior iliac spine to the umbilicus, its centre being along the line at McBurney's point (Figure 72.11). If better access is required, it is possible to convert the gridiron to a Rutherford Morison incision (see below) by cutting the internal oblique and transversus muscles in the line of the incision.

In recent years, a transverse skin crease (Lanz) incision has become more popular, as the exposure is better and extension, when needed, is easier. The incision, appropriate in length to the size and obesity of the patient, is made approximately 2 cm below the umbilicus centred on the mid-clavicular–mid-inguinal line (Figure 72.12) When necessary, the incision may be extended medially, with retraction or suitable division of the rectus abdominis muscle.

When the diagnosis is in doubt, particularly in the presence of intestinal obstruction, a lower midline abdominal incision is to be preferred over a right lower paramedian incision. The latter, although widely practised in the past, is difficult to extend, more difficult to close and provides poorer access to the pelvis and peritoneal cavity.

Rutherford Morison's incision is useful if the appendix is para- or retrocaecal and fixed. It is essentially an oblique muscle-cutting incision with its lower end over McBurney's point and extending obliquely upwards and laterally as necessary. All layers are divided in the line of the incision.

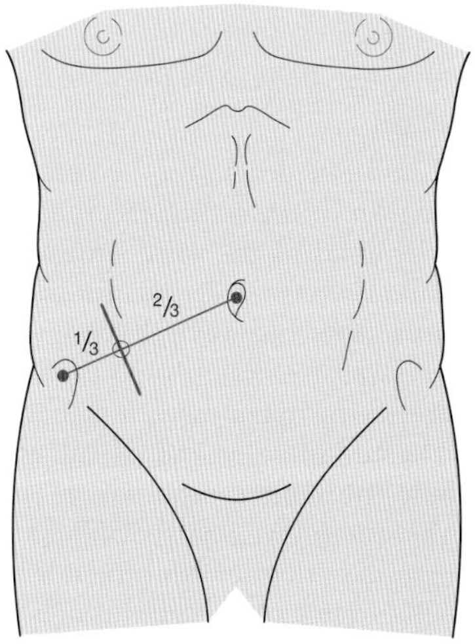

Figure 72.11 Gridiron incision for appendicitis, at right angles to a line joining the anterior superior iliac spine and umbilicus, centred on McBurney's point (courtesy of Professor M Earley, FRSCI, Dublin, Ireland).

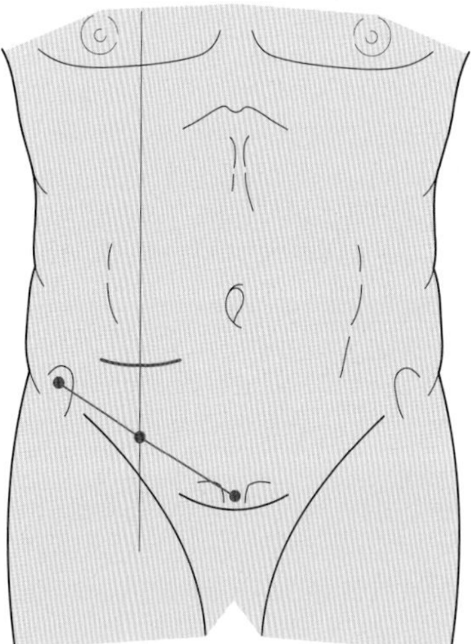

Figure 72.12 Transverse or skin crease (Lanz) incision for appendicitis, 2 cm below the umbilicus, centred on the mid-clavicular–mid-inguinal line (courtesy of Professor M Earley, FRSCI, Dublin, Ireland).

Thomas George Morton, 1835–1903, surgeon, Philadelphia, PA, USA.
Lewis Linn McArthur, 1858–1934, surgeon, St. Luke's Hospital, Chicago, IL, USA.
James Rutherford Morison, 1853–1939, Professor of Surgery, The University of Durham, Durham, UK.
Otto Lanz, 1865–1935, surgeon, Amsterdam, The Netherlands.

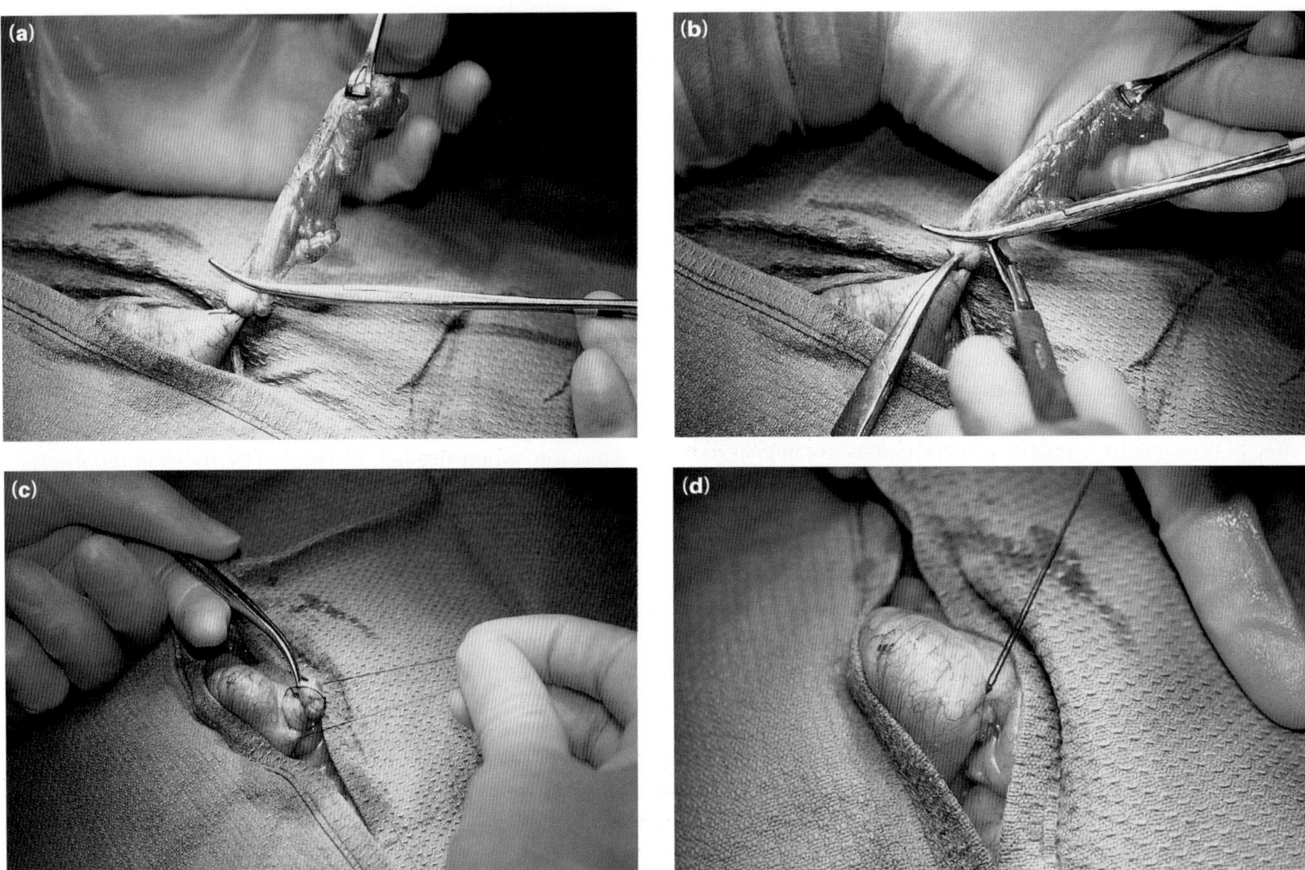

Figure 72.13 Appendicectomy. (a) The mesoappendix divided between artery forceps and ligated. (b) The appendix crushed and ligated at its base and about to be divided. (c) 'Z' suture inserted prior to inversion of the appendiceal stump. (d) The appendiceal stump inverted, the 'Z' suture having been tied.

REMOVAL OF THE APPENDIX

The caecum is identified by the presence of taeniae coli and, using a finger or a swab, the caecum is withdrawn. A turgid appendix may be felt at the base of the caecum. Inflammatory adhesions must be gently broken with a finger, which is then hooked around the appendix to deliver it into the wound. The appendix is conveniently controlled using a Babcock or Lane's forceps applied in such a way as to encircle the appendix and yet not damage it. The base of the mesoappendix is clamped in artery forceps, divided and ligated (Figure 72.13a). When the mesoappendix is broad, the procedure must be repeated with a second or, rarely, a third artery forceps. The appendix, now completely freed, is crushed near its junction with the caecum in artery forceps, which is removed and reapplied just distal to the crushed portion. An absorbable 2/0 ligature is tied around the crushed portion close to the caecum. The appendix is amputated between the artery forceps and the ligature (Figure 72.13b). An absorbable 2/0 or 3/0 purse-string or 'Z' suture may then be inserted into the caecum about 1.25 cm from the base (Figure 72.13c). The stitch should pass through the muscle coat, picking up the taeniae coli. The stump of the appendix is invaginated (Figure 72.13d) while the purse-string or 'Z' suture is tied, thus burying the appendix stump. Many surgeons believe invagination of the appendiceal stump is unnecessary.

METHODS TO BE ADOPTED IN SPECIAL CIRCUMSTANCES

When the caecal wall is oedematous, the purse-string suture is in danger of cutting out. If the oedema is of limited extent, this can be overcome by inserting the purse-string suture into more healthy caecal wall at a greater distance from the base of the appendix. Occasions may arise when, because of the extensive oedema of the caecal wall, it is better not to attempt invagination.

When the base of the appendix is inflamed, it should not be crushed, but ligated close to the caecal wall just tightly enough to occlude the lumen, after which the appendix is amputated and the stump invaginated. Should the base of the appendix be gangrenous, neither crushing nor ligation should be attempted. Two stitches are placed through the caecal wall close to the base of the gangrenous appendix, which is amputated flush with the caecal wall, after which these stitches are tied. Further closure is effected by means of a second layer of interrupted seromuscular sutures. An alternative but more costly option when the appendix base is compromised is to resect the appendix with a cuff of healthy caecum using a single firing of a linear stapling device.

William Wayne Babcock, 1872–1963, surgeon, Philadelphia, PA, USA.
Sir William Arbuthnot Lane, 1856–1943, surgeon, Guy's Hospital, London, UK.

RETROGRADE APPENDICECTOMY

When the appendix is retrocaecal and adherent, it is an advantage to divide the base between artery forceps. The appendiceal vessels are then ligated, the stump ligated and invaginated, and gentle traction on the caecum will enable the surgeon to deliver the body of the appendix, which is then removed from base to tip. Occasionally, this manoeuvre requires division of the lateral peritoneal attachments of the caecum.

LAPAROSCOPIC APPENDICECTOMY

The most valuable aspect of laparoscopy in the management of suspected appendicitis is as a diagnostic tool, particularly in women of childbearing age. The placement of operating ports may vary according to operator preference and previous abdominal scars. Typically, a pneumoperitoneum is established using an open infraumbilical approach. This umbilical port serves as the camera port with two working ports inserted under direct vision, the first suprapublically and second in the left lower quadrant. An alternative to this standard multiport approach is single incision laparoscopic appendicectomy (SILA) using a single multiple access port inserted at the umbilicus. SILA is associated with longer operating times and has not been shown to offer an advantage with respect to postoperative pain or hospital stay when compared with standard techniques, but may have a superior cosmetic outcome. Irrespective of the approach, the operator stands to the patient's left and faces a screen placed at the patient's right. A moderate Trendelenburg tilt with elevation of the right side of the operating table improves exposure and assists delivery of loops of small bowel from the pelvis. The appendix is found in the conventional manner by identification of the caecal taeniae and is controlled using a laparoscopic tissue-holding forceps. Occassionally, it is necessary to divide the peritoneal attachments and mobilise the caecum in order to adequately expose the appendix. By elevating the appendix, the mesoappendix is then displayed. A dissecting forceps, hook or scissors diathermy is used to dissect the mesoappendix (Figure 72.14a) and expose the appendicular vessels, which may be coagulated or ligated using a clip applicator (Figure 72.14b). The appendix, free of its mesentery, can be ligated at its base with an absorbable loop ligature (Figure 72.14c) or a linear stapling device, divided (Fig. 72.14d) and removed in a

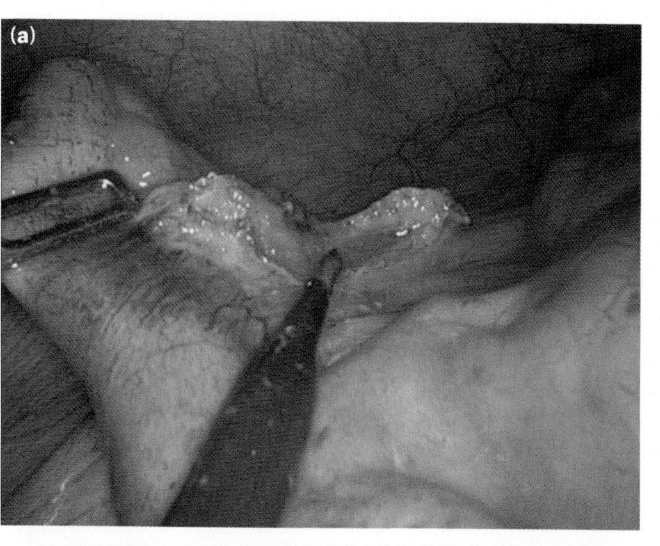
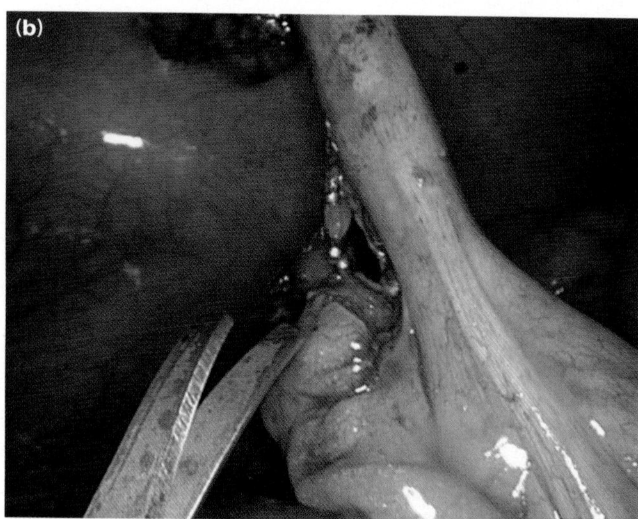
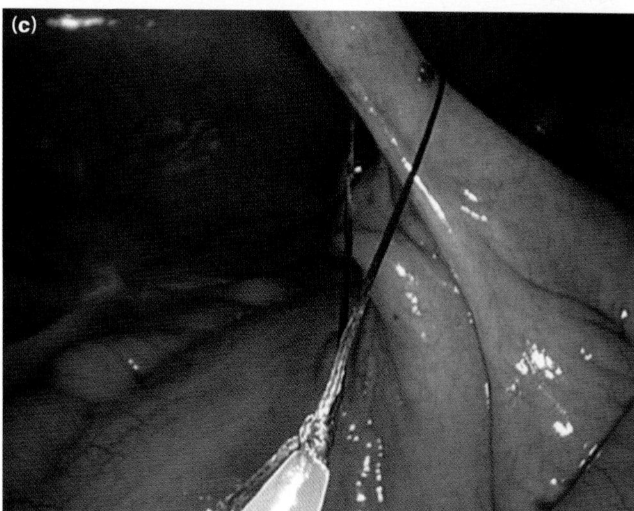
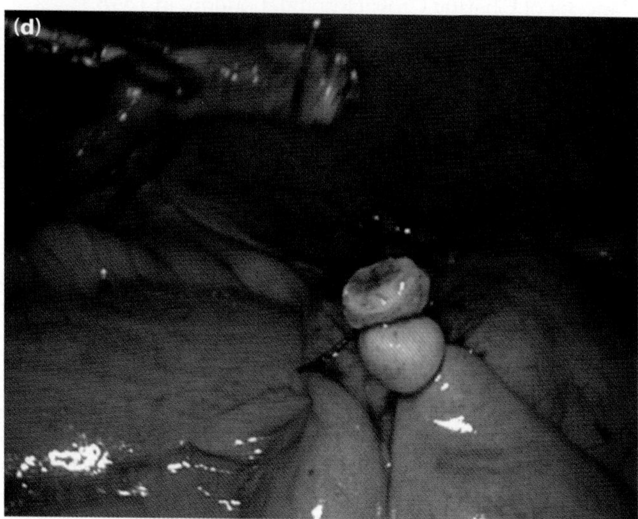

Figure 72.14 Laparoscopic appendicectomy. (a) Hook diathermy dissection of the mesoappendix. (b) The appendicular artery, ligated with clips, is divided. (c) The appendix base is ligated with absorbable ties. (d) Appendicectomy complete.

specimen bag through one of the operating ports. It is not usual to invert the stump of the appendix. Absorbable sutures are used to close the fascia at the umbilicus and at any port sites greater than 5 mm, and the small skin incisions may be closed with subcuticular sutures.

Problems encountered during appendicectomy

A NORMAL APPENDIX IS FOUND

This demands careful exclusion of other possible diagnoses, particularly terminal ileitis, Meckel's diverticulitis and tubal or ovarian causes in women. It is usual to remove the appendix to avoid future diagnostic difficulties, even though the appendix is macroscopically normal, particularly if a skin crease or gridiron incision has been made. A case can be made for preserving the macroscopically normal appendix seen at diagnostic laparoscopy, although approximately one-quarter of seemingly normal appendices show microscopic evidence of inflammation.

THE APPENDIX CANNOT BE FOUND

The caecum should be mobilised, and the taeniae coli should be traced to their confluence on the caecum before the diagnosis of 'absent appendix' is made.

AN APPENDICULAR TUMOUR IS FOUND

Small tumours (under 2.0 cm in diameter) can be removed by appendicectomy; larger tumours should be treated by a right hemicolectomy (see below).

AN APPENDIX ABSCESS IS FOUND AND THE APPENDIX CANNOT BE REMOVED EASILY

This eventuality is rare in the era of modern diagnositic imaging. Percutaneous drainage of the abscess and intravenous antibiotic treatment is to be preferred. If found at operation, the abscess should be drained and intravenous antibiotics administered. Very rarely in the face of a frankly necrotic appendix, a caecectomy or partial right hemicolectomy is required. (The first recorded operation for an appendix abscess was by Henry Hancock of Charing Cross Hospital, London, in 1848.)

Appendicitis complicating Crohn's disease

Occasionally, a patient undergoing surgery for acute appendicitis is found to have concomitant Crohn's disease of the ileocaecal region. Providing that the caecal wall is healthy at the base of the appendix, appendicectomy can be performed without increasing the risk of an enterocutaneous fistula. Rarely, the appendix is involved with the Crohn's disease. In this situation, a conservative approach may be warranted, and a trial of intravenous corticosteroids and systemic antibiotics can be used to resolve the acute inflammatory process.

Appendix abscess

Failure of resolution of an appendix mass or continued spiking pyrexia usually indicates that there is pus within the phlegmonous appendix mass. Ultrasound or abdominal CT scan may identify an area suitable for the insertion of a percutaneous drain. Rarely this is unsuccessful and laparotomy though a midline incision is indicated.

Pelvic abscess

Pelvic abscess formation is an occasional complication of appendicitis and can occur irrespective of the position of the appendix within the peritoneal cavity. The most common presentation is a spiking pyrexia several days after appendicitis; indeed, the patient may already have been discharged from hospital. Pelvic pressure or discomfort associated with loose stool or tenesmus is common. Rectal examination reveals a boggy mass in the pelvis, anterior to the rectum, at the level of the peritoneal reflection. Pelvic ultrasound or CT scan will confirm. Traditionally, treatment has been through transrectal drainage under general anaesthetic; however, increasing availablity of radiologically guided percutaneous drainage has reduced the need considerably.

Management of an appendix mass

If an appendix mass is present and the condition of the patient is satisfactory, the standard treatment is the conservative Ochsner–Sherren regime. This strategy is based on the premise that the inflammatory process is already localised and that inadvertent surgery is difficult and may be dangerous. It may be impossible to find the appendix and, occasionally, a faecal fistula may form. For these reasons, it is wise to observe a non-operative programme but to be prepared to operate should clinical deterioration occur.

Summary box 72.6

Criteria for stopping conservative treatment of an appendix mass

- A rising pulse rate
- Increasing or spreading abdominal pain
- Increasing size of the mass

Careful recording of the patient's condition and the extent of the mass should be made and the abdomen regularly re-examined. It is helpful to mark the limits of the mass on the abdominal wall using a skin pencil. A contrast-enhanced CT examination of the abdomen should be performed and antibiotic therapy instigated. An abscess, if present, should be drained radiologically. Temperature and pulse rate should be recorded 4-hourly and a fluid balance record maintained. Clinical deterioration or evidence of peritonitis is an indication for early laparotomy. Clinical improvement is usually evident within 24–48 hours. Failure of the mass to resolve should raise suspicion of a carcinoma or Crohn's disease. Using this regime, approximately 90% of cases resolve without incident. The need for interval appendicectomy in this

Albert John Ochsner, 1858–1925, Professor of Clinical Surgery, The University of Illinois College of Medicine, Chicago, IL, USA.
James Sherren, 1872–1945, surgeon, The London Hospital, London, UK.

cohort is much debated. The great majority of patients will not develop recurrent appendicitis; however; recently published studies have identified higher than expected rates of underlying appendiceal neoplasm in those patients who do go on to interval appendicectomy, particularly those patients over the age of 40. At the very least, follow-up CT should be performed to ensure complete resolution of findings and patients should undergo colonoscopy.

Postoperative complications

Postoperative complications following appendicectomy are relatively uncommon and reflect the degree of peritonitis that was present at the time of operation and intercurrent diseases that may predispose to complications.

> **Summary box 72.7**
>
> Check-list for unwell patient following appendicectomy
>
> - Examine the wound and abdomen for an abscess
> - Consider a pelvic abscess and perform a rectal examination
> - Examine the lungs – pneumonitis or collapse
> - Examine the legs – consider venous thrombosis
> - Examine the conjunctivae for an icteric tinge and the liver for enlargement, and enquire whether the patient has had rigors (pylephlebitis)
> - Examine the urine for organisms (pyelonephritis)
> - Suspect subphrenic abscess

Wound infection

Wound infection is the most common postoperative complication, occurring in 5–10% of all patients. This usually presents with pain and erythema of the wound on the fourth or fifth postoperative day, often soon after hospital discharge. Treatment is by wound drainage and antibiotics when required. The organisms responsible are usually a mixture of gram-negative bacilli and anaerobic bacteria, predominantly *Bacteroides* species and anaerobic streptococci.

Intra-abdominal abscess

Approximately 8% of patients following appendectomy will develop a postoperative intra-abdominal abscess. In an era of hospital discharge 24–48 hours following appendectomy, patients should be advised prior to discharge that a spiking fever, malaise and anorexia developing 5–7 days after operation is suggestive of an intraperitoneal collection and that urgent medical advice should be obtained. Interloop, paracolic, pelvic and subphrenic sites should be considered. Abdominal ultrasonography and CT scanning greatly facilitate diagnosis and allow percutaneous drainage (Figure 72.15). Laparotomy should be considered in patients suspected of having intra-abdominal sepsis but in whom imaging fails to show a collection, particularly those with continuing ileus.

Ileus

A period of adynamic ileus is to be expected after appendicectomy, and this may last a number of days following removal of a gangrenous appendix. Ileus persisting for more than 4 or 5 days, particularly in the presence of a fever, is indicative of

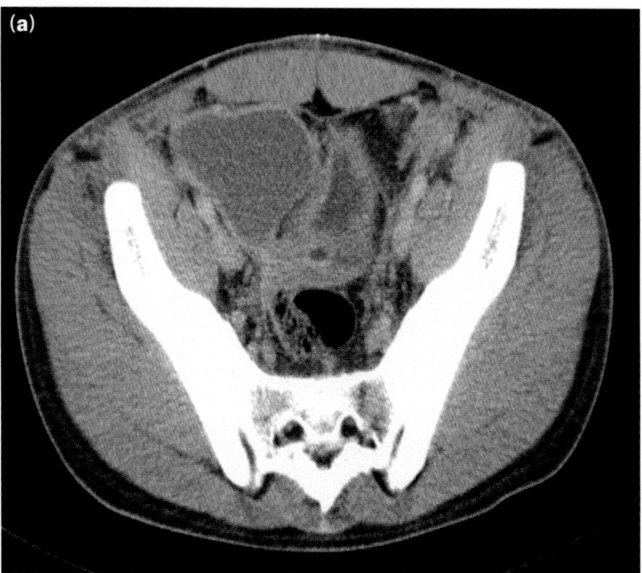

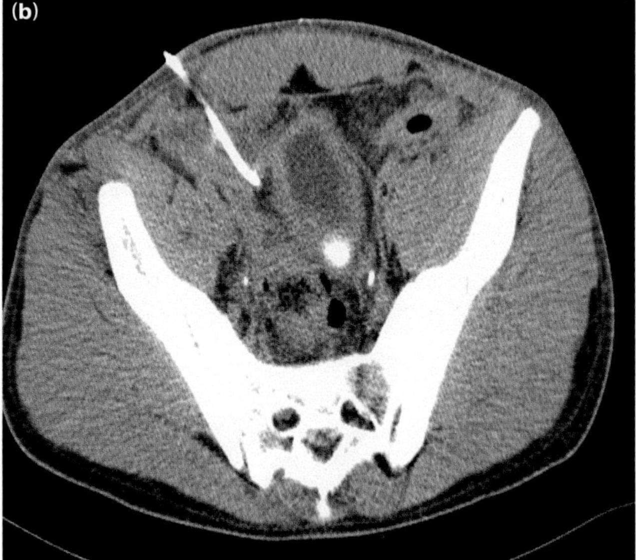

Figure 72.15 (a) Rim enhancing collection in the right iliac fossa, 1 week following open appendicectomy for perforated appendicitis. (b) Successful radiological drainage with resolution of the abscess (courtesy of Dr P MacMahon, FRCR, Dublin, Ireland).

continuing intra-abdominal sepsis and should prompt further investigation (see above). Rarely, early during postoperative recovery, a Richter's type of hernia may occur at the site of a laparoscopic port insertion and may be confused with a post-operative ileus. A CT scan is usually definitive.

Respiratory

In the absence of concurrent pulmonary disease, respiratory complications are rare following appendicectomy. Adequate postoperative analgesia and physiotherapy, when appropriate, reduce the incidence.

Venous thrombosis and embolism

These conditions are rare after appendicectomy, except in the elderly and in women taking the oral contraceptive pill. Appropriate prophylactic measures should be taken in such cases.

Portal pyaemia (pylephlebitis)

This is a rare but very serious complication of gangrenous appendicitis associated with high fever, rigors and jaundice. It is caused by septicaemia in the portal venous system and leads to the development of intrahepatic abscesses (often multiple). Treatment is with systemic antibiotics and percutaneous drainage of hepatic abscesses as appropriate. A screen for underlying thrombophilia should be considered.

Faecal fistula

Leakage from the appendicular stump occurs rarely, but may follow if the encircling stitch has been put in too deeply or if the caecal wall was involved by oedema or inflammation. Occasionally, a fistula may result following appendicectomy in Crohn's disease.

Adhesive intestinal obstruction

This is the most common late complication of appendicectomy. At operation, a single band adhesion is often found to be responsible. Occasionally, chronic pain in the right iliac fossa is attributed to adhesion formation after appendicectomy. In such cases, laparoscopy is of value in confirming the presence of adhesions and allowing division.

RECURRENT ACUTE APPENDICITIS

Rarely, inflammation of the appendix may present as a chronic condition characterised by recurrent episodes of lower abdominal pain. Recurrent appendicitis is thought to arise as a consequence of incomplete self-limiting obstruction of the appendix lumen (Figure 72.16). The attacks vary in intensity and may occur every few months, and the majority of cases ultimately culminate in severe acute appendicitis. If a careful history is taken from patients with acute appendicitis, many remember having had milder but similar attacks of pain. The appendix in these cases is thickened and shows fibrosis indicative of previous inflammation (Figure 72.17).

NEOPLASMS OF THE APPENDIX AND PSEUDOMYXOMA PERITONEI

Neoplasms of the appendix are found in 1% of appendicectomy specimens, with the vast majority being an incidental finding. Most tumours involving the appendix may be classified as either carcinoid or epithelial, with the latter group accounting for approximately three-quarters of all cases.

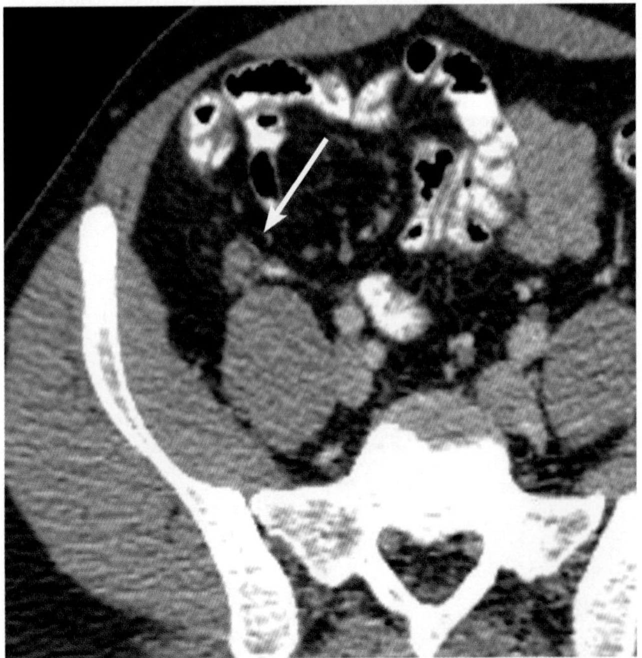

Figure 72.16 Axial computed tomography in a 20-year-old male with recurrent lower abdominal pain, demonstrating some fatty submucosal deposition in a thickened mildly enlarged appendix but without surrounding inflammatory change (arrow), findings suggestive of chronic appendicitis (courtesy of Dr P MacMahon, FRCR, Dublin, Ireland).

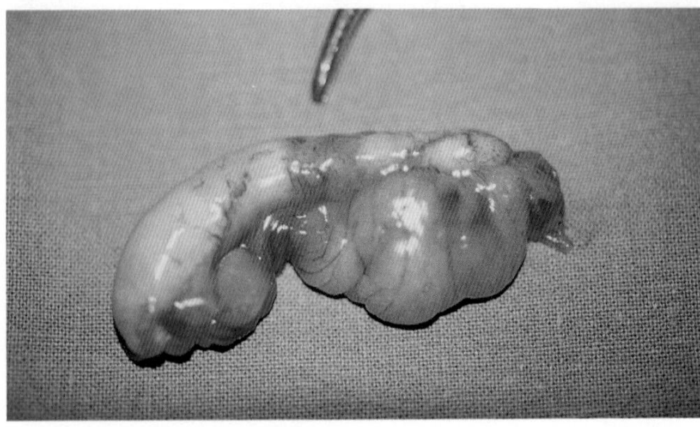

Figure 72.17 Excised appendix showing the point of luminal obstruction with distal fibrosis.

August Gottlieb Richter, 1742–1812, lecturer in Surgery, Göttingen, Germany.

Carcinoid tumour (synonym: argentaffinoma):

Carcinoid tumours arise in argentaffin tissue (Kulchitsky cells of the crypts of Lieberkühn) and are most common in the vermiform appendix. Carcinoid tumour is found once in every 300–400 appendices subjected to histological examination. In many instances, the appendix had been removed because of symptoms of subacute or recurrent appendicitis. The tumour can occur in any part of the appendix, but it is frequently found in the distal third. The neoplasm feels moderately hard and, on sectioning the appendix, it can be seen as a yellow tumour between the intact mucosa and the peritoneum. Microscopically, the tumour cells are small, arranged in small nests within the muscle and have a characteristic pattern using immunohistochemical stain for chromogranin B (Figure 72.18). Unlike carcinoid tumours arising in other parts of the intestinal tract, carcinoid tumour of the appendix rarely gives rise to metastases.

Treatment

Appendicectomy has been shown to be sufficient treatment unless the caecal wall is involved, the tumour is 2 cm or more in size or involved lymph nodes are found, when right hemicolectomy is indicated.

Epithelial tumours of the appendix:

Epithelial neoplasms are found in 0.6% of appendicectomy specimens. Numerous classifications systems have been proposed leading to much confusion and difficulty when comparing treatment modalities and outcomes. Recently, following a modified Delphi consultation process, a group of international experts proposed an updated classification system for appendiceal epithelial neoplasms (Carr). Tumours may be classified as mucinous or non-mucinous (intestinal type) and according to the degree of cytologic atypia and architectural features (infiltrative versus pushing invasion) (*Table 72.3*). Goblet cell carcinoid, a rare tumour of the appendix, which shows both gland forming and neuroendocrine features, has now been reclassified as goblet cell tumour and may be of a mucinous or non-mucinous subtype. The relevance of appendiceal epithelial tumours, particularly when of the mucinous subtype (Figure 72.19), lies in their propensity to disseminate causing the syndrome known as pseudomyxoma peritonei (PMP).

TABLE 72.3 Classification of epithelial neoplasia of the appendix (adapted from Carr *et al.*, 2016).

Adenoma (tubular, tubulovillous, villous)	
Serrated polyp	
Non-mucinous adenocarcinoma	
Mucinous neoplasm	Low-grade appendiceal mucinous neoplasm (LAMN)
	High-grade appendiceal mucinous neoplasm (HAMN)
	Mucinous adenocarcinoma
Adenocarcinoma with signet ring cells (<50%)	
Signet ring (>50%) carcinoma	

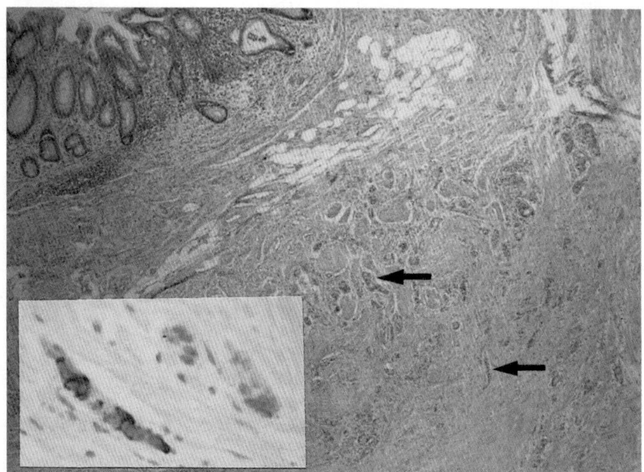

Figure 72.18 Carcinoid tumour. A small incidental carcinoid tumour of the appendix. The tumour cells infiltrate the muscle arranged in small nests and trabeculae (arrows). Tumour cells are small and have inconspicuous nuclei. Inset: higher magnification of an immunohistochemical stain for chromogranin B shows a strong positive reaction (brown) of tumour cells (courtesy of Dr P Kelly, FRCPath, Dublin, Ireland).

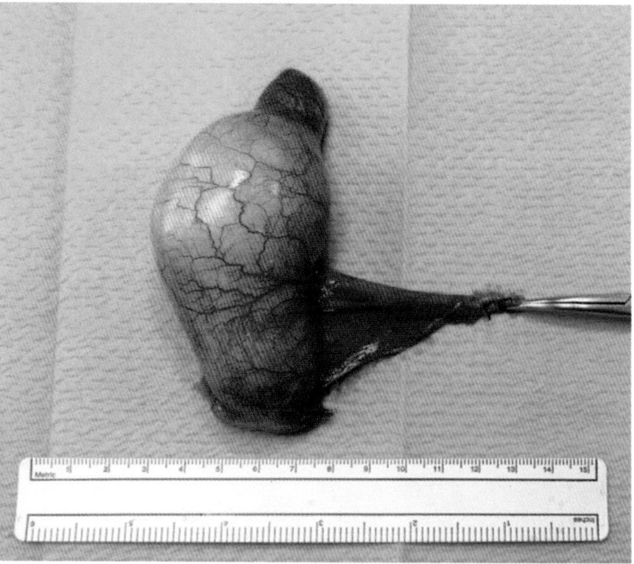

Figure 72.19 Low-grade appendiceal mucinous neoplasm with mucoceole formation that had redistributed causing secondary low-grade mucinous carcinoma peritonei, mainly of the ovary.

Johann Nathaniel Lieberkühn, 1711–1756, physician and anatomist, Berlin, Germany, described these glands in 1745.

Pseudomyxoma peritonei

PMP is a rare condition typified by progressive peritoneal tumour deposits, mucinous ascites, omental cake and ovarian involvement in females (Figure 72.20). The vast majority of cases arise as a result of perforation of a mucinous appendiceal tumour. This association was first described by Fraenkel in 1901. Patients typically present with progressive and massive abdominal distension, anorexia and symptoms of bowel dysfunction. The condition is invariably fatal without intervention. Traditionally, PMP was thought to have an incidence of one per million per year, but it is now thought to be at least double that. The overall risk of developing pseudomyxoma following removal of an appendix harbouring epithelial tumour is approximately 9%, with the risk varying according to the tumour subtype and the mode of presentation. Following removal of a non-mucinous neoplasm the risk of PMP is as low as 3%, while it may be as high as 30–50% in the case of a mucinous adenocarcinoma of the appendix. PMP is classified according to the degree of cytological atypia within the peritoneal deposits (Table 72.4) and its grading may differ from that of the causative appendiceal tumour.

TABLE 72.4 Classification of pseudomyxoma peritonei (adapted from Carr *et al*., 2016).

Acellular mucin
Low-grade mucinous carcinoma peritonei
High-grade mucinous carcinoma peritonei
High-grade mucinous carcinoma peritonei with signet ring cells

TREATMENT – APPENDICEAL EPITHELIAL TUMOUR WITHOUT PMP

In patients with an incidental finding of an epithelial neoplasm and no current evidence of established PMP, subsequent treatment is dependent on the degree of cytological atypia within the primary tumour and the estimated future risk of developing PMP.

Patients with low-grade epithelial neoplasms and no evidence of mucin or epithelial cells beyond the appendix are thought to be at low, but not negligible, risk of future PMP development. A colonoscopy should be performed to exclude associated colonic epithelial lesions and patients entered into

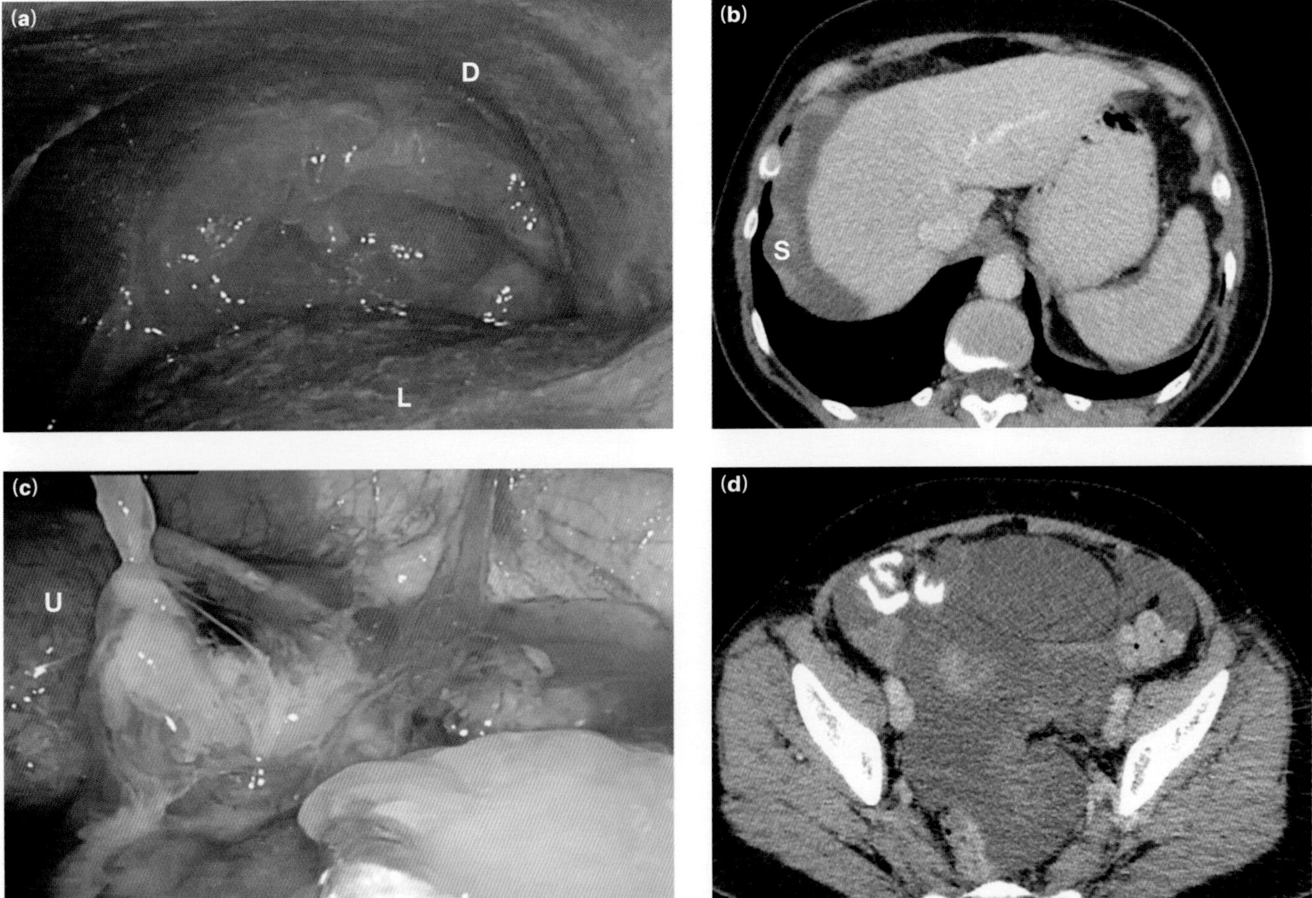

Figure 72.20 Pseudomyxoma peritonei secondary to a high-grade mucinous neoplasm of the appendix as seen at laparoscopy and computed tomography (CT). (a, b) Mucinous tumour of the right hemidiaphragm (D) and liver capsule (L) causing characteristic scalloping (S) at CT. (c, d) Mucinous tumour filling the pelvis posterior to the uterus (U) with the corresponding CT findings (courtesy of Dr C Cronin, FRCR, Dublin, Ireland).

a surveillance protocol for at least 5 years. Surveillance may take the form of clinical review, annual low-dose abdominopelvic CT scan and appendix-related tumour markers (CEA, CA 199, CA 125).

Patients with high-grade tumour, invasive adenocarcinoma or goblet cell tumour and/or those with epithelial cell containing mucin outside the appendix are at higher risk of nodal involvement and subsequent development of PMP. According to current paradigms, such patients should be approached in a similar fashion to patients with established PMP and consideration given to right hemicolectomy with prophylactic regional (right parietal) peritonectomy, omentectomy and intraperitoneal chemotherapy. Consideration should also be given to performing bilaterral salpingo-ophorectomy, although in patients of childbearing age the decision making is complex.

TREATMENT - ESTABLISHED PMP

The standard accepted treatment for established PMP is cytoreductive surgery (CRS) combined with heated intraperitoneal chemotherapy HIPEC (Sugarbaker). This approach combines multiple peritonectomy procedures with multivisceral resections as required to achieve a complete surgical clearance of the tumour (complete cytoreduction), which is augmented by HIPEC to eradicate presumed residual microscopic disease. The combined operation can take in excess of 10 hours and may require total abdominopelvic peritonectomy, greater and lesser omentectomy, bilaterral salpingo-ophorectomy, hysterectomy, cholecystectomy, splenectomy, partial gastrectomy, colectomy and anterior resection of the rectum. The largest reported series of CRS/HIPEC for PMP comes from Basingstoke, UK (Moran). In their experience involving more than 1000 patients, a complete cytoreduction was achieved in approximately 75% of patients with the remainder undergoing maximal tumour debulking. Although a potentially morbid procedure, in experienced centres the operative mortality rate following CRS/HIPEC is less than 2% with major postoperative morbidity occuring in 15% of patients. Following a complete cytoreduction 5- and 10-year survival rates of 87% and 70%, respectively, can be achieved. Poorer outcomes are seen in males, patients with elevated tumour markers and following resection of tumour showing high-grade or invasive features.

FURTHER READING

Andersen BR, Kallehave FL, Andersen HK. Antibiotics versus placebo for prevention of postoperative infection after appendicectomy. *Cochrane Database Syst Rev* 2005; Issue 3, Art. No. CD001439.

Ansari N, Chandrakumaran K, Dayal S *et al*. Cytoreductive surgery and hyperthermic intraperitoneal chemotherapy in 1000 patients with perforated appendiceal epithelial tumours. *Eur J Surg Oncol* 2016; **42**(7): 1035–41.

Berry J, Malt RA. Appendicitis near its centenary. *Am J Surg* 1984; **2000**: 567–75.

Carr NJ, Cecil TD, Mohamed F *et al*. (2016) A consensus for classification and pathologic reporting of pseudomyxoma peritonei and associated appendiceal neoplasia. The Results of the Peritoneal Surface Oncology Group International (PSOGI) Modified Delphi Process. *Am J Surg Pathol* 2016; **40**: 14–26.

Ingraham AM, Cohen ME, Bilimoria KY *et al*. Effect of delay to operation on outcomes in adults with acute appendicitis. *Arch Surg* 2010; **145**: 886–92.

Kim K, Kim YH, Kim Sy *et al*. Low-dose abdominal CT for evaluating suspected appendicitis. *N Engl J Med* 2012; **366**: 1596–1605.

Murphy EMA, Farquharson SM, Moran BJ. Management of an unexpected appendiceal neoplasm. *Br J Surg* 2006; **93**: 783–92.

National Surgical Research Collaborative. Multicentre observational study of performance variation in provision and outcome of emergency appendicectomy. *Br J Surg* 2013; **100**: 1240–52.

Salminen P, Paajanen H, Rautio T *et al*. Antibiotic therapy vs appendectomy for treatment of uncomplicated acute appendicitis. The APPAC randomized clinical trial. *JAMA* 2015; **313**: 2340–8.

Sauerland S, Jaschinski T, Neugebauer EA. Laparoscopic versus open surgery for suspected appendicitis. *Cochrane Database Syst Rev* 2010; CD001546.

van Rossem CC, Bolmers MD, Schreinemacher MH *et al*. Prospective nationwide outcome audit of surgery for suspected acute appendicitis. *Br J Surg* 2016; **103**: 144–51

Wright GP, Mater ME, Carroll JT *et al*. Is there truly an oncologic indication for interval appendectomy? *Am J Surg* 2015; **209**: 442–6.

Paul H. Sugarbaker, contemporary, surgeon, Washingon DC, USA
Brendan J. Moran, contemporary, surgeon, Basingstoke, UK

Chapter 73

The rectum

Learning objectives

To understand:

- The anatomy of the rectum and its relationship to surgical disease and its treatment
- The pathology, clinical presentation, investigation, differential diagnosis and treatment of diseases that affect the rectum

To appreciate:

- That carcinoma of the rectum is common and can present with symptoms similar to benign disease. Careful evaluation is required
- The principles involved in the management of rectal pathologies

ANATOMY

Surgical anatomy

The rectum begins where the tinea coli of the sigmoid colon join to form a continuous outer longitudinal muscle layer at the level of the sacral promontory. The rectum follows the curve of the sacrum, and ends at the anorectal junction. The puborectalis muscle encircles the posterior and lateral aspects of the junction, creating the anorectal angle (normally 120°). The rectum has three lateral curvatures; the upper and lower are convex to the right, and the middle is convex to the left. On the luminal aspect, these three curves are marked by semicircular folds (Houston's valves).

The adult rectum is approximately 12–18 cm in length and is conventionally divided into three equal parts: the upper third, which is mobile and has a peritoneal covering anteriorly and laterally; the middle third, where the peritoneum covers only the anterior and part of the lateral surfaces; and the lowest third, which lies deep in the pelvis below the peritoneal reflection.

The lower third of the rectum is separated by distinct fascial layers from the prostate/vagina anteriorly (Denonvilliers' fascia), and from the coccyx and lower two sacral vertebrae posteriorly (Waldeyer's fascia) (*Table 73.1*). These fascial layers are surgically important as they act as barriers to malignant invasion and form the anatomical envelope for total mesorectal excision (TME) to achieve complete oncological clearance of rectal cancer.

Summary box 73.1

Anatomy of the rectum

- The rectum measures approximately 15 cm in length
- It is divided into lower, middle and upper thirds
- The blood supply consists of superior, middle and inferior rectal vessels
- The lymphatic drainage follows the blood supply. The principal route of drainage is upwards along the superior rectal vessels to the para-aortic nodes, although the lower rectum can drain to lymphatics along the lateral pelvic side walls

TABLE 73.1 Anatomical relations of the rectum.

	Relation
Anterior	Bladder Seminal vesicles and prostate (males) Denonvillier's fascia (males) Pouch of Douglas and rectovaginal septum (females) Uterus and cervix (females) Ureters
Lateral	Lateral ligaments and middle rectal artery Obturator internus muscle and side wall of pelvis Pelvic autonomic plexus Levator ani muscle
Posterior	Sacrum and coccyx Waldeyer's fascial condensation Superior rectal artery and lymphatics Hypogastric nerves

John Houston, 1802–1845, physician, City of Dublin Hospital and Lecturer in Surgery, Dublin, Ireland.
Charles Pierre Denonvilliers, 1808–1872, Professor of Anatomy and later of Surgery, Paris, France.
Heinrich Wilhelm Gottfried Waldeyer-Hartz, 1836–1921, Professor of Pathological Anatomy, Berlin, Germany.

Embryology

The embryological hindgut forms the upper rectum, while the lower rectum is derived from the cloaca and is surrounded by extraperitoneal connective tissue. The primitive gut tube is suspended dorsally by a mesentry throughout its length, to form the mesorectum. The muscular layers of the rectum are derived from the mesenchyme that accompanies the endodermal part of the anorectum, with the inner circular layer preceding the outer longitudinal layer in the 7th week of embryonic development.

The levator ani muscles and external anal sphincter muscles form within the surrounding mesenchyme and grow to make contact with each other and with bundles of smooth muscle cells from the outer longitudinal layer of the rectal wall. A layer of undifferentiated mesenchyme separates the rectal muscle layers from the levator ani muscle and the muscle layer of the future anal canal.

Blood supply

The superior rectal artery is the direct continuation of the inferior mesenteric artery and is the main arterial supply of the rectum (Figure 73.1). The arteries and their accompanying lymphatics lie within the loose fatty tissue in the mesorectum, surrounded by a sheath of connective tissue (the mesorectal fascia). The middle rectal artery arises on each side from the internal iliac artery and passes to the rectum in the lateral ligaments. It is usually small and often only present on one side, and divides into several branches. The inferior rectal artery arises on each side from the internal pudendal artery as it enters Alcock's canal. It hugs the inferior surface of the levator ani muscle as it crosses the roof of the ischiorectal fossa to enter the anal muscles.

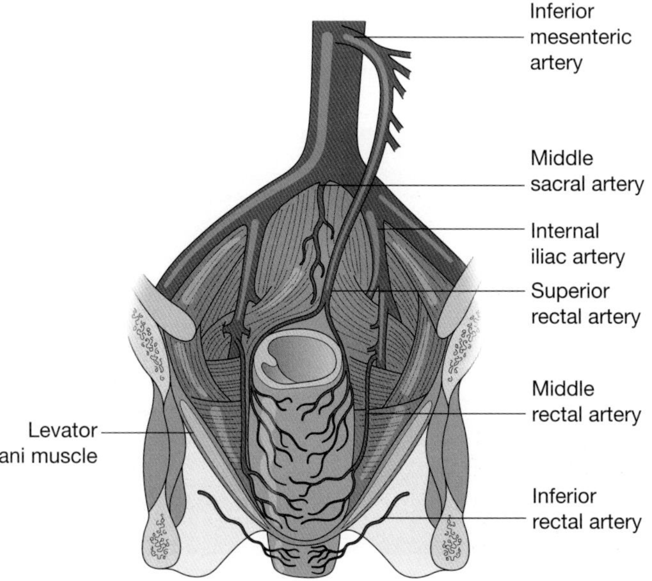

Figure 73.1 Blood supply to the rectum. The main blood supply comes from the superior rectal arteries, supplemented by middle rectal arteries in 20% of cases. The inferior rectal arteries are derived from the pudendal vessels and supply the anal canal and lower rectum.

Venous drainage

The superior haemorrhoidal veins draining the upper half of the anal canal above the dentate line pass upwards to become the rectal veins; these unite to form the superior rectal vein, which later becomes the inferior mesenteric vein. This forms part of the portal venous system and ultimately drains into the splenic vein. Middle rectal veins exist but are small, unimportant channels unless the normal paths are blocked.

Lymphatic drainage

The lymphatics of the rectal mucosa communicate freely with those of the muscle layers. The usual drainage flow is upwards, and only to a limited extent laterally and downwards. For this reason, surgical clearance of malignant disease concentrates mainly on achieving wide resection of proximal lymph nodes. However, if the usual upward routes are blocked, for example by metastatic disease, the flow can reverse and it is possible to find involved lymph nodes on the side walls of the pelvis (along the middle rectal vessels) or even in the inguinal region (along the inferior rectal artery).

CLINICAL FEATURES OF RECTAL DISEASE

Symptoms

Rectal diseases are common and can occur at any age. The symptoms of many of them overlap. In general, inflammatory conditions affect younger age groups, while tumours occur in the middle-aged and elderly.

Summary box 73.2

Main symptoms of rectal disease

- Fresh bleeding per rectum
- Altered bowel habit with loose stool
- Mucus discharge
- Tenesmus
- Prolapse
- Proctalgia (pain)

Bleeding

This is often painless and bright red in colour and should be carefully investigated at any age.

Altered bowel habit

Early morning stool frequency (spurious diarrhoea) is a symptom of rectal carcinoma, while blood-stained, frequent, loose stools characterise the inflammatory diseases.

Discharge

Mucus and pus are associated with rectal inflammation.

Tenesmus

Often described by the patient as 'I feel I want to go but nothing happens', this is normally an ominous symptom of rectal cancer, but can occur with other rectal conditions and is a common symptom of rectal prolapse.

Prolapse

This usually indicates either mucosal or full-thickness rectal wall protrusion from the anus. Internal prolapse or intussusception refers to a telescoping of the rectum into itself without protrusion from the anus.

Pain: 'proctalgia'

This is usually a severe and episodic pain resulting from spasm of the levator ani muscle. It may last for a few seconds to minutes then recur, or it can be constant.

Signs

To examine the rectum the patient is most conveniently positioned in the left lateral (Sims) position.

Inspection

Visual examination of the anus precedes rectal examination, to exclude the presence of anal disease, e.g. fissure or fistula. Evidence of rectal prolapse or abnormal pelvic floor descent can be elicited by asking the patient to strain.

Digital examination

The index finger used with gentleness and precision remains a valuable test for rectal disease (Figure 73.2). The anal sphincters are assessed for anatomical integrity, resting tone and squeeze. In females, a rectocoele may be palpable as a herniation of the anterior rectal wall into the vagina. Tumours in the lower and middle thirds of the rectum can usually be felt. On removal, the finger should be examined for mucus, pus or blood. It is useful to note the normal, as well as the abnormal, findings on digital examination e.g. the prostate in the male. Digital findings can be recorded as intraluminal (e.g. blood, pus), intramural (e.g. tumours, granular areas, strictures) or extramural (e.g. enlarged prostate, uterine fibroids). Intramural lesions can be described as fixed, tethered or mobile.

Proctoscopy

This procedure can be used to inspect the anus, anorectal junction and lower rectum. A lubricated proctoscope is inserted through the anus to provide views of the lower rectum and anal canal (Figure 73.3). Biopsy can be performed of any suspicious areas, provided it is above the sensitive anoderm. Proctoscopy is particularly useful for assessing the presence of haemorrhoids.

Sigmoidoscopy

In the past, the sigmoidoscope was a rigid stainless steel instrument of variable diameter and normally 25 cm in length, but this has been replaced by disposable plastic instruments. The rectum must be empty for proper inspection. Direct inspection of the rectal mucosa may alert the clinician to inflammation or tumours. This procedure can be performed in the outpatient setting.

FLEXIBLE SIGMOIDOSCOPE

This is used as a supplement to rigid sigmoidoscopy or when views proximal to the rectum are required (Figure 73.4). The lower bowel needs to be cleaned out with preliminary enemas. In addition to the rectum, the whole sigmoid colon up to the splenic flexure is within visual reach. Flexible sigmoidoscopy is indicated to investigate underlying causes of fresh rectal bleeding or other bowel symptoms when full visualisation of the colon by colonoscopy is not required.

Summary box 73.3

Examination of the rectum

- Visual inspection of the perineum
- Digital examination
- Proctoscopy
- Sigmoidoscopy – rigid and/or flexible

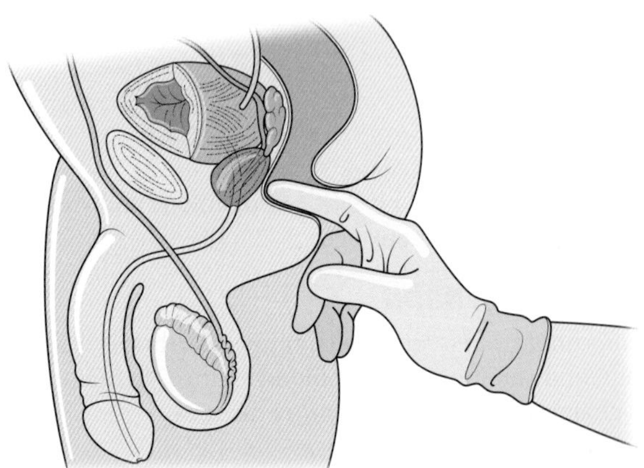

Figure 73.2 Digital rectal examination in the male. Assessment of the anal sphincter complex, lower rectum and prostate.

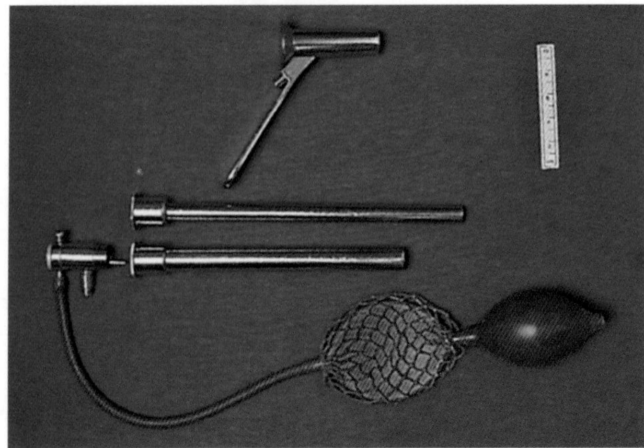

Figure 73.3 Above: proctoscope for visualisation of the anorectum. Below: rigid sigmoidscope for visualisation of the rectum.

James Marion Sims, 1813–1883, gynaecological surgeon, the State Hospital for Women, New York, NY, USA, introduced this position to give access to the anterior vaginal wall during operations for the closure of vaginovesicular fistulae.

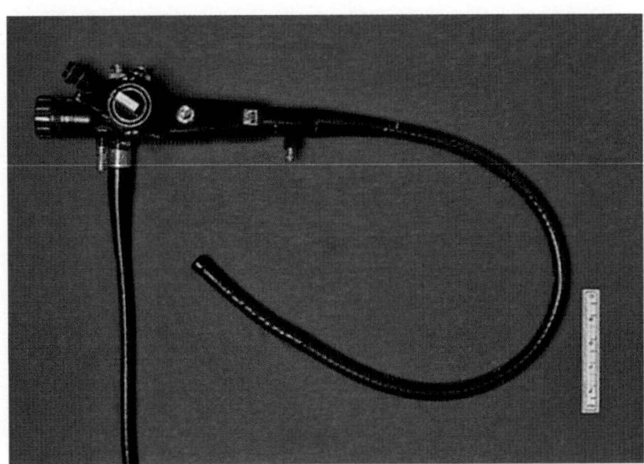

Figure 73.4 Flexible sigmoidoscope.

INJURIES

The rectum or anal canal may be injured in a number of ways, all of which are uncommon:

- by falling in a sitting posture onto a pointed object;
- penetrating injury (including gunshots) to the buttocks;
- sexual assault or sexual activity involving anal penetration;
- by the fetal head during childbirth, especially forceps-assisted.

Diagnosis

The anus should be inspected and the abdomen palpated. If abdominal rigidity or tenderness is present, early laparoscopy or laparotomy is indicated. A water-soluble contrast enema may help in delineating the injury, but a computed tomographic (CT) scan is often preferred and will provide additional information on other pelvic injuries, such as accompanying urethral injury.

Treatment

The rectum is examined under general anaesthetic with a finger and a sigmoidoscope. If penetrating injury is confirmed, laparotomy or laparoscopy is required. If an intraperitoneal rupture of the rectum is found, the perforation is closed with sutures and the rectum defunctioned with a stoma. In the event that the rectal injury cannot be repaired, a Hartmann's procedure may need to be performed. If the rectal injury is below the peritoneal reflection, wide drainage from below is indicated, with rectal washout and a defunctioning colostomy. Care must be taken to preserve sphincter function during debridement of the perineal wounds. Antibiotic cover must be provided against both aerobic and anaerobic organisms.

FOREIGN BODIES IN THE RECTUM

The variety of foreign bodies that have found their way into the rectum is hardly less remarkable than the ingenuity displayed in their removal (Figure 73.5). The difficulty lies in the creation of a vacuum effect when trying to extract the object through the anus. If insurmountable difficulty is experienced in grasping any foreign body in the rectum, laparotomy is usually necessary. The object can be pushed from above into the assistant's fingers in the rectum, or removed by means of a rectotomy in a proximal area of the rectum. If there is considerable laceration of the mucosa, a temporary colostomy is advisable.

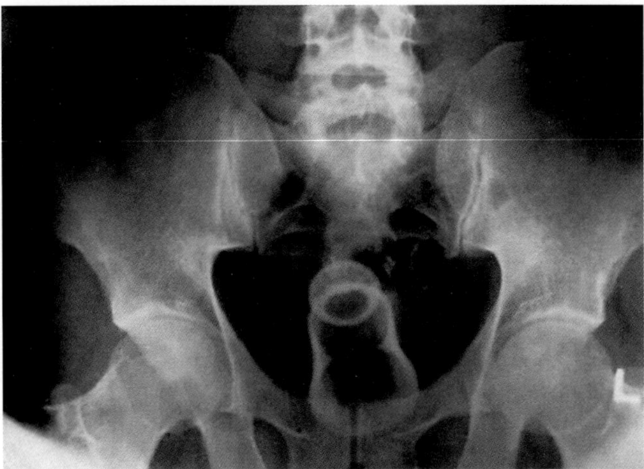

Figure 73.5 Foreign body in rectum as seen on plain abdominal x-ray.

Summary box 73.4

Injuries to the rectum are serious and invariably require surgery

- A temporary colostomy is often necessary
- There is a serious risk of associated necrotising fasciitis, and broad-spectrum antibiotics are mandatory
- There may be associated bladder or urethral damage

PROLAPSE

Mucosal prolapse

The mucous membrane and submucosa of the rectum protrude outside the anus for approximately 1–4 cm. When the prolapsed mucosa is palpated between the finger and the thumb, it is evident that it is composed of no more than a double layer of mucous membrane. This distinguishes mucosal prolapse from full-thickness prolapse where the entire rectal wall exits from the anal canal.

In infants

The direct downward course of the rectum, due to the as-yet undeveloped sacral curve, predisposes infants to this condition.

In children

Mucosal prolapse often commences after an attack of diarrhoea, or from loss of weight and consequent loss of fat in the ischiorectal fossa. It may also be associated with cystic

Summary box 73.5

Rectal prolapse

- It may be mucosal or full thickness
- If full thickness, the whole wall of the rectum is included
- It commences as a rectal intussusception
- In children, the prolapse is usually mucosal and should be treated conservatively
- In the adult, the prolapse is often full thickness and is frequently associated with incontinence
- Surgery is necessary for full-thickness rectal prolapse
- The operation is performed either via the perineum or via the abdomen

fibrosis, neurological disorder, Hirschsprung's disease, rectal polyps and maldevelopment of the pelvis.

In adults

The condition in adults is often associated with third-degree haemorrhoids, when it is referred to as mucohaemorrhoidal prolapse (Figure 73.6). In the female, a torn perineum, and in the male straining from urethral obstruction, predispose to mucosal prolapse. In old age, both mucosal and full-thickness prolapse are associated with weakness of the sphincter mechanism. Partial prolapse may follow an operation for fistula-in-ano where a large portion of muscle has been divided. Here, the prolapse is usually localised to the damaged quadrant and is seldom progressive.

Treatment

IN INFANTS AND YOUNG CHILDREN

- **Digital repositioning**. The parents are taught to replace the protrusion, and any underlying causes are addressed.
- **Submucosal injection or banding**. If digital repositioning fails after a 6-week trial, injection of 5% phenol in almond oil or rubber band ligation is carried out under general anaesthetic (Figure 73.7).

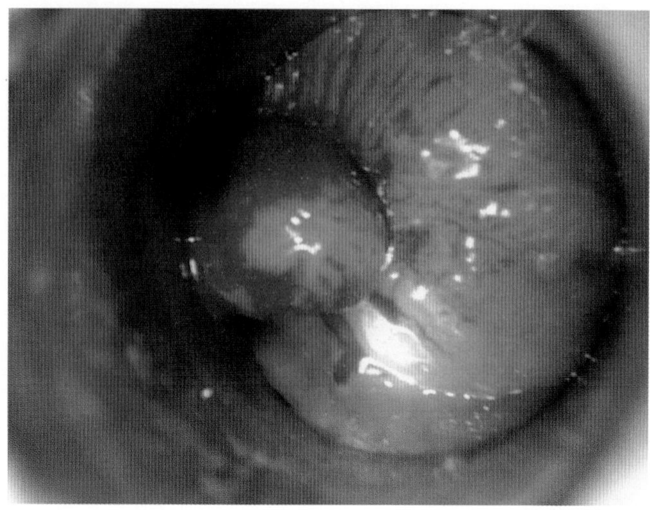

Figure 73.7 Through a proctoscope, a rubber band is applied to an area of mucohaemorrhoidal prolapse.

IN ADULTS

- **Local treatments**. Submucosal injections of phenol in almond oil or the application of rubber bands may be successful in cases of mucosal prolapse.
- **Excision of the prolapsed mucosa**. When the prolapse is unilateral, the redundant mucosa can be excised or, if circumferential, an endoluminal stapling technique or internal Delorme's procedure can be used.

Full-thickness prolapse

Complete rectal prolapse (synonym: procidentia) is less common than the mucosal variety. The protrusion consists of all layers of the rectal wall and is usually associated with a weak pelvic floor and/or chronic straining. The prolapse is thought to commence as an intussusception of the rectum, which descends to protrude outside the anus. The process starts with the anterior wall of the rectum, where the supporting tissues are weakest, especially in women. It is more than 4 cm and commonly as much as 10–15 cm in length (Figure 73.8). On

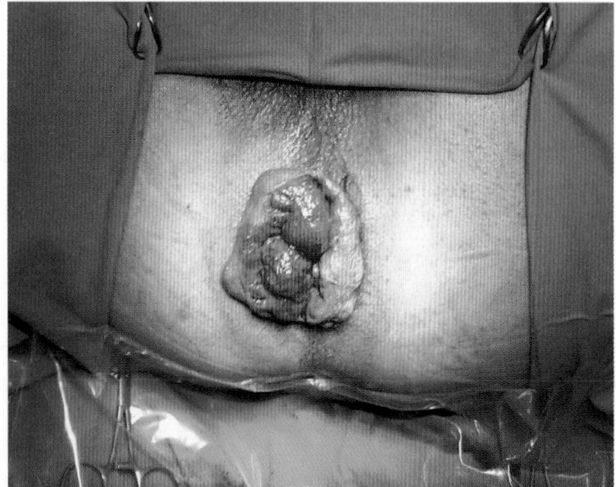

Figure 73.6 Mucohaemorrhoidal prolapse of the anorectum.

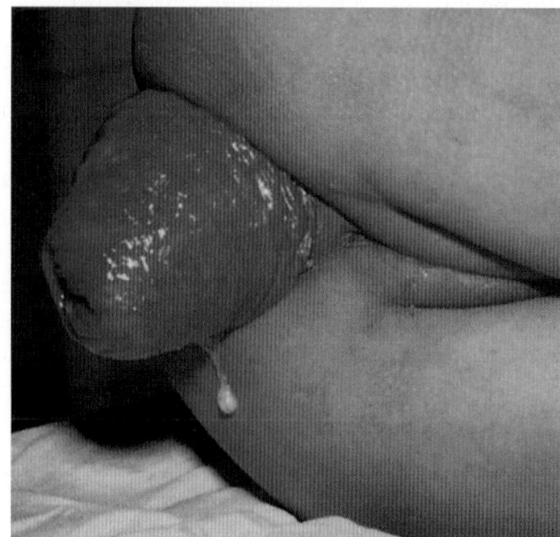

Figure 73.8 Full-thickness rectal prolapse. The whole bowel wall protrudes through the anus.

palpation between the finger and thumb, the prolapse feels much thicker than mucosal prolapse, and consists of a double thickness of the entire wall of the rectum. Any prolapse over 5 cm in length will contain anteriorly, between its layers, a pouch of peritoneum. When large, the peritoneal pouch may contain small intestine or bladder. The anal sphincter is characteristically patulous and gapes widely on straining to allow the rectum to prolapse. Complete prolapse is uncommon in children but may occur as a result of malnutrition. In adults, it can occur at any age, but it is more common in the elderly and sometimes in patients with anorexia nervosa. Women are affected six times more often than men, and it is commonly associated with other pelvic organ prolapse. In approximately 50% of adults, faecal incontinence is also a feature. Complications of rectal prolapse include rectal ulceration and bleeding, incontinence and even incarceration with strangulation of the rectum.

Differential diagnosis

In the case of a child with abdominal pain, the anus should be examined to exclude rectal prolapse as a cause. This should also be distinguished from intussusception protruding from the anus.

Treatment

Surgery is required for full-thickness rectal prolapse, and the operation can be performed via a perineal or abdominal approach. Abdominal operations can be by an open or laparoscopic approach. Abdominal rectopexy, either laparoscopic or open, has a lower rate of recurrence (<10%), but when the patient is elderly and very frail a perineal operation is usually safer, and if necessary can be performed under regional anaesthetic blockade. As an abdominal procedure risks damage to the pelvic autonomic nerves, resulting in possible sexual dysfunction, a perineal approach may be preferred in young men.

PERINEAL APPROACH

These procedures have been used most frequently:

- **Thiersch operation**. In this procedure, a steel wire, or silastic or nylon tape, is placed around the anal canal. It has become largely obsolete owing to problems with chronic perineal sepsis, anal stenosis and obstructed defaecation.
- **Delorme's operation**. In this procedure, the rectal mucosa is stripped circumferentially from the rectum over the length of prolapse (Figure 73.9). The underlying muscle is plicated with a series of sutures, so that the rectal muscle is concertinaed towards the anal canal. The excess rectal mucosa is excised and a mucosal anastomosis performed. The resulting effect is to reduce the prolapse as a plicated ring of muscle above the anal canal. This operation may be preferred in patients with short segment full rectal prolapse, but recurrence rates are high, in the region of 30% over 5 years.

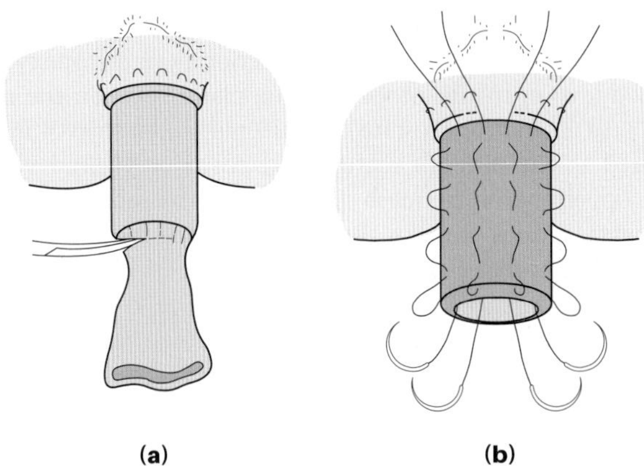

Figure 73.9 Delorme's procedure for rectal prolapse. (a) The mucosa is stripped from the muscular gut tube. (b) Interrupted sutures are used to plicate the muscular gut tube and reduce the prolapse. The operation is concluded by suturing the mucosa. Redrawn with permission from Keighley MRB, Williams NS. *Surgery of the anus, rectum and colon*. London: WB Saunders, 1999.

- **Altemeier's procedure**. In this procedure, the rectum is prolapsed through the anal canal and a full-thickness resection performed, incorporating any associated colonic prolapse. Restoration of colorectal continuity can be performed by either a hand-sewn or stapled anastomosis. This is the procedure of choice in patients presenting with incarcerated and strangulated prolapse. It is a good alternative perineal procedure to the Delorme's operation, particularly following recurrence. However, it is often complicated by poor bowel control with faecal soiling secondary to loss of the rectal reservoir. Recurrence rates range from 0 to 20%.

The advantages of a perineal approach include minimal postoperative pain, early mobility and low levels of morbidity. However, given the higher recurrence rates when compared with the abdominal operations, it is best reserved for patients at high risk of complications when undergoing a major operation.

ABDOMINAL APPROACH

The principle of all abdominal operations for rectal prolapse is to fix the rectum in its normal anatomical position. Many variations have been described, including inserting a sheet of polypropylene mesh between the rectum and the sacrum, hitching up the rectosigmoid junction with a Teflon sling to the front of the sacrum, or simply suturing the mobilised rectum to the sacrum using four to six interrupted nonabsorbable sutures – so-called 'sutured rectopexy'. Currently, the technique is most often performed laparoscopically, reducing the operative trauma, limiting the time in hospital and broadening its indication for higher-risk patients.

As an abdominal rectopexy may lead to severe constipation, some surgeons recommend combining this procedure

Karl Thiersch, 1822–1895, Professor of Surgery, Leipzig, Germany.
Edmond Delorme, 1847–1929, Professor of Surgery, Val-de-Grace Military Hospital, Paris, France.
William Altemeier, 1910–1983, Professor of Surgery, Cincinnati, USA.

with resection of the sigmoid colon, so-called 'resection rectopexy'. Recently, a laparoscopic anterior mesh rectopexy has gained favour. In this procedure, the plane between the rectum and vagina (or prostate) is dissected, and a strip of mesh sutured to the anterior rectum and posterior vaginal vault. The upper end of the mesh is secured to the sacral promontory with sutures or tacks, thus re-suspending the rectum and preventing prolapse (Figure 73.10).

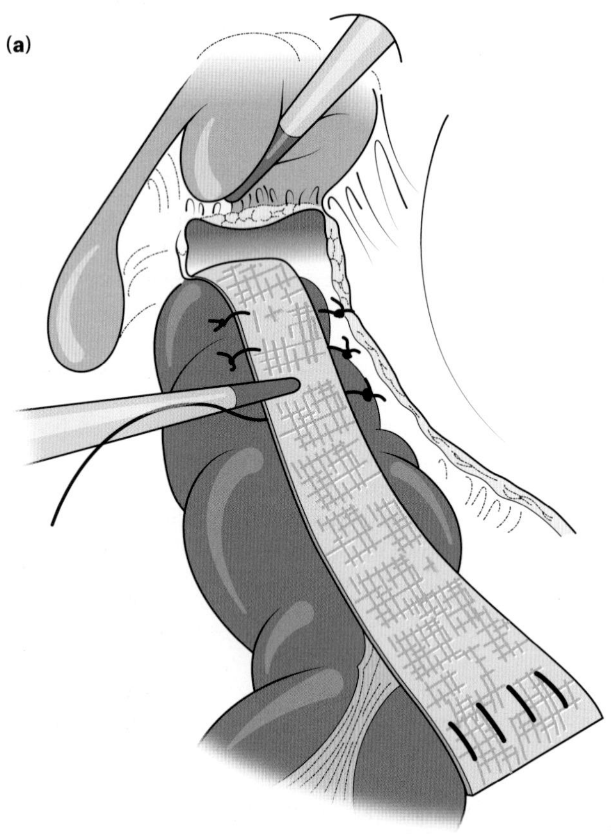

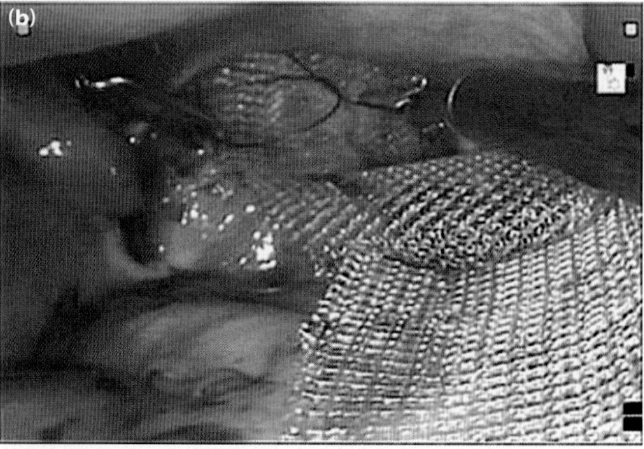

Figure 73.10 (a) Laparoscopic ventral mesh rectopexy: a prosthetic mesh is sutured to the front of the lower rectum and used to resuspend the rectum by securing the proximal end of the mesh to the sacral promontory. (b) Intraoperative image of a robotic ventral mesh rectopexy showing suturing of the mesh to the anterior rectum after dissection of the rectovaginal septum.

RECTAL EVACUATION DISORDER, RECTAL INTUSSUSCEPTION AND SOLITARY RECTAL ULCER SYNDROME (SRUS)

Rectal evacuation disorder (RED) is becoming a more commonly diagnosed problem and is complex in aetiology and treatment. Symptoms consist of a difficulty in emptying despite persistent straining and a feeling of incompleteness in the process. Rectal intussusception is often a component of RED whereby the rectal wall infolds on itself to produce an internal prolapse during straining. Solitary rectal ulcer syndrome may also be another associated manifestation of RED. Classically, SRUS takes the form of an ulcer on the anterior wall of the rectum, situated around 8 cm from the anal verge. In this form, it can be mistaken for rectal carcinoma or inflammatory bowel disease, particularly Crohn's disease. It may heal, leaving a polypoid appearance. Proctographic studies may indicate accompanying rectal intussusception or anterior rectal wall prolapse. Histology will confirm the diagnosis. The condition is difficult to treat. Symptomatic relief from bleeding and discharge may sometimes be achieved by controlling any associated straining with recoordination of defaecation using biofeedback therapy. Transanal stapled resection of the intussusception (STARR procedure) or resuspension of the rectum by abdominal rectopexy may be beneficial. In rare cases, rectal excision may be required with or without stoma.

PROCTITIS

The patient is usually middle-aged and complains of defaecatory frequency with the passage of loose motions, often with blood mixed in the stools. Inflammation is sometimes limited to the rectum; in other cases, it is associated with a similar condition in the colon (proctocolitis). The inflammation can be acute or chronic. Although the patient has a frequent, intense desire to defaecate, the amount of faeces passed at any time is small. Acute proctitis is usually accompanied by malaise and pyrexia. On rectal examination, there may be tenderness and blood on the glove. Proctoscopy is seldom sufficient and sigmoidoscopy is the more valuable method of examination. If the diagnosis is confirmed, colonoscopy with multiple biopsies is mandatory to determine the extent of the inflammatory process. Skilled pathological assessment is required to establish and classify the underlying pathology. Stool cultures should be sent routinely to exclude infective causes. If biopsy and histology are unable to establish an underlying inflammatory aetiology, the condition is frequently termed non-specific proctitis, but may herald a subsequent diagnosis of inflammatory bowel disease (ulcerative colitis or Crohn's disease).

Treatment is usually medical and tailored to the underlying pathology. Non-specific colitis may be self-limiting, but treatment with topical 5-aminosalicylic acid (5-ASA) compounds in the form of suppositories or foam enemas is usually effective. In resistant cases, oral steroids may have to be used.

Summary box 73.6

Proctitis

- May be non-specific or related to a specific infective agent
- Non-specific proctitis usually remains confined to the distal bowel, but can involve the proximal colon
- Symptoms include defaecatory frequency, loose stools, bleeding and tenesmus
- Endoscopic assessment with biopsy is required to establish the diagnosis
- Treatment usually involves medical management

Ulcerative proctocolitis

Proctitis is present in most cases of ulcerative colitis, and the degree of rectal involvement may influence the type of operative procedure (see Chapter 70).

Proctitis due to Crohn's disease

Crohn's disease can occasionally affect the rectum, although classically it is spared. Sigmoidoscopic appearances differ from those in non-specific proctitis. The inflammatory process tends to be patchy rather than confluent, and there may be fissuring, ulceration or even a cobblestone appearance. Rectal Crohn's disease is often associated with severe perineal disease characterised by fistulation, fissuring and haemorrhoids. Coexistent disease is often present in the rest of the colon or small bowel, or both.

Radiation proctitis

Radiation therapy is used in the treatment of cervical, prostate and rectal cancers. It can produce acute radiation proctitis with bleeding, pain, diarrhoea and defaecatory frequency. Most symptoms settle within a few weeks, but some patients develop chronic proctitis with symptoms appearing months or even decades after the radiation exposure.

Proctitis due to specific infections

Clostridium difficile

An acute form of proctocolitis caused by infection with *Clostridium difficile* can follow broad-spectrum antibiotics. A membrane can sometimes be seen on sigmoidoscopy ('pseudomembranous' colitis).

Bacillary dysentery

The appearance is that of an acute purulent proctitis with multiple small, shallow ulcers.

Amoebic dysentery

The infection is more likely to be chronic, with exacerbations after a long period of symptom improvement. Proctoscopy and sigmoidoscopy are not painful. The appearance of an amoebic ulcer is described in Chapter 70.

Tuberculous proctitis

This is nearly always associated with active pulmonary tuberculosis or tuberculous ulceration of the anus. Submucous rectal abscesses burst and leave ulcers with an undermined edge. A hypertrophic type of tuberculous proctitis occurs in association with tuberculous peritonitis or tuberculous salpingitis. This type of tuberculous proctitis requires biopsy for confirmation of the diagnosis.

Gonococcal proctitis

Gonococcal proctitis occurs in both sexes as the result of rectal coitus and, in the female, from direct spread from the vulva. In the acute stage, the mucous membrane is hyperaemic, and thick pus can be expressed as the proctoscope is withdrawn. In the early stages, the diagnosis can be readily established by bacteriological examination but, later, when the infection is mixed, it is more difficult to recognise. Systemic treatment is so effective that local treatment is unnecessary.

Lymphogranuloma venereum

The modes of infection are similar to those of gonococcal proctitis but, in the female, chlamydial infection spreading from the cervix uteri via lymphatics to the pararectal lymph nodes is common. The proctological findings are similar to those of gonococcal proctitis. The diagnosis of lymphogranuloma venereum should be suspected when the inguinal lymph nodes are greatly enlarged, although nodal enlargement may be subsiding by the time proctitis commences.

Acquired immunodeficiency syndrome

Acquired immunodeficiency syndrome (AIDS) due to human immunodeficiency virus (HIV) may present with a particularly florid type of proctitis. In such patients, unusual organisms including cytomegalovirus (CMV), herpes simplex virus and parasites such as *Cryptosporidium* are often found.

'Strawberry' lesion of the rectosigmoid

This results from infection by *Spirochaeta vincenti* and *Bacillus fusiformis*. The leading symptom is diarrhoea, often scantily blood stained. Occasionally, the diagnosis can be made by the demonstration of the specific organisms in the stools. More often, sigmoidoscopy is required. The characteristic lesion is a thickened, somewhat raised mucosa, with superficial ulceration in the region of the rectosigmoid. The inflamed mucous membrane oozes blood at numerous pinpoints, giving the appearance of an over-ripe strawberry. A swab should be taken and examined for Vincent's and fusiform organisms. Swabs from the gums and throat are also advisable.

Jean Hyacinthe Vincent, 1862–1950, Professor of Epidemiology, Val-de-Grace Military Hospital, Paris, France.

Rectal bilharziasis

Rectal bilharziasis is caused by *Schistosoma mansoni*, which is endemic in many tropical and subtropical countries, and particularly in the Nile Delta. In stage 1, a cutaneous lesion develops at the site of entrance of the cercariae (parasites of freshwater snails). Stage 2 is characterised by pyrexia, urticaria and a high eosinophilia. Both these stages are frequently overlooked. Stage 3 results from deposition of the ova in the rectum (much more rarely in the bladder; Chapter 77) and is manifested by bilharzial dysentery. On examination in the later stages, papillomas are frequently seen. The papillomas, which are sessile or pedunculated, contain the ova of the trematode, the life cycle of which resembles that of *Schistosoma haematobium*. Untreated, the rectum becomes festooned, and prolapse of the diseased mucous membrane is usual. Multiple fistulae-in-ano are prone to develop.

The primary treatment is systemic and should be undertaken by a specialist in tropical medicine. When the papillomas persist in spite of treatment, they should be treated by local destruction.

Proctitis due to herbal enemas

This is a well-known clinical entity to those practising in tropical Africa. Following an enema consisting of a concoction of ginger, pepper and bark, administered by a traditional healer, a virulent proctitis sets in. Pelvic peritonitis frequently supervenes. Not infrequently, a complete gelatinous cast of the mucous membrane of the rectum is extruded. Very large doses of morphine, together with antibiotics, often prevent a fatal outcome if commenced early. Temporary colostomy is often advisable.

RECTAL POLYPS

The rectum, along with the sigmoid colon, is the most frequent site of polyps (and cancers) in the gastrointestinal tract. Adenomatous polyps of the colon and rectum have the potential to become malignant. The chance of developing invasive cancer is enhanced if the polyp is more than 1 cm in diameter. Removal of all polyps is recommended to allow complete histological diagnosis and exclude carcinoma. This is best done using endoscopic biopsy or snare polypectomy techniques. If one or more rectal polyps are discovered on sigmoidoscopic examination, a colonoscopy must be performed because further polyps are frequently found in the colon.

The rectum shares the same spectrum of polyps as the colon. Polyps are described in terms of their appearance (pedunculated, sessile, flat) or histological composition (tubular, villous, tubulovillous).

Polyps relevant to the rectum

Hyperplastic polyps

These are small, pinkish, sessile polyps, 2–4 mm in diameter and frequently multiple. They are common and generally harmless.

Tubular adenomas

Tubular adenomas, or mixed tubulovillous adenomas, are the most common type of polyp. They have the potential to turn malignant, particularly if over 1 cm in diameter.

Villous adenomas

These have a characteristic frond-like appearance. They may be very large, occupying much of the circumference of the rectum. These tumours have an increased tendency to become malignant. Rarely, the profuse mucus discharge from these tumours, which is rich in potassium, causes electrolyte and fluid losses (Figure 73.11).

Serrated adenomas

These polyps are more commonly found in the right colon, but may be present in the rectum. They are typically sessile lesions that have a distinct microscopic architecture and can give rise to cancers through an alternative 'serrated' pathway.

Familial adenomatous polyposis

This autosomal dominant inherited condition is characterised by the development of multiple rectal and colonic adenomas around puberty. It is due to mutation in the adenomatous polyposis coli (*APC*) gene, allowing genetic testing in the 75% of families in which a mutation can be identified. A colonoscopy and biopsy will confirm the diagnosis. As this condition is premalignant, total colectomy is usually recommended within 10 years of disease onset. This may take the form of pan-proctocolectomy with permanent ileostomy. Rectal preservation may be an option if the rectal polyp load is not too severe, with colectomy and ileorectal anastomosis, but continuous rectal surveillance for synchronous polyps will

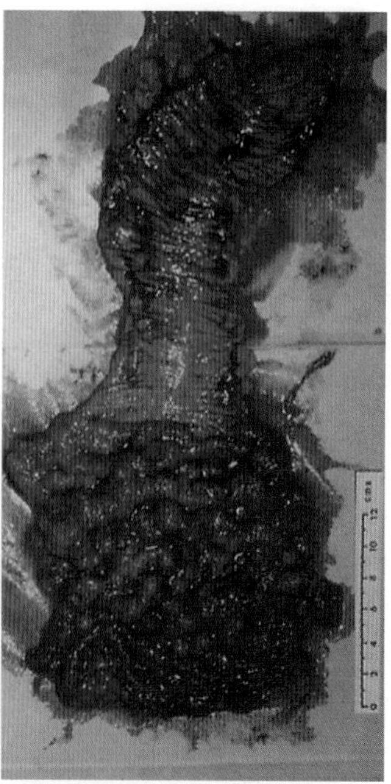

Figure 73.11 Large villous adenoma that occupied the lower half of the rectum and caused hypokalaemia.

Theodor Maximillan Bilharz, 1825–1862, Professor of Zoology, Cairo, Egypt.

be required. The alternative, if restoration of gastrointestinal continuity is desired, is to undertake restorative proctocolectomy with ileal pouch–anal anastomosis (see Chapter 70).

Inflammatory pseudopolyps

These are oedematous islands of mucosa. They are usually associated with colitis in the UK, but most inflammatory diseases (including tropical diseases) can cause them. They are more likely to cause radiological difficulty, as the sigmoidoscopic appearance is usually associated with obvious signs of active or quiescent inflammation.

Juvenile polyp

This is a bright red, glistening pedunculated sphere ('cherry tumour'), which is found in infants and children. Occasionally, it persists into adult life. It can cause bleeding, or pain if it prolapses during defaecation. It often separates itself, but can be removed easily with forceps or a snare. A solitary juvenile polyp has virtually no tendency to malignant change, but should be treated if it is causing symptoms. It has a unique histological structure with large mucus-filled spaces covered by a smooth surface of thin rectal cuboidal epithelium (Figure 73.12). The rare autosomal dominant inherited syndrome juvenile polyposis does carry an increased risk of malignancy. It is characterised by multiple polyps and a positive family history.

Treatment of rectal polyps

All polyps should be biopsied or removed for histological analysis to exclude cancer. A range of techniques can be used to remove rectal polyps, dependent on their size and location. The majority of polyps less than 1 cm in size are benign and are amenable to endoscopic polypectomy. Polyps greater than 1 cm in size have a 10% chance of harbouring a malignancy. Submucosal infiltration with saline or colloid solution can give an indication of invasive malignancy, with cancers exhibiting tethering to submucosal tissues and failing to 'lift'. Most polyps of 2 cm in size or less can be safely removed by endoscopic mucosal resection (EMR) (Figure 73.13). Larger polyps are more difficult to remove by EMR and may require a transanal procedure, such as transanal endoscopic microsurgery (TEMS).

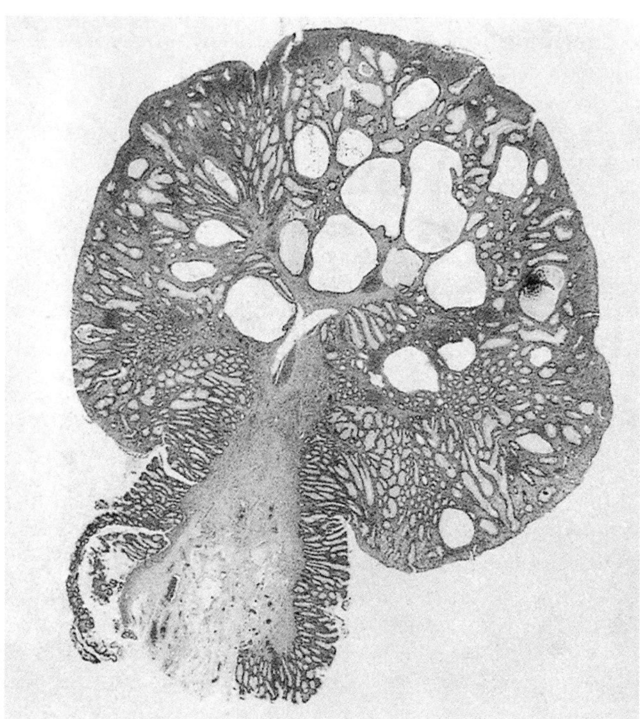

Figure 73.12 Microscopic appearance of a juvenile polyp.

Summary box 73.7

Polyps in the rectum

- Adenomas are the most frequent histological type
- Villous adenomas may be extensive and undergo malignant change more commonly than tubular adenomas
- All adenomas must be removed to avoid malignant change
- All patients must undergo colonoscopy to determine whether further polyps are present
- Most polyps can be removed by endoscopic techniques, but sometimes major surgery is required

BENIGN RECTAL LESIONS

Endometrioma

Endometrioma is rare and may be misdiagnosed as a carcinoma. The focus of the ectopic endometrial tissue produces either a constricting lesion of the rectosigmoid or a tumour invading the rectum from the rectovaginal septum. The latter variety gives rise to a tender submucous elevation of the rectal wall. Endometrioma usually occurs between 20 and 40 years of age. Dysmenorrhoea and rectal bleeding (particularly coinciding with the menses) are the main symptoms. On sigmoidoscopy, endometriosis involving the rectosigmoid junction usually presents as a stricture, with the mucous membrane intact. Hormonal manipulation is the first-line therapy, but sometimes total abdominal hysterectomy and bilateral salpingo-oophorectomy and even bowel resection are required. The laparoscopic approach for resecting deep rectal endometriosis is becoming popular. Isolated endometrial deposits may be treated by diathermy ablation or local 'discectomy' incorporating the rectal wall.

Haemangioma

Haemangioma of the rectum is an uncommon cause of serious haemorrhage. The symptoms may mimic ulcerative colitis, and the diagnosis is often delayed, or it may be mistaken for a carcinoma. Selective angiography and embolisation may be helpful, but excision of the rectum is sometimes required.

Gastrointestinal stromal tumour (GIST)

Smooth-muscle tumours of the rectum are rare. If the mitotic rate is high, and if there is variation in nuclear number, size

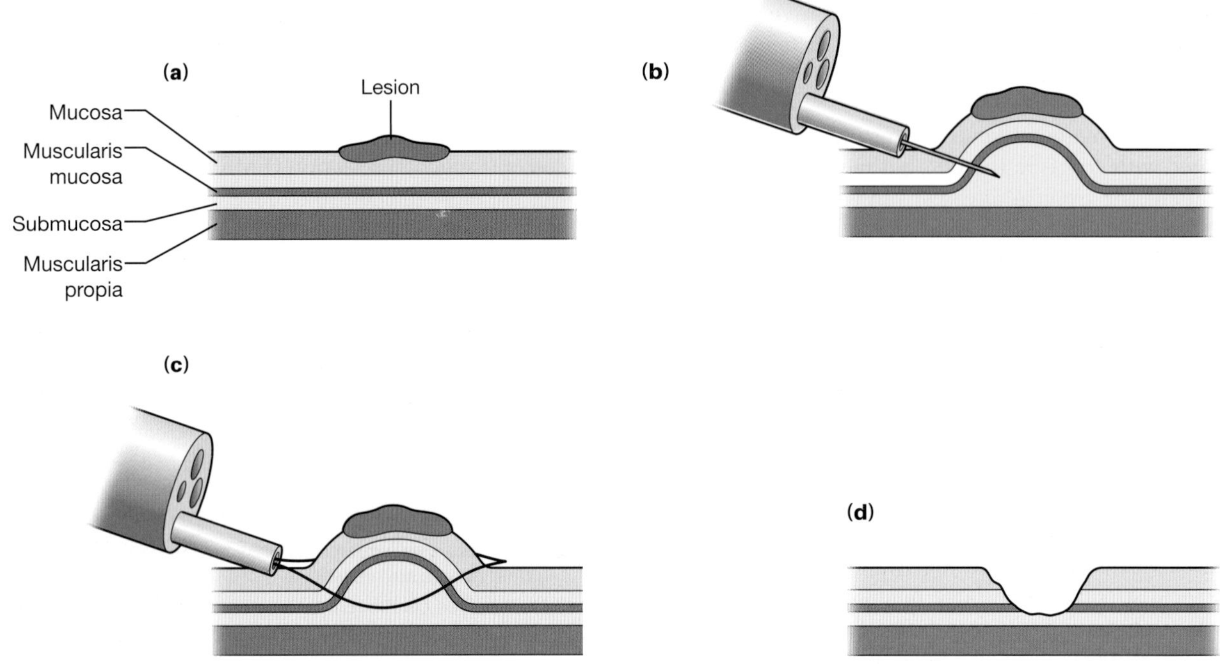

Figure 73.13 Endoscopic mucosal resection. The polyp is identified (a) and infiltration performed (b) to lift it from the underlying muscle layer. A diathermy snare is passed over the raised lesion (c) to achieve complete excision (d).

and shape, hyperchromasia and frequent bizarre cells, these tumours are likely to metastasise. In these circumstances, they should be classified as malignant gastrointestinal stromal tumours (formerly leiomyosarcomas). The uncertainty in their behaviour means that treatment should, whenever possible, be radical excision.

Neuroendocrine tumours

Neuroendocrine tumours (NET) of the rectum comprise 19% of all gastrointestinal NET. They are classified into well-differentiated (grades 1 and 2) and poorly differentiated (grade 3) tumours. Both tumour mitotic index and Ki-67 expression are important factors for histopathological classification. Grade 3 tumours include both small- and large-cell NET. The majority of rectal NET are grade 1, also known as carcinoid tumours, with relatively good prognosis. These tumours are usually small (1–2 cm), solitary and clinically indolent. On the contrary, poorly differentiated grade 3 NETs are rare but very aggressive and metastasise at an early stage, with reported incidence of between 0.1 and 3.9% of all colorectal malignancies. Treatment of NET depends on the size of the tumour, its depth of invasion and the presence or absence of metastasis. Small lesions (1 cm) can often be treated locally, either endoscopically or transanally. However, larger lesions (>2 cm) require formal oncological resection. Adjuvant therapy is indicated only for metastatic disease.

CARCINOMAS

Globally, colorectal cancer is the second most common malignancy, affecting more than 1 million people every year and resulting in around 715,000 deaths. It is the second most common cancer in women and the third most common cancer in men, being the fourth most common cause of cancer death after lung, stomach, and liver cancer. In Western countries the incidence is rising, with an overall 14% increase since the 1970s, but with the largest increase (20%) seen in males. Risk factors include diet, obesity, smoking and lack of physical exercise. Most colorectal cancers are due to old age, with around 60% of cases affecting patients 70 years or older. The rectum is the most frequently involved site, accounting for approximately one-third of the cancers.

Pathogenesis

Colorectal cancer originates from premalignant precursor lesions in the epithelial lining of the colon or rectum in a stepwise progression that results in increasing dysplasia due to an accumulation of genetic abnormalities. In spontaneous colorectal cancer, as compared to hereditary cancers, this is referred to as the adenoma–carcinoma sequence. More than 75–95% of colorectal cancers occur in people with little or no genetic risk. People with inflammatory bowel disease are at an increased risk, which increases with the duration of the disease, and accounts for 2% of cancers each year. Those with a family history in two or more first-degree relatives have a two- to three-fold greater risk of disease and this group accounts for about 20% of all cases. A number of genetic syndromes are also associated with higher rates of colorectal cancer. The most common is hereditary nonpolyposis colorectal cancer (HNPCC or Lynch syndrome), which accounts for 3% of people with colorectal cancer. Other syndromes include Gardner syndrome and familial adenomatous polyposis (FAP).

The most common abnormality found in colorectal cancer is mutation in the Wnt signaling pathway, which increases cell signalling activity. The mutations can be inherited or acquired. The most commonly mutated gene is the *APC* gene, which results in accumulation of the β-catenin protein. β-catenin activates the transcription of various proto-oncogenes that are responsible for normal cell renewal and differentiation, but when overexpressed can cause cancer. Many other mutations, other than in the Wnt signaling pathway, are found in colorectal cancer, and include mutations in the *TP53* gene that controls normal cell division and death, and mutations in genes responsible for programmed cell death, such as the gene encoding transforming growth factor (TGF)-β and *DCC* (deleted in colorectal cancer). Other genetic abnormalities include overexpression of oncogenes, including genes encoding the proteins KRAS (Kirsten rat sarcoma homologue), RAF (rapidly accelerated fibrosarcoma) and PI3K (phosphoinositide 3-kinase), which lead to increased cell proliferation, and inactivation of tumour suppressor genes, such as *PTEN* (phosphatase and tensin homologue), which normally inactivates the PI3K signalling pathway.

In addition to gene mutations, colorectal cancers frequently exhibit epigenetic alterations – cellular or physiological effects resulting from external or environmental factors that switch genes on or off. Epigenetic alterations can affect hundreds of genes and include changes in the expression of microRNAs (miRNA), hypermethylation or hypomethylation of CpG islands of protein-encoding genes, and alterations in histones and chromosomal architecture, all of which can influence gene expression.

Clinical features

Carcinoma of the rectum can occur early in life, but the age of presentation is usually above 55 years, when the incidence rises rapidly. Often, the early symptoms are so insignificant that the patient does not seek advice for 6 months or more, and the diagnosis is often delayed in younger patients as the symptoms are attributed to benign causes. Initial rectal examination and a low threshold for investigating persistent symptoms are essential.

Summary box 73.8

Early symptoms of rectal cancer

- Bleeding per rectum
- Tenesmus
- Early morning diarrhoea

Bleeding

Bleeding is the earliest and most common symptom. Typically, the bleeding is bright red in colour and painless. It can be mixed with the motions or separate in the toilet bowel. It can be indistinguishable from haemorrhoidal bleeding, which is the most common differential diagnosis, particularly in younger patients.

Tenesmus

The patient experiences a sensation of needing to evacuate the rectum but is unable to pass a motion. This is an important early symptom and is almost invariably present in patients with tumours of the lower half of the rectum. The patient may endeavour to empty the rectum several times a day (spurious diarrhoea), often with the passage of flatus and a little blood-stained mucus ('bloody slime').

Alteration in bowel habit

There is frequently a change in bowel habit, with a tendency to more frequent defaecation and the passage of looser stool. A patient who has to get up early in order to defaecate, or one who passes blood and mucus in addition to faeces ('early-morning bloody diarrhoea'), is usually found to be suffering from carcinoma of the rectum. Although a change to looser stools is more common, patients with a stenosing carcinoma at the rectosigmoid junction may complain of increasing constipation.

Pain

Pain is a late symptom, but pain of a colicky character may accompany advanced tumours of the rectosigmoid, owing to a degree of obstruction. Advanced cancers invading outside the mesorectum may infiltrate the prostate or bladder anteriorly or the sacral plexus posteriorly, giving rise to severe, intractable pain.

Weight loss

Weight loss is also a late symptom and is almost always associated with metastatic disease.

Investigation

Abdominal examination

Abdominal examination is normal in early cases. Occasionally, in patients with stenosing tumours at the rectosigmoid junction, signs of subacute large bowel obstruction may be present, with abdominal distension. If large-volume liver metastases are present, an enlarged liver may be palpable along with other signs, such as cachexia. Occasionally, it may be possible to elicit ascites if there is widespread peritoneal dissemination.

Rectal examination

In many cases where the neoplasm is situated within 7–8 cm of the anal verge it can be felt on digital rectal examination as an elevated, irregular and hard endoluminal mass. When the centre ulcerates, a shallow depression will be felt with raised and everted edges. An attempt should be made to determine whether the neoplasm is mobile, tethered or fixed, and to estimate the distance of the lower margin from the top of the anal sphincter complex: these factors are important in assessing resectablility and methods of reconstruction following excisional surgery. In females, a vaginal examination may be useful if involvement of the posterior vaginal wall is suspected. Digital rectal examination also affords the opportunity to evaluate the anal sphincter complex, which is important in cases where resection and low anastomosis are being considered.

Rigid sigmoidoscopy

Rigid sigmoidoscopy can be performed in the outpatient clinic and is useful to identify the neoplasm and possibly obtain biopsies. However, it requires the rectum to be empty of faeces and may require a prior rectal enema, which may not be practical in the outpatient setting. As colonoscopy is almost always required to visualise the whole colorectum, it is often easier and safer to obtain biopsies at this time.

Colonoscopy

A colonoscopy is required in most patients to exclude a synchronous tumour, be it an adenoma or carcinoma. If a proximal adenoma is found, it can be conveniently snared and removed via the colonoscope. If a synchronous carcinoma is present, the operative strategy is likely to change. If a full colonoscopy is not possible, for example where there is a stenosing cancer, a CT colonography or barium enema can be performed.

Differential diagnosis

Many colorectal lesions can give rise to diagnostic difficulty. For example, it may be difficult to distinguish an inflammatory stricture or amoebic granuloma on macroscopic appearance. Similarly, endometriomas, carcinoid tumours and solitary rectal ulcers can be mistaken for adenocarcinoma. Benign adenomas can be distinguished from malignant lesions based on the appearance of their mucosal 'pit-patterns', as highlighted with the 'dye-spray' colonoscopy technique. Biopsy and histological analysis remain the mainstay of diagnosis, accepting that there may be diagnostic limitations caused by sampling errors due to small biopsy samples being unrepresentative of the larger lesion.

Summary box 73.9

Diagnosis and assessment of rectal cancer

All patients with suspected rectal cancer should undergo:

- Digital rectal examination
- Full colorectal visualisation preferably by colonoscopy with biopsy or computed tomography (CT) colonography or barium enema

All patients with proven rectal cancer require staging by:

- Imaging of the chest, abdomen and pelvis, preferably by CT
- Local pelvic imaging by magnetic resonance imaging and/or endoluminal ultrasound

Types of carcinoma spread

Local spread

Local spread occurs circumferentially rather than in a longitudinal direction. After the muscular coat has been penetrated, the growth spreads into the surrounding mesorectum, but is initially limited by the mesorectal fascia. If penetration occurs anteriorly, the prostate, seminal vesicles or bladder become involved in the male; in the female, the vagina or the uterus is invaded. In either sex, if the penetration is lateral, a ureter may become involved, while posterior penetration may reach the sacrum and the sacral plexus. Downward spread for more than a few centimetres is rare.

Lymphatic spread

Lymphatic spread from a carcinoma of the rectum above the peritoneal reflection occurs almost exclusively in an upward direction. Below that level, the lymphatic spread is still upwards, but when the neoplasm lies within the field of the middle rectal artery, primary lateral spread to the pelvic wall lymphatics occurs in around 20% of cases. Downward spread is exceptional, with drainage along the subcutaneous lymphatics to the groins being confined, for practical purposes, to the lymph nodes draining the perianal rosette and the epithelial lining of the distal 1–2 cm of the anal canal.

Metastasis at a higher level than the main trunk of the superior rectal artery occurs late in the disease. A radical operation should ensure that the high-lying lymph nodes are removed by ligating the inferior mesenteric artery at its origin from the aorta. Atypical and widespread lymphatic permeation can occur with highly undifferentiated neoplasms.

Venous spread

The principal sites for blood-borne metastases are liver (34%), lungs (22%) and adrenals (11%). The remaining 33% are divided among the many other locations where secondary carcinomatous deposits tend to lodge, including the brain.

Peritoneal dissemination

This may follow penetration of the peritoneal coat by a high-lying rectal carcinoma.

Stages of progression

Dukes classified carcinoma of the rectum into three stages (Figure 73.14).

Dukes' staging

- A: The growth is limited to the rectal wall (15%). The prognosis is excellent (>90% 5-year survival).
- B: The growth extends to the extrarectal tissues, but without metastasis to the regional lymph nodes (35%). The prognosis is reasonable (70% 5-year survival).
- C: There are secondary deposits in the regional lymph nodes (50%). These are subdivided into C1, in which the local pararectal lymph nodes alone are involved, and C2, in which the nodes accompanying the supplying blood vessels to their origin from the aorta are involved. This does not take into account cases that have metastasised

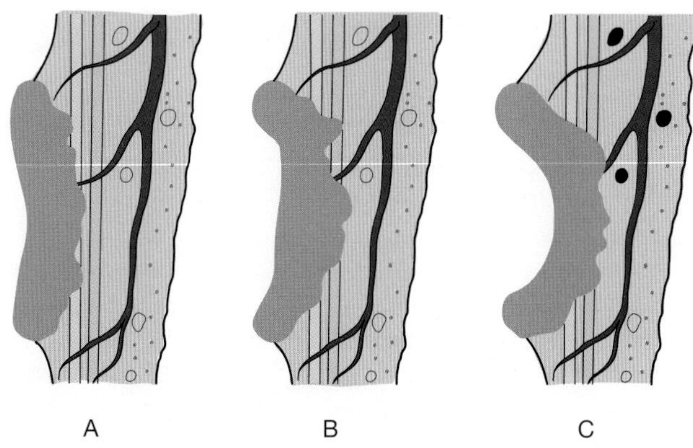

Figure 73.14 Dukes' original classification of colorectal cancer. A: the cancer is confined to the submucosa. B: the cancer penetrates the muscularis propria. C: involvement of the draining lymph nodes.

beyond the regional lymph nodes or by way of the venous system. The prognosis is poor (40% 5-year survival).

A stage D is often included, which was not described by Dukes. This stage signifies the presence of widespread metastases, usually hepatic. Other staging systems have been developed (e.g. Astler–Coller, TNM) to improve prognostic accuracy, with the tumour–node–metastasis (TNM) classification now recognised internationally as the optimum staging classification.

TNM staging - 'radiological staging'

Pretreatment magnetic resonance imaging (MRI) is the evaluation of choice in rectal cancer, helping to guide both surgical and oncological management.

T represents the extent of local spread:

- TX: primary tumour cannot be assessed;
- T0: no evidence of primary tumour;
- Tis: carcinoma *in situ* – intraepithelial or invasion of lamina propria;
- T1: tumour invades submucosa;
- T2: tumour invades muscularis propria;
- T3: tumour invades through the muscularis propria into pericolorectal tissues;
- T4a: tumour penetrates to the surface of the visceral peritoneum;
- T4b: tumour directly invades or is adherent to other organs or structures.

N describes nodal involvement:

- NX: regional lymph nodes cannot be assessed;
- N0: no regional lymph node metastasis;
- N1: metastasis in 1–3 regional lymph nodes:
  - N1a: metastasis in 1 regional lymph node
  - N1b: metastasis in 2–3 regional lymph nodes
  - N1c: tumour deposit(s) in the subserosa, mesentery or nonperitonealised pericolic or perirectal tissues without regional nodal metastasis;
- N2: metastasis in 4 or more regional lymph nodes:
  - N2a: metastasis in 4–6 regional lymph nodes
  - N2b: metastasis in 7 or more regional lymph nodes.

M indicates the presence of distant metastases:

- M0: no distant metastasis;
- M1: distant metastasis:
  - M1a: metastasis confined to one organ or site (for example liver, lung, ovary, non-regional node)
  - M1b: metastases in more than one organ/site or the peritoneum.

Histological grading

In the great majority of cases, carcinoma of the rectum is an adenocarcinoma, derived from malignant transformation of the columnar rectal epithelium. The more the tumour cells retain normal shape and arrangement (well-differentiated), the less aggressive the behaviour. Conversely, the more cells of an undifferentiated type, the more aggressive the behaviour. Other poor prognostic features include vascular and perineural invasion, the presence of an infiltrating (rather than pushing) margin and tumour budding. In a small number of cases, the tumour is a primary mucoid carcinoma. The mucus lies within the cells, displacing the nucleus to the periphery, like the seal of a signet ring. Signet-ring carcinomas are rapidly growing, metastasise early and have a poor prognosis.

Summary box 73.10

Pathology and staging of rectal cancer

- Tumours are adenocarcinomas and are well, moderately or poorly differentiated
- They spread by local, lymphatic, venous and transperitoneal routes
- Circumferential local spread is the most important and dictates management
- Lymphatic spread follows the blood supply of the rectum in a cephalad direction via the superior rectal vessels to the para-aortic nodes, but in low rectal cancer can also involve the lateral pelvic lymph nodes
- The TNM classification is the internationally recognised staging system

Treatment

Surgical excision of the tumour is the conventional management option, provided this can be achieved with clear oncological margins and acceptable risk of morbidity and mortality. However, the management of rectal cancer has become increasingly complex, because of the various surgical techniques available and the range of neoadjuvant and adjuvant options. As a result, the management of rectal cancer needs to be within the multidisciplinary team setting, involving surgeons, radiologists, oncologists, pathologists and specialty nurses.

Before treatment can be planned, it is necessary to assess:

- the fitness of the patient;
- the extent of spread of the tumour.

Assessment of spread should include CT of the chest, abdomen and pelvis to exclude distant metastases (Figure 72.15). Ultrasonography of the liver and a chest radiograph

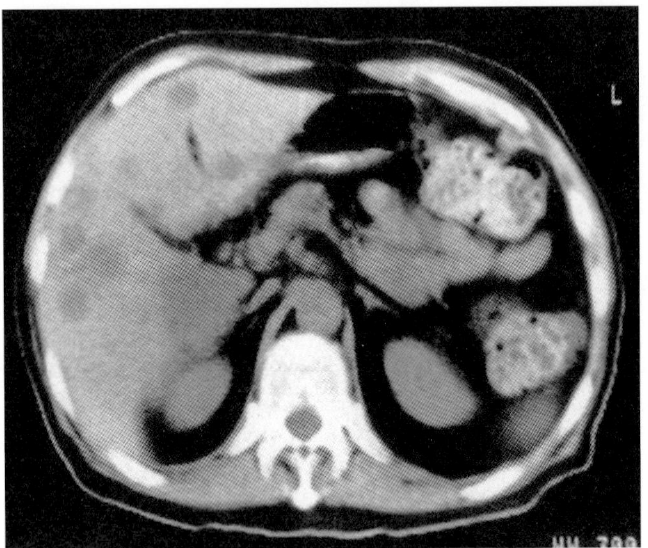

Figure 73.15 Computed tomography scan of the abdomen in a patient with rectal cancer, showing multiple liver metastases.

are decreasingly used alternatives. Positron emission tomography (PET) scanning can be helpful in identifying metastases if imaging is otherwise equivocal.

Endoluminal ultrasound, performed using a probe placed in the rectal lumen, can be used to assess the local spread of low rectal cancers (Figure 73.16), and is particularly useful in patients being considered for transanal endoluminal excision. CT is not particularly accurate in local staging; this is usually performed using MRI, which allows assessment of the circumferential resection margin and lymph node status (Figure 73.17).

Principles of surgical treatment

Radical excision of the rectum, together with the mesorectum and associated lymph nodes, should be the aim in most cases. In the presence of widespread metastases, other means of palliation should be considered, such as endoluminal stenting or

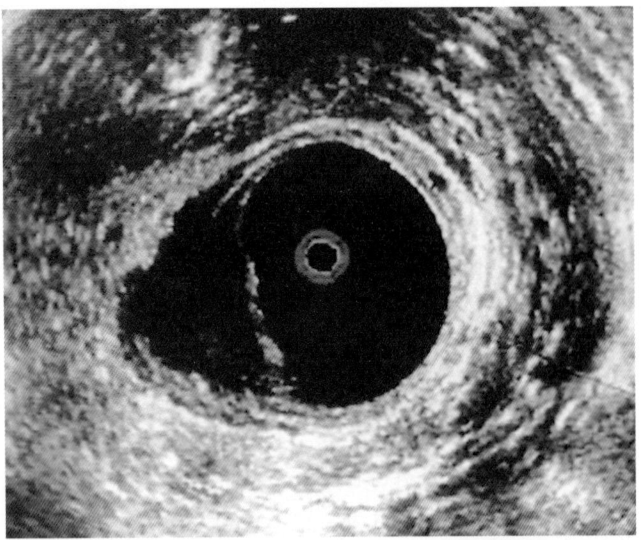

Figure 73.16 Endorectal ultrasound. The probe is in the rectal lumen and shows a rectal tumour invading through the rectal wall.

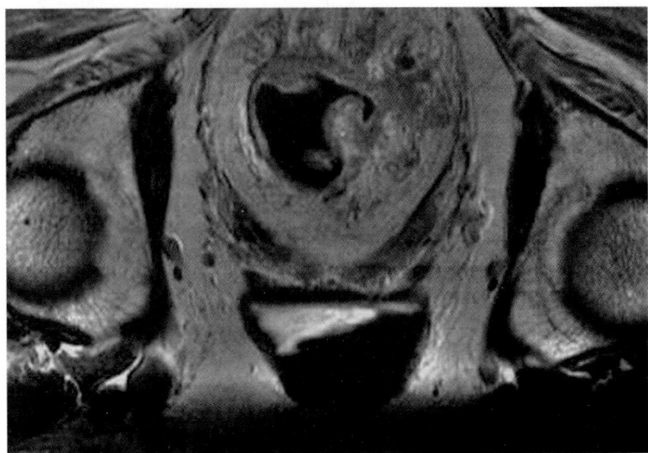

Figure 73.17 Magnetic resonance imaging scan of the pelvis showing extensive T3 rectal cancer involving the left mesorectum.

external beam radiotherapy, although there may still be a role for palliative resection. The presence of liver metastases does not necessarily rule out the feasibility of cure: the results of surgery for liver metastases have greatly improved, with long-term survival being achieved in over a third of patients.

When a tumour appears to be locally advanced (i.e. invading a neighbouring structure or threatening to breach the circumferential resection margin), the use of neoadjuvant (preoperative) radiotherapy or chemoradiotherapy is usually considered. Long-course chemoradiotherapy is given as 5 fractions of radiotherapy combined with chemotherapy over a 6-week period. The aim is to down-stage the cancer and increase the chances of a complete resection with clear oncological margins. Alternatively, preoperative 'short-course' (5 days) radiotherapy can be used if the resection margins are not threatened but the cancer is still at high risk for local recurrence (e.g. peri-rectal lymph node involvement).

Increasingly, there is a trend for 'watch-and-wait' management in cancers that have shown a complete clinical response to long-course chemoradiotherapy (about 20%). If there is no evidence of residual cancer on clinical examination, biopsy or radiological imaging, patients are offered intense surveillance in the hope that they may have been cured of the disease and spared the morbidity of resectional surgery. Some 30% of cases will recur on a 'watch-and-wait' policy, but most can be salvaged by surgical resection.

There is also growing enthusiasm for 'organ-preserving' surgical techniques in early T1 and even T2 cancers with good prognostic features. This usually involves full-thickness excision of the cancer using TEMS (Figure 73.18). Alternative 'organ-preserving' techniques involve the use of brachytherapy and contact radiotherapy, but these are currently reserved for patients unfit for radical resection, or as a means of palliation.

When radical excision is possible, the aim should be to restore gastrointestinal continuity and continence by preserving the anal sphincter whenever feasible. A sphincter-saving operation (anterior resection) is usually possible for tumours whose lower margin is ≥2 cm above the anorectal junction. Although removal of the rectum and anus with a permanent

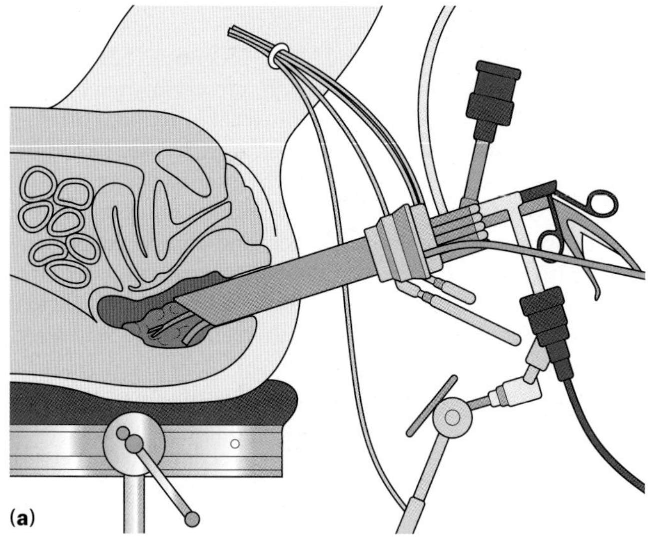

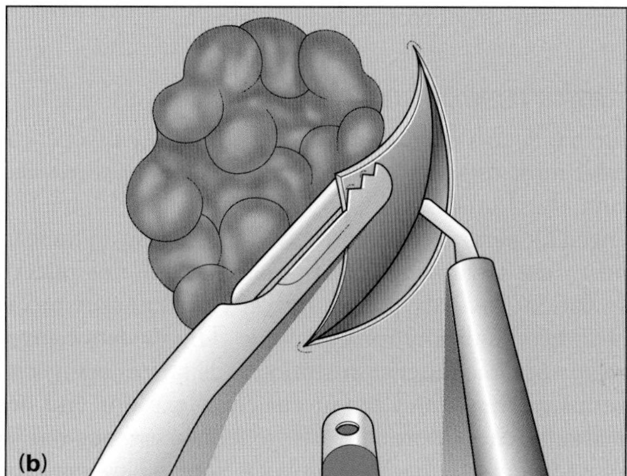

Figure 73.18 Transanal endoscopic microsurgery. **(a)** An operating sigmoidoscope is inserted through the anal canal to visualise the lesion and enable passage of a laparoscope and instruments. **(b)** A full-thickness local excision is performed. The defect is closed or, alternatively, may be left open if the peritoneum is not breached.

colostomy (abdominoperineal excision) was often required for tumours of the lower third of the rectum in the past, the introduction of the stapled anastomosis and chemoradiotherapy down-staging has enabled many more patients to be treated by a sphincter-saving procedure. The principles of anterior resection involve radical excision of the cancer along with its complete mesorectal envelope, combined with high proximal ligation of the inferior mesenteric lymphovascular pedicle. Once the left colon and rectum have been mobilised, the distal rectum is divided at least 1 cm (and preferably more) below the distal cancer margin and the specimen removed. Rectosigmoid cancers and those in the upper third of the rectum are removed by 'high anterior resection', in which the rectum and mesorectum are taken to a margin of at least 3 cm distal to the tumour, and a colorectal anastomosis is performed. For tumours in the middle and lower thirds of the rectum, complete removal of the rectum and mesorectum is required, i.e. total mesorectal excision (TME). Restoration of continuity is usually performed using a stapling technique, which might involve an end-to-end, side-to-end or colopouch construction in low cancers (Figure 73.19). The retention of at least a part of the rectum in high anterior resection results in better postoperative function, with less risk of anterior resection syndrome, a condition characterised by defaecatory urgency, incontinence and incomplete evacuation, secondary

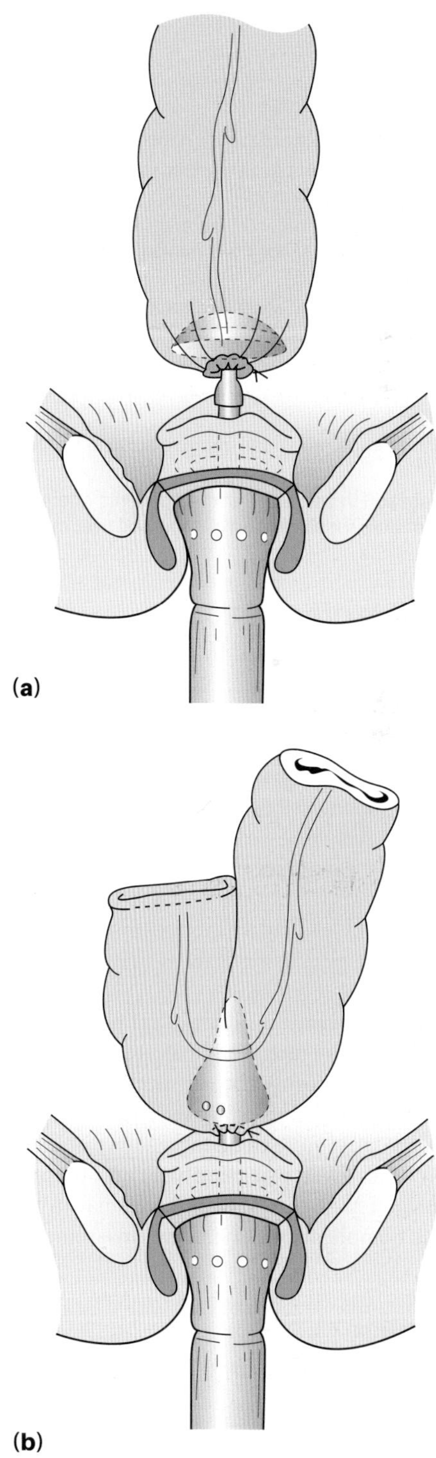

Figure 73.19 Low anterior resection by the double stapling method. The rectum has been excised, and the distal anorectal stump has been transected with a transverse stapling device. A circular stapling gun is used to construct **(a)** a straight low coloanal anastomosis, or **(b)** a colopouch–anus anastomosis.

to removal of the normal rectal reservoir. In cancers situated below the peritoneal reflection it is usual practice to defunction the anastomosis with a temporary stoma because of the higher risk of anastomotic leak. Although a defunctioning stoma does not prevent anastomotic leak, it does mitigate against septic complications should a leak occur.

Summary box 73.11

Surgery for rectal cancer

- Surgery is the mainstay of curative therapy
- The primary resection consists of rectal resection performed by total mesorectal excision
- Most cases can be treated by anterior resection, with the colorectal anastomosis being achieved with a circular stapling gun
- A smaller group of low, extensive tumours require an abdominoperineal excision with a permanent colostomy
- Preoperative radiotherapy with or without chemotherapy can be used to down-stage the cancer and reduce local recurrence
- Adjuvant chemotherapy can improve survival in node-positive disease
- Liver resection in carefully selected patients offers the best chance of cure for single or well-localised liver metastases

Preoperative preparation

The bowel is usually prepared by mechanical cleansing using a combination of diet, purgatives and enemas to reduce intraoperative contamination and the risk of surgical site infection. This approach is now used more selectively, with many surgeons reserving full bowel preparation for those undergoing a low anterior resection.

All patients should see a stoma care nurse preoperatively and be sited for a temporary or permanent ileostomy or colostomy. They must also be counselled as to the complications of the procedure, and particularly about the risks of pelvic autonomic nerve damage causing bladder and sexual disturbance, especially impotence in males.

Prophylactic systemic antibiotics are usually given perioperatively to reduce the risk of surgical site infection. In Europe, this usually takes the form of broad-spectrum antibiotics given intravenously at induction of anaesthesia. In the USA, antibiotic prophylaxis is more frequently administered as a course of oral antibiotics given preoperatively, and there is some evidence to suggest that this may be beneficial in reducing the risk of septic complications, including anastomotic leak.

Summary box 73.12

Preoperative preparation

- Counselling and siting of stomas
- Correction of anaemia and electrolyte disturbance
- Group and save of blood
- Bowel preparation
- Deep vein thrombosis prophylaxis
- Prophylactic antibiotics

Local operations

Early rectal cancers (T1 and good prognosis T2) may be amenable to local transanal excision, preserving much of the rectal reservoir and therefore near normal function. Histological analysis of the specimen is then used to assess the adequacy of excision with respect to the probability of positive lymph nodes being left behind. This may range from 10% in T1 cancers to 20% in T2 cancers and clinical judgement, along with in-depth conversation with the patient, is required to determine whether local excision has achieved a sufficient chance of oncological cure or whether a further radical resection is required.

Local excision is usually performed with one of the commercially available transanal laparoscopic systems or with equipment modified from taTME procedures (see below). A full-thickness excision of the lesion is performed and the defect closed with sutures or else left open. There is a limit to the height of lesion that can be resected, with more proximal lesions in the upper rectum being difficult.

Anterior resection

There has been a move to extend sphincter-saving operations to treat most tumours of the middle and lower thirds of the rectum, thus lowering the abdominoperineal excision rate and the need for permanent colostomy. There is also an increasing trend to use laparoscopic techniques for anterior resection, with patient benefits including less pain, quicker recovery from surgery and improved cosmesis. The evidence suggests that laparoscopic anterior resection is as safe as open surgery in terms of short- and long-term complications and oncological outcomes. More recently, robotic assistance has been employed with the da Vinci robotic surgical system (Intuitive Surgical Inc., Sunnyvale, CA, USA) (Figure 73.20). Although this adds significant cost to the procedure, there may be some benefit in terms of a reduced need to convert to open surgery, and therefore more patients benefiting from a minimally invasive approach. The operation performed is the same whether the procedure is undertaken by open, laparoscopic or robotic surgery, with the difference being in the extent of abdominal access trauma (laparotomy wound versus 'keyhole' incisions).

In open surgery, a midline abdominal incision is made and full laparotomy performed to detect synchronous pathologies, including evidence of intra-abdominal cancer spread. The sigmoid and descending colon are freed by dividing the peritoneal reflection on the left side, and mobilised to the midline on their mesentery, protecting the left ureter and testicular/ovarian vessels. The splenic flexure is mobilised to gain sufficient left colonic length to allow tension-free colorectal anastomosis. Rectal dissection is performed in the embryological planes (total mesorectal excision, TME) with preservation of the autonomic nerves, which course over the pelvic brim (sympathetic nerves) and exit from the pelvic plexuses (parasympathetic nerves) to supply the pelvic floor, and the urogenital organs (Figure 73.21). Once rectal dissection has reached the anorectal junction (low anterior resection), or at least 3 cm below the cancer (high anterior resection), the rectum is divided, usually with the aid of a stapling device.

(a)

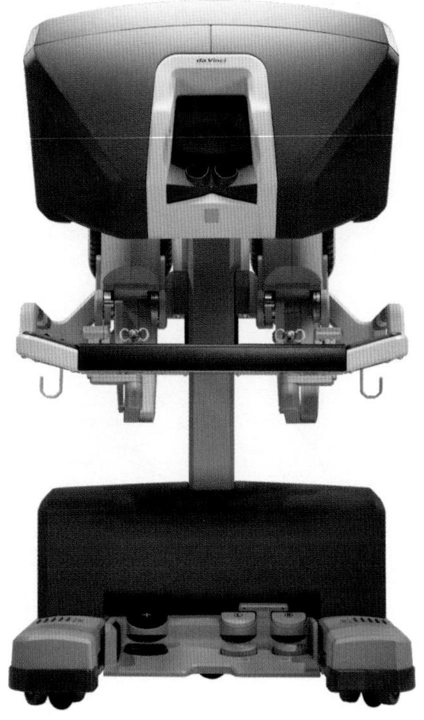

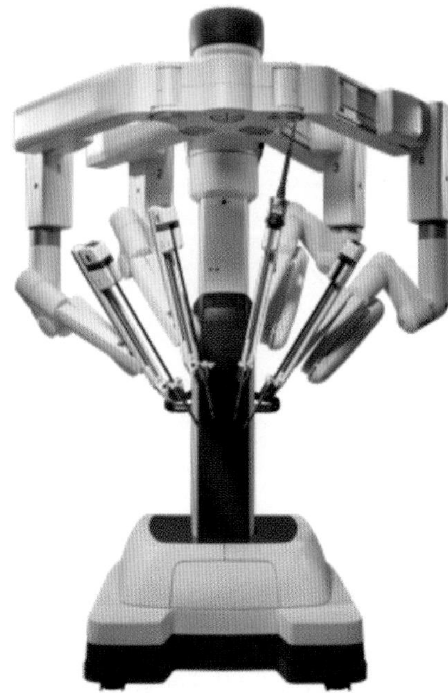

Figure 73.20 da Vinci Xi Robotic Surgical System: (a) surgeon console; (b) patient cart. Reproduced with kind permission from Intuitive Surgical Inc. http://www.intuitivesurgical.com/company/media/images/da-vinci-xi/

The mesocolon is divided at the site of the proposed division of the colon and the trunk of the inferior mesenteric artery is ligated and divided at its origin from the aorta (high-tie). Resection of the specimen is completed by division of the bowel at the point to be used for the proximal anastomosis.

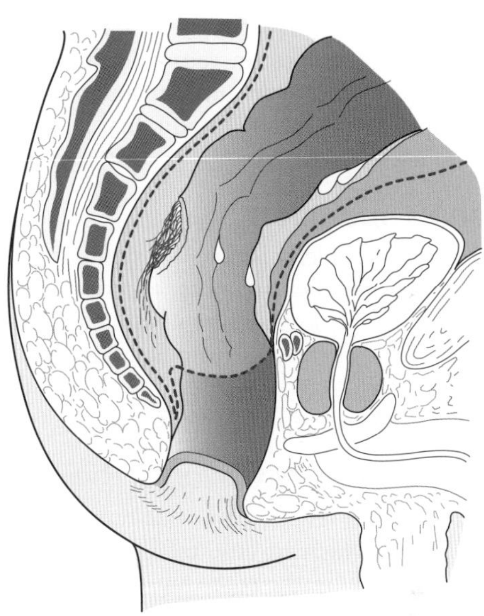

Figure 73.21 Plane of dissection for total mesorectal excision.

Restoration of bowel continuity is usually achieved by means of a stapled anastomosis. The simplest way of achieving this is by using a 'double stapling' technique, whereby a stapling gun is passed transanally to anastomose the stapled ends of the proximal colon and rectal stump. Alternatively, a 'single stapled' anastomosis may be performed in which purse-string sutures are applied to the proximal colon and rectal stump and anastomosed using a single firing of a staple gun inserted transanally. In cases where the anastomosis is very low (coloanal anastomosis) it may be necessary to perform a hand-sewn anastomosis.

Laparoscopic and robotic anterior resection follow the above general principles, but with abdominal access through the use of four or five abdominal ports and carbon dioxide pneumoperitoneum. The dissection usually follows a medial-to-lateral approach, i.e. dissection and high ligation of the vascular pedicle followed by lateral mobilisation of the colon, then rectal resection. A small laparotomy wound is still required to extract the specimen, unless transanal specimen extraction is possible, and restoration of bowel continuity is performed by the usual stapling techniques.

Transanal total mesorectal excision (taTME)

There is growing interest in reducing the trauma of anterior resection by undertaking total endoluminal excision of the rectum: transanal TME (taTME). This builds on the principles of laparoscopic surgery, with an air-tight anal device used to provide transanal insufflation and access for laparoscopic instruments. The operation proceeds by placing a purse-string suture below the distal level of the tumour and incising the bowel wall to enter the mesorectal plane. Dissection then proceeds using a 'bottom-up' approach to accomplish TME. It is usual for this procedure to be undertaken as a combined operation, with synchronous 'top-down' laparoscopic resection by an abdominal operator who mobilises the left colon, takes down the splenic flexure and does some of the upper rectal dissection.

Initial results have shown that taTME is safe, with short-term oncological outcomes, in terms of pathological quality of the resection specimen and circumferential resection margins, comparable to those of traditional laparoscopic and open techniques.

Hartmann's operation

This is an option in elderly and frail patients in whom there is concern about poor anal sphincter function and postoperative incontinence or the viability of an anastomosis. Colorectal excision follows the same principles as outlined above, but the rectal stump is stapled closed and the proximal colon exteriorised as a permanent end colostomy.

Abdominoperineal excision of the rectum

This operation is still required for some tumours of the lower third of the rectum which are unsuitable for a sphincter-saving procedure. Traditionally, the procedure was performed by two surgeons operating simultaneously, one via the abdomen and the other via the perineum, with the patient in the Trendelenburg lithotomy position. More recently, there has been a shift to completing the abdominal procedure first (with the patient in the Lloyd-Davies position, in which the legs are in supports set lower than the lithotomy position), and then placing the patient either in a prone jack-knife or Lloyd-Davies position and completing the operation via the perineum. The aim is to produce a complete resection of the rectum and mesorectum along with cylindrical excision of the extralevator component. This achieves wide excision at the level of the pelvic floor, increasing complete resection rates and reducing local perforation and the risk of local recurrence.

The abdominal procedure is carried out laparoscopically or via a midline laparotomy, and is performed in the same way as an anterior resection, except that dissection stops before the pelvic floor is reached (at the level of the seminal vesicles in men or the cervix in women), to avoid 'coning down' onto the tumour at the level of the pelvic floor. Perineal dissection is achieved through a circumanal incision which is deepened into the ischiorectal fossae and out towards the attachment of the levator muscles to the pelvic side wall (Figure 73.22). The dissection is extended posteriorly by incising Waldeyer's fascia, which is a thick condensation of pelvic fascia lying between the rectum and the sacrum. Some surgeons routinely remove the coccyx to improve access and surgical margins. Anteriorly, the plane between the rectum and the prostate in the male or between the rectum and the vagina in the female is developed, with particular care to avoid the membranous urethra in the male. A catheter within it should be palpated so that it can be avoided. The posterior wall of the vagina can be excised with the rectum if an advanced anterior tumour is present. Resection is completed when the perineal dissection reaches the abdominal dissection, with the specimen retrieved through the perineal wound. An end colostomy is formed in the left iliac fossa and the wounds closed with drains to the pelvis.

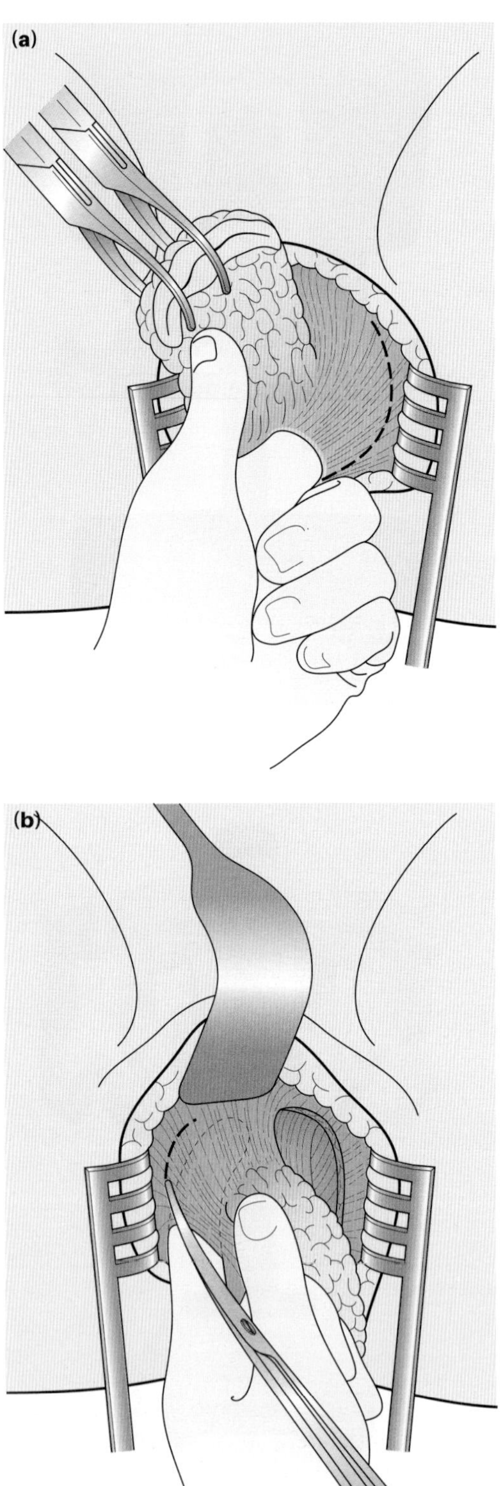

Figure 73.22 (a, b) Separation and division of the pubococcygeus and puborectalis muscles in the course of the perineal phase of an abdominoperineal excision of the rectum. Redrawn with permission from Keighley MRB, Williams NS. *Surgery of the anus, rectum and colon*. London: WB Saunders, 1999.

Friedrich Trendelenburg, 1844–1924, Professor of Surgery successively at Rostock (1875–1882), Bonn (1882–1895) and Leipzig (1895–1911), Germany. The Trendelenburg position was first described in 1885.
Oswald Vaughan Lloyd-Davies, 1905–1987, surgeon, St Mark's Hospital and The Middlesex Hospital, London, UK.

Endoluminal stenting

An increasingly used alternative for patients with an obstructing carcinoma is placement of an endoluminal stent, which can be done endoscopically, often with fluoroscopic guidance. This can either be used as a palliative procedure, or to relieve obstruction and permit elective rather than emergency surgery to be undertaken. Only rectosigmoid and upper rectal tumours are suitable for stenting, because stent impingement on the anorectum in low cancers causes symptoms of tenesmus.

Palliative colostomy

This is indicated only in cases giving rise to intestinal obstruction, or where the rectal cancer is not resectable. It can be performed by either an open or laparoscopic approach. In some cases a defunctioning colostomy is required in advanced cancers to prevent obstruction during down-staging chemoradiotherapy.

More extensive operations

When carcinoma of the rectum has spread to contiguous organs, the radical operation can often be extended to remove these structures *en bloc*. Thus, in the male, in whom spread is usually to the bladder or prostate, a cystectomy or prostatectomy may be required in combination with anterior resection to achieve complete oncological clearance. In the female, the uterus acts as an oncological barrier, preventing spread from the rectum to the bladder. Accordingly, a hysterectomy can be undertaken in addition to excision of the rectum. Pelvic evisceration for carcinoma of the rectum is usually only justifiable when the surgeon is confident that the cancer can be completely removed with negative resection margins.

Pelvic exenteration

The aim is to remove pelvic organs involved in the malignant process, and may involve a partial exenteration (posterior exenteration, including rectum and posterior vagina/uterus) or complete (including rectum and urogenital organs) (Figure 73.23). Exenteration may be necessary for advanced local disease, but more commonly for disease recurrence. It involves a large excision of the pelvic floor, leaving a sizeable perineal defect that has to be reconstructed using a plastic surgical procedure. Rectus abdominus or gluteal flaps can be used to fill the empty pelvis. Special care must be taken to suture the perineal skin accurately, and to avoid pressure necrosis by nursing the patient on alternate sides. Excision of the bladder will require the formation of an ileal conduit in addition to a colostomy.

Liver resection

Single or multiple well-localised liver metastases can now be resected with relatively low mortality and morbidity. Provided the patients are carefully selected, a reasonable long-term survival rate can be achieved (approximately 40%). Such surgery is usually carried out in a specialised liver unit, and may be performed synchronously at the time of anterior resection or else as a delayed procedure.

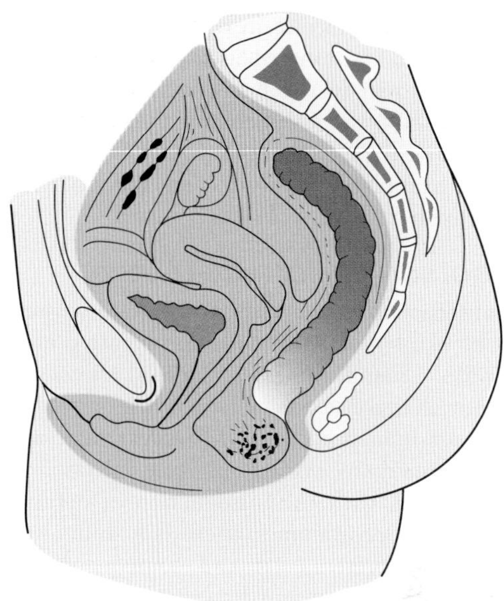

Figure 73.23 Radical pelvic exenteration, indicating the extent of the dissection and the viscera removed (shaded dark pink). Redrawn with permission from Keighley MRB, Williams NS. *Surgery of the anus, rectum and colon*. London: WB Saunders, 1999.

Radiotherapy

Adjuvant radiotherapy is now commonly used in the treatment of rectal cancer. It may be given preoperatively (neoadjuvant) and less commonly postoperatively (adjuvant). In the neoadjuvant setting, radiotherapy is used to either 'sterilise' the operative field in cancers with suspected lymphovascular involvement, or to down-stage locally advanced cancers with threatened circumferential resection margins. In the former instance, radiotherapy is often given as a 'short course' over 5 days with immediate surgery some 7–10 days later. On occasion, short-course radiotherapy can be combined with a delay before surgery (up to 12 weeks) to allow cancer regression. When radiotherapy is used to down-stage a cancer, it is often combined with chemotherapy (chemoradiotherapy) and given over a period of 6 weeks with a 6-week recovery period before surgery. Some 20% of cancers treated with chemoradiotherapy will show a complete pathological response, with a further 25–30% showing a partial response. Unfortunately, it is not yet possible to determine prior to treatment which patients will respond and therefore to tailor treatment accordingly.

Occasionally, radiotherapy is used to palliate unresectable cancers that are causing symptoms due to pain, obstruction or bleeding.

Alternative radiotherapy regimens include the Papillon technique in which intracavity radiation is directed to the cancer in the form of 'contact radiotherapy' or else delivered by brachytherapy techniques. To date, the application of these techniques has been restricted to selected cases, usually in patients unfit for more radical surgery.

Chemotherapy

Chemotherapy is either given in combination with radiotherapy (chemoradiotherapy) to down-stage a cancer prior to surgical resection, or else in the postoperative setting to reduce the risk of disseminated disease. 5-Fluorouracil (5-FU) based regimens remain the first-line therapy and are associated with a 10% improvement in disease-free survival in patients with node-positive rectal cancer. Second-line therapies include oxaliplatin and irinotecan, and biological agents such as cetuximab.

Results of surgery for rectal cancer

In specialised centres, the resectability rate for rectal cancer may be as high as 95%, with an operative mortality of less than 5%. Overall, the 5-year survival rate is about 50% and has not changed appreciably over the last decade. Survival rates are influenced by TNM/Dukes' stage, with node-positive patients doing worse than those with node-negative lesions. However, with the introduction of national bowel cancer screening programmes, there is a shift to an earlier stage of disease presentation and consequently improved survival.

LOCAL RECURRENCE

Local recurrence after rectal excision is a major problem. The patient may be asymptomatic with recurrence diagnosed as part of a surveillance programme, including regular measurements of blood carcinoembryonic antigen (CEA) and cross-sectional radiological imaging. The presence of symptoms is often a poor prognostic feature. Persistent pelvic pain, which may radiate down the legs, is indicative of nerve root involvement and will preclude further surgery. Bladder symptoms may occur or there may be fistulating disease onto the perineum. Most local recurrences are situated extrarectally and are therefore not readily diagnosed on endoscopy examination and biopsy. CT and MRI scan are the best means for detecting local recurrence, but PET-CT is increasingly being used to differentiate metabolically active cancer recurrence from metabolically inactive scar tissue. Local recurrence rates vary between 2 and 25% and are higher after abdominoperineal excision than after sphincter-saving resection. High quality primary surgery with preservation of the mesorectal 'package' and a clear circumferential resection margin are the most important factors in preventing local recurrence.

Overall, 80% of local recurrences develop within 2 years following surgery, and are very difficult to treat. If the patient is radiotherapy naïve then preoperative chemoradiotherapy will be beneficial. Surgical exenteration offers the only hope of cure and may involve a partial sacrectomy, with significant morbidity.

FURTHER READING

Cancer Research UK, Cancer Statistics. www.cancerresearchuk.org/health-professional/cancer-statistics/statistics-by-cancer-type/bowel-cancer

Fearon ER, Vogelstein B. A genetic model for colorectal tumorigenesis. *Cell* 1990; **61**(5): 759–67.

Hanahan D, Weinberg RA. Hallmarks of cancer: the next generation. *Cell* 2011; **144**(5): 646–74.

Keighley MRB, Williams NS (eds). *Surgery of the anus, rectum and colon*, 3rd edn. London: WB Saunders, 2008.

Phillips RKS (ed.). *A companion to specialist surgical practice: colorectal surgery*, 4th edn. London: Elsevier, 2009.

Valenti V, Schmoll H-J, van de Velde CJH (eds). *Multidisciplinary management of rectal cancer*. Berlin: Springer-Verlag, 2012.

Wolthuis AM, Bislenghi G, de Buck van Overstraeten A, D'Hoore A. Transanal total mesorectal excision: Towards standardization of technique. *World J Gastroenterol* 2015; **21**(44): 12686–95.

Chapter 74

The anus and anal canal

Learning objectives

To understand

- The anatomy of the anus and anal canal and their relationship to surgical disease and its treatment
- The pathology, clinical presentation, investigation, differential diagnosis and treatment of diseases that affect the anus and anal canal
- That anal disease is common and its treatment tends to be conservative, although surgery may be required
- That any damage to the anus, including too aggressive or inappropriate surgery, may render the patient permanently disabled

ANATOMY AND PHYSIOLOGY

Surgical anatomy

The anal canal commences at the level where the rectum passes through the pelvic diaphragm and ends at the anal verge. The muscular junction between the rectum and anal canal can be felt with the finger as a thickened ridge – the anorectal 'bundle' or 'ring'.

Anal canal anatomy

The anorectal ring

The anorectal ring marks the junction between the rectum and the anal canal (Figure 74.1). It is formed by the joining of the puborectalis muscle (Figure 74.2), the deep external sphincter, conjoined longitudinal muscle and the highest part of the internal sphincter. The anorectal ring can be clearly felt digitally, especially on its posterior and lateral aspects.

The puborectalis muscle

Puborectalis, part of the funnel-shaped muscular pelvic diaphragm, maintains the angle between the anal canal and rectum and hence is an important component in the continence mechanism (Figure 74.2). The muscle derives its nerve supply from the sacral somatic nerves, and is functionally indistinct from the external anal sphincter. The position and length of the anal canal, as well as the angle of the anorectal junction, depend to a major extent on the integrity and strength of the puborectalis muscle sling. It gives off fibres that contribute to the longitudinal muscle layer.

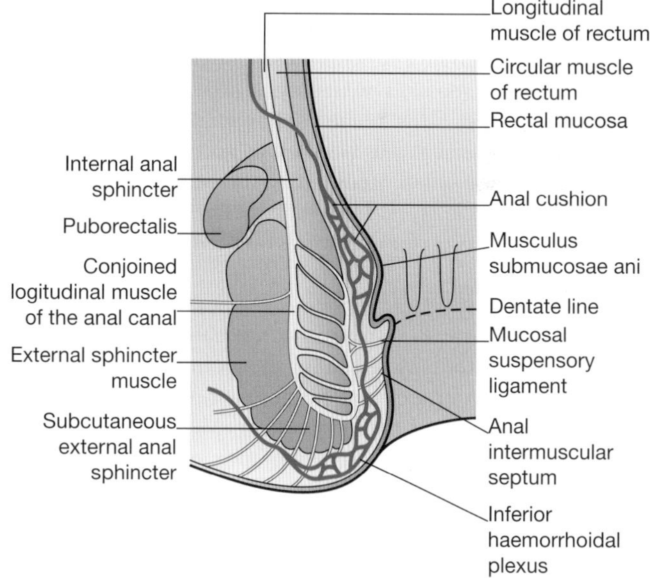

Figure 74.1 Relevant anatomy of the anus. (Redrawn with permission from Mann CV. *Surgical treatment of haemorrhoids*. London: Springer, 2002.)

The external sphincter

The external sphincter forms the bulk of the anal sphincter complex and, although traditionally it has been subdivided into deep, superficial and subcutaneous portions, it is a single muscle (Goligher), which is variably divided by lateral extensions from the longitudinal muscle layer. Some of its fibres are attached posteriorly to the coccyx, whereas anteriorly they fuse with the perineal muscles. Being a somatic voluntary muscle, the external sphincter is red in colour and is innervated by the pudendal nerve.

John Cedric Goligher, 1912–1998, Professor of Surgery, University of Leeds, Leeds, UK.

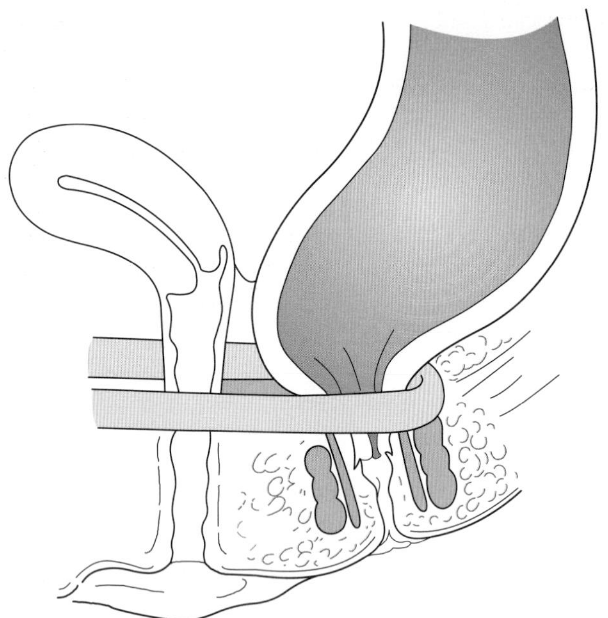

Figure 74.2 The disposition of the puborectalis muscle. Note how it maintains the rectoanal angle.

The intersphincteric plane

Between the external sphincter muscle laterally and the longitudinal muscle medially exists a potential space, the intersphincteric plane. This plane is important as it contains intersphincteric anal glands (see below) and is also a route for the spread of pus, which occurs along the extensions from the longitudinal muscle layer. The plane can be opened up surgically to provide access for operations on the sphincter muscles.

The longitudinal muscle

The longitudinal muscle is a direct continuation of the smooth muscle of the outer muscle coat of the rectum, augmented in its upper part by striated muscle fibres originating from the medial components of the pelvic floor. Most of the muscle continues caudally before splitting into multiple terminal septa that surround the muscle bundles of the subcutaneous portion of the external sphincter, to insert into the skin of the lowermost part of the anal canal and adjacent perianal skin. Milligan and Morgan named the most medial of these septa, passing around the inferior border of the internal sphincter, the 'anal intermuscular septum'. As it descends, however, it gives off fibres that pass medially across the internal sphincter to reach the submucosal space, and laterally across the external sphincter and ischiorectal space to reach the fascia of the pelvic side walls. As well as providing a supportive mesh for the anal canal and other muscular components, its ramifications provide potential pathways for the spread of infection. During defaecation, its contraction widens the anal lumen, flattens the anal cushions, shortens the anal canal and everts the anal margin; subsequent relaxation allows the anal cushions to distend and thus contribute to an airtight seal.

The internal sphincter

The internal sphincter is the thickened (2–5 mm) distal continuation of the circular muscle coat of the rectum, which has developed special properties and which is in a tonic state of contraction. This involuntary muscle commences where the rectum passes through the pelvic diaphragm and ends above the anal orifice, its lower border palpable at the intersphincteric groove, below which lie the most medial fibres of the subcutaneous external sphincter, and separated from it by the anal intermuscular septum. When exposed during life, it is pearly-white in colour and its circumferentially placed fibres can be seen clearly. Although innervated by the autonomic nervous system, it receives intrinsic non-adrenergic and non-cholinergic (NANC) fibres, stimulation of which causes release of the neurotransmitter nitric oxide, which induces internal sphincter relaxation.

The epithelium and subepithelial structures

The pink columnar epithelium lining the rectum extends through the anorectal ring into the surgical anal canal. Passing downwards the mucous membrane becomes cuboidal and redder in colour (Figure 74.3), whereas above the anal valves it is plum coloured. Just below the level of the anal valves there is an abrupt, albeit wavy, transition to stratified squamous epithelium, which is parchment coloured. This wavy junction constitutes the dentate line. The dentate line is a most important landmark both morphologically and surgically, representing the site of fusion of the proctodaeum and postallantoic gut, and being the site of the crypts of Morgagni (synonym: anal crypts, sinuses). The latter are small pockets between the inferior extremities of the columns of Morgagni through which anal ducts that communicate with deeper placed anal glands open into the anal lumen. The squamous epithelium lining the lower anal canal is thin and shiny and is known as the anoderm; it differs from the true skin in that it has no epidermal appendages, i.e. hair and sweat glands. At the dentate line, the anoderm is

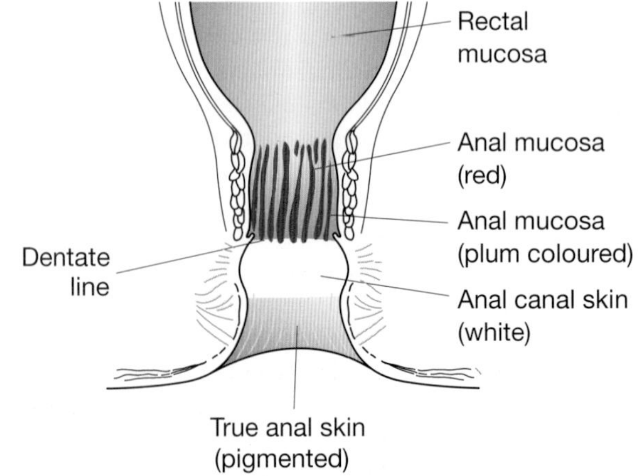

Figure 74.3 The lining membrane of the anal canal (after Sir Clifford Naunton Morgan, London).

Edward Thomas Campbell Milligan, 1886–1972, surgeon, St Mark's Hospital, London, UK.
Sir Clifford Naughton Morgan, 1901–1986, surgeon, St Mark's Hospital and St Bartholomew's Hospital, London, UK.

attached more firmly to deeper structures. The mucosa and submucosa above the dentate line is uneven and thrown into folds, the so called anal cushions. There are variations in the numbers and positions of these cushions but there are usually three, corresponding to those seen in later life. These are described classically as occupying the left lateral, right posterior and right anterior positions, and they continue proximally as the primary rectal foldings. Secondary foldings (the rectal columns of Morgagni) lie both over and between the primary folds. This area is the caudal limit of the so-called epithelial transitional zone, below which the stratified squamous epithelium is richly innervated by sensory nerve endings serving several modalities including touch, pain and temperature. The bulk of the anal cushions themselves, situated in the upper part of the anal canal, receive only visceral afferent innervation and, although there is perception of stretching, sensitivity to noxious stimuli is much more blunted than distally.

Between the epithelial layer and the internal sphincter lies the submucosa, consisting of vascular, muscular and connective tissue supportive elements. From the longitudinal muscle, medial extensions cross the internal anal sphincter and form part of the supporting meshwork of the submucosa, blending with the true submucosal smooth muscle layer and thereby supporting the mucosa itself. Parks described the increased density of fibres that insert into the mucosa of the anal crypts at the level of the dentate line, termed the 'mucosal suspensory ligament'. One feature of this structure is that it separates the superior (portal) and inferior (systemic) haemorrhoidal plexuses; another, is that the mucosa is more firmly tethered to underlying tissues at this level than above. It is important to appreciate that the meshwork of supporting tissues (muscle fibres and connective tissue) within the subepithelial space is intimately linked to deeper structures within the anal sphincter complex, including the internal sphincter, longitudinal muscle layer and external anal sphincter, and indeed structures beyond the sphincter complex. With age, the smooth muscle component of this mesh is reduced and muscle fibres are gradually replaced with fibroelastic connective tissue, which in turn becomes fragmented.

Blood supply

In addition to the meshwork support of the lining of the anal canal, the subepithelial space contains venous dilatations supported by the same fibroelastic connective tissue and smooth muscle scaffolding. Debate has centred on the nature of the vascular component of haemorrhoids, but the seminal anatomical studies of Thomson have clarified this issue. Venous dilatations are seen in the submucosa both above and below the level of the dentate line; they are much more numerous above although tend to be larger below. The historical description of the blood supply to the upper anal canal as constant, with bifurcation of the main trunk of the superior rectal artery into right and left branches and with subsequent division of the former into anterior and posterior divisions, thereby determining the sites of haemorrhoids around the anal circumference, was questioned by Thomson. He demonstrated that the divisions of the superior rectal artery were not constant and that, furthermore, the anal submucosa in a proportion of his specimens received a blood supply from the middle and inferior rectal arteries. He was also able to show the presence of free communications between tributaries of the superior, middle and inferior rectal veins, as well as tiny direct arteriovenous communications with the submucosal venous dilatations. These communications have been shown both histologically and radiologically, and the oxygen tension of the blood contained within the venous dilatations (as well as the colour) is more arterial than venous.

Venous drainage

The anal veins are distributed in a similar fashion to the arterial supply. The upper half of the anal canal is drained by the superior rectal veins, tributaries of the inferior mesenteric vein and thus the portomesenteric venous system, and the middle rectal veins, which drain into the internal iliac veins. The inferior rectal veins drain the lower half of the anal canal and the subcutaneous perianal plexus of veins; they eventually join the internal iliac vein on each side.

Lymphatic drainage

Lymph from the upper half of the anal canal flows upwards to drain into the postrectal lymph nodes and from there goes to the para-aortic nodes via the inferior mesenteric chain. Lymph from the lower half of the anal canal drains on each side, first into the superficial and then into the deep inguinal group of lymph glands. However, if the normal flow is blocked, e.g. by tumour, the lymph can be diverted into the alternative route.

Summary box 74.1

Anal canal anatomy

- The internal sphincter is composed of circular, non-striated involuntary muscle supplied by autonomic nerves
- The external sphincter is composed of striated voluntary muscle supplied by the pudendal nerve
- Extensions from the longitudinal muscle layer support the sphincter complex
- The space between sphincters is known as the intersphincteric plane
- The superior part of the external sphincter fuses with the puborectalis muscle, which is essential for maintaining the anorectal angle, necessary for continence
- The lower part of the anal canal is lined by sensitive squamous epithelium
- Blood supply to the anal canal is via superior, middle and inferior rectal vessels
- Lymphatic drainage of the lower half of the anal canal goes to inguinal lymph nodes

Giovani Battista Morgagni, 1682–1771, Professor of Anatomy, Padua, Italy, for 59 years. He is regarded as the founder of morbid anatomy.
Sir Alan Guyatt Parks, 1920–1962, surgeon, St Mark's Hospital and the London Hospital, London, UK.
William Hamish Fearon Thomson, surgeon, The Gloucestershire Royal Infirmary, Gloucester, UK.

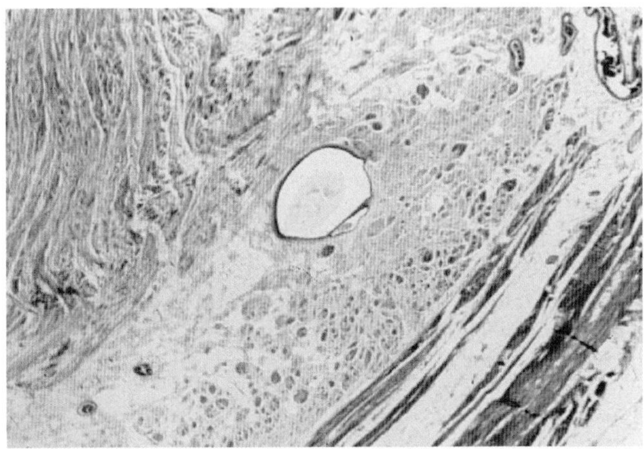

Figure 74.4 Intersphincteric anal gland lying between the voluntary muscle of the external sphincter and the longitudinal muscle. The internal sphincter is also seen. (Reproduced with permission from Nicholls RJ, Dozois RR. *Surgery of the colon and rectum*. Edinburgh: Churchill Livingstone, 1997.)

The anal glands

Anal glands (which are not vestigial remnants of sexual scent glands) may be found in the submucosa and intersphincteric space (Figure 74.4), and normally number between 0 and 10 in an individual. They drain via ducts into the anal sinuses at the level of the dentate line. Not all sinuses have a duct draining into them and, occasionally, more than one gland can discharge into the same sinus. Their function is unknown although they secrete mucin (distinct from that secreted by the rectal epithelium), which perhaps lubricates the anal canal to ease defaecation. The importance of intersphincteric anal glands is that they are widely considered to be the potential source of anal sepsis, either acute, presenting as perianal, ischiorectal or even pelvic sepsis, or chronic, presenting as a cryptoglandular (non-specific) anal fistula.

EXAMINATION OF THE ANUS

Careful clinical examination will be diagnostic in the vast majority of patients complaining of anal symptoms, but it requires a relaxed patient who is informed of what the examination will entail, a private environment, a chaperone (for the security of both parties) and good light. Most commonly, the patient is examined in the left lateral (Sims) position with the buttocks overlying the edge of the examination couch and with the axis of the torso crossing, rather than parallel with, the edge of the couch. Alternatively, in younger patients, the prone jack-knife or knee–elbow positions may be used (Figure 74.5). The examining couch should be of sufficient height to allow easy inspection and access for any necessary manoeuvres. A protective glove should be worn.

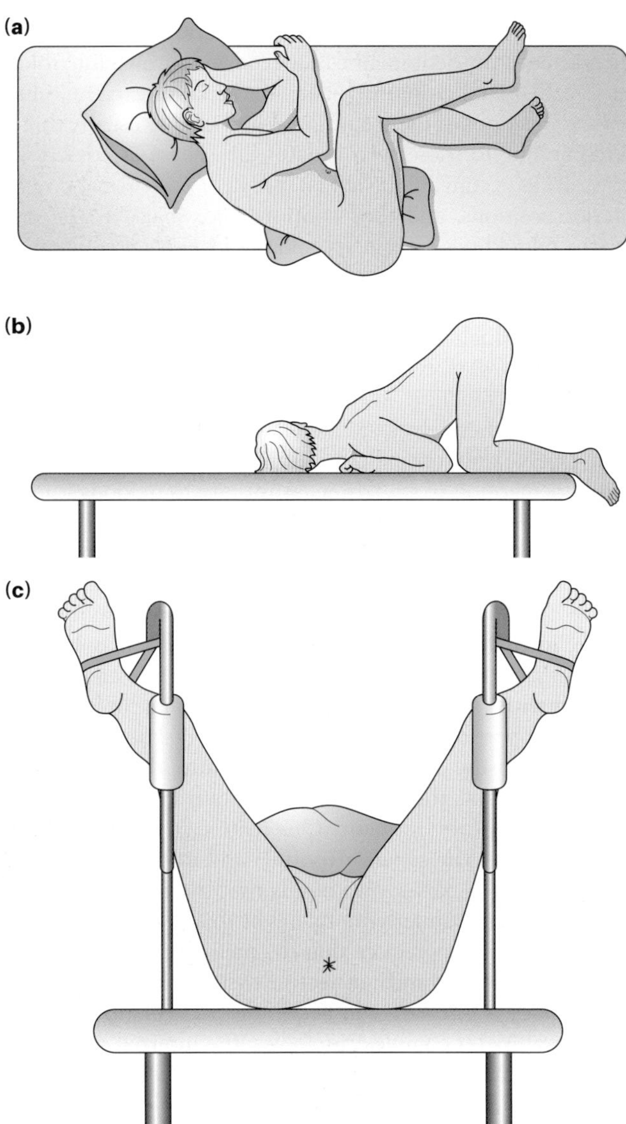

Figure 74.5 (a) The left lateral; (b) knee–elbow and lithotomy (c) positions for examination. (Redrawn with permission from Mann CV. *Surgical treatment of haemorrhoids*. London: Springer, 2002.)

Inspection

The buttocks are gently parted to allow inspection of the anus and perineum: the presence of any skin lesions and whether they are confined to the perineum or evident elsewhere on general examination, e.g. psoriasis, lichen planus, or on genital examination, e.g. warts, candidiasis, lichen sclerosus et atrophicus, the vesicles of herpes simplex virus (HSV); evidence of anal leakage; whether the anus is closed or patulous; and the position of the anus and perineum at rest and on bearing down (the latter may reveal prolapse of haemorrhoids or even the rectum). Pain on parting the buttocks, perhaps

James Marion Sims, 1813–1883, gynaecological surgeon, the State Hospital for Women, New York, USA, introduced this position to give access to the anterior vaginal wall during operations for the closure of vesicovaginal fistulae.

together with the presence of a sentinel tag, may indicate the presence of an underlying fissure, but may also prompt the need for examination under anaesthesia to exclude more suspicious pathology, for example squamous cell carcinoma of the anal canal.

Digital examination with the index finger

With an adequately lubricated index finger, the soft tissues around the anus are palpated for induration, tenderness and subcutaneous lesions. The index finger is then introduced gently into the anal canal along its posterior aspect. At the apex of the canal, the sling of puborectalis is felt posteriorly; supralevator induration feels bony hard and is more easily appreciated if unilateral. The posterior surface of the prostate gland with its median sulcus can be palpated anteriorly in male patients; in female patients, the uterine cervix can be palpated. The presence of any distal intrarectal, intra-anal or extraluminal mass is recorded. Sphincter length, resting tone and voluntary squeeze are assessed. On withdrawal, the examining finger is inspected for the presence of mucus, blood or pus and to identify stool colour.

Proctoscopy

Proctoscopy, performed with the patient in the same position, allows a detailed inspection of the distal rectum and anal canal (Figure 74.6). Minor procedures can also be carried out through this instrument, e.g. treatment of haemorrhoids by injection or banding (see below) and biopsy. Asking the patient to bear down on slow withdrawal of the proctoscope may reveal a descending intussusception.

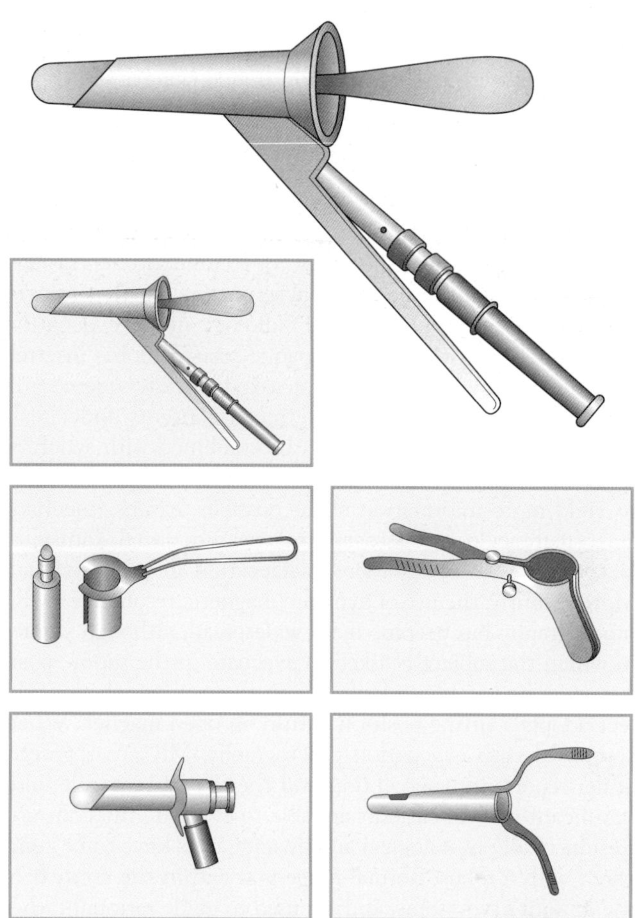

Figure 74.6 Various types of proctoscope. (Redrawn with permission from Mann CV. *Surgical treatment of haemorrhoids*. London: Springer, 2002.)

Sigmoidoscopy

Although sigmoidoscopy is strictly an examination of the rectum (see Chapter 73), it should always be carried out even when an anal lesion has been confirmed. Rectal pathology, e.g. colitis or carcinoma, is frequently associated with an anal lesion, e.g. fissure or haemorrhoids. Not infrequently, rectal pathology is found that is independent of the anal lesion and which requires treatment.

Summary box 74.2

Examination of anal canal

- A rectal examination is essential for any patient with anorectal and/or bowel symptoms – 'If you don't put your finger in, you might put your foot in it'
- A proctosigmoidoscopy is essential in any patient with bowel symptoms, and particularly if there is rectal bleeding

PHYSIOLOGICAL ASPECTS OF THE ANAL SPHINCTERS AND PELVIC FLOOR, AND SPECIAL INVESTIGATIONS

Anal continence and defaecation are highly complex processes that necessitate the structural and functional integrity of the cerebral, autonomic and enteric nervous systems, the gastrointestinal tract (especially the rectum) and the pelvic floor and anal sphincter complex, any of which may be compromised and lead to disturbances of function of varying severity. The sphincter mechanism provides the ultimate barrier to leakage and its integrity can be assessed fairly simply and objectively in the physiology laboratory (Swash and Henry). Perineal position and degree of descent on straining (markers of pelvic floor and pudendal nerve function) can be quantified, and functional anal canal length, resting tone (reflective predominantly of internal sphincter activity) and squeeze increment (reflective of external sphincter function)

Michael Swash, formerly Professor of Neurology, St Bartholomew's and The Royal London Hospital, London, UK.
Michael Meldrum Henry, surgeon, The Chelsea and Westminster Hospital, London, UK.

can be measured by a variety of simple manometric techniques (Figure 74.7). The structural integrity of the sphincters can be visualised with endoluminal ultrasound (Figure 74.8), and neuromuscular function can be measured by assessment of conduction velocity along the pudendal nerve on each side, or, more painfully, by needle electromyogram (EMG) studies (Figures 74.9 and 74.10). In the elderly especially, but also in younger patients, disorders relating to rectal sensorimotor dysfunction can lead to 'overflow' of rectal contents through what may be an otherwise normal sphincter. The dynamics of defaecation can also be assessed radiologically by evacuation proctography, in which radio-opaque pseudostool is inserted into the rectum and the patient asked to rest, squeeze and then bear down to evacuate the rectal contents under real-time imaging. Proctography can be combined with synchronous EMG and pressure studies (Williams) (Figure 74.11) to yield more information about possible reasons (mechanical (rectocoele, intussusception) or functional (anismus, lack of effort)) for disordered defaecation in an individual. More recently, the use of dynamic magnetic resonance (MR) proctography has become more widespread, although studies in which the subject is asked to evacuate in the supine position may be less physiological than those in which the subject adopts a sitting position within an open magnet. When compared with evacuation proctography, MR proctography under-reports intussusception and the size of rectocele; also significantly fewer patients are able to evacuate the contrast. Results of all physiological and imaging tests have to be compared with a robust normal range and within the context of the patient's symptoms, and are used to guide rational rather than empirical treatment strategies.

(a)

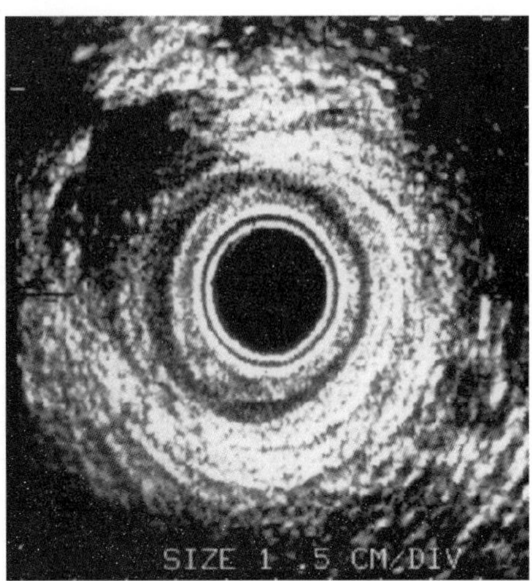

(b)

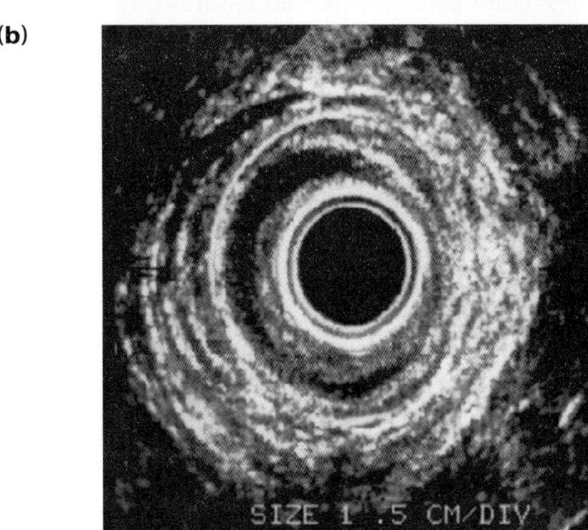

Figure 74.8 Endoanal ultrasonography: (a) external anal sphincter defect caused by obstetric injury; (b) internal anal sphincter defect postsphincterotomy.

CONGENITAL ABNORMALITIES

Early in embryonic life there is a common chamber – the cloaca – into which the hind gut and the allantois open. This endodermlined chamber is separated from the surface ectoderm of the embryo by the cloacal membrane. The cloaca becomes divided into two parts, dorsal (rectum) and ventral

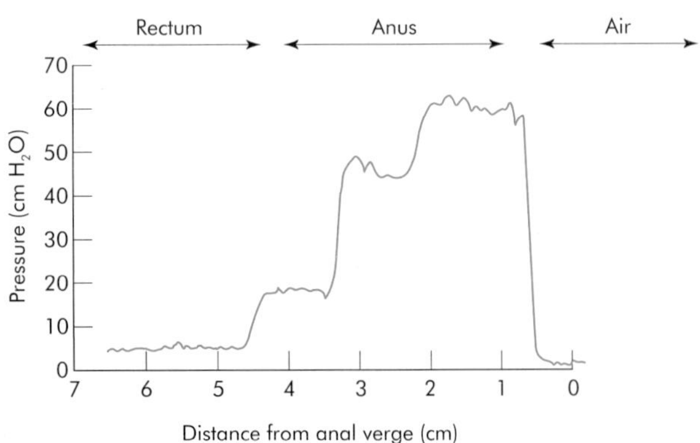

Figure 74.7 A typical, normal 'pull-through' manometric study of the anal canal (3.5 cm long; maximal pressure approximately 60 cmH_2O).

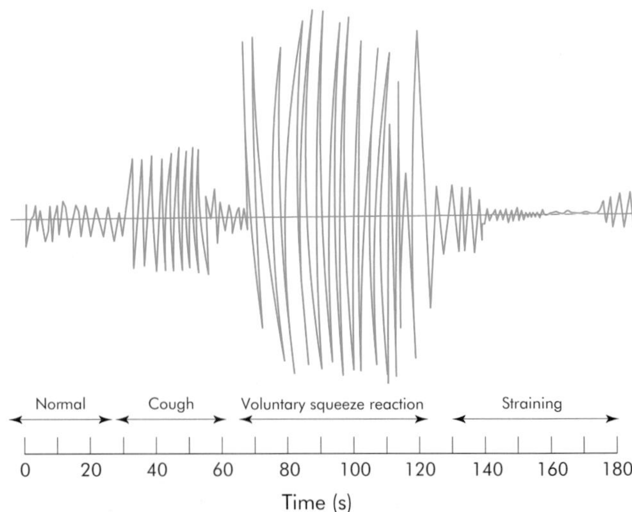

Figure 74.9 A typical, normal electromyographic study of the external sphincter during various activities.

Norman Stanley Williams, contemporary, Emeritus Professor of Surgery, St Bartholomew's and the Royal London Hospital, London, UK.

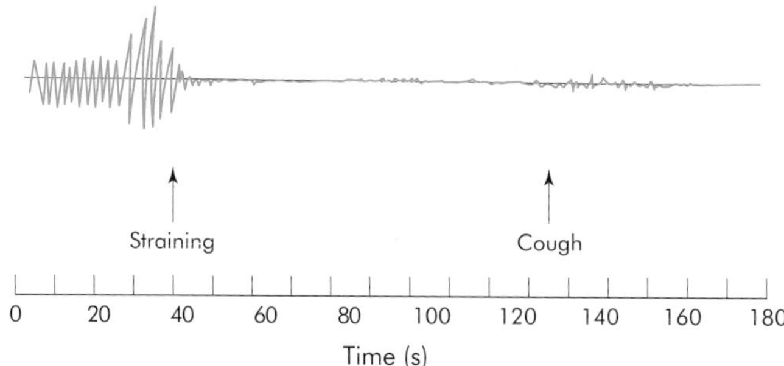

Figure 74.10 An electromyographic study of the external sphincter showing prolonged inhibition on straining and absent cough reflex. This is typical of a denervated patulous sphincter.

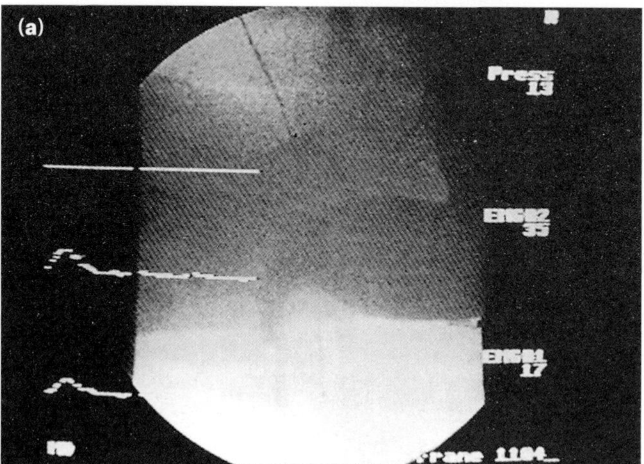

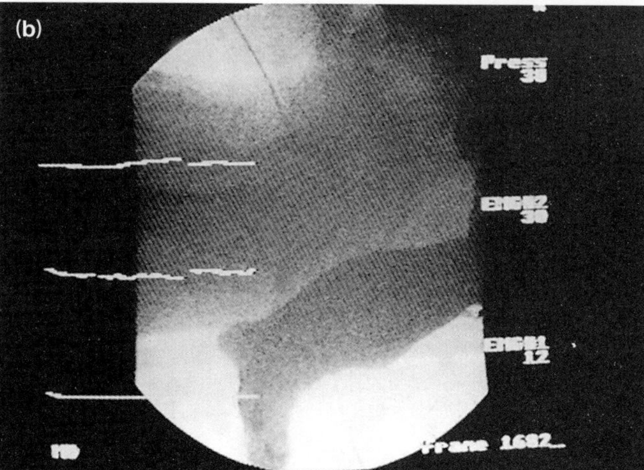

Figure 74.11 Integrated dynamic proctography: (a) at rest; (b) during evacuation. Visualisation of the rectum is achieved using barium-impregnated 'synthetic stool'. The effects of straining and evacuation on the electromyographic activity of the sphincter muscles and intrarectal pressure can be simultaneously recorded (Williams).

(urogenital sinus), by the downgrowth of a septum. The dorsal part of the cloacal membrane, known as the anal membrane, is thus composed of an outer layer of ectoderm and an inner layer of endoderm. Resorption of this anal membrane by the eighth week of embryonic life creates the anal canal.

Imperforate anus

Imperforate anus (strictly, it should be anal 'agenesis' or 'atresia') has historically been divided into two main groups – high and low – depending on the level of termination of the rectum in relation to the pelvic floor. Treatment and prognosis are influenced by any associated abnormalities of the sacrum and genitourinary systems. In both sexes, low defects embrace rectoperineal fistula (Figure 74.12), covered anus and anal

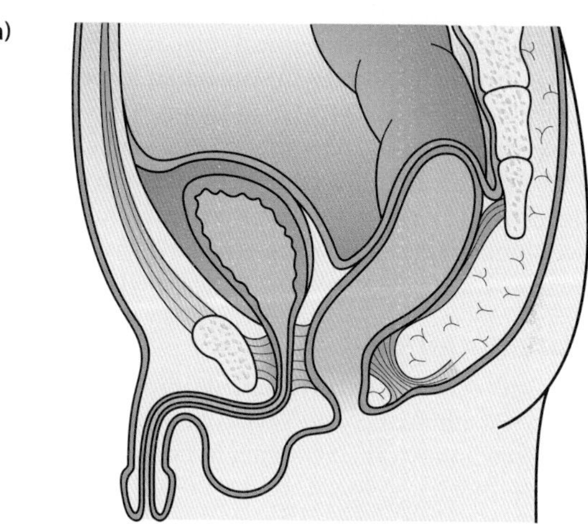

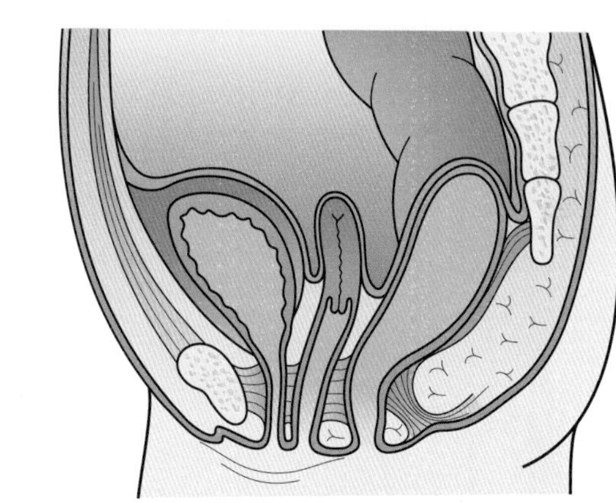

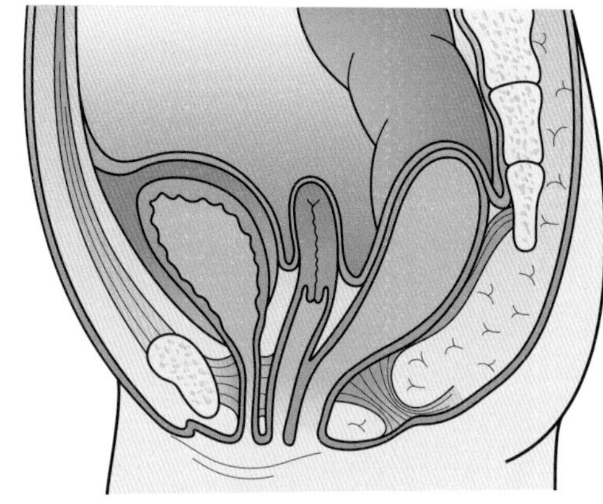

Figure 74.12 Low anorectal malformations: (a) rectoperineal fistula in a boy; (b) rectoperineal fistula in a girl (anterior anus); (c) rectovestibular fistula. (Courtesy of Alberto Pena and Springer-Verlag. From Pena A. *Atlas of surgical management of anorectal malformations*. Copyright Springer-Verlag, 1990.)

Alberto Pena, contemporary, Professor of Pediatric Surgery, Schneider Children's Hospital, New York, NY, USA.

membrane. The most frequent defect in boys with imperforate anus is one in which the distal rectum is sited within the puborectalis sling but terminates as a fistula into the bulbar urethra (Figure 74.13) (see also Chapter 9, Figure 9.32) or prostatic urethra above the main anal sphincter complex. Boys with a fistula into the bladder neck (a high defect) have the poorest prognosis because of the underdevelopment of the sacrum and pelvic and anal musculature. The most common defect in girls is a rectovestibular fistula, in which the fistula opens into the posterior vestibule (not the vagina) (Figure 74.12). The finding of a single perineal orifice indicates a persistent cloaca in which the rectum, vagina and urinary tract form a confluence (Figure 74.13); the longer the common channel, the greater the likelihood of more complex defects, including vaginal and uterine septation, duplication or atresia. An anterior anus, although not imperforate, is not fully located within the sphincter mechanism and is regarded as part of the spectrum of anorectal malformations (Figure 74.12).

Clinical management

Careful perineal examination will usually provide the most important clues about the neonate's type of malformation. The presence of meconium on the perineum indicates a low defect and meconium in the urine is evidence of a urinary tract fistula. During the first 24 hours, the baby should receive intravenous fluids and antibiotics, and should be evaluated for associated congenital anomalies. By 24 hours, the distal limit of air within the rectum, seen on a lateral prone radiograph, indicates the distance between the rectal stump and perineum (Figure 74.14).

Treatment

Low anomalies with a perineal fistula can be treated by an anoplasty. More complex malformations require early colostomy, with definitive repair performed several months later. This may involve posterior sagittal anorectoplasty (PSARP, Pena), with or without transabdominal mobilisation of the left colon and division of any communication with the urinary tract. In girls with a cloaca and long common channel, urinary and vaginal reconstruction is also required. Postoperatively, a programme of anal dilatation is instituted, and any residual colostomy is closed at a later date. Ultimate bowel function (voluntary bowel movements, continence, constipation) is related to the type of anorectal abnormality and the presence of associated defects, especially sacral.

(a)

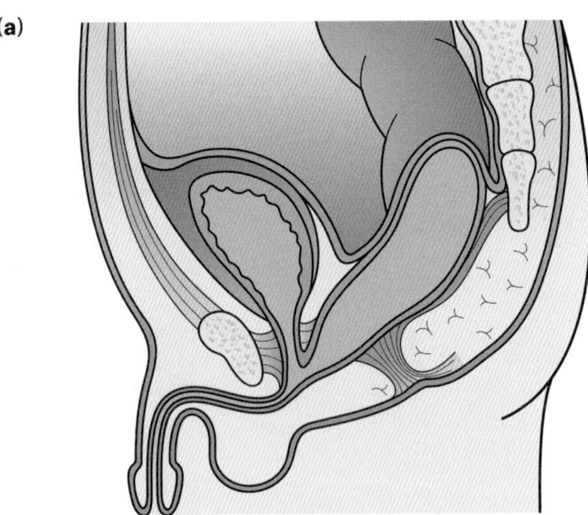

(b)

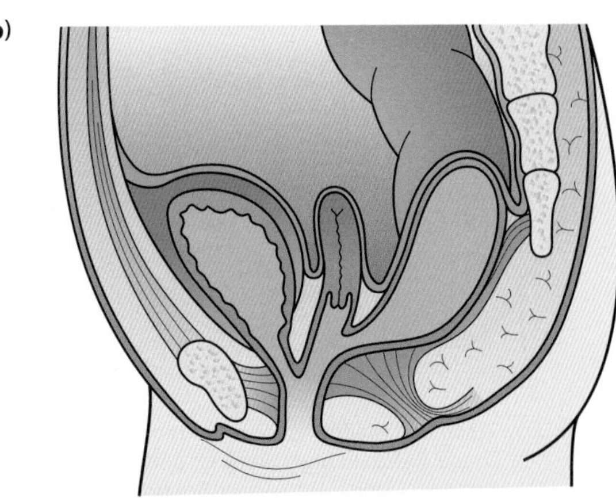

Figure 74.13 More complex anorectal malformations: (a) rectobulbar fistula; (b) cloacal malformation. (Courtesy of Alberto Pena and Springer-Verlag. From Pena A. *Atlas of surgical management of anorectal malformations*. Copyright Springer-Verlag, 1990.)

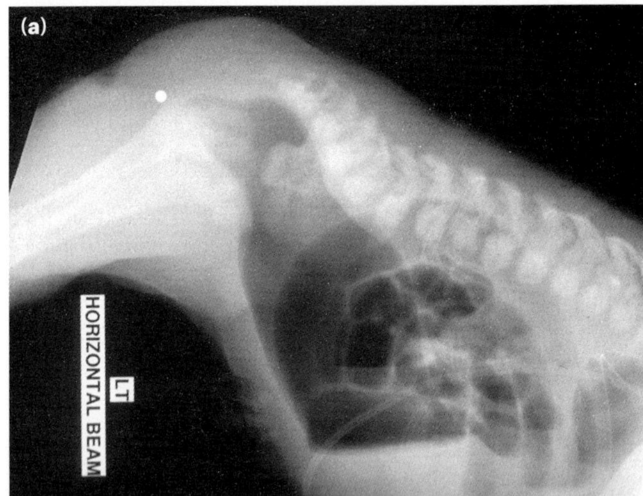

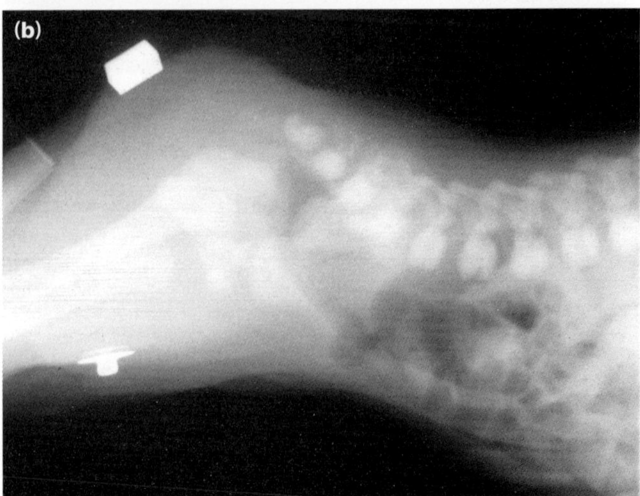

Figure 74.14 Lateral prone shoot-through radiograph of a neonate with (a) low and (b) high anorectal malformation. A radio-opaque marker has been placed on the anal dimple (courtesy of Mark D Stringer, Leeds, UK).

Summary box 74.3

Imperforate anus

- A rare congenital disorder
- Classified as being high or low depending on the site of the rectal termination in relation to the pelvic floor
- Low defects: relatively easy to correct but prone to constipation
- High defects: more difficult to correct and prone to faecal incontinence

Postanal dermoid

The space in front of the lower part of the sacrum and coccyx may be occupied by a soft, cystic swelling – a postanal dermoid cyst. Hidden in the hollow of the sacrum it is unlikely to be discovered unless a sinus communicating with the exterior is present or it develops as a result of inflammation. Such a cyst usually remains asymptomatic until adult life, when it is prone to becoming infected. Exceptionally, because of its size, it gives rise to difficulty in defaecation. The cyst is easily palpable on rectal examination.

Differential diagnosis

Especially in a child, an anterior sacral meningocele must be excluded. This enlarges when the child cries and is frequently associated with paralysis of the lower limbs and incontinence. When a discharging sinus is present, a postanal dermoid will probably be mistaken for a pilonidal sinus or even an anal fistula. Pressure over the sacrococcygeal region with a finger in the rectum may cause a flow of sebaceous material, and injection of contrast media followed by radiography reveals a bottle-necked cyst in front of the coccyx.

Treatment

Treatment involves complete excision of the cyst and, if present, the sinus. In the case of large cysts, it is necessary to remove the coccyx to gain access. The coccyx should also be removed *en bloc* in any child with a presacral dermoid because of the risk of sacrococcygeal teratoma.

Postanal dimple (synonym: fovea coccygea)

A dimple in the skin beneath the tip of the coccyx, sometimes amounting to a short blind pit, is noticed from time to time in the course of a clinical examination and is of no consequence.

Pilonidal sinus

The term pilonidal sinus describes a condition found in the natal cleft overlying the coccyx, consisting of one or more, usually non-infected, midline openings, which communicate with a fibrous track lined by granulation tissue and containing hair lying loosely within the lumen. A common affliction amongst the military, it has been referred to as 'jeep disease'.

Aetiology and pathology

Although acquired theories of development are better accepted than the more historical congenital theories, exact mechanisms of development are speculative. Evidence that supports the theory of the origin of pilonidal sinuses as acquired, can be summarised as follows:

- Interdigital pilonidal sinus is an occupational disease of hairdressers, the hair within the interdigital cleft or clefts being the customers'. Pilonidal sinuses of the axilla and umbilicus have also been reported.
- The age incidence of the appearance of pilonidal sinus (82% occur between the ages of 20 and 29 years) is at variance with the age of onset of congenital lesions.
- Hair follicles have almost never been demonstrated in the walls of the sinus.
- The hairs projecting from the sinus are dead hairs, with their pointed ends directed towards the blind end of the sinus.
- The disease mostly affects men, in particular hairy men.
- Recurrence is common, even though adequate excision of the track is carried out.

It is thought that the combination of buttock friction and shearing forces in that area allows shed hair or broken hairs which have collected there to drill through the midline skin, or that infection in relation to a hair follicle allows hair to enter the skin by the suction created by movement of the buttocks, so creating a subcutaneous, chronically infected, midline track. From this primary sinus, secondary tracks may spread laterally, which may emerge at the skin as granulation tissue-lined, discharging openings. Usually, but not invariably (when diagnosis may be confused with anal fistula or hidradenitis suppurativa), the sinus runs cephalad. Carcinoma arising in chronic pilonidal disease has been described but is exceedingly rare.

Clinical features

The condition is seen much more frequently in men than women, usually after puberty and before the fourth decade of life, and is characteristically seen in dark-haired individuals rather than those with softer blond hair (Oldham). Patients complain of intermittent pain, swelling and discharge at the base of the spine but little in the way of constitutional symptoms. There is often a history of repeated abscesses that have burst spontaneously or which have been incised, usually away from the midline. The primary sinus may have one or many openings, all of which are strictly in the midline between the level of the sacrococcygeal joint and the tip of the coccyx.

Conservative treatment

As the natural history of the condition is usually one of regression, in those whose symptoms are relatively minor, simple

A jeep is a small military, general purpose, vehicle with hard springing, which gives its occupants a very bouncy ride when driven over rough terrain.
James Bagot Oldham, 1899–1977, surgeon, the United Liverpool Hospitals, Liverpool, UK.

cleaning out of the tracks and removal of all hair, with regular shaving of the area and strict hygiene, may be recommended.

Treatment of an acute exacerbation (abscess)

If rest, baths, local antiseptic dressings and the administration of a broad spectrum antibiotic fail to bring about resolution, the abscess should be drained through a small longitudinal incision made over the abscess and off the midline, with thorough curettage of granulation tissue and hair. This procedure may or may not be associated with complete resolution.

Surgical treatment of chronic pilonidal disease

The multitude of surgical procedures advocated to eradicate pilonidal disease, combined with the lack of prospective trials, attests to the lack of overall superiority of one method over the others. Time spent off work and perceived recurrence rates, but more usually surgeon preference, influence the choice of method, which includes the laying open of all tracks with or without marsupialisation, the excision of all tracks with or without primary closure and the excision of all tracks and then closure by some other means designed to avoid a midline wound (Limberg procedure, Z-plasty, Karydakis procedure (Figure 74.15)). Bascom's procedure involves an incision lateral to the midline to gain access to the sinus cavity, which is rid of hair and granulation tissue (Figure 74.16), and excision and closure of the midline pits (Figure 74.17). The lateral wound is left open (Figure 74.18). Irrespective of procedure, postoperative wound care is important and centres around elimination of hair (ingrown, local or other) from the wound. The search for an ideal surgical treatment modality for pilonidal disease is still ongoing, the most essential characteristic being tension-free healing.

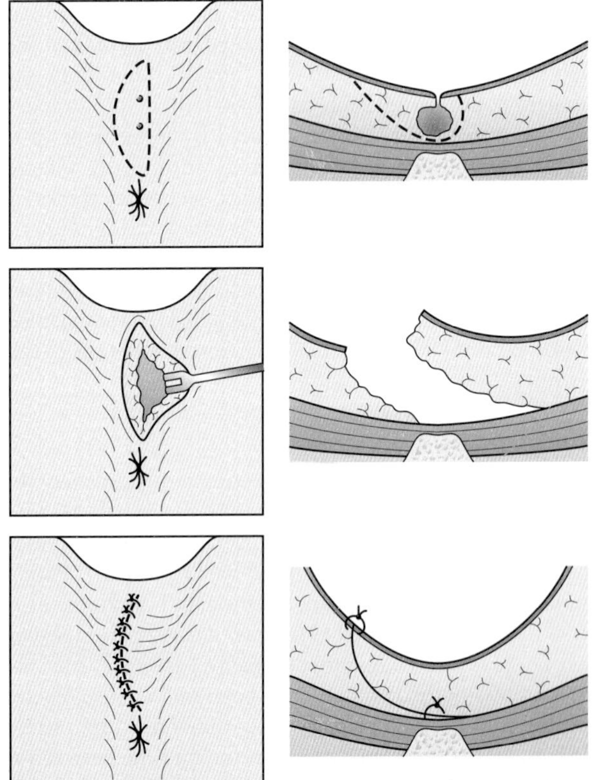

Figure 74.15 Karydakis's operation for pilonidal sinus. A semilateral incision is made around the sinus complex, the diseased component excised and the flap mobilised to allow tension-free closure of the wound off the midline. (Reproduced with permission from Nicholls RJ, Dozois RR. *Surgery of the colon and rectum*. Edinburgh: Churchill Livingstone, 1997.)

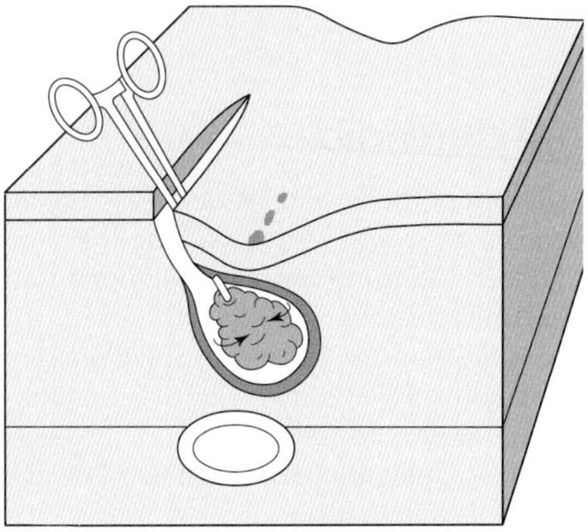

Figure 74.16 Bascom's technique for pilonidal sinus: 1.

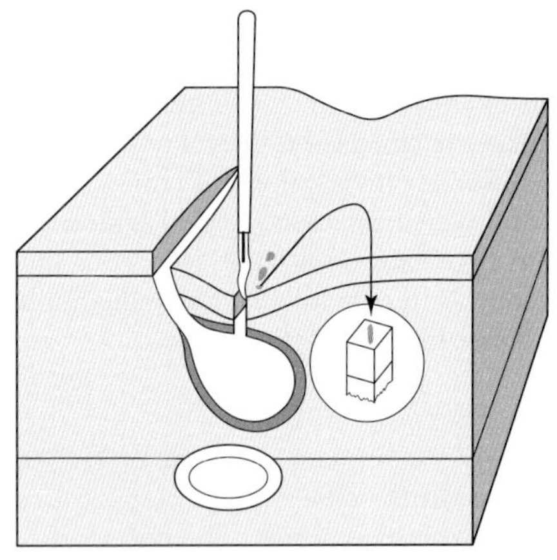

Figure 74.17 Bascom's technique for pilonidal sinus: 2.

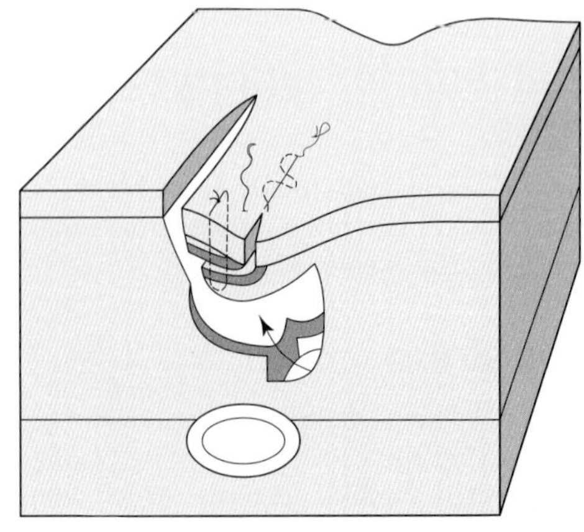

Figure 74.18 Bascom's technique for pilonidal sinus: 3.

Col Dr George E Karydakis, surgeon, Athens, Greece.
John U Bascom, 1925–2013, American surgeon, formerly of Eugene, OR, USA.

Recurrent pilonidal sinus

Three possibilities account for this disappointment:

- part of the sinus complex has been overlooked at the primary operation;
- new hairs enter the skin or the scar;
- there is persistence of a midline wound caused by shearing forces and scarring; in this situation, revisional surgery may include re-excision followed by wound closure and obliteration of the natal cleft, either by myocutaneous rotational buttock flap or cleft closure (Bascom).

ANAL INCONTINENCE

Aetiology

As continence is dependent upon the structural and functional integrity of both the neurological pathways and the gastrointestinal tract, the risk factors for anal incontinence are many. Patients complaining of the involuntary loss of rectal contents require a comprehensive assessment of the nature and severity of symptoms; past history, especially of gastrointestinal disease, neurological conditions, obstetric events and anal surgery; and careful clinical examination (in the elderly, incontinence is often one of overflow secondary to rectal impaction, and proctitis may lead to such an irritable rectum that even the strongest sphincter is occasionally overwhelmed). A combination of history and examination will usually be diagnostic, but special investigations are then usually required to clarify the exact cause, including exclusion of an underlying malignancy, and to direct management.

Sphincteric causes of incontinence may be classified as structural, in which there is disruption (or atrophy) of part of the sphincter muscles, neuropathic (previously termed idiopathic), in which the nerve supply to the sphincters is damaged, usually by chronic straining or complicated vaginal delivery (prolonged second stage), or a combination of the two. The commonest causes of sphincteric disruption are obstetric damage, anal surgery (following haemorrhoidectomy, dilatation or sphincterotomy for anal fissure, and fistulotomy for anal fistula) and trauma (including anal intercourse, forced or otherwise).

In general, conservative measures to reduce symptoms are employed initially. These may be in the form of stool bulking or constipating agents, nurse-led bowel retraining including specific biofeedback programmes, or anal plugs, which expand within and thus seal the anal canal. Failure of such measures and severity of symptoms may result in selection for surgery.

Summary box 74.4

Causes of anal incontinence

Congenital/childhood

- Anorectal anomalies
- Spina bifida
- Hirschsprung's disease
- Behavioural

Acquired/adulthood

- Diabetes mellitus
- Cerebrovascular accident
- Parkinson's disease
- Multiple sclerosis
- Spinal cord injury
- Other neurological conditions:
  - Myotonic dystrophy
  - Shy–Drager syndrome
  - Amyloid neuropathy
- Gastrointestinal infection
- Irritable bowel syndrome
- Metabolic bowel disease
- Inflammatory bowel disease
- Megacolon/megarectum
- Anal trauma
- Abdominal surgery:
  - Small bowel resection
  - Colonic resection
- Pelvic surgery:
  - Hysterectomy
  - Rectal excision
- Pelvic malignancy
- Pelvic radiotherapy
- Rectal prolapse
- Rectal evacuatory disorder:
  - Mechanical, e.g. rectocoele, intussusception
  - Functional, i.e. pelvic floor dyssynergia
- Anal surgery:
  - Haemorrhoidectomy
  - Surgery for fistula
  - Surgery for fissure
  - Rectal disimpaction
- Obstetric events

General

- Ageing
- Dependence of nursing care
- Obesity
- Psychobehavioural factors
- Intellectual incapacity
- Drugs:
  - Primary constipating and laxative agents
  - Secondary effects

Operations to reunite divided sphincter muscles

In situations in which there is a discrete disruption of the sphincters, the ends of the divided muscle are found and reunited by a double overlap repair (Figure 74.19). Short-term results are good, with reports of 75–80% improvement in symptoms at first follow–up. This reduces with time to 50% or less 5–10 years after surgery.

Operations to reef the external sphincter and puborectalis muscle

If the sphincter muscles are stretched and patulous (as they often are in old age and in cases of rectal prolapse) they may

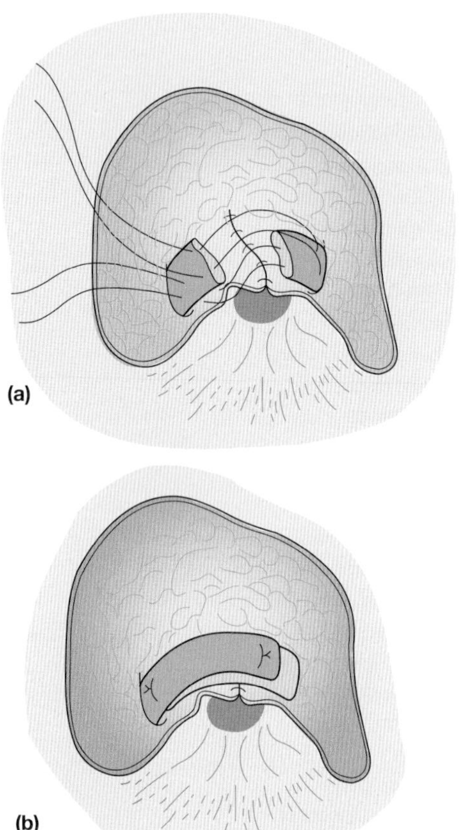

Figure 74.19 Direct sphincter repair in which (a) the sphincter defect is excised and (b) the remaining muscle is overlapped. (Redrawn with permission from Mann CV, Glass RE. *Surgical treatment of anal incontinence*. New York: Springer, 1991.)

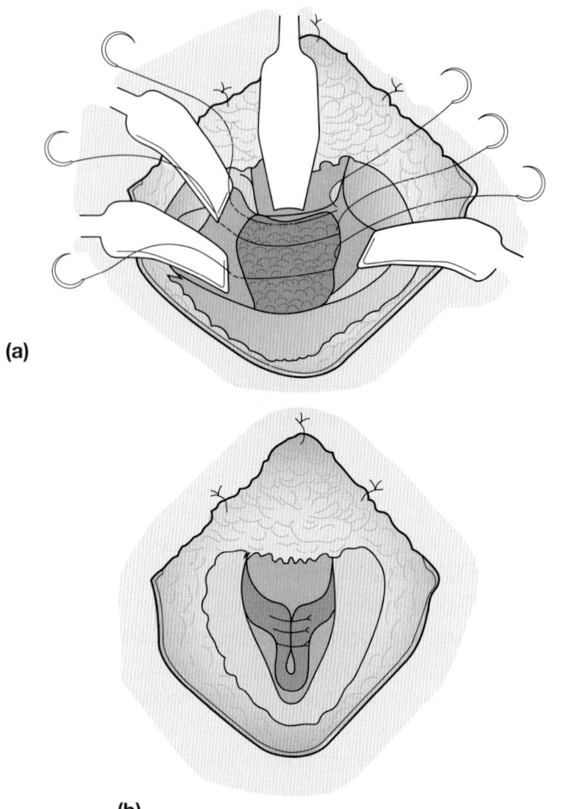

Figure 74.20 Postanal repair in which (a) the sphincter muscle is plicated posterior to the anal canal, thus restoring the anorectal angle; (b) the completed repair. (Redrawn with permission from Mann CV, Glass RE. *Surgical treatment of anal incontinence*. New York: Springer, 1991.)

be tightened by a postanal repair, which, through the use of darns of absorbable material to narrow down and plicate the external sphincter and the puborectalis sling (Figure 74.20), aims to recreate the anorectal angle and to restore length to the anal canal and strength to the anal sphincter. The approach is usually through the intersphincteric plane. The operation is now much less popular because long-term outcomes have been reported as poor.

Operations to augment the anal sphincters

If the degree of sphincter disruption or weakness is such that restoration of function cannot be achieved by direct means, the sphincter can be augmented by using muscle transposed from nearby (gluteus maximus or gracilis) or by using an artificial sphincter. Transposition of the gracilis muscle around the anal canal is followed by electrical stimulation, with conversion from a fast-twitch to a less fatiguable slow-twitch muscle by an implanted pacemaker (Williams) (Figure 74.21). Because of its magnitude this technique is performed only in highly selected and motivated patients, most of whom have had more conventional treatment that has failed to cure their incontinence; it is effective in approximately 60% of patients in the long term. A simpler means of augmenting the sphincter, developed initially for urinary incontinence, is the placement of an inflatable silastic cuff around the anal canal. When evacuation is required the cuff is deflated by squeezing a small balloon positioned in the scrotum or labia, the balloon being attached to a subcutaneous reservoir (Figure 74.22). However, because this device is a foreign body that exerts pressure on the bowel wall, erosion and infection have been found to be common problems. To reduce the risk of septic complications the operation should be covered by antibiotics active against both aerobic and anaerobic organisms. A newer magnetic sphincter (Fenix) is being implanted as part of a national trial in the UK (Safari trial; Fenix versus sacral nerve stimulator), the results of which should be available within the next 2 years. Paradoxically, all of these methods used to treat incontinence may be associated with difficulties in rectal evacuation.

Again, as a result of prior use in urinary incontinence, sacral nerve stimulation has been used to treat faecal incontinence, with encouraging short- and medium-term results. Rather than any direct action on sphincter strength, this technique appears to work by sensorimotor neurophysiological modulation of the hindgut through electrical stimulation of the sacral nerve roots via a needle positioned through one of the posterior sacral foramina (Figure 74.23). The advantage of this technique is its relatively non-invasive nature, causes no additional damage to the sphincter, as well as the fact that its effects can be tested by temporary stimulation

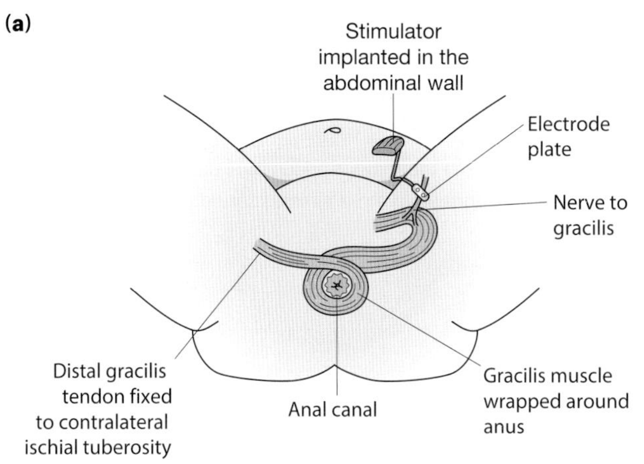

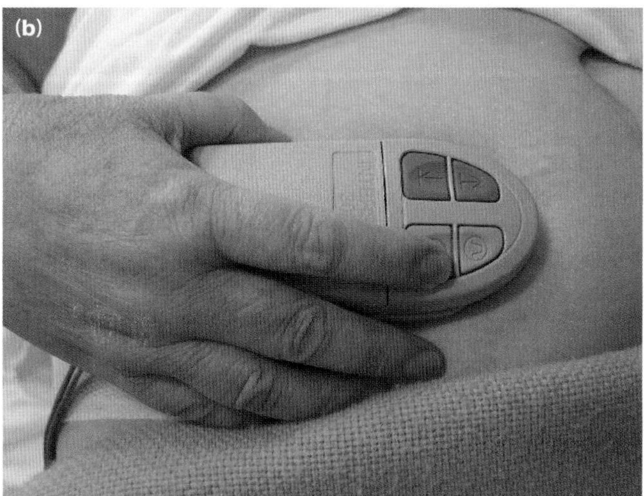

Figure 74.21 (a) The electrically stimulated gracilis neosphincter or dynamic graciloplasty. (b) Hand-held radiotelemetry controller, which allows the patient to turn the stimulator on and off.

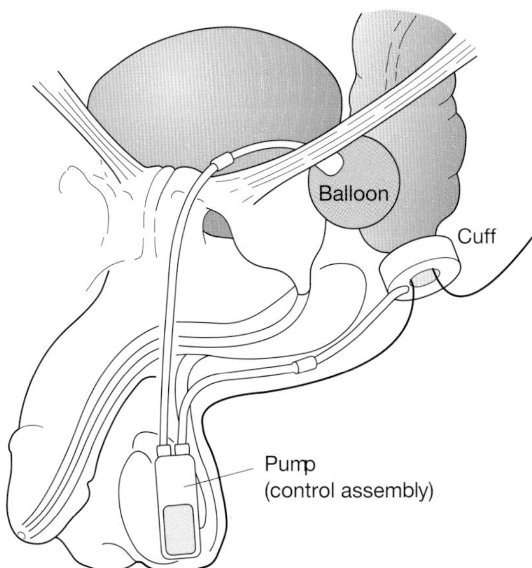

Figure 74.22 Artificial bowel sphincter. A cuff is placed around the anal canal. An inflatable pump control assembly is placed in the scrotum and the balloon reservoir is placed under the symphysis pubis.

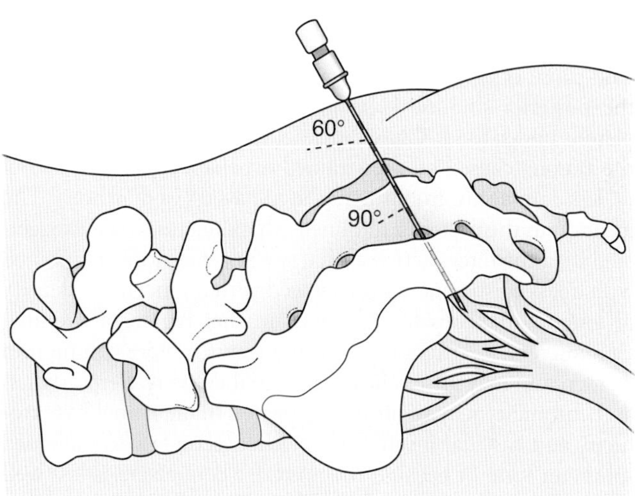

Figure 74.23 Diagram showing the placement of the electrode through a sacral foramen in sacral nerve stimulation.

using an external stimulator before the expensive permanent pacemaker is implanted. A much cheaper and less invasive novel technique to treat faecal incontinence, again mediated through neuromodulation, is percutaneous posterior tibial nerve stimulation (PTNS). Results from a prospective comparative study suggest that there is no benefit in faecal incontinence over placebo effect .

For some patients, and in those in whom quality of life remains poor despite attempts at restoring continence, a colostomy can provide relief from a condition that is both disabling and socially isolating.

ANAL FISSURE

Definition

An anal fissure (synonym: fissure-*in-ano*) is a longitudinal split in the anoderm of the distal anal canal (Figure 74.24), which extends from the anal verge proximally towards, but not beyond, the dentate line.

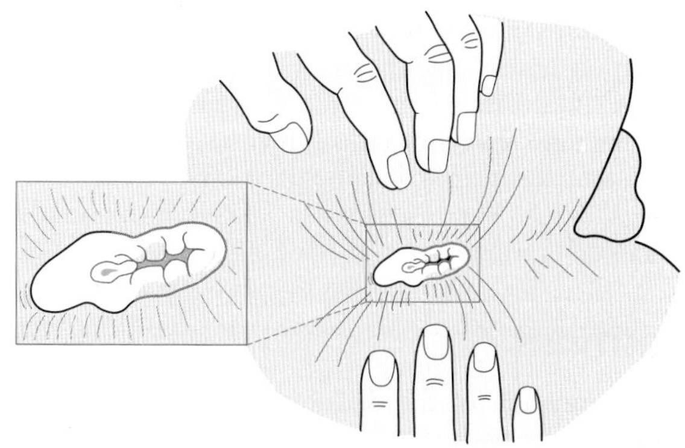

Figure 74.24 The appearance of an anal fissure. If the buttocks are gently parted, the presence of an anal fissure can usually be detected as an ulcer of variable depth with the skin tag and an anal papilla. (Redrawn with permission from Keighley MRB, Williams NS. *Surgery of the anus, colon and rectum*, 2nd edn. Philadelphia: WB Saunders, 1999.)

Aetiology

The cause of an anal fissure, and particularly the reason why the posterior midline is so frequently affected, is not completely understood. Classically, acute anal fissures arise from the trauma caused by the strained evacuation of a hard stool or, less commonly, from the repeated passage of diarrhoea. The location in the posterior midline perhaps relates to the exaggerated shearing forces acting at that site at defaecation, combined with a less elastic anoderm endowed with an increased density of longitudinal muscle extensions in that region of the anal circumference. Anterior anal fissure is much more common in women and may arise following vaginal delivery. Perpetuation and chronicity may result from repeated trauma, anal hypertonicity and vascular insufficiency, either secondary to increased sphincter tone or because the posterior commisure is less well perfused than the remainder of the anal circumference.

Clinical features

Although simple epithelial splits, acute anal fissures are, because of their location involving the exquisitely sensitive anoderm, characterised by severe anal pain associated with defaecation, which usually resolves spontaneously after a variable time only to recur at the next evacuation, as well as the passage of fresh blood, normally noticed on the tissue after wiping. Chronic fissures are characterised by a hypertrophied anal papilla internally and a sentinel tag externally (both consequent upon attempts at healing and breakdown), between which lies the slightly indurated anal ulcer overlying the fibres of the internal sphincter. When chronic, patients may also complain of itching secondary to irritation from the sentinel tag, discharge from the ulcer or discharge from an associated intersphincteric fistula, which has arisen through infection penetrating via the fissure base. Although most sufferers are young adults, the condition can affect any age, from infants to the elderly. Men and women are affected equally. Anterior fissures account for about 10% of those encountered in women (and many of these may occur postpartum) but only 1% in men. A fissure sited elsewhere around the anal circumference or with atypical features should raise the suspicion of a specific aetiology, and the inability to be able to conduct an adequate examination in the clinic should prompt early examination under anaesthesia, with biopsy and culture to exclude Crohn's disease, tuberculosis, sexually transmitted or human immunodeficiency virus (HIV)-related ulcers (syphilis, *Chlamydia*, chancroid, lymphogranuloma venereum, HSV, cytomegalovirus, Kaposi's sarcoma, B-cell lymphoma) and squamous cell carcinoma.

Treatment

After confirmation of the diagnosis in the clinic or under anaesthesia, with exclusion of secondary causes of anal ulceration, conservative management should result in the healing of almost all acute and the majority of chronic fissures. Emphasis must be placed on normalisation of bowel habits such that the passage of stool is less traumatic. The addition of fibre to the diet to bulk up the stool, stool softeners and adequate water intake are simple and helpful measures. Warm baths and topical local anaesthetic agents relieve pain; however, providing patients with anal dilators is usually associated with low compliance and consequently little effect. The mainstay of current conservative management is the topical application of pharmacological agents that relax the internal sphincter, most commonly nitric oxide donors (Scholefield); by reducing spasm, pain is relieved, and increased vascular perfusion promotes healing. Such agents include glyceryl trinitrate (GTN) 0.2% applied two to three times per day to the anal margin (although this may cause headaches) and diltiazem 2% applied twice daily. An alternative medical treatment is Botox (10–100 units) in either divided or a single dose. The cure rate using any of these options is approximately 50% although the headache rate with GTN ointment has been reported to be as high as 30%, which limits its acceptability by patients.

Summary box 74.5

Anal fissure

- Acute or chronic
- Ischaemic ulcer in the midline of the anal canal
- Ectopic site suggests a more sinister cause

Symptoms:

- Pain on defaecation
- Bright-red bleeding
- Mucus discharge
- Constipation

Operative measures

Historically, under regional or general anaesthesia, forceful manual (four- or eight-digit) sphincter dilatation was used to reduce sphincter tone; however, this was achieved in an uncontrolled fashion with potential disruption at multiple sites of the internal (and even external) sphincter. The risk of incontinence following this procedure has now made it unpopular, although more conservative controlled stretching is still practised in young men with very high sphincter tone.

Fissure healing can also be achieved by a posterior division of the exposed fibres of the internal sphincter in the fissure base, but this is associated with prolonged healing, as well as passive anal leakage thought mainly to be due to the resulting keyhole gutter deformity; however, it may be indicated if there is an associated intersphincteric fistula.

Lateral anal sphincterotomy

In this operation, the internal sphincter is divided away from the fissure itself – usually either in the right or the left lat-

Burrill Bernard Crohn, 1884–1983, gastroenterologist, Mount Sinai Hospital, New York, NY, USA.
Moritz Kaposi, 1837–1902, Professor of Dermatology, Vienna, Austria, described pigmented sarcoma of the skin in 1872.
John Howard Scholefield, contemporary, Professor of Surgery, The University of Nottingham, Nottingham, UK.

eral positions (Notaras). The procedure can be carried out using an open or a closed method, under local, regional or general anaesthesia, and with the patient in the lithotomy or prone jack-knife position. The distal internal sphincter is palpated with a bivalved speculum at the intersphincteric groove. In the closed method, a small longitudinal incision is made over this, and the submucosal and intersphincteric planes are carefully developed to allow precise division of the internal sphincter with a knife or scissors to the level of the apex of the fissure; the wound is then closed with absorbable sutures. Alternatively, either plane can be entered using a scalpel (no. 11 blade), with the blade advanced parallel to the sphincter and then rotated such that the sharp edge faces the internal sphincter, which can then be divided along its distal third. Pressure should be applied to the wound for a few minutes to prevent haematoma formation. In the open technique, the anoderm overlying the distal internal sphincter is divided longitudinally to expose the sphincter, which is divided, and the wound is closed with absorbable sutures. Although the fissure needs no specific attention, problematic papillae and external tags can be excised concomitantly.

Early complications of sphincterotomy include haemorrhage, haematoma, bruising, perianal abscess and fistula. Despite low recurrence rates, the most important complication is incontinence of a variable nature and severity, which may affect up to 30% of patients, particularly women, who have weaker, shorter sphincter complexes and in whom there may already have been covert sphincter compromise incurred by childbirth.

Anal advancement flap

The recognition of the risk to continence following internal sphincterotomy has led some to advocate a different approach, especially in women and those with normal or low resting anal pressures, developed from the treatment of anal stenosis. After excision of the edges of the fissure and, if necessary, its base overlying the internal sphincter, an inverted house-shaped flap of perianal skin is carefully mobilised on its blood supply and advanced without tension to cover the fissure, and then sutured with interrupted absorbable sutures (Figure 74.25). The patient is maintained on stool softeners and bulking agents postoperatively, and usually also on topical sphincter relaxants; minor breakdown of one anastomotic edge does not herald ultimate failure. The technique appears to work irrespective of sphincter hypertonicity or patient gender.

Summary box 74.6

Treatment of an anal fissure

- Conservative initially, consisting of stool-bulking agents and softeners, and chemical agents in the form of ointments designed to relax the anal sphincter and improve blood flow
- Surgery if above fails, consisting of lateral internal sphincterotomy or anal advancement flap

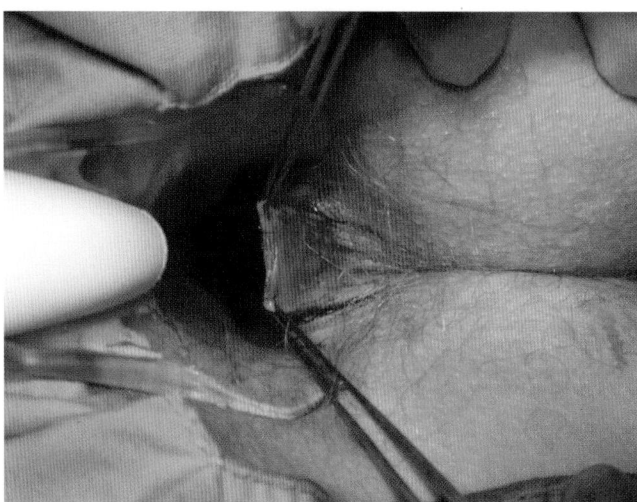

Figure 74.25 Mobilised skin flap prior to suturing intra-anally over the debrided and freshened posterior fissure base.

Hypertrophied anal papilla

Anal papillae occur at the dentate line and are remnants of the ectodermal membrane that separated the hindgut from the proctodaeum. As these papillae are present in 60% of patients examined proctologically, they should be regarded as normal structures. Anal papillae can become elongated, as they frequently do in the presence of an anal fissure. Occasionally, an elongated anal papilla may be the cause of pruritus. An elongated anal papilla associated with pain and/or bleeding at defaecation is sometimes encountered in infancy. Haemorrhage into a hypertrophied anal papilla can cause sudden rectal pain. A prolapsed papilla may become nipped by contraction of the sphincter mechanism after defaecation. Occasionally, a red oedematous papilla is encountered, with local pain and a purulent discharge from the associated crypt. This condition of 'cryptitis' may be cured by laying open the mouth of the infected anal gland and excising the papilla. Troublesome papillae may be simply excised.

Proctalgia fugax

This problem is characterised by attacks of severe pain arising in the rectum, recurring at irregular intervals and apparently unrelated to organic disease. The pain is described as cramp-like, often occurs when the patient is in bed at night, usually lasts only for a few minutes and disappears spontaneously. It may follow straining at stool, sudden explosive bowel action or ejaculation. It seems to occur more commonly in patients suffering from anxiety or undue stress, and it is also said to afflict young doctors. The pain may be unbearable – it is possibly caused by segmental cramp in the pubococcygeus muscle. It is unpleasant and incurable but is fortunately harmless and gradually subsides. If patients have frequent attacks, they may benefit from amitryptiline. Salbutamol inhalers have been

Mitchell James Notaras, surgeon, Barnet General Hospital, Barnet, UK.

suggested as treatment for acute attacks. A more chronic form of the disease has been termed the 'levator syndrome' and can be associated with severe evacuatory dysfunction. Biofeedback techniques have been used to help such patients; in the past, some surgeons tried severing the puborectalis muscle, but this can cause incontinence and should never be carried out. If this is being consider an acceptable alternative is Botox into the puborectalis muscle.

HAEMORRHOIDS

The prevalence of haemorrhoids when patients are assessed proctoscopically far outweighs the prevalence of symptoms, and the term should only be used when patients have symptoms referable to them. Occasionally, patients with portal hypertension develop rectal varices, but these should not be confused with haemorrhoids as the consquences may be disastrous. Internal haemorrhoids (Greek: *haima* = blood, *rhoos* = flowing; synonym: piles, Latin: *pila* = a ball) are symptomatic anal cushions and characteristically lie in the 3, 7 and 11 o'clock positions (with the patient in the lithotomy position). In addition, haemorrhoids may be observed between the main pile masses, in which case they are internal haemorrhoids at the secondary position. External haemorrhoids relate to venous channels of the inferior haemorrhoidal plexus deep in the skin surrounding the anal verge and are not true haemorrhoids; they are usually only recognised as a result of a complication, which is most typically a painful solitary acute thrombosis. External haemorrhoids associated with internal haemorrhoids ('interoexternal piles') result from progression of the latter to involve both haemorrhoidal plexuses, and are best thought of as being external extensions of internal haemorrhoids. Secondary internal haemorrhoids arise as a result of a specific condition, although the mechanisms involved may be the same as those involved in the formation of primary internal haemorrhoids. The most important cause, albeit relatively uncommon, is carcinoma of the anorectum (Figure 74.26) but there may be other causes, which may be categorised as follows:

- local, e.g. anorectal deformity, hypotonic anal sphincter;
- abdominal, e.g. ascites;
- pelvic, e.g. gravid uterus, uterine neoplasm (fibroid, carcinoma of the uterus or cervix), ovarian neoplasm, bladder carcinoma;
- neurological, e.g. paraplegia, multiple sclerosis.

Primary internal haemorrhoids

Theories of development

PORTAL HYPERTENSION AND VARICOSE VEINS

Misconceptions concerning the vascular anatomy of the anal canal (specifically the lack of appreciation of communications between portal and systemic systems and the 'normality' of venous dilatations) led to theories of development of primary internal haemorrhoids that lasted for several centuries. Man's upright posture (we know little about haemorrhoidal problems in animals), lack of valves in the portal venous system and raised abdominal pressure were thought to contribute to the development of anal varicosities. If raised portal venous pressure were indeed the cause, one would expect a high incidence in subjects suffering from portal hypertension; however, although such patients have a higher incidence of anorectal varices, these are a separate anatomical and clinical entity from haemorrhoids, which are seen no more frequently than in those without cirrhosis, portal hypertension and oesophageal varices.

OTHER VASCULAR CAUSES

Historically, some considered haemorrhoids to be haemangiomatous or to result from changes in the erectile tissue that forms part of the continence mechanism, such as hyperplasia of the 'corpus cavernosum recti'.

INFECTION

Repeated infection of the anal lining, secondary to trauma at defaecation, has been postulated as a cause of weakening and erosion of the walls of the veins of the submucosa. This hypothesis is difficult to accept, as one of the truly incredible properties of the anal canal is its resistance to infection, as well as the ability of its mucosa to heal after surgical intervention despite the torrent of microorganisms passing over it.

DIET AND STOOL CONSISTENCY

Much emphasis has been placed on the role of constipation in the development of haemorrhoids and, indeed, much of the management of sufferers involves attempts to 'normalise' bowel habits. A fibre-deficient diet results in a prolonged gut transit time, which is associated with the passage of smaller, harder stools that require more straining to expel. The presence of a hard faecal mass in the rectum could obstruct venous

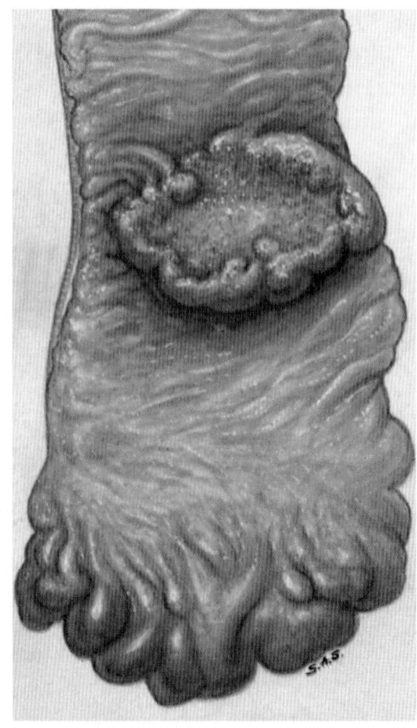

Figure 74.26 Carcinoma of the rectum associated with haemorrhoids, a not infrequent diagnostic pitfall.

return, resulting in engorgement of the anal veins with the act of straining at stool or sitting for prolonged periods on the lavatory with a relaxed perineum, causing a disturbance of vascular flow. However, the epidemiological pattern of constipation is different from that of haemorrhoidal disease and, indeed, an association has been demonstrated between haemorrhoids and diarrhoeal disorders.

ANAL HYPERTONIA

The association between raised anal canal resting pressure and haemorhoids is well known, but whether anal hypertonia causes symptoms attributable to haemorrhoids or whether anal cushion hypertrophy causes anal hypertonia is a subject of debate. The fact that surgical haemorrhoidectomy restores resting pressures to the normal range is not absolute evidence that the pile masses themselves are the cause of the hypertonia. It should be remembered, however, that there are a significant proportion of patients who suffer haemorrhoidal symptoms in whom the anal canal is relatively patulous, and there is mucosal prolapse, which is associated with perineal descent and pudendal neuropathy.

AGEING

In contrast to the anal cushion of early life, with age, the supporting structures show a higher proportion of collagen than muscle fibres and are fragmented and disorganised. Presumably, these changes arise over time with continued use of the anal canal for defaecation; however, similar changes are noted histologically in surgically excised haemorrhoids in younger patients.

CURRENT VIEW

Shearing forces acting on the anus (for a variety of reasons) lead to caudal displacement of the anal cushions and mucosal trauma. With time, fragmentation of the supporting structures (a normal consequence of ageing but perhaps accelerated in those with haemorrhoids) leads to loss of elasticity of the cushions such that they no longer retract following defaecation.

Clinical features

Bleeding, as the name haemorrhoid implies, is the principal and earliest symptom. The nature of the bleeding is characteristically separate from the motion and is seen either on the paper on wiping or as a fresh splash in the pan. Very rarely, the bleeding may be sufficient to cause anaemia. Pain is not commonly associated with the bleeding and its presence should make the clinician alert to the possibility of another diagnosis; however, pain may result from congestion of pile masses below a hypertonic sphincter. Some patients describe the feeling of 'passing ground glass' as they are defaecating and itching is another common symptom. Piles associated with bleeding alone are called first-degree haemorrhoids.

Patients may complain of true 'piles', lumps that appear at the anal orifice during defaecation and which return spontaneously afterwards (second-degree haemorrhoids), piles that have to be replaced manually (third-degree haemorrhoids) (Figure 74.27) or piles that lie permanently outside (fourth-degree haemorrhoids). By this stage there is often a significant cutaneous component to the pile masses, which arise through repeated congestion and oedema. In addition to the main symptoms of pain and prolapse, patients may complain of anal irritation, which may occur as a result of mucus secretion from the caudally displaced rectal mucosa, minor leakage through a now imperfect anal seal or difficulties in cleaning after defaecation because of the irregularity of the anal verge.

Summary box 74.7

Haemorrhoids: clinical features

- Haemorrhoids or piles are symptomatic anal cushions
- They are more common when intra-abdominal pressure is raised, e.g. in obesity, constipation and pregnancy
- Classically, they occur in the 3, 7 and 11 o'clock positions with the patient in the lithotomy position
- Symptoms of haemorrhoids:
  - Bright-red, painless bleeding
  - Mucus discharge
  - Prolapse
  - Pain only on prolapse

Complications

Profuse haemorrhage is not rare. The bleeding mainly occurs externally but it may continue internally after the bleeding haemorrhoid has retracted or has been returned. In these circumstances the rectum is found to contain blood.

Summary box 74.8

Four degrees of haemorrhoids

- First degree – bleed only, no prolapse
- Second degree – prolapse but reduce spontaneously
- Third degree – prolapse and have to be manually reduced
- Fourth degree – permanently prolapsed

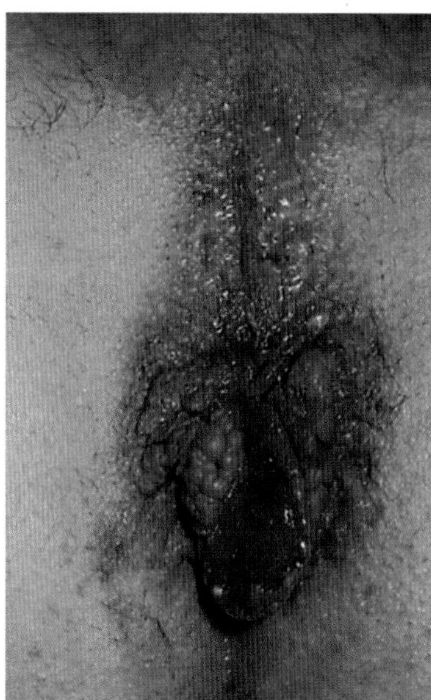

Figure 74.27 Third-degree haemorrhoids (courtesy of CV Mann, The Royal London Hospital, London, UK).

Summary box 74.9

Complications of haemorrhoids

- Strangulation and thrombosis **(Figure 74.28)**
- Ulceration
- Gangrene
- Portal pyaemia
- Fibrosis

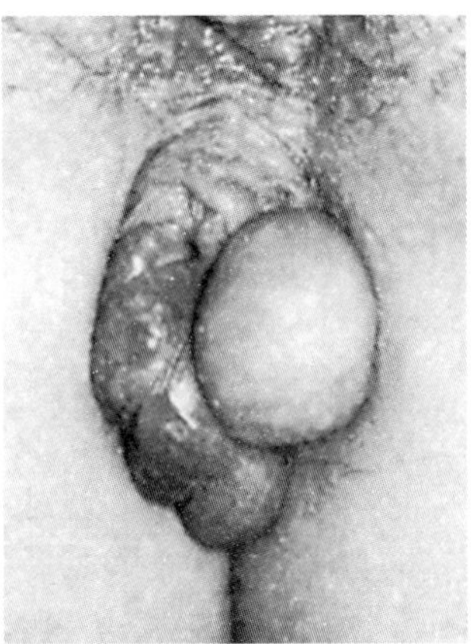

Figure 74.28 An attack of piles. Prolapsed strangulated piles, as commonly seen, on the left. A less common mass on the right with fibrofatty covering.

TREATMENT OF COMPLICATIONS

Strangulation, thrombosis and gangrene. In these cases, it was formerly believed that surgery would promote portal pyaemia. However, if adequate antibiotic cover is given from the start, this is not found to be so, and immediate surgery can be justified in some patients. The other risk if surgery is performed at this stage, that of postoperative stenosis, has resulted in many surgeons adopting a conservative approach, reviewing the situation much later and carrying out haemorrhoidectomy only if necessary. Besides adequate pain relief, bed rest with frequent hot baths and warm or cold saline compresses with firm pressure usually cause the pile mass to shrink considerably in 3–4 days (the author's preference is shrinkage through external application of small bags of frozen peas combined with the use of topical anaesthetic agents). An anal dilatation technique has in the past been used as an alternative treatment to surgery for painful 'strangulated' haemorrhoids. However, because of the risk of incontinence this is no longer advised.

Severe haemorrhage. The cause usually lies in a bleeding diathesis or the use of anticoagulants. If such causes are excluded, a local compress containing adrenaline solution, with an injection of morphine and blood transfusion if necessary, will usually suffice. However, after adequate blood replacement, ligation and excision of the piles may be required.

Management

Exclusion of other causes of rectal bleeding, especially colorectal malignancy, is the first priority. In the absence of a specific predisposing cause, important measures include attempts at normalising bowel and defaecatory habits: only evacuating when the natural desire to do so arises, adopting a defaecatory position to minimise straining, and the addition of stool softeners and bulking agents to ease the defaecatory act. Various proprietary creams can be inserted into the rectum from a collapsible tube fitted with a nozzle, at night and before defaecation. Suppositories are also useful.

In those with first- or second-degree piles whose symptoms are not improved by conservative measures, injection sclerotherapy (Mitchell), the submucosal injection of 5% phenol in arachis oil or almond oil, may be used. Any invasive treatment, however, must be with full agreement of the patient, who should be informed of the potential risks of such interventions. The aim is to create fibrosis, cause obliteration of the vascular channels and hitch up the anorectal mucosa. With the awake patient in the left lateral position and under direct vision with a proctoscope, about 5 mL of sclerosant is injected into the apex of the pile pedicle (Figure 74.29) using a disposable needle and syringe (Figure 74.30). The procedure is repeated for each pile and the patient reassessed after 8 weeks; if necessary, the injections are repeated. Pain upon injection means that the needle is in the wrong place and should be withdrawn. Injections that are too superficial are heralded by the rapid bulging of the musosa, which turns white; this leads to superficial ulceration but rarely serious septic sequelae. However, injections placed too deeply can have disastrous consequences, including pelvic sepsis, prostatitis, impotence and rectovaginal fistula.

For more bulky piles, banding has been shown to be efficacious, but it is associated with more discomfort. The Barron's bander is a commonly available device used to slip tight elastic bands onto the base of the pedicle of each haemorrhoid (Figure 74.31). The bands cause ischaemic necrosis of the piles, which slough off within 10 days; this may be associated with bleeding, about which the patient must be warned. As with sclerotherapy, three piles may be treated at one session, and the process may be repeated after several weeks if necessary. The techniques of cryotherapy (Lloyd Williams) and infrared photocoagulation (Leicester) are not often used nowadays.

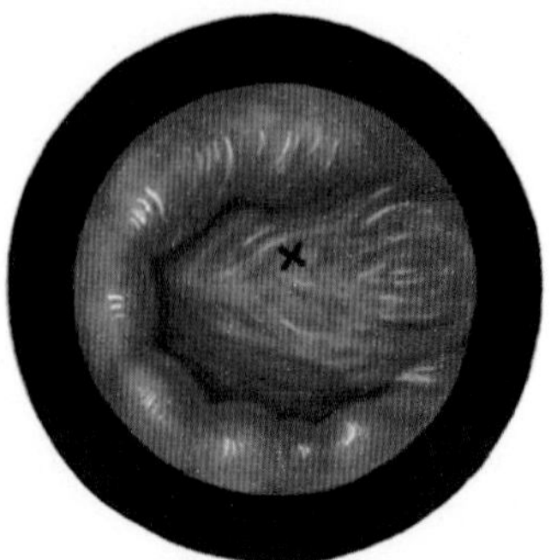

Figure 74.29 Correct site (cross) for injecting a haemorrhoid (after WB Gabriel, London, UK).

Clinton Mitchell, of Illinois, IL, USA was the first to use carbolic acid for injecting haemorrhoids. Itinerant irregular practitioners exploited the method.
John Barron, surgeon, Chicago, IL, USA.
William Bashall Gabriel, 1893–1975, surgeon, St Mark's Hospital and the Royal Northern Hospital, London, UK.
Kenneth Lloyd Williams, d. surgeon, The Royal United Hospitals, Bath, UK.
Roger James Leicester, formerly surgeon, St George's Hospital, London, UK.

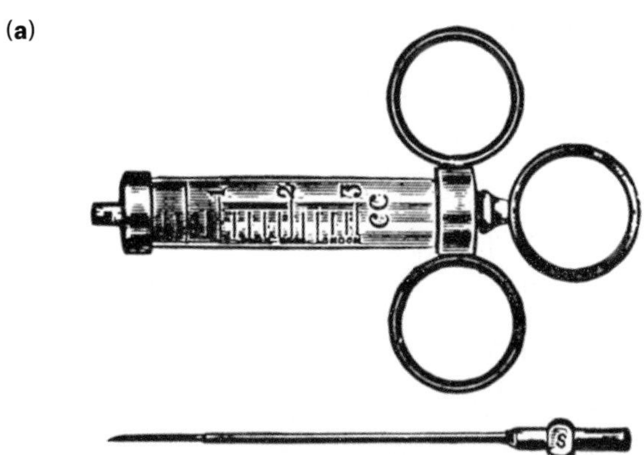

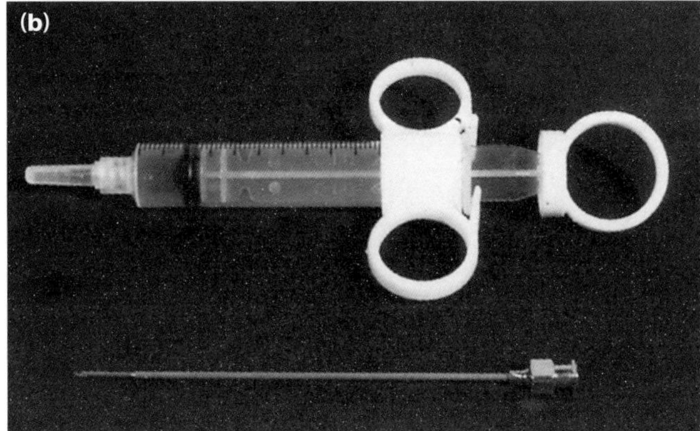

Figure 74.30 Gabriel's syringe (a) has now been replaced by disposable syringes (b).

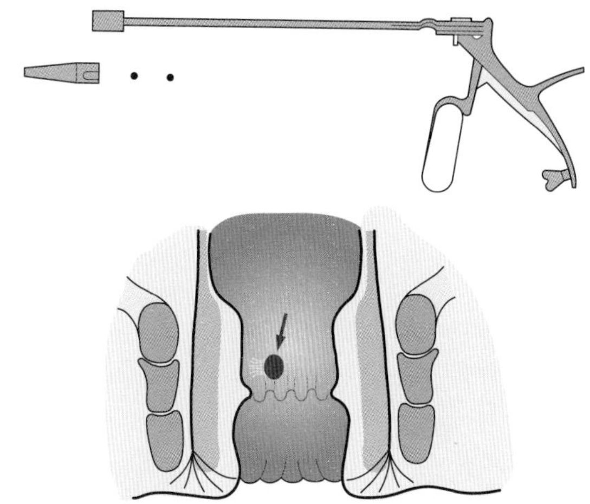

Figure 74.31 Barron's banding apparatus, with the appearance of a typical 'banded' haemorrhoid.

Operations

INDICATIONS

The indications for haemorrhoidectomy include:

- third- and fourth-degree haemorrhoids;
- second-degree haemorrhoids that have not been cured by non-operative treatments;
- fibrosed haemorrhoids;
- interno-external haemorrhoids when the external haemorrhoid is well defined.

If there is any doubt about the diagnosis of haemorrhoids, examination under anaesthesia and, if indicated, biopsy, are necessary. The other strong indication for surgery is haemorrhoidal bleeding sufficient to cause anaemia. Beyond these, the indications summarised above are more relative than absolute, because in these situations surgery aims simply to improve symptoms and, of course, is not without risk. For instance, elderly multiparous women with hypotonic sphincters who are just continent before haemorrhoidectomy may find that the procedure results in frank incontinence, a far worse condition than that for which they originally sought help.

TECHNIQUE

It is usual for the patient to have been taking stool softeners in the days before surgery and a preoperative enema to empty the rectum is administered. The procedure is usually performed under general or regional anaesthesia with the patient in the lithotomy or prone jack-knife position. The perianal skin is shaved and a formal examination performed. Haemorrhoidectomy can be performed using an open or a closed technique. The open technique is most commonly used in the UK and is known as the Milligan–Morgan operation – named after the surgeons who described it. The closed technique is the popular technique in the USA. Both involve ligation and excision of the haemorrhoid, but in the open technique the anal mucosa and skin are left open to heal by secondary intention, and in the closed technique the wound is sutured.

- **Open technique**. The anoderm and subcutaneous tissues between the pile masses may be injected with dilute adrenaline (1:300 000 dilution) to reduce bleeding and aid preservation of the skin bridges left following excision. Artery forceps are applied to the skin-covered external components of the piles and traction exerted to reveal the internal components, which are also grasped by artery forceps. When held out by the assistant these pairs of artery forceps form a triangle (Figure 74.32a). The operator takes the left lateral pair of artery forceps in the palm of the hand and places the extended forefinger in the anal canal to support the internal haemorrhoid. In this way traction is applied to the skin of the anal margin. With scissors or cutting diathermy, a V-shaped cut is made through the skin and those fibres inserting into it around the skin-holding artery forceps. Traction by both operator and assistant, combined with careful dissection, will expose the lower border of the internal sphincter. The dissection proceeds up the anal canal, with the sides of the mucosal dissection converging towards the pile apex and with the internal sphincter visible and separate from the dissected pile (Figure 74.32b). A transfixion ligature of strong Vicryl is applied to the pedicle at this level (Figure 74.32c), the pile is excised well distal to the ligature and, after ensuring haemostasis, the ligature is cut long. Each haemorrhoid is dealt with in this manner, taking care to leave mucocutaneous bridges. If there are

(a)

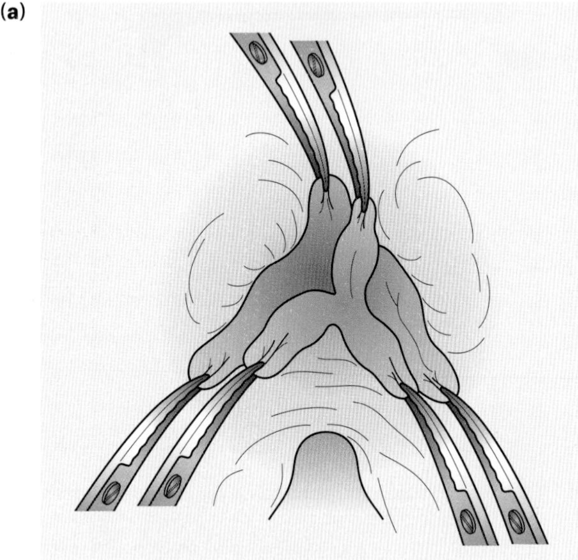

(b)

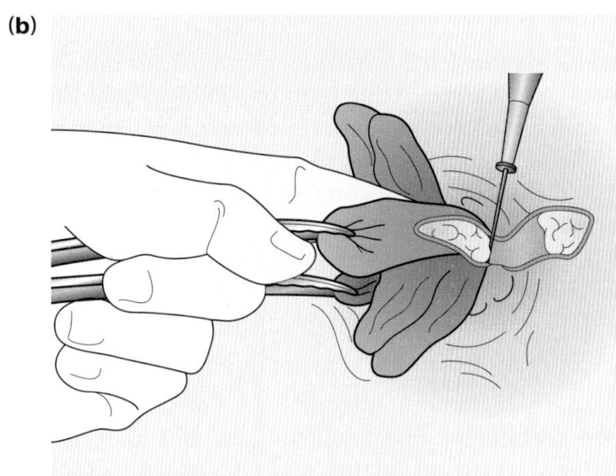

(c)

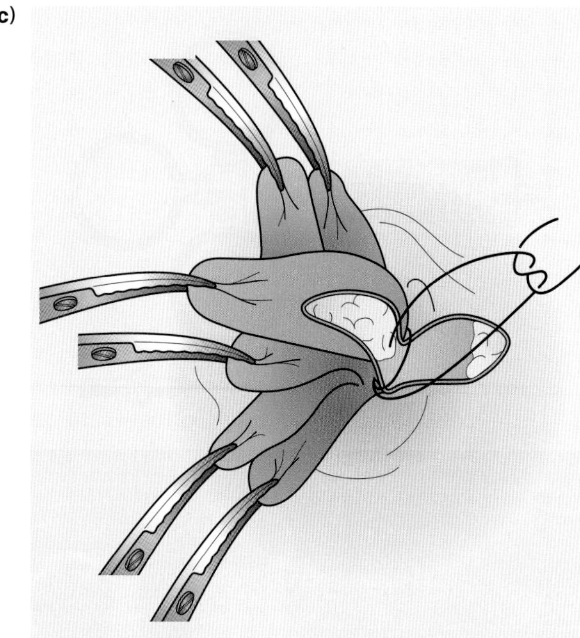

Figure 74.32 Ligation and excision of haemorrhoids. Open technique: (a) the artery forceps have been applied; (b) dissection of the left lateral pedicle; (c) transfixion of the pedicle. (Reproduced with permission from Nicholls RJ, Dozois RR. *Surgery of the colon and rectum*. Edinburgh: Churchill Livingstone, 1997.)

significant secondary haemorrhoids under these bridges they can be filleted out by scissor dissection. Haemostasis must be absolute at the end of the procedure, when a soft absorbable anal dressing is inserted. The margins of the skin wounds are trimmed so as not to leave overhanging edges (Figure 74.33). Bleeding subcutaneous arteries having been secured, the areas denuded of skin are dressed with three pieces of petroleum jelly gauze. A pad of gauze and wool and a firmly applied T-bandage complete the operation.

- **Closed technique**. The haemorrhoid is excised, together with the overlying mucosa, as illustrated in Figure 74.34. The haemorrhoid is dissected carefully from the underlying sphincter and haemostasis is achieved. The pedicle is transfixed and ligated with 3/0 Vicryl or Dexon. Any residual small haemorrhoids should be removed by filleting them out after undermining the edges of the cut mucosa. The mucosal defect is then closed completely with a continuous suture, using the same stitch that was employed to ligate the haemorrhoid pedicle. The remaining haemorrhoids are excised and ligated in a similar fashion, ensuring that there are adequate mucosal and skin bridges between each area of excision to avoid a subsequent stenosis.

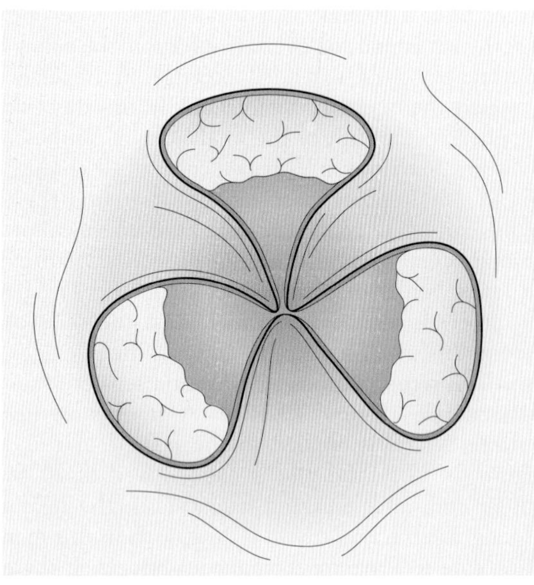

Figure 74.33 The appearance of the anus at the conclusion of the operation. (Note that to avoid stricture formation it is necessary to ensure that a bridge of skin and mucous membrane remains between each wound.) 'If it looks like a clover the trouble is over, if it looks like a dahlia, it is surely a failure.' (Reproduced with permission from Nicholls RJ, Dozois RR. *Surgery of the colon and rectum*. Edinburgh: Churchill Livingstone, 1997.)

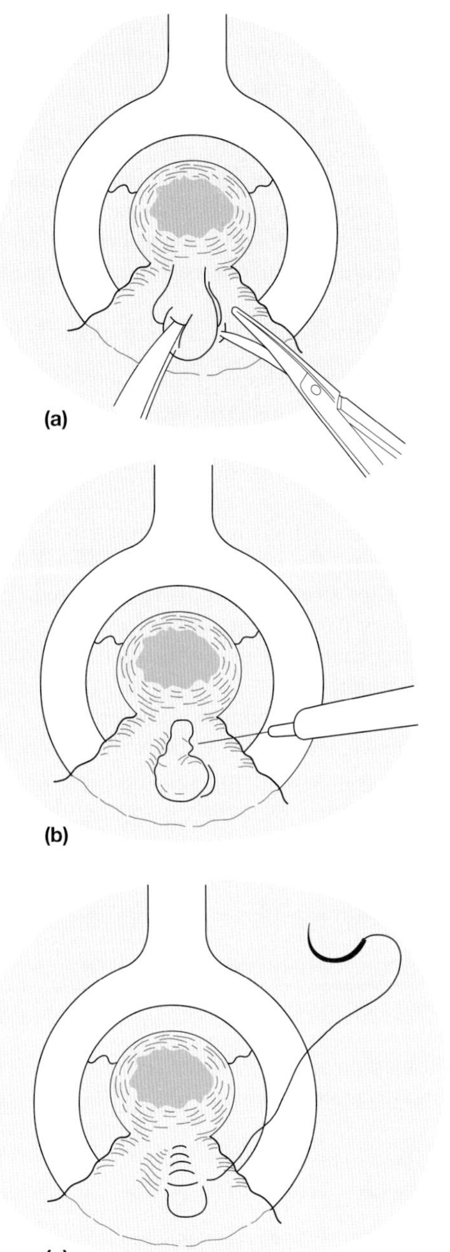

Figure 74.34 Closed technique of haemorrhoidectomy: (a) the haemorrhoidal tissue is excised; (b) bleeding is controlled by diathermy; (c) the defect is closed with a continuous suture after first undermining the anoderm on each side. (Redrawn with permission from Keighley MRB, Williams NS. *Surgery of the anus, colon and rectum*, 2nd edn. Philadelphia: WB Saunders, 1999.)

- **Stapled haemorrhoidopexy**. With the aim of symptom relief but preservation of the anal cushions, the technique of stapled haemorrhoidopexy (Longo), which utilises a purpose-designed stapling gun (PPH, Ethicon Inc.), has also been described and is widely used in Europe. This procedure excises a strip of mucosa and submucosa (together with the vessels travelling within them) circumferentially, well above the dentate line. Activation of the gun also simultaneously repairs the cut mucosa and submucosa by stapling the edges together (Figure 74.35). This procedure is quick to perform, and controlled trials suggest that it is less painful and less traumatic than conventional haemorrhoidectomy and, at least in the short term, it seems to be equally efficacious. However, evidence is emerging that the technique is associated with higher recurrence rates than following conventional haemorrhoidectomy, and associated with more additional surgery. The patient, after counselling, may or may not choose to accept a higher recurrence rate to take advantage of the short-term benefits.

TRANSANAL HAEMORRHOIDAL DEARTERIALISATION (THD) OR HAEMORRHOID ARTERY LIGATION OPERATION (HALO)

For the treatment of second- and third-degree haemorrhoids, some have recently advocated transanal Doppler-guided ligation of those vessels feeding the haemorrhoidal masses, to which others have added suture 'mucopexy' to deal with any prolapse. Long-term outcomes are unknown, but recurrence rates for fourth-degree haemorrhoids (certainly when additional procedures are not incorporated) are high. However, the complication rate and postoperative pain scores are better than with conventional surgery

Summary box 74.10

Treatment of haemorrhoids

- Symptomatic – advice about defaecatory habits, stool softeners and bulking agents
- Injection of sclerosant
- Banding
- THD /HALO/ haemorrhoidopexy
- Haemorrhoidectomy

POSTOPERATIVE CARE

In these days of economic stringencies, the patient is discharged from hospital within 1–2 days of the operation. In many countries, the procedure is often performed on a day-care basis. The patient is instructed to take two warm baths each day and is given a bulk laxative to take twice daily, together with appropriate analgesia. There is some evidence that a 5-day course of oral metronidazole may reduce pain. Dry dressings are applied as necessary, a sterile sanitary towel usually being ideal. The patient is seen again 3–4 weeks after discharge and a rectal examination is performed. If there is evidence of stenosis, the patient is encouraged to use a dilator.

POSTOPERATIVE COMPLICATIONS

Postoperative complications may be early or late. Early complications include pain, which may require opiate analgesia; retention of urine, especially in men, which rarely may need

Antonio Longo, contemporary, surgeon, Sicily, Italy.

(a)

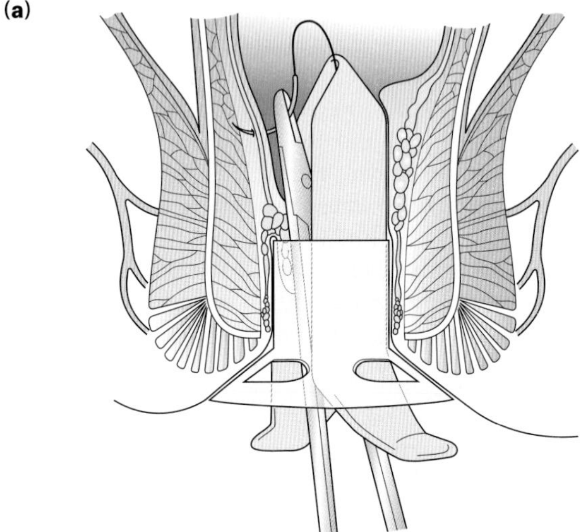

(b)

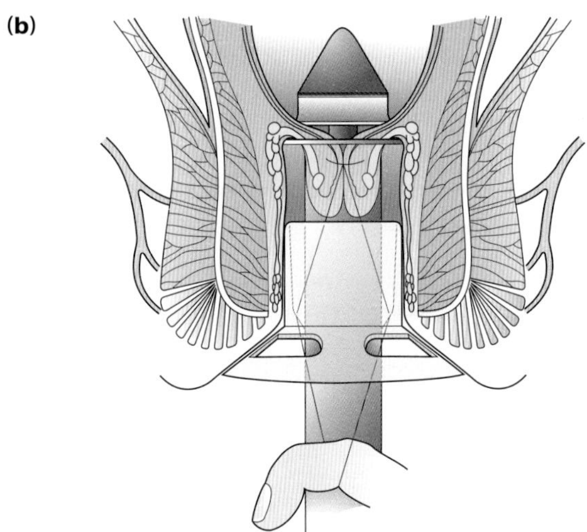

(c)

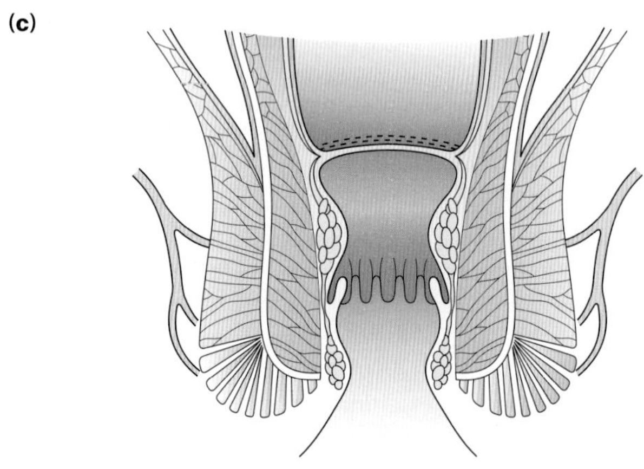

Figure 74.35 Stapled haemorrhoidectomy: (a) the purse-string suture is placed several centimetres above the dentate line; (b) the anvil of the fully opened stapling gun is inserted endoanally so that it is above the purse-string suture, which is then tied around the shaft of the gun. The gun is closed and fired; (c) after firing, a 3–4 cm strip of mucosa and submucosa containing the haemorrhoids is excised and the mucosal edges are simultaneously stapled together.

relief by catheterisation; and reactionary haemorrhage, which is much more common than secondary haemorrhage. The haemorrhage may be mainly or entirely concealed but will become evident on examining the rectum. If persistent following adequate analgesia, the patient must be taken to the operating theatre and the bleeding point secured by careful diathermy or under-running with a ligature on a needle, care being taken to avoid damage to the internal sphincter. Should a definite bleeding point not be found, the anal canal and rectum are packed.

Late postoperative complications include:

- **Secondary haemorrhage**. This is uncommon, occurring about the seventh or eighth day after operation. It is usually controlled by morphine but, if the haemorrhage is severe, an anaesthetic should be given and the bleeding controlled.
- **Anal stricture**, which must be prevented at all costs. A rectal examination at the postoperative review will indicate whether stricturing is to be expected. It may then be necessary to give a general anaesthetic and dilate the anus. After that, daily use of the dilator should give a satisfactory result.
- **Anal fissures and submucous abscesses**.
- **Incontinence**, especially if there has been inadvertent damage to the underlying internal sphincter. Although uncommon, this is obviously a very serious problem that is difficult to treat.

Summary box 74.11

Complications of haemorrhoidectomy

Early

- Pain
- Acute retention of urine
- Reactionary haemorrhage

Late

- Secondary haemorrhage
- Anal stricture
- Anal fissure
- Incontinence

External haemorrhoids

A thrombosed external haemorrhoid relates anatomically to the veins of the superficial or external haemorrhoidal plexus and is commonly termed a perianal haematoma. It presents as a sudden onset, olive-shaped, painful blue subcutaneous swelling at the anal margin and is usually consequent upon straining at stool, coughing or lifting a heavy weight (Figure 74.36). The thrombosis is usually situated in a lateral region of the anal margin. If the patient presents within the first 48 hours, the clot may be evacuated under local anaesthesia. Untreated it may resolve, suppurate, fibrose and give rise to a cutaneous tag, burst and the clot extrude, or continue bleeding. In the majority of cases, resolution or fibrosis occurs. Indeed, this condition has been called 'a 5-day, painful, self-curing lesion' (Milligan).

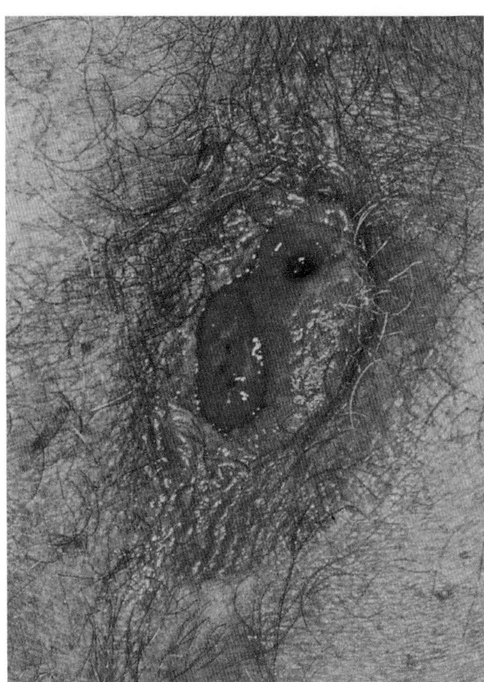

Figure 74.36 A thrombosed external haemorrhoid that has burst. There is also a mucosal prolapse, which is separate from the cutaneous lesion.

PRURITUS ANI

This is intractable itching around the anus, a common and embarrassing condition. Usually, the skin is reddened and hyperkeratotic and it may become cracked and moist.

Causes

The causes are numerous. A useful mnemonic is 'pus, polypus, parasites, piles, psyche':

- **Lack of cleanliness**, excessive sweating and wearing rough or woollen underclothing.
- An **anal or perianal discharge** that renders the anus moist. The causative lesions include an anal fissure, fistula-*in-ano*, prolapsed internal or external haemorrhoids, genital warts and excessive ingestion of liquid paraffin. A mucous discharge is an intense pruritic agent and a polyp can be the cause.
- A **vaginal discharge**, especially caused by *Trichomonas vaginalis* infection.
- **Parasitic causes**. Threadworms should be excluded, especially in young subjects. Children suffering from threadworms should wear gloves at night, lest they scratch the perianal region and are reinfested with ova by nail biting – 'parasites lost, parasites regained'. Scabies and pediculosis pubis may infest the anal region.
- **Epidermophytosis** is a common cause, especially if the skin between the toes is also infected; microscopic and cultural examinations are essential. Half-strength Whitfield's ointment quickly gives relief and is the sheet anchor of treatment.
- **Allergy** is sometimes the cause, in which case there is likely to be a history of other allergic manifestations, such as urticaria, asthma or hay fever. Antibiotic therapy may be the precipitating factor.
- **Skin diseases** localised to the perianal skin: psoriasis, lichen planus and contact dermatitis.
- **Bacterial infection**, such as intertrigo resulting from a mixed bacterial infection. Erythrasma caused by *Corynebacterium minutissimum* is responsible for some cases and its presence is detected by ultraviolet light, which induces a pink fluorescence.
- A **psychoneurosis**. It is alleged that in a few instances neurotic individuals become so immersed in their complaint that a pain–pleasure complex develops, the pleasure being the scratching. Possibly this is true, but such a syndrome should not be assumed without firm grounds for coming to this conclusion.
- **Diabetes** can sometimes present with pruritus ani, and the urine should be tested in all patients.

Treatment

The cause is treated. Symptomatic treatment includes the following:

- **Hygiene measures**. Cotton wool should be substituted for toilet paper. Soap is avoided and replaced by water alone, and the area pat-dried rather than rubbed. These measures alone, combined with wearing cotton underwear and the application of calamine lotion or zinc and castor oil, are all that is necessary to cure some cases. If there is much anal hair trapping the moisture and discharge, shaving can be very helpful.
- **Hydrocortisone**. In patients with dermatitis, and only in patients with dermatitis, the topical application of 0.5% or 1% prednisolone cream is often beneficial; sometimes after discontinuation of the therapy, the pruritus is liable to return, in which case 5% lidocaine hydrochloride (Xylocaine) ointment can be substituted for a time.
- **Strapping the buttocks** keeps moist opposing surfaces apart but is not well tolerated. If the moistness originates from anal discharge, a cotton wool anal plug will seal the anal orifice.

Operative treatment

This may be necessary for a concomitant lesion of the anorectum that is thought to initiate or contribute to the pruritus. Otherwise, surgery is not indicated.

Arthur Whitfield, 1867–1967, Professor of Dermatology, Kings College Hospital, London, UK. Whitfield's ointment is 'compound ointment of benzoic acid'.

Summary box 74.12

Pruritus ani

- Common
- Numerous causes including skin diseases, parasites (threadworm), anal discharge, allergies, diabetes
- Treat the cause if possible
- Symptomatic treatment is the mainstay

ANORECTAL ABSCESSES

Aetiology

Acute sepsis in the region of the anus is common. A fundamental distinction that has to be made is whether the sepsis is in that area by chance (simple boil, skin appendage infection) or whether it has arisen as a consequence of the presence of the anorectum, specifically the anal glands. Overall, anorectal sepsis is more common in men than women, although infections with skin-type organisms (and thus unrelated to fistula) are evenly distributed. The cryptoglandular theory of intersphincteric anal gland infection (Parks) holds that, upon infection of a gland, pus, which travels along the path of least resistance, may spread caudally to present as a perianal abscess, laterally across the external sphincter to form an ischiorectal abscess or, rarely, superiorly above the anorectal junction to form a supralevator intermuscular or pararectal abscess (depending on its relation to the longitudinal muscle), as well as circumferentially in any of the three planes: intersphincteric/intermuscular, ischiorectal or pararectal supralevator (Figure 74.37). Sepsis unrelated to anal gland infection may occur at the same or at other sites (Figure 74.38), including submucosal abscess (following haemorrhoidal sclerotherapy, which usually resolve spontaneously), mucocutaneous or marginal abscess (infected haematoma), ischiorectal abscess (foreign body, trauma, deep skin-related infection) and pelvirectal supralevator sepsis originating in pelvic disease. Underlying rectal disease, such as neoplasm and particularly Crohn's disease, may be the cause. Similarly, patients with generalised disorders, such as diabetes and acquired immunodeficiency syndrome (AIDS), may present with an anorectal abscess; in these patients, abscesses may run an aggressive course.

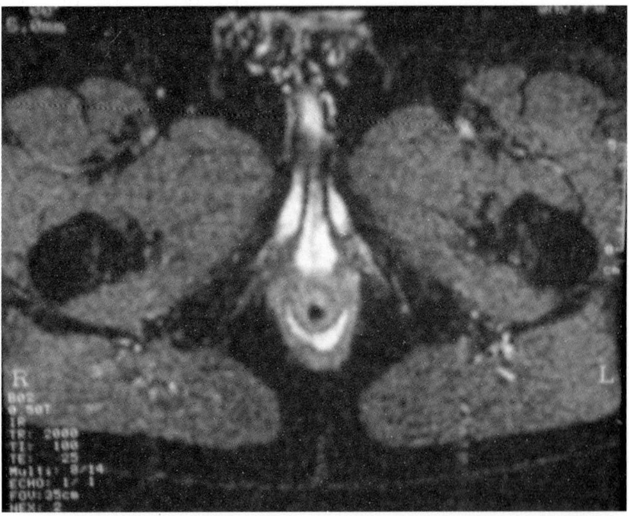

Figure 74.37 Axial magnetic resonance imaging scan (STIR sequence) showing posterior horseshoe spread of sepsis within the intersphincteric space.

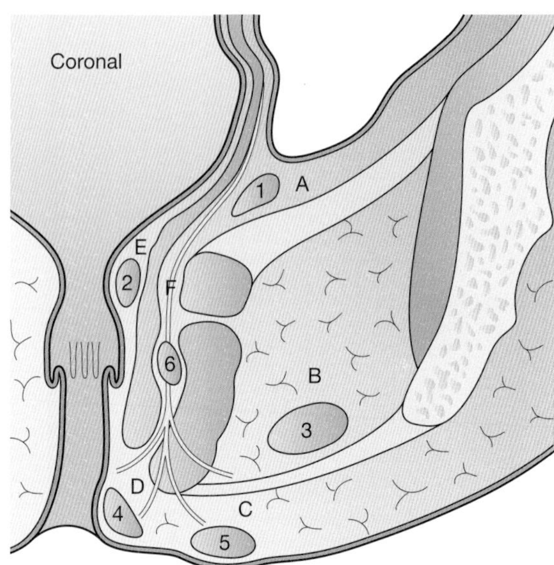

Figure 74.38 Diagram showing the spaces in relation to the anus and types of anorectal abscess in coronal section: A, pelvirectal supralevator space; B, ischiorectal space; C, perianal or superficial ischiorectal space; D, marginal or mucocutaneous space; E, submucous space; F, anorectal intermuscular (intersphincteric) space; 1, pelvirectal supralevator abscess; 2, submucous abscess; 3, ischiorectal abscess; 4, marginal abscess; 5, perianal abscess; 6, intersphincteric abscess. (Reproduced with permission from Nicholls RJ, Dozois RR. *Surgery of the colon and rectum*. Edinburgh: Churchill Livingstone, 1997.)

Presentation

A perianal abscess, confined by the terminal extensions of the longitudinal muscle, is usually associated with a short (2–3 day) history of increasingly severe, well-localised pain and a palpable tender lump at the anal margin. Examination reveals an indurated hot, tender perianal swelling. Patients with infection in the larger fatty-filled ischiorectal space, in which tissue tension is much lower, usually present later, with less well localised symptoms but more constitutional upset and fever. On examination, the affected buttock is diffusely swollen with widespread induration and deep tenderness. If sepsis is higher, deep rectal pain, fever and sometimes disturbed micturition may be the only features, with nothing evident on external examination but tender supralevator induration palpable on digital examination above the anorectal junction.

Caspar Bartholin, (Secundus), 1655–1709, Professor of Medicine, Anatomy and Physics, Copenhagen, Denmark, described these glands in 1677.
William Cowper, 1666–1709, London surgeon, described these glands in 1697.

Differential diagnosis

The only conditions with which an anorectal abscess is likely to be confused are abscesses connected with a pilonidal sinus, Bartholin's gland or Cowper's gland.

Management

Management of acute anorectal sepsis is primarily surgical, including careful examination under anaesthesia, sigmoidoscopy and proctoscopy, and adequate drainage of the pus. For perianal and ischiorectal sepsis (with an incidence of 60% and 30%, respectively), drainage is through the perineal skin, usually through a cruciate incision over the most fluctuant point, with excision of the skin edges to deroof the abscess (Figure 74.39). Pus is sent for microbiological culture (Grace) and tissue from the wall is sent for histological appraisal to exclude specific causes. With a finger in the anorectum to avoid creation of a false opening, the cavity is carefully curetted. A gentle search may be made for an underlying fistula if the surgeon is experienced, and, if obvious, a loose draining seton may be passed; injudicious probing in the acute stage is, however, potentially dangerous and may lead to a much more difficult situation. Unless by highly experienced hands, immediate fistulotomy should not be performed. After irrigation of the cavity, the wound is lightly tucked; antibiotics are prescribed if there is surrounding cellulitis and especially in those less resistant to infection, such as diabetics. If the pus subsequently cultures skin-type organisms, there will be no underlying fistula and the patient can be reassured. If gut flora are cultured, it is likely, but not inevitable, that there is an underlying fistula.

The management of supralevator sepsis is dependent upon its exact anatomy (within or outside the rectal wall) and its origin. Sepsis originating in pelvic disease necessitates appropriate management of the underlying cause (appendiceal, gynaecological, diverticular, Crohn's disease, malignancy), although intrarectal drainage may be apt to avoid creation of an extrasphincteric fistula. Cephalad extension of an intersphincteric fistula can be safely drained into the rectum, whereas supralevator extension of a transsphincteric fistula should be drained via the skin of the buttock. Rarely, a colostomy may be necessary to control severe sepsis, especially in the immunocompromised individual.

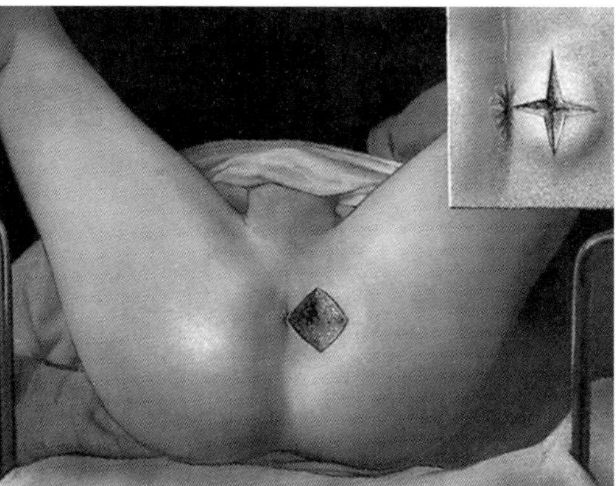

Figure 74.39 Incision of an ischiorectal abscess. The cavity is explored and, if septa exist, they should be broken down gently with a finger and the necrotic tissue lining the walls of the abscess removed by the finger wrapped in gauze. It is wise to biopsy the wall and send the pus for culture. Nothing further is done at this stage.

Summary box 74.13

Anorectal abscess

- Usually produces a painful, throbbing swelling in the anal region. The patient often has swinging pyrexia
- Subdivided according to anatomical site into perianal, ischiorectal, submucous and pelvirectal
- Underlying conditions include fistula-*in-ano* (most common), Crohn's disease, diabetes, immunosuppression
- Treatment is drainage of pus in first instance, together with appropriate antibiotics
- Always look for a potential underlying problem

FISTULA-*IN-ANO*

Aetiology

A fistula-*in-ano*, or anal fistula, is a chronic abnormal communication, usually lined to some degree by granulation tissue, which runs outwards from the anorectal lumen (the internal opening) to an external opening on the skin of the perineum or buttock (or rarely, in women, to the vagina). Anal fistulae may be found in association with specific conditions, such as Crohn's disease, tuberculosis, lymphogranuloma venereum, actinomycosis, rectal duplication, foreign body and malignancy (which may also very rarely arise within a longstanding fistula), and suspicion of these should be aroused if clinical findings are unusual. However, the majority are termed non-specific, idiopathic or cryptoglandular, and intersphincteric anal gland infection is deemed central to them.

Presentation

For reasons that are unknown, non-specific anal fistulae are more common in men than women. The overall incidence is about 9 cases per 100 000 population per year in western Europe, and those in their third, fourth and fifth decades of life are most commonly affected. Patients usually complain of intermittent purulent discharge (which may be bloody) and pain (which increases until temporary relief occurs when the pus discharges). There is often, but not invariably, a previous episode of acute anorectal sepsis that settled (incompletely) spontaneously or with antibiotics, or which was surgically drained. The passage of flatus or faeces through the external opening is suggestive of a rectal rather than an anal internal opening.

Roger Hew Grace, formerly Professor of Colorectal Surgery, The Royal Wolverhampton Hospital, Wolverhampton, UK.

Classification

The most widespread and useful classification of anal fistulae is that proposed by Parks, based on the centrality of intersphincteric anal gland sepsis (the internal opening is usually at the dentate line), which results in a primary track whose relation to the external sphincter defines the type of fistula and which influences management (Figure 74.40). Classifications based simply on level are less practical because they mean different things to different people, although the description of a fistula as high, indicating a high risk of incontinence if laid open, or low, with a lower but still some risk to function, is often used. Similarly, 'simple' and 'complex' are commonly used adjectives – complexity may be endowed by the level at which the primary track crosses the sphincters, the presence of secondary extensions or the difficulties faced in treatment. The vast majority of fistulae are intersphincteric or trans-sphincteric.

Intersphincteric fistulae (45%) do not cross the external sphincter (bar, for the purist, the most medial subcutaneous fibres running below the distal border of the internal sphincter); most commonly they run directly from the internal to the external openings across the distal internal sphincter, but may extend proximally in the intersphincteric plane to end blindly with or without an abscess, or enter the rectum at a second internal opening.

Trans-sphincteric fistulae (40%) have a primary track that crosses both internal and external sphincters (the latter at a variable level) and which then passes through the ischiorectal fossa to reach the skin of the buttock. The primary track may have secondary tracks arising from it, which often reach the roof of the ischiorectal fossa, which may rarely pass through the levators to reach the pelvis and which may spread circumferentially (horseshoe). Circumferential spread of sepsis may occur in the intersphincteric and pararectal planes, as well as in the ischiorectal plane.

Suprasphincteric fistulae are very rare, are thought by some to be iatrogenic and are difficult to distinguish from high-level trans-sphincteric tracks (for which, fortunately, management strategies are similar). Extrasphincteric fistulae run without specific relation to the sphincters and usually result from pelvic disease or trauma.

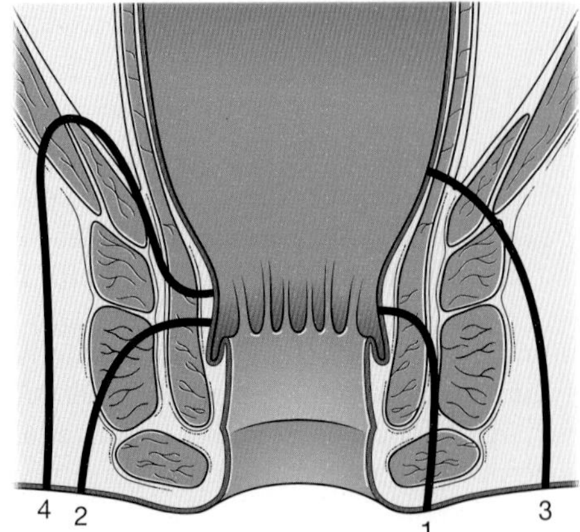

Figure 74.40 Types of anal fistula (Parks' classification): 1, intersphincteric; 2, trans-sphincteric; 3, suprasphincteric; 4, extrasphincteric primary tracks.

Clinical assessment

A full medical (including obstetric, gastrointestinal, anal surgical and continence) history and proctosigmoidoscopy are necessary to gain information about sphincter strength and to exclude associated conditions. The key points to determine are the site of the internal opening; the site of the external opening(s); the course of the primary track; the presence of secondary extensions; and the presence of other conditions complicating the fistula. Palpable induration between external opening and anal margin suggests a relatively superficial track, whereas supralevator induration suggests a primary track above the levators or high in the roof of the ischiorectal fossa, or a high secondary extension. Intersphincteric fistulae usually have an external opening close to the anal verge. Goodsall's rule (Figure 74.41), used to indicate the likely position of the internal opening according to the position of the external opening(s), is helpful but not infallible. The site of the internal opening may be felt as a point of induration or seen as an enlarged papilla. Probing in an awake patient is painful, unhelpful and can be dangerous. Full examination under anaesthesia should be repeated before surgical intervention. Dilute hydrogen peroxide, instilled via the external opening, is a very useful way of demonstrating the site of the internal opening; gentle use of probes (Figure 74.42) and a finger in the anorectum usually delineates primary and secondary tracks and their relations to the sphincters. Any concerns about fistula topography at clinical examination or examination under anaesthesia (more common after previous unsuccessful surgery) should prompt further investigations before surgical intervention.

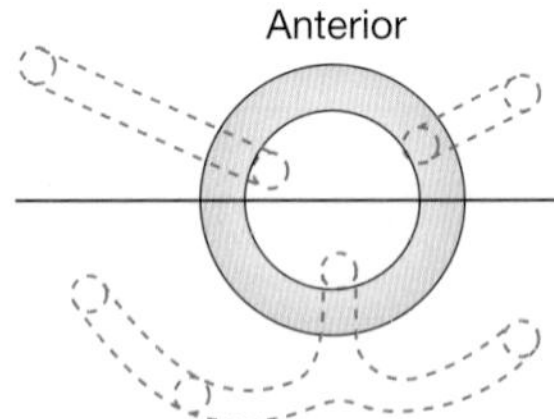

Figure 74.41 Goodsall's rule.

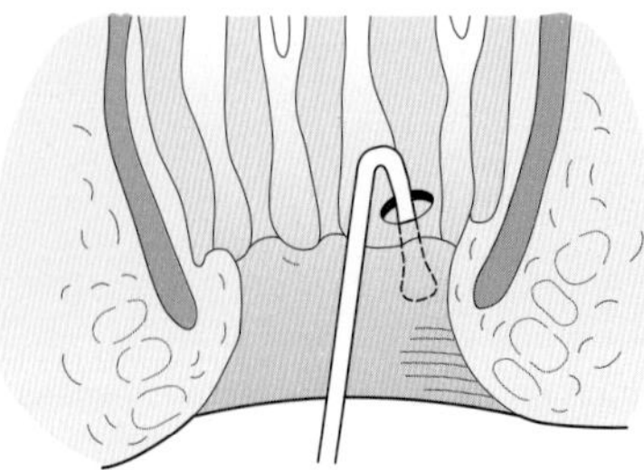

Figure 74.42 Retrograde probing of an anal canal sometimes reveals the internal orifice of the fistula.

David Henry Goodsall, 1843–1906, surgeon, St Mark's Hospital, London, UK.

Special investigations

A successful outcome after fistula surgery requires an accurate assessment of the fistula itself, the sphincter through which it passes and patient expectations (especially in terms of risk to continence). Clinical examination will give some indication of functional anal sphincter length, resting tone and voluntary squeeze; these may be more objectively assessed by manometry, whereas endoanal ultrasound gives useful information about sphincter integrity – the knowledge so gained may well influence surgical strategy. Endoanal ultrasound, especially with hydrogen peroxide, can also be used to delineate fistulae, although definition of sepsis outside or above the sphincters is limited by the probe's focal range and scarring makes interpretation difficult. Nonetheless, ultrasound, which is more accurate than clinical examination, is useful to determine whether a fistula is relatively straightforward or not. MRI is acknowledged to be the 'gold standard' for fistula imaging but it is limited by availability and cost and is usually reserved for difficult recurrent cases. The great advantage of MRI is its ability to demonstrate secondary extensions, which may be missed at surgery and which are the cause of persistence (Figure 74.43). Fistulography and computed tomography (CT) both have limitations but are useful techniques if an extrasphincteric fistula is suspected.

Surgical management

Patients with minimal symptoms, especially if they have compromised sphincters, may be managed expectantly. Eradication of sepsis requires surgery, the aim of which must be balanced with the preservation of continence. Most fistulae are relatively straightforward to deal with; however, a minority are extremely problematic and are not the realm of the 'occasional proctologist'. The multitude of strategies advocated attests to these difficult situations; comparisons between techniques are difficult to make because of the heterogeneity of patient groups, the variability in classification, the inapplicability of certain techniques in some situations, inadequate reporting of functional outcomes, inadequate follow-up and surgeon preference over-riding entry into prospective randomised trials.

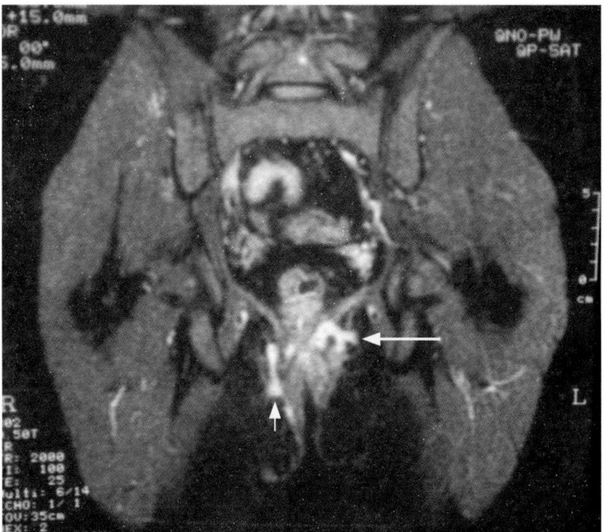

Figure 74.43 Coronal magnetic resonance imaging scan (STIR sequence) demonstrating a primary track running up the right ischiorectal space (short arrow), which then crosses the sphincters to open into the anal canal just below the puborectalis. However, there is a blind secondary extension (long arrow) passing to the contralateral side in the roof of the left ischiorectal fossa (and involving the levators), which was missed at surgery and which was the cause of fistula persistence.

Fistulotomy

That the fistulous track must be laid open from its termination to its source was a rule promulgated by John of Arderne more than 600 years ago. Fistulotomy, or laying open, is the surest way of getting rid of a fistula, but, by definition, it involves division of all those structures lying between the external and internal openings. It is therefore applied mainly to intersphincteric fistulae and trans-sphincteric fistulae involving less than 30% of the voluntary musculature (but not anteriorly-placed fistulae in women); however, even then, it is not immune to postoperative defects in continence. After full examination under anaesthesia in the lithotomy or prone jack-knife position, during which the internal opening should have been identified, a grooved fistula probe is passed from the external to the internal opening (Figure 74.44), the amount of sphincter below and above the probe is noted and, if indicated, the track is laid open over the probe. Granulation tissue is curetted and sent for histological appraisal and the wound edges are trimmed. Secondary tracks, often identified as granulation tissue that persists despite curettage, should be laid open or drained. Marsupialisation reduces wound size and speeds up healing. Primary tracks crossing the external sphincter more deeply have been managed with good outcomes by fistulotomy and immediate reconstitution of the divided muscle – failure to eradicate all sepsis and subsequent breakdown of the repair, however, are very problematic. Alternatively, a staged fistulotomy may be carried out in which secondary tracks are laid open and only part of the sphincter enclosed by the primary track is divided, with the remainder encircled by a loose seton. After sufficient time for healing of the wound and fibrosis, the seton-enclosed track is divided at a second stage.

Fistulectomy

This technique involves coring out of the fistula, usually by diathermy cautery; it allows better definition of fistula anatomy than fistulotomy, especially the level at which the track crosses the sphincters and the presence of secondary extensions. If the sphincteric component of the fistula is deemed low enough to allow safe fistulotomy, then this may proceed (at the expense of longer healing times than conventional fistulotomy). If laying open is not advisable, then the sphincteric component can be managed by another method.

John of Arderne, 1307–1390, was the first English surgeon of note. He practised at Newark-upon-Trent, Nottinghamshire and, from 1370, in London, UK. He described his operation for the treatment of fistulae in about 1376.

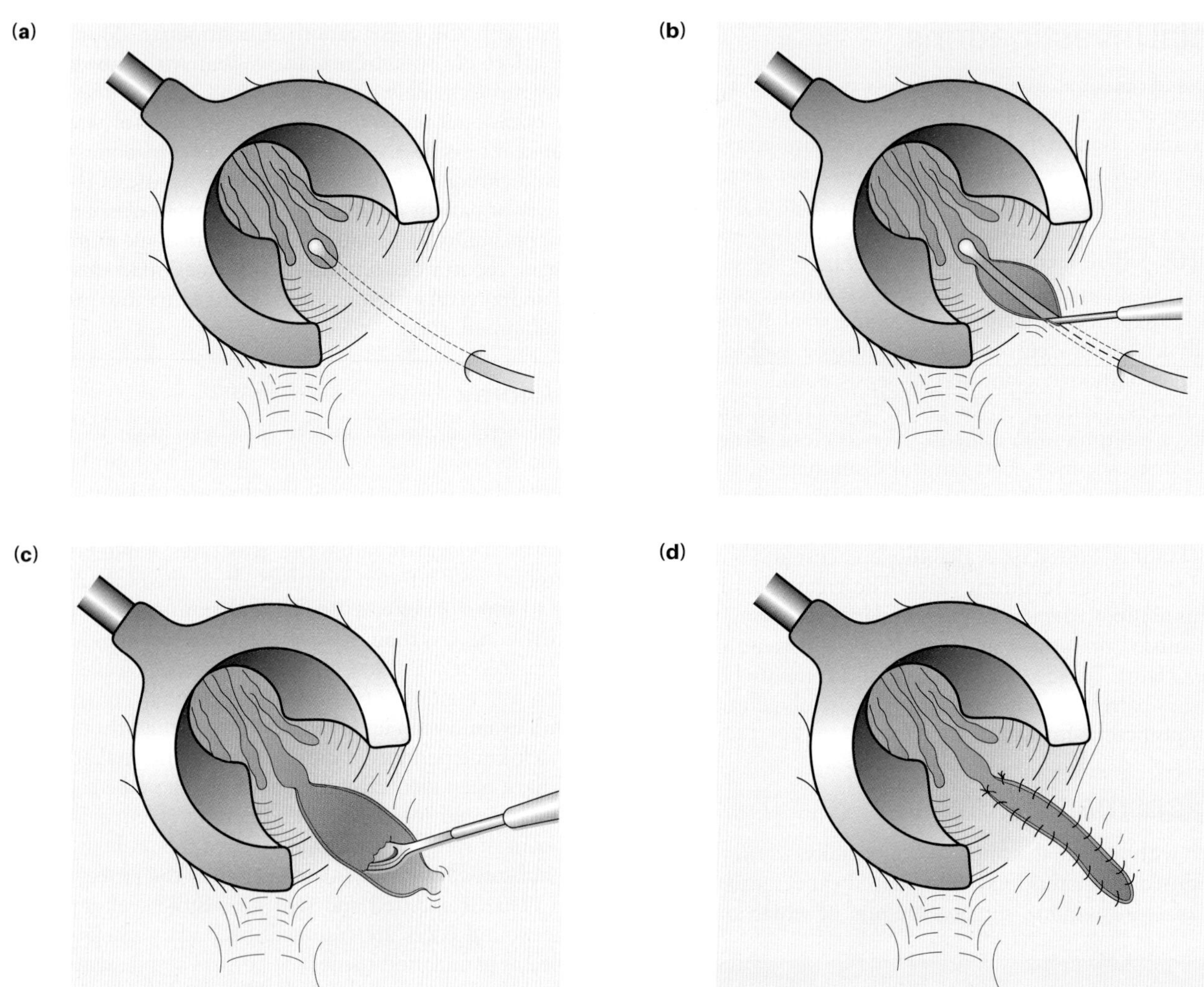

Figure 74.44 Fistulotomy. A grooved probe is passed from the external to internal openings (a) and the track laid open over the probe (b). The track is curetted to remove granulation tissue (c), the edges of the wound are trimmed and the wound may then be marsupialised (d). (Reproduced with permission from Nicholls RJ, Dozois RR. *Surgery of the colon and rectum*. Edinburgh: Churchill Livingstone, 1997.)

Ligation of intersphincteric fistula tract

Ligation of intersphincteric fistula tract (LIFT) was first described in 2006 for trans-sphincteric fistulae. The technique involves disconnection of the internal opening from the fistula tract at the level of the intersphincteric plane and removal of the residual infected glands without diving any part of the sphincter complex. The tract is then ligated and divided, the internal part is removed and the external part of the track is curretted out and drained. Hence it is a sphincter-preserving procedure, thereby maintaining continence. Success in terms of healing have been quoted at anything from 47% to 95%.

Setons

Setons (Latin: *seta* = bristle) have been used in a variety of ways in fistula surgery and it is important for surgeons to be clear about what they are trying to achieve in a particular situation. **Loose** setons are tied such that there is no tension upon the encircled tissue; there is no intent to cut the tissue. A variety of materials have been used but the seton should be non-absorbable, non-degenerative and comfortable. **Tight** or **cutting** setons are placed with the intention of cutting through the enclosed muscle.

USES OF LOOSE SETONS

- For **long-term palliation** to avoid septic and painful exacerbations by establishing effective drainage; most often in Crohn's disease and in those with problematic fistulae not wishing to countenance the possibility of incontinence.
- Used **before 'advanced' techniques** (fistulectomy, advancement flap, cutting seton); acute sepsis and secondary extensions are eradicated and a loose seton is passed across the sphincteric component of the primary track to simplify the fistula and allow fibrosis.
- As part of a **staged fistulotomy**.
- As part of a therapeutic strategy to **preserve the external sphincter** in trans-sphincteric fistulae. Secondary tracks in the ischiorectal fossa are laid open. Access to the site

where the primary track crosses the external sphincter may sometimes necessitate division of the anococcygeal ligaments to reach the deep postanal space. The internal sphincter is laid open to the level of the internal opening (or higher if there is a cephalad intersphincteric extension) to eradicate the presumed source and the sepsis in the intersphincteric space. A seton is then passed along the residual track around the denuded external sphincter and tied loosely, and the wounds are dressed. Initial postoperative management includes daily wound irrigation and light wound redressing. The seton is left in place for 3 months and, if there is evidence of good healing, simply removed. Such a strategy certainly protects against the consequences of external sphincter division, with an incidence of healing in the short term of 50–60%.

USES OF CUTTING SETONS

Cutting setons aim to achieve the high fistula eradication rates associated with fistulotomy, but without the degree of functional impairment endowed by division of the sphincters at a single stage. The enclosed muscle is gradually severed ('cheese wiring through ice') such that the divided muscles do not spring apart, and the site of the fistula track is replaced by a thin line of fibrosis as it is brought down. Some recommend prior internal sphincter division, others incorporation of the internal sphincter within the cutting seton. A variety of seton material has been used, either elastic and 'self-cutting' or non-elastic and tightened at intervals, with the sphincter being divided at varying speeds. In eastern parts of the world the same aim has been achieved by chemical cautery using an Ayurvedic method, known in India as Kshara sutra, in which a specially prepared seton thread burns through the enclosed tissue. This out-patient method has been shown to be equivalent to one-stage fistulotomy in patients with intersphincteric and distal trans-sphincteric fistulae.

Advancement flaps

When the sphincter complex is not too indurated and adequate intra-anal access can be obtained, the advancement flap technique can be employed, which aims to preserve both anatomy and function. The principles are prior elimination of acute sepsis and secondary tracks, with ideally a direct track from internal to external openings; coring out of the entire track; and closure of the communication with the anal lumen with an adequately vascularised flap consisting of mucosa and internal sphincter, sutured without tension to the anoderm, well distant from the site of the (excised) internal opening. Modifications include flap orientation (proximally or distally based) and thickness (mucosal, partial or full-thickness internal sphincter), and treatment of the external wound.

Biological agents

The functional consequences of fistulotomy and the poorer eradication rates of sphincter-preserving techniques has led to a search for agents that essentially plug and seal the track and allow ingrowth of healthy tissue to replace it. Intuitively, success must depend on the biomaterial itself and the environment into which it is placed. The poor long-term results of fibrin glue probably result from its relatively rapid resorption, and thus inadequate time for host tissue incorporation. The variable short-term results associated with porcine small intestinal submucosa may reflect early extrusion, premature degradation within an infected field, or the protocol advocated for its use, which does not include meticulous eradication of secondary extensions, or the lining of the primary tack itself, whether epithelial or granulation tissue. Cross-linked porcine dermal collagen has also, more recently, been studied, but only short-term outcomes (albeit optimistic) are known. Research into biological agents must continue.

Summary box 74.14

Anorectal fistulae

- Are common and may be simple or complex
- Are classified according to their relationship to the anal sphincters
- May be associated with underlying disease such as tuberculosis or Crohn's disease
- Laying open is the surest method of eradication, but sphincter division may result in incontinence

HIDRADENITIS SUPPURATIVA

This is a chronic suppurative condition of apocrine gland-bearing skin, which is found in the axillae, submammary regions, nape of the neck, groin, mons pubis, inner thighs and sides of the scrotum, as well as the perineum and buttocks, and is a source of considerable physical and psychological morbidity. There is no confirmatory test or specific characteristic for diagnosis, which makes definition difficult. Acne, pilonidal sinus and chronic scalp folliculitis may coexist with hidradenitis suppurativa in the condition 'follicular occlusion tetrad'.

Pathology

Occlusion of gland ducts leads to bacterial proliferation, gland rupture and spread of infection and epithelial components into the surrounding soft tissue and to adjacent glands. Secondary infection (with *Staphylococcus aureus*, *Streptococcus milleri* and anaerobes) causes further local extension, skin damage and deformity, with multiple communicating subcutaneous fistulae. There is some evidence that the disease may be related to a relative androgen excess.

Presentation

The condition is not seen before puberty and rarely presents after the fourth decade of life. Overall, it is three times more

The Ayurvedic method is derived from the Ayurveda, the most ancient system of Hindu medicine, whose origin is ascribed to Brahma and dates from circa 1400 to 1200BC.

common in women than men, although anogenital disease is more common in men, and obesity is a common association. When affecting the perineum, lesions begin as multiple raised boils, with recurrent lesions within the same vicinity leading to sinus tract formation, bridged scarring and multiple points of discharge. Rarely, it may involve the anal canal anoderm but it does not extend above the dentate line or involve the sphincter muscles themselves.

Differential diagnosis

In the early stages distinction from furunculosis can be difficult. Crohn's disease, cryptoglandular fistula, pilonidal sinus, tuberculosis, actinomycosis, lymphogranuloma venereum and granuloma inguinale must be considered when later stages present.

Treatment

In the early stages, general measures, including weight reduction and antiseptic soaps, may be helpful. Antibiotics may induce remission but often the disease relapses and progresses, at which point surgery is indicated. Inadequate treatment may lead to prolonged morbidity, but any surgery should be less debilitating than the condition. Surgical intervention ranges from simple incision and drainage of acute sepsis to radical excision of all apocrine gland-bearing skin. Careful laying open of all tracts, possibly as a staged procedure according to anatomical location, is an option that appeals to many patients. Radical excision requires closure by skin graft or rotation flap and, occasionally, a defunctioning colostomy to allow healing.

CONDYLOMATA ACCUMINATA (ANAL WARTS)

There is increasing evidence that sexually-transmitted infection with human papillomavirus (HPV) forms the aetiological basis of anal and perianal warts, anal intraepithelial neoplasia (AIN) and squamous cell carcinoma of the anus. In areas of the world where sexual promiscuity (especially anal intercourse) is more common, and in immunocompromised individuals (HIV-infected individuals and transplant recipients), there have been dramatic increases in the incidence of these conditions over the last 30 years, most importantly of AIN and anal cancers. Similar virally-induced changes have been noted in the genital tracts of women (vulval intraepithelial neoplasia (VIN), cervical intraepithelial neoplasia (CIN) and cancers). It is essential to examine all areas of the genitalia and perineum in an affected person as there is often a field change with the virus affecting any squamous epithelium in that area. There are over 170 subtypes of HPV, but certain subtypes (16, 18, 31, 33) are associated with a greater risk of progression to dysplasia and malignancy. Squamous cell carcinoma (SCC) is associated with HPV (especially subtypes 16, 18, 31 or 33).

Condylomata accuminata is the most common sexually-transmitted disease encountered by colorectal surgeons and is most frequently observed in homosexual men. Associated warts on the penis and along the female genital tract are common.

Presentation

Many are asymptomatic but pruritus, discharge, bleeding and pain are usual presenting complaints. In the early stages, examination reveals separate pinkish-white warts close to the anal margin and also often on the anoderm within the distal anal canal. Later, the warts enlarge, coalesce and carpet the skin. Rarely, relentless growth results in giant condylomata (Buschke–Löwenstein tumour), which may obliterate the anal orifice. The diagnosis is aided by aceto-whitening upon application of acetic acid but confirmed by biopsy, which will also indicate the presence or absence of dysplasia.

Treatment

Because of the field effect endowed by viral skin infection, long-term resolution can be problematic. Careful serial application of 25% podophyllin to discrete warts on the perianal skin is often used; however, it cannot be used intra-anally. Surgical excision under local, regional or general anaesthesia involves raising and separating the lesions with local infiltration of dilute adrenaline, which allows more accurate scissor or electrocautery excision to maximise the preservation of normal skin.

ANAL INTRAEPITHELIAL NEOPLASIA

AIN (Figure 74.45) is a multifocal virally-induced dysplasia of the perianal or intra-anal epidermis, which is associated with HPV (most frequently subtypes 6, 11, 16 and 18; subtypes 6 and 11 are most often associated with warts and early AIN, whereas subtypes 16 and 18 account for more than 75% of anal cancers). The prevalence is <1% of the population

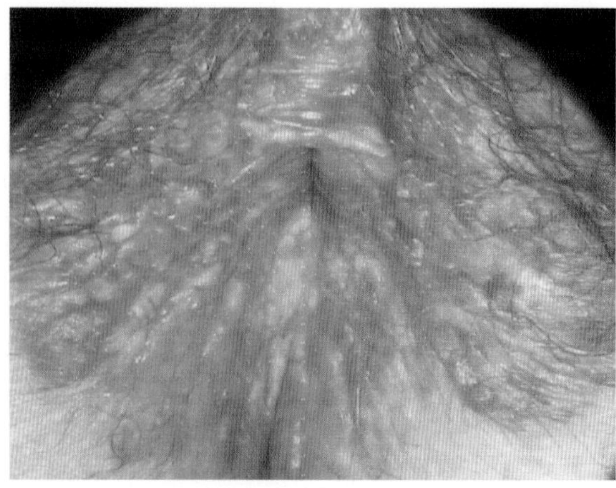

Figure 74.45 Extensive anal intraepithelial neoplasia, which extends intra-anally.

Abraham Buschke, 1868–1943, German dermatologist.
LW Löwenstein described this condition in 1939.

with a rising incidence especially in those areas where anoreceptive intercourse and HIV are prevalent. At-risk groups include patients with HIV as well as immunocompromised patients, women with a history of other genital intraepithlieal neoplasia (VIN and CIN) and patients with extensive anogenital condylomata. Patients may be asymptomatic and the diagnosis is often a histological surprise, although increasing numbers in high-risk groups are picked up on anal cytology. It is classified according to the degree of dysplasia on biopsy into AIN I, AIN II and AIN III, according to the lack of keratocyte maturation and extension of the proliferative zone from the lower third (AIN I) to the full thickness of the epithelium (AIN III), in the same manner as cervical or vulval dysplasia. The natural history is uncertain but progression from AIN II to AIN III to invasive carcinoma has been observed, notably in the immunocompromised. The term Bowen's disease should probably be avoided.

Presentation

Around 10% of AIN lesions are diagnosed by the pathologist after excision of abnormal skin lesions. Low-grade lesions may be raised and similar to anal condylomata; however, AIN III lesions are more often flat and may be white, grey, purple or brown in colour. Ulceration would suggest progression to invasive anal carcinoma. Patients' symptoms include pruritis, pain, bleeding and discharge. AIN is present in 28–35% of excised anal warts. Approximately 10% of AIN III lesions will progress to anal carcinoma at 5 years. Regression of AIN III rarely occurs, but AIN I and AIN II may regress. The association between AIN III and carcinoma is strengthened by the findings of AIN III in 80% of anal cancer biopsies.

Diagnosis and management

A high index of suspicion and targeted biopsy yields the diagnosis, whereas multiple (mapping) biopsies give an indication of the extent and overall severity of the disease. AIN II and III should be regularly monitored clinically and, if necessary, by repeat biopsy to exclude invasive disease. Specialised centres may offer colposcopy of the anus (anoscopy) utilising 5%acetic acid with Lugol's iodine to assess *in vivo* the dysplastic areas of the anus. The affected areas show up white and can be biopsied. Focal disease may be excised and local excision is effective for lesions <30% of the circumference of the anus. More widespread disease can be dealt with surgically by wide local excision and closure of the resultant defect by flap or skin graft, with or without covering colostomy (especially if there is intra-anal disease). However, for a condition with uncertain malignant potential, this approach should be used with caution as it carries with it significant morbidity. It is important to remember that female patients are at risk of other anogenital intraepithlieal neoplasia; it is recommended that those with AIN III have a yearly cervical smear test.

Topical imiquimod, 5% or oral retinoids have some effect on the progression of dysplasia and can cause regression by at least two histological grades. Other newer options may include anti-HPV treatment; vaccination may reduce the incidence long term.

NON-MALIGNANT STRICTURES – ANAL STENOSIS

Spasmodic

An anal fissure causes spasm of the internal sphincter. Rarely, a spasmodic stricture accompanies secondary megacolon, possibly as a result of the chronic use of laxatives.

Organic

Anal stenosis is a rare but serious complication of anorectal surgery, 90% are seen after haemorrhoidectomy. Other causes included trauma, inflammatory bowel disease, radiation treatment, sexually-transmitted disease, tuberculosis and some skin conditions, e.g scleroderma.

Postoperative stricture

This sometimes follows a haemorrhoidectomy performed incorrectly. Removal of excess anoderm and mucosa without adequate skin bridges can lead to scarring and structuring. Stenosis can be seen after stapled haemorrhoidopexy (0.8–5%) and low coloanal anastomoses, especially if a stapling gun is used, but these are really low rectal stenoses.

Irradiation stricture

This is an aftermath of irradiation and is particularly seen after chemoradiation for anal carcinoma, when a wide are of skin and anoderm are irradiated. It can be seen after irradiation for any pelvic tumours.

Senile anal stenosis

A condition of chronic internal sphincter contraction is sometimes seen in the elderly. Increasing constipation is present, with pronounced straining at stool. Faecal impaction is liable to occur. The muscle is rigid and feels like a tight rubber ring. There is no evidence of a fissure-*in-ano*. The treatment is dilatation at frequent intervals.

Lymphogranuloma inguinale

This is by far the most frequent cause of a tubular inflammatory stricture of the rectum and 80% of the sufferers are women. Frei's reaction is usually positive. This variety of rectal stricture is particularly common in black populations and may be accompanied by elephantiasis of the labia majora. In the early stages, antibiotic treatment may lead to cure. In advanced cases, excision of the rectum is required.

John Templeton Bowen, 1857–1941, Professor of Dermatology, Harvard University Medical School, Boston, MA, USA, described this intradermal precancerous skin lesion in 1912.

Wilhelm Sigmund Frei, 1885–1943, Professor of Dermatology, the State Hospital, Spandau, Berlin, who later settled in New York, NY, USA, described his test for lymphogranuloma inguinale in 1925.

Inflammatory bowel disease

Stricture of the anorectum may complicate Crohn's disease and, in this instance, the stricture is annular and often more than one is present. These stenoses are characterised by transmural scarring and inflammation. Occasionally, an anal stricture may occur in ulcerative colitis. Until a biopsy is obtained, a carcinoma should be suspected if a stricture is found.

Endometriosis

Endometriosis of the rectovaginal septum may present as a stricture. There is usually a history of frequent menstrual periods with severe pain during the first 2 days of the menstrual flow.

Neoplastic

When free bleeding occurs after dilatation of a supposed inflammatory stricture, carcinoma should be suspected (Grey Turner) and a portion of the stricture should be removed for biopsy. Sometimes in these cases, repeated biopsies show inflammatory tissue only. If, however, the symptoms show a marked progression, malignancy should be strongly suspected.

Clinical features

Increasing difficulty in defaecation is the leading symptom. The patient finds that increasingly large doses of aperients are required and, if the stools are formed, they are 'pipe-stem' in shape. In cases of inflammatory stricture, tenesmus, bleeding and the passage of mucopus are superadded. Sometimes the patient comes under observation only when subacute or acute intestinal obstruction has supervened.

Rectal examination

The finger encounters a sharply-defined shelf-like interruption of the lumen. If the calibre is large enough to admit the finger, it should be noted whether the stricture is annular or tubular. Sometimes this point can be determined only after dilatation. A biopsy of the stricture must be taken. Often the examination will be painful and needs to be performed under general anaesthesia when biopsies and gentle, graduated dilatation may be undertaken.

Treatment

Before starting treatment it is important to ascertain the cause of the stricture. If associated with Crohn's disease an anoplasty is contraindicated. Non-operative treatment is recommended for mild stenosis. The use of stool softeners and fibre supplements helps aid the passage of stools.

Prophylactic

The passage of an anal dilator during convalescence after haemorrhoidectomy greatly reduces the incidence of postoperative stricture. Efficient treatment of lymphogranuloma inguinale in its early stages should lessen the frequency of stricture from that cause.

Dilatation

Anal dilatation can be performed under general anaesthesia and then, by the patient, using an anal dilator. For anal and many rectal strictures, dilatation at regular intervals is all that is required.

Anoplasty

For severe anal stenosis, an anoplasty is used to replace loss of anal tissue. The stricture is incised and a rotation or advancement flap of skin and subcutaneous tissue replaces the defect and enlarges the anal orifice (Figure 74.46). This technique is particularly useful for postoperative strictures.

Colostomy

Colostomy must be undertaken when a stricture is causing intestinal obstruction and in advanced cases of stricture complicated by fistulae-*in-ano*. In selected cases, this can be followed by restorative resection of the stricture-bearing area. If this step is anticipated, a loop ileostomy is constructed.

Rectal excision and coloanal anastomosis

When the strictures are at, or just above, the anorectal junction and are associated with a normal anal canal, but irreversible changes necessitate removal of the area, excision can be followed by a coloanal anastomosis, with good functional results.

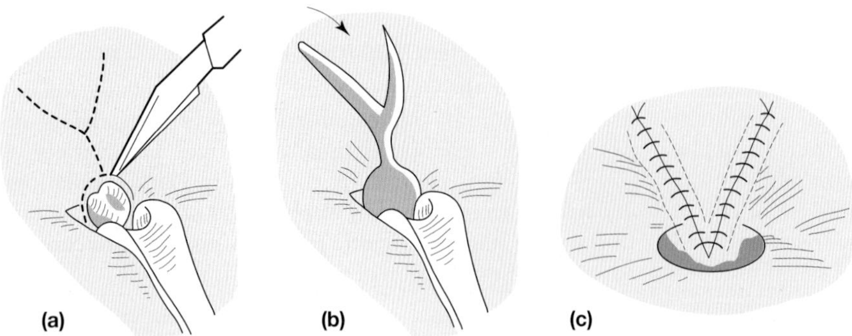

Figure 74.46 (a–c) Y–V advancement flap for anal stenosis.

George Grey Turner, 1877–1951, Professor of Surgery, University of Durham, Durham (1927–1934) and then at the Postgraduate Medical School, London, UK (1934–1945).

Summary box 74.15

Benign anal stricture

- May be spasmodic or organic
- May be iatrogenic, e.g. after haemorrhoidectomy or repair of imperforate anus
- Biopsy must be taken to rule out malignancy
- Can usually be managed by regular dilatation
- Severe anal stenosis may require surgical treatment by an anoplasty

MALIGNANT TUMOURS

Malignant lesions of the anus and anal canal

Anal malignancy is rare and accounts for less than 2% of all large bowel cancers. The crude incidence rate is 0.65 per 100 000. Those arising below the dentate line are usually squamous, whereas those above are variously termed basaloid, cloacogenic or transitional. Collectively they are known as epidermoid carcinomas, and account for >70% of anal malignancies; management and prognosis is similar for this group. Adenocarcinomas are the next commonest. Other tumours include melanoma, lymphoma, and sarcoma.

Squamous cell carcinoma

Although rare, the incidence of anal SCC is rising, with a direct association with HPV infection, AIN and immunosuppression. In the UK in 2012, there were over 1200 new anal cancer cases, with a male:female ratio of 1:2 and 307 deaths from anal cancer. Anal SCC is associated with HPV (especially subtypes 16, 18, 31 or 33) in 70–90% of cases (Figure74.47). Patients at increased risk are those with HIV infection, recipients of organ transplants (renal transplant patients have a 100-fold increased risk) and those with a past history of cancers at 'sexually accessible' sites (usually genital). Pain and bleeding are the most common symptoms and the disease is thus often initially misdiagnosed as a benign condition, highlighting the need for a level of suspicion and adequate examination. A mass, pruritus or discharge is less common. Advanced tumours may cause faecal incontinence by invasion of the sphincters and, in women, anterior extension may result in anovaginal fistulation. On examination, anal margin tumours look like malignant ulcers. There may be associated HPV lesions. Anal canal tumours are palpable as irregular indurated tender ulceration. Sphincter involvement may be evident.

MANAGEMENT

Historically, early anal margin tumours were treated by local excision and anal canal tumours by abdominoperineal excision of the rectum. Nowadays, primary treatment is by chemoradiotherapy (combined modality therapy (CMT); Nigro), the chemotherapy usually including a combination of

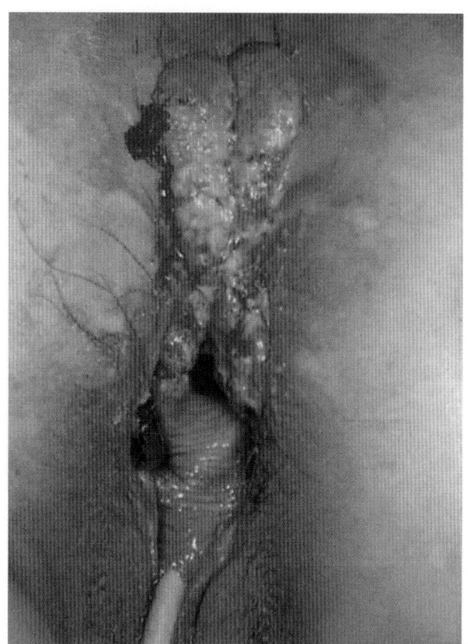

Figure 74.47 Neglected papillomas of the anus that have become malignant.

5-fluorouracil (5-FU) with mitomycin C or cisplatin. Metastases are rare at presentation (5%) and treatment is aimed at local control. Initial staging involves a clinical examination and biopsy of the primary tumour as well as examination of inguinal nodes. Local staging is by MRI scanning and CT is used to assess lungs and abdomen for metasatic spread. Positron emission tomography (PET) CT may help in equivocal inguinal node assessment. The surgeon has an important role in management: initial diagnosis is surgical; small marginal tumours are still best treated by local excision; radical surgery is indicated in those with persistent or recurrent disease following CMT; and a defunctioning stoma may be indicated for those in whom treatment and disease regression is associated with radionecrosis, incontinence or fistula. Despite good results with chemoradiotherapy, 20–25% of patients will have local disease relapse. After thorough assessment, these patients may require radical abdominoperineal resection, including excision of the posterior wall of the vagina in 70% of women and reconstruction of the perineum using myocutaneous flaps.

Other anal malignancies

Adenocarcinomata within the anal canal are usually extensions of distal rectal cancers. Rarely, adenocarcinoma may arise from anal glandular epithelium or develop within a long-standing (usually complex) anal fistula; treatment is as for low rectal cancers (i.e. abdominoperineal excision of the rectum (APER) with or without previous radiotherapy or chemoradiotherapy) but prognosis is less good. Melanocytes can be found in the transitional zone of the anal canal. Malignant melanoma of the anus is very rare and usually presents as a bluish-black soft mass that may mimic a thrombosed external

Norman D Nigro, 1912–2009, surgeon, Wayne State University, Detroit, MI, USA.

pile, although it may be amelanotic (Figure 74.48). The prognosis, irrespective of treatment, is extremely poor. Perianal Paget's disease is exceedingly rare.

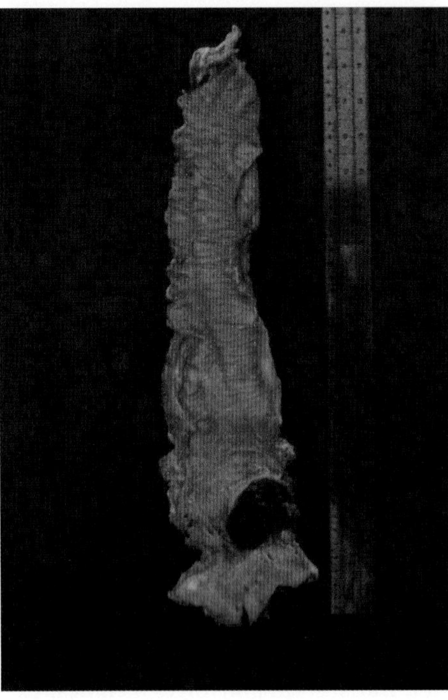

Figure 74.48 Malignant melanoma of the anal canal (courtesy of Mr B Thomas, Kalushi, Zambia).

Summary box 74.16

Anal cancer

- Uncommon tumour, which is usually a squamous cell carcinoma
- Associated with human papilloma virus
- More prevalent in patients with human immunodeficiency virus infection
- May affect the anal verge or anal canal
- Lymphatic spread is to the inguinal lymph nodes
- Treatment is by chemoradiotherapy in the first instance
- Major ablative surgery is required if the above fails

FURTHER READING

Chu CS, Pfister DG. Opportunities and challenges: human papillomavirus and cancer. *J Natl Compr Canc Netw* 2017; **15**(5S): 726–9.

Cross KL, Massey EJ, Fowler AL *et al.* The management of anal fissure: ACPGBI position statement. *Colorectal Dis* 2008; **10** Suppl 3: 1–7.

Geh I, Gollins S, Renehan A *et al.* Association of coloproctology of Great Britain & Ireland (ACPGBI): Guidelines for the management of cancer of the colon, rectum and anus (2017) – Anal Cancer. *Colorectal Dis* 2017; **19** Suppl 1: 82–97.

Keighley MRB, Williams NS, *Surgery of the anus, rectum and colon*, 3rd edn. Philadelphia: Saunders, 2008.

Williams JG, Farrands PA, Williams AB *et al.* The treatment of anal fistula: ACPGBI position statement. *Colorectal Dis* 2007; **9** Suppl 4: 18–50.

Sir James Paget, 1814–1899, surgeon, St Bartholomew's Hospital, London, UK, described this disease in 1874.

PART 12

Genitourinary

75 Urinary symptoms and investigations 1374
76 Kidneys and ureters 1398
77 The urinary bladder 1423
78 The prostate and seminal vesicles 1456
79 Urethra and penis 1477
80 Testis and scrotum 1497
81 Gynaecology 1513

Chapter 75

Urinary symptoms and investigations

Learning objectives

- To understand the significance of pain relating to urinary tract pathology
- To understand the difference between renal pain and ureteric colic
- To understand the definitions of common lower urinary tract symptoms
- To be able to select the appropriate diagnostic tests to establish a diagnosis of urinary tract disease

PAIN

Pain is a common urological symptom and can be due to pathology in any of the component parts of the urinary tract. **Pain passing urine** is called **dysuria** and refers to the discomfort localised to the outlet of the bladder which is experienced during voiding – typically described as a sensation akin to passing razor blades or glass. Most commonly, dysuria is due to an infection in the lower urinary tract but can be a symptom of more serious pathology such as bladder cancer or carcinoma in situ (CIS) of the bladder especially in an older male smoker with haematuria.

Renal pain is usually caused by distension of the renal capsule and is felt as a constant, gnawing pain in the loin/renal angle. **Ureteric colic** (often incorrectly referred to as renal colic) is different from renal pain and is typified by the lateralised, colicky pain experienced by someone who has a ureteric calculus. Ureteric colic can radiate to the groin or lower still to the testicle/labium but does not radiate to the back of the leg. Ureteric colic can be caused by something other than a stone in the ureter, such as a blood clot or, rarely, a sloughed renal papilla. If the history is carefully taken, it will be apparent that some patients simultaneously experience both ureteric colic and renal pain.

Disease processes in the bladder, e.g. infection or inflammation, can produce **suprapubic pain**. Suprapubic bladder pain, which is experienced when the bladder is full and is relieved by micturition, is typical of interstitial cystitis, an idiopathic benign inflammatory disorder of the bladder typically seen in middle-aged females (see Chapter 77).

Testicular pain is a common symptom in men, especially in early middle-age. Sudden severe testicular pain in younger men (<40 years old) should be treated as a medical emergency and the patient assessed so that a diagnosis of acute testicular torsion can be excluded. The time interval from the onset of pain to the diagnosis of suspected testicular torsion should not influence whether scrotal exploration is performed as torsion/detorsion may be occurring and the testis may still be salvageable after a delayed time interval. Hydrocoeles and epididymal cysts usually do not cause significant pain but can have an increasing pressure effect as they enlarge. A dragging sensation in the scrotum which gets worse towards the end of the day is typical of the discomfort associated with a varicocoele, often on the left side. Typically, testicular tumours in young males are not associated with significant pain. Investigation of testicular pain in the young adult male/middle-aged male is frequently negative, resulting in a highly unsatisfactory diagnostic label of 'idiopathic testicular pain' which is subsequently managed with the input of other clinicians, most commonly pain management specialists. Patients undergoing vasectomy are routinely counselled of the approximate 10% risk of testicular pain in the short term following surgery but more importantly the 1% chance of chronic testicular pain in the longer term.

Perineal pain is often a feature of a complex of symptoms typically seen in middle-aged men who, by a process of exclusion, are diagnosed as suffering from acute or chronic

Summary box 75.1

Pain from the urinary tract

- Renal pain is not synonymous with renal colic
- Renal colic is a misnomer and should be referred to as ureteric colic
- Renal pain can be distinguished from ureteric colic by careful history taking
- Renal pain and ureteric colic may be experienced simultaneously
- Ureteric colic may radiate to the groin/testicle/labium
- Ureteric colic does not radiate to the chest or the back of the leg

prostatitis. With prostatitis, perineal pain may be accompanied by suprapubic pain, low back pain which radiates to the legs, penile pain as well as frequency of micturition and dysuria. Perineal pain is an ominous symptom after previous treatment for a pelvic malignancy, often signifying recurrent pelvic disease.

LOWER URINARY TRACT SYMPTOMS (LUTS)

The International Continence Society (ICS) provides the internationally accepted definitions for symptoms relating to lower urinary tract function:

- **Frequency** is the complaint by the patient who considers that he/she voids too often during the day. The patient may report needing to void more frequently than is their usual habit or more frequently than they consider is socially acceptable.
- **Nocturia** is the complaint that the individual needs to wake at night at least once to void.
- **Strangury** is a sensation of constantly needing to void. Typically, the patient describes having to stand/sit for long periods with the sensation that micturition is imminent. Strangury is most commonly due to a lower urinary tract infection (UTI).
- **Urgency** is a sudden compelling desire to pass urine which is difficult to defer.
- **Urge incontinence (UI)** is involuntary urinary leakage, often large volume, immediately preceded by the sensation of urgency. Urgency and episodes of urge incontinence are often associated with an overactive bladder or a bladder neuropathy.
- **Stress incontinence** is involuntary urinary leakage which occurs when the intra-abdominal pressure rises. This is most common in females who have had vaginal deliveries who describe small-volume urinary leakage associated with activity such as coughing, laughing, sneezing or exercising.
- **Nocturnal enuresis** is involuntary loss of urine during sleep. A common cause in an elderly male is chronic retention of urine with overflow incontinence.
- **Hesitancy** is the term used when an individual describes difficulty in initiating micturition, resulting in a delay in the onset of voiding after the individual is ready to pass urine. This can be several seconds to several minutes and is often a symptom of bladder outlet obstruction.
- **Reduced urinary stream** is usually reported compared with previous performance or in comparison with the performance of others. This is often a symptom of bladder outlet obstruction.
- **Intermittency** is the term used when the individual describes urine flow which stops and starts, on one or more occasions, during micturition.
- **Straining** is the muscular effort used in order to initiate, maintain or improve the urinary stream.
- **Incomplete emptying** is the sensation that at the end of micturition bladder fullness persists.
- **Post micturition dribble (PMD)** is the term used when an individual describes the involuntary loss of urine immediately after he/she has finished passing urine. This is a common symptom in the ageing male when the bulbar urethra fails to empty itself of urine at the completion of micturition. PMD is a symptom which is not usually remedied by a transurethral resection of the prostate.

In general terms, LUTS are classified as either **storage LUTS** (frequency, nocturia, urgency and UI); **voiding LUTS** (hesitancy, a reduced stream, straining) or **post-micturitional LUTS** (incomplete emptying and PMD). Storage LUTS result from failure of the bladder to act as a functioning reservoir for urine and are commonly seen in patients with an overactive bladder or a bladder neuropathy. Voiding and post-micturitional LUTS are commonly seen in males with bladder outlet obstruction (BOO); however, a male with BOO may also have storage LUTS as the thickened detrusor muscle resulting from outlet obstruction becomes overactive, resulting in the combination of symptoms. The term 'prostatism' is now obsolete. LUTS are frequently investigated with urodynamics (see below).

Summary box 75.2

Lower urinary tract symptoms (LUTS)

- Are classified as storage, voiding or post-micturitional
- Storage LUTS are frequency, nocturia, urgency and urge incontinence
- Storage LUTS are typical of an overactive bladder
- Voiding LUTS are hesitancy, a reduced stream and straining
- Voiding LUTS are typical of bladder outlet obstruction
- Some patients may have storage and voiding LUTS in combination
- Are often investigated with urodynamics

HAEMATURIA

Haematuria occurs when there is blood in the urine. This is now classified as visible haematuria (VH) or non-visible haematuria (NVH). Older terminology referred to macroscopic (or frank or gross) haematuria and microscopic (or dipstick) haematuria. Enquiry should be made about the timing of the blood in relation to the urinary stream; initial (urethral pathology), throughout the stream (bladder or upper tracts), or terminal (bladder neck or prostatic pathology), as well as degree of haematuria and its frequency. A patient with haematuria should be investigated regardless of whether they are taking anticoagulant therapy. The concern for the urologist is that the haematuria, especially if painless, is due to an underlying neoplasm of the urinary tract, usually a bladder or renal tumour. Causes of haematuria include **T**rauma, **I**nfection and **N**eoplasm (think of TIN) at all levels of the urinary tract. Haematuria in association with loin pain and a palpable loin mass defines the classic triad of symptoms and signs of a renal tumour although this triad is seen in less than 10% of patients presenting with a renal tumour.

Apart from young females with a proven UTI, most patients with haematuria, whether visible or non-visible, will be investigated urgently at a haematuria clinic where they will have a renal ultrasound scan (USS) and a flexible cystoscopy as a minimum. The cancer detection rate depends on the degree of haematuria, being approximately 20% in those patients with visible haematuria but very much lower in those with non-visible haematuria (<5%).

Summary box 75.3

Haematuria

- Nowadays, is classified as visible haematuria (VH) or non-visible haematuria (NVH)
- A list of potential causes for haematuria can be rapidly generated by considering trauma (**T**), infection (**I**) and neoplasm (**N**) at all levels of the urinary tract from kidney to urethra
- Haematuria is investigated with a renal USS and a flexible cystoscopy as a minimum

Discolouration of the urine

Many drugs and foodstuffs have been reported to produce abnormal discolouration of the urine. Most colours have been reported but the most frequently encountered clinically are red/orange and brown. Clearly, haematuria is the commonest cause for red urine; however, the presence of haem in the urine also produces red discolouration and generates a positive dipstick test. Red urine discolouration due to haemoglobinuria may present in haemolytic disorders such as 'march haematuria', classically seen in dehydrated soldiers after prolonged marching. Likewise, myoglobinuria due to myocyte destruction, e.g. caused by rhabdomyolysis after crush injury, can also result in red discolouration of the urine. Disordered haem production, seen in porphyria, can result in red discolouration that may change to brown or purple with exposure to sunlight. Several medications can cause red/orange discolouration of the urine, most commonly rifampicin, isoniazid or phenazopyridine with tears and other bodily fluids generally also discoloured. Others include chlorpromazine, thioridazine, senna and laxatives containing a phenolphthalein component. Consumption of large quantities of beetroot can result in red discolouration of the urine. This discolouration is due to the excretion of betalain (betacyanin) pigments such as betanin. There is no direct genetic influence and no single gene variant that differentiates excreters from non-excreters.

The commonly used antibiotics nitrofurantoin and metronidazole can lead to the urine being discoloured brown. Brown urine due to high-circulating bilirubin is also a feature of obstructive jaundice.

LESS COMMON URINARY SYMPTOMS

Haematospermia

This refers to blood, which can be bright red or a brown colour, seen in the seminal fluid. It is most commonly due to benign inflammatory change in the prostate but occasionally can be the presenting symptom of a prostate cancer. A digital rectal examination (DRE) should be performed alongside a prostate-specific antigen (PSA) test and a transrectal US (TRUS) should be considered. In most cases, haematospermia is self-limiting.

Pneumaturia

This is air, or more correctly gas, in the urine. Patients typically describe frothy urine, bubbles in the urine or a stream which intermittently stops then starts again. The commonest cause is an underlying colovesical fistula, usually due to primary pathology in the rectum or sigmoid colon.

'The urethral syndrome'

In this condition, typically seen in young females, symptoms suggestive of a UTI are reported but with negative bacteriology. It is sometimes remedied by a simple cystoscopy and urethral dilatation.

SYMPTOMS RELATED TO THE EXTERNAL GENITALIA

Testis

A testis may be absent from the scrotum in patients with undescended or ectopic testes.

In boys <5 years, a common cause of testicular pain and swelling is a torted hydatid of Morgagni (appendix testis). Often in these young males the scrotal skin is transparent enough to allow visualisation of a small, bluish swelling at the superior pole of the testis. In a young male suspected of having a testicular torsion, examination of the **normal** i.e. **contralateral** testis may reveal a horizontal lie or 'clapper bell testis', raising the level of clinical suspicion. If torsion is suspected, immediate testicular exploration is mandatory and if confirmed, **bilateral** testicular fixation is performed.

Patients with Klinefelter's syndrome typically have bilateral small, firm testes in addition to the other signs typical of this condition.

A hydrocoele is an accumulation of fluid between the testis and the tunica vaginalis and in the younger male can be associated with a patent processus vaginalis. On opening into a hydrocoele, the fluid is typically a yellow colour. A testis which cannot be felt in a tense hydrocoele in the age groups at risk of testis cancer needs to be assessed by USS preoperatively.

Epididymis

Epididymal pathology is rare in the prepubertal male. In the sexually active male, acute epididymitis (often due to chlamydia) with significant pain and swelling needs to be distinguished from acute testicular torsion. If there is any doubt, scrotal exploration is undertaken. Tiny cysts are frequently

Giovanni Battista Morgagni, 1682–1771, Professor of Anatomy, University of Padua, Italy.
Harry Fitch Klinefelter, 1912–1990, American rheumatologist and endocrinologist, first described Klinefelter's syndrome in 1942.

detected in young males undergoing testicular USS but in the vast majority of patients these do not require attention.

Epididymal cysts can form similar scrotal swellings to hydrocoeles but can be distinguished by the fact that the testis can often be felt separately. They contain clear or white fluid. Both hydrocoeles and epididymal cysts transilluminate on clinical examination.

Genitourinary tuberculosis (TB) can result in bilateral nodular induration of the epididymes.

Spermatic cord

Ten per cent of males have a left-sided varicocoele and a smaller left testis. Masses are occasionally found associated with the spermatic cord, which on removal are found to be lipomas, mesotheliomas or sarcomas.

Prepuce (foreskin)

Phimosis occurs when the distal foreskin is tight and will not allow the foreskin to retract. **Paraphimosis** occurs when a poorly retractile foreskin becomes trapped in the retracted state and cannot be replaced. Significant oedema of the foreskin results, making replacement of the foreskin increasingly difficult. Depigmentation and scarring of the distal prepuce occurs in **balanitis xerotica obliterans (BXO)**.

Penis

Peyronie's disease is an idiopathic condition in which fibrosis develops in the corpora cavernosa of the penis. The 'plaque' of Peyronie's fibrosis is usually palpable in the midline anywhere from the base of the penis to just behind the corona. It gives rise to painful angulation of the penis on erection.

Penile fracture occurs when there is trauma to the erect penis. Classically, there is an audible crack and immediate penile detumescence and the patient presents with gross bruising of the penile shaft skin.

Glans penis

In the younger male, **genitourinary warts** due to human papilloma virus (HPV) infection may be observed. In the older male, red raised patches on the glans penis or the inner aspect of the prepuce due to **Zoon's balanitis** or CIS (**erythroplasia of Queyrat** or **Bowen's disease**) are distinguished only on penile biopsy.

Urethra

Hypospadias occurs when there is failure of the urethra to completely close on the ventral aspect and **epispadias** occurs when there is failure of closure on the dorsal surface. A **urethral diverticulum** in a female can be a cause for recurrent UTIs and is notable for its capacity to fill and empty at cystoscopy. A **urethral caruncle** is a minor prolapse of the urethral mucosa in a female and usually requires no treatment.

INVESTIGATION OF URINARY SYMPTOMS

Blood tests

Screening blood tests

Initial blood tests in a patient with potentially serious urinary tract pathology often start with screening blood tests such as full blood count (FBC) and urea and electrolytes (U&E). Anaemia accompanied by a diagnosis of a urinary tract malignancy is an adverse prognostic feature of renal cell carcinoma (RCC).

Serum biochemistry

Modern assessment of biochemical renal function not only involves reporting of serum levels of urea, creatinine and electrolytes but, in addition, involves the reporting of the estimated glomerular filtration rate (eGFR). Creatinine is an end-product of muscle catabolism and suffers from the disadvantage that eGFR can be wide ranging for a given serum creatinine level. For example, a serum creatinine level of 1.5 mg/dL (132 μmol/L) may correspond to a GFR from approximately 20 to 90 mL/min/1.73 m^2. eGFR is nowadays recommended as the optimal method of reporting renal function in many countries. The Modification of Diet in Renal Disease (MDRD) study equation uses age, gender, race and standardised serum creatinine to estimate the GFR. When patients with a urological cancer are being considered for nephrotoxic cisplatin-based systemic chemotherapy, in general terms, the eGFR needs to be 50 mL/min or greater.

Patients with calculous disease routinely have serum calcium and uric acid levels checked to rule out a metabolic predisposition to stone formation.

Serum alkaline phosphatase may be elevated in patients with bone metastases due to a urological malignancy and is commonly seen in men with disseminated prostate cancer.

Summary box 75.4

Biochemical assessment of renal function

- eGFR is increasingly reported along with urea and creatinine as it is more informative of true renal function
- With both kidneys functioning normally, an individual has approximately 6 times the renal function needed to remain off dialysis
- Serum creatinine will remain normal with unilateral renal pathology but a normally functioning contralateral kidney

---

François Gigot de La Peyronie, 1678–1747, French surgeon.
Johannes Jacobus Zoon, 1902–1958, Professor of Dermatology, University of Utrecht, the Netherlands, described Zoon's balanitis in 1952.
Louis Auguste Queyrat, 1856–1933, French dermatologist, described erythroplasia of Queyrat in 1911.
John Templeton Bowen, 1857–1940, American dermatologist, described Bowen's disease.

Tumour markers

Serum tumour markers are utilised in patients with prostate and testis cancer. As of 2017, no serum tumour markers exist in routine clinical practice for renal or bladder cancer.

Prostate-specific antigen

PSA is a glycoprotein produced by prostatic epithelial cells. It is responsible for liquefaction of seminal fluid and allows spermatozoa to swim freely. As a consequence of altered architecture of the prostate in conditions such as benign prostatic hyperplasia (BPH) and prostatitis as well as prostate cancer, PSA enters the bloodstream and is detected by a blood test. The commonly used PSA assays measure the total amount of PSA. PSA levels can be influenced by certain drugs, most notably 5-α-reductase inhibitors such as finasteride and dutasteride used to treat men with LUTS, but also by aspirin, statins and thiazide diuretics. The PSA needs to be multiplied by 2 in men who have been on a 5-α-reductase inhibitor for at least 6 months to give an approximation of the true PSA value. The PSA test can be significantly influenced by an active or recent UTI and the true PSA level only returns to baseline 6 weeks after treatment and eradication of an infective episode.

Summary box 75.5

Prostate-specific antigen

- Is not significantly altered by digital rectal examination
- Can be significantly altered by a UTI
- After an infective episode takes 6 weeks to return to baseline values
- Is artificially lowered in men taking 5-α-reductase inhibitors (finasteride, dutasteride)

In clinical practice, age-adjusted PSA values have been used for many years (*Table 75.1*), but recently have been called into question as they are highly variable and may reflect differences in demographics and clinical characteristics of a particular population.

The two largest randomised PSA-based screening trials, the European Randomised Study of Prostate Cancer (ERSPC) and the Prostate, Lung, Colorectal and Ovarian (PLCO) Study, have evaluated PSA testing among men aged 55–69 years with the indication for a biopsy being a PSA ≥3 ng/mL. Recommended prostate biopsy referral values are being realigned to the evidence emerging from these two studies. The new recommended referral value for men aged 50–69 years is 3 ng/mL. Further diagnostic evaluation should consider the man's history of comorbidities, ethnicity, family history and abnormal DRE findings prior to biopsy.

A large UK-based clinical study of serum PSA as a tool for identifying asymptomatic men with prostate cancer has recently reported 10-year outcome data (ProtecT trial). At present, screening men in the UK for prostate cancer using regular PSA testing is not routinely performed but men interested in having a PSA test can request this from their family practitioners.

Risk prediction models have been developed in recent years to assist clinicians and patients in predicting prostate cancer diagnosis, stage and prognosis. A number of these risk assessment tools are available online as a decision aid for an individual man to evaluate his own risk of prostate cancer. These include the Prostate Cancer Prevention Trial (PCPT) Risk Calculator and the ERSPC Risk Calculator.

For men newly diagnosed with prostate cancer, PSA assists with risk (of disease progression) stratification. It is also a useful marker of response to treatment and of disease recurrence after treatment.

PSA derivatives

Raised serum levels of PSA in men with BPH and prostatitis decrease the specificity of the PSA blood test as a cancer marker. In an effort to improve specificity of testing, PSA derivatives and PSA kinetics have been used but to date have had little impact in assisting with clinical decision making.

FREE PSA (FPSA), COMPLEXED PSA (CPSA) AND FREE/TOTAL PSA (F/TPSA)

Total PSA detectable in the serum consists of proteolytically active free PSA and complexed PSA. Free PSA constitutes 5–40% of total PSA and cPSA 60–95%. 60–90% of cPSA is bound to α-1-antichymotrypsin, 10–20% to α-2-macrogobulin and 1–5% to α-1-protease inhibitor. A lower percentage fPSA has been associated with prostate cancer and many studies have indicated its value in reducing the

TABLE 75.1 Age-specific reference ranges for prostate-specific antigen (PSA) values.

Age range (years)	PSA reference range (ng/mL)		
	Oesterling *et al.*[1]	Dalkin *et al.*[2]	DeAntoni *et al.*[3]
40–49	0.0–2.5 ng/mL	–	0.0–2.4 ng/mL
50–59	0.0–3.5 ng/mL	0.0–3.5 ng/mL	0.0–3.8 ng/mL
60–69	0.0–4.5 ng/mL	0.0–5.4 ng/mL	0.0–5.6 ng/mL
70–79	0.0–6.5 ng/mL	0.0–6.3 ng/mL	0.0–6.9 ng/mL

[1]Oesterling JE, Jacobsen SJ, Chute CG *et al.* Serum prostate-specific antigen in a community-based population of healthy men. Establishment of age-specific reference ranges. *JAMA* 1993; **270**(7): 860–4.
[2]Dalkin BL, Ahmann FR, Kopp JB. Prostate specific antigen levels in men older than 50 years without clinical evidence of prostatic carcinoma. *J Urol* 1993; **150**(6): 1837–9.
[3]DeAntoni EP, Crawford ED, Oesterling JE *et al.* Age- and race-specific reference ranges for prostate-specific antigen from a large community-based study. *Urology* 1996; **48**(2): 234–9.

number of negative prostate biopsies performed. Studies have varied in the threshold of percentage fPSA used, with cut-offs of 22%, 15% and 10% reported to be of clinical utility. Recent studies have indicated that there are, in fact, 3 forms of fPSA: inactive PSA, known as proPSA, and 2 other forms; BPSA (nicked PSA) and intact PSA (iPSA). BPSA and iPSA have been associated with benign disease of the prostate while proPSA has been found in prostate cancer tissue.

HUMAN KALLIKREIN-2 (HK2)

PSA in prostatic tissue, namely pPSA, is converted to mature PSA via activation of HK2 induced by a physiological process occurring in seminal fluid. HK2 is a protein belonging to the kallikrein family closely related to PSA and is a potential prostate cancer tumour marker.

PROSTATE HEALTH INDEX (PHI)

PHI is a mathematical equation demonstrating the probability of prostate cancer. The equation is formulated as $p2PSA/fPSA \times \sqrt{tPSA}$. p2PSA is an isoform of fPSA. Higher PHI values have been associated with an increased probability of prostate cancer.

PSA kinetics

PSA DENSITY (PSAD)

This factors in the volume of the prostate and assumes contributions to the total PSA of normal prostate epithelium, BPH or prostate cancer to be 0.1 ng/mL, 0.3 ng/mL and 3.5 ng/mL. In clinical practice, PSAD has been found not to have a significant role.

PSA VELOCITY

PSA velocity (ng/mL/yr) has been defined as the annual absolute increase in tPSA. In the past, a velocity of >0.75 ng/mL/yr compared with baseline in those men with a PSA in the range 4–10 ng/mL has been considered suspicious but currently there is no consensus concerning a useful threshold.

PSA DOUBLING TIME

This is defined as the number of months it takes for a baseline PSA to double. It is clinically useful in determining the need for treatment initiation in men undergoing active surveillance and watchful waiting for prostate cancer and for determining the need for further treatment once first-line therapy has failed.

Other possible prostate cancer biomarkers

Recently, two promising urinary ribonucleic acid (RNA) biomarkers, prostate cancer antigen-3 (PCA-3) and the fusion gene TMPRSS2:ERG, have emerged.

Testis tumour markers

There are three serum tumour markers routinely used in the management of men with suspected testis cancer: alpha fetoprotein (αFP), beta human chorionic gonadotropin (βHCG) and lactate dehydrogenase (LDH). These markers sometimes provide insight into the likely histological subtype of germ cell tumour present and, in addition, contribute to the prognostication of testis cancer patients into good prognosis, intermediate prognosis and poor prognosis groups using a classification devised by the International Germ Cell Cancer Collaborative Group (IGCCCG) (see Chapter 80).

Urine-based tests

Urinalysis

Patients in both primary and secondary care settings will very often be screened for significant disease with a urine dipstick test. Urine is dipped with a stick on which there is a series of small chemical-containing pads designed to detect, typically, glucose, bilirubin, ketones, the specific gravity, blood, pH, protein, urobilinogen, nitrites and leucocyte esterase through colour changes which are detected using a bench-top analyser. A trace of blood on dipstick testing should be regarded as a negative test and should not prompt further evaluation of the patient.

Mid-stream specimen of urine (MSU)

A MSU is used to establish the diagnosis of a UTI and primarily allows identification of the responsible urinary pathogen and selection of the most appropriate antibiotic. Most MSUs will be processed in 2 stages with initial urine microscopy followed by urine culture only if appropriate. Normal urine contains small numbers of white blood cells (WBCs) and epithelial cells as indicated:

Normal values	
WBC	($0–40 \times 10^6$/L)
Epithelial cells	($0–55 \times 10^6$/L)

Early-morning urine (EMU)

EMU samples are sent on 3 consecutive days for Ziehl–Neelsen (ZN) staining and culture for acid-fast bacilli if genitourinary TB is suspected. Culture results take 6 weeks.

Voided urine cytology

Voided urine cytology is performed when a urinary tract malignancy, usually a urothelial carcinoma, is suspected, particularly in the setting of a normal cystoscopy. The test has the disadvantage of a high false-negative rate. Approximately 15% of low-grade transitional cell carcinomas produce positive voided urine cytology compared with approximately 50% of high-grade transitional cell tumours.

Endoscopy

Cystoscopy

To further evaluate urinary symptoms, the entire lining of the urinary tract can be directly visualised from the urethra and bladder (using a cystoscope) to the ureter and renal pelvis

Franz Ziehl, 1859–1926, German bacteriologist and a professor in Lübeck, Germany.
Friedrich Carl Adolf Neelsen, 1854–1898, German pathologist and professor at the Institute of Pathology, University of Rostock, Germany.

(semi-rigid ureteroscope), and finally the renal calyces (flexible ureteroscope). Cystoscopy can be undertaken either as a flexible cystoscopy (Figure 75.1) using local anaesthesia or rigid cystoscopy (Figures 75.1 and 75.2), preferably under a general anaesthetic. Telescopes with different fields of view are available (0°, 12°, 30° and 70° lenses are commonly used). In the operating theatre, most endoscopic procedures, including cystoscopy, require the urology stack (Figures 75.3 and 75.4). Insertion of the cystoscope sheath in some centres is performed with the obturator inserted rather than the telescope, which is then switched with the obturator once in the bladder.

Flexible cystoscopy is relatively poorly tolerated in young males. In the male, visualisation of the urethra during flexible cystourethroscopy is often completed on withdrawal of the scope providing there is no stricture in the urethra. Flexible cystoscopy can be performed as a rapid turnover procedure in the outpatient clinic. It is principally a diagnostic tool but a few minor procedures can be accomplished using the flexible cystoscope, such as insertion/removal of ureteric stents, small biopsies and diathermy/laser of small bladder lesions. The tip of most flexible cystoscopes deflects down 90° and upwards/backwards through 180° giving a 270° field of view. Full backward deflection of the flexible cystoscope allows what is referred to as the 'J manoeuvre' permitting excellent visualisation of the bladder neck region.

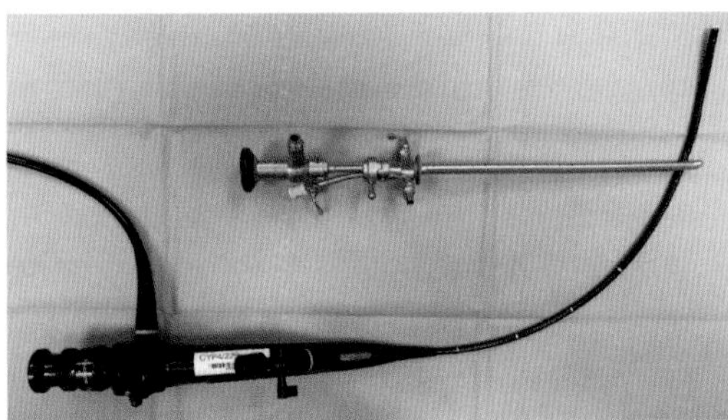

Figure 75.1 A rigid cystoscope (above) assembled with the telescope inside the outer sheath, demonstrating the working channel with the white plastic nipple below the light attachment. Below is the flexible cystoscope that simply needs to be connected to a light source and irrigation and is ready to use.

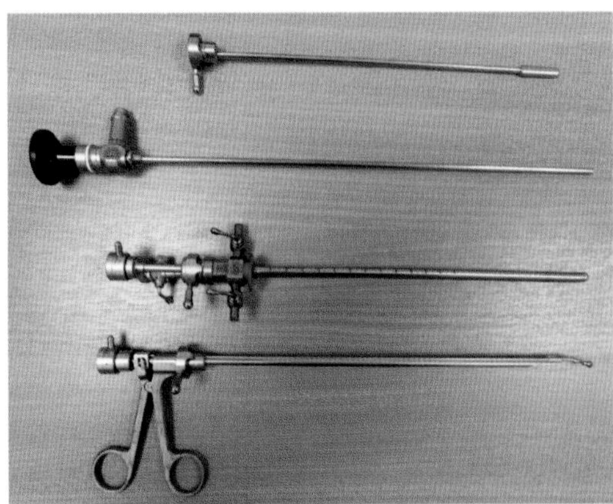

Figure 75.2 The components of a rigid cystoscope. From above down: the obturator for insertion into the outer sheath used in blind insertion of the cystoscope sheath – usually in females; the telescope to which the light cable is attached; the outer sheath containing 2 taps for irrigation and outflow with the bridge with a working channel for guidewires and ureteric catheters already engaged; cold cup biopsy forceps that will accommodate the telescope and fit down the outer sheath.

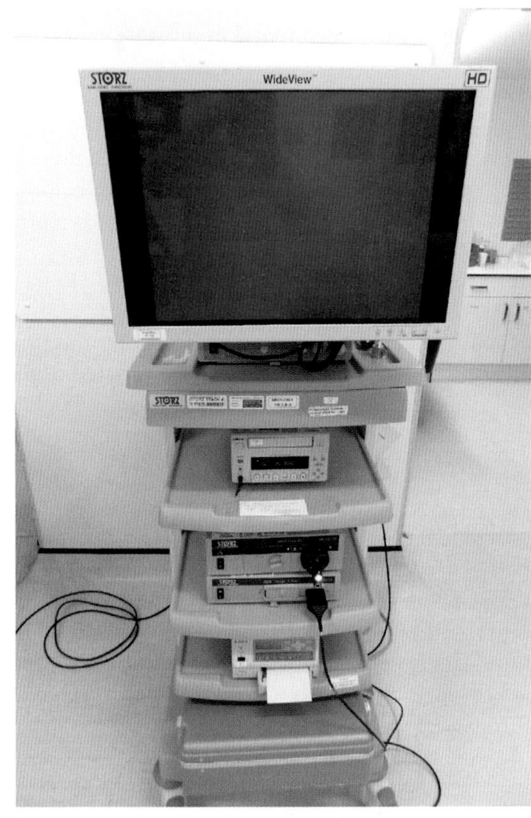

Figure 75.3 The urology 'stack'. In this stack, from above down, are the monitor (often on a telescopic arm), a video recording device, the light source which is on the camera to connect to the endoscope and a printer for capturing images. The endoflator (used for laparoscopic urological procedures) is hidden by the monitor in this image.

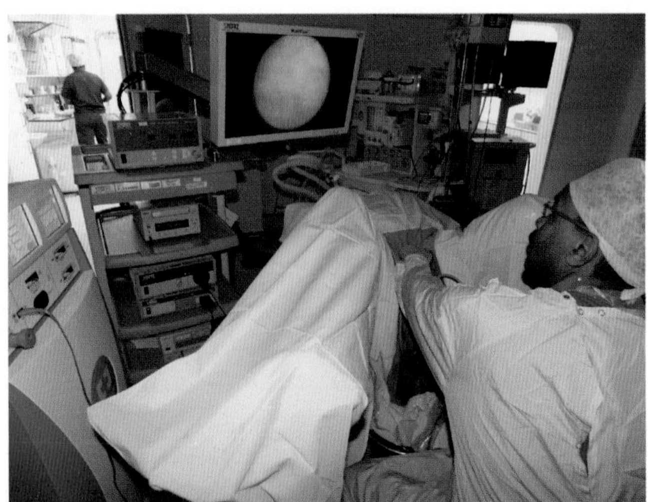

Figure 75.4 The urology stack in use in a patient under general anaesthetic about to undergo a transurethral resection of a bladder tumour.

More can be achieved with a rigid cystoscope under general anaesthetic (GA), especially in relation to instrumentation of the ureters.

In an effort to improve the diagnostic accuracy of cystoscopy, technological advances have produced narrow band imaging (NBI) and photodynamic diagnosis (PDD) combined with cystoscopy.

NBI is an optic enhancement technique which filters the white light into two different bandwidths, including blue (415 nm) and green (540 nm) spectrum. In the NBI mode, the light is strongly absorbed by haemoglobin and only penetrates the tissue superficially, which increases the identification of small capillaries and superficial tissue structures. Since bladder tumours are vascular structures, the tumours appear in brown or green colour against a white background using NBI (Figure 75.5).

With PDD, 60 to 90 minutes before the PDD procedure, a solution containing a drug with fluorescent properties is instilled into the bladder. The drug preferentially accumulates in rapidly proliferating cells such as tumour cells.

During the PDD procedure, the bladder is examined in blue light. The accumulated drug in the tumour cells is spectrally excited by this blue light and emits a pink fluorescence. The tumour cells are highlighted pink and stand out against the normal bladder tissue, which keeps its blue appearance (Figure 75.6). Bladder tumours and areas of CIS are easier to identify compared with white light cystoscopy.

Figures 75.7–75.13 show some normal anatomy as well as some of the pathology seen in the urethra and bladder on cystourethroscopy.

Summary box 75.6

Cystoscopy

- Can be performed either with a rigid cystoscope under general anaesthetic or a flexible cystoscope under local anaesthetic
- Flexible cystoscopy is principally a diagnostic procedure
- The diagnostic accuracy of cystoscopy has recently been improved by techniques such as NBI and PDD

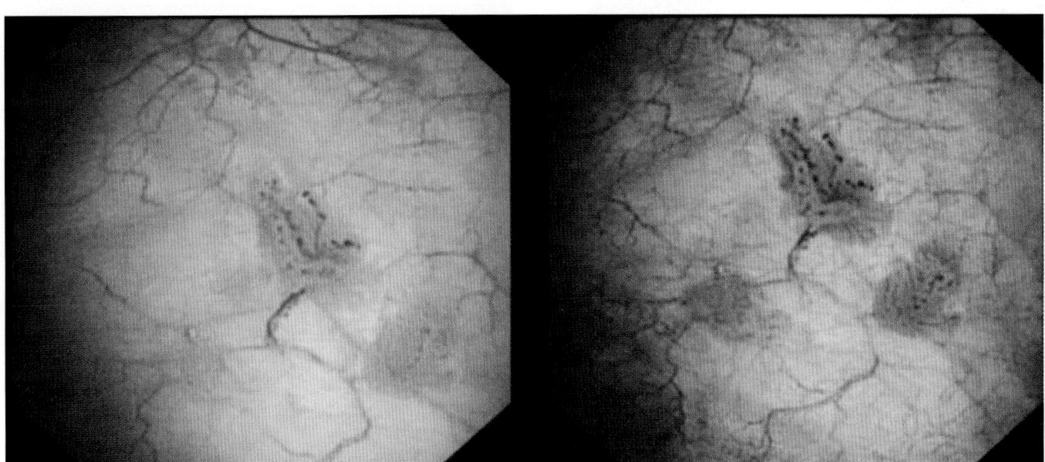

Figure 75.5 Enhanced detection of bladder tumour using narrow band imaging (NBI) (left image, white light; right image, NBI).

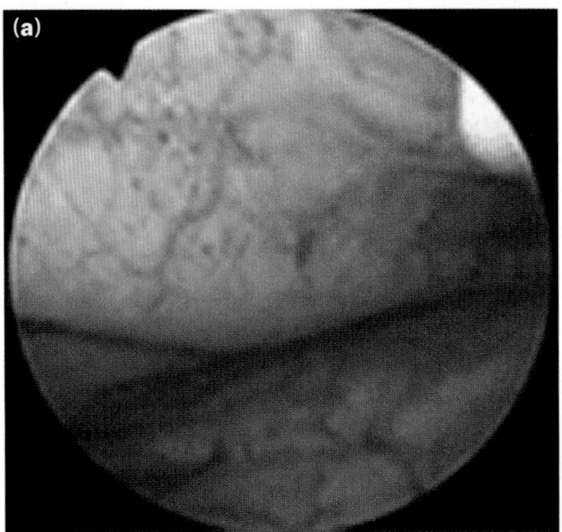

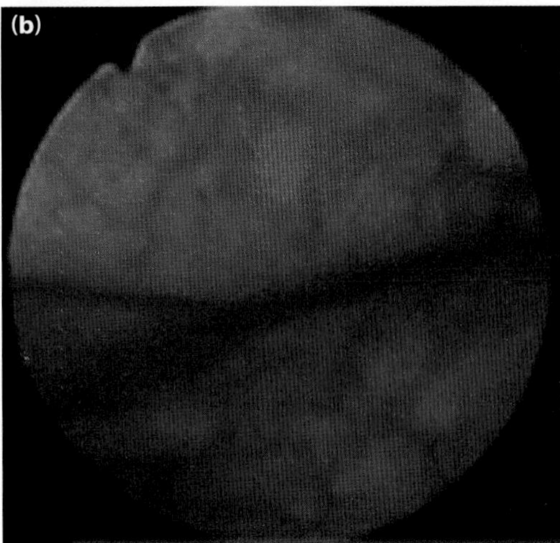

Figure 75.6 Enhanced detection of bladder tumour using photodynamic diagnosis (PDD): **(a)** white light; **(b)** blue light, PPD.

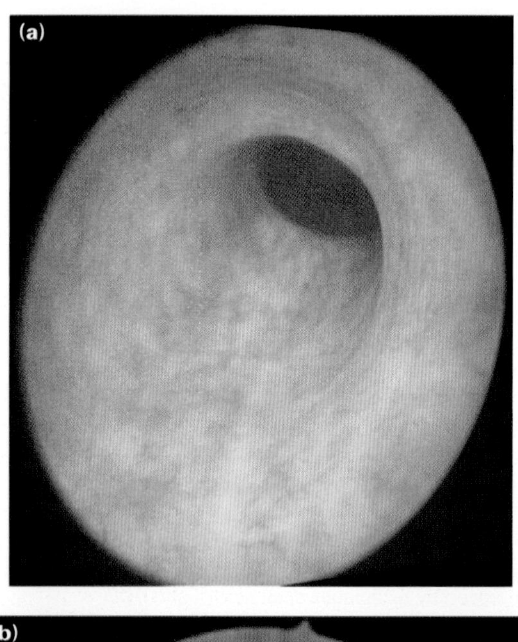
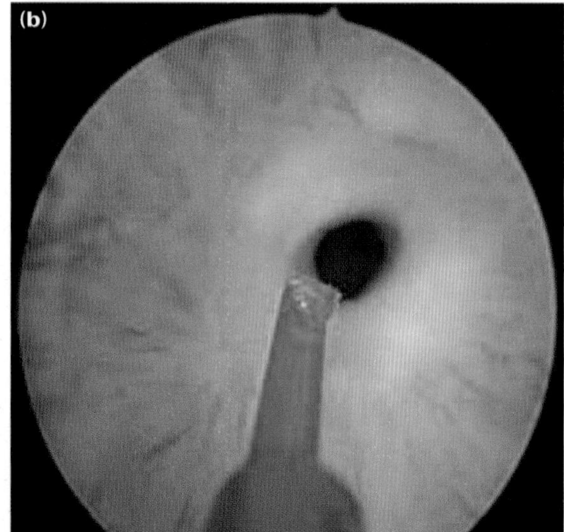
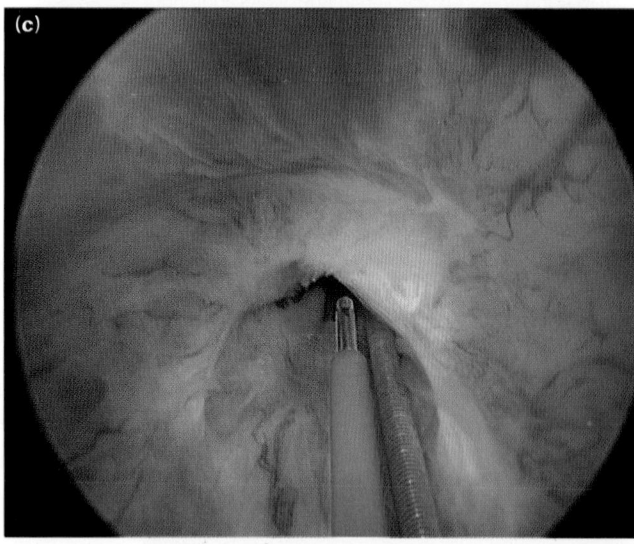

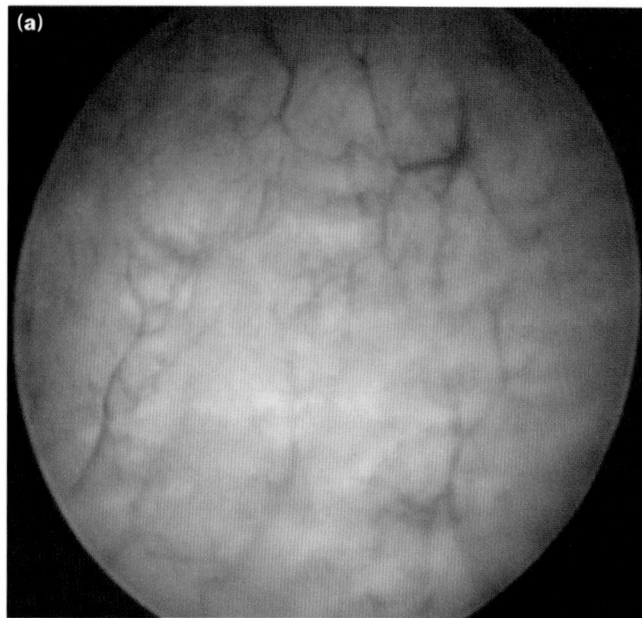
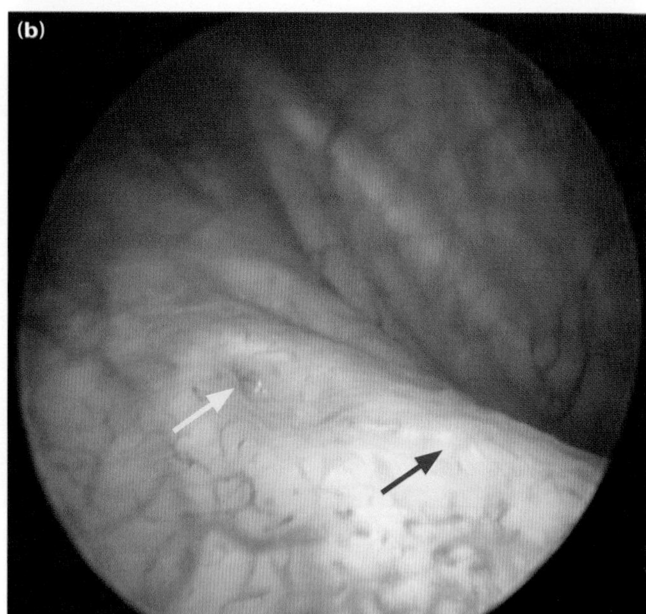

Figure 75.8 **(a)** The appearance of normal bladder mucosa on cystoscopy. **(b)** A normal right ureteric orifice (yellow arrow) at the end of the interureteric bar (red arrow) seen on cystoscopy.

Figure 75.7 **(a)** A normal urethra on urethroscopy. **(b)** A urethral stricture seen on urethroscopy. **(c)** A urethrotomy being performed for a urethral stricture using a laser fibre; the procedure is being performed over a green guidewire that has been inserted into the bladder to ensure the lumen of the urethra is not lost (photograph courtesy of Douglas F Milam, MD).

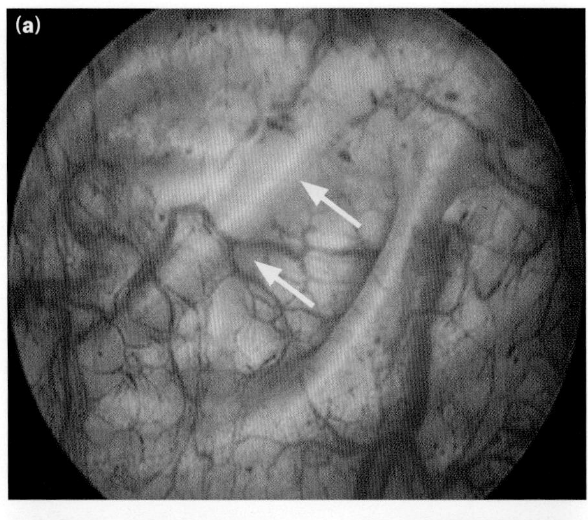

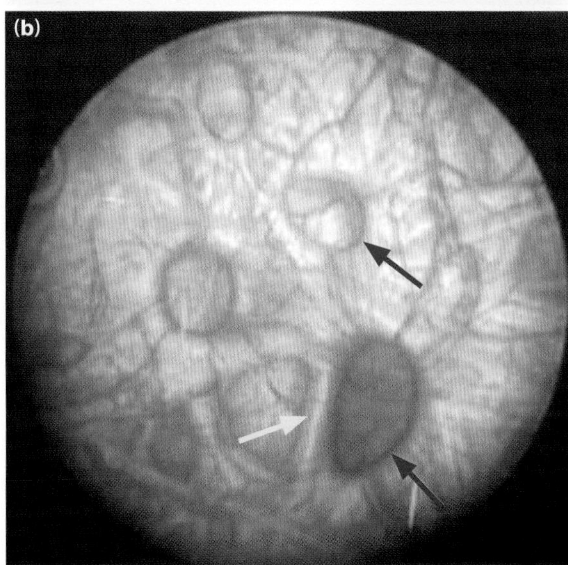

Figure 75.9 (a, b) Bladder wall trabeculation (yellow arrows) and saccules (red arrows) seen on cystoscopy. (Image (a) courtesy of The Center for Reconstructive Urology, CA, USA.)

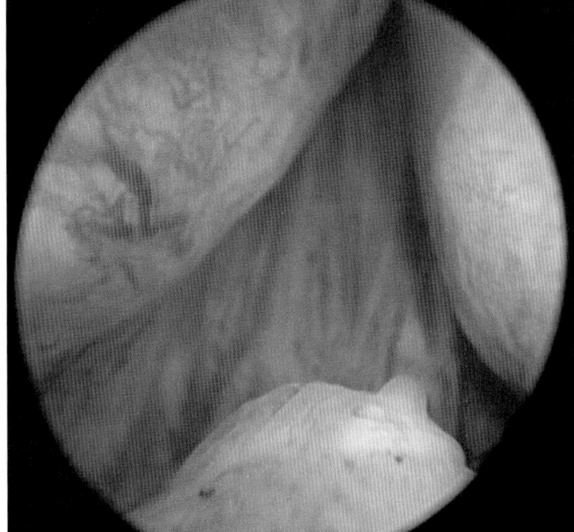

Figure 75.10 An endoscopic view of the prostatic urethra with the veru montanum at 6 o'clock and the bulging right and left lobes of the prostate.

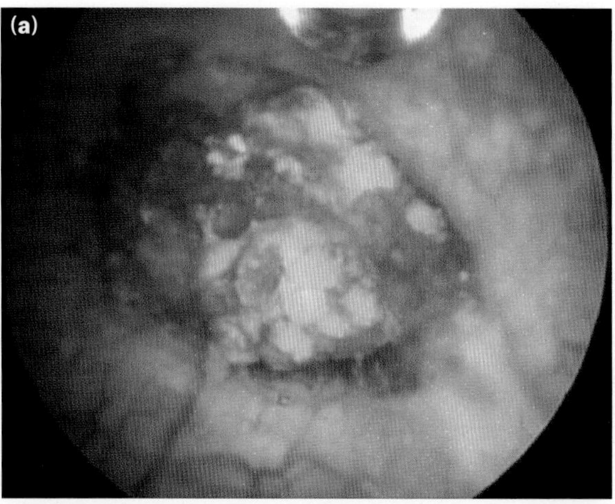

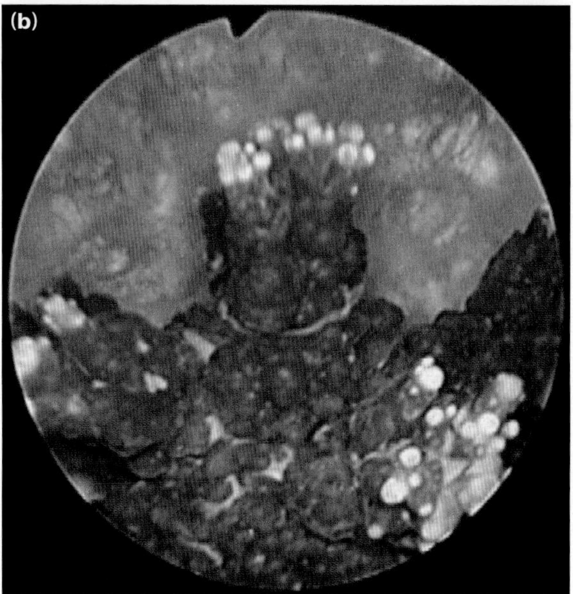

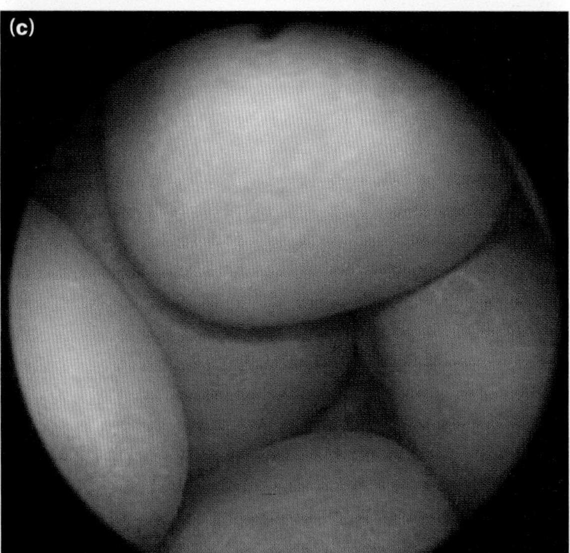

Figure 75.11 Bladder calculi seen on cystoscopy. Stones may be single (a, b) or multiple (c). The stone in (b) has a characteristic shape and is referred to as a 'jack' stone. (Image (b) reprinted with permission from Medscape Drugs & Diseases (http://emedicine.medscape.com/), 2017, available at: http://emedicine.medscape.com/article/2120102-overview.)

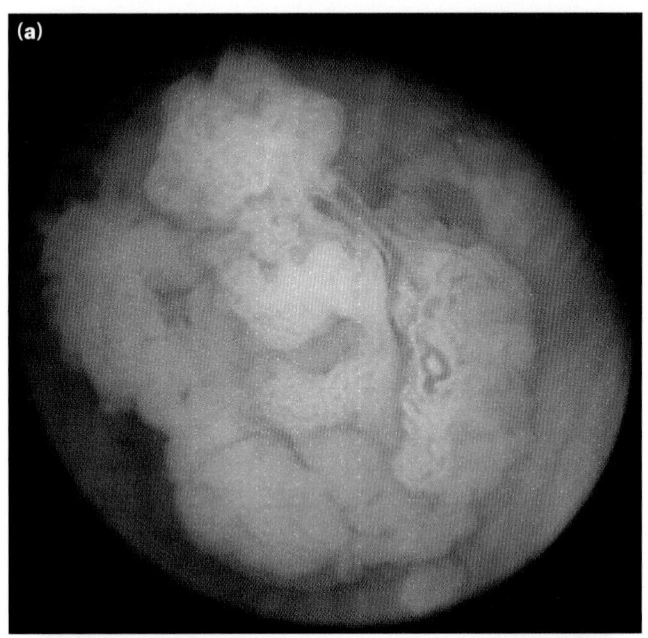

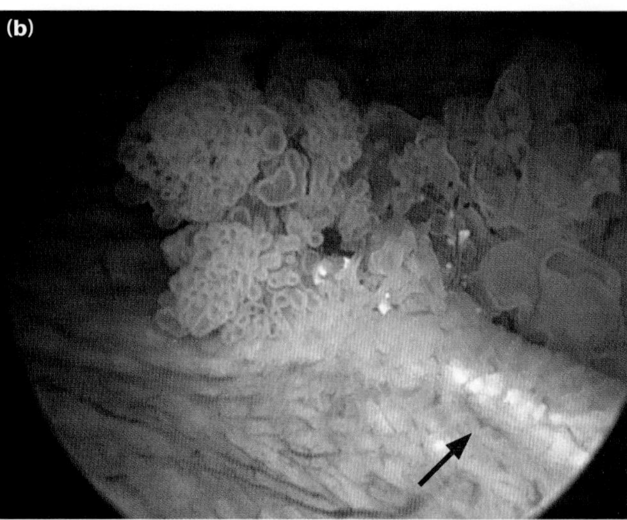

Figure 75.12 (**a, b**) Papillary bladder tumours seen at cystoscopy. (**b**) This illustrates the proximity of the tumour to the right ureteric orifice (arrow) (courtesy of Tim Nathan). Bladder tumours frequently arise close to ureteric orifices.

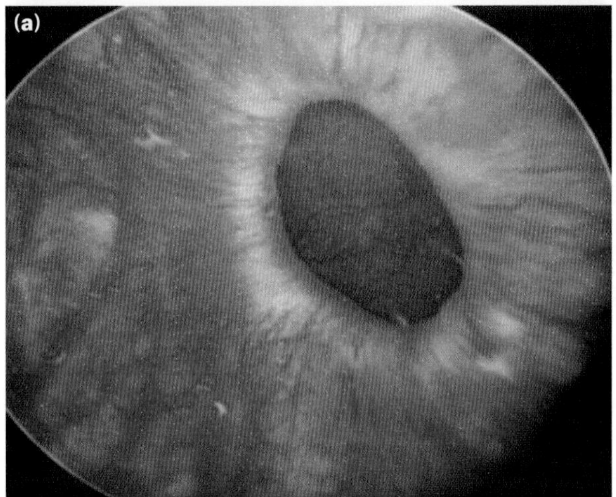

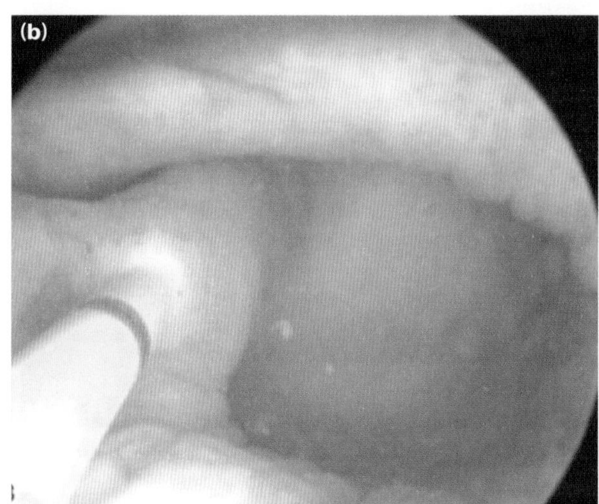

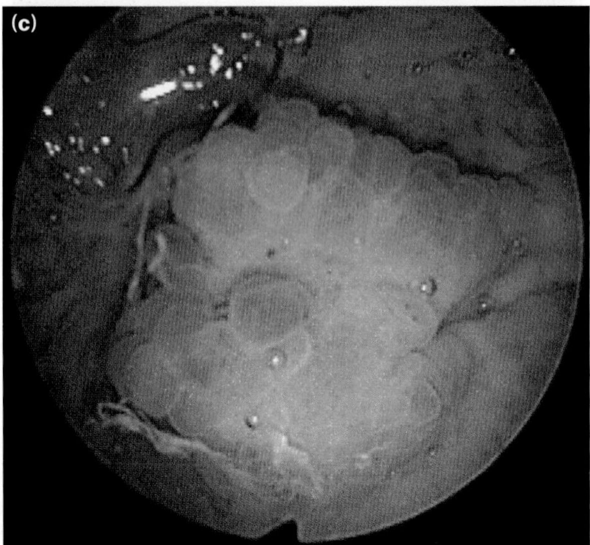

Figure 75.13 (**a**) Bladder diverticulum. (**b**) A paraureteric diverticulum with a ureteric catheter in the left ureteric orifice. (**c**) The raised inflammatory lesion on the left side of the bladder typical of the site of a colovesical fistula with strands of colonic mucus.

CYSTOSCOPY AND RETROGRADE URETEROGRAMS

In patients in whom ureteric pathology is suspected (often stones or tumours), retrograde studies of the entire ureter and renal pelvis can be performed by insertion of a fine ureteric catheter into the ureteric orifice (via a cystoscope) followed by the injection of contrast material retrogradely into the ureter in an effort to confirm the diagnosis. Overexuberant injection of contrast can result in extravasation of contrast material into the retroperitoneum, especially when there is ureteric obstruction.

Ureteroscopy

Ureteroscopy can be performed as both a diagnostic procedure and a therapeutic procedure. A rigid or semi-rigid ureteroscope can be used in the ureter as far as the renal pelvis but to inspect or operate on the renal pelvis or renal calyces, a flexible ureteroscope is, generally, needed (Figure 75.14). The procedure is most often performed when pathology, commonly stones, strictures or tumours of the ureter, is suspected. The insertion of each of these instruments is facilitated by the use of a guidewire in the ureter and in most cases the ureter is best first outlined with radio-opaque contrast material using an image intensifier.

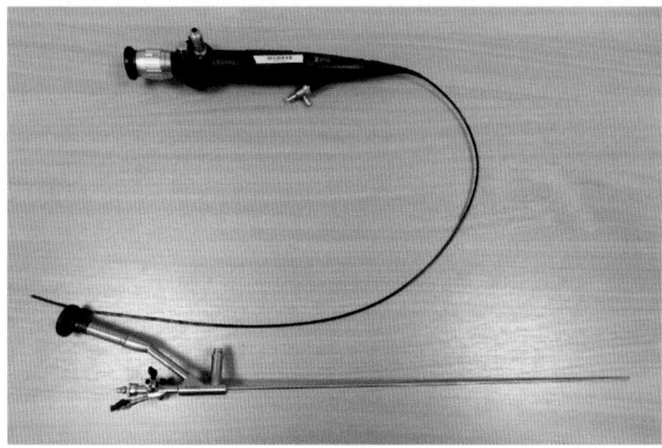

Figure 75.14 Examples of a flexible ureteroscope (above) and a semi-rigid ureteroscope (below).

Radiology

Urinary tract ultrasound scan (USS) (Figure 75.15)

Renal USS is used frequently in the investigation of patients with urinary problems and, in addition to selected use, is used to screen patients with recurrent UTIs and patients with both visible and non-visible haematuria. USS is extremely useful in the detection of hydronephrosis and can be used at the bedside to detect this in the emergency setting. It is useful in detecting renal parenchymal cysts, tumours, renal scarring, and angiomyolipomas (AML) as well as stones. Stones classically produce an acoustic shadow but USS is not the most sensitive imaging modality for detecting renal stones and some stones can be missed on USS. USS is the imaging modality most frequently used to assist with the insertion of a percutaneous nephrostomy (PCN), often placed by a radiologist when there is an obstructed (and/or infected) renal collecting system. USS is sometimes used to further characterise renal lesions detected by other modalities such as computed tomography (CT) or magnetic resonance imaging (MRI) and is a useful adjunct in clarifying whether some lesions on CT/MRI are haemorrhagic cysts or solid renal lesions.

USS is not particularly good for assessing ureters unless there is significant dilatation of the ureter or sizeable pathology in the ureter such as a stone. Soft tissue lesions in the ureter are difficult to detect by USS. USS can be used to detect pathology in the bladder and the bladder is routinely assessed in addition to the kidneys by USS in the haematuria clinic. USS can detect filling defects in the bladder in keeping with bladder tumours and, in addition, can detect bladder calculi, a thickened, trabeculated bladder wall in patients with bladder outlet obstruction and large bladder diverticula, and can be used to determine the residual volume after micturition.

In addition, USS is frequently employed to investigate men with scrotal swellings and has a role to play in the assessment of urethral stricture disease.

Summary box 75.7

Ultrasound scan

- Is frequently used to screen patients with suspected urological pathology
- Is frequently part of a haematuria clinic protocol
- Is an excellent method to detect hydronephrosis
- Can be performed at the bedside in the critically ill patient
- Recently has been combined with contrast enhancement in certain settings such as in the assessment of renal cysts

Transrectal ultrasound scan (TRUS)

TRUS is often performed in conjunction with biopsy of the prostate. Some manufacturers produce USS machines dedicated to USS of the prostate as shown in Figure 75.16. Most prostatic USS is performed using biplanar probes which give transverse as well as sagittal views of the prostate (Figure 75.17). The majority of men undergoing a TRUS and prostate biopsy have the procedure on account of a raised PSA or an abnormal digital rectal examination (DRE) or both. A bridging plan is needed for those patients on oral anticoagulant therapy. Patients can be biopsied while continuing on aspirin therapy. Patients require antibiotic prophylaxis with a regime such as ciprofloxacin orally in the hour before the procedure and IV gentamicin immediately before the procedure is undertaken. Patients are counselled concerning the risk of complications such as a UTI (5%), septicaemia (1%), haematuria, blood per rectum and haematospermia which can be prolonged. Prior to any biopsies, local anaesthetic is infiltrated around the apex of the prostate under USS guidance. During TRUS, a distinct peripheral zone (PZ) and transition zone (TZ) are evident (Figure 75.17); the volume of the prostate can be estimated and biopsies are taken if indicated. If the procedure is being performed for a raised PSA and the prostate looks normal on TRUS, systematic biopsies will be taken

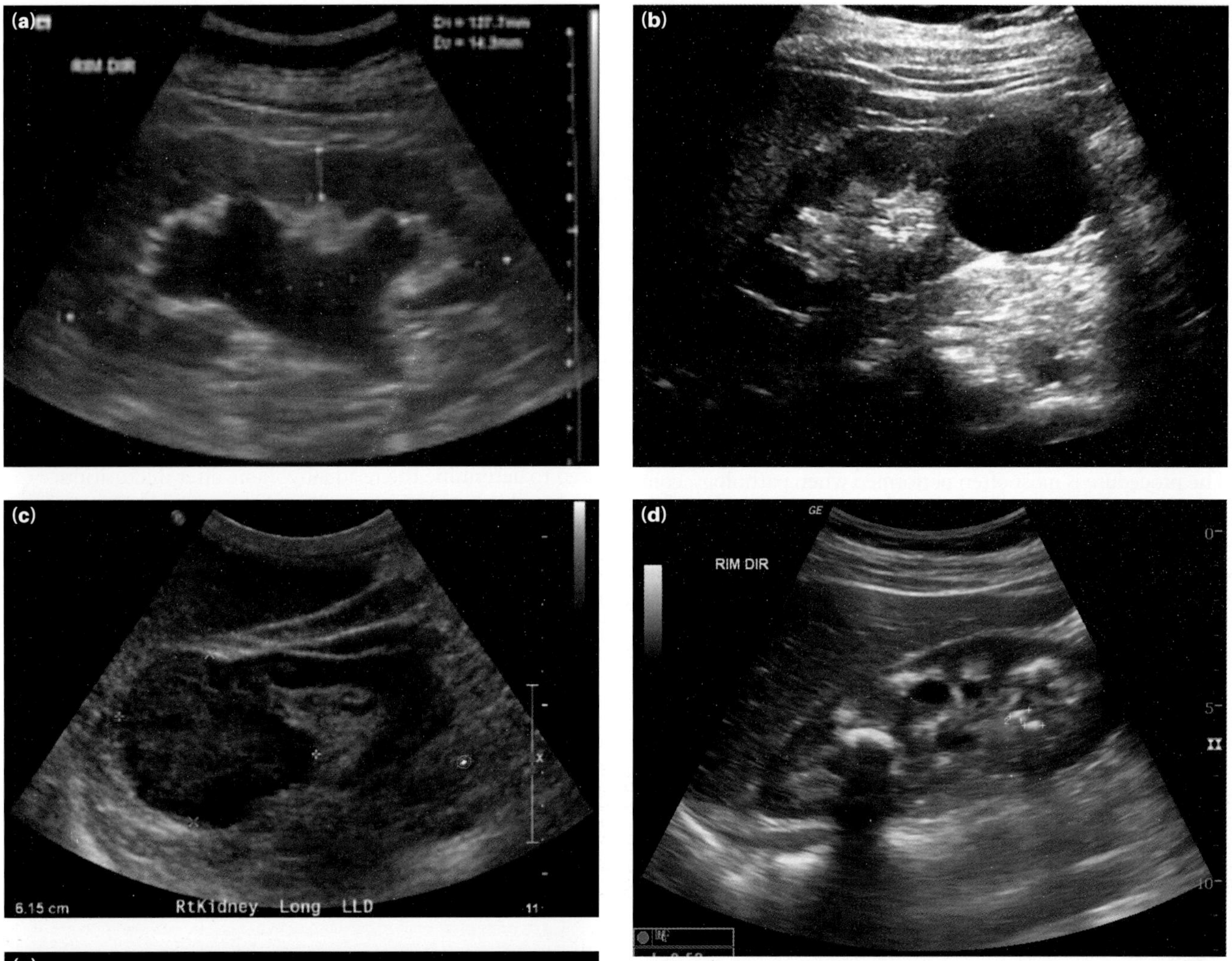

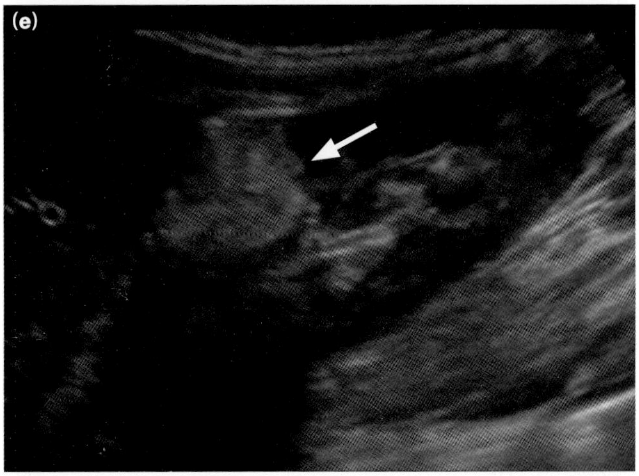

Figure 75.15 Ultrasound scan showing: (a) hydronephrosis (courtesy of Dr Bruno Di Muzio, Radiopaedia.org, rID: 21885); (b) renal cyst (courtesy of Dr Ian Bickle, Radiopaedia.org, rID: 21139); (c) renal tumour (courtesy of Wendy Boller); (d) medullary sponge kidney with renal calculi – note the stone gives rise to an acoustic window (courtesy of Dr Bruno Di Muzio, Radiopaedia.org, rID: 12141); (e) angiomyolipoma (arrow).

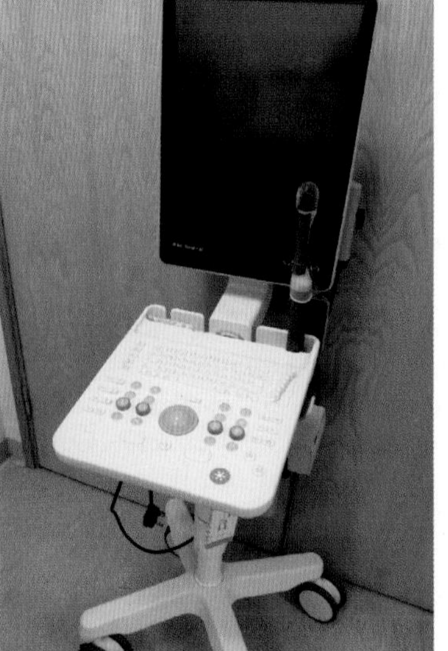

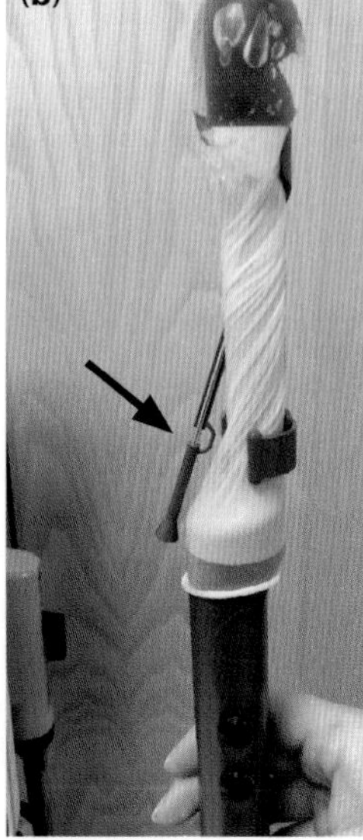

Figure 75.16 (a) A portable machine dedicated to prostatic ultrasound scanning. (b) A close-up view of the transrectal probe demonstrating the diagonal channel through the probe for the biopsy needle (arrow).

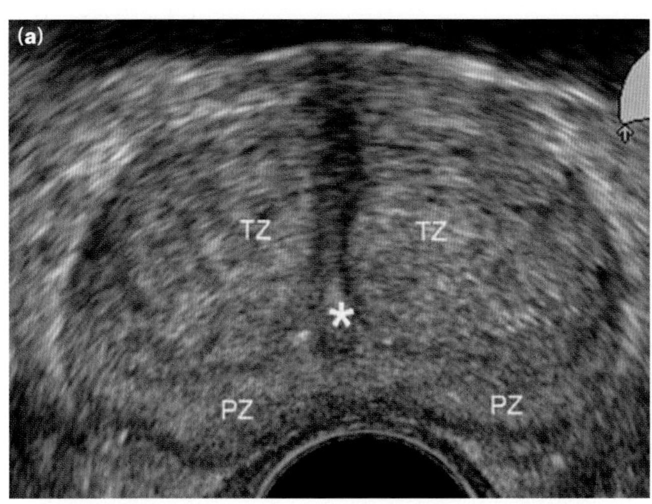

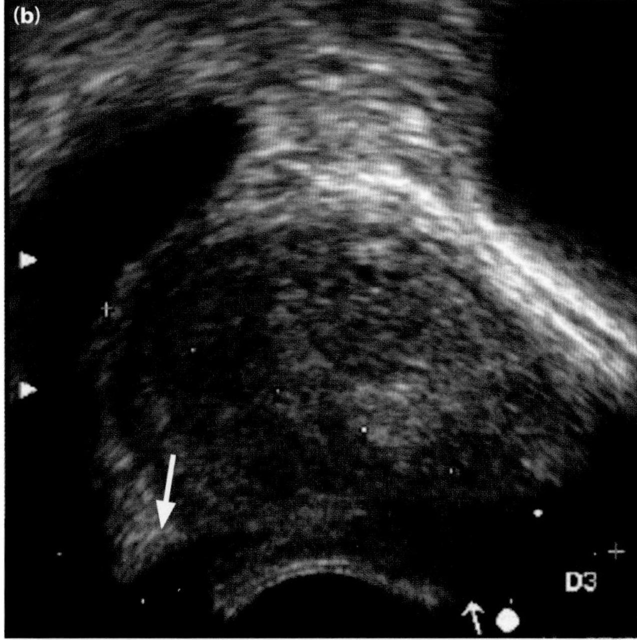

Figure 75.17 Views of the prostate on a transrectal ultrasound scan. (a) On the transverse image, the normal prostate demonstrates an anterior transition zone and a posterior (cow-horn-shaped) peripheral zone. (b) On the sagittal image the bladder is seen above the prostate (arrowheads) as well as the seminal vesicles (arrow).

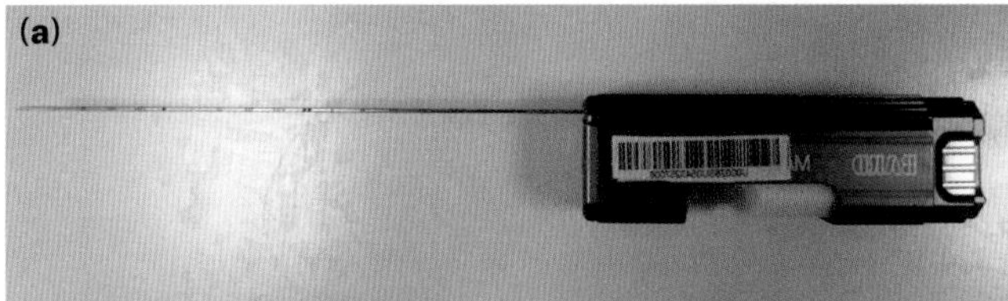

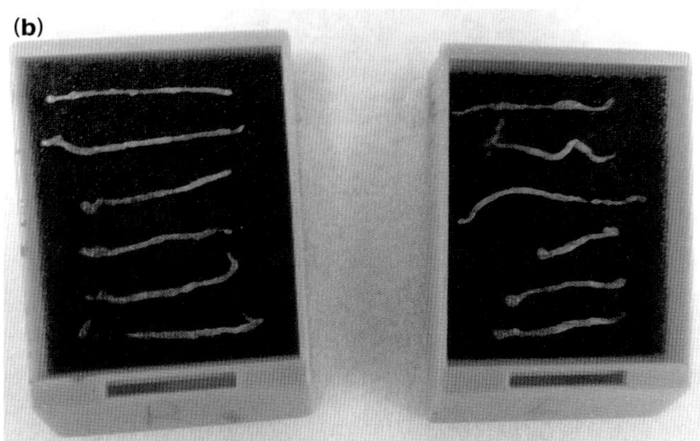

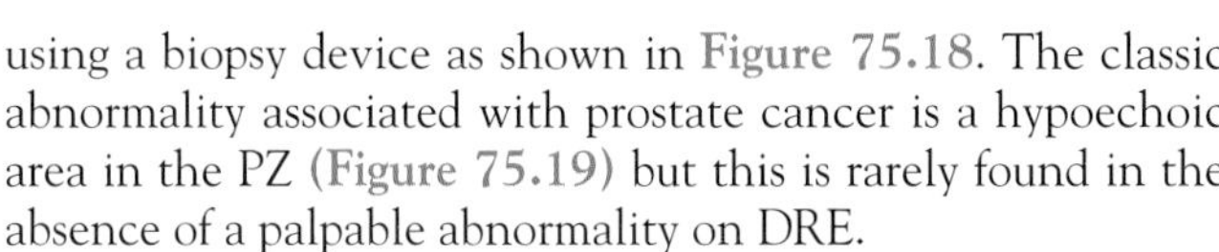

Figure 75.18 (a) A biopsy device used for prostatic biopsy. (b) Biopsy cores taken from right and left prostatic lobes during transrectal ultrasound scanning.

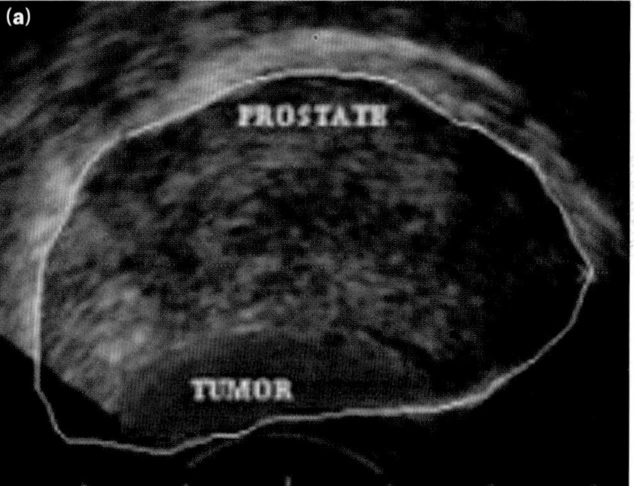

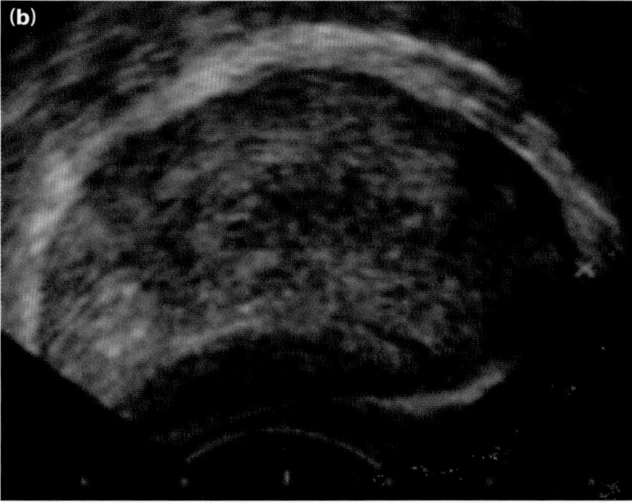

Figure 75.19 (a, b) A transverse image of the prostate on transrectal ultrasound scanning demonstrating the classic hypoechoic lesion in the peripheral zone, typical of a cancer.

using a biopsy device as shown in Figure 75.18. The classic abnormality associated with prostate cancer is a hypoechoic area in the PZ (Figure 75.19) but this is rarely found in the absence of a palpable abnormality on DRE.

Transperineal template biopsies of the prostate

Transperineal template biopsies of the prostate (TPTBP) are increasingly used clinically and although they have not yet replaced TRUS-guided prostate biopsies as a first-line test, they may do this in the future. Currently, TPTBP are used to further evaluate men with a negative TRUS-guided prostate biopsy in whom the PSA trend remains suspicious, or younger men for whom a diagnosis of low-risk prostate cancer has been made and where it is important to exclude more significant disease in other parts of the prostate (most notably in the anterior aspects of the gland) not easily accessible via the transrectal route. TPTBP are usually performed under GA although there are reports that they can be done under local anaesthetic (LA). Typically, around 36 biopsies are obtained during TPTBP including from anterior aspects of the prostate which are impossible to sample during TRUS. TPTBP has a much lower risk of sepsis than TRUS-guided biopsies.

Summary box 75.8

Prostate biopsies

- TRUS has been the traditional method of guiding prostate biopsies
- TRUS-guided biopsies are increasingly being replaced by transperineal template biopsies of the prostate
- TPTBP have a much lower sepsis risk than TRUS biopsies
- TRUS biopsies are usually performed under local anaesthesia
- TPTBP are usually performed under general anaesthesia

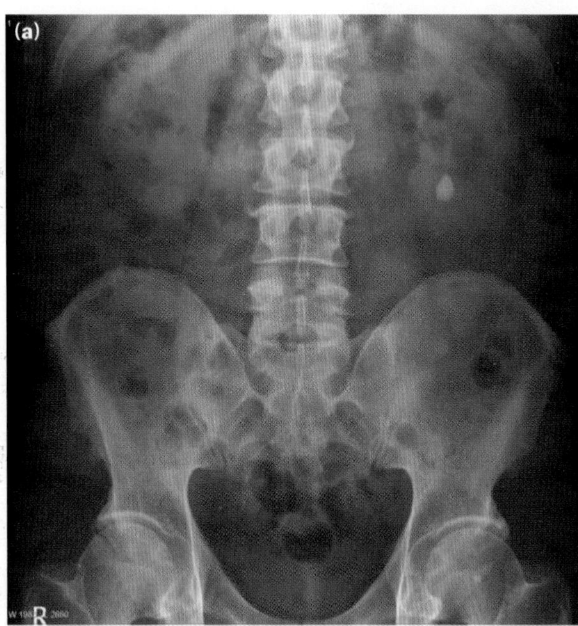

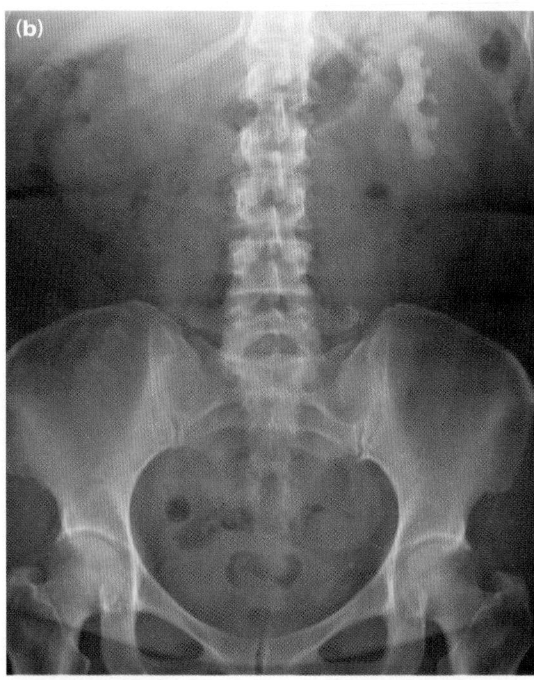

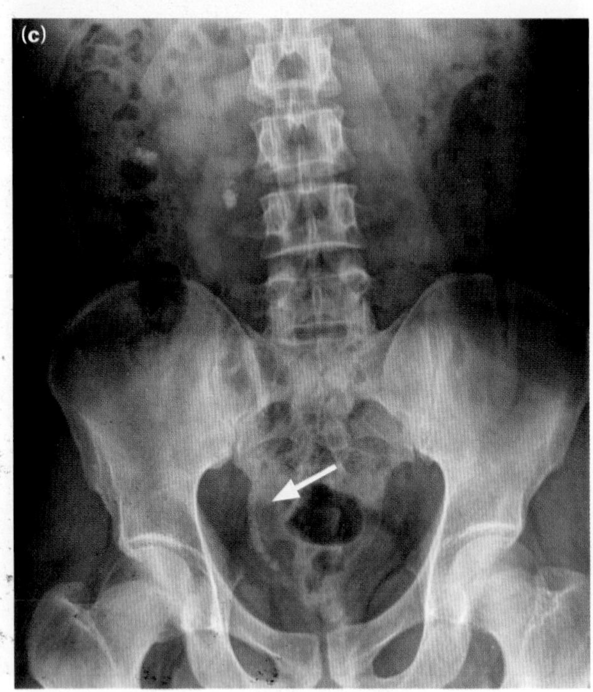

Figure 75.20 (a) Left lower pole renal stone on plain KUB x-ray (courtesy of Prof Frank Gaillard, Radiopaedia.org, rID: 12555). (b) A staghorn calculus in the left kidney (courtesy of Dr Natalie Yang, Radiopaedia.org, rID: 9733). (c) Right lower pole calculi and steinstrasse in the distal right ureter (arrow) (courtesy of Dr Ali Abougazia, Radiopaedia.org).

KUB x-ray (Figure 75.20)

This is a plain x-ray of the abdomen and pelvis that includes the regions of the body occupied by the **K**idneys, **U**reters and **B**ladder. In fact, not a huge amount is learned about these organs in the absence of pathology. In the normal setting, soft tissue outlines of the kidneys are commonly seen but normal ureters and bladder will not be seen. The commonest indication for a KUB is to screen patients for the presence of urinary tract calculi. Patients who have had a CT scan resulting in the diagnosis of a urinary tract calculus often have a supplementary KUB to determine if plain x-ray can be used in the subsequent follow-up of the patient. Phleboliths (thrombosed, calcified veins in the pelvis) can easily be mistaken for distal ureteric stones by the novice. KUB is also frequently used in the management of patients undergoing extracorporeal shockwave lithotripsy (ESWL) for urinary tract stones, to assess the outcome of treatment and to determine whether further treatment is necessary. Finally, a KUB is often used to check for correct positioning of a double-J ureteric stent.

Intravenous urography (IVU)

This is infrequently used nowadays and its primary indication in the investigation of patients with suspected urinary tract calculi has been superseded by non-contrast CT.

Computed tomography (CT) scan

A non-contrast CT scan is now the imaging modality of choice in the investigation of a patient with suspected urinary tract calculi (Figure 75.21a). Angiomyolipomas of the kidney have a characteristic appearance on CT (Figure 75.21b). Other variations of the CT scan include a contrast CT, a contrast CT with a urographic phase and a triple-phase CT.

A contrast CT scan of the chest/abdomen and pelvis is frequently used to stage patients with renal tumours (Figure 75.22), muscle-invasive bladder cancer and young men with testicular cancer. CT is less frequently used in men with prostate cancer but does have a role to play when lymph node disease is being assessed prior to treatment.

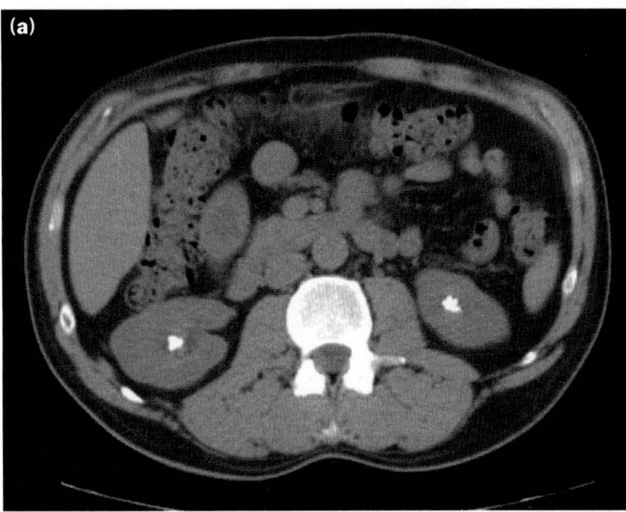

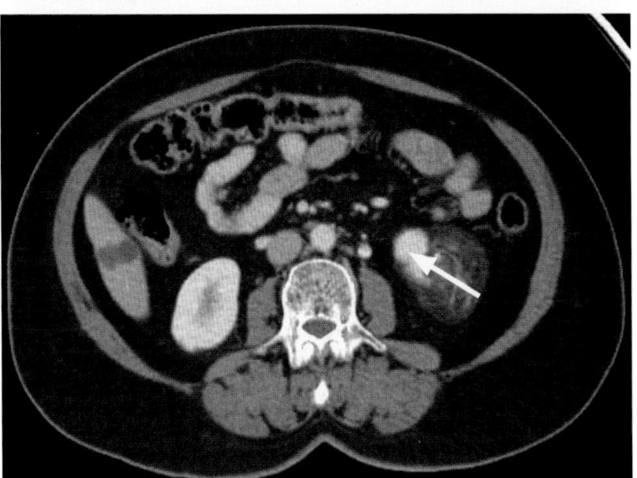

Figure 75.21 **(a)** A non-contrast computed tomography (CT) scan demonstrating bilateral renal calculi (courtesy of Dr Jeremy Jones, Radiopaedia.org, rID: 6211). **(b)** A contrast CT demonstrating a left renal angiomyolipoma with its characteristic content of fat (arrow).

Summary box 75.9

Diagnosis of urinary tract stones

- Intravenous urography is obsolete in diagnosing urinary tract stones
- Non-contrast computed tomography scan is now the technique of choice for this diagnosis

In 1986, a classification of renal cysts based on CT criteria known as the Bosniak classification was devised. Nowadays, this classification can also be applied to MR imaging.

The Bosniak classification of renal cystic masses (Figures 75.23 and 75.24) is as outlined:

I Simple benign cysts with hairline thin walls (Figure 75.24a). The cysts do not contain septations, calcifications or solid components. There are no enhancing soft tissue components.

II Benign cystic lesions (Figure 75.24b). The cysts may have hairline thin septations with fine calcifications in the walls. Minimal enhancement of the hairline thin smooth wall may be seen. No enhancing soft tissue components are present. Non-enhancing high-attentuation cysts <3 cm in size are included.

IIF Complex cysts requiring follow-up imaging. These cysts are more complex and do not fit into category II or III. These cysts have an increased number of hairline septations or mild thickening of the wall and/or septations. No enhancing soft tissue components are present.

III Indeterminate masses (Figure 75.24c). The cystic lesions have thickened walls and septations that are irregular. The cyst walls or septations demonstrate enhancement.

IV Malignant cystic masses (Figure 75.24d). Thick and irregular walls and septations may be present but enhancing soft tissue components are seen, independent of wall or septal enhancement.

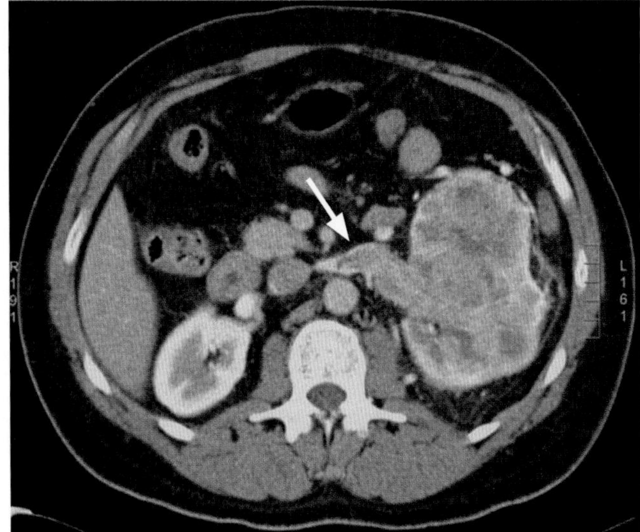

Figure 75.22 Computed tomography scan demonstrating a large left renal tumour with involvement of the left renal vein (arrow) (courtesy of Dr Laughlin Dawes, Radiopaedia.org, rID: 35937).

Morton A Bosniak, 1929–2016, Professor of Radiology, New York University (NYU) Langone School of Medicine, NY, USA.

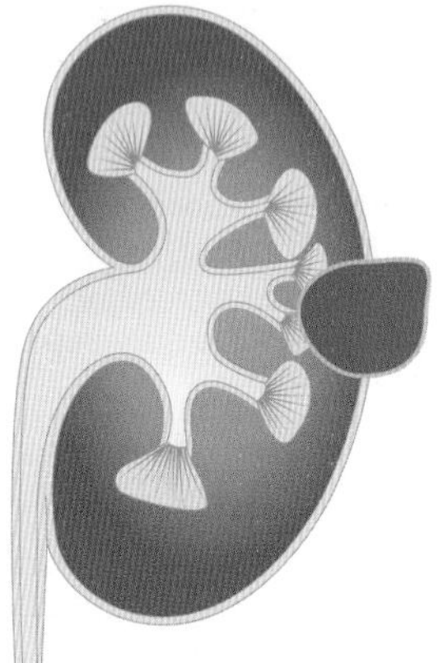

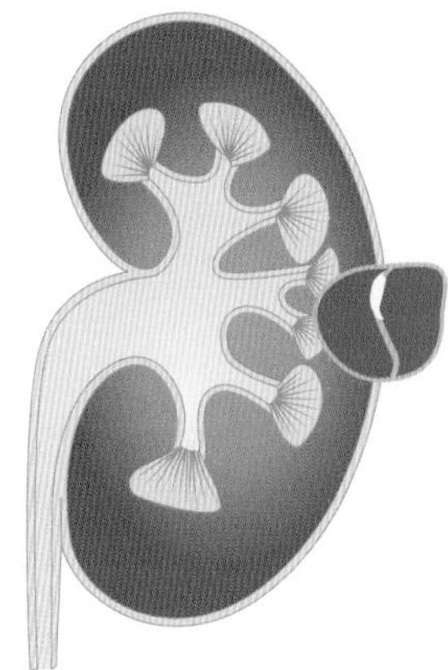

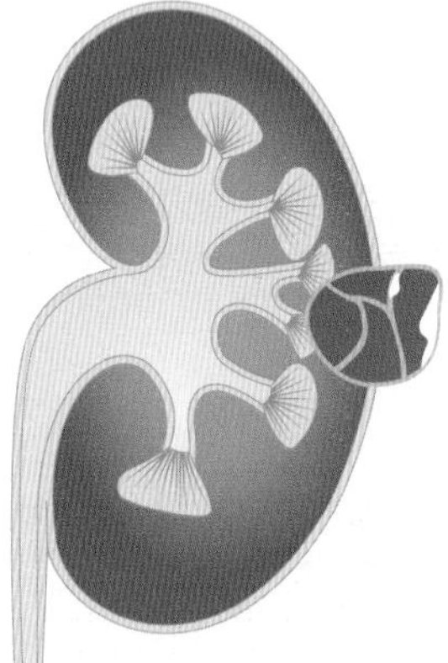

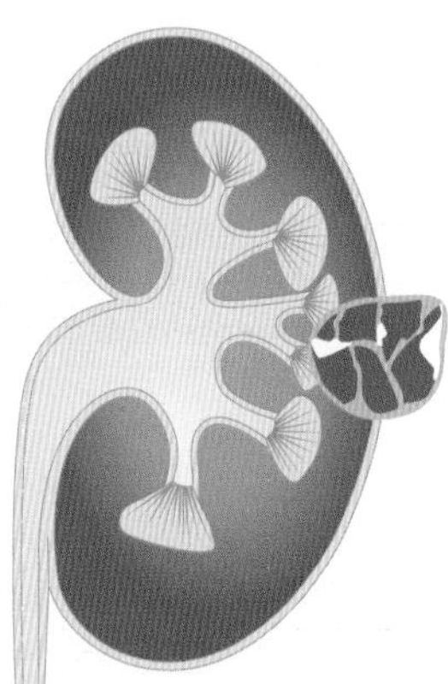

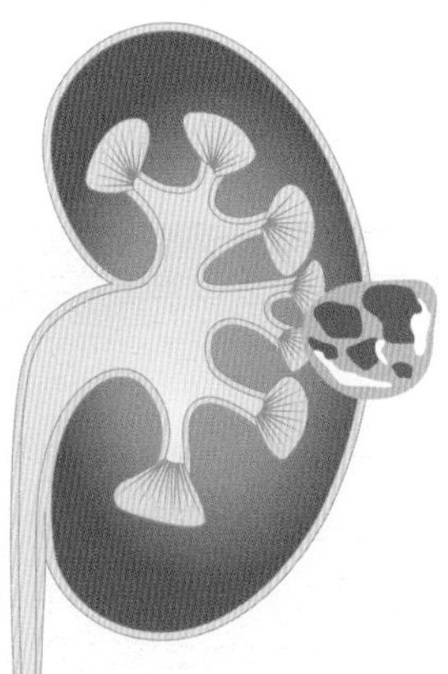

Figure 75.23 Bosniak classification of renal cysts.

Category I and II cysts do not require treatment and do not require follow-up imaging. Category IIF (F indicating need for follow-up) do require further imaging but the duration of this is uncertain. Some authors have suggested 1–2 years but others recommend longer. Category III cysts have a risk of malignancy of 30–100% and should undergo a biopsy to identify those patients requiring surgery. Category IV 'cysts' have an incidence of malignancy of 67–100% and surgical removal should be considered.

Magnetic resonance imaging (MRI)

MRI scanning has a significant role to play, either on its own or as an adjunct to other cross-sectional imaging modalities, in the staging of a number of urological cancers, but it has a central role in the investigation of men suspected of having prostate cancer. Modern MRI techniques in prostate cancer imaging apply the principles of multiparametric MRI (mpMRI), utilising anatomical imaging with standard MRI techniques (T1- and T2-weighted images) and functional imaging such as diffusion-weighted imaging (DWI) (for water molecules motion assessment) and dynamic contrast-enhanced (DCE) imaging (for tissue perfusion assessment after intravenous contrast administration) (Figure 75.25). The advantage of mpMRI is that multiple imaging parameters are combined to assign a degree of suspicion that a clinically significant cancer is present. A 5-point scoring system, called PI-RADS (Prostate Imaging-Reporting and Data System), is used to assign a likelihood (from 1: benign to 5: highly suspicious) that prostate cancer is present within the abnormality detected on mpMRI of the prostate.

mpMRI has a crucial role in the detection and localisation of cancer in men with a persistently elevated PSA but negative previous TRUS biopsy and in men with what is thought to be small-volume, low-risk (of progression) prostate cancer detected on TRUS biopsy who are considered for active surveillance to ensure a significant cancer has not been overlooked for biopsy. The identification of suspicious abnormalities on mpMRI allows subsequent targeted biopsy using novel technologies that utilise MRI during biopsy, and has a major impact on management. Increasingly however, MRI–TRUS fusion biopsies are being performed in a similar manner to TRUS biopsy, with MRI images imported into the specialised workstation to guide biopsy during TRUS.

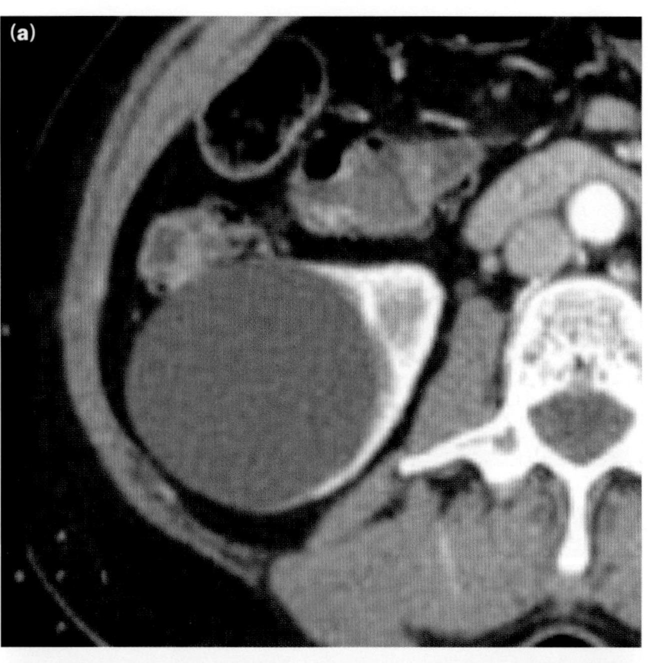

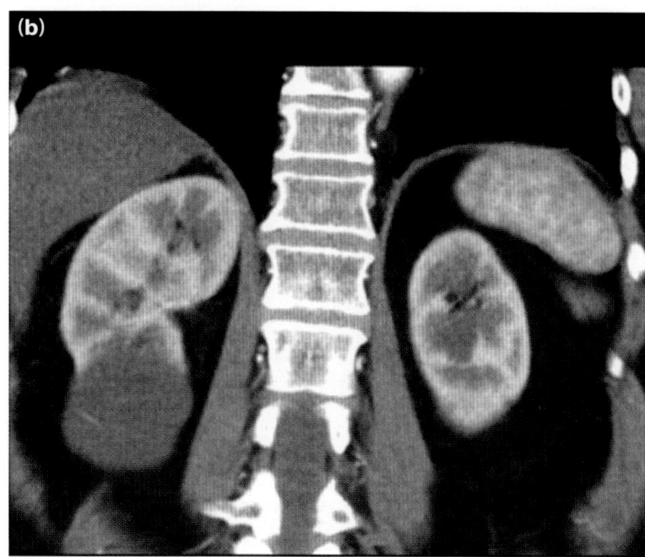

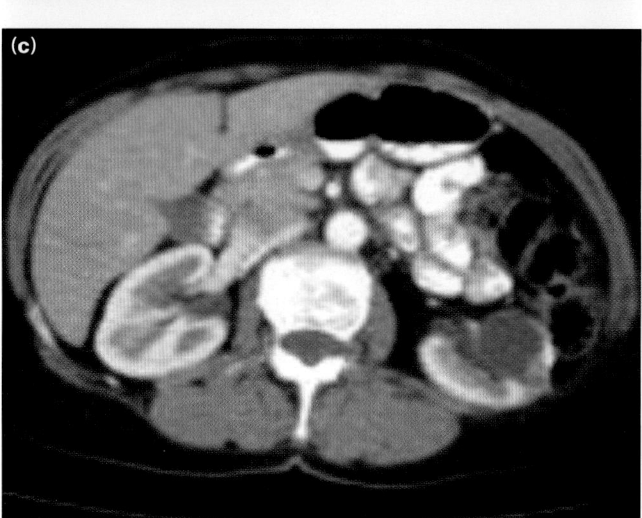

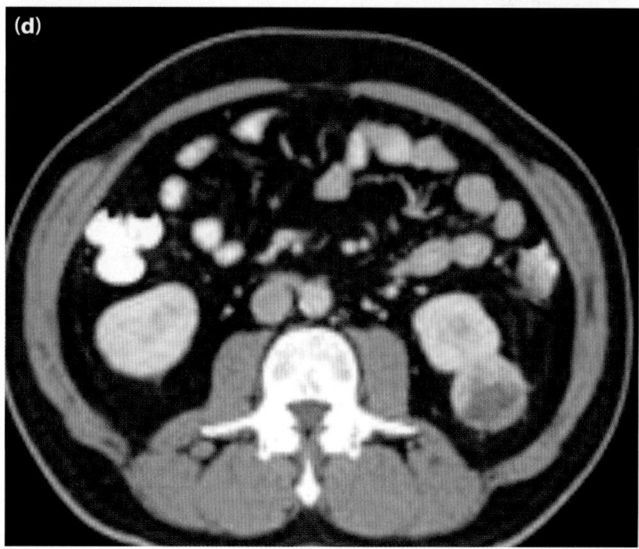

Figure 75.24 Computed tomography scans: (**a**) Bosniak I cyst (courtesy of Dr David Cuete, Radiopaedia.org, rID: 27479). (**b**) Bosniak II cyst (courtesy of Dr Andrew Dixon, Radiopaedia.org, rID: 23404). (**c**) Bosniak III cyst (courtesy of Dr Roberto Schubert, Radiopaedia.org, rID: 17536). (**d**) Bosniak IV cyst/mass (courtesy of Dr Ian Bickle, Radiopaedia.org, rID: 23525).

Summary box 75.10

Magnetic resonance imaging (MRI)

- Is used to stage many urological cancers
- Multiparametric MRI has a significant role in the assessment of men with suspected prostate cancer
- mpMRI is increasingly used prior to prostate biopsy
- Pre-biopsy MRI permits selection of biopsy technique (TRUS v. TPTBP)
- Pre-biopsy MRI assists with targeting of biopsies

SPECT/CT and PET/CT

Single photon emission computed tomography (SPECT) and positron emission tomography (PET) are nuclear medicine imaging techniques that provide metabolic and functional information, unlike CT and MRI. They have both been combined with CT and MRI to provide detailed anatomical and metabolic information. Whereas, initially, separate machines were used to image the patient and the images were then fused, recent technological advances allow the one machine to acquire both sets of data.

Radionuclides used in PET scans are substances that are normally utilised by the particular organ/tissue of interest during metabolism, such as glucose, carbon or oxygen, attached to a radioactive substance. The most common radionuclide in clinical use is FDG (2-fluoro-2-deoxy-d-glucose).

PET/CT looks promising as a tool for the detection of distant metastases in bladder cancer. To date the technique has not been used frequently in those patients with renal cancer. In men with testis cancer, it is recommended in the follow-up of patients with seminoma with any residual mass.

Choline PET/CT using either 11C-choline or 18F-

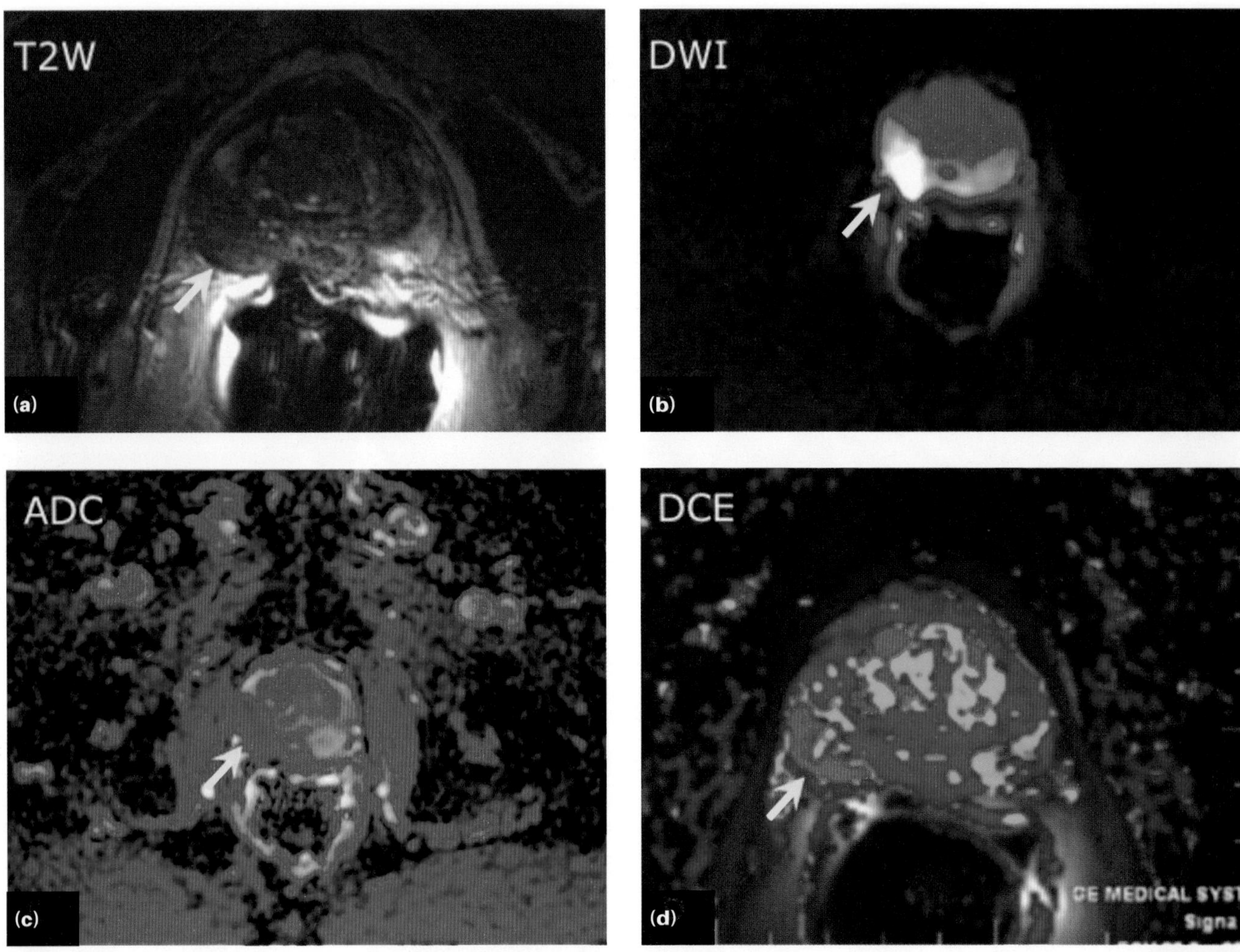

Figure 75.25 Multiparametric magnetic resonance images of a patient with prostate cancer. (a) T2-weighted. (b) Diffusion weighted (DWI). (c) Apparent diffusion coefficient (ADC). (d) Dynamic contrast enhanced (DCE). The tumour appears dark on the axial T2-weighted image (arrow); the corresponding area shows restricted diffusion on the DWI and ADC images as well as abnormal contrast enhancement on the DCE axial image (abnormal red colour coding of the tumour). (Images courtesy of Janet Cochrane Miller, Radiology Rounds, Massachusetts General Hospital.)

choline as the radiotracer have been increasingly used, especially in the assessment of metastatic disease in men with prostate cancer who have failed primary treatment and may be candidates for salvage therapy (Figure 75.26). A new radiotracer for PET/CT, 18F-fluciclovine, was approved by the Food and Drug Administration (FDA) in May 2016 for the diagnosis of suspected prostate cancer recurrence after primary therapy.

Bone scan (Figures 75.27 and 75.28)

A bone scan is most frequently used in patients with a urological malignancy when other imaging suggests there may be bone metastases present. It is also used in the routine staging of patients with high-risk prostate cancer, although there is a <5% chance of a bone scan being positive until the PSA is >40 ng/mL.

Dimercaptosuccinic acid (DMSA) renogram (Figure 75.29)

Tc-99m DMSA is a technetium radiopharmaceutical used in renal imaging to evaluate renal structure, especially in the paediatric population where it is used to detect renal scarring. DMSA is selected for evaluation of the renal cortex as it binds to proximal convoluted tubules in the renal cortex with slow renal excretion. This results in higher concentration and hence higher resolution on imaging. In addition, it allows better assessment of differential (split) renal function.

Diethylene-triamine-penta-acetate (DTPA) renogram

Tc-99m DTPA is another technetium radiopharmaceutical used in renal imaging. Previously it was used frequently in patients suspected of having a ureteropelvic junction (UPJ) obstruction but it has largely been superseded by the mercaptoacetyltriglycine (MAG3) renogram in such cases.

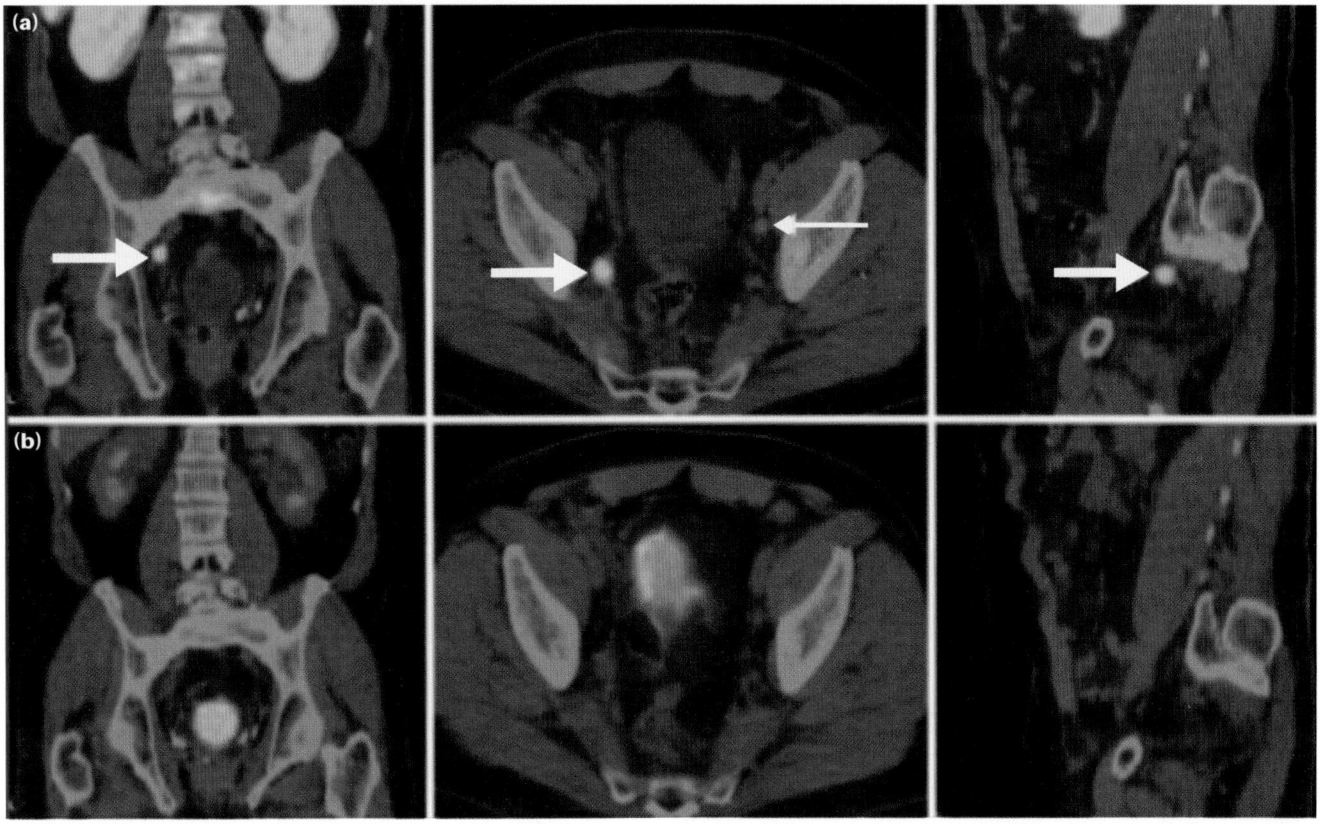

Figure 75.26 Fifty-five-year-old patient with increasing prostate-specific antigen level, 27 months after radical prostatectomy. Coronal (left), axial (middle) and sagittal (right) fused image projections of positron emission tomography/computed tomography (PET/CT) scans. (a) Focal 11C-choline uptake in right (large arrow) and left (thin arrow) iliac region revealed lymph node involvement. (b) This was not observed with 18F-FDG PET. (Courtesy of Hussein Farghaly.)

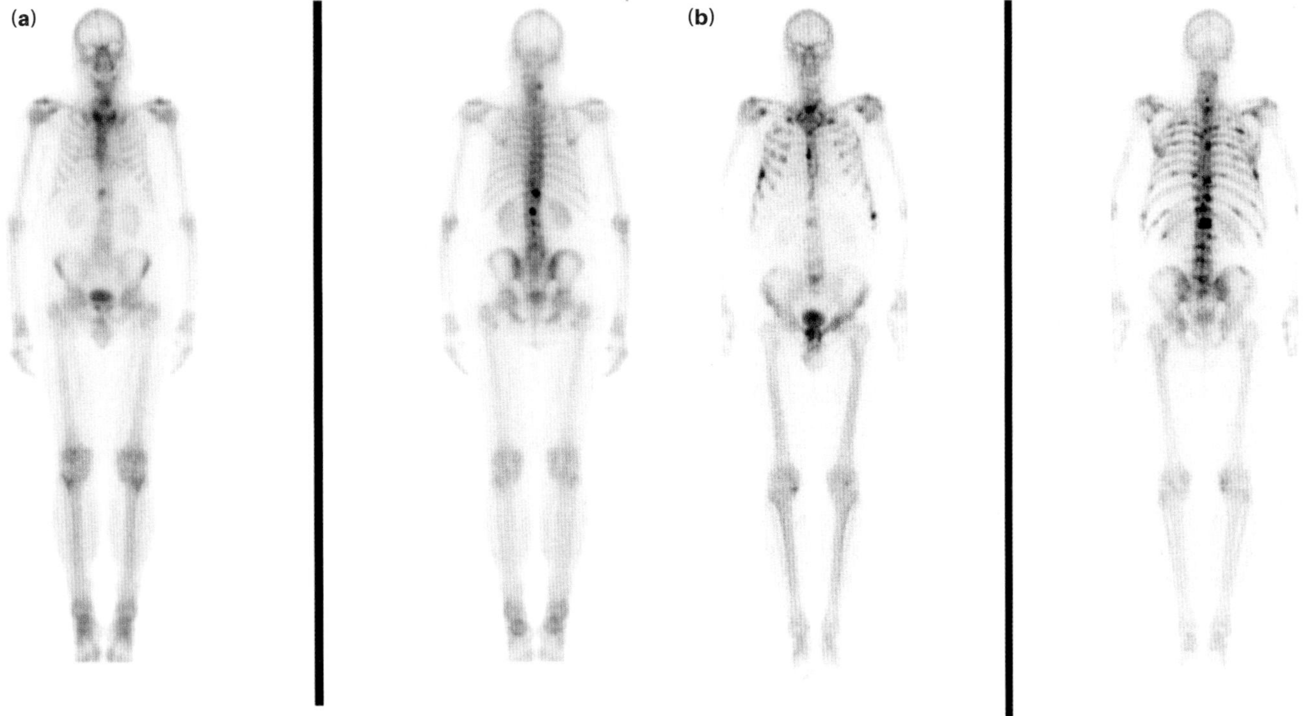

Figure 75.27 Bone scan from patient with (a) low-volume and (b) high-volume metastatic prostate cancer.

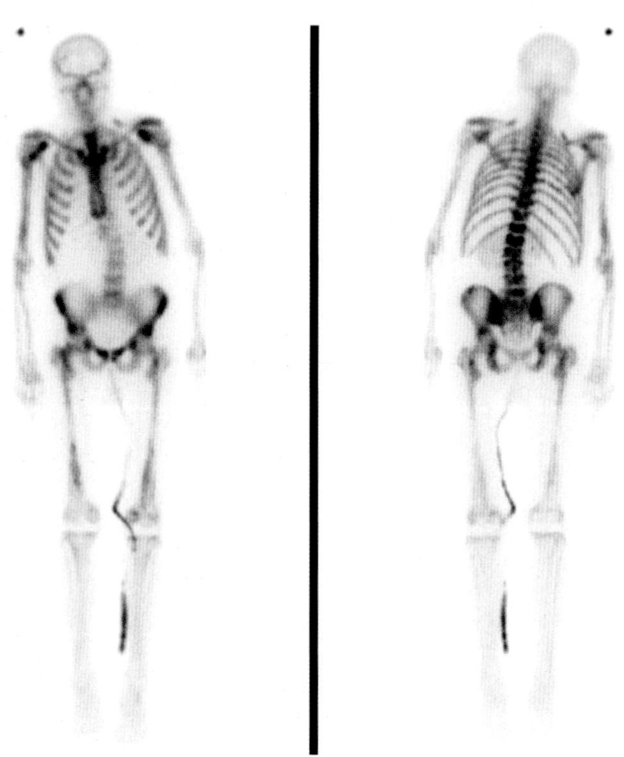

Figure 75.28 Superscan with intense tracer uptake throughout the skeleton.

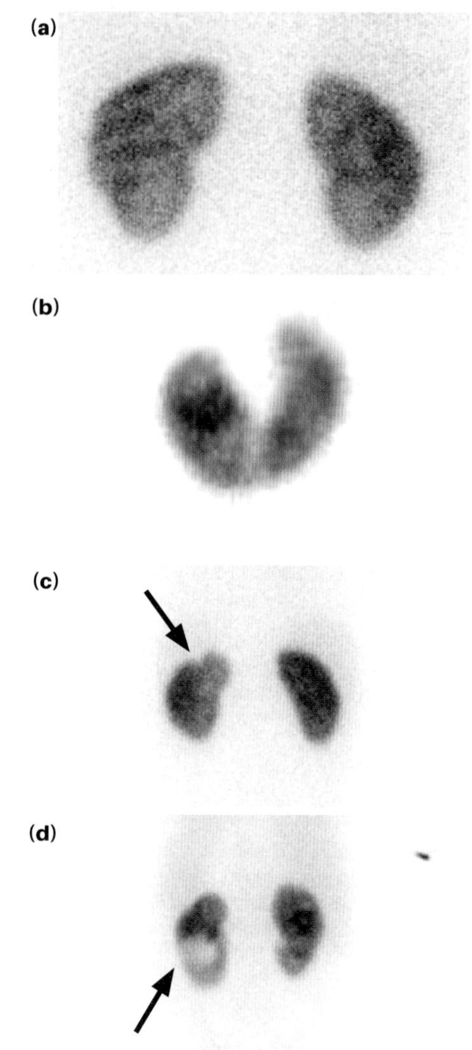

Figure 75.29 Dimercaptosuccinic acid scans. (a) Normal kidneys. (b) Horseshoe kidney. (c) Focal renal scarring (arrow). (d) Renal tumour (arrow).

MAG3 renogram (Figures 75.30 and 75.31)

Tc-99m MAG3 is now the radiopharmaceutical of choice used in the assessment of patients with suspected upper urinary tract obstruction such as UPJO.

The shape of the renogram curve (following subtraction of background activity) is dependent on MAG3 uptake from the circulation to the kidney and secondly MAG3 elimination from the kidney into the bladder.

Classically, the normal MAG3 renogram curve has three phases (Figure 75.30):

1 The curve rises steeply upwards following intravenous tracer injection. This is indicative of the speed of tracer injection and its delivery to the kidneys (i.e. renal vascular supply).
2 A more gradual slope which represents renal handling of MAG3 (renal uptake by tubular secretion and glomerular filtration) and peaks between 2 and 5 minutes. The time taken for the curve to peak following tracer injection is referred to as Tmax. This may be delayed in patients with renovascular insufficiency, renal failure and obstruction.
3 Commences after the peak. It is associated with the emergence of tracer in the bladder and represents elimination (but also delivery) of tracer from the kidney.

After 3 minutes, both elimination and uptake are in competition, but the former subsequently dominates. It is this elimination curve that is dependent on the upper tract urodynamics. Renogram curves of a number of normal and pathological conditions are shown in Figure 75.31.

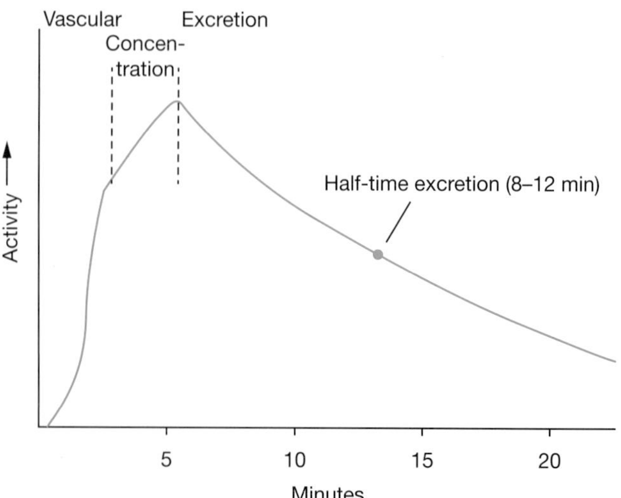

Figure 75.30 The three principal phases of a mercaptoacetyltriglycine renogram curve.

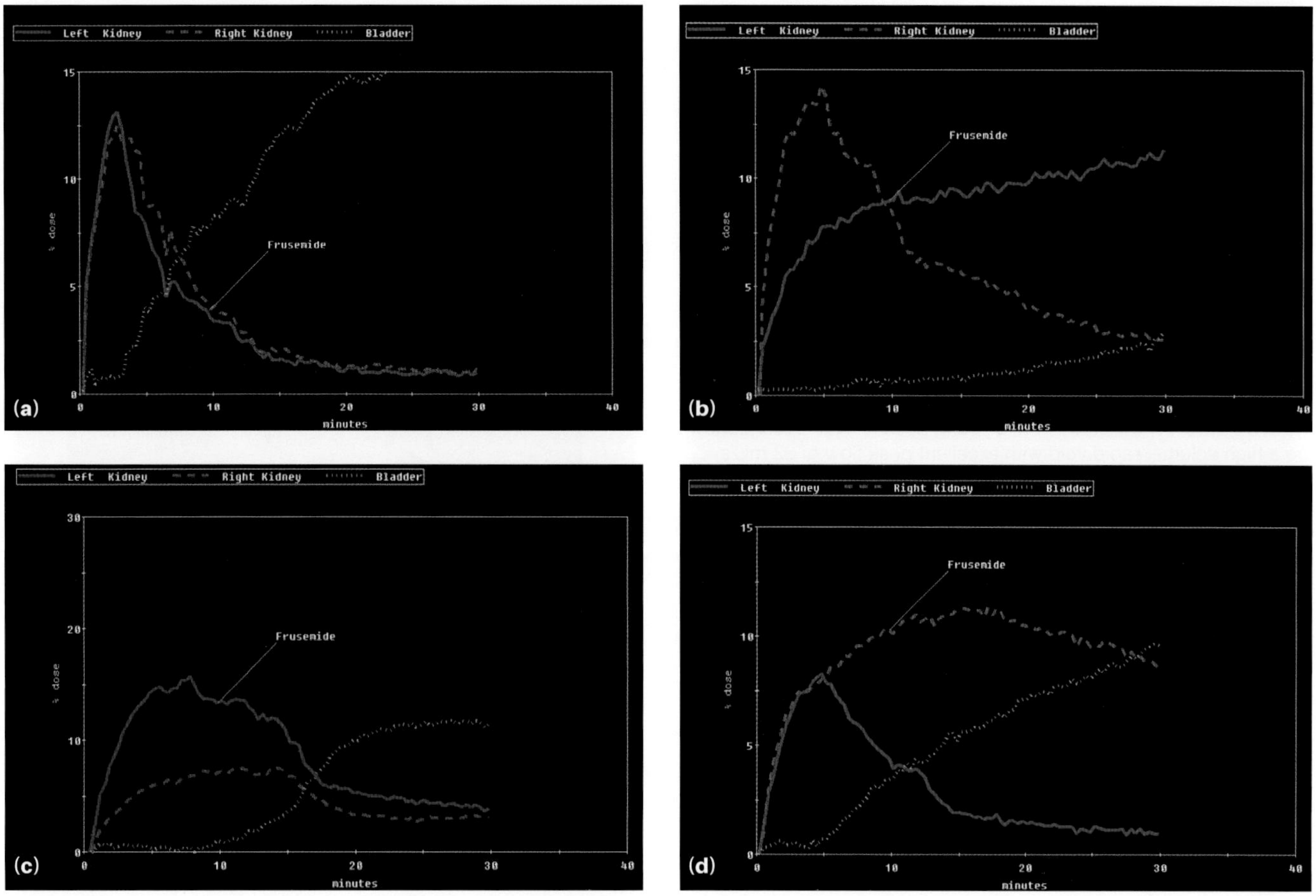

Figure 75.31 Curves from a series of mercaptoacetyltriglycine renograms. (a) Normal excretion. (b) An obstructed left system. (c) Bilateral dilated non-obstructed systems. (d) A partially obstructed right system.

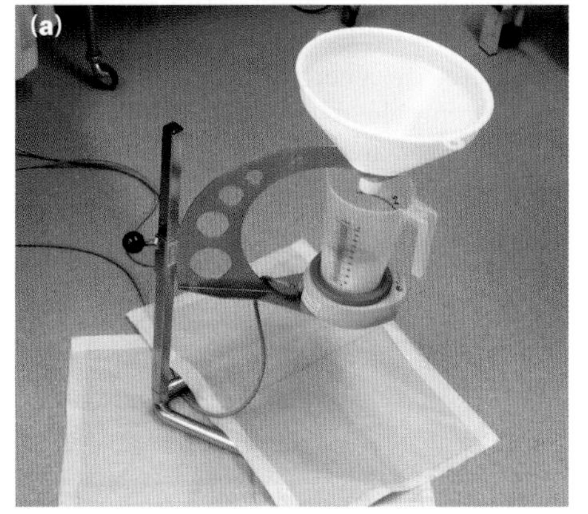

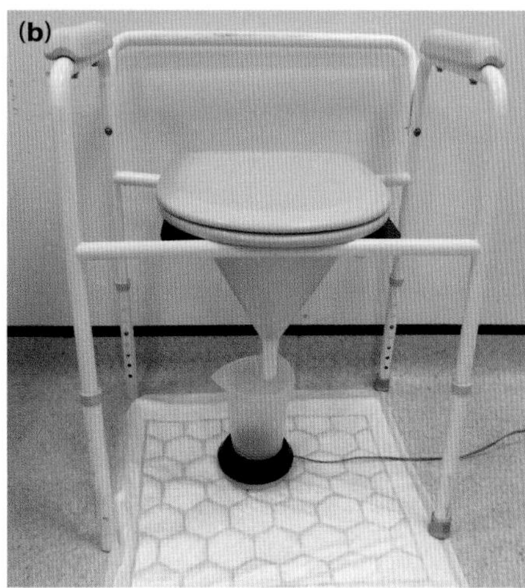

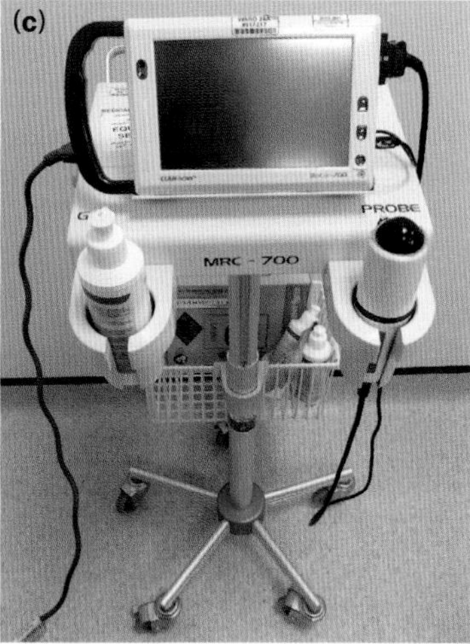

Figure 75.32 (a) A flow meter for use in males. (b) A flow meter for females. (c) An ultrasound scanning device for measuring residual bladder volumes after micturition.

Bladder function assessment

Flow rate and US residual urine

Men with LUTS and females with recurrent UTIs or LUTS are frequently investigated with a **flow rate** and a **US residual urine** at the first clinic appointment (Figures 75.32–75.34). A peak flow rate (Q_{max}) in excess of 15 mL/s suggests significant bladder outlet obstruction is not present whereas a flow rate of <10 mL/s suggests BOO is present. A very low flow rate with a very protracted pattern of voiding is suggestive of a urethral stricture. Caution is required when interpreting the significance of a single high US residual volume and repeated tests often give a more representative picture of the degree of bladder emptying.

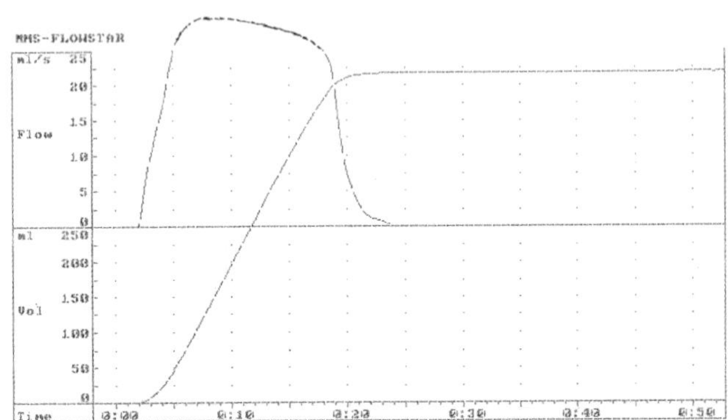

Figure 75.33 A flow study from a young healthy male patient showing a high volume, rapid void with excellent peak flow of 32 mL/s.

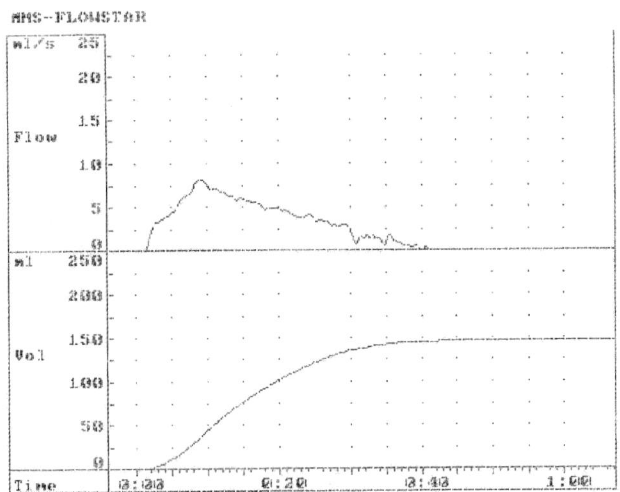

Figure 75.34 A flow study performed by a patient with bladder outlet obstruction showing a very reduced peak flow of urine (8.1 mL/s).

Urodynamics

A urodynamic evaluation provides information about bladder pressure and urine flow and as a consequence has been referred to as a pressure/flow study. A device for urodynamic assessment is shown in Figure 75.35. During urodynamics, fine catheters (or a dual-lumen catheter) are inserted through the urethra into the bladder to allow bladder filling and to record the intravesical pressure. The test is commonly performed to investigate male patients with LUTS and female patients with LUTS or incontinence. It is also commonly used in those patients with a suspected bladder neuropathy. There are 2 phases to the test; a filling phase during which fluid is instilled into the bladder at a constant rate, and a voiding phase when the patient is asked to void. Involuntary rises in the intravesical (detrusor) pressure during the filling phase with or without a desire to void are classical of an overactive bladder (Figure 75.36). High intravesical pressure during voiding with a reduced flow rate is typically seen in a man with bladder outlet obstruction (Figure 75.37). An atonic bladder (no detrusor activity) is seen in diabetic neuropathy and in some patients following abdominoperineal excision of the rectum when damage to the pelvic nerve plexus has occurred. Detrusor-sphincter dyssynergia, when coordinated contraction of the detrusor muscle in conjunction with relaxation of the external sphincter, necessary to permit normal voiding, is lost, is often seen in neurological conditions such as multiple sclerosis (MS).

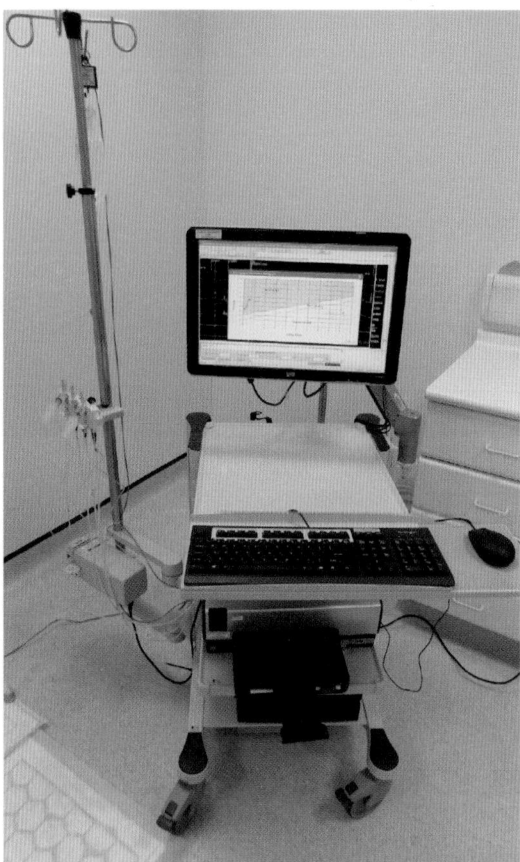

Figure 75.35 A modern urodynamic machine.

Specialised centres have facilities for ambulatory urodynamics when pressure/flow studies can be performed over several hours. A non-invasive system for urodynamics assessment, based on a small penile cuff and avoiding insertion of a catheter into the bladder, has been developed for males.

Summary box 75.11

Assessment of bladder function

- Simple tests are a flow rate and a US residual urine estimation
- Urodynamics provides a pressure/flow profile
- Urodynamics requires fine catheters to be inserted into the bladder and usually the rectum
- Urodynamics can assist with the selection of patients for surgery such as transurethral resection of the prostate (TURP) or anti-incontinence surgery
- A non-invasive technique in males using a penile cuff has a limited clinical role

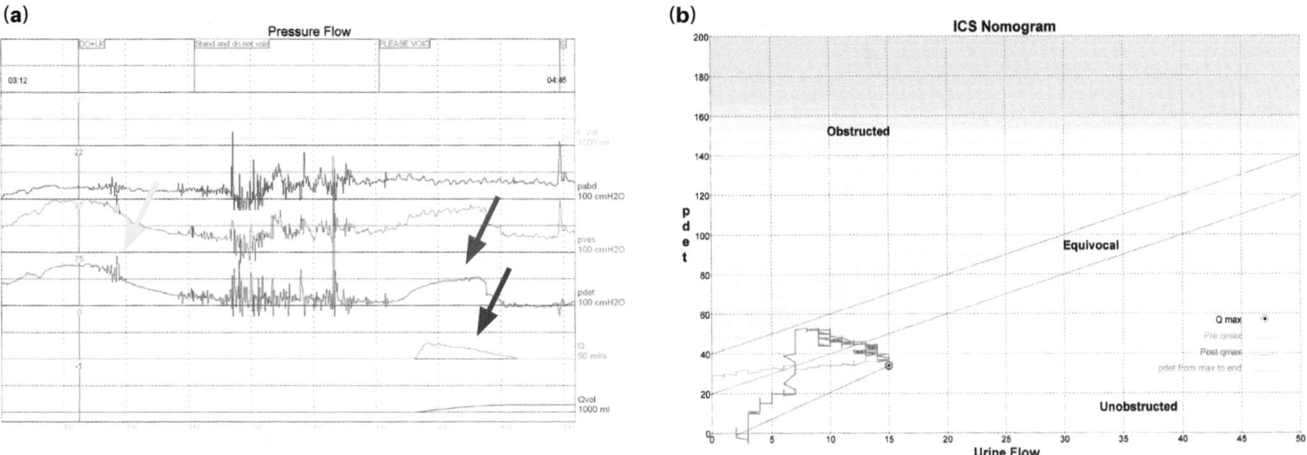

Figure 75.36 A urodynamic outcome (a) in a patient with an overactive bladder, demonstrating a rise in detrusor pressure during filling (yellow arrow), normal detrusor pressure during voiding (red arrow) and a good urinary flow (blue arrow). The Abrams-Griffiths nomogram (b) shows the patient is not obstructed.

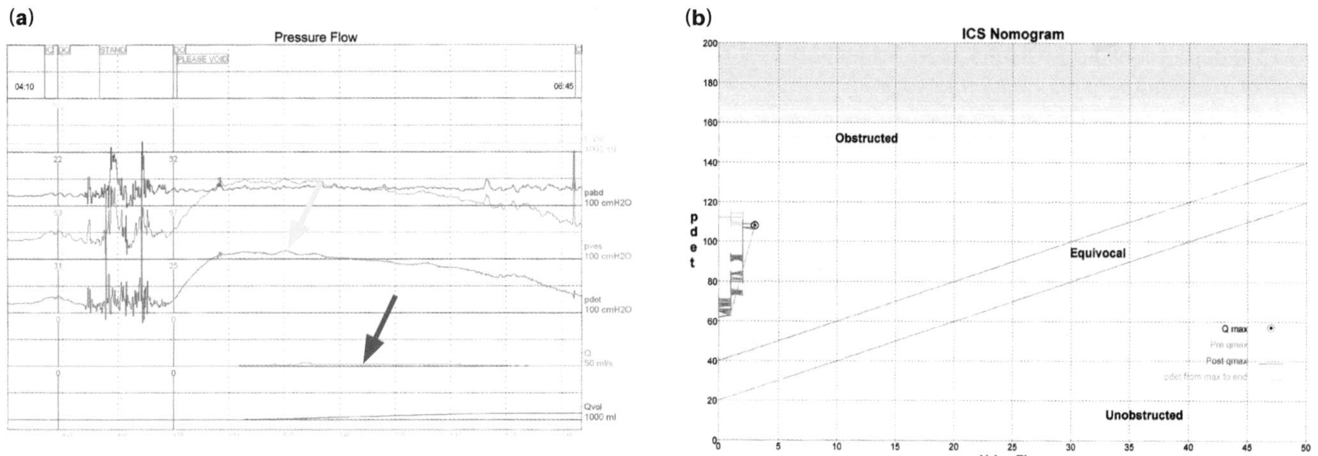

Figure 75.37 A urodynamic outcome (a) in a patient with bladder outlet obstruction, demonstrating a rise in detrusor pressure during voiding (yellow arrow) and a reduced urinary flow rate (red arrow). The Abrams-Griffiths nomogram (b) shows the patient is obstructed.

FURTHER READING

Kaisary AV, Ballaro A, Pigott K. *Lecture notes: Urology*, 7th edn. Hoboken: Wiley-Blackwell, 2016.
McAninch JW, Lue TF. *Smith & Tanagho's general urology*, 18th edn. New York: Lange, 2012.
Wein AJ, Kavoussi LR, Partin AW, Peters CA. *Campbell–Walsh urology*, 11th edn. Amsterdam: Elsevier, 2016.

Paul Abrams, contemporary, Professor of Urology, University of Bristol Medical School, Bristol, UK.
Derek Griffiths, contemporary, professor. He is a physicist who has applied physics to urology, especially urodynamics, in several major centres.

Chapter 76

Kidneys and ureters

Learning objectives

To recognise and understand:

- Important congenital abnormalities of the upper urinary tract
- Important cystic diseases of the kidney
- The management of sepsis in the upper urinary tract
- The pathophysiology of renal stone formation
- The management of urinary tract calculi
- The aetiology, presentation and surgical management of obstruction to the upper urinary tract
- The management of open and closed trauma to the kidney and ureter
- Important renal neoplasms and their presentation
- Surgery of upper urinary tract tumours

SURGICAL ANATOMY

The kidneys are surrounded by a distinct, well-defined envelope of perinephric fat. Nephrectomy is facilitated by staying at the true margin of the perinephric fat envelope. The perinephric fat is 'whiter' than colonic mesenteric fat as observed during a laparoscopic nephrectomy. At the renal hilum, the first structure encountered (i.e. the uppermost) is the renal vein, then the renal artery and lastly the renal pelvis. The right renal vein is much shorter than the left renal vein. The left renal vein is occasionally retroaortic. The right adrenal vein and right gonadal vein drain into the inferior vena cava (IVC) whereas the left adrenal and gonadal veins drain into the left renal vein. Gonadal veins can easily be confused for ureters – these structures are distinguished by pinching the ureter which contracts (vermiculation).

EMBRYOLOGY (FIGURE 76.1)

The urinary tract is formed from the cloaca and intermediate mesoderm in parallel with the early differentiation of the metanephric blastema which will ultimately form the kidney.

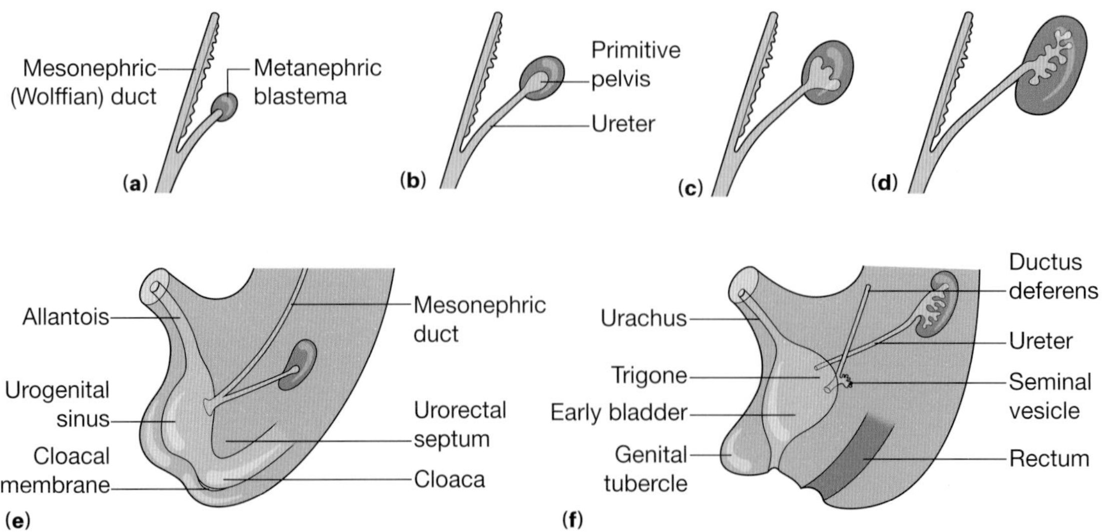

Figure 76.1 Development of the urinary tract. **(a-d)** The growth and development of the primitive ureter and pelvis, with elongation and branching of the ureteral tip and the formation of the calyces. The kidney ascends continuously as the fetus grows. **(e)** During weeks 5–6 of gestation, the cloaca grows and develops. **(f)** During weeks 8–9, the urogenital sinus grows and develops into the bladder and outflow tract.

In the 6-week-old embryo, the mesonephric (Wolffian) duct and the paramesonephric (Müllerian) ducts run in parallel. By week 7, in the male, the Müllerian duct starts to regress, and the Wolffian duct will eventually develop into the epididymis and the caudal part of the vas deferens. In the female, the Müllerian ducts fuse to form the uterovaginal cord which will develop into the vagina. As the urogenital tract develops, there is simultaneous development of the fetal kidney. The ureteric bud arises from the distal end of the Wolffian duct as an unbranched diverticulum and invades the adjacent metanephric mesenchyme, initiating the branching collecting system within the primitive kidney. If the ureteric bud fails to develop, the kidney will not form. Renal development is controlled by the function of a number of transcription factors including PAX-2 and WT1.

Summary box 76.1

Embryology

- Kidney develops from the metanephros
- Ureter sprouts from the mesonephric duct
- Mesonephric duct regresses in females
- Paramesonephric duct regresses in males

CONGENITAL ABNORMALITIES

Unilateral renal agenesis

Complete absence of one kidney occurs in 1 in 500–1000 births and results from failure of connection between the metanephric blastema and the ipsilateral ureteric bud. This condition is an autosomal dominant trait with incomplete penetrance. Typically, there is an absent ipsilateral ureter and the ipsilateral hemi-trigone is missing in the bladder. The remaining kidney is usually hypertrophic but may also be dysplastic. In addition, the ipsilateral testis and vas deferens are usually absent and in some patients the adrenal gland on the affected side is missing as well. Females with the condition may have an absent ovary or Fallopian tube. Renal agenesis is different from renal aplasia where there is a small dysplastic kidney.

Bilateral renal agenesis

Bilateral renal agenesis is incompatible with life. It is associated with pulmonary hypoplasia and Potter's facies due to oligohydramnios.

Multicystic disease

This results from congenital severe renal dysplasia in which the kidney is composed of a mass of various-sized cysts in a loose stroma. If bilateral it is incompatible with survival. It occurs in approximately 1 in 4500 births. It is mostly diagnosed on a prenatal ultrasound scan (USS) and is apparent as a palpable mass in the newborn. Previously, this was surgically excised but nowadays is treated conservatively as there is a tendency for the cystic kidney to regress. Atresia of the ipsilateral ureter is usual and contralateral pelvi-ureteric junction (PUJ) obstruction is common.

Ectopic kidney/crossed renal ectopia

The fetal kidney arises in the pelvis and ascends to attain its normal position. If this process fails to any degree, the kidney ends up being in a lower-than-normal position. During their ascent, the renal pelvis also rotates from facing anteriorly to facing more medially. The most common anomaly is for the renal pelvis to face anteriorly and the more ectopic the kidney, the more severe is the rotational abnormality. In the majority of cases of renal ectopia, both kidneys are fused. In crossed renal ectopia (Figure 76.2), both kidneys are fused and are on the same side – one of the ureters, therefore, crosses the midline to enter the bladder on the correct side of the trigone.

Horseshoe kidney

In a horseshoe kidney (Figures 76.3 and 76.4), the two renal units are low lying and the lower poles fuse to form an isthmus. Further ascent of the fused kidneys is prevented by the inferior mesenteric artery. This condition is detected in 1 in 1000 autopsies and has a male preponderance (2:1). Horseshoe kidneys have an unpredictable vascular supply from nearby major vessels. Horseshoe kidneys are prone to reflux, obstruction and stone formation.

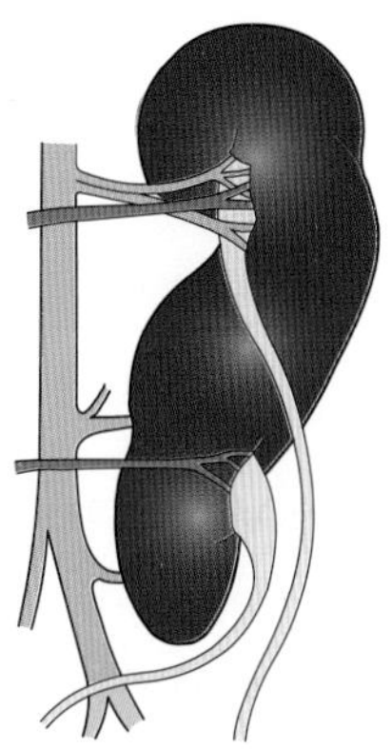

Figure 76.2 Crossed renal ectopia.

Kaspar Friedrich Wolff, 1733–1794, Professor of Anatomy and Physiology, St Petersburg, Russia, described the mesonephric duct and body in 1759.
Johannes Peter Müller, 1801–1858, German physiologist, described these ducts in 1830.
Gabriele Falloppio, 1523–1562, Italian anatomist and physician.
Edith Louise Potter, 1901–1993, American physician, described Potter's facies in 1946.

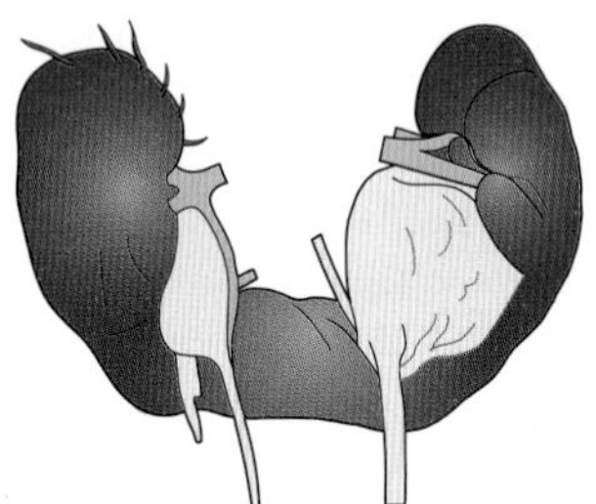

Figure 76.3 Horseshoe kidney. Note the ureters passing in front of the fused lower poles.

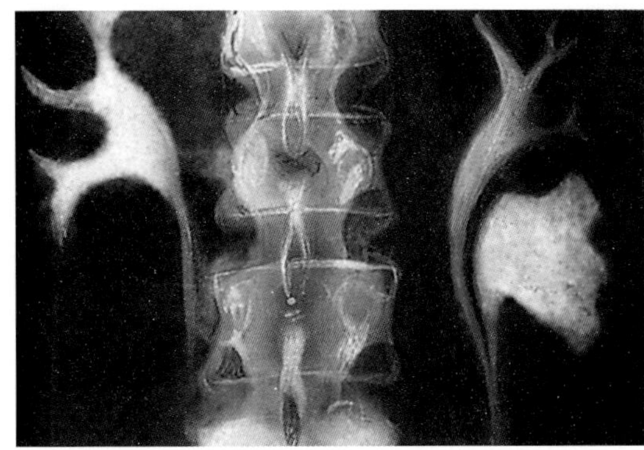

Figure 76.5 Urogram showing a left kidney with double pelvis.

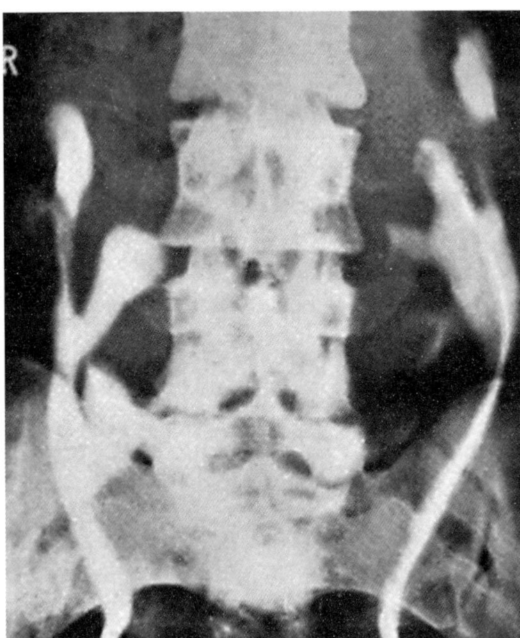

Figure 76.4 Urogram of a horseshoe kidney. Only rarely are all the calyces directed towards the spinal column.

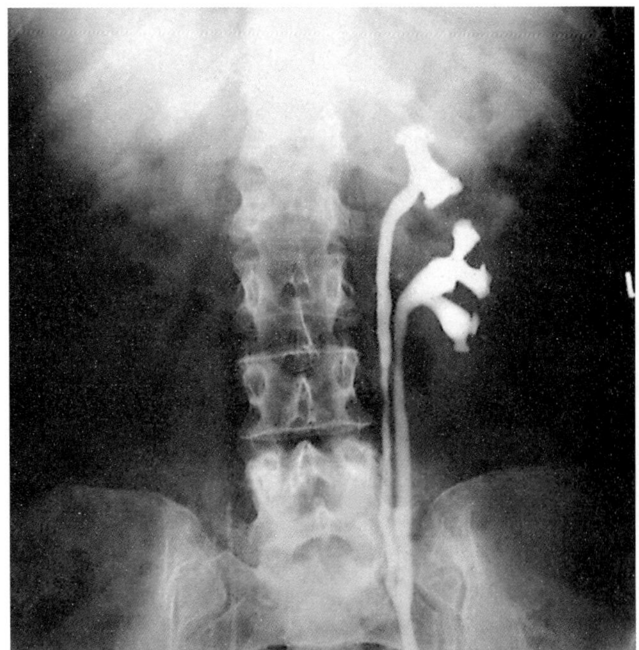

Figure 76.6 Retrograde ureterogram showing a double ureter on the left.

Summary box 76.2

Horseshoe kidneys

- Are prone to pelvi-ureteric junction obstruction, infection and stones
- Can have anomalous vasculature which needs to be considered when planning surgery

Duplex renal pelvis and ureter (Figures 76.5 and 76.6)

Duplication of the ureter and renal pelvis is a common anomaly, with an incidence of approximately 1 in 150 births. Unilateral duplication is six times more common than bilateral and the left side is more commonly involved. The condition is more common in girls and the detection of duplication in a patient increases the risk in a sibling to 1 in 8.

Incomplete duplex ureters with a Y ureter arise if the ureteric bud bifurcates after its initial development from the mesonephric duct. Complete ureteric duplication occurs when there are 2 separate ureteric buds – one in the normal position and the other in a low position. The normal bud ends in the correct site in the trigone of the bladder and is non-refluxing. The lower bud, which will drain the lower pole of the kidney, ends in the bladder with a more laterally placed ureteric orifice with a short submucosal tunnel. The lower pole ureter is, therefore, often associated with vesico-ureteric reflux (VUR).

If there are 2 ureteric buds and the second bud arises from a high position, the upper ureter is incorporated into the bladder, ending more distally and medial to the normal one. Thus, the upper pole ureter ends ectopically and due to obstruction or dysplasia is often associated with severe scarring of the upper pole moiety.

When detected in adults the condition is usually asymptomatic but children with duplex ureters often have VUR. Spontaneous resolution of VUR is less common in patients with duplex ureters compared with patients with single ureters.

Summary box 76.3

Duplex ureters

- Incidence 1 in 150
- Unilateral more common than bilateral
- More common in girls
- Can be complete or incomplete
- In children are associated with vesico-ureteric reflux

Summary box 76.4

Ectopic ureters

- Usually associated with duplex ureters
- More common in females
- Drain the upper pole of the kidney
- May cause incontinence in females
- Never cause incontinence in males

Ectopic ureters

Ectopic ureters are almost always associated with ureteric duplication and 10% are bilateral. There is a female:male ratio of 7:1. As indicated above, the ectopic ureter drains the upper pole of the kidney and inserts into the bladder more distally than normal and towards the bladder neck. In females, the ectopic ureter opens either into the urethra below the sphincter (Figure 76.7) or into the vagina. A female who voids normally but who has dribbled urine for as long as she can remember is typical of the patient with an ectopic ureter. In the male, the opening of the ureter is above the external urethral sphincter so the patient is continent. An ectopic ureteric orifice in a male at the apex of the trigone, in the posterior urethra, in a seminal vesicle or in an ejaculatory duct is likely to be functionally abnormal and infection is common.

A severely diseased or atrophic moiety is effectively treated by partial nephrectomy. A refluxing ureter may need re-implanting. An ectopic ureter in a female often drains hydronephrotic and chronically infected renal tissue and is best excised. Rarely, the incontinence can be cured and renal function preserved by re-implanting the ureter into the bladder.

Ureterocoele

A ureterocoele is a cystic enlargement of the intramural ureter, probably due to atresia of the ureteric orifice. Ureterocoeles affect females more often than males (4:1) and 10% are bilateral. The condition occurs almost exclusively in Caucasians. Similar to ectopic ureters, ureters with ureterocoeles frequently drain the upper pole and are often associated with dysplastic or non-functional renal tissue. In childhood, they usually present with infection. When large, they can obstruct the bladder neck or even the contralateral ureteric orifice. In adults, ureterocoeles typically present with stones in the lower ureter. The classic sign of a ureterocoele on excretion urography was of a 'cobra head' (Figure 76.8) but intravenous urography (IVU) is relatively infrequently undertaken nowadays. On cystoscopy, a bulging, translucent swelling involving the ureteric orifice is typical which fills with and empties of urine with ureteric peristalsis (Figure 76.9). The treatment of simple ureterocoeles is surgical excision with re-implantation of the ureter. Endoscopic incision is a relatively straightforward method of releasing a stone stuck in a ureterocoele but may result in subsequent ureteric reflux. Advanced unilateral cases with hydronephrosis or pyonephrosis may mean that nephrectomy is indicated.

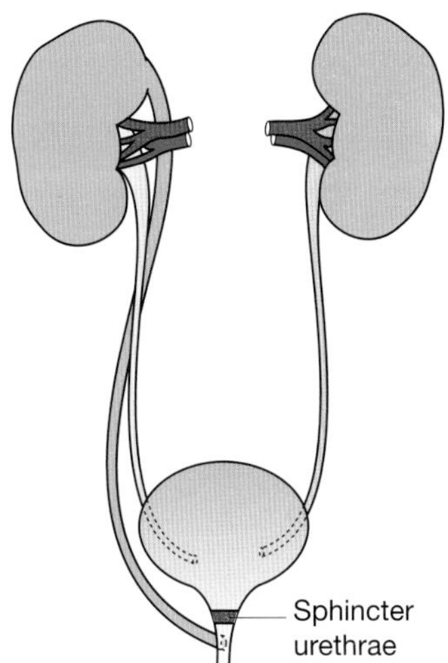

Figure 76.7 In women, one ureteric orifice may open below the sphincter, causing intractable incontinence of urine.

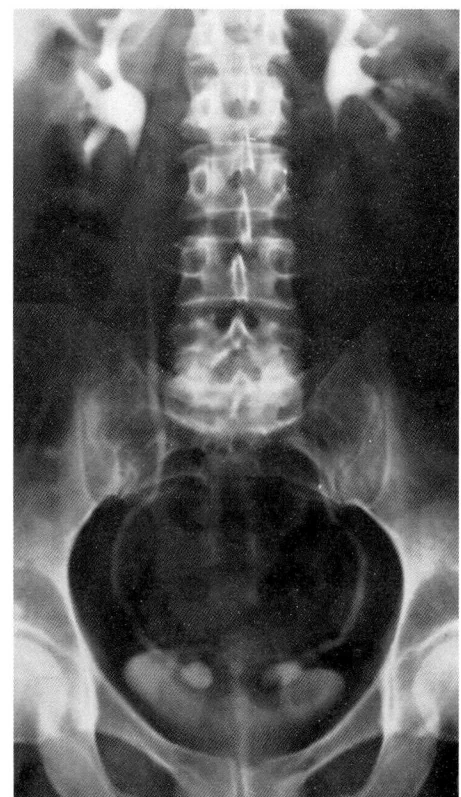

Figure 76.8 Cobra head appearance of a ureterocoele.

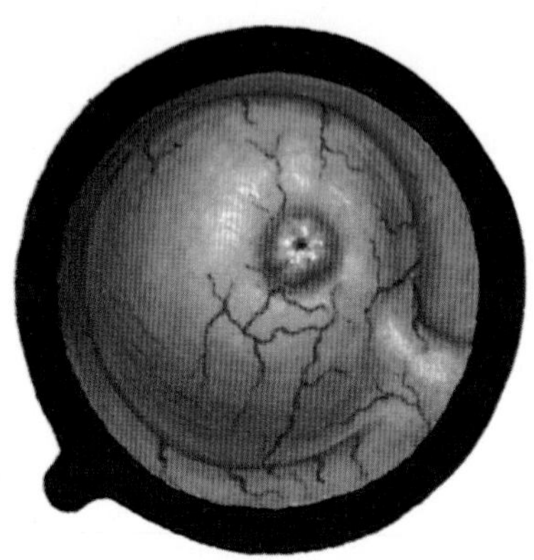

Figure 76.9 Ureterocoele on cystoscopy.

Congenital megaureter

In this uncommon condition, there is ureteric dilatation with or without obstruction. It may be bilateral and associated with other congenital abnormalities. The ureteric orifice looks normal on cystoscopy and a ureteric catheter passes easily. Most cases of megaureter with obstruction present in childhood with severe infections. Renal stones can easily form in the dilated systems. The exclusion of obstruction is often established only by an antegrade pressure-flow study (Whitaker test) in which a nephrostomy tube is placed in the renal pelvis and fluids infused at a rate of 10 mL/min.

Retrocaval ureter

Rarely, the right ureter passes behind the inferior vena cava rather than lying to its right side. This can lead to obstruction and the need to surgically move the ureter to lie anterior to the IVC.

Autosomal dominant polycystic kidney disease (ADPKD)

This is a multisystem disorder characterised by multiple bilateral renal cysts associated with cysts in other organs such as the liver, pancreas and arachnoid membranes. It is a genetic condition caused by mutation in one of two different genes (*PKD1* and *PKD2*) and is expressed in an autosomal dominant pattern, with variable expression. The ADPKD proteins, now known as polycystin-1 and polycystin-2, play a critical role in the normal function of the primary cilium that is essential to maintaining the differentiated phenotype of tubular epithelium. ADPKD occurs worldwide and in all races, with a prevalence of genetically affected individuals at birth of 1:400 to 1:1000. The disease does not usually manifest before the age of 30 years and in some patients it is never diagnosed.

Renal USS is used for pre-symptomatic testing of at-risk individuals. At least 3 (unilateral or bilateral) renal cysts and 2 cysts in each kidney are sufficient for a diagnosis of at-risk individuals aged 15–39 years.

The differential diagnosis of ADPKD includes autosomal recessive PKD, tuberous sclerosis complex, von Hippel–Lindau disease, renal cysts and diabetes syndrome (RCAD), orofaciodigital syndrome type 1, medullary sponge kidney and simple renal cysts.

Clinical manifestations of ADPKD are divided into renal and extrarenal.

Renal manifestations

RENAL SIZE

Renal size increases with age and renal enlargement eventually occurs in 100% of patients with ADPKD, resulting in some patients in a flank or abdominal mass. Cysts contain clear fluid, thick brown material or coagulated blood. Less florid examples are encountered unexpectedly at laparotomy or on abdominal imaging.

PAIN

Pain is commonly a dull loin ache. Haemorrhage into a cyst causes a more acute severe pain, as does passing a calculus from the diseased kidney.

HAEMATURIA AND CYST HAEMORRHAGE

Visible haematuria occurs in up to 40% of patients with ADPKD over the course of the disease. Cyst haemorrhage is a frequent complication with or without haematuria, depending on whether the cyst communicates with the collecting system.

URINARY TRACT INFECTION AND CYST INFECTION

Urinary tract infection is common in ADPKD but its incidence may have been overestimated as sterile pyuria is common in these patients.

NEPHROLITHIASIS

Renal stones occur in approximately 20% of patients with ADPKD. Most stones are composed of uric acid or calcium oxalate or both. Uric acid stones are more common in ADPKD than in stone formers without ADPKD. Stones can be difficult to diagnose on imaging in ADPKD on account of cyst wall and parenchymal calcification.

HYPERTENSION

Hypertension is the most common manifestation of ADPKD and a major contributor to renal disease progression and cardiovascular morbidity and mortality. After the age of 20 years, most patients are hypertensive.

Robert H Whitaker, former urologist, now lecturer at the University of Cambridge, Cambridge, UK.
Eugen von Hippel, 1867–1939, Professor of Ophthalmology in Göttingen, Germany, first described angiomas in the eye in 1904.
Arvid Vilhelm Lindau, 1892–1958, Swedish pathologist, described angiomas of the cerebellum and spine in 1927.

END-STAGE RENAL DISEASE

In most patients, renal function is maintained within normal limits until the 4th to 6th decade of life. Up to 80% of patients are alive with preserved renal function aged 50 years. Men tend to progress to renal failure more rapidly and require renal replacement therapy at a younger age than women. In recent years, a greater understanding of the pathophysiology of ADPKD has led to clinical trials of novel agents such as vasopressin antagonists, somatostatin analogues and mTOR inhibitors to prevent cystogenesis, cyst expansion and declining renal function.

Extrarenal manifestations

POLYCYSTIC LIVER DISEASE

Hepatic cysts are rare in children with ADPKD but thereafter their frequency increases with age. Cysts are usually asymptomatic but symptoms may occur due to a mass effect or due to cyst complications.

INTRACRANIAL ANEURYSMS

Intracranial aneurysms occur in approximately 10% of patients with ADPKD.

VALVULAR HEART DISEASE

Mitral valve prolapse is the most common valvular abnormality and has been demonstrated in up to 25% of patients with ADPKD by echocardiography.

Summary box 76.5

Autosomal dominant polycystic kidney disease

- Autosomal dominant condition
- Cysts may also occur in liver, pancreas and arachnoid membrane
- Usually does not manifest before 30 years of age
- Clinical manifestations are divided into renal and extrarenal
- Hypertension is the most common clinical manifestation
- Renal function declines after the 4th to 6th decade of life
- Men tend to progress to renal failure more rapidly than women

INFECTIONS

Urinary tract infections (UTIs) more commonly involve the lower urinary tract and are significantly more common in females. Infection at any level in the urinary tract is classified as uncomplicated or complicated. A complicated UTI is defined as an episode of infection with an increased risk of serious complications or treatment failure. Complicated UTIs may require different treatment type and duration compared with uncomplicated UTIs.

Acute pyelonephritis

Infection of the kidney (pyelonephritis) can arise in two ways:

- **Haematogenous infection** from a primary site in the tonsils, carious teeth or from cutaneous infections, particularly boils or a carbuncle. Renal tuberculosis occurs by bloodborne spread from lymph nodes in the neck, chest or abdomen.
- **Ascending infection** in the urinary tract is the most common route, and is most likely to occur when there is vesico-ureteric reflux. Urinary stasis and the presence of calculi are common contributory factors.

Acute pyelonephritis is more common in females, especially during childhood, at puberty, after intercourse and during pregnancy. Acute pyelonephritis is suggested by fever (temperature >38°C), rigors, flank pain, nausea and vomiting, and costovertebral angle tenderness. Cystitis symptoms may or may not be present. Symptoms may vary from a mild illness to a severe illness with septic shock, renal failure and a threat to life. Pyuria is almost always present. Both urine and blood are sent for culture. Imaging of the kidney is necessary in the hospitalised patient to rule out pyonephrosis, perirenal abscess and obstruction of the collecting system by renal calculi. A renal USS is often the imaging modality employed initially when the diagnosis is suspected. Alternatively, a contrast-enhanced computed tomography (CT) scan can be used and typically shows decreased opacification of the affected parenchyma, typically in patchy, wedge-shaped or linear distribution.

Escherichia coli and other gram-negative organisms are commonly responsible. In *E. coli* and streptococcal infections, the urine is acidic. *Proteus* and staphylococci split urea to form ammonia, which makes the urine alkaline and promotes the formation of calculi.

Summary box 76.6

Pyelonephritis

- More common in women
- Can be associated with septicaemia
- Associated with pyuria
- Should be treated initially with broad-spectrum antibiotics
- Is potentially fatal, especially if associated with obstruction of the urinary tract

Pyelonephritis complicating pregnancy

Pyelonephritis most often presents between 20 and 28 weeks of gestation with malaise, fever, loin pain and rigors. Not all women will have had lower urinary tract symptoms and pyelonephritis can also manifest in pregnancy as acute abdominal pain or may be detected only after presentation with premature labour. Pyelonephritis is more common in pregnant women with an underlying urological abnormality or diabetes and more often affects the right kidney, probably because the ureter is often more dilated on that side. Pyonephrosis and perirenal abscess are rare complications but should be suspected when treatment fails. Under such circumstances, a renal USS is indicated.

Hans Christian Gram, 1853–1938, Danish bacteriologist, developed Gram staining in 1884.

Urinary infection in childhood/ vesico-ureteric reflux

Symptomatic UTI occurs in 3–5% of girls and 1–2% of boys. In the age-group <3 months, it is more common in boys and in the age-group >1 year, it is more common in girls. The commonest underlying cause is urinary stasis due to VUR, detrusor-sphincter dyssynergia, poor bladder emptying habit or constipation. Other causes of stasis include stones, outlet obstruction or secondary to a neurological disorder such as spina bifida. It is recommended that all children be investigated after their first confirmed UTI.

The most important outcome of a UTI in a child is renal scarring secondary to renal parenchymal inflammation. Scarring can be detected (on IVU) in up to 20% of children who have had a UTI and can be detected in up to 37% of children if assessed with a dimercaptosuccinic acid (DMSA) scan. The maximal renal inflammatory response to infection is seen at 3–5 days, hence the need for prompt antibiotic treatment. Between 10 and 20% of children with renal scarring will develop hypertension. Chronic pyelonephritis (CPN) with renal failure is the commonest reason for renal transplant in children <19 years in the UK. VUR occurs in 1–2% of the asymptomatic paediatric population but in 30–40% of children with a UTI and is apparent in 90% of children with renal scarring on an IVU.

VUR is graded as follows:

- Grade I: reflux into the ureter.
- Grade II: reflux into the ureter and renal pelvis.
- Grade III: reflux is associated with mild/moderate dilatation on an IVU.
- Grade IV: additional blunting of fornices.
- Grade V: absent papillary impressions.

VUR is confirmed by a micturating cystogram and a DMSA scan is used to assess the degree of renal scarring. Grades I–III generally resolve spontaneously. Surgery (ureteric re-implantation, periureteric injections of Teflon or collagen) should be considered if episodes of acute PN recur despite antibiotic therapy or if severe reflux is accompanied by a surgically correctable malformation.

Summary box 76.7

Urinary tract infections (UTIs) in children

- In children > 1 year, more common in girls
- Principal cause is urinary stasis
- All children should be investigated after a single UTI
- VUR occurs in 30–40% of children with a UTI
- Renal scarring is a possible long-term consequence

Renal cortical abscess (carbuncle), corticomedullary abscess and perirenal abscess

A **renal cortical abscess** (carbuncle) is usually caused by *Staphylococcus aureus*, which reaches the kidney by haematogenous spread. A renal carbuncle is most commonly seen in diabetics, intravenous drug abusers, those debilitated by chronic disease and patients with acquired immunodeficiency. A **renal corticomedullary abscess**, in contrast, usually results from an ascending UTI in association with an underlying urinary tract abnormality, such as obstructive uropathy or VUR, and is usually caused by common uropathogens such as *E. coli* and other gram-negative bacilli. Such abscesses may extend deeply into the renal parenchyma, perforate the renal capsule and form a perirenal abscess. Treatment with antibiotics without drainage may be effective if the abscess is small and if the underlying urinary tract abnormality can be corrected. However in many cases, percutaneous drainage of pus is required to stabilise the patient. Two percutaneous drains may be needed, one to drain the perirenal collection and a second to decompress the collecting system of the kidney in the presence of obstruction. Formal open drainage of the abscess may be necessary if the pus is too thick to be drained by the percutaneous route.

Patients usually present with pyrexia, back or abdominal pain and costovertebral tenderness but they may have no urinary symptoms or findings if the abscess does not communicate with the collecting system, as often occurs with a cortical abscess. The clinical presentation may be insidious and non-specific. CT scan is the investigation of choice to establish the diagnosis and location of a renal or perirenal abscess. Empiric antibiotic therapy should be broad and cover *S. aureus* and other uropathogens causing complicated UTI.

Emphysematous pyelonephritis

Emphysematous pyelonephritis is a fulminant, necrotising, life-threatening variant of acute pyelonephritis caused by gas-forming organisms, including *E. coli*, *Klebsiella pneumoniae*, *Pseudomonas aeruginosa* and *Proteus mirabilis*. Up to 90% of cases occur in diabetic patients and urinary tract obstruction may be present. Symptoms are suggestive of pyelonephritis and there may be a loin mass. Gas can be detected on a plain film, on USS or more probably on a CT scan. Intravenous broad-spectrum antibiotics and percutaneous catheter drainage with relief of obstruction may be adequate for the less severely ill patient, but nephrectomy may be needed in the most severely ill patients with this condition.

Xanthogranulomatous pyelonephritis (XGP)

This is a poorly understood, uncommon but severe chronic destructive granulomatous inflammation of the renal

Theodor Escherich, 1857–1911, Professor of Paediatrics, Vienna, Austria, discovered the bacterium coli commune in 1886.
Theodor Albrecht Edwin Klebs, 1834–1913, German-Swiss Professor of Pathology.

parenchyma associated with obstruction and infection of the urinary tract. Patients with XGP are typically middle-aged women and have chronic symptoms such as flank pain, pyrexia and malaise. Flank tenderness, a palpable mass, and irritative voiding symptoms are common. The urine culture is usually positive for *E. coli*, other gram-negative bacilli or *S. aureus*. CT generally shows an enlarged, non-functioning kidney, often the presence of calculi and low-density masses (xanthomatous tissue) and, in some cases, involvement of adjacent structures. It can sometimes be difficult to distinguish XGP from neoplastic disease. Nephrectomy is usually the definitive treatment for the condition but is made more technically challenging the more the kidney is adherent to adjacent structures.

Tuberculosis (TB) of the urinary tract

Genitourinary tuberculosis (GUTB) accounts for 14% of non-pulmonary cases of TB. It is caused by dissemination of the organism through the bloodstream and is thus always secondary TB. There is either reinfection or reactivation of old TB.

Blood-borne organisms are deposited close to the glomeruli causing an inflammatory reaction. Macrophages react and granulomas are formed. If bacterial multiplication is checked, fibrous tissue is formed but if it is unchecked, tubercles result with later caseous necrosis. The healing process produces fibrous tissue and then calcium deposition follows. The lesions will eventually slough causing tuberculous bacilluria. The disease spreads through the collecting system and once a calyx is stenosed it is rare for the communication to be restored. Hypertension is rarely seen except when there is extensive renal destruction.

Involvement of the ureter is an extension of renal TB commonly seen at the vesico-ureteric junction.

Involvement of the bladder is again secondary to renal disease. It is seen around the ureteric orifice as inflammation, then bullous granulations and later as ulcers. It then progresses to the muscle which is replaced by fibrous tissue. Tubercles are infrequent.

Involvement of the testis is usually secondary to epididymitis. Spread to the epididymis is usually blood-borne.

The diagnosis is confirmed on a tuberculin test, or at least 3 consecutive early-morning specimens of urine are examined for acid-fast bacilli with a Ziehl–Neelsen stain and subsequently cultured.

CT is the most sensitive modality for visualising renal calcifications and CT urography is more sensitive at identifying all manifestations of renal tuberculosis:

- **Early:**
  - papillary necrosis (single or multiple) resulting in uneven caliectasis.
- **Progressive:**
  - multifocal strictures can affect any part of the collecting system;
  - generalised or focal hydronephrosis;
  - mural thickening and enhancement;
  - poorly enhancing renal parenchyma, either due to direct involvement or due to hydronephrosis.
- **End-stage:**
  - progressive hydronephrosis results in very thin parenchyma, mimicking multiple thin-walled cysts;
  - amorphous dystrophic calcification eventually involves the entire kidney (known as putty kidney).

Treatment involves short-course therapy as fewer organisms are involved compared with pulmonary TB and drugs tend to concentrate in the urine. Drugs such as pyrazinamide, isoniazid and rifampicin are used. Surgery for GUTB is increasing because although chemotherapy can successfully eradicate bacteria, the complications of infection remain. Surgery entails excision of dead tissue, e.g. partial nephrectomy or nephrectomy, and reconstructive surgery, e.g. for ureteric strictures, mainly distal ureteric, and surgery to the bladder such as augmentation cystoplasty.

Summary box 76.8

Genitourinary tuberculosis (TB)

- Is always either re-infection or reactivation of old TB
- Is a cause of sterile pyuria
- Spreads from the kidney to involve the distal ureters and bladder around the ureteric orifices
- Treatment involves short-course therapy
- Surgery is increasing for this condition

STONES

Aetiology

There are very many causes for urinary tract stone disease which can be classified into the following groups:

- idiopathic calcium urolithiasis;
- hypercalcaemic disorders;
- renal tubular syndromes;
- uric acid lithiasis;
- enzyme disorders;
- secondary urolithiasis;
- other factors.

Idiopathic calcium urolithiasis

In this condition, there is unexplained hypercalciuria but a normal serum calcium distinguishes this condition from primary hyperparathyroidism. It is classified as renal (more common in children) or absorptive (more common in adults). This is present in approximately 70% of patients with urinary tract stones. It often coexists with minimal hyperoxaluria, hyperuricosuria, inhibitor deficiency and incomplete renal tubular acidosis.

Franz Ziehl, 1857–1926, German bacteriologist and professor in Lübeck, Germany.
Friedrich Carl Adolf Neelsen, 1854–1894, German pathologist and professor at the Institute of Pathology, University of Rostock, Germany.

Hypercalcaemic disorders

PRIMARY HYPERPARATHYROIDISM

A parathyroid adenoma or chief cell hyperplasia results in overproduction of parathormone leading to increased synthesis of 1,25-dihydroxycholecalciferol which increases intestinal calcium absorption, renal tubular reabsorption and bone resorption. This is found in <5% of patients with radio-opaque stones. In the past, urologists sometimes performed the parathyroid surgery for their patients with renal stones but this is rarely the case nowadays.

PROLONGED IMMOBILISATION

With this, hypercalcaemia and hypercalciuria result from bone resorption.

MILK-ALKALI SYNDROME

The ingestion of large quantities of calcium, vitamin D and alkali may result in hypercalcaemia, alkalosis and possible renal impairment. The alkalosis compromises renal excretion of calcium, promoting hypercalcaemic-induced soft-tissue calcification (nephrocalcinosis and nephrolithiasis).

SARCOIDOSIS

The non-caseating granulomata produce 1,25-dihydroxycholecalciferol.

OTHER CAUSES

These include disseminated neoplastic disease, Cushing's disease and hyperthyroidism.

Renal tubular syndromes

RENAL TUBULAR ACIDOSIS (RTA)

There are 3 types of RTA but only type I is associated with stone formation, which is due to hypercalciuria and low urinary citrate excretion. Stones are composed of mainly pure calcium phosphate and nephrocalcinosis can occur.

CYSTINURIA

This results from an inherited defect (autosomal recessive) of amino acid transport in renal tubules and the gastrointestinal tract involving cystine, ornithine, lysine and arginine (COAL or COLA). Cystine stones are often multiple, are very hard and are radio-opaque. Family members should be screened with a sodium cyanide–nitroprusside test.

Uric acid lithiasis

Uric acid stones account for approximately 5–10% of urinary tract stones. Patients with uric acid stones either excrete excessive amounts of uric acid or have excessively acid urine and uric acid remains undissociated and insoluble at pH <5.5. Uric acid is an end-product of purine metabolism. Dietary purine and protein excesses may increase urinary uric acid excretion. Extensive cellular turnover in myeloproliferative diseases or in those receiving chemotherapy may result in increased uric acid production. Uric acid stones can also occur in patients with normal serum uric acid levels (idiopathic uric acid lithiasis). Low urine volume may contribute to uric acid stone disease, such as in patients with inflammatory bowel disease and ileostomies. Uric acid stones are hard, smooth, often multiple and are multifaceted. Pure uric acid stones are radiolucent but most uric acid stones contain some calcium and are consequently faintly radio-opaque.

Enzyme disorders

PRIMARY HYPEROXALURIA

This is an autosomal recessive disorder of glyoxalate metabolism. With type I there is a deficiency of alanine:glyoxalate aminotransferase, and with type II a deficiency of D-glycerate dehydrogenase. These enzyme deficiencies lead to an increased production of endogenous oxalate which results in nephrocalcinosis and nephrolithiasis. This condition often presents in childhood.

XANTHINURIA

This is a rare inherited deficiency of xanthine oxidase. Stone formation in these patients can be precipitated by allopurinol, a xanthine oxidase inhibitor.

2, 8-DIHYDROADENINURIA

This is an inherited deficiency of adenine phosphoribosyl transferase.

Secondary urolithiasis

SECONDARY HYPEROXALURIA

Increased oxalate absorption may occur after small bowel resection, or in patients with inflammatory bowel disease or chronic pancreatitis or who have a jejunoileal bypass. This results either from excess fat in the gut binding calcium, hence reducing the calcium available to bind oxalate, or exposure of colonic mucosa to bile salts with detergent properties increases its permeability to charged ions, including oxalate.

DIETARY EXCESS

Rhubarb, spinach, tea, cocoa, chocolate and pepper commonly increase urinary oxalate.

INFECTION

Urease-producing organisms, e.g. *Proteus*, *Pseudomonas* and *Staphylococcus*, break down urea to produce ammonia and CO_2. The urine becomes alkaline which promotes formation of struvite calculi (magnesium ammonium phosphate) which can grow to form a staghorn calculus. *E. coli* never causes struvite stones.

OBSTRUCTION AND STASIS

Delayed crystal washout leads to aggregation and stone formation.

MEDULLARY SPONGE KIDNEY

Up to 20% of patients with calcium stones may have this condition.

Harvey Williams Cushing, 1869–1939, American neurosurgeon, described Cushing's disease in 1912.

URINARY DIVERSION

These patients develop stones due to a combination of infection, acidosis and sometimes stasis.

DRUGS

Several drugs, commonly used, can increase the risk of stone formation. Acetazolamide stimulates renal tubular acidosis. Allopurinol may precipitate xanthine stones. Thiazide diuretics can result in uric acid stone formation.

Other factors

Other factors include:

- geography;
- climatic and seasonal factors;
- water intake;
- diet;
- occupation: especially sedentary jobs in hot environments.

Clinical features

Patients with acute ureteric colic pain represent one of the 3 common emergency admissions seen on urology wards (the other 2 being acute urinary retention and haematuria). Approximately 50% of patients present between the ages of 30 and 50 years. There is a slight male preponderance. Patients describe ureteric colic-type pain but may, in addition, describe renal pain (see Chapter 75 for the distinction between these two types of pain). Visible haematuria is rarely present but dipstick haematuria is a frequent accompaniment to the pain, such that if a patient does not have detectable dipstick haematuria other diagnoses need to be seriously considered – this is especially true in the elderly male presenting for the first time with pain suggestive of a urinary tract stone, in whom a leaking abdominal aortic aneurysm should always be considered and discounted. On account of the fact that other serious pathology can be wrongly attributed to a urinary tract stone, the diagnosis of a urinary tract calculus needs to be confirmed at the earliest opportunity with a non-contrast CT scan. A supplementary plain x-ray is often performed to assess if the stone(s) are radio-opaque and if plain x-rays can be used in the follow-up of a patient who is expected to pass a stone spontaneously. There are 5 recognised narrowings in the ureter which may present obstacles to a stone's passage through to the bladder and these are the PUJ, the point at which the ureter crosses the bifurcation of the common iliac artery, and 3 areas involving the distal ureter (Figure 76.10). Ninety percent of stones <5 mm in maximal dimension are likely to pass successfully. Controversy exists about the value of medical expulsive therapy using agents such as α-blockers and calcium channel blockers (such as nifedipine), with significant variation in whether they are routinely used to facilitate the passage of ureteric calculi.

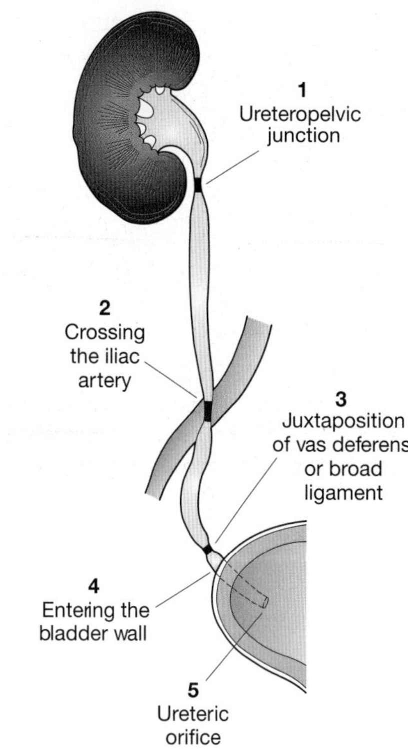

Figure 76.10 Normal anatomical narrowings (1–5) of the ureter.

> **Summary box 76.9**
>
> **Urinary stones**
>
> - The commonest urinary tract stones are calcium oxalate
> - Stones are best diagnosed on a non-contrast computed tomography kidney–ureter–bladder (KUB)
> - Most stones <5 mm will pass spontaneously
> - Medical expulsive therapy remains controversial
> - Indications for surgical intervention are persistent pain, obstruction and infection

Stone management

The management of urinary tract stones can be subdivided depending on whether the patient presents in the emergency or elective setting.

Emergency setting

A CT scan confirms the diagnosis and, as indicated above, small stones (<5 mm), especially in the distal ureter, are treated expectantly as they are likely to pass spontaneously. Medical expulsive therapy may be considered. The patient is usually given a non-steroidal anti-inflammatory drug such as diclofenac for pain relief and observed for further episodes of pain, but also temperature, pulse, blood pressure and white blood count are monitored for signs of developing infection and the estimated glomerular filtration rate (eGFR) is monitored for signs of a decline in renal function. It should be noted that the eGFR should remain within normal limits in the presence of a normal contralateral kidney with normal function. Frequent episodes of pain, signs of infection or a significant decline in renal function are the usual indications to intervene at an early stage.

In a patient requiring relatively urgent treatment for pain, the options are:

- *In situ* extracorporeal shockwave lithotripsy (ESWL).
- Cystoscopy and insertion of a ureteric stent as a temporising procedure.
- Primary ureteroscopic stone retrieval. Nowadays, the stone is usually treated with lasertripsy.

In a patient who is septic secondary to an obstructing urinary tract calculus, the options are:

- Insertion of a percutaneous nephrostomy (PCN) under local anaesthetic by an interventional radiologist.
- Cystoscopy and insertion of a ureteric stent.

When the patient is grossly unwell, insertion of a percutaneous nephrostomy, after the patient has been adequately resuscitated, is preferable to stent insertion as a ureteric stent may not adequately drain pus from a kidney and a PCN results in less manipulation and has a lower risk of producing septicaemia.

Elective setting

The options for surgical treatment are as follows:

EXTRACORPOREAL SHOCKWAVE LITHOTRIPSY (ESWL, ESL)

This is a non-invasive method of treating urinary tract stones by generating shockwaves outside the body which are focused on the stones. It was first used on a human in Germany in 1980. Different methods of generating shockwaves include spark gap, electromagnetic, piezoelectric and microexpulsive. Shockwaves generated using the spark-gap method need to be coordinated with the patient's electrocardiogram (ECG) to prevent cardiac arrhythmias. Stones can be localised for treatment using either fluoroscopy or USS. This is the common form of treatment these days for renal calculi and stones up to approximately 1.5 cm in size are suitable for this form of treatment. More than one treatment session may be needed to fully treat the stone, especially if it is sizeable. Prophylactic antibiotics are used to prevent infection as stones are often colonised by bacteria. Cystine stones are relatively resistant to ESWL due to their hardness. In addition to infection, ESWL may result in haematuria, parenchymal haemorrhage and even perirenal haematoma. A collection of stone fragments in a ureter after ESWL for a significant renal stone is given the German name of steinstrasse ('street of stones') (**Figure 76.11**). Contraindications to ESWL are obese patients, pregnant patients and patients taking oral anticoagulants.

Summary box 76.10

Extracorporeal shockwave lithotripsy

- Is the commonest method of treating urinary tract stones nowadays
- Several sessions of ESWL may be needed for complete stone fragmentation
- Stone fragments collecting in the distal ureter post ESWL are called Steinstrasse

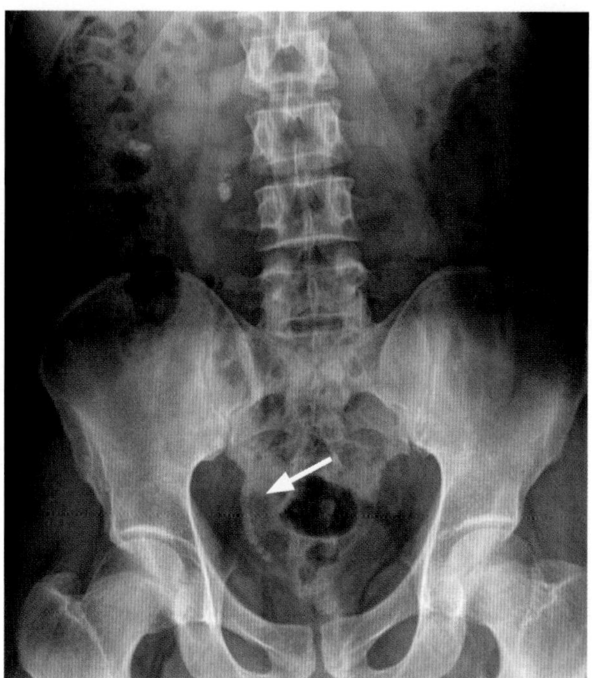

Figure 76.11 Right lower pole calculi and steinstrasse in the distal right ureter (arrow).

URETEROSCOPY

Advances in the design of ureterorenoscopy have rendered the entire urinary tract accessible to endoscopic examination and manipulation. Ureteroscopes are classed as rigid, semi-rigid or flexible. Semi-rigid ureteroscopes are frequently used to directly visualise ureteric calculi (**Figure 76.12**).

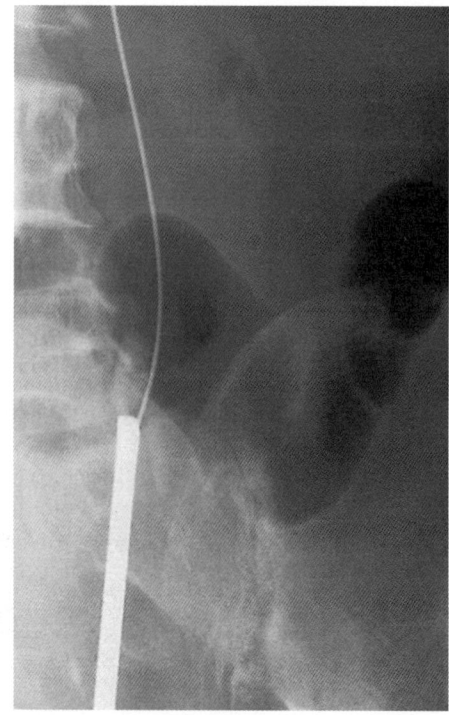

Figure 76.12 Ureteroscopy. X-ray showing a ureteroscope and guidewire in the ureter.

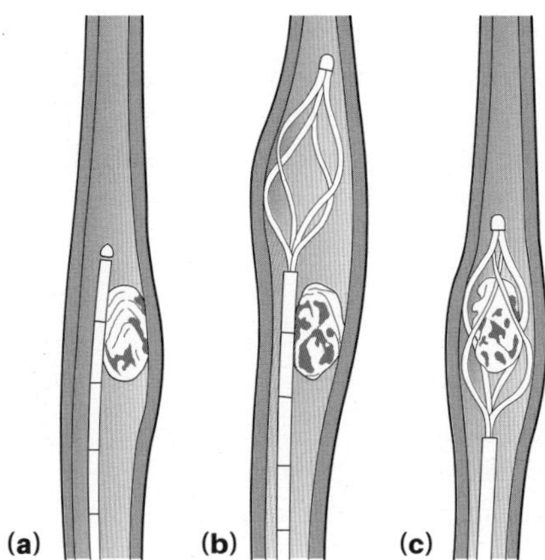

Figure 76.13 Dormia stone-catching basket in use. **(a)** Basket introduced past stone. **(b)** Opened. **(c)** Enclosing stone, ready for withdrawal.

Thereafter, stones are retrieved by either using wire retrieval baskets (if <6 mm and in the distal ureter (Figure 76.13)) or, more commonly, using lithotripsy employing different energy sources (ultrasound, electrohydraulic – rarely used these days, laser, electrokinetic). Stones can also be fragmented using mechanical disintegration using the lithoclast. The most significant complications relate to injury to the ureteric mucosa or wall and include ureteric perforation and extravasation, avulsion of the ureter and ureteric stricture.

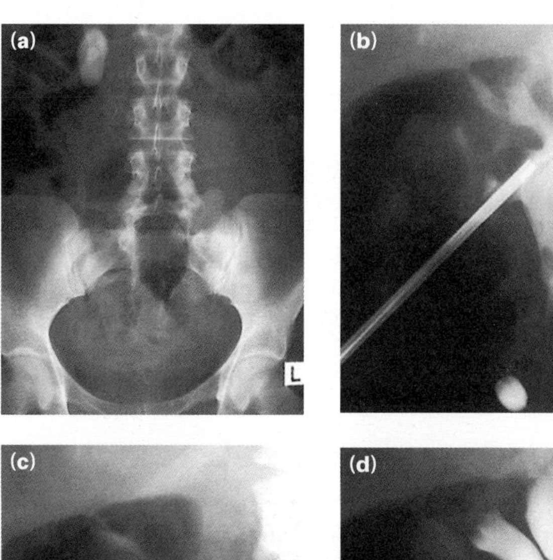

PERCUTANEOUS NEPHROLITHOTOMY (PCNL) (FIGURE 76.14)

Percutaneous nephrolithotomy was performed first in the mid-1970s. It is a technique used to treat larger stones in the renal pelvis or calyces but is sometimes also employed to deal with stones in the proximal ureter. During PCNL, a tract is established into the renal collecting system using ultrasound or fluoroscopic guidance. A series of dilators is used followed by placement of a working sheath into the collecting system through which the stone is visualised and fragmented (using ultrasound, laser or lithoclast). At the conclusion, a nephrostomy tube is left in the kidney for 24/48hrs. As well as for larger stones, PCNL is indicated for:

1. An obstruction: anatomic abnormalities such as PUJ obstruction, calyceal diverticula or ureteric obstruction might prevent the passage of stone fragments after ESWL.
2. Obese patients in whom ESWL is contraindicated.
3. Lower calyceal stones: these are less likely to pass after ESWL.
4. Stone composition: struvite stones need to be completely removed because of associated infection. As previously mentioned, some stones with a very hard composition are difficult to fragment using ESWL, including calcium oxalate monohydrate and cystine stones.

Complications relating to PCNL include:

1. Injury to the spleen, pleura and colon.
2. Haemorrhage from usually the renal parenchyma but also from major renal vessels. If the latter occurs, the treatment of choice is embolisation but, if this doesn't work, nephrectomy very occasionally has to be considered.
3. Sepsis.
4. Extravasation due to rupture of the collecting system.
5. Retained stone fragments.
6. Open surgery to the kidney is sometimes more complicated after PCNL.

OPEN STONE SURGERY

Open stone surgery other than total nephrectomy is incredibly infrequently undertaken in the modern era. In the past, pyelolithotomy, ureterolithotomy and nephrolithotomy with cooling of the kidney were sometimes indicated. A longstanding obstructing calculus can result in chronic inflammatory change in the kidney with substantial if not complete loss of function leading to XGP – see above). Nephrectomy for XGP can be one of the most challenging nephrectomies performed by a urological surgeon as the kidney is often adherent to

Figure 76.14 Percutaneous renal stone removal. **(a)** The stone is in the right renal pelvis. **(b)** Placement of a cannula under radiological control into the renal pelvis and through it a balloon catheter to stop fragments migrating into the upper ureter. **(c)** The stone is disrupted by contact lithotripsy and the fragments have been successfully removed by irrigation. **(d)** A nephrostogram confirms that the renal pelvis is intact.

Enrico Dormia, 1928–2009, Professor of Urology, University of Milan and Chief of the Department of Urology, S Carlo Hospital, Milan, Italy.

many of its surrounding structures. This resulted in the development of the subcapsular nephrectomy for this condition, where the renal capsule is left *in situ*.

Medical treatment of stones

The goal is to prevent further formation of new stones or the further growth of existing stones. Treatment may have to be lifelong. A high fluid intake is advised to prevent supersaturation of the urine, with the aim of producing at least 2.5 L of urine in 24 hours. Dietary excesses need to be eliminated.

Idiopathic calcium lithiasis

An increased fluid intake is advised and correction of dietary excesses of calcium and oxalate. Thiazide diuretics may reduce urinary calcium excretion by increasing fractional calcium reabsorption in the distal nephron. Orthophosphates may be used, which decrease urinary calcium excretion and increase inhibitor activity. Cellulose phosphate given enterally is useful in absorptive hypercalciuria. It is a calcium-binding resin and reduces calcium absorption when taken with meals. Citrate mixtures are useful to increase inhibitor activity in the urine.

Hypercalcaemic disorders

Increased fluid intake may prevent calculus formation, especially in immobilised patients. Oral orthophosphates may be used to decrease urinary calcium excretion. Corticosteroids in sarcoidosis reduce serum calcium. Thiazide diuretics have a role.

Renal tubular acidosis

Sodium or potassium bicarbonate or citrate is given, resulting in an increased renal citrate excretion.

Cystinuria

Potassium citrate is preferred to sodium bicarbonate for this condition. The aim is to increase the urinary pH to 7.5–7.8. D-penicillamine may be used which reacts with cysteine to form a soluble salt that reduces, through competition, the formation of cystine. It is a potentially toxic drug and should only be used if hydration and alkalinisation fail. Adverse effects include rashes, fever, agranulocytosis, arthralgia and lymphadenopathy. 6-mercaptopropionyl glycine (MPG) is an alternative and has fewer side effects. Captopril may be used to lower urinary cystine levels in homozygous cystinuric patients. Dietary methionine (precursor of cystine) restriction is rarely needed.

Uric acid lithiasis

Uric acid stones may be dissolved medically. Urinary pH is increased to 6.5 using sodium bicarbonate or potassium citrate. Allopurinol, a xanthine oxidase inhibitor, may reduce uric acid excretion; once calcium is dissolved this is discontinued and alkalinisation is maintained.

Primary hyperoxaluria

Large doses of pyridoxine reduce urinary oxalate excretion in 20–50% of patients. Neutral orthophosphates may be used to halt the growth of existing calculi.

Enteric hyperoxaluria

Fat restriction is necessary and oral calcium supplements are indicated. Cholestyramine may be used to bind acidic components in the gut lumen, including oxalate. Intestinal bypass may need to be reversed.

Summary box 76.11

Medical treatment of urinary stones

- Aim for urine output of 2.5 L in 24 hours
- Dietary excesses to be corrected
- Specific drugs are available for certain conditions

Stones associated with infection

After surgical removal, antimicrobial prophylaxis should be maintained for 3–12 months. Urinary acidification with ammonium chloride may be used in conjunction. Dissolution of stones with hemiacridrin or Suby G and M solutions is an option.

URINARY TRACT OBSTRUCTION

Obstructive uropathy refers to the structural or functional changes in the urinary tract that impede normal urine flow. **Obstructive nephropathy** refers to the renal disease caused by impaired flow of urine or tubular fluid. **Hydronephrosis** refers to the aseptic dilatation of the urinary tract. Urinary tract obstruction can be classified as either congenital or acquired.

Congenital urinary tract obstruction

Congenital urinary tract obstruction may affect either the upper or lower urinary tract and occurs most frequently in males, most commonly as a result of either posterior urethral valves or pelvi-ureteric junction obstruction. If it occurs early during development, the kidney fails to develop and becomes dysplastic. If obstruction occurs later in gestation and is low grade or unilateral, hydronephrosis and nephron loss will still occur, but renal function may be sufficient to allow survival.

Acquired urinary tract obstruction

Likewise, acquired urinary tract obstruction may affect either the upper or lower urinary tract and can result from either intrinsic or extrinsic causes. Intrinsic causes of obstruction may be intraluminal or intramural.

Causes of upper urinary tract obstruction are summarised in *Table 76.1* and causes of lower urinary tract obstruction are summarised in *Table 76.2*.

Clinical features

Unilateral hydronephrosis

Unilateral hydronephrosis (commonly caused by idiopathic PUJ obstruction or calculus) is more common in women and on the right side.

TABLE 76.1 Causes of upper urinary tract obstruction.

Intrinsic causes	Extrinsic causes
Intraluminal Intratubular deposition of crystals (uric acid, drugs) *Stones* Papillary tissue Blood clots Fungal ball	**Reproductive system** Cervix: *carcinoma* Uterus: *pregnancy*, *tumours*, prolapse, endometriosis, pelvic inflammatory disease Ovary: tumour, cysts Prostate: *carcinoma*
Intramural Functional: pelviureteral or vesicoureteral junction dysfunction Anatomic: tumours (benign or malignant) Infections, granulomas, strictures	**Vascular system** Aneurysms: aorta, iliac vessels Aberrant arteries: pelviureteral junction Venous: ovarian veins, retrocaval ureter
	Gastrointestinal tract Crohn's disease Pancreatitis Appendicitis Diverticulitis Tumours
	Retroperitoneal space Lymph nodes Fibrosis: idiopathic, drugs, inflammatory or IgG4-related disease Tumours: primary or metastatic Haematomas Radiation therapy Surgical disruption or ureteral ligation

The most common causes are in italics. (Adapted from Johnson JJ, Feehally J, Floege J. *Comprehensive clinical nephrology*, 5th edn, Philadelphia: Saunders, 2015, p. 704.)

TABLE 76.2 Causes of lower urinary tract obstruction.

Urethral anatomic causes Urethral strictures: trauma, *postinstrumentation*, infections such as gonococcal urethritis, nongonococcal urethritis, tuberculosis *Posterior urethral valves* Stones Blood clots Periurethral abscess Phimosis Paraphimosis Meatal stenosis
Urethral functional causes Anticholinergic drugs, antidepressants, levodopa
Prostate *Benign prostatic hypertrophy* *Prostatic carcinoma*
Bladder anatomic causes *Bladder cancer* *Schistosomiasis (Schistosoma haematobium infection)* Bladder calculi Bladder trauma, pelvic fracture
Bladder functional causes *Neurogenic bladder:* spinal cord defects or trauma, diabetes, multiple sclerosis, Parkinson's disease, cerebrovascular accidents

The most common causes are in italics. (Adapted from Johnson JJ, Feehally J, Floege J. *Comprehensive clinical nephrology*, 5th edn, Philadelphia: Saunders, 2015, p. 704.)

Presenting features include the following:

- Mild pain or dull aching in the loin, often a dragging heaviness worsened by excessive fluid intake. The kidney may be palpable.
- Intermittent hydronephrosis (Dietl's crisis). Loin swelling is associated with acute renal pain. The pain goes and the swelling disappears when a large volume of urine is passed.
- Antenatal detection in the fetus by USS. Many of these cases are benign, but postnatal investigation is required to detect those with significant PUJ obstruction.

Summary box 76.12

Idiopathic pelvi-ureteric obstruction

- May be asymptomatic
- Can present as intermittent loin pain often exacerbated by a fluid load

Bilateral hydronephrosis

- From lower urinary obstruction: symptoms of bladder outlet obstruction predominate.
- From bilateral upper urinary tract obstruction: idiopathic retroperitoneal fibrosis affects both ureters and idiopathic PUJ obstruction can be bilateral. Symptoms may be referred to one side.
- Hydronephrosis from pregnancy.

Dilatation of the ureters and renal pelves occurs early in pregnancy up to the 20th week. It results from the effects on the ureteric smooth muscle of high levels of circulating progesterone and is part of normal pregnancy. The ureters return to their normal size within 12 weeks of delivery. This physiological condition is associated with an increased liability to infection and there is a possibility that abdominal pain during pregnancy may be erroneously ascribed to ureteric obstruction.

Summary box 76.13

Ureteric dilatation in pregnancy

- Physiological dilatation of the ureter is common in pregnancy

Imaging

Ultrasound scanning (**Figure 76.15**) is the least invasive means of detecting hydronephrosis and is regularly used to diagnose PUJ obstruction *in utero*.

IVU helps only if there is significant function in the obstructed kidney. The extrarenal pelvis is dilated and the minor calyces lose their normal cupping and become 'clubbed'. If the level of obstruction is in doubt, it can help to take follow-up films 36 hours after the contrast has been injected. Contrast slowly diffuses to fill the obstructed system down to the blockage.

Joseph Dietl, 1804–1878, Professor of Pathology and Therapeutics, Krakau, Poland.

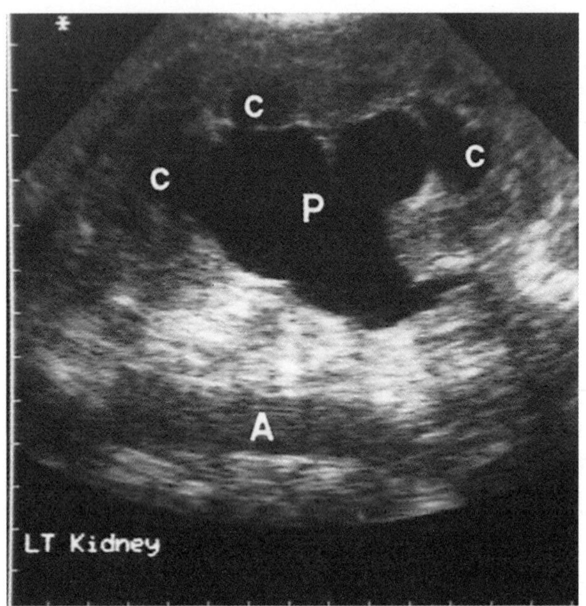

Figure 76.15 Ultrasound of a hydronephrotic kidney. A, artery; C, calyces; P, pelvis.

Isotope renography is the best test to confirm obstructive dilatation of the collecting system. A substance (usually diethylenetriaminepentaacetic acid (DTPA) or MAG-3) is injected intravenously. The DTPA is labelled with technetium-99m, a gamma-ray emitter, so that the passage of 99mTc-labelled DTPA through the kidneys can be tracked using a gamma camera. 99mTc-DTPA is cleared from a normal kidney but stays in the renal pelvis on the obstructed side and is retained even if urine flow is increased by administering frusemide (Figure 76.17).

Very occasionally, a Whitaker test is indicated. A percutaneous puncture of the kidney is made and fluid is infused at a constant rate with monitoring of intrapelvic pressure. An abnormal rise in pressure confirms obstruction. Retrograde pyelography (Figure 76.16) is rarely indicated but will confirm the site of obstruction immediately before corrective surgery.

Summary box 76.14

Imaging

- Obstruction of the ureter is diagnosed by a combination of ultrasound scanning and isotope renography
- An obstructed kidney is worth preserving if it is contributing >20% of total renal function

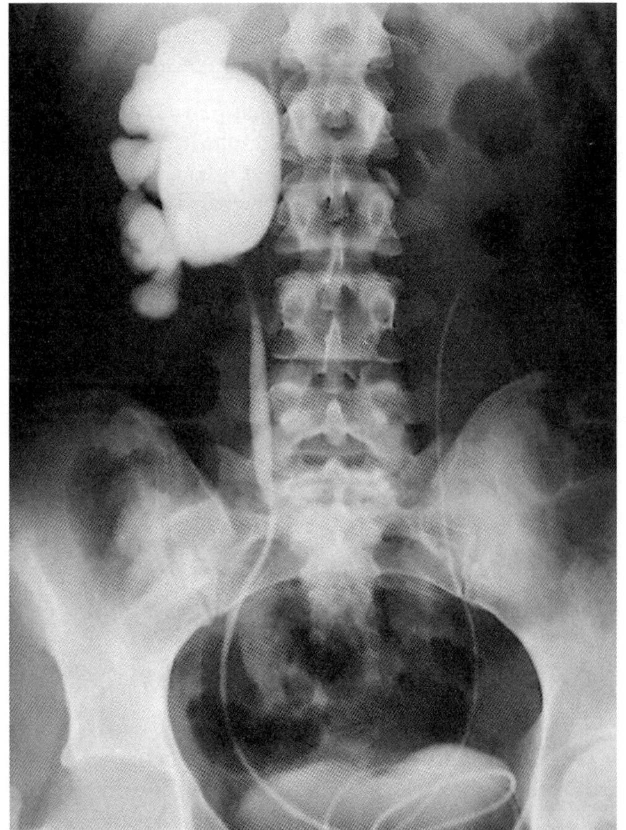

Figure 76.16 Retrograde ureteropyelogram showing hydronephrosis with greatly enlarged pelvis and dilated 'clubbed' calyces.

Treatment

The indications for operation are bouts of renal pain, increasing hydronephrosis, evidence of parenchymal damage and infection. Nephrectomy should be considered only when the kidney has largely lost most of its function (<10% split function). Mild cases should be followed by serial ultrasound scans and operated upon if dilatation is increasing.

Pyeloplasty

In the original Anderson–Hynes open pyeloplasty, the upper third of the ureter and the renal pelvis are mobilised,

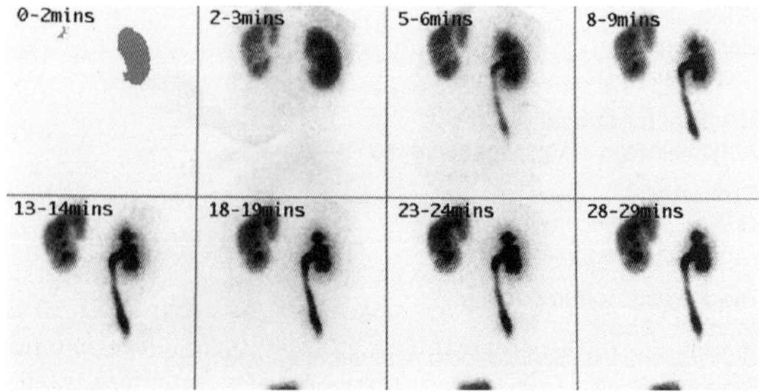

Figure 76.17 Isotope renogram series showing a late accumulation and persistence of radioactivity in the left kidney (the image is a posterior view).

James Christie Anderson, 1899–1984, urologist, The Royal Hallamshire Hospital, Sheffield, UK.

Wilfred Hynes, 1903–1991, plastic surgeon, The Plastic and Jaw Department, The Royal Sheffield Hospital, Sheffield, UK. Anderson and Hynes devised the operation in 1949. It is nowadays done laparoscopically, particularly in children. Robotically assisted laparoscopic dismembered pyeloplasty has also been carried out.

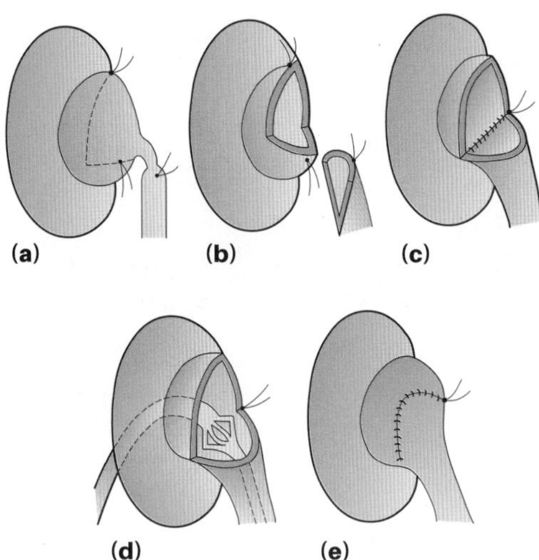

Figure 76.18 (a-e) Anderson–Hynes pyeloplasty.

the ureter is dismembered from the renal pelvis, redundant renal pelvis is excised and a new PUJ is reconfigured (Figure 76.18). A renal vein overlying the distended pelvis can be divided, but an artery in this situation should be preserved to avoid infarction of the renal parenchyma it supplies. The anastomosis is made in front of such an artery if it exists. A ureteric stent is inserted to splint the anastomosis. This type of surgery is now almost universally performed using laparoscopic techniques and in some centres is being performed with robotic assistance. Other surgical procedures have been described to widen the PUJ without dismembering the ureter from the renal pelvis.

Endoscopic pyelolysis

Other endoscopic treatments have been tried to surgically remedy PUJ obstruction including retrograde balloon dilatation, incision of the PUJ using a hot wire over a balloon, laser incision, and percutaneous pyelolysis from above but, in general, these do not produce results equivalent to pyeloplasty.

RETROPERITONEAL PATHOLOGY

Retroperitoneal pathology may result in extrinsic obstruction of the ureters, as can metastases or extension of tumours from the cervix, prostate, bladder, colon, ovary and uterus. Primary tumours of the retroperitoneum, such as lymphomas and sarcomas, can commonly cause obstruction. Obstruction can also result from inflammatory conditions affecting the retroperitoneum such as Crohn's disease and colonic diverticulitis. Less common pathological processes include retroperitoneal fibrosis (RPF), in which thick fibrous tissue 'plaques' extend out from the aorta to encase the ureters and draw them medially. RPF can be idiopathic but can result from inflammatory aortic aneurysms, certain drugs (β-blockers, bromocriptine, methysergide), previous irradiation, trauma or surgery and granulomatous disease (tuberculosis and sarcoidosis).

RPF can be treated medically or surgically. There are reports of favourable outcomes after immunosuppression with high doses of corticosteroids or azathioprine, usually used in combination with bilateral ureteric stents. Alternatively, surgery consisting of ureterolysis (freeing the ureters from the fibrotic plaques) and omentoplasty (transposition of the ureters into the peritoneal cavity in omental wraps) has been shown to have good long-term results. Increasingly, this surgery is being performed laparoscopically with or without robotic assistance rather than as an open surgical procedure.

RENAL TRAUMA

Ten percent of all trauma cases involve the genitourinary tract. This is usually as a result of blunt trauma and the injury is usually self-limiting. Five to 10% of blunt trauma and up to 70% of penetrating trauma are major injuries. Common blunt injuries result often from road traffic accidents, falls, assaults and sporting injuries. Common penetrating injuries are knife or gunshot wounds.

Major renal injury should be suspected with gross haematuria, shock in combination with microscopic haematuria, paediatric renal trauma and penetrating renal injuries. Haematuria may be absent in up to 40% of renal injuries and 24% of pedicle injuries. Renal injuries (Figure 76.19) are classified as follows:

- **Grade I:** contusion or non-enlarging subcapsular perirenal haematoma, and no laceration.
- **Grade II:** superficial laceration <1 cm depth and does not involve the collecting system (no evidence of urine extravasation), non-expanding perirenal haematoma confined to retroperitoneum.
- **Grade III:** laceration >1 cm without extension into the renal pelvis or collecting system (no evidence of urine extravasation).
- **Grade IV:**
  - Laceration extends to renal pelvis or urinary extravasation.
  - Vascular: injury to main renal artery or vein with contained haemorrhage.
  - Segmental infarctions without associated lacerations.
  - Expanding subcapsular haematomas compressing the kidney.
- **Grade V:**
  - Shattered kidney.
  - Avulsion of renal hilum: devascularisation of a kidney due to hilar injury.
  - Ureteropelvic avulsions.
  - Complete laceration or thrombus of the main renal artery or vein.

The indications for radiological assessment are:

- Penetrating injuries.
- Gross haematuria.

Burrill Bernard Crohn, 1884–1983, gastroenterologist, Mount Sinai Hospital, New York, NY, USA, described Crohn's disease in 1932.

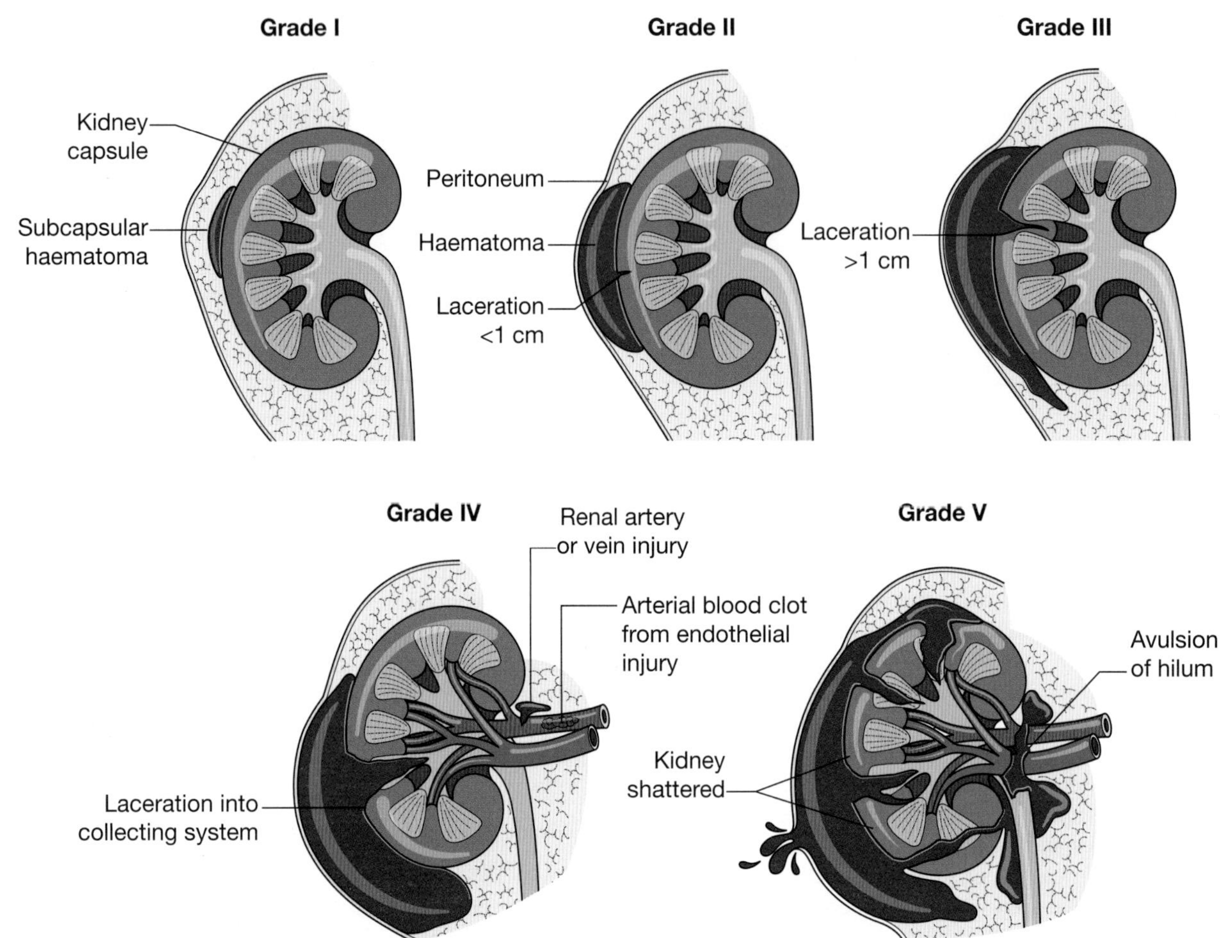

Figure 76.19 Classification of renal trauma.

- Shock in combination with microscopic haematuria.
- Children: in whom the kidneys are much lower and less well protected.

CT scan with contrast is the investigation of choice. It will accurately assess the extent of the injury, showing laceration, extravasation, surrounding haemorrhage and vessel injury. It also shows non-renal injuries and effectively stages renal pedicle injuries. Arterial occlusion is manifest as rim enhancement of the normal renal contour.

The vast majority of cases of blunt renal trauma can be treated conservatively and in one major series only 2.5% of such cases required surgical exploration. Most penetrating injuries from knife or gunshot wounds require renal exploration.

In general, minor and limited major injuries are treated conservatively. Unstable major injuries are best treated with prompt surgical exploration as this lessens the risk of continued bleeding, sepsis and renal loss.

Some patients who have not undergone prior radiological assessment will require an immediate laparotomy and in some patients renal trauma will be encountered unexpectedly during laparotomy. If this occurs, then an on-table intravenous urogram is required. If significant extravasation, non-function, poor opacification or caliceal distortion is found then renal exploration is indicated. An expanding or pulsatile retroperitoneal haematoma should be explored but only after vascular control has been achieved.

Summary box 76.15

Renal trauma

- 10% of trauma cases involve the genitourinary tract
- Blunt trauma is much more common than penetrating trauma
- Most cases of blunt trauma are treated conservatively
- Most penetrating injuries require renal exploration

INJURY TO THE URETER

Rupture of the ureter

This is an uncommon result of a hyperextension injury of the spine. The diagnosis is rarely made until there is swelling in the loin or iliac fossa associated with a reduced urine output. An IVU or contrast-enhanced CT shows extravasation of contrast.

Injury to one or both ureters during pelvic surgery

This occurs most often during vaginal or abdominal hysterectomy when the ureter is mistakenly divided, ligated, crushed or excised. Pre-emptive ureteric catheterisation makes it easier to identify the ureters.

Injury recognised at the time of operation

Ureterovesical continuity should be restored by one of the methods described below unless the patient's condition is poor. Deliberate ligation of the proximal ureter and temporary percutaneous nephrostomy is then the best course until the patient is well enough for a repair.

Summary box 76.16

Ureteric injury during operation

- Surgical trauma during pelvic surgery is the most common cause of ureteric trauma
- Preoperative catheterisation of the ureters makes them easier to protect
- Injuries discovered during surgery should be repaired immediately

Injury not recognised at the time of operation

UNILATERAL INJURIES

There are three possible outcomes:

1. No symptoms. Ligation of a ureter may lead to silent atrophy of the kidney. The injury may be unsuspected until the patient undergoes urological imaging.
2. Loin pain and fever, possibly with pyonephrosis, occur with infection of the obstructed system. Loss of function will be permanent unless obstruction is relieved by promptly inserting a percutaneous nephrostomy.
3. A urinary fistula develops through the abdominal or vaginal wound. The IVU or contrast-enhanced CT shows extravasation with or without obstruction of one or both ureters. Nephrostomies may be inserted and repair postponed until oedema and inflammation have subsided. Early repair is safe if the patient is fit for surgery.

BILATERAL INJURY

Ligation of both ureters leads to anuria. Ureteric catheters will not pass and urgent nephrostomy or immediate surgery is essential.

Repair of the injured ureter

An open repair may be avoidable if a stent will pass the obstruction (*Table 76.3*). If the cut ends of the ureter can be apposed without tension, they should be joined by a spatulated anastomosis over a double pigtail catheter.

If the division is low, the bladder may be hitched and the ureter can be re-implanted. Extra length may be obtained by mobilising the kidney.

In the Boari operation (Figure 76.20), a flap of bladder wall is fashioned into a tube to replace the lower ureter. The disadvantage of implanting the ureter end-to-side into the contralateral ureter (a transureteroureterostomy) is that it risks converting a unilateral injury into a bilateral one.

Nephrectomy may be best when the patient's outlook is poor and the other kidney is normal. When conservation of all renal tissue is vital, replacement of the damaged ureter by a segment of ileum is necessary.

TABLE 76.3 Methods for repairing a damaged ureter.

If there is no loss of length	Spatulation and end-to-end anastomosis without tension
If there is little loss of length	Mobilise kidney
	Psoas hitch of bladder
	Boari operation
If there is marked loss of length	Transureteroureterostomy
	Interposition of isolated bowel loop or mobilised appendix
	Nephrectomy

Summary box 76.17

Repair of ureteric injury

When surgical damage to a ureter is discovered postoperatively:

- Repair need not be delayed
- Ideally surgical repair should be performed by a urologist

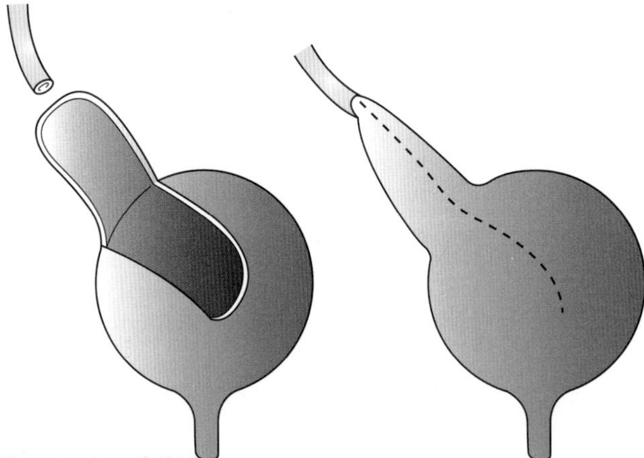

Figure 76.20 Boari operation: a strip of bladder wall is fashioned into a tube to bridge the gap between the cut ureter and the bladder.

Achille Boari, 19th century Italian, urological surgeon from Ferrara, described the technique of a bladder flap in dogs in 1894; it was first performed in a patient in 1936.

VASCULAR PATHOLOGY

Renal artery occlusion/renal infarction

Renal infarction may involve the whole kidney or small areas of the cortex and medulla. The most common presenting symptoms of renal infarction are loin, flank or abdominal pain with nausea and vomiting. Urinalysis often demonstrates microscopic haematuria and proteinuria. Transient or accelerated hypertension may occur secondary to the abrupt release of renin from the infarcted segment. Approximately 25% of cases are asymptomatic. Transient elevation in serum creatinine is not uncommon. When bilateral occlusion of both kidneys or infarction of a single functioning kidney occurs, the patient presents with oliguric or anuric acute kidney injury (AKI). Systemic signs of renal infarction include pyrexia and leucocytosis. CT scan with IV contrast is the best imaging modality for demonstrating areas of renal cortex that are not perfused. The most common causes of renal infarction are trauma, renal artery embolism from cardiac thrombus, and iatrogenic complications of endovascular procedures. Spontaneous renal artery thrombosis or dissection is most often associated with atherosclerotic disease of the aorta or renal arteries, but other vascular causes include fibromuscular hyperplasia, Takayasu's arteritis, polyarteritis nodosa, Marfan's syndrome and Ehlers–Danlos syndrome with associated dissection or aneurysms. Less common causes include hypercoagulable states and inflammatory diseases of the retroperitoneum.

In the setting of renal infarction, a search for the cause of the renal vascular compromise should be undertaken to determine whether it is embolic or thrombotic. Treatment of the infarction itself is usually conservative. If renal artery occlusion is caused by a hypercoagulable state or an embolism from a central source, systemic anticoagulation is indicated. Common sources include atrial fibrillation, atrial or mural thrombi, intracardiac mass and valvular lesions; therefore, echocardiography is indicated.

Renal vein thrombosis

Renal vein thrombosis is rare and primarily observed in children with severe dehydration or in adults with nephrotic syndrome, renal tumours, or hypercoagulable states and after surgery or trauma to the renal vessels. Thrombosis of the longer left renal vein may also involve ureteric, gonadal, adrenal and phrenic branches that drain into the left renal vein. Most patients are treated with systemic anticoagulation.

TUMOURS OF THE KIDNEY

Benign tumours

Adenoma

Pea-like cortical adenomas are occasionally discovered. They are asymptomatic and are benign.

Angioma

Angioma may cause profuse haematuria, often in young adults. The bleeding source may be difficult to diagnose without renal angiography.

Angiomyolipoma

Angiomyolipoma is an unusual tumour of the kidney, often but not always associated with tuberous sclerosis. Its high fat content has a typical appearance on CT. Malignant elements are present in about one-quarter and may metastasise.

Renal cell carcinoma

Renal cell carcinoma (RCC) encompasses a heterogeneous group of cancers derived from renal tubular epithelial cells and is among the 10 most common cancers worldwide, accounting for about 2% of all cancer diagnoses and deaths. The male:female ratio is approximately 2:1. Key advances in histopathological and molecular characteristics of RCC over the past two decades have led to major revisions in its classification. Major subtypes with >5% incidence are clear-cell RCC (ccRCC), papillary RCC (pRCC) and chromophobe RCC (chRCC). ccRCC is the most common subtype and accounts for the majority of deaths from kidney cancer. Indeed, owing to the predominance of clear-cell histology in metastatic disease (83–88%), tumours with non-clear-cell histology have been grouped as 'nccRCC' (*Table 76.4*). Kidney cancer accounts for approximately 84 000 new cases and approximately 35 000 deaths in Europe annually. The median age at presentation is 64 years and when RCC is diagnosed at younger ages (<46 years) the possibility of an underlying hereditary kidney cancer syndrome – which accounts for 3–5% of all RCCs – should be considered (*Table 76.5*). Although overall the incidence rates of RCC are increasing, the mortality rates have levelled off, probably accounted for by increasing incidental detection – from increased use of abdominal imaging – of small renal masses (<4 cm) that are unlikely to have metastasised. The global increase in the prevalence of obesity, an established risk factor, might also play a part in increasing incidence.

Mikito Takayasu, 1860–1938, Japanese ophthalmologist, described Takayasu's arteritis in 1908.
Antoine Bernard-Jean Marfan, 1858–1942, French pediatrician, described Marfan's syndrome in 1886.
Edvard Laurits Ehlers, 1863–1937, Danish dermatologist.
Henri-Alexandre Danlos, 1844–1912, French physician and dermatologist.

TABLE 76.4 Non-clear-cell renal cell carcinomas.

Tumour type	Subtype	Cytogenetic alterations	Genes mutated	Gross appearance	Histological features*
Papillary	Type 1	• Gains of 7, 8q, 12q, 16p, 17 and 20 • Loss of 9p	*MET*	• Mixed cystic or solid consistency • Often whitish in colour and may show haemorrhage and necrosis • Frequently with a well-demarcated pseudocapsule	• Single layer of cuboid tumour cells • Thin, basophilic papillae with scant pale cytoplasm and low nuclear grade • Concentric lamellated calcifications (psamomma bodies) • Foamy macrophage infiltration
	Type 2	• Gains of 8q • Loss of 1p and 9p	• *CDKN2A* • *SETD2* • *NRF2*		• Heterogeneous, thick papillae and eosinophilic cytoplasm, high nuclear grade and pseudostratification • Concentric lamellated calcifications • Foamy macrophage infiltration
Chromophobe	Classic	Loss of chromosomes 1, 2, 6, 10, 13, 17 and 21	• *TP53* • *PTEN*	• Large, well-circumscribed grey to tan-brown coloured tumour • Occasional central scar	• Tumour cells with prominent membrane and pale cytoplasm • Voluminous cytoplasm (cytoplasmic accumulation of acid mucopolysaccharides)
	Eosinophilic				• Large tumour cells with fine eosinophilic granules • Distinct cell borders • Voluminous cytoplasm
MiT family translocation	NA	Recurrent translocations involving Xp11.23 *(TFE3)* or 6p21 (TFEB)	• *TFE3* • *TFEB*	• Yellowish tissue • Often studded by haemorrhage and necrosis	• Papillary or nested architecture • Abundant clear or eosinophilic cytoplasm
Collecting duct	NA	• Losses at 8p, 16p, 1p and 9p • Gains at 13q	Unknown	• Partially cystic • White-grey appearance • Often exhibit invasion into the renal sinus	• Tubulopapillary pattern • Often with cells taking columnar pattern with hobnail appearance • Presence of mucinous material • Desmoplastic stroma
Medullary	NA	Poorly described, but thought to be normal karyotype	*SMARCB1*	• Tan or white appearance • Poorly defined capsule • Extensive haemorrhage and necrosis	• Poorly differentiated, eosinophilic cells • Inflammatory infiltrative cells • Sheet-like or reticular pattern is common
Oncocytoma	NA	• Loss of chromosome 1 and Y chromosome • *CCND1* rearrangement	Mitochondrial genes *(COX1, COX2, MTND4* and *MTCYB)*	• Mahogany colour • Circumscribed • Occasional central scar • Rarely with necrosis	• Polygonal cells with abundant eosinophilic cytoplasm • Uniform, round nuclei

NA, not applicable. *No consensus is currently available that describes the immune infiltration of non-clear-cell renal cell carcinomas. (Adapted from Hsieh JJ, Purdue MP, Signoretti S *et al*. Renal cell carcinoma. *Nat Rev Dis Primers*. 2017; **9**(3): 1–19.)

Risk factors for RCC include:

- age;
- sex;
- obesity;
- hypertension;
- cigarette smoking.

Other medical conditions have been associated with RCC including chronic kidney disease, haemodialysis, kidney transplantation and acquired cystic disease of the kidney (ACDK). Genetic factors also contribute to RCC risk, as evidenced by individuals with a family history of renal cancer having an approximate twofold increased risk. Investigations into familial RCC have uncovered mutations in at least 11 genes (*BAP1, FLCN, FH, MET, PTEN, SDHB, SDHC, SDHD, TSC1, TSC2* and *VHL*), some of which have been implicated in sporadic RCC. A notable example is *VHL*, the mutated gene underlying von Hippel–Lindau disease, which is characterised by a high risk of developing ccRCC.

The classic triad of loin pain, loin mass and haematuria is seen in <10% of patients with a renal tumour. Nowadays, the majority of diagnoses result from incidental findings. This shift is a consequence of the widespread use of USS and CT imaging, performed for other reasons. That said, paraneoplastic

TABLE 76.5 Hereditary syndromes associated with renal cell carcinoma.

Syndrome (phenotype OMIM reference)	Gene (position)	Protein	Incidence of developing a kidney tumour (%)	Median age at diagnosis (years)	Other phenotypic features
Clear cell renal cell carcinoma*					
von Hippel–Lindau disease (193300)	*VHL* (3p25-26)	pVHL	25-45	40	• Haemangioblastoma • Pancreatic neuroendocrine tumours • Pheochromocytoma • Renal cysts • Pancreatic cysts • Ovary cystadenoma • Epididymal cystadenoma
BAP1 mutant disease (also known as tumour predisposition disease; 614327)	*BAP1* (3p21)	BRCA-associated protein	No data	No data	• Breast cancer • Uveal melanoma • Mesothelioma • Other cutaneous melanocytic tumours
SDH-associated kidney cancer (185470, 602413, 602690 and 115310)	*SDHB* (1p36), *SDHC* (lq23) and *SDHD* (llq23)	Succinate dehydrogenase subunits B, C and D	5-15	30	• Paraganglioma • Carotid body tumours • Pheochromocytoma • Gastrointestinal stromal tumour
Papillary renal cell carcinoma					
Hereditary leiomyomatosis and renal cell cancer (150800)[‡]	*FH* (1q43)	Fumarate hydratase	2-21	46	• Uterine leiomyosarcomas • Breast cancer • Bladder cancer • Cutaneous leiomyomas • Uterine leiomyomas
Hereditary papillary kidney cancer (605074)[§]	*MET* (7q31)	Hepatocyte growth factor receptor	No data	<60	No additional features
Multiple tumour types					
Birt-Hogg-Dubé syndrome (135150)[‖]	*FLCN* (17p11.2)	Folliculin	34	50	• Fibrofolliculomas and trichodiscomas • Pulmonary cysts • Pneumothorax
Tuberous sclerosis complex (191100 and 191092)[¶]	*TSC1* (9q34) and *TSC2* (16p13)	Hamartin and tuberin	2-4	30	• Subependymal giant cell astrocytomas • Angiomyolipomas • Renal cysts • Facial angiofibroma • Ungual and periungual fibromas • Hypomelanotic macule • Forehead plaque • Cardiac rhabdomyomas • Connective tissue naevus
Cowden syndrome (also known as multiple hamartoma syndrome; 158350)[#]	*PTEN* (10q23)	Phosphatase and tensin homologue	34	40	• Breast cancer • Endometrial cancer • Thyroid cancer • Prostate cancer • Macrocephaly • Intestinal hamartomatous polyps • Benign skin tumours (multiple trichilemmomas, papillomatous papules and acral keratoses) • Dysplastic gangliocytoma of the cerebellum
Hyperparathyroidism jaw tumour syndrome (145001)**	*HRPT2* (1q31)	Parafibromin	No data	No data	• Parathyroid carcinomas • Uterine carcinomas • Renal cysts and hamartomas • Hyperparathyroidism • Parathyroid gland tumours • Jaw fibromas

OMIM, Online Mendelian Inheritance in Man database. *Familial clear cell kidney cancer with chromosome 3 translocation is another possible syndrome associated with clear cell renal cell carcinoma, but the genetic lesions and associated data are unknown. ‡Main renal cancer type is papillary renal cell carcinoma type 2. §Main renal cancer type is papillary renal cell carcinoma type 1. ‖Main renal cancer types are hybrid tumours, oncocytomas, and chromophobe, papillary and clear cell renal cell carcinomas. ¶Main renal cancer types are angiomyolipomas, epithelioid angiomyolipomas, oncocytomas, and papillary and clear cell renal cell carcinomas; renal cysts also are common. #Main renal cancer types are clear cell, papillary and chromophobe renal cell carcinomas. **Main renal cancer types are mixed tumours (epithelial and connective tissue), papillary renal cell carcinomas and nephroblastomas. (Adapted from Hsieh JJ, Purdue MP, Signoretti S *et al*. Renal cell carcinoma. *Nat Rev Dis Primers*. 2017; **9**(3): 1–19.)

syndromes – symptoms caused by hormones or cytokines excreted by the tumour cells or by an immune response against the tumour – are not uncommon in RCC and symptoms include hypercalcaemia, fever and erythrocytosis.

Summary box 76.18

Renal cell carcinoma (RCC)

- Arises from epithelium of the proximal convoluted tubule
- Frequently detected coincidentally
- Has a male preponderance
- Major subtypes are clear-cell, papillary and chromophobe RCC
- Surgery is the mainstay of treatment for organ-confined disease
- Metastatic disease is treated with tyrosine kinase inhibitors (TKIs) or mTOR inhibitors

Staging (Figure 76.21).

CT imaging with contrast enhancement of the chest, abdomen and pelvis is required for optimal staging. Such imaging enables the assessment of the primary tumour (such as the size and whether the tumour is organ-confined or extends to perinephric fat or the renal hilum), regional spread (lymph node involvement) and distant metastases (including lung, bone and distant lymph nodes). MRI can also provide additional information, especially to determine whether the tumour extends into the vasculature. Bone scan and 18F-FDG PET scan are not recommended for initial staging.

Pathology

In 2016, the World Health Organisation (WHO) classification of RCC was updated from previous (2004) WHO and International Society of Urological Pathology (ISUP) Consensus Conference (2013) systems. At macroscopic level, the cut surface of ccRCC tumours is golden-yellow in colour with frequent haemorrhagic, necrotic and cystic areas (**Figure 76.22**). Microscopically, ccRCC usually consists of tumour cells with clear cytoplasm arranged in nests or tubules surrounded by a rich vascular network. The clear appearance of the cytoplasm is due to the accumulation of glycogen and lipids. The most widely used grading system for ccRCC is the Fuhrman grading system, which defines 4 nuclear grades (1–4) in order of increasing nuclear size, irregularity and nucleolar prominence. The pathologist also often assigns a Leibovich score following nephrectomy – the Leibovich prognostic score runs from 0 to 11 and is based on the tumour's stage, grade, size, involvement of lymph nodes and the presence of tumour necrosis histologically. It should be noted that all RCC types may contain foci of high-grade malignant spindle cells (i.e. sarcomatoid differentiation).

Surgery

Surgical treatment of RCC is related to the clinical stage of the disease and to the general condition of the patient. Although typically reserved for localised disease, nephrectomy can also be used with cytoreductive intent in patients with metastatic

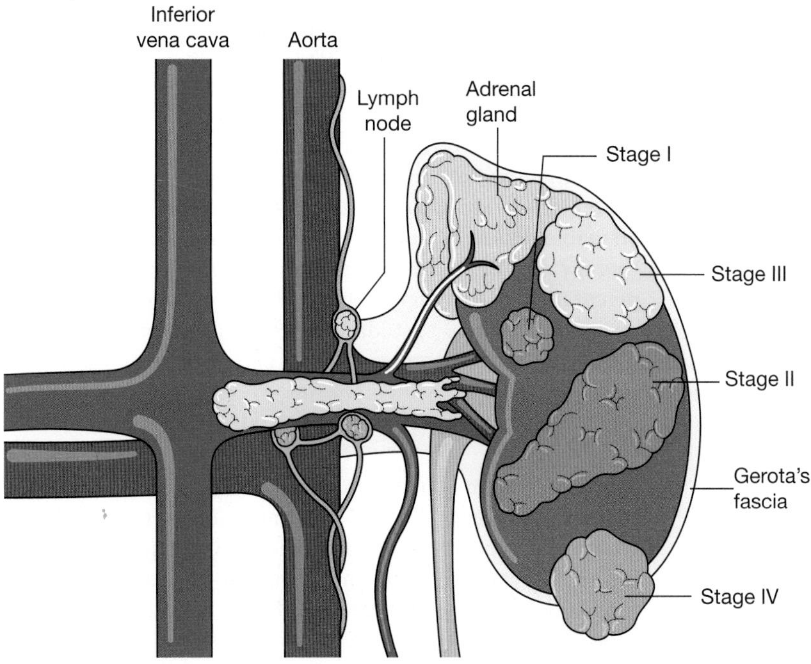

Figure 76.21 Staging renal cell carcinoma is based on size, position and lymph node involvement:
Stage I: tumour <7 cm in the largest dimension, limited to the kidney
Stage II: tumour >7 cm in the largest dimension, limited to the kidney
Stage III: tumour in the major veins or adrenal gland with intact Gerota's fascia, or regional lymph nodes involved
Stage IV: tumour beyond Gerota's fascia

Susan A Fuhrman, American pathologist, described the Fuhrman grading system in 1982.
Bradley C Leibovich, contemproary, Professor of Urology, Rochester, MN, USA.

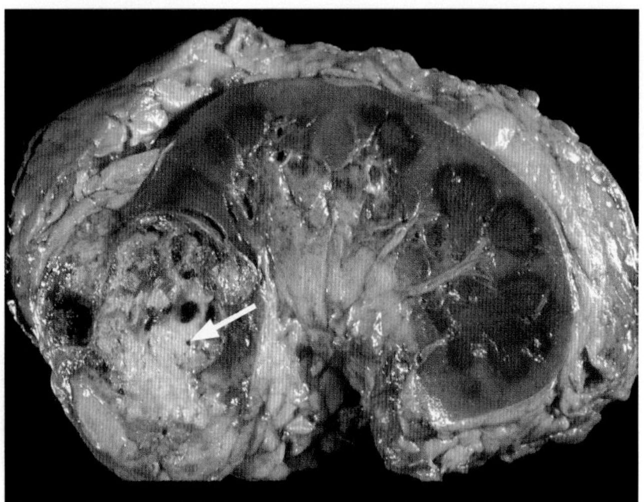

Figure 76.22 A radical nephrectomy specimen containing a renal cell carcinoma (arrow) (courtesy of Dharam M Ramani, MD).

disease, especially if there is substantial disease volume at the primary site but only a low burden of metastatic disease.

PARTIAL NEPHRECTOMY

The goal of partial nephrectomy is to completely remove the primary tumour while preserving the largest possible amount of healthy renal parenchyma. Partial nephrectomy is indicated for patients with a T1 tumour (according to the UICC TNM staging system) and a normal contralateral kidney. Moreover, partial nephrectomy is strongly recommended (imperative absolute indications) in patients with RCC who have only one kidney (anatomically or functionally), in those with bilateral synchronous RCC and in those with von Hippel–Lindau syndrome. Similarly, relative indications include conditions that can impair renal function (e.g. kidney stones, hypertension, diabetes and pyelonephritis). Indeed, partial nephrectomy offers lower renal function impairment and equivalent oncological survival outcomes compared with radical nephrectomy in those with T1 tumours. In the past decade, nephrometry scoring systems (such as the R.E.N.A.L. and PADUA systems) have been proposed to predict the complexity of the partial nephrectomy procedure. Laparoscopic partial nephrectomy (LPN) and robot-assisted partial nephrectomy (RAPN) are the main alternatives to classic open partial nephrectomy (OPN). In the past, cooling of the kidney using crushed ice was frequently employed during partial nephrectomy but this is being used in a more selective fashion in the modern era. Haematuria, perirenal haematoma and urinary fistulas are the most common complications of partial nephrectomy. Less frequent postoperative complications are acute renal impairment and infection.

RADICAL NEPHRECTOMY

Classic radical nephrectomy consists of removal of the kidney, perirenal fat, adrenal gland and regional lymph nodes. However, in patients with a tumour <5 cm in size, located at the inferior pole, the adrenal gland can be spared. Similarly, regional lymph node dissection can be reserved for patients with clinically positive nodes detected by CT or during the surgical procedure. It is performed if possible as a laparoscopic procedure (most stage I and stage II tumours) but if this is not feasible then as an open procedure. Data recently taken from the US National Cancer database support the use of cytoreductive nephrectomy in those with metastatic disease, even while they receive systemic targeted therapies. Indeed, the median overall survival was 17.1 months in cytoreductive nephrectomy patients compared with 7.7. months in the non-cytoreductive nephrectomy group. Patients with renal vein or IVC involvement by tumour but without evidence of metastatic disease remain surgical candidates. Occasionally, nephrectomy and removal of IVC tumour thrombus need to be done in conjunction with cardiothoracic surgeons, using cardiopulmonary bypass techniques for those tumours extending above the diaphragm. Bench surgery and autotransplantation is performed in highly specialised centres for larger tumours in a solitary kidney.

Summary box 76.19

Surgery for renal tumours

- Surgery is the mainstay treatment for organ-confined renal cancer
- Partial nephrectomy is increasingly used for renal tumours <7 cm
- Partial nephrectomy is increasingly performed using robotic assistance
- Cytoreductive nephrectomy (removal of the kidney in the presence of metastatic disease) has a role in patients with a good performance status

Active surveillance and ablative therapies

Active surveillance and ablative therapies, such as radiofrequency ablation (RFA) and cryotherapy, are alternative strategies for elderly patients and/or those with competing health risks and limited life expectancy that render them unsuitable for surgery. Intervention should be considered for growth to >3–4 cm or by >0.5 cm per year.

Ablative technology must be able to completely destroy all viable tumour tissue with no viable tumour left. Both cryotherapy and RFA can be performed using a laparoscopic or percutaneous approach under CT or ultrasound guidance. Available low-quality studies suggest a higher local recurrence rate for ablative therapies than for partial nephrectomy.

Medical management using targeted therapies

The past 10 years have seen the approval of several targeted therapeutic agents for the treatment of metastatic RCC. Given the highly vascular nature of RCCs, it is unsurprising that several therapies are available to exploit this feature. Indeed, tyrosine kinase inhibitors targeting the VEGF (vascular endothelial growth factor) signalling axis that are approved in the first-line and second-line settings for the treatment of metastatic RCC are sorafenib, sunitinib, pazopanib, axitinib, lenvatinib and cabozantinib. In addition, the anti-VEGF monoclonal antibody, bevacizumab, is approved for use with interferon-α. The mTOR inhibitors, everolimus and temsirolimus, are approved as single agents in the second-line setting and in the first-line setting in patients with poor risk status. The average duration of disease control with these drugs is 8–9 months in the first-line setting and 5–6 months in the second-line setting. Most of the phase III RCTs leading to approval of these agents have excluded patients with nccRCC. Many studies are currently investigating combinations of anti-VEGF therapy with a new generation of immunotherapy agents in the form of T cell-immune checkpoint inhibitors such as antibodies against programmed cell death protein 1 ligand 1 (PDL1), which include avelumab and atezolizumab, and antibodies against programmed cell death protein 1 (PD1) which include nivolumab and pembrolizumab.

Summary box 76.20

Targeted therapies for renal cancer

- These include tyrosine kinase inhibitors (TKIs), anti-VEGF monoclonal antibodies and mTOR inhibitors
- The average duration of disease control with these agents is 8–9 months

Upper tract transitional cell carcinoma (UTTCC)

Transitional cell carcinomas of the renal pelves or ureters account for 5–10% of transitional cell tumours of the urinary tract. The risk factors for these tumours are the same as for bladder cancer. Tumours, especially high-grade ones, in the upper urinary tract are often multifocal and associated with carcinoma in situ (CIS). Approximately 5% of patients who have been diagnosed with bladder cancer will, during follow-up, develop a metachronous UTTCC – usually patients with high-grade tumours or CIS of the bladder. Approximately 40% of patients who present with a UTTCC will, at some point, develop a metachronous bladder cancer, hence the need for endoscopic follow-up after the diagnosis of a UTTCC. The incidence of subsequent bladder tumours in these patients has been shown to be reduced by 25% with a single intravesical dose of mitomycin-C around the time of treatment of the UTTCC. UTTCC often presents late with the disease already invading the muscle of the ureter or renal pelvis, involving lymph nodes or already metastatic.

The standard treatment of UTTCC is nephroureterectomy. In most cases, the surgery to mobilise (a) the kidney and (b) the distal ureter is accomplished using different surgical approaches depending on whether the tumour is high up in the renal pelvis or involves the distal ureter. If the tumour is in the renal pelvis, laparoscopic mobilisation of the kidney and ureter can be combined with endoscopic resection of the ipsilateral intramural ureter to allow nephroureterectomy. If the tumour involves the distal ureter, the distal ureter is usually dissected out using a lower midline incision and opening the bladder – with again laparoscopic mobilisation of the kidney which is then delivered through the open incision. A catheter is needed for around 10 days after nephroureterectomy to allow the bladder to heal satisfactorily. Robotic assistance for this operation is likely to continue to develop.

Summary box 76.21

Upper tract transitional cell carcinoma

- Accounts for 5–10% of urothelial carcinomas
- Often presents late with advanced disease
- In the absence of metastatic disease, standard treatment is nephroureterectomy
- Surgical technique is tailored depending on whether the UTTCC is in the upper ureter/renal pelvis or lower ureter

Wilms' tumour (nephroblastoma)

This mixed tumour contains elements from embryonic nephrogenic tissue (Figure 76.23). Nephroblastoma is usually discovered during the first five years of life, usually in one pole of one kidney. Bilateral tumours pose a difficult problem.

Pathology

A rapidly growing tumour is likely to be friable in consistency.

Clinical features

An abdominal tumour grows rapidly in a poorly child. The mass may be very large. Some patients are hypertensive.

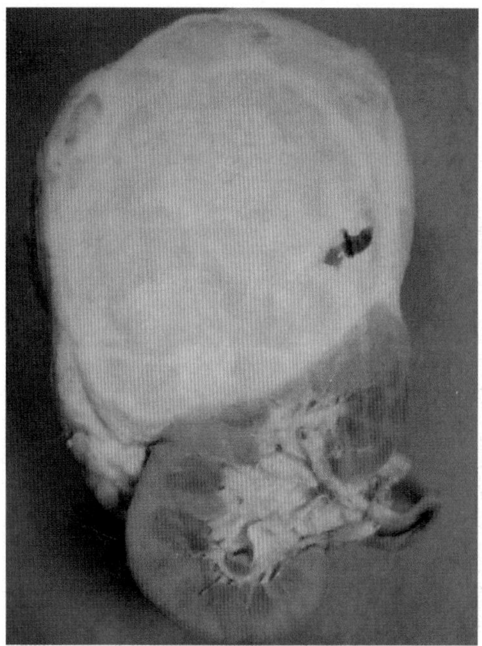

Figure 76.23 Wilms' tumour.

Carl Max Wilhelm Wilms, 1867–1918, German surgeon, described Wilms' tumour in 1899.

Haematuria is an unfavourable symptom denoting extension of the tumour into the renal pelvis.

Imaging confirms a solid space-occupying lesion in the kidney, with or without venous invasion, contralateral disease and distant spread.

Metastasis to the lungs occurs early. Liver, bone and brain metastases are rare. Lymphatic spread is uncommon.

Treatment

These children are best treated in specialist paediatric oncology units. Most unilateral tumours are treated by chemotherapy followed by nephrectomy. Partial nephrectomy may be possible in patients with bilateral disease.

Prognosis

Eighty per cent survive long term with modern chemotherapy and surgery. The prognosis is worse in those with metastases and in older children.

Summary box 76.22

Nephroblastoma (Wilms' tumour)

- Usually presents in the first five years of life
- Typically presents with an abdominal mass
- May cause haematuria, abdominal pain or fever
- Metastasises to the lung
- Is best treated in a specialist paediatric oncology unit

FURTHER READING

Hsieh JJ, Purdue MP, Signoretti S *et al.* Renal cell carcinoma. *Nat Rev Dis Primers*. 2017; **9**(3): 1–19.

Johnson JJ, Feehally J, Floege J. *Comprehensive clinical nephrology*, 5th edn. Philadelphia: Saunders, 2015.

Khan SR *et al.* Kidney stones. *Nat Rev Dis Primers*. 2016; **2**: 1–22.

Chapter 77

The urinary bladder

Learning objectives

To understand:

- The anatomy, vascular supply and innervation of the bladder in relation to function and disease
- The principles of management of bladder trauma, incontinence and fistulae
- The common causes of acute and chronic urinary retention and management
- The different types of bladder cancer and the principles of management

SURGICAL ANATOMY OF THE BLADDER

- It is lined by transitional epithelium covering the connective tissue lamina propria, which contains a rich plexus of vessels and lymphatics.
- When the detrusor muscle hypertrophies, the inner layer, covered by urothelium, stands out, resulting in the appearance of trabeculation.
- Over the trigone is a thin layer of smooth muscle to which the epithelium is closely adherent and which extends as a sheath around the lower ureters and into the proximal urethra.
- Around the male bladder neck is the smooth muscle internal sphincter innervated by adrenergic fibres, which prevents retrograde ejaculation.
- The distal urethral sphincter is a horseshoe-shaped mass of striated muscle that lies anterior and distal to the prostate, or in the proximal two-thirds of the female urethra. It is distinct from the pelvic floor and is supplied by S2–4 fibres via the pudendal nerve and by somatic fibres passing through the inferior hypogastric plexus.

Fascial and ligamentous supports of the bladder

At the posterolateral bladder neck, condensations of fascia pass forward medially and laterally to the ureter to join with the prostatic fascia; this fascia needs to be divided during cystectomy. The puboprostatic ligaments are well-defined condensations of the anterior endopelvic fascia; they stretch from the front of the prostate to the periosteum of the pubis and lie lateral to the dorsal vein complex. The urachus and obliterated hypogastric arteries, together with the folds of peritoneum overlying them, are called the median and lateral umbilical ligaments. Condensations of fascia also occur around the superior and inferior vascular pedicles.

Arteries

The superior and inferior vesical arteries are derived from the anterior trunk of the internal iliac artery. Branches from the obturator and inferior gluteal arteries (and from the uterine and vaginal arteries in females) also help to supply the bladder.

Veins

The veins form a plexus on the lateral and inferior surfaces of the bladder. In males the prostatic plexus is continuous with the vesical plexus, which drains into the internal iliac vein. In females similar large veins are continuous with the vaginal plexus.

Lymphatics

These accompany the veins and drain to nodes along the internal iliac vessels, and then to the obturator and external iliac chains. Some lymphatics pass to nodes that are situated posteriorly to the internal iliac artery (hypogastric nodes).

INNERVATION

The parasympathetic input

The parasympathetic input (Figure 77.1) is derived from the anterior primary divisions of the second, third and fourth

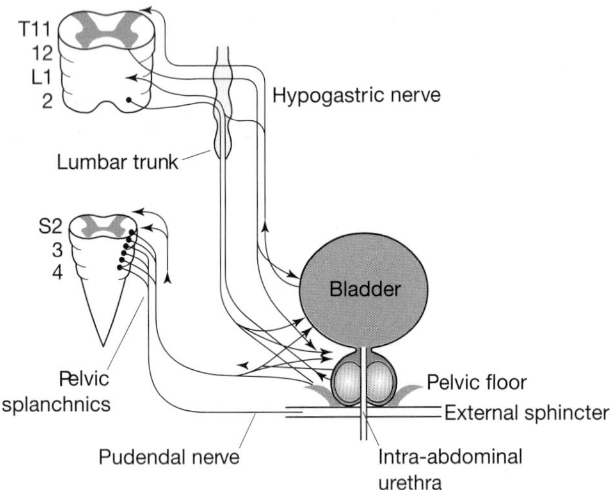

Figure 77.1 The nervous control of the bladder. Micturition is partly a reflex and partly a voluntary act.

sacral segments (mainly S2 and S3). Fibres pass through the pelvic splanchnic nerves to the inferior hypogastric plexus, from where they are distributed to the bladder. The pelvic plexus can be damaged during deep pelvic operations.

The sympathetic input

This arises in the eleventh thoracic to the second lumbar segments; fibres pass via the presacral hypogastric nerve (rather than via the sympathetic chains) to the inferior hypogastric plexus.

Somatic innervation

A somatic innervation passes to the distal sphincter mechanism via the pudendal nerves and also via fibres that pass through the inferior hypogastric plexus.

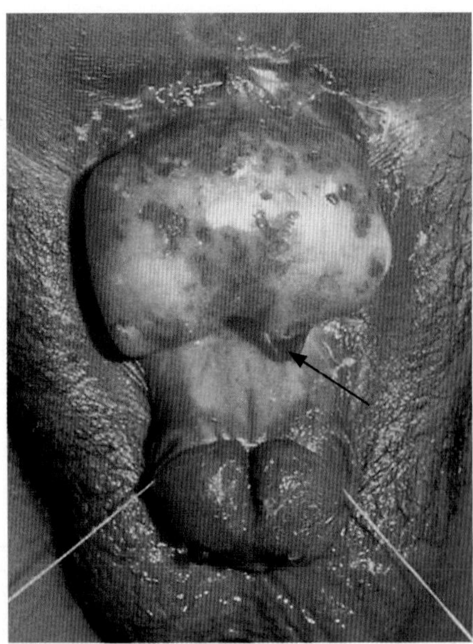

Figure 77.2 Ectopia vesicae in a man. A drop of urine (arrow) is seen at the left ureteric orifice, the corona glandis being retracted by threads (courtesy of GD Adhia, Bombay, India).

Functional aspects

Sympathetic nerves convey afferents from the fundus. Afferents arise from the mucosa, where they respond to touch, temperature and pain, and from the detrusor and lamina propria, where they convey stretch information. Afferents pass via the inferior hypogastric plexus to the posterior roots of S2–4. Some aspects of micturition are centred in the pons, where detrusor contraction is coordinated with inhibition of the distal sphincter. Interruption of this pathway below the pons, with preservation of the sacral cord. is likely to result in a contractile detrusor and tonically active distal sphincter that will not relax during voiding (detrusor–sphincter dyssynergia).

CONGENITAL DEFECTS OF THE BLADDER

Bladder exstrophy

Clinical features

Bladder exstrophy occurs in 1:50 000 births (male:female ratio 4:1) (Figure 77.2). In males, the penis is broad and short, and bilateral inguinal herniae may be present. There is separation of the pubic bones (Figure 77.3). In epispadias alone, the pubes are united and external genitalia are almost normal, although in females the clitoris is bifid (Figure 77.4).

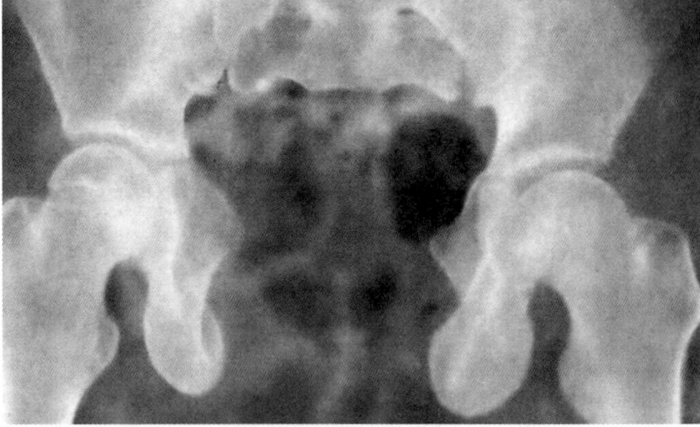

Figure 77.3 Separation of the pubes in a case of ectopia vesicae (courtesy of the late Professor Grey Turner, London, UK).

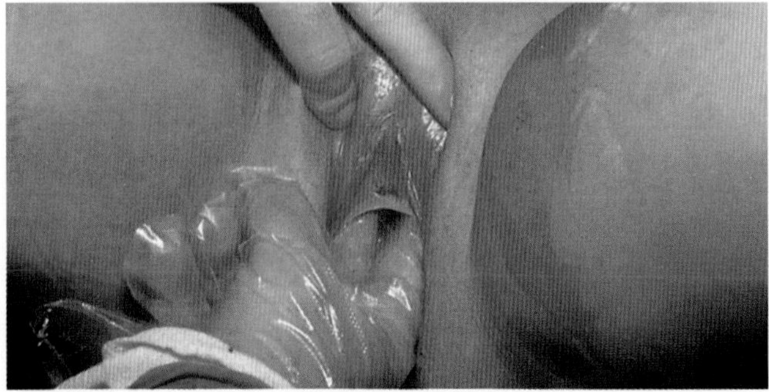

Figure 77.4 Female epispadias showing deficient sphincter and bifid clitoris.

Treatment

The bladder is closed in the first year of life, usually after osteotomy of both iliac bones just lateral to the sacroiliac joints. Later, reconstruction of the bladder neck and sphincters is required. In some patients the reconstructed bladder remains small and requires augmentation. One-stage reconstruction is being practised in some major centres.

Less satisfactorily, urinary diversion can be carried out by means of ureterosigmoid anastomosis, an ileal or colonic conduit, or continent urinary diversion. Long-term complications include: (1) stricture at the site of anastomosis with bilateral hydronephrosis and infection; (2) hyperchloraemic acidosis; and (3) an increased (20-fold) risk of tumour formation (adenoma and adenocarcinoma) at the site of a ureterocolic anastomosis.

BLADDER TRAUMA

Bladder rupture

This can be intraperitoneal (20%) or extraperitoneal (80%) (Figures 77.5 and 77.6). Intraperitoneal rupture is usually secondary to a blow or fall on a distended bladder, and more rarely to surgical damage. Extraperitoneal rupture is caused by blunt trauma or surgical damage. Gross haematuria can be absent. It may be difficult to distinguish extraperitoneal rupture from rupture of the membranous urethra (see Chapter 79). Intraperitoneal rupture is associated with sudden severe pain in the hypogastrium, often accompanied by syncope. The shock subsides and the abdomen distends and there is no desire to micturate. Peritonitis does not follow immediately if the urine is sterile; varying degrees of rigidity are present on examination.

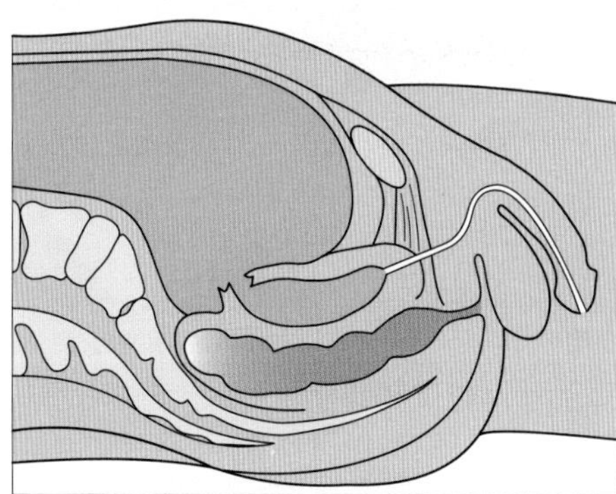

Figure 77.5 Intraperitoneal extravasation of urine.

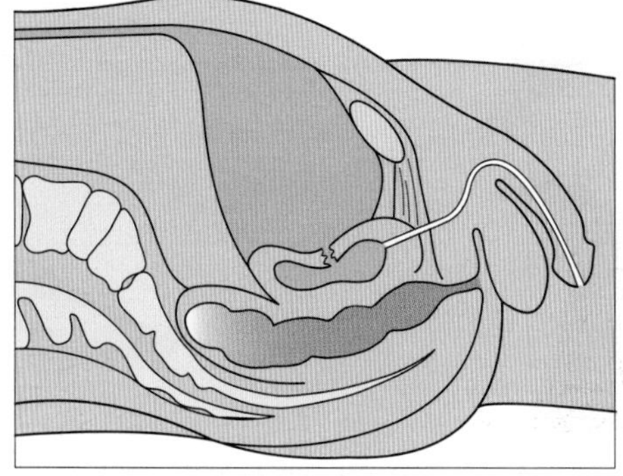

Figure 77.6 Extraperitoneal extravasation of urine.

Investigation

Computed tomography (CT) is ideal. Plain erect radiographs may show a ground-glass appearance (fluid). Intravenous urography (IVU) may confirm a leak. Retrograde cystography will confirm the diagnosis (Figure 77.7). It is important to image the patient after drainage of contrast because the full bladder may mask extravasation.

Treatment of intraperitoneal rupture

A lower midline laparotomy should be performed; the edges of the rent are trimmed and sutured with a single-layer 2/0 absorbable suture. A suprapubic and a urethral catheter are placed. Very rarely, the rupture will be through an unsuspected tumour; a biopsy can be taken before suturing the defect. Laparoscopic approaches are also now being used.

Injury to the bladder during operation

The bladder may be injured in (1) inguinal or femoral herniotomy, (2) hysterectomy and (3) excision of the rectum. If the injury is recognised, the bladder must be repaired and catheter

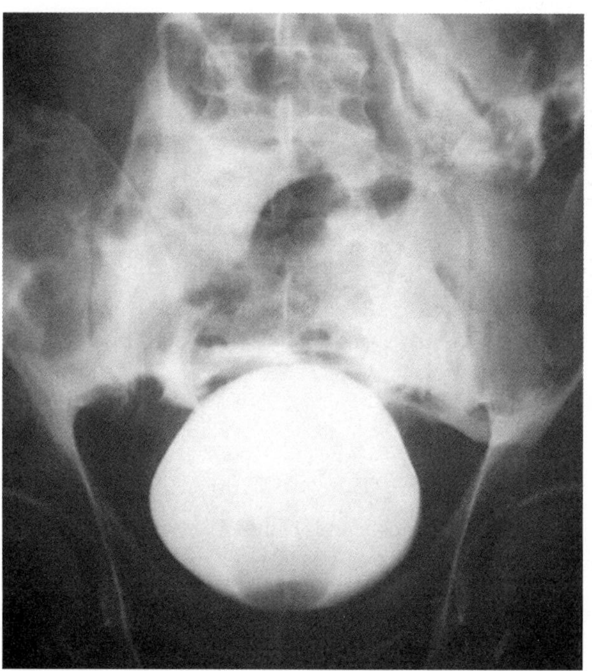

Figure 77.7 Cystogram of a patient who has fallen over and developed severe abdominal pain. Leakage of contrast into the peritoneal cavity is seen.

Summary box 77.1

Bladder trauma

- Intraperitoneal or extraperitoneal
- Suspected if there is trauma and damage to the pelvis
- May be diagnosed by retrograde cystography

drainage maintained for 7 days. If it is not recognised, the treatment is similar to that of rupture of the bladder.

When accidental extraperitoneal perforation of the bladder occurs during endoscopic resection, drainage of the bladder with a urethral catheter and the administration of antibiotics usually suffice. If a mass of extravasated fluid is present it is best to place a small drain through a stab incision. A laparotomy will usually be required if an intraperitoneal perforation is caused by transurethral resection.

Summary box 77.2

Management of bladder trauma

- Extravesical injury – catheter drainage for 10 days
- Intraperitoneal injury – laparotomy, repair and bladder drainage

RETENTION OF URINE (SEE ALSO CHAPTER 78)

Acute retention

There are many possible causes of acute retention of urine.

Summary box 77.3

The most frequent causes of acute retention

Male

- Bladder outlet obstruction (the most common cause)
- Urethral stricture
- Acute urethritis or prostatitis
- Phimosis

Female

- Retroverted gravid uterus
- Bladder neck obstruction (rare)

Both

- Blood clot
- Urethral calculus
- Rupture of the urethra
- Neurogenic (injury or disease of the spinal cord)
- Smooth muscle cell dysfunction associated with ageing
- Faecal impaction
- Anal pain (haemorrhoidectomy)
- Intensive postoperative analgesic treatment
- Some drugs
- Spinal anaesthesia

Clinical features

- No urine is passed for several hours.
- Pain is present.
- The bladder is visible, palpable, tender (Figure 77.8) and dull to percussion.
- Potential neurological causes should be excluded by checking reflexes in the lower limbs and perianal sensation.

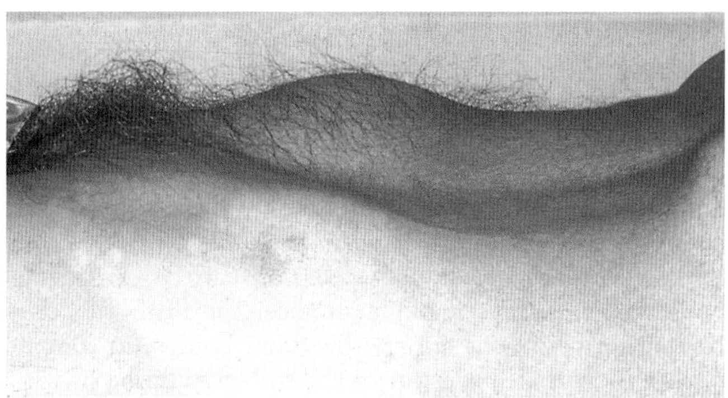

Figure 77.8 Distended bladder in a man who presented with retention of urine.

Treatment

Treatment is to pass a fine urethral catheter (14F – French gauge is defined as the circumference in millimetres) and arrange urological management. Occasionally, in postoperative retention a warm bath can help (Figures 77.9–77.12).

URETHRAL CATHETERISATION

After a thorough hand wash, sterile gloves are donned. The genitalia are cleaned using soapy antiseptic. Lidocaine gel is inserted into the urethra, warning the patient that this may create stinging. The jelly should be massaged posteriorly in an attempt to anaesthetise the sphincter region, and it is of advantage to place a penile clamp for several minutes. A small Foley catheter should be passed while the penis is held

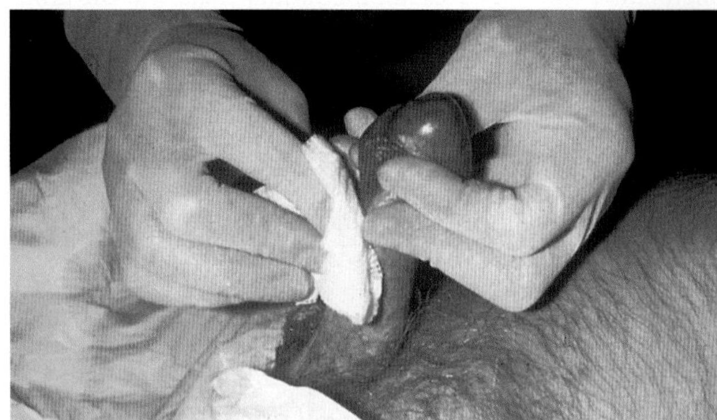

Figure 77.9 Cleaning of the penis before catheterisation.

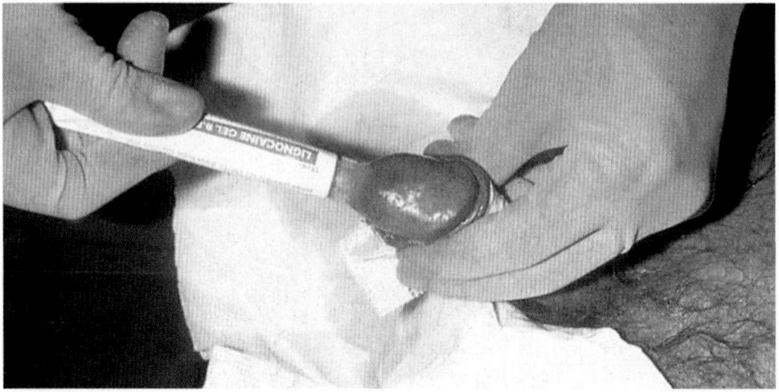

Figure 77.10 Insertion of local anaesthetic before insertion of a catheter.

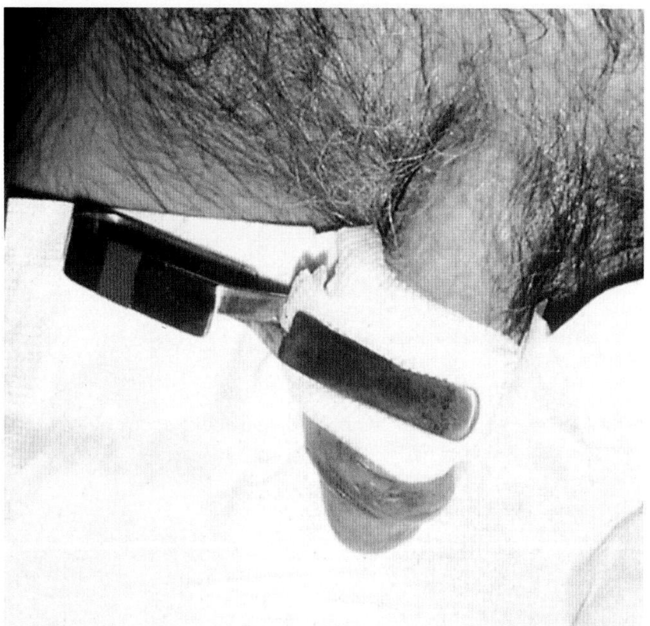

Figure 77.11 The use of a penile clamp to ensure that sufficient time is given to allow the anaesthetic to work before the catheter is inserted.

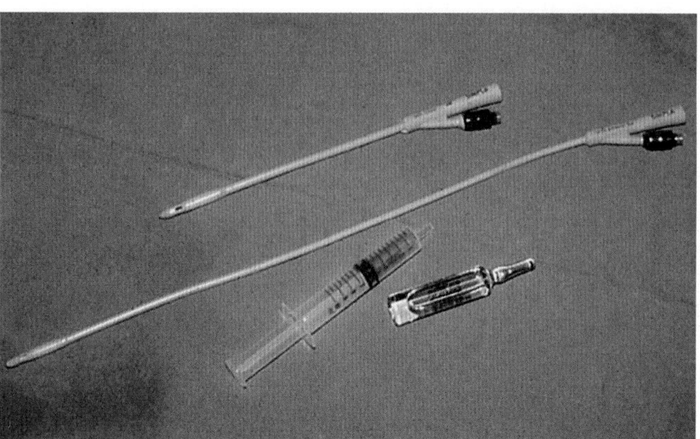

Figure 77.12 A selection of silicone catheters.

taut. In a female patient, the labia should be parted using the middle and index fingers of the left hand, which should not be moved once cleaning has been performed. Provided that a stricture is not the cause, the catheter should pass freely. Once urine begins to drain it is wise to pass a few more centimetres of catheter into the bladder before the balloon is inflated to avoid inflation in the prostate. Force must not be used.

Summary box 77.4

Catheterisation for acute retention of urine

After catheterisation:

- Record the volume of urine drained
- Examine the abdomen to exclude other pathology (rupture of an aortic aneurysm, ureteric colic or diverticulitis can cause confusion)

If the catheter will not pass, it is usually due to poor technique, lack of anaesthesia, traumatisation of the urethra or a urethral stricture. Occasionally, a large prostatic middle lobe may prevent the catheter entering the bladder; sometimes a coudé catheter will pass. If a catheter cannot be passed the following plan should be pursued.

Suprapubic puncture

Suprapubic puncture with commercially available catheters such as Cystofix or Lawrence Add-a-Cath catheters is straightforward provided that the bladder is palpable. The skin, fascia and retropubic space are anaesthetised with 0.5% lidocaine. Correct placement is confirmed by aspiration. A large-bore needle is then placed into the bladder, down which a fine catheter is passed (Cystofix) and then secured in position. The other option is to place a plastic suprapubic trocar and cannula, which has a removable plastic strip on the side. A standard 12F Foley catheter can be passed down the cannula, the balloon is inflated, the cannula is extracted and the strip pulled away from the catheter (Add-a-Cath). If urine cannot be aspirated through the fine-bore needle, passing a suprapubic trocar should not be attempted.

If these devices are not available, a catheter can be placed in the bladder under direct vision through a small incision under local anaesthetic.

Urethral instrumentation

In a patient with a known stricture, an experienced urologist may elect to dilate the stricture or to take the patient to theatre to carry out an optical urethrotomy (see Chapter 79).

Chronic retention

In chronic retention there is no pain. These patients are at risk of upper tract dilatation because of high intravesical tension – they require urgent urological referral. Men with impaired renal function may develop postobstructive diuresis after catheterisation. Such men need careful monitoring, with replacement of inappropriate urinary losses by intravenous saline; they are also at risk of haematuria as the distended urinary tract empties. Often it is several days before full renal recovery occurs.

Retention with overflow

The patient is incontinent with small amounts of urine passing involuntarily from the distended bladder. It usually follows a neglected retention.

Indwelling catheters and closed systems of catheter drainage

The risk of ascending infection is decreased by connecting the catheter to sterile tubing connected to a collecting bag. Irrigations should be avoided unless clot retention occurs. When a catheter has been *in situ* for a few days, some degree

Frederic Eugene Basil Foley, 1891–1966, urologist, Anker Hospital, St Paul, MN, USA.

of urethritis and bacteriuria is likely; changing a catheter then entails risks of severe infection if prophylactic antibiotics are not used (Figure 77.13).

Acute retention due to drugs

A number of drugs can induce retention, including antihistamines, antihypertensives, anticholinergics and tricyclic antidepressants.

The acute neuropathic bladder

1 Immediately after spinal cord injury, 'spinal shock' occurs (see Chapter 25), which may last for days or months. The detrusor cannot contract, the bladder distends and overflow incontinence occurs. Neglected bladder distension will lead to damage to the detrusor, infection and ultimately renal failure. Management is as follows.
2 The bladder must be emptied by aseptic intermittent catheterisation performed two or three times daily or the use of an indwelling urethral catheter on continuous drainage, making sure that the patient has a high urinary output (3 litres per day) to combat infection. Currently, intermittent catheterisation is preferred as soon as the patient's spinal injury is stable.
3 Neurological examination must be performed to assess the level of sensory and motor loss. Ischaemic necrosis of the cord may extend below the upper level of cord injury. When sensory loss below the upper level is total, recovery is unlikely. Incomplete lesions may recover somatic and bladder function.
4 Demonstration of intact bulbocavernosus and anal reflexes indicates that the sacral cord and nerves are intact and that reflex bladder contractions are likely to develop, although they may be insufficient to empty the bladder. If there is persistent total loss of reflexes and perineal sensation then either the sacral cord or the cauda equina is damaged. In such circumstances an acontractile bladder is likely. In cauda equina lesions there may be sensory, motor or mixed loss.
5 Full urodynamic assessment of bladder function should be undertaken when the injury is stable. This allows an accurate assessment of bladder and sphincter activity and will enable decisions to be made about further management; the prime aim is to prevent upper tract damage by promoting good bladder emptying.

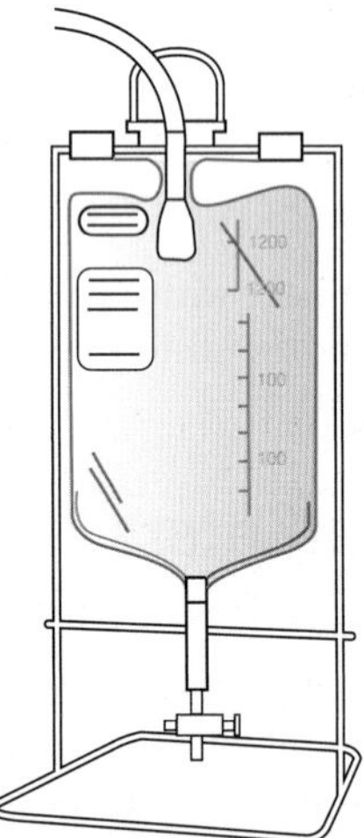

Figure 77.13 Modern Simpla bag used for continuous bladder drainage. (The nurse who is emptying the bag should be wearing disposable gloves to avoid contaminating the hands with organisms.)

Summary box 77.5

Clinical management of spinal injury

- The bladder should be emptied during spinal shock by catheterisation
- Encourage high fluid intake
- Commence intermittent catheterisation
- When the patient is stable undertake full urodynamic evaluation

The following situations represent the typical patterns of bladder function seen after spinal cord injury.

Lesions above T10

Usually leads to an 'upper motor neuron' bladder with reflexes intact but isolated from higher control mechanisms. Such patients are at risk of autonomic dysreflexia.

As a result of detrusor–sphincter dyssynergia, bladder contractions are high pressure and ineffective in producing bladder emptying; the bladder neck is normally open. If left untreated, upper tract dilatation and renal failure may result. Bladder capacity is usually decreased with the development of trabeculation and a typical 'fir-tree' appearance. Patients are incontinent during high-pressure phasic contractions because the sphincter resistance suddenly diminishes.

Some patients with low-pressure bladders that empty may be managed by means of condom drainage. Others will require clean, intermittent, self-catheterisation (CISC), popularised by Lapides. Patients with poor emptying, low bladder capacity and upper tract dilatation require treatment with endoscopic sphincterotomy and condom drainage. Some carefully selected patients may require bladder reconstruction.

Lesions involving the sympathetic outflow (T11, T12, L1, L2)

These patients are usually similar to the group with lesions above T10.

Damage to the sacral centre S2, S3, S4 and cauda equina lesions

Usually leads to a 'lower motor neuron' bladder, also found in spina bifida (myelodysplasia); the detrusor is acontractile. Abdominal straining can produce reasonable emptying but the mainstay is CISC. Some patients may have sensation of filling through the hypogastric nerves if T11 and T12 are intact. The bladder capacity may be good, but some patients have high resting pressures and high increases during bladder filling, which means that there is a risk to the upper urinary tract. The bladder neck is usually open and the distal sphincter mechanisms may be paralysed but of fixed resistance. Vesicoureteric reflux is common and upper tract damage is frequent in neglected cases. Patients who can achieve satisfactory bladder emptying by means of CISC usually have reasonable continence.

Bladder dysfunction after excision of the rectum or radical hysterectomy

Between 10% and 15% of patients undergoing radical rectal excision for cancer sustain damage to the inferior hypogastric plexus, leading to impotence in males and neurogenic bladder dysfunction. This type of bladder dysfunction is similar to the cauda equina lesion. Postoperative retention in other patients may also be caused by simple bladder outlet obstruction. The best plan is to catheterise the patient to allow postoperative recovery and then carry out urodynamic investigation to determine the appropriate treatment.

INCONTINENCE OF URINE

Overall, urinary incontinence occurs in 5% of men and 20% of women. Up to 40% of women over the age of 60 years and 50% of institutionalised elderly patients experience regular episodes of urinary incontinence. Health problems include skin breakdown and depression, and loss of esteem and sexual activity. Continence is dependent on normal mobility and brain function allowing a perception of when it is socially acceptable to void, normal bladder sensation, normal voluntary detrusor contraction producing good bladder emptying, a normally competent sphincter mechanism, which relaxes appropriately during a voluntary detrusor contraction allowing good bladder emptying, and good bladder capacity with normally low pressures during filling. This is clearly a fine balance and several factors can cause incontinence. In children, non-neurogenic incontinence is often associated with other dysfunctional conditions such as infections, constipation, psychological factors, increased fluid intake, intentional misconduct or an overactive bladder. Several investigations are required for diagnosis of urinary incontinence.

Summary box 77.6

Diagnosis of urinary incontinence

The following investigations are required:

- A careful history and physical examination and completion of frequency voiding charts
- Urodynamic testing in most patients and in all patients in whom surgical intervention is proposed
- Urine culture to exclude infection and measurement of serum creatinine

In selected cases IVU is carried out if a ureteric fistula is suspected, although ultrasound examination will often provide adequate details

Urodynamic testing

The key to the practical management of lower urinary tract dysfunction, and particularly incontinence, lies with urodynamic investigation. The principle is to artificially simulate bladder filling and emptying while obtaining pressure measurements (Figure 77.14).

The patient attends with a full bladder and is allowed to void in private to measure the maximum urinary flow rate. After voiding, the residual urine is measured by ultrasound. A pair of catheters or a twin-lumen catheter is passed into the bladder, which allows the bladder to be filled at a rate of 50 mL/min while a continuous recording of intravesical pressure is made. To obtain 'true' detrusor pressure, a second channel is required to assess intra-abdominal pressure, measured by means of a small intrarectal or intravaginal balloon. The bladder is filled until the patient states that the bladder is full. Radiographic screening may be carried out to assess bladder neck closure and urinary leakage during movement or coughing (stress incontinence) or during bouts of phasic detrusor pressure (detrusor instability). The patient is then asked to void at the end of bladder filling after the filling catheter has been removed (Figure 77.15).

The normal bladder will accept approximately 400–550 mL when filled at room temperature at a rate of <50 mL/min. The pressure increase in the bladder should be less than 15 cmH_2O. In addition, phasic pressure increases should not be seen. The normal voiding pressure should not exceed 60 cmH_2O in men and about 40 cmH_2O in women, with a flow rate of between 20 mL/s and 25 mL/s.

Common abnormalities identified during urodynamic testing in incontinence

THE OVERACTIVE BLADDER

Phasic increases in pressure give rise to urgency and urge incontinence (detrusor overactivity; Figure 77.16). This abnormality is found in patients with neurogenic bladder

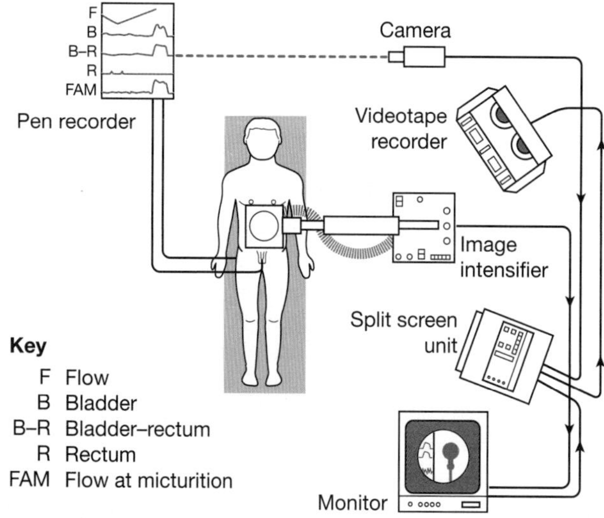

Figure 77.14 Urodynamic study.

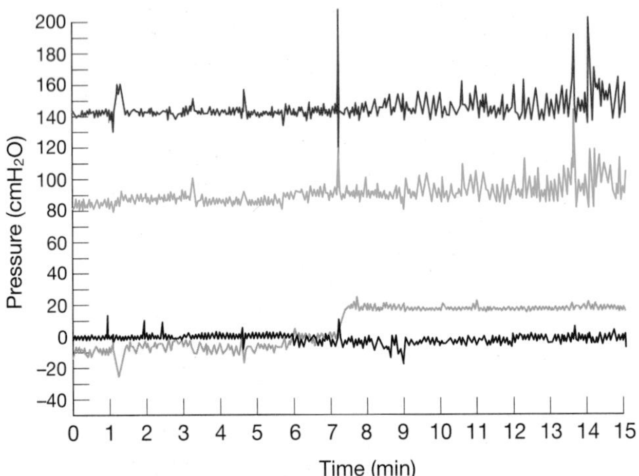

Figure 77.15 A section of an ambulatory, natural-fill urodynamic trace. The rectal pressure is in red, the bladder pressure in blue and the subtracted detrusor trace in black. The orange trace is the output of an electronic nappy, which records urinary leakage. A cough is shown, which results in genuine stress incontinence.

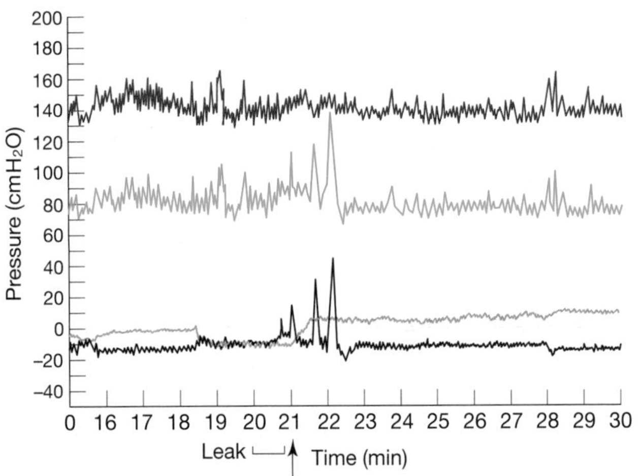

Figure 77.16 A section of an ambulatory, natural-fill urodynamic trace. The rectal pressure is in red, the bladder pressure in blue and the subtracted detrusor trace in black. The orange trace is the output of an electronic nappy, which records urinary leakage. Phasic activity is shown, which is detrusor instability resulting in urge incontinence.

dysfunction, such as in multiple sclerosis (MS) or Parkinson's disease, or after a stroke or spinal injury, when it is known as detrusor hyperreflexia. About 50% of men with bladder outflow obstruction have detrusor instability, and in about half of them the instability resolves after prostatectomy. Idiopathic detrusor overactivity is common and must be distinguished from genuine stress incontinence (GSI) in women before performing bladder neck suspension procedures. In children, overactive bladder symptoms must be carefully investigated and treated with conservative measures before initiating antimuscarinic therapy.

GENUINE STRESS INCONTINENCE

This is defined as urinary leakage occurring during increased bladder pressure when this is solely due to increased abdominal pressure and not to increased true detrusor pressure (see Figure 77.15). It is caused by sphincter weakness.

CHRONIC URINARY RETENTION

Chronic urinary retention with overflow incontinence is recognised by a large residual volume of urine (Figure 77.17) and is usually associated with high pressures during bladder filling.

BLADDER OUTFLOW OBSTRUCTION

Bladder outflow obstruction is associated with increased voiding pressures, often in excess of 90 cmH_2O (Figure 77.18), coupled with low urinary flow rates.

NEUROGENIC DYSFUNCTION

Neurogenic bladder dysfunction may also be identified.

Causes of incontinence

There are various ways of classifying the causes of incontinence.

- **Problems of social control.** Patients with dementia often have incontinence because of uninhibited detrusor hyperreflexia and impaired social perception.
- **Storage problems.** Patients with a small bladder capacity owing to fibrosis (tuberculosis, radiotherapy or interstitial cystitis) can develop incontinence. Patients with a small functional capacity owing to severe detrusor instability, neurogenic dysfunction or infection can develop incontinence.
- **Impairment of emptying.** Patients with chronic retention or neurogenic bladder dysfunction have small functional bladder capacities with detrusor overactivity causing incontinence, despite having large residual volumes of urine.
- **Weak sphincter.** This leads to GSI and can follow surgical procedures such as radical prostatectomy in men.

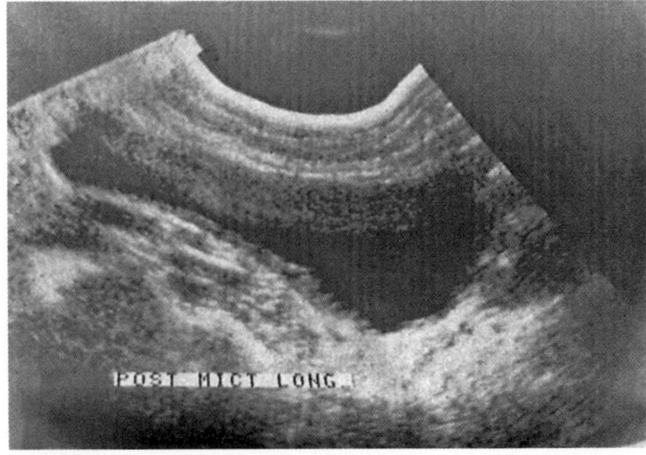

Figure 77.17 An ultrasound scan showing a large postvoid residual urine.

James Parkinson, 1755–1824, general practitioner of Shoreditch, London, UK, published *An essay on the shaking palsy* in 1817.

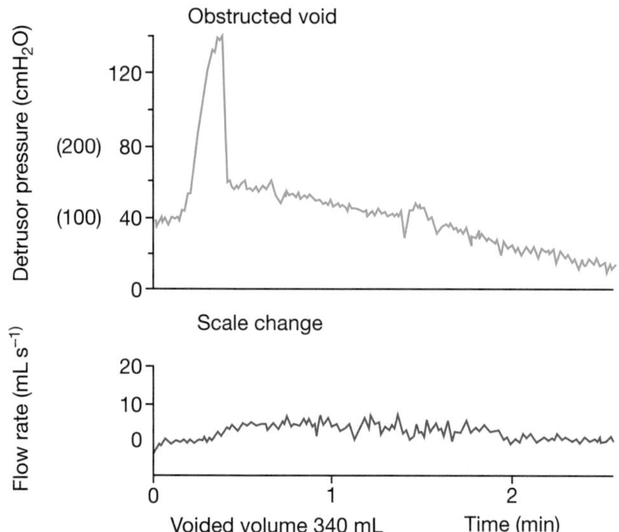

Figure 77.18 A conventional urodynamic trace showing detrusor pressure during voiding. There has been a change of scale because the pressure was so high; voiding pressures are increased with a low flow rate, which is diagnostic of bladder outflow obstruction.

- **Fistulae.** Leakage from fistulae or upper tract duplication with an ectopic ureter.
- **In children**, the causes must be carefully investigated and treated with conservative measures before initiating antimuscarinic therapy.

The common causes may be classified into male, female or mixed-sex groups.

> **Summary box 77.7**
>
> **Uses of urodynamic testing**
>
> - To distinguish genuine stress incontinence (due to sphincter weakness) from detrusor instability in women (see Figure 77.15)
> - For the classification of neurogenic bladder dysfunction
> - To distinguish bladder outflow obstruction from idiopathic detrusor instability in men
> - To investigate incontinence or other lower urinary tract symptoms

Male incontinence

CHRONIC URINARY RETENTION WITH OVERFLOW

This may be due to benign prostatic hypertrophy, carcinoma of the prostate, urethral stricture and, in younger men, hypertrophy of the bladder neck. Examination may reveal that the bladder is distended, and it can be confirmed by ultrasonography. The treatment is discussed in Chapter 78.

POST-PROSTATECTOMY

Post-prostatectomy incontinence may result from injury to the external sphincter mechanism. Treatment should be conservative initially with pelvic floor exercises, and an anastomotic stricture must be excluded. The condition may necessitate insertion of an artificial urethral sphincter (Figure 77.19).

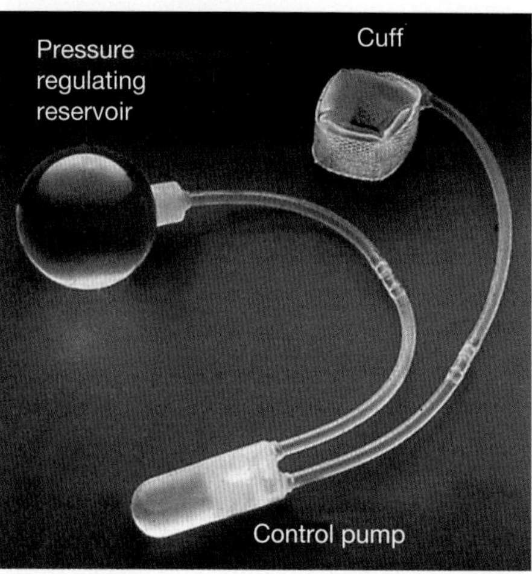

Figure 77.19 The artificial urinary sphincter made by American Medical Systems.

Female incontinence

STRESS INCONTINENCE

The most common cause is GSI although, in some parts of the world, vesicourethral fistulae as a result of neglected labour are common. It is usually found in multiparous women with a history of difficult labour. It can be found in normal young women who indulge in competitive trampolining and in patients with epispadias. The classic symptom is urine loss during coughing, laughing, sneezing or a sudden change of posture. The symptoms may change with the menstrual cycle. The volume of urine loss can be measured during an exercise test, which is performed by putting the patient through a standard set of tests with 300 mL of fluid in the bladder; in GSI the fluid losses usually range from 10 mL to 50 mL. Urinary frequency and urgency are often found in such patients because they try to avoid incontinence by frequent voiding.

Idiopathic detrusor instability can mimic GSI and coexist with it. It is important to make a correct preoperative diagnosis by urodynamic measurements, because the outcome of surgery is suboptimal in women with idiopathic detrusor instability.

Minor-to-moderate stress urinary incontinence can be controlled by pelvic floor exercises. However, if this fails, surgery is indicated. Standard operations include open colposuspension or the use of a minimally invasive approach involving the insertion of a transvaginal tape (TVT procedure).

OPEN COLPOSUSPENSION

This operation is carried out through a Pfannenstiel incision with the patient in the Lloyd-Davies position. The vaginal fascia is identified by sweeping the bladder off the vagina, and three sutures are placed on each side between the vaginal fascia and the iliopubic ligament. A suprapubic catheter is

Hermann Johann Pfannenstiel, 1862–1909, gynaecologist, Breslau, Germany (now Wroclaw, Poland), described this incision in 1900.
Oswald Lloyd-Davies, 1905–1987, surgeon, St Mark's Hospital and the Middlesex Hospital, London, UK.

placed. Voiding difficulties are frequent but usually temporary. It is best to warn women with large bladder capacities and low voiding pressures that this complication may occur and that they may be required to carry out CISC for a period. The operation is very successful for the treatment of GSI, with good results at 1 year in 90% of patients, which are maintained in about 80% of patients at 5 years.

Modifications of bladder neck suspension can also be achieved by minimally invasive approaches such as the transvaginal sling. This technique does reduce both hospital stay and postoperative morbidity.

Incontinence common to both sexes

IDIOPATHIC DETRUSOR OVERACTIVITY

Phasic increases in bladder pressure may occur during filling in otherwise normal patients (idiopathic) or it may be found in neurogenic bladder dysfunction (when it is known as detrusor hyperreflexia) and bladder outflow obstruction. Idiopathic detrusor overactivity may be asymptomatic but usually results in symptoms of frequency, urgency, urge incontinence, nocturia or nocturnal incontinence (enuresis), depending on the severity of the instability. It must be distinguished from GSI and from bladder outflow obstruction before surgical treatment. Infection, tuberculosis or carcinoma *in situ* (CIS) should be excluded. The mainstay of treatment is the use of various anticholinergic medications (oxybutynin and tolterodine). Severe symptoms resistant to conventional conservative treatment, resulting in major impairment of quality of life, may need more aggressive treatment such as enterocystoplasty or the injection of small doses of botulinum toxin (the toxin from *Clostridium botulinum*), known as BoTox, which blocks cholinergic neuromuscular transmission, at least for a time.

AGEING

Ageing can result in smooth muscle cell dysfunction, which can cause combinations of small functional capacity, detrusor overactivity, impaired bladder emptying and symptoms of lower urinary tract dysfunction.

CONGENITAL

Congenital causes include ectopic vesicae and severe epispadias. The abnormal entry of an ectopic ureter distal to the sphincter complex or into the vagina in a female patient should theoretically result in total urinary incontinence. This is discussed in Chapters 9 and 76.

TRAUMA

Trauma, whether from pelvic surgery or associated with pelvic fracture, may result in disruption of the nerve supply to the bladder or urethra, or in fistula formation.

INFECTION

Lower urinary tract infection (UTI) may be sufficient to induce urinary incontinence. A history of frequency, burning and a fever should prompt the diagnosis. Symptoms will usually settle with a course of antibiotics, but in the case of recurrent infection further investigation of the urinary tract will clearly be indicated.

NEOPLASIA

Locally advanced cancers in the pelvis, particularly carcinoma of the cervix in a woman and carcinoma of the prostate in a man, may result in direct invasion of the sphincter mechanism causing incontinence; occasionally, fistula formation may occur in women.

Other causes

CONSTANT DRIBBLING OF URINE COUPLED WITH NORMAL MICTURITION

This occurs when there is a ureteric fistula or an ectopic ureter associated with a duplex system opening into the urethra beyond the urethral sphincter in females or into the vagina. The history is diagnostic, and IVU or ultrasonography may reveal the upper pole segment, which is often poorly functioning. Treatment is by excision of the aberrant ureter and portion of kidney. A ureteric fistula can be difficult to diagnose and its demonstration may require retrograde ureterography and a high degree of suspicion.

NOCTURNAL ENURESIS

This is a condition of young children and young adults. Of course, the time at which children become dry at night varies and, in some, nocturnal enuresis is merely a delayed onset of continence. In others, it persists until late adolescence and is classified into primary and secondary nocturnal enuresis. In children, once neurogenic dysfunction has been excluded, the condition can be associated with other symptoms such as intentional misconduct, infections, constipation and increased fluid intake. These causes must be ruled out before medication is considered.

Primary nocturnal enuresis occurs in patients with nocturnal symptoms alone, which are absent during the day. Often, they have been dry for a period, and the vast majority of patients will eventually become dry. In the meantime, a sympathetic approach to these children is essential. They often respond to a system of rewards using a 'star' chart. In addition, the use of DDAVP (a vasopressin analogue) can produce increased urinary concentration at night with a decrease in nocturnal incontinence. Other treatments include the use of an alarm that wakes the child (or at least the child's parents) when incontinence occurs and medication in the form of an anticholinergic drug such as oxybutynin.

Treatments for incontinence

Treatments are listed below. Management is dependent on making a correct diagnosis.

Management and treatment

After careful assessment and investigation, many cases of incontinence can improve with simple measures such as lifestyle interventions, pelvic floor exercises with biofeedback, bladder training and incontinence devices where necessary. In mixed urge and stress incontinence, the major component has to be treated first.

PROBLEMS OF SOCIAL FUNCTIONING

Patients with dementia may respond to regular toileting. Anticholinergic agents can cause increased confusion in these patients and often, in severe cases, an indwelling catheter is needed.

STORAGE PROBLEMS

Patients with a small bladder capacity because of fibrosis may require augmentation cystoplasty. Detrusor overactivity will require treatment with anticholinergic medication but, in severe cases, particularly in neuropathic patients at high risk of upper tract dilatation, bladder substitution (near-total supratrigonal cystectomy followed by the need for detubularised ileocaecal segment bladder substitution) or augmentation (enterocystoplasty) may be needed. These procedures should be carried out only after careful assessment in units used to dealing with such problems. Patients with very impaired mobility and MS may require ileal conduit diversion. The use of intravesical injections of BoTox has provided good improvements, and it may avoid or delay the need for major surgery.

IMPAIRED BLADDER EMPTYING

Patients with overflow incontinence because of bladder outflow obstruction will usually respond well to prostatectomy. Patients with impaired bladder emptying because of neurogenic bladder dysfunction should be treated in the first place by means of CISC.

WEAK SPHINCTER

Patients with GSI should be treated by means of pelvic floor exercises initially. Duloxetine can be used as medical treatment for GSI. Bulking agents, such as macroplastique, can be used and can provide good temporary solutions. Surgical treatment by means of colposuspension or TVT may be needed. Those with post-prostatectomy incontinence or neurogenic bladder dysfunction may need to be fitted with an artificial urinary sphincter (see Figure 77.19), if they are well motivated and mobile, but careful assessment is required.

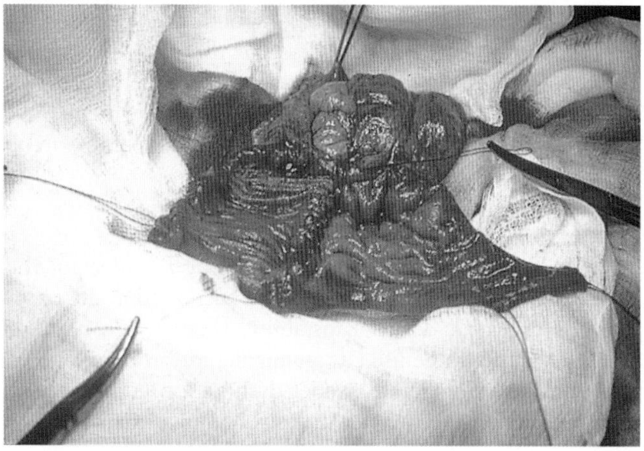

Use of appliances

An indwelling catheter drained constantly into a leg urinal may be a satisfactory solution although, in some instances, diversion via an ileal conduit is necessary. In men, a condom urinary appliance may be satisfactory and can avoid an indwelling catheter.

More major surgical treatments

VARIOUS TYPES OF URINARY DIVERSION

Urinary diversion may be required for the treatment of end-stage incontinence that is not otherwise treatable (see later in this chapter).

BLADDER SUBSTITUTION PROCEDURES

The principle behind these operations is the creation of a low-pressure, large-capacity reservoir, which can be made using any segment of bowel isolated on its vascular pedicle (Figures 77.20–77.22). This is then detubularised by dividing its anti-mesenteric border and suturing this into a plate,

Figure 77.20 A vascularised ileocaecal segment being detubularised.

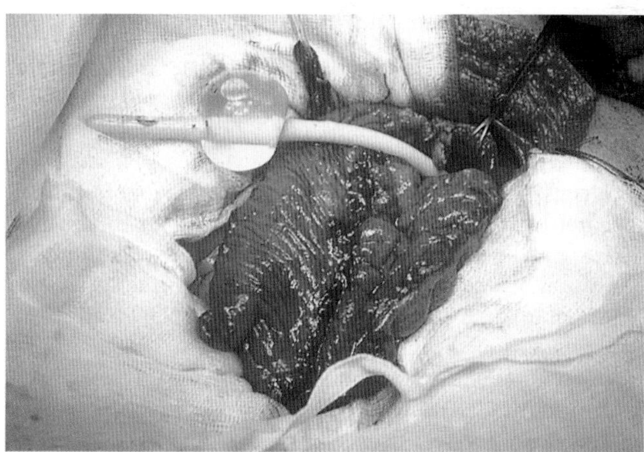

Figure 77.21 An ileocaecal segment being anastomosed to the trigone after near-total cystectomy; the left ureter is about to be implanted by means of a Camay–Le Duc anastomosis.

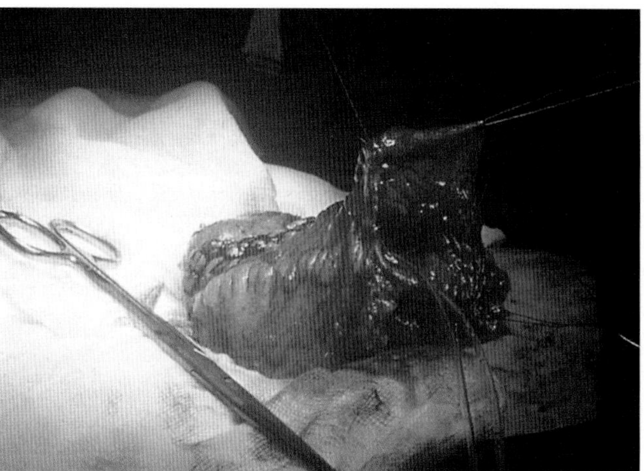

Figure 77.22 A capacious ileocaecal reservoir to be used in a patient requiring bladder substitution. These segments may be used for total bladder replacement, bladder substitution and the construction of continent diversion with a Mitrofanoff-type anti-incontinence mechanism (see later in the chapter).

which is then reconfigured into a spherical structure. This reservoir can then be anastomosed to the bladder remnant after excision of the fundus above the trigone. If necessary, the ureters can be reimplanted into the bowel segment. This new bladder will need to be emptied by means of CISC in up to 30% of cases.

'CLAM' ENTEROCYSTOPLASTY

This procedure was originally described by Bramble for the treatment of nocturnal enuresis. It has been used in the treatment of idiopathic detrusor instability (Figure 77.23). This procedure can also be used as an augmentation procedure in patients with neurogenic bladder dysfunction and a reasonable bladder capacity (approximately 300 mL).

FITMENT OF ARTIFICIAL URINARY SPHINCTER

See Figure 77.19.

Summary

Treatments for incontinence can be summarised as follows:

1 **Conservative** measures such as lifestyle interventions, pelvic floor muscle and bladder training.
2 **Devices for collection**: external penile condom or an indwelling urethral or suprapubic catheter.
3 **Drugs**: to decrease the strength of the bladder neck (e.g. adrenergic blockers); with mixed action on the bladder neck and central nervous system (e.g. tricyclic drugs); to inhibit bladder activity (e.g. anticholinergic drugs). Botulinum toxin A is used in selected patients. Duloxetine can be used as medical treatment for GSI – it is a serotonin–noradrenaline reuptake inhibitor.
4 **Intermittent self-catheterisation**: to improve emptying.
5 **Increasing outlet**: pelvic floor physiotherapy; resistance colposuspension or TVT tapes or slings; periurethral injections of 'bulking agents' such as cross-linked collagen or other particles; use of the artificial urinary sphincter.
6 **Denervation of bladder**: S3 sacral nerve blockade, neurectomy or surgical transection of the bladder to inhibit bladder activity and improve functional capacity. These are rarely used nowadays because of the use of botulinum toxin and the clam cystoplasty or S3 nerve stimulation (see point 7).
7 **Sacral nerve stimulation devices** can improve incontinence. They involve percutaneous insertion of electrodes through the sacral foramina under radiological control and implantation of an electronic stimulator.
8 **Augmentation of bladder**: 'clam' enterocystoplasty, bladder capacity substitution with detubularised bowel segment.
9 **Urinary diversion**: ileal conduit, continent urinary diversion.

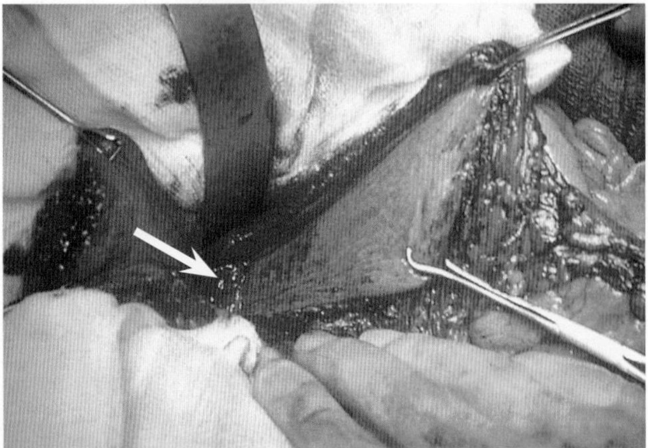

Figure 77.23 A 'clam' cystoplasty being performed. One of the ureteric orifices can be seen with the interureteric bar (arrow); the defect will be filled by a segment of detubularised ileum, performing a bladder augmentation.

BLADDER STONES

Definition

A primary bladder stone is one that develops in sterile urine; it often originates in the kidney. A secondary stone occurs in the presence of infection, outflow obstruction, impaired bladder emptying or a foreign body.

Incidence

Until the twentieth century, bladder stone was a prevalent disorder among poor children and adolescents. As a result of improved diet, especially an increased protein:carbohydrate ratio, primary vesical calculus is rare.

Composition and cystoscopic appearance

Most vesical calculi are mixed. An oxalate calculus is a primary calculus that grows slowly; usually, it is of moderate size and solitary, and its surface is uneven (Figure 77.24). Although calcium oxalate is white, the stone is usually dark brown or black because of the incorporation of blood pigment. Uric acid calculi are round or oval and smooth, and vary in colour from yellow to brown (Figure 77.25). They occur in patients with gout but are also found in patients with ileostomies or bladder outflow obstruction. A cystine calculus occurs only in the presence of cystinuria and is radio-opaque because of its high sulfur content. A triple phosphate calculus is composed of ammonium, magnesium and calcium phosphates and occurs in urine infected with urea-splitting organisms. It tends to grow rapidly. In some instances it occurs on a nucleus of one of the other types of calculus; more rarely it occurs on a foreign body (Figures 77.26 and 77.27). It is dirty white in colour and of chalky consistency.

A bladder stone is usually free to move in the bladder and it gravitates to the lowest part of the bladder. Less commonly, the stone is wholly or partially in a diverticulum, where it may be hidden from view.

Clinical features

Men are affected eight times more frequently than women. Stones may be asymptomatic and found incidentally.

Frank James Bramble, formerly urologist, the Royal Victoria Hospital, Bournemouth, UK.

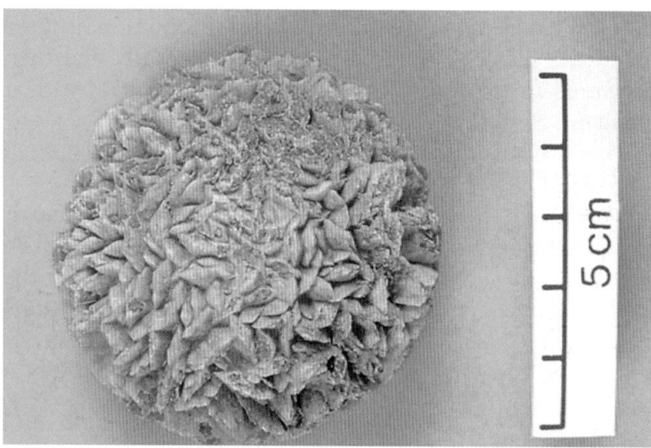

Figure 77.24 A rough bladder stone.

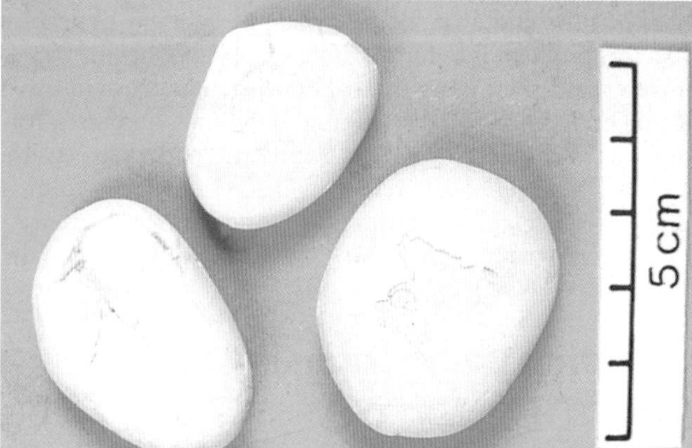

Figure 77.25 Smooth uric acid-type stones.

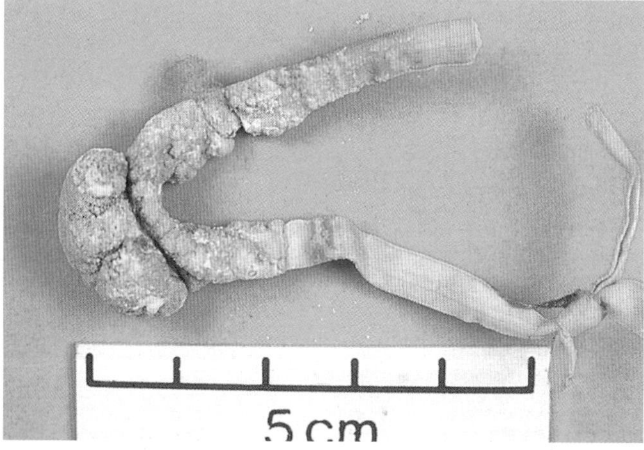

Figure 77.26 Stone on a vaginal sling that had eroded into the bladder.

Symptoms

Frequency is the earliest symptom and there may be a sensation of incomplete bladder emptying. Pain (strangury) is most often found in patients with a spiculated oxalate calculus. It occurs at the end of micturition and is referred to the tip of the penis or the labia majora; more rarely it is referred to

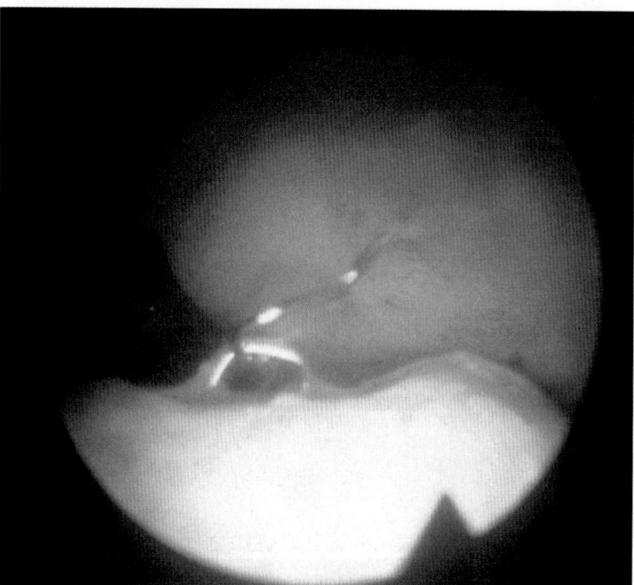

Figure 77.27 Uric acid stones that had formed on metal staples used to construct a colonic bladder augmentation.

the perineum or suprapubic region. The pain is worsened by movement. In young boys, screaming and pulling at the penis with the hand at the end of micturition are indicative of a bladder stone. Haematuria is characterised by the passage of a few drops of bright-red blood at the end of micturition, and is due to the stone abrading the vascular trigone. Interruption of the urinary stream is due to the stone blocking the internal meatus. Urinary infection is a common presenting symptom.

Examination

Rectal or vaginal examination is normal; occasionally, a large calculus is palpable in females. Examination of the urine reveals microscopic haematuria, pus or crystals that are typical of the calculus, e.g. envelope like in the case of an oxalate stone or hexagonal plates in the case of cystine calculi. In most patients the stone is visible on an ultrasound scan or a plain radiograph (Figure 77.28). Imaging of the whole of the urinary tract should be undertaken to exclude an upper tract stone. Nearly all stones can be dealt with endoscopically. In men with bladder outflow obstruction, endoscopic resection of the prostate should be performed at the same time as the stone is dealt with.

Treatment

The cause of the stone should be sought and treated; this may include bladder outflow obstruction or incomplete bladder emptying in patients with neurogenic bladder dysfunction.

Litholapaxy

The blind lithotrite (Figure 77.29) was an early type of minimally invasive technique. Standard management now includes the optical lithotrite, electrohydraulic lithotrite, holmium laser or ultrasound probe (Figure 77.30). Other devices include the stone punch, which is useful for crushing small fragments further so that they can be evacuated with an

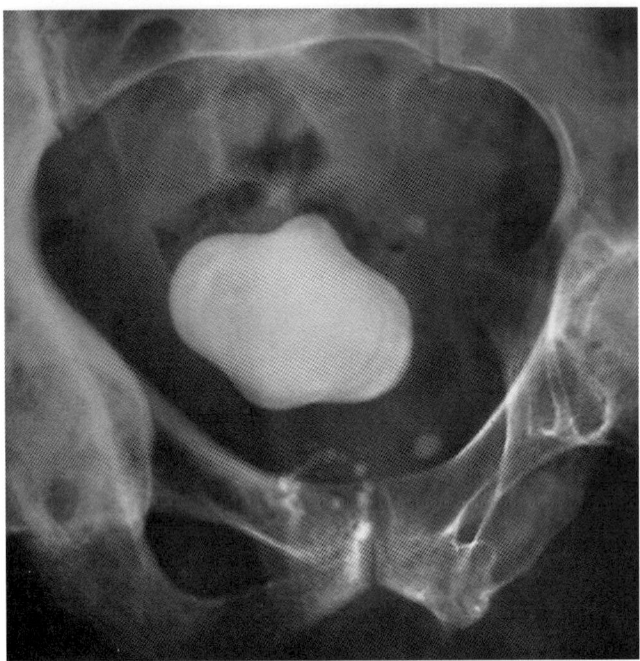

Figure 77.28 Radiograph showing a vesical calculus (no contrast has been used).

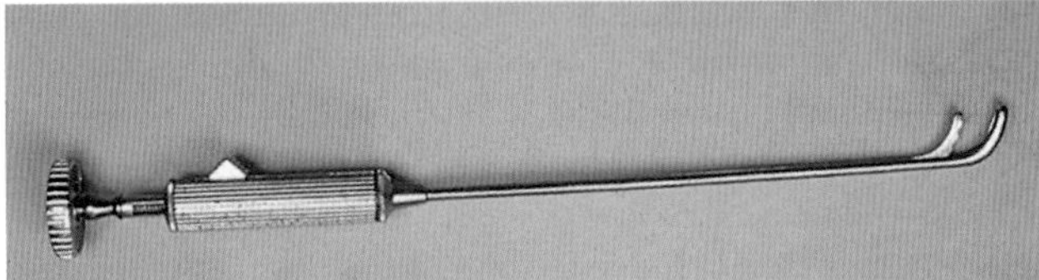

Figure 77.29 'Blind' lithotrite used to crush bladder stones.

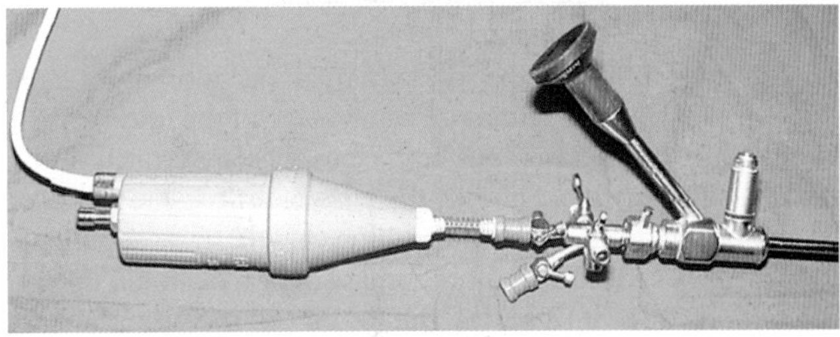

Figure 77.30 An endoscopic ultrasound probe, which is used to fragment bladder or kidney stones.

Ellik evacuator. Contraindications to perurethral litholapaxy are extremely rare and include the following:

- **Urethral**: a urethral stricture that cannot be dilated sufficiently; when a patient is aged below 10 years
- **Bladder**: a contracted bladder
- **Stone characteristics**: a very large stone.

Ultrasound lithotripsy is extremely safe but appropriate only for small stones. Laser lithotripsy with the holmium laser can deal with most large stones. Once small fragments are produced, the optical lithotrite can be used to finish the job. For evacuation of the fragments, fluid (200 mL) is introduced into the bladder. The evacuator, filled with solution, is fitted on to the sheath. The bulb is compressed slowly and then permitted to expand; the returning solution carries with it fragments of stone.

Percutaneous suprapubic litholapaxy

It is possible to insert a needle into the bladder and then pass a guidewire. As in percutaneous nephrolithotomy, Alken metal dilators can be passed over the guidewire to dilate the track and an Amplatz sheath inserted, followed by a large-bore nephroscope. This is the best method to use if it is not possible to carry out litholapaxy per urethram because of a narrow urethra.

Removal of a retained Foley catheter

A retained Foley catheter is usually caused by the channel that connects the balloon to the side arm becoming blocked, usually at the end near the balloon. The best way of dealing with this problem is to further inflate the balloon with 20 mL of water and then burst the balloon percutaneously using a needle under ultrasound screening. If the balloon bursts, it is important subsequently to cystoscope the patient to ensure that any fragments are removed before they can form a foreign body calculus. Cutting off the side arm and attempting to clear the channel with a wire is only occasionally successful.

FOREIGN BODIES IN THE BLADDER

The most common foreign body in the bladder is a fragment of catheter balloon (see above). Occasionally, a foreign body enters through the wall of the bladder, e.g. non-absorbable sutures used in an extravesical pelvic operation. Complications include:

- lower UTI;
- perforation of the bladder wall;
- bladder stone.

Treatment

A small foreign body can usually be removed per urethram by means of an operating cystoscope. Occasionally, a suprapubic approach using the percutaneous insertion of a cystoscope is needed.

DIVERTICULA OF THE BLADDER

Definition

The normal intravesical pressure during voiding is about 35–50 cmH_2O; however, pressures as great as 150 cmH_2O may be reached by a hypertrophied bladder endeavouring to force urine past an obstruction. This pressure causes the lining between the inner layer of hypertrophied muscle to protrude, forming multiple saccules. If one or more, but usually one,

Milo Ellik, b.1905, American urologist.

P Alken, urologist, the University of Heidelberg, Germany.

saccule is forced through the bladder wall, it becomes a diverticulum (Figure 77.31). Congenital diverticula are the result of a developmental defect.

Aetiology of diverticula

Congenital diverticula

These are situated in the midline anterosuperiorly and represent the unobliterated vesical end of the urachus.

Pulsion diverticula

The usual cause is bladder outflow obstruction.

Pathology

The mouth of the diverticulum is situated above and to the outer side of one ureteric orifice. Exceptionally, it is near the midline behind the interureteric ridge. The size varies from 2 cm to 5 cm, but they may be larger. Diverticula are lined by bladder mucosa and the wall is composed of fibrous tissue only (compare with a traction diverticulum). A large diverticulum enlarges in a downward direction and sometimes may obstruct a ureter – probably because of peridiverticular inflammation.

Complications

Recurrent urinary infection

As the pouch cannot empty itself efficiently, there remains a stagnant pool of urine within it. Peridiverticulitis can cause dense adhesions between the diverticulum and surrounding structures. Squamous cell metaplasia and leukoplakia are infrequent complications.

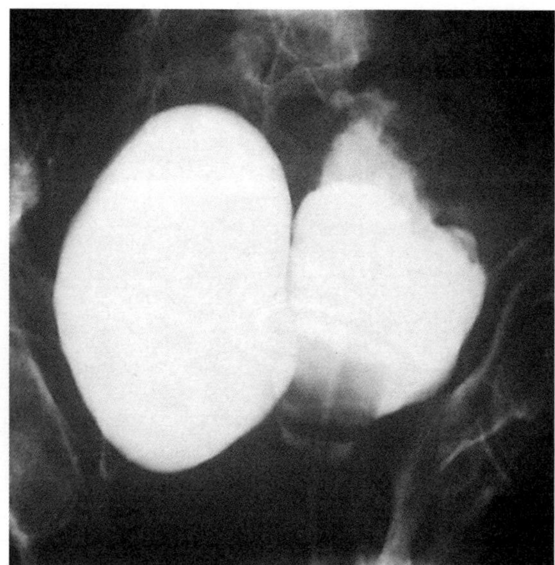

Figure 77.31 Cystogram showing a large diverticulum of the bladder.

Bladder stone

This develops as a result of stagnation and infection. The stone often protrudes into the bladder.

Hydronephrosis and hydroureter

This is extremely rare and is a consequence of peridiverticular inflammation and fibrosis.

Neoplasm

Neoplasm arising in a diverticulum is an uncommon complication (<5%). The prognosis is dependent on the stage of the tumour (see below).

Clinical features

An uninfected diverticulum of the bladder usually causes no symptoms. The patient is nearly always male (95%) and aged over 50 years. Symptoms are those of associated urinary tract obstruction, recurrent infection and pyelonephritis. Haematuria (due to infection, stone or tumour) is a symptom in about 30%. In a few patients micturition occurs twice in rapid succession (the second act may follow a change of posture).

Diagnosis

Diverticula are usually discovered incidentally on cystoscopy or ultrasonography (Figures 77.32–77.34).

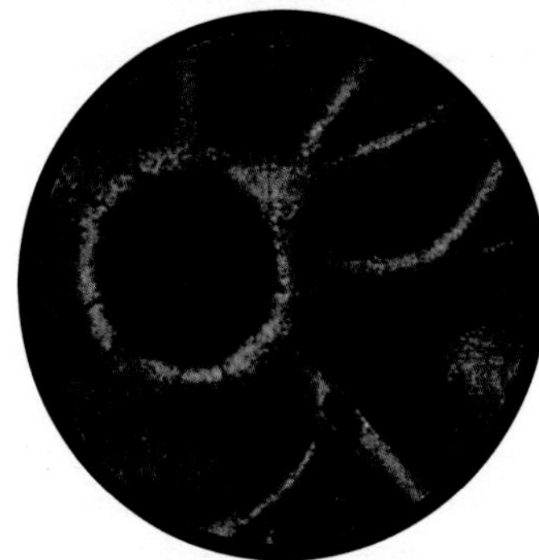

Figure 77.32 Cystoscopic appearance of the orifice of a diverticulum and trabeculation of the bladder.

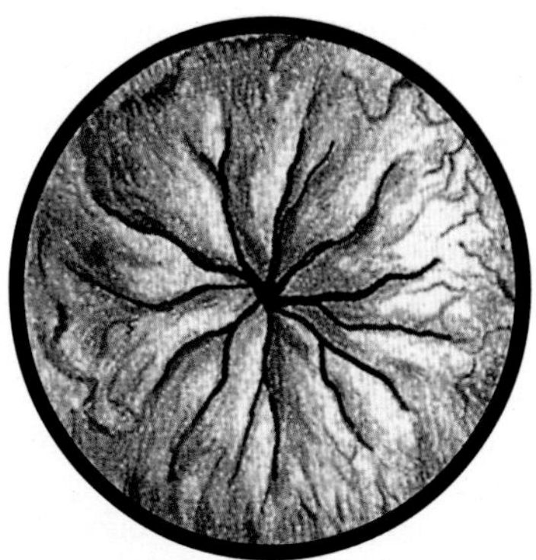

Figure 77.33 Occasional appearance of a diverticulum with inadequate distension of the bladder.

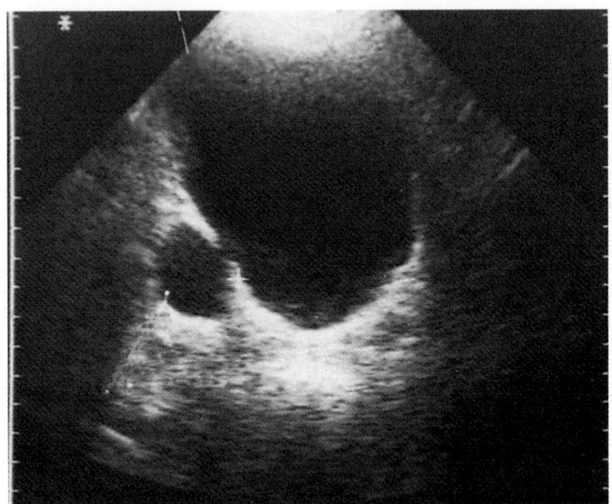

Figure 77.34 Bladder diverticulum demonstrated by ultrasound.

Indications for surgery

Surgery is necessary only for the treatment of complications. Provided that the diverticulum is small and associated outflow obstruction has been dealt with by prostate resection, there is no reason to resect the diverticulum. Even a large diverticulum may not require treatment in the absence of infection or other complications.

Combined intravesical and extravesical diverticulectomy

A ureteric stent is passed up the ureter on the affected side and the anterior bladder wall is exposed through a suprapubic incision. The bladder is incised in the midline and the diverticulum is packed with a strip of gauze. The neck of the diverticulum is separated from the ureter and, when the pouch is free, it is severed from the bladder. The resulting defect is closed in a single layer with 2/0 absorbable sutures. A suprapubic catheter is left in place and an extravesical drain is inserted. An alternative method, if the sac is densely adherent, is to carry the incision in the bladder down to the rim of the diverticular orifice, then to detach the diverticulum together with its fibrous rim. The incision in the bladder is closed and the diverticulum left in position with a corrugated drain placed into it for 2–3 days. The track fibroses rapidly after removal of the drain. If bladder outlet obstruction is present, prostatectomy should be carried out at the same time as the diverticulectomy, using any appropriate method (transurethral resection of the prostate [TURP], laser or open).

Summary box 77.8

Bladder diverticula

- Bladder diverticula are most frequently diagnosed incidentally by cystoscopy or urinary tract imaging
- The presence of a diverticulum – even quite a large one – is not an indication for diverticulectomy unless symptoms or cancer is present

Traction diverticulum (synonym: hernia of the bladder)

A portion of the bladder protruding through the inguinal or femoral hernial orifice occurs in 1.5% of such herniae treated by surgery (Figure 77.35).

URINARY FISTULAE

Congenital urinary fistulae

The causes of congenital urinary fistulae include:

- ectopia vesicae;
- a patent urachus – the presence of a urinary leak from the umbilicus, present at birth or commencing soon after, suggests this diagnosis. In adult life, infection in a urachal cyst may produce a fistula and adenocarcinoma may occur (Figures 77.36 and 77.37). Treatment is by means of excision of the urachal tract and closure of the bladder once distal obstruction has been excluded;
- in association with imperforate anus (see Chapters 9 and 73).

Traumatic urinary fistulae

Perforating wounds, damage not recognised during surgery or poor healing and avascular necrosis after radiotherapy and surgery may lead to fistula formation. Also, clot retention occurring after an open bladder operation may lead to dehiscence of

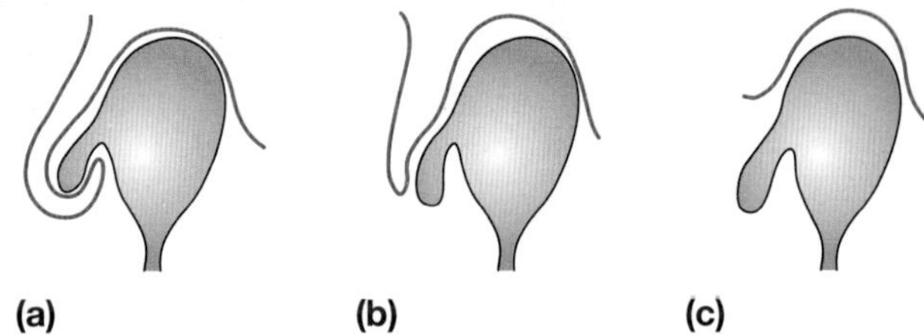

Figure 77.35 (a) Intraperitoneal, (b) paraperitoneal and (c) extraperitoneal hernia of the bladder, in relation to a hernial sac.

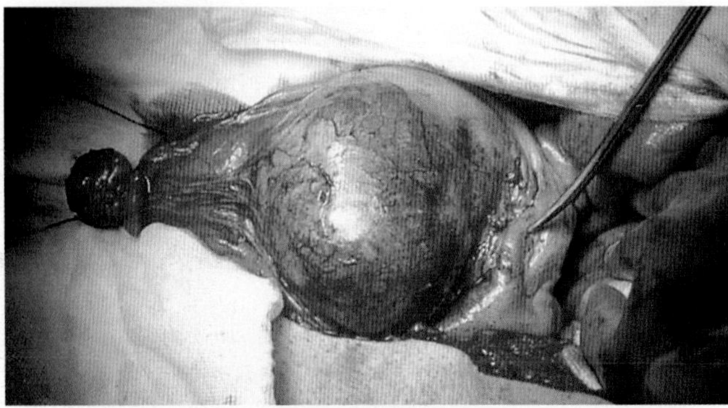

Figure 77.36 An operative photograph showing a large urachal cyst in which adenocarcinoma formation has occurred. A partial cystectomy with total removal of the urachal remnant is about to be carried out.

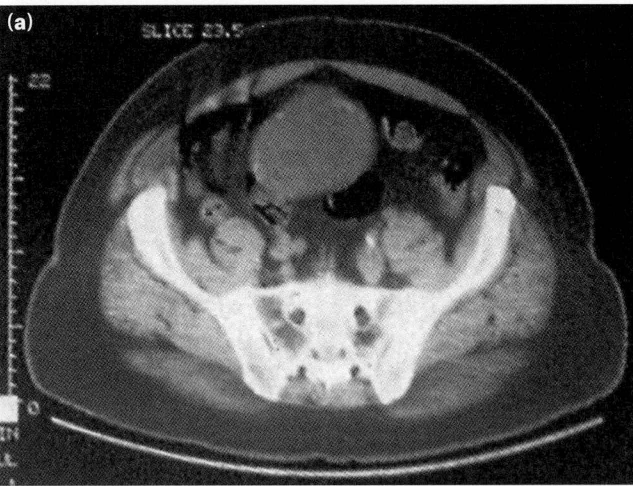

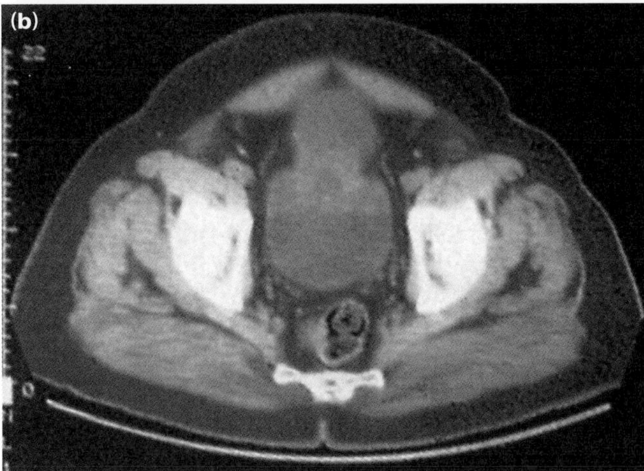

Figure 77.37 (a, b) Computed tomography scans of the same patient as in Figure 77.36, showing a large urachal cyst closely approximated to the dome of the bladder.

the wound and a fistula, which will heal quickly provided that the bladder is kept empty with an indwelling catheter.

Vesicovaginal fistulae

Aetiology

- **Obstetric**. The usual cause is protracted or neglected labour.
- **Gynaecological**. The operations chiefly causing this complication are total hysterectomy and anterior colporrhaphy.
- **Radiotherapy**.
- **Direct neoplastic infiltration**. Exceptionally, carcinoma of the cervix ulcerates through the anterior fornix to implicate the bladder.

When an injury to the bladder is recognised and repaired, leakage is uncommon, but escape of urine will quickly follow if such damage passes unnoticed. However, most vesicovaginal fistulae are the result of ischaemic necrosis of the bladder because of prolonged pressure of the fetal head in obstetric cases. In gynaecological cases, the ischaemia is brought about by grasping the bladder wall in an artery forceps, including the bladder wall in a suture or perhaps even by local oedema or haematoma. Leakage because of tissue necrosis seldom manifests itself before 7 days after the operation. An intractable fistula after radiotherapy for carcinoma of the cervix uteri may arise from avascular necrosis years after the apparent cure of the original lesion.

Clinical features

There is leakage of urine from the vagina and excoriation of the vulva. Vaginal examination may reveal a localised thickening on its anterior wall or in the vault. On inserting a vaginal speculum, urine will be seen escaping from an opening in the anterior vaginal wall.

The 'three-swab test'

The differential diagnosis between a ureterovaginal and vesicovaginal fistula can be made by placing a swab in the vagina and injecting a solution of methylene blue through the urethra; the vaginal swab becomes coloured blue if a vesicovaginal fistula is present. Cystoscopy and bilateral retrograde ureterography provide a more reliable demonstration. IVU should be performed to exclude a coincidental ureterovaginal fistula (ureterovaginal fistula occurs with vesicovaginal fistula in about 10% of cases). Usually, IVU shows some upper tract dilatation resulting from partial obstruction.

Treatment

Just occasionally, conservative management of a vesicovaginal fistula after a hysterectomy, by urethral bladder drainage, is successful; however, most fistulae will require definitive surgical repair. A low fistula (subtrigonal) is best repaired per vaginam. The fistula is exposed, the bladder is closed using absorbable sutures and the vagina subsequently closed with a separate layer. A urethral catheter should be left *in situ* for at least 10 days. For higher (supratrigonal) fistulae a transvaginal approach can be difficult. These patients should always undergo cystoscopy before the repair procedure and bilateral ureterograms performed. For high fistulae a suprapubic approach is the best method in most hands; however, some experts will aim to carry out vaginal closure in most cases that have not involved complex surgery or radiotherapy.

To repair a ureterovaginal fistula, an extraperitoneal approach to the ureter via the previous Pfannenstiel incision is made. Considerable adhesions will be encountered, but the ureter can usually be found above the level of the injury and followed down. Reimplantation into the bladder is often required. Depending on the amount of ureter lost, it may be possible to achieve reimplantation with a psoas hitch procedure. If the gap is too large a Boari flap of anterior bladder wall should be cut and brought over to meet the ureter and a reimplant performed. The most important principle of ureteric reimplantation is that there should be no tension on the repair.

Achille Boari, nineteenth century Italian surgeon.

Fistulae from renal pelvis to skin or gut

Tuberculosis of a kidney may result in a fistula to the duodenum, colon or skin. Similarly, a pyonephrosis may discharge into the gut or on to the skin. Duodenal ulcer involving the pelvis of the right kidney, Crohn's disease involving the renal pelvis or ureter or cases of xanthogranulomatous pyelonephritis may cause fistulae. A longstanding urinoma will occasionally fistulate into the gut.

Fistulae arising from infection

The most common cause is diverticulitis of the colon. Fistulae may also follow Crohn's disease, appendix abscess or pelvis sepsis after acute salpingitis, or pelvic surgery.

The onset of a fistula from diverticular disease may well be treated as a simple urinary infection. The diagnosis can be difficult to make, but on cystoscopy a patch of oedema on the left side of the vault is suggestive and bubbles of gas may be seen (Figure 77.38). A cystogram may reveal the fistula. The passage of gas per urethram in a patient is most suggestive (provided that diabetes resulting in urinary infection with a gas-forming organism is excluded).

Treatment of fistulae caused by diverticular disease

In most patients a single-stage operation is indicated provided that the surgeon is experienced in colonic surgery. At laparotomy, the communication is separated, the hole in the bladder being closed and patched with omentum, and the segment of diseased bowel resected; it is most important to ensure that the left colon and, if necessary, the splenic flexure are fully mobilised to facilitate a tension-free, well-vascularised anastomosis. The bladder is drained by a urethral catheter.

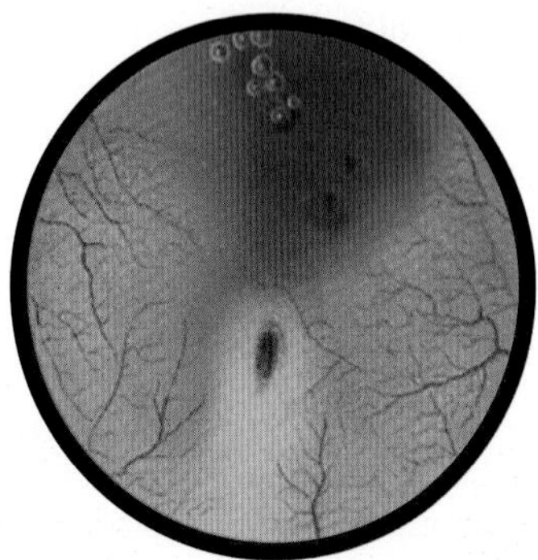

Figure 77.38 Cystoscopic view of a vesicointestinal fistula. Bubbles of gas can be seen issuing from the orifice of the fistula.

Fistulae caused by carcinoma

By the time that a fistula between the bowel and the bladder has developed, the tumour is usually locally advanced but may be operable.

Urethral fistulae in males

These occur as the result of infection above a stricture producing a paraurethral abscess that ruptures into the urethra, allowing extravasation to occur suddenly into the scrotum and perineum. Urine and infection extend into the upper 2.5 cm of the thigh and lower abdominal wall. Widespread cellulitis and tissue necrosis (which may lead to Fournier's gangrene) may occur unless drainage of urine is achieved by suprapubic cystotomy and the tissue planes are freely drained by inguinal and scrotal incisions.

Neoplastic fistulae

Primary bladder tumours very rarely produce fistulae. Involvement of the bladder by tumours of the cervix, uterus, colon and rectum can produce fistulae, as may sarcoma of the small gut. Carcinoma of the prostate rarely produces a rectal fistula. Treatment is difficult and in most cases only palliative relief can be given. It is rarely in the patient's interest to carry out urinary diversion, although minimally invasive techniques such as placement of ureteric stents can be helpful in palliating symptoms.

Summary box 77.9

Fistulae

- A fistula is a communication between two epithelium-lined surfaces
- Most urinary fistulae are vesicovaginal and result from obstetric trauma; an associated ureterovaginal fistulae occurs in about 10% of cases
- A 'three-swab test' is used to aid the diagnosis. An examination under anaesthesia, vaginoscopy, and cystoscopy and intravenous urography should be performed and, if necessary, retrograde ureterography
- Conservative management is rarely successful
- The principles of repair include good exposure, excision of diseased tissue and tension-free vascularised repair in anatomical layers
- Fistulae caused by radiation, cancer and sepsis can be complex with multiple tracts
- The persistence of a fistula on the skin implies the presence of distal obstruction, chronic infection, such as tuberculosis, or a foreign body, such as a stone or non-absorbable ligature

Burrill Bernard Crohn, 1884–1983, gastroenterologist, Mount Sinai Hospital, New York, NY, USA, described regional ileitis in 1932.
Jean Alfred Fournier, 1832–1915, French syphilologist and founder of the Venereal and Dermatological Clinic, Hôpital St Louis, Paris, France.

LOWER URINARY TRACT INFECTION AND CYSTITIS

Infection of the bladder gives rise to symptoms of frequency, urgency, suprapubic discomfort, dysuria and cloudy offensive urine. These symptoms are often known as 'cystitis'. Lower UTIs are much more common in women than in men, particularly in those aged under 50. It should be remembered that a lower UTI is often associated with upper tract colonisation and the presence of associated loin pain, pyrexia, rigors and malaise (these symptoms represent complicated infection and should be taken seriously because serious sepsis can ensue).

Isolated infection

A single episode of lower tract infection occurs frequently in women and is rarely complicated.

Recurrent infection

Recurrent infection may be associated with an underlying predisposing cause or may be a result of bacterial resistance. In healthy women, infection after intercourse can occur without any demonstrable abnormality of the urinary tract. Repeated attacks of UTIs in women, or a single attack in a man or a child of either sex, should always be followed by investigation to discover and treat the cause; sometimes, however, no cause can be found. Asymptomatic bacteriuria is common and investigation may fail to demonstrate any underlying cause.

Infection in men

Although more common in women, the incidence of infection is higher in male infants because underlying urinary tract abnormalities are more frequent. Complicated or recurrent infection in men warrants prompt antibiotic therapy and investigation to exclude an underlying cause.

Infection in pregnancy

The incidence of asymptomatic bacteriuria in pregnant women is twice as high as in non-pregnant women. Simple uncomplicated infection can be treated after urine culture with an appropriate antibiotic that is not contraindicated in pregnancy, such as cephalosporin or ampicillin. Non-responsive infection may require intravenous therapy and an ultrasound scan.

Predisposing causes of urinary tract infection

- Incomplete emptying of the bladder, secondary to bladder outflow obstruction, a bladder diverticulum, neurogenic bladder dysfunction or decompensation of the detrusor muscle.
- A calculus, foreign body or neoplasm.
- Incomplete emptying of the upper tract, dilatation of the ureters associated with pregnancy, or vesicoureteric reflux. In childhood, the mainstay of treatment of vesicoureteric reflux is antibiotic therapy; surgery is reserved for those with recurrent infection despite antibiotics or with severe upper tract dilatation.
- Oestrogen deficiency, which may give rise to lowered local resistance.
- Colonisation of the perineal skin by strains of *Escherichia coli* expressing molecules that facilitate adherence to mucosa.
- Diabetes.
- Immunosuppression.

Avenues of infection

Ascending infection from the urethra is the most common route (see Chapter 79). The organisms originate in the bowel, contaminate the vulva and reach the bladder. The passage of urethral instruments may cause infection in either sex, especially when the bladder contains residual urine (**Figure 77.39**). Other routes are less common and include descending infection from the kidney (tuberculosis), haematogenous spread, lymphogenous spread and spread from adjoining structures (Fallopian tube, vagina or gut).

Bacteriology

Bacterial virulence factors affect the ability of a pathogen to infect the host. The possession of pili (rod-shaped structures) that project from the outer membrane increases adhesiveness.

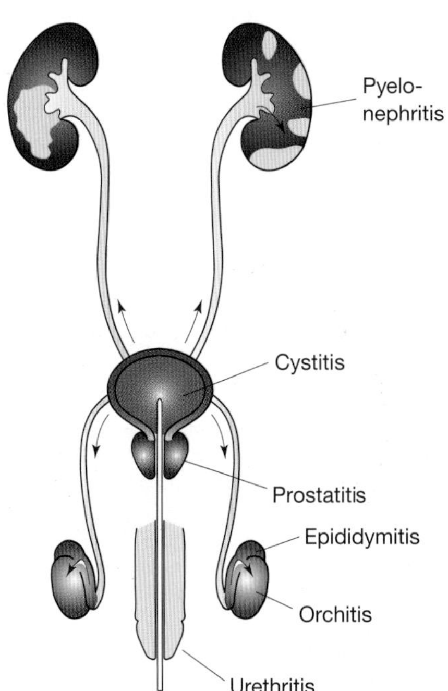

Figure 77.39 Complications liable to follow the changing of a urethral catheter in the presence of urethritis (courtesy of CG Scorer, FRCS, London, UK).

Gabriele Falloppio (Fallopius), 1523–1563, Professor of Anatomy, Surgery and Botany, Padua, Italy.

The type of pilus can be used to classify the pathogen involved. *E. coli* is the most common organism followed by *Proteus mirabilis*, *Staphylococcus epidermidis* and *Streptococcus faecalis*. Infection with other organisms or infection with mixed organisms is found in patients with neurogenic bladder dysfunction or those with a longstanding indwelling urethral catheter. These organisms include *Pseudomonas* and *Klebsiella* spp., *Staphylococcus aureus* and various streptococci. Tuberculous infection is considered below. The presence of pus cells without organisms calls for examination for *Mycobacterium tuberculosis* and *Neisseria gonorrhoeae*. Having eliminated these possibilities, the underlying condition may be abacterial cystitis, CIS, renal papillary necrosis, stones or incomplete treatment of a urinary infection.

Clinical features

These include frequency, pain, haematuria and pyuria. Pyrexia and rigors are not associated with a simple UTI but are a sign of upper tract infection or septicaemia.

Examination

On examination there is tenderness over the bladder. Initial and midstream urine specimens should be collected in males as acute prostatitis may be present (see below), which will lead to threads in the initial specimen. The midstream specimen must be subjected to microscopy and culture, and the sensitivity of any organisms assessed.

Treatment

Treatment should be started immediately and modified if necessary when the bacteriological report is to hand. The patient is urged to drink. Appropriate first-line antibiotics depend on local likely sensitivities but would include trimethoprim or one of the quinolones. Failure to respond indicates the need for further investigation to exclude predisposing factors. It is important to check for associated allergies or other drugs or conditions that might preclude the use of some antibiotics (e.g. concomitant administration of methotrexate and trimethoprim [both inhibit tetrahydrofolate reductase]).

Summary box 77.10

Urinary tract infections (UTIs) in adults

- Isolated UTIs in adults are not infrequent and are more common in women
- Recurrent or complicated infection (haematuria, rigors) warrants appropriate antimicrobial therapy and investigation
- Investigation to exclude a predisposing cause includes urinalysis, microscopy and culture, upper tract imaging and cystoscopy
- *Mycobacterium tuberculosis*, *Neisseria gonorrhoeae* or *Mycoplasma genitalium* should be suspected if pus cells are present but urine culture is negative
- Cancer, especially CIS, masquerading as infection may be diagnosed as abacterial cystitis

Investigation

Investigation may be needed in the male or when recurrent infection occurs. This includes measurement of urinary flow rates and post-void residual urine. IVU, ultrasound scan or CT scanning will usually be carried out together with cystoscopy. Difficult cases may require urodynamic investigation.

SPECIAL FORMS OF LOWER URINARY TRACT INFECTIONS

Acute abacterial cystitis (acute haemorrhagic cystitis)

The patient presents with a severe UTI. Pus is present in the urine but no organism can be cultured. It is commonly sexually acquired but tuberculous infection and CIS must be ruled out. The underlying causative organism may be *Mycoplasma* sp. or herpes simplex virus. Cyclophosphamide can also cause this problem.

Frequency-dysuria syndrome (urethral syndrome)

This consists of symptoms of a lower tract infection but with negative urine cultures. CIS, tuberculosis and interstitial cystitis should be excluded. Most urologists advise patients to adopt general measures such as wearing cotton underwear, using simple soaps, adopting general perineal hygiene measures and voiding after intercourse. Other treatments include cystoscopy and urethral dilatation, although the benefits remain doubtful.

Tuberculous urinary infection

Tuberculous urinary infection is secondary to renal tuberculosis. Early tuberculosis of the bladder starts around the ureteric orifice or trigone, the earliest evidence being pallor of the mucosa due to submucous oedema. Subsequently, tubercles may be seen and, in longstanding cases, there is marked fibrosis and the capacity of the bladder is greatly reduced (**Figure 77.40**).

Treatment

Tuberculous infection usually responds rapidly to antituberculous drugs but occasionally the involved kidney and ureter have to be removed. If the bladder remains of low capacity, patients will have severe symptoms and the upper tracts are at

Theodor Albrecht Edwin Klebs, 1834–1913, Professor of Bacteriology successively at Prague, Czechoslovakia, Zurich, Switzerland, and the Rush Medical College, Chicago, IL, USA.
Albert Ludwig Siegmund Neisser, 1855–1916, Director of the Dermatological Institute, Breslau, Germany (now Wroclaw, Poland).

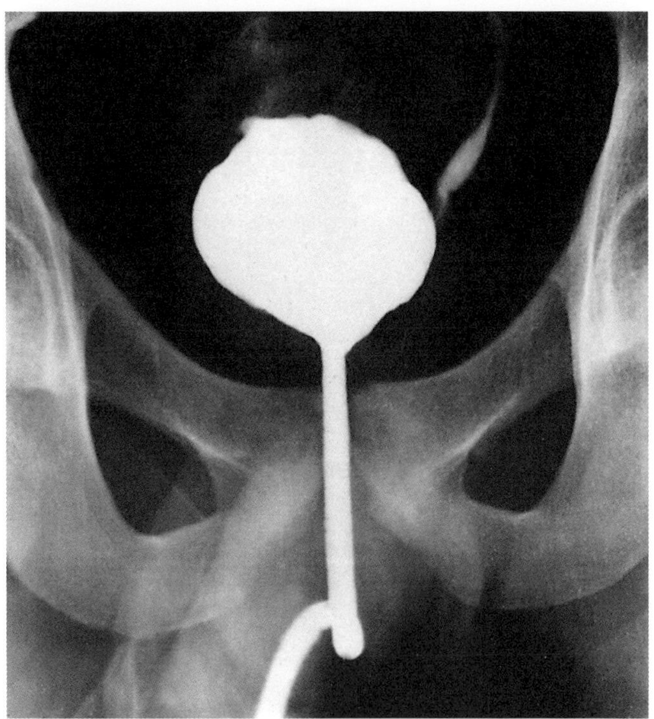

Figure 77.40 Retrograde cystograph showing an exceedingly contracted ('thimble') bladder in a case of tuberculous cystitis.

risk because of high filling pressures and vesicoureteric reflux. Such patients, after appropriate chemotherapy, respond well to bladder augmentation. The ureters may need reimplantation.

BLADDER AUGMENTATION BY ILEOCYSTOPLASTY OR CAECOCYSTOPLASTY

The fibrosed supratrigonal bladder is removed and the bladder augmented with a segment of bowel. This may consist of intact caecum, a detubularised segment of ileum or a detubularised ileocaecal segment (see Figures 77.20–77.22).

Interstitial cystitis (Hunner's ulcer)

For practical purposes, this is confined to women. The first symptom is increased frequency; pain, relieved by micturition and aggravated by jarring and overdistension of the bladder, is another characteristic symptom. In most patients pyuria and urinary infection are absent. Haematuria also occurs. The aetiology remains as obscure as it was when Guy Hunner described the condition in 1914. It consists of a chronic pancystitis, often with marked infiltration with lymphocytes and macrophages. Fibrosis of the vesical musculature and areas of avascular atrophy of the epithelium occur. Ulceration of the mucosa occurs in the fundus of the bladder. In severe cases the bladder capacity is reduced to 30–60 mL. The characteristic linear bleeding ulcer is caused by splitting of the mucosa when the bladder is distended under anaesthesia. Inflammation of all coats of the bladder is present with granulation tissue in the submucosa underlying the ulcer. The muscularis is hypertrophied and the peritoneum in proximity to the area of maximum disease is thickened. The inflammation may involve the trigone, the urethra and, in severe cases, the peritoneum. Pronounced mast cell infiltration is seen but is not specific. It is important to check urinary cytology and to biopsy the mucosa to exclude underlying neoplastic disease.

On cystoscopy the characteristic ulcer is found in the fundus, but it may be absent. This area bleeds readily as the bladder is decompressed. Treatment is difficult and unsatisfactory. Hydrostatic dilatation under anaesthesia may give relief for some months. Instillation of dimethylsulfoxide results in improvement in some patients. Other drugs that have been tried include intravesical heparin, oral ranitidine and steroid therapy. Patients with severe symptoms may well require cystectomy and orthotopic bladder substitution. In patients with severe inflammation involving the trigone and urethra, this operation may not result in complete relief and some type of urinary diversion may be needed.

Alkaline encrusting cystitis

Alkaline encrusting cystitis is rare and is due to urea-splitting organisms causing phosphatic encrustations on the bladder mucosa of elderly women. There are symptoms of a chronic UTI and a plain radiograph shows the bladder outline. The encrustations may be removed by bladder irrigation and the infection treated with appropriate antibiotics.

Cystitis cystica

Under the influence of chronic inflammation the surface epithelium sends down buds, resulting in minute cysts filled with clear fluid, most abundant on the trigone. This is frequently found in patients with recurrent frequency and dysuria.

SCHISTOSOMIASIS OF THE BLADDER (SEE CHAPTER 6)

Geographical distribution

The disease is endemic in Egypt, parts of Africa, Israel, Syria, Saudi Arabia, Iran, Iraq and the shores of China's great lakes. Dwellers of the Nile valley have suffered for centuries. Marshes or slow-running fresh water provide the habitat for the freshwater snail (*Bulinus truncatus*) that is the intermediate host.

Mode of infestation

The disease is acquired through exposure of the skin to infected water, which usually occurs while bathing. The free-swimming, bifid-tailed embryos (cercariae) of the trematode *Schistosoma haematobium* penetrate the skin. Shedding their tails, they enter blood vessels and are swept to all parts of the body but they flourish in the liver where they live on

Guy Leroy Hunner, 1868–1951, gynaecologist, Johns Hopkins Hospital, Baltimore, MD, USA.

erythrocytes and develop into male and female worms. Once sexual maturity has been attained, the nematodes leave the liver and enter the portal vein. The male worm bends into the shape of a gutter (the gynaecophoric canal) into which a female worm nestles, and the pair makes its way towards the inferior mesenteric vein. *Schistosoma haematobium* has an affinity for the vesical venous plexus, which it reaches through the portosystemic anastomotic channels.

Having reached the bladder the female worm eventually enters a submucous venule which is so small that it completely blocks it. It now proceeds to lay about 20 ova in a chain; each ovum is provided with a terminal spine that penetrates the vessel wall. A heavily infected individual passes hundreds of ova a day. If the ova reach fresh water, the low osmotic pressure causes rupture and the ciliated miracidium emerges. To survive, it must reach and penetrate the intermediate snail host within 36 hours. Within the snail's liver, the miracidium enlarges and gives rise to myriads of daughter cysts, which are set free on the death of the snail. A single miracidium begets thousands of cercariae to complete the life cycle.

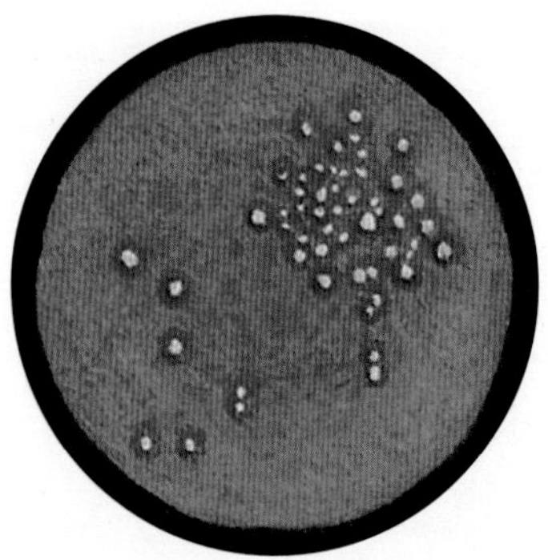

Figure 77.41 Bilharzial tubercles (courtesy of N Makar).

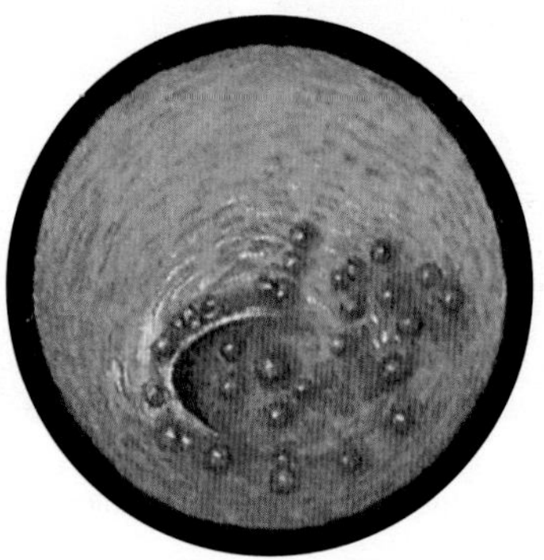

Figure 77.42 Bilharzial nodules (courtesy of N Makar).

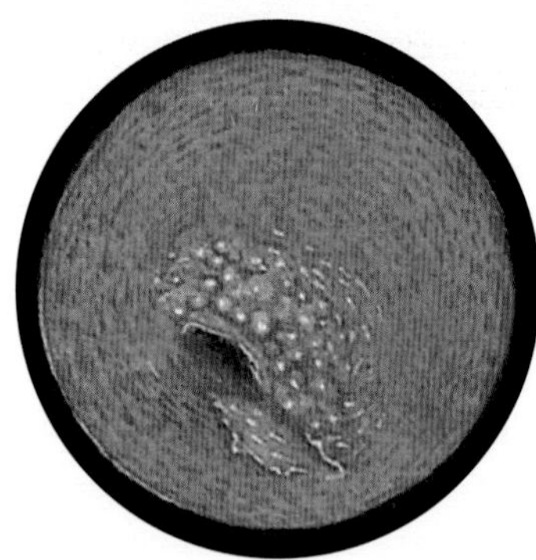

Figure 77.43 'Sandy patches' (courtesy of N Makar).

Clinical features

After penetration of the skin, urticaria lasting about 5 days can occur (swimmer's itch). After an incubation period of 4–12 weeks, a high evening temperature, sweating and asthma, together with leukocytosis and eosinophilia, occur. Usually, an asymptomatic period of several months supervenes before the ova are released, causing the typical early signs and symptoms of intermittent, painless, terminal haematuria. Men are affected three times more frequently than women.

Examination of the urine

The last few millilitres of an early morning urine specimen are collected and centrifuged. Examination on several consecutive days may be required, but a negative result does not exclude bilharziasis, especially in patients no longer resident in bilharzial districts. Antibody detection by enzyme-linked immunosorbent assay (ELISA) using *Schistosoma mansoni* adult microsomal antigen (MAMA) can be performed. The test is positive 1 month after infection and is specific for *Schistosoma mansoni* and *Schistosoma haematobium*.

Cystoscopy

Depending on the length of time for which the disease has remained untreated, cystoscopy will reveal one or more of the following:

1 **Bilharzial pseudotubercles** are the earliest specific appearance of the disease (Figure 77.41).
2 **Bilharzial nodules** (Figure 77.42) are caused by the fusion of tubercles.
3 **'Sandy patches'** are the result of calcified dead ova with degeneration of the overlying epithelium (Figure 77.43).
4 **Ulceration** is the result of sloughing of the mucous membrane containing dead ova (Figure 77.44).
5 **Fibrosis** is mainly the result of secondary infection.
6 **Granulomas**. Bilharzial masses are caused by the aggregation of nodules.
7 **Papillomas** are more pedunculated (Figure 77.45).
8 **Carcinoma** is a common end-result in grossly infected bilharziasis of the bladder that has been neglected for years.

Theodor Maximilian Bilharz, 1825–1862, Professor of Zoology, Cairo, Egypt.
Sir Patrick Manson, 1844–1922, practised in Formosa (now Taiwan), and Hong Kong before becoming physician to the Dreadnought Hospital, Greenwich, London, UK. He is regarded as the founder of Tropical Medicine.

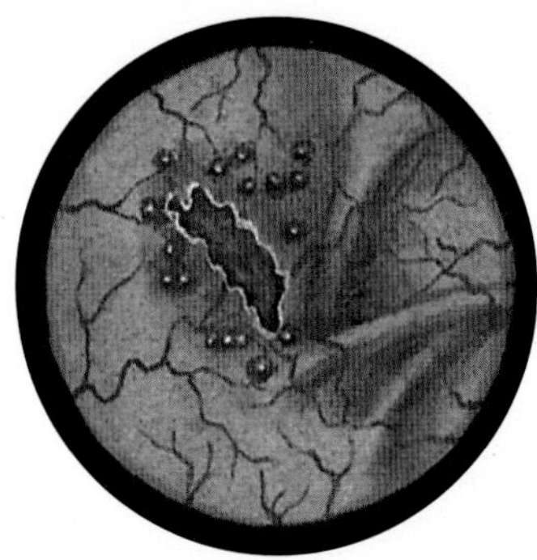

Figure 77.44 Bilharzial ulcer (courtesy of N Makar).

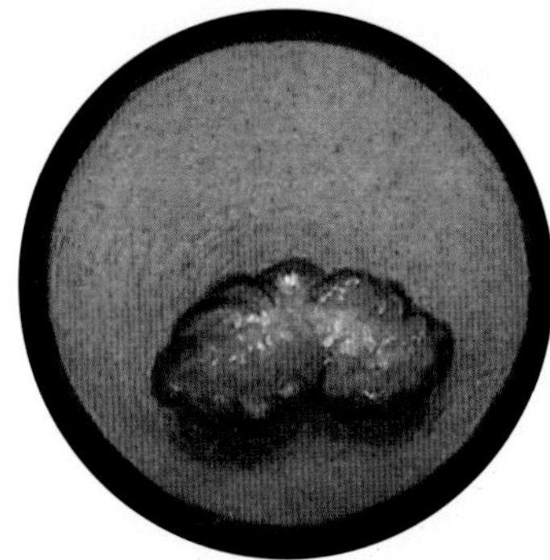

Figure 77.45 Bilharzial papilloma (courtesy of N Makar).

Treatment

Safe and effective drugs are available for the treatment of schistosomiasis, including praziquantel taken in three doses of 20 mg/kg (total 60 mg/kg) 4 hours apart. It takes many months for dead ova to be expelled and, even after repeated courses and healing of the bladder lesion, living bilharzial worms have been found at necropsy in the portal system.

Other complications, requiring specific treatment, include the following:

- urinary calculi;
- stricture of the ureters;
- prostatoseminal vesiculitis;
- fibrosis of the bladder and bladder neck (Figure 77.46);
- bilharzial urethral strictures;
- squamous bladder cancer.

NEOPLASMS OF THE BLADDER

In total, 95% of primary bladder tumours originate in transitional epithelium; the remainder arise from connective tissue (angioma, myoma, fibroma and sarcoma) or are extra-adrenal phaeochromocytomas.

Secondary tumours of the bladder are common and most frequently arise from the sigmoid and rectum, the prostate, the uterus or the ovaries, although bronchial neoplasms may also spread to the bladder.

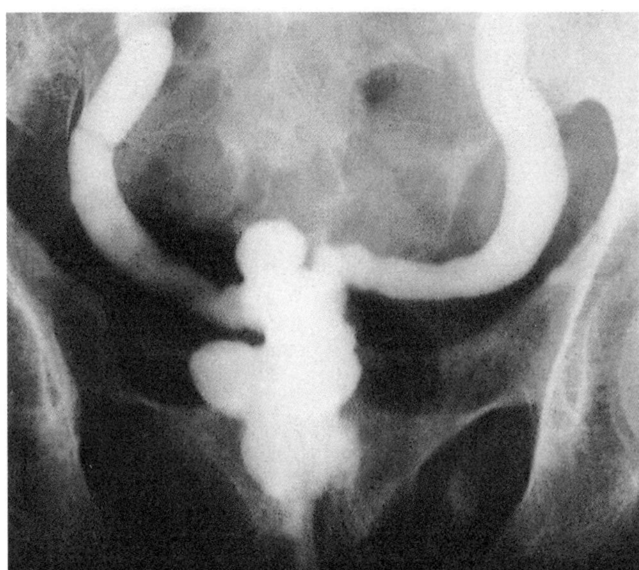

Figure 77.46 Bilharzial contracture of the bladder, with ureteric reflux (courtesy of H Talib, Baghdad, Iraq).

Pathology

Benign papillary tumours

The papilloma consists of a single frond with a central vascular core with villi; it looks like a red sea anemone (Figures 77.47 and 77.48). Inverted papilloma is a condition in which the proliferative cells penetrate under normal mucosa so that the lesion is covered with smooth urothelium. It is benign.

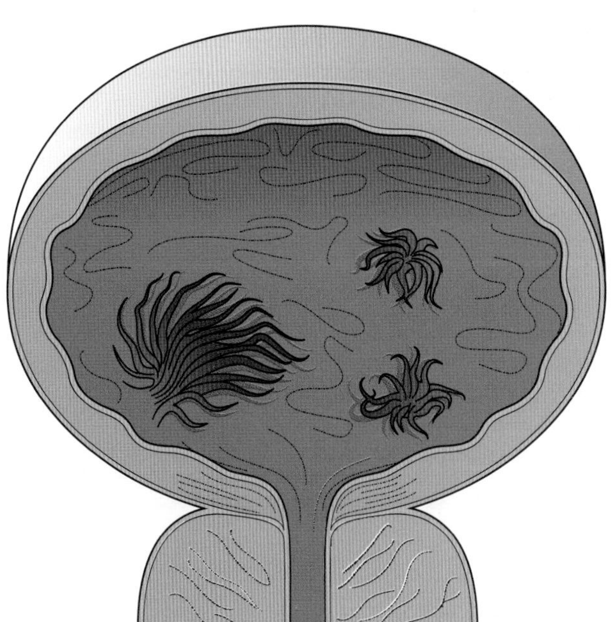

Figure 77.47 Papillary tumour with daughter implantation ('kiss' cancer).

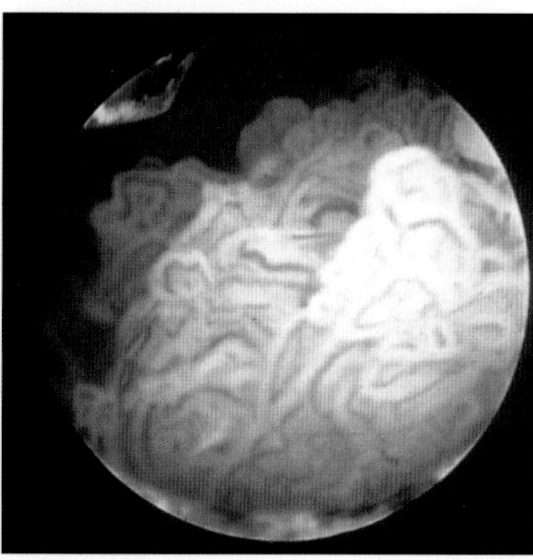

Figure 77.48 Endoscopic photograph of a pTa bladder tumour about to be resected.

CARCINOMA OF THE BLADDER

Histological types of bladder cancer include urothelial, squamous and adenocarcinoma (or mixed, as a result of metaplasia in a transitional cell carcinoma [TCC]). Over 90% are urothelial in origin. Pure squamous carcinoma is uncommon (approximately 5%), except in areas where bilharzia is endemic. Primary adenocarcinoma, which arises from either the urachal remnant or areas of glandular metaplasia, accounts for 1–2% of cases.

Urothelial cell carcinoma

Aetiology

Cigarette smoking is the main aetiological factor (40% of cancers). Occupational exposure to urothelial carcinogens remains common. The first suspicion of a chemical cause for bladder cancer was raised by Rehn in 1895 when he recorded a series of tumours in workers in aniline dye factories. Hueper showed that 2-naphthylamine was carcinogenic in dogs. Subsequent investigation demonstrated that the following compounds may be carcinogenic:

- 2-naphthylamine;
- 4-aminobiphenyl;
- benzidine;
- chlornaphazine;
- 4-chloro-*o*-toluidine;
- *o*-toluidine;
- 4,4′-methylene bis(2-choloroaniline);
- methylene dianiline;
- benzidine-derived azo dyes.

Occupations associated with an increased risk of bladder cancer are:

- textile workers;
- dye workers;
- tyre rubber and cable workers;
- petrol workers;
- leather workers;
- shoe manufacturers and cleaners;
- painters;
- hairdressers;
- lorry drivers;
- drill press operators;
- chemical workers;
- rodent exterminators and sewage workers.

Bladder cancer became a prescribed industrial disease (No. 39) in 1953, and previously exposed workers may be entitled to compensation. Balkan nephropathy is associated with an increased incidence of upper tract urothelial tumours (see Chapter 76).

A series of genetic events has been clearly implicated in cancer formation but is outside the remit of this chapter. Activation of dominantly acting oncogenes such as *ras* and c-*erbB*-1 and -2, and transcription factors such as E2F3, have been reported in bladder cancer, as has the inactivation of tumour-suppressor genes such as *p53*, *p21*, *p16* and the retinoblastoma gene. Activation of many other genes occurs including: those coding for enzymes that dissolve the basement membrane, such as the metalloproteinases (stromelysin, collagenases and elastase), lysosomal enzymes such as the cathepsins and others including urinary plasminogen activators; angiogenic factors (e.g. vascular endothelial growth factor (VEGF]) and other peptide growth factors such as the epidermal growth factor (EGF) and its receptor (EGFR) also have a role to play, as well as the fibroblast growth factor (FGF) and its receptor-3 (FGFR-3) which was found to be altered mostly in non-muscle invasive disease. These changes are common to several tumour types, including prostate cancer. More recently, new approaches through genome-wide association studies allowed the investigation of genetic susceptibility for urothelial cancer. Sev-

Summary box 77.11

Urothelial cell carcinoma of the bladder

- The fourth most common non-dermatological malignancy in men (male:female ratio 3:1)
- Strongly associated with smoking and chemical exposure in western societies
- Strongly associated with *Schistosoma haematobium* infection (bilharzial bladder cancer) in regions where the parasite is endemic
- Reducing in incidence in countries where smoking is decreasing

Ludwig Rehn, 1849–1930, surgeon, Frankfurt am Main, Germany.
The Balkans are the countries that occupy an area in the south-east of Europe. They are south of the Danube and the Sava rivers, and form a peninsula bounded on the east by the Aegean and Black seas, on the west by the Adriatic and Ionian seas, and on the south by the Mediterranean sea.

eral new loci were identified, but, to date, only two, *NAT2* (*N*-acetyltransferase 2) and *GSTM1* (glutathione *S*-transferase Mu 1) have been demonstrated to be consistent germline susceptibility markers. These genetic markers do not yet have sufficient discriminatory ability to be used for clinical decision-making.

Tumour staging and grading

Study of the biological behaviour of TCC of the bladder shows that cancers fall into the three following groups shown in the list. Depth of invasion (T) from the tumour–node–metastasis (TNM) classification and grade (World Health Organization I, II or III) are important factors in planning treatment and determining prognosis in bladder cancer.

- Non-muscle-invasive pTa (see Figure 77.48) and pT1 tumours account for 70% of all new cases; the previous terminology of 'superficial' bladder cancer in this category has now been abandoned; it is important, however, to distinguish 'low-risk' uothelial cancers, which are unlikely to progress, such as well-differentiated (G1) pTa tumours (not invading lamina propria), from 'high-risk' cancers, such as poorly differentiated (G3) pT1 cancers (invading lamina propria), which should be followed up carefully and treated aggressively as necessary. This can be determined by careful histological examination. Single papillary pTa tumours account for a significant proportion of bladder cancers and carry an excellent prognosis.
- Muscle-invasive disease (pT2) accounts for 25% of new cases. Such tumours carry a much worse prognosis because they are subject to local invasion and distant metastasis.
- Flat, non-invasive CIS (primary CIS) accounts for 5% of new cases. Unless diagnosed and treated promptly it carries a poor prognosis. The highest-risk non-muscle invasive cancer is found with multifocal poorly differentiated tumours invading lamina propria (pT1G3) in the presence of CIS.

Summary box 77.12

Bladder cancer staging

- Cystoscopy and resection of tumour with separate resection of the tumour base are essential for accurate analysis of invasion into detrusor muscle
- Bimanual examination should be performed after resection of the tumour
- Complete urinary tract imaging is required using contrast computed tomography (CT) or magnetic resonance (MR) urography. Cross-sectional imaging by CT or MR is essential in high-risk and muscle-invasive disease to stage the tumour, further including lymph node status for metastasis.

Non-muscle invasive bladder cancer

These are usually papillary tumours that grow in an exophytic fashion into the bladder lumen (see Figures 77.47 and 77.48). They may be single or multiple and may appear pedunculated, arising on a stalk with a narrow base, but if the tumours are less well differentiated they are more solid with a wider base. The mucosa around the tumour is often rather oedematous, with angry-looking, dilated blood vessels. These areas may contain *in situ* changes (concomitant CIS).

The urothelium elsewhere in the bladder may appear rather oedematous and velvety; this suggests a generalised 'field change' with the presence of widespread CIS. The most common sites for superficial tumours are the trigone and lateral walls of the bladder.

After initial complete treatment by endoscopic transurethral resection (TURT), patients with pTa or pT1 disease may develop two problems:

1. About 50–70% develop recurrent tumours that may be single or multiple, and the recurrences may occur on one or on many occasions. The recurrent tumours are usually of the same stage or grade as the primary tumour. High-grade multiple tumours with concomitant CIS are most likely to develop recurrent disease.
2. About 15% will develop a recurrent tumour that invades the bladder muscle. The risk of such progression increases with high-grade disease, pT1 disease, multiple primary disease and concomitant CIS. Many urologists now regard the presence of pT1 grade 3 tumours as an indication for offering the patient immediate cystectomy because of the excellent outcome.

This behaviour provides the rationale for performing check cystoscopies. The factors that result in an increased recurrence and progression rate are:

- high grade;
- pT1 disease;
- concomitant CIS;
- multiple primary tumours;
- recurrent disease at the first check cystoscopy 3 months after diagnosis.

Patients presenting with a solitary grade 1 or grade 2 pTa tumour without concomitant CIS, which does not recur within the first 6 months, have an excellent outcome. Patients with recurrent low-grade disease can be treated with intravesical instillations of a chemotherapeutic agent such as mitomycin C or epirubicin, with regular cystocopic check-ups and repeat biopsies, or immunotherapy

Summary box 77.13

Non-muscle-invasive bladder cancer (NMIBC)

- Does not invade the detrusor muscle but can extend to the lamina propria
- Extension to the lamina propria (pT1) is a significant risk factor for progression to invasive disease, especially if associated with high-grade disease and carcinoma *in situ*
- The incidence of recurrence of this disease can be reduced by intravesical chemotherapy and immunotherapy
- High-risk superficial disease (any grade 3 disease) is best managed by bacille Calmette–Guérin immunotherapy followed by radical treatment if disease persists

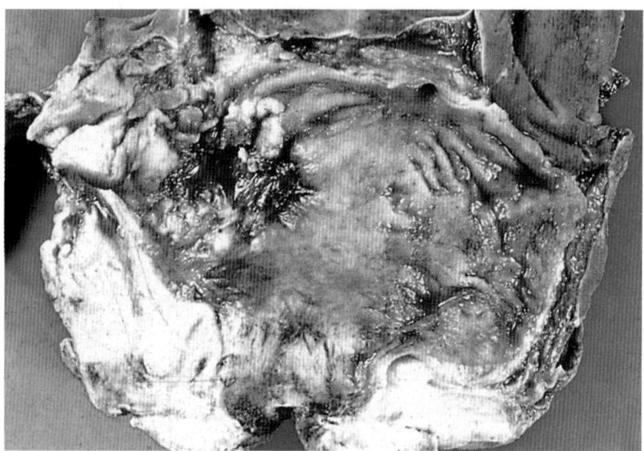

Figure 77.49 Radical cystectomy specimen showing a large solid bladder cancer with total removal of the bladder and prostate.

using regular intravesical instillations of bacille Calmette–Guérin, (BCG) an attenuated form of the anti-tuberculosis vaccine. Patients with high-grade pTa or pT1 disease are at high risk and should be counselled very carefully. The options include immediate cystectomy or a more conservative approach with a course of BCG), followed by careful cystosopic assessment and maintenance instillations. The presence of persistent disease after BCG therapy is a reason for offering cystectomy.

Muscle-invasive bladder cancer

Muscle-invasive tumours are nearly always solid (Figure 77.49), although there may be a low tufted surface. These tumours are often large and broad based, having an irregular, ulcerated appearance within the bladder. The incidence of metastases, whether from lymphatic invasion in the pelvis or blood borne to the lung, liver or bones, is much more common and will cause the death of 30–50% of patients.

> **Summary box 77.14**
>
> Muscle-invasive bladder cancer
>
> - Muscle-invasive bladder cancer (MIBC) should be staged by an accurate bimanual examination performed under anaesthesia before and after resection of the tumour
> - Complete urinary tract assessment should be performed, including CT, MR and IV urography, as well as cross-sectional imaging to identify lymph node involvement and distant spread
> - Radical primary treatment options include radical cystectomy, urinary diversion and thorough lymph node dissection, which tends to be offered as first line, or radical external beam radiotherapy
> - Neoadjuvant chemotherapy improves survival rates as well as adjuvant chemotherapy in some cases, particularly in the presence of nodal and distant disease
> - Locally advanced disease may be downstaged by radiotherapy or chemotherapy to enable salvage cystectomy

In situ carcinoma

The histological appearance of irregularly arranged cells, with large nuclei and a high mitotic index replacing the normally well-ordered urothelium, is known as CIS. It may occur alone (primary CIS) or in association with a new tumour (concomitant CIS), or it may occur later in a patient who has previously had a tumour (secondary CIS). It can be diagnosed only when a biopsy is examined under the microscope. It may cause severe symptoms of dysuria, suprapubic pain and frequency (hence its old name of malignant cystitis). It carries a risk for the patient of developing a malignant muscle-invasive cancer. Without treatment, 50% will die of invasive bladder cancer. It can be treated initially with intravesical BCG, but failure of response is an indication for cystectomy. CIS cannot be treated with external beam radiotherapy

Pure squamous cell carcinoma of the bladder

Squamous cell tumours tend to be solid and are nearly always associated with muscle invasion. This is the most prevalent form of bladder cancer in areas where bilharzia is endemic. Squamous cell tumours may be associated with chronic irritation caused by stone disease in the bladder as a result of metaplasia.

Pure adenocarcinoma

Adenocarcinoma accounts for approximately 1–2% of all bladder cancers. It usually arises in the fundus of the bladder at the site of the urachal remnant. Occasionally, primary adenocarcinomas arise at other sites and probably originate from areas of glandular metaplasia. Such tumours need to be distinguished from secondary cancer, and can be treated with partial cystectomy

CLINICAL FEATURES OF BLADDER CARCINOMA

Painless gross haematuria is the most common symptom and is indicative of a bladder carcinoma until proven otherwise. Often, however, the patient fails to declare the symptom to their GP. The bleeding may give rise to clot formation and clot urinary retention.

Constant pain in the pelvis usually heralds extravesical spread. There is often frequency and discomfort associated with urination. Pain in the loin or pyelonephritis may indicate ureteric obstruction and hydronephrosis. A late manifestation is nerve involvement causing pain that is referred to the suprapubic region, groins, perineum, anus and into the thighs.

Albert Leon Charles Calmette, 1863–1933, and Jean-Marie Camille Guérin, 1872–1961, microbiologists at the Institute Pasteur, at Lille in France, introduced the bacille Calmette–Guérin in 1908.

It is also important to assess the patient as a whole. Many are elderly men who have been lifelong smokers and who have chronic obstructive pulmonary disease or cardiovascular disease. Their suitability for major surgery must be borne in mind.

INVESTIGATION OF BLADDER CARCINOMA

Urine

Urine should be cultured and examined cytologically for malignant cells. This is not a good screening test but a positive result is highly specific, and it is mostly helpful with high-grade disease and CIS. New tests are being developed based on the presence of antigens such as nuclear matrix proteins (NMP22) or mini-chromosome maintenance (MCM) proteins, which may be able to detect new or recurrent tumours, and epigenetic events such as methylated panels of markers or micro-RNA fragments. These tests continue to be under evaluation and are not used routinely.

Blood

Estimation of haemoglobin and the level of serum electrolytes and urea should be carried out.

CT, MR, IV urography or ultrasonography

This should be performed on all patients with painless haematuria. Occasionally, the preliminary film shows a faint shadow of an encrusted neoplasm of the bladder. The most common radiological sign is a filling defect (Figure 77.50). Occasionally, irregularity of the bladder wall may herald the presence of an invasive tumour. Hydronephrosis may occur if a superficial tumour grows up the intramural ureter or direct invasion of the ureteric wall occurs. Ultrasonography should be carried out if the kidney is non-functioning to determine its presence and the possibility of an obstructed system.

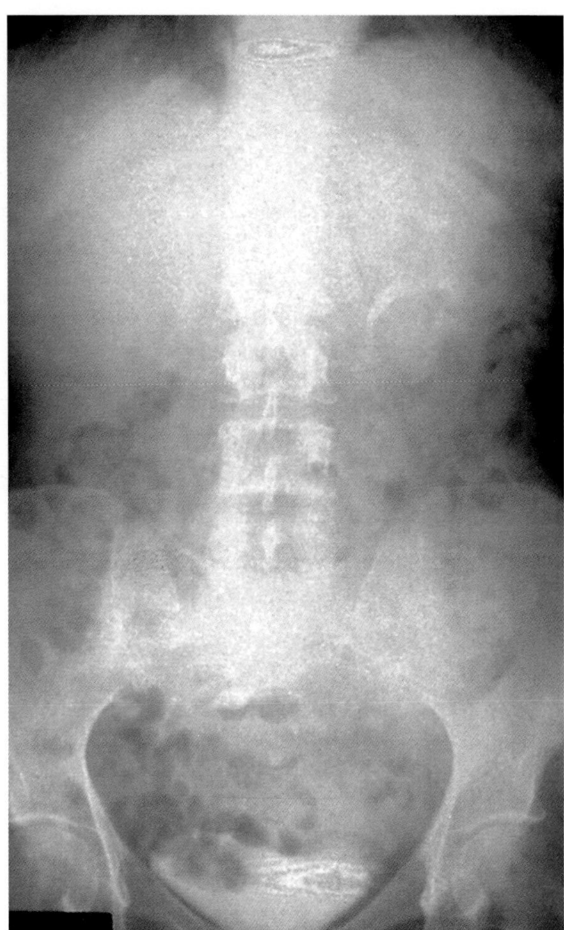

Figure 77.50 Intravenous urography showing a filling defect in the region of the right ureteric orifice.

Cross-sectional imaging

Non-contrast CT and MRI and ultrasonography are now replacing IVU in most centres for the immediate management of patients with gross painless haematuria. For staging when a MIBC is suspected, contrast-enhanced CT is used, ideally before TURT. False-positive pT3 disease can be diagnosed if cross-sectional imaging is carried out soon after TURT. MRI is being used more frequently (Figure 77.51) and can demonstrate lymph node metastasis or muscle invasion.

Cystourethroscopy

Cystourethroscopy is the mainstay of diagnosis and should always be performed on patients with haematuria. It can be carried out with a rigid instrument under general anaesthesia or with a flexible instrument under local anaesthesia. The urethra is inspected at the initial insertion of the instrument (urethroscopy) and the bladder is then examined in a systematic fashion (cystoscopy). Conventional 'white' light cystoscopy has been improved recently by the introduction of photodynamic 'blue' light cystoscopy, which relies on the photosensitiser hexaminolaevulinate. It is now recommended in patients with high suspicion of the disease and negative initial findings and in follow-up of patients with CIS.

Bimanual examination

A bimanual examination with the patient fully relaxed under general anaesthesia should be performed both before and after endoscopic surgical treatment of these tumours. The bladder should be empty. Once there is muscle invasion the differentiation between pT2 and pT3 disease depends on whether a mass is palpable bimanually at the end of the procedure (pT3). When invasion has spread into the prostate in a man or the vagina in a woman it is classified as pT4a. If the tumour is fixed to the lateral pelvic side wall it is staged as pT4b.

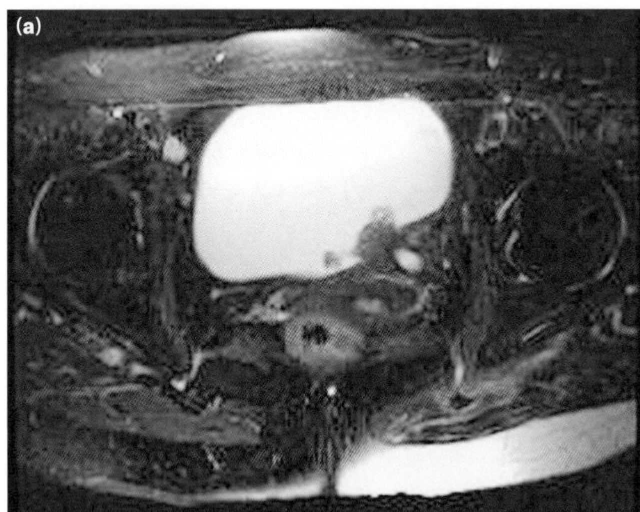

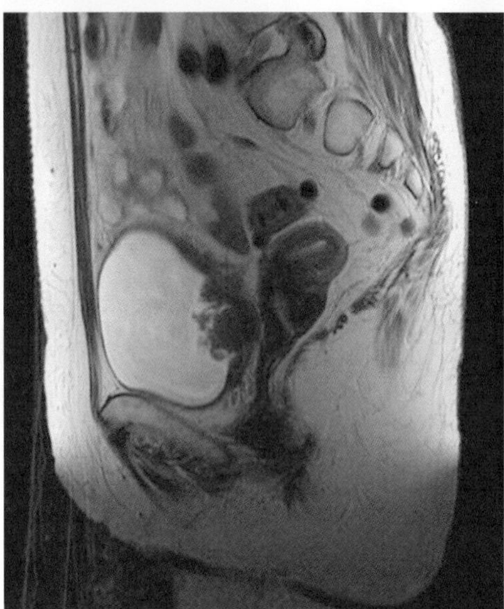

Figure 77.51 (a) Cross-sectional magnetic resonance imaging (MRI) showing a 'cystogram' and a bladder cancer. (b) Cross-sectional MRI showing invasive bladder cancer.

TREATMENT FOR CARCINOMA OF THE BLADDER

Non-muscle invasive tumours

Endoscopic surgery

The tumour should be carefully resected in layers using a resectoscope. The base of the tumour is sent separately for histological examination. Small pinch biopsies are taken near to and distant from the primary lesion when CIS is suspected (inflamed or velvety appearance). After removal of the tumour, two or three further loops of tissue from the base should be sent separately so that the pathologist can accurately determine whether there is lamina propria or muscle invasion. The base of the tumour is then coagulated, so achieving haemostasis. The appearance of pale-yellow glistening fat will indicate a perforation of the bladder. Should this occur before the resection is complete, it may be prudent to stop the resection and leave a catheter in the bladder for a few days. In this instance the procedure could be completed some 2 weeks later. The bimanual examination is repeated at the end of the endoscopic procedure. After these procedures, an irrigating catheter is left *in situ* for 48 hours to prevent clot retention of urine. There is good evidence that a single dose of mitomycin (mitomycin C, 40 mg in 60 mL of fluid) instilled into the bladder before catheter removal decreases the risks of recurrence in patients with pTa and pT1 grade 1 and 2 disease.

Patients with larger solid tumours should have adequate material resected for histological staging and grading. If it is possible and straightforward, the mass of the tumour should be resected as completely as possible – even when pT2 or pT3 disease is suspected.

FOLLOW-UP

Most urologists agree that patients with a single low- or medium-grade pTa tumour can safely be treated by resection alone plus a single instillation of mitomycin, followed up with regular cystoscopies.

The treatment of patients with multiple low- or medium-grade pTa tumours can be by either resection alone or resection followed by a 6-week course of intravesical chemotherapy with mitomycin, doxorubicin or epirubicin.

The treatment of pT1 disease is difficult. Approximately 30% of tumours are understaged at first resection. For this reason, a repeat cystoscopy and resection of the tumour base are advocated within 6 weeks. Some urologists would offer immediate cystectomy to a patient with a high-grade pT1 tumour, particularly if it were multiple or accompanied by CIS, because of the 30–50% risk of progression to muscle invasion. Others will treat such patients by endoscopy followed by immunotherapy with intravesical BCG. The most effective treatment of solitary medium-grade pT1 disease remains uncertain, but a reasonable approach would be endoscopic resection followed by re-resection of the area after 6 weeks, followed by intravesical BCG.

Follow-up cystoscopies are essential; they may be carried out under local anaesthesia with a flexible cystoscope or under general anaesthesia if the urologist feels that the patient is at high risk of recurrence. They should be performed at 3-monthly intervals over the first year; after this the time interval between cystoscopies can be determined according to the presence or absence of further disease. In total, 30% of patients will never develop another tumour so that, if the bladder has remained clear after 2 years, annual inspection may be adequate. For patients who go on to develop multiple recurrences within the bladder at each examination, the cystoscopies need to be maintained at frequent intervals so that the growths can be resected. These patients are at a greater risk of their disease progressing; although intravesical chemotherapy can decrease the recurrence rate, no reduction in progression rates has been found.

Open surgical excision

This should be totally avoided. If by some error a bladder containing a tumour is entered, then the tumour may be removed with a diathermy needle, the base coagulated and the bladder closed. Postoperative radiotherapy to the wound will diminish the chance of tumour implantation.

Muscle-invasive tumours

The treatment of cancer with proven muscle invasion remains a subject for debate. Whatever the modality of treatment employed, few centres have 5-year survival rates of more than 50%. There is a move towards primary surgical treatment in most centres. The use of systemic chemotherapy with a combination of agents – cisplatin, methotrexate, doxorubicin and vinblastine (M-VAC) or cisplatin plus gemcitabine given before (neoadjuvant) radical cystectomy – has been shown to be of benefit. The current evidence is that neoadjuvant chemotherapy improves survival by about 5–7%. There is no good evidence for the use of adjuvant chemotherapy in these patients. Survival from MIBC has not improved over the past two decades, and newer immunotherapy approaches are being evaluated, in particular immune-checkpoint inhibitors with antibodies targeting the programmed cell death 1 ligand 1 (PDL1) pathway with promising results.

Radiotherapy

EXTERNAL BEAM RADIOTHERAPY

External beam radiotherapy is usually given at 60 Gy over a 4- to 6-week period. There is a complete response rate of 40–50%. Unfortunately, some patients do not respond and others exhibit only a partial response, with pTa or pT1 tumour remaining in the bladder, giving rise to a risk of recurrence, and predictive biomarkers of radiosensitivity are emerging to guide therapy, such as the DNA damage-signalling protein MRE11. Patients with residual disease after radiotherapy should be offered 'salvage cystectomy' if they are fit. Proponents of radiotherapy claim that it avoids the need to remove the bladder in some patients and allows men to retain potency. Radiotherapy is not without complications, and during the course of treatment will cause urinary frequency and also diarrhoea. Late complications can leave the bladder contracted and fibrosed, in which case it may need to be removed for palliative reasons. Late complications affecting the rectum should be uncommon, especially if lateral fields of irradiation are employed.

Surgery

PARTIAL CYSTECTOMY

This should be limited to the treatment of small adenocarcinomas of the bladder.

RADICAL CYSTECTOMY AND PELVIC LYMPHADENECTOMY

This is now standard treatment for localised pT2–pT3 disease without evidence of secondary spread or of CIS that has not responded to BCG. However, bladder cancer tends to occur in elderly people, with a median age at diagnosis of 73 years, and radical surgery carries morbidity in this age group; thus patients must be carefully assessed preoperatively. Before contemplating radical surgery to remove the bladder, it is important to have evidence that surgical cure is attainable. Cross-sectional imaging of the pelvis may locally overstage the bladder if a recent resection has been carried out, although the finding of grossly enlarged pelvic, iliac or para-aortic nodes or liver metastases will alter the decision for cystectomy. A bone scan (using technetium-99m [^{99m}Tc]), or bone marrow MRI will help to show whether there is spread to bone, and a chest plain radiograph should be performed to exclude pulmonary metastases, although many centres now perform routine CT imaging of the chest preoperatively and it tends to be more sensitive than plain radiography in detecting small lung lesions.

SURGERY

Alternative drainage for urine is necessary after removal of the bladder. The standard procedure is to perform an ileal conduit diversion. Male patients should be counselled about the onset of erectile impotence and absent ejaculation after the operation, although in some cases the nerve supply for erectile function can be preserved through careful dissection; they should also be told about alternative forms of urinary diversion, which include continent urinary diversions and orthotopic bladder replacement.

Patients should be seen by a stoma care therapist, who will help to advise the patient and will try different ileostomy bags to ensure that the correct site is chosen, avoiding skin creases so that one does not end up with the disaster of a leaking urinary ileostomy. A decision is made about whether the male urethra is to be removed (depending on the estimated risk of recurrence within the urethra); a urethrectomy is usually indicated in patients with primary CIS or those with tumour invading the prostate stroma. Many surgeons are now offering total replacement of the bladder after cystectomy.

The patient should receive prophylactic antibiotics including metronidazole, cefuroxime and amoxicillin, and low-dose heparin or equivalent thromboembolic prophylaxis, including physical means such as stockings and inflatable devices applied to the legs peroperatively to promote venous circulation.

The abdomen is opened through a midline incision extending down to the symphysis pubis. The liver and the retroperitoneum are checked for evidence of metastases, and the operability of the bladder is assessed. A bilateral pelvic lymphadenectomy is performed, removing external iliac nodes, internal iliac nodes and the nodes in the obturator fossae. Some surgeons will remove lymph nodes up to the aortic bifurcation or higher with some evidence of improved long-term oncological outcomes. The vessels passing to the bladder from the side wall of the pelvis are ligated and divided; these include the obliterated hypogastric vessels, the superior vesical artery, the middle vesical veins, and the inferior vesical arteries and veins. The ureters are then divided. The posterior ligaments extending from the pararectal area to the back of the bladder are ligated and divided, and the layer posterior to Denonvilliers' fascia is opened up. The endopelvic fascia is then divided on each side and the puboprostatic ligaments are divided. A ligature is passed between the dorsal vein complex and the urethra, and the former is ligated and divided. The urethra is then mobilised and divided. The ligaments lateral to the prostate are divided and the bladder is removed. In women, the uterus

Charles Pierre Denonvilliers, 1808–1872, Professor of Anatomy, and later of Surgery, Paris, France.

and anterior vaginal wall need to be included. Women must be counselled about the loss of ovarian and uterine function.

An isolated loop of ileum is then prepared on its own mesentery, and continuity of the small bowel restored. The ureters are then implanted into the bowel and the ileostomy is created. Meticulous care must be taken to close all mesenteric windows, thus avoiding internal hernias. If the bladder is to be replaced orthotopically, a reservoir made from detubularised bowel (usually a segment of well-vascularised ileum) is created and anastomosed to the urethra after implantation of the ureters.

More recently, the technique of cystectomy and urinary diversion has evolved using minimally invasive approaches such as robot-assisted surgery, which is being evaluated in some centres, because it may in theory carry advantages including reduced blood loss, improved precision surgery and speedier patient recovery.

The surgical mortality rate associated with cystectomy used to be considerable but is now less than 2%. Late complications include urethral recurrence (about 5–8%), which is increased in the presence of multifocal tumours, CIS and, particularly, invasion of prostatic stroma (Figure 77.52).

Leukoplakia

This condition is simply squamous metaplasia of the bladder. Profuse production of keratin may result in the passing of white particles in the urine. It cannot be treated easily. Localised areas may be resected endoscopically. Diffuse leukoplakia of the bladder is pre-malignant and results in squamous cancer of the bladder. Careful cystoscopic assessment is required and the condition may require cystectomy.

Endometriosis

Endometriosis within the bladder wall is rare but can have the appearance of a vascular bladder tumour or a tumour that contains chocolate-coloured or bluish cysts. The swelling enlarges and bleeds during menstruation. If medical management fails, by means of danazol or luteinising hormone-releasing hormone (LHRH) agonists, further treatment is usually by means of partial cystectomy or full-thickness endoscopic resection, depending on its site. The condition may be part of more widespread disease. Endometriosis is also a cause of ureteric stricture.

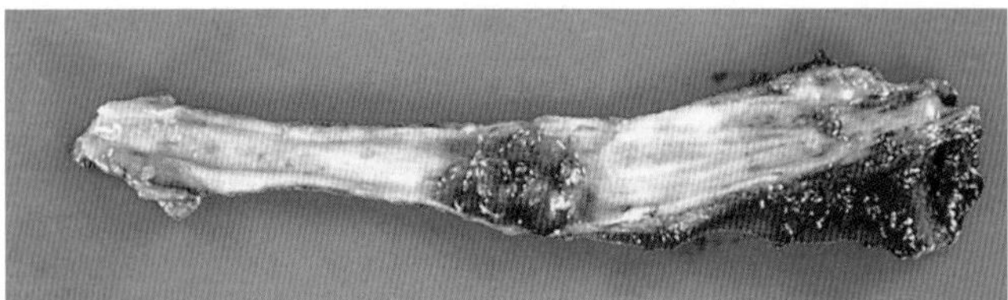

Figure 77.52 Urethrectomy specimen from a patient who has previously undergone a radical cystectomy showing new transitional cell tumour formation in the urethra.

INTERNAL AND EXTERNAL URINARY DIVERSION

Indications

Diversion of the urine may be either a temporary expedient to relieve distal obstruction or a permanent procedure when the bladder has been removed or lost normal neurological control, and in cases of incurable fistula or irremovable obstruction.

Methods of urinary diversion

Temporary methods use prosthetic materials, the most common being a urinary catheter. In elderly patients unfit for prostatectomy, and in some patients with terminal carcinoma of the prostate, an indwelling, silicone, urethral Foley catheter changed every 3 months is a satisfactory method of drainage. A suprapubic placement is an alternative to urethral placement. The major drawback of long-term catheterisation is infection secondary to the associated bacteriuria that invariably develops. Ureteric obstruction can be relieved by placement of internal 'double-J' pigtail ureteric stents, which can remain for 4–5 months but are usually changed every 3 months. As an alternative, a nephrostomy tube, inserted percutaneously by ultrasound and fluoroscopic imaging, is effective when internal stent placement is not feasible.

Permanent urinary diversion

External diversion

ILEAL CONDUIT

Permanent urinary tract diversion is most commonly performed by conduit diversion. The ureters are implanted into a short, isolated segment of ileum (Figure 77.53a) or, less commonly, colon. The conduit diverts the urine onwards to a cutaneous stoma for collection in an ileostomy bag. This form of diversion is well established and associated with a low complication rate of less than 10%. The main complication is ureteroileal stricture, which can be limited by spatulation of the distal ureters and an end-to-end anastomosis as described by Wallace (Figure 77.53a). Stenosis at the ileocutaneous site is less frequent, and a short isoperistaltic conduit limits the formation of a residual urine volume, reducing infection and avoiding the problems of reabsorption of urine. In some cases, when the pelvic area has been subjected to radiation, the lower ureters may be unhealthy; a high division with insertion of the ureters into an ileal loop above the root of the mesentery may then be wiser (Figure 77.54).

The site for the stoma must be chosen before the operation, in consultation with a stoma care therapist; the site is marked indelibly on the skin.

Operative details

A coil of ileum, approximately 15–20 cm long and 30 cm from the ileocaecal valve, with its blood supply intact, is isolated. The left ureter is brought behind the mesorectum. The

David Mitchell Wallace, 1913–1992, urologist, St Peter's Hospital, London, UK.

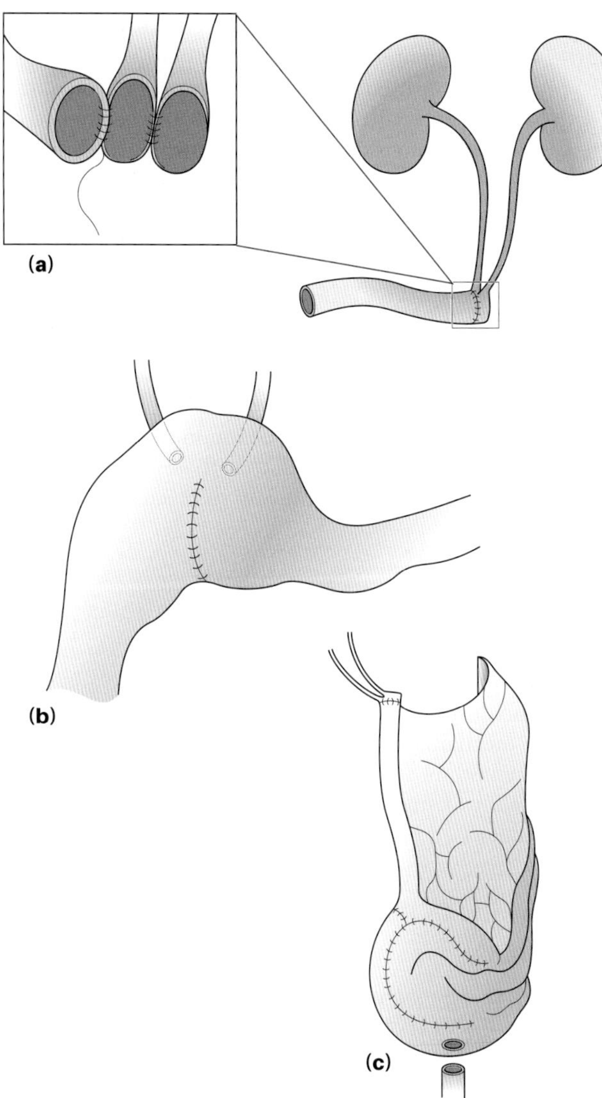

Figure 77.53 Diversion of urine. Favoured methods: (a) ileal conduit; the ureters are spatulated and anastomosed to ileum end to side (insert); (b) ureterosigmoidostomy; (c) ileal neobladder with antireflux long afferent limb.

ureters may be joined to the ileum either end to side or end to end after anastomosing the distal spatulated ureters to form a plate (Wallace). The distal end of the coil is brought out through an incision made at the site identified before operation; a disc of skin and fat is removed, a cruciate incision is made in the fascia and the muscle is split. The stoma is made about 2–3 cm long. It is evaginated initially by means of four sutures passing through the skin, the ileal loop as it passes through the opening and the cut edge of the ileum.

Internal urinary diversion

COLON AND RECTUM

The advantage of diverting urine into the colon is that no collecting apparatus is necessary. Clearly, however, the anal sphincter must be competent. Before ureterosigmoidostomy is undertaken, the patient must prove that he or she can control at least 200 mL of fluid in the rectum. The disadvantage of

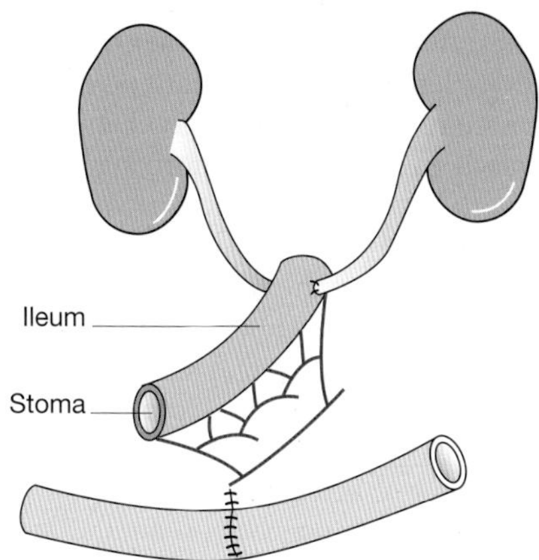

Figure 77.54 Ureteroileostomy (after DM Wallace, FRCS).

the operation is that the renal tract is exposed continuously to infection from the faeces; this can be minimised by constructing an anti-reflux procedure. Various diversions are described; the Mainz II ureterosigmoidostomy creates a cul-de-sac-type, low-pressure reservoir in the sigmoid into which the ureters are placed (see Figure 77.53b). This reduces reflux, and bowel content, although in contact with urine, takes a direct route to the rectum. In the long term, cancer can develop at longstanding ureterocolic junctions (Figure 77.55).

BLADDER RECONSTRUCTION

Over the past decade, several techniques have been developed to allow a near-spherical urinary reservoir to be formed out of various lengths of bowel that are detubularised. These may consist of ileum, ileum and caecum, or sigmoid colon (see Figure 77.53c). The ureters can then be reimplanted in these reservoirs in an anti-reflux manner and the reservoir anastomosed to the membranous urethra in males (see Figures 77.20–77.22). This is indicated only when the urethra can be preserved, with no evidence of tumour at the junction

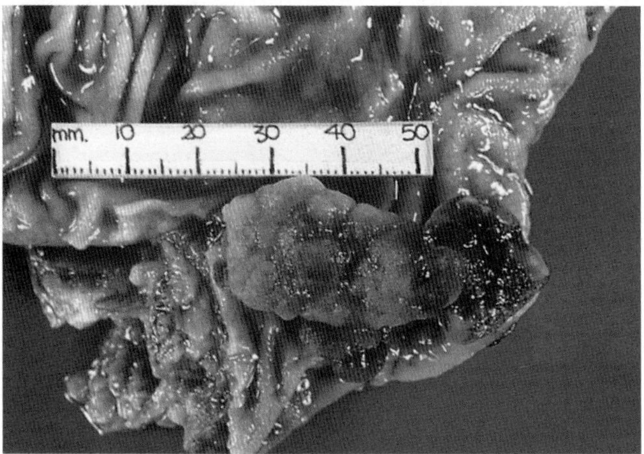

Figure 77.55 An anterior resection of the rectum specimen containing a rectal cancer in a patient aged 18 years who has previously undergone ureterosigmoidostomy for the treatment of bladder exstrophy.

between the urethra and the prostate in males, and bladder neck in females. About 15–30% of patients cannot empty the neobladder completely and will need to perform intermittent self-catheterisation. The results are good after radical cystectomy, particularly in younger well-motivated patients.

CONTINENT URINARY DIVERSION

A similar concept is used in the construction of continent diversions. A urinary reservoir is made as described above and the ureters are attached to the reservoir. A continence mechanism is then made to connect the reservoir to the skin. This is the complication-prone part of the operation. The continence mechanism may be made of an invaginated loop of ileum supported by three rows of staples (Kock pouch) or from the appendix, buried in an anti-reflux manner in a submucosal tube (Mitrofanoff; Figure 77.56). Alternatively, a length of ileum can be made into a tube (of a similar size to the appendix) after excision of the anti-mesenteric ileum, and buried in a submucosal tunnel in an anti-reflux way. Clearly, these operations are complex, with the potential for increased postoperative complications.

BLADDER SUBSTITUTION AND AUGMENTATION

In patients with contraction of the bladder because of tuberculosis or with neuropathic dysfunction and a small bladder capacity, the bladder may need to be augmented. Similar techniques to those used to perform a bladder replacement can be utilised to make a near-spherical pouch from detubularised bowel, which can then be attached to the trigone or bladder neck after a near-total cystectomy (see Figures 77.20–77.22). The ureters are then reimplanted. The facility to provide a continence mechanism must be available if needed in the neuropathic patient. This may comprise an artificial urinary sphincter or a colposuspension in females.

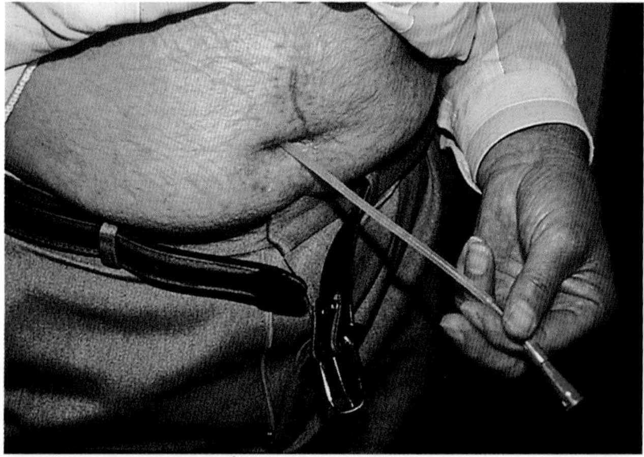

Figure 77.56 A patient with a pT3a bladder cancer who has previously undergone cystoprostatectomy and urethrectomy. A detubularised ileocaecal reservoir has been made with the ureters implanted in submucosal tunnels. The appendix has been implanted within the reservoir in a submucosal tunnel to provide the continence mechanism. The appendix has been brought to the umbilicus and is catheterised 4- to 6-hourly to empty the reservoir.

Complications of internal diversion

Stricture

Ureterosigmoidostomy was first used by Chaput in 1894. Subsequent modifications included those made by Coffey and Grey Turner. In these methods the ureters were cut obliquely and pulled into the gut by a stitch – the ends were not stitched to the gut wall – and stenosis was common. Nesbit, Cordonnier and Leadbetter all recognised that these strictures could be prevented by anastomosing mucosa to mucosa.

Reflux of urine

High-pressure activity within a segment of gut can cause reflux of potentially infected urine at high pressure to the kidneys. In the long term, this can cause renal impairment. The principle of a low-pressure reservoir for both neobladder and ureterosigmoidostomy (Mainz II) reduces this. In addition, an anti-reflux mechanism, used in neobladder construction, is created by anastomosing the ureters to a non-detubularised 20-cm segment of small bowel, which is in continuity with the neobladder (see Figure 77.53c).

Metabolic consequences of internal diversion

Resorption of solutes

This depends upon the following factors: (1) the area of bowel that is exposed to urine, and (2) the length of time that the urine is in contact with the bowel epithelium.

The biochemical changes associated with urinary diversion are due to a combination of reabsorption of chloride and urea and progressively diminishing tubular function as a result of pyelonephritis. Diarrhoea with loss of potassium-containing mucus may exacerbate the loss of potassium. The typical changes of a hyperchloraemic acidosis with potassium depletion occur more frequently with ureterosigmoid diversion than with a colonic and ileal neobladder. When severe, the patient develops loss of appetite, weakness, thirst and diarrhoea. Coma may ensue. Mild acidosis, unrecognised over a long period, produces osteomalacia. Bone pain and even pathological fracture can occur. Renal impairment from pyelonephritis and reabsorption from the mucosa are seen less frequently after ileal or colonic conduit formation, continent urinary diversion or orthotopic bladder substitution. In fact, they are seen very infrequently except in patients with

Nils G Kock, b.1924, Professor of Surgery, the University of Göteborg, Sweden.
Paul Mitrofanoff, b.1934, Professor of Paediatric Surgery, Rouen, France.
Henri Chaput, b.1857, surgeon, La Salpêtrière, Paris, France.
Robert Calvin Coffey, 1869–1933, surgeon, Nashville, TN, USA.
George Grey Turner, 1877–1951, Professor of Surgery, the University of Durham (1927–1934), and at the Postgraduate Medical School, Hammersmith, London, UK (1934–1945).

pre-existing renal impairment and unsatisfactory emptying of the urinary reservoir. Malabsorption can occur with the loss of terminal ileum and small bowel. The loss of terminal ileum can result in vitamin B_{12} deficiency and so monitoring of vitamin B_{12} and folate is recommended after the first year.

TREATMENT

Patients should be instructed to empty the rectum or continent reservoir or neobladder 3-hourly by day. In patients who have undergone ureterosigmoidostomy and in whom acidosis is present, a rectal tube should be inserted at night to drain the urine continuously. The patient should take a mixture of potassium citrate and sodium bicarbonate three times a day (2 g of each, as either crystals or tablets). Regular serum biochemical analyses, including calcium, are required.

Established hyperchloraemic acidosis is usually associated with marked dehydration and the mainstay of treatment is administration of intravenous saline. The patient may be given small doses of sodium bicarbonate to half-correct the pH deficit if it is severe and additional intravenous potassium. This should be coupled with appropriate systemic antibiotic treatment.

Risk of malignancy

There is a risk of cancer developing in bowel used to reconstruct the urinary tract. When the urine is not mixed with faeces, the incidence is small, becoming significant after 15–18 years. The major risk of malignancy was discovered when ureterosigmoidostomy construction enabled free mixing of urine and faeces. The development of sigmoid reservoirs into which the ureters are inserted has reduced this risk.

FURTHER READING

Cardozo L, Staskin DR. *Textbook of female urology and urogynecology*, 4th edn. London: CRC Press, Taylor & Francis Group, 2016.

Hamdy FC, Eardley I. *Oxford textbook of urological surgery*. Oxford: Oxford University Press, 2017.

Scardino PT, Marston Linehan W, Zelefski MJ *et al. Comprehensive textbook of genitourinary oncology*, 4th edn. Philadelphia, PA: Lippincott Williams & Wilkins, 2011.

Wein AJ, Kavoussi LR, Partin AW, Peters CA. *Campbell-Walsh urology*, 11th edn. Philadelphia, PA: Elsevier, 2016.

Chapter 78

The prostate and seminal vesicles

Learning objectives

To understand:

- The relationship of anatomical structure and biochemical function to the development and treatment of benign and malignant disease of the prostate
- The terminology used to describe lower urinary tract symptoms and to know their causes as well as the treatment options available
- Which investigations are appropriate for carcinoma of the prostate
- Clinical staging of carcinoma of the prostate and how staging contributes to the complex decision

EMBRYOLOGY

From the primitive urethra, a series of solid epithelial buds develop and become canalised in a matter of weeks. The surrounding mesenchyme forms the muscular and connective tissue of the gland and has a major role in differentiation (stromal epithelium interactions). Skene's tubules, which open on either side of the female urethra, are the homologue of the prostate.

SURGICAL ANATOMY

The contemporary classification of the prostate into different zones was based on the work of McNeal (Figure 78.1). He showed that it is divided into the peripheral zone (PZ), which lies mainly posteriorly and from which most carcinomas arise, and a central zone (CZ), which lies posterior to the urethral lumen and above the ejaculatory ducts as they pass through the prostate; the two zones are rather like an egg in an eggcup. There is also a periurethral transitional zone (TZ), from which most benign prostatic hyperplasia (BPH) arises. Smooth muscle cells are found throughout the prostate but, in the upper part of the prostate and bladder neck, there is a separate sphincter muscle that subserves a sexual function, closing during ejaculation. Resection of this tissue during prostatectomy is responsible for retrograde ejaculation. The distal striated urethral sphincter muscle is found at the junction of the prostate and the membranous urethra; it is horseshoe shaped with the bulk lying anteriorly and is quite distinct from the muscle of the pelvic floor (Figure 78.1).

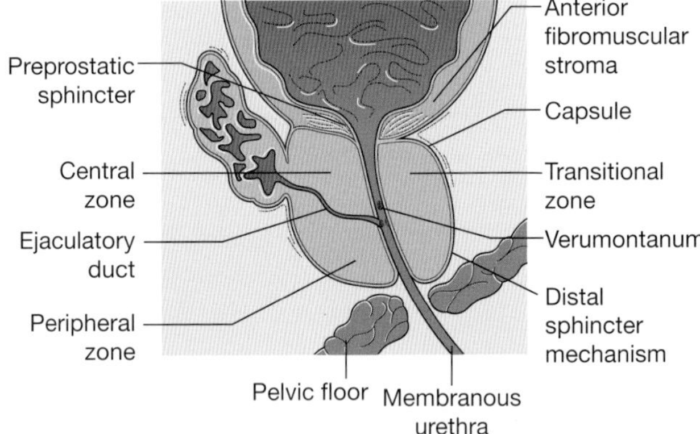

Figure 78.1 Sagittal diagram of the prostate just lateral to the urethra showing the division into the different zones described by McNeal. The transitional zone is the area from which most benign prostatic hyperplasia arises.

The glands of the peripheral zone (Figure 78.2), lined by columnar epithelium, lie in the fibromuscular stroma and their ducts, which are long and branched, open into posterolateral grooves on either side of the verumontanum. The glands of the CZ and TZ are shorter and unbranched. All these ducts, the common ejaculatory ducts and the prostatic utricle open into the prostatic urethra. BPH starts in the periurethral transitional zone and, as it increases in size, it compresses the outer PZ of the prostate, which becomes the false capsule. There is also the outer true fibrous anatomical capsule and external to this lie condensations of endopelvic fascia known

Alexander Johnston Chalmers Skene, 1828–1900, Professor of Gynecology, Long Island Hospital, Brooklyn, New York, NY, USA.

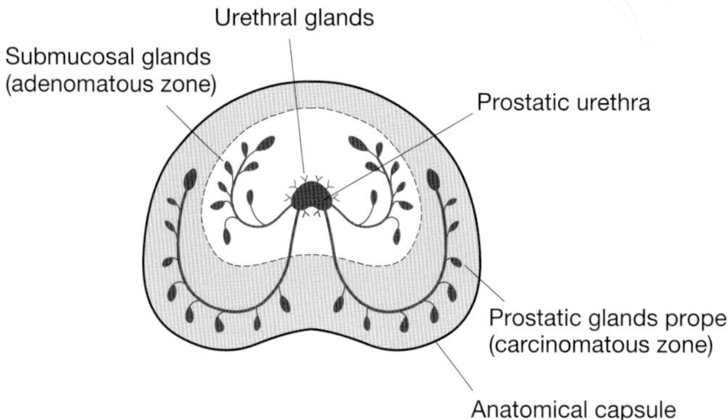

Figure 78.2 A transverse section of the prostate. The peripheral zone is the area from which most prostate cancers arise. The 'adenomatous' zone comprises the central and transitional zones.

as the periprostatic sheath of endopelvic fascia. Between the anatomical capsule and the prostatic sheath lies the abundant prostatic venous plexus. The neurovascular bundles supplying autonomic innervation to the corpora of the penis are in very close relationship to the posterolateral aspect of the prostatic capsule and are at risk of damage during radical cystoprostatectomy or radical prostatectomy; inadvertent diathermy in the region of these nerves may be the cause of uncommon erectile impotence after transurethral prostatectomy.

PHYSIOLOGY

The prostate has a sexual function, but it is unclear how important its secretions are to human fertility. That the normal adult prostate undergoes atrophy after castration was known to John Hunter.

Systemic hormonal influences (endocrine) and local growth factors (paracrine and autocrine)

The growth of the prostate is governed by many local and systemic hormones whose exact functions are not yet known. The main hormone acting on the prostate is testosterone, which is secreted by the Leydig cells of the testes under the control of luteinising hormone (LH), itself secreted from the anterior pituitary under the control of hypothalamic luteinising hormone-releasing hormone (LHRH). LHRH has a short half-life and is released in a pulsatile manner. This pulsatile release is important, as receptors for LHRH will become desensitised if permanently occupied. The administration of LHRH analogues in a continuous, non-pulsatile manner exploits the concept of receptor desensitisation and forms the basis for androgen deprivation therapy in prostate cancer. Testosterone is converted to 1,5-dihydrotestosterone (DHT) by the enzyme 5α-reductase, which is found in high concentration in the prostate and the perigenital skin (type II). Other androgens are secreted by the adrenal cortex, but their effects are minimal in the normal male. Oestrogenic steroids are also secreted by the adrenal cortex and, in the ageing male, may play a part in disrupting the delicate balance between DHT and local peptide growth factors, and hence increase the risk of BPH. Increased levels of serum oestrogens, by acting on the hypothalamus, decrease the secretion of LHRH (and hence LH) and thereby decrease serum testosterone levels. Thus, pharmacological levels of oestrogens cause atrophy of the testes and prostate by means of reductions in testosterone. Other locally acting peptides are secreted by the prostatic epithelium and mesenchymal stromal cells in response to steroid hormones. These include epidermal growth factor, insulin-like growth factors, basic fibroblast growth factor and transforming growth factors alpha and beta. These undoubtedly play a part in normal and abnormal prostatic growth, but as yet their functions are unclear.

Summary box 78.1

Androgenic hormones

- Androgenic hormones, which drive prostate growth, are derived from several sources
- The majority of testosterone (90%) is secreted by the Leydig cells of the testes under the control of luteinising hormone, secreted from the anterior pituitary
- Metabolised adrenal androgen accounts for the remaining 5–10% of testosterone
- Testosterone is converted to 1,5-dihydrotestosterone (DHT) by the enzyme 5a-reductase type II, which is found in high concentration in the prostate and the perigenital skin
- DHT has five times the potency of testosterone

Elaboration and secretion of prostate-specific antigen

Prostate-specific antigen (PSA) is a glycoprotein that is a serine protease. Its function may be to facilitate liquefaction of semen, but it is a marker for prostatic disease. It is measured by an immunoassay and the normal range can differ a little from laboratory to laboratory. There is no real normal upper limit. The levels increase with age, with prostate cancer and with BPH. There are age-related values but, in general, in men aged 50–69 years, a level of about 3–4 ng/mL would prompt a discussion about the need for prostate biopsy. Its level in men with metastatic prostate cancer is usually increased to >30 ng/mL and falls to low levels after successful androgen ablation. Men with locally confined prostate cancer usually have serum PSA levels <10–15 ng/mL. Although PSA is a reliable marker for the progression of advanced disease, it is neither specific nor sensitive in the differential diagnosis of early prostate cancer and BPH, as both diseases are compatible with PSA in the range of 3–15 ng/mL. In summary, about 25% of men with a PSA of 4–10 ng/mL have prostate cancer (i.e. it is not very specific) and about 15–20% of men with a PSA of 1–4 ng/mL have prostate cancer. In general, one would advise men aged

Franz von Leydig, 1821–1908, Professor of Histology successively at Wurzburg, Tubingen and Bonn, Germany.

50–69 years to undergo prostate biopsy if the PSA was more than ~3 ng/mL. The threshold would be lower in younger men with a strong family history. PSA is a useful tumour marker in the postsurgery setting, where a supersensitive assay, with sensitivity to 0.02 ng/mL, facilitates early detection of biochemical recurrence.

BENIGN PROSTATIC HYPERPLASIA

Aetiology

Hormones

Serum testosterone levels slowly but significantly decrease with advancing age; however, levels of oestrogenic steroids are not decreased equally. According to this theory, the prostate enlarges because of increased oestrogenic effects. It is likely that the secretion of intermediate peptide growth factors plays a part in the development of BPH.

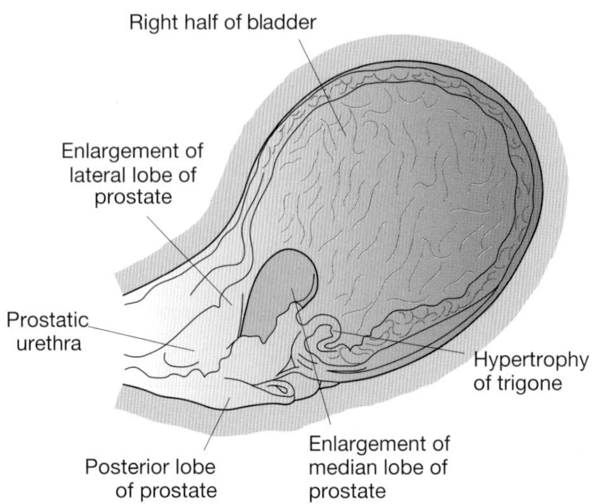

Figure 78.3 Diagram of late-stage bladder outflow obstruction showing enlargement of the prostate from benign prostatic hyperplasia, trabeculation of the bladder with smooth muscle hypertrophy and fibrosis.

Summary box 78.2

Benign prostatic hyperplasia (BPH)

- Occurs in men over 50 years of age; by the age of 60 years, 50% of men have histological evidence of BPH
- Is a common cause of significant lower urinary tract symptoms in men and is the most common cause of bladder outflow obstruction in men >70 years of age

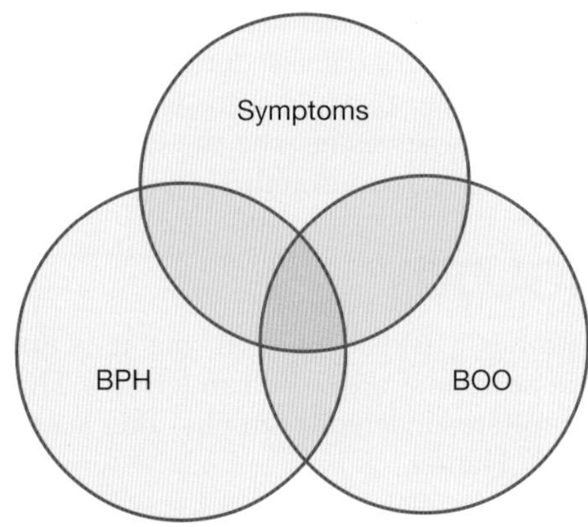

Figure 78.4 Diagrammatic representation of the relation between symptoms of prostatism, benign prostate hyperplasia (BPH) and urodynamically proven bladder outflow obstruction (BOO).

Pathology

BPH affects both glandular epithelium and connective tissue stroma to variable degrees. These changes are similar to those occurring in breast dysplasia (see Chapter 53), in which adenosis, epitheliosis and stromal proliferation are seen in differing proportions. BPH typically affects the submucous group of glands in the transitional zone, forming a nodular enlargement. Eventually, this overgrowth compresses the PZ glands into a false capsule and causes the appearance of the typical 'lateral' lobes.

When BPH affects the subcervical CZ glands, a 'middle' lobe develops that projects up into the bladder within the internal sphincter (Figure 78.3). Sometimes, both lateral lobes also project into the bladder, so that when viewed from within, the sides and back of the internal urinary meatus are surrounded by an intravesical prostatic collar.

Effects of benign prostatic hyperplasia

It is important to realise that the relationship between anatomical prostatic enlargement, lower urinary tract symptoms (LUTS) and urodynamic evidence of bladder outflow obstruction (BOO) is complex (Figure 78.4). Pathophysiologically, BOO may be caused in part by increased smooth muscle tone, which is under the control of α-adrenergic agonists.

Summary box 78.3

Consequences of benign prostatic hyperplasia

- No symptoms, no bladder outflow obstruction (BOO)
- No symptoms, but urodynamic evidence of BOO
- Lower urinary tract symptoms, no evidence of BOO
- Lower urinary tract symptoms and BOO
- Others (acute/chronic retention, haematuria, urinary infection and stone formation)

Anatomically, the effects are as follows:

- **Urethra**. The prostatic urethra is lengthened, sometimes to twice its normal length, but it is not narrowed anatomically. The normal posterior curve may be so exaggerated that it requires a curved catheter to negotiate it. When only one lateral lobe is enlarged, distortion of the prostatic urethra occurs.
- **Bladder**. If BPH causes BOO, the musculature of the bladder hypertrophies to overcome the obstruction and appears

trabeculated (Figure 78.5). Significant BPH is associated with increased blood flow, and the resultant veins at the base of the bladder are apt to cause haematuria.

Lower urinary tract symptoms

In both sexes, non-specific symptoms of bladder dysfunction become more common with age, probably owing to impairment of smooth muscle function and neurovesical coordination. Not all symptoms of disturbed voiding in ageing men should therefore be attributed to BPH causing BOO. Urologists prefer the term LUTS and discourage the use of the descriptive term 'prostatism'.

The following conditions can coexist with BOO, leading to difficulty in diagnosis and in predicting the outcome of treatment:

- idiopathic detrusor overactivity (see Chapter 77);
- neuropathic bladder dysfunction as a result of diabetes, strokes, Alzheimer's disease or Parkinson's disease (see Chapter 77); degeneration of bladder smooth muscle giving rise to impaired voiding and detrusor instability;
- BOO due to BPH.

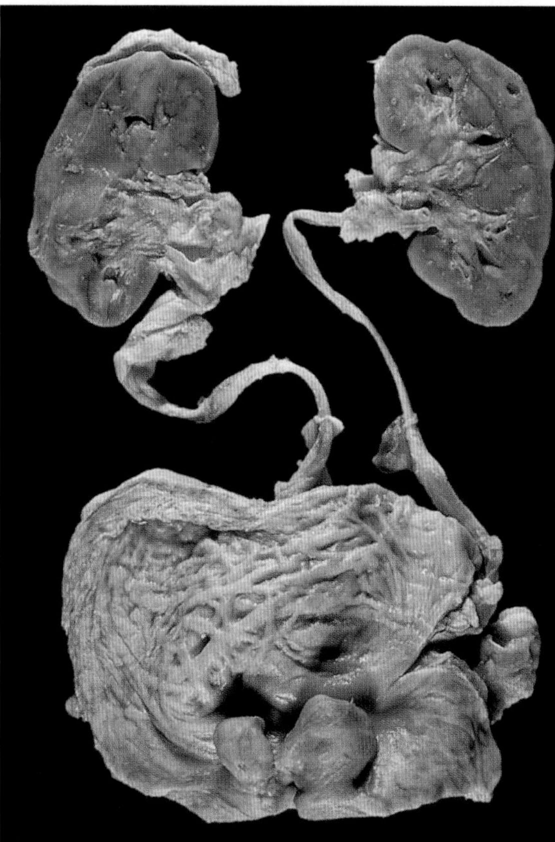

Figure 78.5 Pathological specimen of bladder and kidneys in a case of bladder outflow obstruction caused by benign prostatic hyperplasia. Bladder trabeculation, bilateral hydroureter and hydronephrosis can be seen.

Lower urinary tract symptoms can be described as:

- Voiding:
  - hesitancy (worsened if the bladder is very full);
  - poor flow (unimproved by straining);
  - intermittent stream – stops and starts;
  - dribbling (including after micturition);
  - sensation of poor bladder emptying;
  - episodes of near retention.
- Storage:
  - frequency;
  - nocturia;
  - urgency;
  - urge incontinence;
  - nocturnal incontinence (enuresis).

LUTS are usually assessed by means of scoring systems, which give a semiobjective measure of severity. However, some symptoms do not give an accurate picture of the underlying pathophysiological problem. For instance, a man with severe detrusor instability may void only small volumes and hence he will have a sensation of poor flow because low voided volumes (<100 mL) are associated with low flow rates.

Severe irritative symptoms are usually associated with detrusor instability. Postmicturition dribbling is now known not to be a consequence of BOO and is not usually improved by prostatectomy.

Bladder outflow obstruction

This is a urodynamic concept based on the combination of low flow rates in the presence of high voiding pressures. It can be diagnosed definitively only by pressure–flow studies. This is because symptoms are relatively non-specific and can result from detrusor instability, neurological dysfunction and weak bladder contraction. Even low measured peak flow rates (<10–12 mL/s) are not absolutely diagnostic because, in addition to BOO, weak detrusor contractions or low voided volumes (owing to instability) can be the cause. Nonetheless, flow rates provide a useful guide for everyday clinical management.

Urodynamically proven BOO may result from:

- BPH;
- bladder neck stenosis;
- bladder neck hypertrophy;
- prostate cancer;
- urethral strictures;
- functional obstruction due to neuropathic conditions.

The primary effects of BOO on the bladder are as follows:

- **Urinary flow rates decrease** (for a voided volume >200 mL, a peak flow rate of >15 mL/s is normal (Figure 78.6), one of 10–15 mL/s is equivocal and one <10 mL/s is low (Figure 78.7).

Alois Alzheimer, 1864–1915, neurologist, worked at Heidelberg and Munich before being appointed Professor of Psychiatry at Breslau, Germany (now Wroclaw, Poland).

- **Voiding pressures increase** (pressures >80 cmH_2O are high (Figure 78.8), pressures between 60 and 80 cmH_2O are equivocal and pressures <60 cmH_2O are normal).

The long-term effects of bladder outflow obstruction are as follows:

- The bladder may decompensate so that detrusor contraction becomes progressively less efficient and a residual urine develops.

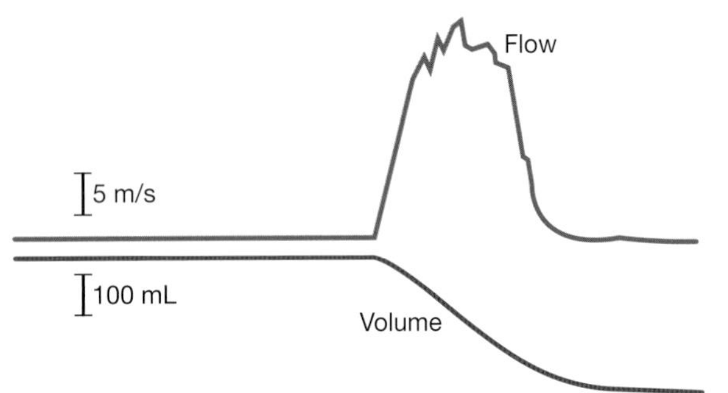

Figure 78.6 Normal flow rate. The voided volume is well in excess of 350 mL, and the maximum flow rate is in excess of 25 mL/s.

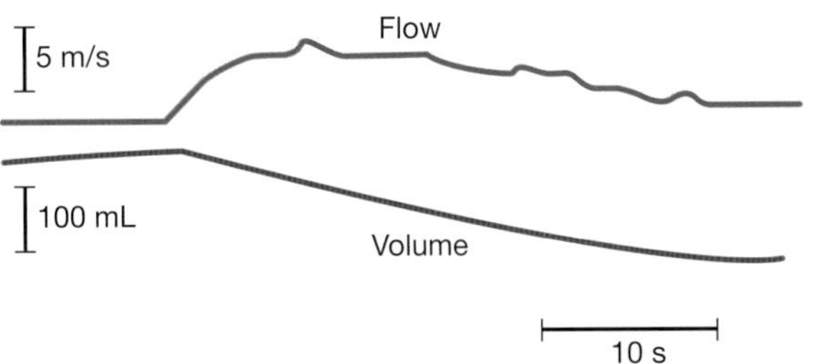

Figure 78.7 Diagram of a low flow rate showing a rather low voided volume of about 200 mL, but with markedly decreased flow rate. Such a flow rate could be caused by a urethral stricture, bladder outflow obstruction or a weak detrusor.

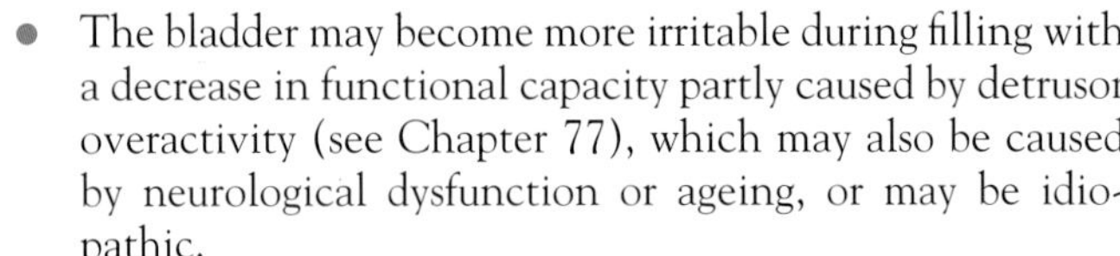

- The bladder may become more irritable during filling with a decrease in functional capacity partly caused by detrusor overactivity (see Chapter 77), which may also be caused by neurological dysfunction or ageing, or may be idiopathic.

Aside from symptoms, the complications of BOO are as follows:

- Acute retention of urine is sometimes the first symptom of BOO. Postponement of micturition is a common precipitating cause; overindulgence in beer and confinement to bed on account of intercurrent illness or operation are other causes.
- Chronic retention. In patients in whom the residual volume is >250 mL or so (Figure 78.9), the tension in the bladder wall increases owing to the combination of a large volume of residual urine and increased resting and filling bladder pressures (a condition known as high-pressure chronic retention). The increased intramural tension results in functional obstruction of the upper urinary tract with the development of bilateral hydronephrosis (Figure 78.10–78.12). As a result, upper tract infection and renal impairment may develop. Such men may present with overflow incontinence, enuresis and renal insufficiency. These symptoms should alert the doctor to the presence of this condition.
- Impaired bladder emptying. If the bladder decompensates with the development of a large volume of residual urine, urinary infection and calculi are prone to develop.
- Haematuria. This may be a complication of BPH. Other causes must be excluded by carrying out an intravenous urography (IVU), cystoscopy, urine culture and urine cytological examination.
- Other than pain from retention, pain is not a symptom of BOO, and its presence should prompt the exclusion of acute retention, urinary infection, stones, carcinoma of the prostate and carcinoma in situ of the bladder.

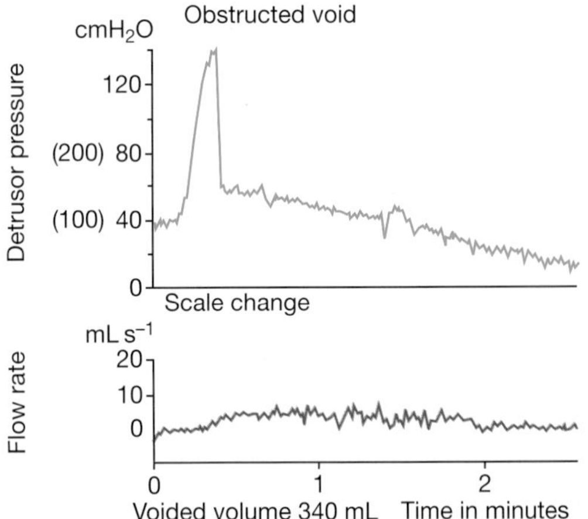

Figure 78.8 Conventional urodynamic trace showing detrusor pressure during voiding. There has been a change in scale because the pressure was so high; voiding pressures are increased with a low flow rate. This is diagnostic of bladder outflow obstruction.

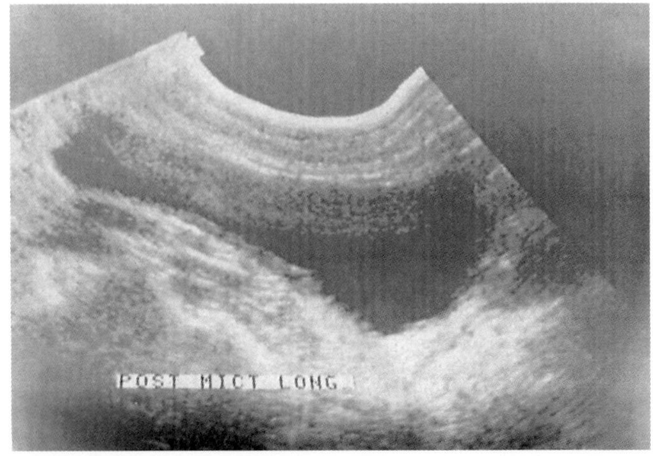

Figure 78.9 An ultrasonogram showing a large postvoid residual urine.

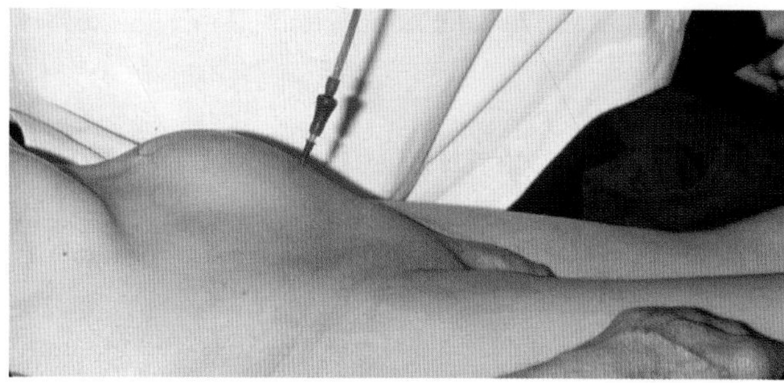

Figure 78.10 Image of an abdomen with high pressure urinary retention.

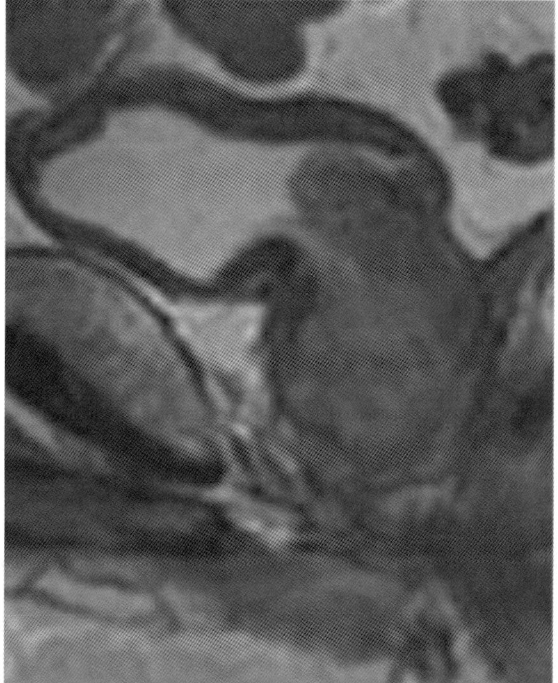

Figure 78.11 Magnetic resonance image showing a median lobe projecting into the bladder and causing bladder outflow obstruction.

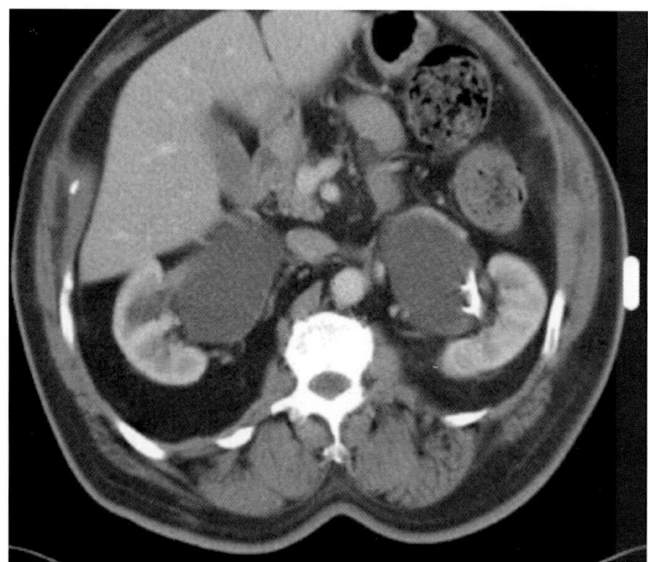

Figure 78.12 Computed tomography scan showing bilateral hydronephrosis as a result of bladder outflow obstruction.

ASSESSMENT OF THE PATIENT WITH LOWER URINARY TRACT SYMPTOMS

History

Symptom score sheets such as the International Prostate Symptom Score (IPSS) assign a score that gives information regarding the severity of symptoms at the outset and changes over time and following intervention. The IPSS assessment should include an assessment of quality of life, which is a reflection of the degree of 'bother' caused by a patient's symptoms. In addition to the IPSS, a frequency–volume diary completed by the patient before attending the clinic is invaluable in revealing fluid intake habits, diurnal variation in outputs and low-volume, frequent voiding. These assessments are routinely performed at lower urinary tract clinics but can be elicited by a thorough clinical history.

Summary box 78.4

Investigations of men with lower urinary tract symptoms

Essential investigations

- Urine analysis by dipstick for blood, glucose and protein
- Urine culture for infection
- Serum creatinine
- Urinary flow rate and residual volume measurement

Additional investigations

- Prostate-specific antigen if indicated
- Pressure-flow studies

Abdominal examination

Abdominal distension is usually normal. In patients with chronic retention, a distended bladder will be found on palpation, on percussion and sometimes on inspection with loss of the transverse suprapubic skin crease. General physical examination may demonstrate signs of chronic renal impairment with anaemia and dehydration. The external urinary meatus should be examined to exclude stenosis and the epididymides are palpated for signs of inflammation.

Rectal examination

In benign enlargement, the posterior surface of the prostate is smooth, convex and typically elastic, but the fibrous element may give the prostate a firm consistency. The rectal mucosa can be made to move over the prostate. Residual urine may be felt as a fluctuating swelling above the prostate. It should be noted that, if there is a considerable amount of residual urine present, it pushes the prostate downwards, making it appear larger than it is. It is not always possible to examine the cranial extreme of the very large prostate per rectum. An inability to get to the prostate base implies a volume of at least 50 mL.

The nervous system

The nervous system is examined to eliminate a neurological lesion. Diabetes mellitus, tabes dorsalis, disseminated sclerosis, cervical spondylosis, Parkinson's disease and other neurological states may mimic prostatic obstruction. If these are suspected, then a pressure–flow urodynamic study should be carried out to diagnose BOO. Examination of perianal sensation and anal tone is useful in detection of an S2 to S4 cauda equina lesion.

Serum prostate-specific antigen

The difficulty here is the uncertain benefit of early detection and radical treatment of prostate cancer – this is dealt with in the section on prostate cancer. Certainly, men should be informed about the test, the risks of the prostate biopsy that might be required and the risks of the detection of a cancer that we are not certain how best to treat, as well as the positive aspects of the early discovery of a small prostate cancer. After suitable counselling, measurement of serum PSA may be helpful. Men in whom a diagnosis of early prostate cancer might influence treatment option (such as those under 70 years or those with a positive family history who might be offered radical treatment) should be offered a PSA measurement. If this is in excess of 2.5–4 ng/mL, then transrectal ultrasound scanning (TRUS) plus transrectal biopsies (12 biopsies taken from six areas) should be considered.

If rectal examination is quite normal with no suspicion of cancer, and if no change in treatment policy would in any case result from the diagnosis of early prostate cancer, then there is little point in the routine measurement of PSA in men with uncomplicated BOO. However, because of the fear of future litigation, many find it easier to offer a PSA test. A variety of online calculators using PSA data from thousands of men involved in clinical trials are available and can be used to calculate the risk of a man having a positive biopsy at a given PSA level.

Flow rate measurement

For this to be meaningful, two or three voids should be recorded using a special flow meter, usually found in urology outpatient clinics and the voided volume should be in excess of 150–200 mL. A typical history and a flow rate <10 mL/s (for a voided volume of >200 mL; see Figure 78.7) will be sufficient for most urologists to recommend treatment. Usually, a flow rate measurement will be coupled with ultrasound measurement of postvoid residual urine.

There are pitfalls in the measurement of flow rates. The machine must be accurately calibrated. The patient must void volumes in excess of 150 mL and two or three recordings are needed to obtain a representative measurement. Decreased flow rates and LUTS may be seen in:

- BOO;
- low voided volumes (characteristically in men with detrusor instability);
- men with weak bladder contractions (low pressure–flow voiding).

Pressure–flow urodynamic studies

Details of these studies are outlined in Chapter 77 (see Figure 77.14). They should be performed on the following patients:

- men with suspected neuropathy (Parkinson's disease, dementia, longstanding diabetes, previous strokes, multiple sclerosis);
- men with a dominant history of irritative symptoms and men with lifelong urgency and frequency;
- men with a doubtful history and those with flow rates in the near normal range (~ or >15 mL/s);
- men with invalid flow rate measurements (because of low voided volumes).

Blood tests

Serum creatinine, electrolytes and haemoglobin should be measured.

Examination of urine

The urine is examined for glucose and blood; a midstream specimen should be sent for bacteriological examination and cytological examination may be carried out if carcinoma in situ is thought possible.

Upper tract imaging

Most urologists no longer carry out imaging of the upper tract in men with straightforward symptoms. Obviously, if infection or haematuria is present, then the upper tract should be imaged by means of intravenous urogram or ultrasound scan.

Cystourethroscopy

Inspection of the urethra, the prostate and the urothelium of the bladder should always be done immediately prior to prostatectomy, whether it is being done transurethrally or by the open route to exclude a urethral stricture, a bladder carcinoma and the occasional non-opaque vesical calculus. The decision of whether to perform prostatectomy must be made before cystoscopy. This should be based on the patient's symptoms, signs and investigations. Direct inspection of the prostate is a poor indicator of BOO and the need for surgery.

Transrectal ultrasound scanning

There is no need to carry this out routinely. Accurate estimation of prostatic size is possible by means of transrectal or transabdominal ultrasound scanning when a very large prostate is suspected.

MANAGEMENT OF MEN WITH BENIGN PROSTATIC HYPERPLASIA OR BLADDER OUTFLOW OBSTRUCTION

Strong indications for treatment (usually prostatectomy) include:

- **Acute retention** (see Chapter 77) in fit men with no other cause for retention (drugs, constipation, recent operation, etc.) (accounts for 25% of prostatectomies).
- **Chronic retention and renal impairment**: a residual urine of 200 mL or more, a raised blood urea, hydroureter or hydronephrosis demonstrated on urography and uraemic manifestations (accounts for 15% of prostatectomies).
- **Complications of bladder outflow obstruction**: stone, infection and diverticulum formation.
- **Haemorrhage**: occasionally, venous bleeding from a ruptured vein overlying the prostate will require prostatectomy to be performed.
- **Elective prostatectomy for severe symptoms**: this accounts for about 60% of prostatectomies. Increasing difficulty in micturition, with considerable frequency day and night, delay in starting and a poor stream are the usual symptoms for which prostatectomy is advised. Frequency alone is not a strong indication for prostatectomy. The natural progression of outflow obstruction is variable and rarely gets worse after 10 years. Severe symptoms, a low maximum flow rate (<10 mL/s) and an increased residual volume of urine (100–250 mL) are relatively strong indications for operative treatment. The exact cut-off for operative or non-operative treatment will depend on careful discussion between the patient and the urologist. Holmium laser enucleation of the prostate (HOLEP) or open prostatectomy should be considered for very large prostates.

Summary box 78.5

Options for treatment of LUTS secondary to BPH

- Conservative measures include watchful waiting in conjunction with fluid restriction and reduction in caffeine intake
- Drug therapy is with a-blockers or, in men with a large prostate, a 5a-reductase inhibitor, or both
- Interventional measures include transurethral resection of the prostate, which remains the 'gold standard'; consider open prostatectomy for large glands

Acute retention

The management of retention is discussed in detail in Chapter 77. Once the bladder has been drained by means of a catheter, the patient's fitness for treatment is determined. If retention was not caused by drugs or constipation, then prostatectomy would usually be the correct management. Unfit men or those with dementia may be treated by means of indwelling prostatic stents or a catheter. Similar comments apply to men with chronic retention once renal function has been stabilised by catheterisation. The role of α-adrenergic drugs followed by a trial of catheter has been tested and found to be successful in certain groups with a short history and a low residual volume of urine, but the recurrence rate becomes cumulatively high. 5alpha-reductase is given to prevent progression of symptoms in men with large (>35 mL) prostates.

Special problems in the management of chronic retention

Men with chronic retention who have relatively low volumes of residual urine and who do not have symptoms suggestive of coexisting infection and with good renal function do not necessarily require catheterisation before proceeding to prostatectomy on the next available list. For those who are uraemic, urgent catheterisation is mandatory to allow renal function to recover and stabilise. Haematuria often occurs following catheterisation owing to collapse of the distended bladder and upper tract, but settles within a couple of days.

Uraemic patients with chronic retention are often dehydrated at the time of admission. Owing to the chronic back pressure on the distal tubules within the kidney, there is loss of the ability to reabsorb salts and water. The result, following release of this pressure, may be an enormous outflow of salts and water, which is known as postobstructive diuresis. It is for this reason that a careful fluid chart, daily measurements of the patient's weight and serial estimations of creatinine and electrolytes are essential. Intravenous fluid replacement is required if the patient is unable to keep up with this fluid loss. These patients are often anaemic and may require a blood transfusion once fluid balance is stabilised (if haemoglobin is <9 g/l).

The general management of retention is discussed in Chapter 77.

Indications for elective treatment in men with LUTS secondary to BPH

Following careful assessment (see section on the assessment of men with LUTS), the following questions should be answered:

- Have they failed a preliminary trial of medical therapy? Commonly, men will have been treated with α-blockers or 5α- reductase inhibitors and will have failed treatment. They are then referred by their general practitioner to the urologist.
- Is BOO present? In many cases, the findings of significant symptoms (assessed by symptom scoring), a benign prostate supplemented by the finding of a low maximum flow rate (<10–12 mL/s for a good voided volume [>200 mL]) will suffice to make a reasonable working diagnosis of BOO. In some men, particularly those with irritative symptoms, suspected neurological disease or those with technically imperfect flow rate measurements, pressure–flow studies will need to be performed.

- How severe are the symptoms and what are the risks of doing nothing? Severe symptoms and a large residual volume of urine will usually require treatment. Men with mild symptoms, good flow rates (>15 ml/s) and good bladder emptying (residual urine <100 mL) may be safely managed by reassurance and review: such patients rarely develop severe complications such as retention in the long term.
- Is the man fit for operative treatment?
- What treatments are available, what are the outcomes and do the side-effects justify treatment?

Treatment

Men with symptoms attending for elective treatment (excluding acute and chronic retention)

CONSERVATIVE TREATMENT

It is in men with relatively mild symptoms, reasonable flow rates (>10 mL/s) and good bladder emptying (residual urine <100 mL) that careful discussion over the merits and side-effects of operative treatment is warranted. Waiting for a period of 6 months after careful discussion of the diagnosis is indicated. After this, a repeat assessment of symptoms, flow rates and ultrasound scan is helpful; many men with stable symptoms will elect to leave matters be. Advice over limiting fluid intake in the evening and careful use of propantheline to help with irritative symptoms is also useful.

DRUGS

In men who are very concerned about the development of sexual dysfunction after transurethral resection of the prostate (TURP), the use of drugs may be helpful. Two classes of drug have been used in the treatment of men with BOO. Alpha-adrenergic blocking agents inhibit the contraction of smooth muscle that is found in the prostate. The other class of drug is the 5α-reductase inhibitors, which inhibit the conversion of testosterone to DHT, the most active form of androgen. These drugs, when taken for a year, result in a 25% shrinkage of the prostate gland. Both groups of drugs are effective; however, α-blockers work more quickly and, although the 5α-reductase inhibitors have fewer side effects, they need to be taken for at least 6 months, and their effect is greatest in patients with large (>50 g) glands. Drug therapy results in improvements in maximum flow rates by about 2 mL/s more than placebo and results in a mild (20%) improvement in symptom scores. TURP, however, results in improvements in maximum flow rates from 9–18 mL/s and a 75% improvement in symptom scores. These drugs are expensive in comparison with their effectiveness, and a significant proportion of men who try these drugs will subsequently undergo TURP. They may be best targeted at men who have failed an initial trial of watchful waiting and who wish to avoid surgery for a period.

OPERATIVE TREATMENT

Apart from the strong indications for operative treatment mentioned above, the most common reason for TURP is a combination of severe symptoms and a low flow rate <12 mL/s. The key is to assess the symptoms carefully and to counsel men about side effects and likely outcome before advising operative treatment.

Counselling men undergoing prostatectomy

Men undergoing prostatectomy need to be advised about the following:

- **Retrograde ejaculation**. This occurs in about 65% of men after prostatectomy.
- **Erectile impotence**. This occurs in about 5% of men, usually those whose potency is waning.
- **Success rate**. On the whole, men with acute and chronic retention do well from the symptomatic point of view. Ninety per cent of men undergoing elective operation for severe symptoms and urodynamically proven BOO do well in terms of symptoms and flow rates. Only about 65% of those with mild symptoms or those with weak bladder contraction as the cause of their symptoms do well. Men with unobstructed detrusor instability do not respond well to TURP. This is the reason for carefully documenting the severity of symptoms and flow rates (supplemented when necessary by pressure–flow studies) before deciding on treatment.
- **Risk of reoperation**. After TURP, this is about 15% after 8–10 years.
- **Morbidity rate**. Death after TURP is infrequent (<0.5%), severe sepsis is found in about 6% and severe haematuria requiring transfusion of more than 2 units of blood occurs in about 3%. After discharge, about 15–20% of men subsequently require antibiotic treatment for symptoms of urinary infection. Risk factors for complications include admission with retention, prostate cancer, renal impairment and advanced age.

Methods of performing prostatectomy

The prostate can be approached (1) transurethrally (TURP), (2) retropubically (RPP), (3) through the bladder (transvesical; TVP) or (4) from the perineum (**Figure 78.13**).

Transurethral prostate surgery

TURP remains the most commonly performed procedure for the surgical correction of BOO. Perhaps the greatest advance in the history of transurethral surgery was marked by the development of the rigid lens system of Professor Harold Hopkins. His lenses, illuminated by a fibreoptic light source, permit unparalleled visualisation of the working field. Men with indwelling catheters, those with recent urinary infection, those with chronic retention or those with prosthetic material or heart valves benefit from prophylactic antibiotics in addition to the standard for clean surgery at induction of anaesthesia.

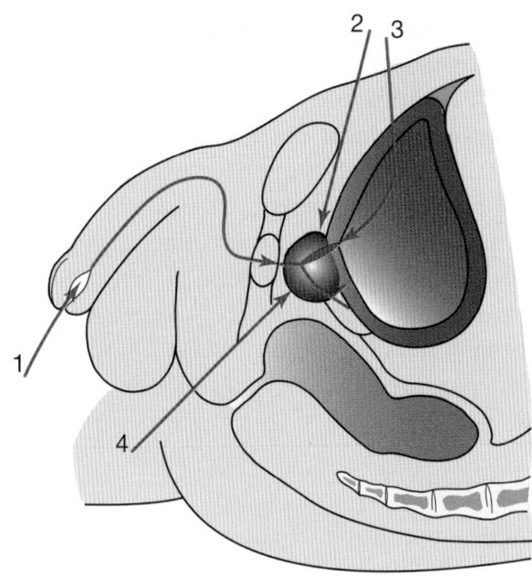

Figure 78.13 The surgical approaches to the prostate. (For key see text.)

Strips of tissue are cut from the bladder neck down to the level of the verumontanum (**Figure 78.14**). Cutting is performed by a high-frequency diathermy current, which is applied across a loop mounted on the hand-held trigger of the resectoscope. Coagulation of bleeding points can be accurately achieved. The 'chips' of prostate are then removed from the bladder using an Ellik evacuator. Resection proceeds at 1 g/minute in experienced hands. The duration of resection for monopolar TURP is limited to 1 hour due to the risk of resorption of water if 1% glycine is used as an irrigant. The advent of bipolar TURP where normal saline is used as an irrigant permits resection of larger prostates. Following TURP, careful haemostasis is performed, and a three-way, self-retaining catheter irrigated with isotonic saline is introduced into the bladder to prevent any further bleeding from forming blood clots. Irrigation is continued until the outflow is pale pink, and the catheter is usually removed on the second or third postoperative day. In men with small prostates or bladder neck dyssynergia or stenosis, it is better to divide the bladder neck and prostatic urethra with a Collings knife.

Laser can be used to evaporate (e.g. Green light laser) or enucleate the prostate (e.g. HOLEP). The advantage of green light laser is that vaporisation is haemostatic and this procedure can be performed even while patients are anticoagulated. HOLEP involves the use of a laser to coagulate any of the small vessels crossing the relatively avascular plane between the peripheral and transitional zones of the prostate while the tip of the cystoscope is used, much like the surgeons finger at Millin's prostatectomy, to enucleate the transition zone adenoma. The enucleated adenoma is pushed into the bladder, where it is morcellated and extracted via the cystoscope. Damage to the external sphincter is avoided provided one uses the verumontanum as a guide to the most distal point of the resection/vaporisation/enucleation.

Retropubic prostatectomy (Millin)

This procedure is rarely performed nowadays as it has been largely superceded by HOLEP. However, where HOLEP is not available or where diverticulectomy or the removal of large stones are required, this open operation may be performed. Using a low, curved transverse suprapubic Pfannenstiel incision, which includes the rectus sheath, the recti are split in the midline and retracted to expose the bladder. With the patient in the Trendelenburg position, the surgeon separates the bladder and the prostate from the posterior aspect of the pubis. In the space thus obtained, the anterior capsule of the prostate is incised with diathermy below the bladder neck, care being taken to obtain complete control of bleeding from divided prostatic veins by suture ligation. The prostatic adenoma is exposed and a finger used to dissect along the avascular plane between the transition and peripheral zones. A wedge is taken out of the posterior lip of the bladder neck to prevent secondary stricture in this region. The exposure of the inside of the prostatic cavity is good, and control of haemorrhage is achieved with diathermy and suture ligation of bleeding points before closure of the capsule over a Foley catheter (inserted per urethram) draining the bladder.

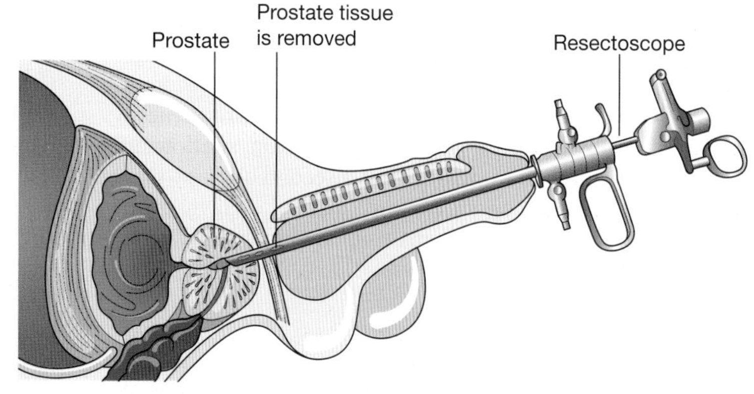

Figure 78.14 For transurethral resection of the prostate the resectoscope is inserted transurethrally. Electric current is passed through a diathermy loop at the end of the instrument. The surgeon moves this back and forth to create a cavity using diathermy to cauterise as they go. The resultant chips are washed out of the bladder intermittently throughout the procedure. A visual image of the operative field is transmitted through lenses running in the middle of the resectoscope. Around this lens, irrigating fluid is instilled and flows out, washing blood away from the operative field. The procedure is complete when an adequate channel has been created through the prostate.

Terence John Millin, 1903–1980, surgeon, The Westminster Hospital, London, UK and Honorary surgeon, All Saints' Hospital for Genitourinary Diseases, London, UK, described the operation of retropubic prostatectomy in 1945. He was regarded as 'the greatest of Irish urologists' and 'the pioneer of the retropubic space'. To facilitate his operation, he devised a self-retaining retractor that goes by his name and the 'boomerang' needle to close the prostatic capsule. He used to be invited all over the world to operate on VIPs. He was a former President of the Royal College of Surgeons in Ireland. He gave up operating at the age of 57 to enjoy his farm in County Wicklow where he died of laryngeal carcinoma. He played international rugby for Ireland.

Transvesical prostatectomy

This operation is very rarely performed nowadays but provides an alternative means by which to enucleate the prostate when BOO is combined with a large bladder stone. The bladder is opened and the prostate enucleated by putting a finger into the urethra, pushing forwards towards the pubes to separate the lateral lobes, and then working the finger between the adenoma and the false capsule (compressed peripheral zone). In Freyer's operation (1901), the bladder was left open widely and drained by a suprapubic tube with a 16-mm lumen in order to allow free drainage of blood and urine. Harris (1934) advocated control of the prostatic arteries by lateral stitches inserted with his boomerang needle. The bladder wall was then closed and the wound drained.

After treatment

Most urologists irrigate the bladder with sterile saline by means of a three-way Foley catheter for 24 hours or so.

Complications

Local

Haemorrhage is a major risk following prostatectomy whatever the surgical approach. Care should be taken in diathermising arterial bleeding points after TURP; they are often better seen when the rate of inflow of fluid is decreased. In the recovery room, one should check that the bladder is draining adequately; if it is not, this may indicate that a clot is blocking the eye of the catheter. The bladder should be promptly washed out using strict aseptic technique. The catheter should be changed by the surgeon. Only rarely is it necessary to return the patient to the operating room.

Secondary haemorrhage tends to occur after the patient has been discharged. All men should be warned about this possibility and given appropriate advice to rest and to have a high fluid intake. It is usually minor in degree but if clot retention occurs, the patient will need to be readmitted, a catheter passed and the bladder washed out.

Perforation of the bladder or the prostatic capsule can occur at the time of transurethral surgery. This usually occurs from a combination of inexperience in association with a large prostate or heavy blood loss. If the field of vision becomes obscured by heavy blood loss, it is often prudent to achieve adequate haemostasis and abandon the operation, swallowing one's pride on the understanding that a second attempt may be necessary. A large perforation with marked extravasation may require the insertion of a small suprapubic drain. Rectal perforation should be extremely rare.

Sepsis

Bacteraemia is common even in men with sterile urine and occurs in over 50% of men with infected urine, prolonged catheterisation or chronic retention. Septicaemia can occur in these patients shortly after operation or when the catheter is removed. Routine use of prophylactic antibiotics is recommended based on local antimicrobial sensitivity profiles. Wound infection following open prostatectomy is common if a urethral catheter has been *in situ* for a number of days before the operation. The most worrying aspect of infection is the early rigor following surgery. If left undetected and untreated, this may progress to frank septicaemia with profound hypotension. A blood culture should be taken and antibiotics given parenterally (e.g. amoxicillin plus cefuroxime, or gentamicin).

Incontinence

Incontinence is inevitable if the external sphincter mechanism is damaged. The bladder neck is rendered incompetent by any prostatectomy and, therefore, an intact distal sphincter mechanism is essential for continence. The verumontanum marks the proximal margin of the external sphincter. If physiotherapy is ineffective, then the only satisfactory treatment is the fitting of an artificial urinary sphincter or a sling to increase the resistance of the urethra. In some patients, detrusor instability contributes to the incontinence. The use of the anticholinergic agents imipramine or duloxetine may help.

Retrograde ejaculation and impotence

Impotence in men with good sexual function before surgery is uncommon, but retrograde ejaculation occurs commonly (>50%) because of disruption to the bladder neck mechanism.

Urethral stricture

This may be secondary to prolonged catheterisation, the use of an unnecessarily large catheter, clumsy instrumentation or the presence of the resectoscope in the urethra for too long a period. These strictures arise either just inside the meatus or in the bulbar urethra. An early stricture can usually be managed by simple bouginage but, later on, it may be necessary to cut the densely fibrotic stricture with the optical urethrotome. The routine use of an Otis urethrotomy prior to TURP reduces the incidence of postoperative stricture.

Bladder neck contracture

Occasionally, a dense fibrotic stenosis of the bladder neck occurs following overaggressive resection of a small prostate. It may be due to the overuse of coagulating diathermy. Transurethral incision of the scar tissue is necessary using laser or diathermy.

Reoperation

It is now well known that, after 8 years, 15–18% of men with BPH will require repeat TURP (the rate after open prostatectomy is about 5%). The reasons include a technically imperfect

---

Sir Peter Johnston Freyer, 1852–1921, Irish born surgeon, performed the first successful prostatectomy in 1900 at St Peter's Hospital for Stone, London, UK. He used to give a running commentary to his visiting surgeons in French and Hidustani.
Samuel Harry Harris, 1881–1937, urologist, Lewisham Hospital, Sydney, NSW, Australia.
Fessenden Nott Otis, 1825–1900, nineteenth century American urologist.

primary procedure and a speculative repeat operation in men with symptoms who are cystoscoped after operation.

General complications

Death occurs in about 0.2–0.3% of men undergoing elective prostatectomy. In very elderly men, in men with prostate cancer admitted as an emergency with acute or chronic retention or in those with very large prostates, the 30-day death rate may be in the order of 1%.

Cardiovascular

Pulmonary atelectasis, pneumonia, myocardial infarction, congestive cardiac failure and deep venous thrombosis are all potentially life-threatening conditions that can affect this elderly and often frail group of men.

Water intoxication

Absorption of water into the circulation at the time of transurethral resection can give rise to congestive cardiac failure, hyponatraemia and haemolysis. Accompanying this, there is frequently confusion and other cerebral events often mimicking a stroke. The incidence of this condition has been reduced since the introduction of isotonic glycine for irrigating during resection, and further still with the development of bipolar TURP where saline is used as an irrigant. The treatment consists of fluid restriction.

Laser treatment of bladder outflow obstruction

A wide range of tissue ablative techniques using hyperthermia and laser energy have been developed and evaluated. These could often be performed as outpatient procedures with little morbidity. However, as experience has grown and high level data has accumulated, several of these techniques have been excluded and others ensconced within the surgical armamentarium in the treatment of BOO. Most successful transurethral alternatives to TURP involve the use of medical lasers.

The different penetrative and haemostatic characteristics render each type of laser most useful for a particular application. The holmium laser does not penetrate deep but is haemostatic, making it useful in sealing the small vessels that are opened on blunt dissection of the Millin's plane using the beak of the cystoscope during HOLEP. This approach involves excision of parts of the prostate using a cutting laser and then morcellating the excised prostate fragments, which fall back into the bladder so that they can be removed. Morbidity with this procedure is low and long-term results suggest that the benefit will be sustained.

The KTP (green light) laser vaporises tissue and has a deeper penetration than holmium, making it suitable for vaporisation of prostate tissue. This has not yet been shown to be as durable as holmium laser treatment or TURP, because the amount of tissue removed is usually less. Vaporisation of the tissue causes minimal bleeding and green light laser has been used to vaporise the prostate of men in whom stopping anticoagulants is dangerous.

Intraurethral stents

These devices (**Figure 78.15**) are possibly helpful in the management of men with retention who are grossly unfit (classified by the American Society of Anesthesiologists as ASA grade IV). These men are rare cases.

BLADDER OUTFLOW OBSTRUCTION CAUSED BY THE BLADDER NECK

Aetiology

This condition usually occurs in men, but can rarely affect children of both sexes and women. It may be due to muscular hypertrophy or fibrosis of the tissues at the bladder neck following TURP.

Clinical syndromes

Owing to muscle hypertrophy or dyssynergia

Marion described a series of cases in which muscular hypertrophy of the internal sphincter in a young person had resulted in the development of a vesical diverticulum or hydronephrosis (Marion's disease or 'prostatism sans prostate'). It is thought that dyssynergic contraction of the smooth muscle of the bladder neck (bladder neck dyssynergia) may account for some cases of BOO.

Owing to fibrosis

The symptoms are similar to those of prostatic enlargement but are a consequence of scarring after TURP or radical prostatectomy (usually compounded by external beam radiotherapy)

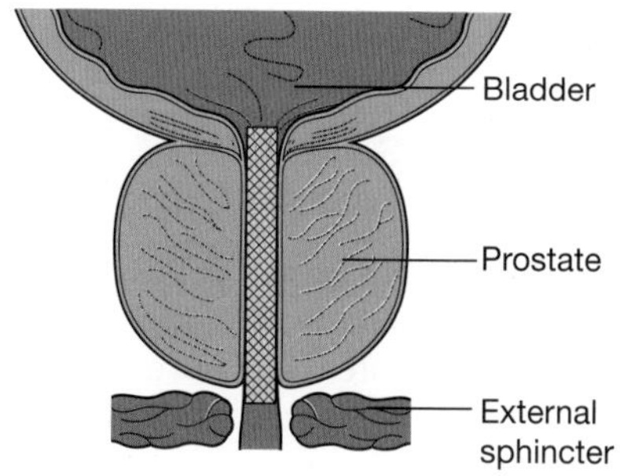

Figure 78.15 Diagram showing one type of prostatic stent *in situ*.

Jean Baptiste Camile Marion, 1869–1932, Professor of Urology, The Faculty of Medicine, Paris, France.

Treatment

The management of these patients depends on achieving an accurate diagnosis. For this, urodynamic investigation is often necessary, which should demonstrate raised voiding pressures and diminished flow rate.

Drugs

The presence of α-adrenergic receptors in the region of the bladder neck and prostatic urethra allows pharmacological manipulation of the outflow to the bladder.

ALPHA-BLOCKING DRUGS

Alfuzosin (2.5 mg b.d. to t.d.s., to a total maximum of 10 mg/day), doxazosin (1 mg nocte, up to a maximum of 8 mg/day), indoramin (20 mg b.d., increased to a total maximum of 100 mg/day in divided doses), prazosin (500 mg b.d., maintenance up to 2 mg/day) and terazosin (1 mg nocte, to a total maximum of 10 mg/day), can be very useful, causing relaxation of the bladder neck. These drugs are not target specific, and patients must be warned of the possibility of postural hypotension, which is usually limited to the first few doses. They can be safely used in combination with anticholinergics to minimise the symptoms of bladder overactivity associated with BOO.

Transurethral incision

Transurethral incision of the bladder neck is the operation of choice. Sometimes symptoms recur, but this is usually due to inadequate division of the fibres of the bladder neck.

Congenital valves of the prostatic urethra

See Chapter 79.

PROSTATIC CALCULI

Prostatic calculi are of two varieties: endogenous, which are common, and exogenous, which are comparatively rare. An exogenous prostatic calculus is a urinary (commonly ureteric) calculus that becomes arrested in the prostatic urethra. Endogenous prostatic calculi are usually composed of calcium phosphate combined with about 20% organic material.

Clinical features

Prostatic calculi are usually symptomless, being discovered on TRUS, on radiography of the pelvis, during prostatectomy or associated with carcinoma of the prostate or chronic prostatitis. In cases associated with severe chronic prostatic infection, the associated fibrosis and nodularity are difficult to differentiate from carcinoma. On radiographs or ultrasound scans, these stones are often seen to form a horseshoe (**Figure 78.16**) or a circle.

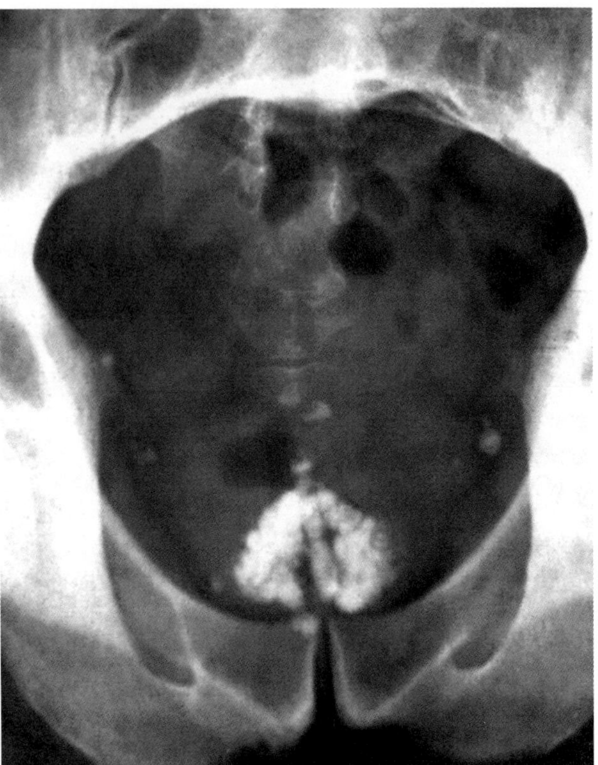

Figure 78.16 Endogenous prostatic calculi.

Treatment of prostatic calculi

Prostatic calculi usually require no treatment.

Conservative measures

Associated chronic prostatic infection may be treated by means of ciprofloxacin or trimethoprim.

Transurethral resection

Transurethral resection will often release small calculi as the strips of prostatic tissue are excised. Others are passed per urethram at a later date.

Corpora amylaceae

Corpora amylaceae are tiny calcified lamellated bodies found in the glandular alveoli of the prostates of elderly men and apes, but not in the prostates of animals lower in the phylogenetic scale than anthropoids. Corpora amylaceae are probably the forerunners of endogenous prostatic calculi.

CARCINOMA OF THE PROSTATE

Carcinoma of the prostate is the most common malignant tumour in men over the age of 65 years. In England and Wales in 2004, 30 000 men were registered and 10 000 died from prostate carcinoma; the corresponding figures in the USA were 260 000 and 35 000, respectively. If histological section of prostates at autopsy is performed, increasingly frequent foci of microscopic prostate cancers are found with increasing age. These foci of prostate cancer have variable potential for progressing clinically to metastatic disease. About 10–15% of younger men who develop prostate cancer have a positive family history of the disease, but the aetiology is unclear.

Throughout the world, rates of microscopic foci of prostate cancer are constant, but rates of clinically evident disease are low in men in Japan and China. Carcinoma of the prostate usually originates in the PZ of the prostate (see **Figure 78.2**), so 'prostatectomy' for benign enlargement of the gland confers no protection from subsequent carcinoma.

Pathology

Serial sections of prostates obtained at routine necropsy demonstrate prostate carcinoma in 25% of men between 50 and 65 years of age. The incidence in men over 80 years is in the region of 70% (Franks). Most of these neoplasms are tiny and (if life had continued) might have remained latent for years.

The following types of prostate cancer occur:

- microscopic latent cancer found on autopsy or at cystoprostatectomy;
- tumours found incidentally during TURP (T1a and T1b) or following screening by PSA measurement (T1c);
- early, localised prostate cancer (T2);
- advanced local prostate cancer (T3 and T4);
- metastatic disease, which may arise from a clinically evident tumour (T2, T3 or T4) or from an apparently benign gland (T0, T1) (i.e. occult prostate cancer).

It should be noted that only the last two groups cause symptoms, and such tumours are not curable. Only screening or the treatment of incidentally found tumours can result in cure of the disease. The problem is that many such tumours would never progress during the patient's lifetime; herein lies the problem with prostate cancer.

Screening for prostate cancer

The cancer detection rate using measurement of PSA is between 2% and 4%, and approximately 30% of men with an elevated PSA will have prostate cancer confirmed by biopsy. Unfortunately, 20% of men with clinically significant prostate cancer will have PSA values within the normal range. There is therefore controversy over the usefulness of PSA alone as a screening procedure. Currently, a number of prospective trials aimed at determining whether or not PSA testing reduces the disease-specific mortality of prostate cancer are under way. At present, in Europe, population-based screening is performed only within the confines of clinical trials.

Summary box 78.6

- The results of several large scale randomised clinical trials evaluating the role of prostate-specific antigen (PSA) screening for prostate cancer suggest that at present screening the entire population with serum PSA is not cost effective as a large number of men must be screened, biopsied and treated in order to prevent each death from prostate cancer.

Histological appearances

The prostate is a glandular structure consisting of ducts and acini; thus, the histological pattern is one of an adenocarcinoma. The prostatic glands are surrounded by a layer of myoepithelial cells. The first change associated with carcinoma is the loss of the basement membrane, with glands appearing to be in confluence. As the cell type becomes less differentiated, more solid sheets of carcinoma cells are seen. A classification of the histological pattern based on the degree of glandular de-differentiation and its relation to stroma has been devised by Gleason. Prostate cancers exhibit heterogeneity within tissue, and so two histological areas of prostate are each scored between 1 and 5. The scores are added to give an overall Gleason score of between 2 and 10; this (and the volume of the cancer) appears to correlate well with the likelihood of spread and the prognosis.

Local spread

Locally advanced tumours tend to grow upwards to involve the seminal vesicles, the bladder neck and trigone and, later, the tumours tend to spread distally to involve the distal sphincter mechanism. Further upward extension obstructs the lower end of one or both ureters, obstruction of both resulting in anuria. The rectum may become stenosed by tumour infiltrating around it, but direct involvement is rare.

Spread by the bloodstream

Spread by the bloodstream occurs particularly to bone; indeed, the prostate is the most common site of origin for skeletal metastases, followed in turn by the breast, the kidney, the bronchus and the thyroid gland. The bones involved most frequently by carcinoma of the prostate are the pelvic bones and the lower lumbar vertebrae. The femoral head, rib cage and skull are other common sites.

Lymphatic spread

Lymphatic spread may occur (1) via lymphatic vessels passing to the obturator fossa or along the sides of the rectum to the lymph nodes beside the internal iliac vein and in the hollow of the sacrum and (2) via lymphatics that pass over the seminal vesicles and follow the vas deferens for a short distance to drain into the external iliac lymph nodes. From retroperitoneal lymph nodes, the mediastinal nodes and occasionally the supraclavicular nodes may become implicated.

Staging using the tumour, node, metastasis (TNM) system (Figure 78.17)

- **T1a, T1b and T1c**. These are incidentally found tumours in a clinically benign gland after histological examination of a prostatectomy specimen. T1a is a tumour involving less than 5% of the resected specimen; these tumours are usually well or moderately well differentiated. T1b is

Donald F Gleason, 1920–2008, pathologist, University of Minnesota, Minneapolis, MN, USA, published The Gleason System in 1966. He spent his last 20 years sailing, baking bread and playing bridge.

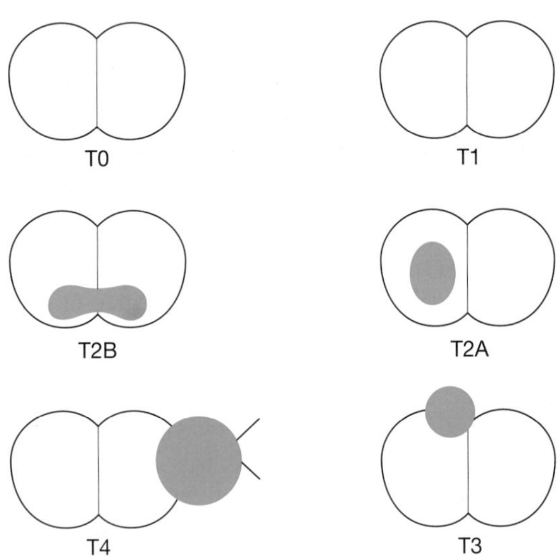

Figure 78.17 Tumour, node, metastasis staging system for prostate cancer.

a tumour involving >5% of the resected specimen. T1c tumours are impalpable tumours found following investigation of a raised PSA.

- **T2a** disease presents as a suspicious nodule (**Figure 78.18**) on rectal examination confined within the prostate capsule and involving one lobe. T2b disease involves both lobes.
- **T3** tumour extends through the capsule (T3a, uni- or bilateral extension; T3b, seminal vesical extension).
- **T4** is a tumour that is fixed or invading adjacent structures other than seminal vesicles – rectum or pelvic side wall.

Summary box 78.7

The natural history of prostate cancer

This depends on the stage and grade of disease:

- T1 and T2

  The progression rate of well-differentiated T1a prostate cancer is very low: 10–14% after eight years. For moderately differentiated tumours, the rate is about 20%

  For T1b and T2 tumours, the rate is in excess of 35%
- T3 and T4 (MO)

  About 50% progress to bony metastases after 3–5 years
- M1

  The median survival of men with metastatic disease is about 3 years

Clinical features

Only advanced disease gives rise to symptoms, but even advanced disease may be asymptomatic. Symptoms of advanced disease include:

- BOO;
- pelvic pain and haematuria;
- bone pain, malaise, 'arthritis', anaemia or pancytopenia;
- renal failure;

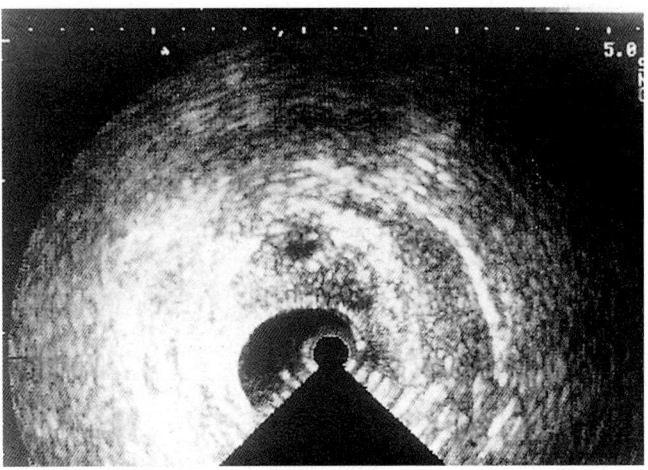

Figure 78.18 Transrectal ultrasound scan of a T2 nodule in the prostate.

- locally advanced disease or even asymptomatic metastases, which may be found incidentally on investigation of other symptoms.

  Early prostate cancer is asymptomatic and may be found:

- incidentally following TURP for clinically benign disease (T1);
- as a nodule (T2) on rectal examination.

Summary box 78.8

The presentation of men with prostate cancer

- Often men are asymptomatic, and detection is by opportunistic PSA testing
- Cancer is detected in men describing lower urinary tract symptoms or may present with symptoms of metastatic disease

Rectal examination

Rectal examination can detect nodules within the prostate and advanced disease. Irregular induration, characteristically stony hard in part or in the whole of the gland (with obliteration of the median sulcus), suggests carcinoma. Extension beyond the capsule up into the bladder base and vesicles (**Figure 78.19**) is diagnostic, as is local extension through the capsule (**Figure 78.20**).

Prostatic biopsy

If there is suspicion of prostate cancer, because of local findings, a raised PSA or metastatic disease, then a prostate biopsy using an automated gun is recommended (**Figure 78.21**). This is usually performed transrectally, although increasingly the transperineal approach is being used. In a standard transrectal biopsy about 12 systematic biopsy cores are obtained as well as biopsy of any suspicious areas. Broad-spectrum antibiotic cover is given to all patients to reduce the incidence of sepsis,

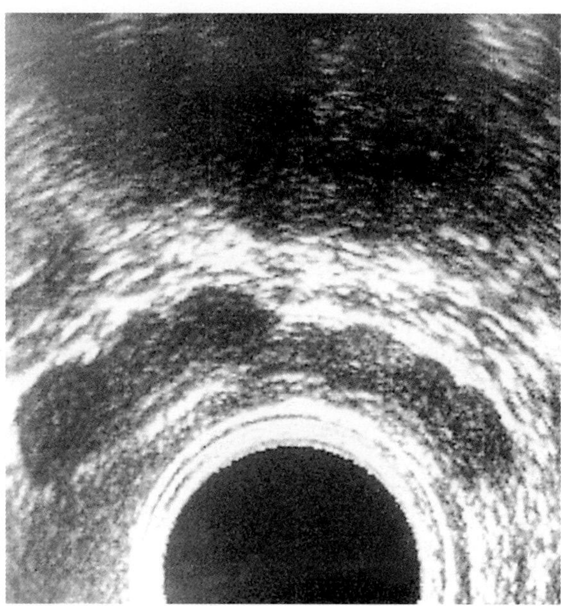
Figure 78.19 Transrectal ultrasound scan showing normal seminal vesicles.

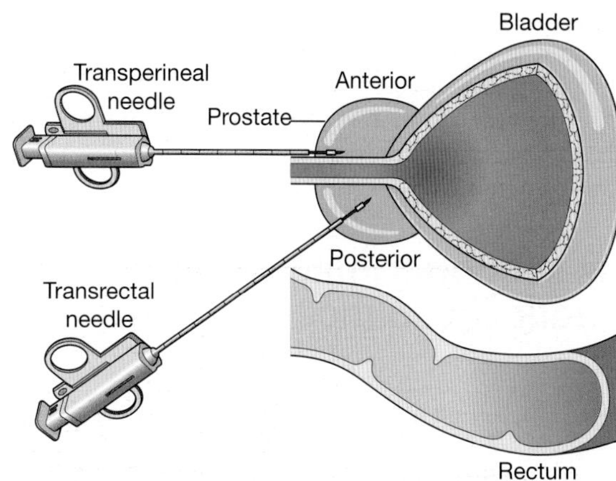

Figure 78.21 The prostate is commonly biopsied by two routes. The biopsy needle can be inserted through skin between the scrotum and anus (perineum) or the rectum. In both cases the passage of the needle is usually guided to the correct place with transrectal ultrasound. Transrectal ultrasound is not good for sampling the anterior prostate, particularly when the prostate is large. Transperineal biopsy is gaining popularity as an alternative to conventional transrectal biopsy.

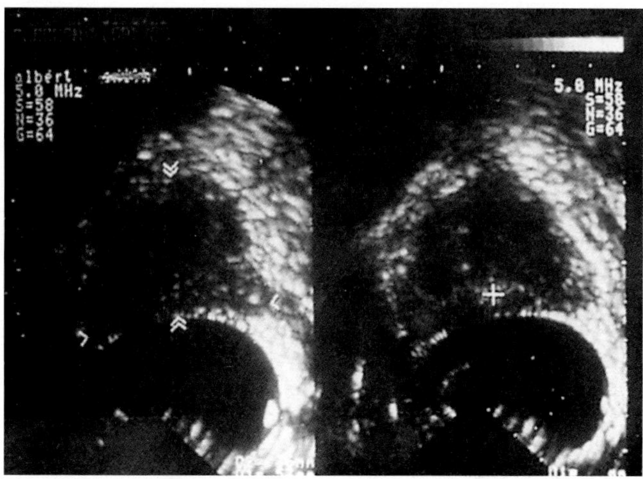
Figure 78.20 Transrectal ultrasound scan showing local extension of a T3 prostate cancer.

which is greater with transrectal than transperineal biopsy. Transperineal biopsy usually involves sedation or general anaesthetic while transrectal biopsy can be performed under local anaesthetic. Increasingly, areas appearing suspicious for prostate cancer on multiparametric magnetic resonance imaging (mp-MRI) can be targeted for biopsy to increase the diagnostic yield.

If there are associated symptoms of BOO, then either:

- a TURP can be performed, which will provide diagnostic material and symptomatic relief; or
- a transrectal biopsy can be carried out. If the diagnosis is positive and there is locally advanced disease, then hormone ablation can provide good symptomatic relief without the need for operation.

General blood tests

These are normal in early disease but, in metastatic disease, there may be leucoerythroblastic anaemia secondary to extensive marrow invasion, or anaemia may be secondary to renal failure. There may be thrombocytopenia and evidence of disseminated intravascular coagulopathy with increased fibrinogen degradation products.

Liver function tests

These will be abnormal if there is extensive metastatic invasion of the liver. Alkaline phosphatase may be raised from either hepatic involvement or secondaries in the bone. These can be distinguished by measurement of isoenzymes or gammaglutamyltransferase.

Prostate-specific antigen

This is discussed earlier in this chapter. It is good at following the course of advanced disease; however, it is lacking in sensitivity and specificity in the diagnosis of early localised prostate cancer. Nevertheless, the finding of a PSA >10 ng/mL is suggestive of cancer and >35 ng/ml is almost diagnostic of advanced prostate cancer. A decrease in PSA to the normal range following hormonal ablation is a good prognostic sign. Following radical prostatectomy the serum PSA should fall to undetectable levels (the limit for detection for modern supersensitive assays is 0.02 ng/mL)

Radiological examination

Radiographs of the chest may reveal metastases in either the lung fields or the ribs. An abdominal radiograph may show the characteristic sclerotic metastases in lumbar vertebrae and pelvic bones (Figure 78.22). The bone appears dense and coarse, and it is sometimes difficult to distinguish the change from that in Paget's disease of bone. Nevertheless, osteolytic metastases are very common in prostate cancer and may coexist with sclerotic ones. Information about the upper urinary tracts can be obtained by excretion urography or ultrasound.

Cross-sectional imaging with magnetic resonance imaging and TRUS

MRI with a high tesla magnet (1.5–3 T) is the most accurate method of staging local disease In order to characterise prostate cancer a combination of imaging sequences must be interpreted (mp-MRI). mp-MRI consists of T2-weighted imaging combined with several functional sequences including diffusion-weighted imaging, perfusion or dynamic contrast-enhanced imaging and spectroscopic imaging. The accuracy of mp-MRI in localising and staging prostate cancer shows a high degree of variation between reporting radiologists. mp-MRI is used preoperatively to assess pelvic lymph nodes as well as local stage, although the sensitivity of mp-MRI to detect small areas of capsular spread is limited, even in the best hands. As well as preoperative staging, mp-MRI plays an important role in active surveillance and localisation of recurrent prostate cancer after surgery. Low-grade tumours are frequently not seen on MRI, which is useful as these low-grade tumours are often clinically insignificant.

Transrectal ultrasound scanning can also be used to stage prostate cancer. Locally extensive disease (T2) can be diagnosed with increased sensitivity by TRUS (see Figure 78.18) compared with rectal examination, but many tumours will still be missed. This problem remains a real one in screening for early prostate cancer; in comparison with breast cancer, with mammography detecting 70–80% of tumours, TRUS plus rectal examination and measurement of PSA will detect only 30–50% of cancers that are known to be present on autopsy studies (although it may detect the larger, more significant cancers).

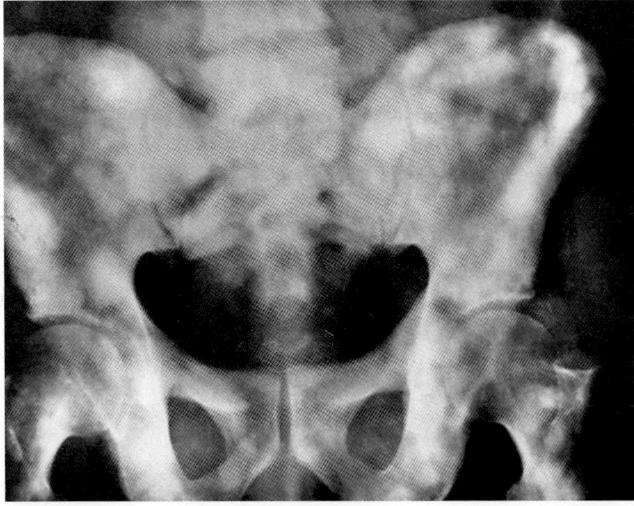

Figure 78.22 Osseous metastases of the pelvic bones in carcinoma of the prostate (courtesy of LN Pyrah, Leeds, UK).

Bone scan

Once the diagnosis has been established, if metastatic spread is suspected (on the basis of a high PSA [>10 ng/mL], locally advanced disease or presence of Gleason 7 or higher) a bone scan should be carried out. If however the PSA is <10 ng/mL, then a bone scan would be performed only on clinical indications. The bone scan is performed by the injection of technetium-99m, which is then monitored using a gamma camera. It is more sensitive in the diagnosis of metastases (Figure 78.23) than a skeletal survey, but false positives occur in areas of arthritis, osteomyelitis or a healing fracture.

Treatment

Patients are counselled on their treatment options based on an estimated risk of a localised cancer spreading and causing death. The strongest risk factors for metastasis are PSA level, Gleason grade and clinical stage.

Early disease

Curative treatment can only be offered to patients with early disease. Low risk prostate cancer (low PSA, small foci of Gleason 6 disease) can be managed by active surveillance. Here, with 3- to 6-monthly digital rectal examination (DRE) and PSA measurement and repeated prostate biopsy, a proportion can safely avoid the toxicity of radical treatment. However, one-third of patients embarking on this approach will require radical treatment within a few years. The options available for T1, T2 or some T3 disease need to take into account patient

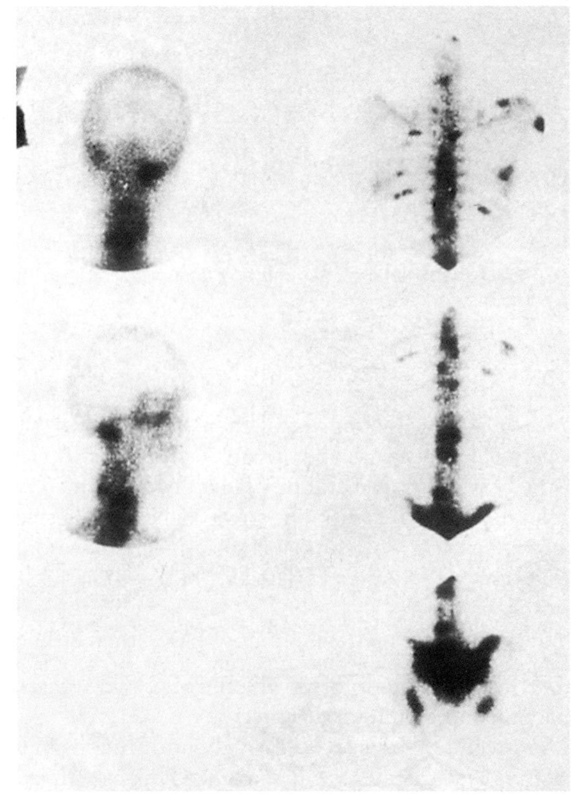

Figure 78.23 Bone scan showing multiple hot-spots suggestive of metastatic disease in a man with prostate cancer.

age, performance status and lifestyle preferences. The treatment of patients with advanced disease (T4 or any nodal or distant metastases) is only palliative.

Summary box 78.9

Treatment and stage

- Treatment options for prostate cancer depend on stage of disease, life expectancy of the patient and patient preference
- Prostate-specific antigen, digital rectal examination and biopsy Gleason grade are used to predict pathological stage
- Localised cancer can be treated by radical prostatectomy, radiation therapy and active monitoring
- Treatment of advanced disease is palliative, and hormone ablation remains the first-line therapy

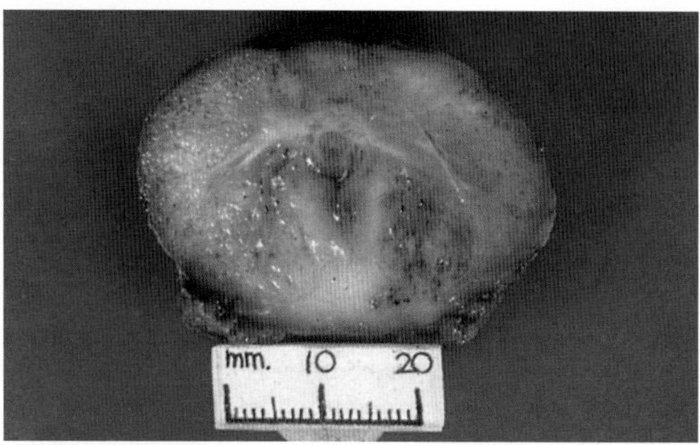

Figure 78.24 Radical prostatectomy specimen for a T2a prostate cancer. Preoperative prostate-specific antigen was 6 ng/mL; postoperative levels remained undetectable at 8 years. The patient is fully continent.

Radical prostatectomy

Radical prostatectomy is suitable for localised disease and should be carried out only in men with a life expectancy of >10 years. A wide excision approach can give clear surgical margins in T3a disease. Exclusion of metastases would require a negative bone scan and MRI of the pelvis. It is a procedure that should be performed only by experienced surgeons when there is a high chance of cure. It results in a high incidence of impotence, but a low incidence of severe stress incontinence (<2%), which may require the fitting of an artificial urinary sphincter or urethral sling. It involves removal of the prostate down to the distal sphincter mechanism in addition to the seminal vesicles (Figure 78.24). The bladder neck is reconstituted and anastomosed to the urethra. Modifications to this operation by Walsh can lead to preservation of the neurovascular bundles that lie behind the prostate. This modification has led to the preservation of erectile function in about 60–70% of cases. Laparoscopic approaches to radical prostatectomy, often with robotic assistance, generate similar oncological results to the open approach with a more rapid recovery.

Radical radiotherapy for early prostate cancer

External beam radiotherapy (EBRT) can be administered in fields that conform to the contours of the prostate, thereby limiting exposure of adjacent tissues. Survival rates following the treatment of T1 and low-volume T2 disease are not greatly different from those following radical prostatectomy, although histological evidence of persistent tumour is found within the prostate in about 30% of treated patients. Patients with locally advanced disease (T3) may be treated by radiotherapy. The treatment requires the patient to attend hospital on a daily basis for between 4 and 6 weeks. Some local complications are inevitable, namely irritation of the bladder with urinary frequency, urgency and sometimes urge incontinence and similar problems affecting the rectum with diarrhoea and, occasionally, late radiation proctitis. Development of erectile dysfunction occurs less frequently than following radical prostatectomy, but is present in up to 30% of cases. EBRT is rendered more effective with a period of neoadjuvant and adjuvant androgen ablation, with its inherent effects on libido.

Brachytherapy

Under transrectal ultrasound guidance, radioactive seeds are permanently implanted into the prostate. A computer program converts accurate ultrasound measurements of the prostate gland to construct a plan of the gland. Under anaesthesia, the patient is placed in the lithotomy position and, according to the template plan, seeds are placed through transperineal needles. The radioisotopes commonly used are iodine-125 and palladium-103. These isotopes deliver an intense, confined radiation dose, which falls off rapidly to spare the surrounding structures. Brachytherapy is gaining widespread acceptance for the treatment of lower grade low-volume T1 disease. A major factor is the reduced peroperative complications and generally low morbidity. Long-term cancer survival results from institutions specialising in the procedure are encouraging.

Advanced disease

There is still debate about the timing of androgen ablation treatment in patients with locally advanced or metastatic disease without symptoms. The options are androgen deprivation at diagnosis or careful review, reserving active treatment for the later development of symptoms. Patients with poorly differentiated disease are at risk of a catastrophic event such as spinal cord compression; in these patients, early androgen ablation can prolong the time to complications. Also, patients with local or general symptoms should be offered androgen deprivation.

Patrick C Walsh, Professor of Urology, Johns Hopkins Hospital, Baltimore, MD, USA, recipient of 2007 National Physician of the Year Clinical Excellence Award.

Orchidectomy

Orchidectomy is performed in advanced disease. In 1941, prostate cancer was shown to be responsive to such treatment by Charles Huggins, the only urologist to win a Nobel Prize. Bilateral orchidectomy, whether total or subcapsular, will eliminate the major source of testosterone production.

Medical castration

Medical forms of androgen ablation have been available since the discovery of stilbestrol. The other commonly available treatments to reduce testosterone levels to the castrate range are LHRH agonists. These agents initially stimulate hypothalamic LHRH receptors but, because of their constant presence (rather than the normal diurnal rhythm), they then downregulate them, resulting in cessation of pituitary LH production and, hence, a decrease in testosterone production. In the first 10 days or so, serum testosterone levels may increase, and it is wise to give flutamide, bicalutamide or cyproterone acetate for this period. LHRH agonists may be given by monthly, 3-monthly or 6-monthly depot injection. Other treatments that block the androgen receptor have become available recently. Cyproterone acetate also has some progestogenic effect, while flutamide and bicalutamide are pure antiandrogen. In general, oral antiandrogen monotherapy has not been shown to be as good as LHRH agonists or orchidectomy. Androgen ablation can be administered in an intermittent fashion governed by serum PSA levels.

Recently agents such as enzalutamide (a second generation androgen receptor blocker), degarelix (an LHRH antagonist), abiraterone (a drug that blocks the production of testosterone from its precursors) and taxane chemotherapy have all been shown to promote survival in metastatic prostate cancer. Many clinical trials are underway to ascertain which drugs should be used in which patients and the therapeutic landscape is changing rapidly.

General radiotherapy

Radiotherapy for symptomatic metastases is an excellent form of palliative treatment, often producing dramatic pain relief in men with hormone-relapsed prostate cancer that can last up to 6 months. When multiple sites are involved, intravenous radiopharmaceuticals such as strontium-89 can be employed. Strontium is a bone-seeking isotope that delivers effective radiotherapy to metastatic areas. It appears to be as effective as hemibody irradiation in the treatment of men with metastatic hormone-relapsed disease; however, the duration of response has been disappointing.

Chemotherapy

Cytotoxic agents in the treatment of these men have proved disappointing, but whether this is because the tumour is inherently insensitive or because these elderly men will not tolerate effective doses is uncertain. Trials of docetaxel and carbitaxel have shown improvements in survival, but only by a few months in end-stage castrate-resistant prostate cancer. Recent data suggest better results when used earlier in the natural history of advanced prostate cancer.

Summary of treatment for carcinoma of the prostate

- **Low risk disease**. For men in their 70s, conservative treatment would usually be the correct approach. Radical surgical treatment might be considered in the younger (<70 years) man with this form of the disease, although even in this group, some men will elect to pursue a conservative course when counselled about risks versus benefits.
- **Intermediate risk disease**. In younger, fitter men (<70 years), this may be treated by radical prostatectomy or radical radiotherapy. Active monitoring remains an option, particularly for more elderly patients towards the lower end of the risk spectrum. In the elderly patient with outflow obstruction, transurethral resection with or without hormone therapy is indicated. The benefit of radical treatment over a conservative approach is likely to be about 25%, given that progression to metastatic disease is of this order of magnitude after 10 years.
- **High risk disease**. These patients are at significant risk of disease progression. Early androgen ablation is favoured if close follow-up is not possible. For the sexually active, a careful conservative approach with the adoption of androgen ablation when symptoms arise is reasonable. Androgen ablation coupled with radiotherapy, perhaps with surgery as part of a multimodal approach, is standard treatment for younger men with T3 disease.
- **Metastatic disease**. Once metastases have developed, the outlook is poor. For patients with symptoms, there is no dilemma; androgen ablation will provide symptomatic relief in over two-thirds of patients. For patients with asymptomatic metastases, the timing of treatment is less clear. Systemic chemotherapy with docetaxel should be considered in younger, fitter men.

PROSTATITIS

In both acute and chronic prostatitis, the seminal vesicles and posterior urethra are usually also involved.

Acute prostatitis

Aetiology

Acute prostatitis is common, but underdiagnosed. The usual organism responsible is *Escherichia coli*, but *Staphylococcus aureus*, *Staphylococcus albus*, *Streptococcus faecalis*, *Neisseria gonorrhoeae* or *Chlamydia* may be responsible. The infection may be haematogenous from a distant focus or it may be secondary to acute urinary infection.

Charles Brenton Huggins, 1901–1997, Canadian born, Professor of Surgery, The University of Chicago, IL, USA, shared the 1966 Nobel Prize for Physiology or Medicine for his discoveries concerning hormonal treatment of prostate cancer.

Clinical features

General manifestations overshadow the local: the patient feels ill, shivers, may have a rigor, has 'aches' all over, especially in the back, and may easily be diagnosed as having influenza. The temperature may be up to 39°C. Pain on micturition is usual, but not invariable. The urine contains threads in the initial voided sample, which should be cultured. Perineal heaviness, rectal irritation and pain on defaecation can occur; a urethral discharge is rare. Frequency occurs when the infection involves the bladder. Rectal examination reveals a tender prostate; one lobe may be swollen more than the other, and the seminal vesicles may be involved. A frankly fluctuant abscess is uncommon.

Treatment

Treatment must be rigorous and prolonged or the infection will not be eradicated and recurrent attacks may ensue. Spread of infection to the epididymides and testes may occur. Prolonged treatment with an antibiotic that penetrates the prostate well is indicated (trimethoprim or ciprofloxacin).

Prostatic abscess

In addition to the foregoing symptoms and signs, the advent of a prostatic abscess is heralded by the temperature rising steeply with rigors. Antibiotics disguise these features. Severe, unremitting perineal and rectal pain with occasional tenesmus often cause the condition to be confused with an anorectal abscess. Nevertheless, if a rectal examination is performed, the prostate will be felt to be enlarged, hot, extremely tender and perhaps fluctuant. TRUS or MRI may aid diagnosis. Retention of urine is likely to occur and, in such men, suprapubic catheterisation is best.

Treatment

The abscess should be drained without delay by perurethral resection (unroofing the whole cavity) or using a needle via the transrectal or perineal route.

Chronic prostatitis

Many urologists find the diagnosis of chronic prostatitis and 'prostatodynia' very difficult, for many men present with perigenital pain, testicular pain, prostatic pain exacerbated by sexual intercourse or pain that apparently renders sexual intercourse out of the question. Psychosexual dysfunction in such patients may be the underlying problem. The diagnosis of chronic prostatitis has to be based on:

- persistent threads in voided urine;
- prostatic massage showing pus cells with or without bacteria in the absence of urinary infection.

Aetiology

This is thought to be the sequela of inadequately treated acute prostatitis. While pus is present in the prostatic secretion, the responsible organism is often difficult to find. Other organisms such as *Chlamydia* species may be responsible for chronic abacterial prostatitis.

Clinical features

The clinical features are extremely varied. Only men with symptoms of posterior urethritis, prostatic pain and perigenital pain accompanied by intermittent fever and pus cells or bacteria in the post-prostatic massage specimen should be diagnosed as having chronic prostatitis.

Diagnosis

The three-glass urine test is valuable. If the first glass with the initial voided sample shows urine containing prostatic threads, prostatitis is present.

Rectal examination of the prostate may be normal or may show a soft, boggy and tender prostate.

Examination of the prostatic fluid obtained by prostatic massage should show pus cells and bacteria.

Urethroscopy may reveal inflammation of the prostatic urethra, and pus may be seen exuding from the prostatic ducts. The verumontanum is likely to be enlarged and oedematous. In many men with the symptoms described above, all investigations are normal.

Treatment

Antibiotic therapy should be administered only in accordance with bacteriological sensitivity tests. Trimethoprim or ciprofloxacin penetrate well into the prostate. If *Trichomonas* or anaerobes are the responsible agent, a rapid response is obtained from administration of metronidazole (200 mg t.d.s. for 7 days to both partners). If *Chlamydia* is suspected, doxycycline is the antibiotic treatment of choice. There is little evidence that prostatic massage helps in eradicating the infection.

Prostatodynia

This diagnosis is made by the presence of perigenital pain in the absence of any objective evidence of prostatic inflammation. Whether the syndrome has any relationship with the prostate is unclear. The syndrome is part of the chronic pelvic pain syndrome spectrum.

TUBERCULOSIS OF THE PROSTATE AND SEMINAL VESICLES

Tuberculosis of the prostate and seminal vesicles is rare and associated with renal tuberculosis. In 30% of cases, there is a history of pulmonary tuberculosis within 5 years of the onset of genital tuberculosis.

Tuberculosis of one or both seminal vesicles may be found when examining a patient with chronic tuberculous epididymitis, no symptoms being referable to the internal genitalia. On rectal examination, the affected vesicle is found to be nodular.

When the prostate is involved, rectal examination reveals nodules in one or both lateral lobes. Patients with tuberculous prostatitis usually present with the following:

- urethral discharge;
- painful, sometimes blood-stained, ejaculation;

- mild ache in the perineum;
- infertility;
- dysuria;
- abscess formation.

Special forms of investigation

Radiography sometimes displays areas of calcification in the prostate and/or the seminal vesicles. Bacteriological examination of the seminal fluid yields positive cultures for tubercle bacilli.

Treatment

The general treatment is that for tuberculosis. If a prostatic abscess forms, it should be drained transurethrally.

SEMINAL VESICLES

Acute seminal vesiculitis

Acute seminal vesiculitis occurs in association with prostatitis. Prior to the antibiotic treatment of gonorrhoea, gonococcal vesiculitis was common.

Chronic seminal vesiculitis

Chronic seminal vesiculitis usually presents with haematospermia and pain on intercourse. TRUS demonstrates the features of distension and thickening and the presence of turbid fluid. The treatment is the same as for chronic prostatitis.

Tuberculous seminal vesiculitis

The clinical features and treatment have been discussed above.

Diverticulum of the seminal vesicle

Diverticulum of the seminal vesicle occurs occasionally. In such cases, the kidney of that side is absent and the diverticulum represents an abortive ureteric bud. It is a cause of persistent infection.

Cyst of the seminal vesicle

A cyst of the seminal vesicle is uncommon and rarely requires treatment. It may be removed by dissection through an incision similar to that for perineal prostatectomy if it is large or giving rise to symptoms.

FURTHER READING

Mundy AR, Fitzpatrick J, Neal DE, George NJ (eds). *The scientific basis of urology*, 3rd edn. London: Informa Healthcare, 2010.

Scardino PT, Linehan WM, Zelefsky MJ, Vogelzang NJ. (2012) *Comprehensive textbook of genitourinary oncology*, 4th edn. Philadelphia: Lippincott Williams & Wilkins,

Wein AJ, Kavoussi LR, Partin AW, Peters CA. *Campbell-Walsh urology*, 11th edn. Philadelphia: Elsevier, 2015.

Chapter 79

Urethra and penis

Learning objectives

To recognise and understand:

- The common congenital abnormalities of the urethra
- The diagnosis and management of urethral trauma
- The diagnosis and management of urethral stricture
- The diagnosis and management of phimosis
- The principles of management of a man with erectile dysfunction
- The common diseases of the penis and urethra and the principles of their surgical management

THE MALE URETHRA

Anatomy

The male urethra is a tubular structure extending from the bladder neck to the external urinary meatus at the tip of the glans penis. It has four components, which are named (from proximal to distal) the prostatic, membranous, bulbar and penile urethra. The prostatic urethra extends from the bladder neck to the verumontanum and is compressed on either side by the lateral lobes of the prostate, giving it a slit-like configuration. The verumontanum is a small hillock of tissue indented at its crown by a pit called the utriculus masculinus, which marks the proximal extent of the external urethral sphincter and is an important landmark for urologists performing transurethral resection of the prostate. The membranous urethra lies just distal to the verumontanum and is located where the urethra penetrates the pelvic floor and it is the usual site of urethral rupture at the time of a pelvic fracture. It is the primary location of continence as a consequence of the surrounding pelvic floor musculature and external urethral sphincter. The bulbar urethra extends from the membranous urethra to the penoscrotal junction and is anteriorly located within the corpus spongiosum. The penile urethra is normally flattened anteroposteriorly but distends when filled with fluid. The urethral lining changes from transitional cell epithelium proximally to stratified squamous cell epithelium distally.

The external urethral sphincter is composed of circular striated muscle within the urethral wall. It is innervated by the pudendal nerve, originating from spinal segments S2, 3 and 4. The bladder neck contributes to maintenance of continence in the man, although its main role is as a genital sphincter that closes at the time of ejaculation. Its innervation originates in the spinal segments T10–12 with sympathetic innervation mediated by release of noradrenaline via alpha adrenoceptors.

Congenital abnormalities

Posterior urethral valves

Posterior urethral valves occur in around 1 in 5000–8000 live male births. The valves are membranes that have a small posterior slit within them, which typically lie just distal to the verumontanum and cause obstruction to the urethra of boys. They function as flap valves and so although they are obstructive to antegrade urinary flow, a urethral catheter can be passed retrogradely without any difficulty.

DIAGNOSIS

Posterior urethral valves need to be detected and treated as early as possible to minimise the degree of renal failure. The presentation varies according to the severity of the obstruction. The more severe the obstruction, the earlier the presentation. Diagnosis is most commonly made antenatally with ultrasound, which demonstrates bilateral hydronephrosis above a distended bladder.

If the diagnosis is not made antenatally, then babies typically present with urinary infection in the neonatal period or with uraemia and renal failure.

Rarely the valves are incomplete and the patient is symptom free until adolescence or adulthood, when again urinary infection or renal impairment can supervene.

Investigation will involve a voiding cystogram, with the dilatation of the urethra above the valves demonstrable on a voiding cystogram (**Figure 79.1**). The bladder is hypertrophied and often shows diverticula. Typically, there is vesicoureteric reflux into dilated upper tracts. The valves themselves can be difficult to see on urethroscopy because the flow of

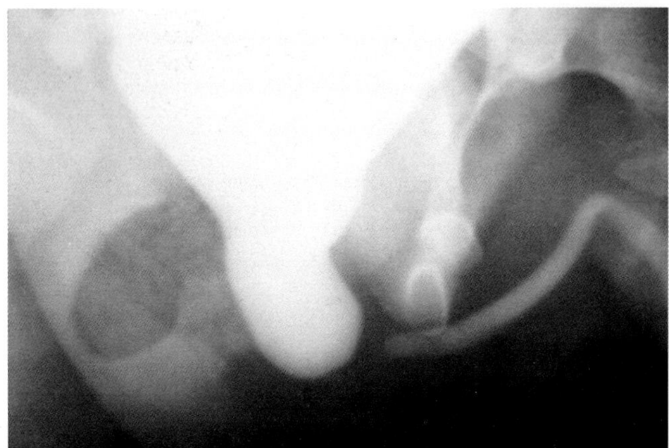

Figure 79.1 A voiding cystogram showing a dilated bladder with a dilated prostatic urethra above an obstruction at the level of the posterior urethral valve.

irrigant sweeps them into the open position. Renal function is usually impaired, albeit to a varying degree, and the extent is further assessed by measurement of ultrasound scanning, which will assess the renal cortical thickness, and renography to assess differential renal function.

TREATMENT

Initial treatment is by catheterisation to relieve the obstruction and to allow the effects of renal failure to improve. Definitive treatment is by endoscopic destruction of the valves with continuing lifelong supportive treatment of the dilated urinary tract, the recurrent urinary infections and the uraemia.

Summary box 79.1

Posterior urethral valves

- Posterior urethral valves are congenital membranes that cause obstruction to the urinary tract in baby boys
- Antenatal ultrasound typically shows urinary tract dilatation
- If not recognised antenatally, they may cause recurrent urinary infection, urinary retention and uraemia
- Treatment is valve destruction accompanied by treatment of urinary infection and renal impairment

Hypospadias (see also Chapter 9)

Hypospadias occurs in around 1 in 200–300 male live births and is the most common congenital abnormality of the urethra. There are three characteristic features. The external meatus opens on the underside of the penis anywhere from just short of the normal site as far back as the perineum, while the ventral aspect of the prepuce is poorly developed (the 'hooded prepuce') and there is usually a ventral deformity of the erect penis (chordee).

Hypospadias is classified according to the position of the meatus (Figure 79.2):

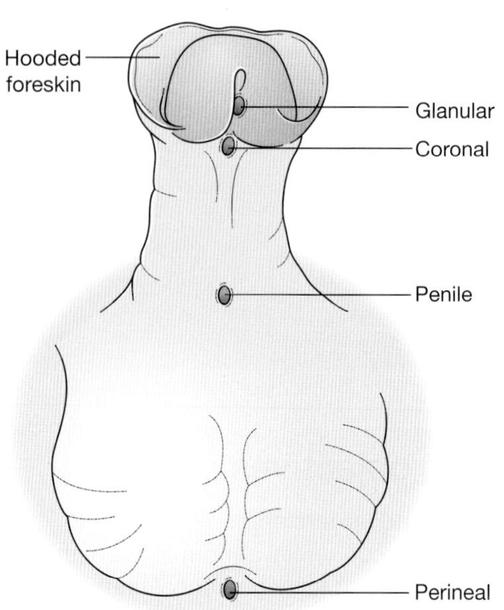

Figure 79.2 Hypospadias classification.

- Glanular hypospadias. The ectopic meatus is placed on the glans penis, but proximal to the normal site of the external meatus, which is marked by a blind pit. Occasionally the two are connected by a channel.
- Coronal hypospadias. The meatus is placed at the junction of the underside of the glans and the body of the penis.
- Penile and penoscrotal hypospadias. The meatus is on the underside of the penile shaft.
- Perineal hypospadias. This is the rarest and most severe abnormality. The scrotum is bifid and the urethra opens between its two halves. In children with severe hypospadias it is important to consider disorders of sexual development, which are usually associated with testicular maldescent and micropenis.

The more severe varieties of hypospadias represent an absence of the urethra and corpus spongiosum distal to the ectopic opening. The absent structures are represented by a fibrous cord, which deforms the erect penis in a downward direction (chordee).

TREATMENT

Hypospadias does not cause either obstruction or urinary tract infection. Surgery is indicated to improve sexual function, to correct problems with the urinary stream and for cosmetic reasons. A variety of plastic surgical procedures have been described to correct the chordee and to re-site the urethral opening. The commonest procedure for distal hypospadias is the 'tubularised incised plate' urethroplasty, while techniques that utilise the foreskin are commonly used for more proximal hypospadias. Circumcision should be avoided, therefore, before the hypospadias has been repaired. Operations for hypospadias are best performed by a paediatric urologist and are typically undertaken before the age of 18 months.

Epispadias

Epispadias is very rare. In penile epispadias, the urethral opening is on the dorsum of the penis and is associated with an upward curvature of the erect penis (Figure 79.3). Epispadias often coexists with bladder exstrophy and other severe developmental defects.

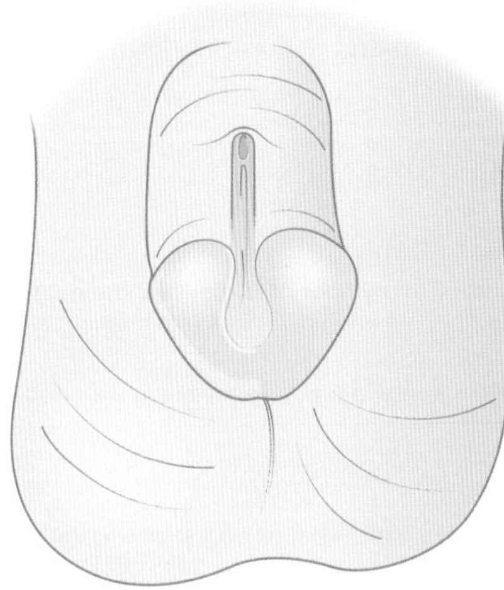

Figure 79.3 Epispadias.

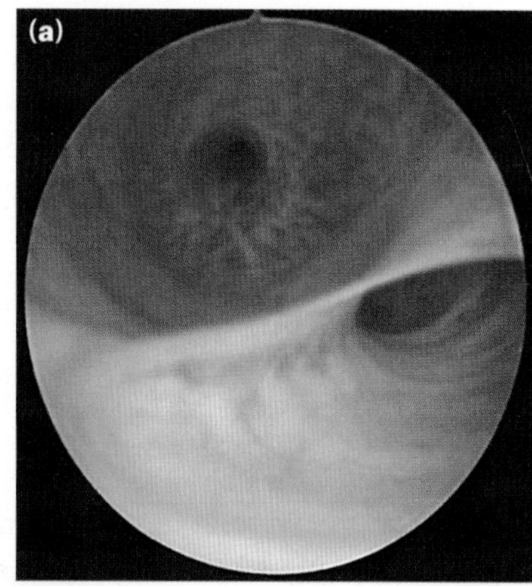

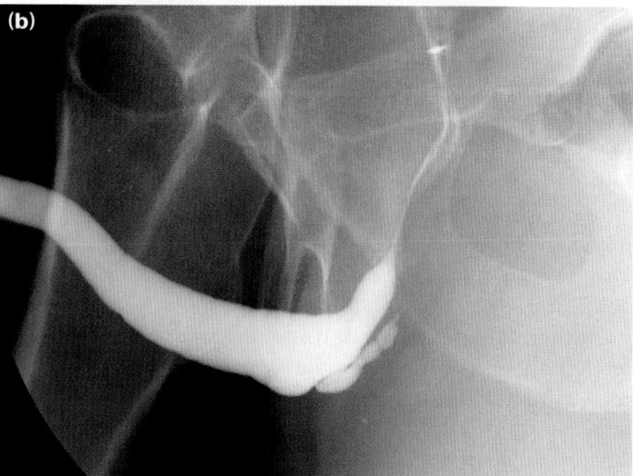

Figure 79.4 Urethral diverticulum. (a) Cystoscopic appearance of a urethral diverticulum. The normal urethra can be seen to extend superiorly to the urethral sphincter, while the blind ending diverticulum is seen inferiorly. (b) Urethrogram showing a urethral diverticulum.

Summary box 79.2

Hypospadias

- Hypospadias is characterised by the combination of a ventrally placed urethral meatus, a hooded foreskin and chordee
- In severe cases with coexisting testicular maldescent and micropenis, consider disorders of sexual development (intersex) as a diagnosis
- Avoid circumcision as the prepuce may be used in procedures to correct the abnormality
- Surgical treatment should be undertaken by a paediatric urologist

Urethral diverticulum

This is usually congenital and represents a partial duplication of the urethra. Acquired cases are uncommon but are sometimes seen as a result of increased intraurethral pressure behind a stricture. Others are caused by the longstanding presence of a foreign body such as a stone or calculus in the urethra. Typically, patients present in adult life with a history of postmicturition dribbling and diagnosis is made at cystoscopy (Figure 79.4a) or via a urethrogram (Figure 79.4b). Treatment is often unnecessary, but they can be treated endoscopically by incising the flap of urethral mucosa between the two lumens or, in severe cases, by excision of the diverticulum.

Injuries to the male urethra

The commonest cause of urethral trauma is that which occurs at the time of instrumentation, either with a catheter or with a cystoscope. Prevention is therefore the most important issue here, with the need for careful urethral instrumentation being paramount. Typically, when such an injury does occur it tends to happen either where the urethra bends or where it narrows. Such injuries initially result in bleeding and typically heal by scarring, which then results in a urethral stricture. The commonest sites of such strictures are the submeatal area, the bulbar urethra or the region of the membranous urethra.

Injuries following external trauma are much less common, but require appropriate and prompt management. The most common sites for such injury are the bulbar urethra and the membranous urethra.

Rupture of the bulbar urethra

There is a history of a blow to the perineum, usually due to a fall astride injury. The bulbar urethra is crushed upwards onto the pubic bone, typically with significant bruising. In the days of sailing ships, the common cause was falling astride a spar and the modern equivalent is seen among workers losing their footing on scaffolding. Cycling accidents, loose manhole covers and gymnasium accidents astride the beam account for a number of cases. Almost certainly King William I of England died in 1087 following a ruptured bulbar urethra. It was written that 'his horse reared in fright at a blazing timber and threw its ponderous rider against the iron of his saddle', suggesting that he ruptured the urethra on the saddle's pommel. He subsequently developed urinary retention and sepsis secondary to infection of the haematoma and he died some days after the accident.

Extravasation of urine is common if the urine is not diverted and the extravasated urine is confined in front of the mid-perineal point by the attachment of Colles' fascia to the triangular ligament and by the attachment of Scarpa's fascia just below the inguinal ligament. The external spermatic fascia stops it getting into the inguinal canals. Extravasated urine collects in the scrotum and penis and beneath the deep layer of superficial fascia in the abdominal wall.

CLINICAL FEATURES

The signs of a ruptured bulbar urethra are perineal bruising and haematoma, typically with a butterfly distribution. There is usually bleeding from the urethral meatus and retention of urine is also typically present.

MANAGEMENT

If the diagnosis is suspected, the patient should be treated with appropriate analgesia and antibiotics should be administered. He should be discouraged from passing urine. A full bladder should be drained with a catheter placed by percutaneous suprapubic puncture using a Seldinger technique (Figure 79.5). This reduces urinary extravasation and allows investigations to establish the extent of the urethral injury. Diagnosis is made by urethrography using water-soluble contrast.

If there is significant extravasation, then the perineal collection should be drained. The suprapubic catheter should remain *in situ* while the bruising and extravasation settle down and a stricture will typically develop at the site of the injury. The optimal treatment is delayed anastomotic urethroplasty after the swelling and bruising have settled down (typically 8–12 weeks later), with excision of the traumatised section and spatulated end-to-end reanastomosis of the urethra.

Summary box 79.3

Bulbar urethral injury

- Suspect urethral injury after blunt perineal trauma when the man cannot void, when there is perineal bruising and when there is blood at the urethral meatus
- Diagnosis is made by urethrography using water-soluble contrast
- The safest initial management is to insert a suprapubic catheter
- Beware of urinary extravasation and sepsis in the perineal haematoma
- Delayed urethroplasty is the preferred definitive management of complete disruptions

Rupture of the membranous urethra

Rupture of the membranous urethra typically occurs in association with a fractured pelvis and may be associated with an extraperitoneal rupture of the bladder. When the pelvis fractures, the membranous urethra is ruptured as it passes through the bony ring of the pelvis. The urethra is elastic at this point, and if the fracture results in only a minor displacement, then the tear may only be partial, but more typically the rupture is complete, such that the two ends are completely displaced,

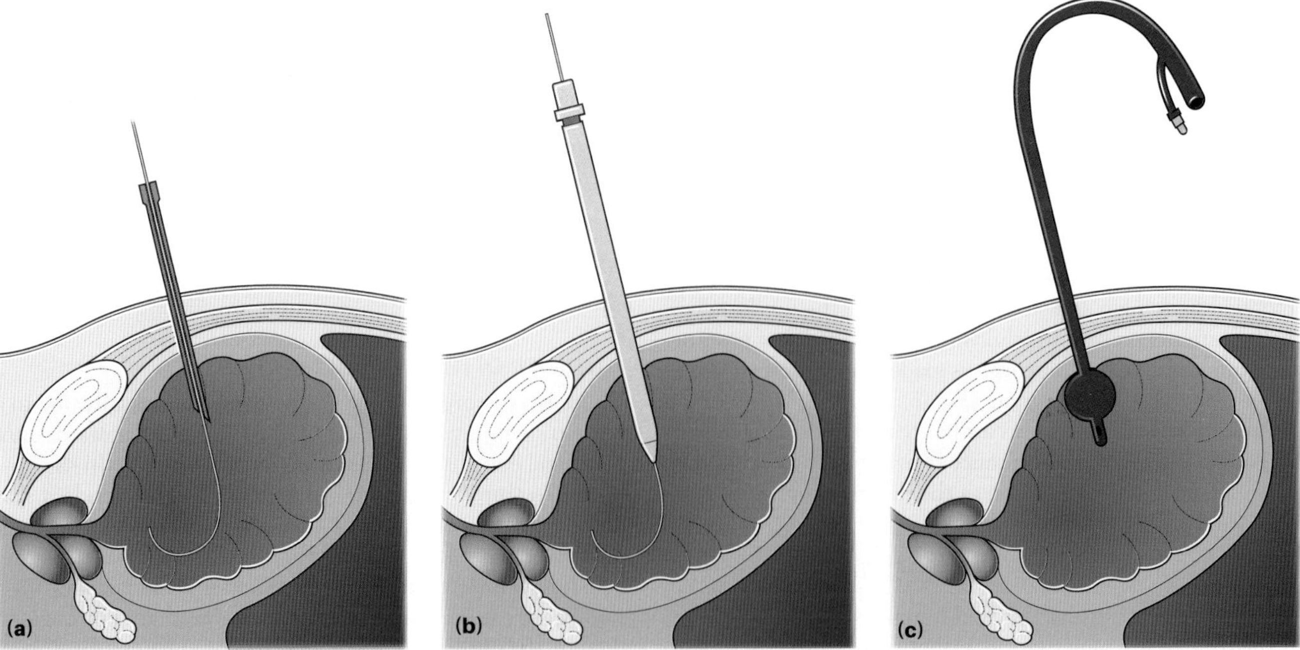

Figure 79.5 (a) Percutaneous puncture of the bladder with passage of a guidewire into the bladder followed by dilatation of the track over the guidewire (b), thereby allowing placement of a catheter into the bladder (c).

Abraham Colles, 1773–1843, Professor of Surgery, The Royal College of Surgeons in Ireland, and surgeon, Dr. Stevens' Hospital, Dublin, Ireland.
Antonio Scarpa, 1747–1832, Professor of Anatomy, Pavia, Italy.
Sven Ivar Seldinger, 1921–1998, Swedish radiologist, introduced the Seldinger technique to obtain safe access to blood vessels and other hollow organs.

with the development of a significant interposing haematoma. About 1–2% of cases of fractured pelvis have an associated urethral injury and such injuries are almost universally seen in men.

CLINICAL FEATURES

The most common causes of pelvic fracture are road traffic accidents, severe crush injuries and falls. Typically there are multiple associated injuries that may be immediately life threatening and the overriding priority is to keep the patient alive by appropriate resuscitation. Under these circumstances the management of the other injuries takes precedence.

The clinical features include urinary retention, blood at the urethral meatus and a high riding prostate on digital rectal examination. There is typically marked bruising of the pubic area, scrotum and penis. If the diagnosis is suspected, a urethrogram performed with water-soluble contrast media is confirmatory (Figure 79.6).

A suprapubic catheter should be inserted as soon as practicable using the Seldinger technique. The distended bladder may be palpable, making suprapubic catheterisation straightforward, but often the bruising and swelling associated with the fracture makes this difficult and ultrasound guidance is required. When suprapubic urinary diversion has been achieved then no further urological management is required until the patient has stabilised.

In the presence of a coexisting extraperitoneal bladder injury, no bladder will be apparent on ultrasound examination, and surgical exploration, bladder repair, suprapubic catheter placement and drainage of the retropubic space is needed.

In a patient with a pelvic fracture who does not have blood at the urethral meatus but who has not yet passed urine (such that there is uncertainty as to whether there is a urethral injury), a single, gentle attempt at catheterization, by an experienced doctor, is permissible. In adults a 16F soft, silicone catheter should be used. If the catheter will not pass or passes and drains only blood, the balloon should not be inflated, but the catheter should be withdrawn and a retrograde urethrogram should be performed.

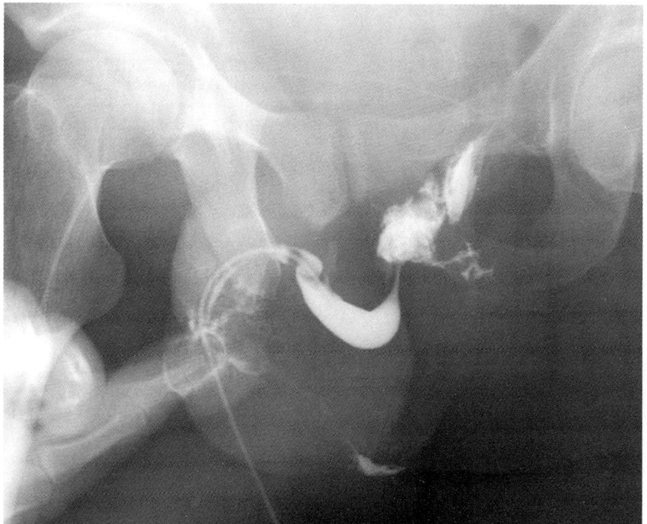

Figure 79.6 An ascending urethrogram demonstrating extravasation of contrast from the membranous urethra at the site of a urethral injury. Note the associated pelvic fracture with disruption of the inferior pubic rami.

COMPLICATIONS

Urethral disruption injury The two ends of the urethra, having been torn apart, become separated by a haematoma. With time, this haematoma resolves and is replaced by fibrosis. This pelvic fracture urethral disruption injury is technically not a stricture of the urethra but is often, erroneously, described as being one. The conventional management of such an injury is delayed surgical reconstruction with excision of the scar tissue and end-to-end anastomosis. This surgery should be delayed until the patient has recovered from any other injuries and is usually undertaken 3–6 months later. It is a highly challenging technical procedure and should be undertaken only in specialist centres. Some surgeons continue to undertake early attempts to realign the urethral ends endoscopically, and while there are some successful reports, most experts feel that there is an increased risk of sepsis, (true) stricture, incontinence and erectile dysfunction (ED).

Urinary incontinence The site of the urethral rupture is at or close to the striated urethral sphincter. If the external urethral sphincter is damaged or destroyed, continence of urine will depend on the bladder neck mechanism. While this is usually adequate to maintain complete continence (only 5–10% of men suffer stress urinary incontinence after urethroplasty), subsequent surgical manoeuvres that destroy the bladder neck (such as transurethral prostatectomy) may cause incontinence.

Erectile dysfunction ED is common after pelvic fracture with urethral injury and is due to damage of either the cavernosal nerves, which innervate the penis, or the penile arteries, which also lie close to the site of the urethral disruption. Indeed, surgical treatment of the urethral disruption can itself cause ED by similar mechanisms. If this does occur, treatment is with an orally active agent such as sildenafil or if that fails, with intracavernosal prostaglandin injections, a vacuum device or a penile implant.

Orthopaedic For management of a fractured pelvis see Chapter 27.

Extravasation of urine This can occur with extraperitoneal rupture of the bladder, pelvic fracture urethral disruption or in the rare cases where the level of the disruption is the prostatic urethra. Urine extravasates in the layers of the pelvic fascia and the retroperitoneal tissues. Treatment is by suprapubic cystostomy. In rare cases where the extravasation persists despite the suprapubic tube, drainage of the retropubic space and definitive repair of the urethral, prostatic or bladder rupture is required.

Summary box 79.4

Pelvic fracture urethral disruption injury

- Suspect the diagnosis in cases of pelvic fracture, when the patient has not voided and when there is blood at the urethral meatus
- If the diagnosis is suspected, a water-soluble urethrogram is needed to confirm the diagnosis
- Initial management is insertion of a suprapubic catheter
- Immediate surgical exploration is needed if there is coexisting rupture of the bladder
- Delayed anastomotic urethroplasty is the preferred definitive management

Urethral stricture

CAUSES

The common causes of urethral stricture are:

- Inflammatory
  - Secondary to urethritis
  - Secondary to balanitis xerotica obliterans (BXO)
- Traumatic
  - Bulbar urethral injury
  - Pelvic fracture urethral disruption injury
- Iatrogenic
  - Secondary to urethral instrumentation including catheterisation and transurethral prostatectomy
  - Secondary to radical prostatectomy
  - Secondary to radiotherapy for prostate cancer
- Idiopathic

PATHOPHYSIOLOGY

Postinflammatory strictures are less common since the introduction of effective antibiotic treatment of gonorrhoea. The stricture is most commonly seen in the bulbar urethra but submeatal strictures also occur. There is infection in the periurethral glands, which persists after inadequately treated gonorrhoea. The infection spreads to cause a periurethritis, which heals by fibrosis. Most strictures appear within 1 year of infection but may not cause difficulty in micturition for some time later.

BXO is a rare condition characterised by fibrosis of the foreskin resulting in phimosis. In around 10% of cases the glans penis is also affected, causing meatal stenosis, and in a proportion of these cases there is also fibrosis and stricturing of the penile urethra. The cause of the condition is unknown, but the strictures produced are typically long and difficult to treat.

Post-traumatic strictures have been discussed previously.

Postinstrumentation strictures follow endoscopy or catheterisation and may affect any part of the urethra. Typically, when such an injury does occur it tends to happen either where the urethra bends or where it narrows. Such injuries initially result in bleeding and typically heal by scarring, which then results in a urethral stricture. The commonest sites of such strictures are the submeatal area, the bulbar urethra or the region of the membranous urethra. Some surgeons recommend prophylactic dilatation or urethrotomy before transurethral prostatectomy in order to try to avoid this complication. Some cases of stricture seem to be due to sensitivity to chemicals from a catheter, but most are the result of a combination of trauma, infection and pressure necrosis.

Bladder neck stenosis can occur following TURP and following radical prostatectomy for the treatment of prostate cancer. If it cannot be managed by dilatation, bladder neck stenosis should be treated by transurethral incision and resection of the stricture, although in the man who has undergone radical prostatectomy, this will result in urinary incontinence.

CLINICAL FEATURES

Symptoms are usually hesitancy of micturition, straining to void and a poor urinary stream. The relative youthfulness of the patient often rules out prostatic enlargement, which characteristically occurs after the age of 50. As the stream becomes narrower, micturition is prolonged and is followed by postmicturition dribbling as a result of urine trickling from the dilated urethra proximal to the stricture. Urinary frequency by day and night is common and is due to incomplete bladder emptying, coexisting detrusor overactivity or urinary infection.

If the stricture is tight enough, the patient will go into acute retention, although this is rare. If this happens, there is a danger that clumsy attempts to pass a urethral catheter will result in a false passage. If a patient has gone into retention because of a urethral stricture, its lumen will be too narrow to pass even a tiny catheter and suprapubic catheterisation is required.

Investigation involves uroflowmetry, urethroscopy, urethrography and ultrasound scanning to assess bladder emptying and to detect any upper tract dilatation. The urinary flow rate is typically prolonged and plateau shaped (Figure 79.7) while urethroscopy allows the stricture to be viewed

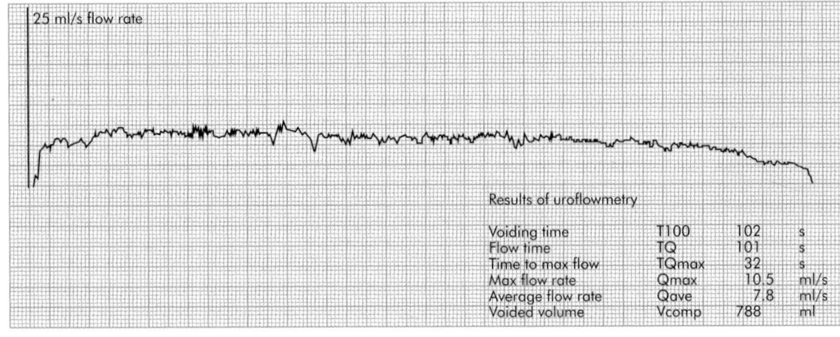

Figure 79.7 Urinary flow rate trace from a patient with a urethral stricture. Note the prolonged flow with the typical plateau shape of the curve.

as a circumferential scar (Figure 79.8). Openings of false passages commemorate previous misguided attempts to pass a urethral catheter. Urethrography using a water-soluble contrast medium will show the extent and severity of the stricture (Figures 79.9 and 79.10).

COMPLICATIONS

The commonest complication of a urethral stricture is urinary tract infections, which usually respond to antibiotic treatment, although there is a tendency for them to recur as a consequence of the increased residual urine within the bladder. Any of the complications of bladder outflow obstruction can occur, including bladder calculi and upper tract dilatation with renal impairment, although the latter is rare. Similarly, retention of urine is also rare and should be treated by suprapubic catheterisation. Rare complications include urethral diverticulum and paraurethral abscess.

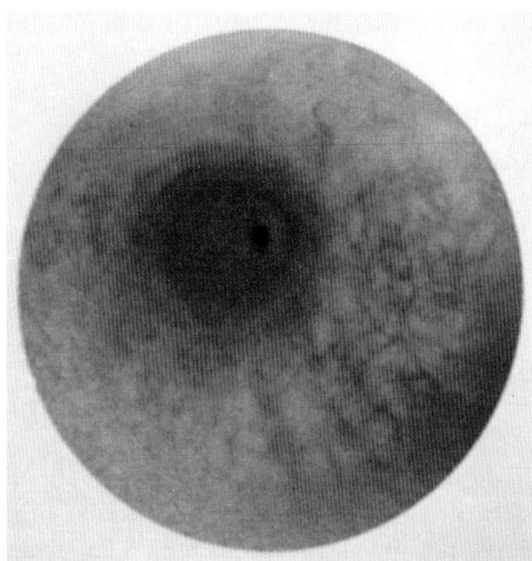

Figure 79.8 Urethroscopic appearance of a urethral stricture.

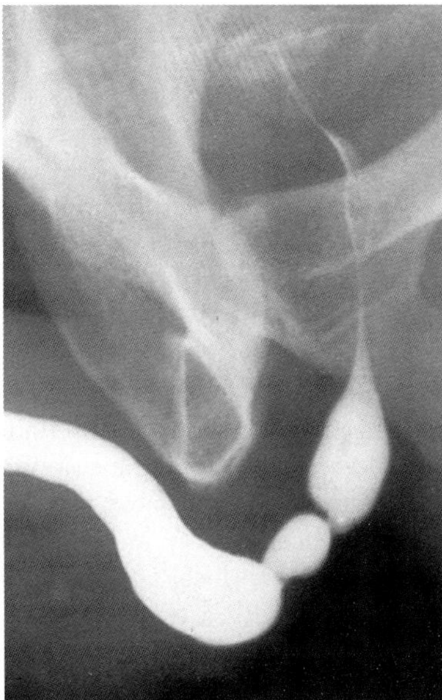

Figure 79.9 Ascending urethrogram showing urethral stricture of the bulbar urethra.

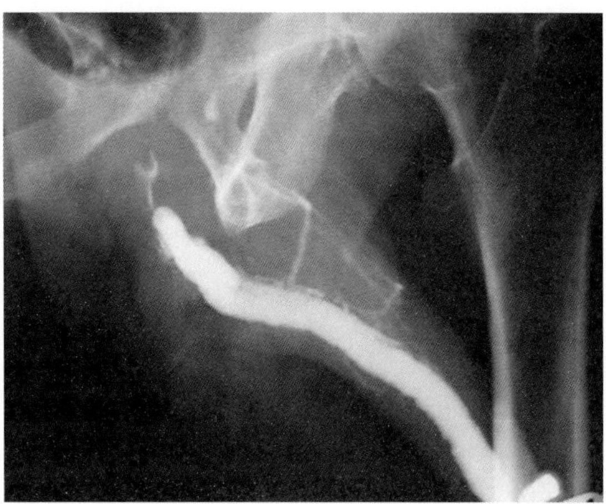

Figure 79.10 Gonorrhoeal stricture of the bulbar urethra. Note that some of the contrast has entered the penile veins.

Summary box 79.5

Diagnosis of urethral stricture

- Suspect the diagnosis of urethral stricture in a young man with poor urinary stream
- Diagnosis is made either by visualisation (urethroscopy) or radiologically (by urethrography)
- Urinary infection should be excluded

TREATMENT

The management of urethral strictures has changed considerably over the past 20 years. The old treatments of urethral dilatation have largely been superceded by endoscopic incision (internal urethrotomy) or by formal reconstruction (urethroplasty). Urethral dilatation still has a place in elderly men with short strictures that recur infrequently and when the stricture is intimately related to the continence mechanism (such as the bladder neck stricture that follows radical prostatectomy). In these patients, occasional dilatation may be preferable to more complex procedures.

In patients with recurrent strictures who are unable or unwilling to undergo urethroplasty, then intermittent self-dilatation with soft hydrophilic catheters on a regular (daily) basis can prevent stricture recurrence, although such self dilatation is needed lifelong.

Short strictures with a clear traumatic history should be treated by urethroplasty since cure rates in excess of 90% can be achieved by excision of the stricture with end-to-end anastamosis.

A conventional therapeutic algorithm, therefore, is to offer an internal urethrotomy to all newly diagnosed strictures (excluding post-traumatic strictures) and to reserve the more major urethroplasty procedures for recurrent strictures.

Urethral dilatation This is the old treatment for stricture. Under aseptic conditions, the urethra is stretched using graduated dilators. With care and gentleness the procedure can be performed under local urethral anaesthesia with lidocaine gel. It is performed 'blind', so there is always a danger of causing a false passage. This is most likely with an inexperienced operator unfamiliar with the complexities of an individual patient's urethra.

Endoscopic (internal) urethrotomy Internal urethrotomy is performed using the optical urethrotome. The stricture is cut under visual control using a knife passed through the sheath of a rigid urethroscope. The stricture is usually cut at the 12 o'clock position, taking care not to cut too deeply into the vascular spaces of the corpus spongiosum that surrounds the urethra. It is possible to get lost when trying to cut a way through a very tight stricture, and this is especially true when there are false passages because of previous dilatation attempts. Accordingly, a guidewire should be passed through to the bladder prior to incision of the stricture in order to establish the true lumen of the urethra. Following urethrotomy a catheter should be left *in situ* for 1–3 days afterwards.

A single urethrotomy seems to give a permanent cure of an uncomplicated stricture in about 50% of patients. Success rates are highest when the stricture is short and when it is present within the bulbar urethra. In contrast, failure rates are highest in long strictures, strictures within the penile urethra and in recurrent strictures. The main complications are infection and bleeding.

Urethroplasty The simplest urethroplasty involves excision of the stenosed length of urethra and reanastomosis of the spatulated cut ends. This operation is possible only if the stricture is relatively short, because there must be no tension at the suture line and it can only be performed where the urethra can be stretched, so it is not possible within the penile urethra. If an end-to-end anastomosis is not feasible, a large number of different surgical procedures can be used to reconstruct the fibrosed urethra. The operations typically utilise free grafts, usually of buccal mucosa, but also occasionally of penile skin, lingual mucosa and bladder mucosa. Buccal mucosa is in plentiful supply (approximately 6–7 cm can be obtained from each cheek), is tough with an excellent vascular plexus, is used to being wet and is associated with minimal donor site morbidity.

Urethroplasty should be considered when the stricture has arisen following trauma and when a stricture has recurred following endoscopic treatment. The actual technique used should depend on the site of the stricture, the length of the stricture and the cause of the stricture. Careful preoperative assessment with ascending and descending urethrography is vital.

Summary box 79.6

Treatment of urethral strictures

- Newly diagnosed strictures are best treated initially by internal urethrotomy, with a high short-term success rate and a 50% long-term success rate
- Intermittent self-dilatation increases the success rate of internal urethrotomy alone
- Urethroplasty should be considered in traumatic strictures and in recurrent strictures
- Urethral dilatation should be considered in strictures closely related to the external sphincter mechanism

Anastomotic urethroplasty has a success rate of around 90% while substitution urethroplasty has a success rate at 10 years of around 80%.

Other conditions of the urethra

Urethral fistula

The most frequent cause of urethral fistula is bursting or incision of a periurethral abscess. If the fistula arises behind a tight stricture, there may be multiple openings (watering-can perineum). A fistula can also follow urethroplasty if there is necrosis of part of the graft or flap. The stricture should be treated, after which case some fistulae heal themselves. Occasionally, formal urethroplasty is indicated.

Urethral calculi

Urethral calculi can arise primarily behind a stricture or in an infected urethral diverticulum. More commonly, the stone is a renal calculus that has migrated to the urethra via the bladder.

CLINICAL FEATURES

Migratory calculi cause sudden pain in the urethra soon after an attack of ureteric colic. There is blockage to the flow of urine and, if the stone is small, the force of the jet will usually expel it from the urethral meatus. Larger stones get stuck and must be removed endoscopically. It is sometimes possible to feel the calculus as a hard lump in the urethra, but if there is doubt the diagnosis is confirmed by urethroscopy.

TREATMENT

A stone lodged within the prostatic urethra should be displaced back into the bladder and treated by lithopaxy or suprapubic cystotomy as if it were a bladder stone. Calculi in more distal parts of the urethra are removed by basketing under vision or fragmented *in situ* using the electrohydraulic or ultrasonic lithotripter. It may be necessary to perform a meatotomy to deliver the stone. Open removal by external urethrotomy is rarely necessary.

Neoplasms

Polyps are a relatively common finding in the prostatic urethra, where they may result from chronic infection. Genital warts acquired by sexually transmitted infection are sometimes found in the anterior urethra as an extension of warts on the skin of the glans penis. Angioma of the urethra is a very rare cause of urethral bleeding.

Bloody urethral discharge without infection should raise the suspicion that the patient has a urethral tumour, although such tumours are rare. Multifocal transitional cell cancers of the bladder are sometimes associated with tumours in the prostatic urethra and occasionally more distally. Although superficial and susceptible to local ablation by diathermy or laser, they are associated with a tendency to distant spread. Squamous carcinoma can develop in an area of squamous metaplasia sometimes seen with a urethral stricture. It carries a poor prognosis even if the patient is treated by radical surgery.

THE FEMALE URETHRA

Anatomy

The female urethra is around 2–3 cm long, extending from the bladder neck to the external urethral meatus. Continence is maintained by the external striated urethral sphincter, which in women extends for almost the whole length of the urethra. There is extra support from the surrounding pelvic floor musculature. In contrast to men, the female bladder neck has little role in the maintenance of continence.

Abnormalities of the female urethra include:

- prolapse;
- stricture;
- Fowler's syndrome (dysfunction of the striated urethral sphincter);
- diverticulum;
- caruncle;
- papillomata acuminata;
- carcinoma.

Prolapse (syn: urethrocele)

Urethroceles reflect weakening of the tissues that hold the urethra in place, causing it to move and to put pressure on the vagina, leading to the prolapse of the anterior distal wall of the vagina. They typically occur in conjunction with prolapse of the bladder into the vagina (cystocele). Prolapse occurs in later life and is usually, in part, due to the trauma of childbirth. Prolapse of the urethral lining also occurs as a congenital abnormality, when it causes discomfort proportional to the degree of prolapse.

Stricture

Urethral strictures are uncommon in women but may follow urethritis or, more commonly, the trauma of a difficult labour. Urinary retention is an occasional consequence and is usually chronic. True strictures in women respond well to urethral dilatation.

Fowler's syndrome

This idiopathic condition, which was described by Fowler and Kirby, is associated with an abnormal myotonic discharge in the striated urethral sphincter that can be detected by sphincter electromyography. It is often associated with polycystic ovaries and causes urinary retention in women and should not be confused with a urethral stricture. Urethral dilatation is ineffective and the retention is best treated by intermittent self-catheterisation. There is some evidence that sacral neuromodulation can be effective.

Diverticulum

Urethral diverticula are more commonly seen in women than in men, but they are still rare. Some seem to be congenital while others are acquired by rupture of a distended urethral gland or injury of the urethra during childbirth. Urine within the diverticulum becomes infected, causing local pain and repeated bouts of cystitis. Purulent urine is discharged if the urethra is compressed with a finger placed in the vagina. Diagnosis is by magnetic resonace imaging (MRI) or by transvaginal ultrasound (Figure 79.11). Excision of the diverticulum through the anterior vaginal wall is effective, but care must be taken not to damage the urethral sphincter.

Caruncle

This is common in elderly women. It presents as a soft, raspberry-like, pedunculated granulomatous mass about the size of a pea, attached to the posterior urethral wall near the external meatus (Figure 79.12). It is composed of highly vascular

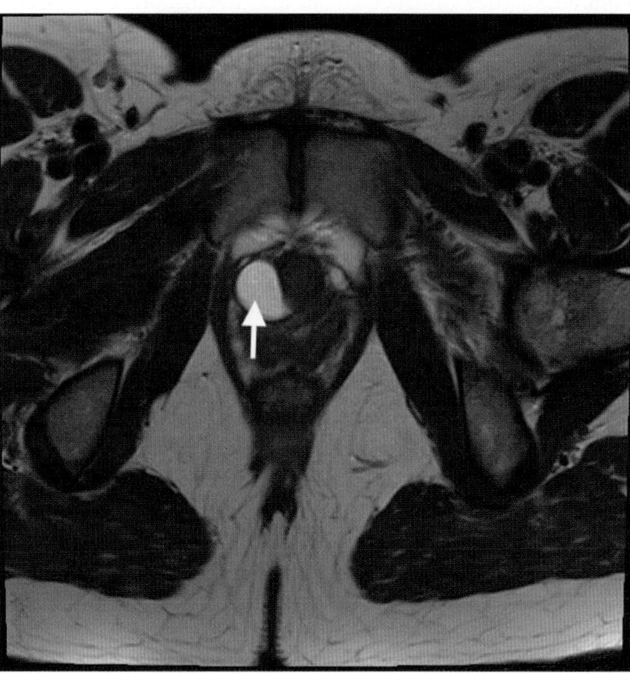

Figure 79.11 A magnetic resonance imaging scan of a urethral diverticulum in a female. The arrow identifies the fluid-filled diverticulum adjacent to the urethra.

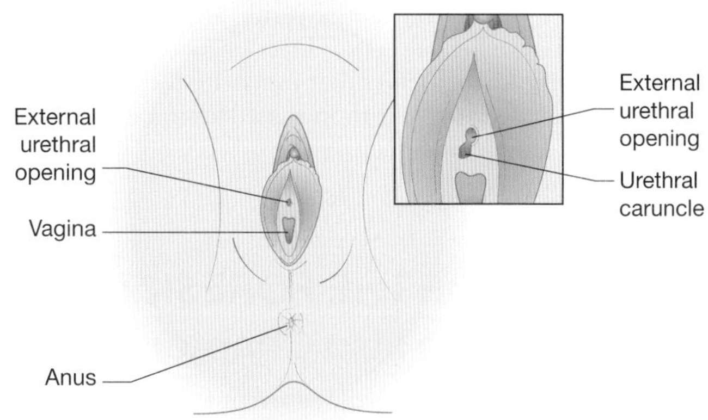

Figure 79.12 A urethral caruncle.

Clare Juliet Fowler, contemporary, Professor of Uroneurology, The National Hospital for Nervous Diseases, Queen Square, London, UK.
Roger Sinclair Kirby, contemporary, Professor of Urology, St George's Hospital, London, UK.

connective tissue stroma infiltrated with pus cells. There may be frequency of micturition and urethral pain afterwards. Occasionally, there is bleeding. A urethral prolapse is less tender and is not pedunculated. Treatment is by excision and diathermy coagulation of the base of the stalk. The patient should be given antibiotics to treat the underlying chronic urethritis.

Papillomata acuminata

Papillomata acuminata are the same as the sexually transmitted warts that occur on the penis. They are treated in the same way. In African women, papillomata acuminata are common and may grow to such a large size during pregnancy that they obstruct labour and necessitate a caesarean section.

Carcinoma of the urethra

This occurs twice as often in women as in men. Whether a caruncle can become malignant is disputed, but caruncles and tumours often occur close together. Malignant swellings of the urethra feel harder than benign ones. Treatment by radiotherapy or radical surgery is often ineffective. The overall prognosis is poor.

THE PENIS

Anatomy

The penis is composed of three tubular structures. The upper two structures, the corpora cavernosa, provide erectile function and are apposed to each other, being anchored posteriorly onto the pubic rami. The third tubular structure is the corpus spongiosum, which contains the urethra and which expands distally to form the glans penis.

The corpora cavernosa have an outer covering of tunica albuginea, which is relatively inelastic and which also forms the septum between them. The tunica albuginea encloses the erectile tissue itself, which has a trabecular structure with a network of sinusoidal spaces lined by endothelium within which the blood pools during erection. The central arterial blood supply (the central penile artery) is a branch of the internal pudendal artery. Erection occurs when the sacral parasympathetic nerves that innervate the penis cause smooth muscle relaxation with increased arterial inflow and dilatation of the sinusoids such that blood accumulates within the trabecular spaces.

DISEASES OF THE FORESKIN

Phimosis (see also Chapter 9)

At birth, the foreskin is normally adherent to the glans penis. These physiological adhesions between the foreskin and the glans penis begin to disappear around the age of 2 years and may persist until 6 years of age or later, giving the false impression that the prepuce will not retract. This condition (sometimes known as physiological phimosis) should not be confused with true phimosis in young boys.

Phimosis in boys

True phimosis is where there is scarring of the prepuce such that it will not retract without fissuring of the foreskin (Figure 79.13). This may result in ballooning of the foreskin during micturition and may also result in infection (balanoposthitis). Rarely, the aperture in the prepuce may be so tight as to cause urinary obstruction.

Phimosis in adults

Scarring in adults occurs as a result of balanitis (inflammation of the glans penis), posthitis (inflammation of the foreskin), or lichen sclerosus et atrophicus (syn: balanitis xerotica obliterans). BXO is an uncommon condition in which the normally pliant foreskin becomes thickened, typically whitish in appearance and forms a constricting band (cicatrix) that prevents retraction (Figure 79.14). BXO may also affect the glans penis (causing meatal stenosis) (Figure 79.15) and the penile urethra (causing urethral stricture). As a consequence it is difficult to keep the penis clean, there may be recurrent attacks of balanitis and there is both a problem with hygiene and, in later life, an increased susceptibility to carcinoma.

Treatment

In a young child with a non-retractile foreskin, no treatment is necessary or appropriate. When the foreskin is mildly scarred, then preputioplasty is possible. For all other cases, circumcision is the appropriate treatment. In cases of BXO, circumcision is often curative, although when the condition affects the glans penis, topical steroid cream may be helpful. In resistant cases, formal meatotomy is necessary. In emergency situations, such as when catheterisation is required, but is impossible, then it is possible to divide the foreskin dorsally under local anaesthetic (a so called dorsal slit).

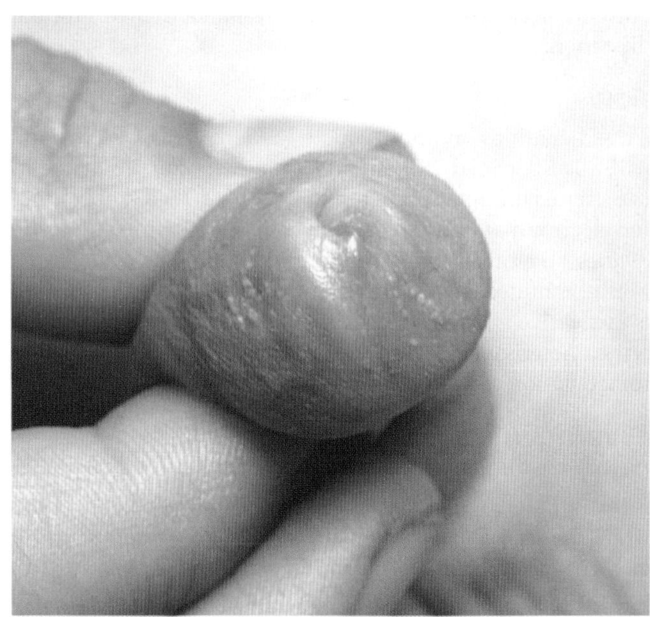

Figure 79.13 Non-retractile foreskin. The patient presented with a recent history of symptoms. Examination reveals thickening and scarring with a true phimosis (picture courtesy of Kim Hutton).

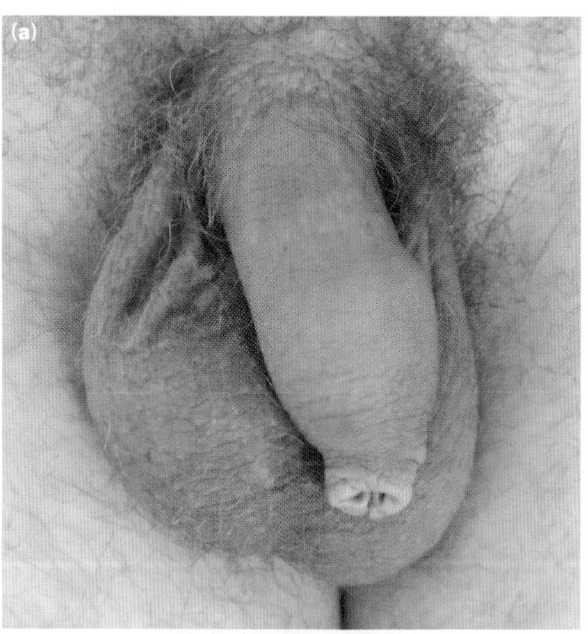

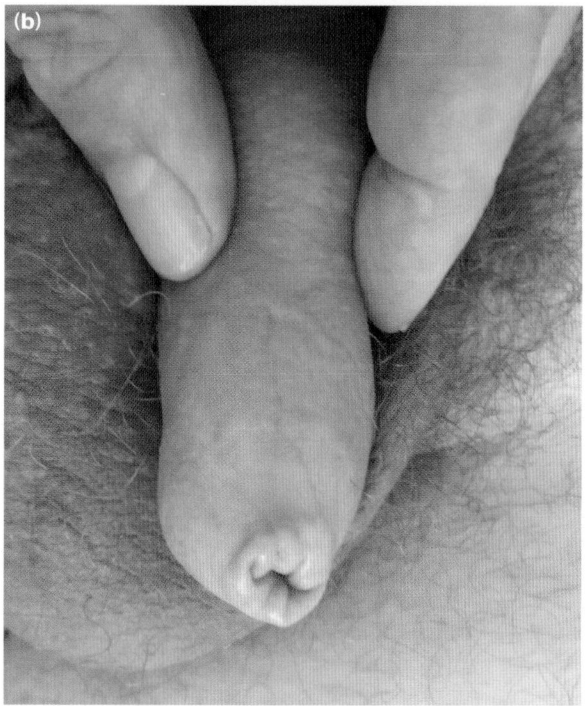

Figure 79.14 Phimosis secondary to balanitis xerotica obliterans. Note the white and thickened appearance of the preputial skin (**a**) with a constriction such that the foreskin cannot be retracted (**b**).

PREPUTIOPLASTY

This is an application of the Heineke-Mikulicz principle whereby the tight ring of the foreskin is divided longitudinally and sewn transversely, thereby allowing retraction of the preserved foreskin. There is a recurrence rate and it is only indicated in mild cases with minimal scarring. If it fails, then circumcision is indicated.

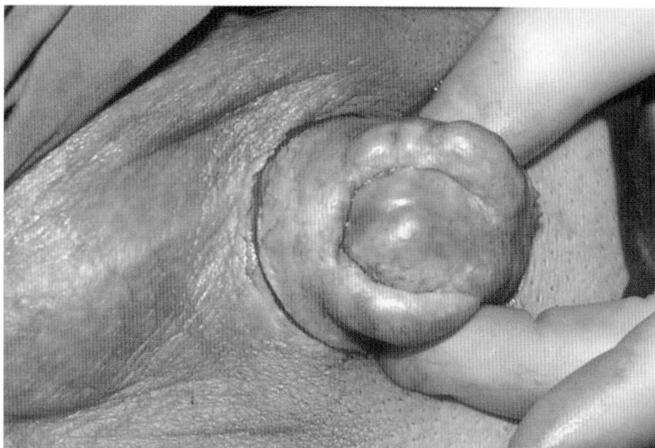

Figure 79.15 Severe balanitis xerotica obliterans causing meatal stenosis, thickened and scarred preputial and penile skin. There was also a severe penile urethral stricture.

CIRCUMCISION

Apparently, circumcision did not originate among the Jewish people; they took the practice either from the Babylonians or from African tribes, probably the latter. It had been practiced in West Africa for over 5000 years.

Indications In infants and young boys, circumcision is most usually performed at the request of the parents for social or religious reasons. Medical indications for circumcision in boys include true phimosis, BXO (rare under the age of 5 years), recurrent attacks of balanoposthitis and recurrent urinary tract infections with an abnormal upper urinary tract.

In adults, circumcision is indicated because of an inability to retract the foreskin for intercourse, for splitting of an abnormally tight frenulum or for recurrent balanitis.

Recently, evidence has emerged that circumcision protects against the spread of human immunodeficiency virus (HIV), and a large scale programme of adult circumcision under the auspices of the World Health Organisation is ongoing in some African countries where HIV is a major health problem.

Technique in an infant Applying a clamp or bone forceps across the prepuce distal to the glans with blind division of the foreskin is to be condemned. To see one boy with partial or total amputation of the glans is enough to realise the folly of this technique. It is far better to perform a proper circumcision under direct vision as in an adult. The Plastibel device can be used in infants (Hollister) and its use is shown in Figure 79.16; the ring separates between 5 and 8 days postoperatively.

Technique in adolescents and adults In adolescents and adults the following method is preferable. The prepuce is held in artery forceps and put on a gentle stretch. Marking the skin with a pen at the level of the corona is essential prior to incision to ensure that excess skin is not removed. A

Walter Hermann von Heineke, 1834–1901, German surgeon and Professor of Surgery in Erlangen.
Jan Mikulicz-Radecki, 1850–1905, Polish surgeon and Director of Surgery in Krakow and Wroklaw.

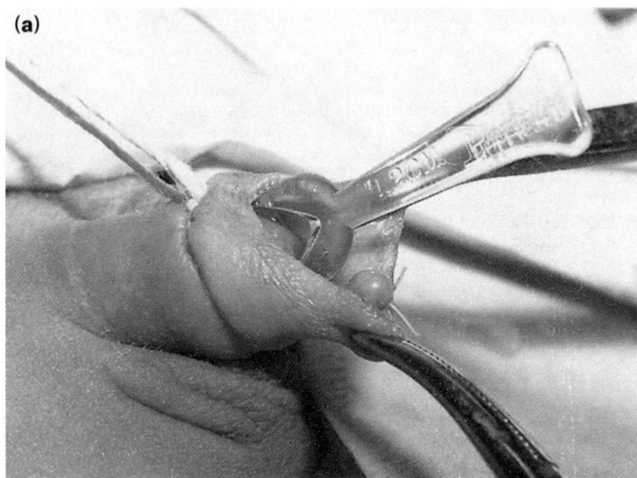

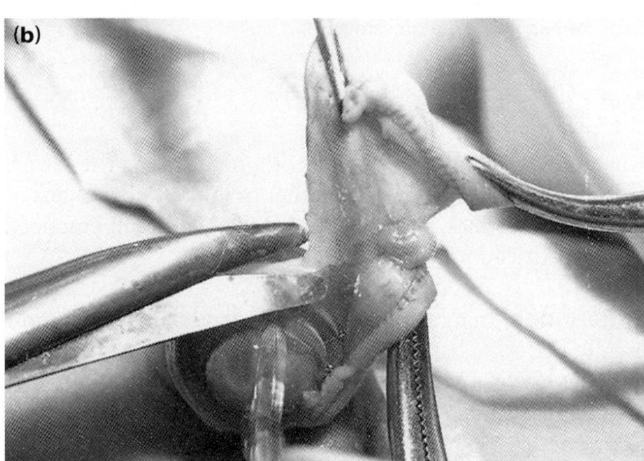

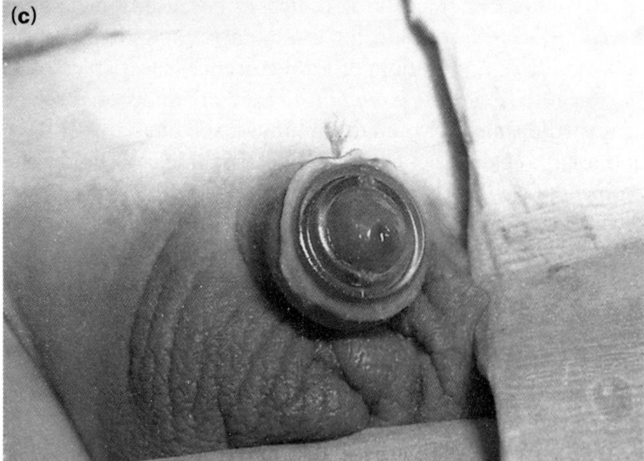

Figure 79.16 The Plastibel (Hollister) device for circumcision in infants. (a) The foreskin is freed and retracted. (b) After the Plastibel device has been slipped into place over the glans penis, the foreskin is ligated over the groove of the bell and redundant foreskin is cut away. (c) This shows the completed operation (courtesy of Professor Asal Y Izzidien Al-Samarrai, King Saud University, Riyadh, Saudi Arabia).

circumferential incision in the penile skin is made at the level of the corona using a knife. The prepuce is then slit dorsally in the midline to within 1 cm of the corona. This converts the foreskin into two flaps connected at the midline anteriorly.

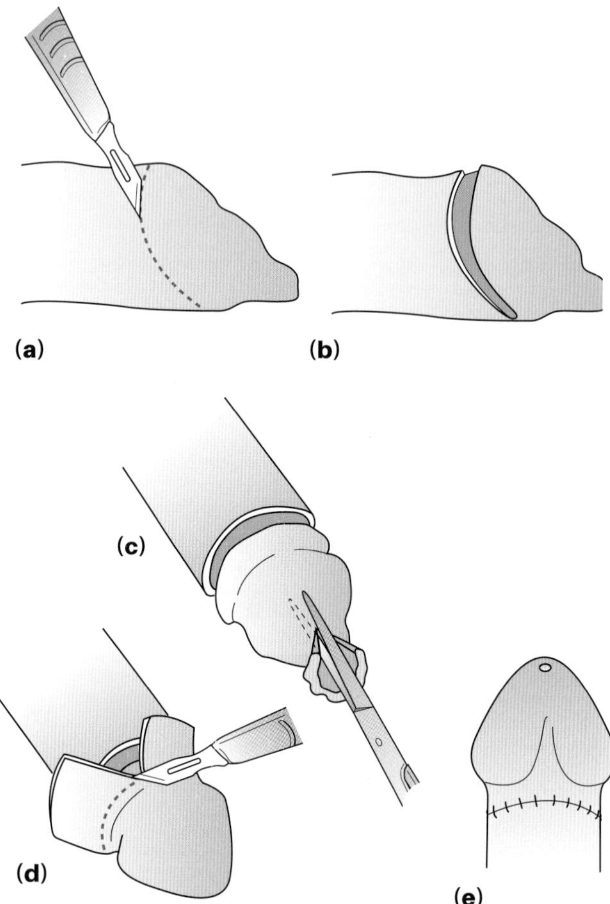

Figure 79.17 (a-e) Stages in circumcision.

When the undersurface of the prepuce has been separated from the glans, the inner layer of each flap is again marked with a pen and then incised with a second circumferential incision, leaving about 0.5 cm of the inner layer of the preputial skin. Cutting the remaining connective tissue completes the excision (Figure 79.17). Monopolar diathermy must be avoided in operations on the penis because there is a danger that the current path will cause coagulation at the base of the penis. Haemostasis is important in circumcision, however, and vessels should be secured with bipolar diathermy or with absorbable ligatures. The cut edges of the skin are approximated using interrupted sutures, making certain that the frenular vessels are ligated.

Summary box 79.7

Circumcision

- Is most commonly performed for cultural reasons
- Is not indicated for failure of retraction caused by congenital adhesions between the glans penis and the prepuce
- Is indicated when there is true phimosis
- Never use monopolar diathermy when performing circumcision

Frenulum breve

Phimosis should not be confused with this condition, where the frenulum is short, such that it causes pain when the foreskin is retracted. Another possible presentation is tearing of the frenulum during sexual activity. Treatment is by frenuloplasty, which utilises the Heineke–Mikulicz principle to 'lengthen' the frenulum.

Paraphimosis

A tight foreskin once retracted may be difficult to return and a paraphimosis results. In this condition, the venous and lymphatic return from the glans and distal foreskin is obstructed and these structures swell, causing even more pressure within the obstructing ring of prepuce. Icebags, gentle manual compression and injection of a solution of hyaluronidase in normal saline may help to reduce the swelling. Such patients can be treated by circumcision if careful manipulation fails. A dorsal slit of the prepuce under local anaesthetic may be enough in an emergency.

Balanoposthitis

Inflammation of the prepuce is known as posthitis; inflammation of the glans is balanitis. The opposing surfaces of the two structures are often involved, hence the term balanoposthitis. In mild cases, the only symptoms are itching and some discharge. In more severe inflammation, the glans and foreskin are red-raw and pus exudes. Treatment is by broad-spectrum antibiotics and local hygiene measures. If there is associated phimosis, then a circumcision is required.

Preputial calculi

Later in life, chronic posthitis may lead to adhesions between the prepuce and the glans and closure of the orifice of the preputial sac. Preputial calculi result from the accumulation beneath a non-retractable foreskin of inspissated smegma, urinary salts or both.

INJURIES OF THE PENIS

Avulsion of the skin of the penis

Entanglement of clothing in rotating machinery is the usual cause. Repair can be effected by burying the shaft of the penis in the scrotum, with subsequent release at the time of a definitive plastic surgical repair. An alternative approach is initial debridement with delayed, but early, skin grafting.

Fracture of the penis

Fracture of the penis is an uncommon accident, usually occurring when the erect penis is bent violently during intercourse. The forced deformity results in a rupture of the tunica albuginea with immediate extravasation of blood from within the penis. There is typically a loud cracking sound with immediate loss of the erection, and the rapid development of a large bruise around the penis and extending onto the scrotum (Figure 79.18). There may occasionally be an associated urethral injury. Optimal management involves early exploration of the penis with surgical repair of the ruptured tunica albuginea.

Strangulation of the penis

Strangulation of the penis by rings placed on the penis, usually for sexual reasons, can cause venous engorgement, which prevents their removal. It may help to aspirate the corpora cavernosa but often the ring must be cut off with a ring cutter or hacksaw.

Other abnormalities of the penis

Erectile dysfunction

ED is failure to attain or maintain an erection. It is a symptom, rather than a condition in itself. It can arise as a consequence of psychological issues, but the commonest cause is vascular disease, and as such ED is associated with diabetes, hypertension, dyslipidaemia and smoking. Other rarer causes include endocrine disease (hypogonadism and prolactin secreting pituitary tumours), neurological disease (multiple sclerosis, spinal cord injury and prolapsed intervertebral disc), iatrogenic damage to the cavernosal nerves due to radical pelvic surgery (e.g. radical prostatectomy, abdominoperineal excision of the rectum and radical cystectomy), neuropathy secondary to pelvic radiotherapy and drug-induced cases (including antihypertensive agents, antidepressants and antipsychotics).

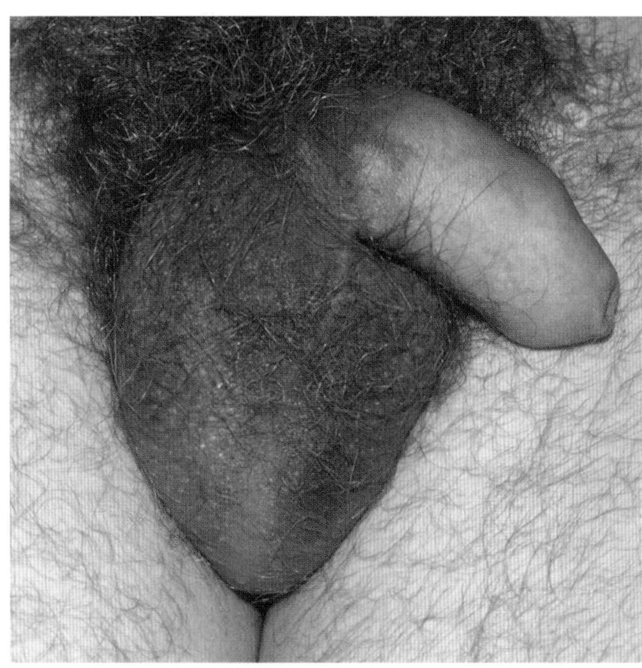

Figure 79.18 Penile fracture. Note the extensive bruising of the penis and scrotum.

Assessment involves confirmation of the diagnosis by taking a careful history, assessing the patient for underlying risk factors and trying to identify the rare case that can be cured as opposed to being treated. Physical examination of the genitalia, measurement of the blood pressure and assessment of the secondary sexual characteristics is required and biochemical assessment of the blood sugar, the serum lipid profile and the serum testosterone is necessary in all cases.

Treatment for most patients involves the use of the phosphodiesterase type 5 inhibitors (such as sildenafil) with intracavernosal injection of alprostadil, vacuum erection devices and penile implants reserved for resistant cases.

Summary box 79.8

Erectile dysfunction

- The commonest cause of erectile dysfunction is atherosclerosis
- Appropriate investigation involves identification of vascular risk factors
- Phosphodiesterase inhibitors are the first line treatment for most men

Peyronie's disease

Peyronie's disease is characterized by penile deformity (Figure 79.19), palpable penile plaques within the penis, ED and pain on erection. The cause is unknown, but probably involves minor injury to the erect penis with secondary microhaemorrhage beneath the tunica albuginea and secondary fibrosis. The latter results in the palpable plaques that can be identified on examination. The plaques may rarely be calcified (Figure 79.20). The presence of these relatively inelastic plaques causes the erect penis to bend, often dramatically, towards the side of the plaque. The commonest direction of deformity is dorsally (towards the abdomen) and the deformity may be so great as to prevent penetrative sexual intercourse.

While the aetiology is uncertain, there is an association with Dupuytren's contracture. The natural history of the condition is that it typically progresses for 18–24 months before stabilising. During this acute (or active) phase of the disease, surgery is not indicated, and a variety of medical treatments have been tried, although none with any good evidence of benefit.

When the disease has stabilised (the chronic or stable phase), the crucial issue is whether the patient is still able to have sexual intercourse. If he can, then no treatment is indicated, while if the deformity prevents penetration, or makes it difficult, then corrective treatment is indicated. Using this criterion, only around a quarter of men require treatment. While injections of collagenase have been recently licensed for this condition, the commonest treatment is surgery with the Nesbitt procedure being the most common procedure. This operation corrects the deformity by plicating the convex side of the deformity, thereby straightening the penis, albeit with some accompanying loss of length.

Summary box 79.9

Peyronie's disease

- Medical treatments during the active phase have little evidence of efficacy
- The disease has two phases: an initial acute phase lasting 12–24 months and a later chronic phase
- There is no effective treatment in the acute phase
- Surgery may be indicated in the chronic phase to correct deformity that interferes with sexual activity
- Surgical treatment will shorten the erect penile length

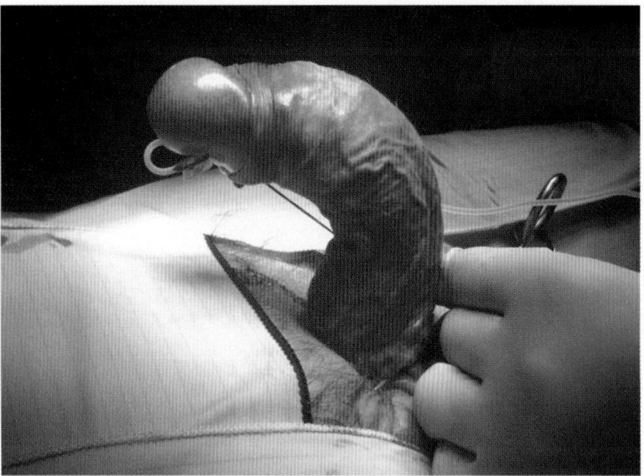

Figure 79.19 An artificial erection obtained perioperatively, demonstrating the dorsal deformity of the erect penis that is typical of Peyronie's disease.

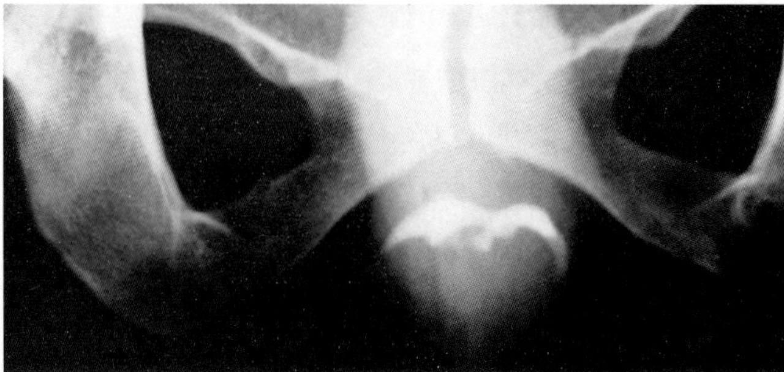

Figure 79.20 Penile calcification in Peyronie's disease (courtesy of Dr SS Rawat, Riyadh, Saudi Arabia).

Francois de la Peyronie, 1678–1747, surgeon to King Louis XIV of France, and Founder of the Royal Academy of Surgery, Paris, France.
Baron Guillaume Dupuytren, 1777–1835, surgeon, Hôtel Dieu, Paris, France, described this condition in 1831.
Reed Nesbitt, urological surgeon, Nashville, TN, USA.

Congenital curvature of the penis

A penile deformity that is similar and analagous to Peyronie's disease is occasionally seen in young men. Called congential curvature of the penis, the urethral length is normal and it typically results in a ventral deformity of the erect penis. If the deformity interferes with sexual activity, then surgery, usually a Nesbit procedure, will straighten the erect penis.

Chordee

Chordee (French = corded) is a fixed bowing of the penis caused by hypospadias or, more rarely, chronic urethritis. Erection is deformed and sexual intercourse may be impossible. Treatment is usually surgical.

Priapism

Priapism means a persistent erection lasting longer than 4 hours and it is a surgical emergency. There are two main types of priapism.

ISCHAEMIC PRIAPISM

Ischaemic or venogenic priapism is the commoner and is due to venous congestion, with consequent thrombosis and ischaemia. The penis remains erect and becomes painful. This is a pathological erection and the glans penis and corpus spongiosum are not involved. The condition is most commonly seen as a side effect of medication, most notably antipsychotic medication and intracavernosal injections, but it can also arise as complication of a hypercoagulable blood disorders such as sickle cell disease or leukaemia. A tiny proportion of cases are caused by malignant disease in the corpora cavernosa or the pelvis.

The clinical features are of a painful erection not involving the glans penis. Blood taken from the penis shows hypoxia, hyercapnoea and acidosis, while Doppler scanning shows an absence of blood flow within the penis.

An underlying cause should be excluded and the patient should be referred for specialist urological care. Treatment is an emergency, since delay beyond 6 hours results in progressive, irreversible damage to the corpus cavernosal tissue with subsequent fibrosis and ED. Aspiration of the sludged blood in the corpora cavernosa is the first-line therapy but if this fails, then intracavernosal injection of phenylephrine (an alpha adrenoceptor agonist) is the next line of therapy. If that proves ineffective, it may be necessary to decompress the penis by creating a shunt between the corpus cavernosum and either the glans penis or the corpus spongiosum. Treatment initiated after 24–36 hours rarely restores normal erectile function.

Summary box 79.10

Ischaemic priapism

- The characteristic clinical features are a painful erection not involving the glans penis
- Blood gas analysis from the penis shows hypoxia, hypercapnoea and acidosis
- Detumescence should be ideally achieved within 6-12 hours to avoid long-term erectile dysfunction

NON-ISCHAEMIC PRIAPISM

This rarer form of priapism arises as a consequence of traumatic damage to the central penile artery, usually as a consequence of blunt perineal trauma. A fistula develops between the artery and the sinusoidal space, which results in a persistent erection that is painless, in contrast to the ischaemic priapism. Blood gas analysis shows the characteristics of arterial blood and Doppler scanning and selective arteriography will demonstrate the fistula (Figure 79.21). Treatment is not an emergency, since there is no ischaemia, and is most appropriate achieved by selective arterial embolisation.

CARCINOMA OF THE PENIS

Penile cancer is rare in the UK, with only around 600 cases being recorded annually. It is much commoner in other parts of the world, most notably South America, where it is one of the commonest cancers.

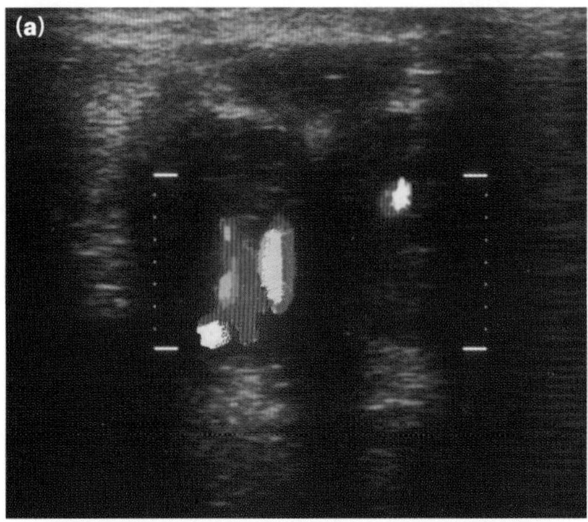

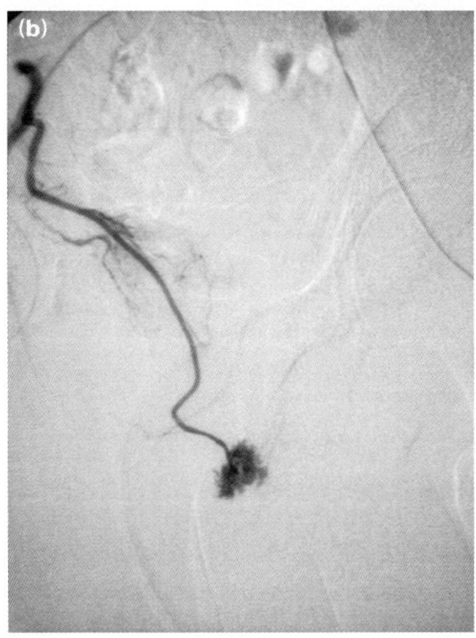

Figure 79.21 (a) Colour Doppler scan of a high flow (non-ischaemic) priapism showing turbulence at the site of the arterial injury. Compare the high unilateral signal (turbulence) with normal contralateral flow. (b) Selective pudendal arteriogram showing the site of the fistula (the arterial blush) between the central penile artery and the corpus cavernosum.

Aetiology

Circumcision soon after birth confers immunity against carcinoma of the penis. Later circumcision does not seem to have the same benefit, with the assumption that smegma is in some way carcinogenic. Human papillomavirus infection (HPV types 16 and 18) is a risk factor, as are BXO and smoking. Phimosis and chronic balanoposthitis are known to be contributory factors, and there are definite precarcinomatous states including leucoplakia of the glans, which is similar to the condition seen on the tongue, and penile intraepithelial neoplasia (PeIN).

Penile intraepithelial neoplasia (carcinoma in situ of the penis, Bowen's disease, erythroplasia of Queyrat)

PeIN is typically seen as a red cutaneous patch on the penis (Figure 79.22). When it occurs on the glans penis, it is known as erythroplasia of Queyrat and when it occurs on the shaft of the penis it is called Bowen's disease. There are several other benign causes of red patches on the penis, and when there is clinical doubt as to the underlying diagnosis a biopsy is indicated. When the diagnosis of carcinoma in situ is confirmed, treatment is by means of topical 5-FU cream, CO_2 laser ablation or surgical excision.

Pathology

Carcinoma of the penis is most typically a squamous cell carcinoma arising in the skin of the glans penis or the prepuce. It may be flat and infiltrating or warty in appearance (Figure 79.23). The former often starts as leucoplakia or PeIN and the latter results from an existing papilloma. Local growth continues for months or years. T1 tumours are confined to the skin, with T2 tumours invading the corpus spongiosum or the corpus cavernosum. T3 tumours invade the urethra and T4 tumours invade adjacent structures. The earliest lymphatic spread is to the inguinal (N1 and N2 disease) and then to the iliac nodes (N3 disease) (Figure 79.24). Distant metastatic deposits are infrequent.

Clinical features

Many patients present late (Figure 79.25), either because of embarrassment or because of misdiagnosis. About 10% of patients are under 40 years of age. By the time the patient presents, the growth is often large and secondary infection causes a foul, bloody discharge. There is typically little or no pain.

Around 50% have inguinal lymph node enlargement at presentation but the nodal enlargement often reflects infection. In many, the prepuce is non-retractile and must be split to view the lesion. A biopsy should be performed to make the diagnosis. Untreated, the whole glans may be replaced by a fungating offensive mass. Later, the inguinal nodes can erode the skin (Figure 79.24) of the groin and in rare cases,

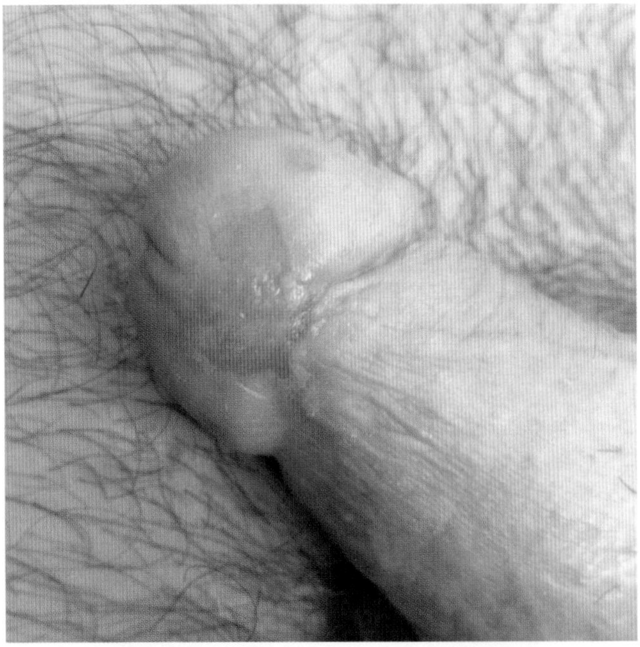

Figure 79.22 Penile intraepithelial neoplasia affecting the glans penis.

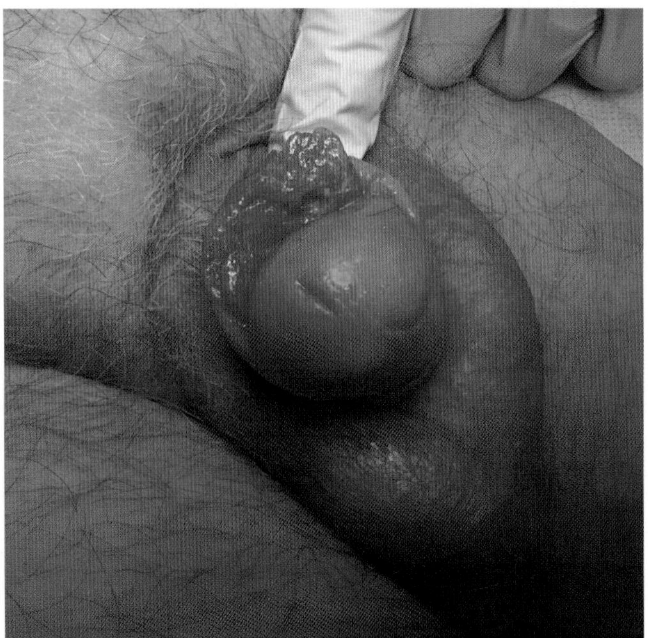

Figure 79.23 A squamous cell cancer arising from the inner aspect of the prepuce.

John Templeton Bowen, 1857–1940, American dermatologist, described this condition in 1912.
Auguste Queyrat, b.1872, dermatologist, Paris, France, described this condition in 1911.

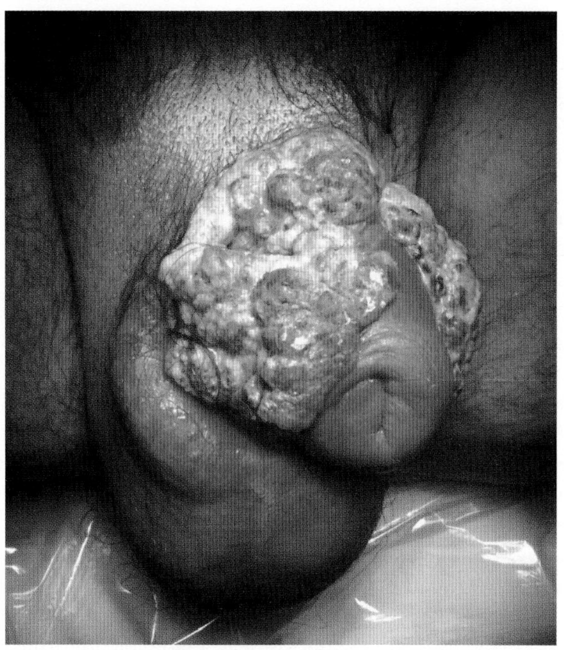

Figure 79.24 A late presenting squamous cell cancer of the penis.

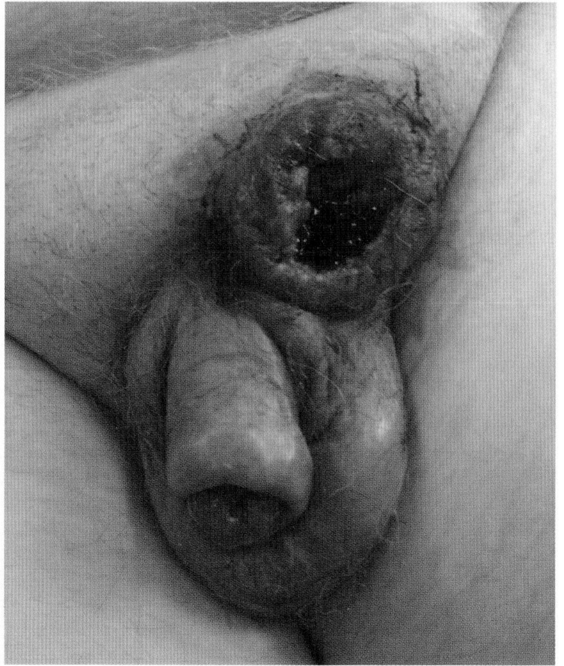

Figure 79.25 A squamous cell cancer of the penis with an ulcerating groin node.

death of the patient can result from erosion of the femoral or external iliac vessels.

Treatment

Management is divided into treatment of the primary tumour and treatment of the inguinal nodes. For the primary tumour surgical excision is the mainstay of treatment, with the traditional view that a 2 cm margin of normal tissue be removed being superceded by a more recent, more conservative view, such that penile preserving surgery with excision of much lower margins of normal tissue are now accepted. Tumours affecting the glans penis require glansectomy, with more advanced tumours requiring partial penectomy. In advanced cases, total penectomy is required with formation of a perineal urethrostomy. Such surgery is indicated even in advanced metastatic disease for reasons of local control.

Treatment of any associated enlarged inguinal lymph nodes should be delayed until at least 3 weeks after local treatment of the primary lesion. Enlargement caused by infection will usually show signs of subsiding with antibiotic treatment. For palpable nodes, ultrasound-guided fine needle aspiration will confirm the diagnosis and a block dissection of both groins should be undertaken. The management of patients where the nodes are not palpable disease involves the use of sentinel lymph node biopsy (SLNB) followed by inguinal node dissection if the SLNB is positive .

Management of the pelvic nodes is controversial. When they are involved on CT scanning, surgery probably has little role, but when the iliac nodes are not enlarged in the presence of N2 disease, the options are observation, pelvic lympadenectomy or radiotherapy. Chemotherapy is relatively ineffective and currently is reserved for palliation in those with metastatic disease. The prognosis for tumours confined to the penis is good with 5-year survival rates in excess of 80%. With nodal involvement the 5-year survival rate falls to around 40%.

Summary box 79.11

Carcinoma of the penis

- A relatively uncommon tumour
- Enlargement of superficial inguinal lymph nodes may be caused by infection or metastatic spread
- Surgery is the mainstay of treatment
- Nodal involvement indicates a poor prognosis

Buschke-Löwenstein tumour

The Buschke–Löwenstein tumour is uncommon. It has the histological pattern of a verrucous carcinoma. It is locally destructive and invasive but appears not to spread to lymph nodes or to metastasise. Treatment is by surgical excision.

Malignant melanoma of the penis

This is an uncommon tumour, with the principles of management being the same as for squamous cell carcinoma. Blood borne metastatic disease is, however, more common.

Abraham Buschke, 1868–1943, dermatologist, Berlin, Germany.
Ludwig Löwenstein, 1885–1959, dermatologist, Berlin, Germany

INFLAMMATION OF THE PENIS AND URETHRA

Urethral discharge

The commonest cause of urethral discharge in men is urethritis and the two commonest causes of urethritis are non-specific urethritis (NSU) and gonococcal urethritis. Other related symptoms include dysuria and urethral pruritis while epididymitis can also be present. A sexual history should be sought, particularly a history of unprotected intercourse, oral sex and anal intercourse. A routine investigative screen includes Gram stain of the discharge, dipstick testing of a urine specimen, culture of a urine specimen and nucleic acid amplification testing (NAAT) of either a urine specimen or a urethral swab. If relevant, the same techniques can be used for vaginal, endocervical, anal and pharyngeal swabs. NAAT is a sensitive way of identifying both gonococcal and chlamydial urethritis. As with all sexually transmitted infections (STIs) the possibility of other infections (such as HIV) should always be borne in mind and, where appropriate, tested for.

Non-specific urethritis (syn: non-gonococcal urethritis)

NSU is a STI that is the commonest cause of urethritis in the Western world. In around 40% of cases it is due to *Chlamydia trachomatis* with other cases being caused by *Ureaplasma urealyticum*, *Trichomonas vaginalis* or *Mycoplasma genitalium*. The causative agent in up to 50% of cases is unknown.

NSU can affect both men and women and asymptomatic infection is common in both. In men, dysuria and a white mucopurulent urethral discharge appear up to 6 weeks after sexual intercourse. Dysuria is usual. The urine appears to be clear but may contain 'threads' or pus cells. Epididymitis is common and urethral stricture is a potential late complication. In women, the condition is usually asymptomatic, although it can present as vaginal discharge or as a form of urethrotrigonitis. It may result in cervicitis or pelvic inflammatory disease.

Exclusion of gonorrheal infection is important. The diagnostic test of choice is NAAT and in men either a urine specimen or a urethral swab can be used, while in women urine, endocervical or vaginal swabs can be used. If testing is positive, then partners should be screened.

The standard treatment regimes are azithromycin as a single dose or doxycycline orally for 7 days. Treatment is usually effective, although relapse is common, especially in men, in whom the prostate may act as a reservoir of infection. It is important to treat both partners as reinfection is probable if this is not done, and re-testing of both partners at 3 months is recommended.

Gonorrhoeal urethritis

Gonorrhoea is a sexually transmitted disease caused by *Neisseria gonorrhoeae* (gonococcus), a gram-negative kidney-shaped diplococcus that infects the anterior urethra in men, the urethra and cervix in women and the oropharynx, rectum and anal canal in both sexes, but especially men. It is transmitted by unprotected sexual intercourse and is the second commonest cause of urethritis in western countries.

Most men have symptoms of urethral discomfort and urethral discharge within a few days of infection. There is often scalding dysuria. In women it is often asymptomatic. There can be mild dysuria or slight urethral discharge, which can go unnoticed by the patient. Cervicitis can occur with about 10% suffering from pelvic inflammatory disease (salpingitis), which, if bilateral, may lead to infertility. A mother may transmit gonorrhea to her newborn during childbirth with the risk that blindness of the child can result. In addition, in both men and women exposed orally or anally, gonococcal infections can cause a predominantly asymptomatic pharyngitis or proctitis.

Traditionally, the diagnosis was made by identification of pus and gonococci in a gram-stained urethral smear with subsequent culture. However, more recently, NAAT, which is more sensitive, has become the norm.

Complications are prevented by effective early treatment. In men complications include posterior urethritis, prostatitis (acute or chronic), acute epididymo-orchitis, periurethral abscess and urethral stricture. Gonococcal arthritis, iridocyclitis, septicaemia and endocarditis are unusual.

Treatment is with antibiotics, with ceftriaxone currently the treatment of choice as a consequence of the increasing prevalence of antibiotic resistance to more traditional antibiotics such as ciprofloxacin or penicillin. Contact tracing is important in controlling the spread of the disease and management is usually by a genitourinary physician. Failure to respond to first-line treatment should raise the possibility of antibiotic resistance or co-infection with chlamydia.

Reiter's disease (syn: sexually acquired reactive arthritis)

Reiter's disease is an autoimmune disease characterised by the triad of urethritis or diarrhoea, conjunctivitis and polyarthritis. Common triggers include chlamydial urethritis, less commonly gonococcal urethritis and diarrhoea secondary to *Salmonella*, *Shigella* or *Campylobacter*. It is an HLA-B27-associated condition. The conjunctivitis (present in around 50%) and arthritis typically occur 1–3 weeks after the primary infection. Diagnosis is made on clinical grounds and treatment is largely symptomatic, although antibiotic treatment of the precipitating infection is important. The urethritis and

Hans Christian Joachim Gram, 1853–1938, Professor of Pharmacology (1891–1900) and of Medicine (1900–1923), Copenhagen, Denmark, described this method of staining bacteria in 1884.
Albert Ludwig Siegmund Neisser, 1855–1916, Director of the Dermatological Institue, Breslau, Germany (now Wroclaw, Poland).
Hans Conrad Julius Reiter, 1881–1969, President of the Health Service and Honorary Professor of Hygiene, Berlin, Germany, described this condition in 1916. He was subsequently convicted of war crimes as a consequence of his involvement in the death of hundreds of inmates in Buchenwald.

conjunctivitis frequently subside after a few weeks but the arthritis may persist for months. Severe anterior uveitis and frequently recurrent attacks suggest a poor outlook.

Periurethral abscess

Periurethral abscesses were once common with high morbidity, but are now rare. Clinical presentation is varied but may include fever, dysuria, urethral discharge and swelling of the penis or scrotum. In untreated cases urethral fistulation can occur and occasionally extensive cellulitis or necrotising fasciitis can occur.

A penile periurethral abscess arises following a gonococcal or chlamydial infection of one of the glands of Littre. There may be delay in diagnosis or a coexisting urethral stricture. There is usually penile swelling with tender induration felt on the underside of the penis, which if left untreated, may discharge externally, often leaving a fistula. Diagnosis can be helped by ultrasound of the urethra. Treatment should include both antibiotic treatment, as for urethritis, combined with surgical drainage into the urethra .

A periurethral abscess in relation to the bulbar urethra is even more uncommon. It may be associated with a urethral stricture, urethral trauma or, rarely, a urethral cancer. The infecting organisms are varied and can include both streptococci and anaerobic organisms. Extravasation of urine is not unusual. There is perineal pain with pyrexia, rigors and tachycardia. Tenderness and swelling rapidly spread from the perineum to the penis and the anterior abdominal wall. Ultrasound scanning and MRI are useful diagnostic aids and treatment with antibiotics are essential. Collections of pus should be drained and the urethra should be defunctioned by a suprapubic urinary catheter.

A chronic periurethral abscess sometimes results from a longstanding urethral stricture (Figure 79.26). The multiple loculi of pus should be drained and the stricture treated. Urethral fistula occurs either spontaneously or as a result of incision of the abscess.

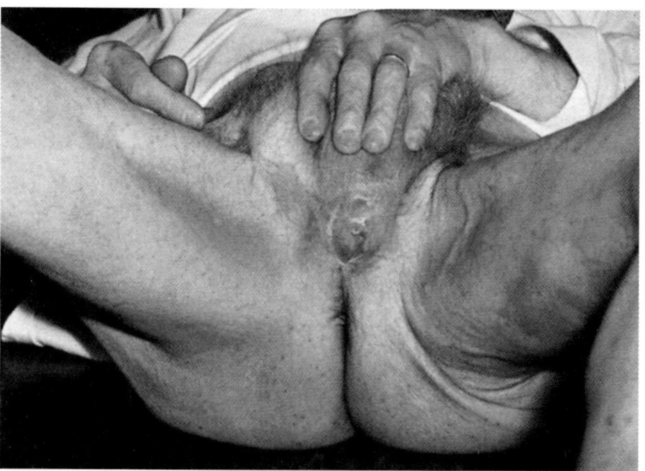

Figure 79.26 Chronic periurethral abscess.

Genital ulcers

The commonest cause of a genital ulcer is genital herpes. Other less common causes include syphilis and chancroid. As with all STIs, the possibilitiy of other infections (such as HIV) should always be borne in mind and, where appropriate, tested for.

Genital herpes

Genital herpes is caused by sexual transmission of the herpes simplex virus (usually HSV-2, occasionally HSV-1). Infection is lifelong with recurrent symptomatic attacks occuring in 50% or more of cases. Pain along the distribution of the sensory nerve, usually the genitofemoral nerve, precedes the eruption by 2 days and may be particularly severe around the anus. A group of tiny vesicles rapidly erodes to form shallow ulcers, which are painful. The first attack occurs around 4 days after exposure and is typically accompanied by fever, myalgia and inguinal lymphadenopathy. In female patients, the ulcers often spread on to the thighs during the attack. Involvement of the urethra may cause retention of urine, which may persist for up to 14 days if there is radiculitis of the S2 and S3 nerve roots.

Diagnosis is made clinically or, when there is doubt, by either cell culture or by polymerase chain reaction (PCR)-based techniques. All primary infections should be treated by oral antiviral agents such as acyclovir or valacyclovir, which have been shown to be effective in treating genital herpes, although they do prevent recurrences.

A child born to a mother with active infection is susceptible to a fatal generalised herpes infection in the neonatal period. Caesarean section should be considered in these circumstances. There is an increased risk of carcinoma of the cervix and annual cytology for life is recommended.

Syphilis

Syphilitic ulcers are typically painless, rubbery and indurated. Caused by the spirochaete *Treponema pallidum*, diagnosis was traditionally achieved by dark-field microscopy, but modern serological techniques are nowadays more appropriate. The incidence of syphilis is increasing since the advent of the retrovirals used to treat HIV in the mid 1990s. Treatment is with long-acting penicillin.

Tropical sexually transmitted infections

Lymphogranuloma veneruem, lymphogranuloma inguinale and chancroid are rare conditions in the Western world. However, they are still relatively common in some resource-poor countries. As with all STIs, the possibilitiy of other infections (such as HIV) should always be borne in mind and, where appropriate, tested for.

Lymphogranuloma venereum

Lymphogranuloma venereum is a sexually transmitted disease caused by *Chlamydia trachomatis* (chlamydia A) types L1–L3

Alexis Littre, 1658–1726, surgeon and lecturer in Anatomy, Paris, France.

and is primarily an infection of the lymphatics and lymph nodes. It can affect both sexes. While it was considered rare in resource-rich countries, some recent outbreaks in Europe have occurred, usually in conjunction with HIV.

The primary lesion is a fleeting, painless, genital papule or ulcer that develops 1–4 weeks after infection and is often unnoticed by the patient. The inguinal glands become enlarged and painful around 2–6 weeks after the primary lesion. The masses of nodes mat together above and below the inguinal ligament to give the 'sign of the groove'. The overlying skin reddens, there may be fluctuance and the mass occasionally ruptures. There may be a proctitis, which can go on to produce a rectal stricture if untreated. Lymphatic obstruction leads to lymphoedema in the perineum and, occasionally, the lower limbs. Urethritis and urethral stricture occur in men.

Diagnosis is confirmed clinically and by the detection of antibodies against the organism. Treatment is by a combination of antibiotics, which may include doxyclycine, azithromycin, erythromycin and ciprofloxacin. The multilocular lymphatic masses should not be incised, although aspiration is permissible to reduce discomfort.

Lymphogranuloma inguinale

This is a chronic and slowly progressive ulcerative tropical disease affecting the genitals and surrounding tissue, but occasionally occurring elsewhere in the body. It is usually sexually transmitted and is caused by *Klebsiella granulomatis* and is most commonly seen among socially deprived people. The incubation period varies greatly but is typically between 7–30 days.

A painless vesicle or indurated papule, usually on the external genitals but occasionally elsewhere on the skin, gradually erodes into a slowly extending ulcer with a beefy-red, granulomatous base. More chronic lesions may become greyish, especially at the edges, where, after months or years, malignant change may develop. The ulcerated area may bleed if touched but is usually surprisingly painless. Without treatment healing is only partial and keloid is common.

Diagnosis is by microscopy of material from the edges of the ulcer, which shows the presence of short gram-negative rods within the cytoplasm of the large mononuclear cells. Treatment is with azithromycin, although doxycycline, erythromycin, trimethoprim/sulfamethoxazole and gentamicin are alternatives.

Chancroid

Chancoid is a sexually transmitted, acute, ulcerative disease caused by *Haemophilus ducreyi*, a gram-negative facultative anaerobe. Following an incubation period of 3–10 days, a soft painful penile ulcer appears and is commonly followed by the development of inguinal lymphadenopathy. Diagnosis is by bacterial culture or by PCR techniques. Antibiotic treatment with ceftriaxone or azithromycin is usually effective therapy.

Condylomata acuminata (syn: genital warts)

Genital warts are caused by infection with HPV and are sexually transmitted. Infection is very common, with only a small proportion of infected patients actually having visible warts.

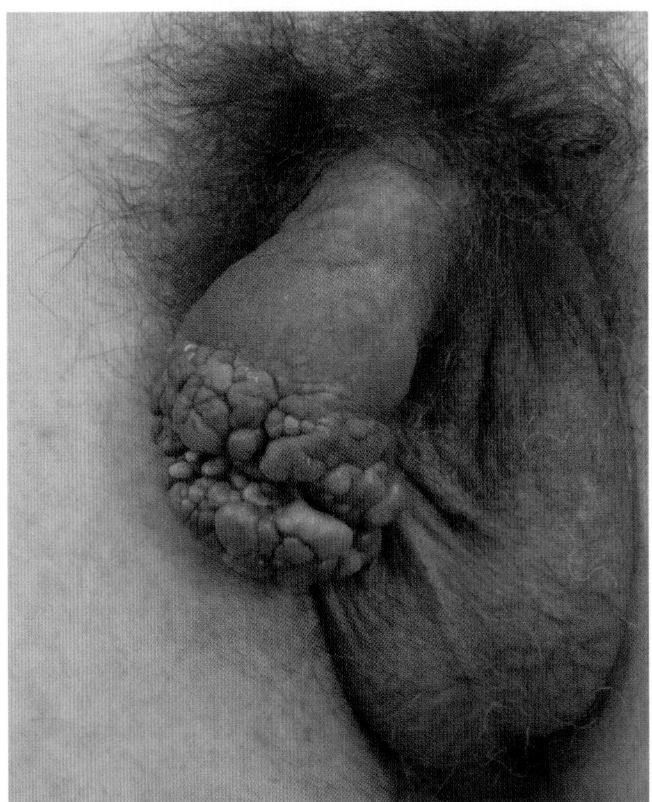

Figure 79.27 Genital warts affecting the outer prepuce. These were treated by radical circumcision.

Most commonly due to HPV types 6 and 11, these viruses do not cause cervical cancer. Ordinary skin warts can occur on the genitals by direct contact with a finger lesion, but they are less moist and soft and less often pedunculated than the genital variety. The lesions most commonly occur under the prepuce in the coronal sulcus but may be found elsewhere, including inside the urinary meatus and on the outer prepuce (**Figure 79.27**). In women, genital warts are most commonly found on the vulva but they may line the vagina and occur on the cervix. Perianal warts are common.

Other associated sexually transmitted diseases should be excluded: in women mainly candidiasis and *Trichomonas* infection and in men syphilis or gonorrhoea. Genital warts may complicate HIV infection.

Treatment is by chemical or physical means. Podophyllin is often effective as a topical application. It is applied to the wart, taking great care to avoid the surrounding skin and washed off after 6 hours or so. An alternative agent is Imidaquod. If chemical methods fail, the warts can be excised or they can be ablated with cryosurgery, electrosurgery or laser. Circumcision is sometimes advised if there are florid lesions under the foreskin.

FURTHER READING

Kaisary AV, Ballaro A, Pigott K. *Lecture notes: urology*, 7th edn. Oxford: Wiley-Blackwell, 2016.

Wein AJ, Kavoussi LR, Partin AW, Peters CA. *Campbell-Walsh urology*, 11th edn. Philadelphia: Elsevier, 2015.

Chapter 80

Testis and scrotum

Learning objectives

- To recognise testicular maldescent and to appreciate the reasons for intervention
- To recognise and manage testicular torsion
- To be able to recognise and understand the management of the common scrotal swellings (varicocoele, hydrocoele and epididymal cysts)
- To recognise and understand the management of testicular tumours
- To understand the treatment options for infertile men

EMBRYOLOGY AND ANATOMY OF THE TESTIS

The testes develop in the retroperitoneum below the kidneys at around the 10th thoracic level. During the 7th week of fetal development, the gubernaculum forms within the folds of the peritoneum. The upper end is attached to the developing testis and the lower end is attached to the fascia between the developing abdominal wall muscles. At the same time an evagination of the peritoneum itself, the **processus vaginalis**, develops adjacent to the gubernaculum and over the subsequent weeks evaginates through the abdominal wall to create the inguinal canal. The processus vaginalis initially picks up fibres of the internal oblique (which become the cremasteric muscle) and then fibres of the external oblique (which become the external spermatic fascia). As it elongates the processus carries with it the gubernaculum, which contains muscle fibres although it is not fully clear what part it plays in testicular descent. What is clear is that the testes lie at the internal inguinal ring at 3 months' gestation and descend to the scrotum between 7 and 9 months. This latter descent into the scrotum is accompanied by shortening of the gubernaculum. Final descent from the external ring to the base of the scrotum takes 4–6 weeks and is usually complete by birth.

The mechanisms that result in testicular descent are poorly understood but probably involve Müllerian inhibiting substance. Maternal chorionic gonadotrophin stimulates growth of the testis and may stimulate its migration. Imperfectly developed testes tend to descend incompletely.

The anatomy of the adult testis reflects its embryonic development. The testicular arteries originate high up in the retroperitoneum from the abdominal aorta just below the renal arteries. The testicular veins drain into the renal vein on the left and the inferior vena cava on the right. For much of their course the testicular artery and vein run parallel to the ipsilateral ureter, for which they may be mistaken during retroperitoneal surgery. Lymphatic drainage also follows this route, such that it is the para-aortic nodes that are the draining lymph nodes, which is important in the assessment and staging of men with testicular cancer.

The epididymis lies on the posterior aspect of the testis and is palpable as a separate structure, with a head, a body and a tail. The seminiferous tubules enter the epididymis at the upper end of the epididymis (the head). From the head, sperm travel through the body and tail of the epididymis to enter the vas deferens at the lower pole of the testis. The vas curves up behind the testis and can be felt above the testis as a firm tubular structure entering the external inguinal ring. In the inguinal canal, the vas deferens is invested by the cremasteric muscle along with the other components of the spermatic cord.

INCOMPLETELY DESCENDED TESTIS (SEE ALSO CHAPTER 9)

Definitions

Incomplete descent of the testis occurs when the testis is arrested in some part of its normal path to the scrotum. An ectopic testis is a testis that is abnormally placed outside this path.

Johannes Peter Müller, 1801–1858, German physiologist and comparative anatomist, first described the paramesonephric (Müllerian) duct.

Incidence

About 4% of boys are born with one or both testes incompletely descended. About two-thirds of these reach the scrotum during the first 3 months of life, but full descent after that is uncommon. The incidence of testicular maldescent at the age of 1 year is around 1%. The condition is sometimes missed in the neonatal period and only discovered later in life. In a few cases, the presence of a hernia, testicular pain or acute torsion directs attention to the abnormality. In 10% of unilateral cases there is a family history.

Pathology

The condition is more common on the right and is bilateral in 20% of cases. In adults, secondary sexual characteristics are typically normal.

The testis may be:

- intra-abdominal; usually lying extraperitoneally just inside the internal inguinal ring;
- intracanalicular; it may or may not be palpable (Figure 80.1);
- extracanalicular; usually at the scrotal neck;
- ectopic; an ectopic testis has taken a non-standard path through the body and has ended up in an unusual location, the commonest site being the superficial inguinal pouch, which lies just inferior and medial to the superficial inguinal ring. Other rarer ectopic sites include the femoral triangle, the root of the penis and perineum.

Incompletely descended testes are often macroscopically normal in early childhood, but by puberty the testis is typically smaller compared with its intrascrotal counterpart. Microscopic changes are apparent from 1–2 years including loss of Leydig cells, degeneration of Sertoli cells and decreased spermatogenesis. The higher the testis, the greater the degree of histological change.

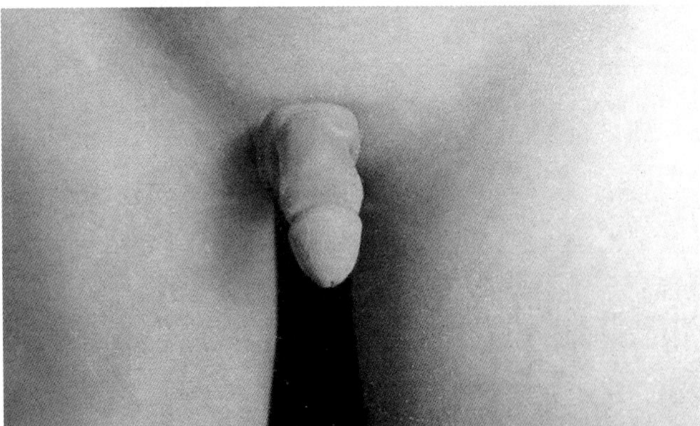

Figure 80.1 Undescended testes in a boy aged 12 years. Note the bilateral undescended testes with the underdeveloped scrotum. In cases of retractile testis, the scrotum is relatively well developed.

Consequences

Infertility

Impaired fertility is a well-recognised consequence of testicular maldescent, with paternity rates around two-thirds of normal for unilateral undescended testes and one-third of normal for bilateral undescended testes. Although there has been a recent tendency to undertake surgical orchidopexy earlier in life, evidence to show that this benefits fertility is currently lacking.

Malignancy

The cancer risk for adults after cryptorchidism in childhood is 5–10 times greater than normal. The commonest cancer is a seminoma, and as with fertility, it is unclear whether early orchidopexy reduces the risk of malignancy. However, if a testicular tumour does develop, it is undoubtedly easier to identify in a testis that is within the scrotum.

Hernia

Around 90% of boys with an undescended testis have a patent processus vaginalis although the incidence of a clinically apparent hernia is much lower.

Testicular torsion

The undescended testis is more prone to testicular torsion, largely as a consequence of a developmental abnormality between the testis and its mesentery.

Summary box 80.1

Undescended testis

- Testes that are absent from the scrotum after 3 months of age are unlikely to descend
- Histological changes in the testis can be seen from 1 year of age
- An incompletely descended testis tends to atrophy as puberty approaches
- Boys with undescended testes are at greater risk of infertility, testicular malignancy, hernia and testicular torsion

Clinical features

When assessing a child with suspected testicular maldesecent, it is helpful to have the boy as relaxed as possible and for him to be examined in a warm room, usually in a supine position. The important differential diagnosis is the so called 'retractile testis'. During childhood the testes are mobile and the cremasteric reflex is active so that in some boys, any stimulation of the skin of the scrotum or thigh causes the testis to ascend and to temporarily disappear into the inguinal canal. When the cremaster relaxes, the testis reappears only to vanish when the scrotal skin is touched again.

In comparison to a true undescended testis, the scrotum of a boy with such a retractile testis is normal as opposed to

Franz von Leydig, 1821–1908, German zoologist and comparative anatomist, discovered the Leydig cells.
Enrico Sertoli, 1842–1910, Italian physiologist, discovered the Sertoli cells of the testis.

underdeveloped, while a retractile testis can be gently milked from its position in the inguinal region to the bottom of the scrotum. A diagnosis of true incomplete descent should be made only if this is not possible.

When the testis is impalpable, ultrasound may be helpful in identifying the intracanalicular testis, while laparoscopy may be needed to differentiate between the abdominal testis and a truly absent testis.

Summary box 80.2

Retractile testis

- Retractile testes should be differentiated from true undescended testes
- This is most easily done with the child relaxed in a warm room
- Retractile testes are more common than true undescended testes
- Retractile testes require no treatment

Surgical treatment

Orchidopexy

Orchidopexy is usually performed before the boy reaches 12 months of age in an attempt to prevent the consequences described earlier. The testis and spermatic cord are mobilised and the testis is repositioned in the scrotum. The operation is performed through a short incision over the deep inguinal ring. The inguinal canal is exposed by division of the external oblique aponeurosis in the direction of its fibres.

Three manoeuvres help to gain the length required to bring the testis down into the bottom of the scrotum. First, the patent processus vaginalis should be indentified, separated and ligated. Second, the coverings of the spermatic cord (including the cremasteric muscle) should be divided and third, lateral fibrous bands just inside the internal inguinal ring should be divided. Although these techniques are usually effective, the tiny vas and testicular vessels are vulnerable to injury. The empty hemiscrotum is stretched with a finger passed into it through the inguinal incision to give enough room for the testis, which is placed in a pouch constructed between the dartos muscle and the skin (Figure 80.2).

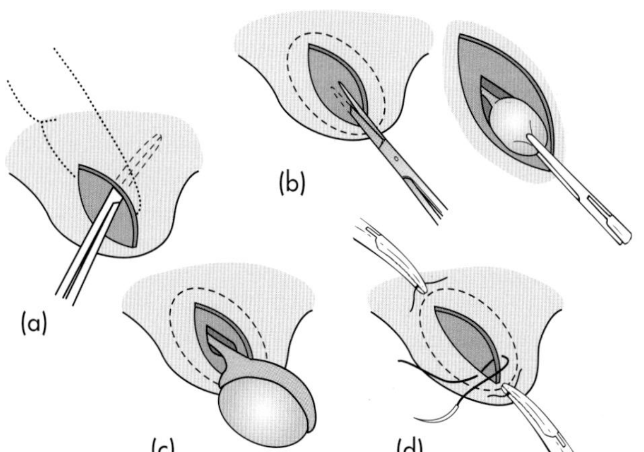

Figure 80.2 The testis is mobilised and retained in a pouch constructed between the dartos muscle and skin.

Failure to bring the testis down

Sometimes for a high undescended testis a two-stage surgical procedure is necessary. The testis is mobilised as far as possible and anchored with a suture and the mobilisation is completed 6 months later. An alternative approach involves initial division of the gonadal artery (which is usually 'tighter' than the vas deferens) such that the testis becomes dependent for its blood supply upon the cremasteric artery. The second stage procedure involves conventional orchidopexy. Orchidectomy should be considered if the incompletely descended testis is atrophic, particularly in the postpubertal boy if the other testis is normal.

INJURIES TO THE TESTIS

The testis can be damaged either by blunt or by penetrating trauma. Injuries can range from simple bruising, through significant intratesticular haematomas to rupture of the tunica albuginea, with very significant collections of blood within the tunica vaginalis (haematocoele) (Figure 80.3). If the tunica ruptures, the blood can track into the groin and perineum.

Careful clinical assessment, together with the use of ultrasound examination, is central to the management of men with a scrotal injury. Ultrasound has excellent sensitivity and specificity in the diagnosis of testicular rupture. If there is testicular rupture, there is good evidence that early surgical exploration, with debridement and repair of the tunica albuginea, is more likely to preserve useful testicular function. Scrotal wall haematomas and injuries without rupture can usually be treated conservatively.

Summary box 80.3

Scrotal trauma

- In cases of scrotal trauma, surgical exploration is indicated when there is testicular rupture or when there is a rapidly expanding scrotal haematoma
- Ultrasound is invaluable in the assessment of the injury

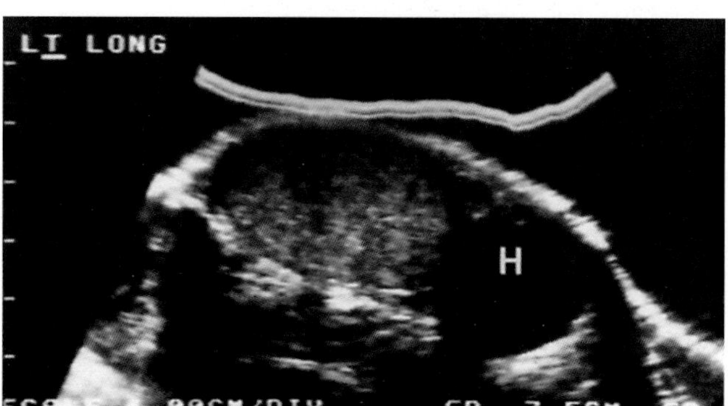

Figure 80.3 Longitudinal scan of a testicle with a haematocoele (H) at the lower pole.

ABSENT TESTIS

'Vanishing' testis describes a condition in which a testis develops but disappears before birth. The most likely cause for this is prenatal torsion. True agenesis of the testis is rarer. Laparoscopy is useful in distinguishing these causes of clinically absent testis from intra-abdominal maldescent.

TORSION OF THE TESTIS

Pathophysiology

Testicular torsion is a condition whereby the testicle twists in such a way that its blood supply becomes compromised. If left untreated the blood flow to the testicle ceases and the testicle dies. Testicular torsion is therefore a surgical emergency and the earlier the surgery to untwist the testis can be undertaken the better the outcome.

Torsion of the testis is uncommon because the normal testis is anchored and cannot rotate. For torsion to occur one of several abnormalities must be present:

- High investment of the tunica vaginalis causes the testis to hang within the tunica like a clapper in a bell (Figure 80.4). This is the most common cause in adolescents and is typically a bilateral abnormality.
- Inversion of the testis. The testis is rotated so that it lies transversely or upside down.
- Separation of the epididymis from the body of the testis permits torsion of the testis on the pedicle that connects the testis with the epididymis (Figure 80.5).

Normally, when there is a contraction of the abdominal muscles, the cremaster contracts as well. In the presence of one of the abnormalities described above, the spiral attachment of the cremaster favours rotation of the testis around the vertical axis. Sudden contraction of the cremasteric muscle, which may be a response to mechanical, sexual or thermic stimulation, may cause a rotational effect on the testis as it is pulled upward. Accordingly, straining on stool, lifting of a heavy weight, sexual activity and sport can all precipitate an episode.

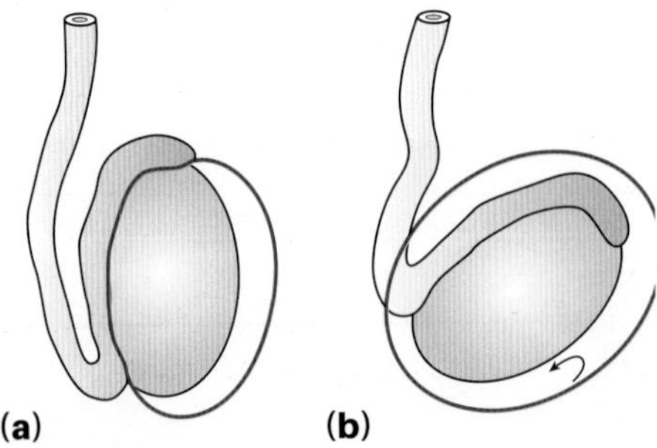

Figure 80.4 Testicular torsion: (a) normal attachment; (b) an abnormally high attachment of the tunica vaginalis predisposes to torsion – the 'bell-clapper'.

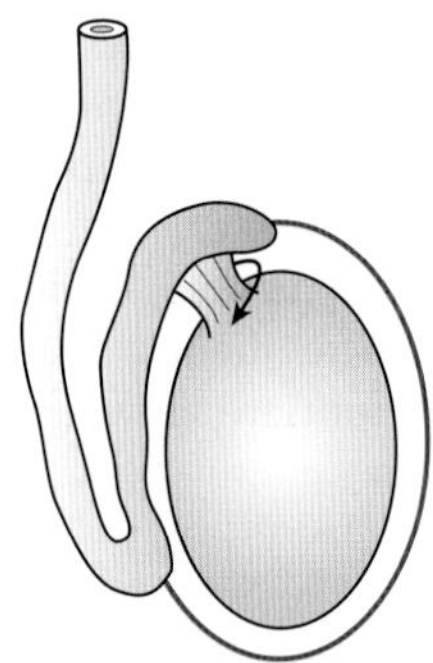

Figure 80.5 Testicular torsion. Separation of the testis from the epididymis – torsion about the pedicle between them.

The two main factors that determine the damage to the testis are the extent of the twist and the duration of the episode. Twists of 720° cause more rapid ischaemia than twists of 360° or less, while if the testis can be untwisted within 6 hours of the torsion taking place there is nearly a 100% chance of testicular salvage compared with a 20% salvage rate if the surgery is delayed for 24 hours.

Occasionally the testis untwists spontaneously without the need for surgical treatment and such episodes of intermittent testicular torsion should be considered as a cause of intermittent testicular pain in adolescents.

Clinical features

Testicular torsion is most common between 10 and 25 years of age, although a few cases occur outside this age range. Typically there is sudden agonising pain in the groin and the lower abdomen and the patient feels nauseated and may vomit. Torsion of a fully descended testis is usually easily recognised. The scrotum is swollen and tender, while the skin is usually not erythematous initially (although it may become so with a prolonged history) and the patient is apyrexial. The testis itself is swollen and tender and seems high within the scrotum, while the tender twisted cord can often be palpated above it. The cremasteric reflex is lost.

Differential diagnosis

Redness of the skin and a mild pyrexia may result in the condition being confused with epididymo-orchitis in the older patient; however, in epididymo-orchitis there will usually be dysuria associated with the accompanying urinary infection. Elevation of the testis reduces the pain in epididymo-orchitis while it makes it worse in torsion.

Torsion of a testicular appendage cannot always be distinguished with certainty from testicular torsion. The most common structure to twist is the appendix of the testis (the pedunculated hydatid of Morgagni). The twisted testicular appendages can sometimes be visible through the scrotal wall as a small dark spot. If the diagnosis is made clinically, then conservative management is possible, but if in doubt then

Giovanni Battista Morgagni, 1682–1771, Professor of Anatomy at the University of Padua, is associated with a number of eponymous structures including the aortic sinus, the appendix testis, the anal columns and the sternocostal triangles. He is regarded as the 'Father of Morbid Anatomy'.

surgical exploration should be undertaken with ligation and amputation of the twisted appendage.

In mumps orchitis, the cord is not particularly thickened and the condition is often bilateral.

Idiopathic scrotal oedema is an oddity that occurs between the age of 4 and 12 years and must be differentiated from torsion. The scrotum is very swollen but there is little pain or tenderness. The swelling is usually bilateral and may extend into the perineum, groin and penis. It is thought to be an allergic phenomenon and occasionally there is eosinophilia. The swelling subsides after a day or so but may recur (Figure 80.6).

Very occasionally, torsion can be convincingly mimicked by a small tense strangulated inguinal hernia compressing the cord and causing compression of the pampiniform plexus.

Management

The management of the case should be determined primarily on clinical grounds. While Doppler ultrasound scanning can confirm the absence of the blood supply to the affected testis, false-positive results can be seen so it is not routinely recommended. If there is any doubt as to the diagnosis, then urgent scrotal exploration is indicated.

Exploration for torsion should be performed through a transverse scrotal incision. If the testis is viable when the cord is untwisted, it should be prevented from twisting again by fixation with three non-absorbable sutures between the tunica albuginea of the testis and the scrotal raphe. The use of absorbable sutures risks the possibility of recurrent torsion at some time in the future. The other testis should also be fixed because the anatomical predisposition is likely to be bilateral. If there is clinical doubt as to testicular viability after detorsion of the testis, then it should be wrapped in a warm swab and observed over a few minutes. If a small incision in the tunica albuginea demonstrates bright red arterial bleeding then the testis may survive. An infarcted testis should be removed – the patient can be counselled later about a prosthetic replacement.

In cases where there is a history of pain for several days, the affected testis will be dead. It is not possible to recover such a testis and although little is gained (other than pain relief) by immediate exploration, it is necessary to fix the contralateral testis.

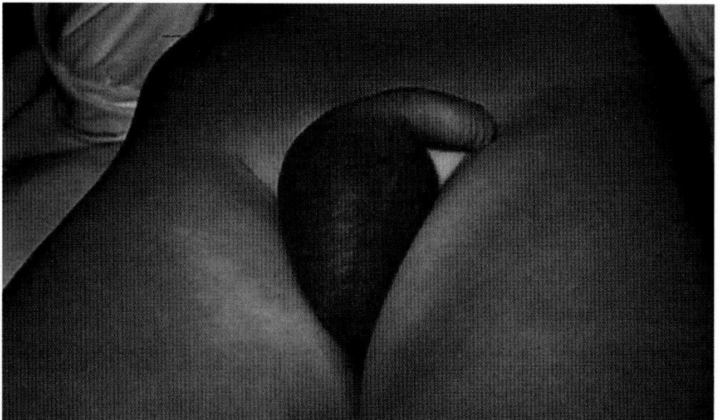

Figure 80.6 Idiopathic oedema of the scrotum.

Summary box 80.4

Testicular torsion

- If the diagnosis of testicular torsion is possible, then surgical exploration is indicated
- Prompt exploration, untwisting and fixation is the only way to save the torted testis
- The patient should be counselled and consented for orchidectomy before exploration
- The anatomical abnormality is bilateral and the contralateral testis should also be fixed
- Three non-absorbable sutures should be used for the fixation of each testis

VARICOCOELE

A varicocoele is a varicose dilatation of the veins draining the testis.

Surgical anatomy

The veins draining the testis and the epididymis form the pampiniform plexus. The veins gradually join each other as they traverse the inguinal canal and at, or near, the inguinal ring, there are only one or two testicular veins, which pass upwards within the retroperitoneum. The left testicular vein empties into the left renal vein while the right empties into the inferior vena cava below the right renal vein. The testicular veins usually have valves near their terminations, but these are sometimes absent. There is an alternative (collateral) venous return from the testes through the cremasteric veins, which drain mainly into the inferior epigastric veins.

Aetiology

Varicocoeles are common, affecting perhaps 15–20% of adult males and 90% are left sided, reflecting the proximal venous anatomy. They are unusual in boys and typically develop during late childhood and adolescence. In some cases, the dilated vessels are cremasteric veins and not part of the pampiniform plexus. The usual cause is absence or incompetence of valves in the proximal testicular vein. While most varicocoeles are idiopathic, obstruction of the left testicular vein by a renal tumour or nephrectomy is a cause of varicocoele in later life; characteristically, in such cases the varicocoele does not decompress in the supine position.

Clinical features

While most varicocoeles are asymptomatic, those that are symptomatic tend to present in adolescence or early

Christian Johann Doppler, 1803–1853, Professor of Experimental Physics, Vienna, Austria, enunciated the 'Doppler Principle' in 1842.

adulthood, when there may be an annoying dragging discomfort that is worse on standing at the end of the day. This presumably reflects distension of the testicular veins. When examined in the erect position, the scrotum on the affected side hangs lower than normal (Figure 80.7); on palpation, with the patient standing, the varicose plexus feels like a bag of worms. There may be a cough impulse. If the patient lies down the veins empty by gravity and this provides an opportunity to ensure that the underlying testis is normal to palpation. In long-standing cases the affected testis is smaller and softer than its fellow, owing to a minor degree of atrophy.

Ultrasonography can be helpful in the diagnosis of small varicocoeles (Figure 80.8), and in older men with an apparently recent onset of varicocoele, ultrasonography of the kidneys is important in excluding a left renal tumour.

Grading of the varicocoele is possible, with a Grade I varicocoele being impalpable (i.e. observed only on ultrasound), Grade II being palpable and Grade III being visible.

Varicocoele and spermatogenesis

Of all the possible causes of primary infertility, oligozoospermia (reduced numbers of sperm in the ejaculate) is one of the most difficult to treat. Because varicocoeles are relatively common, some men with oligozoospermia will have a varicocoele, and it is tempting to blame this for the infertility. Certainly the varicocoele will tend to 'warm' the testis, which is usually around 2.5°C below rectal temperature, and there is conflicting evidence regarding the effect of this temperature difference upon spermatogenesis. Unfortunately, there is little evidence that varicocoelectomy improves semen quality or the rate of conception.

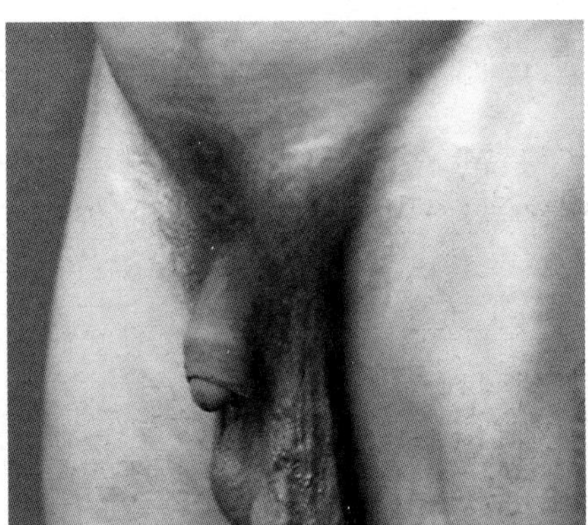

Figure 80.7 Large varicocoele in a pendulous scrotum. Note the left inguinal hernia.

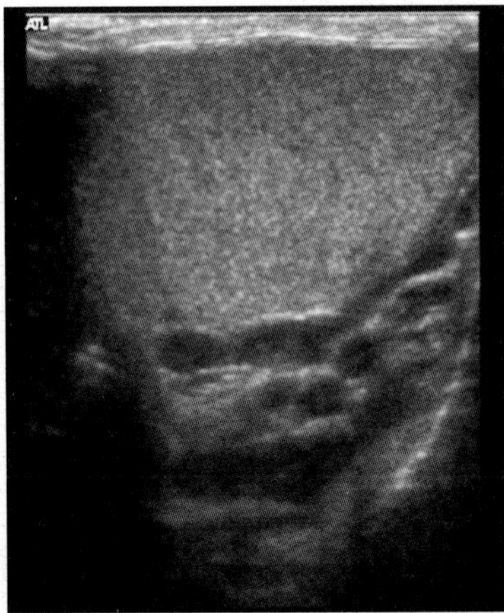

Figure 80.8 Ultrasound of a varicocoele. Note the dilated veins at the lower pole of the testis.

Treatment

Operation is not indicated for an asymptomatic varicocoele. When the discomfort is significant, then percutaneous embolisation of the gonadal veins is the usual first-line intervention. If this is not possible, or if the varicocoele recurs (as it does in around 20% after embolisation), then surgical ligation of the testicular veins is the appropriate treatment, although recurrence can occur even after such surgery.

Summary box 80.5

Varicocoele

- Varicocoele is a common condition and 90% are left sided
- Development of a left-sided varicocoele in later life may indicate the presence of a renal tumour
- They are usually asymptomatic and as such rarely need treatment
- First-line treatment is embolisation in symptomatic cases
- Varicocoeles often recur, even after surgical treatment
- The association of varicocoeles with subfertility is controversial

HYDROCOELE

A hydrocoele is an abnormal collection of serous fluid in a part of the processus vaginalis, usually the tunica vaginalis. Acquired hydrocoeles are primary or idiopathic, or secondary to epididymal or testicular disease.

Aetiology

A hydrocoele can be produced in four different ways (Figure 80.9):

1 By connection with the peritoneal cavity via a patent processus vaginalis (congenital).
2 By excessive production of fluid within the sac, e.g. a secondary hydrocoele.

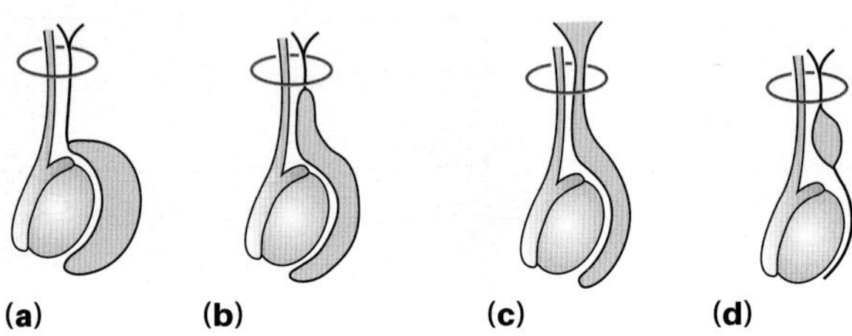

Figure 80.9 (a) Vaginal hydrocoele (very common); (b) 'infantile' hydrocoele; (c) congenital hydrocoele; (d) hydrocoele of the cord.

3 By defective absorption of fluid; this appears to be the explanation for most primary hydrocoeles, although the reason why the fluid is not absorbed is obscure. They are sometimes called vaginal hydrocoeles.
4 By interference with the lymphatic drainage of scrotal structures.

A secondary hydrocoele is most frequently associated with acute or chronic epididymo-orchitis. It is also seen with torsion of the testis and with some testicular tumours. A secondary hydrocoele is usually lax and is typically small: the underlying testis is usually palpable. If a tumour is suspected, the hydrocoele should not be punctured for fear of needle-track implantation of malignant cells. A secondary hydrocoele subsides when the primary lesion resolves.

Clinical features

Examination of a scrotal swelling should be undertaken in both the upright and supine position. The examiner should ask themselves a series of questions. First, is it possible to get above the swelling to palpate a normal cord? For instance, if it is not possible to achieve this, the swelling may represent an inguinal hernia that has entered the scrotum. Second, is the swelling primarily testicular or epididymal or is it enclosing both of those structures? Thirdly, does the swelling transilluminate? In almost all cases of scrotal swelling an ultrasound is a useful adjunct, both in clarifying the nature of the swelling and in determining whether the testis itself is diseased.

A hydrocoele is a swelling that encloses the testis and epididymis such that they may be impalpable, and it is possible to get 'above' it to palpate a normal spermatic cord (Figure 80.10). They are typically translucent.

A primary hydrocoele is seen most commonly in middle and later life, but can also occur in older children. The condition is particularly common in hot countries. Because the swelling is usually painless it may reach a prodigious size before the patient presents for treatment. Be wary of an acute hydrocoele in a young man since there may be a testicular tumour.

In congenital hydrocoele, the processus vaginalis is patent and connects with the peritoneal cavity. The communication is usually too small to allow herniation of intra-abdominal contents. Pressure on the hydrocoele does not always empty it but the hydrocoele fluid may drain into the peritoneal cavity when the child is lying down; thus, the hydrocoele may be intermittent. Ascites should be checked for if the swellings are bilateral.

An encysted hydrocoele of the cord is a smooth oval swelling that lies above the testis near the spermatic cord, which is liable to be mistaken for an inguinal hernia. The swelling moves downwards and becomes less mobile if the testis is pulled gently downwards.

Hydrocoele of the canal of Nuck is a similar condition in females. The cyst lies in relation to the round ligament and is always at least partially within the inguinal canal.

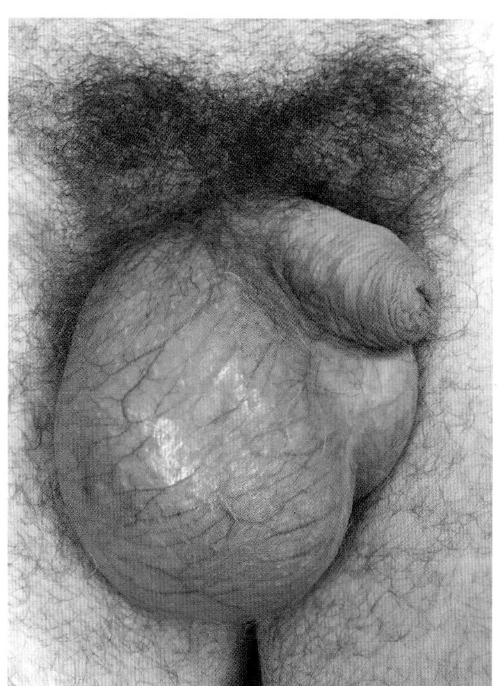

Figure 80.10 A right-sided hydrocoele.

Treatment

Congenital hydrocoeles are treated by herniotomy if they do not resolve spontaneously (see Chapter 9).

Small acquired hydrocoeles do not need treatment. If they are sizeable and bothersome for the patient, then surgical treatment is indicated. Established acquired hydrocoeles often have thick walls. There are three main surgical techniques for hydrocoeles;

- **Plication.** Lord's operation is suitable when the sac is reasonably thin-walled (Figure 80.11). There is minimal dissection and the risk of haematoma is reduced.
- **Eversion.** The sac is opened and everted behind the testis, with placement of the testis in a pouch prepared by dissection in the fascial planes of the scrotum (Jaboulay's procedure) (Figure 80.12).

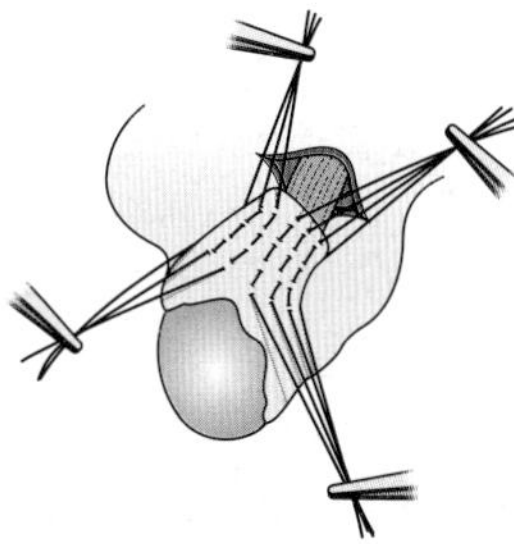

Figure 80.11 Lord's operation. A series of interrupted absorbable sutures is used to plicate the redundant tunica vaginalis. When these are tied, the tunica bunches at its attachment to the testis.

Anton Nuck, 1650–1692, Professor of Anatomy and Medicine, Leiden, The Netherlands.
Peter Herent Lord, contemporary, formerly surgeon, Wycombe General Hospital, High Wycombe, Buckinghamshire, UK.

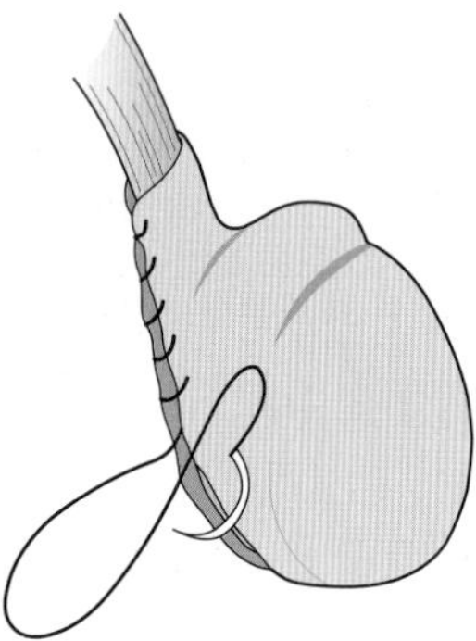

Figure 80.12 Jaboulay's procedure. The hydrocoele sac is everted and anchored with sutures.

- **Excision**. Unless great care is taken to stop bleeding after excision of the wall, haemorrhage from the cut edge is liable to cause a large scrotal haematoma. This approach is not recommended.

Aspiration of the hydrocoele fluid is simple, but the fluid always reaccumulates within a week or so. It may be suitable for men who are unfit for scrotal surgery, although hydrocoele surgery can be undertaken under local anaesthetic. Aspiration can result in bleeding into the hydrocoele sac and haematocoele formation. Injection of a sclerosant, such as tetracycline, is effective but painful.

Summary box 80.6

Hydrocoele

- A hydrocoele is a collection of fluid within the tunica vaginalis
- Primary hydrocoeles surround the testis and transilluminate brightly
- Ultrasound examination is valuable, especially when the testis and epididymis are impalpable
- Hydrocoeles can be treated conservatively unless they are large and symptomatic
- Surgery is the mainstay of treatment
- Testicular malignancy is an uncommon cause of hydrocoele that can be excluded by ultrasound examination

Filarial hydrocoeles and chylocoeles

Filarial hydrocoeles and chylocoeles account for up to 80% of hydrocoeles in tropical countries, where the parasite *Wuchereria bancrofti* is endemic. Filarial hydrocoeles follow repeated attacks of filarial epididymo-orchitis. They vary in size and may develop slowly or very rapidly. Occasionally, the fluid contains liquid fat, which is rich in cholesterol. This is caused by rupture of a lymphatic varix with discharge of chyle into the hydrocoele. In long-standing chylocoeles, there are dense adhesions between the scrotum and its contents. Filarial elephantiasis supervenes in a small number of cases. Treatment is by rest and aspiration. The more usual chronic cases are treated by excision of the sac.

CYSTS ASSOCIATED WITH THE EPIDIDYMIS

There are several types of cyst associated with the epididymis, including epididymal cysts and spermatocoeles.

Epididymal cysts

These are filled with a crystal-clear fluid. They are very common, usually multiple and vary in size at presentation. They represent cystic degeneration of the epididymis. Cysts of the epididymis are usually found in middle age and are often bilateral. The clusters of tense cysts feel like a tiny bunches of grapes that lie posterior to, and quite separate from, the testis. They should transilluminate brilliantly. The diagnosis can by confirmed by ultrasound (Figure 80.13).

Aspiration is useless because the cysts are usually multilocular. If they are causing discomfort they should be excised. While single large cysts can be excised separately, recurrent or multilocular cysts usually require partial or total epididymectomy. Excision should be expected to interfere with the transportation of sperm from the testis on that side and young men should be counselled regarding this.

Spermatocoele

This is a unilocular retention cyst derived from some portion of the sperm-conducting mechanism of the epididymis. A spermatocoele typically lies in the epididymal head above

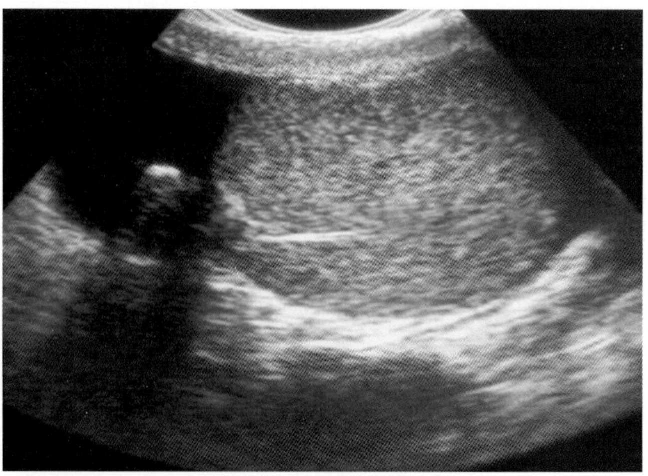

Figure 80.13 Ultrasound of an epididymal cyst.

Mathieu Jaboulay, 1860–1913, Professor of Surgery, Lyons, France.
Edward Gibbon, 1737–1794, the author of '*The decline and fall of the Roman empire*', was greatly embarrassed by a large hydrocoele. The second time that it was tapped it became infected, and Gibbon died a few days later. The hydrocoele was associated with a large scrotal hernia, which had probably been punctured.
Otto Eduard Heinrich Wucherer, 1820–1873, German physician who practised in Brazil.
Joseph Bancroft, 1836–1894, English physician working in Australia.

and behind the upper pole of the testis. It is usually softer and laxer than other cystic lesions in the scrotum but, like them, it transilluminates. The fluid contains spermatozoa and resembles barley water in appearance. Spermatocoeles are usually small and unobtrusive. Small spermatocoeles can be ignored. Larger ones should be excised.

Summary box 80.7

Cysts associated with the epididymis

- Lie posterior to and separate from the testis and they transilluminate
- Diagnosis can be confirmed by ultrasound examination
- Can be treated conservatively unless they are large or uncomfortable

EPIDIDYMO-ORCHITIS

Inflammation confined to the epididymis is epididymitis; infection spreading to the testis is epididymo-orchitis.

Pathophysiology

Infection reaches the epididymis via the vas from a primary infection of the urethra, prostate or seminal vesicles. A general rule is that epididymitis arises in sexually active young men from a sexually transmitted genital infection, while in older men it more usually arises from a urinary infection or may be secondary to an indwelling urethral catheter.

In young sexually active men, the most common cause of epididymitis is now *Chlamydia trachomatis*, but gonococcal epididymitis is still occasionally seen. In older men with bladder outflow obstruction, epididymitis may result from a urinary infection – it is proposed that a high pressure in the prostatic urethra might cause reflux of infected urine up the vasa. Blood-borne infections of the epididymis are less common but may be suspected when there is epididymal infection without evidence of urinary infection; it is presumably the only possible mechanism in men who have previously undergone a vasectomy. Acute epididymo-orchitis can follow any form of urethral instrumentation and it is particularly common when an indwelling catheter is associated with infection of the prostate.

Infection usually starts in the tail of the epididymis and spreads to the rest of the epididymis and occasionally to the testis. Complications include abscess formation, testicular infarction, testicular atrophy, chronic induration and inflammation and infertility.

Clinical features

While there may be initial symptoms of a urinary or a genital infection, such symptoms are not always seen. The development of an ache in the groin and a fever can herald the onset of epididymitis. The epididymis and testis swell and become painful. The scrotal wall, at first red, oedematous and shiny, may become adherent to the epididymis.

Investigation should include a urethral swab, a urine specimen for culture, nucleic acid amplification testing (NAAT) of either a urine specimen or a urethral swab and scrotal ultrasound. Urinalysis will usually show leukocytes and may show a formal urinary tract infection. NAAT is a sensitive way of identifying both gonoccal and chlamydial urethritis. Ultrasound is useful in the initial assessment of epididymitis and will identify abscess formation.

In adolescents, the differential diagnosis is testicular torsion and if there is any clinical doubt as to the diagnosis then testicular exploration should always be performed.

Treatment

Either doxycycline (100–200 mg daily) or a quinolone should be the initial treatment in young men. There should be contact tracing of the partner and treatment if necessary. Antibiotic treatment should continue for at least 2 weeks.

In older men, quinolones are the usual initial treatment, but if there is evidence of systemic sepsis, then intravenous antibiotics directed at urinary pathogens may be valuable. If an organism is isolated from the urine, this simplifies the choice of antibiotic.

All patients should drink plenty of fluid. Local measures including scrotal support and analgesia are helpful. Antibiotic treatment should continue for at least 2 weeks or until the inflammation has subsided. If suppuration occurs, drainage is necessary.

Chronic disease

Chronic non-tuberculous epididymitis usually follows the failure of resolution of an acute episode of epididymitis. Patients typically complain of intermittent episodes of discomfort and the epididymis feels thickened and tender. Treatment involves use of antibiotics (usually quinolones or doxycycline) and anti-inflammatory agents for 4–6 weeks. Epididymectomy or orchidectomy can be considered if there is no resolution, although some patients continue to suffer from pain despite such surgery.

Summary box 80.8

Acute epididymo-orchitis

- In young men usually arises secondary to a sexually transmitted genital infection
- In older men usually arises secondary to urinary infection
- May be a complication of catheterisation or instrumentation of the urinary tract
- May need aggressive treatment with parenteral antibiotics

Tuberculous epididymo-orchitis

Chronic tuberculous epididymo-orchitis usually begins insidiously. The frequency with which the lower pole of the epididymis is involved first indicates that the infection is usually retrograde from a tuberculous focus in the seminal vesicles.

Clinical features

Typically, there is a firm, uncomfortable discrete swelling of the lower pole of the epididymis. The disease progresses until the whole epididymis is firm and craggy behind a normal-feeling testis. There is a lax secondary hydrocoele in 30% of cases, and a characteristic beading of the vas may be apparent as a result of subepithelial tubercles. The seminal vesicles feel indurated and swollen. In neglected cases, a tuberculous 'cold' abscess forms, which may discharge. The body of the testis may be uninvolved for years but the contralateral epididymis often becomes diseased. In two-thirds of cases there is evidence of renal tuberculosis or previous disease. Otherwise, patients typically appear healthy.

The urine and semen should be examined repeatedly for tubercle bacilli in all patients with chronic epididymo-orchitis. A chest radiograph should be performed, as should imaging of the upper urinary tract. Ultrasound will demonstrate a thickened epididymis.

Treatment

Secondary tuberculous epididymitis may resolve when the primary focus is treated. Treatment with antituberculous drugs is less effective in genital tuberculosis than in urinary tuberculosis. If resolution does not occur within 2 months, epididymectomy or orchidectomy is advisable. A course of antituberculous chemotherapy should be completed even if there is no evidence of disease elsewhere.

ORCHITIS

Mumps orchitis, which is the most common form of orchitis, develops in 20–30% of postpubertal patients with a mumps virus infection and it usually develops as the parotid swelling is waning. Evidence of IgM antibodies in the serum supports the diagnosis. The main complication is testicular atrophy, which may cause infertility if the condition is bilateral. Partial testicular atrophy is associated with persistent testicular pain.

Syphilitic orchitis is now uncommon. It can cause bilateral orchitis (which is a feature of congenital syphilis), interstitial fibrosis, which causes painless destruction of the testis, or, rarely, it may lead to a gumma of the testis, which presents as a unilateral slowly growing painless swelling. The latter presentation may be difficult to distinguish from a neoplasm without surgical exploration. Diagnosis is confirmed by serology.

TUMOURS OF THE TESTES

Testicular cancer represents around 1–1.5% of male neoplasms and there is clear evidence of an increased incidence of these tumours in the past 30 years. The vast majority are germ cell tumours and the peak incidence of seminomas is in the 4th decade of life, with the non-seminomatous germ cell tumours (NSGCT) being more common in the 3rd decade of life. They are the commonest form of tumour in young men. Risk factors include a history of testicular maldescent, a history of a contralateral testicular tumour and Klinefelter's syndrome.

Classification and pathology

Tumours of the testis are classified according to their predominant cellular type:

- **germ cell tumours** (90–95%) (these include seminoma, embryonal cell carcinoma, yolk sac tumour, teratoma, and choriocarcinoma);
- **interstitial tumours** (1–2%) (these include Leydig cell tumours);
- **lymphoma** (3–7%);
- **other tumours** (1–2%).

Seminoma

A seminoma typically has a cut surface that is homogeneous and pinkish cream in colour. It appears to compress neighbouring testicular tissue (Figure 80.14). It consists of oval cells with clear cytoplasm and large, rounded nuclei with prominent acidophilic nucleoli. Sheets of cells resembling spermatocytes are separated by a fine fibrous stroma. Active lymphocytic infiltration of the tumour suggests a good host response and a better prognosis. There are two histological variants, one with a more anaplastic appearance and another that is characterised by cells that closely resemble different phases of maturing spermatogonia (spermatocytic seminoma).

Seminomas metastasise mainly via the lymphatics (Figure 80.15) and haematogenous spread is uncommon. The lymphatic drainage of the testes is to the para-aortic lymph nodes near the origin of the gonadal vessels. The contralateral para-aortic lymph nodes are sometimes involved by tumour spread, but the inguinal lymph nodes are affected only if the scrotal skin is involved.

Non-seminomatous germ cell tumours

These tumours may be tiny but can reach the size of a coconut. The smaller tumours may not even distort the tunica albuginea (Figure 80.16). The usual type of teratoma is yellowish in colour with cystic spaces containing gelatinous fluid (Figure 80.17). There are a number of histological types of NSGCT, which may coexist within a single tumour:

- **embryonal carcinoma**: highly malignant tumours that occasionally invade cord structures;
- **yolk sac tumour**: tumours with this component secrete alpha fetoprotein (AFP);

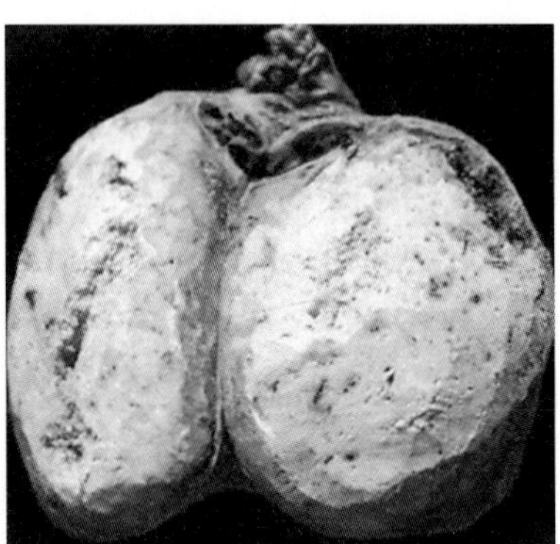

Figure 80.14 Seminoma of the testis.

Harry Fitch Klinefelter, Jr., 1912–1990, American rheumatologist and endocrinologist.

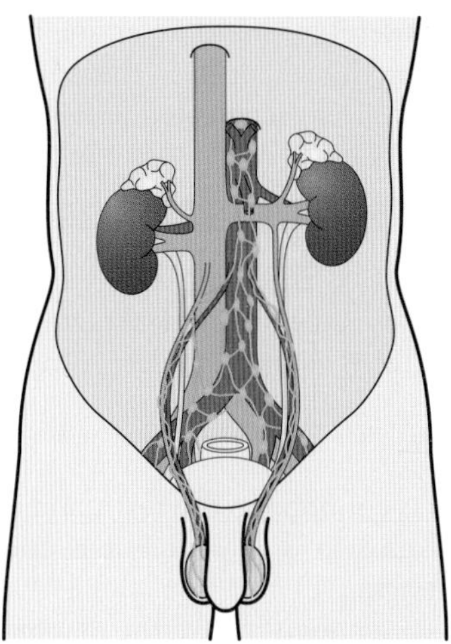

Figure 80.15 Lymphatic drainage of the testes to para-aortic lymph nodes.

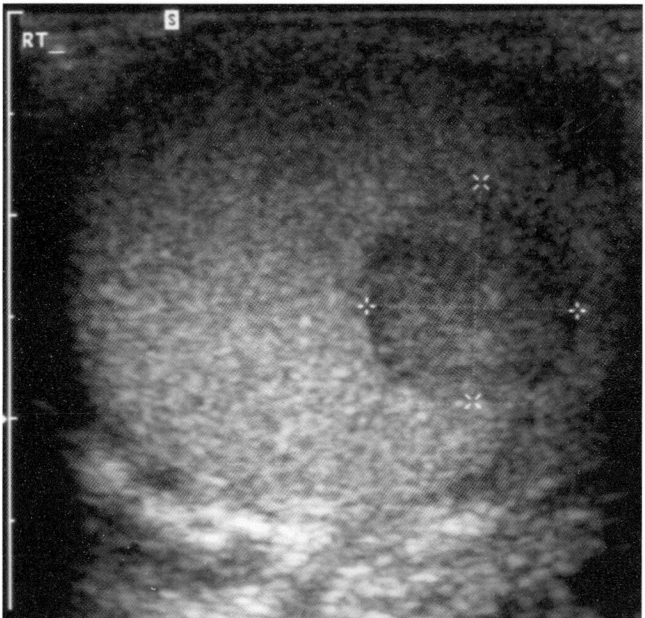

Figure 80.16 Ultrasound of a small intratesticular tumour with minimal distortion of the tunica albuginea.

- **choriocarcinoma**: often produces human chorionic gonadotrophin (hCG). This is a highly malignant tumour that metastasises early via both the lymphatics and the bloodstream;
- **teratoma**: these tumours contain more than one cell type, with components derived from ectoderm, endoderm and mesoderm. Tumours may range from 'mature' with well-differentiated tissue elements, to 'immature' with undifferentiated primitive tissues. All can metastasise.

Interstitial cell tumours

Interstitial cell tumours arise from Leydig or Sertoli cells. A Leydig cell tumour masculinises; a Sertoli cell tumour feminises. They are typically small well-circumscribed tumours with a yellow cut surface. Microscopically, the cells are usually uniform and closely packed. Approximately 10% are malignant.

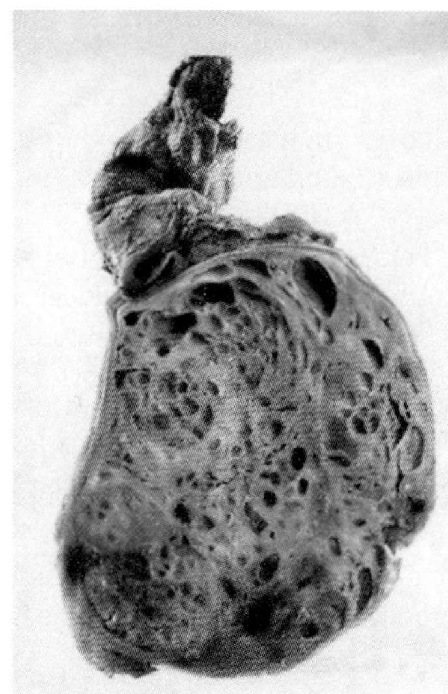

Figure 80.17 Teratoma of the testis – note the solid and cystic areas (courtesy of Dr Keith Simpson, London, UK).

Most prepubertal interstitial cell tumours (which account for around 25% of cases) produce androgens, which cause sexual precocity including prominent external genitalia, suprapubic hair growth and a deep masculinised voice. Regression of the symptoms after orchidectomy may be incomplete. Most postpubertal interstitial cell tumours produce feminising hormones, leading to gynaecomastia, erectile dysfunction, loss of libido and azoospermia.

Clinical features

Usually the patient presents with a painless testicular lump. A sensation of heaviness can occur if the testis is two or three times its normal size, but only a minority of patients experience pain. In a few cases, an episode of trauma calls attention to the swelling. Some cases may simulate epididymo-orchitis and, rarely, some patients present with severe pain and acute enlargement of the testis because of haemorrhage into the tumour. Such cases can occasionally mimic testicular torsion.

Rarely, the predominant symptoms are those of metastatic disease. Intra-abdominal disease may cause abdominal or lumbar pain and the mass may be discovered in the epigastrium. Lung metastases are usually silent, but they can cause chest pain, dyspnoea and haemoptysis in the later stages of the disease. The primary tumour may not have been noticed by the patient, and indeed may be so tiny that it can be detected only by ultrasonography (**Figure 80.16**).

On examination there is an intratesticular solid mass. If present, a lax secondary hydrocoele does not usually obscure the underlying tumour. The epididymis becomes more difficult to feel when it is flattened or incorporated in the growth. The vas is never thickened and rectal examination is normal. Around 5% of cases have gynaecomastia (mainly the NSGCT). Metastatic disease is rarely apparent clinically and is more usually identified by formal staging investigations. In 1–2% of cases the tumour is bilateral at the time of diagnosis.

Investigation and staging

The diagnosis is confirmed by ultrasound scanning of the testis (Figure 80.18), which is also able to assess the contralateral testis. It is a mandatory test in all suspected cases of testicular tumour.

In confirmed cases, staging is an essential step in planning treatment. Blood is taken prior to orchidectomy to measure the levels of tumour markers, which are raised in around 50% of cases. A rise in AFP is seen in around 50–70% of NSGCTs and a rise in hCG is seen in 40–60% of NSGCTs and around 30% of seminomas. When raised, these markers are used to monitor the response to treatment. The mean serum half-lives of AFP and hCG are 5–7 days and 2–3 days respectively, and reassessment of the markers following orchidectomy can indicate whether all the tumour tissue has been removed.

While a chest x-ray will occasionally demonstrate the 'classical' cannon ball metastases (Figure 80.19) computed tomography (CT) of chest, abdomen and pelvis has taken over as the most useful means of detecting metastatic disease and for monitoring the response to therapy. Such imaging is usually undertaken after the affected testis has been removed.

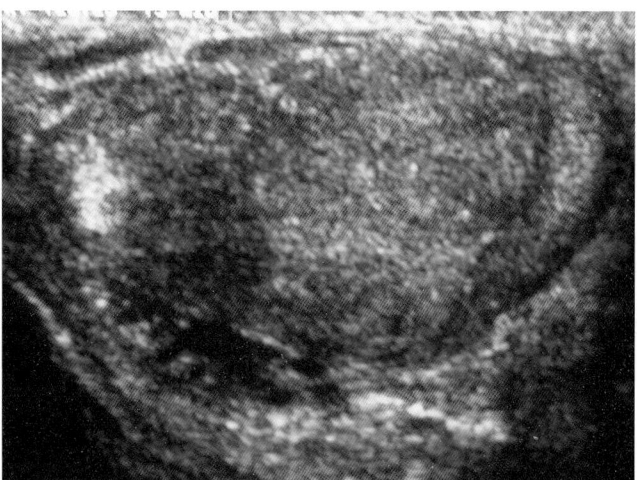

Figure 80.18 Testicular ultrasound: the homogeneous tissue of the testicular teratoma on the left of the image produces multiple ultrasound reflections.

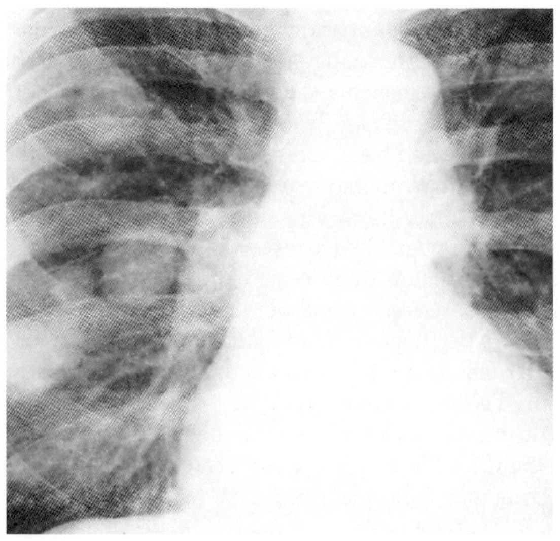

Figure 80.19 Cannon ball metastases from carcinoma of the testis.

Staging of testicular tumours

While TNM staging is the most widely used system for the staging of testicular cancer, the older staging system of Stages I-IV is still considered valuable in determining the treatment options.

The stages are:

Stage I: Tumour is confined to the testis and epididymis.
Stage II: Nodal disease is present but is confined to nodes below the diaphragm.
Stage III: Nodes are present above the diaphragm.
Stage IV: Non lymphatic metastatic disease (most typically within the lungs).

Summary box 80.9

Testicular tumours

- A solid testicular lump that cannot be felt separately from the testis may be a malignant tumour
- Lymphatic spread is to the para-aortic lymph nodes
- Ultrasound is a mandatory investigation in all cases of suspected testicular tumour
- Tumour markers (AFP and hCG) should be measured prior to orchidectomy

Treatment

Scrotal exploration and orchidectomy for suspected testicular tumour

The orchidectomy is undertaken via an inguinal incision. The spermatic cord is displayed by dividing the external oblique aponeurosis and a soft clamp is placed across the cord to stop dissemination of malignant cells as the testis is mobilised into the wound. Rarely, if there is doubt about the diagnosis, the testis should be bisected along its anterior convexity to examine its internal structure. If there is a tumour the cord should be double transfixed and divided at the level of the internal inguinal ring and the testis removed.

Management by staging and histological diagnosis (after orchidectomy)

The treatment of patients with germ cell tumours of the testis is usually successful, even in cases that are advanced at presentation. This largely reflects the excellent response of these tumours to platinum-based chemotherapy and (for seminomatous tumours) to radiotherapy. Indeed in recent years the emphasis of clinical trials has been focused upon the identification of those patients who do **not** need chemotherapy, and who therefore will escape the side effects of treatment.

STAGE I TUMOURS

Seminomas are radiosensitive and for many years adjuvant radiotherapy to the para-aortic nodes was the mainstay of treatment for stage I disease. However, there is also an excellent response to platinum-based chemotherapy, which led to chemotherapy being introduced as the primary treatment for stage I seminoma. However, given that only around 15–20% of men with stage I seminoma have subclinical metastatic disease, current protocols use CT and tumour marker-based surveillance protocols, with chemotherapy being reserved for men who demonstrate relapse.

NSGCTs are not radiosensitive, but they are highly sensitive to combination chemotherapy with bleomycin, etoposide and cis-platinum (so called BEP chemotherapy). Up to 30% of NSGCT patients with stage I disease have subclinical metastases and will relapse if surveillance alone is applied after orchidectomy. Accordingly, some NSGCTs with good prognoses can be managed by surveillance protocols (using regular CT scanning and tumour marker measurement), with the more high-risk cases receiving chemotherapy.

STAGE II-IV TUMOURS

Combination BEP chemotherapy is the mainstay of treatment for stages II–IV seminoma and NSGCT. Retroperitoneal lymph node dissection is sometimes needed in cases of NSGCT when retroperitoneal masses remain after chemotherapy (Figure 80.20). The tissue removed may contain only necrotic tissue, but some patients have foci of mature teratoma or active malignancy. The operation can be formidable if the tumour mass is large, and retrograde ejaculation is likely unless steps are taken to preserve the sympathetic outflow to the bladder neck.

INTERSTITIAL TUMOURS

Most of these tumours are benign (around 80%), so conservative treatment of small lesions with organ-sparing surgery is feasible, if the diagnosis is considered. For larger tumours, orchidectomy is necessary with multimodality treatment for those with the rare malignant forms of these tumours.

Prognosis

The prognosis of testicular tumours depends on several factors, including the histological type and the stage at presentation. For seminoma, if there are no metastases, 90–95% of patients will be alive 5 years after diagnosis. If there are poor prognostic features, the survival rate drops to around 70%. For NSGCTs a 5-year survival rate of more than 90% is achievable in patients with good prognosis tumours, while for more advanced tumours, the 5-year survival rate is about 60%.

Summary box 80.10

Testis tumour staging and treatment

- Tumour markers (AFP and hCG) help to make the diagnosis and to follow the response to treatment
- Computed tomography scanning of chest, abdomen and pelvis is central to the staging of testicular tumours
- Testicular tumours are extremely sensitive to platinum-based chemotherapy
- Prognosis is excellent when the patient is treated with combination chemotherapy in a cancer centre

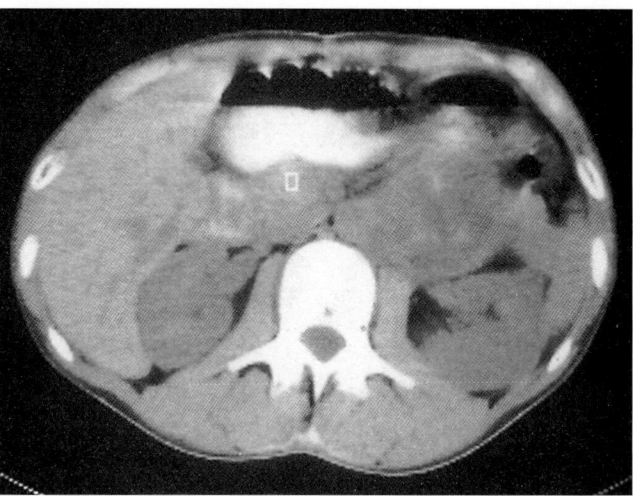

Figure 80.20 Computed tomography scan showing a large residual retroperitoneal mass after chemotherapy.

Testicular tumours in children

These are usually anaplastic teratomas. They occur before the age of 3 years and are often rapidly fatal.

TUMOURS OF THE EPIDIDYMIS

These may be benign mesothelioma or malignant sarcoma or secondary carcinoma. They are extremely rare but should not be forgotten when the patient presents with a non-cystic lump in the epididymis.

THE SCROTUM

Fournier's gangrene

Fournier's gangrene is an uncommon and nasty condition (Figure 80.21) characterised by a polymicrobial infection of the soft tissues of the perineum, external genitalia and perianal region. It is a form of necrotising fasciitis. There is rapid onset of gangrene leading to exposure of the scrotal contents. Although it can occur in conjunction with sepsis of the testis, epididymis or perianal region, an obvious cause is absent in over half the cases. It can arise following minor injuries or procedures in the perineal area, such as a bruise, scratch, urethral dilatation, injection of haemorrhoids or opening of a periurethral abscess. Many patients have concurrent illnesses that diminish their defences, most notably diabetes mellitus and alcoholism.

There is a mixed infection of aerobic and anaerobic bacteria in a fulminating inflammation of the subcutaneous tissues, which results in an obliterative arteritis of the arterioles to the scrotal skin that in turn results in gangrene. The condition can spread rapidly to involve the fascia and skin of the penis, perineum and abdominal wall.

Jean Alfred Fournier, 1832–1915, syphilologist, founder of the Venereal and Dermatological Clinic, Hôpital St Louis, Paris, France.

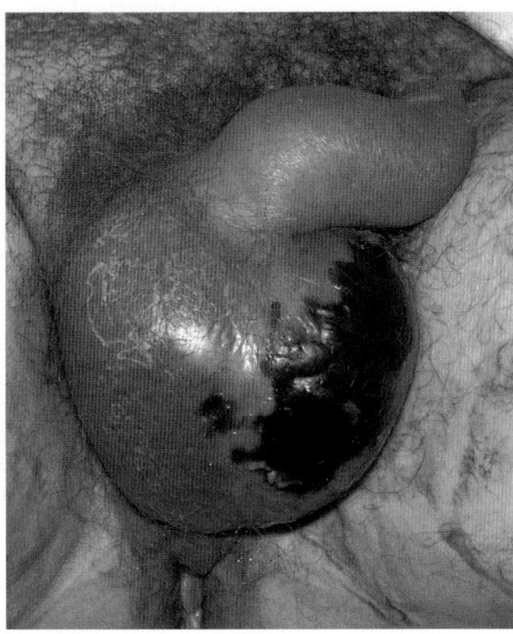

Figure 80.21 Fournier's gangrene with an area of necrotic skin overlying an area of scrotal inflammation.

> **Summary box 80.11**
>
> **Fournier's gangrene**
>
> - Fournier's gangrene requires early and aggressive treatment if the patient is to survive
> - Treatment involves urgent surgical debridement of necrotic tissue in combination with early use of intravenous broad spectrum antibiotics

Clinical features

There is sudden pain in the scrotum associated with prostration, pallor and pyrexia. Cellulitis spreads rapidly (within hours) with small necrotic areas of skin which, if untreated, coalesce to involve the entire scrotal and penile coverings, which may then slough, leaving the testes exposed but healthy. There may be crepitus and a foul-smelling exudate. The patient typically becomes septic and severely unwell in a short period of time

Treatment

Treatment of a case of Fournier's gangrene is a surgical emergency. Initial management involves intravenous fluid resuscitation and early use of broad spectrum intravenous antibiotics. Urgent wide surgical excision of the dead and infected tissue is essential and the extent of the internal necrosis is typically much greater than the external appearances suggest, such that extensive debridement is often necessary. Urinary and faecal diversion may be necessary. Supportive care is essential, because the patients often become severely septic.

Early review of the wounds is helpful to confirm that all dead tissue has been removed, and when the infection has been controlled, vacuum-assisted dressing is helpful, if it is available. If the patient survives the acute episode, skin grafting is often necessary. Despite best therapy, mortality rates as high as 50% are often reported.

Filarial elephantiasis of the scrotum

Filarial elephantiasis of the scrotum is caused by obstruction of the pelvic lymphatics by worms, of which *Wuchereria bancrofti* accounts for 90% of cases. The condition is common in the tropics and is transmitted by mosquitoes. It is often accompanied by superadded infection and lymphangitis, resulting in swelling of the genital skin and skin of the lower limbs. In long-standing cases, the enormously swollen scrotum may bury the penis (Figure 80.22). Associated symptoms and signs include fever, epididymitis, hydrocoele and chyluria. The diagnosis is usually made clinically although immunological testing can be helpful.

Medical treatment involves the use of diethylcarbamazine (DEC), ivermectin and albendazole, with the exact regime depending upon geographical location. Surgical treatment is rarely helpful, although a range of procedures have been devised to remove redundant skin and to reconstruct the enlarged scrotum.

Non-filarial elephantiasis

Elephantiasis can occur in the absence of filariasis, most notably in sub-Saharan Africa. Non-filarial elephantiasis can result from fibrosis of the lymphatics caused by lymphogranuloma venereum, but in many cases it is thought to arise as a consequence of persistent contact with irritant soils.

Sebaceous cysts

Sebaceous cysts are common in the scrotal skin. They are usually small and multiple (Figure 80.23). If troublesome, then surgical excision is necessary.

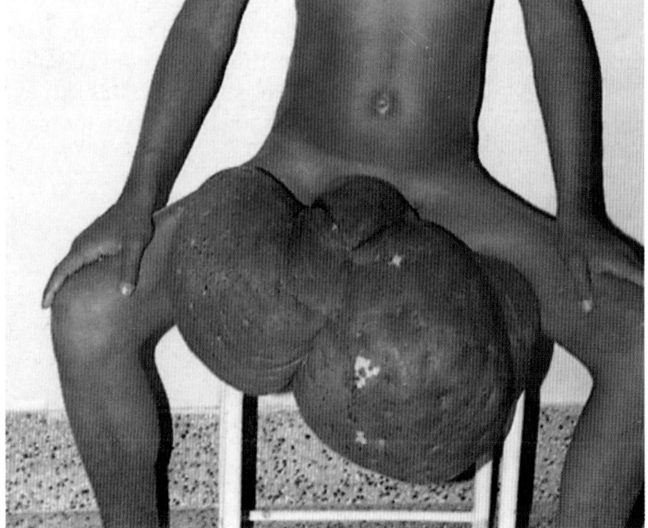

Figure 80.22 Elephantiasis of the scrotum burying the penis (courtesy of Mr S Bhattacharjee, Lucknow, India).

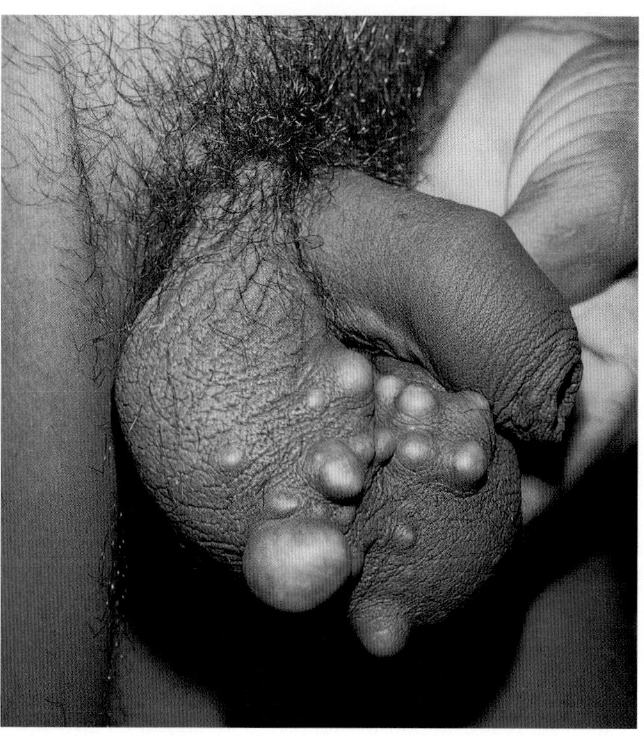
Figure 80.23 Sebaceous cysts of the scrotum (courtesy of Dr R Kaje MS, Jipmer, India).

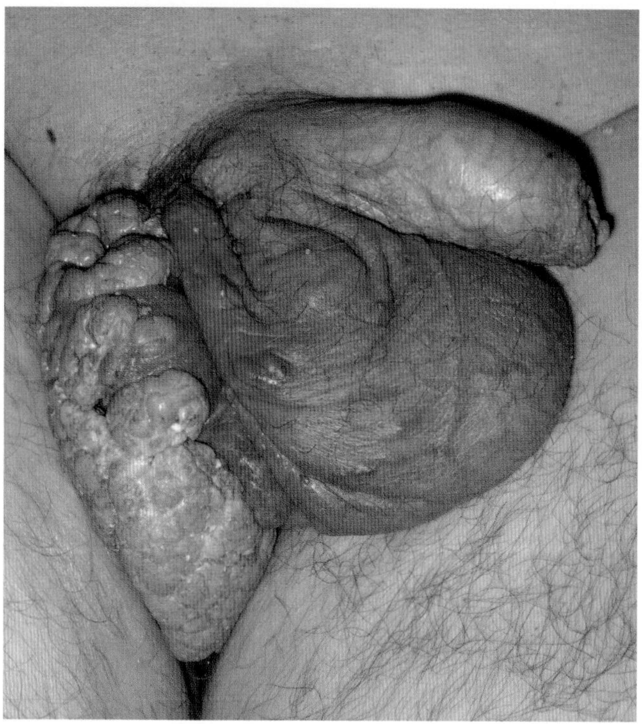
Figure 80.24 Scrotal cancer.

Carcinoma of the scrotum

'Chimney sweeps' cancer' was the first reported occupational cancer (described by Percival Pott in 1775). It is a rare cancer that has also been seen in other workers who come into contact with oil and coal products. Animal studies suggest that aromatic cyclic hydrocarbons are the aetiological factor. Nowadays, this tumour is rarely associated with any obvious aetiological factor. Unlike carcinoma of the penis, carcinoma of the scrotum is almost unknown in India and Asiatic countries.

The growth starts as a wart or ulcer (Figure 80.24) and as it grows it may involve the testis. The tumour should be excised with a margin of healthy skin. The management of the inguinal nodes parallels the management of penile cancer, and if nodal enlargement does not settle with antibiotics following treatment of the primary, then a bilateral groin dissection is indicated.

MALE FACTOR INFERTILITY

For couples of unknown fertility status, approximately 15% are unable to achieve a pregnancy within 1 year. The inability to conceive may be due to female factor infertility, male factor infertility or a combination of these two factors and approximately 20% of cases of infertility are caused entirely by the male factor.

Aetiology

The two main causes of male factor infertility are either primary testicular causes or obstruction at the level of either the vas or the epididymis. A few cases reflect endocrinological abnormalities such as hypogonadism or hyperprolactinaemia. Testicular causes include chromosomal problems (e.g. Klinefelter's syndrome), microdeletions of the Y chromosome, cryptorchidism, mumps orchitis, drugs and radiation damage. In most cases however, the cause is unclear. In these cases, there may be reduced numbers of sperm in the ejaculate (oligozoospermia) or a complete absence of sperm in the ejaculate (azoospermia).

Obstructive causes include congenital absence of the vasa (often in association with cystic fibrosis), surgical damage to the vasa and epididymitis. Azoospermia is inevitable in these cases.

Assessment and investigation

Given the interplay between male and female factors, the man should not be investigated in isolation from his female partner. A careful history is the mainstay of the assessment with a careful search for aetiological factors. Physical examination is usually normal, but occasionally the testes may feel small (suggestive of a testicular cause), the vasa may be absent, there may be evidence of endocrine abnormalities

Percival Pott, 1714–1788, surgeon, St Bartholomew's Hospital, London, UK, described chimney sweeps' cancer of the scrotum in 1775. In those days the chimney sweep's apprentice climbed up inside the chimney.

(gynaecomastia or abnormal hair distribution) or there may be a varicocoele. The relation of any varicocoele to the infertility is controversial and treatment is not usually indicated.

The woman should be also be assessed. It is important to remember that female fertility declines from the age of 35 years in a way that is not true of men. The age of the woman is therefore important and the regularity of menstruation should be confirmed either by temperature testing or by endocrinological testing.

The assessment of the man includes semen analysis, which should be tested within 2 hours of the semen being produced. Two or three samples should be tested. The volume of the ejaculate, the numbers of sperm, their motility and the percentage of abnormal or damaged sperm are all predictive of male fertility. An endocrine screen should be performed including serum testosterone, prolactin, follicle-stimulating hormone (FSH) and luteinising hormone (LH).

Treatment

Sperm counts of less than 15 million sperm per millilitre are defined as oligozoospermia. If there is a reversible cause, it should be treated. However, in many cases, some form of assisted conception is required.

Azoospermia (the complete absence of sperm from the ejaculate) is either due to obstruction of the pathway of spermatozoa from the testis to the ejaculatory ducts or due to severe testicular failure. In the latter the serum FSH is typically raised, while in obstructive cases, the FSH is typically normal. If there is doubt as to the cause, then testicular biopsy is mandated to check for the presence of spermatogenesis, combined with vasography to assess the presence and location of any obstructive lesion. If the site of the obstruction can be identified it may be possible to perform a bypass operation. Unfortunately, even in the best hands, the results of epididymovasostomy are poor.

Assisted conception including *in vitro* fertilisation (IVF) and intracytoplasmic sperm injection (ICSI) has revolutionised the management of male factor infertility regardless of the cause of the problem. In ICSI, spermatozoa harvested from the ejaculate, by aspiration of the epididymis or even from testicular biopsy, can be injected *in vitro* into ova obtained from the mother. Embryos are then transferred into the mother's uterus at the four- to six-cell stage.

Summary box 80.12

Male infertility

- Atrophy of the testis is associated with raised levels of follicle-stimulating hormone in the blood
- Testicular biopsy will show whether azoospermia is a result of obstruction or failure of sperm production
- If spermatozoa can be harvested they can be used in intracytoplasmic sperm injection with a fertility rate of around 30%

Vasectomy for sterilisation

Vasectomy for sterilisation is a common and effective contraceptive procedure. It should be undertaken only after the couple has been carefully counselled. Both partners need to know that the operation is performed to make the man permanently sterile. They should be warned that normal contraceptive precautions should continue until the success of the operation is confirmed by semen analysis performed 12–16 weeks after surgery. They should also be warned of the possibility of spontaneous recanalisation, which may restore fertility unexpectedly and of the possibility of chronic testicular pain that may occur in up to 5% of men.

Vasectomy is easily and painlessly performed under local anaesthetic. The vasa are delivered through tiny bilateral scrotal incisions or through a single midline scrotal incision. For medico-legal reasons it is wise to remove a segment of each vas to prove that it has been successfully divided. Burying the cut ends, fascial interposition or turning them back on themselves helps to prevent them rejoining.

Reversal of vasectomy may not restore fertility even if the surgery is technically successful because of damage to the testis secondary to the vasectomy. Although patency rates of 80% or more are commonly reported, successful fertility rates are much lower, and diminish with increasing delay from the time of vasectomy.

Summary box 80.13

Vasectomy

Counselling before vasectomy should include mention that:

- The operation is not immediately effective and that contraceptive precautions should be continued until there have been two negative semen analyses
- The procedure should be considered irreversible
- Spontaneous recanalisation is rare, but can occur
- There is a risk of chronic scrotal pain postoperatively

FURTHER READING

Kaisary AV, Ballaro A, Pigott K. *Lecture notes: urology*, 7th edn. Oxford: Wiley-Blackwell, 2016.

McDougal WS, Wein AJ, Kavoussi LR, *et al. Campbell-Walsh urology*, 11th edn. Elsevier, 2015.

Chapter 81

Gynaecology

Learning objectives

To understand:

- The pelvic anatomy and reproductive physiology
- The common causes of vaginal bleeding and acute pain in early pregnancy
- The surgical management of acute pelvic inflammatory disease, endometriosis, uterovaginal prolapse, uterine fibroids and ovarian tumours.

ANATOMY

The reproductive structures of the dividing embryo differentiate after the seventh week of development. The gonads, internal and external genitalia consititute the sex organs. In the female, the Müllerian ducts develop into the uterus, Fallopian tubes, cervix and upper third portion of the vagina. The urogenital sinus in turn forms the lower two-thirds of the vagina.

The female external genitalia are described as the vulva, which is bordered by the mons veneris anteriorly and the labiocrural folds posterolaterally. The opposing skin that covers the introitus is known as the labia majora. The labia minora are folds of skin that fuse anteriorly around the clitoris, which contains erectile tissue similar to the penis in the male. The posterior part of the introitus is referred to as the fourcette, and this stretches considerably during childbirth to allow delivery of the baby.

The vagina is an elastic, distensible tube, approximately 6–7 cm in length, passing upwards and backwards from the introitus. The cervix protrudes into the vault of the vagina, dividing it into the anterior, posterior and lateral fornices. Pelvic structures can be felt in the posterior and lateral fornices on bimanual examination, as the vaginal vault sits just below the pouch of Douglas (the area at the bottom of the pelvic cavity bordered by the uterus anteriorly and rectum posteriorly). The urethra and bladder neck sit above the anterior wall of the vagina; the perineal body and rectum behind the posterior wall (Figure 81.1).

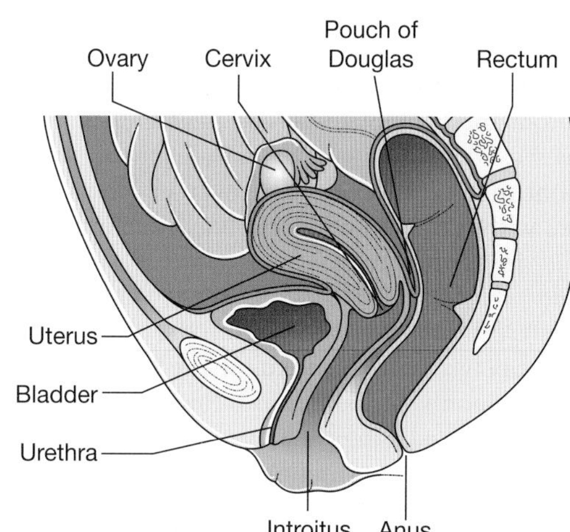

Figure 81.1 Female anatomy.

The uterus consists of a body and a cervix (neck of the uterus), and is an upside-down pear-shaped structure that is flattened anteroposteriorly, giving its cavity a flat, triangular shape. The uterus is supported partly by ligaments attached to the cervix (transverse cervical, pubocervical and uterosacral) consisting of condensed connective tissue. The cervix is a canal, approximately 2–3 cm in length in the non-pregnant woman, connecting the external os, which can be seen on speculum examination, to the internal os, where the cervix enters the uterine cavity. The uterine cavity to cervical length ratio varies through hormonal influences and the developmental phases, with the uterine body increasing in size as puberty progresses.

Johannes Peter Müller, 1801–1858, Professor of Anatomy and Physiology, Berlin, Germany, described the paramesonephric duct in 1825.

Gabriele Falloppio (Falloppius), 1523–1563, Professor of Anatomy, Surgery and Botany, Padua, Italy. He carried out what may have been the first clinical trial in over 1,000 men of the use of condoms to prevent transmission of syphilis.

James Douglas, 1675–1742, anatomist, midwife and physician to Queen Caroline, London, UK, helped expose the fraudulent claims of Mary Toft who, in 1726, famously tricked a number of doctors into believing that she had given birth to rabbits.

The uterine walls are 1–2 cm thick and composed of smooth muscular tissue (myometrium). The uterine cavity is lined with endometrium, a tissue that undergoes cyclical changes in response to ovarian hormones (refer to Reproductive physiology below). The endometrium has both a basal and functional layer. The basal layer lies adjacent to the myometrium and from it develops the functional layer. The basal layer is not shed during menstruation, unlike the functional layer. The functional layer is influenced by oestrogen and progesterone, which thicken it, preparing the lining for implantation. This layer is completely shed during menstruation should conception not occur.

At the uterine fundus, on either side, are the cornua, connecting the uterus to the Fallopian tubes. These are thin, muscular tubes, approximately 10 cm in length. They are divided into four parts: intramural, isthmus, ampulla and the fimbriated opening, which picks up the oocyte following its release at the time of ovulation. The tubes are very narrow in the isthmic and intramural parts but they widen at the ampullary region. Each tube is contained within the upper part of the broad ligament, a fold of peritoneum on either side of the uterus, which also contains blood vessels as well as the round and ovarian ligaments. The fimbriated opening and part of the ampulla, however, are free and closely associated with the ovary on either side. The ovaries are flattened, ovoid structures, approximately 3–4 cm in dimension, suspended from the back of the broad ligament on either side of the pelvic side wall by the ovarian ligament, which originates from the uterine body. The ovarian blood vessels are contained within the infundibulopelvic ligaments, which are continuations of the broad ligament to the pelvic brim on either side.

The cervical canal is located within the centre of the bony cavity of the pelvis, with the uterus pivoted around this point. It is more commonly angled forwards (anteverted), relative to the vagina. It is usually freely mobile, with filling of the bladder or changes in position rotating it backwards. In others, the uterus can be retroverted, as a variation of normal, secondary to either weak ligaments or because the uterus becomes adherent as the result of a disease process such as endometriosis. The uterus may also be angled forwards (anteflexed) relative to the cervix, or backwards (retroflexed), which can be determined through bimanual examination.

In the lean patient the uterine size can also be estimated on palpation. This is usually a subjective assessment outside of imaging modalities. The most common cause of an enlarged uterus, outside of pregnancy, is fibroids (benign tumours of the myometrium) growing inside or outside of the uterus. In the presence of fibroids, the overall size of the uterus is often described in terms of weeks of pregnancy if it expands forwards and upwards into the abdominal cavity, similar to increasing gestational age.

REPRODUCTIVE PHYSIOLOGY

The menstrual cycle is under the control of circulating hormones produced within the hypothalamic-pituitary-ovarian axis and works as part of a negative feedback pathway (Figure 81.2). Gonadotrophin-releasing hormone (GnRH) is produced by the hypothalamus and, in turn, stimulates the pituitary to produce and secrete follicle-stimulating hormone (FSH) and luteinising hormone (LH). FSH and LH act on the ovary (theca and granulosa cells), controlling folliculogenesis (oocyte development) and ovulation. The ovary is responsible for production of the hormones oestrogen, progesterone and androgen. These hormones have an effect on a number of structures within the body, principally the endometrium, which prepares itself to receive a fertilised egg (embryo) during the course of the menstrual cycle. In the first half (proliferative or follicular phase) of the cycle, following menstruation the endometrium starts to regrow or proliferate in response to oestrogen produced by the growing ovarian follicle(s). The endometrium becomes thick and spongy during this phase of the cycle, and is associated with considerable angiogenesis.

Ovulation occurs midcycle, i.e. 14 days prior to the onset of the next menstrual cycle, which is equivalent to day 14 of a 28-day cycle (day 1 defined as the first day of menstruation). After ovulation the remnant follicle is transformed into a corpus luteum, which is responsible for the immediate production of progesterone. During the second half (secretory or luteal phase) of the cycle, the endometrium thickens further under the influence of progesterone in preparation to receive a fertilised ovum.

Fertilisation takes place within the ampullary region of the Fallopian tube, usually within 24 hours after ovulation. The fertilised egg is then transported along the Fallopian tube into the uterine cavity through movement of ciliae and tubal musculature, ideally implanting into the endometrium approximately 5–6 days after ovulation. Through the secretion of human chorionic gonadotrophin (hCG), the corpus luteum is signalled to maintain progesterone production. If fertilisation does not occur, or if the fertilised egg fails to implant, the endometrium is shed as the hCG signal is missing or lost, leading to a fall in progesterone (and oestrogen) levels. Menstruation, (a 'period') lasts on average for 4 days, but can range between 2 and 7 days. Typically, 40 mL of blood is lost during each period; heavy menstruation is described when more than 80 mL of blood loss occurs, which is difficult to assess and can be subjective. The whole process then starts again in the next menstrual cycle.

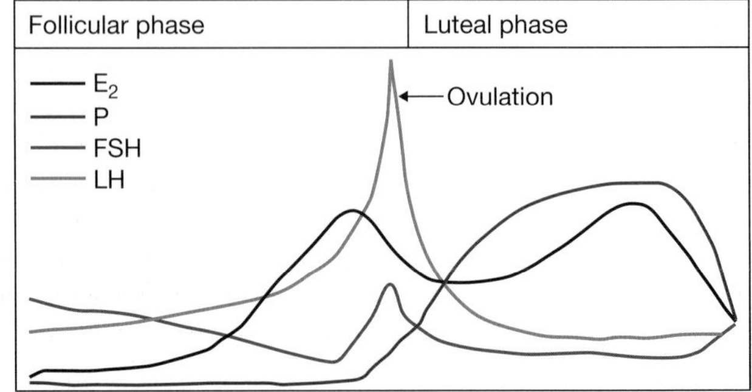

Figure 81.2 Endocrine cycle. E2, oestrogen; FSH, follicle-stimulating hormone; LH, luteinising hormone; P, progesterone.

If fertilisation does occur, the duration of the pregnancy (gestational age) is traditionally calculated from the first day of the last menstrual period (LMP); however, ovulation may occur earlier or considerably later than day 14 and is dependent on the woman's cycle length, or the woman's recollection of the date of the LMP may be incorrect, potentially making calculation of the gestational age on the basis of the LMP alone inaccurate. This explains the alternative practice of calculating gestational age using ultrasound measurements of fetal size, ideally during the first trimester.

VAGINAL BLEEDING IN EARLY PREGNANCY

A miscarriage is defined as the loss of an intrauterine pregnancy at less than 24 weeks' gestation. An early miscarriage refers to pregnancy loss before 12 weeks' gestation ('first trimester'). A late miscarriage refers to pregnancy loss between 12 and 24 weeks' gestation ('second trimester'). Approximately 20% of pregnancies will miscarry. However, this number is highly influenced by maternal age and can reach approximately 50% in a 45-year-old woman.

A miscarriage can be diagnosed on transvaginal ultrasound scan in the absence of a visible fetal heartbeat with a crown–rump length of 7.0 mm or more, or, in the absence of a fetal pole in the presence of a mean gestational sac diameter of 25.0 mm or more.

A miscarriage often begins with painless vaginal bleeding, at which point it is defined as a threatened miscarriage. The bleeding may then become heavier with associated uterine cramps and an opening of the cervical os, at which point it is defined as an inevitable miscarriage. Blood clots and products of conception (i.e. fetal and placental tissue) are passed through the cervical os until the uterus is emptied (defined as a complete miscarriage). If some of the products of conception are retained within the uterus, this is referred to as an incomplete miscarriage. A missed miscarriage occurs when no fetal heart beat can be detected on ultrasound scan, but no clinical signs of a miscarriage as described above are present.

Management of a miscarriage ranges from expectant management to medical or surgical intervention. For medical management, medications such as prostaglandins can be given that support uterine contractions and cervical softening. Surgical management of a miscarriage (SMOM) can be conducted using manual vacuum aspiration under local anaesthesia, or surgically under general anaesthesia. The operation involves passing a plastic suction curette through the cervical opening and into the uterine cavity. A SMOM should be considered in the presence of persistent excessive bleeding, haemodynamic instability, evidence of infected retained tissue or suspected gestational trophoblastic disease. Serious operative complications, which are fortunately rare, include uterine perforation (up to 5 in 1000 women) with the possibility of intra-abdominal trauma (e.g. bowel damage), cervical tears, haemorrhage (risk of needing a blood transfusion is 1–2 in 1000 women) and infection (3 in 100 women). Approximately 5 in 100 women may require a repeat surgical evacuation. In view of the potential risk of organ damage, women should concomitantly be consented for a laparoscopy and laparotomy. Furthermore, anti-D immunoglobulin should be prescribed to all non-sensitised rhesus (Rh)-negative women undergoing surgical treatment for a miscarriage or in cases with excessive bleeding in conservative or medical management of miscarriage.

Vaginal bleeding in early pregnancy may also result from a local cause such as a cervical lesion (which may first manifest itself as bleeding after intercourse) or, rarely, trauma.

VAGINAL BLEEDING IN THE NON-PREGNANT STATE

Bleeding in the non-pregnant state may occur at the time of an expected menstrual period, between periods (intermenstrual bleeding; IMB), after intercourse (postcoital bleeding; PCB) or following the menopause (postmenopausal bleeding; PMB). It may also occur after surgical instrumentation of the uterus and/or cervix, including insertion of an intrauterine contraceptive device (IUCD). The principal causes of uterine or vaginal bleeding in the non-pregnant state can be divided into structural and non-structural (*Table 81.1*) and relationship to menses or coitus (*Table 81.2*).

TABLE 81.1 Structural and non-structural causes of uterine and vaginal bleeding.

Structural	Polyp
	Fibroids (leiomyoma)
	Endometrial hyperplasia
	Malignancy of the genital tract
Non-structural	Coagulopathy, e.g. thrombocytopaenia, von Willebrand's disease
	Ovulatory dysfunction, e.g. polycystic ovary syndrome
	Endometrial, e.g. endometritis
	Iatrogenic, e.g. exogenous sex steroid adminstration, IUCD
	Other, e.g. arteriovenous malformations, chronic renal/hepatic disease

IUCD, intrauterine contraceptive device.

TABLE 81.2 Causes of uterine and vaginal bleeding in the non-pregnant state.

Menstrual	Endometrial polyp/malignancy[a]
	Fibroids
Intermenstrual	Vaginal trauma/malignancy[a]
	Cervical polyp/malignancy
	Endometrial polyp/malignancy[a]
Postcoital	Vaginal malignancy[a]
	Cervical ectropion/polyp/malignancy

[a] These cancers occur principally in postmenopausal women.

Erik Adolf von Willebrand, 1870–1949, physician, Helsinki, Finland.

The mainstay of management is to identify and treat the associated pathology (except in women <40 years of age with heavy menstrual periods in whom malignancy is very rarely found; these women are best managed symptomatically). Investigations include a pregnancy test and ultrasound assessment of the pelvic anatomy (2D/3D ultrasonogram or saline sonogram) as well as an endometrial biopsy of the uterine cavity, either performed under direct vision at hysteroscopy or blindly with a Pipelle® biopsy. Hysteroscopy combined with endometrial biopsy improves the sensitivity and specificity for detection of endometrial pathology compared with either performed alone. A colonoscopy may also be indicated to exclude colorectal pathology as a potential cause for the bleeding. The indications for undertaking an endometrial biopsy are shown in *Summary box 81.1*.

Summary box 81.1

Indications for endometrial biopsy

Endometrial biopsy should be considered in the following women:

- Suspected endometrial pathology
- All women >45 years of age in whom medical treatment has been unsuccessful
- Persistent intermenstrual bleeding
- Endometrial thickness of >4 mm in postmenopausal women or >16 mm in premenopausal women and >7 mm in women with known polycystic ovarian syndrome
- Irregular or unscheduled bleeding while on hormone replacement therapy after the initial 3 months
- Younger women with major risk factors for endometrial hyperplasia/ cancer:
  - Polycystic ovarian syndrome
  - Obesity
  - Treatment with tamoxifen
- Irregular bleeding while on unopposed oestrogen therapy
- Irregular bleeding in high-risk populations, such as family history of endometrial/colon cancer, especially hereditary non-polyposis colorectal cancer

Women taking tamoxifen, a selective oestrogen receptor modulator used in the treatment of breast cancer, represent a special group, as the drug can induce uterine abnormalities in 10–40% of women, such as the development of endometrial polyps, hyperplasia, cancer and, rarely, uterine sarcomas, which are much more aggressive. Tamoxifen treatment results in a doubling of the risk of endometrial cancer after 1–2 years and a quadrupling after 5 years of usage. The relationship is time dependent but dose independent. The risk does not decrease on cessation of treatment. There is no consensus regarding the need for screening and which method to use; the alternative, more common approach, is to investigate only those women who develop abnormal uterine bleeding with tamoxifen use. Aromatase inhibitors such as anastrozole, letrozole and exemestane, also used in the treatment of breast cancer, but whose effects are not mediated via the oestrogen receptor, have been associated with less endometrial pathology than tamoxifen. They may also reverse abnormalities induced by tamoxifen use.

Women known to have Lynch syndrome (hereditary non-polyposis colorectal cancer) and those considered at risk of inheriting a mismatch repair gene abnormality are another special group, as their lifetime risk of developing endometrial cancer is as high as 60%. Unlike sporadic cases of endometrial cancer, which are usually diagnosed during the sixth and seventh decades, the mean age at diagnosis in Lynch syndrome is the fifth decade. However, it appears that the 5-year survival rate in patients with Lynch syndrome associated endometrial cancer is similar to that in women with sporadic disease. International guidelines suggest that these women should be screened annually from the age of 35 years with transvaginal ultrasound to measure the endometrial thickness and with an endometrial biopsy.

Abnormal bleeding can also be caused by invasive carcinoma of the cervix, the incidence of which has been reduced by screening programmes that aim to detect the precancerous state – cervical intraepithelial neoplasia (CIN) – using cervical cytology. In the UK, this is carried out every 3 years in women aged 25–49 years of age, and 5-yearly in women aged 50–64 years. Infection with certain human papillomavirus (HPV) serotypes (16, 18, 31 and 33) is associated with an increased risk of invasive disease. Current vaccination programmes against HPV serotypes are aimed at reducing the incidence of cervical carcinoma. The vaccination is offered to girls aged 12–13 years. Abnormalities in cervical cytology are followed up by microscopic examination of the cervix (colposcopy). CIN may be treated with local ablation (cryocautery, cold coagulation, electrodiathermy or laser) or excision (large loop excision of the transformation zone (LLETZ)).

Menstrual bleeding may be excessively heavy, irregular or frequent in the absence of pathology; this is known as dysfunctional uterine bleeding. The UK's National Institute for Health and Care Excellence (NICE) has suggested a three-step hierarchal treatment approach to the management of heavy menstrual bleeding: (1) medical therapy; (2) minimally invasive uterus-conserving surgey; (3) major surgical procedures. The management plans are individualised for the patient, taking into account the concomitant symptoms and fertility requirements. Medical treatments used to reduce the amount of menstrual blood loss include tranexamic acid, mefenamic acid and the combined or progestin-only oral contraceptive pill (COCP or POP, respectively). It may be necessary to stop the bleeding completely using high-dose progestagens, the COCP taken continuously or a gonadotrophin-releasing hormone (GnRH) analogue with or without add-back hormone replacement therapy (HRT), which induces a menopause-like state. Increasingly, an intrauterine system (IUS) similar to a conventional coil, which releases levonorgestrel, is offered to patients as an alternative; it has the added advantage of being a reliable long-acting reversible contraceptive (up to 5 years). After 1 year of usage, there is a 71–95% reduction in menstrual blood loss with approximately 50% of women becoming amenorrhoeic.

The surgical treatments for excessive bleeding and their principal operative complications are described in *Table 81.3*.

Henry T Lynch, b.1928, Professor of Preventative Medicine, Creighton University, Omaha, NE, USA.

TABLE 81.3 Surgical treatments for excessive vaginal bleeding.

Treatment	Route	Major operative risks
Uterus-conserving surgery:		
• Hysteroscopic polypectomy	Vaginal	Uterine perforation; damage to surrounding organs
• Endometrial ablation	Vaginal	
• Transcervical resection of the endometrium	Vaginal	Fluid overload; thermal injury to surrounding organs
• Focal fibroid destruction (MRI-guided focused ultrasound, radiofrequency ablation)	Transcutaneous	
• Uterine fibroid embolisation	Transcutaneous	
• Uterine artery occlusion	Vaginal/abdominal	Fluid overload; thermal injury to surrounding organs
• Transcervical resection of fibroids	Vaginal	
• Laparoscopic myomectomy	Abdominal	Injury to surrounding organs
• Open myomectomy	Abdominal	Injury to surrounding organs
Non-uterus conserving surgery:		
• Hysterectomy (subtotal or total)	Vaginal/abdominal	Damage to internal organs; fistula formation

MRI, magnetic resonance imaging.

The aim of ablative methods is to reduce the menstrual bleeding by ablating the endometrium down to the basalis layer using electrical, thermal or laser energy. More than 90% of women report a reduction in menstrual blood loss without the need for further treatment at 2 years of follow-up, with 25–35% experiencing amenorrhoea. The criteria for endometrial ablation are described in *Table 81.4*.

TABLE 81.4 Criteria for suitability for endometrial ablation.

Uterus is <10 cm in length (and 14 cm in length for microwave ablation)
Absence of major intrauterine pathology that would distort the uterine cavity
No history of previous endometrial ablation procedures
No evidence of endometritis
Family is complete

A hysterectomy can be carried out by three different routes: vaginally, abdominally or laparoscopically. The route of entry is dependent on a number of factors, including: uterine size; presence of other pathology; mobility and descent of the uterus; history of previous surgery; and skill of the operating surgeon. A total or subtotal (conservation of the cervix) hysterectomy can be performed. No difference in prolapse symptoms, sexual satisfaction or pelvic pain has been reported between the two techniques. Furthermore, it is now recommended that the Fallopian tubes are removed in conjunction with the uterine body, whether the ovaries are conserved or not. The Fallopian tubes have no continued functionality following a hysterectomy, but can be a potential source of malignancy if retained. Conservation or removal of the ovaries is dependent on the woman's age, presence of coexisting pathology and/or risk factors for malignancy.

ACUTE PELVIC PAIN IN EARLY PREGNANCY

Ectopic pregnancy

An ectopic pregnancy refers to a pregnancy that grows outside of the uterine cavity, most commonly within the Fallopian tube, with rarer sites including the ovary, cervix, broad ligament and abdominal cavity. As the ectopic pregnancy grows, the placental tissue can infiltrate the blood vessels surrounding the Fallopian tube, leading to bleeding within the tube and into the peritoneal cavity. Further growth of the ectopic pregnancy can rupture the Fallopian tube, causing significant intraperitoneal blood loss. This constitutes a gynaecological emergency. An ectopic pregnancy occurs in 11 per 1000 pregnancies, and a maternal mortality rate of 0.2 per 1000 estimated ectopic pregnancies. The major risk factors for an ectopic pregnancy are shown in *Summary box 81.2*.

Summary box 81.2

Risk factors for an ectopic pregnancy

- Previous pelvic inflammatory disease
- Smoking
- History of infertility
- Use of an intrauterine contraceptive device
- Previous ectopic pregnancy
- Previous abdominal/pelvic surgery
- Previous tubal surgery, e.g. sterilisation, salpingostomy, tuboplasty
- Endometriosis

An ectopic pregnancy may be suspected on clinical grounds but making the diagnosis can be difficult (*Table 81.5*).

TABLE 81.5 Symptoms and signs of an ectopic pregnancy.

Symptoms	Signs
Abdominal or pelvic pain Vaginal bleeding Gastrointestinal symptoms Dizziness, fainting, syncope Shoulder tip pain Asymptomatic	Pelvic, abdominal and/or adnexal tenderness or fullness Signs of peritonism Cervical motion tenderness (pain on moving the cervix) Tachycardia, hypotension

The presentation of an ectopic pregnancy is very variable and the differential diagnoses include:

- ectopic pregnancy;
- miscarriage;
- urinary tract infection;
- ovarian cyst accident;
- appendicitis.

A transvaginal ultrasound scan should be performed if the diagnosis is suspected. The complete absence of an intrauterine gestational sac with a positive pregnancy test increases the probability of an ectopic pregnancy, unless the pregnancy is not sufficiently advanced for the sac to be seen on ultrasound scan. An ectopic pregnancy is more likely if free fluid is seen in the pouch of Douglas, or an adnexal mass is seen on ultrasound scan.

In equivocal cases, serial measurements of serum beta-human chorionic gonadotrophin (β-hCG) levels, 48 hours apart, can help to establish the diagnosis. A rise in β-hCG levels by at least 63% is more indicative of a viable intrauterine pregnancy. Levels that halve when taken 48 hours apart are more suggestive of a failing pregnancy. Levels that remain static, or show a suboptimal increase or decrease over a 48-hour period, are more likely to be representative of an ectopic pregnancy. Furthermore, a single level above approximately 1500 IU/L, in association with an empty uterus on ultrasound scan, is highly suggestive of an ectopic pregnancy. Laparoscopy can also be used as a diagnostic tool (Figure 81.3); occasionally however, a false-negative diagnosis is obtained, when the pregnancy is not sufficiently advanced and is therefore too small to be seen within the Fallopian tube.

Management of an ectopic pregnancy can be divided into expectant, medical (methotrexate) or surgical treatment. The choice of treatment is dependent on: the haemodynamic stability of the patient; ultrasonographic features of the ectopic pregnancy (presence of free fluid, presence or absence of a fetal heartbeat); serum β-hCG level; and the patient's understanding of the diagnosis, commitment to follow-up and choice.

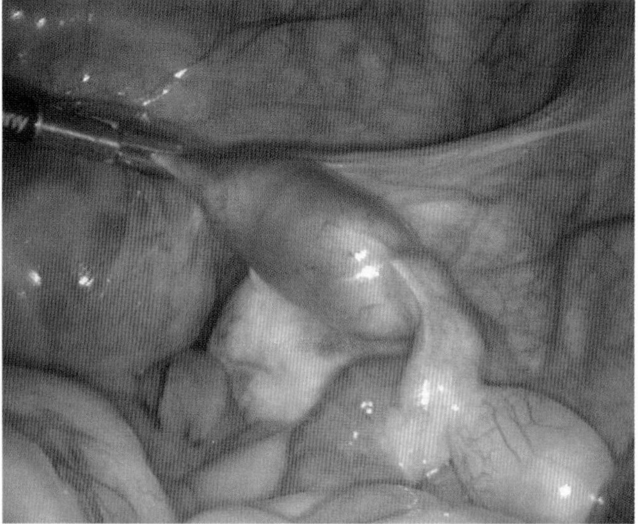

Figure 81.3 Laparoscopy showing an ectopic pregnancy.

Methotrexate is a folic acid anatagonist that interferes with deoxyribonucleic acid (DNA) synthesis. Significant side effects include hepatotoxicity. Further pregnancies should be avoided for a minimum of 3 months following treatment with methotrexate. Careful patient selection is vital. Furthermore, some patients fail to respond to this medication and will require surgical management.

Surgical management occurs in the form of a salpingectomy (removal of the Fallopian tube) or salpingostomy (opening of the Fallopian tube and extraction of the pregnancy tissue). This is ideally performed laparoscopically in the stable patient, as it is associated with shorter operative times, less intraoperative blood loss, shorter hospital stays and similar subsequent intrauterine pregnancy rates. A laparotomy may be required if the woman is haemodynamically unstable. A salpingectomy is the preferential technique in the presence of a contralateral healthy Fallopian tube. A salpingostomy is associated with an 8% risk of persistent trophoblastic tissue, intra-abdominal bleeding and an increased risk of a repeat ectopic pregnancy. These patients are subsequently followed up with monitoring of serum β-hCG levels until a negative result is obtained, to exclude the presence of residual trophoblastic tissue. If a further ectopic pregnancy occurs within the same Fallopian tube, then a salpingectomy is recommended regardless of the condition of the contralateral tube.

The management of non-tubal ectopic pregnancies (e.g. interstitial ectopics, caesarean section scar ectopics) can be complex and associated with more significant complications, such as bleeding and the risk of needing a hysterectomy. These cases are best managed in tertiary centres. The management plan will be guided by the haemodynamic stability of the patient and the location of the ectopic pregnancy, including the expertise of the clinician managing the case.

These patients should be counselled regarding their increased risk of further ectopic pregnancies in subsequent conceptions. In view of this, they are encouraged to present as early as possible in any subsequent pregnancy to establish its location.

INFECTION

The overwhelming majority of cases of pelvic inflammatory disease (PID) are caused by ascending infection, most commonly sexually transmitted, leading to endometritis, salpingitis, tubo-ovarian abscess formation and/or pelvic peritonitis. Rarer causes include spread from other pelvic organs, e.g. the appendix. *Chlamydia trachomatis* is the most common organism responsible for PID; the prevalence of *Neisseria gonorrhoeae* varies depending upon the locality. Other organisms commonly found in the vagina may also be implicated. Risk factors include young age at first sexual activity, a high number of sexual partners and current use of an IUCD; infection may also follow a surgical procedure, e.g. termination of pregnancy.

There are no definitive criteria for making a diagnosis of PID. Most clinicians rely instead upon the presence of one

Albert Ludwig Siegmund Neisser, 1855–1916, Director of the Dermatological Institute, Breslau, Germany, (now Wroclaw, Poland).

or more of the following features, which are suggestive of the diagnosis:

- lower abdominal pain and tenderness, more commonly bilateral;
- deep dyspareunia (pain on intercourse);
- abnormal vaginal bleeding;
- abnormal cervical discharge, commonly purulent;
- cervical excitation and adnexal tenderness;
- fever ≥38°C;
- elevated white blood cells (neutrophils) and platelets.

It should be noted that some patients are asymptomatic or may present with non-specific symptoms, and a high degree of clinical suspicion is needed to avoid a delay in making the diagnosis.

The differential diagnoses include:

- endometriosis;
- urinary tract infection;
- appendicitis;
- gastrointestinal dysfunction;
- ectopic pregnancy;
- ovarian cyst accident.

Raised inflammatory markers (white cell count, neutrophil count and C-reactive protein (CRP)) support the diagnosis. Ultrasound scan assessment of the pelvis can detect the presence of hydrosalpinges and/or a tubo-ovarian abscess. All women with suspected PID should be screened for *N. gonorrhoeae* and *C. trachomatis*; however, an absence of infection does not exclude a diagnosis of PID. *Chlamydia trachomatis* is an intracellular organism; therefore, samples obtained for diagnostic purposes should contain cellular material. If an endocervical swab is to be used to obtain a specimen, then it is important to clean the cervix of excessive discharge before inserting the swab inside the cervical os.

Summary box 81.3

Chlamydia and gonorrhoea testing

There is a need to test women (especially those sexually active under the age of 25 years) who present with:

- purulent vaginal discharge
- postcoital/intermenstrual bleeding
- change in vaginal bleeding pattern
- mucopurulent cervicitis
- inflamed/friable cervix (which may bleed on contact)
- urethritis
- suspected pelvic inflammatory disease
- reactive arthritis

Current guidelines recommend a low threshold for empirical treatment because the consequences of failing to treat acute PID effectively are extremely significant: chronic pelvic pain; infertility; increased risk of an ectopic pregnancy (6%; approximately 10 times higher than the background population); and Fitz-Hugh–Curtis syndrome (an extrapelvic manifestation of PID associated with right upper quadrant pain, most probably resulting from the inflammation of the liver capsule and diaphragm). Approximately 20% of women treated for PID will become infertile, secondary to tubal damage; >50% of tubal factor infertility cases arise from infection secondary to *Chlamydia*; however, interestingly, many of these women do not report a history of PID.

Treatment should be commenced as soon as samples have been obtained for culture, without the need to wait for the results, but changing the antibiotics once the sensitivities become available; it should include a broad-spectrum antibiotic against coliforms and anaerobic species, which are responsible for secondary infection. Contact tracing (a minimum of 6 months within the onset of symptoms) and treatment are essential.

The majority of suspected cases are treated within the community, with a review advised after 72 hours. Hospital admission is advisable if there is doubt about the diagnosis, or if the symptoms/signs are severe. If an IUCD is *in situ*, this is better removed under antibiotic coverage, with adequate counselling regarding pregnancy risk, and emergency contraception prescribed in appropriate circumstances. Counselling should also cover future contraception.

A tubo-ovarian abscess can develop in severe cases of PID; this is where the Fallopian tube and ovary become blended into a single, pus-filled, inflammatory mass, which is usually adherent to the uterus and surrounding bowel. The infection may have progressed from a milder form of PID or, increasingly, it may result from the introduction of infection or bowel damage at transvaginal oocyte aspiration in a patient undergoing *in vitro* fertilisation (IVF). Modern medical practice is to manage the tubo-ovarian abscesses (**Figure 81.4**) conservatively, unless the patient fails to respond to intravenous antibiotics and systemic support. The response is judged to be inadequate if the woman remains systemically unwell, her symptoms do not improve, fever is not reduced, the white blood cell count does not fall and there is no radiological evidence of the abscess becoming smaller. In such circumstances, surgical treatment is necessary, i.e. adhesiolysis and drainage of the abscess, at laparotomy or laparoscopy. As most women with a tubo-ovarian abscess are in the reproductive years, the intention is always to be as conservative as possible at surgery. Rarely, however, if the abscess has ruptured (**Figure 81.5**) and the patient is extremely ill, then a hysterectomy and bilateral salpingo-oophorectomy may become necessary.

Abscess drainage under radiological guidance, e.g. a transgluteal approach via the greater sciatic foramen under computed tomography (CT), is sometimes performed. Transvaginal ultrasound-guided aspiration has also been advocated.

Thomas Fitz-Hugh Jr., 1894–1963, physician, Chief of the Hematological Section, The University Hospital, The University of Pennsylvania, Philadelphia, PA, USA.

Arthur H Curtis, 1881–1955, Professor of Obstetrics and Gynecology, The Northwestern Medical School, Chicago, IL, USA. Fitz-Hugh and Curtis were not the first to describe the syndrome: it was described in 1920 by Stajano, a Uruguyan Professor of Surgery, but the paper was written in Spanish.

Summary box 81.4

Treatment of pelvic inflammatory disease (PID)

- A low threshold for the initiation of empirical treatment for PID is recommended, because of the lack of definitive clinical diagnostic criteria
- Women with suspected PID should be screened for *N. gonorrhoeae* and *C. trachomatis*
- Testing for gonorrhoea should be undertaken with an endocervical specimen, via culture (direct inoculation onto a culture plate or transport of the swab to the laboratory within 24 hours) or using a nucleic acid amplification test (NAAT). Screening for chlamydia should also be from the endocervix, preferably using a NAAT. Taking an additional sample from the urethra increases the diagnostic yield for gonorrhoea and chlamydia. A first-catch urine sample provides an alternative source
- A pregnancy test should be undertaken and screening for other sexually-transmitted infections, such as human immunodeficiency virus and hepatitis
- Out-patient antibiotic treatment should be commenced as soon as the diagnosis is suspected. Treatment should be based on one of the following regimens:
  - Ofloxacin 400 mg orally twice a day + metronidazole 400 mg orally twice a day for 14 days (ofloxacin should be avoided in cases at high risk of gonococcal PID due to increasing resistance against quinolone antibiotics in the UK); or,
  - Ceftriaxone 500 mg intramuscular as a single dose, followed by doxycycline 100 mg orally twice a day + metronidazole 400 mg twice a day for 14 days
- Admission to hospital is appropriate in the following circumstances:
  - Surgical emergency cannot be excluded
  - Clinically severe disease
  - Tubo-ovarian abscess
  - PID in pregnancy
  - Lack of response to oral therapy
  - Intolerance to oral therapy
- In more severe cases, in-patient antibiotic treatment should be based on intravenous therapy, which should be continued until 24 hours after clinical improvement and followed by oral therapy. Recommended regimens are:
  - Ceftriaxone 2 g intravenously daily + doxycycline 100 mg intravenously twice a day (oral doxycycline may be used if tolerated), followed by doxycycline 100 mg orally twice a day + metronidazole 400 mg orally twice a day for a total of 14 days; or
  - Clindamycin 900 mg intravenously three times a day + gentamicin 2 mg/kg loading dose followed by 1.5 mg/kg intravenously three times a day (a single daily dose of 7 mg/kg may be substituted), followed by clindamycin 450 mg orally four times a day to complete 14 days, or doxycycline 100 mg orally twice a day + metronidazole 400 mg orally twice a day to complete 14 days
- Abstinence or the use of barrier contraception is advised until resolution of the condition on repeat testing
- Treatment in the presence of pregnancy should take account of local policies and guidelines with consideration to the treatment's teratogenic potential, but parental therapy is advised secondary to the increased risk of maternal and fetal morbidity
- Surgical drainage of a pelvic abscess may be indicated in the absence of clinical improvement with medical therapy

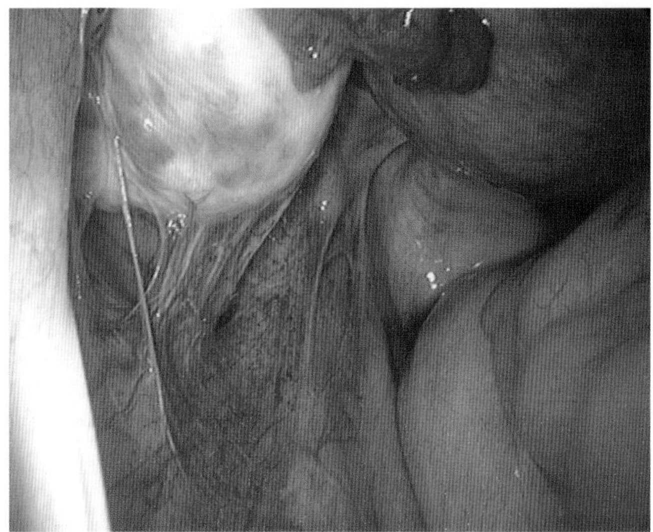

Figure 81.4 Pelvic inflammatory disease.

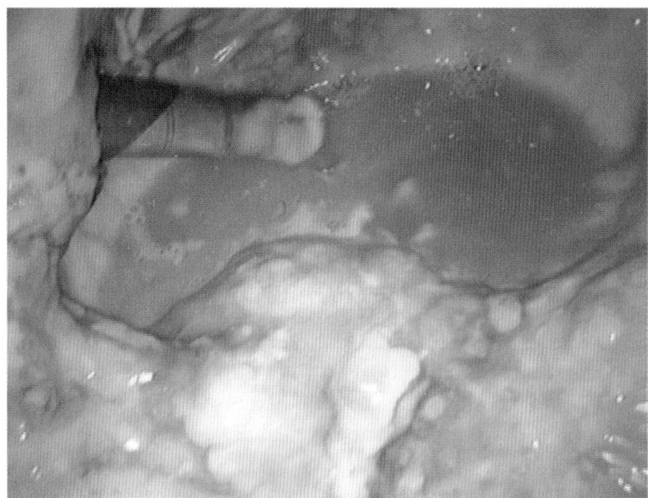

Figure 81.5 Pelvic inflammatory disease with rupture of a pelvic abscess.

It is clearly less invasive and there are claims that the method is as effective as surgery; however, it carries additional risks such as bowel damage and tracking of the infection along the root of entry of the needle.

ENDOMETRIOSIS

Endometriosis is defined as the presence of endometrial-like tissue in extrauterine sites. The most commonly affected sites are the pelvic organs and peritoneum, although distant sites such as the lungs are occasionally affected (resulting in symptoms such as recurrent haemoptysis at the time of menstruation or recurrent pneumothoraxes) (Figure 81.6). The exact pathogonomic mechanism remains elusive, but it is widely believed that most endometriotic lesions develop from retrograde menstruation. It is estimated to affect 5–10% of women mainly of reproductive age, with the incidence reported to be higher in certain subgroups, e.g. women with a history of infertility. Endometriosis may be associated with a number of

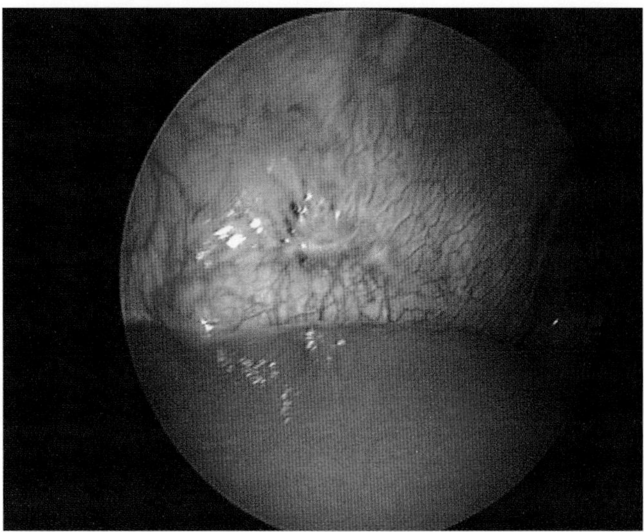

Figure 81.6 Endometriosis seen on the peritoneal surface of the diaphragm.

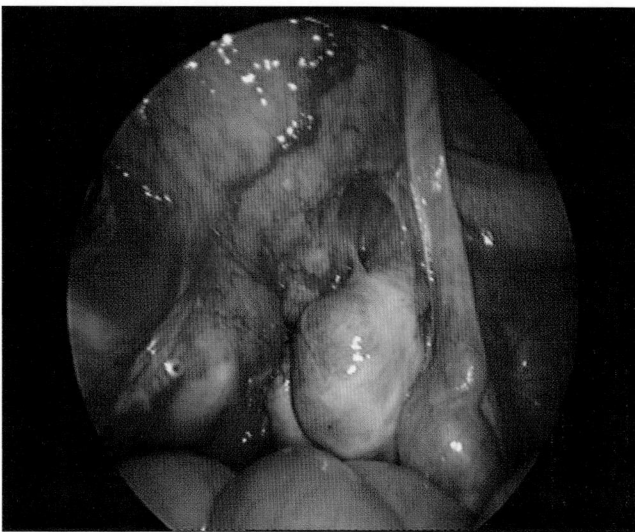

Figure 81.8 Bilateral ovarian endometriosis with pelvic adhesions.

symptoms, but the predictive value of any one symptom or set of symptoms remains uncertain as each can have other causes (e.g. irritable bowel syndrome or interstitial cystitis), with a significant proportion of affected women remaining asymptomatic. The most common symptom is pain. Other symptoms include: cyclical and non-cyclical pain; deep dyspareunia (pain during intercourse); dyschezia (pain on opening the bowels); and dysuria. Many women also suffer from fatigue, haematuria, chronic pelvic pain, infertility and rectal bleeding.

The extent of the disease varies from a few small lesions on otherwise normal pelvic organs to large ovarian endometriotic cysts (endometriomas). There can be extensive fibrosis in structures such as the uterosacral ligaments (Figure 81.7), and adhesion formation causing marked distortion of the pelvic anatomy (Figure 81.8). Disease severity can be assessed by describing the operative findings, or quantitatively using various classification systems, but there is little correlation between such systems and the type or severity of symptoms experienced.

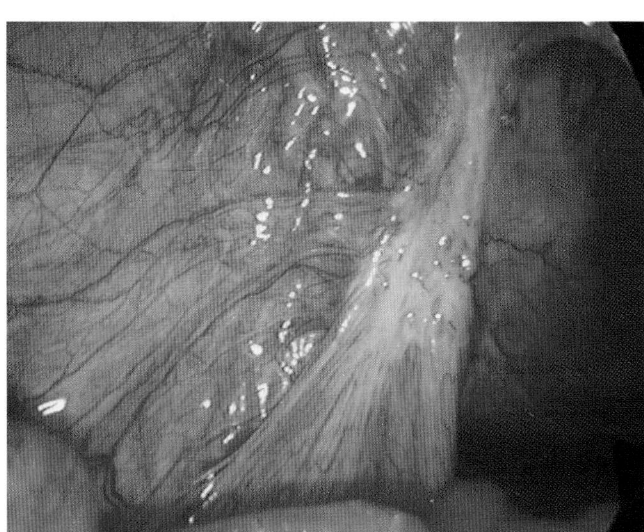

Figure 81.7 Endometriosis seen on the uterosacral ligament.

Endometriosis typically appears as superficial 'powder-burn' or 'gunshot' lesions on the ovaries, serosal surfaces and peritoneum – black, dark-brown or bluish puckered lesions, nodules or small cysts containing old haemorrhage surrounded by a variable extent of fibrosis. Atypical or 'subtle' lesions are also common, including red implants (petechial, vesicular, polypoid, haemorrhagic, red flame-like) and serous or clear vesicles. Other appearances include white plaques or scarring and yellow-brown peritoneal discolouration of the peritoneum. Ovarian endometriomas usually contain thick fluid-like tar. They are distinguishable from simple haemorrhagic ovarian cysts because typically they are densely adherent to the peritoneum of the ovarian fossa. The surrounding fibrosis may involve the bowel. Deeply infiltrating endometriotic nodules represent another disease type. They can extend more than 5 mm beneath the peritoneum and may grow into the uterosacral ligaments, vagina, bowel, bladder or ureters; when such lesions grow into the vagina they may be visible on speculum examination as 'blue-domed' cystic lesions in the posterior fornix. Lesions infiltrating the bowel may mimic cancer in their presentation.

The gold standard for making a diagnosis of endometriosis is through laparoscopy, ideally with histological confirmation; non-invasive diagnostic tools, such as ultrasound scanning, can reliably detect only severe forms of the disease, i.e. endometriomas. Magnetic resonance imaging (MRI) can detect haemosiderin deposits in deeply infiltrating disease.

The treatment options are limited because the cause is uncertain. These include: conservative management; medical management (simple analgesia or hormonal drugs to suppress ovarian function (progestins, the levonorgestrel-IUS)); and surgical management (ablation or excision of endometriotic lesions). Women may require multiple admissions for surgery and/or prolonged treatment with costly drugs that can have problematic side effects. Lastly, endometriosis is associated with an increased risk of ovarian cancer (especially endometrioid and clear-cell types) and non-Hodgkin's lymphoma, which adds to the burden of the disease.

Finding pelvic tenderness, a fixed retroverted uterus, tender uterosacral ligaments or enlarged ovaries on examination is suggestive of endometriosis. The diagnosis is more certain if deeply infiltrating nodules are found on the uterosacral ligaments or in the pouch of Douglas and/or visible lesions are seen in the vagina or on the cervix. The findings may, however, be normal.

For a woman who has completed her family, hysterectomy plus bilateral salpingo-oophorectomy and removal of all of the endometriosis present offers a good chance of cure. However, surgical treatment in a woman who wishes to conceive in the future aims to be as conservative as possible, ensuring in particular that ovarian function is preserved. The aim is to remove all of the endometriotic tissue and restore anatomy to normal by lysing adhesions. The standard (preferably laparoscopic) methods used are ovarian cystectomy and tissue excision or ablation with electrodiathermy, thermal coagulation or laser. The surgical risks include those for any laparoscopic procedure, as well as damage to the ureters and bowel; the risks are increased if deeply infiltrating disease is present, particularly if there is bowel wall involvement. Rarely, infection in an endometrioma will result in the formation of a tubo-ovarian abscess.

UROGYNAECOLOGY

Uterovaginal prolapse

Pelvic organ prolapse refers to the protrusion or displacement of the pelvic organs from their normal anatomical position into or through the vagina to varying degrees (Figure 81.9). It is said to affect up to 40% of women at some time in their

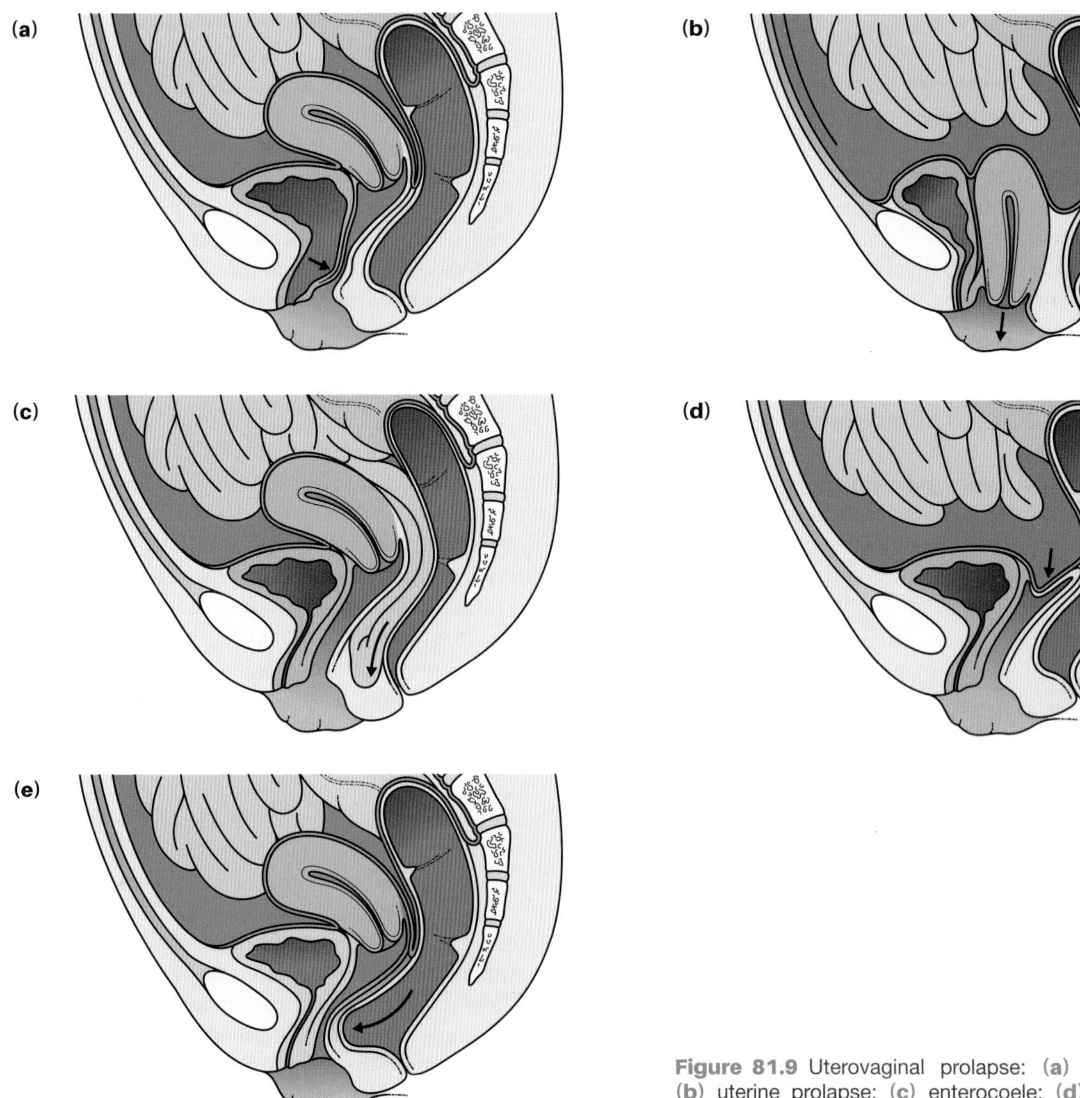

Figure 81.9 Uterovaginal prolapse: (a) urethrocoele/cystocoele; (b) uterine prolapse; (c) enterocoele; (d) vaginal vault prolapse; (e) rectocoele.

Thomas Hodgkin, 1798–1866, curator of the Museum and demonstrator of Morbid Anatomy, Guy's Hospital, London, UK.

lifetime. A prolapse can have a detrimental impact on normal organ performance, including anorectal, urinary and sexual function.

Prolapse is more common in certain groups, including:

- older women;
- parous women, increased parity, prolonged labours, vaginal deliveries;
- obese women;
- sufferers of chronic constipation;
- occupations that involve heavy lifting;
- oestrogen-deficient women;
- women with a family history or genetic risk;
- connective tissue disorders, e.g. Ehlers–Danlos syndrome, Marfan's.

Women with a minor degree of prolapse may be asymptomatic, but with more significant degrees the patient usually complains of a sensation of 'something coming down'. A cystocoele (bladder prolapse) and a cystourethrocoele (prolapse of the bladder and urethra) lead to the sensation of a lump in the vagina, and may be associated with urinary urgency (overactive bladder symptoms) and recurrent urinary tract infections. Uterine descent can lead to a lump in the vagina or a dragging sensation; with complete prolapse of the uterus (procidentia) there may be vaginal discharge, ulceration of the vaginal skin and bleeding. A rectocoele (prolapse of the rectum into the vagina) may cause difficulties with defaecation or a sensation of incomplete emptying, which can be relieved by digital reduction of the prolapse.

The degree of prolapse is graded in terms of descent. Currently, the commonly used grading systems is the Pelvic Organ Prolapse Quantification System (POP-Q).

Non-surgical management of uterovaginal prolapse includes: lifestyle changes (avoidance of constipation); physiotherapy to help strengthen the pelvic floor muscles; HRT for oestrogen deficiency and to help increase tissue strength and elasticity; and vaginal pessaries. There are a number of different pessaries available and they are replaced every 3–6 months, with the ring pessary being the most frequently used. It is inserted between the posterior fornix and the pubic bone. The main complications are vaginal ulceration and infection leading to discharge and bleeding; it is advisable, therefore, to replace the ring frequently.

Surgical management aims to correct the prolapse. The surgical procedures are intended to restore the uterovaginal anatomy and position. They may be carried out using a vaginal or abdominal approach or, increasingly, by a laparoscopic or minimal access approach, with the use of polypropylene mesh to augment weak connective tissue (*Table 81.6*).

TABLE 81.6. Surgical treatments for uterovaginal prolapse.

Condition	Treatment	Complications
Urethrocoele/cystocoele (**Figure 81.9a**)	Traditionally, an anterior vaginal wall repair (anterior colporrhaphy) was performed vaginally. The use of mesh has been utilised but is falling out of favour with the current controversies	Bleeding, infection, fistula formation, voiding dysfunction, unmasking of occult stress urinary incontinence, failure, recurrence
Uterine prolapse (**Figure 81.9b**)	If the patient's family is complete, a vaginal hysterectomy with an anterior vaginal wall repair if necessary can be performed. Uterus-preserving surgery includes: amputation of the cervix with suturing of the transverse cervical ligaments vaginally (Manchester repair); laparoscopic plication of the uterosacral ligaments (McCall suture); or hysteropexy, which may be vaginal (attaching the cervix to the sacrospinous ligaments using non-absorbable sutures) or laparoscopically (using a polypropylene mesh to suspend the uterus to the sacral promontory)	Bleeding, infection, injury to the bladder, bowel or ureters, voiding dysfunction, dyspareunia, failure, recurrence, conversion to a laparotomy. A Manchester repair can specifically be associated with infertility, miscarriage and dystocia
Enterocoele (**Figure 81.9c**)	A similar technique to repair of a hernia is used. The vaginal skin is opened and the hernial sac repaired	Bleeding, infection, rectal or small bowel injury (fistula formation), dyspareunia, failure, recurrence
Vaginal vault prolapse (**Figure 81.9d**)	Sacrospinous fixation performed vaginally: the vault is attached to the right sacrospinous ligament using a non-absorbable suture/mesh, avoiding the rectosigmoid colon on the left. Sacrocolpopexy perfomed abdominally or laparoscopically: the vaginal vault is attached to the sacral promontory using a mesh	Bleeding, infection, injury to the bowel or ureter, unmasking of occult urinary stress incontinence, right buttock pain, sexual dysfunction
Rectocoele (**Figure 81.9e**)	Posterior colperineorrhaphy: the posterior vaginal wall is opened, the rectum returned to its normal position and redundant vaginal skin excised	Bleeding, infection, rectal or small bowel injury (fistula formation), dyspareunia, failure, recurrence

Approximately 30% of women in their lifetime report a recurrence of their symptoms following surgical treatment. This figure increases with subsequent procedures.
The **Manchester repair** was introduced at St Mary's Hospital for Women and Children, Manchester, UK.

Edvard Laurits Ehlers, 1863–1937, dermatologist, Copenhagen, Denmark.
Henri-Alexandre Danlos, 1844–1912, dermatologist, Paris, France.
Antoine Bernard-Jean Marfan, 1858–1942, paediatrician, Paris, France.
Milton Lawrence McCall, 1911–1963, obstetrician, Magee-Womens' Hospital, Pittsburg, PA, USA.

Urinary incontinence

Urinary incontinence is defined as the involuntary leakage of urine. It is said to affect approximately 30% of women, with a higher prevalence seen in older age groups. It can have a significant impact on their quality of life.

Incontinence can be classified into:

- stress urinary incontinence (involuntary leakage of urine secondary to increased intra-abdominal pressure, e.g. coughing, sneezing);
- overactive bladder;
- mixed urinary incontinence (combination of both urge and stress incontinence).

It can result from both functional and anatomical causes, including:

- multiparity;
- vaginal delivery;
- menopause;
- fistulae;
- urethral diverticulum/congenital anomalies, e.g. ectopic ureters;
- immobility, constipation or urinary tract infection;
- neurological disorders, e.g. multiple sclerosis;
- secondary to pelvic masses.

Common symptoms and complaints include:

- frequency (increased frequency of more than 8 times during the day);
- nocturia (increased frequency of voiding more than once a night);
- urgency;
- urinary incontinence with increased coughing;
- altered stream, e.g. slow/intermittent stream or hesitancy;
- incomplete bladder emptying;
- postmicturition dribbling;
- nocturnal enuresis;
- haematuria (in women >40 years of age, additional investigations should be performed to rule out malignancy).

Investigations include:

- urine analysis and mid-stream urine sample for microscopy, culture and sensitivity;
- urodynamics if conservative measures have failed;
- ultrasound kidney, ureters and bladder in cases with recurrent urinary tract infections/haematuria;
- cystoscopy if pathology is suspected.

Management can be divided into conservative methods, medical therapy or surgical intervention (*Table 81.7*). The treatment of choice is dependent on the underlying cause.

Treatments can be combined and are individualised for the patient. Should initial therapy be unsuccessful or repeat procedures be required, then the patients should be discussed within a multidisciplinary team setting.

TUMOURS

Uterine fibroids (leiomyoma)

Fibroids are usually benign, well-circumscribed, smooth muscle tumours of the uterus. Less than 1% of fibroids undergo malignant transformation (leiomyosarcoma). They are more common in certain populations (African-Caribbean women) and vary in size and number. They are typically found in the following locations (**Figure 81.10**):

- **subserosal** – may cause pressure-type symptoms; if pedunculated, they can be difficult to distinguish from an ovarian tumour;

TABLE 81.7. Management options for urinary incontinence.

Method	Techniques	Complications
Conservative	Lifestyle changes (i.e. limit fluid intake, avoid diuretics such as tea/coffee, weight loss) Behavioural modification (i.e. bladder drills) Review of coexistent medications (i.e. diuretics) Pelvic floor exercises (physiotherapy) Bladder catheterisation	Infection
Medical	Antibiotics for a urinary tract infection Topical oestrogen therapy in postmenopausal women with urogenital atrophy Antimuscarinic drug therapy (e.g. oxybutynin (avoid in elderly frail women), tolterodine) Selective β_3 adrenoreceptor agonist (e.g. mirabegron) Serotonin and noradrenaline reuptake inhibitor (e.g. duloxetine) (can be used in stress urinary incontinence when conservative measures have failed and surgical treatment is contraindicated or declined) Desmopressin Intravesical botulinum toxin A/urethral bulking agents (e.g. silicone) Neuromodulation	Dry mouth Repeated procedures
Surgical	Management of pelvic masses Bladder reconstruction (augmentation cystoplasty) Urinary diversion Sling procedures (e.g. transvaginal tapes/transobturator tapes) Burch colposuspension Bladder neck suspension Artificial sphincter Fistulae/ectopic ureter surgical correction	 Dependent on the material used for augmentation Bladder voiding difficulties, organ perforation, de novo incontinence, bleeding, erosion, dyspareunia, suprapubic pain

John C Burch, 1900–1977, gynaecologist, Vanderbilt University, Nashville, TN, USA.

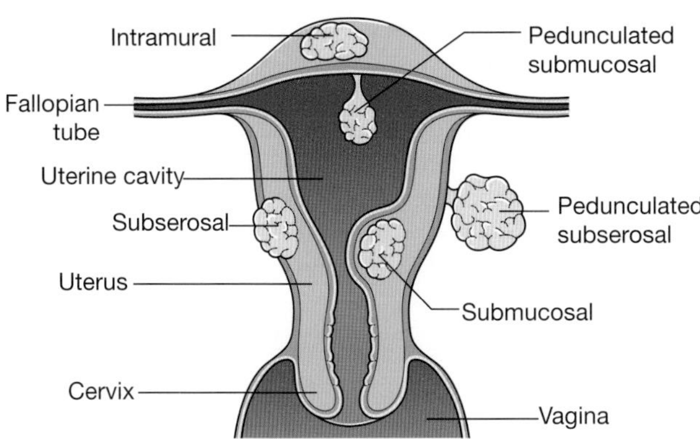

Figure 81.10 Uterine fibroids.

- **intramural** – may similarly cause pressure-type symptoms; associated with infertility and heavy periods;
- **submucosal** – associated with infertility, recurrent pregnancy loss and heavy periods; if pedunculated, may occasionally extrude through the cervical os;
- **rare** – sites include the broad ligament and cervix.

Women with uterine fibroids may present with heavy and/or irregular menstrual bleeding, anaemia, pressure-type symptoms or infertility, especially if the fibroid is distorting the uterine cavity. The pressure-type symptoms include pelvic discomfort, urinary incontinence, frequency and retention, constipation and backache. When large fibroids are present, back pressure may cause or exacerbate varicosities. Although these symptoms are common, it is important to note that some women with fibroids are asymptomatic. Rarely, women may present acutely with pain arising from torsion of a pedunculated fibroid or red degeneration, especially in pregnancy.

A diagnosis can usually be made on bimanual and/or abdominal examination, in the presence of an enlarged uterus with attached swellings. The principal differential diagnosis is an ovarian tumour; in general, if an ovarian tunour is present, the uterus is felt separately on vaginal examination, although not if the structures are adherent to each other. A pelvic ultrasound scan is a good first-line investigation; if not, MRI can be clinically useful (Figure 81.11) but, sometimes, it may be necessary to perform a laparoscopy to distinguish between the two pathologies (Figure 81.12).

Treatment can be divided into: conservative if the woman is asymptomatic; medical to control menstrual bleeding in the form of hormonal manipulation, or newer treatment to shrink the fibroids; or surgical (uterus conserving or nonconserving). The choice of treatment depends upon the woman's age and fertility intentions, the size and number of fibroids as well as their location. Emergency surgical treatment is only required if there is substantial menstrual bleeding or uncontrollable pain; these are rare events.

GnRH agonists aim to shrink the fibroids by inducing a hypo-oestrogenic state. However, this class of drug has the disadvantage that treatment cannot be continued indefinitely because of the associated loss in bone mineral density; in addition, the fibroids tend to regrow to their original size when treatment is discontinued. Ulipristal acetate (Esmya®), a selective progesterone receptor modulator (SPRM), can be used preoperatively to shrink the size of the fibroids through inhibition of cell proliferation. However, these drugs should not be used in conjunction with POP, a progesterone-releasing intrauterine device or the COCP. Uterine artery embolisation (UAE) is becoming increasingly popular as an alternative to surgery. It involves blocking the blood supply to the fibroids using a technique in which particles are embolised into each uterine artery via an angiographic catheter in a similar manner to the well-established technique for treating massive postpartum haemorrhage (Figure 81.13). The aim is to shrink the fibroids, bringing symptomatic relief, i.e. decreased menstrual bleeding and fewer pressure symptoms. This technique has shown more value in the presence of a single large fibroid than in a multifibroid uterus. Complications include arterial injury at the site of catheter insertion, severe pain as a result of uterine ischaemia, infection, ovarian damage

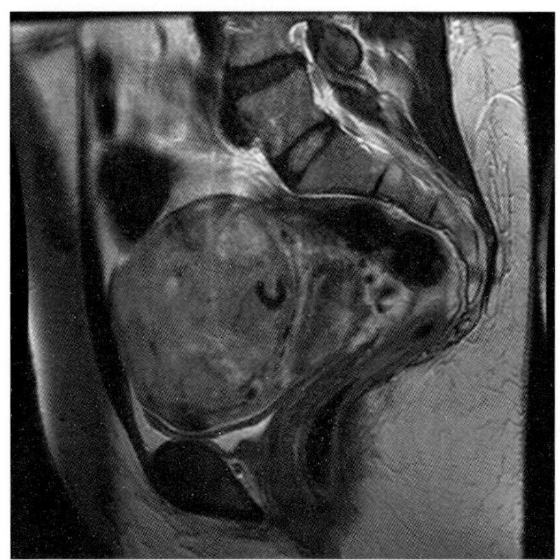

Figure 81.11 Magnetic resonance imaging of uterine fibroids.

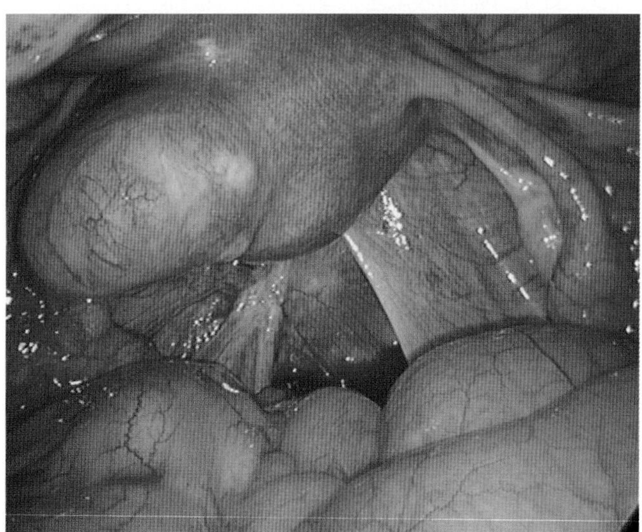

Figure 81.12 Laparoscopic view of a fibroid of the uterine fundus.

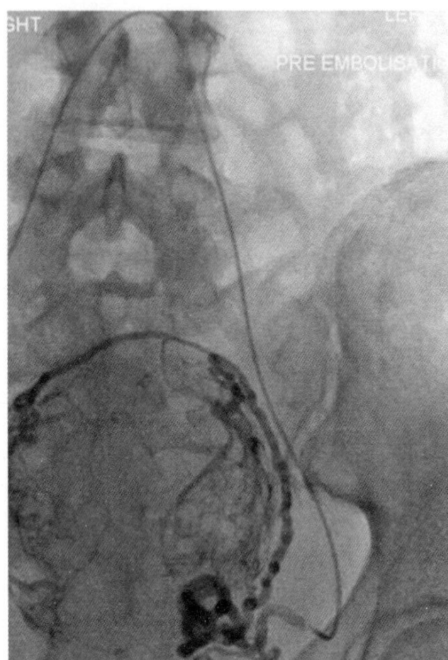

Figure 81.13 Pre-embolisation angiogram showing catheterisation of left uterine artery and blood supply to large fundal fibroid (courtesy of Dr Mark Bratby, Consultant Vascular and Interventional Radiologist, John Radcliffe Hospital, Oxford, UK).

and thromboembolism (a small number of deaths have been reported from uterine infection and pulmonary embolism). There is no consensus regarding the suitability of the technique for women who wish to conceive. Numerous pregnancies have been reported in women who have undergone UAE, but concern still exists regarding the possible adverse effects on the endometrium, myometrial strength and ovarian function, which might affect a woman's chances of conceiving, carrying the pregnancy and delivering normally. Other newer focal fibroid treatments include MR-guided focused ultrasonography, laparoscopic uterine artery occlusion with/without utero-ovarian occlusion, transvaginal Doppler-guided uterine artery occlusion and bipolar radiofrequency ablation (intrauterine ultrasound guided or laparoscopic guided).

A myomectomy (performed through a laparotomy, or increasingly at laparoscopy) involves the removal of pedunculated, subserosal and/or (rarely) intramural fibroids, with closure of the defects left in the uterine wall. Surgical complications include bleeding and damage to surrounding structures, with the risk of conversion to a hysterectomy <1% secondary to uncontrollable blood loss. Fibroids within the uterine cavity can be removed hysteroscopically (transcervical resection of a fibroid (TCRF)); complications include hyponatraemic fluid overload and thermal injury to surrounding structures. This occasionally needs to be performed as a two-stage procedure to avoid the risk of fluid overload and manage the roof of the fibroid, which can protude into the cavity following excision of its base.

Benign ovarian tumour and cysts

Overall, 90% of ovarian tumours are benign, with an increased risk of malignancy in older women: the malignant potential of an ovarian cyst in a premenopausal woman is 1:1000, increasing to 3:1000 at the age of 50 years. Ovarian tumours are subdivided into five main categories according to the World Health Organisation's classification system (*Table 81.8*).

TABLE 81.8 Classification of ovarian tumours.

Epithelial tumours	Represent approximately 75% of all ovarian tumours and 90–95% of ovarian malignancies Further classified by cell type (serous, mucinous, endometrioid, clear cell, transitional cell, epithelial stromal)
Germ cell tumours	Represent approximately 15–20% of all ovarian neoplasms
Sex cord–stromal tumours	Represent approximately 5–10% of all ovarian neoplasms
Metastatic tumours	Represent approximately 5% of ovarian malignancies; usually arise from the breast, colon, endometrium, stomach and cervical cancers
Other/miscellaneous	A small number of other types of neoplasms, which develop from ovarian soft tissue or non-neoplastic processes

The most common solid tumours in young women are cystic teratomas (known more commonly as dermoid cysts), which typically contain a variety of tissues including hair, teeth and bone. Benign ovarian tumours are often asymptomatic and may present incidentally, for example when an abdominal radiograph reveals the appearance of a tooth in the abdomen or pelvis. Conversely, they may present with pain, abdominal swelling and pressure-type symptoms. The pain may result from torsion or bleeding into the cysts. Management will depend on the age of the woman and the characteristics of the cyst. In older women, a conservative approach is reasonable only if the risk of malignancy is low (refer to Ovarian cancer below). In perimenopausal women, the cyst can be followed by serial ultrasound scanning as many will regress. If there is uncontrollable pain, haemodynamic compromise, suspicion of torsion or the cyst does not regress, then surgical management is advised. In most cases this would involve a laparoscopic ovarian cystectomy with conservation of ovarian tissue as the treatment of choice. As the vast majority of oocytes lie within 5 mm of the surface of the ovary, a carefully carried out cystectomy can leave a normally functioning ovary (Figure 81.14).

Ovarian cancer

Ovarian cancer is the sixth most common malignancy in women, behind breast, lung, bowel, uterine cancer and malignant melanoma. In the UK, over 7000 women are diagnosed with ovarian cancer each year. Over 90% of cancers

Christian Johann Doppler, 1803–1853, Professor of Experimental Physics, Vienna, Austria, enunciated the 'Doppler Principle' in 1842.

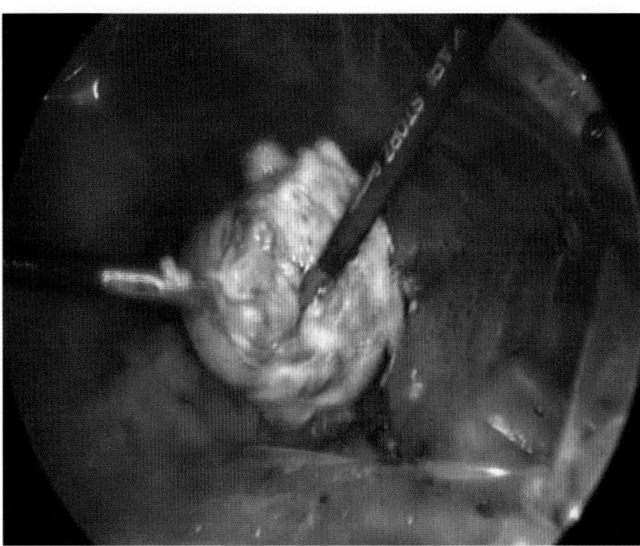

Figure 81.14 Ovarian cystectomy.

Summary box 81.5

Management of benign ovarian cysts

- Commonly, an incidental finding, but may be suggested by symptoms and signs
- A pregnancy test is done to exclude an ectopic pregnancy (however, it is important to note that hCG can also be positive in dysgerminomas and choriocarcinoma)
- Transvaginal ultrasonography (mainstay diagnostic tool) can usually confirm the diagnosis. If the results are indeterminate, MRI or CT imaging may help (MRI is more useful than CT for the assessment of complex cysts/endometriosis). Masses with radiographic characteristics of cancer (e.g. cystic and solid components, surface excrescences, multilocular appearance, irregular shape) require removal
- Tumour markers may help in the diagnosis of specific masses (refer to Ovarian cancer)
- In women of reproductive age, simple, thin-walled cystic adnexal masses of a maximum diameter of 50 mm without characteristics of cancer do not require further investigation unless they persist for more than 3 months. A follow-up scan can be arranged for 4 months to check for resolution. In postmenopausal women, this is conducted every 4 months with cancer antigen 125 (CA-125) levels for 1 year, and if no change is detected, then the women can be discharged
- Perimenopausal women with simple cysts 50–70 mm should undergo annual ultrasound follow-up
- Women with larger cysts (>70 mm) or persistent cysts may benefit from an MRI scan or surgical intervention
- Cyst removal (ovarian cystectomy) is preferrably performed laparoscopically. Cyst aspiration is not recommended as it is associated with a high risk of recurrence. Bilateral salpingo-oophorectomy is preferable for postmenopausal women, if surgery is indicated
- An oophorectomy may become necessary if the cyst cannot be surgically removed from the ovary

arise from the surface epithelium of the ovary (which has the same embryological origins as the peritoneum); the majority arise sporadically rather than secondary to inheritance. The peak incidence is in the age range of 65–69 years. The overall 5-year survival rate is less than 50% because approximately two-thirds of women present with advanced disease.

The common presenting symptoms are:

- abdominal distension and/or pain;
- change in appetite;
- weight gain and increased girth (ascites);
- urinary obstruction.

However, over half of all women present initially to a speciality other than gynaecology, with often vague symptoms caused by metastatic disease, e.g. shortness of breath, gastrointestinal disturbance or a change in bowel habit. Consequently, it is important to include ovarian cancer in the differential diagnosis of any woman presenting with a recent onset of persistent, non-specific, abdominal symptoms (including those whose abdomen and pelvis appear normal on clinical examination).

Ultrasound, more specifically a transvaginal ultrasound scan, is the first-line investigation if an ovarian mass is suspected on clinical grounds. The features suggestive of malignancy on ultrasound include the presence of:

- cyst complexity (number of locules, wall structure, thickness of septae, fluid echogenicity, irregularity, size ≥10 cm);
- solid papillary projections into the cyst (at least four);
- bilateral lesions;
- ascites;
- intra-abdominal metastases;
- strong blood flow.

Serum tumour markers can also be performed to aid diagnosis. CA-125 is a glycoprotein expressed on tissue derived from coelomic and Müllerian epithelia; the normal cut-off value is 35 U/mL. Elevated levels are found in 50% of patients with stage I disease and >90% of those with advanced disease. It primarily detects epithelial ovarian cancers. However, CA-125 is a non-specific marker with raised levels also seen in other cancers, e.g. pancreatic, breast, lung and colon. Levels may also be increased during menstruation; in benign conditions such as endometriosis, PID and liver disease; if ascites or other effusions are present; and after a recent laparotomy. Combining menopausal status, ultrasonographic features and CA-125 measurements using the Risk of Malignancy Index (RMI) algorithm, guides management and helps to identify those patients who require referral to a gynaecological oncologist in a cancer centre. *Summary boxes 81.6 and 81.7* address the basic tests that can be conducted to diagnose ovarian malignancy.

Summary box 81.6

Risk of malignancy index (RMI)

- RMI = U × M × CA-125

  U, ultrasonographic features scoring 1 for each malignant feature (multilocular, solid components, metastases, ascites, bilateral lesions); M, menopausal status with 1 for premenopausal and 3 for postmenopausal; CA-125, CA-125 level in U/mL
- Other tumour markers include lactate dehydrogenase, α-fetoprotein (α-FP), inhibin and β-hCG. They are particularly recommended in women <40 years of age, with a suspected complex ovarian mass, to exclude germ cell tumours

Summary box 81.7

Basic tests on suspicion of ovarian malignancy

- Ultrasonography: findings that suggest cancer include a solid component, surface excrescences, size >5 cm, irregular shape and low vascular resistance on transvaginal Doppler flow studies
- A pelvic mass plus ascites usually indicates ovarian cancer but sometimes indicates Meigs' syndrome (a benign fibroma with ascites and the presence of a pleural effusion)
- CT or MRI is usually carried out before surgery to determine the extent of the cancer
- Tumour markers, including β-hCG, lactate dehydrogenase, α-FP, inhibin and CA-125, CA 19-9, CEA (carcinoembryonic antigen) are measured
- CA-125 is elevated in 80% of advanced epithelial ovarian cancers but may also be mildly elevated in endometriosis, PID, pregnancy, fibroids, peritoneal inflammation and non-ovarian peritoneal cancer

Unfortunately, there are still no effective screening methods for ovarian cancer for the general population. Hence, the preliminary results of the UK Collaborative Trial of Ovarian Cancer Screening are of great interest. The study recruited over 200 000 women, aged 50–74 years, who were randomised to a control arm or one of two screening strategies: primary screening using measurement of serum CA-125 levels followed by transvaginal ultrasound as a second-line test, or transvaginal ultrasound alone. The two screening procedures were similar in terms of sensitivity for all primary ovarian and Fallopian tube cancers, but specificity was higher with combined screening.

There is also no consensus regarding how to screen women who are at high risk for ovarian cancer secondary to a family history, i.e. those with a first-degree relative affected by cancer within a family that meets one of the following criteria:

- two or more individuals with ovarian cancer, who are first-degree relatives of each other;
- one individual with ovarian cancer at any age and one with breast cancer diagnosed at <50 years, who are first-degree relatives of each other (or second-degree relatives if the transmission is paternal);
- one relative with ovarian cancer at any age and two with breast cancer diagnosed at <60 years, who are connected by first-degree relationships (or second-degree relationships if the transmission is paternal);
- a known carrier of relevant cancer gene mutations (e.g. *BRCA1* or *BRCA2*);
- an untested first-degree relative of a predisposing gene carrier;
- three or more family members with colon cancer or two with colon cancer and one with stomach, ovarian, endometrial, urinary tract or small bowel cancer in two generations. One of these cancers must be diagnosed at <50 years (Lynch syndrome);
- an individual with both breast and ovarian cancer.

Some genetic mutations are known to predispose women to ovarian cancer, e.g. *BRCA1* and *BRCA2* and the mismatch repair genes associated with Lynch syndrome families. *BRCA1* mutations confer a 39% lifetime risk of ovarian cancer up to the age of 70 years; the figure for *BRCA2* mutations is 11–17% up to the age of 70 years. The mismatch repair genes confer an increased lifetime risk of ovarian cancer of 9–12%, in addition to the increased risk of endometrial cancer (refer to Vaginal bleeding in the non-pregnant state). Referral to a specialist cancer genetics service is advisable. Women at high risk of ovarian cancer may be offered prophylactic bilateral salpingo-oophorectomy, especially as they may also be at increased risk of breast cancer and there is some evidence to suggest that oophorectomy reduces breast cancer risk in these women. Unfortunately, there is currently no proven role for screening in women at high risk.

Staging (*Table 81.9*) is performed at laparotomy via a midline incision if disease is suspected preoperatively, by:

- careful evaluation of all peritoneal surfaces;
- four washings of the peritoneal cavity: diaphragm, right and left abdomen, pelvis;
- infracolic omentectomy;
- selected lymphadenectomy of the pelvic and para-aortic lymph nodes;
- biopsy and/or resection of suspicious lesions, masses and adhesions;
- random blind biopsies of normal peritoneal surfaces, including that from the undersurface of the right hemidiaphragm, bladder reflection, cul-de-sac, right and left paracolic recesses and both pelvic side walls;
- total abdominal hysterectomy and bilateral salpingo-oophorectomy;
- appendicectomy for mucinous tumours; if a routine appendicectomy results in an intraoperative suspicion of a mucinous tumour, the surgeon should take washings and a biopsy from suspicious area(s).

TABLE 81.9 Staging of ovarian cancer.

Stage I	Growth limited to the ovaries
Stage II	Growth involving one or both ovaries with pelvic extension
Stage III	Tumour involving one or both ovaries with histologically confirmed peritoneal implants outside the pelvis and/or positive retroperitoneal or inguinal nodes. Superficial liver metastases are considered stage III. Tumour is limited to the true pelvis but with histologically proven extension to the small bowel or omentum
Stage IV	Growth involving one or both ovaries with distant metastases. If pleural effusion is present there must be positive cytology to classify a case as stage IV. Parenchymal liver metastasis equals stage IV

Joe Vincent Meigs, 1892–1964, gynaecological surgeon, Massachusetts General Hospital, Boston, MA, USA.

Ovarian cancer is chemosensitive; however, a staging laparotomy and histological findings provide accurate information about prognosis and postoperative therapy. The general principle is cytoreductive surgery followed by combination chemotherapy; only a minority of patients with ovarian cancer need bowel resected during the primary procedure or surgery for recurrent disease. The only exception to this rule is a young woman with stage I disease or a borderline tumour who requests unilateral oophorectomy to conserve her fertility.

Stage IA or IB/grade 1 epithelial adenocarcinoma requires no postoperative therapy. Stage IA or IB/grade 2 or 3 cancers and stage II cancers require six courses of chemotherapy (typically, paclitaxel and carboplatin). Stage III or IV cancer requires six courses of similar chemotherapy. Intraperitoneal chemotherapy or high-dose chemotherapy with bone marrow transplantation is under study. Radiotherapy is used infrequently. Even if chemotherapy results in a complete clinical response (i.e. normal physical examination, normal serum CA-125 and negative CT scan of the abdomen and pelvis), approximately 50% of such patients with stage III or IV cancer will have residual disease. Of patients with persistent elevation of the CA-125, 90–95% will have residual tumour.

Ovarian stimulation with oocyte or embryo cryopreservation has been reported in patients with low-grade tumours (grade IA/B) who wish to preserve their fertility, but the effect of this on the underlying disease is as yet unknown and it must therefore be carried out with caution. Newer techniques include ovarian tissue cryopreservation with the potential risk of cancer reoccurence following autologous transplantation.

FURTHER READING

Cervical screening programme. Available online at: https://www.gov.uk/guidance/cervical-screening-programme-overview.

European Society of Human Reproduction and Embryology (ESHRE) guideline on the management of women with endometriosis. Available online at https://www.eshre.eu/Guidelines-and-Legal/Guidelines/Endometriosis-guideline.aspx

NHS Evidence – women's health. Available online at: http://www.library.nhs.uk/womenshealth.

NICE Guidance on ectopic pregnancy and miscarriage: diagnosis and initial management and heavy menstrual bleeding: assessment and management. Available online at: https://www.nice.org.uk/Guidance/CG154

Prat J, FIGO Committee on Gynecologic Oncology. FIGO Guidelines. Staging classification for cancer of the ovary, fallopian tube, and peritoneum. *Int J Gynaecol Obstet* 2014; **124** (1): 1–5.

RCOG Green-top guidelines on ovarian cysts in postmenopausal women, management of suspected ovarian masses in premenopausal women, pregnancy and breast cancer. Available online at: http://www.rcog.org.uk.

Scottish Intercollegiate Guidelines Network. Management of epithelial ovarian cancer. No. 135. Available online at: http://www.sign.ac.uk/guidelines.

UK National Guideline for the management of pelvic inflammatory disease. British Association for Sexual Health and HIV. Available online at: https://www.bashh.org/documents/3572.pdf

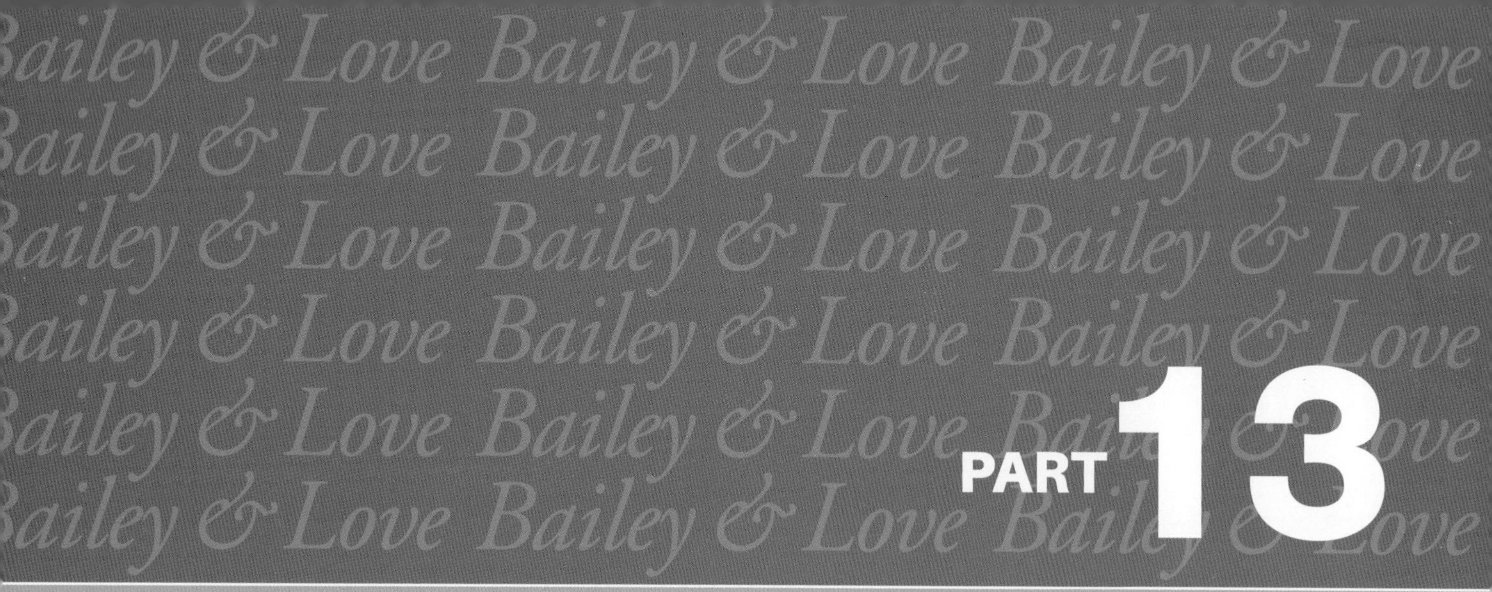

Transplantation

82 Transplantation 1532

Chapter 82

Transplantation

Learning objectives

- To appreciate the immunological basis of allograft rejection
- To know the principles of immunosuppressive therapy
- To be aware of the side effects of non-specific immunosuppression
- To be familiar with the major issues concerning organ donation
- To appreciate the main indications for organ transplantation
- To know the surgical principles of organ implantation
- To be able to give an account of the causes of graft dysfunction
- To know the likely outcomes after transplantation
- To be aware of potential future developments in transplantation

HISTORICAL PERSPECTIVE

Since early times, the idea of tissue and organ transplantation has captured the imagination of successive generations and, over the centuries, numerous fanciful descriptions of successful transplants have been recorded.

The modern era of transplantation began in the 1950s (*Table 82.1*) and relied on surgical techniques for anastomosing blood vessels that had been developed at the start of the twentieth century by Mathieu Jaboulay and Alexis Carrel. The first successful kidney transplant was a living-donor transplant performed between identical twins in 1954 at the Brigham Hospital in Boston by Joseph Murray and colleagues. This, and other kidney transplants between identical twins, demonstrated the technical feasibility of kidney transplantation, but attempts to perform renal transplantation when the donor and recipient were not genetically identical failed because no effective immunosuppressive therapy was available (**Figure 82.1**). Then, in 1959, Schwartz and Dameshek discovered that 6-mercaptopurine had immunosuppressive properties, and Calne showed that azathioprine, a derivative of 6-mercaptopurine, prevented rejection of canine kidney transplants. From the early 1960s, a combination of azathioprine and corticosteroids was used with moderate success in the clinic to prevent graft rejection after kidney transplantation. These chemical agents were sometimes supplemented with a polyclonal anti-lymphocyte antibody.

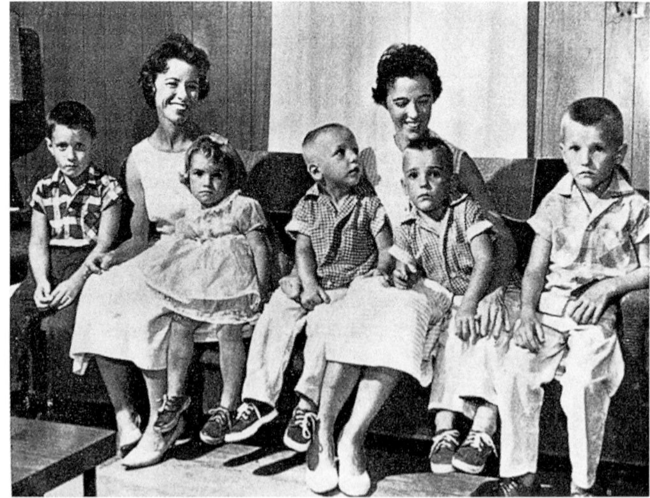

Figure 82.1 One of the early Boston recipients of a kidney transplant from an identical twin, shown here with her twin sister and their children.

Mathieu Jaboulay, 1860–1913, Professor of Surgery, Lyons, France.

Alexis Carrel, 1873–1944, surgeon, Lyons, France, who worked at the Rockefellar Institute for Medical Research in New York, NY, USA. He received the Nobel Prize for Physiology or Medicine in 1912 'In recognition of his works on vascular suture and the transplantation of blood vessels and organs'.

Joseph E Murray, 1919–2012, Professor of Plastic Surgery, Harvard University Medical School, Boston, MA, USA, shared the 1990 Nobel Prize for Physiology or Medicine with E Donnall Thomas for his work on organ and cell transplantation.

Robert S Schwartz, Professor of Medicine, the Tufts University School of Medicine, Boston, MA, USA.

William Dameshek, 1900–1969, American physician and haematologist.

TABLE 82.1 Milestones in organ transplantation.

1954	Joe Murray performed successful kidney transplantations between identical twins (Boston, MA, USA)
1962	Roy Calne demonstrated the efficacy of azathioprine in preventing rejection of kidney allografts (Boston, MA, USA)
1963	Tom Starzl performed the first human liver transplantation (Denver, CO, USA)
1966	Tom Starzl and colleagues used anti-lymphocyte globulin immunosuppression (Denver, CO, USA)
1966	Richard Lillehei and William Kelly performed first human whole organ pancreas transplantation (along with a kidney transplantation) (Minneapolis, MN, USA)
1967	Christiaan Barnard performed the first human heart transplantation (Cape Town, South Africa)
1968	Fritz Derom performed the first human lung transplantation (Ghent, Belgium)
1969	Geoff Collins developed Collins solution – a new kidney preservation solution
1974	David Sutherland and John Najarin performed the first human pancreatic islet transplantation (Minneapolis, MN, USA)
1978	Roy Calne introduced ciclosporin into clinical practice (Cambridge, UK)
1981	Bruce Reitz and Norman Shumway performed the first successful human heart–lung transplantation (Stanford, CA, USA)
1987	Fokert Belzer and colleagues developed University of Wisconsin (UW) solution – a new liver and pancreas preservation solution (Wisconsin, USA)
1988	Rudolf Pichlmayr performed the first splitting of a donor liver for use in two recipients (Hannover, Germany)
1989	Tom Starzl demonstrated clinical efficacy of FK506 (tacrolimus) (Pittsburgh, PA, USA)
1991	Kil Park performed the first living-donor kidney paired exchange to overcome antibody incompatibility (Seoul, South Korea)
1995	Lloyd Ratner and colleagues first described laparoscopic living-donor nephrectomy (Johns Hopkins University, Baltimore, MD, USA)

The ciclosporin era began in the late 1970s after its discovery by Borel at the Sandoz laboratories in Basle and the demonstration, by Calne in Cambridge, UK, of its potent immunosuppressive properties in clinical transplantation. The introduction of ciclosporin was a major advance and ciclosporin (usually given together with azathioprine and steroids) not only improved the results of renal transplantation, but also allowed transplantation of the heart and liver to be undertaken with acceptable results. Organ transplantation is now well established as an effective treatment for selected patients with end-stage organ failure. Kidney, liver, pancreas, heart and lung transplantation are all routine procedures with good outcome, and transplantation of the small intestine is becoming more widely practised. Transplant activity is limited only by the shortage of donor organs.

Summary box 82.1

Definitions

- Allograft: an organ or tissue transplanted from one individual to another
- Alloantigen: transplant antigen
- Alloantibody: transplant antibodies
- HLA: human leukocyte antigen, the main trigger to graft rejection
- Xenograft: a graft performed between different species
- Orthotopic graft: a graft placed in its normal anatomical site
- Heterotopic graft: a graft placed in a site different from that where the organ is normally located

GRAFT REJECTION

Allografts provoke a powerful immune response that results in rapid graft rejection unless immunosuppressive therapy is given. The pioneering studies of Medawar in the 1940s and 1950s firmly established that allograft rejection was due to an immune response and not a non-specific inflammatory response and subsequent studies demonstrated that T lymphocytes play an essential role in mediating rejection.

Allografts trigger a graft rejection response because of allelic differences at polymorphic genes that give rise to histocompatibility antigens (transplant antigens) of which ABO blood group antigens and human leukocyte antigens (HLAs) are the most important.

ABO blood group antigens

The ABO blood group antigens are expressed not only by red blood cells, but also by most other cell types. It is vitally important, for all types of organ allograft, to ensure that recipients do not unintentionally receive a graft that is ABO blood group incompatible otherwise naturally occurring anti-A or anti-B antibodies will likely cause hyperacute graft rejection.

Permissible transplants are from:

- group O donor to group O, A, B or AB recipient;
- group A donor to group A or AB recipient;
- group B donor to group B or AB recipient;
- group AB donor to group AB recipient.

There is no need to take account of rhesus antigen compatibility in organ transplantation.

Jean-Francois Borel, b.1933, research scientist working in Switzerland.
Sir Roy York Calne, Emeritus Professor of Surgery, the University of Cambridge, Cambridge, UK. In 1968 he performed Europe's first liver transplantation. He was associated with the world's first liver, heart and lung transplantation in 1987. He was elected Fellow of the Royal Society in 1974. He is an accomplished painter who has painted many of his transplant recipients and has had exhibitions worldwide.
Sir Peter Brian Medawar, 1915–1987, zoologist and immunologist, Director of the National Institute of Medical Research, London, UK. He shared the 1968 Nobel Prize for Physiology or Medicine with Sir Frank Macfarlane Burnet, for his research into immunological tolerance.

HLA

Allograft rejection (in blood group-compatible grafts) is directed predominantly against HLA – a group of highly polymorphic cell-surface molecules. HLA are strong transplant antigens by virtue of their special physiological role as antigen recognition units for display of antigens from foreign pathogens for recognition by T lymphocytes. Their existence was first demonstrated by Dausset in 1958, through their role in stimulating graft rejection responses, and hence their description as major histocompatibility antigens (MHA).

Summary box 82.2

Human leukocyte antigen (HLA)

- Are the most common cause of graft rejection
- Their physiological function is to act as antigen recognition units
- Are highly polymorphic (amino acid sequence differs widely between individuals)
- HLA-A, -B, -C (class I), and -DR, -DP and -DQ (class II) are most important in organ transplantation

There are two types of HLA molecule: HLA class I and HLA class II (*Table 82.2*). They are broadly similar in structure (Figure 82.2) but have different cell expression profiles. HLA class I antigens are present on all nucleated cells, whereas HLA class II antigens have a more restricted distribution and are expressed most strongly on antigen-presenting cells, such as dendritic cells, macrophages and B lymphocytes. T cells recognize HLA molecules via their T-cell receptor, but full T-cell activation also requires the delivery of an additional or second signal by the interaction of co-stimulatory molecules on the surface of the antigen-presenting cell and T cell (Figure 82.3).

TABLE 82.2 Human leukocyte antigen (HLA) class I and HLA class II molecules.

	Class I	Class II
HLA loci	HLA-A, -B and -C	HLA-DR, -DP and -DQ
Structure	Heavy chain and β_2-microglobulin	α- and β-chain
Distribution	All nucleated cells	B cells, dendritic cells, macrophages

Effector mechanisms of rejection

HLA expressed by graft cells activate T cells and stimulate them to proliferate in response to interleukin-2 (IL-2) and other T-cell growth factors. Activated CD4 T cells, through release of cytokines, play a central role in orchestrating the various effector mechanisms responsible for graft rejection (Figure 82.4). The cellular effectors of graft rejection include cytotoxic CD8 T cells, which recognise donor HLA class I antigens expressed by the graft and cause target cell death through the release of lytic molecules such as perforin and granzyme. Graft-infiltrating CD4 T cells, which recognise donor HLA class II antigens, mediate direct target cell damage and are also able, by releasing proinflammatory cytokines such as interferon-γ, to recruit and activate macrophages that act as non-specific effector cells. Finally, CD4 T cells provide essential T-cell help for B lymphocytes which differentiate into plasma cells and produce alloantibodies that bind to graft antigen and induce target cell injury directly or through antibody-dependent, cell-mediated cytotoxicity.

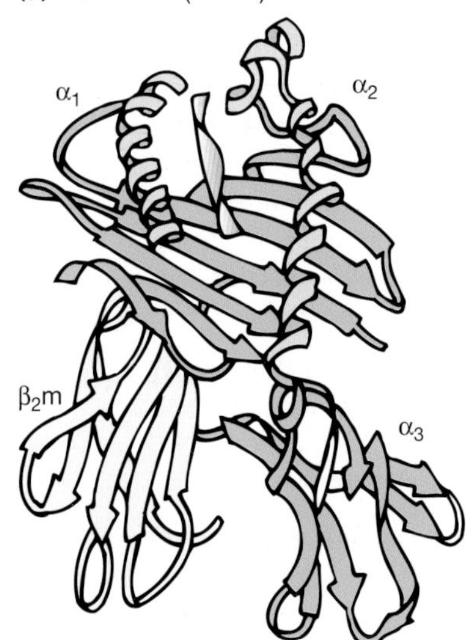

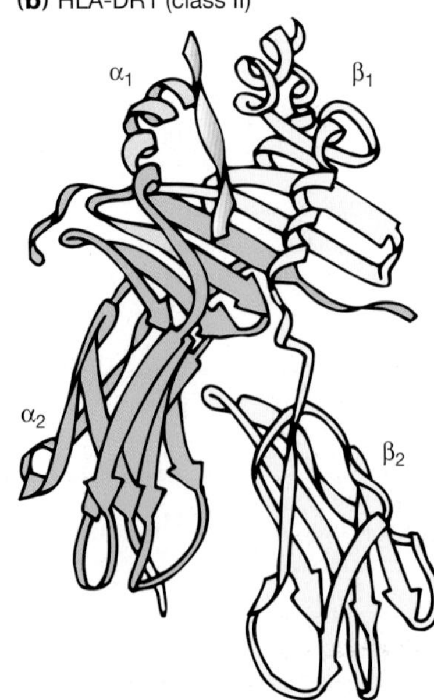

Figure 82.2 The three-dimensional structure of the extracellular domains of human leukocyte antigen (HLA) class I and class II. The α_1 and α_2 domains of class I and the α_1 and β_1 domains of class II form a cleft that is floored by a β-pleated sheet and walled by two α-helices. The cleft binds an antigenic peptide and displays it on the cell surface for recognition by a T lymphocyte. (Redrawn with permission from Stern and Wiley (1994) *Structure* **2**: 245–52.)

Jean Dausset, 1916–2009, French immunologist, Professor of Experimental Medicine at the College of France, Paris, France, shared the 1980 Nobel Prize for Physiology or Medicine with George Snell and Baruj Benacerraf for his discovery of the HLA antigens.

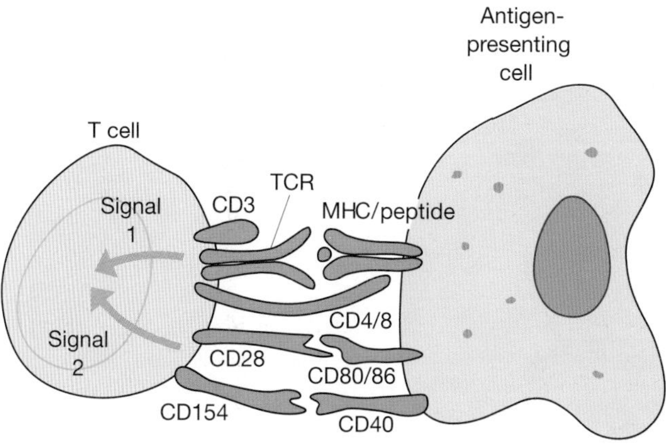

Figure 82.3 Molecular events involved in T-cell activation by an antigen-presenting cell. T-cell activation requires the delivery of two distinct signals to the T cell. The first signal is delivered by ligation of the TCR/CD3 complex with the human leukocyte antigen (HLA)/peptide complex. The second signal is delivered after the interaction between pairs of co-stimulatory molecules such as CD28 with CD80/86 and CD154 with CD40.

Summary box 82.3

Types of graft rejection

- Hyperacute rejection
  - Immediate graft destruction due to ABO or preformed anti-HLA antibodies
  - Characterised by intravascular thrombosis and interstitial haemorrhage
- Acute rejection
  - Usually occurs during first 6 months
  - T-cell dependent
  - May be cell mediated, antibody mediated or both
  - Usually reversible
- Chronic rejection
  - Occurs after first 6 months
  - Most common cause of graft failure
  - Antibodies play an important role
  - Non-immune factors contribute to pathogenesis
  - Characterised by myointimal proliferation in graft arteries leading to ischaemia and fibrosis

Types of allograft rejection

Allograft rejection can be divided into three distinct types:

1 hyperacute rejection (occurs immediately);
2 acute rejection (usually occurs in the first 6 months);
3 chronic rejection (occurs months and years after transplantation).

Allograft rejection manifests itself as functional failure of the transplant and is confirmed by histological examination. Biopsy material is obtained from renal and pancreas grafts by needle biopsy, and from hepatic grafts by percutaneous or transjugular liver biopsy. Cardiac grafts are biopsied by transjugular endomyocardial biopsy and lung grafts by transbronchial biopsy. After small intestinal transplantation, mucosal biopsies are obtained from the graft stoma or more proximally by endoscopy. A standardised histological grading system, termed the Banff classification (named after the Canadian town where the initial scientific workshop was held), defines the presence and severity of allograft rejection after organ transplantation.

Hyperacute rejection

This is due to the presence in the recipient of preformed antibodies against HLA class I antigens expressed by the donor. These arise from a previous blood transfusion, a failed transplant and pregnancy. This type of rejection also occurs if an ABO blood group-incompatible organ graft is performed inadvertently. After revascularisation of the graft, antibodies bind immediately to the vasculature, activate the complement system, and cause extensive intravascular thrombosis, interstitial haemorrhage and graft destruction within minutes and hours. Kidney transplants are particularly vulnerable to hyperacute graft rejection, whereas heart and liver transplants are relatively resistant. It is not clear why the liver is resistant to hyperacute rejection. One factor may be that it is less susceptible to ischaemia than the kidney by virtue of its dual

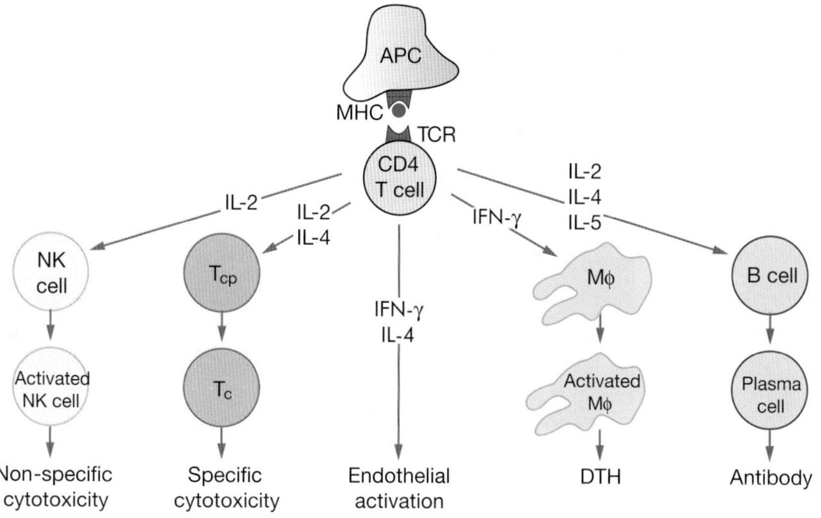

Figure 82.4 The central role of the CD4 T cell in orchestrating the various effector mechanisms responsible for allograft rejection. APC, antigen-presenting cell; DTH, delayed-type hypersensitivity; IFN-γ, interferon-gamma; IL, interleukin; MΦ, macrophage; MHC, major histocompatibility complex; NK, natural killer; Tc, T-cytotoxic cell; Tcp, T-cytotoxic precursor cell; TCR, T-cell receptor.

blood supply: 60% of the hepatic blood supply is derived from the portal vein and 40% from the hepatic artery.

Hyperacute rejection can be avoided by ensuring ABO blood group compatibility and performing a cross-match test on recipient serum to ensure that there are no clinically relevant antibodies directed against HLAs expressed by a prospective kidney donor.

Acute rejection

This usually occurs during the first 6 months after transplantation but may occur later. It is mediated predominantly by T lymphocytes, but alloantibodies may also play an important role. Acute rejection is characterised by mononuclear cell infiltration of the graft (**Figure 82.5**). The mononuclear cell infiltrate is heterogeneous and includes cytotoxic T cells, B cells, natural killer (NK) cells and activated macrophages. Antibody-mediated damage may also be present, as evidenced by the deposition of the complement component C4d within the graft microvasculature (**Figure 82.6**). All types of organ allograft are susceptible to acute rejection (typically occurring in around 20–30% of grafts). Most episodes of acute cellular rejection can be reversed by additional immunosuppressive therapy. Acute antibody-mediated rejection is more difficult to treat effectively and may require plasmaphoresis or immunoadsorption.

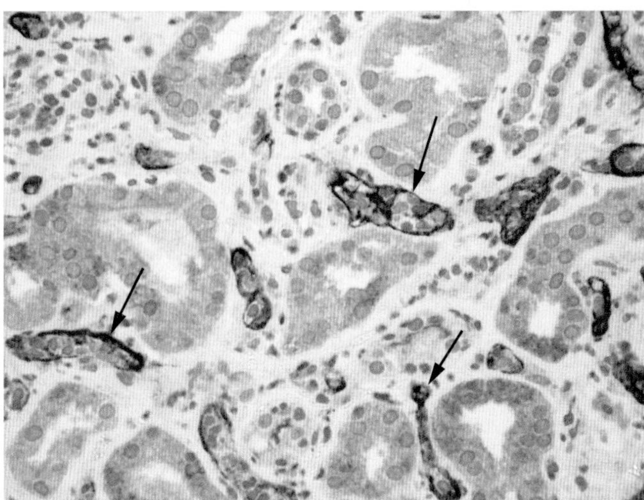

Figure 82.6 Acute antibody-mediated renal allograft rejection. There is widespread staining for the complement component C4d within the peritubular capillaries (arrows), which indicates alloantibody binding to the graft vasculature.

Chronic rejection

This usually occurs after the first 6 months. All types of transplants are susceptible to chronic rejection, and it is the major cause of allograft failure. Interestingly, the liver is more resistant than other organs to the destructive effects of chronic rejection. The pathophysiology of chronic rejection is not well understood, although the underlying mechanisms are immunological, and alloantibodies are thought to be a major cause and cellular effector mechanisms may also contribute. Alloantigen-independent factors also contribute. The risk factors for chronic rejection of a kidney transplant are:

- previous episodes of acute rejection;
- poor HLA match;
- long cold ischaemia time;
- cytomegalovirus (CMV) infection;
- raised blood lipids;
- inadequate immunosuppression (including poor compliance).

The single most important risk factor for chronic rejection after kidney transplantation is acute rejection (with vascular inflammation) and recurrent episodes of acute rejection. As non-immune factors often contribute significantly to the long-term failure of a kidney transplant, the term 'chronic allograft nephropathy' is sometimes used.

The histological picture of chronic rejection after organ transplantation is dominated by vascular changes, with the development of myointimal proliferation in arteries, which results in ischaemia and fibrosis (**Figure 82.7**). In addition to

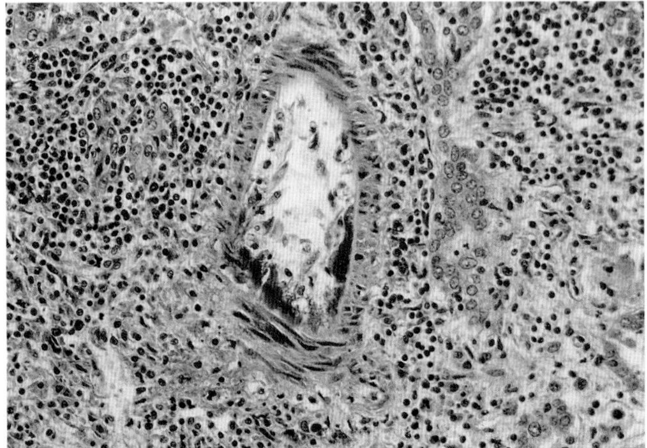

Figure 82.5 Severe acute renal allograft rejection with a heavy mononuclear cell infiltrate and intimal arteritis.

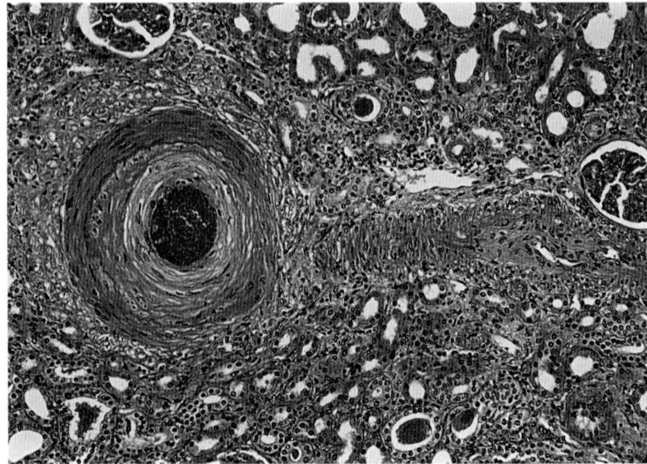

Figure 82.7 Chronic renal allograft rejection. The arteriole shows severe myointimal proliferation and luminal narrowing, resulting in ischaemic fibrosis.

vasculopathy, there are organ-specific features of chronic graft rejection. These are:

- kidney: glomerular sclerosis and tubular atrophy;
- pancreas: acinar loss and islet destruction;
- heart: accelerated coronary artery disease (cardiac allograft vasculopathy);
- liver: vanishing bile duct syndrome;
- lungs: obliterative bronchiolitis.

Chronic rejection causes functional deterioration in the graft, resulting after months or years in complete graft failure. Unfortunately, currently available immunosuppressive therapy has had little effect in preventing chronic rejection.

Graft-versus-host disease

Although the main immunological problem after transplantation is graft rejection, the reciprocal problem of graft-versus-host reaction is occasionally seen after certain types of organ transplantation. Some donor organs (particularly liver and small bowel) contain large numbers of lymphocytes, and these may react against HLAs expressed by recipient tissues, leading to graft-versus-host disease (GVHD). GVHD frequently involves the skin, causing a characteristic rash on the palms and soles. It may also involve the liver (after small bowel transplantation) and the gastrointestinal tract (after liver transplantation). GVHD is a serious and sometimes fatal complication.

HLA MATCHING

HLA molecules are encoded by the major histocompatibility complex (MHC), a cluster of genes situated on the short arm of chromosome 6 (**Figure 82.8**). The HLA class I antigens comprise HLA-A, -B and -C, and the HLA class II antigens comprise HLA-DR, -DP and -DQ. Expression of MHC genes is co-dominant, i.e. the genes on both the maternally derived and the paternally derived chromosomes are expressed. Consequently, an individual may express between 6 and 12 different HLA antigens, depending on the degree of homozygosity (shared genes) at individual loci.

The HLA haplotype inherited from each parent is usually inherited as a complete haplotype, according to simple mendelian genetics (**Figure 82.9**). In deceased donor renal transplantation (but not other types of organ transplantation), attempts are usually made to match the donor and recipient for as many of the relevant HLAs as possible. In addition to reducing the risk of graft loss from rejection, a well-matched kidney allograft that subsequently fails is less likely to cause sensitisation to the HLAs that it expresses. It is particularly important in children and young adults to avoid, where possible, grafts that are mismatched for common HLAs because, if retransplantation is required subsequently, it may be difficult to find an organ donor who does not express the antigens to which the recipient has become sensitised. In terms of organ transplantation, HLA-A, -B and -DR are the most important antigens to take into account when matching donor and recipient in an attempt to reduce the risk of graft rejection (**Figure 82.10**).

HLA matching has a relatively small but definite beneficial effect on renal allograft survival (HLA-DR > HLA-B > HLA-A). Recipients who receive well-matched renal allografts may require less intensive immunosuppression and are also troubled less by rejection episodes. It is common practice to express the degree of HLA matching between the donor and recipient in terms of whether or not there are mismatches at each locus for HLA-A, -B and -DR. A '000 mismatch' is a 'full-house' or complete match, whereas a '012 mismatch' is matched at HLA-A loci, has one mismatched HLA-B antigen and is mismatched for both -DR antigens. Deceased donor kidneys are allocated in some countries, including the UK, by a points system that optimises HLA matching but also takes into account other factors, such as time on the waiting list, sensitisation to HLA antigens and the age relationship between the donor and the recipient. Allocation of organs for transplantation must also take into account the relative size of the donor and recipient. This is not an issue in renal transplantation, and adult kidneys can be readily used for children (and vice versa). However, in the case of heart, lung, liver and

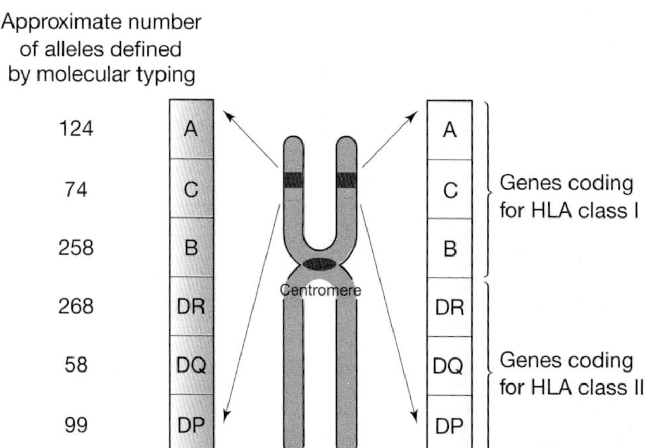

Figure 82.8 The human leukocyte antigen (HLA) system on the short arm of chromosome 6.

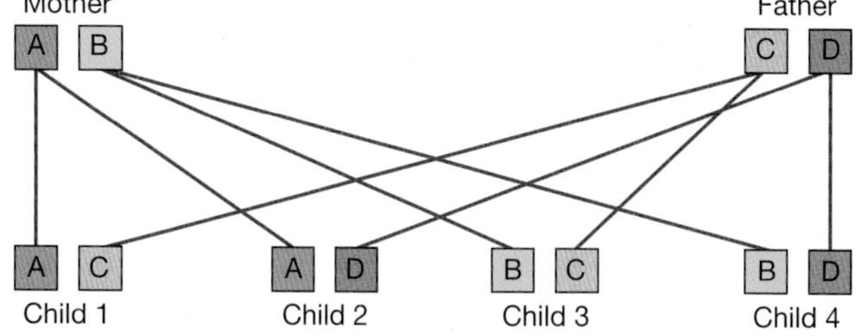

Figure 82.9 Human leukocyte antigen (HLA) inheritance. Children acquire one HLA haplotype (depicted as A–D) from each parent. As shown, child 1 shares one HLA haplotype (haploidentical) with child 2 and child 3, but does not share either haplotype with child 4. The chances that two siblings will share the same parental haplotypes, or that they will share neither HLA haplotype, is one in four. The chance that they will share one HLA haplotype is one in two.

Gregor Johann Mendel, 1822–1884, Austrian monk and naturalist, became Abbot of the Augustinian Monastery at Brunn, former Czechoslovakia and discovered the laws of inheritance by studying the edible pea. In 1865 he described 'dominant' and 'recessive' traits in hybrids. His work passed unnoticed for 35 years.

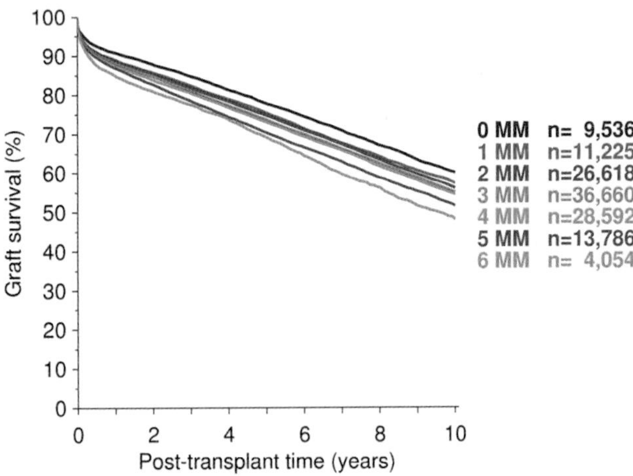

Figure 82.10 Beneficial effect of human leukocyte antigen (HLA) matching (HLA-A, -B and -DR) on first deceased donor renal allograft survival (courtesy of Collaborative Transplant Study, CTC-K-21101-0816). MM, antigen mismatch.

small bowel transplantation, it is important to consider size compatibility between the donor and the recipient. In the case of liver transplants, HLA matching does not confer an advantage and, although it is beneficial in cardiac transplantation, it is not practicable because of the relatively small size of the recipient pool and the short permissible cold ischaemic time.

THE TISSUE-TYPING LABORATORY

Successful organ transplantation requires a close working relationship between the tissue-typing laboratory and the clinical transplant team. The tissue-typing laboratory carries out three key tasks. First, they determine the HLA type ('tissue type') of all potential organ transplant recipients and organ donors. This is achieved by applying polymerase chain reaction (PCR)-based DNA-typing techniques to samples of peripheral blood. Second, they perform a cross-match test to exclude the presence in a recipient of clinically significant circulating antibodies to HLAs expressed by a potential organ donor that would result in rapid or hyperacute graft rejection. This involves incubating recipient sera with donor lymphocytes prepared from either blood or lymphoid tissue. The presence of anti-donor antibodies is detected in a conventional cytotoxic cross-match assay by adding rabbit complement, along with indicator dyes, and visualising target cell death. More often a flow cytometric cross-match is performed as well as, or instead of, a cytotoxic cross-match. Third, the tissue-typing laboratory determines the HLA specificity of circulating anti-HLA antibodies in recipients before and after organ transplantation to guide organ allocation and immunosuppressive therapy. This task has been revolutionised by the availability of solid phase assays, particularly Luminex technology, where patient sera are incubated with a panel of latex beads coated with purified HLA molecules and antibody binding detected by flow cytometric analysis.

Patients on the renal transplant waiting list should be screened for the development of HLA antibodies on a regular basis and especially after potential priming to HLA antigens by blood transfusion.

If, when considering renal transplantation, the cross-match test is strongly positive, transplantation should not proceed, or hyperacute rejection is likely. Antibodies directed against HLA class II antigens, unlike those to HLA class I, do not usually cause hyperacute rejection but are associated with acute rejection and a poor clinical outcome. Patients awaiting heart transplantation are also screened for the presence of HLA antibodies and those with preformed antibodies are subjected to a prospective cross-match test. Although heart allografts rarely undergo hyperacute rejection, transplantation in the presence of a positive cross-match is associated with graft loss from accelerated acute rejection. Even in the presence of a strongly positive cross-match test, liver transplants rarely undergo hyperacute rejection, although long-term survival is reduced.

IMMUNOSUPPRESSIVE THERAPY

A range of different agents are available that act at different sites during T-cell activation to prevent rejection (*Table 82.3* and **Figure 82.11**). They can be classified according to their principal mode of action.

Calcineurin inhibitors (ciclosporin and tacrolimus)

Ciclosporin and tacrolimus are the mainstay of most modern immunosuppressive protocols for organ transplantation. Although structurally distinct, they exert their principal immunosuppressive effect through the same intracellular pathway. Each of the two agents binds within the T cell to a cytoplasmic protein or immunophilin (ciclosporin binds

TABLE 82.3 Immunosuppressive agents.

Agent	Principal mode of action
Corticosteroids	Widespread anti-inflammatory effects
Azathioprine	Prevents lymphocyte proliferation
Mycophenolic acid preparations	Prevents lymphocyte proliferation
Calcineurin inhibitors (ciclosporin/tacrolimus)	Blocks IL-2 gene transcription
mTOR inhibitors	Blocks IL-2 receptor signal transduction
ALG	Depletion and blockade of lymphocytes
Anti-CD25 mAb	Targets activated T cells
Anti-CD52 mAb	Depletion of lymphocytes
Anti-CD20	Depletion of B lymphocytes
CTLA-4Ig	Blocks T-cell costimulation

IL-2, interleukin-2.

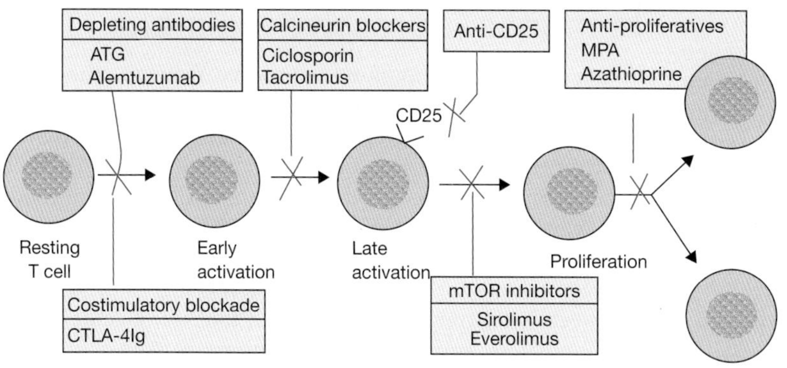

Figure 82.11 Site of action of immunosuppressive agents on T cell. ATG, anti-thymocyte globulin; MPA, mycophenolic acid derivatives; mTOR, mammalian target of rapamycin.

to cyclophilin and tacrolimus to FK-binding protein). The resulting immunophilin–drug complex then blocks the activity of calcineurin (a phosphatase) within the cytoplasm of the T cell. Calcineurin plays a critical role in facilitating the transcription of IL-2, the main T-cell growth factor, and other cytokines after T-cell activation. By blocking cytokine synthesis, ciclosporin and tacrolimus exert a potent immunosuppressive effect. The two agents share a number of side effects, the most notable of which is nephrotoxicity (*Table 82.4*). Ciclosporin sometimes causes cosmetic side effects (hirsutism and gingival hypertrophy) that may be distressing, particularly in younger female recipients. The calcineurin inhibitors (CNIs) have a relatively small therapeutic window. Their immunosuppressive action, as well as their side effects, is dependent on their blood concentration, and monitoring of whole-blood drug levels is an important guide to optimal therapy. Ciclosporin and tacrolimus are broadly equivalent in terms of long-term graft survival but increasing evidence suggests that tacrolimus is more effective in reducing acute rejection. The choice between the two agents depends on the preference of the transplant unit and on individual patient tolerance to the different side effects of the two agents.

TABLE 82.4 Agent-specific side effects of immunosuppressive agents used in organ transplantation (all immunosuppressive agents increase the risk of infection).

Agent	Side effects (not comprehensive)
Corticosteroids	Hypertension, dyslipidaemia, diabetes, osteoporosis, avascular necrosis, cushingoid appearance
Azathioprine	Leukopenia, thrombocytopenia, hepatotoxicity, gastrointestinal symptoms
Mycophenolic acid derivatives	Leukopenia, thrombocytopenia, gastrointestinal symptoms
Ciclosporin	Nephrotoxicity, hypertension, dyslipidaemia, hirsutism, gingival hyperplasia
Tacrolimus	Nephrotoxicity, hypertension, dyslipidaemia, neurotoxicity, diabetes
mTOR inhibitors	Thrombocytopenia, dyslipidaemia, pneumonitis, impaired wound healing
ALG	Infusion reactions, leukopenia and thrombocytopenia
Anti-CD25	Uncommon
CTLA-4Ig	? Increased risk of PTLD
Anti-CD52	Infusion reaction and autoimmune disease
Anti-CD20	Infusion reactions and pulmonary toxicity

ALG, anti-lymphocyte globulin; mTOR, mammalian target of rapamycin; PTLD, post-transplant lymphoproliferative disease.

Antiproliferative agents (azathioprine and mycophenolate)

Lymphocytes are among the most rapidly proliferating cells in the body, and lymphocyte proliferation and clonal expansion are an integral part of the immune response to an allograft. The antiproliferative agents available for immunoprophylaxis are azathioprine and mycophenolic acid preparations (mycophenolate mofetil [MMF] and mycophenolic acid sodium [MPAS]). Azathioprine is converted in the liver to its active metabolite, 6-mercaptopurine, which blocks purine metabolism and thereby inhibits cellular proliferation. Mycophenolic acid (MPA) preparations are more expensive than azathioprine but have largely replaced it as the agent of choice. After ingestion, MMF is converted to its active metabolite MPA. It inhibits the enzyme inosine monophosphate dehydrogenase, which is the rate-limiting enzyme in the de novo pathway of purine nucleotide synthesis. As lymphocytes do not have a salvage pathway for purine synthesis, their ability to proliferate is selectively impaired. The main side effects of azathioprine and MPA are bone marrow suppression and gastrointestinal symptoms.

Steroids

Steroids are an important component of many immunosuppressive regimens. Glucocorticoids are potent anti-inflammatory agents and have wide-ranging effects on the immune response. As a result of their numerous and well-known side effects, some centres attempt to gradually withdraw steroids from patients who have stable graft function after transplantation, but this sometimes precipitates a rejection episode and necessitates recommencement of steroids.

Antibody therapies

Monoclonal antibodies directed against the IL-2 receptor on T lymphocytes (CD25) are commonly given at the time of transplantation to temporarily augment the effects of calcineurin blockade during the early post-transplant period. Their effect lasts for a few weeks only and they lack any significant agent-specific side effects. Polyclonal antibody (antithymocyte globulin [ATG]) and monoclonal antibody preparations (alemtuzumab [anti-CD52 expressed on T cells and dendritic cells]) are also quite widely used as more potent and alternative induction agents. They cause a temporary depletion of circulating lymphocytes that reduces rejection but may lead to an increase in infection and malignancy. In addition to their use as induction agents, antibody preparations may be used to treat acute rejection episodes that fail to respond to steroid therapy.

The monoclonal anti-CD20 antibody (rituximab) depletes B lymphocytes, and is widely used as a component of protocols to enable ABO and HLA antibody-incompatible renal transplantation. It may also be helpful for the treatment of antibody-mediated acute rejection, although its efficacy here is limited because it does not deplete antibody-producing plasma cells.

Mammalian target of rapamycin inhibitors (sirolimus and everolimus)

Sirolimus and its structural analogue everolimus are, similar to tacrolimus, macrolides that bind within T lymphocytes to FK-binding protein. However, their mode of action is completely different to that of both ciclosporin and tacrolimus. They act by inhibiting an intracellular kinase called mammalian target of rapamycin (mTOR) and interfere with intracellular signalling from the IL-2 receptor, arresting T-cell division in the G1 phase. In contrast to CNIs they are not nephrotoxic. However, their side-effect profile includes lymphocele formation, impaired wound healing, an adverse effect on the blood lipid profile, thrombocytopenia and very occasionally pneumonitis. The mTOR inhibitors may have anti-tumour activity and the potential value of this effect in transplant recipients is under investigation. Although the negative effect on wound healing and lymphocele formation limits the immediate use of mTOR inhibitors after transplantation, switching from CNIs to mTOR inhibitors is sometimes used as a strategy to minimise CNI-induced nephrotoxicity.

T-cell co-stimulatory blockers

CTLA-4Ig (belatocept, LEA29Y) is a fusion protein comprising the extracellular domain of CTLA-4 fused to human immunoglobulin (Ig) Fc. It binds to the co-stimulatory ligands CD80 and CD86 expressed on antigen-presenting cells and, as a result, prevents them from delivering the co-stimulatory signals to the T cells that are required for full T-cell activation. It has recently been shown in renal transplantation to provide an effective alternative to CNIs when given by regular intravenous injection, thereby avoiding the metabolic, cardiovascular and nephrotoxic effects of CNIs. Although its future looks very promising, a potential concern is that it may be associated with an increased risk of post-transplant lymphoproliferative disease (PTLD).

Immunosuppressive regimens

When selecting an immunosuppressive regimen, the challenge is to provide levels of immunosuppression that are sufficient to protect the graft from rejection without exposing the recipient to excessive risk from infection and malignancy as a result of non-specific immunosuppression. Immunosuppressive therapy is started at the time of transplantation and is continued indefinitely (as maintenance therapy), although the requirement for immunosuppression is highest in the first few weeks after transplantation when the risk of acute rejection is greatest. Immunosuppressive protocols vary, but all use a combination of immunosuppressive agents acting at different points in the pathway of lymphocyte activation. Most currently include a CNI (ciclosporin or tacrolimus) as the main agent, and this is often supplemented with anti-CD25 monoclonal antibody induction therapy. CNIs are usually combined with an anti-proliferative agent (most often MMF) and steroids, so-called triple therapy. Less often, a CNI is used with an anti-proliferative agent alone or with steroids alone (dual therapy). When there is particular concern about acute rejection, polyclonal or monoclonal antibody preparations are administered followed by a CNI, an anti-proliferative agent and steroids.

Summary box 82.4

Principles of immunosuppression

- Principles are the same for all types of organ transplantation
- Aim is to maximise graft protection with minimum of side effects
- Most regimens are based on calcineurin blockade and include steroids and an anti-proliferative agent
- Need for immunosuppression is highest in the first 3 months but indefinite treatment is needed
- Immunosuppression increases the risk of infection and malignancy

The principles of immunoprophylaxis are similar for all types of organ transplantation. Interestingly, liver grafts seem to be less susceptible to rejection for reasons that are still unclear. The mTOR inhibitors have been shown to be effective immunosuppressive agents for preventing acute rejection after kidney transplantation, and they provide a non-nephrotoxic alternative to CNIs for maintenance therapy. They have a similar safety profile to CNIs in terms of post-transplant infection, but some of their agent-specific side effects are of potential concern and their clinical niche has still to be fully determined. Similarly, the potential role that CTLA-4Ig will find as an alternative to CNIs remains to be seen.

Acute rejection occurs in up to around 30% of transplant recipients but usually responds to a short course of high-dose steroid therapy. If the response to steroids is inadequate or if acute rejection recurs, acute rejection can often be treated successfully by recourse to anti-lymphocyte globulin (ALG) therapy.

COMPLICATIONS OF IMMUNOSUPPRESSION

As well as the agent-specific side effects already mentioned, the immunosuppressive agents used in organ transplantation cause non-specific immunosuppression and increase the risk of both infection and malignancy.

Summary box 82.5

Side effects of non-specific immunosuppression

- Infection
  - Transplant recipients are at high risk of opportunistic infection, especially by viruses
  - Bacterial and fungal infections are also common
  - Risk of infection is greatest during the first 6 months
  - Chemoprophylaxis is important for high-risk patients
  - Viral infection may result from reactivation of latent virus or from primary infection
  - Cytomegalovirus is a major problem
  - Pre-transplant vaccination against community-acquired infection should be considered
- Malignancy
  - Most types of cancer are more common after transplantation (approximately twofold)
  - Recipients, especially children, are at risk of post-transplant lymphoproliferative disease
  - There is a very high risk of squamous cancer of the skin and recipients should have a regular skin review

Infection

Transplant recipients receiving immunosuppressive therapy are at high risk from opportunistic infection, especially by viruses. Opportunistic infection is a potential problem in all transplant recipients, but those receiving aggressive immunosuppressive therapy are most at risk. Chemoprophylaxis is important in high-risk recipients, and early recognition followed by prompt and aggressive treatment of infection is essential in all transplant recipients. Pre-transplant vaccination against community-acquired infections should be considered.

Bacterial infection

The risk of bacterial infection is highest during the first month after transplantation. Transplant recipients are, similar to any patient undergoing major surgery, at risk of bacterial infections in the wound, respiratory tract and urinary tract. It is standard practice to give a broad-spectrum antibiotic to cover the perioperative period as prophylaxis against wound infection and possible bacterial contamination of the donor organ. The risk of bacterial infection is greatest in transplant recipients who are critically ill before or after surgery, and are in the intensive care unit with indwelling catheters and lines. After recovery from surgery, the risk of bacterial infection is much reduced. Tuberculosis is a concern in patients who have previously had mycobacterial infection and in patients from the Indian subcontinent, and it is usual to give them chemoprophylaxis for a period of 6–12 months after transplantation.

Viral infection

The risk of viral infection is highest during the first 6 months after transplantation and the most common problem is CMV infection. CMV disease may arise because of either reactivation of latent infection or primary infection that can be transmitted by an organ from a CMV-positive donor. Recipients at most risk from CMV infection are those who are CMV seronegative (i.e. those who have not been infected previously with CMV) and receive an organ from a CMV-seropositive donor (about half of all UK donors are CMV seropositive). Unfortunately, matching seronegative donors with seronegative recipients is not practicable. Without prophylaxis, CMV disease typically presents at 4–8 weeks with a high swinging fever, lethargy and leukopenia. The severity of the disease is variable and the clinical picture depends on the organ system most affected. It may present as:

- pneumonia
- gastrointestinal disease
- hepatitis
- retinitis
- encephalitis.

Severe CMV disease is potentially fatal. Prophylaxis for CMV consists of administration of antiviral agents, most commonly valganciclovir; aciclovir and valaciclovir are cheaper but less effective alternatives. A diagnosis of active CMV infection is confirmed by PCR to detect viral DNA in whole blood, and by histological examination of biopsy material. Treatment is with antiviral agents (either oral valganciclovir or intravenous ganciclovir), and is more effective when given pre-emptively on the basis of increased viral load detected by quantitative PCR analysis of peripheral blood.

Herpes simplex virus (HSV) infection is common after transplantation and is usually due to reactivation of latent infection. It causes mucocutaneous lesions around the mouth and sometimes the genitalia. These usually respond to topical treatment with aciclovir, but in severe cases systemic antiviral therapy is needed. Disseminated HSV infection is rare.

BK virus is emerging as an important cause of graft dysfunction after renal transplantation. Infection with BK virus is almost universal during childhood, with latent infection in the epithelium of the urinary tract. Immunosuppression causes lytic BK virus replication with graft involvement in 1–5% of renal transplants. The only effective treatment is to reduce the level of immunosuppression to allow natural immune mechanisms to regain control of the virus.

Herpes zoster infection, as a result of reactivation of latent varicella-zoster virus, occurs more frequently in transplant recipients and should be treated with systemic antiviral therapy. Primary varicella-zoster virus infection (chickenpox) is potentially very serious in immunosuppressed patients but is relatively uncommon because most adults have acquired immunity.

Fungal infection

Pneumocystis jiroveci (previously designated *Pneumocystis carinii* and wrongly classified as a protozoa) is one of the more important fungal infections after transplantation. It occurs during the first few months and presents with respiratory symptoms. The diagnosis is made by examination of bronchoalveolar lavage fluid or lung biopsy material for evidence of fungal infection (**Figure 82.12**). Chemoprophylaxis is highly effective and usually continued for up to 6 months after transplantation.

Other types of invasive fungal infections are uncommon in renal transplant recipients but infection with *Candida* or *Aspergillus* spp. is more common after other types of organ transplantation. Fungal infection usually occurs in the first 3 months after transplantation, and early diagnosis and aggressive treatment are essential to avoid fatal infection.

Malignancy

After transplantation, there is an increased risk of developing most types of malignant disease but the risk is particularly high for those types of tumour in which viral infection plays an aetiological role. The increased risk of malignancy is particularly high for skin cancer and PTLD. Most of the skin cancers seen are squamous cell carcinomas, but basal cell carcinoma and malignant melanoma are also more common than in the general population. The risk of skin cancer after transplantation rises with age and exposure to sunlight, and it has been predicted that 50% of transplant recipients will develop a skin malignancy within 20 years of transplantation. Patients must be warned of this risk before they undergo transplantation and be advised to take precautions to protect their skin from excessive sunlight. They should undergo regular review of their skin to detect early malignancy, and when malignant lesions occur they must be treated promptly and aggressively.

PTLD is an abnormal proliferation of B lymphocytes, usually in response to Epstein–Barr virus infection. The condition presents in a variety of ways including as an infectious mononucleosis-type illness or lymphadenopathy, or with involvement of extranodal sites such as the tonsils, gastrointestinal tract, lung, liver or the transplanted organ (**Figure 82.13**). PTLD occurs in around 1–3% of kidney and liver transplant recipients and the incidence is considerably higher in children. Those patients at most risk are those who have received aggressive immunosuppression. PTLD is a serious condition with an overall mortality rate of up to 50%. If it is identified at an early stage, reduction or cessation of immunosuppressive therapy may cause disease regression and result in a cure. Chemotherapy is often given and antiviral therapy, surgery and radiotherapy may also have a role in treating established disease. Disseminated PTLD and central nervous system (CNS) involvement have a very poor prognosis.

Transplant recipients also have a 300-fold increased risk of developing Kaposi's sarcoma, although this malignancy is still very uncommon after transplantation.

ORGAN DONATION

The number of organs required to satisfy the needs of transplantation far exceeds the number of donor organs available. In the case of renal transplantation in the UK there are approximately 6000 patients waiting for transplantation,

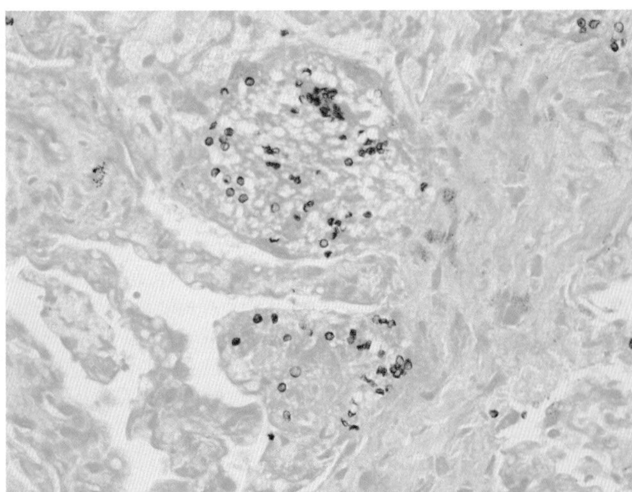

Figure 82.12 Transbronchial lung biopsy from a renal allograft recipient with *Pneumocystis jiroveci* pneumonia. The silver stain used reveals fungal cysts, each containing several intracystic bodies or spores, distributed widely within the biopsy material.

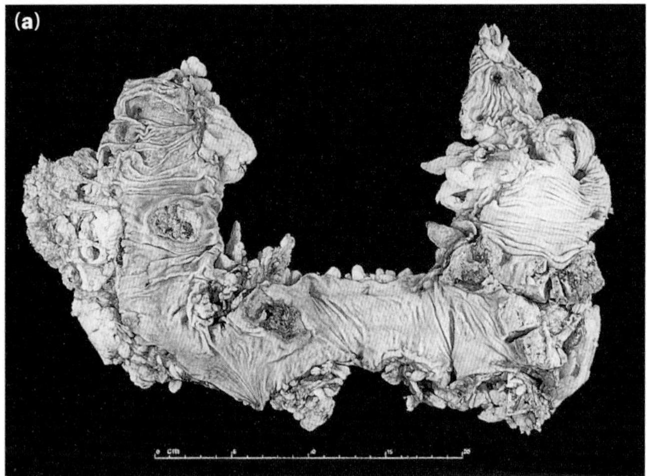

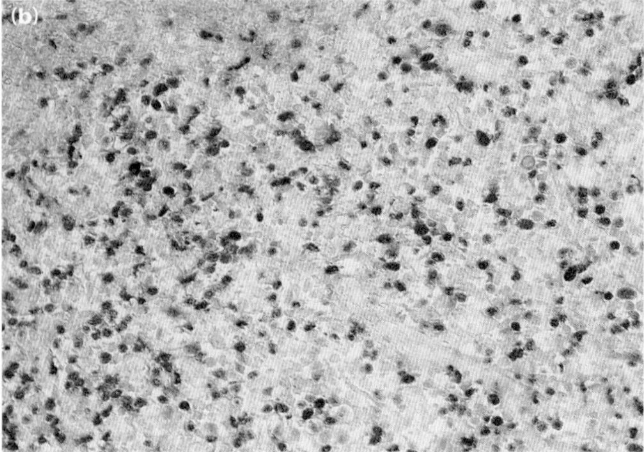

Figure 82.13 **(a)** Intestinal post-transplant lymphoproliferative disease (PTLD). Note multiple lesions in the terminal ileum and colon. **(b)** Atypical B lymphocytes stained positive with a probe for Epstein–Barr virus DNA (courtesy of C Watson, R Chavez-Cartaya and D Wight).

but only around 3000 transplantations performed annually, which has led to a median waiting time for transplantation of around 3 years. Similar shortages exist for liver and pancreas transplantation. For cardiothoracic organs the shortage is even worse and not all patients who might benefit from transplantation are listed.

Organs may be obtained from living donors or from deceased donors (DD) and DD may be either brain-stem-dead, heart-beating donors (donation after brain death or DBD donors) or donation after circulatory death (DCD) donors. Living donation is limited to donation of the kidney and, to a much lesser extent, liver or lung lobe. DBD donors provide most of the organs for transplantation for all organ types, although DCD donors provide an increasing number of kidneys, livers, pancreas glands and lungs for transplantation. The approach to referral and consent for organ donation varies between countries. Some have 'required request' or 'required referral' systems in place, where all patients dying in intensive care settings have to be referred for their potential suitability to be organ donors assessed. Some countries (e.g. Austria and Spain) have an 'opt-out' or 'presumed consent' system, where the assumption is made that individuals wished to donate their organs for transplantation unless they specifically registered their objection before death. There is debate about whether such a policy alone increases organ donation and a concern expressed by some that individuals who may not have wanted to become organ donors may fail to opt out before death, and that conflict may occur with relatives and next of kin who may oppose organ donation.

Summary box 82.6

Overcoming the shortage of organs for transplantation

- Maximising donation after brain-death (DBD) donation
- Use of marginal DBD deceased donors
- Use of donation after circulatory death (DCD) donor
- Increased use of split-liver transplantation
- Increased living donor kidney (and liver) transplantation

Donation after brain death donors

Most DD organs are obtained from patients in whom brain-stem death has been diagnosed. Such donors were previously called 'heart-beating deceased donors' and in most brain death results from stroke or traumatic head injury. Brain death occurs when severe brain injury causes irreversible loss of the capacity for consciousness combined with the irreversible loss of the capacity for breathing. In most countries, it is accepted that the condition of brain death equates in medical, legal and religious terms with death of the patient. The concept of brain death arose through necessity in the management of patients with irreversible brain damage on life support when there was no prospect for recovery. It was not in the interest of such patients, their relatives or the hospital in which they were being treated to delay their inevitable demise by continuing with futile life support. Acceptance of the concept of brain death had major implications for organ transplantation because it allowed the possibility for removal of viable organs from brain-dead patients before their circulation failed.

In the UK and many other countries, brain death is defined in terms of permanent functional death of the brain stem as neither consciousness nor spontaneous respiration is possible in the absence of a functional brain stem. A diagnosis of brain-stem death should be considered only when certain preconditions have been met. The patient must have suffered major brain damage of known aetiology, be deeply unconscious and require ventilatory support. Particular care must be taken to ensure that muscle relaxant agents and drugs with known CNS depressant effects are not contributing to the clinical picture. Hypothermia, profound hypotension, and metabolic or hormonal conditions that may contribute to CNS depression and confound the diagnosis of brain-stem death must also be excluded. When the necessary preconditions have been satisfied, formal clinical assessment of the brain-stem reflexes can be undertaken (*Table 82.5*). The UK guidelines state that the tests should be performed on two separate occasions by two clinicians experienced in this area. At least one of the two clinicians should be a consultant and neither should be connected with the transplant team. The time that must elapse between the two sets of brain-stem tests is not specified in the guidelines and is determined on the basis of clinical judgement. In the UK, there is no requirement to perform electrophysiological or brain perfusion studies to aid the diagnosis of brain-stem death. Particular care is required in the diagnosis of brain-stem death in neonates and infants.

Donation after circulatory death donors

The number of potential DBD donors has remained relatively static or even declined as a result of changes in neurosurgical practice and improved road safety. To address the rising demand for organ transplantation there has been a major trend towards increasing use of organs from DCD donors.

TABLE 82.5 Clinical testing for brain-stem death.

Absence of cranial nerve reflexes	Pupillary reflex
	Corneal reflex
	Pharyngeal (gag) and tracheal (cough) reflex
	Oculovestibular (caloric) reflex
Absence of motor response	The absence of a motor response to painful stimuli applied to the head/face and the absence of a motor response within the cranial nerve distribution to adequate stimulation of any somatic area is an indicator of brain-stem death. The presence of spinal reflexes does not preclude brainstem death
Absence of spontaneous respiration	After pre-ventilation with 100% O_2 for at least 5 minutes, the patient is disconnected from the ventilator for 10 minutes to confirm absence of respiratory effort, during which time the arterial Pco_2 level should be >8 kPa (60 mmHg) to ensure adequate respiratory stimulation. To prevent hypoxia during the apnoeic period, O_2 (6 L/min) is delivered via an endotracheal catheter

DCD donors can be grouped according to the Maastricht classification as follows:

- category 1: dead on arrival at hospital;
- category 2: resuscitation attempted without success;
- category 3: 'awaiting cardiac arrest' after withdrawal of support;
- category 4: cardiac arrest while brain dead;
- category 5: cardiac arrest and unsuccessful resuscitation in hospital.

Maastricht categories 1, 2 and 5 donors are sometimes referred to as uncontrolled DCD donors. The warm ischaemic time of organs from these three categories of donor is usually longer and less predictable than in the case of categories 3 and 4 (controlled) donors. Most DCD donor organs used for transplantation in the UK, USA and several other European countries are from controlled (category 3) donors who have died in intensive care after planned withdrawal of futile cardiorespiratory support.

Kidneys may be also be recovered from carefully selected patients who are dead on arrival at the hospital or who have died after unsuccessful resuscitation. In Spain and France most DCD kidneys are obtained from uncontrolled donors.

Evaluation of the deceased donor

After a deceased donor has been referred to the transplant team with a view to organ donation, the general suitability of the potential organ donor must be carefully assessed. Particular care must be taken to assess the donor from the point of view of transmissible infectious agents and malignancy. The medical history should be scrutinised and evidence sought of risk factors for human immunodeficiency virus (HIV) and hepatitis B and C virus infection, such as intravenous drug abuse. The presence of Creutzfeldt–Jakob disease is an absolute contraindication to organ donation. Organs from HIV-infected donors should not be used for transplantation, except sometimes in recipients who are already infected by HIV. Hepatitis B infection (in most countries) and active systemic sepsis, e.g. major abdominal infection, are contraindications to donation. The presence of malignancy within the past 5 years is usually an absolute contraindication to organ donation with the exceptions of primary tumours of the CNS, non-melanotic tumours of the skin and carcinoma *in situ* of the uterine cervix. If there are no general contradictions to organ donation, consideration is then given to organ-specific selection criteria.

As a result of the high demand for donor organs there has been a progressive relaxation in the organ-specific selection criteria. The chronological age of the donor is less important than the physiological function of the organs under consideration for transplantation.

The organs to be donated should generally be free from primary disease. Potential kidney donors should have a reasonable urine output and relatively normal serum urea and creatinine, although acute terminal elevations are acceptable. Liver donors should not have hepatic disease, although impaired liver function tests are common in deceased donors and do not necessarily preclude donation. Heart donors should have a normal electrocardiogram and, in doubtful cases, echocardiography may be necessary. For lung donors the chest radiograph and gas exchange should be satisfactory, and bronchial aspirates should be free from fungal and bacterial infection. Elevations of blood glucose and serum amylase are not uncommon in deceased donors and do not preclude pancreas donation. The use of organs from suboptimal or 'marginal' deceased donors has increased markedly in an attempt to address the demand for transplantation. The definition of a marginal donor depends on the organs being considered for transplantation and varies between countries. In the case of kidney transplantation an extended criteria donor is defined in the USA as a donor age >60 years or one between the ages of 50 and 60 years with two of the following: hypertension, death from stroke and a terminal creatinine >132 mmol/L. Organs from 'marginal donors' generally lead to less satisfactory transplant outcomes than those from standard donors.

Organ recovery from deceased donors

In DBD donors, once brain-stem death has been confirmed, management of the donor is aimed at preserving the functional integrity of the organs to be recovered. Brain-stem death produces profound metabolic and neuroendocrine disturbances, leading to cardiovascular instability. Careful monitoring and management of fluid balance is essential. Vasopressin is often given to allow reduction or cessation of catecholamine pressors and, along with DDAVP, to treat diabetes insipidus. Donors are also usually given methylprednisolone to aid fluid and metabolic management, together with triiodothyronine (T_3) to help cardiovascular stability.

Recovery of multiple organs from a DBD donor requires cooperation between the thoracic and abdominal surgical teams. A midline abdominal incision and median sternotomy are used to obtain access. After dissection of the organs to be recovered, they are perfused *in situ*. The heart is perfused with cold cardioplegia solution via a cannula in the ascending aorta and the lungs are perfused via a cannula in the pulmonary artery. The abdominal organs are perfused with chilled organ preservation solution via an aortic and portal cannula. Blood and perfusate are vented from the left atrial appendage and the inferior vena cavae. This produces rapid cooling of the organs, reduces their metabolic activity and preserves their viability. Additional surface cooling of the abdominal organs may be achieved by application of saline ice slush. The heart and lungs are excised simultaneously with the liver and pancreas, followed by the kidneys, either en bloc or separately. The extent to which the abdominal organs are dissected before cold flush depends on the preference of the surgical team. Some surgeons perform minimal dissection before cold perfusion and complete the dissection

Maastricht is a city in the province of Limburg, in The Netherlands.

of the abdominal organs *in situ* or on the back table after the organs have been removed en bloc. During recovery of the liver, care is taken to ensure that, if there is an aberrant hepatic artery arising from the superior mesenteric artery, it is included in the aortic patch. An adult donor liver cannot be transplanted into a child because of the size mismatch, and there are insufficient deceased paediatric donor livers available for transplantation. One solution is to undertake split-liver transplantation, which was first performed by Pichlmayr in 1988. The liver from a deceased donor is split and the left lobe or left lateral segments are used for a child and the right lobe for an adult recipient (**Figure 82.14**).

When removing the donor kidneys care is taken to ensure that any polar renal arteries are included on an aortic patch with the renal artery (**Figure 82.15**). In older kidney donors with atherosclerosis the aortic segment may be too diseased to use as an arterial patch, and the donor renal artery and any polar arteries are divided shortly after their origin and, if necessary, reconstructed before implantation (**Figure 82.16**). In the case of the pancreas, a Y graft of donor iliac artery is excised and used to reconstruct the divided splenic and superior mesenteric arteries of the graft before implantation (**Figure 82.17**).

In DCD donors there is an inevitable period of warm ischaemia (up to 45 minutes is acceptable) between the diagnosis of death (cardiorespiratory arrest) and cold perfusion of the organs. The aim during organ recovery is to minimise the period of warm ischaemia, although the approach used differs according to whether the donor is a controlled or uncontrolled DCD donor. It is important to note that only around 50% of all patients considered as potential controlled DCD donors have a cardiorespiratory arrest within the period of time (usually 3 hours) considered practicable for the surgical team to stand by for organ recovery. After cardiorespiratory arrest there is an obligatory 'hands off' period before certification of death of at least 5 minutes, before the surgical procedure for organ recovery can begin. If not already in the operating theatre, the DCD donor is transferred immediately to the operating room and the abdomen opened to allow rapid cannulation of the aorta and cold perfusion of the organs to be recovered. In the case of uncontrolled DCD donors the warm ischaemic time can be minimised by rapid insertion of a double balloon catheter introduced into the aorta via a femoral cut-down and used to cool the kidneys *in situ* by chilled perfusate preferably within 30 minutes of circulatory arrest (**Figure 82.18**). This allows time to gain consent from relatives for organ donation to proceed if it is not already available and to assemble the surgical team for organ recovery.

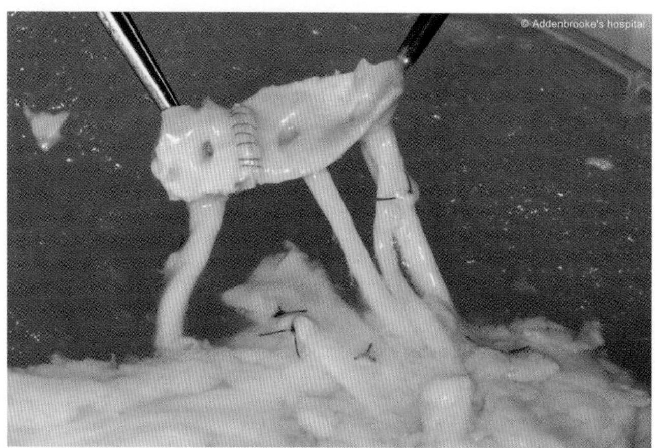

Figure 82.15 Deceased donor kidney with multiple renal arteries on an aortic patch. The aortic patch has been shortened to limit the length of the anastomosis needed when joining the donor patch to the side of the recipient external iliac artery (Medical Photography, Addenbrooke's Hospital).

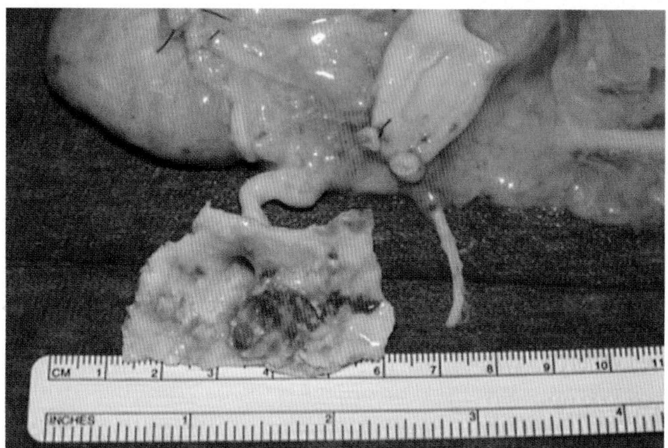

Figure 82.16 Deceased donor kidney from elderly (>70 years) donor illustrating the technical challenges of using kidneys from marginal donors. The aorta shows severe atherosclerosis with extensive plaque formation and ulceration, and is not suitable for use as an aortic patch. A lower polar artery has already been divided. The two arteries can be joined together before implantation or implanted separately.

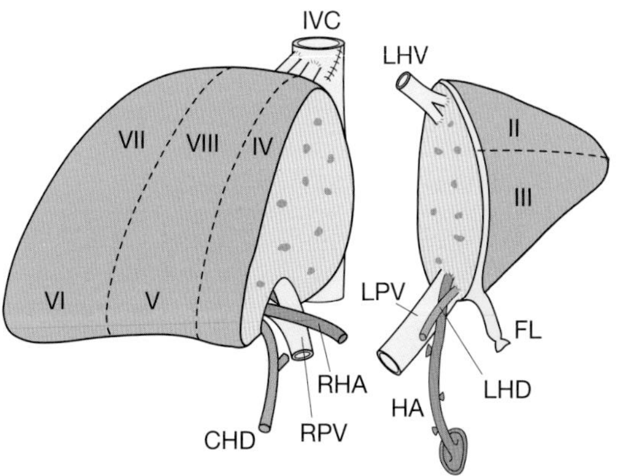

Figure 82.14 An adult liver may be split (according to Couinard's segments) so that the left lateral segment (segments II and III) can be transplanted into a child and the right lobe (together with segment IV) can be transplanted into an adult. CHD, common hepatic duct; FL, falciform ligament; HA, hepatic artery (on aortic patch); IVC, inferior vena cava; LHD, left hepatic duct; LHV, left hepatic vein; LPV, left portal vein; RHA, right hepatic artery; RPV, right portal vein.

Rudolph Pichlmayr, 1932–1997, surgeon, Hannover, Germany.

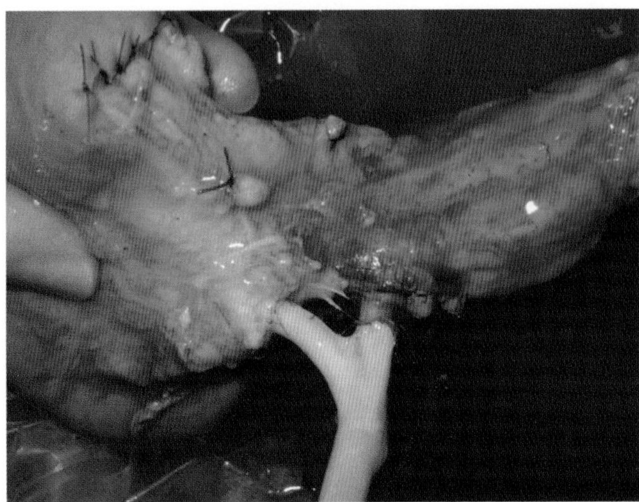

Figure 82.17 Donor pancreas viewed from the posterior aspect after preparatory bench surgery. The duodenal component of the graft has been sutured closed proximally and distally, and a Y graft of donor iliac artery used to reconstruct the divided splenic and superior mesenteric arteries. The bile duct (ligated) and portal vein are anterior and not seen in this view.

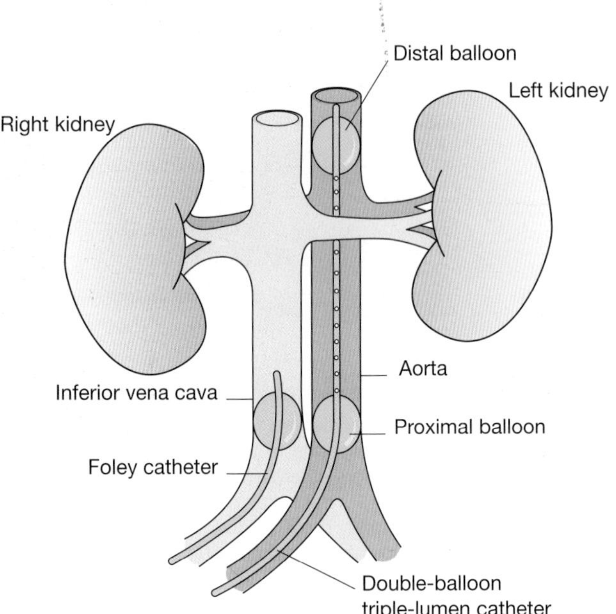

Figure 82.18 *In situ* perfusion of kidneys in a non-heart-beating donor (donation after cardiac death [DCD]). A double-balloon aortic catheter is introduced through a groin incision and 10–15 litres of chilled preservation solution is administered. The perfusate is vented through a Foley catheter introduced into the femoral vein.

After removal from the donor, the organs may undergo a further flush with chilled preservation solution before they are placed in double or triple sterile bags and stored at 4°C by immersion in ice, while they are transported to the recipient centre and await implantation. Once the donor organs have been excised, samples of donor spleen and mesenteric lymph nodes are obtained for confirmation of tissue type and use in the cross-match test.

Various organ preservation solutions are available for flushing organs before cold storage. They all contain impermeants to limit cell swelling, buffers to counter acidosis and electrolytes, the composition of which reflects that of intracellular rather than extracellular fluid. Commonly used preservation solutions include University of Wisconsin (UW) solution and Euro-Collins solution, but there are many others. The use of UW solution (*Table 82.6*) (developed by Belzer and colleagues in Wisconsin, USA) is particularly effective for liver grafts, and after perfusion with UW solution the liver can be stored safely for up to 24 hours. The length of time for which an organ can be stored before transplantation varies depending on the type of organ (*Table 82.7*). Although minimising the duration of organ storage is important for all organs, it is essential that organs from DCD donors be transplanted with the minimum possible cold storage time. Most organs for transplantation are stored by static cold storage in an icebox. However, there is a recent trend towards storing deceased donor kidneys by pulsatile machine perfusion,

TABLE 82.6 Composition of University of Wisconsin (UW) solution.

Component	Amount
Potassium lactobionate (mmol/L)	100
Sodium phosphate (mmol)	25
Magnesium sulphate (mmol)	5
Adenosine (mmol/L)	5
Allopurinol (mmol/L)	1
Glutathione (mmol/L)	3
Raffinose (mmol/L)	30
Hydroxethyl starch (g/L)	50
Insulin (U/L)	100
Dexamethasone (mg/L)	8
Potassium (mmol/L)	135
Sodium (mmol/L)	35
Osmolality (mosmol/L)	320
pH	7.4

TABLE 82.7 Maximum and optimal cold storage times (approximate).

Organ	Optimum (hours)	Safe maximum (hours)
Kidney	<18	36
Liver	<12	18
Pancreas	<10	18
Small intestine	<4	6
Heart	<3	6
Lung	<3	8

(Assuming zero warm ischaemic time and organs obtained from a non-marginal donor.)

The University of Wisconsin is at Madison, WI, USA.
Fokert O Belzer, 1931–1995, surgeon, Madison, WI, USA.

where the kidneys are placed inside a purpose-designed perfusion machine that pumps cold preservation solution through the renal artery in an attempt to reduce ischaemic injury. Machine perfusion can be started immediately after kidney recovery or as soon as practicable thereafter, and is usually continued until the time of implantation. The benefit of machine perfusion over simple cold storage is currently the subject of considerable debate.

Living kidney donors

Living-donor renal transplants account for around 30% of the total renal transplant activity in the UK, but in some countries (notably the Scandinavian countries and the USA) this figure is much higher (>50%). The justification for living-donor renal transplantation is based on the shortage of deceased donor transplants and the superior results obtained. Traditionally, most living-donor transplants were between genetically related individuals. However, living-donor kidney transplantations performed between genetically unrelated individuals also fare better than even well-matched deceased donor grafts, and this observation gave rise to a steady increase in living-unrelated kidney transplantation activity, usually between spouses or partners. It is essential to ensure that, in all cases of living donation, the prospective donor is fully informed and free from coercion to donate, and that the risk to the donor is small. In the UK, all living-donor transplants (irrespective of whether they are or are not genetically related) require prior approval by the Human Tissue Authority (HTA). An independent person (one not associated with the transplant team) approved by the HTA must provide confirmation to the HTA that the donor and recipient understand the implications of the proposed operation and that there is no evidence of coercion or financial inducement.

Live donation should proceed only after prospective donors have undergone rigorous assessment to ensure that they are suitable. Before the donation, it is essential to perform imaging (usually magnetic resonance angiography or computed tomography-guided angiography), to delineate the anatomy of the arterial supply to the kidneys. If the left kidney has a single renal artery (10% of kidneys have two or more renal arteries), it is usually chosen for transplantation because the longer left renal vein simplifies the transplant operation. The presence of multiple renal arteries does not necessarily preclude donation, although implantation of living-donor kidneys with multiple renal arteries may increase the chances of vascular complications developing after implantation.

Live donor nephrectomy was historically undertaken either through a loin incision and retroperitoneal approach or through a midline abdominal incision and transperitoneal approach. In most transplant units, nephrectomy is now undertaken laparoscopically (totally laparoscopic or hand assisted). Laparoscopic nephrectomy is associated with less wound pain in the donor, allows more rapid mobilisation after surgery and reduces hospital stay. Initial concerns that kidneys removed by the laparoscopic technique may have more ureteric complications after implantation have proven unfounded. After removal from the donor the kidney is flushed immediately with chilled organ preservation solution (Figure 82.19). The mortality rate for live donation is less than 0.05%, and around half of reported deaths are due to pulmonary embolic disease, so it is essential to ensure prophylaxis to reduce deep-vein thrombosis (DVT). The major complication rate after live donor nephrectomy is <5%: potential complications include haemorrhage requiring blood transfusion or surgery, infection (chest, abdomen, renal tract and wound), damage to an intra-adominal viscus, adverse reaction to drugs and anaesthetic agents, and DVT and pulmonary embolus. In the long term, kidney donors may be at increased risk from hypertension and donors should have their blood pressure and urine checked annually.

Around 35% of potential living donor transplant recipients will be ABO blood group incompatible with their intended donor and until recently this precluded transplantation. However, there are now two potential solutions to this problem. The first is 'paired exchange' where incompatible donor/recipient pairs exchange kidneys between pairs to allow ABO-compatible transplantation (Figure 82.20).

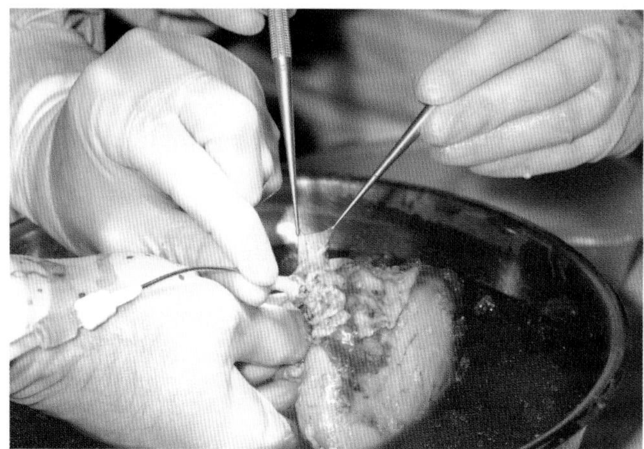

Figure 82.19 After removal from the donor, the kidney is flushed with chilled organ preservation solution and, if necessary, stored briefly on ice until transplanted into the recipient.

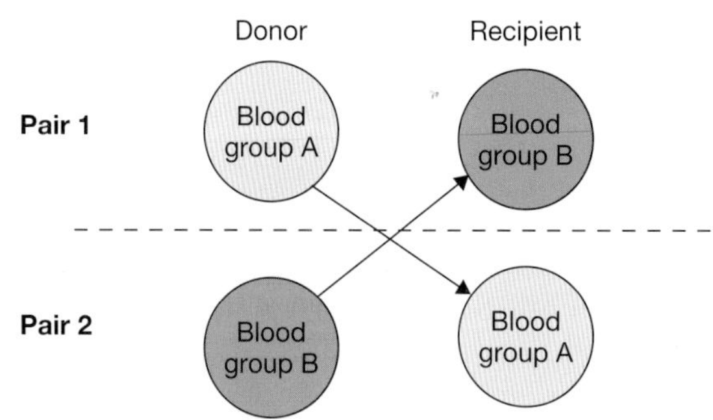

Figure 82.20 Paired living-donor kidney transplantation. Paired donation allows patients with willing but blood group-incompatible donors to be transplanted by pairing them with other incompatible donor–recipient pairs. In the example shown, the two willing donors are incompatible with their intended recipient (blood groups A to B and B to A) but by paired donation each recipient can receive an ABO-compatible kidney transplant (blood groups A to A and B to B).

Recruitment of more than two pairs to facilitate 'pooled donation' increases the likelihood of matching donors with compatible recipients and, although such schemes pose considerable logistical challenges, they are now operating successfully in several countries. An alternative approach is to transiently deplete ABO antibodies from potential recipients by passing their blood through special absorption columns or by performing plasmaphoresis along with administration of pre-transplant immunosuppressive agents (**Figure 82.21**). Perhaps surprisingly, graft outcome after desensitisation is similar to that after paired donation. Both paired donation and antibody depletion strategies are also potentially applicable to recipients in whom HLA antibodies preclude transplantation from an intended living donor, but graft survival after depletion of HLA antibodies is lower than when the recipient receives a kidney from an HLA antibody-compatible donor.

Living liver donors

Living donor liver transplantation is now undertaken in a number of transplant centres worldwide and is relatively common practice in some countries where deceased donation is not practised for cultural or religious reasons, notably Japan and Korea. The concept was first pioneered to allow children to receive the left lobe or left lateral segment from an adult donor and has been very successful. It has now been extended to adult-to-adult live liver transplantation (**Figure 82.22**). The majority of such transplants require a right liver lobe to provide adequate hepatic function. For adult-to-adult live liver donation, the donor procedure has a reported mortality rate of around 0.5% and a major complication rate of up to 15%. One of the more common donor complications is bile leak.

Living donors: other organs

Occasionally, living donors have provided segments of pancreas, small bowel and lung for transplantation, but this is more controversial. In the USA, living-donor, combined kidney and segmental pancreas transplantation has been undertaken to treat people with type 1 diabetes with end-stage renal disease. In occasional patients, living-donor small bowel transplantation has been performed using a small bowel graft, which comprises a length of around 1.5 m of ileum. Finally, a small number of living-donor segmental lung transplantations have been performed. To provide sufficient pulmonary tissue without compromising the donor, it is necessary to use segments from two different donors for each recipient. The ethical issues raised by living donation for extrarenal organs are understandably complex.

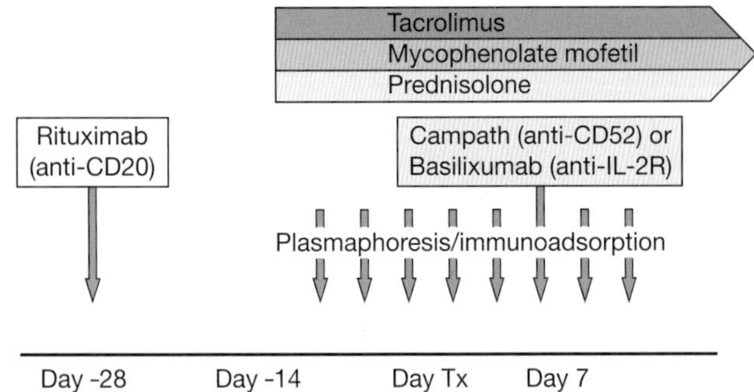

Figure 82.21 Typical desensitisation protocol for ABO or human leukocyte antigen (HLA) antibody-incompatible live-donor kidney transplant.

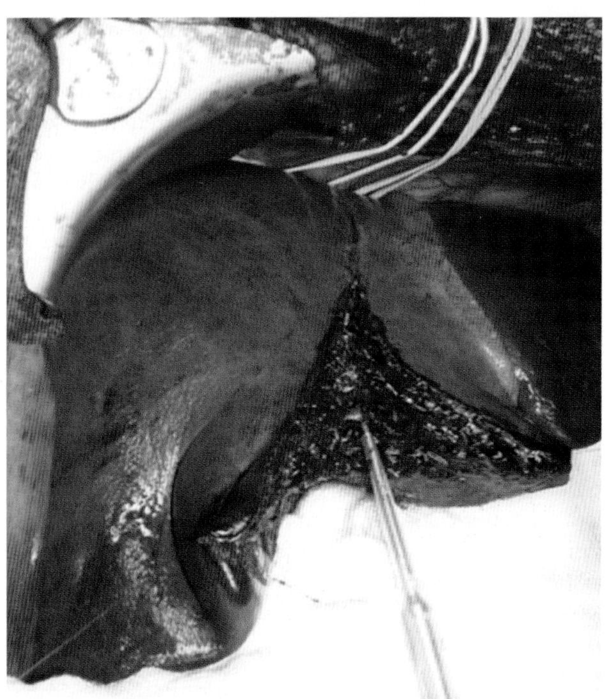

Figure 82.22 Living donor hepatectomy. A CUSA (cavitron ultrasonic aspirator) is being used to divide the right and left lobes of the liver so that the right lobe can be transplanted into an adult recipient.

Resumption of function after organ transplantation

It is crucial that, after a heart, lung or liver transplantation, the transplanted organ resumes satisfactory function immediately. If primary non-function occurs, the only option is rapid re-transplantation. After kidney, pancreas or small bowel transplantation, immediate graft function is desirable but not vital. Kidneys obtained from DCD donors invariably suffer a variable degree of ischaemic damage, and delayed graft function is more common (typically 50% for category 3 DCD donors) than for kidneys obtained from DBD deceased donors (typically 25%). Irreversible ischaemic necrosis occasionally occurs and the graft never functions adequately (primary non-function). However, graft survival results for kidneys from controlled DCD kidneys are similar to those obtained from DBD deceased donors. Livers obtained from DCD donors have an increased incidence of primary non-function and biliary complications, including biliary anastomotic strictures, bile leak and ischaemic cholangiopathy.

Summary box 82.7

Factors determining organ function after transplantation

- Donor characteristics
  - Extremes of age
  - Presence of pre-existing damage in transplanted organ
  - Haemodynamic and metabolic instability
- Procurement-related factors
  - Warm ischaemic time
  - Type of preservation solution
  - Cold ischaemic time
- Recipient-related factors
  - Technical factors relating to implantation
  - Haemodynamic and metabolic stability
  - Immunological factors
  - Presence of drugs that impair transplant function

KIDNEY TRANSPLANTATION

Patient selection

Renal transplantation is the preferred treatment for many patients with end-stage renal disease because it provides a better quality of life for them than dialysis. Transplantation releases patients from the dietary and fluid restrictions of dialysis and the physical constraints imposed by the need to dialyse. Transplantation is also more cost-effective than dialysis and improves patient survival.

In the UK, around 100 people per million of the population develop end-stage renal disease, and the incidence increases with age. The causes of end-stage renal disease are numerous and include the following:

- glomerulonephritis;
- diabetic nephropathy;
- hypertensive nephrosclerosis;
- renal vascular disease;
- polycystic kidney disease;
- pyelonephritis;
- obstructive uropathy;
- systemic lupus erythematosus;
- analgesic nephropathy;
- metabolic disease (oxalosis, amyloid).

Sometimes, the primary cause of end-stage renal disease is uncertain. For renal transplantation, as for other types of organ transplantation, careful patient selection is essential. Before acceptance as suitable candidates on the transplant waiting list, a transplant surgeon and nephrologist should formally assess all patients. A significant number of patients are likely to be considered unsuitable for renal transplantation because of major comorbid disease, especially cardiovascular disease. In the UK, around 30–40% of the dialysis population are on the waiting list for renal transplantation.

The nature of the primary renal disease does not generally affect the decision to proceed to transplantation. Many of the glomerulonephritides (especially IgA, focal segmental glomerulosclerosis, and mesangiocapillary glomerulonephritis types I and II) may recur in a kidney transplant, and sometimes can lead to early graft failure (especially focal segmental glomerulosclerosis). In the case of primary oxalosis, combined kidney and hepatic transplantation is usually undertaken to eliminate the metabolic defect and thereby prevent early graft failure from the formation of further oxalate stones.

The age of patients with end-stage renal failure accepted for dialysis has gradually risen over the last two decades, and in the UK the mean age of patients starting dialysis is around 70 years. There is no absolute upper age limit to renal transplantation, but inevitably older patients (aged >65 years) are less likely to be considered suitable candidates because of major cardiovascular and other comorbid diseases.

A careful assessment of comorbid disease that might significantly reduce the chances of successful outcome after transplantation is essential. Rigorous evaluation of the cardiovascular system is particularly important. Cardiovascular disease is very common in the dialysis population, especially those with diabetes, and is the major cause of death after transplantation. Before listing patients for transplantation, it is important to ensure that their urinary tract is functional and that there is no need for corrective urological surgery. Only when there is intractable renal sepsis or very large polycystic kidneys that intrude into both iliac fossae is native nephrectomy required before transplantation (**Figure 82.23**). Finally, the prospective transplant recipient must be deemed able to cope with the psychological consequences of transplantation and likely to comply with immunosuppressive therapy.

Summary box 82.8

Evaluation of potential recipients for organ transplantation

- Evaluation undertaken by appropriate multidisciplinary team including surgeon and physician
- Determine presence of comorbid disease
- Exclude malignancy and systemic sepsis
- Evaluate against organ-specific criteria for transplantation
- Determine probable ability to cope psychologically with transplant and comply with immunosuppression
- Evaluate need for any preparative surgery needed to facilitate transplantation
- Optimise recipient condition before transplantation

Immunosuppressive therapy impairs the protective response to both malignancy and infection. Consequently, pre-existing malignancy is an absolute contraindication and, even after curative treatment, transplantation should not usually be considered for at least 3 years. Similarly, the presence of active infection is a contraindication to transplantation.

Technique of renal transplantation

The transplant kidney is placed in the iliac fossa, in the retroperitoneal position, leaving the native kidneys *in situ*. After induction of general anaesthesia, a central venous line and

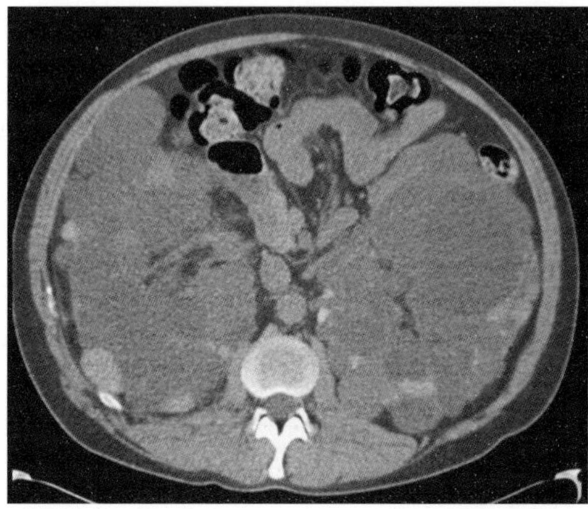

Figure 82.23 Computed tomography scan of a patient with very large polycystic kidneys that extend well into both iliac fossa. The patient requires removal of one of the polycystic kidneys to make room for a subsequent renal transplant. Nephrectomy should be performed several weeks before transplantation.

a urinary catheter are inserted. It is helpful to distend the bladder with saline containing methylene blue to allow it to be identified with certainty before ureteric implantation. A curved incision is made in the lower abdomen and, after dividing the muscles of the abdominal wall, the peritoneum is swept upwards and medially to expose the iliac vessels. These are dissected free so that they can be controlled with vascular clamps. The kidney is then removed from ice and the donor renal vein is anastomosed end to side to the external iliac vein. The donor renal artery on a Carrel patch of donor aorta is anastomosed end to side to the external iliac artery (**Figure 82.24a**). If the donor renal artery lacks an aortic patch, as in the case of a living-donor transplant, it may be preferable to anastomose the donor artery end to end to the recipient internal iliac artery (**Figure 82.24b**). While the vascular anastomoses are being undertaken, the kidney is kept cold by application of topical ice.

After completion of the venous and arterial anastomoses, the vascular clamps are removed and the kidney is allowed to reperfuse with blood. The ureter, which is kept reasonably short to avoid the risk of distal ischaemia, is then anastomosed to the bladder (**Figure 82.25**). This is achieved by direct implantation of the ureter into the dome of the bladder with a mucosa-to-mucosal anastomosis, followed by closure of the muscular wall of the bladder over the ureter to create a short tunnel, the Lich–Gregoir technique. A double-J ureteric stent should be left *in situ*, to reduce the risk of urine leak or early obstruction, and removed after several weeks by cystoscopy. If the donor ureter is too short to reach the bladder, the native ureter can be divided and the distal segment anastomosed to the ureter or renal pelvis of the donor kidney. The proximal segment of the native ureter can usually be ligated and the native kidney left *in situ* without causing a problem. Before closing the transplant wound, it is very important to ensure that the kidney is lying in a satisfactory position without kinking or torsion of the renal vessels. In small children receiving an adult donor kidney, the abdomen is opened through a midline incision and the graft is placed intra-abdominally with anastomosis of the renal vessels to the aorta and vena cava.

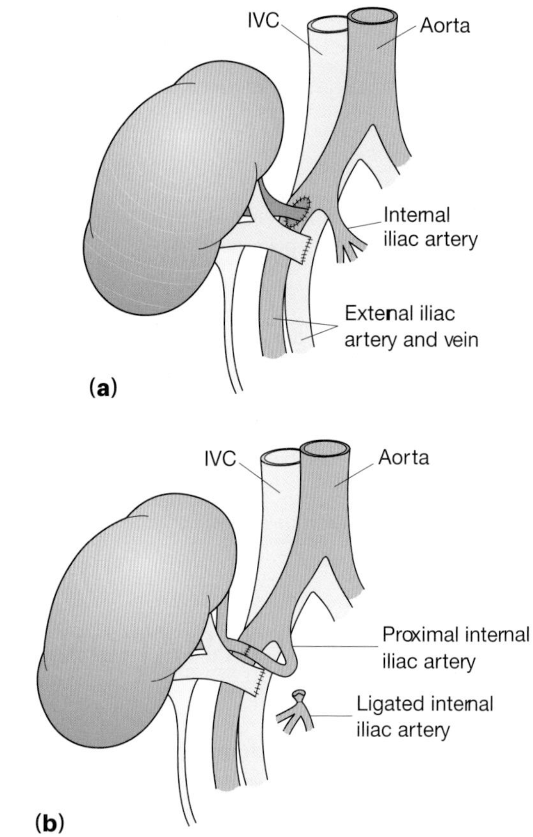

Figure 82.24 Implantation of renal allograft: (**a**) the renal artery on a Carrel patch is anastomosed to the external iliac artery; (**b**) the renal artery is anastomosed end to end to the internal iliac artery. IVC, inferior vena cava.

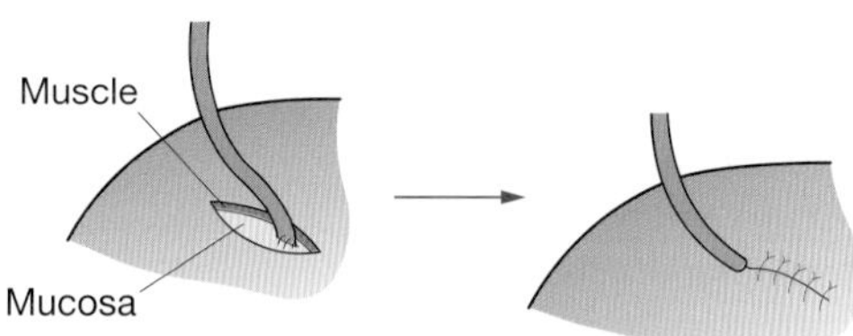

Figure 82.25 Ureteric implantation by direct anastomosis to a small cystomy: Lich–Gregoir technique.

Technical complications

Vascular complications

The incidence of vascular complications after renal transplantation is quite low. Renal artery thrombosis occurs in approximately 1% of cases. Renal vein thrombosis is more common

Robert Lich Jr, urologist, Louisville, KY, USA.
Willy Gregoir, Chef de Clinique Urologique, Brussels, Belgium 1962–1987.

(up to 5% of cases) and, although sometimes due to technical error, the aetiology is often uncertain. It presents during the first week after transplantation with sudden pain and swelling at the site of the graft. The diagnosis is confirmed by Doppler ultrasonography. Urgent surgical exploration is indicated, and in most cases transplant nephrectomy is required. The incidence of renal vein thrombosis can be minimised by giving low-dose heparin or aspirin prophylaxis. Renal artery stenosis usually presents late (often years) after transplantation with increasing hypertension and decreasing renal function. It may occur in up to 10% of grafts and is diagnosed by angiography. Renal artery stenosis is best treated by angioplasty, but if angioplasty fails or is not technically possible then the condition can be treated successfully by open surgery and vascular reconstruction.

Urological complications

Urological complications occur in around 5% of patients in the early post-transplantation period, but their incidence can be reduced markedly by leaving a temporary ureteric stent *in situ*. Urinary leaks result from technical errors at the ureteric anastomosis or because of ureteric ischaemia. They present with discomfort and leakage of urine from the wound and usually require surgical intervention and reimplantation of the ureter into the bladder or anastomosis of the transplant ureter to the ipsilateral native ureter. Obstruction of the transplant ureter may occur early or late. Causes of obstruction include technical error, external pressure from a haematoma or lymphocele and ischaemic stricture. Ureteric obstruction presents with painless deterioration in graft function and is confirmed by demonstrating hydronephrosis and ureteric dilatation on ultrasound examination. Initial treatment is by percutaneous anterograde nephrostomy and insertion of a stent. Some ureteric strictures may be amenable to treatment by balloon dilatation but most are best treated by surgical intervention, reimplanting the donor ureter into the bladder or anastomosing it to the native ureter.

Lymphocele

Peri-transplant lymphoceles are usually asymptomatic, but occasionally they become large enough to cause ureteric obstruction or oedema of the ipsilateral leg. Initial treatment is usually by ultrasound-guided percutaneous drainage. In the case of large or recurrent lymphoceles, surgical intervention may be needed to drain a persistent lymphocele into the peritoneal cavity, and this can often be achieved by an ultrasound-guided laparoscopic approach.

Investigation of graft dysfunction

Graft dysfunction during the early postoperative period is a common problem. Possible causes are:

- acute tubular necrosis;
- arterial/venous thrombosis;
- urinary leak/obstruction;
- CNI toxicity;
- hyperacute/accelerated acute rejection.

Summary box 82.9

Causes of allograft dysfunction

- Early
    - Primary non-function (irreversible ischaemic damage)
    - Delayed function (reversible ischaemic injury)
    - Hyperacute and acute rejection
    - Arterial or venous thrombosis of the graft vessels
    - Drug toxicity (e.g. calcineurin inhibitor toxicity)
    - Infection (e.g. cytomegalovirus disease in graft
    - Mechanical obstruction (ureter/common bile duct)
- Late
    - Chronic rejection
    - Arterial stenosis
    - Recurrence of original disease in graft (glomerulonephritis, hepatitis C)
    - Mechanical obstruction (ureter, common bile duct)

Delayed graft function (defined as the need for dialysis post-transplantation) as a result of acute tubular necrosis occurs in around 25% of kidneys from DBD and up to 50% of kidneys from DCD donors, but is uncommon (<5%) after living-donor transplantation. Often, recipients produce significant volumes of urine from their native kidneys, making the diagnosis of delayed graft function more difficult. The incidence of delayed function can be minimised by optimising donor management before kidney procurement and reducing the cold ischaemia time by avoiding unnecessary delay before implantation. As a first step in the management of early graft dysfunction, the urinary catheter should be irrigated in case it is occluded by a blood clot. Hypovolaemia, if present, should be corrected with the aid of central venous pressure (CVP) monitoring. A Doppler ultrasound examination of the graft is the single most important investigation because it allows exclusion of vascular thrombosis and urinary obstruction as causes of graft dysfunction. Renal radionuclide scanning provides information on renal perfusion and excretion and may be helpful but is used infrequently. If graft dysfunction is still present after several days, it is usual to perform an ultrasound-guided needle biopsy of the kidney to ensure that graft rejection is not present, and then to repeat the investigation every week or so until graft function occurs. CNI toxicity may cause graft dysfunction and it is important to monitor CNI blood levels to avoid nephrotoxicity. Acute tubular necrosis usually resolves within the first 4 weeks of transplantation, but a small number of grafts (<5%) suffer primary non-function (i.e. never function).

Allograft dysfunction developing late (>1 month after transplantation) may be due to:

- acute/chronic rejection;
- drug toxicity;
- ureteric obstruction (lymphocele/ureteric stricture);
- recurrent disease;
- urinary tract infection.

Blood levels of ciclosporin or tacrolimus are assessed to ensure that they are not unduly elevated, and ultrasound examination of the graft is performed to determine whether ureteric obstruction is present. If obstruction is detected, it is further investigated by percutaneous anterograde urography and treated as outlined above. If there is uncertainty about the cause of graft dysfunction, a transplant biopsy should be performed to establish whether allograft rejection is present.

Outcome after transplantation

The results of organ transplantation are generally defined in terms of patient and graft survival. Patient survival after deceased donor renal transplantation is >95% at 1 year and >85% at 5 years. Graft survival is around 90% at 1 year and 80% at 5 years. Graft survival after a second transplant is only marginally worse than after a first graft. After living-related kidney transplantation, overall graft survival is around 95% at 1 year and 85% at 5 years. Graft survival after transplantation can also be expressed in terms of the half-life of the graft. The half-life of grafts obtained from living donors is substantially longer than that of DD grafts:

- deceased donor grafts, 13 years;
- living-unrelated grafts, 16 years;
- living-haploidentical grafts, 17 years;
- living-identical sibling grafts, 27 years.

Summary box 82.10

Outcome after transplantation

- Transplantation improves the quality and duration of life in most recipients
- Transplant outcome has improved progressively over the last two decades and continues to improve
- Improved outcome is due to better immunosuppression, organ preservation, chemoprophylaxis and technical advances
- Graft survival after kidney, liver and heart transplantation is >90% at 1 year and >80% at 5 years
- The results of lung and small bowel transplantation are less good
- Chronic rejection is the most common cause of graft failure after all types of solid-organ transplant
- Recurrence of the original disease necessitating transplantation may also lead to graft failure
- Death with a functioning transplant from cardiovascular disease is relatively common
- Up-to-date transplant outcomes for the different organs can be found at the online national and international transplant databases (see end of chapter for website addresses)

If a kidney transplant fails late after transplantation, the graft can often be left *in situ* and immunosuppression stopped, but transplant nephrectomy may be indicated if the graft is causing symptoms. The operation is undertaken via the original wound, but the kidney is dissected free from the renal capsule and delivered into the wound. The renal vessels are then ligated and divided, leaving behind the original vascular anastomosis.

In addition to graft survival, it is important to consider the extent to which transplantation improves the physical and mental wellbeing of the patient and allows them to lead a satisfactory social life. In the case of a kidney, as in other types of solid organ transplant, successful transplantation undoubtedly leads to a substantial improvement in quality of life. However, although some recipients return to a normal or near-normal life, others fare much less well and, for the group overall, the quality of life after transplantation falls short of that seen in normal healthy individuals. Renal transplantation is best regarded, therefore, as an effective form of therapy rather than a complete cure.

PANCREAS TRANSPLANTATION

Successful pancreas transplantation restores normal control of glucose metabolism and obviates the need for insulin therapy in patients with diabetes mellitus. Improved control of blood glucose levels in diabetes reduces the progression of secondary complications such as retinopathy, peripheral vascular disease and nephropathy. However, in considering the indications for pancreas transplantation, these advantages have to be weighed carefully against the risks posed by both the transplantation procedure itself and the immunosuppressive therapy required to prevent graft rejection. For most patients with diabetes, the additional risks associated with pancreas transplantation and immunosuppression are such that the operation can be justified only when kidney transplantation for diabetic nephropathy is also being undertaken. The additional risks of pancreas transplantation relate to the transplantation operation itself and the need for enhanced immunosuppressive therapy compared with kidney transplantation alone. In the USA, around a half of all patients with diabetes undergoing kidney transplantation also receive a pancreas transplant. In most cases, the kidney and pancreas are obtained from the same donor, so-called simultaneous pancreas and kidney (SPK) transplantation. Pancreas transplantation is sometimes performed in patients who have already undergone successful kidney transplantation, pancreas-after-kidney (PAK) transplantation. Occasionally, pancreas transplantation alone (PTA) can be justified to treat life-threatening diabetic complications such as hypoglycaemic unawareness.

Careful patient selection is essential to avoid excessive mortality and morbidity. The procedure is usually reserved for those patients with type 1 diabetes who are relatively young (aged <60 years) and do not have advanced coronary artery disease or advanced peripheral vascular disease. Investigation of the heart's response to stress, either using echocardiography or nuclear medicine imaging is usual.

Surgical technique

The whole pancreas gland together with a segment of duodenum is transplanted, essentially as pioneered by Lillehei in 1966. SPK transplantation is usually performed through a midline incision (**Figure 82.26**). The pancreas graft is placed intraperitoneally in the pelvis, usually on the right, and the

Richard Lillehei, surgeon, the University of Minnesota, Minneapolis, MI, USA.

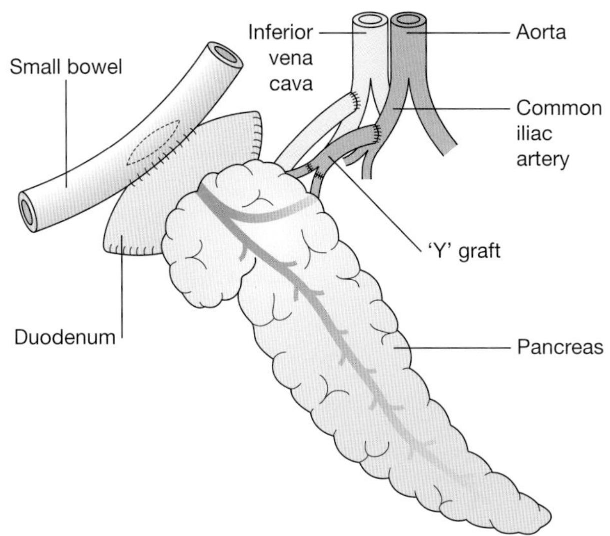

Figure 82.26 Pancreas transplantation operation with enteric drainage of the exocrine secretion via a duodenoenterostomy. A 'Y' graft using donor iliac artery is usually used to reconstruct the divided splenic and superior mesenteric arteries of the graft before implantation.

kidney graft is placed on the left side. The donor vessels of the pancreas graft are anastomosed to the recipient iliac vessels and the exocrine secretions are most commonly dealt with by anastomosing the graft duodenum to the small bowel (enteric drainage) often via a Roux-en-Y loop, although the duodenum may sometimes be anastomosed to the bladder (urinary drainage). The pancreas graft functions immediately after revascularisation, although supplementary insulin may be required for a few days. Technical complications usually occur early and include vascular thrombosis of the graft (5%) and duodenal anastomotic leaks. Graft pancreatitis is very common, but usually mild and unlikely to need intervention. Wound infection occurs in up to 10% of patients, and intra-abdominal infection is relatively common. The specific complications of enteric drainage include intra-abdominal sepsis and adhesive small intestinal obstruction. Bladder drainage of the exocrine pancreas may result in the following complications:

- bladder/duodenal anastomotic leaks;
- cystitis (owing to effect of pancreatic enzymes);
- urethritis/urethral stricture;
- reflux pancreatitis;
- urinary tract infection;
- haematuria;
- metabolic acidosis (due to loss of bicarbonate in the urine).

Urinary drainage of the pancreas has the advantage that urinary amylase levels can be used to monitor for graft rejection. However, after bladder drainage, urinary complications are common, and in around 20% of cases their severity necessitates conversion to enteric drainage. Most centres now prefer primary enteric drainage after SPK transplantation. Acute rejection after SPK transplantation is relatively common (10–20%) and if detected early responds to treatment with steroids. Biopsy confirmed that acute renal allograft rejection may be a surrogate for pancreas rejection, but acute rejection of the kidney or pancreas graft may occur in isolation. Serum lipase and amylase levels are useful indications of pancreas graft inflammation of which acute rejection is one cause. Elevation of blood glucose level is a late feature of acute rejection and often indicates the process is beyond reversal.

Results of pancreas transplantation

The principal aim of pancreas transplantation is to prolong life in patients with diabetes who otherwise have a high mortality at 10 years after receiving a kidney transplant alone. It also provides freedom from insulin treatment and improves quality of life.

The results of pancreas transplantation have improved significantly over the last decade. After SPK transplantation, the 1-year patient survival rate is greater than 95% and the 1-year graft survival rates for pancreas and kidney grafts are 85 and 95%, respectively. Most deaths are due to cardiovascular complications or overwhelming infection. Patient and kidney graft survival after SPK transplantation in patients with diabetic nephropathy is at least as good as after kidney transplantation alone in this group. The results of PTA are not as good as after SPK transplantation (1-year pancreas graft survival rate of 75%) because acute rejection is more difficult to monitor in the absence of a kidney allograft.

Transplantation of isolated pancreatic islets

Treatment of diabetes by transplantation of isolated islets of Langerhans is a more attractive concept than vascularised pancreas transplantation because major surgery and the potential complications of transplanting exocrine pancreas are avoided. Pancreatic islets for transplantation are obtained by mechanically disrupting the pancreas after injection of collagenase into the pancreatic duct. The islets are then purified from the dispersed tissue by density-gradient centrifugation and can be delivered into the recipient liver (the preferred site for transplantation) by injection into the portal vein. Until recently, human islet transplantation had been performed intermittently and with very disappointing results. However, in 2000, Shapiro and colleagues in Edmonton, Canada, reported success with islet transplantation in seven patients with type 1 diabetes. Sequential islet transplantation from two or three donor pancreas glands was required to produce insulin independence and, although the long-term success is less than initially hoped for, some patients remained free from exogenous insulin and other units are now undertaking islet transplantation with variable results.

As an alternative to preventing islet rejection through immunosuppressive therapy, attempts have been made to protect isolated islet cells from rejection by encapsulating them inside semipermeable membranes. The protective

Paul Langerhans, 1847–1888, Professor of Pathological Anatomy, Freiberg, Germany, described the islets in 1869.
Andrew Mark James Shapiro, Chairman of Clinical Research in Transplantation, CHRI/Wyeth Canada, Edmonton, Alberta, Canada.

membranes are designed with a pore size that allows insulin to pass through but prevents antibodies and leukocytes from reaching the islets, thereby avoiding the need for immunosuppressive therapy. A major attraction of this approach is that islets isolated from animals can be used and bioartificial pancreas grafts containing xenogeneic islets are currently under evaluation.

LIVER TRANSPLANTATION

Starzl first attempted liver transplantation in 1963 and, by 1967, had achieved prolonged survival. The first liver transplant performed outside the USA was performed in Cambridge, UK by Calne in 1968. Throughout the 1970s, liver transplantation remained a hazardous procedure that frequently failed. However, since then, the results have progressively improved as a result of better patient selection, improved immunosuppression and chemoprophylaxis, better organ preservation, refinements in the surgical technique, and advances in per- and postoperative management.

Indications and patient selection

The indications for liver transplantation fall into four groups:

1 cirrhosis;
2 acute fulminant liver failure;
3 metabolic liver disease;
4 primary hepatic malignancy.

The most common indication for transplantation is chronic liver failure. In adults the most common causes are alcoholic liver disease, viral liver disease (hepatitis C in Europe and the USA, and hepatitis B in some other countries), non-alcoholic steatohepatitis, primary biliary cirrhosis and sclerosing cholangitis. In children, who account for around 10–15% of all liver transplantations, biliary atresia is the most common indication for transplantation. Acute fulminant liver failure requiring transplantation on an urgent basis accounts for approximately 10% of liver transplant activity and is usually viral or drug induced (e.g. paracetamol overdose in the UK). There are a variety of metabolic diseases for which transplantation offers the prospect of cure, including Wilson's disease, oxalosis and familial amyloid polyneuropathy. Primary hepatic malignancy is more common in patients with cirrhosis, especially virally induced disease, and may be best treated by transplantation because the field changes in the cirrhotic liver predispose to further primary malignancies. Cholangiocarcinoma has a high recurrence rate and is seldom an indication for liver transplantation.

Technique of liver transplantation

A transverse abdominal incision with a midline extension is usually made and the diseased liver is mobilised (**Figure 82.27**).

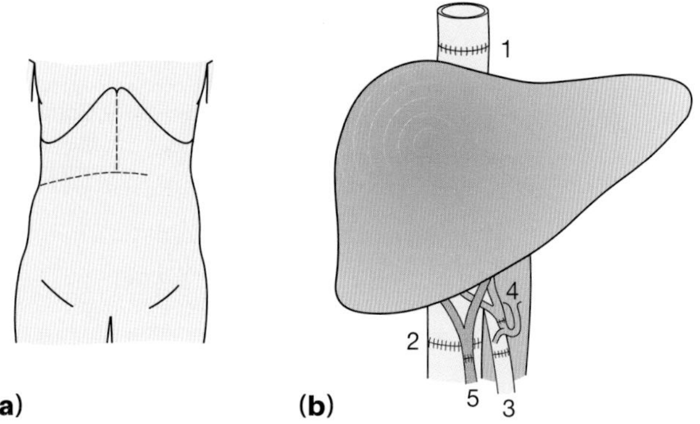

Figure 82.27 (**a**) Incision used for liver transplantation; (**b**) completed implantation. The anastomoses, in order of performance, are: (1) suprahepatic cava; (2) infrahepatic cava; (3) portal vein; (4) hepatic artery; (5) bile duct.

As a result of portal hypertension, the recipient hepatectomy is often the most difficult part of the operation, especially if there has been previous upper abdominal surgery. The common bile duct is divided, as is the hepatic artery. The inferior vena cava is clamped and divided above and below the liver, and the portal vein is clamped and divided, allowing the recipient liver to be removed. Occlusion of the vena cava and portal vein results in a reduction in cardiac output and may necessitate the use of venovenous bypass. The bypass circuit delivers blood from the inferior vena cava and/or portal vein and back to the heart via a cannula inserted into the internal jugular vein. After placing the donor liver in position, the supra- and infrahepatic caval anastomoses are performed. The portal vein and the hepatic arterial anastomoses are then completed and the graft is re-perfused. Finally, biliary drainage is re-established usually by a duct-to-duct anastomosis (without the use of a T-tube). It may be necessary, for example in recipients with biliary atresia or sclerosing cholangitis, to reconstruct the biliary drainage by a bile-duct-to-Roux-loop anastomosis. An alternative caval preservation technique of liver transplantation allows the recipient liver to be removed without cross-clamping the vena cava and the donor liver to be implanted using a 'piggy-back' technique on to the recipient hepatic veins, or using a side-to-side cavo-cavoplasty.

Many patients undergoing liver transplantation are extremely ill, and the surgery involved can be very technically demanding. Optimal perioperative management is crucial to a successful outcome and presents a major challenge. Blood loss during and after the transplantation procedure can be very considerable, and management of coagulopathy is particularly important. Coagulation is assessed repeatedly throughout the transplantation period and corrected with appropriate clotting factors if required. Many centres routinely use thromboelastography to perform dynamic assessment of coagulation.

Thomas Earl Starzl, Professor of Surgery, Pittsburgh, PA, USA.
Samuel Alexander Kinnier Wilson, 1878–1936, Professor of Neurology, King's College Hospital, London, UK, described this condition in 1912.

Technical complications

Haemorrhage

Meticulous haemostasis during the transplantation operation is important in order to minimise the risk of early haemorrhage. It may be necessary, occasionally, to pack the peri-transplant area for 2–3 days to achieve adequate haemostasis when there is diffuse oozing despite correction of coagulopathy. Evacuation of extensive peri-hepatic haematoma may be required to avoid secondary infection.

Vascular complications

Hepatic artery thrombosis may occur spontaneously or as a result of acute rejection and is more common in children and in adults with primary sclerosing cholangitis. It may present as a rise in serum transaminase levels, unexplained fever or bile leak. Doppler ultrasonography or angiography is used to confirm the diagnosis, and urgent re-transplantation is usually required. Portal vein thrombosis is rare and presents with the features of portal hypertension. Hepatic vascular occlusion often presents with increasing ascitic fluid losses over the postoperative period. A cavogram with hepatic vein pressure studies should be undertaken to confirm the diagnosis, and insertion of vascular stents, surgical correction or re-transplantation may be required to treat the problem.

Biliary complications

Biliary leaks are now relatively uncommon and biliary stenosis is the more common problem. It usually occurs within the first few months of transplantation and is managed by endoscopic dilatation and stenting or by surgical correction.

Outcome after liver transplantation

The outcome after liver transplantation depends on the underlying liver disease and the best results are seen in patients with chronic liver disease (Figure 82.28). Patients undergoing transplantation as a result of acute liver failure have a higher mortality in the early post-transplantation period because of multiorgan failure, but those who make a satisfactory recovery have very good long-term liver allograft survival. Conversely, patients transplanted for tumour have a very good early outcome but ultimately fare much less well because of recurrent malignancy. Patients receiving a liver transplantation after hepatitis B or hepatitis C infection may develop graft failure as a result of recurrent viral disease. However, the availability of improved antiviral therapy has largely eliminated this problem in recipients with hepatitis B infection and in the near future is expected to do so in those with hepatitis C infection.

SMALL BOWEL TRANSPLANTATION

Progress in small bowel transplantation has lagged behind that of other types of organ transplantation but it is now a well-established therapy for highly selected recipients. Intestinal transplants stimulate a particularly strong graft rejection

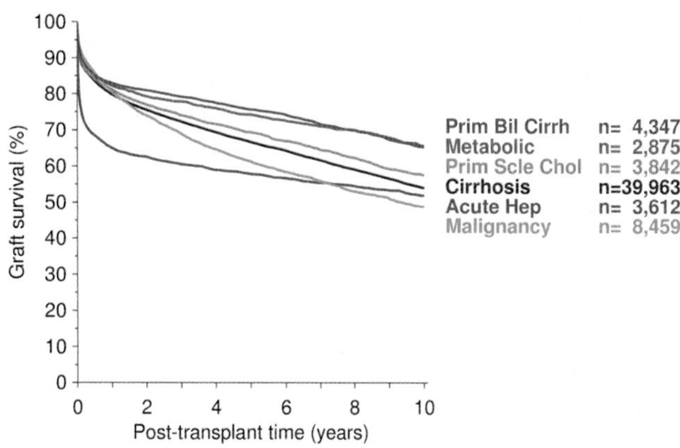

Figure 82.28 Outcome after liver transplantation according to the initial liver disease. Patients transplanted for acute liver disease have a higher early mortality but good long-term outcome. Patients transplanted because of liver tumour have a good initial outcome but survival continues to decline progressively (courtesy of Collaborative Transplant Study, L-75101-0816). Bil, biliary; Cirrh, cirrhosis; Chol, cholangitis; Hep, hepatitis; Scle, sclerosing.

response, probably because the small intestine contains very large amounts of lymphoid tissue. Moreover, ischaemia and rejection increase intestinal permeability and allow translocation of bacteria from the lumen of the bowel. Added to this, the operation is often complex and is made technically difficult because of repeated previous abdominal surgery. Consequently, graft rejection and infection remain major problems after small bowel transplantation and the results obtained are inferior to those seen after other types of organ transplantation. Small bowel transplantation is a treatment option for patients with intestinal failure requiring long-term parenteral nutrition. Intestinal failure may result from short bowel syndrome after resection of the intestine or from intestinal dysfunction. Conditions that may give rise to intestinal failure include the following:

- intestinal atresia;
- necrotising enterocolitis;
- volvulus;
- disorders of motility;
- mesenteric infarction;
- Crohn's disease;
- trauma;
- desmoids tumours.

As a result of the substantial risks associated with small bowel transplantation, the procedure is considered only for those patients in whom long-term total parenteral nutrition (TPN) has failed, usually because venous access has become impracticable or because of frequent life-threatening line sepsis. The need for small bowel transplantation is estimated at around 0.5–1.0 patients per million of the population. Previously 50% of cases were children but improvements in parenteral nutrition have reduced the role of small bowel transplantation in children.

Small bowel transplantation may be carried out as an isolated procedure, performed together with a liver transplantation or undertaken as a component of a multivisceral transplantation. When possible, isolated small bowel transplantation is undertaken because patient survival is higher.

A small bowel transplant from a deceased donor comprises the entire small bowel, and may include the ascending colon in the graft. The superior mesenteric artery of the graft (with an aortic patch) is anastomosed to the recipient aorta, and the superior mesenteric vein is anastomosed to the inferior vena cava or to the side of the portal vein. The proximal end of the small bowel graft is anastomosed to the recipient jejunum or duodenum. The distal end of the graft is anastomosed to the side of the colon (with a loop ileostomy) or is fashioned as an end-ileostomy. A gastrostomy tube (to overcome delayed gastric emptying) and a feeding jejunostomy tube are inserted.

About 10–20% of all patients who require small bowel transplantation have cholestatic liver disease secondary to TPN and require combined liver and small bowel transplantation. When combined liver and small bowel transplantation is carried out, the two grafts are transplanted en bloc. The donor aorta is fashioned into a conduit including the superior mesenteric and coeliac arteries and anastomosed to the recipient aorta. There is no requirement for a portal vein anastomosis and venous drainage is exclusively by the inferior vena cava (**Figure 82.29**).

Multivisceral or 'cluster' transplants may be necessary in the case of large desmoid tumours when excision of both the small bowel and adjacent organs is required, when there has been extensive thrombosis of the splanchnic vessels and for generalised disorders of gastrointestinal motility.

The 1-year graft survival rate after small bowel transplantation is about 80% for both isolated small bowel transplantation and combined liver and small bowel transplantation. After 3 years, the graft survival rate is around 70% after isolated small bowel transplantation and 50% after multivisceral transplantation. Most of the mortality after small bowel transplantation is due to sepsis and multiorgan failure. The risk of infection after small bowel transplantation is heightened by the additional requirements for immunosuppression in order to control graft rejection. This accounts for the relatively high incidence of lymphoproliferative disease (around 10%) observed in patients who have undergone small bowel transplantation. As a result of the large amount of donor lymphoid tissue transplanted, GVHD may be an added complication. Despite the hazards, small bowel transplantation offers patients with intestinal failure a chance to lead an active life free from the constraints of long-term nutritional support.

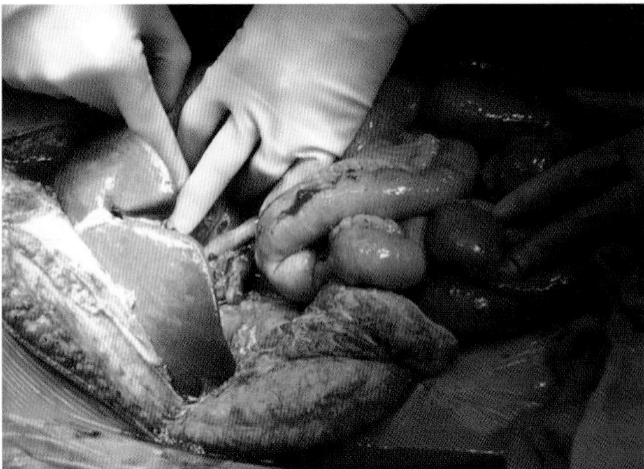

Figure 82.29 Combined liver and small bowel transplant in an adult shortly after reperfusion of the grafts. The small bowel is well perfused via the superior mesenteric artery anastomosed to the aorta on a patch along with the coeliac axis, and the venous blood drains into the portal vein via the superior mesenteric vein.

THORACIC ORGAN TRANSPLANTATION

Heart transplantation

Dr Christiaan Barnard performed the first human heart transplantation in Cape Town, South Africa, in 1967. The operation was based on the experimental work of Lower and Shumway in Stanford, and Shumway subsequently went on to pioneer successful cardiac transplantation in the clinic. Heart transplantation is now considered an effective treatment for selected patients with end-stage cardiac failure. The most common indications for heart transplantation are ischaemic heart disease and idiopathic cardiomyopathy, but other indications include valvular heart disease, myocarditis and congenital heart disease.

Transplantation is considered only in patients with end-stage heart disease that has failed to respond to all other conventional therapy and when predicted survival without transplantation is only 6–12 months. Transplantation is usually limited to patients under the age of 65 years who do not have irreversible damage to other organ systems. The preoperative assessment is rigorous, and measurement of pulmonary vascular resistance is mandatory because when it is raised the perioperative mortality is high.

Technique of heart transplantation

A median sternotomy is performed and the patient is given systemic heparin, placed on cardiopulmonary bypass and cooled to 29°C. After cross-clamping the aorta, the recipient heart is excised at the mid-atrial level. The donor heart is then prepared and the left atrium is opened by making incisions (**Figure 82.30**) in the posterior wall, between the orifices of the pulmonary veins, to create an atrial cuff. The left and then right atrial anastomoses are performed and the pulmonary and aortic arterial anastomoses are then completed (**Figure 82.31**). The patient is then rewarmed and weaned from cardiopulmonary bypass. Occasionally, heterotopic cardiac transplantation is undertaken, when the donor heart is placed adjacent to and augments the recipient's own heart.

Christian Neethling Barnard, 1922–2001, Professor of Cardiac Surgery, the University of Cape Town, Cape Town, the Republic of South Africa.
Richard Rowland Lower, contemporary, thoracic surgeon, Richmond, VA, USA.
Norman Edward Shumway, 1923–2006, cardiothoracic surgeon, Stanford University School of Medicine, Palo Alto, CA, USA.

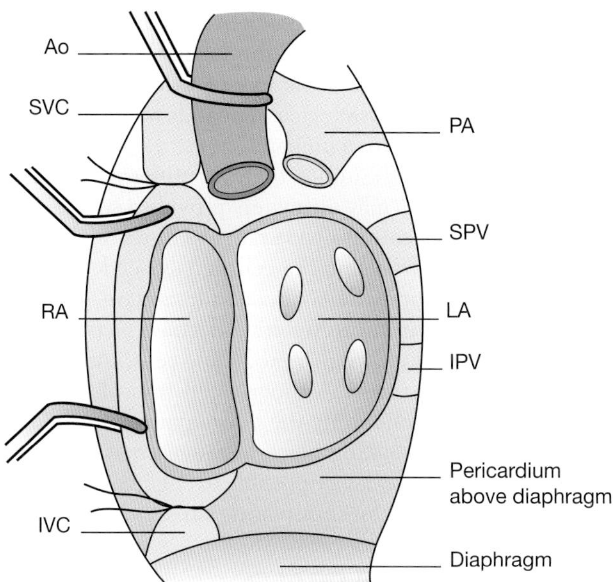

Figure 82.30 Recipient cardiectomy. After median sternotomy, the recipient is placed on cardiopulmonary bypass. Venous cannulae for bypass are sited in the superior vena cava (SVC) and inferior vena cava (IVC) via punctures in the right atrium (RA), and oxygenated blood is returned via a cannula in the ascending aorta (Ao). The diseased recipient heart is excised, leaving behind cuffs of right and left atria (courtesy of J Dunning). PA, pulmonary artery; IPV/SPV, inferior/superior pulmonary veins; LA, left atrium.

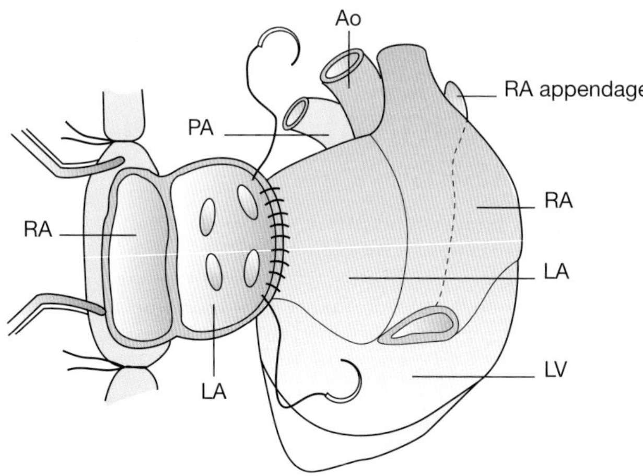

Figure 82.31 Implantation of the donor heart. The donor left atrium is opened by an incision connecting the four pulmonary veins, excising the central portion. The left atrial anastomosis is performed, starting at the lateral wall of the donor and continuing inferiorly and superiorly, concluding with the interatrial septum. The right atrial anastomosis is performed matching the recipient atrium by an incision towards the donor right atrial appendage (dotted line), which avoids the sinus node at the cavoatrial junction. Finally, the pulmonary artery and aortic anastomosis are completed. Abbreviations as for Figure 82.30; LV, left ventricle.

Heart-lung, single-lung and double-lung transplantations

Pulmonary transplantation became a clinical reality when Dr Bruce Reitz performed the first successful combined heart–lung transplantation in 1981. Combined heart–lung transplantation is still sometimes performed, usually in patients with pulmonary vascular disease in whom there is cardiac dysfunction due to congenital (e.g. Eisenmenger's syndrome, in which the left-to-right shunt is reversed owing to pulmonary hypertension) or acquired cardiac dysfunction. For most patients with end-stage pulmonary disease, however, single- or double-lung transplantation has now replaced heart–lung transplantation. Lung transplantation is more economical in terms of organ use, although, if heart–lung transplantation is undertaken for isolated respiratory disease, the healthy native heart can be used for transplantation, the so-called 'domino procedure'. Heart–lung transplantation is performed through a median sternotomy, taking particular care to avoid injury to the phrenic, vagus and recurrent laryngeal nerves during excision of the recipient heart and lungs. The recipient right atrium and aorta are divided as for orthotopic cardiac transplantation and the donor heart–lung block readied for implantation, incising the right atrium from the divided inferior vena cava. An end-to-end tracheal anastomosis is performed and the right atrial and aortic anastomoses are performed as for cardiac transplantation.

Single- and double-lung transplantation are effective therapies for selected patients with end-stage chronic lung disease, in whom declining lung function limits life expectancy despite optimal medical therapy. Common indications are pulmonary fibrosis, pulmonary hypertension, emphysema and cystic fibrosis. Single-lung transplantation can be performed for pulmonary fibrosis. Single-lung transplantation is performed through a posterolateral thoracotomy and double-lung transplantation through a bilateral thoracotomy or median sternotomy. During lung transplantation, the donor pulmonary veins on a left atrial cuff are anastomosed to the recipient left atrium. Next, the bronchial anastomosis and the pulmonary arterial anastomosis are completed. Cardiopulmonary bypass is usually required if pulmonary hypertension is present. Dehiscence of the airway anastomosis used to be common after heart–lung and lung transplantation, but improvements in organ preservation and surgical technique have dramatically reduced the incidence of this often fatal complication to <5%. Late airway stenosis at the bronchial anastomosis due to ischaemia occurs in around 10% of bronchial anastomoses and is treated by dilatation.

Outcome after thoracic organ transplantation

The 1- and 5-year graft survival rates after heart transplantation are around 85% and 70%, respectively. The results after

Bruce Arnold Reitz, thoracic surgeon, Stanford University School of Medicine, Palo Alto, CA, USA.
Victor Eisenmenger, 1864–1932, German physician.

heart–lung and lung transplantation are less good, with 1-year graft survival rates of around 75% and 5-year survival rates of around 50%.

FUTURE PROSPECTS

The two major problems in organ transplantation are:

1 chronic graft rejection and the side effects of non-specific immunosuppression;
2 the shortage of organs for transplantation.

New immunosuppressive agents that have fewer or different agent-specific side effects than existing therapy are likely to enter clinical practice and there is continuing research into the development of non-invasive biomarkers (in urine or blood) that will allow early diagnosis of graft rejection. A long-standing goal in organ transplantation has been the development of strategies for inducing specific immunological tolerance. Transplantation tolerance would eliminate the need for long-term, non-specific, immunosuppressive agents, leaving the immune system intact for defence against infection. It has long been possible to induce transplant tolerance in experimental animals with a variety of preconditioning regimens that often involve pre-treatment schedules using donor bone marrow cells or donor antigen. So far, however, there is no clinically applicable strategy for inducing transplant tolerance.

Summary box 82.11

Future developments in transplantation

- Novel immunosuppressive agents
- Non-invasive biomarkers for early diagnosis of graft rejection
- Donor-specific immunological tolerance
- Xenotransplantation
- Stem cell medicine and tissue engineering

The demand for human organs for transplantation is so great that deceased donors can never satisfy it. Many consider that the solution is to perfect xenotransplantation, and there is general agreement that the pig is the most suitable source of xenogeneic organs. However, all humans have preformed antibodies directed against carbohydrate antigens expressed by pig organs, and these cause hyperacute rejection. The dominant carbohydrate antigen responsible is gal-1, 3α-gal. Progress has been made towards circumventing hyperacute xenograft rejection and pigs that have been genetically engineered not to express the gal-1, 3α-gal antigen have been produced. However, organs from genetically modified pigs are still rejected within a few weeks by primates, despite the use of potent immunosuppressive agents. In addition to the complex immunological problems posed by xenotransplantation, there is a risk that pig organs may transmit infectious agents, and there is particular concern about the risks posed by the porcine endogenous retrovirus (PERV). Last, there are unanswered questions about the extent to which pig organs are able to fulfil the physiological demands required of them after transplantation into a human.

Finally, looking to the future, there is optimism that human pluripotent stem cells may ultimately provide a source of tissue transplants for treating a wide range of diseases. Attempts are now under way to define the cell signals needed to guide human embryonic and adult-induced pluripotent stem cells to differentiate *in vitro* into functional tissue of the desired cell type. These include insulin-producing cells, cardiac myocytes and neuronal tissue. Although cell transplantation is the initial goal, by combining the developments in stem cell medicine with those taking place in tissue engineering and biomaterials it may one day be possible to engineer more complex vascularised grafts for transplantation.

FURTHER READING

Clavien PA, Trotter J (eds). *Medical care of the liver transplant patient*, 4th edn. Oxford: Wiley-Blackwell, 2006.

Hricik D (ed.). *Primer on transplantation*, 3rd edn. Oxford: Wiley-Blackwell, 2011.

Morris PJ, Knechtle SJ (eds). *Kidney transplantation: principles and practice*, 7th edn. Philadelphia, PA: WB Saunders, 2008.

Oniscu G, Forsythe J. Abdominal organ retrieval and transplantation bench surgery. Oxford: Wiley-Blackwell, 2013.

Rainer WG, Sutherland DER. Transplantation of the pancreas. New York: Springer, 2011.

Vigneswaran W, Garrity E. Lung transplantation: principles and practice. Boca Raton, FL: CRC Press, 2015.

WEBSITE ADDRESSES FOR SELECTED NATIONAL AND INTERNATIONAL TRANSPLANT DATABASES

European Liver Transplant Registry: www.eltr.org
NHS Blood and Transplant: www.nhsbt.nhs.uk
United Network for Organ Sharing (USA): www.unos.org
Collaborative Transplant Study (Europe): www.ctstransplant.org
Scandiatransplant: www.scandiatransplant.org

REFERENCES/WEBSITES FOR USEFUL CLINICAL GUIDELINES IN ORGAN TRANSPLANTATION

UK guidelines for living-donor kidney transplantation: www.bts.org.uk
UK guidelines on CMV in transplantation: www.bts.org.uk
UK guidelines on solid organ transplantation from DCD donors: www.bts.org.uk
Antibody incompatible transplantation: www.bts.org.uk
Kidney Disease: Improving global outcomes (KDIGO): www.kdigo.org
International Society for Heart and Lung Transplantation: http://www.ishlt.org

Appendices

1 Common instruments used in general surgery 1560

2 Fundamental principles in the operating theatre and the importance of global health 1563

Appendix 1

Common instruments used in general surgery

This is a list of some of the instruments used in open (as opposed to minimal access surgery) 'general surgery' with information on how they are used and about the people associated with them. It is hoped that this information will help the general surgical trainee answer questions on operative surgery in postgraduate examinations.

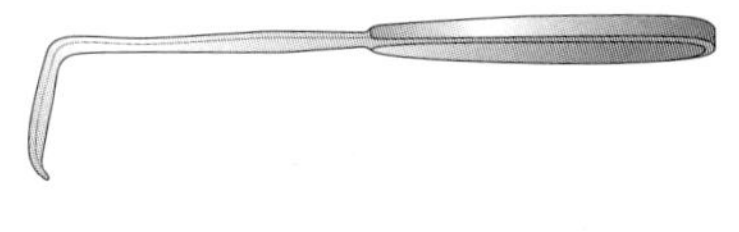

Langenbeck retractor. This small general purpose retractor is useful for holding open wounds, as in an open appendicectomy. They are often used in pairs (one in each of the assistant's hands). They stay in position best if the handles are lifted slightly so that the tips lock in under the fascia. The width of the lip of the retractors varies. Bernhard Rudolf Konrad von Langenbeck (1810–1887) was Professor of Surgery successively at Kiel and Berlin, Germany. He performed the first internal fixation of a femoral neck fracture in 1850.

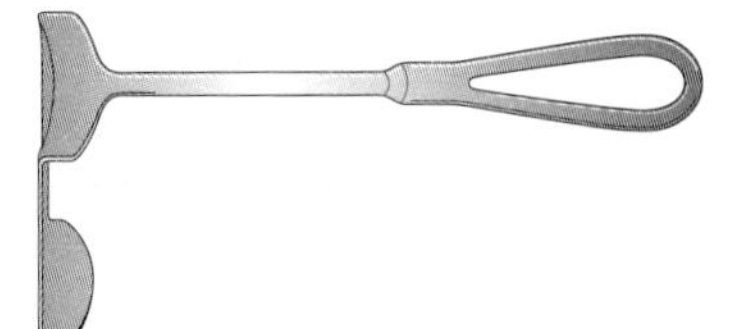

Morris retractor. This is a big retractor which is useful for giving maximum exposure in large incisions such as those used in the abdomen. It can be used to improve visibility on one side of an incision (by pulling firmly in that direction); so is valuable during the initial phase of a laparotomy. Sir Henry Morris (1844–1926) was a surgeon at the Middlesex Hospital, London, UK.

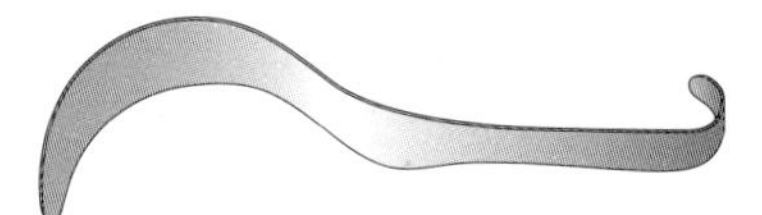

Deaver retractor. This retractor is specifically designed for holding the liver up out of the way during a cholecystectomy. It needs to be used carefully to avoid damaging the liver. Some surgeons protect the liver with an abdominal pack before placing the blade on top. John Blair Deaver (1855–1931) was Professor of Surgery at the University of Pennsylvania Medical School, Philadelphia, PA, USA. He also described a paramedian incision for appendicectomy.

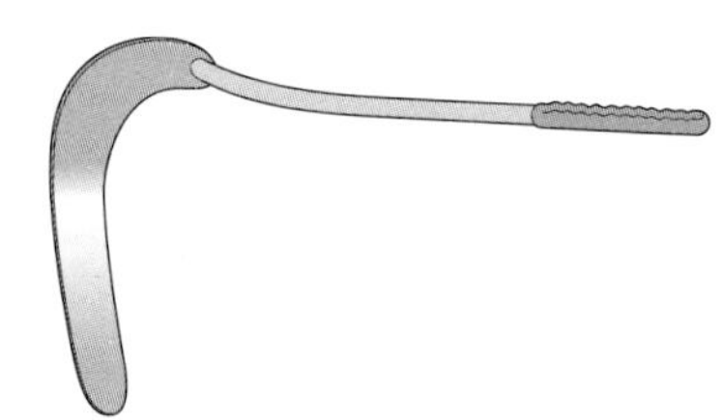

Dyball retractor. Used in major abdominal surgery to retract deeper parts of the abdominal wall or the bladder or the uterus while operating on the rectum and entering the rectovesical or rectouterine pouch. It has a lip at the bottom of the blade to prevent slippage. Care should be taken if it is used to retract the liver in operations in the region of the right upper quadrant as it may damage the liver parenchyma. Brennan Dyball was a distinguished West Country surgeon from Exeter. He also excelled as a carpenter and motor mechanic. He died in 1934 at the age of 62 leaving a great professional legacy to the Royal Devon and Exeter Hospital.

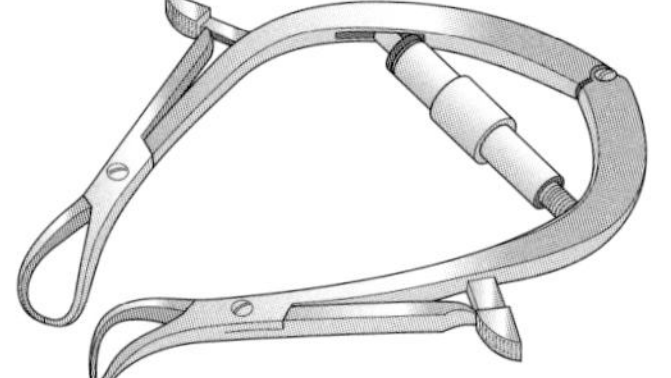

Joll retractor. This is a self-retaining retractor used in thyroid surgery. After making the collar incision and raising the lower and upper flaps fully, this retractor is then inserted. The two clips on the upper and lower edges are attached to the skin preferably with a swab over the skin edge. The central segment is then unscrewed to separate the two edges to obtain full exposure. Cecil Augustus Joll was a surgeon in London who first qualified as a dentist. He was regarded as 'a brilliant technician and an extraordinarily versatile surgeon' who operated on conditions 'from knees to necks and stomach to perineum'. A keen ornithologist, he was a connoisseur of all things good – furniture, pottery, food, wines and cigars. He died in 1945 at the age of 59.

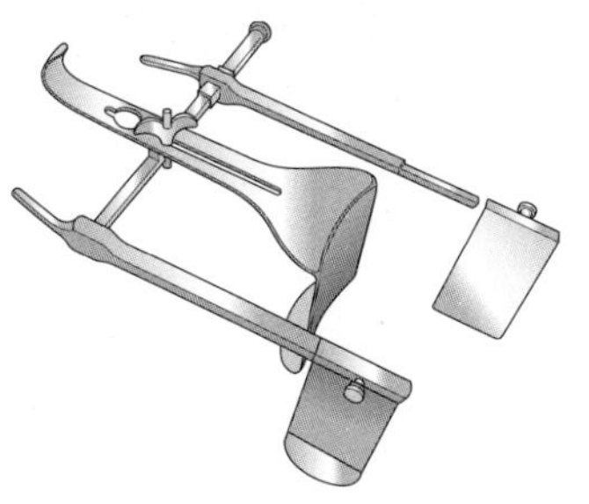

Goligher retractor. This is a self-retaining retractor used in operations on the sigmoid colon and rectum, such as anterior resection and upper end of abdominoperineal resection. Once the abdomen has been opened and laparotomy performed, the patient is placed head down and all the small bowel is packed to the upper end of the abdomen. The retractor is then inserted with the side blades to separate the edges of the abdominal wall. The central blade is then inserted to keep the small bowel well tucked away from the operation site. All three blades come in different widths to fit in with the patient's build. John Cedric Goligher (1912–1998), Ulsterman by birth, Professor of Surgery at Leeds, his contributions to colorectal surgery in the world have been legendary. His operating theatres at Leeds General Infirmary 'have been the Mecca for surgeons from all over the world'. His book, *Surgery of the Anus, Rectum and Colon*, was regarded as the ultimate authority on the subject and had five editions.

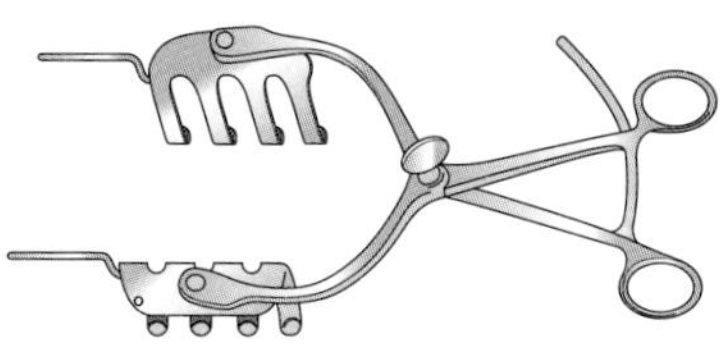

St Mark's perineal retractor. This is used for the perineal part of an abdominoperineal resection. After making the perineal incision and adequate dissection of the perineal wound, the retractor is inserted. As the dissection proceeds, the retractor has to be repositioned. The pointed ends are directed towards the front. St Mark's Hospital, Harrow, UK, is recognised as a national and international referral centre for intestinal and colorectal disorders. It was founded in a small room in No. 11 Aldersgate Street. Established in 1854 on City Road in Hackney as St Mark's Hospital for Fistula and other Diseases of the Rectum. It was so named as it was opened on St Mark's Day, 25 April. In 1994, it moved to its present site in Harrow.

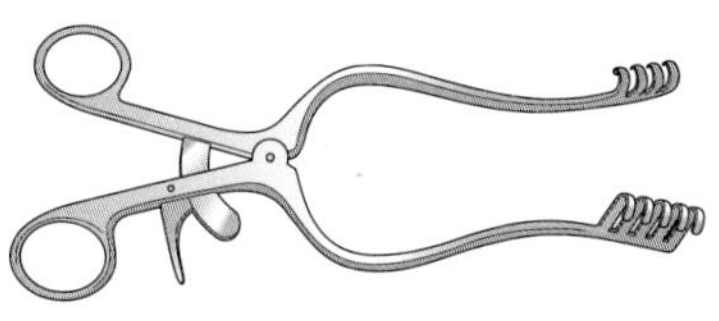

Travers retractor. This is a self-retaining retractor used for intermediate-type operations, such as heriorrhaphy, groin dissection for varicose veins and femoral embolectomy. It retracts skin and subcutaneous tissues; as the incision is deepened, the retractor has to be repositioned. If used incorrectly, it can traumatise the skin. For longer incisions, two such retractors may be used, one at each end of the incision for good exposure. Benjamin Travers (1783–1858) was a surgeon to the London Infirmary for Disease of the Eye (now Moorfields Ophthalmic Hospital). He is regarded as the first general hospital surgeon in England to devote himself specially to disease of the eye. He later became surgeon to St Thomas's Hospital and Vice-President and President of Royal College of Surgeons of England and a Fellow of the Royal Society. As an operator, he was regarded as clumsy and nervous. He had 'exquisite polish of manners, took off his hat and acknowledged salutes more elegantly than any contemporary dandy'.

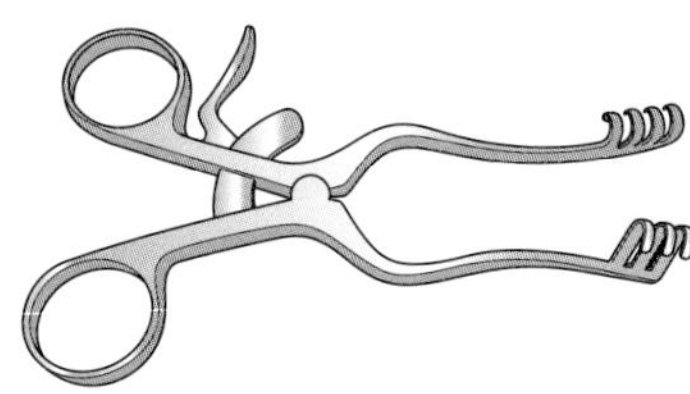

West retractor. Used in a similar manner to the Travers retractor, this is ideal for minor procedures under local anaesthetic where the surgeon is operating without an assistant, e.g. lymph node biopsy, temporal artery biopsy. After making the incision and undermining the edges, the retractor is then inserted and the jaws are prised open gently. Charles Ernest West (1873–1951) 'aural surgeon' of St Bartholomew's Hospital is credited with devising this retractor. It is possible that he got the idea from Franz Weitlaner, an Austrian physician who published the first description of his retractor in the *Vienna Clinical Review* in 1905. He became known as 'the great spreader of surgery'. It would be safe to presume that the present retractor is West's modification of Weitlaner's spreader.

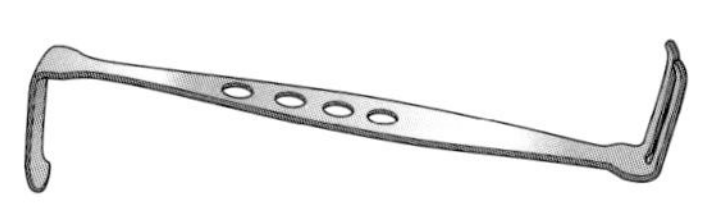

Czerny retractor. This is a double-ended retractor used to retract wound edges for intermediate-type procedures. One end has a blade with a lip which helps to retract without the edge slipping. The other end has two prongs and helps to retract the ends of an incision. When using it, a slight upward tilt gives a better exposure. It is used where a Langenbeck retractor can also be used, but the lip here is broader making it more versatile. Vincenz Czerny (1842–1915) was Professor of Surgery at Freiberg and Heidelberg in Germany. He was a disciple of Theodor Billroth. He was the originator of the concept of multidisciplinary management in cancer.

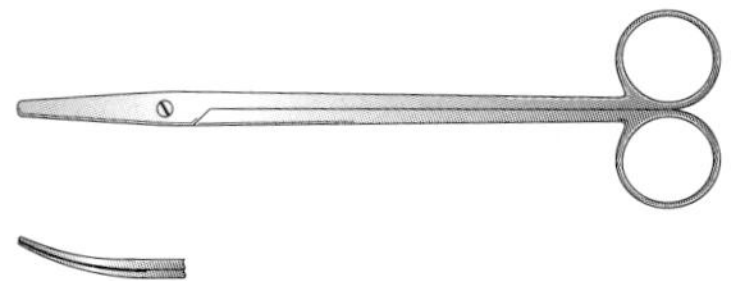

McIndoe scissors are used by surgeons to perform dissection respecting anatomical planes. The closed blades are inserted into a fascial plane, and then gently opened. The tissue to be divided can then be seen clearly and divided without risk of damage to vital structures. Sir Archibald Hector McIndoe (1900–1960) was a plastic surgeon at St Bartholomew's Hospital, London, and the Queen Victoria Hospital, East Grinstead, UK. He was born in New Zealand (cousin of Harold Gillies) and became a consultant plastic surgeon to the RAF during the Second World War. He supervised the rehabilitation of badly disfigured airmen who later formed the Guinea Pig Club.

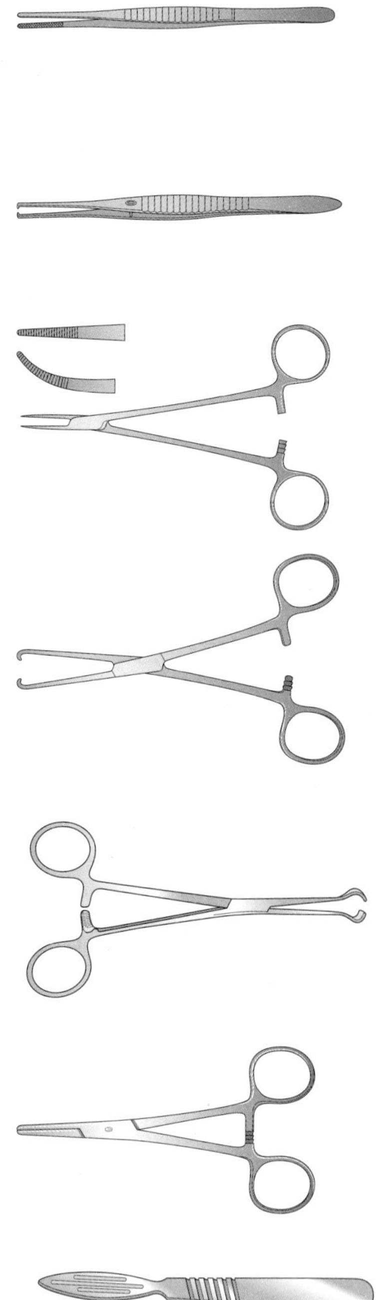

DeBakey forceps allow the surgeon to grasp tissues firmly while minimising damage to the tissue held in the jaws of the forceps. They are useful for holding vessel walls in vascular surgery. Michael Ellis DeBakey (1908–2008) was Professor of Surgery at Baylor University College of Medicine, Houston, TX, USA. He was the first to successfully implant an artificial heart; he also performed the first successful carotid endarterectomy.

Gillies forceps have teeth and are ideal for holding tough tissues, such as skin. Sir Harold Gillies (1882–1960) was a plastic surgeon at St Bartholomew's Hospital, London, UK. He was born in New Zealand (cousin of Archibald McIndoe) and became one of the founders of British plastic surgery. He originated the tubed pedicle flap.

Adson forceps are non-toothed, and so are ideal for holding delicate tissues, such as bowel. Alfred Washington Adson (1887–1951) was Professor of Neurosurgery at the Mayo Clinic, Rochester, MN, USA. He was one of the first to use sympathectomy for the treatment of hypertension, and cervical sympathectomy for Raynaud's syndrome.

Allis forceps are used to hold soft tissues for a long period while minimising tissue damage. Using the ratchet they can be locked on to tissue, such as bowel, and can be used to provide gentle traction. Oscar Huntington Allis (1836–1921) was a surgeon at the Presbyterian Hospital, Philadelphia, PA, USA.

Babcock forceps. This is used to grasp any part of the bowel. The jaws are atraumatic and cause minimal tissue damage. Used commonly in appendicectomy to grasp the appendix and deliver it out of the wound. Care is taken when using it not to perforate the inflamed appendix. William Wayne Babcock (1872–1963), Professor and Head of the Department of Surgery at the Temple University School of Medicine, Philadelphia for 40 years. 'He was the inventor of the acorn-shaped vein stripper, introduced the alloy steel wire sutures, wire mesh in hernia repairs, and zinc chloride in the treatment of osteomyelitic sinus'.

Spencer Wells forceps. These were one of the first ratchet forceps ever designed and are still very useful. They are often used in pairs for clamping an artery before dividing it. The cut ends of the artery are then tied off, and the forceps removed (carefully!). Sir Thomas Spencer Wells (1818–1897) was a surgeon at the Samaritan Free Hospital for Women and Children, London, UK. He was one of the earliest surgeons to make use of anaesthetics in operation.

Kocher dissector. This is used during a thyroidectomy to dissect the upper pole of the thyroid. The instrument is blunt and therefore the surgeon is highly unlikely to inadvertently damage the superior thyroid artery or the external laryngeal nerve. It is used to dissect the superior pedicle, the superior thyroid artery. Once it has been isolated, the dissector is pushed under the pedicle. A tie is then put through the eye of the dissector which at this stage doubles up as an aneurysm needle. The pedicle is thus tied three times as close to the gland as possible. With the dissector under the tied pedicle, a fine knife is now used to cut leaving two ties in the patient. The presence of the dissector under the pedicle prevents any damage to the underlying structures. Emil Theodor Kocher (1841–1917), Professor of Surgery at Berne, Switzerland, was awarded the Nobel Prize for Physiology or Medicine in 1909 for his work on the thyroid. The first surgeon to be a Nobel Laureate.

ACKNOWLEDGEMENTS

With thanks to Steven Kerr, Librarian, Royal College of Surgeons of Edinburgh.

Fundamental principles in the operating theatre and the importance of global health

INTRODUCTION

Historically, operating theatres were designed to encourage large audiences of observers. Surgeons often wore their outdoor clothes and no consideration was given to sterility. The outcomes of surgery were less than satisfactory.

The modern operating theatre, safety checks, accepted theatre etiquette and theatre instrument sterilisation process have made a significant positive impact on outcomes after surgery.

A basic knowledge of the principles of theatre design, theatre etiquette and sterilisation are important for surgeons, aiding them to work with the 'flow' in theatres, preserve the sterile field, and communicate effectively with other members of the theatre and sterilisation team. This fundamental knowledge is applicable in a global setting.

PRINCIPLES OF THEATRE DESIGN

Optimisation of location and spaces

When building new operating theatres, both the principle of locating the operating theatre away from passing traffic (at a terminal location) and the concept of maintaining optimum 'patient flow' should be considered. Operating theatres are often co-located near wards and the intensive care unit to minimise transfer time, thereby increasing efficiency and productivity in the theatre.

Operating theatres should have both easy access to sterile services and sufficient space for all necessary equipment to be stored. The concept of good 'flow' should be extended to staff (in the location of their changing, rest and office areas) and surgical equipment (to and from sterile services).

A reception area for patient safety checks, an area for the patient to be anaesthetised (this may be done in a separate anaesthetic room or in the operating theatre itself) and a recovery area must be included in the theatre design.

The importance of the sterile surgical field

The principle of maintaining the sterile surgical field is at the heart of theatre design. To maintain this field, clean and contaminated areas of the theatre complex are separated into 'zones'. Although there are different individual designs, the principle of minimising the risk of cross-contamination between the 'clean' and 'dirty' zones remains.

Materials used to construct operating theatres should be smooth and easy to clean. Doors disrupt airflow and should be kept closed whenever possible. Sliding doors (electrically operated) cause less airflow disruption than swinging doors. Doors (when closed) and windows should be sealed.

Operating theatres should be large enough for the purpose for which they are used. There should be sufficient space to allow those 'circulating' to move freely without risk of contaminating the sterile surgical field. Modern operating theatres often have a 'modular' design where commonly used equipment is stacked together and mounted on movable gantries to improve cleaning and reduce clutter.

After surgery, contaminated instruments and equipment are physically isolated and removed from the clean to the contaminated zone, where the waste is disposed of and instruments decontaminated and reprocessed for sterilisation. This is often through the use of a 'dirty' corridor.

Theatre air and ventilation

Specialised ventilation in the operating theatre aids in the maintenance of clean and dirty zones because airborne bacteria are prevalent. Between 5000 and 55 000 skin particles laden with bacteria are shed each minute by each individual in the operating room.

Positive pressure ventilation forces airflow from clean to contaminated areas with 15–25 theatre air exchanges taking place per hour using conventional ventilation systems. These systems deliver atmospheric filtered air with positive pressure (15–25 N/m^2) through a downward displacement over the operating table. This ventilation allows for clearance of airborne particles, bacteria and waste anaesthetic gases. Ventilation ducts allow contaminated air to be expelled from the operating theatre.

Ultra-clean ventilation systems use high-efficiency particulate air (HEPA) filters that remove 99.9% of particulate matter >0.3 μm in diameter (bacteria are 0.5 μm). They also use vertical laminar airflow over the operating table to minimise turbulence, reduce contamination at the surgical site (horizontal laminar air flow is less effective (Salvati *et al.* 1982)). Laminar airflow theatres have an air exchange every 2–3 minutes.

The operating lights disturb the laminar airflow and are optimally placed to either side of the operative wound with 0.6 m between the lights to minimise obstruction to the vertical airflow (Refaie *et al.* 2015). Temperature in the operating theatre should be between 18 and 25°C.

STERILISATION

Preoperative checks

When equipment is taken from storage for use, careful checking of the instrument packaging must be carried out. Care must be taken to ensure that the instrument set is complete, without torn packaging, and has undergone sterilisation within the recommended time.

Postoperative checks

After the instruments have been used, they must go through decontamination. This process is standardised and includes cleaning the instruments thoroughly with water immediately after use. Staff involved in this decontamination should wear personal protection. In addition to using water, mechanical agitation aided by chemical cleansing and heat are all needed. Instruments can be decontaminated by hand (for delicate instruments) or in industrial washers.

After decontamination, instruments are checked for damage, sharpened and otherwise maintained. Broken or damaged instruments are replaced. This process is helped by the surgeon during the final step of the surgical safety checklist, when all instrument issues are noted. After maintenance, the instruments are packaged into sets and double wrapped before sterilisation.

Sterilisation for most instruments is carried out in a steam autoclave. For some equipment gas sterilisation is used. Accurate documentation of the sterilisation procedure, expiry dates, the contents of packaged sterile instruments, and missing or damaged instruments on labels before storage is imperative.

THEATRE ETIQUETTE AND INFECTION CONTROL

Personnel factors

At the start of an operating list, it is important, as part of the team brief, for each member of the team to introduce him- or herself. For members of staff arriving after the start, it is important to introduce themselves to the theatre practitioner in charge of the operating theatre at the outset. Behaviour and discipline of staff are a key aspect in the maintenance of patient safety and adequate infection control.

Scrub staff will wear a hat, mask with visor or protective glasses. They will then don a sterile gown and use a closed-glove technique to don their sterile gloves. It is also important that other members of the circulating team take account of universal precautions, including the use of non-sterile gloves when handling or transferring a patient and consideration of the use of masks and protective glasses. Careful handling of sharps is paramount.

Staff clothing is also important. It acts as an effective barrier against the spread of infection. Each operating theatre suite will have specific policies that should be adhered to. The principles are that within the clean zone of the operating theatre all staff must wear scrubs. These scrubs should not be worn in dirty zones if the member of staff is to walk back into the clean zone. If scrubs are soiled, these should be changed for a fresh pair. Hair should be covered by an appropriate hat.

Many policies state that masks should be worn when sterile instruments are opened or in the presence of an open wound. In contaminated surgery, some policies allow for surgeons to dispense with the mask, but consideration must be given for personal protection from fluids on to the face. Both mask visors and/or protective goggles protect the eyes from potential cross-contamination from the patient.

Shoes used in the operating theatre should have a solid covering over the dorsum of the foot, enclosing the toes, and not have multiple holes. This is protection in case sharp instruments fall to the floor, resulting in foot injuries. Shoes should be cleaned after every case to ensure that there is no cross-contamination.

Environmental factors

A number of different skin disinfectant surgical preparation fluids have been described in either an aqueous or an alcoholic base. The antiseptic is normally iodine based (e.g. Betadine) or chlorhexidine based. Chlorhexidine comes in two concentrations – 0.5% or 2% weight:volume (w/v) – and a number of different trials have shown the latter to be the most effective.

Surgical drapes that are used to isolate the surgical wound will be resistant to mechanical stress, impenetrable to liquids and ideally absorbent. Depending on the hospital situation, disposable or reusable drapes can be used if they fit these criteria. The use of incision drapes has some advantages, but recent evidence has shown that those incision drapes that are impregnated with iodine are more effective at reducing the skin bacterial load than non-iodine-impregnated drapes.

The number of people in the operating theatre also increases the risk of contamination of the sterile field. The number should be kept to the minimum. At least 1 metre must be kept between non-scrubbed staff and any sterile instrument tray or the operating table. Non-scrubbed staff should never pass between the sterile instrument tray and the operating table with the patient on it. When the doors are opened to the operating theatre a disturbance is made to the ventilation system. The number of times the doors are opened during the operation should be kept to the minimum. This often requires a high level of advance planning to ensure that all the necessary equipment is available at hand in the operating theatre.

GLOBAL HEALTH AND SURGERY

The previous sections identify fundamental principles relating to surgery wherever it is practised around the world. By way of contrast, in Chapter 33 the differing surgical options for spinal surgery in different global settings were highlighted.

In the last two decades, the interest in global health has notably increased. There are many reasons for this. First, there is better global communication, such that what happens in one part of the world is known almost instantaneously in the rest of the world. Second, there is an increased understanding that the world is a small place, and that the health needs of the poorest in the planet should be the concern of the whole planet. Global health as a concept started with the treatment of medical and infectious diseases such as malaria and tuberculosis (TB), but in the last few years there has been an increasing interest in global surgery. In 2013 the *Lancet* journal commissioned a group of surgeons, health planners, health economists and politicians to prepare a report on the state of surgery in the world. It was published in 2015 (Meara *et al.* 2015) and has been a major influence in world surgery, with five key messages that clarify the levels of disparity in surgical services globally; however, it ends with a strong economic argument for the surgeons of the world to engage with the global need.

The five key messages from the *Lancet* Commission

5 billion people cannot access safe, affordable surgery when needed

The World Health Organization (WHO) has previously stated that 2 billion people had no access to surgery. This is true, but when one adds a quality measure to the surgery available, and also an affordability measure, the number of people who cannot access surgery for themselves or their family within a reasonable time period is increased to 5 billion, which is most of the people on the planet.

143 million more surgical procedures are needed each year

This is the number of operations needed to bring the world up to a reasonable standard of surgery.

33 million individuals and families face catastrophic expenditure each year paying for surgery and anaesthesia

This figure is in fact higher if one adds the incidental expenses associated with having surgery, such as transport and accommodation for family members during the operation. The annual total then rises to US$81 million.

Investing in surgery is affordable, saves lives and promotes economic growth

The cost of improving surgical services across the world to a satisfactory level over the next 15 years is enormous, and has been estimated at US$350 billion, or just over US$20 billion per year. However, the cost of not investing in surgery is many times higher at US$12.3 trillion over 15 years, or US$820 billion a year because of lost economic growth resulting from untreated surgical conditions. **Figure 1** shows the estimated economic loss due to untreated surgical conditions. The graph clearly shows that untreated cancer and trauma are the two big causes of such economic loss.

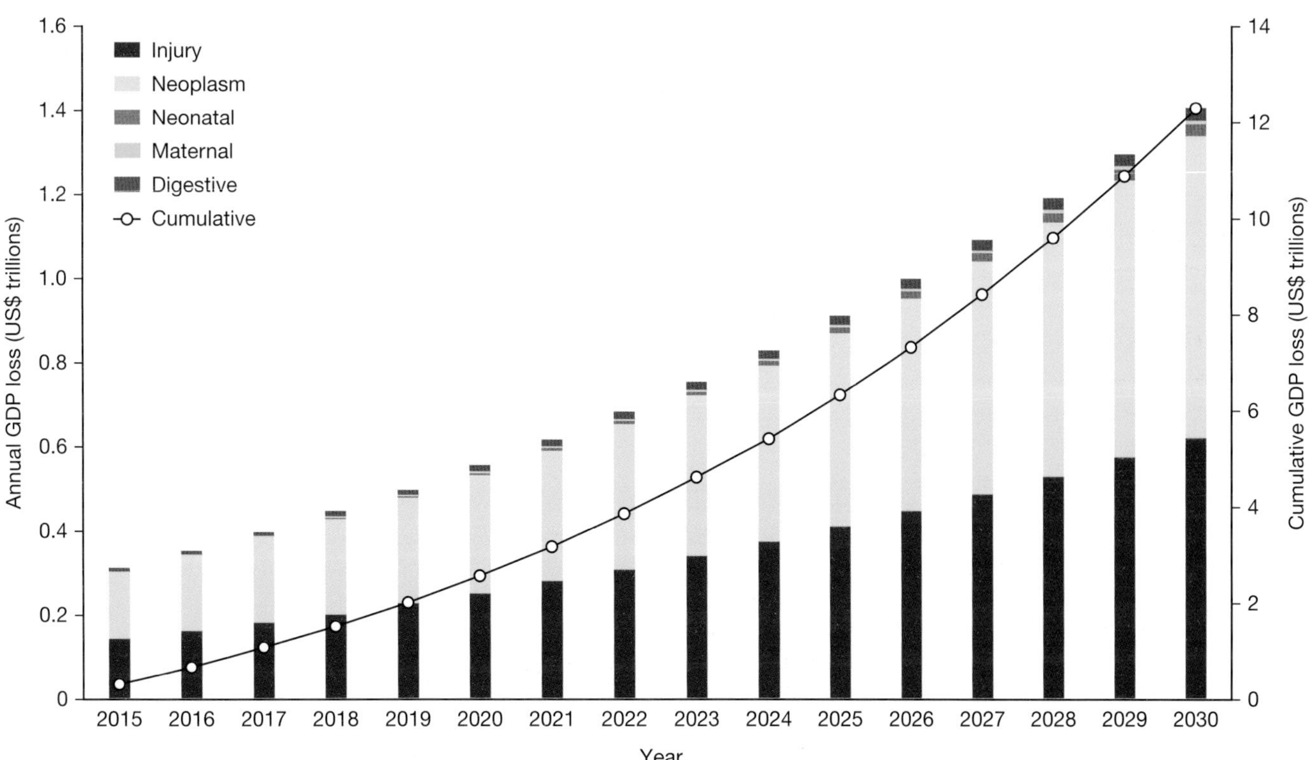

Figure 1 The graph illustrates the estimated economic loss due to untreated surgical conditions; untreated cancer and trauma represent the two largest causes of such economic loss (with permission of Meara *et al.* 2015).

Surgery is an indivisible, indispensable part of health care

This is a message that is directed more to health planners and public health teams. Surgery has in the past been seen as a minor and expensive part of a country's health plan. Most public health interventions are measured in terms of disability-adjusted life-years (DALYs) averted. The methodology involves calculating how much it costs to avert 1 year of suffering due to a disability. When measured in these terms, surgery competes well with the treatment of malaria and TB. The fact that surgery saves lives, surgery changes lives and surgery is a boost to the economy should encourage health planners to put surgery in the essential group of services in any national health strategy.

References and further reading

Booth C. Operating room principles: environment. In: Porteous M, Bauerle S (eds), *Techniques and principles for the operating room*. Stuttgart: Thième, 2010: pp 45–56.

Meara JG, Leathe AJ, Haganda I *et al*. Global surgery 2030: evidence and solutions for achieving health, welfare, and economic development. *Lancet* 2015; **386**: 569–624.

Refaie R, Jameson S, Reed M. Prevention of periprosthetic joint infection. J Trauma Orthop 2015; 3: 50–2. Video: www.youtube.com/user/orthopodresearch

Salvati EA, Robinson RP, Zeno SM, Koslin BL, Brause BD, Wilson PD. Infection rates after 3175 total hip and total knee replacements performed with and without a horizontal unidirectional filtered air-flow system. *J Bone Joint Surg* 1982; **64A**: 525–35.

Van Rie I. Operating room principles: instrumentation. In: Porteous M, Bauerle S (eds), *Techniques and principles for the operating room*. Stuttgart: Thième, 2010: pp 58–67.

Index

Note: Page references in *italic* refer to figures or tables.

eABCD protocol, 323–6
abdomen
  abscesses, 1055–7
  anatomic extent of, *365*
  differences in paediatric/adult, 119, *120*
  examination, 1019–21
    auscultation, 1021
    hernia sites, 1021
    inspection, 1019–20
    palpation, 1020–1
    percussion, 1021
  history of symptoms, 1016–17
  pressure within, 1022
abdominal aortic aneurysm (AAA)
  asymptomatic, 961
  incidence, 961
  investigations, 213, 961, 961–6, *962*
  repair, 265, 961–4
    endovascular, 962–4
    open surgery, 961–2
    postoperative complications, 965–6
  rupture, 964–5
  symptomatic, 965
abdominal compartment syndrome, 380, 1045
abdominal examination
  acute pancreatitis, 1223
  intestinal obstruction, 1286, 1296
  intussusception, 1287
  LUTS (male), 1461
  rectal cancer, 1329
abdominal masses, 1020–1
abdominal pain, 1017
  abdominal wall movement, 1020
  acute appendicitis, 1302–3
  acute in children, 130–2
  acute non-specific, 130
  after laparoscopic surgery, 115
  gallstones, 1018–19, 1199
  intestinal obstruction, 1285–6
  large intestine, 1258
  palpation, 1020
  patient observation/review, 1021
  in peritonitis, 1050
  sites of, 1019
abdominal paracentesis, 1053, 1059, 1166
abdominal reflex, superficial, 472–3
abdominal trauma, 372–6, 1061
  blast, 431
  categories, 372
  children, 123–4
  CT imaging, 207, *208*
  investigation, 372–3
  pancreas, 1220–1
  retroperitoneum, 376
  specific organs, 373–6
  spleen, 123, *208*, 374
  stomach, 375
abdominal wall
  anatomy, 1022
  closure, 86
  cutaneous fistula, 1045
  defects, 135
  incisions, 86
  infections, 1044–5
  innervation, 1018
  necrotising fasciitis, *30*, 50
  neoplasms, 1045
  transplant, 649
  varicose veins, 983
abdominoperineal excision of rectum, 1336
abductor pollicis brevis, 446, 469
abductor pollicis longus, tenosynovitis (De Quervain's disease), 443, 469, 507–8
Aberdeen knot, 95
ABO blood groups, 21, *22*
  organ transplantation, 1533, 1547–8
Abrams–Griffiths nomogram, *1397*
abscesses
  abdominal, 1055–7
  amoebic, 57–60, 1169
  anorectal, 1362–3
  appendix, 1312
  bone, 204, 587–8, 589
  brain, 656–7
  breast, 866–7
  'cold', 77–8
  collar-stud, 78, 757
  colonic diverticula, 1274
  epidural, 481
  liver, 1168–9
  lungs, 937
  orbit, 721–2
  pancreas, 1227–8
  parapharyngeal, 737
  pelvic, 1055, 1312
  perirenal, 1404
  peritonsillary (quinsy), 735–6
  periurethral, 1495
  prostatic, 1475
  psoas, 1065
  renal cortical, 1404
  renal corticomedullary, 1404
  retropharyngeal, 737
  sinus/fistula formation, 48
  surgical, 47–8
  tubo-ovarian, 1519–20
abuse, children, 138
acalculous cholecystitis, 1200
acanthamoeba, 677
access to surgery, 1565
acetabular index, 571
acetabulum, 511
  augmentation, 570–1
acetazolamide, 1407
achalasia, 223, 1095–9
Achilles tendon
  examination, 460
  rupture, *382*, 383, 403, 468, 529
  tendinosis, 529
  tenotomy, 578
achondroplasia, 564–5
acid burns, *622*, 632
  oesophagus, 1075–6
acidosis
  hyperchloraemic, 1454–5
  lactic, 12, *14*, 17
acinar cells, 1212
acne rosacea, 603
AcoRD guidance, 165
acoustic neuromas, 666–7, *706*, 715–16
acral lentiginous melanoma, 610
acrocyanosis, 967–8
acromial spur, 489, *491*
acromioclavicular joint
  arthritis, 489, 495
  injury, 469
ACTHoma, 849
actinic (solar) keratoses, 606
Actinomyces, 56
Actinomyces israelii, 1249
actinomycetoma, 71, 72, 73, 74
actinomycin D, *156*
actinomycosis
  abdominal, 1249
  breast, 867
activated partial thromboplastin time (APTT), 258
activated protein C, 987
acute coronary syndromes (ACS), 889
acute peripancreatic fluid collection, 1226
acute phase protein response, *4*, 7–8
acute traumatic coagulopathy (ATC), 18, 427
adalimumab, 1245, 1269
adamantinoma, *542*
Adams forward bend test, 472, *581*
Addison's disease, 13, 844
adductor pollicis, 446
  weakness, 502
adductor pollicis brevis, 446
adenitis, mesenteric, 1062
adenocarcinoma
  anal canal, 1371
  bladder, 1448
  duodenum, 1141
  gastro-oesophageal junction, 1132
  histology, 239, 241
  lung, 925
  nose/sinuses, 724
  oesophagus, *1083*, *1086*, 1087
  small bowel, 1250
adenoid cystic carcinomas, 724, *778*
adenoidectomy, 732–3
adenoids, enlarged, 732
adenoma–carcinoma sequence, 1261
adenomas
  adrenal glands, 839
  colorectal, 1259, 1261
  duodenal, *233*
  duodenal villous, 1141
  kidneys, 1416
  liver, 1172
  parathyroid glands, 826–30
  pituitary, 665–6, 841, 842
  rectum, 1326

salivary glands, 777–8, *784*, *787*, *788*, *790*, *793*
thyroid follicular, 816
adenoma sebaceum (tuberous sclerosis/Bourneville disease), 602–3
adenomatous polyposis coli (APC) gene, 1259, 1261, 1329
adenomatous polyps, large intestine, 1259, 1261
adhesions, 1049, 1060–1
after appendicectomy, 1314
causes, 1283
intestinal obstruction, 1060, 1283
pathophysiology, 1060
pelvic, 1521
prevention, 1060–1
treatment, 1292
adhesive capsulitis (frozen shoulder), 492, *493*
adjuvant therapies, 151–3
breast cancer, *155–7*, 877–9
colorectal cancer, 1266
oesophageal cancer, 1093–4
pancreatic carcinoma, 1237
adnexa, 592–3
adolescents
fractures, growth plate, 387
hip dysplasia, 568, 570
tendon injuries, 464
adrenalectomy, 847–8
Conn's adenoma, 841
Cushing's syndrome, 842
laparoscopic, 847–8
open, 848
adrenal glands
acute insufficiency, 844
anatomy, 838
chronic insufficiency, 844
embryology, 839
function, 839
ganglioneuroma, 847
histology, 839
hydatid cyst, 65
hyperaldosteronism, 840–1
incidentaloma, 839–40
metastases, 842
neuroblastoma, 847
phaeochromocytoma, 839, 844–7, 857, 936
primary insufficiency (Addison's disease), 844
resection, 847–8
tumours, in MEN 1 syndrome, 856, 857
adrenaline (epinephrine), 3, 839
adrenal vein catheterisation, selective, 840–1
adrenocortical carcinoma, 843
adrenocortical suppression, 260
adrenocorticotrophic hormone (ACTH), 3, 4, 839
excess, 841–2, 844
insufficiency, 844
tumours secreting, 666
α-adrenoreceptor blockers, 846
bladder outflow obstruction, 1468
BPH, 1464
Adson forceps, 1562
Advance Decisions, 173
Advanced Trauma Life Support (ATLS), 312, 322, *365*
advancement flaps, 641, *642*
anal, 1353, 1370
adverse events, reporting, 181–2
aerobic glycolysis (Warburg effect), 142
inhibitors, *158*
Afghanistan war, 426
aflatoxins, *146*
aflibercept, *158*
agenesis, renal, 1399
AIDS
ENT system, 738
gastritis, 1116
intestinal complications, 1249, 1273
proctitis, 1325
see also HIV infection
aircraft
conflict zones, 425
major disasters, 411
air cysts (bullae), lungs, 937
air embolism, 956
air enema, 129
airway
burns, 618, 620–1
children, 120, 122
dysfunction in craniofacial anomalies, 687, 688
foreign body, 132
obstruction, 924–5
postoperative obstruction, 292
preoperative assessment, 261, *262*
airway management
burns patient, 620–1, *629*
cleft lip/palate, 691
emergency procedures, 744–9
general anaesthesia, 271–2
maxillofacial trauma, 323, 355, *356*
severe trauma, 323
alanine transaminase (ALT), 1155
albendazole, 63, 66, 1169
albumin, serum, 7, 279
Alcock's canal, 1319
alcohol use
and acute pancreatitis, 1222
associated cancers, *145*, 760, 1086
and chronic pancreatitis, 1230
and hepatocellular carcinoma, 1173
aldosterone, 9, 839
aldosterone:cortisol ratio (ACR), 841
alemtuzumab, *157*
alfuzosin, 1468
alimentary tract, duplications, 136
alkali burns, *622*, 631–2
oesophagus, 1075–6
alkaline encrusting cystitis, 1443
alkaline phosphatase (ALP), 826, 1155, 1471
alkalosis, 128, 1130
Allen's test, 443, *444*, 890
allergies, 1017, 1361
Allis forceps, 1562
Allison hiatus hernia repair, *1079*
allografts, 649–50
rejection, 1533–7
allopurinol, 1407
alpha fetoprotein (AFP), 483, 667, 1506, 1508
ALPPS procedure, 1172
Altemeier's procedure, 1323
Alvarado score, *1307*
alveolar bone grafting, 698–9
Alzheimer's disease, 1459
amaurosis fugax, 954–5
amazia, 865
American Cancer Society (AJCC) cancer staging, 148, *149*
American Society of Anaesthesiologists (ASA) scoring system, 263, *264*
American Spinal Injury Association (ASIA), spinal injury evaluation, 341, *342*
aminoglycosides, 56
aminosalicylates, 1245
5-aminosalicylic acid (5-ASA), 1245, 1269, 1324
amoebiasis, 57–60, 1272–3
colonic ulcers, 1272
intestinal, 1272–3
liver abscess, 58, 1169
pathogenesis, 57–8
treatment, 59–60
amoeboma, 58, 60, 1272
amoxicillin, 56, 1009
ampicillin, 56
AMPLE mnemonic, 381
ampulla of Vater, 1188, 1207, 1213, *1214*
adenoma, 1234
carcinoma, 1234, *1235*, 1236, 1237
amputation, 957–60
above knee, 957, 959
below knee, 957, 958–9
blast trauma, 432
complications, 960
diabetic foot, 559
distal, 957
mycetoma, 74, *75*
phantom limb pain, 276
postoperative care, 959–60
through knee, 959
transmetatarsal, 957
amylase, serum, 77, 1051, 1214, 1223, 1228
anaemia
haemolytic, 1183–4
preoperative management, 258–9
anaesthesia
day case surgery, 304
ground rules, *270*
history, 269
intravenous agents, *269*
local, 273–5
minimising myocardial ischaemia, 265
monitoring, 273
muscle relaxation, 272, *273*
perivenous tumescent, 978
preparation, 270
rapid sequence induction, 270
total intravenous (TIVA), 270
ventilation, 272–3, 1563
anaesthetist, role of, 269
anal advancement flap, 1353
anal canal
anatomy, 1339–40
blood supply, 1341
congenital abnormalities, 1345–7
embryology, 1344–5
epithelium and subepithelial structures, 1340–1
examination, 1342–3
injuries, 1321
lymphatic drainage, 1341
malignant tumours, *155*, 1371–2
venous drainage, 1341
anal cancer, *155*, 1371–2
anal continence, 1343–4
anal dilatation, 1356, 1370
anal fissure, 1351–3
analgesia
after laparoscopic surgery, 115
burns, 626
chronic pancreatitis, *1231*
day case surgery, 304, *305*
end-of-life care, 173
lung resection, 933–4
lymphoedema, 1008, 1009
peritonitis, 1052
sports injuries, 470
thoracotomy, 931
anal glands, 1342
infection, 1362
anal hypertonia, 1355
anal incontinence, 1349–51
after haemorrhoid treatment, 1360
assessment, 1344
causes, 1349
treatment, 1349–51
anal intraepithelial neoplasia (AIN), 1368–9
anal papillae, hypertrophy, 1353
anal sphincters
artificial, 1350, *1351*
assessment, 1344, *1345*
augmentation, 1350–1
examination, 1343
external, 1319, 1339
internal, 1340
spasm, 1369
internal sphincterotomy, 1352–3
intersphincteric plane, 1340
repair, 1349–50
anal stenosis, benign, 1369–70

anal stricture, benign, 1360, 1369–70, *1371*
anal veins, 1341
anal warts, 1368
anaphylaxis, 13
anaplastic carcinoma, thyroid, *816*, 817, 820
anastomoses
 bowel, 97–9
 laparoscopic, 99
 oesophagogastric, 1093
 stapling devices, 96
 vascular, 99
anastrozole, *156*, 878, 1516
Anderson–Hynes pyeloplasty, 1412–13
androgen ablation, *156*, 1473, 1474
androgenic hormones, 1457
androgen insensitivity syndrome (testicular feminisation), 124
aneurysmal bone cyst, 541, *542*
aneurysms
 abdominal aorta, *see* abdominal aortic aneurysm
 classification, 960
 clinical features, 960
 ectactic, 960
 femoral artery, 966
 hepatic artery, 1163, *1163*
 iliac artery, 966
 intracranial, 658–9, 1403
 popliteal artery, 966
 splenic artery, 1179, *1180*
 thoracic aorta, 908–9
angina, 257, 889
angiodysplasia, 1276
angioectasia, colon, 231
angioembolisation, 209, *319*, 365, 378
angioendothelioma, malignant (angiosarcoma), 615
angiofibroma
 juvenile, 719
 nasopharynx, 733
angiogenesis, tumours, 140
angiography
 arteriovenous malformation, 661, 662
 liver disease, 1159
 parathyroid, 828
 pelvic injuries, *319*
 subarachnoid haemorrhage, 659, 660
 upper GI tract, 1113
angioma
 kidney, 1416
 venous, 993, *994*
angiomyolipoma (AML), 1385, *1386*, 1416
angiosarcoma, *146*, 615
angiosomes, 593, *594*
angiotensin I/II, 839
angular deformities, knee, 454
ankle
 anatomy, 524
 clinical examination, 457–62
 fractures, 401–2
 fusion (arthrodesis), 528
 instability, 460–1, 530
 movements, 458–9, 524
 osteochondral lesions, 531
 reconstructive surgery, *645*
 rheumatological disease, 529
 sports injuries, 468
 sprains, 468
 synovitis, 531
 total replacement (TAR), 528
ankle–brachial pressure index (ABPI)
 arterial disease, 945–6, *947*
 lymphoedema, 1009
 venous ulcers, 985
ankylosing spondylitis, 261, 481
 spinal fractures, 348
 spinal surgery, 481, *482*
ankylosis, elbow, *499*
annuloplasty, 898, 899
anoderm, 1340–1
anoplasty
 anal stricture, 1370
 imperforate anus, 1346
anorectal abscesses, 1362–3
anorectal malformations, 136–7, 1345–7
anorectal ring, 1339
anosmia, 664
antalgic gait, *437*, *453*
antenatal diagnosis, cleft lip and palate, 691
anterior (accessory) saphenous vein (ASV), 969–70
anterior cruciate ligament (ACL), 454, 455, *518*, 519
 injuries, 520–1
 reconstruction, 521
anterior draw test
 ankle stability, 461
 knee stability, 455, *456*
anterolateral thigh (ALT) flap, 769, 771, *774*
anthropometry, 279–80
antibiotic prophylaxis, 53
 acute severe pancreatitis, 1225
 cholecystecomy, 1202
 colorectal surgery, 1263–4
 gastrointestinal endoscopy, 219–20
 heart valve surgery, 896
 rectal cancer surgery, 1334
 splenectomy, 1187
antibiotics
 acute osteomyelitis, 556
 appendicitis, 1308
 causing urine discolouration, 1376
 Crohn's disease, 1245
 gallstone disease, 1200
 gas gangrene, 420
 H. pylori eradication, 1114
 intestinal obstruction, 1290
 lower urinary tract infections, 1442
 lymphoedema, 1009
 military wounds, 433
 MRSA, 44
 necrotising fasciitis, 419
 osteomyelitis, 552
 ototoxicity, 714
 pelvic inflammatory disease, *1520*
 peritonitis, 1049, 1052, 1053
 prostatitis, 1475
 septic arthritis, 554, 586–7
 surgical infections, 55–6
 torso trauma, 380
antibodies, cell surface antigens, *157*
antibody therapies, immunosuppression, 1539–40
anti-CD20 antibody (rituximab), *157*, 1540
anticholinergic agents, 1433
anticoagulants
 DVT management, 990
 'novel', 990
anticoagulation
 day case surgery, 304
 endoscopy patients, 220–1
 heart valve surgery, 896
 preoperative, 258, 260–1
anticonvulsants, 261, 276
antidiuretic hormone (ADH/ vasopressin), 9, 13
antiepileptic drugs, brain tumours, 663
antigen presenting cells, 1534, *1535*
anti-motility drugs, 284
antipituitary hormone drugs, 277
antiplatelet drugs
 endoscopy, 220–1
 peripheral arterial disease, 948
 preoperative withdrawal, 261
anti-tetanus globulin (ATG), 417–18
antithyroid drugs, 812, 815
antrectomy, 1080, 1123
antrochoanal polyp, 733
anus, imperforate, 136–7, 1345–7
AO (Arbeitsgemeinschaft für Osteosynthesefragen) classification, 349, 386–7
aorta
 cannulation, 884–5
 dissection, 909–11
 thoracic, rupture, 366, 369–70
aortic aneurysms
 abdominal, *see* abdominal aortic aneurysm
 thoracic, 908–9
aortic bifurcation, embolus, 954
aortic coarctation, 906
aortic enteric fistula, 966, 1129
aortic pulsations, 1020
aortic valve
 anatomy, 894
 replacement, 902
 transcatheter implantation (TAVI), 902
aortic valve disease, 899–902
 regurgitation, 900–2
 stenosis, 899–900
aortofemoral bypass, 949, 950–1
aortoiliac occlusion, 943, *944*
 reconstructive surgery, 949, 950–1
Apert syndrome, *687*, 689, 701
Apfel score, *299*
apical ectodermal ridge, 561
apixaban, 990
apocrine glands, 593
apoptosis, 242
 cancer cell evasion, 140, 249
 inducers of, *157*, *158*
appendicectomy
 children, 130
 conventional, 1309–10
 laparoscopic, 1309, 1311–12
 postoperative complications, 1313–14
 problems encountered during, 1312
 retrograde, 1311
appendices epiploicae, 1258
appendicitis
 acute, 1301–8
  aetiology, 1301–2
  clinical diagnosis, 1302–3
  differential diagnosis, 1304–7
  investigation, *21*, 211, 1307, *1308*
  non-operative management, 1308
  pathology, 1302
  special features, 1304
  surgery, *see* appendicectomy
 children, 130
 diagnosis, 211, *212*
 gangrenous, 1302, 1304
 investigation, 1307, *1308*
 peritonitis in, 1302, 1308
 recurrent acute, 1314
 role of omentum, 1061
 scoring systems, 1307
appendicolith (faecolith), 1301–2
appendicostomy, antegrade colonic enema, 137
appendicular artery, 1300
appendix
 abscess, 1312
 'absent', 1312
 anatomy, 1299–300, 1304
 carcinoid tumours, 1315
 epithelial tumours, 1315–17
 mass, 1312–13
 mesentery (mesoappendix), 1300, 1301
 microscopic anatomy, 1300–1
 pelvic, *1299*, 1304
 postileal, *1299*, 1304
 retrocaecal, *1299*, 1304
appendix testis (hydatid of Morgagni), 126, 1376, 1500
apprehension test
 patellar, 456–7
 shoulder instability, 450, 496
aprotinin, 1225
aqueous humour, 673
arachnoid cyst, 667
arcade of Struthers, 501
areola, 860
aresenic trioxide, *157*
argentaffin (Kulchitsky) cells, 1300, 1315

argentaffinoma, 1315
argon plasma coagulation (APC), 231, 1171
Arnold–Chiari malformation, 484, 668
aromatase inhibitors, *156*, 878, 1516
arrhythmias
  after CABG, 891
  postoperative, 294
  preoperative management, 258, 265
arterial blood gases, 256, 918
arterial bruit, 944
arterial dissection
  aorta, 909–11
  cerebral, 336
arterial injuries
  neck, 756
  thoracic aorta, 366, 369–70
arterial stenosis/occlusion
  acute, 953–6
  chronic, 942–52
arteriotomy, closure, 99
arteriovenous fistula, 966–7
arteriovenous malformations (AVMs), 658, 661–2
arteritis, 967–8
  temporal, 683, 967
arthritis
  sexually-acquired reactive (Reiter's disease), 681, 1494–5
  in ulcerative colitis, 1267
  see also osteoarthritis; rheumatoid arthritis; septic arthritis
arthrodesis
  ankle, 528
  elbow, 499
  hand joints, 505, 506
  hip, 515
  knee, 521
  shoulder, 495
arthrography, MRI, 201–2, 496, *497*
arthrogryposis multiplex congenita (AMC), 564
arthroplasty
  extremity fractures, 393–4
  joint infection following, 554–6
  see also hip replacement; knee replacement; shoulder replacement
arthroscopy
  hip, 515
  knee, 521
  shoulder, *491*
articles
  analysis, 167–8
  publishing, 168
articular cartilage, imaging, 201–2
artificial limb, 960
asbestos exposure, *146*, 922
ascariasis, 60–2
  bile/pancreatic ducts, 60, *61*, 62, 1205, 1207
  intestinal obstruction, 60–1, 1282–3
  treatment, 61–2
ascites, 1057–9, 1166
  chronic liver disease, 1058, 1166
  chylous, 1003, 1013, 1059
  clinical features, 1058
  congestive heart failure, 1058
  investigation, 1058
  pancreatic, 1228
  pathophysiology, 1057
  treatment, 1058–9, 1166
ASEPSIS wound score, *48*
aseptic surgery, 43
Ashkenazi Jewish populations, 880–1, 1241
asiatic cholangiohepatitis, 62–3, 1207
aspartate transaminase (AST), 1155
aspirin, *158*, 221
  preoperative withdrawal, 261
assisted conception, 1512
Aster–Coller staging, *149*
asthma, 259
astrocytomas, 664–5
ataxia–telangiectasia, *145*
ataxic gait, *437*
atelectasis, *293*
atherosclerosis, 887
  carotid stenosis, 951–2
  mesenteric/coeliac vessels, 1254
  peripheral arterial disease, 945, 947
Atlanta classification, acute pancreatitis, 1223
atlantoaxial instability, 346
atlantoaxial ligaments, *339*
atlantoaxial subluxation (AAS), 481
atlas
  anatomy, *338*
  fractures, 346
atracurium, *273*
atresia
  biliary, 135–6, 1196–7
  duodenal, 133–4, 1293–4
  oesophageal, 133
atrial fibrillation, 258, 265
atrial flutter, *258*
atrial myxoma, 911–12
atrial septal defect (ASD), 905, 907
  closure, 907
  types, 907
atrophie blanche, 973
attorney, power of, 173
audiometry, 705–6, 712–13
  evoked-response, 712
audit, clinical, 161–2, 175, 185–6
Auerbach's plexus, 1067, 1095, 1107, 1296–7
auscultation, abdomen, 1021
autoantibodies, thyroid, 802–3, 808
autocannibalism, 8–9
autoimmune disease
  gastritis, 1115
  oesophagus, 1100–1
  pancreatitis, 1230
  thyroiditis, 821–2
autoimmune haemolytic anaemia, acquired, 1183
autonomic dysreflexia, 354
autonomy, patients, 170–1
autopsy, 251
avascular necrosis (AVN)
  carpal bones, 508–9
  femoral head, 512–13, *571*
  osteochondroses showing radiographic appearance of, *571*, *572*
  proximal femoral epiphysis (Legg–Calvé–Perthes disease), 571–3
axillary artery, cannulation, 885
axillary lymph nodes, 860–1
axillary nerve, injury, 448
axillary vein
  compression, 991–2
  thrombosis, 992
axiltinib, *156*
axis
  anatomy, *338*
  odontoid fractures, 346–7
  traumatic spondylolisthesis (hangman's fracture), 347, *348*
axonotmesis, 385
Ayurvedic method, 1367
azathioprine, 1245, 1269, 1532, *1538*, 1539

Babcock's forceps, *1229*, 1310, 1562
Babinski response, 473
Bacille Calmette–Guérin (BCG), intravesical, 1447, 1448, 1450
Bacillus fusiformis, 1325
back pain
  children, 583
  epidemiology, 471
  investigations, 474
  malignancy, 544–5
  non-spinal causes, *472*
  patient history, 472
  physical examination, 472–3
  red flags, *472*, *583*
backslab, 390
bacteraemia, 50–1, 53, *54*
  after prostatectomy, 1466
  GI endoscopy, 219
bacteria, large intestinal flora, 46–7, 1048–9
bacterial infections
  biliary tract, 1168
  lower urinary tract, 1441–2
  mastitis, 866–7
  peritonitis, 1049, 1053
  sialadenitis, 786
  surgical, 44–7
  see also named bacteria
bacterial overgrowth, 1255–6
bacterial translocation, 46–7, 288
bacterial virulence factors, 1441
Bacteroides spp., 45, 50, 56, 1049
β-adrenergic blocking drugs, thyrotoxicosis, 813, 815
Baker's cyst, 989
balance disorders, 714–15
balanitis xerotica obliterans (BXO), 127, 1377, 1482, 1486, *1487*
balanoposthitis, 127, 1489
Balkan nephropathy, 1446
ballet dancers, injuries, 466
ballistic injuries, 315, 428
  see also gunshot wounds
ballistics, 427–8
balloon catheter, percutaneous transluminal angioplasty, 948–9
balloon dilatation, achalasia, 1098
balloon tamponade, oesophageal varices, 1164
bandaging, four-layer system, 984–5
banding, haemorrhoids, 1356, *1357*
band ligation
  mucohaemorrhoidal prolapse, 1322
  oesophageal varices, 222, 1164
bands, intestinal obstruction, 1283
Bankart's lesion, 496, *497*
BAP1 mutant disease, *1418*
Barcelona Clinic Liver Group staging system, 1174, *1174*
barefoot walking, 1005
bariatric surgery
  complications, 1150–1
  cost effectiveness, 1145–6
  eligibility criteria, 1146
  follow-up, 1151
  laparoscopic, 1147
  'metabolic/diabetes' surgery, 1145
  outcomes, 1145, 1151
  rationale, 1145
  RCTs, 1145, 1147
  service setup, 1146–7
  types of operation, 1147–50
barium enema
  amoebiasis, 59
  caecal volvulus, 1290
  colorectal cancer, 1263
  Hirschsprung's disease, 136
barium studies
  peptic ulcers, *1117*, *1118*
  radiation doses, *192*
  roundworm infestation, 60, *61*
  small bowel obstruction, *193*
  tuberculosis, 80
barium swallow, 730, *1068*
  achalasia, 1097–8
  pharyngeal pouch, 739
Barlow test, 568
barotrauma, oesophagus, 1072–3
Barrett's oesophagus, 221, 224, 233, 241–2, 1077, 1081–3, 1087
Barron's banding, 1356, *1357*

basal cell carcinoma (BCC), 604–5, *616*
eyelids, 674
basal cell naevus (Gorlin) syndrome, *145*, 595
basal cell papilloma (seborrhoeic keratosis), 599
Bascom's technique, 1348
base deficit, 17
basketball, 466
Bassini's operation, 1032
Batson's venous plexus, 537
batteries, ingestion, 132, 1072
Battle's sign, 332, 333
β-catenin protein, 1329
B-cell lymphomas, 1251
Beahrs' triangle, 802
bed sores, 953
see also pressure sores
beetroot, urine discolouration, 1376
Beger procedure, 1227, 1232
Behçet's disease, 681
Bell's palsy, 715
Belsey mark IV operation, *1079*
Bence Jones proteins, 545
benign paroxysmal positional vertigo, 714
benign prostatic hyperplasia (BPH), 1456, 1458–60
assessment, 1461–2
bladder outlet obstruction, 1459–60, *1461*
indications for prostatectomy, 1463
LUTS, 1459
management, 1463–7
Bentall's operation, 909
benzodiazepines, *219*, 1111
benzpyrones, 1011
benzylpenicillin, 56
Berry's ligament, 802, 813
best practice, 186
beta-thalassaemia, 1183
betel nut, 760
bevacizumab, *157*, *158*, 1420
bias, clinical studies, 164–5
bicalutamide, *156*, 1474
bicarbonate (HCO_3), in GI secretions, *281*
biceps muscle
injuries, 469
long head rupture, 469, 495–6
Bier's block, 275, 632
bile, 1155, 1189, 1190
vomiting, 1123
in children, 128, 134
bile ducts, 1188, *1189*
benign tumours, 1207–8
cancer (cholangiocarcinoma), 1167, 1208–9
dilation, 1157–8
injuries, 184, 1203–4
stones, 228, 1204–5, *1206*, *1216*
stricture
after cholecystectomy, 1204
after liver trauma, 1163
benign, 1206
investigation, *1206*
malignant, 1208, 1209
bile peritonitis, 1052, *1053*
bile salts, 283, 1241
bilharziasis, *see* schistosomiasis
biliary atresia, 135–6, 1196–7
classification, 1196, *1197*
clinical features, 1196
treatment, 1197
biliary colic, 1017, 1018–19
imaging, 212–13
biliary dilatation, 228
biliary tract
anatomy, 1188–9
ascending bacterial infection, 1168
congenital abnormalities, 1168, 1195–8
cystic disease, 1197–8
imaging, 1190–5
intraoperative, 1194–5
injuries
classification, *1204*
iatrogenic, 184, 1203–4
traumatic, 374
tumours, 1207–11
biliopancreatic diversion (BPD), *1147*, 1149
bilirubin, 1155, 1206
Billroth I gastrectomy, 1120, 1123
Billroth II gastrectomy, 1118, 1120–1, 1221
bimanual examination, bladder cancer, 1449
bimaxillary osteotomy, 701, *702*
Biobrane®, 630
bioelectrical impedence analysis (BIA), 280
bioengineering, 650
see also tissue engineering
biofeedback, constipation, 1279
biofilm, 550
biological dressings, 985
biomarkers, bone and joint infection, 550
biomedical scientists (BMSs), 236
biopsy
bone, 545–6
breast, 862–3
endometrium, 1516
lung, 928–9, 930
prostate, 1385, 1387, 1470–1
rectal (amoebiasis), *1272*
sentinel node
breast cancer, 877
malignant melanoma, 612
thyroid, 809
bipolar electrosurgery devices, 104
birthmarks, 613
Birt–Hogg–Dubé syndrome, *1418*
birth order, and hip dysplasia, 567
Bismuth–Corlette classification, cholangiocarcinoma, 1209, *1210*
bisphosphonates, 485, 567, 826, 831
bite wounds, 27, 138, 363
bivalirudin, 990
Bjork flap, 745–6
BK virus, 1541
β-lactamases, 43, 44, 56
extended spectrum, 43, 45
bladder
anatomy, 1423
calculi, 1383, 1434–6
cystoscopy, 1379–85
denervation, 1434
descent through inguinal/femoral hernia, 1030, 1438
diverticulae, *1384*, 1436–8
endometriosis, 1452
exstrophy, 1424–5, *1453*
foreign bodies, 1434, *1435*, 1436
function assessment, 1395–7
innervation, 1423–4
neck, disorders causing obstruction, 1467–8
neuropathic, 1428–9
in children, 131
normal cystoscopy, *1382*
overactivity, 1429–30, 1432, 1460
treatment, 1433
urodynamics, 1396, *1397*
pain, 1374
papillary tumours, *1384*, 1445, *1446*
reconstruction, 1453–4
removal (cystectomy), 1451–2
schistosomiasis, 1443–5
small capacity, 1430, 1433
substitution/augmentations procedures, 1433–4, 1443, 1454
trauma, 375–6, 1425–6, 1466, 1481
wall trabeculation, 1383
bladder cancer, 1446–55
adenocarcinoma, 1448
causes, *146*
chemotherapy and biological agents, *155*
clinical features, 1448–9
imaging, *194*
in situ carcinoma, 1448
investigation, 1449, *1450*
muscle-invasive, 1448
treatment, 1451–2
non-muscle invasive, 1447–8
treatment, 1450–1
squamous cell carcinoma, 1448
staging and grading, 1447
treatment, 1450–2
urinary diversion, 1452–5
urothelial cell carcinoma, 1446–7
bladder outflow obstruction (BOO)
flow rate assessment, 1395, *1396*
male, 1459–60
bladder neck pathology, 1467–8
in BPH, 1458–9, 1463–7
urodynamic studies, 1396, *1397*, 1430, *1431*, 1460, 1462
blast, 429–30
blast injuries, 430–3
blast lung, 430
bleeding
gastrointestinal, in endoscopy, 220
punctate, *635*
bleomycin, *155*
blind loop syndrome, 1255–6
blisters, burn wounds, 631
Blom–Singer valve, *753*
blood
autologous, 21
donation, 20
viscosity, 945
blood clots, evacuation, 114
blood gases, 256, 918
blood groups, 21–2
organ transplantation, 1533, 1547–8
blood loss
classification, 19
see also haemorrhage
blood pressure
postoperative, 293–4
shock, *14*, 15
trauma, 323–4
see also hypertension; hypotension
blood products, 20–1
blood substitutes, 23
blood tests
extremity trauma, 384
oesophageal cancer, 1089
peritonitis, 1051
preoperative, 256
prostate cancer, 1471
urinary disorders, 1377–9
blood transfusion, 20–3
blood/blood products, 20–1
complications, 22–3
history of, *20*
indications for, 21
massive, 427
preoperative, 258–9
transfusion reactions, 22
blood volume, 19
Bloom syndrome, *145*
Blount's disease, 576
blue naevus, 601, *602*
blunt trauma, 314–15, 1061
diaphragm, 370
liver, 1161
renal, 1413–14
Boari operation, 1415
body composition, after injury/critical illness, 8–9
body mass index (BMI), 260
calculator, *303*
and day surgery, 303–4
and nutritional status, 279
obesity, 1144
thresholds for bariatric surgery, 1146
body proportions, at various ages, *316*

body temperature
after trauma, 317
children, 119–20
postoperative, 299
body weight, children, *120*
Boerhaave's syndrome, 1072–3, 1075
bolus obstruction, intestines, 1282
bone, biopsy, 545–6
bone cyst
aneurysmal, 541, *542*
simple, 541, 546
bone disease
aggressive, 202–3
metabolic, 205, 485
bone grafting
alveolar, 698–9
oral cavity cancers, 771, 773, 774, *774–5*
bone healing, 25, 388, 394
direct, 388
indirect, 388
pathological fractures, 548
bone metastases, 537, 547–8
breast cancer, *534*, 881
common sites of, *538*
pathological fracture, 407
prostate cancer, 1382, *1383–4*, 1471–2, 1474
scintigraphy, *199*
thyroid carcinoma, *817*
treatment, 547–8
tumours commonly metastasising, *534*
bone mineral density, 205, 474, 825, 833
bone-morphogenetic protein-4 (BMP4), 37
bone remodelling, 388
bone scans, 474
hyperparathyroidism, 825, 833
metabolic bone disease, 205
prostate cancer, 1392, *1393–4*, 1472
spinal osteoblastoma, 480
bone tumours, 535–44
chondrogenic, 539–41
classification, 535
classification by site, *542*
evaluation and investigation, 544–6
giant cell, 541, *542*
osteogenic, 538–9
pathological fractures, 406–7
spine, 480
staging, 543
treatment, 546–7
boretezomib, *156*
Bosniak classification (renal cysts), 1389–90
botulinum toxin
anal fissure, 1352
cerebral palsy, 585
detrusor overactivity, 1432
lower oesophageal sphincter, 223, 1099
sphincter of Oddi, 1233
Bouchard's nodes, *443*, 506
Bourneville disease (adenoma sebaceum), 602–3
boutonnière deformity, *443*, *504*
bowel anastomoses, 97–9
extramucosal technique, 97–8
two-layer technique, 97, 98
bowel habit alteration
colorectal cancers, 1262, 1319, 1329
inflammatory bowel disease, 1017
bowel injury, blast, 431
bowel preparation, 98, 1263, 1334
bowel sounds, 1021
intestinal obstruction, 1286
Bowen's disease, 606, 607, 1492
bow legs, 563, 576
boxing injuries, 469
brachial plexopathy, neonatal, 586
brachial plexus block, 274
brachycephaly, 668
brachytherapy
oesophageal cancer, 1095
prostate cancer, 1473
bradycardia, 294
B-RAF protein, 612
brain abscess, 656–7
brain death, 671, 1543
brain herniation, 328–9, 331, 333
brain injury
deaths, 364
minor/mild, 329–30
moderate and severe, 330–7
timeline of management, 312, *313*
brain tumours, 663–7
aetiology, 662, 663
chemotherapy and biological agents, *155–6*
in children, 667
classification, 662, *663*
glioma, 664–5
meningioma, 665
metastatic, 663, 664, 665
pituitary, 664, 665–7
presentation, 662–3, 664
branchial cyst, 753–4
branchial fistula, 754
BRCA1; *BRCA2* genes, *144*, 880–1, 1528
breast
aberrations of normal development and involution (ANDI), 868–9
abscesses, 866–7
actinomycosis, 867
anatomy, 860–1
changes throughout life, 868
congenital abnormalities, 865
cysts, *861*, 868, 869
diffuse hypertrophy, 865
duct excision, 865, 868
fibroadenoma, 868, 870
fistula, 867, 868
galactocoele, 869
inflammatory, 866–8
injuries, 866
investigation of symptoms, 861–3, *871*
lumps, 863, 869
male, disorders of, 69–70, 871, 882, 1507
needle biopsy/cytology, 862–3
nipple disorders, 863–5, 873
pain (mastalgia), 869
phyllodes tumour, 870
reconstruction, 879–80
sarcoma, 882
tuberculosis, 867
breast carcinoma, 871–81
aetiological factors, 871–2
clinical presentation, 873–4
diagnosis, 861–3
ductal, 872
familial, *144*, 880–1
follow-up, 879
genetics, *144*, 871, 880–1
Her2-positive, 249, 872, 878
and HRT, 871, 881
inflammatory, 872
in situ, 872–3
lobular, 872
local spread, 873
lymphoedema, 879, 1005
male breast, 871, 882
metastases, *534*, 548, 873, 881, 882
oestrogen receptor status, 872
pathology, 872–3
phenomena of lymphatic obstruction, 879
and pregnancy, 881
prognosis, 875
risk in benign disease, 871
screening, 880
sentinel node biopsy, 877
staging, 874, *875*
treatment, 875–9
adjuvant systemic therapy, *155–7*, 877–9
advanced disease, 881
costs, *158*
multidisciplinary team, 875
radiotherapy, 877
surgery, 875–7
breastfeeding, 871
breathing, mechanics, 914–15
breech presentation, 567
Breslow thickness, 611, 612
bridge plating, *393*
British Association for Parenteral and Enteral Nutrition, 280
British Journal of Surgery (BJS), 168
British Obesity and Metabolic Surgery Society (BOMSS), 1145, *1151*
British Society of Gastroenterology, 218
brittle bone disease, 566–7
Brodie's abscess, 589
bromocriptine, *156*, 869
bronchial tree, anatomy, 914, *915*
bronchiectasis, 936
bronchioalveolar carcinoma (BAC), 925
bronchodilators, 266
bronchogenic cyst, 936
bronchoplastic lung resection, 933
bronchopleural fistula, 933
bronchoscope, fibreoptic intubating, 271, *272*
bronchoscopy, 923–4
flexible, 923, *924*
lung cancer, 928
oesophageal cancer, 1089
rigid, 924
Brown Kelly syndrome, 740
Brown-Sequard syndrome, 353
brown tumours, 825
Brugia spp., 63
bruising, periorbital, 332, 359, 362
bruits
aortic and iliac, 1021
arterial, 1021
Brunner's glands, 1108, 1141
buccal mucosa, squamous cell carcinoma, 772
Budd–Chiari syndrome, 991, 1057, 1058, *1156*, 1166–7
Buerger's disease, 967, 990
bullae, lungs, 937
bunion, 458, 525
bupivacaine, *273*
buprenorphine, 276
Burhenne technique, 1205, *1206*
Burkitt's lymphoma, 1251
burns
airway and respiratory injury, 617, 618, 620–1
analgesia, 626
assessment, 621–2
causes and likely depth, *622*
chemical, 631–2, 679–80
children, 624
circumferential, 619, 624–5
contamination, 625
contractures, 32
depth, 622, *623*
diathermy, 103
dressings, 625–6
electrical, 631, *632*
extent, 619, 621
eye, 679–80
fluid resuscitation, 622–4
healing, 630–1
immediate care, 620–1, 628
incidence, 617
infection, 627, 630–1
inflammatory and circulatory changes, 618–19
metabolic poisoning, 618, 621
minor/outpatient, 628, 630
nursing care, 627
nutritional support, 626–7
psychological impacts, 627
radiation, 632
surgery for acute, 627–8, *629–30*
treatment, 624–6
burns unit, admission criteria, *620*

Burow's triangles, 641, *642*
bursae, sports injuries, 464
bursitis, olecranon, 500–1
burst fractures
cervical, 348
decompression, *345*
lumbar spine, *345*, *350*
Busche–Löwenstein tumour, 1368, 1493
buserelin, *156*
business performance methodology, 187–8
buttocks, strapping, 1361
button batteries, ingestion, 132, 1072

CA 19-9, 1167, 1208, 1211, 1235
CA-125, 1527, 1528, 1529
cABCDE protocol, 323–6
cabergoline, *156*
caecocystoplasty, 1443
caecum, 1258, 1259, 1299–300
carcinoma, *1262*, 1264, 1306
volvulus, 1288, 1289–90, 1295
café-au-lait spots, 595, 596, 600
Caisson disease, 512
calcaneonavicular bar, *563*
calcaneus, fractures, 208, 402
calcimimetics, 831, 834, 835
calcineurin inhibitors (CNI), 1538–9, 1540
calciphylaxis, 833–4
calcitonin, 802, 825, 826, 845
medullary thyroid carcinoma, 820
calcium
daily requirements, 281
homeostasis, 824–5
soft-tissue deposits, 833
supplementation, 831
see also hypercalcaemia; hypocalcaemia
calcium channel antagonists, 967, 1099
calcium receptor gene (*CAST*), 832
calcium sensing receptor (CaR), extracellular, 831
calculi
bladder, *1383*, 1434–6
pancreatic duct, *1216*, *1217*, 1231–2
parotid gland, 787
preputial, 1489
prostatic, 1468
renal, *see* renal calculi
submandibular salivary glands, 780–1
urethral, 1484
calf muscle pump, 971
Calne, Sir Roy York, 1533
calorie requirements, 282
Calot's triangle, 1188, *1189*
dissection, 1202, 1203
Campbell de Morgan spots, 613, *614*
camptodactyly, 580
Campylobacter jejuni, 1248, 1272
canal of Nuck, 1503
cancer
bone, 202–3
causes, 143
diagnosis and classification, 147–8
environmental causes, *145*–6
gene changes, 249
histological diagnosis, 238–41
inherited syndromes associated with, *144*–5
non-surgical treatment, 150–4
pain management, 276–7
'precision medicine', 251
prevention, 143, 146
radiation-induced, *145*, 191
screening, 146–7
staging, 148, *149*, 213, 251
tumour growth, 142–3
see also named cancers; tumours
cancer cells, 139–42
dissemination and implantation, 141
cancer-en-cuirasse, 873–4, 879
cancer management, 143
end-of-life care, 159
multidisciplinary teams, 148, *149*
palliative therapy, 150, 158–9
cancer surgery
metastatic disease, 150
primary disease, 150
principles, 148–50
candidiasis
chronic hyperplastic, 763
oesophageal, 1103–4
Cantlie's line, 1155
capacitance coupling, 103
capacity, 173, 267
capecitabine, *155*
capillaries, lymphatic, 995–6
capillary haemangioma, 613
orbit, 676
capillary pressure, 1057
capillary refill time, 14, 943–4
capillary vascular malformations, 613
capitellum, osteochondritis dissecans, *500*
capsule endoscopy, 226–7, 1244
carbapenems, 56
carbimazole, 812, 813, 815
carbohydrate, daily requirements, 282
carbon monoxide toxicity, 618
carboplatin, *155*
carboxyhaemoglobin, 618, 621
carbuncle, renal, 1404
carcinoembryonic antigen (CEA), 1172, 1228, 1266
carcinogens, urothelial, 1446
carcinoid syndrome, 854, 855, 1251
carcinoid tumours
appendix, 1315
pancreas, 849
small bowel, 853, 1250–1
stomach, 1130
carcinoma, histology, 239, 240
carcinomatosis peritonei, 1059
cardiac arrest, after cardiac surgery, 912–13
cardiac failure
ascites, 1058
high-risk patients, 265
cardiac isoenzymes, 888
cardiac massage, internal, 912–13
cardiac output
after cardiac surgery, 892
aortic stenosis, 900
monitoring, 17
shock, *14*
cardiac surgery
cardiac arrest following, 912–13
valvular heart disease, 894–5
see also coronary artery bypass grafting
cardiac tamponade, 123, 367–8, 911
cardiectomy, transplant recipient, 1556, *1557*
cardiogenic shock, 13
cardioplegic solutions, 885
cardiopulmonary bypass circuit, 895
cardiopulmonary bypass (CPB), 884–6
cardiopulmonary resuscitation (CPR), and emergency thoracotomy, 371
cardiopulmonry exercise testing, 257, 264–5, 888
cardiovascular disease, preoperative management, 256–8
cardiovascular system complications, 293–4
Carney complex, 911
Caroli's disease, 1168, 1197
carotid arteries, injuries, 756
carotid artery stenosis, 662, 946, 951–2
carotid body tumour (chemodectoma), 711, 757–8
carotid cavernous fistula, 661–2
carotid duplex scan, 265
carotid endarterectomy, 662, 951, *952*
indications, 265, 952
carpal bones
avascular necrosis, 508–9
fractures, 396–7
instability, 397
carpal tunnel syndrome, 508
Carpentier–Edwards annuloplasty, 898, 899
cartridge, structure, 427
caruncle, urethral, 1377, 1485–6
Casanova test, 833
case-controlled study, *164*
cassava (tapioca), 76, 1230
castration, medical, 1474
casts, 390–1
Sarmiento patella tendon below knee, 406
catabolism
burns patient, 626–7
post-trauma, 5–7, 279
cataract surgery, 683
catecholamines, 839
excess, 845
cationic trypsinogen gene (*PRSS1*), 1222, 1230
Catterall classification, 572
cauda equina, *340*
cauda equina syndrome, 475–6, 1428–9
cavernomas, 662
cavernous sinus thrombosis, 721
cavitron ultrasonic aspirator (CUSA), *1548*
CD4 T cells, 1534
ceftriaxone, *1520*
cell seeding techniques, 39–40
cell surface antigens, antibodies against, *157*
cellulitis, 48–9, 597
periorbital, 722
pinna, *707*
central venous access, 287
central venous pressure (CVP), 16
centre–edge (CE) angle, 571
cephalosporins, 56
cerebral blood flow (CBF), 328
cerebral contusions, 336
cerebral palsy, 584–5
classification, *584*
cerebral perfusion pressure (CPP), 328, *337*
cerebral vasospasm, 660
cerebritis, 656, *657*
cerebrospinal fluid (CSF)
analysis in SAH, 659
disorders of flow, 655
drainage, 654, 655
excessive production, 653, 655
flow pathways, 653
leaks, 362
rhinorrhoea, 717
volume, 653
cerium nitrate, 625
cervical canal, 1514
cervical cancer, *146*, 1516
chemotherapy and biological agents, *155*
cervical intraepithelial neoplasia (CIN), 1368, 1516
cervical lymphadenitis, tuberculosis, 77–8, 757
cervical lymph nodes, 800–1
anatomy, 728–9, 764
metastatic disease, 729, 764
resection, 758–9
cervical rib, 939, 952, 992
cervical smear specimen, 238
cervical spine
anatomy, 338–9, 338–40
clinical examination, 439–40
degenerative disorders, 474–5
immobilisation, 323, 340
injuries, 345–9
assessment, 340–2
associated with head injury, 332
functional outcomes, *353*

imaging, 342–4
management, 344–5
subaxial spine, 348, *349*
upper spine, 345–8
instability, 261
lordosis, 439, *440*, 471
movement, 440
nerve root entrapment, 440
stability, 339
cervical sympathectomy, 968
cervicothoracic junction injury, 338–9
cervix, anatomy, 1513, 1514
cetuximab, *157*, *158*
CFTR gene, 1216, 1230
Chagas' disease, 1095, 1104, *1298*
chalazion, *see* meibomian cyst
chalmoogra oil, 70
Chance fractures, 350–1
chancroid, 1496
Charcot foot, 528, 532–3
Charcot–Leyden crystals, 60
Charcot–Marie–Tooth disease, 458, 531
Charcot retaining orthotic walker (CROW), 533
Charcot's triad, 1168, 1205
Charles procedure, 1012
checklists, surgical safety, 182–4
cheilectomy, 527
chemical burns, 631–2, 679–80
oesophagus, 1075–6
chemicals
associated with bladder carcinoma, 1446
associated with cancers, *146*, 1208
chemodectoma (carotid body tumour), 711, 757–8
chemoradiotherapy
anal cancer, 1371
oesophageal cancer, 1094
pancreatic cancer, 1238–9
principles, 157–8
rectal cancer, 1337–8
chemotherapy, 154–8
adjuvant, 151–3
anal malignancy, 1371
bladder cancer, 1451
breast cancer, 878–9
classes of drugs, *155–7*
colorectal cancer, 1266
colorectal liver metastases, 1173
gastric cancer, 1139
neuroblastoma, 847
oesophageal cancer, 1093
ovarian cancer, *155*, 1529
pancreatic cancer, 1237, 1238
prostate cancer, 1474
rectal carcinoma, 1337–8
targeted, 154, *157–8*
renal cell carcinoma, 1420–1
Chernobyl nuclear disaster, 816
chest drain, 100, 920, *921*
pneumothorax, 919–20, *921*
post-pneumonectomy, 933
thoracotomy, 931
underwater sealed, 100, 366
chest pain, oesophageal disease, 1069, 1077
chest radiography
aortic disruption, *369*
aortic stenosis, 900
congenital diaphragmatic hernia, 939
inhaled foreign body, *132*
lung cancer, 926, 928
mitral regurgitation, 896
mitral stenosis, 897–8
pectus excavatum, 939
perforated peptic ulcer, 1125
peritonitis, 1051, *1054*
pneumoperitoneum, 210–11
post-pneumonectomy, *934*
preoperative, 256, 259
pulmonary hydatid disease, 67
retrosternal goitre, *803*
rolling hiatus hernia, 1084
testicular cancer metastases ('cannon ball'), *1508*
trauma, 205, 366, 372
chest trauma, 375–81, 938
children, 122–3
'deadly dozen', *367*
chest wall
burns injuries, 621
congenital abnormalities, 939–40
tumours, 938
chest wound, sucking, 366
Chiari malformations, 668
Chiari I, 668
Chiari II, 484, 668
Chicago Classification, *1096*
chief cells, 1107, *1108*
Chilaiditi's syndrome, 210
child abuse, 138
children
acute abdominal pain, 130–2
age terminology, *119*
ankle and foot abnormalities, 577–80
appendicitis, 1303, 1304, 1308
differential diagnosis, 1304–5
atherosclerosis, 887
basic physiological data, *120*
body proportions, *316*
body temperature, 119–20
brain tumours, 667
burns, 624
cleft lip and palate, 688–700
congenital adrenal hyperplasia, 844
congenital and developmental skeletal abnormalities, 564–6
congenital hearing loss, 712
congenital malformations, 132–8
abdominal wall, 135
alimentary tract duplications, 136
anorectal, 136–7
biliary system, 135–6
diaphragmatic hernia, 133
Hirschsprung's disease, 136
intestinal atresias, 133–4, *135*
oesophageal atresia, 133
urinary tract, 137–8
craniofacial anomalies, 686–8
Crohn's disease, 1243
epiglottitis, 743
examination, 121
fluid administration, 120–1
fractures, 403–6
growth plate, 387
hernias
inguinal, 124, 1032
midline, 127
hip abnormalities
DDH, 567–71
slipped upper femoral epiphysis (SUFE), *382*, 404–5, 573–5
idiopathic thrombocytopenic purpura, 1182–3
inguinoscrotal disorders, 124–6
intussusception, 129–30, 1283–4
differentiation from appendicitis, 1304
treatment, 1293
knee and lower leg abnormalities, 575–7
laryngotracheobronchitis (croup), 743
limb development, 561
limping, 568, 589
metabolic bone disease, 566–7
necrotising enterocolitis, 138
neuroblastoma, 138, 847
neuromuscular conditions, 583, *584*
nocturnal enuresis, 1432
non-accidental injuries (NAI), 138, 311, 315, 316, 330, 589–90
normal limb variants, 562–4
oncology, 138
operative surgery, 121–2
long-term outcomes, 122
techniques, *122*
parotitis, 786
penile disorders, 126–7
primary lymphoedema, 1002
primary peritonitis, 1053
pyloric stenosis, 127–8
retinoblastoma, 676
safeguarding, 138
spinal deformities, 581–3
stridor, 742–3
swallowed/inhaled foreign bodies, 132, 743–4
testicular tumours, 1509
trauma, 122–4
umbilical hernias, 1036–8
upper limb abnormalities, 580–1
vomiting, 128, 134
Wilms' tumour, 138, *152*, *156*, 832, 1421–2
see also infants; neonates
Child–Turcotte–Pugh (CTP) classification, 1156–7, 1175
China, cancer incidence, 1086, 1131
Chlamydia spp., prostatitis, 1475
Chlamydia trachomatis, 1049, 1306, 1495–6, 1505, 1518–19
chloramphenicol, 82
chlorhexidine, 1564
chlorine, in GI secretions, *281*
'choke' vessels, 593, *594*
cholangiocarcinoma, 1167, 1208–9, *1210*
cholangiography
percutaneous transhepatic, 1159, 1193–4
perioperative, 1194, *1195*
cholangiohepatitis, Asiatic (clonorchiasis), 62–3, 1207
cholangioscopy, 1158–9
cholangitis, 1205
ascending, 1168
immunoglobulin G4-related, 1207
primary sclerosing, *1159*, 1167, *1167*, 1206–7, 1208
cholecystectomy, 1202–5
common bile duct injury, 184
complications, 1203–5
gallbladder polyps, 1211
gallstone disease, 1200
indications, 1203
laparoscopic, 1202
late symptoms, 1204–5
open, 1202–3
cholecystitis
acalculous, 1200
acute, 212–13, 1018, 1199
severity grading, 1200
emphysematous, 1190, *1191*
Salmonella, 1201–2
cholecystitis glandularis proliferans, 1201
cholecystohepatic duct, 1196
cholecystojejunostomy, 1237
cholecystokinin (CCK), 1214
cholecystitis, acute, differential diagnosis, *1199*
choledochal cysts, 1197–8
choledochojejunostomy, 63
choledocholithiasis, post-cholecystectomy, 1204–5
choledochoscopy, 1194
choledochotomy, 1205, *1206*
cholelithiasis, *see* gallstones
cholescintigraphy, 192, 1192, 1204, 1232
cholesterosis (strawberry gallbladder), 1201
chondroblastoma, 540–1, *542*
chondromatosis, synovial, 500
chondrosarcoma, *536–7*, 541
clear cell, 541, *542*
treatment, 546
chordee, 1491
choriocarcinoma, 1507
choroid, melanoma, 676–7
chromoendoscopy, 233
chromogenic *in situ* hybridisation (CISH), 247

chromogranin A, 852, 853
Chvostek's sign, 831
chylocoeles, 1504
chylolymphatic cyst, 1063
chylothorax, 1013
chylous ascites, 1003, 1013, 1059
chyluria, 1003, *1004*, 1013
ciclosporin, 1245, 1269, 1533, 1538–9
Cierny and Mader classification, 557–8
cinacalcet, 831, 834
CINAHL, *163*
ciprofloxacin, 220
circle of Willis, aneurysms, 658, 659
circular stapling devices, 96, *97*
circumcision, 126–7, 1487–8
  in adolescents/adults, 1487–8
  diathermy, 103
  indications, 127, 1487
  in infants, 1487
  and penile carcinoma, 1492
cirrhosis, 1206
  ascites, 1058, 1166
  portal hypertension, 1163–6
  primary biliary, 1167–8
cis-platinum, *155*
c-kit oncogene, 1140, 1251
clam cystoplasty, 1434
clamps, vascular, 99
clarithromycin, 1114
claudication
  intermittent, 943, 947
  spinal, 476
claudication distance, 943
Clavian–Dindo system, 292
clavicle
  fracture, 400
  lateral end excision, 495
clavulanic acid, 56
claw hand, 69
claw toes, 69, *458*
clean intermittent self-catheterisation (CISC), 1428–9
clear cell carcinoma, *241*
clear cell chondrosarcoma, 541, *542*
cleft lip and palate, 688–700
  aetiology, 686, 688–9
  airway management, 691
  alveolar bone grafting, 698–9
  antenatal diagnosis, 691
  cleft lip alone, 688, 689, 697–8
  dental issues, 695, 696
  feeding, 691
  hard palate, 690, *691*
  hearing problems, 694–5
  incidence, 687, 688
  primary surgery, 692–4
  secondary surgery, 695–8
  soft palate, 689–90
  speech problems, 695
clindamycin, 420, 1009, *1520*
Clinical-aEtiology-Anatomy-Pathophysiology (CEAP) classification, 974
clinical audit, 161–2, 175, 185–6
clinical microsystems, 180
clinical outcomes, 185–6
clinical research
  article analysis, 167–8
  differentiation from audit, 161, *162*
  ethics, 166, 174
  identifying a topic, 162–3
  integrity, 166
  presenting and publishing, 168
  project design, 163–6
  qualitative *vs* quantitative, 164
  regulation, 165, 174
  regulatory approvals, 166
  statistical analysis, 166–7
  study protocol, 165
  study types, 164
clinodactyly, 580
cloaca, 1344–5
  persistent, 1346
clonality analysis, 247, *248*, 249
clonorchiasis, 1207
Clonorchis sinensis, 62–3, 1208
clopidogrel, *220*, 948
Clostridium difficile, 44
  antimicrobials effective against, 56
  infection control, 52
  proctitis, 1325
  pseudomembranous colitis, 44–5, 1269, 1273
Clostridium perfringens, 44, 45, 49–50, 420, 1049
Clostridium septicum septicaemia, 1307
Clostridium tetani, *45*, 50, 417
ClosureFast™, 978
clothing, operating theatre, 1564
clotting screen, 256
clubbing, 926
club foot (congenital talipes equinovarus), 577–9
club hand, radial, 580
coagulopathy
  acute traumatic, 427
  during/following transfusion, 22–3
  trauma-induced, 18
co-amoxiclav, 56
coarctation of the aorta, 906
Cobb angle, 482, 582
cocaine, topical, 274
cochlea, 703–5
cochlear duct, 703, *704*
cochlear implant, 712
Cochrane Collaboration, 163, 168
Cochrane Library, *163*, 168
Codman's triangle, 73
coeliac disease, 1255
coeliac plexus block, 277
coiling, 659, 660
cold injuries, 422, 632, 953, 954
colectomy
  colorectal cancer, 1264–5
  diverticular disease, 1276
  nutritional consequences, 283
  subtotal in ulcerative colitis, 1270
Coleman's block test, 460
colic
  biliary, 1017, 1018–19
  intestinal obstruction, 1285–6
  renal/ureteric, 213, 1017, 1305, 1374, 1407
colitis
  C. difficile, 44–5, 1269, 1273
  Crohn's, 1242, 1271–2
  indeterminate, 1271
  infective, 1269, 1272–3
  ischaemic, 1276–7
  see also ulcerative colitis
'collagen disease', 1024
collar and cuff, 391–2
collateral circulation, 942, *943*, 954
collateral ligaments, knee, 454–5, *518*, 519
Colles' fascia, 1480
Colles' fracture, 398
Collis gastroplasty, 1081
Collis–Nissen operation, 1081
colloid cyst, 667
colloid fluids
  burns patient, 624
  composition, *281*
coloanal anastomosis, 1370
colocutaneous fistula, 1274
colon
  acute obstruction, 1294–5
  anatomy, 1258–9
  angioectasia, 231
  benign tumours, 1259–61
  Crohn's disease, 1271–2
  diversion of urine into, 1453
  diverticular disease, 1273–6
  duplicated, 136
  functions, 283, 1259
  injuries, 375
  ischaemia, after AAA repair, 965–6
  perforation, 232, 1274
  pseudo-obstruction, 1297–8
  stricture, malignant, 1281
  transit times, 283
  volvulus, 1284–5, 1288, 1290
colonic polyps
  children, 131
  endoscopic resection, 230–1, 232
colonoscopy, 229–32
  appendicitis, *1301*
  colorectal cancer, 1262–3
  complications, 231–2
  Crohn's disease, 1244
  diverticular disease, 1274–5
  indications, *230*
  practical performance, 229–30
  rectal cancer, 1330
  therapeutic, 230–1
  ulcerative colitis, 1268
  virtual CT, 1263
colorectal cancer, 142, 1261–6
  adjuvant therapy, 1266
  aetiology and risk factors, 1261, 1268, 1328
  chemotherapy and biological agents, *155*, *157*
  clinical features, 1017, 1262
  distribution by site, *1262*
  epidemiology, 1261, 1328
  follow-up, 1266
  hereditary non-polyposis (HPCC), *144*, 1260–1
  investigation, 1262–3
  malignant obstruction, 231
  metastatic disease, *195*, 1172–3, 1262, 1266
  molecular testing, 250–1
  pathology, 1261
  prognosis, 1266
  risk in adenomas, 1259
  risk in ulcerative colitis, 1268
  screening, 230, 1263
  spread, 1262
  staging systems, *149*, 1262
  surgery, 1263–5
    emergency, 1265
    laparoscopic, 1265
    postoperative care, 1265
colostomies, 1277–8
  anal stricture, 1370
  bags/appliances, 1277
  colon injury, 375
  complications, 1043, 1278
  end, 1277, *1278*, 1336
  loop, 1277
  rectal cancer, 1336, 1337
colour duplex scanning, 946
colovaginal fistula, 1274
colovesical fistula, 1274, 1275–6
colposuspension, open, 1431–2
combined modality therapy (CMT), 1371
common bile duct (CBD), 1188
  ascariasis, 60, *61*, 62
  imaging, 213, *1159*
  in liver resection, 1170
  malignant stricture, *1217*
  obstruction, *1193*
  relation to pancreatic duct, 1213, *1214*
  stones, 1204–5, *1206*, *1216*
communication
  healthcare workers, 182
  and patient safety, *178*, 181
comorbidity, day surgery, 302
compartment pressure monitoring, 406
compartment syndrome, 28
  abdominal, 380, 1045
  acute postoperative, 85
  acute arterial occlusion, 955–6
  causes, 408, 422
  crush injuries, 422
  diagnosis, 382–3, 408
  limb, 382, 408, 955–6
  postoperative, 298
compensatory anti-inflammatory response syndrome (CARS), 3
competence, 181
complaints, patient/carer, 181–2
complications, *see* postoperative complications
compression
  lymphoedema, 1009–10

pneumatic, 1010
varicose veins, 977
venous leg ulcers, 984–5
compression garments, 1010
compression hosiery, 977
compression injury, liver, 373
compression plating, *390*
compressive neuropathies
foot, 533
median nerve, 443, 508
ulnar nerve, 501–2, 508
computed-integrated surgery (CIS), 108
computed tomography (CT), 195–6, *197*
abdominal aortic aneurysm, *961–2*
abdominal hernias, 1026
abdominal trauma, 373
children, 123
advantages, 196
amoebiasis, 59
angiography (CTA), 213
extremity trauma, *197*, *383*, 384
aortic disruption, *369*
aortic dissection, 910
aortoiliac stent-graft, *964*
appendicitis, 211, *212*, *1301*, 1307, *1308*
recurrent, *1314*
arthrography, 202
ascites, 1058
biliary tract, 1190, 1192
bone tumours, *536*
bowel obstruction, 210
brain abscess, 656, *657*
cholangiocarcinoma, *1209*
colonic diverticular disease, 1274
colorectal cancer, 1263
Conn's adenoma (adrenal gland), 840, *841*
Crohn's disease, 1244
disadvantages, 196
diverticulitis, 212
ear, 706
enterocutaneous fistula, *1256*
extremity trauma, 384, 396
FNA guidance, 928–9
GISTs, *1140*
glioblastoma multiforme, *664*
hydatid disease, 65, 66, *1169*
hydronephrosis in BOO, *1461*
intestinal obstruction, 1289
ischaemic heart disease, 888
kidneys, ureter, bladder (KUB), 213
leiomyosarcoma, 994
liver, 1158
abscess, *1168*
colorectal metastases, *1173*, 1266
injury, *1162*
lung cancer, 926, 928
lymphoedema, 1006
mediastinal cyst, 936
mesenteric cyst, *1064*
multidetector (MDCT), 1062
multiphase (4D-CT), 828
oesophageal cancer, *1086*, 1090, 1091
oesophageal perforation, *1073*
optic nerve meningioma, *684*
oral cancer, 766
orbital abscess, 721–2
osteomyelitis, 551
pancreas, 1215, *1216*
pancreatic carcinoma, 1215, *1216*, 1235
pancreatic trauma, 1220
pancreatitis, 212, *1051*, 1224, 1226–7, 1231
paranasal sinuses, 717, *721*
parathyroid glands, 828
pelvic abscess, *1056*
peritonitis, 1051, *1054*
with PET (PET-CT), 1091, 1112, *1113*
pharynx, larynx, neck, 730
polycystic kidney disease, *1550*
principles, 195–6
pulmonary embolism, 989
pulmonary hydatid disease, 68
radiation doses, 191, *192*, 196, 317
retroperitoneal mass, *1509*
spinal osteoblastoma, *480*
spine, 474
spiral, *962*, *964*, 1158
spleen, 1178, *1179*, *1180*
stomach, 1112
subarachnoid haemorrhage, 659
subphrenic abscess, 1056, *1057*
thoracic trauma, 366
thymoma, 935
thyroid, 803, *804*
thyroid eye disease, *675*
trauma, 207–8, 317, 324
head injury, *197*, 207, 330
maxillofacial, 357–8, 358, 361, 362
spinal, 343, *350*
ulcerative colitis, 1268–9
urachal cyst, *1439*
urinary tract, 1389–90, *1391*
virtual colonoscopy, 1263
whole body scan, 317, 324
concussion, 330
condylar hyperplasia, 701
condylomata acuminata, 1368, 1486, 1496
confidence intervals, 167
confidentiality, 174
conflict surgery
contrasts with civilian surgery, 424
damage control, 426–7
decision making, 427
ethical and legal issues, 424–5
medical evacuation, 425
medical support roles, 425
patterns of injury, 425–6
principles, 426
weapon effects, 427–8
congenital adrenal hyperplasia (CAH), 844
congenital diaphragmatic hernia, 133
congenital heart disease, 902–8
acyanotic, 906–8
aetiology, 903
aortic stenosis, 899
cyanotic, 904–6
diagnosis, 903
incidence, 903
congenital hypertrophy of the retinal pigment epithelium, 1259
congenital malformations, 132–8
congenital vertical talus, 579
congestive heart failure, ascites, 1058
Congo red stain, 244
'coning', 329, 654
conjunctivitis, 680–1
connective tissue disorders, 967, 1251–3
Conn's adenoma, 839, 840–1
conscious level, shock, *14*
Consolidated Standards of Reporting Trials (CONSORT), 167–8
constipation, 1278–9
children, 131
drugs causing, *1278*
and haemorrhoids, 1354–5
illnesses associated with, *1278*
intestinal obstruction, 1286, 1296
investigation, 1278–9
treatment, 1279
contraceptive pill, 260, 1516
contractures
spinal cord injury, 354
wounds, 32, 628, *629*, *635*
contralateral stretch test, 442
contrast enhanced ultrasound scanning (CEUS), 1158
contrast media, hazards, 191
contrast radiology, upper GI tract, 1111
conus medullaris, *340*
Cooley's anaemia, 1183–4
Coombs' test, 1183
coracoacromial ligament, 490
cordotomy, percutaneous anterolateral, 277
cornea, 672
abrasions and ulceration, 677, 681
burns, 679–80
grafting, 677
inflammation (keratitis), 681
corona phlebectatica, 972
coronary angiography
ischaemic heart disease, 888–9
valvular heart disease, 898, 900
coronary arteries
anatomy, 886–7
calcification (calcium score), 888
stenoses, 888–9
coronary artery bypass grafting (CABG), 886–93
conduit selection, 890
indications for, 889
minimal access, 893
mortality rates, 892
off-pump, 893
operation, 890–1
postoperative complications, 891–2
postoperative recovery, 891
preoperative assessment, 890
surgical outcomes, 893
coronary stents, 886, 889
thrombosis risk, 257
coronary vein, 1106
corpora amylaceae, 1468
Corrigan's sign, 901
corticospinal tracts, 340
corticosteroids
adverse effects, bone infarction, *198*
Crohn's disease, 1245
delayed healing, 46
facet joint injections, 474
foraminal epidural injections, 474
immunosuppressive regimens, 1539
intra-articular injections, shoulder, 490, *491*, 492, 493, 495
pruritus ani, 1361
spinal cord injury, 345
sports injuries, 470
ulcerative colitis, 1269
corticotrophin-releasing factor (CRF), 3
corticotrophin-releasing hormone (CRH), 839
cortisol, 3, 4, 13, 839
deficiency, 844
excess, 841–2, 843
Corynebacterium minutissimum, 1361
cost-effectiveness, targeted cancer therapies, 154, *158*
cough impulse, 1025, 1031
coughing, 915
Couinaud's segments, 1154, *1545*
Courvoisier's sign, 1199–200, 1205, 1208, 1234–5
Cowden syndrome, *144*, 663, *1418*
Craig's test, *562*
cranial nerves
facial, 363, 715, 789, 790–2, *792*, *793*
oculomotor, 672
optic, *672*, *673*
submandibular gland excision, 783
supplying ear, 705
trigeminal, 672, 705
vagus, 727, 810, 814, 1107
craniofacial anomalies, 686–8
diagnosis, 687
epidemiology, 687
management, 687–8
types, 686
craniofacial fractures, *323*, 362
craniopharyngioma, *683*

craniosynostosis, 668, 669, 687–8
  types of, 668, 669
craniotomy
  risks of, 671
  subarachnoid haemorrhage, 659–60
  trigeminal neuralgia, 670
cranium bifidum, 667
C-reactive protein, 551
creatine kinase, 419, 888
credentialing, 181
cremasteric reflex, 1498
crepitus, 383, 952
Creutzfeldt–Jakob disease (CJD), 215, 671, 1544
Crew Resource Management (CRM) training, 177
cricoid cartilage, 725, *726*, 727
  injury, 755–6
cricothyroidotomy, 749
critical care, 263, 266–7
critical limb ischaemia, 943, 949
Crohn's disease, 46, 225, 227, 616, 1241–8
  aetiology, 1241–2
  appendicitis in, 1312
  clinical features, 1243
  colitis, 1242, 1271–2
  epidemiology, 1241
  extraintestinal manifestations, 1243, *1244*
  fistulas, 1045, 1243, 1440
  indications for surgery, 1246
  investigations, *193*, *196*, 212, 1243–5
  Montreal classification, 1243
  nutrition, 1242, 1246
  oesophagitis, 1104–5
  pathogenesis, 1242
  pathology, 1242–3
  perianal, 1243, 1247–8, 1363, 1370
  proctitis, 1325
  small bowel stricture, 1242, 1246, 1282
  terminal ileitis, 1305
  treatment
    medical, 1245–6
    surgical, 1246–8
  vs ulcerative colitis, *1243*, *1268*
cross-matching, 22
cross-sectional study, *164*
croup, 743
Crouzon syndrome, 687, 701
cruciate ligaments, knee, 454, 455–6, *518*, 519
  injuries, 520–1
  reconstruction, 521
crush injuries, 28, 420–2
  liver, 1162
crush syndrome, 421–2
cryoprecipitate, 21
'cryptitis', 1353
crypts of Lieberkühn, 1250, 1267
crypts of Luschka, 1188
crystalloid fluids, burn patient, 624
crystalloid solutions, composition, *281*
CTLA-4Ig, 1540
cubital tunnel, ulnar nerve compression, 500–1
cubitus valgus, 447
cubitus varus, 447
Cullen's sign, 1019–20, 1223
Cushing's adenoma, 839
Cushing's disease, 841
Cushing's syndrome, 841–2, 843
  ACTH-dependent, 841
  ACTH-independent, 841
Cushing's triad, 328–9
cutaneous (keratin) horn, 606
cutis aplasia congenita, 615
cyanogenic glycosides, 76
cyclo-oxygenase-2 (COX-2), 4
  inhibitors, 1115
cyclophosphamide, *155*
cyclophosphamide, methotrexate and 5-fluorouracil (CMF), 878
cylindroma (turban tumour), 603
cyproterone acetate, *156*, 1474
cystadenoma (hydrocystadenoma), 603
cystectomy, bladder cancer, 1451–2
cysterna chyli, 995
cystgastrostomy, 1229
cystic duct, 1188
  absence, 1196
  low insertion, 1196
cystic fibrosis, 1219, 1294
cystic hygroma, 754–5
cystic myxomatous degeneration, 967
cystine stones, 1406, 1408, 1434
cystinuria, 1406
  treatment, 1410
cystitis
  acute abacterial (acute haemorrhagic), 1442
  alkaline encrusting, 1443
  definition, 1441
  interstitial (Hunner's ulcer), 1443
  tuberculous, 1442–3
cystitis cystica, 1443
cyst of Moll, 674
cystocoele, *1522*, *1523*
cystography
  bladder rupture, 1425
  tuberculous cystitis, *1443*
cystoscopy, 1379–85
  bladder cancer, 1449
  bladder diverticulum, *1437*
  flexible, 1380
  minor procedures, 1380
  narrow band imaging, 1381
  photodynamic diagnosis, 1381
  rigid, 1380
  schistosomiasis, 1444–5
  ureterocoele, 1401, *1402*
  vesicointestinal fistula, *1440*
cysts
  branchial, 753–4
  breast, *861*, 868, 869
  epididymal, 1374, 1376–7, 1504–5
  ganglion, 509, 528
  hydatid, 64–7, 1169, *1169*
  intracranial in children, 667
  liver, 1168
  lung, 937
  mediastinum, 936
  minor salivary glands, 776
  ovary, 1526, *1527*
  renal, *1386*, 1389–90, *1391*
  sebaceous, 598–9, 1510, *1511*
  seminal vesicle, 1476
  skin and soft tissue, 598–9
  spleen, 1178–9, *1179*
  Stafne bone, 780
  sublingual glands, 779
  thyroglossal duct, 755
  thyroid, 809–10
  urachal, 1438
cyst of Zeis, 674
cytogenetics, 247–8
cytokeratins, 245–6
cytokines
  endogenous antagonists, 4
  proinflammatory, 3, 7–8, 47, 1242
cytology
  microscopy, 242, *243*
  sample adequacy, 243
  samples, 238
  specimen processing, 238
  specimens, 235
  vs histology, *243*
cytomegalovirus (CMV), 246, 247, 1104, 1541
cytopoiesis, 1178
cytoreductive surgery
  ovarian cancer, 1529
  pseudomyxoma peritonei, 1317
cytosine arabinoside, *155*
Czerny retractor, 1561

dabigatran, *221*
dabrafenib, 612
dacarbazine, *156*
Dacron grafts, 949, 950, *951*
dacryocystitis, 674
daily water balance, 280
DAIR strategy, 556
damage control resuscitation (DCR), 20, 379, 427
damage control surgery (DCS), 318–19, 326, *327*, 378–80
  conflict zones, 426–7
  disaster zones, 413–15
  indications for, *379*
  principles, *414*
danazol, 869, 1452
Dandy Walker malformations, 668
dapsone, 70
data, statistical, 167
databases, research, 163
data collection, 165
da Vinci robotic surgical system, 1334, *1335*
daVinci system, 109
day case surgery
  advantages, 301
  discharge, 304, 306, *307*
  elective, 305
  emergency, 306
  models of care, 301–2
  patient pathway, 301, 306
  perioperative management, 304–5
  preoperative assessment, 304
  selection criteria, 302–4
DDH, *see* developmental dysplasia of the hip
deaths
  head injuries, 328
  preventable, 178
  RTAs, 310, *311*
  traumatic causes, 364
Deaver retractor, 1560
DeBakey classification (aortic dissection), 910
DeBakey forceps, 1562
debridement, 26, 27, 415–16
deceleration injuries, 1161
decellularised scaffolds, 38–9
decongestive lymphoedema therapy, 1008
decortication, 923
deep brain stimulation, 670, 671
deep fascial space infection, hand, 504
deep vein thrombosis (DVT), 986–91
  after hip replacement, 517–18
  differential diagnosis, 989
  lymphoedema, *1000*, 1005
  postoperative, 296
  risk of, 260
  treatment, 990
defaecating proctography, 1278, 1344
defaecation
  difficulty, 1324, 1370
  obstructed, 1278
  see also constipation
degarelix, 1474
degloving injuries, 27–8, *325*
dehiscence of Killian, 1101
dehydration
  children, 120
  gastric outlet obstruction, 1130
  intestinal obstruction, 1286
dehydroepiandrosterone (DHEA), 839
dehydroepiandrosterone sulphate (DHEAS), 839
Delaire technique and sequence, 692
delayed ischaemic neurological deficit, 660–1
delirium, postoperative, 295
Delorme's operation, 1323
Delphinian nodes, 800–1
dementia patients, 1430, 1433, 1459, 1462, 1463
de Musset's sign, 901
Denonvilliers' fascia, 1318, 1451
dental anomalies, cleft lip/palate, 695, 696
dental injuries, 357, 363
dental occlusion, jaw deformities, 701, *702*

dentate line, 1340–1
de Quervain's tenosynovitis, 443, 469, 507–8
de Quervain's thyroiditis, 822
dermatomes, abdominal wall, 1018
dermatome (skin harvesting), 639–40
dermis, 592, 634
  artificial, 628, *630*
dermo-epidermal junction, 592, 599
dermoid cysts, 667, 673
  intracranial, 667
  orbit, 673
  ovary, 1526
  postanal, 1347
Descamets stripping endothelial keratoplasty (DSEK), 677
desmoid tumour
  abdomen, 1259
  abdominal wall, 1045
detrusor instability, 1431
detrusor overactivity, 1429–30, 1432, 1460
  treatment, 1433
detrusor–sphincter dyssynergia, 1396, 1424, 1428
developing countries, *see* low-income countries
developmental dysplasia of the hip (DDH), 567–71
dexamethasone suppression, 842
dextrose infusions, 10, 281
dextrose–saline, 624
diabetes insipidus, 666
diabetes mellitus
  cystic fibrosis, 1219
  day case surgery, 302–3
  endoscopy, 219
  fibrocalculous pancreatic, 77
  foot disease, 532–3, 559, 953
  gangrene, 953
  hepatocellular carcinoma, 1173
  pancreatic islet transplantation, 1553
  peripheral arterial disease, 947
  preoperative assessment, 256, 260
  sialadenosis, 796
  type 2, bariatric surgery, 1145
diamorphine, 277
diaphragm, 914–15, 938
  congenital hernia, 133, 938, 939
  injuries, 365, 938
    blunt, 370
    children, 123
    penetrating, 370
  weakness, 1022
diaphyseal aclasis, 539, 565
diarrhoea, post-vagotomy, 1124
diastematomyelia, 484
diathermy, 101–4
  bipolar, 102
  complications, 102–3, 258
  effects, 102
  laparoscopic surgery, 103, 114
  monopolar, 102
  principle, 102
diazoxide, 849–50
diclofenac, suppository, 115
diet
  and appendicitis, 1301
  and breast cancer risk, 871
  coeliac disease, 1255
  and colon cancer, 1261
  and colonic diverticular disease, 1273, 1275
  and constipation, 1279
  and Crohn's disease, 1242
  fat, 282
  and gastric cancer, 1131
  and haemorrhoids, 1354–5
  liver shrinkage, 1146
  oxalate excess, 1408
diethylcarbamazine, 64, 1005
Dietl's crisis, 1411
Dieulafoy's disease, 1128
diffuse axonalinjury, 336
diffusion capacity (DLCO), 917, 918
digastric muscle, 790
diGeorge syndrome, 903
digestion, small intestine, 1241
digestive enzymes
  gastric, 1108–9
  pancreas, 1214
digital rectal examination, 1320
digital subtraction percutaneous angiography (DSA), 946–7
2,8-dihydroadeninuria, 1406
1,5-dihydrotestosterone (DHT), 1457
dilatation
  anal, 1356, 1370
  biliary stricture, 228, 1157–8
  iliac artery stenosis, 948, 950
  oesophageal strictures, 1071
  urethral stricture (male), 1483
diloxanide furoate, 59, 1273
dinaciclib, *158*
diphthermia, 737
diplopia, vertical, 677
dipstick, urine, 1379
disability, assessment in trauma, 325
disasters
  common features, 409
  damage assessment, 410–11
  damage control surgery, 413–16
  definitive management, 416
  factors influencing relief effort, 409–10
  field hospitals, 413, *414*
  handing over, 422
  hospital organisation, 416
  organisation of relief efforts, 410–13
  planning for, 422–3
  specific injuries and conditions, 416–22
  triage, 412, *413*
discharge
  day surgery, 304, 306, *307*
  following head injury, 329–30
  laparoscopic surgery, 116
  requirements, 300
disc herniation
  cervical spine, 474, *475*
  lumbar spine, *198*, 476
  thoracic spine, 475
discitis, 589
discography, provocative, 474, *475*
disc replacement, total, *475*, 476, *477*
distal interphalangeal (DIP) joints, arthritis, *443*, 506
distraction osteogenesis, craniofacial deformity, 688, 691, 702
distributive shock, 13
diuretics, ascites, 1166
divarification of the recti, 1022, *1023*
diverticulae
  bladder, *1384*, 1436–8
  colonic, 1273–6
  gallbladder, 1201
  Meckel's, 131–2, 1044, 1252, *1253*
  oesophagus, 1101–2
  seminal vesicle, 1476
  small intestine, 1251–3
  urethra
    female, 1377, 1485
    male, 1479
diverticulectomy, 1438
diverticulitis
  clinical presentation, 1274
  differentiation from appendicitis, 1306
  fistula formation, 1274, 1275–6, 1440
  imaging, 211–12
  management, 1275
  Meckel's, 1252
DMAIC, 187–8
DNA
  drugs directly damaging, *155–6*
  drugs interfering with synthesis (antimetabolites), *155*
  epigenetic modification, 142, 249
  first described, 139
'dog ear', 86
dopamine, 839
Doppler ultrasound, 17, 194, 203
  peripheral arterial disease, 945–6
  priapism, *1491*
  venous disease, 975–6
Doppman, John L, 826
Dormia stone-catching basket, *1409*
dorsalis pedis pulse, 458, 459
dorsal root entry zone (DREZ) operation, 671
dorsiflexors, testing, 461
dose–response relationships, 150, *151*
dot-in-circle sign, 73
double-balloon endoscopy, 226, 227
double effect, 173
Down syndrome, 132, 133, 136, 689, 708, 903, 907, 1219
doxazosin, 1468
doxorubicin, *155*
doxycycline, 1505
drains/drainage, 99–101, 299
  ascites, 1058, 1059
  basic principles, 100
  chest, *see* chest drains
  image-guided, 100–1
  intraperitoneal abscesses, 1056–7
  laparoscopic patient, 115–16
  pancreatic necrosis, 1227
  pancreatic pseudocyst, 1229
  removal, 101
  T-tube, 100, 101
  value and use of, 100
drapes, surgical, 1564
draw tests
  ankle, 461
  knee, 455, *456*
dressings, *see* wound dressings
drooling, 797
  child, 743
drug history, 1017
drugs
  causing constipation, *1278*
  causing urinary retention, 1428
  causing urine discolouration, 1376
  damaging DNA, *155–6*
  increasing risk of urinary stones, 1407
  influencing PSA levels, 1378
  safe prescribing, 182
  see also named drugs and drug classes
dual X-ray absorptiometry (DEXA) scan, 205, 825, 833
Duchenne muscular dystrophy, 482, 583
ductal carcinoma *in situ* (DCIS), 872, *875*
ductoscopy, 865
ductus arteriosus, 903, 904
  patent, 906
ductus venosus, 903, 904
Dukes' staging, *149*
  colorectal cancer, 1262
  rectal carcinoma, 1330–1
duloxetine, 1433, 1434
dumping, after peptic ulcer surgery, 1123–4
Dunhill procedure, 807
duodenal atresia, 133–4, 1293–4
duodenaljejunal flexure, 1240
duodenal switch (DS), *1147*, 1150
duodenal ulcers, 1117
  aetiology, 1116
  bleeding, 1127–8
  incidence, 1117
  pathology, 1117
  surgery, 1120–3
duodenoileal bypass, single anastomosis with sleeve gastrectomy, 1150
duodenum
  adenocarcinoma, 1141
  adenoma, *233*

anatomy, 1240–1
gastrinoma (Zollinger–Ellison syndrome), 850–2, 1116, 1120, 1141–2
injuries, 375
microscopic anatomy, 1108
neuroendocrine tumours, 1141
obstruction, 1142
peptic ulcer bleeding, 1127–8
physiology, 1108–10
villous adenoma, 1141
Duoderm®, 626, 630
duplex renal pelvis/ureters, 1400, *1401*
duplex scanning
peripheral arterial disease, 946
varicose veins, 975–6
duplications
alimentary tract, 136
hand/digits, *510*, 580
Dupuytren's contracture, 442–3, 506–7, 1065
dural arteriovenous fistulae (DAVFs), 661–2
dural tears, 717
Durkin's compression test, 508
dutasteride, 1378
Dyball retractor, 1560
dyschondrosis, 686
dysmenorrhoea, 1516–17
dysostosis, 686
dyspepsia
H. pylori eradication, 1115, 1117
investigation, 1131
management guidelines, 221
dysphagia, 1069, 1077
in absence of stricture, 1095
oropharyngeal, 1099
sideropenic, 740, 763, 1105
dysplasia
colorectal, 239, *240*, 1267
oral epithelium, 767
dysplasia associated lesions or mass (DALMs), 1267
dyspnoea, risk of postoperative, 916
dysuria, 1374

ear
anatomy, 703–5
congenital anomalies, 706
examination, 705–6
inflammation and infection, 707–8
neoplasms, 708, 711–12
trauma, 706–7, 708
early dumping, 1123–4
early-morning urine (EMU), 1379
early total care (ETC), 318–19
vs damage control surgery, *327*
early warning system, national, 290, *291*
Eaton–Lambert syndrome, 926
eccrine glands, 593
eccrine poroma (papillary syringoma), 603
Echinococcus granulosus, 64, 1169
Echinococcus multilocularis, 64
echocardiography
aortic stenosis, 900
ischaemic heart disease, 888
mitral regurgitation, 896
mitral stenosis, 898
ectopia vesicae (bladder exstrophy), 1424–5, *1453*
ectopic kidney, 1399
ectopic pancreas, 1219
ectopic pregnancy, 1306, 1517–18
ectopic salivary glands, 780
ectopic testis, 1498
ectopic thyroid gland, 936
ectopic ureters, 1401
ectropion, 674, 680, *681*
eczema
lower limb, 973
in lymphoedema, 1008
nipples, 864
education
continuing professional, 174–5
quality improvement, 188
Edwards syndrome, *903*
Ehlers–Danlos syndrome, 908, 1416
Eisenmenger syndrome, 905–6
ejaculation, retrograde, 1466
elastic stable intramedullary nailing (ESIN), 405–6
elbow
anatomy, 498–9
clinical examination, 447–8
distal lateral condylar mass fracture, *382*, 404, *405*
loose bodies, 500, *501*
olecranon bursitis, 500–1
olecranon fracture, 399
osteoarthritis, 499–500
replacement, 500
rheumatoid arthritis, 499
ulnar nerve compression, 501–2
elderly patients
anal stenosis, 1369
appendicitis, 1303, 1304
diverticulitis, 1306
falls, 322
fractures, 311, 320
hip fractures, 318
shock, 15
subdural haematoma, 335
elective surgery
day case, 305
patient journey, 186
electrical injuries, 631, *632*
electrical stimulation, 671
electrocardiography (ECG)
aortic stenosis, 900
hypercalcaemia, 826
hypocalcaemia, 831
ischaemic heart disease, 888
mitral regurgitation, 896
mitral stenosis, 897
myocardial ischaemia, 294
peripheral arterial disease, 945
preoperative, 256, 257, 258
electrocution, diathermy, 102
electroencephalography (EEG), epilepsy, 669
electrolytes
adult daily requirements, 281
in GI secretions, *281*
paediatric requirements, *120*
electromyography (EMG), anal sphincters, 1344, *1345*
electronic information sites, 163
electronic patient records, 180–1
electron microscopy, 245
electrospinning technology, 39
electrosurgery, 101–4
advanced energy devices, 103–4
during laparoscopy, 103, 114
see also diathermy
elephantiasis
endemic (podoconiosis), 1005
filarial, 63, 64, 1510
non-filarial, 1510
Ellik, Milo, 1436
EMBASE, *163*
Emberger syndrome, *1002*
embolectomy, 955
embolisation (therapeutic), 956
angiographic, 209, *319*, 365, 378
cerebral aneurysms, 659, 660
pelvic vein, 986
renal metastases, 547
uterine artery, 1525–6
embolism
acute arterial occlusion, 953–6
air, 956
fat, 956
parasitic, 956
pulmonary, *see* pulmonary embolism
embryology
adrenal glands, 839
anal canal, 1344–5
craniofacial malformations, 686
female reproductive organs, 1513
gallbladder and bile ducts, 1195
kidneys, 1398–9
liver, 1155
lungs, 914
lymphatics, 995
musculoskeletal system, 561
pancreas, 1213
parathyroid glands, 800, 823
peritoneal cavity, 1047
prostate, 1456
rectum, 1319
testes, 1497
thyroid, 800
embryonic stem cells (ESCs), 35–6
emergency surgery
laparoscopic, 116
patient journey, 186
preoperative assessment, 261–2
EMLA (eutectic mixture of local anaesthetics), 274
emollients, 1008
emphysema, surgical, 919
emphysematous pyelonephritis, 1404
empyema
gallbladder, 1200
pleural, 922, 923
subdural, 657–8
encephelocoele, 667, 668
encephalopathy
hepatic, 1156
hyponatraemic, 120
enchondromatosis, *537*, 540, 565–6
enclosed blast, 432
endoanal ultrasound, 1344
endobronchial ultrasound (EBUS), 928, 929
endocarditis
endoscopy patient, 219
prosthetic valves, 895–6
EndoClose, 114
endocrine shock, 13
end-of-life care, 159, 173
endoleaks, 966
endolymph, 703–4
endometrial cancer, *146*, 250, 1516
endometrioma, 1327, 1521
endometriosis, 1520–2
anorectal, 1327, 1370
bladder wall, 1452
histology, *243*
endometrium, 1514
endoprosthesis, bone tumours, *547*
endoscopes
decontamination, 218
standard, *217*
endoscopic mucosal resection (EMR), 224, 230, *231*, 1327, *1328*
endoscopic pancreatic sphincterotomy, 1231, 1233
endoscopic retrograde cholangiopancreatography (ERCP), 227–9, 1158, *1159*, 1192–3, 1217–18
in acute pancreatitis, 1224, 1225
in chronic pancreatitis, 1232–3
complications, 228–9
pancreatic carcinoma, 1217, *1218*, 1235
pancreatitis after, 1222
sclerosing cholangitis, 1206, *1207*
therapeutic, 228
endoscopic ultrasound (EUS), 232
advantages of, 232
biliary tract, 1191
indications, *232*
liver, 1159
oesophageal disease, *232*, 1070, 1090–1
pancreas, 1218–19, 1235
stomach, 1111–12
endoscopy
bladder and urethra, 1379–85

colon, *see* colonoscopy
gastrointestinal
antibiotic prophylaxis, 219–20
anticoagulation, 220–1
capsule, 226–7
consent, 218
double/single balloon, *226*, *227*
equipment, *217*, 218
history of, 216–17
improved imaging, 233
perforations, 225, 1073–4, 1111
risks of, *218*
sedation, 219
small bowel, 225–7
upper tract, 221–5, 1070, 1110–11
oesophageal carcinoma, 1087, 1088
ureters, 1385
endoscopy unit, organisation, 217–18
endothermal ablation, 977
endotoxins, 46–7, 1049
endotracheal intubation, 271–2, 748
endovascular aneurysm repair (EVAR), 962–4
complications, 966
endovascular techniques, 209
endovenous glue, 980
endovenous laser ablation (EVLA), 977–8
comparison with RFA, 978–9
enema
air, 129
antegrade colonic, 137
barium, *see* barium enema
contrast, 59, 136
herbal causing proctitis, 1326
small bowel, 80, 1244
energy requirements, 282
burns patient, 626–7
enhanced recovery after surgery (ERAS), 11, 299–300
colonic surgery, 1265
Enneking staging system, 543
enophthalmos, 361
Entamoeba histolytica, 57, 1169, 1272
enteral nutrition, 284
after laparoscopic surgery, 115
complications, 286
sip feeds, 285
tube-feeding techniques, 284–6
enteritis, infective, 1248–9
Enterobacter spp., 433
enterochromaffin-like (ECL) cells, 1107, 1108, 1115
enterochromaffin-like (ECL) omas, *853*, 854
enteroclysis, 226, 1244–5
enterococci, 44
antimicrobials, 56
glycopeptide-resistant (GRE), 43
Enterococcus faecalis, 56
enterocoele, *1522*, *1523*
enterocolitis, necrotising, 138
enterocutaneous fistula, 1256
enterocystoplasty, clam, 1434
enterogastric reflux, 1115
enterogenous cysts, 1063–4
entropion, 680, *681*
enucleation, eye, 684
enuresis, nocturnal, 1375, 1432
enzalutamide, 1474
eosinophilic gastritis, 1116
eosinophilic granuloma, 541, *542*, *543*
eosinophilic oesophagitis, 1100–1
eosinophils, 241, *242*
epicondylitis
lateral (tennis elbow), 448
medial (golfer's elbow), 448, 464–5
epidermal growth factor receptor (EGFR)
inhibitors, *158*
mutations, 250
epidermal (sebaceous) cysts, 598–9, 1510, *1511*
epidermis, 592, 593, 634
epidermoid carcinoma, 1371
epidermoid cysts, 667
spleen, 1179
epidermophytosis, 1361
epididymal appendage, torsion, 126
epididymis, 1376–7, 1497
cysts, 1374, 1376–7, 1504–5
tumours, 1509
epididymo-orchitis, 126, 1503, 1505–6
chronic, 1505
pathophysiology, 1505
treatment, 1505
tuberculous, 1505
epidural abscess, 481
epidural anaesthesia, 275
epidural opiates, 277
epigastric hernia, 127, 1039
epigastric vessels, inferior, 1029
epigenetics
cancer, 142, 249
colorectal cancers, 1329
epiglottis, *726*, *727*
epiglottitis, acute, 743
epilepsy, 668–70
and day surgery, 303
investigation, 668–9
surgical management, 670
epiphrenic diverticula, 1102, *1103*
epirubacin, 1139
episcleritis, 682
epispadias, 1377, 1424, 1478, *1479*
epistaxis, 719–20
epithelial–mesenchymal transition (EMT), 141
epithelial tumours, appendix, 1315, 1316–17
epithelioma, *616*
calcifying of Malherbe (pilomatrixoma), 602
Epley manoeuvre, 714
Epstein–Barr virus (EBV), 246, *247*, 734, 738
erectile dysfunction, 1489–90
after pelvic fracture, 1481
erlotinib, *156*, *158*
ertapenem, 1308
erysipelas, 596–7
erythrasma, 1361
erythrocyte sedimentation rate (ESR), 544–5, 551
erythroplakia, 762, 767
erythroplasia of Queyrat, 606, *607*, 1377, 1492
escharotomy, 621, 624–5
ESCHAR trial, *165*
Escherichia coli, 45, 51, 56, 550, 1053, 1186, 1248
urinary tract infections, 1403, 1404, 1441–2, 1474
ESPAC-1 study, 1237
ethics, 170–5
conflict surgery, 424–5
informed consent, 171–3
patient autonomy, 170–1
research, 166, 174
stem cell therapy, 35–6
transplantation surgery, 174
ethmoid sinus, 716
infection, 721–2
ethnic variation
acral lentiginous melanoma, 610
breast cancer, 880–1
Crohn's disease, 1241
DDH, 567
gallbladder cancer, 1209–10
sickle cell disease, 1184
see also geographical factors
etomidate, *269*
etoposide, *155*
etrolizumab, 1245
eumycetoma, 71, 72
European Clinical Trials Database, 166
EuroSCORE II, 890
Eustachian tubes, *704*, 725
dysfunction in cleft lip/palate, 694–5
evacuation
conflict zones, 425
major disasters, 413, 423
evening primrose oil, 869
everolimus, *157*, 1420–1, 1540
evidence-based surgery, 168
Ewing's sarcoma, 250, 478, 535, *537*, 542
treatment, 546
excimer laser, 683
exemestane, *156*, 878
exercise, in lymphoedema, 1011
exercise tolerance testing, 257, 264–5, 888
exomphalos, 135
exophthalmos, 675–6
exorbitism, 687
exostoses
ear canal, 708
hereditary multiple, 539, 565
experimental study, *164*
explosions/explosives, 426, 429
explosive formed projectiles (EFPs), 430
extended focused assessment with sonography for trauma (eFAST), 366, 367, 372, *373*
extensor digitorum brevis, 524
extensor pollicis brevis, tenosynovitis, 507–8
extensor pollicis longus, 446
external ear
anatomy, 703
exostoses, 708
otitis externa, 707–8
squamous cell carcinoma, 708
external fixation, 392
advantages, *392*
disadvantages, *392*
indications, 392
external ventricular drain (EVD), 655
extoeing gait, 563
extracorporeal membrane oxygenation (ECMO), 892
extracorporeal shockwave lithotripsy, 1408
extradural haematoma, 312, *313*, 333–4
extremity trauma
compartment syndrome, 408
examination, 381–3
fractures, growth plate, 387
history, 381
injuries easily missed, *382*, 408
investigations, 384–5
major disasters, 416–17
neurological injury, 385
in skeletally immature, 403–6
soft tissue, 385
eye
acute red eye, 680–2
anatomy, 672–3
in craniofacial anomalies, 687, 688
injuries, 677–80
thyroid eye disease, 675–6, *811*
tumours, 676–7
eyelids
anatomy, 672
basal cell carcinoma, 674
burns, 628, 629
ectropion/entropion, 680, *681*
meibomian cysts, 673–4
swellings, 673–4
eye surgery, 683–5
enucleation, 684
eyeball evisceration, 685
laser, 682, 683, 684

face
developmental anomalies, 686–8
cleft lip/palate, 688–700
jaw disproportion, 701, *702*
muscles, 689
skeletal buttresses, 360
squamous cell carcinoma, 607, 608

facet joints, *338*
  injections, 474
facet subluxation, *339*, 348, *349*
facial injuries, 678–9
  airway management, 323
  burns, 628, *629*, 679–80
  major disasters, 417, *418*, *421*
facial nerve
  dissection in parotid surgery, 790–2, *793*
  injuries, 363, 789, 792
  palsies, 715
facies
  Cushing's syndrome, 841
  hippocratic, 1050
  'leonine', 69, *70*
factitious lymphoedema, 1006
faecal incontinence, *see* anal incontinence
faeces, fluid losses, 280, 281
faecolith, 1301–2
Fairbank's test, 456–7
falciform ligament, 1153, 1170
Fallopian tubes
  anatomy, 1514
  ectopic pregnancy, 1517–18
  removal at hysterectomy, 1517
Fallot's tetralogy, 904–5
falls
  elderly, 318, 322
  from a height, 314
false aneurysms, 966
familial adenomatous polyposis (FAP), *144*, 595, 1061
  clinical features and diagnosis, *236*, 1259–60
  duodenal polyps, 1234
  rectal, 1326–7
  surgical treatment, 1260
familial atypical multiple mole-melanoma (FAMM) syndrome, 604
familial hypocalciuric hypercalcaemia, 832
familial retinoblastoma syndrome, *537*
family history
  abdominal symptoms, 1017
  breast cancer, 871
  ovarian cancer, 1528
  rectal cancer, 1328–9
farnesyl transferase inhibitors, *157*
fasciitis, necrotising, 30–1, 50, 419–20, 597–8
fasciocutaneous flaps, 644–5, 646
fasciotomy, 28, 956
  delayed wound closure, 54
FAST, *see* focused assessment with sonography for trauma
fasting
  children, *122*
  metabolic response to, 10, 278–9
fat
  absorption, 1256
  dietary, 282
  digestion, 1241
  as reconstructive tissue, 639
fat burns, *622*
fat embolism, 956
fat mass, 8
fat mobilisation, 10
fat necrosis, breast, 866
fatty acids, 282
feeding, cleft lip/palate, 691
feeding formulae, burns patient, *627*
feeding tubes, 284–5
felon, 503–4
Felty's syndrome, 1184–5
female reproductive system, 1513–15
femoral artery
  aneurysm, 966
  false aneurysm, 966
  superficial, 943
femoral head, 511
  avascular necrosis, 512–13
  blood supply, 511
femoral hernia, 1025, 1034–6
femoral nerve, blockade, 1034
femoral nerve stretch test, 473
femoral osteotomy, varus, 515
femoroacetabular impingement (FAI), 453, 513, 515
  associated with SUFE, *574*, 575
femorodistal bypass, 951
femorofemoral crossover graft, 951
femoropopliteal bypass, 949, 950, 951
femoropopliteal obstruction, *944*
femur
  anteversion, 562
  endoprosthetic replacement, *547*
  fractures
    distal, 401
    paediatric, 405–6
    proximal, 400, *401*
    shaft, 400–1
  osteomyelitis, *551*
  slipped upper (capital) epiphysis, *382*, 404–5, 573–5
fentanyl, 276, 277
Ferguson-Smith syndrome, 595
fertilisation, 1514
fertility (male), 1511–12
  after orchidopexy, 125
  testicular maldescent, 1498
fetal circulation, 903, *904*
fetal stem cells, 36
fibre
  dietary, 1261, 1279, 1301, 1354
  fermentation, 1259
fibrin glue, 1367
fibrinolysis, 1060
fibroadenoma, breast, 870
fibroblast growth factors (FGFs), 561, 833
fibroblasts, 24–5
fibroids, 1514, 1524–6
fibroma, plantar, 506, 531
fibromatosis, diffuse, 1061
fibrosarcoma, 1045
fibrosis
  bladder neck, 1467–8
  intraperitoneal, 1060–1
  nephrogenic systemic, 191
  oral submucous, 763
  retroperitoneal, 1064–5, 1413
fibrous dysplasia, 541–2, *543*, 566
fibular collateral ligament, *518*
fibular flap, osseocutaneous, 771, *772*, *774*
fibular hemimelia, 576
field change ('cancerisation'), 762–3
field hospitals, 413, *414*
Filaria sanguinis hominis, 956
filariasis, 63–4, 1003–5, 1013
  elephantiasis, 63, 64, 1510
  hydrocoele, 1504
finasteride, 1378
fine-needle aspiration cytology (FNAC), 235
  breast lesions, 862–3
  CT-guided, lung cancer, 928–9
  mycetoma, 74
  neck swellings, 731
  oral cancer, 766
  thyroid, 804–5
  thyroid swellings, 808, 809
finger clubbing, 926
fingers
  congenital defects, *510*
  contractures, 32, 507
  deformities in arthritis, *443*, 505–6
  flexor muscles, 445
  mallet, 469
  pulleys, 507
  trigger, 507
firearm injuries, *see* gunshot wounds
firearms, 427–8
first aid, major disasters, 413
First World War, 633
fish bones, 743
'fish tail' deformity, 404
fissure-*in-ano*, 1351–3
fistula-*in-ano*, 1363–7
fistulas
  abdominal wall, 1045
  aerodigestive, 1073
  aortic enteric, 966, 1129
  arteriovenous, 966–7
  branchial, 754
  bronchopleural, 933
  colonic diverticular disease, 1274, 1275–6, 1440
  Crohn's disease, 1045, 1243
  definition, 616
  enterocutaneous, 1256
  faecal post-appendicectomy, 1314
  in imperforate anus, 136–7, 1345–6
  malignant tracheo-oesophageal, 1095
  mammary, 867, 868
  neoplastic, 1440
  pancreatic, 1221
  umbilical, 1045
  urinary tract, 1438–40
    male urethra, 1484
fistulectomy, 1365
fistulotomy, 1365, *1366*
Fitz, Reginald Heber, 1301
Fitz-Hugh–Curtis syndrome, 1049, 1519
fixed flexion deformity
  hip, 451, *452*
  knee, 454
flail chest, 368
flame burns, *622*
flaps, 27, 637, 641–9
  advancement, 641, *642*
  anal advancement, 1353, 1370
  anal fissure treatment, 1367
  anal sphincter augmentation, 1350, *1351*
  axial, 636, 637
  bilobed, *641*, *643*
  bipedicle, *641*
  breast reconstruction, 879, 880
  combined, 646, *647*
  combined local, 644
  composite, 637
  distant, 644–5
  free, 636, 637, 638, 645–6
  limb amputation, 959, 960
  lip reconstruction, 769
  pedicled/islanded, 636, 637, 644–5
  perforator, 637, 645–6
  postoperative care, 646–8
  random, 637
  rhomboid, *641*
  rotation, *641*
  tongue reconstruction, 771
  transposition, *641*, *643*
  V to Y, 641, *642*
  Y to V, *642*, *644*
flat foot (pes planus)
  acquired adult, 530
  causes, *458*
  children, 563
  flexibility tests, 460, *461*
  rigid, 563
flavonoids, 1011
flexible access bio-inspired (FAB) systems, 118
flexible bronchoscopy, 923, *924*
flexible endoscopy, upper GI tract, 1110–11
flexible sigmoidoscopy, 1320
flexor digitorum profundus, 445
flexor digitorum superficialis, *445*
flexor pollicis longus, 446
flexor tendon sheath infection, hand, 504
flow cytometry, 248
flucloxacillin, 56, 1009
fluid
  free intraperitoneal, 207, *208*
  intestinal absorption, 283
  obstructed intestines, 1281, 1288, *1289*
fluid administration
  burns patient, 622–3
  children, 120–1
  crush syndrome, 421

gastric outlet obstruction, 1130
hypercalaemia/ hyperparathyroidism, 826
hyperparathyroidism, 826
peritonitis, 1051
postoperative, 10
shock, 15–16
trauma, 317–18
fluid displacement test, 454
fluid losses, routes of, 280–1
fluid overload, 288
fluids
after laparoscopy, 115
calculation of requirements, 281
intake, 280
osmolarity, 121
tonicity, 121
fluorescein, 28
fluorescein angiography, 683
fluorescent *in situ* hybridisation (FISH), 247
fluoroscopy, 194
5-fluorouracil (5-FU), *155*, 1139, 1173, 1237, 1238, 1371
flutamide, *156*, 1474
foam sclerotherapy, 979–80
focal neurological deficit, brain tumour, 663, *664*
focal nodular hyperplasia, 1172
focused assessment with sonography for trauma (FAST), 123, 206–7, 324, 372, 1160
extended (eFAST), 366, 367, 372, *373*
Fogarty balloon catheter, 955
folate deficiency, 1243–4
Foley catheter, retained, 1436
folic acid supplementation, 1151
follicle-stimulating hormone (FSH), 1514
follicular carcinoma, thyroid, 809, *816*
follicular cyst, rupture, 1306
follicular occlusion tetrad, 1367
follow-up clinic, 300
fondaparinux, 990
fontanelle, raised ICP, 652
foods
bolus impacted in oesophagus, 1072
causing urinary oxalate, 1406
discolouring urine, 1376
intestinal obstruction, 1282
see also diet; nutrition; nutritional support
foot
anatomy, 524, *525*
biomechanics, 525
chondrosarcoma, *536*
clinical examination, 457–62
cutaneous nerve supply, *525*
deformities
congenital, 577–80
leprosy, 69, 70
diabetic, 532–3, 559, 953
entrapment neuropathies, 533
flat, 457, *458*, 460, *461*, 530
forefoot disorders, 525–8
frostbite, 953, *954*
heel pain, 533
hindfoot disorders, 528–9
infection, 531–2
longitudinal arch, 457
lymphoedema, 998
midfoot disorders, 528
movements, 458–9
neurological disease, 531, 533
progression angle, 562
reconstructive surgery, *647*
shape, 457, *458*
sports injuries, 468
stress fractures, 468, 528
tendon disorders, 529–30
tumours, 531
venous drainage, 969
venous pressure, 971
foot abduction orthosis (FAO), 578
football injuries, 465
foot drop, 69, 70
footwear, 458, 525, 527
foramen of Bochdalek, 938, 939
foramen of Luschka, 653
foramen of Magendie, 653
foramen of Monro, 653, 656
foramen of Morgagni, 938
foramen ovale, closure at birth, 903, *904*
foramen of Winslow, 1056, 1161
forced expiratory volume in 1 second (FEV_1), 916–17, 918
forced vital capacity (FVC), 917
forceps, 1562
atraumatic, 99
forearm
fractures, 398–9
testing rotation, 447
foreign bodies
bladder, 1434, *1435*, 1436
ear canal, 707
eye, 677, 679
inhaled, 132, 743–4, 924–5
oesophagus, 132, 1071–2
rectum, 1321
foreskin (prepuce)
disorders, 126–7, 1377, 1486–9
genital warts, 1496
forkhead box subgroup O (FOXO), 5
forward bending test, 441, 472, 581
Foster-Kennedy syndrome, 664
Fournier's gangrene, 50, 419, 597, 1440, 1509–10
fovea coccygea, 1347
Fowler's syndrome, 1485
fractional coronary flow reserve, 257
fractures
ankle, 401–2
AO classification, 386–7
calcaneus, 402
clavicle, 400
description, 385–6
diaphyseal, 394
femur, 400–1
forearm, 398–9
healing, 388, 394, 548
humerus, 399–400
imaging, 200–1, 206, 207, *208*
intra-articular fractures, 394–5
malunion, 394, 404, *494*
metaphyseal, 394
nasal bones, 362, 717
neurovascular injury, 404
olecranon, 399
open, *385*, 407–8
orbit, 356, 360–1, 677–8
in osteogenesis imperfecta, 567
osteoporotic, 349, 395, 406, *407*, 485
pathological, 406–7
radius, distal, 398
scaphoid, 396–7
skull, 207, *323*, 332–3, 356, 362
spinal
cervical spine, 206, 345–9, 485, *486*
imaging, 206, 209
lumbar spine, 209, 351
thoracic, 349
thoracolumbar, 350–1
sports, 464
stress, 464, 468, 528
talus, 402
fracture treatment
holding fragments, 389–94
infection, 556, *557*
reduction, 388–9
risks and benefits, *388*
in skeletally immature, 403–6
fragility fractures, 311, 320
fragility test, 1183
Francis report (2013), 178, 181
freckle (ephelis), 599
free tissue transfer, 637, 638, 645–6
Freiberg's disease (osteochondrosis), 527, *573*, 579
frenulum breve, 1488–9
frequency, 1375
frequency–dysuria (urethral) syndrome, 1376, 1442
fresh-frozen plasma (FFP), 21, 23
Freyer's operation, 1466
Frey procedure, 1232
Frey's syndrome, 792, 794–5
Friedlander curve, 429
Froment's sign, *444*, *446*, 502
frostbite, 422, 632, 953, *954*
frozen section specimens, 238
frozen shoulder (adhesive capsulitis), 492, *493*
Fuhrman grading, 1419
fulguration, diathermy, 102
functional endoscopic sinus surgery (FESS), 723
fundoplication
laparoscopic, 1080
Nissen, *1079*, 1080
fungal infections
ear, 707
military wounds, 433
transplant recipient, 1541–2
fungal toxins, *146*
furosemide, 1166
future liver remnant, 1172

gabapentin, 276
Gabriel's syringe, *1357*
gadolinium-containing contrast agents, 191
gait, 437
extoeing, 563
foot and ankle disorders, 458
in hip disease, *437*, 453
intoeing, 562–3
limping child, 589
toe-walking, 563
types of limp, *437*
gait analysis, cerebral palsy, 584–5
gait cycle, 525
galactocoele, 869
galactorrhoea, 666
Galen, 42
gallbladder
anatomy, 1188–9
cholecystitis glandularis proliferans, 1201
cholesterol polyposis, 1201
cholesterosis (strawberry gallbladder), 1201
congenital abnormalities, 1195–6
distension, 212–13
diverticulosis, 1201
embryology, 1195
empyema, 1200
functions, 1189–90
gas, 1190, *1191*
imaging, 1190–5
intraoperative, 1194–5
palpable, non-tender, 1199–200
physiology, 1189
polyps, 1210
porcelain, 1190, *1190*, 1210
torsion, 1198
gallows traction, 405
gallstones (cholelithiasis), 212, 213, *1157*, 1198–200
after peptic ulcer surgery, 1125
bile ducts, 228, 1204–5, *1206*, *1216*
causes, 1198–9
clinical features, 1018–19, 1199
CT scan, 1192
diagnosis, 1199–200
ERCP, 228, 1158, *1159*
intestinal obstruction, 1282
pancreatitis, 1222, 1224, 1225
pigment stones, 1183, 1199
treatment, 1200
ultrasound, 1191
gamekeepers' thumb, 398, 469, *503*
gamma-glutamyl transpeptidase (GGT), 1155
ganglion
midfoot, 528
wrist, 509

ganglion cells
  congenital absence, 136
  loss, 1095–6
ganglioneuroma, 847
gangrene, 952–3
  arterial insufficiency, 943
  diabetic, 953
  dry, *943*, 952
  Fournier's, 50, 419, 597, 1509–10
  gas, 45, 49–50, 420, 960
  Meleney's, 50, 419
  separation, 952
  synergistic, 50, 419, 597, 1045
  synergistic spreading (necrotising fasciitis), 30–1, 50, 419–20, 597–8
  treatment, 952–3
  venous, 988
  wet, 952
Gardner syndrome, *144*, *236*, 595, 1259
Garrod's knuckle pads, 506, *507*
gas
  free intraperitoneal, 210–11
  intestinal obstruction, 1280–1, 1288
  in urine (pneumaturia), 1376
gas bloat syndrome, 1080
gas gangrene, 45, 49–50, 420, 960
Gasserian rhizolysis, 670
gastrectomy
  Billroth I, 1120, 1123
  Billroth II, 1118, 1120–1
  palliative, 1138
  postoperative complications, 1138–9
  sequelae, 1123–5
  sleeve, *1147*, 1148–9
  subtotal, 1138
gastric acid
  hypersecretion, 1114
  normal secretion, 1108–9
gastric antral vascular ectasia (GAVE), 223
gastric arteries, 1106
gastric banding, 1147–8
  complications, 1150
gastric bypass, *1147*, 1148
  banded Roux-en-Y, 1149
  complications, 1150
  one anastomosis (mini-gastric bypass), 1149–50
gastric cancer, *146*, 1130–9
  aetiology and risk factors, 1131
  after gastric ulcer surgery, 1124
  bleeding, 1128
  chemotherapy, *155*, 1139
  clinical features, 1131–2
  endoscopic procedures, 224, *225*
  in gastric ulceration, 1118
  GISTs, 1139–40
  imaging, *214*
  incidence, 1130–1
  investigations, 1110–13
  lymphoma, 1140–1
  molecular pathology, 1133–4
  operability, 1136
  pathology, 1132–3
  radiotherapy, 1139
  site, 1132
  surgery
    complications, 1138–9
    outlook following, 1139
    palliative, 1138
    relapse following, 1139
    subtotal gastrectomy, 1138
    total radical gastrectomy, 1136–8
gastric emptying studies, 1112–13
gastric lymphoma, 1140–1
gastric metaplasia, 1114
gastric mucosal barrier, 1109, 1114
gastric outlet obstruction, 1129–30
gastric stasis, 1021
gastric ulcers, 222–3, 1117–18
  bleeding, 1127–8
  clinical features, 1118–19
  incidence, 1117
  malignancy in, 1118
  pathology, 1117–18
  surgery, 1123
gastrin, 851, 1107, 1108, *1110*, 1114, 1115
gastrinomas, 849, 850–2, 1116, 1120, 1141–2
gastritis, 1115–16
  autoimmune, 1115
  eosinophilic, 1116
  erosive, 1115, 1128
  H. pylori, 1114, 1115
  lymphocytic, 1116
  phlegmonous, 1116
  reflux, 1115
  stress, 1115
gastroduodenal artery, 1106
gastroduodenoscopy
  peptic ulcers, *1117*, 1119
  video, 1070
  see also oesophagogastroduodenoscopy
gastroenteritis, 131, 1248, 1272–3
gastroenterostomy, 1121, 1123
gastroepiploic arteries, 1106
gastrointestinal (GI) tract
  bacteria, 46–7, 1048–9
  endoscopy, *see* endoscopy
  haemorrhage, 211, 222–3, 1126–9
  injuries, 375
  motility, 1109–10
  perforation, 225, 232, 1019
gastrointestinal secretions, composition, *281*
gastrointestinal stromal tumours (GIST), 154, *156*, 1139–40
  immunohistochemistry, *246*
  molecular testing, 250
  oesophagus, 1084, *1085*
  rectum, 1327–8
  small bowel, 1251
  stomach, 1139–40
gastro-oesophageal junction
  adenocarcinoma, 1132
  endoscopy, *222*
gastro-oesophageal reflux disease (GORD), 1069, 1076–83
  aetiology, 1076
  after oesophagogastric resection, 1094
  children, 128
  clinical features, 1077
  complications, *1078*, 1080–3
  diagnosis, 1077–8
  endoscopic procedures, 221, 223, 1079
  investigations, 1071
  management guidelines, 221
  medical management, 1078–9
  surgical treatment, 1079–80
gastroplasty, Collis, 1081
gastroschisis, 135
gastroscopy, 1110–11
  gastric ulcers, *1118*
  normal stomach, *1111*
gastrostomy, 223–4, 285–6
Gaucher's disease, 1184
G cells, 1107, 1108, 1114, 1115
gefitinib, *156*
gemcitabine, *155*, 1237, 1238
gene expression
  major injury, 4–5
  and radiation, 153
  see also epigenetics
General Medical Council, 175
general practitioner (GP), 300
genetic mutations, detection, 249–50
genetics
  bladder carcinoma, 1446–7
  breast cancer, *144*, 871, 880–1
  cancer, 142, 249
  colorectal cancer, 1261
  Crohn's disease, 1242
  cystic fibrosis, 1219
  familial adenomatous polyposis, *144*, 1259
  Lynch syndrome, 1260
  ovarian cancer, 1528
  primary lymphoedema, 1001–2
  rectal cancer, 1329
  renal cell carcinoma, 1417
genetic testing
  cystic fibrosis, 1219
  MEN 1, 857
genitalia, ambiguous, 844
genital warts, 1486, 1496
genitourinary tuberculosis, 1405
genomic instability, 142
gentamicin, 56
geographical factors
  chronic pancreatitis, 1230
  colonic diverticula, 1273
  Crohn's disease, 1241
  gallbladder cancer, 1209–10
  gastric cancer, 1130–1
  oesophageal cancer, 1086–7
  ulcerative colitis, 1267
germ cell tumours
  chemotherapy and biological agents, *155*
  mediastinum, 935
  ovary, *1526*
  testes, 1506–9
Gerota's fascia, 838, 848
Gerstmann syndrome, *664*
gestational age, calculation, 1515
Giacomini vein, 976
giant cell tumour, 541, *542*, 546
giant condylomata, 1368
giant congenital pigmented naevus (giant hairy naevus), 603–4
gigantism, *1000*
Gillies forceps, 1562
Gilmore's groin, 1034
gladiators, 89
glandular fever (infectious mononucleosis), 738
Glasgow Coma Scale (GCS), 312, 325, 331
  calculation, 325
  head injury classification, *329*
Glasgow outcome score, 337
Glasgow scoring system (pancreatitis), *1224*
glaucoma
  acute angle closure, 682
  secondary, 678
  surgical treatment, 683–4
glenohumeral joint, 488
  instability, 496–8
  osteoarthritis, 493–5
  posterior dislocation, *384*
  rheumatoid arthritis, 493
glenoid labrum, *497*
glioblastoma multiforme, *156*, 664, 665
glioma, 664–5
gliptins, 1222
Glisson's capsule, 1049, 1153
global health, 1564–6
Global Surgical Outcomes Collaboration, 165
globus syndrome, 738
glomus tumours, 614, 711, *712*
glossopharyngeal nerve, 705
glossoptosis, 689, 691
glucagon, 3, 848, 1212
glucagon-like-peptide 1 (GLP-1), 1145
glucagonoma, 849
gluconeogenesis, 279
glucose
  blood levels, 8, 256, 260
  obligatory requirements, 282
glue ear, 709–10
gluten, dietary, 1255
glycaemic control, endoscopy, 219
glyceryl trinitrate, 1352
glycolysis, aerobic (Warburg effect), 142
GnRH agonists, 1525
goblet cell carcinoid tumours, 1315
goitre, 805–7
  aetiology, 805–6
  diagnosis, 807
  diffuse hyperplastic, 806, 807
  nodular, 806, 811, 812
  prevention and treatment, 807

retrosternal, 803, *804*, 807, 810–11, 936
toxic, 811, 812
goitrogens, 806
golfer's elbow, 448, 464–5
golf injuries, 464–5
Goligher retractor, 1561
Gompertzian growth, 142–3
gonorrhoea
pelvic inflammatory disease, 1518–19
proctitis, 1325
testing, *1520*
urethritis, 1494
Goodsall's rule, 1364
Gorlin (basal naevus) syndrome, *145*, 595
goserelin, *156*
gout, 506
gracilis muscle, anal canal transposition flap, 1350, *1351*
graft rejection, 1533–7
acute, 1536
chronic, 1536–7
hyperacute, 1535–6
mechanisms, 1534–5
graft-versus-host disease, 1537
gram-negative bacilli, aerobic, 45
granny knot, 95, 96
granulomas
bladder (bilharzial), 1444
eosinophilic, 541, *542*, *543*
lung, 934
pyogenic, 614
granulomatosis with polyangiitis (Wegener's syndrome), 795
Graves' disease, 810, 811
great saphenous vein (GSV), 969–70
incompetence, 975
stripping, 981
great vessels, transposition, 905
Grey Turner's sign, 1019, *1020*, 1223
GRFoma, *849*
gridiron incision, 1309
groin pain, 467
grommets, 710
Gross Motor Function Classification, 584
growth hormone (GH), 3
tumours secreting, 666
growth plate injuries, 403
classification, 387
guarding, abdominal, 1020, 1050
Guillain–Barré syndrome, 75–6
Guinea Pig Club, 628
gunshot wounds
assessment of extent, 428, *429*
management, 428–9
mechanisms of injury, 315, 427–8
military, 426, *426*, 428–9
radiography, 372
thorax, 370, *372*
Gustilo and Anderson classification (open fracture), 385, 407
gut failure, 46–7
gut mucosal permeability, 1242
Guyon's tunnel syndrome, 508
gynaecomastia, 69–70, 882, 1507

Hadfield's operation, 865, 868
haemangiomas, 612–13
capillary, 613
liver, 1171–2
orbit, *676*
rectum, 1327
spleen, 1185
haemangiosarcoma, 1185
haematemesis, 1075, 1126–9
haematocoele, 1499
haematocrit, 281
haematoma, 27
breast, 866
ear, 706–7
extradural, 312, *313*, 333–4
pelvic, 376
prevertebral, *342*
rectus sheath, 1023
retroperitoneal, 964, *965*
subdural, 334–5
thigh (thigh bruise), 27, 467
urethral disruption injury, 1481
haematopoiesis, 1178
haematopoietic tumours, 538
haematospermia, 1376
haematuria, 1375–6
benign prostatic hyperplasia, 1460
bladder cancer, 1448
causes, 1375
classification, 1375
polycystic kidney disease, 1402
renal stones, 1407
haemoglobin, glycated (HbA1c), 256, 260, 302
haemoglobin levels
in haemorrhage, 19
indication for transfusion, 21
haemoglobin S (HbS), 1184
haemoglobinuria, 1376
haemolytic anaemias, 1183–4
Haemophilus ducreyi, 1496
Haemophilus influenzae, 56, 587, 709, 743, 922, 1186, 1187
haemoptysis, 923–4
haemorrhage, 18–20
acute pancreatitis, 1228
after thyroidectomy, 815
day case surgery, 305
degree and classification, 19
exsanguinating external, 323
gastrointestinal, 211
colonic diverticula, 1274
colonic polypectomy, 232
peptic ulcers, 222–3
upper tract, 1126–9
haemorrhoids, 1355–6
intracerebral, 661
laparoscopic surgery, 113–14
liver surgery, 1171
management, 19–20
maxillofacial trauma, 355
pathophysiology, 9–10, 18
pelvic injuries, 209, 324, 365, 376–8
postoperative, 295–6
primary, 19
reactionary, 19, 305
retrobulbar, 361
revealed and concealed, 18–19
secondary, 19
shock, 13, 18
subarachnoid, 335, 658–61
subconjunctival, 359, 680
surgical, 19
tonsillectomy, 736–7
trauma, 323–4
torso, 365
variceal, 1163–6
haemorrhoidal veins, superior, 1319
haemorrhoid artery ligation operation (HALO), 1359
haemorrhoidectomy, 1357–9
complications, 1359–60, 1369, 1370
haemorrhoidopexy, stapled, 1359, *1360*, 1369
haemorrhoids, 1354–61
causes, 1354–5
clinical features, 1355
complications, 1355–6
external, 1360, *1361*
four degrees, *1355*
management, 1356–9
postoperative care, 1359
postoperative complications, 1359–60, 1369, 1370
primary internal, 1354–60
rectal prolapse, 1322
strangulation, 1356
haemosiderosis, 973, *974*, 984
haemostasis
liver transplant, 1555
liver trauma, 1161–2
thyroidectomy, 814, 815
haemothorax, 366
management, 368
massive, 368
Hageman factor, 618–19
Haglund's prominence, 460
hair cells, 704–5
hair follicles, 593
lesions, 602–3
Hallpike test, 714
hallux rigidus, 526–7
hallux valgus, *458*, 525–6
halo brace, 345
halo naevus, 600
hamartomas
lung, 934
spleen, 1178
hammer toe, *458*, 527
hamstring injury, 467
hand
bony deformities, 443
clinical examination, 442–6, 502
congenital anomalies/ malformations, 509, *510*, 580
deformity in leprosy, 69, 70
function, 502
imaging, 503
infections, 503–4
innervation, *443*
joint replacements, 506
movements, 444–5
muscle wasting, 443, 502, 508
osteoarthritis, *504*, 506
rheumatoid arthritis, *443*, 504–5
sports injuries, 469, *470*
swelling and stiffness, 503
transplantation, 649
trauma, *28*
Hand–Schuller–Christian disease, 541
hand washing, 43, 52
hangman's fracture, 347, *348*
Hansen's disease, *see* leprosy
hard palate
anatomy, 690, *691*
cleft, 690, *691*
squamous cell carcinoma, 774
harmonic scalpel, 104
Hartmann's procedure, 1265, *1275*, 1295, 1321, 1336
Hartmann's solution, 281, 624, 1290
Hashimoto's disease (autoimmune thyroiditis), 821–2
Hasselbach's triangle, 1030, 1033
Hasson port, 112
Hawkin's impingement test, 489
Hayflick hypothesis, 140
HDAC inhibitors, *157*
headache
brain tumours, 663
'thunderclap', 659
head injury
annual mortality, 328
associated cervical spine fracture, 332
cerebral contusions, 336
classification, 329
concussion, 330
CT scanning, *197*, 207, 357–8
diffuse axonal injury, 336
discharge criteria, 329–30
extradural haematoma, 312, *313*, 333–4
hearing loss, 713
intracranial pressure, 328–9, 336
medical management, 336–7
meningitis following, 656
minor and mild, 329–30
non-accidental, 330
outcomes and sequelae, 337
pituitary dysfunction, 337
primary survey, 331–2
secondary survey, 332
seizures, 337
subarachnoid haemorrhage, 335
head and neck cancers
causes, *145*, *146*
cervical lymph node disease, 758–9
chemotherapy agents, *155*, *157*
larynx, 751–2

lymphomas, 741
nasopharynx, 733–5
non-surgical treatment, *152*
oral, *see* oral cavity cancer
oropharynx, 740–1
staging, 764
healing, *see* bone healing; wound healing
healthcare workers
communication, 182
and patient safety, *178*, 180
Health Research Authority (HRA), 161
hearing aid, bone conduction, 711
hearing loss
brain tumour, 664
cleft lip/palate, 694–5
congenital sensorineural, 712
noise exposure, 713, *714*
presbycusis, 712–13
sudden sensorineural, 713
hearing tests, 705–6
heart
coronary artery anatomy, 886–7
development, 903, 904
masses, 911–12
surgical approaches, 884, 931
thrombus, 911
transplantation, 1556–8
valve anatomy, 894
heart block, 258
heartburn, 1077
heart disease, *see* congenital heart disease; ischaemic heart disease; valvular heart disease
heart–lung transplantation, 1557
heated intraperitoneal chemotherapy (HIPEC), 1317
Heberden's nodes, *443*, 506
heel pain, 533
Heerfordt's syndrome, 795
Heimlich manoeuvre, 132, 744
Heineke–Mikulicz pyloroplasty, 1122
Heineke–Mikulicz strictureplasty, 1247, *1248*
Heinrick's safety pyramid, 179
Heinz bodies, 1178, 1183
Helicobacter pylori, *146*, 246, 1076, 1113–15, 1140
eradication regimes, 1114–15, 1119–20
and gastric cancer, 1131
gastritis, 1114, 1115
peptic ulcers, 1116, 1117
helicopters, 411
Heller–Dor operation, 1099
Heller's myotomy, 1098–9
hemianopia
bitemporal, 664
homonymous, 664
hemiarthroplasty, shoulder, 400, 493, *494*
hemicolectomy
left, 1264–5
right, 1264
hemifacial microsomia, 686, *687*, 702
hemihepatectomy, 1170
hemiplegia, epilepsy, 670
hemispherectomy, anatomical, 670
hemivertebrae, *581*
Henoch–Schönlein purpura, 131, 1283, 1288, 1305
heparin, *221*, 258, 989, 990
hepatectomy, 1169–71
hepatic artery, 1153
aneurysm, 1163, *1163*
common, 1154
tortuous, 1188–9
thrombosis, 1555
hepatic duct, common, 1154, 1188
hepatic encephalopathy, 1156
hepatic veins
inferior, 1154
right, 1154
thrombosis, 1166–7
hepatitis, amoebic, 58
hepatitis, viral, 51–2, 1173
hepatitis B, 51, 1173
hepatitis C, 51, 1173
and hepatocellular carcinoma, 1173
organ donation, 1544
universal precautions, 52
hepatocellular carcinoma, 1173–5
hepatoma, *145*, *146*
Her2 gene, 249, 250
breast cancer, 250, 872, 878
gastric cancer, 1139
herbal enemas, causing proctitis, 1326
Herceptin®, 873, 878, 1139
hereditary haemorrhagic telangiectasia (Osler's disease), 719, 720
hereditary leiomyomatosis and renal cell cancer, *1418*
hereditary multiple exostoses (diaphyseal aclasis), 539, 565
hereditary non-polyposis colorectal cancer (HNPCC), *144*, 663, 1260–1, 1329
endometrial cancer, 1516
hereditary papillary kidney cancer, *1418*
hereditary spherocytosis, 1183
hernias
abdominal
anatomical causes, 1023
common principles, 1024
examination, 1025
history and diagnosis, 1025
investigations, 1025–6
management, 1026
mesh repairs, 1027–9
pathophysiology, 1023–4
sites, *1029*
surgical approaches, 1026–7
diaphragmatic, 133, 938, 939
epigastric, 1039
femoral, 1025, 1034–6
gluteal, 1044
hiatus, 1076, *1078*, 1081, 1083–4
incisional, 1026, 1039–41, 1287
inguinal, 124, 1029–34
internal (small intestines), 1282
irreducible, 1024, 1026
laparoscopy port site, 115, 1023, 1291
lumbar, 1042–3
management, 1026
mesh repairs, 1027–9
midline, 127
obstructed, 1024
obturator, 1043–4
omentum, 1061
parastomal, 1043, 1255, 1278
perineal, 1043
reducible, 1024
sciatic, 1044
scrotal, 1030, 1031
spigelian, 1024, 1041–2
sportsman's, 1034
strangulated, 1024, 1038
traumatic, 1043
umbilical, 1036–8
ventral, 1028, 1036
herniation syndromes, 328–9
herniogram, 1026, 1032
herniorrhaphy, 1032
herniotomy, 1032
herpes simplex virus
corneal ulcers, 677, 681
genital infections, 1495
oesophagitis, 1104
transplant recipient, 1541
herpes zoster virus, 681, 715, 1541
Herring classification, 572
heterografts (xenografts), heart valves, 895
Heuter–Volkmann principle, *561*
hiatus hernia
Allison repair, *1079*
paraoesophageal (rolling), 1083–4
sliding, 1076, *1078*, 1081
Hickman lines, 287
HIDA scanning, 1192, 1204, 1232
hidradenitis suppurativa, 595–6, 1367–8
pathology, 1367
presentation, 1367–8
hidradenoma, 603
highly active antiretroviral therapy (HAART), 52
high-pressure injection injuries, 28–9
high-risk patient
critical care, 266–7
factors contributing to risk, 262–3
identification, 263–5
minimising impact of surgery, 266
optimisation, 265–6
risk management, 263
high-tension electrical injuries, 631, *632*
Hilgenreiner's line, 569
Hill procedure, *1079*
Hill–Sach's lesion, 496
Hilton's law, 573
Hinchey classification, diverticulitis, *1274*
hindgut, embryology, 1319, 1344–5
hip
anatomy, 511
arthrodesis, 515
arthroscopy, 515
biomechanics, 511–12
clinical examination, 451–3
developmental dysplasia, 567–71
dislocation, cerebral palsy, 585
fixed flexion deformity, 451, *452*
fractures, 400, *401*
movements, 451–2
septic arthritis, *553*, 586, *587*
hip disease
avascular necrosis, 512–13
children, 589
femoroacetabular impingement (FAI), 453, 513, 515
gait disturbance, *437*, 453
inflammatory arthritis, 515
osteoarthritis, *437*, 513–14
Hippocrates, 42
hippocratic facies, 1050
hip replacement
bearing surfaces, 516
complications, 517–18
femoral component materials, 516
implant fixation, 516–17
infection, 554–6
osteoarthritis, 514, *515*
outcomes, 515–16
principles and design, 516
revision, 518
surgical approaches, 517
total, 515–18
hip screw, dynamic, 400, *401*
hip spica, 405
Hirschsprung's disease, 136, 1096
histamine, 1107, 1108, *1109*, *1110*
histamine receptor (H_2-receptor) antagonists, 1108, 1119, 1127
histology
deeper levels, 244
electron microscopy, 245
frozen section, 238
light microscopy, 242, *243*
sample adequacy, 243
special stains, 244–5
specimen processing, 236–8
specimens, 235
vs cytology, *243*
histopathology
bone infections, 552
intestinal tuberculosis, 79
mycetoma, 74
typhoid, 82

histopathologist, *237*
history taking
  abdominal symptoms, 1016–17
  extremity trauma, 381
  musculoskeletal disease, 436
  preoperative, 254–5
  shoulder disorders, 489
  spinal injuries, 341
  sports injuries, 463
  trauma, 315–16
  traumatic brain injury, 330–1
HIV infection, 51–2
  associated cancers, *146*
  circumcision in, 1487
  ENT system, 738
  intestinal complications, 1249, 1273
  and organ donation, 1544
  sialadenitis, 787
  transmission
    and circumcision, 127
    needle-stick injuries, 52
  universal precautions, 52
hoarseness, causes, 749, *750*
Hodgkin's disease, 147, 596, 741, 872, 882, 1182, 1185, 1251
Hoffmann's sign, 473
Holman–Miller (antral) sign, 719
Holmes–Adie pupil, 331
holmium laser enucleation of the prostate (HOLEP), 1463, 1465, 1467
Holt–Oram syndrome, 903
Homans' procedure, 1011–12
Homans' sign, 296
homeostasis, 2–3
home parenteral nutrition (HPN), 1257
homovanillic acid (HVA), 847
Hopkin's rod, 731
hormone replacement therapy (HRT), 260
  and breast cancer, 871, 881
  hyperparathyroidism, 831
hormone therapy
  breast cancer, *156*, 878
  prostate cancer, *156*, 1474
Horner's syndrome, 672, 1087
horseshoe kidney, 1399, *1400*
hospital acquired infection (HAI), 45, 47
Houston's valves, 1319
Howell–Jolly bodies, 1178
HRPT2 gene, 835
human chorionic gonadotrophin (hCG), 256, 1507, 1508, 1514, 1518
human factors, 176–7
human herpes virus 8 (HHV8), 246
human kallikrein-2 (HK2), 1379
human leucocyte antigens (HLAs), 1534
  matching in organ transplantation, 1537–8
human papillomavirus (HPV), *146*, 760, 1368
  anal intraepithelial neoplasia, 1368–9
  anal SCC, 1371
  anal warts, 1368
  cervical cancer, 1516
  genital warts, 1496
  oral SCC, 760
  oropharyngeal carcinoma, 740–1
  penile cancer, 1492
Human Tissue Authority (HTA), 1547
humerus
  chondrosarcoma, *536*
  distal lateral condylar mass fracture, *382*, 404, *405*
  distal (supracondylar) fracture in children, 403–4
  proximal fractures, 400
  proximal malunion, *494*
  shaft fractures, 383, 399–400
  thyroid carcinoma metastases, *817*
Hunner's ulcer (interstitial cystitis), 1443
Hürthle cell tumours, 818, 827
Hutchinson's melanotic freckle, 609, *610*
Hutchinson's sign, 610
hydatid disease, 64–8
  biliary, 1207
  liver, 65–7, 1169, *1169*
  pulmonary, 67–8
hydatid of Morgagni, 126, 1376, 1500
hydrocephalus, 586, 653–6
  aetiology, 653–4
  normal pressure, 654
  spina bifida, 484
  treatment, 655–6
hydrocoele, 63, 64, *124*, 125, 1376
  aetiology, 1502–3
  clinical features, 1374, 1503
  congenital, *124*, 125, 1503
  secondary, 1503
  treatment, 1503–4
hydrocolloid dressings, 625–6, 630
hydrocortisone
  intravenous, 844
  oral, 844
  pruritus ani, 1361
hydrocystadenoma (cystadenoma), 603
hydrofluoric acid, 632
hydrogel scaffolds, 39, 40
hydrogen cyanide, 618
hydronephrosis, 137, 213
  bilateral, 1411
  bladder outflow obstruction, 1460, *1461*
  causes of lower tract, *1411*
  causes of upper tract, *1411*
  imaging, 1411–12
  treatment, 1412–13
  ultrasound scan, *1386*
  unilateral, 1410–11
hydroureter, 213
21-hydroxylase deficiency, 844
1,25-hydroxyvitamin D, 825, 833
hygiene, and pruritus ani, 1361
hyperbaric oxygen (HBO), 420
hypercalcaemia, 825–6
  causes, *826*
  familial hypocalciuric, 832
  in hyperparathyroidism, 825–6
  renal calculi, 1406
hypercalciuria, 1405–6
hyperchloraemic acidosis, 1454–5
hypercortisolism, 841–2, 843
hypergastrinaemia, 1114, 1115
hyperglycaemia
  parenteral nutrition, 288
  postoperative, 4, 8
hyperhidrosis, 72, 595, 968
hyperlaxity syndrome, *458*
hypermetabolism, 3, *4*, 5, 6, 279
hyperoxaluria, 1406
hyperparathyroidism
  familial syndromes, 831–2
  lithium-induced, 831
  persistent, 836
  primary (pHPT), 825–32, 857, 858, 1406
  recurrent, 836–7
  secondary, 833–5
  tertiary, 835
hyperparathyroid-jaw tumour syndrome (HPT-JT), 832, *1418*
hyperplasia, 241
hypersplenism, 1180, 1184, *1184*
hypertension
  hyperaldosteronism, 840
  phaeochromocytoma, 845
  polycystic kidney disease, 1402
  postoperative, 294
  preoperative assessment, 257
hyperthermia, malignant, 272, *273*
hyperthyroidism, 13, 811–16
  eye disease, 675–6, *811*
hyphaema, 678
hypocalcaemia
  after parathyroid surgery, 831
  after thyroid surgery, 815, 816
hypochloraemic alkalosis, 128, 1130
hypochlorhydria, 1114, 1115
hypoglossal nerve, 782, 785
hypokalaemia
  intestinal obstruction, 1286
  primary hyperaldosteronism, 840
hyponatraemia
  children, 121
  encephalopathy, 120
  subarachnoid haemorrhage, 660–1
hypoparathyroidism
  after thyroid surgery, 815
  permanent, 830–1
hypoperfusion, occult, 18
hypopharynx
  anatomy, 726
  tumours, 741–2
hypospadias, 126, 1377, 1478, *1479*
hypotension
  permissive, 964
  postoperative, 293–4
  trauma/haemorrhage, 323–4
hypothalamus, 3, *4*
hypothenar wasting, 443
hypothermia, 10
  in CPB, 885
  postoperative, 299
  in trauma, 317
hypothesis, 162
hypothyroidism, 13, 802, 812, 822
hypovolaemia, trauma, 324
hypovolaemic shock, 13, 352, 368
hypoxaemia, postoperative, 292–3
hysterectomy
  bladder dysfunction after, 1429
  endometriosis, 1522
  excessive vaginal bleeding, 1517
  vesicovaginal fistula, 1439

iatrogenic injuries
  bile ducts, 184, 1203–4
  bladder, 1425–6, 1466
  colon perforation, 232
  male urethra, 1479, 1482
  pancreas, 1221
  upper GI endoscopy, 225
  ureters, 1415
idelalisib, *157*
idiopathic intracranial hypertension (IIH), 655
idiopathic thrombocytopenic purpura (ITP), 1182–3
ifosfamide, *155*
i-Gel airway, 271
i-Knife, 118
ileal conduit, 1452–3
ileal transposition, 1150
ileitis, Crohn's, 1242, 1305
ileoanal anastomosis, 1270–1
ileoanal pouch, 1270–1
ileocaecal valve, 1256
ileocolic artery, 1264
ileocystoplasty, 1443
ileorectal anastomosis, 1260, 1271
ileosigmoid knotting (compound volvulus), 1285
ileostomy, 1254–5, 1270
  end, 1254
  loop, 1254
ileum
  anatomy, 1240
  atresia, 1293–4
  neuroendocrine tumours, 854–5
  resection, 283–4
  terminal, *1240*, 1241
    Crohn's disease, 1242, 1305
ileus
  after appendicectomy, 1313–14
  gallstone, 1282
  meconium, 134, 1219, 1294
  paralytic, 297, 1296–7
  see also intestinal obstruction

iliac artery
  anatomy, 1034–5
  aneurysm, 966
  stenosis, 944, 948, 950
iliac crest graft, 771, 773, *774*, *778*
iliac vein, 1034–5
iliopsoas, 511
Ilizarov fixator, *557*
imaging
  abdominal aortic aneurysm, 213
  bowel ischaemia/infarction, 211
  bowel obstruction, 210
  hazards, 191
  head injury, 330
  image interpretation, 190, *191*
  inflammatory processes, 211–13
  in major trauma, 205–8
  oncology, 213–15
  orthopaedic surgery, 200–5
  renal colic, 213
  requesting, 190
  soft-tissue mass lesions, 203
  spinal injuries, 342–4
  see also individual imaging modalities
imatinib, 154, *156*, 1140, 1251
imetelstat, *158*
imidaquod, 1496
immersion injuries, 422
immobility, 11, 1006, 1406
immune system
  in major burns, 619
  response to injury, 3, *4*
  role in cancer, 141
immunoglobulins, 1176–7
immunohistochemistry, *243*, 245–7
  infections, 246
  tumour pathology, 245–6
immunosuppression, surgical infections, 46
immunosuppressive therapy
  complications, *1539*, 1541–2
  modes of action, *1538*
  principles, *1540*
  regimens, 1540
  transplantation, 649–50, 1538–41
immunotherapy agents, *157*, 1421
imperforate anus, 136–7, 1345–7
impetigo, 596
impingement
  femoroacetabular, 453, 513, 515
  shoulder, 449, 489
impotence, after prostatectomy, 1466
improvised explosive devices (IEDs), 426, 430, 432
IMRAD format, 168
incidentaloma, 839–40
incisional hernia, 1026, 1039–41, 1287
inclusion cysts, peritoneal, 1060
incontinence, *see* anal incontinence; urinary incontinence
indocyanine green (ICG), 1007
indoramin, 1468
induced pluripotent stem cells (iPSCs), 36–7
infants
  appendicitis, 1304
  definitions, *119*
  hip dysplasia, 567–71
  hypertrophic pyloric stenosis (IHPS), 127–8
  intussusception, 1283–4, 1293
  mastitis, 865
  postural abnormalities, 564
  preoperative care, 259
  rectal prolapse, 1321
infection control
  burns, 627, 630–1
  theatre, 52, 1563–4
infections
  after splenectomy, 1186–7
  foot, 531–2, 559
  hand, 503–4
  intracranial, 656–8
  joints, *see* joint infections
  liver, 1168–9, 1173
  military wounds, 432–3
  oesophagus, 1103–4
  skin, 596–8
  spinal, 481
  surgical, *see* surgical infections
  transplant recipients, 1541–2
  wounds, *see* wound infections
  see also specific infections
infectious mononucleosis (glandular fever), 738
inferior vena cava filter, 990
inferior vena cava (IVC), 1153, 1154, 1398
  injuries, 1162
  in liver resection, 1170
  retrocaval ureter, 1402
infertility, male factor, 1511–12
inflammation
  imaging, 211–13
  major burns, 618–19
  microscopic features, 241, *242*
  systemic response syndrome, 3, 47, 51, 1223
  tumour-related, 142
inflammatory bowel disease, 212, 1017, 1241, 1266–72
  anal stricture, 1370
  Crohn's disease, *46*, 225, 227, 616, 1241–8, 1271–2
  risk of malignancy, 1268
  symptoms, 1017, 1267
  ulcerative colitis, 1206, *1207*, 1267–71
infliximab, 1269
information technology, patient records, 180–1
informed consent, 171–3, 181, 267
  capacity, 173, 267
  endoscopy, 218
  surgeon's notes, 172
  transplantation surgery, 174
infrared radiation, 594
inguinal canal, anatomy, 1023, 1029–30
inguinal hernias, 1029–34
  causes, 1023, 1029
  children, 124
  classification, 1031
  congenital, 1029
  contralateral, 1031
  diagnosis, 1031
  direct, 1039
  indirect, 1030
  investigations, 1032
  management, *158*, 1032–4
  sliding, 1030
inguinal (Poupart's) ligament, 1029
inhalation injury, 618
inhaled particles, causing cancers, *146*
injection injuries, high-pressure, 28–9
injection sclerotherapy, 1356, *1357*
injury prevention, 320
Injury Severity Score (ISS), 310
inner ear, 703–5
inotropic drugs, 16, 892
in situ hybridisation, 247
Institute of Medicine (IOM), *Crossing the Quality Chasm*, 176
instruments
  forceps, 1562
  Kocher dissector, 1562
  McIndoe scissors, 1561
  retractors, 1560–1
  sterilisation, 1564
insulin, 848
insulin infusion, 8, 10
insulin-like growth factor-1 (IGF-1), 3
  inhibitors, *158*
insulinoma, 848–50, 857, *1216*
insulin resistance, 6, 8, 288
Integra®, 628, 630
Integrated Research Administration System (IRAS), 166
integrins, 141
intensive care outreach services (ICORS), 267
intensive care unit (ICU)
  acute pancreatitis, 1225
  role, 263, 266–7
interdigital pilonidal sinus, 1347
interferon alpha-2b, *157*
interleukin-2 (IL-2), 1534
intermaxillary fixation, 358
intermittent claudication, 943, 947
intermittent cross-clamp fibrillation, 885
internal carotid artery
  giant aneurysm, 660
  occlusive disease, 662
internal iliac artery, embolisation, 956
International Humanitarian Law, 424–5
international normalised ratio (INR), 220, *221*, 258
International Prostate Symptom Score (IPSS), 1461
internet, research databases, 163
interscalene block, 274
interspinous ligament, *338*
interstitial cell tumours, testes, 1507
interstitial cystitis, 1443
interstitial fluid (ISF), 995, 997
intervertebral disc, *338*
  herniation
    cervical, 474, *475*
    lumbar, *198*, 476, *477*
    thoracic, 475
  total replacement, *475*, 476, *477*
intervertebral foramen, 471
intestinal atresias, 133–4
intestinal failure, 46–7, 1555
intestinal hormones, 1241
intestinal obstruction
  acute in newborn, 1293–4
  adynamic, *1280*, 1296–8
  causes, 60–2, *1280*, 1282–5
  classification, 1280
  clinical features, 1285–8
  colonic diverticula, 1274
  congenital causes, *137*
  dynamic, 1280, 1285
  imaging, 1288–90
  Meckel's diverticulum, 1252
  parasites, 60–1, 1282–3
  pathophysiology, 1018–19, 1280–1
  postoperative, 1292
  pseudo-obstruction, 1297–8
  radiography, *193*
  recurrent caused by adhesions, 1292
  strangulation, 1281, 1286–7
  symptoms, 1017
  treatment
    large intestines, 1294–6
    small intestines, 1290–4
  vs appendicitis, 1306
intestinal perforation
  colonic diverticula, 1274
  colonic polypectomy, 232
  imaging, 210–11
  typhoid, 82–3, 1248
intestinal permeability, 1242
intestinal resection, fluid and nutritional consequences, 283–4
intestines
  atresia, 1293–4
  blast injury, 431
  intussusception, 129–30, 1283–4
  ischemia, reperfusion injury, 1291
  in major burn injuries, 619
  malrotation, 134, *135*, 1284–5, 1300
  tuberculosis, 78–81

  - vascular anomalies, 1276–7
  - viability assessment, 1291
  - volvulus, 1284–5
- intoeing gait, 562–3
- intra-abdominal pressure, raised, 380
- intra-aortic balloon pump, 892
- intracranial pressure (ICP)
  - normal values, 328
  - raised, 328–9, 652–3
    - brain tumours, 663
    - clinical features, 652
    - control, 336
    - in craniofacial malformations, 688
    - head injury, 328–9, 336
    - idiopathic, 655
    - investigation, 653
- intracytoplasmic sperm injection (ICSI), 1512
- intraductal papillary mucinous neoplasms (IPMNs), 1234
- intradural tumours, 480–1
- intramedullary nails, *390*, 392–3
  - elastic stable (ESIN), 405–6
- intraosseous infusion, 122
- intrathecal baclofen pumps (ITB), *584*
- intrauterine contraceptive device (IUCD), 1515, 1519
- intravenous cannulae, children, 122
- intravenous drug use, *553*
- intravenous urogram, *192*, 193, *194*, 1389
  - bladder cancer, 1449
- intubation
  - burns patient, 620, *629*
  - fibreoptic, 748
  - severe trauma, 323
- intussusception
  - children, 129–30, 1283–4
  - clinical features, 1287
  - differential diagnosis, 1287–8
  - imaging, 1289
  - pathology, 1284
  - rectal, 1324
  - treatment, 1293
- inverted papillomas, 723–4
- investment, surgical services, 1565
- iodine, 805, 813
- ionising radiation, 594
  - associated cancers, *145*
  - biological effects, 191
  - and breast cancer, 871–2
  - doses from CT scanning, 191, *192*, 196, 317
  - doses from radiographs, *192*, 861
  - injuries, 632
  - legislation, 191–3
  - proctitis, 1325
  - risks of, 191, 317
  - thyroid tumours, 816
- Ionising Radiation (Medical Exposure) Regulations (IRMER), 191–2
- ipilumumab, *157*, *158*
- Iraq war, 426
- iridotomy, laser, 682, 684
- irinotecan, *155*
- iritis, 678
- iron deficiency
  - after gastrectomy, 1124
  - dysphagia, 740, 763, 1105
- irritable bowel syndrome (IBS), 1017, 1279
- Isaacson, Peter Gersohn, 1140
- ischaemia
  - chronic small intestinal, 1254
  - mesenteric, 956, 1061, 1253–4
  - myocardial, 265, 294
- ischaemia–reperfusion syndrome, 13
- ischaemic colitis, 1276–7
- ischaemic heart disease (IHD), 887–9
  - clinical manifestations, 887
  - indications for surgery, 889
  - investigations, 888–9
  - pathophysiology, 887
  - preoperative care/assessment, 257, 890
  - risk factors, *887*
  - surgical risk management, 265
- ischaemic limb
  - acute, 955–6
  - chronic, 943–52
  - critical, 943, 949
- ischiorectal abscess, 1362, *1363*
- islets of Langerhans, 848, 1212, 1219
  - transplantation, 1553
- isotope renogram, 1392–4, *1395*, 1404, 1412
- itching, burn wounds, 631
- Ivor Lewis operation, 1092, 1093

- Jaboulay's operation, 1503–4
- jackhammer (nutcracker) oesophagus, 1099–100
- Jack's test, 460, *461*
- Japan, gastric cancer, 1130–1, 1136–7, 1139
- jaundice
  - after cholecystectomy, 1203
  - bile peritonitis, 1052
  - imaging, 213
  - neonatal, 135, 1196
  - pancreatic carcinoma, 1234
- javelin throwers, 465
- jaw, developmental abnormalities, 701, *702*
- jaw tumour syndrome, hyperparathyroid, 832
- Jehovah's Witness, 173, 259
- jejunostomy, 283, 286
- jejunum, 1241
  - atresia, 134, 1293–4
  - diverticulae, 1251–2
  - neuroendocrine tumours, 854–5
- Jenkins' rule, 1041
- Jobe's test, 449, 450
- Johansen step technique, 768–9
- Johne's disease of cattle, 1242
- Joint Advisory Group (JAG), UK, 217
- joint contractures, release, *584*
- joint disease, imaging, 201–2
- joint effusions, 204
- joint fractures, 394–5
- joint infections
  - children, 586–7
  - complications, 588–9
  - imaging, 204, *205*
  - implant-related, 554–6
  - native joint, 553–4
- joint laxity, generalised, 498
- joints, assessment of movement, 438–9
- Joll retractor, 1560
- journals, peer-reviewed, 167–8
- J pouch, 1271
- jugular venous pressure (JVP), 255
- junctional naevus, 599
- junctional zones, torso, 364–5
- juvenile polyp, rectum, 1327

- Kanavel's cardinal signs, 504
- Kaposi's sarcoma, 52, *146*, 615, 738
  - chemotherapy and biological agents, *155*
  - conjunctiva, 680
  - lymphoedema, 1005
- Karydakis procedure, 1348
- Kasai procedure, 135, 1197
- kayaking, 467
- *KCNJ5* gene, 840
- Keinböck's disease, 508–9
- Keller's excision arthroplasty, 526
- keloid scars, 31, 815
- keratin horn, 606
- keratinocytes, 592, 634
- keratitis, 677, 681
- keratoacanthoma, 606
- Kerlix®, 630
- ketamine, 269
- ketone production, 279
- Ki67, 245, 246
- kidneys
  - anatomy, 1398
  - benign tumours, 1416
  - calculi, 213, 825, *1386*, 1405–7
  - congenital abnormalities
    - agenesis, 1399
    - duplex renal pelvis/ureter, 1400
    - ectopic/crossed renal ectopia, 1399
    - horseshoe kidney, 1399, *1400*
    - multicystic disease, 1399
  - embryology, 1398–9
  - enlargement, 1402
  - infarction, 1416
  - injury
    - acute postoperative, 294–5
    - preoperative management 259,
  - medullary sponge, *1386*, 1406
  - parathyroid hormone actions, 825
  - polycystic disease, 1402–3, 1549, *1550*
  - renal cell carcinoma, 547, 548, 1416–21
  - scarring, 1404
  - transitional cell carcinoma, 1421
  - trauma, 1413–14
  - Wilms' tumour (nephroblastoma), 138, *152*, *156*, 832, 1421–2
- kidneys, ureters and bladder (KUB) X-ray, 1388
- kidney transplantation
  - first successful, 1532
  - graft dysfunction, 1551–2
  - graft rejection, 1535–7
  - hyperparathyroidism after, 835
  - living donor, 1547–8
  - organ donation, 1542–8
  - organ recovery (deceased donor), 1544–7
  - outcomes, 1552
  - with pancreas transplant, 1552
  - patient selection, 1549
  - technical complications, 1550–1
  - technique, 1549–50
- Kienbock's disease, *573*
- Kiesselbach's plexus, 717, 719
- Killian's dehiscence, 738
- *Kingella kingae*, 587
- Kirschner wires (K-wires), 389, 392, 398, 399
  - indications for, *392*
- *Kit* gene, 154, 249
- *Klebsiella* spp., 45, 56, *937*, 1442
- *Klebsiella granulomatis*, 1496
- *Klebsiella pneumoniae*, 1404
- Klinefelter's syndrome, 882, 1376, 1506, 1511
- Klippel–Feil syndrome, 489
- Klippel–Trenaunay syndrome, 972, 991, *1000*
- knee
  - anatomy, 518–19
  - arthrodesis, 521
  - arthroscopy, 521
  - biomechanics, 519
  - clinical examination, 453–7
  - dislocation, *382*, 383
  - giving way, 467, 468
  - instability, 468
  - joint replacement, 521–3
  - locking, 467
  - meniscal injuries, 456, 467
  - movement, 454, 519
  - osteoarthritis, 519–20
  - osteotomy, 521
  - paediatric metaphyseal corner injury, *590*
  - soft tissue disorders, 520–1
  - sports injuries, 465, 466, 467–8
  - through-knee amputation, 959
  - varus deformity, 454, 521
  - *see also* patella
- knee angle, 563
- knee–ankle–foot orthosis (KAFO), *564*

knee–elbow position, 1342
knee pain
  children and adolescents, 575–6
  patellofemoral, 467–8
knock-knees, 563
knot tying, 94–5, 96
Kocher dissector, 1562
Kocher manoeuvre, 850
Koch's postulates, 42–3
Kock pouch, 1454
Köhler's disease, *573*, 580
Kras mutations, *248*, 249, 250, 1261
Krukenberg's tumours, 1135
Kshara sutra, 1367
KTP (green light) laser, 1467
Kulchitsky cells, 1250, 1300, 1315
Kupffer cells, 1155, 1172
Kussmaul's sign, 911
kyphoplasty, 485
kyphosis
  in ankylosing spondylitis, 481, *482*
  normal thoracic, 471
  Scheuermann's, 483, 582

Lachmann test, 455
lacrimal canaliculi, injuries, 678
lacrimal gland
  anatomy, 672
  tumours, 675
lacrimal sac, mucocoele, 674–5
lactate, 17, 326, *327*
lactic acidosis, 12, *14*, 17
lactiferous ducts, 860
Ladd's procedure, 134
lag screw, *393*
lag test, 454
Lancet Commission, 1565–6
Lane's forceps, 1310
Langenbeck retractor, 1560
Langerhans' cells, 592
Langer's lines, 85–6, 636
laparoscopic surgery, 86–9
  abdominal trauma, 373
  adrenalectomy, 847–8
  anastomoses, 99
  anterior mesh rectopexy, 1324
  appendicectomy, 1309, 1311–12
  bariatric surgery, 1147
  benefits, *87*
  cholecystectomy, 1202
  colorectal cancer, 1265
  diathermy, 103, 114
  discharge, 116
  emergency situations, 116
  fundoplication, 1080
  hernia repair, 1026, 1033
    epigastric hernia, 1039
    femoral hernia, 1036
    incisional hernia, 1040–1
    inguinal hernia, 1033
    umbilical hernia, 1038
  liver resection, 1170–1
  natural orifice (NOTES), 117, 118
  operative problems, 113–14
  patient positioning, 85, 266
  pneumoperitoneum creation, 112
  port-site hernias, 115, 1023, 1291
  postoperative care, 114–16
  preoperative problems, 112–13
  principles of safe, *87*
  risks of complications, 266
  single incision, 117
  splenectomy, 1186, *1186*
  stapling devices, 97
  training, 117–18
  trocar insertion, 87–9, 112
  trocar site haemorrhage, 114
laparoscopy
  gallbladder carcinoma, *1211*
  gastric cancer, *1110*, 1112
  liver disease, 1160
  oesophageal cancer, 1089–90
  uterine fibroids, *1525*
lapatinib, *156*
lap-belt injuries, 351
large intestine
  amoebiasis, 57–60, 1272–3
  anatomy, 1258–9
  bacteria, 46–7, 1048–9
  benign tumours, 1259–61
  malignant tumours, *see* colorectal cancer
  obstruction, *see* intestinal obstruction
  physiology, 1259
  volvulus, 1284–5
laryngeal mask airway, 271, 748
laryngeal nerves
  recurrent, 727, 801–2
    identification in thyroidectomy, 813–14
    intraoperative monitoring, 814
    paralysis after thyroidectomy, 815
  superior, 727, 815
laryngectomy, 752–3
laryngitis
  acute, 750
  chronic, 750
laryngoscope, paediatric, 120
laryngoscopy, *728*, 731
  thyroid assessment, 809
laryngotracheobronchitis (croup), 743
larynx
  anatomy, 727, *728*
  examination, 729, 731
  functions, 727, *728*
  imaging, 730
  injuries, 755–6
  papillomata, 750
  tumours, 751–2
  venous oedema, 815
Lasègue's straight leg raise test, 441–2, 473
Laser Assisted Bile duct Exploration by Laparo-endoscopy for choledocholithiasis (LABEL), 118
laser treatments
  eye surgery, 682, 683, 684
  oesophageal cancer, 1094
  prostate, 1463, 1465, 1467
  varicose veins, 977–9
last menstrual period (LMP), 1515
late dumping, 1124
latissimus dorsi flaps, *645*, *647*
  breast reconstruction, 879, *880*
lavage
  peritoneal, 373
  pulsed jet, 27
laxatives, 1279
leadership, healthcare, 188
lead time bias, 146–7
lean body mass, 8
lean manufacturing principles, 187
ledderhosen disease, 506, 531
Le Fort fractures, 360
left anterior descending artery (LAD), 886, *887*
left internal mammary artery (LIMA) graft, 890, *891*
left ventricular failure, 265
Legg–Calvé–Perthes disease, 571–3
leg length discrepancy, 452–3, 514
leg ulcers, *see* venous leg ulcers
Leibovich score, 1419
leiomyoma
  uterine (fibroids), 1514, 1524–6
  vein wall, 994
leiomyosarcoma
  oesophagus, *1085*
  uterine, 1524
  vein wall, 994
lens, subluxation, 678
lentigo, 599
lentigo maligna melanoma, 609, *610*
lenvatinib, *156*
leprosy, 68–71, 882
Leriche's syndrome, 943
letrozole, *156*, *158*, 878
Letterer–Siwe disease, 541
leukaemia
  acute promyelocytic, *156*
  causes, *145*, *146*
  chronic myeloid, *156*
  hairy-cell, *157*
  splenomegaly, 1182
  treatment, *152*, *155*, *156*, *157*
leukoplakia, 761–2
  bladder, 1452
  hairy, 738
  management, 767
  proliferative verrucous, 763
  speckled, 762, 767
leuprolide, *156*
levator ani muscles, 1319, 1320
'levator syndrome', 1354
levobupivacaine, *273*
Leydig cells, 1457, 1498
Leydig cell tumours, 1507
Lich–Gregoir technique, 1550
Lichtenstein's repair, 1032, 1033
lifestyle factors, associated with cancers, *146*
Li–Fraumeni syndrome, *144*, 663, 880
ligament injuries
  grading, *464*
  sports, 464
ligaments of Cooper, 860, 1035
ligament of Treitz, 221
ligamentum teres, *511*
ligament of Wrisberg, *518*
Ligasure system™, 104
ligation of intersphincteric fistula tract (LIFT), 1366
lighting, operating theatre, 1563
lignocaine, *273*, 274
limb ischaemia
  acute, 955–6
  chronic, 943–52
  critical, 943, 949
limb malformations, congenital, 564–6
limb reduction procedures, 1011–12
limb revascularisation, 326
limbs
  development, 561
  normal variants of growth/ development, 562–4
limb salvage
  bone tumours, 546–7
  extremity trauma, 416–17
limb swelling
  differential diagnosis, *1000*
  see also lymphoedema
limb transplantation, 649
limb volume measurement, 1007
limp, childhood, 589
linea alba, 1022
  hernia through, 1039
  stretching, 1022, *1023*, 1037–8
lingual nerve, 782, 785
linsitinib, *158*
Linxian, China, 1086
lipase, serum, 1223
lipid storage disease, 1184
lipodermatosclerosis, 973, 984, 986
lipodystrophy, 595
lipoedema, 1006
lipofilling, 639
lipoma, 544, 936
  retroperitoneal, 1065
lipomyelomeningocoele, 667, 668
lipoproteins, plasma, 1241
liposuction, 1011
lips
  mucous retention cyst, *776*
  reconstruction surgery, 769
  tumours, 765, 767–9, 777
Lisch nodules, 595
Lisfranc fracture–dislocation, *197*, 402–3, 524
Lisfranc's ligament, 403
lithium, 261
  hyperparathyroidism, 831
litholapaxy, 1435–6
lithotomy position, 1342

lithotripsy, 1409, 1436
lithotrite, blind, 1435, *1436*
liver
  abscess
    after trauma, 1162
    amoebic, 57–60, 1169
    pyogenic, 1168, *1168*
  acute failure, 1155–6
  anatomy, *215*, 1153–5
  bile production, 1189
  blood supply, 1153
  chronic disease, 882, 1156–7, 1166–8
  embryology, 1155
  fatty, 1157
  functions, 1155
  hydatid cyst, 65–7, 1169, *1169*
  imaging, 1157–60
    hepatocellular carcinoma, 1174
  infections, 1168–9, 1173
    treatment, *1173*
  metastases, *195*, 214, *215*, 1112, *1158*, *1160*
    colorectal cancer, 1173, *1173*, 1262, 1266
    oesophageal cancer, 1089
  packing, 1161
  palpation, 1021
  response to injury, 4, 7–8
  simple cysts, 1168
  trauma, 208, 373–4, 1160–3, *1162*
    in children, 123
  tumours, 1169–75
    ablation, 1171
    benign, 1171–2
    hepatocellular carcinoma, 1173–5
    metastases, 1172–3
    surgical approach, 1169–71
  venous drainage, 1154
liver disease
  polycystic, 1403
  preoperative management, 259
liver flukes, 1207, 1208
liver function tests (LFTs), 256, 1155
  oesophageal cancer, 1089
  prostate cancer, 1471
  TPN, 288
liver transplantation, 1554–5
  in acute liver failure, 1156
  after variceal haemorrhage, 1166
  for ascites, 1166
  cholangiocarcinoma, 1209
  hepatocellular carcinoma, 1175
  indications and patient selection, 1554
  living donor, 1548
  organ donation, 1542–8
  outcomes, 1555
  recovery from deceased donor, 1545
  technical complications, 1555
  technique, 1554
living donor transplantation, 1547–8
Lloyd-Davies position, 1336
lobectomy, 932
local anaesthesia, 273–5
locking screws, 392
lockjaw (tetanus), 417–18, *419*
Loeffler's syndrome, 60
log-rolling, 325–6, 341
lonafarnib, *157*
London Blitz, 421
long head of biceps, rupture, 469, 495–6
longitudinal muscle, anal canal, 1340
longitudinal study, *164*
long saphenous vein (LSV), grafts, 890, *891*, 949
loose bodies
  elbow, 500, *501*
  peritoneal, 1060
lordosis
  cervical spine, 439, *440*, 471
  lumbar spine, *440*, 441, 471
Lord's operation, 1503
low back pain
  discogenic, 476
  epidemiology, 471
  patient history, 472
  physical examination, 472–3
  see also back pain
lower limb
  axes, 519
  compartments, 524
  compartment syndrome, 382, 408, 955–6
  length discrepancy, 452–3, 514
  neurological examination, *473*
  oedema, 972–3
  paediatric orthopaedics, 575–7
  venous anatomy, 969–70
lower motor neurone (LMN) lesions, 473
lower oesophageal sphincter (LOS), 1067–8, 1076, *1077*
  botulinum toxin injection, 223, 1099
  incompetence, 1100
  non-relaxing, 1097, 1098
  postprandial transient relaxations, 1076
lower urinary tract symptoms (LUTS), 1375
  BPH, indications for treatment, 1463–4
  investigation
    blood tests, 1377–9
    endoscopy, 1379–85
    urine-based tests, 1379
  male, 1459
    assessment, 1461–2
  post-micturitional, 1375
  storage, 1375
  voiding, 1375
low-income countries
  patient safety, 180
  spinal care, 485–7
low molecular weight heparin (LMWH), *221*, 258, 989, 990
Ludwig's angina, 756
Luer connection, 748
Lugol's iodine, 815
lumbar hernia, 1042–3
lumbar puncture, subarachoid haemorrhage, 659
lumbar spine
  clinical examination, 441–2
  disc herniation, 476
  fractures, *345*, 351
  lordosis, *440*, 441, 471
lumbar sympathectomy, 276, 968
lumps
  breast, 861–3, 869, *871*
  history and examination, 438
  neck, 753–5
lunate, avascular necrosis, 508–9
lunate dislocation, 397
Lund and Browder chart, 621
Lundh test, 1214
lung cancer, 925–34
  causes, 143, *145*, *146*
  chemotherapy and biological agents, *155*, *156*
  clinical features, 925–6
  histological classification, 925
  investigations, 926–30
  molecular testing, 250
  pathological types, 925
  pleural effusion, 921, 922
  risk factors, 925
  screening, *158*
  surgical management, 931–4
  survival rates, 926, 928
lung disease
  obstructive, 917
  restrictive, 917
lung resection, 932–4
  broncoplastic, 933
  complications, 933–4
  metastases, 934
lungs
  abscess, 937
  anatomy, 914
  benign tumours, 934
  biopsy, 928–9, 930
  blast injury, 430
  fetal development, 914
  fluid losses, 280
  functional assessment, 916–18
  hydatid disease, 67–8
  inhalation injury, 618
  metastases, 214, 934
  sequestration, 937
  transplantation, 1557
  tuberculosis, 937
luteinising hormone (LH), 1457, 1514
luteinising hormone-releasing hormone (LHRH), 1457
  agonists, 869, 878, 1452, 1474
lymph
  transport, 996
  volume, 997
lymphadenitis
  acute, 996–7
  cervical, 77–8, 756, *757*
  lymphoedema, 1005
  mesenteric, 1062
  tuberculosis, 77–8, 757
lymphadenopathy, paratracheal, *928*
lymphangiography
  direct, 1006, *1007*
  filariasis, *1004*
  primary lymphoedema, 1003, *1004*
lymphangiomas, 999
lymphangions, 996
lymphangiosarcoma, 879, 999–1000
lymphangitis, 49, 597, 1005
  acute, 996–7
lymphatic bypass, 1011
lymphatic drainage, manual, 1009
lymphaticovenular anastomosis, 1011
lymphatic system
  anal canal, 1341
  anatomy and physiology, 995–6
  bladder, 1423
  development, 995
  gallbladder, 1189
  imaging, 1006–7
  rectum, 1319
  stomach, 1107, 1135–6
  thyroid, 800–1
lymph nodes
  axillary, 860–1
  cervical
    adenitis, 77–8, 756–7
    anatomy, 728–9, 800–1
    dissection, 758–9, *784*, 785, 819
    metastases, 729, 764
  groin, 1031
  mediastinal, 922, 929–30, 936
  mesenteric, 855, 1062
  resection
    gastric cancer, 1137–8
    neck, 758–9, 767, *784*, 785, 819
    oesophageal cancer, 1092
  retropharyngeal, 727
  thorax, 914, *915*
  tumour infiltration, 213–14
lymphocoele, 1013
  peri-transplant, 1551
lymphocytic gastritis, 1116
lymphoedema, 997–1000
  acute inflammatory episodes, 1008–9
  after breast cancer treatment, 879, 1005
  and chronic venous insufficiency, 1005–6
  conditions mimicking, 1006
  definition, 997
  investigation, 1006–7
  malignancies associated with, 999
  management, 997, 1007–12
  pathophysiology, 997–8
  primary, 998, 1001–3
  risk factors, 998, 999
  scope of clinical problem, 997
  secondary (acquired), 998, 1003–6

severity classification, 997
symptoms and signs, 997, 998–9
lympho-fluoroscopies, 1007
lymphogranuloma inguinale, 1325, 1369, 1496
lymphogranuloma venereum, 1325, 1495–6
lymphomas
causes, *145*, *146*
classification, 147
cutaneous T cell, *157*
gastric, 1140–1
head and neck, 741, 761
mediastinum, 935–6
molecular testing, 250
pancreas, 1238
salivary glands, *789*
in Sjögren's syndrome, 796
small bowel, 1251
spleen, 1185
thyroid, 816–17, 821
treatment, *152*
chemotherapy and biological agents, *155*, *157*
lymphorrhoea, 1008
lymphoscintigraphy, 1006
lymph trunks, 996
Lynch syndrome, 251, 1260–1, 1329, 1516

Maastricht classification, 1544
McBurney's point, 1303, 1309
McCune Albright's syndrome, 566, 600
McFarlane staging, 843
McIndoe scissors, 1561
McKeown operation, 1092, 1093
McMurray's test, 456
macrophages, 24, 1178
macula, 673
macular disorders, 683
mafenide acetate cream, 625
Maffucci syndrome, *537*, 540, 565
Magenstrasses and Mill operation, 1148
magnesium, requirements, 281
magnetic resonance angiography (MRA), 197, *199*, 213, 947
magnetic resonance cholangiopancreatography (MRCP), 197, *198*, 1215, *1216*
ascariasis, 60–1
cholangiocarcinoma, 1208, *1209*
chronic pancreatitis, 1231
gallstone, 1192, *1193*
hydatid disease, 66
magnetic resonance imaging (MRI), 197–8
advantages, 197, *199*
anal fistula, 1365
anatomical hemispherectomy, 670
arthrography, 201–2, 496, *497*, 503
benign prostatic hyperplasia, *1461*
bone infections, 204
bone tumours, *536*
brain abscess, 656, *657*
brain tumours, *664*, *665*, 683, *684*
breast, 862
cardiac, 888
contraindications, 474
Crohn's disease, 1244–5
cross-sectional, bladder cancer, 1449, *1450*
diffusion weighted, 197–8
disadvantages, 198, *199*
ear, 706
enterography, 212, 1244–5
femoral head osteonecrosis, 512, *513*
HIV-associated parotitis, 787
knee, 520
liver, 191
liver disease, 1158
lymphoedema, 1006–7
multiparametric (mpMRI), 1390, *1392*
mycetoma, 73
myelofibrosis, *1185*
oesophageal cancer, 1090
oral cancer, 766
osteomyelitis, 551
pancreas, 1215, *1216*
paranasal sinus carcinoma, *724*
parathyroid glands, 828
parotid gland tumours, *788*, *790*
phaeochromocytoma, 845–6
pharynx, larynx, neck, 730, *731*
pituitary gland, 842
principles, 197
proctography, 1344
rectal cancer, *1332*
shoulder, 489, *490*
skier's thumb, *503*
spinal, 338–9, 343, 474
stomach, 1112
synovitis, 201
thyroid lymphoma, *821*
trauma, 209
extremities, 385
urethral diverticulum, *1485*
urinary tract, 1390
uterine fibroids, *1525*
venous angioma, 993, *994*
major adverse cardiovascular events (MACE), 257
major histocompatibility complex (MHC), 1537
malabsorption, 1255–6
bacterial overgrowth, 1255–6
bowel resection, 283
coeliac disease, 1255
cystic fibrosis, 1219
maladie de Roger, 908
malaria, 1180, 1181, 1187
malignant melanoma, 608–12
anus, 1371–2
choroidal, 676–7
cytology, *240*
epidemiology, 608–9
familial cutaneous, *145*
management, *156*, *157*, 611–12
molecular testing, 250
pathophysiology, 609
penis, 1493
premaligant lesions, 603, 604
staging, 611
malignant transformation, 141, 142
malleolar flare, 972
mallet finger, 469
mallet toe, 458, 527
Mallory-Weiss syndrome, 1075, 1128
malnutrition, 46, 260, 796
malnutrition universal screening tool (MUST), 280
malrotation with volvulus, 134, *135*, 1284–5
mammalian target of rapamycin (mTOR) inhibitors, *157*, 1420–1, 1540
mammography, 861, 880
mandible
advancement surgery, 688
fractures, 358–9
prognathism, *700*, *701*
reconstruction, 771, *772*, 773
underdevelopment, 688, 701
Mangled Extremity Severity Score (MESS), 416
mannitol, 421
manometry
anorectal, 1278, 1343–4
oesophagus, 1068, *1069*, 1070–1, 1078, 1098
Mantoux test, 78
MANTRELS score, *1307*
marathon runners, 467
Marfan syndrome, *458*, 901, 903, 908, 909, 1416
Marion's disease, 1467
Marjolin's ulcer, 29, 605, 984
martial arts, 466
Masaoka staging (thymoma), 935
Massive Transfusion Protocols, 427
mastalgia, 869
mast cells, degranulation, 619
mastectomy
breast reconstruction, 879–80
lymphoedema after, 999
procedures, 876
mastitis
bacterial, 866–7
of infants, 865
periductal (duct ectasia), 867–8
mastoiditis, 709
maxilla
advancement surgery, 696, 699, *700*, 701, *702*
fractures, 360
reconstruction, 774, 778
underdevelopment, 701, *702*
maxillary alveolus, cancer, 774
maxillectomy, 774, *775*, 778
maxillofacial trauma
airway management, 323, 355, *356*
assessment, 356–8
bone, 356
craniofacial, *323*, 362
emergency assessment/ treatment, 355–6
imaging, 357–8
major disasters, 417, *418*, *421*
mandible, 358–9
maxillary fractures, 360
naso-orbito ethmoidal fractures, 362
orbital fractures, 360–1
panfacial, 362–3
soft tissue, 356, 363
teeth, 363
zygomatico-orbito complex fractures, 359
May–Thurner syndrome, 991
mean arterial pressure (MAP), 328, *337*
Meckel's diverticulum, 131–2, 1044, 1116, 1282, 1304
excision, *132*, 1253
features, 1252, *1253*
meconium ileus, 134, 1219, 1294
meconium peritonitis, 134
MED16383, *157*, *158*
media, in major disasters, 412
medial canthal ligament, injury, 362
medial sural artery perforator (MSAP) flap, 769
median nerve
compressive neuropathy, 443, 508
hand, *443*
mediastinal lymph nodes
assessment, 929–30
metastases, 922, 936
mediastinitis, oesophageal perforation, 1074
mediastinoscopy, 929, *930*
mediastinotomy, 929–30
mediastinum, 935–6
displacement, 367
injuries, 365
parathyroid adenoma, 830
primary tumours, 935–6
surgical approaches, 935
widened, 369
medical errors
common causes, 178
operative, 184
prevalence, 178
Medicines and Health Care products Regulatory Agency (MHRA), 166
Mediterranean fever, periodic, 1055
MEDLINE, 163
medullary sponge kidney, *1386*, 1406
medullary thyroid carcinoma, *816*, 820–1
in MEN, 856, 858
MEFV gene, 1055
'megaoesophagus', 1096, *1097*
megaureter, congenital, 1402

meibomian cyst (chalazion), 673–4
  curettage, 685
meibomian glands, 672
Meige syndrome, *1002*
Meigs' syndrome, 1058
Meissner's corpuscles, 592
Meissner's plexus, 1067, 1107, 1297
MEK inhibitors, *157*
melaena, 1126–9
melanin, 592, 594
melanin spots, 1250
melanocytes, 592
melanoma
  acral lentiginous, 610
  amelanotic, 610
  desmoplastic, 610
  nodular, 609
  superficial spreading, 609
  see also malignant melanoma
MELD score, 1157
Meleney's synergistic gangrene, 50, 419, 597
Ménétrier's disease, 1116
Menière's disease, 714
meningiomas, *197*, 480–1, 665, 684
meningitis, 656
  tuberculous, 658
meningococcal septicaemia, 588, *589*, 598
meningocoele, 484, 667
menisci, 518
  discoid, 575
  examination, 456
  tears, 456, 467, 518–19, *520*
meniscus (crescent) sign, 67
menstrual cycle, 1514–15
menstruation, 1514
  dysfunctional bleeding, 1516–17
Mental Capacity Act (2005), 173, 267
6-mercaptopurine, *155*, 1245, 1532, 1539
Mercedes–Benz sign, 1190
Merkel cells, 592
Merkel cell tumour, 612
mesenchymal stem and stromal cells (MSCs), 35
mesenteric artery
  inferior, 1258, 1319
  superior, 1153, 1241, 1258
    occlusion, 1253
mesenteric artery occlusion, 952, 956, 1253
mesenteric ischaemia, 956, 1061, 1253–4
mesenteric lymph nodes
  metastases, 855
  tuberculous adenitis, 1062
mesenteric vein, superior, 1241
mesentery
  cysts, 1062–4
  injury, 1061
  misty, 1062
  tumours, 1064
mesh hernia repairs, 1027–9
mesh rectopexy, 1324
mesoappendix, 1300, 1310
mesothelioma, *146*, 922
metabolic bone disease, 205, 485
metabolic equivalent tasks (METs), 263–4
metabolic response to starvation, 10, 278–9
metabolic stress response, 3–7, 279
  ebb and flow model, 5–6
  mediators, 3–5
metacarpophalangeal (MCP) joints
  contractures, 507
  ulnar drift, 505
meta-iodobenzylguanidine (MIBG) SPECT, 846
metaphyseal fractures
  distal radius, 403, *404*
  treatment, 394
metaplasia, 241–2
  bladder, 1446, 1448, 1452
  gastric, 1114
  oesophagus, 241–2, 1081–3
metastases
  adrenal glands, 842
  bone, *see* bone metastases
  'cannon ball' in testicular carcinoma, 1508
  cerebral, 663, *664*, *665*
  colorectal cancer, *195*, *1158*, 1172–3, 1262
  formation of, 141
  imaging, *195*, *199*, 214, *215*
  liver, *195*, 214, *215*, 1089, 1112, *1160*, 1172–3
  lung, 934
  lymph nodes
    melanoma, 612
    mesenteric, 855
    neck, 729, 758–9
  ocular, 676
  ovary, *1526*
  peritoneal, *1211*
  prostate cancer, 1471–2, 1474
  spinal, 478
  surgical resection, 150
metatarsalgia, 527–8
metatarsophalangeal (MTP) joints, 460
  dislocation, *382*
  first
    deformities, *458*, 525–7
    fusion, 526, *527*
  rheumatological disease, 529
metatarsus adductus, 562, *563*
metformin, *158*
methotrexate, *155*, 1518
metopic synostosis, *687*
metronidazole, 56, 59, 559, 1272–3, 1475
Meyerding classification (spondylolisthesis), *478*, *479*
'Mickey Mouse' sign, 976
microbiology, surgical infections, 44–7
microcephaly, 668
microdiscectomy, 476
microdochectomy, 865
microscopy, light, *237*, 242–3
microsurgery, 645–6
microtome, 236, *237*
microvascular free flaps, oral reconstruction, *774–5*
micturition, control, 1424
middle ear
  anatomy, 703, *704*
  disorders of, 708–12
midface fractures, 355, 356
midface retrusion, correction, 696, 699, *700*
mid-stream specimen of urine (MSSU), 1379
migraine, vestibular, 715
migrating motor complex, 1109
Milan criteria, 1175
milia, 598
'milieu intérieur', 2
military wounds, 49
  blast injuries, 430–2
  gunshot, 426, *426*, 428–9
  infection, 432–3
milk-alkali syndrome, 1406
Milligan–Morgan operation, 1357
Milroy's disease, 1001
Milwaukee classification, 1232, *1233*
minimal access surgery
  coronary artery bypass, 893
  future directions, 117–18
  oesophagectomy, 1092–3
  parathyroidectomy, 829–30
  thyroid, 814
  see also laparoscopic surgery; robotic surgery
Mirels score, *548*
Mirizzi syndrome, 1203
miscarriage, 1515
miserable malalignment syndrome, 562
mismatch repair (MMR) gene mutations, 249–51
mitogen-activated protein kinase (MAPK), 612
  inhibitors, 154, *157*
mitomycin C, *155*, 1421, 1450
mitosis, drugs interfering with, *155*
mitotane, 843, 846
MitraClip®, 899
mitral valve
  anatomy, 894
  disease, 896–9
    ischaemic, 889
    prolapse, 1403
    regurgitation, 896–7
    stenosis, 897–9
  repair, 898, 899
  replacement, 899
Mittelschmerz, 1306
mixed venous oxygen saturation, 17–18
Mohs' micrographic surgery, 605, 674
Molders' click, 462
molecular diagnosis, 247–51
  GISTs, 250
  lymphoma, 250
  and prognosis, 251
  soft-tissue tumours, 250
  and tumour staging, 251
moles (naevi), 599–602
Mondor's disease, 867
Mongolian spot, 601
monoclonal antibodies
  Crohn's disease, 1245–6
  renal cell carcinoma, 1420–1
  transplantation, 1539–40
  ulcerative colitis, 1269
Monro Kellie doctrine, 328–9
Montgomery's glands, retention cyst, 864
Montgomery's tubercles, 860
Morgagni hernia, 938, 939
morphine, oral, 276, 277
Morris retractor, 1560
Morton's neuroma, 462, 527–8
mosquito, filariasis transmission, 63
mouth opening, assessment, 261, *262*
movement
  assessment, 438–9
  descriptive terms, *438*
movement disorders, 670
moya moya disease, 662
mucinous tumours
  appendix, 1315, 1316
  pancreas, 1234
mucocoele, lacrimal sac, 674–5
mucohaemorrhoidal prolapse, 1322
mucosa-associated lymphoid tissues (MALT), 725, 1140
mucous cysts, 509
mucous retention cysts, *776*, 779
Muir and Barclay formula, 624
Müllerian ducts, 1399, 1513
Müller's muscle, 672
Müller's sign, 901
multidisciplinary teams
  bariatric surgery, 1146
  breast cancer treatment, 875
  cancer management, 148, *149*
  pain management, 276, 277
multilayer lymphoedema bandaging (MLLB), 1009–10
multiple endocrine neoplasia type 1 (MEN 1), *144*, 856–7
  adrenals, 856, 857
  anterior pituitary, 856, 857
  epidemiology, 856
  genetic screening, 857
  operative therapy, 857
  pancreas/duodenum, 848, 849, 851, 1141–2
  parathyroids, 826, 830, 832, 856, 857
multiple endocrine neoplasia type 2 (MEN 2), 856, 857–8
  familial medullary thyroid carcinoma, 856, 858
  type 2a, *144*, 820, 832
  type 2b, *144*, 856, 857
multiple myeloma, 538, 544
  treatment, *156*, 547

multiple organ dysfunction syndrome (MODS), 15, *47*, 51
multiple sclerosis, 1430
mumps, 786
  orchitis, 1501, 1506
murmurs
  aortic regurgitation, 901
  aortic stenosis, 900
  mitral regurgitation, *897*
  mitral stenosis, 897
Murphy's sign, 213, 1018, 1199, 1303
muscle, ultrasound scanning, 195
muscle injuries, sports, 464
muscle power, grading, *438*
muscle relaxants, 272, *273*
muscle wasting
  hands, 443, 502, 508
  stress response, 6–7
muscular dystrophy, 482, 583, 586
musculoskeletal disease, history taking, 436
musculoskeletal examination
  ankle and foot, 457–62
  elbow, 447–8
  hand and wrist, 442–6
  hip joint, 451–3
  knee, 453–7
  look, feel, move, 437–9
  shoulder, 448–50, *451*
  spine, 439–42
musculoskeletal system
  development, 561
  normal variants, 562–4
mutation analysis, 247, *248*
mutation detection, 249–50
myasthenia gravis (MG), 935
mycetoma, 71–5, 937
mycobacterial infections
  hand, 504
  musculoskeletal, 559–60
  salivary glands, 795
  see also leprosy; tuberculosis
Mycobacterium leprae, 43, 68
Mycobacterium paratuberculosis, 1242
Mycobacterium tuberculosis
  drug resistance, 560
  drug therapy, 560
  see also tuberculosis
mycophenolate, 1539
mydriasis, 331
myelodysplastic syndrome, *157*
myelofibrosis, spleen, 1185, *1185*
myeloma, *157*, 538, 544
myelomeningocoele, 484, 667
myelopathy, cervical, 475
mylohyoid muscle, 782, *783*
myocardial infarction (MI)
  CABG following, 889
  perioperative risk assessment, 265, 915
  surgery following, 257, 265, 915
myocardial injury, blunt, 370
myocardial ischaemia
  minimising in surgery, 265
  postoperative, 294
myocardial perfusion scanning, 888
myocardial protection, 885
myocutaneous flaps, *594*, 644–5
  free transfer, 645–6
  postoperative care, 646–8
myoglobinuria, 421, 631, 1376
myomectomy, 1526
myometrium, 1514
myopathy, critical illness, 7
myositis ossificans, 470
myotomy
  endoscopic, 1099
  Heller's, 1098–9
myxoedema, 802
  pretibial, 1006
myxoma, atrial, 911–12

nadolol, 813
naevi
  atypical (dysplastic), 604
  blue, 601, *602*
  compound, 599
  giant congenital pigmented, 603–4
  halo, 600
  intradermal, 599
  junctional, 599
  of Ota and Ito, 601–2
  spider, 614
  spindle cell, 600
  Spitz, 599–600
  strawberry (capillary haemangioma), 613
naevus sebaceous of Jadassohn (tricholemmoma), 602
naevus spilus, 600–1
nails
  infections, 503–4
  melanoma, 610
narrow band imaging, 233
nasal bones
  anatomy, 716
  fractures, 362, 717
nasal deformity, cleft lip/palate, 699, *700*
nasal microdebrider, 723
nasal polyps, 722–3
nasal septum
  anatomy, 716
  deformity, 718
  perforation, 718–19
nasogastric tubes, 285
nasojejunal tubes, 286
nasolacrimal duct, 672
nasopharynx
  anatomy, 725, *726*
  tumours, 733–5
National Confidential Enquiry into Surgical Deaths (NCEPOD), 266–7
National Institute for Health Care Excellence (NICE), 174, 256
  bariatric surgery guidance, 1146
  dyspepsia/GORD guidance, 221
  head injury guidelines, *330*
  lung cancer referral guidance, *928*
  lung cancer treatment guidance, *932*
  peripheral arterial disease guidance, 948
  trauma guidance, 313
National Institute for Health Research (NIHR), 164
National Research Ethics Service, *162*
National Spinal Injuries Centre (UK), 352
natural orifice transluminal endoscopic surgery (NOTES), 117, 118
nausea
  postoperative, 298–9, 304, *305*
    laparoscopic surgery, 115
navitoclax, *158*
neck
  anatomy, 728–9
  examination, 729
  lumps, 753–5
  root (base) injuries, 364
  secondary carcinoma, 729, 758
  trauma, 755–6
neck dissection, 758–9
  classical radical (Crile), 758, 785
  modified radical, 759
  oral cavity cancer, 767
  selective, 759
  submandibular gland tumours, *784*, 785
  suprahyoid, *784*
  thyroid cancer, 819
necrosectomy, pancreatic, 1227
necrosis, microscopy, 239
necrotising enterocolitis, 138
necrotising fasciitis, 30–1, 50
  causes, 30, 419, 597
  clinical signs, *30*, 419, 597
  management, 419–20, 597–8
necrotising otitis externa, 707–8
necrotising sialometaplasia, 778
needles, suture, 94, 95
needle-stick injuries, 52
Neisseria gonorrhoea, 1442, 1494, 1518–19
Neisseria meningitidis, 598, 1186, 1306
Nelson's syndrome, 842
neoadjuvant therapy
  oesophageal cancer, 1093–4
  rectal carcinoma, 1332
neonates
  acute intestinal obstruction, 1293
  bone and joint infections, 587–8
  brachial plexopathy, 586
  cystic hygroma, 754–5
  definition, *119*
  hip dysplasia, 568, 569, *570*
  intravenous fluids, *121*
nephrectomy
  calculus, 1409–10
  live kidney donor, 1547–8
  partial, 1420
  radical, 1420
  renal cell carcinoma, 1420
nephroblastoma (Wilms' tumour), 138, *152*, *156*, 832, 1421–2
nephrogenic systemic fibrosis, 191
nephrolithiasis, *see* renal calculi, 1402
nephrolithotomy, percutaneous, 1409
nephrometry scoring systems, 1420
nerve blocks, 274–5
nerve grafts, 637
nerve healing, 25
nerve injury
  extremity trauma, 383, 385, 400
  inguinal hernia repair, 1034
  surgery, 85
  thyroidectomy, 815
  varicose vein surgery, 982
nerve monitoring, thyroidectomy, 814
nerve regeneration, 25
nerve roots, *439*, 471
  compression, 476
nerve sheath tumours, 666–7
nerve stimulation procedures, 276
Nesbitt procedure, 1490
netball injuries, 466
neural tube defects, 483–4, 667–8
neurinomas, 856
neuroblastoma, 138, 847
neuroendocrine cell system, 852–3
neuroendocrine response to injury, 3–4
neuroendocrine tumours
  cytology, *240*
  duodenum, 1141
  immunohistochemistry, 246, *247*
  lung, 925
  rectum, 1328
  relative organ distribution, *853*
  small bowel, 854–5
  stomach, 853–4
neurofibromas
  orbit, 673
  spinal, 481
neurofibromatosis, 594–5
  incidence, *687*
  type 1 (NF1), *145*, 481, 595, 600, 663, 845
  type 2 (NF2), *145*, 481, 663
neurogenic shock, 352
neurogenic tumours, mediastinum, 936
neurological deficit, head injury, 331–2
neurological disease
  foot, 531
  mimicking prostatic obstruction, 146, 1462

neurological examination
  lower limb, *473*
  sensory testing, 438
  spinal disorders, 472–3
  upper limb, *473*
neurolysis, cancer pain, 277
neuromuscular disorders, 583–6
  brachial plexopathy, 586
  cerebral palsy, 584–5
  management principles, 583
  muscular dystrophy, 482, 586
  polio, 75–6, 583, 586
  spina bifida, 586
  surgical procedures, *584*
neuropathic bladder, 1428–9
  in children, 131
neuropathic foot, 532–3
neuropathic (neurogenic) pain, 275, *276*, 354
neurosurgery
  functional, 668–71
  paediatric, 667–8
  vascular, 658–62
neurosurgical centres, 336, *337*
neurotmesis, 385
neutrophils, 241, *242*
Never events, 184
newborn and infant physical examination (NIPE) guidelines, 568
next-generation sequencing (NGS), *248*, 249
nifedipine, 967, 1099
nil by mouth (NBM), 259
nilutamide, *156*
nimodipine, 660
nipple, 860
  cracked, 863
  discharges, 864–5
  Paget's disease, 864, 873
  reconstruction, 879–80
  retraction, 863, *864*
  supernumerary, 863
niraparib, *158*
Nissen fundoplication, *1079*, 1080
nitric oxide (NO), 3–4
nitrogen, urinary losses, 7, 8–9
nitrous oxide anaesthesia, 271, 919
nivolumab, *157*
nociceptive pain, 275, *276*
nocturia, 1375
nocturnal enuresis, 1375, 1432
NOD2/CARD15 gene, 1242
node of Cloquet, 1035
noise exposure, 713, *714*
non-accidental injury (NAI), 311, 589–90
  factors raising suspicion, 138, 316, *590*
  fractures, *590*
  head, 330
non-governmental organisations (NGOs), disaster relief, 411
non-Hodgkin's lymphoma (NHL), 147, 741, *789*, 1251, 1522
Nonne–Milroy disease, *1002*
non-seminomatous germ cell tumours (NSGCT), 1506–9
non-steroidal anti-inflammatory drugs (NSAIDs), 221, 276, 1115, 1116, 1120
Noonan syndrome, *903*, 1001
noradrenaline (norepinephrine), 839
nose
  anatomy, 716–17
  packing, 719–20
  reconstructive surgery, *643*, *648*
  trauma, 717–18
  tumours, 723–4
nuclear factor kappa B (NFkB), *5*
nuclear medicine, 199–200
  bone scans, *see* bone scans
  head and neck cancers, 766
  hepatobiliary, 192, 1204, 1232
  lymphoscintigraphy, 1006
  octreotide scan, 855
  parathyroid, 827
  radiation exposure, *192*
  renograms, 1392–4, *1395*, 1412
  strengths, *200*
  thyroid, 804
  trauma, 385
  weaknesses, *200*
nucleic acid amplification testing (NAAT), 1505
nursing care, burns patient, 627
Nuss procedure, 939
nutrition
  following bariatric surgery, 1151
  and goitre, 805
  and hypercalcaemia, *826*
  and intestinal resection, 283–4
  requirements, 281–3
nutritional assessment, 279–80
nutritional deficiencies
  after peptic ulcer surgery, 1124
  after total gastrectomy, 1139
  and oesophageal cancer, 1086
nutritional support, 284–8
  burns patient, 626–7
  chronic pancreatitis, *1231*
  Crohn's disease, 1246
  gastrostomy, 285–6
  head injury, 337
  multidisciplinary teams, 288
  oesophagectomy, 1093
  parenteral, 286–8
  perioperative, 260
  short bowel syndrome, 1256–7
  tube feeding, 284–6

obesity
  acute appendicitis in, 1304
  associated cancers, *146*
  breast cancer risk, 871
  central, *841*
  and day surgery, 303–4
  definition, 1144
  epidemic, 1144
  hepatocellular carcinoma, 1173
  laparoscopic surgery, 112–13
  and oesophageal cancer, 1087
  preoperative care, 260
  surgery, *see* bariatric surgery
Obesity Surgery Mortality Risk Score (OS-MRS), 1146
observational study, *164*
obstructive shock, 13
obstructive sleep apnoea, 732
  and bariatric surgery, 1146
  children, 732
  craniofacial anomalies, 688
  obesity, 260
obturator hernia, 1043–4
obturator test, 1303
occipital condyle fracture, 345
occipitoatlantal dislocation, 345–6
occult hypoperfusion, 18
Ochsner–Sherren regime, 1312
Octopus® stabiliser, 893
octreotide, 284, 1124, 1129, 1237, 1251
octreotide scan, 855
ocular coherence tomography (OCT), 683
oculomotor nerve, 672
odontoid (dens), *338*
  fractures, 346–7
odynophagia, 370, 1069, 1077
oedema
  lower limb, 972–3
  visceral, 9–10
oesophageal cancer, *1083*, 1085–95
  adenocarcinoma, *1083*, *1086*, 1087
  in Barrett's oesophagus, 1082–3, 1087
  causes, *145*, *146*
  chemotherapy and biological agents, *155*
  clinical features, 1087
  geographical variation, 1086–7
  investigation, 1088–91
  involving gastric cardia, 1087, *1089*, 1091
  neoadjuvant therapy, 1093–4
  non-surgical treatments, 1094
  palliative treatment, 1094–5
  pancreatic cancer, 1238–9
  pathology and aetiology, *1083*, 1085–6
  spread of, 1088, 1089
  squamous cell carcinoma, 1085–7, 1092
  staging, 1088–9
  stent placement, 224, *225*, 1094
  surgery, 1092–3
  tissue specimen, *236*
  tracheo-oesophageal fistula, 1095
  treatment principles, 1091–2
oesophageal motility disorders, 1095
  achalasia, 1095–9
  in autoimmune disease, 1100–1
  classification, *1095*, *1096*
  functional pain, 1095
  oesophageal body, 1099–101
  pharyngeal/oesophageal diverticula, 1101–2
  pharyngo-oesophageal junction, 1099
oesophageal speech, 753
oesophagectomy, 1092–3
oesophagitis
  Candida albicans, 1103–4
  Crohn's, 1104–5
  eosinophilic, 1100–1
  reflux, 1076, *1078*
oesophagogastric junction
  adenocarcinoma, 1132
  endoscopy, *222*
oesophagogastroduodenoscopy (OGD), 221–5
  complications, 224–5
  indications, 221
  peptic ulcer disease, 222–3, *1117*, 1119
  therapeutic procedures, 221–4
oesophagojejunostomy, 1136, *1137*
oesophagoscopy, 1087, 1088
oesophagus
  anatomy, 1067
  Barrett's, 221, 224, 233, 241–2, 1077, 1081–3, 1087
  benign tumours, 1084, *1085*
  cancer, *see* oesophageal cancer
  congenital abnormalities, 133
  congenital atresia, 133
  corrosive injury, 1075–6
  diverticula, 1101–2
  drug-induced injury, 1076
  foreign bodies, 132, 1071–2
  infections, 1103–4
  injuries, 370
  investigations, *1069*, 1070–1
  jackhammer (nutcracker), 1099–100
  Mallory-Weiss tear, 1075, 1128
  normal squamous mucosa, *1077*
  pain, 1095
  perforation, 1072–4
    in endoscopy, 225, 1073–4
    pathological, 1073
    spontaneous, 1072–3
    treatment, 1074
  pH recording, 1071, 1078
  physiology, 1067–9
  replacement, 1076
  Schatzki's ring, 1102–3
  shortening, 1081
  sideropenic dysphagia, 740, 763, 1105
  strictures
    Barrett's oesophagus, 1082
    corrosive injury, 1075, *1076*
    dilatation, 1071
    reflux-induced, *1078*, 1080
  surgical approaches, 1092
  symptoms of disease, 1069
  thermal recanalisation, 1071
  varices, 222, 1126, 1127
    haemorrhage, 1163–6
  webs, 1105
oestrogen, 1514
office-based care, 301–2

off-pump coronary artery bypass grafting (OPCAB), 893
ofloxacin, *1520*
olaparib, *158*
olecranon bursitis, 500–1
olecranon fracture, 399
Olgilvie's syndrome (colonic pseudo-obstruction), 1297–8
oligodendroglioma, *198*
oligohydramnios, 567
Ollier disease, *537*, 540, 565, 566
omentum
  fat necrosis, 1225
  functions, 1061
  torsion, 1061
oncogenes, 140, 249
open disclosure, 181
open reduction and internal fixation (ORIF)
  mandibular fractures, 358
  maxillary fractures, 360
operating list, 267
operating table
  patient positioning, 84
  transfer to and from, 84
operating theatre
  air and ventilation, 1563–4
  etiquette, 1564
  infection control, 52, 1564
  location and spaces, 1563
  sterile surgical field, 1563
  surgical safety, 182–4
operation planning, trauma, 319–20
opiates, *219*, 276, 277
Opisthorchis viverrini, 1208
opportunistic infections, 47
  postsplenectomy (OPSI), 1187
Opsite® sandwich, 379
optic nerve, 672, 673
  meningioma, *684*
oral cavity
  anatomy, 760–1
  minor salivary glands, 776–8
  trauma, 357, 363
oral cavity cancer
  anatomical sites, 761
  buccal mucosa, 772
  clinical features, 764–5
  epidemiology, 760
  field change, 762–3
  floor of mouth, 771
  hard palate/maxillary alveolus, 774
  investigations, 765–7
  lips, 765, 767–9
  mandibular alveolus, 772–3
  pathology, 761
  premalignant conditions, 763, 767
  retromolar pad, 774
  second primary tumours, 762
  staging, 764
  tongue, *765*, *766*, 769–71
  treatment, 767
oral contraceptive pill, 260, 1516
oral hypotonic solutions, 283
oral submucous fibrosis, 763
Oram, Samuel, 903
orbicularis oculi, paralysis, 69
orbit
  anatomy, 673
  bruising, 332, 359, 362
  complications of rhinosinusitis, 721–2
  dermoid cysts, 673
  fractures, 356, 360–1, 677–8
  neurofibroma, 673
  swellings, 673, 675–6
    cellulitis, 675, 722
orchidectomy
  prostate cancer, 1474
  testicular maldescent, 1499
  testicular tumours, 1508
orchidopexy, 125, 1499
orchitis, 1506
  mumps, 1501
organ of Corti, *704*
organ donation, 1542–8
  after brain death, 1543
  after circulatory death, 1543–4
  evaluation of deceased donor, 1544
  living donors, 1543, 1547–8
  organ recovery, 1544–7
organ perfusion, monitors, 17
organ preservation solutions, 1546
orogastric tube, laparoscopic surgery, 115
oropharynx
  anatomy, 726
  disorders, 735–41
  examination, 729
  tumours, 740–1
orotracheal tube, 271, *272*
orthodontic treatment, 695
orthognathic surgery, 696, 699, *700*, 701–2
orthopaedic wool, 984
Ortolani test, 568
os calcis, fractures, 402
Osgood–Schlatter disease, 575
Osler's disease, 719, 720
osseous flaps, 646
ossicles, 703, *704*
osteitis fibrosa cystica, 825
osteoarthritis (OA)
  elbow, 499–500
  foot and ankle, 528
  gait abnormalities, *437*
  hand, *504*, 506
  hand deformity, *443*
  hip, *437*, 513–14
  knee, 519–20
  shoulder, 493–5
osteoblastoma, 480, 539
osteochondritis dissecans (OCD)
  elbow, 500
  knee, 575
osteochondromas, 539–40, 565
osteogenesis imperfecta (brittle bone disease), 566–7
osteoid osteoma, 538–9, *542*
  treatment, 546
osteomas
  nasal skeleton, 723
  orbit, *675*
osteomyelitis
  acute, 556, *557*
  antibiotic therapy, 552
  children, 587–9
  chronic, 556–9
  complications, 588–9
  diagnosis, 551–2
  epidemiology, 549
  frontal bone (Pott's puffy tumour), 657, *658*, 722
  imaging, 204, *205*
  management, 552
  microbiology, 550
  pathology, 550, 587–8
  pyogenic vertebral, 481
osteophytes, *494*, 495
osteoporosis
  after spinal cord injury, 354
  fractures
    intra-articular, 395
    limb, 406, *407*
    spinal compression, 349
  imaging, 205
  spine, 349, 485
osteoradionecrosis, 775
osteosarcoma, 535, 539
  distal femur, *203*, *535*
  parosteal, 539
  treatment, 546
osteotomies
  in ankylosing spondylitis, 481, *482*
  around the hip, 515
  hallux valgus treatment, 525–6
  knee, 521
  pelvic in DDH, 570, 571
osteotomy, bimaxillary, 701, *702*
otalgia, referred, 705
otitis externa, 707–8
otitis media
  acute, 708–9
  chronic, 710–11
  cleft lip/palate, 694–5
  with effusion (glue ear), 709–10
otosclerosis, 711
otoscope, *705*
ototoxicity, 714
Otovent® device, 710
Ottawa ankle rules, 468
outcome indicators, 185
outcomes, spinal cord injuries, 353
outpatient parenteral antibiotic therapy (OPAT), 552
ovarian cancer, *155*, 1526–9, 1529
ovarian cysts, 1526
  management, 1526, *1527*
  torsion, 1306
ovarian tissue cryopreservation, 1529
ovarian vein, incompetence, 985, 986
ovaries
  anatomy, 1514
  benign tumours, 1526
  endometriosis, 1521
ovulation, 1514
oxalate, urinary, 1406
oxaliplatin, *155*
oxycodone, 276
oxygenation, children, 122
oxygen saturation, 918
  mixed venous, 17–18
oxygen therapy, burns patient, 620, 621
Oxyuris vermicularis, 1302

P13K inhibitors, *157*
p53 gene, 140, *144*, 249, 880, 1261, 1329
pacemakers, diathermy, 103, 258
Pacinian corpuscles, 592
packed red blood cells, 21
packing
  liver injury, 1161–2
  nasal, 719–20
  pancreas, 1227
Paget–Schrötter disease, 992
Paget's disease, 407, 535, *537*
  extramammary, 603
  nipple, 864, 873
pain
  abdominal, *see* abdominal pain
  after laparoscopic surgery, 115
  amputations, 960
  back, *see* back pain
  breakthrough, 277
  breast (mastalgia), 869
  chest, 1069, 1077
  knee, 467–8, 575–6
  lymphoedema, 1008
  neuropathic, 275, *276*, 354
  oesophagus, 1095
  sympathetic nervous system activity, 276
  syndromes, 670–1
  types of, 275, *276*
  urological, 1017, 1305, 1374–5
painful arc test, 449, *450*
pain management
  benign disease, 276
  chronic pain, 275–6
  double effect, 173
  malignant disease, 276–7
  neurosurgical, 670–1
  WHO ladder, 276
palate
  anatomy, 690, *691*
  benign tumours, 777, *778*
  cleft, *see* cleft lip and palate
  squamous cell carcinoma, 774
palbociclib, *158*
palliative care, 150, 158–9
  domains and interventions, *159*
  gastric surgery, 1138
  life and death issues, 173
  oesophageal cancer, 1094–5
  pancreatic carcinoma, 1237–8
palpation
  abdomen, 1020–1
  liver, 1021
  spleen, 1021
pampiniform plexus, 1501
'pan', 760
Pancoast's syndrome, 926

pancreas
abscess, 1227–8
anatomy, 1212–14
calcifications, *1218*, 1231
congenital anomalies, *1213*, 1219–20
development, 1213
effusion, 1228
endocrine tumours, 848–52, 857
exocrine function tests, 1214
fistula, 1221
hydatid cyst, 65
imaging, 1215–19
injuries, 375, 1220–1
necrosis, 1226–7
non-functional endocrine tumours, 852
physiology, 1214
pseudocysts, *1216*, 1221, 1228–9
sphincterotomy, 228
transplantation, 1552–4
isolated islets, 1553–4
organ recovery from deceased donor, 1545, 1546
results, 1553
surgical technique, 1552–3
pancreas divisum, *1213*, 1219
pancreatic ascites, 1228
pancreatic carcinoma, 1233–9
adjuvant therapies, 1237
ampullary, 1234, *1235*, 1236, 1237
chemotherapy and biological agents, *155*, *156*
clinical features, 1234–5
endoscopic ultrasound, *1218*
ERCP, 1217
incidence, 1233
investigation, 1235
neoadjuvant therapy, 1238–9
palliation, 1237–9
pancreatic fluid histology, *1218*
pathology, 1234
risk factors, *1233*
surgical decisions, 1235–6
surgical resection, 1236–7
pancreatic duct, 1213, *1214*
accessory (Santorini), 1213, 1221
stones, *1216*, *1217*, 1231–2
stricture, 1230, 1231
pancreatic necrosectomy, 1227
pancreatitis, 1221–33
acute, 212, 1017, *1051*, 1221–30, 1306
aetiology, 1222
categories, 1221–2
clinical presentation, 1222–3
complications, 1226–9
incidence, 1222
investigation, 1223–5
management, 1225
mechanism of injury, 1221
outcomes and follow-up, 1229–30
severity assessment, 1223–4
after ERCP, 228–9
autoimmune, 1230
chronic, *1215*, 1217, *1218*, 1230–2
ERCP, 1217, *1218*, 1232–3
hereditary, 1222, 1230
tropical chronic, 76–7, 1230
pancreatoduodenectomy, 1236–7
pylorus-preserving (PPPD), 1236–7
Whipple's procedure, 375, 1141, 1209, 1236
panfacial fractures, 362–3
Panner's disease, 500, *573*
pannus, 504, 505
panobinostat, *157*
pantalar fusion, 528
pantaloon hernia, 1030
paper-based records, 180–1
papillary carcinoma, thyroid, *809*, *816*, 817, 818
papillary muscle, 894
papillary syringoma (eccrine poroma), 603
papillary tumours, bladder, *1384*, 1445, *1446*
papillary warts (verruca vulgaris), 599
papilloedema, *652*, 659
papillomas
bile ducts, 1207–8
bladder (bilharzial), 1444, *1445*
laryngeal, 750
nasal, 723–4
nipple, 863
papillomata acuminata, female urethra, 1486
Papillon technique, 1337
Pap stain, 238
paracentesis
ascites, 1059, 1166
peritonitis, 1053
paracetamol, 115, 276, *1156*
paradoxical respiration, 368
parafibromin immunohistochemistry, 836
paraganglioma
familial syndrome, 845
vagal, 758
paralytic ileus, 297, 1296–7
clinical features, 1297
management, 1297
post-appendicectomy, 1313–14
varieties, 1297
paranasal sinuses
anatomy, 716–17
endoscopic surgery, 723
imaging, 717
tumours, *146*, 724
parapharyngeal abscess, 737
parapharyngeal space, 726–7
paraphimosis, 1377, 1489
parastomal hernias, 1043, 1255, 1278
parathyroidectomy
hypoparathyroidism after, 830–1
persistent hyperparathyroidism, 836
primary hyperparathyroidism, 829–30
recurrent hyperparathyroidism, 836–7
secondary hyperparathyroidism, 834–5
subtotal, 834
parathyroid glands
adenoma, 826–30
anatomy, 823–4
autotransplantation, 834
carcinoma, 832, 835–6
embryology, 800, 823–4
hyperplasia in MEN 1 syndrome, 857
imaging, 826–8
insufficiency following thyroid surgery, 815
reimplantation in thyroidectomy, 814
role in calcium regulation, 824–5
see also hyperparathyroidism; hypoparathyroidism
parathyroid hormone (PTH)
functions of, 824–5
in parathyroid carcinoma, 836
venous sampling, 828
parathyroid hormone-related protein (PTHrP), 845
parathyromatosis, 836–7
paratyphoid, 1248, 1273
paraumbilical hernia, 1037, *1038*
parenteral nutrition, 286
complications, 287–8
home (HPN), 1257
short bowel syndrome, 1256–7
venous access, 286–7
parietal cells, 1107, 1108, *1109*, 1115
Parinaud's syndrome, 652
parity, and breast cancer risk, 871
Parkes–Weber syndrome, 991
Parkinson's disease, 670, 1430, 1459
Parkland formula, 624
Parks procedure, 1270–1
paronychia, 503
parotid duct, injuries, 363
parotidectomy, 789–92
complications, 792–7
extracapsular dissection, 792, *793*
radical, 792, *794*
superficial, 789–92
parotid gland
anatomy, 785
inflammatory disorders, 786–7
tumours, 787–9
parotitis, 786, 787
Parry–Romberg disease, 615
patella
biomechanical role, 519
dislocation, 468
fractures, 401
tracking, 456, 576
patella alta, 457
patellar apprehension, 456–7
patellar tap test, 454
patellar tendon, 457
rupture, 457
tendinosis, 465
traction apophysitis (Osgood–Schlatter disease), 575–6
patellofemoral joint, examination, 456–7
patellofemoral pain, 467–8
patent ductus arteriosus, 906
Paterson–Kelly syndrome, 740, 763, 1105
Patey mastectomy, 876
pathological fractures, 406–7
healing, 548
metastatic bone disease, 548
simple bone cyst, 541, *542*
pathology department, 234
patient advocacy, 182
patient-centred approach, 181
patient journey, 186–7
day-case surgery, 301, 306
elective surgery, 186
urgent surgery, 186
patient positioning
anal examination, 1342
laparoscopic surgery, 85, 266
safety, 84–5
thoracotomy, 930, *931*
patient records, 180–1
Patient Reported Outcome Measures (PROMs), 164
patient safety, 177–84
concept underlying, 179, *180*
diathermy use, 102–3
incident causes, 178
incident definitions, *178*
incident prevalence, 178
Never events, 184
patient positioning, 84–5
Safety II approach, 184
strategies, 180–1
and surgeon, 182–4, *185*
Paul–Bunnell test, 735, 738
Paul–Mikulicz procedure, 1295, *1296*
Pavlik harness, 569, *570*
peak expiratory flow rate (PEFR), 916
peau d'orange, 63, 873, *874*, 879
pectus carinatum (pigeon chest), 940
pectus excavatum, 939
peer review, research, 165–6
peer-reviewed journals, 167–8
pelvic abscess, 1055, 1312
pelvic binder, 323, 324
pelvic congestion syndrome, 985–6
pelvic exenteration, rectal cancer, 1337
pelvic fractures, 376–8
angiography protocol, *319*
assessment, 325, 326, 377–8
classification, 377
haemorrhage, 324, 365, 376–7, 378
imaging, 206, 378
management, 209, 378
'open-book', 378

urethral injury (male), 1480–1
pelvic inflammatory disease (PID), 1306, 1518–20
causes, 1518
diagnosis, 1518–19
treatment, 1519–20
pelvic inlet, 376
pelvis
anatomy, 376–7
spastic cerebral palsy, 585
pelvi-ureteric junction (PUJ), obstruction, 1410–13
pembrolizumab, *157*, *158*
penetrating injuries
abdomen, 372, 373–4
liver, 373, 1160, 1161
mechanisms of injury, 314–15
neck, 756
oesophagus, 073
radiographic markers, 372
renal, 1413–14
thorax, 368, *372*, 938
penicillins, 43, 55–6, 419, 420
penile intraepithelial neoplasia (PeIN), *1492*
penis
anatomy, 1486
chordee, 1491
congenital curvature, 1491
disorders in children, 126–7
inflammatory disorders, 1494–6
Peyronie's disease, 506, 1377, 1490
priapism, 1491
trauma, 1377, 1489
tumours, 1491–3
causes, *146*
Penrose drains, 1227
pen sliding test, 443
pentoxifylline, 985
pepsin, 1108
pepsinogen, 1107
peptic stricture, 1077, *1078*
peptic ulcers, 1116–26
aetiology, 1116
bleeding, 222–3, 1127–8
clinical features, 1118–19
duodenal, 1116, 1117
failure to heal, 1120
gastric, 1117–18
investigation, 1119
medical treatment, 1119–20
perforation, 1019, 1048, 1125–6, 1305
pre-pyloric, 1118
pyloric, 1118
recurrent after surgery, 1123
sequelae of surgery, 1123–5
sites, 1116
stress, 1128
surgical treatment, 1120–3
peptide hormones, 1109, *1110*
percutaneous coronary intervention (PCI), 886, 889
percutaneous endoscopic gastrostomy (PEG), 223–4, 285–6
percutaneous nephrolithotomy (PCNL), 1409
percutaneous posterior tibial nerve stimulation (PTNS), 1351
percutaneous suprapubic litholapaxy, 1436
percutaneous transgastric cystgastrostomy, 1229
percutaneous transhepatic cholangiography (PTC), 1159, 1193–4
percutaneous transluminal angioplasty (PTA), 948–9
perforation
hollow organ, 210–11, 1019
intestinal
colonic diverticula, 1274
imaging, 210–11
in polypectomy, 232
typhoid, 82–3, 1248
oesophagus, 225, 1072–4
peptic ulcers, 1125–6
upper GI tract in endoscopy, 225, 1073–4, 1111
perforator ligation, 982
perianal abscess, 48
perianal Crohn's disease, 1243, 1247–8, 1363, 1370
pericardial effusion, 911
pericardial tamponade, 123, 367–8, 911
pericardiocentesis, 368, 911
pericarditis, 911
constrictive, 1058
pericardium, malignant infiltration, 911
perihepatitis, 1049
perilunate dislocation, *382*, 397
perilymph, 703, 704
perineal dissection, rectal cancer surgery, 1336
perineal hernia, 1043
perineal pain, 1374–5
periodic acid–Schiff (PAS) stain, 244
periodic familial Mediterranean fever, 1055
perioperative mortality, 262, 266–7
risk assessment, 915
periorbital bruising, 332, 359, 362
peripheral arterial disease
acute, 953–6
amputation, 957–60
chronic, 942–52
clinical features, 943–4
co-morbidity, 945
investigations, 945–7
non-surgical management, 947–9
risk of cardiovascular event, 947
risk factors, 945, 947
surgical management, 949–52
diabetes, 947, 953
renal artery stenosis, *942*
peripherally-inserted central venous catheter (PICC) line, 287
peripheral nerves
compression, 443, 501–2, 508, 533
injuries, 383, 400
leprosy, 68–9
spinal roots, *439*
tumours, 758
peripheral sensorimotor neuropathy (PSN), 953
peristalsis, visible, 1286
peritalar release, 578
peritendonitis, 463
peritoneal lavage, 373
peritoneum
embryology, 1047
functions, 1047–8
gallbladder metastases, *1211*
inclusion cysts, 1060
innervation, 1018
loose bodies (mice), 1060
tumours, 1059–60
peritonitis, 1048–52
in appendicitis, 1302, 1308
bile, 1052, *1053*
causes, 1048
clinical features, 1050
diagnosis, 1050–1
diffuse (generalised), 1049–50
localised, 1049, 1050
management, 1051–2
microbiology, 1048–9
periodic (familial Mediterranean fever), 1055
primary pneumococcal, 1053
prognosis, 1052
sclerosing encapsulating, 1061
spontaneous bacterial, 1053
tuberculous, 1053–4
periurethral abscess, 1495
perivenous tumescent anaesthesia, 978
periventricular leucomalacia (PVL), 584
Perkins line, 569, 585
peroneal tendons, 458, 461–2
subluxation, 529–30
tendinosis, 529
peroneus longus, 461–2
personalised (precision) medicine, 150
Perthes (Legg–Calvé–Perthes) disease, 571–3
pes cavus, 457, *458*, 531
pes planus, 457, *458*, 460
Peutz–Jeghers syndrome, *144*, 221, 599, *1233*, 1250, 1284
Peyer's patches, 82, 129, 1062, 1241, 1282
Peyronie's disease, 506, 1065, 1377, 1490
Pfannenstiel incision, 1431
Pfeiffer syndrome, 687
phaeochromocytoma, 839, 936
aetiology, 844–5
clinical features, 845
diagnosis, 845–6
malignant, 846
MEN 1 syndrome, 856, 858
pathology, 845
in pregnancy, 846–7
treatment, 846
Phalen's test, *444*, *445*, 508
phantom limb, 960
pharyneal pouch (Zenker's diverticulum), 738–40, 1101–2
pharyngo-oesophageal junction disorders, 1099
pharyngoscopy, 731
pharynx
anatomy, 725–7
examination, 729, 731
oedema, 744
phenoxybenzamine, 846
phenytoin, brain tumour seizures, 663
phimosis, 1377, 1486
children, 127, 1486
'physiological', 1486
treatments, 1486–8
phlebectomy, 982
phleboliths, 1388
phlegmasia alba dolens, 988
phlegmasia cerulea dolens, 988
phlegmonous gastritis, 1116
phosphate, serum, 826, 833
phosphate binders, 834
phosphate calculi, 1434
'phrenic' pain, 1050
Phrygian cap, 1195
phyllodes tumour, 870
physiotherapy, burns patient, 627
phytobezoars, 1282
Pick's disease, 1058
Pierre Robin sequence, 689, 691, 701
pigeon chest, 940
pigmented villonodular synovitis (PVNS), 531
pigment gallstones, 1183, 1199
pilomatrixoma, 602
pilonidal sinus, 1347–9
pilosebaceous cysts, 599
pinna
cellulitis, *707*
haematoma, 706–7
piperacillin, 56
pituitary, 3, *4*
pituitary apoplexy, 666
pituitary function, traumatic brain injury, 337
pituitary–thyroid axis, 802
pituitary tumours, *664*, 665–7
adenoma, 841, 842
chemotherapy agents, *156*
in MEN 1 syndrome, *856*, 857
prolactinoma, *156*, 665–6
plagiocephaly, 668
plantar fascia, 524
plantar fasciitis, 533
plantar fibroma, 506, 531
plant toxins, 76, *146*
plasma proteins, 624
plaster casts, 390–1
Plaster of Paris, 390
Plastibel (Hollister) device, *1488*
plastic and reconstructive surgery
breast and nipple, 879–80

burns, 627–8, *629–30*
complex areas, 648–9
flaps, 637, 641–9
history, 633
implants and prosthetics, 638–9
lip cancer, 768–9
oral tumours, 770–1, 772, 773, 774, *774–5*, 778
scope, 635–6
skin grafts, 634–5, 636–7, 639–41
skin substitutes, 637
tissue expansion, 637–8
tongue, 770–1
toolbox, 635
vacuum-assisted closure, 638
vascularised composite allografting, 649–50
platelets, wound healing, 24
platelet transfusions, 21
plate and screw fixation, 392, *393*, 399
pleomorphic adenoma
minor salivary glands, 777–8
parotid gland, 787, *788*, *790*, *793*
submandibular gland, *784*
plethysmography, 1007
pleura, 918–19
infection and empyema, 922, *923*
pleural effusion, 921–3
cytology, *243*
exudates/transudates, 921
malignant, 921, 922, 926
pancreatitis, 1223
surgical management, 922–3
pleural fluid, physiology, 918, 921
pleural space, gases, 919
pleurectomy, 921
pleurisy, 1305
pleurodesis, 921, 922
Plummer–Vinson syndrome, 740, 763, 1105
pneumaturia, 1376
Pneumocystis jiroveci, 1541–2
pneumonectomy, 932–4
pneumonia
lobar, 1305
Pneumocystis jiroveci, 1541–2
postoperative, 293
pneumoperitoneum, 210–11
laparoscopy, 112
pneumothorax, 205, 919–21
imaging, 205, 207
management, 920–1
open (sucking chest wound), 368
recurrence, 919
spontaneous, 919
tension, 292, 366, 367, 919
in children, 122–3
podoconiosis, 1005
podophyllin, 1496
pointing sign, 1303
poliomyelitis, 75–6, 583, 586
pollutants, associated with cancers, *146*
polyarteritis nodosa, 1416
polyclonal antibody, 1540
polycystic kidney disease, 1402–3, 1549, *1550*
polycystic liver disease, 1168
polymazia, 865
polymerase chain reaction (PCR), 247, *248*
polyps
antrochoanal, 733
colonic, 230–1, 232
children, 131
gallbladder, 1210
gastric, 1130
intestinal, 1259
nasal, 722–3
rectal, 1326–7
endoscopic mucosal resection, 1327, *1328*
juvenile, 1327
urethra, male, 1484
vocal folds, 749–50
polytetrafluoroethylene (PTFE) arterial graft, 949, *951*
Ponseti method, 578, *579*
popliteal artery
aneurysm, 944, 966
thrombolysis, 956
popliteal pulse, 944
popliteal vein, 969, 970
entrapment, 991–2
porcine small intestinal mucosa, 1367
porencephalic cysts, 667
porphyria, 1184
porta hepatis, 1153
portal gastropathy, 1129
portal hypertension, 1106, 1129, 1163–6
and haemorrhoids, 1354
splenomegaly, 1184, *1184*
portal pyaemia, 1314
portal vein, 1153, 1154, 1241
thrombosis, 1165–6, 1228
porto-enterostomy, Kasai, 135–6, 1197
port site herniation, 115, 1023, 1291
port-wine stain (capillary vascular malformation), 613
positive end expiratory pressure (PEEP), 273
positron emission tomography (PET), 200, 214, *215*
with CT (PET/CT), 1091, 1112, *1113*, 1391–2, *1393*
FDG, 214, *215*, 551, 766, 926–7, 929, 1159–60
ischaemic heart disease, 888
liver, 1159–60
lung cancer, 926–7
oesophageal cancer, 1091
oral cancer, 766
stomach, 1112, *1113*
thyroid, 803
POSSUM score, 264
post-anal dermoid, 1347
post-anal dimple (fovea coccygea), 1347
post-cholecystectomy syndrome, 1204
post-concussive syndrome, 330
postcricoid tumours, 741–2
posterior cruciate ligament (PCL), 454, 455–6, *518*
posterior fossa malformations, 668
posterior sagittal anorectoplasty, 1346
posterior urethral valves, 137–8, 1410, 1477–8
post-micturition dribble, 1375
postoperative care
amputee, 959–60
colorectal cancer, 1265
discharge and follow-up, 300
drainage, 99–101, 299
enhanced recovery, 299–300
follow-up, 300
hip replacement, 517–18
immediate, 290
laparoscopic surgery, 114–16
lung resection, 933–4
observations, 290, *291*
plastic and reconstructive surgery, 646–8
standards, 290
tracheostomy, 747
wounds, 299
postoperative complications
abdominal surgery, 297–8
intestinal obstruction, 1292
amputation, 960
appendicectomy, 1313–14
bleeding, 295
central nervous system, 295
cholecystectomy, 1203–5
classification, 292
day case surgery, 304–5
diathermy, 102–3, 258
ERCP, 228–9
gastrectomy, 1138–9
haemorrhoids, 1359–60
hip replacement, 517–18
laparoscopic surgery, 266
lung resection, 933–4
nausea and vomiting, 298–9, 304, *305*
neck surgery, 298
neurosurgery, 298
orthopaedic surgery, 298
plastic surgery, 298
pressure sores, 297
renal and urinary system, 294–5
respiratory system, 292–3
splenectomy, 1186–7
thoracic surgery, 298
thyroid surgery, 815–16
total knee replacement, *522*
tracheostomy, 747, *748*
urinary retention, 295, 1429
vascular surgery, 298
wound dehiscence, 297
post-thrombotic syndrome (PTS), 984, 986, 990, *1000*, 1005
post-transplant lymphoproliferative disease (PTLD), 1542
post-traumatic reactions, 627
post-traumatic syringomyelia, 354
potassium, 281, *281*, 840
Pott's puffy tumour, 657, 722
pouch–anus anastomosis, *1271*
pouch of Douglas, 1513, 1518, 1522
pouchitis, 1271
Power's ratio, 346
prasugrel, *220*
praziquantel, 63, 66, 1169, 1445
prazosin, 1468
'precision medicine', 251
pregabalin, 276
pregnancy
appendicitis, 1304
breast carcinoma, 881
duration, 1515
early loss, 1515
ectopic, 1306, 1517–18
phaeochromocytoma in, 846–7
pyelonephritis, 1403
ureters/renal pelves dilatation, 1411
urinary tract infection, 1441
preherpetic pain, 1306
Preiser's disease, 508–9
premalignant lesions
oesophagus, 241–2, 1081–3
oral, 763, 767
skin, 603, 604
preoperative assessment, 254–6
airway, 261, *262*
anaemia, 258–9
cardiovascular disease, 256–8
cholecystectomy, 1203
coagulation disorders, 260
day case surgery, 304
emergency surgery, 261–2
endocrine and metabolic disorders, 260
gastrointestinal disease, 259
hepatocellular carcinoma, 1175
high-risk patient, 262–8
history taking, 254–5
investigations, 256
lung cancer treatment, 931–2
medical examination, 255–6
neurological and psychiatric disorders, 260–1
rectal carcinoma surgery, 1331–2
renal disease, 259
respiratory disease, 259
splenectomy, 1185
UTI, 260
preoperative preparation
bowel, 98, 1263, 1334
fasting, 10
skin, 52, 1564
prepuce, *see* foreskin
preputioplasty, 1487
presbycusis, 712–13
prescribing, safety, 182
pressure sores, 29–30, 297, 615–16, 953

prevention in surgery, 84
spinal cord injuries, 340, 354
staging system, *29*
preterm infant
definition, *119*
fluids, *121*
pretibial myxoedema, 1006
priapism, 332, 1491
PRICE protocol, 468, *470*
prilocaine, *273*
primary biliary cirrhosis, 1167–8
primary hyperaldosteronism (PHA/Conn's syndrome), 840–1
primary hyperparathyroidism (pHPT), 825–32
diagnosis, 826–8
hypercalcaemia, 825–6
management, 829–31
in MEN 1, 830, 857
in MEN-2, 858
pathology, 826
presentation, 825
renal stones, 1406
primary sclerosing cholangitis (PCS), *1159*, 1167, *1167*, 1206–7, 1208
primary survey
head injury, 331–2
severe trauma, 323–6
primum non nocere, 177
Pringle's manoeuvre, 374, *374*, 1161, 1171
probability (*P*-values), 167
process measures, 185
processus vaginalis, 124, 125, 1497
patent, 125, 1023, 1032, 1376, 1503
procidentia (complete rectal prolapse), 1322–4
proctalgia, 1320
proctalgia fugax, 1353–4
proctitis, 1267, 1324–6
proctocolectomy
and ileostomy, ulcerative colitis, 1270–1
restorative with ileal pouch–anal anastomosis (RPC), 1260, 1270–1
proctography, 1278, 1344, *1345*
proctoscopy, 1320, 1343
professionalism, 181
professional performance
monitoring, 174–5
quality improvement, 186–8
progesterone, 1514
prognathism, *700*, *701*
prolactin, 3
prolactin inhibitors, 869
prolactinomas, *156*, 665–6
prolapse
rectal, 1288, 1320, 1321–4
urethra, 1485, *1522*, 1523
uterovaginal, 1522–3
pro-opiomelanocortin (POMC), 844
propofol (di-isopropyl phenol), 269
propranolol, 813, 815
proptosis, 361, *673*, 675–6
propylthiouracil, 812
prostanoids, 4
prostate
abscess, 1475
anatomy, 1456–7
benign hyperplasia, *see* benign prostatic hyperplasia
biopsy, 1385, 1387, 1470–1
transperineal template (TPTBP), 1387–8
TRUS, 1385, 1387
calculi, 1468
embryology, 1456
physiology, 1457–8
ultrasound imaging, 1385–7
prostate cancer, 1468–74
chemotherapy and biological agents, *155–6*
clinical features, 1470
early diagnosis, 1462
epidemiology, 1468–9
histological classification, 1469
investigation, 1470–2
bone scans, 1392, *1393–4*, 1472
MRI scanning, 1390, *1392*
pathology, 1469
risk prediction models, 1378
screening, 1469
spread of, 1469
staging, 1469–70
treatment
advanced disease, 1473–4
early disease, 1472–3
prostatectomy, 1473
tumour markers, 1378–9
prostatectomy
in BPH, 1463
reoperation, 1466–7
complications, 1431, 1466–7
counselling, 1464
indications for in LUTS/BOO, 1464
radical, 1473
retropubic, 1465
transperineal, *1465*
transurethral (TURP), 1464–5
transvesical, 1466
prostate health index, 1379
prostate-specific antigen (PSA), 1378–9, 1457–8, 1462
age-specific reference ranges, *1378*
derivatives, 1378–9
drugs influencing, 1378
kinetics, 1379
levels in prostate cancer, 1378, 1457, 1471
measurement in LUTS/BPH, 1462
use in screening, 1378, 1469
prostatic plexus, 1423
prostatitis, 1474–5
acute, 1474–5
chronic, 1475
prosthetic valves
biological, 895
dysfunction and complications, 895–6
endocarditis (PVE), 895–6
mechanical, 258, 895
protease inhibitors, *156*
protein
daily requirements, 282
metabolism in stress response, 6–7
total body mass, 8–9
protein turnover, 8
Proteus spp., 56, 481, 1403, 1442
Proteus mirabilis, 1404
prothrombin complex concentrates, 21
proton pump, 1107, 1108
proton pump inhibitors, 284, 1077–9, 1114, 1119
proto-oncogenes, 249
provocative discography, 474, *475*
proximal femoral focal deficiency (PFFD), 564
proximal interphalangeal (PIP) joints
arthritis, *443*, 506
contractures, 507
prucalopride, 1279
pruritus ani, 1361, *1362*
pseudarthrosis, congenital of tibia, 576, *577*
pseudoachalasia, 1097
pseudocysts
pancreas, *1216*, 1221, 1228–9
spleen, 1179, *1179*
Pseudomonas spp., 45, 56, 433, 559, 1442
Pseudomonas aeruginosa, 56, 708
pseudomyxoma peritonei, 1059–60, 1316
classification, *1316*
treatment, 1317
pseudo-obstruction, intestinal, 1297–8
pseudopolyps, inflammatory, 1327
pseudotumour cerebri (idiopathic intracranial hypertension), 655
psoas abscess, 1065
psoas sign, 1303
psoriatic arthritis, 506
psychiatric medications, 261
psychoneurosis, pruritus ani, 1361
psychosocial interventions, *159*
ptosis, 672
bilateral, 675–6
pubic bones, separation, 1424
publication, research, 168
Pubmed, *163*
Pubmed Central, *163*
puborectalis muscle, 1318, 1339, 1343
puerperal sepsis, 43
pulmonary contusion, 370–1
pulmonary embolism, 292, 296, 986–91
investigations, 988–9
prophylaxis, 989, 990
treatment, 990
Wells criteria, 989
pulmonary function tests, 916–18
pulmonary hypertension, VSD, 908
pulmonary sequestration, 937
pulmonary stenosis, 904
pulmonary venous drainage, total anomalous, 905
pulse rate, shock, *14*
pulses
aortic, 1020
arterial disease, 944
extremity trauma, 383, 404
lower limb, 458, *459*
waterhammer, 901
PUMA 560, 108
puncture wounds, 27
pupil examination, head injury, 331
purpura fulminans, 598
pus
joint, 586–7
staphylococcal, *44*
pyelonephritis
acute, 1305, 1403
chronic, 1404
emphysematous, 1404
in pregnancy, 1403
xanthogranulomatous, 1404–5
pyeloplasty, 137, 1412–13
pylephlebitis, 1314
pyloric mucosal diaphragm, 1130
pyloric stenosis
adult, 1129, 1130
infantile hypertrophic, 127–8
pyloric stricture, dilation, 223, *224*
pyloromyotomy, Ramstedt's, 128
pyloroplasty, Heineke–Mikulicz, 1122
pylorus-preserving pancreatoduodenectomy (PPPD), 1236–7
pyoderma gangrenosum, 596
pyogenic granuloma, 614
pyogenic infections, spine, 481
pyogenic liver abscess, 1168
pyonephrosis, 1403, 1440
pyrexia
appendicitis, 1303
intestinal obstruction, 1286
postoperative, 296–7
surgical infection, *54*
pyuria, 1403

quadriceps
lipoma, 544
rupture, 383, 467
tears, 467
quality improvement, 185–8
investment and education, 188
pathway, 187–8
pioneers of, *186*
tools used, *187*
quality measures, 185
Quincke's sign, 901
quinolones, 1505
quinsy, 735–6

radial artery, coronary artery bypass graft, 890
radial club hand, 580
radial forearm free flap, *774–5*
radial head, congenital dislocation, 580, *581*
radial nerve
  hand, *443*
  injuries, 383, 400
radiation, *see* ionising radiation; ultraviolet radiation
radiation proctitis, 1325
radicular artery of Adamkiewicz, 471
radiculopathy, cervical, 473, 474
radiofrequency ablation (RFA)
  Barrett's oesophagus, 1083
  liver tumours, 1171
  renal carcinoma, 1420
  varicose veins, 978–9
radiography
  abdominal wall hernia, 1025
  cervical spine, 342–4
    dynamic imaging, 343
  checking radiographs, *191*
  chest, *see* chest radiography
  current legislation, 191–3
  extremity trauma, 384
  gallbladder, 1190, *1191*
  hazards of, 191
  hip, avascular necrosis, 512, *513*
  intestinal obstruction, 1288–90
  KUB, 1388
  major trauma, 205–6
  mammography, 861, 880
  oesophagus, 1070
  peritonitis, 1051
  pharynx, larynx, neck, 730
  principles, 193–4
  prostate cancer, 1471–2
  responsibilities, *192*
  shoulder, 489
  spine, 474
  typical radiation doses, *192*
  wasteful use, *192*
radioiodine, 812, 819–20
radiologist, 190
radiology, intervention, 380
radionuclide imaging
  see nuclear medicine
  biliary tract, 1192
  gallbladder, 1192, 1204
  ischaemic heart disease, 888
  spleen, 1178
  thyroid, 804, 808
radiotherapy, 153–4
  bladder cancer, 1451
  breast carcinoma, 877
  combined with chemotherapy, 157–8
  five 'Rs', 154
  gastric cancer, 1139
  oesophageal cancer, 1094
  oral cancer, 767, 775
  processes involved in, 153
  prostate cancer
    advanced disease, 1474
    early disease, 1473
  rectal carcinoma, 1337
radioulnar synostosis, 580
radius
  distal fractures, 398
    paediatric, 403, *404*
  shaft fractures, 398–9
RAF inhibitors, *157*
Ramirez's component separation technique, 1041
Ramsay Hunt syndrome, 715
ramucirumab, *158*
randomised controlled trials (RCTs)
  bariatric surgery, 1145, 1147
  definition, 164
randomised studies, 164–5
Ranson score, acute pancreatitis, *1224*
ranula, 779
rapid sequence induction (RSI), 270
Ravitch procedure, 939
Raynaud's disease, 967
Raynaud's syndrome, 967
reactionary haemorrhage, 19, 305
rebound tenderness, 1020
rectal arteries, 1319, 1341
rectal biopsy, amoebiasis, *1272*
rectal bleeding, 1319, 1329
  children, 131–2
  rectal carcinoma, 1329
rectal carcinomas, 1328–38
  chemotherapy, 1337–8
  chemotherapy and biological agents, *155*
  clinical features, 1329
  differential diagnosis, 1330
  epidemiology, 1328
  investigation, 1329–30
  local recurrence, 1338
  neoadjuvant therapy, 1332
  pathogenesis, 1328–9
  radiotherapy, 1337
  stages of progression, 1330–1
  surgery
    abdominoperineal excision, 1336
    anterior resection, 1332–3, 1334–6
    bladder dysfunction, 1429
    extensive, 1337
    liver resection, 1337
    local, 1334
    patient assessment, 1331–2
    preoperative preparation, 1334
    principles of, 1332–4
    results of, 1338
  types of spread, 1330
rectal evacuation disorder, 1324
rectal irrigation, 1279
rectal prolapse, 1320, 1321–4
  children, 131, 1321–2
  full-thickness, 1322–3
  mucosal, 1321–2
  surgical treatment, 1323–4
  vs intussusception, 1288
rectal veins, 1319, 1341
rectobulbar fistula, 1346
rectocoele, *1522*, *1523*
rectoperineal fistula, 1345–6
rectopexy
  abdominal, 1323–4
  perineal, 1323
rectourethral fistula, 137
rectovestibular fistula, *1345*, 1346
rectum
  adenoma, 1259
  benign lesions, 1327–8
  blood supply, 1319
  discharge, 1319
  diversion of urine into, 1453
  embryology, 1319
  examination, 1320
    anal stricture, 1370
    digital, 1320
    prostate disease, 1461, 1470, *1471*
    rectal cancer, 1329–30
    sigmoidoscopy, 1320, 1330
    in spinal injury, 332
  foreign bodies, 1321
  injuries, 375, 1321
  lymphatic drainage, 1319
  pain (proctalgia fugax), 1353–4
  polyps, 1326–7
  surgical anatomy, 1318
  symptoms and signs of disease, 1319–20
  varices, 1354
  venous drainage, 1319
rectus abdominis muscle, 1022, *1023*
rectus abdominus free flap, 771, *774*
rectus sheath, haematoma, 1023, 1306
recurrent laryngeal nerve (RLN), 727, 801–2
  identification in thyroidectomy, 813–14
  intraoperative monitoring, 814
  paralysis after thyroidectomy, 815
5α-reductase, 1457
5α-reductase inhibitors, 1378, 1464
refeeding syndrome, 288
reflux gastritis, 1115
reflux oesophagitis, 1076, *1078*
refusal of treatment, 170–1, 173, 259
regional anaesthesia, 274–5
regorafenib, *156*
regurgitation, 1069, 1077
  risk in surgery, 259
rehabilitation
  limb fractures, 394
  spinal injuries, 353
  sports injuries, 470
Reissner's membrane, 703, *704*
Reiter's disease, 681, 1494–5
relief efforts, major disasters, 409–13
remote presence systems, 118
renal artery
  occlusion, 1416
  organ donor, 1550
  stenosis, *942*, 952
    balloon dilatation, 949
renal calculi, 213, 825, *1386*, 1402
  aetiology, 1405–7
  clinical features, 1407
  management, 1407–10
renal cell carcinoma, 1416–21
  ablative therapies, 1420
  clear cell, 1416, 1419
  diagnosis, 1417, 1419
  hereditary syndromes associated with, 1416, *1418*
  incidence, 1416
  medical management, *156*, *157*, 1420–1
  metastases, 547, 548
  non-clear-cell, 1416, *1416*
  pathology, 1419
  risk factors, 1417
  staging, 1419
  surgery, 1419–20
renal colic, 213, 1017, 1305, 1374, 1407
renal cysts, *1386*, 1389–90, *1391*
renal failure
  after AAA repair, 966
  end-stage, 1403, 1549
  polycystic kidney disease, 1403
renal function
  contrast media, 191
  raised intra-abdominal pressure, 380
  response to injury, 9
  shock, 12
renal injuries, 375–6, 1413–14
renal scarring, 1404
renal secondary hyperparathyroidism, 833–5
renal tubular acidosis, 1406
renal vein
  anatomy, 1398
  thrombosis, 1416
renin–angiotensin–aldosterone axis, 9, 12, 839, 840
renography, isotope, 1392, *1394*, 1404, 1412
reperfusion injury, 13, 421
  crush syndrome, 421
  intestinal obstruction, 1291
reproductive physiology, female, 1514–15
Rescue and Preparedness in Disasters (RAPID), 411
Research Ethics Committee (NHS), 166
resection margins
  bone tumours, *546*
  malignant melanoma, 611
  soft tissue tumours, *545*, 548
respiratory disease, preoperative care, 259
respiratory failure, high-risk patients, 265–6
respiratory rate, shock, *14*
resternotomy, emergency, 912
resting energy expenditure, 279
rest pain, 943

resuscitation, 15–18
  assessment of response to, 326, *327*
  cardiac arrest after cardiac surgery, 912–13
  damage control (DCR), 20, 379, 427
resveratrol, *158*
reticular vein, 972, 973
retina
  anatomy, 673
  detachment, 683, 683
  dialysis, 678, 679
retinal artery, occlusion, 682, 954–5
retinal haemorrhages, 678, 679
retinal vein, occlusion, 682
retinoblastoma, *144*, 676
RET proto-oncogene, 136, *144*, 856, 857, 858
retractors, 1560–1
retrobulbar haemorrhage, 361
retrognathia, 688, 701
retrograde ureterogram, 1385
retrograde ureteropyelogram, 1411, *1412*
retrograde urethrogram, 206
retroperitoneum
  abscess, 1065
  fibrosis, 1064–5, 1413
  haematoma, 964, 965
  injuries, 376
  tumours, 1065–6, 1414, 1509
  zones, 376
retropharyngeal abscess, 737
retropharyngeal space, 727
retroviruses, in stem cell therapy, 36–7
rhabdomyoma, 912
rhabdomyosarcoma, *156*
rhesus system, 21, 22
rheumatoid arthritis (RA)
  arteritis, 967
  atlantoaxial subluxation, 481
  elbow, 499
  foot, 529
  hand, *443*, 504–5
  preoperative care, 261
  shoulder, 493
  wrist synovitis, 201
rhinophyma, 603
rhinoplasty, cleft lip/palate, 699, *700*
rhinosinusitis
  acute, 720–2
  chronic, 722–3
rib hump, 581
rib notching, 906
ribs
  children, *119*
  fractures, 366, 368
Richter's hernia, 115, 1024, 1281, 1286, 1291, 1314
rickets, 566, *567*
  biliary, 1196
rifampicin, 560
rifles, 428
right coronary artery (RCA), 886–7
right ventricular hypertrophy, 904
rigidity, abdomen, 1020
Rigler's triad, 1282
Ringer's lactate solution, 373, 624
ring fixator, *390*, 392, *393*
risk assessment
  bariatric surgery, 1146
  major thoracic surgery, 915–16
  patient safety, 179
Risk of Malignancy Index, 1527
risk management
  clinical, 181
  high-risk patient, 263
  tissue analysis, 235–6
rituximab, *157*, 1540
rivaroxaban, 990
road traffic accidents (RTAs), 310–11
  fatalities, 310, *311*
  head injuries, 328
  mechanisms of injury, 313, 314
  seatbelt injuries, 123, 351, 1061
  severe injuries, *325*
  survivors, 310–11
  total casualties, 310
robotic surgery, 108–10
  benefits, 108–9
  disadvantages, 116
  future development, 118
  image-guided, 108
  rectal cancer, 1334, *1335*
  systematic overview, 110
  teleoperated, 108
  thyroid, 814
rocuronium, 272, *273*
rodent ulcer, *see* basal cell carcinoma
ronaciclib, *158*
ropivacaine, *273*
rotator cuff
  anatomy, 488
  calcific tendinitis, 493
  tears, 202, 491–2, *494*
  tendonitis, 469, 490, *491*
round ligament, 1029
roundworm, *see* ascariasis
Roux-en-Y choledochojejunostomy, 63, 1204
Roux-en-Y gastrectomy, 1121, 1124, 1126
Roux-en-Y gastric bypass, 1148
Roux-en-Y oesophagojejunotomy, 1136, *1137*
Roux-en-Y pancreatojejunostomy, 1221
Rovsing, Neils Thorkild, 1303
Rovsing's sign, 1303
rowing injuries, 465
Royal College of Radiologists (RCR), 191
rucaparib, *158*
rugby injuries, 465
rule of 2's, 384
runners, injuries, 467
running, 525
Rutherford Morison's incision, 1309
Rutherford Morison's pouch, 1056

sacral nerve blockade, 1434
sacral nerve stimulation, 1279, 1350–1, 1434
sacroiliac joint, 377
sacroiliitis, 1267
safeguarding, 138
sagittal synostosis, *687*
St Mark's perineal retractor, 1561
saline
  hypertonic, 624
  normal, 281
saliva, composition, *281*
salivary glands
  ectopic tissue, 780
  minor, 776–8
  sublingual, 778–9
  submandibular, 780–5
  tumours, *789*, *793*
Salmonella enteritidis, 1248, 1273
Salmonella typhi, 82–3, 1201–2, 1248, 1273
Salmonella typhimurium, 1201–2
salmonellosis, 1248, 1273
salmon patch, 613
salpingectomy, 1517, 1518
salt, dietary, 1131
Salter–Harris fractures, 387, 403
sample size, clinical studies, 164
saphena varix, 972, *973*, 975, 1031
saphenofemoral junction (SFJ), 969, 975
  competence assessment, 976
  ligation, 981
saphenopopliteal junction (SPJ), 970
  ligation, 981–2
saphenous nerve, injury, 982
saphenous veins, 969–70
  incompetence, 975
  long vein grafts, 890, *891*, 949
  stripping, 981–2
sarcoidosis, 795, 1406
sarcomas
  breast, 882
  chemotherapy and biological agents, *155–6*
  Ewing's, 542
  retroperitoneal, 1065–6
  soft-tissue, *537*, 548
Savage's decompressor, 1291
Savary–Guillard bougie dilators, 223
scaffolds, tissue engineering, 38–40
scala vestibuli, 703, *704*
scald burns, *619*, *622*, *628*
scalpel blades, sizes/shapes, 85
scaphocephaly, 668, 669
scaphoid
  avascular necrosis, 508–9
  fracture, *382*, 396–7
scapula, 488
Scarf osteotomy, 525–6
Scarpa's triangle, 1043
scars
  avoidance, 31–2
  burns patient, 628, *629*
  keloid, 31, 815
  limbs, 382
  prior abdominal surgery, 112, 1023
  thyroid surgery, 815
Schatzki's ring, 1102–3
Scheuermann's kyphosis, 483, 582
Schistosoma haematobium, 1182, 1443–4
Schistosoma mansoni, 1182, 1326, 1444
schistosomiasis, *146*
  bladder, 1443–5
  geographical distribution, 1443
  mode of infection, 1443–4
  rectal, 1326
  splenomegaly, 1182
  treatment, 1445
Schlemm's canal, 673
Schober's test, 472
Schwann cells, 594, 758
schwannomas, 481, 758, 936
  vestibular, 666–7, *706*
sciatica, 476
sciatic nerve, tests, 441–2
sclera, 672
scleritis, 682
scleroderma, oesophagus, 1100
sclerosing encapsulating peritonitis, 1061
sclerotherapy
  haemorrhoids, 1356, *1357*
  oesophageal/gastric varices, 1164
  varicose veins, 979–80
scoliosis, 581–2
  classification, *581*
  congenital, 482
  functional, 441
  idiopathic, 482, *483*, 581–2
  neuromuscular, 482, *484*
  structural, 441
Scottish Improvement Hub, 187
screening
  breast carcinoma, 880
  cancer, 146–7
  colorectal cancer, 230, 1262
  lung cancer, *158*
  prostate cancer, 1378, 1469
  using histology/cytology, 243
screw fixation, *390*, 392, *393*
scrotal hernia, 1030, 1031
scrotum
  acute, 125–6
  carcinoma, 1511
  elephantiasis, 1510
  Fournier's gangrene, 50, 1509–10
  idiopathic oedema, 1501
  sebaceous cysts, 1510–11
  trauma, 1499
scrubs, 1564
SDH-associated kidney cancer, *1418*

seatbelt injuries, 351, 1061
children, 123
sebaceous (epidermal) cysts, 598–9
scrotal skin, 1510, *1511*
sebaceous glands, 593
seborrhoeic keratosis (basal cell papilloma), 599
secondary survey, 326
sedation, gastrointestinal endoscopy, 219, 1111
Seddon classification, 385
seed ganglion, 509
segmentectomy, lung, 932
seizures
after head injury, 337
brain tumours, 662–3
Seldinger technique, 1480
selective dorsal rhizotomy (SDR), *584*
selective oestrogen receptor antagonists (SERMs), 485, 831
selective progesterone receptor modulator (SPRM), 1525
seliciclib, *158*
selumetinib, *157*
seminal vesicles
cyst, 1476
diverticulum, 1476
normal ultrasound, *1471*
prostate cancer spread, 1469
tuberculosis, 1475, 1506
seminal vesiculitis, 1476
seminiferous tubules, 1497
seminomas, 1498, 1506, 1508–9
Sengstaken–Blakemore tube, 374, 1127, 1129, 1164, *1164*
sensory testing, 438, 443
sentinel node biopsy
breast carcinoma, 877
malignant melanoma, 612
sepsis, 51
acute pancreatitis, 1226–7
after prostatectomy, 1466
catheter-related, 288
definitions, *51*
intraperitoneal, 1055–7
management, 266
metabolic response, 279
septicaemia
meningococcal, 588, 589, 598
post-splenectomy, 1186
septic arthritis
children, 586–7
clinical predictors, *587*
complications, 588–9
epidemiology, 549
foot/ankle, 531–2
implant-related, 554–6
native joint, 553–4
septic shock, 13, 18
septorhinoplasty, cleft lip/palate, 699, *700*
sequestration, bone infections, 550, *551*
seroma, 1026, 1034
serous cystadenomas, 1234
serrated adenomas, 1326
Serratia spp., 433
Sertoli cells, 1498
Sertoli cell tumours, 1507
service delivery
bariatric surgery, 1146–7
paediatrics, 138
service evaluation, *162*
service investment, 1565
sesamoid injuries, 527
sestamibi scan, parathyroid glands, 827
setons, anal fistula, 1366–7
Sever's disease, 580
sex cord-stromal tumours, ovary, *1526*
sexually-transmitted infections
genital herpes, 1495
gonorrhoea, 1325, 1494, 1518–19
tropical, 1495–6
see also AIDS; HIV infection
shared-care model of chronic disease, 1151
SHELL model, 177
Shigella, 433, 1248, 1273
shock
classification, 13–15
clinical features, *14*
definition, 12
haemorrhagic, 18–20
hypovolaemic, 13, 352, 368
multiple organ failure, 15
neurogenic, 352
pathophysiology, 12–13
resuscitation, 15–18
resuscitation end points, 18
severity, 14–15
spinal trauma, 352
unresuscitatable, 15
short bowel syndrome, 283, 1256–7
short-stay surgery, 302
shotguns, 428
shoulder
anatomy, 488
arc of motion, 490
arthrodesis, 495
clinical examination, 448–50, 448–51, *451*, 489
congenital abnormalities, 488–9
dislocation, 469, 496–8
habitual, 498
posterior, *382*, *384*, 497, *498*
recurrent traumatic, 496
frozen (adhesive capsulitis), 492, *493*
hemiarthroplasty, 400, 493, *494*
history taking, 489
imaging, 489
impingement syndrome, 449
instability, 449–50
atraumatic, 497–8
osteoarthritis, 493–5
pain, 489, 490
after laparoscopic surgery, 115
replacement, 493, *494*
reverse geometry, 492
rheumatoid arthritis, 493
rotator cuff disorders, 202, 469, 490–2, *494*
sports injuries, 469
Shouldice repair, 1032
shrapnel, 431
shunts
surgical, variceal haemorrhage, 1165
transjugular intrahepatic portosystemic (TIPSS), 1058–9, 1129, 1164, *1165*
ventriculoperitoneal, 586, 655–6
sialadenitis
acute ascending bacterial, 786
granulomatous, 795
submandibular, 780, *781*
sialadenosis (sialosis), 795–6
sialolithiasis, 780–1, 787
sialometaplasia, necrotising, 778
sialorrhoea, 797
sickle cell disease, 1184
sideropenic dysphagia, 740, 763, 1105
sigmoid colon
carcinoma, *1262*, *1263*, 1264–5
volvulus, 1284–5, 1288, 1295–6
sigmoidoscopy
amoebiasis, 58
anal lesions, 1343
colorectal cancer, 1262–3
flexible, 1320, *1321*
rectal examination, 1320, 1330
rigid, 1320, 1330
sigmoid volvulus, 1295
ulcerative colitis, 1268
Silastic prosthesis (nasal septum), 718–19
silicone sheet, fenestrated, 625
silver nitrate solution, 625
silver sulphadiazine cream, 625, 630
Simmond's test, 460, 468
Sims position, 1342
simulation, laparoscopy, 117
simultaneous pancreas and kidney (SPK) transplant, 1552–3
Singapore Statement on Research Integrity, 166
single anastomosis duodenoileal bypass with sleeve gastrectomy (SADI-S), 1150
single incision laparoscopic appendicectomy (SILA), 1311
single incision laparoscopic surgery (SILS), 117
single-photon emission computed tomography (SPECT), 846, 1391
sinus
abscesses, 48
definition, 616
pilonidal, 1347–9
sinusitis, *see* rhinosinusitis
sinus tarsi syndrome, 458
sip feeding, 284
Sipple's syndrome, 856
sirolimus, 1540
Sister Mary Joseph's nodule, 1044, *1045*, 1135
Sistrunk procedure, 755, 1011
Six Sigma methodology, 187
Sjögren's syndrome, 787, 796, 1100
skeletal muscle, protein degradation, *4*
Skene's tubules, 1456
skew foot, 457
skiers, injuries, 466
skier's thumb, 398, 469, *503*
skin
adnexa, 592–3
benign lesions/tumours, 599–604
blood supply, 593, *594*, 634
congenital/genetic disorders, 594–5
congenital wounds, 615
cysts, 598–9
functions, 594
hair follicle lesions, 602–3
infections, 596–8
malignant lesions/tumours, 604–12
manifestations of generalised disease, 595–6
radiation damage, 594
structure, 592–4, 634
tension lines, 85–6, 636
thickness, 593
vascular lesions, 612–15
skin adhesive strips, 96
skin cancer
basal cell carcinoma, 604–5
causes, *145*
malignant melanoma, 608–12
premalignant lesions, 603–4
squamous cell carcinoma, 605–8
transplant recipient, 1542
skin care, lymphoedema, 1008–9
skin examination
foot, 458
musculoskeletal disorders, 437, 438
skin flaps, 27
see also flaps
skin grafts, 27, 634–5, 636
composite, 636
failure, 640
full-thickness, 635, 636, 640
harvesting, 639–40
infections, 54
split-thickness, 28, 634–5, 636, 639–40
survival, 635
skin incisions, 85–9
abdominal, 86
factors in planning, 85–6
laparoscopic surgery, 86–7, 88
skin preparation, 52, 1564
skin substitutes, 637

skull deformities, craniosynostosis, 668, 669, 687–8
skull fractures, 207
  depressed, 333
  with facial fractures, *323*, 356, 362
  reconstructive surgery, *645*
  skull base, 332, 333
  skull vault, 332–3
skull tongs, *344*
sleep apnoea, 732
  and bariatric surgery, 1146
  children, 732
  in craniofacial anomalies, 688
  obese patient, 260
sleeve gastrectomy, *1147*, 1148–9
  complications, 1150
  and ileal transposition, 1150
slipped upper femoral epiphysis (SUFE), *382*, 404–5, 573–5
slit ventricle syndrome, 655
small bowel enema, 80, 1244
small cell lung cancers, 925, 926
small intestines
  anatomy, 1240–1
  atresia, 133–4, 1293–4
  endoscopy, 225–7
  enterocutaneous fistula, 1256
  infective enteritis, 1248–9
  injuries, 375
  internal herniation, 1282
  malabsorption, 1255–6
  motility, 283
  neuroendocrine tumours, 854–5
  obstruction, *193*, 210, 1018, 1060
    adhesions, 1060, 1283
    bands, 1283
    internal hernia, 1282
    strictures, 1282
  physiology, 1241
  pseudo-obstruction, 1297
  resection, effects of, 283–4, 1256–7
  strictures, 79, 80, 1242, 1282
  transplantation, 1555–6
  tuberculosis, 78–81
  tumours, 1249–51
  vascular anomalies, 1253–4
  volvulus, 1288
small saphenous vein (SSV), 970
  incompetence, 975
  stripping, 981–2
small stomach syndrome, 1123
Smith's fracture, 398
smoking
  associated cancers, *145*, 751
  and bladder cancer, 1446
  and Crohn's disease, 1242
  lung cancer risk, 925
  and oesophageal cancer, 1086
  and oral cancer, 760
  and peptic ulcers, 1116
  and ulcerative colitis, 1267
SNAP mnemonic, 1256
snow blindness, 679
snowboarding injuries, 466
snuff box, anatomical, 397, 444, *445*
social functioning, urinary continence, 1430, 1433
social history, 1017
sodium
  dietary requirements, 281
  dietary restriction, 1059
  in GI secretions, *281*
  hyponatraemia, 120, 121, 660–1
sodium iodide, 815
soft palate
  cleft, 689–90
  erythroplakia, *762*
soft-tissue infections, necrotising, 30–1, 419–20, 597–8
soft-tissue tumours, 544
  evaluation and investigation, 544–6
  treatment, *545*, 548
soil-borne disease, 50, 71
soleal sinusoids, 971
solitary rectal ulcer syndrome, 1324
solute resorption, urinary diversion, 1454–5
somatic cells, 34–5
somatostatin, 848, 855, 1107–8, 1109
somatostatin analogues, 284, 1124, 1129, 1225, 1237, 1251
somatostatinoma, *849*
somatostatin receptor scintigraphy, 855
Sonde endoscopy, 225–6
sorafenib, *156*
Southampton wound grading system, *48*
Southwick slip angle, 574
Souttar tube, 1094
spaces of Disse, 995–6
spastic diplegia, 584–5
spastic gait, *437*
spasticity, spinal cord injury, 354
specialised pro-resolving mediators (SPM), 4
specialist centres
  neurosurgical, 336
  spinal cord injuries, 352
speech, 727
  cleft lip/palate, 695
  oesophageal, 753
  rehabilitation after laryngectomy, 752–3
speech therapy, 749
spermatic cord, 1377
spermatocoele, 1504–5
sperm counts, 1512
spherocytosis, hereditary, 1183
sphincter of Lütkens, 1188
sphincter of Oddi, 228, 1188, 1189, 1207, 1214, 1232
  dysfunction (SOD), 1222, 1232–3
spider naevi, 614
spigelian hernia, 1024, 1041–2
spina bifida, 483–4, 583, 586, 615, 667
  meningocoele, 484, 667
  myelomeningocoele, 484, 667
spina bifida occulta, 667
spinal anaesthesia, 275
spinal canal, 471
spinal claudication, 476
spinal cord, neuroanatomy, 339–40
spinal cord injury (SCI)
  assessment, 332
  associated complications, 354
  contusion, *348*
  epidemiology, 352
  incomplete, 353
  outcomes and prognosis, 353
  pathophysiology, 352–3
  specialist centres, 352
spinal disorders
  degenerative, 474–6
  infections, 481
  inflammatory spondyloarthropathies, 261, 348, 481, *482*
  investigation, 474, *475*
  neurological examination, 472–3
  physical examination, 472–3
  spondylolisthesis, 478
  spondylolysis, 476–7
spinal dysraphism, 484
spinal fusion, 476, *477*
spinal immobilisation, 340
spinal injuries
  in ankylosing spondylitis, 348
  cervical spine, 345–9
  children, 122
  decompression, 345
  diagnostic imaging, 342–4
  history, 341
  imaging, 200
    MRI, 209
    radiographs, 206
  lumbar spine, *350*, 351
  management, 344–5
  neuropathic bladder, 1428–9
  patient assessment, 340–1
  physical examination, 341, *342*
  spinal realignment, 344–5
  stabilisation, 345
  thoracic, 349, *350*
  thoracolumbar, *344*, 350–1
spinal nerve roots, *439*, 471
  compression, 440, 476
spinal shock, 352, 1428
spinal stability, 339
spinal stenosis, 476
spinal surgery
  costs of, 485
  global issues, 485–7
  lumbar disc disease, 476, *477*
spindle cell naevus, 600
spindle cells, *246*
spine
  anatomy, 338–9, 471
  clinical examination, 439–42, 472–3
  deformities, 472, 482–3, 581–3
  developmental abnormalities, 483–5
  imaging, 474, *475*
    in low-income countries, 485, *486*
  mobility testing, 472
  osteoporosis, 349, 485
  tumours, 478, 480–1
SPINK1, 1230
spinothalamic tracts, 340
Spirochaeta vincenti, 1325
spirometry, 916, *917*
spironolactone, 841, 1166
Spitz naevus, 599–600
splanchnic nerves, 1241, 1258
spleen
  abscess, 1180, *1180*
  anatomy, 1176, *1177*
  congenital abnormalities, 1178–9
  functions, 1177–8
  infarction, 1179, *1180*
  investigation, 1178
  neoplasms, 1185
  palpation, 1021
  physiology, 1176–7
  rupture, 1180
  trauma, *208*, 374
    in children, 123
splenectomy, 374, 1185–7
  haemolytic anaemias, 1183, 1184
  idiopathic thrombocytopenic purpura, 1182–3
  indications, 1185
  laparoscopic, 1186, *1186*
  open, 1185–6
  pancreatic cancer surgery, 1236
  postoperative complications, 374, 1186–7
  trauma, 374
splenic artery, 1176, *1177*
  aneurysm, 1179, *1180*
splenic flexure, carcinoma, 1264
splenic vein, 1176, *1177*
  thrombosis, 1165–6, 1228
splenomegaly, 1180–5
splenunculi, 1178
splints
  burn injuries, 628
  limb fracture, 390–1
spondyloarthropathy, inflammatory, 261, 481, *482*
spondylolisthesis, 478, *479*, 582
spondylolysis, 476–7, 582
spontaneous bacterial peritonitis (SBP), 1053
sports injuries
  bursae, 464
  by individual sport, 464–7
  by regions of symptoms, 467–9
  diagnosis, 463
  fractures, 464
  ligaments, 464
  muscles, 464
  rehabilitation, 470
  tendons, 463–4
  treatment, 470
sportsman's hernia, 1034
Sprengel's shoulder, 488–9
spring ligament, 530

Spurling's test, 440
sputum cytology, 927
SpyGlass™, 1158–9
squamous cell carcinoma (SCC)
anal canal, 1371
arising in venous ulcer, 605, 984
bladder, 1448
cervical lymph nodes, 758, 759
in chronic osteomyelitis, 558
cutaneous, 605–8
external ear, 708
histology, 240, *241*
hypopharynx, 741–2
in situ (Bowen's disease), 606, 607, 1492
middle ear, 711
nose/sinuses, 724
oesophagus, 1085–7, 1092
oral
anatomical sites, 761
buccal mucosa, 772
clinical features, 761–2, 764–5
epidemiology, 760
field change and second primary tumours, 762–3
floor of mouth, 771, *772*
investigations, 765–7
lips, 767–9
mandibular alveolus, 772–3
palate, 774
pathology, 761
post-treatment management, 775
premalignant lesions, 763, 767
staging, 764
tongue, 769–70
oropharynx, 740–1
penile, 1492–3
squeeze test, 461
Stafne bone cyst, 780
staghorn calculus, *1388*, 1406
staging
adrenocortical carcinoma, 843
breast cancer, 874, *875*
cancers, 148, *149*, 213
gastric cancer, 1134–5
hepatocellular carcinoma, 1174
lung cancer, 926, *927*
malignant melanoma, *611*
molecular testing, 251
oesophageal cancer, 1088–9
oral cancers, 764
ovarian cancer, 1528
pressure sores, *29*
rectal carcinoma, 1330–1
renal cell carcinoma, 1419
testicular tumours, 1508
thymoma, 935
thyroid carcinomas, 819
standards of excellence, 174–5
Stanford classification (aortic dissection), 910
stapedotomy, 711
stapes, *704*, *711*
otosclerosis, 711
Staphylococcus aureus, 44, 532, 559, 587, 1442
bone and joint infections, 554
methicillin-resistant (MRSA), 43, 44, 56, 532, 588
antimicrobials, 56
parotitis, 786
pneumonia, *293*
renal carbuncle, 1404
spinal infection, 481
Staphylococcus epidermidis, 44, 518, 896, 1442
stapled haemorrhoidopexy, 1359, *1360*, 1369
stapling, pharyngeal pouch, 739–40
stapling devices, 96–7
Starling's forces, 971, 996
starvation, 8, 10, 278–98
statins, 948, 1222
statistics, 166–7
steatorrhoea, 283, 1219, 1234, 1256
Steinberg classification, 512, *513*
steinstrasse, 1408
stem cells, 34, 35–8, 1558
adult/somatic, 35
embryonic, 35–6
fetal, 36
induced pluripotent (iPSCs), 36–7
in vitro differentiation, 37–8
Stemmer's sign, 998
Stener lesion, 398, 469
stented valves, 895, 902
stent-graft, aorta, 963, *964*
stents
aorta, 370, 963, *964*
biliary, 228, 1237
biliary/duodenal in pancreatic cancer, 1237, *1238*
colon, 231, 1295
coronary, 257, 886
oesophageal, 224, *225*, 1074, 1094
peripheral arterial disease, 948–9
rectal cancer, 1337
thoracic aorta, 370, 910–11
urethral, 1467
stercoliths, 1282
sterile surgical field, 1563
sterilisation, male, 1512
sternoclavicular joint, 488
sternocleidomastoid muscle, 790, *791*
sternotomy, median, *371*
Stewart–Treves' syndrome, 999
stilboestrol, *146*
stitch granuloma, 815–16
stomach
blood supply, 1106–7
cancer, *see* gastric cancer
GISTs, 1139–40
injuries, 375
investigations, 1110–13
lymphatics, 1107, 1135–6
microscopic anatomy, 1107–8
nerves, 1107
neuroendocrine tumours, 853–4
outlet obstruction, 1129–30
physiology, 1108–10
polyps, 1130
variceal haemorrhage, 1163–6
stomal stenosis, 1296, *1297*
stomas, 1254–5, 1277–8
bags and appliances, 1254–5, 1277–8
children, *119*, 122
complications, 1043, 1255, 1278
large intestines, 1277–8
small intestines, 1254–5
tracheal, 752–3
urinary diversion, 1452–3
stone-catching basket, *1409*
stones, *see* calculi; gallstones
stools
consistency, 1354–5
fluid losses, *280*, 281
'redcurrant jelly', 129
Stoppa's operation, 1034
straight leg raise test, 441–2, 473
strangulation
haemorrhoids, 1356
hernias, 1024, 1038, 1287
intestinal obstruction, 1281, 1286–7
penis, 1489
strangury, 1375
Strasberg classification, *1204*
strawberry gallbladder, 1201
'strawberry' lesion, rectosigmoid, 1325
strawberry naevus, 613
Streptococcus, 44
b-haemolytic, 44, 559
Streptococcus faecalis, 44, 56, 1442
Streptococcus milleri, 922
Streptococcus pneumoniae, 709, 896, 1186
Streptococcus pyogenes, 30, 44
Streptococcus viridans, 786
stress fractures, 464, 468, 528
stress-free perioperative care, 2
stress gastritis, 1115
stress ulceration, 1128
strictures
anal, 1243, 1360, 1370
biliary, 228, 1163
colonic, 231
Crohn's disease, 1242
treatment, 1246, 1247, *1248*
oesophageal/pyloric, 223, *225*
oesophagus, 1071, 1075, *1076*, *1078*, 1080
small bowel, 79, 80, 1242, 1246, 1282
urethra
female, 1485
male, 1466, 1482–4
stridor, 742–3
'string sign' (Kantor), 1244
stroke
care costs, *158*
following CABG, 892
haemorrhagic, 661
minor/TIAs, 951, 954–5
postoperative, 294
preoperative care, 260–1
stroke test, 454
strontium-89 radiotherapy, 1474
Struma valley, 805
struvite calculi, 1406, 1409
stye (hordeolum), 674
stylomastoid artery, 791
subacromial impingement, 490, *491*
subarachnoid haemorrhage (SAH), 335, 658–61
grading, 659
management, 659–61
perimesencephalic, 658
traumatic, 335
subclavian artery, stenosis, 952
subclavian line, infraclavicular, 287
subclavian steal syndrome, 952
subconjunctival haemorrhage, 359, 680
subdural empyema, 657–8
subdural haematoma, 334–5, 335
subhepatic abscesses, 1056–7
sublingual glands, 778–9
submandibular glands, 780–5
excision, 781–3
inflammatory disorders, 780, *781*
stone formation, 780–1
stricture, 780
tumours, 783–5
submucosal plexus of Meissner, 1107
submucous resection, 718
subphrenic abscess, 1055–7
subtalar joint, 459, 460, 524
succussion splash, 1021
sucking chest wound, 366, 368
Sucquet–Hoyer canals, 614
sugammadex, 272
Sugarbaker technique, 1059–60
sulcus sign, *498*
sunitinib, *156*
sunsetting, 652
supermicrosurgery, 646
supracondylar humeral fractures, 403–4
suprapubic catheter, 1480, 1481
suprapubic pain, 1374
supraspinatus
tendon calcification, 493
trauma, *202*, 491
supraspinous ligament, *338*
sural nerve neurapraxia, 982
'surfer's ear', 708
surgeons, global distribution, 485, 486
surgeon's knot, 95, 96
surgical emphysema, 919
surgical infections
antimicrobial treatment, 55–6
colonic surgery, 1265
'decisive period', 46
history, 42–4
microbiology, 44–7
prevention, 52–5

reduced resistance, 46–7
sources, 45–6
surgical site (major and minor), 47–50
systemic, 50–1, 53, *54*
viral, 51–2
surgical proficiency, 184
Sushruta, 633
suture materials, 89–91
absorbable, 90, 93
characteristics, 90–1
non-absorbable, *92*
sutures
alternatives, 96–7
barbed, 91
bowel anastomoses, 98
continuous, 91
interrupted, 91
knot tying, 94–5, 96
mattress, 91, *94*
minimising marks, 32
needles, 94
postoperative removal, 299
reducing incisional hernia risk, 1041
siting, 91
subcuticular, 94
vascular anastomoses, 99
suxamethonium, 272, *273*
swab, retained, *183*
swallowing, 726
assessment, 726, 1068, *1069*
difficult/painful, 1069
physiology, 1067–9
restoration in oesophageal cancer, 1091
swan neck deformity, *443*, *504*
sweat glands, 593
lesions, 603–4
sweating, gustatory (Frey's syndrome), 792, 794–5
sweat test, 1219
Swedish Obese Subjects (SOS) study, 1145
'Swelling' acronym, *438*
swimmer's itch, 1444
swimming injuries, 466
Swiss cheese model, 179
sympathectomy, 968
symptom relief, cancer, *159*
synacthen test, 842
syndactyly, *580*
syndrome of inappropriate antidiuretic hormone (SIADH), 337
synergistic effect, 158
synergistic gangrene, 30–1, 50, 1045
synovectomy, rheumatoid hand, 505
synovial chondromatosis, 500
synovitis
ankle, 531
imaging, 201
wrist, *195*, *201*
syphilis, 616, 1495
orchitis, 1506
syringomyelia, 484–5
post-traumatic, 354
systemic inflammatory response syndrome (SIRS), 51
acute pancreatitis, 1223
definitions, *51*, 1223
pathogenesis, 47, 51
systemic lupus erythematosus (SLE), 967
systemic sclerosis, 1100
systems thinking, 188

tachycardia, 14, 294
tacrolimus, 1538–9
taenia coli, 1258, 1300
Taenia echinococcus, 956
Takayasu's arteritis, 967, 1416
talipes equinovarus, congenital, 577–9
talus
congenital vertical, 579
fractures, *382*, 402
tamoxifen
breast cancer, *156*, *158*, 878, 881
endometrial cancer risk, *146*, 1516
mastalgia, 869
tapentadol, 276
tapeworm, dog, 64, 1169
targeted therapies, 154, *157–8*
cost-effectiveness, 154, *158*
renal cell carcinoma, 1420–1
tarsal coalition, 563, 579
tarsal tunnel syndrome, 533
tarsometatarsal (TMT) joint
anatomy, 524
examination, 458–9, 460, 461
injuries, *197*, 402–3, 524
taxanes, *155*, 1474
Taylor spatial frame, 392, *393*
tazobactam, 56
T-cell activation, allograft rejection, 1534, *1535*
T-cell co-stimulatory blockers, 1540
T-cell-immune checkpoint inhibitors, 1421
T-cell lymphomas, 1251
team working, 180, 182
tears, 672
technetium 99 (Tc99m) scanning
gallbladder, 1192, 1204, 1232
thyroid, 804
trauma, 385
urinary tract, 1392, *1394*, 1404, 1412
teeth, injuries, 357, 363
teicoplanin, 56
telangiectasia
hereditary haemorrhagic (Osler's disease), 719, 720
lower limb, 972, *973*, 975
telecanthus, traumatic, 362
telesurgery, 108
telomeric shortening, 140
temozolomide, *156*
temporal arteritis, 683, 967
temporal bone, fractures, 713–14
temsirolimus, *157*, 1420–1
tendinosis
Achilles, 529
peroneal tendons, 529–30
tendon disorders
hand, 504, 505, 507–8
lower limb, 529–30
rheumatoid arthritis, 504–5, 529
rotator cuff, 469, 490, *491*, 493
tendon grafts, 637
tendon injuries
Achilles, *382*, 383, 403, 468, 529
healing, 25, 27
sports, 463–4
tendonitis, calcific, 493
tendon transfers, 531, *584*
tenesmus, 1319–20, 1329
tennis elbow, 448
tennis injuries, 465
Tenon's capsule, 684
tenosynovitis, extensor (wrist), *195*
tension pneumothorax, 292, 366, 367, 919
children, 122–3
management, 367, 919
teratoma, testes, 1507
terazosin, 1468
terminal ileitis, 1242, 1305
Terson's syndrome, 659
testes
absence, 1500
anatomy, 1497
descent, 124, 1023, 1029–30, 1497
ectopic, 1498
embryology, 1497
incomplete descent, 125, 1497–9
injuries, 1499
lymphatic drainage, 1506, *1507*
pain, 1374, 1376
torsion, 1498, 1500–1
children, 125–6
vs appendicitis, 1306
tumours, 1498, 1506–9
children, 1509
testicular artery, 1497
injury, 1034
testicular veins, 1497, 1501
testosterone, 1457
tetanus, 50, 417–18, *419*
tethered cord syndrome, 667
tetralogy of Fallot, 904–5
thalassaemia, 1183–4
thalidomide, *157*
theatre etiquette, 1564
thenar muscles, 446
wasting, 443, 508
Thessaly's test, 467
thiazide diuretics, 1407
Thiersch operation, 1323
thigh, bruise, 467
thigh–foot angle, *562*, 563
thiocyanates, 806
6-thioguanine, *155*
thiopentone, *269*
thiopurine methyltransferase (TPMT), 1245
Thomas splint, 391
Thomas's test, modified, 451, *452*, 514
Thompson procedure, 1012
Thompson's test, 460, 468
thoracic aorta
aneurysms, 908–9
disruption, 366, 369–70
thoracic duct, 995
injuries, 756
thoracic outlet syndrome, 939, 991–2
thoracic spine
clinical examination, 440–1
disc herniation, 475
fractures, 349, *350*
thoracic surgery
emergency, 371
postoperative care, 298
thoracic trauma, 365–71, *372*, 938
thoracolumbar junction injury, 338–9
thoracolumbar spine, fractures, *344*, 350–1
thoracoscopy, video-assisted (VATS), 370, 922–3, 931, 934
Thoracoscore, 915
thoracotomy, 930–1
anterior, 931
emergency, 371, 931
lung cancer, 930–1
survival rates, *371*
threadworms, 1361
three-glass urine test, 1475
three-swab test, 1439
thromboangiitis obliterans (Buerger's disease), 967, 990
thrombocytopenic purpura, idiopathic (ITP), 1182–3
thrombocytosis, post-splenectomy, 1186
thromboelastography (TEG), 1161
thromboembolism
after hip replacement, 517–18
after SCI, 354
postoperative, 296
preoperative care, 260
prosthetic valves, 895
risk in endoscopy, 220
risk factors, *260*
thrombolysis, 955, 956, 990
thrombophilia, 260, 987
thrombophlebitis, 287, 990–1, 1005
thrombophlebitis migrans, 990
thrombosis
axillary vein, 992
cavernous sinus, 721
coronary stent, 257
deep vein, *see* deep vein thrombosis (DVT)
haemorrhoids, 1360, *1361*
hepatic venous, 1167–8
portal vein, 1165–6

superior mesenteric artery, 1253
thrombus
abdominal aortic aneurysm, 961, *962*
acute arterial occlusion, 953–6
aortic bifurcation, 954
cardiac, 911
through-the-scope (TTS) balloons, 223, 231
thumb
examination, 446
trigger, 507, *580*
ulnar collateral ligament injury (gamekeepers'/skier's thumb), 398, 469, 503
Thunderbeat S™, 104
thymectomy, primary hyperparathyroidism, 830
thymoma, 935
thyroglobulin, 800, 802
measurement after thyroid cancer surgery, 820
thyroglossal duct cysts, 755
thyroid
anatomy, 800–2
core biopsy, 809
cysts, 809–10
discrete swellings (nodules), 807–8
toxic, 811, 812
ectopic tissue, 936
embryology, 800
enlargement, 805–11
goitre, 805–7
retrosternal, 803, *804*, 807, 810–11, 936
toxic, 811, 812
histology
autoimmune thyroiditis, *821*
follicular carcinoma, 818
medullary carcinoma, 820
normal, 800, *801*, 811
thyrotoxicosis, 811, *812*
imaging, 803–4
neoplasms, *145*, 816–21
aetiology, 816
benign, 816
clinical features, 817
diagnosis, 817
follicular carcinoma, 809, *816*
malignant lymphoma, 816–17, 821
medullary carcinoma, *816*, 820–1, 856
papillary carcinoma, 809, *816*, 817, 818
prognosis, 818–19
relative incidence, *816*
surgical treatment, 819
undifferentiated (anaplastic) carcinoma, *816*, 817, 820
physiology, 802–3
surgery, 298, 810, 813–14
indications for, 810
thyroid cartilage, trauma, 755–6
thyroidectomy
alternative surgical techniques, 814
Graves' disease, 810
hyperthyroidism, 812, 813
indications for, 810
Kocher dissector, 1562
new technology, 814
postoperative complications, 815–16
retrosternal goitre, 811
in simple goitre, 807
subtotal, 807, 812, 815
surgical technique, 813–14
thyroid neoplasms, 810, 819
in thyrotoxicosis, 812, 813
thyroid eye disease, 675–6, *811*
thyroid function tests, 802, 808
thyroiditis
autoimmune (chronic lymphocytic), 821–2
granulomatous (de Quervain's), 822
Riedel's, 822
thyroid-stimulating antibodies, 802
thyroid-stimulating hormone (TSH), 802
thyrotoxic crisis (storm), 815
thyrotoxicosis, 13, 811–16
drug and radioiodine treatment, 812, 813
eye disease, 675–6, *811*
surgical treatment, 810, 812, 813–16
thyroid histology, 811, *812*
thyroxine, 802
after thyroid surgery, 819
in hyperplastic goitre, 807
replacement after thyroidectomy, 815
thyroxine-binding globulin (TBG), 802
thyroxine-binding prealbumin (TBPA), 802
tibia
axis, 519
congenital pseudarthrosis, 576, *577*
high osteotomy, 521
torsion
external, 562
internal, 563
tibial fractures
articular, 396
closed, 382
diaphyseal, 394, *395*
infections, 556, *557*
plateau, 401
shaft, 401
shaft in children, 406
tibialis anterior, 461
tendinosis, 528
tibialis posterior, 461
tibialis posterior tendon
failure, 530
transfer, 531
tibial nerve, posterior, 69
tibia vara, 576
tibiofemoral angle, 563
tibiofemoral dislocation, 383
tibiofibular stability, distal, 461
ticagrelor, *220*
ticarcillin, 56
Tietze Syndrome, 869
Tillaux's sign, 1063
tilt test, 461
timeline principle, 312–13
Tinel's sign, 502, 508
Tinel's test, *444*, *445*
tinidazole, 59
tinnitus, 713
tipifarnib, *157*
tissue analysis
autopsy, 251
malignancy diagnosis, 238–41
microscopy, 242, *243*
non-neoplastic/inflammatory conditions, 241, *242*
reasons for, 234–5
specimen adequacy, 243
specimen processing, 236–8
tissue specimens, 235–6
tissue blocks, 236, *237*, 244
tissue engineering, 650
challenges, 40
future directions, 41
potential applications, 33–4, 650
safety concerns, 40
scaffolds, 38–40
science underpinning, 34
sources of cells, 34–8
tissue implantation, 40
tissue expansion, 628, 637–8
tissue glue, 96
tissue oedema, 10
tissue perfusion, 10
lactate levels, 326, *327*
monitoring, 17
reduced, 18
tissue plasminogen activator (tPA), 422, 990
tissue typing, 1537–8
tissue-typing laboratory, 1538
tobacco use
associated cancers, *145*, 751
and oral malignancy, 760
see also smoking
tobramycin, 56
toes
congenital curly, 579
first
hallux rigidus, 526–7
hallux valgus, 525–6
lesser toe deformities, 458, 527
'too many toes' sign, 457, 461
Tokyo Consensus Guidelines, acute cholecystitis, *1200*
tongue
hairy leukoplakia, 738
leukoplakia, 761–2, 767
neurinomas, 856
reconstruction, 770–1
squamous cell carcinoma, *765*, *766*, 769–71
tonsillectomy, 736–7
tonsillitis
acute, 735
chronic, 736
tonsils, 726
'too many toes' sign, 457, 461
topical anaesthetics, 274
torsion
omentum, 1061
ovarian cyst, 1306
testicular, 125–6, 1306, 1376, 1498
tibial, 562, 563
torso, junctional zones, 364–5
torso trauma
abdominal, 372–6
antibiotics, 380
damage control surgery, 378–80
deaths, 364
interventional radiology, 380
mechanisms of injury, 364–5
non-operative management, 380
pelvis, 376–8
thoracic, 365–71, *372*, 938
torsion, testes, 1500–1
torticollis, congenital, 582
total anomalous pulmonary venous drainage (TAPVD), 905
total circulatory arrest, 885
total contact cast, 533
total hip replacement, 515–18
total intravenous anaesthesia (TIVA), 270, 304
total knee replacement, 521–3
totally extraperitoneal (TEP) hernia repair, 1033
total mesorectal excision (TME), 1334–5
total parenteral nutrition (TPN), 286–8
toxic shock syndrome, 30
Toyota Production System, 187
trabecular artery, 1177
trabeculectomy, 683–4
trace elements, 282–3
trachea
deviation, 366, 367
obstruction, 924–5
oesophageal cancer invasion, 1089
wounds, 756
tracheal dilator, 745
tracheal stoma, 752–3
tracheobronchial injuries, 370
tracheo-oesophageal fistula
malignant, 1095
oesophageal atresia, 133
tracheostomy
complications, 747, *748*
elective, 745–6
emergency, 744–5
indications for, *744*
percutaneous, 747
tracheostomy tubes, 747
trachoma, 677
traction
cervical spine, *344*
limb fractures, 391–2, 405
training
endoscopy, 217
ethics and, 174–5
laparoscopic surgery, 117–18

trametinib, *157*, 612
tranexamic acid, 324
transabdominal preperitoneal (TAPP) hernia repair, 1033, 1042
transanal endoluminal microscopic surgery (TEMS), 1332, *1333*
transanal stapled resection of intussusception (STARR), 1324
transanal total mesorectal excision (taTME), 1335–6
transbronchial needle aspiration (TBNA), 928
transcapillary escape rate (TER), 7
transcatheter aortic valve implantation (TAVI), 902
transcervical resection of fibroid (TCRF), 1526
transdifferentiation, 40
transforming growth factor-alpha (TGF-α), 1116
transforming growth factor-beta (TGF-β), 4
transfusion, *see* blood transfusion
transient ischaemic attacks (TIAs), 951, 954–5
transitional cell carcinoma
  bladder, 1446
  upper urinary tract, 1421
transitional cell papilloma, nasal, 723–4
transjugular intrahepatic portosystemic stent shunts (TIPSS), 1058–9, 1129
  ascites, 1166
  variceal haemorrhage, 1164, *1165*
transluminal angioplasty, 948–9
transperineal template biopsies of the prostate (TPTBP), 1387–8
transplantation
  clinical guidelines, 1558
  combined liver and small bowel, 1556
  composite tissues, 649–50
  ethics, 174
  future prospects, 1558
  graft rejection, 1533–7
  history of, 1532–3
  HLA matching, 1537–8
  immunosuppressive therapy, 1538–41
  informed consent, 174
  international databases, 1558
  kidney, 835, 1549–52
  liver, 1156, 1166
  living donor, 1547–8, 1553–4
  milestones, *1533*
  organ donation, 1542–8
  organ function after, 1548, *1549*
  pancreas, 1545, 1552–4
  simultaneous pancreas and kidney, 1552
  small bowel, 1555–6
  thoracic organs, 1556–8
  tissue-typing laboratory, 1538
transposition of the great vessels, 905
transrectal ultrasound (TRUS), 1385–7, 1462, 1470, *1471*
transtracheal ventilation, 748–9
transurethral resection of prostate (TURP), 298
  complications, 1466–7
  indications in LUTS, 1464
  reoperation, 1466–7
  surgical technique, 1464–5
transverse abdominis muscle (TRAM) flap, 879, *880*
transversus abdominis plane block (TAP), 274
trapezius myocutaneous flap, *644*
trastuzumab (Herceptin), *157*, *158*, 873, 878, 1139
Traube's sign, 901
trauma
  bladder, 1425–6
  causing lymphoedema, 1005
  children, 122–4
  ear, 706–7, 708
  early total care (ETC), 318–19, *327*
  extremity, *see* extremity trauma
  gallbladder/biliary tree, 1198
  history, 315–16
  imaging, 200–1, 205–8
  liver, 123, 208, 373–4, 1160–3, *1162*
  major
    identification, 322
    imaging, 205–8
    primary survey, 323–6
  pancreas, 1220–1
  penis, 1377, 1489
  physiological response to, 3–7, 317–18
  rectum/anal canal, 1321
  renal, 1413–14
  splenic injury, 1180
  surgical, *see* iatrogenic injuries
  testes, 1499
  ureters, 376, 1414–15
  venous, 992–3
trauma assessment, 313–17
  hidden factors, 315–17
  initial, 318
  mechanisms of injury, 313–15
    response to, 320
  obvious injuries, 315
  patient factors, 315, *316*, 317, 320
  primary survey, 323–6
  secondary survey, 326
trauma-induced coagulopathy (TIC), 18
trauma management
  local protocols and guidelines, 319
  operation planning, 319–20
  timeline, 312–13
trauma team, 318, 322, *323*
Travers retractor, 1561
Treacher Collins syndrome, 687, 689, 701, 708
tremor, flapping, 1156
trench foot, 422
Trendelenburg gait, *437*
Trendelenburg positioning, 266, 792
Trendelenburg test, 452, *453*, 514
Treponema pallidum, 1495
triage
  categories, *412*
  major disasters, 412
triage tags, 412, *413*
triangular fibrocartilage complex (TFCC), 202, 503
trichobezoars, 1282
trichoepithelioma, 602
tricholemmal (pilosebaceous) cysts, 599
tricholemmoma, 602
trick movements, 383
tricyclic antidepressants, 276, 277
trigeminal nerve, 672, 705
trigeminal neuraligia, 670
trigger digit, 507, *580*
trigger thumb, 507, *580*
triglycerides, long-chain (LCTs), 282
trigonocephaly, 668, 669
tri-iodothyronine (T_3), 802
tripartite risk assessment, 915–16
trocar insertion
  previous abdominal surgery, 112
  technique, 87–9
trocar site haemorrhage, 114
Troisier's sign, 1135
Trojani system, 544
trophic ulceration, 69–70
tropical pancreatitis, 76–7, 1230
tropical sexually transmitted infections, 1495–6
tropical splenomegaly, 1182
troponin testing, 265, 888
Trousseau's sign, 831, 1132
truncal vagotomy, 1121–2, 1125
  and antrectomy, 1223
trunk asymmetry, 472
Trypanosoma cruzi, 1095
T-tube drains, 100, 101
tube-feeding techniques, 284–5
tubercles, bladder (bilharzial), 1444
tubercle of Zuckerkandl, 802
tuberculoma, 658
tuberculosis, 77–81, 559–60, 588
  breast, 867
  central nervous system, 658
  cervical lymphadenitis, 77–8, 757
  diagnosis, 78
  drug-resistant, 560
  epididymo-orchitis, 1505–6
  foot, 532
  hand, 504
  hyperplastic, 1248–9
  intestinal, 1248–9
  mesenteric lymphadenitis, 1062
  miliary, 658
  peritonitis, 1053–4
  proctitis, 1325
  prostate, 1475–6
  pulmonary, 937
  renal, 1440
  salivary glands, 795
  seminal vesicles, 1476, 1506
  small intestines, 78–81
  splenomegaly, 1182
  transplant recipient, 1541
  treatment, 560
  ulcerative, *616*, 1248
  urinary tract, 1405, 1442–3
tuberous sclerosis, 602–3, 912, 1001, *1418*
tubo-ovarian abscess, 1519–20
tubular adenomas, rectum, 1326
tumourigenesis, 249
  tissue engineering, 40
tumour markers, 1378
  Ca 19-9, 22, 1167, 1208, 1211, 1235
  CA-125, 1527, 1528, 1529
  human kallikrein-2 (HK2), 1379
  prostate-specific antigen (PSA), 1378–9
  testis, 1379
tumour necrosis factor alpha (TNF-α), 619
tumour, nodes, metastases (TNM) staging, 148, *149*, 213, 240
  colorectal cancer, *1262*
  gastric cancer, 1134–5
  laryngeal cancer, *752*
  lung cancer, 926, *927*
  oesophageal cancer, 1088–9
  oral cavity cancer, 764
  rectal carcinoma, 1331
tumour predisposition disease, *1418*
tumours
  adrenal glands, 841, 842, 843, 857
  angiogenic competence, 140
  bile ducts, 1207–9
  bone, *see* bone tumours
  cardiac, 911–12
  chest wall, 938
  eye, 676–7
  gallbladder, 1209–11
  growth of, 142–3
  hypercalcaemia, *826*
  larynx, 751–2
  liver, 1169–75
  mesentery, 1064
  metastatic, *see* metastases
  neck (primary), 757–8
  ovary, 1526–9
  paediatric, 138
  pancreas, 848–52
  parathyroid glands, 835–6
  penis, 1491–3
  retroperitoneum, 1065–6, 1414, 1509
  salivary glands
    minor, 777–8

parotid, 787–9
sublingual, 779
submandibular, 783–5
small intestines, 1249–51
spinal, 478–81
testes, 1506–8
thyroid, *145*, 816–21
venous, 993–4
tunica vaginalis, 1029
turban tumour, 603
turbinates, 716
turf toe, 468, 527
Turner syndrome, 903, 906, 1001
tympanic membrane, 703, *704*
blast rupture, 430, 432
perforation, 708, *709*
ventilation tube (grommet), 710
typhilitis, 1307
typhoid, 82–3
gallbladder, 1201–2
intestinal, 1248, 1273
tyrosine kinase inhibitors, 154, *156*, 1420

ubiquitin–proteasome pathway, 7
ulcerative colitis, 1267–71
acute colitis in, 1267–8, 1269
aetiology, 1267
cancer risk, 1268
distinguishing from Crohn's disease, *1243*, *1268*
epidemiology, 1267
extraintestinal manifestations, 1267
indications for surgery, 1269
investigations, 1268–9
medical treatment, 1269
pathology, 1267
primary sclerosing cholangitis in, 1206, *1207*
proctitis, 1325
severity classification, 1267
surgical treatment, 1270–1
ulcers
amoebic, 57, 58, 1272
arterial insufficiency, 943
bladder (bilharzial), 1444, *1445*
characteristic edge shapes, *616*
definition, 616
diabetic foot, 532
genital, 616, 1495
peptic, 222–3, 1019, 1048
trophic, 69–70
venous, *see* venous leg ulcers
ulna, shaft fractures, 398–9
ulnar collateral ligament injury, thumb, 398, 469, 503
ulnar drift, *443*, 505
ulnar nerve
compression in cubital tunnel, 501–2
compression in Guyon's canal, 508
hand, *443*
ultrasonic dissector, 1170
ultrasound, 194–5
abdominal aortic aneurysm, *961*
abdominal wall hernias, 1025–6
advantages, 194–5, *196*
amoebiasis, 58–9
appendicitis, 1307
biliary tract, 1191
bililary system, 213
bladder diverticula, *1438*
breast, 861–2
cholecystitis, 212–13
contrast enhanced (CEUS), 1158
DDH assessment, 568, 569
disadvantages, 195, *196*
duodenal atresia, 133, *134*
endoanal, 1344, 1365
endobronchial (EBUS), 928, 929
endorectal, 1332
endoscopic, *see* endoscopic ultrasound
epididymal cyst, 1504
extremity trauma, 384
eye
choroidal melanoma, *677*
retinal detachment, 683
FAST, 123, 206–7, 324, 372, 1160
hip effusion, 586
hydronephrosis, 1411, *1412*
intraoperative, insulinoma, 850
joint disease, 201, 202
laparoscopic, biliary tract, 1195
lithotripsy, 1436
liver, 1157–8
major trauma, 206–7
miscarriage diagnosis, 1515
mycetoma/actinomycetoma, 73
oesophageal cancer, 1089
oral cancer, 766
ovarian cancer, 1527
pancreas, 1215
panoramic, 195
parathyroid glands, 827–9
regional anaesthesia guidance, 274
roundworm infestation, 60, *61*
soft-tissue mass lesions, 203
stomach, 1111–12
testicular tumours, *1507*, *1508*
thyroid, 803, 808, 817
transrectal (TRUS), 1385–7, 1462, 1470, *1471*
transvaginal, 1515, 1527, *1527*
urinary tract (USS), 1385
varicocoele, 1502
ultraviolet (UV) radiation
corneal injury, 679
skin cancers, *145*, 594, 604, 608
umbilical hernia, 127, 1023, 1036–8
umbilicus
chronic infection, 1044
fistula, 1044
malignancy, 1044, *1045*
patent urachus, 1044
skin discolouration around, 1019–20
trocar insertion, 87–9
uncal herniation, *329*, 331
underbody blast, 432
unicoronal synostosis, 687
United Nations (UN), relief agencies, 411
University of Wisconsin solution, 1546
upper limb
congenital anomalies, 580–1
neurological examination, *473*
sports injuries, 469, *470*
see also parts of upper limb
upper motor neurone (UMN) lesions, 473
upper oesophageal sphincter (UOS), 1067, *1069*
upper tract transitional cell carcinoma, 1421
urachal cyst, 1438
urachus, patent, 1044, 1438
urea and electrolytes, 256
urease-producing organisms, 1406
ureteric bud, 1399, 1400
ureterocoele, 1401, *1402*
ureterogram, retrograde, 1385
ureteroileostomy, 1452, *1453*
ureteropyelogram, retrograde, 1411, *1412*
ureteroscopy, 1385
calculi management, 1408–9
ureterosigmoidostomy, 1453
complications, 1454–5
ureterovaginal fistula, 1439
ureters
congenital megaureter, 1402
dilation in pregnancy, 1411
duplex, 1400, *1401*
ectopic, 1401, 1432
injury, 376, 1414–15
repair, 1415
retrocaval, 1402
urethra
bladder cancer recurrence, 1452
caruncle, 1377, 1485–6
diverticulum, 1479, 1485
female
abnormalities, 1485–6
anatomy, 1485
carcinoma, 1486
male
anatomy, 1477
calculi, 1484
congenital anomalies, 126, 137–8, 1477–8, *1479*
dilatation, 1483
fistula, 1440, 1484
injuries, 1479–82
neoplasms, 1484
stricture, 1466, 1482–4
urethral sphincters
artificial, 1431
distal striated, 1423, 1456, 1477
urethral syndrome, 1376, 1442
urethritis
gonococcal, 1494
non-specific (non-gonococcal), 1494
Reiter's disease, 1494–5
urethrocoele, 1485, *1522*, 1523
urethrogram
retrograde, 206
urethral injury, *1481*
urethral stricture, *1483*
urethroplasty, urethral stricture, 1484
urethroscopy, urethral stricture, *1483*
urethrotomy, endoscopic (internal), 1484
urgency, 1375
uric acid stones, 1406, 1434, *1435*
urinalysis
dipstick test, 1379
early-morning urine, 1379
male lower urinary tract symptoms, 1462
mid-stream specimen, 1379
preoperative, 256
voided urine cytology, 1379
urinary catheterisation
laparoscopic surgery, 115
neuropathic bladder, 1428
peritonitis, 1052
suprapubic, 1480, 1481
urinary diversion, 1433, 1452
bladder cancer, 1452–4
bladder exstrophy, 1425, *1453*
complications, 1425, 1454–5
continent, 1454
external, 1452–3
internal, 1453–4
risk of malignancy, 1455
urinary flow rates, 1395, *1396*
bladder outflow obstruction, 1395, *1396*, 1459, *1460*, 1462
men, 1459, *1460*, 1462
normal, *1396*
urethral stricture, 1482
urinary incontinence, 1429–34
female, 1431–2, 1524
male, 1431
after prostatectomy, 1431, 1466
overflow, 1421, 1430, 1433, 1460
urethral rupture, 1481
stress, 1375, 1430, 1431, 1433
treatment, 1432–4
urge, 1375
urinary retention, 1426–9, 1463
acute, 1426–7
in BPH, 1460, *1461*
management, 1463
chronic, 1421, 1427, 1430, 1433, 1463
drugs inducing, 1428
postoperative, 295, 1429
urinary ribonucleic acid (RNA) biomarkers, 1379
urinary stream, reduced, 1375
urinary tract
calculi
bladder, 1383, 1434–6
causes, 1405
imaging, 1388

kidneys, 213, 825, *1386*, *1388–9*, 1405–7
renal, 1405–10
endoscopy, 1379–85
fistulae, 1438–40
malformations, 137–8, 1424–5, 1432, 1477–9
obstruction, 1410–13
pain, 1017, 1305, 1374–5
radiology, 1385–95
trauma, 375–6, 1413–14
tuberculosis, 1405, 1442–3
urinary tract infection (UTI), 1441–2
acute abacterial cystitis, 1442
alkaline encrusting cystitis, 1443
avenues of infection, 1441
bacteriology, 1441–2
in children, 127, 131, 1404
cystitis cystica, 1443
frequency–dysuria (urethral) syndrome, 1376, 1442
interstitial cystitis (Hunner's ulcer), 1443
in men, 1441
polycystic kidney disease, 1402
postoperative, 295
predisposing factors, 1441
in pregnancy, 1441
preoperative care, 260
recurrent, 1441
treatment, 1442
tuberculous, 1442–3
upper tract, 1403–5
urinary incontinence in, 1432
urine
blood (haematuria), 1375–6, 1460, 1524
discolouration, 1376
dribbling, 1401
postvoid residual, 1395, 1430, 1460
urine examination, schistosomiasis, 1444
urine output
fluid resuscitation, 624
healthy adult, *280*
postoperative, 294–5
shock, *14*
urodynamic studies, 429, *430*
bladder outflow obstruction, 1396, *1397*, 1430, *1431*, 1460, 1462
bladder overactivity, 1396, *1397*
indications in men, 1462
urogenital remnant, 1063
urography
intravenous, *192*, 193, *194*
ureterocoele, 1401
urology stack, 1380
urticaria, schistosomiasis, 1444
uterine artery embolisation, 1525–6
uterine bleeding, 1515–17
uterovaginal prolapse, 1522–3
uterus
anatomy, 1513–14
fibroids, 1514, 1524–6
utriculus masculinus, 1477
uvea, 672–3
uveitis, 681

V600E BRAF mutation, 154
vaccination
human papillomavirus, 1516
splenectomy, 1187, 1236
tetanus, 50, 417–18
VACTERL syndrome, 580
vacuum-assisted closure, 30, 416, 638, *639*
vagal body tumour, 758
vagal nerve stimulation, 670
vagina, anatomy, 1513
vaginal bleeding
early pregnancy, 1515
non-pregnant state, 1515–17
vaginal vault prolapse, *1522*, *1523*
vagotomy
highly selective, 1122, 1123
sequelae, 1123–5
truncal, 1121–2, 1123, 1125
vagus nerve, 727, 810, 1107
monitoring in thyroid surgery, 814
valgus cut angle, 519
valgus stress test, 455, 456
Valsalva manoeuvre, 1020
value, concept of, 185
valves of Heister, 1188
valvulae conniventes, 1241, 1258
valvular heart disease, 893–902
antibiotic prophylaxis, 53, 896
aortic valve, 899–902
polycystic kidney disease, 1403
preoperative management, 258
surgical options, 894–5
vancomycin, 56
vanillylmandelic acid (VMA), 847
varices
anorectal, 1354
gastric, 1129
management of bleeding, 1163–6
oesophageal, 222, 1126, 1127
varicocoele, 1377, 1501–2
varicography, 976
varicose veins, 972, 974–82
complications of surgery, 982
epidemiology, 974
investigation, 975–6
management, 976–7
adjunctive surgical techniques, 982
compression, 977
endothermal ablation, 977
endovenous glue, 980
laser ablation, 977–8
open surgery, 981–2
radiofrequency ablation, 978–9
sclerotherapy, 979–80
recurrence, 982, 983
symptoms and signs, 974–5
varicosities, pelvic, 985–6
varus deformity
elbow, 447
knee, 454, 521
varus femoral osteotomy, 515
vasa brevia, 1106
vascular access
children, 122
parenteral nutrition, 286–7
trauma, 323
vascular endothelial growth factor C (VEGF-C), 1001, *1002*
vascular endothelial growth factor (VEGF)
antibodies targeting, 1420–1
inhibitors, *158*
vascular endothelial growth factor (VEGF) receptor-3 (VEGFR-3), 1001
vascular injuries
extremity trauma, 383
liver trauma, 1162
veins, 992–3
vascular interventional radiology, 209
vascular invasion, tumour cells, *239*
vascularised composite allografting (VCA), 649–50
vascular malformations
cerebral, 661–2
omtestome, 1276–7
skin, 613
vascular resistance, shock, *14*
Vascular Society Quality Improvement Programme (VSQIP), 162
vas deferens, 1497
vasectomy, 1374, 1512
Vaseline gauze, 625, 630
vasoactive intestinal polypeptide (VIP), 845
vasodilation, 10
vasopressin, *see* antidiuretic hormone (ADH)
vasopressor therapy, 16
vasospastic disorders, 967–8
Vaughan Jackson syndrome, 505
vecuronium, *273*
vedolizumab, 1245, 1269
vein of Galen malformations, 661
vein patch, 99
veins
congenital anomalies, 991
cystic degeneration, 994
entrapment syndromes, 991–2
injuries, 992–3
lower limb, 969–70
neck, 367, 368
repair and replacement, 993
total blood volume, 970
veliparib, *158*
velopharyngeal incompetence, 695
vemurafenib, 154, *157*, 612
vena cava, injuries, 1162
venae commitantes, 969
venetoclax, *158*
venoarteriolar reflex (VAR), 1001
venography, ascending, 989
venous disease
classification, 974
prevalence, 969
venous hypertension, 983
causes, *971*
clinical features, 972–4
management, 984–5
pathology, 971–2
venous leg ulcers, 29, 973, *974*, 982–5
causes, *29*, 983
clinical features, 984
investigation, 984
mixed, 983, 985
pathophysiology, 983
prevention of recurrence, 985
prognosis, 985
venous malformations, 993, *994*
venous reflux, 975–6
and lymphoedema, 1005–6
venous thromboembolism, 986–91
aetiology, 986–7
diagnosis, 987–8
investigations, 988–9
pathology, 987
prophylaxis, 989, 990, 1263
risk factors, 986, *987*
venovenous bypass, 1162
ventilation
anaesthesia, 272–3, 1563
transtracheal, 748–9
ventricular aneurysm, 889
ventricular assist device (VAD), 892
ventricular fibrillation (VF), 912
ventricular septal defect (VSD), 904, 907–8
ventricular septal rupture, 889
ventricular tachycardia, 912
ventriculomegaly, 654
ventriculoperitoneal (VP) shunts, 586, 655–6
complications, 655–6
shunt valves, 655
ventriculostomy, endoscopic third ventricle, 656
vermiculation, 1019
vernal conjunctivitis, 680
Verres needle, 112
vertigo, benign paroxysmal positional, 714
verumontanum, 1477
vesical arteries, 1423
vesical plexus, 1423
vesico-intestinal fistula, 1440
vesico-ureteric reflux (VUR), 131, 1404
grading, 1404
vesico-urethral fistulae, 1431
vesicovaginal fistula, 1439
vestibular labyrinth, 705
vestibular neuronitis, 714
vestibular schwannoma, 666–7, *706*, 715–16
vibration white finger, 967
Vibrio spp., 433
Victoria, Queen, 269

video-assisted thoracoscopic surgery (VATS), 922–3
  empyema debridement, 923
  lung/lymph node biopsy, 930
  lung resection, 931, 934
  mediastinal tumour, 936
  pleural effusion drainage, 922
  pneumothorax, 921
videofluoroscopy, 726
video gastroduodenoscopy, 1070
video-gastroscope, *1110*
villous adenomas, rectum, 1326
vinblastine, *155*
vincristine, *155*
VIPoma, *849*
viral infections, 51–2
  associated cancers, *146*
  hepatitis, 51–2, 1173
  parotid gland, 786
  transplant recipient, 1541
viral oncogenes (*v-onc*), 140
Virchow's triad, 986
virilisation, 844
visceral oedema, 9–10
visceral pain, 1018, 1258
visual loss
  arterial occlusion, 954–5
  painless, 682–3
Vitallograph, 917
vital signs
  children, *120*
  postoperative, 290, *291*
vitamin B12
  absorption, 283, 1241
  deficiency, 1124, 1243, 1256
vitamin D, *158*, 825, 831
vitamin K, 1163
vitamins, 282
  supplementation after bariatric surgery, 1151
vocal folds, 727, *728*
  nodules, 749, *750*
  palsy, 751
  polyps, 749–50
vocal rehabilitation, 752–3
voice change, after thyroidectomy, 815
voided urine cytology, 1379
voiding pressures, bladder outflow obstruction, 1430, *1431*, 1460
Volkmann's ischaemic contracture, 404, 422
volleyball, 466
volume loading, crush syndrome, 421
volume loss, 9–10, 13
volume procedures, as day surgery, 305
volvulus, 134–5, 1284–5
  caecal, 1288, 1289–90, 1295
  causes, 1284–5
  clinical features, 1288
  compound, 1285
  imaging, 1289–90
  sigmoid colon, 1284–5, 1288, 1290
  small intestine, 1288
volvulus neonatorum, 1284, 1288, 1290
vomiting
  after peptic ulcer surgery, 1123
  bilious in children, 128, 134
  cyclic in children, 1307
  gastric outlet obstruction, 1130
  intestinal obstruction, 1286
  Mallory-Weiss syndrome, 1075
  postoperative, 298–9, 304, *305*
  spontaneous oesophageal perforation, 1072–3
von Hippel–Lindau (VHL) syndrome, *145*, 845, 1220, *1418*, 1420
von Recklinghausen disease, *see* neurofibromatosis type 1 (NF1)
vorinostat, *157*
V to Y flap, 641, *642*
vulval intraepithelial neoplasia (VIN), 1368

Wada test, 669
Waldeyer's fascia, 1318, 1336
Waldeyer's ring, 725, *726*, 761
walking cycle, 525
Wallerian degeneration, 25, 385
Warburg effect, 142
warfarin
  endoscopy patient, *221*
  venous thromboembolism, 990
warm ischaemic time, 1545
Warthin's tumour, *789*
warts
  anal, 1368
  genital, 1486, 1496
  papillary (verruca vulgaris), 599
water balance, daily, 280
Waterhouse–Friderichsen syndrome, 844
water intoxication, in transurethral prostatectomy, 1467
'water-lily' sign, 68
water plethysmography, 1007
Weber–Christian disease, 1062
Weber–Fergusson incision, 774, *775*
wedge compression fractures, 349
wedge resection, lung, 932
weight loss
  after bariatric surgery, 1145
  lifestyle change, 1144
weight training, 467
Wells criteria, 988, 989
West retractor, 1561
Wharton's duct, 780
Whipple's procedure, 375, 1141, 1209, 1236
Whipple's triad, 848
Whitaker test, 1412
white cell counts (WBC)
  bone/joint infections, 551, 553
  primary pneumococcal peritonitis, 1053
whole blood, 20
whole body CT scanning, 317, 324
whole-gut transit time, 1278, *1279*
Williams syndrome, *903*
Wilms' tumour (nephroblastoma), 138, *152*, *156*, 832, 1421–2
Wiltse classification (spondylolisthesis), *478*
windlass mechanism, 524
Windlass test, 460, *461*
wingless-type (Wnt) pathway, mutations, 561, 831, 1329
withdrawal of treatment, 173
Wolfe grafts, 635, 636, 640
Wolffian duct, 1063, 1399
Wolff's law, *561*
World Anti-Doping Agency (WADA), 470
World Cancer Research Fund, 143, 146
World Federation of Neurological Surgeons (WFNS), SAH grading, 659
World Health Organization/Revised European–American Lymphoma (WHO/REAL) system, 147
World Health Organization (WHO)
  analgesic ladder, 276
  surgical safety checklist, 182–3
worms
  appendix, 1302
  biliary, 1205, 1207
  intestinal obstruction, 60–1, 1282–3
  roundworm (ascariasis), 60–2, 1282–3
  threadworm, 1361
wound closure, 89–97
  negative pressure (vacuum-assisted), 30, 416, 638, 639
  temporary in DCS, 379
wound dehiscence, 297
  risk factors, *297*
wound dressings
  biological, 985
  burns, 625–6, 630
  venous ulcers, 985
wound healing, 634
  abnormal, 25–6
  burns, 630–1
  contractures, 32, 635
  delayed, 46, *54*, 89
  factors influencing, *24*
  infected wounds, 53–5
  normal phases of, 24–5
  primary intention, 89
  scarring, 31–2
  secondary intention, 89
  specific tissues, 25
  tertiary intention, 89
wound infections
  after appendicectomy, 1313
  following CABG, 892
  following colonic surgery, 1265
  postoperative, 53–5, 299
  prevention, 52–3
  scoring systems, 47, *48*
  thyroid surgery, 815
wound management
  acute wounds, 26–7
  debridement, 26, 27, 415–16
  necrotising fasciitis, 419
  postoperative, 299
wounds
  acute, 26–9
  bites, 27
  blast, 431, 433
  chronic, 29–30
  congenital, 615
  contamination, 416
  degloving, 27–8
  gunshot, 315, 370, 372, 426, 427–9
  neck, 755–6
  punctures, 27
  'sucking' entry, 49
  tidy *vs* untidy, 26
wrist
  clinical examination, 442–6
  congenital malformations, 509, *510*
  fractures, 396–7
  ganglion, 509
  instability, 397–8
  osteoarthritis, 506
  synovitis, *195*, *201*
  total replacement, 505
Wuchereria bancrofti, 63, 1003–4, 1504, 1510

xanthinuria, 1406
xanthogranulomatous pyelonephritis, 1404–5, 1409
xenotransplantation, 1558
xeroderma pigmentosum, *145*, 595
xerostomia, 797–8

Yersinia enterocolitica, 1248, 1305
yersiniosis, 1248
yolk sac tumour, 1506
Y to V flaps, *642*, *644*, 1370

Z deformity, thumb, *443*
Zenker's diverticulum (pharyngeal pouch), 738–40, 1101–2
Zollinger–Ellison syndrome, 850–2, 1116, 1120, 1141–2
zone of polarising activity (ZPA), 561
Zoon's balanitis, 1377
Z-plasty, 32, 628, *641*
zygomatico-orbito complex fractures, 359